(See Chapter 8 for listing according to human response patterns)

Activity Intolerance

Activity Intolerance, High Risk for

Adjustment, Impaired

Airway Clearance, Ineffective

Anxiety

Aspiration, High Risk for

Body Image Disturbance

Body Temperature, High Risk for Altered

Breastfeeding, Effective

Breastfeeding, Ineffective

Breastfeeding, Interrupted

Breathing Pattern, Ineffective

Cardiac Output, Decreased

Caregiver Role Strain

Caregiver Role Strain, High Risk for

Communication, Impaired Verbal

Conflict, Decisional (Specify)

Conflict, Parental Role

Constipation

Constipation, Colonic

Constipation, Perceived

Coping, Defensive

Coping, Family-Ineffective: Compromised

Coping, Family-Ineffective: Disabling

Coping, Family: Potential for Growth

Coping, Individual, Ineffective

Denial, Ineffective

Diarrhea

Disuse Syndrome, High Risk for

Diversional Activity Deficit

Dysreflexia

Family Processes, Altered

Fatigue

Fear

Fluid Volume Deficit

Fluid Volume Deficit, High Risk for

Fluid Volume Excess

Gas Exchange, Impaired

Grieving, Anticipatory

Grieving, Dysfunctional

Growth and Development, Altered

Health Maintenance, Altered

Health Seeking Behaviors (Specify)

Home Maintenance Management, Impaired

Hopelessness

Hyperthermia

Incontinence, Bowel

Incontinence, Functional

Incontinence, Reflex

Incontinence, Stress

Incontinence, Total

Incontinence, Urge

Infant Feeding Pattern, Ineffective

Infection, High Risk for

Injury, High Risk for

Knowledge Deficit (Specify)

Mobility, Impaired Physical

Noncompliance (Specify)

Nutrition, Altered: Less than Body Requirements

Nutrition, Altered: More than Body Requirements

Nutrition: Potential for More than Body Requirements, Altered

Oral Mucous Membrane, Altered

Pain

Pain, Chronic

Parenting, Altered

Parenting, High Risk for Altered

Peripheral Neurovascular Dysfunction, High Risk for

Personal Identity Disturbance

Poisoning, High Risk for

Post-Trauma Response

Powerlessness

Protection, Altered

Rape-Trauma Syndrome

Rape-Trauma Syndrome: Compound Reaction

Rape-Trauma Syndrome: Silent

Role Performance, Altered

Self Care Deficit:
    Bathing/Hygiene
    Feeding
    Dressing/Grooming
    Toileting

Self Esteem, Chronic Low

Self Esteem Disturbance

Self Esteem, Situational Low

Self Mutilation, High Risk for

Sensory/Perceptual Alterations (Specify) (visual, auditory, kinesthetic, gustatory, tactile, olfactory)

Sexual Dysfunction

Sexuality Patterns, Altered

Skin Integrity, Impaired

Skin Integrity, High Risk for Impaired

Sleep Pattern Disturbance

Social Interaction, Impaired

Social Isolation

Spiritual Distress

Suffocation, High Risk for

Swallowing, Impaired

Therapeutic Regimen, Ineffective Management of (Individuals)

Thermoregulation, Ineffective

Thought Processes, Altered

Tissue Integrity, Impaired

Tissue Perfusion, Altered (Specify Type) (renal, cerebral, cardiopulmonary, gastrointestinal, peripheral)

Trauma, High Risk for

Unilateral Neglect

Urinary Elimination, Altered

Urinary Retention

Ventilation, Inability to Sustain Spontaneous

Ventilatory Weaning Response, Dysfunctional

Violence, High Risk for: Self-Directed or Directed at Others

▼ *Sorensen and Luckmann's*

▼ *Basic Nursing*

▼ *A Psychophysiologic Approach*

▼ *Third Edition*

▼ *Sorensen and Luckmann's*

▼ *Basic Nursing*

▼ *A Psychophysiologic Approach*

▼ *Third Edition*

VEROLYN BARNES BOLANDER, M.S., R.N.
Associate Professor
University of Texas Medical Branch School of Nursing
Galveston, Texas

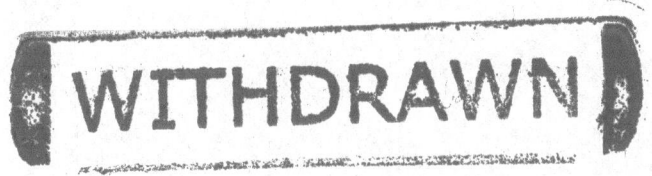

W.B. SAUNDERS COMPANY
A Division of Harcourt Brace & Company
Philadelphia London Toronto Montreal Sydney Tokyo

W.B. SAUNDERS COMPANY
A Division of Harcourt Brace & Company

The Curtis Center
Independence Square West
Philadelphia, Pennsylvania 19106

Library of Congress Cataloging-in-Publication Data

Sorensen and Luckmann's basic nursing : a psychophysiologic approach.
—3rd ed. / Verolyn Barnes Bolander [editor]
  p.   cm.
  Rev. ed. of: Basic nursing. [2nd ed. / edited by] Karen Creason
Sorensen, Joan Luckmann. 1986.
  Includes index.
  ISBN 0-7216-4013-3
  II. Sorensen, Karen Creason. III. Luckmann, Joan. IV. Basic nursing.
  [DNLM: 1. Nurse-Patient Relations. 2. Nursing Care. WY 100 S713 1994]
RT44.S594 1994
610.73—dc20
DNLM/DLC   93-21589

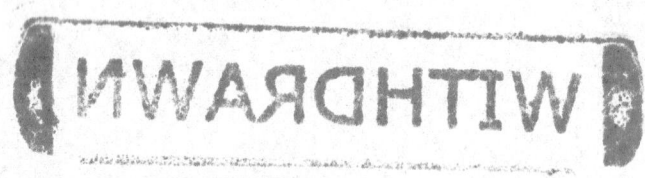
The editor and publisher gratefully acknowledge permission to reproduce the following photographs: Unit photograph for Unit 1 courtesy of The Alan Mason Chesney Medical Archives of The Johns Hopkins Medical Institutions; Unit photograph for Unit 4 from Jarvis, C. (1991). *Physical examination and health assessment*. Philadelphia: W. B. Saunders; Unit photographs for Units 6, 8, and 9 from Black, J. M., & Matassarin-Jacobs, E. (1993). *Luckmann and Sorensen's Medical-Surgical Nursing: A Psychophysiologic Approach* (4th Ed.). Philadelphia: W. B. Saunders.

SORENSEN AND LUCKMANN'S BASIC NURSING:
A PSYCHOPHYSIOLOGIC APPROACH   ISBN 0-7216-4013-3

Last digit is the print number: 9   8   7   6   5   4   3   2   1

For Aunt Pearl
Pearl Wehlan 1876–1953

▼ *Contributors*

Marsha Howell Adams, DSN, RN
Capstone College of Nursing
University of Alabama
Tuscaloosa, Alabama
Health Assessment
Assisting with Diagnostic Procedures

Elizabeth Arnold, PhD, RN, CS
University of Maryland
Baltimore, Maryland
Communication Within Groups

Verolyn Barnes Bolander, MS, RN
University of Texas Medical Branch
Galveston, Texas
Changing Concepts of Health, Disease,
and Health Care
Human Needs
Infection Control
Preventing Back Injury
Preventing Complications of Immobility
Meeting Mobility Needs

M. Eloise Boortz, RN,C, MS
Formerly University of Texas
Medical Branch
Galveston, Texas
Administering Medications
Administering Intravenous Therapy

Kay K. Chitty, EdD, RN
University of Tennessee at Chattanooga
Chattanooga, Tennessee
Delivery Systems, Finance, and Policy
in Health Care

Leslie Ann Clark, RN, MSN
University of California San Diego
Medical Center
San Diego, California
Facilitating Relief from Pain

Sherill Nones Cronin, PhD, RN,C
Bellarmine College
Louisville, Kentucky
Meeting Respiration Needs

Eleanor McElhenry Crowder, PhD, RN
The Pennsylvania State University
University Park, Pennsylvania
Historical Introduction to Nursing

Jeanette Daly, PhD, RN
Oaknoll Retirement Residence
Iowa City, Iowa
Meeting Bowel Elimination Needs

Barbara Dancy, RN, PhD
University of Illinois at Chicago
Chicago, Illinois
Culture and Ethnicity

Susan C. deWit, MSN, RNCS
El Centro College
Dallas, Texas
Promoting Hygiene

Diane C. Dodaro-Surrusco, MSN, RN
Mount Saint Mary College
Newburgh, New York
Meeting Urinary Elimination Needs

Kathleen M. Driscoll, MS, JD, RN
University of Cincinnati
Cincinnati, Ohio
Legal and Ethical Aspects of Nursing
Consumer Rights and Health Care Re-
sponsibilities

Michele J. Eliason, RN, PhD
University of Iowa
Iowa City, Iowa
Conception Through Childhood

Carol Diane Epstein, MSN, CS, CCRN
Case Western Reserve University
Cleveland, Ohio
Applying Research to Nursing
Practice Boxes

Marilyn Frenn, RN, PhD
Marquette University
Milwaukee, Wisconsin
Health Promotion in the Community

Susan Garnett-Nell, RN, MSN, CNOR
Harris Methodist Fort Worth
Fort Worth, Texas
Perioperative Nursing

Helen Harkreader, PhD, RN
Austin Community College
Austin, Texas
Providing Physical Protection and Body
Support

Linda F. Heffernan, RN, MSN, JD
Concordia–West Suburban College of
Nursing
Oak Park, Illinois
Assessing Vital Signs

Virginia Hopkins, RN, EdD
University of Texas Medical Branch
Galveston, Texas
Promoting Spiritual Health

Sharon S. Hudacek, RN, EdD, CS
University of Scranton
Scranton, Pennsylvania
Promoting Rest and Sleep

Patricia Iyer, RN, MSN, CNA
Patricia Iyer Associates and Med
League Support Services
Stockton, New Jersey
*The Nursing Process: The Basis for
Nursing Care*
Nursing Assessment
Nursing Diagnosis
Planning
Implementation
Evaluation

**Marguerite McMillan Jackson, RN,
MS, CIC, FAAN**
University of California San Diego
Medical Center
San Diego, California
Infection Control

Carolyn Jarvis, RN,C, MSN, FNP
Illinois Wesleyan University
Bloomington, Illinois
Assessing Vital Signs

Jennifer E. Jenkins, MBA, RN, CNAA
Vanderbilt University School of Nursing
Nashville, Tennessee
*Delivery Systems, Finance, and Policy
in Health Care*

Esperanza Villanueva Joyce, EdD, RN
University of Texas Health Sciences
Center
San Antonio, Texas
Stress and Adaptation

Laurel Kersten, RN, PhD
University of Colorado Health Sciences
Center
Denver, Colorado
Meeting Respiration Needs

Priscilla W. Koester, MSN, RN, CS
University of Texas Medical Branch
Galveston, Texas
Meeting Nutritional Needs

Carol Ann Lammon, RN, MSN, CS
University of Alabama
Tuscaloosa, Alabama
Health Assessment
Assisting with Diagnostic Procedures

Dorothy M. Lanuza, PhD, RN, FAAN
Loyola University Chicago
Chicago, Illinois
Homeostasis and Biologic Rhythms

Judith Kline Leavitt, RN, MEd, FAAN
Transformations
Ithaca, New York
*Delivery Systems, Finance, and Policy
in Health Care*

Susan Lewis, RN, CS, PhD
Department of Veterans Affairs
Medical Center
Louisville, Kentucky
Psychosocial Assessment

Barbara Bryan Logan, PhD, RN, FAAN
Clemson University
Clemson, South Carolina
Culture and Ethnicity

Patricia Lynch, RN, MBA
University of Washington
Seattle, Washington
Infection Control

Sally L. Maliski, RN, MS
University of North Carolina, Chapel Hill
Chapel Hill, North Carolina
Coping with Loss and Grief

Barbara G. Mason, EdD, RN,C
University of Texas Medical Branch
Galveston, Texas
Midlife Through Late Adulthood

Diana J. Mason, RN,C, PhD, FAAN
Beth Israel Medical Center
New York, New York
*Delivery Systems, Finance, and Policy
in Health Care*

Gail C. McCain, PhD, RN
Children's Hospital Medical Center
Cincinnati, Ohio
The Family

Noreen McDonough, RN, MSN
Southern Union State Junior College
Wadley, Alabama
Hospital Admission and Discharge

Anne M. McMahon, MSN, RN
Marquette University
Milwaukee, Wisconsin
Health Promotion in the Community

Delois Meyer, RN, MN, CCRN
William Jewell College
Liberty, Missouri
Meeting Sensory/Perceptual Needs

Carolyn O. Morse, RN, MSN, ONC
Austin Community College
Austin, Texas
*Providing Physical Protection and Body
Support*

Giovanna B. Morton, EdD, MSN, RN
Marshall University
Huntington, West Virginia
Psychosocial Assessment

Michele Nanchoff-Glatt, RN, MN
The University of Calgary
Calgary, Alberta
Enhancing Self-Concept

Bonita Ann Pilon, DSN, RN, CNAA
Vanderbilt University
Nashville, Tennessee
*Box 5–6. Comparisons Between the
Canadian and the United States Health
Care Systems*

Barbara C. Rynerson, MS, RN,C
University of North Carolina at Chapel
Hill
Chapel Hill, North Carolina
Promoting Sexual Health

Mary Lou Shannon, EdD, RN
University of Texas Medical Branch
Galveston, Texas
Caring for Persons with Wounds

Carol E. Smith, PhD, RN
University of Kansas
Kansas City, Kansas
Teaching and Learning

Claudia C. Straub, RN, MSN
Galveston College
Galveston, Texas
Cardiopulmonary Resuscitation

Mary Anne Sweeney, RN, PhD
University of Texas Medical Branch
Galveston, Texas
Documenting Care

Daria Virvan, RN, MSN, CS
Health Care for the Homeless
Washington, District of Columbia
*Therapeutic Communication: The
Nurse-Client Interaction*

Bernadette White, RN, MSN
University of Nebraska
Omaha, Nebraska
Maintaining Fluid and Electrolyte Balance

Jill E. Winland-Brown, EdD, RN
Florida Atlantic University
Boca Raton, Florida
Adolescence and Early Adulthood

Bonnie S. Worthington-Roberts, PhD
University of Washington
Seattle, Washington
Meeting Nutritional Needs

Deborah K. Zastocki, RN, MA, EdM
Fairleigh Dickinson University
Teaneck, New Jersey
Home Care Nursing

Nancy Bateman Zweig, EdD, RN, CS
Mount Saint Mary College
Newburgh, New York
Meeting Urinary Elimination Needs

▼ *Contributors*
to the Second Edition

Mary X. Britten, RN, EdD
Decker School of Nursing
SUNY-Binghamton
Binghamton, New York

Ruby Monson Englund, MN, RN
Seattle Pacific University
Seattle, Washington

Barbara Innes, RN, EdD
Seattle Pacific University
Seattle, Washington

Carol Sue Ivory-Carline, RN, MN, CRRN
Hospital Liaison Nurse
Group Health Cooperative of Puget Sound
Seattle, Washington

Rosemary Craig Kelly, BSN, RN, RRT, RCP
Sharp Memorial Hospital
San Diego, California

Margaret M. McMahon, RN, MN CEN
Clinical Director
Emergency Department
Tacoma General Hospital
Tacoma, Washington;
Clinical Instructor
University of Washington
Seattle, Washington

Laura M. Murphy, JD
Seattle, Washington

Sarah J. Sanford, RN, MA, CNAA, FAAN
Chief Executive Officer
American Association of Critical-Care Nurses
Aliso Viejo, California

R. Jack Stephenson, JD
Seattle, Washington

▼ *Reviewers*

Connie Austin, RN, MAEd, MSN
School of Nursing
Azusa Pacific University
Azusa, California

Diane M. Black, RN, MS
South Suburban College
South Holland, Illinois

Eileen E. Bolcer, MSN, RN
Schoolcraft College
Livonia, Michigan

Dianne M. Booth, RN, MSN
Golden West College
Huntington Beach, California

Eleanor F. Brown, MSN, RN, C
Macon College
Macon, Georgia

Carole Broxson, RN, PhD
Sinclair Community College
Dayton, Ohio

Paula A. Bugay, MSN, RN, CS
Del Mar College
Corpus Christi, Texas

Filomena Cañalita-Flores, RN, PhD
California State University, Fresno
Fresno, California

Madolyn J. Cutter, MS, RN
Texas Woman's University
Denton, Texas

Mary de Meneses, RN, EdD
Southern Illinois University at
Edwardsville
School of Nursing
Edwardsville, Illinois

Julia C. Dent, BSN, MEd, EdS
Brunswick College
Brunswick, Georgia

Katherine H. Dimmock, EdD, MSN, RN
Indianapolis, Indiana

Patricia Ann Durham-Taylor, RN, MSN, EdS
Truckee Meadows Community College
Saint Mary's Hospital
Reno, Nevada

Sandi Emerson, RN, MSN
Truckee Meadows Community College
Reno, Nevada

Jane H. Freeman, EdD, RN
Jacksonville State University
College of Nursing
Jacksonville, Alabama

Mary Dolores Garcia, PhD, RN, C
Del Mar College
Corpus Christi, Texas

R. Aurora Garcia, RN, MSN
San Antonio College
San Antonio, Texas

Dickie H. Gerig, RN, MS
Grayson County College
Denison, Texas

Patricia E. Green, RN, MSN, MA
Victor Valley Community College
Victorville, California

Edythe (Lyn) Greenberg, PhD, RN, FNP
University of Texas Health Science
Center, Houston
School of Nursing
Houston, Texas

Milly Gutkoski, MN, RN, C
Montana State University
College of Nursing
Bozeman, Montana

J. Taylor Harden, PhD, RN, C
School of Nursing
University of Texas Health Science
Center at San Antonio
San Antonio, Texas

Carol J. Higashi, MSN, EdD, RN
San Joaquin Delta College
Stockton, California

Doris Hoerdeman, RN, MSN
The Methodist Medical Center of Illinois
School of Nursing
Peoria, Illinois

Sue Holcomb, RN, BA, MEd
Retired, Angelina College
Lufkin, Texas

Dorothy N. Holley, RN, MSN
Baltimore City Community College
Baltimore, Maryland

▼ *Foreword*

It is a great honor to be asked to write the Foreword to *Sorensen and Luckmann's Basic Nursing: A Psychophysiologic Approach*, third edition. As I reviewed the outline and content for the new *Basic Nursing*, I was pleased and impressed by the excellent changes that Verolyn Bolander has made in the book's overall organization and format. Aspects of Bolander's new edition that I particularly like are:

▶ The breakdown of the book into two major parts: "Concepts Basic to Nursing" and "Skills Basic to Nursing."
▶ The addition of individual chapters on the family, culture and ethnicity, health promotion in the community, hospital admission and discharge, home care nursing, communication within groups, documenting care, preventing back injury, and assisting with diagnostic procedures.
▶ The allocation of an entire unit to the nursing process, and a separate chapter corresponding to each step of the nursing process.
▶ The development of a new unit, "Applying Nursing Skills to Meet Psychosocial Needs."

It was 1975—almost two decades ago—when Karen Sorensen and I started writing the *first* edition of *Basic Nursing: A Psychophysiologic Approach*. At that time, the learning needs of nursing students were quite different from the needs of students today. Although nursing students have always faced tremendous challenges, students in the 1990s are required to be more knowledgeable and sophisticated than were students in the past.

Currently, it is not enough for students to simply learn the basics of nursing. Students must now grasp the many complex physiologic and psychosocial concepts that support those basics. Today it is not enough for students to just talk to clients. Students must now communicate therapeutically with people from different cultures, different lifestyles, different religions, and different ethnic backgrounds. They must master the skills involved in research and documentation, in teaching and leadership. They must learn how to give quality care in hospitals and in homes, in crowded cities and in the wilderness.

The third edition of *Sorensen and Luckmann's Basic Nursing* is constructed to teach students *what they must know* to successfully practice nursing in the 1990s. I want to thank Verolyn Barnes Bolander for undertaking the difficult task of revising *Sorensen and Luckmann's Basic Nursing*. I want to thank her for preparing a revision that will help nursing students, instructors, and graduates give comprehensive care to people with complex needs and problems. Finally, I want to express my gratitude that the revised *Sorensen and Luckmann's Basic Nursing* is now available to teach future generations of nurses, and to guide them in their quest for knowledge, skill, and excellence.

JOAN LUCKMANN, RN, MA

▼ *Preface*

Many years ago, when I initially picked up Luckmann and Sorensen's first medical-surgical nursing text, I was enchanted by a book that presented nursing in a way that no other text had. I enjoyed reading it and went on to enjoy their first basic nursing text and then the second edition of that text. Ultimately, I used all of their editions, at one time or another, to teach students in an associate degree nursing program, a generic baccalaureate program, and an RN-to-BSN program. As a part of different teaching teams, I have attempted to use other texts at various times but have always returned to the authoring team that first showed me that *reading about* nursing can sometimes be as exciting and wonderful as *doing* nursing.

When I picked up that original book, I could never have foreseen that I might one day edit a text that those authors had written. Attempting to follow in their footsteps has been an unforgettable challenge. As this book goes to press, I can only hope that the third edition of *Sorensen and Luckmann's Basic Nursing: A Psychophysiologic Approach* is appreciated by the students of today as much as the earlier editions were enjoyed by the students of previous years.

The intent of the third edition is to continue to present basic nursing information with a strong emphasis on the psychophysiologic aspects of the client of nursing. To strengthen this content, material has been added to help to prepare the beginning nursing student for a career that will hardly be started as we enter the 21st century. New content in this edition reflects the fact that the nurse provides increasingly complex care for groups of clients as well as for individuals, and that the nurse is carrying out the work of nursing in the home and in agencies other than the hospital.

Organization

The text is organized into two parts: a discussion of concepts and a discussion of skills. Concepts presented include those important to an understanding of the nursing profession: the nursing process; normal human growth and development; characteristics of individuals, families, and groups; and health and illness in various health care settings. Skills are divided into those required for communication; those required of anyone prior to working in a health care setting (infection control, preventing back injury, and CPR); those used for assessment; and those used for intervention in biologic and psychosocial problems.

Content Changes

Much of the content from the second edition has been rearranged, and some chapters and sections of chapters have been combined. Of course, this edition has been completely updated to thoroughly integrate the very latest in NANDA diagnoses and CDC guidelines. Also included are the latest nutritional requirements, CPR guidelines, ethical codes, AHCPR pressure ulcer guidelines, and other standards and guidelines that affect the daily practice of professional nurses. Some of the new material presented in this edition includes the following:

▶ Expanded coverage of nursing history.
▶ Expanded coverage of the nursing process, including an entire unit devoted to the nursing process with one chapter covering each step. Additionally, wherever pertinent following the nursing process chapters, the steps of the nursing process are thoroughly integrated in each chapter. Much attention is devoted throughout the text to discussions of the appropriate use of nursing diagnoses, according to the latest North American Nursing Diagnosis Association (NANDA) taxonomy.
▶ Expanded coverage of growth and development from two chapters in the second edition to three chapters in the current edition.

- New chapters on the family and on culture and ethnicity.
- A new chapter on health promotion in the community that introduces the reader to the concepts of health promotion and to the community as a health care setting before introducing the student to the experience of illness and to the hospital setting.
- A new chapter on hospital admission and discharge planning that draws together the client and the nurse in the hospital setting. This chapter is designed to introduce the reader to the hospital setting just as the new client would be introduced to it. It orients the reader to the hospital layout, to the way nursing care is organized in the hospital setting, and to the nursing unit, with its furniture and accessories.
- A new chapter on home care nursing that follows the client, after discharge from care in a centralized agency, to care in the home.
- A new chapter on communication within groups that separates out and expands material that had previously been a part of the chapter on therapeutic interaction.
- A new chapter on documenting care that has drawn together and updated material that had been spread throughout several chapters in the second edition. This chapter also contains guidelines for verbal reporting (such as end-of-shift reporting) and verbal communication over the telephone.
- A new chapter that focuses on prevention of nurse back injury. This is not merely the "body mechanics" material that is common to all fundamentals texts. It is material that is separated out in order to focus on the prevention of injury to the nurse's back, because this is material that is now the focus of much in-service education and orientation training in hospitals. Owing to the large number of back injuries each year, it is material that many hospitals insist their employees and students master before they are allowed to practice within the agency.
- A completely updated cardiopulmonary resuscitation chapter that conforms to the latest American Heart Association guidelines.
- A new chapter on assisting with diagnostic procedures.
- New chapters on enhancing self-concept, promoting sexual health, and promoting spiritual health that have been added to a new unit on applying nursing skills to meet psychosocial needs.

Approaches

Major theories and models continue to be presented throughout the discussions of nursing concepts.

Skills are presented in the order in which they are likely to be encountered in a real hospital situation. That is, they begin in the hospital setting, with the client who is very sick and who cannot even move without help, and teach the reader how to safely position and move the person. The next skills chapter discusses how to help the client to get up and move (with

and without ambulation aids) and includes methods to help the client regain full vigor with the use of strenuous exercise. The following chapter covers special cases in which clients or their body tissues require special protection and support measures, including the use of restraints. Having mastered the care of clients at all levels of physical ability and mobility, the student is ready to provide nursing care to clients at all these levels. Hygiene care is presented, followed by skills that promote rest and sleep; relieve pain; and meet needs for nutrition, fluid and electrolytes, bowel and urinary elimination, and respiration.

Following these general chapters, specific interventions are reviewed, including those in chapters on administering medications and administering IV therapy. Many of the skills discussed earlier are needed for an understanding of the two chapters that discuss care of persons with wounds and perioperative nursing care. Finally, five chapters present skills that help meet higher level, psychosocial needs.

Features

Readers will appreciate the continued use of the highlight boxes that were first used by Sorensen and Luckmann to signal especially important information. Highlighted material now appears in color. Readers will also be able to rely on the continued inclusion of scientific principles to help in understanding and to guide practice.

What were called *Interventions* in earlier editions are now termed *Procedures* as a means of signaling that these nursing behaviors are only a few of the interventions that nurses provide. Included among the book's *Procedures* are 36 step-by-step, numbered Procedures, with a scientific rationale or comment included for each step. Approximately 35 variations in these procedures are also provided. More than 120 additional procedures are described in the text narrative, and over 20 additional procedures are depicted in Figures and Boxes.

Newly added features include:

- The use of color to highlight important information in illustrations.
- A glossary.
- A set of broadly worded objectives that serve to provide a brief overview of the content in each chapter.
- A list of **Key Terms** for each chapter, with the use of boldface print to highlight these terms when they are defined in the text and to indicate that they are also defined in the new glossary.
- Detailed discussion of nursing diagnoses in special **Nursing Diagnosis Profiles** throughout the text to assist the reader in making a differential diagnosis.
- Ten new **Scientific Principles and Related Nursing Interventions** tables that appear in selected clinically oriented chapters.
- **Case Studies** in each clinically oriented chapter to show application of the nursing process to the material in the chapter.

▶ **Applying Research to Nursing Practice** boxes in selected chapters.

▶ Summaries of the main points in all chapters.

Terminology

In keeping with the original authors' abiding respect for the person, this edition has continued to refer to the individual served by the nurse as a person, individual, or client except where historical references or citations from other sources demanded use of the term "patient." Likewise, use of sexist terminology has been avoided, even when doing so has led to the awkward "his/her" construction. When extensive use of "he/she" would have made the material too difficult to follow, such as in certain procedures, the nurse was sometimes referred to as "he" and the client as "she," and at other times these pronouns were reversed.

Teaching and Learning Package

With this Third Edition, *Basic Nursing: A Psychophysiologic Approach* is accompanied for the first time with a full ancillary package to assist students and instructors.

▶ **Instructor's Manual.** To help instructors use a variety of teaching methods, a brand new Instructor's Manual includes both direct and indirect teaching strategies, the latter intended to develop student's critical thinking skills. Group activities, paper assignments, suggestions for clinical assignments, and resource referrals are also included in the Instructor's Manual. In addition, the Instructor's Manual contains a testbank of over 700 items (with correct answers and rationale) and the answers, with discussion, to the case studies from the Student Study Guide.

▶ **Student Study Guide.** More than just a workbook, the Student Study Guide (making its debut with this edition of *Basic Nursing*) helps engage the student in learning more than just the "facts" about nursing. A variety of learning exercises will help the student not only to absorb and prioritize the appropriate information but also to begin to apply it to different situations. In particular, client case studies are included for each clinical chapter of the textbook. Answers for the case studies are given in the Instructor's Manual; all other answers are provided in the Student Study Guide itself, so students can quickly check their responses. The Student Study Guide begins with an extremely helpful discussion of study skills and test-taking strategies. Critical thinking, focused relaxation, and sample test questions with explanatory strategies will help students improve their learning for this and all their other course work in nursing.

▶ **Performance Checklists.** Checklists for over 150 skills that are presented in this edition of *Basic Nursing* are provided in a separate book for sale to students. These checklists do not simply repeat the steps of a skill but identify the critical behaviors that would be evaluated to determine safe and proficient execution of the skill.

▶ **Transparencies.** The transparency set includes 100 color and black-and-white acetate transparencies for classroom projection. These were selected by practicing fundamentals instructors for the usefulness of their content in classroom teaching. The set also includes over 50 masters ready for you to create transparencies at your own discretion. The Transparencies for *Basic Nursing, 3rd Edition* are available to adopters of the textbook.

▶ **Computerized Testbank.** The testbank printed in the Instructor's Manual is also available on W. B. Saunders Company's propriety software, ExaMaster. As with the transparencies, the computerized testbank is available only to adopters of the textbook.

VEROLYN BARNES BOLANDER

▼ Acknowledgments

I owe my deepest gratitude to those closest to me, for all they have done to help throughout the long process of completing this text. My profound thanks goes to Gary Mills for helping the most for the longest period of time and in too many ways to enumerate; to my son Jeffery David Bolander for his patience and understanding the many times I could not be there for him; to my son John Dunay Bolander for his unforgettable acceptance when I could not be there for him on the one, all-important day he asked for; to my sister, Terryl Paiste, for helping to sustain me with her editorial guidance, rare wit, broad shoulders, and timely personal advice; to my mother, Hazel Barnes, for bearing with me on the far too many occasions when she missed something because I could not take her to it while she, so many times, readily dropped everything she was doing in order to help me find a needed reference; and to my friend Virginia Hopkins, who was there encouraging me through thick and thin.

My sincere appreciation also goes to the administration and my teaching colleagues at the School of Nursing at The University of Texas Medical Branch, especially to my Department chairperson and mentor, Phyllis Kritek, and my Co-Lead Teacher, David Crowther; to the administration and my nursing peers at Baywood Hospital; to the reviewers of and contributors to this edition, their significant others, and their secretarial assistants; to Yvette Viator, who typed much of the manuscript; to my students past and present, who taught me what it is that nursing students want to know; to Marilyn Bradley, who never let me forget how to laugh; to those who contributed photographs and other work to this edition; and to the reference librarians Mary Vaughn and Alex Bienkowski, who provided ready assistance at the Moody Medical Library.

Very special recognition is due to Karen Creason Sorensen and Joan Luckmann and to the editors and staff of W. B. Saunders Company, without whom this edition could never have been.

VEROLYN BARNES BOLANDER

▼ *Contents in Brief*

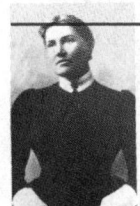

Part I   CONCEPTS BASIC TO NURSING, 1

Unit 1
The Evolving Profession of Nursing   3

Chapter 1
Historical Introduction to Nursing   5
Eleanor L. M. Crowder

Chapter 2
Changing Concepts of Health, Disease, and Health Care   25
Verolyn Barnes Bolander

Chapter 3
Legal and Ethical Aspects of Nursing   43
Kathleen Driscoll

Chapter 4
Consumer Rights and Health Care Responsibilities   65
Kathleen Driscoll

Chapter 5
Delivery Systems, Finance, and Policy in Health Care   87
Jennifer E. Jenkins, Kay K. Chitty, Diana J. Mason, and Judith Leavitt

Unit 2
The Nursing Process   107

Chapter 6
The Nursing Process: The Basis for Nursing Care   109
Patricia W. Iyer

Chapter 7
Nursing Assessment   117
Patricia W. Iyer

Chapter 8
Nursing Diagnosis   129
Patricia W. Iyer

Chapter 9
Planning   143
Patricia W. Iyer

Chapter 10
Implementation   157
Patricia W. Iyer

Chapter 11
Evaluation   165
Patricia W. Iyer

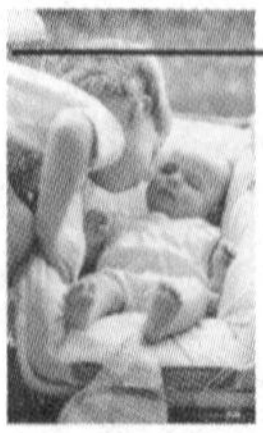

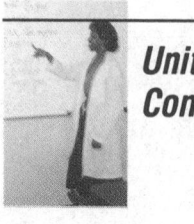

Unit 3
Growth and Development   175

Chapter 12
Conception Through Childhood   177
Michele Eliason

Chapter 13
Adolescence and Early Adulthood   209
Jill Elizabeth Winland-Brown

Chapter 14
Midlife Through Late Adulthood   227
Barbara G. Mason

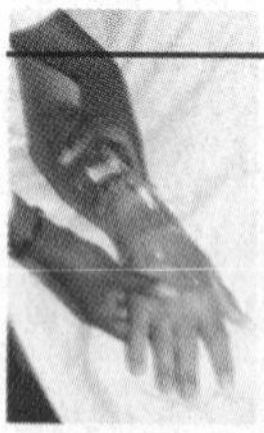

Unit 4
Characteristics of Persons
Served by the Nurse   247

Chapter 15
Human Needs   249
Verolyn Barnes Bolander

Chapter 16
Stress and Adaptation   267
Esperanza Villanueva Joyce

Chapter 17
Homeostasis and Biologic Rhythms   299
Dorothy M. Lanuza

Chapter 18
The Family   321
Gail C. McCain

Chapter 19
Culture and Ethnicity   331
Barbara Dancy and Barbara Logan

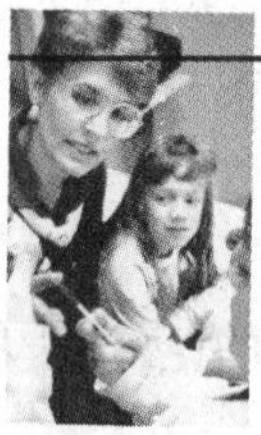

Unit 5
Health, Illness, and Health Care
Settings   343

Chapter 20
Health Promotion in the Community   345
Marilyn Frenn and Anne McMahon

Chapter 21
The Illness Experience   363

Chapter 22
Hospital Admission and Discharge   381
Noreen McDonough

Chapter 23
Home Care Nursing   399
Deborah Zastocki

Part II   SKILLS BASIC TO NURSING, 417

Unit 6
Communication Skills   419

Chapter 24
Therapeutic Communication: The Nurse-Client
Interaction   421
Daria Virvan

Chapter 25
Communication Within Groups   451
Elizabeth Arnold

Chapter 26
Teaching and Learning   467
Carol E. Smith

Chapter 27
Documenting Care   483
Mary Anne Sweeney

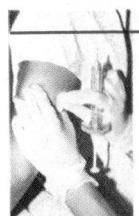

Unit 7
Skills Required for Safe Practice
503

Chapter 28
Infection Control 505
Marguerite M. Jackson, Patricia I. Lynch, and Verolyn Barnes Bolander

Chapter 29
Preventing Back Injury 539
Verolyn Barnes Bolander

Chapter 30
Cardiopulmonary Resuscitation 555
Claudia C. Straub

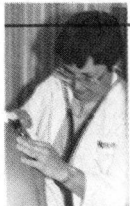

Unit 8
Assessment Skills
583

Chapter 31
Assessing Vital Signs 585
Carolyn M. Jarvis and Linda Heffernan

Chapter 32
Psychosocial Assessment 627
Susan Lewis and Giovanna B. Morton

Chapter 33
Health Assessment 649
Marsha Adams and Carol Lammon

Chapter 34
Assisting with Diagnostic Procedures 703
Carol Lammon and Marsha Adams

Unit 9
Therapeutic Skills
727

Chapter 35
Preventing Complications of Immobility 729
Verolyn Barnes Bolander

Chapter 36
Meeting Mobility Needs 805
Verolyn Barnes Bolander

Chapter 37
Providing Physical Protection and Body Support 847
Carolyn Morse and Helen Harkreader

Chapter 38
Promoting Hygiene 891
Susan C. deWit

Chapter 39
Promoting Rest and Sleep 947
Sharon S. Hudacek

Chapter 40
Facilitating Relief From Pain 967
Leslie Ann Clark

Chapter 41
Maintaining Fluid and Electrolyte Balance 999
Bernadette White

Chapter 42
Meeting Nutritional Needs 1049
Bonnie S. Worthington-Roberts and Priscilla W. Koester

Chapter 43
Meeting Bowel Elimination Needs 1125
Jeanette Daly

Chapter 44
Meeting Urinary Elimination Needs 1155
Diane Dodaro-Surrusco and Nancy Zweig

Chapter 45
Meeting Respiration Needs 1203
Laurel Kersten and Sherill Nones Cronin

Chapter 46
Administering Medications 1255
M. Eloise Boortz

Chapter 47
Administering Intravenous Therapy 1307
M. Eloise Boortz

Chapter 48
Caring for Persons with Wounds   1335
Mary Lou Shannon

Chapter 49
Perioperative Nursing   1403
Susan Garnett-Nell

Unit 10
Applying Nursing Skills to Meet Psychosocial Needs   1445

Chapter 50
Enhancing Self-Concept   1447
Michele Nanchoff-Glatt

Chapter 51
Meeting Sensory/Perceptual Needs   1469
Delois Meyer

Chapter 52
Promoting Sexual Health   1487
Barbara Rynerson

Chapter 53
Promoting Spiritual Health   1509
Virginia L. Hopkins

Chapter 54
Coping with Loss and Grief   1533
Sally Maliski

Appendix 1
Universal Precautions   1559

Appendix 2
American Nurses' Association Standards of Clinical Nursing Practice   1560

Appendix 3
Nursing's Agenda for Health Care Reform   1562

Glossary   1571

Index   1599

▼ *Contents in Detail*

Part I   CONCEPTS BASIC TO NURSING, 1

Unit 1
The Evolving Profession of Nursing   3

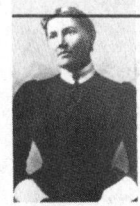

Chapter 1
Historical Introduction to Nursing   5

The Evolving Definition of Nursing   6

Nightingale's Definition of Nursing, 6 ▼ Henderson's Definition of Nursing, 7 ▼ American Nurses' Association's Definition of Nursing, 7 ▼ Canadian Nurses Association's Definition of Nursing, 7

The Image of Nursing   7

Nursing and the Image of Women, 7 ▼ Nursing and Religious Orders, 9 ▼ The Image of Contemporary Nursing, 10

Nursing Practice   10

Early Development of Nurses' Roles, 10 ▼ Major Settings for Contemporary Nursing Practice, 10 ▼ Clinical Specialization, 13 ▼ Standards of Nursing Practice, 14 ▼ Patients/Clients/Consumers, 15

Nursing Education   15

Early Schools, 15 ▼ Wars and Changing Patterns of Nursing Education, 16

The Nursing Profession   18

Early Collaborative Efforts of Nurses, 18 ▼ Developing a

Professional Career, 18 ▼ Expanded Roles for Nurses, 19 ▼ Professional Organizations, 21

Chapter 2
Changing Concepts of Health, Disease, and Health Care   25

Health and Disease: Changing Definitions and Viewpoints   26

The Problem of Defining Health and Disease, 26 ▼ Models of Disease and Health, 27

Concepts of Health Promotion and Disease Prevention   30

Prevention, 30 ▼ Health Promotion Versus Disease Prevention, 31

Therapeutic Activities   31

Primary Prevention Activities, 32 ▼ Secondary Prevention Activities, 34 ▼ Tertiary Prevention (Rehabilitation) Activities, 37 ▼ Health Promotion Activities, 39

Chapter 3
Legal and Ethical Aspects of Nursing   43

Ethics, Morals, and Values   44

Types of Ethical Theories, 44 ▼ Ethical Principles, 46 ▼ Codes of Ethics, 47 ▼ Ethical Decision Making in Nursing, 48

Law and Its Sources   48

Constitutional Law, 49 ▼ Case Law, 50 ▼ Statutory Law, 50 ▼ Administrative Law, 51

Types of Law   51

Civil and Criminal Law, 51 ▼ Procedural and
Substantive Law, 51 ▼ Tort Law, 52 ▼ Contract Law,
57 ▼ Licensure Laws, 59

What is Good?   61

Chapter 4
Consumer Rights and Health Care Responsibilities   65

The Nature of Rights and Responsibilities   66

**Statutory and Professional Statements of Health Care
Consumer Rights   67**

**Consumer Rights, Health Care Provider
Responsibilities, and Personal Choice   68**

Informed Consent, 70 ▼ Forgoing Life-Sustaining
Measures, 74 ▼ Reproductive Rights, 76

**Consumer Rights and Health Care Provider
Responsibilities in Health Care Facilities   77**

Long-Term Care Facilities, 77 ▼ Facilities for the
Mentally Ill and Developmentally Disabled, 78

**Consumer Rights, Health Care Provider
Responsibilities, and Health Care Resources   81**

Organ Transplantation, 81 ▼ Access to Health Care, 84

Chapter 5
Delivery Systems, Finance, and Policy in Health Care   87

Health Care Delivery Systems   88

Types of Health Care Services, 88 ▼ Health Care
Agencies and Personnel, 89

Health Care Finance   95

The Price of Health Care, 95 ▼ Methods of Payment for
Health Care, 96 ▼ Cost Containment, 97 ▼ The
Economics of Nursing Care, 98

Health Care Policy and Politics   99

Policy Defined, 99 ▼ Politics Defined, 103 ▼ Politics,
Policy, and Values, 104 ▼ Spheres of Political Action,
104

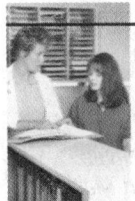

Unit 2
The Nursing Process   107

Chapter 6
The Nursing Process: The Basis for Nursing Care   109

The Five Steps of the Nursing Process   110

Assessment, 110 ▼ Diagnosis, 110 ▼ Planning,
110 ▼ Implementation, 111 ▼ Evaluation, 111

Attributes of the Nursing Process   112

A Systematic Approach, 112 ▼ Interrelated and Fluid
Steps, 112 ▼ A Person-Centered Process,
113 ▼ Emphasize Feedback, 113 ▼ Facilitates
Creativity, 113 ▼ The Foundation of Nursing
Practice, 113

Problem Solving and the Scientific Method   113

Unlearned Problem Solving, 113 ▼ Trial-and-Error
Problem Solving, 113 ▼ The Scientific Method of
Problem Solving, 113

**The Modified Scientific Method Used by Health Care
Professionals   113**

Chapter 7
Nursing Assessment   117

Definition, Purpose, and Data Sources   118

Typical Data Base, 118 ▼ Data Gathering, 119 ▼
Subjective and Objective Data, 119 ▼ Sources of Data,
119 ▼ Confidentiality of Data, 120

**Factors That Influence the Nature of the Data
Base   120**

Urgency of the Situation, 120 ▼ Nurse's Knowledge
and Skills, 121 ▼ Perspective of the Nurse, 121

Methods of Assessment   121

Review of the Clinical Record, 121 ▼ Interview,
121 ▼ Nursing History, 121 ▼ Physical Assessment,
122 ▼ Formats for the History and Physical
Examination, 122 ▼ Psychosocial Assessment,
126 ▼ Consultation, 126 ▼ Review of the
Literature, 126

Chapter 8
Nursing Diagnosis   129

Nursing Diagnosis Defined and Explored   130

The Diagnostic Process   130

Step One: Analysis and Interpretation, 131 ▼ Step Two:
Making and Validating Inferences, 131 ▼ Step Three:
Comparing Cues and Clusters of Cues with Defining
Characteristics, 131 ▼ Step Four: Identifying the
Related Factors, 131 ▼ Step Five: Documenting the
Nursing Diagnosis, 132

Human Response Patterns   132

Functional Health Patterns   134

**Documentation of the Actual Nursing
Diagnosis   134**

Variations of the Diagnostic Statement **136**

Guidelines for Writing an Actual Nursing Diagnosis **138**

Write the Diagnosis in Terms of the Person's Response Rather than Nursing Need, 138 ▼ Use "Related to" Rather than "Due to" or "Caused by" to Connect the Two Parts of the Statement, 138 ▼ Write the Diagnosis in Legally Advisable Terms, 138 ▼ Write the Diagnosis Without Value Judgements, 138 ▼ Avoid Reversing the Parts of the Statement, 138 ▼ Avoid Using Single Cues in the First Part of the Statement, 139 ▼ The Two Parts of the Statement Should Not Mean the Same Thing, 139 ▼ Express the Related Factor in Terms that Can Be Changed, 139 ▼ Do Not Include Medical Diagnoses in the Nursing Diagnostic Statement, 139 ▼ State the Diagnosis Clearly and Concisely, 140

Collaborative Problems **140**

Implications of Nursing Diagnoses **141**

Legal Aspects of a Nursing Diagnosis, 141 ▼ Critical Thinking and Errors in the Diagnostic Process, 141 ▼ Implications of Nursing Diagnosis for Nursing Practice, 141

Chapter 9
Planning   *143*

Setting Priorities **144**

High-Priority Nursing Diagnoses, 144 ▼ Medium-Priority Nursing Diagnoses, 144 ▼ Low-Priority Nursing Diagnoses, 144 ▼ Mutual Negotiation of Priorities, 145

Developing Specific Outcomes **145**

Verification of Outcomes, 145 ▼ Realistic Outcomes, 145 ▼ Acceptable Outcomes, 146 ▼ Consistent Outcomes, 146

Setting Time Frames **146**

Identifying Interventions **146**

Types of Nursing Interventions, 146 ▼ Characteristics of Nursing Interventions, 147

The Nursing Care Plan **147**

Student Nursing Care Plans, 148 ▼ Individually Developed Nursing Care Plans, 148 ▼ Standardized Nursing Care Plans, 148 ▼ Teaching Plans, 151 ▼ Practice Guidelines, 151 ▼ Case Management Care Plans, 151 ▼ Computerized Nursing Care Plans, 154

Chapter 10
Implementation   *157*

Skills Used During Implementation of Nursing Care **158**

Cognitive Skills, 158 ▼ Interpersonal Skills, 158 ▼ Technical Skills, 158

Responsibilities in Implementation of Nursing Care **158**

Reviewing the Planned Interventions for Appropriateness, 159 ▼ Scheduling and Organizing the Interventions, 162 ▼ Collaborating with Other Team Members, 162 ▼ Supervising and Delegating Nursing Care by Other Members of the Nursing Team, 162 ▼ Providing Direct Nursing Care, 162 ▼ Providing Counseling, 163 ▼ Involving the Client in Health Care, 163 ▼ Teaching the Client and Family, 163 ▼ Making Referrals to Other Health Care Professionals, 163 ▼ Documentating Nursing Care Provided, 163

Chapter 11
Evaluation   *165*

Definitions and Purposes of Evaluation **166**

Steps in the Evaluation Process **166**

Step 1: Refer to the Client's Planned Outcomes, 166 ▼ Step 2: Evaluate the Client's Condition and Compare Actual Outcomes with Expected Outcomes, 166 ▼ Step 3: Summarize the Results of the Evaluation, 169 ▼ Step 4: Identify Reasons for Client's Failure, If Indicated, to Achieve Expected Outcomes, 169 ▼ Step 5: Take Corrective Action to Modify the Plan of Care as Necessary, 169 ▼ Step 6: Document the Evaluation of the Client's Achievement of Outcomes and the Modification, If Any, of the Plan of Care, 169

Evaluation: Additional Applications **170**

Malpractice Suits, 170 ▼ Performance Evaluations, 171 ▼ Nursing Research, 171 ▼ Quality Improvement, 171

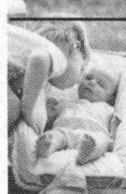

Unit 3
Growth and Development   *175*

Chapter 12
Conception Through Childhood   *177*

Principles of Growth and Development **179**

Major Principles of Physiologic Growth and Development **180**

Normal Physiologic Development Proceeds in Three Directions, 180 ▼ Physiologic Growth and Development Occur in a Predictable Pattern, 181 ▼ Processes of Physiologic Development Occur in a Predictable Sequence, 181 ▼ Physiologic Growth and Development Occur When "Readiness" Has Been Reached, 181 ▼ Physiologic Development Is the Result of a Combination of Maturational and Learning Factors, 181 ▼ Each Stage of Physiologic Development Is

Different from the One Before, 181 ▼ Each State of Physiologic Development Depends on Growth in Previous Stages, 181

Physiologic Systems that Regulate Growth and Development   181

Regulation of Growth and Development by Genetic Inheritance, 181 ▼ Regulation of Growth and Development by the Nervous System, 182 ▼ Regulation of Growth and Development by the Endocrine System, 182

Interactional Factors that Influence Development   182

Adaptation, 182 ▼ Motivation, 182 ▼ Learning and Socialization, 182 ▼ Individual Differences, 184

Psychosocial Theories of Human Development   184

Contributors to Psychodynamic Theories, 185 ▼ Contributors to Cognitive Theories, 186 ▼ Contributors to Behavioral Theories, 189 ▼ Summary of Psychosocial Theories of Human Development, 190

Conception Through Childhood   190

Prenatal Period   190

Conception, 190 ▼ Germinal Stage of Development, 190 ▼ Embryonic Stage of Development, 191 ▼ Fetal Stage of Development, 191 ▼ Major Health Concerns, 191 ▼ Role of the Nurse, 191

Neonatal Period   192

Physical Development and Change, 192 ▼ Head and Body, 192 ▼ Reflexes, 193 ▼ Care of the Newborn Infant, 193 ▼ Psychosocial Development, 194 ▼ Self-Concept and Self-Image, 194 ▼ Cognitive and Intellectual Development, 194 ▼ Communication, 194 ▼ Relationships and Roles, 194 ▼ Bonding and Family Relationships, 194 ▼ Establishing Trust, 194 ▼ Values and Beliefs, 195 ▼ Major Health Concerns, 195 ▼ Role of the Nurse, 195 ▼ Apgar Scale, 195 ▼ Brazelton Neonatal Behavior Assessment Scale, 195

Infancy   196

Physical Development and Change, 196 ▼ Psychosocial Development, 196 ▼ Self-Concept and Self-Image, 196 ▼ Cognitive and Intellectual Development, 196 ▼ Communication, 196 ▼ Relationships and Roles, 197 ▼ Expressing Emotions, 197 ▼ Establishing Trust, 197 ▼ Values and Beliefs, 198 ▼ Major Health Concerns, 198 ▼ Role of the Nurse, 198

Early Childhood   198

Physical Development and Change, 199 ▼ Weight Gain, 199 ▼ Sleep, 199 ▼ Motor Skills, 199 ▼ Eating Patterns, 199 ▼ Developing Toilet Independence, 199 ▼ Psychosocial Development, 199 ▼ Self-Concept and Self-Image, 199 ▼ Cognitive and Intellectual Development, 200 ▼ Communication, 200 ▼ Play, 200 ▼ Developing Autonomy, 200 ▼ Developing Initiative, 201 ▼ Developing Self-Control, 201 ▼ Values and Beliefs, 201 ▼ Major Health Concerns, 201 ▼ Role of the Nurse, 202 ▼ Health Screening and Assessment, 202 ▼ Health Education, 202

School Age   202

Physical Development and Change, 203 ▼ Physical Growth Patterns, 203 ▼ Eating Patterns and Sleep, 203 ▼ Psychosocial Development, 203 ▼ Self-Concept and Self-Image, 203 ▼ Cognitive and Intellectual Development, 203 ▼ Communication, 203 ▼ Relationships and Roles, 204 ▼ Family Relationships, 204 ▼ Sibling Relationships, 204 ▼ Peer Relationships, 204 ▼ Values and Beliefs, 204 ▼ Major Health Concerns, 204 ▼ Role of the Nurse, 204 ▼ Health Screening and Assessment, 204 ▼ Health Education, 205

Child Abuse   205

Risk Factors for Child Abuse, 206 ▼ Age, 206 ▼ Sex, 206 ▼ Family Size, 206 ▼ Family Intactness, 206 ▼ Childhood Sexual Abuse, 206

Chapter 13
Adolescence and Early Adulthood   209

Adolescence   210

Physical Development and Change   210

Musculoskeletal Changes, 210 ▼ Reproductive Changes, 211

Psychosexual Development   211

Psychosocial Development   211

Self-Concept and Self-Image, 211 ▼ Cognitive and Intellectual Development, 212 ▼ Relationships and Roles, 212

Values and Beliefs   213

Moral Development, 213 ▼ Spiritual Values, 213

Major Health Concerns   214

Pregnancy, 214 ▼ Substance Abuse, 214 ▼ Acquired Immune Deficiency Syndrome (AIDS) and Sexually Transmitted Diseases (STDs), 215 ▼ Eating Disorders, 215 ▼ Tobacco Use, 215 ▼ Depression and Suicide, 215

Role of the Nurse   215

Health Screening and Assessment, 215 ▼ Health Education, 216

Early Adulthood   220

Physical Development and Change   220

Musculoskeletal System, 220 ▼ Reproductive System, 220

Psychosexual Development   220

Psychosocial Development **220**

Self-Concept and Self-Image, 220 ▼ Cognitive and Intellectual Development, 220 ▼ Relationships and Roles, 220

Values and Beliefs **222**

Moral Development, 222 ▼ Spiritual Values, 222

Major Health Concerns **222**

Lifestyle, 222 ▼ Environment, 223 ▼ Acquired Immune Deficiency Syndrome (AIDS), 223 ▼ Date (Acquaintance) Rape, 223

Role of the Nurse **223**

Health Screening and Assessment, 223 ▼ Health Education, 224

Chapter 14
Midlife Through Late Adulthood **227**

Midlife **228**

Physical Development and Change **228**

Psychosexual Development **228**

Psychosexual Changes in Women, 228 ▼ Psychosexual Changes in Men, 229

Psychosocial Development **229**

Self-Concept and Self-Image, 229 ▼ Cognitive and Intellectual Development, 230 ▼ Relationships and Roles, 231

Values and Beliefs **233**

Major Health Concerns **233**

Lifestyle, 233 ▼ Genetics, or Familial Characteristics, 233 ▼ Workplace or Place of Residence, 233 ▼ Cultural and Ethnic Influences, 234

Role of the Nurse **234**

Health Screening and Assessment, 234 ▼ Health Education, 234

Late Adulthood **235**

Physical Development and Change **235**

Psychosexual Development **236**

Deterrents to Sexual Expression in Late Adulthood, 236 ▼ Sexuality in Older Adults, 237

Psychosocial Development **237**

Self-Concept and Self-Image, 237 ▼ Cognitive and Intellectual Development, 237 ▼ Relationships and Roles, 238

Values and Beliefs **240**

Major Health Concerns **241**

Personal Losses, 241 ▼ Psychosocial Losses, 241 ▼ Depression, 241 ▼ Medication Use and Misuse, 242 ▼ Environment, 242 ▼ Lifestyle, 242

Role of the Nurse **242**

Health Screening and Assessment, 242 ▼ Health Education, 242

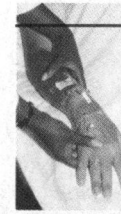

Unit 4
Characteristics of Persons Served by the Nurse **247**

Chapter 15
Human Needs **249**

People as Living Systems **250**

General Systems Theory **250**

Living Systems and Adaptations **251**

Human Needs **253**

Problems of Unmet Needs **256**

Helping People with Unmet Needs **257**

The Need to Understand the Self During Health and Illness **258**

The Self and Integration and Wholeness, 258 ▼ The Self and Individuality and Uniqueness, 259 ▼ The Self and Autonomy, 259 ▼ The Self and Personal Values, 259 ▼ The Self and Self-Actualization, 260 ▼ The Self, Introspection, and Time, 260 ▼ The Self and Emotional Conflict, 261 ▼ The Self and Other "Selves," 261 ▼ The "Public Self" and the "Private Self," 262 ▼ Self-Concept, 262 ▼ Individual Self and Universal Self, 263 ▼ The Self and Significant Others, 264

Needs, the Self, and Nursing Care **264**

Chapter 16
Stress and Adaptation **267**

Stress, Stressors, and Stress Responses **268**

Difficulties in Defining Stress, 268 ▼ Defining Stressors and Stress Responses, 269

Theoretical Models of Stress **272**

Selye's General Theory of Stress, 272 ▼ Holmes and Rahe's Model Relating Life Change to Illness, 274 ▼ Lazarus's Model of Stress and Coping, 274

Concept of Adaptation **276**

Levels of Adaptation, 277 ▼ Characteristics of Adaptation, 278

Concept of Crisis **279**

Maturational and Situational Crises, 280 ▼ Characteristics of Crises, 280 ▼ Crisis Intervention, 281

Assessment   281

Stressors, 282 ▼ First Line of Defense Against Stressors: Present Status, 283 ▼ Initial Psychophysiologic Stress Response Indicators, 283

Nursing Diagnosis   286

Planning   287

The Client, 288 ▼ Significant Others, 288 ▼ Community Resources, 288 ▼ The Nurse, 288

Nursing Intervention   288

Second Line of Defense Against Stressors: Self-Help, 288 ▼ Managing Stress Reduction, 291 ▼ Coping with Actual Crisis, 291

Evaluation   291

Third Line of Defense Against Stressors: Professional Help, 292 ▼ Failure of Stress Reduction: Chronic Disease, 292

Stress, Adaptation, and Crisis: Implications for Nurses   292

Caring for Hospitalized Persons, 292 ▼ Stress of Caring for Ill People, 294

Chapter 17
Homeostasis and Biologic Rhythms   299

The Study of Homeostatic Mechanisms   300

Physiologic and Psychologic Homeostasis   301

Maintenance of Physiologic Homeostasis   301

Major Regulators of Physiologic Homeostasis, 302 ▼ Mechanisms of Physiologic Homeostasis, 304 ▼ Failure of Homeostatic Mechanisms, 310

Chronobiology   311

Rhythmic Cycles and Frequencies, 311 ▼ Circadian Rhythms, 311 ▼ Clinical Applications of Chronobiologic Principles, 314

Nursing Implications Related to Homeostasis and Biologic Rhythms   314

Biofeedback, 315 ▼ Assessment, 315 ▼ Nursing Diagnosis, 316 ▼ Planning, 317 ▼ Nursing Intervention, 317 ▼ Evaluation, 318

Chapter 18
The Family   321

Family Diversity   322

Family-Centered Care   323

Frameworks for Understanding the Family   323

General Systems Theory, 323 ▼ Structural-Functional Theory, 323 ▼ Developmental Theory, 324 ▼ Nursing Theories, 324

The Family in Health and Illness   325

Health Promotion and Maintenance, 325 ▼ Impact of Illness on the Family, 325

Assessment   326

Nursing Diagnosis   326

Planning   327

Nursing Intervention   327

Evaluation   329

Chapter 19
Culture and Ethnicity   331

Culture   333

Material Culture and Nonmaterial Culture, 333 ▼ Socialization, 333 ▼ Subcultures, 333 ▼ Acculturation, 333 ▼ Assimilation, 334 ▼ Cultural Sensitivity and Stereotyping, 334

Ethnicity   334

Ethnic Pluralism, 334 ▼ Behavioral Ethnicity, 334 ▼ Ideologic Ethnicity, 334 ▼ Intraethnic Variations, 334 ▼ Ethnocentrism, 334 ▼ Ethnic Conflicts, 334

Race   335

Differentiation Among Racial Groups, 335 ▼ Race as a Legal-Cultural Phenomenon, 335 ▼ Race as an Economic Phenomenon, 335 ▼ Race as a Political Phenomenon, 335 ▼ Racial Prejudice, 335

Minority Status   335

Social Class   336

Differential Health Status Among Cultural, Ethnic, and Racial Groups   336

Chronic Diseases, 336 ▼ Mortality Rates, 337 ▼ Excess Mortality, 337 ▼ Life Expectancy, 337 ▼ Mental Disorders, 338 ▼ Suicide, 338

Variations in Health Behaviors Among Cultural, Ethnic, and Racial Groups   338

Help-Seeking Processes, 338 ▼ Use of Mental Health Services, 338 ▼ Access to Health Services, 339

Managing Cultural, Ethnic, and Racial Differences   339

Self-Awareness, 339 ▼ Cultural Competence, 339

Culture, Ethnicity, Race, and the Nursing Process: Assessment   341

Cultural, Ethnic, and Racial Factors Relevant to the Assessment, 341 ▼ Conducting the Assessment, 341

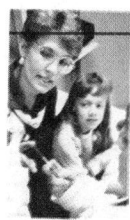

Unit 5
Health, Illness, and Health Care Settings   *343*

Chapter 20
Health Promotion in the Community   *345*

Concepts and Terms   346
Health and Wellness, 346 ▼ Health Protection,
346 ▼ Health Promotion, 347

Nursing's Focus on Health   347

Health Goals for the Year   347

Factors that Influence Health   348
External Factors that Influence Health, 348 ▼ Internal
Factors that Influence Health, 349

Models of Health Behavior   350
Health Belief Model, 351 ▼ Health Promotion Model,
351 ▼ A Framework for Health Promotion, 351

Working with Individuals to Promote Health   353

Nursing Strategies for Health Promotion   353
Role Modeling, 353 ▼ Acting as a Change Agent,
353 ▼ Setting Priorities, 356 ▼ Using Principles of
Behavior Modification, 356 ▼ Promoting Holistic Health,
358 ▼ Collaborating with Other Health Care
Providers, 358

**Working with Families, Groups, and Communities to
Promote Health   358**
Family Health Promotion, 358 ▼ Health Promotion
Within Groups, 359 ▼ Targeting At-Risk Groups in
Communities, 360 ▼ Evaluating Responses to Health
Promotion Programs, 361

Health Public Policy   361

Chapter 21
The Illness Experience   *363*

Stages of the Illness Experience   365
Transition, 365 ▼ Acceptance, 365 ▼
Convalescence, 365

Seeking Assistance   365
Responses to Initial Cues About Illness, 365 ▼ Factors
Affecting Initial Responses to Illness, 366

Reactions to Confirmed Illness   367
Uncertainty, 367 ▼ Anxiety, 367 ▼ Shock,
367 ▼ Denial, 368 ▼ Anger, 368 ▼ Information
Seeking, 368 ▼ Shame, 368 ▼ Isolation, 368 ▼ Fear,
369 ▼ Depression, 369 ▼ Mood Swings,
369 ▼ Powerlessness, 369 ▼ Altered Body Image, 370

Roles of the Ill Person   373
Sick Role, 374 ▼ Impaired Role, 374

Chronic Illness   374
Individual Responses to Chronic Illness, 374 ▼ Family
Support During Chronic Illness, 376

Quality of Life   376

Meeting Human Needs During Illness   377

Chapter 22
Hospital Admission and Discharge   *381*

Health Care Organizations   382
Classifications of Organizations, 382 ▼ The Hospital,
383 ▼ Nursing Care Models, 385

The Client   388
Client Expectations, 388 ▼ Client Anxiety,
388 ▼ Orienting the Client, 389

Assessment   392
Preventing Liability, 393 ▼ Documenting
Admission, 394

Nursing Diagnosis   394

Planning   395

Nursing Intervention   395

Evaluation   395

The Discharge Process   395

Chapter 23
Home Care Nursing   *399*

History of Home Care Nursing   400
Development of Home Care Nursing in Europe,
400 ▼ Development of Home Care Nursing in the
United States, 400

Terminology of Home Care Nursing   401

**Social, Technologic, Economic, and Regulatory
Developments in Home Care Nursing   401**
Medicare and Medicaid, 401 ▼ Diagnosis-Related
Groups, 402

Scope of Home Care Services   402
Types of Care Providers, 402 ▼ Individuals Requiring
Home Care, 404

Home Care Nursing Practice   405
A Model for Home Care Nursing Practice, 405 ▼ Goals
of Home Care Nursing, 405 ▼ Case Management,
405 ▼ Legal and Ethical Issues in Home Care Nursing
Practice, 406

Assessment   **407**

Nursing Diagnosis   **409**

Planning   **409**

Nursing Intervention   **409**

Clinical Skills, 409 ▼ Teaching, 410 ▼ Counseling, 410 ▼ Coordination of Care, 410

Evaluation   **412**

Case Study   **413**

Part II   SKILLS BASIC TO NURSING, 417

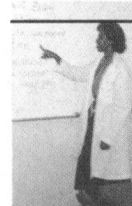

Unit 6
Communication Skills   419

Chapter 24
Therapeutic Communication: The Nurse-Client Interaction   421

The Therapeutic Relationship   **422**

Phases of the Therapeutic Relationship, 423 ▼ Improving the Therapeutic Relationship Through Process Recordings, 424

Elements of the Therapeutic Relationship: the Nurse, the Client, and Communication   **425**

Elements of Communication, 425 ▼ Theories Concerning the Nurse, the Client, and Communication, 427

Types of Communication   **429**

Verbal Communication, 429 ▼ Nonverbal Communication, 430

Facilitating Effective Therapeutic Communication   **434**

Nursing Attitudes that Promote Communication, 434 ▼ Action-oriented Characteristics, 435

Techniques that Impair Therapeutic Communication   **436**

Techniques that Enhance Therapeutic Communication   **436**

Techniques Often Helpful at the Beginning of an Interaction, 440 ▼ Techniques Often Helpful as an Interaction Progresses, 444 ▼ Techniques Often Helpful in Keeping Communication Clear, 444 ▼ Techniques that Can Help the Client Gain Increased Self-Awareness, 445 ▼ Techniques Helpful When Contact with Reality is Impaired, 446 ▼ Techniques Often Helpful Near the End of an Interaction, 446 ▼ One Technique that Must Occur Throughout the Interaction: Active Listening, 447

Effective Communication with Different Groups   **447**

Developmental Differences, 447 ▼ Cultural Differences, 447 ▼ Gender Differences, 447 ▼ The Hearing Impaired, 447 ▼ The Visually Impaired, 448 ▼ The Dying, 448

Chapter 25
Communication Within Groups   451

The Nature of Groups   **452**

Characteristics of Groups, 452 ▼ Primary and Secondary Groups, 453

Types of Groups Found in Health Care Settings   **453**

Therapeutic Groups, 453 ▼ Task (Work) Groups, 455 ▼ Educational Groups, 455

Group Dynamics and Group Process   **455**

Concepts Related to Group Dynamics, 455 ▼ Concepts Related to Group Process, 459

Group Leadership   **462**

Leadership Development, 462 ▼ Leadership Styles, 462

Strategies for Effective Group Communication   **463**

Barriers to Effective Group Interactions, 463 ▼ Constructive Confrontations, 464

The Group as Change Agent   **465**

Group Decision Making   **465**

Decision-Making Strategies, 465 ▼ Steps in the Decision-Making Process, 466

Chapter 26
Teaching and Learning 467

Domains of Learning 468

Perceptual Domain, 469 ▼ Cognitive Domain, 469 ▼ Affective Domain, 470 ▼ Psychomotor Domain, 470

Understanding the Individual Learner 471

Assumptions that Characterize Adult Learning, 471

Principles of Learning 472

Factors that Facilitate Learning, 472 ▼ Factors that Hinder Learning, 474

Principles of Teaching 474

What to Teach, 474 ▼ When to Teach, 475 ▼ How to Teach, 475

Assessment 475

Client Characteristics, 475 ▼ Level of Education, 475 ▼ Cultural Awareness, 476 ▼ Psychologic/ Physiologic Considerations, 476 ▼ Socioeconomic Considerations, 477

Nursing Diagnosis 477

Planning 477

Planning Concepts Related to Learning/Teaching Theory, 477 ▼ Learning Objectives, 478 ▼ Additional Learning Objectives, 478

Nursing Intervention 478

Enhancing Client's Motivation to Learn, 478 ▼ Developing Content and Learning Activities, 479

Evaluation 480

Short-Term Learning, 480 ▼ Long-Term Learning, 480

Chapter 27
Documenting Care 483

The Client Record 484

Historical Issues in Recording, 484 ▼ Purposes of the Client Record, 484 ▼ Guidelines for Documentation, 485 ▼ Current Problems in Recording, 485

Common Documentation Systems 488

Narrative Charting, 488 ▼ Flowcharts and Other More Structured Formats, 490 ▼ The Problem-Oriented Record System, 490 ▼ FOCUS Documentation, 492 ▼ PIE Charting, 494 ▼ Charting by Exception, 495 ▼ CORE Documentation, 495

Methods of Documentation 495

Hand-Written Records, 495 ▼ Dictated and Recorded Records, 496

Verbal Reporting 498

Automated Information Systems 498

Future Trends 499

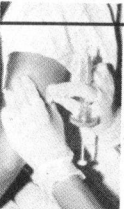

Unit 7
Skills Required for Safe Practice 503

Chapter 28
Infection Control 505

Promoting Microbial Safety 506

Infection Control in Historical Perspective 507

Process of Infectious Disease 509

Infectious Agents, 509 ▼ Infection Risk, 511 ▼ Nosocomial Infections, 511

Breaking the Chain of Infection 512

Infectious Agents, 512 ▼ Reservoir, or Source, of Infection, 512 ▼ Portal of Exit, 513 ▼ Mode of Transmission, 513 ▼ Portal of Entrance, 513 ▼ Susceptible Host, 513

Nursing Process and Infection Control 513

Assessment, 514 ▼ Nursing Diagnosis, 514 ▼ Planning, 515 ▼ Nursing Intervention, 515 ▼ Evaluation, 535

Chapter 29
Preventing Back Injury 539

Selected Physics Principles 540

Stability of Objects, 540 ▼ Use of Leverage, 542 ▼ Motion, 542

Guidelines for Correct Body Mechanics 542

Correct Body Alignment, 542 ▼ Effective Body Movement, 542

Chapter 30
Cardiopulmonary Resuscitation 555

Historical Perspective on Methods of Resuscitation 556

Cardiopulmonary Arrest 557

Normal Cardiopulmonary Function, 557 ▼ Failure of the Respiratory System, 557 ▼ Failure of the Cardiovascular System, 557 ▼ Clinical and Biologic Death, 558 ▼ Recognition of Cardiopulmonary Arrest, 558

Basic Life Support 559

Sequence of Cardiopulmonary Resuscitation, 559 ▼ Two-Person Rescue, 564 ▼ Performance Errors and Problems in Cardiopulmonary Resuscitation, 569

Infant and Child Resuscitation 570

Newborn Resuscitation, 570 ▼ Causes of Infant and Child Respiratory Arrest, 570 ▼ Establishing an Airway, 571 ▼ Signs of Successful Ventilation, 571 ▼ Chest Compressions, 571 ▼ Compressions Mnemonic, 571

Complications of Cardiopulmonary Resuscitation   571

Termination of Basic Life Support   574

Advanced Life Support   574

Helping Significant Others   574

Survivors of Cardiopulmonary Arrest   575

Foreign Body Airway Obstruction   575

Recognition of Foreign Body Airway Obstruction, 576 ▼ Management of Obstructed Airway, 576

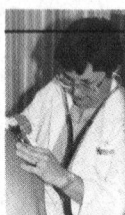

Unit 8
Assessment Skills   583

Chapter 31
Assessing Vital Signs   585

Vital Signs as the Building Blocks of Assessment   586

Assessment of Temperature   587

Heat Production, 587 ▼ Heat Loss, 587 ▼ Regulation of Body Temperature, 588 ▼ Normal Ranges for Body Temperature, 589 ▼ Measuring Body Temperature, 591 ▼ Alterations in Body Temperature, 598

Assessment of Pulse   602

Basic Cardiovascular Physiology, 602 ▼ Pulse Sites, 603 ▼ Pulse Rate, 605 ▼ Pulse Rhythm, 607 ▼ Pulse Force (Pulse Quality), 608

Assessment of Respiration   608

Basic Pulmonary Physiology, 608 ▼ Control of Respiration, 608 ▼ Techniques for Assessing Respiration, 609 ▼ Quality of Respiration, 609 ▼ Rate and Depth of Respirations, 610 ▼ Patterns of Respiration, 611 ▼ Significant Characteristics in Respiratory Assessment, 611

Assessment of Blood Pressure   612

Physiology of Arterial Pressure, 612 ▼ Blood Pressure Equipment, 614 ▼ Blood Pressure Measurement Techniques, 615 ▼ Blood Pressure Measurement in Infants and Children, 619 ▼ Errors in Blood Pressure Measurement, 619 ▼ Interpreting Abnormal Blood Pressure Findings, 619

Nursing Responsibility in Communicating Findings   621

Special Procedures Using Electronic Monitoring   621

The Cardiac Monitor, 621 ▼ The Doppler, 621 ▼ The Pulse Oximeter, 621 ▼ The Arterial Line, 622 ▼ Hemodynamic Pressure Monitoring, 624 ▼ Care of the Person Being Monitored, 624

Chapter 32
Psychosocial Assessment   627

Purpose of Psychosocial Health Assessment   628

Obtaining a Psychosocial Health Assessment   629

The Interview Process, 629 ▼ Data-Collecting Skills, 630 ▼ Components of Psychosocial Health Assessment, 630

Data Analysis   636

Physiologic Dimension, 636 ▼ Psychologic Dimension, 636 ▼ Social and Cultural Dimension, 643 ▼ Spiritual Dimension, 645

Chapter 33
Health Assessment   649

The Health History   650

Principles of History-Taking   650

Major Components of a Health History   651

Chief Complaint, 651 ▼ Present Illness, 651 ▼ Past Health History, 652 ▼ Family Health History, 652 ▼ Personal and Social History, 652 ▼ Systems Review, 652

Physical Assessment   653

Preparation for Physical Assessment   653

Purpose, 653 ▼ Equipment Needed, 653 ▼ Techniques, 655 ▼ Promoting Client Comfort During Physical Assessment, 657

Conducting the Physical Assessment   658

Vital Signs, 658 ▼ Height and Weight, 659 ▼ General Appearance, 659 ▼ Mental Status and Speech, 660 ▼ Integument, 661 ▼ Head and Neck, 665 ▼ Chest, 676 ▼ Abdomen, 685 ▼ Genitals and Rectum, 688 ▼ Extremities, 691 ▼ Motor System, 692 ▼ Sensory System, 693

Postexamination Activities   701

Documentation   701

Chapter 34
Assisting with Diagnostic Procedures   703

Nursing Responsibilities Related to Medical Diagnostic Procedures   704

Nursing Responsibilities Before the Diagnostic Procedure   705

Prepare the Person and Significant Others, 705 ▼ Obtain Informed Consent, 706 ▼ Schedule the Test, 706 ▼ Prepare the Person Physically, 706 ▼ Prepare the Equipment, 707 ▼ Transport the Person to the Examination Room and Significant Others to Waiting Area, 707

Nursing Responsibilities During the Diagnostic Procedure   707

Support the Person During Diagnostic Testing, 707 ▼ Collect Baseline Assessment Data and Continue to Evaluate the Client, 707 ▼ Assist with the Diagnostic Procedure, 707

Nursing Responsibilities After the Diagnostic Procedure   707

Provide Postprocedure Care and Comfort Measures, 707 ▼ Notify the Family/Significant Others of Procedure Completion, 707 ▼ Process Specimens, 708 ▼ Clean or Dispose of Equipment, 708 ▼ Document the Procedure, 708

Diagnostic Procedures Across the Life Span   708

Diagnostic Procedures and the Infant, 709 ▼ Diagnostic Procedures and the Toddler, 709 ▼ Diagnostic Procedures and the Preschooler, 709 ▼ Diagnostic Procedures and the School-Age Child, 709 ▼ Diagnostic Procedures and the Adolescent, 709 ▼ Diagnostic Procedures and the Adult, 709 ▼ Diagnostic Procedures and the Elderly, 709

Special Considerations for Diagnostic Procedures on an Outpatient Basis   710

Assessment by Radiographic Procedures (X-rays)   710

Upper Gastrointestinal Series, 711 ▼ Small Bowel X-ray Series, 711 ▼ Lower Gastrointestinal Series or Barium Enema, 711 ▼ Cholecystogram, 711 ▼ Intravenous Pyelogram, 713 ▼ Angiogram, 714 ▼ Myelogram, 714 ▼ Bronchogram, 714 ▼ Computed Tomography, 714 ▼ Magnetic Resonance Imaging, 714

Assessment by Radioactive Materials   715

Assessment by Laboratory Studies   716

Blood Studies, 719 ▼ Specimens for Culture, 719 ▼ Urine Studies, 719 ▼ Aspiration Studies, 719

Assessment of Electrical Impulses   721

Electrocardiogram, 721 ▼ Electroencephalogram, 722 ▼ Electromyogram, 722

Assessment by Endoscopy   723

Bronchoscopy, 723 ▼ Esophagogastroduodenoscopy, 725 ▼ Proctosigmoidoscopy, 725 ▼ Colonoscopy, 725 ▼ Cystoscopy, 725

Assessment by Ultrasonography   725

Assessment by Pulmonary Function Studies   725

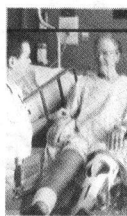

Unit 9
Therapeutic Skills   727

Chapter 35
Preventing Complications of Immobility   729

Assessment   730

Review of Anatomy and Physiology, 730 ▼ General Mobility Level, 733 ▼ Range of Motion of Spine and Extremities, 735 ▼ Effects of Immobility, 741

Nursing Diagnosis   757

Planning   757

Nursing Intervention   757

Examining Bedrest, 757 ▼ Equipment for Positioning, 758 ▼ Positioning the Immobilized Client, 769 ▼ Equipment to Assist in Transferring the Immobilized Client, 769 ▼ Transferring the Immobilized Client, 796 ▼ Additional Nursing Interventions to Prevent Disuse Phenomena, 797

Evaluation   797

Case Study   800

Chapter 36
Meeting Mobility Needs   805

Assessment   806

Causes of Immobility, 806 ▼ Responses of the Body to Immobility, 806 ▼ Assessing Readiness for Mobility, 806

Nursing Diagnosis   810

Planning   810

Nursing Intervention   813

Exercises, 813 ▼ Progressive Mobilization, 823 ▼ Assistive Ambulation Devices, 829 ▼ Promoting Fitness for the Mobile Person, 839

Evaluation   842

Case Study   843

Chapter 37
Providing Physical Protection and Body Support   847

Clients Who Require Protective and Supporting Devices   848

Clients with Orthopedic Disorders, 848 ▼ Clients with

Neuromuscular Disorders, 849 ▼ Clients with Behavioral and Neurologic Disorders, 850

Assessment   850

General Considerations, 850 ▼ Considerations Related to the Application of Restraints, 852

Nursing Diagnosis   853

Planning   854

Nursing Intervention, 854 ▼ Binders, 854 ▼ Bandages, 858 ▼ Antiembolism Hosiery, 863 ▼ Sequential Compression Devices, 863 ▼ Casts, 865 ▼ Bracing and Splinting, 870 ▼ Traction, 873 ▼ Movement Devices, 879 ▼ Restraints, 880 ▼ Suicide Precautions, 886

Evaluation   887

Case Study   887

Chapter 38
Promoting Hygiene   891

Hygiene Care in Perspective   893

Individual Variations in Hygiene Practices, 893 ▼ Territoriality, 893

General Hygiene Care   894

Assessment, 894 ▼ Nursing Diagnosis, 894 ▼ Planning, 894 ▼ Nursing Intervention, 896 ▼ Evaluation, 896

Elimination Hygiene   896

Bedpans and Urinals, 897 ▼ Assessment, 898 ▼ Nursing Diagnosis, 898 ▼ Planning, 898 ▼ Nursing Intervention, 898 ▼ Evaluation, 900

Assisting with Handwashing   900

Maintaining Oral Health   900

Oral Cavity Alterations, 901 ▼ Assessment, 902 ▼ Nursing Diagnosis, 904 ▼ Planning, 904 ▼ Nursing Intervention, 904 ▼ Evaluation, 908

Hygiene for the Eyes   908

Assessment, 908 ▼ Nursing Diagnosis, 909 ▼ Planning, 909 ▼ Nursing Intervention, 909 ▼ Evaluation, 911

Hygiene for the Ears   911

Assessment, 911 ▼ Nursing Diagnosis, 911 ▼ Planning, 912 ▼ Nursing Intervention, 912 ▼ Evaluation, 912

Hygiene for the Nose   912

Assessment, 912 ▼ Nursing Diagnosis, 913 ▼ Planning, 913 ▼ Nursing Intervention, 913 ▼ Evaluation, 913

Skin Hygiene   913

Skin Structure and Function, 913 ▼ Self-Care of the Skin, 914 ▼ Skin Integrity, 915 ▼ Assessment, 916 ▼ Nursing Diagnosis, 916 ▼ Planning, 917 ▼ Nursing Intervention, 917 ▼ Evaluation, 925

Perineal Care   925

Perineal Area, 925 ▼ Principles of Perineal Care, 926 ▼ Assessment, 926 ▼ Nursing Diagnosis, 926 ▼ Planning, 926 ▼ Nursing Intervention, 926 ▼ Evaluation, 929

Nail and Foot Care   929

Assessment, 929 ▼ Nursing Diagnosis, 929 ▼ Planning, 929 ▼ Nursing Intervention, 929 ▼ Evaluation, 930

Hair Care   930

Hair Structure and Function, 931 ▼ Assessment, 931 ▼ Nursing Diagnosis, 931 ▼ Planning, 931 ▼ Nursing Intervention, 931 ▼ Evaluation, 934

Cosmetic Care as Hygiene   935

Comfort and Cleanliness in Bed   935

Bed Linens, 935 ▼ Assessment, 935 ▼ Nursing Diagnosis, 941 ▼ Planning, 941 ▼ Nursing Intervention, 942 ▼ Evaluation, 943

Case Study   943

Chapter 39
Promoting Rest and Sleep   947

Nature of Sleep   948

Rapid Eye Movement Sleep, 948 ▼ Non-Rapid Eye Movement Sleep, 949 ▼ Sleep Cycle, 950 ▼ Circadian Rhythms, 950

Sleep Disorders   951

Disorders of Excessive Somnolence, 951 ▼ Disorders of Initiating and Maintaining Sleep, 952

Assessment   954

Subjective Data, 954 ▼ Objective Data, 955

Nursing Diagnosis   955

Planning   955

Nursing Intervention   958

Back Massage, 958 ▼ Sleeping Aids, 958

Evaluation   963

Case Study   964

Chapter 40
Facilitating Relief From Pain   967

What is Pain?   968

Acute Versus Chronic Pain, 968 ▼ Somatic, Visceral, and Sympathetically Maintained Pain, 968 ▼ Phantom

Pain, 969 ▼ Referred Pain, 969 ▼ Pain and Suffering, 969

Pain Transmission and Pain Modulation   971

Opiate Receptors, 971 ▼ Endogenous and Exogenous Opioids, 971 ▼ Pain Modulation in the Peripheral Nervous System, 972 ▼ Early Theories of Pain Transmission, 972 ▼ Recent Theories of Pain, 972

Assessment   973

Assessment of Acute Pain, 973 ▼ Assessment of Chronic Pain, 973 ▼ Tolerance, Dependence, and Addiction, 974 ▼ Assessment of Pain in the Elderly, 975 ▼ Assessment of Pain in Children, 975 ▼ Sociocultural Aspects of Pain Assessment, 977 ▼ Pain Assessment Tools, 978

Nursing Diagnosis   978

Planning   978

Nursing Intervention   979

Pain and Loss of Control, 980 ▼ Pharmacologic Interventions, 981 ▼ Psychologic Interventions, 984 ▼ Nonpharmacologic Interventions Directed by the Client, 985 ▼ The Team Approach, 986 ▼ Physical Interventions, 987 ▼ Patient-controlled Analgesia, 988 ▼ Epidural Analgesia, 988 ▼ Transcutaneous Electrical Nerve Stimulation, 991 ▼ Alternative Routes of Opioid Therapy, 991 ▼ Biofeedback, 992 ▼ Neuroablation, 992 ▼ Interventions for Children, 992 ▼ Documentation of Interventions, 992

Evaluation   992

Case Study   993

Chapter 41
Maintaining Fluid and Electrolyte Balance   999

Body Water   1001

Total Body Water, 1001 ▼ Water Distribution, 1001 ▼ Water Balance, 1001 ▼ Minimal Water Requirements, 1002

Electrolytes and Plasma Proteins   1002

Chemistry of Electrolytes and Plasma Proteins, 1002 ▼ Functions of Electrolytes and Plasma Proteins, 1005 ▼ Measuring Fluids and Electrolytes, 1005 ▼ Electrolyte Concentrations in the Body's Fluid Compartments, 1009

Movement of Fluid and Electrolytes   1010

Fluid and Electrolyte Transport Between the Intracellular and the Extracellular Fluid, 1010 ▼ Fluid Transport Between the Vascular and Interstitial Compartments, 1011

Fluid and Electrolyte Balance   1013

Neuroendocrine System as a Homeostatic Regulator, 1013 ▼ Gastrointestinal Tract as a Homeostatic Regulator, 1017 ▼ Renal System as a Homeostatic Regulator, 1017 ▼ Cardiovascular System as a Homeostatic Regulator, 1018

Acid-Base Balance   1018

Mechanisms of Acid-base Regulation, 1019 ▼ Failure of Acid-base Regulation, 1020 ▼ Risk Factors for Fluid, Electrolyte, and Acid-base Imbalances, 1021

Assessment   1022

Client History, 1033 ▼ Physical Assessment, 1034

Nursing Diagnosis   1035

Planning   1035

Nursing Intervention   1035

Recording Intake and Output, 1036 ▼ Regulating Diet, 1036 ▼ Regulating Oral Fluid Intake, 1038 ▼ Administering Medications, 1038 ▼ Administering Tube Feedings, 1041 ▼ Monitoring Intravenous Therapy, 1042

Evaluation   1043

Case Study   1043

Chapter 42
Meeting Nutritional Needs   1049

Basic Concepts of Good Nutrition   1050

Structure and Function of the Gastrointestinal Tract, 1050 ▼ Calories, Body Weight, and Nutrients, 1052 ▼ Recommended Dietary Allowances and Dietary Guidelines, 1057

Popular Concerns About Diet and Health   1062

Food Additives, 1062 ▼ Natural and Organic Foods, 1062 ▼ Vitamin, Mineral, and Food Supplements, 1063 ▼ Special Foods, 1065 ▼ Vegetarianism, 1065

Assessment   1066

Food and Dietary Records, 1066 ▼ Physical Assessment, 1066 ▼ Feelings About Diet Changes, 1067 ▼ Factors that Influence Food Intake, Dietary Patterns, and Nutritional Status, 1069

Nursing Diagnosis   1076

Planning   1078

Nursing Intervention   1079

Managing Diet Therapy, 1080 ▼ Maintaining or Improving the Appetite, 1089 ▼ Increasing Ingestion of the Appropriate Diet, 1090 ▼ Increasing Digestion, 1091 ▼ Increasing Absorption, 1093 ▼ Maintaining Nutrition When Gastrointestinal Function is Impaired, 1094

Evaluation   1118

Case Study   1119

Chapter 43
Meeting Bowel Elimination Needs   1125

Structure and Function of the Gastrointestinal Tract   1126

Assessment   1127
Taking the History, 1127 ▼ Psychologic Factors Affecting Bowel Elimination, 1127 ▼ Physiologic Factors Affecting Bowel Elimination, 1128 ▼ Physical Assessment, 1129 ▼ Diagnostic Tests to Locate and Identify Bowel Elimination Problems, 1131

Nursing Diagnoses   1132

Planning   1132

Nursing Intervention   1133
Bowel Management, 1133 ▼ Stimulating Bowel Evacuation, 1135 ▼ Constipation Management, 1143 ▼ Impaction Management, 1144 ▼ Diarrhea Management, 1145 ▼ Flatulence Reduction, 1146 ▼ Bowel Incontinence Care, 1147 ▼ Bowel Training, 1148 ▼ Ostomy Care, 1150

Evaluation   1152

Case Study   1152

Chapter 44
Meeting Urinary Elimination Needs   1155

Anatomy and Physiology of the Urinary System   1156
Urinary Structures and Related Functions, 1156 ▼ Changes of the Urinary Tract with Aging, 1158

Maintaining Normal Urinary Elimination   1158
Fluids and Exercise, 1158 ▼ Urinary Elimination During Illness, 1159 ▼ Teaching About Urinary Elimination, 1160

Assessment   1160
Physiologic Factors, 1160 ▼ Personal Factors, 1161 ▼ Psychosocial Factors, 1161 ▼ Cultural Factors, 1161 ▼ Medications, 1161 ▼ Trauma, 1161 ▼ Difficulties with Urinary Elimination, 1162 ▼ Problems with Urinary Elimination, 1163 ▼ Urine Characteristics, 1165 ▼ Routine Urine Testing, 1166 ▼ Urine Specimens, 1168 ▼ Diagnostic Tests for Urinary Dysfunction, 1169

Nursing Diagnosis   1169
Altered Urinary Elimination, 1169 ▼ Urinary Incontinence, 1170 ▼ Urinary Retention, 1171

Planning   1171
Altered Urinary Elimination, 1171 ▼ Urinary Incontinence, 1173 ▼ Urinary Retention, 1175

Nursing Intervention   1176
Altered Urinary Elimination, 1176 ▼ Urinary Incontinence, 1178 ▼ Urinary Retention, 1181

Evaluation   1199
Altered Urinary Elimination, 1199 ▼ Urinary Incontinence, 1199 ▼ Urinary Retention, 1199

Case Study   1200

Chapter 45
Meeting Respiration Needs   1203

Overview of the Respiratory System   1204
Normal Structure, 1204 ▼ Normal Function, 1205 ▼ Control of Breathing, 1205 ▼ Factors that Affect Breathing, 1206

Respiratory Disorders   1206
Hypoventilation, 1206 ▼ Hyperventilation, 1208 ▼ Hypoxemia and Hypoxia, 1208

Working as Part of the Health Care Team   1208

Assessment   1209
Taking a Respiratory History, 1209 ▼ The Chest Examination, 1210 ▼ Laboratory and Diagnostic Studies, 1213

Nursing Diagnosis   1218

Planning   1218

Nursing Intervention   1219
Basic Respiratory Therapeutic Measures, 1221 ▼ Measures to Maintain Airway Patency, 1239

Evaluation   1249

Case Study   1252

Chapter 46
Administering Medications   1255

General Principles of Medication Administration   1256
The Role of the Nurse, 1256 ▼ The Role of the Physician, 1257 ▼ The Role of the Pharmacist, 1258 ▼ Rights and Responsibilities of Persons Receiving Medications, 1258 ▼ Legal and Ethical Aspects of Medication Administration, 1258 ▼ Scientific Principles Concerning Medications, 1260 ▼ Routes of Administration, 1260 ▼ Effects of Medication, 1260 ▼ Medication Delivery Systems, 1261 ▼ Medication Orders, 1261 ▼ Computing and Timing Dosages, 1262 ▼ Safety Measures for Medication Administration, 1263

Assessment   1264
Physiologic Factors, 1264 ▼ Psychosocial Factors, 1265 ▼ Special Needs, 1266

Nursing Diagnosis   1266

Planning   1267

Nursing Intervention **1267**

Teaching Self-Care to Persons Receiving Medications, 1267 ▼ Using Judgment in the Administration of Medications, 1267 ▼ Administering Oral Medications, 1267 ▼ Administering Topical Medications, 1273 ▼ Administering Parenteral Medications, 1280

Evaluation **1295**

Case Study **1304**

Chapter 47
Administering Intravenous Therapy   *1307*

Indications for Intravenous Therapy **1308**

Intravenous Solutions **1308**

Blood Transfusions, 1311 ▼ Parenteral Hyperalimentation, 1312 ▼ Equipment for Intravenous Therapy, 1313 ▼ Complications of Intravenous Therapy, 1326

Assessment **1328**

Nursing Diagnosis **1328**

Planning **1330**

Nursing Intervention **1330**

Percutaneous Venipuncture, 1330 ▼ Maintaining the IV System, 1330

Case Study **1332**

Evaluation **1333**

Chapter 48
Caring for Persons with Wounds   *1335*

Normal Skin Integrity **1336**

Layers of Skin, 1337 ▼ Elements of Soft Tissue, 1337 ▼ Alterations in Skin and Soft Tissue Due to Aging, 1338 ▼ Assessment of Skin and Soft Tissue, 1338

Classification of Wounds **1339**

Surgical or Traumatic Wounds, 1340 ▼ Open or Closed Wounds, 1340 ▼ Full-Thickness and Partial-Thickness Wounds, 1341 ▼ Noninfected, Contaminated, Infected, or Dirty Wounds, 1341 ▼ Wounds and Blood-borne Transmissible Infectious Diseases, 1344 ▼ Chronic Wounds: Pressure Ulcers, 1345

Wound Healing **1354**

Phases of Wound Healing, 1354 ▼ Factors Affecting Wound Healing, 1357 ▼ Local Factors in Wound Healing, 1358 ▼ Systemic Factors in Wound Healing, 1358 ▼ Wound Closure, 1359 ▼ New Therapies for Wound Care, 1362

Assessment **1363**

Initial Assessment, 1363 ▼ Ongoing Assessment, 1365

Nursing Diagnosis **1365**

Planning **1366**

Nursing Intervention **1367**

Management of Wounds, 1367 ▼ Applications of Heat or Cold, 1386

Evaluation **1397**

Case Study **1397**

Chapter 49
Perioperative Nursing   *1403*

Basic Concepts **1404**

Purposes and Types of Surgery, 1404 ▼ Phases of the Surgical Experience, 1407

Roles and Responsibilities of the Surgical Team **1409**

The Person Undergoing Surgery **1410**

Profile of the Surgical Candidate, 1410 ▼ Psychophysiologic Alterations from Surgery, 1410 ▼ Developmental Considerations in Perioperative Nursing, 1412

Legal Implications of Surgery **1412**

Perioperative Phase **1413**

Admission to the Health Care Facility, 1413 ▼ Assessment, 1413 ▼ Nursing Diagnosis, 1420 ▼ Planning, 1421 ▼ Nursing Intervention, 1421 ▼ Evaluation, 1428

Intraoperative Phase **1428**

Assessment, 1428 ▼ Nursing Diagnosis, 1428 ▼ Planning, 1429 ▼ Nursing Intervention, 1429 ▼ Evaluation, 1432

Postoperative Phase **1434**

Assessment, 1434 ▼ Nursing Diagnosis, 1434 ▼ Planning, 1434 ▼ Nursing Intervention, 1435 ▼ Evaluation, 1440

Case Study **1440**

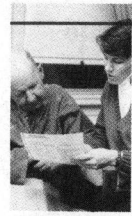

Unit 10
Applying Nursing Skills to Meet Psychosocial Needs   1445

Chapter 50
Enhancing Self-Concept   *1447*

Theories of Self-Concept and Self-Esteem **1448**

Historical Overview of the Concept of Self, 1449 ▼ Contemporary Theories of Self-Esteem, 1449

Research on Self-Concept   **1450**

Early Research, 1450 ▾ Relationship Between Illness and Caregivers, 1450 ▾ Problems with Research on Self-Esteem, 1451

A Family Systems Nursing Approach to Self-Esteem   **1452**

Self-Concept Across the Family Life Cycle   **1452**

Adults, 1452 ▾ Families with Infants and Young Children, 1453 ▾ Families with School-Age Children, 1453 ▾ Families with Adolescents, 1454 ▾ Middle-Aged Families, 1454 ▾ Aging Families, 1454

Assumptions About the Nursing Care of People with Low Self-Esteem   **1455**

Assessment   **1456**

Assess the Problem of Low Self-Esteem, 1456 ▾ Assess the Impact of Low Self-Esteem, 1457 ▾ Assess the Context in Which Low Self-Esteem Occurs, 1457 ▾ Assess Beliefs Related to Self-Esteem, 1457 ▾ Assess Solutions Attempted to Enhance Self-Esteem, 1458 ▾ Assess Exceptions to the Problem of Low Self-Esteem, 1458 ▾ Rating Scale Assessment Questions, 1459

Nursing Diagnosis   **1459**

Planning   **1461**

Nursing Intervention   **1461**

Validating and Affirming the Client's Experiences, 1461 ▾ Commending the Client, 1462 ▾ Advising and Informing the Client, 1462 ▾ Redefining Normality to Highlight the Client's Strengths, 1462 ▾ Normalizing the Client's Responses to Events, 1462 ▾ Asking Future-Oriented Questions, 1463 ▾ Implementing Bibliotherapy, 1463 ▾ Making Behavioral Assignments, 1463 ▾ Conducting "Research" on Self-Esteem, 1463 ▾ Implementing "Pretending Interventions," 1464 ▾ Suggesting Narrative Tasks, 1464 ▾ Promoting Positive Self-Talk, 1464

Evaluation   **1464**

Case Study   **1465**

Chapter 51
Meeting Sensory/Perceptual Needs   **1469**

Sensation/Perception   **1470**

Neurophysiology of Sensation/Perception, 1470 ▾ Factors Affecting Sensation/Perception, 1471 ▾ Alteration in Sensory Stimuli, 1471 ▾ Alteration in Perception, 1473

Assessment   **1474**

Persons at Risk for Sensory/Perceptual Alteration, 1474 ▾ Nursing History, 1475 ▾ Physical Assessment of Sensory Deficit, 1475 ▾ Symptoms of Sensory/Perceptual Alterations, 1475

Nursing Diagnosis   **1476**

Planning   **1476**

Nursing Intervention   **1476**

Sensory Deficits, 1476 ▾ Preventing Sensory/Perceptual Alterations in the Hospitalized Child, 1479 ▾ Sensory Deprivation, 1479 ▾ Sensory Overload, 1480 ▾ Communication with a Client with Sensory/Perceptual Alteration, 1480

Evaluation   **1483**

Case Study   **1483**

Chapter 52
Promoting Sexual Health   **1487**

Sexual Growth and Development   **1488**

Physiology and Sexuality, 1488 ▾ Psychosocial Development and Sexuality, 1492 ▾ Cultural Components of Sexuality, 1495

Sexual Function   **1495**

Sexuality and Sexism in Nursing   **1497**

Nurse-client Relationships, 1497 ▾ Interprofessional Relationships, 1499

Sexuality and the Client's Health Status   **1499**

Assessment   **1499**

General Physical Assessment, 1500 ▾ Assessment of the Client's Sense of Self as a Sexual Being, 1500 ▾ Assessment of the Client's Sexual Roles and Relationships, 1500 ▾ Assessment of Sexual Function, 1500 ▾ Gathering the Sexual History, 1500

Nursing Diagnosis   **1501**

Planning   **1502**

Nursing Intervention   **1503**

Culturally Sensitive Interventions, 1504 ▾ Problems that Can Interfere with Sexuality, 1504

Evaluation   **1504**

Case Study   **1505**

Chapter 53
Promoting Spiritual Health   **1509**

Concepts of Spirituality and Spiritual Care   **1510**

Holistic Care, 1510 ▾ Nurses' Role in Spiritual Care, 1511

Universality of Spirituality   **1511**

Historical Perspectives, 1511 ▾ Cultural Factors, 1511 ▾ Societal Influences, 1512

Spirituality and Religion   1512

Spiritual Needs   1512

Need for a Sense of Meaning and Purpose, 1512 ▼ Need for Love and Relatedness, 1512 ▼ Need for Forgiveness, 1513 ▼ Need for Hope, 1513

Spiritual Development Throughout the Life Span   1513

Religious Development, 1513 ▼ Psychosocial Development, 1513 ▼ Faith Development, 1514 ▼ Developmental Stages, 1514

Major World Religions   1515

Hinduism, 1515 ▼ Judaism, 1516 ▼ Christianity, 1517 ▼ Buddhism, 1517 ▼ Islam, 1522 ▼ Other Religious Groups, 1522

New Age Spiritualism   1522

Agnosticism and Atheism   1523

Resources for Clients Needing Spiritual Care   1523

Prayer, 1523 ▼ Sacred Writings, 1523 ▼ Clergy, 1524

Practices to Promote Your Own Spiritual Health   1524

Know Yourself, 1524 ▼ Recognize the Role of Faith, 1524 ▼ Meditate, 1524 ▼ Practice Guided Imagery, 1524 ▼ Pursue Aesthetic Experiences, 1524

Assessment   1525

Nursing Diagnosis   1526

Planning   1526

Nursing Intervention   1526

Evaluation   1528

Case Study   1529

Chapter 54
Coping with Loss and Grief   *1533*

Grief and Loss, 1534

Definitions, 1534 ▼ Forms of Loss, 1535 ▼ Physiologic Effects of Grief, 1535 ▼ Developmental Perspectives on Loss and Grief, 1536 ▼ Cultural Perspectives on Loss and Grief, 1537

Theories of Dying and Grief   1538

Theories of Death and Dying and the Hospice Movement, 1538 ▼ Theories of Grief and Grieving, 1541 ▼ Cautions About Stage and Phase Theories, 1543

The Nurse and Loss and Grief   1543

Assessment, 1544 ▼ Nursing Diagnosis, 1547 ▼ Planning, 1547 ▼ Nursing Intervention, 1551 ▼ Evaluation, 1554

Case Study   1555

Appendix 1
Universal Precautions   *1559*

Appendix 2
American Nurses' Association Standards of Clinical Nursing Practice   *1560*

Appendix 3
Nursing's Agenda for Health Care Reform   *1562*

Glossary   *1571*

Index   *1599*

▼ Special Features

▼

▼

▼

▼

PROCEDURES

PROCEDURE

28–1 Hand Washing...................... 518
29–1 Lifting an Object From the Floor....... 547
29–2 Placing a Lift Sheet Under the Client ... 547
29–3 Shoulder Lift Procedure for Moving a Helpless Person in Bed 549
29–4 Emergency Carries.................... 551
30–1 Cardiopulmonary Resuscitation 565
31–1 Measurement of Body Temperature 594
31–2 Assessing the Radial and Apical Pulses 606
31–3 Measuring Blood Pressure at the Brachial Pulse Site 616
35–1 Moving a Helpless Person in Bed 770
35–2 Positioning a Helpless Person in Bed... 775
35–3 Transferring a Helpless Person from the Bed 785
36–1 Passive Range-of-Motion Exercises 817
36–2 Teaching a Person to Sit on the Side of the Bed and "Dangle" 824
36–3 Assisting with Ambulation.............. 830
38–1 Complete Bed Bath.................... 919
38–2 Making an Occupied Bed 935
39–1 Back Massage 960
41–1 Recording Intake and Output.......... 1003
42–1 Serving Food and Assisting with Feeding 1092
42–2 Insertion of Nasogastric or Nasoenteric Tube 1104
42–3 Irrigation of Gastrointestinal Tubes 1112
43–1 Preparing and Administering a Normal Saline Enema (NSE) 1138
44–1 Female and Male Urethral Catheterization........................ 1181
45–1 Administering Oxygen 1229
45–2 Suctioning the Tracheobronchial Tree .. 1245

PROCEDURE

46–1 Administering Oral Medications 1270
46–2 Administering Intradermal Injections.... 1293
46–3 Administering Subcutaneous Injections............................. 1296
46–4 Administering Intramuscular Injection, Including Air Lock and Z-Track Techniques............................ 1298
47–1 Percutaneous Venipuncture (for Blood Collection, IV Infusion, and Saline or Heparin Lock) and Discontinuing an IV Line............................... 1316
47–2 Administering Intravenous Medications 1321
48–1 Irrigation of Wound.................... 1368
48–2 Applying Dry Sterile Dressing 1371
48–3 Applying Wet Sterile Dressing.......... 1374
48–4 Applying Hydrocolloid Dressings 1378

Additional Procedures Described in Text

CHAPTER

16 Using guided imagery.................. 290
22 Orienting the client to the hospital setting............................... 389
22 Discharging a client 395
26 Teaching by demonstration 479
28 Donning a clean gown................. 517
28 Opening a sterile package 529
28 Opening and pouring sterile liquids...... 530
28 Adding sterile supplies to a sterile field ... 530
28 Sterile gloving (open method)........... 531
28 Removing contaminated gloves.......... 531
28 Donning a mask 533
28 Removing a mask 533
28 Completing a surgical hand scrub........ 533

CHAPTER

28 Drying after a surgical hand scrub........ 533
28 Donning a sterile gown and gloving (closed method)..................... 534
28 Removing a contaminated gown and gloves................................ 534
30 Establishing ventilation with mouth-to-mouth respiration 561
30 Other rescue breathing methods......... 562
30 Two-person CPR..................... 564
30 Changing rescuer roles................ 568
30 Finger sweeps and interventions for foreign body airway obstruction in infants and children 577
31 Measuring apical-radial pulses 603
31 Using palpation to estimate systolic blood pressure 615
31 Measuring blood pressure at the thigh 615
31 Using the flush method of measuring blood pressure in a newborn or small infant 619
31 Using a Doppler to obtain pulse and blood pressure readings............... 621
35 Making trochanter rolls................ 767
37 Applying an arm sling................. 856
37 Applying a roller bandage (with circular turns) 859
37 Applying an elastic bandage (with spiral turns, spiral reverse turns, figure-of-eight turns, spica turns, and recurrent turns).... 861
37 Applying a stockinette and tube-gauze 862
37 Applying an Unna boot 863
37 Applying sequential compression hosiery.. 863
37 Using a JED sled..................... 879
38 Placing and removing the bedpan........ 899
38 Assisting with a urinal................. 900
38 Assisting with tooth brushing........... 905
38 Assisting with tooth flossing............ 906
38 Brushing dentures 907
38 Cleaning the eyes during bathing 909
38 Removing an eye prosthesis............. 909
38 Cleansing an eye socket 910
38 Reinserting an eye prosthesis........... 910
38 Inserting contact lenses 910
38 Removing hard contact lenses........... 910
38 Inserting a hearing aid earmold......... 912
38 Assisting with showering and bathing..... 916
38 Making a mitt........................ 918
38 Providing male and female perineal care.. 927
38 Cleaning and trimming nails............ 929
38 Assisting with hair care................ 930
38 Caring for tangled or matted hair 931
38 Shampooing the hair with the client on the side of the bed.................... 932
38 Shampooing the hair with the client on a stretcher............................ 932
38 Shampooing the hair in bed............. 932
38 Shaving.............................. 933
38 Making an orthopedic bed.............. 942
38 Making a surgical bed................. 942
42 Administering a tube feeding through an oral or nasogastric tube................ 1110

CHAPTER

42 Administering a tube feeding through a gastrostomy tube or jejunostomy tube..... 1114
43 Collecting a stool specimen.............. 1130
43 Collecting a specimen to check for pinworms 1130
43 Administering a hypertonic enema........ 1142
43 Administering a retention enema.......... 1142
43 Placing a rectal tube................... 1147
43 Administering a return flow (Harris flush) enema 1147
43 Irrigating a colostomy 1151
44 Testing specific gravity with a urinometer 1167
44 Labeling urine specimens 1168
44 Collecting a routine urine specimen....... 1168
44 Collecting a clean-catch or midstream urine sample 1168
44 Collecting a sterile urine specimen from an indwelling catheter.................. 1168
44 Collecting a timed urine specimen 1169
44 Applying a condom catheter............. 1175
44 Removing an indwelling catheter.......... 1190
44 Teaching a client to perform intermittent self-catheterization.................... 1194
44 Bladder irrigation (closed and open methods)............................ 1196
45 Inserting an oral airway................. 1240
45 Inserting a nasopharyngeal airway......... 1241
45 Oropharyngeal or nasopharyngeal suctioning........................... 1243
46 Applying topical medications 1274
46 Applying aerosols...................... 1275
46 Applying patches 1275
46 Inserting a rectal or vaginal suppository ... 1276
46 Instilling nose drops................... 1277
46 Instilling eye drops 1277
46 Administering eye ointment.............. 1277
46 Irrigating the eye 1278
46 Instilling ear drops.................... 1278
46 Irrigating the external auditory canal 1278
46 Irrigating the vagina 1278
46 Preparing medication from an ampule..... 1287
46 Preparing medication from a vial......... 1291
47 Changing IV tubing and IV bags 1332
47 Changing IV tubing without changing the IV bag 1332
47 Changing the client's gown without disrupting an IV system................. 1333
48 Applying hot water bottles............... 1391
48 Applying disposable chemical hot packs... 1391
48 Applying electric heating pads 1391
48 Applying Aqua K pads.................. 1391
48 Applying heat cradles.................. 1391
48 Applying infrared or gooseneck lamps 1392
48 Applying chemical counterirritants 1392
48 Applying hot compresses 1393

CHAPTER

48 Applying hydrocollator packs 1393
48 Assisting with sitz baths................ 1394

CHAPTER

48 Giving contrast baths 1394
48 Applying normal or chemical cold packs .. 1394
48 Applying ice bags or ice collars 1394
48 Applying hypothermia blankets 1395
48 Applying cold compresses 1395
48 Applying tepid baths, tepid sponges,
   alcohol sponges, ice, and aerosol sprays
   to promote cooling 1395
49 Teaching a client to splint an incision
   when coughing 1422
49 Removing hair prior to surgery 1424
49 Preparing a client on the day of surgery ... 1425
49 Transporting a client to surgery 1428
49 Preparing a client's room as a postoperative
   unit 1428
54 Providing postmortem care 1554

Additional Procedures Described in Figures and Boxes

28 Donning sterile gloves 532
28 Scrubbing (stroke method) 534
28 Gloving oneself (closed technique) 537
30 Determining whether cardiopulmonary
   arrest has occurred 560

CHAPTER

30 Opening an obstructed airway 561
30 Identifying correct hand positions for
   chest compressions 564
30 Infant and child CPR 573
30 Action steps for complete airway
   obstruction 577
30 Thrust techniques for a conscious or
   unconscious choking victim 578
35 Using a Surgilift 784
37 Applying antiembolism hosiery 864
37 Using a restraining hold 881
37 Applying a soft limb restraint by using a
   clove hitch knot 882
38 Removing soft contact lenses 910
38 Bathing an infant 924
44 Teaching Kegel exercises 1159
45 Helping a person to cough effectively 1224
45 Teaching pursed-lip breathing 1238
45 Teaching diaphragmatic breathing 1238
47 Administering medications by slow IV
   push with heparin or saline locks 1314
47 Administering a large volume of
   medication with heparin or saline locks ... 1315
48 Applying and removing adhesive tape 1362

APPLYING RESEARCH TO NURSING PRACTICE BOXES

Validating Nursing's Worth Through Historical
   Research 11
Evaluation: The Forgotten Step of the Nursing
   Process 173
... But Names Can Never Hurt Me? 184
Cocaine-exposed Newborns Have Distinctive
   Cry Patterns 194
Promoting Self-Esteem in Early Teens 217
Measuring Circadian Rhythms in Older Adults ... 316
Helping Care Givers Cope with High-Tech
   Home Care 402
Tailoring Your Teaching to Fit Your Clients 476
Double Bagging is a Procedure of the Past 520
When Performing Cardiopulmonary
   Resuscitation, Keep Both Hands on the Bag .. 575
Recognizing the Importance of Subjective Data
   in Assessing Bronchial Asthma 651
Preventing Confusion to Promote Self-Care
   Among Hospitalized Elderly Clients 807
Preventing Pressure Ulcers 743
Understanding the Feelings of Clients Wearing
   a Halo Brace—and Helping Them to Cope .. 879
Deciding Whether to Get Post-MI Clients Out of
   Bed During Bedmaking 942
Critically Ill Children Need Their Sleep 953
Using Psychologic Preparation to Alleviate the
   Pain of Chest Tube Removal 984

Using Swedish Massage to Relieve Cancer
   Pain 987
Accurately Detecting Dehydration in Elderly
   Clients 1032
Can Feeding Tubes Handle Metamucil? 1109
Timing Bowel-Training Programs for Clients
   with Strokes 1149
Diagnosing and Intervening for Urinary
   Incontinence 1173
Evaluating the Effect of Complex Medication
   Regimens on Compliance among Elderly
   Clients 1259
Avoiding Simultaneous Infusion of Incompatible
   IV Drugs 1311
Determining Risk for Pressure Ulcers on the
   Basis of Nutritional Status 1350
Preventing Complications of the Lithotomy
   Position 1430
Enhancing Self-Concept by Helping Clients
   Work with the Patterns of a Chronic Illness .. 1451
Promoting Sexual Health After Ostomy
   Surgery 1503
Matching Spiritual Care to Spiritual Needs 1525
Helping Families Cope with Sudden Death in
   the Emergency Department 1553

CASE STUDIES WITH CARE PLANS

Stress and Adaptation........................ 295
Home Care Nursing........................... 413
Preventing Complications of Immobility........ 800
Meeting Mobility Needs....................... 843
Providing Physical Protection and Body
  Support 887
Promoting Hygiene 943
Promoting Rest and Sleep.................... 964
Facilitating Relief from Pain 993
Maintaining Fluid and Electrolyte Balance 1043
Meeting Nutritional Needs.................... 1119
Meeting Bowel Elimination Needs.............. 1152

Meeting Urinary Elimination Needs 1200
Meeting Respiration Needs.................... 1252
Administering Medications 1303
Administering Intravenous Therapy 1332
Caring for Persons with Wounds 1397
Perioperative Nursing 1440
Enhancing Self-Concept...................... 1465
Meeting Sensory/Perceptual Needs 1483
Promoting Sexual Health..................... 1505
Promoting Spiritual Health 1529
Coping with Loss and Grief 1555

NURSING DIAGNOSIS PROFILES

Anxiety.................................... 287
Altered Family Processes.................... 328
Health-Seeking Behaviors (specify) 360
Impaired Home Maintenance Management 408
High Risk for Disuse Syndrome................ 456
Impaired Physical Mobility 811
High Risk for Violence: Self-directed or
  Directed at Others....................... 854
Self-Care Deficit, Bathing/Hygiene 895
Self-Care Deficit, Dressing/Grooming 895
Sleep Pattern Disturbance................... 957
Pain....................................... 979
Chronic Pain 980
Fluid Volume Deficit........................ 1036
Fluid Volume Excess........................ 1037
Altered Nutrition: More than Body
  Requirements............................ 1077
Altered Nutrition: Less than Body
  Requirements............................ 1078

High Risk for Altered Nutrition: More than Body
  Requirements............................ 1079
Constipation............................... 1132
Stress Incontinence 1170
Urinary Retention 1171
Ineffective Airway Clearance 1218
Impaired Gas Exchange...................... 1219
Impaired Tissue Integrity 1366
Fear....................................... 1421
High Risk for Infection...................... 1429
Situational Low Self-Esteem 1460
Sensory/Perceptual Alterations (specify Visual,
  Auditory, Kinesthetic, Gustatory, Tactile,
  Olfactory)............................... 1477
Altered Sexuality Patterns................... 1502
Spiritual Distress (Distress of the Human
  Spirit).................................. 1526
Anticipatory Grieving........................ 1550
Dysfunctional Grieving 1551

SCIENTIFIC PRINCIPLES TABLES

TABLE

28–4 Selected Scientific Principles and
         Related Nursing Interventions for
         Maintaining a Sterile Field 528

29–1 Selected Scientific Principles and
         Related Nursing Interventions for
         Body Mechanics..................... 544

35–5 Selected Scientific Principles and
         Related Nursing Interventions for
         Positioning and Moving Immobilized
         Client 782

36–3 Selected Scientific Principles and
         Related Nursing Interventions for
         Assistive Ambulation................ 840

37–4 Selected Scientific Principles and
         Related Nursing Interventions for
         Immobilizing Devices (Casts and
         Braces) 872

TABLE

38–1 Selected Scientific Principles and
         Related Nursing Interventions for
         Promoting Hygiene.................. 941

44–2 Selected Scientific Principles and
         Related Nursing Interventions for
         Persons with Indwelling Urethral
         Catheters.......................... 1190

45–9 Selected Scientific Principles and
         Related Nursing Interventions to Assist
         Effective Coughing 1224

45–11 Selected Scientific Principles and
         Related Nursing Interventions for Safe
         Oxygen Administration 1232

45–16 Selected Scientific Principles and
         Related Nursing Interventions for
         Meeting Respiration Needs........... 1251

▼ *Sorensen and Luckmann's*

▼ *Basic Nursing*

▼ *A Psychophysiologic Approach*

▼ *Third Edition*

Concepts Basic to Nursing

Part

I

▼ The Evolving Profession of Nursing

The Individual
Profession of
Nursing

Chapter 1

▼ Historical Introduction to Nursing

> *Those who cannot remember the past are condemned to repeat it.*
>
> **George Santayana**

▼ CHAPTER OUTLINE

THE EVOLVING DEFINITION OF NURSING
    Nightingale's Definition of Nursing
    Henderson's Definition of Nursing
    American Nurses' Association's
        Definition of Nursing
    Canadian Nurses' Association's
        Definition of Nursing
THE IMAGE OF NURSING
    Nursing and the Image of Women
    Nursing and Religious Orders
    The Image of Contemporary
        Nursing
NURSING PRACTICE
    Early Development of Nurses'
        Roles
    Major Settings for Contemporary
        Nursing Practice

    Clinical Specialization
    Standards of Nursing Practice
    Patients/Clients/Consumers
NURSING EDUCATION
    Early Schools
    Wars and Changing Patterns of
        Nursing Education
    Nursing Education Today
THE NURSING PROFESSION
    Early Collaborative Efforts of
        Nurses
    Developing a Professional Career
    Expanded Roles for Nurses
    Professional Organizations

▼ KEY TERMS

American Nurses'
  Association
Bellevue Training School
Boston Training School
Canadian Nurses
  Association
Connecticut Training
  School for Nurses

Henderson, Virginia
International Council of
  Nurses
National League for
  Nursing
National Student Nurse
  Association, Inc.
Nightingale, Florence

Nightingale School at St.
  Thomas Hospital,
  London
Nursing
Nursing Standards
Nutting, Mary Adelaide
Robb, Isabel Hampton
Sigma Theta Tau

▼ LEARNING OBJECTIVES

After studying this chapter, you should be able to

1. *Trace the evolution of definitions of nursing.*
2. *State the American Nurses' Association's definition of nursing.*
3. *Trace the changing image of nursing.*
4. *Identify positive and negative qualities currently associated with a career in nursing.*
5. *Compare nursing roles in the formative stages of formal nursing education in the United States with nurses' roles existing today.*
6. *Describe the three major settings for contemporary nursing practice.*
7. *List the four factors that have most influenced the shape of nursing education.*
8. *Identify the earliest schools of nursing in London and in the United States.*
9. *Describe how nursing education changed as a result of wars.*
10. *Contrast the three most commonly encountered types of educational programs for the generic preparation of Registered Nurses.*
11. *Discuss the variety of educational opportunities available for registered nurses after generic preparation.*
12. *Discuss the contributions made by early nursing leaders, such as Florence Nightingale, Isabel Hampton Robb, Mary Adelaide Nutting, Lillian Wald, and Lavinia Dock.*
13. *Identify the means by which an organization may be accepted as a profession.*

Nursing has been practiced since the beginning of human history, whenever the first person cared for another who was sick or injured. Nursing practice has been carried out in a variety of forms throughout the ages. Organized nursing in the United States had its roots in the Civil War, but not until 1873 were the first formal schools of nursing established in the United States. Nursing today is a dynamic field enriched by the traditions of the past and challenged by profound changes in society and health care.

In this opening chapter you will look at definitions of nursing, evolving images of nursing, nursing practice, nursing education, and nursing as a profession—all with an eye on how the present grew out of the past. How nursing continues to develop in the face of contemporary challenges depends not only on how we understand the traditions of the past but also in large part on the behavior of the nurses of today and tomorrow—in other words, on you.

To put a historical perspective on today's nursing profession is to see how often nursing's problems are merely old problems with new names. One example is the "entry into practice" issue, the ongoing debate about the appropriate level of education for a beginning professional nurse. Some argue that the basic level of education should be a baccalaureate degree, while others strongly oppose that as a requirement. This controversy can be traced to the beginning of formal nursing education, when it was thought of as a choice between the "trained versus the untrained nurse."[55]

At the time of the advent of formal nursing education in the United States, large numbers of practical nurses considered themselves nurses by virtue of their experience in caring for sick friends, neighbors, and others for pay. One of the few arenas of employment open to the women who graduated from the early nursing schools was private duty nursing, usually performed in people's homes. Consequently, competition arose between the existing practical (untrained) nurses and those who had graduated from training schools.

Another example of the repetition of problems in nursing's history is the recurring shortage of nurses. These shortages often have many similarities, though each one stems from a different cluster of specific events.

Understanding nursing history can give you a perspective on contemporary developments and a sense of pride about our traditions, our extraordinary practitioners, and our invaluable contributions to society.

THE EVOLVING DEFINITION OF NURSING

For most of our history, no one was concerned about a definition of nursing. Nurses did whatever needed to be done for those in their care. Such caring embodied activities including cleaning, cooking, and flower arranging, as well as more typical direct nursing care activities. Over the years, however, as more para-professionals and technicians moved into the health care arena, nursing began to try to discern what part of health care was and is unique to nursing.

For a definition of nursing, it was logical to look to **Florence Nightingale,** the founder of modern nursing and a prolific writer on the subject.

Nightingale's Definition of Nursing

Quite ahead of her time in many things, Florence Nightingale advocated a philosophy of nursing that incorporated total care. Nightingale said nurses were to care for the entire person, not the illness alone, and she meant that the nurse should look at both the person and the person's environment. She recommended use of flowers to cheer, a pet to distract, and, for comfort, one bed for day and another for night.[52] She did not want the nurse to perceive the person only as "a fracture," "a gun-shot wound," or "a fever," but rather as a human being with an illness.

The most often-quoted definition of nursing attributed to Nightingale is to "put the patient in the best condition for nature to act upon him."[6] These words appear, however, on page 75 of her 76-page *Notes on Nursing*. On page 6 of that document she says:

I use the word nursing for want of a better. It has been limited to signify little more than the administration of medications and the application of poultices. It ought to signify the proper use of fresh air, light, warmth, cleanliness, quiet, and the proper selection and administration of diet—all at the least expense of vital power to the patient.[6]

"The proper use of fresh air, light, warmth, cleanliness, quiet, and the proper selection and administration of diet—all at the least expense of vital power to the patient" is a definition of nursing that reflects not only Nightingale's own philosophy, but also the temper of the time. The absence of technology available to health care workers of that day left little to be done but to manipulate the environment. The results Nightingale achieved at Scutari during the Crimean War speak for themselves. By merely manipulating the environment and diet, she lowered the mortality rate from 42.7 per cent to 2.2 per cent.[18] In spite of the scientific breakthroughs, such as knowledge of antiseptics and general acceptance of the germ theory, Nightingale maintained that the criteria set forth in her definition were all that were needed.

Henderson's Definition of Nursing

In 1966, **Virginia Henderson,** one of the first nursing theorists to write a generally accepted definition of nursing and a framework for nursing care, said:

The unique function of the nurse is to assist the individual, sick or well, in the performance of those activities contributing to health or its recovery (or to peaceful death) that he would perform unaided if he had the necessary strength, will or knowledge. And to do this in such a way as to help him gain independence as rapidly as possible.[38]

Henderson's overt mention of caring for well individuals and the dying sets her definition apart: Neither health concepts nor caring for the dying person were in the mainstream of nursing school curricula when her definition was published.

Although public health nurses have always been concerned with health, most nurses trained and worked in hospitals caring for the sick, where nursing them back to health was part of the nurse's role and teaching them about health was not. Specific concepts about caring for the dying individual are a relatively new phenomenon resulting from Kübler-Ross's work published in 1969.[44] The concepts of health and caring for those who are dying are now an integral part of nursing school curricula. Henderson's definition is still widely accepted.

American Nurses' Association's Definition of Nursing

The American Nurses' Association, the national organization for registered nurses in the United States, has accepted different definitions of nursing over the years, reflecting the changing role of the nurse as well as the nurse's changing relationship with other professions, most notably medicine. The current definition of nursing was accepted in 1980:

Nursing is the diagnosis and treatment of human responses to actual or potential health problems.[6]

The ANA definition of nursing is deliberately broad. Reflecting changes in the theory of nursing developed during the 1970s, it legitimizes nursing diagnoses and distinguishes nursing diagnoses from medical diagnoses (see Chapter 6). Because each state has its own licensing law for nursing, such a broad, yet comprehensive definition allows much latitude.

Much like a nursing philosophy, a definition of nursing can provide an umbrella under which nurses practice their profession. A definition can also explain the unique function of nursing to those outside the profession.

Canadian Nurses Association's Definition of Nursing

The Canadian Nurses Association also encourages the use of a theoretical model for nursing:

Nursing practice can be defined generally as a dynamic, caring, helping relationship in which the nurse assists the client to achieve and maintain optimal health. The nurse fulfills this purpose by applying knowledge and skills from nursing and related fields using the nursing process, the substance of which is determined by a conceptual model(s) for nursing.[15]

The authors of this definition qualify it by saying a definitive definition of nursing would be derived by the nurse depending on which one conceptual model of many, was chosen to guide that nurse's practice.

THE IMAGE OF NURSING

The image of nursing has varied throughout our history. As a profession in today's society, nursing seeks to clarify and improve its image so that the work and its practitioners can receive just recognition from both the health care system and the larger society.

Nursing and the Image of Women

Nursing, as a part of the woman's role in caring for her family, has been part of human existence since the beginning of time. An injured or ill person has often required care by others. Throughout history those individuals recognized for their special nursing ability acquired their skills by either trial and error or intuition.

Whenever useful remedies were discovered, they were passed down from mother to daughter.

The identification of nursing activity with the mother (and therefore with women) is apparent in the English use of the same word "nurse" to refer both to a woman breastfeeding her infant and to the person who cares for or watches over the sick. Many issues related to the image of nursing stem from the identification of nursing with so-called feminine aspects of human character: caring, compassion, and obedience. Unfortunately, this image has not been universally perceived over time. By the 19th century, nursing for hire was not highly esteemed; the negative attitude was reflected by the English novelist Charles Dickens, who introduced the two "nurses" Betsy Prigg and Sairey Gamp in his novel *Martin Chuzzlewit*. Sairey is by far the more mentioned of the two nurses. She was an obese,

drunken, uncouth woman from the dregs of society. Dickens later said he believed his portrayal of Sairey was accurate at the time. Since his serialized novels were very widely read, the image he portrayed tended to be indelibly imprinted into the minds of readers, thereby reinforcing a very negative image of nurses.[24]

The image of Florence Nightingale, on the other hand, was that of a national heroine. Nightingale's significant accomplishments in caring for wounded soldiers during the Crimean War made her the antithesis of Sairey and Betsy. Yet when Nightingale introduced her training school for nurses in 1860, she knew that she faced the formidable task of overcoming images such as those Dickens portrayed. Students were carefully chosen and closely supervised to be certain the image they displayed was one of which Nightingale approved.

Box 1–1. As We Were: Florence Nightingale — The Founder (1820–1910)

She was the lady with the lamp. She was the lady with the brain.

A. G. GARDINER

At an early age, Florence Nightingale demonstrated that she was not pleased with the round of parties, teas, and formal visiting expected of women in her social class. "I craved for some regular occupation for something worth doing instead of frittering time away on useless trifles."[71] Armed with an incredible education, even by today's standards, Nightingale made it her goal to learn as much as she could about hospitals and nursing. When traveling, she toured hospitals and charitable institutions to observe the architecture and the activities of the people working there. In 1850, she stopped at Kaiserwerth, Germany for 2 weeks to observe the school for deaconesses operated by Pastor Theodor Fleidner and his wife Frederika. She later returned to Kaiserwerth to study nursing for 3 months.[58] Her travels and the two experiences at Kaiserwerth were the extent of her nursing education.

Nightingale riveted the attention of the British public with her leadership of nurses during the Crimean War, in which her official title was Superintendent of the Female Nursing Establishment of the English General Hospitals in Turkey.[71] Faced with appalling conditions of filth, inappropriate and insufficient rations, and inadequate facilities, Nightingale and her band of 40 nurses turned the situation around, reducing mortality significantly. Through her frequent reports, the British public had a heightened consciousness of the need for reform in the management of health care in the British military.

After the war, she organized what is generally considered the first formal training school for nurses, which opened in 1860, financed with money donated to a fund by a grateful British public.[9] She was only indirectly involved in its management once it opened, however, and spent more of her time writing.[9] Among her works is *Notes on Nursing: What It Is and What It Is Not*, privately printed in 1859 and published in 1860. A facsimile edition is readily available and worthy of reading.

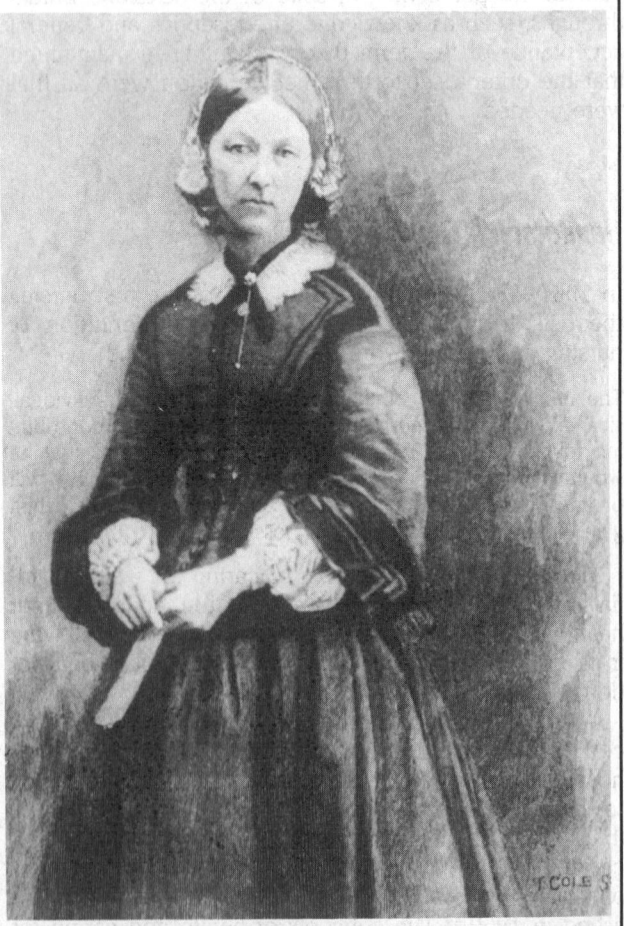

Florence Nightingale. (From The National Library of Medicine, Bethesda, MD.)

The **Nightingale School at St. Thomas Hospital, London,** was the prototype for the earliest training schools for nurses in the United States, thus influencing nursing education in North America. In addition, she had widespread influence on hospital construction, sanitation measures, and reform of the British Army medical establishment.

Since Florence Nightingale, the image of the nurse has continued to evolve. Beatrice and Philip Kalisch have written frequently on the development of nursing's image. After an extensive examination of popular literature, film, and television, they have described the development of nursing's image and have identified several phases prevalent during the past 130 years. These are described in Table 1–1.

Nursing and Religious Orders

In the history of western civilization over the last thousand years, certain religious orders played an important role in the care of the sick and injured, as members of these orders fulfilled their mission to shelter the homeless and care for orphans and ill people. Their association with the Christian religion, its principles and ideals, was the source of much that formed the image of nursing through the centuries.

In France, for instance, the Daughters of Charity of St. Vincent de Paul, founded in 1633, was a noncloistered religious order that ministered to the sick in their homes as well as in hospitals. In the United States, the Daughters of Charity, as well as many other religious orders, were instrumental in founding and maintaining numerous clinics, infirmaries, and hospitals throughout the country.

Although the image of nursing through the ages has been predominantly female, men have also made significant contributions to organized nursing. During the Middle Ages, religious orders involved in caring roles included those formed by men as well as by women. Religious crusaders during the 11th to 13th centuries needed care for those who fell to disease or injury during their military campaigns. The Knights Hospitalliers of St. John was one of the most famous orders to provide such care during that period. Originally established to oversee the hospital in Jerusalem, the Knights soon established other hospitals for pilgrims needing

TABLE 1–1. Evolving Image of Nurses from Florence Nightingale Through the 1970s

Image	Features
Angel of Mercy (Nightingale's era through World War I)	Nurse as a saintly, self-sacrificing, and virtuous woman devoted to her clients. Nurses' efforts during the Spanish-American War and World War I reinforced this image and blended it with a sense of heroic patriotism
Girl Friday (World War I through the 1920s)	Nurse as subordinate of physician, more focused on romance or marriage than on the work of nursing. In media representations of the period, romance, marriage, or both often develop either between the nurse and the doctor she served or between the nurse and the person for whom she cared
Heroine (1930s through World War II)	Nurse as courageous individual, "brave, rational, dedicated, decisive, humanistic, and autonomous." Unlike the image of World War I, the nurse's heroism was associated with a budding sense of commitment and professionalism rather than personal saintliness
Wife and mother (World War II through the mid-1960s)	Nurse as wholesome, feminine, supportive, and patient. In films and romance novels of the period, the nurse's family roles take priority over the professional role as a nurse. The esteem given to physicians increased over this period with the rapid development of medical breakthroughs; as a result, the image of working nurses took on an even more pronounced subservience to the scientific superiority of the physician
Sex object (1960s and 1970s)	Nurse as manifestation of female sexuality. The revolution in sexual morals that took place during this period affected the nurse's image. Films and novels exploited the possibilities of sexual involvement that seemed (to the authors of these works and their audiences) to be an aspect of the nurse's work situation

Data from Kalisch, P.A., & Kalisch, B.J. (1987). *The Changing Image of the Nurse.* Menlo Park, California: Addison-Wesley.

help along the road to that city.[28] The Alexian Brothers organized in the 14th century as a group of laymen who would care for those stricken with bubonic plague and bury those who succumbed to the disease. They later formed an order under Augustinian rule using St. Alexius as their patron saint. Their order is still active.[40]

The Image of Contemporary Nursing

Although the tradition of men in nursing is old and honorable, males today form approximately 3 per cent of the total number of nurses in the United States.[53] Because of this great disparity in the numbers of men and women and because of the vastly different perceptions that society still holds of men and women in the workplace, men in nursing may have different concerns with respect to their public image than do female nurses. Nevertheless, given the disparity in numbers of men and women in nursing, it would still seem to be true that, as an early nursing leader, Lavinia Dock, stated, "The status of nursing . . . depends on the status of women."[26] The feminist movement of the 1960s and 1970s has affected the relationship between women and the world of work, as well as the relationship between men and women themselves. These shifting relationships are bound to have a continuing effect on the perception of nurses and nursing in the society at large.

Several studies have been conducted to learn how nursing is currently perceived by society. Positive qualities attributed to nursing include career security, intellectual application, caring for people, and academic and scholastic achievement. Negative qualities associated with a nursing career, whether true or not, include lack of independent decision making, less safety in the workplace, less financial reward, and less respect and appreciation than is offered in other careers.[30,46] While nursing's image in some segments of society may be improving,[45] each nurse must still take responsibility for fostering a positive image through personal practice and conduct.

Studies indicate that when the general public has personal acquaintance or professional contact with nurses, it helps them avoid the negative stereotypes built up through history and to see nurses as educated, conscientious, caring professionals.[45,49]

NURSING PRACTICE

Early Development of Nurses' Roles

During the American Civil War, nurses' roles were not defined, and volunteer nurses did what they felt was needed to carry out their mission. Nursing included setting up and maintaining a laundry, gathering food from the civilian population, writing letters home for sick and wounded soldiers, guarding the liquor, sitting with the dying, and assisting in surgeries, which were usually amputations.[1,8,11,14,57] Acquiring, preparing, and serving food was a major responsibility and was often performed under extreme scarcity and hardship.

With the advent of formal nursing education, needed to overcome the long-standing negative image of nursing, the nurse and physician became the only health care providers who came in contact with the patient. The nurse did everything that the physician did not do, and this meant that nursing encompassed a broad range of activities.

During the formative stages of formal nursing education, student nurses provided the bulk of nursing care in most hospitals, with only the superintendent (director of nursing) and perhaps a few head nurses as graduate nurses. This practice of nursing students providing the bulk of nursing care continued in diploma schools of nursing well into the 1950s.

Thus, with few exceptions, when student nurses graduated, they had to do what they could to find employment outside the hospital setting. Only a few exceptional students, once graduated, were hired to be superintendents or head nurses in hospitals from which they graduated or in other hospitals hoping to open schools of nursing.

Superintendents in these schools were responsible both for overseeing all nursing care and for teaching the students. Their role encompassed two distinct roles in contemporary nursing: the nurse administrator (by whatever title chosen and used in different health care organizations) and the nurse educator, found predominantly in schools of nursing. The value of the trained nurse was soon recognized, and other distinct nursing roles evolved by the dawn of the 20th century. Those roles were private duty nursing, visiting/public health nursing, industrial nursing, and military nursing.

Major Settings for Contemporary Nursing Practice

In today's health care system, the activities of nursing span an extremely broad range. Some nurses, for example, may seem to be more and more involved in assisting with highly technologic medical care to the exclusion of anything else. Yet while all nurses are not involved in direct client care, they are indirectly contributing to that care in some way. Nurses are also performing their activities in myriad settings.

HOSPITALS

In 1991, the American Nurses' Association published *Nursing's Agenda for Health Care Reform.*[4] Although this document advocated the movement of the bulk of client care into community settings, the most common setting for nursing care is still in hospitals, also referred to as acute care settings. In these settings nurses are responsible for rendering care 24 hours a day, 7 days a week. Nurses work in any number of specialty areas, such as intensive care units, obstetrical departments (including labor and delivery, nurseries, and post-partum), surgical departments, the operating room, and medical units. The acuity level of people admitted to

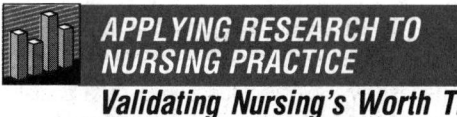

APPLYING RESEARCH TO NURSING PRACTICE
Validating Nursing's Worth Through Historical Research

Fairman, J. (1992). Watchful vigilance: nursing care, technology, and the development of intensive care units. *Nursing Research,* 41(1), 56–60.

▼▼▼

Until now, little has been known about the development of nursing practice within the intensive care units that emerged during the 1950s. The historical nursing research described in this article was conducted at the Center for the Study of the History of Nursing, based at the University of Pennsylvania School of Nursing.

Prior to the development of the intensive care unit, nurses traditionally provided specialized care to unstable persons by intensive observation and by the triage method; that is, grouping the physiologically unstable in one area of the hospital ward. When hospital administrators and physicians recognized the value of these nursing strategies, the intensive care unit was specifically designed and designated for the care of critically ill persons. Although critically ill persons were finally located in one place, the knowledge required to care for these people was not made available to these pioneer nurses. As a result, critical care nurses actively identified the kinds of knowledge necessary for nursing practice and shared this information with other nurses.

Initially, nurses and physicians "traded" different kinds of knowledge. Nursing observations of the critically ill person's condition were offered in exchange for the physician's knowledge of physiology and interpretation of data. This strategy set the stage for the eventual organization of formalized nursing knowledge specific to the care of the critically ill.

Applications for Practice

The wise utilization of intensive observation and triage is a hallmark of excellence in nursing practice. Lessons gained from historical nursing research identify successful ways of gaining and applying nursing knowledge to clinical practice today.

hospitals is generally very high and demands intensive nursing care from caring, well-educated, well-organized, cost-conscious nurses.

Besides delivering care ordered by physicians, nurses assess their clients, make nursing diagnoses, plan and deliver nursing care, and coordinate care with other departments of the hospital. Nurses also help plan for each person's discharge from the hospital and evaluate the results of nursing care given (see Unit 2). In addition, professional nurses supervise paraprofessionals, such as licensed practical nurses and nurse aides, as prescribed by law.

AMBULATORY CARE SETTINGS

Nurses working in ambulatory care settings care for people who are not confined to the health care setting.

These individuals come to settings such as doctors' offices, clinics (such as family-planning and well-baby clinics), and counseling centers. In general, ambulatory clients come in for treatment of minor illnesses or injuries and for counseling. Rehabilitation care, hospice care, and respite care are also frequently located in ambulatory care settings. Such settings are usually, although not always, operated during daylight hours and closed on weekends.

COMMUNITY/PUBLIC HEALTH SETTINGS

When Nightingale formalized her notion of nursing, she envisioned public health, then called district nursing, to be an occupation for better-educated women from the upper strata of society. Since Nightingale's time, public health nursing has taken several specialized forms.

Visiting Nursing. Visiting nursing is one form of public health nursing, and it too has evolved for some time. In the United States, visiting nursing was initiated in 1877, when trained nurses were sent into the homes of the poor by the Women's Branch of the New York City Mission.[42] Several other organizations put nurses in dispensaries and to work doing health teaching. The most successful visiting nurse project was initiated at the Henry Street Settlement by Lillian Wald and Mary Brewster in 1893 on New York City's Lower East Side. Beginning as a visiting nurse enterprise, the settlement house soon greatly expanded its scope of nursing and related activities.[59,63,64,69]

In the beginning, the two nurses sought out patients. Before long their neighbors heard of their services and came to them. The nurses provided what services they could and sought medical advice from physicians, when necessary. As the news of their activities spread, physicians began referring patients to them as well.

As health departments became part of city, county, and state governments, they, too, were involved in the health of the public. City and county health departments sent out visiting nurses to care for individuals and families in their homes. They also held clinics for impoverished citizens. The American Red Cross used visiting nurses in its Rural Nursing Service.[10]

Home health nursing is today's version of visiting nursing and is a major force in the growing area of delivering care to individuals in their homes. As the cost of in-hospital care has spiraled upward, and as other financial factors have shortened the average hospital stay, home health nursing has been an important resource for many clients. Visiting nurses are now caring for and directing the care of home-bound persons, some of whom are severely ill. This calls for skills only nurses working in hospitals once needed. The need to possess such skills is a new phenomenon.

The rapid rise in cases of acquired immune deficiency syndrome (AIDS) has also resulted in a renewed need for home care services. In 1984, the Visiting Nurse Association and Hospice of San Francisco organized the first program of home care services for persons with AIDS. These organizations were followed the next year by the Visiting Nurse Service of New York, which now operates the world's largest home care pro-

Box 1-2. Home Health Nursing in the 1890s and 1990s

The home health nurse of 1890 was embodied in the private duty nurse acting as a private agent or as visiting nurse. The private duty nurse generally worked a 24-hour day, sleeping whenever she could. Her term of employment could be from several days to, in some situations, years. In the latter case, it was usually as a companion. Her duties included care of the ill person and in many instances involved other duties such as cooking. If the client was the mother of the household, the nurse's role could include the whole range of activities the mother would have done.

The private duty nurse's clients generally were those with communicable diseases or with trauma from accidents. Childbirth also took place at home, and the nurse would assist at the birth and then care for mother and infant for several weeks afterward.

Surgery was commonly performed in the home. In such cases nurses set up for and assisted with the surgery, sometimes administering the anesthetic. The nurse then monitored the client during recovery from anesthesia and cared for the client postoperatively.

The visiting nurses of the 1890s visited patients who comprised their case load, performing whatever services were deemed necessary. The range of activities was exhaustive; care included bathing to cleanse or to decrease fevers, cooking, teaching, administering medications, and manipulating the environment. The nurse returned to visit as frequently as was deemed necessary. She also functioned as a social worker, referring patients to physicians or agencies where necessary.

The home health nurse of the 1990s is employed by one of numerous home health agencies and is part of a complex team. Because governmental policies have greatly reduced the length of hospital stays, these agencies have increased significantly. The nurse visits clients who have been referred to the agency by physicians, other health care professionals, neighbors, family, friends, or in some instances, the clients themselves.

In the home health arena the nurse's roles include assessor, caregiver, referral agent, case manager, coordinator, teacher, and client advocate. Nurses make decisions about problems that must be addressed by a professional nurse, a paraprofessional, a nurse's aide, or the client's family. A key responsibility is teaching the family to assume as much of the care as possible.

The acuity level of ill persons in the home has increased significantly. Consequently, nurses skilled in critical care are highly sought to fill the role of home health care nurse. Home health nurses are part of an interdisciplinary team including physical therapists, speech therapists, occupational therapists, social workers, and dietitians. The nurse can also be a clinical specialist concentrating on caring for a specific type of client.

gram for persons with AIDS and averages more than 900 clients a day.[68] Nursing activities in the home can include assessment and management, evaluating the adequacy of nutrition, health teaching for the client and family, and coordinating the services and resources necessary for the client's care.

School Nursing. School nursing was initiated when Lillian Wald became appalled at the number of children sent home or barred from attending public school because of minor ailments. She believed that, with nurses in attendance, children with minor maladies could be kept in school. As a result, she initiated school nursing on a trial basis in 1902. The experiment proved an unqualified success.

"During the month of September, 1902, 10,567 children had been sent home from the New York schools, while in September, 1903, with a school nurse in attendance, there were only 1,101 exclusions."[42]

Nursing in school systems, be they private or public, varies considerably by locale. Generally, in schools, nurses do such things as monitor the health of children, check compliance with immunization policies, teach health, and make referrals to physicians and agencies. *Nursing's Agenda for Health Care Reform*, however, calls for moving nursing practice out of acute care settings and into community settings, such as workplaces and schools.[4] Consequently, we can expect to see a dramatic change in the way school nursing is practiced.

Occupational Health Nursing. Occupational health nursing, previously known as industrial nursing, was initiated in 1888, when Betty Moulder was employed by some coal-mining companies in Pennsylvania to care for coal miners and their families. In the same period, Ada Mayo was hired to care for people in several Vermont villages, most of whom were employed by the Vermont Marble Company.[3] Before the turn of the century, several New York department stores had initiated the practice of using industrial nurses to care for sick employees in their homes.[3] Industrial nursing expanded significantly during World Wars I and II to care for the large number of employees in the greatly expanded industries needed to support the war effort.

Today, occupational health nursing is an important part of industry. Rather than caring for employees and their families in their homes, occupational health nurses care for injured employees and are concerned with health teaching, health promotion, and safety within the work place. They are also responsible for identifying potential hazards that could result in illness or injuries to employees.

Nursing Homes and Extended-Care Facilities. The burgeoning of the aged population, coupled with homemakers now working outside the home, has left no one to care for many frail or ill elderly at home. Although only a minority of elderly are institutionalized, the numbers of facilities needed to care for them has increased significantly over the last decade. The care of elderly persons in these settings presents a tremendous challenge to nurses. Such institutions typically have a

---

Box 1–3. As We Are: Keeta Lewis — School Nursing for Children and Families

School nursing for children with developmental problems is a relatively new area of nursing practice . . .

As a school nurse, I work in an early intervention program with infants and toddlers from birth through 3 years old who have developmental delays or specific disabilities. People are often surprised that this population and their families are served in a school setting. Many see this role as nontraditional. School nursing for children with developmental problems is a relatively new area of nursing practice, one for which there is little preparation available in graduate or other educational programs.

As a nurse in the hospital, I had observed infants and small children with a variety of developmental delays and realized that their caregivers desperately needed information. I wanted to work with these children and their families outside the hospital setting. The value of early intervention, as I saw it, was the potential for positive long-term outcomes.

Each year I have seen an increasing variety in the structures of the families I serve. There are traditional families, single-parent families, alternative lifestyle families, and families in which one or both parents are mentally or physically disabled. A growing number of families have little or no health insurance. The lifestyle or high-risk behaviors of some families may predispose their young children to HIV, syphilis, or hepatitis. Frequently, I see young children who are neglected or sexually, physically, or mentally abused.

Many of the children I work with are prenatally drug-exposed (PDE). One of the things I do in the program is visit the homes of these children to obtain a health history and physical assessment for the infant and to observe family interactions. One child, Sunshine, was 2 months old, extremely irritable, and crying through much of the day and night. She rarely attempted eye contact and avoided the gaze of others. She did not like to be held and was unable to soothe herself or be soothed. Because of increased mus-

cle tone, she was difficult to cuddle. Her sucking reflex was poor, making it difficult to feed her, and she had a severe reflux and diarrhea. Some of these typical PDE characteristics place the infant-caregiver relationship at risk and also jeopardize the infant's development.

As I observed and assessed Sunshine and other PDE infants for 7 years, I became aware of the need for a simple means of assessing this population. With this awareness and the encouragement of my family and colleagues, I developed an assessment protocol to identify the atypical neurobehavioral characteristics of PDE infants from birth to 12 months of age. The protocol allows the clinician and caregiver to describe the individual infant's strengths and weaknesses, give priority to the infant's needs, and develop intervention strategies. I continued to develop this protocol in my MSN program and in my doctoral work. I hope the Lewis Protocol will make a difference in the children and their families' lives and will give them an early opportunity for a successful and happy quality of life.

Health and education are two public services that can have a great impact on children's lives. The link between the two needs to be well understood: to learn, children need to be healthy both physically and mentally. School nursing services have been providing this link for almost 100 years. By working with children, families, and teachers, school nurses detect social and health problems that interfere with learning, and they discover options and opportunities for effective interventions. With more and more school nursing specialists prepared at the graduate level and with the dramatic changes in the North American educational system, school health will continue to present exciting challenges and rewards for nurses.

---

high ratio of non-professional nursing personnel to registered nurses. The registered nurse spends most of the time planning and coordinating care and supervising paraprofessionals.

The level of care given to residents differs between nursing homes and extended-care facilities. The former give custodial care. The latter are staffed and supplied with the resources to provide skilled nursing care. As the acuity of illness of these elderly persons changes, there is frequent transferring of residents from one type of agency to another, requiring the nurse's diligent attention to continuity of care.

Military Nursing. Female nurses were first used formally in the military in the United States as contract nurses during the Spanish-American War, in 1898. A total of 1563 nurses served during that short war.[42] The formation of the Army Nurse Corps in 1901 was a direct result of the success of use of those trained nurses; the establishment of the Navy Nurse Corps in 1908 was an indirect result. Nurses have been an integral part of the military ever since.

New Settings for Nursing Practice. In virtually every setting where the physical and psychosocial well-being

of individuals is a vital interest, nurses will be found. Some nurses practice as lawyers, as expert witnesses assisting lawyers, as elected representatives, as legislative aides advising representatives, and as consultants to health care agencies and financial institutions. Traveling nurses contract with a traveling nurse bureau and work wherever they are sent for contracted periods of time. Nurse-midwives work in some hospitals and as self-employed professionals doing home deliveries. Churches are beginning to hire parish nurses to serve the members of their congregations.

One reason for nursing shortages is that nurses are invaluable assets in many settings. Consequently, even with a steadily increasing number of nurses in the workplace, their number is frequently insufficient to meet the demands.

Clinical Specialization

Clinical specialization in nursing has historical roots in the earliest days of modern nursing but has recently grown in importance partly in response to increasing specialization in medicine.[37] As medicine has specialized and the use of technology for care has increased,

Box 1–4. As We Are: Peter Ungvarski—The Challenge of Experiential Learning

. . . nurses will ensure that their clients are well cared for, even under the most adverse circumstances.

As I approach my thirtieth year as a professional nurse, I sometimes wonder what life would have been like if I had chosen another profession. It is with the utmost confidence that I conclude that had I not chosen to be a nurse, my life would have been quite boring. If I were to ascribe a theme to my life's chosen work, it would be the constant challenge of experiential learning.

As a new graduate in 1964, I chose to work on a medical-surgical ward at Bellevue Hospital in New York City. Not just any medical-surgical ward, but a prison ward. My experiences there taught me the values of nursing the disenfranchised in our society.

In 1966 I decided to "join the Navy and see the world." I went from New York City to Philadelphia. However short the distance, it was just as well I was close to home, because as a newly appointed ensign in the U.S. Navy Nurse Corps I found caring for young Marine amputees my own age quite stressful. With time I learned the invaluable lesson of focusing on individual capabilities and not dwelling upon disabilities. With the escalation of the war in Viet Nam, I eventually received orders overseas and was a charge nurse of an aeromedical evacuation unit at the U.S. Naval Hospital in Guam. My time spent caring for wounded Marines and sailors taught me the rewards of esprit de corps and the important role nurses played in the military during a time of war. We not only nursed our troops but also represented mothers and fathers, sisters and brothers, and all that was "back home."

Upon my discharge from the Navy, both curious and concerned about the growing problem of drug addiction, I went to work in a drug addiction rehabilitation program. It was there that I learned that the plan of care developed by nurses, doctors, and others really belonged to the client and not the person writing the care plan. I learned that setting health care goals must be done by the nurse with the person receiving care. I learned that the label "noncompliant" was an excuse used by health care professionals to avoid dealing with the behaviors at hand. There are definite reasons why people don't comply with care plans and instructions.

Until the early 1980s, the major portion of my career was spent in the area of critical care. I was challenged by the continuous need to learn new procedures and to use new equipment to enhance care. Caught up in the maze of tech-

nology, resuscitation advances, and new drugs, I eventually became aware of an emerging paradox. Death was no longer viewed as an inevitable consequence of life, but rather a failure on the part of health care professionals. I found myself crying at a person's bedside not because the person had died but because our resuscitation efforts failed.

In 1981, in my quest for learning, I began working in hospice care. It was in this area that I met the extraordinary clinicians, both nurses and doctors, of my career. It was the first time I truly experienced the interdisciplinary team in action. I realized that nursing involved not only the person in the bed but also the family. Most of all I learned symptom control and comfort measures that would and should be practiced in any setting. Imagine my amazement when I discovered that the main principle is allowing the person to control the pain (by preventing recurrence) rather than allowing the pain to control the person. I learned that nurses' and doctors' fear of the patient becoming addicted was not only unfounded but also cruel.

When the AIDS epidemic began, I was confronted with caring for those with diseases I had never encountered. I found myself spending endless hours in the library learning about *Pneumocystis carinii* pneumonia and Kaposi's sarcoma and reviewing the literature on caring for immunocompromised clients. My interest in nursing people with HIV diseases and AIDS carried me through the 1980s and into the 1990s in various settings, including hospice, critical care, acute care, research, and finally home care.

It appears that I am back where I started, nursing the disenfranchised, homosexual and bisexual men, injecting drug users, racial and ethnic minorities, and the poor. I've had the privilege of lecturing nurses across the United States, in Europe, and the Caribbean and have been consistently impressed by nurses' dedication and commitment to caring for people with HIV and AIDS. I learned that nurses will ensure that their clients are well cared for, even under the most adverse circumstances.

Would I do it all again? Most definitely, and I wouldn't change anything. For all the positive and negative experiences I've encountered in nursing, I've learned a great deal about making people feel safe and comfortable and how to help them make their choices in life.

---

caring for the ill has become more complicated and has required nurse specialization. Nurses specialize in their practice depending on the type of client, the setting, or both. A nurse can also specialize without a formal educational program by working in a specialized area and undertaking independent study, or by taking continuing education courses, although these means do not lead to certification in any specialty.

Some nurses choose to specialize in the care of clients of a particular type or those with a particular health problem. Within the hospital, for example, nurses often choose to specialize in the care of adults, children, pregnant women, cancer patients, or people

with neurologic problems. Clients are often segregated in separate units of the hospital or in hospitals dedicated to particular conditions or level of care. For instance, the intensive care units, operating room, or emergency department of a hospital often will have nurses who are specially trained for practice in such settings.

Standards of Nursing Practice

Setting standards for nursing practice was done as an effort to delineate nursing activities more clearly. Nursing standards have undergone an evolutionary process. The ANA implemented their development in the late 1960s, with the first published in 1973. The latest version was in 1991:

In defining the role of **nursing standards,** the ANA states: Standards are authoritative statements by which the nursing profession describes the responsibilities for which its practitioners are accountable. Consequently, standards reflect the values and priorities of the profession.[5]

In addition to the overriding *Standards of Clinical Nursing Practice,* which appears in the appendices to this text, the ANA has also published standards for specialty practice, teaching, and administration. The Canadian Nurses Association has developed *Standards for Nursing Practice,* which are shown in Box 1–5. Some specialty organizations have also published standards of which practicing nurses should be aware. When a malpractice suit is filed against a nurse, professional standards are used as one criterion to determine whether the nurse was negligent.

Patients/Clients/Consumers

Over the last several decades the term applied to the people for whom nurses care has been evolving. At one time all people cared for by nurses were referred to as patients no matter the setting. The term, however, implied being sick. As nurses moved into settings where they were caring for essentially healthy people or where the presenting illness was perceived as an episodic phenomenon, the term no longer seemed appropriate.

The use of the term *client* evolved to be applied, in general, to those people not confined to institutions. As nurses moved into private practice and charged for their services, the term client seemed more appropriate. It reflects a relationship like that of a lawyer and a person who engages legal services.

Box 1–5. Canadian Nurses Association Standards for Nursing Practice

These four standards are necessarily interdependent and interrelated.

Standard I	Nursing practice requires that a conceptual model(s) for nursing be the basis for that practice.
Standard II	Nursing practice requires the effective use of the nursing process.
Standard III	Nursing practice requires that the helping relationship be the nature of the client-nurse interaction.
Standard IV	Nursing practice requires nurses to fulfill professional responsibilities.

From Canadian Nurses Association (1987). *A definition of nursing practice. Standards for nursing practice.* Ottawa: Canadian Nurses Association.

The term *consumer* was used as early as 1974 by Freymann when he spoke of a "rational consumer contract."[33] Freymann pointed out that patients are really consumers of health care and as such have the power to exert some kind of influence on that care. In 1978, Kohnke wrote of "the nurse's responsibility to the consumer."[43]

Today, while hospitals and physicians refer to health care consumers as patients, it is becoming more and more acceptable for nurses to refer to their charges as clients. This is true in any health care setting and regardless of the person's health status.

NURSING EDUCATION

Formal nursing education has been shaped by numerous factors. Wars, the most notable of all catalysts for social change, the educational system in general, and the status of women have all contributed in their own ways to shaping nursing education. Some of the most influential factors have been the leadership exerted by nurses in the vanguard during the formative stages of modern nursing. These include Florence Nightingale, **Mary Adelaide Nutting, Isabel Hampton Robb,** and others. Generally, nursing leaders during the formative period of formal nursing education were a cohesive group who worked together to shape nursing as they envisioned it.

Early Schools

NIGHTINGALE SCHOOL AT ST. THOMAS HOSPITAL, LONDON

The school generally considered the first formal school of nursing was Nightingale's school of nursing at St. Thomas Hospital in London. Nightingale opened her school against some opposition on the part of physicians.[71] Her initial goal was to educate nurses who would go on to ". . . take posts in hospitals and public institutions . . ."[71] Nightingale did not personally oversee the school but rather delegated that responsibility to Mrs. Wardroper, who had been the Matron at St. Thomas for some time. Money contributed by the British public to the Nightingale Fund for her noble wartime services enabled her to establish the school as a financially independent entity. Although the school was on precarious footing during its early years, ultimately it became a very successful and prominent nursing school.[9]

People who wanted to establish nursing schools in the United States in the early 1870s consulted Nightingale about the operation of such schools. Consequently, she had considerable influence on the establishment of some of the earliest schools opened here.

THE FIRST THREE AMERICAN SCHOOLS

The year 1873 is generally credited as the date that the first three formal training schools for nurses opened in the United States. The impetus for the founding of the schools lies in the American Civil War. Volunteer nurses during that period demonstrated that good nursing care made a difference. Consequently, after the war, some of the women who had been active as nurses diverted their attention to social reform, and improving the conditions in civilian hospitals became a "cause." They saw improved nursing care as the cornerstone of hospital improvement and to that end they exerted their energies.[7,35]

Those first three U.S. training schools were the **Bellevue Training School,** the **Connecticut Training School for Nurses** at the New Haven State Hospital, and the **Boston Training School.** The superior nursing care provided by the students in the training schools was soon recognized, and nursing schools began opening in a geometric progression.

The initial period of training was 1 year but gradually lengthened to 2 then 3 years, where it stayed until the 1950s, when radical changes in the education of nurses caused considerable variation in the length of nursing education programs.

The rapid extension of nursing schools into most hospitals, even those unable to provide an adequate training, caused the nursing leadership considerable concern. As a result, nursing leaders banded together to form the earliest national nursing organizations in the United States. Their goal was to bring about reform. Their continuing concerns were the impetus for numerous studies of nursing education.

Wars and Changing Patterns of Nursing Education

Just as wars have affected society at large, they have had a profound effect on nursing in the United States.

THE CIVIL WAR

Although some data point to the use of untrained nurses on a contract basis to the army during the Revolutionary War,[62,66] the use of volunteer nurses during the Civil War is widely documented. After the firing on Fort Sumter, President Lincoln called for 75,000 volunteers for the militia. In addition to the male volunteers, hundreds of northern women also volunteered. From that number, 100 women were selected to take a short course in "nursing" at Bellevue Hospital.[23]

Because of the large volume of northern women volunteers, the Secretary of War appointed Dorothea Dix as the superintendent of women nurses. She was well known as a humanitarian reformer among the mentally ill and as a person of considerable organizational skills.[65] Dedicated women who were refused entry into service as nurses through Miss Dix served in other ways. Large numbers of women joined the U.S. Sanitary Commission, and still others just showed up at hospitals and served.

Women in the south were also involved in volunteer nursing endeavors, but they did not have the strong organizational support that the northern nurses had. The lack of organization did not hamper their efforts to serve, however, and some opened hospitals in their homes. The northern blockade of southern ports intensified the privations that these nurses endured in trying to help the sick and wounded.[22]

Many diaries of volunteer nurses from both sides of the conflict still exist. They detail the bravery, creativity, and political astuteness of the Civil War volunteers.

WORLD WAR I

Even before the entry of the United States into World War I, three years after it erupted in Europe, American nursing leaders were concerned about nursing resources. Their overriding concern was to be able to provide an ongoing supply of trained nurses if the United States became embroiled in the war. Patriotism inspired nurses to enroll in the Red Cross Nursing Service, the recruiting mechanism for service in the military. Their departure from the civilian sector threatened to leave civilian nursing needs unmet.

In addition to recruiting larger numbers of young women into civilian training schools, the collective nursing leadership devised two creative schemes to mitigate possible shortages of trained nurses for the military: the Army School of Nursing and the Vassar Training Camp. The Vassar Training Camp was conducted on the campus of Vassar College during the summer of 1918. More than 400 women with college degrees were recruited into nursing. They got their preliminary training during that summer, then went into existing schools of nursing that had agreed to participate in the scheme.[42]

The Army School of Nursing was opened in 1918, with Annie Goodrich as its head. The students got their training in various military hospitals. The school continued until 1932 when lack of funds forced its closure.[67]

WORLD WAR II

As with the first World War, the collective nursing leadership was concerned with a potential shortage of nurses during World War II. The military services required considerable nursing personnel, so that a concern was the potential of depleting the ability to meet civilian nursing needs. Schools of nursing were asked to increase their enrollments as much as possible. Refresher courses were initiated to bring back into the work force nurses who had dropped out of nursing. In addition, the federal government appropriated large sums of money to support nursing education. Even with these measures, a nursing shortage still existed. As a result, legislation was passed establishing the Cadet Nurse Corps.

The law provided that schools of nursing wishing to participate would receive full reimbursement for the students' tuition, books, and uniforms and full maintenance from the federal government. In addition, the students were given monthly stipends and street uniforms of the corps. The scheme proved to be immensely popular, educating 125,000 nurses before it was terminated in 1948.[43]

After the war, the Serviceman's Readjustment Act (G. I. Bill) was passed into law; among other provisions, the law provided funds for veterans to return to school. Many nurses took advantage of the opportunity to return to school to earn college degrees. This trend began a new era in nursing education.

Nursing Education Today

LPN/LVN EDUCATION

The titles for licensed practical nurse and licensed vocational nurse vary throughout the United States. Different areas use different titles, but in general, education for LPNs or LVNs is approximately 1 year of training beyond high school.[51] Control of licensure lies with each state.

The shortage of nurses during and after World War II led to increased use of LPN/LVNs and the opening of schools to train these nurses. LPN/LVNs practice under the supervision of a registered nurse or physician.

GENERIC PREPARATION FOR RNs

Three educational routes prepare nurses to take the National Council for Licensing Examination–Registered Nurse (NCLEX–RN) to become a registered nurse.

Diploma. The oldest educational route for registered nurses is the hospital setting, where after approximately 3 years the graduate is awarded a diploma from the hospital. This 3-year time frame, however, is beginning to vary throughout the country. Between 1873 and 1952 this setting for nurse education predominated. In recent years the number of such programs has decreased significantly.

Associate Degree. Nurses educated at the associate-degree level receive the degree after 2 years' matriculation. Community colleges predominate in this form of education, although some 4-year colleges and universities also offer the associate degree in nursing.

Associate degrees in nursing were envisioned and initiated by Mildred Montag in 1952 as a research project at Teachers College, Columbia University. Her purpose was twofold: to educate nurses more efficiently than in a 3-year diploma school and to promote entry of registered nurses into the workplace more rapidly. Placing students in community colleges also put them into institutions of higher education rather than hospitals, which had generally been considered service institutions. Associate-degree programs proved to be very popular. They now graduate more nurses than any other form of nurse education.

Baccalaureate Degree. The baccalaureate degree in nursing had its formative roots in postgraduate programs that became popular around the turn of the century. Nurses who wanted to specialize or who believed they had inadequate preparation in some area of nursing often sought out "postgraduate" courses in hospitals offering them. Some of the specialty areas available were operating room, lying-in (maternity), and pediatrics. Unfortunately, the courses were primarily service to the hospital rather than actual advanced education.[42]

The earliest endeavor to make nursing education part of a college setting was the establishment of the Hospital Economics Course in 1899 at Teachers College, Columbia University. As Robb said,

The aim of the course is to fit persons who are already trained nurses for the responsible duties of superintendent of hospitals and principals of training schools for nurses.[60]

Originally, the nurses matriculating through the course did not receive an academic degree. In 1916 the baccalaureate degree was first awarded on successful completion of the program.

In 1923, after a large study of nursing, the *Goldmark Report* was published. One of its recommendations was the reiteration that schools of nursing be put into the mainstream of higher education.[36] In response, the first autonomous collegiate school of nursing was opened in 1924 at Yale University with funding from the Rockefeller Foundation. The pilot program, initiated in 1924, was so successful that in 1929 the Foundation awarded Yale a million dollar endowment to make it a permanent school of nursing.[42] In 1928 the school elevated its entrance requirement to a baccalaureate degree, thus making the generic nursing degree a master's degree.[42] In spite of this early and successful experiment in collegiate nursing education, such a pattern was slow in gaining favor.

BEYOND GENERIC PREPARATION

When registered nurses decided to seek a baccalaureate degree, many colleges and universities would grant them 2 years of college credit for their 3 years of education in a hospital diploma program. Thus the nurses had to take, for the most part, only another 2 years of college to earn a baccalaureate degree. During the 1950s, however, when the number of baccalaureate programs slowly began to increase, the nursing literature contained numerous articles about how best to structure nursing programs in college settings; Murchison's article, "A Four-Year Basic Collegiate Program" is only one of these.[50] In some university hospitals, students with 2 years of collegiate education prior to matriculating at the university hospital school of nursing would be granted a baccalaureate degree from the university owning the hospital.[13]

RN to BSN. Today, many nurses holding diplomas and associate degrees are finding it difficult to advance professionally without a baccalaureate degree. Generally, the baccalaureate nursing curriculum is concentrated in the last 2 years of the educational experience, building on 2 years of lower-division liberal arts courses. In the past, because the associate degree and diploma programs have philosophical bases different from the baccalaureate-granting institutions, many registered nurses found getting a baccalaureate degree very laborious. Consequently, many RN-to-BSN programs have been established, the goal being to build on the RN's strengths yet provide the education to fill in the deficits.

Because many master's programs in nursing will not admit nurses without a baccalaureate in nursing, the

RN-to-BSN programs are providing a needed service to RNs wishing to go on to graduate study in the future. Because of the large numbers of RNs without baccalaureate degrees, the American Association of Colleges of Nursing is recommending more flexibility to assist RNs with a diploma or an associate degree to move into a baccalaureate program and work toward a baccalaureate degree.[2]

Graduate Education. Graduate education for nurses has taken many forms and remains broad and diverse. Originally, with few exceptions, advanced degrees were earned outside nursing. Since the advent of the Nurses Training Act in 1964, however, the number of graduate programs in nursing has increased significantly, both at the master's and at the doctoral levels.[19]

These programs vary considerably. Master's programs prepare nurses for a variety of roles. Master's preparation for clinical specialties and practitioner programs is clinically focused. Master's education preparing nurses for doctoral study is theoretically focused and usually requires the student to write a thesis. An increasing number of individuals already holding baccalaureate and higher degrees in fields outside nursing are choosing to enter nursing for many reasons. Consequently, programs have been developed to grant a "generic" master's degree in nursing, as Yale has done since 1928.

Other nursing master's programs are offering joint or dual degrees with other disciplines; one such program combines a master's in nursing with one in business or public affairs. The former is of particular interest to those nurses planning to work in administrative roles.

Nurses wishing to pursue a career in nursing education, especially in 4-year colleges and universities, generally need a doctorate. Nurses with doctoral degrees outside nursing, in areas such as education, anthropology, and physiology, are still hired as faculty members and bring much to a nursing faculty. More and more universities, however, are seeking nurses with nursing doctorates. The most common are the Doctor of Philosophy (PhD) and the Doctor of Nursing Science (DNS). Philosophically, these nursing doctoral degrees are supposed to differ, but research has demonstrated that the different programs have more similarities than differences.

Continuing Education. Some states now require evidence of continuing education (CE) for nurses in order to renew their licenses. In such states specific providers of CE are approved by the state board of nursing. Educational institutions and private organizations providing such education offer CE courses and programs. Some hospitals also have in-service programs approved so they may grant CE credit.

Some CE programs are 1- to 3-day programs for which continuing education units are awarded. One continuing education unit (CEU) is awarded for one contact hour in a continuing education program. CEUs can be awarded for other educational experiences such as enrolling in courses toward a degree, presenting papers, and writing articles. In states requiring mandatory CE, it behooves nurses to keep careful records of CEUs received.

THE NURSING PROFESSION

The status of nursing as a bona fide profession has been a topic of discussion for many years. Extant data do not reveal that Nightingale set out to establish a profession of nursing, but, in the United States we have much evidence that early leaders of nursing wanted to establish professional status for nursing. Exactly what is meant by the term *profession* is much disputed. In a study of ten definitions of the term by authors from numerous disciplines, one researcher found very little congruence.[20]

Although definitions vary, many agree that a profession has a code of ethics and a professional organization and that it provides a needed service to society. Nursing meets those criteria.

Whether or not others choose to put nursing within the ranks of a profession, nurses do.

Early Collaborative Efforts of Nurses

From the time emerging nursing leaders met at the Chicago World's Fair and established the American Association of Superintendents of Training Schools for Nurses (the forerunner of the National League for Nursing), they worked together to try to shape the emerging profession. Abundant data demonstrate their collaborative relationships. In the history of nursing, the names Hampton (later Mrs. Robb), Nutting, Wald, Dock, and others appear repeatedly. Wald's work at the Henry Street Settlement involved Dock directly and was a clinical experience in public health for students at Teachers College headed by Nutting. While some contemporary researchers believe these women charted an elitist path not subscribed to by most other nurses,[48] their wisdom and efforts set nursing on the path followed by many nurses in the following years. Not only did they work to establish the superintendents' group and the Associated Alumnae (the forerunner of the American Nurses' Association), but they also worked to establish the International Council of Nurses. Eventually, the establishment of the *American Journal of Nursing* in 1900 was a joint effort both in its financing and in its publishing.

Developing a Professional Career

Whereas some individuals enter nursing with a clear idea of where they want to go and what they want to do with their professional careers, many are not so decisive. Many enter with the altruistic idea that they want to "serve people" by being a "bedside nurse." They do not realize that there are numerous ways to achieve those goals.

In today's world, with few exceptions, a baccalaureate degree is needed to advance within nursing, and most teaching and management positions now call for an education beyond the baccalaureate level. The National League for Nursing, the national accrediting body

Box 1-6. As We Were: Isabel Hampton Robb (1860-1910)—Paradigm of Professionalism

No monument of marble nor tablet of brass will be more enduring than the spirit which Isabel Adams Hampton imbred into her first school for nurses.

B. MELOSH

Isabel Adams Hampton was born in 1860 in Welland, Ontario, Canada, the fourth of seven children.[54] After first attending public school, she attended St. Catherine's Collegiate Institute where she earned a teaching certificate.[17, 54] After teaching school for about 3 years, she entered Bellevue Hospital Training School for nurses in 1881, graduating 2 years later.

Immediately after graduation, she worked as a substitute superintendent of nurses at Woman's Hospital in New York for a short period.[17] Hampton then left to go to Rome to work with former fellow students at St. Paul's House, caring for British and American travellers for 18 months.[54]

Upon her arrival home, the position of superintendent of nurses at the Illinois Training School for Nurses at Cook County Hospital, Chicago, was offered to her. Her leadership ability soon became apparent as she implemented educational innovations at the training school. There she stopped the exploitative practice of sending students out of the hospital to do private duty, with the hospital collecting the fees. A graded program of study was introduced, and the practice affiliations with other hospitals was initiated to round out the students' hospital experiences. She resigned from this position in 1889 to accept the position of superintendent of nurses and principal of the school of nursing at Johns Hopkins Hospital in Baltimore, Maryland.[45]

Hampton established that school upon a sound base that readily gained recognition for excellence. In 1894, she resigned to marry Dr. Hunter Robb, a physician. Mary Adelaide Nutting, who had been in the first class admitted to the school, assumed her position. Some of her colleagues, especially Lavinia Dock, were quite distraught at Hampton's marriage, fearing that they would lose a very capable ally in the fight to elevate the status of nursing, but such was not the case. Atypical for the Victorian age, Isabel Hampton Robb remained active in nursing in volunteer capacities after she married and moved to Cleveland, Ohio.[55]

Isabel Hampton was instrumental in establishing the American Society of Superintendents of Training Schools (the forerunner of the National League for Nursing). In 1896, as Mrs. Robb, she helped organize the Nurses Associated Alumnae of the United States and Canada (the forerunner of the American Nurses' Association), in 1900, she helped found

the International Council of Nurses.[54] She was also instrumental in helping organize the Hospital Economics Course at Teachers College, Columbia University, in 1899. She left behind a legacy of commitment to the elevation of nursing education that had lasting impact.

She died an untimely death at age 50 years. While walking with a friend, she abruptly stepped away to avoid an oncoming speeding vehicle and was crushed between two trolley cars. Speculations abound about what she might have accomplished had she lived as long as her cohorts.

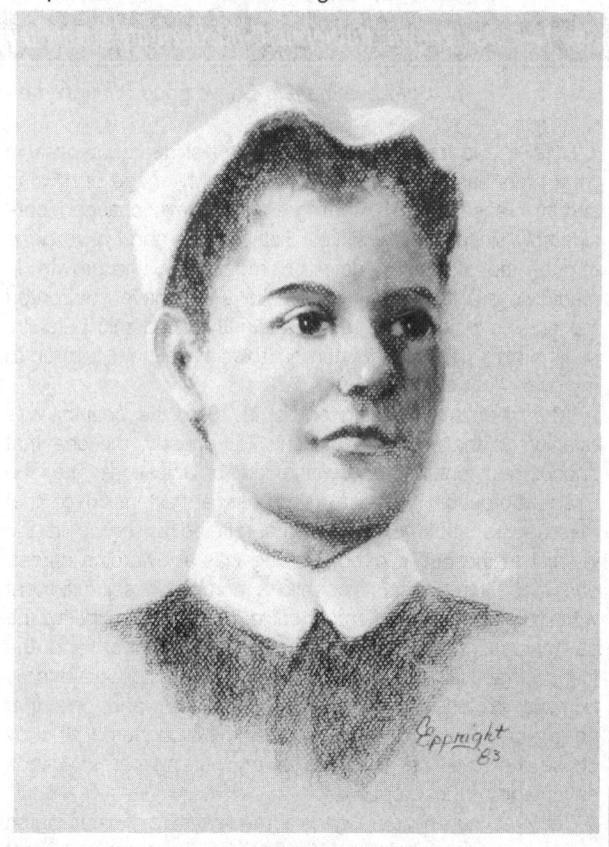

Isabel Adams Hampton Robb. (From The Southwest Center for Nursing History, University of Texas at Austin School of Nursing, Austin, Texas.)

for nursing schools, requires that nurse educators in diploma, associate-degree, and baccalaureate-degree settings have master's degrees in nursing rather than a related field. Consequently, nurses are wise to seek counsel when making career decisions about the best path to follow in preparation for a chosen role.

In many organizations, even midmanagement positions require a master's degree. The complexity of being the top nursing administrator has increased significantly in the last decade, and many nurses in such positions find that a master's in business administration (MBA) is invaluable.

Expanded Roles for Nurses

Expanded roles for nurses are not a new phenomenon. Because the earliest trained nurses in the United States learned in hospitals to give bedside care to patients but were often left, after completing their training, to find their own employment, nurse registries evolved as employment clearing houses. The registries united nurses with clients or clients' families desiring private-duty nurses, and private service became the largest field of employment for nurses. The role of the private-duty nurse was not defined. Consequently, nurses did what was needed to be done to care for the people in their care.

Nurses continued to expand their role in industry, after their entry into this area in 1888.[3] Nurses also expanded their efforts in social services. Lillian Wald and her nurses at the Henry Street Settlement were the backbone of visiting and school nursing and embraced work that today is largely done by social workers.[69]

The contemporary phenomenon of expanded nursing roles has its genesis in the 1960s when Loretta Ford initiated a pediatric nurse practitioner program at the University of Colorado. The concept evolved as a response to a need, as some areas experienced gaps in service. The concept was quick to catch on, and practitioner programs were initiated in both degree and nondegree settings. Practitioners will be in increased demand as *Nursing's Agenda for Health Care Reform* is implemented, moving clients from tertiary to community settings.[4]

Clinical specialization typically focuses on a population, such as adults, children, and older adults, or on a clinical area such as maternity, oncology, enterostomies, and cardiac rehabilitation. Preparation for clinical specialization can take place in degree-granting institutions at the master's level or by self-study through continuing education combined with on-the-job learning.

Nurse managers and administrators have changed their roles since assuming responsibilities as superintendents of the earliest schools of nursing. Originally, they were superintendent over both the school of nurs-

---

Box 1–7. As We Are: Katherine C. McDermott—New Directions in Clinical Research

Both nursing and I have gone through the process of definition, redefinition, and growth.

Nursing and I have evolved over the last quarter century in what I feel has been a shared process. My image of nursing and my reasons for becoming a nurse have changed considerably since the late sixties. Both nursing and I have gone through the process of definition, redefinition, and growth. In many ways, the issues and questions that have confronted the nursing profession, such as identity, academic pursuits, patient care issues, and nursing roles have been similar to my own.

When I entered nursing school in 1965, the country was listening to the message of John F. Kennedy, the one that encouraged public service through organizations like the Peace Corps or VISTA. Nursing was an extension of that message, a noble profession that offered a service in the interest of the public good. Nursing was a rewarding career, one that offered attractive options combining self-fulfillment with practicality. Self-fulfillment could be realized by being the patient's advocate, the care giver, the comforter, and the friend. Practically speaking, nursing was a geographically portable profession, domestically functional, and one that permitted women to leave or enter the work force as they chose. For the first 10 years of my nursing career, I took advantage of these options.

I entered nursing as a general medical/surgical staff nurse at a university-based teaching hospital. Then, as a clinical care coordinator in an urban medical center, my role was to facilitate the opening of a new female medical unit. In a California community hospital, I was a team leader on one of the first clinical units to use computerized care plans. I became a public health and education coordinator in a child care center, a counselor in a comprehensive women's health care center, a specialist in a coronary care unit, and an emergency room nurse.

The first ten years of my career were varied and rewarding, but I was still trying to identify a place in the profession that was uniquely me. In 1978 that opportunity presented itself when I was hired as a research nurse to work in the medical biochemistry laboratory of a renowned research university. In that environment, I began to see where I wanted to go in my career. The field was called clinical research, and in the late 1970s it was an unexplored area for nurses. The research focus of this laboratory was in diabetes mellitus. It was very exciting to see how basic research could affect care and the management of chronic conditions. My responsibilities as a research nurse clinician were varied and included assisting with protocol development, caring for clients on those protocols, developing educational materials, instituting nursing guidelines and policies for clients participating in research protocols, and participating in basic laboratory experiments. During this period I published my first article.

The experience I gained during those four years prepared me for the next step in my career. For the last 10 years, I have been practicing as a clinical research coordinator and oncology clinical nurse specialist (CNS) at Memorial Sloan-Kettering Cancer Center. This position has been the most challenging, the most professionally rewarding, the most personally satisfying, and the most "uniquely me" role that I have had during my nursing career.

Cancer affects three of every four families in the United States and is the second leading cause of death among adults and young children. As a CNS in the area of oncology clinical research, I practice in an advanced role. I am able to offer clients protocols that include state-of-the-art technology and then assess the impact of that research on nursing responsibilities. This role includes the preparation, guidance, and education of the nursing staff caring for people who are on research protocols. Clinical research also affords nurses who participate as members of research teams the opportunity to use assessment, technical, psychosocial, and intellectual skills to advance and contribute to quality care.

The reasons for my becoming a nurse, practicality and self-fulfillment, in the final analysis are not the same as the reasons I choose to stay in the profession. What motivates me now is that nursing is a challenging profession, one that offers diversity, stimulates both personal and professional growth, and gives one the satisfaction of making differences and contributions to the quality of care.

Oncology nurses take these qualities a step further by assuming leadership roles that create and provide quality-of-life services for people with cancer and their families. It is a truly rewarding speciality within a profession offering a variety of opportunities.

ing and the nursing service of the hospital. Today, the complexity of nursing practice and education make these separate and ever-expanding roles.

Professional Organizations

Professional organizations are among the most visible and most powerful means by which a group impresses society with its professional status.

Nursing is well served by its many professional associations.

NATIONAL LEAGUE FOR NURSING

At the Chicago World's Fair in 1893, numerous congresses convened. One was an International Congress of Charities, Corrections, and Philanthropy, which included a section on hospitals and nursing.[27] Seventy-two superintendents of nursing schools were invited, and eighteen gathered at the Congress. They formed the first national organization of nurses: The American Society of Superintendents of Training Schools for Nurses. Their overriding goal was to standardize nursing education, including such aspects as the length of the training period and admission requirements. Two other goals were "to promote fellowship of members, . . . and to further the best interests of the nursing profession."[31]

In 1912, the organization's name was changed to the National League for Nursing Education (NLNE). In 1952, as part of a plan to consolidate many special-interest nursing organizations, the NLNE, the National Organization of Public Health Nurses (NOPHN), and the Association of Collegiate Schools of Nursing (ACSN) all merged to become the National League for Nursing (NLN).

Today, the **National League for Nursing,** headquartered in New York City, is a nonprofit national coalition of individuals and agencies working to improve nursing education and practice so that the quality of health care throughout the nation will be enhanced. Membership is open to non-nurses as well as nurses, and their many activities include the accreditation of nursing schools. Many graduate schools of nursing require graduation from an NLN-accredited school for admission.

AMERICAN NURSES' ASSOCIATION

From the outset, members of the superintendents' organization recognized the need for the members of the grass roots of nursing also to have an organization. Because many training schools for nurses already had alumnae associations in place, the logical step was to federate them into a larger organization. In 1897, alumnae associations of various hospital schools of nursing were brought together in a single organization named the Nurses' Associated Alumnae of the United States and Canada.[32] New York state law did not permit the incorporation of an organization from two countries, so "and Canada" was dropped from the name.

The stated objectives for the organization were "to establish and maintain a code of ethics; to elevate the standard of nursing education; to promote the usefulness and honor, the financial and other interests of the nursing profession."[32] In 1911, the name of the organization was changed to the American Nurses' Association (ANA). With the merger of various nursing associations in 1952, the National Association of Colored Graduate Nurses (NACGN) merged with the ANA.

The **American Nurses' Association,** formerly headquartered in Kansas City, Missouri, and recently moved to Washington, D.C., is the national professional association for registered nurses in the United States. It is a federation of constituent associations in all 50 states, the District of Columbia, Guam, and the Virgin Islands. Individual nurses are members of their state nurses' associations (SNA). The ANA represents nurses and nursing in various ways. They include but are not limited to lobbying at the federal level for health care programs and increased monies for nursing research and educational programs, working for improved work conditions for nurses, and collaborating with other nursing organizations and governmental agencies on health care and nursing issues.

Membership in the ANA automatically gives a nurse membership in the International Council of Nurses. *American Nurse* is the association's national organ.

CANADIAN NURSES ASSOCIATION

The **Canadian Nurses Association** (CNA), the national organization of Canadian nurses, was founded in 1908 and is a federation of 11 provincial or territorial member associations. The CNA represents Canadian nursing to other national and international organizations, provides leadership on issues related to nursing and health care, influences national policy, and promotes quality in nursing education, practice, research, and administration.

INTERNATIONAL COUNCIL OF NURSES

In 1899, Mrs. Bedford Fenwick, a British nurse, laid the groundwork for the International Council of Nurses (ICN). Fenwick was in charge of forming a program on nursing within a section of professional women gathered as part of the International Council of Women. She and Isabel Stewart presented a resolution to form a group of nurses with international representation.[26] Dock states that its purpose was "to bring together in international union, nurses who, in their home lands, had developed or who were endeavoring to develop, *professional self government*" [the emphasis is Dock's]. She went on to say, "In other words, the International stood for emancipation."[26] Even though the first Congress in 1901 was held in the United States, American nurses were not accepted for membership until 1905.[32]

The **International Council of Nurses** is an organization that meets every 4 years. These quadrennial meetings are called "Congresses," and when they are in session, the organization is called the International Congress of Nurses. The purpose of the ICN is to foster international relationships and provide a forum for international concerns to be aired.

Box 1–8. As We Were: Mary Adelaide Nutting (1858–1948)—Innovator in Education

A profession cannot rise above the character of those who practice it.

M.A. NUTTING

Mary Adelaide Nutting was born in Quebec, Canada, in 1858. Although the family was not wealthy, it placed high value on good education academically as well as in the arts.

In 1884, when her mother became quite ill, Nutting provided much of her care, which aroused a personal interest in nursing.[16] By chance she read that Johns Hopkins University was founding a school of nursing, with Isabel Hampton, also Canadian, as the superintendent of nurses and head of the training school. Nutting applied for admission and was accepted. At the age of 31 years, she entered nurses training in October 1889 and graduated in June, 2 years later.

While she was still a student, Isabel Hampton recognized Nutting's potential and did much to shape her career.[39] Two years after graduation, she became Hampton's assistant, and when Hampton left to marry, Nutting was appointed to the superintendency.

Nutting introduced many invocations into the training school. She eliminated stipends, increased the length of the probationary period, and initiated scholarships.[39] With Dr. William Osler's help, she expanded the library considerably[16] and expanded the nursing course to 3 years, making the school recognized as one of the best schools in the country.

Nutting was instrumental in helping form many nursing organizations, serving in many capacities in the process. Included in the long list of organizations she helped organize are the organizational forerunners of the National League for Nursing and the American Nurses' Association, the International Council of Nurses, and the Hospital Economics Course at Teachers College, Columbia University. She held numerous offices and served on many committees in all the organizations.

Nutting was also a prolific writer. In 1912 she published a profound report entitled *The Educational Status of Nursing.* The document was a strong indictment against the exploitation of young women in nursing schools throughout the country, as well as the appalling state of nursing education at the time. She also collaborated with Lavinia Dock to publish a four-volume history of nursing.

In 1907 she took charge of the Hospital Economics Course at Teachers College, Columbia University, where she became the first nurse to hold the rank of professor. She retired from the University in 1925. Even in retirement she received many prizes in recognition of her previous work.[29]

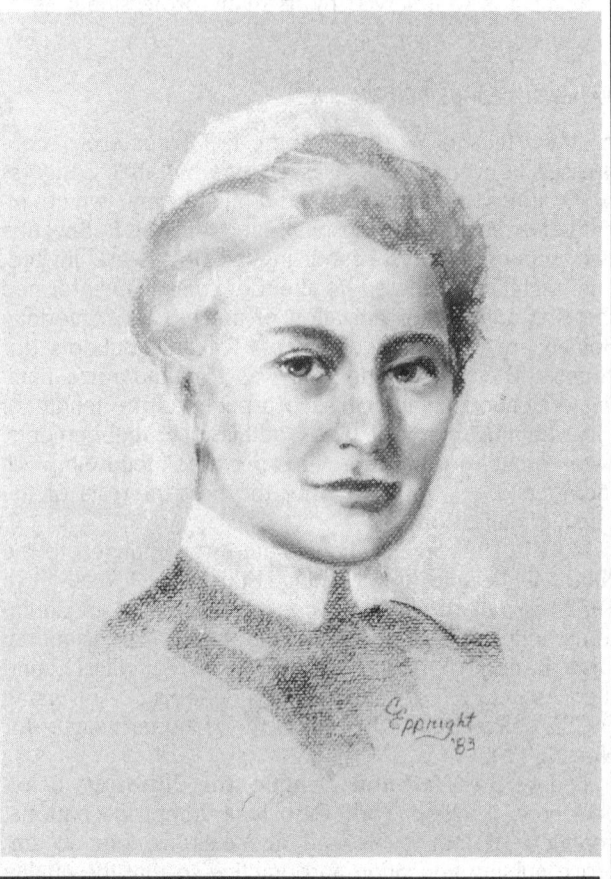

Mary Adelaide Nutting. (From The Southwest Center for Nursing History, University of Texas at Austin School of Nursing, Austin, Texas.)

SIGMA THETA TAU

Sigma Theta Tau is an international nursing honor society committed to excellence in nursing. Founded in 1922 by six student nurses at Indiana University Training School for Nurses, it has expanded to more than 160,000 members. More than half of its active members hold master's and doctoral degrees.[12]

The organization's purposes are to "recognize superior achievement, recognize the development of leadership qualities, foster high professional standards, encourage creative work, [and] strengthen commitment to the ideals and purposes of the profession." [70] In addition to the prestige that comes with being a member, other benefits of membership are the opportunity to apply for research grants and subscriptions to *Image,*

the organization's research journal, and *Reflections*, its news journal.

NATIONAL STUDENT NURSE ASSOCIATION

The **National Student Nurse Association, Inc.,** is the national organization for students enrolled in schools of nursing. Active membership is open to both generic students and registered nurses enrolled in undergraduate, state-approved schools of nursing. The organization is financed and run by students, except for the paid staff in the headquarters office in New York City.

The bylaws list several functions. In essence they are to influence education, nursing practice, and health care; to recruit and encourage active participation of its members in health-related and social issues; and to promote collaborative relationships with the American Nurses' Association, National League for Nursing, and International Council of Nurses. Active participation in the organization is an excellent opportunity for students to meet others throughout the country and to become socialized into organizational processes.

CLINICAL SPECIALTY ORGANIZATIONS

Organizations for specialties in nursing are diverse and numerous. They exist for such specialties as nurse-midwives, black nursing faculty in higher education, pediatric oncology, and I.V. nurses. Each year, the April issue of the *American Journal of Nursing* contains complete listings of nursing organizations, including their addresses, telephone numbers, and a contact person by name.

Summary

- Florence Nightingale, Virginia Henderson, the American Nurses' Association, and the Canadian Nurses' Association are among those who have contributed to the evolving definition of nursing.
- The American Nurses' Association currently defines nursing as, ". . . the diagnosis and treatment of human responses to actual or potential health problems."[6]
- Nursing has historically been associated with the image of women and with the principles and ideals of the Christian religion.
- Kalisch and Kalisch found that the popular media portrayed nurses as "angels of mercy," "girl Friday," "heroines," "wife and mother," and "sex objects."
- A career in nursing is perceived by society to have the positive qualities of security, intellectual application, caring for people, and academic and scholastic achievement along with the negative qualities of lack of independent decision making, less safety in the workplace, less financial reward, and less respect and appreciation.
- At the time of the Civil War, nurses' roles were ill defined, but by the dawn of the 20th century the roles were private duty nurse, visiting/public health nurse, industrial nurse, and military nurse.
- Contemporary nursing practice takes place mainly in hospital, ambulatory care, and community/public health settings, but nurses may be found in virtually every setting where the physical and psychosocial well-being of individuals is a vital interest.
- Formal nursing education has been shaped most by early leaders in nursing, wars, the educational system in general, and the status of women.
- Important early schools of nursing were the Nightingale School at St. Thomas Hospital in London and the first American schools.
- Some major changes in nursing education occurred as a result of the large number of nurses needed in times of war.
- Registered nurses are most frequently educated in one of three types of generic programs: diploma, associate degree, and baccalaureate.

- A variety of opportunities are available for education beyond the generic preparation, and continuing education is mandatory in a growing number of states.
- The profession of nursing was shaped by the early efforts of nursing leaders such as Nightingale, Hampton Robb, Nutting, Wald, Dock, and others.
- Professional organizations are among the most visible and most powerful means by which a group impresses society that it has achieved professional status.

Bibliography

1. Alcott, L.M. (1960). *Hospital sketches* (edited by Bessie Z. Jones). Cambridge, Massachusetts: The Belknap Press of Harvard University Press.
2. American Association of Colleges of Nursing (1993). *Position statement on educational articulation* (draft). Washington, D.C.
3. American Association of Industrial Nurses (1976). *The nurse in industry*. New York.
4. American Nurses' Association (1991). *Nursing's agenda for health care reform*. Kansas City, Missouri.
5. American Nurses' Association (1991). *Standards of clinical nursing practice*. Kansas City, Missouri.
6. American Nurses' Association (1980). *Nursing: A social policy statement*. Kansas City, Missouri.
7. Austin, A.L. (1975). Nurses in American history: wartime volunteers — 1861–1865. *American Journal of Nursing*, 75, 816–818.
8. Austin, A.L. (1971). *The Woolsey sisters of New York*. Philadelphia: American Philosophical Society.
9. Baly, M.E. (1986). *Florence Nightingale and the nursing legacy*. London: Croom Helm.
10. Bigbee, J.L., & Crowder, E.L.M. The Red Cross Rural Nursing Service: an innovative model of public health nursing delivery. *Public Health Nursing*, 2, 109–121.
11. Boyden, A.L. (1914). *War reminiscences. A record of Mrs. Rebecca R. Pomeroy's experience in war-times*. New York: Neal Publishing Company.
12. Brown, B. (1989). *A brief history of Sigma Theta Tau*. Unpublished paper.
13. Brown, B. (1975). *The historical development of the University of Texas System School of Nursing: 1890–1975*. Unpublished doctoral dissertation, Baylor University, Waco, Texas.
14. Bucklin, S.E. (1869). *In hospital and camp: A woman's record of thrilling incidents among the wounded in the late war*. Philadelphia: J.E. Potter & Company.
15. Canadian Nurses' Association (1987). *A definition of nursing practice/standards for nursing practice* (p. iii). Ottawa, Ontario, Canada.
16. Christy, T.E. (1969). Portrait of a leader: Adelaide Nutting. *Nursing Outlook*, 17(1), 20–24.
17. Christy, T.E. (1969). Portrait of a leader: Isabel Hampton Robb. *Nursing Outlook*, 17(3), 26–29.
18. Cohen, I.B. (1984). Florence Nightingale. *Scientific American*, 250(3), 128–137.
19. *Congressional Record*, August 12, 1964.
20. Crowder, E.L.M. (1985). Historical perspectives of nursing's professionalism. *Occupational Health Nursing*, 33, 184–190.
21. Crowder, E.L.M. (1979). *The evolution of diploma curricula of three schools of nursing in Texas: an historical treatment*. Unpublished doctoral dissertation, University of Texas, Austin, Texas.
22. Cumming, K. (1975). *The journal of Kate Cumming: A Confederate nurse*. Savannah, Georgia: The Beehive Press.
23. Dannett, S.G.L. (ed.) (1959). *Nobel women of the North*. New York: Thomas Yoseloff.
24. Dickens, C. (1982). *Martin Chuzzlewit* (rev. ed.). Oxford: Clarendon Press.
25. Dickens, C. (1956). *Mrs. Gamp* (a facsimile of the author's prompt copy). New York: The New York Public Library.

26. Dock, L.L., & Stewart, I.M. (1925). *A short history of nursing* (p. 338). New York: G.P. Putnam's Sons.

27. Dolan, J.A. (1978). *Nursing in society: A historical perspective.* Philadelphia: W.B. Saunders Company.

28. Dolan, J.A., et al. (1983). *Nursing in society: A historical perspective.* Philadelphia: W.B. Saunders.

29. Donahue, M.P. (1988). Mary Adelaide Nutting: 1858–1948. In Bullough, V., et al. (eds.). *American nursing: A biographical dictionary* (pp. 244–247). New York: Garland Publishing Company.

30. Fagin, C.M. (1992). President's message. *Nursing and Health Care,* 13, 208.

31. *First Annual Report of the American Society of Superintendents of Training Schools for Nurses, 1894* (1987). Harrisburg, Pennsylvania: Harrisburg Publishing Company.

32. Flanagan, L. (1976). *One strong voice.* Kansas City, Missouri: American Nurses' Association.

33. Freymann, J.G. (1974). *The American health care system: Its genesis and trajectory* (p. 328). Baltimore: Williams & Wilkins.

34. Gardiner, A.G. (1908). *Prophets, priests and kings* (p. 15). London: Alstoon-Rivers, Ltd.

35. Giles, D. (1949). *A candle in her hand.* New York: G.P. Putnam's Sons.

36. Goldmark, J. (1923). *Nursing & nursing education in the United States.* New York: Macmillan.

37. Hamric, A.B. (1989). History and overview of the CNS role. In Hamric, A.B., & Spross, J.A. (eds.). *The clinical nurse specialist in theory and practice* (pp. 3–18). Philadelphia: W.B. Saunders.

38. Henderson, V. (1966). *The nature of nursing* (p. 15). New York: Macmillan.

39. Johns, E., & Pfefferkorn, B. (1954). *The Johns Hopkins Hospital School of Nursing, 1889–1949.* Baltimore: Johns Hopkins Press.

40. Jones, M.V.H. (Spring 1989). The Alexian Brothers: Nursing as a man's profession. *American Association for the History of Nursing Bulletin,* 9–12.

41. Kalisch, P.A., & Kalisch, B.J. (1987). *The changing image of the nurse.* Menlo Park, California: Addison-Wesley.

42. Kalisch, P.A., & Kalisch, B.J. (1986). *The advance of American nursing* (2nd ed). Boston: Little, Brown.

43. Kohnke, M. (1978). The nurse's responsibility to the consumer. *American Journal of Nursing,* 78, 440–442.

44. Kübler-Ross, E. (1969). *On death and dying.* New York: Macmillan.

45. Lippman, D.T., & Ponton, K.S. (1989). Nursing's image on the university campus. *Nursing Outlook,* 37(1), 24–27.

46. May, F.E., et al. (1991). Public values and beliefs toward nursing as a career. *Journal of Nursing Education,* 30, 303–310.

47. McIsaac, I. (1910). Personal recollections of Isabel Adams Hampton Robb—teacher and friend, 1886–1910. *American Journal of Nursing,* 11, 13–15.

48. Melosh, B. (1982). *"The physician's hand." Work culture and conflict in American nursing.* Philadelphia: Temple University Press.

49. Mendez, D., & Louis, M. (1991). College students' image of nursing as a career choice. *Journal of Nursing Education,* 30, 311–319.

50. Murchison, I. (1952). A four-year basic collegiate program. *American Journal of Nursing,* 52, 481–482.

51. National League for Nursing (1989). *Practical nursing career.* New York.

52. National League for Nursing (1991). *Nursing datasource 1990; Vol. III: The silent few: Men and minorities in nursing education.* New York: National League for Nursing Press.

53. Nightingale, F. (1859). *Notes on nursing: What it is and what it is not.* London: Harrison.

54. Noel, N. (1988). Isabel Adams Hampton Robb: 1860–1910. In Bullough, V., et al. (eds.). *American nursing: A biographical dictionary* (pp. 274–276). New York: Garland Publishing Company.

55. North, F.H. (1882). A new profession for women. *Century Magazine, the Quarterly,* 25, 38–47.

56. Nutting, M.A. (1926). *A sound economic basis for schools of nursing* (p. 231). New York: G.P. Putnam's Sons.

57. Pember, P.Y. (1879). *A southern woman's story.* New York: G.W. Carlton & Company.

58. Poplin, I.S. (1988). *A study of the Kaiserwerth Deaconess Institutes Nurses Training School in 1850–1851: Purposes and curriculum.* Unpublished doctoral dissertation, The University of Texas, Austin, Texas.

59. Reznick, A.E. (1973). *Lillian D. Wald: The years at Henry Street.* Unpublished doctoral dissertation, University of Wisconsin, Madison, Wisconsin.

60. Robb, I.H. (1900). Hospital economics. *American Journal of Nursing,* 1, 29.

61. Santayana, G. (1922). *The life of reason* (2nd ed.). New York: C. Scribner's Sons.

62. Selevan, I.C. (1975). Nurses in American history: The Revolution. *American Journal of Nursing,* 75, 592–594.

63. Siegel, B. (1983). *Lillian Wald of Henry Street.* New York: Macmillan.

64. Silverstein, N.G. (1985). Lillian Wald at Henry Street, 1893–1989. *Advances in Nursing Science,* 7(1), 1–2.

65. Stein, A.P. (1988). Dorothea Lynde Dix: 1802–1887. In Bullough, V., et al. (eds.). *American nursing: A biographical dictionary* (pp. 89–91). New York: Garland Publishing.

66. Stimpson, J.C. (1925). Earliest known connection of nurses with Army hospitals in the United States. *American Journal of Nursing,* 25, 18.

67. Suspension of the Army School of Nursing (1931). *American Journal of Nursing,* 31, 1058.

68. Ungvarski, P.J., & Nokes, K.M. (1992). Community-based and long-term care. In *HIV/AIDS: A Guide to Nursing Care* (2nd ed.). Philadelphia: W.B. Saunders Company.

69. Wald, L.D. (1915). *House on Henry Street.* New York: Holt.

70. Widmer, C.L. (1972). Sigma Theta Tau: golden anniversary. *Nursing Outlook,* 20, 786–788.

71. Woodham-Smith, C. (1951). *Florence Nightingale, 1820–1910.* New York: McGraw-Hill.

▼ Changing Concepts of Health, Disease, and Health Care

There is a healthy way to experience disease as well as a constantly challenging way to be healthy

Marilyn Frank-Stromborg, et al.

▼ CHAPTER OUTLINE

HEALTH AND DISEASE: CHANGING
   DEFINITIONS AND VIEWPOINTS
      The Problem of Defining Health and
      Disease
      Models of Disease and Health
CONCEPTS OF HEALTH PROMOTION AND
   DISEASE PREVENTION
      Prevention

Health Promotion Versus Disease
   Prevention
THERAPEUTIC ACTIVITIES
      Primary Prevention Activities
      Secondary Prevention Activities
      Tertiary Prevention (Rehabilitation)
      Activities
      Health Promotion Activities

▼ KEY TERMS

Acupressure
Acupuncture
Adaptive model
Ayurveda
Biopsychosocial model of
   disease
Chiropractic treatment
Color therapy
Diagnosis
Ecologic approach
Eudemonistic model of
   health
Evolutionary model
Germ theory

Health (World Health
   Organization definition)
Health belief model
Health-illness continuum
Health promotion model
Herbalism
High-level wellness
Holistic view of humans
Homeopathy
Humoral theory of
   medicine
Medical model
Naturopathy
Osteopathy

Physiatrist
Prescriptions
Primary prevention
Prognosis
Reflexology (zone therapy)
Role performance model
Secondary prevention
Shiatsu
Social cognitive theory
Spiritual healing
Tertiary prevention
Therapeutic touch
Western medicine
Yoga

▼ **LEARNING OBJECTIVES**

After studying this chapter, you should be able to

1. *Describe selected models of health and disease.*
2. *Differentiate among strategies used for disease prevention and health promotion.*
3. *Discuss the purpose of the health belief model in primary prevention.*
4. *Explain selected biomedical treatments.*
5. *Identify selected alternative therapies.*
6. *Discuss the use of social cognitive theory and the health promotion model in health promotion activities.*

If you could be granted 10 wishes, what would your wishes be? Probably, like most people, high on your list would be a wish to attain or continue with a healthy life. People long for freedom from pain, for the joy that accompanies a healthy body and mind, for the opportunity to live in harmony with their environment, and for a long and productive life. To promote the dream of health, endless hours and millions of dollars have been spent on biomedical research. Hospitals and other health care facilities have been built and expanded. Schools for health practitioners and administrators have grown. In fact, so much growth has occurred in the last few decades that health care is currently one of the top industries in the United States. Despite these advances, our dream of mental and physical health for all people has remained just that—a dream. Yet it is a dream worth pursuing because of the effects of disease on individuals and on society.

The relative presence or absence of disease is both a personal and a societal problem. It is a personal problem because a person's ability to work, to be productive, to love, and to play are all related to that individual's mental and physical health. It is a societal problem because the illness of one person can adversely affect significant other people (e.g., family, friends, and colleagues).

Moreover, if the disease or injury is serious or disabling, a person may be forced to depend on significant others or on society for financial support and physical care. In addition, some diseases may spread from one person to another, possibly disrupting the social order. The great epidemics of the past—influenza, smallpox, and bubonic plague—have immobilized and even decimated entire populations.

To offset these problems, a variety of social institutions have developed over the centuries. Governments pass laws to control disease and to fight pollution. Public health services promote sanitation and prevent and treat communicable diseases. Private insurance and government programs finance health care services. In addition, philosophers and clerics attempt to explain disease and death and offer comfort to those afflicted. Health care professionals attempt to treat disease and thereby alleviate mental and physical suffering, and to promote health as a means of improving the quality of life.

Because of the universal nature of disease and its far-reaching personal and social consequences, thoughtful individuals have always asked questions about disease. Some of the most important questions are these: What is disease and why does disease exist? What is health in relation to disease? What impact does disease have on the individual and on society? To what extent do societal pressures on an individual cause disease? How can health care services best be delivered to all people?

In this chapter we explore these questions, all of which are central to an approach to health care that incorporates all parts of a person's life. Our exploration includes some information that is theoretical and speculative. Researchers are only beginning to study health, disease, and health care in a manner that is holistic and yet precise. As human beings, we continue to explore ourselves as physical, emotional, intellectual, and social organisms struggling to adapt and remain healthy in a challenging and sometimes harsh environment. Our explorations must begin with an attempt to define the concepts of health and disease.

HEALTH AND DISEASE: CHANGING DEFINITIONS AND VIEWPOINTS

Health and disease are not static conditions. Rather, they are vital concepts that are subject to continuous evaluation and change.

In the not-so-distant past, disease was often defined as "an absence of health," and health was defined as "an absence of disease"—definitions that were not enlightening. Some authorities saw disease and health as states of physical discomfort or well-being. Unfortunately, such narrow viewpoints caused researchers and health care professionals to disregard the emotional and social components of health and illness. Broader definitions of health and disease have taken into account many aspects of disease causation and health maintenance such as psychologic, social, and biologic factors. Despite efforts to characterize these concepts, however, universal definitions for health and illness do not exist. Table 2–1 lists some definitions of health and disease based on various viewpoints.

The Problem of Defining Health and Disease

It is difficult to derive a universally acceptable definition for the terms health and disease because health and disease are concepts that often elude strict, objec-

TABLE 2-1. *Definitions of Health and Disease*

Viewpoint	Health	Disease
Epidemiologic	A state in which the host has remained resistant to pathogenic agents in the environment	A state resulting from the susceptibility of the host to pathogenic agents in the environment
Ecological	The product of a harmonious relationship between people and their environment	The product of a non-adaptive maladjusted relationship between people and their environment
Sociologic	Conformity to that physical or behavioral state that is considered normal (or modal in statistical terms) within a particular group	Deviancy from that physical or behavioral state that is considered normal within a particular group
Consumer	A commodity or an investment that can be purchased	An abnormal condition that can be treated, controlled, and possibly cured through the purchase of health care services

tive standardization. That is, they are subjective states difficult to "measure." People define these terms according to personal value systems that are influenced by culture, socioeconomic status, age, knowledge, and preexisting states of health or disease. Indeed, we all have our own definitions of health and disease based on our individual life experiences.

No clear line exists between health and disease. Today we view these as relative concepts and not as separate absolutes. It is helpful to imagine health and disease as a graduated scale we term the **health-illness continuum,** a range of well-being from excellent health through wellness and illness to death. Excellent health appears at one end of the continuum, death at the other end, and the status of most people lies somewhere in between. Moreover, a person's position on the health-illness continuum varies from year to year, day to day, and hour to hour owing to the impact of life events on the person and the process of aging (Fig. 2-1).

Let us look at some case examples to illustrate these points. Examine each one and ask yourself, Who is sick? Who is well? Where would each be placed on the health-illness continuum?

▶ A business executive has experienced two serious heart attacks yet continues to function satisfactorily on the job.
▶ A middle-aged individual has an aortic aneurysm (a localized ballooning of the largest artery due to a weakness in the vessel wall) but does not know it.

This condition is often symptomless but is nevertheless life-threatening.
A college student occasionally consumes large quantities of alcohol, a practice approved by the school peer group.
A young boy of Tristan da Cunha, an island in the South Atlantic, is a powerful swimmer and mountain climber even though he is infested with worms, a condition he ignores because it is so common on his island.
A woman living in Los Angeles suffers from congestion on smoggy days, a condition to which she has become accustomed.

Each of these people views disease and health according to individual values. Thus, they may define disease by considering whether they can continue to work, play, or study; whether signs and symptoms are present or absent; whether a state of discomfort is short or prolonged; whether a problem is physical, mental, or social. Their definitions of health and disease vary according to personal values, peer group, cultural background, and social class.

One widely used definition of **health** is the World Health Organization (WHO) concept:

Health is a state of complete physical, mental, and social well-being and not merely the absence of disease or infirmity.

This definition has been both praised and criticized for its all-inclusive nature. On the one hand, the WHO definition excels because it includes the psychologic and social aspects of health as well as the physical. The WHO definition therefore places the concept of health into the broad context of human life. On the other hand, critics point out that the WHO definition is imprecise and unrealistic and that the word "complete" establishes expectations of a state of perfection so rarely attained that hope of attaining it can lead only to disappointment.

Models of Disease and Health

In addition to defining health and disease, philosophers and health care experts have developed paradigms or models to explain these abstract concepts. Health professionals use these models as bases for providing health care.

EARLY MODELS

Supernatural Causation. Ancient theories of disease often focused on supernatural causes. A person fell ill as a result of invasion by a spirit or the casting of an evil spell by an unfriendly sorcerer. Some cultures viewed illness as a punishment for displeasing the gods or breaking a societal taboo. Even now, some cultures continue to believe in spirit possession and supernatural causes of disease. Have you ever experienced a feeling of devastation as a result of disease (perhaps you were badly injured in an automobile accident, suf-

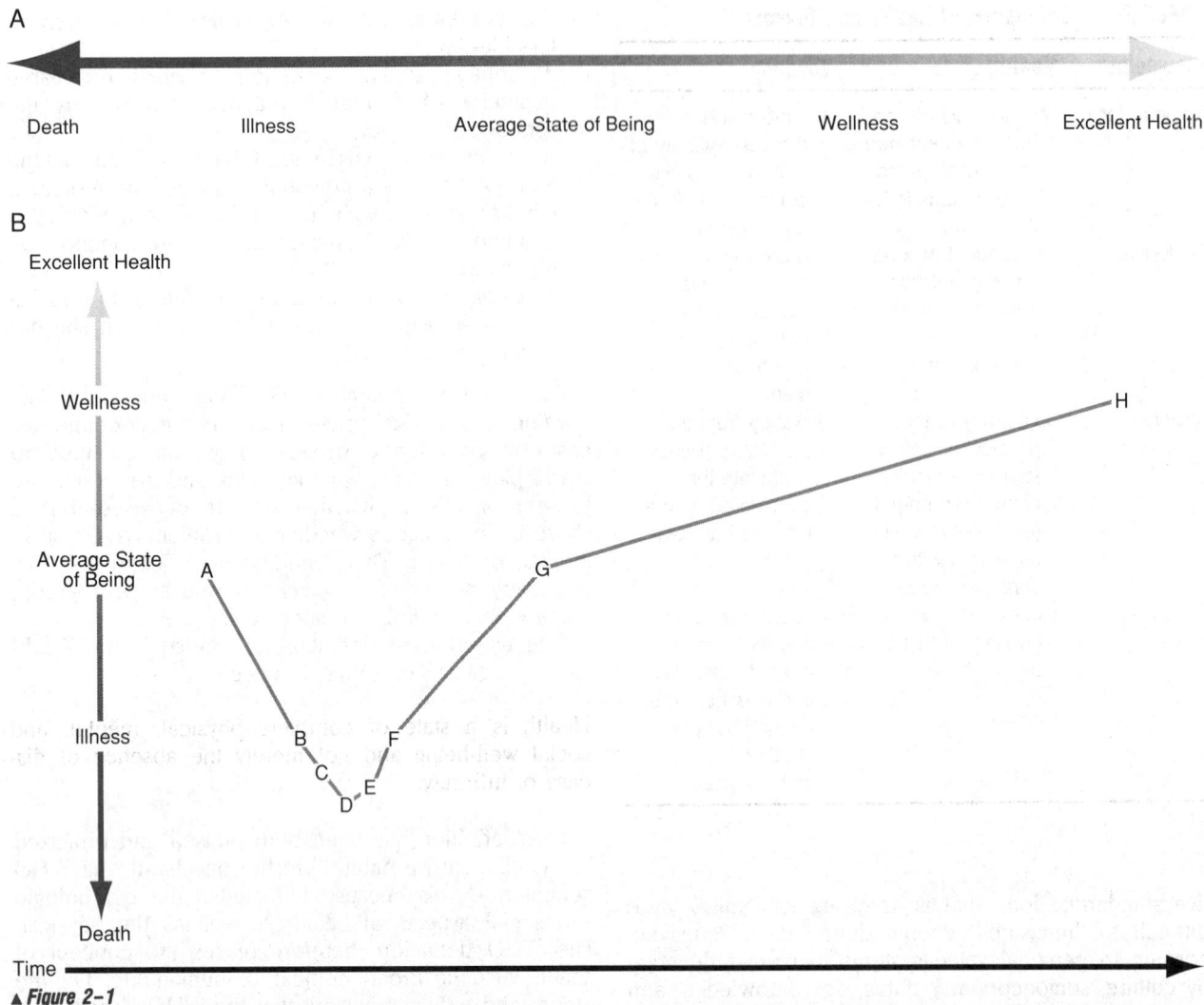

A

Death   Illness   Average State of Being   Wellness   Excellent Health

B

Excellent Health

Wellness

Average State of Being

Illness

Death

Time

▲ *Figure 2–1*

A, The health-illness continuum on a horizontal axis, as usually depicted. At any particular point in time, a person's health status may be placed on the health-illness continuum to represent the individual's level of wellness. *B*, A health-illness continuum on a vertical axis that allows the plotting of a person's level of wellness over time. Consider a person in an average state of being who will later develop a breast lump. At point A on the continuum, no lump or other illness is present, but the person is not particularly a model of health. At point B, during a routine examination, a breast lump is discovered. At point C, the client becomes more and more anxious as a mammogram is done and surgery is scheduled for a biopsy of the lump. Point D occurs during surgery, when the blood pressure and other vital signs drop as a response to general anesthesia. The body is invaded by a needle in the vein and by the surgeon's scalpel during creation of a surgical opening for removal of the lump. In the recovery room, at point E after surgery, the client has a dressing over her surgical wound, has an I.V. in place in her arm, and is beginning to experience pain even though the untoward effects of anesthesia have not yet worn off. At point F, three days after surgery, the I.V. has been removed; the surgical wound is beginning to heal; the client is up and around; and her anxiety is relieved by a negative biopsy report. Three months after surgery, at point G, the surgical wound is still pink, and the client hardly thinks about it. She has resumed all normal activities and is now doing monthly breast self-examinations. One year later, at point H, the breast incision is barely discernible, breast self-examinations have been done routinely, the client has reduced dietary fat and caffeine intake and has begun to take 2-mile walks each day in an effort to improve overall health. Musculature is firmer, and cardiovascular tone is improved over that of the previous year.

fered abuse at the hands of an alcoholic parent, or even withstood the loss of a loved one due to a terminal illness)? In such instances, there is a tendency to ask, What did I do to deserve this? It is natural to ask whether God or fate is punishing us for some of our misdeeds. When we do ask these questions, we are attributing illness to a supernatural force. We ask even though we are intelligent, rational beings, and we understand that it was the inflammatory response in the appendix, the fractures in the bones, or the cancer in the liver that caused us to suffer so much misery.

The ancient theory of supernatural causation is alive and well.

The Greek Humoral Theory. The ancient Greek theory of the four humors guided medical practice for centuries. The **humoral theory of medicine** was a belief that the four humors (body liquids or semifluids) were phlegm, blood, black bile, and yellow bile and that these humors corresponded with the four qualities of cold, heat, dryness, and moisture. These vital elements existed in various quantities in the body, and when the equilibrium among them was disrupted, disease resulted. Treatments were designed to reestablish humoral equilibrium. For example, when a person was thought to have an excess of blood, the person underwent bloodletting.

The Body Machine and the Mind-Body Dichotomy of Descartes. Another theory of disease viewed the human body as a machine and disease as the result of a defective part. The basis of the theory originated with René Descartes, a 17th-century French philosopher who envisioned each person as a well-functioning "body machine." He and other philosophers viewed the body as an entity that can be divided and analyzed by studying its parts. Physicians, influenced by Descartes, reasoned that if disease were caused by a malfunctioning of the body machine or by a defective part, the cure for disease was simply to repair or remove that part or parts. Thus, the rationale for surgery as treatment is based on Descartes' ideas, as are many other medical procedures.

In addition to the body machine concept, this philosophy split humans into two entities, mind and body. This mind-body dichotomy (known as Cartesian dualism) greatly influenced the medical model of disease, in which treatment for diseases of the body and treatment for diseases of the mind became separate and distinct. This separation was unfortunate because it served as a barrier to our perception of humans in their wholeness.

The Germ Theory. Scientific discoveries of the 19th century gave rise to the **germ theory** of disease (the belief that microorganisms cause infectious diseases). The germ theory became popular after Pasteur, Koch, and others demonstrated that microorganisms cause certain diseases. This model of disease led to research into treatments designed to destroy germs within the human body. It also changed the focus from treatment to prevention through such measures as vaccination and sanitation.

CURRENT MODELS

The Biomedical Model. Today, the biomedical model, or medical model, based on Descartes' mechanistic concepts of the body machine, is still used to explain illness and define treatments. The **medical model** is the belief that diseases can be understood merely as physiologic processes. The mind-body dichotomy, or concept of dualism, dividing a person into body and mind, has contributed to the idea that the body can be understood entirely in physical terms. According to this model, disease results from such physiologic disturbances as genetic imperfections, biochemical imbalances, and damage from physical agents (e.g., irradiation) or biologic agents (e.g., bacteria). The biomedical model has been criticized for deemphasizing the psychosocial component of disease causation. Yet it was the use of this model that provided evidence of the link between stress in general (whether biologic, psychologic, environmental, or social in nature) and biochemical changes that can lead to both physical and emo-

tional disorders. This model continues to be the basis for much research.

Using the biomedical model, Western medicine has achieved unparalleled success in combating disease. For decades, it seemed the advantages provided by such miraculous drugs as anesthetic agents, vaccines, insulins, antibiotics, and vitamins would one day conquer all diseases. René Dubos, however, assured us that this would never be the case.

The Ecological Approach of Dubos. Dubos, the man responsible for gramicidin (the first clinically useful antibiotic), used an **ecological approach** (the study of living things as they exist in their natural environment) to study microbes in their natural environment. With his studies, Dubos was able to predict that microbes would adapt to drugs used against them and would develop resistant strains. He began to study humans in their natural environment and concluded that freedom from disease was impossible because of the continuous need for humans to adapt to an ever-changing environment in which new diseases would continue to arise.

His solution to this problem was not to develop stronger and stronger chemicals to control microbial disease but, rather, to make humans healthier so they could resist disease. Dubos said that health was not some state of vigor, of freedom from disease, or even of long life. He proposed that being healthy ". . . means you can function, do what you want to do and become what you want to become."[18]

Dunn's Model of High-Level Wellness. Dubos published his beliefs about health in 1959. That same year, Halbert Dunn published a classic article defining **high-level wellness** as ". . . an integrated method of functioning which is oriented toward maximizing the potential of which the individual is capable, within the environment where he is functioning."[9]

Dunn's model describes health as an emerging process rather than a static state (Fig. 2-2). With this model, you can plot an individual's health along a horizontal axis that represents a continuum from an extreme near death to an extreme of peak wellness. You can also plot the individual's environment along a vertical axis that represents environmental extremes from very unfavorable to very favorable. Using Dunn's model to plot an individual's health and environment, you can place the individual in one of four quadrants, the most ideal of which is high-level wellness in a favorable environment.

Other Current Models. In part, Dunn viewed health as being at various places on a health-illness continuum that includes high-level wellness at the peak. Others proposed a eudemonistic model of health that focuses only on the peak level. The **eudemonistic model of health** is a model that defines health as an ideal state of vibrant, exuberant well-being in which the person experiences positive effects such as happiness, good concepts of the self, sound relationships with others, and an optimal ability to think and act.

Others began to conceptualize health more in the manner of Dubos, as less than some ideal but allowing

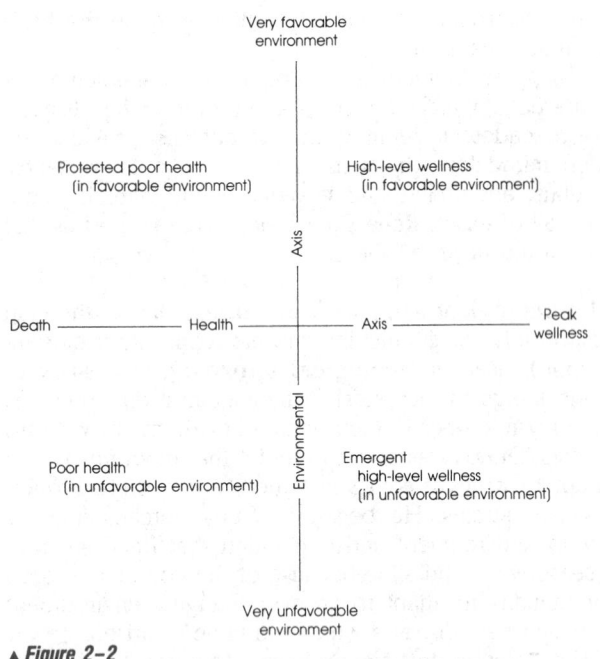

Very favorable
environment

Protected poor health
(in favorable environment)

High-level wellness
(in favorable environment)

Axis

Death —————— Health ——— Axis ——————— Peak
wellness

Environmental

Poor health
(in unfavorable environment)

Emergent
high-level wellness
(in unfavorable environment)

Very unfavorable
environment

▲ *Figure 2–2*

Dunn's health grid, its axes and quadrants. (From U.S. Department of Health, Education, and Welfare, Public Health Service, National Office of Vital Statistics.)

the greatest ability to survive. For Dubos and others, health meant the greatest ability to adapt to stressors in the internal and external environment (the **adaptive model**). For others, health meant the greatest ability to perform one's expected activities (the **role performance model**). For still others, it meant the greatest ability to survive long enough to pass along one's genes (the **evolutionary model**). These are but some of the models available to explain health and disease.

MODELS USED BY NURSES

Nurses use models as a basis for understanding and providing care to individuals, families, groups, and the larger society. You will encounter various models as you progress through your nursing studies; and many of them have been created by nurses. As you practice nursing, you will use one or more of the known models as they exist in the literature or you will take an eclectic approach and use parts of several models you find useful. One day you may even contribute your own model to the growing body of nursing literature that helps to make up the known information about health, disease, and health care.

Most nursing models are holistic in nature. The **holistic view of humans** is the view that the human person is a whole with at least biologic, psychologic, and social parts and that the whole is more than the sum of its parts. One of the simplest holistic models is the **biopsychosocial model of disease.** This model represents a recognition that mind and body continuously interact with each other; that the total person constantly interacts with the external, social environment; and that an illness in the biologic, psychologic,

or social realm can cause disease in the other realms as well. Thus, a physical illness can cause mental depression, which in turn can affect significant others in the person's environment. Mental illness can cause a breakdown in physical health because of poor nutrition, inadequate rest, and so on. Societal instability or stress can cause personal illness, both mental and physical. Likewise, the illness of one member of a close social network can adversely affect the health and functioning of others within that network.

More complex models add one or more concepts to the biopsychosocial model. Cultural, spiritual, linguistic, and other concepts are added as they are believed to be important to an understanding of humans and their health or disease status. For example, you may use a biopsychosociocultural model. Such additions are attempts to describe the nature of humans in their fullness, their wholeness.

CONCEPTS OF HEALTH PROMOTION AND DISEASE PREVENTION

Before the ways in which nurses and others use models in health care are discussed, it is helpful to understand the concepts of health promotion and disease prevention. Traditionally, modern health care systems have used three strategies for providing health care. These strategies are based on the biomedical model that defines health as the absence of disease. The three strategies are (1) primary prevention, (2) secondary prevention, and (3) tertiary prevention. Many health care systems have added an additional strategy, health promotion, aimed at increasing health, not merely preventing disease.

Prevention

Primary prevention refers to strategies used for persons who are considered to be free from disease. The main goal of primary prevention is to prevent illness. Strategies used to meet this goal for individuals and groups include measures such as counseling to prevent unhealthy effects of stress, teaching how to improve sanitation and prevent the spread of disease, and immunizing against infection.

Secondary prevention refers to strategies used for people in whom disease is present. The disease may not yet cause symptoms and may have been discovered only through routine screening (such as a small breast lump that is found by a routine mammogram), or the disease may be a severe illness that causes a great deal of discomfort and disability (such as a severe pelvic fracture that requires emergency surgery). The goal of secondary prevention is to halt or reverse the disease process in order to prevent further disability or death. The strategy used to meet this goal is to treat the disease at the earliest possible moment in its progression.

Tertiary prevention refers to strategies used to restore the physically or emotionally disabled person to the highest level of physical and mental health possible for that individual. Rehabilitation is an integral part of tertiary care. The three major goals of rehabilitation are to (1) protect the person from further disability; (2) strengthen and support the person in the use of remaining abilities; and (3) assist the individual to adapt physically, psychologically, and socially to permanent disabilities.

Health Promotion Versus Disease Prevention

Nola Pender, a noted researcher and author, has helped clarify the difference between strategies that promote health and those that treat disease. She described health promotion strategies as behaviors ". . . directed toward sustaining or increasing the individual's level of well-being, self-actualization, and personal fulfillment."[34] Health-promoting behaviors are related to individual lifestyle and personal choices and include efforts to increase physical activity and fitness; improve nutrition; enhance mental health; plan families; decrease use of tobacco, alcohol, and other drugs; and prevent mental disorders and violent, abusive behavior.[33]

Keeping the concepts of health promotion and disease prevention clearly differentiated is difficult. The main reason for this difficulty is that not all health care providers use the same models of health and disease. Because they conceptualize health and disease differently, many health care providers define health promotion and disease prevention differently as well. For example, the U.S. government uses a biomedical model and conceives of disease prevention and health promotion as three separate types of strategies: (1) disease prevention, (2) health promotion, and (3) health protection. Each of these types of strategies uses both disease prevention activities and health promotion activities, but the three types are differentiated more according to who provides the care, who receives the care, and what the goals of care are.[33] Table 2–2 outlines this model.

This textbook uses the terms *health promotion* and *disease prevention* as they are used by most nurses.

We refer to health promotion activities as activities that help to move the person along the health-illness continuum toward a higher level of wellness, and we refer to disease prevention activities as activities that help prevent the person from moving toward the illness end of the continuum.

Both health promotion and disease prevention may be used with any person, regardless of the person's place on the health-illness continuum. Note that the strategies of health promotion and disease prevention are not used strictly for individuals but pertain to activities that are equally useful to individuals, families, groups, and communities. Tables 2–2 and 2–3 compare the U.S. government's use of these terms with their use throughout this text.

THERAPEUTIC ACTIVITIES

With a general understanding of the different strategies used in the three levels of prevention versus the strategies used in health promotion, you can more easily understand some of the more specific approaches used in health care today.

TABLE 2–2. *Primary Disease Prevention, Health Promotion, and Health Protection as Described by the U.S. Government in Its National Objectives for the Year 2000*[33]

Strategy	Provider	Care Recipients	Goals of Care	Examples of Care
Primary prevention	Clinical personnel	Individuals	Disease prevention	Counseling, screening, immunizations, chemoprophylactic measures (medications that prevent disease)
Health promotion	Educational and community-based programs	Individuals	Improving individual lifestyles by influencing personal choices made in a social context	Encouraging good nutrition, exercise, physical fitness, and mental health and discouraging the use of tobacco, alcohol, drugs, and violent and abusive behavior
Health protection	Community/ government organizations	Larger population groups	Health protection and disease prevention through environmental or regulatory measures	Fostering occupational health and safety, environmental health, food and drug safety, and oral health

TABLE 2–3. *A Nursing Approach to Health Promotion and Disease Prevention*

Strategy	Provider	Care Recipients	Goals of Care	Examples of Care
Health promotion	Nurses	Individuals, families, groups, and communities	Achievement of the highest possible level of wellness on the health-illness continuum	Teaching nutrition, encouraging exercise, promoting fitness
Disease prevention	Nurses	Individuals, families, groups, and communities	Least possible movement toward the illness end of the health-illness continuum	Counseling to decrease stress, teaching hygienic practices, encouraging immunizations

Primary Prevention Activities

Activities directed at preventing the occurrence of disease have probably been around since the beginnings of humanity. For example, the first time human beings strapped animal furs on their feet before stepping out of their caves to hunt for hours (or days) in the snow, they were practicing disease prevention. When people first cast out lepers in an attempt to isolate themselves from those with the disease they most dreaded, they were attempting disease prevention. When the first person deliberately exposed herself to cowpox to prevent the much more virulent disease of smallpox, she was attempting an early form of immunization. Surely you could think of many more examples of measures humans have taken to prevent disease. Our history is rife with them.

Preventing disease is usually preferable to attempting to treat those suffering from its consequences. Preventive medicine is, therefore, an important part of any health care system. The prevention of disease depends to a large extent on commitment by health care recipients and providers. A person must commit to actions that meet the goal of disease prevention even when alternatives seem more pleasant, less difficult, or less costly. Health care workers must be prepared to provide accurate information about actions to take for achieving the goals of disease prevention. Accurate information about disease prevention is abundant; so is inaccurate information. Important for nurses engaged in primary prevention are sorting out the differences between facts and fallacies, remaining aware of the latest research findings, and presenting the best information to those in need of it.

If the nurse uses a holistic approach, multiple strategies may be used to prevent disease. Box 2–1 lists activities aimed at primary prevention in the biologic, psychologic, social, and cultural realms. Prevention activities often require a person to take an action, for example, going to a support group to see what it is like or changing to a better diet.

THE HEALTH BELIEF MODEL

One model particularly appropriate for predicting whether a person will take a given action in relation to disease prevention is Rosenstock's health belief model.

Irwin Rosenstock is given the most credit for developing and testing the **health belief model** for predicting human behavior in relation to health (Fig. 2–3). This model is based on the assumption that several factors can contribute to a person's taking a recommended action. In this case, the recommended action is a measure designed to prevent a disease (disease X).

If a person is to take an action to prevent disease X, the person should perceive (1) that he or she is susceptible to disease X, (2) that disease X is serious enough to necessitate the required preventive action, and (3) that the required action will be of benefit in preventing disease X. Even these perceptions do not guarantee that the preventive behavior will occur. These perceptions must be weighed against what the person perceives to be barriers to the preventive action. As Rosenstock said, "An individual may believe that a given action will be effective in reducing the threat of disease, but at the same time see that action itself as being inconvenient, expensive, unpleasant, painful, or upsetting. These negative aspects of health action serve as *barriers* to action and arouse conflicting motives of avoidance."[27]

Other variables, termed modifying factors in Rosenstock's model, also influence the way a person perceives the benefits and barriers of the preventive action. Modifying factors include demographic, sociopsychologic, and structural variables. Examples are listed in Figure 2–3. These modifying factors can strengthen the perception of either the benefits or the barriers to cause the person to move toward the recommended preventive action or away from it.

In addition to perceived benefits and perceived barriers to the preventive action, another factor that may move the person toward the preventive behavior is a trigger, or "cue to action." Cues to action may be internal (such as physical signs or symptoms) or external (such as communications from the mass media, from health care providers, or from significant others). If the person is unable to decide about the preventive action because the benefits and barriers appear approximately equal, the cue to action may add just enough additional incentive to bring about the behavior necessary to prevent disease X.

For an example of the health belief model, let us look at the case of Mrs. Dodds. Mrs. Dodds knew the flu season was about to arrive (in this case, disease X was the flu). She knew that the flu was, as usual, a new

Box 2–1. Nursing Activities that Promote Primary Prevention

Biologic Realm

Supporting public health programs such as measures to prevent water-borne infections

Teaching sanitation measures, such as safe food handling and preparation, safe practices related to elimination, and safe care of an infected person in the household, since others are at risk of becoming infected with a communicable disease.

Assisting in prophylaxis (prevention) of infectious diseases through immunization programs, such as immunizations against diphtheria, pertussis (whooping cough), tetanus, measles, mumps, rubella (German measles), polio, influenzas, and other communicable diseases.

Participating in epidemiologic studies (the studies of disease frequency and distribution in various populations) related to disease prevention.

Participating in programs believed to lower the incidence of certain diseases, for example, encouraging low-fat diets to prevent breast cancer, low-cholesterol diets to prevent heart disease, and decreased tobacco use to prevent oral and lung cancer.

Supporting programs believed to prevent accidents, such as programs to help increase seatbelt use or increase safety in the home and workplace.

Counseling people regarding nutritional needs in order to prevent dietary deficiencies.

Psychologic Realm

Promoting the mental health of individuals through activities such as teaching stress reduction and relaxation techniques.

Referring high-risk individuals to specific sources of support for their needs (e.g., support groups for persons experiencing high stress levels).

Promoting the mental health of groups by supporting programs to help prevent behaviors that could become addictive (e.g., tobacco, alcohol, and drug use).

Sociocultural Realm

Supporting programs to prevent social problems such as child abuse, homelessness, and criminal activities that victimize the helpless.

Serving as advocate for others in their spiritual beliefs when these are needed as a source of strength (see Chapter 53).

Counseling families and groups regarding effective means of communication and mutual support.

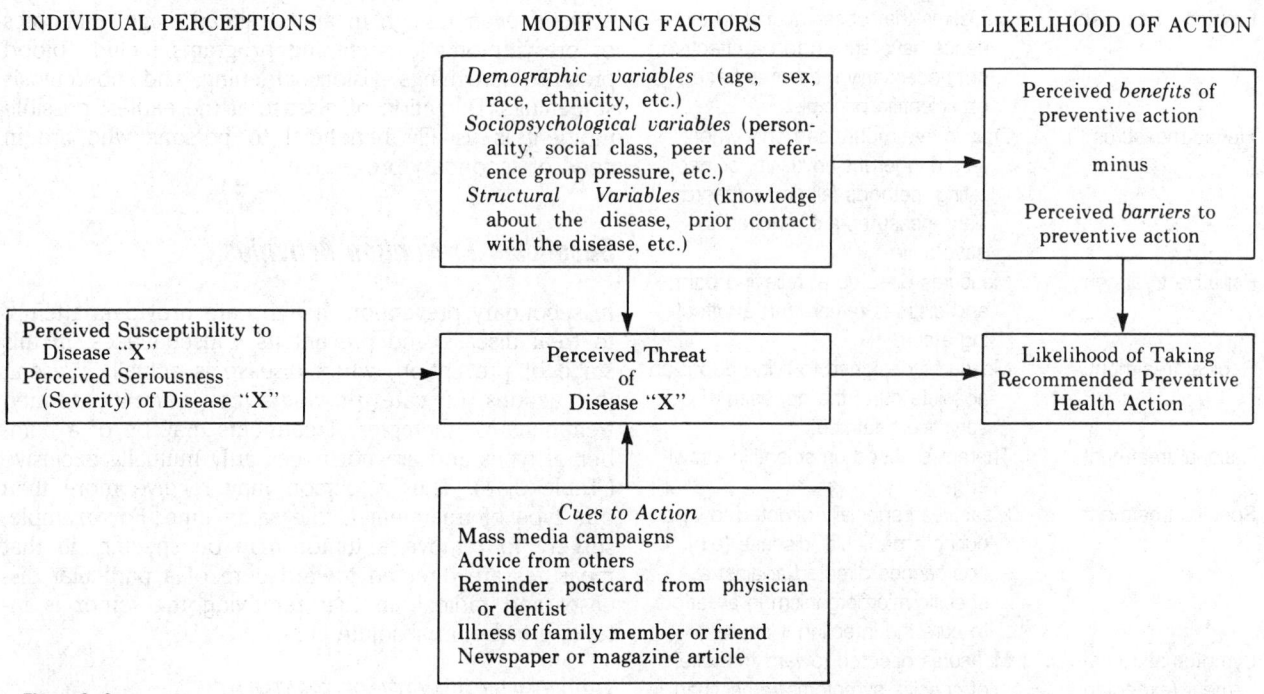

INDIVIDUAL PERCEPTIONS   MODIFYING FACTORS   LIKELIHOOD OF ACTION

Demographic variables (age, sex, race, ethnicity, etc.)
Sociopsychological variables (personality, social class, peer and reference group pressure, etc.)
Structural Variables (knowledge about the disease, prior contact with the disease, etc.)

Perceived *benefits* of preventive action

minus

Perceived *barriers* to preventive action

Perceived Susceptibility to Disease "X"
Perceived Seriousness (Severity) of Disease "X"

Perceived Threat of Disease "X"

Likelihood of Taking Recommended Preventive Health Action

Cues to Action
Mass media campaigns
Advice from others
Reminder postcard from physician or dentist
Illness of family member or friend
Newspaper or magazine article

▲ *Figure 2–3*

The health belief model (From Becker MH, Drachman RH, and Kirscht JP: A new approach to explaining sick-role behavior in low-income populations. *American Journal of Public Health* 64[3]: 206, 1974).

strain to which she had no immunity (i.e., she was susceptible). She had heard on the news that this particular flu strain was particularly virulent and that everyone should get a flu shot (i.e., the disease was serious enough to necessitate preventive action). She knew from previous experience that flu shots worked (i.e., the required action would be of benefit in preventing the disease). Considering only this information, you might conclude that Mrs. Dodds would get a flu shot. Instead, she had "a strange feeling that something terrible would happen" if she got the immunization. She had had these intuitive feelings before and was quite frightened because sometimes her intuition was correct (a barrier to the preventive action and a conflicting motive of avoidance).

Regarding modifying factors, we find that demo-

graphic variables had no particular effect on her decision about the health action. Mrs. Dodds's age (40 years), sex (female), race (Caucasian), ethnicity (Polish heritage), and other demographic variables were all such that she was not in a particularly vulnerable group. Her middle-class peers all valued disease prevention and pressured her to get the injection. She agreed that she should. Her very close friend, Dorothy, however, believed Mrs. Dodds had "psychic ability" and pressured her to listen to her own "inner feelings." As a result, the sociopsychologic variables tended to both encourage and discourage the health action. Mrs. Dodds had also lived through two particularly bad flu epidemics, had suffered miserably with the flu on at least one occasion, and had even seen people die from this disease. Therefore, the structural variables tended to encourage her toward the health action.

In short, Mrs. Dodds was certain she needed the flu shot but terrified of getting it. The benefits and barriers to action were of approximately equal weight. Finally, her niece, a registered nurse, encouraged her, stressed the importance of the injection, and offered to drive her to a clinic where both of them could get their shots at the same time. Her niece's offer provided cues to action. In the balance between the benefits and barriers, the cues to action tilted the scales, and Mrs. Dodds got her immunization.

SCREENING

In addition to working in many ways to prevent illness in healthy individuals, nurses also screen people who appear to be healthy. Presymptomatic screening programs are an attempt to discover cases of actual disease. In such cases, the disorder may be in an early stage of development or may be one that is not yet evident, even though in an advanced stage. Examples of presymptomatic screening programs include blood pressure screenings, vision screening, and tuberculosis screenings. Detection of disease at the earliest possible moment is usually beneficial to persons who are in need of secondary prevention.

Secondary Prevention Activities

In secondary prevention, health care providers attempt to treat disease and prevent its consequences. In this stage of prevention, when disease is actually present, the actions of care providers are correctly termed treatments or therapies. Treatments may be of a number of types and are not necessarily mutually exclusive (Table 2–4). Thus a person may receive more than one type of treatment at the same time. For example, surgery to remove a tumor may be specific, in that measures are directed toward cure of a particular disease, and radical, in that removing the tumor is intended to be an absolute cure.

THE BIOMEDICAL MODEL OF TREATMENT

Most frequently, treatments for disease are prescribed by physicians (Box 2–2) using what is known as West-

TABLE 2–4. Terms Describing Types of Treatment

Type of Treatment	Purpose of Therapy
Causal treatment	Measures directed at removing the cause of a disorder
Conservative treatment	The withholding of medical or surgical measures until treatment is clearly indicated; treatment designed to prevent the debilitation that could be caused by heroic methods; or treatment to conserve body organs by preventing radical surgery unless it is demonstrated to be necessary
Curative treatment	Measures directed at eradicating the person's disorder by healing the existing disease
Empirical treatment	Measures that observation and experience have shown to be effective, not necessarily measures based on scientific principles
Heroic measures	Drastic treatment used only when less dangerous, invasive, or debilitating methods fail and extraordinary measures are required to save a life
Palliative treatment	Measures directed at relieving pain and distress rather than at effecting a cure
Radical treatment	Measures designed to bring about an absolute cure; the opposite of conservative treatment
Rational treatment	Therapies based on scientific knowledge
Specific treatment	Measures especially directed toward curing a particular disease (e.g., approaches directed against a specific microorganism in an effort to cure the infection it causes)
Symptomatic treatment (expectant treatment)	Measures directed toward the relief of specific symptoms rather than toward a cure (e.g., treatment to relieve fever, pain, cough)

ern medicine. **Western medicine,** the modern, scientific medicine usually practiced according to the biomedical model, has traditionally been divided into surgery and medicine, which includes less invasive procedures. Invasive procedures are those in which a body cavity is entered or body tissue is damaged. The type of practitioner the client consults often determines the treatment received. For example, a person with a lower back pain might consult a neurosurgeon and receive back surgery, an orthopedic surgeon and receive either back surgery or traction, a family practitioner and receive an order for traction and muscle relaxant medication, or a psychiatrist and receive an analysis of why the person's stress is evidenced in back pain.

Most treatments done in health care facilities today are classified as either medical or surgical. Some specialty areas, however, have traditionally combined medicine and surgery, as warranted by the consumer's disease process (e.g., eye, ear, nose, and throat services or obstetrics and gynecology services) or by the client's developmental level (e.g., pediatric services or gerontologic services).

Both medicine and surgery have flourished during the past 150 years. The use of anesthesia, which began about the mid-19th century, allowed tremendous advances in surgery. Other pharmaceuticals have provided hitherto undreamed-of cures and treatments in the field of medicine. Medicine and surgery have both advanced because of the availability of computers and other technology not in existence 50 years ago. Only within the past few decades, for example, have we been able to provide multiple organ transplants and surgical joint replacements and prevent their rejection by the body. These are but a few examples of the many newer

treatments now available. Many are used in combination with older treatments, thereby expanding the biomedical field. For the most part, in some form or other, many common therapies have been around since before recorded history.

Nutritional (Diet) Therapy. Nutritional considerations are universally accepted as important in the treatment of disease. Changes in the amounts, types, or manner of preparation of various foods are common measures used alone or in conjunction with other treatments. Sometimes dietary change is needed only temporarily; sometimes change is necessary for the remainder of the person's life. Because nutrition is so important to health, nurses are expected to be knowledgeable in the area of diet therapy. Clinical dietitians specialize in nutrition and serve as expert resources for nurses and for other members of the health care team (see Chapter 42).

Pharmaceutical (Medication) Treatments. Since primitive times, herbs, minerals, and animal parts have been concocted and given to the ill for help in treating disease. These precursors of pharmaceuticals were sometimes worn, sometimes rubbed onto the skin, and sometimes eaten or drunk.[2] Today, they have been almost completely replaced by manufactured chemical compounds that make possible many of the cures now available. The person who cannot be cured can often be treated symptomatically or comforted by a drug. Pharmaceuticals, although they cannot do everything and although they sometimes even cause health problems, have become a mainstay of modern medical practice.

Nurses are expected to give pharmaceuticals to ill persons and to be knowledgeable about what they have given (see Chapter 46). Understanding medications is quite difficult because the pharmaceutical industry has made available a tremendous number of drugs, with new ones continually placed on the market. Pharmacists can be extremely helpful resources for nurses and other members of the health care team.

Physical Medicine. In the history of the treatment of disease, physical medicine is probably as old as the use of drugs. Physical medicine has traditionally used physical agents to treat disease. Among these are water, heat, light, massage (rubbing), and exercise. In modern times, the practitioners of physical medicine use exercise, massage, and the application of heat and other forms of energy by electrical current, diathermy, ultraviolet therapy, and hydrotherapy to treat disease. Sometimes the exercises performed prepare the individual for work or activities of daily living (the goals of occupational therapy). Sometimes the exercises are focused more on leisure activities and help repair the ailing mind as well as the body (the goals of recreational therapy). These other therapies still come under the heading of physical medicine.

A physician who specializes in physical medicine is a **physiatrist.** Non-physicians who work in this area of

---

Box 2–2. Physicians and Professional Nurses

Physicians

Although licensing laws vary from state to state, physicians are generally licensed to make a **diagnosis** (establishment of the cause and nature of a disease), determine a **prognosis** (a prediction of the probable outcome of a disease), and write **prescriptions** (orders for medications and treatments or procedures). Physicians are legally allowed to cut and penetrate the human body and to pronounce death. Physicians treat disease. The persons they treat are termed patients.

Professional Nurses

Nursing license laws also vary by state, but generally professional nurses provide care to individuals, families, groups, and communities of people to promote, maintain, or restore health. Nurses work as colleagues with physicians, sometimes functioning in a dependent role and sometimes functioning independently. Nurses manage the care of a person's health. The persons they treat are termed clients.

medicine are physical therapists, occupational therapists, recreational therapists, and others, depending on their area of practice. Nurses work with various therapists from the realm of physical medicine to greater or lesser extents, depending on their area of nursing practice. For example, nurses who work in an orthopedic unit work with physiotherapists more than do nurses who work in a psychiatric unit, where recreational or occupational therapists tend to predominate.

Radiation Therapy (Radiotherapy, Nuclear Medicine). Radiation therapy is a natural offshoot of physical therapy. Both disciplines use radiant energy. The radiation used in physical therapy, however, is fairly safe, nonionizing radiation. The radiation used in radiation therapy penetrates deeply into human tissue and can cause changes in the structure of body cells. It is used for treatment of malignancies as well as for diagnostic purposes.

Inhalation (Respiratory) Therapy. Inhalation therapy focuses on the delivery of gases for therapeutic purposes. Oxygen and mixtures of oxygen and room air are given to individuals to improve oxygen levels in their blood. Gases may be provided under varying pressures and by a number of different methods (see Chapter 45). Because nurses frequently work with persons who receive inhalation therapy, they must be knowledgeable about the safe use of gases.

Psychiatric Therapies. Psychiatric therapies focus on correcting psychosocial problems. Techniques vary but include biologic measures such as medication administration, psychologic measures such as psychoanalysis or other forms of individual therapy, and social measures such as family therapy or group therapy.

Physicians who practice psychiatry are psychiatrists. Psychologists are practitioners who have advanced education and training but are not physicians. Both psychiatrists and psychologists can provide valuable insight into behaviors of the persons who are in the care of nurses. Both can also provide support to nurses who are under high levels of stress, but only psychiatrists can prescribe medication and treatment. Psychiatric nurses and other psychiatric health care providers use their knowledge of psychiatric principles to care for persons in a variety of settings including, but not limited to, mental health centers.

ALTERNATIVES TO TRADITIONAL MEDICINE

Colonial Times. Western medicine did not always enjoy the high regard that it does today. Less than 200 years ago, the first U.S. president was literally bled to death by his physicians (1799). The heroic measures of blistering, bleeding, and purging that were used on George Washington to treat what was probably a strep throat were based on the humoral model of medicine used in ancient Greece. In colonial times, humoral medicine was practiced by physicians with the highest standing among their peers and the best education and training available.

Along with these esteemed, university-educated practitioners of the medical arts, of whom there were actually few, were other practitioners: unschooled "surgeons" who "doctored" because they said they could; physicians who learned by the apprenticeship system and practiced by empirical methods; barbers who pulled teeth, did surgery, and let blood as needed; outright quacks who were out to take advantage of the sick; and ministers and other educated lay people who were well schooled in the medical (humoral) theory of the day. Nursing had not yet been established as a helping profession, but some religious orders and others who did charitable work provided comfort to the poor who were sick. For the most part, only those who had no home and family to provide better care entered a hospital or other institution when they were sick.

Common people could call on any of the medical practitioners of the day but often relied on relatives, friends, and neighbors with whom they traded herbal "kitchen remedies" like they traded recipes for food. Another source of help for the lay public was the written word. One of the most helpful books of the colonial period was a collection of many "receipts" (remedies) to be used for treating some 780 conditions that were listed in alphabetical order. This popular little book, *Primitive Physick: or an Easy and Natural Method of Curing Most Disease,* by John Wesley, founder of the Methodist Church, remained in print for approximately 200 years.[2]

Throughout the years between colonial times and the present day, millions of immigrants came to the United States from all over the world, bringing medications and treatments from their homelands to use as their parents had before them. The treatments brought from other lands consisted of orthodox medical treatments as well as folk remedies from their country of origin. The immigrants learned about treatments used by Native Americans and by other immigrants who had come before them. Some mutual adoption of treatments occurred on the part of both the newcomers and those who had been here much longer.

The Nineteenth Century. During the 1800s, as the industrial age began in earnest, several groups became concerned about the unhealthy minds and bodies of the populace and advocated methods of improving general health. Some of these groups grew into nationwide health movements that pressed for individual changes in lifestyle and for reform of some practices that threatened the health of the general public. Women took important parts in these health movements, and nurses often served in leadership roles. In general, they advocated fresh air, exercise, healthy diets, bathing, and temperance. They also sought to end social evils such as slavery and the filthy industrial slums that bred crime and poverty.

In relation to the treatment of disease, an occasional 19th-century herbalist, physician, or other lay practitioner of medicine developed a theory of healing that did not fit the orthodox medical practice of the day. When their medical practices were judged by the public to be empirically useful, these theories became popular, and the practitioners remained in business but were considered "irregulars."

Some irregulars had large followings at one time or another. One was Samuel Thomson (1769–1843), a nearly illiterate, self-taught purveyor of herbal remedies that were based on his "system" of botanic remedies and whose followers were called Thomsonians. Another was Samuel Hahnemann (1755–1843), a well-educated physician who theorized that a minute dose of a drug (e.g., one millionth of a grain) could effect a cure. His followers were called homeopaths. Sylvester Graham (1794–1851) was another irregular, a minister who advocated a healthy way of life that included fresh air, exercise, and a diet with plenty of fresh fruit, vegetables, and coarsely ground whole-wheat bread. He is now remembered most for his graham crackers.

As the 19th century progressed, the regular medical practitioners of the day came to accept some of the practices of healthy living advocated by those in health movements. They began to prescribe exercise, diet, and sanitary practices. "Heroic medicine" was gradually replaced by less drastic treatments, and some of the irregulars faded from sight or adopted more of the practices of the regular medical practitioners.

The Modern Era. As medicine entered the 20th century, the mainstream medical establishment developed methods that improved the classification, diagnosis, and treatment of diseases. The U.S. government assisted in regulating medical practice by both orthodox practitioners and irregulars, and the general population became better educated about health care practices.

Today, we have available a variety of alternative health care practices. Some we have inherited from as long as 5000 years ago, some from our own grandparents, others from lands at great distances from our own. Compared with the modern Western medicine available in the U.S., some of these treatments seem completely alien. Yet they have been, and continue to be, accepted by many health care consumers. Some common alternative health care practices are defined in Table 2–5.

Nurses should be aware that these or other alternative health care practices may be being practiced by individuals who are, at the same time, using the biomedical treatment offered by their physician.

Often the use of these practices continues without the knowledge of physicians, who believe they are providing the only treatment for the ill person.[19] Nurses who are aware that their clients are using alternative practices are in an excellent position to judge the therapeutic value of these practices and to reinforce the use of safe and effective remedies in their overall plan of care for the clients or to caution against unsafe practices, as necessary.[3] For example, in your nursing career you may find some clients rely on meditation or prayer and that your support of these practices strengthens the clients' resolve to continue with painful but necessary treatments and that their prayer or meditation even lessens their pain. On the other hand, you may find that one of these clients also has a belief that drinking sea water is "good for what ails you" while

this same client is on a low-salt diet for treatment of a heart condition. Openness to and support of your clients' beliefs and alternative practices should place you in a position of trust so that you will be believed when you have to explain why certain practices may be harmful.

Prayer and meditation are alternative therapies common to many people of diverse backgrounds, so that you probably feel comfortable with clients who use these approaches. Some alternative practices, however, may sound foreign to you. Many are closely bound to one cultural group or another, and your particular culture may hold different ideas about what is or is not therapeutic. Yet if you are able to keep an open mind about the practices that your clients find helpful, you may learn a great deal from the diverse persons in our multicultural society.

Tertiary Prevention (Rehabilitation) Activities

After an acute illness, some individuals are left with residual mental or physical impairments that restrict their ability to function in a manner usually considered to be within the normal range. Other individuals develop impairments as a result of chronic illness. These persons need assistance to prevent their tendency to move more toward the illness end of the health-illness continuum. They also require rehabilitation to assist them to move, to the greatest extent possible, toward the wellness end of the health-illness continuum.

The scope of health problems experienced by individuals who can benefit from rehabilitation services is wide ranging. It includes cardiac, respiratory, orthopedic, burns, cancer, addictive, and neuromuscular problems. Such health problems can occur on either a time-limited or a chronic basis.

The unique goals and needs of the individual determine the members of the rehabilitation "team" required. The participants in the rehabilitation process always include the individual needing rehabilitation and the person or persons who can provide the particular services needed. An individual's ability to achieve rehabilitation goals may relate to the availability of not only a specialized health care team but also a support network of significant others. Those people can often offer the kind of support that keeps this person motivated and self-confident enough to persist with a rehabilitation program.

The more complex the needs and goals of the individual, the greater the number of health care professionals involved in the process. The potential members of the rehabilitation team and their general area of responsibility will depend on the problems to be addressed. A typical team for a person with a neuromuscular disorder, such as cerebral palsy, might include the members shown in Table 2–6. Each member of the team should consider the biologic, psychologic, educational, social, and vocational needs of the disabled individual while working with the person to meet the goals of tertiary prevention.

Coordination of efforts is an essential component of a successful rehabilitation program. Lack of coordina-

TABLE 2-5. Alternative Practices Sometimes Used Together with Western Medicine

Alternative Practice	Therapeutic Method
Acupressure	A noninvasive technique that applies the pressure of the practitioner's fingers to acupuncture sites to cure or ameliorate diseases.
Acupuncture	A technique based on an ancient Chinese belief that the entire universe is composed of two types of energy: the positive yang, which contracts and stimulates, and the negative yin, which sedates and expands. Health is believed to exist when equilibrium between yang and yin in the vital life force *(c'hi)* moves along meridians as it flows through the human body. Disease is believed to result from an imbalance of yang and yin in the *c'hi*. Acupuncture is believed to restore balance. Long, fine needles are introduced through the skin at specific acupuncture sites, along the meridians, to cure diseases associated with each site. In the past, the needles were often twirled; now they may be stimulated with a weak electrical current.
Ayurveda (a 4000-year-old Sanskrit word meaning "the science of life")	An ancient tradition of Indian medicine derived from a belief that the body is created from the flow of the mind. In this tradition, each cell of the body contains intelligence, and the mind has control over all diseases. The body and mind interact through techniques such as meditation.
Chiropractic treatment	A system of healing that is based on the belief that malalignment of the spinal column causes the vertebral bones to place pressure on nerves and cause symptoms such as pain and loss of function. Treatment consists of spinal manipulations (adjustments), spinal traction, and applications of heat to the spinal area.
Color therapy	A therapy, dating back to ancient Egypt, in which colored light is used to treat disease. Red, orange, and yellow are considered hot colors; blue, indigo, and violet are considered cool colors; green is believed to be a balancing color. Color therapy is based on the belief that each color of the rainbow has a vibration level that corresponds with a similar vibration in one of the seven *chakras* (body centers). Red, for example, corresponds with the base of the spine and mediates physical imbalances such as yeast infections, fluid retention, and problems of the sciatica, colon, bladder, urethra, and male reproductive tract. Research has shown that exposure to certain colors does affect humans in a number of ways and that color can cause changes in behavior and emotions.
Herbalism	The use of leaves, flowers, stems, or roots of plants to heal illness. Medicinal herbs were, at one time, selected on the basis of "signatures"; that is, the appearance of a plant supposedly indicated its utility in medicine (e.g., a heart-shaped leaf might be good for a disease of the heart). Generally, use of herbs was and continues to be based on empirical evidence of efficacy.
Homeopathy	A system of treatment based on the belief that large doses of drugs that produce symptoms of a disease in healthy individuals will cure the same symptoms when administered in minute amounts to sick persons. This theory is often called "like cures like."
Naturopathy	A system of healing that does not use drugs or other unnatural treatments. Naturopathy relies on cleansing and restoration of the body through the use of natural forces such as air, light, heat, water, and massage.
Osteopathy	A system of medicine, founded by Dr. Andrew Taylor Still (1828–1917), based on the belief that health depends on the body's ability to rectify itself against toxic conditions when it has satisfactory nourishment and favorable environmental circumstances. Osteopathic physicians use manipulation to restore the body's structural and functional balance, and they use medicine and surgery to repair any internal or external abnormalities of the system.
Reflexology (zone therapy)	A therapy developed by Dr. William Fitzgerald in approximately 1913, but that harkens back to the ancient Chinese treatment of acupressure. Reflexology relies on the application of pressure to certain body parts to relieve symptoms at distant sites and in specific organs. Pressure points used in reflexology are primarily in the hands and feet.
Shiatsu	An ancient Japanese therapy based on maintaining and restoring the flow of energy *(ki)* in the human body. Like acupressure, shiatsu (literally, "finger pressure") uses the application of rhythmic pressure at certain points along the body meridians to relieve symptoms of disease. Shiatsu is used to help maintain health as well as to prevent disease.
Spiritual healing	The use of prayer or other religious rituals such as the "laying on of hands," visiting of shrines, or bathing in holy waters to promote healing. Spiritual healing sometimes involves a person (healer) considered to have special gifts derived from a higher power and is sometimes done without the intervention of another person.

TABLE 2–5. Alternative Practices Sometimes Used Together with Western Medicine Continued

Alternative Practice	Therapeutic Method
Therapeutic touch	A method used to diagnose and relieve symptoms in ill persons by using the hands, much like the ancient Christian "laying on of hands." Touching was rediscovered as a therapeutic modality in the 1970s by Delores Krieger, who taught nurses to think of the human body according to ancient Eastern beliefs as a flow of energy and to use their hands to feel for blocks in the energy flow. Blocks can, for example, be indicated by increased areas of heat. To heal, nurses lay their hands on the areas of blocked flow and concentrate on restoring the energy needed.
Yoga (derived from the Sanskrit word *yuj* for yoking or joining)	A way of life that combines mental and physical exercises to bring the mind and body into balance and prepare the person for union with the higher spiritual power in an ultimate state of being.

tion can lead to confusion for the person with a disability, who may lose confidence and fail to meet rehabilitation goals. In settings where the rehabilitation team has many members, weekly meetings are often held to coordinate the rehabilitation program with an individual. This process includes assessing progress or lack of progress toward goals and changing the program as necessary. The nurse serves a vital function in coordinating the efforts of the health care team.

Health Promotion Activities

THE NURSE'S ROLE

Promotion of health must begin with clients at their individual level of wellness on the health-illness continuum. Any existing disease must be treated to restore health to the highest possible level. Clients must also be protected from additional disease by preventive actions, when this is feasible. Disease treatment and pre-

TABLE 2–6. Potential Members of the Rehabilitation Team and their Principal Functions

Team Member	Principal Function(s)	Team Member	Principal Function(s)
Nurse	Advocate for the person with disability and significant others	Social worker	Assesses and develops resources for income, equipment, and housing
	Coordinates team		Provides information related to transportation and recreational resources
	Prevents complications		
	Maintains normal body functions	Psychologist	Provides intelligence and psychologic testing
	Provides psychosocial support and health teaching		
Personal physician—family practitioner or specialist	Manages medical problems		Asseses motivation, values, and response to disability
Physiatrist—physician specializing in physical medicine and rehabilitation	Tests physical functioning		Assists the person and significant others with coping
	Determines functional goals	Dietitian	Assesses and provides for nutritional needs
	Supervises rehabilitation process		
Physical therapist	Strengthens muscles		Makes sure foods are appropriate based on swallowing and physical abilities
	Maintains mobility		
	Develops new means of ambulation	Rehabilitation engineer	Develops adaptive equipment for severely disabled so some level of functioning can be maintained
Occupational therapist	Develops functional living skills, e.g., activities of daily living, household maintenance, child care		
		Recreational therapist	Assists person with resocialization and community reentry
Speech pathologist	Treats swallowing, speech, and communication disorders		Teaches leisure activities and architectural barrier problem-solving
Vocational rehabilitation counselor	Tests for vocational aptitudes, skills, and interests		
	Initiates job placement and acts as liaison between employer and person		

vention can occur at the same time that health promotion activities are occurring. For example, you may some day be providing nursing care to individuals who are about to undergo heart surgery. In such cases, you may

▶ Teach them how to turn, cough, and deep breathe to help in preventing postoperative complications.
▶ Prepare them for surgery by listening to their concerns and helping them to express and deal with their anxieties. Research has shown that clients will have less pain in the postoperative period if their anxiety is reduced before surgery.
▶ Teach them the importance of the low-fat, low-cholesterol, low-sodium diet the physician has ordered for help in preventing further cardiac problems.
▶ Discuss with them the plans they have to begin a healthier life, including exercising regularly after surgery.
▶ Answer their questions about a support group they may be thinking of joining after surgery, so they have some social contacts with others who understand their illness and will support their plans to improve their general cardiovascular fitness.
▶ Assist them to verbalize their unspoken fears about possible changes in their bodies or their sexuality.

These are common nursing activities. What are the specific actions that promote health (as opposed to preventing disease)? These are actions that help people to move toward that definition of health put forth by the World Health Organization: ". . . a state of complete physical, mental, and social well-being. . . ." Examples of health-promoting activities are listed in Box 2–3.

Box 2–3. Examples of Health-Promoting Activities

Biologic Realm

Eating a balanced, healthy diet
Taking sufficient fluid
Exercising regularly
Getting adequate, regular rest and sleep
Eliminating wastes regularly through the bladder and bowels

Psychologic Realm

Finding satisfying (stimulating, rewarding) work
Finding regular times for play
Using moderation in work and play
Exploring new things
Creating

Social Realm

Communicating well with others
Expressing love and closeness appropriately

CHANGING BEHAVIORS

Much of the work that a nurse does in health promotion is teaching, modeling, or otherwise supporting and encouraging clients to change unhealthy behaviors to healthy behaviors. Two models, Bandura's social cognitive theory and Pender's health promotion model, help explain how people change their behaviors. Both are particularly pertinent to health promotion.

Social Cognitive Theory. In 1977, Albert Bandura formulated what he originally termed social learning theory. This theory, now called **social cognitive theory,** states that all behavior changes depend on a person's belief in self-efficacy (the ability to successfully perform the new behavior). Belief in self-efficacy can be learned by positive or negative personal experiences or by examples provided by others.

In addition to beliefs about self-efficacy, each person has beliefs about whether a new behavior will lead to a desired outcome. According to Bandura, behavior change depends more on expectations of one's self-efficacy than on any expectations regarding outcomes. For example, a sedentary person may believe that beginning to exercise for a half hour each day can lead to increased muscle strength. Whereas increased muscle strength (the expected outcome) may be desirable, the behavior (a half hour of daily exercise) may or may not occur, depending on the belief in self-efficacy, here a belief in the ability to successfully complete a half hour of exercise each day.

The Health Promotion Model. Still another model concerned with the changing of behavior is the health promotion model developed and tested by Nola Pender et al. The **health promotion model** is used to predict the likelihood of a person's engaging in health-promoting behaviors. It is based on Bandura's social cognitive theory as well as on Rosenstock's health belief model (see Fig. 2–3). Whereas the health belief model focuses on the behaviors that prevent illness, the health promotion model focuses on health promotion without consideration of beliefs about illness (Fig. 2–4).

According to the health promotion model, seven cognitive/perceptual factors reflect an individual's beliefs. Together, these beliefs help determine the likelihood of the person's engaging in specific health-promoting behaviors. These factors include the importance of health, perceived control of health, perceived self-efficacy, definition of health, perceived health status, perceived benefits of health-promoting behaviors, and perceived barriers to health-promoting behaviors.

As with the health belief model, the health promotion model incorporates the effects of modifying factors, including demographic characteristics. Additional modifying factors in the health promotion model include biologic characteristics, interpersonal influences, and situational and behavioral factors. Cues to action are the same as those in the health belief model.

As you continue your study of nursing, you will find other models that will be helpful to you in your understanding of health care. For example, growth and de-

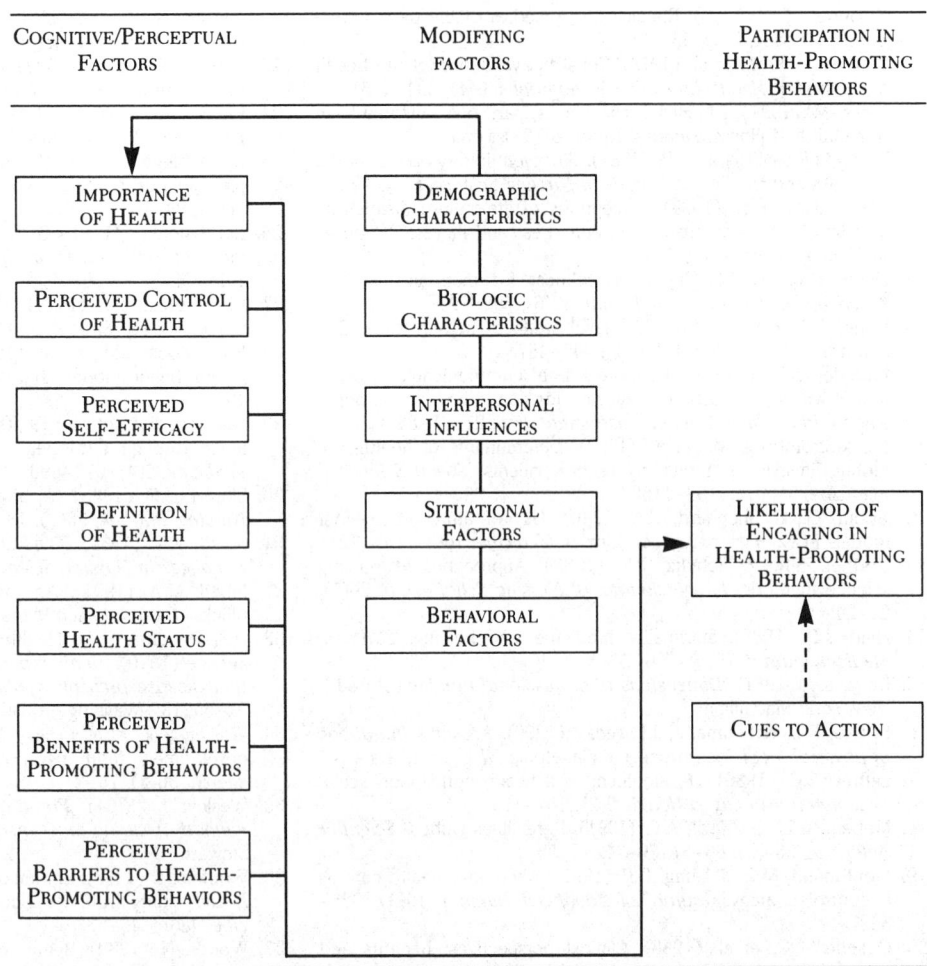

COGNITIVE/PERCEPTUAL FACTORS   MODIFYING FACTORS   PARTICIPATION IN HEALTH-PROMOTING BEHAVIORS

IMPORTANCE OF HEALTH

PERCEIVED CONTROL OF HEALTH

PERCEIVED SELF-EFFICACY

DEFINITION OF HEALTH

PERCEIVED HEALTH STATUS

PERCEIVED BENEFITS OF HEALTH-PROMOTING BEHAVIORS

PERCEIVED BARRIERS TO HEALTH-PROMOTING BEHAVIORS

DEMOGRAPHIC CHARACTERISTICS

BIOLOGIC CHARACTERISTICS

INTERPERSONAL INFLUENCES

SITUATIONAL FACTORS

BEHAVIORAL FACTORS

LIKELIHOOD OF ENGAGING IN HEALTH-PROMOTING BEHAVIORS

CUES TO ACTION

▲ *Figure 2-4*

Pender's Health Promotion Model (From Pender NJ et al: Predicting health-promoting lifestyles in the workplace. *Nurs Res* 39[6]: 331, 1990).

velopment models are presented in Unit 3. Together, these models can inform your practice of nursing and guide the care you provide clients.

Summary

▶ Models of health and disease have progressed from a focus on superstition through a focus on the individual to a focus on the wholeness of persons in relation to their environment and to society. Models include supernatural causation, the Greek humoral theory, the body machine and the mind-body dichotomy, the germ theory, the medical model, the ecological approach, the model of high-level wellness, the biophyschosocial model, and others.

▶ Disease prevention may be primary, secondary, or tertiary. Health promotion is a newer concept. Primary prevention is aimed at people who are free from disease. Secondary prevention involves strategies to halt or reverse the disease process. Tertiary prevention is designed to restore health, physically or emotionally, to the greatest degree possible. Health promotion is aimed at sustaining or increasing well-being.

▶ The health belief model is particularly appropriate for use in predicting human behavior in relation to disease prevention.

▶ A partial list of biomedical treatments for secondary prevention includes causal, conservative, curative, empirical, heroic, palliative, radical, rational, specific, and symptomatic (expectant) treatment.

▶ A partial list of alternative therapies includes acupressure, acupuncture, ayurveda, chiropractic, color therapy, herbalism, homeopathy, naturopathy, osteopathy, reflexology (zone therapy), shiatsu, spiritual healing, therapeutic touch, and yoga.

▶ The health promotion model builds on the health belief model and on social cognitive therapy to explain behavior changes in health promotion activities. The health promotion model helps predict the likelihood of a person's engaging in health-promoting behavior. The model draws on social cognitive theory, which states that behavior change depends on a person's belief in self-efficacy.

Bibliography

1. Bandura, A. (1977). Self-efficacy: toward a unifying theory of behavioral change. *Psychological Review,* 84(2), 191–215.
2. Bolander, V.R. (1983). A preliminary examination of John Wesley's *Primitive physick. The Bookman,* 10(4), 3–10.

3. Bolander, V.R. (1988). Rheumatism remedies of the past. *Orthopaedic Nursing*, 7(2), 53–58.

4. Cummings, K.M., et al. (1978). Construct validation of the health belief model. *Health Education Monographs*, 6(4), 394–405.

5. Davis, M. (1991). P1: Health and illness, part 1: A personal view of health and illness. *Nursing Times*, 87(22), i–viii.

6. Dixon, J.K., & Dixon, J.P. (1984). An evolutionary-based model of health and viability. *Advances in Nursing Science*, 6(3), 1–18.

7. Dixon, J.P., et al. (1989). Perceptions of life-pattern disintegrity as a link in the relationship between stress and illness. *Advances in Nursing Science*, 11(2), 1–11.

8. Dunn, H.L. (1959). High-level wellness for man and society. *American Journal of Public Health*, 49(6), 786–792.

9. Dunn, H.L. (1959). What high-level wellness means. *Canadian Journal of Public Health*, 50(11), 447–457.

10. Enderle, J.D. (1991). A discrete-time communicable disease model with a stochastic contact rate for nonhomogeneous populations. *Biomedical Sciences Instrumentation*, 27, 77–88.

11. Frank-Stromborg, M., et al. (1990). Determinants of health-promoting lifestyle in ambulatory cancer patients. *Social Science & Medicine*, 31(10), 1159–1168.

12. Godin, G., & Shephard, R.J. (1990). Use of attitude-behaviour models in exercise promotion. *Sports Medicine*, 10(2), 103–121.

13. Gortner, S.R., & Schultz, P.R. (1988). Approaches to nursing science methods. *Image: Journal of Nursing Scholarship*, 20(1), 22–24.

14. Hiatt, J.F. (1986). Spirituality, medicine, and healing. *Southern Medical Journal*, 79(6), 736–743.

15. Kelly, L.Y. (1981). *Dimensions of professional nursing* (4th ed.). New York: Macmillan.

16. Kottke, F.J., & Lehmann, J.F. (eds.) (1990). *Krusen's handbook of physical medicine* (4th ed.). Philadelphia: W.B. Saunders.

17. Laffrey, S.C. (1986). Development of a health conception scale. *Research in Nursing & Health*, 9(2), 107–113.

18. Moberg, C.L., & Zanvil, A.C. (1991). René Jules Dubos. *Scientific American*, 264(5), 66–67, 70–74.

19. Montbriand, M.J., & Laing, G.P. (1991). Alternative health care as a control strategy. *Journal of Advanced Nursing*, 16(3), 325–332.

20. Ockene, J.K., et al. (1988). Clinical perspectives: benefits and costs of lifestyle change to reduce risk of chronic disease. *Preventive Medicine*, 17(2), 224–234.

21. Pender, N.J. (1990). Expressing health through lifestyle patterns. *Nursing Science Quarterly*, 3(3), 115–122.

22. Pender, N.J., et al. (1990). Predicting health-promoting lifestyles in the workplace. *Nursing Research*, 39(6), 326–332.

23. Pender, N.J., et al. (1988). Development and testing of the health promotion model. *Cardiovascular Nursing*, 24(6), 41–43.

24. Price, S.A., & Wilson, L.M. (1986). *Clinical concepts of disease processes* (3rd ed.). New York: McGraw-Hill.

25. Riebschleger, J.L. (1991). Families of chronically mentally ill people: siblings speak to social workers. *Health & Social Work*, 16(2), 94–103.

26. Rosenstock, I.M. (1988). Adoption and maintenance of lifestyle modifications. *American Journal of Preventive Medicine*, 4(6), 349–352.

27. Rosenstock, I.M. (1974). Historical origins of the health belief model. *Health Education Monographs*, 2(4), 328–335.

28. Rosenstock, I.M., et al. (1988). Social learning theory and the health belief model. *Health Education Quarterly*, 15(2), 175–183.

29. Sandroff, D.J., et al. (1990). Meeting the health promotion challenge through a model of shared responsibility. *Occupational Medicine*, 5(4), 677–690.

30. Shaver, J.F. (1985). A biopsychosocial view of human health. *Nursing Outlook*, 33(4), 186–191.

31. Smith, J.A. (1981). The idea of health: a philosophical inquiry. *Advances in Nursing Science*, 3(3), 43–50.

32. Smith, M.A. (1991). Age and health perceptions among elderly blacks. *Gerontological Nursing*, 17(11), 13–19.

33. U.S. Department of Health and Human Services, Public Health Service (1990). *Healthy people 2000: National health promotion and disease prevention objectives*. (DHHS Publication No. PHS 91–50213.) Washington, DC: U.S. Government Printing Office.

34. Walker, S.N., et al. (1987). The health-promoting lifestyle profile: development and psychometric characteristics. *Nursing Research*, 36(2), 76–81.

35. Wesley, J. (1764). *Primitive physick: Or an easy and natural method of curing most disease* (12th ed.). Philadelphia: Andrew Stewart.

36. Wolffers, I. (1988). Limitations of the primary health care model. A case study from Bangladesh. *Tropical & Geographical Medicine*, 48(1), 45–53.

37. Woods, N. (1989). Being healthy: conceptualizations of self-care: toward health-oriented models. *Advances in Nursing Science*, 12(1), 1–13.

38. Woods, N.F., et al. (1988). Being healthy: women's images. *Advances in Nursing Science*, 11(1), 36–46.

▼ Legal and Ethical Aspects of Nursing

It is not, what a lawyer tells me I may do; but what humanity, reason, and justice, tell me I ought to do.

Edmund Burke

▼ CHAPTER OUTLINE

ETHICS, MORALS, AND VALUES
    Types of Ethical Theories
    Ethical Principles
    Codes of Ethics
    Ethical Decision Making in Nursing
LAW AND ITS SOURCES
    Constitutional Law
    Case Law
    Statutory Law

    Administrative Law
TYPES OF LAW
    Civil and Criminal Law
    Procedural and Substantive Law
    Tort Law
    Contract Law
    Licensure Laws
WHAT IS GOOD?

▼ KEY TERMS

Administrative law
Assault
Autonomy
Battery
Beneficence
Case law
Civil law
Common law
Constitutional law
Contract
Criminal law
Defamation
Duty-oriented ethical
  theory
Ethics

False imprisonment
Fidelity
Goal-oriented ethical
  theory
Intuitionist ethical theory
Invasion of privacy
Justice
Law
Liability
Libel
Licensure
Malpractice
Morals
Negligence

Nonmaleficence
Parentalism
Patient privilege
Prima facie case
Privacy
Procedural law
Rights-oriented ethical
  theory
Slander
Standard of care
Statutory law
Substantive law
Tort law
Values

Nurses often wonder, "What approach in my relationship to my client will achieve the most good?" A quick response indicates a superficial appreciation of the question. The more reflective response means examining options for achieving good according to various systematic sets of criteria or principles. This analysis occurs before decision making. Ethical theories provide the systematic sets of criteria for decision making. Ethical principles are important concepts to consider when ethical dilemmas arise.

Nurses frequently voice concerns about their legal liability. When nurses voice these concerns, they are actually asking, "What is the risk of my being sued for negligence or malpractice as a result of my nursing decisions in this situation?" Nurses who view the threat of malpractice suits as the sole source of legal influence on their practice have a narrow perspective. A broader view of law is that law reflects societal choices about the ordering of relationships among persons in that society. Thus, the law affects nurses not only in their relationships with their clients but also in their relationships with their employers, other nurses, other health care providers, and the public.

The law attempts to create orderly relationships in a society and to make decisions that will be good for society as a whole. Thus, law and ethics become intertwined. A law can be viewed as ethical or unethical. The United States and Canada, however, place a high value on human rights as moral good, so that law in both countries largely reflects a rights-oriented ethical framework. To start thinking about the relationship between ethics and law, consider Box 3–1 and Figure 3–1.

ETHICS, MORALS, AND VALUES

Knowing the derivation of the term "ethics" can help you understand its meaning. Ethics derives from the Greek word "ethos," which refers to "customs, habitual usages, conduct, and character."[18] The term "morals" derives from the Latin word "mores" for custom or habit. Thus, **morals** are the ethical customs of a society or ethical habits of a person.

Both terms also imply goodness, worthiness, or desirability. Thus, an action or motive described as good, worthy, or desirable is termed moral or ethical, whereas an action or motive described as bad, unworthy, or undesirable is considered unethical or immoral.[18] **Ethics** is a system or code of morals and is a discipline that seeks to formulate and systematically justify responses to moral dilemmas.[8] Ethical principles and theories are the bases for justifying the various responses to moral dilemmas.

Values refer to an individual's personal assignment of worth to an action or idea. Because each value has its assigned worth, values can be ranked. Individuals hold values with respect to many aspects of life; some examples are economic, aesthetic, and moral values. Moral beliefs reflect personal and societal choices about values that represent good, worthy, or desirable actions. The values of a society influence personal values.

Ethical theories provide a systematic approach to decision making about "what, all things considered, ought to be done in a given situation." A different conclusion about what achieves "good" results from each ethical theory rank ordering a similar set of concepts—goals, duties, and rights. Box 3–2 shows how values influence moral choices and demonstrates the application of ethical theories and principles. Ethical dilemmas cannot be resolved by applying technical expertise or scientific research because the choices are value laden.

Types of Ethical Theories

Various ethical theories provide helpful guidelines for decision making, but each set of guidelines has both

Box 3–1. Examining the Relationship Between Ethics and Law

Problem

State law prohibits smoking by employees, visitors, and clients in a state-run hospital. You are a nurse caring for a client with cardiac disease who insists he can relax only if he can smoke at least five times a day. Is the law ethical or unethical?

Analysis

The person with cardiac disease values relaxation with a cigarette over a healthy lifestyle. Valuing relaxation creates a moral belief that smoking is a good, worthy, or desirable action. In turn, the ethical system his actions reflect is a rights-oriented system that values the ethical principle of autonomy. From this client's perspective, the law is unethical.

On the other hand, you, as the nurse caring for this person, recognize the dangers of passive smoking. You appreciate the client's valuing relaxing with a cigarette over personal health, but you value the health of the many others who may be harmed by this smoking over the client's personal desire for relaxation. The ethical system you reflect is a goal-oriented system that incorporates the ethical principle of justice for many over the rights of one. From your perspective, the law is ethical.

The Ethical Dilemma

Your ethical dilemma can be framed as the right of one versus the rights of many or as the goal of one over the goal of many.

Choice

Will you let your client smoke, or will you enforce the law?

Box 3–2. Values in Conflict and Ethical Dilemmas

A client has been in a coma for several months. One group of nurses supports the family, which wishes to discontinue life-sustaining measures. Another group of nurses believes the measures should be continued. Thus, one group values the preservation of life no matter what level of thinking or feeling the client possesses. The second group values the preservation of life only if that life will include the ability to think and feel. The first group ranks preserving life as a value higher than thinking or feeling. The second group does not value preserving life unless thinking and feeling are possible. Together, the groups represent the struggle of a society to define when nonlife is of higher value than life.

Each group views its approach as moral, that is, good, worthy, and desirable. The first group reflects a duty-oriented ethical approach that life must be preserved at all costs. The second group may be reflecting a rights-oriented approach that permits a person to choose nontreatment or a goal-oriented approach that would shift health care resources to those who retain functional capability.

advantages and disadvantages. Figure 3–2 illustrates the structure of specific types of ethical theories.

DUTY-ORIENTED ETHICAL THEORIES

A **duty-oriented ethical theory** is a system of ethical thinking having the concept of duty or obligation as a foundation. Duties are strict obligations that take primacy over rights and goals. Keep in mind, however, that each duty has a corresponding right. For example, if the nurse has a duty to keep confidential personal information, then the client has a right to privacy.

Duty-oriented theories are advantageous in homogeneous societies in which each person holds the same values. A duty-oriented theory would work well in a tribal society because it is easier to share values and therefore moral beliefs among a small group of people. A disadvantage of a duty-oriented theory is determining how to rank duties. For example, a nurse may be torn between a duty to support life and a duty to prevent suffering. Duty-oriented theories ignore consequences. For example, the outcome of prolonged suffering could be ignored by honoring the duty to prolong life.

RIGHTS-ORIENTED ETHICAL THEORIES

A **rights-oriented ethical theory** is a system of ethical thinking having the concept of rights as a foundation. Rights-oriented theories assign the highest value to rights, so that duties and goals flow from rights. From a rights-oriented perspective, you would first look to the client's right to privacy. Flowing from that right to privacy would be your duty to keep health care information confidential to achieve the goal of encouraging clients to communicate information freely.

A pluralistic society like the United States can remain

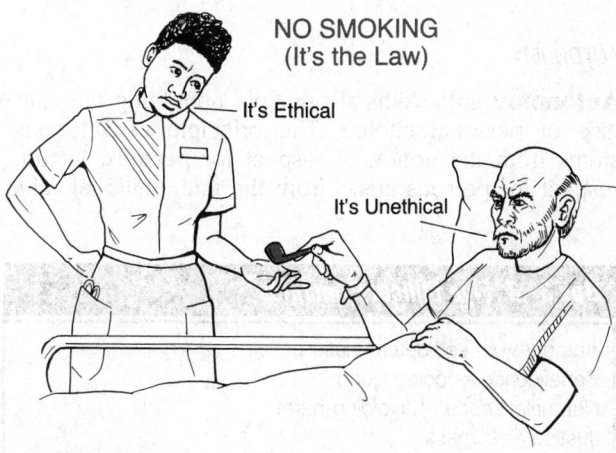

NO SMOKING
(It's the Law)

— It's Ethical

It's Unethical

▲ Figure 3–1

Questions of law and ethics.

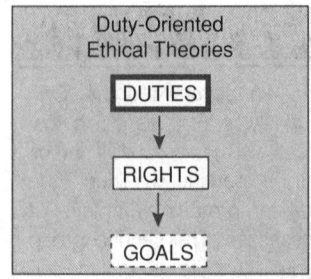
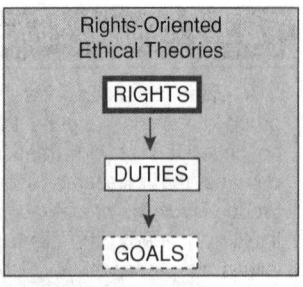
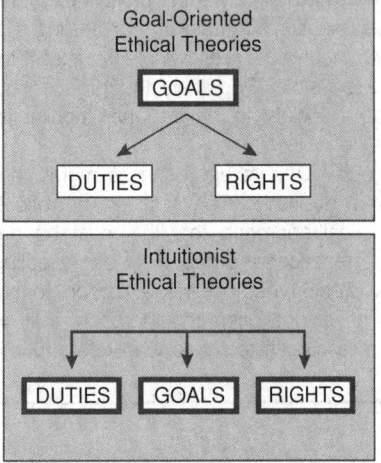

▲ *Figure 3–2*

Structures of four types of ethical theories.

cohesive because the foundation of the society is a set of fundamental rights for all citizens. Like duty-oriented theories, which fail to rank duties, however, rights-oriented theories may be weak because rights are not ranked. This lack of rank ordering presents a problem when rights conflict. For example, persons have a right to be free from government intrusion into their homes. However, is it ethical to infringe on this right with child abuse protection laws? That choice has been made in American society because society has set a greater value on the child's right to protection than on the individual's right to be free from intrusion.

GOAL-ORIENTED ETHICAL THEORIES

A **goal-oriented ethical theory** is a system of ethical thinking having the concept of maximizing the overall good as its foundation. Goal-oriented theories suggest that good choices result from concern with the consequences of actions. For example, the theory known as utilitarianism states that choices that are good maximize the happiness or welfare of society as a whole.[8]

What ethical choices can nurses make that will maximize societal welfare? In today's environment of health care reform, nurses might choose to support changes that will provide basic preventive and treatment services for all. Providing both prevention and treatment could be viewed as maximizing the welfare of society.

The flaw of a goal-oriented ethical theory is its failure to consider the principle of justice.[43] For example, despite the fact that basic health care would be provided to all, a reformed system could cause some persons who might contribute greatly to society to suffer. For example, a person with great potential might be denied a bone marrow transplant if that procedure were not part of the basic health care package.

INTUITIONIST ETHICAL THEORY

An **intuitionist ethical theory** is a system of ethical thinking that balances goals, rights, and duties according to the situation. Philosophers espousing this theory argue that humans innately know good from bad and that, through intuition, duties, goals, and rights can be balanced. However, this approach also has failings. Most significant is the question, "How can one be certain one's intuition is correct?"

For example, some nurses might argue that it is intuitively correct in a basic health care package to supply bone marrow transplants for the young because they have the most potential to contribute to society. Others might argue that it is intuitively correct to withhold expensive technologies from all basic health care packages so that preventive care can be maximized and all persons have the opportunity to live out life to their maximum potential. Here the right of health care, the duty to provide health care, and the goals to be achieved in the distribution of health care resources are balanced. However, who can determine which of these intuitively derived results is the correct choice when health care resources are scarce?

Ethical Principles

Another approach to examining ethical choices is to evaluate them in light of the incorporation of recognized ethical principles such as those defined in Box 3–3. Each is not necessarily applicable in all situations involving ethical choices, nor is the list exhaustive.

Ethical principles in and of themselves do not form a comprehensive ethical theory.[7] Each may be used in resolving ethical dilemmas in relation to discussion of duties, rights, and goals. In ethical dilemmas, these principles can be in conflict with each other.

AUTONOMY

Autonomy is the ethical principle upholding the exercise of personal choice. The principle of autonomy stems from the notion of respect for persons. In turn, respect for persons arises from the unconditional value

Box 3–3. Five Ethical Principles

Autonomy = self-determination
Beneficence = doing good
Nonmaleficence = avoiding harm
Justice = fairness
Fidelity = commitment

placed on persons because they have the capacity to act morally and make rational choices.[7] Because of the capacity for choice, persons ought not be treated as things and used as means to achieve the ends of other individuals. In other words, persons then have the right to make their own decisions free of external control. The singular constraint is that decisions must be made within the limits of morality.

One can view the concept of truth telling, or veracity, as deriving from autonomy because persons must have facts to make life decisions. The principle of autonomy will thus be violated when a health care provider, believing a person will be harmed by knowing the truth, acts parentalistically and withholds information about the person's health status. For example, a nurse who did not tell a requesting client the results of a blood pressure reading would violate that client's autonomy.

The principles of privacy and confidentiality stem from the principle of autonomy. **Privacy** is the right to be free from intrusion into one's personal affairs. For example, an individual is free to choose to disclose or not disclose the nature of an illness, and privacy is invaded when disclosure occurs without permission. Confidentiality is the ethical principle upholding the practice of safeguarding personal information. Clients should be able to rely on the nurse to share health care information only with other health care providers legitimately concerned about the client's health care.

BENEFICENCE

The principle of **beneficence** is the ethical principle of upholding doing good. Sometimes beneficence incorporates avoidance of harm. Doing good, preventing harm, and removing harm are the essence of the nurse's obligation to clients. Doing good will occur when the nurse provides care according to standards. Preventing harm occurs when, for example, the nurse questions a physician's incorrect medication dosage and the order is changed. The nurse might remove harm by stopping the administration of blood that is causing an adverse reaction. In these examples, beneficence does not conflict with autonomy.

Parentalism can be thought of as an exaggerated form of beneficence that achieves good at the expense of autonomy. Parentalism means acting as a parent to do good for a client despite the client's ability to make decisions. For example, the nurse might inform a postoperative client who is in pain that a particular postoperative complication will occur if the client does not walk. The nurse may thus manipulate the person to walk. Here the nurse is using deception by giving a false impression that exercise must take precedence over pain relief. Besides manipulation, coercion—using threats—to obtain a client's cooperation is another parentalistic approach to acting for the client's good. Rational persuasion, in which both nurse and client are regarded as equals, is an ethically acceptable approach to beneficence. For example, you could explain the benefits of walking and the risks of remaining sedentary rather than tell a client that a complication will occur.

NONMALEFICENCE

Literally translated, the principle of **nonmaleficence** means not inflicting harm on a person. For example, the nurse is responsible for not abandoning a client when the nurse disagrees with the client's ethical choice. Some nurses, for example, do not wish to care for persons having abortions. If no other nurse is present to provide care, the nurse must stay with the client.

JUSTICE

Justice is the ethical principle that upholds giving people their due and treating them fairly. Inherent in the term "justice" is the notion of equality. The principle of justice is not easily applied and does not provide specific guidelines by which to measure equality. Are all persons equal for all purposes, or are persons to be regarded primarily as individuals and equal to each other only in some respects?

The problem of distribution of scarce resources always raises questions of justice. Consider the distribution of health care resources. Will not some persons be more deserving than others, despite inequality in personal financial resources, because the talents they have to offer society are greater? Suppose a lottery system were used to allocate scarce beneficial medication for a fatal disease. Consider that in such a system the developer of the medication might go untreated. Would justice be served?

FIDELITY

Fidelity is the ethical principle upholding commitment or the keeping of promises. Nurses, both collectively as a profession and personally as individuals, make commitments as caregivers to provide their services. That commitment encompasses the provision of care according to ethical principles. Nursing care will honor autonomy, do good, avoid harm, and be justly distributed. Nursing will honor truth telling, protect individuals from invasion of their privacy, and keep confidential health care information. In this sense, fidelity is the all-inclusive principle for all professionals.

Keeping such promises poses difficulties. Honoring autonomy will be difficult, for example, when families insist a family member should not know a fatal diagnosis. Doing good, such as providing sufficient guidance about aftercare, can be difficult when a client's hospital stay seems cut short by guidelines dictating length of hospitalization. Avoiding harm may be difficult when the care of two clients seems to call for equal priority, and the nurse has time for only one client. Justice may not seem served when home care can be reimbursed for one person but not for another client with similar needs.

Codes of Ethics

The preamble to the American Nurses' Association (ANA) Code for Nurses with Interpretive Statements notes that nurses make clinical judgments based on

---

Box 3–4. American Nurses' Association Code for Nurses

1. The nurse provides services with respect for human dignity and the uniqueness of the client unrestricted by considerations of social or economic status, personal attributes, or the nature of health problems.
2. The nurse safeguards the client's right to privacy by judiciously protecting information of a confidential nature.
3. The nurse acts to safeguard the client and the public when health care and safety are affected by the incompetent, unethical, or illegal practice of any person.
4. The nurse assumes responsibility and accountability for individual nursing judgments and actions.
5. The nurse maintains competence in nursing.
6. The nurse exercises informed judgment and uses individual competence and qualifications as criteria in seeking consultation, accepting responsibilities, and delegating nursing activities to others.
7. The nurse participates in activities that contribute to the ongoing development of the profession's body of knowledge.
8. The nurse participates in the profession's efforts to implement and improve standards of nursing.
9. The nurse participates in the profession's efforts to establish and maintain conditions of employment conducive to high-quality care.
10. The nurse participates in the profession's effort to protect the public from misinformation and misrepresentation and to maintain the integrity of nursing.
11. The nurse collaborates with members of the health professions and other citizens in promoting community and national efforts to meet the health needs of the public.

Reprinted with permission from *Code for Nurses with Interpretive Statements,* © 1985, American Nurses Association, Washington, D.C.

"consideration of consequences and universal moral principles." [1] The preamble refers to essential ethical principles, and the code provides guidelines with respect to the care of individuals and for accountability to individuals, to the profession, and to society (Box 3–4). The International Council of Nurses Code for Nurses and the Canadian Nurses Association Code of Ethics for Nursing reflect beliefs similar to the ANA Code for Nurses (Box 3–5).

The ANA Code speaks of respect for human dignity without consideration of personal, socioeconomic, or health status characteristics. The code specifically mentions safeguarding privacy by maintaining confidentiality of information. The code promises to safeguard individuals from incompetent, unethical, or illegal practice, thus supporting reporting provisions in nurse practice acts. The code also espouses nurses' responsibility for individual actions. Nurses promise to maintain competence in practice, and the code makes nurses responsible for seeking consultation when needed and know-

ledgeably delegating responsibility for nursing care. The code supports nurses' participation in nursing research, the development of nursing standards, and the efforts of nurses to create conditions of employment conducive to quality nursing care. The code acknowledges responsibility to the public to prevent misinformation and misrepresentation of nursing. The code supports collaborative efforts with other health professionals to meet the health needs of the public.

To the extent that the code prescribes activities for individual nurses, it can be considered reflective of duty-oriented ethical theory because the profession is a generally cohesive group that can agree on standards for action.

Although the code, along with its interpretive statements, is an impressive professional document, it provides only general guidelines and cannot resolve nurses' ethical dilemmas in a particular situation.

For example, when a client with acquired immune deficiency syndrome (AIDS) tells the nurse he will not tell his sexual partner of the diagnosis but will continue to have unprotected sexual relations, is the nurse obligated to keep the information confidential? What are the limits of confidentiality as an ethical concept? The code does not provide those answers.

Another example of a specific dilemma concerns the nurse who regularly handles antineoplastic agents but now wishes to conceive a child, is pregnant, or is breastfeeding. Is that nurse still obligated to care for cancer clients despite known reproductive risks associated with handling antineoplastics? Is it ethical to ask for transfer to other duties at these times?

Ethical Decision Making in Nursing

The study of ethics will not provide certain answers. What the study of ethics will do is provide nurses with a reasoned approach to thinking about ethical dilemmas. For instance, can beneficence as the withholding of information ever be justified over truth telling? How is justice served when two clients have equally compelling claims to nursing care? Does one look to a rights-oriented, duty-oriented, goal-oriented, or intuitionist approach in deciding how to handle an ethical problem?

Ethical decision making in nursing practice requires determining facts, identifying the ethical problem, analyzing options by applying ethical theories and principles, and making choices. Because health care is ideally delivered by a team, many ethical decisions should be team based. That team includes not only nurses and other health providers but also clients and families.

LAW AND ITS SOURCES

Webster's dictionary defines **law** as the "body of rules or principles, prescribed by authority or established by custom, which a state, community, society, or the like

Box 3-5. Canadian Nurses Association Code for Nurses

Clients

Value I: Respect for Needs and Values of Clients

A nurse treats clients with respect for their individual needs and values.

Value II: Respect for Client Choice

Based upon respect for clients and regard for their right to control their own care, nursing care reflects respect for the right of choice held by clients.

Value III: Confidentiality

The nurse holds confidential all information about a client learned in the health care setting.

Value IV: Dignity of Clients

The nurse is guided by consideration for the dignity of clients.

Value V: Competent Nursing Care

The nurse provides competent care to clients.

Nursing Roles and Relationships

Value VI: Nursing Practice, Education, Research and Administration

The nurse maintains trust in nurses and nursing.

Value VII: Cooperation in Health Care

The nurse recognizes the contribution and expertise of colleagues from nursing and other disciplines as essential to excellent health care.

Value VIII: Protecting Clients from Incompetence

The nurse takes steps to ensure that the client receives competent and ethical care.

Value IX: Conditions of Employment

Conditions of employment should contribute in a positive way to client care and the professional satisfaction of nurses.

Value X: Job Action

Job action by nurses is directed toward securing conditions of employment that enable safe and appropriate care for clients and contribute to the professional satisfaction of nurses.

Nursing Ethics and Society

Value XI: Advocacy of the Interests of Clients, the Community and Society

The nurse advocates the interests of clients.

Value XII: Representing Nursing Values and Ethics

The nurse represents the values and ethics of nursing before colleagues and others.

Value XIII: Responsibilities of Professional Nurses' Associations

Professional nurses' organizations are responsible for clarifying, securing and sustaining ethical nursing conduct. The fulfillment of these tasks requires that professional nurses' organizations remain responsive to the rights, needs and legitimate interests of clients and nurses.

Reprinted with permission from Code of Ethics for Nursing, 1991, Canadian Nurses Association, Ottawa, Canada.

recognizes as binding on its members."[39] Law is the force that orders relationships in a society. Nurses' privilege of practicing nursing creates special legal relationships between nurse and client, between nurse and employer, and among nurses and other health care providers. Box 3-6 provides an overview of law and its sources. The principal substantive areas of the law that affect nurses are tort law and contract law. Nursing practice acts are statutory law, and regulations passed by boards of nursing are administrative law.

Constitutional Law

Constitutional law is the principal foundation of American law. The first 10 amendments to the United States Constitution, the Bill of Rights, form the core of individual rights. **Constitutional law** is the body of law defining and limiting government powers and protecting the rights of citizens. Constitutional law develops when persons or groups bring a lawsuit that challenges how the constitution has been applied.

The Constitution guarantees religious freedom, freedom of assembly, freedom of speech, freedom of the press, and freedom from unwarranted intrusion by government into personal choices. The Fifth Amendment states that individuals cannot be deprived of life, liberty, or property without due process of law. The Fourteenth Amendment applies the Fifth Amendment to the individual states. States can expand individual rights in state constitutions. The Canadian Constitution includes the Canadian Charter of Human Rights. The charter is similar to the United States Bill of Rights.[50]

Box 3-6. Overview of the Law

LAW—a body of guidelines governing relationships of individuals in a society arising from what that society decides best permits that society to function—somebody holds power to enforce the law.

Law as It Applies to Citizens

Civil | *Criminal*

(Standard of proof is preponderance of the evidence)

(Standard of proof is clear and convincing evidence)

(Standard of proof beyond a reasonable doubt)

Potential cost to defendant is money damages or (a) doing something he would rather not or (b) not doing something he would like to do

Potential cost to defendant is deprivation of liberty

Law as Balance of Power

Case Law | *Statute* | *Administrative*

(Judiciary) called common law

(Legislature)

(Executive) called regulations

Affected persons can question in court the constitutionality of statutory law and can question congruency of administrative law (regulations) with the intent or scope of the governing statute

Law from a Lawyer's Perspective

Substantive | *Procedural*

Refers to what legal theory is being tested, e.g., negligence or contract law

Refers to the process to be followed in the judicial system as a plaintiff moves forward with a complaint

The Constitution with its Amendments is the underpinning of American law.

Copyright 1993 by Kathleen M. Driscoll, R.N., M.S., J.D. Reprinted by permission.

Case Law

American law evolved from the English tradition of case law **(common law). Case law** is judge-made law. Case law achieves consistency when one judge follows another's reasoning in a subsequent case, so that one case acts as a precedent for another. Leading cases are cases in which the law changes direction.

Individuals cannot go to a court just to find out what the law is. First, there must be a disagreement among persons. The facts must also present a **prima facie case;** that is, the facts must establish the legal elements necessary to a lawsuit. For example, plaintiffs in a malpractice case must indicate that the nurse had a duty of care to a person, that arguably the nurse breached the duty to provide the expected standard of care, and that as a result of the breach the person was harmed.

Statutory Law

Statutory law is law created by state legislatures or the United States Congress. State codes and the United States code are contained in multivolume sets of books.

A bill is a proposed new or revised statute. Proposed laws reflect current societal concerns. For example, in the early 1990s, state and federal initiatives in the legislative arena included proposals for revising the health care system. Nurses, as both citizens and health care professionals, have an opportunity to influence the development of statutory law. Two ways to exert this influence are writing or meeting with state legislators or members of Congress. Nurses can support, oppose, or suggest changes in proposed laws.

The development of statutory law is a lengthy process that includes compromise of the various perspectives of interested parties.

Compromise may be personal or professional. On a personal level, the nurse as citizen desires a cost-efficient and outcome-effective health care system. Legislation to achieve this goal may mean giving up ready personal access to some health care technology. On a professional level, the nurse is interested in a system that will recognize and reward the full potential of nursing's ability to contribute to an effective health care system. Nurses would like to see nurse practitioners become entry points for persons seeking health care, but medicine will be interested in maintaining its power as gatekeeper to the health care system. If nurses wish to become gatekeepers in the system, the interests of both professions will need to be balanced.

How does a bill become a law? Bills need to be passed by both houses at the state and federal level. Conference committees, in which representatives of both houses meet, often negotiate a final bill. That final bill must also take into account the concerns of the executive branch of government, lest a governor or the president veto the bill. Sometimes legislators are aware there are insufficient votes to override a veto, but a bill will be passed simply to make a legislative statement in opposition to the position of the executive branch.

With a few exceptions, Canada's legislative process is similar to that of the United States. For example, legislation with respect to marriage, divorce, and criminal law are the responsibility of the federal Parliament, and the provinces legislate on other matters. At the federal level in Canada, only members of one house, the House of Commons, are elected. The Senate is appointed by the Prime Minister of Canada. Provincial legislatures have only one house. The party receiving the largest number of votes in an election forms the provincial government, and the party with the next largest number of votes becomes the official opposition party.[50]

Administrative Law

In the United States, the agencies of the executive branch of government administer legislation. The Department of Health and Human Services, the Department of Labor, and the Department of Education are examples of federal agencies that administer health care law. At the state level, agencies concerned with health include departments of health, mental health, and licensing boards. Administrative agencies develop regulations to guide the application of statutory law. **Administrative law** consists of rules and regulations of federal or state agencies effective only after a process of review and comment by affected persons or groups. Administrative agencies have staff with the professional expertise to develop regulations.

Administrative agencies must develop regulations that are reasonable; that is, they may not be arbitrary or capricious. Because regulations flow from statutes, they must also be consistent with the intent of the legislature. State and federal agencies finalize regulations only after a review and comment period that follows due process. Due process requires notice of proposed regulations to affected persons and a period of opportunity for comments of support or comments suggesting revisions.

For example, the historically significant Baby Doe regulations reflected input from the American Medical Association, which opposed any federal intervention in treatment decisions. On the other hand, the American Academy of Pediatrics suggested mandatory infant care review committees. The final regulations reflected a compromise position. Infant care review committees were suggested but not mandatory.

Affected persons can challenge regulations in court. The American Hospital Association (AHA), for example, challenged regulations affecting infant care treatment decisions that were proposed under the Rehabilitation Act. The AHA argued the Rehabilitation Act did not reflect statutory authority. The court agreed, saying that Congress did not intend the Rehabilitation Act to apply to these decisions.[10] Court challenges to regula-

tory law exemplify how the executive, legislative, and judicial branches of government can be intertwined.

In Canada, administrative law is defined as statutes that apply to the functioning of administrative agencies. An administrative agency need not be a governmental body. For example, in Canadian provinces, the nursing professional association, not the state board of nursing, regulates nursing practice.

TYPES OF LAW

Civil and Criminal Law

Civil law is the ordering of relationships among persons and groups whose violation results in monetary damages or the obligation to take or refrain from a specific action. Thus, if as a nurse you are found to have breached a duty of care to a person who is harmed by that breach, you will have to pay money to compensate the person for the loss. If you are insured, payment of that judgment will come from the insurance company. If uninsured, your personal assets may be lost.

In civil law, the plaintiff and defendant confront each other. A plaintiff is the person or persons bringing a lawsuit. A defendant is the person or persons against whom a lawsuit is brought.

Criminal law punishes behavior that threatens the integrity of society and may warrant the deprivation of personal liberty. In criminal law, society, in the person of the state or federal prosecuting attorney, takes on the role of plaintiff. If you, as a nurse, physically assault a client or even threaten assault and appear to have the means to carry out that threat, you may be judged to be acting criminally. Unjustifiably restraining a person or threatening to restrain a person can constitute a criminal act.

The law requires varying levels of evidence. In civil law, the jury determines whether the plaintiff or defendant has the preponderance of evidence. In criminal law, the jury must determine the evidence against the defendant and establish guilt beyond a reasonable doubt. The law uses an intermediate level of evidence by which a determination that law has been violated may result in deprivation of a highly private right. This level of evidence is called clear and convincing evidence. Thus, parents cannot be deprived of the right to care for their children when abuse or neglect is suspected without clear and convincing evidence. Clear and convincing evidence of a person's wishes has also been termed necessary to discontinue life-sustaining measures.

Procedural and Substantive Law

Procedural law governs the legal process. Procedural law sets forth the process of developing a case under both civil and criminal law. State and federal codes of civil and criminal procedures provide direction for selection of the proper court, notice of a suit, gathering of evidence before trial, and presentation of evidence at trial.

Procedural law contrasts with **substantive law** in that the latter is the legal theory under which a case is brought (e.g., tort or contract law). Tort law is the substantive law of a negligence or malpractice suit. Contract law is the substantive law of an employee wrongful discharge suit.

Tort Law

Tort law is that area of substantive law that recognizes that individuals, in their relationships with each other, have a general duty to take care to avoid injuring others. For example, a building contractor has a general duty to build a structure that will not collapse and injure persons; a driver has a duty to drive in such a manner that others will not be harmed; and a nurse has a duty to deliver care in such a manner that individuals do not suffer harm. Legal duties of care may be violated both unintentionally and intentionally.

UNINTENTIONAL TORTS—NEGLIGENCE AND MALPRACTICE

Negligence is the unintentional tort of acting or failing to act as an ordinary, reasonable, prudent person with resulting harm to the person to whom the duty of care is owed.

The legal elements of negligence consist of duty, breach of duty, causation, and harm or injury.

The duty of care owed is the standard of care. For professionals, the law defines the **standard of care** as what a reasonable, prudent practitioner with similar education and experience would do or not do in similar circumstances. **Malpractice** is the term for professional negligence. As Figure 3–3 illustrates, you can successfully defend yourself in a lawsuit if you adhere to the expected standards of care for nurses.

Even for professionals, the law uses the term "negligence" when questions are raised about duties that are obvious. For example, you, as a nurse, have a clear obligation to put side rails up on infant's crib. A jury would know this duty without explanation from an expert. On the other hand, a jury would not know that administering potassium to a client who lacked renal function did not meet the expected standard of care. When fulfillment of duties requires the specialized education of a nurse, the term "malpractice" is used. Administering the potassium might result in your being guilty of malpractice. A plaintiff's attorney would use an expert witness to testify to the standard of care.

Applying the Standard of Care. In what other situations might your nursing judgment be called into question? You might need to determine when to restrain a person, what constellation of symptoms constitutes the need to notify the physician, and to whom nursing responsibilities can safely be delegated. Box 3–7 lists sources for establishing the standard of care.

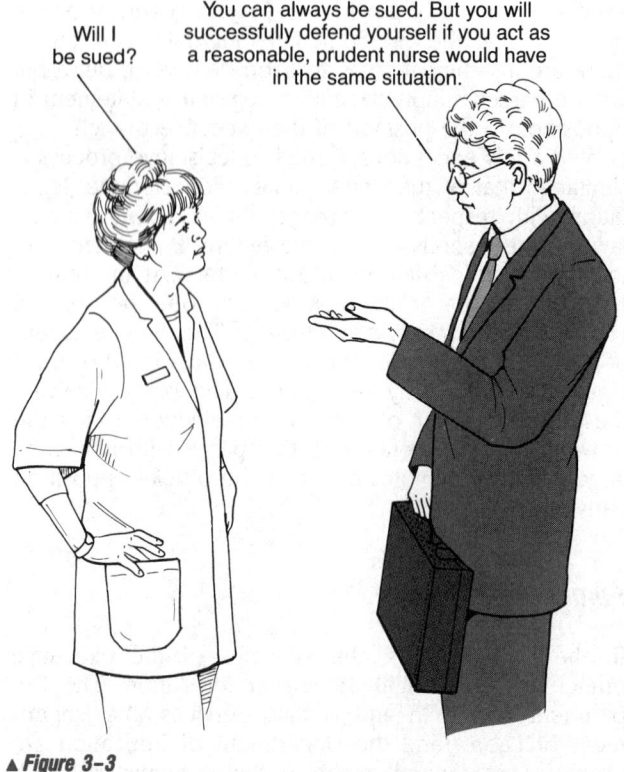

Will I be sued?

You can always be sued. But you will successfully defend yourself if you act as a reasonable, prudent nurse would have in the same situation.

▲ **Figure 3–3**

How to defend yourself successfully in a lawsuit.

Expected Standards of Care. Nursing has a basic body of knowledge for which all nurses are responsible. Thus, any nurse may be expected to provide essential care in areas of medical-surgical, psychiatric, and maternal-child care. Essential care is a minimally safe level of care. Crucial to basic practice is knowing when to seek consultation about care. Just as a family practitioner in medicine should seek consultation when basic treatments do not alleviate a particular set of symptoms, so should the generalist nurse seek consultation when common nursing interventions do not achieve positive outcomes. Experience is also a component of the standard of care, and over time, even the generalist nurse will be expected to draw on a broader

---

Box 3–7. Sources of Nursing Standards of Care

Practice and Educational Program Guidelines of State Boards of Nursing

Joint Commission on Accreditation of Health Care Organizations

American Nurses' Association and state nursing association standards

Specialty nursing organization standards

State and federal laws, regulations, and guidelines

Health care facility policy and procedure

Relevant nursing literature

base for making nursing judgments and applying nursing interventions.

The specialist nurse will have gained expertise in a particular area through both experience and defined education. Formal recognition of specialist expertise can occur through institutional career ladders or professional certification programs.[20] The specialist nurse will be held to a higher standard of care.

Student nurses are held to the minimum standard of care required of the generalist. Thus, it is critical that students not engage in nursing interventions until they have learned those interventions and have been appropriately supervised in their practice.

Several options for action or inaction may be reasonable and prudent in any given set of circumstances. Remember that practice standards change with the development of knowledge in a profession.

A good example is practice regarding use of restraints. In the past, restraint devices were commonly used whenever threats to patient safety were foreseeable. Today, use of alternatives to such devices are encouraged. Competent clients and their families may also elect to waive use of physical restraints.

Health care facilities must have policies and procedures consistent with the currently accepted standard of care. In the past, this standard was generally that of the local community. Ready access to professional literature and opportunities for other types of continuing education both within and outside health care facilities have led courts to adopt national standards of care.[25]

DOCUMENTING THE STANDARD OF CARE

Documentation links professional and legal accountability, so that legal accountability—meeting the standard of care—occurs when professional accountability occurs. Any form of documentation that can demonstrate reasonable and prudent carrying out of the nursing process will suffice for professional accountability.

Check list, narrative, and computer documentation are all appropriate. In any client information system, remember to record time of client encounters, actions taken, evaluation of those actions, and the signature or other notation indicating the name of the nurse who took the actions. For example, if a nurse checks an intravenous (IV) site, the nurse should record time, whether the IV is intact or adverse responses have occurred, actions taken for adverse responses, and the nurse's name.

In any client information system, facts should precede judgments or opinion about client status.

In this example, redness and edema around IV insertion site are facts. IV infiltration is the judgment or opinion based on the facts. The change in IV site to the left forearm is the action taken. IV fluids absorbed on schedule is the evaluation.

Anyone can record in the client medical record, but health care facility policy may permit only licensed personnel to do so. When such a policy exists, information reported by a nursing assistant should indicate the nursing assistant as the source of the information. When nursing judgments must be based on reported data, the nurse should verify that data by personally observing the client.

Nurses often make judgments based on conversations. Just as it is important to document observations that are the basis for nursing actions, so too conversations that lead to nursing actions should be recorded. For example, you may determine in a conversation that a client misunderstands medication times or does not appreciate the nature of an invasive surgical procedure. In the first instance, corrective education can occur. In the second instance, the physician should be called to explain the procedure further. (See Chapter 4 for more information about informed consent.)

Good Samaritan Laws and the Standard of Care. All states and several Canadian provinces have Good Samaritan laws. These laws state that health care providers, including nurses, will be immune from lawsuit for providing assistance at the site of an emergency unless the care provided is grossly negligent.

Willfully or knowingly ignoring obvious needs at the site of an emergency would constitute gross negligence.

For example, suppose you stop at the scene of an accident and fail to stem the flow of blood from a severed artery. That failure would be an example of gross negligence. In effect, Good Samaritan laws ask that care provided be reasonable under the circumstances. Stemming the flow of blood from an artery would be expected in an emergency outside a health care facility; providing IV fluids would not be expected.[40,64]

Health care providers often wonder whether they must stop at the scene of an accident. In most states and all Canadian provinces with Good Samaritan statutes, the health care provider has no legal obligation to assist at the scene of an emergency. In 1989 five states did include a legal duty to rescue in their Good Samaritan statute.[40]

Whether ethics or law motivates you as a nurse to begin care at the scene of an emergency, you have a legal duty to remain at the scene until care can be turned over to emergency units that can safely transport victims to a health care facility.

Lawsuits. What if you are sued? What are the steps in a lawsuit? These are listed in Box 3-8. If you are sued, your attorney will be your ally in your defense. The attorney will provide guidance regarding your appearance, demeanor, and responses to the opposing side's questioning. Remember that a strong plaintiff's case will generally avoid a trial and end in a settlement. A weak plaintiff's case risks a trial. A trial may also occur when the facts or the standard of care is clearly at issue. A

Box 3–8. Steps in a Lawsuit

1. Client believes an injury resulted from a nurse's practice.
2. Client seeks the advice of an attorney.
3. Client's attorney has nurse expert review client's record to provide opinion as to whether the defendant nurse violated the standard of care.
4. If nurse expert's opinion states the standard of care was violated, a lawsuit is begun.
5. Period of discovery begins. Statements are taken from the defendant nurse, any actual witnesses, the nurse expert, other health care providers as necessary, and the client (now the plaintiff). Information is also obtained about health care facility policy and procedure.
6. Trial
7. Judgment
8. Possible appeals

(A settlement may occur any time after a lawsuit is begun.)

---

strong defendant's case may result in motions to dismiss the case.

Professional Liability Coverage. **Liability** is a legal obligation to pay damages, perform or refrain from a specific action, or suffer a criminal penalty. Professional liability insurance shields the nurse's personal assets in the event of a judgment that the nurse has been negligent.

There are two types of liability insurance. Claims-made insurance covers claims brought during the period the policy is in force. A lawsuit brought several years after a negligent act has occurred will not be covered by a claims-made policy if you are uninsured at the time the lawsuit is initiated. Occurrence insurance covers claims if a policy was in force at the time the alleged negligence occurred. The insurance thus protects you whether or not you are still insured when a lawsuit is brought.

Nurses should check to determine whether their insurance is a claims-made or occurrence policy. A nurse carrying a claims-made policy who retires or drops out of the work force should maintain liability insurance by purchasing a tail policy. The tail policy will cover the nurse if a lawsuit is subsequently brought. Nurses working in newborn and pediatric settings need particularly long periods of coverage because, in most states, children injured through negligence can bring actions up to the time they reach the age of majority plus the normal statute of limitations period for negligence in that state. This special exception to negligence statutes of limitation permits the child to seek redress for injury if the parents have not done so earlier.

Health care facilities may tell nurses that it is unnecessary to carry personal professional liability insurance because the health care facility will cover them and the nurse will usually be sued as an employee of the health care facility. However, individuals are also liable for their own actions, and nurses can always be personally sued.

Because personal suit is always a possibility, nurses need individual malpractice insurance.

There are other reasons for carrying personal malpractice insurance. If a judgment is taken against a health care facility because of a nurse's negligence, the health care facility may lawfully seek reimbursement from the nurse through the process of indemnification. Indemnification is the act of protecting someone from loss. In this case, the protected party would be the health care facility or its insurer who would be protected from the nurse's negligence. Another reason for carrying personal malpractice insurance is that nurses can practice independently. Wrong advice given to a neighbor that results in harm may be construed as nursing practice, and the nurse may be sued personally. In that event, the employing facility cannot shield the nurse's assets with the facility's professional liability insurance.

In the United States, members of the ANA can obtain but must pay for coverage through insurance plans sponsored by the association or by private insurers.[34] The Canadian nurse does not pay extra for malpractice insurance. The insurance is a benefit of belonging to the nursing professional association.

Canadian nurses launched their own self-insurance fund when they discovered that 98.2 per cent of nurse malpractice insurance premiums payments represented insurance company profits.[12,53]

The threat of losing malpractice insurance led to the ANA's establishing a claims data base for the purpose of creating a loss history so that malpractice insurance will be appropriately priced.[14]

Practices That Control Lawsuits. Mechanisms for controlling lawsuits and the rising cost of insurance began to evolve in the mid-1970s. Their impetus came from a malpractice crisis that led to risk management and quality-of-care programs as efforts to improve practice. Risk management is the process of identifying areas of risk, estimating and financing loss, preventing and controlling risk.[71] Because it focuses on avoiding financial loss to a health care facility, risk management is clearly economically oriented. Quality programs, on the other hand, focus on the health care provider's ethical, professional, and legal obligation to make efforts to maintain and, more recently, improve the standard of care.[69]

Today health care facilities have designated persons responsible for risk management and quality assurance. Both are required for facilities to be accredited by the Joint Commission on Accreditation of Health Care Organizations. As a nurse, you should regard your facility's offices for both risk management and quality assurance as resources.

Risk Management. Identified areas of risk include not only exposure to malpractice claims but also employee injury and client lost-property claims. The risk manager bases purchase of insurance, facility self-insurance, or a combination of these on an estimation of future risk based on the cost of past claims.

Important strategies for risk prevention are staff education, policy and procedure development, and incident reports. For example, education about the use of new equipment is an effort to reduce risk of harm to persons from its inappropriate use. Development of documentation policy and procedures that ensure that relevant information appears in the medical record can prevent harm resulting from inappropriate care.

Incident reports or variance reports, as incident reports have lately been termed, act both as a source for identifying risk and as a risk prevention measure. Reports can be used as illustrations to educate staff about approaches to avoiding risk. In fact, the reports often seek suggestions from the reporting person as to how the situation might have been avoided. Reports can also be used to identify areas for development of new or refined policy and procedures.

As a nurse, you must realize that incident reports should be written not only when actual harm has occurred to a patient, visitor, or staff member but also when a set of circumstances might have caused harm.

Medication errors are a good example. For example, one nurse may hand another an ampule of the correct medication, leading the administering nurse to believe that all rather than part of the ampule is the correct dosage. The client may not be harmed, but investigation of the occurrence should lead to reinforcement of the safe practice of preparing one's own medications.

Incident reports need not be written only by persons involved in the circumstances. The reports may also be written by persons who discover the circumstances. For example, a nurse on a subsequent shift may discover that an IV fluid has been running at the wrong rate. The nurse who discovers the incorrect rate may write the incident report.

Does short staffing call for an incident report? If not, how can instances of short staffing be handled? First, as a nurse, you need to realize that facilities are staffed on the basis of expected demand for services. When demand exceeds expectations, nurses must first seek back-up assistance. If this help cannot be forthcoming, the nurse's next option is to provide only essential care. You may also want to cut off the admission of additional clients to the unit.

When nurses perceive understaffing of a unit to be chronic, however, each instance must be documented and reported to nursing administration so that administration has an opportunity to remedy the situation. When no response occurs, the nurse has an ethical duty to by-pass regular channels of communication to be sure that upper-level administration has been made aware of the problem. Risk management employees can provide support and direction to the nurse when the nurse believes understaffing situations create unnecessary risks to client safety. The nurse must remember, however, that risk-free situations are impossible. If every nurse cared for only two clients, both might experience cardiac arrest at the same time and

Box 3-9. Measures to Diminish the Risk of a Lawsuit

1. Do an accurate nursing assessment. (Know your client.)
2. Follow up on laboratory reports.
3. Document timely and thoroughly during the course of care (document, document, document).
4. Do not alter the chart. (Avoid even the appearance of negligence.)
5. Read the nurse's notes, the laboratory reports, and the physician's progress notes.
6. Do not promise the impossible to clients.
7. Do not ignore a dissatisfied client. (Maintain communication and exercise courtesy. Make sure you maintain good client relations.)
8. Do not point fingers when something goes wrong. State the facts. (Facts in incident reports should match those in the medical record.)
9. Do not overreach your training and ability. (Stay within the limits of your experience.)
10. Know your institution's policies and procedures.

only one be resuscitated. Box 3–9 lists measures nurses can take to diminish the risk of lawsuits.

Controlling risk is the converse of preventing risk. Controlling risk occurs after an adverse event. When failure to follow the standard of care has resulted in harm, health care facilities, in an effort to ward off a lawsuit, may offer to pay health care bills incurred as a result of that harm. For example, the facility may absorb the cost of surgery to remove a sponge or pay laboratory bills and transportation costs for a person whose digitalis levels must be monitored because of an inadvertent overdose.

Health Care Facility Quality Programs. Quality programs monitor, evaluate, and take action to improve care using preestablished criteria. Criteria may specify professional practice or client outcomes or both. Several types of quality programs are used by both nurses and other health care providers.

Quality-assurance programs look to achieve preset standards of nursing care. For example, notation in the client record might state that the client had been taught and successfully demonstrated the ability to self-administer insulin. Continuous quality-improvement programs focus on improving client outcomes. Outcomes must be measurable. For example, an indicator related to a client outcome might be the number of diabetic clients with their disease in control as determined by blood glucose levels. Once the current number of stable clients is established, actions are taken to increase that number.

Total quality-management programs focus on responding to identified client needs. The focus of these programs is customer satisfaction. In health care facilities, customers include not only clients but also staff and visitors. Efforts to meet staff needs for prompt laboratory results, visitor needs for flexible visiting hours, and client needs for planned periods of rest from therapy are all examples of total quality management.

In current practice, you will find both unit-based and total facility–based quality-assurance (quality improvement, quality management) programs. These programs are important because they ultimately influence standards of care.

INTENTIONAL TORTS

Negligence and malpractice are not intentional acts in the sense that no professional consciously sets out to violate the standard of care to cause harm to another. Under both Canadian and United States law, however, nurses are vulnerable to another set of legal actions under tort law. These are intentional torts.

Because one person cannot enter the thoughts of another, how can a determination be made that an action is intentional? That determination is made by looking at the actions themselves. Actions include both words and conduct. When an action is "substantially certain" to cause an effect, it becomes intentional.[55] Unlike negligence, harm need not occur; the intent to cause harm is enough to establish the tort.

Professional liability insurance does not shield the assets of the nurse sued for an intentional act.

Moreover, a finding for the plaintiff may mean the nurse must pay not only compensatory damages for any harm, which may be minimal, but also punitive damages because of the intentional nature of the act. See Box 3-10 for five intentional torts that a nurse might commit.

Assault and Battery. Assault and battery are torts that may fall under civil or criminal law. **Assault** is the act of threatening when one apparently has the capability of carrying out the threat. A nurse who threatens to do or not do something to or for a client—and who clearly has the capability of carrying out the threat—may be guilty of assault. For example, a nurse who threatens not to take a nursing home resident to the bathroom unless the person finishes a sufficient amount of a meal is committing an assault. **Battery,** on the

other hand, is unwanted touching. For example, surgery carried out without consent, as in the removal of an appendix when only gallbladder removal appeared on the consent form, is battery. Touching to move a competent person—one who is able to make decisions—from bed to chair when the person has refused is also battery.

In nursing practice, a nurse might also have occasion to sue a client for assault and battery. A client who is capable of understanding the consequences of actions but who threatens to harm a nurse or actually does so can be sued by the nurse. If the client is incapable of reasoned actions, however, as may be the case with some psychiatric clients, the nurse's recovery may be limited to workers' compensation.

False Imprisonment. If you restrain a client without making a reasoned judgment as to the need for restraint, the client may bring an action for false imprisonment. **False imprisonment** is the unlawful detention of a person. To demonstrate false imprisonment, the client must merely show that no reasonable means of exiting the environment was available. Thus, the client does not need to be physically restrained. False imprisonment can occur when a person is threatened with detention in a health care environment if the bill is not paid and when persons not mentally ill are confined in mental hospitals.

Defamation. Defamation is intentional use of the spoken or written word to injure the reputation of another. For example, if you as the nurse falsely include on the client record that a person has a history of mental illness, you would be regarded as making a defamatory statement. Because it is written communication intended to injure the reputation of another, your statement would be termed **libel.** Libel is written defamation. If the statement were spoken to someone other than the client, the defamatory oral communication would be termed **slander.**

Defamatory statements may injure the reputation of another but can be defended if they are true. Thus, a nurse who reports an incompetent practitioner to a state board of nursing with intent that is not personal malice but professional accountability will not be guilty of defamation. Neither will an employer who honestly and without malice indicates to a potential employer that a nurse's performance has been poor.

Invasion of Privacy. Invasion of privacy is making public the private affairs of a person without the person's consent. Well-known, public persons have less right to privacy than ordinary individuals. Thus, if the president is found to have cancer, even though he would like that information to remain confidential, the public nature of his position would preclude an action for invasion of privacy should a newspaper learn of and publish the fact. Invasion of privacy differs from defamation because, even though the information is true, an action may still be brought forward.

Charges of invasion of privacy can be avoided by obtaining a client's consent to use a photograph, tape recording of a conversation, or videotape recording of

---

Box 3-10. Five Intentional Torts a Nurse Could Commit

Assault = words or actions that lead a client to perceive a threat of harm.
Battery = unwanted touching.
False imprisonment = unwarrantedly confining a client with no reasonable means of exit available.
Defamation = making a false statement to injure the reputation of a client, visitor, or other health care provider.
Invasion of privacy = making public the private affairs of a person without the person's consent.

the client's actions and conversation. The consent should specify how the photograph, tape recording, or videotape will be used. If, as a nurse, you obtain permission for use of a videotape recording for presentation to facility staff or nursing students, you will need to obtain an additional consent for the videotape recording to be used in a presentation at a national nursing conference.

HANDLING CLIENT AND PROVIDER INFORMATION

Confidentiality Versus Patient Privilege. Confidentiality can best be regarded as an ethical obligation to share health care information about a person only with other persons who need to know the client's health status. As an ethical concept, confidentiality incorporates the notion of respect for persons. **Patient privilege** is the statutory protection and restriction of communication of personal health care-related information. Patient privilege means that information essential to the provision of health care cannot be shared with others unless the patient waives the privilege.

Patient privilege can pose a problem in states with laws regulating driving under the influence when the suspected drunk driver is injured in an accident. Because of injury, health care needs may take precedence over law enforcement authorities' administering of Breathalyzer tests. A physician may then measure the blood alcohol level to determine the person's status for treatment. In a subsequent lawsuit for negligence, the driver can invoke patient privilege to prevent having the blood test introduced as evidence.

A plaintiff in a malpractice case automatically waives any patient privilege with respect to the introduction of the medical record, including blood alcohol levels. For the law to allow otherwise, the health care provider's defense could be compromised.

Because in many states privileged communication applies only to the physician, the nurse may not be in the same position as the physician with respect to patient privilege. A nurse who knows about a blood alcohol level may be required to testify or face a contempt of court charge.

Reporting Laws. For the safety of their citizens, states permit invasion of personal privacy when there is a compelling state interest. The reporting of child abuse, gunshot wounds, and incompetent professional practice are all instances in which invasion of privacy can be justified. Drawing the line between compelling state interest and a simple desire to know, however, can be difficult. Current controversies illustrating this difficulty include mandatory human immunodeficiency virus (HIV) testing of certain classes of persons, voluntary versus mandatory disclosure of HIV status, and disclosure of positive HIV status to potentially affected parties, such as the affected person's spouse.

Human Immunodeficiency Virus Testing. Mandatory HIV testing of health care workers and hospital clients is currently controversial. The risk of transmission of HIV from health care worker to client is small; the risk of transmission from client to health care worker is larger but still regarded as insufficient in extent to warrant the cost of mandatory testing.[5,27]

Many view mandatory disclosure of HIV status as a more effective approach because it appeals to the sense of professional responsibility held by most health care workers. Professional responsibility in many cases, however, conflicts with the HIV-infected professional's economic well-being and is thus a disincentive to voluntary reporting. The recent reluctance of the United States surgeon general to promulgate guidelines for HIV-infected professionals to participate in certain procedures is in part a response to that concern. Instead, many states are suggesting that local panels familiar with the actual functional status of the professional govern practice for these persons.

Mandatory disclosure of HIV-positive status to spouses or sexual partners is difficult to enforce. To disclose without the consent of the affected person is to violate the ethic of confidentiality. Not to disclose when the affected party refuses to do so violates the opposing duty ethic that the health care professional must "do no harm" when clients are put at unwarranted risk because of their ignorance.

Currently, AIDS and AIDS-related complex are reportable conditions in most states, and records of positive HIV test results may be kept in state health department laboratories. Test results may be either anonymous or confidential. In anonymous testing, the client is known only by a number. In confidential testing, client identity is known, but confidentiality is maintained.

Abuse and Neglect of Children and the Elderly. To encourage reporting of child and elder abuse, states provide immunity from civil and criminal prosecution for good-faith reporting. Good-faith reporting means the reporting person had reason to believe child abuse was occurring even if child abuse or neglect is not eventually found.

Gunshot Wounds. Because a gunshot wound may be the result of a felony, mandatory reporting of gunshot wounds is consistent with state laws that require citizens to report felonies. A felony is a crime punishable by 1 year or more in jail.

Contract Law

A **contract** consists of an offer to provide goods or services and an acceptance of the offer by another in return for some sort of consideration, usually monetary payment. In the delivery of health care, individuals contract with health care facilities, health care providers, and insurers. Nurses may contract with employing facilities or, acting as entrepreneurs, offer their services to individuals. If accepted, such offers also result in contracts.

CONSUMER CONTRACTS

Clients, as consumers of care, enter into contracts with health care providers and health care facilities. Providers and facilities offer care. When consumers accept that care, a contract is created. This contractual relationship creates the facility's and the nurse's duty of care, one of the elements that must be established in a lawsuit for negligence or malpractice.

The creation of the contract obligates the health facility or provider to provide care. In turn, the consumer agrees to pay for the care. These are the duties of provider and consumer.

The benefit—or in legal terms, consideration—received by the consumer is treatment for an actual or potential health problem. The consideration for the provider or facility is payment for the service. When individuals enter a health care facility, they sign a form in the admissions office that creates a contract.

An individual entering a provider's office, submitting the insurance card, or indicating how one will pay for services initiates contractual negotiations. The consumer's offer can be refused. For example, many physicians do not currently accept Medicaid or Medicare payments. Thus, a person who has only Medicaid or Medicare as a source of payment would not be able to create a contract with a non-Medicaid or non-Medicare provider.

Individuals entering an emergency department may not be capable of expressing their desire for care. A duty to care for the person is then implied by the person's presence in the department. United States law provides that a person cannot be discharged or transferred to another facility unless it is safe to do so.[23] As an emergency room nurse, you might have to act as an advocate for clients and ensure that this law is not violated.

Insurance companies, Medicare, and Medicaid are called third-party payors. They are neither the giver nor the receiver of health care but have a duty to both giver and receiver to pay for all or a portion of the care. The extent of their obligation is dictated by the terms of the insurance contract or, in the case of Medicare and Medicaid, the legislation and rules governing payment.

NURSE-EMPLOYER CONTRACTS

Legal aspects of the nurse-employer relationship are governed by a number of laws, some of which are listed in Box 3–11.

Type of Employment

At-Will Employment. At-will employment refers to any employment that the employer can terminate at any time with or without cause. Because most staff

nurses work as employees of nonunionized health care facilities, they are at-will employees. Incompetence, insubordination, and abuse of clients are reasons for a nurse to lose a job with cause. An administrative decision to close a unit would be reason for termination of employment without cause.

Personal Contract Employment. Nurse administrators may have an employment contract that specifies employment for a period of time. Although their compensation levels are higher, these nurses run the risk that the contract for personal services will not be renewed when the contract terminates.

Union Contract Coverage. Nurses working in unionized settings have a formal grievance process that permits an opportunity to challenge any negative action, such as a reprimand, suspension, or dismissal from employment, taken against the employee. Without a union contract, the nurse may have access to a grievance process but only if the employer so chooses.

Union contracts may provide some measure of, but not total, job security. For example, the union contract may provide that nurses first laid off are those first called back or that nurses on a unit about to be closed must be offered the opportunity to retrain in an area in which staffing needs remain.

Most collective bargaining agreements also give nurses rights to participate in defining how they will carry out their professional responsibilities. Thus, under union contract terms, staff nurses will have opportunities to participate on committees, such as quality-improvement and policy and procedure committees, that deliberate aspects of care delivery.

In the United States, state nurses associations, rather than trade service unions, are more likely to negotiate for staff nurse participation in setting practice standards.[49] A 1987 AHA report and a 1988 study show that more than 60 per cent of contracts were negotiated by state nurses associations and 26 per cent were negotiated by trade service unions. A recent United States Supreme Court decision preserves nursing's right to bargain as a distinct unit rather than be incorporated in a unit with other health care providers. In 1987 the AHA reported that 14.8 per cent of nurses were working under union contracts. Many Canadian nurses are also unionized.

Civil Service Employment. Nurses working in civil service have, by far, the greatest measure of job security. Termination for cause requires a due process hearing and includes rights of appeal to the courts.

Unemployment Compensation

Unemployment compensation laws reflect social policy that individuals receive financial support while they search for work.

Compensation generally acts as a financial cushion when economic downturns in an industry trigger loss of a job.

Box 3–11. Laws That Affect the Nurse as Employee

Labor laws	Workers' compensation
Civil service laws	Civil rights laws
Unemployment compensation	Worker safety laws

Nurses whose employment is terminated without cause may receive unemployment compensation. Nurses dismissed for cause cannot collect unemployment compensation. Nurses may challenge a denied claim for unemployment compensation in an agency administrative hearing and ultimately in court.

Workers' Compensation. The workers' compensation law ensures that nurses suffering work-related injuries or illnesses will have both medical benefits and compensation for permanent partial and total disability and temporary partial and total disability. The system is a substitute for the tort system of compensation. Under the tort system, workers trade off the certainty of the lower level of compensation offered through workers' compensation for the uncertain, although potentially larger, recovery available through the tort system. Employers' workers' compensation rates are based on the number of claims filed by employees. This rate setting represents policy supporting workplace safety.

For workers' compensation to apply, injury must occur in the course of employment.

Thus, a nurse who shops at a mall during lunch hour and is injured in an automobile accident leaving the parking lot would probably not be recognized as injured in the course of employment. The same nurse would, however, receive compensation if being in the mall parking lot were part of a job that required accompanying a group of residents from the retirement home where the nurse was employed.

To receive compensation, nurses need to be conscientious about reporting injuries such as needle sticks, so that they can be tested for HIV at the time of injury. Later conversion to HIV-positive status can then be traced to the work injury. Back injuries are the most common work-related injury for nurses and should be similarly reported.

Civil Rights Laws. Since 1964, Title VII of the Civil Rights Act has provided for equal employment opportunity on the basis of ethnicity, race, and gender.[13] The Pregnancy Discrimination Act modified Title VII to extend that same opportunity to pregnant women.[52] Recent key case law has emphasized equal employment opportunity. In the case *United Automobile Workers v. This case,* the United States Supreme Court ruled that women could not be excluded from work environments where they were exposed to lead on the basis of potential hazard to the health of a fetus.[72] The Court found a company policy clearly discriminatory because it did not extend to men. This extension did not occur despite evidence that the reproductive systems of men were also affected by exposure to lead.

This case can be viewed in two ways. Some would say that the ruling bodes ill for children because it emphasizes the rights of the mother over the health of the fetus. Others say it will encourage industry to take steps to increase levels of protection for all workers by enforcing the use of protective measures. Enforcement of protective measures should alleviate industry concern that workers will sue if a child can be proven

damaged by workplace exposure to toxic substances. To date, that situation has not arisen, but it is precisely that circumstance that Johnson Controls sought to avoid with its discriminatory policy.[70]

The Rehabilitation Act of 1973 placed affirmative obligations to employ the disabled on programs receiving federal funding.[56] Recent law, the American with Disabilities Act of 1990, extends that obligation to almost all employers.[2] The act permanently excludes only employers with 15 or fewer employees. The social policy underlying the new law is employment of the disabled to reduce dependence on public monies for health care and other welfare programs. The law assures the disabled nurse of accommodation to disability in the workplace.[48]

Worker Safety Standards. The federal Occupational Safety and Health Administration (OSHA) concerns itself with worker safety in private industry. For this reason, it applies to most of the health care industry, with the exception of public employers. Some states apply OSHA and their own workplace standards to public employment settings as well.

OSHA addresses worker safety in three ways. First, OSHA issues guidelines on areas of concern. Guidelines in and of themselves are not legally enforceable. OSHA may choose to enforce those guidelines under its general duty clause, but it can do so only when a hazard is common knowledge in the industry. Second, OSHA can issue emergency temporary standards if a substance poses a "grave danger" to health. Third, OSHA can issue a full-blown standard. The second and third approaches are enforceable as administrative law.[73]

Two areas of OSHA concern are of particular importance to nurses. These are the guidelines on handling cytotoxic agents and, more recently, the OSHA Blood-Borne Pathogen Standard (BBPS). As evidence of health hazards related to handling cytotoxic drugs has increased, OSHA has enforced its guidelines under the general duty clause. More recently, OSHA has promulgated the BBPS.[9] The standard covers all workers with exposure to blood or other potentially infectious material and obviously applies to nurses.

Under the standard, health care facilities must determine exposures, have an exposure control plan, and develop a procedure for evaluating exposure incidents. Nurses and other health care providers must have orientation and training to the standard. The standard includes universal precautions and requires the facility to offer free hepatitis B vaccinations. The standard also covers management of waste, contaminated laundry, and housekeeping requirements.[3,4]

Licensure Laws

Licensure is the statutory-based privilege to practice a profession intended to protect the public from harm as well as establish an exclusive practice area for that profession. The movement for licensure of nurses had its origins in the late 19th century. Nurses who campaigned for licensure believed that graduates of various programs should pass the same examination as a means of ensuring the quality of their educational programs.[11]

TYPES OF LICENSURE LAWS

Permissive Licensure. The term "registered nurse" originated during the period from 1903 to 1938. Persons completing educational programs and a recognized test could be registered with the state.

Registration statutes were known as permissive licensure laws. Persons could still practice nursing without being registered but could not call themselves registered nurses.

Mandatory Licensure. Mandatory licensure began in 1938 with passage of New York State's law. Moving from permissive to mandatory licensure required that nursing be defined so that persons practicing unlawfully could be identified. The development of practical or vocational nursing as a second level of nursing practice was the impetus for mandatory licensure. States differentiated these levels of nursing practice by stating registered nurses used "substantial specialized judgment and skill," whereas practical nurses did not require the "substantial specialized" level of knowledge, skill, and judgment. In 1955 an ANA Model Practice Act included a disclaimer that the practice of nursing was not the practice of medicine. The disclaimer read that nursing did not include "any acts of diagnosis or prescription of therapeutic or corrective measures." The quoted phrase is the definition of practice commonly used in medical practice acts.[31]

Current and Evolving Concerns About Nursing Licensure. Because of the changing nature of health care delivery during the 1950s, 1960s, and 1970s, the disclaimer quickly became outdated. Nurses began making what had previously been called medical judgments in both intensive care and primary care nursing. An early example was the coronary care nurse who learned to diagnose arrhythmias. In primary care, nurse practitioners diagnosed and managed common health problems. By 1976 another model act did not include the disclaimer. Because the disclaimer appeared in many state practice acts, however, and because licensure is an attempt to differentiate one profession from another, concerns continued that nurses would be charged with practicing medicine without a license.

Nurse practice act or regulatory change in the 1970s and 1980s offered two ways to attempt to alleviate the concern that nurses might be charged with the unlicensed practicing of medicine. The first route was to change definitions of nursing practice so that they incorporated what had come to be known as advanced practice roles in nursing. The second route was to recognize separately advanced practice as another level of practice. The second approach could be accomplished by either statutory or regulatory change.

Remember that licensing laws are intended to protect the public, but they also carve out practice territory.

Although nurses think of their practice as distinct from medicine—and much of nursing practice can be identified as such—there always remains an area of overlap with medical practice that is legally useful to recognize in order to ward off unnecessary lawsuits. Both the general definition and the specific recognition of advanced practice afford this protection for nurses. At the same time, they protect the interests of individuals in obtaining health care along a spectrum, without gaps created by professional territorial disputes.

A key 1983 decision in Missouri supported practice expansion under a broad definition.[30] Specific recognition of advanced practice within licensure laws, however, has the disadvantage of creating potential territorial practice disputes within the profession of nursing itself. Permitting use of advanced practice titles like nurse practitioner only after the nurse passes a certification examination offers a solution that avoids potential territorial turf wars within nursing.

PRACTICE ACT PROVISIONS COMMON TO STATES

The United States Constitution does not empower the federal government to license occupations. Nurse practice acts therefore do vary somewhat, and nurses moving from state to state must obtain licenses in and familiarize themselves with the nurse practice act of each new state. Although definitions of practice may differ from state to state, some features of practice acts are common to most states (Box 3–12).

Practice acts empower state nursing boards to guide education and practice through the development of state regulations. Thus, a state may require specific educational preparation for nursing faculty or curriculum content. Nursing boards give approval for nursing programs. They do not accredit programs. Accreditation is a function of the nursing profession carried out by the National League for Nursing.

By regulation, a state may also more specifically define the scope of a level of practice. One example is the extent of responsibility a licensed practical nurse may assume for IV fluid administration.

State statutes outline violations of the practice act. Practicing without a license is always a violation of the nurse practice act. Common practice act provisions that will subject a licensed nurse to disciplinary action

---

Box 3–12. Some Provisions of Nurse Practice Acts Common to Many States

Definitions of registered nursing and licensed practical nursing or vocational nursing
Powers of the state board
Provisions for punishing practicing without a license
Violations of the practice act that may lead to discipline of license holders
Due process rights of the nurse who is alleged to have violated disciplinary provisions of the practice act
Provision for peer assistance programs

include (1) practicing incompetently, (2) violating client safety, (3) having a felony conviction, (4) committing a misdemeanor in the course of practice, and (5) abusing drugs to the extent that practice is impaired.

With acknowledgment of the widespread extent of substance abuse among health care professionals, many state practice acts now contain provisions that provide suspension of disciplinary actions for substance-abusing (impaired) nurses. The suspension of action is contingent on their ongoing compliance with a drug rehabilitation program that is approved and monitored by peer assistance programs of state nursing associations.

Peer assistance programs use volunteer state nursing association members to develop, with the impaired nurse, a contract of compliance with a treatment and monitoring program.

The nurse who successfully complies with the program — determined by random drug tests — returns to the practice setting. The peer assistance volunteer reports for disciplinary action nurses who violate the terms of the contract to the state nursing board.

Peer assistance programs result in an exception to the mandatory reporting of practice act violations by certain persons or groups, including employers and state nursing associations. Provisions for mandatory reporting of practice act violations, such as child abuse reporting laws, include the provision that reports made in good faith are immune from civil and criminal liability.

TYPES OF STATE DISCIPLINARY ACTIONS

Nurses who violate state practice acts are generally subject to three categories of disciplinary action. The first is a reprimand and may consist simply of a letter admonishing the nurse to cease the activity that has called the license into question. The second level of discipline is suspension of the license to practice. The third level of discipline is revocation of the license to practice.

The nurse accused of violating the practice act may challenge that accusation. Practice acts provide that the nurse have an administrative hearing to defend himself or herself against the accusation.

The hearing may be conducted by a hearing officer, a member or members of the state board who act as hearing officers, or the full state board. Findings in the case will be reported to the full state board for action against the nurse's license or dismissal of the charges. If action is taken against a license, the nurse may then appeal the action in a court of law. This right of judicial appeal recognizes the importance to the nurse of the privilege of licensure.

Licensure to practice nursing is not a right but a societal privilege. That privilege is secure only as long as the nurse demonstrates competence and moral integrity.

CANADIAN LICENSURE

In Canada, licensure power belongs to the provinces, and the provincial nursing associations administer the licensing laws. Mandatory licensure has only recently been achieved in the province of British Columbia.[28] Advanced practice has recently been an issue in both British Columbia and Ontario with respect to nurse-midwifery.[45]

WHAT IS GOOD?

What is good for your client? What is good from an ethical perspective? What is good from a legal perspective? Remember that the discipline of ethics never ceases to explore what "ought to be done" to achieve good in your professional relationships. Remember that law is the current and ever-evolving embodiment of a society's definition of "good" ordering of human relationships. Studies of law and ethics are important building blocks in the foundation of your professional nursing practice.

Summary

- Law and ethics are intertwined.
- Ethics is a discipline that seeks to formulate and systematically justify responses to moral dilemmas.
- Ethical theories are based on duties, rights, goals, and intuition.
- The five main ethical principles include the concepts of autonomy, beneficence, nonmaleficence, justice, and fidelity.
- Codes of ethics for nurses provide broad guidelines but not clear resolutions of ethical dilemmas.
- Ethical decision making in nursing practice requires determining facts, identifying the ethical problem, analyzing options by applying ethical theories and principles, and making choices.
- Law should be thought of as the force that orders relationships in a society. Law reflects the primary ethical perspective of a society.
- Sources of law are constitutions, legal cases, statutes, and regulations.
- Types of law include civil and criminal law and procedural and substantive law.
- Practice standards change with the development of knowledge in a profession.
- Practices that discourage lawsuits include risk management and health care facility quality programs.
- Intentional torts that nurses should be aware of include assault, battery, false imprisonment, defamation, and invasion of privacy.
- Both clients and nurses contract with health care facilities. Clients contract for the provision of medical and nursing care. Nurses contract with health care facilities as employees. Most nurses are at-will employees and work in settings without union contracts.
- Licensure laws protect the public through the disci-

plinary provisions of state nurse practice acts. Licensure laws also define nurses' scope of practice.

▶ Although specific definitions for advanced practice may reduce the risk of illegal overlap of nursing with medical practice, they can result in territorial practice disputes within the profession of nursing.

▶ A number of provisions of nurse practice acts are common among states. These provisions include the power of state boards to regulate practice, approve nursing education programs, and discipline license holders. Most state boards of nursing support peer assistance programs that suspend disciplinary actions against substance-abusing nurses if they successfully participate in a rehabilitation program.

▶ Law is the current and ever-evolving embodiment of a society's definition of "good" ordering of human relationships.

Bibliography

1. American Nurses Association. (1985). *Code for nurses with interpretive statements*. Kansas City, MO: American Nurses Association.
2. Americans with Disabilities Act, Pub. L. No. 101-336, 104 Stat 327 (July 26, 1990).
3. Barlow, R., & Handelman, E. (1992). OSHA's final bloodborne pathogen standard: part I. *AAOHN Journal*, 40, 502–567.
4. Barlow, R., & Handelman, E. (1992). OSHA's final bloodborne pathogen standard: part II. *AAOHN Journal*, 41, 8–15.
5. Barnes, M., Rango, N., Burke, G.R., & Chiarello, L. (1990). The HIV infected health care professional: employment policies and public health. *Law, Medicine & Health Care*, 18, 311–330.
6. Batey, M.V., & Holland, J.M. (1983). Impact on structural autonomy accorded through state regulatory policies on nurses' prescribing practices. *Image*, 15, 84–89.
7. Beauchamp, T.L., & Walter, L. (1982). *Contemporary issues in bioethics* (2nd ed.). Belmont, CA: Wadsworth.
8. Benjamin, M., & Curtis, J. (1992). *Ethics in nursing* (3rd ed.). New York: Oxford University Press.
9. Bloodborne Pathogen Standard, 29 C.F.R., S1910.1030 (1992).
10. Bowen v. American Hospital Association, 106 S. Ct. 2101 (1986).
11. Bullough, B. (1980). *The law and the expanding nurse role* (2nd ed.). New York: Appleton-Century-Crofts.
12. Business of nursing: professional liability protection: created by nurses for nurses. (1990, May). *The Registered Nurse*, p. 27.
13. Civil Rights Act, 28 U.S.C. S 1971, 1975a–1975d, 2000a–2000b-6, 78 Stat 241 (1964).
14. Claims data base. (1990, April). *The American Nurse*, p. 22.
15. Cushing, M. (1986). How courts look at nurse practice acts. *American Journal of Nursing*, 86, 131–132.
16. Cushing, M. (1987). When the courts define nursing: what it is, what it does. *American Journal of Nursing*, 87, 773–774.
17. Cushing, M. (1988). The legal side: dealing with details. *American Journal of Nursing*, 88, 955–957.
18. Davis, A.J., & Aroskar, M.A. (1983). *Ethical dilemmas and nursing practice* (2nd ed.). Norwalk, CT: Appleton-Century-Crofts.
19. Definitions adopted for standards, guidelines. (1991, March). *The American Nurse*, p. 11.
20. delBueno, D. (1988). The promise and reality of certification. *Image*, 20, 208–211.
21. Dick, D., Harris, B., Lehman, A., & Savage, R. (1986). Getting into the act: a Canadian nurse's experience. *International Nursing Review*, 33, 165–170.
22. Donabedian, A. (1966). Evaluating the quality of medical care. *Milbank Memorial Fund Quarterly*, 44, 166–203.
23. Emergency Medical and Active Labor Treatment Act, COBRA, Pub. L. No. 99-272, S 9121, 42 U.S.C.A. S 1395dd (1986).
24. Feutz, S.A. (1988). Legal insights: nursing work assignments: rights and responsibilities. *Journal of Nursing Administration*, 18(4), 9–11.
25. Gaskin v. Goldwasser, 166 Ill. App. 3d 996, 117 Ill. Dec. 734, 520 N.E.2d 1085 (Ill. App. 45th Dist., 1988).
26. Gillman, S.L., & Hirsch, D.L. (1991). Civil rights for handicapped workers. *The Brief*, 20(4), 16–21, 43.
27. Gostin, L. (1990). The HIV infected health care professional: public policy, discrimination and patient safety. *Law, Medicine & Health Care*, 18, 303–310.
28. Government approves changes to nurses act: new legislation requires mandatory registration of all B.C. nurses. (1988, July-August). *RNABC News*, pp. 6–8.
29. Greenlaw, J. (1981). Understaffing: living with the reality. *Law, Medicine & Health Care*, 9(5), 23–24, 33.
30. Greenlaw, J. (1984). Commentary: *Sermchief v. Gonzales* and the debate over advanced practice legislation. *Law, Medicine & Health Care*, 12(1), 30–31, 36.
31. Greenlaw, J. (1985). Nursing law and ethics: definition and regulation of nursing practice: an historical survey. *Law, Medicine & Health Care*, 13, 117–121.
32. Heath, S.W., & McArthur, J. (1991). Risk management: reducing the incidence of medication errors. *The Provider*, 16(3), 29–32.
33. Holden, L.M. (1989). Quality, standards, and criteria: a physician and nurse perspective. *Journal of Nursing Quality Assurance*, 3(2), 27–33.
34. Insurance crisis eases for nurse practitioners; experts foresee "no problem" for staff nurses. (1987). *American Journal of Nursing*, 87, 1503–1504, 1512–1514.
35. Kane, R., & Kane, R.L. (1988). Long term care: variations on a quality assurance theme. *Inquiry*, 25, 132–146.
36. Kraus, G.P. (1986). *Health care risk management*. Owings Mills, MD: National Health Publishing.
37. Kuyper, A. (1991). Patient counseling by pharmacy personnel: a risk management perspective. *The Provider*, 16(3), 32–35.
38. Legal services. (1988, November–December). *RNABC News*, p. 9.
39. *The living Webster: Encyclopedic dictionary of the English language*. (1975). Chicago: English Language Institute of America.
40. Maher, V.F. (1989). Your legal guide to safe nursing practice. *Nursing '89*, 19(11), 34–41.
41. McCarty, P. (1991, September). Worker safety must be priority. *The American Nurse*, p. 26.
42. Mehlman, M.J. (1990). Assuring the quality of medical care: the impact of outcome measurement and practice standards. *Law, Medicine & Health Care*, 18, 368–384.
43. Munson, R. (1983). *Intervention and reflection: Basic issues in medical ethics* (2nd ed.). Belmont, CA: Wadsworth.
44. Northrop, C.E. (1986). Legal outlook: unprofessional conduct and licensure revocation. *Nursing Outlook*, 34, 48.
45. Nurse midwifery: the first step. (1988, March–April). *RNABC News*, pp. 10–13.
46. Ohio Nurses Association v. Ohio Board of Nursing, 44 Ohio St. 3rd (1989).
47. Smith, M.A. (ed.). *The Oxford dictionary of quotations* (2nd ed.). (1955). London: Oxford University Press.
48. Parmet, W.E. (1990). Discrimination and disability: the challenges of the ADA. *Law, Medicine & Health Care*, 18, 331–344.
49. Pettengill, M.M. (1990). Collective bargaining: impact on nursing. In Chaska, N.L. (ed.). *The nursing profession: Turning points* (pp. 454–463). St. Louis: C.V. Mosby.
50. Philpot, M. (1985). *Legal liability & the nursing process*. Toronto, Ontario, Canada: W.B. Saunders.
51. A political legacy. (1987, September–October). *RNABC News*, pp. 28–30.
52. Pregnancy Discrimination Act, 42 U.S.C. S2000 e(K), 92 Stat 2076 (1978).
53. Professional liability: a successful year of self-protection for Canadian nurses. (1989). *The Canadian Nurse*, 85(5), 26–29.
54. The professional responsibility clause: a new tool for the professional nurse. (1989, September–October). *RNABC News*, pp. 19–20.
55. Prosser, W.L. (1971). *Handbook of the law of torts*. St. Paul, MN: West Publishing.
56. Rehabilitation Act, 29 U.S.C., S701–709, 720–724, 730–732, 740, 741, 750, 760–764, 770–776, 87 Stat 355 (1973).
57. Rozovsky, L.E., & Rozovsky, F.A. (1986). Case comment: *Pike v. Peace Arch District Hospital*. *Canadian Critical Care Nursing Journal*, 3(2), 18–20.

58. Rozovsky, L.E., & Rozovsky, F.A. (1986). Nurses under legal attack. *Canadian Operating Room Nursing Journal,* 4(4), 11–12.

59. Rozovsky, L.E., & Rozovsky, F.A. (1987). Critical care, AIDS and the law. *Canadian Critical Care Nursing Journal,* 4(2), 16–17.

60. Rozovsky, L.E., & Rozovsky, F.A. (1987). Dividing the responsible pie. *Canadian Critical Care Nursing Journal,* 4(3), 16–17.

61. Rozovsky, L.E., & Rozovsky, F.A. (1987). The operating room nurse, AIDS and the law. *Canadian Operating Room Nursing Journal,* 5(2), 31, 33–34.

62. Rozovsky, L.E., & Rozovsky, F.A. (1988). Dismissing an employee without the legal hassles. *Canadian Operating Room Nursing Journal,* 6(6), 12–13.

63. Rozovsky, L.E., & Rozovsky, F.A. (1988). Incident reports and the law. *Canadian Critical Care Nursing Journal,* 5(4), 20–21.

64. Rozovsky, L.E., & Rozovsky, F.A. (1989). The nurse as "Good Samaritan." *Canadian Operating Room Nursing Journal,* 7(3), 20–21.

65. Rozovsky, L.E., & Rozovsky, F.A. (1990). Legal implications of high tech surgery. *Canadian Operating Room Nursing Journal,* 8(2–3), 15–16.

66. Selby, T. (1991, November–December). RN copes with HIV infection: she was infected while providing emergency care. *The American Nurse,* pp. 1, 39.

67. Sermchief v. Gonzales, 660 S.W.2d 683 (Mo. banc, 1983).

68. Shaw, G.J., & Bransford, W.L. (1991). From disabled to enabled: new law extends rights of handicapped in employment. *American Bar Association Journal,* 77(2), 70, 72.

69. Springhouse Corp. (1992). *Nurse's handbook of law and ethics.* Springhouse, PA: Springhouse Corp.

70. Stewart, D.O. (1991). Supreme court report: unleaded. *American Bar Association Journal,* 77(6), 38–40.

71. Tan, M.W., & McDonough, W.J. (1990). Risk management in psychiatry. *Psychiatric Clinics of North America,* 13(1), 135–147.

72. U.A.W. v. Johnson Controls, Inc., 111 S.Ct.1196, 113 L.Ed. 2d 158 (1991).

73. U.S. Congress, Office of Technology Assessment. (1985). *Reproductive health hazards in the workplace* (OTA-BA-266). Washington, DC: U.S. Government Printing Office.

74. Waithe, M.E., & Ozar, D.T. (1990). The ethics of teaching ethics. *Hastings Center Report,* 20(4), 17–21.

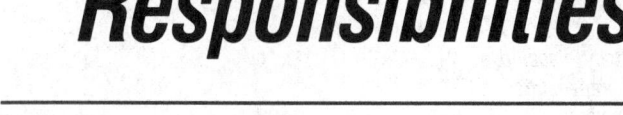

▼ Consumer Rights and Health Care Responsibilities

Chapter

4

▼ *Liberty means responsibility. That is why most people dread it.*

▼ **George Bernard Shaw**

▼

▼

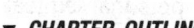

▼ CHAPTER OUTLINE

THE NATURE OF RIGHTS AND
   RESPONSIBILITIES
STATUTORY AND PROFESSIONAL
   STATEMENTS OF HEALTH CARE
   CONSUMER RIGHTS
CONSUMER RIGHTS, HEALTH CARE
   PROVIDER RESPONSIBILITIES, AND
   PERSONAL CHOICE
   Informed Consent
   Forgoing Life-Sustaining Measures
   Reproductive Rights

CONSUMER RIGHTS AND HEALTH CARE
   PROVIDER RESPONSIBILITIES IN
   HEALTH CARE FACILITIES
   Long-Term Care Facilities
   Facilities for the Mentally Ill and
      Developmentally Disabled
CONSUMER RIGHTS, HEALTH CARE
   PROVIDER RESPONSIBILITIES, AND
   HEALTH CARE RESOURCES
   Organ Transplantation
   Access to Health Care

▼ KEY TERMS

Active involuntary
   euthanasia
Active voluntary
   euthanasia
Advance directive
Assent
Best interests
Certification
Durable power of attorney
   for health care

Earned right
Ethical right
Fundamental right
Informed consent
Legal guardian
Legal right
Licensure
Living will
Moral right

Passive voluntary
   euthanasia
Presumed consent
Required request
Responsibility
Right
Routine inquiry
Surrogate

What are the individual rights of health care consumers? Do some consumers of health care have more rights than others? If so, what characteristics make these consumers different? Does the facility providing health care affect the rights of the consumer? Is health care a right?

This chapter examines health care consumer rights and the corresponding responsibilities of nurses and other health care providers. Fundamental to an appreciation of the content of this chapter is an appreciation of the nature of rights. Thus, the chapter first discusses rights and the historical origins of the consumer rights movement.

The concept of personal choice underpins the first section of the chapter. Rights focused on are informed consent to treatment and research, forgoing life-sustaining measures, and reproductive rights. In relation to personal choice, the chapter emphasizes distinctions between adults and minors and between adults and other persons whose decision-making capability may be impaired. The chapter next discusses rights of consumers in long-term care and facilities for the mentally ill and developmentally disabled. The focus then moves to a discussion of health care resources. Here the text examines legal and ethical concerns in relation to organ transplants. Next the chapter reviews concerns about access to health care.

The nurse of the future cannot practice in ignorance of individual rights. Neither can the nurse ignore health care professional and health care facility responsibility to respect rights. Problems of access to health care resources fall within the nurse's concern. Indeed, the nurse must assume professional responsibility for acting as an advocate for both individual and societal rights to effective and available health care.

All the rights discussed in this chapter have some basis in law. Because law represents a society's choices about what achieves good, these legal rights are also moral and ethical rights. As moral rights, they represent the ethical customs of American and Canadian societies. Because the law of both societies has it roots in rights, they represent ethical rights based in a rights-oriented ethical framework (see Chapter 3).

Although each society acknowledges certain rights in its laws, all members of each society may not support those rights. These differences stem from the value system and moral perspective of individuals and families, from cultural or religious perspectives, and from the ethical system of the individual contrasting with that of society. A clear example is the moral division over a woman's right to terminate a pregnancy. In America, this is a societal legal right justified by prevailing moral-ethical perspective. For many health care consumers, however, the right may be a legal right but is not a moral right justifiable by their personal ethical perspective.

THE NATURE OF RIGHTS AND RESPONSIBILITIES

Similar to physics — in which every action has a reaction — in law and ethics the right of one person or group creates a responsibility for another person or group. Here the rights of health care consumers create responsibilities for health care providers, including nurses.

A **right** is a claim one person has to a responsibility or duty on the part of another person. Rights and responsibilities can be both legal and moral. A **legal right** is a claim one person has to a responsibility or duty on the part of another person that is enforceable by law. A **moral right** is a claim one person has to a duty or responsibility on the part of another person that is more likely to be honored when both persons base their actions in the same ethical theory or system. Moral rights consistent with a society's laws are legally enforceable. You can think of an **ethical right** as a right based in a particular ethical framework. A **responsibility** is a duty or obligation of one person with respect to another person.

Rights can also be regarded as both fundamental and earned rights. A **fundamental right** is a basic right shared by all human beings; for example, rights to food, clothing, and shelter. An **earned right** is a right that stems from the performance of certain activities. In United States society, a history of employment is the key that unlocks the federal government's responsibility to provide health care benefits for the elderly under Medicare. Canada, on the other hand, provides universal health care without any prerequisites.

STATUTORY AND PROFESSIONAL STATEMENTS OF HEALTH CARE CONSUMER RIGHTS

The consumer rights movement had its historic roots in the ground swell of rights activities that occurred in the 1960s. The legacy of that decade included landmark civil rights legislation and health care rights legislation for both the poor—Medicaid—and the elderly—Medicare. The rights momentum continued through the 1970s. Later, federal legislation provided individuals with legal redress for age discrimination in hiring[1] and supported both modification of public areas and assurances from public employers and educational institutions that handicapped persons would not suffer discrimination. The Occupational Safety and Health Act (1970)[59] legislated a safe workplace. In the late 1980s, the rights of long-term care residents were recognized under the Omnibus Budget Reconciliation Act (OBRA).[65]

State legislation also frequently identifies consumer rights. These include rights as a research subject,[58] as a consumer of mental health services,[62] and as a resident in long-term care settings.[61]

In addition to this flourishing of consumer legal rights, many professional organizations published statements supporting rights for health care consumers. One that received much attention was the 1973 American Hospital Association's (AHA) Patient's Bill of Rights. In 1992 the AHA published an updated version (Box 4–1). The following paragraphs outline the recognition of many of these rights in both law and practice.

Right to "Considerate and Respectful Care." The right to considerate and respectful care undergirds not only the AHA Patient's Bill of Rights but also both the American Nurses Association's (ANA) code of ethics for nurses. Respect is also a fundamental concept in both duty-oriented and rights-oriented ethical frameworks.

Rights to Obtain Complete and Current Information Concerning Diagnosis, Treatment, and Prognosis and to Information Necessary to Give Informed Consent. Rights to obtain complete and current information concerning diagnosis, treatment, and prognosis and to information necessary to give informed consent include rights to opportunities to discuss and request information, to know the general plan of care, to know the identities of caregivers—including students—, and to know the known immediate and long-term financial implications of treatment choices.

Right to Have an Advance Directive. The 1992 bill specifies a right to have an advance directive and the responsibility of the hospital to advise individuals of their rights under state law and hospital policy. This right reflects case and statutory law development relevant to use of life-sustaining measures.

Rights to Consideration of Privacy and Confidential Treatment of Communication and Records. Rights to consideration of privacy and confidential treatment of communication and records support the legal concept of privacy and the ethical principle of confidentiality. The 1992 version of the bill, however, notes that requirements, such as suspected abuse and public health hazards, may override these rights.

Right to Review Medical Records. The 1992 version includes a person's right to review medical records and also to receive an explanation of information unless the law restricts record access.

Right to Reasonable Responses to Requests for Services. The right to reasonable responses to requests for services is now embodied in law in the United States in the Emergency Medical Treatment and Active Labor Act of 1986, known as the Anti-Dumping Act. The act requires hospitals to treat persons requesting services. Transfer to another facility must be based only on medical need.[34]

Right to Information about Business Relationship of the Hospital to Other Health Care Facilities, Educational Institutions, and Other Health Care Providers or Payers. The 1992 version of this bill specifies the person's right to information about the *business* relationship of the hospital to other health care facilities, educational institutions, and other health care providers or payers. Recent legislation constrains physician rights to refer clients to health care facilities—including laboratories and radiography facilities—in which they have a personal financial interest.[47]

Right to Consent to or Decline Participation in Human Subjects Research. Legal support of the right to consent to or decline participation in human subjects research stems from the National Research Act of 1974, which sets forth conditions that must be met to engage in research on human subjects.[57]

Right to Continuity of Care. Support for the right to continuity of care has been embodied in the emphasis on discharge planning during the 1970s and 1980s. In the 1990s, planning with a systems orientation is further refining this process.

Right to be Informed About Hospital Policies Related to Care and About Hospital Charges and Available Payment Methods. The bill focuses on the responsibility of the hospital to inform individuals not only of policies related to care but also of hospital charges and available payment methods. Clients can also expect hospitals to inform them of resources for resolving their care concerns and financial disputes. Examples of these resources are ethics committees and patient representatives. These practices reflect the increasing customer service orientation of hospitals.[48]

Box 4–1. The American Hospital Association's Patient's Bill of Rights

Bill of Rights*

1. The patient has the right to considerate and respectful care.

2. The patient has the right to and is encouraged to obtain from physicians and other direct caregivers relevant, current, and understandable information concerning diagnosis, treatment, and prognosis.

   Except in emergencies when the patient lacks decision-making capacity and the need for treatment is urgent, the patient is entitled to the opportunity to discuss and request information related to the specific procedures and/or treatments, the risks involved, the possible length of recuperation, and the medically reasonable alternatives and their accompanying risks and benefits.

   Patients have the right to know the identity of physicians, nurses, and others involved in their care, as well as when those involved are students, residents, or other trainees. The patient also has the right to know the immediate and long-term financial implications of treatment choices, insofar as they are known.

3. The patient has the right to make decisions about the plan of care prior to and during the course of treatment and to refuse a recommended treatment or plan of care to the extent permitted by law and hospital policy and to be informed of the medical consequences of this action. In case of such refusal, the patient is entitled to other appropriate care and services that the hospital provides or transfer to another hospital. The hospital should notify patients of any policy that might affect patient choice within the institution.

4. The patient has the right to have an advance directive (such as a living will, health care proxy, or durable power of attorney for health care) concerning treatment or designating a surrogate decision maker with the expecta-

tion that the hospital will honor the intent of that directive to the extent permitted by law and hospital policy.

   Health care institutions must advise patients of their rights under state law and hospital policy to make informed medical choices, ask if the patient has an advance directive, and include that information in patient records. The patient has the right to timely information about hospital policy that may limit its ability to implement fully a legally valid advance directive.

5. The patient has the right to every consideration of privacy. Case discussion, consultation, examination, and treatment should be conducted so as to protect each patient's privacy.

6. The patient has the right to expect that all communications and records pertaining to his/her care will be treated as confidential by the hospital, except in cases such as suspected abuse and public health hazards when reporting is permitted or required by law. The patient has the right to expect that the hospital will emphasize the confidentiality of this information when it releases it to any other parties entitled to review information in these records.

7. The patient has the right to review the records pertaining to his/her medical care and to have the information explained or interpreted as necessary, except when restricted by law.

8. The patient has the right to expect that, within its capacity and policies, a hospital will make reasonable response to the request of a patient for appropriate and medically indicated care and services. The hospital must provide evaluation, service, and/or referral as indicated by the urgency of the case. When medically appropriate and legally permissible, or when a patient has so re-

Box continued on following page

Right to Know What Hospital Rules and Regulations Apply to the Person's Conduct as a Patient. The right to know what hospital rules and regulations apply to the person's conduct as a patient has become reality as hospital rules and regulations have been shared with consumers. The increasing customer service orientation of hospitals has also led hospitals to share with consumers what they can expect from hospital personnel.[48]

Both health care providers and consumers have responsibilities in relation to consumer rights. The revised AHA *A Patient's Bill of Rights* recognizes a variety of client responsibilities, including providing and requesting information, accommodating to the needs of others in the hospital, and recognizing the impact of life style on personal health. This balancing scheme must be kept in mind throughout the discussion of rights.

CONSUMER RIGHTS, HEALTH CARE PROVIDER RESPONSIBILITIES, AND PERSONAL CHOICE

Who can make personal choices about health care? Persons who have reached the age of 18 years and who are capable of decision making can make decisions for themselves. What if you are unsure whether an adult can make health care decisions? In that case, you need to obtain an evaluation. This evaluation will usually be done by a psychiatrist or psychiatric nurse.

If it is determined that an adult is unable to make health care decisions, a suitable substitute decision maker must be found. **Surrogate** is the term for a substitute decision maker. There are three types of surrogates. First, many states have laws that provide for an order of decision making within a family. The order might be spouse, children of legal age, parents, and siblings. A second type of surrogate is the holder of a

---

Box 4–1. The American Hospital Association's Patient's Bill of Rights (Continued)

Bill of Rights*

quested, a patient may be transferred to another facility. The institution to which the patient is to be transferred must first have accepted the patient for transfer. The patient must also have the benefit of complete information and explanation concerning the need for, risks, benefits, and alternatives to such a transfer.

9. The patient has the right to ask and be informed of the existence of business relationships among the hospital, educational institutions, other health care providers, or payers that may influence the patient's treatment and care.

10. The patient has the right to consent to or decline to participate in proposed research studies or human experimentation affecting care and treatment or requiring direct patient involvement, and to have those studies fully explained prior to consent. A patient who declines to participate in research or experimentation is entitled to the most effective care that the hospital can otherwise provide.

11. The patient has the right to expect reasonable continuity of care when appropriate and to be informed by physicians and other caregivers of available and realistic patient care options when hospital care is no longer appropriate.

12. The patient has the right to be informed of hospital policies and practices that relate to patient care, treatment, and responsibilities. The patient has the right to be informed of available resources for resolving disputes, grievances, and conflicts, such as ethics committees, patient representatives, or other mechanisms available in the institution. The patient has the right to be informed of the hospital's charges for services and available payment methods.

The collaborative nature of health care requires that patients, or their families/surrogates, participate in their care. The ef-

fectiveness of care and patient satisfaction with the course of treatment depend, in part, on the patient fulfilling certain responsibilities. Patients are responsible for providing information about past illnesses, hospitalizations, medications, and other matters related to health status. To participate effectively in decision making, patients must be encouraged to take responsibility for requesting additional information or clarification about their health status or treatment when they do not fully understand information and instructions. Patients are also responsible for ensuring that the health care institution has a copy of their written advance directive if they have one. Patients are responsible for informing their physicians and other caregivers if they anticipate problems in following prescribed treatment.

Patients should also be aware of the hospital's obligation to be reasonably efficient and equitable in providing care to other patients and the community. The hospital's rules and regulations are designed to help the hospital meet this obligation. Patients and their families are responsible for making reasonable accommodations to the needs of the hospital, other patients, medical staff, and hospital employees. Patients are responsible for providing necessary information for insurance claims and for working with the hospital to make payment arrangements, when necessary.

A person's health depends on much more than health care services. Patients are responsible for recognizing the impact of their life-style on their personal health.

---

*These rights can be exercised on the patient's behalf by a designated surrogate or proxy decision maker if the patient lacks decision-making capacity, is legally incompetent, or is a minor.

Reprinted with permission of the American Hospital Association, Copyright 1992.

---

durable power of attorney for health care decision making. Third, a court-appointed legal guardian may act as a surrogate. A **legal guardian** is a person appointed by a court to make decisions about personal or financial affairs of a person when clear and convincing evidence demonstrates that the person is unable to do so for himself or herself. Generally, persons may be incapable of decision making for three reasons. First, persons may lapse into unconsciousness. Second, dementia may disturb thinking processes to the point at which information cannot be rationally acted on. Third, the person may have always been incapable of making decisions, as with persons suffering severe and profound mental retardation.

A word of caution is in order. Even an adult with a legal guardian may still be able to indicate wishes re-

garding health care. For example, a person may be able to indicate by gestures and other behavior that he or she wants a tube removed. Legal guardians, as surrogate decision makers, have a responsibility for attempting to determine these wishes. Family and holders of durable powers of attorney are also responsible for making decisions as the person would have wished. If the person can no longer demonstrate any indication of wishes and the surrogate has little information about health care wishes, previous lifestyle may provide clues to the surrogate as to the appropriate decision. The surrogate may also decide for or against treatment on the basis of whether the benefits outweigh the burdens.

Parents are the natural legal guardians of their children. Parents must make decisions based on the best interests of their child. The term **best interests** means that the benefits of a decision outweigh the burdens. Judgments that parents are neglectful may arise from decisions that demonstrate parents do not have in mind the best interests of their children. Courts will then appoint legal guardians for the children until the parents have gained or regained the capability to make decisions in their children's best interest.

What about children of divorce? The parent who has legal custody is the decision maker. In cases of joint custody, both parents should share in the decision making.

Persons are not legally competent to consent to treatment until they reach the age of legal majority—18 years. However, because many persons younger than 18 years can be considered capable of understanding the nature of invasive procedures, their risks and consequences, rights-oriented ethical practice dictates that mature minors be involved in this decision making.

In addition to ethical responsibility to involve minors in decision making, there are also legal exceptions. One exception occurs when a minor becomes emancipated from the control of their parents through marriage. Another occurs when minors make reproductive decisions. You should know, however, that many state abortion laws place limitations on this right. Minors who have children may make decisions for their children. Minors who live with parents—even those with children of their own—may, however, be totally subject to parental decision making regarding their health in areas other than their reproductive health.

In some states, minors receiving government support through aid to dependent children programs—even though living with parents—may make health care decisions for themselves. However, as is the case for adults, emergency treatment of minors may proceed when time does not permit or providers are unable to contact parents or other designated surrogates for permission to treat. Nurses should acquaint themselves with their state laws regarding decision making for minors so nurses can support minors' rights to informed consent. Box 4–2 lists health care decision makers.

Can health care providers make decisions about a person's health care? The answer is "no." A health care provider has an advisory role. In the case of an adult, the provider must honor the client's decision. In situations in which health care providers believe parents are not making decisions in their child's best interest, providers can challenge the parents' decision in court. Consultation with a health care facility bioethics committee can often resolve differences between families and providers. Consultation can thus be a useful approach to avoiding a legal action.

Conflict resolution through consultation is one function of a health care facility bioethics committee. Bioethics committees may also educate facility staff and consumers of care about ethical concerns in health care. Some bioethics committees also develop facility policies that involve ethical concerns. Examples are informed consent policies and policies addressing use of life-sustaining measures. As a nurse, your responsibility is to familiarize yourself with these policies so you can act as an advocate for your client.

Informed Consent

INFORMED CONSENT TO TREATMENT

The consumer's right to informed consent evolves from the common law of battery, an intentional tort that provides damages for unconsented touching. A 1914 New York State case first applied this legal concept to invasive procedures.[89]

The law of informed consent applies only to invasive procedures. Examples are surgery, diagnostic studies such as cardiac catheterizations, and therapeutic procedures such as insertion of hyperalimentation catheters.

Components of Informed Consent to Treatment. Informed consent is the process of providing clients information about (1) the nature and purpose of a treatment or procedure, (2) the expected outcomes and probabilities of success, the material risks, the benefits, and the consequences, (3) alternatives to the procedure and supporting information, and (4) the effect of no treatment or no procedure, including the effect on the prognosis and material risks associated with no treatment (Box 4–3). If an undisclosed risk occurs about which the consumer should have received information from the health care provider, the consumer may bring a lawsuit based on lack of informed consent. The law governing informed consent is similar in both Canada and the United States.[84-86]

Legal Standards for Informed Consent to Treatment. The law recognizes one of three standards for determining the information the consumer needs to know to give informed consent. The first provides information based on what other health care providers customarily give consumers. This is called the professional standard and is biased in favor of health care

---

Box 4–2. Health Care Decision Makers

- ▶ Adults of legal age
- ▶ Parents of children
- ▶ Minors according to state law
- ▶ Court-appointed legal guardians of children or adults
- ▶ Holders of durable powers of attorney
- ▶ Order of surrogates identified by state statute

Box 4–3. Legal Components of Informed Consent

- ▶ Nature and purpose of treatment or procedure
- ▶ Risks and benefits
- ▶ Alternatives
- ▶ Effect of no treatment

TABLE 4-1. Legal Standards Used to Determine the Content of Information the Consumer Needs in Order to Give Informed Consent

Standard	Description
Professional	What the physician believes the consumer should know
Subjective	What the particular consumer believes the consumer should know
Objective	What a reasonable person believes the consumer should know

professionals. The second asks that information meet the needs of the particular health care consumer. This standard is known as the subjective standard and is biased in favor of the consumer who stands to gain damages if any unknown risk is suffered. The third asks that information be sufficient to permit a reasonable person in similar circumstances to make a judgment about whether to accept or refuse care. This standard is known as the objective standard. This last standard is accepted by the majority of states as fairest to both parties in a lawsuit because a jury composed of noninvolved persons would make this judgment (Table 4-1).

Canterbury v. Spence (1972)[13] is a leading case for the law of informed consent. In that case, the neurosurgeon informed the person of the usual risks of surgery—that is, infection and hemorrhage—but failed to inform the individual of the risk of paralysis with the anticipated spinal surgery. The client sued and recovered damages when the risk materialized.

Your Responsibility in Informed Consent to Treatment

In the past and often in current practice, nurses have taken responsibility for getting the consent form signed before invasive procedures. In carrying out this activity, nurses are *not* obtaining informed consent, they are merely witnessing the signature of the patient on a form. State statutory law governing informed consent assigns to the physician the role of informing the patient about invasive procedures.

Should the nurse have any part in obtaining informed consent? From a risk management perspective, the answer is "yes." It can be helpful for the nurse to be present when the physician explains the procedure because the client may be anxious and may not initially grasp the physician's information. If the nurse is present, he or she can explain terms the physician used when questions about the procedure later arise. However, when a client asks questions or seeks further information about medical diagnoses, prognoses, and risks, the nurse should contact the physician to address the client's concerns. Addressing those concerns will assure the physician that he or she has truly obtained informed consent. The nurse can always and should always give information about nursing care. For exam-

ple, the nurse should provide an explanation of preoperative and postoperative nursing care.

You, as a nurse, will not always be present during the physician's informed consent conversation with the client. The reason for this is that these conversations generally occur in the physician's office before admission to the hospital or outpatient facility. The fact that the conversation occurs outside the health care facility does not diminish the nurse's ethical responsibility to notify the physician when a person raises concerns about the procedure that indicate the individual needs more information to give truly informed consent.

What about other information for consumers? Generally, no law requires that informed consent be obtained before a provider prescribes a medication. Similarly, a nurse generally need not, by law, provide information about the purpose of a medication. To provide information is good professional practice because the giving of information acts as an invitation to the consumer to participate in and share control of personal health care. Sharing control respects the consumer as a person. Communication of this information to clients is also good risk management because possessing the information may lead the consumer to early identification of harmful side effects. The law requires this information be provided only when doing so becomes a part of the usual and customary standard of nursing care.

Today nursing has assumed responsibility for providing medication information, nutrition information, and other health-related information. Consumers have come to expect this as a right. Your practice should reflect this growing responsibility. You will want to ensure that you are professionally responsible so that you are legally accountable to your clients.

You should know that information sharing is gradually becoming the usual and customary standard of care.

An example of information sharing that has become the standard of care is advising persons who are taking antihistamines not to operate heavy machinery.

Withdrawal of consent to both invasive and noninvasive procedures can occur at any time and need not be in writing. Thus, a person can withdraw consent to surgery just before receiving anesthesia for an operative procedure. The preoperative medication alone does not ordinarily result in a person becoming incapable of decision making. Withdrawal of consent can be either verbal or nonverbal. A patient who makes an arm unavailable for withdrawal of blood is indicating lack of consent for this procedure.

Informed Consent and the Treatment of Infants. Treatment for infants born with handicaps was the subject of major legal controversy in the early 1980s. An Indiana case precipitated the controversy when parents of an infant born with Down's syndrome and an esophageal fistula refused surgical treatment to correct the defect. Although pediatricians, who were in ethical conflict with the parents' decision, sought a court order for treatment, the infant died before the case could be heard. Immediate reaction at the federal level led to the issuance of a notice to health care providers that Section 504 of the Rehabilitation Act of 1973 — the law addressing discrimination against handicapped persons — applied to newborns. Regulations under this law required posting of notices in delivery, maternity, pediatric, and nursery units that stated "Discriminatory failure to feed and care for handicapped infants in this facility is prohibited by law."[38] Later, these regulations were defeated on the basis that the Rehabilitation Act was never intended to apply to the treatment of infants.[11]

Congress remedied the concerns about infant treatment by amending the Child Abuse and Prevention Act. Rules enacted under that amendment expanded the definition of child abuse to include the withholding of medically indicated treatment that would be likely to be effective in ameliorating or correcting conditions. Treatment includes appropriate nutrition, hydration, and medication.

Although nutrition, hydration, and medication may *never* be withheld, corrective procedures may be withheld under three conditions: first, if the infant is chronically and irreversibly comatose; second, if the treatment would merely prolong dying, not be effective in ameliorating or correcting all life-threatening conditions, or otherwise be futile; or third, when the survival of the infant and the treatment itself would be inhumane.[22]

An appendix to the rules suggests hospital ethics committees can be helpful in arriving at decisions, but the congressional amendment did not mandate their existence.

INFORMED CONSENT TO RESEARCH

Origins of Informed Consent to Research. Legal requirements for consent to research on human subjects derive historically from a series of situations that abused a person's right to choose whether or not to participate in research. Abuse of human subjects during the Nazi regime in Germany led to the Nuremberg Code. The Nuremberg Code is an international agreement that supports adult participation in research only with informed consent. It does not mention children. The later Helsinki Agreement provides guidelines for children as subjects of research.[52]

The Nazi regime was not alone in abusing human rights. In the United States, an originally well-intentioned study of the treatment of syphilis among African-Americans in southern states that began in the 1920s ran out of private supporting funds with the Depression.[97] The government took over the study, but all subjects did not receive sufficient treatment to cure their syphilis, although they believed they had. The study, which continued through the 1970s, became merely a chronicle of the course of the disease until a former government employee blew the whistle.

This study, coupled with reports of a study that permitted institutionalized developmentally disabled children to be subjected to conditions that led to infection with hepatitis without the knowledge or consent of their parents, led to legal reform. In the United States, this reform was the National Research Act.[57] Canada's Medical Council has developed guidelines for human subjects research in that country.[39]

Legal Rights of Human Subjects in Research. Today in the United States any human subject involved in federally funded research (and parents in the case of a minor) must be informed of the purpose and the risks and benefits of the study. Many facilities by institutional policy extend the scope of review of their institutional review boards (IRBs) to both privately funded and unfunded research studies. Exceptions to the review process include surveys and observational studies that meet the criteria listed in Box 4–4.[18]

Remember that the law requires informed consent to research. Under a rights-oriented ethical framework, ethical practice also requires informed consent.

Similar to withdrawing consent to treatment, subjects of research can withdraw consent at any time during the course of the study without fear of losing access to appropriate treatment. Furthermore, subjects in the study must be provided with the name of a person to contact if they believe they have been injured in the research process.

Rules of confidentiality protect consumers from unauthorized release of information from their medical records. The law requires that information obtained during a research study receive equivalent protection. Grouping individual data so that individuals cannot be identified is one way to protect confidentiality. Coding data, keeping data in a locked file, limiting access to data, and destroying data that are no longer needed also protect subjects from identification.

Members of research review boards focus their review on the informed consent process. They look for sufficient explanation of, and evidence of an under-

---

Box 4–4. Research Exempt From the Institutional Review Board Review Process

1. Surveys, interviews, and observational studies that:
   a. Lack sensitive subject areas.
   b. Record responses in a manner that cannot identify subjects directly or through identifying characteristics.
   c. Do not include responses that could reasonably place the subject at risk of criminal or civil liability or be damaging to the subject's financial standing or employability.
2. Research involving normal educational practices or educational testing.
3. Generally research involving use of existing data sets.

From *Code of Federal Regulations* S. 46.101 (b) (1981, amended 1983)

standing of, the risks or discomforts of the research, provisions for dealing with risks that actually occur, and documentation of the informed consent process. Federal regulations have special provisions for more vulnerable populations such as children, pregnant women, and prisoners.[19-21] Risks to the fetus are the concern with pregnant women. In fact, one reason offered for the lack of research on premenopausal women has been the ever present possibility of a pregnancy. With prisoners, the concern is the possibility of coerced participation.

Children capable of understanding procedures must give assent to involvement in research. **Assent** is the agreement of a child to participate in research based on the child's understanding of the purpose, risks, and benefits of the research. The child's assent plus the parent's or legal guardian's consent is necessary to participation in a study. This provision acknowledges the child's legal incompetency to consent because he or she is younger than 18 years. On the other hand, the provision recognizes that children progress in their level of maturity and understanding of choices in their own lives. Federal law sets forth circumstances of risk under which children may participate in research. Table 4–2 presents categories of research risk, along with the related consent process and justification for each level of risk.

Your Responsibility in Informed Consent to Research. Why should every nurse be concerned about informed consent rights of research subjects? Is not research unusual except in large medical centers?

Every nurse should be concerned about informed consent to research. Why? Nurses themselves are the subjects of research. Nurses can be readily identified through membership in professional associations. Nurses are a largely female population. All these characteristics make them a ready source of subjects to fill the gap of research data on women's health. As both consumers and providers of health care, nurses appreciate the importance of health. Thus, they are also likely to be ready volunteers for research.

Of course, it is not true that all research is conducted in major medical centers. In the future, that is even less likely to be the case, particularly as the health care system begins to evaluate outcomes of provider practices across both a broad spectrum of providers and wide geographic areas. So you are at the very least likely to participate in an evaluation of your own practice outcomes.

It is also quite possible that you will be working with persons who already are or who have potential to be participants in research. The exponentially increasing amount of research in the discipline of nursing is one reason. A second is that the advent of computerized data and ability to store large quantities of data make larger study populations possible. Therefore, supporting consumers in exploring the question of whether or not to participate in a research project will be part of your practice. You may also have opportunities to participate in both the review and approval processes for research protocols. You may also identify deviations from protocol that violate consumer rights and call for advocacy action by you.

TABLE 4–2. Risk Categories, Consent Process, and Justification for Risk for Research Involving Children as Human Subjects

Category	Consent	Justification
Minimal risk	▶ Consent of parents ▶ Assent of child	
Greater than minimal risk but prospect of direct benefit to subject	▶ Consent of parents ▶ Assent of child	▶ Anticipated benefit as favorable as available alternatives
Greater than minimal risk but no prospect of direct benefit to subject	▶ Consent of parents ▶ Assent of child	▶ Risk only a minor increase over minimal risk ▶ Intervention similar to what is expected in actual or expected medical, dental, psychologic, social, or educational situations ▶ Intervention likely to yield generalizable knowledge of vital importance for understanding or ameliorating the subject's condition
Research not otherwise approvable that offers opportunity to alleviate a serious problem affecting health or welfare of children	▶ Consent of parents ▶ Assent of child ▶ Consultation by the Secretary of Health and Human Services with panel of experts and public review	▶ Presents reasonable opportunity of further understanding, preventing, or alleviating a serious problem affecting the health or welfare of children. ▶ Must be conducted with sound ethical principles ▶ Must fulfill the necessary consent requirements

From *Code of Federal Regulations* S. 46.404, S. 46.405, S. 46.406, S. 46.407 (1983)

Forgoing Life-Sustaining Measures

BACKGROUND LAW

Questions about the legality of forgoing life-sustaining measures began to be answered with the decision in the 1976 *Quinlan* case.[73] The *Quinlan* decision permitted Karen Ann Quinlan to be removed from a respirator at the request of her father, who was acting as her guardian. The case began to answer specifically two important questions: (1) What measures are considered life-sustaining technology? (2) Who can speak for a person unable to speak for herself or himself about removal of life-sustaining measures? Additional questions about how, where, and when life-sustaining measures might be removed have been answered by further case law development. Legislation has addressed these questions through brain death, durable power of attorney for health care, and living will legislation.

The *Quinlan* case was the first to consider removal of a respirator. From then through 1986, ethicists and lawyers debated whether the removal of nutritional support devices could also be legally and ethically supported. The 1986 landmark *Brophy* case was the first to support their withdrawal.[12] In that case, the court called nutritional support devices medical treatment. Given the medical treatment label, the court said the person had the same right to refuse this treatment—even though beneficial—as any other medical treatment.

Early on, courts recognized the right to refuse cardiopulmonary resuscitation as a life-sustaining measure.[31] Renal dialysis has also been specifically supported in case law.[92]

Courts and ethicists generally regard both withholding and withdrawal of life-sustaining measures as ethical equivalents.

THE DECISION-MAKING PROCESS

People Remaining Capable of Decision Making. Table 4–3 shows that, as for informed consent to treatment and research, persons who remain capable of decision making can always make decisions about use of life-sustaining measures. This is true even if the person is 99 years old. Families and physicians cannot and should not make decisions about use of life-sustaining measures for individuals capable of making their own decisions.[37,76,89]

TABLE 4–3. Appropriate Decision Makers Concerning Life-Sustaining Measures for Clients with Various Capabilities and Wishes

Capability	Wishes	Appropriate Decision Maker
Capable	▶ Known or unknown	▶ Client
Now incapable	▶ Known	▶ Client
Now incapable	▶ Unknown	▶ Surrogate
Always incapable	▶ Unable to be known	▶ Surrogate

Remember that even persons who have a legal guardian may still be able to understand the nature of decisions about treatment and use of life-sustaining measures. The same holds true for persons involuntarily committed to facilities for treatment of mental illness. Although they may be a threat to the health or welfare of themselves and others, they may still be able to understand the consequences of treatment decisions and be capable of participating in this decision-making process.

Obviously, with mentally ill persons and persons with legal guardians, their decision-making capability must be carefully scrutinized when they elect to refuse beneficial treatment.

People Who Earlier Expressed Their Wishes. Persons may have earlier expressed their wishes about use of life-sustaining measures either in conversations with family, friends, and health care providers or in formal documents called advance directives. An **advance directive** is a written document expressing a person's wishes about use of life-sustaining measures or appointing a surrogate decision maker when he or she can no longer make decisions. Some advance directives serve both purposes.

Earlier Verbally Expressed Wishes. Written documents are always preferable to verbally expressed wishes regarding the use of life-sustaining measures. The reason for this is that written documents more likely provide clear and convincing evidence of a person's desires. Case law acknowledges verbal wishes but indicates that written documents carry greater weight.

Living Wills. **Living wills** are written documents that state a person's own wishes regarding the use of life-sustaining measures when a person becomes incapable of expressing his or her wishes. All states do not have legislation that creates legal recognition for living wills. However, even without living will legislation, these documents deserve respect from health care providers and family members. This is because the documents represent the personal wishes of the individual and should, therefore, not be taken lightly.

Durable Powers of Attorney. A **durable power of attorney for health care** is a written document that gives power to another person—generally a trusted friend or family member—to make health care decisions for a person when the person becomes incapable of making health care decisions. They are regarded as expressing the wishes of the person giving the power of attorney under the assumption that the person has discussed health care issues and wishes with the person to whom the power of attorney is given. Some durable power of attorney statutes incorporate living will features. Ohio's statute, for example, provides that specific language regarding refusal of nutritional support devices be included.[60]

Durable powers of attorney are always supported by state law. States may have statutes supporting durable powers of attorney that include power to make decisions about financial and other decisions including health care. Other states require a person to execute separate durable powers of attorney—one for health care and one for all other matters.

Operation of Living Wills and Durable Powers of Attorney for Health Care. Both living wills and durable powers of attorney for health care require witnesses who generally must meet certain qualifications. These include *not* being an heir or beneficiary in a will of the person creating the directive. Witnesses must also be at least 18 years of age.

Health care facilities may have a conflict of interest with the person creating the document. This is because clients pay for services from health care facilities, and the facility may therefore have an interest in either continuing provision of services to continue receiving payment or discontinuing services so a higher paying customer client can be admitted. For this reason, employees of facilities may be prohibited from acting as witnesses.

When do advance directives go into effect? Besides the condition of the person being incapable of decision making, both living wills and durable powers of attorney may become operational only when the treating, and often a second, physician determines that a person is terminally ill. The usual definition of terminal illness is an illness for which further treatment is futile. In fact, recently, this has led physicians to raise the ethical question of whether they have a duty to treat a terminally ill person even when the person requests medically futile therapy.[28]

People with No Express Wishes. What happens when a person is incapable of decision making and that person has no advance directive? How then are individual rights considered in decision making?

Historically, these decisions were made by physician and family. Society made the assumption that, with the input of each, decisions would be made that reflected the person's own desires. In situations in which all family members were in agreement, a comfortable decision-making process could occur. In the rare case in which agreement did not occur, approaches to achieving consensus were sought within the supporting framework of the health care facility by approaching client relations personnel, clergy, and ethics committees. Courts were used only as a last resort.

Today, the historic framework is still that most often used when persons have not expressed their wishes about use of life-sustaining measures. When no family exists, the legal guardian must make the decision based on the best interests of the client when unable to determine what the person might have desired.

Problems often arise when a person is in a persistent vegetative state. This often occurs after brain damage has occurred or after an unsuccessful attempt at cardiac resuscitation. The person frequently has not expressed his or her desires regarding the use of life-sustaining measures. The person is not regarded as terminally ill because he or she can live for a long period of time.[24] State statutes may make provision for dealing with this state in which the person has no thinking capability and can be kept alive only with nutritional support.

People Always Incapable of Decision Making. When a person has always been incapable of decision making, decisions can be made by the physician and family. These situations are different in that a benefits versus burden analysis must be engaged in by the physician and family. The decision must be based on their perception of what this person in such circumstances would choose for himself or herself. Parents may do this for children; others may do so for the always mentally incapable.

At least two courts have dealt with the latter circumstance. A Massachusetts court in 1977 required that a court order be obtained for an institution to withhold chemotherapy from an institutionalized, mentally retarded man whose prospects for benefit from therapy were minimal.[96] There was no family. However, in New York State another retarded man was given blood transfusions for bladder cancer, even though his caring legal guardian—his mother—refused. The court saw the transfusions as a temporary benefit to his status, a position supported by staff of the institution where he resided.[94]

UNITED STATES STATE AND FEDERAL LAW AFTER CRUZAN

In the *Cruzan* decision, the United States Supreme Court upheld the right of an individual to refuse life-sustaining measures under the federal constitution's liberty right. The Court also held that a state could legally require an evidentiary standard of clear and convincing evidence of the person's wishes to honor that right (see Chapter 3).[25]

The Court's decision in *Cruzan* influenced many state legislatures that had previously hesitated to pass living will legislation and to amend or create durable power of attorney statutes that included health care decision making. Obviously, a written document is the easiest route to establishing the clear and convincing evidentiary standard. The *Cruzan* case also influenced the passage of federal legislation. This legislation, called the Patient Self-Determination Act or Danforth Amendment, affects many facilities providing care including hospitals, long-term care facilities, and managed-care organizations.[69] The legislation requires that facilities

▶ Ask whether a person has executed a living will or durable power of attorney, or both, on admission
▶ Give information about state law regarding such documents
▶ Educate the public and facility staff about advance directives
▶ Inform patients about hospital policy regarding advance directives

ASSISTED SUICIDE

Withholding life-sustaining measures at a person's request is termed **passive voluntary euthanasia.** On the other hand, **active voluntary euthanasia** is performing an act at a person's request that results in the death of the person. Active voluntary euthanasia is assisted suicide. The act is a crime in many states. A Michigan physician's role in assisting the suicide of several persons has drawn national attention to this potential role for physicians and, perhaps, other health care providers. The state of Washington recently defeated a referendum vote to permit terminally ill persons to request and receive physician aid in dying. Fear of progression down the slippery ethical slope to active involuntary euthanasia—performing an act that results in the death of a person without his or her consent—was believed to be the reason for the Washington referendum defeat.[51]

A utilitarian ethical perspective can arguably support taking the path to active involuntary euthanasia. However, active involuntary euthanasia can be regarded as violating the principle of autonomy and respect for persons. In assisted suicide, the person violates respect for themselves as a person. Assisted suicide also violates the ANA Code for Nurses in its call for caring for all persons regardless of status.[3]

YOUR RESPONSIBILITY IN DECISIONS ABOUT FORGOING LIFE-SUSTAINING MEASURES

As a nurse, you will care for many terminally ill persons. As each comes to terms with the end of life, you may be the person with whom they share their concerns about life-sustaining treatments. It is important that you make them aware that choices about life-sustaining measures are their right. Even though in many instances you will be repeating information they have already received under the Patient Self-Determination Act, you will want to remind them of the approaches to legally expressing their wishes in your state. Talking about use of life-sustaining measures may signal a readiness to execute a living will or durable power of attorney for health care. Remind individuals to give a copy of these documents to their attending physician.

You will also want to encourage clients to discuss their wishes with family members and with their attending physician. This step can lead to the avoidance of conflicts when decisions must actually be made.

Remember that conversations with consumers and communications with other providers about use of life-sustaining measures should be documented in the clients' records.

Documentation in the client record can also set the stage to avoid later conflicts. Last, review the policy and procedure of your health care facility regarding use of life-sustaining measures so that you can interpret the policy to your clients.

Because assisted suicide will continue to receive national attention, nurses, at a minimum, need to track this social policy debate. Active involvement in the debate may also be a choice.

Reproductive Rights

ABORTION

The 1973 United States Supreme Court decision in *Roe v. Wade* gave women the right to make a decision to abort a pregnancy. In the first trimester, the woman must make her decision in consultation with her physician. In the second trimester, the state may regulate facilities where abortions are conducted. In the third trimester, the state's interest in the fetus is considered to override the woman's right to terminate a pregnancy.[80] *Roe v. Wade* limited third-trimester pregnancy terminations to situations in which the life of the mother was endangered. From the outset, *Roe v. Wade* has been controversial and subject to legal attack.

Legally, the right to abort a pregnancy is rooted in the right to privacy. This right, not specifically enunciated in the Constitution's Bill of Rights, is inferred from the First, Fourth, and Fifth Amendments. Because the privacy right is not clearly specified, some legal scholars argue its existence. Thus, a Supreme Court majority against that right could eliminate the right to choose to terminate a pregnancy. Over time, *Roe v. Wade* has been narrowed by several decisions. Thus, states are free to regulate the right to abort a pregnancy by regulations that may include waiting periods, consent by a minor's parents or a judge, and regulation of facilities providing abortions. In 1992, the United State Supreme Court reaffirmed support for regulatory constraints but stopped at requiring the father's consent to abort the pregnancy.[71]

In *Rust v. Sullivan* (1991), the United States Supreme Court supported regulations that precluded federally funded clinics from engaging in abortion counseling.[88] Although some see the case as supporting the rights of legislators to set federal policy, others view it as infringement on First Amendment free-speech rights. Subsequent action by the Department of Health and Human Services lifted the gag order imposed by the case but only for physicians. However, because nurses are the primary counselors in clinics, political pressure forced legal action to lift the order for nurses and other providers as well.[36]

Until 1988, Canadian law prohibited abortions unless a committee of three hospital physicians certified that the pregnancy would endanger the life or health of the woman if carried to term. When these conditions were met, however, Canada's universal health insurance did pay for abortions. A 1988 decision declared unconstitutional a provision of Canada's Criminal Code making unauthorized abortions a criminal act. Although the criminal penalty no longer exists, the decision does not require Canadian hospitals to provide abortions without the certification of three physicians. Physicians must also obtain privileges to perform abortions.[23]

CONTRACEPTION AND STERILIZATION

As mentioned earlier, the underpinning law of *Roe v. Wade* is a series of decisions applying the right to privacy. The first declared unconstitutional a Connecticut law that forbade the sale of contraceptives.[43] Subsequent case law provided accessibility to contraceptives for minors.[33] In some states, case law also addressed the right of a woman to seek a tubal ligation without the consent of her husband, a right reflected in the 1992 Supreme Court decision on abortion.

PREGNANCY AND SUBSTANCE ABUSE

In 1988, 1 in 10 infants was born exposed to cocaine. One newspaper poll reflected society's outrage at that figure; 71 per cent of persons were in favor of criminal penalties for pregnant women who abused illegal drugs. Forty-five per cent favored prosecution of women who used only tobacco or alcohol.[27]

Courts have left criminalization of the conduct of pregnant substance-abusing women up to legislatures. Although Illinois criminalized drug abuse under its child protection legislation, no massive ground swell of public opinion has caused this to occur in other states. Instead, courts have found this behavior sufficient to apply child abuse and neglect statutes.[87] This may result in the infant being separated from the mother at birth. Infants are then placed by the state in the custody of a trusted care giver, often a close relative.

Persons supporting criminalization of drug abuse believe it is not inconsistent with treatment for substance abusers.[77] However, opponents believe criminalization will result in women refusing to be honest about substance abuse. Opponents believe in increasing health services to pregnant women, including treatment of substance abuse.[68]

YOUR RESPONSIBILITY IN REPRODUCTIVE DECISIONS

Most nurses in their practice encounter women of childbearing age. It is important for you to be aware of these reproductive rights of female consumers of health care in order to teach and counsel them. It is particularly important for you to be aware of the provisions of abortion laws in your state with respect to the rights of minors. Contraceptive use is a decision a minor can make independently. Abortion may require the consent of parents or a court and a waiting period.

What if your personal value system is in conflict with some contraceptive measures and with abortion? Your best choice is to avoid an area of practice such as community health or maternity nursing, where clients will frequently have health care needs in relation to contraception and abortion. Otherwise, you will have to assure yourself that other nurses are available to provide guidance and counseling in these areas. Before you are hired, it will be important for you to let the agency know about your potential value conflicts so arrangements can be made for others to provide this care. You can, of course, choose to practice in these areas in a health care facility that is supportive of your moral stance.

As a nurse, you also need to examine your value system in relation to women who engage in substance abuse while pregnant. When you cannot provide supportive care to these affected women, you should seek a work site more consistent with your beliefs.

CONSUMER RIGHTS AND HEALTH CARE PROVIDER RESPONSIBILITIES IN HEALTH CARE FACILITIES

Long-Term Care Facilities

The rights of persons living in long-term care facilities are an important concern because the population is vulnerable as a result of dependence on others for the basic needs such as nutrition, exercise, sleep, rest, and socialization. The long-term care population includes not only the elderly but also persons suffering disability incurred at an earlier stage in life. Federal, state, and local laws are the embodiment of public policy that influences the rights of persons living in these settings. The certification process for receiving Medicare and Medicaid funding and state and local long-term care facility licensure laws clearly reflect this influence.

CERTIFICATION AND LICENSURE

How do certification and licensure protect this vulnerable group of persons? **Certification** is the process of review to determine whether a care facility meets standards of care at a level sufficient to qualify for payment by Medicare or Medicaid. **Licensure** is a process of review to determine whether a care facility meets standards of care at a level sufficient to continue operation regardless of source of payment. Licensure standards may be more or less strict than Medicare or Medicaid payment standards.

The Medicare and Medicaid certification processes have, since the late 1960s, attempted to ensure quality of care in long-term care settings. In addition, state and local licensure laws have also attempted to ensure that quality when facilities did not seek payment from Medicare and Medicaid sources. Medicare and Medicaid payment standards, however, remain influential even when facilities do not receive payment through these sources because they set the standard for the long-term care industry.

When Medicare and Medicaid reimbursements were based on per diem rates, some profit-making facilities skimped on the nutritional quality of food to cut costs and increase profits. The certification process changed to respond to this and other similar concerns. In the mid-1980s, the certification process began to provide for actual observation of care. This approach replaced mere review of client records and facility policies and procedures.

Unlike Joint Commission on Accreditation of Health Care Organization visits, certification and licensure visits are unannounced. Thus, the surveyor is more likely to view care as it is actually provided on a daily basis. To enhance this likelihood, surveyors take only a brief period of time to organize their visits before beginning observations in actual care areas. Not only is care observed, but surveyors also ask residents who are able to communicate verbally about the quality of care they receive.

The certification process in long-term care facilities will next move to an outcome-oriented approach that is consistent with current trends in acute care health facilities. The Omnibus Budget Reconciliation Acts (OBRAs) of 1987 and 1989 are the enabling legislation supporting this approach to the individual's right to quality care in long-term care settings.

RESIDENT RIGHTS

Under OBRA legislation, residents of long-term care facilities have specified rights when they reside in Medicare- and Medicaid-certified facilities. Individual states may also have legislation supporting resident rights.[65]

Control over Property and Funds. Under Medicaid, residents of long-term care facilities have a designated amount per month available to them for personal spending. Facilities must have a procedure for distribution of these funds to the resident at reasonable times. In many facilities, social workers assume this responsibility. Private-pay clients who are capable of doing so may retain responsibility for their own financial affairs or elect to give a power of attorney to a trusted person, usually a friend or family member.

Freedom from Restraint, Safety Provisions, and Quality Care. OBRA 1987 regulations emphasized reduction in the use of both physical and chemical restraints in long-term care settings. The law makes these restraints permissible only when necessary to treat the person's medical symptoms. Restraints may not be imposed for discipline purposes or for the convenience of the staff. Consistent with the law, facilities have adopted procedures that call for residents or their decision-maker surrogates to consent or refuse restraints.

To meet Medicare and Medicaid standards, many facilities must now upgrade to meet resident safety rights. This is because the law now calls for safety provisions in the physical environment such as emergency power systems, call systems, and preventive maintenance activities.

Another significant change triggered by OBRA is training nursing assistants working in long-term care facilities. The law provides for training requirements, including competency testing, for first-time nursing assistants. Experienced nursing assistants must pass the competency examination. In addition, the law mandates quarterly continuing education requirements. All nursing assistants must also be on file with a state agency. This may be the responsibility of the state board of nursing. Training requirements are an effort to upgrade the quality of nursing care in long-term facilities.

Another quality enhancement in facilities reimbursed by Medicare and Medicaid is the nationwide uniform resident assessment system. The system includes a minimum data set on each resident plus triggers for additional assessment when the minimum data set identifies problems. The system, based on a pilot study, will be further revised in the future.

The law also encourages long-term care facilities to set up quality-assurance programs that look to continuous quality improvement. For residents, this is another mechanism to ensure their right to receive quality care. For facilities, the reward will be recertification visits every 2 years rather than every year.

Other Rights. OBRA emphasizes that long-term care residents retain all their rights as citizens. The right to vote is an example. Access to their records is also a right under OBRA. Other rights include the right to privacy, confidentiality, filing grievances about care without fear of reprisal, and self-administration of medications if a determination of competency is made by staff. Residents also have a right to participate in their plan of care.

The long-term care industry, because of its high degree of regulation, clearly affords individuals more legal rights than those available in the acute care system. In the latter system, rights are much more dependent on the ethical stance of providers of care. Box 4–5 lists the rights addressed by OBRA of 1987.

YOUR RESPONSIBILITY IN LONG-TERM CARE FACILITIES

Staff members of long-term care facilities look to nurses to take a leadership role as advocates for residents by taking responsibility to recognize and support residents' rights. That responsibility includes being personally aware of residents' rights, ensuring that residents understand their rights, and responding to residents' requests for exercise of their rights.

Beyond responsibility to individual residents, the nurse also has a responsibility for creating a facility climate that ensures that certification and licensure standards of care are consistently met. That climate prevails when staff members feel empowered to strive to continually maintain and improve standards of care—when they view a high level of care as their responsibility and within their control. The nurse's leadership fails when staff regard certification and licensure standards as outside forces of control that are meaningful only when a review process is imminent.

Facilities for the Mentally Ill and Developmentally Disabled

In the late 1970s and early 1980s, the individual rights of the mentally ill and developmentally disabled expanded dramatically. Today these individuals can

Box 4–5. Rights of Residents In Long-Term Care Facilities

1. A dignified existence
2. Self-determination and communication with and access to persons and services inside and outside the facility.
3. Protection and promotion of rights by the long-term care facility in relation to:
   a. Exercise of rights
      1) as a resident of the facility and as a citizen or resident of the United States
      2) freedom from interference, coercion, discrimination, and reprisal from the facility in exercising his or her rights
      3) if legally adjudicated incompetent exercise of rights by the person appointed under State law to act on the resident's behalf
      4) if not legally adjudicated incompetent exercise of rights by a legal-surrogate designated in accordance with State law
   b. Notice of rights
      1) oral and written information in language the resident understands of his or her rights and all facility rules and regulations governing resident conduct and responsibilities
      2) resident or legal representative has the right to
         a) access within 24 hours to clinical records on oral or written request
         b) photocopies of records within 2 working days advance notice to the facility
      3) full information in language the resident can understand of his or her total health status, including but not limited to his or her medical condition
      4) the right to refuse treatment, and to refuse to participate in research
      5) information for persons receiving Medicaid about items for which the person may or may not be charged and information when changes occur in relation to personal charges
      6) information about facility services and related charges and whether or not covered by Medicare
      7) a written description of legal rights
         a) manner of protection of personal funds
         b) requirements and procedures for establishing eligibility for Medicaid
         c) posting of client advocacy groups
         d) statement that resident may file a complaint with the State survey and certification agency concerning resident abuse, neglect, and misappropriation of resident property
      8) name, specialty, and way of contacting the physician responsible for his or her care
      9) display in the facility written information and communicate orally and in writing to applicants for admission information on application for Medicare and Medicaid, and how to receive refunds for previous payments covered by these benefits
      10) inform resident; consult with resident's physician; communicate with resident's legal representative or interested family member when there is
         a) an accident involving the resident which results in injury and has potential for requiring physician intervention
         b) a significant change in the resident's physical, mental, or psychosocial status
         c) a need to alter treatment significantly
         d) a decision to transfer or discharge the resident from the facility
            (and notification to resident or legal representative of change in roommate, change in resident's rights)
   c. Protection of resident funds
      1) resident may manage his or her own financial affairs and the facility may not require residents to deposit their personal funds within the facility
      2) the facility may manage, safeguard, and account for resident funds on written authorization of the resident
      3) funds in excess of $50.00 must be deposited in an interest bearing account
      4) accounting must be according to accepted accounting principles and the facility must
         a) preclude commingling with facility funds
         b) make the financial record available quarterly
      5) the facility must notify a resident on Medicaid if funds available to him or her reach $200.00 less than the resource limit and if the amount in the account plus other exempt resources reaches the amount that may result in the resident's losing eligibility for Medicaid.
      6) facility must convey remaining funds of a deceased resident to the individual or court administering the person's estate
      7) the facility must purchase a surety bond to assure the security of personal funds
      8) the facility may not charge personal funds for items or service for which payment is made under Medicare or Medicaid
   d. Free choice
      The resident has the right to choose:
      1) a personal attending physician
      2) be fully informed in advance about treatment and care and of any changes that may affect the resident's well-being
      3) to participate in planning care and treatment or changes in care and treatment
   e. Privacy and confidentiality
      The resident has the right to personal privacy and confidentiality of personal and clinical records
      1) personal privacy includes accommodations, medical treatment, written and telephone communications, personal care, visits, and meetings of family and resident groups

Box continued on following page

Box 4–5. Rights of Residents in Long-Term Care Facilities (Continued)

2) the resident may approve or refuse the release of personal and clinical records to any individual outside the facility except when the resident is transferred to another facility or record release is required by law

f. Grievances

A resident has the right to

1) voice grievances without discrimination or reprisal including furnished or omitted treatment

2) prompt efforts by the facility to resolve grievances including those with respect to the behavior of other residents

g. Examination of survey results

A resident has the right to

1) examine the results of the most recent survey of the facility

2) receive information from agencies acting as client advocates and be afforded the opportunity to contact these agencies

h. Work

A resident has the right to

1) refuse to perform services for the facility

2) perform services for the facility if he or she chooses, when

a) the facility documents the need or desire for work in the plan of care

b) the plan specifies the nature of the services performed and whether they are voluntary or paid

c) compensation for paid services is at or above the prevailing rates, and

d) the resident agrees to the work arrangement described

i. Mail

The resident has the right to

1) send and promptly receive mail that is unopened

2) have access to stationery, postage, and writing implements at the resident's own expense

j. Access and visitation rights

1) The resident has the right and the facility must provide immediate access to any resident by the following:

a) a representative of the Secretary of the Department of Health and Human Services

b) a representative of the State

c) the resident's individual physician

d) the state long-term care ombudsman

e) the agency responsible for the protection and advocacy system for developmentally disabled individuals

f) the agency responsible for the protection and advocacy system for mentally ill individuals

g) subject to the resident's right to withdraw consent, to immediate family or other relatives

h) subject to reasonable restrictions and the resident's right to withdraw consent, others who are visiting with the consent of the resident

2) The facility must provide reasonable access to any resident by any entity or individual that provides health, social, legal, or other services to the resident, subject to the resident's right to deny or withdraw consent at any time

3) The facility must allow representatives of the state ombudsman to examine a resident's clinical records with the permission of the resident or the resident's legal representative consistent with state law

k. The resident has the right to have reasonable access to the use of a telephone where calls can be made without being overheard.

l. The resident has the right to retain and use personal possessions, including some furnishings, and appropriate clothing, as space permits, unless to do so would infringe upon the rights or health and safety of other residents.

m. The resident has the right to share a room with his or her spouse when married residents live in the same facility and both spouses consent to the arrangement.

n. An individual resident may self-administer drugs if the interdisciplinary team has determined the practice is safe.

o. The resident has the right to refuse a transfer within the facility if the purpose of the transfer is to relocate

1) a resident of a skilled nursing facility to a distinct part of the facility that is not a skilled nursing facility (refusal to transfer does not affect the individual's eligibility or entitlement to Medicaid)

2) from the distinct part of the facility that is a nursing facility to a distinct part that is a skilled nursing facility

From *Federal Register*, Vol. 56, No. 187, September 26, 1991 *Code of Federal Regulations*, Part 483, Subpart B, S. 483.10.

▶ Challenge involuntary commitments in courts and have regularly scheduled court review of initially justified commitments

▶ Refuse psychotropic medication

▶ Receive treatment in the least restrictive environment

COMMITMENT PROCEEDINGS AND REVIEW OF INVOLUNTARY COMMITMENTS

Until recently, the mentally ill and developmentally disabled had little ability to protect themselves from involuntary commitment to institutions. Courts routinely ordered such commitments, often on simply the word of family or friend and a concurring physician. The physician was often the family physician and therefore subject to bias in favor of family rather than advocate for the person whose behavior was subject to question.

New laws that attempt to remedy this bias do not tilt entirely in favor of the individual. Persons judged imminently dangerous to themselves or others may still be involuntarily hospitalized without a court order but must have a commitment hearing in court within a relatively short period of time: days, not weeks or months. At the commitment hearing, the person has the right to be present in court and be represented by an attorney to challenge the commitment. Physicians and family members or other concerned persons supporting the commitment may also present their testimony. Judges make the decision for or against commitment based on the evidence presented.[4,6]

When commitment is ordered, that commitment must be regularly reviewed at intervals specified by state statutes. Typically, review would occur in 1 month, 3 months, 6 months, and every 6 months thereafter. Initial hearings and reviews represent public policy that seeks to preclude persons from being unjustifiably labeled as mentally ill and from being confined for treatment long after the need has ceased to exist.[91]

USE OF PSYCHOTROPIC MEDICATIONS

When psychotropic medications were first introduced in the late 1950s, the socially negative consequences of their physical side effects were unforeseen. These effects included awkward facial and bodily movements that labeled a person as mentally ill. Concerns then arose about the practice of forcibly medicating the mentally ill because the side effects of the medications could be viewed as worse than the mental illness itself.[46] This led to law that supports refusal of psychotropic medications, even for involuntarily committed patients, unless an emergency situation exists.

An emergency is defined as a person's being an immediate threat of harm to self or others.[50,75,81]

A corollary to the mentally ill individual's right to refuse psychotropic medication is the right to receive information about the side effects of the medications. In this respect, the law mirrors the responsibility of physicians to provide information to persons so that they can make a decision about whether to consent to invasive physical procedures.

TREATMENT IN THE LEAST RESTRICTIVE ENVIRONMENT

The third change provides both the mentally ill and the developmentally disabled with the right to individual treatment plans that provide for care in the least restrictive environment. The law developed from a Pennsylvania case: *Romeo v. Youngberg* (1980).[82] In this case, the restrictive environment included shackling a mentally retarded person. This case and others have led facilities to also examine circumstances that lead to seclusion as a treatment for mentally ill persons.[8,9] Like the law governing use of restraints in long-term care facilities, it is of foremost importance that the treatment be used for therapy rather than simply the convenience of the staff.

NURSING RESPONSIBILITIES IN FACILITIES FOR THE MENTALLY ILL AND DEVELOPMENTALLY DISABLED

The nurse's first responsibility is to be aware of the client's legal rights. The nurse's ensuing responsibility is to follow through on the client's rights with nursing actions that ensure implementation of those rights.

Because interdisciplinary care characterizes treatment of the mentally ill and developmentally disabled, the nurse will act as advocate for client rights as a member of a health care team. The nurse brings to the team a knowledge of the client that derives from the unique data base of regular and frequent encounters with clients. This is true when care is institutionally based. The nurse increasingly maintains that advantage when clients are followed at home and in group home settings.

To team deliberations, the nurse brings first-hand knowledge of client behaviors that indicate readiness for discharge and release from involuntary commitment. The nurse is also in a unique position to identify behaviors that indicate when restrictive measures such as seclusion should be initiated. The nurse can also identify behaviors that indicate that those restrictive measures should be terminated. The nurse also has opportunities to identify behaviors that lead to emergency situations in which clients put themselves or others at risk. This puts the nurse in a unique position to identify interventions that have worked successfully to avoid escalation of those situations to the emergency level.

Careful attention to responsibility for documentation of the nurse's observations and interventions puts the nurse in a unique position to take additional responsibility for raising questions as to which interventions produce desirable outcomes. Attempts to answer those questions acknowledge the ultimate right of clients to have care that will permit effective coping with their mental illness or developmental disability.

CONSUMER RIGHTS, HEALTH CARE PROVIDER RESPONSIBILITIES, AND HEALTH CARE RESOURCES

Organ Transplantation

What are organ donor rights? What are recipient rights? What approaches has the law used to facilitate donation of organs? These questions are important because organ transplants result in increasingly longer survival times, and some, like bone marrow transplants, offer the possibility of a normal life span. The answers to these questions depend on the critical fact that organ availability has never been able to meet the demand.[79]

UNIFORM ANATOMICAL GIFT ACT

The National Conference of Commissioners on Uniform State Laws adopted the Uniform Anatomical Gift Act in 1968. Since that time, all states have developed versions of the act. The Uniform Anatomical Gift Act provided for donations by persons capable of decision making who are of legal age, designated types of donees such as hospitals and teaching institutions, and introduced the concept of the donor card as evidence of the person's desire to make an anatomical gift.

A 1987 amendment to the Uniform Anatomical Gift Act eliminated the need for witnesses to the donor card, made the gift irrevocable and not subject to overriding by next of kin at death, provided that persons not wishing to donate organs may affirmatively assert that right in writing, and expanded the list of persons who can make donations at death in the absence of the decedent's own expression of wishes.[79] These amendments have not been adopted by all states.

INCREASING THE DONATION OF ORGANS

The donation of organs is a right held by individuals when they are alive but becomes operational only at death. However, because the body is legally treated as property at death, the wishes of a person in life to donate organs at death can be overridden by next of kin who assume custody of the body at death. Relatives may have difficulty accepting the wishes of the person and may also be repelled by the thought of mutilating the deceased person. For these reasons, they may refuse to donate organs. To overcome this problem, the law has developed a number of approaches to increase organ donation.

Presumed Consent. Many European countries use the concept of presumed consent for organ donations. **Presumed consent** is a method of increasing donation of organs by assuming a person wishes to donate organs unless the person has clearly expressed a desire to the contrary. The approach makes it unnecessary to approach families of persons with requests for donation at a time when their decision-making capabilities may be colored by bereavement.

Required Request and Routine Inquiry. United States law has generally assumed an intermediate stance, with states passing routine inquiry or required request legislation. **Routine inquiry** is a method of encouraging donation of organs that calls for inquiry on hospital admission as to whether the person has indicated the desire to be an organ donor. Under these laws, paramedics, police, and firefighters may also have a legal duty to make a reasonable search for documentation of organ donor status.

Required request is an approach to encouraging organ donation that mandates that health care facilities develop a process for requesting organ donation from appropriate family members at the time of the potential donor's death or when death is anticipated. When the person's wishes are known, that information becomes an important consideration in the consent process.

In the OBRA of 1986, Congress required hospitals receiving Medicare and Medicaid funds to develop written protocols for identifying potential organ donors.[64] The protocols must also provide reasonable assurance that families will be offered the option of donation and that the regional organ procurement organization is notified. Because few hospitals do not receive Medicare and Medicaid funding, this federal law, in effect, mandates required request even in states without such laws.

As indicated previously, however, the person's desires are only a consideration, not an enforceable right. Some states have enacted laws that permit donation of certain tissues—such as corneas—when next of kin have given no actual notice of objection.

Requiring Donation of Organs by Relatives. Can related individuals be required to donate organs? Adults capable of decision making cannot be required to donate organs.

What about children and other persons incapable of personal decision making? Courts have taken a mixed approach. A Kentucky court determined a retarded child would be more traumatized by the death of his brother than by any ill effect he might suffer from the organ donation.[95] On the other hand, a Wisconsin court found no benefit would accrue a retarded individual if he donated a kidney to a brother with whom he had no relationship.[70]

A 1990 Illinois Supreme Court decision found it not in the best interest of twin half brothers to be tested as potential bone marrow donors to a half brother with whom they had no contact and with whom they were related only through their father, with whom they also had no contact.[26] A court has agreed that parents have the right to consent to kidney transplantation from one identical twin to the other using the rationale of negligible risks to donor and recipient.[44] Thus, the answer to the question about children and other persons incapable of decision making is not clear-cut, although the quality and kind of relationship influence the decision of the court.

SHARING INFORMATION ABOUT DONOR AND DONEE

Can organ donors' families know the identity of the recipients of the organs? This is a complex area of law involving the confidentiality of patient records, the duty of physicians and hospitals to patients, and the privacy of donors and donees.

Bylaws of the United Network for Organ Sharing (UNOS) permit sharing of information about donors only with potential donee institutions, not individual recipients. This information sharing does not include specific identification such as names and social security numbers. Information sharing about donors and donees may be permitted by some state laws. To avoid unwarranted breaches of confidentiality, persons involved would have to consent to this information sharing.

DISTRIBUTING ORGANS AND FINANCING ORGAN TRANSPLANTATION

Given organ scarcity, how is the distribution of organs organized? What laws influence the distribution of organs? Can organs be bought? Who pays for organ transplants?

The National Organ Transplant Act of 1984 created the federal Task Force on Organ Transplantation and the Organ Procurement and Transplantation Network. The nationally based Organ Procurement and Transplantation Network authorizes financial assistance to

---

Box 4–6. Responsibilities of Organ Procurement Organizations

Responsibilities of the Organ Procurement and Transplantation Network

▶ Authorize financial assistance to regional organ procurement organizations.
▶ Maintain a registry of recipients.
▶ Use a computerized matching system.

Responsibilities of Regional Organ Procurement Organizations

▶ Establish procurement agreements.
▶ Educate public and professionals.
▶ Procure, preserve, and allocate organs according to established protocols.
▶ Coordinate with other procurement agencies.

---

procurement organizations, maintains a registry of potential recipients, and uses a computerized matching system so that organs can be fairly distributed. The Department of Health and Human Services awarded the contract for network operations to the UNOS, which had previously operated a computerized matching program.[79] At present, the UNOS also maintains a scientific registry to gather statistical information on organ recipients. The National Organ Transplant Act makes the sale of organs for profit a criminal act.

Organ procurement organizations (OPOs) are regionally based organizations responsible for establishing procurement agreements with hospitals in their service areas; educating public and professionals; procuring, preserving, and allocating organs according to established protocols; and coordinating activities with other organ procurement agencies. The responsibilities of national and regional OPOs are compared in Box 4–6. OPOs and hospitals performing transplant procedures must abide by UNOS policies. The Health Omnibus Programs Extension Act of 1988 extended OPO responsibilities to require OPOs to log 50 donors per year, perform appropriate testing to prevent transmission of acquired immune deficiency syndrome, and establish a voluntary bone marrow registry.

The 1988 act also funds immunosuppressive therapy. Since 1972, Medicare coverage had been available for kidney dialysis, kidney transplantation, and kidney procurement. In 1986, Medicare began to cover liver transplantation under specific circumstances, and in 1987 Medicare extended coverage to heart transplantation.[79] Other insurers have begun to fund transplants because the procedures have become "less experimental" in nature.[29]

ALLOCATING ORGANS

What characteristics are considered in positioning a potential organ recipient on a waiting list? Because the organ supply does not meet the demand, persons responsible for organ allocation must address the ethical principle of justice. Age as a criterion has received less consideration because success of transplantation has escalated at both ends of the age spectrum. Patient compliance after the transplant is always a consideration. Ability to return to work, improved quality of life, and lengthened life span may also be considered.

When an organ becomes available, who on the waiting list receives that organ? UNOS guidelines for extrarenal transplants include considerations of blood type, size, medical urgency, geographic location, and waiting time. For kidney transplants, controversy currently exists over whether waiting time should be weighted more heavily than tissue type. The reason for this is the success of cyclosporine decreasing the need for highly matched kidneys. UNOS guidelines further require that, when any organ becomes available, it first be offered within the service area of the OPO, then in the UNOS region, and then within a 500-mile radius of the hospital.[29]

Ethical concerns have also been raised in relation to the racial distribution of organs as initial evidence raises questions about UNOS's policy of awarding points for histocompatibility seeming to bias distribution in favor of Caucasian recipients. A lower organ donation rate also exists among African Americans.[5]

The use of anencephalic infants as organ donors is also an issue. These infants do not meet current definitions of brain death because brainstem function exists and therefore mechanical support for respiration is unnecessary.[14] Right-to-life groups argue that redefining brain death statutes to include anencephalic infants would, like assisted suicide, begin to support active voluntary euthanasia. In this case, parental consent would make the act voluntary.

Others argue that establishing legal guidelines for diagnosis, parental voluntary choice, review of decisions by ethics committees, and review of disputed decisions by courts would ensure an ethically sound process.[67] UNOS has taken the position that society is not ready yet to clearly make this decision.[29]

YOUR RESPONSIBILITY IN ORGAN TRANSPLANTATION

Nurses touch the lives of both donors and recipients of organ transplants. Nurses' responsibilities may include assisting with the sensitive conversations between provider and family when the possibility of organ donation must be raised. Responsibilities also include assisting the recipient in exploring the feelings that stem from dealing with the reality that another person needed to die in order for him or her to live.

The nurse's technical expertise in provision of the specialized care required for all transplant recipients is essential to the success of any transplant team. On the other hand, the nurse sitting on a transplant recipient selection committee has the responsibility for bringing both nursing wisdom and concerns to those deliberations.

Access to Health Care

As this chapter is being written, the United States has committed itself to change its health care system to one that will be accessible to all its citizens regardless of financial means. When the United States achieves this goal, the country will mirror opportunities of developed countries throughout the world. Like Canada, all citizens will have access to a health care package that includes preventive as well as illness care. In effect, the nation will have created a right to health care not tied to employment or some status such as level of poverty.

Access to care will not ensure that care occurs. First, potential consumers of care will need to be responsible for taking advantage of this new opportunity. However, nurses know that lack of availability of financial resources is not the only barrier to accessing health care. Every day community health nurses note that lack of transportation, working hours, difficulty finding substitute care givers for children and the elderly, and lack of trust and respect for health care providers serve as deterrents to accessing health care. Other deterrents are more personal. They include lack of appreciation of the benefits of healthy behaviors, lack of faith in self to incorporate healthy behaviors in one's lifestyle, valuing the satisfactions of the moment over the long-term commitment required to maintain health, and perhaps just having a different view of what particular type of health care is desirable.

The removal of financial barriers to access provides nurses with the opportunity to work in partnership with consumers of care to remove the remaining barriers and perhaps redefine health care need. To paraphrase George Bernard Shaw, others may not desire the same things, so do not do unto others as they would do unto you. First, determine what they want and need. Again to paraphrase, the new freedom of access does not fail to bring with it new responsibilities.

Rights and responsibilities move in tandem. One cannot exist without the other. As a nurse educated to provide nursing care services and to be a critical player on the health care team, you are responsible for assisting in the implementation of consumer rights. It is important that you apply both the legal and ethical, as well as the clinical, bases of knowledge to your responses to consumers. Drawing on those legal and ethical perspectives helps set you apart as a professional health care provider.

Summary

- ▶ Types of rights include ethical, legal, moral, fundamental, and earned rights.
- ▶ Health care consumer rights began to be acknowledged in law and in organizational statements beginning in the 1960s. Acute care for the elderly and a broad spectrum of care for the impoverished began to be reimbursed. Workplace law affecting hiring and safety was initiated. The law eventually recognized residents' rights in long-term facilities. Rights first enunciated in the AHA's Patient's Bill of

Rights eventually became customarily acknowledged — though not always legally recognized — rights.
- ▶ A key consumer right is informed consent. The components of informed consent to treatment always include (1) the nature of the treatment or procedure, (2) the risks, benefits, and consequences, (3) alternatives to the procedure and supporting information, (4) the effect of no treatment or no procedure, including the effect on the prognosis and material risks associated with no treatment.
- ▶ Physicians are legally required to obtain informed consent to invasive procedures. However, as members of the health care team, nurses should take responsibility for dealing appropriately with consumer concerns about procedures that legally require informed consent. Nurses should (1) identify when a consumer desires to withdraw consent to a treatment or procedure, (2) be aware of legal limitations on the decision of parents and guardians in the care of infants, (3) inform consumers about medications administered, treatments, and other interventions carried out by nurses, and (4) support use of facility bioethics committees when decision-making conflicts occur.
- ▶ The prime concern of the institutional review boards that examine research proposals is protecting human subjects from unwarranted risks. Protection of subject identity is another concern in review of research. All federally funded research must follow federal regulations. Privately funded research frequently adopts these guidelines.
- ▶ Every person has a right to refuse life-sustaining measures. Persons who become incapable of expressing their wishes may have evidenced that right in conversations with family and friends or through an advance directive: a living will or durable power of attorney for health care. When persons have never expressed their wish or have always been incapable of such decision making — as in the case of those who are severely mentally retarded — surrogate decision makers must do their best to decide in the persons' best interests or as they believe the persons would have decided had they been capable.
- ▶ The *Cruzan* decision influenced federal and state legislation to recognize legally a person's right to forgo life-sustaining measures.
- ▶ Nurses have a responsibility to make persons aware of their right to forgo life-sustaining measures. Nurses need to be aware of facility policy and procedure on life-sustaining measures. Documenting client decisions in the client's record is a critical responsibility.
- ▶ The right of a woman to terminate a pregnancy under *Roe v. Wade* continues. However, the right has been modified by many state laws to require that minors obtain the consent of their parents or, when this may result in harm to the minor, of a court. The modifications to the right to terminate a pregnancy are inconsistent with law that permits minors free access to contraceptives. The law has

consistently upheld the right of women to make reproductive decisions without the consent of their spouse or sexual partner.

▶ Because substance abuse can harm a fetus, controversy exists over the treatment of pregnant substance abusers.

▶ Rights of residents of long-term care facilities are protected by certification and licensure procedures.

▶ In long-term care facilities, the nurse has a responsibility to recognize and support residents' rights by being personally aware of rights, ensuring that residents understand their rights, and responding to residents' requests for exercise of rights. The nurse also has a responsibility to ensure that certification and licensure standards are consistently met between periods of review.

▶ The mentally ill and developmentally disabled can challenge involuntary commitments in court, can refuse psychotropic medication, and have a right to treatment in the least restrictive environment.

▶ The nurse should act as an advocate to ensure that those rights are honored. As a member of an interdisciplinary team, the nurse is in a unique position to identify interventions that succeed or do not succeed with clients. Thus, the nurse can make an important contribution to enhancing clients' effective coping with their illness or disability.

▶ Legal and ethical concerns in organ transplantation revolve around the acquisition and allocation of organs.

▶ Nurses have a responsibility to discuss organ donation with families, explore feelings of recipients of organs, provide technical expertise on the transplant team, and serve on transplant recipient selection committees.

▶ The creation of a United States health care system that is financially accessible to everyone will not diminish the responsibility of the nurse to continue efforts to remove other personal and socioeconomic barriers to care.

Bibliography

1. Age Discrimination in Employment Act Pub. L. 90-202, Dec. 15, 1967, Stat. 602 (rev. 1978 & 1986).
2. American Hospital Association. (1972). *A patient's bill of rights* (rev. 1992). Chicago, IL: American Hospital Association.
3. American Nurses Association. (1985). *Code for nurses with interpretive statements.* Kansas City, MO: American Nurses Association.
4. Appelbaum, P.S. (1984). Is the need for treatment constitutionally acceptable as a basis for civil commitment? *Law, Medicine & Health Care, 12*(4), 144–149.
5. Arnason, W.B. (1991) Directed donation: the relevance of race. *Hastings Center Report, 2*(6), 13–19.
6. Arboleda-Florez, J., & Holly, H. (1984). How Alberta psychiatrists view commitment criteria and the problem of predicting dangerousness. *Canadian Journal of Psychiatry, 29*, 38–41.
7. Baker, F.M. (1987). Competent for what? *Journal of the National Medical Association, 79*, 715–720.
8. Betemps, E.J., Somoza, E., & Buncher, C.R. (1993). Hospital characteristics, diagnoses, and staff reasons associated with use of seclusion and restraint. *Hospital and Community Psychiatry, 44*, 367–371.
9. Betemps, E.J., Buncher, C.R., & Oden, M. (1992). Length of time spent in seclusion and restraint by patients at 82 VA medical centers. *Hospital and Community Psychiatry, 43*, 912–914.
10. Boland, R. (1990). Recent developments in abortion law in industrialized countries. *Law, Medicine & Health Care, 18*, 404–418.
11. Bowen v. American Hospital Association, 106 S Ct 2101 (1986).
12. Brophy v. New England Sinai Hospital, 398 Mass. 417, 497 N.E.2d 626 (1986).
13. Canterbury v. Spence, 464 F.2d 772 (1972).
14. Capron, A.M. (1987). Anencephalic donors: separate the dead from the dying. *Hastings Center Report, 17*(1), 5–9.
15. Cate, F., & Gill, B. (1991). *The patient self-determination act: Issues and opportunities.* Washington, DC: Annenberg Washington Program in Communications Policy of Northwestern University.
16. Chervernak, F.A., & McCullough, L.B. (1991). Justified limits on refusing intervention. *Hastings Center Report, 21*(2), 12–18.
17. Clayton, E.W. (1987). From *Rogers* to *Rivers:* The rights of the mentally ill to refuse medication. *American Journal of Law and Medicine, 13*, 7–52.
18. Code of Federal Regulations, S.46.101 (1981).
19. Code of Federal Regulations, S. 46.401–S.46.408 (1983).
20. Code of Federal Regulations, S.46.201–S.46.203 (1975), S.46.204–S.46.205 (1975, amended 1978), S.46.206 (1975, amended 1981), S.46.207–S.46.209 (1975, amended 1975).
21. Code of Federal Regulations, S.46.301–S.46.304 (1978), S.46.305 (1978, amended 1981), S.46.306.
22. 45 Code of Federal Regulations, S1340 (b)(2) (1984).
23. Cohen, S.S. (1990). Health care policy and abortion: a comparison. *Nursing Outlook, 38*(1), 20–25.
24. Cranford, R. (1988). The persistent vegetative state: the medical reality (getting the facts straight). *Hastings Center Report, 21*(2), 36–46.
25. Cruzan v. Director, Missouri Dept. of Health, 497 U.S. 110 S Ct 2841 (1990).
26. Curran v. Bosze, No. 70501 (Ill S. Ct., 1990).
27. Curriden, M. (1990). Holding mom accountable. *American Bar Association Journal, 76*(3), 50–53.
28. Daniels, N. (1991). Duty to treat or right to refuse? *Hastings Center Report, 21*(2), 36–46.
29. Davis, F.D. (1989). Organ procurement and transplantation. *Nursing Clinics of North America, 24*, 823–836.
30. Davis v. Hubbard, 506 F. Supp. 915 (1980).
31. Delio v. Westchester County Hospital, 516 N.Y.S.2d 677 (A.D. 2 Dept. 1987).
32. In re Dinnerstein, 6 Mass. App. 466, 380 N.E.2d 134 (Ct. App., 1978).
33. Eisenstadt v. Baird (1972) 405 US 438, 31 L Ed 2d 349, 92 S Ct 1029.
34. Emergency Medical and Active Labor Treatment Act, COBRA, Pub. L. No. 99-272, S 9121, 42 U.S.C.A. S 1395dd (1986).
35. Federal family planning program set to expand after 12-year stall. (1993, March). *The Nation's Health,* p. 5.
36. Family planning groups try again to block "gag rule". (1992, May–June). *The Nation's Health,* p. 5.
37. In re Farrell, 108 N.J. 335, 529 A.2d 404 (1987).
38. 48 Federal Register 9630, 1983.
39. Freedman, B., Fuks, A., & Weijer, C. (1993). In loco parentis: minimal risk as an ethical threshold for research upon children. *Hastings Center Report, 23*(2), 13–19.
40. Freedman, B., & Glass, K.C. (1990). Weiss v. Solomon: A study in institutional responsibility for clinical research. *Law, Medicine & Health Care, 18*(4), 395–403.
41. In re Gardner, 534 A.2d 947 (Maine 1987).
42. Gostin, L. (1991). Ethical principles for the conduct of human research: population-based research and ethics. *Law, Medicine & Health Care, 19*, 191–201.
43. Griswold v. Connecticut (1965) 381 US 479, 14 L Ed 2d 510, 85 S Ct 1678.
44. Hart v. Brown, 289 A.2d 386 (Conn., 1972).
45. Health Omnibus Programs Extension Act of 1988, Pub.L.No. 100-607, S401, 102 Stat. 3048, 3114 (1988).
46. Inoue, F. (1979). Adverse reactions of antipsychotic drugs. *Drug Intelligence and Clinical Pharmacy, 13*, 198–208.

47. Inspector General v. The Hanlester Health Network, Nos. C-186 through C-192, C208, and C213, Department of Health and Human Services, Departmental Appeals Board, Civil Remedies Division, March 1, 1991.

48. Katz, J., & Greene, E. (1992). *Managing quality: A guide to monitoring and evaluating nursing services.* St. Louis: Mosby-Year Book.

49. Katz, R.J. (1972). *Experimentation with human beings.* New York: Russell Sage Foundation.

50. *In re* K.K.B., 609 P.2d 747 (Oklahoma, 1980)

51. Kowalski, S. (1993). Assisted suicide: where do nurses draw the line? *Nursing & Health Care,* 14(2), 70–76.

52. Lee, L.L. (1991). Ethical issues related to research involving children. *Journal of Pediatric Oncology Nursing,* 8(1), 24–29.

53. McCarthy, C.R., & Porter, J.P. (1991). Confidentiality: the protection of personal data in epidemiological and clinical research trials. *Law, Medicine & Health Care,* 19, 238–241.

54. Medical Research Council of Canada. (1987). *Guidelines on research involving human subjects.* Ottawa, Ontario, Canada: Minister of Supply and Services.

55. Miller, T.E. (1990). Public policy in the wake of *Cruzan:* a case study of New York's health care proxy law. *Law, Medicine & Health Care,* 18, 360–367.

56. National Organ Transplant Act of 1984, Pub. L.No.98-507, 98 Stat. 2339 (1984).

57. National Research Act Pub. L. 93-348, July 12, 1974, 88 Stat. 342.

58. N.Y. Public Health Law S2440-2446 (McKinney).

59. Occupational Safety and Health Act Pub. L. 91-596, Dec. 29, 1970, 84 Stat. 1590.

60. Ohio Revised Code S.1337.17.

61. Ohio Revised Code (LTC)

62. Ohio Revised Code (Mental Health) (1990) 497 US 502, 111 L Ed 2d 405, 110 S Ct 2972.

63. Ohio v. Akron Center for Reproductive Health (1990) 497 US 502, 111 L. Ed 2d 405, 1105 Ct 2972.

64. Omnibus Budget Reconciliation Act of 1986, Pub. L. No. 99-509, S9318, 100 Stat 1874 (1986).

65. Omnibus Budget Reconciliation Act of 1987, Pub. L. No. 100-203, Dec. 22, 1987, 101 Stat. 1330.

66. *The Oxford dictionary of quotations* (2nd ed.). (1955). London: Oxford University Press.

67. Paliokas, K.L. (1989). Anencephalic newborns as organ donors: an assessment of "death" and legislative policy. *William and Mary Law Review,* 31, 197–239.

68. Paltrow, L. (1989). Fetal abuse: should we recognize it as a crime? No. *American Bar Association Journal,* 75(8), 39.

69. Patient Self Determination Act

70. *In re* Guardianship of Pescinski, 67 Wis. 2d 4, 226 N.W.2d 180 (Wis., 1975).

71. Planned Parenthood of Southeastern Pennsylvania v. Casey, 60 U.S.L.W. 4795, 1992 WL 142546 (U.S.Pa).

72. Presser, S., & Presser, A.L. (1991). At issue: first Amendment: what will be the impact of Rust v. Sullivan? *American Bar Association Journal,* 77(8), 32–33.

73. *In re* Quinlan, 70 N.J. 10, 355 A.2d 647, *cert. denied sub nom* Garger v. New Jersey, 429 U.S. 992 (1976), *overruled in part, In re* Conroy, 98 N.J. 321, 486 A.2d 1209 (1985).

74. Rehabilitation Act of 1973, 29 U.S.C., S701-709, 720-724, 730-732, 740, 741, 750, 760-764, 770-776, 87 Stat 355 (1973).

75. Rennie v. Klein, 653 F.2d 836 (1981).

76. *In re* Requena, 213 N.J. Super. 475, 517 A.2d 886 (Super. Ct. Chan. Div.), *aff'd,* 213 N.J. Super. 443, 517 A.2d 869 (Super. Ct. App. Div., 1986) (per curiam).

77. Robertson, J. (1989). Fetal abuse: should we recognize it as a crime? Yes. *American Bar Association Journal,* 75(8), 38.

78. Robertson, J.A. (1991). Second thoughts on living wills. *Hastings Center Report,* 21(6), 6–9.

79. Rodgers, S.B. (1989). Legal framework for organ donation and transplantation. *Nursing Clinics of North America,* 24, 837–850.

80. Roe v. Wade, 410 U.S. 113 (1973).

81. Rogers v. Okin, 478 F. Supp. 1342 (D. Mass. 1979), *aff'd in part, rev'd in part,* 634 F. 2d 650 (1st Cir. 1980), *vacated sub nom* Rogers v. Mills 457 U.S. 291 (1982), *opinion on certified issues sub nom.* Rogers v. Commissioner of Dept. of Mental Health, 390 Mass. 489, 458 N.E.2d 308 (1983), *opinion on remand sub nom.* Rogers v. Okin, 239 F.2d 1 (1st Cir. 1984).

82. Romeo v. Youngberg, 644 F.2d 147 (1980), *cert. granted,* 101 S. Ct. 2313.

83. Rouse, F. (1990). Where are we heading after *Cruzan? Law, Medicine & Health Care,* 18(4), 353–359.

84. Rozovsky, L.E., & Rozovsky, F.A. (1986). Consent and marital status—the legalities. *Canadian Operating Room Nursing Journal,* 4(3), 19–20.

85. Rozovsky, L.E., & Rozovsky, F.A. (1987). Should nurses be involved in consent? *Canadian Critical Care Nursing Journal,* 4(1), 8–9.

86. Rozovsky, L.E., & Rozovsky, F.A. (1990). Consent to treatment: four legal myths. *Canadian Critical Care Nursing Journal,* 7(1), 15–16.

87. *In re* Ruiz, 27 Ohio Misc. 2d 31 (Ct. Comm. Pleas, 1986).

88. Rust v. Sullivan (1991, US) 114 L Ed 2d 233, 111 S Ct 1759.

89. Satz v. Perlmutter, 362 So.2d 160 (Fla. Dist. Ct. App. 1978), *aff'd,* 379 So.2d 359 (Fla., 1980).

90. Schloendorff v. Society of New York Hospitals, 211 N.Y. 125, 105 N.E. 92 (1914).

91. Schwartz, H.I., Appelbaum, P.S., & Kaplan, R.D. (1984). Clinical judgments in the decision to commit. *Archives of General Psychiatry,* 41, 811–815.

92. Scofield, G.R. (1991). Is consent useful when resuscitation isn't? *Hastings Center Report,* 21(6), 28–36.

93. *In re* Spring, 380 Mass. 629, 405 N.E.2d 115 (1980).

94. *In re* Storar, 52 N.Y.2d 363, 420 N.E.2d 64, 438 N.Y.S.2d 266, *cert. denied,* 454 U.S. 858 (1981).

95. Strunk v. Strunk, 445 S.W.2d 145 (Ky. Ct. App., 1969).

96. Superintendent of Belchertown State School v. Saikewicz, 373 Mass. 728, 370 N.E.2d 417 (1977).

97. Thomas, S.B., & Quinn, S.C. (1991). Public health then and now: the Tuskegee syphilis study, 1932 to 1972: implications for HIV education and AIDS risk education programs in the black community. *American Journal of Public Health,* 81, 1498–1505.

98. Uniform Anatomical Gift Act of 1968 SS 1-11, 8A U.L.A. 30 (1989); Uniform Anatomical Gift Act of 1987 SS 1-17, 8A U.L.A.2 (1989).

99. Weber, G. (1993). Tips on implementing the Patient Self Determination Act. *Nursing & Health Care,* 14(2), 86–91.

100. Webster v. Reproductive Health Services (1989) 492 US 490, 106 L Ed 2d 410, 109 S Ct 3040.

101. Yeasavage, J.E. (1984). A study of mandatory review of civil commitment. *Archives of General Psychiatry,* 41, 305–308.

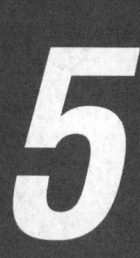

Chapter 5

▼ Delivery Systems, Finance, and Policy in Health Care

▼ *. . . government has a special obligation to ensure that the public interest is served by whatever measures are adopted.*

**Institute of Medicine
1988**

▼ CHAPTER OUTLINE

HEALTH CARE DELIVERY SYSTEMS
    Types of Health Care Services
    Health Care Agencies and
      Personnel
HEALTH CARE FINANCE
    The Price of Health Care
    Methods of Payment for Health
      Care

Cost Containment
    The Economics of Nursing Care
HEALTH CARE POLICY AND POLITICS
    Policy Defined
    Politics Defined
    Politics, Policy, and Values
    Spheres of Political Action

▼ KEY TERMS

Chaplain
Cost containment
Diagnosis-related group
Dietitians
For-profit agency
Health Care Financing
  Administration
Health maintenance
  organizations
Laboratory technologists
Medicaid

Medicare
Not-for-profit agency
Occupational therapists
Pharmacists
Physical therapists
Preferred provider
  organizations
Primary care
Professional review
  organizations
Proprietary agency

Radiologic technologists
Rehabilitation
Respiratory technologists
Secondary care
Social worker
Tertiary care
Workers' compensation

▼ *LEARNING OBJECTIVES*

After studying this chapter, you should be able to

1. *Describe the goals of the health care delivery system.*
2. *List the ways in which health care agencies are classified.*
3. *Describe the members of the health care team.*
4. *Discuss the roles of nurses in the health care team.*
5. *Explain changes in health care financing during the past 50 years.*
6. *Describe how cost containment in health care spending came about.*
7. *Contrast prospective payment and retrospective payment.*
8. *Identify factors that will continue to cause changes in the health care system.*
9. *Explain why nurses need to become knowledgeable about policy and politics.*
10. *List spheres of influence for nurses' political action.*

The health care delivery system in the United States has traditionally been a system of illness care delivery. The system is complex, and negotiating through it can be difficult for clients. Health care is also extremely expensive, with multiple types of financing. The technology and sophisticated procedures available in the United States are the best in the world, but many people have lacked access to even the most basic care. The health care system is in a state of change.

Encouraging signs indicate that the system may be different in the future. Experts predict that reform will take place before the year 2000, early in the careers of today's students.

HEALTH CARE DELIVERY SYSTEMS

The very words "health care delivery system" speak to the coming change in addressing health and illness needs of clients in the 21st century. Most planners believe that one of the essential parts of an improved health care system will be an emphasis on prevention and the active participation of clients in their own health choices. Whereas scientists will continue to search for and find cures to many illnesses, health care services will increasingly emphasize holistic care, which means treating the whole person, not just the diseased part. Another prediction is that health care professionals and government officials will work together to return the environment to a healthier balance, thus reducing pollution-related disease.

The U.S. government has taken an important first step. In 1990, a consortium of nearly 300 national health organizations, the United States Public Health Service, and state health departments together drafted goals and objectives for improving the health of the nation's citizens by the year 2000. The resultant report, *Healthy People 2000: National Health Promotion and Disease Prevention Objectives*, sets out three main goals, as outlined in Box 5–1. How well these goals are met will be determined by the commitment of health care providers, citizens, and government officials (elected and appointed) to achieve desired health outcomes through effective use of the political process.

Types of Health Care Services

The four major types of health services are health promotion, illness prevention, diagnosis and treatment, and rehabilitation and long-term care.

HEALTH PROMOTION

Health promotion services help people remain healthy, prevent diseases and injuries, and promote healthier lifestyles. These services require clients' active participation and cannot be performed solely by a health care provider. Health promotion services are based on the assumption that clients who participate in certain lifestyle changes are likely to avoid heart attacks, lung cancers, and other lifestyle-related diseases.

Prenatal classes are one example of health promotion services. By learning good nutritional habits, an expectant mother can take care of both herself and her baby during pregnancy and after delivery. Good nutrition increases the chances of a normal pregnancy and the birth of a healthy baby. Other examples include aerobic exercise classes and smoking cessation classes aimed at increasing the health of an individual's cardiovascular and respiratory systems.

ILLNESS PREVENTION

Illness prevention depends on the identification of risk factors. Risk factors are characteristics that increase a person's chances of developing a specific disease or condition. When risk factors, such as a family history of

---

Box 5–1. *Healthy People 2000 Goals*

1. Increase the span of healthy life for Americans
2. Reduce health disparities among Americans
3. Achieve access to preventive services for all Americans

▼▼▼

From U.S. Department of Health and Human Services (1990). *Healthy people 2000: National health promotion and disease prevention objectives.* Washington, DC.

heart disease, are identified, illness prevention services assist clients in reducing the impact of those risk factors on their health and well-being. These services also involve the clients' active participation.

Prevention services differ from health promotion services in that they address health problems *after* risk factors are identified; whereas health promotion services seek to *prevent* development of risk factors. For example, a health promotion program might teach the detrimental effects of alcohol and drugs on the person's health for preventing the person from using alcohol and drugs. Illness prevention services would be used when the client has been using alcohol or drugs and is at risk for developing health problems as a result. In reality, the boundary between health promotion and illness prevention is often blurred. Box 5–2 lists samples of activities in these two areas.

DIAGNOSIS AND TREATMENT

Our health care system has traditionally placed heavy emphasis on diagnosis and treatment. Early diagnosis, detecting disease as soon as the first signs occur, has been the focus of most physicians' efforts. Modern technology has enabled the medical profession to refine the act of diagnosing illnesses and disorders and to treat them more effectively.

Health care technology has allowed physicians to cure illnesses and disorders that have plagued humans for thousands of years. As a result, much human suffering has been avoided, and newer scientific advances permit many tests and treatments to be performed noninvasively, or without cutting into the body. Among these new developments are ultrasound, which examines unborn fetuses for determining whether they are developing normally, and lithotripsy, which disintegrates kidney stones so they can be expelled in the

urine. The future promises more "high-tech" noninvasive technologies.

Yet high-tech services can also cause clients to feel dehumanized when the care givers focus on machines rather than on people. Nurses should remember that clients benefit most when they understand their diagnoses and treatments and can be active participants in the development and implementation of their own treatment plans.

REHABILITATION AND LONG-TERM CARE

Rehabilitation comprises services that help restore the client to the fullest possible level of function and independence after injury or illness. Rehabilitation programs deal with conditions that leave patients with less than full functioning, such as strokes, broken bones, or severe burns. Both clients and their families must be active participants if care is to be successful.

Rehabilitation services should begin immediately after the client's condition has stabilized after an injury or the onset of illness. These services may be provided in institutional settings such as hospitals, in special rehabilitation facilities, in long-term care facilities such as nursing homes, and in the home and the community. The objectives are to assist clients to achieve their potential and to return them to a level of functioning that permits them to be contributing members of society again.

Health Care Agencies and Personnel

The health care delivery system consists of hospitals, clinics, associations, and home health care agencies. These provide any or all of the four major types of health care services: health promotion, illness prevention, diagnosis and treatment, and rehabilitation and long-term care. Hospitals are the most complex health care institutions, and hospital organization will affect the place of nursing in the hospital structure.

Although much health care is delivered in hospital settings, many other agencies are involved in the entire health care delivery system. Organizations that deliver care can be classified in several ways: as governmental or voluntary agencies, as not-for-profit or for-profit agencies, and as health care services providing a specific level of care.

GOVERNMENTAL, OR PUBLIC, AGENCIES

Many governmental, or public, agencies contribute to the health and well-being of our citizens. All are primarily supported by taxes, administered by elected or appointed officials, and tailored to the needs of the communities served.

Local Agencies. Local agencies serve one community, one county, or a few nearby counties. These agencies provide services to both paying and nonpaying citizens. Public health departments are examples of local governmental agencies found in almost every county in the nation. All citizens, whether or not they can pay, are

---

> ### Box 5–2. Illness Prevention and Health Promotion Activities
>
> #### Illness Prevention
>
> Periodical histories/physicals
> Identification of familial/environmental risk factors
> Community health programs
> Promotion of healthy lifestyles to counteract risk factors
> Occupational safety programs (use of eye guards for work that endangers the eyes)
> Environmental safety programs (proper disposal of hazardous waste)
> Legislation that prevents injury/disease (seat restraint laws)
>
> #### Health Promotion/Maintenance
>
> Health education programs (prenatal classes)
> Exercise programs
> Health fairs
> Wellness programs (worksite/school)
> Proper nutrition
> Learning how to balance one's life

eligible for health care through local public health departments. These services usually include immunizations, prenatal care and counseling, well-baby and child clinics, sexually transmitted disease clinics, tuberculosis clinics, and others. Public health nurses sometimes make home visits as well.

State Agencies. State health agencies oversee programs that affect the health of citizens across the state. Examples of state governmental health agencies include state departments of health and environment, departments that regulate and license health professionals such as state boards of nursing, and those that administer Medicaid insurance programs for the poor. These agencies are not typically involved in providing direct care. Instead, they support local agencies that do provide direct care.

Federal Agencies. Federal agencies focus on the health of all the nation's citizens. They promote and conduct health and illness research, provide funding to train health care workers, and assist communities in planning health care services. They also develop health programs and services and provide financial and personnel support to staff them. They establish standards of practice and safety for health care workers and conduct national health education programs on subjects such as the benefits of not smoking, prevention of infectious diseases, and need for prenatal care. Federal agencies include the United States Public Health Service, the National Institutes of Health, the United States Department of Health and Human Services, the Occupational Safety and Health Administration, and the Centers for Disease Control.

In addition, the federal government operates hospitals providing direct care to active-duty military personnel and veterans. A little known but important branch of the United States Public Health Service is the Indian Health Service, which provides health care to Native Americans who live on federal reservations.

VOLUNTARY, OR PRIVATE, AGENCIES

Citizens often voluntarily support agencies working to promote or restore health. When an agency providing health care is supported by private volunteers, it is called a voluntary or private agency. Support is generally through private donations, although many of these agencies apply for governmental grants to support some of their activities.

Voluntary agencies often begin when a group of individuals band together to address a health problem. All their services may initially be performed by volunteers. Later, they may obtain enough donations to hire personnel, staff an office, and expand services. They may be able to secure ongoing funding through grants or organizations like the United Way. Examples of voluntary health agencies are the Visiting Nurses Association, American Heart Association, Hospice, the American Cancer Society, and the Mental Health Association.

NOT-FOR-PROFIT AND FOR-PROFIT AGENCIES

Another way to classify health service delivery is by what is done with the income earned by the agency. A **not-for-profit agency** is one that uses profits to pay personnel, improve services, advertise services, provide educational programs, or otherwise contribute to the mission of the agency. A common misconception is that not-for-profit agencies do not ever make a profit. The reality is that they may make profits, but the profits must be used for the improvement of the agency. Most voluntary agencies are not-for-profit, as are many private hospitals.

For-profit, or **proprietary, agencies,** on the other hand, are health care organizations that may distribute profits to partners or shareholders. The number of for-profit health care agencies has mushroomed over the past decade. Health care is big business and has the potential to be very profitable.

For-profit agencies include numerous home health care companies that send nurses and other health personnel to care for clients at home. There are also several large national chains of for-profit hospitals, such as Hospital Corporation of America.

LEVEL OF HEALTH CARE SERVICES PROVIDED

A third way health care services are classified is by the level of health care services provided.

Primary Care Services. Services provided at the point at which a client first enters the health care system are considered **primary care.** This point may be a student health clinic, health centers in the community, an emergency department, physicians' offices, nurse practitioners' clinics, health clinics at work, and many more. Aydelotte[2] defined the major goals of the primary health care system as providing

► entry into the system
► emergency care
► health maintenance
► long-term care
► treatment of temporary malfunctioning that does not require hospitalization

In addition to treating common health problems, primary care centers are, for many citizens, where much prevention and health promotion take place. Box 5-3 lists examples of primary care agencies.

Secondary Care Services. Agencies providing **secondary care** prevent complications from disease, treat temporary dysfunction requiring hospitalization, evaluate long-term care for clients who may need treatment changes, and provide counseling and therapy not available in primary care settings.[2] Hospitals have traditionally been associated with secondary care.

In addition to hospitals, agencies that provide secondary health services are the home health care agencies, ambulatory care agencies and surgical centers. These agencies offer skilled personnel, easy access,

Box 5-3. Examples of Primary Care Agencies

Ambulatory Care Centers

Ambulatory care centers provide a variety of services ranging from diagnostic to therapeutic; nurse practitioners and clinical nurse specialists may have pivotal roles in providing services in these centers.

Crisis Centers and Hotlines

Hospitals and communities typically offer services to assist citizens experiencing things like suicide, acquired immune deficiency syndrome, herpes, abuse, and psychiatric crisis. Hotlines generally provide information and support. Crisis centers may provide telephone hotlines, direct counseling, limited first aid, ongoing support, and guidance.

Day Care Centers

Formerly thought of for children only, day care centers now also serve the elderly and medically/emotionally impaired. Usually open during daytime hours, some may offer extended hours when there is a need. Respite care for families who need a break from caring for family members in the home or who need help while they work is also provided.

Employment Settings

As managers and employees recognize the benefits of healthy employees, nurses are much in demand to run employee health clinics at the worksite. Services may include histories/physicals, health teaching/promotion, health screens and occupational safety programs.

Home Health Care Agencies

Home health care agencies are a fast-growing service. Nurses and other health care team members (social workers, physical therapists, respiratory therapists, pharmacists, and others) render services traditionally provided in both the home and hospital; even acute care services (home ventilators, intravenous therapy, chemotherapy) are provided.

Managed Care Organizations

To hold down health care costs, many businesses use managed care organizations to provide health care to employees at a prearranged fee; examples of these are

HMOs: Health maintenance organizations are group health agencies providing basic and supplemental services to enrollees at a fixed rate; clients generally may not have much choice as to which physician will care for them; preventive care is stressed.

PPOs: Preferred provider organizations are groups of physicians/hospitals that provide services at a discounted rate; the client chooses which physician in the group they wish to see.

IPAs: Independent practice organizations are "middlemen" in the system; clients pay the IPA for services at a fixed rate, and the IPA pays the providers; profits are shared with the providers, and losses are absorbed by the IPA.

Neighborhood Health Centers

Neighborhood health centers are usually found in areas where citizens are underserved, financially stressed, and at risk; a variety of health care workers provide basic health care and social services support. A recent addition to this category is the health care center run primarily by volunteers to provide health services to the "working poor" (those who have jobs but cannot afford health care insurance).

Physicians' Offices

In general, people seek the services of the physician when they are ill; nurses working in these settings register clients, give medications, take vital signs, assist with examinations, and provide information and education.

Support Groups

Support groups assist individuals with ongoing coping and lifestyle changes. Reach for Recovery assists women who have had mastectomies, Alcoholics Anonymous helps alcoholics stop drinking through a 12-step program; the Dream Machine helps children who are terminally ill have one of their wishes come true; some of these are well funded by agencies, and others are purely voluntary.

---

convenient parking, compact equipment and monitoring systems, medications and anesthesia services, and a financial reimbursement program that rewards shorter lengths of stay and home/community care. The trend toward providing community-based secondary care is expected to continue well into the next century.

Tertiary Care Services. Tertiary care comprises services provided to acutely ill clients, those requiring long-term care, and those needing rehabilitation. Tertiary care also includes provision of care to the terminally ill. Tertiary care usually involves many health professionals working together on multidisciplinary teams to design treatment plans. Agencies providing tertiary care include specialized hospitals such as trauma centers and specialized pediatric centers, long-term care facilities (skilled nursing, intermediate care, and supportive care), rehabilitation centers, and hospices (where care is provided to the terminally ill and their families in the hospital, in the home, or in special centers).

HOSPITAL STRUCTURE AND ORGANIZATION

Institutional structure is the way an agency is organized to do what it is intended to do. The institutional structure of most hospitals includes a governing body; typically, it is a board of trustees, also called a board of directors.

Hospital Governance. In the past, board members were often chosen from two groups: community philanthropists who were expected to donate generously to the facility and physicians who practiced there. Boards were large, met infrequently, and had mainly ceremonial functions.

As the health care environment became more complex, board members were chosen to represent various business and political interests of the community. They were expected to bring knowledge and expertise from the larger business world and to have an appreciation and understanding of hospital operations. Boards now tend to be smaller and carry significant responsibility for the mission of the hospital, the quality of services provided, and the financial status of the organization. Boards are not involved in the day-to-day running of the hospital, but they are responsible for establishing policies governing operations and for ensuring that the policies are executed.

The chief executive officer is the individual responsible for the hospital's overall operation on a daily basis. The chief executive officer usually has a master's degree in business or hospital administration. The responsibilities of the chief executive officer include making sure that the hospital runs efficiently, is cost-effective, and carries out the policies established by the board. The chief executive officer usually sits on the board of trustees.

The Medical Staff. A hospital's medical staff (physicians) may be either employees or independent practitioners. In either case, they must be granted privileges by the board of trustees before they can see clients at that particular institution. They may not simply decide to admit patients to a hospital. First, they must submit evidence that they are qualified and competent and must show periodically that they have kept their skills and knowledge updated.

Medical staffs are usually organized by service (e.g., department of surgery, department of medicine, department of pulmonary medicine). The actions of the medical staff must be approved by the board of trustees, to whom the physicians are responsible. A chief of staff is usually elected by the entire medical staff. Together with the chiefs of the various services, the chief of staff makes important decisions regarding medical policy for the institution. Bylaws govern these activities.

The Nursing Staff. The top nurse in a hospital is known as the nurse executive, vice president for nursing, or director of nursing. Once excluded from decision making, nurse executives of today are often members of the board of trustees. Many hospitals now consider the nurse executive and the chief of the medical staff to be of equal stature.

The educational preparation for nurse executives includes a master's degree in nursing administration or business administration. Nurse executives are responsible for overseeing all the nursing care provided in the hospital and serving as clinical leaders as well as administrators. Nurse executives supervise the largest group of hospital employees, the nursing staff.

The nursing staff consists of all the registered nurses, licensed practical/vocational nurses, and nursing assistants employed by the department of nursing. They are usually organized according to the units on which they work. The typical nursing unit consists of a nurse manager or head nurse, several assistant managers, and a number of registered nurses, licensed practical/vocational nurses, and nursing assistants.

Registered nurses are the direct, bedside care givers. They are responsible for planning and delivering care to a group of clients. They are also responsible for supervising licensed practical/vocational nurses and unlicensed personnel. Staff nurses are the backbone of hospital nursing.

Each nursing unit has its own budget and staff for which the nurse manager is responsible. The nurse manager is also a communication link between the nursing staff and the next level, middle management. Between the nurse executive and the nurse manager of a unit are middle-management nurses, known as clinical directors or supervisors. They have responsibility for multiple units, whereas the nurse manager is responsible for one. Clinical directors serve as the communication link between the nurse managers and the nurse executive.

Some nurses employed in hospitals have neither direct client care responsibilities nor management responsibilities. They include nurse educators, nurse researchers, clinical nurse specialists, and infection control nurses. Nurses in these roles support direct-care nurses and serve as resources to them.

Hospital Support Personnel. Hospitals employ far more than doctors and nurses. Doctors, nurses, and all the other individuals who work with clients are called the health care team, or interdisciplinary team. They are supported in their work by a number of other departments such as dietary, housekeeping, and laundry.

THE HEALTH CARE TEAM

In addition to nurses, dozens of health care workers serve from time to time on interdisciplinary health care teams.

Physicians. Physicians have completed 4 years of college and 3 to 4 years of medical school and have been licensed by a state board of medical examiners. Most physicians have also completed a residency in a hospital setting. Many do postgraduate work in a specialty area.

Physicians are responsible for the medical diagnosis and medical therapies designed to restore health. Increasingly, physicians are specializing in an area of medicine and see only patients with that particular problem. As a result, one patient may have five or more doctors, each treating a different body system. Whereas physicians have traditionally been involved mainly in restorative care, many are coming to recognize the value of illness/injury prevention and health promotion.

Dietitians. Many patients, particularly in hospitals, require management of their nutritional intake as part of the healing process. Others need to know how to prepare and eat a healthy diet. **Dietitians,** sometimes called nutritionists, are experts about the way diet (oral or intravenous) may affect a client's recovery and promote and maintain health. Dietitians have baccalaureate or higher degrees and may have completed internships. They focus on the therapeutic value of foods and on teaching people about therapeutic diets.

Pharmacists. Pharmacists are professionals who prepare and dispense medications, instruct clients and other health care workers about the medications, monitor the use of controlled substances such as narcotics, and work to reduce medication errors. The number and complexity of drugs available today require special education and training in their preparation, dispensing, and monitoring and in the evaluation of actions and effects on clients.

Pharmacists must earn at least a bachelor's degree in pharmacy. Depending on state licensing requirements, pharmacists may also be required to do an internship. Pharmacists are an integral part of the interdisciplinary team. They administer intravenous medications and nutrition (antibiotics, cancer drugs, and liquid nutrients) in hospitals and homes. They serve and support physicians, nurses, and patients.

Paramedical Personnel. Other personnel are educated to assist the physician in the diagnosis of a client's problems. This connection with medicine identifies them as "paramedical" staff.

Laboratory technologists handle client specimens such as blood, sputum, feces, urine, and body tissues to be examined for cancer or other abnormalities. Laboratory technologists carefully subject these body substances to various tests that will help determine whether the client needs treatment. Technologists have at least a bachelor's degree and are often assisted by laboratory technicians, who have 2-year degrees. They must pass a licensing examination before they can practice.

Radiologic technologists perform procedures necessary for taking x-rays and other images for diagnostic purposes. Although clients still need routine x-rays, technology in this field has become sophisticated. Subspecialties such as computed axial tomography, magnetic resonance imaging, and positron emission tomography have developed. These are all ways of "seeing" what is going on inside the body without surgery. In fact, the term applied to the field, "diagnostic imaging," reflects its expansion beyond techniques based solely on x-rays or radiography. All require specially educated technicians who operate multimillion-dollar equipment. Although some radiologic technologists are still trained on the job, most are educated in formal programs lasting 1 to 4 years. They must be registered with the state in which they practice.

Respiratory Technologists. Acutely ill or injured patients often require assistance in breathing. **Respiratory technologists** carry out procedures and operate equipment that assists clients in breathing. Respiratory technologists operate ventilators, oxygen therapy devices, and intermittent positive-pressure breathing machines. They also perform some diagnostic procedures such as pulmonary function tests and, in some facilities, blood gas analyses. With the increase in respiratory care in the home and community, these health care team members are working closely with home health care agencies and community health care centers. They must complete either a 2-year or a 4-year educational program. In some states, they must also complete an internship.

Social Workers. The psychosocial impact of illness and injury on patients and their families can often be profound. Financial problems may arise if a breadwinner cannot work or if insurance benefits are inadequate. Interruption of the normal family relationships may produce family crises. Lack of knowledge about community support systems may hinder discharge of a client from the hospital.

The **social worker** is a professional specifically educated to assist clients and their families with social challenges. Social workers hold either a bachelor's or master's degree. They serve as liaisons between hospitalized clients and the resources and services available in the community.

Therapists. Several types of therapists help clients with special challenges. **Physical therapists,** or physiotherapists, assist clients in regaining the maximal possible physical activity and strength. They focus on assessing pre-illness or injury function, current damage, and potential for recovery. They then develop a long-term plan for gradual return to function through exercise, rest, heat application, and hydrotherapy. Physical therapists, who have a minimum of a bachelor's degree, also supervise physical therapy assistants, who hold associate degrees.

Occupational therapists work with physical therapists to develop plans to assist clients in resuming the activities of daily living after illness or injury. They may help clients learn to cook, take care of their own hygiene, or drive a specially equipped car with the physical capacity left to them. In addition, they assist clients in learning skills to return to previous employment or retrain clients for new employment options. Occupational therapists hold at least bachelor's degrees.

Chaplains. Chaplains are pastoral care providers who offer spiritual support for clients and their families. Full-time chaplains are employed in some agencies, especially those affiliated with a specific religion. Some hospitals provide religious services. All chaplains are prepared to refer clients to clergy of their own faith.

Administrative Support Personnel. All organizations include essential administrative functions: payroll, billing, filing insurance claims, filing forms, paying bills, system support, and others. These activities require considerable time. When they are managed by administrative staff, the clinical staff is freed to concentrate on direct client care services.

The administrative staff ensures that the operations of the facility run smoothly and that clinicians have the resources necessary to meet the client's needs. They also educate the clinical staff about the financial realities of the environment and work with the staff to find ways to provide quality care at least cost.

Nurses' Roles. Nurses fulfill a number of roles on the health care team. They are perhaps the most flexible of health professionals and carry out a number of functions well.

Provider of Care. Nurses provide direct, hands-on care to clients in all health care agencies and settings. They take an active role in illness prevention and health promotion and maintenance. They offer health screenings; home health care services; and an array of health care services in schools, workplaces, clinics, doctors' offices, and other settings. They are instrumental in achieving the high survival rates in trauma centers and newborn intensive care units.

Provision of direct care also requires management skills. The bedside staff nurse must manage the care of a group of clients, decide priorities, assign staff members to clients, and accomplish all activities during an 8- or 12-hour period. Nurses are also involved in case management, or managed care, in which they review client cases and coordinate services so that quality care can be achieved at the lowest cost. With health care costs escalating, managed care is one way of distributing scarce resources to the greatest number of clients.

Educator. Nurse educators teach clients and families, the community, other health care team members, students, businesses, and government. In hospital settings as client/family educators, nurses provide information about illnesses and teach about medications, treatments, and rehabilitation needs. They help clients understand how to deal with the life changes necessitated by chronic illnesses. When necessary, nurses also teach how to adapt care to the home setting.

In community settings, nurses offer classes in injury/illness prevention and health promotion. Often these classes are jointly taught with other health care team members. For example, a nutritionist and a nurse may teach a group of expectant parents to prepare and feed their infants. Nurses have a responsibility to understand and teach how the health or dysfunction of the environment may affect both the short- and long-term health of the community.

Nurses also serve as teachers of the next generation of nurses. Nursing students need educators who set high standards and ideals and also help students understand how to make the ethical choices that all health care providers must make.

Counselor. People who experience illness or injury often have strong emotional responses, and the relationship between mind and body is critical to promotion of and restoration to health. As counselors, nurses provide basic counseling and support to clients and their families.

The nurse's role as counselor often overlaps the roles of social workers, psychiatrists, spiritual advisors, and mental health specialists. Because nurses spend more time with clients, they have opportunities to respond to the emotional needs of clients as they occur.

Using therapeutic communication techniques, nurses encourage people to discuss their feelings, explore possible options and solutions to their unique problems, and choose the best alternatives for action (see Chapter 24). They also serve as bereavement counselors with terminally ill clients and their families. Nurses may, with advanced education and certification, provide psychotherapy services, which extend beyond the basic counseling role.

Collaborator. With so many health care workers involved in providing care, collaboration among the professions is important. An important role for nurses is working with others to ensure that everyone has the same client outcomes in mind. Collaboration requires that nurses understand and appreciate what other health professionals have to offer. They must also be able to interpret to others the nursing needs of clients.

An often-overlooked collaborative function is collaboration with clients and families. In planning nursing care, clients should always be involved to the full extent of their interests and abilities.

Involving clients and their families in the plan of care from the very beginning is the best way to ensure their cooperation, enthusiasm, and willingness to work toward the best outcomes.

Change Agent. When changes are needed in the nursing system, nurses themselves can serve as agents of change. Most professional nursing education programs include change theory as part of their management courses, and graduates are prepared to become change agents in their work settings. The role of change agent requires a combination of tact, energy, creativity, and interpersonal skills. People often resist change, particularly if they are comfortable with the "old way" and believe it works.

Client Advocate. Because hospitals and the entire health care system are so complex, clients sometimes "fall through the cracks." Others need someone to help them negotiate the way through the system. They need to know how to cut through the levels of bureaucracy and red tape to get what they need when they need it.

Nurses who value client self-determination, that is, client independence and decision making, often serve as client advocates. In this role, nurses sometimes help clients cut through the system when it is in the client's best interests and no one else will be harmed by doing so. Nurse advocates realize that policies are important and govern most situations well but that rules occasionally can be broken. For example, special care units often have strict visiting hours. Family members may be allowed to see the client only for 10 minutes each hour. If a client is not expected to live, however, the nurse, serving as a client advocate, will allow the family members more generous visitation than the rules provide.

HEALTH CARE FINANCE

Most Americans believe that health care is a right, not a privilege. President George Bush, in his 1992 State of the Union address, affirmed that belief with his statement, "Good health is every American's right." In spite of this affirmation by the highest elected official in the nation, the statistics are disturbing.

An estimated 35.7 million Americans have no health insurance,[15] and millions more are underinsured.[6] In 1991, health care consumed 17 per cent of the gross national product, more than any other entity. More than $2 billion per day is spent on medical care in the United States, a staggering amount.

During 1990, employee health care benefits consumed 26 cents of every dollar of business profits.[7] General Motors alone spent $3.2 billion, more than it spent on steel, to provide health coverage for employees, their dependents, and retirees.[6] All of these figures are expected to increase, and if this trend is allowed to continue until the year 2010, one third of all national resources will be spent on health care.

Nurses and nursing practice are profoundly affected by financial issues. It is therefore necessary to understand the overall economic context in which nursing care is provided.

The Price of Health Care

In pre–health insurance days, when people paid their own medical bills, doctors and hospitals set their fees with some sensitivity to what patients could pay. When costs were high, patients complained. But health insurance created a system that lowered sensitivity to price as a concern of most health care consumers because they paid only a small portion of the real costs; a third party (the insurance company) paid the rest.

PRIVATE INSURANCE

In 1943, the Internal Revenue Service ruled that people did not have to pay income tax on health benefits paid by their employers. During the same period, World War II caused the government to impose wage controls to keep the wartime economy stable. As a result, employer-paid health benefits became a new way employers could reward employees without violating wage controls. When states chose to grant tax-exempt status for hospital- and physician-owned private insurance companies, such as Blue Cross and Blue Shield, these private insurers grew dramatically. By 1960, two thirds

of nonelderly Americans had private health insurance, mostly paid for by employers.

PUBLIC INSURANCE

The growth of private insurers did not solve the problem of paying for health care for the unemployed and the elderly, and many continued to receive inadequate care. In 1965, Congress approved two public insurance programs to cover these groups: Medicare, which is mainly for the elderly, and Medicaid, which is for the poor and certain disabled people. They were designed to protect citizens who were uninsured by employers and unable to afford their own private health insurance. At that time, a unique public-private partnership system of insurance that would care for all seemed to be in place. Unfortunately, that partnership was far from a coordinated system and began to display some major flaws.

RETROSPECTIVE REIMBURSEMENT AND RISING COSTS

Originally, both public and private insurance plans were based on after-the-fact, or retrospective, reimbursement. This method meant that when Mrs. Johnson went to the hospital with pneumonia, a request for reimbursement for whatever services were rendered (chest x-rays, blood work, physical examinations, antibiotic therapy) was sent to the insurer. Depending on the terms of her insurance policy and the level of Mrs. Johnson's deductible (the portion she was to pay personally), the hospital was reimbursed for much or even most of the charges. Retrospective reimbursement originally meant the out-of-pocket cost of services to insured consumers of health care was extremely low. Because neither the physicians, who ordered health care, nor the consumers (clients) were concerned about cost, the demand for health care services became virtually insatiable, driving costs up dramatically.[31]

From 1960 to 1983, state and federal government spending for health care nearly doubled, rising from 5.3 per cent of the gross national product to 10.8 per cent.[18]

One of the reasons for the rise in costs is the development and use of new technologies. New technologies are extremely costly: a single x-ray machine can cost $250,000, and more advanced types of diagnostic imaging machines can cost up to $2 million each. In 1991, a single dose of a drug used to treat heart attacks cost $2500 per dose.[6] Box 5–4 itemizes a sampling of medical charges in 1991.

The United States has experienced increases in both the elderly and the uninsured populations. Members of both groups desire and require increasing amounts of health care, creating additional cost escalation. Another reason for increasing costs is that expanding employment opportunities for health care personnel outside hospitals has caused shortages of such personnel in hospitals and nursing homes. These shortages, in turn, have resulted in increased salary and benefit costs.

The result of upwardly spiraling costs, fueled by technology and demographic changes, is that health care costs accounted for 17 per cent of the gross

---

Box 5–4. Some Examples of Medical Charges, 1991

▶ Annual cost of human growth hormones for a child with a severe deficiency: $20,000
▶ Coronary bypass surgery for a 50-year-old man: $49,000
▶ Cost of a Bufferin tablet for a patient in a psychiatric hospital: $3.75
▶ Price of a modified radical mastectomy: $7900
▶ One day's intensive care for a crack baby: $2000
▶ A 50-minute session with an elite psychotherapist: $160
▶ Delivery of a baby by cesarean section: $7500

▼ ▼ ▼

Data from Castro, J. (1991). Condition: Critical. *Time,* November 25, 1991, 34.

---

national product in 1991. Unable to pay for employees' health care, some employers have left the system and insured their own employees (called self-insurance), scaled back or eliminated health benefits, or passed more and more of the costs of insurance on to employees. In 1989, 78 per cent of all labor union strike activity was stimulated by employers' eliminating previously provided health care benefits.[14]

An estimated 35.7 million Americans, three fourths of whom are full-time workers and their dependents, have no health insurance.[15] In 1990, more than 100 million people were either underinsured or unable to pay their portion of the coverage available to them.

Methods of Payment for Health Care

Five major methods of payment for health services are in use today: personal payment, workers' compensation, Medicare, Medicaid, and private insurance.

PERSONAL PAYMENT

Personal payment for services is the least common method. Few people can afford out-of-pocket payment for more than the most basic health services. At today's prices, an illness or injury severe enough to require hospitalization can quickly exhaust a family's financial reserves, forcing them into bankruptcy. Generally, only those people without access to some form of private group insurance or public insurance rely on personal payment.

WORKERS' COMPENSATION

Workers' compensation is a system that varies from state to state but generally insures only workers who are injured on the job. Workers' compensation usually covers both treatment for injuries and weekly payments during the time the worker is absent from work for injury-related causes. In the case of accidental death, the worker's family receives compensation. Companies are required by law to contribute to a compensation fund from which money is withdrawn when accidental injuries or deaths occur.[4]

MEDICARE

Medicare, or Title XVIII of the Social Security Act, is a nationwide federal health insurance program established in 1965. Medicare is available to people age 65 years and over, regardless of the recipient's income. It also covers certain disabled individuals and people requiring dialysis or kidney transplants. Medicare has two separate but coordinated programs. The first, known as Part A, is a hospitalization insurance program. Part B is a supplementary medical insurance program that covers visits to physicians' offices and other outpatient services. Although Medicare was originally intended to be a no-cost or low-cost program for the elderly, the cost of participating in Medicare has steadily risen. Ironically, many elderly people, including groups already underserved, such as rural populations,[12] find they cannot afford to participate in Medicare. Moreover, Medicare's limited scope of services emphasizes institutional care in hospitals and skilled nursing facilities. Little Medicare reimbursement is directed toward management of chronic illness and functional disabilities, which are among the elderly's most pressing needs.[12]

MEDICAID

Medicaid, or Title XIX of the Social Security Act, is a group of jointly funded federal-state health insurance programs for low-income, elderly, blind, and disabled individuals. It, too, was established in 1965. There are broad federal guidelines, but states have some flexibility in how they administer the program. People must meet eligibility requirements determined by each state. Eligibility depends on income and varies from state to state. Rates of payment also vary; some states provide far higher payments than others do. The amount the federal government contributes to Medicaid varies from a minimum of 50 per cent of total costs to a maximum of 75 per cent. The differences in eligibility and payment rates lead to wide variations in the level of care provided to the poor in different states. Unlike those on Medicare, people who receive Medicaid are not required to pay any fees to participate. Table 5–1 highlights the similarities and differences in the Medicare and Medicaid programs.

PRIVATE INSURANCE

Private insurance, also called voluntary insurance, is a system in which periodic payments, or insurance premiums, are paid by insured individuals or their employers, or the cost of premiums is shared between individuals and employers. Premiums are paid into the insurance plan, and specified health care benefits are covered as long as the premiums are paid. Early in the development of private insurance, many treatments were covered only if they were performed in an inpatient (hospital) setting. This feature tended to drive up the cost of services. Today, most insurers stipulate that

TABLE 5–1. Facts about Medicare and Medicaid

	Medicare	Medicaid
Source of funds	Federal government	Federal and state governments
Administrator	Federal government	State governments
Eligibility	People over 65 years	Poor and disabled
Level of benefits	Same nationwide	Varies from state to state
Payment by recipients?	Required	Not required
Coverage	Hospitalization, outpatient care, no prescriptions or optical care	Comprehensive, including prescriptions and optical care

costs of hospitalization are reimbursable only if treatment cannot be performed on an outpatient basis. In 1988, 73 per cent of Americans with medical insurance were covered through employers.[15]

Cost Containment

Spiraling health care costs have caused both public and private insurers to examine their practices and to institute a variety of measures designed to reduce health care costs. This initiative is referred to as **cost containment.**

The 1970s saw attempts to control health care costs through legislation designed to regulate costs and monitor the quality of care. Comprehensive health-planning agencies and certificates of need were two mechanisms used. Some states also practiced rate setting, in which the state set limits on reimbursements. Yet costs continued to rise. Retrospective payment for Medicare and Medicaid had become uncontrollable. It was apparent that basic changes in payment mechanisms were required. Box 5–5 contains information about the dramatic increases in costs to taxpayers of Medicare and Medicaid since they were implemented in 1967.

Through legislation passed in 1982, the federal government changed the payment method for Medicare from the retrospective system to a prospective payment system based on diagnosis-related groups. Prospective payment was designed to create a more competitive environment and resulted in an emphasis on efficiency, cost-effectiveness, and financial accountability. It also stimulated competition among health care providers. For the first time, providers had incentives to operate in a cost-effective manner.

Entire governmental agencies have been created to monitor and administer cost-containment programs. Private insurers have also instituted cost-containment measures.

FEDERAL COST-CONTAINMENT PROGRAMS

The Health Care Financing Administration administers federal cost-containment programs. Two principal federal cost-containment programs are professional review organizations and diagnosis-related groups. Each is designed to limit costs by defining standards of treatment.

The Health Care Financing Administration. The **Health Care Financing Administration** is a federal cost-containment agency created to administer the Medicare and Medicaid programs. Briefly stated, the goals of the Health Care Financing Administration are

▶ to develop and establish standards for ensuring that quality care is rendered to recipients of Medicare and Medicaid
▶ to improve the efficiency and responsiveness of Medicare and Medicaid and to promote beneficiary awareness
▶ to enforce standards for hospitals, nursing homes and other long-term care facilities, laboratories, clinics, and other health care facilities

Professional Review Organizations. Professional review organizations oversee and review every Medicare hospital admission to make sure clients meet criteria for hospitalization and that their health care needs

---

Box 5–5. Medicare and Medicaid Costs, 1967 and 1991

Facts About Medicare

Costs in first full year (1967)	$ 5 billion
Costs in 1991	$110 billion
Those helped	All elderly, regardless of family resources

Facts About Medicaid

Costs in first full year (1967)	$ 2.3 billion
Costs in 1991	$158.7 billion
Those helped in 1980	65% of the poor
in 1991	40% of the poor

Medicaid is the fastest-growing spending program in the United States.

▼ ▼ ▼

Data from Health care expenditures and other data: an international compendium from the Organization for Economic Cooperation and Development. *Health Care Financing Review.* (1989). Annual supplement, 111–195.

cannot be met on an outpatient basis or in a community-based setting. Professional review organizations also monitor all Medicare clients' lengths of stay. If a client is hospitalized longer than the professional review organization determines is appropriate or if procedures are performed that the professional review organization determines are unnecessary, the hospital is denied reimbursement for the extra days and the unnecessary procedures.[11] Hospitals are therefore careful about whom they admit, how long they allow clients to stay, and what procedures are performed while clients are hospitalized.

Diagnosis-Related Groups. Diagnosis-related groups (DRGs) are categories that represent all known disease entities classified according to medical diagnosis. Each disease is combined with similar diseases into nearly 500 DRGs for Medicare reimbursement. For each DRG, the Medicare system has predetermined a fair price for hospital services. This price represents the amount the hospital is paid by Medicare to treat clients in that particular DRG. If the hospital's costs exceed the preestablished reimbursement rate, the hospital loses money. If it is able successfully to treat the client for less than the established reimbursement rate, the hospital can keep the excess. DRGs are one example of a prospective payment system.

PRIVATE COST-CONTAINMENT PROGRAMS

Private insurers have benefited from federal cost-containment initiatives because private reimbursement rates tend to be established at the same level the federal government uses for reimbursing hospitals for Medicare DRGs. Two additional types of programs designed to lower health care costs have been established by private insurers.

Preferred Provider Organizations. Preferred provider organizations are groups of physicians or institutions to which insurance companies direct their policyholders for care. These providers have agreed to provide services at somewhat lower-than-usual cost. Policyholders are provided a list of "preferred providers" from whom to choose. If they choose to use providers not on the list, they usually must pay a larger share of the costs of care.

Health Maintenance Organizations. Health maintenance organizations are networks or groups of providers who agree to provide certain basic health care services for a single predetermined yearly fee. The voluntarily enrolled participants in health maintenance organizations pay the same regardless of the amount and kind of services they actually receive. Health maintenance organizations benefit financially when their clients stay well. Therefore, they have an incentive to promote health maintenance and prevention of illness in their enrolled participants.

The Economics of Nursing Care

THE COST OF NURSING SERVICES

Traditionally, nurses have been unconcerned with the cost of care, believing all patients were entitled to high-quality nursing care regardless of ability to pay. Until fairly recently, few efforts were made to determine the actual cost of nursing care. The average hospital bill included the cost of nursing services in the general category of "room rate" (much as hotels include the cost of maid service in the price of a room). In the past, the hospital census (number of clients) was used to determine the number of nurses needed. This method worked fairly well when payment was retrospective. With the advent of prospective payment, however, hospitals had to determine their staffing needs more efficiently.

Health care providers have long recognized that different clients require different amounts of nursing time, depending in large part on how sick they are. Conner, working at Johns Hopkins Hospital in 1960, developed a classification system that identified clients' needs for nursing care in quantitative terms. It was a new idea that client needs were quantifiable, were predictable, and could help hospitals determine the need for nursing resources. For the first time, client needs, as opposed to hospital census, could be used as criteria for determining the number of nurses needed.[10] Since that time, different classification systems have been developed; most depend on client acuity, or degree of illness and the resultant amount and complexity of nursing care required.

Initiatives called "costing nursing services" are under way to determine precisely the cost of nursing care. It is believed that this will solve one dilemma of contemporary nurses who find themselves torn between two conflicting goals: their own desire to provide comprehensive care regardless of cost, and the pressure from financial managers to provide only services reimbursable under insurance regulations.

In the past, the assumption was that the cost of nurses was a major part of hospital costs. Tough economic times therefore meant that the first cost-reduction efforts were aimed at nursing. Since 1983, many researchers have undertaken to determine the actual costs of nursing care. Studies by the American Nurses' Association Center for Nursing Research found that nursing accounts for only 20 to 28 per cent of the costs of hospitalization for two thirds of DRGs examined.[23] This finding places nursing in a stronger position than it has enjoyed in the past. Costing nursing services and developing standardized reimbursements based on cost will enhance the ability of nurse managers to control nursing resources and negotiate for a fair share of hospital financial resources.

THE IMPACT OF COST CONTAINMENT ON NURSING CARE

When the drive to provide high-quality nursing care meets the constraints of cost containment, something has to give. What nurses hope, as both providers and consumers of health care, is that quality has not and will not suffer because of emphasis on "the bottom line." Yet hospitals face hard financial realities, and 68 per cent of nurses practice in hospitals.[5] To stay in business, hospitals must make at least enough money to pay personnel costs, maintain buildings and equipment, and pay suppliers of goods and services.

The financial vitality of a hospital depends in large measure on attracting physicians who will use that hospital's inpatient and outpatient services in providing medical care to their clients. A 1991 study done for the American College of Healthcare Executives examined the factors that influence physicians to seek affiliation with hospitals. When asked to rank factors, a panel of physicians ranked "quality of nursing staff" as the number-one factor affecting this choice.[1] If attracting physicians is essential to financial stability and depends in large measure on the quality of the nursing staff, attaining or maintaining quality nursing care is critical to the survival of hospitals.

HEALTH CARE POLICY AND POLITICS

In 1992, the United States and South Africa were the only two industrialized nations without universal access to health care for all citizens.[16] Even though 1990 health care expenditures averaged $2354 per person, infant mortality ranked 22nd—lower than many countries with far fewer national resources. Two thirds of inner-city children under 4 years of age did not have the full series of immunizations to protect them from preventable childhood diseases.[16]

The United States has no established minimum set of health services available to the entire population, but neither does it have a maximum.[30] Some people cannot pay for even the most basic services, whereas others can afford any procedure, no matter how expensive.

The reform of health care delivery in the United States has become a topic of national discussion, most obviously during the presidential campaign of 1992. The Canadian health care system, although often held up as a model for others, is also the subject of debate over problems of escalating costs and system inefficiencies.[19] The debate in the United States over the direction reform should take must grapple with some basic social and cultural dilemmas:[15]

▶ Is health care a right to which all citizens are entitled, or is it a commodity to be distributed at prices determined by the market?
▶ If greater involvement of government is necessary to reform the health care system, how can this involvement be reconciled with the traditional American belief in limited government and individual freedom?
▶ If access to health care is to be guaranteed to all citizens, including the poor and unemployed, are the American people willing to increase their tax burden to achieve this goal?

These and other social and cultural dilemmas complicate plans to model a new health care system on Canada's or any other nation's. Many industrialized nations do better than the United States in achieving higher standards of health at a lower cost to the nation (Table 5-2). Differences in culture and politics will need to be considered, however, in reforming the U.S. health care system or adopting one imported from abroad.

Professional nursing is prepared to address the questions surrounding health care financing. Other policy issues will confront nurses throughout their professional careers, not only on the national level but also in such arenas as the workplace and the community. When nurses are confronted with these issues, political action may frequently be called for.

An increasing number of nurses recognize that political action is an appropriate part of professional nursing practice. Yet research concerning nurses' attitudes toward politics and political behavior suggests that many nurses continue to be involved in political action in limited ways, expressing their views largely by voting.[8,26] Research further suggests that the dissonance between nurses' attitudes and behaviors related to political activism may be due to their need to develop political knowledge and skills.

The development of political skills is based on an understanding of what policy is and how it is made. Nurses need no longer just react to policy—they can shape it in a variety of ways and in a variety of places, not the least of which are the places where they work. Policy and politics can be explicitly related to bedside nursing. For example, the nurse who is caring for the elderly client who has had bypass surgery needs to understand that this nurse-client interaction is occurring within the context of a "health" care system that is really an "illness" care system. Health care financing ensures that the bypass surgery will be funded but does not fund programs to assist the client to quit smoking, to exercise, or to learn to cope with stress. Furthermore, the length of the client's stay in the hospital is driven by reimbursement mechanisms that reward hospitals for discharging the client as early as possible. Whereas early discharge may be a laudable goal, it can obstruct recovery if there is not enough time for sufficient client teaching for self-care at home.

Policy Defined

Policy is "the principles that govern action directed towards given ends."[28] It is "a consciously chosen course of action (or inaction) directed toward some end."[17] It is a plan, direction, or goal for action. Policy encompasses the choices that a society, segment of society, or organization makes regarding its goals, priorities, and allocation of resources. It is "authoritative decision making."[27]

There are different kinds of policy.

▶ Public policy is policy formed by governmental bodies (e.g., legislation passed by Congress and the regulations written from that legislation). Public policy related to sexual harassment, for example, might

TABLE 5-2. Comparison of National Health Care Systems (as of July 18, 1991)

Country	Access	Costs	Finance
Canada	Canada provides health care for all its citizens through a national health insurance program operated by the provincial governments; primary care providers are evenly distributed, and specialists are concentrated in "centers of excellence"	Canada spends about 8.6% of GNP on health care; physicians are paid on a fee-for-service basis with rates negotiated annually with the provincial governments; hospitals have global annual budgets set by the provincial governments	The Canadian federal and provincial governments share the financing of health costs; the federal share comes primarily from income taxes, as does the provincial share
Great Britain	Great Britain provides health care for all its citizens through a government-operated national health service	Great Britain spends 6.1% of GNP on health care; the government operates the hospitals and employs hospital-based physicians with a budget based on allocations by Parliament; general practitioners are paid on the basis of government-set rates	89% of the financing of health care in Great Britain is from general federal revenues; 9% is from an employee-employer contribution fund; the final 2% is from direct client payment
Japan	Japan provides access to health care for all its workers and their families through an employer-mandated health insurance program; all other citizens are covered through a national health insurance program	Japan spends 6.7% of GNP on health care; the Health Ministry sets rates for private and public providers on a fee-for-service basis; it operates a utilization review system; providers can, in some cases, charge more than the government rate, but this overcharge must be paid out-of-pocket	About 60% of health costs in Japan come from the employment-based health program that is financed through an 8–9% payroll tax split by the employee and employer; 30% comes from local taxes, with the final 10% from direct client payment
Sweden	Sweden provides access to health care for all its citizens through an almost completely government operated national health service program	Sweden spends 9% of GNP on health care; 95% of physicians are employed by County Councils that operate the health system locally; hospitals are run by either local or area agencies with budgets based on the medical needs of the area	60% of the financing for Sweden's health system is from a proportional wage tax of 13.5%; 35% of costs are covered by general federal revenues; the remainder are paid for through direct client fees
South Africa	South Africa did not guarantee health care for all of its citizens, but the Post-Apartheid health policy act will implement a private-public partnership for health care delivery with emphasis on access and affordability	South Africa spends 6.4% of its GNP on health care; there is an intense privatization of physicians, and there is no strict government regulation of private fees	N/A
Australia	Australia provides a public health plan that covers all citizens; also available to supplement the public plan is a national private plan as well as numerous other independent private plans	Australia spends 7.2% of its GNP on health care costs; the responsibility for health services is given to the individual states, which differ in their administration of services	Australia levies a 1.25% income tax on citizens above a fixed income to finance the public Medicare and Medibank Private systems
United States	Access to health care is not a right in the U.S.; Medicaid covers 17 million low-income people; Medicare covers 30 million senior citizens and 2 million people with disabilities; private insurance, usually employment-based, covers 137 million people; 37 million Americans are uninsured	The U.S. spends 10.9% of GNP on health care (11.2% in 1987); most providers are private with little rate setting (Medicaid; Medicare for hospital services, and a few private insurance companies); hospital care consumes about one half of health costs, and physician services another one quarter	Private insurance pays 31% of health costs; Medicare, financed through a 3.5% payroll tax and premiums, pays 17% of health costs; Medicaid pays 10% and is funded jointly by federal and state taxes; other government programs pay 14%; direct patient payments pay 25%; private sources pay the remaining 3%

From Citizen Action, 1120 19th St. NW, Suite 630, Washington, DC 20036.
GNP, gross national product.

Administration	Benefits	Quality
The Federal Ministry of Health sets standards and approves provincial government annual plans; providers are primarily private, but provincial governments set rates after negotiating with physicans; the government also sets global hospital budgets annually	The same benefits are provided as in Sweden (Sweden has the most comprehensive benefits package and is used as the standard for comparison in this category), except that eye care is not covered and dental care is limited	The infant mortality rate improved from 13.5 deaths/1000 births in 1975 to 7.9 in 1986, ranking Canada third in this chart; life expectancy rose from 74.3 years in 1975 to 75 in 1986, ranking Canada in a tie for fourth in this chart
The Secretary for Social Services oversees the health system; it sets fees for private general practitioners; it sets hospital budgets and employs hospital physicians; input comes from regional, district, and community boards	The same benefits are provided as in Sweden, except dental care is limited	The infant mortality rate improved from 14.3 deaths/1000 births in 1975 to 8.8 in 1986, ranking Great Britain in a tie for fourth in this study; life expectancy rose from 73.4 in 1975 to 75 in 1986, ranking Great Britain in a tie for fourth in this study
The Minister of Health and Welfare oversees both the employer-mandated health program (two thirds of population) and the National Health Insurance program (all others); it sets fees for public hospitals, clinics, their physicians, and the majority of facilities that are private	The same benefits are provided as in Sweden, except paramedical treatment, eye care, and psychiatric care are not covered and dental care is limited	The infant mortality rate improved from 9.3 deaths/1000 births in 1975 to 5.2 in 1986, ranking Japan first in this study; life expectancy rose from 75.5 in 1975 to 76 in 1986, ranking Japan in a tie for second in this study
The Ministry of Health and Social Affairs oversees 23 county councils and three municipal boards, elected every 3 years, that employ physicians and operate hospitals and clinics; six medical regions operate specialized facilities	Sweden covers hospital (tests, lab work, nonelective surgery), physician services, preventive care, home care and nursing home care, prescription drugs, dental care, eye care, paramedical services, and psychiatric care	The infant mortality rate improved from 8.3 deaths/1000 births in 1975 to 5.9 in 1986, ranking Sweden second in this study; life expectancy rose from 75.5 in 1975 to 77 in 1986, ranking Sweden first in this study
The Department of National Health and Population Development is responsible for administering and regulating the South African health system	N/A (the Republic of South Africa emphasizes preventive medicine and primary care)	The infant mortality rate is 13 deaths/1000 births for whites and 57 for blacks; life expectancy is 71 years for whites and 62 for blacks; given these data, South Africa could not be ranked in this study
The national Commonwealth Government appoints two ministers to the Portfolio of Community Services and Health who are responsible for the budgetary and policy decisions for the states; health services are delivered by local government, semivoluntary agencies, and profit-making nongovernmental organizations	The public plan covers all public hospitals and physician services; supplemental private insurance covers eye care, psychiatric and rehabilitative services, and other services varying by the insurance plan	Infant mortality improved from 14.3 deaths/1000 births in 1975 to 8.8 in 1986, ranking Australia in a tie for fourth in this study; life expectancy rose from 72.7 in 1975 to 76 in 1986, ranking Australia in a tie for second in this study
The federal government sets hospital rates and standards for Medicare; states set rates and regulate Medicaid; over 1500 private insurers set their own regulations; physicians are mostly private; only 5% of hospitals are public; the U.S. health system can best be described as a *non*-system.	Private plans vary, but few compare with Sweden's; Medicare does not cover dental, eye, and preventive care or paramedical services and limits psychiatric, drug, and long-term care; Medicaid recipients can have fuller coverage, but few states take advantage of all options	The infant mortality rate improved from 16.1 deaths/1000 births in 1975 to 10.4 in 1986, ranking the U.S. sixth, or last, in this study; life expectancy rose from 73.5 in 1975 to 74 in 1987, ranking the U.S. fifth, or last, in this study

Box 5–6. Comparisons Between the Canadian Health Care System and the United States Health Care System

As discussion and debate over health care reform intensify, there is increasing comparison of the United States health care system with the Canadian system. Some individuals suggest that the Canadian model be adopted in the United States. Others are very much opposed to such a transformation.

The Canadian health care program is universal, comprehensive, publicly funded (with no financial access barriers to care), and privately delivered. All citizens are covered for all medically necessary services through a federal-provincial health insurance system. The United States system is not universal, comprehensive, or publicly funded except for Medicare and Medicaid enrollees (32 million and 17 million, respectively). These enrollees are subject to financial means tests (Medicaid) and copayment/deductible access barriers (Medicaid and Medicare). The majority of United States citizens (137 million) have private health insurance, largely financed through employers (82 per cent). Coverage varies widely, from minimal to comprehensive. Premium rates, copayments, and deductibles also vary by policy type.[2] An estimated 37 million Americans have no health insurance whatsoever.[4]

Canadian federal-provincial funding arrangements vary across provinces, and administration and control of the program are unique within each province and the two territories. Provinces are single-source payers for both hospital and physician expenditures. Control is centralized and the role of private insurance companies is limited by law. In the United States, private insurers are highly influential in the health care system, covering more than 50 per cent of the population. Control in the United States is dispersed over multiple-payer sources, making control of resources much more difficult.

Using a centralized control approach, each Canadian province (and territory) prospectively determines each hospital's global budget for the coming year. A global budget is the total or lump sum amount the hospital will receive for its services. Hospitals themselves determine the distribution of allocated funds within the institution. No deficit spending is permitted; hospitals must live within their budgets. Methods for adjusting the global budget vary by province. In Ontario (the most populated province), the Ministry of Health makes adjustments based on inflation, workload, approved new programs or expansion of existing programs, and increases in the cost or volume of certain services such as dialysis, oncology, neonatal intensive care, and cardiovascular surgery.[4] Within these constraints, hospitals must serve everyone who seeks care.

Provincial governments also negotiate reimbursement rates with medical associations, and the governments set fees prospectively. Five provinces (which contain 80 per cent of the population) control aggregate physician expenditures through a threshold approach. If physician expenditures within the province exceed what was budgeted because of increased volume of client services, provinces can recoup their losses by adjusting future reimbursement rates downward or by paying current fees at a discount. This approach affects the total amount of money available to the medical

profession for reimbursement and indirectly affects individual physician income.[2]

Like other provinces, Quebec negotiates expenditure targets for the total physician group; however, the province sets individual physician income targets as well. There are imposed ceilings on the quarterly gross billings of individual physicians, and if a physician exceeds the ceiling, he or she is reimbursed at only 25 per cent of the allowable rate for additional care delivered. The Ministry of Health also reimburses new physicians in rural areas at a higher rate than those opening practices in urban areas, thereby influencing the geographic distribution of care.[2]

Clearly, the Canadian government at the provincial level has much tighter control over health care expenditures than do the multiple payers in the United States. Other system-wide comparison data are displayed in the following table.

Selected Comparisons of United States and Canadian Health Care Systems

	Canada	United States
Health care as a percentage of GNP	8.7 [1988]	11.2 [1987]
Per capita expenditures (U.S.$)	$1556 [1989]	$1973 [1987]
Length of stay (days)	8.1 [1988]	7.1 [1987]
Cost per hospital stay (U.S.$)	$2014 [1988]	$3532 [1987]
Cost per day (U.S.$)	$243 [1988]	$500 [1987]
Beds per 1000 population	7.1 [1986]	5.4 [1986]
Occupancy rate	83.8% [1988]	68.4 [1987]
Ratio of physicians to population	1:486 [1985]	1:418 [1985]

GNP, Gross National Product.

Satisfaction surveys have indicated that 95 per cent of Canadians surveyed preferred their own health care system over a United States model, whereas only 37 per cent of United States citizens surveyed preferred the United States system over the Canadian model.[1] Health status indicators for 1982 to 1984 reveal that Canada's infant mortality rate and age-standardized death rate for all causes were lower than those for the United States and that life expectancy at birth for males and females was slightly higher in Canada.[2] All data on expenditures and health status outcomes provide support for the apparent success of the Canadian model.

Can or should the United States replicate such a model? There is strong debate over the feasibility of replicating the Canadian system in the United States. Canada has only one tenth the population (25 million versus 241 million) and only seven provincial and two territorial government structures in addition to the federal level. In contrast, there are 50 state governments with which the federal government would have to negotiate funding formulas in the United States. Moreover, people in the United States hold a substantially different view of the government's role in the lives

---

Box 5–6. Comparisons Between the Canadian Health Care System and the United States Health Care System (Continued)

of citizens. Canadians expect government to design, implement, and support social programs.[2] In the United States there is much more emphasis on individual accountability and noninterference by government. The second critical factor that may prevent adoption of a Canadian model in the United States is the political environment. Congress and state legislatures are under heavy influence of special interest groups. A movement toward a centralized, single-payer system in the United States would likely trigger intense opposition from hospital, physician, and health insurance lobbies, among others.

Finally, barriers to change may arise from among United States citizens who are adequately insured and receive health care "on demand." Shifting from the current open-ended system to a resource-controlled system would mandate care delivery on an "as needed" basis. Citizens would wait for elective services in some cases. In the current system, primarily those uninsured (37 million) and underinsured United States citizens (19 million Medicaid plus unknown numbers of privately insured persons) are denied services or are subject to delayed services because of a lack of resources needed to provide services in a timely manner. Under a single-payer, centralized control system, all citizens would, in theory, be treated equitably within the

health care system. Ability to pay would no longer separate the "haves" from the "have nots." Although many from both groups would welcome such a redistribution of health care resources, United States citizens would have to modify their expectations of health care services. As in Canada, there may be a gradual shift to a single-payer system, and this shift may begin at the state level. The United States must resolve these issues in this decade, or face a possible collapse of the current system.

▼ ▼ ▼

1. Blendon, R. J. (1989). Three systems: A comparative survey. *Health Management Quarterly, 11,* 2–10.
2. Rakich, J. S. (1991). The Canadian and U.S. health care systems: Profiles and policies. *Journal of the American College of health-care Executives, 36*(1), 25–42.
3. U.S. Department of Commerce, 1989. *Statistical abstract of the United States, 1989.* Washington, D.C.: Author.
4. U.S. Department of Health and Human Services, 1989. *National medical expenditure survey: A profile of uninsured Americans, research findings 1.* Publication No. PHS 89-3443. Washington, D.C.: Author.

By Bonita Ann Pilon, DSN, RN, CNAA, Assistant Professor, Specialty Director, Nursing Administration Graduate Program, Vanderbilt University, Nashville, Tennessee.

---

be a law passed by Congress that defines sexual harassment as an act of discrimination that will result in financial penalties to institutions that receive federal funds, such as hospitals and home health care agencies, that tolerate such behavior.

▶ Social policy pertains to the directives that promote the welfare of the public. For example, the state writes regulations mandating that job-training programs for women on welfare include procedures for dealing with work-related sexual harassment. This law could be viewed as a policy that promotes the welfare of women.

▶ Health policy includes the directives and goals for promoting the health of citizens (e.g., the town council might believe that victims of sexual harassment should be provided with counseling services to assist them in coping with the experience and passes legislation authorizing such services).

▶ Institutional policies are those governing workplaces (e.g., what the institution's goals will be and how it will operate, how the institution will treat its employees, and how employees will work). A hospital might, for example, develop and promote a policy that prohibits sexual harassment in the institution and includes a grievance process for reporting and handling claims.

▶ Organizational policies are the rules governing and positions taken by organizations, such as a state nurses' association. For example, a state nurses' association might pass a resolution that identifies sexual harassment as an issue of importance to nurses in the workplace and call for the development of workshops to help nurses prevent and address sexual harassment in the workplace.

Policy is shaped by politics, beginning with the determination of the issues to consider for policy statements and continuing through decisions regarding the evaluation of outcomes.

Politics Defined

Politics is often associated with negative images—smoke-filled rooms, deals made by power brokers, bribes, unethical compromises, pork barreling, bureaucracies, vote buying, and abuses of power such as sexual harassment. These images arise from newspaper headlines about scandals in local, state, and federal government. The negative associations are highly visible and leave the impression that all politics are tainted, if not dirty and unethical.

Yet politics is, in fact, a neutral term. It means influencing; specifically, it means influencing the allocation of scarce resources. It is a process by which one influences the decisions of others and exerts control over situations and events. It is a means to an end.

Politics is thus a term associated with conflicting values. It is a necessary part of operating where multiple interest groups are competing for scarce resources, whether they are money, time, supplies, personnel, or access to information. Whether the perception of politics is negative or positive depends largely on

▶ an individual's own biases, experiences, and knowledge of politics
▶ how the game of politics is played (i.e., the system in which politics is operating and what rules have been established as acceptable within that system)
▶ whether the goals or ends are important
▶ whether one has a vision for different ways of influencing and is in a position to change the rules of the system

This last variable is one that nurses, as members of a profession that continues to be represented predominantly by women, must address. Do nurses want to participate in political processes that are too often corrupt and oppressive, or should nurses play a leadership role in transforming political systems?

Politics, Policy, and Values

The development of policy is a value-laden process, beginning with determining the problems that become issues and including who will implement and evaluate policy. Policy making is a complex process, seldom straightforward, but it is a dynamic process that reflects the values of those involved. When values are in conflict, as they often are when interests are diverse, politics will come into play.

Nursing's values are often in conflict with the dominant values of society.[9,21] Nursing emphasizes caring and connectedness.[3,32]

When women and nurses are not at the policy tables in significant numbers, the policies that result often do not support the health and development of women, families, and communities.

Consider the following examples:

▶ A coalition of women's organizations, female scientists, and legislators brought to the public's attention that most of the federally funded research in this country excluded women. The body of biomedical knowledge used to treat both men and women therefore may not be accurate when it is applied to women. The coalition worked to develop a policy mandating that federally funded research include women as subjects. In addition, efforts are under way to emphasize research on women's health.
▶ Whereas the U.S. government has made much of valuing the family, the United States has a record of being the only industrialized country without policies that support workers' taking leaves of absence from their jobs to care for ill children or elders. This responsibility often falls to women, even though most women hold paid jobs.
▶ Prenatal care in this country costs approximately $1500 per mother. Because prenatal care is not guaranteed, some women receive little or no prenatal care and deliver very low birthweight infants who require immediate, prolonged care in neonatal intensive care units. This intensive care is mandated and costs between $25,000 and $200,000 per infant, depending on the length of hospitalization. The infant can be sent home without a guarantee that the mother will receive the support she needs to provide for the infant or that the infant will receive the developmental support and special education that may be needed.
▶ In a thorough review of research and demonstration projects aimed at improving the odds for high-risk children and families, Schorr notes that the successful programs have repeatedly shown that this risk can be reduced through comprehensive, intensive, and responsive services with "staffs with the time and skill to establish relationships based upon mutual respect and trust."[25] Such humanistic approaches to health and social problems are rarely embraced by policymakers, who will unflinchingly fund costly missiles, biomedical diagnostic equipment, high-tech care, or new hospitals. As Schorr notes,

In today's world, social policy can significantly strengthen or weaken a family's ability to instill virtue in its children. . . . It lies within our reach, before the end of the twentieth century, to change the futures of disadvantaged children. The children who today are at risk of growing into unskilled, uneducated adults, unable to help their own children realize the American dream can, instead, become productive participants in a twenty-first-century-America whose aspirations they will share. The cycle of disadvantage that has appeared so intractable can be broken.[25]

Public policy is about choices. These choices are based on values that come into play in the political dynamics of policy making.

Spheres of Political Action

Although politics and policy are usually associated with government, nurses have other spheres for political action: the workplace, professional organizations, and the community. These four spheres are interconnected and overlapping.

WORKPLACE

Bedside client care is a political endeavor. The kind and quality of health care a client receives and the choice of provider who gives it are political issues that involve the resources of money, time, equipment/supplies, and personnel. Workplace policies are important in addressing questions such as the following:

▶ Who has authority for budgeting and procuring unit supplies?
▶ Are visiting hours limited?
▶ Is there a policy on client self-medication?
▶ Is there a policy on the routine assessment of vital signs?

▶ Who is responsible for ensuring that the client's diet is appropriate and that the client is able to eat what is served?

▶ How does the institution decide what client teaching is appropriate, and who should do the teaching?

Nurses have the knowledge and the power to ensure that client care policies truly serve clients' best interests. They can work toward this goal both as advocates for individual clients and as coauthors with other professionals of policies that govern the entire institution.

GOVERNMENT

Government provides society with a legal definition of nursing, nursing's scope of practice. Government influences reimbursement systems for health care and nursing services, and to a great extent, it determines who will get what kind of health care. For a client receiving Medicaid or Medicare, governmental policies determine how much the hospital is paid for the client's care and whether rehabilitation or home care is provided.

In the early 1990s, government decided whether women could receive full information about reproductive rights and who could provide that information. Governments are setting policies about where smoking may take place, where alcohol and smoking may be advertised, what health services are available in schools, whether schools should distribute condoms to prevent the spread of acquired immune deficiency syndrome, what resources are available to communities for low-income housing development and maintenance, whether education of children will be a top priority, and whether families will be supported in their efforts to care for sick children or frail elders at home. Government often influences which health problems will be researched and targeted for government funding and support.

PROFESSIONAL ORGANIZATIONS

Professional organizations are instrumental in shaping the practice of nursing (e.g., developing standards of practice, lobbying for progressive changes in the scope of nurses' practice, and playing a role in collective action in the workplace). They are an increasingly significant force in the development of health policy. Recent years have seen an unprecedented collaboration on issues of mutual concern among nursing organizations through the TriCouncil for Nursing (American Nurses' Association, National League for Nursing, American Association of Colleges of Nursing, and the American Organization of Nurse Executives) and the National Federation of Specialty Nursing Organizations. Two notable examples of this collaboration include nursing's efforts to defeat the registered care technician proposal of the American Medical Association in the late 1980s and the development of Nursing's Agenda for Health Care Reform, a policy statement on national health care.

COMMUNITY

In years past, leaders such as Lillian Wald viewed the community as more than a practice site (see Chapter 1). Communities are social units with a variety of interest groups, community activities, health and social problems, and resources for solving problems. The community can be one's neighborhood, or it can be the international connections that will characterize the 21st century. The other three spheres of influence — workplace, government, and professional organizations — are an integral part of the community. As members of a community, we have responsibility to promote the welfare of the community and its members. In turn, the community's resources can be invaluable assets to health promotion and health care delivery. Government officials, hospital administrators, clients, corporate managers, presidents of private and public organizations — all players who can effect change in health policy — are affiliated with at least one community, the one in which they live. When nurses become visible in the affairs of their communities, they represent an entire profession. Community networks can be called on to support nursing agendas.

Likewise, nursing should be called on to support the agendas of communities trying to develop a better place in which to live. Nurses are involved in the PTA, senior citizen councils, community-planning boards, advocacy and civic organizations, and business groups. They can be instrumental in organizing and mobilizing communities on issues such as recycling, environmental cleanup, and safety.

Understanding the health care system in which nurses work is a professional responsibility of every nurse. With the active discussion of health care taking place on a national level, nursing will face many complex and significant policy issues. Facing these issues will require political reflection and action from nurses, both individually and collectively. It is incumbent on every nurse to realize that caring includes such activities as

▶ voting for policymakers who support humanistic policies

▶ joining professional organizations that work to shape nursing and health care

▶ working with other nurses to transform the places in which health care is provided

▶ participating in the improvement of our neighborhoods and communities

Summary

▶ The health care delivery system is a complex system that provides illness prevention, health promotion and maintenance, diagnosis and treatment, and rehabilitative and long-term care.

▶ Health care agencies are classified as governmental or voluntary, for-profit or not-for-profit, or according to level of care provided.

▶ The interdisciplinary health care team consists of an array of professionals. Each member has an important part to play in ensuring the best client outcomes.

▶ Nurses often serve as liaisons between the health care system and clients and their families. In doing so, they use a variety of roles—such as provider, educator, counselor, collaborator, change agent, and client advocate—in meeting clients' needs.

▶ Health care financing in the United States has changed dramatically during the past 50 years, from a system dominated by personal payment to one dominated by third-party payment. This change has created basic economic disequilibrium in health care.

▶ Medicare and Medicaid programs, begun in 1965, created a serious financial drain on federal and state budgets. In response, cost-containment efforts were begun by the federal government in the 1970s.

▶ Retrospective payment, or reimbursement for the cost of services rendered, was replaced in 1982 by prospective payment, by which health care providers are reimbursed at a set rate depending on the client's diagnosis, regardless of the actual costs of treatment.

▶ Despite profound changes already in place, the health care system is likely to undergo more significant changes in the future as policymakers address rising costs and increasing demand for quality care.

▶ To influence coming changes in the health care system in the United States, nurses need to become knowledgeable about policy and politics and promote values, like caring and connectedness, that reflect the values of the nursing profession.

▶ Nurses can exert influence in four spheres of political action: government, the workplace, professional organizations, and the community.

Bibliography

1. American College of Healthcare Executives (1991). *The future of healthcare: Physician and hospital relationships.* Author.
2. Aydelotte, M.K. (1983). The future health care delivery system in the United States. In Chaska, N.L. (ed.). *The nursing profession: A time to speak.* New York: McGraw-Hill.
3. Benner, P., & Wrubel, J. (1988). *The primacy of caring.* Menlo Park, CA: Addison-Wesley.
4. Black, H.C. (1988). *Black's law dictionary.* St. Paul, MN: West Publishing.
5. Bocchino, C.A. (1990). An interview with Kathryn M. Mershon. *Nursing Economics,* 8(4), 219–228.
6. Castro, J. (1991). Condition: Critical. *Time,* Nov. 25, 1991, 34–42.
7. Cuniff, J. (1991). Soaring health costs need brake. *Chattanooga News-Free Press,* Jan. 31, 1991, B-5.
8. Daffin, P.N. (1988). Similarities and differences in political expectations and participation among nurses in clinical practice, education, and administration. Unpublished doctoral dissertation, University of Alabama at Birmingham.
9. Davis, G.C. (1988). Nursing values and health care policy. *Nursing Outlook,* 36(6), 289–292.
10. DiVestea, N. (1985). The changing health care system: an overview. In Shaffer, F.A. (ed.). *Costing out nursing: Pricing our product.* New York: National League for Nursing.
11. Dougherty, C.J. (1989). Cost containment, DRGs, and the ethics of health care. *The Hastings Center Report,* 19(1), 5–7.
12. Gale, B.J., & Steffl, B.M. (1992). The long-term care dilemma: what nurses need to know about Medicare. *Nursing & Health Care,* 13(1), 34–41.
13. Holzemer, W.L. (1990). Quality and cost of nursing care: is anybody out there listening? *Nursing & Health Care,* 11(8), 412–415.
14. Horine, M. (1990). Assuring access to quality care. *Pension World,* 26(9), 26–28.
15. Iglehart, J.K. (1992). The American health care system: introduction. *New England Journal of Medicine,* 326(14), 962–967.
16. Johnson, P.A. (1990). A national health insurance program: a nursing perspective. *Nursing & Health Care,* 11(8), 416–429.
17. Kalisch, B.J., & Kalisch, P.A. (1982). *Politics of nursing.* Philadelphia: J.B. Lippincott.
18. Lampe, S. (1987). *Costing hospital nursing services: A review of the literature.* Washington, DC: U.S. Department of Health and Human Services.
19. Laschinger, H.K.S., & McWilliam, C.L. (1992). Health care in Canada: the presumption of care. *Nursing & Health Care,* 13(4), 204–207.
20. Little, C. (1992). Health for all by the year 2000: where is it now? *Nursing & Health Care,* 13(4), 198–203.
21. MacPherson, K. (1987). Health care policy, values and nursing. *Advances in Nursing Science,* 9, 1–11.
22. Manion, J. (1990). *Change from within: nurse intrapreneurs as health care innovators.* Kansas City, MO: American Nurses' Association.
23. McKibben, R.C. (1985). *DRGs and nursing care.* Kansas City, MO: American Nurses' Association Center for Research.
24. National Commission on Nursing (1981). *Initial report and preliminary recommendations.* Chicago: The Hospital Research and Educational Trust.
25. Schorr, L. (1989). *Within our reach: breaking the cycle of disadvantage.* New York: Doubleday.
26. Small, E.B. (1989). *Factors associated with political participation of nurses.* Unpublished doctoral dissertation, North Carolina State University.
27. Stimpson, M., & Hanley, B. (1991). Nurse policy analysts. *Nursing & Health Care,* 12(1), 10–15.
28. Titmus, R.M. (1975). *Social policy: An introduction.* New York: Pantheon Books.
29. U.S. Department of Health and Human Services (1990). *Healthy people 2000: National health promotion and disease prevention objectives.* Washington, DC: Author.
30. Ward, D. (1990). National health insurance: where do nurses fit in? *Nursing Outlook,* 38(5), 206–207.
31. Ward, J.W. (1988). *An introduction to health care financial management.* Owings Mills, MD: Rynd Communications for National Health Publishing.
32. Watson, J. (1990). The moral failure of the patriarchy. *Nursing Outlook,* 38(2), 62–66.

The Nursing Process

▼ The Nursing Process: The Basis for Nursing Care

▼ *It is possible to fly without motors, but not without knowledge and skill.*

Wilbur Wright

▼ CHAPTER OUTLINE

THE FIVE STEPS OF THE NURSING
  PROCESS
    Assessment
    Diagnosis
    Planning
    Implementation
    Evaluation
ATTRIBUTES OF THE NURSING PROCESS
    A Systematic Approach
    Interrelated and Fluid Steps
    A Person-Centered Process
    Emphasizes Feedback

Facilitates Creativity
    The Foundation of Nursing Practice
PROBLEM SOLVING AND THE SCIENTIFIC
  METHOD
    Unlearned Problem Solving
    Trial-and-Error Problem Solving
    The Scientific Method of Problem
      Solving
THE MODIFIED SCIENTIFIC METHOD
  USED BY HEALTH CARE
  PROFESSIONALS

▼ KEY TERMS

Assessment
Evaluation
Implementation

Nursing diagnosis
Nursing intervention
Nursing process

Outcomes
Planning

The nursing process is one of the most important nursing subjects you will ever study. It is significant because it forms the foundation for nursing education, for nursing practice and research, and consequently for your career in professional nursing. Throughout your life as a health care professional, you will use the nursing process daily as you care for individuals and their significant others. What, then, is the nursing process, and what makes it the cornerstone of nursing practice?

Essentially, a *process* is a series of planned steps, methods, or operations that produce a particular result. We speak of the process of making something, performing activities, traveling, working, and so forth.

The **nursing process** is a series of planned steps and actions directed at meeting the needs and solving the problems of people.

More specifically, the nursing process is systematic problem solving. It is a scientific method adapted to the often unpredictable conditions of human life and applied to human beings who have unmet needs.

The nursing process is a five-step process. The steps are assessment, diagnosis, planning, implementation, and evaluation. As you study Figure 6–1, observe that assessment consists of the collection and analysis of data and leads to the next step, the formulation of the nursing diagnosis. When the nursing diagnosis is developed, the nurse establishes the plan of care. Implementation (also referred to as intervention) follows. Evaluation is the last step of the nursing process. Figure 6–1 shows the nursing process to be continuous, with no absolute beginning or end. Evaluation of how well the person achieved the outcomes leads not only to further data collection but also to a redefinition of the person's problems and to the planning of new interventions.

THE FIVE STEPS OF THE NURSING PROCESS

Assessment

During the **assessment** phase, you collect information about the person. This includes data about the person's physical and psychosocial status. Data are obtained through interviews, observation, physical assessment, review of the medical record, and discussion with the family or significant other. The initial collection of data occurs when the person enters the health care system. A nurse will assess the person and record this information on a document called the admission assessment or data base. However, assessment is an ongoing process that occurs whenever the nurse interacts with the person. Subsequent assessments are recorded on progress notes and flowsheets.

Diagnosis

The assessment data are used to identify the person's nursing diagnoses. Diagnoses are formulated by sorting, organizing, and analyzing the assessment data. A **nursing diagnosis** is "a clinical judgment about individual, family or community responses to actual or potential problems/life processes. Nursing diagnoses provide the basis for selection of nursing interventions to achieve outcomes for which the nurse is accountable." [5] This definition will be expanded in Chapter 8.

During the diagnosis phase, you will develop nursing diagnoses. The specific components of the nursing diagnosis are discussed in Chapter 8. A historical overview of nursing diagnosis is presented in Box 6–1. Diagnoses are usually recorded in a variety of places, including the plan of care and the progress notes.

Planning

Once the person's nursing diagnoses are identified, you begin **planning** the care to be provided. You may review the nursing literature as the plan of care is developed. Current articles and textbooks can contain invaluable information that can be used to tailor the plan to the needs of the person. The plan of care includes three components:

▶ Nursing diagnoses
▶ Outcomes
▶ Interventions

Outcomes are statements that describe the behavior the person will display if the nursing diagnosis is resolved. For example, if the person has lost weight because the dentures do not fit properly, the outcome may be stated as "will gain 5 pounds within 1 month."

Nursing interventions are the specific actions that you will perform to help the person achieve desired outcomes. In the example mentioned, the nurse may encourage the person to see a dentist to have the dentures refitted. In addition, the nurse may arrange for

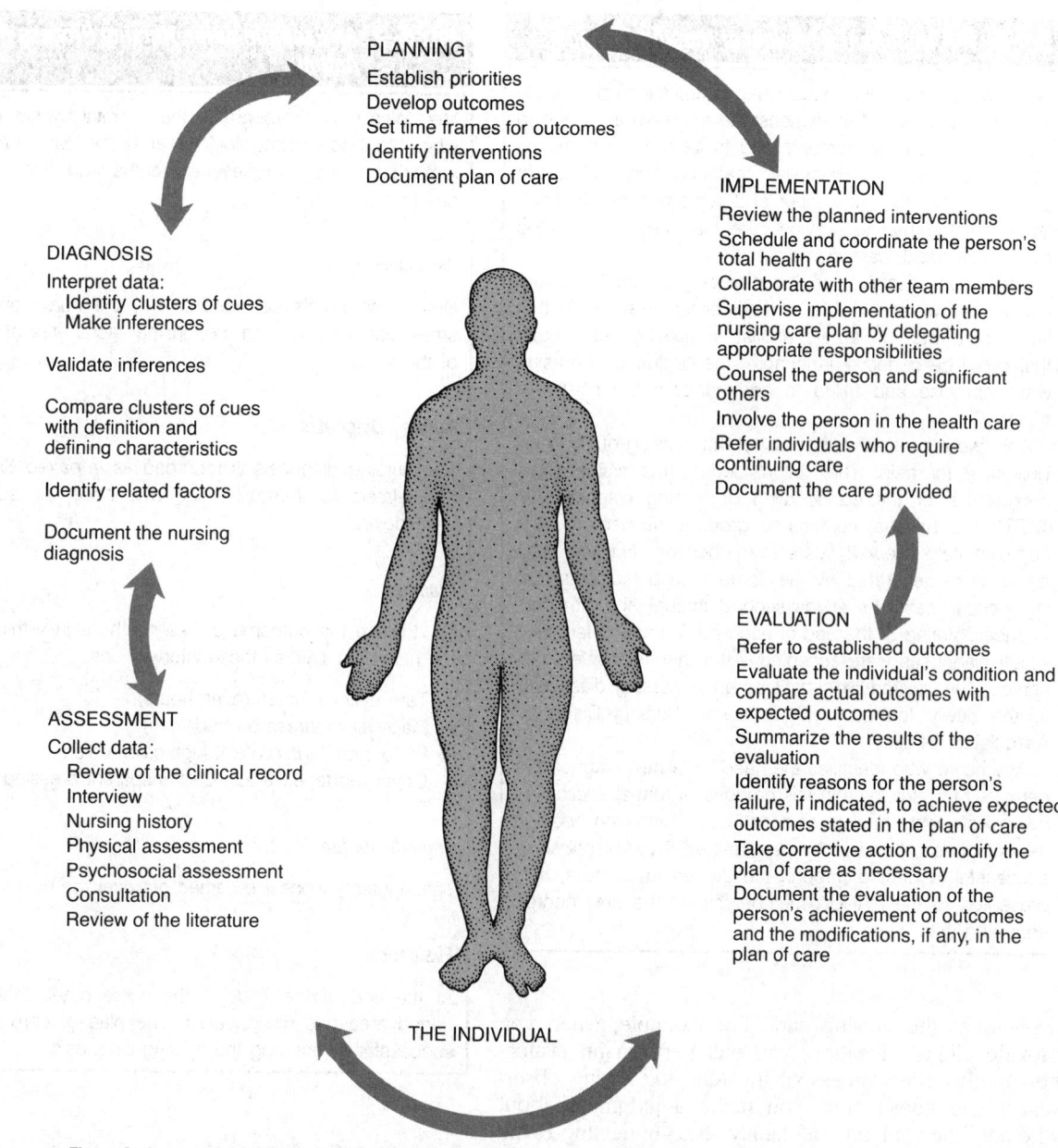

PLANNING
Establish priorities
Develop outcomes
Set time frames for outcomes
Identify interventions
Document plan of care

IMPLEMENTATION
Review the planned interventions
Schedule and coordinate the person's total health care
Collaborate with other team members
Supervise implementation of the nursing care plan by delegating appropriate responsibilities
Counsel the person and significant others
Involve the person in the health care
Refer individuals who require continuing care
Document the care provided

DIAGNOSIS
Interpret data:
    Identify clusters of cues
    Make inferences

Validate inferences

Compare clusters of cues with definition and defining characteristics

Identify related factors

Document the nursing diagnosis

EVALUATION
Refer to established outcomes
Evaluate the individual's condition and compare actual outcomes with expected outcomes
Summarize the results of the evaluation
Identify reasons for the person's failure, if indicated, to achieve expected outcomes stated in the plan of care
Take corrective action to modify the plan of care as necessary
Document the evaluation of the person's achievement of outcomes and the modifications, if any, in the plan of care

ASSESSMENT
Collect data:
    Review of the clinical record
    Interview
    Nursing history
    Physical assessment
    Psychosocial assessment
    Consultation
    Review of the literature

THE INDIVIDUAL

▲ *Figure 6–1*

Diagram of the nursing process. The nursing process consists of five steps: assessment, diagnosis, planning, implementation, and evaluation. The purposes are to maintain health, prevent illness, promote recovery, restore wellness and maximal function, and provide support in peaceful death. Note that the nursing process is a cyclical, problem-solving method that allows for change. When the evaluation step indicates that some problems are unresolved or are unidentified, the process continues with data gathering, problem identification, and so forth.

the person to eat soft foods that can be easily chewed. The plan of care is documented in a variety of ways. The traditional format is a nursing care plan, although newer formats are emerging.

Implementation

The **implementation** phase consists of the provision of nursing care. It involves

► administering direct care
► supervising the care provided by others, such as nursing assistants

► teaching
► counseling
► identifying the need for referrals (such as to a home health care agency)
► carrying out orders of health care providers

The implementation phase is documented on flow-sheets and progress notes.

Evaluation

The nurse is responsible for evaluating the care that has been provided by making a judgment about the effec-

---

Box 6-1. A Historical Overview of Nursing Diagnosis

In the early 1970s, two nurses had a chance to participate in a project designed to demonstrate the team approach to client care. Two requirements had to be met for participation in the project: (1) client data that were collected had to be coded for computer input and retrieval, and (2) each team member had to provide care that was not provided by another health care discipline.

The nurses assigned to the project grew frustrated because they were not able to meet either criterion. At that time, there was no agreed-on list of nursing phenomena that could be coded. Furthermore, the language of nursing was imprecise and failed to communicate the nature of nursing.

The two nurses asked the School of Nursing of St. Louis University for help. Their efforts led to the first national conference for the classification of nursing diagnoses in 1973.[6] The national conference group continued to meet approximately every 2 years from then on. Nursing diagnoses were generated by the conference participants during working sessions at the second through the fifth conferences. Voting at the end of each conference determined which diagnoses were accepted. After the fifth conference, nurses were invited to submit potential nursing diagnoses to the newly formed North American Nursing Diagnosis Association (NANDA).

Any nurse who identifies the need for a new diagnosis is permitted to participate in this process. A formal application now exists that consists of submitting information about a new diagnosis, followed by peer review. If the diagnosis is successful in getting through the screening process, it is presented to the NANDA membership at the next conference and then voted on.

Box 6-2. An Example of the Nursing Process in Action

Mrs. Westin was brought to the hospital by her daughter, who had been caring for her at home. Mrs. Westin has remained in bed for several months and has developed pneumonia.

Assessment

During the admission assessment, the nurse observes a small reddened, broken area in the sacral area at the base of the spine.

Nursing Diagnosis

The nursing diagnosis is recorded as *Impaired Skin Integrity* related to immobility, as evidenced by sacral skin breakdown.

Planning

To achieve the outcome of healing the skin within a week, the nurse establishes these interventions:

▶ Turn every 2 hours (even hours).
▶ Place air mattress on bed.
▶ Encourage high-protein, high-calorie diet.
▶ Cover reddened area with transparent dressing.

Implementation

These interventions are carried out over the next week.

Evaluation

At the end of the 7 days, the nurse notes that the reddened area has disappeared. The plan of care has been successful in resolving the nursing diagnosis.

---

tiveness of the nursing care. For example, when you provide client education, you will perform an evaluation of the effectiveness of the teaching. Using observation and questioning, you make a judgment about whether the person or family has understood the teaching.

Evaluation is an ongoing process that occurs whenever you have contact with the person. It consists of reviewing the appropriateness of the nursing diagnoses, outcomes, and interventions. On the basis of the discussions that are made during the evaluation phase, you may change the plan of care or continue as originally planned. Your conclusions about the progress of the person in achieving the outcomes are recorded in the progress notes and on flowsheets.

Box 6-2 provides a clinical example of the five steps of the nursing process in action.

ATTRIBUTES OF THE NURSING PROCESS

The five basic steps of the nursing process are broken down into multiple smaller steps, as shown in Figure 6-1. As you study this model of the nursing process, note the following attributes.

A Systematic Approach

The nursing process provides a systematic approach for nurses to assist clients. The purposes of the nursing process include maintenance of health, prevention of illness, promotion of recovery, restoration of wellness and maximal function, and support in peaceful death.

Interrelated and Fluid Steps

The steps of the process are interrelated. Also, the arrows uniting the steps flow back and forth within the system, emphasizing that the system is fluid rather than static. The nursing process is easiest to conceive of as an open process. One step builds on the next and is dependent on the preceding step. For example, diagnosis flows from the assessment and leads to planning. Continual use of the nursing process will help the beginning nurse develop more skills and experience in meeting the person's needs. In time, the nurse will be able to move rapidly and efficiently between the steps of the nursing process.

A nurse may remove a dressing (implementation) and assess the condition of the incision while simultaneously teaching the person about the signs and symptoms of infection (implementation). On the basis of the person's responses, the nurse will evaluate the effectiveness of the teaching. During the process of implementing the plan of care, the nurse may need to return to the planning phase and restate the outcomes or change the interventions.

A Person-Centered Process

The person is at the center of the process. The nurse involves that person in each step of the nursing process, from assessment through evaluation.

Emphasizes Feedback

Feedback is emphasized; for example, the results of step 5 (evaluation of the intervention) are fed back into the system, leading to a revision of the care plan as needed.

Facilitates Creativity

The nursing process allows maximal creativity on the part of the nurse as well as maximal use of education and skills.

The Foundation of Nursing Practice

The nursing process forms the foundation for nursing practice. It defines nursing practice in state practice acts and is used to organize nursing textbooks and state nursing board exams.

PROBLEM SOLVING AND THE SCIENTIFIC METHOD

The foundation of the nursing process is helping people meet needs through effective problem solving. As will be emphasized in Unit 4, the goal of the nursing process is to maintain a state of equilibrium. When needs are unmet, illness results. Nurses help people cope with stressors and adapt to changes in their lives. The nursing process is used to help clients achieve homeostasis. It is a deliberative, logical problem-solving approach that forms the framework for nursing practice. It defines the role of the nurse as you and the person together determine the need for nursing care.

There are three common methods of problem solving. The method of choice depends on the nature of the problem and on the experience, skill, energy, and intelligence of the problem solver. Common methods

of problem solving (arranged from the least to the most sophisticated processes) are as follows.

Unlearned Problem Solving

Unlearned problem solving involves mechanical reflexive reactions to problems. Unlearned problem solving is used by lower animals to solve problems of obtaining food or shelter and by humans in startling new situations. For example, if a person touches something hot, a reflexive reaction will be withdrawal of the hand from the heat source.

Trial-and-Error Problem Solving

Trial-and-error problem solving involves testing possible solutions without forethought and without recording the outcome (i.e., which solutions fail and which succeed). In this form of problem solving, the solver does not know why certain actions work whereas others fail. This method means guessing, and guessing by nurses can be dangerous to the people for whom they care. If the trial solution works, the person is lucky. If the solution fails, the results can be life-threatening.

The Scientific Method of Problem Solving

The scientific method is a logical and systematic procedure for solving problems. Scientific problem solving is an outgrowth of Western civilization and is the foundation of much of our medicine and technology. The scientific method can be broken down into the following seven steps:

▶ Recognition of the general problem, including defining the problem and developing hunches about its basis and solution.
▶ Collection of data from all relevant sources.
▶ Formulation of a hypothesis, or theory, which is an attempt to assign meaning to the data.
▶ Preparation of a plan for testing the hypothesis.
▶ Testing the hypothesis.
▶ Interpretation of test results and acceptance or rejection of the hypothesis.
▶ Termination of the study or modification of the plan, on the basis of further data collection.

For accurate results to be ensured, the problem solver must carefully record the data, hypotheses, initial plan, test results, evaluation, and modification of the plan.

THE MODIFIED SCIENTIFIC METHOD USED BY HEALTH CARE PROFESSIONALS

Health care professionals use a modified form of scientific problem solving in working with clients. In Table 6-1, the classic scientific problem solving method and the nursing process are compared.

Nurses must modify the scientific method when

TABLE 6-1. Comparison Between the Classic Scientific Method of Problem Solving and the Nursing Process

Classic Scientific Method	Nursing Process
Collecting data from all relevant sources	**Assessment** Developing data base ▶ Nursing history ▶ Psychosocial assessment ▶ Physical examination ▶ Review of laboratory test findings ▶ Review of diagnostic studies ▶ Consultation
Formulating a hypothesis	**Diagnosis** ▶ Analyzing and interpreting the nursing data; making inferences ▶ Defining the person's problems and stating the impact of these problems on the person's life situation
Preparing a plan for testing the hypothesis	**Planning** ▶ Stating the person's expected outcomes ▶ Review of the literature ▶ Developing plan of care, including outcomes and interventions
Testing the hypothesis	**Implementation** ▶ Administering or supervising nursing care ▶ Teaching the person ▶ Making referrals ▶ Carrying out orders
Interpreting test results and evaluating the hypothesis	**Evaluation** ▶ Reviewing the progress in relation to the expected outcomes ▶ Recording the person's progress on the chart ▶ Evaluating nursing diagnoses and interventions and determining whether the outcomes are being achieved
Terminating the study or modifying the plan of action on the basis of further data collection	Terminating, modifying, or continuing nursing care plan, depending on findings from the evaluation process

working with people. There are several reasons for this modification. First, scientists and health care professionals typically work in different *environments* and have different *goals*. The scientist works in a laboratory, experimenting under controlled conditions with various chemicals, apparatus, or laboratory subjects. Typically, the scientist is searching for new knowledge, which may be esoteric or theoretical. In contrast, nurses usually work in health care facilities, clinics, offices, schools, and private homes. Their goals are to help individuals solve immediate and long-range problems and to prevent further problems from arising.

Second, scientists and health care professionals work within *different time frames*. Scientists sometimes take years to gather data, plan changes, and evaluate results. Nurses obviously have limited time to work on an individual's problem before it *must* be resolved. For example, a child suffering from severe vomiting and diarrhea must be treated *promptly*, or dehydration and other problems develop. In this situation, the staff cannot spend days or even hours gathering data about the child's symptoms. Instead, they must start corrective action immediately.

A third reason that health care professionals must modify the scientific method is scientists have far greater *control* over their work than do nurses. For example, when a scientist in a controlled setting places a group of subjects on an experimental reducing diet, the researcher can be certain that the subjects will eat only the foods allowed on the diet. Because food intake is rigidly monitored, the subjects will have no food source available other than that provided within the controlled setting. If these individuals fail to lose weight, the scientist knows that the diet is at fault and not the people on the diet. On the other hand, when a nurse teaches a person about a reducing diet, there is no guarantee that the person will follow the diet after going home. If the person fails to lose weight, the nurse cannot know for certain whether the problem lies with the effectiveness of the diet, the teaching technique used, or the individual's failure to follow the diet. Furthermore, the nurse cannot control another person's eating behavior. For some health care professionals, this lack of control in the clinical situation can be frustrating.

Differences in the *complexity* of their tasks creates the fourth difference between the scientist's and the health care professional's approach to problem solving. The scientist typically can choose to work on *one* problem at a time. When one problem is solved, the next may be addressed. Because nurses work with human beings, they must apply problem-solving techniques to numerous interrelated problems at once. An ill person usually has both physical and psychologic problems and may face economic and family troubles. Furthermore, medical interventions may themselves produce complications; for example, many medications have side effects almost as severe as the condition for which they are prescribed. Thus, for nurses, the question is not What problem shall I solve? but *Which problem shall I work on first?*

Summary

▶ The nursing process is a series of planned steps and actions directed at meeting the needs and solving the problems of people.

▶ The nursing process consists of five steps: assessment, diagnosis, planning, implementation, and evaluation.

▶ A variety of sources and methods are used to collect data.

▶ Assessment data are used to develop nursing diagnoses.

▶ A nursing diagnosis is a clinical judgment about individual, family, or community responses to actual or potential problems/life processes. Nursing diagnoses provide the basis for selection of nursing interventions to achieve outcomes for which the nurse is accountable.

▶ The nursing care plan is established during the planning phase.

▶ Nursing care is provided during the implementation phase of the nursing process.

▶ During evaluation, the nurse makes a judgment about the effectiveness of nursing care.

▶ The nursing process is systematic, consisting of interrelated steps, and focuses on the person receiving the care. The nurse uses creativity and feedback to proceed through the nursing process, which is the foundation of nursing practice.

▶ As an open and flexible system, it allows you to use a modified scientific problem-solving method for assisting the person to achieve homeostasis.

▶ Problem solving can be unlearned, trial-and-error, and scientific.

▶ The nursing process has both important similarities and differences, compared with the scientific method of problem solving.

▶ Continued use of the nursing process will help the beginning nurse develop more skills and experience in meeting the person's needs. In time, you will be able to move rapidly and efficiently among the steps of the nursing process.

Bibliography

1. Christensen, P., & Kenny, J. (1990). *Nursing process, application of conceptual models.* St. Louis: C.V. Mosby.
2. Henderson, V. (1987). Nursing process: a critique. *Holistic Nursing Practice,* 1(3), 7–18.
3. Iyer, P., et al. (1991). *Nursing process and nursing diagnosis* (2nd ed.). Philadelphia: W.B. Saunders.
4. McHugh, M. (1987). Has nursing outgrown the nursing process? *Nursing 87,* 17(8), 50–51.
5. NANDA News (1990). *Nursing Diagnosis,* 1(3), 124–128.
6. Warren, J., & Hoskins, L. (1990). The development of NANDA's nursing diagnosis taxonomy. *Nursing Diagnosis,* 1(4), 162–167.

Chapter 7

▼ Nursing Assessment

▼

You can observe a lot just by watchin'.

Yogi Berra
Quoted in Eric Hodgin's Episode

▼ CHAPTER OUTLINE

DEFINITION, PURPOSE, AND DATA
  SOURCES
    Typical Data Base
    Data Gathering
    Subjective and Objective Data
    Sources of Data
    Confidentiality of Data
FACTORS THAT INFLUENCE THE NATURE
  OF THE DATA BASE
    Urgency of the Situation
    Nurse's Knowledge and Skills
    Perspective of the Nurse

METHODS OF ASSESSMENT
    Review of the Clinical Record
    Interview
    Nursing History
    Physical Assessment
    Formats for the History and
      Physical Examination
    Psychosocial Assessment
    Consultation
    Review of the Literature

▼ KEY TERMS

Data base   Data gathering   Functional health patterns

DEFINITION, PURPOSE, AND DATA SOURCES

Assessment is considered to be the first step in the nursing process and influences all of the remaining steps.

Assessment is the organized, systematic, and continuous process of collecting data from a variety of sources.

This step in the nursing process is performed to analyze the person's health status. Data are gathered during assessment to identify nursing diagnoses and select appropriate outcomes and interventions. Registered nurses perform assessments. Other nursing personnel, such as licensed practical/vocational nurses and nursing assistants, may collect data that will assist the registered nurse in performing an assessment. For example, the nursing assistant may take vital signs (data collection) that may reveal an elevated temperature. It is the responsibility of the registered nurse to perform a more detailed assessment. In the presence of an elevated temperature, the registered nurse may assess the skin for warmth, sweating, redness, swelling, drainage, rash, or other signs that may help the nurse interpret the temperature elevation.

The information that is collected during assessment is called the data base.

A **data base** is defined as a series of pieces of information about an individual and significant others that is used to identify strengths and unmet needs and to establish the plan of care.

The data base is also used as the basis for comparing the person's status before and after the plan of care is implemented. Assessment consists of collecting and communicating information through the nursing interview, review of the clinical record, physical and psychosocial assessment, consultation with other health care professionals, and review of the literature.

Typical Data Base

A typical data base may include some or all of the following types of information:

▶ *Demographic information,* such as age, address, and place of birth
▶ *Present symptoms and concerns*

▶ *Reaction to illness* and *expectation and goals* regarding the outcome of health care
▶ Client *profile,* including a description of the person and a typical day's activities
▶ *Social and cultural history,* including a description of the client's occupation, education, significant others, and spiritual and social affiliations
▶ *Medical history,* including previous hospitalizations, surgeries, and illnesses; medications taken; chronic health problems; and allergies
▶ *Interpersonal and communication patterns and skills*
▶ *Coping strategies*
▶ *Self-care abilities,* including the ability to perform activities of daily living such as feeding, bathing, dressing, grooming, toileting, and walking and the ability to transfer from a bed to a wheelchair, toilet, or chair
▶ *Mental and emotional status,* including reactions to real or perceived stressors; general affect or mood; self-concept; body image; thought processes (ordered, disordered, or rational); interests and motivations; willingness to take risks; nonverbal communication (posture, hand motions, facial expressions); awareness of feelings and the manner of managing those feelings; and orientation to time, place, and person
▶ *Substance abuse,* such as use of mood-altering chemicals including street drugs and alcohol, abuse of prescription drugs and over-the-counter drugs, and addiction to tobacco and caffeine
▶ *Environmental factors,* including the person's home living environment for such factors as the presence of running water, stairs, and so forth and assistive devices required, such as walkers, canes, hearing aids, and glasses
▶ *Educational needs,* such as knowledge deficits revealed through the interview process or by observation
▶ *Discharge planning factors,* such as where the person will go after discharge from a health care facility and with whom the person will live; knowledge of community resources; and accessibility of transportation, shopping, and health care facilities
▶ *Biophysical factors,* including review of relevant major body systems
▶ *Laboratory and diagnostic tests*

Additional pieces of data may be added to the preceding factors. For example, prenatal care will be part of the data base when a laboring woman is admitted to a hospital. A pediatric data base may include the prenatal and obstetric history, immunizations, observations about parent-child interaction, relationship with peers, and developmental growth.

Data Gathering

In addition to forming the data base, **data gathering** is used during assessment to follow the progress of the person, to serve as a basis for evaluating the effectiveness of nursing care, and to help redefine problems as they change over time.

Types of data gathered for these purposes include information about the normal and abnormal patterns of the individual, including changes in elimination habits; vital sign patterns; increases or decreases in activity; and change in symptoms, mental status, or emotional status. Thus, assessment is a continuous process that does not end at the time of admission to a health care facility or at the first contact the nurse has with the person. The assessment process is used to collect information each time the nurse interacts with the person. Data gathering does not include interpretation or analysis of the information gathered. Interpretation of data and the deriving of conclusions constitute the second step of the nursing process: nursing diagnosis.

Subjective and Objective Data

The data gathered should include two kinds of statements: what the individual says (subjective data), and what the health practitioner observes about the person (objective data). It is important to distinguish between objective and subjective data and to validate or check both types of data against each other before including them in the data base.

SUBJECTIVE DATA

Subjective data, or "symptoms," are basically what individuals *tell you* they are experiencing, feeling, seeing, hearing, or thinking.

The following statements are examples of subjective data:

"I feel very depressed today."
"I don't feel like eating or doing anything."
"I feel very warm. In fact, I think I may have a fever."
"I haven't moved my bowels in days. I must be getting constipated."

Subjective data are usually noted by the nurse when the nursing history is obtained. They are also gathered during daily contacts with the person. In recording subjective data, write *exactly* what the individual says. For example, it is correct to chart: Mrs. Jones stated "I feel depressed today." It is incorrect to write: "Mrs. Jones appears depressed today." The latter is *your impression* of how she feels rather than a statement made by her.

OBJECTIVE DATA

Objective data, or "signs," are information about the person obtained by the nurse through observations—listening to the person's chest through a stethoscope; palpation of body parts; feeling the person's skin for warmth, dryness, or moistness; smelling the breath for the odor of alcohol. The following are examples of recorded objective data:

"Mrs. Jones crying. Refused breakfast tray. Drank a few sips of water."
"Skin warm and dry to touch. Temperature 38°C orally."
"No bowel movements recorded for 3 days. Hard mass of stool felt on digital rectal examination."

Objective data are usually gathered during the physical examination or psychosocial assessment. However, objective data gathering is also a *continuous* process requiring daily, hourly, or even minute-to-minute updating.

Signs and symptoms, subjective and objective data are all considered to be cues identified through observation, interview, or statements made by the person (subjective data). Nurses use these cues to formulate nursing diagnoses and plan care. This is discussed further in the next chapter.

VALIDATION OF DATA

When gathering objective and subjective data, be sure to validate the data by checking what the person says against your own observations. For example, consider how subjective data are checked with objective data. If Mr. Johnson says, "I feel very warm, I think I may have a fever," you should validate the subjective statement with objective data. For example, feel his skin and take his temperature to see if indeed he does have a fever. If he says, "I feel constipated," check the chart for the last recorded bowel movement and perform a digital rectal examination for the presence of a fecal mass.

It is also necessary to validate objective data with subjective data. For instance, if you observe that a person has a forlorn expression, is tearful, and is anorectic (lacks appetite), *check this observation* with the individual. You might say to the person, "You seem depressed today. I notice you've been crying and you didn't touch your tray." The individual may confirm your observation or may deny it. In the latter case, the individual might say "I'm *not* depressed. I'm in pain! That's why I'm crying and why I can't eat." If you had failed to validate these observations, you would have misinterpreted the behavior.

Validation of both subjective and objective data is the cornerstone of accurate diagnosis.

Sources of Data

There are two major sources of data: primary and secondary. A *primary* source is the client. Data may be obtained through formal or informal interviewing, direct observation of behaviors, or physical examination. *Secondary* sources include the following:

▶ The person's significant others, such as family, friends, and business associates
▶ Clinic documents, developmental documents, charts from former hospitalizations, previous care plans, current hospital documents, medical and nursing histories, and current care plans
▶ Laboratory and diagnostic reports
▶ Other members of the health care team—physician, social workers, psychiatrist, dietitian, physical therapist, and other nurses
▶ Medical and nursing literature, notes from classes and lectures, and educational films and tapes

The subjective data that the individual (primary source) supplies are an invaluable part of the data base. For this reason, encourage people to participate in the data-gathering process whenever possible. However, some factors influence one's ability to act as a willing and reliable source of data. Factors to evaluate are summarized in Box 7–1 and include the following:

▶ Desire and need for medical and nursing care
▶ Previous illness
▶ Language and communication skills. The person who speaks only Spanish will have difficulty communicating with English-speaking personnel. The person who has suffered a stroke may not be able to speak.
▶ Age. An infant or very young person obviously cannot act as a reliable data source.
▶ Physical condition. Very ill persons, highly sedated persons, or those in great pain are often unable to speak coherently.
▶ Mental condition. A person who has a very low IQ or who is disoriented as to time, place, or person cannot give reliable data.
▶ Emotional state. A depressed person may be unable or unwilling to speak. Someone in a manic (extremely excited) state may be unable to give information.
▶ Fears concerning diagnosis. People who have a great dread of cancer might consciously or unconsciously withhold information that they fear would indicate the presence of cancer.
▶ Fears concerning legal implications or possible job loss. An airline pilot may fear loss of employment if symptoms indicate a substance abuse problem.
▶ Fear of supplying data that could lead to painful or embarrassing examinations or treatments. A woman may minimize menstrual problems because she dreads undergoing a pelvic examination.
▶ Fear of criticism by significant others. A young adult with a sexually transmitted disease may be reluctant to discuss sexual contacts because this information could adversely affect relationships.

Confidentiality of Data

Most people will give information about themselves, family members, and friends if they know that the in-

---

> **Box 7–1. Factors that Influence Reliability of Data Sources**
>
> Desire and need for medical and nursing care
> Previous illness
> Language and communication skills
> Age
> Physical condition
> Mental condition
> Emotional state
> Fears concerning the diagnosis
> Fears concerning legal implications or possible job loss
> Fear of supplying data that could lead to painful or embarrassing examinations or treatments
> Fear of criticism by significant others

formation will remain *confidential*. No matter what the potential benefit of data collecting, it is still an intrusion into personal lives and feelings. In a health care facility or clinic, individuals are asked to tell strangers about their lives, problems, fears, and most intimate feelings. Before you ask people to lower defenses and discuss themselves honestly, guarantee that you will respect their privacy and that their statements will be read and discussed only by the professionals directly concerned with their care. Honor this commitment by not sharing sensitive information with your classmates, and do not ever discuss people in public areas such as elevators and coffee shops. The nurse should also be careful in disposing of written information about people that has been used in providing care, such as class assignments and data carried in the pocket while in a clinical area. At times, people are hospitalized for reasons that they want to keep private, such as for substance abuse problems. The nurse must maintain the confidentiality of information about the person.

FACTORS THAT INFLUENCE THE NATURE OF THE DATA BASE

The amount, nature, and source of information for the data base depend on many factors. Some of these factors are identified in the following.

Urgency of the Situation

When an individual is in a life-threatening situation, data gathering focuses on the immediate problem. For example, a person is rushed into the emergency department after a motor vehicle injury. Quickly, the nurse and physician work together to assess injuries. The person will be asked about how the accident occurred, if there are any allergies or other medical conditions that are going to require care, and so on. Later, after the immediate injuries have been treated, a more detailed assessment can be performed. Compare this with the type of assessment that would be performed when an elderly person is admitted to a long-term care facility. In this situation, there is more time to obtain a detailed data base. The long-term care nurse is more likely to focus on the person's abilities to perform activities of daily living, the family relationships, and the person's risk for falls and skin breakdown.

Nurse's Knowledge and Skills

The abilities of the nurse will influence the type of assessment that is performed. A novice nurse often has difficulty sorting out the types of data that should be collected in certain situations. The inexperienced nurse is often fearful of missing some significant piece of data. A new graduate expressed it this way: "Since I am new, I may not notice something, or let something go wrong on a patient, not report it and then cause him further problems."[1] The nurse should focus on the information that is most directly related to the person's nursing care needs. This can be accomplished by (1) setting priorities for the types of data to be collected, (2) obtaining sufficient data, (3) obtaining information in a timely fashion, and (4) using resources such as nursing literature and proficient nurses to expand your knowledge base.

Perspective of the Nurse

The assessment process will also be influenced by the nurse's perspective. For example, a medical-surgical nurse will expect that a postoperative patient will experience some incisional pain. When a surgical patient complains of pain, the nurse should ask for a description of the pain, including intensity, duration, and location. This will help ensure that the nurse has not overlooked signs of a serious complication, such as sudden chest pain.

METHODS OF ASSESSMENT

The type of data collected is influenced by a variety of factors, including the urgency of the situation and the nurse's knowledge, skills, and perspective.

Box 7–2 summarizes the ways of assessing the client. The methods of data gathering are listed in this order for purposes of discussion. In actual practice, the order depends on the clinical situation. The beginning nurse must practice each method of assessment to gain skill and proficiency. One of the hallmarks of the experienced nurse is the ability to combine the assessment steps. For example, the nurse can obtain the nursing history while performing parts of the physical assessment. During the interview, the types of responses offered by the person will provide clues to the psychosocial status. The ability to combine assessment methods comes with experience.

Box 7–2. Step 1 of the Nursing Process: Assessment

Assessment Methods

Review of the clinical record
Interview
Nursing history
Physical assessment
Psychosocial assessment
Consultation
Review of the literature

Review of the Clinical Record

Often the nurse has access to information collected by other members of the health care team. If the person is in an acute care facility, these data may include laboratory tests; x-ray results; progress notes from the physicians, social service, physical therapy, and dietary; and so on. The clinical record contains valuable information that helps the nurse focus on the important assessment information.

Interview

The nursing interview (formal and informal) is a valuable data collection method. You need to be proficient and comfortable using communication skills and interviewing techniques. The process of obtaining accurate information through interviewing depends greatly on the skill and sensitivity of the interviewer as well as on the willingness or ability of the person to provide the necessary information. The interview is discussed in further detail in Unit 8.

Nursing History

Assessment serves a few major purposes. First, it allows the nurse to systematically obtain and record the health history. Second, it provides insight into the major areas of concern. This information helps the nurse focus on specific aspects of the physical assessment. For example, if the client states she is having difficulty breathing, the nurse will do a thorough assessment of breath sounds. Nursing histories have a different focus from the medical history collected by the physician. The medical history concentrates on the person's symptoms of illness and the disease progression. It includes (1) the chief complaint, (2) the client profile, (3) the history of the present illness, (4) the medical history, (5) the social history, (6) the genetic family history, and (7) a review of body systems.

In contrast, the *nursing* history focuses on the client's *perception* of illness and the psychologic, physical, and emotional responses to illness. The history explores the individual's reactions to current problems, presenting symptoms, and previous health problems.

By obtaining a thorough nursing history, you gain insight into how people meet basic human needs.

A complete history will reveal *which* needs the person is unable to meet and *why* these particular needs remain unfulfilled. By applying a solid knowledge base and by interviewing the person in a thoughtful, sensitive manner, you will learn what is of greatest concern to the individual. By knowing what causes or contributes to a certain problem, you can identify the areas both you and the individual need to explore in depth.

Taken by a skilled interviewer, the nursing history is a valuable assessment tool. Essentially, the nursing history

- provides the focus for the physical assessment that will be performed by the nurse
- is part of the first stage of the nursing process and provides a basis for planning care
- establishes an information base on which the nursing diagnosis and plan of care are built
- allows the nurse to investigate health status problems commonly associated with certain populations; for example, signs of abuse, presence of certain injuries, problems with medications, and concerns related to recent life changes are commonly noted to be present in the elderly client
- initiates a helpful relationship with the person and provides the opportunity to share mutual expectations regarding health care
- allows the nurse to observe the person's verbal and nonverbal communication and general behavior
- allows the person the opportunity to discuss personal feelings or fears and current problems
- reveals the person's past, present, and potential ability/inability to meet basic human needs
- helps the person remember events and symptoms that have been forgotten or repressed
- provides a written format in which to record biophysical and psychosocial information

Physical Assessment

On admission to a health care facility, a person is examined by the physician and by the nurse. The physician often performs a physical assessment to diagnose illness. The nurse performs a physical assessment to identify the person's needs and to plan care. For example, an elderly woman falls on the ice and fractures her hip. The physician diagnoses the fracture and prepares her for surgery. The nurse notes that the woman has poorly fitting dentures that have created lesions in her mouth. This problem will influence the woman's ability to eat, frequency of mouth care, and comfort level. The nurse will use this information and other assessment data to plan the woman's care.

Today, nurses routinely conduct physical assessment in health care facilities, clinics, schools, and people's homes.

After the initial physical examination, the nurse should assess the hospitalized person's physical condition daily or more frequently, depending on the person's condition.

Be systematic in your approach. Because a methodic approach enables clinicians to assess a person quickly and thoroughly, educators and health care professionals have devised methods for systematic inspection and examination.

More information on physical assessment is provided in Unit 8.

Formats for the History and Physical Examination

The format or assessment tool for collecting the nursing history and performing the physical examination will be selected by the health care facility in which you work. The use of an assessment tool helps ensure that the nurse systematically collects information by following a structured format.

There are three commonly used formats for collecting assessment data, including body systems approach, functional health patterns approach, and human response patterns approach.

BODY SYSTEMS APPROACH

The traditional approach is a body systems approach (Box 7–3). Using this method, the nurse observes and records data about each of the body systems, such as the neurologic, musculoskeletal, and integumentary system. Use of the body system approach has some drawbacks. First, it tends to be an incomplete data base. This format does not usually permit the nurse to collect all of the information needed to perform a holistic nursing assessment. In addition, it is difficult to develop nursing diagnoses from a body systems approach. Therefore, there is a strong trend toward the use of nursing models, such as functional health patterns or patterns of unitary person (defined later). Wake[4] surveyed approximately 1000 members of the American Organization of Nurse Executives in 1989. She found that the prevalence of the body systems assessment format was projected to decline to 37 per cent by 1992. Forty-eight per cent of those surveyed projected they would be using functional health patterns by 1992. The human response patterns format was expected to be used by 12 per cent of the respondents by 1992.

FUNCTIONAL HEALTH PATTERNS APPROACH

As nurses became more sophisticated in the use of nursing diagnoses, they identified the need for a formal nursing diagnosis system. The **functional health patterns** format, developed by Marjorie Gordon, organizes data collection into 11 categories of information (Box 7–4). These categories or patterns describe a sequence of behavior over time. Sequences of behavior, rather than isolated events, are the data used for making clinical judgments. Assessment of health patterns permits

Box 7–3. Body Systems Approach to Assessment

General Appearance

▶ *Observations*—age, sex, race, height, weight, nutritional status, development

Vital Signs

▶ Temperature
▶ Pulse (rate)
▶ Respirations
▶ *Blood pressure*—supine, sitting, right and left arms

Neurologic System

▶ Level of consciousness
▶ *Skull*—size, contour, symmetry, color, pain, tenderness, lesions, edema
▶ *Eyes*—acuity, visual loss, glasses, contacts, prosthesis, diplopia, photophobia, color vision, pain, burning, eyelid ptosis, edema, styes, exophthalmos, extraocular movement, position and alignment, strabismus, nystagmus, conjunctival color, discharge, vascular changes, corneal reflex, scleral color, vascularity, jaundice, pupils: size, shape, equality, reaction to light
▶ *Neck*—symmetry, movement, range of motion, masses, scars, pain, stiffness, lymph nodes: size, shape, mobility, tenderness, enlargement
▶ *Reflexes*—Deep tendon reflexes, Babinski, posturing

Musculoskeletal System

▶ *Activity level*—prescribed, actual, range of motion
▶ *Extremities*—size, shape, symmetry, temperature, color, pigmentation, scars, hematoma, bruises, rash, ulceration, numbness, paresis, swelling, prosthesis, fracture
▶ *Joints*—symmetry, active and passive mobility, deformities, stiffness, fixation, masses, swelling, fluid, bogginess, crepitation, pain, tenderness
▶ *Muscles*—symmetry, size, shape, tone, weakness, cramps, spasms, rigidity, tremors
▶ *Back*—scars, sacral edema, spinal abnormalities, kyphosis, scoliosis, tenderness, pain

Respiratory System

▶ *Nose*—smell, nasal size, symmetry, flaring, sneezing, deformities, mucosal color, edema, exudate, bleeding, furuncles, pain, tenderness, sinus pain
▶ *Chest*—size, shape, symmetry, deformities, pain, tenderness, expansion, crepitation, tactile fremitus
▶ *Trachea*—deviation, scars
▶ *Breathing patterns*—rate, regularity, depth, ease, use of accessory muscles, cyanosis, clubbing
▶ *Sounds*—normal, adventitious, intensity, pitch, quality, duration, equality, vocal resonance

Cardiovascular System

▶ *Cardiac patterns*—rate, rhythm, intensity, regularity, skipped or extra beats, point of maximal impulse, bruits, thrills, murmurs, rubs

▶ Precordial movements, neck veins, right and left cardiac borders, pacemaker

Gastrointestinal System

▶ *Mouth and throat*—odor, pain; ability to speak, bite, chew, swallow, taste; tongue: size, shape, protrusion, symmetry, color, hydration, markings, ulcers, burning, swelling, coating; gums: color, edema, bleeding, retraction, pain; teeth: number, absence, caries, caps, dentures, sensitivity to heat or cold; gag reflex, throat soreness, cough, sputum, hemoptysis
▶ *Abdomen*—size, color, contour, symmetry, fat, muscle tone, turgor, hair distribution, scars, umbilicus, striae, rashes, distention, abnormal pulsations, sounds: absent, hypoactive, hyperactive; tenderness, rigidity, free fluid, liver border, air bubble, splenic dullness, air rebound, muscle spasm, masses, guarding, pain
▶ *Rectum*—pigmentation, hemorrhoids, excoriation, rashes, abscess, pilonidal cyst, masses, lesions, tenderness, pain, itching, burning

Renal System

▶ *Urinary patterns*—amount, color, timing, odor, sediment, frequency, urgency, hesitancy, burning, pain, dribbling, incontinence, hematuria, nocturia, oliguria, change in stream, enuresis, flank pain, polyuria, retention, stress incontinence, bladder distention

Reproductive System

▶ *Male*—*penis:* discharge, ulceration, pain, size, prepuce; *scrotum:* size, color, nodules, swelling, ulceration, tenderness, pain; *testes:* size, shape, swelling, masses, absence
▶ *Female*—labia majora and minora, urethral and vaginal orifices, discharge, swelling, ulcerations, nodules, masses, tenderness, pain, pruritus, Pap smear, menstrual flow, menopause
▶ *Breasts*—contour, symmetry, color, shape, size, inflammation, scars; masses: location, size, shape, mobility, tenderness, pain; dimpling, swelling; nipples: color, discharge, ulceration, bleeding, inversion, pain; axillae: nodes, enlargement, tenderness, rash, inflammation

Integumentary System

▶ *Color*—pink, pale, red, jaundice, mottled, blanched, cyanotic
▶ *Patterns*—pigmentation, vascularity, temperature, texture, turgor, lesions (type, color, size, shape, distribution), bruises, bleeding, scars, edema, dryness, ecchymoses, masses (size, shape, location, mobility, tenderness), odors, petechiae, pruritus, bruises, bleeding, scars, edema

▼ ▼ ▼

From Iyer, P.W., et al. (1991). *Nursing process and nursing diagnosis* (2nd ed.). Philadelphia: W.B. Saunders.

Box 7–4. Functional Health Patterns Approach to Assessment

Health Perception—Health Management

▶ Description of health (usual, current), preventive measures, previous hospitalizations and expectations of current hospitalization, description of illness (onset, cause), prior treatment (including compliance, anticipated self-care problems)

Nutritional-Metabolic

▶ Usual daily food and fluid intake, appetite, food restrictions or preferences, food supplements, recent weight change; swallowing, chewing, feeding problems

Elimination

▶ *Bowel*—usual time, frequency, color, consistency, assistive devices (laxatives, suppositories, enemas), constipation, diarrhea
▶ *Bladder*—usual frequency; problems with frequency, urgency, burning, retention, incontinence, dribbling, dysuria, polyuria; assistive devices
▶ *Skin*—condition, color, temperature, turgor, lesions, edema, pruritus

Activity-Exercise

▶ Usual daily/weekly activities, occupation, leisure-exercise patterns, limitations in ambulation, bathing, dressing, toileting, dyspnea, fatigue

Sleep-Rest

▶ *Usual sleep pattern*—bedtime, hours, sleep aids; problems falling asleep, staying asleep, feeling rested

Cognitive-Perceptual

▶ *Sensory deficits*—hearing, sight, touch; problems with vertigo, heat or cold sensitivity, ability to read or write

Self-Perception

▶ Major concerns, health goals, self-description, effects of illness on self-perception; factors contributing to illness, recovery, health maintenance

Role-Relationship

▶ *Communication*—language; clear and relevant speech, expression, understanding
▶ *Relationships*—living arrangements, support system, family life, complaints (parenting, relatives, abuse, marital problems)

Sexuality-Reproductive

▶ Changes anticipated or experienced because of condition (fertility, libido, erection, pregnancy, contraception, menstruation)

Coping—Stress Tolerance

▶ Decision making (independent, assisted), major life changes (past, future, desired), stress management (eat, sleep, take medication, seek help), comfort/security needs

Value-Belief

▶ Sources of strength, meaning, religion (importance, type, frequency of practice), recent changes in values, beliefs, needs during hospitalization

Physical Assessment

▶ General appearance, weight, and height
▶ Eyes: appearance, drainage, pupils, vision
▶ Mouth: mucous membranes, teeth
▶ Hearing: acuity, aids
▶ Pulses: rate, rhythm, volume
▶ Respirations: rate, quality, sounds
▶ Blood pressure
▶ Temperature
▶ Skin color, temperature, turgor, lesions, edema, pruritus
▶ Functional ability, dominant hand, use of arms, legs, hands, strength, grasp, range of motion, gait, use of aids, weight bearing
▶ Mental status, orientation, memory, affect, eye contact

▼▼▼

From Iyer, P.W., et al. (1991). *Nursing process and nursing diagnosis* (2nd ed.). Philadelphia: W.B. Saunders.

---

the nurse to identify functional patterns (client strengths) and dysfunctional patterns or nursing diagnoses.[2] Nursing diagnoses are grouped into these patterns and are discussed further in Chapter 8. The nurse must collect information about all of the patterns to make a complete assessment.

HUMAN RESPONSE PATTERNS APPROACH

In the 1980s, the North American Nursing Diagnosis Association developed a conceptual framework initially called the "patterns of unitary person" and later changed to the "human response patterns." This approach divides a person's health status into nine human response patterns: exchanging, communicating, relating, valuing, choosing, moving, perceiving, knowing, and feeling (Box 7–5). Guzzetta et al.[3] have been active in developing assessment tools based on the human response patterns. Nurses are referred to their work for samples of forms useful in a variety of clinical settings. The human response patterns are discussed further in Chapter 8.

Box 7–5. Human Response Patterns Approach to Assessment

Exchanging

A human response pattern involving mutual giving and receiving

- *Cardiac*—apical rate, rhythm, point of maximal impulse, blood pressure (sitting, supine, standing, right and left)
- *Cerebral*—level of consciousness, pupils, eye opening, best verbal response, best motor response
- *Peripheral*—pulses, skin temperature, color, capillary refill, clubbing, edema
- *Skin integrity*—rashes, petechiae, abrasions, lesions, bruises, surgical incisions, other
- *Oxygenation*—respiratory rate, rhythm, depth, use of accessory muscles, dyspnea including precipitating factors, orthopnea, splinting, cough, sputum color/amount/consistency, breath sounds, history of smoking
- *Physical regulation*—lymph nodes, temperature
- *Nutrition*—eating patterns, number of meals per day, special diet, food preferences/intolerances, food allergies, caffeine intake, appetite changes, nausea/vomiting, condition of mouth/throat, height, weight, ideal body weight, alcohol use
- *Elimination*—usual bowel habits, alterations from normal, constipation, diarrhea, incontinence; bowel sounds; usual urinary habits, alterations from normal, incontinence, retention, urine color/consistency/odor
- *Safety*—risk for falls

Communicating

A human response pattern involving sending messages

- Read/write/understand English, other languages, impaired speech, other forms of communication

Relating

A human response pattern involving establishing bonds

- *Relationships*—marital status, age/health of significant other, number of children/sex/ages, role in home, financial support, occupation, job satisfaction/concerns, physical/mental energy expenditures, sexual relationships, physical difficulties/effects of illness on sexuality
- *Socialization*—quality of relationships with others, client's description, significant other's description, staff observations, verbalization of aloneness

Valuing

A human response pattern involving the assigning of relative worth

- Religious preference, important religious practices, spiritual concerns, cultural orientation, cultural practices

Choosing

A human response pattern involving the selection of alternatives

- *Coping*—client's/significant other's usual problem-solving methods, client's/significant other's method of managing stress, client's affect, physical manifestations, available support systems
- *Participation*—compliance with past/current health care regimens, willingness to comply with future health care regimen
- *Judgment*—decision-making ability, client's perspective, others' perspectives

Moving

A human response pattern involving activity

- *Activity*—history of physical disability, limitations in daily activities, verbal reports of fatigue/weakness, exercise habits
- *Rest*—hours slept per night, feeling rested on awakening, sleeping aids, difficulty falling/remaining asleep
- *Recreation*—leisure activities, social activities
- *Environmental maintenance*—size and arrangement of home/stairs/bathroom, safety needs, home responsibilities
- *Health maintenance*—health insurance, regular checkups, medications prescription/availability
- *Self-care*—client's ability to feed, bathe, dress, and toilet self
- *Meaningfulness*—verbalizes hopelessness, verbalizes/perceives loss of control
- *Sensory-perception*—history of restricted environment, impaired vision, glasses, impaired hearing, hearing aid, body position/motion, taste, touch, smell, reflexes

Perceiving

A human response pattern involving the reception of information

- *Self-concept*—client's description of self, effects of illness/surgery on self-concept
- *Meaningfulness*—verbalizes hopelessness, verbalizes/perceives loss of control
- *Sensory perception*—history of restricted environment, vision impaired, glasses, contact lenses, prosthesis, auditory impaired, hearing aid, body position/motion, taste, touch, smell, reflexes

Knowing

A human response pattern involving meaning associated with information

- *Current health problems* (client's/significant other's perception)
- *Health history*—previous illnesses/hospitalizations/surgery; diseases of heart, peripheral vascular systems,

Box continued on following page

Box 7–5. Human Response Patterns Approach to Assessment (Continued)

lungs, liver, kidneys; cerebrovascular disorders, rheumatic fever, thyroid, others
▶ *Current medications*—name, dosage, frequency, action
▶ *Risk factors*—hypertension, hyperlipidemia, smoking, obesity, diabetes, sedentary lifestyle, stress, alcohol use, oral contraceptives, family history
▶ *Readiness*—perception/knowledge of illness/tests/surgery, expectations of therapy, misconceptions, readiness to learn, requests for information, educational level, learning barriers
▶ *Orientation*—level of alertness, orientation to person/place/time, appropriate behavior/communication
▶ *Memory*—intact, recent only, remote only

Feeling

A human response pattern involving the subjective awareness of information

▶ *Pain/discomfort*—onset, duration, location, quality, radiation, associated/aggravating/alleviating factors
▶ *Emotional integrity/status*—recent stressful life events, fears, anxiety, grieving, source, physical manifestations

▼ ▼ ▼

Modified from Iyer, P.W., et al. (1991). *Nursing process and nursing diagnosis* (2nd ed.). Philadelphia: W.B. Saunders.

Psychosocial Assessment

The psychosocial assessment is an important component of the assessment process. It takes as much skill and sensitivity to note a person's mood, manner, and speech as it does to observe skin changes.

In assessing psychosocial status, include the following areas: general appearance and behavior, sensorium, and mental dysfunction. Assessment of *general appearance and behavior* includes assessment of motor ability, language ability, writing ability, and sensory function. Assessment of *sensorium* includes assessment of level of consciousness, orientation, attention span, memory, cognitive abilities, general knowledge, intellectual level, emotional state, and life situation. Assessment of *mental dysfunction* focuses on assessment for mental disorders. For additional information on psychosocial assessment, see Chapter 32.

Consultation

Consultation is an important way to test the validity of your assessment and enlarge your knowledge base.

What resource people are available to you for consultation?

Experts provide detailed information about certain *specific aspects* of the person's condition. For example, nurses frequently discuss the medical diagnosis and symptoms with the physician, the person's dietary restrictions with a nutritionist, and financial concerns with the social worker. In the example of the woman with mouth lesions, the nurse may request a consultation with a dentist to confirm that the dentures have caused the problem. You may also want to consult other health care professionals who have interacted with the person to see if their assessment validates your own observations.

As stated, the person's *significant others* also supply important data. Indeed, consulting with significant others is essential for understanding the individual's home and lifestyle.

Other sources include old medical documents, current health documents, and care plans from earlier hospitalizations. When reviewing health documents, study the medical and nursing histories, laboratory studies, progress and nursing notes, and entries from consultants (neurologists, psychiatrists, physical therapists, and clinical specialists).

Review of the Literature

You will need to review the literature during assessment and throughout the nursing process. A thorough literature search for information about the person's diagnosis, symptoms, medications, functional disabilities, and rehabilitation serves several purposes.

First, the literature presents a "textbook picture" of the general condition with which you can compare the person's actual experiences. Second, selected readings help you to expand your knowledge of the medical diagnosis and nursing diagnosis. In addition, reviewing

---

Box 7–6. American Nurses' Association Standard for Assessment

The nurse collects client health data.

Measurement Criteria

1. The priority of data collection is determined by the client's immediate condition or needs.
2. Pertinent data are collected by use of appropriate assessment techniques.
3. Data collection involves the client, significant others, and health care providers when appropriate.
4. The data collection process is systematic and ongoing.
5. Relevant data are documented in a retrievable form.

▼ ▼ ▼

Reprinted with permission from *Standards of clinical nursing practice* (1991). Washington, DC: American Nurses' Association.

nursing literature provides you with insights for making *your own diagnosis* of the client's problems and their causation. Finally, a careful survey of current reading creates a solid theoretical basis for planning and evaluating nursing intervention.

Nurses are professionally accountable for maintaining up-to-date nursing knowledge.

When you review the literature, begin with a general textbook that provides basic information about health and illness. Next, consult journal articles and specialized textbooks. They will give you more specific information, and they often present research findings that are relevant to your client's situation. Finally, take advantage of the health science or nursing library services. Many libraries have audiovisual and computerized learning packages that cover a wide range of clinical topics. The librarian can assist you in obtaining computerized literature searches and other resource materials available through interlibrary loan arrangements.

Nurses play a pivotal role in coordinating client care. The ability of nurses to detect abnormalities is therefore essential. Accordingly, the American Nurses' Association has established a standard of nursing assessment (Box 7–6).

Summary

▶ Assessment data are categorized into subjective and objective data and obtained through primary and secondary sources.

▶ Many factors influence the nature of the data base, including the urgency of the situation, the nurse's knowledge and skills, and the perspective of the nurse.

▶ Assessment information is collected in a variety of ways, including review of the clinical record, interviewing, history taking, and physical and psychosocial assessment.

▶ Physical assessment skills are used to identify a person's needs.

▶ Admission assessment forms and data bases are structured in a variety of formats.

▶ Psychosocial assessment provides an important dimension of information about the person.

▶ Consultation with other professionals and review of the literature add to the knowledge base of the nurse.

▶ The American Nurses' Association has established a standard and measurement criteria for assessment.

Bibliography

1. Andrews, C. (1987). Orientation: graduate's preparation of initiation. *Nursing Management,* 18(11), 110–111.
2. Gordon, M. (1987). *Nursing diagnosis: Process and application* (2nd ed.). New York: McGraw-Hill.
3. Guzzetta, C., et al. (1989). *Clinical assessment tools for use with nursing diagnosis.* St. Louis: C.V. Mosby.
4. Wake, M. (1990). Nursing care delivery systems: status and vision. *Journal of Nursing Administration,* 20(5), 47–51.
5. White, N., et al. (1990). Promoting critical thinking skills. *Nurse Educator,* 15(5), 16–19.

▼ *Nursing Diagnosis*

▼ *I reckon that being ill is one of the great pleasures of life, provided
one is not too ill and not obliged to work until one is better.*

▼

Samuel Butler
The Way of All Flesh

▼

▼

▼ CHAPTER OUTLINE

NURSING DIAGNOSIS DEFINED AND
  EXPLORED
THE DIAGNOSTIC PROCESS
    Step One: Analysis and
      Interpretation
    Step Two: Making and Validating
      Inferences
    Step Three: Comparing Cues and
      Clusters of Cues with Defining
      Characteristics
    Step Four: Identifying the Related
      Factors
    Step Five: Documenting the
      Nursing Diagnosis
HUMAN RESPONSE PATTERNS
FUNCTIONAL HEALTH PATTERNS
DOCUMENTATION OF THE ACTUAL
  NURSING DIAGNOSIS
VARIATIONS OF THE DIAGNOSTIC
  STATEMENT
GUIDELINES FOR
WRITING AN ACTUAL NURSING
  DIAGNOSIS
    Write the Diagnosis in Terms of
      thePerson's Response Rather
      than Nursing Need
    Use "Related to" Rather than "Due
      to" or "Caused by" to Connect
      the Two Parts of the Statement

    Write the Diagnosis in Legally
      Advisable Terms
    Write the Diagnosis Without Value
      Judgments
    Avoid Reversing the Parts of the
      Statement
    Avoid Using Single Cues in the
      First Part of the Statement
    The Two Parts of the Statement
      Should Not Mean the Same
      Thing
    Express the Related Factor in
      Terms that Can Be Changed
    Do Not Include Medical Diagnoses
      in the Nursing Diagnostic
      Statement
    State the Diagnosis Clearly and
      Concisely
COLLABORATIVE PROBLEMS
IMPLICATIONS OF NURSING DIAGNOSES
    Legal Aspects of a Nursing
      Diagnosis
    Critical Thinking and Errors in the
      Diagnostic Process
    Implications of Nursing Diagnosis
      for Nursing Practice

▼ Key Terms

Collaborative problems
Cues
Defining characteristics
Diagnostic cues
High-risk nursing
  diagnosis

Inferencing
Life processes
North American Nursing
  Diagnosis Association
  (NANDA)

Related factors
Risk factors
Wellness diagnosis

Making nursing diagnoses is an indispensable and high-level intellectual skill that you will develop and practice throughout your professional life. Nursing diagnoses are applicable to all strata of clients. Depending on your area of nursing, you will apply nursing diagnostic skills to individuals, families, groups, or even entire communities.

Because the nursing diagnosis culminates the assessment phase, it is the pivotal step in the nursing process. Without accurate nursing diagnoses, there is no point in progressing to the other stages of the nursing process, for there will be no basis for planning care or intervention or for evaluating the outcome of nursing intervention.

Today it is recognized that diagnosis is *not* the exclusive domain of the physician or even of health care professionals. If a diagnosis is "essentially an inference about a state that is undesirable," then lawyers, social workers, police detectives, and auto mechanics all make diagnoses. Clearly, nurses share with these experts from other fields the common diagnostic skills associated with uncovering problems and finding their cause, such as gathering facts, organizing data, analysis of data, seeking patterns, and stating conclusions. It is the drawing and stating of conclusions that has relevance to our present discussion of diagnosis.

NURSING DIAGNOSIS DEFINED AND EXPLORED

Nursing diagnosis is a complex concept to define. Nursing diagnoses are *not* medical diagnoses, although there are similarities between the two. Nursing diagnoses are *similar* to medical diagnoses in that the same basic methods underlie both processes: obtaining the person's history, performing the physical examination, organizing the data base, and analyzing the data obtained. Both nurses and physicians need similar skills to make diagnoses: communication skills, physical assessment skills, observational skills, and intellectual skills.

On the other hand, nursing diagnoses *differ* from medical diagnoses in their focus and consequently in their specific goals and objectives. Physicians are primarily involved in diagnosing disease and its underlying pathologic processes. Physicians examine people to learn the source of their symptoms and the metabolic,

chemical, or pathologic structural changes resulting from the disorder.

A physician may examine a person with chest pain and formulate a medical diagnosis of myocardial infarction (heart attack). The nurse may assess the same person and identify several nursing diagnoses. These diagnoses could relate to specific problems or responses such as pain, fear, ineffective denial, and so on.

Both medical and nursing diagnoses are necessary and valid. To develop a person's total diagnostic picture, nurses and physicians must work together as well as independently. Also, they must communicate their findings to one another.

The North American Nursing Diagnosis Association (**NANDA**—an organization formed in the 1980s to promote the development of and education about nursing diagnosis) has identified three types of nursing diagnoses: actual, high-risk, and wellness diagnoses. In 1990, NANDA accepted a definition of an actual nursing diagnosis.

A nursing diagnosis is a clinical judgment about individual, family, or community responses to actual or potential health problems/life processes. Nursing diagnoses provide the basis for selection of nursing interventions to achieve outcomes for which the nurse is accountable.[16]

High-risk and wellness nursing diagnoses are defined and described later in the chapter.

THE DIAGNOSTIC PROCESS

During the assessment process, you gather a large amount of information about the person. These data must be sorted, organized, analyzed, and interpreted for a nursing diagnosis to be made. As discussed in Chapter 7, the admission assessment helps organize the data and ensure that the important points are assessed. Depending on the format of the data base, you will collect information according to major body systems, human response patterns, or functional health patterns.

Step One: Analysis and Interpretation

Diagnosis, which is summarized in Box 8–1 in relation to assessment, begins with analysis and interpretation of the data. Interpretation is based on cues and inferences. **Cues** are subjective or objective pieces of information obtained through assessment. **Diagnostic cues** are clinical evidence that describes a cluster of behaviors or signs and symptoms that represent a diagnostic label. Diagnostic cues are concrete and measurable through observation or client/group reports and are separated into major and minor. In the diagnosis step, the nurse sorts through the cues and selects the ones that are relevant. Extraneous information not directly related to the cues is put aside. Several cues are grouped together to form a cluster.

The potential for making an accurate nursing diagnosis increases when you use a cluster of cues rather than a single cue.

For example, suppose you see a person grimacing. This facial expression (cue) could have a variety of meanings, including anger, disagreement, or pain. However, when you see the person grimacing, rubbing his chest, and moaning, this cluster of cues leads to the conclusion that the man is experiencing pain.

Step Two: Making and Validating Inferences

The process of assigning meaning to a cue or cluster of cues is **inferencing.** Theory, experience, intuition, and validation are used to make an inference. Whenever possible, you should validate the inference with the person, such as by asking "Are you in pain?" Textbooks, articles, and other health care professionals can also validate or verify the inference.

Step Three: Comparing Cues and Clusters of Cues with Defining Characteristics

The next step in the diagnostic process involves comparing the cluster of clinical cues with the definition and defining characteristics of a nursing diagnosis. The definition of a diagnosis provides a clear, precise description. It delineates the meaning of the diagnosis and helps differentiate the diagnosis from similar diagnoses. Some of the nursing diagnoses are closely related, and you may need to use the definition to select the more applicable diagnosis. For example, fear and anxiety have similar defining characteristics, but their definitions differ. According to Taptich,[18] anxiety is defined as the state in which an individual experiences a vague uneasy feeling, the source of which is often nonspecific or unknown. Fear is defined as the state in which the individual experiences feelings of dread related to an identifiable source perceived as dangerous. The definition of these two diagnoses indicates how they differ.

Defining characteristics are also used to select the most appropriate diagnosis.

Defining characteristics are clinical cues that cluster as manifestations of a nursing diagnosis.[16] Defining characteristics are categorized as major and minor. Major defining characteristics are present 80 to 100 per cent of the time when a person is experiencing a particular nursing diagnosis. Minor defining characteristics may be present 50 to 79 per cent of the time but increase your confidence that you are making the correct diagnosis.[16]

Box 8–2 illustrates the major and minor defining characteristics for colonic constipation. The designation of major and minor characteristics is a new trend in nursing diagnosis language. You will note that not all information on nursing diagnoses includes this concept.

There are a number of nursing diagnosis handbooks available that provide information about each nursing diagnosis that has been approved by NANDA for clinical testing. These handbooks typically provide a definition, defining characteristics, and related factors or risk factors. Use the definition and defining characteristics to determine whether there is a match and to verify that the person is experiencing the nursing diagnosis you have identified. When you have found the best match, you still have not made a complete diagnosis. There is more to the process.

Step Four: Identifying the Related Factors

Identification of the related factors is the next step in the diagnostic process.

Related factors are conditions or circumstances that can cause or contribute to the development of a diagnosis.

Related factors can be environmental, physiologic, psychosocial, or spiritual factors that contribute to the development of the problem. The factors should be changeable through nursing intervention. A medical diagnosis, therefore, is not an appropriate related fac-

---

Box 8–1. Step 2 of the Nursing Process: Diagnosis	
Assessment	**Diagnosis**
Collect data:	Interpret data:
Review of the clinical record	Identify clusters of cues
Interview	Make inferences
Nursing history	Validate inferences
Physical assessment	Compare clusters of cues
Psychosocial assessment	with definition and defining characteristics
Consultation	Identify related factors
Review of the literature	Document the nursing diagnosis

Box 8–2. Examples of Defining Characteristics

Colonic Constipation

Definition

The state in which an individual's pattern of elimination is characterized by hard, dry stool that results from a delay in passage of food residue

Defining Characteristics	Related Factors
Major	Less than adequate
	Fluid intake
Decreased frequency	Dietary intake
Hard, dry stool	Fiber intake
Straining at stool	Physical activity
Painful defecation	Immobility
Abdominal distention	Lack of privacy
Palpable mass	Emotional disturbances
	Chronic use of medication
Minor	and enemas
	Stress
Rectal pressure	Change in daily routine
Headache	
Appetite impairment	
Abdominal pain	

▼▼▼

From Taptich, B.J., et al. (1989). *Nursing diagnosis and care planning.* Philadelphia: W.B. Saunders.

Box 8–3. Examples of Related Factors

Impaired Verbal Communication

Definition

The state in which an individual experiences a dysfunction in ability to verbalize appropriately or interpret the meaning of words

Defining Characteristics	Related Factors
Difficulty with phonation	Altered thought processes
Disorientation	Auditory impairment
Dyspnea	Effects of
Flight of ideas	Surgery
Inability to	Trauma
Find words	Inflammation
Identify objects	Physical barrier
Modulate speech	Intubation
Name words	Tracheostomy
Speak dominant language	Respiratory embarassment
Lack of desire to speak,	Speech pattern dysfunction
speak in sentences	Inability to read or write
Incessant verbalization	Ineffective listening skills
Loose association of ideas	Language barrier
Stuttering/slurring	Psychologic barriers
	Anxiety
	Fear

▼▼▼

(Modified from Taptich, B.J. et al. (1989). *Nursing diagnosis and care planning.* Philadelphia: W.B. Saunders.

---

tor. Box 8–2 lists related factors associated with colonic constipation. In contrast to defining characteristics, usually only a few related factors from the list are applicable. For example, a non–English-speaking person may have the nursing diagnosis of impaired verbal communication, which is defined in Box 8–3. Of the related factors listed, "language barrier" is the most applicable one.

Step Five: Documenting the Nursing Diagnosis

The last step in the diagnostic process is the documentation of the nursing diagnosis. The list of NANDA-approved nursing diagnoses should be referred to for developing the diagnostic statement. The list of NANDA-approved diagnoses may be organized in a variety of ways: alphabetically (inside back cover) or in a classification system that groups diagnoses into categories. Human response patterns and functional health patterns are two commonly used classification systems.

HUMAN RESPONSE PATTERNS

In work that spanned 4 years, a group of nursing theorists developed a way of organizing nursing diagnoses. The intent of their work was a classification system (taxonomy) that would sort and group diagnoses. The result of this collaboration was called Taxonomy 1, which was accepted at the seventh NANDA conference. The taxonomy classified all accepted nursing diagnoses into nine human response patterns. Taxonomy 1 was renamed Taxonomy 1R (Box 8–4) when more diagnoses were accepted at subsequent conferences. Although a draft of Taxonomy II was presented at the NANDA conference in 1990 and nine new diagnoses were added in 1992, Taxonomy II has not yet been published. The taxonomy is not based on the philosophy of any one theorist. The use of a taxonomy has the following benefits:

▶ The taxonomy provides a framework for organizing existing diagnoses.
▶ Gaps or omissions in the framework suggest the need for the development of additional diagnoses.

Box 8-4. North American Nursing Diagnosis Association Taxonomy 1R

Exchanging

A human response pattern involving mutual giving and receiving

1.1.2.1	Nutrition, Altered: More than Body Requirements
1.1.2.2	Nutrition, Altered: Less than Body Requirements
1.1.2.3	Nutrition, Altered: Potential for more than body requirements
1.2.1.1	Infection, High Risk for
1.2.2.1	Body Temperature, High Risk for Altered
1.2.2.2	Hypothermia
1.2.2.3	Hyperthermia
1.2.2.4	Thermoregulation, Ineffective
1.2.3.1	Dysreflexia
1.3.1.1	Constipation
1.3.1.1.1	Constipation, Perceived
1.3.1.1.2	Constipation, Colonic
1.3.1.2	Diarrhea
1.3.1.3	Incontinence, Bowel
1.3.2	Urinary Elimination, Altered
1.3.2.1.1	Incontinence, Stress
1.3.2.1.2	Incontinence, Reflex
1.3.2.1.3	Incontinence, Urge
1.3.2.1.4	Incontinence, Functional
1.3.2.1.5	Incontinence, Total
1.3.2.2	Urinary Retention
1.4.1.1	Tissue Perfusion, Altered (specify type) (renal, cerebral, cardiopulmonary, gastrointestinal, peripheral)
1.4.1.2.1	Fluid Volume Excess
1.4.1.2.2.1	Fluid Volume Deficit
1.4.1.2.2.2	Fluid Volume Deficit
1.4.1.2.2	Fluid Volume Deficit, High Risk for
1.4.2.1	Decreased Cardiac Output
1.5.1.1	Gas Exchange, Impaired
1.5.1.2	Airway Clearance, Ineffective
1.5.1.3	Breathing Clearance, Ineffective
*1.5.1.3.1	Inability to Sustain Spontaneous Ventilation
*1.5.1.3.2	Dysfunctional Ventilatory Weaning Response (DVWR)
1.6.1	Injury, High Risk for
1.6.1.1	Suffocation, High Risk for
1.6.1.2	Poisoning, High Risk for
1.6.1.3	Trauma, High Risk for
1.6.1.4	Aspiration, High Risk for
1.6.1.5	Disuse Syndrome, High Risk for
1.6.2	Protection, Altered
1.6.2.1	Tissue Integrity, Impaired
1.6.2.1.1	Oral Mucous Membrane, Altered
1.6.2.1.2.1	Skin Integrity, Impaired
1.6.2.1.2.2	Skin Integrity, High Risk for Impaired

Communicating

A human response pattern involving sending messages

2.1.1.1	Communication, Impaired Verbal

Relating

A human response pattern involving establishing bonds

3.1.1	Social Interaction, Impaired
3.1.2	Social Isolation
3.2.1	Role Performance, Altered
3.2.1.1.1	Parenting, Altered
3.2.1.1.2	Parenting, High Risk for Altered
3.2.1.2.1	Sexual Dysfunction
3.2.2	Family Processes, Altered
*3.2.2.1	Care Giver Role Strain
*3.2.2.2	Care Giver Role Strain, High Risk for
3.2.3.1	Parental Role Conflict
3.3	Sexuality Patterns, Altered

Valuing

A human response pattern involving the assigning of relative worth

4.1.1	Spiritual Distress

Choosing

A human response pattern involving the selection of alternatives

5.1.1.1	Individual Coping, Ineffective
5.1.1.1.1	Adjustment, Impaired
5.1.1.1.2	Defensive Coping
5.1.1.1.3	Denial, Ineffective
5.1.2.1.1	Family Coping, Disabling, Ineffective
5.1.2.1.2	Family Coping, Compromised, Ineffective
5.1.2.2	Family Coping: Potential for Growth
*5.2.1	Management of Therapeutic Regimen (Individuals), Ineffective
5.2.1.1	Noncompliance (specify)
5.3.1.1	Decisional Conflict (specify)
5.4	Health-Seeking Behaviors (specify)

Moving

A human response pattern involving activity

6.1.1.1	Physical Mobility, Impaired
*6.1.1.1.1	Peripheral Neurovascular Dysfunction, High Risk for
6.1.1.2.1	Fatigue
6.1.1.3	Activity Intolerance, High Risk for
6.2.1	Sleep Pattern Disturbance
6.3.1.1	Diversional Activity Deficit
6.4.1.1	Home Maintenance Management, Impaired
6.4.2	Health Maintenance, Altered
6.5.1	Self-Care Deficit, Feeding
6.5.1.1	Swallowing, Impaired
6.5.1.2	Breastfeeding, Ineffective
*6.5.1.2.1	Breastfeeding, Interrupted
6.5.1.3	Breastfeeding, Effective
*6.5.1.4	Infant Feeding Pattern, Ineffective

Box continued on following page

Box 8–4. North American Nursing Diagnosis Association Taxonomy 1R (Continued)

6.5.2	*Self-Care Deficit, Bathing/Hygiene*
6.5.3	*Self-Care Deficit, Dressing/Grooming*
6.5.4	*Self-Care Deficit, Toileting*
6.6	*Growth and Development, Altered*
*6.7	*Relocation Stress Syndrome*

Perceiving

A human response pattern involving the reception of information

7.1.1	*Body Image Disturbance*
7.1.2	*Self-Esteem Disturbance*
7.1.2.1	*Self-Esteem, Chronic Low*
7.1.2.2	*Self-Esteem, Situational Low*
7.1.3	*Personal Identity Disturbance*
7.2	*Sensory/Perceptual Alterations* (specify) (visual, auditory, kinesthetic, gustatory, tactile, olfactory)
7.2.1.1	*Unilateral Neglect*
7.3.1	*Hopelessness*
7.3.2	*Powerlessness*

Knowing

A human response pattern involving the meaning associated with information

8.1.1	*Knowledge Deficit* (specify)
8.2	*Thought Processes, Altered*

Feeling

A human response pattern involving the subjective awareness of information

9.1.1	*Pain*
9.1.1.1	*Pain, Chronic*
9.2.1.1	*Grieving, Dysfunctional*
9.2.1.2	*Grieving, Anticipatory*
9.2.2	*Violence, High Risk for: Self-directed or directed at others*
*9.2.2.1	*Self Mutilation, High Risk for*
9.2.3	*Post-Trauma Response*
9.2.3.1	*Rape-Trauma Syndrome*
9.2.3.1.1	*Rape-Trauma Syndrome: Compound Reaction*
9.2.3.1.2	*Rape-Trauma Syndrome: Silent Reaction*
9.3.1	*Anxiety*
9.3.2	*Fear*

---

* New diagnoses approved in 1992.

▶ The taxonomy promotes research efforts into nursing diagnoses.

▶ The diagnoses provide a language for communication of nursing knowledge and retrieval of information.

▶ The taxonomy offers a coding system to facilitate computerization of nursing documentation.

FUNCTIONAL HEALTH PATTERNS

In the 1980s, Marjory Gordon developed functional health patterns, as described in Chapter 7. The functional health patterns approach is another system for organizing nursing diagnoses. Box 8–5 lists the nursing diagnoses that fit into each of the 11 functional health patterns. Functional health patterns differ from Taxonomy 1R in that they do not use numbers to show the relationship of diagnoses within the pattern. However, some nurses find the titles of the patterns to be less abstract than the nine human response patterns.

DOCUMENTATION OF THE ACTUAL NURSING DIAGNOSIS

Each of the three types of nursing diagnosis is written differently. The first part of an actual diagnosis, the human response, comes from the NANDA list whenever possible. (Because the list continues to grow every 2 years, it is not considered to be complete.) The NANDA list contains qualifiers or adjectives that clarify the nursing diagnoses (Table 8–1) and precede the human response.

The second part of the nursing diagnosis is the related factor. It is linked to the human response with the words "related to," abbreviated in this text as R/T. The words "related to" demonstrate that there is a relationship between the first two parts of the diagnosis; this implies that if one part changes, the other will also.

The third part of the statement consists of the pertinent defining characteristics. They are linked to the second part with the words "as evidenced by," abbreviated AEB in this text. Figure 8–1 summarizes the three components of an actual nursing diagnosis. The three-part actual nursing diagnosis has been referred to as the PES format: Problem (or human response), Etiology (related factors), and Signs and Symptoms (or defining characteristics). Some nurses argue that the inclusion of the third part of the statement helps clarify the basis for formulating the nursing diagnostic statement. Other nurses write the actual diagnosis as a two-part statement, saying that the defining characteristics are documented in the data base, flow sheets, or other parts of the medical record.

Box 8-5. Functional Health Patterns

Health Perception-Health Management Pattern

Health Maintenance, Altered
Protection, Altered Therapeutic Regimen, Ineffective Management of
Noncompliance (specify)
Infection, High Risk for
Injury, High Risk for
Trauma, High Risk for
Poisoning, High Risk for
Suffocation, High Risk for
Health-Seeking Behaviors (specify)

Nutritional-Metabolic Pattern

Nutrition, Altered: High Risk for More than Body Requirements
Nutrition, Altered: More than Body Requirements
Nutrition, Altered: Less than Body Requirements
Breastfeeding, Effective
Breastfeeding, Ineffective
Breastfeeding, Interrupted
Infant Feeding Patterns, Ineffective
Aspiration, High Risk for
Swallowing, Impaired
Oral Mucous Membrane, Altered
Fluid Volume Deficit, High Risk for
Fluid Volume Deficit (1)
Fluid Volume Deficit (2)
Fluid Volume Excess
Skin Integrity, High Risk for Impaired
Skin Integrity, Impaired
Tissue Integrity, Impaired
Body Temperature, High Risk for Altered
Thermoregulation, Ineffective
Hyperthermia
Hypothermia

Elimination Pattern

Constipation
Constipation, Perceived
Constipation, Colonic
Diarrhea
Incontinence, Bowel
Urinary Elimination, Altered Patterns of
Incontinence, Functional
Incontinence, Reflex
Incontinence, Stress
Incontinence, Urge
Incontinence, Total
Retention, Urinary

Activity-Exercise Pattern

Activity Intolerance, High Risk for
Dysfunctional Ventilatory Weaning Response
Inability to Sustain Spontaneous Ventilation
Peripheral Neurovascular Dysfunction, High Risk for
Activity Intolerance
Physical Mobility, Impaired
Disuse Syndrome, High Risk for

Fatigue
Self-Care Deficit, Bathing/Hygiene
Self-Care Deficit, Dressing/Grooming
Self-Care Deficit, Feeding
Self-Care Deficit, Toileting
Diversional Activity Deficit
Home Maintenance Management, Impaired
Airway Clearance, Ineffective
Breathing Pattern, Ineffective
Gas Exchange, Impaired
Decreased Cardiac Output
Tissue Perfusion, Altered (specify type) (renal, cerebral, cardiopulmonary, gastrointestinal, peripheral)
Dysreflexia
Growth and Development, Altered

Sleep-Rest Pattern

Sleep Pattern Disturbance

Cognitive-Perceptual Pattern

Pain
Pain, Chronic
Sensory/Perceptual Alterations (specify) (visual, auditory, kinesthetic, gustatory, tactile, olfactory)
Peripheral Neurovascular Dysfunction, High Risk for
Unilateral Neglect
Knowledge Deficit (specify)
Thought Processes, Altered
Decisional Conflict (specify)

Self-perception-Self-concept Pattern

Fear
Anxiety
Hopelessness
Powerlessness
Body Image Disturbance
Personal Identity Disturbance
Self-Esteem Disturbance
Self-Esteem, Chronic Low
Self-Esteem, Situational Low

Role-Relationship Pattern

Grieving, Anticipatory
Grieving, Dysfunctional
Role Performance, Altered
Care Giver Role Strain
Care Giver Role Strain, High Risk for
Social Isolation
Social Interaction, Impaired
Relocation Stress Syndrome
Family Processes, Altered
Parenting, High Risk for Altered
Parenting, Altered

Box continued on following page

Box 8–5. Functional Health Patterns (Continued)

Parental Role Conflict
Communication, Impaired Verbal
Violence, High Risk for: Self-directed or directed at others

Sexuality-Reproductive Pattern

Sexual Dysfunction
Sexuality Patterns, Altered
Rape-Trauma Syndrome
Rape-Trauma Syndrome: Compound Reaction
Rape-Trauma Syndrome: Silent Reaction

Coping–Stress Tolerance Pattern

Individual Coping, Ineffective
Defensive Coping

Denial, Ineffective
Adjustment, Impaired
Post-Trauma Response
Family Coping: Potential for Growth
Family Coping, Compromised, Ineffective
Family Coping, Disabling, Ineffective

Value-Belief Pattern

Spiritual Distress (Distress of the Human Spirit)

▼ ▼ ▼

From Kim, M., et al. (1993). *Pocket guide to nursing diagnosis* (5th ed.). St Louis: Mosby.

VARIATIONS OF THE DIAGNOSTIC STATEMENT

As stated earlier, there are three types of nursing diagnoses: actual, high-risk, and wellness diagnoses.

A **high-risk nursing diagnosis** is a clinical judgment that an individual, family, or community is more vulnerable to development of the problem than are others in the same or a similar situation. High-risk nursing diagnoses include risk factors that guide nursing interven-

tions to reduce or prevent the occurrence of the problem.[16]

Risk factors identify behaviors, conditions, or circumstances that render an individual, family, or community more vulnerable to a particular problem than others in the same or a similar situation. There are no signs and symptoms (defining characteristics) for high-risk diagnoses because they represent potential, not actual, problems. Therefore, high-risk diagnoses are written as two-part statements.

Example *High-Risk for Injury: Fall* R/T fatigue and altered gait.[16]

Box 8–6 illustrates a high-risk nursing diagnosis as it would appear in a nursing diagnosis handbook.

The third type of nursing diagnosis focuses on wellness or areas of strength in the person. The key concept that links wellness nursing diagnoses to the defini-

TABLE 8–1. Suggested Qualifiers for Nursing Diagnoses

Qualifier	Definition
Altered	A change from baseline
Impaired	Made worse, weakened, damaged, reduced, deteriorated
Depleted	Emptied wholly or partially, exhausted of
Deficient	Inadequate in amount, quality, or degree; defective; not sufficient; incomplete
Excessive	Characterized by an amount or quantity that is greater than is necessary, desirable, or useful
Dysfunctional	Abnormal, incomplete functioning
Disturbed	Agitated, interrupted, interfered with
Ineffective	Not producing the desired effect
Decreased	Lessened; lesser in size, amount, or degree
Increased	Greater in size, amount, or degree
Acute	Severe but of short duration
Chronic	Lasting a long time, recurring, habitual, constant
Intermittent	Stopping and starting again at intervals, cyclic
Potential for enhanced	(For use with wellness diagnoses) Enhanced is defined as made greater, to increase in quality, or more desired

From NANDA News (1990). *Nursing Diagnosis*, 1(3), 124.

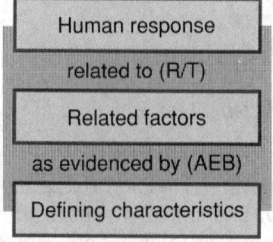

Example:
Colonic Constipation R/T less than adequate fluid intake AEB hard, dry stool

▲ *Figure 8–1*

The three components of an actual nursing diagnosis.

Box 8–6. Example of a High-Risk Nursing Diagnosis

High Risk for Aspiration

Definition

The state in which an individual is at risk for entry of gastrointestinal secretions, oropharyngeal secretions, solids, or fluids into tracheobronchial passages

Risk Factors

Reduced level of consciousness
Depressed cough and gag reflex
Presence of tracheostomy or endotracheal tube
Gastrointestinal tubes
Tube feedings
Medication administration
Situations hindering elevation of upper body
Increased gastric residue
Decreased gastrointestinal motility
Delayed gastric emptying
Impaired swallowing
Facial, oral, or neck surgery or trauma
Wired jaw

▼▼▼

Modified from Taptich, B.J., et al. (1989). *Nursing diagnosis and care planning.* Philadelphia: W.B. Saunders.

Box 8–7. Examples and Definitions of Wellness Diagnoses

Effective Breastfeeding

Definition

The state in which a mother-infant dyad/family exhibits adequate proficiency and satisfaction with breastfeeding behaviors

Family Coping: Potential for Growth

Definition

The state in which the family effectively manages adaptive tasks involved with a health challenge and exhibits desire for enhanced growth

Health-Seeking Behaviors

Definition

The state in which an individual in stable health is actively seeking ways to alter personal health habits or the environment to move toward a higher level of health (stable health status is defined as age-appropriate illness prevention measures achieved, client reports good or excellent health, and signs and symptoms of disease, if present, are controlled)

▼▼▼

Modified from Taptich, B.J., et al. (1989). *Nursing diagnosis and care planning.* Philadelphia: W.B. Saunders.

tion of a nursing diagnosis is that a nursing diagnosis is a clinical judgment about individual, family, or community responses to actual or potential health problems (life processes). Life processes may consist of normal stages of growth and development or situational crises, such as major changes in lifestyle.

Wellness diagnoses focus on the nurse's role in promoting health and prevention of illness. A **wellness diagnosis** is defined as a clinical judgment about an individual, family, or community in transition from a specific level of wellness to a higher level of wellness.[16]

In 1990, NANDA suggested the term "potential for enhanced" as a qualifier. Enhanced is defined as "made greater, to increase in quality, or more desired." Wellness diagnoses are to be stated as one-part statements.

Example *Potential for Enhanced Parenting*

Box 8–7 provides examples of wellness diagnoses. Table 8–2 summarizes the three types of nursing diagnoses.

TABLE 8–2. Summary of the Three Types of Nursing Diagnoses

Type of Diagnosis	Components	Format of Diagnostic Statement	Example
Actual	Definition	Human response	*Colonic Constipation* R/T lack of privacy, AEB hard, dry stool
	Defining characteristics	Qualifier	
	Related factors	Related to related factors	
		As evidenced by defining characteristics	
High-risk	Definition	Human response	*High Risk for Aspiration* R/T impaired swallowing
	Risk factors	High risk for	
		Related to risk factors	
Wellness	Definition	Potential for enhanced, or human response	*Effective Breastfeeding*
	Defining characteristics		

GUIDELINES FOR WRITING AN ACTUAL NURSING DIAGNOSIS*

The guidelines apply to the development of a two-part actual nursing diagnosis and are reproduced with modifications from Iyer et al.[12]

Write the Diagnosis in Terms of the Person's Response Rather than Nursing Need

The first part of the diagnostic statement identifies the person's response to health or illness. Therapeutic or functional needs, such as "needs frequent turning" or "needs coughing and deep breathing," describe nursing interventions rather than client responses and should not be included in the diagnostic statement.

Examples

Stella Blackwell is a 45-year-old client who has a nasogastric tube after surgery. She tells her nurse that she is thirsty and that her mouth and lips are dry. The nurse recognizes that the client "needs additional fluids" and communicates this response in the diagnostic statement "*Fluid Volume Deficit* R/T decreased oral intake."

Incorrect	Correct
Needs Suctioning because she has many secretions	*High Risk for Aspiration* R/T excessive oral secretions
Needs Frequent Rest Periods because of shortness of breath	*Fatigue* R/T persistent shortness of breath

---

Use "Related to" Rather than "Due to" or "Caused by" to Connect the Two Parts of the Statement

The first and second parts of the diagnostic statement should always be linked by the words "related to" (R/T). This identifies a relationship between the human response and the related factors, which implies that if one part of the diagnosis changes, the other part may change also.

Example

Incorrect	Correct
High Risk for Injury caused by change in mental status	*High Risk for Injury* R/T change in mental status

---

* Modified from Iyer, P.W., Taptich, B.J., & Bernocchi-Losey, D. (1991). *Nursing process and nursing diagnosis* (2nd ed.). Philadelphia: W.B. Saunders.

Write the Diagnosis in Legally Advisable Terms

A diagnostic statement such as "*Impaired Skin Integrity* R/T infrequent turning" is not legally advisable. This statement implies negligence or blame that may not be accurate and can create potential legal problems for the health care personnel. This statement could be better phrased as "*Impaired Skin Integrity* R/T prolonged immobility." The therapeutic nursing orders would be similar in both instances, but the second statement is factual and does not imply fault.

Examples

Incorrect	Correct
High Risk for Injury R/T inadequately maintained skin traction	*High Risk for Injury* R/T hazards of skin traction
Ineffective Airway clearance R/T excessive sedation	*Ineffective Airway Clearance* R/T effects of sedation

---

Write the Diagnosis Without Value Judgments

Nursing diagnoses should be based on objective and subjective data collected and validated in conjunction with the client or significant other. The behavior of the client should not be judged by the nurse's personal values and standards. Use of words such as inadequate, poor, and unhealthy in diagnostic statements frequently implies value judgments.

Examples

Incorrect	Correct
Altered Parenting R/T poor bonding with child	*Altered Parenting* R/T prolonged separation from child
Impaired Home Maintenance Management R/T poor housekeeping habits	*Impaired Home Maintenance Management* R/T lack of knowledge regarding home safety measures

---

Avoid Reversing the Parts of the Statement

Remember that the first part of the diagnostic statement identifies the human response and suggests outcomes. The second part of the statement defines the related factors and suggests nursing interventions. Reversing the clauses may result in unclear communication about the client's response and its contributing factors, which makes the writing of appropriate outcomes and nursing interventions difficult.

Examples	
Incorrect	**Correct**
Sensory Overload R/T sleep pattern disturbance	*Sleep Pattern Disturbance* R/T sensory overload
Decreased Caloric Intake R/T altered nutrition: Less than body requirements	*Altered Nutrition: Less Than Body Requirements* R/T decreased caloric intake

Examples	
Incorrect	**Correct**
Inability to Feed Self R/T feeding problems	*Feeding Self-Care Deficit,* RT pain in fingers
Ineffective Family Coping, Disabling, R/T inability to handle client's illness	*Ineffective Family Coping, Disabling,* R/T lack of support systems

Avoid Using Single Cues in the First Part of the Statement

The first part of the diagnostic statement is derived from a cluster of signs and symptoms observed by the nurse during the assessment of the client. An isolated cue is not a nursing diagnosis, but it may provide information to help define the response. Inaccurate diagnoses may occur if the nurse focuses on an isolated sign or symptom rather than on the entire clinical picture.

Example
William Ward, an elderly client admitted to a nursing home, has a history of lung problems. The nurse observes that he is restless. Writing the diagnosis as "*Restlessness* R/T Change in Environment" suggests that restlessness is the response. In fact, the presence of restlessness may be a cue to other responses, such as ineffective airway clearance, altered coping, or fear.

A number of the approved diagnoses may appear to be isolated cues because of their one-word titles (pain, fear, anxiety). Remember that these are diagnostic terms that refer to a phenomenon that has a number of defining characteristics. For example, some of the characteristics for the diagnosis of pain include increased blood pressure, pulse, and respiratory rate; reports of pain; clutching of the painful area; and facial mask of pain.

The Two Parts of the Statement Should Not Mean the Same Thing

In some instances, diagnostic statements are written in which the two parts are almost identical. Examine this statement: "*Ineffective Airway Clearance* R/T inability to clear airway." Both parts of the statement have the same meaning. This is confusing and may result in difficulties when the nurse attempts to determine appropriate nursing interventions for the related factor. The diagnosis should be written "*Ineffective Airway Clearance* R/T retained secretions."

Express the Related Factor in Terms that Can Be Changed

Keep in mind that the diagnostic statement identifies actual or potential client responses. These responses and the factors that contribute to their existence should be changeable by interventions that are within the realm of nursing practice.

Examples
Shelby Donovan is a 6-year-old who is 2 days postoperative after an appendectomy. She is crying and points to the incisional area and says, "My tummy hurts." The diagnosis "*Pain* R/T surgical incision" is not accurate because nursing intervention cannot change the presence of a surgical incision. This can be restated as "*Pain* R/T the effects of surgery." Nursing interventions may relieve the effects of surgery—pain, immobility, anxiety, nausea.

Incorrect	**Correct**
Caregiver Role Strain R/T death of previous care giver	*Caregiver Role Strain* R/T lack of respite and recreation for care giver
Dysfunctional Grieving R/T death of spouse	*Dysfunctional Grieving* R/T perceived loss of security

Do Not Include Medical Diagnoses in the Nursing Diagnostic Statement

The nursing diagnostic statement differs from the medical diagnosis, because it reflects the essence of nursing rather than medical practice.

Examples	
Medical Diagnosis	**Nursing Diagnosis**
Identifies a specific illness	Identifies an actual or potential response to the illness
Clinical manifestations suggest medical need	Responses suggest a nursing need
Implies associated medical interventions	Implies associated nursing interventions.

The following examples compare medical and nursing diagnoses that might be found in the same client.

Examples

Medical Diagnosis	Nursing Diagnosis
Hepatitis	*Ineffective Individual Coping* R/T prolonged isolation
Diabetes mellitus	*Knowledge Deficit (Foot Care)* R/T inability to retain information
Cancer	*Altered Oral Mucous Membranes* R/T effects of chemotherapy
Myocardial infarction	*Ineffective Denial* R/T fear of disability

As identified previously, the medical diagnosis suggests medical interventions; therefore, its use is inappropriate in either of the two parts of the nursing diagnostic statement.

Examples

Incorrect	Correct
Ineffective Breathing Pattern R/T emphysema	*Ineffective Breathing Pattern* R/T retained secretions
Congestive Heart Failure R/T failure to take medications	*Noncompliance (Cardiac Medications)* R/T lack of knowledge about action and correct dosage

State the Diagnosis Clearly and Concisely

Nursing diagnostic statements should be clear and concise; confusing and wordy statements tend to obscure the nurse's focus.

Example

Kathleen Inman, the mother of a premature infant, reveals that she feels that *she* caused her premature labor. "I wouldn't be in this mess if I hadn't lifted that heavy can of paint—that's why my labor started." The client states that she is concerned about her 2-year-old son because she spends a great deal of time at the hospital. She also indicates that she sees very little of her husband, which has created tension in their marriage.

The following are examples of diagnostic statements that could be written for this client.

Incorrect	Correct
Altered Interactions Between Husband and Wife and Mother and 2-Year-Old Son R/T mother's hospital-visiting patterns	*Altered Family Processes* R/T mother's hospital-visiting patterns
Ineffective Individual Coping R/T belief that she caused the onset of premature labor by lifting heavy paint can on day of delivery	*Ineffective Individual Coping* R/T feelings of guilt

Neither of the incorrect examples shown is clear or concise. Although the client's comments are cues that suggest disrupted family interactions and feelings of guilt, it is not necessary to include her entire statements in the nursing diagnoses.

Clear and concise diagnostic statements facilitate communication and allow the nurse to concentrate on the client's response and the related factors. This approach promotes quality, individualized nursing care.

Example

Laura Wilson, age 38, is admitted to an acute care facility with a diagnosis of multiple sclerosis. She has developed a urinary tract infection and a high fever and will be receiving intravenous antibiotics. During the admission assessment, Laura begins to cry and says, "I feel so dependent. I can't dress myself any more. I hate to rely on my mother for help. It is becoming very difficult for her to care for me. Her blood pressure is out of control." Laura states that she has been unable to eat much over the last week because she had no appetite. After the nurse finishes assessing Laura, Mrs. Wilson pulls the nurse aside. "I don't know what to do," she says. "It is getting too hard to pick up Laura. I'm getting too weak to manage her."

Identify three actual nursing diagnoses and one high-risk diagnosis.

Actual Diagnoses

Anxiety R/T feelings of helplessness, AEB (as evidenced by) tearful statements of dependency.

Caregiver Role Strain R/T care giver's health impairment, AEB history of high blood pressure.

Altered Nutrition: Less than Body Requirements R/T anorexia, AEB reports of decreased intake.

High-Risk Diagnosis

High Risk for Trauma R/T decreased mobility.

COLLABORATIVE PROBLEMS

Collaborative problems are certain physiologic complications that nurses monitor for detection of their onset or changes in status.

Nurses manage collaborative problems using both physician-prescribed and nursing-prescribed interventions. You make independent decisions for both collaborative problems and nursing diagnoses. However, in nursing diagnoses, nurses prescribe the treatment for achieving the desired outcome. When collaborative problems exist, treatment is prescribed by both nurses and physicians. Collaborative problems involve primarily nurses' monitoring for the onset and change in status of physiologic complications. These complications are usually related to disease, treatments, trauma, diagnostic studies, or medications. Examples of collaborative problems include stress fractures, gastrointestinal bleeding, hyperglycemia, seizures, hypertension, and air embolism.

Not all physiologic complications are collaborative problems. Nurses can prevent some physiologic complications, such as infections from incisions and catheters, contractures, some types of incontinence, and pressure ulcers.[5]

IMPLICATIONS OF NURSING DIAGNOSES

Legal Aspects of a Nursing Diagnosis

The validity of a nursing diagnosis is strengthened when you follow the systematic diagnostic process described earlier in the chapter.

Nurses are legally responsible for carrying out the diagnostic process accurately.

The law is most concerned with the implications of the nursing diagnosis. Incorrect diagnoses may lead to inappropriate nursing interventions. When a client is injured and initiates a lawsuit, lawyers, judges, and juries will ask the following questions:

▶ Did the nurse correctly diagnose the client's problem?
▶ What consequences should have followed the diagnosis?
▶ Did they occur in this case?
▶ In assessing, diagnosing, and implementing, did the nurse follow the appropriate standards?[8] Standards are found in nursing literature and are published by major nursing organizations such as the American Nurses' Association and the American Association of Critical Care Nurses. The American Nurses' Association Standard relating to the diagnosis phase of the nursing process is shown in Box 8–8. Standards are discussed in more detail in Chapter 11.

Critical Thinking and Errors in the Diagnostic Process

When standards are not followed and the nurse does not correctly follow the diagnostic process, the nurse may not use appropriate critical thinking. Critical thinking is "an investigation whose purpose is to explore a situation, phenomenon, question or problem to arrive at a hypothesis or conclusion about it that integrates all available information and can therefore be convincingly justified."[13] Today's complex health care environment requires nurses to be able to think critically to be safe and effective. Faulty critical thinking can result in errors in the diagnostic process.

> ### Box 8–8. American Nurses Association Standard for Nursing Diagnosis
>
> The nurse analyzes the assessment data in determining diagnoses.
>
> **Measurement Criteria**
>
> 1. Diagnoses are derived from the assessment data.
> 2. Diagnoses are validated with the client, significant others, and health care providers, when possible.
> 3. Diagnoses are documented in a manner that facilitates the determination of expected outcomes and plan of care.
>
> ▼ ▼ ▼
>
> Reprinted with permission from *Standards of clinical nursing practice* (1991). Washington, DC: American Nurses' Association.

You may arrive at an incorrect diagnosis by committing a diagnostic error. Errors occur when you do not move beyond the data to their meaning. For example, a student took the blood pressure of a man who had hypertension. Over the course of a few hours, the blood pressure progressively dropped from 180/100 to 90/50. The student commented to the instructor, "His blood pressure is finally coming down to normal." Alarmed, the instructor entered the room and found the man in a state of shock. In this situation, the student did not understand the implications of the data or take appropriate action based on the blood pressure readings.

Errors occur when there is a mismatch between the data and the nursing diagnosis. This may occur when the nurse does not gather enough data to match the defining characteristics of the nursing diagnosis. For example, a student nurse was assigned to a woman with asthma. When she found the client was having difficulty breathing, she assumed that the client was anxious. As a way of demonstrating her concern for the client, the student held her hand and said a prayer out loud. The administration of oxygen, elevating the head of the bed, and additional medications would have been more effective immediate interventions.

Implications of Nursing Diagnosis for Nursing Practice

Nursing diagnosis language provides nurses with a method for describing behavior of concern to nurses. This language is documented on the client's medical records in the form of nursing care plans and progress notes. During change-of-shift report and walking rounds, nurses use a common terminology to discuss the client. Research can provide information on the most frequently seen nursing diagnoses in certain populations or types of nursing practice. With the increasing use and acceptance of nursing diagnoses, nursing is demonstrating its unique contributions to health care.

Summary

▶ A nursing diagnosis is a clinical judgment about individual, family, or community responses to actual or potential health problems/life processes. Nursing diagnoses provide the basis for selection of interventions to achieve outcomes for which the nurse is accountable.

▶ Cues and inferences are used in the diagnostic process.

▶ Clusters of cues are compared with the defining characteristics of the nursing diagnosis.

▶ Related factors, the second component of the nursing diagnosis, are conditions or circumstances that can cause or contribute to the development of a diagnosis.

▶ The list of nursing diagnoses can be organized alphabetically, in functional health patterns, or according to human response patterns.

▶ Actual nursing diagnoses can be written as a two-part statement, consisting of the human response and the related factor, or with the addition of a third part, the defining characteristics.

▶ A high-risk diagnosis is a clinical judgment that an individual, family, or community is more vulnerable to development of the problem than are others in the same or a similar situation.

▶ A wellness diagnosis is a clinical judgment about an individual, family, or community in transition from a specific level of wellness to a higher level of wellness.

▶ Guidelines for documenting the nursing diagnoses make it easier to write clear statements.

▶ Collaborative problems are certain physiologic complications that nurses monitor for detecting their onset or changes in status.

▶ You are legally responsible for developing accurate diagnoses.

Bibliography

1. Allen, C. (1989). Incorporating a wellness perspective for nursing diagnosis in practice. In Carroll-Johnson, R. (ed.). *Classification of nursing diagnoses, proceedings of the eighth conference.* Philadelphia: J.B. Lippincott.
2. Aydelotte, M., & Peterson, K. (1987). Nursing taxonomies—state of the art. In McLane, A. (ed.). *Classification of nursing diagnoses: Proceedings of the seventh conference.* St. Louis: C.V. Mosby.
3. Bell, E. (1991). Debate: a strategy for teaching critical thinking. *Nurse Educator*, 16(2), 6–7.
4. Carlson, J.H., et al. (1991). *Nursing diagnosis: A case study approach.* Philadelphia: W.B. Saunders.
5. Carpenito, L.J. (1991). *Nursing care plans and documentation.* Philadelphia: J.B. Lippincott.
6. del Bueno, D. (1990). Experience, education and nurses' ability to make clinical judgments. *Nursing & Health Care,* 11(6), 290–293.
7. *Development/submission criteria and guidelines for proposed nursing diagnoses* (1990). North American Nursing Diagnosis Association, handout at ninth conference.
8. Fortin, J., & Rabinow, J. (1979). Legal implications of nursing diagnosis. *Nursing Clinics of North America,* 14(3), 553–561.
9. Fredetta, S. (1988). Common diagnostic errors. *Nursing Educator,* 13(3), 31–35.
10. Gordon, M. (1987). *Nursing diagnosis: Process and application* (2nd ed.). New York: McGraw-Hill.
11. *Guidelines for submission of proposed diagnoses* (1992). St. Louis: North American Nursing Diagnosis Association.
12. Iyer, P., et al. (1991). *Nursing process and nursing diagnosis* (2nd ed.). Philadelphia: W.B. Saunders.
13. Kurfiss, J.G. (1988). *Critical thinking: Theory, research, practice and possibilities.* ASHR-ERIC Higher Education Report No. 2. Washington, DC: Association for the Study of Higher Education.
14. Lunney, M., & Svitlik, B. (1988). Educating nurse diagnosticians. *Nurse Educator,* 13(1), 24–29.
15. Miller, M., & Malcolm, N. (1990). Critical thinking in the nursing curriculum. *Nursing & Health Care,* 11(2), 67–73.
16. NANDA News (1990). *Nursing Diagnosis,* 1(3), 124–128.
17. Sheppard, K. (1989). Evaluation of the NANDA taxonomy as an assessment guideline in an oncology setting. In Carroll-Johnson, R. (ed.). *Classification of nursing diagnoses.* Philadelphia: J.B. Lippincott.
18. Taptich, B., et al. (1989). *Nursing diagnosis and care planning.* Philadelphia: W.B. Saunders.
19. Tribulski, J. (1988). Nursing diagnosis: waste of time or valued tool? *RN,* 15(12), 30–34.
20. Warren, J., & Hoskins, L. (1990). The development of NANDA's nursing diagnosis taxonomy. *Nursing Diagnosis,* 1(4), 162–167.

Chapter 9

 Planning

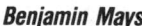

The tragedy of life doesn't lie in not reaching your goal. The tragedy lies in having no goal to reach.

Benjamin Mays

▼ CHAPTER OUTLINE

SETTING PRIORITIES
    High-Priority Nursing Diagnoses
    Medium-Priority Nursing Diagnoses
    Low-Priority Nursing Diagnoses
    Mutual Negotiation of Priorities
DEVELOPING SPECIFIC OUTCOMES
    Verification of Outcomes
    Realistic Outcomes
    Acceptable Outcomes
    Consistent Outcomes
SETTING TIME FRAMES
IDENTIFYING INTERVENTIONS
    Types of Nursing Interventions

Characteristics of Nursing
    Interventions
THE NURSING CARE PLAN
    Student Nursing Care Plans
    Individually Developed Nursing
      Care Plans
    Standardized Nursing Care Plans
    Teaching Plans
    Practice Guidelines
    Case Management Care Plans
    Computerized Nursing Care Plans

▼ KEY TERMS

Case management
Independent interventions

Interdependent
  interventions
Nursing care plan

Practice guidelines
  (protocols)

After studying this chapter, you should be able to

1. Explain the priority-setting process.
2. Describe nursing outcomes.
3. Discuss the establishment of time frames for accomplishment of outcomes.
4. Describe nursing interventions.
5. Contrast the various methods for documenting the nursing care plan.

In Chapter 6 we presented an overview of the nursing process and expanded on the roles of assessment and nursing diagnoses in Chapters 7 and 8, respectively. In this chapter the planning phase of the nursing process is discussed.

The goal of planning care is to make the best possible use of resources to help the person achieve the desired outcomes.

The plan of care establishes priorities and guides the efforts of the person and their significant other, the nurses, and other members of the health care team.

Planning begins with the *review of the nursing diagnoses*. Accurate nursing diagnoses enable you to accomplish the following four purposes of the planning phase:

▶ To set priorities
▶ To develop outcomes and designate deadlines (times and dates) for their accomplishment
▶ To formulate a plan of action
▶ To write the nursing care plan

In slightly different terms, these four purposes may be identified as essential elements of the planning phase, as shown in Box 9–1.

Box 9–1. Step 3 of the Nursing Process: Planning

Assessment	Diagnosis	Planning
Collect data	Interpret data	Establish priorities
Review the clinical record	Identify clusters of cues	Develop outcomes
Interview	Make inferences	Set time frames for outcomes
Nursing history	Validate inferences	Identify interventions
Physical assessment	Compare clusters of cues with definition and defining characteristics	Document plan of care
Psychosocial assessment		
Consultation	Identify related factors	
Review the literature	Document the nursing diagnosis	

SETTING PRIORITIES

The first step in planning nursing care is to decide which nursing diagnoses require immediate attention and which ones are less threatening. Nursing diagnoses are ranked as having high, medium, or low priority.

High-Priority Nursing Diagnoses

High-priority nursing diagnoses are those that are life-threatening and require immediate action. Examples of high-priority nursing diagnoses include *High Risk for Aspiration* and *High Risk for Violence—Self-directed or directed at others*. In emergency and critical care situations, people can develop several high-priority nursing diagnoses at the same time.

Medium-Priority Nursing Diagnoses

Medium-priority nursing diagnoses do not directly threaten a person's life, although they may result in unhealthy physical or emotional consequences. For example, *Impaired physical mobility* may lead to collaborative problems or complications such as pneumonia, pressure ulcers (bed sores), contractures, and depression. These complications can develop into serious problems, especially when combined.

Low-Priority Nursing Diagnoses

Low-priority nursing diagnoses are problems that a person can handle with minimal assistance. These problems may not be of low priority in terms of significance to the individual but are assigned a lower priority in comparison with life-threatening problems. Some of the wellness nursing diagnoses defined in Chapter 8 might be low-priority nursing diagnoses in a given situation.

When setting priorities, remember that basic survival needs must be met before higher-level needs can be realistically considered. Problems that involve "higher needs," such as self-esteem or self-actualization needs, have low priority if the person is critically ill. As high-priority problems are resolved, medium- and low-priority problems become higher in priority. Priorities change daily or even hourly as the person's condition improves or worsens.

Nursing diagnoses provide the framework for establishing outcomes for care.

Outcomes may be defined for many different aspects of the person's health status. When establishing priorities, consider the following list of aspects of health (not in order of priority):

▶ Physiological status—changes in vital signs, skin integrity, weight, and laboratory values
▶ Psychosocial status—patterns of communication, relationships, attitudes, mood, coping, and social functioning
▶ Functional measures—mobility, activities of daily living, and other self-care abilities
▶ Knowledge—application of knowledge and skills, compliance with health care regimen, readiness to learn
▶ Symptom control—the presence or absence of pain, fatigue, nausea and diarrhea
▶ Home maintenance—functioning of the family in the home environment, family roles, and living environment
▶ Safety—prevention of injuries[13]

Another consideration in setting priorities for problems is the individual's perception of the situation. Whenever possible, include the person in the priority setting and management of problems. Such input provides insight and a necessary point of view that may differ significantly from your assessment of priority needs.

Mutual Negotiation of Priorities

Mutual negotiation of priorities helps to assure that the person has input into the decision-making process. People are often more willing to comply with suggested therapies when they are treated with respect and allowed to maintain some control over their care. Other factors that may influence priority setting include:

▶ Size and availability of nursing staff
▶ Accessibility of equipment and other resources
▶ Cost of needed services and the person's financial situation
▶ Approximate time needed to resolve problems
▶ Type of care facility (acute care, chronic, or rehabilitative)

DEVELOPING SPECIFIC OUTCOMES

The next step in the planning process is to develop outcomes specific to each nursing diagnosis. The term *outcome* reflects a focus on the observable, measurable changes in a person's health status. Outcomes are replacing the older terms of nursing goals or objectives.

Outcomes are concrete descriptions of the type of behavior the person will display if the plan of care has been successful.

They must be clear, concise, client-centered, specific, and measurable. They should direct interventions to achieve the desired changes and measure the effectiveness of those interventions.

The following is an example of a nursing diagnosis with its outcome:
NURSING DIAGNOSIS: *Constipation* R/T decreased oral intake, as evidenced by absence of stools
OUTCOME: Resumes normal bowel pattern within 3 days

Notice that the outcome is linked to resolution of the human response in the nursing diagnosis.

In order to determine if the constipation has disappeared, you will have to note whether the person has resumed a normal pattern of elimination. You can determine the individual's normal pattern by asking the person.

Verification of Outcomes

By using measurable verbs in outcomes, you can verify the achievement of the outcome. Examples of measurable verbs are:

administers	has an increase in
demonstrates	identifies
has a decrease in	performs
has an absence of	states

Examples of verbs that are *not* measurable by observation are:

accepts	knows
appreciates	understands

In addition to being accurate and well stated, outcomes must be (a) realistic, (b) acceptable to the person, and (c) consistent with the plans of the entire health care team.

Realistic Outcomes

Realistic outcomes are based on a review of the entire data base and the medical/nursing diagnoses. As you consider possible outcomes, carefully evaluate the person's disabilities, resources, and unique life circumstances. For example, one outcome for a middle-aged person with heart disease is to increase tolerance to physical exercise. Next you must think about how this individual can safely meet the outcome. For example, it is unrealistic and dangerous to expect this person to jog for a mile on the first morning of an exercise program. He or she *eventually* may be able to jog a mile without cardiovascular symptoms, but to try to do so immediately could prove difficult. A realistic objective might be to expect people to walk one full block every morning at their own pace for the first week, two blocks the second week, and so forth, until they gain the stamina to walk briskly or to jog a mile.

Acceptable Outcomes

If outcomes are to be acceptable to the client, they must be planned not only for the person but *with* the person. Establishing outcomes with the person can favorably affect treatment outcomes. The nurse is able to assist people in setting more realistic outcomes for what can be expected with their illnesses and treatment regimens.[3] The outcomes the nurse identifies must be acceptable to the person because it is the *person* and not the nurse who must live with the goals —often for a long time. According to Carnevali, the person often signals disenchantment with the plan of care in the following ways:[5]

▶ A lack of enthusiasm for ideas or activities
▶ An absence of questions
▶ Nodding compliance
▶ Failure to take any initiative
▶ Failure to contribute any ideas about how to fit actions or desires into the proposed plan
▶ Expressions of guilt at failure to comply

To elicit people's enthusiastic participation in the program of care, listen to their concerns, talk frankly, negotiate, and sometimes compromise. Many people welcome the opportunity to be more actively involved in decision making. This tends to lessen the person's feeling of loss of control and dependency that may be generated by the health care system.

In addition, it helps to involve *family* and *friends* in setting outcomes. Significant others are often responsible for carrying out the nursing plan following discharge. They may be more willing to continue the therapeutic regimen at home if they understand its rationale and if they have had input into the decision-making process.

Consistent Outcomes

Finally, to assure that outcomes are consistent with the plans of the entire team, consult with the physician and other members of the health care team about their plans for the person. Whenever possible, team members (nurse, physician, physical therapist) need to coordinate their aims and plans for the person.[17]

SETTING TIME FRAMES

You can communicate to others the outcome that is to be accomplished with wording that will let others know when it has been achieved. As indicated in our sample outcome, it is essential to determine a realistic *deadline or time frame* for the accomplishment of outcomes. Specifying the date for meeting an outcome reflects your *best judgment* about the time needed to reverse the alteration. This judgment is based on your knowledge about the problem, the person's condition, the support systems, and the necessary nursing interventions. Setting time frames requires critical thinking and judgment.

Additionally, time frames

▶ motivate people to strive toward their goals; they give purpose and meaning to nursing intervention
▶ provide the person (and you) with a sense of accomplishment
▶ "pace" nursing care, focusing on continued progress
▶ signal the nurse to evaluate the achievement of the outcome

Unmet outcomes indicate that either the time frames were unrealistic or the outcomes need to be modified, as will be described further in Chapter 11. Beginning students sometimes find it difficult to know what is realistic when setting time frames. As your knowledge base and experience increase, you will become proficient in setting realistic outcomes. Box 9–2 presents the ANA standard that summarizes the important points about establishing outcomes.

IDENTIFYING INTERVENTIONS

This step in the planning phase involves selecting actions that enable the person to achieve the outcomes and to resolve the related factor in the nursing diagnosis. These selected actions or strategies are called nursing interventions.

Nursing interventions have been named nursing actions, activities, approaches, and orders.

Types of Nursing Interventions

Nursing interventions are nursing actions that focus on assisting people to cope successfully with problems and to achieve the outcome. Nursing interventions are classified as *independent* and *interdependent*.

Box 9–2. ANA Standard for Outcome Identification

The nurse identifies expected outcomes individualized to the client.

Measurement Criteria

1. Outcomes are derived from the diagnoses.
2. Outcomes are documented as measurable goals.
3. Outcomes are mutually formulated with the client and health care providers, when possible.
4. Outcomes are realistic in relation to the client's present and potential capabilities.
5. Outcomes are attainable in relation to resources available to the client.
6. Outcomes include a time estimate for attainment.
7. Outcomes provide direction for continuity of care.

▼ ▼ ▼

Reprinted with permission from *Standards of clinical nursing practice* (1991). Washington, DC: American Nurses Association. © 1991.

INDEPENDENT INTERVENTIONS

Independent interventions involve carrying out the *nursing interventions* written on the nursing care plan. The basis for independent nursing interventions is the *nursing diagnosis*. These actions *do not* require a physician's order.

Independent nursing interventions evolve logically from the identification of problems that *nurses* are qualified to treat by law and by educational preparation.

INTERDEPENDENT INTERVENTIONS

Interdependent interventions are those performed by nurses *in collaboration* with other members of the health care team. For example, you may work with the physician in setting up a teaching program for people with similar problems. When establishing the program, you might delegate tasks to other health care professionals. You may ask the nutritionist to teach nutritional aspects to clients, you may arrange for the occupational therapist to demonstrate how to perform activities of daily living (ADLs) utilizing aids that minimize dysfunction, or you may ask the community health nurse to provide information about services available after discharge from the health care facility. Interdependent actions enable nurses to coordinate interventions in order to maximize knowledge and skills from various disciplines for the benefit of the client. In addition, an interdisciplinary approach is time efficient. Interdependent interventions may also include functions nurses perform in *implementing the medical regimen*, for example, administering prescribed nursing schedules or other criteria that will make the medical treatment of more benefit to the client.

Another way of conceptualizing nursing interventions has been suggested by Bulechek and McCloskey.[4] They have worked to further define nursing interventions, and they argue that interventions should be viewed as nurse-initiated or physician-initiated. They define a nursing intervention as follows:

A nursing intervention is any direct care treatment that a nurse performs on behalf of a client. These treatments include nurse-initiated treatments resulting from nursing diagnoses, physician-initiated treatments resulting from medical diagnoses, and performance of the daily essential functions for the client who cannot do these.

Typically, nurse-initiated interventions include such actions as counseling, teaching, relaxation training, mouth care, bathing, turning, feeding, and assisting with ambulation. Typical physician-initiated treatments include actions such as administration of medications and blood, dressing changes, performing prescribed medical treatments, drawing blood, administration of IV fluids, and obtaining specimens. Daily essential functions characteristically include answering the phone, opening mail, watering flowers, bed making, serving trays, and obtaining equipment. Increasingly, ancillary health care workers such as nursing assistants or unit hostesses are being used to perform these activities. Chapter 10 will focus specifically on how interventions are selected and implemented.

Characteristics of Nursing Interventions

A complete, well-written nursing intervention is composed of five components:

- ▶ *Date*
- ▶ *Specific action verb,* such as instruct, place, supervise, compliment, and observe. Occasionally a modifier, such as actively, softly, or gently helps clarify the verb
- ▶ *Prescribed activity,* such as "Keep shaver and mirror within easy reach"
- ▶ *Time units or frequencies,* such as "Supervise periods of ambulation q 2 h throughout day"
- ▶ *Signature* of nurse writing the intervention

Additionally, to enable the person to attain the outcome by alleviating the related factor, the nursing interventions must be:

- ▶ Consistent with the nursing care plan and the medical regimen
- ▶ Planned on the basis of problem-solving techniques and scientific principles
- ▶ Therapeutically safe and effective
- ▶ Individualized to treat each related factor
- ▶ Geared to use appropriate health facility resources, e.g., staff, specialists, equipment
- ▶ Developed to maximize the person's resources, strengths, and capabilities
- ▶ Scheduled to coincide with the person's needs for rest, activity, food, sleep, recreation, and other activities
- ▶ Organized to allow the person and significant others to participate in the therapeutic program
- ▶ Geared to enable the individual to perform *self-care* activities and to learn how to avoid complications and setbacks
- ▶ Continuously updated to reflect changes in the person's condition and situation
- ▶ Consistent with current nursing practice
- ▶ Planned to provide continuity of care

THE NURSING CARE PLAN

The **nursing care plan** is a written plan that communicates the nursing diagnoses (actual, high-risk, and/or wellness), the outcomes, and nursing interventions.

Nurses develop a nursing care plan to accomplish the following purposes:

- ▶ Provides a detailed guide for nursing care
- ▶ Individualizes nursing care
- ▶ Provides a source of information and a line of communication for nursing team members
- ▶ Fosters continuity of care

- ► Coordinates the efforts of all nursing team members
- ► Provides for individual and family participation in the nursing care plan
- ► Outlines a program for health education of individuals and significant others
- ► Encourages adequate discharge planning
- ► Provides a source of information for quality improvement and research

Box 9–3 presents the planning standard of the American Nurses' Association.

As you care for people in various health care facilities, you will discover a variety of nursing care plan formats. The documentation of the plan of care is also changing as federal, state, and accrediting agencies examine and modify their standards.

The most common formats for care plans include student nursing care plans, individually developed nursing care plans, standardized nursing care plans, practice guidelines, critical path or case management care plans, and computerized nursing care plans.

Student Nursing Care Plans

Each school of nursing has a care plan format adopted by or developed by the faculty for student use. Because student plans are used as learning tools, they are usually more comprehensive and detailed than the care plans utilized by graduate staff nurses. Student care plans focus heavily on documenting signs and symptoms and providing the rationale for specific nursing interventions. This information is no less important to the graduate nurse. However, the experienced nurse is capable of high-level assessment and synthesis of data, which are still step-by-step processes for the student.

Box 9–3. ANA Standard for Planning

The nurse develops a plan of care that prescribes interventions to attain expected outcomes.

Measurement Criteria

1. The plan is individualized to the client's condition or needs.
2. The plan is developed with the client, significant others, and health care providers, when appropriate.
3. The plan reflects current nursing practice.
4. The plan is documented.
5. The plan provides for continuity of care.

▼▼▼

Reprinted with permission from *Standards of clinical nursing practice* (1991). Washington, DC: American Nurses Association. © 1991.

Individually Developed Nursing Care Plans

The individually developed care plan is the most traditional and oldest method of documenting the plan of care. It typically consists of three columns, which are labeled, according to the setting, as nursing diagnoses or problems, outcomes or goals, and nursing interventions or orders. Additional columns may be added to the format to include a spot for the date and initials of the nurse who developed the plan, the date for the outcome achievement, and the date the nursing diagnosis was resolved (Table 9–1).

Individual care plans are intended to focus on the specific needs of the person and are to be updated as the person's condition changes.

The individually developed care plan, like the other formats for the plan of care, is usually combined with a Kardex. A Kardex is an abbreviated form that contains (1) basic demographic information about the person, such as name, age, sex, medical diagnoses, surgical procedures, and physician's name, and (2) basic care information, such as type of bath, frequency of vital signs, allowable activity, ordered treatments, and so on.

ADVANTAGES

The advantages of individually developed care plans include their specificity to a particular person. They contain only the pertinent nursing diagnoses, outcomes, and interventions.

DISADVANTAGES

The primary disadvantage of individually developed care plans is the time-consuming aspect of the development process. Also, as is true with the other formats for care plans, the individually developed care plan may not accurately reflect the person's current problems if it has not been updated.

Standardized Nursing Care Plans

Printed care plans, known as standardized care plans, are developed commercially or by an individual health care facility. They direct nursing care for people with specific medical diagnoses (e.g., myocardial infarction), with certain nursing diagnoses such as pain or anxiety, or who are undergoing special procedures, such as cardiac catheterization. These care plans are typed, preprinted, duplicated, and made available to the appropriate units in the health care facility.

The format is designed to leave space for the nurse to individualize the care plan by filling in specific related factors associated with the nursing diagnosis, adding deadlines to the outcomes, and clarifying the interventions with additional details (Table 9–2).

For example, the interventions could be individualized by adding frequencies, amounts, times, and the client's preferences.

TABLE 9-1. Sample of an Individually Developed Nursing Care Plan for a Client with Pneumonia

Date/Initials	Nursing Diagnosis	Planning: Expected Outcomes	Implementation: Nursing Interventions	Date Resolved
	Airway Clearance, Ineffective, R/T increased production of viscous secretions, dehydration, fatigue, decreased energy level	Breath sounds WNL within 72 hours	a. Monitor breath sounds b. Administer humidified O_2 at 4L/min via mask c. Encourage/assist client to cough and deep breathe using splinting as necessary q2h d. Assist with and monitor effects of chest physiotherapy and breathing treatments e. Maintain adequate hydration: 1500 cc days, 1000 cc evenings, 500 cc nights f. If client unable to cough, suction prn g. Utilize artificial airway as needed h. Administer and monitor effects of expectorants, antibiotics	

Modified from Iyer, P.W., et al. (1991). *Nursing process and nursing diagnosis* (2nd ed.). Philadelphia: W.B. Saunders.

TABLE 9-2. Sample of a Standardized Nursing Care Plan for a Client with Total Hip Replacement

Nursing Diagnosis	Planning: Expected Outcomes	Implementation: Nursing Interventions
Skin Integrity, High Risk for Impaired, R/T decreased mobility	No evidence of skin breakdown at time of discharge	a. Initiate turning schedule; turn q _2_ h (specify) *even hrs* b. Inspect skin for redness, swelling, and breakdown c. Keep skin clean and dry at all times d. Relieve pressure on both heels with bilateral heel protectors e. Initiate pressure-relieving devices (eggcrate air mattress, air fluidized bed, gel, pad) Specify *air mattress* f. ~~instruct to use overbed trapeze to shift weight q____~~ g. Monitor protein and fluid intake

Modified from Iyer, P.W., et al. (1991). *Nursing process and nursing diagnosis* (2nd ed.). Philadelphia: W.B. Saunders.

THE CHAMBERSBURG HOSPITAL

LESSON III
DIABETIC LESSON PLAN

CONTENT	INFORMATION SOURCE	DATE TAUGHT	NURSE INITIALS	PATIENT ACCOMPLISHMENT BY DISCHARGE	DATE ACTION ACHIEVED	NURSE INITIALS
A. MEDICATION Insulin - Facts						
*a. Type and strength	Start Pack Given			Explain how insulin is stored.		
*b. Onset/Peak/Duration	Flipchart Pages 25-34			State type of insulin used, dosage and time to be given.		
*c. How Stored - Expiration Date	Booklet					
*d. When Administered	Pages 18-21			Explain need for site rotation.		
e. Parts of Syringe				Select appropriate injection sites.		
*f. Reading Syringe				Correctly draw insulin into syringe.		
*g. Injection Sites				Accurately administer own injection.		
*h. Rotation of Sites				Discuss proper disposal of syringes.		
*i. Cleansing of Skin						
*j. Drawing Up Procedure						
*k. Injecting Procedure						
*l. Sterile Technique						
m. Disposal of Needles						
n. Mixing of Insulin						

B. DISCHARGE PLANNING   Family member taught ( ); Outpatient Class Referrals ( ); Diabetic Association ( )

INSTRUCTOR OR PATIENT COMMENTS:

NURSE INITIALS AND SIGNATURES

*Critical Information   Use N/A for items that are not applicable.

▲ Figure 9-1

Sample of teaching plan. (Courtesy of Chambersburg Hospital, Chambersburg, PA.)

ADVANTAGES

The advantages of standardized care plans are the reduced amount of writing needed to record routine nursing interventions and help to the staff by highlighting necessary interventions. Standardized care plans are usually developed by a group of nurses who use their collective expertise and experience to produce a well-researched tool. These types of plans are particularly helpful to nurses who may be asked to work in an unfamiliar area.

DISADVANTAGES

The disadvantages include the concern that nurses may use standardized care plans without individualizing them for a particular person. Many of the nursing diagnoses, outcomes, and interventions may not be applicable. However, unless the nurse follows the agency's format for eliminating the nonapplicable sections, it will be assumed that the full care plan is to be followed. This assumption may be questioned if the nurse's care is examined, such as in a malpractice suit. Standardized care plans also may tend to be long. Frustrated by the amount of time it takes simply to read them, some nurses have not found them to be helpful. This problem can be reduced by developing concise standardized care plans that contain only the essential information.[16]

Teaching Plans

Teaching plans are a specialized form of nursing care plan. Individually developed teaching plans may be handwritten or computer-generated for individuals with complex teaching needs. An agency may have a variety of standardized teaching plans prepared for people with commonly seen teaching needs — for example, newly diagnosed diabetic person (Figure 9–1), post-myocardial infarction client, new parent. The nurse modifies the standard teaching plan as needed and uses the form to document the outcome of the teaching.

Practice Guidelines

Practice guidelines, also called **protocols,** specify nursing management of broad clinical issues like maintenance of skin integrity, phases of hospitalization such as postoperative care, or interdependent clinical issues — for example, management of a person receiving a certain type of potent medication, such as cardiac medications given intravenously in the intensive care units.

Whereas the standardized care plan or individually developed care plan contains information about a variety of nursing diagnoses, the practice guideline typically addresses one issue, problem, or nursing diagnosis.

Like standardized care plans, practice guidelines are usually developed by experts and reviewed by a group of nurses for validity. When a practice guideline ad-dresses an interdependent clinical issue that includes both medical and nursing management of a particular concern, physician committee review of the medical orders is usually needed. For example, a hospital may develop a practice guideline that describes the use of lidocaine, a drug used to control irregular heart beats in the Emergency Department or Critical Care Units. Portions of the practice guideline will contain medical orders for the changes in the dosage of the medication based on the person's response, and other portions will address the nursing management of the person receiving the medication. These plans illustrate the manner in which health care professionals collaboratively manage treatment.

Practice guidelines are used commonly in short stay areas of a hospital, such as Emergency Departments and Post-Anesthesia Care Units. In these areas the practice guideline may be used alone as the primary plan of care. Certain commonalities exist among people in these areas, making it possible to manage their care according to practice guidelines. For example, all people recovering from anesthesia have certain common needs that are addressed by the post-anesthesia care unit nurses. It is not necessary to develop an individually written plan in order to care for people who stay in this area on the average of only 2 hours.

ADVANTAGES

The advantages of practice guidelines are similar to those of standardized care plans. They clearly specify well-researched and agreed-upon management of certain problems or issues. Once the initial work of developing the practice guideline is completed, their use saves much time by quickly transmitting information that does not need to be documented for each person for whom it is applicable. Unlike standardized care plans, practice guidelines are not considered standards. They are suggested guidelines for care and are not designed to establish a mandatory standard that must be followed.

DISADVANTAGE

The main disadvantage of practice guidelines, like that of standardized care plans, is the temptation to follow uncritically the interventions without individualizing them for a particular person. No prepared plan of care, no matter what its format, replaces the judgment and critical thinking of the nurse.

Case Management Care Plans

Case management is a method of delivering care that has evolved from the emphasis on decreasing the length of stay in hospitals and the focus on achieving timely client outcomes. Case management is designed to organize care to achieve certain specific outcomes within a time frame permitted by the reimbursement system.

CRITICAL CARE PATH - PNEUMONIA
DAY #1

	2	3	4	5	6	7	8	9	10	11

Admission via ER
Assess Resp. Status
—Lung Sounds
deep breath

ABG's-may need to
be repeated
O₂ if indicated
Record V.S.

ABG's to determine
home O₂ therapy

Discharge
2 weeks after disch.
possible Legionella
Blood screen

Labs
CBC w/ diff
SMA15
Lytes
Blood Cultures
U.A./C.S.
If applicable:
CCU Labs

Repeat CBC if
elevated

Tests
EKG
CXR
Sputum-gram stain &
culture
AFB

IV for antibiotic-
Monitor IV
Diet-encourage p.o.
fluids based on
assessment

Dietary consult if
needed

Remove IV or INT
needle

Pt. should be eating
meals w/ minimal
assistance

Monitor I.O.

Stop I.O. monitoring

Review diagnostic
process w/ pt. & the
family

Assess mental &
functional status

Assess mobility OOB
to chair (Possible
P.T. consult)

Amb. in room

Amb. in room

Amb. lgth of hallway
w/ assistance

Amb. hallway w/
assistance

Amb. hallway w/
minimal assistance

Ambulate independ-
ently

Social Serive Consult

Assess bowel
function

Provide rest periods
for patients

Assess skin integrity-
if pt. is at risk, apply
A.P.P. in bed.

Assess hearing

Assess anxiety level

Reassure patient
Assess level of
understanding of
diagnostic process-
Pt/Family/Sig. Other

Education-Pt/Family/
Sig. Other RE:
medication, diet,
signs & symptoms of
diarrhea, temp.

▲ *Figure 9–2*

Sample of a critical path derived from a case management plan. (Courtesy of St. Peter's Medical Center, New Brunswick, NJ.)

```
            CliniCom Medical Center - QA        03/11/90 22:03
                                                      Page: 1
                    ACTIVE CARE PLAN
            From 03/11/90 00:00  To 03/11/90 22:00
            -------------------------------------------
```

Active Care Plan Module

```
  Date       Freq NURSING DIAGNOSIS
03/11(AMJ)         7.Anxiety
                      Defining Characteristics:
03/11(AMJ)            -  wringing of hands
03/11(AMJ)            -  expressing insecurity
                      Related to
03/11(AMJ)            -  addition to family
                      Goals:
03/11(AMJ)   Q8H      -  Patient demonstrates ability to use techniques to
                         reduce anxiety.
                         Target Date: 15-mar-1990
                      Interventions:
03/11(AMJ)   PRN      -  Assist with coping techniques: relaxation - slow,
                         deep breathing.
03/11(AMJ)   PRN      -  Assist with coping techniques: diversional
                         activities.

03/11(AMJ)         3.Respiratory Function, Alt in: airway clearance ineffective
                      Defining Characteristics:
03/11(AMJ)            -  change in respiratory rate
03/11(AMJ)            -  inability to expectorate, cough
03/11(AMJ)            -  shortness of breath
                      Related to
03/11(AMJ)            -  excess thick secretions
03/11(AMJ)            -  inability to cough effectively
                      Secondary to
03/11(AMJ)            -  edema
03/11(AMJ)            -  bronchospasm
                      Goals:
03/11(AMJ)   Q8H      -  Patient is able to expectorate secretions
                         effectively.
                         Target Date: 15-mar-1990
                      Interventions:
03/11(AMJ)   Q4H      -  Assist patient with effective coughing and deep
                         breathing.
Care Providers:
JONES, ANNE (AMJ) NRN
```

```
0500-A          Name: SMITH, CHARLEY B. MD: SILVER,JOHN
Sex: M Age: 40 Adm: 10/28/89 13:45 Patient Id: 456456456 Med Rec No: 654654654
```

LAST PAGE

SMITH, CHARLEY B.   ACTIVE CARE PLAN   PERM

▲ Figure 9-3

Sample of computerized care plan. (Courtesy of CliniCom Inc., Boulder, CO.)

The case management plan is a standardized care plan that consists of nursing diagnoses, outcomes, deadlines, nursing interventions, and physician interventions.

The plan is developed collaboratively by nurses, physicians, and other health care professionals and is reviewed and individualized for a particular person. The comprehensive case management plan is often summarized in the form of a critical path or patient outcome timeline. The one-page critical path (Figure 9–2) identifies the events that must occur at specific times to achieve an appropriate, reimbursable length of stay.

Critical paths can improve quality of care by

- allowing health care professionals to share knowledge with each other
- educating clients by thoroughly explaining the treatment plan
- permitting comparison of outcomes or results of various treatment methods
- identifying and reinforcing steps critical to the desired outcome[6]

ADVANTAGES

The advantages of this system of documenting the plan of care relate to the ease of identifying the appropriate steps in achieving the outcomes. Resources of the nursing staff and hospital are used more effectively as they become directed at moving the person through the hospitalization. The person is actively involved in reviewing the plan of care. Nurses are given more authority to make changes in the system to facilitate the achievement of outcomes.

DISADVANTAGES

The disadvantages to the case management approach refer primarily to the great deal of planning needed to implement this method of delivering care. It may be difficult in some instances to gain the cooperation of physicians in defining how to manage certain types of clients and to collaborate with nurses on a professional level.[10] In addition, certain people will have preexisting conditions or complications that will prevent the achievement of outcomes at specified time periods. These deviations are called variances and are documented and analyzed as part of the case management system.

Computerized Nursing Care Plans

Many software vendors have developed computerized nursing care plans (Figure 9–3) and critical paths. The software can be tailored to the needs of the health care institution and to the population it serves.

ADVANTAGES

Computerization of care planning has many advantages including

- legibility
- reduction in the amount of time needed to develop and update the plan
- access to plans developed by expert clinicians
- ability to collect information about groups of patients for research

DISADVANTAGES

The disadvantages of computerized care planning are like those associated with standardized care plans. Their use requires a critical analysis of a preexisting plan to ensure that it is appropriate and current.

Summary

- The planning phase of the nursing process is used to set priorities, develop outcomes and designate deadlines, formulate a plan of action, and document the plan of care.
- High-priority nursing diagnoses are addressed before low-priority ones.
- Outcomes are clear descriptions of the type of behavior the person will exhibit if the plan of care is successful and the human response is resolved.
- Outcomes must be realistic, acceptable to the person, and consistent with the plans of the entire health care team.
- It is essential to establish a realistic time frame for accomplishment of outcomes.
- Nursing interventions are concrete actions that enable the nurse to help the person achieve the outcomes.
- Nursing interventions are documented with the date and signature of the nurse, action verb, description of prescribed activity, and time units or frequencies.
- The planning phase of the nursing process can be documented in a number of different formats.
- Increasingly, software programs are being developed and marketed to assist nurses in the documentation of the care planning process.
- No matter what type of program is available, the language of nursing diagnosis, outcomes, and interventions is used in the creation of the plan of care.

Bibliography

1. American Nurses Association (1988). *Nursing case management.* Kansas City, MO: American Nurses Association.
2. Blount, B. (1990). The documentation maze: finding the right path. *Journal of Nursing Staff Development,* 6(1), 21.
3. Bulechek, G., & McCloskey, J. (1992). *Nursing interventions,* (2nd ed.). Philadelphia: W.B. Saunders.
4. Bulechek, G., & McCloskey, J. (1989). Nursing interventions: treatments for potential nursing diagnoses. In Carroll-Johnson, R. (ed.) *Proceedings of the eighth conference.* Philadelphia: J.B. Lippincott.
5. Carnevali, D. (1983). *Nursing care planning: Diagnosis and management* (3rd ed.). Philadelphia: J.B. Lippincott.
6. Critical paths—a pre-existing tool ready-made for TQM implementation (1992). *QI/TQM,* January 1–2, 4.
7. Etheredge, M. (1989). *Collaborative care: Nursing case management.* Chicago: American Hospital Publishing, Inc.

8. Ferguson, G., et al. (1987). The effect of nursing care planning systems on patient outcomes. *Journal of Nursing Administration,* 17(9), 30–36.

9. Gould, E. (1987). Standardized home health care plans: a quality assurance tool. In Fisher, K., & Gardner, K. (eds.). *Quality and home health care: Redefining the tradition.* Chicago: Joint Commission on Accreditation of Health Care Organizations.

10. Iyer, P., et al. (1991). *Nursing process and nursing diagnosis* (2nd ed.). Philadelphia: W.B. Saunders.

11. Lang, N., & Marek, K. (1990). The classification of patient outcomes. *Journal of Professional Nursing,* 6(3), 158–163.

12. Loveridge, C., et al. (1988). Developing case management in a primary nursing system. *Journal of Nursing Administration,* 18(10), 36–39.

13. Marek, K. (1989). Outcome measurement in nursing. *Journal of Nursing Quality Assurance,* 4(1), 1–9.

14. McFarland, G., & McFarlane, E. (1989). *Nursing diagnosis and intervention: Planning for patient care,* St. Louis: Mosby.

15. Sovie, M. (1989). Clinical nursing practices and patient outcomes: evaluation, evolution and revolution. *Nursing Economics,* 7(2), 79.

16. Taptich, B., et al. (1989). *Nursing diagnosis and care planning.* Philadelphia: W.B. Saunders.

17. Yura, H., & Walsh, M.B. (1983). *The nursing process; Assessing, planning, implementing and evaluation* (4th ed.). Norwalk, CT: Appleton-Century-Crofts.

18. Zander, K. (1988). Nursing case management. *Journal of Nursing Administration,* 18, 23–30.

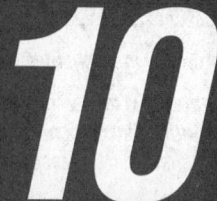

Chapter 10

Implementation

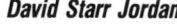

Wisdom is knowing what to do next. Skill is knowing how to do it. Virtue is doing it.

David Starr Jordan

▼ CHAPTER OUTLINE

SKILLS USED DURING IMPLEMENTATION
OF NURSING CARE
    Cognitive Skills
    Interpersonal Skills
    Technical Skills
RESPONSIBILITIES IN IMPLEMENTATION
OF NURSING CARE
    Reviewing the Planned
      Interventions for Appropriateness
    Scheduling and Organizing the
      Interventions
    Collaborating with Other Team
      Members

Supervising and Delegating Nursing
    Care by Other Members of the
    Nursing Team
Providing Direct Nursing Care
Providing Counseling
Involving the Client in Health Care
Teaching the Client and Family
Making Referrals to Other Health
    Care Professionals
Documenting Nursing Care
    Provided

▼ KEY TERMS

Clinical nurse specialists   Interventions, dependent

SKILLS USED DURING IMPLEMENTATION OF NURSING CARE

The implementation phase of the nursing process draws heavily on the cognitive, interpersonal, and technical skills of the nurse. Decision making, observation, and communication are significant skills, enhancing the success of action. These skills are utilized with the client, the nurse, nursing team members, and health team members.[10]

Cognitive Skills

The nurse uses cognitive or intellectual skills during the implementation phase of the nursing process. These skills include problem solving, decision making, critical thinking, and innovation. As you prepare to administer nursing care, a review of the planned interventions will utilize your cognitive abilities. You use intellectual skills to implement the plan of care to meet the client's needs. For example, before helping a patient get out of bed for the first time after surgery, you might consider these factors:

▶ When was the last time the person received pain medication? Is the person comfortable now?
▶ Does the person know how to use deep breathing and relaxation techniques that help facilitate the movement from the bed to the chair?
▶ How large is the person? How strong is the nurse? How much equipment needs to be moved? For example, are there IV poles or drainage bags? Does the nurse need to get additional staff to help move the person?
▶ What time is it now? Does the person want to be sitting in a chair for the next meal or for visiting hours? Will you be available to help the person back to bed when needed?

These are examples of the kinds of decision-making skills that are components of cognitive skills. Creativity is employed when you use innovative approaches to implement nursing care.

Interpersonal Skills

Verbal and nonverbal communication skills are utilized when you interact with the person, significant others, and other members of the health care team. These skills are often crucial in the successful implementation

of nursing care. They have a major impact on the person's perception of the quality of nursing care. People often judge nurses not by our technical skills alone but by whether we are kind, concerned, and caring. Your ability to use effective interpersonal skills when communicating with physicians, social workers, and other personnel will also affect the success of the implementation phase. Beginning nurses are often intimidated by the apparent expertise of other members of the health care team and need time and experience to become more comfortable in communicating with others. The ability to teach or counsel clients and interact with others is a skill that improves with practice. It is essential that you be able to use cognitive skills to solve problems and make decisions and use interpersonal skills to implement those decisions.

Technical Skills

Psychomotor or technical skills are the third major category of skills used during implementation of nursing care. These skills are used whenever you manipulate a piece of equipment, prepare an injection, or change a dressing. Both cognitive and interpersonal skills are called upon during the performance of technical skills. For example, after a nurse prepares an injection for a young child, cognitive skills are used to determine the appropriate site. Interpersonal skills are helpful in obtaining the cooperation of the child. Nurses often find that when technical skills are unfamiliar, it is difficult to incorporate the cognitive and interpersonal components. For example, when a student nurse gives an injection for the first time, it is hard to use interpersonal skills to put the client at ease since the student's anxiety level is high. When the nurse is comfortable with the technical or psychomotor task, it is easier to focus on communication with the client. Box 10–1 summarizes the three types of skills used during implementation.

RESPONSIBILITIES IN IMPLEMENTATION OF NURSING CARE

Implementation is *action oriented*. It is your professional responsibility to (a) carry out the nursing care yourself as the primary nurse; (b) delegate certain interventions to appropriate nursing or allied health professionals (such as nursing assistants and occupational

Cognitive (Intellectual) Skills

Problem solving
Decision making
Critical thinking
Innovation

Example: A nurse calculates how to integrate the special diet needed by a Puerto Rican woman with the requirements for a high-protein, low-carbohydrate diet.

Interpersonal Skills

Verbal communication
Nonverbal communication
Teaching
Counseling
Conveying caring

Example: A nurse comforts a toddler who is hospitalized with croup by holding the child in the nurse's lap.

Technical (Psychomotor) Skills

Preparation, adjustment of equipment
Pouring/drawing up medication
Making beds
Changing dressings and so on

Example: A nurse places an air mattress on a bed and inflates the mattress.

therapists); and (c) carry out physician orders, thereby integrating medical therapy into the overall care plan.

Nursing care is implemented to assist people in achieving the outcomes established in the plan of care, to prevent disease and illness by promoting wellness, to restore functioning, and to facilitate coping with illness.

The major responsibilities in implementing nursing care include

▶ Reviewing the planned interventions for appropriateness
▶ Scheduling and organizing the interventions
▶ Collaborating with other team members
▶ Supervising and delegating nursing care by other members of the nursing team
▶ Providing direct nursing care
▶ Providing counseling
▶ Involving the client in health care
▶ Teaching the client and family
▶ Making referrals to other health care professionals
▶ Documenting nursing care provided

Box 10-2 illustrates how the components of the implementation phase fit within the nursing process.

Reviewing the Planned Interventions for Appropriateness

The first phase of implementation involves reviewing the planned interventions. Cognitive skills are used to choose the appropriate nursing interventions. Although as a student you may prepare a nursing care plan before seeing a person for the first time, frequently changes in the person's condition or circumstances will alter the plan. You will be faced with the need to choose new nursing interventions.

CHOOSING THE APPROPRIATE NURSING INTERVENTION

Developing a *plan of action* is a two-step process. The first step is to develop interventions. The second step is to select the *best* intervention for a particular individual.

Develop Interventions. Develop as many possible interventions for the person's problems as you can. Generating different options is advantageous in at least three ways. First, if one option fails to solve the problem, interventions can be tried and one of them may succeed. In addition, having a pool of interventions readily available protects the individual from gaps in nursing care resulting from a lack of possible interventions. Finally, researching various interventions enables you to develop creative approaches to care rather than relying on a few basic routines and procedures.

How are interventions developed? Interventions are generated through processing information and using creativity. The specific ways in which interventions are developed are given in Box 10-3. Ideally, the consideration of numerous interventions results in a creative solution to the diagnosis. To arrive at such a solution, you must feel free to think in new ways and express different ideas, even if those ideas seem unrealistic and far-fetched. Only by considering the *entire range* of possible solutions can you hope to select the one most likely to resolve the nursing diagnosis.

Select the Best Intervention. The next step is to analyze the interventions and choose the one that seems best. In most nursing care situations, the best approach is the one promising the greatest benefit with the least risk. To select such an intervention, systematically examine all the available options. Ask yourself the following questions and try to answer them objectively:

▶ Has this type of intervention been used before in a similar situation? If so, what were the results?
▶ Will this particular intervention enable the person to meet outcomes within the proposed time limits?
▶ Does this intervention take into consideration the person's age, sex, lifestyle, attitudes, religious and cultural traditions, social resources, and coping abilities?
▶ Is this intervention acceptable to the individual and family?
▶ Is the intervention realistic? Are equipment, staff time, staff size, and other resources adequate?

Box 10-2. Step 4 of the Nursing Process: Implementation

Assessment	Diagnosis	Planning	Implementation
Collect data 　Review of the clinical record 　Interview 　Nursing history 　Physical assessment 　Psychosocial assessment 　Consultation 　Review of the literature	Interpret data 　Identify clusters of 　　cues 　Make inferences Validate inferences Compare clusters of 　cues with definition 　and defining character- 　istics Identify related factors Document the nursing 　diagnosis	Establish priorities Develop outcomes Set time frames for outcomes Identify interventions Document plan of care	Review the planned inter- 　ventions Schedule and coordinate 　the person's total 　health care Collaborate with other 　team members Supervise implementation 　of the nursing care 　plan by delegating ap- 　propriate responsibili- 　ties Counsel the person and 　significant others Involve the person in the 　health care Teach the client and fam- 　ily as needed Refer individuals who re- 　quire continuing care Document the care pro- 　vided

---

▶ What might be some undesirable consequences if this intervention is selected? Would this particular solution bring more problems in its wake?

Remember that all decisions concerning human problems carry some risk of being the "incorrect" decision.

Some uncertainty underlies all aspects of providing care. If your chosen approach does not give you the results you expected, review the interventions you considered earlier, develop some new approaches, and select another intervention for testing and evaluation. If this solution also fails, proceed through the planning process again. The next chapter addresses evaluation

of the plan of care and modification of the approach in further detail.

CRITERIA FOR CHOOSING INTERVENTIONS

An alternative method of selecting nursing interventions is suggested by Bulechek and McCloskey.[4] They believe that nurses use six criteria to choose an intervention: (1) desired client outcome; (2) characteristics of the nursing diagnosis; (3) research base associated with the interventions; (4) feasibility of successfully implementing the intervention; (5) acceptability of the interventions to the client; and (6) capabilities of the nurse.

Desired Client Outcome

The primary consideration in selecting a nursing intervention is to identify one that will facilitate moving the client toward the desired outcome.

Judging the intervention begins in the planning phase of the nursing process. However, as you implement care and encounter unanticipated situations, you will select new interventions. For example, the nurse entered Frank Watson's room with the intention of teaching him how to get out of bed and into the wheelchair for the first time since his leg was amputated below the knee. Mrs. Watson said to the nurse, "Can you show me how to help you? I need to learn what to do with this chair so I can help Frank at home." The nurse used this opportunity to instruct Mrs. Watson to help move Frank toward the outcome of being able to get out of bed into a wheelchair.

Box 10-3. Specific Ways to Develop Interventions

▶ Recall ways in which you handled a similar nursing diagnosis in the past.

▶ Consider the nursing diagnosis from various angles and in different ways.

▶ Imagine how you would *ideally* like to see the nursing diagnosis resolved.

▶ Discuss the interventions with the person and family to hear their ideas on solutions to resolving the nursing diagnosis.

▶ Talk with a colleague, or meet with a group of colleagues, and "brainstorm" possible solutions to the diagnosis.

▶ Obtain expert advice and recommendations.

▶ Review current literature.

Characteristics of the Nursing Diagnosis. The nature of the nursing diagnosis is also an important consideration. The primary objective of nursing intervention is to facilitate the person's progress toward achieving the outcome.

Actual Nursing Diagnosis

Nursing interventions are directed toward alleviating the related factor in the nursing diagnosis.

If the related factor is correctly identified and the nursing intervention is effective in changing it, the outcome can be achieved. This improvement can be measured by a favorable change in the defining characteristics of the nursing diagnosis (Table 10–1). In the example of "*Constipation* R/T decreased oral intake, as evidenced by absence of stools," increasing the oral intake may be effective in alleviating the problem. The improvement will be observable when the defining characteristic, absent stools, is no longer present, and the person achieves the outcome of a normal pattern of elimination.

High-Risk Nursing Diagnosis. As defined in Chapter 8, a high-risk nursing diagnosis is a clinical judgment that an individual, family, or community is more vulnerable to develop the problem than others in the same or similar situation.

A person with a high-risk nursing diagnosis has a potential problem. The nursing interventions in this case are directed toward altering or eliminating the risk factors, if possible.

For example, a person who has had surgery has the diagnosis of high risk for infection. As you wash your hands, you will be assisting the person in avoiding the development of an infection. In some instances you may be unable to alter the risk factors. For example, certain physiological factors cannot be changed, such as prematurity, infancy, being elderly, decreased immune responses, and altered mental status. In these situations, nursing interventions are directed toward protecting the person by trying to prevent a problem from occurring. For example, a person may have the nursing diagnosis of "*High Risk for Falls* R/T history of previous fall." You cannot change the fact that the person has fallen previously, but you can promote safety by implementing a falls prevention program.

Wellness Nursing Diagnosis. As you will recall from Chapter 8, a wellness diagnosis is a clinical judgment about an individual, family, or community in transition from a specific level of wellness to a higher level of wellness.

Nursing interventions are directed toward maximizing one's strengths and assisting the person in moving to a higher level of wellness.

For example, a person with the nursing diagnosis of *Health Seeking Behaviors* may ask you for information on how to reduce cholesterol levels. You may provide information on dietary changes and on the benefits of exercise.

Research Base Associated with Interventions. Nursing researchers have been active since the early 1960s in producing research to validate and direct nursing practice. Some aspects of nursing care have been extensively researched, such as reduction in pressure on skin. Other areas are still relatively untested.

Feasibility of Successfully Implementing Interventions. Many factors are used to judge the feasibility of the interventions. You will need to consider the overall plan of care in relation to treatments being provided by other health care professionals. For example, if a person is supposed to walk three times a day, you will want to determine the time of the scheduled physical therapy. With this knowledge, you can plan the ambulation without tiring or overwhelming the person.

In addition to taking into account the overall plan of care, you will also need to consider the availability of resources such as staffing, time, and costs associated with the interventions. Critical paths, which have been developed based on the available resources, will provide guidance in judging the feasibility of interventions.

Acceptability of the Interventions to the Client

Whenever possible, involve the person in establishing the outcome and selecting the interventions.

The individual's beliefs and cultural values will influence the acceptability of the interventions. The person will need information in order to make an informed choice between the various options. In addition, involving the individual helps decrease some of the sense of helplessness that many hospitalized people feel.

Capabilities of the Nurse. As Benner's classic research indicates, not all nurses practice at the same level.[3] As nurses progress from novice through the ex-

TABLE 10–1. Relationship Between Parts of the Nursing Diagnosis and the Nursing Process

Components of Actual Nursing Diagnosis	Use of Components of Nursing Diagnosis During Nursing Process
Human response	Used by nurse to identify outcomes for care
R/T Related factor	Used by nurse to identify interventions to eliminate or modify related factor
as evidenced by Defining characteristics	Used by nurse to judge when nursing diagnosis has been resolved

pert stage, interventions may vary. The nurse's knowledge base, experience, and skills will influence the choice of interventions. It is important for the novice and beginning nurse to recognize those situations in which it is necessary to seek help from other nurses.

Once you have completed the first phase of implementation, that of reviewing the planned interventions, you will activate the other components of implementation:

▶ Scheduling and organizing
▶ Collaborating
▶ Supervising
▶ Counseling
▶ Involving the person in care
▶ Teaching
▶ Making referrals, and
▶ Documenting

Scheduling and Organizing the Interventions

Specific coordinating activities include (a) meeting with other health care team members to plan and organize care; (b) scheduling the person's activities, e.g., scheduling appointment with dietitian, determining the best time for physical or occupational therapy, and scheduling rehabilitation exercises (Box 10–4); (c) discussing the person's progress with significant others; (d) consulting with the physician; and (e) arranging for discharge and long-term needs.

Scheduling and coordinating nursing care require time management skills. You will be involved in balancing the requirements of several people, including several patients and health care practitioners. As you become more comfortable with providing nursing care, you will be better able to organize your day and address the needs of many people.

Collaborating with Other Team Members

You will not be the primary nurse for every person in your clinical area. Therefore, communication with and collaboration among team members are essential. You may be involved with conferring with **clinical nurse specialists.** These valuable resource people are nurses prepared at the master's level who possess expertise in specific clinical specialties (e.g., oncology, critical care). Staff nurses should also consult *each other* as

professional colleagues, so that nursing as a profession is strengthened. Collaboration with other professional nurses also improves the quality of nursing care.

Supervising and Delegating Nursing Care by Other Members of the Nursing Team

As a professional, you will delegate appropriate responsibilities to the person, significant others, and other team members. The delegation of nursing care is based on six elements, as defined by the Joint Commission of Accreditation of Healthcare Organizations:

▶ The complexity of the individual's condition and nursing care needs
▶ The stability of the person's status
▶ The complexity of the assessment required to care for the person properly, including the knowledge and skills needed by the nursing staff member in order to complete the assessment
▶ The type of technology or equipment employed in providing nursing care
▶ The degree of supervision required by the nursing staff member based on the nurse's level of competence
▶ The availability of supervision[2]

Delegation of nursing care also depends on the job description and legal limitations of the scope of practice of other team members. For example, a registered nurse could not ask a nursing assistant to give a dose of intravenous medication. Table 10–2 illustrates a sample assignment based on these factors.

Providing Direct Nursing Care

Nursing interventions may be independent or interdependent, as discussed in Chapter 8. They may also be dependent.

TABLE 10–2. Sample Assignment

Client	Assigned to
George Wilson, 79, Alzheimer's disease, awaiting nursing home placement	Sue Jackson, Nursing Assistant
Barbara Tratler, 32, first day post-op after knee surgery, has a PCA (patient-controlled analgesia) pump	Betty Lewis, Registered Nurse
Robert Langley, 28, unstable diabetic, requires teaching concerning blood glucose monitoring	Cindy Eberle, Registered Nurse
Sarah Keane, 93, sacral decubiti, needs decubitus care	Tim Frey, Licensed Practical Nurse

Box 10–4. Schedule for a Hospitalized Person

8:30	Breakfast
9:30	Bath
10:00	Out of bed to chair
11:00	Return to bed
12:00	Lunch
1:00	Visit by dietitian to discuss food preferences
2:30	Visit by discharge planner
4:00	Trip to physical therapy

Dependent interventions are carried out based on the physician's orders. These include activities such as medication administration, providing IV fluids, offering a specific type of diet, and activity orders.

In some instances, there are standing orders that direct the care of the client. Standing orders are typically developed when the facility is caring for a group of people with clearly identified and anticipated needs. For example, an obstetrician may use standing orders for the care of a woman after a normal vaginal delivery. The Coronary Care Unit may have standing orders to guide the care of people admitted with chest pain. Both dependent interventions and standing orders must be evaluated carefully to be sure they are appropriate for the person. Fatigue, distraction, or lack of knowledge may lead to a physician giving an improper order. You are legally responsible for questioning physicians' orders that are inappropriate or inaccurate. For example, you are expected to know the expected dose of a medication and question improper doses.

Providing Counseling

Counseling in *acute* situations may require crisis intervention techniques (see Chapter 16). Counseling also helps individuals with *long-term chronic illness* and disabilities to come to terms with their condition. In this case, encourage people to verbalize fears or concerns by establishing a warm, nonthreatening atmosphere.

Counseling also involves helping people *cope successfully* as they pass through the *various developmental stages* of a normal life: childhood, adolescence, pregnancy, childbearing, retirement. In this case, the counselor not only discusses the person's problems at different developmental stages but also talks about the many normal changes that occur as a person performs life's developmental tasks.

This type of assistance involves helping people identify stresses and develop effective techniques for managing stress. You will find it useful to teach concepts of progressive relaxation and guided imagery to manage stress (Chapter 16). In addition, these techniques are sometimes used when pain is present.

Involving the Client in Health Care

There is a strong trend toward offering the client choices to enhance the acceptability of the outcomes and interventions. Clients and, to the degree considered necessary or desirable by the client, family members have a right to be informed about and involved in the provision of nursing care.[2]

Teaching the Client and Family

Teaching is a vital part of implementing the care plan and promoting change. Because of its tremendous importance, teaching is discussed in detail in Chapter 26.

Box 10–5. ANA Standards for Implementation

The nurse implements the interventions identified in the plan of care.

Measurement Criteria

1. Interventions are consistent with the established plan of care.
2. Interventions are implemented in a safe and appropriate manner.
3. Interventions are documented.

Reprinted with permission from *Standards of clinical nursing practice* (1991). Washington, DC: American Nurses Association. © 1991.

Making Referrals to Other Health Care Professionals

Referrals are written on special forms, made over the phone, or requested in person. Most health care agencies have a referral procedure to simplify the transfer of information from one health care facility or department to another. Clients are typically referred to dietitians, social workers, psychiatrists, clergy, physical therapists, occupational therapists, and various organizations such as Alcoholics Anonymous, clinics, nursing homes, rehabilitation centers, or public health nursing departments. Referrals must be made thoughtfully and carefully. Mutually negotiating needs and outcomes *with* the person will help you make referrals that are necessary and that the person desires, or at least accepts.

Documenting Nursing Care Provided

During and after implementation of care you will record information in the medical record. This information includes data, observations, interventions, and your evaluation of the effectiveness of care. Documentation is covered in greater detail in Chapter 27. Box 10–5 presents the American Nurses' Association standards on the implementation phase of the nursing process.

Summary

▶ The ultimate intent of the implementation phase is the use of strategies to help the person achieve the outcomes. By providing focused and planned care, you use your cognitive, interpersonal, and technical skills to assist the person.

▶ The major responsibilities of nursing care involve reviewing the planned interventions, scheduling, organizing, collaborating, supervising, providing direct care, counseling, teaching, referring, and documenting.

▶ Prior to implementing care, the nurse reviews the appropriateness of the interventions that were selected.

▶ Nurses use six criteria for selecting interventions, including consideration of the desired outcome, the characteristics of the nursing diagnosis, the research base associated with the interventions, the feasibility of successfully implementing the intervention, the acceptability of the intervention to the client, and the capabilities of the nurse.

▶ Nurses often schedule and coordinate the person's total health care regimen.

▶ A variety of team members collaborate to provide care.

▶ The nurse considers several factors when delegating care.

▶ Nurses use independent, interdependent, and dependent interventions to provide direct nursing care.

▶ Counseling skills are useful to help people cope with illness and developmental issues.

▶ People are involved in their health care through being consulted when planning and implementing interventions and in receiving education about how to manage their health needs.

▶ Nurses refer people to a variety of resources.

▶ Documentation is performed both during and after the implementation of care.

Bibliography

1. American Nurses Association (1991). *Standards of clinical care.* Washington, DC: American Nurses Association.
2. *AMH scoring guidelines* (1992). Oakbrook Terrace, IL: Joint Commission on Accreditation of Health Care Organizations.
3. Benner, P. (1984). *From novice to expert.* Menlo Park, CA: Addison-Wesley Publishing Company.
4. Bulechek, G., & McCloskey, J. (1992). Nursing interventions (2nd ed.). Philadelphia: W.B. Saunders.
5. Bulechek, G., & McCloskey, J. (eds.) (1992). Symposium on nursing interventions. *Nursing Clinics of North America,* June.
6. Bulechek, G., & McCloskey, J. (1989). Nursing interventions: treatments for potential nursing diagnoses. In Carroll-Johnson, R. *Proceedings of the eighth conference.* Philadelphia: J.B. Lippincott.
7. Iyer, P. (1991). New trends in charting. *Nursing 91,* January, 48–50.
8. Iyer, P., & Camp, N. (1991). *Nursing documentation: A nursing process approach.* St. Louis: Mosby Year Book.
9. McCloskey, J., & Bulechek, G. (1992). *Nursing interventions classification.* St. Louis: Mosby Year Book.
10. Yura, H., & Walsh, M. (1983). *The nursing process: Assessing, planning, implementing and evaluation* (4th ed.). Norwalk, CT: Appleton-Century-Crofts.

▼ Evaluation

It is a bad plan that can't be changed.
Publilius Syrus: *Maxims*

▼ CHAPTER OUTLINE

DEFINITIONS AND PURPOSES OF
   EVALUATION
STEPS IN THE EVALUATION PROCESS
      Step 1: Refer to the Client's
         Planned Outcomes
      Step 2: Evaluate the Client's
         Condition and Compare Actual
         Outcomes with Expected
         Outcomes
      Step 3: Summarize the Results of
         the Evaluation
      Step 4: Identify Reasons for
         Client's Failure, If Indicated, to
         Achieve Expected Outcomes

      Step 5: Take Corrective Action to
         Modify the Plan of Care as
         Necessary
      Step 6: Document the
         Evaluation of the Client's
         Achievement of Outcomes and
         the Modification, If Any, of the
         Plan of Care
EVALUATION: ADDITIONAL APPLICATIONS
      Malpractice Suits
      Performance Evaluations
      Nursing Research
      Quality Improvement

▼ KEY TERMS

Performance Evaluation   Quality improvement

▼ LEARNING OBJECTIVES

After studying this chapter, you should be able to:

1. Distinguish between assessment and evaluation.
2. Identify the sequential steps in evaluation.
3. List at least two additional uses of evaluation.

DEFINITIONS AND PURPOSES OF EVALUATION

Evaluation involves the use of nursing judgment in identifying the client's responses to nursing care and the success of the plan in achieving the outcomes. This phase of the nursing process focuses heavily on the process of determining whether the client has achieved these outcomes as stated in the plan of care.

Evaluation is not the same as assessment, although the terms are often incorrectly interchanged.

Assessment involves data gathering for the purposes of deriving a nursing diagnosis and forming a plan. Therefore, the assessment phase consists of gathering information about the existing problems and strengths of the person. The evaluation step of the nursing process uses your knowledge and skills to make a *clinical judgment* about the achievement of outcomes (Table 11–1). During evaluation, you compare the current status of the person with the expected outcomes. When you evaluate the person, you make a decision about how well the person achieved the outcomes and whether the plan of care should be continued, modified, or discontinued.

As a part of professional accountability, nurses are answerable to themselves as practitioners, to individuals and significant others, to physicians and others who participate in giving care, to the agencies in which they practice, and to the community. The use of evaluation helps fulfill the nurse's duty to act in a professionally responsible way.

Ideally, evaluation is an ongoing process that takes place on a continuing basis throughout your interactions with the client. It may occur as frequently as every few minutes when a person is critically ill or as infrequently as daily, weekly, or monthly, depending on the setting. When evaluation is performed on an ongoing basis, it is called formative evaluation. For example, an instructor in a school of nursing who evaluates students after each clinical experience is performing a formative evaluation. The end of the semester evaluation is a summative evaluation that examines the overall performance of the student. Summative evaluation is performed when nurses evaluate how well clients have met several outcomes, as might occur when a person is discharged from a facility.

STEPS IN THE EVALUATION PROCESS

The evaluation process has six steps when evaluation is used to determine whether the person achieved the expected outcomes. These steps are listed in the evaluation column of Box 11–1.

Step 1: Refer to the Client's Planned Outcomes

As described in Chapter 9, the planning phase involves establishing clear, objective, and measurable outcomes. These outcomes are documented on the plan of care in the form of an individually developed, standardized or computerized care plan, critical path, or practice guideline. These stated outcomes become the criteria for evaluating whether or not the outcome has been achieved.

The first step of the evaluation process involves referring to the outcomes in order to make comparisons with the client's current status.

Step 2: Evaluate the Client's Condition and Compare Actual Outcomes with Expected Outcomes

This step of the evaluation process involves gathering data about the person's current status and comparing the observable actual outcomes with the planned outcomes. There are two components to this step: (1) evaluate the person's physiological and behavioral responses and the degree to which they conform to the expected outcomes outlined in the nursing care plan, and (2) evaluate the nursing care plan itself.

EVALUATE THE CLIENT'S RESPONSES

To evaluate the client's responses, you can do the following: review expected outcomes; observe physiologic and behavioral responses; and compare actual responses and expected outcomes.

TABLE 11–1. Documentation of Achievement of Outcomes

Examples of Behavior to Be Evaluated	Outcome of Plan of Care	Evaluative Statement Documented by Nurse	Achievement of Outcome
Response to prn medication within 1 hour of administration, with the exception of long-acting prns such as laxatives and antidiarrheals	Verbalizes relief of pain within 1 hour of receiving pain medication	"Verbalized relief of pain 45 min after injection of morphine."	Outcome has been achieved
	Verbalizes relief of nausea and vomiting within 1 hour of receiving antiemetics	"Vomiting subsided 1 hour after received Compazine."	Outcome has been achieved
Response to activity following changes in activity or progression of activity	Ambulates within room without dyspnea by 6/11	"Able to walk from bed to bathroom without getting dyspneic."	Outcome has been achieved
Tolerance to treatments as appropriate and especially a change in response	Able to tolerate being flat without c/o (complaints of) dyspnea by 9/10	"Unable to tolerate having head of bed lowered from 90° to 45°. Became short of breath."	Outcome has not been achieved
Response to oxygen therapy or respiratory care	Is free of respiratory distress by 7/12	"15 min after nasal oxygen was applied, skin became pink and less dusky."	Outcome has been achieved
Tolerance to diet following changes in diet or advancement of diet, and in presence of food intolerance	Tolerates advancement of diet to regular diet by 3/19 without vomiting	"Consumed all of full liquid lunch, stated she was hungry and wanted more solid food."	Outcome has been achieved
Client complaints or concerns, and your response to their needs	(Outcomes will be individualized to person's needs)	"Became calmer after being encouraged to ventilate her anxiety about her children."	Outcome has been achieved
Ability to perform activities of daily living, particularly those that may influence discharge planning	Is independent in bathing and ambulation by time of discharge	"Unable to wash self independently owing to left-sided weakness."	Outcome is not being achieved
		"Was able to walk unassisted yesterday but now requires a walker to ambulate to bathroom."	Outcome is not being achieved
Other elements of response specific to client's psychological, emotional, or educational needs	No evidence of incisional infection throughout hospitalization	"Incision shows no signs of infection."	Outcome has been achieved
	By time of discharge, verbalizes feelings about loss of hand	"Is beginning to show signs of being able to cope with the loss of his left hand."	Outcome has been achieved
	Following teaching, is able to correctly prepare and administer own insulin	"Able to draw up and inject insulin using correct technique."	Outcome has been achieved

Review Expected Outcomes. *Review* the written plan of care for the *expected outcomes* and their *projected dates* for accomplishment. As discussed in Chapter 10, expected outcomes must express in clear, measurable terms exactly what the person should feel like, look like, and act like once the problem is re-solved or is progressing toward resolution. In addition, well-stated outcomes indicate those *clinical manifestations* that result from therapy.

Observe Physiologic and Behavioral Responses. *Observe* the person's physiologic and behavioral re-

Box 11–1. Step 5 of the Nursing Process: Evaluation

Assessment	Nursing Diagnosis	Planning	Implementation	Evaluation

Collect data
  Review of the clinical record
  Interview
  Nursing history
  Physical assessment
  Psychosocial assessment
  Consultation
  Review of the literature
	Interpret data:
	  Identify clusters of cues
	  Make inferences
	Validate inferences
	Compare clusters of cues with definition and defining characteristics
	Identify related factors
	Document the nursing diagnosis
		Establish priorities
		Develop outcomes
		Set time frames for outcomes
		Identify interventions
		Document plan of care
			Review the planned interventions
			Schedule and coordinate the person's total health care
			Collaborate with other team members
			Supervise implementation of the nursing care plan by delegating appropriate responsibilities
			Counsel the person and significant others
			Involve the person in the health care
			Teach the client and family as needed
			Refer individuals who require continuing care
			Document the care provided
				Refer to established outcomes
				Evaluate the individual's condition and compare actual outcomes with expected outcomes
				Summarize the results of the evaluation
				Identify reasons for the person's failure, if indicated, to achieve expected outcomes stated in the plan of care
				Take corrective action to modify the plan of care as necessary
				Document the evaluation of the person's achievement of outcomes and the modifications, if any, in the plan of care

sponses. *Physiologic* responses include clinical measurements such as vital signs, skin condition, and loss or gain in body weight. *Behavioral* responses include both verbal statements and nonverbal activities.

Compare Actual Responses and Expected Outcomes. *Compare* the person's actual responses with the expected outcomes and *look for discrepancies*. For example, suppose the plan of care states that by 3/21 Mr. Grim will wash his hands and face after meals, by 3/18 he will request assistance to change his underclothes when soiled, and so on. If by 3/21 you find that Mr. Grim is indeed washing his hands and face after meals and asking for assistance to change his underclothes when soiled, you know that the expected outcomes and projected dates were realistic and that the nursing orders accomplished their intent. On the other hand, if you evaluate his progress at frequent intervals between 3/18 and 3/21 and find that his personal hygiene is *not* improving and is even growing worse, then you have objective data that he is not meeting the objectives of the care plan. You also know that the care plan (in particular the outcomes, projected dates,

and nursing interventions) needs to be reviewed, revised, and reimplemented.

Involve the person and significant others in the evaluation process. Discuss the success or failure of the plan of care. Determine whether the outcomes the person achieved were the ones that were anticipated according to the person. With a shortened length of stay in acute care facilities, many people are going home still feeling sick, or they may feel worse than they expected they would at the time of discharge. Part of your job is to help people identify achievable outcomes and help them understand that some of their expectations may be unrealistic.

EVALUATE THE PLAN OF CARE

The nursing care plan needs frequent and careful reevaluation. Questions you must ask yourself are: Is the care plan complete? Does it clearly communicate this person's nursing diagnoses, outcomes, and nursing interventions? Is it realistic? Is it helping the person reach the outcomes? Is it completely up to date? Is it being revised as necessary in keeping with the changes in the individual's needs?

Step 3: Summarize the Results of the Evaluation

Once the person's progress has been assessed, the next step is to summarize the findings from the evaluation process. Possible outcomes of the evaluation procedures are as follows:[9]

▶ The person's nursing diagnosis is *resolved:* the person has achieved the expected outcome by the projected date.

▶ The person's nursing diagnosis has *not* been resolved and the expected behaviors have *not* been demonstrated.

▶ *New* nursing diagnoses are evident. These may have been identified from untoward changes in the person's condition; more astute observations of the person's clinical condition and further research on the part of the nursing staff; and the therapy program (i.e., hospital-acquired infections).

▶ The *nursing diagnosis is in error.* Some problems are wrongly labeled, or the related factors (pointing to causation) are incorrect.

If the individual's actual nursing diagnoses have all been resolved and the outcomes have been achieved, you will focus on the prevention of potential problems (high-risk diagnoses) and the support of healthy behaviors (wellness diagnoses).

On the other hand, if evaluation reveals that problems remain unresolved and new problems are developing, it is essential to proceed to step 4 of the evaluation process.

Step 4: Identify Reasons for Client's Failure, If Indicated, to Achieve Expected Outcomes

There are numerous reasons why individuals fail to achieve the outcomes formulated in the nursing care plan: (1) an erroneous, incomplete assessment; (2) inappropriate interventions; (3) uncooperative attitudes on the part of the person; (4) conflicts between the person and/or significant others and the nursing staff; (5) conflicts between the nursing staff and the medical staff; (6) conflicts between the person and significant others; (7) failure by the person, significant others, or the staff to follow the plan of care; and (8) faulty or inadequate implementation of the plan.

As you research the reasons *why* the person has not met the outcomes, attempt to be as objective as possible about the person, the nursing staff, the plan, and yourself. Also try to accept the fact that no plan is perfect and no nursing action is infallible. Most plans of care and clinical situations require careful evaluation, problem and error identification, and modification before all or even most of a person's problems can be resolved.

Step 5: Take Corrective Action to Modify the Plan of Care as Necessary

The nursing care plan is modified when (1) the person has not met the outcomes and new interventions are needed, (2) the person's condition has changed, or (3) the nursing staff have gained new insights into the person's background and behavior and have new approaches that may be effective in helping the person achieve the outcomes.

To modify the plan of care, you may need to (1) reassess the person's current status, strengths, and deficiencies; (2) develop new nursing diagnoses; (3) draw up fresh outcomes; (4) update and implement new nursing interventions; and (5) evaluate, once again, the person's progress under the revised plan of care. This cycle of activity continues until the person finally achieves the realistic outcome that has been mutually negotiated between the nurse and the person.

Step 6: Document the Evaluation of the Client's Achievement of Outcomes and the Modification, If Any, of the Plan of Care

PROGRESS NOTES

It is your professional responsibility to record your judgments about how the person is progressing. Progress notes or nurses' notes will contain this information for other members of the health care team. Your professional accountability is not satisfied simply by documenting on the clinical record. Unexpected, ominous, and significant failures to achieve the established outcomes would be reported to the appropriate health care team member. For example, Carrie Young, age 47, had abdominal surgery yesterday. She requested medication for pain, which you provided an hour ago. She informed you that she is still having severe pain. She states that the pain is now in her chest. You note that she is pale and diaphoretic (perspiring profusely) and has a rapid, weak pulse. Suspecting that she needs to be seen immediately by a physician, you place a call to her surgeon. It is determined that Carrie is having a myocardial infarction, and she is transferred to the Intensive Care Unit.

MODIFYING THE PLAN OF CARE

The second component of documentation involves changing the plan. Care plans are modified on paper by crossing off the resolved nursing diagnosis, outcomes, and interventions. Depending on the policy of the agency, a line may be drawn through the entries or a yellow highlighter used. When a nursing diagnosis is still present but the outcomes or interventions need to be modified, only the applicable sections are changed (Box 11–2).

The nursing process is a continuous cyclical process that results in the achievement of client outcomes. Evaluation is the ongoing planned process of compar-

Box 11–2. Modification of Nursing Care Plan

Example

Linda Dote was admitted to the hospital after an argument in which her husband fractured her ribs and ruptured her spleen. On the second day after admission the nurse helped Linda set an outcome of being able to work out a plan to move out of her home permanently. During discussions Linda continued to say, "Part of me wants to leave him and part of me is afraid to try to make it on my own. I've never lived alone. I'm afraid I would be lonely."

On the fourth day of her hospitalization, Linda's husband showed up with a dozen red roses and promises of never hitting her again. Although the nurse explained to her that this is a predictable phase in the cycle of violence, Linda was unwilling to listen. "Don't you see? He promised he wouldn't hurt me. I think he really means it this time."

Recognizing that Linda was now uninterested in moving out, the nurse gave her written information on the local shelter for battered women. The nurse said, "Linda, you may need this information some day. You will be protected at the shelter and will have a chance to think while your husband cools off." Linda replied, "I am sure I will never need this phone number but I will keep it — just in case."

Nursing Diagnosis	Outcome	Interventions
Decisional Conflict (separation from husband) R/T fear of loneliness	~~By the time of discharge identifies a plan for alternative living arrangements~~	~~1. Assist client to identify alternative living arrangements~~ ~~2. Encourage client to verbalize feelings~~

	Revised Outcome	Revised Interventions
	By the time of discharge is able to describe how to contact shelter	3. Provide client with phone number of shelter 4. Assist client to identify advantages of temporarily utilizing shelter

The nurse in this example determined that Linda was not ready to achieve the outcome of planning a move into her own apartment. Since the nursing diagnosis was appropriate, the nurse revised the outcome and interventions to reflect a different strategy for assisting Linda.

From Iyer, P., et al. (1981). Nursing process and nursing diagnosis (2nd ed.). Philadelphia: W.B. Saunders.

Box 11–3. ANA Standard for Evaluation

The nurse evaluates the client's progress toward attainment of outcomes.

1. Evaluation is systematic and ongoing.
2. The client's responses to interventions are documented.
3. The effectiveness of interventions is evaluated in relation to outcomes.
4. Ongoing assessment data are used to revise diagnoses, outcomes, and the plan of care, as needed.
5. Revisions in diagnoses, outcomes, and the plan of care are documented.
6. The client, significant others, and health care providers are involved in the evaluation process, when appropriate.

Reprinted with permission from *Standards of clinical nursing practice* (1991). Washington, DC: American Nurses Association. © 1991.

ing the person's status with the expected outcomes. When progress is not being made to move the client toward the outcomes, the client and nurse must revise the plan of care. Box 11–3 presents the American Nurses Association Standard on Evaluation.

EVALUATION: ADDITIONAL APPLICATIONS

Evaluation is an essential, ongoing component of the nursing process. It is used in many other nursing activities. Malpractice suits, performance evaluations, research, and quality improvement use nursing knowledge to measure something in comparison with a standard.

Malpractice Suits

A nursing standard is a statement that establishes the desired behaviors or activities of nursing and other health care personnel. Many professional groups develop standards to define how professionals should perform their responsibilities. The standards of nursing practice, which have been integrated into the last five chapters, were established by the American Nurses Association. Several specialty nursing organizations have published standards, including the Emergency Nurses Association, the Association of Operating Room Nurses, the American Association of Critical Care Nurses, and so on.

Standards are also established by what is customary or general practice. For example, in the case cited earlier in which the postoperative client developed chest pain, it would be an expected standard of care for the nurse to notify the physician. Standards are used to determine whether a particular professional performed in the customary manner. Suppose the nurse did not notify the physician of the chest pain, and there was a delay in diagnosis of a myocardial infarction that resulted in the client's death. If a malpractice suit resulted from this outcome, the standard of care or expected behavior by the nurse would be used to determine whether the nurse acted appropriately.

Therefore, standards are used in our legal system when institutions and people are accused of malpractice.

Performance Evaluations

A **performance evaluation** is a set of measureable observable statements used to determine how a student or graduate nurse compares with the expected behavior or standard (Fig. 11–1). Job descriptions incorporate standards of professional behavior and form the basis for evaluating a nurse's performance. In some settings, the nurse manager is responsible for completing the performance evaluation of the staff nurses. In other areas, the staff nurses evaluate each other (peer review). Performance evaluations become a part of the person's employee file and are considered at the time of raises or promotions.

Nursing Research

EVALUATING NURSING DIAGNOSES

Clinical research allows nurses to evaluate the validity of nursing practice. In the past, much of nursing was based on trial and error. With the focus on nursing research that began in the 1960s, nursing researchers have been making progress in validating nursing diagnoses, outcomes, and interventions. For example, nursing research is used to identify nursing diagnoses that should be added to the North American Nursing Diagnosis list. Data are collected to identify the new diagnoses' defining characteristics and related factors. Existing diagnoses may be modified based on research.

EVALUATING OUTCOMES

Outcomes are also evaluated through nursing research. A Rhode Island study showed that outcomes of residents in nursing homes were linked to factors such as insufficient staffing, high turnover of nurses, overuse of urinary catheters, and low rates of skin care. When these factors were present, there appeared to be more negative patient outcomes, or residents were less likely to improve.[1]

EVALUATING NURSING INTERVENTIONS

Research studies evaluate nursing interventions. Research is undertaken to examine the usefulness of certain interventions and to identify the strategies that are not effective. For example, a study published in 1991 demonstrated that it was not necessary to give heparin subcutaneously in the abdomen for maximum effective-

ness. This finding challenged the common practice of using the abdomen as the preferred site.[3]

One of nursing's challenges is to ensure that findings of research are integrated into practice.

Quality Improvement

Also called total quality management (TQM) or continuous quality improvement (CQI), quality improvement (QI) focuses on evaluating and improving the delivery of care. In the early 1990s, health care organizations began modifying the industrial model of QI. The Joint Commission on Accreditation of Healthcare Organizations, whose standards influence much of the activities of hospitals, began requiring QI in 1992. **Quality improvement** is

- ▶ a systematic approach for improving the effectiveness of an organization while reducing costs
- ▶ based on an underlying assumption that every process can be improved
- ▶ a continuous process that evaluates the needs and expectations of customers and searches for better ways to meet those needs
- ▶ a long-term commitment that drives the philosophy of the organization

QUALITY ASSURANCE AND INDIVIDUAL PERFORMANCE

Quality improvement is gradually replacing quality assurance (QA). Developed in the mid-1980s, QA put a great deal of emphasis on evaluating the performance of individual practitioners. Standards were used to determine whether people were doing their jobs. This approach is now referred to as "searching for the bad apple." Quality assurance fell short of making dramatic improvements within organizations. In the late 1980s, we gradually realized that most people want to do their jobs well and are quite capable. However, the majority of problems occurring within a health care facility are due to problems in the system and are not due to incompetent people. For example, a physician becomes angry when the results of a laboratory test are not on the record the next day. The system problems that could contribute to the missing results include:

- ▶ The laboratory technician came to draw the blood but the client was not in the room, **or**
- ▶ The technician tried to draw the blood but missed the vein, and there was no system in place to notify someone to try to draw the blood later, **or**
- ▶ The machine required to perform the blood test was broken and the repair person was on vacation, **or**
- ▶ The only person who knew how to run this test was off duty, **or**
- ▶ The test had been run but the results were placed on the chart of a person who had the same first and last name as the client.

All these factors illustrate systems issues that ultimately lead to an unhappy customer, the physician.

UNION HOSPITAL
Performance Evaluation

Page 1 of 7

JOB TITLE: _____ REGISTERED NURSE _____ DATE: _____

MAIN DUTIES:
- Makes an accurate assessment of patient's nursing needs upon admission and on an ongoing basis.

    YES ___ NO ___ NEEDS IMPROVEMENT ___

- Demonstrates ongoing assessment skills that are reflected in care rendered and nursing documentation.

    YES ___ NO ___ NEEDS IMPROVEMENT ___

DIAGNOSIS:
- Analyzes patient data and formulates appropriate nursing diagnoses.

    YES ___ NO ___ NEEDS IMPROVEMENT ___

PLANNING:
- Plans appropriate nursing interventions by applying current scientific principles and knowledge.

    YES ___ NO ___ NEEDS IMPROVEMENT ___

- Determines severity of patient's problems and prioritizes patient care.

    YES ___ NO ___ NEEDS IMPROVEMENT ___

- Develops a teaching plan for patient and/or significant other based on the patient's needs as identified through ongoing assessment and evaluation to prepare patient for discharge.

    YES ___ NO ___ NEEDS IMPROVEMENT ___

- Delegates responsibility for healthcare activities to other members of nursing staff based on needs of patient, capabilities of staff, degree of supervision needed and technology used in patient's care.

    YES ___ NO ___ NEEDS IMPROVEMENT ___

▲ Figure 11–1

Sample performance evaluation. (Courtesy of Union Hospital, Union, NJ.)

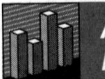

APPLYING RESEARCH TO NURSING PRACTICE

Evaluation: The Forgotten Step of the Nursing Process

Hurst, K., Dean, A., & Trickey, S. (1991). The recognition and non-recognition of problem-solving stages in nursing practice. *Journal of Advanced Nursing, 16,* 1444–1455.

▼ ▼ ▼

Hurst, Dean, and Trickey examined whether nurses are able to identify the steps of the nursing process when presented with written descriptions of real-life incidents related to problem solving. The researchers asked 116 nurses to read seven scenarios, each one missing a stage of the nursing process. The researchers then interviewed the nurses to determine whether they were able to identify each of the stages of the nursing process, as well as the missing one. Of the total sample, 71% successfully recognized *Assessment.* Fifty-one percent were able to identify *Diagnosis* (problem identification). Whereas 55% recognized *Planning,* the largest number of nurses (87%) commented on the presence of *Implementation.* In contrast, only 44% commented on the presence of *Evaluation.* When the description of the evaluation process was deliberately omitted from the vignettes, only 21% of the nurses recognized the missing step.

Applications for Practice

Findings from this well-designed study suggest that some nurses might focus primarily on the detection of problems and on the hands-on intervention aspect of problem solving. In practice, you must purposefully explore how information about your clients has been processed. When an important aspect of the nursing process, such as evaluation, has been neglected, you should consciously devote more attention to it. Although nurses may perceive that the assessment and implementation steps of the nursing process are more active and useful, in practice one must recognize and use the *whole* nursing process.

QUALITY IMPROVEMENT AND TEAMWORK

Quality improvement uses data to identify problems and measure improvements. Teams of health care professionals from many departments work together to improve the organization. For example, a team might try to reduce the amount of time it takes to admit a new client, to improve the delivery of hot meals of the correct type of diet to the right person, or improve the medication administration system to decrease medication errors.

To correct the problem of missing results of laboratory tests, a team of people might consist of a physician, a nurse, and a laboratory technician. This team would systematically analyze all the activities that occur from the time an order for a laboratory test is written to the time the results are available to the physician. The steps would be examined to determine how to eliminate delays or opportunities for mistakes to occur.

Quality improvement is grounded on the concept that improved quality can reduce costs. Much money and time are wasted in correcting mistakes.

For example, a nurse who has not received enough training in inserting intravenous needles may be required to start an IV. When the nurse is unsuccessful on the first or second try, equipment and time have been wasted. In addition, the person who is being repeatedly stuck is left with an unfavorable impression of the skills of the nurse.

IDENTIFYING THE NEEDS OF INTERNAL AND EXTERNAL CUSTOMERS

Quality improvement acknowledges that there are many customers, both internal and external to the organization. A customer is someone who receives goods or services. In this perspective, internal customers are the personnel within a facility, such as physicians and employees in other departments. External customers are clients, regulatory agencies, insurance companies, and so on. Just as you hear "the customer is always right," so you will hear that QI tries to identify and satisfy the needs of customers.

The emphasis on teamwork, reducing costs, and satisfying customers requires a long-term commitment. The top management in an organization must be knowledgeable about quality improvement and be willing to stick to its principles in the face of resistance to change. Quality improvement offers exciting opportunities to evaluate and improve health care.

Summary

▶ Assessment involves data gathering, whereas evaluation consists of making judgments about the achievement of outcomes.

▶ The evaluation process has six steps.

▶ Clear, measurable outcomes are needed in order to make an evaluation. The first step is to refer to these.

▶ The second step consists of evaluating both the person's responses and the plan of care.

▶ The next step involves summarizing the results of the evaluation by making a determination of the degree to which the person's nursing diagnoses are resolved.

▶ There may be several reasons for a person's inability to achieve the expected outcomes. These should be identified during the fourth step.

▶ During the fifth step, the plan of care must be modified as needed to help the person achieve the outcomes.

▶ Professional accountability requires documentation and appropriate reporting of your evaluation of the person's status.

▶ Evaluation may be used in malpractice suits, staff performance evaluations, research, and quality improvement.

Bibliography

1. Characteristics of nursing homes that affect resident outcomes (1991). *Journal of Aging & Health,* 3(4), 427–454.
2. Critical paths—a pre-existing tool ready-made for TQM implementation (1992). *QI/TQM,* January 1–2, 4.
3. Fahs, P., et al. (1991). The abdomen, thigh and arm as sites for subcutaneous sodium heparin injections. *Nursing Research,* 40(4), 204–207.
4. Hegvary, S. (1991). Issues in outcomes research. *Journal of Nursing Quality Assurance,* 5(2), 1–6.
5. Iyer, P. (1991). Thirteen charting rules to keep you legally safe. *Nursing 91,* 21(6), 40–44.
6. Iyer, P. (1991). Six more charting rules to keep you legally safe. *Nursing 91,* July, 34–39.
7. Krenz, M. (1989). Linking nursing diagnosis, QA and nursing standards. *Journal of Advanced Medical Surgical Nursing,* 1(3), 53–61.
8. Martin, C. (1990). NAQAP position paper: the role of QI in health care QA. *Journal of Quality Assurance,* Nov/Dec, 12–16.
9. Patterson, C. (1988). Standards of patient care: the Joint Commission focus on nursing quality assurance. *Nursing Clinics of North America,* September, 625–638.
10. Quality, thy name is nursing care, CEOs say (1989). *Hospitals,* February 5, 32.
11. Schroeder, P. (1991). *Encyclopedia of nursing standards.* Rockville, MD: Aspen.
12. Yura, H., & Walsh, M.B. (1983). *The nursing process; Assessing, planning, implementing and evaluation* (4th ed.). Norwalk, CT: Appleton-Century-Crofts.

Growth and Development

Unit

3

▼ *Conception Through Childhood*

The child's great task is "freeing himself from the parents, for only after this detachment is accomplished, can he cease to be a child and so become a member of the social community."

Sigmund Freud

Listening to girls and women speaking about themselves . . . . I heard conceptions of self and morality that implied a different way of thinking about relationships, one that often had set women apart from the mainstream of Western thought because of its central premise that self and others were connected and interdependent.

Carol Gilligan

▼ CHAPTER OUTLINE

PRINCIPLES OF GROWTH AND
  DEVELOPMENT
MAJOR PRINCIPLES OF PHYSIOLOGIC
  GROWTH AND DEVELOPMENT
    Normal Physiologic Development
      Proceeds in Three Directions
    Physiologic Growth and
      Development Occur in a
      Predictable Pattern
    The Processes of Physiologic
      Development Occur in a
      Predictable Sequence
    Physiologic Growth and
      Development Occur When
      "Readiness" Has Been Reached
    Physiologic Development Is the
      Result of a Combination of
      Maturational and Learning
      Factors
    Each Stage of Physiologic
      Development Is Different from
      the One Before
    Each Stage of Physiologic
      Development Depends on Growth
      in Previous Stages

PHYSIOLOGIC SYSTEMS THAT REGULATE
  GROWTH AND DEVELOPMENT
    Regulation of Growth and
      Development by Genetic
      Inheritance
    Regulation of Growth and
      Development by the Nervous
      System
    Regulation of Growth and
      Development by the Endocrine
      System
INTERACTIONAL FACTORS THAT
  INFLUENCE DEVELOPMENT
    Adaptation
    Motivation
    Learning and Socialization
    Individual Differences
PSYCHOSOCIAL THEORIES OF HUMAN
  DEVELOPMENT
    Contributors to Psychodynamic
      Theories
    Contributors to Cognitive Theories
    Contributors to Behavioral Theories
    Summary of Psychosocial Theories
      of Human Development

▼ **CHAPTER OUTLINE**

CONCEPTION THROUGH CHILDHOOD
Prenatal Period
CONCEPTION
GERMINAL STAGE OF DEVELOPMENT
EMBRYONIC STAGE OF DEVELOPMENT
FETAL STAGE OF DEVELOPMENT
MAJOR HEALTH CONCERNS
ROLE OF THE NURSE
Neonatal Period
PHYSICAL DEVELOPMENT AND CHANGE
   Head and Body
   Reflexes
   Care of the Newborn Infant
PSYCHOSOCIAL DEVELOPMENT
   Self-Concept and Self-Image
   Cognitive and Intellectual
      Development
   Communication
RELATIONSHIPS AND ROLES
   Bonding and Family Relationships
   Establishing Trust
VALUES AND BELIEFS
MAJOR HEALTH CONCERNS
ROLE OF THE NURSE
   Apgar Scale
   Brazelton Neonatal Behavior
      Assessment Scale
Infancy
PHYSICAL DEVELOPMENT AND CHANGE

PSYCHOSOCIAL DEVELOPMENT
   Self-Concept and Self-Image
   Cognitive and Intellectual
      Development
   Communication
RELATIONSHIPS AND ROLES
   Expressing Emotions
   Establishing Trust
VALUES AND BELIEFS
MAJOR HEALTH CONCERNS
ROLE OF THE NURSE
Early Childhood
PHYSICAL DEVELOPMENT AND CHANGE
   Weight Gain
   Sleep
   Motor Skills
   Eating Patterns
   Developing Toilet Independence
PSYCHOSOCIAL DEVELOPMENT
   Self-Concept and Self-Image
   Cognitive and Intellectual
      Development
   Communication
   Play
   Developing Autonomy
   Developing Initiative
   Developing Self-Control
VALUES AND BELIEFS
MAJOR HEALTH CONCERNS

ROLE OF THE NURSE
   Health Screening and Assessment
   Health Education
School Age
PHYSICAL DEVELOPMENT AND CHANGE
   Physical Growth Patterns
   Eating Patterns and Sleep
PSYCHOSOCIAL DEVELOPMENT
   Self-Concept and Self-Image
   Cognitive and Intellectual
      Development
   Communication
RELATIONSHIPS AND ROLES
   Family Relationships
   Sibling Relationships
   Peer Relationships
VALUES AND BELIEFS
MAJOR HEALTH CONCERNS
ROLE OF THE NURSE
   Health Screening and Assessment
   Health Education
CHILD ABUSE
RISK FACTORS FOR CHILD ABUSE
   Age
   Sex
   Family Size
   Family Intactness
CHILDHOOD SEXUAL ABUSE

▼ **KEY TERMS**

Conceptus	Extinction	Nägele's rule	Readiness	Subconscious
Conscious	Growth	Placenta	Reinforcer	Superego
Development	Id	Psychosexual theory	Response cost	Unconscious
Ego	Libido	Punishment	Socialization	

▼ **LEARNING OBJECTIVES**

After studying this chapter, you should be able to

1. Explain basic principles underlying human growth and development.
2. Define the role of motivation, learning, socialization, and individual difference factors in human growth and development.
3. Explain characteristics of major theories of human psychosocial development.
4. Describe rates and patterns of physical growth and cognitive and psychosocial development in the neonatal, infancy, early childhood, and school-age stages of development.
5. Identify patterns of child abuse and characteristics of abused or neglected children.

▼ PRINCIPLES OF GROWTH AND DEVELOPMENT

As the opening quotations illustrate, there is no agreement about the goals or desired outcomes of human growth and development. The study of development is a relatively new field and one that is still evolving. The purpose of this chapter is to outline some of the well-accepted principles of growth and development, to present some of the theoretical perspectives on human psychosocial development, and to describe developmental processes for humans from prenatal life to puberty. Chapter 13 will present adolescent and young adult development, and Chapter 14, middle age and older adulthood.

The human life span can be interpreted in a number of ways. One way is *linear,* or a straight line — assuming that life begins with conception, continues through birth, childhood, adolescence, and adulthood, and ends with death. Some people do not believe in a fixed beginning or ending and consider the linear approach too simplistic. An alternative view of human life is a *cyclic* one, which views life as a series of cycles through which all living beings evolve. Cycles may be repeated at different points in the life span. Some cultures believe in reincarnation and constant evolution of life forms. In Western society, there may be times when a person's sense of identity changes. For example, the young child's primary source of identity may come from the same-sex parent. The adolescent redefines identity separate from the family of origin. An adult may alter his or her sense of identity if a major career change is made in midlife.

There is value in various views of human development. Theories provide a way of organizing complex human developmental factors into smaller, more understandable units. Theories are developed for convenience but they do not necessarily reflect objective reality. They provide ways to understand human behavior but are not rigid, inflexible rules. In nursing practice, clinicians incorporate many aspects of different theories into their day-to-day work and may work with clients who have diverse points of view. Respect for alternative world views and theories different from your own is important.

Development was defined by Bronfenbrenner (1989) as "a set of processes through which properties of the person and the environment interact to produce constancy and change in the characteristics of the person over the life span."[3]

Development affects growth patterns in all domains: physical, cognitive, and psychosocial. *Physical maturation* refers to development related to genetic factors (heredity) and resulting in biologic growth processes such as height, weight, and brain size. The term *maturation* is often used interchangeably with *development.* The acquisition of knowledge, values, and specific skilled behaviors through formal and informal channels such as experience, trial and error, or direct training is called *learning.* Developmental changes throughout life enable human beings to function at increasing levels of complexity. Development never ends. **Growth** refers primarily to physical changes and results from the proliferation of cells, growth of cells, and maintenance or replacement of cells. Cell growth and proliferation occur primarily early in development, the first 15 to 18 years of life, whereas maintenance and replacement growth are daily processes that occur at a stable rate throughout life.

This chapter is divided into three sections: the physiologic principles of development, an overview of developmental theories of psychosocial growth and development, and a review of development from prenatal life up to puberty. Nurses need to understand "normal" growth and development for a number of reasons. First, nurses need to understand human behavior and identify nursing needs of people at different developmental stages. Second, normal behaviors or growth patterns should not be mistaken for disease or disorder and vice versa. For example, the elderly adult who shows signs of depression should not be assumed to be undergoing normal aging. Finally, effective nursing strategies can be applied only when nurses understand appropriate developmental needs. Stranger anxiety in the 12-month-old child is a "normal" developmental phase or stage, and nurses need to accommodate to it rather than consider it a problem.

Individual differences should be appreciated.

What is considered normal varies by historical time period, age, and culture. Even within the same time period and culture, there is considerable variation in what are considered normal rates and patterns of development.

A good example of wide variation in American culture is the proliferation of family forms. Macklin and Rubin,[20] in a book on contemporary families, present separate chapters on each of the following kinds of families: single head of household, nonmarital heterosexual cohabitation, single-parent families, voluntarily childless, divorced and remarried families, dual-career, dual-work families, commuter marriage, gay and lesbian families, open marriage/multilateral relationships, multigenerational families, and communes. In the 1990s, the "traditional" nuclear family consisting of two parents and at least two children is no longer the most common family form.

It is easier to study the processes of growth and development by focusing attention on particular human characteristics or specific functions than by considering the entire human being as an integrated being. Nevertheless, all the separate parts of the person work together in harmony. People are complex, unique individuals who are also parts of families, social groups, and societies. The number of variables that influence development is staggering. For convenience's sake, growth and development are often divided into two overlapping categories: physiologic and psychosocial (Figure 12–1).

Physiologic development includes physical size, growth patterns, bodily functioning, and states of illness and health. *Psychosocial* development includes a vari-

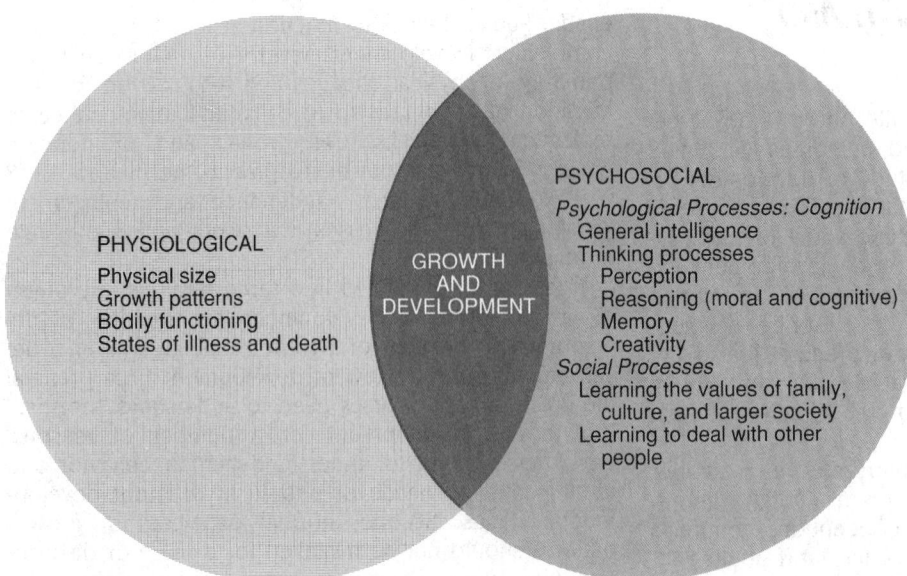

PHYSIOLOGICAL

Physical size
Growth patterns
Bodily functioning
States of illness and death

GROWTH AND DEVELOPMENT

PSYCHOSOCIAL

Psychological Processes: Cognition
General intelligence
Thinking processes
Perception
Reasoning (moral and cognitive)
Memory
Creativity
Social Processes
Learning the values of family,
  culture, and larger society
Learning to deal with other
  people

▲ *Figure 12–1*

Categories of growth and development.

ety of psychologic and social developmental processes. Psychologic development includes cognition—a complex human characteristic consisting of general intelligence as well as specific thinking processes such as perception, judgment, reasoning (moral and cognitive), memory, and creativity. Social development includes learning the values of the family, culture, and larger society and learning to deal with other people effectively.

Although discussed separately, development in both areas occurs simultaneously, and development in one area affects development in the other area. The following section describes universal principles that underlie the processes of physiologic growth and development.

MAJOR PRINCIPLES OF PHYSIOLOGIC GROWTH AND DEVELOPMENT

Major principles of physiologic growth and development are summarized in Box 12–1.

Normal Physiologic Development Proceeds in Three Directions

Normal physical growth and development proceed in three directions: cephalocaudal, proximodistal, and general to specific.

CEPHALOCAUDAL GROWTH AND DEVELOPMENT

Physiologic growth and development proceed in a cephalocaudal manner: from head to feet. For example, in the neonate, head control develops before control of the hands, and the arms develop faster than the legs.

PROXIMODISTAL GROWTH AND DEVELOPMENT

Proximal physical coordination (closer to the body's midline) matures before distal functions (farther away

from the midline). For example, babies can make sophisticated facial expressions long before they learn to control their hands.

MATURATION OF GENERAL TO SPECIFIC SKILLS

Generalized skills mature faster than specific skills, or simple functions mature before complex functions. For example, gross motor skills precede fine muscle coordination. A baby uses a palmar grasp (grasps objects with the whole hand) before using a pincer grasp (thumb and forefinger). When learning a new skill as an adult, such as tennis, we learn the general concepts and basic strokes before mastering the finer points like the serve.

Box 12–1. Major Principles of Physiologic Growth and Development

▶ Normal physiologic growth and development proceed in three directions: cephalocaudal, proximodistal, and general to specific.
▶ Physiologic growth and development usually occur in a predictable pattern, but the rate of development may vary considerably.
▶ The processes of physiologic development occur in a predictable sequence.
▶ Physiologic growth and development occur when "readiness" has been reached.
▶ Physiologic development is the result of a combination of maturational and learning factors.
▶ Each stage of physiologic development is different from the one before it.
▶ Each stage of physiologic development depends on growth in previous stages.

Physiologic Growth and Development Occur in a Predictable Pattern

Growth and development usually occur in a predictable pattern, but the rate of development may vary considerably. Times of rapid growth (spurts) alternate with times of slower growth (plateaus). The timing of growth spurts and plateaus varies somewhat for each person. Most children grow rapidly in infancy, then grow slowly until age 10 to 12 years, then have another period of rapid growth. Individual variations in rate of development are affected by differences in the genetic blueprint, the environment, and the interaction of genetics and environment. For example, one child may experience a growth spurt at the age of 10 years whereas another child does not "spurt" until age 13 years. The first child's growth spurt may last for 10 months, then plateau, while the second child may grow rapidly for 20 months before reaching a plateau.

The Processes of Physiologic Development Occur in a Predictable Sequence

The processes of development are in a predictable sequence. For example, children sit before they walk and say single words before sentences. The timing of the skill may vary because of environmental influences or genetic factors, but in general the process has a consistent sequence.

Physiologic Growth and Development Occur When "Readiness" Has Been Reached

Readiness refers to physiologic, cognitive, or emotional preparedness for some task.

Readiness implies that a critical period for learning may occur, when the child is "ready." Physical maturation is one of the determinants of readiness. A child cannot gain bladder control until the sphincters of the bladder are mature and until the child can understand the parent's instruction to urinate in a toilet. The environment is also important, and if no one teaches the child to use a toilet, the skill will not develop.

Physiologic Development Is the Result of a Combination of Maturational and Learning Factors

Development is the result of a combination of maturational and learning factors. For example, a child will not be able to walk until the physiologic maturity (control of the leg muscles, good vision, balance) is present. However, physiologic readiness alone is not sufficient. The child will not walk if kept in a crib all the time and never given the opportunity to walk. The environmental factors that influence achievement of developmental skills include opportunity to learn, culture, ethnic background, race, religion, and socioeco-

nomic class. However, the basic maturational processes remain the same regardless of the environment.

Each Stage of Physiologic Development Is Different from the One Before

Each stage of development is different from the one before or after it. Children of adolescent age differ from infants both in degree of development and in qualitative differences in their abilities. The particular characteristics of each child's intellectual, moral, or personality development differ according to developmental stage. For example, the type of logic used to solve problems differs in young children and older children and adults. The interpretation of how and why these changes occur differs in the various theories. Theories of psychosocial development are discussed later in this chapter.

Each Stage of Physiologic Development Depends on Growth in Previous Stages

Each stage of development depends on growth in previous stages. The major tasks of one stage must be at least partially achieved before the individual can go on to the next stage or sequence of developmental tasks.

PHYSIOLOGIC SYSTEMS THAT REGULATE GROWTH AND DEVELOPMENT

Human growth and development are guided by physiologic "blueprints" that affect all aspects of human life. The major systems that regulate growth and development are genetics, the nervous system, and the endocrine system. Of course, all these systems are overlapping and function simultaneously.

Regulation of Growth and Development by Genetic Inheritance

All the cells in the human body contain 46 chromosomes, in 23 pairs. The first 22 are the *autosomes* and the last pair are the sex *chromosomes* (XX for females and XY for males). Each chromosome carries several thousand genes, consisting of coiled DNA strands that code genetic information. Although all the cells in the body have the same chromosomes, only the germ cells (reproductive cells: sperm in males and eggs, or ova, in females) are involved in reproduction. When egg and sperm cells are produced, the chromosome complement is split in half so that the cell contains only 23 chromosomes. In this way, offspring receive half their genes from their mother and half from their father.

The genetic code serves as the physiologic blueprint for future growth and development and allows learning to occur. The genetic code sets parameters for physical and cognitive development, but the environment can influence the actual attainment of physical skills and learning.

For example, a child may be born with a genetic potential for high intelligence. However, if raised in an environment with improper nutrition and a lack of stimulation, the IQ may reach only the average range. Some human traits that are known to have a strong genetic component include height, weight, intelligence, temperament, and some psychologic disorders (such as alcoholism and depression).

Regulation of Growth and Development by the Nervous System

The nervous system regulates all body functions. The central nervous system consists of the brain and spinal cord and is the "higher" control center. The peripheral nervous system, consisting of the nerves to and from the internal organs, skin, muscles, and glands, is the operating system. If the nervous system is compromised in any way, "normal" growth and development are much more difficult to achieve. Children who have sustained some nervous system injury before or during birth (often diagnosed as cerebral palsy or CP) often have a much slower course of development. However, they achieve motor milestones in the same sequence as other children—they sit before standing and stand before walking, and so on. The nervous system is immature at birth and develops slowly over the course of childhood and adolescence. Maturation of the nervous system is necessary for higher levels of cognitive development to occur.

Regulation of Growth and Development by the Endocrine System

A variety of glands secrete chemical substances called hormones into body tissues or the bloodstream and make up the endocrine system. The function of hormones is to control the activities of certain organs and body tissues by turning certain receptor cells off and on. The major endocrine glands that affect growth and development are highlighted in Figure 12–2. The *pituitary* controls the activity of other endocrine glands and regulates the basal metabolic rate. The *parathyroids* regulate calcium and phosphorus and the normal excitability of the nervous system. The *adrenals* maintain salt and water balance and create physical responses to emotional stimuli. The islets of Langerhans of the *pancreas* regulate blood sugar levels. The *thyroid* influences physical growth and maintains an appropriate energy level. The *gonads* (*ovaries* and *testes*) influence sexual development and functioning and reproduction.

The endocrine glands can have a major influence on growth and development. For example, if the islets of Langerhans of the pancreas do not produce insulin, an individual cannot adequately break down glucose into the energy source needed to "feed" the body. As a result, growth is inhibited. Some of the hormones secreted by the endocrine glands influence emotional responses. The adrenal glands underlie the fight-or-flight response to extreme stress. If female sex hormones are lacking, a girl may not experience puberty. One of the sex hormones, testosterone, has been linked to aggressive behavior in some studies.

The aforementioned concepts are primarily physiologic in nature, and normally we do not have conscious control over them. Some factors are the result of the interaction between physiologic processes and the environment, over which we have some control. These are called "interactional" factors.

INTERACTIONAL FACTORS THAT INFLUENCE DEVELOPMENT

Some of the other factors that affect an individual's development and are dependent on both physical and psychosocial factors are adaptation, motivation, learning, socialization, and individual differences.

Adaptation

The body has many methods of adapting to its immediate environment. Some of these adaptation processes are purely physiologic, such as producing antibodies to fight off a bacterial infection, or sweating when the body temperature becomes too high. Physiologic processes of adaptation are sometimes called *homeostatic*. Other adaptation methods are cognitive, such as the infant using the sucking reflex to explore the environment; or psychosocial, such as developing a sense of trust in an environment in which needs are met promptly. Adaptation ensures survival.

Motivation

Motivation is a force or a process that initiates or explains behavior. Behaviors can be motivated by physical or psychosocial factors singly or in combination. Behaviors are initiated to satisfy needs or correct deficiencies. Theories of development vary widely in their ideas about what motivates human behavior. Some theories, such as Freud's, suggest that there are internal life energies that motivate behavior. Others, such as Skinner's, suggest that behavior is often motivated by "rewards" in the environment. Some motivations, such as the hunger drive, are purely physiologic in infancy, but through developmental processes and learning come to be influenced by the environment. The adult eats for many reasons other than just hunger. Most physiologic drives or motivations come to be influenced by the environment to some extent.

Learning and Socialization

Infants are born with a repertoire of reflexes, such as sucking and sneezing, that ensure survival. Very early,

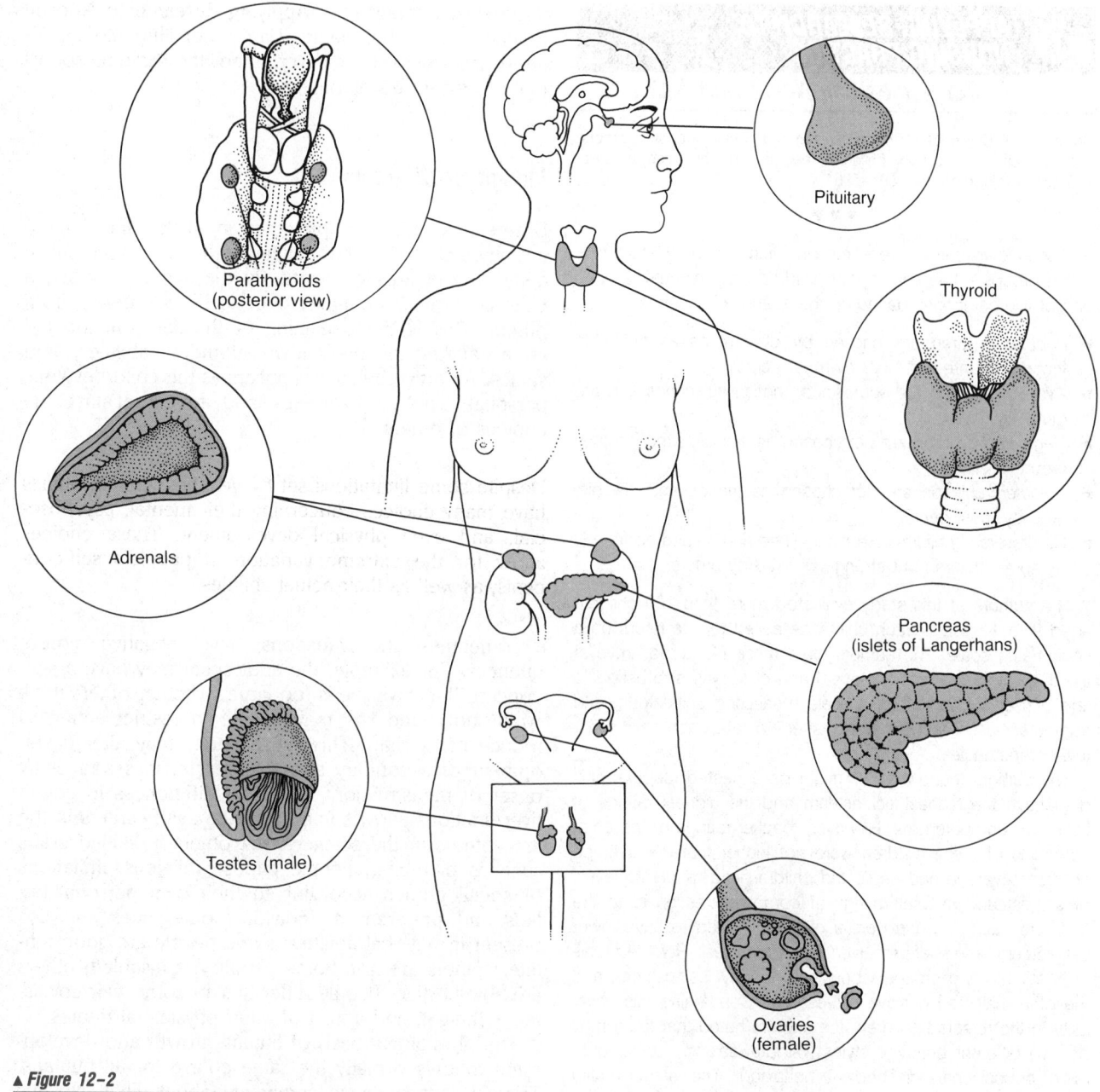

▲ **Figure 12-2**

The major endocrine glands that affect growth and development.

the infant learns increasingly complex behaviors that take the place of most reflexes in the survival of the organism. Some reflexes, such as the eyeblink, continue through the life span, but reflexes alone cannot protect people in a hostile environment.

Learning is a complex process by which people gain knowledge and skills. Learning occurs in a number of ways: from direct experience with the environment, by a system of rewards and punishments, and/or by observing and imitating others.

Socialization is a particular form of learning by which individuals learn the rules, attitudes, and norms of the social group in which they live (society). Socialization is regulated by positive and negative feedback

from significant others in the society. The most important social groups involved in socialization vary somewhat according to the child's age. For the infant and young child, the primary social group is the family (the basic caretaking unit). For older children and adolescents, peers (others of approximately the same age and socioeconomic class) become a major source of socialization. Children are also influenced by racial, ethnic, and religious subcultures. Adults are regulated more directly by society as a whole, through powerful institutions such as education, the legal system, and religious or other spiritual organizations; socioeconomic status; the military; and leisure activities (country clubs, collegiate sports, and so on). Socialization promotes acceptance within the social group. The person who is ignored or rejected by the social group may have al-

Boivin, M., & Begin, G. (1989). Peer status and self-perception among early elementary school children: the case of the rejected child. *Child Development, 60,* 591–596.

APPLYING RESEARCH TO NURSING PRACTICE
···But Names Can Never Hurt Me?

▼ ▼ ▼

Sociometric research—research on interpersonal relationships within groups—has shown that children can be classified into one of five categories based on the attitudes of their peers:

▶ *Popular* children are chosen by classmates as desirable friends and are well liked by most peers.
▶ *Average* children are sometimes chosen as friends and are generally liked.
▶ *Neglected* children are not chosen as friends, although they are not disliked.
▶ *Rejected* children are not chosen as friends and are disliked by most peers.
▶ *Controversial* children are highly liked and valued as friends by some children but strongly disliked by others.

The authors of this study evaluated more than 200 children aged 9 to 11 years. Each child was asked to rate peers on a sociometric scale. The authors used these ratings to arrive at the five categories listed above. Each child was also asked to rate himself or herself on a scale measuring self-esteem and competencies. Teachers were asked to rate each child's actual competencies.

The authors found that, as might be expected, *popular* children have the highest self-esteem and the highest ratings of their own competencies. However, teacher ratings of the competencies of these children were not higher than for *average* children. *Average* and *neglected* children had moderate levels of self-esteem and self-ratings of competencies equal to the teachers' ratings. *Controversial* children tended to have lower self-esteem and self-perceived competencies. *Rejected* children fell into two groups: about half had low self-esteem, and the other half had positive self-esteem. Concerning this variability in the rejected children, the authors noted that there may be two different behavior styles: withdrawal and "acting out" (silly, oppositional, disobedient behavior). The authors also noted that some rejected children may have had positive experiences outside the classroom that maintained their self-esteem and their sense of competency.

Applications to Practice

Social status among peers appears to be related to self-esteem, although the relationship is not always in the direction expected. Variables unrelated to peers seem to be influential. These variables may include family support, religious or other institutional support, and cultural values and beliefs.

Rather than viewing children isolated from their social contexts, nurses need to consider the peer status of child clients. Peer status may be observed directly on a nursing unit or assessed via interviews with child and parent(s). Children who are neglected or rejected may be at risk for later stress-related disorders.

tered development (see Applying Research to Nursing Practice: ". . . But Names Can Never Hurt Me?"). Altered development, however, is not the same as abnormal or deviant development.

Individual Differences

Differences among people occur in all domains, including physical growth and abilities, self-concept, cognitive abilities, and artistic talents. By the age of 2 years, a child achieves a strong sense of "self" as different from others. This is the beginning of the self-concept, the understanding of one's own attitudes, abilities, and values. Assertive behavior appears as the child develops personal likes and dislikes and rebels against the choices of others.

Despite some limitations set by genetics, human beings have many choices concerning their mental, psychosocial, and even physical development. These choices allow for the extreme variation in people's self-concepts, as well as their actual abilities.

Sometimes the variations have negative consequences. For example, the adolescent may have a self-concept that says she is too large (whether others think so or not), and she may decide to restrict eating to reduce her weight. This subsequently may alter development of secondary sexual characteristics and delay onset of menstruation. Individual differences in cognitive functions allow some people to seek careers in the arts, others in the sciences, yet others in skilled crafts such as plumbing. People choose religious affiliations or social groups according to their own personal beliefs and preferences. Individual differences are also present in physical abilities: some people are good athletes; others are not. Some people are disabled; others are able-bodied. People differ in skin color, hair consistency, height, and a host of other physical attributes.

The physiologic basis of human growth and development follows virtually the same course for all humans. There is not as much agreement about what explains psychosocial development. Some of the best-known theories are described next.

PSYCHOSOCIAL THEORIES OF HUMAN DEVELOPMENT

Many theories attempt to explain human behavioral development. No single theory can explain all aspects of human development. Many of these theories have been criticized for their emphasis on white, middle-class, male individuals. The theories presented here have all made valuable contributions to the study of human development, even though they all have limitations. The theories are grouped into three categories: psychodynamic, cognitive, and behavioral.

Contributors to Psychodynamic Theories

Psychodynamic theories recognize the presence of different levels of awareness: conscious, subconscious, and unconscious. **Conscious** awareness involves feelings and thoughts of which a person is aware. The **subconscious** includes thoughts and feelings that the person is not aware of at the moment, but that can be brought to awareness easily. Finally, the **unconscious** contains thoughts and feelings that are unavailable to awareness, such as those that are repressed. In these theories, the person is primarily a passive being to whom psychic events "happen." Two of the best-known psychodynamic theorists, Freud and Erikson, have suggested explicit stages of human development.

FREUD

Sigmund Freud has been called the father of modern psychiatry because of his efforts to study the processes of the mind, or psyche. He developed the process of *psychoanalysis,* a set of techniques such as word associations, dream analysis, and hypnosis that attempt to identify unconscious thoughts and feelings by examining dreams, slips of the tongue, and childhood memories. From the information gathered on many people that Freud saw in therapy over the course of several years, he developed a theory of psychosexual development.

Individuals Are Motivated by the Basic Instincts of Eros and Destruction. In Freud's **psychosexual theory,** individuals are motivated by two basic instincts: Eros (sex, love, self-preservation, unity with others) and destruction (aggression, hate, death). The force or energy of Eros is called the **libido,** which has often been associated with a sex drive. However, it can be broadly defined as the motivating force of all positive behavior. Freud thought that the accumulation of libido is uncomfortable and that people strive to release this energy (experience catharsis).

Id, Superego, and Ego. According to Freud, three structures make up the human personality: the *id,* the *superego,* and the *ego.* Freud described the id as "the dark, inaccessible part of our personality . . . a chaos, a cauldron full of seething excitations."[9] The **id** is most influential in the earliest developmental stages of childhood and is manifest through thoughts, desires, and sensations. The id is governed by the pleasure principle, the drive to obtain pleasure and avoid pain.

The **ego** operates according to the reality principle and develops when the id cannot always be satisfied. The ego ensures survival. It negotiates among the demands of the id for pleasure, the superego's moralistic judgments, and the realities of the situation. It allows the individual to make decisions.

The **superego** is the last to develop and is the conscience, the moral dimension of the personality. Experiences and interactions with the environment allow the child to learn right from wrong. Authority figures, such as parents and teachers, are important conveyors of moral information. The entire process of socialization highly influences superego development.

Defense Mechanisms. Another important aspect of Freud's theory is the concept of *defense mechanisms.*

Freud thought that people need to protect their fragile egos by distorting reality. Common defense mechanisms include *regression,* or returning to a behavior pattern common to an earlier stage of development; *repression,* or blocking anxiety-producing memories from the conscious mind; *projection,* attributing one's own negative thoughts or feelings to another; and *sublimation,* or channeling socially undesirable impulses into acceptable activities.

Defense mechanisms are not necessarily bad or indicative of personality problems unless they are used to extreme. See Chapter 16 for more on defense mechanisms.

Freud's Five Stages of Development. Freud proposed five stages of development: (1) oral stage, (2) anal stage, (3) phallic stage, (4) latency stage, and (5) genital stage. He thought the first few years of life were the most crucial for personality development, and that development essentially ended with the onset of young adulthood. Freud suggested that excessive energy-tensions are focused on certain areas of the body in different stages of childhood (Table 12–1). If the child fails to resolve the crisis of the current stage, the personality becomes *fixated* (immobilized) at that stage, and problems may be reflected in adult personality styles.

Although other theories have tended to supplant much of Freud's developmental theory, it still has historical value and provides an alternative view of human development as a complex, intrapsychic process. Of particular value were Freud's ideas about the unconscious and the defense mechanisms.

ERIKSON

Erik Erikson adapted some of Freud's ideas into a theory that is more *psychosocial* than *psychosexual.* Erikson focused on the ego, the structure of the personality that protects the individual and is reality based. According to Erikson, physical maturation opens up new psychologic possibilities for the child and greater social demands. The ego tries to meet these new demands of the body and the environment.

Erikson's theory describes eight stages that span infancy to late adulthood. He viewed each individual to be in a life cycle in a "community of life cycles"— meaning that the child is surrounded by significant others who are also passing through life cycles. Each stage has a major crisis. The crisis can be resolved to some degree, or not resolved. If the crisis is resolved in a positive manner, the individual is ready to deal with the next crisis and healthy development occurs. Each stage builds somewhat on the stage(s) before, so success at one stage influences the degree of success

TABLE 12–1. Summary of Freud's Theory of Psychosexual Development

Stage	Age Range	Energy Focus	Selected Characteristics
ORAL	Birth to 18 months	Mouth	▶ Needs must be met quickly ▶ Governed by id, pleasure principle ▶ Fixation can lead to eating disorders, alcohol/drug addiction, smoking, self-centeredness, dependency, unrealistic optimism
ANAL	18 months to 3 years	Anus, rectum	▶ Learning to control bowel and bladder ▶ Ego begins to develop ▶ Fixation can lead to stinginess, hoarding, overcleanliness, explosive personality, or stubbornness
PHALLIC	3 to 5 years	Genitalia	▶ Boys: Oedipus complex (attraction to mother, father seen as rival), castration anxiety ▶ Girls: Electra complex (attraction to father, mother as rival), penis envy ▶ Resolution leads to identification with same-sex parent ▶ Fixation can lead to problems with sexual identity or to seeking a mate who is a parent figure
LATENCY	6 to 12 years	Intellectual and play activities	▶ Sexual feelings are repressed ▶ Calmest period of childhood ▶ Fixation can lead to a constricted, narrow world view, difficulty identifying with peers, and lack of social skills
GENITAL	13 years to adulthood	Genitalia	▶ Separates from family and transfers sexual attraction to nonfamily member of opposite sex ▶ Fixation can lead to an inability to form intimate relationships or lack of strong sense of personal identity

likely at subsequent stages. However, Erikson believed that it is never too late to resolve any of the crises. Table 12–2 outlines Erikson's eight stages of development.

HAVIGHURST

Robert Havighurst proposed a series of developmental tasks that people of different ages must achieve in order to have happy and satisfying lives. The tasks progress from simple, basic requirements of infants, such as learning to eat solid foods, to the more com-

plex tasks of adults, such as selecting a mate. Havighurst's stages cover the entire life span. They are more descriptive than explanatory. Havighurst's developmental tasks for people of different ages are listed in Table 12–3.

Contributors to Cognitive Theories

Cognitive theories are concerned primarily with the development of thinking and reasoning skills and are less concerned with personality/emotional development. In

TABLE 12–2. Summary of Erikson's Theory of Psychosocial Development

Approximate Age	Stage of Development	Crisis	Successful Resolution of Crisis
Birth to 18 months	Infancy	Trust vs. Mistrust	Ability to trust others and a sense of one's own trustworthiness; a sense of hope
18 months to 3 years	Early childhood	Autonomy vs. Shame and doubt	Self-control without loss of self-esteem; ability to cooperate and to express one's needs
3 to 5 years	Late childhood	Initiative vs. Guilt	Realistic sense of self; ability to evaluate one's own behavior
6 to 12 years	School age	Industry vs. Inferiority	Feelings of competence, self-esteem
12 to 20 years	Adolescence	Identity vs. Role diffusion	Clear sense of self and direction of one's own life; plans for the future
18 to 25 years	Young adulthood	Intimacy vs. Isolation	Capacity to make commitments to work and relationships
25 to 65 years	Adulthood	Generativity vs. Stagnation	Creativity; productivity; ability to guide the next generation
65 years to death	Old age	Integrity vs. Despair	Acceptance of the accomplishments of one's life

TABLE 12–3. Summary of Havighurst's Developmental Tasks

Developmental Stage	Major Achievements
Infancy and Early Childhood	Walking, talking, eating independently
	Appropriate elimination patterns
	Learning gender role expectations
	Relating to others appropriately
Middle Childhood	Physical skills for recreation and activities of daily living
	Positive self-concept
	Relating to peers
	Developing sense of morals, values
	Achieving academic skills
Adolescence	Increased problem-solving abilities
	Mature peer relationships
	Higher level of morals/values
	Adapting to bodily changes
	Preparing for adult roles in career and family
	Achieving independence from parents
Young Adulthood	Assuming family roles
	Managing home and career
	Assuming civic responsibilities
	Acquiring social networks
Middle Adulthood	Maturation of family roles; children leave home, aging parents
	Maintaining career; civic, economic responsibilities
	Adjusting to changes of aging
Older Adulthood	Adjusting to physical and mental changes of aging
	Adjusting to changing social roles such as retirement, loss of spouse and friends
	Possible changes in living arrangements

these theories, the person is an active agent seeking out new experiences in his or her environment. Piaget is the most famous of the cognitive theorists. Kohlberg also offers a cognitively oriented stage theory that focuses on moral development.

PIAGET

Jean Piaget's theory of cognitive (intellectual) development is based on the observation that children's behavior and thought processes are qualitatively different at different ages.

Cognitive development is motivated by the process of *adaptation* or learning strategies to cope with changes in the environment.

Schemata. *Schemata* (singular is schema) are basic cognitive units organized into categories that make sense of the world. For example, the infant may categorize objects as pleasant to suck and unpleasant to suck. Preschool-age children can divide animals into discrete categories such as cats, dogs, and fish. Older children further refine the categories to include differ-

ent kinds of cats and fish. Schemata are developed and refined by the processes of assimilation and accommodation.

Assimilation. *Assimilation* is the process of incorporating new information into an existing schema without needing to alter the schema. For example, the infant learns that throwing a rattle while sitting in a car seat has the same result as throwing the rattle from a highchair.

Accommodation. *Accommodation* is the process of changing an existing schema to match the demands of the environment. Now the infant must adjust arm movements in order to throw the rattle out of the crib. The simultaneous processes of assimilation and accommodation allow adaptation to take place.

Intelligence is a form of adaptation in which, with experience, higher levels of thinking and problem-solving abilities are achieved. In infants, schemata are mostly physical sensations, based on reflex behaviors (such as sucking), but these "primitive" schemata are refined and come to include cognitive concepts. Intelligence grows from the use of primitive strategies to the use of differing levels of logical reasoning. Young children use a less efficient form of logic, referred to as transductive (they generalize from one specific fact to another). Older children use inductive or deductive logic, a more "scientific" way of thinking.

Piaget's Four Stages of Cognitive Development. Piaget described four stages of cognitive development: (1) sensorimotor, (2) preoperational, (3) concrete operational, and (4) formal operational thought. Each stage has unique characteristics. A stage both derives from and transforms previous stages so that no regression is possible. Piaget suggested that the stages are universal (occur in all cultures) and invariant (must proceed in the order he specified). Piaget's theory spans only the years from birth to adolescence. Table 12–4 describes these stages in detail.

KOHLBERG

Piaget offered a framework for how children learn rules. Lawrence Kohlberg extended Piaget's theory to the development of moral reasoning.

Development of Moral Reasoning. Moral development refers to a pattern of beliefs and values about what constitutes appropriate human behavior. Moral thinking includes rules about how one should behave. The rules are specific to a given culture and are taught, formally and informally, by the process of socialization. Kohlberg believed that a child is born *amoral*, without a sense of right or wrong, but with the cognitive structures needed to learn moral reasoning. Moral behavior develops in a series of stages. It is influenced by cognitive development and by interaction with significant others and cultural institutions such as schools, religion, and the media. Kohlberg outlined three levels of moral development: preconventional, conventional, and post-

TABLE 12-4. Summary of Piaget's Stages of Cognitive Development

Stage	Approximate Ages	Method of Learning	Major Accomplishments/Limitations
Sensorimotor	0 to 24 months	Exploring the environment using the senses: touch, taste, smell, hearing, seeing	Starts with reflexes, which gradually become purposeful movements Learns to separate self from environment Delayed imitation Object permanence—things continue to exist even when out of sight Beginning of verbal language
Preoperational	2 to 7 years	Trial and error	Symbolic play—understanding that objects can stand for other objects, ideas Egocentric—unable to take another person's viewpoint Cannot sort objects by more than one characteristic Cannot conserve (understand that things remain the same even if their material is rearranged) Transductive reasoning—from one specific fact to another specific fact
Concrete operations	7 to 11 years	Concrete experiments	Operations—manipulation of objects or their internal representations Concrete—here and now Addivity—can add things together Reversibility—can subtract Decentration—can focus on more than one aspect of a problem Conservation—not fooled by rearrangement of matter Recognizes importance of rules
Formal operations	12 to 18 years	Systematic, logical reasoning	Capable of abstract thought Uses hypothetical-deductive reasoning Can generate many possible solutions to a given problem

TABLE 12-5. Summary of Kohlberg's Theory of Psychosocial Development

Level and Stage	Defining Right and Wrong	Typical Behaviors
Level I. Preconventional		
Stage 1 Punishment and obedience orientation	Do not do anything for which you might be punished.	Avoids punishment
Stage 2 Concern with satisfying own needs	Doing the right thing means getting something out of it. It is also when there is an equal exchange so that both parties gain.	If you don't get caught, it's OK
Level II. Conventional		
Stage 3 "Good boy, good girl" orientation	"Being good" is the goal for moral behavior.	Tries to live up to expectations of significant others
Stage 4 The law-and-order orientation	The law, the rules, are right.	Follows rules in rigid manner
Level III. Postconventional		
Stage 5 The social contract	Moral behavior results in the greatest amount of good for the greatest number of people in the society.	Follows rules, but only when they lead to greatest good for society
Stage 6 The universal "good"	Universal principles that transcend even the rules of a given society. The individual is obligated to live by these principles, which include justice and equality of human rights.	True to personal sense of justice and universal human rights

conventional. Each level contains two stages that are universal and invariant in sequence. Table 12–5 lists the main characteristics of each level and stage.

Challenge to Kohlberg's Theory. Kohlberg's theory (and by extension, those of Freud and some of the moral philosophers) has been challenged recently on a number of points. For example, some argue that Kohlberg's stages may not be universal and that there may be major cultural differences in moral reasoning. The achievement of Kohlberg's highest level of development seems to be associated with higher education and living in a complex, technologic society. Even in the United States, only about 20 per cent of adults achieve postconventional reasoning. Another problem is the lack of direct correspondence between moral reasoning on a test and actual moral behavior.

Finally, Gilligan noted that Kohlberg's original research included only male subjects.[12,13] Later, when Kohlberg used his method with women, he suggested that women often had "inferior" moral development. Gilligan and others have found that many women follow a different course of moral development because of the strong gender-role socialization present in our society. Because of the role women are socialized to take in nurturing and caring for others, women grow up to value relationships more than individual achievements. This line of research has enhanced our thinking about moral reasoning by considering the possibility that there may be alternative but equally valid ways of reasoning in persons in our diverse culture.

Contributors to Behavioral Theories

Behavioral theories promote the environmental view of learning: that individuals acquire knowledge through their senses and are influenced by rewards or punishments. There are no identifiable stages of development. Instead, children steadily increase the amount of knowledge and skills that they possess. The three major classes of behavioral theories are classical conditioning associated with Pavlov, operant conditioning associated with Skinner, and social learning theory associated with Bandura.

PAVLOV

The Russian physiologist Ivan Pavlov first described a behavior pattern he observed in his research on the digestive system of dogs. In a number of experiments, he put food in the mouths of dogs, which resulted in a reflex behavior of salivation. After several trials, his mere presence in the room caused the dogs to salivate. He discovered that by pairing an event that causes a reflexive response with a second event that does not cause the reflex, like the sound of a bell, subjects could be "conditioned" to respond to the second event. Classical conditioning has been shown to be associated with many fears and phobias. The most famous example was John Watson's experiment with a young child named Albert. The child, who previously played with a rabbit without fear, became "conditioned" to fear the rabbit after only a few trials of pairing presentation of the rabbit with a loud noise.

SKINNER

B.F. Skinner described a different type of conditioning. The main principle of operant conditioning is that behavior that is rewarded will be repeated. The converse is also true; behavior that is not rewarded will not be repeated. Figure 12–3 shows the different forms of reinforcement proposed by Skinner. A **reinforcer** is an event that follows a behavior and increases the likelihood that the behavior will be repeated. Reinforcers can be positive, such as administering money, stickers, or praise, or they can be negative, such as removing an unpleasant event. An example of negative reinforcement might be to allow the child to stop washing dishes every evening as a reward for washing the family car once a week.

Response cost refers to removing a pleasant reinforcement, such as taking away television privileges. A **punishment** is an aversive event that follows a behavior and decreases the likelihood that the behavior will be repeated. Punishment has many undesirable side effects; it does not tell the child what is appropriate behavior, only what not to do. Sometimes punishment elicits resentment and an urge to get revenge. And it may elicit fear. Punishment can include a frown, a harsh word, or physical pain or discomfort. If punishment is used, it should immediately follow the undesirable behavior and be done in an unemotional manner. Skinner noted that the most effective means of eliminating undesirable behavior is by **extinction,** or stopping a reinforcement (ignoring).

Principles of operant conditioning have been used to shape or change people's behavior. Using principles of operant conditioning to change behavior is called *behavior modification.*

BANDURA

Albert Bandura extended Skinner's theory to suggest that children can learn by observing other people being rewarded or punished. In other words, learning did not have to be direct but could be vicarious. Children

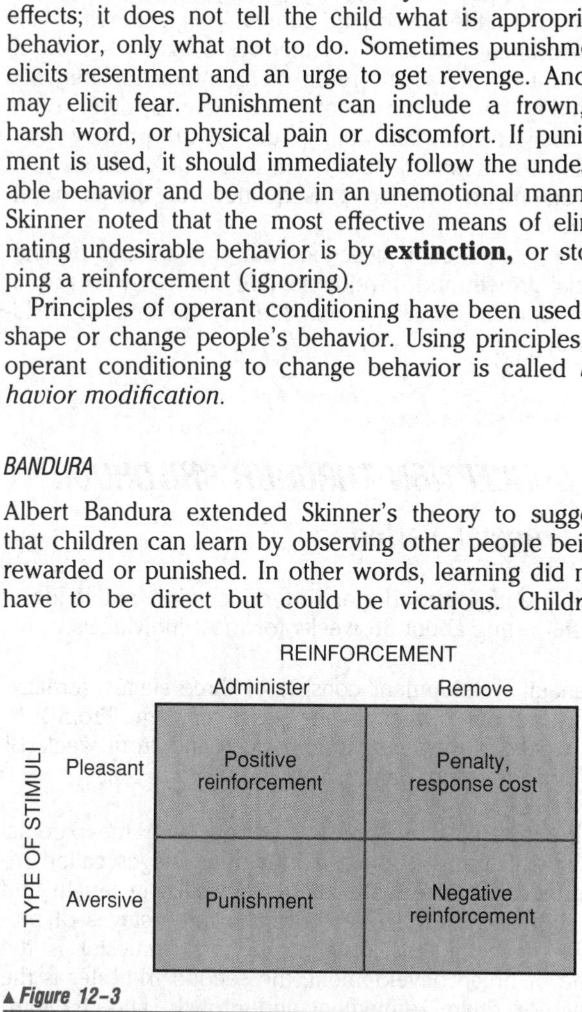

| | REINFORCEMENT | |
	Administer	Remove
Pleasant	Positive reinforcement	Penalty, response cost
Aversive	Punishment	Negative reinforcement

(TYPE OF STIMULI)

▲ *Figure 12–3*

Types of reinforcement in operant conditioning proposed by Skinner.

observe others—parents, teachers, peers, media characters—and actively decide who to imitate.

Social learning theory recognizes the influence of cognitive factors on behavior because children selectively imitate some behaviors of some people and then evaluate the effects of their own behavior.

Social learning theory also differs from other behavioral models by suggesting that the child is an active agent in the environment rather than a passive recipient of rewards or punishments.

Summary of Psychosocial Theories of Human Development

Although the foregoing theories of psychosocial development are quite varied, they share some common features. First, development occurs in an orderly sequence. The lower level (simpler) tasks must be achieved before higher level (complex) tasks are possible. Tasks build upon each other. Failure at any task potentially produces problems or delays in learning or development. Second, human beings have a basic motivation to grow and develop, whether the motivation is internal to the person or comes from rewards in the environment. Most of the theories suggest that development occurs as the result of an interaction between heredity and environment. The theories differ on a number of important points, such as the primary motivation for human behavior, the major tasks or crises of development, and the consequences of altered development.

The next section describes the physical and psychosocial growth and development of children who vary in development from prenatal life to the end of childhood.

▼ CONCEPTION THROUGH CHILDHOOD

▼ Prenatal Period

The prenatal period starts at conception and ends at birth, lasting about 38 weeks for most individuals.

Prenatal development consists of three stages; fertilization to about 2 weeks is the *germinal* stage. From 2 to 12 weeks is the *embryonic* period, and from week 12 to birth, the *fetal* period.

Pregnancy is the prenatal period from the parents' perspective and is divided into three stages called trimesters. Trimesters are about 12 weeks in length and do not correspond directly to the three stages of prenatal development. Roughly, the first trimester is the time of organ development, the second trimester is the time for organ refinement and growth, and the third trimester involves primarily growth of the central nervous system and deposit of body fat.

CONCEPTION

Conception, or fertilization, is the process by which an ovum from a female and a spermatozoon from a male fuse to produce a single-celled organism that consists of 23 chromosomes from the mother and 23 from the father. The single-celled zygote duplicates itself by cell division (mitosis) as it travels down the fallopian tubes, where most fertilizations take place. The zygote takes 3 to 4 days to reach the uterus and another day or two to implant in the wall of the uterus. A human infant, the umbilical cord, fetal membranes, amniotic fluid, and the fetal side of the placenta all develop from the zygote. These parts are known as the **conceptus** (products of conception). The developing infant is connected to the placenta by the umbilical cord, which contains two arteries and one vein. The **placenta** is the vital link between the mother's system and the unborn child. It delivers oxygen and nourishment to the fetus and removes waste products. The placenta also offers some protection to the fetus from infections by filtering out large molecules such as bacteria. The *fetal membranes* surround the developing infant and create the amniotic sac, a fluid-filled chamber that protects the baby and allows movement.

The dating of a pregnancy is an imprecise estimate of the expected date of birth of the baby (or babies). **Nägele's rule** is the most common method. Take the first day of the last menstrual period (LMP), subtract 3 months, and then add 7 days. However, if the woman's cycle is irregular or if she was using oral contraceptives, Nägele's rule may not provide a very accurate prediction of the date of the birth. Later in the pregnancy, a more accurate estimate may be obtained using ultrasound.

Accommodating a new life requires enormous adaptations in the mother's physical and emotional responses. Pregnancy is considered a major change in a woman's life: she must stop considering herself as a childless woman and start considering herself as a mother. The 1980s saw an explosion of new reproductive technologies. Previously, conception occurred as a result of sexual intercourse between a woman and a man. Now there are many options for reproduction, including artificial insemination (husband or donor insemination), extrauterine conception, and surrogate motherhood. These changes in reproduction are altering our views of motherhood in many ways.

GERMINAL STAGE OF DEVELOPMENT

In the first 2 weeks of development, the rapidly dividing ball of cells is called a zygote. Once implanted in the wall of the uterus, cells cluster on one side of the zygote to form the embryonic disk from which the baby will develop. The disk quickly differentiates into two layers; the endoderm forms internal organs and the ectoderm forms the skin, hair, sensory organs, and the nervous system. Later, a middle layer appears, which forms the inner layer of skin, muscles, the circulatory system, and skeleton.

EMBRYONIC STAGE OF DEVELOPMENT

During the second stage, the implanted zygote matures into an embryo. The germinal and embryonic periods are very crucial times for physical development, and the zygote/embryo is vulnerable to many types of risk factors. Spontaneous abortion (or miscarriage) occurs in 30 to 50 per cent of all pregnancies, most often in the first 12 weeks. The causes of the miscarriage may include chromosome abnormalities, defective sperm or egg, abnormalities of the placenta or umbilical cord, or major birth defects. Many women are unaware of the pregnancy for the first few weeks of development, a time when developing organs are very susceptible to *teratogens* (any chemical or physical factor that may adversely affect an embryo or fetus). Some of the environmental influences known to affect prenatal development adversely are listed in Box 12-2. Many embryos do not survive the embryonic period.

FETAL STAGE OF DEVELOPMENT

The developing being is called a fetus from 12 weeks until birth. The fetal period is a time of rapid growth and development. All the body parts are formed but continue to grow. The fetus starts to move in utero at about 8 weeks, but often the movements cannot be felt by the mother until 17 to 20 weeks. The time when the mother can feel movements is referred to as *quickening*. About one in ten fetuses will survive if born at 28 weeks. The survival rate improves to one in three if the fetus is born at 32 weeks. The ability to survive outside the uterus is called *viability*.

Box 12-2. Some Environmental Influences on Prenatal Development

Maternal Illnesses	**Prescription Medications**
Rubella	Phenytoin (Dilantin)
Toxoplasmosis	Retinoic acid (Tretinoin)
Diabetes	Warfarin sodium (Coumadin)
Seizure disorders	

Legal Substances	**Maternal Injury**
Nicotine	Battery
Alcohol	Accidents

Ilicit Substances	**Poor Nutrition**
Cocaine	Undernutrition
Heroin	Poorly balanced diet
Marijuana	

MAJOR HEALTH CONCERNS

The prenatal period is a very hazardous time that many fetuses do not survive. The major causes of miscarriage and stillbirth are chromosome disorders and congenital birth defects.

Some of the birth defects are caused by exposure to environmental agents that are toxic to the embryo or fetus (see Box 12-2). During the embryonic period, the major effects of teratogens are on the developing organ systems and thus result in physical birth defects. During the fetal period, the most common teratogenic effects are on growth and brain development.

Recently, the media have focused much attention on the problems of prenatal drug exposures. Since 1973, we have known that alcohol use during pregnancy is related to significant birth defects. These birth defects include a pattern of growth deficiency (height, weight, and head circumference), a characteristic facial appearance, central nervous system dysfunctions such as lowered intelligence, hyperactivity, or learning disabilities, and the presence of other major or minor birth defects.[1] Nicotine exposure is related to lowered birth weight and probably to attention deficit disorder in childhood.[18] Cocaine exposure during pregnancy does not appear to cause such a striking pattern of physical problems as alcohol does. Instead, the most dramatic effects are on newborn states of arousal. The cocaine-exposed baby is often irritable, unable to tolerate stimulation in the environment, and may cry unconsolably.[4] Little is known yet about the long-term effects of cocaine on infant and child development. Other drugs such as heroin and marijuana can also adversely affect development, and all drugs (including alcohol and nicotine) are associated with a higher risk for miscarriage and stillbirth.

In addition to avoiding known teratogens, a pregnant woman should also do positive things for herself and her baby, such as maintaining a healthy diet, engaging in moderate exercise, avoiding stress, and relaxing. Prenatal care has been associated with a better outcome for all women and children, but particularly for those from disadvantaged circumstances.[25] Healthy mothers have a greater chance of having healthy babies. However, even under the best circumstances, about 3 per cent of infants are born with some kind of birth defect.

ROLE OF THE NURSE

During the prenatal period, the nurse's primary responsibility is in assessing for possible risk factors and guiding mothers to healthy lifestyles. Nurses need to take detailed family histories to identify the risk for genetic disorders and obtain environmental risk histories to identify possible teratogenic exposures. Mothers at risk need good education and may need referrals to smoking cessation clinics, prenatal clinics, substance abuse rehabilitation programs, or dietary counseling programs.

▼ Neonatal Period

The first 28 days after birth are called the *neonatal* period.

The first 24 hours after birth are the most crucial, and infant mortality is at its highest rate in the first day after birth.

The neonate makes some major changes in adjusting to life outside the uterus. The environment changes from a wet, dark, relatively quiet place with little sensory stimulation to a bright, air-filled, stimulating environment. The temperature of the uterus is relatively constant. Once outside, the neonate must rely on its own body temperature regulation system. The neonate must adapt to a new method of receiving nourishment, changing from a passive to an active agent. Perhaps the most important adaptation of all is learning to respond to other human beings in the environment. Developmental tasks of the neonatal period are listed in Box 12–3.

PHYSICAL DEVELOPMENT AND CHANGE

Head and Body

A neonate's head is proportionately large and makes up about one fourth of the entire body length. A neonate's eyes are usually blue or gray at birth and may not assume their mature color for several months. The eyes may become red or swollen if silver nitrate is used to prevent or treat gonorrheal infections (required in many states). A visual inspection of the newborn's body reveals a number of features:

▶ *Lanugo,* a fine downy hair, may cover the neonate's body at birth but disappears within 2 weeks.
▶ *Vernix caseosa,* a white, cheeselike substance, covers the body at birth and protects the fetus' skin in utero. It washes off easily after birth.
▶ *Milia* (small, white pimples) on the face are due to immature sebaceous glands and disappear quickly.
▶ *Icterus neonatorum,* a mild jaundice, manifests as a yellowish tint to the skin between the second and third day. The jaundice occurs because of excess red blood cells, since the neonate has some extra blood cells from the mother and the placenta. As those extra cells break down, mild jaundice results.
▶ *Mongolian spots* (flat blue, gray, or purple spots on the skin) across the buttocks are normal, especially in children of Asian or Southern European descent.

Box 12–3. Developmental Tasks of the Neonatal Period

▶ Adapt to life outside of mother's body.
▶ Strive to have needs met.
▶ Develop methods for dealing with environmental stimuli.
▶ Form attachments to caregivers.

They disappear in most children by the age of 5 years.
▶ *Cephalhematoma,* a collection of blood that results from ruptured blood vessels between the skull bones and membranes surrounding them, may appear as a bruise. Cephalhematoma is not a serious problem and disappears without treatment in 2 to 3 weeks.
▶ *Caput succedaneum* is a raised, swollen area on the head that forms when there is a long or difficult labor, or when forceps are used. It usually resolves within a few days. Caput succedaneum and cephalhematoma require no treatment and are never aspirated (fluid removed with a needle), since the risk for infection is very high.

During a vaginal delivery, considerable molding (movement of the skull bones to fit through the birth canal) occurs. The bones of the skull are soft in the neonate but gradually *ossify* (harden due to calcium deposits) during childhood. Soft tissue gaps between the bones are called *fontanelles.* Eventually the bones fuse together and close the gaps. The posterior fontanelle, which is approximately 0 to 2 cm in diameter at its largest and has a triangular shape, usually closes by 2 to 3 months of age. The diamond-shaped anterior fontanelle, 3 to 4 cm long by 2 to 3 cm wide at its largest, actually may increase in size for a short time but then decreases after 6 months and is completely closed by 18 months.

Figure 12–4 shows the location and shape of the fontanelles. When the infant is in a quiet state, the fontanelles should be even with the surrounding skin. Fontanelles may bulge somewhat when the infant is crying, coughing, or vomiting, but this is temporary. A fontanelle that bulges over an extended period of time could indicate increased intracranial pressure and needs to be investigated immediately. A depressed fontanelle is often a sign of dehydration. Parents need to be taught that the fontanelles cannot be damaged by washing or gentle touching. However, vigorous shaking

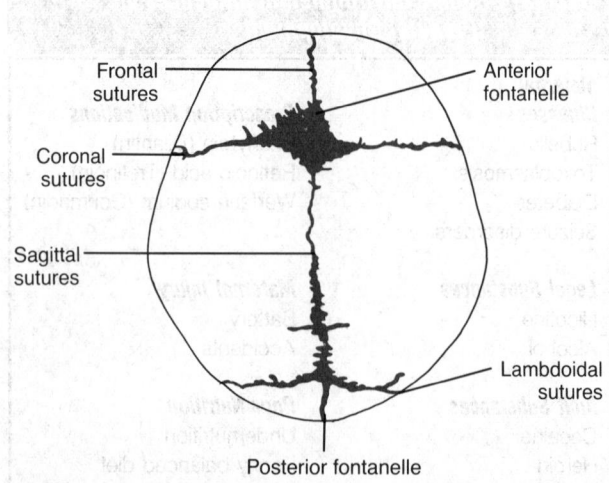

Frontal sutures
Anterior fontanelle
Coronal sutures
Sagittal sutures
Lambdoidal sutures
Posterior fontanelle

▲ *Figure 12–4*

Location and shape of the fontanelles.

TABLE 12-6. Neonatal Reflexes That Normally Disappear

Reflex	Description	Disappears at
Babinski	When a foot is stroked, the neonate hyperextends the toes and fans toes outward.	6 to 9 months
Sucking	When an object is placed in the mouth, the neonate sucks.	9 months
Grasp	When a finger is placed in the palm or base of the toes, the fingers or toes grasp it.	2 months
Moro	When the infant's head is dropped backward, the neonate extends all four limbs, then flexes the limbs.	3 months
Fencing	If the neonate's head is turned quickly to one side, the baby extends the limbs on the same side and flexes the limbs on the opposite side.	2 months

or bouncing of the baby can be dangerous, resulting in shaken baby syndrome. The exposed brain tissue can be bruised by the jostling.

Reflexes

Reflexes are involuntary physical responses that serve to protect, aid in survival, or stimulate human interaction. Many initial reflexes disappear and are replaced by learned responses. Table 12-6 lists some of the transient reflexes found in neonates. Neonates also have protective reflexes that persist throughout life, such as the eyeblink, gag, yawn, stretch, and hiccough reflexes. If a reflex does not disappear when it should, that is a sign of possible central nervous system dysfunction. By the same token, a neonatal reflex that reappears later in life is also a sign of central nervous system dysfunction.

Care of the Newborn Infant

The neonate requires some specific physical care in the first few weeks of life.[5] The umbilical stump needs daily cleaning with soap and water and alcohol wipes. It usually heals in about a week. Little bleeding of the stump should occur after the first day.

Some male children are circumcised (the foreskin of the penis is surgically removed), for religious or personal reasons of the family. If the baby is circumcised, direct parents to clean the penis thoroughly with soap and water every day and observe for signs of infection.

Neonates sleep most of the time, usually in the same curled position they maintained in utero (the fetal position). They wake only to satisfy needs. Most neonates establish a pattern of waking every 3 to 4 hours for nourishment and sleep a total of 18 to 22 hours per day. There is still considerable debate among health care professionals whether it is better to feed babies on demand or try to put them on a schedule.

Table 12-7 lists the normal ranges of physical growth and vital signs starting at birth.[27] The growth charts are divided by sex, since there are some differences in growth patterns in boys and girls. Boys tend to be larger in the first year of life, and girls are larger in late childhood. There are little or no differences in vital signs by sex.

TABLE 12-7. Normal Physical Development and Vital Signs for Children

	Birth	6 Months	12 Months	2 Years	4 Years	6 Years	12 Years
Physical Development							
Girls							
Weight (kg)	3.23	7.21	9.53	11.8	15.96	19.52	41.53
Height (cm)	49.9	65.9	74.3	86.8	101.6	114.6	151.5
Head Circumference (cm)	34.0	42.0	45.5	48.0	50.0	50.0	53.0
Sleep Needs (hours)	18–22	20	18	12 + nap	11–12	11	9
Caloric Needs (per kg)	115	105	100	100	85	85	48
Boys							
Weight (kg)	3.27	7.85	10.15	12.34	16.69	20.69	39.78
Height (cm)	50.5	67.8	76.1	86.8	102.9	116.1	149.7
Head Circumference (cm)	34.0	44.0	46.5	49.0	50.0	52.0	54.0
Sleep Needs (hours)	18–22	20	18	12 + nap	11–12	11	9
Caloric Needs (per kg)	115	105	100	100	85	85	60
Vital Signs							
Resting Pulse	100–180	80–150	80–150	70–110	70–110	70–110	55–90
Respirations	35	30	30	25	23	21	19
Temperature (°C)	36–37.7	37.7	37.7	37.2	37.0	37.0	36.6
BP Systolic	70–75	65–125	70–100	75–100	80–120	85–115	80–120
BP Diastolic	30–50	40–90	40–90	40–90	45–85	50–60	50–70

PSYCHOSOCIAL DEVELOPMENT

Self-Concept and Self-Image

One of the earliest developmental tasks of neonates is to learn to distinguish self from others. This allows for later development of a self-concept.

Cognitive and Intellectual Development

Neonates are capable of learning from the moment of birth (and probably begin learning in utero). At birth, they have intact sensory abilities in vision, hearing, and touch, and primarily use reflex behaviors such as sucking and grasp to explore their environments.

However, the opportunities for learning in the first month of life are limited by the neonates' sleeping patterns. They are awake, alert, and capable of learning only about 10 per cent of the day.

Memory skills begin to develop early. Memory is often assessed by two different kinds of tasks. *Recall* memory requires that an individual retrieve some information on demand. *Recognition* memory merely requires the knowledge that one has seen, heard, or felt this information before. Recognition memory is easier to assess in the nonverbal infant than is recall memory. Research shows that infants can recognize the sound of their mother's voice, the smell of their mother's breast-pads, and some simple visual images. Thus, some memory abilities are present at birth and increase with exposure to the environment.

Communication

Neonates communicate without words (prelingual). Crying is the main way that neonates express discomfort. Other forms of communication appear later; for example, cooing sounds begin around 1 month, and repetitions of vowel sounds when the baby is content appear soon after. Some nonverbal methods of communication occur as well, such as increased body movements, changes in breathing patterns and skin color, and facial expressions. Caretakers usually learn to discriminate among these signals to meet the neonates' needs. Distinct crying patterns in neonates exposed to cocaine prenatally are described in Applying Research to Nursing Practice.

RELATIONSHIPS AND ROLES

Bonding and Family Relationships

Bonding, or attachment, is the process of forming relationships with significant others, usually the primary caretaker.

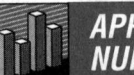

APPLYING RESEARCH TO NURSING PRACTICE

Cocaine-Exposed Newborns Have Distinctive Cry Patterns

Lester, B.M., Corwin, M.J., Sepkoski, C., Seifer, R., Peuker, M., McLaughlin, S., & Golub, H. (1991). Neurobehavioral syndromes in cocaine-exposed newborn infants. *Child Development, 62,* 694–705.

▼ ▼ ▼

Researchers in Providence, Rhode Island, compared newborn cry patterns in 80 infants exposed prenatally to cocaine and 80 infants not exposed to any drug prenatally. Cries were tape recorded on the second day after delivery, following a heel "stick" for routine blood tests or a flick of the heel administered by the researcher. These recorded cries were analyzed with a special computer program that measured the acoustic properties of the cry. Properties measured included the length of the crying spells, the intensity and loudness, the pitch, and the amount of "noise" (a combination of several different sounds within the cry pattern).

The cocaine-exposed babies had two patterns of abnormal cries. The first pattern, due to the direct effects of cocaine on the baby's nervous system, was an excessively long, high-pitched cry. The second was a quieter but more turbulent (noisy) crying pattern and seemed to be related to low birthweight. Both types of cries were present in each baby with prenatal cocaine exposure. Both types of crying patterns may be distressing for parents.

Applications to Practice

If the infant is directly affected by cocaine, the long, high-pitched cry pattern may be a short-term problem that may resolve without treatment. The crying pattern associated with low birthweight may persist longer, and nurses may need to provide parents with coping strategies.

Bonding is the most important psychosocial task of the neonate and infant and strongly influences later emotional development.

Bonding occurs when the child and the caretaker(s) look, touch, and pay attention to each other. They learn each other's signals. Caretakers need to have physical contact with their baby as soon as possible after birth to facilitate this bonding process. This is more difficult for sick or premature infants, but parents can be shown how to interact with the fragile or incubator-bound infant. Although some researchers maintain that the first few hours or days after birth are a crucial period for bonding, others believe that strong bonds can occur even if caretaker and infant are not together at birth.

Establishing Trust

Bonding is a first step toward the development of trust (see Erikson), but the removal of discomfort is also important. Infants are aware when they are uncomfortable, and they want immediate relief (see Freud). When discomforts are promptly removed and needs are met quickly, the infant builds a sense of trust in the world.

VALUES AND BELIEFS

In the neonatal period, nurses will be primarily concerned with the caretakers' moral and spiritual beliefs. Different cultures and religions vary in conceptions of the newborn infant's moral capacity. Some believe the neonate is neutral, with no sense of morality; others believe infants are born into sin. Respect for diverse opinions is important.

MAJOR HEALTH CONCERNS

Box 12–4 lists the leading causes of death in the neonate, as well as the leading health concerns for those who survive the first month of life.[14] The causes of death are primarily related to birth complications. Thus, the best treatment is prevention—education and counseling during the prenatal period and even before pregnancy begins. Good preparation for parenting can also help avoid some of the common health problems of neonates. If caregivers are well educated about infant nutritional needs and physical care, their infants will be healthier. Some parents will need information about programs such as WIC (Women, Infants, and Children) that provide food for low-income families.

ROLE OF THE NURSE

Apgar Scale

The most common method of assessing neonatal status is the Apgar scale (Table 12–8). An Apgar score is taken at 1 minute after birth and again at 5 minutes after birth. The total possible score is 10; a neonate with a score of 7 or higher is usually in good condition. If the score is less than 7, the baby is at risk. Scores below 4 indicate serious risks.

Brazelton Neonatal Behavioral Assessment Scale

A more sophisticated assessment tool for the neonate is the Brazelton Neonatal Behavioral Assessment Scale, which measures four dimensions of newborn abilities: interaction with others, motor behaviors, physiologic control, and response to stress. The Brazelton may be used if there is suspicion that the neonate is having problems. The Brazelton also may be used as a teaching tool to demonstrate newborn behaviors to inexperienced or high-risk caregivers. Examples of items on the Brazelton include moving a brightly colored object in front of the neonate and observing visual tracking, test-

---

Box 12–4. Leading Health Problems and Leading Causes of Death in the Neonatal Period

Leading Health Problems

Infections
    Middle ear
    Digestive tract
    Respiratory tract
Problems related to nutrition
    Inadequate nutrition
    Food allergies
    Poor eating
    Overfeeding

Leading Causes of Death

1. Conditions arising in the perinatal period
2. Congenital anomalies
3. Sudden infant death syndrome (SIDS)
4. Low birthweight/prematurity
5. Respiratory distress syndrome
6. Intrauterine hypoxia and birth asphyxia
7. Influenza/pneumonia

---

ing for symmetry of motor reflexes, and observing the neonate's use of social cues.

Nurses need to know their local referral sources so they can recommend appropriate help when babies do not pass screening tests. In most states, area education agencies have programs for developmentally delayed infants.

Table 12–9 provides some nursing implications for the care and health education of neonates.

TABLE 12–8. Apgar Scale

	Score		
	0	**1**	**2**
Appearance (skin color)*	pale, blue	body pink, extremities dusky	pink
Pulse (heart rate)	absent	slow (< 100)	normal (> 100)
Grimace (reflex response)			
Catheter in nose	no response	grimace	cough, sneeze
Slap on foot	no response	grimace	cries
Activity	limp	flexion of extremities	active movement
Respirations	absent	slow, irregular, weak cry	strong, regular cry

* For infants with darker skin, check mucous membranes.

TABLE 12-9. Nursing Implications for the Neonatal Period

Nursing Assessment	Possible Nursing Implications
Physical Development	
Growth measurements	Teach caregivers appropriate child care techniques and warning signs of illness/distress. Provide anticipatory guidance about normal physical growth and development. Monitor infants with risk factors identified by assessment
Temperature regulation	
Eyes	
Umbilical stump	
Reflexes	
Sleep patterns	
Eating and elimination patterns	
Fontanelles	
Vital signs	
Cognitive Development	
Home environment	Counsel parents on stimulating infant activities and toys. Talk to infants frequently
Alertness	
Psychosocial Development	
Infant-caretaker interaction	Stress the importance of touch and eye contact in forming attachment. If infant and caregivers are separated, encourage as much contact as possible. Help parents identify cry patterns and anticipate child's needs
Communication of needs	

▼ Infancy

The infancy period extends from 1 to 18 months and is a time of extremely rapid growth and change. Box 12-5 summarizes the developmental tasks of infancy.

PHYSICAL DEVELOPMENT AND CHANGE

Table 12-7 gives physical developmental guidelines and normal vital signs for infants. An infant spends more time awake and alert than a neonate but still sleeps about 18 hours per day at 4 months of age and about 14 hours per day at 12 months. Most infants sleep through the night by 3 to 6 months. Active sleep (REM, or rapid eye movement, sleep) accounts for about half their sleep time and is characterized by considerable movement and facial grimacing. Quiet sleep (non-REM) becomes more prevalent after 6

Box 12-5. Developmental Tasks of Infancy

- ▶ Gain control over body movement.
- ▶ Adjust to adults' schedule (feeding, elimination, sleep).
- ▶ Develop an ego.
- ▶ Develop trust in the environment.
- ▶ Learn to communicate needs.
- ▶ Begin to develop self-care skills (feeding, toileting, dressing).
- ▶ Explore the environment using the senses.

---

months and is characterized by low muscle tone and little movement. When babies are awake, they cycle between active alert stages (when most learning occurs), drowsiness, and distress.

The bones of the skull may still be affected by position. If the baby is left lying in the same position for too long, the head may flatten. Teach parents to place infants in a variety of positions for sleep.

Table 12-10 shows the usual developmental sequence of infant motor skills. Infant motor development is rapid. The average child can sit unaided by age 6 months, which allows greater use of both hands. Infants walk at 9 to 16 months, allowing them to explore a much larger environment. Thus, physical development enhances cognitive development.

However, the increase in mobility that comes with refinement of motor development puts the infant at greater risk for injury. Infants and toddlers are prone to falls and susceptible to poisoning (from opening cupboard doors and tasting any products they may find).

Parents need education about making their homes and automobiles safe for their children. Box 12-6 gives suggestions for increasing the safety of their environments.

PSYCHOSOCIAL DEVELOPMENT

Self-Concept and Self-Image

Rudimentary self-awareness grows from a sense of being different from others, asserting one's own likes and dislikes. Infants show highly individual preferences early.

Cognitive and Intellectual Development

Infants begin learning from the moment of birth. They are exposed to sensory experiences and gain control over their physical environment as the maturation process proceeds. One of the primary intellectual goals of infancy is to achieve the concept of *object permanence* (see Piaget). Infants need to realize that an object or person that is out of sight continues to exist. Infants cannot know that they are separate from objects or other people until object permanence develops. One sign that this process of permanence has developed is when infants show separation anxiety and fear of strangers. They have learned to trust and recognize the primary caretaker(s) and prefer to be with that person or persons. Separation anxiety is also evidence of improved memory skills, as the infant must be able to remember familiar people.

Communication

Communication begins as *prelinguistic,* or without words, and consists of cries, coos, smiles, gestures,

TABLE 12-10. Development of Infant Motor Skills

Motor Skill	Age in Months				
	3	6	9	12	18
Head control	Can lift head when prone	Holds head steady when sitting	Good head control		
Grasping	Briefly holds objects; carries objects to mouth	Use of thumb in grasping	Coordinated eye-hand activities	Handedness determined	
Sitting	Sits only with support	Brief sitting unaided	Sits alone steadily; good trunk control	Can sit from standing position	
Crawling/creeping			Crawling—trunk touches floor	Creeping—trunk raised	
Standing				Stands while holding on	
Walking					Walks and begins to run

whimpers, and laughter. Caretakers must learn to interpret accurately the infant's communication, such as distinguishing between a hunger cry and a colicky cry. Through interaction with significant others in the environment, speech (verbal communication) gradually develops, and prelinguistic forms of communication decrease in use. There is wide variability in speech and

language development, but single words usually appear at about 8 to 10 months, and two-word phrases ("give me," "Daddy go") at 12 to 18 months. Receptive skills, the ability to understand what someone says, develop faster than expressive skills. Infants can follow simple verbal directions even before they can speak words clearly. There is still some debate as to how speech and language skills develop. The two extreme views suggest that either infants are born with innate language-processing abilities, or infants learn speech from hearing it in the environment and imitating the sounds they hear. The "true" process is probably some combination of genetic and environmental factors.

RELATIONSHIPS AND ROLES

Expressing Emotions

Infants express emotions through generalized responses; they smile, laugh, kick, cry, or wiggle when they feel happy, angry, or frustrated. Because of their lack of verbal skills, we really cannot know exactly what specific emotions they may be feeling. We do know, however, that responding to an infant's needs promptly leads to better emotional adjustment later in life.

Establishing Trust

Positive experiences build trust. Trust is developed in many ways; through having needs met quickly, and as the child matures, through increasing physical competency. Psychosocial competence increases as an infant gains control over the environment. Having a secure attachment with one or more caretakers is an important component of trust. In the beginning, the sense of trust is usually associated with family.

Box 12-6. Increasing the Safety of the Child's Environment

The Home

Maintain fire extinguishers and smoke alarms.
Cover electrical outlets.
Turn down the temperature on the water heater.
Keep handles of pans on the stove turned inward.
Keep poisonous fluids and medicines in locked cabinets.
Put gates at the tops of stairs and across fireplaces.

The Child

Use only fire-retardant clothing.
Do not allow the child to run with food in his or her mouth.
Teach basic safety rules as early as possible.

The Car

Put the child in a car seat or seat belt *every time*.
Attach toys to the car seat for entertainment.

The Yard/Neighborhood

Supervise outdoor play until safety rules are well learned and demonstrated.
Put fences around pools.
Teach children about poisonous plants and berries.
Put helmets on children before bicycling.

VALUES AND BELIEFS

The infant is exposed to the moral values and spiritual beliefs of the caretakers and extended family from the time of birth. However, infants lack the cognitive skills needed to understand these values.

MAJOR HEALTH CONCERNS

Box 12–7 lists the leading health problems and causes of death in infancy. In infancy, accidental deaths are related to motor vehicle accidents, particularly when infants are not constrained in safe car seats. Infants are also prone to falls and accidents in the home (from chewing electrical cords, suffocating on food when they are allowed to run while eating, and drowning).

ROLE OF THE NURSE

Health assessment of the infant includes knowing normal infant physical growth and development patterns and checking for developmental milestones. The Denver Developmental Screening Test (DDST-2) is a screening tool used by many pediatric nurses to identify children at risk. The DDST screens development in communication skills, personal-social skills, gross motor skills, and fine motor skills.[8]

Hospitalization and visits to medical clinics can be stressful for children and their caretakers. Both the illness or injury and the alien environment with its numerous strangers contribute to heightened stress.

Several researchers have noted that children's conceptions of their own bodies and adaptation to illness and hospitalization vary according to their stage of cognitive development.

In the infant, the perception of illness relates to the degree of discomfort and pain. Since the primary developmental tasks of infancy are attachment and development of trust, the presence of the parents or primary caretakers is of the utmost importance. Most nursing interventions in this age group focus on parents, since adults can inadvertently transmit their own feelings of fear, anxiety, and guilt to the infant. Teaching parents to provide as much of the care in the hospital for their own children keeps them more involved in their child's recovery and enhances the relationship they already have with the child. Introducing strangers to provide intimate care may increase stress on the infant.

Table 12–11 lists some nursing implications for the care of the infant, and for health education with caregivers.

▼ Early Childhood

A child aged 18 months to 3 years has a particular, precarious, waddling gait, hence the name "toddler." The child of age 3 to 5 years is often called a preschooler. Toddlers and preschoolers are often grouped together in the developmental period called "early childhood." Developmental tasks of early childhood are summarized in Box 12–8.

Box 12–7. Leading Health Problems and Leading Causes of Death in Infancy

Leading Health Problems

Infections
    Middle ear
    Digestive tract
    Respiratory tract
Problems related to nutrition
    Inadequate nutrition
    Food allergies
    Poor eating
    Overfeeding

Leading Causes of Death

1. Congenital anomalies
2. Sudden infant death syndrome (SIDS)
3. Short gestation and low birthweight
4. Respiratory distress syndrome
5. Maternal complications of pregnancy

Data from U.S. Department of Health and Human Services, Public Health Service (1990). Healthy People 2000: National health promotion and disease prevention objectives (DHSS Publication No. PHS 91-50213, Washington, D.C.: U.S. Government Printing Office.

TABLE 12–11. Nursing Implications for Infancy

Nursing Assessment	Possible Nursing Implications
Physical Development	
Growth	Provide anticipatory guidance for
Sleep patterns	normal infant development. Avoid
Eating and eliminating	"milk bottle" syndrome—putting
patterns	infant to bed with sweet fluids that
Motor development	can decay early teeth. Stress the
Fontanelles/head	wide range of "normal" develop-
shape	ment
Tooth development	
Immunizations	
Vital signs	
Cognitive Development	
Alertness	Developmental delay may first mani-
Reaction to strangers	fest as a dull, uninterested baby.
and caretakers	Encourage considerable verbal in-
Communication	teraction with baby
Psychosocial Development	
Attachment	Faulty attachment may be a risk fac-
Expression of emotions	tor for abuse, neglect, infant emo-
	tional disturbance. Fussy, irritable
	baby difficult to parent

Box 12–8. Developmental Tasks of Early Childhood

- ▶ Increase social skills.
- ▶ Increase in coordination and physical strength.
- ▶ Develop self-control and initiative.
- ▶ Achieve autonomy in self-care skills.
- ▶ Communicate as social interaction, not just to express needs.
- ▶ Start learning "right" and "wrong" (develop a super-ego).
- ▶ Form a healthy self-concept.

PHYSICAL DEVELOPMENT AND CHANGE

Weight Gain

Birthweight generally quadruples by age 2 years, then weight gain slows somewhat. Toddlers gain an average of 4 to 5 pounds between ages 2 and 3 years. Most 2-year-olds are about 3 feet tall and grow another 3 to 4 inches in the next year. By age 3 to 5 years, children grow in a slow, steady pattern. Weight increases at about 5 pounds or less a year. Young children lose that plump baby appearance as their height growth is greater than weight gain, giving them a taller, thinner appearance. All primary (or deciduous) teeth are usually present. See Table 12–7 for normal growth parameters and vital signs.

Sleep

Most toddlers require a daytime nap of 1 to 2 hours and need about 12 hours of sleep per night. Children aged 3 to 4 years old may not sleep during the day but require 9 to 12 hours of sleep at night. They usually benefit from quiet rest times during the day. Preschoolers often develop bedtime rituals such as prayers, stories, being tucked in, snacks, or music. Many parents report that getting their young child to bed is a real chore. Children enjoy the attention of adults and evening activities and are often reluctant to miss any fun. However, it is important to maintain routine sleep hours.

Motor Skills

Motor skills are becoming increasingly complex, enabling the child to run, jump, and throw and catch objects. By 5 years of age, able-bodied children can run, balance on their tiptoes, skip, hop on one foot, climb, and ride a tricycle. These are gross motor skills. The fine motor skills, which require eye-hand coordination, are refined throughout childhood. The fine motor skills include dressing and undressing (buttoning and unbuttoning clothing, zipping, and tying shoelaces), and cutting, pasting, coloring, and writing. It is important that children get practice and encouragement with these activities. If they do not have experience, they

will not master the skills. The increased autonomy and advanced motor skills in combination with limited cognitive reasoning abilities put the young child at risk for accidents. Box 12–6 provides suggestions for a safer environment.

Eating Patterns

Children in the early childhood period eat much the same kinds of foods as adults do but in smaller quantities. Because of the young child's high activity level and physical growth needs, between-meal snacks are necessary. Preschoolers may show temperamental eating habits, such as refusing particular foods or demanding only certain foods (peanut butter sandwiches or hot dogs). They are extremely variable in appetite and may eat voraciously one day and hardly anything the next day. It is important to look at overall eating patterns from week to week rather than patterns from day to day. Poor eating patterns may be due to excessive between-meal snacking, unrealistic expectations of parents, tooth pain or decay, sibling rivalry, physical illness or fatigue, or a behavioral control issue (such as exercising autonomy).

Developing Toilet Independence

Establishing independence in bowel and bladder elimination (toilet training) is a major task of early childhood.

Like other developmental tasks, toileting requires an interaction of physical, intellectual, and psychosocial development for success. Physical development of muscle control of sphincters combines with the child's desire to please parents or other caretakers, and the ability to understand the requests of the caretaker to eliminate in a certain way. By the age of 2 to 2.5 years, children have greater physiologic awareness of when they need to eliminate, the sphincter control to wait for a brief time, and the communication skills to ask for help. Bowel control is usually achieved before bladder control. Most children achieve daytime control before nighttime control. In general, the later toilet training begins, the faster it is accomplished.

PSYCHOSOCIAL DEVELOPMENT

Self-Concept and Self-Image

Self-concept refers to people's awareness of their own characteristics, abilities, and values, and how they are different or similar to others. Self-esteem refers to the value the child places on self-identified characteristics. Self-concept is one aspect of the overall identity, or the integration of self-knowledge and value with the values of the larger culture. Children acquire an identity via a developmental process. First, they learn their names, their gender, their race, and other obvious traits. Then they learn the meanings that these categories have in their particular culture or family. Research on black children living in poverty has enhanced our thinking about this developmental process of identity development. Much of the research with young African-American children indicated that they have a positive self-concept but would select white playmates and teachers when given a choice. At first this was interpreted to mean that African-American children acquired a self-hatred related to their race very early. Further research revealed, however, that young children do not have the cognitive capacity to understand racism. Instead, they had noticed that white people were often preferred in their environment; their teachers were mostly white, the media showed whites in a positive light, and African-American characters in the media were missing or portrayed negatively. Thus, their early socialization told them to select white companions and teachers. Race awareness and understanding of racism mature much later.[26]

Gender identity (an awareness of one's own sex) also begins in this period and is complete around 6 years of age. Along with gender identity, gender role expectations—a sense of the appropriate behavior for a member of each gender—develops. Some cultures have strong attitudes about appropriate sex roles while others do not. Self-concept in the young child is largely egocentric and in a primitive state of evolution.

Cognitive and Intellectual Development

The young child is in Piaget's preoperational stage of development and can use mental representations (via language) to refer to people or objects that are not actually present. This ability allows the child to defer imitation and engage in symbolic play, while it lays the groundwork for logical reasoning. There are many limitations to preoperational thought. Young children tend to *centrate* or focus on only one aspect of a problem and ignore other important aspects. They lack *conservation*, the ability to recognize that two things equal in size remain equal even if their shape or form is changed (such as pouring water from a tall thin glass to a short squat glass). Young children are also somewhat *egocentric* and have difficulty accepting the point of view of another. Their logical reasoning skills are *transductive*, that is, they generalize from one specific fact to another specific fact. For example, 4-year-old Melissa met 1-year-old Todd and asked him what his name was. Later, she told her mother, "He didn't have a name because he can't talk." The combination of transductive logic and egocentrism makes trying to reason with a preschooler frustrating.

Memory development in the young child increases as the child gains vocabulary and experience with the environment. The memory skills of the child are hampered primarily by a lack of strategies. Young children often use rehearsal (saying it over and over) but few more effective strategies. They are also poor at judging their own memory abilities (metamemory), and will grossly overestimate how much they can remember.

Communication

Toddlers are in a rapid stage of speech and language acquisition. They may have unique words that only their caregivers understand but increasingly use speech and language skills to communicate their needs *(social speech)*. They also exhibit a lot of *private speech*, or talking to themselves as they play. This private speech later becomes internalized into thought. A preschooler asks questions—why, what, where, when, who, and how. They may not be satisfied with your answer and will ask again and again. It is important to encourage talking and asking questions. Speech development matures into adult form by early childhood. By age 4 to 5 years, the speech is fairly grammatical, and sentences consist of 6 to 8 words. Many children still have mild difficulties pronouncing all the speech sounds (such as W and L) correctly, but their speech is understandable. Speech may not reach an adult level of intelligibility until the age of 7 or 8 years. Language development progresses with an increase in vocabulary and understanding. Children learn new words and language concepts (under, over, before, later) through concrete experiences. Language development is influenced strongly by cognitive development, and both speech and language development depend upon a stimulating environment that allows children to explore.

Play

Play is the focus of most of the child's waking hours. Piaget stated that play is the work of the child. Very young children play alone. Then they engage in "parallel play," in which the children are playing alongside each other but are not interacting. Finally, they learn to play cooperatively with others.

Play serves many purposes: socializing with others, developing solitary skills, and enhancing cognitive development.

Piaget suggested that play progresses from simple functional play (shaking a rattle), which was primarily sensorimotor, to constructive play (building), to dramatic play (pretending), and finally, to games with rules (cognitive and morals-building play). Physical play helps build coordination and muscle strength as well as imagination and creativity.

Developing Autonomy

Young children have a much broader social and physical world than the infant because they are more mobile and able to communicate with others. A sense of themselves as separate beings has developed. Children with a secure sense of trust feel confident in exploring and experimenting with new things in the environment. Toddlers are becoming autonomous, and with increasing autonomy comes assertive behavior. They want to

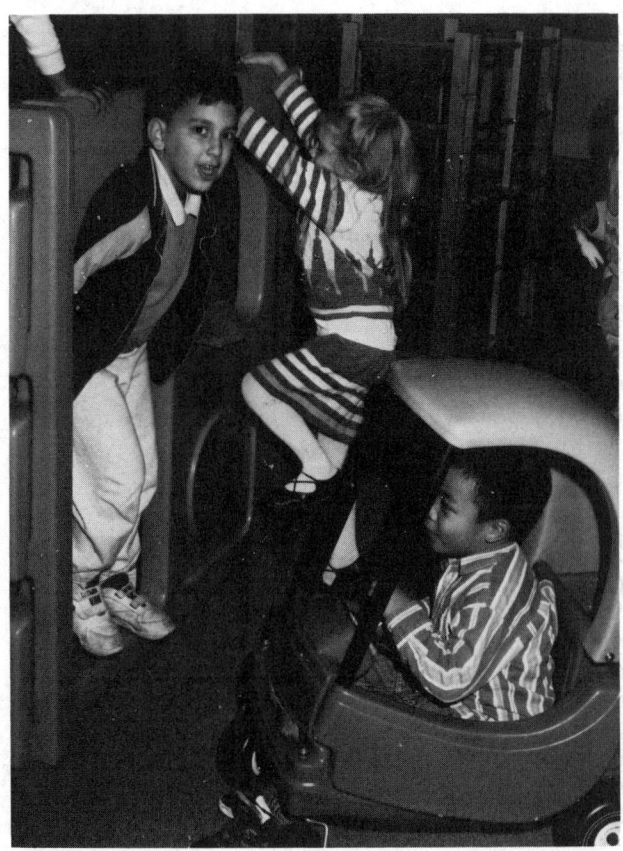

▲ *Figure 12-5*

In early childhood, playing with others becomes very important.

be independent and make their own decisions sometimes. Caretakers can provide choices. For example, they can ask "Do you want to take a bath now or after Mr. Rogers?" They should not offer a choice they do not have available or do not want the child to choose.

The toddlers' behavior can seem difficult to parents and other caretakers for a number of reasons, including their independence, dawdling, and apparent negativism. *Independence* develops out of an increased sense of autonomy. *Dawdling* is when children become preoccupied with interesting things and forget what they are supposed to be doing. *Negativism* is also related to growing autonomy and results when a child asserts personal likes and dislikes. These are "normal" behaviors of the young child. Rephrasing requests in the form of a choice may have more success.

Developing Initiative

Children with some degree of trust and autonomy are ready for initiative (see Erikson). *Initiative* is the ability to begin and carry out an activity without much adult guidance. Children need to be encouraged to plan and carry out independent activities. If children are criticized for their efforts, a sense of guilt may develop and seriously affect self-esteem. Caretakers can be encouraged to avoid punishment and criticism whenever pos-

sible. Focusing on the positive is far more effective (see the section on operant conditioning). Punishment should be reserved for activities that are dangerous.

Developing Self-Control

A child of preschool age develops socially acceptable patterns of behavior via the process of socialization. Socially acceptable behaviors include manners, customs, and rituals, such as the appropriate ways to interact with various others, especially with family members and other caretakers; learning to eat independently and with the appropriate tools and utensils; developing regular and routine sleeping patterns; self-care such as dressing, toileting, and general cleanliness; and participating in household tasks. These skills are enhanced through play activities.

VALUES AND BELIEFS

The preschool years lay the groundwork for moral and spiritual development. Most theorists believe that children are initially amoral, or without knowledge of right and wrong. They learn morals (or mores) from significant others, peers, television, books, and so on. Spiritual beliefs come from teachings by significant others and formal or informal religious training, and are highly related to moral development. Feedback (both positive and negative) from significant others, as well as individual cognitive development, influences a child's moral and spiritual development. Young children tend to rely on authority figures for information about good and bad. If mother says it, it must be right. They also evaluate their own behavior by the consequences. If they were punished, the behavior must have been wrong. Therefore, young children may engage in behaviors if they know they will not be caught. If not punished, the behavior is not wrong.

MAJOR HEALTH CONCERNS

Box 12-9 lists the leading causes of death in children aged 1 to 4 years. In early childhood, when judgment is impaired by immature cognitive processes, the child is in danger in the home. There are poisonous substances in the cupboards, sharp objects in drawers, and dangerous electrical receptacles that look like the perfect place to put the sharp object. The young child explores the environment and learns by trial and error. Sometimes the errors are life-threatening.

The major health concerns that arise in early childhood often revolve around achievement of developmental milestones. Parents may wonder about their child's vision or hearing. If the child is not speaking clearly, parents may consult nurses about speech and language development.

Parents often consult with nurses about day care issues for their children. About 75 per cent of women

---

Box 12–9. Leading Causes of Death in Children Aged 1–4 Years

- ▶ Unintentional injuries
- ▶ Congenital anomalies
- ▶ Cancer

---

work outside the home in the 1990s and need good child care. According to Zigler and Hall, about 26 per cent of children receive in-home care, 18 per cent go to day care centers, and 56 per cent are in family day care (several children cared for in someone's private home).[29] Although there are strict requirements for day care centers, the other two options are largely unregulated and vary widely in their quality.

Results of research on the short- and long-term effects of day care on child adjustment are mixed. However, most studies show that quality day care has no detrimental effects, and may be beneficial for many children.

Zigler and Hall provide some guidelines for evaluating day care. Nurses should keep in mind that the exposure to many other children leads to increased risk for infections.

ROLE OF THE NURSE

Health Screening and Assessment

The DDST can be used with the young child as well as infants. It provides a gross estimate of developmental progress. Since speech and language development is often a concern of parents, nurses should know when and where to refer children for speech and language evaluations. Some rules of thumb about normal speech development to guide the decision of when to refer are listed in Table 12–12.

Children should be referred to a speech/language clinician at any age if they show hypernasality, hyponasality, an excessively monotonous voice, or consistent hoarseness.

TABLE 12–12. Rules of Thumb for Normal Speech Development

Age of Accomplishment	Task
2 years	Points to body parts
	Says two-word phrases
3 years	Asks simple questions
	Uses short sentences
	Speaks intelligibly to family
4 years	Has few or no episodes of dysfluency (stuttering)
	Speaks intelligibly to strangers
6 years	Has no articulation errors

Health Education

Young children are egocentric and do not have good logical reasoning skills. They are also seeking control over their environment (autonomy). Preschoolers often view illness as punishment for bad behavior and have a "magical" belief that adults could cure them if they wanted to. They subscribe to the *contagion view*—that illness is caused by contact with sick others. Preschoolers have a very limited understanding of internal organs.

Table 12–13 provides nursing implications for care and health education of children in the early childhood period.

▼ School Age

According to Freud and Erikson, the school-age years (ages approximately 6 to 12 years) are the most peaceful and calm times of childhood. Freud's latency period described a time of rapid socialization and self-discovery. Erikson described school age as a time for industry, or developing productivity. School age can be calm years for children who have had healthy physical and psychosocial development in earlier years. However, if earlier developmental periods were stressful and developmental tasks were not successfully

TABLE 12–13. Nursing Implications for Early Childhood

Nursing Assessment	Possible Nursing Implications
Physical Development	
Growth	Encourage parents to wait until after age 2 years to begin toilet training. Accident prevention is essential: encourage parents to safeguard the home and car. Encourage parents to teach the child basic safety rules
Sleep patterns	
Eating patterns	
Bowel and bladder control	
Vital signs	
Motor development	
Safety of environment	
Dental status	
Immunizations	
Cognitive Development	
Delayed imitation	Speech development has a wide range of normal, but the child should be monitored closely if the child falls behind expectations. Encourage parents to play with children and to provide plenty of opportunity for active play. Encourage parents to model moral behavior
Symbolic play	
Speech and language	
Play patterns	
Moral development	
Psychosocial Development	
Autonomy	Advise parents to give the child choices when possible and encourage child to be independent and resourceful. Encourage parents to avoid criticism and punishment
Initiative	
Independence	

achieved, school-age children may have problems. With societal changes such as the younger age of dating and the move from the junior high model to middle schools, the preadolescent child has taken on some adolescent characteristics earlier than in previous decades. Box 12–10 summarizes the developmental tasks of school age.

PHYSICAL DEVELOPMENT AND CHANGE

Physical Growth Patterns

Physical growth patterns are slow and steady throughout most of the school-age period but vary in individual children based on genetic and environmental influences. See Table 12–7 for average height and weight. A *growth spurt* occurs prior to puberty, at age 10 years for girls and 12 years for boys, on average. By 12 years of age, the brain is adult sized, although not of adult maturity since myelinization (the insulating layer of fat on nerves that enhances nerve impulse transmission) is not complete. Average vital signs for children in the school-age period are summarized in Table 12–7.

At age 5 or 6 years, the primary or deciduous teeth begin to fall out and are replaced by permanent teeth. All the permanent teeth except the third molars (which do not erupt until young adulthood) are present by the age of 12 to 13 years.

Children's body proportions begin to approximate those of adults. They lose the rounded abdomen, the back and shoulders straighten; all the bones lengthen, and calcium deposits cause them to harden. The facial bones alter somewhat and sinuses enlarge, giving the face an adult appearance.

Neuromuscular development combined with experiences and training gives children increasing coordination and strength throughout the school-age years. Exercise enhances both cognitive and neuromuscular development.

Children explore their world with their bodies. They climb trees, swing from bars, and run in fields of grass. Exercise is particularly important for children who tend to spend considerable time in sedentary activities such as watching television, reading, or playing video games. Lifestyle patterns of diet and exercise are established in childhood, so prevention activities need to be targeted at school-age children (but certainly must include their parents to be successful). Childhood is also a time when obesity may first become a problem.

Eating Patterns and Sleep

Because of the energy needs of active play and exercise, school-age children need plenty of food. See Table 12–7 for specific caloric needs by age. Nutrition is also important in achieving normal growth and for good attention and concentration at school.

Most school-age children do not sleep during the day and require 9 to 11 hours of sleep per night.

PSYCHOSOCIAL DEVELOPMENT

Self-Concept and Self-Image

Industry refers to a sense of competence and mastery over the environment. Success, primarily in the social and academic worlds of the school, is important for achieving industry and developing positive self-esteem. Children need to be provided with challenging, interesting tasks within their ability level to ensure more success than failure. School-age children tend to compare their performance with others and become more competitive. If children experience much failure or feel that their performance is less than that of peers, they can develop a feeling of inferiority. If this inferiority becomes deeply ingrained, they may experience low self-esteem, give up easily, and become socially withdrawn.

Cognitive and Intellectual Development

School-age children are "concrete" and need to focus on the here and now. In Piaget's terminology, they are "*operational*" or able to use symbols to carry out mental activities. They are gradually gaining *conservation* skills, the recognition that objects do not change even if their form is altered. An understanding of time concepts develops. At 6 years, a child understands about the past and the future, but does not have a clear understanding of time. For example, the child may know that first there is Christmas, then her birthday, even though the birthday is in April. Most school-age children are focused on the present. They become concerned with punctuality but often lose track of time and arrive home late. By the age of 12 years, a child can keep time obligations. Concepts of space develop from experience with the child's own body in space as well as the physical layout of the home and neighborhood. By the end of school age, the child understands the concept of the "world," space, and time. These are quite abstract concepts for younger children to grasp.

Communication

School-age children use speech and language skills mostly for communication. Their self-talk is internalized as thought and they are less likely to play with sounds than younger children. They have well-developed vocabularies and adult speech patterns. By this time, culture has influenced communication skills. Communication styles may vary even within people who speak the same language. They may have dialects or accents, use body language and gestures differently, and have different rhythms of speech.

Learning to communicate by reading and writing are the major academic tasks. However, 5 to 10 per cent of children have some degree of learning disabilities that affect school performance.

Early signs of learning disability include delayed speech and language development and mild speech problems, difficulty following directions, difficulty in learning the names of colors or the alphabet, short attention span, poor memory, and letter or word reversals. If the child has difficulty mastering the basics of academics, self-esteem may suffer. Thus, early recognition and treatment of learning disabilities is crucial. Nurses can be resources to caretakers about normal speech, language, and cognitive development as well as about referral sources for evaluation of learning disabilities.[28] Nurses can also be "culture brokers" who help clients from other cultures communicate within the health care system.

According to Kohlberg, school-age children are "conventional" moral reasoners. Early in the school-age period, children focus on external controls. If they are punished, their behavior must be bad. They learn to obey rules in order to get rewarded. Young children focus more on consequences of behavior than intentions. They reason that if you do only a little damage, it is not as bad as if you do a lot of damage. By the end of the school-age period, children begin to consider the intentions of the action.

RELATIONSHIPS AND ROLES

Family Relationships

Family attachments and relationships still affect trust, autonomy, and self-esteem. Parents and siblings continue to exert much influence on the child's socialization. In the past, there was much debate about birth order, whether first borns were different from later borns, and the influence of being in a large family versus a small family. Much of the research has been unclear on these issues, but some conclusions can be made. Parents do learn by experience and may be more effective parents with later born children than with first borns. Children may have different "statuses" and interactional styles within the family due to birth order. The first born has more exposure to an adult-only world, whereas later borns have other children to contend with. First borns may be given greater responsibilities for child care of later borns.

Sibling Relationships

Siblings are often providers of affection, counselors, leaders, protectors, and parent substitutes.[6] Sometimes sibling relationships are the most significant attachments in a child's life and may help the child survive severe traumas such as abuse by a parent or loss of a parent.

Peer Relationships

Going to school extends a child's world considerably and allows for greater self-sufficiency. Children learn about alternative family patterns from friends who may have single parents, two heterosexual parents, multigenerational households, or gay or lesbian parents, and so on. School-age children often play in loose groups or "gangs" but often have a "best" friend.

A best friend relationship helps develop interpersonal communication skills, social interactions, and the ability to compromise.

VALUES AND BELIEFS

Children learn about the spiritual beliefs of their culture and learn specifics about prayer, rites, sacraments, chanting, meditation, and so on. By the end of school age, fantasy beliefs are replaced by logical reasoning, paralleling changes in cognitive development from magical, transductive thinking to the use of deduction and induction. Moral reasoning is characterized by a desire to be a "good" boy or girl, and the idea that rules are absolute and unchangeable.

MAJOR HEALTH CONCERNS

Box 12-11 summarizes the major causes of death in children aged 5 to 14 years. School-age children have the lowest rates of mortality and serious illnesses of any age group.[7] Accidents of school-age children are more likely to be related to independent activities of the child, such as bicycling and skateboarding. The more independent child is at higher risk for accidental death and injury. The main concerns that parents report during this period are related to developmental delays or deviations rather than illnesses.

ROLE OF THE NURSE

Health Screening and Assessment

Since the primary concerns of the school-age period are not physical illnesses but school learning or behavioral concerns, nurses need to educate themselves about these problems. Warning signs of a learning disability might include the following: history of numerous middle ear infections as a young child, mild speech problems, difficulty learning rote memory tasks (the alphabet letters or the letter sounds), mild clumsiness, especially of fine motor activities such as handwriting, and difficulties learning to read, write, spell, or do mathematics.

Health Education

School-age children have a much better understanding of the insides of their bodies than young children do and often subscribe to a *"germ theory"* and the concept of contamination (that germs rather than people transmit illness). They may fear loss of control over their bodies and are concerned about the disruption illness causes in their lives—missing school and friends. Because they are concrete thinkers, school-age children do well with demonstrations of procedures on models or use of films and storybooks to describe illnesses and procedures. The following sections offer some ways of making the experience less traumatic for children and their significant others.

PREPARING CHILDREN FOR HOSPITALIZATION

The best preparation begins when the child is healthy or uninjured. Hospital or clinic tours can be scheduled for children for whom no hospitalization is planned, such as elementary school classes, or scout troops. Then if an emergency admission or a scheduled hospitalization becomes necessary, the child has been prepared under less stressful conditions. Siblings will also be prepared to adjust better to their brother's or sister's hospitalization.

Encourage children to ask questions about hospitalization and illness and do not become impatient if they ask the same questions repeatedly. Since young children are egocentric, try to explain the hospitalization from the child's point of view. What is important for adults may not be important for children. The young child may need to know whether mother can stay overnight rather than what the visiting hours are.

WHILE CHILDREN ARE HOSPITALIZED

Parental Role. When a child is hospitalized, the whole family is affected. Parents will continue to be the primary caregivers, even when the child is in the hospital. Parents play a crucial role in their child's adjustment to hospitalization and to the recovery process. If the parents feel guilt (that they should have recognized the symptoms earlier or prevented the accident) or extreme anxiety, these negative feelings may be transmitted to their children. Nurses need to help parents work through negative feelings. One way to decrease the anxiety is to involve parents in direct care. Most young children under stress or discomfort would rather have their parent bathe or dress them than a stranger.

Most pediatric units encourage one or both parents to stay with their children as much of the time as possible.

Establishing Trust. Honesty is very important in establishing a supportive and trusting relationship with young patients and their families. When explaining procedures, use language appropriate to the child's developmental level and use as many audiovisual aids as possible. Show the child what equipment will be used and turn it on so they can hear the noise it makes. For example, show the child how noisy the cast saw is, but how it stops working if it touches skin. Give choices whenever you can ("Would you like me to change your dressing now or after your bath?"). Try to be present during doctors' rounds so that you can answer questions or explain what the physician means.

Children (and adults, too) often show some behavioral regression when they are hospitalized. For example, the 2-year-old may return to thumb sucking or the 6-year-old may use baby talk. Bedwetting is quite common. Nurses should be nonjudgmental and explain to parents that these regressions are usually temporary.

Play Therapy to Reduce Stress. Some researchers have investigated the uses of play for hospitalized children and suggest that play may reduce stress.[16] Playing with medically oriented toys may be "doing the work of worry." Hospital playrooms could be stocked with play stethoscopes, hospital dollhouses, wheelchairs, anatomic dolls, and so on. In addition, familiar toys from home offer a sense of continuity and comfort. Nurses may be able to establish a positive relationship with a distrustful child by participating in play. Play can also be used to educate and inform children about procedures.

Siblings of Hospitalized Children. The siblings of hospitalized children often experience considerable stress as well. They often feel left out, abandoned, uninformed, or frightened by their brother's or sister's illness. Siblings may be moved from one household to another by well-intentioned parents who do not want to overburden any of their friends or relatives. Whenever possible, it is best to keep siblings together in one setting where they can feel safe. If possible, they should be allowed to visit their sibling or talk on the phone regularly. Siblings need honest explanations about the brother's or sister's condition.

Table 12–14 summarizes nursing implications for school-age children.

▼ CHILD ABUSE

Some caregiver-child relationships are stressful and may result in abuse or neglect. Serious physical, sexual, and psychologic abuse of children has increased in U.S. society, presumably due to greater stresses in families related to poverty, drugs, alcohol addictions, crowded conditions, and a host of other factors. Child abuse is often cyclical and intergenerational. A parent who was

TABLE 12–14. Nursing Implications for School Age

Nursing Assessment	Possible Nursing Implications
Physical Development	
Sleep patterns Eating patterns Vital signs Dental status Motor development Exercise Immunizations Overall health	Remind parents that immunizations must be up-to-date before school registration can occur. Encourage parents to promote active play and discourage excessive sedentary activities such as watching TV and playing video games. Urge parents to help their children establish good eating patterns
Cognitive Development	
Conservation skills Speech and language School achievement Moral development	Encourage parents to take steps to ensure that school is a positive environment. If the child dislikes school, parents should investigate the reasons; learning disabilities and social problems may emerge. Stress to parents that children look to significant adults and peers outside the family as role models
Psychosocial Development	
Industry Relationships/friendships Self-esteem	Failures at school or in peer relationships or family stress may result in low self-esteem. Avoid criticism and punishment

abused as a child learned unhealthy family patterns and lacks knowledge of child development and parenting. This adult may abuse his or her own children.

RISK FACTORS FOR CHILD ABUSE

Many studies have tried to identify risk factors for child abuse and neglect. Friedrich and Einbender summarized these as follows.[10]

Age

Younger children are more likely to be found in Emergency Department admissions. They speculated that younger children, because of their greater dependency, are more frustrating to care for, are less able to defend themselves, and are physically more fragile. However, children of all ages can be abused.

Sex

Most studies find no differences in the percentages of boys and girls who are victims of child abuse in gen-

eral. However, there are still more reports of sexual abuse of girls than boys.

Family Size

In about one third to one half of families, more than one child is abused. This is contrary to the idea that one child is the family scapegoat.

Family Intactness

Twice as many children from single-parent homes are reported to be abused than is true of children from two-parent homes. This finding may be related to economic status, as 50 per cent of single-parent homes are below the poverty level.

Most of the research indicates that families under stress are at high risk for child abuse and neglect. Economic status is the greatest predictor of abuse.[10]

Parents who abuse their children are often socially isolated, have low self-esteem, and have recently had a major life change (loss of job, move to new location, divorce, and so on).

Research on recurrence of abuse suggests that over 50 per cent of reported cases will have at least one future occurrence of child abuse, with younger children at higher risk than older children. The consequences of abuse on children can be extensive and long-term and can include serious emotional maladjustment, low self-esteem, behavioral insecurity and withdrawal, lowered intelligence test scores, and lowered school achievement (from neurologic damage, emotional damage, or both). Children who were sexually abused may have significant difficulties in establishing intimate relationships when they become adults. There is a link between childhood sexual abuse in females and later eating disorders, drug/alcohol abuse, and emotional problems.[15]

Children with special needs seem to be particularly vulnerable to abuse. Research has found that children who were born prematurely and children with birth defects or mental retardation are at a much higher risk for abuse and neglect than the general population of healthy children.[11] Special needs children may deviate from their parents' expectations and may place greater demands for care on their families.

Box 12–12 summarizes possible indicators of child abuse and neglect, including physical and behavioral symptoms.

CHILDHOOD SEXUAL ABUSE

Childhood sexual abuse includes a wide variety of coercive sexual activities. Perpetrators of sexual abuse are often close relatives, such as the father, stepfather, older brother, or mother but may be nonfamily members as well, such as neighbors, babysitters, or teachers. Many research studies have demonstrated long-

---

Box 12–12. *Warning Signs of Possible Child Abuse and Neglect*

Warning Signs in Children

Signs of Possible Neglect

Frequent lack of supervision
Torn, dirty clothing
Tooth decay
Absenteeism
Poor dental hygiene

Signs of Possible Physical Abuse

Bruises in various stages of healing
Burns
Passivity, excessive shyness
Repeated trips to the Emergency Department
Fear of adults
Anxiety

Signs of Possible Sexual Abuse

Presence of any sexually transmitted disease
Vaginal bleeding
Unusual sexual knowledge or behavior for age
Withdrawn manner, shyness, depression
Reluctance to change clothes for gym
Poor peer relationships

Warning Signs in Parents

Signs of unmet emotional needs
Poor relationship with own parents
Unrealistic expectations for children
Lack of skills for coping with stress

---

term effects on mental health when sexual abuse is not identified or treated.[24]

Nurses are mandatory reporters of child abuse and must report the situation to appropriate social services immediately. Sometimes it is necessary to remove the child from the home to ensure safety. The treatment for child abuse must be instituted quickly for both child and abuser, and the treatment must be ongoing and comprehensive.

Summary

- ▶ The human life span may be interpreted as linear or cyclical.
- ▶ Normal growth and development proceed from head to feet, proximal to distal, and general to specific; all in a predictable pattern but at variable rates among different individuals.
- ▶ Timing of developmental skills depends upon maturational readiness and environmental opportunities.
- ▶ Development occurs in stages, and each stage rep-

resents a task that must be accomplished before successful progression to the next step.
- ▶ The genetic code sets the parameters for physical and cognitive development.
- ▶ Maturation of the nervous system is necessary for higher levels of development to occur.
- ▶ The endocrine glands have a major influence on growth and development.
- ▶ Interactional factors that influence growth and development include adaptation, motivation, learning, socialization, and individual differences.
- ▶ Major theories important in growth and development include: Freud's psychosexual stages, Erikson's psychosocial stages, Havighurst's developmental tasks for different ages, Piaget's cognitive stages, Kohlberg's moral stages, Skinner's behavioral theories, and Bandura's social learning theory.
- ▶ The prenatal period progresses from conception to birth and is marked by great hazards, so that many fertilized eggs do not survive this 38-week period.
- ▶ The nurse's role during the prenatal period is to assess for possible risk factors and to guide mothers to healthful lifestyles.
- ▶ The neonatal period consists of the first 28 days after birth and is marked by: highest infant mortality during the first 24 hours following birth, distinctive physical features, prelingual communication, bonding as the most important psychosocial task of the stage, and birth complications as the major cause of death.
- ▶ The Apgar score and the Brazelton Neonatal Behavioral Assessment Scale are two of the tools used to assess neonates.
- ▶ Infancy extends from 1 month to 18 months of age and is a time marked by rapid growth and change, mobility and refinement of motor development, greater risk for injury, awareness of being different from others, learning to gain control over the physical environment and understanding object permanence, beginning of verbal speech progressing to two-word phrases, the establishment of trust, and accidents in motor vehicles and in the home as major causes of death.
- ▶ Toddlers (18 months to 3 years) and preschoolers (3 to 5 years) are in the early childhood development period, which is marked by a gain in height with loss of "baby fat"; increasing competence at performing motor skills; bowel and bladder control at approximately age 2 to 2.5 years; the development of identity concerning name, gender, race, and other obvious traits; the preoperational stage of cognitive development and transductive reasoning; rapid speech and language development; play as the focus of most waking hours; the development of autonomy; the development of more and more trust until the child is ready to develop initiative; development in the preschool child of socially acceptable behaviors with dependence upon authority figures for decisions about what is good and what is bad; and dangers in the home and environment as the young child explores these areas.
- ▶ In school-age children, development is marked by

rapid socialization, self-discovery, industry, and productivity; rapid growth spurts; increasing coordination and strength; high-energy needs of play and exercise requiring plenty of food; competition with increasing sense of positive self-esteem gained by successes in school; intellectual development at the concrete level with gradual understanding of conservation and, by age 12 years, a grasp of some abstract concepts; well-developed vocabularies and adult speech patterns; learning to communicate by reading and writing; "conventional" moral reasoning; important relationships with family, siblings, and peers; and the lowest rates of mortality and serious illnesses of any age group.

▶ Child abuse and neglect result from stresses in the home, and abuse is often cyclical and intergenerational.

Bibliography

1. Abel, E. (1984). *Fetal alcohol syndrome and fetal alcohol effects.* New York: Plenum.
2. Boivin, M., & Begin, G. (1989). Peer status and self-perception among early elementary school children: the case of the rejected child. *Child Development,* 60, 591–596.
3. Bronfenbrenner, U. (1989). Ecological systems theory. *Annals of Child Development,* 6, 187–249.
4. Chasnoff, I. (1986). *Drug use in pregnancy: Mother and child.* Boston: MTP Press Limited.
5. Cohen, S.M., et al. (1991). *Maternal, neonatal, and women's health nursing.* Springhouse, PA: Springhouse.
6. Craft, M.J., & Denehy, J.A. (1990). *Nursing interventions for infants and children.* Philadelphia: W.B. Saunders.
7. Foster, R.L.R., et al. (1989). *Family-centered nursing care of children.* Philadelphia: W.B. Saunders.
8. Frankenberg, W.K., & Dodds, J.B. (1990). *Revised Denver Developmental Screening Test.* Denver: University of Colorado.
9. Freud, S. An outline of psychoanalysis. In Strachey, J. (ed. & translator). (1964). *The standard edition of the complete psychological works of Sigmund Freud.* London: Hogarth.
10. Friedrich, W.N., & Einbender, A.J. (1983). The abused child: a psychological review. *Journal of Clinical Child Psychology,* 12, 244–256.
11. Garbarino, J., et al. (1987). Special children—special risks: The maltreatment of children with disabilities. New York: de Gruyter.
12. Gilligan, C. (1982). *In a different voice.* Cambridge, MA: Harvard University Press.
13. Gilligan, C., et al. (1988). *Mapping the moral domain.* Cambridge, MA: Harvard University Press.
14. Haggerty, R. (1986). The changing nature of pediatrics. In Krasnegor, N.A., et al. (eds.). *Child health behavior.* New York: Wiley.
15. Hurley, D. (1991). Women, incest, and alcohol. *Journal of Studies on Alcohol,* 52(3), 253–268.
16. Kampe, E. (1990). Children in health care: when the prescription is play. In Klugman, E., & Smilansky, S. (eds.). *Children's play and learning.* New York: Teacher's College Press.
17. Kohlberg, L. (1984). *Essays on moral development.* San Francisco, CA: Harper & Row.
18. Kristjansson, E.A., et al. (1989). Maternal smoking during pregnancy affects children's vigilance performance. *Drug and Alcohol Dependence,* 24, 11–19.
19. Lester, B.M., et al. (1991). Neurobehavioral syndromes in cocaine-exposed newborn infants. *Child Development,* 62, 694–705.
20. Macklin, E.D., & Rubin, R.H. (1983). *Contemporary families and alternative lifestyles.* Beverly Hills, CA: Sage.
21. Magrab, P.R. (1984). *Psychological and behavioral assessment: Impact on pediatric care.* New York: Plenum.
22. Miller-Jones, D. (1988). The study of African-American children's development. In Slaughter, D.T. (ed.). Black children and poverty: a developmental perspective. New Directions for Child Development, No. 42, 75–92.
23. Papalia, D.E., & Olds, S.W. (1989). *Human development.* New York: McGraw-Hill.
24. Patton, M.Q. (1991). *Family sexual abuse: Frontline research and evaluation.* Newbury Park, CA: Sage.
25. Schorr, L.B. (1988). *Within our reach: Breaking the cycle of disadvantage.* New York: Doubleday.
26. Spencer, M.B. (1988). Self-concept development. In Slaughter, D.T. (ed.). Black children and poverty: a developmental perspective. *New Directions in Child Development,* No. 42, 59–72.
27. Whaley, L.F., & Wong, D.L. (1987). *Nursing care of infants and children.* St. Louis: Mosby.
28. Williams, J., & Eliason, M.J. Nursing interventions for parents of children with learning disabilities. Iowa City, IA: The University of Iowa College of Nursing (unpublished manuscript).
29. Zigler, E., & Hall, H.W. (1987). Day care and its effects on children: An overview for pediatric health professionals. *Developmental and Behavioral Pediatrics,* 9, 38–46.

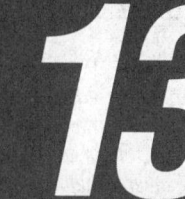

 ## ▼ *Adolescence and Early Adulthood*

▼ *Make the most of yourself for that is all there is to you.*
Ralph Waldo Emerson

▼ CHAPTER OUTLINE

ADOLESCENCE
PHYSICAL DEVELOPMENT AND CHANGE
    Musculoskeletal Changes
    Reproductive Changes
PSYCHOSEXUAL DEVELOPMENT
PSYCHOSOCIAL DEVELOPMENT
    Self-Concept and Self-Image
    Cognitive and Intellectual
      Development
    Relationships and Roles
VALUES AND BELIEFS
    Moral Development
    Spiritual Values
MAJOR HEALTH CONCERNS
    Pregnancy
    Substance Abuse
    Acquired Immune Deficiency
      Syndrome (AIDS) and Sexually
      Transmitted Diseases (STDs)
    Eating Disorders
    Tobacco Use
    Depression and Suicide
ROLE OF THE NURSE
    Health Screening and Assessment
    Health Education

EARLY ADULTHOOD
PHYSICAL DEVELOPMENT AND CHANGE
    Musculoskeletal System
    Reproductive System
PSYCHOSEXUAL DEVELOPMENT
PSYCHOSOCIAL DEVELOPMENT
    Self-Concept and Self-Image
    Cognitive and Intellectual
      Development
    Relationships and Roles
VALUES AND BELIEFS
    Moral Development
    Spiritual Values
MAJOR HEALTH CONCERNS
    Lifestyle
    Environment
    Acquired Immune Deficiency
      Syndrome (AIDS)
    Date (Acquaintance) Rape
ROLE OF THE NURSE
    Health Screening and Assessment
    Health Education

▼ *KEY TERMS*

Apocrine sweat glands   Ethgender   Menarche
Egocentricity   Family of origin   Pubescence (Puberty)

Opinions vary as to when adolescence begins. This chapter considers adolescence as the period of development between the onset of puberty and young adulthood, which usually encompasses the ages of 13 to 19 years. Early adulthood begins around the age of 20 years and may continue into the early thirties. We all recognize that some young adults are still adolescent in behavior while some teenagers have already accomplished their developmental tasks and are ready for more adult challenges. Since age is relative, once specific tasks are accomplished persons are ready to progress to the next stage regardless of chronologic age.

Adolescence is marked by profound changes, not only in accelerated physical growth but also in cognitive ability, social expectations, and personality development. As a result, the adolescent faces many choices that distinguish adolescence as a unique stage in human development on the way to independence.[31]

Young adulthood is marked by the person's assumption of an independent lifestyle with financial independence, separate from the family of origin. The young adult has a sense of direction and responsibility, has clear-cut goals, and is ready to make a personal commitment to another individual.

▼ ADOLESCENCE

PHYSICAL DEVELOPMENT AND CHANGE

Table 13–1 summarizes physical changes that occur during adolescence.

Musculoskeletal Changes

During adolescence, a growth spurt takes place, beginning about age 10.5 to 11 years in girls and 12.5 to 13 years in boys. In both sexes, this growth continues for about 2.5 years. Prior to this growth spurt, adolescents will have reached 75 to 80 per cent of their adult height and about 50 per cent of their adult weight.[14] Boys may grow about 8 inches, mainly in the trunk region, whereas girls grow slightly less during their growth spurt.

The peak of this growth spurt is about age 14 years for boys and age 12 years for girls.[38] Although adult stature for African-Americans and whites eventually equalizes, during the growth spurt in adolescents African-Americans attain a greater proportion of their adult stature earlier than do whites.[14] For this period of time the adolescent may appear clumsy and uncoordinated because of an increase in skeletal growth accompanied by a temporary delay in the development of muscle growth.

TABLE 13–1. Summary of Physical Changes Occurring During Adolescence

Girls	Boys
Growth Spurt	
Ages 10–14	Ages 12–16
38 pounds	42 pounds
9⅝ inches	9⅝ inches
Cardiovascular System	
Pulse	
Slows to 75–90 beats/min	Slower rate
Blood Pressure	
120/76	130/76
	Higher systolic pressure
Respiratory System	
16–20 respirations/minute	Greater volume, greater vital capacity, increased respirations
Gastrointestinal System	
Stomach capacity increases	Similar changes
Intestines grow in length	
Stomach and intestinal muscles become stronger	
Liver attains adult size	
Urinary System	
Bladder capacity increases	May void up to 1500 ml daily
Musculoskeletal System	
Fat distribution over thighs, breasts, and buttocks because of estrogen production	Amount of fat decreases as body energy focuses on bone and muscle due to androgen production

From Jarvis, C. (1992). *Physical examination and health assessment.* Philadelphia: W.B. Saunders.

Reproductive Changes

PUBESCENCE

The period of **pubescence (puberty)** is the two-year period that marks the physical changes that accompany the beginning of sexual maturity. Until this adolescent spurt, the gonads and external genitalia grew very slowly. Now the gonads and external genitalia mature, owing to an increased production of sex hormones by the testes in boys and the ovaries in girls, as well as some adrenal cortex hormones in both sexes. All individuals produce both male and female sex hormones, but males produce more testosterone and females produce more estrogens.[1]

Pubescence in Girls. The appearance of pubic hair is the first sign that a young girl is beginning pubescence. This is followed by the beginning of the growth of her breasts, and then the development of hips. Soon after these changes, she will begin to menstruate as her production of female hormones becomes cyclical.[1] The average age of the **menarche,** or the beginning of cyclic menstrual function, is around 12 years. African-American females tend to reach the menarche earlier than whites and develop secondary sexual characteristics earlier.[14] During puberty the ovaries begin to enlarge and will increase in size to about 20 times greater than that at birth. The ovaries will lose their smooth surface and will take on a "cobbled" appearance.[38] Girls will also develop axillary hair.

Pubescence in Boys. When a young boy begins pubescence, his penis and testes increase in size, and he also develops pubic and axillary hair. His voice will become lower and louder due to an enlarged larynx and lengthening of the vocal cords.[1]

Exocrine Glands. Probably one of the most outwardly distressing marks during pubescence is the development of acne if it occurs. During this time, the sweat glands become active or hyperactive and begin secreting fatty substances that may result ultimately in acne as well as an increased body odor. The specialized **apocrine sweat glands** found under the arms and around the genital area are active during this time and respond to emotional stimuli during adolescence. Because adolescents may not be used to perspiration, this may be an additional stressor during this period.

PSYCHOSEXUAL DEVELOPMENT

While adolescents are experiencing major physical developmental changes during puberty, probably the most distressing and yet exciting area for them is their psychosexual development. It is distressing because it may be embarrassing to develop physically "overnight." It is exciting because they now consider themselves on the path to adulthood.

Persons who progress through this phase in a healthy atmosphere and develop healthy sexual attitudes will have a healthy self-image.

It is normal behavior at this stage of development for adolescents to question what is normal and what is not. Masturbation is common at this stage for both boys and girls. Individuals may feel that this is abnormal and question their "normality" and therefore worry about being homosexual.[17] Self-recognition of homosexuality may surface during adolescence; when it does, individuals usually acknowledge this within themselves by the age of 17 years.[41]

PSYCHOSOCIAL DEVELOPMENT

Self-Concept and Self-Image

A major task during adolescence is that of identity formation. From the beginning of adolescence to approximately age 18 years, the individual develops a strong sense of personal identity through experimenting with different roles.[32] During this period, adolescents begin to develop the capacity to be intimate, which is more formally developed during the young adult years (Box 13–1).

PROCESS OF DEVELOPING IDENTITY

The process of developing identity involves interpersonal relatedness. The adolescent's crisis over identity follows the sequential developmental tasks of Erikson up to this point, which are trust, autonomy, initiative, and industry. Identity development during the adolescent years is evolving and includes experiencing love and romance, sexual experimentation, and intense friendships.[30] The strength that emerges in adolescence is the capacity to be intimate. The foundation for interpersonal relatedness was laid in the formative years, and now the adolescent looks to peers for reinforcement of intimacy. If you can remember your adolescent years, you will remember the many conflicts that you experienced. Adolescents are just getting used to their many physical changes related to growth and puberty, and now have to adjust to many social expectations, including dating.

Many stressors are present in dating situations concerning the person's decisions to progress from hand-

---

Box 13–1. Developmental Tasks of Adolescence

► Achieve a stable identity.
► Establish independence.
► Assume adult sex roles.
► Select a vocation or career.

Data from Humphrey, P. (1982). The adolescent. In Hill, P.M., and Humphrey, P. (eds.). *Human growth and development throughout life.* New York: John Wiley and Sons.

holding to kissing, to becoming more intimate. Early dating usually involves groups with boys and girls participating in activities without selecting a specific partner. Once the adolescent feels comfortable with both sexes, "double dating" may be initiated, or the individual may begin dating one person. For the majority of adolescents, dating activities usually revolve around school, sports activities, visits to the local mall, or movies. In economically deprived areas, teens still congregate together and socialize at local establishments. They usually "hang out" in a group with both sexes rather than date as individuals.

The role confusion that adolescents experience is overcome by the identity recognition that results from a healthy environment and is nourished by the family unit. Parents must be supportive to assist the adolescent to establish an identity without being overprotective, which may stifle identity formation.

If adolescents are not successful in their search for identity, identity diffusion results: these individuals will feel self-conscious, doubt themselves, and question their roles in life.[1]

ETHGENDER AND THE DEVELOPMENT OF SELF-CONCEPT

Other factors affect the development of self-concept. One of these additional factors is **ethgender,** which considers the effects of the combination of race and gender. In a study of almost 7000 participants in grades 7 through 12, a question was asked regarding how intelligent individuals felt they were in comparison to others their age.[20] Within each race or ethnic category, the general tendency was for lower perceived intelligence levels for girls than for boys. This study did find that Asian girls had fairly positive estimates of their intelligence. Another finding regarding self-satisfaction was that the white male group was not the most satisfied with self, but the Chicano group was very satisfied with self.[20]

Cognitive and Intellectual Development

STAGE OF FORMAL OPERATIONS

By the time individuals reach adolescence, according to Piagetian theory, they have the ability to reach the stage of formal operations. This is the last stage of cognitive development and the highest level of intellectual functioning. The transition to this stage begins at the age of 11 or 12 years; it takes 3 to 5 years for the adolescent to feel confident and establish a sound sense of self-esteem.

The majority of persons in this stage have developed a sense of time and can think in the past, present, and future.

With the development of formal operational thought, persons can understand symbolic meaning, such as the double meaning of jokes. They can also reason inductively as well as deductively.[23]

Adolescents in this stage are able to think of a particular circumstance and conceive many different consequences that might possibly occur. Thinking is both from the real to the possible and from the possible to the real. The ability to think abstractly means that the individual no longer learns solely from experience but also may learn vicariously. When asked the meaning of the statement: People who live in glass houses shouldn't throw stones, school age children will give a concrete answer, such as, "The window will break." When asked the same question, adolescents may respond, "If you aren't willing to accept criticism, don't offer any."

Because the use of formal operational thought is a new capability, adolescents need practice and reinforcement. Also, because the skill is not perfected, the use of formal operational thought is often situational and may be influenced by the adolescent's emotions. It may not be utilized when a person lacks experience or confidence.[31] We must not assume that all adolescents use formal operational thought all the time.

DEVELOPMENT OF EGOCENTRISM

Piaget also recognized that adolescence is one of three periods in which egocentrism is being developed.[1] Persons at this stage feel that everyone is looking at them, listening to them, and paying attention to what they believe in. Adolescents are very idealistic and feel that others agree with them. They may have difficulty with those in authority or with peers who criticize them. Eventually, this **egocentricity** of adolescence is taken over by the reasoning process as a component of formal operational thought.

Relationships and Roles

ASSUMING THE ADULT ROLE

One of the developmental tasks that the adolescent accomplishes while progressing to young adulthood is the assumption of adult roles. Adolescents experiment with clothing, hair, and, for girls, makeup, to adopt the adult role. Although their appearance may appear outrageous to some, it is all a part of the process of trying out adult roles.[14] The peer group will also influence the choice of clothing and mannerisms.

Adolescents may also experiment with jobs during this time and "job hop" from one place to another. Teenagers are exposed to a variety of roles and interact in a variety of settings with many different individuals. Not only are their communication skills enhanced but they also have an awareness of many different job positions and responsibilities.

FAMILY RELATIONSHIPS

Fewer than half the children born today will reach the age of 18 having lived continuously with both parents. This affects the adolescent's relationships with everyone he or she comes in contact with. In almost every family relationship, regardless of the makeup of the family, teenagers seem to question all authority as a "rite of passage." Even when adolescents seem to agree internally with the rules, it is almost expected that they will argue with those in authority. At times the person behaves in an adult manner and accepts responsibility, and at other times acts like a child. While this is very confusing for parents, it is also disturbing to the adolescents themselves. This identity crisis that faces all teens results in their struggle to assert themselves and progress to becoming persons with their own identity.

PEER RELATIONSHIPS

Friendships play an important role in an adolescent's life. Having friends means that teenagers are accepted, liked, and respected for who they are. The adolescent's identity and self-concept are tested and influenced through these social interactions.[31] Peer groups provide support for adolescents in their search for identity. The advent of formal operational thought allows the adolescent to see situations from the other's perspective. Achieving this perspective leads to the development of social responsibility.[31] The adolescent's social status with peers has both immediate and long-term effects. By fostering positive relationships with peers, the adolescent's self-image will be enhanced.

Peer groups may focus around common interests, such as skateboarding, tennis teams, or church groups. They may be solely a result of physical location and encompass neighborhood groups.

Adolescents at this age may also be influenced by peer pressure: when one group member begins to smoke or experiment with drugs or alcohol, others in the group may follow suit. Not until teenagers have developed their own identity do they have the ability to assert their own independence and step away from this type of peer group pressure.

Peers also play an important role in the social educational process of one another. Many teenagers are reluctant to discuss issues with parents related to smoking and sexual concerns like wet dreams. They turn to their peers or get information wherever they can — movies, television, or magazines. Information may be accurate or inaccurate, but adolescents have such a quest for answers that they often believe what they see, hear, or read.

COMMUNITY ROLES

First Job. Adolescents work for a variety of reasons. Certainly they enjoy the extra money that is earned, but also they obtain satisfaction from earning it themselves. Employment is also seen as part of the transition from school to "real life" employment. It offers both discipline and responsibility and provides social experiences outside the home or school. During the academic year, many seniors work 20 hours per week.[11] For some adolescents, work is not a choice: they work for the added income that helps their family survive.

In a study of 1105 adolescents, 83 per cent had a job outside the home at least once a week for pay. The majority obtained their first job at the age of 12 years or younger. Gender differences related to when individuals started to work did not exist.[22]

Volunteer Work. Parents can help adolescents assume social responsibility by encouraging their children to get involved in some type of volunteer work, either through church, school, or community agencies. This may also assist in helping the person through the egocentricity that is apparent in adolescence.

VALUES AND BELIEFS

Moral Development

An important task during the adolescent years is the development of a personal value system. With the development of formal operational thought, the adolescent is now able to consider moral issues in a more progressive, sophisticated manner. According to Kohlberg's developmental stages of moral judgment, after the age of 10 years persons change their way of thinking regarding moral situations and progress through several stages of moral development (see Table 12–5 in Chapter 12.)[18]

In early adolescence, the majority of teenagers are in the stage of reciprocity, which is stage two in the first level of preconventional thinking. Adolescents at this stage will return favors because it is expected of them, and they will also expect a favor in the future. Stage two is mainly a stage of self-interest. The next level is the Conventional Level of Moral Reasoning, and stage three signifies approval and harmony. At this stage, persons do what is "expected" of them as a member of a group. Maintaining the expectations of that group takes precedence regardless of the consequences of their actions. They are trying to maintain their reputation of being "one of the crowd." If adolescents at this stage in their development get in with the wrong crowd, they will display behavior that is expected of them from their group members, regardless of the outcome.

When exploring choices to take in moral dilemmas, gender differences continue to exist. Boys are more likely than girls to focus on self, whereas girls are more likely to focus on relationships.[16]

Spiritual Values

Many religions recognize the transition from childhood to adulthood with rites of confirmation, such as the Jewish faith with bar mitzvahs and bat mitzvahs.[1] It is common at this stage of development for adolescents to seek out and explore different varieties of the spiritual experience.[31]

Box 13–2. Leading Causes of Death in Adolescence

1. Automobile accidents
2. Suicide*
3. Homicide*
4. Poisonings
5. Drownings

*Some authorities interchange #2 and #3.

MAJOR HEALTH CONCERNS

Adolescents are at high risk for many health problems that can lead to death or illness. Box 13–2 lists the leading causes of death, and Box 13–3 lists leading causes of illness in adolescents.

Pregnancy

Teenage pregnancy is one of the major school health problems in the United States today.[29]

Because adolescence is a normal developmental crisis and pregnancy is a situational crisis, the psychologic stress is compounded when these two crises are combined.[14] Many factors contribute to an unplanned pregnancy. Peer pressure to engage in intercourse when not prepared or an inadequate sex education may result in a pregnancy. Other potential factors prior to pregnancy include:

▶ Girls have a significant psychosocial difficulty, such as occurs at school or in family relationships.
▶ Students experience difficulty in school, and many repeat grades.
▶ The teen's parents experience marital problems.
▶ Family communications are strained.
▶ The teens have prior experience with someone being pregnant — either their parents, a sibling, or a friend.
▶ Family violence is common.
▶ Drug and alcohol abuse within the family is a common thread.

Box 13–3. Leading Causes of Illness in Adolescence

▶ Illness related to trauma
▶ Mental health problems (depression and substance abuse)
▶ Sexually transmitted diseases
▶ AIDS
▶ Eating disorders

▶ They have known and dated the father of the baby for at least a year.[6,29]

School health programs need to focus on both prevention and intervention related to teen pregnancies. Prevention needs to be focused on all adolescents, not only those who are at risk, whereas interventions can be focused on pregnant adolescents.

When a teenager becomes pregnant, it seems that in most cases the father of the baby is "out of the picture." However, adolescent fathers can provide emotional and social support for the adolescent mother and the baby that her parents may not be able to offer. One study found that two thirds of adolescent fathers were very supportive and still involved with pregnant teens both during and after the delivery.[6] The adolescent father is going through many of the same dilemmas that the mother is going through and cannot be ignored. Health professionals need to include the fathers in counseling sessions and assist the boys in assuming as much responsibility as they are willing to accept.

Substance Abuse

Adolescence is a time of experimentation with life. It follows that sometimes teenagers will also experiment with alcohol, marijuana, other more potent inhalants, or even mood-altering oral medications as well as injectable medications.

In the United States, the percentage of high school seniors who have tried alcohol has gradually tended to decrease from 93.2 per cent in 1980 to 89.5 per cent in 1990. The percentage trying marijuana decreased from 60.3 per cent to 40.7 per cent during these same years. Inhalant experimentation rose from 11.9 per cent to 18.0 per cent in the same student group between 1980 and 1990.[13]

Adolescents experiment with alcohol and drugs for many reasons. They may feel insecure or anxious, and drugs give them confidence by releasing some inhibitions. Others may feel more mature by engaging in "adult" behaviors or may be rebelling against their parents. While many parents feel that using a substance once is considered an experiment, we know that "once" with some of these substances can kill. Many famous actors and actresses are now appealing to youths to discourage experimenting with crack cocaine even once. Drug abuse by minors may be a sign of some deeper psychologic disturbance and should be identified as soon as possible so treatment options can be explored.

In a study of 654 male high school students that examined the relationship of shyness and sociability to use of illicit substances, it was found that shy male adolescents were significantly more likely to use illicit substances compared with those who were not shy.[28]

Acquired Immune Deficiency Syndrome (AIDS) and Sexually Transmitted Diseases (STDs)

Because adolescents experiment with sex and drugs and may engage in high-risk behaviors, they are at risk for exposure to a viral infection resulting in the acquired immune deficiency syndrome (AIDS) as well as other sexually transmitted diseases (STDs). About 21 per cent of young adults diagnosed with AIDS were infected when they were teenagers.[15] In a Planned Parenthood poll, 57 per cent of teenagers admitted to having sexual intercourse by the age of 17 years. However, when asked about the use of condoms, only 47 per cent of the boys and 25 per cent of the girls reported using them.[12]

Because of adolescents' feelings that AIDS and STDs "happen to other people" and they are therefore "exempt," the majority of adolescents do not take precautionary measures when engaging in sexual activities.

When adolescents are asked regarding the use of condoms, they state that they may use them to avoid pregnancy without any thought that they may also prevent the AIDS virus and STDs.

Eating Disorders

Anorexia nervosa and bulimia nervosa are two eating disorders that have many things in common and may first occur in adolescence. Teenagers with either disorder have an intense fear of being fat, are not satisfied with their physical appearance, and feel that thinness is associated with happiness.

Anorexia Nervosa. Adolescents with anorexia nervosa look into a mirror and see a fat person. They then begin to diet, feeling that this is how they can control their bodies. Dieting becomes an obsession. Prior to this condition, most of these individuals were seen as having been responsible and successful. Once the disorder emerges, they become obsessed. They are angry at others for not accepting their choices in diet habits and become almost hostile. Many of these adolescents have a family history of eating disorders and substance abuse.[24] The majority of anorectics are teenage girls.[1]

Bulimia Nervosa. Clients with bulimia nervosa go on binges. They eat whatever they can get their hands on, usually in secret. Then they feel guilty about the possible weight gain and try to purge their bodies by forcing themselves to vomit. In addition to the family problems associated with anorexia, these adolescents seem to be more isolated and to have more special meanings attached to food and eating.[24]

Tobacco Use

The use of smokeless tobacco, such as snuff and chewing tobacco, has increased in schools. This may be due to the role modeling of baseball heroes. In addition, many teenagers prefer smokeless tobacco to smoking because they think it is safer than smoking cigarettes. While an increased risk of oral cancer has been documented from the use of both forms of tobacco—cigarettes as well as smokeless tobacco—many other health risks are present. These range from dental caries to the low-birthweight infants whose mothers used any tobacco products during pregnancy.[3] Adolescents need to be educated regarding the risks of tooth decay, lip cancer, and effects to unborn babies, to mention a few hazardous consequences of using tobacco products. Ideally, adolescents should be educated regarding these issues before they use them for the first time, thus avoiding addiction, if possible.

Depression and Suicide

There is a known link between depression and suicide.

In a study using the Beck Depression Inventory of 366 "normal" high school students between the ages of 13 and 19 years, 31 per cent were mildly to clinically depressed.[9]

In this study there were no gender differences among the early adolescent group. In the middle adolescent group, more girls than boys were mildly and clinically depressed.[9] Another study found that half of the 80 students in the sample had an average depression score that was equivalent to a clinical population with mild depression.[4] The majority of adolescents who attempt suicide are not receiving inpatient psychiatric treatment.[39] Depression must be identified and treated, because these teenagers are out there just waiting to "explode" (Figure 13–1).

Although more teenage girls attempt suicide than boys, boys are more successful at succeeding. This is probably related to the fact that boys choose violent means when attempting suicide while teenage girls tend to use an overdose of drugs.[19]

ROLE OF THE NURSE

Health Screening and Assessment

DEPRESSION

When you are performing an assessment, one area of concern that you should discuss with adolescents is depression. Depression is the most common characteristic of those who attempt or succeed in committing suicide. As a nurse, you should ask all adolescents undergoing a complete health assessment whether they have ever been depressed or had thoughts of suicide. Sometimes teenagers are relieved to have someone broach the subject and welcome the opportunity to talk about their feelings; they did not feel comfortable bringing up the subject themselves.

Depressed adolescents are vulnerable, have a sense of hopelessness and despair, and have decreased

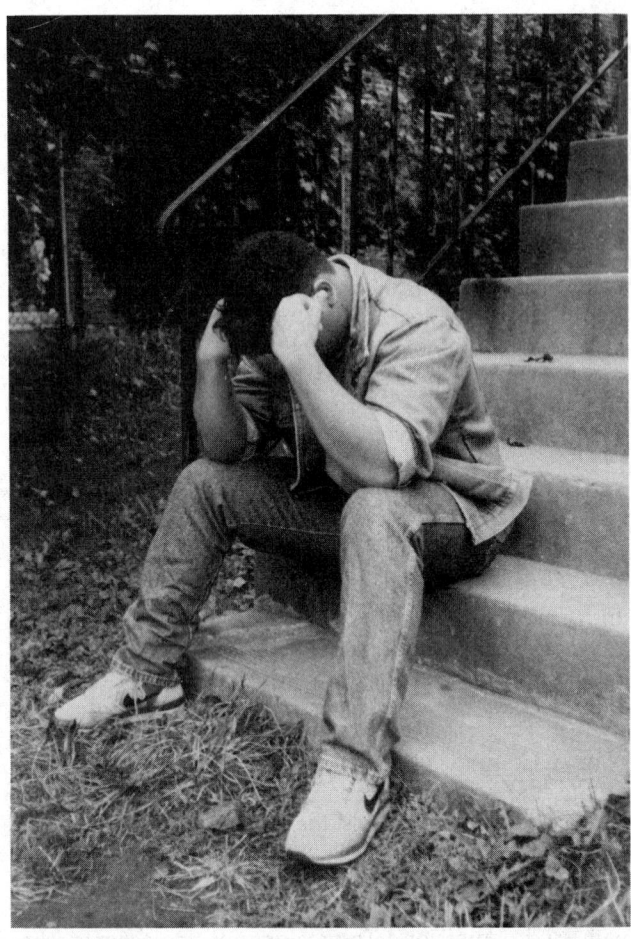

▲ *Figure 13–1*

Depression is a leading problem in adolescence.

adaptive coping mechanisms to deal with everyday stressors. Some of the signs that may indicate thoughts of suicide include

▶ an unusual degree of withdrawal
▶ severe hopelessness
▶ talk of death
▶ an increase in substance abuse
▶ giving away personal belongings
▶ sudden cheerfulness in a previously depressed person[14]

Depression is usually developed over a period of time and not as the result of one particular situation.[44] A risk assessment tool that will identify depression might be utilized with adolescents to prevent suicide attempts. If teens at high risk for suicide are identified, you can make a concerted effort to initiate preventive strategies. Screening and prevention programs that identify and deal with depression will improve the adolescent's development of coping strategies for dealing with perceived hopeless situations. You can refer the teen to a counseling center that will assist in identifying the adolescent's strengths and weaknesses. Both the client and health professional can then work on a treatment plan. The ultimate goal is that of improving

the adolescent's chance of making it to young adulthood.

HIGH-RISK SEXUAL BEHAVIORS

Another area of concern that needs to be addressed during your initial screening and assessment of adolescents is in the area of safe sex. This topic needs to be explored with adolescents whether or not they are currently engaged in sexual activity. With adolescents becoming sexually active at an earlier age, habits regarding condom use need to be developed so that they become routine and expected behaviors. While not condoning their behavior, you do need to discuss the use of condoms with all teenagers you come in contact with. STDs are approaching epidemic proportions and need to be eliminated.

One in seven teenagers has had a sexually transmitted disease.[2]

The four most prevalent and problematic of these are gonorrhea, syphilis, urethritis, and herpes simplex Type II. Education is the key to prevention, but if teenagers suspect that they may have a sexually transmitted disease, they need to know where they can be diagnosed and treated in a confidential manner. Confidentiality needs to be stressed so that if teenagers suspect possible exposure they are aware that they can receive treatment without permission of their parents. You would want to encourage them to discuss this with their parents, but they must know that this is their choice.

Health Education

ANTICIPATORY GUIDANCE

When adolescents enter the health care system, the first person they usually encounter is a nurse. You, as the nurse, may have the opportunity to do a complete health history and physical on these clients or only talk to them for a moment. Anticipatory guidance is essential to help prepare adolescents and their families for life events that will occur during this period. Discussions should include physical as well as psychologic changes that are taking place. Topics may include sexual concerns, smoking, drug use, stress, depression, and others. Healthy habits related to nutrition and exercise also need to be addressed, as well as the prevention of accidents through the use of seat belts, helmets, and so on.

PROMOTING GOOD NUTRITION

Dietary Habits and Adolescent Growth. Adolescents' food habits are influenced by peers, families, the media, and other psychosocial factors. A challenge exists for health professionals to take all these into consideration when counseling individuals about their dietary habits. With the growth spurt that adolescents experience comes an increased need for energy in the

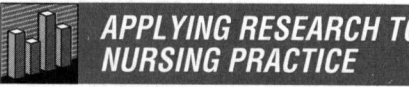

Pletsch, P.K., Johnson, M.K., Tosi, C.B., Thurston, C.A., & Riesch, S.K. (1991). Self-image among early adolescents: revisited. *Journal of Community Health Nursing, 8*(4), 215–231.

▼▼▼

APPLYING RESEARCH TO NURSING PRACTICE

Promoting Self-Esteem in Early Teens

Community health nurses and school nurses often work with early adolescents who are in the process of accomplishing a tremendous number of developmental tasks. These nurses may provide counseling to early adolescents to assist them in the psychologic, physical, cognitive, and social transitions needed for progression to full adolescence. During this transition, some aspects of self-image may be threatened.

The investigators sought information that would assist nurses in planning for the health and developmental needs of middle school children and their families. Responding to a questionnaire that measured 12 different aspects of self-image, nonwhite students scored higher than white students only in the areas of *body self-image* and *family relationships*. Of 349 middle school students, girls scored higher than boys in only one area, that of *educational goals*. In contrast, boys' scores were higher for all other areas of self-image, including *mastery of the external world, impulse control*, and *social relationships*.

Applications for Practice

In spite of progress toward gender and socioeconomic equality, girls still need help in developing a sense of pride and a sense of celebration about their maturing bodies, so that their self-image can continue to flourish. Community health and school nurses should assess the developmental needs of early adolescent girls and incorporate interventions that promote female self-image. For example, the greater emphasis girls placed on educational goals can be reinforced by organizing career days and discussions with female professionals from the community. Special support is needed for early teens from African-American, Asian, Hispanic, and Native American cultural backgrounds.

form of nutrients. Dietary habits are extremely important at this stage because they influence future patterns of eating. Adolescents' complexions may be affected, which in turn may affect their self-image. Weight gain at this point may be extremely hard to reduce in the future if the adolescent is not engaged in some type of strenuous activity.

In a study of 160 15-year-old girls, it was found that breakfast was the meal most often missed.[25]

Need for Acceptance and the Development of Eating Disorders. The need for acceptance by others is very strong during adolescence. While many teenagers are relatively well-nourished and in good health, others become preoccupied with their self-image. Be-

cause of media concentration on thin, blue-eyed blondes, teenagers that do not fit this stereotype may experience a lowered self-esteem and try to correct their perceptions of themselves with an eating disorder. You need to begin educating them on what anorexia nervosa and bulimia nervosa mean and what the effects of starvation or poor dieting are on their physiologic and psychologic well-being.

Teenagers may seem knowledgeable regarding nutrition, yet their perception of themselves interferes with proper eating habits. If an adolescent will keep a diary of foods eaten during the day, the activities engaged in, and the feelings at the time, you will be able to put together a picture of why the individual eats what and when. Sitting together discussing this might give the adolescent some insight about the behavior.[24] Because of the psychologic makeup of teenagers with eating disorders, you almost become a confidant and must know when to refer clients for professional help.

Dietary Deficiencies During Adolescence. Calcium and iron are two of the common elements deficient in adolescent diets. Foods that are high in these need to be encouraged and made a part of the daily routine. Supplemental calcium and iron could be taken, but a healthy diet that includes recommended daily requirements should suffice. A protein deficiency may exist along with an iron deficiency because the teenager may be drinking sodas instead of milk and replacing meals with snacks.

Dietary Teaching. When you have the opportunity to do some diet instruction with teenagers, you'll want to discuss the importance of developing good eating habits. Since teens often frequent fast-food restaurants, you might also include a discussion about which entrées at each one may include healthy food. It would also be the perfect time to talk about the high caffeine content of many carbonated beverages. During this discussion, you might share the daily nutritional requirements, which include:

▶ 2800 calories for males
▶ 2200 calories for females
▶ 45 to 60 grams of protein
▶ 1200 mg of calcium
▶ 4000 to 5000 IU of vitamin A
▶ 50 to 60 mg of vitamin C
▶ 400 IU of vitamin D
▶ 18 mg of iron[8]

PROMOTING ACTIVITY AND EXERCISE

During adolescence, teens are susceptible to multiple injuries resulting from sports activities, because their musculoskeletal systems are not fully developed. Injuries also occur at a more frequent rate during this period, because the person may be uncoordinated owing to an increased skeletal growth with a temporary lag in the development of muscle growth. The two most common types of injuries are acute injuries involving sprains and strains and injuries resulting in an overuse syndrome.[14] As a nurse, you can be very effective in preventing these injuries, or at least recognizing the syndromes early enough to prevent further damage to the musculoskeletal system.

You can do several things to prevent acute injuries. First, make sure that the adolescent athlete has been physically cleared to participate in sports activities and that participation will not aggravate a preexisting organic problem. The second thing is to emphasize proper stretching and warm-up exercises prior to sports activities. Proper conditioning cannot be overemphasized.

Overuse syndromes result when the adolescent athlete participates in excessive activities without proper conditioning. The person will usually stop the activity when pain occurs and by doing so will prevent the possibility of damage to the musculoskeletal system. Resumption of physical activity should be gradual, and a conditioning program should be suggested.

DISCOURAGING SUBSTANCE ABUSE

Research has shown that shy males may turn to psychoactive substances to alleviate their discomfort in social situations. If health professionals recognize and treat shyness, future problems with drugs may be prevented. This is not to say that shyness is "abnormal," but it should be examined in a social context. Drug treatment programs could also emphasize the development of social skills and incorporate strategies that will focus on these personality factors.[28]

Many adolescents need to confide in someone. You may be a "sounding board" because you are an uninvolved third party. As the nurse, you need to encourage open lines of communication between parents and teens and stress the need for active listening. Unless your role is one of counseling, you need to recognize when to refer teens and parents for family counseling.

PROMOTING AIDS PREVENTION AND PROMOTING SAFE SEX

In a recent study conducted with students in an urban high school, students stated that schools became the major source of learning about AIDS. A pretest was administered one month prior to instruction, with a posttest given one week following teaching. Before the instruction was received regarding knowledge about AIDS, only one half the students felt that schools were a source of learning about AIDS.[21]

Until an AIDS vaccine or cure becomes available, the best strategy to prevent the spread of HIV infection is prevention. Prevention can best be accomplished through education. Schools are probably the major source of information about AIDS. Instruction should include basic information, fallacies, and myths about AIDS, as well as individual attitudes and beliefs regarding persons with AIDS. Universal precautions should be stressed, then several situations could be presented for student discussion about how they would handle them. Adolescents' knowledge regarding the disease, as well as behavior and attitudes, needs to be addressed at this

age so that these persons do not grow up to become "ignorant adults at risk for AIDS."[21]

There is a great need for health education about sexually transmitted diseases (discussed in the health screening section). Teenagers are usually afraid to discuss fears of possibly being infected with the AIDS virus or STDs with peers and certainly parents. A teenager who suspects possible exposure to someone with the AIDS virus needs to know how to proceed in getting confidentially tested.

Teens need to be informed about the early symptoms of sexually transmitted diseases. These usually include a discharge from the vagina or penis or a lesion in the genital area. This is also an opportunity to discuss ways to protect themselves, which include abstinence from sex, making informed choices about partners, and safer sexual practices.[9] While most teenagers are aware of condoms and their use in preventing the spread of AIDS and STDs, few are aware of the proper technique of applying them (Figure 13–2). This is a perfect opportunity to demonstrate the application of a condom, either with an anatomic model of a penis or with a banana.

PROMOTING RESPONSIBLE PARENTING

Although teenagers in America are not more sexually active than those in comparable nations, adolescent pregnancy has reached epidemic proportions, with approximately one of ten teenagers becoming pregnant.[40] Two computer games have been developed that simulate life experiences, designed to foster more responsible reproductive attitudes. Each game gives adolescents a chance to make important choices without suffering the consequences of making the wrong choice. *Baby Game* is an interactive computer game that simulates

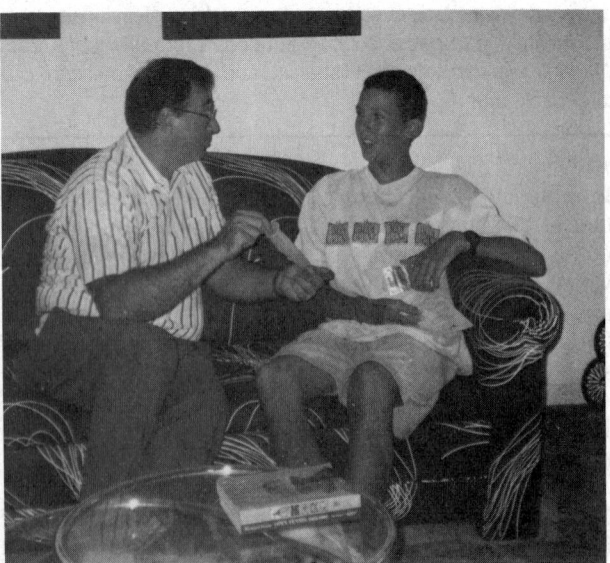

▲ *Figure 13–2*

Safe sex and proper application of condoms should be an open topic of conversation.

parenting responsibilities, and *Romance* is a game that simulates responsible choices regarding sex and contraception.[40]

Whenever a teenager is having either a thorough assessment or simply completing a physical form, a nonjudgmental sexual history should be included. This matter-of-fact attitude may show the adolescent that concerns and questions regarding sex are normal, that you are not shocked, and that you are willing to discuss whatever is bothering the individual.

Adolescents need to be knowledgeable about the available methods of contraception. Certainly abstinence needs to be mentioned first, with its 100 per cent success rate in preventing pregnancy! You may also want to discuss briefly the rhythm method, diaphragms, cervical caps, condoms, chemical contraceptives, and the oral contraceptive (the pill) for females. You would want to recommend to female adolescents that if they are sexually active or considering it, they should have an initial gynecologic examination and discuss contraceptives with the nurse practitioner or physician.

If the atmosphere for this very confidential personal matter is conducive, the adolescent may feel comfortable in discussing this information with you; other similar personal topics may come up that might have an impact on the teenagers' health practices.

PROMOTING SAFETY

Encouraging Seat Belt Use

In a study of 541 minority adolescents with an average age of 15 years, seat belt use was reported by almost half the individuals and no use or intermittent use was reported by slightly more than half. Those adolescents who did not use seat belts or used them intermittently were significantly more depressed, had family problems and problems in school, and in general felt dissatisfied with their lives.[36]

Nurses can play a pivotal role in preventing or lessening injuries as a result of accidents that occur during adolescence. Automobile accidents are the leading cause of death during this period. In all encounters with adolescents and parents, you should stress the importance of wearing seat belts. Acting as role models and wearing them ourselves is the very least we should do. Although it is seldom helpful to "preach" to teenagers, we can help prevent drinking and driving through promotion of responsible driving behaviors, such as supporting Students Against Drunk Drivers (SADD), encouraging "designated drivers," and promoting other such programs for teens.

Encouraging Helmet Use. Adolescents who drive dirt bikes and motorcycles need to be encouraged to wear helmets. Most accidents involving these vehicles result in serious head injuries in persons who choose not to wear helmets. Many accidents are caused or intensified by the adolescent's use of alcohol or drugs prior to the accident. Most students have seen movies in school related to the effects of driving while drinking. We

need to reinforce to parents and peers the necessity of confiscating adolescents' car or motorcycle keys if they are under the influence of alcohol or drugs.

Encouraging Safe Diving. Head and spinal cord injuries causing death or permanent disability occur every year to adolescents who dive into shallow water and strike their heads on the bottom. Water safety classes need to stress the importance of assessing the depth of any water before persons dive into pools or lakes. Injuries to the head and neck also occur when teenagers run into the ocean, dive into waves, and strike their heads on the sandy bottom. This practice needs to be discouraged. The phrase *feet first* was originated to remind persons to avoid diving into unknown waters.

Promoting Responsible Handling of Weapons. Hand guns or other weapons in a household need to be kept in a locked drawer, or else the proper handling of them should be demonstrated to children before adolescence. Death and severe injuries may occur when adolescents find weapons in the home and pretend to use them on friends without realizing that they are actually loaded. We all should assume that all weapons are loaded and handle them accordingly.

PROMOTING SELF-CARE

The need for health promotion programs geared to adolescents is of prime importance because teenagers are formalizing behavioral decisions and practices that will influence their health habits the rest of their life. We must exhort all clients to assume more responsibility for their own health choices and decisions. Programs involving adolescents need to emphasize skills that promote psychologic as well as social growth.[31] Not all adolescents have achieved mature abstract thinking; they often believe they are infallible or invulnerable. Therefore education is of primary importance to this age group.

Peer education is probably the most effective means for imparting information to teenagers. Education by peers has the greatest impact on adolescents, since they accept other teenagers as role models and try to emulate those they admire and respect. Adolescent support groups can capitalize on the teenagers' tendency to seek out peers for information.

Unfortunately, sometimes the information they receive is incorrect. One way to circumvent this problem is to have nurses screen individuals and educate motivated adolescents who could assist with teaching their peers. A health promotion program would then have the advantage of both the knowledge of the nurse and the effectiveness of peer teaching.[10] Educational programs that focus on psychologic as well as social skills seem to enforce health-enhancing lifestyles by adolescents. With promotion of adolescent wellness, the vulnerability to the psychosocial factors that assist in the adoption of health-compromising behaviors can be reduced.

When persons feel good about themselves and care for themselves as persons, they are more interested in taking care of their bodies and taking responsibility for their own well-being. These are the adolescents who will use seat belts, keep dental appointments, use condoms. By instilling self-pride and self-responsibility in adolescents, nurses hope they will grow up to be responsible adults and influence their peers.

▼ EARLY ADULTHOOD

PHYSICAL DEVELOPMENT AND CHANGE

Musculoskeletal System

By young adulthood, persons have reached their mature skeletal size, with the exception of weight and muscle mass. The skeletal growth is accomplished with the completion of calcified epiphyseal lines that prevent any further skeletal growth. This may be as early as the midteens or as late as the early twenties. However, weight and muscle mass may fluctuate greatly throughout a person's life, depending on diet and exercise.

During young adulthood, persons are at their peak functioning level for most of the body systems.

▶ Muscle tone and strength peak between ages 20 and 30 years.
▶ Cardiovascular system peaks around age 20 years.
▶ The brain continues its developmental process until age 25 years.
▶ Visual acuity peaks around age 20 years.
▶ Hearing acuity peaks in adolescence.
▶ Male libido peaks between ages 15 and 20 years.
▶ Female libido peaks between ages 26 and 40.[1,27]

Reproductive System

Attaining the capacity for reproduction is one of the most complex and creative tasks of any species. For young adults, having children may be the first confrontation with an adult role and adult responsibilities. The reproductive systems of both men and women are fully mature by their twenties, and these are the best years for reproducing offspring.[1] However, some young couples may choose to delay pregnancy and child rearing until their careers are established.

PSYCHOSEXUAL DEVELOPMENT

Although the sex drive peaks in men between the ages of 15 and 20 years, for women the peak is between 26 and 40 years.[27] A teenager may have been sexually intimate during adolescence, but usually not until the individual is a young adult can a sexual commitment to one other person be made. At this age, the young adult is usually aware of both the emotional and financial responsibilities involved in either the commitment to a relationship or a beginning family.

PSYCHOSOCIAL DEVELOPMENT

Self-Concept and Self-Image

Erikson's theory of psychosocial development views *intimacy* as the young adult's developmental task that follows the adolescent's task of identity development (Box 13–4). Both identity and intimacy continue to develop and mature during the stage of young adulthood. Young adults view intimacy as relating closely to others and not strictly as sexual relationships. The young adult reaches out to make a personal commitment to another person.[1] Intimacy encompasses cognitive, affective, and behavioral components and applies to all types of relationships, whether friendships or those involving sexual relationships.[30]

Cognitively, young adults can begin to know the other, to enter that person's world and see things from the other's view. Affectively, they begin to experience empathy and can appreciate what the other is feeling. In behavior, young adults experience romantic and physical relationships and can begin making a commitment to another.[30]

Cognitive and Intellectual Development

Brain development continues into the twenties. Creativity and productivity probably reach their peak in young adulthood.[27] Most young adults reached the capacity for formal operational thought during their adolescent years. Now is the time for them to practice and reinforce operational thought in adult situations. Achievement motivation encompasses the need to learn and do well. The young adult combines cognitive ability with achievement motivation when determining formal educational programs and career goals.

Relationships and Roles

FAMILY RELATIONSHIPS

Young adulthood implies maturity; often persons question whether they feel competent to make "adult" decisions. Often young adults state that they would like to be back in the childhood role and have decisions made for them so they don't have to accept the responsibility of making wrong choices. If a wrong choice is made, they would then have the luxury of blaming the person who made the choice for them, rather than assuming responsibility for self.

Box 13–4. Developmental Tasks of Early Adulthood

▶ Begin an occupation
▶ Select a mate and establish a relationship
▶ Start a family
▶ Raise children
▶ Manage a home

As young adults become more mature, more distance is placed between them and their **family of origin** (the family into which a person is born)—both cognitive distance as well as possible geographic distance. They depend less on their parents regarding many decisions. In addition, young adults depend less on their parents for financial and emotional needs. As they mature, they accept responsibility for themselves in all aspects. As part of maturity, they recognize that they must first care for themselves completely before they can assume care for others.

MAKING A COMMITMENT

The decision to marry or cohabit is usually given much thought in young adulthood. Parental pressures to marry are less than they were a decade ago, and many young couples are living together to try to understand the level of commitment that a long-term relationship might command.

Marriage is a universal concept in all societies. There are many reasons for deciding to marry, which include

▶ love
▶ companionship, support
▶ a sexual partner
▶ to meet others' expectations
▶ to have children
▶ economic security
▶ prestige[27]

PARENTING

Deciding to become parents usually depends on whether or not the young adults have accomplished their developmental tasks. Pregnancy and parenthood also depend on adequate physical, psychologic, and social development that allows the couple to deal with the requirements of this developmental period. Having children outside of marriage is not as taboo as it once was. When young women get pregnant today, they have many choices. It is not unusual for a young woman to choose to raise her child alone and not be disowned by her parents, as might have happened years ago.

However, with the increase in education available regarding birth control measures, most young adults plan for parenthood, and it is a joyous occasion. With the addition of a baby in the relationship, the couple now becomes a family that takes on its own growth and development. Children place a stress on the marriage and a strong foundation should exist prior to having children. Many young adults feel that children will help bind the marriage together, without understanding the additional stressors that will be present. Deciding to become parents takes a commitment from both potential parents and a willingness to share and openly discuss decisions related to family matters. Persons caught up in thinking about a baby may not have considered the economic responsibility that accompanies childbirth and parenting. Although providing specific advice about financial matters is not a nursing responsibility, an open discussion of infants' needs may lead to a dialogue about economic responsibility that had not been addressed before.

COMMUNITY ROLES

Young adults today are very much aware of global environmental concerns, and many respond by becoming active in community organizations that address global caring. Recycling is becoming commonplace and expected. Young adults feel a social responsibility to maintain the environment for future generations.

Almost half of all adults (more than a 23 per cent increase in a two-year period) volunteer their time to charitable organizations. Volunteering gives added meaning to life and seems to help adults appreciate what they have more.[5] Charitable organizations are also social groups that enable persons to meet others with common interests, as well as to work toward worthwhile organizational objectives. Some social service organizations are Big Brothers–Big Sisters, American Red Cross, Lions Club, Junior League, and Jaycees.

CAREERS

The career choice of young adults may be influenced by peers, parents, teachers, or personal experiences. Young adults may be concerned mainly with income, or with the prestige of a certain profession or job. It is unfortunate that a person must choose a career or start on an educational path while still so young and lacking in experience in a particular field that they do not know all the pros and cons. While young adults are making career choices, they should be exposed to other individuals in their choice of career who might guide them and give them honest input about the benefits and pitfalls of their life's work.

Persons at the age of 18 years might consider the military as a career. When you encounter young adults who have not made a career choice, you might recommend that they approach each branch of the service. Several career aptitude tests might determine hidden potential and interests. One of the services might offer some schooling in that identified area and offer to send the person to their desired geographical location.

It is an economic reality that the majority of families today are two-income families, and family togetherness has become relegated to weekends. Many young adults today are rediscovering the joys of home life, basic values, and family togetherness. There seems to be a shift to pursuing a simpler life with deeper meaning.[5] Even though it represents loss of income, many young mothers are choosing to work only part-time, are working in the home, or are participating in a job-sharing program in which two individuals fill one full-time job position. Just as some women find great satisfaction in a career outside the home, some fathers are choosing to remain at home and are finding much satisfaction in caring for the children.

SOCIAL AND LEISURE TIME

More young adults than ever before are participating in leisure and sports activities. Some reasons for spending time in these activities include

- awareness of benefits of exercise
- motivation for personal fitness
- release of stress, anxiety
- an additional outlet for making personal and professional contacts

Many activities are structured, such as participation on a tennis team, in aerobic classes, and so on. Other unstructured activities, such as bicycling, gardening, swimming, and walking, accomplish the same results.

VALUES AND BELIEFS

Moral Development

As persons encounter and discuss more situations and dilemmas in their personal, social, and moral life, they progress sequentially through Kohlberg's stages of moral development. Individuals can comprehend reasoning at one stage higher than their own. Because of this, persons can integrate arguments and reasoning from others into their being and thus progress to the next stage of moral reasoning.[18] The majority of adults reason at the conventional level, which emphasizes doing what is expected and maintaining the social order of the community.

Some young adults, however, progress to higher stages of moral reasoning and use principled thinking at the Postconventional Level in their decision making related to ethical, personal, or moral dilemmas. Persons at this level rely on principles such as autonomy, beneficence, justice, dignity, and fidelity in arriving at decisions for difficult dilemmas, rather than being influenced by others.

Spiritual Values

A study of 1960 young adults found that spiritual/religious values were positively correlated with community service.[37]

When young adults move away from their parents, they typically change their attendance habits related to church activities. Whether it is because of disinterest, rebellion, or a change in values is not clear. After the person has asserted his or her independence and established a routine, by the late twenties there is often a renewed interest in religion.[27] One study of almost 17,000 young adults found that although there was a decline in the attendance at formal religious services, there was no decline in the importance of religion to individuals.[33]

MAJOR HEALTH CONCERNS

Major health concerns in early adulthood focus on prevention of the leading causes of death (Box 13–5) and illness (Box 13–6).

Box 13–5. Leading Causes of Death in Early Adulthood
1. Accidents 2. Cancer 3. Heart disease

Lifestyle

ALCOHOL USE

Alcohol remains the number one drug in the country today.

Alcohol abuse exceeds the amount of abuse of all other drugs.[1] Now that young adults are of legal drinking age and it is accepted as a social custom, some persons at first will experiment with the freedom of drinking. They may arrange to meet at Happy Hour or for a drink after work as part of their new social life. With the many other responsibilities that young adults face, this will be a phase that most go through. Some, however, may develop a drinking problem that will surface later.

USE OF OTHER "RECREATIONAL" DRUGS

The freedom of young adulthood, along with the stress and pressures of feeling the need to be productive, may cause some individuals to experiment with drugs either for the first time or as a carryover from adolescence. Marijuana is the most commonly used illegal drug, although in some states it is now legal to use it and to possess it in small quantities for personal use.[1] Persons who are against the legalization of marijuana feel that its use leads to abuse of other drugs, such as cocaine. These other addictive drugs are commonly referred to as "recreational" drugs. The psychologic dependence and continued use of recreational drugs may ruin the young adult's personal and social relationships and professional career as well as financial stability.

Box 13–6. Leading Causes of Illness in Young Adulthood
▶ Illness related to trauma ▶ Psychologic illness (drug and alcohol abuse and stress-related disorders) ▶ Preexisting chronic conditions ▶ Cancer ▶ High blood pressure

STRESS

Stress is a major component of many illnesses that affect young adults. By learning strategies for dealing with stress early in life, young adults may lengthen their life span. Many strategies exist to cope with stress. Some of these include exercise, assertiveness training to learn to manage anger appropriately, relaxation therapy, and guided imagery.

Environment

The home and work environment may contain many stressors and pollutants. Stressors may induce physical as well as emotional or mental stress, as discussed in the previous section.

POLLUTANTS

Pollutants include noise pollution as well as the more typical environmental pollutants such as asbestos, smoke, and chemical fumes. Public health nurses can assist with identifying pollutants in the home environment if they make home visits. Once a pollutant is identified, you can suggest ways to diminish or eliminate the offending agent. If you have no control over the pollutant's removal, as in the case of asbestos, you might refer the individual to an appropriate authority.

Occupational health nurses have the opportunity to identify pollutants that are present in the work environment. Ideally, all these pollutants should be reduced or eliminated in order to make the work environment safe and conducive to productivity.

OTHER WORK HAZARDS

A major risk factor related to the work environment concerns safety. Many organizations and companies have inadequate training or orientation programs. In their desire to make a good impression early in the job, young adults may rush to accomplish a task without following or even knowing about safety precautions. This may result in accidents. The Occupational Safety and Health Administration (OSHA) is an agency that was established to develop and enforce job safety and health regulations. Many companies still have industrial hazards; therefore, young adults need to recognize the importance of following safety guidelines and stress to others the benefits of a safe work environment.

Acquired Immune Deficiency Syndrome (AIDS)

Young adults, as a group, still tend to be impulsive regarding sexual activity. While they admit to hearing about AIDS daily, their attitudes are similar to those of adolescents: they think that AIDS "happens only to other people." In a survey of 750 individuals with an average age of 20 years, respondents were asked about any changes in sexual behavior as a result of a fear of AIDS. Only a third of those surveyed reported actually changing their sexual behavior in this regard. However, these results could indicate that these young adults already practiced safe sex and therefore did not see the need to change their practice.[34]

Date (Acquaintance) Rape

Date rape, or acquaintance rape, has been present for decades. In a study conducted at one college campus, 34 per cent of 518 female students reported experiencing unwanted sexual contact; 20 per cent, unwanted attempted intercourse; and 10 per cent, unwanted completed intercourse.[43] This was probably a low, conservative estimate.

Other experts guess that one in four women will be raped in her lifetime. They also estimate that less than 10 per cent will report the assault, and less than 5 per cent of the rapists will go to jail.

Incidents of rape by nonstrangers and the reporting of them have never been accurately accounted for. Some of the reasons that women do not report rape by acquaintances are that they

▶ cannot believe they were "taken advantage" of by someone they knew and have trouble admitting it even to themselves
▶ are reluctant to label the incident as rape
▶ are afraid that they will get a "bad reputation"
▶ may think that parents and friends will not believe them
▶ may feel partly at fault—for not saying "no" in a firm enough voice
▶ may feel that they protested too late—that the intimacy got out of hand
▶ know that they will continue seeing this person and will not be able to face him if the incident is reported
▶ may have been intimate with the person on prior occasions involving consent

Rape may also occur within a marriage or a partnership if one partner is not willing to engage in intercourse at a particular time and is forced to do so by the other partner. Rape is an act of violence and is usually the result of maladaptive responses to psychologic tensions.

ROLE OF THE NURSE

Health Screening and Assessment

During the young adult years, clients are ripe to learn. They experience many different developmental milestones, such as the first job in their career, meeting a life mate, marriage, and parenthood. Although these are normal developmental tasks, persons' coping abilities vary, and some of these experiences may place stress on young adults as well as on their relationships.

You may be the first person to encounter these clients in health settings. Therefore you might be able to assess for successful coping strategies related to stress and how the young adult is dealing with everyday dilemmas. If a problem exists, you can then direct the clients to the appropriate resource.

Because malignant neoplasms are a leading cause of both illness and death in young adults, you should teach all clients the seven warning signs of cancer:[35]

- ▶ **C**hange in bowel or bladder habits
- ▶ **A** sore that does not heal
- ▶ **U**nusual bleeding or discharge
- ▶ **T**hickening or lump in breast or elsewhere
- ▶ **I**ndigestion or difficulty in swallowing
- ▶ **O**bvious change in wart or mole
- ▶ **N**agging cough or hoarseness

You should recommend that women have a Pap smear, beginning at the age of 20 years, and at least every 3 years thereafter. Breast self-examination should be taught to all persons and you should encourage women to perform it on a monthly basis. In addition, men should be taught how to perform a monthly testicular self-examination.

Health Education

PROMOTING GOOD NUTRITION

The eating patterns established in adolescence carry over into young adulthood. If the person was headed toward unhealthy habits and developed anorexia or bulimia, the condition will continue until recognized, diagnosed, and treated. Until the young adult recognizes that a problem exists, treatment will be ineffective.

Education should focus on maintaining healthy eating habits, as many of the leading causes of death are linked to diet. Young adults are probably not as active as they were as adolescents, and if the same level of food consumption continues, their weight will probably increase.

To maintain one's adequate weight, caloric intake must be balanced with energy expenditure. If the client is overweight or underweight, either caloric intake or energy expenditure needs to be increased. Discussion should mention the pros and cons of crash diets and diet centers but focus on a healthy diet using the basic four food groups and food exchanges for dieting.

Heart disease is one of the leading causes of death in adults. High blood pressure is a major cause of illness in young adults.[9] Nurses should discuss the benefits of avoiding foods high in cholesterol and fat and the judicious use of salt.

General guidelines to follow are given in Chapter 42.

PROMOTING ACTIVITY AND EXERCISE

The patterns of physical exercise established during the young adult years tend to become a way of life and assist in the maintenance of a healthy body. Additionally, exercise on a regular basis, such as 30 minutes three times a week, will affect cardiovascular health favorably, reduce stress, and assist in maintaining an ideal weight. You might also discuss other benefits of physical exercise, which include ways to interact socially, promoting a sense of well being, and feeling good about one's self.

DISCOURAGING SUBSTANCE ABUSE

The drug abuses of young adults often continue to be related to peer pressure regarding illicit drugs, such as marijuana and cocaine. In addition, many persons take over-the-counter (OTC) medications. Sleeping pills or depressants assist the person in falling asleep, then a stimulant may be needed to get the person functioning again. This cyclical pattern may become habit-forming. Often young adults do not realize that OTC medications may be just as psychologically addicting as illicit drugs.

When taking a health history on young adults and asking questions regarding current medications, be sure to also ask questions about their use of OTC medications. Many clients feel that health professionals are asking only about prescribed medications when asking about current medications.

PROMOTING SAFE SEX AND AIDS PREVENTION

Education on the prevention of HIV infection remains the number one priority to prevent the spread of AIDS since no vaccine or cure is available. A receptive population for this education is susceptible persons on the college campus. Young adults are still experimenting with their sexuality, and it is crucial to reach this group regarding attitudes toward AIDS and knowledge about AIDS. A study conducted in 1990 found that, after an AIDS program on campus, students' attitudes toward AIDS were more positive and their knowledge about AIDS had increased.[7]

When young adults become involved in a one-to-one relationship, they may no longer feel the need to practice safe sex. As a health professional, you might encourage them to continue to do so for several reasons. A person may have been infected with the AIDS virus many years ago, before the current relationship, and may unwittingly transmit the virus to another. An infected pregnant woman can transmit the AIDS virus to her child even if she has no symptoms.

Health professionals need to stress that the AIDS virus is not highly contagious but is transmitted by intimate sexual contact and the exchange of bodily fluids, exposure to infected blood, and transmission from an infected woman to her fetus. Nurses should discuss universal precautions with all clients with whom they come in contact.

Young adults are just as susceptible to STDs as adolescents are. The same education regarding ways to protect themselves, which include abstinence from sex, making informed choices about partners, and safer sexual practices, needs to be imparted to this age group as well. Reviewing the benefits of condom usage with young adults is just as essential as with all sexually active persons.

PROMOTING SAFETY

A study conducted in 1990 investigated the effects of alcohol in simulated driving conditions. Thirty-six male and female social drinkers (18 of each sex) were randomly assigned to conditions while driving sober or under the influence of alcohol and tested at different blood alcohol levels. Young adults who drank drove faster, made more mistakes, and perceived themselves to be more capable than they actually were. Men in both groups took more risks and engaged in more dangerous driving than women.[26]

Typically, accidents involving young adults are very similar to those involving adolescents. To prevent or lessen the injuries from accidents, see this section in the first part of this chapter.

PROMOTING SELF-CARE

Many young adults do not regularly visit a physician for routine health checkups because of lack of health insurance and a limited income. Only when problems occur do some clients enter the health care system. Although most Americans agree that access to quality care should be a guaranteed right for all citizens, this is a public policy issue that will not be addressed here.

You, as a health care provider, may be the first contact person for young adults entering the system with health concerns. By gaining their trust, you can be effective in discussions regarding self-care and suggest resources available to assist them. Many agencies and programs are under-utilized because young adults are not aware of their existence or how to gain access to them. You may be in a position to match clients with appropriate agencies and programs to enable persons to receive care they might not have sought otherwise.

For young families experiencing pregnancy and early parenthood, you are in an excellent position to provide information on how to have a healthy pregnancy and a healthy baby.

Summary

▶ Adolescence is a time marked by: musculoskeletal, reproductive, and endocrine changes; pubescence and sexual awakenings; the developmental task of achieving identity; cognitive development at the stage of formal operations; family stresses during the struggle for self-assertion; important ties with peers; progression through several stages of moral development; exploration of different varieties of spiritual experiences; major risk factors for death, including auto accidents, suicide, homicide, poisoning, and drowning; the possibility of pregnancy, substance abuse, AIDS, eating disorders, tobacco use, and depression and suicide

▶ The role of the nurse includes health screening for depression and for high-risk sexual behaviors; health education with anticipatory guidance; and promotion of good nutrition, activity, exercise, safety, and responsibility

▶ Early adulthood is a time marked by: physical maturation and the capacity for reproduction; the developmental task of achieving intimacy; peak creativity and productivity; more responsibility for all aspects of the self; marriage and parenting; a feeling of social responsibility; educational and career choices; social and leisure activities; moral reasoning at the Conventional Level with some adults; progressing to the Postconventional Level; major risk factors for death, including accidents, cancer, and heart disease; the possibility of alcohol use, drug abuse, stress-related illnesses, safety hazards at work, AIDS, and date rape

▶ The role of the nurse includes screening for stress and malignancies; educating about nutrition and health; promoting activity and exercise; discouraging substance abuse; preventing AIDS; and promoting safety and self-care

Bibliography

1. Berger, K.S. (1988). *The developing person through the life span* (2nd ed.). New York: Worth Publishers, Inc.
2. Bloome, A. (1988). Acquired immune deficiency syndrome in childhood. *Public Health*, 102(2), 97–106.
3. Boyle, R. (1989). Adolescent knowledge of smokeless tobacco's health consequences. *Health Education*, 20(4), 35–38.
4. Brightman, B.K. (1990). Adolescent depression and the susceptibility to helplessness. *Journal of Youth and Adolescence*, 19(5), 441–449.
5. Castro, J. (1991). The simple life. *Time*, 137(14), 58–63.
6. Cervera, N. (1991). Unwed teenage pregnancy: family relationships with the father of the baby. *Families in Society: The Journal of Contemporary Human Services*, 72(1), 29–37.
7. DiPasquale, J.A. (1990). HIV infection—an educational program on prevention for college freshmen. *Cancer Nursing*, 13(3), 152–157.
8. Edelman, C.L., & Mandle, C.L. (1990). *Health promotion throughout the lifespan*. St. Louis: C.V. Mosby.
9. Ehrenberg, M.F., et al. (1990). The prevalence of depression in high school students. *Adolescence*, 25(100), 905–912.
10. Gillis, A. (1988). Promoting health among teenagers. *International Nursing Review*, 35(1), 10–12.
11. Green, D.L. (1990). High school student employment in social context: adolescent's perceptions of the role of part-time work. *Adolescence*, 25(98), 425–434.
12. Harris, L., and Associates, Inc. (1986). *American teens speak: Sex, myths, T.V. and birth control* (pp. 66–67). New York: Planned Parenthood Federation of America, Inc.
13. Hoffman, M.S. (ed.) (1992). *The world almanac and book of facts*. New York: Pharos Books.
14. Humphrey, P. (1982). The adolescent. In Hill, P.M., & Humphrey, P. (eds.). *Human growth and development throughout life*. New York: John Wiley and Sons.
15. Janke, J. (1989). Dealing with AIDS and the adolescent population. *Nurse Practitioner*, 14(11), 35–36.
16. Johnston, D.K., et al. (1990). Adolescent's moral dilemmas: the context. *Journal of Youth and Adolescence*, 19(6), 615–622.
17. Karshmer, J.F. (1989). Human sexuality. In Birckhead, L.M. *Psychiatric/mental health nursing—The therapeutic use of self* (pp. 549–566). Philadelphia: J.B. Lippincott.
18. Kohlberg, L. (1981). *The philosophy of moral development* (vol. 1). San Francisco: Harper and Row.
19. Lamb, M. (1990). The suicidal adolescent. *Nursing*, 20(5), 72–76.
20. Martinez, R., & Dukes, R. (1991). Ethnic and gender differences in self-esteem. *Youth and Society*, 22(3), 318–338.
21. Miller, L., & Downer, A. (1988). AIDS: What you and your friends need to know—a lesson plan for adolescents. *Journal of School Health*, 58(4), 137–141.
22. Mortimer, J.T., et al. (1990). Gender and work in adolescence. *Youth and Society*, 22(2), 201–224.

23. Murray, F.B. (1990). The conversion of truth into necessity. In Overton, W.F. (ed.). *Reasoning, necessity, and logic: Developmental perspectives* (pp. 183–203). Hillsdale, NJ: Lawrence Erlbaum Associates.
24. Muscari, M.E. (1988). Effective nursing strategies for adolescents with anorexia nervosa and bulimia nervosa. *Pediatric Nursing,* 14(6), 475–481.
25. Newell, G.K., et al. (1990). Self-concept as a factor in the quality of diets of adolescent girls. *Adolescence,* 25(97), 117–128.
26. Oei, T.P., & Kerschbaumer, D.M. (1990). Peer attitudes, sex, and the effects of alcohol on simulated driving performance. *American Journal of Drug Alcohol Abuse,* 16(1 & 2), 135–146.
27. Owen, B.D. (1982). The young adult. In Hill, P.M., & Humphrey, P. (eds.). *Human growth and development throughout life.* New York: John Wiley and Sons.
28. Page, R.M. (1990). Shyness and sociability: a dangerous combination for illicit substance use in adolescent males? *Adolescence,* 25(100), 803–806.
29. Palmone, S., & Shannon, M. (1988). Risk factors for adolescent pregnancy in students. *Nursing,* 14(3), 241–245.
30. Paul, E.L., & White, K.M. (1990). The development of intimate relationships in late adolescence. *Adolescence,* 25(98), 375–397.
31. Petosa, R. (1989). Adolescent wellness: implications for effective health education programs. *Health Values,* 13(5), 14–20.
32. Reiff-Ross, E. (1982). Psychosocial theories relating to human growth and development. In Hill, P.M., & Humphrey, P. (eds.). *Human growth and development throughout life.* New York: John Wiley and Sons.
33. Rodgers, W.L., & Bachman, J.G. (1988). *The subjective well-being of young adults.* Michigan: The University of Michigan.
34. Roscoe, B., & Kruger, T.L. (1990). AIDS: Late adolescents' knowledge and its influence on sexual behavior. *Adolescence,* 25(97), 39–48.
35. Rubin, P. (ed.) (1983). *Clinical oncology: A multidisciplinary approach* (6th ed.). Rochester, NY: American Cancer Society.
36. Schickor, A., et al. (1990). Seat belt use and stress in adolescents. *Adolescence,* 25(100), 773–779.
37. Serow, R.C., & Dreyden, J.I. (1990). Community service among college and university students: individual and institutional relationships. *Adolescence,* 25(99), 553–566.
38. Sinclair, D. (1989). *Human growth after birth.* Oxford: Oxford University Press.
39. Spirito, A., et al. (1990). Social skills and depression in adolescent suicide attempters. *Adolescence,* 25(99), 543–552.
40. Starn, J., & Paperny, D. (1990). Computer games to enhance adolescent sex education. *MCN; American Journal of Maternal Child Nursing,* 15(4), 250–253.
41. Troiden, R.R. (1988). Homosexuality development. *Journal of Adolescent Health Care,* 9(1), 105–113.
42. Varcarolis, E.M. (1990). *Foundations of psychiatric–mental health nursing.* Philadelphia: W.B. Saunders.
43. Ward, S.K., et al. (1991). Acquaintance rape and the college social scene. *Family Relations,* 40(1), 65–71.
44. White, G.L., et al. (1990). Development of a tool to assess suicide risk factors in urban adolescents. *Adolescence,* 25(99), 655–662.

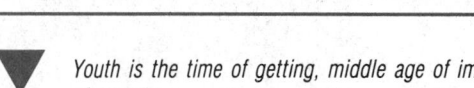

Midlife Through Late Adulthood

Chapter 14

> Youth is the time of getting, middle age of improving and old age of spending . . .
>
> **Anne Bradstreet**

▼ CHAPTER OUTLINE

MIDLIFE
PHYSICAL DEVELOPMENT
  AND CHANGE
PSYCHOSEXUAL
  DEVELOPMENT
    Psychosexual
      Changes in
      Women
    Psychosexual
      Changes in Men
PSYCHOSOCIAL
  DEVELOPMENT
    Self-Concept and
      Self-Image
    Cognitive and
      Intellectual
      Development
    Relationships and
      Roles
VALUES AND BELIEFS
MAJOR HEALTH
  CONCERNS
    Lifestyle

Genetics, or
  Familial
  Characteristics
Workplace or Place
  of Residence
Cultural and Ethnic
  Influences
ROLE OF THE NURSE
  Health Screening
    and Assessment
  Health Education

LATE ADULTHOOD
PHYSICAL DEVELOPMENT
  AND CHANGE
PSYCHOSEXUAL
  DEVELOPMENT
    Deterrents to
      Sexual
      Expression in
      Late Adulthood
    Sexuality in Older
      Adults

PSYCHOSOCIAL
  DEVELOPMENT
    Self-Concept and
      Self-Image
    Cognitive and
      Intellectual
      Development
    Relationships and
      Roles
VALUES AND BELIEFS
MAJOR HEALTH
  CONCERNS
    Personal Losses
    Psychosocial
      Losses
    Depression
    Medication Use
      and Misuse
    Environment
    Lifestyle
ROLE OF THE NURSE
  Health Screening
    and Assessment
  Health Education

▼ KEY TERMS

Ageism
Ego integrity

Empty nest syndrome
Generativity

Sandwich generation

Greater survival rates and reduced birth rates are changing the United States from a society focusing on children and adolescents to one that is focusing on adults: young, middle-aged and older. Because of better lifestyles, increased living standards, better nutrition, and increased medical knowledge and technology, Americans can expect to spend 50 to 60 years as adults.

Today, adults of all ages are healthier, more educated, and in better economic positions than previous generations were. The elderly seem younger than ever, and the middle-aged group keeps expanding their upper age limits.

▼ MIDLIFE

The midlife years generally are designated as those between ages 40 and 65 years. Almost 60 million Americans, or one fourth of the population, are considered middle-aged.[63] They earn most of the money, pay most of the bills and taxes, are very influential in their careers, and are most productive in terms of social and civil responsibility.

The midlife years are frequently thought of as the years of many life changes. Children grow up and move away, marital relationships strengthen or weaken, and parents may die or become dependent. Men and women begin noticing physical changes; hair becomes gray, bald spots may appear, weight increase becomes common, and wrinkles appear.

In general, the changes of the middle years are gradual, and there can be vast individual differences in appearance and behavior among people of the same chronologic age. Some people in their early forties are just marrying; others are becoming grandparents. Some midlife people have a number of health problems while others concentrate on the healthy life, emphasizing diet, exercise, and physical fitness.

Life begins at 40 for some; for others it is the beginning of the end.

PHYSICAL DEVELOPMENT AND CHANGE

The physical signs of aging start to become apparent during the middle years. At some point, most people begin to feel such symptoms as muscle or joint stiffness, decreased energy, weight gain (middle-age spread), slight hearing loss, and a need for reading glasses. The physical changes of aging are gradual. Not all people age alike, and different body parts age at different rates.

How quickly one ages physically may depend partly on the stresses and strains that one experiences. Psychosocial crises can take their toll on a person's stamina. Economic status can play a major role in the process of aging. People in lower financial stratas tend to have poorer nutrition, a higher incidence of disease, more years of hard physical labor, and less money to spend on health and beauty aids. Table 14–1 summarizes some of the physiologic changes that may occur during the middle years.

PSYCHOSEXUAL DEVELOPMENT

The reproductive changes that occur at midlife need not affect sexual activity. With an interested and stimulated partner, both men and women can remain sexually active throughout this part of their lives and into the older adult years.

Psychosexual Changes in Women

The end of the female reproductive cycle is marked by menopause. Menopausal symptoms vary from woman to woman. Most women experience very minor effects; a few experience almost traumatic psychologic and physical symptoms. Menopause historically has been considered a negative experience. The stereotypical menopausal woman has been portrayed as being irritable, depressed, forgetful, and emotionally labile. In reality, the only signs and symptoms that can be truly

TABLE 14-1. Summary of Possible Physical Changes of Midlife

System	Characteristics and Changes
Integumentary	Skin elasticity and moisture decrease. Loss of subcutaneous fat results in less turgor. Wrinkles and looseness of skin begin to appear. The more the skin has been exposed to sun throughout the years, the more pronounced skin changes will be. Hair begins to thin and turn gray. Body contours change as fatty tissue becomes redistributed, particularly for those who lead sedentary lifestyles.
Cardiovascular	The ability of the heart to contract decreases. Blood vessels become less elastic. Blood pressure may increase. Varicosities appear.
Respiratory	Vital respiratory capacity remains unchanged unless respiratory illnesses occur. People who do not exercise may notice a decline in breathing capacity as lung tissues lose their elasticity.
Genitourinary	In general, renal filtration and disposal of waste remain normal. Some women may begin experiencing stress incontinence related to weakening bladder and sphincter muscles.
Gastrointestinal	A low-bulk diet combined with a sedentary lifestyle can lead to diminished motility in the gastrointestinal tract. Constipation may become a problem. A decrease in gastric juices may bring complaints of acid indigestion.
Musculoskeletal	Bone density and mass progressively decrease, particularly in women after menopause. Calcium loss begins in the later midlife years, and some adults may experience a decrease in height and a vertebral hump. Degenerative joint disease may afflict some people in the extremities as well as the back. Muscular status depends on amount and type of exercise. Lack of exercise can lead to a decrease in general muscle tone and weak abdominal muscles.
Endocrine	Menopause occurs between ages 40 and 55 years in women. Production of ovarian estrogen and progesterone ceases. Some secondary sexual characteristics may regress. Men may experience gradual changes in sexual response as testosterone levels plateau or decline. Spermatogenesis continues. A decline in basal metabolism rate may cause a decrease in physical work capacity, energy, and endurance. It also may cause an increase in weight if caloric intake is not reduced.
Neurologic	Central nervous system has no major changes. After age 50 years, a small loss of neurons may begin.
Sensory	A decline in visual acuity (presbyopia) begins in the late forties. The lens of the eye becomes less elastic, and eyes lose the ability to focus on near images clearly. Presbycusis, or a decrease in auditory acuity, begins to occur, particularly for high frequencies. There may be a diminished sense of taste, particularly to salt and sweet foods.

associated with menopause are hot flashes, perspiration, and a gradual cessation of the menses.

Women in midlife are likely to be faced with many major changes in their lives, such as children leaving home, divorce, illness or death of parents, and illness or death of spouse. Research has shown that menopausal symptoms are worse in women who experience recent loss or recent marital or psychosocial stress.[19] Psychosocial symptoms experienced during menopause may be associated with other concurrent life events.

Many women find that the end of their menses comes as a welcome relief. They report that their sex life remains the same or may even improve, particularly since there is no threat of pregnancy. For other women, menopause is equated with aging: loss of beauty, youth, sex appeal, and usefulness.

Psychosexual Changes in Men

Midlife men do not experience the same dramatic physical sexual changes as women. Some may experience a gradual waning of sexual interest and activity. As with women, men in midlife also experience many psychosocial stresses—competition with younger men in the workplace and on social levels, confrontations with teenage children's identity crises, assumptions of new financial burdens. Chronic illnesses may appear.

Midlife is often a time of transition for men. For many it is a time to reexamine one's life and for some to make radical changes. These events can be traumatic and can interfere with sexual functioning. For the first time in their lives, many men begin experiencing problems with ejaculation, decreased libido, and impotence.

PSYCHOSOCIAL DEVELOPMENT

Self-Concept and Self-Image

The developmental stage associated with middle adulthood is Erikson's stage of **generativity** versus stagnation. Generativity implies productivity and creativity for self as well as others. Generative people expand interests and responsibilities. They are involved and accept leadership roles in their careers, communities, social

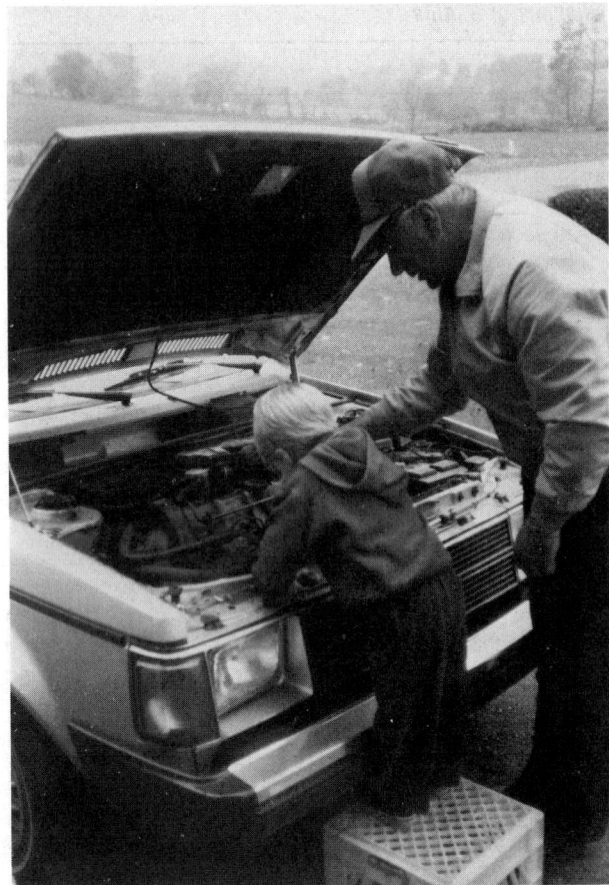

▲ *Figure 14-1*

Middle adults take interest in future generations. This grandfather takes the time to let his grandson help with automobile maintenance.

They are aware of no longer being young and of being mortal. However, they still have a zest for life and a feeling of being young.

Many become very active in exercise and diet programs. They are interested in maintaining their health and beauty, and they dress and groom themselves appropriately for their age and position in life. People who learned to adapt to stress and change in earlier periods of life usually can handle midlife changes successfully. Midlife crises that may occur in one's forties usually are followed by a period of restabilization and mellowing in the fifties.

Cognitive and Intellectual Development

Continuous learning is found throughout adulthood. The middle-aged adult processes new information and learns new skills easily. Cognitive ability is at a high point. Many feel that persons make their greatest contributions to society during their fourth and fifth decades.

REFINEMENT OF COGNITIVE PROCESSES DURING MIDDLE AGE

According to Piaget, cognitive processes such as abstract reasoning, problem-solving, and intellectual growth reach a stable operational stage at adolescence and continue to be refined during adulthood. Studies that have assessed these abilities across the life span find that results are similar for young and middle-aged adults, with few changes occurring until late old age. [53] Cognitive variability in middle age usually is related to the psychosocial aspects of one's personality. A person's intellectual functions in middle age are very dependent on motivation, education, experience, occupation, intellectual activity, and intellectual stimulation.

ADULT EDUCATION

Today, with the increase in emphasis on adult education, the middle-aged person is frequently seen back in the classroom. Many women are beginning careers for

and religious activities, politics, and cultural and artistic efforts. They are concerned with creating something that will be lasting and worthwhile for future generations. The generative person has a sense of parenthood and takes pride in guiding the next generation (Figure 14-1). This means caring about children as well as assisting them to become independent young adults.

Stagnation implies being static; not growing. People who are stagnant tend to be egocentric, nonproductive, self-indulgent, and impoverished. Some experience early invalidism. Others regress to inappropriate youthfulness in behavior and appearance. Infidelity sometimes occurs.

Midlife adults can experience both generativity and stagnation to some degree (Box 14-1). Some middle adults find it difficult to deal with the aging process. They may experience various types of midlife crises. Goals that were established earlier in life may not have been met. Relationships with spouse, children, friends, and colleagues may change unexpectedly and take unanticipated directions.

Middle-aged adults who accept that not all their dreams may come true usually have a better self-image.

the first time at midlife. Some men and women want to change their professions or occupations in order to achieve greater personal satisfaction. Rapid technologic changes and new professional developments frequently make one's knowledge and skills obsolete. Middle-aged adults enjoy the process of learning and, for many, going back to school becomes a leisure-time activity. Those contemplating retirement may want to expand their repertoire of skills and knowledge to make their retirement years more productive and interesting.

Relationships and Roles

FAMILY RELATIONSHIPS

During the middle years, relationships with children, spouses, and parents undergo many changes. Middle-aged persons see themselves as neither young nor old but somewhere in between. They feel a responsibility to the generations on either side of them. Often they are referred to as the "sandwich generation."

Relationships with Children. Midlife adults in their forties and early fifties are often parents of teenagers, an experience filled with crises, ambiguities, and pleasant, proud moments. Midlife parents grew up in a world of different values and expectations; a slower-paced, less affluent, simpler society. Their children are growing up in an era in which the mass media help set standards and expectations about behavior, some of which may be counter to parental teaching or wishes. Conflict between the generations is common and usually arises over differences in perception. Parents often perceive their adolescents as having excessive, unrealistic demands for independence, and children perceive their parents' behavior as being overprotective. For those families who can maintain open communication during this time, the generation gap becomes minimal. Parents become role models, and children grow and develop in a positive manner.

When the children leave home to enter college, get married, or begin a career or profession, the parental role changes. Parents who have been overinvolved or excessive in their identification with their children may have difficulty adjusting to this. They may experience feelings of depression, sadness, and loss, a condition commonly referred to as the **"empty nest syndrome."**

In some instances adult children return to the empty nest after a period of being on their own. The majority of reasons for return are economic: the high cost of living, inflation, high unemployment, rise in cost of education, rise in cost of child care. Other children return for emotional support following broken marriages and romances.

Over 400 mothers of young adults in 23 states were surveyed regarding adult children moving back home for an extended period of time. More than 10 per cent of them stated that their adult children had come home again for stays of 3 months to 2 years or longer.[24]

Spousal Relationships. Many midlife couples find the postparental years to be the happiest years of their marriage. They now experience privacy and freedom that they have not had for years. There are fewer money worries, and there is time to become reacquainted as individuals and to share favorite activities. Their relationship becomes redefined as lovers or companions rather than as parents. If the marriage has been basically good during the parenting years, now it becomes better than ever.

Divorce in Midlife. If the marriage has undergone difficulties over the years, midlife is the time when it usually breaks up. The divorce rate is very high among middle adults, as is the rate of remarriage. In fact, the divorce rates peak at age 44 years.[63] Over the years, the middle-aged couple may have drifted apart instead of growing closer together. As the children leave, a major bond may be broken. Time becomes empty. Sexual relationships may have grown stale. The wife may feel neglected; the husband may feel nagged. They may be bored with each other. Loss of youth, reproductive changes, unfulfilled dreams and expectations, all can lead to marital strife and eventual divorce.

Both men and women find divorce difficult and depressing. For the men, custody decisions, visitation arrangements, and child support are often a source of distress. The midlife woman finds financial changes and loneliness to be the most difficult aspects of divorce, particularly if she is experiencing the empty nest syndrome and grew up with the notion that marriage was forever. Many midlife women are not prepared to support themselves financially to the same degree that their husbands did. It is estimated that the average woman's standard of living declines by 73 per cent with divorce and the man's increases by 42 per cent.[69] Many divorced midlife women are bitter and disappointed, feeling that they have wasted years of their lives promoting and caring for their husbands and children when they could have been developing their own skills and interests.

Remarriage can have its unique stresses. Second marriages at midlife are usually package deals. The new spouse also may be divorced or widowed. The package may include teenage children, elderly parents, and other relatives who may or may not be accepting of the new spouse. There also may be an ex-spouse or the fond memory of a deceased one.

Spousal Abuse. A problem often associated with divorce is spousal abuse. In most cases spousal abuse is physical abuse of a woman by her husband or male partner. Often the abuse is psychologic as well. Men also can be victims of spousal abuse, particularly if they are not the dominant partner in the relationship or if they are ill or handicapped.

Spousal abuse occurs in every social and economic group as well as in every race and adult age group.

More than one million women seek medical assistance for injuries caused by battery each year.[55] The causes of wife abuse are many and varied. Researchers have studied the behavior and responses of both abusers and abused. Neither fit into any neat categories. In many instances spousal abuse is not reported. The abused partner remains silent because of embarrassment, shame or guilt, terror, or demoralization. Services and centers for abused people are available in most communities. Prevention of spousal abuse requires societal attitude changes and enforcement of laws as well as personal and family counseling.

Grandparenting. The average age for becoming a first-time grandparent is somewhere between 49 and 53 years. Today's grandfathers and grandmothers are active in the workplace and very much involved in the community. Grandparents vary in the amount of interaction they have with their grandchildren (Box 14–2). Becoming a grandparent often improves relationships with older children.

Relationships with Aging Parents. At some time during the middle years, relationships with parents change. The middle-aged children suddenly notice that their parents have grown old, and they look at them more objectively and with more warmth and affection. Relationships and roles are redefined. Some aging parents now may need to turn to their children for assistance with financial, psychosocial, or physical problems. Others may not, preferring to remain as independent as possible. The death of a parent is a reality during midlife.

A role reversal occurs when aging parents become physically or mentally incapacitated, or when they become financially dependent upon their middle-aged children. This role reversal is emotionally significant for both children and parents. It is often the cause of much psychologic tension. Daughters, especially, feel "sandwiched" (the **sandwich generation**) between caring for children (teenagers and young adults) and dealing with aging parents. The parents may be in-laws.

Often middle-aged daughters feel caught between the generations with no time to take care of themselves.

Even though American society tends toward nuclear families, the bonds between generations are very strong. The generations may live in different households, but they are linked by mutual aid and affection. The elderly are not isolated from their adult children.

In a national study of older people and their families, 70 per cent of older persons with children reported that they received aid from their children; 70 per cent reported that they gave help to their children and grandchildren; and 50 per cent gave aid to their great-grandchildren.[59]

COMMUNITY RELATIONSHIPS

Civic Responsibilities. People in midlife see themselves in terms of their positions in the community as well as their career or family. Because of their accomplishments, many middle adults are elected or appointed to status or authority positions such as school board member, member of a religious institutional board, officer of an organization, or political leader.

Volunteerism is an important part of civic responsibility. Most volunteer work still is done by women working in such activities as garden clubs, hospital auxiliaries, charitable organizations, political parties, and religious groups. However, today's midlife women increasingly are seeking careers, elected offices, and part-time positions for which they are paid. Volunteerism is on the decline.

Careers. During the middle years, men and women are usually at the peak of their careers. Most people have accumulated wisdom and experience in their chosen fields and have attained seniority status or positions of power. There is a great deal of job satisfaction, and sense of identity is closely linked with occupation.

Social/Leisure Time. After the children leave home, many middle adults find themselves with free time. Some take an early retirement and the amount of free time expands even more. Leisure-time activities in the middle years are many and varied. Some spend their time rather conservatively: watching television, eating out, socializing with friends and neighbors, attending cultural, religious or sports events, gardening, and participating in activities with family members. Many develop and pursue hobbies or do-it-yourself projects. For those who can get extended periods of time away from the job or who are retired, enjoyable leisure-time pursuits include travel, fishing, hunting, and camping.

Not all adults in their forties and fifties have unlimited leisure time. Many are still tied up with long work weeks, may have to do work-related tasks at home, or take on a second job to supplement the income from the first (Figure 14–2). Although the middle years usually bring an increase in income, they may also bring an increase in expenses. Children may be going to college; a divorced daughter or son may be coming home; an aging parent may become a financial burden.

Box 14–2. Styles of Grandparenting

▶ *Formal grandparents*—interested in their grandchildren but offer no advice; separate themselves from the child-rearing role

▶ *Fun-seeking grandparents*—have an informal, playmate role with grandchildren; enjoy them as a source of leisure

▶ *Distant grandparents*—only see grandchildren on special occasions: birthdays, holidays, religious observances

▶ *Parent-surrogate grandparents*—take on the caregiving responsibilities for grandchildren, a role especially played by grandmothers when mother works or is incapacitated due to poor health or drug addiction

▶ *Reservoir of wisdom grandparents*—pass on special skills, knowledge, and family history to grandchildren and their parents

---

Data from Neugarten, B.L., & Weinstein, K.D. (1968). The changing American grandparent. In Neugarten B.L. (ed.). *Middle age and aging.* Chicago: University of Chicago Press.

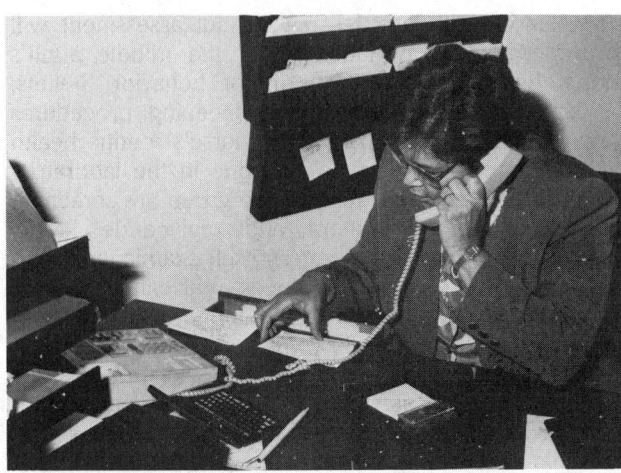

▲ *Figure 14-2*

Many middle adults work long hours.

VALUES AND BELIEFS

Much of what people value and believe develops early in life. Some values may be altered or changed during the adult years, particularly when one is involved in parenting or in the pursuit of a career. The middle years offer a time to review one's value system. Often this is done when an illness or crisis occurs. Some values may be discarded; others may be added. Basically, in midlife one becomes satisfied with one's own value system.

MAJOR HEALTH CONCERNS

Lifestyle

The major risks to good health in the middle years are related to lifestyle, particularly nutrition, exercise, smoking, and the use of alcohol. The degree of stress that accompanies one's lifestyle and the quality of the environment also can be influential. Many of the leading causes of death are preventable at this age, either entirely or in part, by a change in lifestyle or social norms. According to the U.S. Department of Health and Human Services, behavioral changes have saved many lives in the past two decades.[65] Declines of 40 per cent in coronary artery disease and 50 per cent in stroke can be directly linked to reduced rates of cigarette smoking, lower blood cholesterol, and increased control of high blood pressure. Decreased deaths from motor vehicle accidents can be linked to increased seat belt use, lower rates of alcohol use, and changes in speed limits on highways.

Genetics, or Familial Characteristics

In addition to lifestyle, genetics or familial characteristics may be a risk factor for some middle-aged adults.

Box 14-3. Leading Health Problems in Midlife

- ▶ Arthritis
- ▶ Hypertension
- ▶ Chronic sinusitis
- ▶ Orthopedic impairments
- ▶ Hearing impairments
- ▶ Heart disease
- ▶ Hay fever, allergic rhinitis
- ▶ Hemorrhoids
- ▶ Chronic bronchitis
- ▶ Diabetes

Data from the National Center for Health Statistics, 1986.

Chronic diseases such as diabetes, hypertension, glaucoma, heart disease, arteriosclerosis, obesity, and alcoholism tend to run in families (Box 14-3). Certain malignancies such as breast cancer and colorectal cancer also seem to be linked to families. For people who have family histories of these illnesses, preventive measures are extremely important. Certain eating patterns, especially excessive consumption of fats, are linked with breast and colon cancer as well as heart disease. Obesity is associated with hypertension, diabetes, heart disease, stroke, and some cancers. It also can be a factor in the development of osteoarthritis of some joints. Cigarette smoking is a major risk factor for heart disease, stroke, and lung cancer. Alcohol is a major factor in many motor vehicle accidents, homicides, and suicides. Alcohol abuse is responsible for many fatal liver diseases. (See Box 14-4 for leading causes of death in midlife.)

Workplace or Place of Residence

The workplace or place of residence may be a risk factor for the health of many middle-aged adults. Noise, air pollution, and extreme temperatures can have direct effects on health. Irreversible hearing loss can occur because of prolonged exposure to high-intensity sounds. Prolonged noise has been associated with headaches, nervousness, and insomnia. Polluted air has a direct correlation with the incidence of respiratory diseases.

Stress can be a part of the workplace. Stress can lead to the development of physical disease or mental disorders. Stressors can be physical or psychologic and can be within the workplace or within the individual.

Box 14-4. Leading Causes of Death in Midlife

- ▶ Heart disease
- ▶ Cancer
- ▶ Cerebrovascular accident (stroke)
- ▶ Liver disease
- ▶ Accidents (including motor vehicle)

Data from the National Center for Health Statistics, 1985.

Cultural and Ethnic Influences

The predominant minority populations in the United States are the African-Americans, Hispanic-Americans, Asian-Americans, and Native Americans and Alaskan Natives. Within each of these ethnic or racial groups are many subgroups, each with differences in beliefs and practices. Asian-Americans speak over 30 different languages and have as many different cultures. The Hispanic-American group is made up of people with roots in Mexico, Puerto Rico, Cuba, Central and South America, and the Caribbean. African-Americans living in the rural South have very different beliefs and practices than do African-Americans living in a northern inner city. Socioeconomic factors can make a big difference among members of the same minority or ethnic group. It is very important that nurses recognize their own ethnic beliefs and practices as well as those of their clients.

Health practices and definitions of health vary with minorities and may be totally different from those of the white health care provider. In some minority groups, being pleasantly plump is more beautiful than being thin. Many Hispanics and Asians practice herbal medicine. Native Americans may prefer traditional health care from their own tribal medicine people. Language differences are barriers to health care for a big proportion of the Hispanic population as well as some of the Asian peoples.

Health problems also vary with minority groups. A major problem of the middle-aged African-American man is hypertension. Diabetes is more common among black middle-aged women, particularly if they are overweight. Middle-aged Hispanic men are heavy smokers. It is common for middle-aged Mexican-American women to be overweight.

Big risk factors for Native Americans are alcohol use and obesity. Cirrhosis and diabetes are the two leading chronic illnesses of Native Americans. Smoking rates among Asian immigrant men are extremely high. The incidence of tuberculosis is especially high in Asian immigrants. Tuberculosis is the leading cause of death in many Asian countries.

A major risk factor for most minorities, particularly those with low incomes, is not receiving early, routine, and preventive health care.

ROLE OF THE NURSE

One of the major goals of the nurse working with middle-aged adults is the promotion of health care measures and behaviors that will improve their quality of life during the midlife years and into the future. Strategies that can be used for achieving this goal are health assessment and screening, health education, and the promotion of self-care and personal responsibility for health.

Health Screening and Assessment

The purpose of health assessment and screening is to obtain an overview of the middle-aged client's health status and health practices. A careful assessment will give the nurse information about the middle adult's biopsychosocial being: patterns of behavior, beliefs, perceptions, and values. Some screening procedures may be included as a part of the nurse's routine health assessment. Others have to be done in the laboratory setting. Recommended for this age group are screening procedures for cholesterol and triglyceride levels, breast cancer (especially breast self-examination and mammography), colorectal cancer, oral cancer, hypertension, diabetes, cervical and uterine cancer (especially in postmenopausal women), lung cancer, glaucoma, and hearing loss.

A mental health assessment is very important in midlife. This period of life includes many stresses and stressors. The nurse needs to help the middle adult client identify these so that behaviors that can become health risks may be prevented. The health assessment opens up many opportunities for the nurse to provide health teaching and counseling.

Health Education

Health education programs are effective means of changing behavior and lifestyle. Teaching is a primary function of nursing and should occur in all health care settings. It can be accomplished on an individual or group basis. Today, many middle-aged adults want to be active participants in their health care. They want health care information that is relevant to them and that will allow them to be involved in health care decision making.

PROMOTING GOOD NUTRITION

Weight management for the adult in midlife can be a serious problem. The middle-aged adult has a lower metabolic rate and leads a more sedentary lifestyle than the young adult. Unfortunately, eating habits tend to remain the same. The 1988 Surgeon General's Report on Nutrition and Health[55] found that for the two out of three Americans who neither smoked or consumed alcohol, eating patterns were the factors that affected their long-term health prospects the most. Nutritional problems that affect many middle-aged Americans revolve around eating too many foods high in saturated fats and cholesterol and too few that are high in dietary fiber (Figure 14-3).

The nurse can be very effective in assisting the middle-aged adult to maintain a healthy diet and weight. A comprehensive diet assessment should be followed by nutritional education, which includes such recommendations as: eat a variety of foods, choose a diet low in fat and cholesterol, choose a diet with plenty of fruits, vegetables, and grains, and use sugar, salt, and sodium in moderation. If the middle-aged person is having difficulty losing weight or maintaining a healthy diet, the nurse could suggest behavior modification programs or support groups such as Weight Watchers.

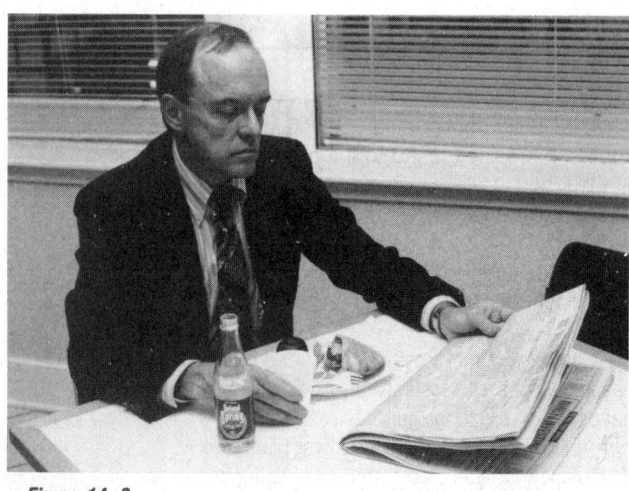

▲ Figure 14-3

Middle-aged adults should eat foods low in saturated fats and cholesterol and high in dietary fiber.

PROMOTING EXERCISE AND REST

Regular physical activity increases life expectancy and helps prevent and manage chronic diseases such as coronary heart disease, hypertension, diabetes, and osteoporosis. Physical activity helps manage depression and is essential to any weight loss program. In spite of all these benefits, many middle-aged Americans do not engage in any regular physical activity.

Nurses need to focus on the physical activity patterns of their middle-aged clients. A good assessment will help suggest physical activities that fit in with a client's lifestyle and promote cardiorespiratory fitness, build muscle strength and endurance, and assist with weight control and relief of stress. Activity should not be unduly strenuous. Walking for about 30 minutes a day is an excellent exercise activity that will fit in with most lifestyles and will produce measurable health benefits. Physical activity should be balanced with sleep, rest, and relaxation. Teaching the middle-aged person a few good relaxation techniques may be very useful in helping relieve some of the stresses of midlife.

PROMOTING SAFETY

Accidents or unintentional injuries are the third leading cause of adult death in the United States. Approximately one half of these deaths are due to motor vehicle accidents, many of which are alcohol-related. Work-related injuries account for another large proportion of accidental deaths. Electrical shocks, falls, burns, and eye injuries are among the most prevalent injuries.

Many of the accidents that cause injuries to middle-aged adults are preventable. Many occur in the home and are due to such factors as faulty electrical wiring, tools and equipment that do not work, poor lighting in hallways, throw rugs, and loose or nonexistent handrails on stairways and in bathtubs. Recreational accidents are common in middle age, particularly with the increase in leisure time and discretionary income. This includes accidental injuries with handguns and rifles. As health educators, nurses can initiate safety programs and safety measures for midlife adults in both the home and workplace.

▼ LATE ADULTHOOD

The period of late adulthood begins around the age of 65 years, the traditional age of retirement. In the United States, over 12 per cent of the population is 65 years of age or over, and the numbers keep growing. There are now more than 30 million persons in late adulthood, 40 per cent of whom are over the age of 85 years. Some people refer to this phenomenon as the "graying of America."

Late adulthood has an age span of 30 years. Because of this and the increasing number of older adults, there is a growing trend to categorize late adulthood into subgroups; the young-old (ages 65 to 74 years), the middle-old (ages 75 to 84 years), and the old-old (over age 85 years). Some people categorize older adults according to functional status: the "frail elderly" and the "able elderly."

Classifying older people is misleading. Throughout life, people become more diverse as they age, and people in late adulthood are more heterogeneous than in any other age period.

The majority of older persons are reasonably healthy, although the rate of illness in the elderly is higher than that of other age groups. Eighty-six per cent have at least one chronic disease, and most suffer from more than one.[40] Studies have shown that the majority of older people (up to age 82 years) consider themselves to be in good-to-excellent health. These same studies indicate that self-assessment of health status in older adults correlates highly with actual measures of health status.[40] Older adults are very concerned about health and social issues, particularly those that directly affect them. Health promotion and wellness activities are becoming more popular as most elderly search for a new and better way to age.

PHYSICAL DEVELOPMENT AND CHANGE

Aging is a normal developmental process. The exact physiologic mechanisms that cause it are unknown. There are changes in all organ systems, but the rate of change varies and is very individualistic. Of the many theories of aging, none has been universally accepted. Aging is a complex process, influenced by many factors—heredity, nutrition, disease, and socioeconomic circumstances. Certain factors seem to hasten the aging process: physical and psychologic inactivity, attitudes of hopelessness and depression, diet and eating habits, smoking, and abuse of alcohol and other drugs. Some of the physiologic changes that may occur with normal aging are outlined in Table 14-2.

TABLE 14–2. Summary of Possible Physical Changes of Late Adulthood

System	Characteristics and Changes
Integumentary	Skin becomes less elastic, drier, and more fragile. Subcutaneous fat is lost, causing wrinkles, lines, and sagging. "Age spots" appear in areas exposed to the sun. Bruises occur easily. Scalp, axillary, and pubic hair thins and whitens. Women may develop facial hair. Perspiration lessens. Hair in nose and ears becomes evident.
Cardiovascular	Cardiac output decreases; systolic and diastolic blood pressures increase. Vessels lose their elasticity and become narrower as fatty plaque and calcium deposits build up. Heart valves are less flexible. Vessels in head, neck, and extremities are more prominent.
Respiratory	Residual volume increases and vital capacity is lowered. Efficiency of lungs decreases owing to reduction of alveoli and loss of elasticity. Loss of elasticity and ciliary action may cause reduced cough response and ineffective gas exchange.
Genitourinary	Renal function slows because of loss of nephron units. Renal blood flow slows. Fluid and electrolyte balance becomes fragile. Bladder muscles weaken, and some stress incontinence may occur. The prostate becomes enlarged in most men. Women experience atrophy of the genitals: vaginal secretions decrease and vaginal epithelium becomes thin. Ovaries and fallopian tubes atrophy.
Gastrointestinal	Many older people suffer loss of teeth due to poor dental care and diet. The amount of saliva and esophageal motility may decrease. Digestive juices decrease in amount, and absorption decreases owing to atrophy of intestinal cells. Reduced muscle tone and decreased peristalsis may cause a problem with constipation.
Musculoskeletal	Changes may include kyphosis, enlarged joints, flabby muscles, and decreased height. Skeletal mass decreases, and bones become porous and brittle. Mobility may decrease if exercise is not taken.
Endocrine	Thyroid gland activity may decrease, causing less alertness, less activity, and more susceptibility to cold. Basal metabolism is reduced. Testosterone, estrogen, and progesterone secretions decrease. The pancreas may have a delayed and insufficient release of insulin.
Neurologic	Reduction in the velocity of nerve impulses may cause a decrease in reaction time and movements. Changes in sleep pattern may occur, with frequent awakenings.
Sensory	Presbyopia (farsightedness) continues. Peripheral vision may be narrowed. Lens of eye yellows, causing an alteration in color perception. Depth perception may become distorted. There is poor accommodation to dark. Hearing loss (presbycusis) occurs, particularly for high frequencies. Cerumen often accumulates in the middle ear. Sense of smell is reduced. Sense of taste is less acute. Temperature regulation and pain perception are less efficient.

PSYCHOSEXUAL DEVELOPMENT

The personal and emotional needs of older adults are very similar to those of younger adults and include the need for intimacy and sexual expression. There is no strict correlation between age and sexual activity. Individuals in old age retain the same sexual interests and the same patterns of sexual behavior as they did throughout the earlier years of their lives. However, there often is a loss of opportunity for sexual expression because of loss of partner, change in health status, or lack of privacy.

Deterrents to Sexual Expression in Late Adulthood

LOSS OF PARTNER

Loss of partner is the primary reason for the discontinuation of sexual activity for many older women. Almost 70 per cent of women over the age of 75 years are either widowed or divorced. In contrast, most men over the age of 75 years (70 per cent) are married.[63] Old social mores may also contribute to the lack of a partner for older women. Older women feel inhibited to take the initiative in dating, to marry a younger man, or to engage in extramarital sex.

CHRONIC HEALTH PROBLEMS AND MEDICATIONS

Chronic health problems and medications are often a deterrent to sexual activity in old age. Stiff and painful arthritic joints can make sexual activity difficult. Medications may cause a decrease in libido and impotency. Emotional responses to chronic illnesses may affect sexual functioning. The presence of cardiovascular disease or stroke may cause both partners to be reluctant about engaging in sexual activity for fear of causing an exacerbation of the disease or death. Some older persons who really do not enjoy sexual activity may use chronic disease as an excuse to give it up.

LACK OF PRIVACY

Lack of privacy can be a real deterrent to sexual activity in late adulthood, particularly for those who live with younger family members or in institutions. Many younger family members find it difficult to accept the fact that their elderly parents or grandparents are still sexually active. Many nursing homes seem to disapprove of sexual expression; not only is there a lack of privacy, there are no double beds. Some institutions still find an excuse to separate husbands and wives upon admission, interrupting sleeping patterns that couples may have had for 40 or 50 years.

Sexuality in Older Adults

There are many myths and stereotypes regarding sexual activity in old age: women lose all desire for sex after menopause; old people are too unattractive to be sexually appealing; old age brings impotence; and most older people do not enjoy sexual relations. Stereotypes and myths occur because of lack of knowledge on the part of the general public as well as older people themselves.

Sexuality for older people is more than the physical sexual act. It includes affection, warmth, concern, and sharing between people. Older people desire and need intimacy. They need physical closeness and affection. Feeling wanted and important to someone else promotes security and emotional well-being. A meaningful relationship is very necessary in older age to help counteract the many physical, psychologic, and social losses that older people experience.

PSYCHOSOCIAL DEVELOPMENT

Few, if any, universal changes in personality are caused by the aging process. There may be a difference in focus and an increase in cautiousness, but basically there is continuity in an individual's personality over time.[40,45]

Self-Concept and Self-Image

Most older people are psychologically healthy. Erikson states that the developmental task for older adults is to achieve a sense of **ego integrity** versus one of despair. Establishing ego integrity includes reviewing one's life, interpreting past experiences in relation to self-concept, and perceiving and accepting one's life as meaningful and whole. There is a sense of satisfaction that people have lived life to the best of their abilities. The process of establishing ego integrity allows one to accept the inevitability of death without fear. Without ego integrity, the older individual experiences despair. Despair represents a sense of incompleteness: life has been too short, meaningless, and futile. Time has run out and death is feared.

Self-concept continues to develop throughout the life span (Box 14–5). One's self-concept is a combination of the way one perceives changes in body structure

> ## Box 14–5. Developmental Tasks of Late Adulthood
>
> ► Adjust to decreases in physical strength and health
> ► Adjust to retirement and reduced income
> ► Adjust to death of spouse and other loved ones
> ► Establish an explicit affiliation with one's own age group
> ► Adjust and adapt to social roles in a flexible way
> ► Establish satisfactory living arrangements

and function plus a reflection of other's perceptions. It is a person's total sense of self. The obvious changes in appearance and bodily function that come with aging make it necessary for the older person to adjust to a different body image. Most older people can do this successfully.

Some older people deny the changes of aging and make the same demands on their body as they did when they were younger. They become preoccupied with achieving a youthful appearance and invest in cosmetic surgery, miracle drugs, and expensive treatments in an attempt to stay forever young. Others exaggerate the aging process and may restrict their activity and lifestyle unnecessarily. Often this occurs when family roles change or switch. It also may happen when older people are subjected to or believe in some of the stereotypes and myths of aging. Health status is an important determinant of self-concept and morale in old age.

Cognitive and Intellectual Development

Cognitive abilities in old age seem to be related to use. Older adults' ability to learn, think, and remember can be stimulated by exercises and activities that demand the use of mind and memory. Intellectual processes such as reasoning and abstract thinking remain the same throughout life unless they are affected by physical or mental deterioration. Creativity does not decline with age. History is filled with examples of people who composed or created works of art after the age of 70 years.

MEASURING INTELLIGENCE IN LATE ADULTHOOD

Measuring intelligence is very difficult in late adulthood because so many variables can interfere with the testing procedures: state of health, educational background, sensory deficits, and test-taking skills. It also is very difficult to find measurement tools that are not biased in favor of younger people.

ABILITY TO LEARN IN LATE ADULTHOOD

The ability to learn is not seriously altered by aging. Older people do have a slowing of response time, so more time may be needed to perform tasks and process information. Perception is vital to learning. If older people have poor eyesight or a diminished sense of hearing, they may not perceive information correctly.

Sometimes older people have difficulty learning new tasks, especially if one requires unlearning an old one first. Older people learn best if the material is relevant and they are motivated to learn. The same is true for younger people.

MEMORY IN OLDER ADULTS

Memory may be altered with age. Memory is a vital part of learning and may account for some difficulty in the learning ability of older adults. A distinction is made between short-term and long-term memory. Short-term memory deals with the initial reception of information. If information is fed in too fast, some will fail to register or be wiped out by newer information. Many older people have difficulty with their short-term memory. Long-term memory refers to the storage of material and the recall of past events. Long-term memory does not appear to be affected by age.

The memory loss that occurs with old age is usually related to difficulty in organizing material and to a general slowing down that causes old people to need a longer period of time to process information and to retrieve it from storage in the brain. Older people who experience problems with day-to-day cognitive functions, such as recalling names, words, dates, phone numbers, and daily chores, can use devices such as lists, notes, and calendars, or practice cognitive aids such as imagery, word associations, cues, and mnemonics.

Relationships and Roles

FAMILY RELATIONSHIPS

The family is the primary source of social support for older people. Nearly 94 per cent of people over the age of 65 years have living family members.[32,66] Today's families frequently span three and four generations. Although some older people live in the residences of their children or other family members, most prefer living in their own homes. This allows them to maintain their privacy and a sense of independence. Also, differences in lifestyles and expectations are not always conducive to healthy family relationships. Most elderly people live within a half hour's drive of at least one family member, and contact with children and other family members is frequent.

Relationships with Adult Children, Grandchildren, and Siblings. The relationship between the elderly and their adult children can be complex but mutually satisfying. Adult children help their older parents in many ways: household management, financial assistance, socialization, aid during illness, transportation, and emotional support to help with the multiple losses and changes of aging. In fact, approximately 80 per cent of persons over age 75 years who have functional disabilities are assisted by their families.[32,66] Most adult children would be willing to have their elderly parents move in with them if the need arose. Often, the assistance of family members is the determining factor in whether an older person is institutionalized or stays at home in the community.

Support within families goes in both directions. Elderly parents often serve as the source for the family values, and teach the younger members norms, traditions, and skills. Elderly parents can provide affection and emotional support. Sometimes they also provide financial support.

The relationship between siblings becomes very strong in late life. Sibling rivalry generally decreases with advancing age. The bond between sisters is especially strong. Relationships between siblings are very important for those older people who have no spouse, children, or grandchildren.

Relationships Between Older Couples. Marital relationships in late life are interdependent. Married couples who are still together in late life have usually either worked out their differences over the years or have learned to live with them. Successful marriages in late adulthood are characterized by more equality of partners. The traditional male/female sex roles associated with such tasks as household chores, family finances, and organizing social activities become blurred. Values and beliefs are shared, and there is a strong bond of companionship. In fact, the major reason for remarriage in late life for both men and women is a desire for companionship. Most older people who remarry choose someone they have previously known, someone with similar interests and background. A few older couples choose to live together but not marry. This is primarily because of economic and inheritance restrictions. Late-life marriages are more likely to end in death than divorce.

Life events can have an impact upon the quality of the marital relationship. The major events are retirement, change in residence, and change in the health of one spouse. The illness of one partner puts a great burden on the other one. Usually, the well partner tries to care for the ill one as well as assume all the responsibilities of keeping the household together. The stress is sometimes too much, resulting in depression, anger, or illness for the caregiver partner.

The concept of couples in old age includes gay and lesbian partners. Approximately 10 per cent of the older population have chosen this sexual orientation and lifestyle. Many feel that this population is at risk because health care providers lack information and sensitivity to their concerns.[10]

Widows and Widowers. The death of a spouse brings a host of emotional and practical problems. Women are affected more than men. For those women whose only career was wife and mother, widowhood may mean loss of status, income, and old friendships. For the most part, once the initial grief has subsided, widows adjust very well. Usually they find companionship with other widows and learn to live independently. They interact with others as a single person.

A recent study asked a group of women ages 67 to 92 years what resources helped them adjust successfully to unavoidable losses, such as the loss of a significant person. Responses included such inner resources as a belief in oneself, determination, sense of humor, and faith in God. External resources included family and friends, meaningful work, and activities such as gardening or playing a musical instrument.[67]

Loss of spouse seems to be particularly difficult for men, as evidenced by higher early mortality rates after the death of the spouse and higher remarriage rates. Most men do not know where to turn for help when widowed; many find it difficult to ask for help. Marriages within the first 18 months after the spouse's death often end in divorce.[2,16]

Family Caregivers. Most family members who care for their ill or frail elderly relatives are women. Usually, they are wives, daughters, or sisters. Men who are primary caregivers usually receive assistance from daughters or wives, especially for the "hands-on" type of care.[39] Caregivers who are spouses or siblings most often are elderly persons themselves, and their physical, emotional, and social health care can be seriously affected by providing care.

Wives are the highest-risk group. They usually are living alone with their husbands and receive very little assistance with the daily caregiving. Often they are in the process of grieving, particularly if the husband is incapacitated with dementia. The emotional burdens of feeling alone, isolated, and without time for oneself are the greatest risks. Rates of depression are extremely high in this group.

A study of predictors of depression among wife caregivers found that caregiver health and attitude were the two highest predictors of depression. Spouse caregivers reported significantly more physician visits and poorer health than adult children caregivers. They also had a negative attitude toward asking for help. Spouses generally believed caregiving was their own responsibility, and that they should be able to do it without assistance.[56]

Middle-aged daughters are another vulnerable group of caregivers. Just as they are receiving some freedom from the responsibilities of childrearing and have an opportunity to begin new ventures, they become faced with dependent parents and a new set of demands. Most daughters are willing to assume the responsibilities of caregiving despite the physical, emotional, and financial cost. Compared with male caregivers, women are more likely to quit their jobs or reduce their hours of employment to provide care.[7]

Care for the family caregivers is an important part of community health nursing. Nursing interventions should include instruction in nursing care skills, information about available resources and support groups, and encouragement to care for themselves in terms of nutrition, sleep, exercise, and respite. The necessity of leaving the care situation to seek respite and relaxation periodically should be stressed strongly.

The stress on caregivers, especially the emotional strain, may cause families to institutionalize their older relatives. Probably the most difficult decision a family must make is placing a parent in a nursing home. Institutionalization is a very emotional event for all family members and is usually a last resort, precipitated by either the illness or death of the family caregiver or a severe family strain.

In some cases caregiving stress can lead to elder abuse. The extent of elder abuse is unknown. Forms of elder abuse are listed in Box 14–6.

It is estimated that over one million elderly Americans are the victims of abuse and that only one in five cases is reported.

Spouses and sons are most often the abusers. Elderly victims may fail to report abuse because they feel intimidated by the abuser or because they love the family member too much to report the person. A growing number of states have passed laws requiring professionals to report elder abuse. Adult Protective Services is the state or county agency that becomes involved in cases of elderly abuse or neglect.

COMMUNITY INTERACTIONS WITH OLDER ADULTS

Most communities have informal support systems that become natural helping networks for their older citizens. These support groups include friends and neighbors, religious organizations, service organizations, grass roots support groups for health-related problems (e.g., Reach to Recovery, support for new widows, stroke group), community watch organizations, hobby groups, and senior citizen clubs. The assistance received from many of these community groups is similar to that provided by family and is utilized especially by elderly people who have no living relatives.

Living Arrangements. The majority of older Americans own their own homes. Most of the young-old live in their homes with a spouse or a significant other, such as a friend, an adult child, or a sibling. After the age of 75 years, most elderly persons live alone in their own residences. Only 5 per cent of elderly people at

---

Box 14–6. Forms of Elder Abuse

▶ *Physical abuse*—Violence that results in bodily harm. Includes sexual abuse. May also include physical injury from restraints or confinement
▶ *Psychologic abuse*—The infliction of mental anguish; verbal assaults, name calling, threats, forced isolation, frightening, demeaning, treating as a child
▶ *Material abuse*—The illegal or unethical exploitation or use or both of an elderly person's money or property
▶ *Active neglect*—The intentional withholding of food, drugs, or assistive aids such as false teeth, glasses, or hearing aids; deliberate abandonment
▶ *Passive neglect*—An unintentional failure to care for a dependent older adult. May be the result of inadequate skills or knowledge, or the incapacitation of the primary caregiver. May be related to a lack of understanding of the necessity for prescribed or essential services

any one time live in institutions like nursing homes or hospitals. Other living arrangements for older people include condominiums, group homes, public housing, and mobile homes. Special retirement communities are popular places for people to move to in their later years.

There are problems associated with older people living in their own homes. Poverty is prevalent among the older generation. Older people may own their own homes but be unable to maintain or repair them. They may not be able to pay the utility bills. If they want to move, they may not be able to find a buyer for their house or afford the moving costs. Crime in the neighborhood can be a problem for older homeowners. Annual housing surveys have revealed that for many elderly, crime is of more personal concern than income or health.[32]

Transportation. Automobiles have a special significance for older people. They are equated with freedom and independence. The loss of a driver's license can be devastating. Many older people avoid freeways and take circuitous routes to make sure that they do not have even a minor accident. Many states require special testing before reissuing a license to anyone over the age of 70 years.

Public transportation is not always available for older people. Buses and subways in some urban areas may be physically hazardous or dangerous. Many older people, particularly in rural areas, have to depend on friends and relatives. Lack of transportation presents many problems for older adults and may contribute to poor nutrition, lack of health care, and social withdrawal.

Retirement. In 1935, Congress established the Social Security Act which arbitrarily set the age of 65 years as the age of retirement. Even though Congress banned this mandatory retirement age in 1970 (at the request of senior citizens' groups), the majority of employed people still retire at age 65. Professionals and people who are self-employed or own their own businesses are inclined not to retire unless necessary. Many of these people find a great deal of pleasure and sense of satisfaction in their work. Many equate their identity with their professional position.

Many people look forward to retirement with relief. They have never found fulfillment in their work and now no longer have to endure the constraints of full-time employment. They now have an opportunity for choices. Probably the most powerful factors in retirement satisfaction are health status, sufficient income, and the option to continue working if one wants to.

Retirement may occupy 30 or more years of a person's life. It is almost another developmental stage. Retirement can bring problems as well as pleasures. Most large companies now offer retirement planning programs that help employees with financial planning as well as issues such as role change, use of time, relocating, relationships with spouse, and the social impact of not working. Many older people, after a few years of retirement leisure, seek part-time jobs. Others

become active as volunteers or pursue creative hobbies. People react differently to retirement, depending upon such factors as retirement income, personal hobbies or interests, and whether or not they enjoyed their occupation.

Resources and Services. Most communities offer many types of resources and services for their elder citizens. Local offices on aging, commissions on retirement education, libraries, religious institutions, health departments, and radio and television stations can provide assistance to older people to learn about available community resources and services.

VALUES AND BELIEFS

The majority of older people value conformity, loyalty, and social order. They follow the social rules of conduct and respond to other's expectations. Often this means responding to society's view of aging. Unfortunately, there are many negative attitudes and prejudices about aging and the elderly, most of which are related to fear and lack of knowledge about growing old. These prejudices have been termed **"ageism,"** and their effects can be seen in all facets of our society. Individuals who are not highly valued in a society have fewer opportunities for employment and health care. They may be abused by family and friends, unjustly labeled, and segregated. Ageism can cause older persons to have negative views about themselves.

American society is composed of many subcultures, and many older people counteract the negative values of ageism through their identification with an ethnic group. Strong identification with an ethnic group can enhance role and status for the elderly even when being a member of that ethnic minority group may mean being at greater risk for economic insecurity and poorer health status. For instance, older relatives are held in high esteem by the Hispanic cultures, and it is expected that children will care for their elderly parents. A study of informal support networks found that Hispanic elderly had consistently higher levels of interaction and greater support from their children than either white or black Americans. The elderly in Pacific-Asian communities have a special support system. Many live in closely knit ethnic neighborhoods that are centers for leisure activities and delivery of services. Many underutilize Medicare and Medicaid because they rely on non-Western medicine or family and friends to help them with their health problems.[32]

Many elderly African-Americans have a greater sense of satisfaction with their lives than do elderly white Americans who have better living conditions. This is attributed to the spiritual orientation of many African-Americans, plus the support of their extended families and their religious institutions. Older black women are often regarded as a source of strength in African-American communities. Family bonds are especially strong among Jewish-Americans, who have strong positive feelings for their elderly. Jewish communities have shown leadership in developing community and institutional services for their elderly.

Box 14–7. Leading Health Problems in Late Adulthood

- ▶ Arthritis
- ▶ Osteoporosis
- ▶ Incontinence
- ▶ Visual and hearing impairments
- ▶ Dementia

Data from U.S. Department of Health and Human Services (1990). *Healthy people 2000: National health promotion and disease prevention objectives.* Washington, DC: U.S. Government Printing Office.

MAJOR HEALTH CONCERNS

The primary health care goal for people over the age of 65 years centers on quality of life rather than quantity of life. Promoting health in late adulthood is directed toward improving or maintaining activity and independence. Many people think that health problems in old age are inevitable. However, many are preventable or can be controlled. Leading health problems of the elderly are listed in Box 14–7.

The nurse can play an influential role in the health and well-being of older clients.

Chronic illness is a major problem for older people and a major source of disability. Most older people have at least one chronic illness, which they have learned to live with. The elderly experience fewer acute illnesses than younger age groups. However, acute illnesses in late life usually last longer and are more severe. Leading causes of death in the elderly are both acute and chronic. They are listed in Box 14–8.

There are many detrimental factors in the physical and mental health of older adults. Personal losses, adverse medication effects, the environment, and personal lifestyles all are risk factors that can affect functional independence and quality of life.

Personal Losses

Personal losses can be both physical and psychosocial. Physical changes and limitations, such as muscle weak-

---

Box 14–8. Leading Causes of Death in Late Adulthood

1. Heart disease
2. Cancer
3. Cerebrovascular accident (stroke)
4. Chronic obstructive pulmonary disease (COPD)
5. Pneumonia

Data from U.S. Department of Health and Human Services (1990). *Healthy people 2000: National health promotion and disease prevention objectives.* Washington, DC: U.S. Government Printing Office.

---

ness, unsteady gait, altered sense of balance, and decreased vision and hearing, often lead to falls. Falls are one of the most threatening events for older people. One third of all people over the age of 65 years experience at least one fall per year. Falls can precipitate many disabling complications, most of which result in loss of independence. Many falls are fatal. Risk factors for falls can be identified (Box 14–9).

Psychosocial Losses

Psychosocial losses can result from life events such as death of a spouse or close friends, retirement, relocation (especially to nursing homes), and chronic illness or disability. These life events can bring losses in social status, financial well-being, friends, physical health, self-confidence, and self-esteem. Some life events can cause social isolation, resulting in loneliness and depression.

Depression

Depression is the most common mental health problem in late adulthood. It is estimated that from 10 per cent to 65 per cent of older persons suffer from this illness. Depression may have been a lifelong problem for some elderly; for others it is a new experience. Depression is

---

Box 14–9. Risk Factors for Falls in the Elderly

- ▶ Environmental hazards, such as poor lighting, clutter, uneven stair and sidewalks, slick floors, loose rugs, stools, and pets
- ▶ Problems with walking, such as limited ability to correct imbalances while transferring or walking, gait disturbances, or the need for assistive devices
- ▶ Improperly fitted shoes or slippers
- ▶ Sensory deficits, such as decreased vision or hearing
- ▶ Physical conditions that cause loss of consciousness, such as orthostatic hypotension and syncope
- ▶ Cardiac arrhythmias
- ▶ Peripheral neuropathies
- ▶ Muscle weakness
- ▶ Central nervous system disorders, such as seizure disorders, Parkinson's disease, or multiple sclerosis
- ▶ History of falling
- ▶ Diseases that alter cognitive ability, such as excessive use of alcohol, dementias, confusion, and strokes
- ▶ Polypharmacy or use of a single drug that increases instability, interferes with coordination, causes postural hypotension or confusion, or generally interferes with the client's sense of reality and orientation
- ▶ Client's belief that the caregiver resents calls for assistance

Data from Ross, J.E.R. (1991). Iatrogenesis in the elderly. *Journal of Gerontological Nursing, 17*(9), 19–23; and Ebersole, P., & Hess, P. (1990). *Toward healthy aging: Human needs and nursing response* (3rd ed.). St. Louis: C.V. Mosby.

of particular concern in this age group because it is a risk factor for suicide. Men aged 65 through 74 years have the highest suicide rate in the United States.[17]

Medication Use and Misuse

Medication misuse can be a risk to the physical and mental health of older adults. Because of their many health problems, older adults consume a greater number and variety of prescription medications than other age groups do. They also frequently self-medicate themselves with over-the-counter drugs such as analgesics, laxatives, antihistamines, and antacids. The physiologic changes that come with aging can affect the way the older body processes medications. Older adults are at an increased risk for adverse drug reactions and drug interactions.

Environment

The environment can be a risk factor for older people. Relocation to residences that are devoid of familiar belongings and furnishings can be extremely stressful. Colors, patterns, floor coverings, odors, noise, and constant, strong, or dim lighting are just a few environmental factors that can affect an older person's health. Personal environments conducive to wellness are safe, comfortable, and functional and compensate for physical limitations. They allow for the enjoyment of nature and beauty and offer opportunities to give and receive affection. They include areas for privacy. Many elderly, particularly those living in institutions, do not have a personal environment that contains these necessities.

Lifestyle

Through the years, people's lifestyles continue to put them at risk for health problems. Changing that lifestyle, even in old age, can benefit health and quality of life. Changing diet habits, losing weight, and cutting down on sodium and sugar intake can help keep chronic diseases such as hypertension and diabetes under control and reduce the risk of contracting others. Smoking cessation programs are important for older people. Studies have shown that when older people quit smoking they reduce the risk of heart disease, improve their circulation and respiratory function, and increase their life expectancy.[65] Increased physical activity can reduce the risk for osteoporotic fractures and improve balance, strength, and coordination. Increased levels of physical activity have been associated with reduced incidences of such chronic diseases as heart disease, cancer, diabetes, and depression.

ROLE OF THE NURSE

Because of their diversity and unique needs, older adults present a challenge to nursing. Their health status is influenced by a wide range of physical and psychosocial factors, and their nursing care is given in a variety of settings. Maintaining independence and maintaining a high level of wellness are the underlying themes in the care of older people. Independence is very important to maintaining quality of life during late adulthood.

Assisting older people to experience a healthy aging process requires the nurse to assume many roles: caregiver, counselor, health educator, coordinator of health care services, and advocate. Advocacy is an important component of nursing care for the elderly, particularly the frail elderly. An advocate is one who defends, pleads, or acts on behalf of another person or on behalf of a cause. Ebersole and Hess consider advocacy to be necessary for persons who cannot recognize or articulate their own needs.[16] They identify the following as examples of advocacy action:

▶ Finding physicians who are interested in long-term care of the elderly
▶ Interacting with physicians and other health care workers regarding therapeutic care and options for care
▶ Promoting the individuality of clients in institutional settings and making their unique needs known
▶ Helping the client and family decide on whether to die at home or in an institution
▶ Acting as an ombudsman and spokesperson for the elderly to state and federal legislators

Health Screening and Assessment

An accurate and comprehensive assessment is a very important part of the nursing care of older adults. To do an effective assessment, the nurse must be aware of the normal physical and psychologic changes that accompany aging. A comprehensive health assessment for the older adult should include an appraisal of the physical health, mental health, social resources, and economic resources. For many, it should also include an assessment of activities of daily living (ability to bathe, dress, toilet, transfer, and feed themselves and degree of continence). Instrumental activities of daily living (ability to use telephone, prepare meals, manage finances, and so on) may need to be included. The latter two assessments provide quantitative data regarding a person's ability to function or live independently. Health-screening procedures are a part of any comprehensive assessment program. Those that are appropriate for older persons and which the nurse should encourage include vision, hearing, dental, blood pressure, mammography, and examination for skin, cervical, and colorectal cancers. Laboratory tests should include screening for cholesterol, blood sugar, hematocrit and creatinine levels, fecal occult blood, hyperthyroidism, and urinalysis.

Health Education

Counseling and health education are effective means of promoting health in the older generation. Studies have shown that when educated about health practices, older people have higher levels of compliance and behavior change than those in other age groups.[32]

PROMOTING GOOD NUTRITION

Malnutrition is a particular problem for older persons. It is not a problem restricted to the very poor or to a single ethnic group, although lack of money often is a major contributing factor. Decreased sense of taste and smell, decreased appetite, poor food choices, lack of cooking facilities, lack of transportation, social isolation, alcohol and drug abuse, and physical limitations are all factors that can contribute to malnutrition in the elderly. A thorough nutritional assessment should precede any educational program so that nutritional counseling can be tailored to individual clients. The client should be informed about available resources in the community, such as Meals on Wheels and senior citizen centers that provide socialization as well as nutritionally balanced meals.

PROMOTING ACTIVITY AND EXERCISE

Physical activity is a key ingredient for healthy aging. Exercise not only improves physical fitness, it also contributes to emotional well-being. There are many obstacles to being physically active in old age: stiff joints, decreased energy level, hypotension, lack of motivation. Each older person should be individually counseled and no formal exercise program begun without a physical examination. Exercise can be a part of an older person's regular activities of daily living. Many senior citizen centers now are instituting exercise and physical fitness programs.

Psychologic activity or mental stimulation is also vital to the well-being of older adults. Arts, crafts, educational courses, games, and care of pets can be therapeutic activities to help the older mind maintain its functioning.

PROMOTING SLEEP AND REST

Older persons need to maintain a balance between activity and sleep or rest in order to rejuvenate themselves. Older people generally need 5 to 7 hours of sleep over a 24-hour period. Often older people have difficulty sleeping in long blocks of time, and many develop routine periods during the day for naps or rest. Older people sleep less soundly, and sleep is frequently interrupted by muscle cramps, nocturia, or environmental noises.

Older persons frequently turn to drugs to help them sleep. This should be discouraged, particularly if they are using addictive depressant drugs. Simple insomnia can be assisted by such activities as reading in the middle of the night, listening to the radio or watching television, drinking warm milk, and reducing daytime naps. Persistent sleep disturbances may be due to physical or emotional disturbances, which should be evaluated by a physician.

PROMOTING SAFETY

Older adults are at special risk for safety. Sensory deficits such as reduced peripheral vision, altered depth perception, poor hearing, decreased sense of smell, loss of taste, reduced tactile sensations, and slower response and reaction times contribute to falls, burns, food poisoning, and other accidents. Older people should be encouraged to perform safety checks of their homes periodically, particularly the kitchen, bathrooms, stairs, and halls.

Medications can be hazardous. Teaching the older adult safe use of medications is essential. Outdated medications should be discarded. Safety practices should be encouraged, such as not taking medications in the dark, pouring liquid medications away from the label, and putting special marks on the labels of medicines that are similar in appearance. Older adults should learn the names of their medications, what they look like, and their side effects. They should keep a list of all their current prescription and over-the-counter medications, and take it with them whenever they visit physicians, dentists, or optometrists.

PROMOTING GOOD MENTAL HEALTH

"Good mental health practices throughout one's lifetime promote good mental health in late life," writes Eliopoulos.[18] Independence, a positive self-concept, and involvement in activities and decision making contribute to positive mental health in older adults. Maintaining friendships and family relationships and having someone to confide in and share with help decrease the effects of loss, change, and loneliness. Loneliness affects millions of individuals over the age of 65 years and has been called an emotional state worse than anxiety. It is particularly intense in elderly persons. Interventions for loneliness usually center on involvement in activities that shift attention from self to meeting the needs of others. Such activities as foster grandparent programs, the Retired Seniors Volunteer Program, volunteer companionship programs, and the use of pets can be successful means for establishing feelings of relatedness.[3] It is very important that older people be involved in programs or groups in which they receive formal or informal psychosocial support. Older people need the opportunity to share feelings, make new friends, and enhance their feelings of self-esteem.

Summary

▶ Those at midlife are between ages 40 and 65 years; experience physical changes that are gradual and highly individualized; experience reproductive changes that may have positive or negative effects on sexual activity; are at a high point in their cognitive ability; are in Erikson's stage of generativity versus stagnation; are often responsible for their teenage or young adult children as well as for their aging parents; are often in their postparental years, which years may be their happiest, but this is also a peak time for divorce; may experience spousal abuse as a result of life stresses; are often grandparents. The average age for becoming a grandparent is between 49 and 53 years; are often open to taking on civic responsibilities as well as enjoying the peak of their careers; often have increased leisure time after their children leave the nest; and are at risk for disorders associated with lifestyle, particularly disorders related to poor nutrition, lack of exercise, smoking, and alcohol use.

▶ The major role of the nurse in working with the middle-aged is to promote health care measures and behaviors that improve the quality of life. This includes screening procedures, identification of stressors, health teaching, and counseling.

▶ Those in late adulthood are age 65 years or older; are reasonably healthy, although 86 per cent have at least one chronic disease; age at highly individualized rates; may experience changes in sexual expression due to loss of a partner, chronic health problems, or lack of privacy; are mostly psychologically healthy; are in Erikson's stage of ego integrity versus despair; retain cognitive abilities in relation to their continued use; usually contact their children and other family members frequently; may be in long-standing, interdependent relationships or may be widowed; may need help with care from middle-aged children; may experience elder abuse related to the stresses on the caregiver; may receive help from community support systems; may retire, may continue to work, or may become more involved in volunteer work or hobbies; may suffer the prejudice of ageism; seek quality of life rather than quantity; and experience risk factors for ill health, including personal losses, adverse medication effects, and environmental and personal lifestyle risks.

▶ Nursing care is directed toward maintaining quality of life in late adulthood.

▶ Counseling and health education are effective means of promoting health in the elderly.

Bibliography

1. Alford, D.M. (1982). Tips for teaching older adults. *Nursing Life*, 2(5), 60–63.
2. American Association of Retired Persons (1988). Volunteer program seeks out widowers for special project. *AARP News Bulletin*, 29(1), 11.
3. Austin, A.G. (1989). Becoming immune to loneliness; helping the elderly fill a void. *Journal of Gerontological Nursing*, 15(9), 25–28.
4. Baillie, V., et al. (1988). Stress, social support, and psychological distress of family caregivers of the elderly. *Nursing Research*, 37(4), 217–222.
5. Behler, D., & Tippett, T. (1986). Middle adulthood. In Edelman, C., & Mandle, C.L. (eds.). *Health promotion throughout the lifespan* (pp. 518–536). St. Louis: C.V. Mosby.
6. Braudis, E.M. (1986). Late adulthood. In Edelman, C., & Mandle, C.L. (eds.). *Health promotion throughout the lifespan* (pp. 537–567). St. Louis: C.V. Mosby.
7. Brody, E.M. (1990). *Women in the middle: Their parent-care years.* New York: Springer Publishing Company.
8. Campbell, J.C. (1989). A test of two explanatory models of women's responses to battering. *Nursing Research*, 38(1), 18–23.
9. Carson, V.B. (1989). Spiritual development across the life span. In Carson, V.B. (ed.). *Spiritual dimensions of nursing practice.* Philadelphia: W.B. Saunders.
10. Deevey, S. (1990). Older lesbian women: an invisible minority. *Journal of Gerontological Nursing*, 16(5), 35–37.
11. Dellasega, C. (1989). Health in the sandwich generation. *Geriatric Nursing*, 10(5), 242–243.
12. DeLucci, M.F., et al. (1989). The Men's Adult Life Experiences Inventory: an instrument for assessing developmental concerns of middle age. *Psychological Reports*, 64(2), 479–485.
13. Douglass, R.L. (1988). *Domestic mistreatment of the elderly: Towards prevention* (3rd printing). Washington, DC: American Association of Retired Persons.
14. Duffy, M.E. (1988). Determinants of health promotion in midlife women. *Nursing Research*, 37(6), 358–362.
15. Dychtwald, K. (1986). *Wellness and health promotion for the elderly.* Rockville, MD: Aspen Publishing Co.
16. Ebersole, P., & Hess, P. (1990). *Toward healthy aging: Human needs and nursing response* (3rd ed.). St. Louis: C.V. Mosby.
17. Eliopoulos, C. (1987). *Geronotological nursing* (2nd ed.). Philadelphia: J.B. Lippincott.
18. Eliopoulos, C. (1990). *Health assessment of the older adult* (2nd ed.). Redwood City, CA: Addison-Wesley.
19. Engel, N.S. (1987). Menopausal stage, current life change, attitude toward women's roles, and perceived health status. *Nursing Research*, 36(6), 353–357.
20. Erikson, E. (1950). *Childhood and society.* New York: Norton Company.
21. Fogel, C.I., & Lauver, D. (1990). *Sexual health promotion.* Philadelphia: W.B. Saunders.
22. Freiberg, K.L. (1987). *Human development: A life-span approach* (3rd ed.). Boston: Jones & Bartlett Publishers.
23. Gaynor, S.E. (1990). The long haul: the effects of home care on caregivers. *Image*, 22(4), 208–212.
24. Gross, Z.H. (1985). *And you thought it was all over: Mothers and their adult children.* New York: St. Martins/Marek.
25. Gunter, L.M., & Kolanowski, A.M. (1986). Promoting healthy lifestyles in mature women. *Journal of Gerontological Nursing*, 12(4), 6–13.
26. Hamilton, G.P. (1989). Preventing elder abuse: using a family systems approach. *Gerontological Nursing*, 15(3), 21–26.
27. Havighurst, R.J., & Orr, B. (1972). *Developmental tasks and education* (3rd ed.). New York: David McKay.
28. Heckheimer, E.F. (1989). *Health promotion of the elderly in the community.* Philadelphia: W.B. Saunders.
29. Hogan, S. (1990). Care for the caregiver: social policies to ease their burden. *Gerontological Nursing*, 16(5), 12–17.
30. Hogstel, M.O. (1990). *Geropsychiatric nursing.* St. Louis: C.V. Mosby.
31. Hogstel, M.O., & Gaul, A.L. (1991). Safety or autonomy: an ethical issue for clinical gerontological nurses. *Journal of Gerontological Nursing*, 17(3), 6–11.
32. Hooyman, N.R., & Kiyak, H.A. (1991). *Social gerontology* (2nd ed.). Boston: Allyn and Bacon.
33. Janz, M. (1990). Clues to elder abuse. *Geriatric Nursing*, 11(5), 220–222.
34. Johnston, L., & Gueldner, S.H. (1989). Remember when . . . ? Using mnemonics to boost memory in the elderly. *Journal of Gerontological Nursing*, 15(8), 22–26.
35. Kahn, A.P., & Holt, L.H. (1987). *Midlife health.* New York: Facts on File Publication.
36. Levkoff, S.E., et al. (1987). Differences in the appraisal of health between aged and middle-aged adults. *Journal of Gerontology*, 42(1), 114–120.
37. Maas, M., et al. (1991). *Nursing diagnoses and intervention for the elderly.* Redwood City, CA: Addison-Wesley.
38. Malasanos, L., et al. (1990). *Health assessment* (4th ed.). St. Louis: C.V. Mosby.
39. Mathew, L.J., et al. (1990). Exploring the roles of men caring for demented relatives. *Journal of Gerontological Nursing*, 16(10), 20–25.
40. Matteson, M.A., & McConnell, E.W. (1988). *Gerontological nursing: Concepts and practice.* Philadelphia: W.B. Saunders.
41. Matthieson, V. (1989). Guilt and grief: when daughters place mothers in nursing homes. *Journal of Gerontological Nursing*, 15(7), 11–15.

42. Miller, C.A. (1990). *Nursing care of older adults*. Glenview, IL: Scott, Foresman and Company.
43. Miller, M.P. (1991). Factors promoting wellness in the aged person: an ethnographic study. *Advances in Nursing Science*, 13(4), 38–51.
44. Murray, R., & Zentner, J. (1979). *Nursing concepts for health promotion* (2nd ed.). Englewood Cliffs, NJ: Prentice-Hall.
45. Neugarten, B. (1973). Adult personality: a developmental view. In Charles, C. & Looft, W. (eds.). *Readings in psychological development through life*. New York: Holt, Rinehart and Winston.
46. Neugarten, B.L., & Weinstein, K.D. (1968). The changing American grandparent. In Neugarten, B. (ed.). *Middle age and aging*. Chicago: University of Chicago Press.
47. Nolan, J.W. (1986). Developmental concerns and the health of midlife women. *Nursing Clinics of North America*, 21(1), 151–159.
48. O'Neill, C., & Sorensen, E.S. (1991). Home care of the elderly: a family perspective. *Advances in Nursing Science*, 13(4), 28–37.
49. Oriol, W.E. (1990). The struggle for older women's economic equity is still uphill. *Perspective on Aging*, 19(5), 4–8.
50. Pallett, P.J. (1990). A conceptual framework for studying family caregiver burden in Alzheimer's type dementia. *Image*, 22(1), 52–58.
51. Papalia, D.E., & Olds, S.W. (1978). *Human development*. New York: McGraw-Hill.
52. Patsdaughter, C.A., & Killien, M. (1990). Developmental transitions in adulthood: mother-daughter relationships. *Holistic Nursing Practice*, 4(3), 37–46.
53. Perlmutter, M., & Hall, E. (1985). *Adult development and aging*. New York: John Wiley & Sons.
54. Piaget, J. (1952). *The origins of intelligence in children*. New York: International Universities Press.
55. Public Health Service (1988). *The Surgeon General's report on nutrition and health*. DHHS Pub. No. (PHS) 88-50210. Washington, DC: U.S. Department of Health and Human Services.
56. Robinson, K.M. (1989). Predictors of depression among wife caregivers. *Nursing Research*, 38(6), 359–363.
57. Schank, M.J., & Lough, M.A. (1989). Maintaining health and independence of elderly women. *Gerontological Nursing*, 15, 8–11.
58. Schorr, J.A., et al. (1991). Health patterns in aging women as expanding consciousness. *Advances in Nursing Science*, 13(4), 52–62.
59. Shanas, E. (1980). Older people and their families: the new pioneers. *Journal of Marriage and the Family*, 42, 9–14.
60. Skinner, B.F. (1983). *Enjoy old age: A program of self management*. New York: Warner Books.
61. Spitze, G., & Logan, J. (1990). More evidence on women (and men) in the middle. *Research on Aging*, 12, 182–198.
62. Thomas, J.L. (1992). *Adulthood and aging*. Boston: Allyn and Bacon.
63. U.S. Bureau of the Census (1988). *Statistical abstract of the United States* (108th ed.). Washington, DC: U.S. Government Printing Office.
64. U.S. Congress, Office of Technology Assessment (1990). *Preventive health services for Medicare beneficiaries: Policy and research issues*, OTA-H-416. Washington, DC: U.S. Government Printing Office.
65. U.S. Department of Health and Human Services (1990). *Healthy people 2000: National health promotion and disease prevention objectives*. Washington, DC: U.S. Government Printing Office.
66. U.S. Senate Special Committee on Aging (1988). *Aging America: Trends and projections*. Washington, DC: U.S. Government Printing Office.
67. Wagnild, G., & Young, H.M. (1990). Resilience among old women. *Image*, 22(4), 252–255.
68. Weiler, K. (1989). Financial abuse of the elderly. *Gerontological Nursing*, 15(8), 10–15.
69. Weitzman, L.J. (1985). *The divorce revolution: The unexpected social and economic consequences for women and children in America*. New York: Free Press.
70. Wells, R.G. (1990). The hot flash: answering patients' pleas for help. *Senior Patient*, 2(6), 24–27.
71. Whall, A. (1990). Geropsychiatry: using mental health principles as we age. *Journal of Gerontological Nursing*, 16(10), 40–41.
72. Willits, F.K., & Crider, D.M. (1988). Health rating and life satisfaction in the later middle years. *Journal of Gerontology*, 43(5), S172–S176.

Characteristics of Persons Served by the Nurse

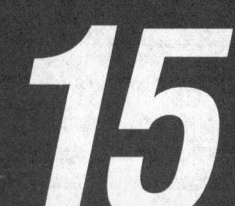

▼ *Human Needs*

Chapter *15*

A man travels the world over in search of what he needs . . . .
George Moore

▼ CHAPTER OUTLINE

PEOPLE AS LIVING SYSTEMS
GENERAL SYSTEMS THEORY
LIVING SYSTEMS AND ADAPTATION
HUMAN NEEDS
UNMET NEEDS
HELPING PEOPLE WITH UNMET NEEDS
THE NEED TO UNDERSTAND THE SELF
   DURING HEALTH AND ILLNESS
      The Self and Integration and
        Wholeness
      The Self and Individuality and
        Uniqueness

The Self and Autonomy
The Self and Personal Values
The Self and Self-Actualization
The Self, Introspection and Time
The Self and Emotional Conflict
The Self and Other ''Selves''
The ''Public Self''
Self-Concept
Individual Self and Universal Self
The Self and Significant Others
NEEDS, THE SELF, AND NURSING CARE

▼ KEY TERMS

General systems theory
  (GST)
Hierarchy
Holistic nursing care
Human need theory

Input
Need
Output
Self
Self-actualization

Self-perception
Subsystem
Suprasystem
System

▼ LEARNING OBJECTIVES

After studying this chapter, you should be able to

1. *Explain why nursing is both a science and an art.*
2. *Discuss general systems theory (GST) as it applies to nursing.*
3. *Describe needs theory according to Maslow, Orem, and Yura and Walsh.*
4. *Describe how unmet needs can result in illness.*
5. *List seven general obstacles to need satisfaction.*
6. *Explain the three major ways nurses help satisfy unmet needs.*
7. *Describe how an understanding of the various characteristics of the self help the nurse improve nursing care for both sick and well individuals.*

Nursing involves intense and sometimes long-term interaction with people who are threatened, who are suffering, who are dying. We care for people who are asking questions for which there are no answers. We are able to do this because of the nature of nursing. The profession of nursing is both a science and an art. But what is science and what is art? A science involves a systematic approach to knowledge. In a science, information is categorized and organized within a clearly defined framework. An art involves the conscious application of both learned skills and creative imagination to a particular medium of expression, be it a musical composition, a painting, or a person.

Nursing is a science that deals with human needs and related health problems. The science of nursing is built upon a systematic step-by-step method of problem solving called the nursing process (see Chapter 6). Your studies in the biologic and social sciences and in the humanities are directed toward helping you apply the nursing process to people with unmet needs and to those who can achieve higher levels of health. Much of your nursing education is directed toward helping you learn this indispensable method of assessing, diagnosing, planning, implementing, and evaluating. Your success as a nurse is based in large part on how consistently and how accurately you use the nursing process.

Systematic problem solving is the cornerstone of modern nursing practice.

Nursing is a practical science. We use what we learn to bring positive change into the lives of the people for whom we care. We use research, theories, and facts to help us understand human needs and the pathologic processes that block the satisfaction of needs, thus creating problems.

More than a science, nursing is the art of meeting human needs. The art of nursing involves the skillful and creative application of the nursing process to the solution of human problems. Like other arts, nursing requires skill, imagination, dedication, and love of the work. The nursing art involves giving care that is based on scientific principles but founded in human caring.

Like any art, the practice of nursing requires great sensitivity. To limit ourselves to the science of nursing and ignore the art is to violate the meaning and spirit of nursing.

Nursing meshes science and art in the care of a person's totality: body, mind, and spirit. Nurses provide **holistic nursing care** (the provision of biologic, psychologic, and sociocultural care to persons so that they are treated as a human whole). Nurses cannot limit themselves to technical care. We cannot divide nursing care into physical and psychologic components. The only nursing care worth giving is complete care that approaches each person as a unique, respected human being.

Because nursing is holistic, we take care of developing persons who are physical, intellectual, spiritual, emotional, and social beings. As we care for people, we apply the art and science of nursing to meet individual human needs, solve human problems, and promote physical and psychosocial health.

In this chapter, we explore human nature and focus on human needs. We discuss systems theory that enables us to examine the interrelatedness of organ systems within the body and of people within society. We also explore theories concerning human needs. An understanding of human needs is important because unmet needs can result in illness.

PEOPLE AS LIVING SYSTEMS

Scientists and philosophers, nurses and physicians are always searching for unifying concepts with which to correlate the individual psychophysiologic, social, and cultural dimensions of human existence. One way to integrate these various facets into a unified whole is to use the systems approach.

GENERAL SYSTEMS THEORY

General systems theory (GST) refers to the use of a hierarchical method of studying and talking about phenomena. The theory was developed by Ludwig von Bertalanffy during the late 1930s. GST was meant to provide a common language and a set of common concepts to assist scientists from diverse disciplines to speak to and learn from each other. Since its conception, this theoretical construct has been applied to many disciplines: nursing, management theory, engineering, physics. Systems theory is a framework used to study planets, cultures, organisms, subatomic particles, and so forth.

In essence, a **system** is a set consisting of integrated, interacting parts that function as a whole (e.g., a human being, an elephant, a computer, a truck, a birdhouse, a rosebush). Systems can be open or closed. An open system exchanges matter, energy, and information with other systems and with the environment. An open system maintains itself in a steady state. All living systems are open systems. A closed system does not interact with its environment. There are no totally closed systems. Some systems, however, are more closed than others.

For example, a high school education system may be considered an open system where students come and go each day from the time they enter as freshmen until their graduation as seniors, where teachers use paper and chalk as matter from the environment, where the furnace obtains fuel oil from the environment to heat for warmth, where the principal purchases information from outside by hiring teachers and buying books, and where the students expel old papers and other trash into the environment.

The school building in summer, used only for an occasional meeting, may also be considered an open system, with parts that interact and exchange matter, energy, and information with the environment. Phones ring; lights go on and off; and doors open and close. However, this system is less an open system than the educational system that uses a good deal of matter and energy to teach students.

An abandoned school building, on the other hand, would more nearly resemble a closed system because very little or no matter, energy, or information would be exchanged with the environment.

All living systems have an internal environment (internal milieu) as distinguished from the external environment (external milieu) that surrounds them. This internal milieu is created by boundaries that separate living systems from the external milieu. For example, a human being's boundary consists of the skin and mucous membranes.

The maintenance of the internal milieu is essential for life.

The three major functions of the internal milieu are to (1) help the living system adjust to changes in the external environment, (2) prevent the intrusion of noxious substances that disturb the function of the system, and (3) enable the system to exchange vital substances with the external environment. Any breakdown or disruption of this internal environment can destroy the living system.

According to systems theory, systems exist in a **hierarchy** (a grading or ranking of members of a group in order of relative importance). A system consists of **subsystems,** subsets of a system, sets of integrated, interacting parts that, together with one or more other subsystems, make up a system. For example, the solar system is composed of planets, each of which is a subsystem. A subsystem could also have its own subsystems of interacting, integrated parts. For example, a

planet, as one subsystem of the solar system could be composed of a core, mantel, and crust as its subsystems). Likewise, the human body may be viewed as a system, with the various organs as its subsystems. Each organ, in turn, is composed of subsystems of interacting tissues; each tissue is composed of subsystems of interacting cells. We could even break these subsystems down into their subsystems and find cells composed of subsystems of atoms and atoms composed of subsystems of subatomic particles.

Each system is a part of a larger system known as a **suprasystem,** a collection of two or more systems into a larger system. For our solar system, the suprasystem is the Milky Way galaxy, and the suprasystem for all of the galaxies is the universe. In the same way, human beings are both systems and parts of a suprasystem consisting of a group of significant others, who in turn are part of a suprasystem consisting of a group of the larger community. The suprasystem for many communities is the larger society, which is part of the suprasystem made up of all humanity. Humanity then belongs to a suprasystem that includes all other living species in the biosphere (Figure 15-1).

A system meets goals by interacting with its environment and through the interaction of its subsystems. Therefore, communication between systems and within a system is essential. Effective communication involves the processes of input, feedback, and transformation. **Input** is the general systems theory term for the movement of matter, energy, or information from the environment into a system. The input is either meaningful or meaningless, helpful or unhelpful, useful or nonuseful. Before a system can interpret or use this input, the input must sometimes be transformed. For example, food must be digested before the body can use it. Systems also produce **output,** the general systems theory term for the movement of matter, energy, or information out of a system and into the environment. Some of this output is fed back into the system to correct or modify further output from the system. This process is called feedback.

The basic goal of a system is to maintain a state of equilibrium or homeostatic balance. A state of balance must exist both within the system and between the system and its external environment. The system uses input, transformation, output, and feedback to accomplish this goal. Unfortunately, this balance is elusive and ever-changing.

LIVING SYSTEMS AND ADAPTATION

To maintain homeostatic balance, all living systems must have the capacity to adapt themselves internally to changes in the external environment. This ability enables the living system to escape harm, minimize injury, cope with stress, and restore internal balance once this balance is lost. The late Hans Selye, an authority on stress theory, wrote that "adaptability is probably the most distinctive characteristic of life."[36] Indeed, Selye equated adaptability with life and the loss of adaptability with death.

People, then, can be viewed as systems composed of

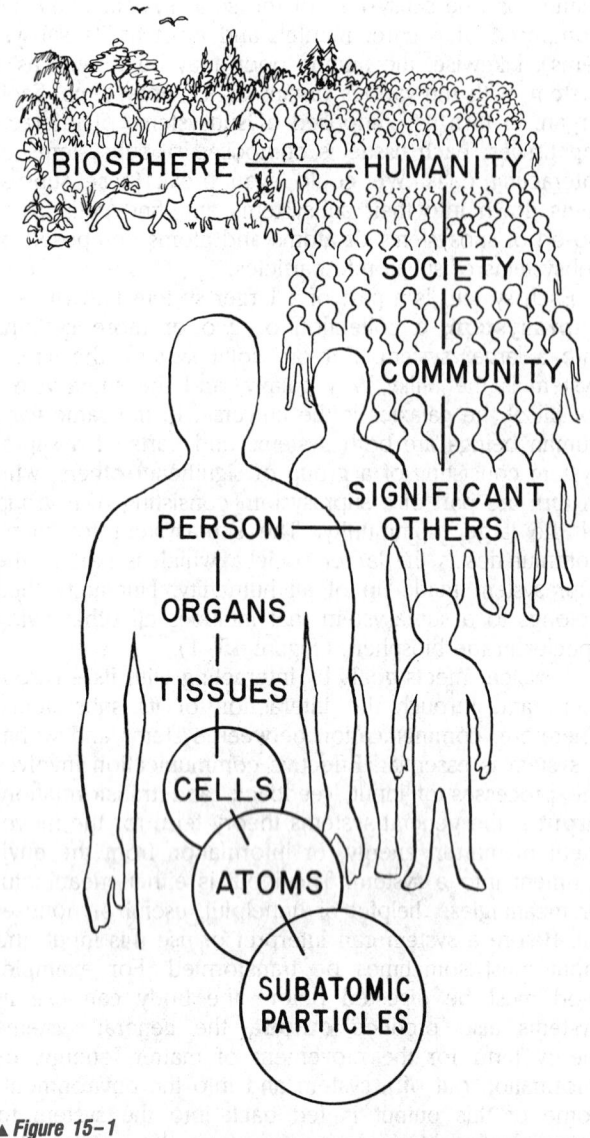

▲ *Figure 15–1*

A person is a natural, living system composed of increasingly smaller subsystems known as organs, tissues, cells, atoms, and subatomic particles. A person is also one part of increasingly larger suprasystems known as significant others, communities, societies, humanity, and the biosphere.

subsystems that maintain the internal milieu of the body. When people are in a state of equilibrium, or homeostatic balance, their internal environments are stable despite demands from the external environment. Not only must people maintain physiologic equilibrium (e.g., fluid and electrolyte balance, balance between food intake and energy expenditure), but they must also be in psychologic equilibrium.

To maintain homeostasis, people must satisfy basic physiologic requirements for oxygen, water, nutrients, and so forth. Moreover, adaptation to the external environment depends on an individual being able to meet basic sociocultural needs for shelter, security, safety, and belonging. When these vital needs are not met, the human system breaks down. Without therapeutic inter-

vention, a severely disrupted human system collapses and dies.

The ultimate goal of nursing is to help individuals regain and maintain psychophysiologic and sociocultural equilibrium.

Achievement of this nursing goal is based on an intricate series of steps. The first step is assessment of the total human system and subsystems in terms of (a) internal organ and system function and interaction, and (b) interaction of the total organism with the external environment and the larger suprasystems.

When caring for people, ask yourself the following questions:

▶ Do the individual's body and mind seem to be functioning together as an integrated system? If not, psychosomatic illness or somatopsychic illness may develop. In *psychosomatic* illness, physical symptoms are emotional in origin. In *somatopsychic* illness, physical symptoms result in emotional problems.

▶ Are the body systems operating together as an integrated whole? If not, an imbalance in one system (e.g., the cardiovascular system) can cause an imbalance in another system (e.g., the renal system).

▶ Are the subsystems intact and working in concert? For example, is the person's gastrointestinal tract functioning properly to absorb ingested food? Is the person eating and drinking adequate amounts to sustain activity and cell function? Is the cardiovascular system delivering sufficient oxygen to cells?

▶ Is the person functioning adequately within other systems? Are positive, supportive relationships available to the person? Is the person's societal role consistent with self-image and personal expectations? Holistic nursing care requires recognizing the role of the person within the context of broader systems such as family, community, society, and culture.

▶ Are feedback mechanisms intact? For example, is the brain receiving and sensing stimuli from peripheral receptors and using the information to adapt to its internal and external environment? On the psychosocial level, is the person receiving feedback from other people to verify feelings or to adjust behavior?

▶ Is the human system able to meet basic needs essential to homeostatic balance? Does the person have adequate food, clean air to breathe, sufficient rest, shelter, a support system of significant others, and so on?

▶ What internal and external stressors or demands are challenging the system? To what extent are these demands disturbing the balance and function of the system? How well is the system adapting to the demands?

▶ Is the person receiving adequate information from the environment? Is the person able to transform this input into meaningful or useful information or substances?

▶ Is the system self-regulatory? Does the person's system automatically maintain itself physiologically? Or does the individual require medication, surgical procedures, or other therapeutic support to function?

▶ Has the system been disrupted by disease? Is the person no longer able to meet needs arising from illness? To what extent does the person require nursing intervention to meet basic human needs?

Your plan of care for restoring balance to a person with a disrupted system depends on answers to these broad questions and on your analysis of this information. To be holistic, nursing intervention must address the person as a total system.

To practice holistic nursing, appreciate each person as a total individual. Be aware of each person's interaction with other individuals and with broader systems such as the group or culture in which the person lives. Take time to appreciate the complex interrelationships among body systems and between body and mind. Recognize that basic needs must be met so that people can function as integrated systems.

HUMAN NEEDS

A **need** is a requirement or a lack. All people have certain fundamental needs that they strive to satisfy. These needs are both physical (e.g., the need for oxygen and food) and psychologic (e.g., the need to be loved or to feel respected). The relative importance of each need depends on the individual. The relative value of each need is influenced by such things as personal expectations, societal and cultural influences, physical health, and the person's level of psychophysiologic development.

Basic needs unite people by identifying just what makes us human. People are bonded to one another because we share the same needs. A wealthy person and an impoverished person, despite vast differences in lifestyle, each understand what it means to be hungry. Both must eat to maintain life. An elderly woman dying of cancer in Israel and a young man dying of cancer in Canada both understand the need to be free from pain. Our ancestors who endured hunger and cold felt the need for food and shelter. They needed the warmth and security of a group to survive a hostile environment. Today we have the same basic needs as they did.

Psychologists, nurses, and philosophers have crystallized the concept of human needs into theories to explain human behavior.

Human need theory is the doctrine that all persons have certain requirements essential for maintaining life and health.

Abraham Maslow is an important example of a human needs theorist. Maslow, a psychologist, developed one of the earlier theories based on human needs. His hierarchy of human needs is well known to psychology and nursing students.

His scheme presents five levels of needs:

1. Physiologic needs: food, air, water, temperature, elimination, rest, pain avoidance

2. Safety needs: safety, security, protection, and freedom from fear, anxiety, and chaos

3. Belongingness and love needs: love, belonging, closeness

4. Esteem needs: esteem of others, self-esteem

5. Self-actualization: the process of making maximal use of one's abilities and potential

Maslow organized human needs according to this hierarchy to emphasize the relationships among them. He pointed out, for example, that people must fulfill physiologic needs before attempting to address safety needs. Likewise, safety needs must be satisfied before a person can fulfill love needs, and so on. However, Maslow also emphasizes that although the lower needs (e.g., the physiologic needs) must be satisfied if life is to continue, the higher needs also have survival value —a fact that health professionals sometimes forget. In this context, Maslow states:

Living at the higher level means greater biological efficiency, greater longevity, less disease, better sleep, appetite, etc. The psychosomatic researchers prove again and again that anxiety, fear, lack of love, domination, etc., tend to encourage undesirable physical as well as undesirable psychological results. Higher need gratifications have survival value and growth value as well.[21]

Clearly, some needs require immediate and constant gratification (e.g., respiratory needs); some needs can be temporarily postponed (e.g., food and sleep); and still other needs can be postponed indefinitely (e.g., sexual needs). Although need gratification can be postponed or modified for varying periods, the needs are still present.

The means by which we satisfy needs become more divergent as we move up the hierarchy. The mechanisms by which people fulfill the basic need for oxygen, for example, do not vary greatly. Everyone must draw sufficient oxygen into the lungs, where it is diffused into the alveolar capillaries and transported to all body cells. Yet the means by which a person achieves self-actualization is highly individualized. To become self-actualized an author writes, an athlete competes, a scientist performs research.

Several years after Maslow first described his theory, Richard Kalish adapted it and added another "level" of needs (Figure 15–2.) The "new" fifth level fits in between the physiologic and safety needs. Note that it includes sexual needs and the need for activity, exploration, manipulation, and novelty.

Many nursing theorists base their frameworks on human needs. One group of nurses, for example, ranked Maslow's subcategories of human needs to establish priorities for nursing intervention (Box 15–1.)

Dorothea Orem bases her theory of nursing on the concept of self-care. Orem groups human needs into three categories: (1) universal self-care requisites, (2) developmental self-care requisites, and (3) health-deviation self-care requisites. The first two categories represent basic human needs; the last group identifies needs arising from illness.

1. Universal self-care requisites are common to all human beings during all stages of the life cycle, ad-

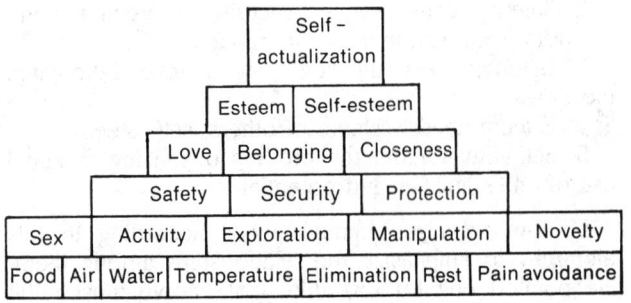

		Self–actualization		
	Esteem		Self-esteem	
	Love	Belonging	Closeness	
	Safety	Security	Protection	
Sex	Activity	Exploration	Manipulation	Novelty
Food	Air	Water	Temperature	Elimination	Rest	Pain avoidance

▲ *Figure 15–2*

Maslow's hierarchy of human needs, as adapted by Kalish. (From Kalish, R.A. (1982). *The psychology of human behavior* (5th ed.). Monterey, CA: Brooks/Cole Publishing Company.)

justed to age, developmental state, and environmental and other factors. Universal self-care requisites are associated with life processes and with the maintenance of the integrity of human structure and functioning.[24]

Examples of universal self-care requisites or needs include maintenance of sufficient intake of air, water, and food; maintenance of elimination processes; maintenance of a balance between rest and activity; maintenance of a balance between time spent alone and social interaction; prevention of hazards and promotion of safety; and development of a realistic self-concept.

2. Developmental self-care requisites are associated with human developmental processes and with conditions and events occurring during various stages of the life cycle (e.g., prematurity, pregnancy) and events that can adversely affect development.[24]

Box 15–1. Priority Ranking of Maslow's Subcategories of Human Needs

Physiologic Needs

Oxygen, circulation
Water-salt balance
Food balance
Acid-base balance
Waste elimination
Normal temperature
Sleep, rest, relaxation
Activity, exercise
Energy
Comfort
Stimulation
Cleanliness
Sexuality

Safety Needs

Protection from physical harm
Protection from psychologic threat
Freedom from pain
Stability
Dependence
Predictable, orderly world

Belongingness Needs

Love and affection
Acceptance
Warm, communicating relationships
Approval from others
Unity with loved ones
Group companionship

Self-Esteem Needs

Sense of value, usefulness
High evaluation of self
Adequacy
Self-reliance
Goal achievement
Mastery and competence in skills
Independence
Endurance

Esteem-from-Others Needs

Recognition
Dignity
Appreciation from others
Importance, influence
Reputation of good character
Attention
Status
Dominance over others

Self-Actualization Needs

Personal growth and maturity
Awareness of potential
Increased learning
Full development of potential
Improved values
Religious, philosophic satisfaction
Increased creativity
Increased reality perception and problem solving abilities
Less rigid conventionality
Less of the familiar, more of the novel
Greater satisfaction in beauty
Increased pleasantness
Less of the simple, more of the complex

From Campbell, C. (1978). *Nursing diagnosis and intervention in nursing practice* (p. 15). New York: John Wiley and Sons.

Developmental self-care requisites can be broken down into two subcategories. The first category includes the need to promote the processes of development during fetal life, birth, childhood, adolescence, pregnancy, and adulthood. The second category emphasizes the need to prevent untoward conditions that can affect development, such as educational deprivation, loss of significant others, poor health, a disability, oppressive living conditions, or terminal illness.

3. Health-deviation self-care requisites are associated with genetic and constitutional defects and human structural and functional deviations, their effects, and medical diagnosis and treatment.[24]

Health-deviation self-care requisites arise from disease, injury, disfigurement, disability, and medical care itself (iatrogenic illness).

Yura and Walsh, two prominent nurse theorists, emphasize that the principal role of the nurse is to meet human needs by utilizing the nursing process. They point out that "the nurse's function is to assess the existence and extent of illness or wellness."[42] Assessment, in turn, serves as a framework for diagnosing, planning, implementing, and evaluating health and nursing care. Box 15–2 lists the needs that nurses assess and try to meet. Note that Yura and Walsh divide needs into two groups: (1) human needs for the individual client, and (2) human needs for the family and community.

Box 15–2. Basic Human Needs Amenable to Nursing Intervention

Human Needs for Individual Client	*Human Needs for the Family and Community*
Acceptance of self and others, by others	*Survival Needs*
Activity	activity
Adaptation, to manage stress	adaptation, to manage stress
Air	air
Appreciation, attention	effective perception of reality
Autonomy, choice	elimination
Beauty and esthetic experiences	fluids
Belonging	interchange of gases
Challenge	nutrition
Conceptualization, rationality, problem solving	protection from excessive fear, anxiety, and chaos
Confidence	rest and leisure
Effective perception of reality	safety
Elimination	sensory integrity
Fluids (intake)	skin integrity
Freedom from pain	sleep
Humor	structure, law, and limits
Interchange of gases	*Closeness Needs*
Nutrition (intake)	acceptance of self and others
Personal recognition, esteem, respect	appreciation, attention
Protection from excessive fear, anxiety, and chaos	belonging
Rest and leisure	confidence
Safety	humor
Self-control, self-determination, responsibility	personal recognition, esteem, respect
Self-fulfillment, to be, to become	sexual integrity
Sensory integrity	tenderness
Sexual integrity	to love and be loved
Skin integrity	wholesome body image
Sleep	*Freedom Needs*
Spiritual integrity	autonomy, choice
Structure, law, and limits	beauty and esthetic experiences
Tenderness	challenge
Territoriality	conceptualization, rationality, problem solving
To love and be loved	freedom from pain
Value system	self-control, self-determination, responsibility
Wholesome body image	self-fulfillment, to be, to become
	spiritual experience
	territoriality
	value system

From Yura, H., & Walsh, M.B. (1983). *The nursing process: Assessing, planning, implementing, evaluating* (4th ed., pp. 136–137). Norwalk, CT: Appleton-Century-Crofts.

PROBLEMS OF UNMET NEEDS

People must meet basic needs to survive and to grow and develop. Ideally, people meet their needs independently, within their personal and sociocultural milieu. When most of a person's needs are met, that person is then in a state of homeostatic balance, or equilibrium. Although some human needs are not portrayed in Figure 15–3, it does show many needs of concern to nurses. Note that Figure 15–3 illustrates a person we will call John who is temporarily in a state of psychophysiologic balance and consequently healthy. Because John's needs for food and fluid intake are met, the need for proper elimination is met. The need for adequate nutrition, fluid and electrolyte balance, and healthy elimination are thus in equilibrium. Moreover, John is fortunate in that he is meeting his needs for safety, sleep, and rest. Also, he is currently adapting satisfactorily to life's stressors. Because basic needs have been satisfied, John now has the time and energy to address the need for self-actualization. Although poems have been written in foxholes, creativity blooms most fully when a person has satisfied basic needs.

When needs go unmet, disequilibrium and eventual illness result. In nursing terminology, the unmet need develops into a problem. Nurses and other health care professionals intervene to help people satisfy these needs and consequently resolve problems. To illustrate this idea, imagine this scenario. John has developed a severe gastrointestinal upset due to a flu virus. Before developing the flu, John was preparing for an important business meeting and had been overworking and eating "on the run." He became tired physically and emotionally. John was failing to meet his need for rest and adequate nutrition. He was therefore in a state of mild psychophysiologic imbalance. This imbalance, in turn, predisposed John to developing a serious case of flu.

Now John has multiple unmet needs that are creating problems in meeting still other needs (Figure 15–4). Because of the flu, John is vomiting and also has severe diarrhea. These manifestations have further upset his need for adequate nutrition. Needs for normal elimination and fluid and electrolyte balance are adversely affected. Because John is up all night running to the bathroom, the need for sleep and rest suffers. Also, because of his acute illness, John, a fastidious person, finds it hard to meet his need for hygiene. Under these conditions, the need for sexuality is diminished and self-actualization is temporarily halted. If John continues to be unable to eat, drink fluids, or sleep, he will need health care professionals to help him meet his basic needs.

Although we realize that unmet needs bring problems, the question is, why are needs not met? Obstacles to need satisfaction include:

▶ Physiologic obstacles: illness, fatigue, pain, immobility. In John's case, a need for rest and better nutrition made him susceptible to a viral infection. The gastrointestinal infection, in turn, hampered John's efforts to satisfy his needs for nutrition, elimination, fluid and electrolyte balance, and so forth.

▶ Emotional obstacles: anxiety, excitement, fear. Anxiety, for instance, can result in loss of appetite, thus thwarting satisfaction of nutritional needs. In John's case, anxiety about his job disturbed his nutrition.

▶ Intellectual obstacles: lack of information, knowledge, and understanding. A person must know how to meet needs. For instance, a person who knows nothing about basic nutritional requirements may eat a diet that lacks essential nutrients. This diet in turn may disrupt elimination, fluid and electrolyte balance, and so on.

▶ Social obstacles: strained interpersonal relationships, fear of another person, feeling intimidated by others, shyness, an inadequate social network. For example, when people feel shy, fearful, and alone, they may not be sufficiently assertive to meet their needs for such things as sexuality and belonging.

▶ Environmental obstacles: extremes in environmental temperatures, unfamiliar surroundings (such as a hospital), air pollution.

▶ Personal obstacles: habits, beliefs, values, and life experiences of the person. For example, a person with a rigid view of available options may be unable to explore new and more effective ways of meeting needs.

▶ Cultural obstacles: values, beliefs, practices, and habits particular to a group of people. In some cultural groups, for example, strong sexual taboos hinder satisfaction of sexual needs.

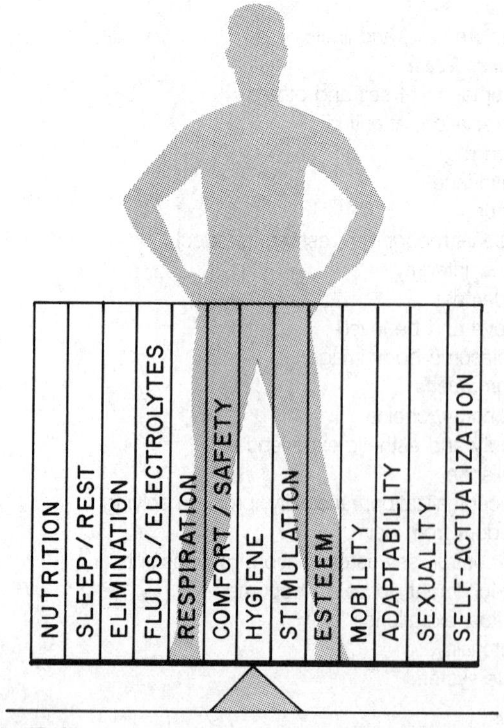

▲ *Figure 15–3*

A person in homeostatic balance with basic needs met.

NUTRITION | SLEEP / REST | ELIMINATION | FLUIDS / ELECTROLYTES | RESPIRATION | COMFORT / SAFETY | HYGIENE | STIMULATION | ESTEEM | MOBILITY | ADAPTABILITY | SEXUALITY | SELF-ACTUALIZATION

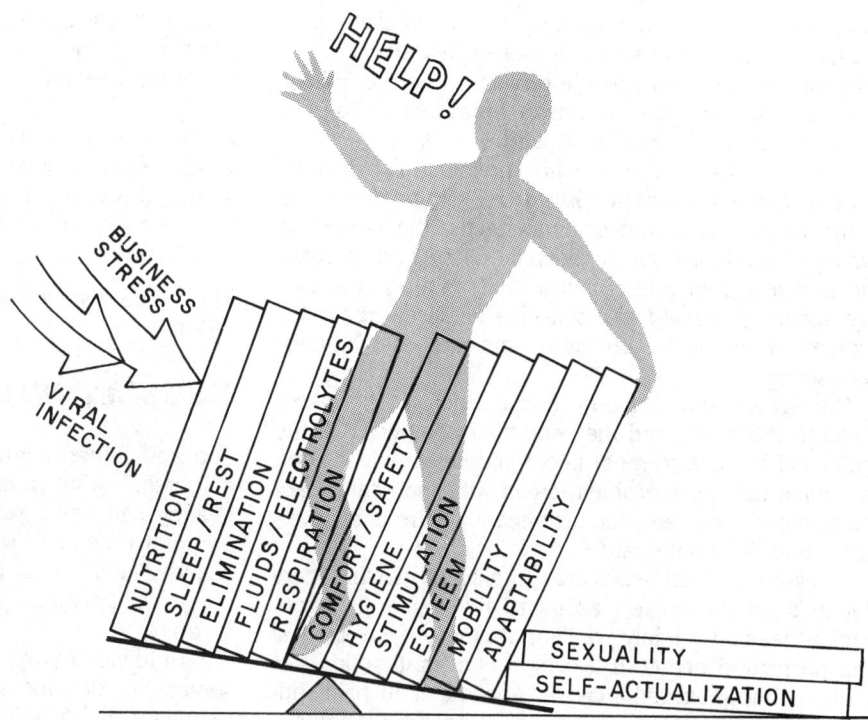

▲ *Figure 15–4*

A person in homeostatic imbalance with some basic needs unmet.

HELPING PEOPLE WITH UNMET NEEDS

Nurses help people satisfy unmet needs and solve problems in three major ways.

Nurses help people who are temporarily or permanently dependent on others to meet their basic psychophysiologic needs. For example, some people are so ill that they need a mechanical ventilator to breathe. Others can receive fluid only by intravenous infusion. Many people rely on nurses to turn, feed, and bathe them.

Nurses help people attain a state of optimal independence so that they can care for themselves as much as possible and meet their own needs. One of the most important aspects of nursing is rehabilitation, which involves assisting people to attain their maximal potential for a satisfying life.

Nurses help prevent the development of unmet needs and problems by helping people remove or diminish obstacles to need satisfaction. Nurses accomplish this goal primarily through the learning/teaching process (Chapter 26) and through appropriate referrals. For instance, you can help people satisfy the need for good nutrition by providing them with pamphlets on nutrition, working out a dietary plan with them, or making a referral to the dietitian for further education and counseling.

Recall that human needs exist in a hierarchy. Nursing care is based on this hierarchy. For example, people who are critically ill are usually cared for in an intensive care unit (ICU). In an ICU, nursing intervention primarily focuses on helping critically ill people satisfy physiologic needs. For example, if a person is admitted with uncontrolled bleeding, the first priority is to stop

the hemorrhage, replace fluids, and save the person's life. Nurses administer powerful medications, whole blood, plasma, and other fluids to sustain adequate circulation. They monitor and administer oxygen therapy to maintain sufficient respiration. Nursing care, however, does not stop at this physiologic level.

When the client with uncontrolled bleeding stabilizes, nurses focus their attention on other unmet needs. Perhaps this person is in pain resulting from surgery, trauma, or medical and nursing therapies. Nurses then intervene by positioning the person comfortably, by turning the person gently, or by administering pain medications. The individual is also at risk for infection. Hence, nurses use medical and surgical aseptic techniques and administer antibiotics to prevent or combat possible infection.

Having satisfied the basic physiologic needs and the need for safety and relief from pain, nurses can then address love and belonging needs. They may arrange to have significant others visit the person. They use their own therapeutic communication skills to establish and foster a supportive, caring relationship with the individual.

The client who has become stronger is transferred from the ICU. Nurses on the general medical-surgical unit continue to help the individual with physiologic needs. In time, they assist the person to ambulate. Having lost a great amount of blood, the person may be very weak and need assistance and encouragement to begin sitting on the side of the bed, then transferring from bed to chair, then ambulating down the hall. Perhaps the period of immobility has altered bowel habits, resulting in constipation. To deal with this problem, nurses encourage (a) intake of fluids and high-fiber foods, and (b) ambulation, which stimulates peristalsis and strengthens muscles used in defecation. In addition, nurses must provide privacy when the individual attempts to have a bowel movement—thereby meeting a prescribed cultural need.

These nurses also deal with the person's "higher" needs. Nurses encourage visits from significant others. If the client has unmet spiritual needs, the nurse can arrange for a visit from the hospital chaplain or perhaps the person's own priest, minister, or rabbi. If the person seems depressed, the sensitive nurse discusses the problem with the health care team and recommends counseling.

Throughout the person's hospitalization, the nurse looks to the future and the person's discharge. Will the individual be able to meet needs independently? If not, the nurse discusses problem areas with the health care team, the person, and the significant others and develops a plan for home care.

In essence, then, sensitive, intelligent nursing care depends on the nurse's ability to recognize all unmet human needs. Certainly we cannot ignore basic survival and protection needs. If a person is cyanotic (skin has a bluish hue), oxygen may be needed; if in pain, administration of analgesics may be necessary; if unconscious, protection from biologic and physical dangers is essential.

On the other hand, the needs for love, stimulation, and esteem are equally important. Surgery can partially repair a broken body following an accident, but it cannot repair a scarred and distorted body image. The need for self-esteem cannot be ignored once the surgery is over. Immobilized people can deteriorate both mentally and physically if their needs for mental stimulation and physical movement are not met. The loss of a significant other and of the accompanying love and security are sometimes followed by the development of cancer.[3]

People requiring nursing care want to do more than just exist. Too frequently, nursing care is directed only at the survival needs. We all desire and need novelty, love, and esteem. We all need to strive for self-actualization. Even people who are dying want to live their last moments with dignity. We all want to live a full life despite our limitations.

THE NEED TO UNDERSTAND THE SELF DURING HEALTH AND ILLNESS

According to Maslow, the need for self-actualization is a person's highest need. **Self-actualization** is the highest state of being, the full realization of the individual's potential.

It is our human need to understand ourselves that continuously moves us toward meeting our highest need—the need for self-actualization.

We can understand various characteristics of the self by reviewing representative studies of philosophers, so-ciologists, psychologists, psychiatrists, and nurses. Understanding these characteristics of the self helps us better understand

▶ the persons we call our clients
▶ ourselves as persons
▶ the ways we, as nurses, can better help meet the needs of our clients in both their health and their illnesses

The characteristics we will discuss are listed in Box 15–3.

The Self and Integration and Wholeness

The **self** is the union of all the elements that comprise a person's individual and particular make-up. The healthy self has a sense of personal integration or coherent wholeness. There is within each of us a recognizable "self." It is the part of each of us that thinks about what we said or did and about what we will say or do.

As individuals we each strive to come to know ourselves. We develop a sense or a feeling about the kind of person we are. To some extent we create the kind of person we are. We reach a consciousness about ourselves, our values, and our life directions. We develop our own values, thoughts, and opinions from the variety of ideas and life patterns that surround us. Part

---

Box 15–3. Some Characteristics of the Self

The healthy self has a sense of personal integration or coherent wholeness.
Each self is individual and unique from others.
The healthy self strives to maintain some autonomy: i.e., a sense of uniqueness.
The self is largely determined and recognized by the values it assumes.
The healthy self is characterized by energy directed toward self-actualization:

(a) Some of the values and goals people seek vary from culture to culture and from person to person.
(b) Individuals vary in their ability to become aware of deeper levels of the self and to gain insight or self-awareness.
(c) The self is simultaneously composed of sameness and change.

The self is capable of introspection and is aware of time.
The healthy self is not entirely free from emotional conflicts or symptoms of illness.
Even though individual "selves" are separate from one another, it is possible to form bonds with others.
The self is composed of a "public self" and a "private self."
Self-concept is founded on perceptions of oneself. At times we perceive ourselves differently from the way others perceive us.
Beyond concepts of the "individual self" are broader, deeper concepts of the "universal Self."

of the process is to consider the contradictions and inconsistencies of life. We evaluate our own behavior against the values of the outer world, and we make choices for ourselves.

Getting to know oneself is a process of introspection (looking within). Sometimes the process is peaceful; sometimes it causes anxiety. We each do it in an attempt to achieve an inner sense of order and meaning. It is difficult to live with too much disorder. We need to feel related to our inner and outer universes. We need to feel that we can predict to some extent what our universes are like and can understand them. It is uncomfortable to experience ourselves as impulsive, erratic, lacking in direction, or buffeted by fate. We need to believe that there is meaning, direction, and wholeness in who we are and what we do.

An individual who is ill needs a sense of order and personal integration as much as a healthy individual does. Nurses can help people who are ill maintain order by preventing surprises and preparing them for what will be happening. This preparation is done in small ways, for it is mainly in small ways that we order our lives. For example, you should tell a hospitalized person about the general routine of the hospital. Allow the individual to participate in making time decisions, such as "Would you like your bath early this morning or later?" If a person is waiting for professional attention, let the person know what time frame is operating. Keep the person informed of any changes that occur. Often the "small things" get forgotten in a busy schedule. This is unfortunate because the small things make the difference between helpful and unhelpful experiences for the person requiring care.

Some people become confused or disoriented and lose the important sense of personal integration. When confusion occurs, help orient the person to establish a sense of order and personal integration.

The Self and Individuality and Uniqueness

Each self is individual and unique. This fact helps make life the interesting experience that it is. It also produces difficulties in interaction with others, because we cannot always predict what another person is like or how another person will behave. Individual uniqueness brings with it an interesting uncertainty!

Why is each individual unique? How has such uniqueness come about? We can think of every organism and each part of every organism as consisting of the interaction of at least three indispensable factors: time, heredity, and environment. Time is the life span in which to grow and develop. Growth and development are guided by the blueprint of heredity and the experiences created by the environment. Each individual or organism embodies a unique combination of these factors.

Nurses can expect and even enjoy differences in people. As a nurse you will not necessarily like everybody you meet. However, you may find that one of nursing's most rewarding aspects is meeting many different people. An appreciation of individuality and a

conscious effort to allow it to flourish contribute to the quality of nursing care.

The Self and Autonomy

The healthy self strives to maintain some autonomy, a sense of uniqueness, independence, and the ability to function independently. For this reason, a person does not always conform to social expectations. Although we all want to know others and to be like them to some extent, a healthy person also wants to maintain individuality. We enjoy the idea of establishing our independence. We are each most comfortable when we are able to respect our own "selves" and to become our own friend.

People try to maintain their autonomy even if they are ill, and nurses frequently experience evidence of this fact. Clients do not like to conform to enforced ways of behaving (and neither do nurses!). Autonomy expresses itself in various preferences that reach nurses as innumerable requests—requests that express a wish to be treated individually. No one wants to be thought of as part of a nameless, faceless group in which the individual ceases to exist. No one wants to be thought of as a "gallbladder," a "bland diet," or "room 214." These are depersonalizing terms that should be replaced with the names of individuals. Always take time to personalize nursing care. This is done in small ways that may have important results.

Individual requests directed to a nurse are important. They are important to the person who asks, even though they may seem minute and unimportant to others. Bids for autonomy may sound like this: "These vegetables are overcooked. I like mine crisp." "I don't want a spread on my bed." "I don't care if it is not visiting hours, I am expecting company." "I don't like iced water. I want a cup of warm water." "My roommate wants the window open. I want it closed." "I want my medicine early."

Whenever possible, people should have control over their environments and experiences. Sometimes a nurse needs to mediate between the need for some conformity and the equally important need for personal autonomy. Meeting individual preferences enhances comfort and reinforces a person's sense of autonomy.

The Self and Personal Values

The self is largely determined and recognized by the values it assumes. Ultimately the search for oneself is an individual responsibility. Although we can be supported by others, no one but ourselves can tell us who we are. The self we choose to be stems to a large extent from our values. We choose what values we will live by. From all the possible values we might embrace, we select those by which we will live. We choose values that we believe are "better than" others. Our values may or may not conform to those of the people around us. Perhaps our values are valid, and perhaps they are not. At times, values transcend the evidence of proof.

Our identity is ultimately founded on the values we assume because our values determine our goals and our goals define our identity (i.e., our "self"). Our values may change at times. Our values are not what we say but rather what we do.

The value system of individual nurses influences nursing practice. Personal values may not influence how nurses talk about their practice, but these values are directly reflected in their actual practice. Nurses may say they value and respect individual differences, but the manner in which they treat people who are different shows what their true values are.

Nurses must be able to tolerate ideas and values that are different. Eiseley has said, "On the world island we are all castaways so that what is seen by one may often be obscure to another."[9] It is the task of nurses to try to understand the obscure. It is their privilege to come to know differing visions of life on this "world island." For example, two nurses heard their client, Mrs. Rains, say that she believed in reincarnation. Both nurses had only a vague idea of the meaning of this word. One nurse talked further with Mrs. Rains and found that her client believed that each person lives a series of lives as different people in order to learn and grow more and more toward a state of spiritual perfection. The nurse who failed to stay for this talk went away thinking, "That Mrs. Rains is some kind of a kook who believes that, when she dies, she will come back as a frog or something." The first nurse had a clearer vision of her client's values. The second nurse continued to be misinformed.

The Self and Self-Actualization

The healthy self is characterized by energy directed toward self-actualization. To move toward self-actualization is to strive to develop potentialities and to become a better person. To be self-actualized is to be comfortable and happy with oneself, to be creative and secure, to be spontaneous. A healthy self has energy for this process despite all the calls life has on our energy supply. Conflicts are part of life, and it takes energy to resolve conflicts. The healthy self is able to cope with difficulties and still have energy for a productive life and the enjoyment of pleasure.

Some principles that help us understand ourselves as we move toward self-actualization are:

▶ *Some of the values and goals people seek vary from culture to culture and from person to person.* In spite of the diversity of cultural and personal goals, people everywhere strive toward self-actualization. They strive to fulfill their potentials, to grow and to achieve as much as they can. Growth is not possible without encountering conflict. The healthy individual attempts to learn from conflict and go on to achieve higher levels of self-actualization.

▶ *Individuals vary in their abilities to become aware of deeper levels of the self and to gain insight or self-awareness.* Although many people recognize

the importance of understanding oneself (i.e., developing self-awareness), not everyone is able to work to attain it.

▶ *The self is simultaneously composed of sameness and change.* We remain the same people, recognizable to ourselves and to others, even though we change physically and psychologically.

I was a moment ago; I am part of the past. Yet it is I who now am, who then was. Though I passed with time, I did persist.[39]

We are able to remain ourselves while undergoing change. We remain the same and yet change, in a nebulous manner. This makes tracking and understanding the elusive self difficult.

Lack of energy is a general symptom of physical and mental illness. The body is often weak and fatigued when combating physical stresses and illness. The mind is likewise weary. People lack energy when they are experiencing mental stress and anxiety. When one is ill, however, the drive toward self-actualization does not necessarily stop. A nurse's responsibility is to help ill people continue to fulfill their potentials and to grow and achieve as much as they can within limitations imposed by their conditions. People can grow and learn from periods of stress and change. They do not usually become emotionally and psychologically immobilized or cease being themselves because they are ill or disabled.

Likewise, nurses can learn from the times of stress they experience as individuals. They, too, can take hold of the potential for self-actualization contained in both personal and professional life.

The Self, Introspection, and Time

The self is capable of introspection and is aware of time. We each have a unique consciousness. Loren Eiseley[9] describes human beings as having evolved into something unique—a "dream animal." Unlike the rest of the animal world (as far as we know), we can escape the eternal present into a knowledge of past and future. It is possible for us to imagine tomorrow, remember yesterday, and dream about how things might be. This consciousness can bring us joy or sorrow, depending on how we choose. We can choose to think of good times and dream future dreams, or we can imagine terror and suffering. Through our unique consciousness we can become morbidly preoccupied with the past, or the future, to the point of becoming ill. Or we can become so introspective that we shut out the rest of the world. On the other hand, we can choose to focus on the positive and create our own peace and security.

The self is not "found"; it is "achieved" through introspection (i.e., looking within). Many people speak of finding themselves as if, quite by accident, they had stumbled upon something lost. The self is ever-present, although it may be present behind a variety of masks. The self is ever-evolving and ever-becoming. It is evanescent and appears as reflections of its parts. What it represents, at any given time, is the life achievement of the individual. We do not lose our old self; we outgrow it and achieve something more.

It is through the baffling ability of introspection that we can become aware of our own consciousness. We can perceive ourselves in the act of perceiving. We can see ourselves seeing ourselves! We can question ourselves and what our existence is all about. That part of the "self" that watches our self *is* the self.

The healthy self uses introspection for growth and better self-understanding — striving for maximal achievement. Introspection generally serves to guide us in the best direction. We can transcend time, which means we can learn from the past and plan for the future. We have the opportunity to use time creatively, in a constructive effort for self-actualization.

Because we are aware of the passage of time, we are also able to see our own development through past, present, and future. We can choose to use this knowledge constructively. Many people find that the most positive life emerges by keeping the self mostly in the present. The present is exactly where reality lies. Rollo May states

It is by no means as easy as it may look to live in the immediate present. For it requires a high degree of awareness of one's self as an experiencing "I".... But the more awareness one has — that is, the more he experiences himself as the acting, directing agent in what he is doing — the more alive he will be and the more responsive to the present moment. Like self-awareness itself, this experiencing of the quality of the present can be cultivated.[22]

Illness often brings uncertainty and therefore may be a time of introspection. Often a person needs and wants to think out loud and talk to others. At times that "other" may be a nurse. It is natural to want to talk. What is unnatural for people needing health care is that those around them at a time of crisis or concern may not be familiar significant others. It is difficult and in some ways "unnatural" to talk with strangers about issues that are often deeply personal.

Through introspection, a person may become aware of inner feelings. Through communication, others can learn something of a person's feelings and concerns. Nursing consequently requires skills in communication. It is necessary that a nurse put people at ease. This requires sensitivity to both verbal and nonverbal communication (see Chapter 24). Furthermore, a nurse must be able to talk with people from diverse backgrounds. Speaking simply and slowly enhances clarity of communication. Avoid complicated terms or professional jargon.

Nurses also need to consider the self and time. It is not time in itself that is important, but the quality and meaning of time. Each of us has considerable control over the quality of our time. Nurses can choose to enhance the quality of the time they spend with people requiring care. Whether a nurse is with a person for 1 minute or for 8 hours, the quality of the relationship that develops (e.g., the nurse's caring attitude and willingness to listen) significantly influences the quality of the time spent. Each of us must determine for ourselves how much we "give" to the time we spend with others.

A nurse may grudgingly "put in time" or may attentively, helpfully, and creatively spend time with another.

Another aspect of time is that the present is really all that any of us has. Although the past and future are important, we live in the present. Occasionally, people (both consumers and care providers) view illness as a time away from life — as if life were suspended in time.

A nurse can help people become constructive agents of their time. However, a nurse caring for a terminally ill person may see the person's future as brief and thus may tend to negate the importance of the present. Terminally ill people, maybe more than anyone else, need the comfort, warmth, and security of a caring person in the present. They want the quality of their present life to be meaningful. The dying are still living; only the dead are dead. The dying live in present time, as they have always lived, and as we all live!

The Self and Emotional Conflict

The healthy self is not entirely free from emotional conflicts or symptoms of illness. A certain amount of imbalance, conflict, or illness is a natural part of life. The healthy self is able to live with and resolve conflicts and not be overwhelmed or immobilized by them. Stress and conflict produce some mental disequilibrium, even in the healthy self.

Conflict and illness are normal life experiences. Because nurses often care for people who are not healthy and adjusted, viewing imbalances in their proper perspective can be helpful. Recognize imbalances that are temporary and view them as such. Also recognize imbalances that are permanent and accept the fact that they cannot be reversed. In both situations, look for and support the strengths that individuals have and prevent further impairments.

The Self and Other "Selves"

Even though individual "selves" are separate from one another, it is possible to form bonds with others. Self-knowledge and communication are the means we use to reach out to others. We examine our own experiences and try to relate them to those of others. Likewise, we look at the experiences of others and try to relate them to our own. How are the experiences similar? How do they differ? Why do they differ? We try to understand our awareness of ourselves and others to "make sense of" our interpersonal world.

An ability to communicate with others is essential to the healthy self. Communication is a bond with others. It is our means of feeling less like separate planets pursuing our individual orbits and more like a united galaxy. The philosopher Karl Kaspers wrote, "The individual cannot become human by himself. Self-being is only real in communication with another self-being. Alone, I sink into gloomy isolation — only in community with others can I be revealed in the act of mutual discovery."[18]

Our interpretation of the feelings and behavior of

others is largely subjective but we can find common bonds with other people. We all work within the limitations of subjectivity. Thus, when a person says "I am miserable and I have a lot of pain" or "The physician told me this morning I have cancer," a nurse cannot truthfully say "I know how you feel." A nurse can, however, draw on personal experience and look for common bonds of experience to understand the feelings of others. To use a phrase of Loomis, the nurse and "patient" can, in the purest sense, "resonate together."

To "resonate" with another human being is to know that when you speak you are heard by him. The echoes that reverberate to you in his voice are rich with the sounds of your own concern. Similarly, your own voice, echoing back to him, has been affected by what you have heard him say and what you felt that he believed.[19]

A nurse who can communicate at this level is a person who understands "humanness." Such a nurse is an "idea person" as well as a "fact person." If we deal with separate facts, we fail to see the relationships between them. If we think only of separate people, we fail to recognize the bonds that unite them. A factual approach to nursing is oriented toward objects (e.g., medications, hypodermics, dressings). On the other hand, the nurse who works with "ideas" recognizes that consciousness, subjectivity, and communication are instruments for health and that the "self" of each nurse is an instrument that can be therapeutically applied.

The "Public Self" and the "Private Self"

The self is composed of the "public self" (the "me" I show to others) and the "private self" (the "me" I keep to myself or to a few significant others). We are each aware that our public self is often not the same as our private self, because we frequently disguise our private self when in the company of others. Often, if we want, we can decide what our public self will be. As individuals we are isolated from others in the sense that we can never become another person and no one can become us. We can present a part of ourselves to others, but we cannot give our self-perception (the way we see ourselves from the inside) to others.

Because of the existence of a public self and a private self, we develop a consciousness of ourselves as separate from other people, that is, feelings of otherness. (We are not suggesting that there is no such thing as spiritual unification.) Others may come and go. We remain with our self. From within our physical form we experience the mixtures of life's individual joys and sadnesses. This separateness of the self makes some people feel helpless and insignificant. For others it is a source of strength and completeness.

The healthy self is able to accept the division between the public and private self and the accompanying sense of separation. In the healthy self the public and private self are fairly similar—certainly consistent. Separateness from others is balanced by life experiences that can be shared. These shared experiences become bonds that unite people (e.g., in the areas of spirituality, culture, social networks, social groups, and roles). Thus, even though we are separate and see things from our own point of view, we can communicate with others. To communicate accurately and to establish bonds, we must each know and be comfortable with our own private selves.

Occasionally we are brought to the realization that we really didn't know someone at all. All we saw was the public self. For a vivid illustration, read the poem "Richard Cory" by Edwin Arlington Robinson.[31]

Just as you may not appear to others as you think you appear, so the people you care for may not appear to you as they think they do. A man may think he is calm when, in fact, he looks apprehensive to others. A woman may think she isn't irritable when she seems very short-tempered to others. A man may think you know he feels faint as he stands by an examining table when you really cannot tell that he feels this way. A physician may think she appears calm when she actually looks very pressured to others. You may think you do not seem hurried, but you make the people you are with feel rushed.

As people and as nurses, we strive to see both the public and private sides of ourselves. We also need to distinguish between the public and private selves of people we care for. Just as we understand that our own public behavior does not always express our private feelings, so we must grasp the same thing about the behavior of others. Skill in verbal communication and sensitivity to and awareness of nonverbal communication are necessary if we are to see glimpses of a veiled private self behind a public mask.

The private self is separate from other selves. By understanding this separateness, a nurse can empathize with those who are feeling lonely, isolated, and alienated. Illness, misfortune, and suffering can make people realize how separate they are from other people. They are in pain; they face death; they are frightened. But the world goes on. And no one can assume the pain, death, or fear of others. Nurses, however, can reduce the feelings of isolation through a skilled, comforting presence and by a willingness to allow others to talk about their life situations. This way, pain and fear can be alleviated or at least made easier to bear. The differences between the public and private selves can be reduced, and so a person can feel less alone.

Self-Concept

Self-concept is founded on perceptions of oneself. At times we perceive ourselves differently from the way others perceive us. **Self-perception** is the way one, correctly or incorrectly, believes oneself to be. How fragile one's self-concept is! How easily it is influenced or damaged! Every time we speak of another person we are speaking of a self. The challenge is to see how honestly, accurately, fairly, and kindly we can refer to that self. When describing a person, we must invest as much effort in the description as we would in our own self-description. If others see us differently from our own self-perception, and we see them differently from theirs, we must evaluate ourselves and others cautiously.

How do others describe you? Do they do it in terms of themselves and their needs? In part they do, and you also describe others partially in terms of yourself. The essential element is self-knowledge. Your feelings and perceptions about yourself will serve as your "antenna," your baseline for understanding others.

We perceive ourselves, or think of ourselves, in many different ways. In part we think of ourselves in terms of our feelings, abilities, and actions. Our perceptions evoke feelings about ourselves, and our feelings about ourselves are usually intense. Let us think of our own experience. We each know how easily our feelings may be hurt or how insecure we may feel if our self-image is threatened. We know of self-disappointment as well as dreams of fulfillment. One's feelings about oneself (self-concept) may correspond with truth or reality or they may not. Actually, does truth or reality mean anything in relation to the self, since both our own self and the self of another are primarily subjective experiences? Of more relevance is the fact that our behavior nearly always seems more consistent to ourselves than it does to others who observe it. We all tend to see what we want to see.

We may not be as we think we are. Self-deception may be unrecognized. Often we find that we are part of what we have denied we are. Often, unknown to us, we each possess qualities that we have either disliked or admired in others but thought were absent in ourselves. The consequences are interesting. For example, I may think of myself as friendly while others find me hard to get to know; I may believe I do not do well in a certain activity while others consider that I excel.

Self-knowledge will help each of us over time to obtain a more realistic view of ourselves. Self-knowledge will enable us to understand better how we present ourselves to others. We might also see incongruities between how we appear to others and how we see ourselves. Such insight is essential. Our self-concept greatly influences how we act toward others and how others act toward us.

Gaining self-knowledge is difficult, however, for a number of reasons:

▶ First, seeking self-understanding involves learning about our own unconscious psychologic defenses and coping mechanisms as well as our unconscious motivations. Thus, our vision is often distorted.
▶ Second, it may be difficult to believe facts about ourselves that do not support our own self-image. If we are not able to look at parts of ourselves that displease us, we cannot develop an accurate self-perception.
▶ Third, because the process of looking at ourselves may be uncomfortable at times, we often prefer to focus on the behavior of others. This deflecting of our focus is not usually helpful. Gaining self-understanding precedes the ability to understand others.
▶ Fourth, a reasonably high level of intelligence is required to undertake the rigorous process of self-examination. Language skills, vocabulary, memory, and foresightedness are closely related to intelligence and vary from person to person.

In part, then, the self we can become is determined by our vocabulary and verbal ability, because thinking involves the use of concepts and concepts are often verbal. Therefore, the more concepts individuals are able to develop, the more clearly they can think. Individuals also vary in their ability to think in abstractions. Those who cannot think abstractly have difficulty thinking about the self because the self *is* an abstraction.

Self-knowledge helps one to obtain a realistic view of oneself. There is a desirable balance between self-acceptance and self-rejection. Healthy people achieve a balance (homeostasis or equilibrium) between accepting themselves as they are and rejecting those parts of themselves they wish to change. Gently done, this process can precipitate growth. It is the ability to change, evolve, and be flexible that facilitates growth. Flexibility makes healthy psychologic adaptation possible.

Human beings are not bound to a static existence. Change is ongoing. As life progresses, change occurs. Some changes are beyond our control (e.g., physical aging), whereas others can be made voluntarily (e.g., behavioral change). Fortunately, awareness of oneself can lead to growth in behavior and in personal insights. An individual is not bound always to act the same. People are not static but are always in the process of becoming something more.

Individual Self and Universal Self

Beyond concepts of the "individual self" are broader, deeper concepts of the "universal Self." Many spiritual paths refer to the "Self" (with a capital "S"). This Self is that part of each of us that is beyond the individual self, beyond our personal behavior, even beyond the mind. The Self is that place deep within each of us that is calm and peaceful and is full of joy and hope. It is the place we each recognize as our "own being," as our "private home." It is a unique, special, and personal place, and yet in a mysterious way it is a place we share with all creation.

In a sense our lives are directed to finding that Self and basking in its happiness forever. We each strive to realize that Self in our own ways. Some people do it through meditation and prayer, others through running or some other physical activity, others through selfless service, and still others in artistic creativity. Whatever the avenue, we all know when we are experiencing the essence of ourselves, and we know that it is good. It is the Self that exists in everyone that we can acknowledge, respect, and honor. It is this Self that ultimately makes sense of everything.

Poor health sometimes brings people to a closer consideration of and connection with the Self. People call it by various names (e.g., the Self, God, universal consciousness). Whatever the name, it represents the most valuable and most significant part of an individual. The specific definition and meaning of the Self varies from person to person. Nurses need to recognize that people they care for may experience some connection with their own ultimate reality. To support their needs in a nonjudgmental way is the most helpful approach a nurse can take.

The Self and Significant Others

Interaction with "significant others" (i.e., people who are personally significant in the life of an individual) is very important in the development of oneself. Significant others may include not only one's family but also other people such as friends, peers, and teachers. Never assume you know who another's significant others are. Traditional social networks are changing. Family groups were traditionally categorized into the nuclear family and the extended family. The divisions are not so clear anymore.

NEEDS, THE SELF, AND NURSING CARE

When you have a good grasp of the various selves that make up each unique individual, you will be better prepared to assess your client's needs. In review, as a basis for understanding your client's needs, you may:

▶ Look at your client holistically and assess biologic, psychologic, and sociocultural needs
▶ Use general systems theory and look at your client's needs relative to such concepts as subsystems, suprasystems, input, output, and feedback mechanisms
▶ Use Maslow's hierarchy of needs to help you identify and set priorities for needs according to the five levels he identified
▶ Use another theorist's system, such as that of Orem, to identify needs

You may also take an eclectic approach and consistently use a combination of theories and systems. Your nursing instructors will guide you in your beginning use of these theories and systems, as appropriate for your best learning.

Summary

▶ Nursing is a science because it uses a systematic approach to knowledge, and it is an art because it involves the skillful and creative application of the nursing process in the solution of human problems.
▶ Nurses may correlate the individual psychophysiologic, social, and cultural dimensions of human existence into a unified whole by using general systems theory to understand people.
▶ Maslow identified human needs and placed them in a hierarchy with five levels. Orem identified a different list of needs and grouped them into three categories. Yura and Walsh emphasized that the principal role of the nurse is to meet human needs by using the nursing process.
▶ When needs are unmet, disequilibrium and eventual illness result.
▶ Physiologic, emotional, intellectual, social, environ-

mental, personal, and cultural obstacles may prevent satisfaction of needs.
▶ Nurses help satisfy unmet needs by helping people who are temporarily or permanently dependent meet their basic psychophysiologic needs, helping people obtain an optimal state of independence, and helping people prevent the development of unmet needs and problems.
▶ An understanding of the various characteristics of the self assists the nurse in assessing client needs. Careful assessment is the foundation for applying the nursing process and providing client care.

Bibliography

1. Abiodun, O.A. (1991). The need for a holistic approach to patient care. *East African Medical Journal*, 68(1), 25–28.
2. Bar-Yam, M. (1991). Do women and men speak in different voices? *International Journal of Aging and Human Development*, 32(4), 247–259.
3. Bieliauskas, L.A. (1982). *Stress and its relationship to health and illness*. Boulder, CO: Westview Press.
4. Blasi, A., & Milton, K. (1991). The development of the sense of self in adolescence. *Journal of Personality*, 59(2), 217–242.
5. Briggs, C.D. (1977). *Celebrate yourself*. Garden City, NY: Doubleday.
6. Campbell, C. (1984). *Nursing diagnosis and intervention in nursing practice* (2nd ed.). New York: John Wiley and Sons.
7. Coward, D.D. (1991). Self-transcendence and emotional well-being in women with advanced breast cancer. *Oncology Nursing Forum*, 18(5), 857–863.
8. Diekman, A.J. (1982). *The observing self*. Boston: Beacon Press.
9. Eiseley, L. (1962). *The immense journey*. New York: Time Life, Time Reading Program.
10. Jourard, S. (1968). *Disclosing man to himself*. Princeton, NJ: D. Van Nostrand Company.
11. Jourard, S. (1971). *The transparent self*. Princeton, NJ: D. Van Nostrand Company.
12. Kalish, R.A. (1982). *The psychology of human behavior* (5th ed.). Monterey, CA: Brooks/Cole Publishing Company.
13. Kernis, M.H., et al. (1991). Stability of self-esteem as a moderator of the relation between level of self-esteem and depression. *Journal of Personality and Social Psychology*, 61(1), 80–84.
14. Kersey, D., & Bates, M. (1984). *Please understand me*. Del Mar, CA: Prometheus Nemesis Book Company.
15. King, I.M. (1981). *A theory for nursing: Systems, concepts, process*. New York: John Wiley and Sons.
16. Kirshner, L.A. (1991). The concept of the self in psychoanalytic theory and its philosophical foundations. *Journal of the American Psychoanalytic Association*, 39(1), 157–182.
17. Kleinpell, R.M. (1991). Needs of families of critically ill patients: a literature review. *Critical Care Nurse*, 11(8), 34, 38–40.
18. Levi, A.W. (1967). Existentialism and the alienation of man. In Lee, E., Mandelbaum, M. (eds.). *Phenomenology and existentialism*. Baltimore: Johns Hopkins Press.
19. Loomis, E.A. (1960). *The self in pilgrimage*. New York: Harper and Row.
20. Mann, D.W. (1991). Some philosophical directions towards a simple theory of the self. *Theoretical Medicine*, 12(1), 53–68.
21. Maslow, A.H. (1954). *Motivation and personality*. New York: Harper and Row.
22. May, R. (1953). *Man's search for himself*. New York: W.W. Norton and Company.
23. Ong, B.N. (1991). Researching needs in district nursing. *Journal of Advanced Nursing*, 16(6), 338–347.
24. Orem, D.E. (1980). *Concepts of practice* (3rd ed.). New York: McGraw-Hill Book Company.
25. Patton, W. (1991). Relationship between self-image and depression in adolescents. *Psychological Reports*, 68(3, pt. 1), 867–870.

26. Pelham, B.W. (1991). On confidence and consequence: the certainty and importance of self-knowledge. *Journal of Personality and Social Psychology, 60*(4), 518–530.

27. Prather, H. (1980). *There is a place where you are not alone.* Garden City, NY: Doubleday.

28. Putt, A.M. (1978). *General systems theory applied to nursing.* Boston: Little, Brown and Company.

29. Raskin, R., et al. (1991). Narcissism, self-esteem, and defensive self-enhancement. *Journal of Personality, 59*(1), 19–38.

30. Reed, P.G. (1991). Toward a nursing theory of self-transcendence: deductive reformulation using developmental theories. *Advances in Nursing Science, 13*(4), 64–77.

31. Robinson, E.A. (1976). Richard Cory. In Ellmann, R. (ed.). *The new Oxford book of American verse.* New York: Oxford University Press.

32. Rogers, C. (1961). *On becoming a person.* Boston: Houghton Mifflin Company.

33. Rogers, C. (1980). *A way of being.* Boston: Houghton Mifflin Company.

34. Roy, C., Sr., & Roberts, S.L. (1981). *Theory construction in nursing: An adaptation model.* Englewood Cliffs, NJ: Prentice-Hall.

35. Ryff, C.D. (1991). Possible selves in adulthood and old age: a tale of shifting horizons. *Psychology and Aging, 6*(2), 286–295.

36. Selye, H. (1974). *Stress without distress.* Philadelphia: J.B. Lippincott.

37. Shepard, J.M., & Brooks, K.L. (1991). Self-concept among senior students in four types of nursing education programs. *Nurse Educator, 16*(4), 8–9.

38. Weelis, P. (1967). *The quest for identity.* New York: W.W. Norton Company.

39. Weiss, P. (1967). *Reality.* Carbondale, IL: Inter Varsity Press.

40. Wilson, E.D. (1985). *The discovered self.* Downers Grove, IL: Inter Varsity Press.

41. Yura, H., & Walsh, M.B. (eds.) (1978). *Human needs and the nursing process.* New York: Appleton-Century-Crofts.

42. Yura, H., & Walsh, M.B. (1983). *The nursing process: Assessing, planning, implementing, evaluating* (4th ed.). Norwalk, CT: Appleton-Century-Crofts.

Chapter 16

▼ Stress and Adaptation

> Stress can be fantastic. Or it can be fatal. It's all up to you.
>
> **P.G. Hanson**

▼ CHAPTER OUTLINE

STRESS, STRESSORS, AND STRESS
  RESPONSES
    Difficulties in Defining Stress
    Defining Stressors and Stress
      Responses
THEORETICAL MODELS OF STRESS
    Selye's General Theory of Stress
    Holmes and Rahe's Model Relating
      Life Change to Illness
    Lazarus's Model of Stress and
      Coping
CONCEPT OF ADAPTATION
    Levels of Adaptation
    Characteristics of Adaptation
CONCEPT OF CRISIS
    Maturational and Situational Crises
    Characteristics of Crises
    Crisis Intervention
ASSESSMENT
    Stressors
    First Line of Defense Against
      Stressors: Present Status
    Initial Psychophysiologic Stress
      Response Indicators

NURSING DIAGNOSIS
PLANNING
    The Client
    Significant Others
    Community Resources
    The Nurse
NURSING INTERVENTION
    Second Line of Defense Against
      Stressors: Self-Help
    Managing Stress Reduction
    Coping with Actual Crisis
EVALUATION
    Third Line of Defense Against
      Stressors: Professional Help
    Failure of Stress Reduction:
      Chronic Disease
STRESS, ADAPTATION, AND CRISIS:
  IMPLICATIONS FOR NURSES
    Caring for Hospitalized Persons
    Stress of Caring for Ill People
CASE STUDY

▼ KEY TERMS

Adaptation
Anxiety
Burnout
Coping
Crisis

Cultural adaptation
Defense mechanisms
Maturational crises
Situational crises

Social adaptation
Stress
Stress responses
Stressors

Stress is a universal feeling. All persons have experienced a multitude of uncomfortable subjective emotional and bodily changes that reflect its presence. These feelings and emotions were identified as a part of the concept of stress early in the 20th century by scientists who attempted to crystallize this vague concept into precise scientific terminology. During the first part of this century, physicians such as William Osler and Walter Cannon wrote about stress as a possible cause of illness. By the 1950s, the late Hans Selye, considered the "father of stress theory," was among the first to describe the specific effects of stressors on the physiology and body chemistry of animals. His findings had implications for studying stress in humans. Selye linked stress with certain diseases (e.g., gastric and duodenal ulcers, endocrine disorders, and high blood pressure). Soon it became clear that stress could precipitate many physical and mental illnesses in humans.

Since the mid-1950s, physiologists, biologists, physicians, nurses, psychologists, sociologists, and anthropologists have studied the causes of and responses to stress. Their studies increased our knowledge concerning stress and helped us to develop practical applications of this knowledge in reducing stress. Currently, nurses are specifically educated to observe for psychophysiologic stress responses in themselves and in the persons they care for. They are also taught to use the nursing process to reduce the negative effects of stressors. Even though it is difficult to define stress and almost impossible to measure it quantitatively, the concept of stress remains a cornerstone in the study of health and disease. It is a concept the nurse must understand and work with daily.

STRESS, STRESSORS, AND STRESS RESPONSES

Difficulties in Defining Stress

Stress is difficult to define because

▶ The concept of stress involves several dimensions: (1) the causes of stress; (2) the nature of the stres-

sor; (3) the immediate physical, social, and psychologic responses to stress; and (4) the long-term or permanent physical and mental changes created by stress.

▶ It is often difficult to know whether stress is the cause or the consequence of certain events.

▶ The term "stress" is used differently by experts from various disciplines. A physiologist describes stress through its physiologic correlates (e.g., an elevation of blood pressure), whereas a psychologist defines stress as anxiety. Engineers and physicists use the terms "stress" and "strain" in relationship to solid bodies. In physics and engineering, stress can be quantitatively measured, whereas in human relationships, stress can be only described.

▶ The concept of stress has been popularized by the lay press, who further obscure and confuse its meaning.

In this chapter, **stress** is considered the process of adjusting to circumstances that disrupt, or threaten to disrupt, a person's equilibrium.[46,74] Here is an example: Mary has traveled 7 hours in a bus from Houston to El Paso, Texas. The bus is not air-conditioned, and the person next to her has a body odor that indicates he has not had a bath for several days. By the time she reaches El Paso, Mary is hot, dizzy, tired, depressed, and irritable. This scenario demonstrates that stress involves a relationship between people and their environments, more specifically, between stressors and stress reactions. The problem of defining stress is due in part to the difficulty in distinguishing between sources of stress and responses to stress. Events and situations (such as the uncomfortable bus ride) to which people must adjust are sources of stress. Stress reactions are the physical, psychologic, and behavioral responses (such as the nausea, nervousness, and tiredness) that people display in times of stress. As a stressful situation (such as the long bus ride) continues, these reactions may themselves become sources of further stress. To a considerable degree, the experience of stress depends on the circumstances in which the stress occurs and on each person's physical and psychologic characteristics. Stress is therefore not a specific occurrence but a process. Understanding the process of stress requires attention to sources of stress, to the mediating factors that make people more or less sensitive to stressors, and to the differences among stress responses.

Defining Stressors and Stress Responses

STRESSORS

In this chapter, the term "stressors" is used for sources of stress, and the term "stress response" is used for reactions to stress. **Stressors** are agents or factors that challenge the adaptive capacities of an organism or person. These forces place a strain on the person, resulting in a stress response and possibly illness.

Stressors are beneficial or harmful depending on the individual (or organism), the total situation, the intensity of the stressor, and the person's coping responses.

Examples of stressors are

▶ attacks by bacteria, viruses, or parasites
▶ competitive sports
▶ trauma (injury, burns, assaults, electric shock)
▶ inadequate food, warmth, protection
▶ disruptive social and family relationships
▶ conflicting social and cultural expectations
▶ unmet basic needs (e.g., hunger, sexual desires)
▶ normal changes in physiologic function (e.g., puberty, menstruation, pregnancy, menopause)
▶ pathologic changes caused by disease or injury
▶ imagined threats of injury (sources of stress do not have to be based in reality)
▶ anticipated stressful events (e.g., an important social event, an examination, a courtroom hearing, or a painful diagnostic test)
▶ geographic relocation (even a welcome change of residence, travel)
▶ war and social unrest
▶ social isolation
▶ natural disasters (earthquakes, floods)
▶ planned therapeutic programs (dieting, physical therapy, psychotherapy)
▶ activities of everyday life (e.g., entertaining, driving on a freeway)
▶ positive situations that nonetheless bring momentous change (e.g., marriage, having a baby, graduation from college)

STRESS RESPONSES

Stress responses are physiologic and psychologic reactions to stress. Physiologic stress responses include reactions such as changes in cardiovascular function, increased gastric secretion, tremor, and loss of sphincter control. Psychologic responses include such reactions as anxiety and depression and the use of defense mechanisms such as denial or repression. A stress response is not a static event, nor does it occur in isolation from other responses. The manner in which an individual responds to stressful situations is mediated by (1) personality, (2) perception of the stressor, and (3) resources for coping.

Stressors and stress reactions have been studied in many settings: laboratories, disaster situations, military training centers, battle situations, preliterate cultures, modern city streets, and health care facilities.

General conclusions drawn from studies of stress include the following:

▶ A stress response may result from any one of many different stressors
▶ Most people tend to avoid such stressors as injury, temperature extremes, and pain
▶ Different people respond to the same stressor in a variety of ways
▶ Almost all individuals react in similar ways to extreme stressors (e.g., catastrophic events)
▶ The same person may develop a stress response to one critical situation but not to another critical situation
▶ The intensity and duration of the stress response depend on the experiences, socialization patterns established during childhood, and the meaning of the situation to the person
▶ Humans endeavor to adapt to stressors (e.g., environmental cold and heat) and to satisfy basic needs by deliberately modifying the environment (e.g., clothing, housing, medicines)
▶ Challenge from a stressor is beneficial under certain conditions. For example, mountain climbing is stressful, but for the properly trained person, it is an invigorating experience. Likewise, an absence of stressors can be harmful in that it results in boredom and lack of personal growth

Whether our stress responses are successful or not, they are often means of defending us from stressors.

Physiologic Defenses. There are several types of physiologic defenses. Two examples are the unbroken skin and intact immune system that protect us against the onslaught of viral and bacterial stressors. Note in Figure 16–1 that other physiologic defenses include genetic make-up, nutritional status, and general physical condition. For example, an infection may develop more readily in a malnourished person who receives a cut than in a well-nourished, well-exercised individual who receives a more serious injury.

Psychologic Defenses. The ability to respond adaptively to stress depends on previous experience with the stressor, formal education, support systems, intellectual capabilities, tendency toward anxiety, lifestyle, and economic status. In addition, "hardiness" is a personality trait that defends a person against stressors. The hardy person believes that (1) life has meaning, (2) people can influence the environment, and (3) change is a challenge. Hardy people survive slum upbringings, concentration camps, wars, and the like with mind and body intact.[42,95]

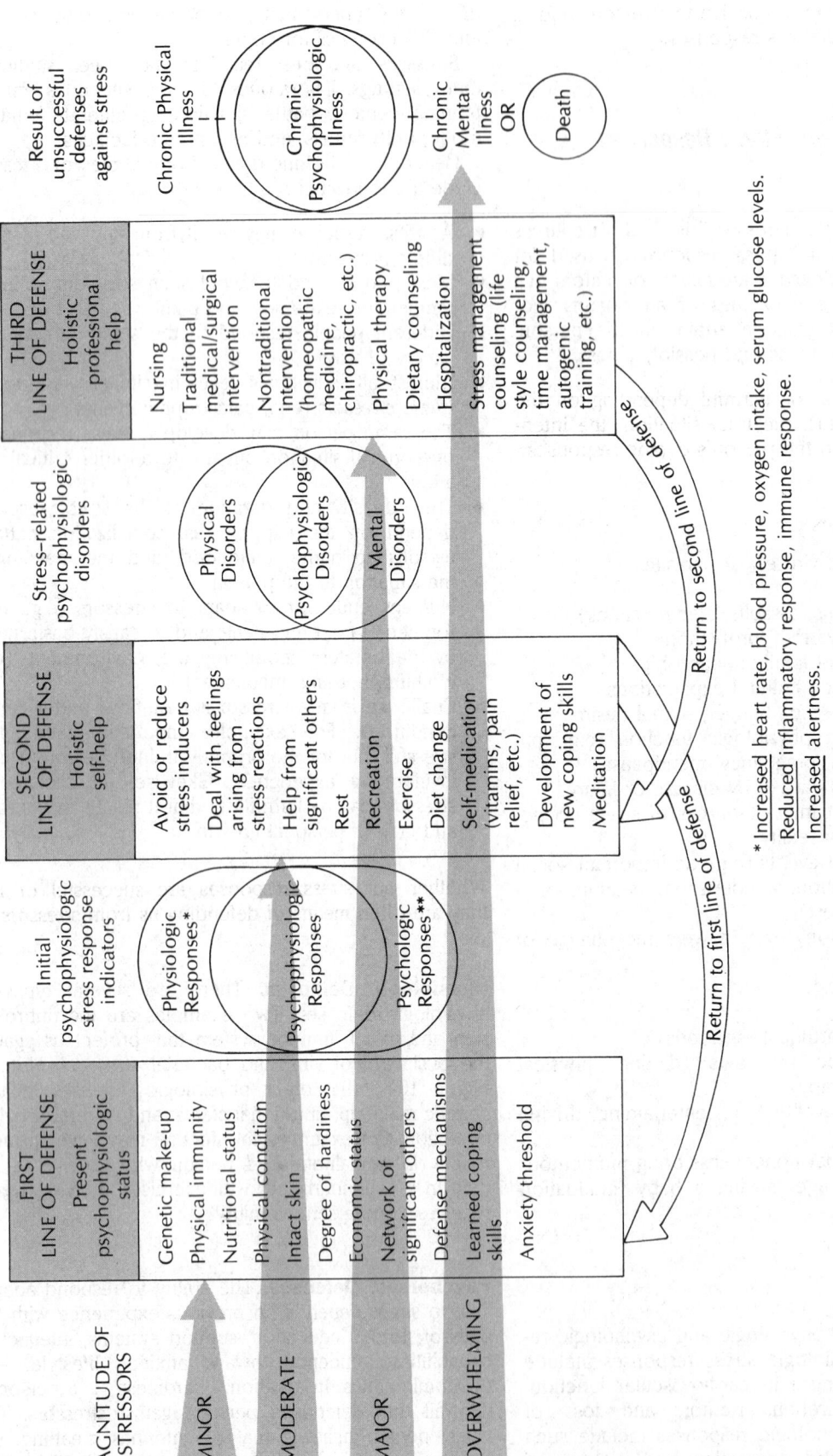

▲ *Figure 16–1*

A "working" model of stress. The magnitude of a stressor depends on the person's perception of and vulnerability to the stressor. The first, second, and third lines of defense summarize some specific means by which people defend themselves against stressors. A successful defense halts the stressor and prevents it from overwhelming the person. Psychophysiologic stress response indicators and stress-related psychophysiologic disorders result when stressors are able to penetrate lines of defense. Note that ideally the development of new defense mechanisms and coping behaviors is fed back to the second and then to the first line of defense. Thus, new behaviors and ways of reacting to stressors ultimately become a part of the person's customary behavior and lifestyle. (From Dudley, D.L., & Welke, E. (1977). *How to survive being alive.* New York: Doubleday.)

People who are responding adaptively to stress are coping. **Coping** means adjusting to or solving internal and external challenges. People learn new coping responses throughout their lives. Coping measures help us resist and master stressors. Also, once we master a stressor by using a particular coping response, that coping skill becomes part of our inner armor or first line of defense, and we are able to use it again in a similar situation. Thus, coping responses can be viewed as the immunology of emotion.[19,24,26]

Coping responses may be grouped into three major types on the basis of the ways they help us deal with potential and actual stressful situations:

▶ Responses that change the situation from which a potentially stressful experience arose
▶ Responses that control the meaning of the situation before it can elicit a stress response
▶ Responses that control the stress reaction after it has developed[60]

Lazarus described five models of coping:[46]

▶ Information seeking from ourselves and from others
▶ Direct action (e.g., walking away from a tense situation or confronting a person with whom you are having a disagreement; by using direct action, you deal directly with the stressor)
▶ Inhibition of action (e.g., not pounding your fist on the table even though you are very angry; by inhibiting your action, you protect yourself from unhelpful responses)
▶ Seeking social support from significant others or other appropriate sources
▶ Use of intrapsychic defense mechanisms

Defense mechanisms are unconscious psychologic and behavioral strategies that help protect a person from anxiety. We develop defense mechanisms throughout our lives. Typically, we use those defenses that have worked successfully in the past to solve problems and regulate emotions. When defense mechanisms work correctly, they both reduce anxiety and decrease the secretion of stress hormones, thereby protecting the person against a serious stress response.

Adequate self-esteem and self-respect are necessary for health. We all use defense mechanisms, especially in stressful situations, to maintain and improve our self-concept.

Defense mechanisms are not used deliberately. They almost always operate at an unconscious level. These mechanisms tend to be self-deceptive; that is, they work by masking or disguising our true motives from ourselves or by denying the existence of impulses, actions, or memories that might be anxiety-provoking. Therefore, defense mechanisms protect us from anxiety by distorting perception, memory, action, motivation, and thinking. In addition, they partially or completely block out disturbing ideas.

We can assess and understand more clearly the fears and concerns of people in our care if we can identify their defense mechanisms and coping patterns. Table 16-1 outlines some common defense mechanisms and examples that you may see used. The most commonly used mechanisms are denial, selective inattention, and isolation.[12]

Defense mechanisms are essential for mental health. Used properly, established defense mechanisms provide a strong first line of defense against stressors and contribute to psychologic growth and development. If used inappropriately or excessively, however, defense mechanisms can result in disruptive, unhappy life patterns. You need advanced education and experience before you can identify the pathologic use of defense mechanisms.

Defense mechanisms, although helpful to the individual, often evoke feelings of retaliation or retreat in others. Other people may react negatively to the person, thus intensifying the stress. Therefore, if you become upset when people in your care use defense mechanisms, you intensify their anxiety rather than reduce it. Assess your own coping behavior, and recognize that your own defense mechanisms can create problems for the people in your care and for your co-workers. Labeling behaviors as "defense mechanisms" can be harmful. Do not use the term defense mechanism in such a way that it results in the labeling of people. For example, remarks such as "He is a defensive person" are inappropriate.

When we say a certain behavior is a defense mechanism, we are speaking theoretically. Behavior labeled as a defense mechanism in one situation may not be used as a defense mechanism in another situation.

Although it is possible to describe defense mechanisms and behavior, we often cannot identify or understand the specific needs that make the person rely on these mechanisms. Therefore, never directly challenge a person's defenses. Rather, recognize the behavior as protecting the individual from anxiety reactions. Although a person's behavior may seem maladaptive to you, defense mechanisms serve adaptive purposes for that person. Without them, anxiety might be overwhelming.

There are no clear boundaries between various defense mechanisms. When an individual reacts to stress, the behavior is often a combination of several mechanisms. Defense mechanisms normally conserve emotional energy. An individual who has chronically low self-esteem, however, may use so much energy for defense mechanisms that little energy remains for use in constructive self-realization. This possibility is also true for the person experiencing illness. Illness produces frustrations, conflicts, and anxiety. In trying to ward off anxiety caused by illness and to retain a satisfactory self-concept, a person may overuse certain defense mechanisms, thus taxing mental energy and flexibility. Also the person may find that certain mechanisms that helped with adaptation during wellness fail in illness. Recognize that illness and confinement in a care facility are stressful. Therefore, expect that individuals may

TABLE 16–1. Selected Defense Mechanisms

Defense Mechanism	Description	Examples in Nursing Care
Rationalization	Assigning logical reasons or plausible excuses for what we have done impulsively or for motives that we do not wish to acknowledge; serves to maintain self-respect and prevents feelings of guilt	A male client is extremely rude and demanding; he thinks to himself that it is all right for him to behave this way because he is sick; he thus excuses his behavior.
Projection	Attributing to others exaggerated amounts of undesirable qualities that we have but do not wish to recognize in ourselves	The rude, demanding individual may not recognize his behavior; instead he thinks the nurse is behaving in this way, thus projecting his feelings onto her; actually her behavior is misinterpreted by him, because she has not been rude or demanding.
Repression	Involuntarily excluding from conscious awareness unacceptable ideas, impulses, or events; serves to protect us from being aware of anxiety-producing situations	A mother does not understand how her child received multiple bruises that are suspected to be related to child abuse by the father (when it is believed that she actually witnessed the abuse)
Suppression	Consciously putting unacceptable ideas, impulses, or events out of mind; the material can readily be recalled	An individual has been told by her physician that she has to undergo surgery; this thought is upsetting to her; she leaves the physician's office and says to herself, "I won't think about it now; I'll do some shopping instead."
Denial	Unconsciously refusing to acknowledge to oneself a known fact that is uncomfortable to accept; not consciously lying to oneself	An individual is proved to have cancer and is told the diagnosis by her physician; the patient does not consciously admit to herself that she has cancer; she denies the diagnosis.
Selective/inattention	Excluding from awareness those situations that provoke anxiety	A student is being evaluated by her nursing instructor. She fails to hear the comments about where she needs to improve and cannot understand why her grade is less than perfect.
Reaction formation	A forbidden motive or behavior is denied, and the individual develops behavior displaying the opposite motive	A woman wants an abortion but decides against it. When her daughter is born, she is a "perfect" mother and joins child protection and anti-abortion groups to help crusade against any actions against children or the unborn.
Sublimation	The "socialization of energy" by diverting unacceptable impulses into socially accepted behavior	An individual is angry because he was hit by a car and is hospitalized. He is missing work and his wife is home taking care of their three children. He directs his "anger energy" into pounding designs into leather and selling the purses, wallets, and so on that he makes. He sends home the small amount of money he makes and thus has a sense of contributing to his home and family.

react to these situations by using defense mechanisms that result in mental, physical, and emotional fatigue.

The notion of defense mechanism is based on the theories of Sigmund Freud. The concept of coping is broader and more generally useful.

THEORETICAL MODELS OF STRESS

Recent developments in the field of stress owe a great deal to the pioneer work of scholars such as Hans Selye, Thomas Holmes, Richard Rahe, and Richard Lazarus. Selye's model emphasized the physiologic components of stress, in particular the body's attempts to deal with stressors by means of adaptive hormones.

Studies by Holmes and Rahe concentrated on the effects of life changes on health and illness. Lazarus focused on the role of cognition and appraisal in stress. These theoretical models are not meant to be all inclusive, but they offer a starting point for the understanding of the concept of stress, anxiety, crisis, and adaptation.

Selye's General Theory of Stress

In the late 1930s and 1940s, Selye performed the first extensive studies on stress responses.[69-74] In 1950, he published his now-famous *The Physiology and Pathology of Exposure to Stress*.[69] This massive treatise described his general theory of stress and influenced

TABLE 16-1. Selected Defense Mechanisms (Continued)

Defense Mechanism	Description	Examples in Nursing Care
Displacement	Redirection of emotion or behavior from the original objects or person to a more acceptable substitute object	A hospitalized client hopes to go home but is told by her physician that she cannot be discharged. The person is angry but does not want to appear angry at the physician; the rest of the day she is short tempered with the nurse. She thus displaces her anger from the physician to the nurse.
Regression	Returning to an earlier level of emotional adjustment; an unconscious process	A person is usually quite self-sufficient when he is feeling well; however, with his illness he becomes somewhat more dependent than his physical condition necessitates; thus, he returns to an earlier level of dependency.
Introjection	Unconsciously adopting the personality characteristics of another individual whom the subject admires—the opposite of projection; not consciously trying to be like someone else	Two individuals with multiple sclerosis share a room in the hospital for several weeks; one admires the other very much and over a period of time her attitude toward her illness becomes similar to that of the friend she admires.
Identification	Unconsciously endeavoring to relate the self to another person or group	A young boy admires his older brother, who is going off to fight in a war. The boy joins the scouts so he can wear a uniform and he spends his time "playing army."
Isolation or depersonalization	Removing feeling from what one perceives as stressful	A nursing student stoically faces a painful dressing change and is doing a good job even though the client screams in agony.
Compensation	A conscious or unconscious attempt to overcome real or imagined inferiorities by developing one special ability or trait	A person who feels he is too short to be accepted at sports develops the ability to play the piano so well that he is always "the hit of the party."

stress research throughout the world. Selye defined stress as a physiologic phenomenon:

Stress—in biology, the nonspecific response of the body to any demand made upon it. For general orientation, it suffices to keep in mind that by stress the physician means the common results of exposure to any stimulus. For example, the bodily changes produced whether a person is exposed to nervous tension, physical injury, infection, cold, heat, x-rays, or anything else are what we call stress.[74]

Selye defined a nonspecific response as one that nonselectively affects most, if not all, of a system. Thus, when he wrote of the "nonspecific response of the body" to stimuli, he meant that the entire body tries to adjust to any specific agents that place demands on it. Agents that place demands on the body and precipitate stress he termed stressors. For example, exposure to extreme heat or cold acts as a specific stressor to which the body adapts by either shivering (in the case of cold) or perspiring (in the case of heat). Although the specific responses to these stressors are different (shivering vs. perspiring), heat and cold are nonetheless similar in that they promote a nonspecific response. In other words, they force the total body (nervous system, skin, blood vessels) to perform adaptive functions to return the organism to its previous state of balance.

On an emotional level, the body also responds nonspecifically to stressful events. These events can be perceived as either joyful or distressing. For example, a stress response can be as powerful at a person's wedding as at a loved one's funeral. In both cases, the body responds as a whole, nonspecifically, to specific events.

According to Selye, the stresses to which a person is exposed throughout life cause "wear and tear," which produce physical and psychologic signs of aging. Although Selye once labeled stress and aging as the same phenomenon, he later believed aging to be the result of stress. Stress responses continue throughout life.

As Selye emphasized, "Complete freedom from stress is death."

Selye became interested in formulating a general theory of stress and disease causation when he was a medical student. He noted that most diseases are characterized by only a few specific signs and that almost all maladies share common signs and symptoms. Common manifestations of illness include weight loss, fatigue, malaise, aches and pains, and gastrointestinal upsets. In other words, he observed that almost all sick people, regardless of diagnosis, shared some of the same general pathologic responses. Initially, Selye called this phenomenon the "syndrome of just being sick." Later he renamed it the stress syndrome or general adaptation syndrome (GAS). Furthermore, he suggested that certain hormones, called adaptive hormones, are released during stress responses. He theorized that these hormones created the symptoms seen in all ill people. From his observations, Selye concluded that stress plays a role in every disease process regardless of causation.

According to Selye, the GAS appears whenever an organism is subjected to long-continued stress. Some manifestations of GAS include adrenal gland stimulation and release of adrenocortical hormones, gastrointestinal ulcers, and lymph gland atrophy (shrinkage). Stressors that cause GAS are nonspecific and include trauma, infection, burns, severe cold, and emotional upsets.

In addition to the body's systemic response to stress, Selye proposed that the body also adapts to local stressors. He named this local response the local adaptation syndrome (LAS). LAS takes place within a single organ or specific area. Inflammation is an example of LAS.

Selye suggested that both the GAS and the LAS develop in three distinct stages: (1) alarm, (2) resistance, and (3) exhaustion. These three phases are elaborated in Figure 16–2.

Selye theorized that adaptation plays a role in every disease. He also stated that faulty adaptation in itself can cause disease. Selye named these "derailments" of the adaptive syndrome the diseases of adaptation.

According to Selye, these maladies are not due to any specific pathogen but instead are a direct result of a faulty response to a stressor. Usually, adaptation involves a balance of defense and submission on the part of the body. However, when the body overdefends itself, Selye suggested, excessive proinflammatory hormones are released and such problems as arthritis, allergy, and asthma develop. When the body underdefends itself, excessive antiinflammatory hormones are released, and overwhelming infection or ulcers result.

Holmes and Rahe's Model Relating Life Change to Illness

Over the centuries, philosophers and scientists theorized that life change and illness were related. These

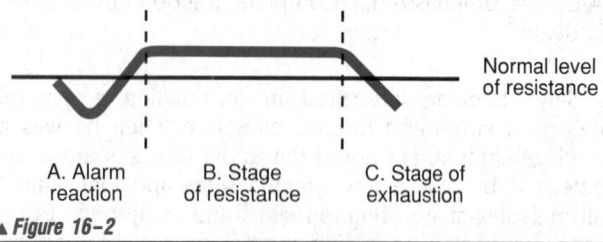

▲ Figure 16–2

The three phases of the general adaptation syndrome (GAS). *A*, Alarm reaction. The body shows the changes characteristic of the first exposure to a stressor. At the same time, its resistance is diminished, and if the stressor is sufficiently strong (severe burns, extremes of temperature), death may result. *B*, Stage of resistance. Resistance results if continued exposure to the stressor is compatible with adaptation. The body signs characteristic of the alarm reaction virtually disappear, and resistance rises above normal. *C*, Stage of exhaustion. After long-continued exposure to the same stressor, to which the body had become adjusted, adaptation energy is eventually exhausted. The signs of the alarm reaction reappear, but now they are irreversible, and the individual dies. (From Selye, H. (1974). *Stress without distress*. Philadelphia: J.B. Lippincott.)

theories were largely unsubstantiated until about 25 years ago, when Thomas Holmes and Richard Rahe began studying the relationship between change and illness.

Change is a form of stress requiring both psychologic and physical adaptations. Adapting to change consumes a person's energy beyond that needed to maintain a "steady state" of life. Holmes and Rahe documented that adapting to many significant changes in a short period leaves a person overextended and more susceptible to illness.

Holmes and Rahe began their studies using a questionnaire called the Schedule of Recent Experience, in which they asked respondents to list major life changes. Later, they asked respondents to assign numerical values to those major life changes on the basis of their significance to the respondent. From this information, Holmes and Rahe developed the Social Readjustment Rating Scale (SRRS), a ranking of major life events according to life change units (LCU) (Fig. 16–3). The death of a spouse, for example, is worth 100 LCUs (and ranks highest as a stressor), whereas a vacation is worth only 13 LCUs.

By obtaining life change scores from thousands of people, Holmes and Rahe explored the link between the amount of change in a person's life and subsequent illness. They discovered that the higher a person's life change score, the greater the likelihood that an illness would subsequently develop.

Assessment tools like the SRRS provide a general impression of the stressors in a person's life. In fact, a great deal of research with such tools has suggested that the more stressors a person experiences in a short period of time (1 to 2 years), the more likely that physical illness, mental disorders, or other stress responses will follow. This conclusion is based in large measure on the fact that most persons who suffer from certain physical illnesses or mental disorders report having experienced one or more major stressors just before their disorders appeared.[36,37] Does this mean that you can predict the stress problems in a person's life just by using the SRRS? No. Many people with high scores on the SRRS do not subsequently experience serious problems. In addition, low scores do not guarantee a life free of the dangers of stress. Why? One reason is that mediating factors, such as how the individual perceives and copes with each stressor, play an important role in determining the impact stressors will have on each individual. The Lazarus model attempts to explain this further.

Lazarus's Model of Stress and Coping

Lazarus and associates[30,46] stated that stress encompasses "any event in which environmental or internal demands (or both) tax or exceed the adaptive resources of an individual, social system or tissue system."[46] The Lazarus model emphasizes that cognitive appraisal is central in determining what is stressful and

Rank	Life Event	Life Change Units	Your Score	Rank	Life Event	Life Change Units	Your Score
1	Death of spouse	100	____	23	Son or daughter leaving home	29	____
2	Divorce	73	____	24	Trouble with in-laws	29	____
3	Marital separation	65	____	25	Outstanding personal achievement	28	____
4	Jail term	63	____	26	Wife begins or stops work	26	____
5	Death of close family member	63	____	27	Begin or end school	26	____
6	Personal injury or illness	53	____	28	Change in living conditions	25	____
7	Marriage	50	____	29	Revision of personal habits	24	____
8	Fired at work	47	____	30	Trouble with boss	23	____
9	Marital reconciliation	45	____	31	Change in work hours or conditions	20	____
10	Retirement	45	____	32	Change in residence	20	____
11	Change in health of family member	44	____	33	Change in school	20	____
12	Pregnancy	40	____	34	Change in recreation	19	____
13	Sex difficulties	39	____	35	Change in church activities	19	____
14	Gain of new family member	39	____	36	Change in social activities	18	____
15	Business readjustment	39	____	37	Mortgage or loan less than $10,000	17	____
16	Change in financial state	38	____	38	Change in sleeping habits	16	____
17	Death of close friend	37	____	39	Change in number of family get-togethers	15	____
18	Change to different line of work	36	____	40	Change in eating habits	15	____
19	Change in number of arguments with spouse	35	____	41	Vacation	13	____
20	Mortgage over $10,000	31	____	42	Christmas	12	____
21	Foreclosure of mortgage or loan	30	____	43	Minor violations of the law	11	____
22	Change in responsibilities at work	29	____			TOTAL	____

Scoring
Add up your score. If your total for the year is under 150, you probably won't have any adverse reaction. A score 150–199 indicates a "mild" problem, with a 37 percent chance you'll feel the impact of stress with physical symptoms. From 200–299, you qualify as having a "moderate" problem with a 51 percent chance of experiencing a change in your health. A score of over 300 could really threaten your well-being.

▲ *Figure 16–3*

Social Readjustment Rating Scale (SRRS). (Adapted from Holmes, T.H., & Rahe, R.H. (1967). The social readjustment rating scale. *Journal of Psychosomatic Research,* 11(2), 213.)

in coping with stress. Lazarus also pointed out that one of the major problems in defining stress is that emotions have been treated as causes of stress responses rather than as effects of these responses.

According to Lazarus, both stress and coping are processes, not events.

Both change over time, partly as a result of interaction between the two processes. In the process of coping, the individual shapes as well as responds to a demand or stress. Coping may change the person's appraisal of the stressful experience and thus may influence what happens next.[37,46]

Figure 16–4 illustrates the basic theoretical framework underlying Lazarus's work. Note that major elements of this model are demands, primary appraisal of the demands, secondary appraisal, stress, coping, emotions, and reappraisal.[86,87]

Demands confronting an individual may be internal (e.g., adolescence, pregnancy, menopause) or external/environmental (e.g., extreme heat, cold).

Primary appraisal of the demands is a cognitive or intellectual process by which people evaluate the demand in terms of its significance in their lives. Thus, we ask ourselves the following: Is the demand irrelevant? Is it benign or positive? Is it stressful? According to Lazarus, we appraise everything that happens to us. For example, if you live in an apartment house, you may frequently hear the garage door open. Most of the time, the sound is irrelevant. The comings and goings of others in the apartment house usually do not concern you. However, if you are waiting for your roommate to come home and celebrate your birthday with you, the sound is probably positive. On the other hand, if you have had a fight with your roommate, the sound of the garage door opening is stressful.

At the point of *secondary appraisal*, individuals evaluate their coping options and resources in relation to their first appraisal, if they perceived the original

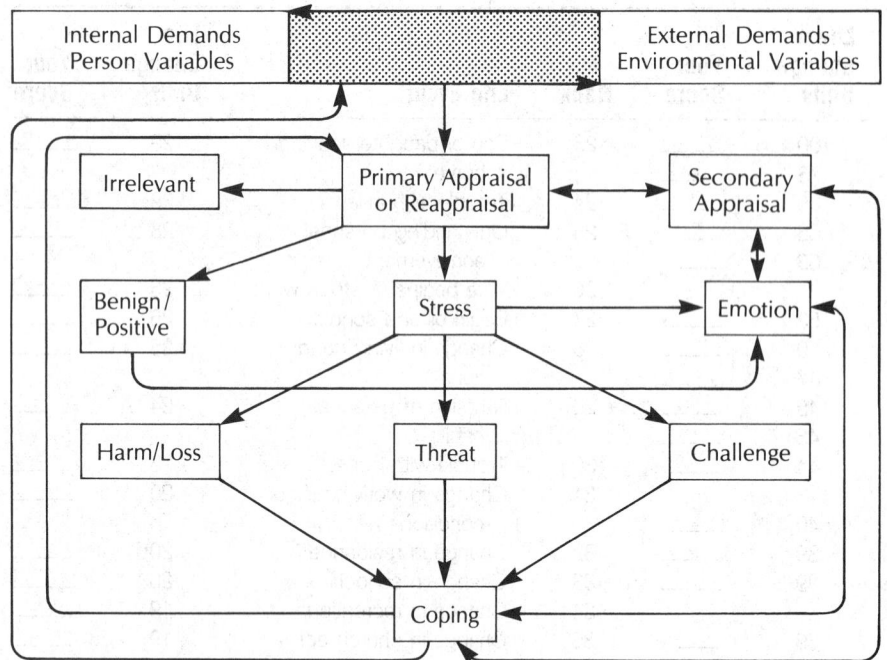

▲ **Figure 16–4**

Lazarus stress and coping paradigm. (From Trygstad, L. (1984). *Stress and coping in psychiatric nursing.* Unpublished dissertation, University of California, San Francisco Medical Center.)

demand as stressful. For instance, you would reevaluate the sound of the garage door only if you perceived the opening of the garage door as a threat. The secondary appraisal leads to an emotional response (fear, anger, pleasure). In addition, because the secondary appraisal provides more information about your coping responses and about the situation, the primary appraisal may change. For example, if you have had a fight with your roommate, you evaluate your coping options in relation to the mood of your roommate. If your roommate is extremely angry and much larger than you, you might be afraid and elect to leave. If your roommate comes in the door in a surprisingly good mood, you may then change your first appraisal to one of a benign or even positive nature. Thus, your emotion may be one of pleasure.

According to Lazarus, *stress* occurs when a person's adaptive responses are less than required by environmental or internal demands (or both).

As broadly defined by Lazarus, *coping* mechanisms are "efforts to manage environmental and internal demands and conflicts among demands."[46] Coping mechanisms are methods for managing the demand and the emotions elicited by it. These methods are based on both the primary and the secondary appraisals. Individuals activate their coping options to deal with conditions involving harm or loss, threat, and challenge (e.g., will coping with the demand result in personal growth and development?).

Emotions are positive feelings (elation, love) and negative feelings (anger, depression, anxiety) that arise in response to the secondary appraisal and the process of coping. In the case of threat, the degree of discrepancy between the perceived degree of threat and the person's perceived available coping options accounts for the emotion the person feels and that person's reactive behavior. For example, if a person feels cor-

nered or outnumbered in a situation, the individual reacts with fear, anger, or aggression and as a result fights or flees.

In *reappraisal*, individuals reevaluate the demand based on feedback from their attempts to cope with it. The initial anger or fear a person feels in a situation may dissipate once the individual elicits more information, uses coping skills, and then, on reevaluation, discovers that the threat is reduced or was perhaps incorrectly perceived in the first place.

Observe that this model is cyclic. It represents a continuous process of appraising and coping with demands or stress. In essence, Lazarus emphasized the changing nature of life. Perceptions of demands or stressors change with information, and once coping activities are initiated, the person must continually reevaluate the situation as it changes in response to the act of coping with the demands that can lead to stress.

CONCEPT OF ADAPTATION

The word "adapt" comes from the Latin word *adaptare,* meaning "to adjust." **Adaptation** is thus the adjustment of an organism to changes in its environment. Adaptation is the ultimate goal of coping. In fact, it can be viewed as long-term coping. Biologists and behavioral scientists have shown that whenever people encounter stressors from any source, they attempt to adapt to them. If adaptation is successful, balance is maintained or restored. If adaptation is faulty, people become ill. Then they must adapt to illness. Adaptation is of vital concern to nurses and physicians, who cope daily with the adaptive changes that illness forces on people.

Because adaptation is characteristic of all living things, it has been studied in many disciplines, ranging from plant biology to psychiatry. In its most comprehensive sense, the notion of adaptation includes the whole range of protection adjustments from the simplest motor action to the most complex interaction between individuals or entire nations. It involves the simple responses of single-cell organisms as well as complex human behaviors.

As Selye aptly stated, "The great capacity for adaptation is what makes life possible on all levels of complexity. It is the basis of homeostasis and of resistance to stress . . . . Adaptability is probably the most distinctive characteristic of life."[72]

Adaptation is one characteristic that separates living organisms from inanimate objects. Human adaptation is more complicated than adaptation among less complex organisms, and it involves more than a simple biologic process. Instead, we respond to the environment with our bodies, intellects, and emotions.

Levels of Adaptation

Human adaptation occurs at three main levels: (1) physiologic or biologic, (2) psychologic, and (3) sociocultural. In daily life, these three levels are interrelated.

PHYSIOLOGIC LEVEL OF ADAPTATION

Physiologic, or biologic, adaptation involves compensatory changes that occur within the body in response to increased or altered demands made on the body.

For example, consider Ted Creighton. Mr. Creighton, at age 42, realized that he had been leading a sedentary, unhealthy lifestyle. He decided to begin a jogging program. Consequently, he experienced physical strain during his first exercise sessions. He felt exhausted and experienced muscular soreness and aching. However, he continued to follow the recommended jogging schedule, increasing his efforts a little every day, and eventually was able to jog quite a distance at a moderate rate without undue strain. His muscles, heart, and lungs gradually increased in strength and functional efficiency, adapting to the additional demands placed on these organs. As most frequently happens with exercise, the immediate stress seemed negative, but the long-term benefits were quite positive.

The body's reaction to invading microorganisms also illustrates physiologic adaptation to stress. We resist attacks by such stressors as viruses and bacteria by becoming immune to them. Immunity may be either inherited or acquired. When it is inherited, the individual is naturally resistant to certain organisms. When it is acquired, immunity develops as a result of previous contact with an organism. This contact involves having the infectious disease and overcoming it or being inoculated against it. With acquired immunity, then, the body adapts to the presence of disease by producing protective antibodies. Humans thus acquire an immunity to specific diseases.

In physiology, adaptation is sometimes described as a decrease in the intensity of a sensation resulting from steady-state stimulation or continuous responses. Olfaction provides a good example of adaptation. For instance, when we come into contact with a noxious odor, we are immediately offended. If we remain in contact with this odor (steady-state stimulation), however, we become accustomed to it rather quickly. Gradually, intensity of sensation decreases until we are oblivious to the odor.

PSYCHOLOGIC LEVEL OF ADAPTATION

Psychologic adaptation involves adjusting our attitude toward a psychologically stressful situation so that we are better able to cope with it. To accomplish this adjustment, we might use defense mechanisms or learn new behaviors (e.g., relaxation techniques) for coping with the stressor.

Modes of psychologic adaptation can be healthy or unhealthy. Consider, for example, John and Jim, both first-year nursing students and dormitory roommates. John is an affable person, but his constant chatter drives Jim crazy. Jim is a tolerant person, but he is also a serious student and finds he just cannot get any work done in his room when John is around. Jim has spoken to the dorm's head resident about the possibility of moving, but changing rooms is not possible. The dormitories, already overcrowded, have waiting lists. In addition, no one else in Jim's building expressed interest in switching places with him. So because Jim cannot move and John cannot be quiet, Jim spends more of his study time in the library. When in his room, he frequently wears his stereo earphones to tune in his favorite music while tuning out John.

Recognizing that the situation with John was potentially disruptive, Jim temporarily altered his attitude and lifestyle patterns in such a way that he felt more comfortable in an uncomfortable situation. Of course, there were alternatives. Jim could have lost his temper and argued with John. He could have lost sleep over the situation. He could have allowed the stress to foment until he became ill. Instead, Jim adapted.

In trying to adapt to a stressful situation, some individuals may adapt in a manner that may temporarily function to relieve anxiety and physiologic discomfort but that ultimately is not in their best interest. For example, consider Martha's case of unhealthy adaptation. Martha is a 14-year-old, middle-class, high school freshman. All of her life, she has maintained a high grade point average, has been considered a loyal friend, and has been a source of pride for her parents. Martha strives to be the best at whatever she does, including controlling her personal appearance. So driven is she, in fact, that she is slowly starving herself to death. Martha has anorexia nervosa. Fearful of unwanted fat and, most of all, the loss of her parents' love and admiration, Martha is dieting her life away. Although Martha's behavior is maladaptive, it protects her and should not be tampered with by unskilled persons. Her adaptation appears to be harmful. Nonetheless, it is the most successful adaptation that she can make at the time. It may be the only way that Martha can feel any control over her life.

Individuals adapt to stressors to the best of their ability at the time. Coping behavior may not always seem appropriate. However, it is always purposeful.

SOCIOCULTURAL LEVEL OF ADAPTATION

Social adaptation is the adjustment of an individual's actions and conduct to the norms, conventions, beliefs, and pressures of various groups. Families, professional societies, labor unions, social clubs, and sororities are but a few examples of the wide assortment of groups that demand our involvement and commitment. **Cultural adaptation** means adjustment of an individual's behavior to the concepts, ideas, traditions, and institutions of a culture. Examples of cultural groups include racial groups, geographic groups (e.g., American, European), and certain religious groups.

As an illustration of sociocultural adaptation at the group level, consider your own experience as a student preparing to become a professional nurse. When you first entered your school of nursing, you were exposed, almost immediately, to a new set of ethics that you had to accept, to a new vocabulary that you had to learn, and to certain standards of performance that you had to achieve. All these demands perhaps seemed overwhelming at first. Furthermore, your initial experiences with sick people may have been overshadowed by a sense of uncertainty, nervousness, and even fear. Gradually, however, over time, you began to adapt by learning to speak the language of nursing and medicine. You should be adopting more and more the values that you were taught, and as time goes on, you will certainly gain the confidence necessary to function effectively in the nursing role.

The longer you remain in nursing, the more natural it will seem to you to be a nurse. Your changed perception will occur because you will have adapted to the nursing profession. You will have become a bona fide member of the group. You may eventually become so well adapted to nursing that you will find it difficult to relate to other professional and social groups. This sense of exclusiveness is a common characteristic of professional societies, and it is one of the dangers of social adaptation. If you find yourself experiencing this exclusion, you will have adapted so exclusively to one group that you have reduced your ability to adapt to others.

In addition to adapting at the group level, nurses are continually called on to adapt at the cultural level. Indeed, nurses may experience cultural shock as their nursing practice brings them into contact with various cultural groups. Also, nurses frequently work with people who are poverty-stricken. For the student nurse who has been raised in a middle-class or professional-class home and neighborhood, the first contacts with severe poverty may be devastating and disturbing. Not all students psychologically survive the challenge of working with very poor people who are ill. Those who do adapt use various coping mechanisms. Some mechanisms, such as developing a hardened attitude or burning out, may be unhealthy. Other students use healthy adaptation. For example, they talk with classmates, discuss the problems of the people in their care with their instructor, develop plans of action with a social worker, face the fact that they may sometimes feel inadequate in the face of so much suffering, and finally begin to set realistic goals for themselves and for those in their care. In time, with experience and personal growth, the student who successfully adapts can work with very poor people and feel accepting and empathic but not shocked and disillusioned.

Remember that when we adapt culturally, we also adapt psychologically and in some instance physiologically. Peace Corps volunteers working in a small African village, for example, must adapt psychologically to new stressful situations. They must also adapt physiologically to a new climate and diet.

TECHNOLOGIC LEVEL OF ADAPTATION

People must also make technologic adaptations. Technologic adaptations are scientific and industrial arts and innovations that people create through the use of their cultural heritage. Technology, an outgrowth of culture, has allowed us to modify and change our surrounding environment and to control many of the stressors that are a natural part of that environment. Unfortunately, modern technology has also created new stressors to which we must adapt (e.g., water, air, and noise pollution).

Health care technology, in particular, has evolved at a tremendous rate over the last decades. As a result, we are making strides in understanding and in gaining control over disease, pain, and death. The successes of health science, however, have not been obtained without a price. Serious philosophic, ethical, and legal dilemmas have evolved as a result of our technologic adaptation. These complex dilemmas serve as stressors to which we must adapt. For example, with increasing use of radioactive materials, we must be concerned with disposal of radioactive waste in the environment. How do we control medical waste? How should technology be used? How do we provide health care for all individuals? Who should control health care decisions? These are some of the important questions that have evolved as a result of our technologic adaptation. Answering them requires more adaptation still.

Characteristics of Adaptation

All human adaptive mechanisms (whether physiologic, psychologic, or cultural) have common characteristics.

All adaptive mechanisms attempt to maintain optimum physical and chemical conditions within the system or organism. The process of maintaining a fairly steady internal environment is called homeostasis (see Chapter 17). Adaptation is a dynamic process. Individuals do not passively submit to environmental or internal stressors. Such internal stimuli as hunger and thirst result in our actively seeking food and water. When external stressors (e.g., fires, battle conditions, extreme weather, an attack by an animal or another person) threaten us, we can flee from them, block them from consciousness (e.g., by fainting), or actively struggle against them.

When individuals adapt to change or to stress, they tend to adapt as total organisms. In other words, adaptation does not occur exclusively at any one level of human experience. Rather, it embraces all levels—physiologic, psychologic, sociocultural, perhaps even technologic. Thus, when you became a nursing student, you probably had to adapt physiologically to the greater workload, to the long hours of study, and to the muscular exertion required for lifting and moving people. You had to adapt intellectually to the new and different subject matter and emotionally to the responsibilities and problems of giving care. At the sociocultural level, you had to adjust to the ethics, norms, and subculture of the nursing profession. At the technologic level, you had to adapt to new equipment.

Adaptation has limitations. Although adaptive mechanisms and behavior exploit human potential, they also operate within the limitations of that individual's genetic make-up, general physical condition, intelligence, and emotional stability. For example, people cannot flap their arms and fly away from danger like birds, nor can they remain submerged in water indefinitely like fish. We must adapt within the confines of human nature or through technologic innovations (e.g., use of an airplane, scuba diving equipment). Adaptive responses are much more limited in number and scope at the physiologic level than they are at the social and psychologic levels. For instance, blood sugar, oxygen content, and internal body temperature can fluctuate only within certain narrow limits and still be consistent with life. On the other hand, many adaptive solutions are available in emotional or social difficulties. Even in these circumstances, however, the number of possible solutions is finite.

Adaptation occurs over time. The individual who has sufficient time can adapt better to stress than can the individual who must adapt quickly. For example, the body is able to adapt to gradual blood loss. Individuals with a slowly bleeding peptic ulcer can lose quite a bit of blood without symptoms of shock because blood loss occurs over a prolonged period. Under these conditions, the bone marrow increases red blood cell production to compensate for the blood loss. In contrast, the body adapts less adequately to rapid blood loss. Consequently, persons experiencing sudden hemorrhage from trauma may suffer shock, as evidenced by rapid pulse, low blood pressure, and restlessness. If the body is unable to compensate quickly and appropriate emergency measures are not taken swiftly, the shock may become irreversible, and death may result. Thus, time is an important factor in adaptation.

Adaptability varies from individual to individual. Flexible individuals who respond readily to change and who use a wide range of compensatory mechanisms are more adaptable than those who lack these qualities. Consequently, they are more likely to survive stressful situations and change than are individuals who react to life challenges in a rigid, limited manner. Physical illnesses challenge people's adaptive capabilities. For example, people with incapacitating diseases, such as severe heart problems, may be called on to change their occupation and lifestyle. These changes may be demanded of them at a time in their lives when they are least able to make sweeping modifications. Unless these individuals are given reassurance and guidance in planning the future, they may be unable to adapt to a new way of living.

Adaptation makes us less sensitive to some stimuli and more sensitive to other stimuli. For example, when we are listening to a lecture that has great interest or importance for us, we focus on what the speaker is saying. We may not notice that the person sitting next to us is whispering or coughing. We become selective in our attention.

Selye suggested that "an essential feature of adaptation is the elimination of stress to the smallest area capable of meeting the requirements of the situation."[72] To exemplify this limiting process, Selye discussed the inflammatory process. Inflammation is a local reaction to injury characterized by heat, pain, redness, and swelling. The injury may result from microorganisms, irritants, or allergens. Inflammation barricades infected or irritated areas of tissue from those areas that are healthy. This localization allows white blood cells to deal more effectively with the insult. Localization also prevents injury from spreading throughout the body.

Adaptive responses may be adequate to meet stress or to change and reestablish homeostatic balance, but adaptive mechanisms may also be inadequate, excessive, inappropriate, or stressful in themselves. Inflammation, for example, can serve adequately as an adaptive function but can also be inadequate, so that the body is overwhelmed by the invading organisms. An inflammatory process can also be excessive and inappropriate. If, for example, the irritant is not a dangerous microbe but a harmless pollen, then inflammation acts as an excessive and inappropriate adaptive mechanism. Inflammation, in this case, is not aiding the individual. Instead, it is creating unnecessary pathologic changes that do not serve any protective purpose.

Although it is usually helpful, adaptation itself can be stressful. For example, although inflammation is useful, it is also stressful because it causes physiologic changes that result in heat, swelling, and pain. These uncomfortable symptoms demand a response and therefore are stressful.

CONCEPT OF CRISIS

Unlike stress, which continuously exists in our lives, a crisis is a sporadic phenomenon that interrupts our existence dramatically. Bircher attempted to define a crisis in general terms:

What is a crisis? It is a decisive moment or turning point, a situation in which turns of events and decisions determine whether the results will be for better, or for worse. A crisis is a challenge, an opportunity for learning and growth. It is a subjective experience in which old ways of doing things no longer assure success and survival.[7]

Gerald Caplan, an authority in crisis theory, concluded that a crisis develops "when a person faces an obstacle to important life goals, that is, for a time, insurmountable through the utilization of customary methods of 'problem solving.' A period of disorganization ensues, a period of upset, during which many abortive attempts at a solution are made."[12]

Obstacles to life goals produce periods of disorganization and disturbance typically called crises. We define a **crisis** as disequilibrium in a steady state, occurring when the usual problem-solving strategies are ineffective. Examples of crises include the following:

▶ Sudden death of a family member
▶ Severe family discord
▶ Spouse or child abuse
▶ Serious accidents
▶ Military combat
▶ Loss of a limb
▶ Loss of a job with severe financial ramifications
▶ Rape or attempted rape
▶ Natural disasters (e.g., tornadoes)
▶ Disasters caused by people (e.g., forest fires)

In each of these situations, people suffer abrupt interruptions in the normal routine of life; in each case, disequilibrium occurs. Furthermore, because crises are not everyday events, people usually have not developed problem-solving methods for dealing with them. During this chaotic period, people may frantically try to solve the problem through trial and error.

If people survive a crisis either by solving the problem or by adapting to it, they may emerge mentally healthier. Emotional growth may have occurred because of the ordeal. On the other hand, people who do not satisfactorily "work through" a dilemma will find it more difficult to deal with future problems. Ultimately, the outcome of resolution of a crisis (for better or for worse) depends on the individual's perception of life and on the available resources (e.g., significant others, health care professionals, a minister).

Maturational and Situational Crises

Crises may be categorized as maturational or situational. **Maturational crises** are predictable, stressful events that occur during each person's developmental process and for which the person has no coping skills. Severe stress at each stage of development interferes with mastery of developmental tasks. In infancy, childhood, adolescence, and adulthood, events that may lead to crisis are usually related to family and peer relationships. For example, at approximately 2 years of age, children are expected to learn to control their bladder and bowel functions. They learn that they can please their parents if they are successful but may earn their displeasure if they are not. They have no previous experience with mastery of their sphincters, do not know how to gain control as expected at this stage of development, and begin to feel a great deal of stress as they face this maturational stage. They are in a maturational crisis. As they learn to control elimination, they will solve the crisis of this stage and will not experience another maturational crisis until the next developmental stage. Because individual growth occurs in stages, it is possible to anticipate maturational events that may create disequilibrium and thus assist the individual in dealing with the crisis of each stage. Expected maturational events, for example, include the first day of school, first date, marriage, childbirth, and death of a parent.

Situational crises are usually sudden, unexpected stressful events that happen to an individual at any point in life and that cannot be controlled by the individual. Divorce, death, war, and natural disasters such as floods or tornadoes are examples of events that can lead to a situational crisis. Situational crises usually cannot be predicted, and anticipatory guidance cannot be offered. Early identification and intervention, however, can assist the individual to cope with the crisis. Self-help groups such as rape crisis centers have been developed to assist individuals to cope with specific events that precipitate a situational crisis.

Characteristics of Crises

Characteristics of crises include the following key points:

▶ Crisis is a universal experience. Crises develop among individuals of all races, cultures, and socioeconomic levels.
▶ A crisis is usually time limited. It typically is resolved (it is hoped with success) within 4 to 6 weeks.
▶ Almost all crises develop in a predictable manner.

Caplan outlined the four developmental phases of a crisis as follows:

1. When a serious problem or threat develops, people become increasingly tense as they attempt to use their usual problem-solving techniques.

2. People grow more upset with each failure of their usual coping methods, and they enter a state of disequilibrium.

3. As tensions continue to build, people mobilize all internal and external resources to restore equilibrium. At this stage, the problem may be reevaluated and attacked from a new angle, or the problem may be distorted and viewed as unsolvable.

4. If the problem is not resolved, emotional pressures continue to build, and people become completely disorganized or immobilized because of severe anxiety or depression.

Like anxiety, crisis exists on a continuum. Note in Figure 16–5 that crisis begins with the potential crisis state, then proceeds through precrisis, immediate crisis, and intermediate and advanced crisis states before developing into a full crisis state. Note, too, that anyone is susceptible at the potential crisis state. At full crisis, however, individuals at risk are those who have failed at all attempts to solve their problems, who believe all available problem-solving resources have been used, and who do not obtain relief from their stress.[10,12,39]

Crises tend to occur in cycles, with one crisis following another. For example, people who have been in-

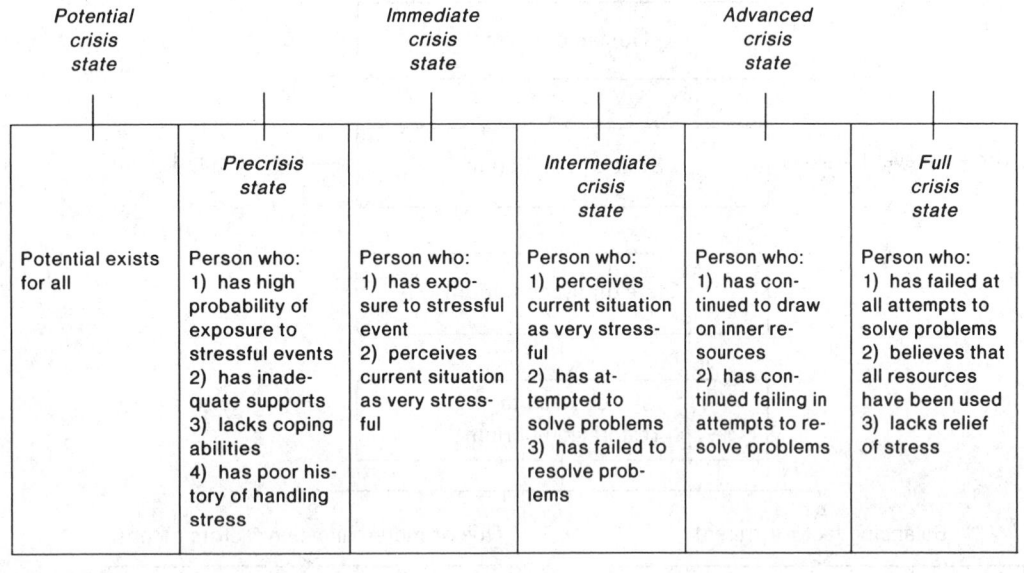

▲ **Figure 16-5**

Crisis continuum. (From Brownell, M.J. (1984). The concept of crisis: its utility for nursing. *Advances in Nursing Science: Crisis Intervention*, 6(4), 1. Reprinted with permission of Aspen Systems Corporation.)

volved in serious automobile accidents are usually hospitalized. Hospitalization may threaten a person's job and financial stability. If married, the spouse may be forced to work overtime, thus disrupting family cohesiveness. Consequently, serious behavioral problems may develop in the children. Thus, as the old saying goes, "troubles never come singly."

People undergoing crisis are often highly susceptible to the influence of other individuals in their environment. Thus, the individuals in crisis are usually quite responsive to crisis intervention by others.

Crisis Intervention

REACTIONS TO CRISES

People in crisis display typical psychologic and physiologic reactions. Immediate reactions to a critical problem include fear, anxiety, anger, panic, the drive to act, and heightened tension. All these responses suggest an emergency with activation of the "fight-or-flight" mechanism. Within hours to days after the onset of a crisis, a person may become confused, depressed, immobilized, and unable to make decisions. These responses are not helpful and in fact prevent satisfactory resolution of the problem.

COPING WITH POTENTIAL CRISES

Personal problems, even serious ones, do not have to culminate in a crisis. Crises are preventable. According to Aguilera, whether a situation develops into crisis depends on three factors: (1) the individual's perception of the problem or event, (2) available situational supports, and (3) coping mechanisms.[1,2]

Note in Figure 16-6 that if a person undergoing a stressful event perceives the situation realistically and

has adequate situational support (e.g., significant others with whom to discuss the problem) and adequate coping mechanisms (e.g., ways of reducing tension by expressing anger or frustration), the problem will probably be resolved and crisis averted. On the other hand, if one or more factors are missing, the problem may not be resolved, and a crisis could develop.

ASSESSMENT

The basis for competent professional care to protect and promote health is a thorough assessment of the individual's health status. Assessment involves collection of physiologic, psychologic, and sociocultural data that may assist us in determining what is creating an imbalance in the individual's present state of health. Nurses help people appraise and cope with the stressors in their lives. To do so, we must assess people's perceptions of and vulnerability to stressors, responses to stressors, and coping resources. In addition, we must plan nursing interventions to help people cope with stress responses and stress-related illnesses. The more we understand the underlying dynamics of stress, the better we can prevent harmful stress responses or stress-related psychophysiologic disorders in ourselves and others.

The ultimate goal of stress management is to adapt to stressors, not succumb to them.

Dudley and Welke[26] designed a "working" model of stress (see Fig. 16-1) based on the notion that the impact of a stressor on an individual depends on that person's perception of the stressor and vulnerability to it. Vulnerability, in turn, depends on the person's psychophysiologic defenses and coping mechanisms

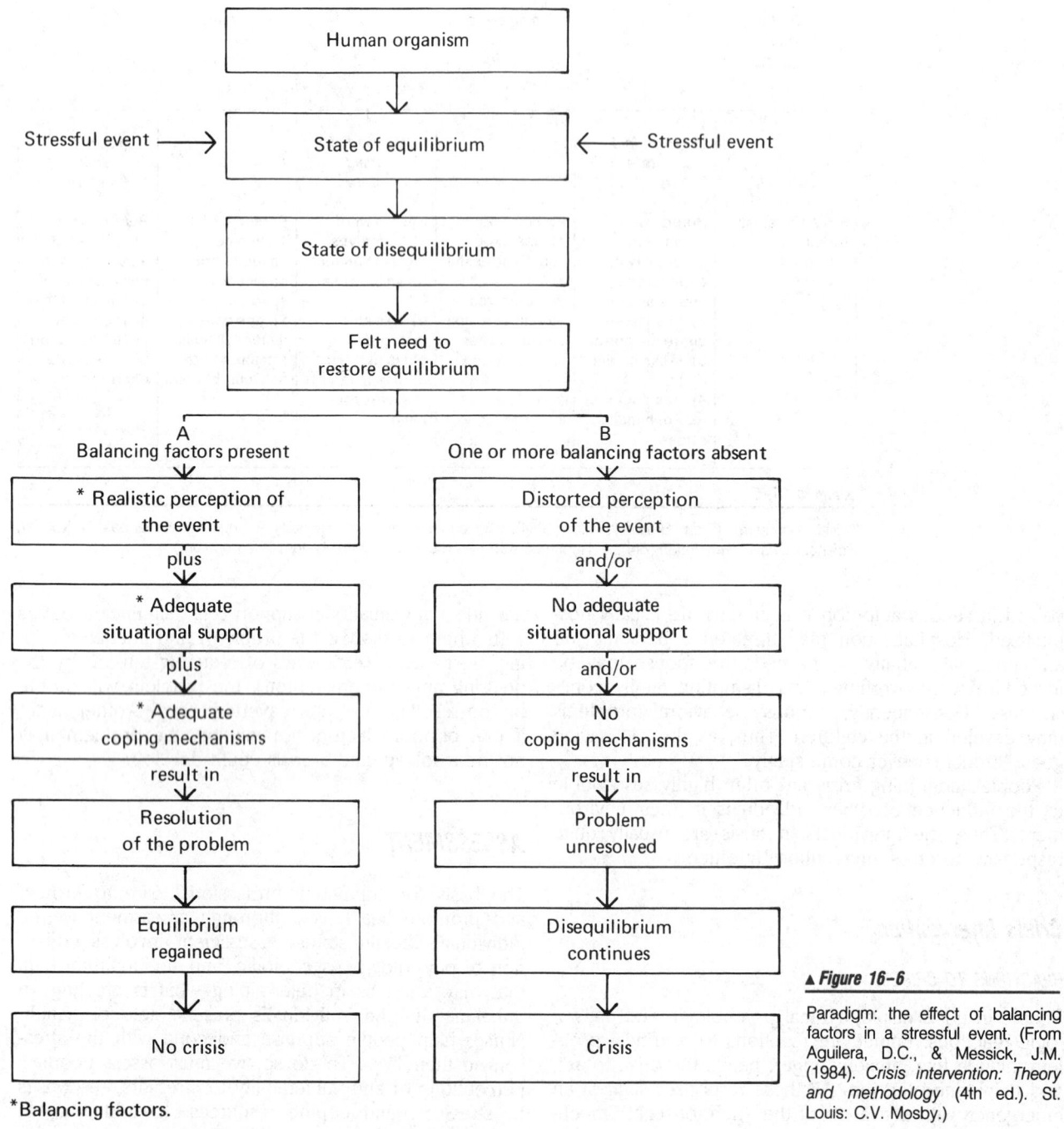

*Balancing factors.

▲ *Figure 16-6*

Paradigm: the effect of balancing factors in a stressful event. (From Aguilera, D.C., & Messick, J.M. (1984). *Crisis intervention: Theory and methodology* (4th ed.). St. Louis: C.V. Mosby.)

against stressors. People with inadequate defenses and coping mechanisms suffer severe stress responses and even illness. On the other hand, individuals with strong natural defenses do not perceive most stressors as major or even moderate. Still other people have fewer natural defenses but are willing to develop and experiment with new coping skills. By using new coping skills, these individuals may emerge from a stressful situation with a sense of mastery that they carry over to new situations. For this reason, the model is not linear but involves feedback as the person learns to cope with new stressors. Let us now consider each aspect of the model and its implications for nursing.

Stressors

Recall that stressors are agents or factors that challenge the adaptive capacities of an individual. These agents place a strain on the person, resulting in a stress response and possibly illness. Stressors may be environmental, internal, imagined, or anticipatory. In addition, stressors are perceived by an individual as minor, moderate, major, or overwhelming. The magnitude of the stressor depends on the individual's unconscious and conscious perception and cognitive appraisal of the event. Thus, for one person, flying in an airplane is a minor stressor, whereas for another person it is an overwhelming stressor.

As Lazarus pointed out, it is not the major problems and life changes that are overwhelming for most people. Rather, it is the everyday hassles that finally push us to the breaking point.

Part of assessment is determining the cause of the precipitating event that led to the individual's request for help. By listening to the "last straw," you can assess the critical issues that are problematic to the person.

First Line of Defense Against Stressors: Present Status

Our first line of defense against internal and external stressors is the present status of our physical and psychologic defenses.

Initial Psychophysiologic Stress Response Indicators

Note in Figure 16–1 that when a person perceives that a stressor is overwhelming or the first line of defense against the stressor is weak, the stressor can provoke a psychophysiologic stress response. Although the psychologic and physiologic components of the stress response are connected, we can separate them for purposes of discussion. When collecting your data during assessment, however, remember that, in reality, mind and body continuously interact with each other. Distressing physiologic symptoms trigger anxiety and other emotions, which in turn trigger more distressing physiologic symptoms.[38,70,74,76]

PHYSIOLOGIC RESPONSES TO STRESSORS

Clues about the physical and emotional stress reactions of other people come from behavioral stress responses, that is, from changes in how people look, act, or talk. Emotional responses usually show up in facial expressions or other nonverbal communications (e.g., perspiration, a shaky voice, tremors, or spasms in facial or other muscles may be indicators of physiologic stress responses). Posture can also provide information about stress. Consider a person who has come home from work after being fired and who is fully dressed but is curled up in bed, in a fetal position, with face covered, window blinds drawn, and door closed. This person's posture signals a stress reaction, and this scenario helps to demonstrate that, as people attempt to escape stressors, unusual behaviors may be observed. Some people quit their jobs, drop out of school, run away from home, or commit suicide to escape stressors.

In response to stressors, the body alerts itself physiologically for "fight or flight." Major physiologic responses to stressors include the following:

- ▶ Increased heart rate (tachycardia) as a result of the release of epinephrine (adrenalin)
- ▶ Increased blood pressure resulting from (1) vasoconstriction (resulting from the effects of epinephrine and norepinephrine); (2) increased cardiac output; (3) increased shunting of blood toward vital organs and away from the gastrointestinal tract and other nonvital organs; (4) increased sodium and water retention resulting from the release of mineralocorticoid hormones, which results in increased blood volume; and (5) decreased blood to the kidneys and increased secretion of renin caused by release of norepinephrine
- ▶ Increased oxygen intake as a result of faster, deeper respirations and dilation of bronchi (extreme anxiety can sometimes produce shallow respirations)
- ▶ Increased serum glucose levels resulting from (1) release of glucocorticoid hormones; and (2) gluconeogenesis (synthesis of glucose from noncarbohydrate substances such as amino acids)
- ▶ Decreased inflammatory and immune responses
- ▶ Pupil dilation caused by release of epinephrine, which allows us "to see more" in emergencies
- ▶ Reduced peristaltic action caused by the release of epinephrine
- ▶ Increased alertness resulting from increased sympathetic nervous system stimulation (three signs of increased alertness are quickened movements, greater muscular tension, and a greater startle sensitivity). By becoming more alert when faced with a stressor, we prepare for "fight or flight."

The hypothalamus, a vital structure in the brain, coordinates the physiologic activities and orchestrates the release of stress hormones. In Figure 16–7, note the role the general adaptation syndrome plays in the body's response to stressors. Note that, in general, the cardiovascular system is stimulated and the gastrointestinal system is inhibited during a stress response. Be aware that these stress responses are not under conscious control.

When stressors are less than overwhelming, homeostasis, or physiologic balance, is usually restored. When the stress is overwhelming, however, physiologic mechanisms go awry, and disease or death results.

In the early stages of human evolution, the "fight-or-flight" response was important to human survival. Most often, today, this response occurs in situations that are unrelated to survival.

PSYCHOLOGIC RESPONSES TO STRESSORS: ANXIETY

When we perceive that we must confront a major stressor, we prepare for "fight or flight," a series of physiologic responses. The emotional components of fighting or fleeing are anger or rage and anxiety or fear. As nurses, we deal with both anger and anxiety in people. Of these two, the more common emotional response to life's stressful demands is anxiety, and nurses work daily with anxious people.

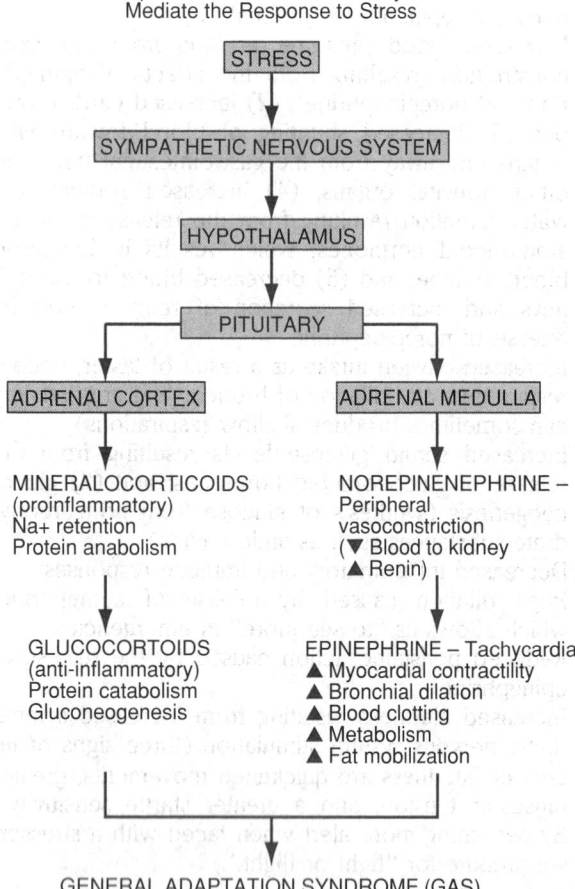

Principal Neuroendocrine Pathways that Mediate the Response to Stress

STRESS

SYMPATHETIC NERVOUS SYSTEM

HYPOTHALAMUS

PITUITARY

ADRENAL CORTEX — ADRENAL MEDULLA

MINERALOCORTICOIDS
(proinflammatory)
Na+ retention
Protein anabolism

NOREPINENEPHRINE –
Peripheral
vasoconstriction
(▼ Blood to kidney
▲ Renin)

GLUCOCORTOIDS
(anti-inflammatory)
Protein catabolism
Gluconeogenesis

EPINEPHRINE – Tachycardia
▲ Myocardial contractility
▲ Bronchial dilation
▲ Blood clotting
▲ Metabolism
▲ Fat mobilization

GENERAL ADAPTATION SYNDROME (GAS)

Stage 1.   ALARM REACTION
Enlargement of adrenal cortex
Enlargement of lymphatic system
Increase in hormone levels

Stage 2.   RESISTANCE
Shrinkage of adrenal cortex
Lymph nodes closer to normal size
Hormone levels sustained

Stage 3.   EXHAUSTION
Enlargement/dysfunction of
  lymphatic structures
Increase in hormone levels
Depletion of adaptive hormones

A stress syndrome, termed the General Adaptation Syndrome, by Hans Selye, evolves in three stages. Stages 1 and 2 are continuously repeated throughout a lifetime cycle. If resistance cannot be sustained, exhaustion (Stage 3) with its altered psychophysiologic functioning, occurs.

▲ **Figure 16–7**

Physiologic responses to stress: General Adaptation Syndrome (GAS). (From Smith, M.J., & Selye, H. (1979). Effects of stress, reducing the negative. Reprinted with permission from the *American Journal of Nursing,* 79(10), 1953–1964. Copyright 1979, American Journal of Nursing Company.)

Because it arises from the frustrations and conflicts of life, anxiety has always been part of human existence. **Anxiety** is apprehension, dread, foreboding, or uneasiness that is not related to an identifiable source of danger. Anxiety differs from fear. Although we ex-

perience the same feelings with fear as with anxiety, our feelings stem from different sources.

With fear, the source of danger is recognized and can be identified. With anxiety, it is not.

Both anxiety and fear arise in the same part of the brain, and both cause the "fight-or-flight" response. The two emotions differ because of their source. Other distinctions between anxiety and fear are as follows:

- ▶ Anxiety is concerned with the future; fear is concerned with the present.
- ▶ Anxiety is vague in character; fear is definite.
- ▶ Anxiety is the result of psychologic conflict; fear is the result of a specific threat to biologic integrity.
- ▶ Anxiety does not always make sense; fear is rational.

Generally, anxiety makes us feel uncomfortable. Such feelings are usually a mix of physical and mental states. We are aware of feeling nervous or uneasy. We may also experience various physiologic reactions (e.g., diarrhea). As uncomfortable as anxiety is, we usually cannot identify its exact cause, and the confusion is all the more distressing. People experience anxiety in certain situations and not in others, and a situation may provoke anxiety in a person one time but not another time. In this case, the meaning of the situation for the person has changed, probably because of reappraisal.

Anxiety varies with an individual's perception, which in turn depends on a person's psychosocial make-up, education, degree of maturity, and life experience. Figure 16–8 presents an example of how perception contributes to anxiety.

Anxiety has many causes.

Generally, situations of frustration, conflict, or stress that threaten the physical or mental security of an individual produce anxiety. Because illness is physically as well as mentally taxing, sickness produces anxiety. Hence, ill people are usually uncomfortable emotionally as well as physically.

Physiologic threats are recognized more easily than threats to a person's mental well-being. For instance, life-threatening physiologic disorders have distinct manifestations. Infections or injury have obvious signs and symptoms. Identifying psychologic threats, however, is more difficult. We must remember to be as sensitive to the anxiety a sick person experiences as we are to signs of physical disease.

Anxiety may be communicated.

People may communicate their anxiety both verbally and nonverbally. A person's voice may shake or break, pitch may change, and speed may fluctuate. A tense posture, nervous movements, sweat, or a "wide-eyed" appearance hint, nonverbally, at anxiety, and, like a bad cold, anxiety can spread from one person to another. One anxious person can make others anxious. An anxious nurse can communicate anxiety to coworkers and to those receiving care.

Anxiety can be assessed.

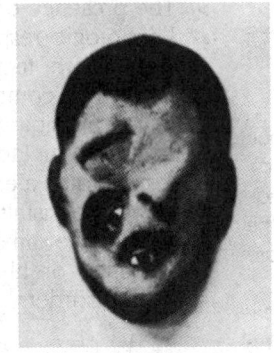
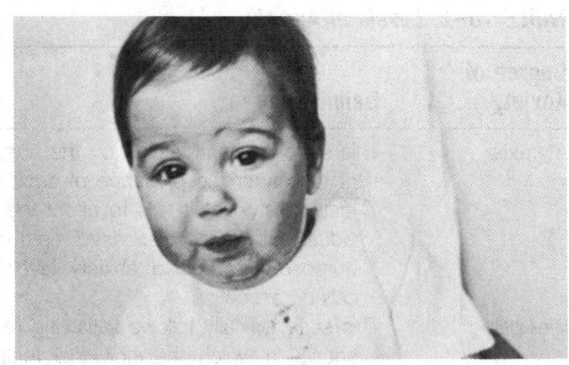

▲ *Figure 16–8*

Perceptual distortion and anxiety. Violation of perceptual expectancies makes the baby of about 8 months of age express anxiety when he sees the distorted mask at left. At an earlier period, before he learned what the human face is supposed to look like, he might have smiled at the mask. (From Kagan, J., et al. (1984). *Psychology: An introduction* (5th ed.). New York: Harcourt Brace Jovanovich.)

Anxiety can be assessed by analyzing its intensity, appropriateness, duration, and somatic symptoms. We can conceptualize the intensity of anxiety by viewing it on a continuum, ranging from ataraxia to panic. Table 16–2 defines the levels of anxiety.

As our level of anxiety increases, we become increasingly unable to understand what is happening to us and what is expected of us.

Because the extremely anxious person easily misunderstands what is said, remember to keep your communication with anxious people clear and brief. Repeating statements is helpful because anxious people tend to forget easily. Nonverbal movements may aid in clarifying communication. Remember also that the anxious person needs an opportunity to discuss feelings with a calm, nonjudgmental person.

Assess the appropriateness of anxiety, and remember that appropriate anxiety serves a useful, adaptive purpose. Students, for example, tend to lack the appropriate motivation to study unless they are mildly anxious, but excessive anxiety has a disintegrative effect. It can immobilize the person or lead to panic, making appropriate goal-directed behavior impossible. On the other hand, apathy or the absence of anxiety also makes goal-directed behavior impossible.

Also assess the duration of the person's anxiety. Most people can tolerate even intense levels of anxiety for brief periods, but our bodies cannot tolerate severe anxiety for sustained periods. Sustained anxiety can lead to chronic physical or mental illness or both, if the condition is not controlled by self-help measures or professional intervention. When working with an anxious individual, gear questions to the length of time the person has been feeling anxious. Is being anxious a chronic state, or is the person's anxiety related to a specific individual or situation?

Finally, remember to assess the somatic symptoms that anxiety generates; some of these physiologic effects are anorexia, nausea, vomiting, abdominal cramps, and diarrhea. In addition, people may feel flushed, perspire excessively, or experience chest pain. Some individuals urinate more often. Anxiety can produce dysmenorrhea and frigidity in women. Men may become impotent. In some instances, aching muscles or joints, backache, and headache are also attributable to anxiety.

Each individual experiences different somatic reactions to anxiety. One person may experience mainly gastrointestinal symptoms, whereas another may typically notice cardiovascular symptoms. If the anxiety is short lived, (i.e., successfully dealt with), these effects do not cause harm. Sustained or chronic anxiety, however, eventually causes disease by keeping the body in an abnormal state.

Although anxiety produces physiologic symptoms, do not assume automatically that anxiety is the sole basis for these symptoms or bodily responses. For example, anxiety may or may not be a contributing factor in the causation of headache. Only a thorough assessment can identify the specific cause of a symptom. Furthermore, if anxiety does prove to be a significant factor, remember that the symptom is out of the individual's conscious control. The pain experienced from a headache caused by anxiety may be as intense as that of a headache resulting from a brain tumor.

STRESS-RELATED PSYCHOPHYSIOLOGIC DISORDERS

Physical or mental illness develops if (1) a person's defenses are overwhelmed by stressors, (2) a person is unaware of the significance of a stress response and chooses to deny or ignore it; (3) a person is either unwilling or unable to engage in self-help activities; or (4) a person overuses defense mechanisms. For example, some people pass through a period of denial and psychologic withdrawal when exposed to major stressors (e.g., death of a loved one). These responses are temporarily helpful during the early phases of grief, but they are harmful if the grief goes unresolved after a long period.

According to some estimates, stress-related problems account for nearly 80 per cent of all visits to physicians' offices. The financial cost of stress-related illness is high. For example, lowered productivity by employees as a result of stress-related physical illnesses accounts for a loss of at least $60 billion each year. Stress-induced mental dysfunction accounts for a loss of $17 billion annually.[38]

Various studies linked family crises with the onset of streptococcal infection, increased use of medical services, and complications of pregnancy. Tuberculosis has been shown to occur after the death of a spouse. Parental illness has followed the death of a child. Stress has been identified as a factor in cardiovascular disease, ulcers, and cancer.

TABLE 16-2. Levels of Anxiety

Degree of Anxiety	Definition
Ataraxia	This state is characterized by the absence of anxiety or the presence of such minimal anxiety that it fails to affect the individual. (Note: Medications given for the purpose of reducing anxiety levels are called "ataractics.")
Well-being	This state typically follows satisfying experiences, in which the individual feels relaxed, comfortable, and happy. Minimal anxiety exists, but the individual is not excessively alert. This level of anxiety is believed to be healing.
Mild anxiety (1+)	This attentive, gentle level of anxiety is useful and is experienced by most productive, healthy persons. Mild anxiety is an asset to successful adaptation in life. Perception becomes keener. The person is in a state conducive to learning and is able to solve problems.
Moderate anxiety (2+)	This intermediate, tempered level of anxiety can take on the qualities of either mild or severe anxiety. At its lower levels, moderate anxiety heightens productivity and abilities. At higher levels, a person may use selective inattention, thus being unaware of ongoing activities but noticing those pointed out by an observer.
Severe anxiety (3+)	This painful level of anxiety is not useful and hence requires intervention. Severe anxiety consumes most of an individual's energy, inhibiting the physiologic powers of restoration. The person does not notice what is going on and is unable to do so even if activity is pointed out.
Panic (4+)	This frightening, violent, disintegrating, overpowering anxiety causes the individual to lose control. Such anxiety is not frequently encountered but is critical when it does occur. Panic is a severe state of psychologic disequilibrium and cannot be endured for long. During panic, people distort situations and events and are unable to comprehend them in a realistic way. Panic eliminates the ability to maintain goal-directed activity.

Therefore, when assessing a client for stress, you will assess for such factors as the following:

▶ Stressors impinging on the individual (the Social Readjustment Rating Scale—see Fig. 16–3—can be a valuable assessment tool for such purposes)
▶ The presence of maturational crises (see Chapters 12–14 for a review of developmental crises at each stage of growth and development)
▶ The presence of situational crises
▶ Physiologic responses to stressors, including behavior, posture, facial expressions, and other verbal and nonverbal communications of emotion, as well as major physiologic indicators of the "fight-or-flight" response, including increased pulse, blood pressure, respirations, alertness, and serum glucose levels; decreased peristalsis; and pupil dilation
▶ The level of anxiety (ranging from ataraxia to panic)
▶ Presence or history of stress-related psychophysiologic disorders.

NURSING DIAGNOSIS

Many nursing diagnoses relate to stress, but anxiety is the most pertinent example of the stresses of life. Anxiety, fear, dread, and panic—and their associated signs and symptoms, which result from the "fight-or-flight" response—are all important factors in several nursing diagnoses. These related causes of stress can be quite confusing but do point to the importance of anxiety in the lives of human beings. The two most important nursing diagnoses you may make for anxious individuals are as follows:

▶ *Anxiety* (see Nursing Diagnosis Profile 16–1)
▶ *Fear*

In other nursing diagnoses, anxiety may be a related factor. Each of the nursing diagnoses in Box 16–1 could be followed by the words "related to anxiety." Thus, *Anxiety* may be the first part of the nursing diagnosis for an anxious individual, or it may be the second part of the nursing diagnosis. In fact, the word "anxiety" need not appear in a nursing diagnosis statement every time you observe signs and symptoms of anxiety in a person. The individual may have another problem that requires nursing intervention, one for which anxiety is but one of the defining characteristics. For example, anxiety may be a defining characteristic in the following nursing diagnoses:

▶ *Fluid Volume Excess*
▶ *Impaired Social Interaction*
▶ *Ineffective Denial*
▶ *Decisional Conflict* (specify)
▶ *Sensory/Perceptual Alteration* (specify)
▶ *Altered Thought Processes*
▶ *Pain*
▶ *Anticipatory Grieving*
▶ *High Risk for Violence*
▶ *Posttrauma Response*
▶ *Rape-Trauma Syndrome* (all types)

Anxiety can also alter a person's life in ways that create difficulties and can therefore lead to other defining characteristics. Anxiety may serve as

▶ an internal cue to which some persons respond with *Altered Nutrition: More Than Body Requirements* or *Altered Nutrition: Potential for More Than Body Requirements*
▶ a mental factor that leads to decreased fluid intake

NURSING DIAGNOSIS PROFILE

Anxiety

Definition. A vague uneasy feeling whose source is often non-specific or unknown to the individual

Classification. Feeling 9.3.1

Defining Characteristics. Defining characteristics may be divided into subjective symptoms or experiences only the client can describe and objective signs that can be observed and sometimes measured by the nurse or others.

Subjective symptoms described by anxious persons include feelings of being jittery, shaky, apprehensive, fearful, scared, distressed, rattled, worried, and other states that are synonymous with feeling anxious. Anxious persons also express concerns of a general nature (e.g., about a change of life events or about a fear of unspecific consequences). In relation to possible life events, they describe themselves as feeling inadequate, uncertain, and painfully and persistently helpless.

Objective signs include the effects of sympathetic nervous system stimulation (e.g., increased cardiac output and increased peripheral vasoconstriction resulting in increased blood pressure and a rapid pulse and respiration). Other sympathetic nervous system effects include pupil dilation, elevated blood glucose levels, hand tremors, and increased perspiration. As the client experiences the "fight-or-flight" response, the nurse can observe behavioral changes such as increased wariness with facial tension, poor eye contact, and a tendency to glance about; restlessness with extraneous movements such as foot shuffling, quivering vocalizations, insomnia, and a tendency to focus on the self.

Sample Related Factors. Anxiety may be related to any threat to the individual's physical or psychologic integrity, including the following:

▶ Unconscious conflicts about essential values or goals of life
▶ Threat to the self-concept
▶ Threat of death
▶ Threat to or change in health status, role functioning, environment, or interaction patterns
▶ Situational or maturational crises
▶ Interpersonal contagion
▶ Unmet needs

Concept Description. This diagnosis refers to the state in which a person experiences a threat to a sense of well-being so that the person feels in peril. The individual is unsure about what

exactly the danger is, however, and cannot actually express the fear of what may be the outcome. The person senses only that the threat is potentially overwhelming and must be avoided or overcome. At the same time, the person feels powerless to deal with the threat and is painfully apprehensive about it.

Examples. Depending on the specific assessment data, this diagnostic category could be applicable in the following situations, among others:

▶ A nursing student who has a low test average and who knows she must make a grade of at least 97% on the final examination if she is to pass her course. She knows that nothing in the testing room will physically harm her, and she knows that failure to pass a test or even failure to pass the course will in no way threaten her life. Yet she experiences the same physical and psychologic feelings as if someone were pointing a loaded gun at her head. Her diagnosis might be *Anxiety* R/T threat to self-concept.
▶ A 20-year-old female who has been planning her wedding for the past 8 months and who has spent over $15,000.00 of her father's money on the festivities to come but who suddenly feels a total panic at the thought of marrying her lifelong sweetheart. Her diagnosis might be *Anxiety* R/T maturational crisis.

Related/Similar Nursing Diagnoses. *Anxiety* should be distinguished from the nursing diagnosis *Fear*. *Anxiety* is very similar to *Fear* in that the source of discomfort stems from the same area of the brain and the "fight-or-flight" mechanism is activated in both instances so that the actual physical responses are identical.

The main difference between the experiences of anxiety and fear is that the person experiencing fear is able to identify the object of fear and the person experiencing anxiety is unsure about the source of these feelings. Other differences stem from this difference. The person who experiences anxiety feels that this emotion is irrational and feels more helpless because both fight and flight are impossible. The feeling is within the person and cannot be overcome or escaped. The person who experiences a rational fear of a specific, dreaded object, which is external, has the option to fight or to flee and thus does not feel so helpless.

---

with resulting *Fluid Volume Deficit* or *High Risk for Fluid Volume Deficit*
▶ a mental status change that leads to blood pressure variations and *Decreased Cardiac Output*
▶ an internal risk factor leading to a *High Risk for Injury*
▶ a basis for feelings of inadequacy that can lead to parental role conflict
▶ evidence of alterations in mood that can lead to *Spiritual Distress*

The nursing process applies to both anxiety and other forms of stress.

PLANNING

In assisting the client to control stressors, the nurse should plan for the healthiest possible outcomes. In general, as independently as possible, the person will be able to do the following:

▶ Deal with the stressful problem
▶ Deal with the feelings engendered by the problem
▶ Reduce the physiologic arousal of stress[86]

(The case study shows how these general outcomes can be applied to a specific client.) Who will help

---

Box 16-1. Nursing Diagnoses for Which Anxiety May Be a Related Factor

Altered Nutrition: Less Than Body Requirements
Constipation
Colonic Constipation
Diarrhea
Ineffective Breathing Pattern
Impaired Verbal Communication
Social Isolation
Altered Role Performance
Altered Parenting
High Risk for Altered Parenting
Sexual Dysfunction
Altered Sexuality Patterns
Altered Family Processes
Ineffective Family Coping
Compromised Family Coping
Ineffective Individual Coping
Noncompliance
Fatigue
Sleep Pattern Disturbance
Altered Health Maintenance
Ineffective Breastfeeding
Bathing/Hygiene Self-Care Deficit
Dressing/Grooming Self-Care Deficit
Toileting Self-Care Deficit
Body Image Disturbance
Personal Identity Disturbance

---

ensure these outcomes? Resources include the client, the client's significant others, community resources, and the nurse.

The Client

As much as possible, individuals must make decisions so they can increase their sense of control over their own health care. The nurse must be judicious, however, because urging decision making before a person is ready can lead to increased, possibly intolerable levels of stress. The ultimate goal is to have the person independently managing stress. The nurse must plan to teach the person to use all the resources available to manage stress.

Significant Others

A strong, supportive network of significant others can help a person weather life's difficulties. A significant other may be a parent, a spouse, a child, a best friend, or a pet. Encourage individuals to confide in those close to them. Help those who are lonely to reach out and bring new people into their lives. When feeling anxious, talking with an empathic person, perhaps one who has been through a similar experience, is beneficial.

The effects of social support on stress have been heavily researched. The results imply that social support is a powerful modifier of potentially negative stress effects. In addition, social support facilitates coping with life's demands. Research indicates that individuals with social support have less somatic (physical) illness, increased mental health,[14] and longer lives.[84]

Community Resources

Help your client to understand that, when in need of information concerning a specific problem, it is wise to seek information from appropriate resources (e.g., a professional counselor or an organization devoted to helping people with certain problems). For some people, a religious affiliation is a source of comfort. For others, personal growth groups, assertiveness training, encounter groups, and other self-help organizations prove useful.

The Nurse

The nurse assists the individual in planning for stress management by helping to strengthen ties with significant others, making referrals to community resources, and teaching the client to manage stress. Obviously, the optimum time for planning occurs before a person becomes hospitalized as a result of stress. To teach stress management after a person has suffered a stroke or some other health-related problem is, in many ways, too late. Plan to teach stress management before the person becomes hospitalized. To accomplish this goal, you must regard the nurse's role as extending beyond the health care facility.

Nurses are role models. People look to nurses for example of healthy lifestyles.

You do not have to be in a formal setting or in a therapeutic relationship to teach stress management. First, plan to teach stress management by example. If you look fit and exude vitality and enthusiasm, people will notice and may want to imitate you in diet, exercise patterns, and so on. You can also be available as a significant other to those around you who are feeling stressed. Associates will listen to your recommendations for stress control if you seem to have your own life and health under control.

NURSING INTERVENTION

Second Line of Defense Against Stressors: Self-Help

Some stress responses may be so distressing that they demand the person's attention. For example, physiologic responses that demand attention include heart palpitations, difficulty breathing, nausea, and loss of appetite. One disturbing psychologic response is severe anxiety or panic. If responses of this magnitude develop, the aware person uses and develops self-help measures to counter and control stress reactions, thereby reducing the chance of developing an acute or chronic illness.

Three methods of stress management identified by Trygstad are as follows:

▶ Deal with the problem by identifying the source of the problem, changing the situation, changing your perception, and changing your response.
▶ Deal with the feelings engendered by the problem by identifying, acknowledging, experiencing, and expressing feelings.
▶ Reduce the physiologic arousal of stress by resting, engaging in physical exercise, relaxing, eating properly, smoking less, and using relaxation techniques.[86]

You will want to apply the essentials of stress management to your own life and to your work with people who are experiencing stress responses.

DEALING WITH THE PROBLEM

Perhaps the first step in handling a stressor is to identify its source. Identification helps reduce the powerlessness we often feel while in the grip of a stress response.

It is often possible to pinpoint the source of a stressor by asking a few general self-assessment questions. For example, ask yourself, or have the person you are caring for ask, the following:

▶ Is the stress related to work, to home, or to a relationship?
▶ Are too many demands being made at home, on the job, or at school?
▶ Is it impossible to get enough rest?
▶ Is the possibility of a serious illness a concern?
▶ Has a distressing situation occurred recently that has not been adequately resolved?
▶ Are there events coming up in the future that are anxiety provoking?
▶ Are many life changes going on at one time?

If the answer to one or several of these questions suggests a possible source, then take the second step and deal with the stressor. You can try to change the situation, and if change is not entirely possible, at least alter your perception of the situation and your response. For example, if you feel overwhelmed with your studies, changing the situation by quitting school is rarely appropriate. Instead, change your perception of the problem and your response. When you feel overburdened, look at each assignment separately rather than as one large mountain of work, and tackle each task one at a time. Develop a reasonable schedule. Make small but important changes in your situation by eliminating superfluous tasks. Also you might apply for a scholarship or loan so that you do not have to work in addition to going to school.

If a person for whom you are providing care feels overburdened with responsibilities at home, suggest a change in the situation by delegating tasks. If the person feels guilty about delegation, point out that no one person should assume all the housekeeping tasks. In this way, you help change the person's self-perception of a martyr who must shoulder all the burdens of home alone. The person's response to housework may also change after requesting help without feeling guilty.

Recognizing stressors and acting on them early, instead of denying them and allowing them to grow, are essential to mental and physical health.

DEALING WITH FEELINGS

Feeling "stressed" can manifest itself in anxiety, frustration, anger, or other emotions.

The first step in handling feelings of stress is assessment. What feeling is being experienced? What is its source? It is not always easy for people to identify what they are feeling at a particular time or why they are feeling as they do. Therefore, encourage self-assessment. Specifically look at what happened to precipitate the feeling. Did a friend make an unkind remark? Did the person fail a major examination or make a mistake at work? What somatic responses accompanied the feeling (upset stomach, tears, palpitations)? Under what circumstances did the feeling dissipate (e.g., did you discuss the problem with a friend who helped you to see the humorous side of the situation)?

Once the feeling has been identified, it is important for the person to acknowledge it. For instance, if you feel very angry with a client who is not complying with your instructions, you need to acknowledge to yourself that you are angry. Acknowledging anger can be difficult. The idealized view of nursing is that nurses are always kind and helpful and never irritated or angry. In reality, we all become angry at times, and that anger needs to be acknowledged and expressed in an appropriate way.

For example, imagine that you are taking care of Mr. Jones, who suffers from severe arthritis. Mr. Jones sometimes expresses his anger, frustration, and pain by leveling harsh criticisms at the nurses. Today you are taking care of Mr. Jones, and he is in a bitter mood. As you give him his bath, you can feel yourself becoming angrier as he becomes more caustic. Finally, with your stomach in knots, you excuse yourself for a minute and leave the room. You realize that you must help Mr. Jones deal with his frustrations, but first you must deal with your own! You take a few deep breaths and try to relax. You review in your mind what you have learned about pain and the many ways people try to cope with it. You may take time to talk with your instructor or other nurses who care for Mr. Jones. As you discuss how you feel, you sense your anger is decreasing. Soon you feel able to return to Mr. Jones. In time, as you work with Mr. Jones and grow to know him and as he comes to trust you, it may be possible to help this person express his feelings more appropriately.

REDUCING THE PHYSIOLOGIC AROUSAL OF STRESS

General Methods of Stress Reduction. Poor physical condition lowers our resistance to stressors and makes us more vulnerable to serious stress responses. Peak physical condition, on the other hand, means stamina, the necessary reserves to withstand an attack of stressors, and protection against unpredictable periods of life change. Exercise not only works toward physical fitness but also relieves stress and tension.

Keeping fit is one of the best self-help mechanisms for coping with stress.

Because certain foods seem to magnify stress responses, dietary changes can help manage stress. Substances such as caffeine, alcohol, sugar, preservatives, and certain food flavorings and colorings can cause adverse psychophysiologic responses. For example, too much caffeine increases blood pressure, causes tachycardia, and induces "nervousness." Excessive alcohol can have serious short- and long-term effects on mind and body. Good nutrition strengthens that first line of defense against stress.

Cigarette and pipe smoking also can increase stress responses. Nicotine increases epinephrine and norepinephrine secretion, which results in increased heart rate, blood pressure, and oxygen consumption. To control stress responses, smokers need to stop smoking or at least to control smoking by modifying the amount smoked per day.

Behavioral coping strategies such as time management (e.g., part-time vs. full-time job) can assist in decreasing stress levels. Stress also can be dissipated through relaxation exercises, controlled breathing techniques, or meditative approaches such as yoga, Zen, or transcendental meditation.

In progressive relaxation, the patient is taught first to tense and then to relax groups of voluntary muscles in a systematic manner: first the feet, then the lower legs, the thighs, and so on up to the trunk and arms to the face. This process helps the person learn to control tension in the muscles, thus leading to reductions in heart rate and blood pressure and creating mental and emotional calmness.

Forms of personal recreation, such as reading, listening to music, or taking walks, are also practical methods for dealing with stress.

Biofeedback Training. Biofeedback training uses the concept of feedback to help individuals monitor and control automatic physiologic functions (e.g., blood pressure, heart rate). Biofeedback is a technique that is still evolving but has been found to be effective in stress reduction.

Biologists have traditionally divided physiologic functions into two distinct group: voluntary functions, which are governed by the conscious mind (e.g., motor skills and speech) and involuntary functions (sometimes called visceral functions). Involuntary functions are governed by the autonomic nervous system and operate automatically without the individual's awareness or control. Among involuntary functions are temperature regulation, brain wave activity, and cardiovascular function.

Within the last decade, the concept of feedback has been applied with considerable success to the behavioral regulation of the so-called involuntary biologic functions (hence, the term biofeedback). As a result, the rigid dichotomy between voluntary and involuntary physiologic functions is gradually disintegrating. Scientists now believe that, with biofeedback training, people may learn to self-regulate such body functions as blood pressure and heart rate. As a result, people can learn to avoid disease.

Biofeedback training is a scientifically planned program that trains selected subjects to control one or more "involuntary" functions. While in the program, the person may learn to regulate blood pressure, heart rate, brain waves, skin temperature, and muscle tension. Biofeedback training involves (a) attaching the subject to electronic monitoring equipment; (b) monitoring a particular physiologic function (e.g., heartbeat); (c) "feeding back" selected information about that function (e.g., increases or decreases in heart rate) to the subject by pictures, sounds, and so on; and (d) rewarding the person for learning to control that function.

Biofeedback training is used by some clinicians to treat hypertension, lower back pain, tension headache, and insomnia when these symptoms are due to anxiety and muscle tension. In addition, biofeedback training is used on a more limited basis to treat the following:

▶ Neuromuscular disorders such as paralysis and muscle spasticity;
▶ Epilepsy, which is caused by a disturbance in the electrical activity of the brain and which is characterized by seizures; and
▶ Phobias, which are mental disorders characterized by the extreme fear of or aversion to certain conditions (e.g., high places), objects (e.g., cars), or persons

Guided Imagery. Guided imagery is a method of enhancing relaxation and comfort by suggesting that a person relax and picture himself or herself in a certain pleasant scene; experience sights, sounds, smells, and other sensations associated with the scene; and feel the comfort and relaxation associated with the scene and experiences. At first, the nurse guides the person in this imagery, but after learning the method, the individual may independently concentrate on the pleasant image and experience reduced anxiety without the nurse's guidance. Similar techniques can also be used to help a person control pain and other unpleasant sensations.

Guided imagery involves the following steps:

1. Begin the session with the person lying in bed or seated in a chair.

2. Ask the person to assume a position as comfortable as possible, one in which the person might even fall asleep.

3. Sit near the person and speak slowly and soothingly as you provide guidance in the person's thought processes.

4. Try to elicit images that are pleasant, relaxing, and associated with positive physical sensations.

One example of an image is the following scenario.

Picture yourself on a warm fall evening. You are in a wagon on its way home from a hay ride. You are dressed in comfortable clothing and are lying back against a soft pile of hay, looking up at the vast black sky with its millions of stars and its huge harvest moon. You are there among many friends, and all of you have been singing old songs. Now it is mostly quiet as one friend plays a guitar. As the two horses pulling the wagon slowly plod toward home, the wagon below you sways slightly as it moves along the road. You smell the odor of hay mixed with a slight smell of the horse, and it is very pleasant out there in the warm, fresh air. Every now and then you hear a wheel creak, and feel a soft breeze blow across your face and feel yourself so relaxed and so happy. The wagon transports you slowly through the night toward home, and you are at peace with your friends and all the world. You are rocked gently and you feel your eyelids grow heavy with sleep. As you ride along, so relaxed, so pleasant, your eyelids grow heavier and heavier, and you feel yourself floating pleasantly. You begin to fall asleep and as you sleep, you have very, very pleasant dreams.

Managing Stress Reduction

Despite the benefits of these self-help measures, keep in mind that the mechanisms for reducing stress can promote stress as well. For example, if a person embarks on an exercise program to regulate stress, the novelty of exercise to the unprepared body can be jolting. Likewise, an extreme change in diet (e.g., a low-calorie diet to reduce weight) can be physiologically upsetting.

Self-help mechanisms used for reducing stress must be applied with moderation.

Help persons who are under stress to assess their lifestyles and coping responses. Help people engage in self-care and make the lifestyle changes to control stress and prevent stress-related disorders.

Coping with Actual Crisis

Crisis intervention begins with an initial assessment of the individual and the circumstances that led to the crisis. Next, armed with knowledge about the person and precrisis events, the nurse plans and prescribes proper intervention. At this point, the intent is simply to return the individual to a precrisis state rather than to make major changes in the person's character and lifestyle.

Now the stage is set for actual intervention. According to Aguilera, crisis intervention should help the individual to do the following:

▶ Understand the nature of the crisis, the nature of the events that precipitated the crisis, and the relationship between the two;

▶ Examine conscious feelings concerning the crisis as well as feelings the individual may have suppressed; and

▶ Reenter the social world if the person has retreated from others because of grief or depression.

After crisis intervention, resolution of the crisis begins. Crisis management should include planning. At this point, the nurse reinforces coping responses that the person successfully used to reduce tension and anxiety in the past. The nurse also helps the individual develop new coping skills to deal with the present crisis. Newly learned coping strategies used for the present crisis can then be incorporated into the body's defense system for future use, preferably long before a situation reaches another crisis state.

To help the person develop these new coping strategies, you might make appropriate referrals to other professionals or agencies that can be of assistance as needed for the immediate crisis. Federal, state, and community organizations such as the American Red Cross help people deal with major crises, such as floods and hurricanes. Other sources of assistance are more available for assistance on a day-to-day basis. The client should understand that such sources of assistance will often be available in the future to prevent another crisis from arising. You might, for example, refer the person to sources of assistance for food, shelter, employment, child care, medical care, and so forth as needed by the individual. You can also assist the individual in dealing with stress. Skills that will remain useful as a means of helping to cope in the future include guided imagery and other relaxation techniques.

As you progress in your nursing education, you will learn more about sources of assistance to which you can refer clients and about more specific methods you can use when assisting clients to help themselves to cope. Your early experience is just a beginning.

EVALUATION

Nursing evaluation includes assessing the degree to which the interventions were effective in assisting the person to reduce anxiety or stress. With effective interventions, the person should have taken measures to reduce identified sources of stress, and the person's anxiety should be reduced to a moderate (2+) level or below. Physiologic measurements of stress (e.g., pulse and blood pressure readings) should be within the normal range or approaching normal limits. Perhaps more important, the person should have new coping skills necessary to be able to independently manage stress that occurs in the future.

With ineffective interventions and continued high levels of stress, the person may show evidence of serious illness.

Third Line of Defense Against Stressors: Professional Help

As illustrated in Figure 16–1, once serious illnesses develop, the individuals must reach out beyond self-help to the health care professional. At this point, drug therapy, hospitalization, physical therapy, crisis intervention, or psychotherapy may be needed.

Within the therapeutic setting—be it a hospital, clinic, or home—it is hoped that people will learn coping skills they can incorporate into their lifestyles once the illness is under control.

Third-line defenses are crucial. Beyond this point, unchecked stress could lead to chronic physical or mental illness and even death.

Failure of Stress Reduction: Chronic Disease

If professional help is not sought in time or it is inadequate, chronic diseases may develop that are sometimes a direct result of the continued stress (e.g., ulcerative colitis or chronic depression and anxiety). These conditions then act as stressors in themselves, burdening the individual still further. When a stressor is overwhelming and all defenses fail, death results.

STRESS, ADAPTATION, AND CRISIS: IMPLICATIONS FOR NURSES

Caring for Hospitalized Persons

When stressors cause illness, the illness in itself becomes a stressor. When illness is so serious that hospitalization is required, hospitalization compounds the stress of illness. As a result, the person faces escalating psychologic and physiologic stressors.

Volicer and Bohannon studied specific causes of stress responses in hospitalized people. The Hospital Stress Rating Scale measures stress caused by hospitalization (Table 16–3). Note the similarities between this assessment tool and the one developed by Holmes and Rahe (see Table 16–2). According to Volicer, the greater the magnitude of stress scale events reported, the greater the number of problems described by the subjects of the study on discharge (e.g., increased pain and slower recovery).[90]

Cohen and Lazarus extensively studied how people cope with illness and hospitalization. They presented five major coping tasks for the ill person:

▶ Reduce harmful environmental conditions and enhance prospects of recovery.
▶ Tolerate or adjust to negative events and realities.
▶ Maintain a positive self-image.
▶ Maintain emotional equilibrium.
▶ Continue satisfying relationships with others.[16]

Several nursing interventions help the hospitalized person master coping tasks. First, help the person reduce harmful environmental conditions within the care facility and thus enhance prospects of recovery. For many people, a hospital is a frightening place filled with unfamiliar people. Take time to orient the individual to the facility's schedule for meals, visitors, physician's rounds, nursing routines, and religious services. Introduce the individual to roommates. Support the person and significant others.

Also reduce iatrogenic problems (i.e., problems that arise as a result of treatment, medication, or hospitalization). For example, so often nurses and other health care workers forget that rest promotes healing. Medications, treatments, and even surgery cannot replace rest as a vital therapeutic intervention. Yet the schedule for routine nursing care and meals in many health care facilities completely overlooks this need. It is not unusual for a hospitalized person who has been awake, restless, and anxious all night and who finally falls asleep at 4:30 a.m. to be awakened at 5:00 a.m. to be weighed or have vital signs checked. This schedule benefits the facility, not the person. Therefore, keep these factors in mind and try to work for the convenience and comfort of the person in your care.

Help the person adjust to the realities of current health status. The hospitalized person often experiences fears, real or imagined. Recognize these fears, accept them, and help the person cope with them. The nurse, by acting as a sounding board, can allay fears and soften reality. Talking things out not only provides catharsis for the individual but also gives the nurse valuable information and insight into the person. Discussion also provides the person with insight into himself or herself and perhaps a greater sense of control.

Help the person maintain a positive self-image. Remember that the hospitalized person frequently is dependent, an uncomfortable status for most adults. Be prepared to give additional emotional support as needed. While hospitalized, people often feel a loss of identity. For example, we view ourselves as individuals on the basis of the clothes we wear, our diet, our daily routine, and the like. Often residents in a hospital wear the same hospital gown, almost everyone eats a regular diet, and an entire ward of clients is expected to go to sleep and wake up at the same time every day. To help affirm a person's identity, talk with respect and warmth. When permitted, allow the person to wear regular clothes, read until sleepy, or sleep late some mornings. These interventions reinforce the person's self-image and help speed recovery.

Assist people in maintaining emotional equilibrium by helping them cope with the hospital experience. For example, most people are nervous when they must undergo a crucial diagnostic test or uncomfortable procedure. Some people fear that they will lose control or experience intolerable pain. Take time to explain what will happen during tests and procedures and how they can cooperate and assist. Allow clients to verbalize questions and concerns.

Help clients continue to have satisfying relationships with others by encouraging them to relate to the staff,

TABLE 16–3. Hospital Stress Factors

Factor	Stress Scale Events	Assigned Rank
Unfamiliarity of surroundings	Having strangers sleep in the same room with you	01
	Having to sleep in a strange bed	03
	Having strange machines around	05
	Being awakened in the night by the nurse	06
	Being aware of unusual smells around you	11
	Being in a room that is too cold or too hot	16
	Having to eat cold or tasteless food	21
	Being cared for by an unfamiliar doctor	23
Loss of independence	Having to eat at different times than you usually do	02
	Having to wear a hospital gown	04
	Having to be assisted with bathing	07
	Not being able to get newspapers, radio, or TV when you want them	08
	Having a roommate who has too many visitors	09
	Having to stay in bed or the same room all day	10
	Having to be assisted with a bedpan	13
	Not having your call light answered	35
	Being fed through tubes	39
	Thinking you may lose your sight	49
Separation from spouse	Worrying about your spouse being away from you	20
	Missing your spouse	38
Financial problems	Thinking about losing income because of your illness	27
	Not having enough insurance to pay for your hospitalization	36
Isolation from other people	Having a roommate who is seriously ill or cannot talk with you	12
	Having a roommate who is unfriendly	14
	Not having friends visit you	15
	Not being able to call family or friends on the phone	22
	Having the staff be in too much of a hurry	26
	Thinking you might lose your hearing	45
Lack of information	Thinking you might have pain because of surgery or test procedures	19
	Not knowing when to expect things will be done to you	25
	Having nurses or doctors talk too fast to use words you can't understand	29
	Not having your questions answered by the staff	37
	Not knowing the results or reasons for your treatments	41
	Not knowing for sure what illnesses you have	43
	Not being told what your diagnosis is	44
Threat of severe illness	Thinking your appearance might be changed after your hospitalization	17
	Being put in the hospital because of an accident	24
	Knowing you have to have an operation	32
	Having a sudden hospitalization you weren't planning to have	34
	Knowing you have a serious illness	46
	Thinking you might lose a kidney or some other organ	47
	Thinking you might have cancer	48
Separation from family	Being in the hospital during holidays or special family occasions	18
	Not having family visit you	31
	Being hospitalized far away from home	33
Problems with medications	Having medications cause you discomfort	28
	Feeling you are getting dependent on medications	30
	Not getting relief from pain medications	40
	Not getting pain medication when you need it	42

Adapted from Volicer, B. J., et al. (1977). Medical-surgical differences in hospital stress factors. *Journal of Human Stress* 3, 3. Reprinted by permission of Opinion Publications, Inc., and the author.

to roommates, and to their significant others. Remember to support significant others as well as the hospitalized individual. Encourage friends and family to visit, and plan your interventions around their visits. By showing compassion, understanding, and concern for the person's significant others, you reinforce those valuable relationships.

Stress of Caring for Ill People

As we have said, illness is stressful for most people. Because ill people look to the nurse to reduce stress, alleviate pain, give comfort and support, and provide selfless service, caring for the sick is also demanding and stressful. Many nurses work a lifetime without becoming physically exhausted and emotionally drained. Others burn out early in their career and either leave the nursing profession or continue to work in nursing but without enthusiasm or interest. What causes a person who was once excited about being a nurse to gradually become indifferent, even callous to the needs of sick people?

BURNOUT: WHAT CAUSES IT AND WHY ARE NURSES VULNERABLE?

What is professional burnout, what are its causes, what are its signs, and how can you prevent it from damaging your career?

Burnout is a condition of physical and emotional exhaustion experienced as a result of job stressors related to caring for the ill and the troubled. Burnout is described by Maslach as "a syndrome of emotional exhaustion, depersonalization, and reduced personal accomplishment that can occur among individuals who do 'people work' of some kind. It is a response to the chronic emotional strain of dealing extensively with other human beings, particularly when they are troubled, ill or having personal problems."[48]

If being idealistic and doing "people work" puts a person at risk for developing burnout, nurses are clearly vulnerable. People who enter the nursing profession tend to be idealistic and altruistic. When you ask nursing students why they want to be a nurse, the answer often is "I want to help people." However, if the idealistic student graduates and finds it impossible to apply what has been learned in the classroom, disillusionment results. When workloads are too heavy, demands are too great, and nursing care suffers, ideals clash head on with reality. The resulting disappointment and failed personal expectations are the breeding ground for burnout in nurses.

SIGNS OF BURNOUT

In the early stages of burnout, nurses recognize that they are not performing up to standard but may not understand why. They may not realize that overwork can produce not only physical exhaustion but emotional exhaustion as well. Because nurses have high expectations for themselves, they sometimes blame themselves rather than the work situation for an emotional "slump." Self-blame and guilt brewing inside the person may later erupt in numerous self-destructive ways.

Behavioral indicators of burnout include decreased productivity and quality of job performance, frequent mistakes or acts of poor judgment, forgetfulness, reduced attention to detail, preoccupation, reduced creativity, loss of interest, absenteeism, and lethargy. Some physical signs of burnout are elevated blood pressure, increased muscle tension, slumped posture, tension headache, upset stomach, change in appetite, and restlessness. Emotional indicators include irritability, depression, withdrawal, emotional outbursts, hostile and aggressive behavior, paranoia, and feelings of worthlessness.[65]

Burnout results from the hopelessness and helplessness that people feel when they try to achieve the unachievable. Signs of burnout indicate that the exhausted persons are trying to protect themselves from further psychologic exhaustion.

PREVENTING BURNOUT

Preventing burnout requires many of the same coping skills we use to combat reactions to any stressor. Recognition of the problem is a first step, followed by self-help measures (including use of available sources of support) and, if necessary, professional counseling.

To better illustrate how to fight burnout, let us look at an example. Jean G. recently graduated with honors from a nursing program. She was highly regarded by instructors for her careful attention to the needs of sick people. After graduation, Jean took a position as a night nurse at a large city hospital. Because she had satisfied her clinical requirements at a small private hospital, Jean was not prepared for the unrealistic workload she now faced every night. In addition, Jean was asked to "float" from one ward to another and therefore had difficulty learning names of each sick person for whom she cared, let alone providing for individual needs. Time passed, and the work situation worsened as disgruntled staff members quit one by one. Then one day Jean noticed that she was beginning to feel tired and sluggish and blasé about her work. She also began to suffer from almost daily tension headaches. People would want to talk with her about their pain or fears, and whereas Jean once made time for such talks, now she felt too rushed. At home, Jean found that she was irritable. More and more she wanted to sleep. Finally, two of her former classmates told Jean they were worried because they felt that she might be "burning out."

At first, Jean denied the fact she was suffering early burnout. Gradually, however, she accepted that it was true and that she must change her attitude and life. Jean remembered back to a course she took in stress management. She recalled that when you face difficult internal or external demands, you should (1) deal with the problem, (2) deal with your feelings, and (3) reduce the magnitude of the stress responses by appropriate activities.

With these steps in mind, Jean requested a change to day shift and she asked to be assigned to one ward. When there was insufficient nursing staff to meet needs, Jean decided she would be assertive and request help. She also joined a nurses' support group. With her colleagues, Jean explored her feelings, in particular her unrealistic expectations of herself as a nurse. She came to accept that she was human and fallible and that she could only do her best and no more. Jean also made changes in her daily routines. She joined an exercise class, which included both aerobics and yoga. Then, too, Jean infused some fun into her life by spending more time with her friends.

Jean continued to use these self-help measures until they became a habit and a natural part of her daily life. In time, not only did she practice nursing successfully, but she grew as a person in the process. If she continues to practice stress management, her life will be full and satisfying because it will be based on self-awareness and self-care.

To care for others, you must first care for yourself. To help others deal successfully with life's demands, you must practice stress management in your own life.

CASE STUDY

The Client

One month ago, Nancy Sanchez, a middle manager for a large accounting firm, was seen by the occupational nurse for heart "palpitations" and a "fluttery feeling" in her chest. These symptoms first occurred when she was working at her high-pressure job and she feared she was "having a heart attack."

The company physician saw Mrs. Sanchez and ruled out any physical causes for her symptoms but did note that she was 15 pounds overweight and had slightly high blood pressure. The physician's orders included the following:

▶ Low-sodium, low-cholesterol, 1400-calorie diet
▶ Weekly blood pressure checks
▶ See Tom Walker, R.N., for assessment, diet counseling, and stress reduction techniques

At 2:00 p.m., October 14, a partial listing of Tom Walker's assessment findings for Mrs. Sanchez included the following:

▶ 35-year-old, slightly obese female
▶ Height = 58 inches; weight = 145 lbs.
▶ Skin intact, warm, and ivory in color
▶ Temperature = 36.7 °C; blood pressure = 150/92; pulse = 76; respirations = 24
▶ Complained of being "very tired lately" and suffering from daily headaches for past 3 weeks
▶ Stated she loves her job but has been under increased stress during the past 2 months because of the demands of her new position within the company

One month has passed since her initial visit. The following represents part of a nursing care plan written for her at the time she was assessed and the current evaluation of outcomes that were expected at that time.

CARE PLAN

3:00 p.m., October 14

Nursing Diagnosis	Planning: Expected Outcomes	Implementation: Nursing Interventions	Evaluation
Anxiety R/T change in role functioning	By 9:00 a.m., November 14: 1. Demonstrates ability to deal with job stressors in a healthier manner; AEB limiting work to 40 hours/week	Discuss with client the potential sources of her job-related stress. Once specific sources of stress have been identified, assist client in deciding how to change situation (e.g., delegating minor tasks, eliminating superfluous tasks).	9:00 a.m., November 14 Understands that she works too much States she works less overtime now but still exceeds 40 hours/week States she negotiated with her supervisor for an early vacation

Care Plan continued on following page

CARE PLAN (Continued)

3:00 p.m., October 14

Nursing Diagnosis	Planning: Expected Outcomes	Implementation: Nursing Interventions	Evaluation
	2. Deals with anxiety in a healthier manner; AEB identifying her anxious feelings and taking steps to deal with them	Assist client in identifying her own anxiety by asking her to identify the feeling, its source, and her responses to the feeling	Now admits that she had been denying her feelings of anxiety
		Assist client in acknowledging her feeling and accept this as a common experience that can be dealt with appropriately	
		Teach appropriate ways to deal with anxiety (e.g., be aware of the feeling, take a break from the anxiety-provoking situation, seek support persons, use coping skills that have been helpful in the past)	Spends more time with close friends in the evening States she feels better physically and mentally
	3. Demonstrates reduced physiologic arousal in work setting; AEB blood pressure below 145/90, other vital signs within normal limits	Teach exercises to improve general physical fitness (e.g., aerobic exercises)	Weight = 141 lbs. Temperature = 36.6 °C Pulse = 72 Respiration = 20 BP = 144/88
		Teach progressive relaxation exercise to be performed for 20 minutes each day	
		Teach about low-sodium, low-cholesterol, 1400-calorie diet	
		Teach to avoid caffeine, alcohol, sugar, and preservatives	
		Discuss biofeedback training as a potential means of learning to control stress	

Summary

- Stressors are sources of stress; the stress response refers to reactions to stress.
- Selye defined stress from a physiologic focus and described the general adaptation syndrome and local adaptation syndrome; Holmes and Rahe developed a social readjustment rating scale to quantify stressors; Lazarus emphasized the cognitive in appraising and coping with stress.
- Adaptation refers to the adjustment of an organism to changes in its environment.

▶ A crisis may be maturational or situational but is always a disequilibrium in a steady state, occurring when usual problem-solving strategies are ineffective.

▶ To assess the person in stress, assess stressors impinging on the individual (including crises), physiologic responses to stressors, the level of anxiety, and the presence of stress-related physiologic disorders.

▶ The most pertinent nursing diagnosis for the anxious client is *Anxiety*.

▶ The nurse should plan with the client to deal with the stressful problem, deal with the feelings engendered by the problem, and reduce the physiologic arousal of stress.

▶ Useful nursing interventions for the person experiencing stress include identifying the source of stress; acknowledging and dealing with client feelings; and teaching the importance of such stress reduction methods as fitness, dietary changes, and reduction in caffeine, alcohol, and tobacco intake. Additional nursing interventions that may be used include improving time management skills, using relaxation exercises, assisting with biofeedback training, providing guided imagery, and (when needed) providing crisis intervention.

▶ Crisis intervention includes making appropriate referrals and helping the client to develop new, effective coping strategies.

▶ Stress reduction interventions can be evaluated by noting measures the client has taken to reduce identified sources of stress, a reduction in the level of anxiety, physiologic measurements of stress approaching or within normal limits, and the acquisition of new effective coping skills.

▶ To help others deal successfully with life's demands, you must practice stress management in your own life.

Bibliography

1. Aguilera, D. C. (1990). *Crisis intervention: Theory and methodology* (6th ed.). St. Louis: C.V. Mosby.
2. Aguilera, D. C., & Messick, J. M. (1984). *Crisis intervention: Theory and methodology* (4th ed). St. Louis: C.V. Mosby.
3. Albrecht, T. L., & Halsey, J. (1991). Supporting the staff nurse under stress. *Nursing Management*, 22(7), 60–61, 64.
4. Aldwin, C. M. (1991). Does age affect the stress and coping process? Implications of age differences in perceived control. *Journal of Gerontology*, 46(4), 174–180.
5. Alley, N. M., & Foster, M. C. (1990). Using self-help support groups: a framework for nursing practice and research. *Journal of Advanced Nursing*, 15(12), 1383–1388.
6. Benner, P. E., & Wrubel, J. (1989). *The primacy of caring: Stress and coping in health and illness*. Menlo Park, CA: Addison-Wesley.
7. Bircher, A. U. (1972). Mankind in crisis: an application of clinical process to population—environmental issues. *Nursing Forum*, 11(1), 10–33.
8. Brown, G. W., & Harris, T. O. (1989). *Life events and illness*. New York: Guilford Press.
9. Brown, J. D. (1991). Staying fit and staying well: physical fitness as a moderator of life stress. *Journal of Personality and Social Psychology*, 60(4), 555–561.
10. Brownell, M. J. (1984). The concept of crises: its utility for nursing. *Advances in Nursing Science: Crisis Intervention*, 6(4), 10–21.
11. Calarco, M. M., & Krone, K. P. (1991). An integrated nursing model of depressive behavior in adults. Theory and implications for practice. *Nursing Clinics of North America*, 26(3), 573–577.
12. Caplan, G. (1964). *Principles of preventative psychiatry*. New York: Basic Books.
13. Caplan, G. (1984). Mastery of stress: psychosocial aspects. *American Journal of Psychiatry*, 138(4), 413–420.
14. Cobb, S. (1976). Social support as a moderator of life stress. *Psychosomatic Medicine*, 38(5), 300–314.
15. Cohen, F., & Lazarus, R. S. (1979). Coping with the stresses of illness. In Stone, G. C., Cohen, F., & Adler, N. E. (eds.) *Health Psychology*. San Francisco: Jossey-Bass.
16. Cohen, G. D. (1991). Anxiety and general medical disorders. In Salzman, C., & Lebowitz, B. D. (eds.). *Anxiety in the elderly*. New York: Springer.
17. Croyle, R. T., & Hunt, J. R. (1991). Coping with health threat: social influence processes in reactions to medical test results. *Journal of Personality and Social Psychology*, 60(3), 382–389.
18. Dang, S. (1990). When the patient is out of control. *RN*, 53(10), 57–58.
19. Davis, M., & Eshelman, E. R. (1982). *The relaxation and stress reduction workbook*. Oakland, CA: New Harbinger Publications.
20. DeLaune, S. C. (1991). Effective limit setting. How to avoid being manipulated. *Nursing Clinics of North America*, 26(3), 757–764.
21. Dellasega, C. (1990). Coping with caregiving. Stress management for caregivers of the elderly. *Journal of Psychosocial Nursing and Mental Health Services*, 28(1), 15–16, 19–22.
22. Der, D. F., & Lewington, P. (1990). Rational self-directed hypnotherapy: a treatment for panic attacks. *American Journal of Clinical Hypnosis*, 32(3), 160–167.
23. Dimsdale, J. E. (1982). Helping patients cope. *Consultant*, 22, 171.
24. Dolan, J. T. (1991). *Critical care nursing: Clinical management through the nursing process*. Philadelphia: F.A. Davis.
25. Dossey, B. (1991). Awakening the inner healer. *American Journal of Nursing*, 91(8), 30–32, 34.
26. Dudley, D. L., & Welke, E. (1977). *How to survive being alive*. New York: Doubleday.
27. Durham, E., & Frost-Hartzer, P. (1991). Relaxation therapy works. *RN*, 54(8), 40–42.
28. Easton, S. (1990). Learn to relax and counter stress. *Occupational Health*, 42(6), 172–174.
29. Endler, N. S., & Edwards, J. (1982). Stress and personality. In Goldberger, L. & Breznitz, S. (eds.). *Handbook of stress: Theoretical and clinical aspects* New York: Free Press.
30. Fine, S. B. (1991). Resilience and human adaptability: who rises above adversity? 1990 Eleanor Clarke Slagle Lecture. *American Journal of Occupational Therapy*, 45(6), 493–503.
31. Hanna, B. D. (1991). Stress in the head nurse role. *Nursing Management*, 22(10), 120.
32. Hanson, P. G. (1985). *The joy of stress*. Kansas City, MO: Andrews, McMeel and Parker.
33. Harbison, J. (1991). Clinical decision making in nursing. *Journal of Advanced Nursing*, 16(4), 404–407.
34. Hillarad, J. R. (ed.). (1990). *Anxiety disorders in manual of clinical emergency psychiatry*. Washington, DC: American Psychiatric Press.
35. Holden, L. C. (1988). Effects of relaxation with guided imagery on surgical stress and wound healing. *Research in Nursing and Health*, 11(4), 235–244.
36. Holmes, T. H., & Rahe, R. H. (1967). The social readjustment rating scale. *Journal of Psychosomatic Research*, 11(2), 213–218.
37. Holroyd, K. A., & Lazarus, R. S. (1982). Stress, coping and somatic adaptation. In Goldberger L., & Breznitz, S. (eds.). *Handbook of stress: Theoretical and clinical aspects*. New York: Free Press.
38. Hopping, B. (1980). Physiological response to stress: a nursing concern. *Nursing Forum*, 19(3), 259–269.
39. Infante, M. S. (1982). *Crisis theory: A framework for nursing practice*. Reston, VA: Reston Publishing.
40. Johnston, M., & Wallace, L. (1990). *Stress and medical procedures*. Oxford, England: Oxford University Press.
41. King, J. V. (1988). A holistic technique to lower anxiety: relaxation with guided imagery. *Journal of Holistic Nursing*, 6(1), 16–20.

42. Kobasa, S. C. (1979). Stressful life events, personality and health: an inquiry into hardiness. *Journal of Personality and Social Psychology*, 37(1), 1–11.

43. Koontz, E., Cox, D., & Hastings, S. (1991). Implementing a short-term family support group. *Journal of Psychosocial Nursing and Mental Health Services*, 29(5), 5–8, 10.

44. Kramer, N. A. (1990). Comparison of therapeutic touch and casual touch in stress reduction of hospitalized children. *Pediatric Nursing*, 16(5), 483–485.

45. Kunkler, J., & Whittick, J. (1991). Stress-management groups for nurses: practical problems and possible solutions. *Journal of Advanced Nursing*, 16(2), 172–176.

46. Lazarus, R. S., & Forlman, S. (1984). Coping and adaptation. In Gentry, W. D. (ed.). *Handbook of behavioral medicine*. New York: Guilford Press.

47. Lim, M. (1990). Ki Aikido: a solution to stress—Yetter's comment. *British Dental Journal*, 168(11), 428–429.

48. Maslach, C. (1982). *Burnout: The cost of caring*. Englewood Cliffs, NJ: Prentice Hall.

49. Mayer, J. D., et al. (1991). A broader conception of mood experience. *Journal of Personality and Social Psychology*, 60(1), 100–111.

50. McKerracher, B. (1990). How to lend support in a crisis. *Nursing*, 20(11), 62–64.

51. Musolf, J. M. (1991). Easing the impact of the family caregiver's role. *Rehabilitation Nursing*, 16(2), 82–84.

52. Nicholson, L. G. (1990). Stress management in nursing. *Nursing Management*, 21(4), 53–55.

53. Nolan, M. R., et al. (1990). Stress is in the eye of the beholder: reconceptualizing the measurement of career burden. *Journal of Advanced Nursing*, 15(5), 544–555.

54. Noshpitz, J. D., & Coddington, R. D. (eds.). (1990). *Stressors and the adjustment disorders*. New York: Wiley.

55. Nowack, K. M. (1989). Coping style, cognitive hardiness, and health status. *Journal of Behavioral Medicine*, 12(2), 145–158.

56. O'Connell, K. A. (1991). Why rational people do irrational things. *Journal of Psychosocial Nursing and Mental Health Services*, 29(1), 11–14.

57. Olsen, E. (1990). Beyond positive thinking. *Journal of Nursing Administration*, 20(5), 11–12.

58. Ormel, J., & Schaufeli, W. B. (1991). Stability and change in psychological distress and their relationship with self-esteem and locus of control: a dynamic equilibrium model. *Journal of Personality and Social Psychology*, 60(2), 288–299.

59. Pasquali, E. A. (1990). Learning to laugh: humor as therapy. *Journal of Psychosocial Nursing and Mental Health Services*, 28(3), 31–35.

60. Pearlin, L. (1984). Stress and coping mechanisms. *AMWA*.

61. Puntil, C. (1991). Integrating three approaches to counter resistance in a noncompliant client. *Journal of Psychosocial Nursing and Mental Health Services*, 29(2), 26–30.

62. Richardson, S. F., & Petrarca, D. V. (1990). Educating nurses in health promotion. *Journal of Nursing Education*, 29(8), 351–354.

63. Robinson, L. (1990). Stress and anxiety. *Nursing Clinics of North America*, 25(4), 935–943.

64. Sadow, D., & Ryder, M. (1990). Anxiety reduction. Lessons that benefit students and patients. *Journal of Psychosocial Nursing and Mental Health Services*, 28(9), 29–30.

65. Schneider, S. (1982). Curing burnout while you work. *Nursing Life*, 2(5), 38–43.

66. Schroeder, P. (1991). *Monitoring and evaluation in nursing*. Gaithersburg, MD: Aspen Publishers.

67. Scully, R. (1980). Stress in the nurse. *American Journal of Nursing*, 80(5), 912–915.

68. Seifert, P. C., & Grandusky, R. J. (1990). Nursing diagnoses. Their use in developing care plans. *ADORN Journal*, 51(4), 1008–2021.

69. Selye, H. (1950). *The physiology and pathology of exposure to stress: A treatise based on the concepts of the general adaptation syndrome and the disease of adaptation*. Montreal: Acta.

70. Seyle, H. (1956). *The stress of life*. New York: McGraw-Hill.

71. Selye, H. (1974). *Stress without distress* Philadelphia: J.B. Lippincott.

72. Seyle, H. (1976). *Stress in health and disease*. Reading, MA: Butterworths.

73. Selye, H. (ed.). (1980). *Selye's guide to stress research*. New York: Van Nostrand Reinhold.

74. Selye, H. (1982). History and present status of the stress concept. In Goldberger, L., & Breznitz, S. (eds.). *Handbook of stress: Theoretical and clinical aspects*. New York: Free Press.

75. Smith, F. B. (1991). Three ways to manage stress. *Nursing*, 21(2), 130, 132.

76. Smith, W. H. (1990). Hypnosis in the treatment of anxiety. *Bulletin of the Menninger Clinic*, 54(2), 209–216.

77. Sparaks, S. M., & Taylor, C. M. (1991). *Nursing diagnosis reference manual*. Springhouse, PA: Springhouse Corp.

78. Speck, B. J. (1990). The effect of guided imagery upon first semester nursing students performing their first injections. *Journal of Nursing Education*, 29(8), 346–350.

79. Spielberger, C. D., & Sarason, I. G. (eds.). (1989). *Stress and anxiety*. New York: Hemisphere.

80. Steeves, R. H., et al. (1990). Nurses' interpretation of the suffering of their patients. *Western Journal of Nursing Research*, 12(6), 715–729; 729–731.

81. Steinmetz, J., et al. (1980). *Managing stress before it manages you*. Palo Alto, CA: Bull Publishing.

82. Stevenson, S. (1991). Heading off violence with verbal de-escalation. *Journal of Psychosocial Nursing and Mental Health Services*, 29(9), 6–10.

83. Swayze, S. (1991). Helping them cope. *Journal of Psychosocial Nursing and Mental Health Services*, 29(5), 35–37.

84. Syme, S. F., & Berkman, L. F. (1979). Social networks, host resistance, and mortality: a nine year follow-up study of Alameda county residents. *American Journal of Epidemiology*, 109(2), 186–204.

85. Tauschke, E., et al. (1990). Psychological defense mechanisms in patients with pain. *Pain*, 40(2), 161–170.

86. Trygstad, L. (1980). Simple new ways to help anxious patients. *RN*, 43, 28–32.

87. Trygstad, L. (1984). *Stress and coping in psychiatric nursing* (unpublished doctoral dissertation). University of California at San Francisco Medical Center.

88. Varcarolis, E. M. (1990). *Foundations of psychiatric mental health nursing*. Philadelphia: W.B. Saunders.

89. Vingerhoets, A. J., & Van Heck, G. L. (1990). Gender, coping and psychosomatic symptoms. *Psychological Medicine*, 20(1), 125–135.

90. Volicer, B. J., & Bohannon, M. W. (1975). A hospital stress rating scale. *Nursing Research*, 24(5), 352–359.

91. Wakeman, J. R., & Mestayer, R. F. (1985). Stress-related disorders. *Postgraduate Medicine*, 77(6), 189–191, 194–196.

92. Watson, M., et al. (1991). Relationships between emotional control, adjustment to cancer and depression and anxiety in breast cancer patients. *Psychological Medicine*, 21(1), 51–57.

93. Wheatley, D. (1990). The stress profile. *British Journal of Psychiatry*, 156, 685–688.

94. White, N. E., et al. (1990). Promoting critical thinking skills. *Nurse Educator*, 15(5), 16–19.

95. Whitley, G. G. (1989). Anxiety. Defining the diagnosis. *Journal of Psychosocial Nursing and Mental Health Services*, 27(10), 7–12.

96. Woolfolk, R. L., & Lehrer, P. M. (1984). Clinical applications. In Woolfolk, R. L., & Lehrer, P. M. (eds.). *Principals and practice of stress management*. New York: Guilford Press.

97. Woolley, N. (1990). Crisis theory: a paradigm of effective intervention with families of critically ill people. *Journal of Advanced Nursing*, 15(12), 1402–1408.

98. Zachariae, R., et al. (1990). Effect of psychological intervention in the form of relaxation and guided imagery on cellular immune function in normal healthy subjects. An overview. *Psychotherapy and Psychosomatics*, 53(1), 32–39.

▼ *Homeostasis and Biologic Rhythms*

Chapter 17

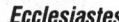

▼ *There is a season for everything and a time for every purpose under heaven; A time to be born and a time to die; A time to plant and a time to reap . . .*

Ecclesiastes

▼ CHAPTER OUTLINE

THE STUDY OF HOMEOSTATIC
  MECHANISMS
PHYSIOLOGIC AND PSYCHOLOGIC
  HOMEOSTASIS
MAINTENANCE OF PHYSIOLOGIC
  HOMEOSTASIS
    Major Regulators of
      Physiologic Homeostasis
    Mechanisms of
      Physiologic Homeostasis
    Failure of Homeostatic Mechanisms
CHRONOBIOLOGY
    Rhythmic Cycles and Frequencies

    Circadian Rhythms
CLINICAL APPLICATIONS OF
  CHRONOBIOLOGIC PRINCIPLES
NURSING IMPLICATIONS RELATED TO
  HOMEOSTASIS AND BIOLOGIC
  RHYTHMS
    Biofeedback
    Assessment
    Nursing Diagnosis
    Planning
    Nursing Intervention
    Evaluation

▼ KEY TERMS

Autonomic nervous
  system
Biofeedback training
Chronobiology
Circadian rhythms
Circannual rhythms
Endocrine system
Feedback

Homeostasis
Homeostatic mechanisms
Hormones
Infradian rhythms
Milieu intérieur
Jet lag syndrome
Negative feedback

Overshoot
Physiologic homeostasis
Positive feedback
Psychologic homeostasis
Set point
Target tissues
Ultradian rhythms

After studying this chapter, you should be able to

1. *Define the concept of homeostasis.*
2. *Identify the body systems that serve as regulators of homeostasis.*
3. *Contrast psychologic equilibrium and psychologic disequilibrium.*
4. *List requirements for maintenance of physiologic homeostasis.*
5. *Describe the characteristics of physiologic homeostatic mechanisms.*
6. *Describe the means by which physiologic homeostatic mechanisms may be disrupted.*
7. *Explain chronobiology in human life and its clinical applications.*
8. *Explain biofeedback.*
9. *Discuss how the nurse assesses homeostasis.*
10. *List examples of nursing diagnoses appropriate for persons with problems in homeostasis.*
11. *State the main outcome for a nursing diagnosis of Relocation Stress Syndrome.*
12. *Identify nursing interventions appropriate for a person with a nursing diagnosis of* Relocation Stress Syndrome.
13. *State how to evaluate nursing interventions for a person with a nursing diagnosis of* Relocation Stress Syndrome.

For generations scientists believed that constancy and stability were fundamental characteristics of life. Today, we recognize that the essence of life is change and instability. For an organism to preserve its life, it must adapt satisfactorily to change. In addition, it must maintain a degree of internal stability in the face of a variable and stressful environment. Over thousands of years, this need to maintain stability forced living organisms to develop internal mechanisms for automatically maintaining balance despite constant threats to equilibrium. Processes of self-regulation that preserve an organism's ability to adapt to stressors while maintaining inner balance are called **homeostatic mechanisms.** A vital form of adaptation, homeostatic mechanisms operate at all levels of life, regulating biologic functioning and counteracting change and imbalance.

THE STUDY OF HOMEOSTATIC MECHANISMS

Although the scientific study of homeostatic regulation is relatively new, the concept of a need for physiologic balance has existed for centuries. Hippocrates, known as the father of medicine, conceived of health as the result of a balance or harmony between individuals and their environment. In the middle of the 19th century, the French physiologist Claude Bernard was impressed with the relative stability and resistance to change of the **milieu intérieur** (internal milieu or environment) of living organisms.[4] He believed that life and health depended upon the constancy and stability of the circulating fluids of the body and that compensatory reactions occurred in response to change, resulting in a return from a perturbed state to a steady state.

Later, Walter Cannon was similarly impressed with the resistance of the internal environment of living organisms to both internal and external changes. He expanded Bernard's concepts by describing self-regulation processes and negative feedback systems, which work to produce compensatory and anticipatory adjustments in maintaining the constancy of the internal environment in spite of changes.[7] Cannon coined the term **homeostasis** from the Greek words *homoios,* meaning "like," and *stasis,* meaning "standing." In his classic text, *The Wisdom of the Body,* Cannon wrote

The constant conditions which are maintained in the body might be termed equilibria. That word, however, has come to have fairly exact meaning as applied to relatively simple physio-chemical states, in closed systems, where known forces are balanced. The coordinated physiological processes which maintain most of the steady states in the organism are so complex and so peculiar to living beings—involving as they may the brain and nerves, the heart, lungs, kidneys and spleen, all working cooperatively—that I have suggested a special designation for these states, homeostasis. The word does not imply something set and immobile, a stagnation. It means a condition—a condition which may vary, but which is relatively constant.[7]

Cannon viewed homeostasis as a type of dynamic equilibrium rather than a static condition. His use of the term *homeostasis* was applied mainly to systems related to the fight-or-flight response associated with emotional arousal and the self-regulation of such internal physiologic processes as

► body temperature
► blood pressure
► blood glucose concentration
► water and electrolyte balance
► hydrogen ion (pH) balance
► muscle tone
► blood oxygen and carbon dioxide levels

Today the concept of homeostasis has applications wider than simply explaining physiologic and emotional processes. Currently, the notion of homeostasis is used to explain perceptual and cognitive processes, instinctive behavior, genetics, growth, and even intellect and creativity. In addition, the concept of homeostasis encompasses not only the automaticity of homeostatic mechanisms but also the rhythmicity of changes within the internal environment of human beings.

Although earlier theories emphasized knowledge of anatomy, physiology, and the psychosocial realms of living organisms, it is now becoming increasingly apparent that time is also significant. Virtually all physiologic and psychosocial variables are known to vary rhythmically over time, and many of these rhythms are closely interwoven, that is, they vary together or inversely. Thus, when considering the concept of homeostasis, it is important to remember that ". . . the constancy of the internal milieu waxes and wanes with a . . . rhythm."[32] The study of internal rhythms, or "body clocks," of organisms from single cells to human beings is called **chronobiology.**

PHYSIOLOGIC AND PSYCHOLOGIC HOMEOSTASIS

Physiologic homeostasis is the maintenance of a relatively stable and constant internal dynamic equilibrium. The internal environment is composed primarily of fluid, which is divided into extracellular fluid (ECF), which is found outside cells, and intracellular fluid (ICF), found inside cells. The ECF is what Bernard referred to when he coined the term *interior milieu.* The ECF provides essentially all cells with the same environment of nutrients, such as glucose, fatty substances, and amino acids, as well as other constituents, such as oxygen.[14] Because cell function depends upon internal equilibria, the internal environment must be maintained within narrow limits, for if it becomes physiologically unbalanced, the individual becomes ill. If the physiologic imbalance of the internal environment is severe and remains uncorrected, death ensues.

Although homeostasis may seem simple in theory, in reality it is quite complex. Homeostatic mechanisms govern body functions through a multitude of interrelated control mechanisms. Therefore, an imbalance in one system (e.g., the cardiovascular system) can cause disequilibria in other systems (e.g., the renal and adrenocortical systems). A dynamic homeostatic balance, then, is the basis for health, whereas homeostatic imbalances underlie disease.

Returning the ill person to homeostatic balance is the ultimate goal of all nursing care.

The concept of homeostasis also refers to emotional equilibrium (balance) and disequilibrium (imbalance). **Psychologic homeostasis** is a state of equilibrium characterized by a satisfying self-concept, emotional balance, and harmonious interactions with the environment.

Recall those days when you have felt especially good about yourself. During those times, you probably experienced a satisfying self-concept, felt emotionally balanced, and had relatively harmonious interactions with your environment. What was your life like during those periods?

Typically, a person who is in a state of emotional balance has

- a harmonious relationship with the environment
- a stable physical environment (e.g., a safe and relatively comfortable living situation, adequate food)

- life experiences that are consistent with the individual's self-concept or self-image
- healthy relationships (i.e., the ability to love and experience love, as well as to maintain close and supportive relationships with significant others)
- work or study that is interesting and fulfilling
- a sense of interdependence with others
- good physical health
- adequate economic means
- enjoyable creative and recreational outlets
- a sense of hope for the future

People with consistently good mental health may have had a stable psychologic environment from infancy onward and thereby developed the capacity to trust and love others early in life.

On the other hand, when people view themselves negatively, a state of psychologic imbalance, or disequilibrium, may be experienced. They usually feel out of step with the environment and perceive other people — even friends — as remote and distant. What causes this disequilibrium?

Emotional disequilibrium can be triggered by many factors, such as a sense of loss of control or a threat to self-image.

Emotional disequilibrium can be triggered whenever a person feels loss of control. Failing a major examination, losing a job, being reprimanded by a supervisor, having a serious argument with a loved one, or being hospitalized are examples of stressors that can lead to emotional as well as neuroendocrine imbalances.

Emotional imbalance also develops when one's self-image is threatened. For example, a professional dancer's self-image might be based on having graceful movements and the capacity for strenuous physical activity. The dancer who suffers a severe injury that limits movement may experience a devastating blow to self-image, which then may precipitate emotional imbalance. Resolution of the crisis and a return to emotional balance depends upon support from significant others, appropriate health care, and sometimes professional counseling. The person's learned coping skills play an important role in returning to emotional equilibrium.

MAINTENANCE OF PHYSIOLOGIC HOMEOSTASIS

To maintain physiologic homeostasis, the body must meet basic physiologic requirements for oxygen, water, and nutrients including electrolytes and tissue-building materials. Therefore, a sufficient supply of these elements must be available in the environment. The body must also have the appropriate mechanisms for using these elements under varying conditions. For example, pulmonary ventilation increases during exercise to accommodate the body's need for more oxygen. Providing additional oxygen depends on healthy lungs and adequate circulation of blood. In addition, the body must be able to store certain basic nutrients; for example, glucose is stored as glycogen for use during periods of exercise or fasting. Finally, to remain in balance, the body must be able to eliminate waste products and quantities in excess of basic requirements. For instance, if a person takes in certain water-soluble vitamins in excess of what is needed, the body excretes the excess, thereby avoiding toxic build-up of these substances.

Homeostasis depends also upon physical integrity, so the body must be kept whole and in good repair. Mechanisms that protect the body from injury (e.g., blinking to guard the eye from foreign particles or objects) or that repair damage (e.g., clotting to prevent blood loss from a cut blood vessel) promote physical integrity.

Furthermore, homeostasis depends upon sociocultural and behavioral factors. Malnutrition, drug addiction, or air pollution, for example, upset physiologic balance by altering the body's chemical balance. Similarly, certain emotional states, such as fear, anxiety, or hostility, as well as psychologic conditions, such as depression or irregular behavioral patterns of rest and activity, also affect physiologic balance.

Major Regulators of Physiologic Homeostasis

The major homeostatic regulators are the nervous and endocrine systems. Because the nervous system and endocrine system complement one another in promoting homeostasis, the two systems are often linked and called the neuroendocrine system. In addition, the gastrointestinal (GI), cardiovascular, and renal systems also promote homeostatic balance as they respond to signals from the neuroendocrine system. In reality, all healthy systems and organs work together to maintain a balanced interior milieu.

Although virtually all systems in the body are involved in homeostatic regulation, the cardiovascular, respiratory, GI, biliary, and renal systems play particularly important roles.

The cardiovascular system pumps oxygen and nutrients to cells and removes carbon dioxide and other waste products from them. The respiratory system controls the exchange of oxygen and carbon dioxide. Oxygen is necessary for metabolism and energy production. In conjunction with the nervous system, the respiratory system regulates the concentration of carbon dioxide in the extracellular fluid (ECF), which in turn controls hydrogen ion (pH) balance. Under normal circumstances, the GI tract is the sole route of intake for fluids and electrolytes, thus performing an important role in regulating fluid and electrolyte balance. The concentration of glucose in the blood is primarily regulated by the liver, kidney, and pancreas. The kidneys, by their excretory and reabsorptive mechanisms, regulate not only fluid balance but also the ECF concentrations of hydrogen, sodium, potassium, phosphate, calcium, and other ions. In addition, the kidneys excrete and/or reabsorb many byproducts of carbohydrate, fat, and protein metabolism.

AUTONOMIC NERVOUS SYSTEM

The **autonomic nervous system** (ANS) is a portion of the nervous system consisting of the sympathetic and parasympathetic systems and primarily controlling involuntary body functions; that is, it operates automatically or without conscious control. The ANS (Figure 17–1) regulates visceral activities (i.e., activities of smooth muscle, cardiac muscle, and glands) and is itself regulated by centers in the brain (e.g., the cerebral cortex, the hypothalamus, and the medulla oblongata). The ANS is composed of two major divisions: the sympathetic, or thoracolumbar, and the parasympathetic, or craniosacral, systems, which usually affect body functions in opposite ways. For example, parasympathetic stimulation increases GI motility, whereas sympathetic stimulation decreases GI motility.

Under stressful conditions, the sympathetic nervous system initiates a series of physiologic responses that may be grouped together as the fight-or-flight response.[7] This response makes the individual more alert and prepared to fight or flee. The parasympathetic nervous system has an opposite effect and often exerts its major influence during periods of rest. When the body is in homeostatic balance, the parasympathetic division is more dominant, but the sympathetic division still supplies sufficient input to maintain the balance. Under extreme stress, the sympathetic nervous system predominates and enables the individual to gather the necessary energy for either battle or flight.

ENDOCRINE SYSTEM

The **endocrine system** consists of several glands and other tissues that discharge their hormone secretions directly into the bloodstream. While each hormone-secreting gland or tissue is separate and has its own unique function, they also can act interdependently as an organ system.

The endocrine system (Figure 17–1) includes the following glands:

▶ the pineal, which secretes melatonin, a hormone with a major role in circadian rhythmicity
▶ the anterior pituitary (i.e., anterior hypophysis), which secretes adrenocorticotropic hormone (ACTH), follicle-stimulating hormone (FSH), luteinizing-hormone (LH), prolactin (luteotropic hormone: LTH), thyroid-stimulating hormone (TSH), and growth hormone (GH)
▶ the posterior pituitary, which secretes oxytocin and the antidiuretic hormone (ADH)
▶ the thyroid, which secretes thyroxine (T_4) and triiodothyronine (T_3) from the follicular cells and calcitonin from the parafollicular cells
▶ the parathyroids, which secrete the parathyroid hormone (PTH)
▶ the adrenals, including the adrenal medulla, which secrete catecholamines (epinephrine and norepinephrine), and the adrenal cortex, which secretes primarily cortisol (hydrocortisone) and aldosterone
▶ the islets of Langerhans in the pancreas, whose A cells secrete glucagon and whose B cells secrete insulin

HOMEOSTASIS: The tendency of biologic organisms to maintain constant conditions in the internal environment

MAJOR HOMEOSTATIC REGULATORS:

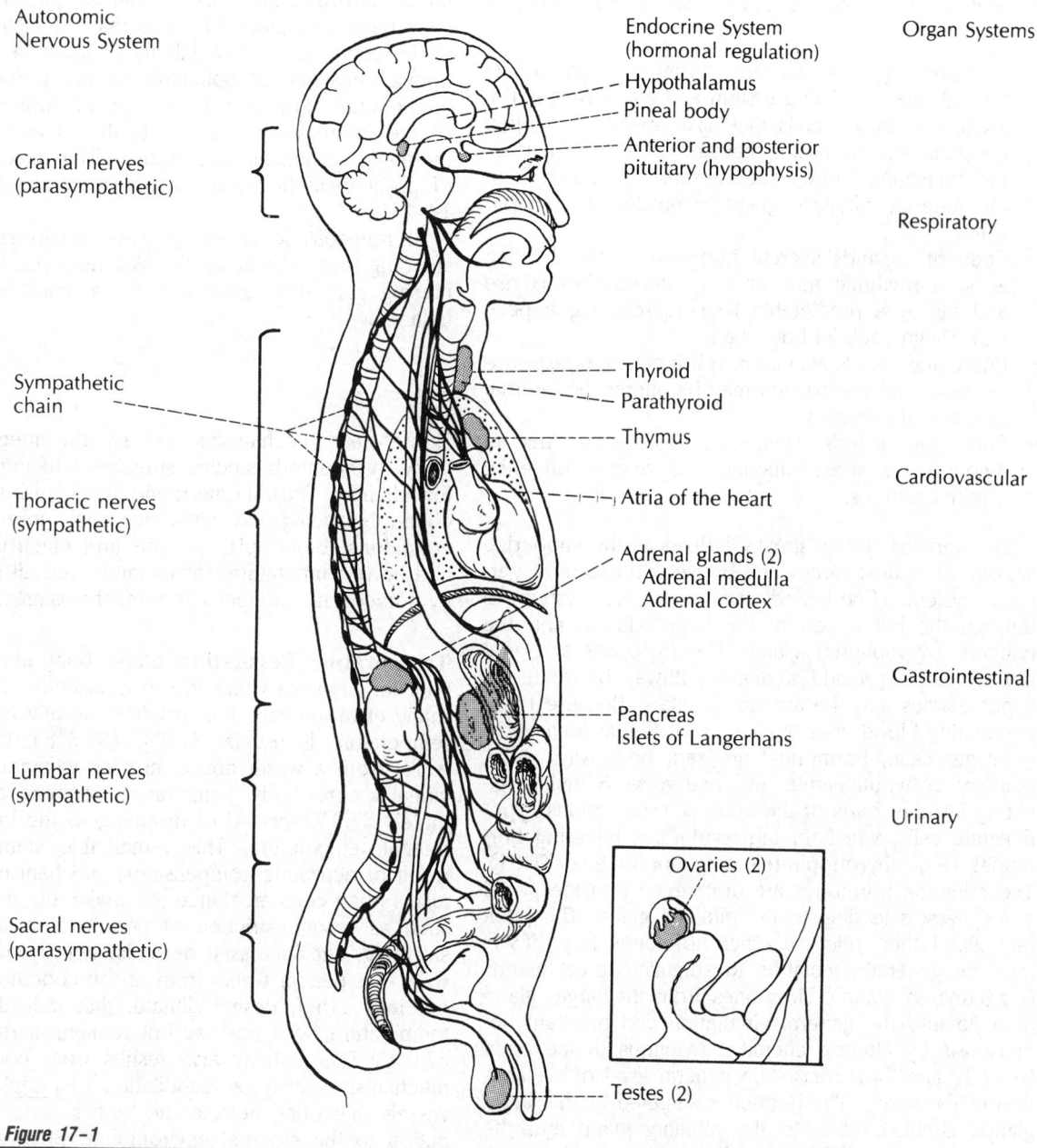

Autonomic
Nervous System

Endocrine System
(hormonal regulation)

Organ Systems

— Hypothalamus
— Pineal body

— Anterior and posterior
pituitary (hypophysis)

Cranial nerves
(parasympathetic)

Respiratory

Sympathetic
chain

— Thyroid
— Parathyroid

— Thymus

Thoracic nerves
(sympathetic)

Cardiovascular

— Atria of the heart

Adrenal glands (2)
Adrenal medulla
Adrenal cortex

Gastrointestinal

— Pancreas
Islets of Langerhans

Lumbar nerves
(sympathetic)

Urinary

Ovaries (2)

Sacral nerves
(parasympathetic)

— Testes (2)

▲ *Figure 17–1*

Physiologic homeostasis: the maintenance of a relatively stable and constant dynamic equilibrium of the internal environment.

▶ the ovaries, which secrete estrogens and progesterone
▶ the testes, which secrete testosterone

Recent evidence indicates that the atria of the heart may also be considered an endocrine gland because these structures secrete a hormone, atrial natriuretic factor or peptide (ANF or ANP), which has diuretic, natriuretic, and vasorelaxant activities.[9,20]

Hormones are chemical substances secreted by endocrine glands or tissues directly into the bloodstream to act as messengers linking one body system with an-

other, thereby regulating and integrating many body functions.

Hormones are transported through the circulatory system to other cells, where they produce physiologic effects. Thus, they act as relatively discrete chemical messengers, creating an intricate chain of communication that links one body system with another. Hormones regulate various metabolic processes, such as reactions to stressors and maintenance of homeostasis. In its communicative and integrative roles, the endocrine system resembles the nervous system. Neural effects, however, usually have a more rapid onset and are shorter lived and more localized.

Although each endocrine gland possesses its own attributes, all endocrine glands share the following characteristics:

▶ Endocrine glands secrete hormones that travel through the circulating system and affect **target tissues,** specialized cells that have specific receptors for particular hormones that are carried to them by the circulating blood) (e.g., the release of TSH from the anterior pituitary gland stimulates the thyroid gland).

▶ Endocrine glands secrete hormones cyclically, that is, in a rhythmic manner (e.g., cortisol levels rise and fall in a predictable fashion, reaching a peak and trough each 24-hour day).

▶ Endocrine glands also secrete hormones in response to need, and the pattern may be altered by internal or external stressors.

▶ Endocrine glands secrete hormones in minute · amounts, yet these amounts can readily influence bodily functions.

The nervous system greatly influences the endocrine system. The most direct link between the central nervous system (CNS) and the endocrine system is through the interaction of the hypothalamus and the pituitary (hypophysis) gland. The hypophyseal portal blood vessels provide a direct pathway between the hypothalamus and the anterior pituitary. Because these connecting blood vessels have capillaries at both ends, messages (e.g., hormones) are sent both ways, from pituitary to hypothalamus and vice versa. Stimuli originating in other parts of the body activate various hypothalamic cells, which in turn synthesize releasing hormones (e.g., thyrotropin-releasing hormone, or TRH). The releasing hormones are discharged into the portal blood vessels leading to the pituitary gland. The pituitary gland then releases other hormones (e.g., TSH) into the general circulation to stimulate target glands (e.g., thyroid gland). Hormones from the target gland then go into the general circulation and maintain homeostasis by altering chemical reactions in the body (e.g., T_4 and T_3 increase the general level of metabolism of the body). The hormones secreted by the target glands circulate back to the pituitary gland and the hypothalamus to inhibit further hormone secretions.

Mechanisms of Physiologic Homeostasis

Homeostatic regulators control numerous physiologic processes, including those involved in

▶ water, sodium, hydrogen ion (pH), potassium, calcium, and phosphate balance
▶ regulation of blood oxygen and carbon dioxide levels
▶ body temperature regulation
▶ control of blood pressure

Examples of homeostatic imbalance abound in the medical-surgical literature because all illness results from disturbances, often minute, within the body's internal environment. These internal imbalances may have been precipitated by disturbances in the external environment (e.g., unavailability of water or certain nutrients; presence of pollutants in water, food, or air; temperature extremes). Correction of these imbalances of the internal environment is the basis for medical therapy and nursing intervention. The major elements of physiologic homeostasis are summarized in Figure 17–1.

All homeostatic devices possess certain traits. Understanding these characteristics will help you in planning nursing care that restores and maintains homeostatic balance.

COMPENSATION

Homeostatic mechanisms preserve the integrity of the body by counterbalancing stressors and compensating for change. Thus, homeostatic mechanisms assist by counterbalancing any variation from normal optimal conditions. Blood pH, glucose and electrolyte levels, and body temperature, for example, are all maintained by homeostatic compensatory mechanisms.

Temperature Regulation. Stable body temperature is vital for organisms that live in constantly changing climatic environments. For instance, normal human body temperature is usually 37.0°C (98.6°F). If a person walks from a warm house into icy weather, that individual's core body temperature remains at approximately 37.0°C instead of dropping to the low environmental temperature. This remarkable stability is the result of activating compensatory mechanisms (mechanisms that counterbalance or make up for change), such as vasoconstriction of peripheral blood vessels, shivering, and increased muscular activity. In the same way, if a person walks from an air-conditioned house out into a hot, desert climate, that individual's body temperature does not rise but remains fairly steady at 37.0°C. This stability also results from compensatory mechanisms, such as vasodilation of peripheral blood vessels that bring heat to the body's surface for dissipation to the external environment. Because of these temperature-stabilizing mechanisms, human beings are able to adapt to changing climates and maintain remarkably constant internal temperatures.[23]

Compensatory Growth. Cell proliferation and organ and tissue hypertrophy (enlargement) also illustrate the compensatory nature of homeostasis. For example, the red blood cell count gradually rises in response to increased demands for oxygen, and muscle hypertrophies in response to vigorous and prolonged exercise. The spleen and lymphatic organs enlarge when infectious organisms invade the body. Moreover, when a kidney is severely damaged or removed, the remaining kidney increases in size to perform the work of both kidneys. If hardened arteries (arteriosclerosis) increase the workload of the heart, the left ventricle enlarges to overcome increased arterial blood vessel resistance and to maintain adequate circulation.

SELF-REGULATION

Fortunately for us, homeostatic mechanisms automatically attempt to correct any deviation from what is normal for the individual. As Cannon[7] explained,

Without homeostatic devices, we should be in constant danger of disaster, unless we were always on the alert to correct voluntarily what normally is corrected automatically. With homeostatic devices, however, that keep essential bodily processes steady, we as individuals are free from such slavery—free to enter into agreeable relations with our fellows, free to enjoy beautiful things, to explore and understand the wonders of the world about us, to develop new ideas and interests, and to work and play, untrammeled by anxieties concerning our bodily affairs.

Homeostasis grants us the opportunity for a creative life rather than a bare existence that continually focuses on consciously adapting to changes, both large and minute.[23] Yet only the healthy individual enjoys the privilege of a body that is essentially self-regulating. When severe illness strikes, physiologic homeostatic mechanisms lose their automatic corrective responses to deviation. At this point, the health care team attempts to regulate the normally self-adjusting physiologic functions by, for example, administering intravenous fluids or medications, and using technologic devices such as hypothermia blankets and ventilators, or performing surgical procedures.

The main objective of a homeostatic mechanism is to minimize the difference between how a system should behave ideally and how it is behaving in reality.

A system is a complex set of interacting parts. Homeostatic mechanisms maintain a given system within controlled limits through feedback loops and the exchange of information and energy with the internal or external environment. If there is too much or too little of a substance (e.g., blood glucose), homeostatic mechanisms initiate changes to return that substance to a point within a normal range through a process called feedback.

Feedback is a process that feeds some of the output of a system back into the system as input. This input of information then influences the behavior of the system and its subsequent output. Feedback may be negative or positive. Negative feedback inhibits further change, whereas positive feedback encourages or stimulates change. Figure 17–2 illustrates the essential differences between the two feedback systems.

Thermostat-Like Negative Feedback Mechanisms. Negative feedback is feedback that leads to the initiation of a series of changes that negate and attempt

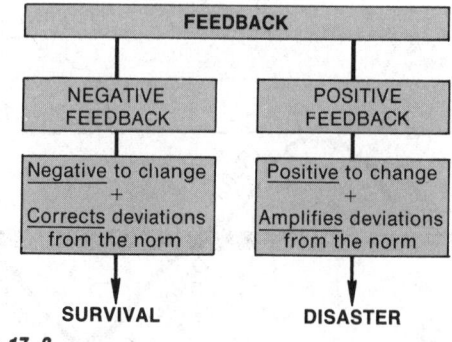

▲ *Figure 17–2*

Negative and positive feedback mechanisms.

to correct any radical change from the norm, either toward excess or deficiency. Negative feedback thus inhibits further change from the norm, as illustrated in Figure 17–3.

To understand how negative feedback operates within the body, we use models and analogies, such as comparing a home-heating system that is regulated by a thermostat with biologic regulator mechanisms.

Many negative feedback systems are thermostat-like in their operation. Thermostat-like regulators are distinguished by two features. First, these mechanisms operate by correcting deviations from a predetermined goal or set point. The **set point** is the optimal level or concentration above or below which the negative feedback system will inhibit or enhance the output. For example, low hormone concentration results in negative feedback signals that lead to stimulation of further hormone secretion. The second feature of thermostat-like regulators is that they appear to have the following components:

▶ A receptor, which receives input from the internal or external environment
▶ A central integrator (e.g., thermostat), which senses a deviation from the set point
▶ An effector, which attempts to correct the deviation

Thus, whenever the system detects an error or deviation, it activates responses to correct the deviation and return to the set point.

Negative Feedback and Temperature. An obvious example of thermostat-like regulators is the type of thermostat found in homes (Figure 17–4A). If the thermostat is set at 22°C (72°F) but the temperature of house or room registers only 18°C (65°F), receptors in the thermostat feed information to the integrator, which is also in the thermostat. A small deviation from the set point is allowable within a limited range, but if the deviation becomes too great, the thermostat stimulates the furnace (effector) to produce more heat. Once the heat turns on, the temperature in the house may in-

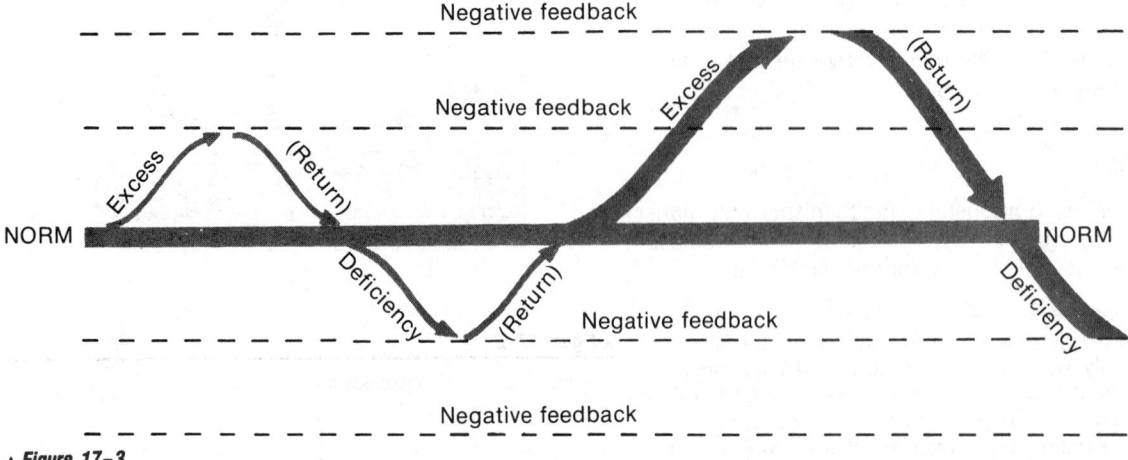

▲ **Figure 17–3**

Negative feedback redirecting body processes toward a normal range.

▲ **Figure 17–4**

Control of temperature with a set point mechanism. *A,* House temperature. *B,* Body temperature.

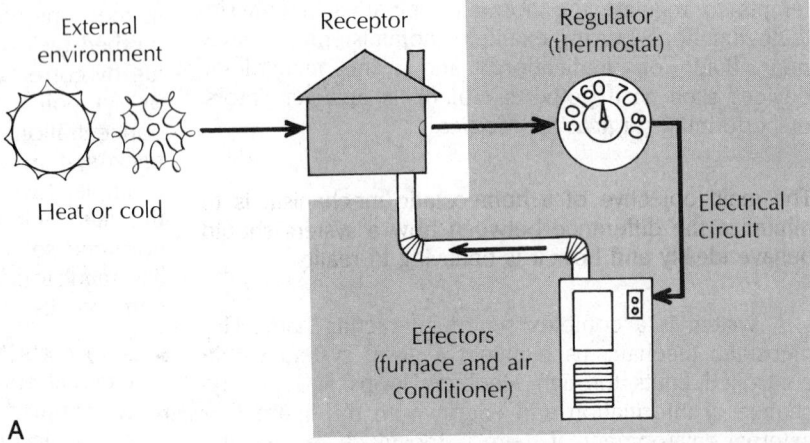

A

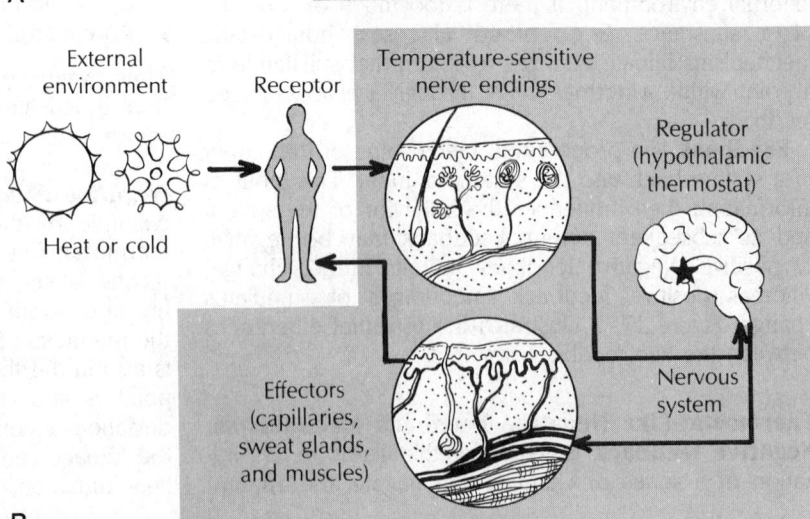

B

crease to as much as 23° to 24°C (74° to 75°F); that is, the deviation will now be in excess of the set point. When the elevated temperature is sensed by the thermostat, the furnace will shut off until the house again becomes too cool. If the system is working properly, the house will remain at approximately the same temperature indefinitely, despite outdoor weather conditions.[23]

The temperature control system within the body is a very good example of thermostat-like regulation. The thermostat that controls body temperature is located within the hypothalamus. Operating by negative feedback, the hypothalamic thermostat keeps the body temperature steady at a set point of around 37.0°C (98.6°F), despite environmental conditions. Figure 17–4A and B compares body temperature regulation with a house thermostat. Many researchers now believe that in some cases of temperature elevation resulting from infection or toxic substances, the set point is changed. Hence, the body attempts to maintain an elevated temperature.

Although set points may change secondary to pathologic processes and overwhelming stress (the primarily neuroendocrine response to stressors), normal fluctuations in physiologic variables also occur. Researchers now point out that the concept of homeostasis must incorporate changes that occur with chronobiologic rhythms.[32]

Negative Feedback and Body Weight. Another illustration of thermostat-like control and set points is a theory of weight regulation, which states that body weight and fat are maintained at a genetically predetermined or preferred level by feedback control. Again, the theory suggests that mechanisms transmit signals from the periphery to the hypothalamus, the central controller.[16] The hypothalamus then processes the information and transmits signals that adjust food intake or energy expenditure. The body automatically balances food intake, physical activity, and metabolism to sustain this level of body weight. Moreover, the body inclines toward a specific "ideal" weight, which is the weight at which an individual functions most comfortably. Unfortunately, what the body determines as an ideal weight may directly conflict with what fashion or the individual decrees is ideal. Therefore, after a regimen of appreciable weight loss or gain, the body returns to its "ideal" weight unless the person maintains constant vigilance over food intake and exercise.

Rangelike Negative Feedback Mechanisms. Unlike body temperature, which has a relatively stable set point of 37.0°C (98.6°F), numerous other negative feedback mechanisms, such as those involved in the control of blood glucose and hormone levels, are rangelike and are characterized by a set point that continually but moderately fluctuates within a range of normal limits. The controls of blood glucose and hormone levels are set points that operate within a range depending upon the time of day and other factors (e.g., diet, time of meals).

Negative Feedback and Blood Glucose Levels. The negative feedback mechanism for blood glucose operates within the normal range of approximately 80 to 100 mg/dl. Following a meal, blood glucose rises rapidly. At this point there is a discrepancy between the normal range and the actual glucose level. As a result, signals related to the elevated glucose levels are sent to the pancreas and result in increased insulin secretion. Insulin moves glucose into muscles or into the liver for storage as glycogen. As the blood glucose level returns toward the normal range, insulin secretion is blunted; if the glucose level falls below the normal range, insulin secretion may be inhibited and glucagon release initiated.

In the same way, when exercise and metabolic demands increase the cellular need for glucose, glucose blood levels fall as glucose is taken up and used by the cells. With negative feedback, detection of the low glucose levels results in glucagon release and insulin inhibition from the pancreas. Glucagon accelerates the breakdown of liver glycogen to glucose, which in turn raises the blood glucose level until it is again within the normal range. Cortisol, a glucocorticoid from the adrenal cortex, and the catecholamines from the adrenal medulla also play a prominent role in glucose homeostasis.

Negative Feedback and Blood Hormone Levels. Hormone levels are controlled by negative feedback. For example, consider the interrelationships of the hypothalamus, the anterior lobe of the pituitary gland, and the adrenal cortex (Figure 17–5). The hypothalamus releases corticotropin-releasing hormone (CRH), which stimulates the anterior pituitary to secrete ACTH. ACTH is then transported through the circulatory system to the adrenal glands and stimulates the adrenal cortex to secrete cortisol and, to some extent, aldosterone, a mineralocorticoid. Elevated cortisol levels initiate the negative feedback system to inhibit additional CRF and ACTH release, and then cortisol levels gradually fall to within the normal range, which is partially determined by the time of day. If blood cortisol levels become sufficiently low, the hypothalamic-pituitary-adrenal system is stimulated to secrete ACTH and CRH, again raising the cortisol levels.

Positive Feedback Mechanisms. Unlike negative feedback, **positive feedback** is a response to stimuli that results in intensifying the initiating stimuli, leading the organism away from the normal state (Figure 17–6). Except for a few instances, positive feedback tends to be disruptive for biologic systems. The original error or imbalance, rather than being corrected, is repeated or intensified, thus compounding the problem. Consequently, severe injury, illness, or even death may result unless the positive feedback is corrected.

Although most homeostatic mechanisms are based on negative feedback, some biologic organisms can tolerate limited positive feedback. Cyclic changes in female reproductive hormones exemplify this type of system. In this instance, FSH and LH stimulate the

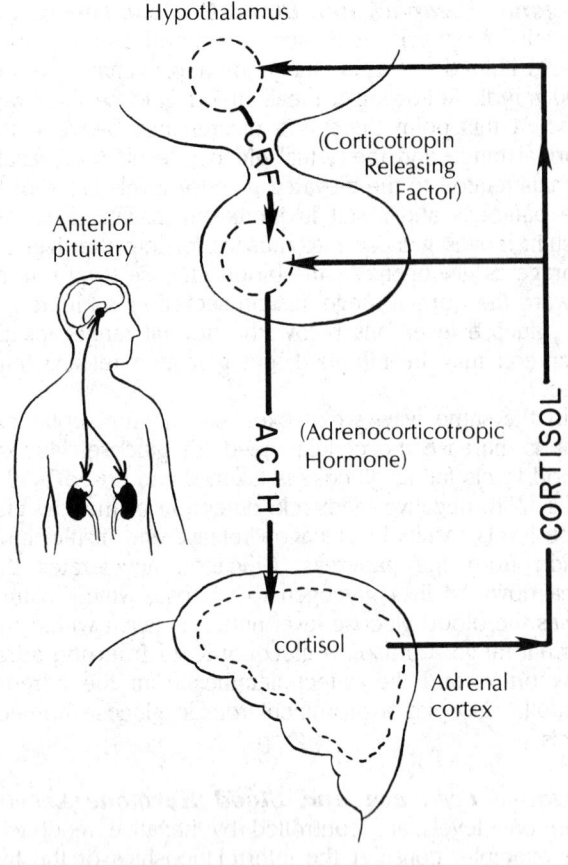

Anterior pituitary

(Corticotropin Releasing Factor)

CRF

ACTH

(Adrenocorticotropic Hormone)

CORTISOL

cortisol

Adrenal cortex

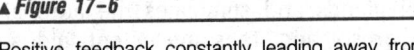

▲ *Figure 17–5*

Regulation of cortisol secretion.

▲ *Figure 17–6*

Positive feedback constantly leading away from the norm.

development of the ovarian follicle, which secretes estrogens. High levels of estrogens indirectly stimulate the secretion of LH. This positive feedback mechanism produces a sudden rise of LH, thus triggering ovulation and the formation of the corpus luteum, which secretes progesterone, a hormone that inhibits LH secretion.

Note that the positive feedback cycle breaks after a certain point; that is, feedback is limited. Continued positive feedback causes an uncontrolled, increasing deviation from the norm. Living organisms can tolerate positive feedback only if it is limited.

COMPLEMENTARY PROCESSES

Many body processes are influenced by several feedback systems, all of which must complement each other. Cortisol secretion by the adrenal cortex is one example of the complementary process of negative feedback. Cortisol secretion increases blood cortisol levels, and these elevated levels activate a negative feedback mechanism that then inhibits both the hypothalamus and the anterior pituitary gland.

NORMAL DEVIATIONS

The concept of homeostatic balance represents an ideal, but every self-regulating system incorporates some deviation or error from what is optimal or normal for that system. Control, after all, can be achieved only through adjustment of the error.

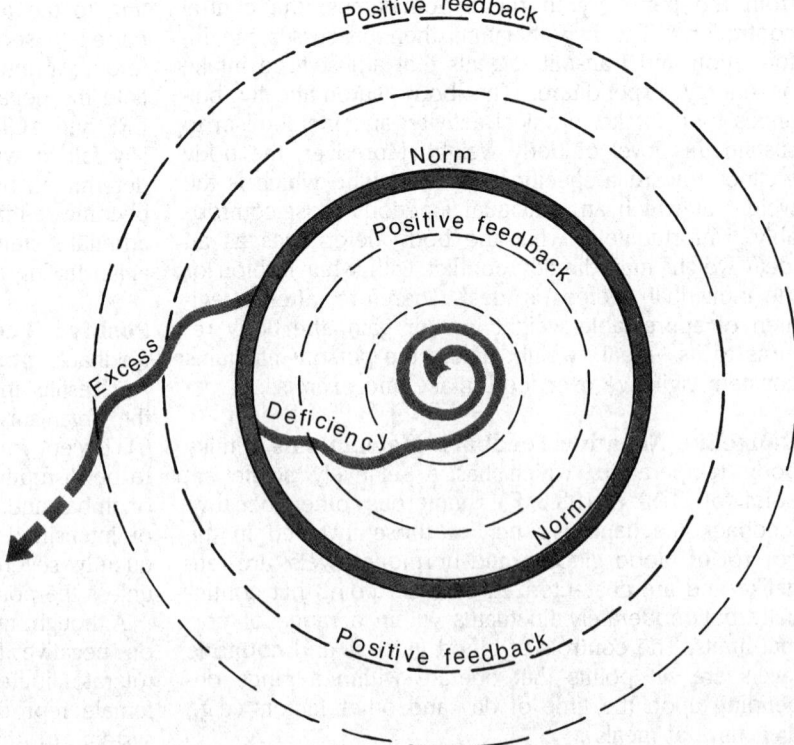

Positive feedback

Norm

Positive feedback

Excess

Deficiency

Norm

Positive feedback

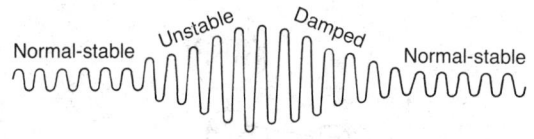

▲ *Figure 17-7*

Types of fluctuations.

HOMEOSTATIC FLUCTUATIONS

Homeostatic mechanisms always fluctuate to some degree. When an error is detected in a homeostatic system, the system tries to correct the error. Yet the system is imperfect in its correction efforts. A time lag may exist between the moment the error is detected and the moment corrective action is started, and as a result of this time lag, the system may **overshoot** or overcompensate during attempts at system self-correction to achieve homeostasis.

This overshooting, in itself, is an error. Consequently, after another time lag, the system again readjusts and so overshoots in the opposite direction.* Overshooting in opposite directions creates fluctuations as the system attempts to correct itself and return to a normal range. If the fluctuations increase in magnitude, unstable changes develop and may cause the system to lose its self-correcting mechanism. If, on the other hand, fluctuations are damped or decrease in magnitude, then the system can return to normal function (Figure 17-7). Fluctuations normally occur within narrow limits.

Some overshooting is unavoidable because homeostatic systems continually adjust to new stressors. If a homeostatic system is not too badly disturbed by a stressor, it returns to its former status. If a system is severely disturbed, however, it may either break down entirely or go on to a completely new steady state. In the latter case, the system will stabilize, but at a different set point or range. If the fluctuations become too great, the organism is threatened.

Homeostatic Fluctuations in Hemorrhagic Shock.
Control of arterial blood pressure (BP) and the stressor of hypovolemic (low blood volume) hemorrhagic shock is one example of fluctuations and deviations in a negative feedback system. If BP falls precipitously as a result of hemorrhage, the pressure receptors primarily in the carotid arteries, heart, and lungs detect a change from the norm and send signals to the cardiovascular centers in the brainstem. To compensate for the changes in volume and BP, the sympathetic nervous system is activated and hormones that promote water and sodium retention are secreted.

The stimulation of the sympathetic nervous system results in constriction of primarily peripheral blood ves-

sels, an increase in the pumping action of the heart, and an increase in cardiac contractility in an effort to provide an adequate cardiac output and to increase BP. The low blood volume associated with acute blood loss causes blood flow to be shunted to the heart and brain and away from other less essential organs, such as kidneys, lungs, skin, and the GI system.

The resulting decrease in blood flow to the kidneys stimulates the release of renin and the activation of the renin-angiotensin system, which then produces two substances, angiotensin II and III. Angiotensin II and III then stimulate further vasoconstriction, resulting in an increase in BP. Angiotensin II and III also stimulate the adrenal cortex to release aldosterone, which leads to sodium retention and potassium excretion by the kidneys. The retention of sodium leads to an increase in serum osmolarity that is sensed by the osmoreceptors in the hypothalamus and leads to the secretion of ADH from the posterior pituitary gland. The overall effect of these hormonal changes is an increase in blood volume due to water and sodium retention.[37]

If, however, the person receives emergency care and bleeding is controlled before blood loss becomes too great, vasoconstriction and effects of compensatory mechanisms to correct blood volume will lead to an increase in BP and cardiac output. Eventually, the person's vital signs will return to a normal range. If compensatory mechanisms fail, however, a condition such as hemorrhagic shock becomes progressive and may reach an irreversible stage resulting in death.[18]

Even when the body's compensatory efforts to return to a normal range are working, overcompensation may occur, and BP may rise to a level greater than it was before the bleeding began. The body then senses this error, and initiates new responses to lower BP again. The new compensatory responses may persist beyond the normal point, causing BP again to become too low. The body then detects yet another error. Under these conditions, BP continues to overshoot between high and low extremes. If the fluctuations become too unstable and wild, the system may break down. Fortunately, most fluctuations within the human body are readily dampened; that is, their range diminishes as a result of compensatory reactions. Therefore, these types of unstable BP fluctuations are usually dampened, and BP either returns to the level that preceded the upset or readjusts to a new norm.

Limitations of Homeostatic Mechanisms.
All self-regulating homeostatic mechanisms, however complex and sophisticated, have limitations. Rapid growth and change, severe stressors, reduction in adaptive energy, or damage to the system lead to one or all of the following consequences: (1) a continued but inadequate performance of the mechanism, leading eventually to an overdriven system; (2) interruption of the mechanism; or (3) a complete breakdown of negative feedback control, resulting in death. Negative feedback mechanisms typically disintegrate in conjunction with uncontrolled positive feedback.

---

* Note the difference between overshooting and positive feedback. Positive feedback goes continually *away* from the norm. Overshooting means moving *back and forth* around the norm.

Failure of Homeostatic Mechanisms

OVERDRIVEN SYSTEMS

When compensatory reactions are inadequate, the result can be an overdriven system. One example is blood glucose regulation. Recall that in normal blood glucose regulation, levels must remain within certain limits; if these limits are exceeded, glucose is converted to glycogen and stored in the liver. This homeostatic mechanism depends upon insulin and glucagon. When an insulin deficiency exists, as in diabetes mellitus, glucose is not oxidized and stored properly. Thus, blood glucose levels remain high. If the blood levels get too high (> 180 mg/dl), the kidney excretes glucose in the urine. Urinary glucose also pulls water with it by osmosis, thus resulting in dehydration. Abnormal glucose excretion, in turn, leads to such compensatory mechanisms as a craving for sweets, increased urinary output, and thirst. In cases of severe insulin deficiency, the diminished entrance of glucose into the cells leads to the inability of the body to function. The person's system becomes overdriven, and the result is irreparable organ and tissue damage.

INTERRUPTIONS OF HOMEOSTATIC MECHANISMS

Some diseases interrupt and thereby disrupt homeostatic mechanisms. Cancer, for example, appears to disrupt the normal regulation of cell division. In general, the physical crowding of cells as they divide (i.e., cellular density) naturally inhibits, through negative feedback, the further growth of cells. This regulation is impaired in malignant cells, and instead they multiply in an uncontrolled and uncoordinated manner. Lack of negative feedback on abnormal cell division apparently causes unrestrained proliferation of malignant cancer cells (Figure 17–8).

RAPID AND COMPLETE BREAKDOWN OF HOMEOSTASIS

One example of rapid and complete breakdown of negative feedback compounded by positive feedback is a person with severe, biventricular (i.e., left and right) heart failure that is unresponsive to treatment. Heart failure is a condition in which the heart is unable to meet the metabolic needs of the body. Many factors may lead to heart failure (e.g., cardiac overload due to excessive volume, high BP, or loss of cardiac functional tissue).[14] Regardless of the underlying cause, the failing heart becomes overloaded and so weak that it cannot pump an adequate amount of blood out with each contraction. The result is a decrease in cardiac output, an increase in the amount of blood remaining in the heart, an increase in pressure within the heart, and subsequent dilatation (short-term) or hypertrophy (long-term) of cardiac muscle.

The decreased cardiac output results in activation of compensatory mechanisms that increase cardiac output. One compensatory response to the decreased cardiac output, initiated by the volume receptors, is the transmission of a signal activating the sympathetic ner-

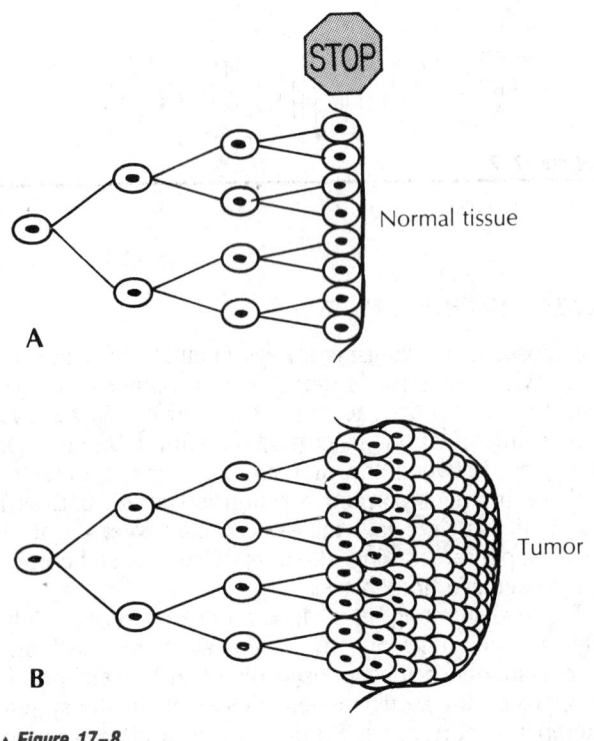

▲ **Figure 17–8**

Cancer cell proliferation.

vous system and leading to an increase in heart rate, peripheral vasoconstriction, and shunting of blood from less essential organs to the heart and brain. In addition, other homeostatic mechanisms (e.g., stimulation of the renin-angiotensin-aldosterone system and ADH secretion) are activated, which leads to water and sodium retention, resulting in increased circulating volume and increased venous return to the heart.

Because the problem is the inability of the heart to pump effectively, the vasoconstriction only adds to the problem by increasing the peripheral resistance that the heart must work against to pump the blood. The weakened heart is faced not only with increased resistance but also with increased volume. The heart becomes more dysfunctional, and fluid retention, as evidenced by edema, becomes increasingly severe. The compensatory mechanisms eventually fail, with an increase in both left and right ventricular pressures and dilatation of these chambers. Blood backs up from the left side of the heart, and plasma accumulates in the interstitial fluid of the lungs, interfering with gas exchange of oxygen and carbon dioxide.

If the problem is not corrected, blood backs up in the right side of the heart, causing congestion and edema of the venous system (e.g., jugular vein distention, engorgement of the liver, edema of the lower extremities). As biventricular heart failure progresses, cardiac output continues to drop; cardiac muscle contractions continue to become weaker; and mechanisms leading to vasoconstriction and water and sodium retention continue to operate. This vicious cycle, unless stopped, is repeated until negative feedback breaks down totally. The muscle contraction of the heart fails; heart activity stops; and death results.

Severe biventricular heart failure illustrates positive feedback in that the resulting decreased cardiac output exerts a stimulating effect on the control mechanism, causing the responses of the system to increase continuously. The continuous reinforcing of the original error results in a breakdown of the system. When negative feedback mechanisms break down and positive feedback is uncontrolled, the result is increasing deviation from the norm, leading to death.

CHRONOBIOLOGY

Chronobiology, the study of biologic rhythms that regulate bodily functions and behavior, is an area of research involving the clinical significance of homeostasis and feedback. This area of study has important implications for health care. Biologic rhythms are found at all levels of the hierarchy of living organisms, from a single cell to a complex organism, such as a human being. Rhythms are either exogenous (i.e., resulting from a passive response to environmental periodic stimuli) or endogenous (i.e., self-sustaining and originating within an organism). The changes in the tides in response to changes in the phase of the moon is one example of an exogenous rhythm. Endogenous rhythms are of greatest relevance to human beings.

Great interest has been focused on finding anatomic sites and neurophysiologic mechanisms related to endogenous rhythms. Current information reveals that endogenous rhythms are driven by two or more major pacemakers, or biologic clocks.[3,29,30] One, the suprachiasmatic nucleus (SCN) located in the anterior hypothalamus, is believed to be the pacemaker that drives the cycles of sleeping and waking, skin temperature, plasma growth hormone levels, urinary calcium excretion, and slow wave sleep.[30] The location of other pacemakers that generate the rhythms for core body temperature, plasma cortisol, urinary potassium excretion, and rapid eye movement (REM) sleep have not yet been identified.[30]

To understand biologic rhythms, you need to know some of the factors that influence the expression of endogenous rhythms. The timing of the rhythm's peak, or *acrophase* (maximum value), and the *trough* (lowest value) can be synchronized by cues from periodic changes in the environment, such as the alternation of light and dark cycles. A predominant stimulus, which synchronizes the rhythm, is called a *Zeitgeber*. The most important Zeitgeber for lower animals is thought to be the alternating light and dark cycle. While light is a very important stimulus, social interactions (e.g., social events, home routines) and rest and activity schedules related to school, work, or other activities of daily living are considered the most important stimuli for human beings.[6] Figure 17–9 shows the relationship among the period, amplitude, and frequency of a cycle.

Rhythmic Cycles and Frequencies

Rhythms are categorized according to their frequency, which may range from less than a second to several years.[8] Rhythmic cycles shorter than 24 hours, such as sleep cycles, are called **ultradian rhythms.** Rhythmic cycles longer than 24 hours, such as the menstrual cycle, are called **infradian rhythms.** Rhythm cycles that occur over a period of a year are called **circannual rhythms.** The most frequently investigated cycles in human beings are **circadian rhythms,** which occur with a frequency of approximately 24 hours and are thought to be adaptive mechanisms that enable individuals to adjust to their temporal environment. The word *circadian* comes from the Latin words *circa* (around) and *dies* (day). To understand circadian rhythms, you need to become familiar with terms that describe these rhythms. Table 17–1 defines some of the major terms.

Circadian Rhythms

Almost all physiologic variables exhibit rhythmicity. Rhythms of approximately 24 hours, circadian rhythms, are thought to be in synchrony when a person is healthy.

Since almost all measurable physiologic variables exhibit rhythmicity, their normal range and the time of day when the measurements are made must be taken into consideration when assessing clients' physiologic data. Disorders of circadian rhythms have been reported to be associated with illness[17,25,28,32] and aging.[38,43]

BODY TEMPERATURE RHYTHMS

Body temperature was one of the first physiologic variables known to have a rhythmic variation. As early as the 18th century, it was known that body temperature varies approximately 0.5°C to 1.0°C (1.5°F) between sleeping and waking. Since then, the circadian rhythm of body temperature has been shown to be an endogenous rhythm that can persist in the absence of normal environmental Zeitgebers, such as light-dark variation. The body temperature of day-active adults usually begins to rise shortly before or just after awakening, reaches a peak in late afternoon or early evening, and then declines to its lowest level during the time of

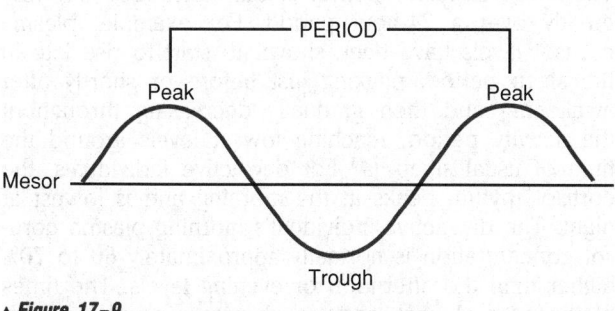

▲ *Figure 17–9*

The relationship among the period, amplitude, and frequency of a cycle.

TABLE 17–1. Basic Terms Used in Describing Rhythms

Term	Definition
Period	The time interval between recurrences of peak phases of the rhythm
Rhythm	Regularly occurring, oscillating process that has a peak and a trough
Endogenous rhythms	Rhythms originating within the organism
Exogenous rhythms	Rhythms that exist in response to periodic stimuli outside the organism (e.g., movement of the tides in response to the phases of the moon)
Acrophase	Time of occurrence of rhythm peak
Amplitude	The difference between the maximum (peak) or minimum (trough) and the rhythm mean (mesor)
Cycle	The shortest part of a rhythm that repeats itself indefinitely
Mesor	Rhythmic mean
Peak	The maximum response of the rhythm studied
Trough	The minimum response of the rhythm studied
Zeitgeber (synchronizer)	The predominant stimulus that synchronizes the expression of a rhythm (e.g., alternation of light and dark)
Desynchronization	The loss of synchrony between or among two or more previously temporally related rhythms. For example, a temporal association normally occurs between normal body temperature and certain aspects of performance rhythms. If an individual abruptly changes the sleep/wake cycle, these rhythms will temporarily be out of synchrony with each other
Free-running	An endogenous rhythm that continues in the absence of entraining environmental time cues (i.e., Zeitgebers)
Phase-shift	An advance or delay of a rhythm along the time axis. The peaks and troughs occur earlier or later in time, while the rhythm remains the same

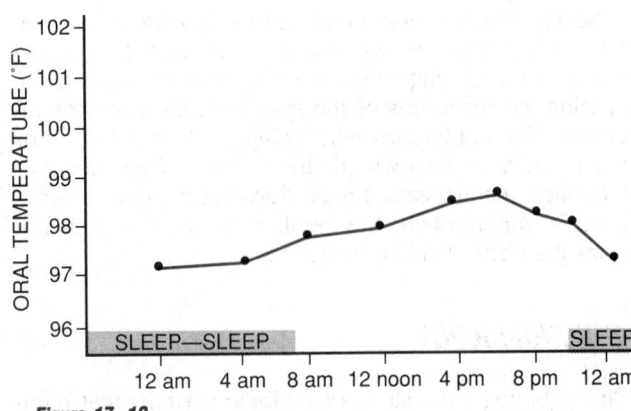

▲ *Figure 17–10*

Circadian rhythm of oral temperature of a day-active individual. (From Lanuza, D.M. (1976). Circadian rhythms of mental efficiency and performance. *Nursing Clinics of North America,* 11[4], 584.)

mately 6 PM in day-active individuals.[39] For example, a temperature of 37.4°C (99.2°F) at 6 AM, when a day-active individual's temperature normally is low, indicates that the client is running a low-grade fever and needs to be monitored for further temperature elevations. A 37.4°C temperature at 6 PM for an individual with this type of sleep-wake pattern, however, would not be a cause of concern.

BLOOD PRESSURE RHYTHMS

Circadian variations in systolic, diastolic, and mean arterial BP have been reported, with the lowest readings for day-active individuals occurring at night and the highest readings occurring during the day, in the morning or early afternoon.[44] Diurnal (day versus night) BP rhythms with higher values during the day and lower values at night have been demonstrated in normotensive and hypertensive individuals.[36] Deviations from this type of rhythmic pattern (e.g., loss of nocturnal decline) have been reported in patients with left ventricular hypertrophy (enlarged heart)[47] and in postoperative cardiac transplant patients.[26] The relevance of these altered rhythms to the patient's health is currently being investigated.

HORMONAL RHYTHMS

The blood concentration of certain hormones may vary greatly over a 24-hour period. For example, plasma cortisol levels have been shown to start to rise late in the sleep period, peaking just before or shortly after awakening and then gradually decreasing throughout the activity period, reaching lowest levels around the time of usual sleep.[27,46] For day-active individuals, the cortisol rhythm peaks in the morning and is lowest at night. The day-active individual's morning plasma cortisol concentration is normally approximately 60 to 70% higher than the afternoon or evening levels. The times of the cortisol peak and trough are reversed in night-active individuals. Therefore, the time when the blood sample is drawn should be noted, and the client's

usual sleep (Figure 17–10). It has been suggested that people who awaken early and retire early (larks) tend to have temperature patterns that rise and peak earlier than people who prefer to awaken later in the day and go to bed later (owls). Mood states and some performance patterns have been reported to be temporally associated with patterns of body temperature, so that the peaks for these variables occur about the same time as the temperature peak.

Measuring body temperature, an index of a client's state of health, is one of the most frequently performed nursing procedures. Normally, the best time to screen for fevers is to schedule temperature measurements at the peak of the temperature circadian cycle, approxi-

sleep-activity pattern should be considered when reporting laboratory test results.

Plasma cortisol adult values are

▶ 0700 to 0900 hr = 6 to 25 $\mu g/dl$
▶ 1500 to 1700 hr = 2 to 18 $\mu g/dl$

URINARY VOLUME AND ELECTROLYTE EXCRETION RHYTHMS

Urine output (volume, electrolytes, and so on) is greatest in the morning to midday and lowest during the night in day-active individuals. This rhythmic pattern holds true even when people drink fluids around the clock, indicating that these rhythms are not dependent on fluid intake, although the times of peaks and troughs may be reversed by reversing sleep-wake patterns. Urinary volume and electrolyte excretion rhythms are the result of many physiologic processes (e.g., glomerular filtration rate, tubular reabsorption rate), but the major factor is thought to be osmotic load, that is, the changing rate of excretion of urinary solids.[8] Urinary electrolytes, such as sodium, potassium, chloride, and calcium, are all excreted in small amounts in the morning, reaching a peak around late morning or early afternoon.[22] In addition, urine flow is controlled in part by plasma levels of ADH, which are lower in the recumbent position and higher when sitting or standing.

CELL DIVISION RHYTHMS

The rate of cell replacement roughly approximates the rate of cell damage and erosion. Cell division is more rapid, however, during certain hours of a 24-hour period than at others. For example, the division of skin cells, which require constant replacement, occurs primarily during our deepest hours of sleep—roughly between midnight and 4 AM.[40] This nightly period of non-neuronal cellular renewal may be one of the functions of sleep.

SLEEP-WAKE RHYTHMS

Sleep Cycles. Nearly one third of an individual's life is spent sleeping. Yet, only in the last 60 years has much progress been made in sleep research. Sleep has been found to be developmental and species-specific. In human beings, sleep patterns may vary greatly among individuals, but they remain remarkably the same for each individual. Sleep is composed of two distinctly different types of sleep: nonrapid eye movement (NREM—Stages I, II, III, and IV) and rapid eye movement (REM) sleep. NREM alternates with REM sleep in a cyclic manner.

A sleep cycle is approximately 90 minutes, with most people averaging about four to six cycles per night. Fluctuations in sleep cycles may be part of the 90-minute basic rest-activity cycles that occur during the waking state and could account for fluctuations in alertness and drowsiness.[21]

Psychosocial, physiologic, and environmental factors that disrupt sleep-wake cycles also demand a readjustment of circadian rhythms.

Sleep Deprivation. Whereas sleep deprivation may occur during both REM and NREM sleep, REM sleep deprivation is most common. It occurs whenever the sleep period is shortened, as is often the case when a person is hospitalized. Most medications that affect sleep usually decrease REM sleep. The deprivation of REM sleep may result in emotional lability, irritability, difficulty in concentrating, hyperactivity, and increased appetite.[35] Although sleep deprivation may be detrimental, maintaining a regular circadian pattern of sleep may be more important to waking efficiency than the actual number of hours slept.[45]

DISRUPTION OF CIRCADIAN RHYTHMS

Circadian rhythms may be disrupted by physiologic and emotional stressors, as well as by abrupt changes in sleep-wake patterns. The physiologic and emotional changes that may disrupt biologic rhythms include

▶ physical illness (e.g., high fevers, head injury)
▶ mental illness (e.g., bipolar depression)
▶ drugs and toxins (e.g., barbiturates)
▶ minimal or absent time cues (e.g., people who are immobilized, placed in isolation because of communicable disease, or treated in intensive care units may experience serious disturbances of body rhythms similar to those affecting astronauts in space)

Social and environmental changes that abruptly disrupt usual sleep-wake cycles also demand a readjustment of circadian rhythms.

Jet Travel. Jet lag syndrome is a complex of symptoms that occurs after jet travel across four or more time zones when the traveler attempts to adapt too rapidly to the new time zone with its different light-dark cycle and time of social activities. Jet lag syndrome is characterized by irritability, fatigue, hunger and sleepiness at inappropriate times, and difficulties sleeping at appropriate times.[24]

Shift Rotation. Rotating work shifts also disrupt circadian rhythms by forcing workers to adjust continually to new eating, sleeping, and social patterns. Some of the major consequences of a shift worker's inability to adjust to changing sleep-wake cycles are alterations in the quality and quantity (decrease in sleep length by 2 to 4 hours) of sleep, persistent fatigue, behavioral change, and decreased performance.[2,45] Rotating shift workers report higher incidences of fatigue, nervousness, and inadequate sleep than do fixed-shift workers.[2] A National Institute for Occupational Safety and Health (NIOSH) report found that nurses on rotating shifts had more occupational injuries than their fixed-shift colleagues.[41]

The difficulties experienced by individuals working the night shift are thought to be caused by their efforts to work when they have had little sleep and their body temperature and performance capabilities are at their lowest levels. Therefore, it is not surprising that the incidence of single-vehicle accidents and performance errors is higher between 3 AM and 5 AM than at any other time of day.[15] Shift-work schedules are believed to be factors in the Three Mile Island nuclear reactor accident,[11] as well as the accident at Chernobyl.

Chronic disruption of the circadian rhythm in shift workers is thought to be a potential cause of illness and pathology, such as cardiovascular conditions and GI disorders.[33] For example, the incidence of colitis and gastroduodenitis was found to be higher in shift workers than in nonshift workers.[10]

Hospitalization or Institutionalization. When individuals enter a health care facility, jail, or military setting, they are forced to fit into a rigid time schedule over which they have little control. In a health care facility, especially an intensive care setting, the times for eating, sleeping, and socializing are typically dictated by the rules at the unit rather than by the needs and desires of the people who are hospitalized. In addition, the medications or treatments that patients receive may blunt the individual's ability to respond to environmental time cues. Moreover, the environment may lack circadian time cues.[6] Unfortunately, hospitalized people are forced to accommodate to a new schedule and environment at the same time that they are struggling with stressors associated with illness.

Individuals who experience an abrupt change in their sleep and activity patterns vary in their rate of adjustment. Some persons adapt rapidly, others slowly, and others not at all. Also, the rhythms of specific physiologic and psychologic variables adjust to time changes at different rates. Some cardiovascular rhythms adjust to a new time schedule within a few days, whereas readjustment of adrenal hormonal rhythm patterns may require a week or more.[27] Having to adjust to rapid time changes is a challenge. Occasionally, the stress associated with this process may be so great that biologic rhythms that usually are temporally related become dissociated from one another, resulting in a sense of a loss of well-being and possibly illness.

CLINICAL APPLICATIONS OF CHRONOBIOLOGIC PRINCIPLES

The application of chronobiologic principles to health care is still in its early stages. In the future, our growing knowledge of biologic rhythms will probably be employed in a number of practical ways.

UNDERSTANDING THE NATURE OF DISEASE

The study of circadian rhythms can help us understand the nature of disease.[32,42] Chronopathology, which is the study of the time factor associated with symptoms and disease, uses knowledge of a circadian rhythm of susceptibility and focuses on the cyclical nature of certain physical (e.g., asthma) and mental disorders (e.g.,

bipolar depression). Population circadian rhythms have been demonstrated for the occurrence of myocardial infarctions, strokes, and sudden cardiac deaths.[34,42]

Chronopathology can help elucidate the nature of disease and the influence of circadian rhythms on symptoms associated with illness.

ENHANCING THE ACCURACY OF DIAGNOSTIC TESTING

A knowledge of circadian rhythms could be used to revolutionize diagnostic testing in the laboratory. Almost all measurable physiologic variables (e.g., levels of cortisol, growth hormone, and urinary electrolytes) are known to ebb and flow with the body's inner clock. Therefore, the time of day that specimens are obtained for laboratory tests is important.

In most clinical settings, laboratory specimens are generally collected in the morning rather than at other times over a 24-hour period. The test results are then compared with standard laboratory normal values, which have typically been established without consideration of circadian rhythm fluctuations. As a result, the reported comparison of the blood or urine data may be inaccurate.[12] Medical laboratories of the future will probably consider the effects of rhythmic cycles on blood and urinary constituents when analyzing test results.

IMPROVING THE TREATMENT OF DISEASE

Knowledge of circadian rhythm could also be useful in the treatment of disease. A number of illnesses, such as certain sleep disorders, depressive conditions, or endocrine diseases, may be manifestations of circadian rhythm disorders. Additionally, the body may be more susceptible to some diseases at certain times during the circadian cycle than at others. Recent evidence has shown a circadian rhythm in the incidence of morbidity and mortality.[34]

New scientific evidence indicates that circadian rhythms also influence the absorption rate, effectiveness, and toxicity of drugs. This exciting new area of research is called chronopharmacology,[1] and its focus is to determine the appropriate time to administer medications or treatments (e.g., radiation therapy) to get the most effective response with the fewest side effects, using the lowest possible dosage. In particular, this finding has implications for the administration of cancer chemotherapy.[19]

NURSING IMPLICATIONS RELATED TO HOMEOSTASIS AND BIOLOGIC RHYTHMS

Moore-Ede[31] suggests that Cannon's initial formulation of the concept of homeostasis, which focused on compensatory mechanisms in response to changes that have already occurred, needs to be extended. This researcher argues that the human body is not limited to reactive responses but is capable of initiating responses in anticipation of regularly occurring, predictably timed circumstances. For example, body temperature and cortisol levels begin to rise as if in anticipation of waking.

Knowledge about homeostasis and biologic rhythms has many implications for nursing care. Because nurses deliver around-the-clock care, nurses have many reasons and opportunities to play an important role in homeostasis, biologic rhythm, and biofeedback research. The number of nurses conducting research related to homeostasis and circadian rhythms is increasing, but more work is needed.

Remember the following:

▶ Self-regulating systems can break down as a result of extreme stress, a reduction in energy, or damage to part of the system.
▶ Biologic rhythms are upset by numerous factors, including toxins, drugs, surgery, and time changes.
▶ Disturbances in rhythmic cycles result in a loss of a sense of well-being and possibly illness.
▶ Illness is a result of disturbances within the body's internal environment (neuroendocrine function, fluid and electrolyte balance, circadian rhythms) that are frequently precipitated by disturbances arising from the external environment (pollutants, viruses).
▶ Understanding how people adapt adequately to stress and how they normally maintain homeostatic balance will promote better understanding of faulty adaptation and deviations from homeostasis that occur in illness.

Biofeedback

Biofeedback is an area of research that uses the concepts of homeostasis and feedback. Physiologists have traditionally categorized functions as voluntary and involuntary. Voluntary functions, such as motor skills and speech, are governed by the conscious mind. Involuntary biologic functions are governed primarily by the autonomic nervous system (ANS) and can operate automatically without the individual's awareness or control (e.g., temperature regulation, brain wave activity, and cardiovascular function).

Within the last 20 years, the concept of feedback has been applied with considerable success to behavioral and physiologic regulation. Information about the so-called involuntary biologic functions is fed back to the individual so that the person can develop an awareness of them and learn to control certain physiologic responses (hence, the term *biofeedback*). In other words, the individual is taught to be sensitive to the language of body cues and develop cognitive control.[48] In this way, the rigid dichotomy between voluntary and involuntary physiologic functions is gradually disintegrating. Scientists now believe that with biofeedback training, people may learn to use their minds to self-regulate certain body functions and avoid disease.

Biofeedback training is a process that involves using feedback methods to teach individuals to be sensitive and aware of body cues so that they can cognitively control certain involuntary physiologic functions.

Biofeedback training is a scientifically planned program that trains selected individuals to control one or more involuntary functions.[48] Awareness and use of the mind/body interaction is the key to the success of biofeedback training. This treatment technique provides information or feedback to help individuals monitor and control automatic physiologic functions, such as BP, heart rate, brain waves, skin temperature, and muscle tension, normally considered involuntary. Biofeedback, as a treatment technique, is still evolving.

Individuals can be taught awareness of the mind-body interaction and to use biofeedback to control certain physiologic processes. Biofeedback is used by some clinicians to treat hypertension, lower back pain, tension headache, chronic pain, insomnia, stress, and anxiety. In addition, biofeedback training is used on a more limited basis to treat conditions such as neuromuscular disorders (e.g., paralysis and muscle spasticity); epilepsy, a condition characterized by brief episodes of sudden excessive electrical activity of the brain resulting in seizures (e.g., motor, sensory, reflex); and disturbances in cerebral function and consciousness.

Assessment

To assess whether a client is able to maintain normal physiologic homeostasis, including biologic rhythmicity, you may note whether the client

▶ has available a sufficient supply of basic physiologic requirements (oxygen, food, water, and electrolytes)
▶ has appropriate mechanisms for using these requirements, storing them for future use when necessary, and eliminating wastes (has adequate function of body systems)
▶ has the ability to maintain physiologic integrity (has normally functioning processes that protect the body from injury and that repair the body when physical damage has occurred)
▶ has a satisfying self-concept
▶ is emotionally balanced
▶ has relatively harmonious interactions with the environment, including others in society
▶ can appropriately compensate for any variations from those conditions that are normal and optimal for the individual

Human beings must maintain homeostasis to survive on all levels, from the cellular level to the entire human organism. Also, problems in homeostatic regulation can become evident in all interactions between the person and the environment. Therefore, assessment of homeostasis involves the use of biologic, psychologic, social, and cultural measurements.

Although the nervous system and the endocrine system work together to control much of human homeostasis, not only the neuroendocrine system must be assessed. Rather, any assessment tool that can measure changes from the individual's normal range of responses and behaviors is a tool that can help in assessment of homeostasis.

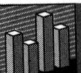

APPLYING RESEARCH TO NURSING PRACTICE
Measuring Circadian Rhythms in Older Adults

Mason, D.J., & Tapp, W. (1992). Measuring circadian rhythms: actigraph versus activation checklist. *Western Journal of Nursing Research*, 14(3), 358–379.

▼▼▼

Most research on circadian rhythms has been carried out on young and middle-aged adults. However, older adults show different patterns of circadian rhythms. There are two ways to interpret these different patterns: (1) Either they represent a deviation from the standard determined to be "normal" for all age groups, or (2) they reflect a normal developmental phenomenon of healthy aging.

To determine which interpretation is correct, it is necessary to have reliable ways of measuring circadian rhythms. Mason and Tapp therefore examined the accuracy and precision of two instruments designed to measure circadian rhythms: the Ambulatory Monitoring Actigraph and the Activation-Deactivation Adjective Checklist. The Actigraph is an electronic instrument that measures and logs movement at 1-minute intervals. The Activation-Deactivation Checklist is a form on which participants described and recorded changes in general energy during wakeful periods.

In the study, 11 older adults, aged 60 to 83 years, used both the Actigraph and the Activation-Deactivation Checklist. In addition, each participant kept a sleep-wake diary that provided information about times of awakening, getting out of bed, daytime naps, and sleep onset. The nurse researchers found that the Actigraph, which provided a daily set of 1440 data points per person, was more accurate and precise than the checklist. Study participants also preferred the Actigraph over the checklist, which required more active participation by the elderly subjects. However, the combination of instruments was more useful to the researchers than any single instrument.

Applications for Practice

Until reliable means for measuring circadian rhythms in older adults become more widely used, keep an open mind about the meaning of your assessment findings. In practice, you will observe that activity-rest patterns in older adults may be different from those of other age groups. As you assess your clients, be careful to determine whether the patterns that you observe are normal for the clients, or whether they represent an alteration that requires further exploration.

A familiar assessment tool is the sphygmomanometer that is used for measuring blood pressure. Determination of a person's blood pressure, at intervals over time, can show normal homeostatic responses to the anxiety of pending surgery, to the effects of anesthesia on the cardiovascular system during surgery, and to the pain experienced at intervals during the early postoperative period. Additional homeostatic measurements may be taken from each body system. For example, the following measurements might indicate alterations in homeostasis:

▶ Immunologic responses to infection, such as an increased white blood cell count
▶ Hormonal responses to stress, such as an increased blood cortisol level
▶ Gastrointestinal responses to dehydration, such as constipation
▶ Sensory responses to changes in light exposure, such as pupillary constriction in bright light
▶ Renal system changes in responses to excess fluid intake, such as increased urinary output

You can certainly identify many more biologic measurements that show homeostatic mechanisms in action. In addition, there are numerous tests for psychologic homeostasis, including measurements of social and cultural responses and behaviors.

Nursing Diagnosis

The concept of homeostasis encompasses many biologic, psychologic, and sociocultural processes. Therefore, a large number of nursing diagnoses relate to homeostasis.

There is no one specific nursing diagnosis that pertains only to homeostasis. In fact, there are only a few nursing diagnoses that do not pertain to homeostasis in one way or another.

Following are just a few examples of nursing diagnoses that indicate homeostasis is altered.

▶ *Altered Nutrition: Less than Body Requirements* R/T inability to ingest nutrients secondary to poor body image
▶ *High Risk for Infection* R/T immunosuppression and insufficient knowledge to avoid exposure to pathogens
▶ *Ineffective Thermoregulation* R/T fluctuating environmental temperature
▶ *Constipation* R/T lack of fluid intake
▶ *Functional Incontinence* R/T muscular weakness and lack of timely assistance to the bathroom facilities
▶ *Fluid Volume Excess* R/T excess fluid intake
▶ *High Risk for Injury* R/T recent visual impairment and lack of knowledge of hospital environment
▶ *Social Isolation* R/T inability to engage in satisfying social relationships secondary to anxiety
▶ *High Risk for Altered Parenting* R/T lack of available role model and lack of knowledge
▶ *Impaired Adjustment* R/T incomplete grieving
▶ *Decisional Conflict* R/T unclear personal values
▶ *Sleep Pattern Disturbance* R/T external environmental changes

These nursing diagnoses and many more relate in some way to homeostatic mechanisms. All are amenable to nursing intervention. Yet another nursing diagnosis, *Relocation Stress Syndrome*, is made after completing a physical and psychosocial assessment and

NURSING DIAGNOSIS PROFILE

Relocation Stress Syndrome

Definition. Physiologic and/or psychosocial disturbances as a result of transfer from one environment to another.

Classification. Moving 6.7

Defining Characteristics. Major defining characteristics, which must be present for this nursing diagnosis to be made, include a change in environment accompanied by the psychologic symptom(s) of anxiety, apprehension, depression, loneliness, or (in elderly persons) increased confusion. Minor defining characteristics that might be present include the physical signs or symptoms of sleep disturbance, change in eating habits, gastrointestinal disturbances, and weight change. Minor psychosocial signs or symptoms include verbalization of unwillingness to relocate, verbalization of being concerned/upset about transfer, unfavorable comparison of post/pre-transfer staff, increased verbalization of needs, dependency, insecurity, lack of trust, vigilance, restlessness, sad affect, and withdrawal.

Sample Related Factors. Sample related factors include those that might have led up to the decision to transfer, including past, concurrent, and recent losses (such as losses of a spouse or other close support person or losses of a home, money, or property), impaired psychosocial health status, or decreased physical health status. Other related factors might relate more to untoward events occurring before, during, or soon after the time of the move. Examples might include history and types of previous transfers, little or no preparation for the impending move, losses involved with the decision to move (loss of support persons or belongings that might not have been lost except for the decision), moderate-to-high degree of environmental change, and lack of an adequate support system throughout the process of moving.

Concept Description. *Relocation Stress Syndrome* can occur whether the person moves across the country, across town, or to a different room within a health care facility. It is the stressors involved in the change that cause this unhappy response in the individual. The more stressors involved with the decision to move and with the actual move, the more likely the person is to have a negative response. Moving is not always a negative stress. The person might, in fact, look forward to the move with a great deal of anticipation, but even positive stress can lead to inability of the person to adjust adequately. Much depends on the total amount of stress in the person's life and on the adaptability of the person.

Examples. Depending on the specific assessment data, this diagnostic category could be applicable in the following situations, among others:

▶ The wife of a corporate manager who must move to another state because her husband has been transferred
▶ The child of a newly divorced mother who is taking her child and is moving back with her own parents until she is financially able to provide independently for her child
▶ An elderly widow who is no longer able to maintain her home and feels she must move into a nursing home

Related/Similar Nursing Diagnoses. This nursing diagnosis should be differentiated from the diagnoses of *Anxiety* or *Powerlessness*. Although the person who experiences *Relocation Stress Syndrome* may feel anxious or powerless, these feelings are but symptoms of *Relocation Stress Syndrome*. If your client's feelings of anxiety or powerlessness can be related to other causes, the additional nursing diagnoses of *Anxiety* and/or *Powerlessness* should be made. If these emotions stem only from the *Relocation Stress Syndrome*, however, only the latter nursing diagnosis is appropriate.

---

noting specific defining characteristics, including an environmental move accompanied by at least one physical or psychosocial problem from among a list of specific signs and symptoms related to the move (see Nursing Diagnosis Profile).

Planning

For any nursing diagnosis, planning means identifying expected outcomes. The main outcome for the nursing diagnosis *Relocation Stress Syndrome* is that the person adapts to (or adequately copes with) the new environment, as evidenced by diminished psychologic or physical symptoms. When planning, you must identify the specific psychologic or physical symptoms experienced by the individual client. These include any defining characteristics for this nursing diagnosis that are experienced by the client (see Nursing Diagnosis Profile). For example, "adequately adapts to new environment, as evidenced by decreased complaints of loneliness, of inability to sleep, and of decreased appetite."

Nursing Intervention

Nursing and medical interventions, if appropriate and timely, aid the body in returning to homeostatic balance, either to the same level or to a new "steady state," which may be irreversible but is still functional. Typically, reestablishing and maintaining a person's physiologic balance requires the provision of the necessary elements (e.g., nutrients, fluids, medications, rest, and psychologic support) for good health.

The person's circadian rhythms, which include the sleep-wakefulness pattern, should be taken into consideration when monitoring and evaluating BP, body temperature, and laboratory test results and when carrying out such interventions as client teaching or physical therapy. Disruptions of a person's circadian rhythms can be minimized by preventing sleep loss and sleep pattern irregularity, maintenance of a regular wake-up schedule, regular meal times, and time orientation.

Interventions for a nursing diagnosis of *Relocation Stress Syndrome* involve assisting the individual to cope with the move. Some helpful interventions include the following:

▶ assess the client's perception of the situation
▶ monitor physical and psychosocial responses to the situation
▶ identify the client's coping mechanisms
▶ establish a supportive, caring relationship with the client
▶ encourage the client to discuss feelings about the situation
▶ listen to and accept the client's feelings
▶ assist the client to look at alternative ways to cope with the situation
▶ refer the client to appropriate resources, as needed
▶ provide relaxation and comfort measures, such as a back rub
▶ teach the client general relaxation techniques

Evaluation

As with all interventions, evaluation for interventions planned to address *Relocation Stress Syndrome* means comparing actual to expected outcomes. To evaluate whether the individual has been able to adapt adequately to the new environment, you must look for evidence that the specific psychologic and/or physical symptoms experienced as part of the syndrome have been decreased or no longer exist. For example, when comparing the person with your baseline assessment, you may find that the person who previously complained of feeling lonely, being unable to sleep, and having a decreased appetite no longer voices such complaints. Instead, you may find that the person is engaging in satisfying social relationships in the new environment, has increased food consumption to normal levels, has regained lost weight, and is sleeping 8 full hours each night, as was the pattern before the relocation.

Summary

▶ Homeostasis is the maintenance of a relatively stable and constant dynamic equilibrium of the internal environment.
▶ Two major homeostatic regulators are the nervous system, primarily the autonomic nervous system, and the endocrine system, which work together as the neuroendocrine system.
▶ Psychologic equilibrium is manifested by feelings of positive self-image, emotional balance, and being in harmony with the environment; psychologic disequilibrium is manifested by negative self-perception and feeling out of step with the environment and with other people.
▶ To maintain physiologic homeostasis, the body must meet basic needs for oxygen, water, and nutrients. In addition, the body must be able to store certain nutrients and eliminate waste products and excess quantities of basic requirements.

▶ Homeostatic mechanisms are characterized by (1) being compensatory, (2) being self-regulatory, (3) being primarily negative feedback processes, (4) exhibiting some degree of deviation, (5) having limitations, and (6) working together in regulating a single physiologic process.
▶ Homeostatic mechanisms can be disrupted when the system is overdriven, is interrupted by illness, or completely breaks down as accelerated positive feedback ensues.
▶ Almost all physiologic variables exhibit a rhythm. Rhythms vary in frequency. Chronobiology is a field of study that may lead to improved understanding of disease, enhancing the accuracy of diagnostic testing and improving the treatment of disease.
▶ Biofeedback training involves educating an individual through feedback to become aware of and learn to control certain involuntary physiologic variables.
▶ Assessment of homeostasis involves the use of biologic, psychologic, social, and cultural measurements.
▶ There is no one specific nursing diagnosis that pertains only to homeostasis. An example of one nursing diagnosis that pertains to homeostasis is *Relocation Stress Syndrome*.
▶ The main outcome for the nursing diagnosis of *Relocation Stress Syndrome* is that the person adapts to (or adequately copes with) a new environment as evidenced by diminished psychologic or physical symptoms.
▶ Nursing interventions for a diagnosis of *Relocation Stress Syndrome* involve assisting the individual to cope with the move.
▶ To evaluate whether the individual with *Relocation Stress Syndrome* has been able to adapt adequately to the new environment, you must look for evidence that the specific psychologic and/or physical symptoms experienced as part of the syndrome have been decreased or no longer exist.

Bibliography

1. Aherne, G.W. (1989). An introduction to chronopharmacology. In Arendt, J., et al. (eds.). *Biological rhythms in clinical practice* (pp. 8–19). London: Wright.
2. Akerstedt, T. (1987). Sleep/work disturbances in working life. In Ellingson, R.J., et al. (eds.). *The London Symposia* (pp. 360–363). (EEG Suppl. 39.) New York: Elsevier Science.
3. Aschoff, J., & Wever, R. (1976). A multioscillatory system. *Federation Proceedings*, 35, 2326–2332.
4. Bernard, C. (1949). *An introduction to the study of experimental medicine.* (Translated by H.C. Greene.) New York: Henry Schulman, Inc.
5. Binkley, S. (1990). *The clockwork sparrow: Time, clocks, and calendars in biological organisms.* Englewood Cliffs, New Jersey: Prentice-Hall.
6. Campbell, I.T., et al. (1986). Are circadian rhythms important in intensive care? *Intensive Care Nursing*, 1, 144–150.
7. Cannon, W.B. (1967). *The wisdom of the body: Revised and enlarged edition.* New York: W.W. Norton and Company.
8. Conroy, R.T.W.L., & Mills, J.N. (1970). *Human circadian rhythms.* London: J. & A. Churchill.
9. De Bold, A.J. (1986). Atrial natriuretic factor: an overview. *Federation Proceedings*, 45, 2081–2085.
10. di Pietralata, M.M., et al. (eds.). (1990). Digestive disturbances in shift-workers: a clinical statistical investigation. In *Chronobiology:*

Its role in clinical medicine, general biology, and agriculture (pp. 369–377). New York: Wiley-Liss, Inc.

11. Ehret, C.F. (1981). New approaches to chronohygiene for the shift worker in the nuclear power industry. In Reinberg, A., (eds.). *Night- and shift-work. Biological and social aspects* (pp. 263–270). Oxford: Pergamon Press.

12. Felton, G. (1987). Human biologic rhythms. *Annual Review of Nursing Research*, 5, 45–77.

13. Goldstein, D.S. (1990). Neurotransmittors and stress. *Biofeedback and Self-Regulation*, 15(3), 243–271.

14. Guyton, A.C. (1991). Functional organization of the human body and control of the "internal environment." In *Textbook of medical physiology* (8th ed, pp. 2–8). Philadelphia: W.B. Saunders.

15. Harris, W. (1977). Fatigue, circadian rhythm, and truck accidents. In Mackie, R. (ed.). *Vigilance therapy, operational performance, and physiological correlates* (pp. 133–146). New York: Plenum Press.

16. Harris, R.B. (1990). Role of set-point in regulation of body weight. *FASEB Journal*, 4(15), 3310–3318.

17. Healy, D., & Williams, J.M.G. (1988). Dysrhythmia, dysphoria, and depression: the interaction of learned helplessness and circadian dysrhythmia in the pathogenesis of depression. *Psychological Bulletin*, 103, 163–178.

18. Houston, M.C. (1990). Pathophysiology of shock. *Critical Care Nursing Clinics of North America*, 2(2), 143–149.

19. Hrushesky, W.J.M. (1990). Cancer chronotherapy: A drug delivery challenge. In *Chronobiology: Its role in clinical medicine, general biology, and agriculture* (pp. 1–10). New York: Wiley-Liss, Inc.

20. Inagami, T. (1989). Atrial natriuretic factor. *Journal of Biological Chemistry*, 264(6), 3043–3046.

21. Kleitman, N. (1963). *Sleep and wakefulness*. Chicago: University of Chicago Press.

22. Koopman, M.G., et al. (1989). Urinary and renal circadian rhythms. In Arendt, J., et al. (eds.). *Biological rhythms in clinical practice* (pp. 83–98). London: Wright.

23. Langley, L.L. (1965). *Homeostasis*. New York: Van Nostrand Reinhold Company.

24. Lanuza, D.M. (1976). Circadian rhythms of mental efficiency and performance. *Nursing Clinics of North America*, 11, 569–638.

25. Lanuza, D.M. (1993). Circadian rhythm disorders. In Carrieri, V.K., et al. (eds.). *Pathophysiological phenomena in nursing: Human responses to illness* (2nd ed.). Philadelphia: W.B. Saunders.

26. Lanuza, D.M., et al. (1991). Blood pressure and heart rate circadian rhythm changes post cardiac transplantation. *Circulation*, 84(4), (Suppl.II), II-695.

27. Lanuza, D.M., & Marotta, S.F. (1976). Circadian and basal interrelationships of plasma cortisol and cations in women. *Aerospace Medicine*, 45, 864–868.

28. Lanuza, D.M., et al. (1989). Body temperature and heart rate rhythms in acutely head-injured patients. *Applied Nursing Research*, 2, 135–139.

29. Moore, R.Y. (1983). Organization and function of a central nervous system circadian oscillator: the suprachiasmatic hypothalamic nucleus. *Federation Proceedings*, 42, 2783–2789.

30. Moore-Ede, M.C. (1983). The circadian timing system in mammals: Two pacemakers preside over many secondary oscillators. *Federation Proceedings*, 42, 2801–2808.

31. Moore-Ede, M.C. (1986). Physiology of the circadian timing system: predictive versus reactive homeostasis. *American Journal of Physiology*, 250 (Regulatory Integrative Comparative Physiology 19), R735–R752.

32. Moore-Ede, M.C., et al. (1983). Circadian timekeeping in health and disease. Part II, Clinical implications of circadian rhythmicity. *New England Journal of Medicine*, 309, 530–536.

33. Moore-Ede, M.C., & Richardson, G.S. (1985). Medical implications of shift-work. *Annual Review of Medicine*, 36, 607–617.

34. Muller, J.E., et al. (1985). Circadian variation in the frequency of onset of acute myocardial infarction. *New England Journal of Medicine*, 313, 1315–1322.

35. Naitoh, P., et al. (1971). Psychophysiologic changes after prolonged deprivation of sleep. *Biological Psychiatry*, 3, 309.

36. Pickering, T.G. (1990). Diurnal rhythms and other sources of blood pressure variability in normal and hypertensive subjects. In Laragh, J.H., & Brenner, B.M. (eds.). *Pathophysiology, diagnosis, and management* (pp. 1397–1405). New York: Raven Press.

37. Rice, V. (1991). Shock, a clinical syndrome: an update. Part 1. An overview of shock. *Critical Care Nurse*, 11(4), 20–27.

38. Rosenberg, R.S. (1984). Aging and biological rhythms: complaints of insomnia in the elderly. In Hans, E., & Kabat, H. (eds.). *Chronobiology 1982–1988* (pp. 345–349). Paris: S. Karger.

39. Samples, J.F., et al. (1985). Circadian rhythms: Basis for screening for fever. *Nursing Research*, 34(6), 377–379.

40. Scheving, L.E. (1959). Mitotic activity in the human epidermis. *Anatomical Record*, 135, 7–14.

41. Smith, M.J. (1979). *Occupational injury rates among nurses as a function of shift schedule*. Washington, D.C.: National Institute for Occupational Safety and Health Publications.

42. Smolensky, M.H. (1983). Aspects of human chronopathology. In Reinberg, A., & Smolensky, M.H. (eds.). *Biological rhythms and medicine* (pp. 131–209). New York: Springer-Verlag.

43. Smolensky, M.H., & D'Alonzo, G.E. (1988). Biologic rhythms and medicine. *American Journal of Medicine*, 85, 34–36.

44. Smolensky, M.H., et al. (1976). Circadian rhythmic aspects of human cardiovascular function: a review by chronobiologic statistical methods. *Chronobiologia*, 3, 337–371.

45. Taub, J.M., & Berger, R.J. (1973). Performance and mood following variations in the length and timing of sleep. *Society for Psychophysiological Research*, 10, 559–570.

46. Van Cauter, E. (1989). Endocrine rhythms. In Arendt, J., et al. (eds.). *Biological rhythms in clinical practice* (pp. 23–49). London: Wright.

47. Verdecchia, P., et al. (1990). Circadian blood pressure changes and left ventricular hypertrophy in essential hypertension. *Circulation*, 81, 528–536.

48. Zolten, A.J. (1989). Constructive integration of learning theory and phenomenological approaches to biofeedback training. *Biofeedback & Self-Regulation*, 14(2): 89–99.

The Family

No matter how many communes anybody invents, the family always creeps back.

Margaret Mead

▼ CHAPTER OUTLINE

FAMILY DIVERSITY
FAMILY-CENTERED CARE
FRAMEWORKS FOR UNDERSTANDING
   THE FAMILY
      General Systems Theory
      Structural-Functional Theory
      Developmental Theory
      Nursing Theories

THE FAMILY IN HEALTH AND ILLNESS
   Health Promotion and Maintenance
   Impact of Illness on the Family
ASSESSMENT
NURSING DIAGNOSIS
PLANNING
NURSING INTERVENTION
EVALUATION

▼ KEY TERMS

Blended family
Extended family

Family
Nuclear family

Single-parent family

The discipline of nursing defines the **family** as the basic social unit in which human behavior occurs in relation to health.

The basic family unit is composed of individuals who continuously interact with each other and with an environment that includes other persons. From a nursing perspective, the major goal of the family is to seek, maintain, and restore health for members of the family unit. The family seeks, maintains, and restores health through adaptation to environmental influences on health and illness. Nursing views the family as a unit with the capacity for change and growth toward optimal health status.

The family may be the *context* for nursing care provided to an individual, or the family as a whole may be the *unit* of care. Throughout its history, nursing practice has promoted caring for individuals within the context of their families. Nurses who are educated as generalists are taught to care for individuals within a family context. Selected graduate nursing education programs prepare nurses for advanced practice roles in which nursing care is provided to the family as a unit. For example, master's programs in psychiatric mental health nursing prepare nurse specialists to care for family units with interpersonal problems requiring family therapy. This chapter focuses on the family as the context for nursing care of individuals.

FAMILY DIVERSITY

Nurses recognize that there is a great diversity of family types in the United States. Men and women who live together may or may not be married and may or may not have children. Single adults may be heads of households composed of children and grandparents. Divorce and remarriage may reconstitute non–blood-related adults and children into new family units. Gay and lesbian adult couples may be parents to their own biologic children from previous heterosexual marriages, or they may adopt children.[1]

Many different family compositions exist in American culture. A **nuclear family** consists of a husband and wife and their biologic children. In contrast, a **blended family** consists of a husband and wife who have children from previous marriages and their own biologic children who all live together. Traditionally, an **extended family** consists of husband, wife, children, grandparents, and other blood relatives such as aunts, uncles, and cousins who live together. Although extended families do not live together as frequently as in the past, they do still provide emotional support, child care, and financial assistance for family members.

Single-parent families (families of one or more children headed by only one parent) are more common today than in the past, as 50 per cent of children in the United States will live with only one parent for some part of their lives. Most commonly in the past, a single-parent family resulted from death, desertion, or divorce. Currently, unmarried women have the option to choose artificial insemination to experience pregnancy and bring children into their lives. Women who choose this method to become pregnant and bear children as single parents are commonly over age 35 years and have established careers and secure incomes. In contrast, teenage mothers constitute a growing percentage of single parents in the United States. Teen pregnancy is associated with poverty, lack of social support, and poor pregnancy outcomes.

Gay and lesbian couples desire to be recognized as families. These couples have sought to have their marriages and family status recognized by religious groups, business, and government. Currently, gay and lesbian couples seek medical and other benefits for each other, like the benefits extended to heterosexual married couples.

Nursing also recognizes that different cultural backgrounds influence family adaptation in health and illness. The two largest minority groups in the United States are African-American and Hispanic families. Studies of African-American families have reported the existence of strong extended family relationships, involvement with church, and shared parenting by mothers and fathers.[17] In Hispanic families, individualism is secondary to family concerns; extended families are highly cohesive, and religion is important as a coping resource.[6] These family characteristics may serve to support African-American and Hispanic family members in times of illness. Conversely, poverty and related inadequate health care for many in these minority groups may impose special health problems. For example, a proportionately higher number of low birthweight infants are born to African-American families.[16]

FAMILY-CENTERED CARE

A nursing perspective of the family includes an understanding of the philosophy of family-centered care. This philosophy is based on the premise that the family unit affects the care, treatment, and recovery of both physical and mental illness for its members. While nursing care is most often focused on the individual, it is important to recognize that there is a family response to the health or illness needs of family members. The family's response must be considered when providing care to an individual family member. For example, immunization for a child is a health-promoting behavior. When the family is unable or unwilling to comply with the recommended immunizations, intervention with adult family members is required.

Putting a philosophy of family-centered care into practice requires that the nurse view both the individual and the individual's family members as legitimate recipients of nursing care.

During hospitalization of an individual child, adult, or older person, family members have a need for information about the individual's illness and treatment, access through visitation, and the opportunity to participate in care of their loved one. For example, family members provide the majority of home care to dependent older persons in the United States and Canada.[9,32] When hospitalization occurs for these dependent persons, the focus of care must be on both the older persons and their family caregiver. Because these older persons are dependent on their family caregivers, it is essential to exchange information with the caregivers to provide for continuity in care after hospital discharge.

FRAMEWORKS FOR UNDERSTANDING THE FAMILY

To understand families and integrate this information into nursing care for individuals, it is helpful if nurses have a working knowledge of the theoretical frameworks for study of the family. The most commonly used frameworks for family study include general systems, structural-functional, and developmental theories. Selected nursing theorists have also addressed the family.

To help in your understanding of each of these theories, it may be helpful to consider the Cox family. The Cox family is a traditional nuclear family. Mr. Larry Cox is a 41-year-old African-American engineer who is married and has two children. His 41-year-old wife works as a substitute elementary school teacher. His 14-year-old daughter's major interest is her horse, which is boarded at a local stable. Mrs. Cox drives her daughter to the stable every day after school. Mr. Cox's 10-year-old son is involved in baseball and soccer, and Mr. Cox coaches both sports. Mr. Cox's mother is a retired widow who lives independently in her own home about 5 miles from her son. Mr. Cox has two adult brothers who also live in the same community. Mrs. Cox's parents are retired and active and also live in the same community as the Cox family. Mr. Cox has been treated for hypertension since graduation from college at age 22 years. Recently, his physician diagnosed Mr. Cox with diabetes mellitus and admitted him to the local hospital for stabilization on insulin and for diabetic teaching.

General Systems Theory

General systems theory defines family as an open system, a unit of goal-directed and interacting parts.[4] Open systems are constantly being stimulated by and reacting to environmental stimuli. The environment includes those factors outside the family system.

The goal is for the family system to adapt to its environment.

For adaptation to occur, the family system's boundaries must be open. Open boundaries allow for family members to interact and exchange information with the community outside the family. Systems theory focuses on adaptation and system maintenance. Using a systems theoretical framework, the family with an ill family member is viewed as an open system interacting with the health care system, reacting and adapting to information and intervention from health care providers.

For example, as a family system, Mr. Cox and his wife have accepted reading material on diabetes mellitus from Mr. Cox's nurse. The nurse encourages them to read the information and ask questions. Mr. and Mrs. Cox share with each other the feeling that the nurse seems to recognize their worry and lack of knowledge about diabetes, and they plan to discuss some questions with her. In this example, the Cox family system is opening the boundaries to the nurse and trying to adapt to the new diagnosis of diabetes mellitus through acquisition of knowledge.

Structural-Functional Theory

Structural-functional theory defines the family as a societal institution.[30] Examples of other societal institutions are educational, governmental, economic, and religious. The structure of a family refers to the composite of family members and how their positions or roles are defined. Family structure for a traditional nuclear family includes husband-father, wife-mother, son-brother, and daughter-sister. Traditional family functions include provision of economic resources, reproduction, socialization of children, and meeting affective needs for family members.

The goal is for the family to contribute to the maintenance of society by fulfilling its functions.

Within a structural-functional framework, illness of one family member would present a threat to family unit maintenance. Illness would require changes in role functions to accomplish family unit maintenance if the ill family member was not able to fulfill the usual role activities.

For example, while Mr. Cox is in the hospital, Mrs. Cox has to do the yard work that Mr. Cox usually took care of on a regular basis. She delegates mowing the lawn to their son and cleaning the pool to their daughter. Mrs. Cox also is finding it more difficult to please her mother-in-law. Grandmother Cox no longer drives and Mr. Cox's routine had been to stop by her house every day. Her mother-in-law has taken to telephoning her and complaining about being neglected since her son is in the hospital. Mrs. Cox is stressed by the demands of trying to work, visit her mother-in-law, take care of her children, and visit her husband in the hospital. In this example, Mrs. Cox is experiencing some success and some stress as she tries to adapt her role to take on role functions usually fulfilled by Mr. Cox.

Developmental Theory

Developmental theory describes the family as it develops through several stages in its own life cycle.[13] The family life cycle begins with marriage, and subsequent stages are identified as families with young children, school-age children, and adolescents; children leaving the family; retirement; and death. This theory assumes that all adults marry and have children.

At each stage, the family has tasks it must accomplish in order to proceed through the life cycle.

For example, it is a family task that adult children leave the family and start their own families. Using a developmental framework, the family with an ill adult child may become arrested at the particular stage in the life cycle when adult children are expected to leave the parental home. That is, an adult child who has a life-threatening physical illness, chronic illness, or mental illness may remain dependent on the family and not be able to leave the family and live independently.

In the Cox family example, their developmental stage is the family with school-age children. One of many family developmental tasks during this period is maintaining family ties with relatives. During Mr. Cox's hospitalization, Mrs. Cox requests that one of Mr. Cox's brothers visit his mother every day. She asks her own parents to stay with her children in the evenings when she visits her husband in the hospital. In this way, she not only maintains family ties but also uses relatives to support her during this time of stress.

Nursing Theories

Nursing theories were developed with a primary focus on the individual. While they are not specifically family theories, selected nurse theorists have addressed the family (Table 18–1).

NEUMAN'S CONCEPT OF THE FAMILY

Neuman defines the family as a system within society.[29]

The goal is for the family system to maintain itself in an optimal state of health.

Nursing's role is to intervene to reduce stressors related to the family's health status. Applying Neuman's concept in the example of the Cox family, the nurse would try to reduce stress related to Mr. Cox's new diagnosis of diabetes mellitus by providing education to the family about the illness and its management. The nurse might provide education through the provision of written information, discussion, and answering questions about diabetes mellitus.

ROY'S CONCEPT OF THE FAMILY

Roy defines the family as an adaptive system.[35] Stimuli from individual family members' needs and from the

TABLE 18–1. Nursing Theories Applied to the Study of Families

Theorist	Definition of Family	Goal for Family
Neuman	A system within society	For the family system to maintain itself in an optimum state of health
Roy	An adaptive system	To promote family system adaptation toward "survival, continuity, and growth"
King	A social system	For the family to influence individuals in growth and development and in progressing from dependence in childhood to interdependence in adulthood
Rogers	An energy field in continuous process with environmental fields	For family maintenance and promotion of family well-being through restructuring of family and environmental fields

external environment have an impact on the family system. The family system internally processes input through "supporting, nurturing, and socializing."

The goal is to promote family system adaptation toward "survival, continuity, and growth."

The nurse's role is to participate with the family in processing and adapting to stimuli affecting the family system. Applying the Roy concept to the example of the Cox family, the nurse listens to Mrs. Cox talk about how "difficult" her mother-in-law has been because Mr. Cox cannot visit her every day since he has been hospitalized. The nurse helps her plan strategies for dealing with the family stresses, such as asking what other family members might also visit Mr. Cox's mother, at least for the time that he is hospitalized.

KING'S CONCEPT OF THE FAMILY

King defines the family as a social system and an interpersonal system of interacting individuals.[24]

The goal for the family is to influence individuals in growth and development, and in progressing from dependence in childhood to interdependence in adulthood.

Nursing's role is to assist families through nurse-family interactions that clarify and provide information necessary for goal setting and problem resolution related to family health. Applying King's concept to the Cox family example, the nurse meets with Mr. and Mrs. Cox to discuss and plan for necessary changes in their lifestyle related to diabetes mellitus. As the nurse reviews dietary guidelines related to diabetes mellitus, the Coxes identify the importance of regular, well-balanced meals in diabetic management. They verbalize that their current lifestyle practices such as skipping meals and not having regular meal times are areas they will need to change.

ROGERS' CONCEPT OF THE FAMILY

Rogers defines the family as an energy field in continuous process with environmental fields.[34] She views the family as an irreducible whole that cannot be understood solely by knowledge about the individual family members.

The goal of the family is maintenance and promotion of family well-being through restructuring of family and environmental fields.

An application of Rogers' concept to the Cox family example would have the nurse consider the family's well-being and assist the family members to plan how they might, for example, increase their time for exercise by sharing activities they enjoy.

THE FAMILY IN HEALTH AND ILLNESS

Health Promotion and Maintenance

As the basic social unit in which health behaviors occur, the family may foster or hinder health promoting behaviors.[37] Family lifestyle practices related to nutrition, exercise, and sleep habits directly influence individual family members. For example, an obese family member wishing to lose weight will be much more successful if the family member responsible for food shopping and preparation is knowledgeable and willing to provide the low calorie diet[36] and if other family members support the desire to change.

Whether family members receive preventive medical and dental care depends on family resources and attitudes.[26] Enough money is needed if a family is to take advantage of preventive health care services. Adult family members must value and be knowledgeable about the benefits of preventive health practices, such as cleaning of teeth or screening for hypertension, in order for the family to participate in these practices.

Nursing practice addresses health promotion for the family in hospital, community, and home settings. Nurses may provide health screening services and provide education about health-promoting behaviors. For example, school nurses might provide information to parents and children about prevention of substance abuse. In a clinic or physician's office, the nurse might teach family members how to take a blood pressure measurement in order to monitor a hypertensive family member in the home.

Impact of Illness on the Family

When a family has a member with a serious illness or a member undergoing a major surgery, all family members may experience anxiety and stress. Research has documented this experience as similar for families whose members have had cardiac surgery,[18] myocardial infarction,[3] and cancer.[8]

The stress and anxiety of serious illness is exacerbated by hospitalization of the ill member. Family members worry about the severity of the illness and the suffering and possible death of their family member.[21] As a result of these worries, family members report feelings of fear, helplessness, vulnerability, uncertainty, frustration, and depression.[25,41] Responses from family members of hospitalized adults include needs for information about their hospitalized family member's condition, reassurance that the person is receiving high-quality care, and hope for the family member's recovery.[27,33] There is much evidence that parents of hospitalized children suffer significantly from stress and anxiety.[14,23,42] Further, mothers' anxieties may be transmitted to their hospitalized children.[22] A study of siblings of hospitalized children found their stress manifested as feeling deprived of parental time and having decreased food intake, nervousness, and trouble with concentration.[10]

Nursing practice that incorporates a philosophy of family-centered care can do much to allay the anxieties of family members of hospitalized individuals. Consideration of family members' worries and needs are legitimate nursing activities. The nurse, for example, might assist a mother to remain in her child's hospital room throughout the night. You can often help most just by listening and caring.

Families who have a member with a chronic illness experience stress related to diagnosis, special care needs, and long-term management. On receiving a diagnosis of a chronic or life-threatening illness for a child, parents and grandparents may respond with shock, disbelief, and denial.[39]

The special care needs and long-term management for chronically ill children have significant effects on their families, including increased time and energy expenditure for physical care, decreased time for leisure activities, isolation, and fear of complications or equipment failure.[2,11,12] Career advancement may be curtailed for many parents because additional time must be spent with the child at the expense of work. Parents also report that they spend less time with and pay less attention to their healthy children. Repeated and extended hospitalizations for children with long-term disabilities are stressful and anxiety-provoking for their parents.[19] A financial burden may result from extended hospitalization and continuous medical expenses related to the care of children with special needs and chronic illnesses.[2,22,28]

Less study has been done of chronic illness in adults and how this affects the family. Spouses of chronically ill adults have responded with depression, anxiety over role changes in the marital relationship, and guilt.[15,38] Families who provided home care for a relative with cancer were stressed by physical care requirements and fears for their family member.[20] Children of chronically ill adults with multiple sclerosis have evidenced feelings of lower family cohesiveness and higher conflict among family members.[31]

Because persons live longer today after the onset of chronic disease, adult children provide more home care to elderly parents. This care is most often provided by daughters and daughters-in-law. Providing this care affects the caregiver and her family. Research has shown that individual caregivers may suffer depression, anxiety, frustration, and exhaustion. The family unit experiences disruption in lifestyle, privacy, and income.[5] Family responses to chronic illness are similar, regardless of whether the chronically ill individual is a child, spouse, or older person.

Nursing practice addresses family management of chronically ill individuals. Nursing activities involve teaching special care procedures, making referrals for support services, helping obtain equipment, and providing emotional support. These nursing activities occur in a variety of settings, including acute care hospitals, long-term facilities, and client homes.

ASSESSMENT

Assessment information needed about a family includes noting the composition of the family (including which family members live together), the quality of their relationships, and the health status of family members. The nurse often will obtain family information from one individual. The person who gives information about the family may be the individual receiving nursing care or another member of the family.

Composition of a family can be determined by asking a question such as, "Who are the members of your family?" Once this has been determined, a follow-up question might be "Of these persons you identify as your family, who lives together?" To assist in understanding the relationship among family members, the nurse, as a routine part of family assessment, draws a genogram (Figure 18–1). A genogram is a family tree diagram that clearly depicts family relationships and major health problems over three or more generations. The nurse might also ask, "How does your family get along together?" and "Are you satisfied with how you and your family get along?" Issues about family health can be approached with a question such as "Does anyone in your family have health problems or illnesses?" (See Chapter 33, "Health Assessment," for a list of body systems that can be reviewed to help the person recall family health problems.) The responses to these questions provide the nurse with information about family structure, functioning, satisfaction, and members' health.

As an example of how the nurse begins to assess a family, let us consider the family of Mrs. Bessie Mueller. The nurse calls Mrs. Bessie Mueller into an examining room in Medical Clinic. The nurse notes the following information on Mrs. Mueller's medical record: white, female, 86 years old, widowed, diagnosed 5 years ago with progressive Alzheimer's disease, and lives with a daughter. The nurse settles Mrs. Mueller into an examining room and asks her the purpose of her visit. Mrs. Mueller does not respond. Her 55-year-old daughter, Mrs. Mary Fields, tells the nurse her mother is here ". . . to have her blood checked and get a prescription refilled." A nursing assistant takes Mrs. Mueller to the laboratory to obtain a blood specimen.

During the time Mrs. Mueller is gone from the room, the nurse talks with Mrs. Fields. The nurse asks who the other members in the family are. Mrs. Fields responds that she has been divorced for 20 years and that her father, Mr. Mueller, died 30 years ago. Her 25-year-old unmarried daughter, her mother, and she live together in her house. The nurse asks how well they get along together. Mrs. Fields starts to cry and tells the nurse that it is difficult to deal with her mother as she is increasingly disoriented and she can no longer be left alone. Mrs. Fields says, "I have to find some help." In talking with Mrs. Fields, the nurse has begun to assess the family composition, role responsibilities, and family satisfaction.

NURSING DIAGNOSIS

Nursing diagnoses related to families address family functioning and coping (e.g., *Altered Family Processes, Ineffective Family Coping: Disabling; Ineffective Family Coping: Compromised;* and *Family Coping: Potential*

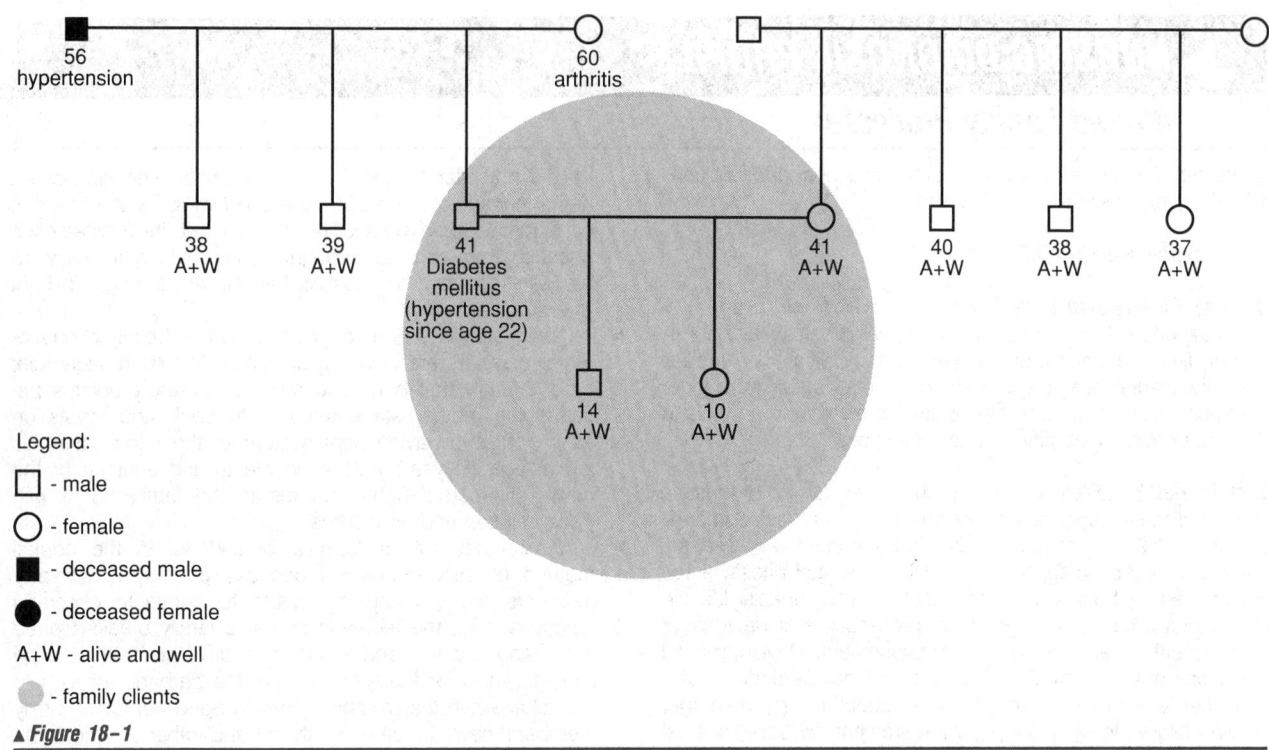

Legend:

☐ - male

○ - female

■ - deceased male

● - deceased female

A+W - alive and well

⬤ - family clients

▲ *Figure 18–1*

The Cox family genogram.

for Growth). Families may display dysfunctional behavior due to illness, unique life circumstances, or developmental transitions. Family dysfunction may be a temporary or a chronic situation. See the Nursing Diagnosis Profile for a discussion of *Altered Family Processes*.

In the Fields-Mueller example, the family's diagnosis would be *Altered Family Process R/T* the stresses of progressive illness in a family member. Specifically, the increasing dependence of Mrs. Mueller on her daughter has altered their former relationship. Mrs. Fields now finds herself in a caregiver role for her mother. The intensity of this new 24-hour caregiver responsibility is causing psychologic and social stress for Mrs. Fields, who has little patience with her mother. Her mother is responding by withdrawing more than usual.

PLANNING

After a family nursing diagnosis has been identified, the nurse works with the family to define expected outcomes. These should help resolve any expressed family problems or needs.

The nurse's role is to ensure that family members talk together and come to agreement on expected outcomes.

Strategies to achieve these outcomes must also be mutually agreed upon in order to help ensure success.

In the Fields-Mueller family example, the nurse helps Mrs. Fields explore options for help in caring for her mother. Their planning results in two possible options that Mrs. Fields agrees to try. First, Mrs. Fields will discuss with her daughter the possibility of the daughter providing supervision for her grandmother one hour each evening so Mrs. Fields can take a "time out." Second, Mrs. Fields' church provides visitors to "shut-ins," and she will try to arrange for one of the visitors to stay with her mother a few hours every week so she can get out of the house. The expected outcome is that, with help caring for her mother, Mrs. Fields will state that she feels less stressed and better able to function.

NURSING INTERVENTION

As discussed in the Family-Centered Care section, nursing interventions related to families include more than providing nursing care to an ill family member. The nurse must respond to the needs of the family as a whole. The nurse may be instrumental in bringing family members together to work on family issues. Nursing interventions often include physical care, emotional support, education, and referral.

In the case of the Fields-Mueller family, nursing interventions that help reduce stress include support, provision of information about resources, and referral. Support is accomplished by listening and helping Mrs. Fields problem-solve about how to care for her mother and still have some time for herself. The nurse offers support to Mrs. Fields by listening to her and by responding, "This must be very difficult for you." The

NURSING DIAGNOSIS PROFILE

Altered Family Processes

Definition. The state in which a family that normally functions effectively experiences a dysfunction

Classification. Relating 3.2.2

Defining Characteristics. A family may exhibit temporary dysfunction when it is unable to meet the physical, emotional, and/or financial needs of its members. Additionally, families who experience temporary dysfunction may suffer from poor communication, may lack the ability to express feelings, and may be unable to identify and use resources.[7]

Sample Related Factors. Factors that alter family processes include disease, special life circumstances, or developmental transitions. When a family member is confronted with disease, the result may be diagnosis of a chronic or fatal illness, surgical or medical treatments, and hospitalization. Special life circumstances that may alter family processes include loss of employment, death, divorce, or imprisonment. Developmental transitions also alter family processes and include addition of a new family member through birth, adoption, or marriage; grown children leaving home; and retirement. Disease, special life circumstances, or developmental transitions may interfere with the physical, emotional, and financial well-being for all family members.

Concept Description. Altered family processes are temporary dysfunctions in how family members relate to one another, enact their roles, and function within the family. The existence of the aforementioned related factors may place stress on family members and change how they relate to one another, resulting in poor communication or conflict. Family members may be physically or emotionally unable to fulfill their family roles, such as going to work or caring for children. When a family member's functioning is temporarily impaired, all other family members are affected. Some causes of altered family processes may result in positive adaptation, such as to the birth of a new baby. Other causes of altered family processes, such as imprisonment, may invoke stress for family members. Adaptation in this case may be more difficult and cause prolonged distress in the family.

Examples. Depending on the specific assessment data, this diagnostic category would be applicable in the following situations, among others:

▶ A family in which members who usually communicate well are now failing to communicate clearly because of some stress on the family system; e.g., two family members stop speaking to each other after they argue over who should be invited to a wedding; a young wife accuses her husband of not loving her now that she is pregnant because he did not offer to take her out to dinner (she did not tell him she wanted to go but expected him to "just know it"); or a middle-aged couple fail to iron out their differences because their son has brought home a daughter-in-law to live with them and the husband is refusing to "fight in front of a stranger."

▶ A family that is failing to attain its goals because one or more members are unwilling or unable to fulfill a usual role; e.g., a family that begins to suffer monetary problems because the mother starts refusing to cook and insists on eating out and having parties catered; the father loses his job at age 50 years and is unable to find another; or the newly divorced daughter returns to the family home with three children and no income.

▶ A family that suffers from a breakdown in the normal method of daily operations because one or more family members are unwilling or unable to complete expected functions; e.g., the teen-age son in a family breaks his leg in a skiing accident and is unable to drive his mother to the store to shop for food, to take out the garbage, or to help his father when the plumbing gets stopped up. Other family members have to take on these and other functions he usually tends to, and they also have to help him until he is able to get around better.

Related/Similar Nursing Diagnoses. Several nursing diagnoses might be confused with the diagnosis of *Altered Family Processes*. These similar diagnoses include *Ineffective Family Coping: Compromised*; *Ineffective Family Coping: Disabling*; *Family Coping: Potential for Growth*; and *Altered Parenting*. Carpenito recommends the use of the diagnosis *Altered Family Processes* in lieu of *Ineffective Family Coping: Compromised* and *Family Coping: Potential for Growth* until nursing research can validate and differentiate the Family Coping diagnoses from the Family Processes diagnosis.[7] Currently, there is overlap in the related factors for these diagnoses.

However, a clear distinction can be made between *Altered Family Processes* and *Ineffective Family Coping: Disabled*. *Ineffective Family Coping: Disabled* is applicable when a family member's response to stress results in abuse or neglect within the family. The factors that trigger such ineffective coping responses may arise from substance abuse or psychiatric disorders. When ineffective family coping occurs within a family, the result may be bodily harm or psychologic trauma to one or more family members and legal arrest and/or imprisonment for the abuser (e.g., *Ineffective Family Coping* R/T wife abuse). The diagnosis of *Altered Parenting* is similar to *Altered Family Processes* but specifically focuses on a parent's temporary inability to provide physical, emotional, or financial support for the development and nurturing of a child or children (e.g., *Altered Parenting* R/T recent divorce).

---

nurse shares information about community resources by telling Mrs. Fields of a local retirement center that has a day program for persons with Alzheimer's disease. Mrs. Fields expresses an interest in the program and the nurse gives her the name and telephone number of the director. The nurse asks Mrs. Fields if a community health nurse could visit and talk with her, her daughter, and mother. Mrs. Fields expresses appreciation for this suggestion, and the nurse completes the referral.

EVALUATION

When the nurse includes family members in nursing care, it is important to evaluate individual as well as family outcomes. In evaluating the interventions with the Fields-Mueller family, the nurse provides follow-up with Mrs. Fields. Two weeks following Mrs. Mueller's clinic visit, the nurse telephones Mrs. Fields to evaluate how she is managing. Mrs. Fields reports that her daughter is giving her an hour of "time out" every evening except Friday and Saturday nights when she dates her steady boyfriend. The church "shut-in" visitors are going to visit Mrs. Mueller every Sunday afternoon for 2 hours. Mrs. Fields has not yet contacted the Alzheimer's program but tells the nurse that she will within the next week. Mrs. Fields reports that the public health nurse visited once and that it was ". . . so good to have someone to talk with who understands Alzheimer's." She reports that, because she feels less stress, she has more patience with her mother, and her mother seems to respond better to everyone.

Summary

▶ There is a great diversity of family types in the United States. Examples include the nuclear family, blended family, extended family, and single-parent family.

▶ Family-centered care requires that the nurse view the individual and family members as legitimate recipients of nursing care.

▶ The nurse may be helped to understand families by having a working knowledge of various theoretical frameworks that relate to families. Major frameworks include general systems theory, structural-functional theory, developmental theory, and several nursing theories.

▶ Family behaviors can affect the health of each family member, and an illness of an individual family member can have an impact on the rest of the family.

▶ Family assessment should provide information about the family's structure, functioning, satisfaction, and members' health.

▶ Nursing diagnoses related to families address family functioning and family coping.

▶ The nurse works with the family to help members define expected outcomes.

▶ Family nursing interventions often include support, provision of information about resources, and referrals.

▶ It is important to evaluate individual as well as family outcomes expected.

Bibliography

1. Adams, B.N. (1988). Fifty years of family research. *Journal of Marriage and the Family,* 50(1), 5–18.
2. Aradine, C. (1978). Development of toddlers with long-term tracheostomies (Doctoral Dissertation, University of Michigan, 1978). *Dissertation Abstracts International,* 39, 48098.
3. Bramwell, L., & Whall, A. (1986). Effect of role clarity and empathy on support role performance and anxiety. *Nursing Research,* 35, 282–287.
4. Broderick, C., & Smith, J. (1979). The general systems approach to the family. In Burr, W.R., et al. (eds.). *Contemporary theories about the family* (Vol. 2, pp. 112–129). New York: Free Press.
5. Brody, J. (1985). Parent care as normative family stress. *Gerontologist,* 25, 19–28.
6. Carillo, C. (1982). Changing norms of Hispanic families; implications for treatment. In Jones, E.E., & Korchin, S.J. (eds.). *Minority mental health.* New York: Praeger.
7. Carpenito, L.J. (1992). *Nursing diagnosis; Application to clinical practice* (4th ed.). Philadelphia: J.B. Lippincott.
8. Cassileth, B.R., et al. (1986). Factors associated with psychological distress in cancer patients. *Medical and Pediatric Oncology,* 14, 251–254.
9. Chappell, N.L. (1991). Living arrangements and sources of caregiving. *Journal of Gerontology,* 46(1), 51–58.
10. Craft, M.J., et al. (1985). Behavior and feeling changes in siblings of hospitalized children. *Clinical Pediatrics,* 24(7), 374–378.
11. Deatrick, J., & Knalf, K.A. (1990). Management behaviors: day-to-day adjustments to childhood chronic conditions. *Journal of Pediatric Nursing,* 5(1), 15–22.
12. Deatrick, J., et al. (1988). The process of parenting a child with a disability: normalization through accommodations. *Journal of Advanced Nursing,* 13, 15–21.
13. Duvall, E.M. (1977). *Family development* (5th ed.). Philadelphia: J.B. Lippincott.
14. Eberly, T.W., et al. (1985). Parental stress after the unexpected admission of a child to the intensive care unit. *Critical Care Quarterly,* 8(1), 57–65.
15. Ekberg, J., et al. (1986). Spouse burnout syndrome. *Journal of Advanced Nursing,* 11, 161–165.
16. Epstein, M. (1987). Major causes of neonatal mortality and morbidity. In Taeusch, H.W., & Yogman, M.W. (eds.). *Follow-up management of the high risk infant* (pp. 15–20). Boston: Little, Brown.
16a. Fielding, J.E., & Williams, C.A. (1991). Adolescent pregnancy in the United States: a review and recommendations for clinicians and research needs. *American Journal of Preventive Medicine* 7 (1), 47–52.
17. Friedman, M.M. (1990). Transcultural family nursing: application to Latino and Black families. In Bell, J.M., et al. (eds.). *The cutting edge of family nursing* (pp. 51–65). Calgary, Alberta, Canada: Family Nursing Unit Publications.
18. Gortner, S.R., et al. (1985). After cardiac surgery: monitoring recovery by telephone. American Heart Association Abstracts No. 389. *Circulation,* 72(4), III-98.
19. Hayes, V., & Knox, J. (1984). The experience of stress in parents of children hospitalized with long-term disabilities. *Journal of Advanced Nursing,* 9(4): 333–341.
20. Hinds, C. (1985). The needs of families who care for patients with cancer at home: are we meeting them? *Journal of Advanced Nursing,* 10(6), 575–581.
21. Hodovanic, B.H., et al. (1984). Family crisis intervention program in the medical intensive care unit. *Heart and Lung,* 13, 243–249.
22. Jacobs, P., & McDermott, S. (1989). Family caregiver costs of chronically ill and handicapped children: method and literature review. *Public Health Reports,* 104, 158–163.
23. Kidder, C. (1989). Reestablishing health: factors influencing the child's recovery in pediatric intensive care. *Journal of Pediatric Nursing,* 4, 96–103.
24. King, I. (1983). King's theory of nursing. In Clements, I.W., & Roberts, F.B. (eds.). *Family health: A theoretical approach to nursing care* (pp. 177–188). New York: John Wiley & Sons.
25. King, S.L., & Gregor, F.M. (1985). Stress and coping in families of the critically ill. *Critical Care Nurse,* 5, 48–51.
26. Kviz, F., et al. (1985). Mothers' health beliefs and use of well-baby services among a high risk population. *Research in Nursing and Health,* 8, 381–387.
27. Mathis, M. (1984). Personal needs of family members of critically ill patients with and without brain injury. *Journal of Neurosurgical Nursing,* 16, 37–44.
28. McCain, G.C. (1990). Parenting growing preterm infants. *Pediatric Nursing,* 16, 467–470.
29. Neuman, B. (1983). Neuman's theory of nursing. In Clements, I.W., & Roberts, F.B. (eds.). *Family health: A theoretical ap-*

proach to nursing care (pp. 239–254). New York: John Wiley & Sons.

30. Parsons, T., & Bales, R.F. (1955). *Family, socialization, and interaction process*. Glencoe, IL: Free Press.
31. Peters, L.C., & Esses, L.M. (1985). Family environment as perceived by children with a chronically ill parent. *Journal of Chronic Diseases*, 38(4), 301–308.
32. Phillips, L.R. (1989). Elder-family caregiver relationships. *Nursing Clinics of North America*, 24(3), 795–807.
33. Price, D.M., et al. (1991). Critical care needs in an urban teaching medical center. *Heart and Lung*, 20, 183–188.
34. Rogers, M. (1983). Neuman's theory of nursing. In Clements, I.W., & Roberts, F.B. (eds.). *Family health: A theoretical approach to nursing care* (pp. 219–228). New York: John Wiley & Sons.
35. Roy, C. (1983). Roy's theory of nursing. In Clements, I.W., & Roberts, F.B. (eds.). *Family health: A theoretical approach to nursing care* (pp. 255–278). New York: John Wiley & Sons.
36. Saltzer, E., & Golden, M. (1985). Obesity in lower and middle socioeconomic status mothers and their children. *Research in Nursing and Health*, 8, 147–153.
37. Schwenk, T., & Hughes, C. (1983). The family as patient in family medicine: rhetoric or reality? *Social Science Medicine*, 17, 1–16.
38. Sexton, D., & Munro, B. (1985). Impact of a husband's chronic illness (COPD) on the spouse's life. *Research in Nursing and Health*, 8, 83–90.
39. Shapiro, J. (1983). Family reactions and coping strategies in response to the physically ill or handicapped child: a review. *Social Science Medicine*, 17, 913–931.
40. Stryker, S. (1964). The interactional and situational approaches. In Christensen, H. (ed.). *Handbook of marriage and the family* (pp. 125–171). Chicago: Rand McNally & Co.
41. Titler, M.G., et al. (1991). Impact of adult critical care hospitalization. Perceptions of patients, spouses, children, and nurses. *Heart and Lung*, 20, 174–182.
42. Wyckoff, P.M., & Erickson, M.T. (1987). Mediating factors of stress on mothers of seriously ill hospitalized children. *Children's Health Care*, 16, 4–12.

Chapter 19

▼ # Culture and Ethnicity

We hold these truths to be self-evident, that all men are created equal, that they are endowed by their Creator with certain inalienable Rights, that among these are Life, Liberty and the pursuit of Happiness.

The Declaration of Independence
July 4, 1776

▼ ## CHAPTER OUTLINE

CULTURE
    Material Culture and Nonmaterial
      Culture
    Socialization
    Subcultures
    Acculturation
    Assimilation
    Cultural Sensitivity and
      Stereotyping
ETHNICITY
    Ethnic Pluralism
    Behavioral Ethnicity
    Ideologic Ethnicity
    Intraethnic Variations
    Ethnocentrism
    Ethnic Conflicts
RACE
    Differentiation Among Racial
      Groups
    Race as a Legal-Cultural
      Phenomenon
    Race as an Economic Phenomenon
    Race as a Political Phenomenon
    Racial Prejudice
MINORITY STATUS

SOCIAL CLASS
DIFFERENTIAL HEALTH STATUS AMONG
  CULTURAL, ETHNIC, AND RACIAL
  GROUPS
    Chronic Diseases
    Mortality Rates
    Excess Mortality
    Life Expectancy
    Mental Disorders
    Suicide
VARIATIONS IN HEALTH BEHAVIORS
  AMONG CULTURAL, ETHNIC, AND
  RACIAL GROUPS
    Help-Seeking Processes
    Use of Mental Health Services
    Access to Health Services
MANAGING CULTURAL, ETHNIC, AND
  RACIAL DIFFERENCES
    Self-awareness
    Cultural Competence
CULTURE, ETHNICITY, RACE, AND THE
  NURSING PROCESS: ASSESSMENT
    Cultural, Ethnic, and Racial Factors
      Relevant to the Assessment
    Conducting the Assessment

▼ ## KEY TERMS

Acculturation
Assimilation
Behavioral ethnicity
Cultural competence
Cultural diversity
Cultural sensitivity
Culture

Ethnic humanism
Ethnic pluralism
Ethnicity
Ethnocentrism
Ethnoscience
Excess mortality
Ideal cultural behavior

Ideologic ethnicity
Intraethnic variation
Manifest cultural behavior
Material culture
Nonmaterial culture
Racism
Subculture

▼ *LEARNING OBJECTIVES*

After studying this chapter, you should be able to

1. *Define culture and its major components: material culture, nonmaterial culture, subculture, cultural sensitivity, and cultural diversity.*
2. *Discuss ethnicity in terms of behavioral ethnicity, ideologic ethnicity, intraethnic variations, and ethnocentrism.*
3. *Describe racism as a legal-cultural, political, and social phenomenon.*
4. *Explain minority status as it relates to ethnicity, racial status, and economic status.*
5. *Describe the impact of poverty on the health of ethnic groups.*
6. *Compare the health status—chronic diseases, mortality rate, excess mortality, life expectancy, mental disorders, and suicide—among ethnic groups.*
7. *Describe ethnic variations in seeking health care.*
8. *Identify strategies the nurse can use to manage cultural and ethnic differences.*
9. *Explain how the nurse can best assess clients of diverse backgrounds.*

What would it be like for you to be alone and suddenly seriously ill in a foreign country? Unaware of the culture and marginally fluent in the language, you would undoubtedly experience some anxiety about what to expect and about how to clearly communicate your symptoms. The different culture of the foreign country as well as the diverse backgrounds of the physicians and nurses there might evoke some preconceived beliefs and emotions within you. In turn, consider what preconceived beliefs and emotions might be evoked within the people of the foreign culture while they are caring for you. Also, contemplate in what ways your interactions with these people could be influenced by your, and their, preconceived beliefs and emotions.

The social unrest of the 1960s and 1970s heightened the public's awareness of ethnic and cultural differences between people and of the need to bridge gaps brought about by these differences. There was an explosion of knowledge reflected in the professional literature. In the nursing profession, there was considerable emphasis on recognizing the special health care needs of members of different ethnic, racial, and cultural groups and on developing ways of meeting these unique needs. Ideas that appeared in books and articles in that era are still relevant today.

Bullough and Bullough[4] addressed the relationships among ethnicity, poverty, and health care. They showed that ethnicity combined with poverty resulted in greater morbidity: the poorer ethnic families, including Appalachian whites, experienced the greater health problems.

Madeline Leininger, a nurse-anthropologist, has been in the forefront of the transcultural nursing movement since the 1960s and 1970s. She advanced the **ethnoscience** approach,[19] which she viewed as a scientific method of studying the unique ways of life of particular cultural groups. This approach accurately documents people's behaviors as well as their perceptions and interpretations of such behaviors and of life around them. An appropriate method of obtaining this in-depth information is through the ethnographic approach, a face-to-face interview method. It is the preferred data-gathering technique for obtaining information about the unique ways of life of cultural groups. Open-ended questions are used so that people can give full descriptions of their experiences and of their own thoughts, feelings, and behaviors concerning particular subjects.

Branch[3] described **ethnic humanism** as a humanistic perspective that focuses on the strengths and resources of all ethnic groups, on the blending of traditional and Western healing practice, and on client participation in health care. Branch challenged the nursing profession to adopt this view in educating nursing students. According to Branch, this view is a necessary ingredient for the provision of safe, effective nursing care and for the improvement of health services for people of diverse ethnic backgrounds. Adoption of the ethnic humanistic view includes the following:

▶ Emphasis on the strengths and resources of all ethnic groups
▶ Commitment to a holistic perspective, that is, the blending of traditional and Western healing practices
▶ Acceptance of consumers' participation in decisions that affect their welfare
▶ Being accountable to ethnic communities of color[3]

Branch[3] contends that certain ethnic groups fail to receive safe, effective nursing or medical care when cultural and ethnic differences are ignored. This is likely to occur when the patterns of the dominant culture are recognized as the only correct ways of life.

Spector[34] examined cultural diversity in the context of health and illness and focused on differences between clients' and providers' perceptions of health and illness. Spector's findings are presented in Box 19–1.

Nursing authors have continued to address cultural and ethnic differences in society and changes that are necessary in the health care delivery system to provide health care that is both accessible and acceptable to all segments of the population. In this chapter, these issues are addressed. An overview of basic concepts including race, minority, and social class is presented; specific health-related examples of the importance of culture, ethnicity, and race follow the overview.

CULTURE

The concept of culture has been central in the field of anthropology. Cultural anthropologists have contributed to our understanding of the concept of culture through their systematic studies of peoples of different lands. Nurses who have studied anthropology and focused on culture have contributed a great deal to our understanding of the concept and have increased our awareness of how culture influences health and illness.

Leininger,[19] a nurse-anthropologist, described **culture** as an umbrella term used to denote the accumulation of human experiences that evolve into a way of life for a group of people.[19]

These experiences over several generations culminate into specified lifestyles—the way a group of people conduct their lives. Culture is reflected in peoples' social institutions and creations: their art, tools, equipment, traditions, customs, religion, language, dress, food, beliefs, values, attitudes, stereotypes, and prejudices.[19] Culture provides strategies for dealing with environmental demands; that is, the social traditions and customs delineate solutions to problems with which people are confronted in their everyday existence.[19] Because the social traditions and customs are shared within the group, they dictate and predict expectations as well as behavioral patterns within the group. In addition to providing solutions, culture also provides goals and the mechanism for devising innovative strategies for new challenges.[19]

Material Culture and Nonmaterial Culture

Material culture is the sum of the tangible items produced by people in a cultural group, such as tools, equipment, furniture, and clothes.[19] **Nonmaterial culture** is the sum of the intangible products of a cultural group, such as religion, legal systems, values, and attitudes.[19] Both material and nonmaterial culture are created by men and women to assist them in coping with their environment. Culture also has been discussed in terms of manifest and ideal cultural behavior.[19] **Manifest cultural behavior** consists of behavioral patterns that can be readily observed and identified by individuals who are considered to be outsiders. **Ideal cultural behavior** is a set of behavioral patterns that people in the culture believe to be desirable but do not practice.

Socialization

Culture is not a static process but rather a dynamic process that is constantly evolving. It is not a biologic trait inherited through the genes. It is learned through socialization.

Socialization is the systematic process of transmitting material and nonmaterial culture from one generation to the next generation.[19,40] Socialization occurs through social interaction primarily by the use of language and by understanding and integrating what has been learned.[40] Consequently, culture is the sum total of learned behaviors of a group of people.

Subcultures

A **subculture** is a smaller group within a culture. Subcultures have unique ways of living that distinguish them from the larger or dominant culture.[19] **Cultural diversity** is the term used to convey that there are differences among cultures as well as between subcultures and the dominant culture. Although the subculture's customs, traditions, and beliefs are different from those of the dominant culture, this does not connote that their customs, traditions, and beliefs are inferior. These subcultures must be assessed and evaluated on the basis of their customs, traditions, and beliefs that have evolved over time, not those of the dominant culture. However, there is a tendency to view one's own culture as the standard all other people should strive to achieve and by which all people should be judged.[8]

Cultural relativity holds that there are no superior or inferior cultures and that no scales exist to measure the value of different cultures.[8] Cultures must be assessed on their own merit independently of other cultures.

Cultural differences exist not only across divergent groups of people but also within a group of people who share the same cultural background. Within a specific group, there can be intragroup differences based on socioeconomic status, degree of acculturation, and life cycle stage.

Acculturation

Acculturation is the degree to which one culture has adopted the traditions, customs, and beliefs of another culture, thereby increasing the similarities between the two cultures.

Assimilation

Assimilation is the process whereby individuals from a subculture adopt the dominant culture.[8]

Cultural Sensitivity and Stereotyping

It is necessary to be cognizant of the cultural background of a group of people and intragroup differences that exist. This requires **cultural sensitivity,** the awareness of cultural generalizations and intragroup differences, as well as the avoidance of stereotypes.

Stereotyping is the process of placing labels on people and treating everyone in a specific cultural group as if all individuals and families within a culture are similar in every possible way.[8]

The term *culture* is sometimes used interchangeably with the term *ethnicity*.

ETHNICITY

Focus on ethnicity and ethnic differences in the health and social sciences literature originated primarily from studies of the early migration of Europeans to the United States. Although there are many definitions of **ethnicity,** the term is generally used to describe a group of people within a larger society who share a social and cultural heritage that is passed on from generation to generation. This group of people is identified as having cultural and historical uniqueness, including a common ancestry, a shared historical past, and a cultural focus on one or more of the following symbolic elements: phenotypic features (physical contiguity), language or dialect, religion, kinship patterns, and nationality.[10]

Ethnic Pluralism

The United States and Canada are made up of a variety of ethnic groups. **Ethnic pluralism** is the term used to describe a larger culture within which several different ethnic groups have maintained distinct subcultures. Ethnic groupings have been a structural part of the United States and Canada since the beginning of their histories. Within both countries, early immigrants formed ethnic communities that provided congenial associations and opportunities for socialization.

It has generally been held to be true that as older immigrants become more acculturated into the larger society—as they learn the language, manners, and customs of the larger dominant culture—they move up the socioeconomic ladder and out of ethnic communities. Their upward mobility leaves behind space for new ethnic communities to be formed for newly arriving immigrants. Old and new immigrants maintain varying levels of their cultural heritage. To delineate the extent to which ethnic group members maintain their cultural and ethnic traditions within the larger society, Howard[10] defined behavioral and ideologic ethnicity.

Behavioral Ethnicity

Behavioral ethnicity refers to situations in which ethnic customs are practiced systematically and members are well socialized into the traditional customs and values of the ethnic group.

Ideologic Ethnicity

Ideologic ethnicity is the voluntary rather than systematic practice of ethnic customs. These customs are therefore not central to the individual's life.

All people belong to an ethnic group, but ethnic identity is maintained at varying degrees along a continuum of behaviors that ranges from behavioral ethnicity to ideologic ethnicity. Some people are well assimilated, whereas others maintain a distinct ethnic subculture.

Intraethnic Variation

Whereas people share ethnic norms, values, and standards of behavior, each individual is nevertheless unique.

Usually much variation exists within ethnic groups. This **intraethnic variation** is defined as the existence of cultural differences within groups. Howard[10] identified several factors that contribute to intraethnic variations: advanced education, several generations removed from immigrant status, estrangement from ethnic and family network, immigration experienced at an early age, urban residence, and restricted visits to country of origin.

Ethnocentrism

Ethnocentrism is the belief that one's own ethnic beliefs, customs, and attitudes are the correct ones and are better than those of others. Other ethnic groups' customs, behaviors, and attitudes are viewed as different, immoral, or inferior. For example, in the United States, standards of beauty are based on height and weight that may be unrealistic for people from other cultures. In one culture, being short and plump may be viewed as more attractive than being tall and slender. Ethnocentrism makes a group unaware of the fact that its customs and ideas may appear strange or bizarre to people of other ethnic backgrounds.

Ethnic Conflicts

Despite the view that American society is a "melting pot," assimilation has not occurred to the extent that all ethnic groups have come together to share a common culture and to have equal access to all opportunities. Many conflicts still exist among some ethnic groups and between some ethnic minority groups and the white majority groups. For example, some Native Americans, Hispanics, Asian-Americans, and African-Americans have not been well integrated into mainstream American society and do not have equal access to opportunities and resources, including health care.

RACE

Differentiation Among Racial Groups

Race is an ubiquitous yet vague concept[40] that is often defined in terms of a person's physical characteristics, namely, skin color, hair type, and facial features. The heavy reliance on physical characteristics for differentiating among racial groups is a problem because no one physical characteristic can reliably be used to distinguish among different races.[5,42] In addition, various physical characteristics do not always coexist in a given person.[42] For example, within a given racial group, skin color can and does vary widely. Additionally, a person can have dark skin and straight hair or very light skin and kinky hair. Also, physical characteristics that are shared do not reliably dictate the cultural or behavioral patterns of people. People with similar physical characteristics may have different cultural beliefs and traditions.[42]

The validity of race as a biologic concept is questionable.[42] Genetic analyses support the view that racial groups are more similar to other racial groups than they are different.[5,42] Research findings based on personality traits also support the view that there is more variability within a particular racial group than between racial groups.[42]

The number of races reported to be *Homo sapiens* has ranged from three to 40 and is basically defined by an arbitrary process, which again makes the scientific validity of race dubious. Some have suggested that the concept of race should be deleted and replaced with the term *ethnic group*.[40]

Race as a Legal-Cultural Phenomenon

Whereas race was originally believed to be a biologic phenomenon, it is now considered to be a legal-cultural phenomenon,[42] a political phenomenon, and a social phenomenon that defines a group of people.[5] Historically, the concept of race was an important economic factor that helped to shape the structure of society.[5]

Race as an Economic Phenomenon

In the 18th and 19th centuries, certain Caucasians used the concept of race for their own economic advancement. Their success was ensured through **racism,** the belief in the superiority of one's own race over other races. That is, to acquire land and a consistent pool of free labor and systematically deny economic success to other races, it was necessary to create an ideology based on the biologic superiority of the Caucasian race over other racial groups. Because all "Third World" peoples (people of developing nations, especially those of Asia and Africa) were viewed as inferior, as less than human, these Caucasians could rationalize their exploitation and destruction of other racial groups for the purpose of taking their lands, wealth, and people.[5,17]

In the 18th and earlier part of the 19th century, to acquire land in the new world, many European settlers warred with the Native Americans. Some were even guilty of committing torture and genocide against Native Americans. These European settlers justified their attack on the Native Americans by rationalizing that the Native Americans were heathen who deserved to be exploited. At the same time, the European settlers' growing desire for free labor could not be met entirely by Native Americans, and indentured servants, and slavery grew as an institution.

Race As a Political Phenomenon

The ideology of racism has been supported by the legal system. Throughout history, the United States government legally took land from Native Americans, reneged on treaties, and confined Native Americans to reservations.[17] Laws were passed that defined African individuals as slaves for life and as property with no rights. After the abolition of slavery, some states passed laws forbidding social interaction between the Caucasian and the African races. These laws became known as Jim Crow laws and successfully legalized segregation. Then, in the late 19th century, the United States government passed immigration acts that prohibited the immigration of nonwhites—Chinese, Japanese, Indian.[17]

Racial Prejudice

Racism led to racial prejudice, the phenomenon of covertly or overtly denying racial groups equal access to opportunities to achieve economic success and the blaming of their failure to achieve on their "racial inferiority." The blaming of the individual or the individual's culture successfully camouflaged the true reasons for failure to achieve and hindered effective problem solving.

Since the 1950s, laws have been passed to help ensure desegregation and ensure civil rights for all. However, some racism still exists in the United States today. Whether it takes a subtle or more blatant form, it threatens the fabric of our society.

MINORITY STATUS

Minority is another term that has been used to refer to ethnic groups or subcultures (Figure 19–1). In the early history of the United States, minority status was based

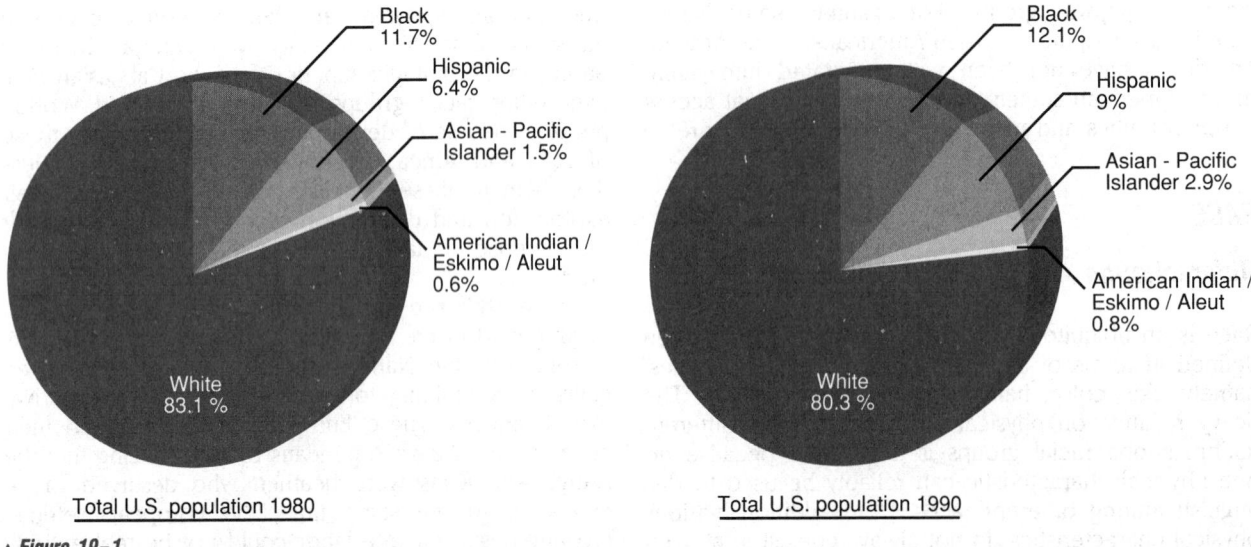

▲ **Figure 19–1**

Percentages of persons identifying themselves as belonging to a particular cultural/ethnic/racial group in 1980 and 1990. (Data from U.S. Bureau of the Census, U.S. Department of Commerce.)

mostly on religion, but in the 20th century, racial and economic factors became the most often used means of designing minority status.[4] In contemporary society, ethnicity and minority status are overlapping concepts that interact with socioeconomic class and poverty issues to significantly affect an individual's health status, health behaviors, and use of health services.

SOCIAL CLASS

Like culture and ethnicity, the term *social class* has varying definitions and meanings. Generally, social classes are hierarchical divisions of social groups with each member of society assigned to a specific group on the basis of caste, rank, or economic worth. Movement among classes ranges from fairly free to impossible, depending on the society. In the United States, we informally recognize classes mostly on the basis of economic status and speak of upper class, middle class, and lower class.

With class membership based mostly on economic status, ethnicity and racial status serve as less important barriers to movement from lower to higher classes. However, many persons in the lower classes of U.S. society are members of specific ethnic groups and have little hope of upward mobility. In fact, persistent poverty has become a way of life for a group of poor, inner-city residents, primarily African-Americans and Hispanics, who are experiencing ethnic segregation and spatial isolation.[23] Wilson[37] indicates that inner-city neighborhoods are characterized by increased rates of joblessness, out-of-wedlock births, families headed by women, and welfare dependency. Poverty has been cited as the primary reason for these conditions.

This concentration of ethnic minorities in urban poverty areas has great implications for nurses because these individuals are likely to have the greatest need for health care services. Unfortunately, they are likely to have the lowest access because of their inability to pay and their lack of knowledge or "savvy" for dealing with the increasingly complex health care system.

DIFFERENTIAL HEALTH STATUS AMONG CULTURAL, ETHNIC, AND RACIAL GROUPS

Health status has been shown to differ dramatically among ethnic groups. A brief discussion of chronic diseases, mortality rates, excess mortality, life expectancy, mental disorders, and suicide follows. Keep in mind that any highly consistent pattern of nongenetic differential mortality and morbidity existing between ethnic groups is primarily an environmental or social phenomenon. Most people exposed to the same environment will experience similar diseases at similar rates. Nelson[26] concluded from his study of three ethnic groups that a complex interaction among cultural factors, life events, and socioeconomic status influences health care behavior and attitudes. In a study that investigated the association of health with income and race, Satariano[32] found that health was associated more strongly with income than with race. The results of a study by Ulbrich et al.[35] revealed that one's socioeconomic status and race interact to produce psychologic symptoms of distress. Finally, employment was found to have a profound effect on people's perceptions of their health status: the employed individuals had better perceived health than did unemployed individuals.[1]

Chronic Diseases

Approximately three fourths of deaths in the United States are caused by chronic diseases. Fifty per cent of deaths caused by chronic diseases are due to heart disease; one third are due to malignant neoplasms.

Mortality due to chronic diseases is 0.33 to 2.8 times greater for African-Americans than for Caucasians, especially for diabetes mellitus, nephritis/nephrosis, heart disease, cerebrovascular disease, cancer, chronic liver disease, and cirrhosis.[36]

In the United States, certain diseases are associated with persons in one ethnic group more than with persons in another ethnic group.

Following are the results of some studies that show health and disease patterns among some of the ethnic groups in the United States. In a study of the health status of Hispanic-Americans in Arizona, Krikman-Liff and Mondragon[14] found that Hispanics experienced lower health status and poorer access to health care than Caucasians did and that Spanish-speaking Hispanics experienced lower health status and poorer access to health care than did their Hispanic counterparts who spoke English. They concluded that English-speaking Hispanics are more assimilated into the American culture, are better educated than those speaking exclusively Spanish, and also experience higher health status.

More than 13,000 Asian-Americans participated in a study to determine the cardiovascular risk factors for Asian-Americans in northern California.[15] Those Asian-Americans volunteering to have physical examinations defined themselves as Chinese, Filipino, Japanese, and other.

In terms of obesity, Chinese men and women had the lowest adjusted mean body mass index, whereas Filipino men and women had the highest. However, obesity tended to be a problem for all Asian-American men.

Hypertension appeared to be a special problem for Filipino men and women, whereas hypercholesterolemia was a problem for all Asian-Americans, with the Japanese men and women having the highest rate.

Smoking tended to be a problem for all Asian-American women, in contrast to their male counterparts. When comparison was made of the four Asian-American ethnic groups, Chinese men and women tended to smoke less than the other three groups did. However, Japanese women were more likely to be smokers than were women in the other three groups.

Kabat et al.[13] compared the smoking habits of African-Americans with those of Caucasians. The prevalence of current smokers was higher among African-Americans than among Caucasians. The African-Americans who were current smokers tended to smoke fewer cigarettes daily, to smoke cigarettes that had higher tar and were mentholated, and to have smoked for fewer years than Caucasians who were current smokers. Romano et al.[31] found that a stressful environment was the most significant contributing factor for smoking behavior among African-Americans living in U.S. cities.

Mortality Rates

In 1986, the mortality rate of Native Americans was higher than the rates for all other racial groups in the United States. Mortality rates for Native Americans were lower for major cardiovascular disease, malignant neoplasms, and chronic obstructive pulmonary disease but were four times higher for tuberculosis, three times higher for chronic liver disease and cirrhosis, two times higher for diabetes mellitus, and almost twice as high for homicide and accidents.

In 1987, the African-American mortality rates, for all causes of death combined, were 52 per cent higher than the Caucasian mortality rates. Again, looking at diseases individually, mortality rates of African-Americans due to homicide were six times that of Caucasians. Rates for African-Americans were more than twice that of Caucasians for nephritis, septicemia, perinatal conditions, and diabetes mellitus. Rates for African-Americans were lower for suicide, chronic obstructive pulmonary diseases, and motor vehicle accidents.

Hispanics, compared with non-Hispanics, have lower mortality rates for most chronic diseases, with the exception of diabetes mellitus and chronic liver disease and cirrhosis.[36]

The mortality rates during the 1984–1986 period for Native Americans and Alaskan natives, compared with all other races in the United States, were higher in all age groups except for infants and adults 55 years and older.[36] Mortality rates in 1986 were higher for African-Americans than for Caucasians in all age groups except the 15- to 19-year age group and the 80-year and older age group.

Excess Mortality

Excess mortality refers to the difference between the number of deaths observed in a group, such as a particular ethnic group, and the number of deaths that would have occurred in that group if it experienced the same death rates for each age and sex as occurred in the general population.

The excess mortality for African-Americans tends to increase by gender; the African-American man suffers more deaths from cerebrovascular disease and cancer than the African-American woman does.[36] The excess mortality of African-American men has progressively increased for almost all major chronic disease in the last 37 years, compared with their Caucasian counterparts. For African-American women, compared with Caucasian women, the excess mortality has decreased somewhat but not disappeared. Any decline in chronic disease mortality has been greater for Caucasians than for African-Americans.[36]

Life Expectancy

Life expectancy rates reflect the health status of different ethnic and racial groups. Caucasian life expectancy exceeded African-American life expectancy by 7.6 years in 1970 and by 6.2 years in 1987. These differences are largely a factor of gender; Caucasian men's life expectancy is 72 years, compared with 65 years for African-American men.[36] An African-American woman's life expectancy is 8.4 years longer than her male counterpart's, whereas a Caucasian woman's life expectancy is 6.7 years longer than that of her male counterpart.[36]

In 1980, the Native American's life expectancy was longer than the life expectancy of the African-American by some 3 years. The Native Americans had a shorter life expectancy than Caucasians did by some 3.3 years in 1980. The Native American's life expectancy has increased dramatically since 1940 from 13.2 years shorter than that of Caucasians to 3.3 years shorter in 1980.[36]

Mental Disorders

The Epidemiologic Catchment Area Program study of 1980–1982 found no significant differences between African-Americans and Caucasians in overall prevalence of mental disorders. There is one exception, however; phobic disorders tended to be diagnosed at a higher rate in African-Americans than in Caucasians. When mental health was analyzed in terms of age, racial differences did emerge for alcohol abuse or alcohol dependence. Younger African-Americans tended not to have histories of alcohol abuse and alcohol dependence to the same degree as Caucasian youths did. Middle-aged and older African-Americans, however, tended to have rates of alcoholism higher than their Caucasian counterparts did. Mexican Americans and non-Hispanic whites differed only in the rate of major depressive disorders; non-Hispanic whites experienced more episodes of major depression. However, Hispanic men tended to have higher rates of alcohol abuse and alcohol dependence than non-Hispanic whites or non-Hispanic African-Americans did. Hispanic women's rates of alcohol abuse and alcohol dependence were lower than those of non-Hispanic white or non-Hispanic African-American women. Drug abuse and drug dependence appeared to be a more serious problem among minorities, especially for African-Americans and Hispanics. For Native Americans, alcohol abuse, alcohol dependence, and suicide are serious mental health problems. The rate of their alcohol problems is twice that of other ethnic groups.[36]

Suicide

The 1986 suicide rates for Caucasians were higher than those for African-Americans in all age groups across both genders. For Native Americans, the suicide rates are higher than those in the general population up to age 45 years. Their rates are twice as high for both genders, compared with the general population.[36]

VARIATIONS IN HEALTH BEHAVIORS AMONG CULTURAL, ETHNIC, AND RACIAL GROUPS

There are several examples in the literature of ethnic and sociocultural influences on health behaviors.

Peoples' ethnic origin may lead them to react in certain ways to varying symptoms or changes in illnesses.

In one of the classic studies of ethnic variations in the manifestation of symptoms conducted in the outpatient clinics of the Massachusetts General Hospital, Zola[41] found differences in the perception of, and concern with, certain types of symptoms among Irish and Italian clients. For example, even when clients had the same disorder, Irish clients, more than Italians, denied pain as a feature of their illness, thus seeming to have higher pain tolerance.

Help-Seeking Processes

In another study, Lin et al.[21] conducted semi-structured interviews to determine help-seeking processes of 48 Caucasians, African-Americans, and Asian-Americans. They found a strong correlation between the persons' ethnicity and their help-seeking processes. Both Asian-Americans and African-Americans involved extended family members in their processes of seeking help a great deal more than did Caucasians. Asians showed the longest delay in seeking professional help, and Caucasians the shortest. Health professionals may interpret delay in help seeking to mean that ethnic minority groups are taking no action about their health condition. This would be an incorrect interpretation because studies clearly show that ethnic group members, particularly minorities, tend to seek advice and other forms of help from informal networks, particularly members of the extended family, before seeking professional help. For instance, in a 1984 study, African-Americans, even when they admitted to having symptoms and health problems, did not seek professional help. This behavior was noted regardless of their income level.[25] Many African-Americans use an informal social network for help with a variety of health and personal problems. The same behavior occurs in other cultures, including Chinese-Americans, and Koreans.

Use of Mental Health Services

In a study of the use of mental health services,[11] Asian-Americans, African-Americans, and Hispanic-Americans varied in their use of mental health services. Asian-Americans tended to use individual outpatient mental health services more often and emergency, inpatient, and case-management mental health services less often than did Caucasians. African-Americans tended to use emergency mental health services more often and case management and individual outpatient mental health services less often than did Caucasians. Hispanic-Americans used case management mental health services more often and emergency mental health services less often than did Caucasians. Both Caucasians and Hispanics tended to use inpatient and individual outpatient mental health services to the same extent.

Access to Health Services

In addition to variations in seeking help and use of health services, some studies showed ethnic differences in access to health services. For example, in a national study, Blendon et al.[2] showed that there is a significant deficit in access to health care (including physician care) among African-Americans, compared with Anglo-Americans. African-Americans were found to underuse medical services, be less satisfied with physician treatment, be more dissatisfied with hospital care, and be more likely to believe that duration of their hospitalization was too short.

With respect to a specific health condition, Satariano et al.[33] found African-American women to be at high risk for the most advanced form of breast cancer at diagnosis. Their risk increases with age, whereas it decreases for Anglo-American women. They concluded that this difference may reflect differences in preventive health practices, delay in seeking medical attention, and differences in recognition and reporting of symptoms. Their study is important in that it shows the need for further research to help us better understand the influences of ethnic as well as socioeconomic differences in preventive health practices. Better understanding of these differences, which clearly exist, would enhance the assessment, planning, and implementation of quality health care to all groups.

MANAGING CULTURAL, ETHNIC, AND RACIAL DIFFERENCES

Self-awareness

To work with individuals, groups, and families from different racial, cultural, and ethnic backgrounds, you first need to understand your own racial, cultural, and ethnic customs and traditions. In the examination and analysis of your own racial, cultural, and ethnic background, you will become more aware of the ways your background has influenced the course of your life and your interaction with people of diverse racial, cultural, and ethnic groups. This self-examination is a crucial part of the nursing assessment process. The questions in Box 19–2 will help you explore the influences of your own ethnic and cultural background.

If you are able to answer the questions in Box 19–2, you are at the first step of becoming more aware of the impact your own racial, cultural, and ethnic beliefs have on your interactions with ethnically diverse clients.

Cultural Competence

Being aware of your own cultural and ethnic background and its influences on your beliefs, behaviors, and interactions with others is a necessary step for being culturally competent.

Cultural competency enables you to provide safe and effective care to people of diverse cultures. A culturally

---

> ### Box 19–2. Exploring Your Own Ethnic and Cultural Background
>
> ► With what ethnic, social, or cultural group do you most closely identify?
> ► In what ways have your racial, cultural, and ethnic beliefs, perceptions, prejudices, and traditions influenced your reactions, behaviors, nursing diagnoses, and interventions?
> ► In what ways can you objectively assist ethnically diverse clients in achieving their optimal health status?
> ► Will you be able to respect the different perceptions and views of ethnically diverse clients as relevant and important?
> ► Can you accept ethnically diverse clients as active, valid participants in their health care?
> ► Will you be able to treat ethnically diverse clients with respect, that is, not belittle them by assuming that you understand their situation and that you know what the correct solutions are?
> ► In what ways can you create a respectful, nonthreatening environment for the ethnically diverse client? This environment should foster open communication and optimal sharing.

competent nurse has knowledge and empathy, communicates effectively, and serves as an advocate for clients.

KNOWLEDGE

Cultural competence requires that you become knowledgeable about the beliefs and values of diverse ethnic groups in the society and their predisposition to certain illnesses and conditions.

Cultural competence does not mean that you need to readily recall details of particular values, customs, and practices of these groups.

You must, however, know how to access relevant information about diverse ethnic groups. Methods of accessing relevant information include talking with your colleagues and other people of diverse ethnic backgrounds and with the client and the family. The information obtained will reflect intraethnic differences because people of any ethnic group will identify with the group's customs and traditions in varying degrees ranging from no identification to maximal identification. These intraethnic differences make it imperative that health care be tailored to the individual and not to preconceived notions about the individual's ethnic background.

Ethnic people in the United States vary in their adherence to traditional beliefs. For example, Chinese immigrants who were born in China and who came to the United States 50 years ago tend to adhere to the traditional beliefs more strongly than do Chinese people who are first- and second-generation Americans, who may be more receptive to Western health practices.[22]

Many Chinese, Hispanics, and Navajo Indians believe that health is a reflection of a balance existing within the person. Often, Chinese believe that health is based on yin and yang, forces that influence the dynamic flow of the universe. Health is the balance of yin and yang, whereas illness is the imbalance of these forces.[22] Many Hispanics also believe that to maintain health, there must be a balance within the body. Navajo Indians often view health as a harmonious balance between mind and body as well as between the person and the environment—family, supernatural forces, and nature. Because of these beliefs, some Chinese may use certain foods and beverages to maintain balance; some Hispanics may drink either hot or cold beverages or eat foods that have "hot" or "cold" properties to enhance balance.

In an ethnographic research of rural African-Americans,[30] it was disclosed that they perceived health to be a gift from "God" uniting mind, body, and spirit. As such, these African-Americans believed that prayer, faith, and the Bible could lead to spiritual, mental, and physical health. Illness, on the other hand, was caused by sin, evil spirits, and the devil. Even though God was identified as the primary healer, these African-Americans did use the Western health system in conjunction with their faith in God.

EMPATHY

Cultural competence (being knowledgeable about health practices, beliefs, values, culture, and ethnicity within and between different groups and being able to provide health services that are acceptable to these groups) requires that you approach clients with an open mind. You must approach them with a desire to understand their perspective and to learn what it is like for them to be in a specific situation. Specifically, you learn from clients about how their ethnic, racial, and cultural backgrounds have influenced their life patterns and current health situation and how conditions such as class and ethnic or racial differences may have affected their health. The client's ethnic, racial, and cultural background as well as any exposure to discrimination or poverty can have an impact on the client's ability to adapt to health care planning and intervention.

COMMUNICATION

To be culturally competent, you need to promote understanding by practicing effective communication. You need to communicate with your clients clearly by sending unambiguous verbal and nonverbal messages, by clarifying the communication styles of ethnic clients, by validating your interpretations of the clients' messages, and by ascertaining their ability to understand and speak English.

Barriers to communications include assumptions about particular ethnic groups; differences in knowledge levels; differences in social class; disparate expectations of the client-nurse relationship; and the use of different words, dialect, or manner of speech as well as the use of different nonverbal communication styles.

The following example illustrates the nurse's failure to communicate adequately with a client.

Mrs. Ríos comes to the family practice clinic with her 10-year-old daughter. She encounters Miss Thomas, the registered nurse working in the clinic. Miss Thomas is assigned to assess the nature of Mrs. Ríos' health problem. Miss Thomas greets Mrs. Ríos. Mrs. Ríos smiles and looks at her daughter. The daughter says, "My mother doesn't speak much English." Miss Thomas asks the daughter to ask Mrs. Ríos why she is here today. As Miss Thomas continues to direct more questions to the daughter, who translates the questions to her mother, Mrs. Ríos becomes visibly upset. Miss Thomas excuses herself and goes to consult with her supervisor. The supervisor recommends that Miss Thomas ascertain Mrs. Ríos' level of understanding of English and her comfort in having her daughter serve as a translator. The supervisor suggests that Miss Thomas use the clinic's bilingual translator if needed.

Miss Thomas learns, in such cases, that she needs to assess the client's abilities to understand and speak English, the client's level of comfort in having a family member serve as translator (thus recognizing generational boundaries), and the client's need to protect family members from worrying about the mother's health problem.

ADVOCACY

Advocating for the client is possible only if it takes place in an atmosphere of mutual trust and respect. To be an advocate, you have to overcome any existing prejudices about poor or ethnic minority clients and avoid judgmental attitudes about their situation. Advocacy involves accurate assessment, which takes into account the client's point of view; incorporation of the client in treatment planning; and provision for outreach and community action.

Client advocacy may require you to work with unfamiliar community agencies or lay practitioners on behalf of the client. It requires understanding the role of informal networks, such as the extended family, friends, and lay practitioners. Oftentimes, people blend their traditional methods of health intervention with services received from the health care system. It is not uncommon for some persons from various cultures to combine the services of lay practitioners with the services of Western physicians.

Advocacy may also require political action—a willingness to communicate the client's health care needs to governmental and other officials who can do something about these needs. As a client advocate, you teach the client and the community to care for themselves, which necessitates recognition and sanctioning of the client's and community's strengths. You cannot ignore political, social, and economic factors that may combine with ethnic and cultural factors to contribute to the client's health status and course of treatment and recovery from illness.

CULTURE, ETHNICITY, RACE AND THE NURSING PROCESS: ASSESSMENT

To be culturally competent and to provide safe and effective care to all clients, you must recognize and address the relevance of culture and ethnicity as integral to the nursing process.

Culture is relevant to all stages of the nursing process, particularly the assessment phase.

Cultural, Ethnic, and Racial Factors Relevant to Assessment

To assess clients of diverse cultural, ethnic, and racial backgrounds, you will need to assess the following:

▶ How the client's background influences the client's perceptions of health and illness, and treatment
▶ How the client's background has influenced his or her help-seeking process
▶ How the client's background is likely to influence his or her interaction with professionals
▶ What impact the client's background will have on treatment, including treatment after discharge

Some questions relevant to assessment include those in Box 19–3.

With respect to the last question in Box 19–3, you may encounter some ethnic groups who value individualism and some who value the family. In such instances, being an advocate for the client may entail working with one member, all, or several members of the extended family. In working with the Navajo Indians, for example, family members must be included in the assessment and intervention.

A cultural profile will add to the comprehensive assessment of your client. Fong[6] has proposed that you (1) assess your client's ability to communicate and to comprehend in English; (2) understand the meanings your client gives to specific nonverbal behavior; (3) elicit your client's ethnic identification and value system; (4) identify your client's dietary habits, specifically foods that are considered special and foods to be avoided; (5) assess the family composition, living arrangement, relationship, goals, and various roles that exist within the family; (6) identify the client's beliefs and practices regarding health and illness; (7) assess the client's educational achievement acquired through formal education and life experiences; and (8) assess the client's religious beliefs.

Conducting the Assessment

In conducting the assessment, you must create a non-judgmental atmosphere in which the clients can feel that their cultural background and beliefs will be respected and appreciated. This nonjudgmental atmosphere will promote trust within the nurse-client relationship.

Only when the client feels that he or she can trust you will the client reveal important information.

In addition to communicating your respect for your client's cultural background verbally and nonverbally, you must explain to your clients the reason you are asking questions about their beliefs. Clients need to know how the information they give you will be used and who will have access to this information.

Summary

▶ Culture denotes the accumulation of human experiences that evolve into a way of life. Culture is categorized as material and nonmaterial. Subcultures are smaller subgroups that have unique lifestyles distinguishing them from the dominant culture. Cultural diversity reflects differences among cultures, whereas cultural sensitivity reflects an awareness of these differences.
▶ Everyone belongs to an ethnic group—a group that shares a social and cultural heritage passed on from generation to generation. Ethnic identity is on a continuum of behaviors ranging from behavioral ethnicity to ideologic ethnicity. Many factors contribute to intraethnic variations. Ethnocentrism denotes accepting your own customs while rejecting the customs of other ethnic groups.
▶ Race is more a legal-cultural, political, and social phenomenon than a biologic phenomenon.
▶ Minority status reflects the relationship between the dominant ethnic group or groups and the less powerful ethnic groups.
▶ Poverty has an impact on the lifestyle of ethnic groups residing in the poor urban communities.
▶ The rates of chronic illnesses, mortality, life expectancy, mental disorders, and suicide differ significantly among ethnic groups.
▶ Ethnicity and socioeconomic status influence health-seeking behavior.

Box 19–3. Questions Relevant to Assessment

▶ What does the client perceive as causing the symptoms and illness?
▶ What words does the client use to describe the symptoms and illness?
▶ What has the client done to resolve the problem?
▶ What folk medicine and lay practitioners have been used to resolve the problem?
▶ What are the client's health care beliefs and practices?
▶ What treatment interventions would the client find acceptable or unacceptable?

▶ The nurse must manage cultural and ethnic differences by developing self-awareness and cultural competence.

▶ Assessment should include an exploration of the effects of the client's ethnic and cultural heritage on the client's understanding and description of the illness, on how the client has attempted to resolve the illness, and on what treatments the client will accept and reject.

Bibliography

1. Ahmad, W.I., et al. (1989). Influence of ethnicity and unemployment on the perceived health of a sample of general practice attenders. *Community Medicine*, 11(2), 148–156.
2. Blendon, R.J., et al. (1989). Access to medical care for Black and White Americans: a matter of continuing concern. *Journal of the American Medical Association*, 261(2), 278–281.
3. Branch M., & Paxton, P. (1976). *Providing safe nursing care for ethnic people of color.* New York: Appleton-Century-Crofts.
4. Bullough, B., & Bullough, V. (1972). *Poverty, ethnic identity, and health care.* New York: Appleton-Century-Crofts.
5. Cooper, R., & David, R. (1986). The biological concept of race and its application to public health and epidemiology. *Journal of Health Politics, Policy and Law*, 11(1), 97–115.
6. Fong, C.M. (1985). Ethnicity and nursing practice. *Topics in Clinical Nursing*, 7(3), 1–10.
7. Ford, E., et al. (1989). Coronary arteriography and coronary bypass survey among Whites and other racial groups relative to hospital-based incidence rates for coronary artery disease: findings from NADS. *American Journal of Public Health*, 79(4), 437–440.
8. Friedman, M. (1990). Transcultural family nursing: application to Latino and Black families. *Journal of Pediatric Nursing*, 5(3), 214–222.
9. Glazer, N., & Moynihan, D.P. (1970). *Beyond the melting pot: The Negroes, Puerto Ricans, Jews, Italians, and Irish of New York City.* Cambridge, MA: MIT Press.
10. Howard, A. (1981). *Ethnicity and medical care.* Cambridge, MA: Harvard University Press.
11. Hu, T., et al. (1991). Ethnic population in public health: services choice and level of use. *American Journal of Public Health*, 81(11), 1429–1434.
12. Hurh, W.M., & Kim, K.C. (1990). Correlates of Korean immigrants' mental health. *Journal of Nervous and Mental Disease*, 178(11), 703–711.
13. Kabat, G.C., et al. (1991). Comparison of smoking habits of Blacks and Whites in a case-control study. *American Journal of Public Health*, 81(11), 1483–1486.
14. Kirkman-Liff, B., & Mondragon, D. (1991). Language of interview: relevance for research of southwest Hispanics. *American Journal of Public Health*, 81(11), 1399–1404.
15. Klatsky, A.L., & Armstrong, M.A. (1991). Cardiovascular risk factors among Asian Americans living in northern California. *American Journal of Public Health*, 81(11), 1423–1428.
16. Kleinman, A. (1980). *Patients and healers in the context of culture.* Berkeley, CA: U.C. Press.
17. Lauren, P.G. (1988). *Power and prejudice: The politics and diplomacy of racial discrimination.* London: Westview Press.
18. Lefley, H.P. (1990). Culture and chronic mental illness. *Hospital and Community Psychiatry*, 41(3), 277–286.
19. Leininger, M. (1978). *Transcultural nursing: Concepts, theories, and practice.* New York: John Wiley.
20. Leininger, M. (1984). Transcultural nursing: an overview. *Nursing Outlook*, 32(2), 72–73.
21. Lin, K., et al. (1982). Sociocultural determinants of help-seeking behavior of patients with mental illness. *Journal of Nervous and Mental Disease*, 170(2), 78–85.
22. Louie, K.B. (1985). Providing health care to Chinese clients. *Topics in Clinical Nursing*, 7(3), 18–25.
23. Massey, D., & Eggers, M. (1990). The ecology of inequality: minorities and the concentration of poverty, 1970–1980. *American Journal of Sociology*, 9(5), 1153–1188.
24. Mayer, W.J., & McWhorter, W.P. (1989). Black/White differences in non-treatment of bladder cancer patients and implications for survival. *American Journal of Public Health*, 79(6), 772–775.
25. Neighbors, H. (1984). Professional help use among Black Americans: implications for unmet need. *American Journal of Community Psychology*, 12(5), 551–566.
26. Nelson, C.W. (1985). Does ethnicity matter? Utilization, responses to medical problems: attitudes and satisfaction in a medically underserved community. *Journal of Mental Health Administration*, 12(1), 34–41.
27. Office of the Federal Register National Archives and Records Administration (1989). *The United States government manual 1989/1990.* Washington, DC: U.S. Government Printing Office.
28. Pilpel, D., et al. (1990). Gross intellectual impairment among non-institutionalized elderly: difficulties in assessment and risk factors. *Journal of Community Health*, 15(3), 209–223.
29. Polednak, A.P. (1991). Cancer incidence in the Puerto-Rican-born population of Long Island, New York. *American Journal of Public Health*, 81(11), 1415–1422.
30. Roberson, M.H.B. (1985). The influence of religious beliefs on health choices of Afro-Americans. *Topics in Clinical Nursing*, 7(3), 57–63.
31. Romano, P.S., et al. (1991). Smoking, social support, and hassles in an urban African-American community. *American Journal of Public Health*, 81(11), 1415–1422.
32. Satariano, W.A. (1986). Race, socioeconomic status, and health: a study of age differences in a depressed area. *American Journal of Preventive Medicine*, 2(1), 1–5.
33. Satariano, W.A., et al. (1986). The severity of breast cancer at diagnosis: a comparison of age and extent of disease in Black and White women. *American Journal of Public Health*, 76(7), 779–782.
34. Spector, R. (1979). *Cultural diversity in health and illness.* New York: Appleton-Century-Crofts.
35. Ulbrich, P.M., et al. (1989). Race, socioeconomic status, and psychological distress: an examination of differential vulnerability. *Journal of Health and Social Behavior*, 30(1), 131–146.
36. United States Department of Health and Human Services (1991). *Health status of minorities and low-income groups* (3rd ed.). Washington, DC: U.S. Government Printing Office.
37. Wilson, W. (1988). The ghetto underclass and the social transformation of the inner city. *The Black Scholar*, 19(3), 10.
38. Woods, N.F., et al. (1988). Being healthy: women's images. *Advances in Nursing Science*, 11(1), 36–46.
39. Zborowski, M. (1952). Cultural components in response to pain. *Journal of Social Issues*, 8, 16–20.
40. Zeitlin, I.M. (1984). *The social condition of humanity: An introduction to sociology.* New York: Oxford University Press.
41. Zola, I. (1966). Culture and symptoms: an analysis of patients presenting complaints. *American Sociological Review*, 31, 615–630.
42. Zuckerman, M. (1990). Some dubious premises in research and theory on racial differences: scientific social and ethical issues. *American Psychologist*, 45(19), 1297–1303.

Health, Illness, and Health Care Settings

▼ Health Promotion in the Community

Chapter 20

> *Wellness is a unique and individualized state for each person. . . .*
> *A wellness lifestyle is the process of working toward that ultimate*
> *state of wholeness and well-being. . . . The process is dynamic*
> *and ever-changing as you evolve throughout life.*
>
> **Patricia A. Swinford**[70]

▼ CHAPTER OUTLINE

CONCEPTS AND TERMS
    Health and Wellness
    Health Protection
    Health Promotion
NURSING'S FOCUS ON HEALTH
HEALTH GOALS FOR THE YEAR 2000
FACTORS THAT INFLUENCE HEALTH
    External Factors that Influence
      Health
    Internal Factors that Influence
      Health
MODELS OF HEALTH BEHAVIOR
    Health Belief Model
    Health Promotion Model
    A Framework for Health Promotion
WORKING WITH INDIVIDUALS TO
  PROMOTE HEALTH
NURSING STRATEGIES FOR HEALTH
  PROMOTION

Role Modeling
Acting as a Change Agent
Setting Priorities
Using Principles of Behavior
    Modification
Promoting Holistic Health
Collaborating with Other Health
    Care Providers
WORKING WITH FAMILIES, GROUPS, AND
  COMMUNITIES TO PROMOTE HEALTH
    Family Health Promotion
    Health Promotion Within Groups
    Targeting At-risk Groups in
      Communities
    Evaluating Responses to Health
      Promotion Programs
HEALTHY PUBLIC POLICY

▼ Key Terms

Aggregate	Community	Self-care
At-risk aggregate	Health education	Social support
Change agent		

Lorenzo, an occupational health nurse, leads an exercise class for employees after work. Felicia, a school nurse, talks with pregnant adolescents about a healthy diet and the effects of smoking, alcohol, and other substances harmful to a developing fetus. Dana, a parish nurse, facilitates a support group for older adults experiencing grief after the death of a spouse. Mai, a home health care nurse, talks with a family about effective ways of coping with stress. Tony, a hospital nurse, talks with adults who have had surgery about the benefits of quitting smoking. What do these nurses have in common? They are all engaged in health promotion.

CONCEPTS AND TERMS

Health and Wellness

Health and *wellness* are closely related terms. Although some authors view them as separate concepts, the terms are used interchangeably in this chapter to refer to the optimal physical, cognitive, psychosocial, and spiritual well-being of the individual, group, or community. As a discipline, nursing has defined health as "a dynamic state of being in which the developmental and behavioral potential of an individual is realized to the fullest extent possible."[1] Health is seen as a resource enabling people to lead socially and economically productive lives.[13]

A key facet of health is being able to function fully and to find self-expression in all the domains of one's life —physical, emotional, social, spiritual, occupational, recreational, and political.

Health Protection

Health protection activities are those that individuals, families, and communities do to protect themselves from disease. Certain diseases may pose a special threat because of a person's age, gender, family history, or other risk factor. Examples of health protection activities that guard against specific diseases include using "safe sex" behaviors to avoid acquired immune deficiency syndrome and other sexually transmitted diseases, receiving immunizations to prevent infectious diseases, using sun blockers to minimize the risk of skin cancer, and drinking fluorinated water to reduce dental cavities. Health protection activities also can minimize the effects of a health problem the individual already has. An example is taking prescribed medications to reduce high blood pressure and prevent worsening of cardiovascular disease. Can you think of other examples?

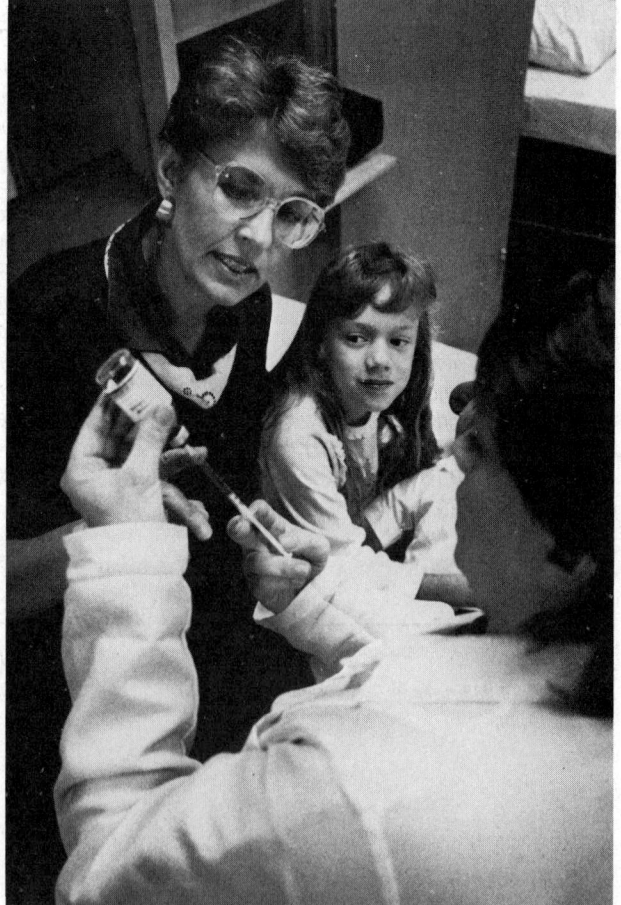

▲ Figure 20–1

Nurses teach families about medications as a way to help them protect their health.

Health Promotion

Health promotion activities are aimed at enhancing the well-being of an individual, family, or group.[27] Most of these activities are continuing behaviors that are integrated into people's daily living. Some examples are eating a well-balanced diet, exercising regularly, maintaining ideal body weight, and developing attitudes that minimize psychologic distress. What other examples can you think of?

Health promotion efforts are focused on promoting self-actualization and integrated functioning among individuals, families, groups, and communities. In this chapter, the term **community** is used to refer to a specific population living in a defined area and having shared institutions, values, and problems. A community may have many *groups,* defined as people who have common goals but interact independently. An **aggregate** is a group of people sharing one or more common characteristics. Some groups within a community are described as **at-risk aggregates**—subgroups of a community that are at increased risk of illness because of some variable, such as living in poverty.

RISK FACTORS

A risk factor is a condition that increases the probability that an individual or group will have a particular disease or injury; most are related to heredity, behavior, or environment. For example, a person's gender is a *heredity*-linked risk factor for many diseases. Working with a harmful substance such as asbestos is a *behavior*-linked risk factor for lung disease. Living in an area where drinking water is contaminated is an *environment*-linked risk factor for many communicable diseases.

HEALTH PROMOTION IN PERSONS WITH DISABILITIES AND ILLNESSES

Although it might seem that health promotion is something well people primarily engage in, persons with disabilities and illnesses also benefit from healthy promotion activities. Adults with disabilities reported perceiving themselves as predominantly healthy, perceiving their health as about the same as or better than that of most people their age. They place strong emphasis on their ability to function and to develop their abilities fully. Individuals with disabilities now live longer and are more fully integrated into the community than was true in the past. Thus, it is increasingly important for nurses to be prepared to respond to the needs for health promotion in *all* clients in the community.[68,69]

Everyone can benefit from health promotion, including persons with illnesses or disabilities.

NURSING'S FOCUS ON HEALTH

Nurses have actively participated in the societal transition from a disease-oriented to a health-oriented system of care. In 1859, Nightingale said that being a nurse is to "have charge of someone's health."[48] More recently, the American Nurses' Association stated, "The core, or essence, of nursing practice is the diagnosis and treatment of human responses to health and to illness."[3] Similarly, the Canadian Nurses' Association said, "Nursing practice can be defined as a dynamic, caring, helping relationship in which the nurse assists the client to achieve and maintain optimal health."[12]

In 1991, Nursing's Agenda for Health Care Reform was launched by more than 50 organizations representing American nurses.[4] This blueprint for changing the American health care system described ways of meeting health objectives set for the year 2000. The proposal identified consumers as the central focus of the health care system and called for making a basic core of essential health care services available to all Americans.

Nurses provide health promotion services where people live, work, and play. Some settings in which they do so are listed in Box 20-1.

Nurses promote health on the basis of the unique ways individuals, families, and communities experience health. We assist people in achieving knowledge, attitudes, and behaviors that are associated with health. We also work to remove the economic, cultural, and political barriers that prevent people from staying healthy.[66]

Our understanding of what it means to promote health within families and communities has grown with technologic advances that have made instant communication possible across the world. Nurses promote health with a global perspective, because actions taken in one part of the world affect health in many other places.

HEALTH GOALS FOR THE YEAR 2000

Nurses collaborate with other health care professionals in working toward health goals. American and Canadian health officials have set goals for achieving health

---

Box 20-1. Settings in Which Nurses Provide Health Promotion Services

- ► Agencies providing health information
- ► Churches and other religious institutions
- ► Clinics
- ► Community health departments
- ► Day care centers
- ► Health and exercise clubs
- ► Homes
- ► Hospitals
- ► Industries and other work settings
- ► Nursing centers
- ► Nursing homes
- ► Nutrition and diet centers
- ► Prisons
- ► Schools
- ► Senior centers

for the populations they serve. The U.S. Department of Health and Human Services set objectives for national health promotion and disease prevention efforts for the decade ending in the year 2000. These objectives, derived from the input of 10,000 contributors, were published in a comprehensive document, *Healthy People 2000*.[76] The report identifies priority areas for health promotion, health protection, and preventive services for four age groups.

To boost American children and adults toward their full potential and functioning, the report *Healthy People 2000* urges achievement of three broad goals:

▶ Increase the span of healthy life for all Americans
▶ Reduce health disparities among Americans
▶ Achieve access to preventive services for all children and adults

Three challenges were identified in achieving health for all Canadians:

▶ Reduce inequities in the health of low- and high-income groups
▶ Increase efforts to prevent injuries, illnesses, chronic conditions, and their resulting disabilities
▶ Enhance people's ability to cope with chronic conditions, disabilities, and mental health problems

FACTORS THAT INFLUENCE HEALTH

As we seek ways to promote health we ask, What characteristics are associated with health? What do people do that keeps them well? What resources do individuals need for optimal health at different stages of their lives? How can we foster healthy families and healthy communities?

Our answers to these questions fall into two broad areas: external factors and internal factors. External factors are those outside of individuals, such as their income, where they live, and other cultural, social, and political factors affecting their health. Internal factors are attitudes, beliefs, and behaviors that influence health.

External Factors that Influence Health

As a nurse involved in health promotion, you need to be concerned with factors beyond people's immediate control that affect their health. Industrial and auto emissions may be contaminating the air people breathe. Food additives may have beneficial or adverse effects. Peeling paint can cause lead poisoning if lead-contaminated dust is ingested. The noise in some occupational settings can damage hearing. Helping people become aware of such factors is important in health promotion and protection.

Health promotion and protection activities stimulate nurses to become involved in the larger world that affects people's health. Political actions by representatives at the city, provincial, state, or national level may affect people's access to health resources, such as health insurance, immunizations, or technology for

diagnosis of health problems. Social and economic factors in the community may affect the availability of jobs, housing, educational materials, and other resources needed for optimal health.

To achieve optimal health, people need access to resources for health protection and health promotion. Accessible health care systems must be available, acceptable, and effective. This means facilities and health care professionals need to be affordable and have values in agreement with those of clients. Effective care leads to improved health outcomes for consumers.

For many, poverty is a factor that is clearly related to limited access to health resources. People's health remains directly related to their economic status. People with low income have a shorter life expectancy, a higher prevalence of disability, and lower levels of almost every dimension of health than do those with higher incomes.[76] The largest group of poor people in the United States is children. Compared with middle-class children, poor Canadian children had almost twice the rate of chronic health problems and more than twice the rate of psychiatric disorders, poor school performance, regular tobacco use, and social impairment.[51]

Although the poor tend to have longer hospitalizations and more physician visits than those with higher incomes do, they tend to have limited use of health promotion resources.[32] In Canada, death rates are consistently higher in the poorest neighborhoods. For example, the rate of injury to children living in the poorest neighborhoods is four times that of children living in the least poor neighborhoods.[18] In addition to higher rates of injuries, when basic needs are not met, health promotion may not be a priority. For example, a woman struggling to provide food and health care for her young children may put off mammography screening for breast cancer for herself. The poor may tend to use emergency room services in place of coordinated, continuous care.

Poor people may encounter a number of barriers to health protection services, such as needing to endure prolonged waiting times at clinics or feeling the stigma of receiving care funded by public assistance. Other barriers include financial constraints, isolation, impaired mobility, and limited transportation.[16] Poverty and limited education often go hand in hand. Health education materials written above the individual's reading level create another barrier.

Some experts say that even if we ensure access to health care, we will improve health outcomes only when we alleviate poverty and the despair, joblessness, and limited education that may accompany it.[25] Proportionately more people in minority groups live in poverty than is true of white Americans.

Even when the effects of poverty are accounted for, disparities in health exist for members of ethnic minorities. African-American babies are twice as likely as are white babies to die before their first birthday. African-Americans and Hispanic-Americans receive less preventive health care, including prenatal care, than does the total population.[76] Compared with white Americans, African-Americans are 1.3 times as likely to die of heart disease, twice as likely to die of stroke, and six times as likely to be murdered.[25] In Canada, cultural groups tend to maintain their identity in what has been called a multicultural mosaic, compared with what some have called the "melting pot" pattern of cultural integration in the United States (see Chapter 19 for an alternative view of the United States as a "melting pot"). Lifestyle behaviors, such as smoking, have not been compared among the Canadian cultural groups. Because diseases such as heart disease and stroke are affected by lifestyle behaviors as well as by genetic factors and access to health care, the impact of ethnicity on rates of death requires further study.

However, the compelling relationships among poverty, ethnicity, and health outcomes require nurses to be aware of political and economic issues that may jeopardize people's health. Policies that influence access to and cost of health care are made by corporations, health insurance providers, and governmental agencies at city, provincial, state, and federal levels.

Nurses are taking leadership in working with policymakers to develop cost-effective alternatives to the present health care system.

This is discussed further in the section Healthy Public Policy.

Internal Factors that Influence Health

As a nurse involved in health promotion, you will need to be concerned with people's behaviors, attitudes, and beliefs. People's everyday behaviors often determine the agents of disease that enter their bodies—for example, tars inhaled in cigarette smoke; saturated fats ingested in the diet; or sound waves at decibel levels harmful to hearing, such as those heard at some concerts and in some work settings. Lifestyle behaviors also help determine which building blocks of health are taken into the body—for example, vitamins, minerals, and other dietary nutrients, or air free of cigarette smoke and other pollutants.

ATTITUDES AND BELIEFS THAT INFLUENCE HEALTH

Attitudes and beliefs influence the development of physical and cognitive attributes and the achievement of genetic potentials. They influence skills in relating to society, skills needed to acquire resources and achieve expression as a self-actualized human being. Attitudes and beliefs also direct thought patterns, responses to stress, self-esteem, and ways of relating to others, all of which have important impacts on mental health and social support systems. Belief systems and spiritual resources are essential for the health of individuals, families, and communities.

BEHAVIORS THAT INFLUENCE HEALTH

What behaviors are most associated with health? Early classic studies demonstrated that eating breakfast, getting 7 to 8 hours of sleep, maintaining proper weight, not smoking, regular physical activity, not eating between meals, and moderate or no use of alcohol were associated with decreased mortality and increased physical health.[8,9] Subsequent studies have demonstrated that maintaining a network of social support and individual hardiness of spirit also contribute to well-being, especially as people grow older, regardless of the types of illness they may experience.[39,57]

Behavioral Risk Factors. A large study of premature deaths among Canadians found that an estimated 50,000 premature deaths (over 50 per cent) could be prevented through control of smoking, hypertension, elevated serum cholesterol, diabetes, and alcohol abuse.[81] Behavioral risk factors are associated with the five major causes of death among adults: cancer, heart disease, stroke, injury, and chronic lung disease. These risk factors are listed in Box 20–2 and discussed in the following.

High-Fat Diet. A diet high in fats has been associated with increased risk of heart disease, breast and colon cancer, and gallbladder disease. A total fat intake of no more than 30 per cent of calories is recommended. Saturated fats, commonly found in animal sources and dairy products, should be no more than 10 per cent of total daily fat intake.

Obesity. Obesity has been associated with high blood pressure, elevated blood cholesterol, diabetes, heart disease, stroke, some cancers, and gallbladder disease. Being overweight has been especially prevalent in some minority groups and in those with low socioeconomic status; it is a problem for one fourth of American adults and an undefined number of Canadians.[76,81]

Sedentary Lifestyle. A sedentary lifestyle appears to be an independent risk factor for coronary artery disease. Regular physical activity, at even a moderate level, can reduce this risk. Physical activity is helpful in preventing and managing hypertension, diabetes, osteoporosis, and obesity. Exercise may also help in relieving depression and improving mood, self-esteem, and anxiety.

Smoking. Smoking increases the risk for heart disease, stroke, and some forms of cancer. Smoking is estimated to be responsible for one in six deaths in the United States and 9000 deaths per year in Canada.[81] In general, smoking rates are higher among African-Amer-

---

Box 20–2. Behavioral Risk Factors

► Consuming a diet high in fats
► Being overweight
► Leading a sedentary lifestyle
► Smoking
► Abusing alcohol
► Abusing drugs
► Not wearing seat belts

icans, Hispanics, blue-collar workers, and people with fewer years of education. Although 45 per cent of those who ever smoked have quit, 50 million Americans still smoke.[76]

Alcohol Abuse. Alcohol abuse is associated with deaths due to motor vehicle accidents, homicides and suicides, cirrhosis of the liver, and esophageal and liver cancers. It is the leading preventable cause of birth defects. It is estimated that 9 per cent of people 21 years of age and older drink more than two alcoholic beverages per day.[76] In Canada, alcohol presents a similar health risk. In one study, binge drinking was reported among 20 per cent of teenagers, with 55 per cent reporting being intoxicated or sick at least once in the previous 6 months.[21]

Drug Abuse. Illicit drugs, mainly cocaine, are associated with about 10 per cent of homicides.[76] In addition to increasing the risk for death due to injury, the effect of drug use is even more devastating when we consider babies affected by cocaine, transmission of AIDS and hepatitis viruses through intravenous drug use, and the breakdown of family relationships associated with chemical dependency. Because cocaine can cause malignant hypertension (high blood pressure), cocaine users are at risk for heart attack and stroke.

Not Wearing Seat Belts. Risk of death due to injury is reduced through use of seat belts. In Canada, motor vehicle accidents are the largest cause of death in children.[18] Although only 42 per cent of motor vehicle passengers used their seat belts in 1987, it is estimated that seat belts saved 4000 lives that year.[76] Seat belts also protected people from disability due to head and other injuries in motor vehicle accidents.

ILLNESS PREVENTION STRATEGIES

Beyond these broad risk factors, individuals need to become aware of illness prevention strategies pertinent throughout their life span. Objectives that relate to developmental levels, as identified in *Healthy People 2000*, are summarized in Table 20–1.

Strategies for health protection throughout the life span include health screenings, immunizations, and age-related education. Age-appropriate health protection schedules should be based on the most recent guidelines of the Centers for Disease Control, National Screening Council, Health and Welfare Canada, and other national associations (e.g., the American Heart Association).

MODELS OF HEALTH BEHAVIOR

What influences behavior? What motivates an individual to embark on an exercise program, limit intake of saturated fats and cholesterol, wear a helmet while cycling, or try alternative responses to life's stresses?

Numerous studies indicate that knowledge, attitudes, and perceptions have a pronounced effect on whether individuals engage in health-promoting behaviors. In general, people are likely to engage in health promotion behaviors when they have sufficient knowledge of what is necessary to promote health, they believe the

TABLE 20–1. Objectives for Health Through the Life Span

Developmental Level	Objectives
Children	Reduce deaths, illness, and disabilities caused by unintentional injuries; continue to increase use of child safety seats
	Reverse the impacts of poverty and high-risk environments: child homicide, lead poisoning, learning disorders, emotional and behavioral problems
Adolescents and young adults	Reduce deaths caused by injuries; three fourths are due to automobile accidents involving alcohol ingestion
	Reduce homicides among African-American men aged 15 to 24 years; for this group, the primary cause of death is homicide, most often committed with a gun
	Reduce deaths due to suicide
	Reduce factors that undermine health: use of tobacco, alcohol, and illicit drugs; unwanted pregnancy; and sexually transmitted diseases, including human immunodeficiency virus infection
Adults aged 25 to 64 years	Reduce leading causes of deaths and disabilities: cancer, heart disease, stroke, injuries, chronic lung disease, liver disease
	Continue altering behavioral risk factors: high blood pressure, fat intake, smoking
Older adults	Reduce leading causes of deaths: heart disease, cancer, stroke, chronic lung disease, pneumonia
	Preserve function and reduce disability associated with chronic problems: arthritis, osteoporosis, incontinence, visual and hearing impairments, dementia
	Increase years of functional independence in activities of daily living
	Reduce social isolation and depression

Adapted from *Healthy people 2000* (1990). U.S. Department of Health and Human Service. Washington, DC: U.S. Government Printing Office.

behaviors are important for maintaining health, and they perceive *themselves* as needing to take those actions to have better health. Often people decide they need to take action when they receive information that the lack of a behavior puts them at risk or that current behaviors could lead them to experience a health problem, such as an elevated blood glucose level or high blood pressure.[6]

Before you can assist individuals in reducing their risk factors and enhancing their quality of life, you need to understand their unique motivations.

Two widely used models of health behavior provide a framework for planning strategies to help people change their health behaviors.

Health Belief Model

According to the health belief model discussed in Chapter 2, individuals' behaviors are greatly affected by their perceptions, or health beliefs.[7,61,63] This model proposes that people's perceptions are influenced by psychosocial variables, such as their age, gender, family experiences, and ethnicity. Cues to action, such as advertisements and anecdotes from friends, also affect perceptions. The concepts underlying this model can be summarized by the equation

$$\text{Motivation} = \text{Reward} - (\text{Perceived cost} + \text{Barriers})^{62}$$

Notice that this model is built around a central assumption of the threat of disease. It is a model of health protection, a model that explains behavior changes as being motivated by a desire to protect oneself from disease. An example of an individual experiencing this type of motivation is the person who wants to quit smoking because of an awareness that smoking increases the likelihood of developing heart disease and cancer.

Take time now to apply the health belief model in looking at Mrs. Carson, a 59-year-old African-American woman who has high blood pressure. She has primary responsibility for two grandchildren, ages 2 and 4 years, who live in her household, along with their mother, who works two jobs. When asked if she takes medication every morning and evening as prescribed for her blood pressure, Mrs. C. says, "Some weeks I do better than others. I try." When asked if she knows that high blood pressure could lead to a stroke, she says, "That would be a long time from now. I have enough to worry about today. That medicine isn't cheap either! And I feel pretty good. I think the medicine makes me tired."

On the basis of the information provided, what do you know about how Mrs. C. perceives (1) her susceptibility to stroke, (2) the severity of high blood pressure, (3) the benefits of the medication, and (4) the barriers to taking the medication? What questions could you ask her to learn more about her perceptions? On the basis of this model, what might increase the likelihood of her taking her medication? Be creative!

The health belief model is not applicable to health promotion activities. Health promotion entails actualizing one's potential for health, beyond freedom from disease. Another limitation of the health belief model is that it does not account for other things that affect behavior, such as habit and environmental influences, apart from perceptions and beliefs.[33] For example, some people choose to diet not for health reasons but because they think they will look better if they lose weight.

Health Promotion Model

Like the health belief model, the health promotion model, which also was presented in Chapter 2, emphasizes the importance of people's perceptions. It says that people's health behaviors depend on their unique perceptions of their health and of the consequences of their actions. This model proposes that individuals' perceptions and beliefs are influenced by modifying factors including their age, hereditary characteristics, family, culture, and socioeconomic status. Health promotion encompasses the whole client and focuses on the following lifestyle behaviors:

▶ Avoiding unhealthy substances
▶ Diet
▶ Exercise/activity/mobility
▶ Healthy relationships
▶ Managing stress
▶ Optimistic outlook on life
▶ Integrated functioning of mind, body, and spirit

Take time now to apply the health promotion model in assessing the health behaviors of Mr. Nakamoto, a second-generation Japanese-American who is consulting a nurse at a Nursing Center about starting an exercise program. Mr. N. is a busy, 38-year-old executive who travels monthly for business. He is 15 pounds over his ideal weight and says he "feels flabby." He has been experiencing headaches, which he attributes to work-related stress. He saw his physician recently for a complete physical and received a "clean bill of health." He has no history of health problems.

On a recent business trip, he noticed a fully equipped exercise room with swimming pool at his hotel. This stimulated his interest in beginning an exercise program. He is interested in types of exercise he can do with his wife and two school-age children on weekends.

With the information provided, which factors from the health promotion model can you begin discussing with Mr. N.? How does each affect the likelihood that he will engage in an exercise program? How could you use this information in planning an exercise program with Mr. N.?

A Framework for Health Promotion

The framework for health promotion presented in Figure 20–2 is a model for promoting health for an entire

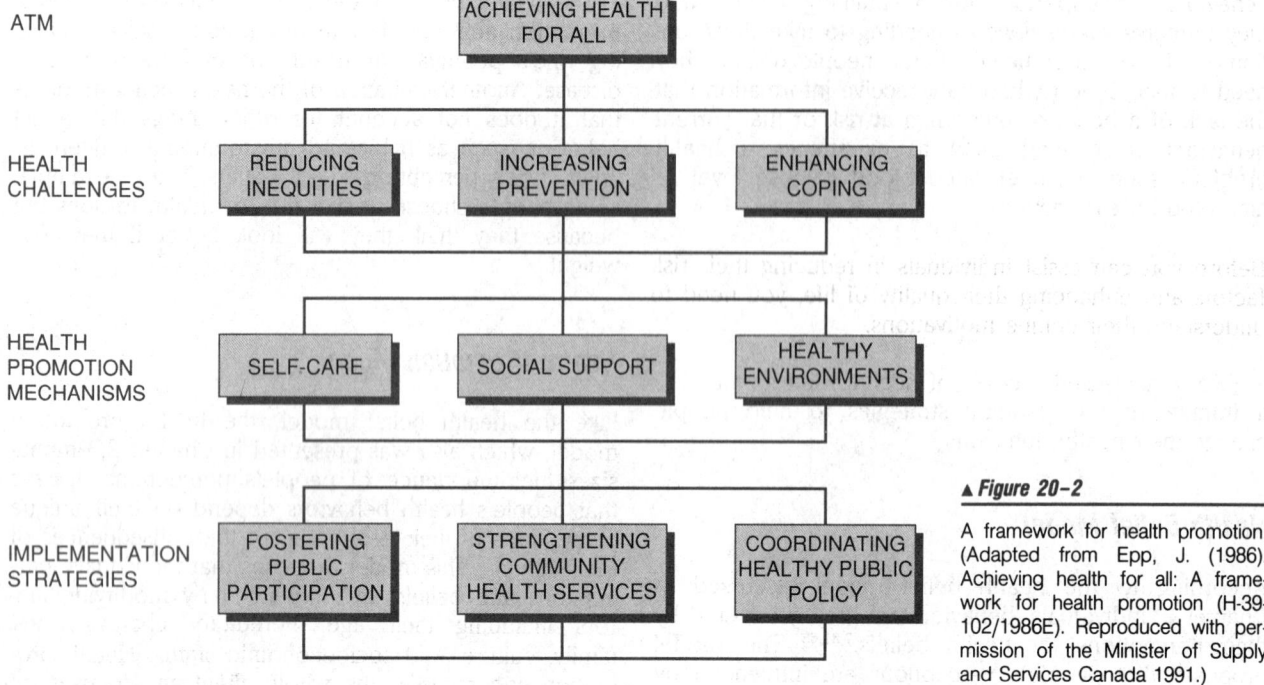

ATM

HEALTH
CHALLENGES

HEALTH
PROMOTION
MECHANISMS

IMPLEMENTATION
STRATEGIES

▲ *Figure 20-2*

A framework for health promotion. (Adapted from Epp, J. (1986). Achieving health for all: A framework for health promotion (H-39-102/1986E). Reproduced with permission of the Minister of Supply and Services Canada 1991.)

nation of people.[20] Although it was developed by Canadian health officers, the framework is applicable to the health challenges facing the United States as well. The model summarizes the following ideas. The *aim* of achieving health for all is not being adequately met by present health care systems, as discussed previously.

The American and Canadian health care systems face three important *challenges*. The first is to reduce inequities in health care and quality of life for high- and low-income groups. The second challenge is to increase prevention efforts, to find more effective ways of preventing injuries, illnesses, and chronic health problems and their resulting disabilities. The third challenge is to enhance people's ability to cope with chronic health deficits, disabilities, and mental health problems. Effective coping allows persons of all ages to live stable, satisfying lives.

HEALTH PROMOTION MECHANISMS

The model proposes three *health promotion mechanisms* that can be applied in meeting the challenges identified.

Self-care. The term **self-care** refers to actions or choices individuals make to promote their own health. Examples include an older person's using a cane or walker to prevent falls, a diabetic person's self-injecting insulin, and a parent's providing a balanced diet for his children. What other examples can you think of?

Social Support. Social support encompasses people's actions to promote one another's health by sharing emotional support, ideas, information, and assistance. Such interactions may occur within families,

neighborhoods, voluntary organizations, or support groups. What are some of the voluntary associations and groups available in your community?

Healthy Environments. A healthy environment is the sum of the physical, social, and economic conditions that preserve or enhance health. This complex area includes homes, work settings, and the purity of air and water as well as education, transportation, and health systems. What news stories have you heard or read recently that illustrate the relationship of environment and health?

STRATEGIES FOR DECISIVE ACTION IN RESPONSE TO HEALTH CHALLENGES

The model recommends three *strategies* for decisive action in response to the health challenges.

Fostering Public Participation. Fostering public participation enables people to act in ways that preserve or enhance their health. Nurses facilitate support groups for persons and families coping with spina bifida, heart attack, Alzheimer's disease, sickle cell anemia, and many other health problems. In what other ways can nurses mobilize people to enhance their health?

Strengthening Community Health Services. Strengthening community health services involves targeting disadvantaged groups for health promotion services and involving people in planning services for their own communities. In both urban and rural areas, nurses are taking leadership in providing prenatal services and well-child services to disadvantaged communities, in providing care and referrals for persons coping with disabilities, and in mobilizing services to maintain elders in their homes. These community health promotion efforts improve quality of life for individuals at all stages of the life cycle.

Coordinating Healthy Public Policy. Public policy includes legal and other decisions that determine how funds and other limited resources are used. As Epp says, "Public policy has the power to provide people with opportunities for health, as well as to deny them such opportunities."[20] Public policy should provide equitable access to health care. The role of nurses in promoting such policy is discussed in the section Healthy Public Policy at the end of this chapter.

WORKING WITH INDIVIDUALS TO PROMOTE HEALTH

The first step in working with people to promote health is assessing their present knowledge, beliefs, and lifestyle behaviors. When you begin talking with someone, you will want to find out what they think is important to promote their health. The Self-test for Health Style presented in Box 20–3 is a sample of a tool that can be used to help people assess their health-related behaviors. Many similar tools, often labeled Health Risk Assessment tools, are available.

Individuals have grown up with unique personal perspectives on how to stay healthy. Nurses can be most successful in promoting health if they work within these individual perspectives. For example, Mr. Green was raised with the idea that eating regular meals is important to health. As his nurse, you can commend him for continuing this practice and then assess the nutritional adequacy of the foods he chooses to eat during his meals.

When people have perspectives about staying healthy that differ from what you have learned as a nurse, it is important to acknowledge their views and seek to understand them. Many people find it difficult to interpret the changing information they hear or read about staying healthy. Your interest in understanding their perspectives can become an opportunity for clarifying misperceptions and providing up-to-date information about effective health practices.

As you continue your discussion with individuals, you will want to find out whether they understand basic self-care practices and have integrated them into a daily routine. Are they aware of behaviors that increase their risk for health problems? Are they engaging in illness prevention strategies appropriate for their age? (Fig. 20–3)

In assessing basic self-care practices, you may ask individuals to describe their usual day. How long do they sleep, how do they relax, and do they feel refreshed. When, where, and with whom do they eat? What does their diet usually include? Are they sexually active, and if so, do they understand and use safe sexual practices? Do they have a regular pattern of physical activity? What hygiene practices, such as toothbrushing and flossing, bathing, and hair and nail care, do they use? As you are talking about their daily routine, it also may be a good time to ask about family and friends, pets, the hobbies or other activities they enjoy, and what is important in their life.

As you complete your assessment, you will consider nursing diagnoses appropriate to the client you are working with. There are important differences in the way you work with your client, depending on the diagnosis you make.

Altered Health Maintenance is a diagnosis you would choose if the client were prevented from pursuing health behaviors, for example, because of disability or lack of resources. If the client does choose to pursue health promotion activities with you, the appropriate diagnosis is *Health-Seeking Behaviors* (specify), as shown in the Nursing Diagnosis Profile.

NURSING STRATEGIES FOR HEALTH PROMOTION

Nurses use a variety of strategies in promoting healthy attitudes and behaviors. Some of these approaches, and the skills necessary for each, are discussed below.

Role Modeling

There are many ways in which you can have a positive impact on the health beliefs and behaviors of individuals. One of the most powerful is by being a role model of good physical, mental, and spiritual health yourself. The adage "Actions speak louder than words" proves true in this aspect of nursing. When you make a balanced diet, sufficient rest, regular exercise, and a positive outlook on life priorities for yourself, you are also becoming a credible and knowledgeable resource for health promotion. People find it easier to accept a message about the benefits of quitting smoking from a nurse who does not smell of cigarette smoke. If you do regular exercise, you know firsthand some of the rewards and barriers associated with such a program. If you read labels in making your own food choices, you can share this skill with others.

Acting as a Change Agent

As a **change agent**—a person who facilitates planned change with an individual or group or within an institution—you can stimulate people to see things in new ways and to try new behaviors, attitudes, and beliefs. Skills used by a change agent are[59]

▶ Inquiring
▶ Helping
▶ Teaching
▶ Supervising
▶ Coordinating
▶ Collaborating
▶ Consulting
▶ Negotiating/bargaining
▶ Confronting
▶ Lobbying

Box 20-3. Self-test for Health Style

Directions: This is not a pass-fail test. Its purpose is simply to tell you how well you are doing in staying healthy. The behaviors covered in the test are recommended for most people. Some of them may not apply to persons with certain chronic diseases or handicaps. Such persons may require special instructions from their physician or other health care professional.

The test has six sections: smoking, alcohol and drugs, nutrition, exercise and fitness, stress control, and safety. Complete one section at a time by circling the number corresponding to the answer that best describes your behavior (2 for Almost Always, 1 for Sometimes, and 0 for Almost Never). Then add the numbers you have circled to determine your score for that section. Write the score on the line provided at the end of each section. The highest score you can get for each section is 10.

Cigarette Smoking	Almost Always	Sometimes	Almost Never
If you never smoke, enter a score of 10 for this section and go to the next section.			
1. I avoid smoking cigarettes.	2	1	0
2. I smoke only low-tar and nicotine cigarettes, or I smoke a pipe or cigars.	2	1	0

Smoking Score: _____

Alcohol and Drugs	Almost Always	Sometimes	Almost Never
1. I avoid drinking alcoholic beverages, or I drink no more than one or two drinks a day.	4	1	0
2. I avoid using alcohol or other drugs (especially illegal drugs) as a way of handling stressful situations or the problems in my life.	2	1	0
3. I am careful not to drink alcohol when taking certain medicines (for example, medicine for sleeping, pain, colds, and allergies) or when pregnant.	2	1	0
4. I read and follow the label directions when using prescribed and over-the-counter drugs.	2	1	0

Alcohol and Drugs Score: _____

Eating Habits	Almost Always	Sometimes	Almost Never
1. I eat a variety of foods each day, such as fruits and vegetables, whole-grain breads and cereals, lean meats, dairy products, dry peas and beans, and nuts and seeds.	4	1	0
2. I limit the amount of fat, saturated fat, and cholesterol I eat (including fat on meats, eggs, butter, cream, shortenings, and organ meats, such as liver).	2	1	0
3. I limit the amount of salt I eat by cooking with only small amounts, not adding salt at the table, and avoiding salty snacks.	2	1	0
4. I avoid eating too much sugar (especially frequent snacks of sticky candy or soft drinks).	2	1	0

Eating Habits Score: _____

Exercise and Fitness	Almost Always	Sometimes	Almost Never
1. I maintain a desired weight, avoiding overweight and underweight.	3	1	0
2. I do vigorous exercises for 15 to 30 minutes at least three times a week (examples: running, swimming, brisk walking).	3	1	0
3. I do exercises that enhance my muscle tone for 15 to 30 minutes at least three times a week (examples: yoga and calisthenics).	2	1	0
4. I use part of my leisure time participating in individual, family, or team activities (such as gardening, bowling, golf, and baseball) that increase my level of fitness.	2	1	0

Exercise and Fitness Score: _____

Stress Control	Almost Always	Sometimes	Almost Never
1. I have a job or do other work that I enjoy.	2	1	0
2. I find it easy to relax and express my feelings freely.	2	1	0
3. I recognize early, and prepare for, events or situations likely to be stressful for me.	2	1	0

Box continued on following page

		Almost Always	Sometimes	Almost Never
4. I have close friends, relatives, or others whom I can talk to about personal matters and call on for help when needed.		2	1	0
5. I participate in group activities (such as church and community organizational activities) or hobbies that I enjoy.		2	1	0

Stress Control Score: _____

Safety

	Almost Always	Sometimes	Almost Never
1. I wear a seat belt while riding in a car.	2	1	0
2. I avoid driving while under the influence of alcohol and other drugs.	2	1	0
3. I obey traffic rules and the speed limit when driving.	2	1	0
4. I am careful when using potentially harmful products or substances (such as household cleaners, poisons, and electrical devices).	2	1	0
5. I avoid smoking in bed.	2	1	0

Safety Score: _____

Your Health Style Scores

After you have figured your scores for each of the six sections, circle the number in each column that matches your score for that section of the test.

Cigarette Smoking	Alcohol and Drugs	Eating Habits	Exercise and Fitness	Stress Control	Safety
10	10	10	10	10	10
9	9	9	9	9	9
8	8	8	8	8	8
7	7	7	7	7	7
6	6	6	6	6	6
5	5	5	5	5	5
4	4	4	4	4	4
3	3	3	3	3	3
2	2	2	2	2	2
1	1	1	1	1	1

Remember, there is no total score for this text. Consider each section separately. You are trying to identify aspects of your lifestyle that you can improve to be healthier and to reduce the risk of illness. So let's see what your scores reveal.

Scores of 9 and 10

Excellent! Your answers show that you are aware of the importance of this area to your health. More important, you are putting your knowledge to work for you by practicing good health habits. As long as you continue to do so, this area should not pose a serious health risk. It is likely that you are setting an example for your family and friends to follow. Because you got a very high score on this part of the test, you may want to consider other areas where your scores indicate room for improvement.

Scores of 6 to 8

Your health practices in this area are good, but there is room for improvement. Look again at the items you answered with a Sometimes or Almost Never. What changes can you make to improve your score? Even a small change can often help you achieve better health.

Scores of 3 to 5

Your health risks are showing! Would you like more information about the risks you are facing and about why it is important for you to change these behaviors? Perhaps you need help in deciding how to successfully make the changes you desire. In either case, help is available.

Scores of 0 to 2

Obviously, you were concerned enough about your health to take the test, but your answers show that you may be taking serious and unnecessary risks with your health. Perhaps you are not aware of the risks and what to do about them. You can easily get the information and help you need to improve, if you wish. The next step is up to you.

▼ ▼ ▼

From U.S. Department of Health and Human Services, Office of Health Information, Health Promotion and Physical Fitness and Sports Medicine (1985). *Health style quiz.* Washington, DC: U.S. Government Printing Office.

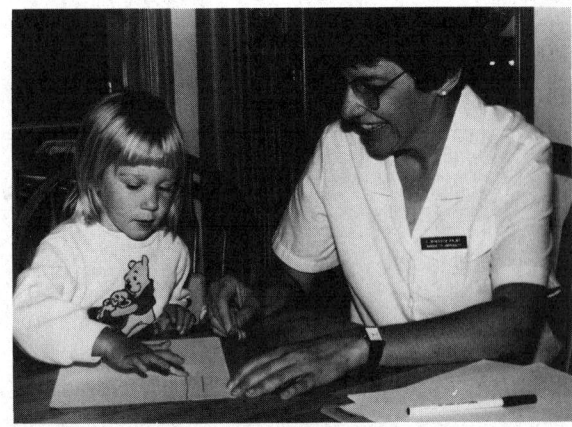

▲ *Figure 20-3*

Health screenings offer the opportunity for teaching to reduce risk factors, early detection of problems, and referral.

▶ Administrating
▶ Reconciling

You have probably had experience in using the first three skills, perhaps in areas unrelated to your nursing education. How could you use inquiring, helping, and teaching to guide individuals in identifying their risk factors?

Health education—education promoting wellness behaviors and the prevention of disease, often focusing on groups and communities—is an integral part of the

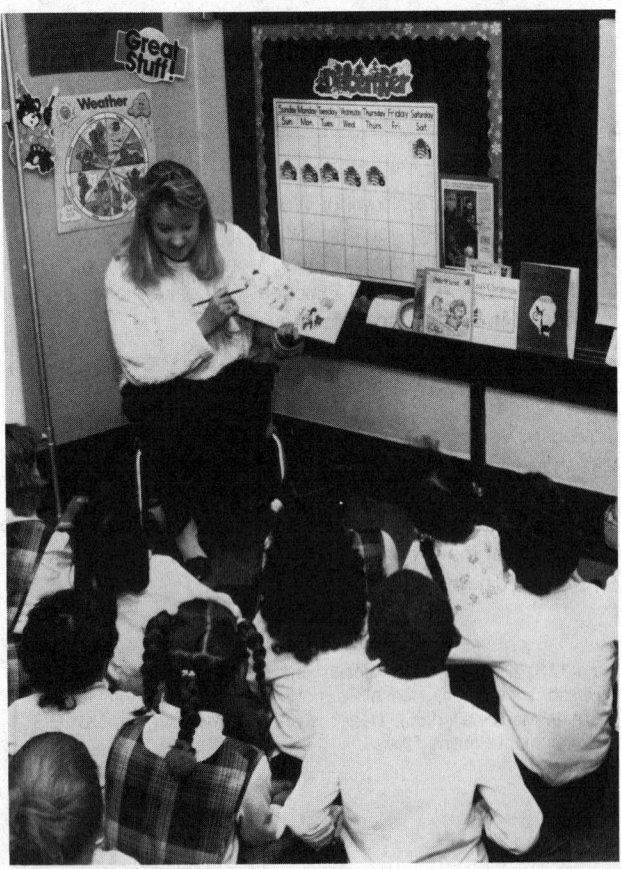

▲ *Figure 20-4*

Health teaching is a useful way to promote health.

nurse's role in health promotion. Nurses apply skills in teaching as they provide information to children and adults, families, groups, and communities (Fig. 20-4). See Chapter 26 for a discussion of teaching and learning.

In health care encounters, every nurse is called on to provide clients and families with an opportunity to learn.[59]

Setting Priorities

The likelihood of succeeding in your attempts to motivate people to adopt a new health behavior is greatly enhanced when you understand their frame of reference. You need to know how they perceive their needs and resources and what value they place on each. The health belief model and the health promotion model discussed earlier can give you a systematic approach for doing this.

You need to set goals that match the value system and needs of your individual client.

For example, Pat is a nurse who works with a group of homeless individuals, many of whom are addicted to intravenous drugs. He knows these people would benefit from yearly physical examinations, nutritious diets, and regular exercise. His priority concern, however, is their risk of contracting AIDS through shared needles and syringes. Pat first gains the confidence of some individuals in the group by helping them get access to care for needs *they* identify as important—treatment for a foot infection and for a tooth abscess, for example. He then works to help them perceive their risk of blood-borne diseases and begin disinfecting their syringes and needles.

Using Principles of Behavior Modification

You can apply principles of behavior modification in providing health counseling and health education for individuals and groups. In attempting to alter individuals' attitudes or beliefs, it is sometimes helpful to get them to first alter a behavior. Suppose, for example, you want to stimulate participants at a student health fair to begin a program of regular exercise. One approach is to give students a pamphlet outlining the benefits of aerobic exercise. Another approach is to have a treadmill, stationary bicycle, and rowing machine available for students to do a trail workout; this experience is likely to stimulate responses such as "That was kind of fun!" or "I didn't know I could do that!" It is likely that success and a sense of satisfaction with the behavior will alter students' attitudes about exercise.

Changes in *behavior* often stimulate changes in *attitudes* or *health beliefs.*

Another tool that is useful for stimulating a change in

behavior is *self-monitoring*. You can instruct clients to keep a log or diary of a specific behavior, such as eating or smoking. An example of a smoking log is shown in Figure 20–5. People who accurately record every cigarette smoked tend to decrease their smoking. The same is true of using a food log to record eating behaviors. For most people, this initial change in behavior will be sustained only if other methods of behavior modification also are used.

Monitoring a behavior has the effect of altering that behavior. This technique is effective for short-term use.

People can alter their health *behaviors* by altering the *antecedents* that precede them or the *consequences* that follow. The circumstances that precede and follow behaviors are important in modifying the behaviors.

Antecedents are factors that tend to stimulate certain behaviors. (Other words for antecedents are "cues" and "triggers.") For example, a coffee break may be a cue for a smoker to light up a cigarette. Getting up in the morning is a cue for toothbrushing for many people. Can you think of other cues to healthy and unhealthy behaviors? People are often unaware of the cues that trigger their behaviors. You can help clients use self-monitoring techniques such as logs and diaries to help them identify their behavioral cues. You can then discuss ways they can alter their cues, for example, by removing high-calorie snack foods from the house, putting an exercise bicycle in front of the television, or getting rid of ashtrays.

If a behavior is followed by pleasant consequences, the individual is likely to repeat or maintain the behavior. Pleasant consequences of behaviors are sometimes called "rewards." Examples include the feeling of relaxation that may accompany smoking or the feeling of stimulation that follows vigorous exercise.

The ABCs of behavior are

Antecedent ⟶ Behavior ⟶ Consequences

When assisting individuals who are working on giving up a harmful behavior that has pleasant consequences, you can teach them to build pleasant experiences into their day to reward successful efforts. The first step is to have them make a list of experiences they perceive as pleasant—a reward list. Everyone's list will be unique. Rewards do not have to be expensive. Taking time out of a busy day to watch a sunset is an example of a "free" reward. It is helpful to place a cost-limit on items on the reward list, to emphasize that price is not important. Allow people some uninterrupted time alone to make a list of 12 rewards. Examples of rewards that people have listed include buying a plant or flower, time for reading a newspaper or chapter of a paperback book, an uninterrupted soak in the bathtub, time to work on a hobby, a special meal, a favorite television show, a movie, a chat on the telephone, and a leisurely walk. You can help people make specific plans

NO.	TIME	NEED	PLACE OR ACTIVITY	WITH WHOM	MOOD OR REASON
1	7:15 am	5	Breakfast - Coffee	Family	Relaxed
2	8:00 am	3	Train - playing cards	Friends	Having fun
3	8:25 am	4	RR Station	Alone	Rushed
4					
5					
6					
7					
8					
9					
10					
11					

▲ *Figure 20–5*

A smoking log. In using such a log, a smoker records the following data about each cigarette smoked: time, rating of craving or perceived need (0–5 scale), circumstances, and mood or reason associated with smoking.

TABLE 20-2. Applying Principles of Behavior Modification

Principle	Example	Using the Principle to Help Change a Health Behavior
Many behaviors are triggered by *antecedents:* feelings, situations, or cues immediately preceding the behavior	Mr. Stanford's overeating is triggered by feeling stressed, seeing high-calorie foods, or being in social situations where food is served	Mr. S. can learn to ▶ cope with stress in other ways ▶ have only low-calorie snacks available ▶ select foods and drinks low in calories and fats
Behaviors associated with pleasant feelings tend to be repeated; behaviors associated with unpleasant feelings tend to be avoided	Ms. Lee tries to ride her stationary bicycle for an hour three to four times a week; lately she's been having trouble "sticking with it"; she feels bored while biking, and has knee pain after 30 minutes of biking	Ms. L. could try ▶ listening to music or watching TV while biking ▶ stopping her exercise when her knee begins to hurt ▶ alternating biking with low-impact aerobic exercise
Behaviors followed by pleasant consequences (rewards) tend to be repeated	Mr. Avati always felt "more relaxed" after a "cigarette break"; now he's trying to quit smoking	Mr. A. can build other pleasant experiences into his day by ▶ going for a walk ▶ carrying low-calorie snacks ▶ taking relaxation breaks ▶ making time for a hobby or family activity

to build rewards from their lists into their days after successful efforts at altering a health behavior.

Table 20-2 summarizes some principles of behavior modification, with some examples of applying them.

Promoting Holistic Health

In helping people to achieve integrated and balanced functioning of body, mind, and spirit, nurses apply the strategies summarized in Table 20-3. You can develop skill in applying each strategy with specific groups of individuals through guided practice with nurses who have this expertise.

Collaborating with Other Health Care Providers

When engaging in health promotion activities, you may collaborate with other health care providers, such as these:

▶ Art therapists
▶ Chiropractors
▶ Epidemiologists
▶ Exercise physiologists
▶ Health educators
▶ Massage therapists
▶ Music therapists
▶ Nutritionists
▶ Occupational therapists
▶ Physical therapists
▶ Physicians
▶ Psychotherapists
▶ Recreational therapists
▶ Respiratory therapists
▶ Speech therapists

Clients may be consulting several health care providers in traditional or nontraditional settings. They may be participating in alternative modalities like yoga, acupuncture, and reiki. Yoga and acupuncture have been found to be useful for stress reduction and healing. Reiki is a form of healing by the laying on of hands. It is important to be open to such alternative ways of promoting health because they may be effective adjuncts to traditional health care for some clients.[67]

WORKING WITH FAMILIES, GROUPS, AND COMMUNITIES TO PROMOTE HEALTH

In addition to working with individuals, you will be working with families, groups of people, and communities to promote health. Although all of these aggregates are composed of individuals, your perspective will change as you consider the broader issues and interactions among the individuals.

Family Health Promotion

Health and illness behaviors are learned within families. Families come in a variety of shapes and sizes. The

TABLE 20-3. Strategies to Strengthen the Whole Person

Strategy	Definition
Relaxation	Techniques to promote the absence of physical, mental, and emotional tension
Imagery	Internal experiences of memories, dreams, fantasies, and visions involving one, several, or all of the senses
Music therapy	Use of music to affect behavior, emotions, and physiology
Play	Enjoyable activity undertaken spontaneously and without specific goals for productivity
Humor	The mental faculty of discovering, expressing, or appreciating wit or comedy
Healthy relationships	Mutual support from one or more nonjudgmental people with whom to share hurts, failures, successes, interests, and excitements; people who help us reach our potential
Therapeutic touch	A process by which energy is transmitted from one person to another with the intention of promoting healing of mind, body, and spirit; the nurse as healer remains centered and mentally focused on healing
Life review	The remembering of significant past events

Data from Dossey, B.M., et al. (1989). *Strategies for strengthening the whole person.* Rockville, MD: Aspen Publishers.

way families function with regard to their health depends on the culture of its members. Each family decides for itself what health care and health promotion activities and priorities will be addressed. When we look beyond individuals to families as the focus of our interventions, we see that the family is instrumental in the development, prevention, and correction of health problems.[14]

Families move through a variety of stages that parallel the development of its members. Each stage has ramifications for the health of family members as well as for healthy family functioning. For example, John and Nancy Bertram, a couple beginning their marriage, may have health promotion concerns regarding choices about sexual expression and reproduction, balancing career interests with home maintenance, and separating from families of origin. On the other hand, Amanda Brown and Florence Green, retired widows who are living together, may have health promotion issues regarding sexual expression and dealing with sexual mores in the community in which they live, maintaining mobility and social activities, coping with personal loss of function, and maintaining their own health while caring for the other person during periods of illness. They also may eventually need help in dealing with health institutions, financing health care, and coping with one another's and their own approaching death in healthy ways.

As a nurse, you will need to assess how adequately the family feels it is functioning as a unit with special regard to its role in health promotion. For example, are parents able to provide healthy role modeling for children? Are resources regarding single parenting available? Are individuals supported by their family and friends in pursuing a healthy lifestyle?

The issues of shape and size of the family, culture, and developmental stage of the family and its members all will affect the range of approaches you discuss with

them to improve their health. Also, how well is the family connected with available community resources, including education and support groups? What ideas might you suggest for enhancing their connection with these resources?

Health Promotion Within Groups

To reach large groups with health promotion messages, new ideas can be introduced in a variety of ways. Mass media are useful for sharing information and changing attitudes. Flyers and press releases to newspapers, radio, and television provide unique ways of reaching people who may not ordinarily use health promotion services.

Interpersonal strategies such as classes, health advocacy groups, and community task forces may be most effective after the ideas have been introduced with mass media strategies. Interpersonal strategies are required to teach, encourage practice, and provide support and positive feedback as well as to promote peer acceptance of new behaviors.[74] The following steps of a program planning process are useful in developing such strategies:[74]

▶ Planning and choosing strategies
▶ Choosing routes and materials
▶ Developing/procuring and pretesting materials
▶ Implementing strategies and tracking audience response
▶ Evaluating effectiveness
▶ Refining the program

As you plan a program, you may wish to consider the unique needs of the group. For example, where do teens learn things they want to know? What do they

NURSING DIAGNOSIS PROFILE

Health-Seeking Behaviors (specify)

Definition. The state in which an individual in stable health is actively seeking ways to alter personal health habits and/or the environment in order to move toward a higher level of health. (Stable health status is defined as age-appropriate illness prevention measures achieved; client reports good or excellent health; and signs and symptoms of disease, if present, are controlled.)

Classification. Choosing 5.4.

Defining Characteristics
Major
Expressed or observed desire to seek a higher level of wellness
Minor
Expressed or observed desire for increased control of health practice
Expressed concern about current environmental conditions or health status
Stated or observed unfamiliarity with wellness community resources
Demonstrated or observed lack of knowledge in health promotion behaviors

Sample Related Factors. Situational/maturational event precipitating desire to take action to promote or maintain health.

Concept Description. Clients' stated desires to pursue health promotion are central to helping them achieve this goal. Some may simply require information about risks to their health and how to reduce them. Others may need help in developing a sense of personal ability or efficacy in promoting their health. It is important to listen carefully both to the desired health behavior and to the client's perceived needs in accomplishing the behavior.

Some clients become aware of environmental health hazards, which leads them to contact a nurse for help in safeguarding their health. For example, a client may notice that only fried foods are available on the cafeteria menu and seek assistance in developing strategies for having healthy options included. Other clients may have identified the need for health promotion but not know where they can find educational materials, a needed health professional, or the necessary social support to accomplish health behavior change.

Examples. Depending on the specific assessment data, this diagnostic category could be applicable to a number of situations, including the following.

▶ *Health-Seeking Behaviors* (healthy diet) R/T desire to decrease fat and salt in diet
▶ *Health-Seeking Behaviors* (exercise) R/T lack of knowledge of safe exercise practices and places
▶ *Health-Seeking Behaviors* (managing stress) R/T lack of assertiveness on the job
▶ *Health-Seeking Behaviors* (healthy environment) R/T lack of a workplace smoking policy

Related/Similar Nursing Diagnoses. When making a diagnosis, you should be able to differentiate between *Health Maintenance, Altered* and *Health-Seeking Behaviors*. These two diagnoses may seem similar on the surface, but they are quite different.

The diagnosis *Altered Health Maintenance* would be appropriate when an individual's health status, developmental disabilities, socioeconomic status, culture, or other barriers prevent the person from identifying, managing, or requesting nursing assistance with health maintenance. In contrast, the diagnosis of *Health-Seeking Behaviors* would be used when an individual in stable health identifies a need for health promotion services to elevate health to an even higher level. The diagnosis of *Health-Seeking Behaviors* (specify) could also be used with a family or group as well as with individuals who seek nursing assistance for increasing their health.

---

see as the most important issues confronting them? Critical to planning effective programs is a clear understanding of the topic to be addressed, what people in the group already know and think about the topic, and what resources are available. When choosing materials and ways to present them, you will also want to consider if there are smaller subgroups within the group to whom you especially wish to target certain information.

What objectives do the groups hope to accomplish? What level of change is feasible to expect? Feedback from the group throughout the planning and implementation phases is essential to program success. Is there a small group with whom you can pretest the materials? Is the information presented in a way they find interesting? Is the reading level appropriate? What suggestions do they have about the content?

Each program is a chance to learn new ways of most effectively working with groups. What teaching materials work best with African-American teens in the central city? How can you effectively share information with adults in rural areas? How can you target your efforts to groups most at risk for health problems?

Targeting At-risk Groups in Communities

If we had unlimited time, energy, and money, we could provide health promotion services at every available opportunity. Because that is usually not the case, we try to provide services where they are most needed.

Health departments at the local, provincial, state, and national levels set objectives and target levels for achievement of health objectives. Efforts are most effective if the nurse involves members of the community in setting the objectives as well as in planning and implementing programs. You can be assisted to target programs effectively by reading available research reports as well as by asking experts in given areas to identify priorities. Experts you may wish to include are consumers and representatives of business, labor, food distribution, housing, cultural, and civic groups. Although these experts are not usually thought of as being distinctly involved in promoting health, they can be helpful in identifying priorities and possible solutions.

Evaluating Responses to Health Promotion Programs

Effective planning includes realistic goal setting. Few programs are 100 per cent effective. Comparative analysis of the effectiveness of similar programs in other settings and with other groups provides useful data by which to evaluate program success.[34]

HEALTHY PUBLIC POLICY

By working through professional organizations and with consumer groups, nurses help create healthy public policy. For example, agriculture policies can be modified to support healthy foods and to end subsidies for tobacco production. These policies will enable many people to promote their health more easily.

Although individuals and groups can accomplish much to promote their own health, even more people can benefit when public policies support an environment conducive to health. For example, most vending machines contain one or two healthy snacks amid 15 or more snacks that are high in fat and salt. What if you worked with others in your school or workplace to increase the availability of healthy snack foods? What would happen if fruit cost less than candy bars and the money earned on the candy subsidized the cost of fruit?

Federal subsidies currently support tobacco growing. What if farm policies were changed to support re-education of tobacco growers in other jobs as well as to provide tobacco farmers with subsidies for planting alternative crops?

Incorporating consumer input and engaging in collaborative negotiation with everyone who has an interest in the policy is vital in planning policy changes. Remember, policies change very slowly and incrementally, so be patient, but do not give up!

Summary

▶ Health is being able to function fully and find self-expression in all the domains of one's life. Health protection involves preventing disease, whereas health promotion involves enhancing well-being. Nurses provide health promotion services where people live, work, and play as well as in traditional health care settings.

▶ External factors (such as income) and internal factors (such as attitudes, beliefs, and behaviors) influence health.

▶ Models of health behavior help nurses and other professionals plan effective strategies to promote health with individuals and communities.

▶ In assessing health, it is important to understand what individuals believe is important in staying healthy and the actions they already are taking to promote health.

▶ Nurses make a positive impact through their own healthy lifestyles, teaching, and assisting with behavior change.

▶ Nurses assess family functioning and health promotion needs and work with groups and communities to target and develop programs that address crucial health needs.

▶ Nurses work through professional organizations and with consumer groups to create healthy public policies that enable many people to live healthier lives.

Bibliography

1. American Nurses' Association (1980). *A social policy statement.* Kansas City: The Association.
2. American Nurses' Association (1987). *The nursing center concept and design.* Kansas City: The Association.
3. American Nurses' Association (1987). *The scope of nursing practice.* Kansas City: The Association.
4. American Nurses' Association (1991). *Nursing's agenda for health care reform.* Washington, DC: American Nurses' Association.
5. Barger, S.E., & Bridges, W.C. (1990). An assessment of academic nursing centers. *Nurse Educator*, 15(2), 31–36.
6. Baumann, L.J., & Keller, M.L. (1991). Responses to threat information. *Image*, 23(1), 13–18.
7. Becker, M.H. (ed.). (1974). *Health belief model and personal health behavior.* Thoroughfare, NJ: Charles B. Slack.
8. Belloc, N.B. (1973). Relationships of health practices and mortality. *Preventive Medicine*, 2(1), 67–81.
9. Belloc, N.B., & Breslow, L. (1972). Relationship of physical health status and health practices. *Preventive Medicine*, 1(3), 409–421.
10. Bulechek, G., & McCloskey, J. (1989). Nursing interventions: treatments for potential nursing diagnoses. In Carroll-Johnson, R.M. (ed.). *Classification of nursing diagnoses: Proceedings of the eighth conference* (pp. 23–30). Philadelphia: J.B. Lippincott.
11. Butterfield, P.G. (1990). Thinking upstream: nurturing a conceptual understanding of the societal context of health behavior. *Advances in Nursing Science*, 12(2), 1–8.
12. Canadian Nurses' Association (1987). *A definition of nursing practice.* Ohawa: The Association.
13. Canadian Nurses' Association (1988). *Health for all Canadians: A call for health-care reform.* Ohawa: The Association.
14. Casey, B.A. (1989). The family as a system. In Bomar, P.J. (ed.). *Nurses and family health promotion* (pp. 37–46). Baltimore: Williams & Wilkins.
15. DiMatteo, M.R., & DiNicola, D.D. (1982). *Achieving patient compliance.* New York: Pergamon Press.
16. Donabedian, A. (1989). Quality of care and the health needs of the elderly patient. In Barondess, J.A., et al. (eds.). *Care of the elderly patient: Policy issues and research opportunities.* Washington, DC: National Academy Press.
17. Dossey, B.M., et al. (1989). *Holistic health promotion: A guide for practice.* Rockville, MD: Aspen Publishers.
18. Dougherty, G., et al. (1990). Social class and the occurrence of traffic injuries and deaths in urban children. *Canadian Journal of Public Health*, 81(3), 204–206.
19. Edwards, N.C., & McMillan, K. (1990). Tobacco use and ethnicity: the existing data gap. *Canadian Journal of Public Health*, 81, 32–35.
20. Epp, J. (1986). *Achieving health for all: A framework for health promotion* (H39-102/1986E). Ohawa: Minister of Supply and Services.
21. Faulkner, R.A., & Slattery, C.M. (1990). The relationship of physical activity to alcohol consumption in youth 15–16 years of age. *Canadian Journal of Public Health*, 81(2), 168–169.
22. Feinstein, D., & Krippner, S. (1988). *Personal mythology: The psychology of your evolving self.* Los Angeles: J.P. Tarcher.
23. Frenn, M., et al. (1989). Lifestyle changes in a cardiac rehabilitation program: the client perspective. *Journal of Cardiovascular Nursing*, 3(2), 43–55.
24. Frenn, M., & Lee, H. (1992). Health maintenance altered. In Gettrust, K., & Brabec, P. (eds.). *Nursing diagnosis in clinical practice: Guides for care planning* (pp. 276–284). Albany, NY: Delmar Publishers.

25. Funkhouser, S.W., & Moser, D.K. (1990). Is health care racist? *Advances in Nursing Science*, 12(2), 47–55.

26. Glanz, K., & Mullis, R.M. (1988). Environmental interventions to promote healthy eating: a review of models, programs, and evidence. *Health Education Quarterly*, 15(4), 395–415.

27. Guidotti, T.L. (1989). Health promotion in perspective. *Canadian Journal of Public Health*, 80(6), 400–405.

28. Hann, M., et al. (1987). Poverty and health: prospective evidence from the Alameda County study. *American Journal of Epidemiology*, 125(6), 989–998.

29. Harper, D.C. (1988). Why health care costs so much. *Personnel Journal*, 67(9), 45–51.

30. Higgins, W. (1988). The economics of health promotion. *Health Values*, 12(5), 39–45.

31. Houldin, A.D., et al. (1987). *Nursing diagnoses for wellness: Supporting strengths*. Philadelphia: J.B. Lippincott.

32. Inforum (1990). Wellness popular, but lags behind primary care. *Hospitals*, 64(5), 14.

33. Janz, N.K. (1988). The Health Belief Model in understanding cardiovascular risk factor reduction behaviors. *Cardiovascular Nursing*, 24(6), 39–41.

34. Kar, S.B. (ed.). (1989). *Health promotion indicators and actions*. New York: Springer.

35. Katz, S., et al. (1983). Active life expectancy. *New England Journal of Medicine*, 309(20), 1218–1224.

36. Lantz, J.M. (1989). Family culture and ethnicity. In Bomar, P.J. (ed.). *Nurses and family health promotion* (pp. 47–54). Baltimore: Williams & Wilkins.

37. Lee, H., & Frenn, M. (1992). Health seeking behaviors (specify). In Gettrust, K., & Brabec P. (eds.). *Nursing diagnosis in clinical practice: Guides for care planning* (pp. 285–288). Albany, NY: Delmar Publishers.

38. Lindberg, S.C. (1987). Adult preventive health screening: 1987 update. *Nurse Practitioner*, 12(5), 19–41.

39. Lubben, J.E., et al. (1989). Health practices of the elderly poor. *American Journal of Health Promotion*, 79(6), 731–734.

40. Maglacas, A.M. (1988). Health for all: nursing's role. *Nursing Outlook*, 36(2), 66–71.

41. Mallinger, K.M. (1989). The American family: history and development. In Bomar, P.J. (ed.). *Nurses and family health promotion* (pp. 37–46). Baltimore: Williams & Wilkins.

42. Matheus, R. (1990). *A parish nurse curriculum*. (Available from Rosemarie Matheus, R.N., M.S.N., College of Nursing, Marquette University, Milwaukee, WI 53233.)

43. McLeroy, K.R., et al. (1988). An ecological perspective on health promotion programs. *Health Education Quarterly*, 15(4), 351–377.

44. Meleis, A.I. (1990). Being and becoming healthy: the core of nursing knowledge. *Nursing Science Quarterly*, 3(3), 107–114.

45. Million-Underwood, S., & Sanders, E. (1990). Factors contributing to health promotion behaviors among African-American men. *Oncology Nursing Forum*, 17(5), 707–712.

46. Mindell, A. (1990). *Working on yourself alone*. London: Arkana.

47. Moccia, P. (1990). Reclaiming our communities. *Nursing Outlook*, 38(2), 73–76.

48. Nightingale, F. (1969 republication of 1859 work). *Notes on nursing: What it is and what it is not*. New York: Dover.

49. North American Nursing Diagnosis Association (1990). *Taxonomy I revised*. St. Louis: The Association.

50. Office of Disease Prevention and Health Promotion, Department of Health Education and Human Services (1991). *Healthy people 2000: National health promotion and disease prevention objectives* (DHHS Publication No. PHS 91–50212). Washington, DC: U.S. Government Printing Office.

51. Offord, D. (1991). Growing up poor in Ontario. *Transition*, (June), 10–14.

52. Opatz, J.P. (1987). *Health promotion evaluation: Measuring the organizational impact*. Stevens Point, WI: A National Wellness Institute Publication.

53. Payne, W.A., & Hahn, D.B. (1989). *Understanding your health*. St. Louis: Times Mirror/Mosby.

54. Pender, N.J. (1987). *Health promotion in nursing practice* (2nd ed.). Norwalk, CT: Appleton & Lange.

55. Pender, N.J. (1987). Health and health promotion: The conceptual dilemmas. In Duffy, M.E., & Pender, N.J. (eds.). *Conceptual issues in health promotion* (pp. 7–23). Indianapolis, IN: Sigma Theta Tau International, Honor Society of Nursing.

56. Philips, B.U. (1988). Epidemiological issues in health promotion and cost containment. *Health Values*, 12(5), 32–38.

57. Pollock, S.E., et al. (1990). Responses to chronic illness: analysis of psychological and physiological adaptation. *Nursing Research*, 39(5), 300–304.

58. Popkess-Vawter, S. (1991). Wellness nursing diagnoses: to be or not to be? *Nursing Diagnosis*, 2(1), 19–25.

59. Rankin, S.H., & Stallings, K.D. (1990). *Patient education: Issues, principles, and practices* (2nd ed.) Philadelphia: J.B. Lippincott.

60. Rooney, E. (1990). Corporate attitudes and responses to rising health care costs. *American Association of Occupational Health Nurses Journal*, 38(7), 304–311.

61. Rosenstock, I.M. (1990). The health belief model: explaining health behavior through expectancies. In *Health behavior and health education: Theory, research, and practice*. San Francisco: Jossey-Bass Publishers.

62. Ryan, P. (1989). Noncompliance. In Thompson, J.M., et al. *Mosby's manual of clinical nursing*. St. Louis: C.V. Mosby.

63. Salazar, M.K. (1991). Comparison of four behavioral theories. *American Association of Occupational Health Nurses Journal*, 39(3), 128–135.

64. Selker, L. (1986). Special implications for special populations: the elderly, the disabled, and the ethnic minorities. *Journal of Allied Health*, 15(4), 310–313.

65. Shannon, I.S. (1990). Public health's promise for the future: 1989 presidential address. *American Journal of Public Health*, 80(8), 909–912.

66. Smith, M.D. (1990). Nursing's unique focus on health promotion. *Nursing Science Quarterly*, 3(3), 105–106.

67. Stein, D. (1990). *All women are healers: A comprehensive guide to natural healing*. Freedom, CA: The Crossing Press.

68. Stuifbergen, A.K., et al. (1990). Barriers to health promotion for individuals with disabilities. *Family & Community Health*, 13(1), 11–22.

69. Stuifbergen, A.K., et al. (1990). Perceptions of health among adults with disabilities. *Health Values*, 14(2), 18–26.

70. Swinford, P.A., & Webster, J.A. (1989). *Promoting wellness: A nurse's handbook*. Rockville, MD: Aspen.

71. Taptich, B.J., et al. (1989). *Nursing diagnosis and care planning*. Philadelphia: W.B. Saunders.

72. Tzuriel, D. (1989). Development of motivation and cognitive-informational orientations from third to ninth grades. *Journal of Applied Developmental Psychology*, 10, 107–121.

73. U.S. Department of Health and Human Services, Office of Health Information, Health Promotion and Physical Fitness and Sports Medicine (1985). *Health style quiz*. Washington, DC: U.S. Government Printing Office.

74. U.S. Department of Health, Education, and Welfare (1989). *Making health communication programs work: A planner's guide* (NIH No. 89–1493). Washington, DC: Public Health Services National Cancer Institute.

75. U.S. Department of Health and Human Services (1989). *United States 1989 and health prevention profile* (PHS 90–1232). Washington, DC: U.S. Government Printing Office.

76. U.S. Department of Health and Human Services (1990). *Healthy people 2000: National health promotion and disease prevention objectives* (PHS 91–50212). Washington, DC: U.S. Government Printing Office.

77. Walker, S.N., et al. (1988). Health-promoting lifestyles of older adults: comparisons with young and middle-aged adults, correlates and patterns. *Advances in Nursing Science*, 11(1), 76–90.

78. Weitzel, M.H., & Waller, P.R. (1990). Predictive factors for health-promotive behaviors in white, Hispanic, and black blue-collar workers. *Family & Community Health*, 13(1), 23–34.

79. Wierenga, M.E. (1991). The smoking cessation process. *Wisconsin Medical Journal*, 90(1), 19–21.

80. Wierenga, M.E., et al. (1990). A descriptive study of how clients make life-style changes. *The Diabetes Educator*, 16(6), 469–473.

81. Wigle, D.T., et al. (1990). Premature deaths in Canada: impact, trends and opportunities for prevention. *Canadian Journal of Public Health*, 81(5), 376–382.

82. Woods, N. (1989). Conceptualizations of self care: toward health oriented models. *Advances in Nursing Science*, 12(1), 1–13.

83. Zimmerman, R.S., & Conner, C. (1989). Health promotion in context: the effects of significant others on health behavior change. *Health Education Quarterly*, 16(1), 57–85.

▼ The Illness Experience

Chapter

21

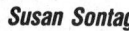

Everyone who is born holds dual citizenship, in the kingdom of the
well and in the kingdom of the sick. Although we all prefer to use
only the good passport, sooner or later each of us is obliged, at
least for a spell, to identify ourselves as citizens of that other place.

Susan Sontag
Illness as Metaphor, 1978

▼ CHAPTER OUTLINE

STAGES OF THE ILLNESS EXPERIENCE
    Transition
    Acceptance
    Convalescence
SEEKING ASSISTANCE
    Responses to Initial Cues About
      Illness
    Factors Affecting Initial Responses
      to Illness
REACTIONS TO CONFIRMED ILLNESS
    Uncertainty
    Anxiety
    Shock
    Denial
    Anger
    Information Seeking
    Shame

    Isolation
    Fear
    Depression
    Mood Swings
    Powerlessness
    Altered Body Image
ROLES OF THE ILL PERSON
    Sick Role
    Impaired Role
CHRONIC ILLNESS
    Individual Responses to Chronic
      Illness
    Family Support During Chronic
      Illness
QUALITY OF LIFE
MEETING HUMAN NEEDS DURING
    ILLNESS

▼ KEY TERMS

Body image
Chronicity
Compliance

Powerlessness
Proprioceptive stimuli
Quality of life

Sick role
Symptom

After studying this chapter, you should be able to

1. *Describe the major stages of the illness experience.*
2. *Discuss the individual's responses to the first signs of illness and the factors affecting those responses.*
3. *List common reactions to confirmed illness.*
4. *Discuss the roles of the ill person.*
5. *Discuss the key issues affecting the person with chronic illness.*
6. *Define quality of life.*
7. *Discuss the ways the nurse can support a person in meeting basic human needs during illness.*

Illness is an unavoidable, common, and normal part of human experience. We have all had at least a cold or the flu, for instance. Although virtually everyone encounters illness at some point, the effects of illness and the day-to-day responses are experienced individually and subjectively in ways that can never be fully communicated to others. For nurses to care *for* ill people, they must care *about* them. They must understand as much as possible about the subjective experiences of ill people in general and their own clients in particular.

Nurses can enrich their understanding by talking to others about their feelings during illness, by reading or watching films of fictional and nonfictional accounts of illness (Box 21–1), and by considering their own encounters with illness. By thoughtful observation, nurses can gain useful insights into typical experiences of illness, the services that ill people require and find helpful, and the reasons ill people behave as they do.

In relating the inner, subjective experiences of the ill person to the external, objective, observed signs of disease, remember that science and philosophy have not yet explained the relationship between mind and body. It may seem simple common sense to remember that an individual's mind and body are always components of an organic whole. We are sometimes tempted, however, to give one priority over the other, often depending on our personal philosophy, our intellectual outlook, and our particular concept of health and disease (see Chapter 2). The fallacy of placing mind over body, for instance, is evident in the way we often attach significance or meaning to illness. For instance, many people believe that illness or injury is a punishment for behavior, as when a person develops lung or throat cancer after years of smoking, is killed while driving drunk, or contracts acquired immune deficiency syndrome through illegal drug use.

More subtly, some have suggested relationships between personality traits or attitudes and susceptibility to certain illnesses or the ability to deal with or overcome illness. Cancer, for example, has been thought to be linked with a personality that represses the expression of strong feelings or to be a response to depressed emotions.[34]

Much exciting research has been conducted on the relationship between illness and affective states such as depression, optimism, and pessimism and also on the relationship between stress and the immune system.

The effects of lifestyle, behaviors, and nutritional choices (such as red meat, sugar, and saturated fat) have also received much research attention. It is important, however, for clients and care givers not to ignore the real physiologic bases of many illnesses. To overemphasize the role of a person's attitude, lifestyle, or behavior in the development of illness can often place an unrealistic burden of responsibility on the ill person.

Some people are more effective than are others in controlling their attitudes and behavior, but their control does not mean that illness is a simple matter of the

---

Box 21–1. Selected Readings on Illness

Broyard, Anatole (1992). *Intoxicated by my illness: And other writings on illness and dying.* New York: Clarkson Potter.

Charmaz, Kathy (1991). *Good days, bad days: The self in chronic illness and time.* New Brunswick, NJ: Rutgers University Press.

Graham, Jory (1987). *In the company of others.* San Diego: Harvest/Harcourt Brace Jovanovich.

Hoffman, Nancy Yanes (1985). *Change of heart: Coronary bypassers tell their experiences.* San Diego: Harcourt Brace Jovanovich.

Mann, Thomas (1924). *The magic mountain.* New York: Alfred A. Knopf.

Monnette, Paul (1988). *Borrowed time: An AIDS memoir.* San Diego: Harcourt Brace Jovanovich.

Morse, Janice M., & Johnson, Joy L. (1991). *The illness experience: Dimensions of suffering.* Newbury Park, CA: Sage.

Sacks, Oliver (1984). *A leg to stand on.* New York: Harper & Row.

Soiffer, Bill (1991). *Life in the shadow: Living with cancer.* San Francisco: Chronicle Books.

Solzhenitzyn, Aleksandr; N. Bethell & D. Burg, trans. (1974). *Cancer ward.* New York: Farrar Straus & Giroux.

Spohr, Betty Baker (1990). *To hold a falling star: A personal memoir of living at home with Alzheimer's disease.* Stamford, CT: Longmeadow.

Tolstoy, Leo; R. Edmonds, trans. (1960). *The death of Ivan Ilyitch.* New York: Penguin Books.

Wheelis, Allen (1992). *The life and death of my mother.* New York: Norton.

individual's choice. Because illness or health is not completely under a person's control, viewing disease as a judgment—of either a specific behavior or a way of living over an entire lifetime—can sometimes become a barrier to effective health care and recovery. To understand the experience of ill people and to use that understanding therapeutically, nurses need a balanced view. Knowing that a disease or disability is a physiologic reality, you can enhance nursing care with an understanding of illness as a profound subjective experience in the mind of the individual.

STAGES OF THE ILLNESS EXPERIENCE

Whereas every person experiences illness in unique ways, the psychologic progress of the experience can fall into three stages: transition, acceptance, and convalescence.

Transition

Illness may begin with vague, nonspecific symptoms that a person initially attempts to deny. A **symptom** is a subjective indication of organic or psychic malfunctioning, or a change in a person's condition that indicates some physical or mental state of disease. The indication is considered subjective because it is the evidence perceived by the patient. When symptoms persist, a person may seek medical consultation but still not admit to being ill. If illness occurs as a sudden crisis, such as a serious accident, stroke, or heart attack, the person may fear that medical help will be either incompetent or not immediately available. Significant others will probably feel shock, disbelief, and denial. Therapeutic interaction with the ill person and significant others is important through the stage of transition.

Acceptance

The stage of acceptance occurs as the person stops denying illness and takes on a "sick role." This stage may be a time of considerable physiologic and psychologic dependence, when the ill person becomes unusually focused on the self. This self-centeredness may be considered a positive response in that the body is permitted to concentrate energy on healing and recovery.

Convalescence

As convalescence (recovery) takes place, a person passes through a transition from illness to health. Usually, the resolution of physical illness precedes the individual's return to normal psychologic and social functioning. If the client's diagnosis is of a chronic or terminal condition, the nurse assists and supports the client and significant others in adjusting their expectations of recovery and "normal" functioning.

SEEKING ASSISTANCE

It is often difficult for a person to seek health care and to undergo diagnostic and treatment procedures. Because health care professionals routinely provide health services, they may sometimes forget that these services may not be routine for the client. Procedures that are unfamiliar are often stressful.

The realization that one needs health care often comes gradually. Sometimes weeks or months may pass between the beginning of a disorder and the seeking of medical help. During this time, the person may experience anxiety and conflict about the illness. People who have delayed seeking health care should not be scolded; instead, they should be treated with support and understanding.

When the person does seek assistance, the apparent symptom is not always the real reason a person seeks help. Physical symptoms are often easier to discuss with a health care professional than are social or interpersonal problems, and so symptoms may simply serve as a starting point for discussion of underlying problems. For example, it may be easier for a person to discuss a headache or backache than to talk about feelings of personal rejection, traumatic abuse, or depression. Even though the physical symptoms may be real, the deeper problems may be the person's true reason for seeking help.

When people are seeking assistance with their health care, nurses often aid them in deciding what kind of help they need and show them where to get it. Nurses, then, are often a bridge between people and other health care professionals such as physicians and specific therapists. Advocacy for the client with these other professionals is an important nursing role.

Responses to Initial Cues About Illness

When a person experiences the first signs of illness, several responses are possible.

No Action or Delayed Action. A person may wait and see, believing that symptoms are not serious enough for professional help to be sought.

Action to Seek Help. A person may take constructive or harmful action. This action may mean seeking help from traditional health care professionals, trying nontraditional therapies, or attempting self-diagnosis and self-treatment. It is common for a person to seek provisional validation from others, discussing the health problem with them to gain confirmation that there is indeed "something wrong" or that their choice of treatment is appropriate.

Vacillation. A person may be ambivalent about seeking help and may vacillate between seeking and not seeking help. The conflict between wanting relief and not wanting to undergo diagnostic and treatment procedures can often be uncomfortable or frightening.

Denial. A person may try to prove that symptoms are not real by continuing or increasing activity, thus denying the illness. The person may refuse to seek help or may consult one health care professional after another in an effort to find someone who will confirm the absence of illness. As a nurse, you need to differentiate between real lack of knowledge (failure to realize that the symptoms represent illness) and the psychologic coping mechanism of denial (denying the presence, or minimizing the severity, of symptoms that indicate illness).

Factors Affecting Initial Responses to Illness

Many variables influence the ways people deal with their initial symptoms or indications of illness. These factors may stem either from the symptoms themselves or from the psychosocial context in which the person experiences them.

SYMPTOM-RELATED FACTORS

Symptom-related factors involve the physical experience of illness. Although physiologic mechanisms are similar among people with a specific condition, responses can vary in a number of ways.

Perceived Symptom Seriousness. People usually seek health care promptly for frightening or dramatic symptoms. Symptoms that are not perceived as serious or incapacitating may be ignored or denied. Often it takes a person some time to determine the seriousness of symptoms, to decide whether treatment is required or whether the symptoms will clear up by themselves, and to understand whether the symptoms are real or imagined.

Ability to Assess Symptom Seriousness. People may not be in a position to evaluate with any accuracy the severity of their own symptoms. They may have a prior disorder that clouds their judgment, such as psychiatric problems, alcoholism or other substance abuse, intellectual disability, confusion or disorientation, or neurologic impairment. The very young or the very old may be unable to understand the seriousness of their symptoms for various reasons. The symptoms themselves may be in their early stages, as is often the case in chronic illness, and therefore not detectable by the person they affect.

Interference with Normal Activities. A person may be more concerned and more likely to seek help if symptoms interfere with the usual activities of daily living. Many people wish to avoid assuming a "sick role" at any cost. Some may perceive symptoms as more serious if they disrupt the lives of others.

Visibility. A person may seek professional help more readily for conspicuous conditions, such as external bleeding, than for less obvious symptoms, such as indigestion.

Frequency, Intensity, Persistence, and Recurrence. The more frequent, annoying, persistent, or constant a symptom or disorder, the more likely a person is to seek professional help.

PSYCHOSOCIAL CONTEXT

The psychosocial context in which a person experiences illness also affects the way in which that person seeks health care. A person's psychosocial context includes family, community, personality, and experience, which interact to influence health and illness. People respond to various components of their psychosocial context.

Pressure from Significant Others. People tend to seek help earlier if they have significant others who are concerned and counsel them to seek professional advice.

Social Characteristics. Social factors such as sex role, age, socioeconomic status, and culture can all affect a person's expectations of health care. For example, some men consider help seeking to be contrary to their self-image of being strong and independent, and so they may avoid seeking health care. Older people may attribute their symptoms to their age and assume they are natural developments and not treatable by health care professionals.

Access to Health Care. A person's ability to get to a health care facility and to obtain the necessary services is an important factor in a person's choice of responses to illness. Some people may be reluctant to enter a complex, time-consuming, degrading, and expensive system. Others may not be willing to go through numerous referrals. Still others may find it difficult to determine the best choice from among various alternatives. For a growing number of people, the financial ability to obtain necessary health care services is a serious problem.

Previous Experience with Health Care. Some people may have had previous unpleasant experiences in seeking health care, either for themselves or for loved ones. Some may be terrified that admission to a health care facility will inevitably result in their death. Their criticism of the health care setting and health care professionals, which may extend to nurses, may or may not be justified. For gaining their trust, it is essential for care givers to exhibit caring and professional behavior. Care givers also need to explore the ill person's feelings about prior experiences in an open and nonjudgmental way.

Loss of Privacy. The psychologic discomfort of physical examination and revealing one's intimate life history may also prevent a person from seeking health care. For some, the physical contact required in a physical examination is embarrassing, intrusive, sexually threatening, or disturbing in some other way. People may fear the pain, exposure, and strangeness that are often part of medical treatments and procedures. What is familiar and routine to health care professionals is often strange to everyone else.

REACTIONS TO CONFIRMED ILLNESS

Each person's reaction to the confirmation of illness is unique. What frightens one person may be inconsequential to another. What may seem trivial to a health care professional may be a major concern to an ill person. People often attribute meanings to illness, and these meanings will greatly affect their responses. An individual's coping patterns, which are usually established during states of health, will often be reflected in the specific behaviors used to deal with illness. For example, a person who responds with extreme behavior to the normal stresses of life will probably exhibit the same kind of responses to the crisis of illness.

Self-concept and philosophy of life also influence a person's reaction to illness. For instance, someone who has always taken a pessimistic view of life may well expect the worst outcome from the illness. Although it is often possible to affect a person's reaction to illness by changing self-concept or personal outlook, that change may require undoing a lifetime of ingrained beliefs and habits. As a nurse, you need to distinguish between appropriate action to change the ill person's outlook and attempts at change that may be ineffective or unfair to the client.

Other factors affecting a person's reaction to illness include the following examples.

► *Age.* An older person who feels content with the achievements and fulfillment of life may be able to accept a serious illness better than a young person might.
► *Socioeconomic status.* People with limited income and no health insurance may incur serious debt because of illness, whereas people with secure finances have less worry.
► *Personal strength.* People with sources of inner strength may handle illness with the same confidence they handle the rest of life.
► *History of past illness.* One's first experience with serious illness may be particularly stressful as one becomes aware of physical vulnerability. Someone who has experienced repeated illness may become exhausted and depressed about facing the ordeal yet again.

Illness is a major life disruption and requires both physical and psychosocial adaptation. People often adapt (or fail to adapt) to illness in the same way they have adapted to other stresses. Adaptation takes time, and an ill person needs support while adapting to the new circumstances. Some reactions may be difficult to handle; others are often a natural part of adapting. You can learn to deal effectively with clients' responses to illness through skillful therapeutic interaction and ongoing observation.

Uncertainty

Uncertainty is an important factor for anyone with an illness. Uncertainty is defined as "the inability to determine the meaning of illness-related events." It takes four forms: (1) ambiguity concerning the state of the illness, (2) complexity regarding treatment and system of care, (3) lack of information about the diagnosis and seriousness of the illness, and (4) unpredictability of the course of the disease and prognosis.[20]

Uncertainty is not necessarily an undesirable state of mind for the ill person. Uncertain events can be evaluated as having possibilities for harmful or positive outcomes. When a person perceives uncertainty as a danger, one of the most important strategies for reducing uncertainty is information seeking from physicians, nurses, and significant others. When a person perceives uncertainty as a positive opportunity, on the other hand, the person often prefers the hope of a positive outcome to the alternative expectation of a negative outcome. Because hope is desirable, you might find that supporting the ill person's uncertainty is beneficial. Before deciding to resolve uncertainty, you need to determine the implications of that uncertainty for the client.

Anxiety

Everyone experiences some degree of anxiety on being confronted with illness, and certain physical and emotional symptoms associated with anxiety should be differentiated from the symptoms of the illness (see Chapter 16). Illness sometimes leads to introspective thoughts about the meaning of life. The ill person may begin to realize that life is short and death inevitable. Such thoughts produce anxiety; for some, this introspection can help uncover personal sources of strength and faith.

Shock

Many people experience a period of shock when they first learn of a diagnosis, especially a serious one. Shocked people feel immobilized, and life seems unreal and dreamlike.

Shocked people are often incapable of thinking clearly or acting rationally. Their behavior may make no sense to themselves or to others. They may act automatically or inappropriately.

A person in shock will seem to be in a protective cocoon and exhibit little feeling. When the shock lessens, however, other emotions like anger, fear, and depression emerge. People in shock need support, protective care, understanding, and advocacy. The nurse is often the care giver who takes on the advocate role.

Denial

A person may deny a health problem and insist that others are wrong. The purpose of denial is often to maintain psychic protection from the overwhelming threat that the illness represents. A person in denial searches for evidence to support this belief and sometimes misquotes a nurse or physician to obtain that evidence. This behavior may provide important self-protection and personal comfort for the client even if an unintended result is the obstruction of care givers' efforts.

Denial occurs in varying degrees. Forgetting is a mild form, as when a person forgets to take prescribed medication. When denial is more extreme, some people push themselves into overexertion or go from one consulting room to another seeking someone who will tell them what they want to hear.

For most people, denial passes naturally as adaptation progresses. Forcing someone to give up denial and face facts may be nontherapeutic; this exposes the person to painful realities and challenges, for which many clients are unprepared. Sometimes denial persists, and a person may die still denying the presence of illness.

Denial is a part of life. We all try to deny unhappiness and suffering at some point in our lives. Although nurses too have experiences they may want to deny, denial does not usually result in good nursing practice. Nurses may sometimes need help in identifying personal tendencies toward denial of pain, death, or fear, which can interfere with competent, caring nursing practice.

Anger

An ill person may feel angry at the impairment of abilities, activities, or sensations that the illness brings about. Sometimes this anger is expressed directly or indirectly toward significant others or the health care worker. Because anger is a difficult emotion to accept, ill people may attribute it to others, using the coping mechanism of projection. Nurses need to understand this projected anger and not take tears, irritability, or other expressions of anger as a personal attack. Of course, if the care a person is receiving could justify anger, tears, or frustration, it is the nurse's responsibility to identify the cause and correct it.

Information Seeking

Ill persons may aggressively seek information because of suspicion, a quest for intellectual control, a need to reduce uncertainty, a sense of protest, or a combination of all these reasons. A person who responds to illness with suspicion may not be denying the truth of the diagnosis but may instead be trying to find reason for doubt. People who tend to be suspicious in other respects will also respond to illness with suspicion. Suspicious people are not necessarily complaining. They are frightened of being hurt or taken advantage of. Suspicious people lack trust and ask a lot of questions. The most effective approach is patience, integrity, and sensitivity in answering all questions.

Many people respond to illness by attempting to learn as much about the disease as they can. Knowledge gives them a sense of mastery to combat the powerlessness that can often result from the serious reduction in physical capability that illness brings. Knowing about the disease and its treatment also allows the client to participate more fully in the decisions regarding treatment alternatives and options such as the care setting. The nurse plays an important role in providing the client with information about the disease and treatment.

Questions can also stem from a protest against the unfairness of disease. "Why me?" "Why did I have to get this?" People who become ill often search for reasons, for the meaning of the illness. Some are content to believe that there are no answers. Others may believe that illness is the consequence of factors such as wrongdoing, destiny, lifestyle, genetic inheritance, personal outlook, or neglect of one's health. Whatever the reasons, many questions about life and death become more focused at times of illness, and the spiritual dimension of life often becomes an important part of nursing care (see Chapter 53).

Shame

People who believe their illnesses to be a punishment may experience shame and guilt. Some people feel ashamed if they develop a disease they consider socially unacceptable, such as worm or lice infestation, a psychiatric problem, or a sexually transmitted disease. Feelings of shame and guilt can diminish a person's self-concept (see Chapter 50).

The attitudes of others toward a person's illness can also provoke shame and guilt. Some illnesses are more threatening than others are and therefore provoke fear. Communicable diseases, particularly acquired immunodeficiency syndrome, are prime examples. Disfiguring conditions such as burns, amputations, or processes that produce odors may frighten or repel others, leading in turn to the ill person's sense of social rejection.

Isolation

Even when the condition does not cause others to withdraw, the ill person can still feel rejected. These feelings may arise in part from the person's separation, by necessity or personal choice, from normal daily activities. When we are not feeling well, the isolation that illness imposes may seem like rejection by others. Chronic illnesses often result in rejection when ill people can no longer engage in accustomed social activities or when the people around them become tired of trying to accommodate a person with illness.

During times of illness, people often become acutely aware of their separateness from others. In fact, sick or well, we are each making our way through life alone to some degree. Social support is vital to all of us, but expressions of care and concern are particularly important to ill people as they experience periods of unaccustomed isolation.

Fear

Fear is an emotional response to a real or imagined harm or unpleasantness. Many specific fears can accompany illness. Some of these are included in Table 21-1.

Some fears develop in childhood and become evident when illness strikes. Other fears arise from a person's past experience or the experiences of significant others. Nurses may use therapeutic communication skills to help the ill person express and understand fears (see Chapter 24). Sometimes, however, barriers to open communication arise between the care giver and the client. These may include a fearful person's hostility and anger or the person's reluctance to risk loss of affection or respect by openly expressing fear.

Depression

Some feelings of withdrawal and depression are normal responses to illness. If they become prolonged or extreme, however, health care providers may have some cause for concern, and the client may need psychiatric referral.

A depressed person typically appears sad, with little emotive expression. Typical behavioral signs include sighing, wringing of hands, slowed speech, weeping, frowning, turned down mouth, loss of appetite, and impaired concentration. Depressed people may neglect personal hygiene. Physiologic signs may include altered bowel function, menstruation, and sexual patterns; unusual weight gain or loss; tightness in the throat and

TABLE 21-1. General and Specific Fears Related to Illness

General Fear	Specific Examples
Fear of harm	Fear of pain, loss of body parts, or mutilation
	Fear of abuse or neglect
	Fear of being punished for past behavior or lifestyle
	Fear of death
Fear of the unknown	Fear of a strange place, such as the health care or treatment facility
	Fear of being the subject of experimental treatments
	Fear of equipment, diagnostic procedures, or treatment regimens
Fear of impaired relations with others	Fear of having one's feelings hurt
	Fear of impersonal treatment
	Fear of being alone or isolated from significant others
	Fear of burdening others

hollowness in the stomach; and insomnia (difficulty sleeping), early morning awakening, nightmares, and other sleep pattern disturbances.

Depression may also become evident as agitated depression with hyperactivity, pacing, and restlessness. Suicide is an extreme manifestation. Whether the signs are mild or severe, health care providers should not take the concerns of depressed people lightly. Again, therapeutic interaction can often help alleviate the fears and concerns that lead to depression.

Once the person has become depressed, treating the depression seriously becomes important. It is not helpful to try to cheer the person up. Forced cheerfulness can lead to further depression and possibly suicide.

Mood Swings

Illness is often accompanied by fluctuations in mood and behavior. Sick people often feel anxious, depressed, discouraged, restless, angry, powerless, dependent, and frustrated. A person's mood may change rapidly, going from laughter to tears in a few moments.

Hospitalized people have additional stresses that may accentuate mood swings. The hospital is a strange place with unknown people and unfamiliar noises. Hospitalized clients are also under almost constant supervision and observation. Anyone's behavior, when observed around the clock, might begin to seem strange, even under normal circumstances.

Ill people become very tired, and their fatigue may increase irritability and mood swings. For ill people, fatigue can result from worries and fears; disrupted sleep; physical immobilization from confinement, traction, or casts; or pain or other physical discomfort such as nausea, vomiting, muscle cramping, irritated skin, or stiff joints.

Although nurses need to accept emotional swings, excessive emotional responses or extreme shifts in behavior or mood may indicate serious emotional difficulties requiring psychiatric help. Careful assessment is therefore critical. Knowing a person's preillness personality is helpful in assessing the effect of the stresses of illness and hospitalization on the person's usual behavior and emotions.

Powerlessness

The experience of illness, which often entails a decrease in physical function, may lead to a sense of lost control over one's body. If the ill individual then enters the complex, technologic environment of medical care, the result may be a further erosion of the sense of control—not only over the body but also over personal destiny. This perceived loss of control is termed **powerlessness.** Powerlessness has been defined as "the state in which an individual experiences the perception that one's own actions will not significantly affect an outcome"; or as "a perceived lack of control over a current situation or immediate happening."[36]

CAUSES AND INDICATORS OF POWERLESSNESS

A sense of powerlessness can result from many aspects of the illness experience. Most significant are usually separation and loss of control. Some examples include (1) loss of control over one's body, as evidenced by involuntary tremors or fecal or urinary incontinence; (2) loss of control over basic self-care needs, which leads to an unaccustomed reliance on others; (3) separation from significant others and other social supports; and (4) facing a serious illness and hospitalization without adequate material and financial supports.

A person can express a sense of powerlessness verbally or through signs of emotions such as apathy, withdrawal, depression, resentment, guilt, anxiety, or anger. Powerlessness can also affect the ill person's participation in personal health care. Possible manifestations of loss of control as a result of illness or injury are inappropriate dependence on others, including health care givers; failure to seek necessary health care information; failure to give relevant information to health care givers; and lack of participation in care activities or decisions.

COMPLIANCE WITH THERAPEUTIC REGIMENS

A client's feelings of powerlessness often lead to the client's ignoring the advice or prescriptions of physicians and other health care providers. Missing appointments or failing to follow a diet, for example, might reflect a person's refusal to surrender control over health and well-being to the external authority of the health care professional.

A person's behavior and willingness to follow the advice or prescription of the health care provider is called **compliance.** In many situations, compliance with health care instructions is an important concern in providing effective care to the client. Some behaviors that indicate compliance include the following:

▶ Taking prescribed medications at recommended dosages and frequencies
▶ Keeping appointments with physician or other health care provider
▶ Following a dietary regimen, such as low salt, no sugar, or high fiber
▶ Changing high-risk behaviors or lifestyles such as smoking, sedentary inactivity, stressful responses to work and environment, or drug or alcohol abuse
▶ Performing routine preventive measures, such as breast self-examination

Many factors can affect compliance, including the ill person's perspective of the illness, cost of treatment, access to care, poor communication, cultural beliefs, and conflicting objectives between health care providers and the individual. As more health care moves to the outpatient and home care setting, where contact between client and health care professional is less frequent, compliance with health care instructions becomes an increasingly important concern. Compliance can be greatly improved by an effective therapeutic relationship between the nurse and client and by a conscious emphasis on client teaching.

Some theorists consider the notion of compliance to be controversial. Usually, they object to the assumption that the health care professional's perception of what is right for the client is necessarily the correct course. For the client to "comply" with a physician's or nurse's instructions, these theorists point out, indicates a power imbalance in which the professional knows best and the client (or "patient") is dependent on the professional's expertise and must passively agree. Critics of the notion of compliance argue for recognition of client autonomy, or the need for clients to make their own decisions about their health.

Altered Body Image

Body image is the dynamic, personal picture of one's own body or physical being. This picture is made up not only of our mental image, or what faces us in the mirror, but also of our feelings and attitudes toward the body. These feelings and attitudes in turn are affected by our accumulated social experiences and interactions with others.

Body image refers not only to the appearance of one's body but also to its boundaries and function. A person senses the body's boundaries and function in part through **proprioceptive stimuli,** sensations from within body tissues (mainly muscles, tendons, and the neural labyrinth) that provide information about the body's position and movement. Any disruption of the body's physiologic function—for instance, disease or trauma affecting the neurologic system—can alter a person's ability to process these stimuli and thus can physiologically alter body image.

Body image further incorporates the interplay of three components: body reality, body ideal, and body presentation.[31] Body reality is the body as it actually exists, with all its strengths and flaws. Body ideal is the way each of us would like our bodies to look and perform. Body ideal is affected by changes in body reality, but distortions of body ideal (as evidenced, for example, by anorexia nervosa or abuse of steroids) can also pose a threat to health. Body presentation is a conscious attempt to reconcile body reality with body ideal. Posture, grooming, gait, speech patterns, exercise, and style of dress are all external ways in which we can alter our body reality to bring it closer to our body ideal.[31]

Body image is an important aspect of self-concept, because the judgments we make about our body affect our self-esteem. Body image can be radically changed by illness. Helping a person successfully integrate these changes into a new sense of self is a key aspect of nursing care. If body image changes are not effectively integrated by the individual, quality of life may suffer.[3]

There is a tendency to categorize people according to physical characteristics. For example, "fat people are jolly or have no control"; "a receding chin indicates weakness"; "certain physical gestures or speech patterns indicate femininity or masculinity." These are all stereotypes or labels that are often unconsciously applied in judging another's appearance. Such labels are part of the larger social environment in which a person forms a body image. Nurses must recognize that they, too, are part of this social environment.

When nurses apply preconceived notions about the meaning of a physical characteristic, they can adversely affect the quality of nursing care. No one should be judged because of a physical characteristic.

DEVELOPMENT OF BODY IMAGE

Body image remains fluid throughout life, gradually developing from before birth through normal growth and maturation. Awareness of internal body structures, however, is less clear than awareness of the body's exterior. During illness, awareness of the body develops mainly through pain and discomfort.

During infancy and childhood, direct explorations of body surfaces and orifices lead to a developing body image. Body protuberances and orifices are important in orienting ourselves to the environment and to the bodies of other people. They help us define our sense of boundaries, which is a basic part of body image. Early sensations of pain, touch, and temperature further contribute to the development of body image, as do movement, play, and comparing oneself with others. Through socialization, children develop attitudes toward body functions such as urination, defecation, and salivation. The attitudes of significant others affect what children learn to view as "clean, good, and pleasing" about the body and what is "bad, dirty, and repulsive." Such attitudes can affect later personality adjustment.

As people grow older, they may develop attachments to certain body parts. For example, one man may highly value his muscular upper torso, and another may prize his strong legs; one woman may be pleased with her small waist, and another likes her shapely hands. If something happens to the body parts a person especially values, the loss is particularly stressful. Some have argued that the intensity of emotional reaction to body changes is influenced by the importance a person attaches to the affected body part more than by the actual severity of the disability.[10]

Body image is particularly important in adolescence, a time of rapid physical change. The adolescent, eager for social acceptance, is usually concerned about developing "normally" and attractively. Many adolescents constantly compare themselves to others. A positive or negative comparison will affect an adolescent's body image and self-esteem.

Some adults in middle age may have difficulty with the aging process and its effect on body image. Western culture tends to value a youthful appearance, and anyone who accepts this cultural value may have difficulty as youth begins to fade. For people of all ages, external objects such as glasses, canes, hearing aids, and wheelchairs often become part of one's body image. Becoming dependent on these objects for the first time in middle or late adulthood, however, can present particular problems of adjustment.

SITUATIONS AFFECTING BODY IMAGE

Disturbances in body image are associated with many physical problems. Physical and psychosocial disorders can distort a person's body image, which makes adjustment necessary. Body image can be affected by an individual's normal growth and development, by surgical changes that the individual chooses to undergo, by diseases or other disorders, by the effects of surgery or trauma, by the effects of drugs, and by the results of not meeting the perceived expectations of society (Table 21–2).

Certain intrusive nursing, diagnostic, or monitoring procedures can be threatening to body image. Procedures such as temperature taking, nasogastric tube insertion, urinary catheterization, injections, enemas, sigmoidoscopy, and dilation and curettage can affect body image not only by piercing the body's boundaries with a foreign object but also by symbolizing the body's dependence on an external force to regain health. This dependence may increase a person's sense of powerlessness.

REACTIONS TO BODY IMAGE CHANGES

A number of factors influence a person's reactions to body image changes. These include (1) the person's coping ability, (2) the reactions of significant others, and (3) the nature and meaning of the threat. Adaptation to body image changes goes on long after the physical changes have occurred, especially if the changes are sudden and undesirable.

Some common reactions to body image changes indicate normal adaptation rather than emotional disorder. These include (1) grief, (2) fear of rejection, (3) anger, and (4) "phantom" sensations of missing body parts. Problem reactions include (1) prolonged denial, (2) severe prolonged depression, and (3) failure to adjust. Problem reactions to body image changes may be reflected by these indications:

▶ Reluctance to meet others, reclusive tendencies
▶ Unwillingness to look into mirrors or to look directly at one's altered body part
▶ Unwillingness to discuss the deformity
▶ Unwillingness to accept corrective surgery, corrective aids, vocational rehabilitation, or other devices that aid rehabilitation
▶ Refusal to leave home for visits, vacations, or even essential activities of daily living
▶ Discontinuance of social relationships that were significant before the body image change
▶ Marital discord or withdrawal from intimacy
▶ Failure to resume normal work activity

Distortion of body image can be reflected in the subconscious mental life. A person may dream of the disfiguring incident or may have a wish-fulfilling dream in which the disfigurement disappears. Sometimes repressed fears surface. People with amputated or separated limbs sometimes become anxious about the way the limb will be disposed of. Sometimes psychotic reactions related to distorted body image follow acute trauma or prolonged disease.

TABLE 21-2. Examples of Alterations Affecting Body Image

Alteration	Examples
Normal situations	Normal growth and development of infant, child, adolescent; normal changes with pregnancy and aging
Elective surgical changes	
Plastic surgery procedures that alter appearance	Facelift, rhinoplasty, scar revision, breast augmentation, liposuction
Alteration of internal body parts with reproductive or sexual significance	Tubal ligation, vasectomy, hysterectomy, abortion
Disease or other disorder	
Loss of body function	Cerebrovascular accident ("stroke"), paraplegia, quadriplegia, laryngectomy, epileptic seizure, bowel/bladder incontinence
Impaired organ function	Myocardial infarction ("heart attack"), asthma attack, pneumonia
Pathophysiologic changes in body size and proportion	Obesity, gigantism, acromegaly, emaciation
Psychopathologic disorders	Schizophrenia, anorexia nervosa, bulimia, hysteria, hypochondriasis
Birth defects or anomalies	Large birthmarks, cleft lip/palate, extra body parts, absence or malformation of body parts or organs
Painful body part	Migraine headaches, chronic pain such as phantom limb pain or disease-related pain
Alterations in skeleton, joints, or muscles	Atrophic and hypertrophic arthritis, systemic lupus erythematosus, osteoporosis
Surgery or trauma	
Loss or change of obvious body part through surgery or trauma	Loss of major body part (limb); loss of sexually characteristic body part (penis, female breast); loss of other obvious body part (eye, hair, teeth); burns; large scars
Surgical loss or change of internal body part	Loss of gallbladder, stomach, or kidney; gastrostomy; colostomy; ileostomy; ureteroenterostomy
Violent physical assaults	Gunshot or knife wound, sexual assault
Drugs	
Side effects of drug therapy	Striated skin, "moon face," loss of hair, hirsutism
Drug-induced states	Results of hallucinogenic drugs, delirium tremens
Social influence	
Sexual performance	Impotence, lack of sexual desire, premature ejaculation, painful coitus
Sociocultural concepts of physical attractiveness and normality	Halitosis; body odor; inability to control flatus; poor hygiene or grooming; deviation from socially influenced norms of body size, weight, and proportion

Adaptation to body image change can proceed through a series of stages:

▶ *Impact:* The initial stage is a stage of shock for both the person and significant others.
▶ *Retreat:* As the shock subsides, the people involved become anxious and tend to withdraw emotionally (or even physically when possible) from the situation. Denial may be a useful coping strategy.
▶ *Acknowledgment:* The person and significant others acknowledge the tragedy and grieve for their losses. Significant others must change their concept of the affected person. Some will be supportive; others will withdraw.
▶ *Reconstruction:* Reconstruction is a period of adjustment to the required change in lifestyle. Adjustment may be adaptation to technical devices or procedures, reorganization of social values, or reintegration of body image.

Responding to changes in body image is easier for

people who have strong coping abilities and the support of significant others than for those who do not. Many small changes in body image, spread out over a long period, may be less threatening to some individuals than one large, sudden change. The nurse needs to be sensitive to the individual's own perception of changed body image. For example, even though thousands of people have adapted successfully to a permanent ostomy, a person facing this experience may express fear and resentment. You need to address these feelings seriously and sensitively.

Shame and embarrassment are common reactions to body image changes, especially if a physical change causes difficulties in performing routine activities. Unfortunately, physical disfigurement and deformity are often viewed with repulsion and rejection. People with physical deformities *are* often rejected by others, and clients may develop a hostile attitude as a result.

People trying to adjust to an altered body image are often anxious. "I look different. Will I be loved and accepted? Am I repulsive and ugly?" Such anxiety may be lessened or relieved by loving and accepting responses from significant others. Strong social support from family and friends can also improve the progress of the person's adjustment to altered body image.[31]

The significance that the person gives to the body image change and its effects greatly influences the ability to adapt. For instance, alterations in body image sometimes occur as a result of long-term confinement to a wheelchair. Because the wheelchair, not the body boundaries, becomes the interface between the body and the environment, the body image boundaries for a person in a wheelchair may become distorted, and judgments about body boundaries may become inaccurate. A person has to deal with the body plus the wheelchair when moving through the environment. In a sense, the body and wheelchair become one unit.

The nature of the injury or loss can make the person's subjective experience of the change differ from what has actually occurred. People with a paralyzed limb (for instance, after a stroke) often feel the limb is gone even though it is still part of the body. Conversely, people who have had a limb amputated feel it is still present through painful or nonpainful sensations —an experience called phantom limb. Phantoms can also occur with removal of other protuberances, such as the nose, teeth, nipples, breast, or penis.

NURSING MANAGEMENT RELATED TO BODY IMAGE CHANGES

Appropriate nursing interventions for people with body image changes are based on accurate assessment, therapeutic interaction, client teaching, and support. Examples of such nursing interventions are shown in Box 21–2.

ROLES OF THE ILL PERSON

A social role is a pattern of expected behavior. We either assume a social role or have it assigned to us, and it then determines the expectations others have of us.

Box 21–2. Examples of Nursing Interventions for People with Body Image Changes

Assessment

▶ Assess to identify the significance of the change to the person. Include assessment of the person's (1) developmental level (age, psychosocial maturity); (2) level of self-esteem and how dependent it is on body image; (3) typical patterns of adjusting to stress; (4) occupation and other life roles; and (5) preparation for body image change.

▶ Assess to identify the significance of the change to others. Include assessment of (1) the ways significant others perceive the person's body image change and (2) sociocultural views of body image change held by the people involved.

▶ Carefully assess the person's emotional state to identify any excessive withdrawal, denial, or depression. Suicide is possible.

Therapeutic Interaction

▶ Therapeutic interaction is important over the short and long term for both the person and significant others. Remember that any negative or judgmental attitudes will be perceived by the person and significant others and will hinder the person's rehabilitation. Encourage people to discuss their feelings.

▶ Touch the person's changed body part in appropriate ways. This provides sensory input that assists body reorientation.

▶ Encourage the person to move. Movement helps build body image by bringing the body into new relationships with itself, others, and the environment. Either passive or active movement of affected parts can provide kinesthetic feedback. When doing passive movements, provide the person with verbal feedback of the movements being performed; for example, "I am lifting your arm off the pillow. I am bending your elbow."

▶ Encourage the person to perform self-care so that love for the body as it now exists can be developed. Self-care directly increases visual, tactile, and proprioceptive stimuli that help a person to know the body again.

▶ Discussions of body image changes that affect sexuality may be helpful when the person is ready. Areas of concern may include (1) ability to reproduce; (2) modifications required for sexual activity; and (3) problems concerning cosmetic appearance. It is often helpful to discuss sexuality with both the person and the sexual partner.

Client Teaching

▶ Whenever possible, people need thorough preparation for procedures that may alter their body image. When change is sudden and traumatic, the shock is usually greater, and more help is usually required.

▶ Prepare significant others for changes in their loved one's body whenever possible.

Support

▶ Encourage the person to gradually look at visible body changes. Be supportive during these times and realize the person is gaining important visual feedback about the body changes.

▶ Assist the person to gain a balanced self-image by not focusing excessively on the changed body part.

▶ Respect the need for privacy.

▶ Show respect for the person's body by helping with hygiene care and performing activities that will enhance the person's appearance.

▶ Encourage interaction with others. It is important to learn to relate to others again. Initial interactions may be difficult for both the person and significant others; if the experiences are positive, they will help in long-term adjustment.

Sick Role

A **sick role** is a pattern of behavior that society generally expects from ill people. Parsons identified four aspects of the sick role that provide a useful, general description, as long as one keeps in mind the wide spectrum of individual variations.[28]

▶ Sick people are exempt from usual social role responsibilities.
▶ Sick people are not morally responsible for taking care of themselves during illness.
▶ Sick people are obliged to desire recovery.
▶ Sick people are obliged to seek competent help.

Depending on the severity of the illness, ill people are often excused from their usual roles related to work, family, or social life. It becomes acceptable, for example, to cancel prearranged appointments. A physician is often called on to provide validation of the need to suspend social responsibilities (e.g., the physician's note excusing a child from school).

People are not considered responsible for taking care of their illness. If someone is sick, it is expected others will provide care. The dependency that can result from relying on others may make the ill person's behavior seem less mature than usual.

Suspension of social roles brings other responsibilities. Ill people are expected to want to get better and to do what is necessary to recover. Caretakers can become frustrated when the ill person refuses to take necessary medication, proper nutrition, or adequate rest. Ill people are expected to cooperate with treatment; when they do not, conflicts may arise.

The ill person may deviate from these prescriptions for the sick role. Some people may not want to recover and will not comply with treatment (their behavior is often termed noncompliance). Others enjoy the secondary gains of power over others, greater dependence, and lessened responsibility and do not wish to give these up by working toward recovery. Still others may not care whether they get better and are submissive, indifferent, withdrawn, uncommunicative, and lacking in enthusiasm and initiative.

Impaired Role

In some situations people are not assigned a sick role, but they are not expected to fulfill normal social roles. They take on an impaired role. Such situations include people who are sick but not seriously or acutely ill with a positive prognosis, disabled, or chronically ill. For example, people who are blind, paraplegic, or living with a disease such as multiple sclerosis may assume an impaired role. People assuming an impaired role often do not consider themselves ill but rather see themselves as restricted physically or psychologically. To avoid the negative connotations of such words as "handicapped," "impaired," or "disabled," professionals are working toward a new vocabulary, using such words as "challenged," to reflect the positive potential in the lives of people with conditions such as these.

An impaired person is expected to behave more normally than a sick person. Independence is encouraged. Some normal social roles are expected. The balance between what is possible and what is not possible is delicate. Helping a person assume the appropriate impaired role is often the task of a rehabilitation program.

The impaired role is common in our society. Many health problems leave people impaired but not ill, able to fulfill most if not all social roles required of them. Indeed, part of the public relations work of many advocacy groups has been to make society aware of the positive potential and worth of those with impaired function. By increasing society's sensitivity, these groups seek to identify and combat discriminatory attitudes and practices that affect people with impairments. Increased wheelchair access in public facilities has been one exemplary result. An important nursing role is to assist people in fulfilling their potential to the maximum of their desire and capability.

CHRONIC ILLNESS

Men and women of industrial societies suffer more from chronic, incurable illnesses than they do from acute disorders. Strauss described chronic illnesses as "long term, uncertain, expensive, often multiple, disproportionately intrusive and they require palliation, especially because they are incurable."[35] Chronically ill people assume an impaired or "at-risk" role rather than a sick role. The long-term nature, or **chronicity,** of an illness affects a person in every possible way—for example, in self-concept, social relationships and roles, sexuality, and independence.

Chronic illness, rather than acute illness, is the leading health problem in the United States.[9] More people are living with illnesses that were formerly fatal; more children are living into adulthood with diseases that were previously considered childhood conditions; and more premature and low-birthweight infants are surviving devastating impairments, some with severe persistent problems and others with virtually no residual effects. Important contemporary social trends will have a continuing effect on the psychosocial aspects of chronic illness care. Some of these are summarized in Table 21-3.

Individual Responses to Chronic Illness

Whatever the diagnosis, people with chronic illnesses tend to share similar psychosocial problems. Their ability to adapt to these problems seems to be independent of their medical diagnosis.[30] Strauss et al. have identified seven major problems typical for chronically ill people and their significant others.[35] Whereas these problems may not be vastly different from the problems of any ill person, for chronically ill people these seven problems do not go away:

▶ Preventing and managing medical crises
▶ Managing prescribed regimens

TABLE 21-3. Contemporary Trends and Implications for Chronic Illness Care

Contemporary Trend	Implications for Health Care
Information society North American society and economy are changing from a focus on industry (production of material goods) to a focus on information (transmission of data and knowledge) with improved electronic and computer technology	▶ Greater availability of health information to clients and health care professionals ▶ Innovative means of monitoring clients at home from remote locations ▶ Better means and increased opportunities for client education
Self-help Increase in people being cared for and receiving services at home and in community agencies outside traditional health care facilities Chronically ill people are increasingly being cared for by family members Growth in number of self-help groups	▶ Greater ability of consumers to carry out complex procedures such as ventilator management and dialysis ▶ Necessity for health care professionals to listen to family members of chronically ill person to identify support needs ▶ Increasing need for client education ▶ Need for health care professionals to teach clients how to manipulate medical and community systems to obtain needed services
High touch and high technology Advances in innovative medical technology (such as drugs, monitoring, and therapeutic devices) and surgical procedures (high technology) necessitate comparable increase in human caring, concern, and psychosocial support (high touch)	▶ Increased life span of persons with diseases previously considered life-threatening, including childhood conditions such as cystic fibrosis ▶ Participation by health care professionals in decisions on use of limited technologic resources, taking into account ethical and advocacy concerns

Information from Hymovich, D.P., & Hagopian, G.A. (1992). *Chronic illness in children and adults: A psychosocial approach.* Philadelphia: W.B. Saunders.

▶ Controlling symptoms
▶ Preventing social isolation
▶ Adjusting to changes
▶ Normalizing daily life
▶ Managing time

PREVENTING AND MANAGING MEDICAL CRISES

Chronic illness proceeds in a relentless, nonacute fashion, but sudden, acute medical crises can also arise. For example, a person with epilepsy may well have the symptoms under control, but the possibility of a sudden convulsion is always present. Chronically ill people and their significant others need to (1) know that crises are likely, (2) know and implement ways of reducing or preventing the occurrence of crises, (3) know the signs of an imminent crisis, and (4) have a plan of action that can be quickly implemented should a crisis occur.

MANAGING PRESCRIBED REGIMENS

Most chronically ill people are prescribed some kind of long-term regimen for management of the illness. Managing chronic illness often requires major life adjustments. Each person's adaptation to a prescribed regimen depends on (1) the difficulty of learning the regimen, (2) the amount of time required, (3) the amount of energy, discomfort, or both that is involved, (4) the regimen's acceptability to other people, (5) the

extent to which the regimen increases social isolation or rejection, (6) the regimen's effectiveness in relieving symptoms, and (7) the expense involved.

CONTROLLING SYMPTOMS

Recurring symptoms of chronically ill people can include pain, nausea, vomiting, decreased mobility, and altered bowel or urinary elimination patterns. The lives of chronically ill people and their significant others must be reordered, sometimes dramatically, so that symptoms can be controlled to allow as normal a lifestyle as possible. These changes can be time-consuming and exhausting. Those involved must learn about the symptoms, including their onset, duration, and severity, and the degree to which they can be controlled. Daily life requires planning so that the person's energy is not depleted and so that required facilities and equipment are always accessible.

PREVENTING SOCIAL ISOLATION

Chronically ill people may withdraw from other people, or other people may reject them. These reactions can precipitate loneliness and depression. Long-term relationships, such as marriages, sometimes end. A reduction in social support may be unavoidable, and professional counseling may be helpful in preventing further erosion.

ADJUSTING TO CHANGES

Some chronic illnesses, such as controlled diabetes, remain relatively stable; others, such as multiple sclerosis, are unpredictable. The more unpredictable and frequent the changes, the more difficult it is for people to make the necessary ongoing adjustments. Chronic illness becomes part of the personal identity of chronically ill people and their significant others.

NORMALIZING DAILY LIFE

Many chronically ill people try to manage their symptoms to make their disabilities or disfigurements less obvious. They may schedule their social engagements only at certain times of day, for instance, or avoid certain locations such as beaches and health spas. The degree to which they are able to mask their condition depends on their social arrangements, the severity of symptoms, and the complexity of prescribed regimens.

MANAGING TIME

For the chronically ill, perception and management of time become altered. Some people find they have too much time, others not enough. Those who must give up cherished activities because of illness may find excessive "free" time. Those who continue with work and social activities, or find acceptable substitutes for those they can no longer pursue, may find that medical regimens and symptom control leave them less time for meeting their commitments. These limitations can be particularly difficult for people trying to continue with a job or profession.

Family Support During Chronic Illness

Essential to providing care for chronically ill people is consideration of family needs.[42] Support from family members or significant others can be crucial to enhancing positive adaptation of the ill person. The nurse can play a crucial role in helping the family identify the most important needs stemming from the demands of illness and in helping the family obtain necessary resources for meeting those needs.

Families provide important support to the ill person in a variety of ways, including access to a supportive spouse, family outlet for expression of feelings, family interactions specifically related to the ill person's self-care, and reassignment of usual household roles and functions. The family can be stressed by these and other activities of caring for the ill person and may need additional resources—both material and emotional—from outside the immediate family unit. The nurse can provide information, opportunities to express fears and concerns, emotional reassurance, and linkage to additional community support systems, all of which can assist the family in maintaining its ability to adjust to and care for the ill person.[42]

QUALITY OF LIFE

People of all ages who have disabling conditions are surviving in increasing numbers. These people need varying amounts of material, functional, and social support, and nurses caring for them will have to consider issues related to quality of life. **Quality of life** is generally the degree to which an individual's continued existence is of significant value to that person. Whether chronically or acutely ill, people want to know how their condition and its treatment will affect their daily lives. The individual's perception of quality of life, both before the disease or disability and after, will have an important effect on treatment choices and on the illness experience.

More specific definitions of the concept of quality of life fall into five broad categories.[5]

▶ *Normal life.* Normal life encompasses the ill person's ability to function at a level comparable to that of healthy people. The standard of comparison in defining quality of life is thus a person who does not have the disability of the ill person. These definitions tend to be a problem in determining who defines "normal" and what importance the ill person attaches to specific aspects of a "normal" life.

▶ *Happiness and satisfaction.* Happiness and satisfaction are related although not synonymous terms. In descriptions of quality of life, happiness is related more to short-term feelings, whereas satisfaction is a longer-term rational judgment of the conditions of one's life. Measuring quality of life from this perspective also depends on the ill individual's perception of the situation.

▶ *Achievement of personal goals.* In considerations of quality of life, achievement focuses on specific goal achievement and on the success or failure the individual experiences in achieving those goals. An important consideration is that goals are those that matter to the individual, not general goals that apply to all people.

▶ *Social utility.* Definitions of quality of life based on social utility involve the usefulness of the individual's life to society at large. Such descriptions place positive value on roles such as parent, physician, responsible citizen, or gainfully employed person. The problem with these definitions of quality of life is that not everyone in a pluralistic society will agree about what is socially useful and the relative values of various roles.

▶ *Natural capacity.* Definitions based on natural capacity focus on the individual's capabilities, both physical and mental, actual and potential. What will the impaired individual be able to do? How much self-care is possible? What degree of mental capacity will the person have? Will communication from others be understandable? Definitions focusing on natural capacity can aid in making treatment choices, such as those concerning severely impaired newborn infants or adults who have suffered traumatic injury and lost almost every ability to function normally.

Each of these groups of definitions is hampered to a degree by a tension between subjectivity and objectivity. Just whose perspective is used in judging quality of life? The individual, the significant others and family members, the medical establishment, the community, and the society at large—all may have a claim in determining the quality-of-life issues that should apply to a particular case, especially in a time when allocation of scarce health care resources has become a critical issue. Although a single definitive answer might not be possible, individual nurses need to be aware that their perceptions of quality of life may differ from those of their clients.[22] Effective nursing care requires a clear understanding of the client's priorities.

The concept of quality of life encompasses many dimensions and addresses broad concerns across the spectrum of life. Table 21–4 presents examples of characteristics that have been used in evaluating quality of life.

Varying criteria concerning quality of life involve a number of nursing implications. The following are important considerations for nurses.

► A person's decisions about quality of life may not agree with the nurse's or anyone else's and will be influenced by personal characteristics, cultural background, belief system, and other individual factors.
► Respecting clients' views about quality of life means respecting their decisions to accept or reject a proposed therapy. If a client rejects treatment because its side effects or outcome would reduce quality of life in an unacceptable way, the nurse needs to accept this decision and not attribute it to a failure in nursing care or to a "bad patient."
► Nurses generally deal only with the disease-related issues concerning quality of life, not overall quality of life. Although nurses can assess both areas, they are not responsible for improving everyone's overall quality of life.

TABLE 21–4. Dimensions of Quality of Life

Area of Life	Specific Indicators
Health and physical functioning	Activity level and mobility
	Physical symptoms
	Sexual activity
	Toxicity of treatment
	Ability to take care of responsibilities
	Participation in recreational activities
Psychologic and spiritual attitudes and responses	Satisfaction with life
	Affect
	Anxiety and stress
	Self-esteem
	Achievement of goals/purpose in life
	Spiritual aspects/religion
	Depression
	Coping
	Creative expression
	Hope
	Enthusiasm for life, fortitude
	Sense of security
	Control over own life
Social and economic involvement	Employment/work (includes social aspects)
	Education
	Financial status, income
	Housing and neighborhood (includes social aspects)
	Friendships and social life
	Social support
	Satisfaction with city and nation
Family relationships	Relationship with spouse
	Relationship with children
	Family happiness

Adapted from Ferrans, C.E. (1990). Quality of life: conceptual issues. *Seminars in Oncology Nursing, 6*(4), 252.

MEETING HUMAN NEEDS DURING ILLNESS

Healthy people satisfy human needs on their own (see Chapter 15 for a discussion of basic human needs). The stress of illness can interfere with the usual ways in which people satisfy basic human needs. Needs to which we hardly give a second thought when healthy —such as breathing, eating, and bowel elimination—can become the center of attention for an ill person. Other needs, such as shelter and a clean bed for a homeless person, may be met during hospitalization when they are not met in the person's "normal" life.

Nursing is required when people are unable to meet needs in their usual fashion. Whereas much of nursing seems to address physiologic or survival level of need, nurses must be concerned with the total picture of a person's needs. Nursing is concerned with the whole person. Nurses must recognize (1) the point at which a basic need is not being met, (2) what effect the unmet need has on the person, and (3) what nursing interventions will be most effective in meeting the need. Table 21–5 summarizes human needs that can manifest themselves during illness and nursing actions for addressing unmet needs.

Nursing is not concerned with physical problems alone. Nursing is concerned with complex people and their life experiences.

Summary

► The stages of the illness experience include transition, acceptance, and convalescence. During transition, a person responds to symptoms; during acceptance, the person acknowledges the illness; during convalescence, the person regains health to the greatest degree possible.

TABLE 21-5. Human Needs During Illness

Expressions of Human Need	Nursing Implications
Survival Needs	
Unmet physiologic (body) needs (e.g., problems of bowel elimination, nausea, pain)	▶ Identifying unmet needs related to body function may be embarrassing for the client. Use therapeutic communication techniques to help client discuss needs clearly and openly. ▶ Some people, unable to distinguish between what is important and what is not, may exaggerate attention to basic functions such as pulses, breathing, or bowel movement. Recognize this behavior as a normal expression of anxiety, listen empathetically, and provide appropriate information.
Stimulation Needs	
Unmet need for novelty, manipulation, exploration, and sexual expression leads to boredom, restlessness, irritability, depression, and even disorientation	▶ Restriction of illness and hospitalization may block expression and satisfaction of some needs (e.g., sexual expression), but evidence of unmet needs may be expressed in disguised form such as jokes and sexual banter. Recognize these expressions for what they are. ▶ Support person's effort to introduce novelty into environment as much as institutional policy will allow.
Safety and Security Needs	
Need for safety and security is disrupted by illness or injury The assault on health makes the ill person feel vulnerable Relocation to the strange environment of a health care facility can increase the sense of insecurity Separation from family or significant others can lead to fear of abandonment and helplessness	▶ Facilitate communication between ill person and family members and significant others. ▶ Provide strong advocacy for client's concerns and needs for support so that it is clear to everyone that the client is not powerless in a strange situation. ▶ Keep ill person well informed to allow sense of control over the circumstances surrounding illness and treatment. Orient the ill person to the physical environment, to procedures being undertaken, and to time frame.

▶ A person's response to the first signs of illness may include a lack of action or delayed action in seeking help, eventual action to seek help, vacillation in seeking help, or denial of the illness. A person's initial response to illness may be a result of the symptoms of illness, the person's perception of the symptoms, or the extent to which symptoms interfere with daily activities. Responses to illness are also influenced by a person's psychosocial context of family, community, personality, and prior experience.

▶ Reactions to confirmed illness include uncertainty, anxiety, shock, denial, anger, information seeking, shame, isolation, fear, depression, mood swings, altered body image, and powerlessness, which may affect compliance with therapy.

▶ People who are ill may assume a sick role, in which they withdraw from an accustomed social role and responsibilities, suspend some degree of self-care, and seek recovery and competent help. With some illnesses, people assume an impaired role, in which

they attain some degree of independence and normal social interaction.

▶ The key issues affecting the person with chronic illness are preventing and managing medical crises, managing prescribed regimens, controlling symptoms, preventing social isolation, adjusting to changes, normalizing daily life, and managing time. Support from family members and significant others is essential for positive adaptation to a chronic condition.

▶ Quality of life is the degree to which an individual's continued existence is of significant value to that person. Quality of life is often defined according to specific criteria: normal life, happiness and satisfaction, achievement of personal goals, social utility, and natural capacity.

▶ Nurses can support a person in meeting basic human needs during illness by recognizing the point at which a need is not being met, determining the effect of the unmet need on the person, and planning nursing interventions to meet the need.

TABLE 21-5. Human Needs During Illness (Continued)

Expressions of Human Need	Nursing Implications
Love and Belonging Needs	
Need for love, belonging, and closeness is threatened by physical or emotional separation from loved ones or by fear that relationships with loved ones will change as a result of health crisis	▶ Identify specifically who are the important people to the person under care, and include those people in interactions with the ill person. ▶ Include significant others in plan of nursing care. ▶ Avoid impersonal treatment of ill person. Nonverbal communication and physical contact within a professional context can help the person feel valued and considered.
Esteem Needs	
Self-esteem can be diminished by the dehumanizing experiences of illness and hospitalization (e.g., separation from familiar objects; common hospital gown; parade of different health care professionals, each performing different tasks) Diminished physical capacity by itself can lessen self-esteem, especially for those whose self-concept is related to physical accomplishments (e.g., athletes) The ill person may also be isolated from normal sources of status and respect	▶ Think of, and refer to, the client as a person and by name, not as a disease or body part (e.g., as "Mrs. Samuels," not as "the gallbladder in 214"). ▶ Always introduce yourself by name to the people you are caring for and to their significant others when you first meet them. ▶ Minimize exposure of a person by proper draping; make physical contact firmly, gently, and professionally.
Self-actualization Needs	
Need to express one's personality and develop one's abilities may be submerged in the dependency resulting from illness Loss of physical abilities (e.g., sight, hearing, mobility, or manual dexterity) may also hamper the development and use of personal talents	▶ The best way for nurses to help people meet their needs for self-actualization is to make sure that the needs lower on the hierarchy are met. ▶ Encourage expressions of individuality. ▶ Times of illness can sometimes bring people closer to their inner selves and to their own spiritual center. Nurses can notice and support these moments of introspection. Referral to a spiritual counselor may sometimes be appropriate.

Bibliography

1. Barry, P.D. (1989). *Psychosocial nursing assessment and intervention* (2nd ed.). Philadelphia: J.B. Lippincott.
2. Bernstein, S.B. (1989). Breaking the vicious circle of noncompliance. *Nursing 89*, 19(1), 74–75.
3. Burns, N., & Holmes, B.C. (1991). Alterations in body image. In Baird, S.B., et al. *Cancer nursing: A comprehensive textbook* (pp. 821–830). Philadelphia: W.B. Saunders.
4. Cohen, A. (1991). Body image in the person with a stoma. *Journal of Enterostomal Therapy*, 18(2), 68–71.
5. Ferrans, C.E. (1990). Quality of life: conceptual issues. *Seminars in Oncology Nursing*, 6(4), 248–254.
6. Gedan, S. (1985). Say goodbye to guilt. *Nursing 85*, 15(Jul), 30.
7. Given, B.A., & Given, C.W. (1989). Compliance among patients with cancer. *Oncology Nursing Forum*, 16(1), 97–103.
8. Hodgin, J.D. (1984). The emotional dynamics of physical illness. *American Family Physician*, 30(Sep), 235.
9. Hymovich, D.P., & Hagopian, G.A. (1992). *Chronic illness in children and adults: A psychosocial approach*. Philadelphia: W.B. Saunders.
10. Klopp, A.L. (1990). Body image and self-concept among individuals with stomas. *Journal of Enterostomal Therapy*, 17, 98–105.
11. Kolton, K.A., & Piccolo, P. (1988). Patient compliance: a challenge to practice. *Nurse Practitioner*, 13(12), 37–50.
12. Lambert, V.A., & Lambert, C.E., Jr. (1985). *The impact of physical illness and related mental health concepts* (2nd ed.). East Norwalk, CT: Appleton & Lange.
13. Lewis, S.A., et al. (1990). *Manual of psychosocial nursing interventions: Promoting mental health in medical-surgical settings*. Philadelphia: W.B. Saunders.
14. Lipkin, M., Jr., & Kupka, K. (eds.). (1982). *Psychosocial factors affecting health*. New York: Praeger.
15. Lund, V.E., & Frank, D.I. (1991). Helping the medicine go down: nurses' and patients' perceptions about medication compliance. *Journal of Psychosocial Nursing and Mental Health Services*, 29(7), 6–9.
16. Martin, H.W., & Prange, A.J., Jr. (1962). The stages of illness—psychosocial approach. *Nursing Outlook*, 10(Mar), 168.
17. McNall, M.C.C. (1989). Healing we cannot explain. *American Journal of Nursing*, 89(9), 1162–1163.
18. Miller, J. (1985). Inspiring hope. *American Journal of Nursing*, 85(Jan), 22.
19. Miller, J.F. (1983). *Coping with chronic illness: Overcoming powerlessness*. Philadelphia: F.A. Davis.
20. Mishel, M.H. (1988). Uncertainty in illness. *Image: Journal of Nursing Scholarship*, 20(4), 225–232.
21. Mishel, M.H. (1990). Reconceptualization of the uncertainty in illness theory. *Image: Journal of Nursing Scholarship*, 22(4), 256–262.
22. Molzahn, A.E., & Northcott, H.C. (1989). The social bases of discrepancies in health/illness perceptions. *Journal of Advanced Nursing*, 14(2), 132–140.
23. Monahan, R.S. (1982). The 'at-risk' role. *Nurse Practitioner* 7(May), 42.
24. Morse, J.M., & Johnson, J.L. (1991). *The illness experience: Dimensions of suffering*. Newbury Park, CA: Sage.
25. Norris, C.M. (1969). The work of getting well. Reprinted in *American Journal of Nursing*, 90(7), 47–50.

26. Northouse, L.L., et al. (1991). Psychologic consequences of breast cancer on partner and family. *Seminars in Oncology Nursing, 7*(3), 216–223.

27. Nyamathi, A., & Shuler, P. (1989). Factors affecting prescribed medication compliance of the urban homeless adult. *Nurse Practitioner, 14*(8), 47–54.

28. Parsons, T. (1951). *The social system.* New York: Free Press.

29. Pike, A.W. (1990). On the nature and place of empathy in clinical nursing practice. *Journal of Professional Nursing, 6*(4), 235–241.

30. Pollock, S.E., et al. (1990). Responses to chronic illness: analysis of psychological and physiological adaptation. *Nursing Research, 39*(5), 300–304.

31. Price, B. (1990). A model for body-image care. *Journal of Advanced Nursing, 15*(5), 585–593.

32. Ruffalo, R.L., et al. (1985). Patient compliance. *American Family Physician, 31*(Jun), 93.

33. Ryder, R.L., & Ridley, M.G. (1990). The place from which the patient comes. *Journal of Professional Nursing, 6*(5), 255.

34. Sontag, S. (1978). *Illness as metaphor.* New York: Farrar, Straus and Giroux.

35. Strauss, A.L., et al. (1984). *Chronic illness and the quality of life.* St. Louis: C.V. Mosby.

36. Taptich, B.J., et al. (1989). *Nursing diagnosis and care planning.* Philadelphia: W.B. Saunders.

37. Turnbull, J.M., & Turnbull, S.K. (1985). Management of specific anxiety disorders in the elderly. *Geriatrics, 40*(Aug), 75.

38. Varricchio, C.G. (1990). Relevance of quality of life to clinical nursing practice. *Seminars in Oncology Nursing, 6*(4), 255–259.

39. Vincent, P. (1975). The sick role in patient care. *American Journal of Nursing, 75*(Jul), 1172.

40. Westbrook, M., & Viney, L. (1982). Psychological reactions to the onset of chronic illness. *Social Science and Medicine, 16*(Aug), 508.

41. When families get together. (1985). *Nursing 85, 15*(Feb), 58.

42. Woods, N.F., et al. (1989). Supporting families during chronic illness. *Image: Journal of Nursing Scholarship, 21*(1), 46–50.

▼ Hospital Admission and Discharge

 It is a bad plan that admits of no modification.
Publilius Syrus, first century, B.C.

▼ CHAPTER OUTLINE

HEALTH CARE ORGANIZATIONS
    Classifications of Organizations
    The Hospital
    Nursing Care Models
THE CLIENT
    Client Expectations
    Client Anxiety
    Orienting the Client

ASSESSMENT
    Preventing Liability
    Documenting Admission
NURSING DIAGNOSIS
PLANNING
NURSING INTERVENTION
EVALUATION
THE DISCHARGE PROCESS

▼ KEY TERMS

Agency
Ambulatory care center
Case method
Clinic
Discharge planning
Dispensary

Extended-care facility
Functional method
Health care organization
   (agency)
Home health agency
Hospice

Hospital
Infirmary
One-to-one method
Primary care method
Team method (team
   nursing)

Some time ago, Mr. Lipski, age 87, balanced himself by leaning his legs against the rung of a ladder for approximately one-half hour when he was trying to repair a broken window. Because his circulation was poor, this trauma to the leg tissues caused severe circulatory problems, and he must now have both legs amputated. Misty Flowers, age 16, has run away from home twice, has been getting poorer and poorer grades at school, and has been drinking and taking large amounts of various types of drugs on a regular basis. This behavior has been occurring since her mother remarried approximately 2 years ago. Today Misty took an overdose of an unknown quantity of mixed drugs and alcohol and lost consciousness. Mary Ann Morris, age 43, holds a high-stress position as an executive in a large company. At various intervals over the past few weeks, she has been experiencing chest pain but has coped with it by using denial. Currently, she is suffering from severe chest pain that she describes as "squeezing," and she is short of breath, pale, cold, and clammy. Within 1 minute she will be clinically dead, and two of her co-workers will be performing cardiopulmonary resuscitation.

What do these three persons have in common? They represent three typical clients who are about to enter the health care system for treatment. Each is at a very different developmental level. Each has a very different health care problem. While in a specific health care agency (hospital), each will receive a very different type of medical treatment. When finally discharged from the agency, each will be referred for a very different type of care.

This chapter examines nursing actions that can best assist clients during their admission to a hospital and discusses the planning necessary for successful outcomes at the time of discharge from the agency. As we look at ways to assist clients entering a health care agency, we will review the various types of health care agencies and note how they are organized and how they provide nursing care.

HEALTH CARE ORGANIZATIONS

Health care organizations (agencies) may be defined as structural and functional units of personnel who provide health services to individuals, families, groups, and society. These agencies can differ in many ways and may be identified by a number of different terms (some of these terms are defined in Box 22–1).

Classifications of Organizations

Organizations may be classified in several ways.

CLASSIFICATION ACCORDING TO FOCUS OF SERVICES

Organizations may be classified according to the focus of the services provided. This classification can generally be divided into those agencies that exist mainly to provide health care and those that exist for another purpose but also include the provision of some health care as part of their services.[26] Among the former are hospitals, hospital-based or free-standing ambulatory care centers, home health agencies, and extended-care facilities. Agencies with a primary purpose other than health care include work settings that provide occupational health services, schools that provide student health services, and prisons that provide infirmaries or dispensaries.

CLASSIFICATION ACCORDING TO TYPE OF SERVICES

Organizations may also be classified according to the type of health services provided.[26] For example, some agencies exist specifically to provide one or a limited number of health services such as diagnostic studies, counseling, formal instruction, surgery, or specific types of nonsurgical treatments such as physical therapy. Other agencies, such as general hospitals, provide a more comprehensive array of services.

CLASSIFICATION ACCORDING TO POPULATION SERVED

Organizations may also be classified according to the population they serve.[26] For example, some agencies exist specifically to meet the health care needs of those in a particular age group such as pediatric, adult health, or geriatric (gerontologic) clients. Agencies might also

> ### Box 22–1. Types of Health Care Organizations
>
> **Agency:** See *health care organization.*
> **Ambulatory care center:** See *clinic.*
> **Clinic:** traditionally, a place where a group of physicians worked together to study and treat persons who were admitted for medical and surgical care. Currently, the term refers to a place where outpatients come for brief treatments or follow-up observations by a group of physicians and other health team members. Hence, such places are now most often called ambulatory care centers.
> **Dispensary:** a place where free or low-cost medications or medical treatments are dispensed.
> **Extended-care facility:** a type of agency that provides long-term medical, rehabilitative, or custodial care (care that focuses on observing and protecting a person rather than providing for a cure).
> **Health care organization (agency):** a structural and functional unit of personnel who provide health services to individuals, families, groups, and society.
> **Home health agency:** a type of agency that provides certain types of health care in the home setting.
> **Hospice:** an agency that provides palliative and supportive care for the dying and support for their families. In medieval times, hospices were guest houses or places of shelter for wayfarers such as pilgrims.
> **Hospital:** an agency that provides medical and surgical care and treatment for the sick and injured and possibly obstetric care for healthy women who are giving birth.
> **Infirmary:** a place where the infirm (the sick, weak, or feeble) are treated. This term may refer to a hospital or to an area within another institution, such as a school or prison, set aside for the infirm.

serve individuals at a particular stage of illness such as those requiring primary, secondary, or tertiary prevention. Others are designed to meet the needs of persons with specific types of health problems, such as communicable diseases, drug addictions, or neuromuscular disorders. Still others exist to meet all of the health care needs of individuals in certain circumstances such as those who belong to a particular health maintenance organization, those in need of home health care, those who are indigent, or those who are dying.

CLASSIFICATION ACCORDING TO SOURCE OF FUNDS

Organizations may also be classified according to their source of funding.[26] Agencies are either profit (proprietary) or nonprofit (not-for-profit) institutions. Proprietary agencies are, like any other private business, financed by private sources, such as the sale of stocks. These agencies receive payment from those who use their services. They must make a profit to stay in business. The Humana Corporation is an example of a proprietary organization that might be familiar to you.

Nonprofit agencies may be voluntary agencies or public (government-operated) agencies. Voluntary agencies are financed by private charitable or religious organizations or by voluntary contributions from those in the surrounding community. They exist to meet the

needs of certain individuals with defined needs. A familiar example is the Shriners Hospitals for burned children. Public agencies receive funding from local, state, or federal governments. When possible, these agencies may also receive payment from those who use their services, but they provide free or low-cost care to those who are unable to pay. Veterans Administration hospitals are examples of federal level public agencies.

As you think about the ways in which health agencies may be classified, you should realize that these classifications are not mutually exclusive. Take, for example, the type of agency that could provide care for all three of the clients mentioned at the beginning of this chapter: an elderly man facing amputation, an unconscious teenager with an overdose, and a middle-aged woman with cardiac pathology. For individuals as sick as these, the organization would have to focus exclusively on providing health care services. Because the three clients have such acute disorders, a hospital would be the best agency to provide for their care (secondary prevention). However, the hospital would have to provide medical, surgical, and psychiatric care, including the emergency services two of the three would require on admission. The hospital would also have to be able to care for adults and teenagers as well as elderly clients. The client's ability to pay would also have to be considered. Because a highly paid executive would probably be well insured, the typical teenager would be insured through a parent's insurance (if the parent were insured), and an elderly person would be eligible for Medicare (and may well have supplemental insurance coverage), none of the three would be highly likely to have to rely on a charitable institution for hospital care. All three might find themselves at a large, nonprofit public university teaching hospital supported by state funding and receiving private grants and endowments. Alternatively, all three might be admitted to a private, proprietary community hospital that provides similar services on a smaller scale.

The Hospital

Hospitals can differ considerably, but they have many aspects in common. They all have some type of administrative organization, some type of functional organization, and some type of structural organization.

HOSPITAL ADMINISTRATIVE ORGANIZATION

Hospital administrative organization refers to the flow of power and responsibility, the chain of command. Several models commonly exist, the most common of which is the traditional hierarchical structure that resembles a pyramid. Figure 22–1 illustrates one example. Be aware that many health care organizations can be quite complex, so that the flow of power and responsibility cannot be entirely depicted by a simple pyramid shape.

HOSPITAL FUNCTIONAL ORGANIZATION

Each agency is made up of distinct components that serve a specific function. They are usually called de-

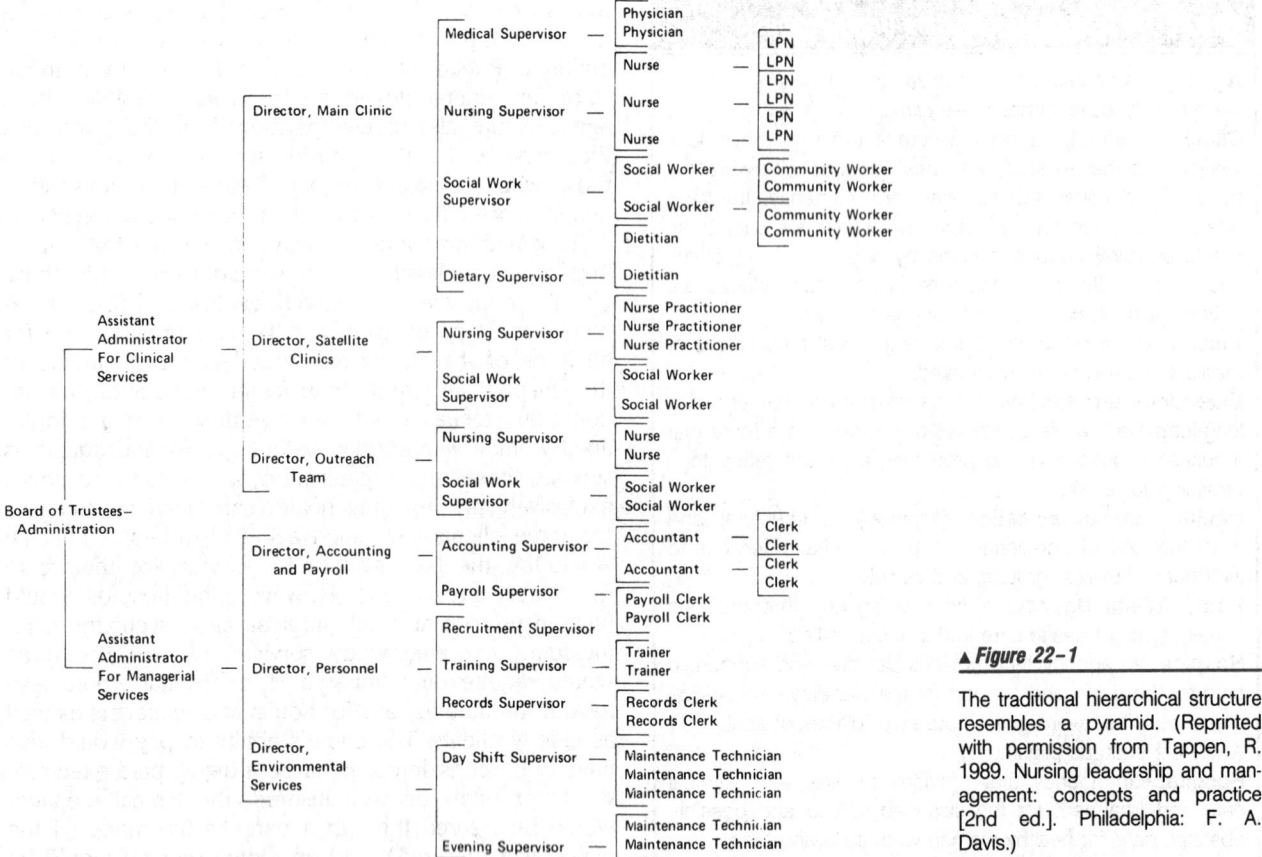

▲ *Figure 22–1*

The traditional hierarchical structure resembles a pyramid. (Reprinted with permission from Tappen, R. 1989. Nursing leadership and management: concepts and practice [2nd ed.]. Philadelphia: F. A. Davis.)

partments or services and may consist of one person or several hundred. Indeed, from agency to agency, each of these functional components can vary considerably in size and importance. Some may not exist in one agency but are vital in another. If present, each should fit within the administrative organization and be visible on the organizational flow chart.

Some departments provide health services or therapies directly to the client. Examples include

▶ Specific departments providing physician and physician's assistant services (such as internal medicine, surgery, psychiatry, obstetrics, gynecology, pediatrics, dermatology, neurology, orthopedics, plastic surgery, oncology, and other departments based on agency goals)
▶ Nursing service
▶ Surgical operating room
▶ Recovery room
▶ Emergency room
▶ Dietary
▶ Pharmacy
▶ Physical medicine (physical therapy, occupational therapy, recreational therapy)
▶ Radiology
▶ Radiation therapy (radiotherapy, nuclear medicine)
▶ Inhalation (respiratory) therapy
▶ Laboratory
▶ Social services
▶ Chaplain services

Other departments exist to provide a service for the client. Although these services may not seem to be directly health related or may not be considered to be a "therapy," they can greatly enhance the client's feelings of well-being. Examples include

▶ Volunteers (to provide such ancillary services as a bookmobile, gift shop, and television rental)
▶ Barber and beauty shops

Still other departments exist to maintain the physical upkeep of the agency (housekeeping, maintenance, laundry); to obtain, retain, and dispose of equipment and supplies used by the system (purchasing, central supply, waste removal); to obtain, retain, and train personnel (personnel, payroll, in-service education); and to handle the flow of information necessary to maintain the system (medical records, billing, telephone operators, secretaries, and clerks).

HOSPITAL STRUCTURAL ORGANIZATION

Hospitals consist not only of departments with various levels of management but also of structural (architectural) divisions with names that can be confusing to the outsider. To make it even more confusing, hospital personnel sometimes refer to these different areas by using abbreviations or jargon unfamiliar to the outsider.

You may have heard the story of a hospital visitor who was looking for her mother. The nurse told her, "I am sure your mother is here somewhere. I saw her on the floor only 5 minutes ago." Of course, the nurse meant "the floor" to be understood as "the unit," but the daughter did not understand hospital jargon and believed that her mother was literally lying on the floor.

Any hospital that is built with more than one story has floors that are usually numbered as is done in any multilevel building. Aside from this one convention, the different structural divisions of a hospital may be named in a manner that is inconsistent from building to building. Many hospitals are built using traditional, square, and rectangular designs, but a good number have been designed that are shaped like the spokes of a large wagon wheel, with each spoke a long hallway with rooms on either side. A large number of round hospitals have also been built with all of the client rooms around the outside edge.

Whatever the building's design, if each floor is large, you may find that it has been divided into two or more areas that may be termed wings or halls. Often these divisions are referred to by floor number and direction, such as 3 east or 9 north. Sometimes, these areas are color coded and are referred to by floor number and color scheme such as 4 green or 7 yellow. Other methods for naming major divisions of a floor are possible, but these two are common.

If each wing or hall is large enough, it may be further divided into two or more nursing units. Each of these divisions probably consists of a number of client rooms as well as additional rooms and areas for use by clients and staff. Additional rooms and areas usually include the nurses' station or desk, medication preparation area, conference room, clean and dirty utility rooms, kitchen or kitchenette, shower or tub room, examination room, treatment room, storage areas, offices, lounge for personnel, lounge for clients and visitors, and rest rooms.

Sometimes, the client rooms within each nursing unit are divided into clusters so that individual nursing teams within each nursing station have their own client rooms assigned to their care. For example, a nursing unit might have a total of 16 rooms divided into 4 clusters of 4 rooms each. Each cluster could also be referred to as a module or a pod. Whether in a cluster or not, each client's room may be a private room for one person, a semiprivate room for two persons, or a ward for three or more persons. Whether a person is in a private room or in a room with others, each has an individual care unit for personal use. An individual care unit consists of the client's bed, other furniture, and devices to be used by the client during the hospital stay. Usually a privacy curtain is available to separate each unit. By convention, these units are referred to as beds, even though they consist of more than simply a bed. According to hospital policy, individual units within a client room may be lettered, numbered, or referred to by some other designation such as position in the room (e.g., "door" or "window" if identified by placement nearest to a certain structure). Thus, depending on policy, your client's individual unit might be in "room 368-2," "room 368-B," or "room 368-window."

Unit or bed designations can be very important because fatal errors can occur if a client is identified by bed placement and is given a medication or treatment meant for someone in a different unit. Never rely strictly on placement for client identification.

To find a certain client in a fairly large and complex hospital, you may have to go to the fourth floor, east wing, yellow nursing unit, third cluster, second room, bed B. In a smaller hospital, you may find a client on the first floor, south hall, seventh room on the right. Obviously, you will need a few minutes to become oriented to each hospital's structural organization. Once you understand how your hospital is organized, you should understand how nursing care is organized for delivery within it. In other words, you will need a basic understanding of the nursing care model in use.

Nursing Care Models

Four nursing care models are commonly used in hospitals and other health care settings. Each agency adopts the model it feels is best suited to its goals and resources. Some agencies combine various aspects from several models to make their own models. Some use one model most of the time but may temporarily switch to another model under certain conditions. No model is perfect for everyone. Each has advantages and disadvantages.

CASE METHOD

The **case method (one-to-one method)** is a method of providing nursing care in which one nurse provides total, comprehensive nursing care to one or more clients. This method is usually used by the private-duty nurse, the community health nurse, the intensive care nurse, and the student nurse when each works alone (Fig. 22-2). The advantages of this method are as follows:

▶ Assignments are easy to make.
▶ Lines of communication are direct.
▶ Care provided is holistic.
▶ The nurse has a good deal of autonomy.
▶ Satisfaction is high for both client and nurse.

Disadvantages of this method are as follows:

▶ It is not the most efficient way of completing some tasks.
▶ It requires more staff members, and more of these must be registered nurses who have a wide range of knowledge and skills.
▶ It usually does not provide around-the-clock care.
▶ It requires more coordination among the many case nurses and the various hospital departments with whom they must interact each day in order to obtain supplies and services.
▶ It may be too costly for most hospitals to use.

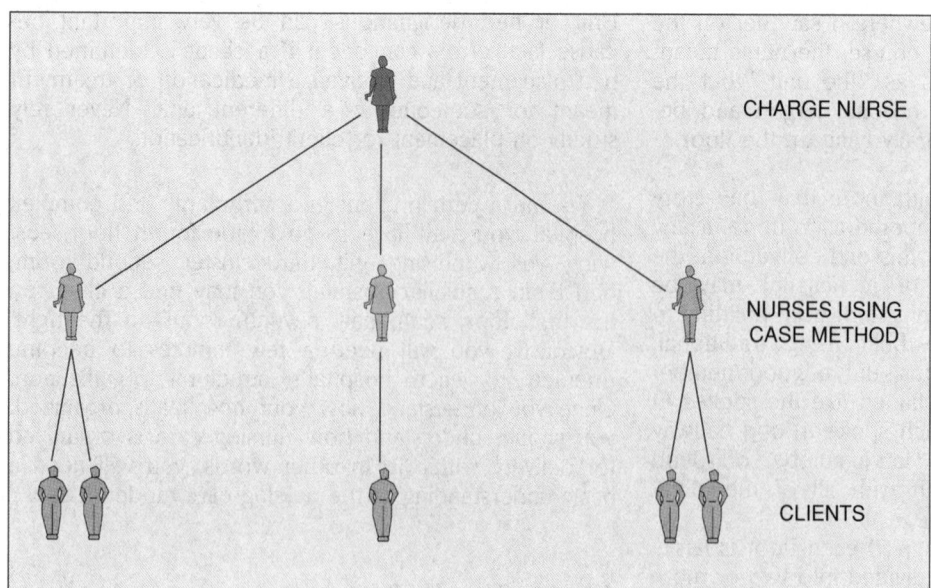

▲ *Figure 22–2*

The case method of providing nursing care, in which one nurse provides total, comprehensive nursing care to one or more clients.

FUNCTIONAL METHOD

The **functional method** is a method of providing nursing care in which one nurse is assigned to do specific tasks for a large number of clients rather than being assigned to complete all tasks for a smaller number of clients. With this method, one registered nurse might be assigned to give medications to all clients; another registered nurse might be assigned to do all treatments; and a licensed vocational or practical nurse might be teamed up with a nurse's aide to provide all hygiene care needed for each client, with each one doing the hygiene care for specific clients, according to each client's need for assistance (Fig. 22–3).

The advantages of this method are as follows:

► Assignments are fairly easy to make.
► Lines of responsibility are clear.

► Because their focus is narrower, workers can gain expertise and skill and can do higher quality work more efficiently and effectively with this method than with any other method.
► More semiskilled and unskilled workers can be used than with the case method.
► This method may be used as a temporary measure when a staff shortage exists and more work must be done by fewer persons.

Disadvantages of this method are as follows:

► The holistic view of the client is lost as care is fragmented.
► Care provided may become rigid, mechanistic, impersonal, and boring.
► The client's psychologic and social needs are often overlooked.

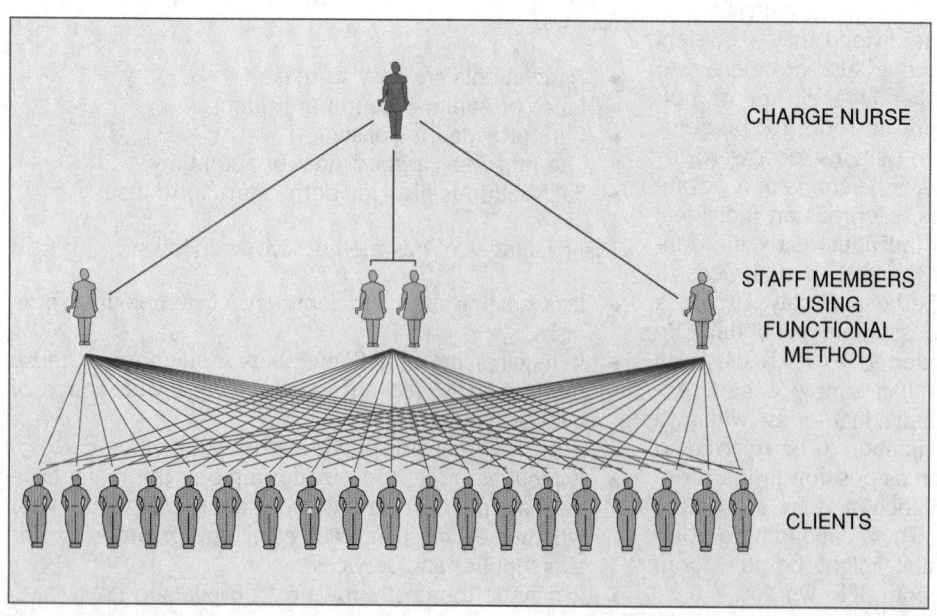

▲ *Figure 22–3*

The functional method of providing nursing care. In this case, one registered nurse has been assigned to give medications to all clients, another registered nurse has been assigned to do all client treatments, and a licensed vocational or practical nurse has been teamed up with a nurses' aide to provide all hygiene care needed for each client.

▶ Satisfaction is generally low for both client and nurse.

TEAM METHOD

With the **team method (team nursing),** groups of nurses and ancillary staff (teams), led by registered nurse team leaders, provide nursing care to groups of clients. With this method, each team leader must be a highly effective, democratic leader with special skills in teaching and communication. Each must teach and lead a larger number of ancillary personnel than with other models of care (Fig. 22–4).

If carried out correctly, this method provides the following advantages:

▶ A higher quality of care may be given with fewer registered nurses than with other methods of delivering care.
▶ Whenever possible, the client is included in planning.
▶ Care provided is comprehensive and holistic.
▶ Satisfaction is generally high for both client and staff.
▶ Morale or team spirit is generally higher compared with other methods of providing care.
▶ Different types and combinations of care methods may be used by the team members.

Disadvantages of the team method are as follows:

▶ Some efficiency is lost compared with the functional method.
▶ Not all registered nurses are as skilled at management, communication, teaching, and democratic leadership as required of team leaders.
▶ Team leaders may not know their individual clients as well as nurses who use other models of care.
▶ A great deal of communication is required, taking time away from actual client care.
▶ This method of care is often done poorly.

PRIMARY CARE METHOD

The **primary care method** is a method of providing nursing care in which one nurse takes responsibility for making the initial nursing assessment, making all nursing diagnoses, planning all nursing care, and ensuring the implementation of the plan for a group of clients 7 days a week, 24 hours a day. The primary nurse is also responsible for evaluating the outcomes of client care. Unlike the nurse who uses the case method of nursing, the primary nurse does not always provide total nursing care but does take responsibility for completing complex nursing tasks and for delegating other tasks to appropriate persons.

When the primary nurse is not available to do and to direct client care, such as on off shifts and on days off, a number of other nurses, referred to as associate nurses, take over the implementation of the primary nurse's plan of care (Fig. 22–5). The advantages of this method are as follows:

▶ The primary nurse has more autonomy than in functional or team nursing.
▶ The primary nurse spends more time in direct client care activities than in coordinating and supervising care done by others.
▶ Nursing care provided is holistic.
▶ Satisfaction is generally high for both client and primary nurse.
▶ Because there is less nurse turnover with this method and because less supervision is required, this is a cost-effective model.

Disadvantages of this method are as follows:

▶ It requires a greater proportion of registered nurses to ancillary staff (an all-registered-nurse staff is ideal).
▶ Not all registered nurses have sufficient knowledge and skills required for this role.
▶ Some ancillary personnel may feel less satisfaction with this model than with other models.

▲ **Figure 22–4**

The team method of providing nursing care. In this case three team leaders each lead a team of four staff members, including registered nurses, licensed vocational or practical nurses, orderlies, and nurses' aides. Each team is responsible for the nursing care of a group of clients.

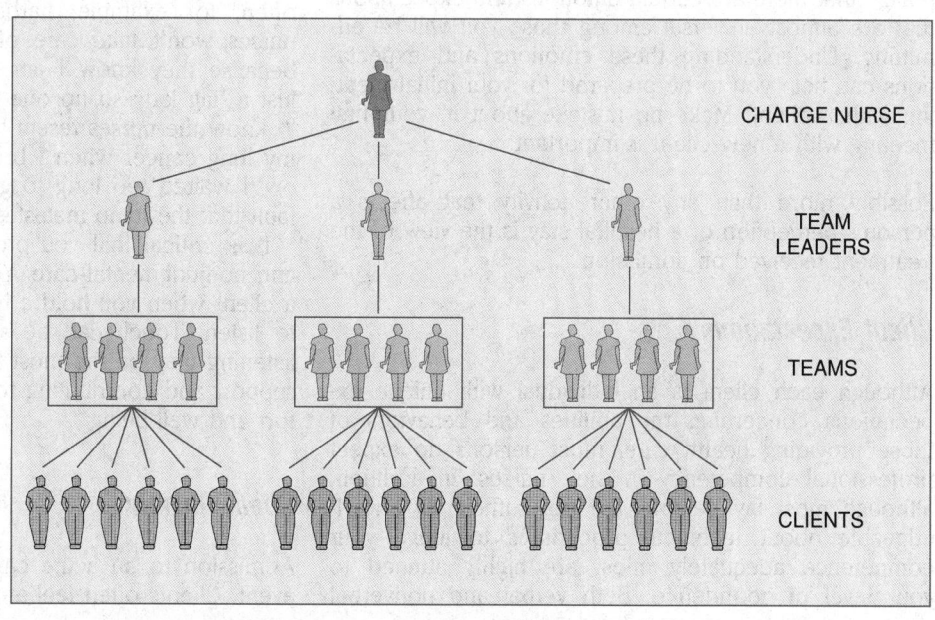

CHARGE NURSE

TEAM LEADERS

TEAMS

CLIENTS

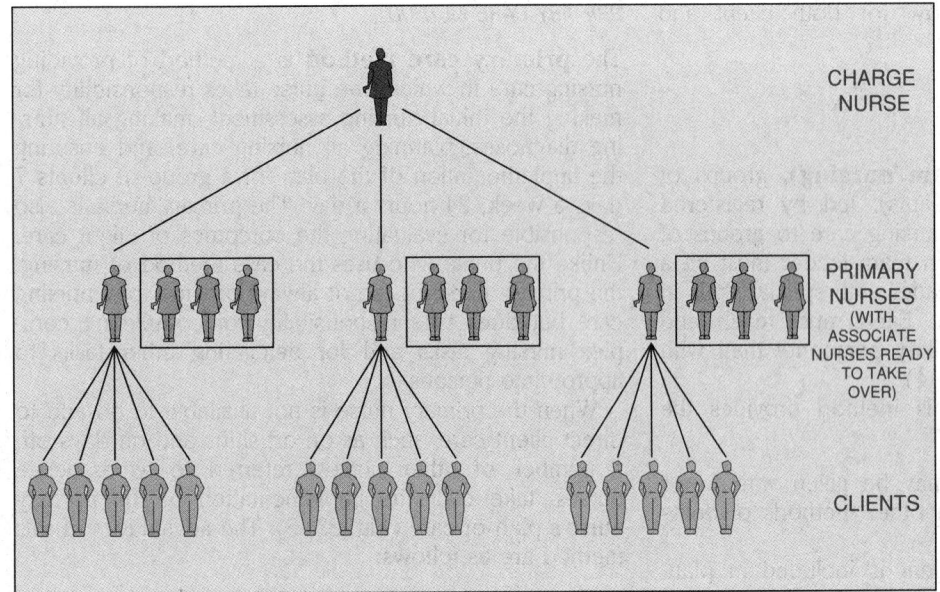

▲ *Figure 22-5*

The primary care method of providing nursing care. Here three primary nurses are each assigned the responsibility for the total nursing care of five clients. Associate nurses (shown in the box next to each primary nurse) are available to take over implementation of the primary nurse's plans on off shifts and on days off.

No matter what nursing care method is used in your agency, each nurse is expected to use the nursing process to plan, implement, and evaluate the nursing care provided. If you have an adequate grasp of how your hospital is organized and the way nurses and other services function within it, you will be better prepared to orient a new client to the facility as part of the admission process. You will have more confidence as you teach and as you answer questions about what to expect during and after the client's stay.

THE CLIENT

Just as you should know about the hospital, you should understand something of the client you will be admitting. Although most persons you admit to a hospital will not be individuals you know personally, you should realize that there are certain emotions and expectations that are almost universal among those you will be admitting. Understanding these emotions and expectations can help you to be prepared for your initial meeting with a client. Make no mistake about it, your first meeting with a new client is important.

Possibly more than any other activity that affects a person's perception of a hospital stay is the view of the treatment received on admission.

Client Expectations

Although each client is an individual with unique expectations concerning the abilities and behaviors of those providing health care, most persons do expect professional competency in their nurses. In addition, although most lay persons are not sufficiently knowledgeable about technical procedures to judge your competence adequately, most are highly attuned to your level of confidence. Both verbal and nonverbal communications can clearly indicate your lack of confidence in your own competence. Comments such as "I've never seen this type of intravenous pump before; I hope nothing goes wrong with it before the head nurse gets back" or "I think I heard your blood pressure correctly that last time I tried" are not statements that engender feelings of trust and security. Confidence in your abilities grows when clients observe that you are carrying out procedures with the deftness and self-assurance that comes only with practice.

Most clients also hope for, and have every right to expect, acceptance and understanding. Clients present themselves to you and depend on you for help in restoring their health or easing their pain. They hope that you will accept them for the persons that they are and that you will not judge them harshly for any part they might have had in causing their own disease or in not seeking professional assistance earlier. Clients often, for example, harbor such thoughts as, "The nurses won't take care of me in the recovery room because they know I am from the prison unit," "I'm just a bag lady so no one will come if I ring my bell," "I know the nurses resent having to take care of me for my lung cancer when I brought it all on by smoking," or "I waited too long to go to the doctor, so it is my fault that the lump metastasized."

It is critical that you provide thoughtful, concerned, and nonjudgmental care. You can give great comfort to a client when you hold a hand or take an extra minute to listen. Touch can be a powerful intervention, and listening may be the most any nurse can do in offering support and contributing to feelings of emotional comfort and well-being.

Client Anxiety

Admission to an acute care setting can be a stressful event. Clients often feel anxiety, although they may not admit this feeling to others or even to themselves. Anxiety stems from the unknown. The client's senses are alert and attuned in this new and threatening atmosphere. A client may also experience anxiety because of a possibility of being placed in a dependent position, having to rely on total strangers, and losing control over decisions that are vital to feelings of comfort and well-being.

Apprehension is increased by hearing unfamiliar sounds and by hearing terms that may sound like a foreign language, by the sight of strange equipment and perhaps by seeing other persons in pain, and by odors that are unfamiliar or that arouse memories associated with painful experiences. At the time of the client's admission, you can be instrumental in reducing feelings of anxiety that stem from such sensory input from the surroundings. For example, you can greatly relieve a client's anxiety by providing a brief orientation to the nursing unit and a more thorough orientation to the individual care unit within the client's room.

For most persons, what is known is much less frightening than what is unknown.

To allay a sense of powerlessness and loss of personal control, you can explain the care to be given and help the client to understand how to be a partner in planning this care. It helps to let the client know that your hospital encourages client participation in daily routines, in determining the care to be provided, and in control of the environment and services provided.

Orienting the Client

ORIENTATION TO THE NURSING UNIT

In many hospitals, new clients are brought to the nursing unit from an admissions area. Usually in the admissions area they have been asked a number of questions about themselves and their insurance coverage and have been given forms to sign for permission for the hospital to give them care. Most often, they have had an identification bracelet applied to their wrist. An identification bracelet usually contains the client's name, room number, hospital number, physician's name, and other information the agency may require, such as a list of allergies.

As each new client arrives on your unit, it may be your assignment to complete the admission process. As you meet the client, you will want to use good techniques of communication. For example, you should smile warmly and shake the person's hand as you repeat his or her name. Begin the orientation to the unit and to nursing care by introducing yourself and explaining your role.

On your way to the client's room, if the person is able to concentrate on the surroundings, point out significant areas that any person (or visitor) might want to know about and add a few words of explanation, as necessary. For example, clients typically need to know the whereabouts of waiting rooms, day rooms, public telephones, water fountains, public rest rooms, the

nurse's desk (station), and their own room in relation to everything else. In addition to these areas on their assigned nursing unit, clients usually like to know the whereabouts of the gift shop and cafeteria, as well as any additional places where they or their visitors may purchase articles such as newspapers, soft drinks, and reading materials.

ORIENTATION TO THE ROOM AND INDIVIDUAL CARE UNIT

The Room and Bathroom. Each client room usually consists of one or more care units and an adjoining bathroom. The client should be oriented to the bathroom and the care unit and should be introduced to any roommates who will share the room.

There is usually only one bathroom per room regardless of the number of care units within each room. In private and semiprivate rooms, each bathroom usually contains one shower, sink, and toilet. In a multibed ward, the bathroom may offer several of each. Bathtubs may be present in the client's bathroom, or the client may have to go to a central bathroom (or tub room) to use a tub. In addition to these familiar facilities, hospital bathrooms also contain grab bars for weak persons to grasp and hold onto for support. These usually take the form of bars on the walls near shower, tub, and toilet. If there is no wall near the toilet, railings or other supporting frameworks may be made available on either side of the bowl. Hospital bathrooms also contain at least one emergency call light so that assistance may be summoned if needed. As part of the orientation to the bathroom, point out this call light and instruct the client about how and when to use it.

The Individual (Basic) Care Unit. The individual care unit consists of a hospital bed, bedside stand, over-bed table, chair, overhead light, suction and oxygen outlets, electrical outlets, a sphygmomanometer, and a nurses' call light (Fig. 22–6). Each unit within a room may also have a locker, a closet, or a set of built-in drawers. Help the client to understand how to work with the furniture and accessories.

Hospital Beds and Side Rails. The three general types of beds currently supplied to acute care settings — manual, hydraulic, and electric — are all capable of adjustment for height from the floor and for positioning to elevate the head, knees, and feet.

Manual Beds. Manual beds require the use of hand cranks or foot pedals to manipulate the bed into desired positions. Hand cranks are used to elevate the head and knee sections of the bed; manual manipulation of a gatch at the foot of the bed is necessary for elevating the foot of the bed; and foot pedals are used to raise the height of the bed from the floor. Manual beds are generally less expensive and are almost free of safety hazards.

The cranks or pedals are usually located at the foot of the bed. To prevent anyone from accidentally injuring a leg on the crank when walking near the bed, crank

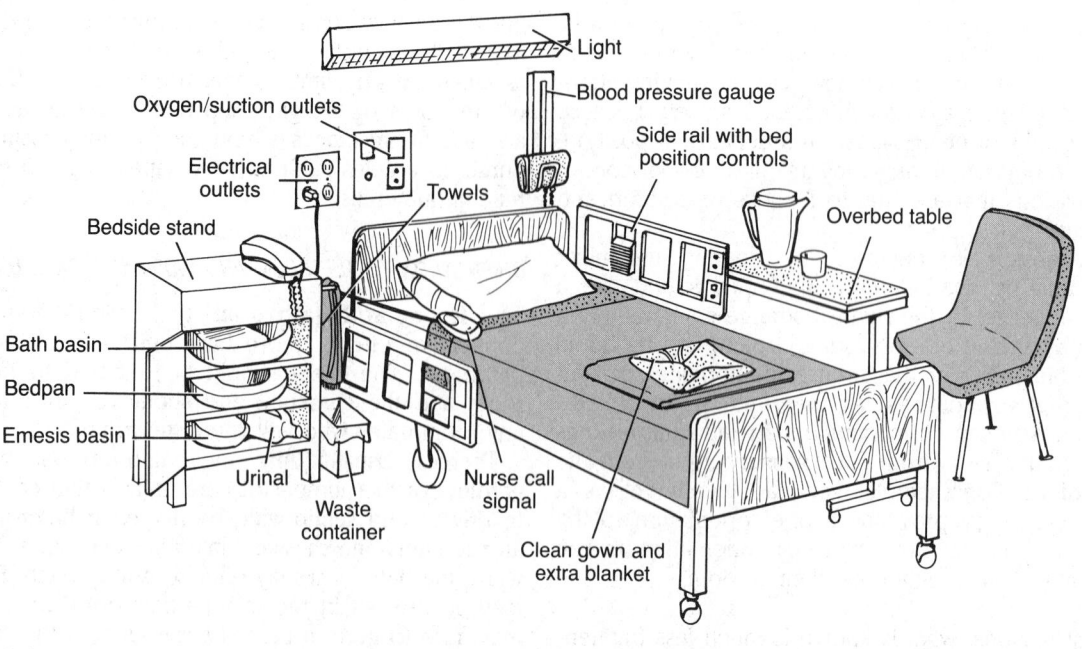

▲ *Figure 22-6*

The individual (basic) care unit consists of a hospital bed, bedside stand, overbed table, chair, overhead light, suction and oxygen outlets, electrical outlets, a sphygmomanometer, and a nurses' call light. To prepare the unit for a new client's arrival, place the bed in the lowest position from the floor with side rails up on one side of the bed, turn the bedding down (open the bed) in preparation for use, provide a gown and extra blanket (if weather necessitates), be certain room temperature is seasonably appropriate and comfortable, assure that the lighting provides a welcome atmosphere, and be sure that supplies are available (new or sterile basins, bedpan, and urinal in bedside stand and filled water pitcher and clean drinking glass nearby, if client condition permits fluids by mouth).

handles should be positioned under the bed when not in use.

Hydraulic Beds. Hydraulic beds function through the use of compressed air fed to the bed system through a hose attached to a wall outlet that supplies compressed air. Manual operation of the bed is also possible through the use of foot pedals, which may be pumped to simulate the wall outlet system of compressed air. These systems are useful in the presence of other electrical equipment.

Electric Beds. Powered by an electric motor, electric beds require an electric outlet to function. An advantage of the electric bed is that it allows control of position by the client. Control switches are generally located for ease of use by the bed's occupant, but they may be "locked out" when conditions warrant.

Authorities have debated the possible hazards associated with the use of these beds in certain areas, such as critical care units, previously thought to be electrically hazardous. Preventive maintenance and up-to-date electrical engineering, however, have allowed the use of electric beds in such areas. (Special beds, frames, and mattresses are discussed in Chapter 35.)

Side Rails. Whatever type of bed used in your hospital, it should have a set of side rails attached (or available for attachment) on both sides of the bed. Side rails are meant to prevent client falls. They come in two main types: full rails and half (short, partial) rails. Full rails run the length of the bed; half rails run only half the

length of the bed. Half rails may be used at the top of the bed only, as shown in Fig. 22-6, or two half rails may be used on each side of the bed with a set near the head of the bed and a set near the foot of the bed. When both sets are up, the effect is the same as having a full set in place. Side rails help prevent the client from rolling out of bed. When half rails are used alone, they may help prevent falls by serving as a railing for the weaker client to hold onto for support when getting into and out of bed. Either type of rail is useful in helping the client change positions.

When orienting your client to the bed, demonstrate how to work the bed controls. If the client is ambulatory, show him or her how to raise and lower the side rails. Present the side rails as useful devices to help in positioning and in "reminding" sleeping clients that they are not at home in a bigger bed. Let the clients know that they are in charge of the rails, so that the rails are less likely to be seen as threatening to client autonomy.

Bedside Stand. The bedside stand is a small cabinet that generally consists of a drawer and a cupboard area with shelves. It is used to store the utensils needed for client care, including the washbasin (bath basin), emesis (kidney) basin, bedpan, and urinal. Bedside stands often have a towel rack on either side or along the back, so bath linens may be kept handy. When orienting the client to the bedside stand, tell him or her that the closets and built-in drawers that are farther away from the bed are better used for storing items that will be used only occasionally, whereas the bedside stand is best for storing personal items that are desired nearby or that will be used frequently, such as soap, shampoo, lotion, mouth care supplies, and other items needed for hygienic care.

Overbed Table. The overbed table consists of a rectangular, flat surface supported by a side bar attached to a wide base on wheels. The height of the table is adjustable. Depending on the model, part of the table surface may conceal a storage compartment and a mirror, which may be useful for less mobile clients. The table may be positioned alongside or over the bed or over a chair.

The table is most frequently used for holding the tray during meals and for holding care items when completing personal hygiene. At other times, it is used by the client as a desk for letter writing or by the nurse for holding supplies during treatments. When orienting the client to the overbed table, show him or her how to open the storage compartment (if any) and how to raise and lower the table. Because this table surface is used so frequently, the client should be told that it is not the best place for keeping things such as flower arrangements that cannot be moved easily.

The Chair. Most basic care units have at least one chair located near the bedside. The chair is for the use of the client, a visitor, or a care provider. Unit chairs are usually of the straight-back variety and may or may not have armrests. Some chairs are actually convertible to single beds that allow more comfortable overnight stays for a client's family member or significant other.

Hospital chairs are usually upholstered in vinyl for ease in cleaning. When placing a client in the chair, it is often helpful to place a sheet or bath blanket over the vinyl to prevent chilling. Additional body covering may also be warranted.

Overhead Light. An overhead (or examination) light is usually placed at the head of the bed, attached to either the wall or the ceiling. A movable lamp may also be available as part of each unit. Lights are useful to the client for reading or doing close work but are also important for nurses during assessments. Lights can be particularly important when specific body areas must be examined or must be clearly visible for treatments. If your individual care units offer more than one light switch, orient the client to the system. In some settings, it is not an infrequent occurrence when a client sets off emergency alarms while trying to turn on a light.

Suction and Oxygen Outlets. Suction is a vacuum created in a tube that is used to pull (evacuate) fluids from the body. Most frequently, it is used to clear upper respiratory tract passages of mucus or fluids, but it may be used in an emergency situation or in an operating room to clear blood from a rapidly bleeding wound.

Because it is a requirement for human life, oxygen is one of the gases frequently used in health care today. Just the opposite of suction, oxygen is delivered under positive pressure. Like suction, oxygen is delivered through a tube.

Suction and oxygen are not needed for every client, but they are needed more frequently now that hospitals are providing care for increasing numbers of acutely ill clients. It can be life threatening when either oxygen or suction is needed and is unavailable. Therefore, both suction and oxygen are becoming standard in each basic care unit. Both are often available through pipes (lines) in the wall, and nurses have access to both by merely opening an adapter that is fitted into an outlet to one line or the other. Suction and oxygen outlets, when available in the unit, are located in the wall at the head of the client's bed. Portable suction and oxygen equipment is available on nursing units that do not have piped-in suction and oxygen available.

Electrical Outlets. Electrical outlets are placed in varying positions in the basic care unit and are almost always available in the wall at the head of the bed. Because some life-saving equipment requires the use of electricity, working electrical outlets are a vital part of the nursing unit. To ensure continuity of care during power outages, all hospitals must have a back-up source of electricity available from a separate generator. Because emergency power generation cannot sustain a complete hospital system during an electrical failure, power is supplied only to certain electrical outlets. These emergency outlets have specific markings to identify them in an emergency. For example, emergency outlets are frequently color coded red.

Sphygmomanometer. The blood pressure gauge is an important assessment tool frequently used by nurses. Although portable sphygmomanometers are available on each nursing unit, many hospitals are supplying this equipment as a part of each basic care unit. When available in each unit, the sphygmomanometer is placed on the wall above the head of the bed.

Call Light. Clients can maintain constant contact with care providers with the call light. Therefore, it may well be the most important accessory at the bedside. All call lights work by turning on a specific light that tells nurses at a distance exactly which client is signaling. Most often, the nurse can answer the light by pressing a button and opening communications over an intercom between the nurses' station and the client's unit. The light may then be turned off at the nurses' desk, or the nurse may go to the client's unit and turn it off.

Some call lights, such as emergency call lights in bathrooms, cannot be turned off from a distance but must be turned off manually at the source of the call.

Because the call light helps the client to maintain control over the environment by enabling him or her to notify the nursing staff of needs, the light's accessibility to the client must always be ensured. When orienting the client to the unit, you must be certain that the client knows how to operate the call light.

Other Accessories. Additional accessories may be available to clients in some hospitals but unavailable or optional in others. Such accessories include telephones, radios, and television. When such accessories are optional, they may be rented or brought in from home.

If they are present in the unit, telephones should be placed where clients can reach them from the bed but where they are not likely to be easily knocked off the table. The same principle applies to radios. Televisions have to be at a distance from the client for best viewing. Most often, they are mounted on the wall or are wheeled in on a stand and left by the wall opposite the head of the bed. The client should have access to a remote control to be able to make desired adjustments.

The controls for televisions, beds, and call lights may all be individual, hand-held controls at the end of separate electrical cords, or they may be combined into one or two hand-held controls. Alternatively, these controls may be built into a push-button system in the bedside stand or in the bed's side rail (see Fig. 22–6). A radio may also be built into the bedside stand or into a side rail. Various combinations exist. You should explain your hospital's system to your new client as part of the orientation to the unit.

ASSISTING THE PERSON TO ADJUST TO THE CLIENT ROLE

If you have prepared the client's basic care unit for the individual's arrival (see Fig. 22–6), the client should have a good initial impression of the unit. If you orient the client to the unit appropriately, the client should have a positive impression of your competence. The person needs some time to settle in and adjust to the client role. If the client is able to change clothing and put away belongings without your assistance, this is a good time to allow these activities. This will give the person an opportunity to look in the drawers, to turn the water on in the bathroom, or to flush the toilet—in other words, to do in privacy some of the little things that we tend to do to make ourselves feel more at home in a strange environment.

Before you leave the client alone to change into a hospital gown, verify the information on the client's identification bracelet (wristband). Accurate information on the client's identification band is absolutely necessary to ensure appropriate care and treatment during hospitalization. Also instruct the person about hospital policies regarding telephone, television, and radio usage; smoking restrictions; visiting hours; meal times; side rails; safe care of valuables; and any other policies the person needs to know. Explain any necessary measures needed for collection of specimens or for monitoring fluid intake and output. Provide for privacy by closing the drapes or blinds, pulling the privacy curtain between units as necessary, and closing the room door as you leave.

ASSESSMENT

As your client is changing into a client gown in preparation for the admission assessment, you may assemble the equipment you will need for the admission assessment, if you have not done so already. Generally speaking, the following equipment is required:

▶ a stethoscope to assess various body systems
▶ a sphygmomanometer to assess blood pressure
▶ a watch with a second hand to assess heart and respiratory rate
▶ a thermometer to assess temperature
▶ specimen containers as needed for admission blood and urine collection
▶ a scale to determine the client's weight and height
▶ appropriate forms or paper and pen to record findings

A nursing admission assessment requires a complete data base to help ensure correct nursing care. Basic data needed include a subjective report of the client's health history and an objective physical assessment. Chapters 31, 32, and 33 provide details concerning the assessment of vital signs and the completion of psychosocial and health assessments. These skills take time to learn and practice to master. You should have had some practice with these assessment skills before you actually use them to admit a client.

All of the data you gather as you assess the client are used to plan care for the client in order to ensure a successful discharge from the hospital. Discharge planning, then, begins on admission.

As you complete your assessment of the client, you should understand that you are concerned with the total needs of the client and that you are gathering information that will help you to plan for the client's future needs. Therefore, your admission assessment must be more extensive than an assessment that is done to identify only immediate needs.[24]

Many clients are admitted with physician's orders. If you have no orders at the time of a client's admission, you must notify the physician of the client's admission and obtain orders. Sometimes, for your client's immediate safety or comfort, you must carry out orders immediately. For example, you may have to start an intravenous line or give a pain medication before you can complete the full assessment. Then, during your assessment, you may find that a client's needs require you to contact the physician for additional orders. These activities, together with a thorough report to the appropriate nurse colleagues, can require approximately 90 minutes for a nurse who works full time as an experienced admission assessment coordinator.[20] If you have less experience with assessment, you will want to allow yourself more time.

As part of the thorough assessment of your clients, you may complete a brief screening procedure to help identify those who are at risk for a prolonged hospital stay and the degree of discharge planning needed. One such screen is the Blaylock Risk Assessment Screen (BRASS). The BRASS lists 10 characteristics that should be assessed; each characteristic has several options that might apply to a given client (Fig. 22–7). Each option has a numerical value. The nurse using this as-

Circle all that apply and total. Refer to the Risk Factor Index.*

Age
0 = 55 years or less
1 = 56 to 64 years
2 = 65 to 79 years
3 = 80+ years

Living Situation/Social Support
0 = Lives only with spouse
1 = Lives with family
2 = Lives alone with family support
3 = Lives alone with friends' support
4 = Lives alone with no support
5 = Nursing home/residential care

Functional Status
0 = Independent in activities of daily living and
    instrumental activities of daily living
Dependent in:
1 = Eating/feeding
1 = Bathing/grooming
1 = Toileting
1 = Transferring
1 = Incontinent of bowel function
1 = Incontinent of bladder function
1 = Meal preparation
1 = Responsible for own medication
    administration
1 = Handling own finances
1 = Grocery shopping
1 = Transportation

Cognition
0 = Oriented
1 = Disoriented to some spheres† some of the
    time
2 = Disoriented to some spheres all of the time
3 = Disoriented to all spheres some of the time
4 = Disoriented to all spheres all of the time
5 = Comatose

Behavior Pattern
0 = Appropriate
1 = Wandering
1 = Agitated
1 = Confused
1 = Other

Mobility
0 = Ambulatory
1 = Ambulatory with mechanical
    assistance
2 = Ambulatory with human assistance
3 = Nonambulatory

Sensory Deficits
0 = None
1 = Visual or hearing deficits
2 = Visual and hearing deficits

Number of Previous Admissions/
Emergency Room Visits
0 = None in the last 3 months
1 = One in the last 3 months
2 = Two in the last 3 months
3 = More than two in the last 3 months

Number of Active Medical Problems
0 = Three medical problems
1 = Three to five medical problems
2 = More than five medical problems

Number of Drugs
0 = Fewer than three drugs
1 = Three to five drugs
2 = More than five drugs

Total Score:

*Risk Factor Index: Score of 10 = at risk for home care resources; score of 11 to 19 = at risk
for extended discharge planning; score greater than 20 = at risk for placement other than
home. If the patient's score is 10 or greater, refer the patient to the discharge planning
coordinator or discharge planning team.
†Spheres = person, place, time, and self.
Copyright 1991 Ann Blaylock

▲ **Figure 22-7**

Blaylock Discharge Planning Risk
Assessment Screen.

sessment tool circles the options most pertinent to the client being assessed and adds up the numerical values to arrive at a total score.[1] Total scores range from 0 to 40. A score less than 10 is low and suggests that the client has a low demand for discharge planning resources. A score of 10 to 19 is moderate and suggests that the client has more complicated problems that will require extensive discharge planning resources but probably will not require institutionalization. A score greater than 19 is high and suggests that the client has vast problems that will require extensive discharge planning resources and will probably require institutionalization or rehabilitation.[1]

Preventing Liability

Part of the admission procedure is to help ensure the safekeeping of the client's belongings as well as to help protect the agency from liability in the event of their loss. You must make note of any clothing or other articles that the client brings or wears to the hospital. Particularly important to note are items of value, such as jewelry or money. Clients are usually discouraged from having more than a few dollars in their possession while they are hospitalized, and they are encouraged to send valuable articles home with a relative or to place them in a special envelope and have them locked in the hospital safe. Many clients will refuse to remove wedding or engagement rings or other items of high sentimental value, and many prefer to wear their watches at all times. Prosthetic devices such as hearing aids and glasses are quite valuable and, of course, must remain with the client. The disposition of all money and articles of value should be recorded in the client's chart. Articles remaining in the client's possession should be so noted.

When describing a client's jewelry, use care not to suggest that it has a certain value. For example, do not describe an engagement ring as having a diamond in a gold setting. Rather, describe it as a ring with a clear stone in a yellow metal band. This description will avoid any problems with a client who might turn in a rhinestone ring for safekeeping on admission and request return of a diamond ring on discharge.

Usually, medications are treated as valuables and either sent home or locked in the hospital safe. Normally, clients should not be allowed to keep medications in their possession because they might take a medication that they are also being given as part of their care and thus receive a double dose. Also their medication may not be compatible with other medications given, and unexpected side effects could occur. In certain cases, however, medications may be left at the client's bedside for self-administration. The physician must write an order for client self-administration of medication, and it must be noted on the chart and elsewhere, according to hospital policy.

Another area of potential liability is related to client injuries. Any signs of preexisting injuries should be noted as part of the assessment and should be carefully recorded. This procedure helps document that the client entered the agency with the injury and did not receive it during hospitalization. Wounds such as bruises, bites, and scratches might be signs of abuse. Wounds such as bedsores might be signs of neglect. Many states have laws that require the reporting of any suspicion of such abuse.

Still another potential area of hospital liability is the possibility of exposing the client to any medications, food, or other materials to which he or she is allergic. To prevent possibly tragic outcomes, all allergies identified during the assessment (or the fact that the client denies allergies) must be posted in prominent places, according to hospital policy. Most often, allergies are listed on the client's chart cover, at specific places within the chart, on any medication records that are kept apart from the chart, and on the client's care plan; they may also be listed on the identification band and in the client's care unit.

Documenting Admission

When you begin (open) a new client's chart, certain forms must be filled out as part of the admission process. Each agency will vary in the type of forms and the style of charting to be used (see Chapter 27 for

examples). Whatever the style of charting, the information to be conveyed in an admission note usually consists of the following:

▶ Date/time admitted
▶ Client age and sex
▶ Room and care unit to which client was admitted
▶ Medical diagnosis
▶ How the person was transported to the unit (ambulatory or via wheelchair, stretcher, or some other conveyance)
▶ Who, if anyone, accompanied the client (family member, police, ambulance crew, parent/guardian, friend, neighbor)
▶ Reason for admission, in the client's own words (e.g., "plastic surgery on my face," "tests for my stomach pain," "a depression I can't seem to shake")
▶ Orientation to unit completed
▶ Vital signs
▶ Physician's notification of admission
▶ Disposition of valuables
▶ Assessment completion
▶ Allergies
▶ Unusual assessment findings (including marks or bruises)
▶ Any teaching done
▶ Any immediate treatments completed
▶ Disposition of any specimens obtained
▶ Your signature

Following is one example:
January, 23/11:00 a.m.—Sixteen-year-old female admitted to room 108, bed 2, via wheelchair from emergency room, with a diagnosis of polydrug abuse and alcohol dependency. Accompanied to unit by mother and maternal aunt. Stated, "They pumped my stomach in the emergency room and sent me up here." Oriented to unit. B/P = 104/68, T = 36.5°C, P = 110, R = 22. Dr. Calhoun notified of admission. Two religious medals sent home with mother. Claims no other valuables. Nursing assessment completed. Denies allergies to any foods, medications, or materials. No unusual marks noted on skin assessment. Urine spec. to lab.—Marilyn Niles, R. N.

In addition to charting, it may be your responsibility to notify other hospital departments of the admission and to let them know about any physician's orders. For example, you may notify the dietary department to order meals, the pharmacy to order medications, or the x-ray department or the laboratory to order diagnostic tests. Be sure to notify these departments of client allergies, as necessary. You may also have to order supplies needed for client care and treatments. For example, you may need additional pillows or suction equipment to attach to the wall outlet.

NURSING DIAGNOSIS

Nurses are in a unique position among care givers in that they are able to gather and assess data concerning the whole client and the full range of client needs.[24]

When your assessment is completed, you will have a good deal of data from the health history and physical assessment. You should also have information from the physician, and you may have input from the client's family or others. As the admitting nurse, it will be at least partially your responsibility to synthesize all of this information into an initial list of nursing diagnoses. In agencies in which team nursing is practiced, this task may be shared with others. In other agencies, formulating nursing diagnoses is usually the responsibility of one nurse.

Often nursing diagnoses are to be written on the special nursing care planning forms, or they may be written into the chart, depending on the style of charting used in your agency. Some agencies provide a check list for indicating nursing diagnoses. Others use computer programs that allow selection from a list so that selections can be printed out to be added to the client's record. (See Chapter 8 for a more detailed discussion of nursing diagnoses.)

PLANNING

Planning is discussed in Chapter 9. Planning done at the time of admission should include discharge planning. **Discharge planning** is a process of anticipating and planning for changing client care needs as the client moves from one level of care to another. For example, you might plan for a client to progress from an intensive care to an intermediate care unit and then to a medical-surgical care unit before transferring to a rehabilitation hospital. Alternatively, you might plan for a client's progression from a surgical unit to a home health care nursing service or to a hospice. Your nursing diagnoses and related outcomes should reflect a view of the future. The ultimate goal is to ensure continuity of care.[24]

A clear idea of the finished picture or goal improves the effectiveness of discharge planning.[24]

You should understand that discharge planning may already have been done when you receive a client for admission because this process is not done only by nurses in hospitals. Instead, discharge planning should be ongoing in all health agencies. For example, you may admit a client to a surgical unit for a second or third reconstructive surgery after a previous hospitalization for acute burn care and a stay at a rehabilitation center. The plan for all of these levels of care should have been initiated by the nurse who admitted the newly burned client. Ongoing planning, with changes according to changing client needs, should have been made by other nurses as the client progressed through different health care agencies and levels.

Actually, discharge planning is not done *for* the client: It is done *with* the client. It involves the client, family, and significant others. Discharge planning, like all nursing care planning, should involve multidisciplinary collaboration. Expert instruction and evaluation can be obtained from other disciplines within the acute care setting. For example, dietary consults can serve as educational resources to the client and significant others in providing for nutritional needs. Physical therapy consults can provide rehabilitative instruction. Social service consults can coordinate activities for multiple needs, including financial advisement, nutritional assistance, and the acquisition of equipment such as hospital beds, wheelchairs, and walkers needed for home use.

If the nursing staff, the interdisciplinary team, and the client, family, and significant others plan well together, discharge planning should

▶ include concern for the client's total well-being
▶ be based on thorough, up-to-date knowledge of available resources
▶ result in mutually agreed-on decisions concerning the most economic and appropriate options for continuing care[24]

Your plan should be written on the chart or separate nursing care plan, depending on your agency policies. Outcomes should be clearly stated and agreed on by all concerned. Usually, as the admitting nurse, your responsibility is to write an initial list of interventions that must be carried out to meet the stated outcomes.

NURSING INTERVENTION

As previously mentioned, some nursing interventions must be carried out immediately on admission to ensure client comfort and safety. Once the admission process has been completed and the plan of care is written out, interventions should be carried out according to the plan of care.

EVALUATION

As evaluation of ongoing care is completed, revision of the discharge plan may be necessary. (See Chapter 11 for a review of the evaluation process.) If the discharge plan is kept up to date, with continual evaluative input, you and the client will be ready and the transition will be smooth when the time comes for client discharge.

THE DISCHARGE PROCESS

When the time comes for discharge from your agency, several final steps should be taken. These include the following:

▶ Obtain a physician's order for dismissal.
▶ Make any final client assessments required for the record.
▶ Finalize any teaching by reiteration of previous teaching.
▶ Verify availability of any required equipment.
▶ Ensure that final arrangements are made regarding the financial aspects of the client's stay at your agency.

▶ Return valuables and medications to the client, as indicated.

▶ Assist with packing personal belongings, and assist the client in dressing as needed.

▶ Provide the client with any written instructions needed for continuation of care, such as date and time of follow-up appointment at a clinic.

▶ Provide the client with any written prescriptions from the physician as required.

▶ Ensure that the client has transportation to home or to the next agency.

▶ Take the client (and all belongings) from the unit to your agency exit. Most agencies require that the client be transported by wheelchair rather than by walking.

▶ Complete all nursing records. This usually includes making a discharge notation that includes written confirmation that all of the above items have been done, as necessary, according to the needs of each client.

▶ Arrange for the unit to be terminally cleaned and readied for the next client.

The final discharge note, when written, may look something like the following:

January, 28/10:00 a.m.—Discharged per wheelchair to care of mother. Alert and oriented ×3 following uneventful 5-day detoxification from drug and alcohol abuse. Accompanied to mother's car. Mother states she will be taking client directly to Sunnylands Drug Rehabilitation Center as planned by her, the client, and the interdisciplinary team.—Marilyn Niles, R. N.

SUMMARY

▶ Health care organizations (agencies) may be classified in several ways, depending on the focus of the services provided, the types of health services provided, the population served, and the source of funds.

▶ Hospitals are health care organizations that may be understood by examining their administrative, functional, and structural components.

▶ The four main nursing care models are the case method, the functional method, the team method, and the primary care method.

▶ Most clients who are admitted to the hospital have certain expectations, often based on past experience, and most are anxious.

▶ Client anxiety may be reduced by a brief orientation to the nursing unit and a more careful orientation to the client care unit.

▶ Client assessment includes obtaining data needed for immediate care and for discharge planning and must attend to preventing liability.

▶ Depending on the nursing care model used, it may be the admitting nurse's sole or shared responsibility to synthesize all assessment data into an initial list of nursing diagnoses.

▶ Planning done at the time of admission should include discharge planning.

▶ Some nursing interventions must be carried out immediately on admission, but all others should be carried out according to the written plan of care established after the client's admission assessment has been completed.

▶ If the discharge plan is kept up to date, with continual evaluative input, client discharge will be smooth.

▶ At the time of final discharge, the process should include only a limited number of nursing activities.

Bibliography

1. Blaylock, A., & Cason, C.L. (1992). Discharge planning: predicting patients' needs. *Journal of Gerontological Nursing*, 18(7), 5–10.
2. Chovaz, C.J. (1992). Communicating with the hearing impaired patient. *Axone*, 13(3), 77–88.
3. Corkery, E. (1989). Discharge planning and home health care: what every staff nurse should know. *Orthopedic Nursing*, 8(6), 18–27.
4. Daly, M.R. (1990). Sensory supports for the visually impaired. *Journal of Ophthalmic Nursing and Technology*, 9(6), 243–244.
5. Dellasega, C., & Shellenbarger, T. (1992). Discharge planning for cognitively impaired elderly adults. *Nursing and Health Care*, 13(10), 526–531.
6. Dugan, J., & Mosel, L. (1992). Patients in acute care settings. Which health-care services are provided? *Journal of Gerontological Nursing*, 18(7), 31–36.
7. Esper, P. (1988). Discharge planning: a quality assurance approach. *Nursing Management*, 19(10), 66–68.
8. Farren, E.A. (1991). Effects of early discharge planning on length of hospital stay. *Nursing Economics*, 9(1), 25–30, 63.
9. Fulton, J. (1988). Acute care of elders. In Burnside, I. (ed.). *Nursing and the aged: A self-care approach* (3rd ed., pp. 897–916). New York: McGraw-Hill.
10. Hamilton, B., & Vessey, J. (1992). Pediatric discharge planning. *Pediatric Nursing*, 18(5), 475–478.
11. Hirsch, C.H., et al. (1990). The natural history of functional morbidity in hospitalized older patients. *Journal of the American Geriatrics Society*, 38(12), 1296–1303.
12. Hunter, J.K. (1992). Making a difference for homeless patients. RN, 55(12), 48–53.
13. Inglehart, A.P. (1990). Discharge planning: professional perspectives versus organizational effects. *Health and Social Work*, 15(4), 301–309.
14. Johannsen, J.M. (1992). Self-care assessment: key to teaching and discharge planning. *Dimensions of Critical Care Nursing*, 11(1), 48–56.
15. Johnson, J. (1989). Where's discharge planning on your list? *Geriatric Nursing*, 10(3), 148–149.
16. North, M., et al. (1991). Discharge planning: increasing client and nurse satisfaction. *Rehabilitation Nursing*, 16(6), 327–329.
17. O'Hare, P.A., & Terry, M.A. (1988). *Discharge planning: Strategies for assuring continuity of care*. Rockville, MD: Aspen Publishers.
18. Owen, J., et al. (1992). Discharge planning in the ICU: a case study. *Critical Care Nurse*, 12(4), 69–72.
19. Packard-Hale, M., & Lancaster, D. (1989). A vital link in continuity of care. *Nursing Management*, 20(8), 32–34.
20. Patrick-Baker, D. (1992). An admission assessment coordinator. *Nursing Management*, 23(1), 46, 48.
21. Pray, D., & Hoff, J. (1992). Implementing a multidisciplinary approach to discharge planning. *Nursing Management*, 23(10), 52–53, 56.
22. Proctor, E., et al. (1992). Patient and family satisfaction with discharge plans. *Medical Care*, 30(3), 262–275.
23. Rhoads, C., et al. (1992). Comprehensive discharge planning: a hospital-home healthcare partnership. *Home Healthcare Nurse*, 10(6), 13–18.
24. Rorden, J.W., & Taft, E. (1990). *Discharge planning guide for nurses*. Philadelphia: W.B. Saunders.

25. Schlemer, B. (1989). The status of discharge planning in intensive care units. *Nursing Management,* 20(7), 88a–88p.
26. Tappen, R.M. (1989). *Nursing leadership and management: Concepts and practice* (2nd ed.). Philadelphia: F.A. Davis.
27. Tuzman, L., & Cohen, A. (1992). Clinical decision making for discharge planning in a changing psychiatric environment. *Health and Social Work,* 17(4), 299–307.
28. Weinberger, B. (1989). Discharge planning: the sooner, the better. *Nursing,* 19(2), 75–76.
29. Wertheimer, D.S., & Kleinman, L.S. (1990). A model for interdisciplinary discharge planning in a university hospital. *Gerontologist,* 30(6), 837–840.
30. Wilson, E.B., et al. (1991). Take a fresh look at discharge planning. *Geriatric Nursing,* 12(1), 23–25.
31. Ziegler, S., et al. (1992). Discharge planning: Collaboration between the community and the acute care hospital. *Journal of Nursing Administration,* 22(10), 8.

▼ *Home Care Nursing*

▼

▼

Home health service is that component of comprehensive health care whereby services are provided to individuals and families in their places of residence for the purpose of promoting, maintaining or restoring health or minimizing the effects of illness and disability.

Evelyn McNamara[23]

▼

▼

▼ CHAPTER OUTLINE

HISTORY OF HOME CARE NURSING
    Development of Home Care
       Nursing in Europe
    Development of Home Care
       Nursing in the United States
TERMINOLOGY OF HOME CARE NURSING
SOCIAL, TECHNOLOGIC, ECONOMIC, AND
  REGULATORY DEVELOPMENTS IN
  HOME CARE NURSING
    Medicare and Medicaid
    Diagnosis-Related Groups
SCOPE OF HOME CARE SERVICES
    Types of Care Providers
    Individuals Requiring
       Home Care
HOME CARE NURSING PRACTICE

    A Model for Home Care Nursing
       Practice
    Goals of Home Care Nursing
    Case Management
    Legal and Ethical Issues in Home
       Care Nursing Practice
ASSESSMENT
NURSING DIAGNOSIS
PLANNING
NURSING INTERVENTION
    Clinical Skills
    Teaching
    Counseling
    Coordination of Care
EVALUATION
CASE STUDY

▼ KEY TERMS

Home care	Skilled nursing	Third-party reimbursement
Public health nursing		

The component of the health care system that provides care in the home has been referred to in the literature as both *home care* and *home health care.* In describing home care, one author[23] says,

Services . . . are . . . made available by an agency or . . . institution, organized for the delivery of health care through the use of employed staff, contractual arrangements or a combination of administrative patterns. These services are provided under a plan of care which includes . . . medical care, dental care, nursing, physical therapy, speech therapy, occupational therapy, social work, nutrition, homemaker, home health aide, transportation, laboratory services, medical equipment and supplies.

Home care nursing cannot simply be described as care rendered in the home.

Home care nursing is comprehensive nursing that is holistically focused on both the individual requiring care and the family or support system.

This type of nursing requires skill in health assessment, health maintenance, health promotion, restorative care, rehabilitative care, and terminal care. The home environment challenges the nurse to be both creative and flexible whether the nurse is practicing as a generalist or has chosen to specialize within the field.

HISTORY OF HOME CARE NURSING

Development of Home Care Nursing in Europe

In Europe, before the efforts of Florence Nightingale, both religious and secular groups were known to provide home nursing care. For example, at the start of the 14th century, women in Belgium, France, Germany, and Switzerland provided home nursing and social work services through the secular order of Beguine. Also, Saint Vincent de Paul organized women in 1617 to visit the sick in their homes. For the most part, however, home care was provided by lower-class, uneducated, and overworked women.[37]

After Nightingale elevated the status of nursing, nurses influenced by the Nightingale school directed and provided skilled nursing care to patients with both acute care and chronic illness needs.[35] Philanthropist William Rathbone founded the first public health nursing association in 1859 in Liverpool, England. The success of the program resulted in the 1889 creation of The Queen Victoria Jubilee Institute. This formal training program for nurses in home care required 3 years of hospital training plus 6 months of postgraduate training in district nursing.[37] In addition to care of the sick, home care nursing included health promotion and illness prevention throughout the life span. This was true in the United States as well as in Europe.

Development of Home Care Nursing in the United States

In the United States, the first home care program was established in Boston in 1796.[11] District nursing was initiated in 1877 when the New York City Mission hired the first visiting nurses. By this time, nurses were becoming known as disciplined, well-bred women. The district nurses cared for people in their homes and instructed families about the care of the sick and about basic hygiene. In 1891, nursing leaders Lillian Wald and Mary Brewster created what was to become the Henry Street Settlement House on the lower east side of New York. The settlement house provided care for the sick without regard to social class. Nursing's primary role in home care was firmly established by Lillian Wald when she founded the Visiting Nurse Service of New York City in 1893. This first American visiting nurse service began the change from voluntary organizations with lay persons supervising nursing care to nursing care under the supervision of nurses. Under Wald's leadership in the 1900s, the district nurse's role expanded to include the general public, not just the poor, and to promote health rather than focus only on illness.

The benefits of Wald's approach were recognized by the Metropolitan Life Insurance Company, which in 1909 began to offer home nursing service for its New York City policyholders. This became the model for full coverage of home services for other insurance companies during the 1920s.[25]

Through increased service to the public, these early 20th century public health nurses continued to enhance their knowledge and skills in bedside care, health promotion, and disease prevention. Through demonstrated leadership and advances in nursing practice, public health nurses received increased professional recognition.

As public health nursing continued to grow, hospital-based home care programs began to reach out more into the community. In 1947, the first of many American hospital-based home care programs was begun at Montefiore Hospital in New York City. Montefiore's program was designed, in part, to respond to the needs of the convalescing and chronically ill and to decrease long hospital stays. By 1958 (in addition to the services of physicians, nurses, and social workers), physical therapy, nutrition, and laboratory services were included in the home care program. Homemaker and housekeeping service supports were also incorporated.[23] During the 1960s, New York Blue Cross developed the "continued care" program to bridge the gap between acute care and home care. The program planned to reduce costs and to promote early hospital discharge. As more programs developed (along with changes in provider structures, roles, and financing), the hospital-sponsored home care programs began competing to serve the same populations that had once been only in the domain of the community health nurse.

At the same time, baccalaureate nursing education required all graduates to understand and use public health principles such as disease prevention and health promotion. Acute care nurses made home visits to discharged patients, and community health nurses visited home patients during acute care admissions.

By the mid-1970s, what had begun as district nursing and evolved to public health nursing came to be community health nursing. Community health nursing's focus was to care for, but was not limited to being in, the community.[36] With this "population perspective," health promotion continued to gain in importance, as did the need to meet the diverse and comprehensive health demands of the community.

As the roles of the *public health* and *community health* nurses evolved, it is notable that each featured health as integral to the nursing model of providing care throughout the health-illness continuum.

TERMINOLOGY OF HOME CARE NURSING

During the evolution of home-based nursing practice, the distinctions among district nursing, public health nursing, community health nursing, and home care or home health nursing often became blurred. To make matters more confusing, these terms have sometimes been used interchangeably in the literature. This chapter uses the term *home care nursing* to refer to the broad scope of nursing practiced within home health care services. This is not meant to discount any qualitative role interpretations implied by the terms *public*

health, community health, or *home health nursing.* For more discussion of the role of the nurse in health promotion in the community, see Chapter 20. In this chapter, **home care** is defined as services for individuals and families in their place of residence for the purpose of treatment of illness, restoration of health, rehabilitation, and health promotion. A home care provider is a person or organization/agency that delivers home care.

Public health nursing, in contrast, refers to population-focused activities designed to improve the quality of life, including physical, mental, and social well-being; prevention of disease; promotion of health; and control of communicable disease consistent with available knowledge and resources at a given time and place.

SOCIAL, TECHNOLOGIC, ECONOMIC, AND REGULATORY DEVELOPMENTS IN HOME CARE NURSING

Historically, people who could afford private care received nursing and medical care at home. The advent of World War II limited the availability of physicians, particularly for home visits. Individuals requiring a physician's care had to seek care at a centralized location, such as the physician's office or the acute care hospital. Because of its efficiency and cost effectiveness, this delivery pattern predominated in health care until the 1980s. While physicians concentrated their efforts in the acute care hospitals, nursing expanded its availability and leadership in providing care in the home.

Medicare and Medicaid

In 1965, the creation of Medicare and Medicaid (Titles XVII and XIX of the Federal Social Security Act) began to change this system. The Medicare and Medicaid acts established specific criteria to be met by home care agencies for reimbursement of their services. Before the 1965 Medicare and Medicaid legislation, ". . . it was not seen as necessary or even appropriate for physicians to direct home care."[25] The introduction of the Medicare and Medicaid legislation created a clear shift to a medical model of practice. The focus became one of disease treatment. For a client to receive reimbursement for home care services, the legislation required that (1) the person be under the treatment of a physician, (2) the physician verify the need for services and write appropriate orders specifying the plan of treatment with frequency and duration of services, and (3) the person be homebound and require skilled care/services. The referring physician, who rarely saw the patient in the home, had to plan, review, and certify that care was necessary. The rich heritage of the nursing model of health promotion and disease prevention was threatened; these services were not reimbursable.

To make matters more difficult, support services

(such as assistance with shopping, meals, and cleaning for the homebound) were discounted. The home care nurse faced the crisis of attempting to find or create other support services to enable the individual to remain at home. For the first time, Medicare also required that home care agencies provide at least one other service in addition to nursing. Up to this point, many visiting nurse associations provided only nursing services. Unable to compete with hospital-based and proprietary agencies offering the complexity and scope of physical therapy, speech therapy, occupational therapy, home health aides, and social services, the smaller nursing agencies were not able to remain in business. Those remaining in the practice of home care nursing faced numerous challenges as the system for delivering care changed.

With these changes in the law, the home care nurse was faced with the need to respond to the individual's and family's needs holistically while practicing under a system in which reimbursement was based on a multidisciplinary approach.

Diagnosis-Related Groups

The next dramatic health care system development occurred in 1983 with the federal government's introduction of the prospective payment system for acute care hospitals. Diagnosis-related groups (DRGs) established a predetermined reimbursement rate for different medical diagnoses for Medicare patients. This system was designed to place constraints on rising health care costs and to provide incentives for hospitals to decrease costs. Before the implementation of DRGs, hospitals received a per diem (daily) rate from Medicare based on the cost of services per hospital day. For each diagnosis, the basic DRG rate was determined by analyzing the cost of (1) the usual hospital resource utilization, (2) a predictable length of stay, and (3) an estimated group of services.[20]

Diagnoses with similarities, particularly of resource consumption, were grouped together. The hospital was allowed to keep the difference in the reimbursement rate if the actual cost of the individual's stay totaled less than the amount reimbursed. The faster the individual was discharged, the greater the potential for the hospital to make a profit. Therefore, under DRGs, hospitals implemented discharge as soon as possible. This early discharge thrust has shifted an increasing number of individuals with more intense and complex care needs (greater acuity) out of acute care hospitals and into their homes. In response, the field of home care was stimulated to develop lower cost and highly technical home-based care.

With DRGs, the 1980s witnessed a shift from institutional care to home and outpatient care. The increasing availability of technology appropriate for use in the home, as well as the impact of regulatory and economic developments, resulted in profound changes in the health care system.

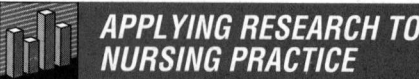

APPLYING RESEARCH TO NURSING PRACTICE

Helping Care Givers Cope with High-Tech Home Care

Smith, C.E. Giefr, C.K., & Bieker, L. (1991). Technological dependency: a preliminary model and pilot of home total parenteral nutrition. *Journal of Community Health Nursing*, 8(4), 245–254.

▼ ▼ ▼

As hospital stays have become shorter, the home care environment has become increasingly technologic. Consequently, care givers at home have faced greater demands in managing more complex equipment. How well have care givers been coping with the challenge of learning new skills? What have been the care giver's problems with dependence on complex technology? In this pilot study, Smith and colleagues interviewed five care givers responsible for administering total parenteral nutrition to a family member. Total parenteral nutrition —a solution containing carbohydrates, proteins, fats, vitamins, and minerals—is administered intravenously to individuals who are unable to meet their nutritional needs through the gastrointestinal tract. In the study, the care givers initially expressed anxiety about managing the intravenous pump that regulates intravenous flow. However, with the assistance of the home care nurse, care givers developed a sense of pride in handling the equipment. These care givers also reported that the nurse had been an important resource for helping them cope with episodes of depression, feelings of social isolation, and the stress of financial burden.

Applications for Practice

These findings suggest that when they are supported by the home care nurse, care givers are able to respond to the challenges of home care. As you prepare clients needing complex home care for discharge from an acute care setting, encourage clients and care givers to work closely with their home care nurses.

SCOPE OF HOME CARE SERVICES

The trend in home care services is one of growing diversity and scope.

The trend has been described as an extension of institutional medical care into the home. Before the widespread availability and acceptance of high technology for home care, individuals requiring sophisticated treatment modalities were hospitalized. With DRGs, the demand for home care services exceeded the supply of available providers. This situation encouraged more providers to begin to offer services.

Types of Care Providers

Organizations like the Visiting Nurse Association were some of the earliest providers of community-based services. Hospital-based home care agencies and governmental agencies, such as the local health departments, were also early providers of home care. Home health aide agencies have entered the field. Home health aide agencies may be a subdivision of a home health agency or the Visiting Nurse Association, or they may be structured as a private agency. These agencies provide home health aide, homemaker, and companion services.

Proprietary (for-profit) organizations, such as major health care corporations, recognized the business opportunities in home care and began to offer complex and comprehensive services. Proprietary temporary staffing agencies also entered the field to supply the much-needed personnel for home care services. In conjunction with other care providers, palliative and supportive care for the terminally ill began to be offered by a growing number of hospice agencies. Durable medical equipment companies and certain retail pharmacies provide medical equipment and supplies, such as walkers, wheelchairs, hospital beds, apnea monitors, and ventilators.

The home care nurse is now confronted with numerous types of providers having varying abilities to offer services.

The home care nurse must develop skill in determining which type of provider is best able to meet the needs of the individual and the family in each situation. Although some providers may offer wellness-oriented services, the majority of providers focus on medically oriented services.

Medically oriented services usually require a physician's order. Home health services include nursing care, social work, physical therapy, respiratory therapy, speech therapy, occupational therapy, registered dietitian counseling, laboratory services, transportation services, and home health aide services. Home care equipment includes the following:

▶ Respiratory therapy equipment (oxygen, mechanical ventilation, apnea monitors, and related treatments)
▶ Nutritional therapies support (oral and enteral feeding supplies)
▶ Medical equipment (beds, wheelchairs, walkers, canes, grab bars, commodes, and pain control systems)
▶ Medical-surgical supplies (supplies related to ostomy, diabetic, wound, incontinence, respiratory, and peritoneal dialysis care)

A separate and growing service component involves nursing and pharmacy in-home infusion therapy (parenteral nutrition, antibiotics, pain control, chemotherapy, and blood administration).[21] Agencies offering high-technology services provide visits 7 days a week, 24 hours a day. Individuals requiring high-technology services present complex needs (Fig. 23–1). The home care nurse must recognize the danger of inappropriate use of equipment and technology for an individual who cannot be safely cared for in the home. It is through the home care nurse's refined assessment skills that safe and effective care is accomplished in the home.

In addition to ensuring quality and safety, the home care nurse evaluates the most cost-effective approach to providing care. Reimbursement issues and financial constraints of the family may require alternative sources for equipment and supplies. Part of the home health nurse's responsibility is to become aware of various religious, charitable, and voluntary organizations that often provide free or lower-cost equipment or that make loans of equipment to those in the population served. The local church or branch of the American

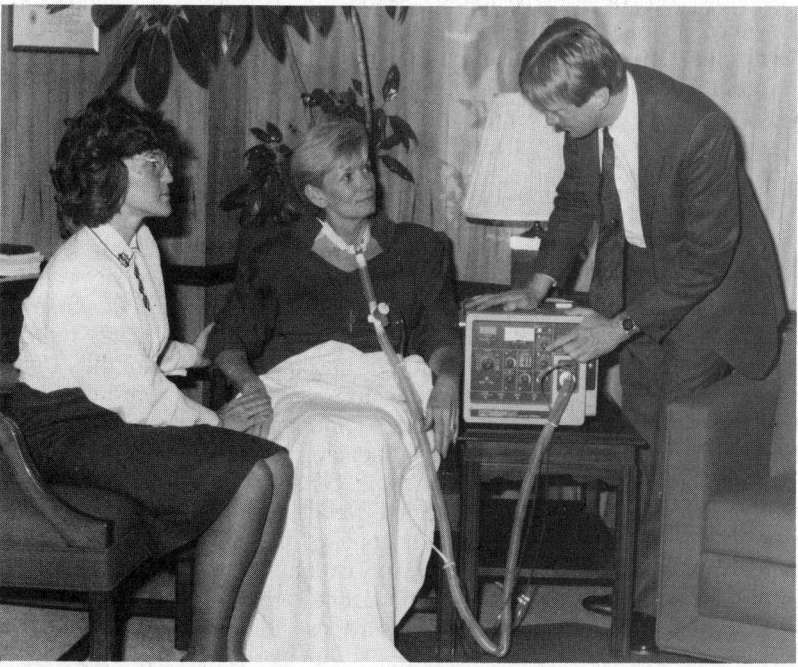

▲ Figure 23–1

Individuals requiring high-technology home care present complex needs. (Courtesy of Ho Med Convalescent Equipment, Inc.)

Cancer Society, for example, can be valuable resources for both equipment and support. A more comprehensive listing of community resources and self-help groups can be found in *Home Care: A Technical Manual for the Professional Nurse*.[30]

Collaboration with other members of the multidisciplinary team can result in home-based adaptations that may negate the need for a more expensive alternative.

Occupational and physical therapists can be particularly helpful in suggesting modifications of routines and households, such as wheelchair ramps, that promote maximal independence in activities of daily living.

The changing nature of government and health care regulations and reimbursement requirements places an increased pressure on home care agencies to improve cost effectiveness (productivity) while increasing documentation, reporting, and quality assurance activities. To be eligible for reimbursement through Title XVII of the Social Security Act, home care agencies must meet certification requirements.

Accreditation, a means of promoting quality by voluntarily meeting national standards, is typically a requirement for receiving third-party reimbursement. **Third-party reimbursement** is defined as payment from sources other than the person receiving care, such as insurance companies or the federal government programs of Medicare and Medicaid. Home care agencies have been subject to accreditation by three boards:

▶ The Joint Commission on Accreditation of Healthcare Organizations, which surveys patient care issues (rights, safety, confidentiality, informed consent, care planning, teaching, and documentation), quality assurance, agency management and administration, equipment management, pharmaceutical services, and personal care/supportive services[17]
▶ The Community Health Accreditation Program, a subdivision of the National League for Nursing, which reviews agency programs and services, organization and administration, and strategic planning and marketing and completes an overall evaluation
▶ The National Home Caring Council, which reviews organization and structure, training requirements, and staffing for homemakers and home health aides[32]

Each action of the multidisciplinary team must be carefully and efficiently orchestrated to ensure that the individual client receives the required care, that the care is accurately documented, and that members of the team effectively communicate to maximize outcomes of care in the most cost-effective manner. As the coordinator of the team or *case manager*, the home care nurse measures the achievements of planned outcomes as a result of home care services. Outcomes such as acquisition of knowledge or skills needed for self-care are considered one of the most significant indicators of quality. Application of the home care nurse's specialized knowledge promotes safe and effective medically oriented services.

As noted earlier, providers of wellness services focus on the health-oriented consumer. Health promotion services frequently are not reimbursed by third-party payers and typically do not require a physician's order. Services and products include health education (such as teaching about nutrition and stress management), self-improvement material, diagnostic screening (such as blood pressure monitoring and blood cholesterol level monitoring), illness prevention (such as assistance with smoking cessation), and promotion of fitness. Services that promote self-care are required by people who need assistance with home maintenance, such as homemaking, housekeeping, chores, and companion services. Selected examples of services required for home maintenance management include meal preparation, food shopping, laundry, and house cleaning. Lack of attention to these activities can result in an unsafe home environment. Homemaking, housekeeping, and companion services assume increasing significance as the population ages and the availability of family members as care givers decreases.

Individuals Requiring Home Care

People of all ages and from varying socioeconomic backgrounds may need a variety of home health care services.

In the course of any day, the home care nurse may see the following:

▶ A new mother and infant for their first postpartum and infant care visit
▶ A chronically ill or high-risk infant requiring oxygen or apnea monitoring
▶ A child requiring long-term mechanical ventilation in a family learning to plan for long-term care needs
▶ An adolescent adjusting to a new diagnosis of type I diabetes mellitus and requiring a plan that includes family support
▶ A person convalescing from surgical interventions who requires assistance with wound management
▶ A person with arthritis who needs to learn to use assistive equipment to maintain independence in the home (Fig. 23–2)
▶ A terminally ill person who needs care to promote quality of life and pain control while at home

Examples of the types of people needing home care services seem endless.

Of those using home care, the elderly (over age 65 years) represent the largest and fastest growing group in the United States. The increased incidence of chronic illness and disability associated with an aging population and the limited availability of care givers are just two reasons for a growing use of home care services by the elderly. Care of the elderly will continue to demand increased emphasis on effective strategies for dealing with such a large and growing subpopulation.

Another important group includes individuals with acquired immune deficiency syndrome, which has had a dramatic effect on the U.S. health care system. As the

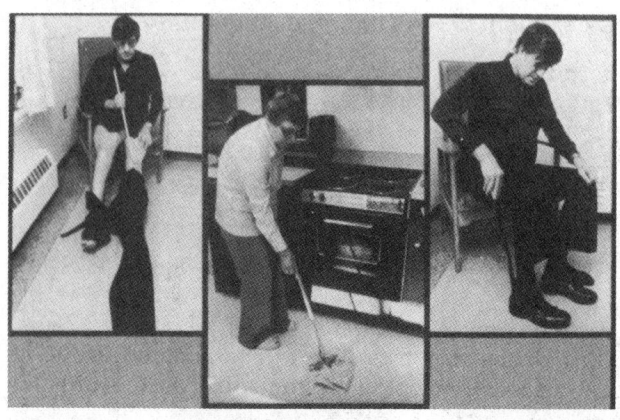

▲ *Figure 23–2*

Individuals requiring home care. Clients with arthritis can learn to use a reaching device through the guidance of a home care nurse. (From the Arthritis Teaching Slide Collection, copyright 1980. Used by permission of the Arthritis Foundation.)

number of people with AIDS increases, the demand for treating these individuals in their homes will increase.

HOME CARE NURSING PRACTICE

Home care nursing is in the process of changing, as is the field of home health care.

The home care nurse generalist cares for individuals from birth to death throughout the health-illness continuum.

To do so, the nurse must use the knowledge and skills required for acute care, chronic illness care, mental health promotion, rehabilitation care, and meeting age-specific needs for preventive care within the community. Home care nursing offers opportunities for clinical subspecialization in areas such as gerontology, maternal-child, diabetes, hospice, and parenteral infusion therapist, to name a few. The home care nurse can use a strong knowledge base and holistic approach to promote the successful use of acute care technology while preventing the creation of a "mini-hospital" milieu in the home. The home care nurse assumes the roles of the technically skilled direct care provider, educator, advocate, collaborator, leader, and case manager.

A Model for Home Care Nursing Practice

Home care nursing practice is built on several theoretical models such as general systems, self-care, and adaptation theories. A unique framework for home care nursing is the Albrecht Nursing Model for Home Health Care (Fig. 23–3). This model assumes that individuals and their families are active, capable, and responsible participants in their care. The model addresses the complex and dynamic relationships among variables in home care. Albrecht used the interaction of structural elements and process elements to predict the outcomes of care.[2] Albrecht defines structural elements as the client, family, provider agency, professional nurse, and health team. The structural elements can be modified by such factors as client classification (acuity), costs, and demand. Interacting with the structural elements are process elements, which are described as the type of care (focus and intensity), coordination of care (case management by the professional nurse), and intervention. Outcomes (the responses to care) are defined as satisfaction, quality of care, cost effectiveness, health status, and self-care capability.[2] This professional nursing model represents a significant step in advancing home care nursing practice and research. In addition to nursing model development, research efforts continue in the development of a widely accepted client classification system that objectively measures the home care recipient's requirements for nursing care.

Goals of Home Care Nursing

Home care nursing practice takes place within an interdisciplinary delivery system. The professional nurse is the manager of care (a case manager) in the individual's home. Collaboration and coordination with other members of the multidisciplinary health care team demand a leadership role by the home care nurse. The home care nurse strives to

▶ restore the person's health and assist the person to return to an appropriate level of functioning
▶ maintain the person's health and preserve the person's functional abilities and independence
▶ promote the person's health and minimize the effects of illness
▶ improve the person's health and help the person achieve a higher level of functioning than previously existed[39]

Case Management

To accomplish these goals, the nurse as case manager must bring the appropriate resources (both personnel and equipment) together in a coordinated plan. In home care nursing, case management requires coordination of all aspects of care and all activities of the multidisciplinary team, usually by a single professional, to ensure care coordination. Case management requires the ability to

▶ function autonomously, make decisions, solve problems, and manage emergency situations in the home
▶ consult, collaborate, coordinate, and direct other health care providers, contracted equipment/service providers, and community resources and to decide when to contact the physician
▶ develop a plan of care to assist the client/family to achieve clearly defined/measurable client-centered

Structural elements ⟶ Process elements ⟶ Outcome elements ⟶

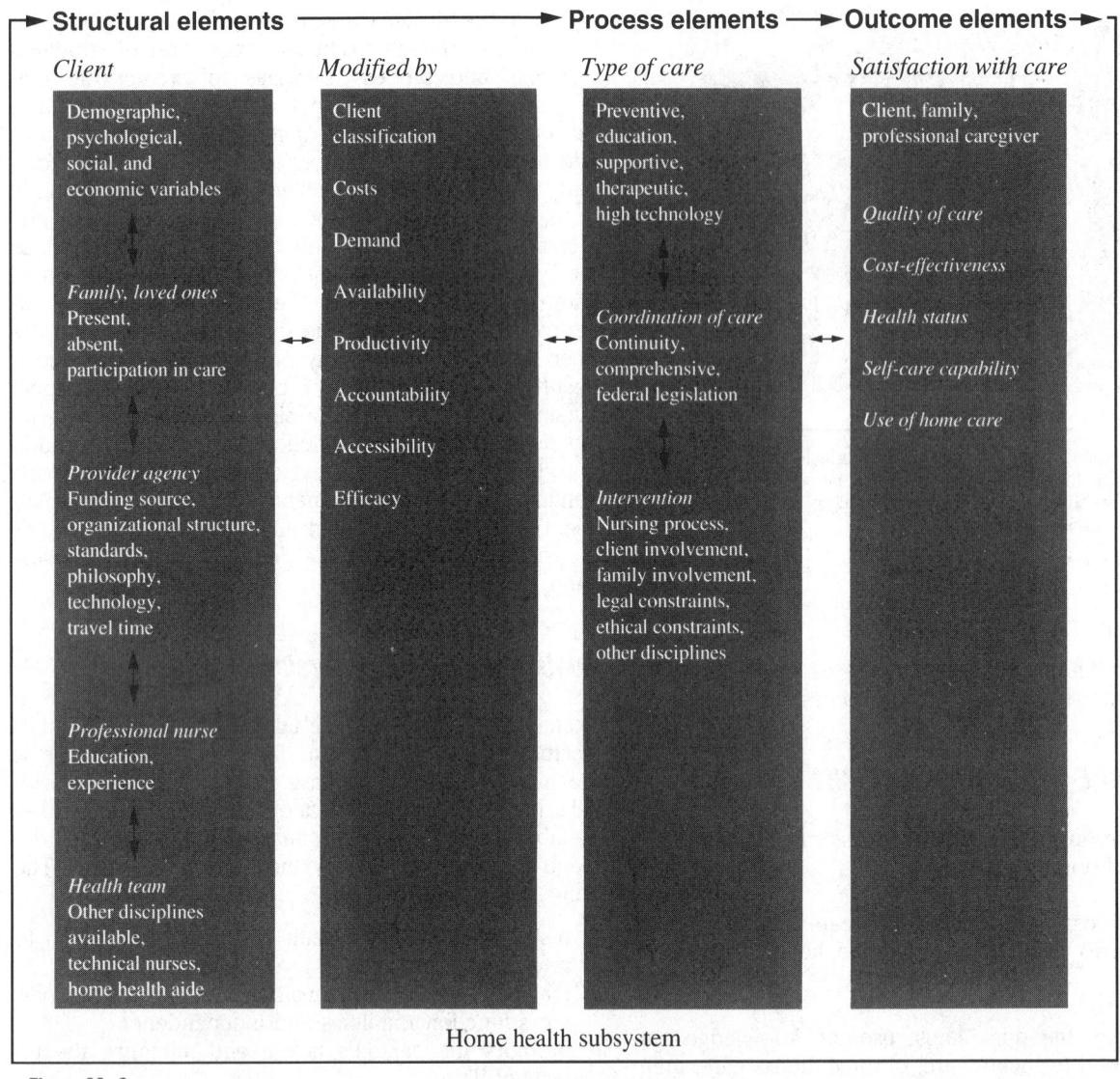

Client

Demographic, psychological, social, and economic variables

Family, loved ones
Present, absent, participation in care

Provider agency
Funding source, organizational structure, standards, philosophy, technology, travel time

Professional nurse
Education, experience

Health team
Other disciplines available, technical nurses, home health aide

Modified by

Client classification

Costs

Demand

Availability

Productivity

Accountability

Accessibility

Efficacy

Type of care

Preventive, education, supportive, therapeutic, high technology

Coordination of care
Continuity, comprehensive, federal legislation

Intervention
Nursing process, client involvement, family involvement, legal constraints, ethical constraints, other disciplines

Satisfaction with care

Client, family, professional caregiver

Quality of care

Cost-effectiveness

Health status

Self-care capability

Use of home care

Home health subsystem

▲ *Figure 23–3*

The Albrecht nursing model for home care nursing. (From Mary Nies Albrecht, Ph.D., RN. The Albrecht Nursing Model for Home Health Care: Implications for Research, Practice, and Education. *Public Health Nursing,* Vol. 7, No. 2, June 1990, pp. 118–126. Model p. 123. Reprinted by permission of Blackwell Scientific Publications, Inc.)

outcomes by an anticipated date (negotiation among the client, family, and nurse is used to determine expectations)

► "think interactionally" (to think in terms of family dynamics)

► implement appropriate protocols for all procedures and equipment used

► communicate verbally (interviewing, teaching, providing feedback) and in writing (documentation of skilled care and client response to care provided by oneself and other health care providers)

► function effectively in regard to cost with an understanding of the economics of legislation and regulatory issues[30]

Legal and Ethical Issues in Home Care Nursing Practice

Nursing practice in home care proceeds according to professional nursing standards; nurse practice acts; licensure requirements; the nurse's educational preparation, clinical experience, and specialization; and the protocols of the employing agency. Each home visit requires the nurse to respond to the unique needs of the individual and family as well as to the unique home situation.

Although the home care nurse engages in case finding and is able to perform assessments independently, a physician's order is required to provide care.

At times, the home care nurse will be the only professional in direct contact with the individual receiving care. The early identification and communication of problems may rest entirely with the nurse.

When the services of additional professionals are needed, the home care nurse must maintain an ongoing dialogue with the members of the multidisciplinary team and the physician to promote continued treatment and coordination of care. In addition to the quality of care issues, careful documentation is required to meet eligibility criteria for reimbursement of home care services. For some families, the home care nurse understands that nursing diagnoses represent identified needs but may not address what is realistic or achievable within the individual and family system.

Home care nurses, like nurses in other practice arenas, confront ethical issues. The home care nurse may be faced with the following situations:

▶ An individual or family unable to comply with the demand for significant psychomotor, cognitive, and emotional commitment required by the client's need for high-technology care
▶ Evaluating the environment as unsafe in relation to the treatment regimen
▶ An inability to provide care while maintaining the quality of life for individuals with chronic and disabling disease processes
▶ The need for premature cessation of services because of financial and reimbursement limitations
▶ Lack of response by the individual and family

The home care nurse assumes the role of advocate in balancing technology and therapeutic interventions. Knowledge of legal and ethical guidelines can be helpful in this role. Refer to Chapter 3 for additional readings concerning legal and ethical issues and guidelines.

As is true in all settings, the nursing process is the foundation for nursing practice in home care nursing.

ASSESSMENT

Assessment is the basis for meeting human needs for both the individual and the family. In the assessment phase, data are collected in a systematic manner through methods such as the interview and nursing history, physical examination, and diagnostic test results.

Assessment includes biopsychosocial and environmental factors as well as functional abilities. The assessment phase identifies biopsychosocial patterns of need.

These patterns are then organized to lead to the identification of nursing diagnoses. Table 23–1 lists areas for assessment.[30] For example, a person who is blind and has been newly diagnosed as having type 1 diabetes mellitus presents with a slightly different set of needs than does a person with vision. In contrast to acute care nursing, in which the nurse is the primary care giver, the person or the family assumes the principal care giver role in the home. Functional abilities and limitations of the individual and the care givers are thus of utmost importance.

TABLE 23–1. Assessment Guidelines for Home Care Nursing

Area	Assessment
Biopsychosocial	Physical assessment of body systems
	Age, sex, developmental level
	Medical diagnoses, nursing diagnoses
	Ethnicity, race, culture, religion, language
	Socioeconomic status, living arrangements
	Support systems, marital relationships, roles of family members/care giver support
	Relationship with health care provider
Environmental	Occupational, job-related issues
	Home and community setting/safety
	Location in the home of stairs and bathroom
	Availability of heating, water, telephone, refrigerator, and stove
Functional Abilities/Limitations	
Psychomotor areas	Sensory impairment
	Mobility, dexterity, use of one or both hands or legs, use of assistive devices
	Physical discomfort
	Body system functioning (impaired) such that it has impact on activity and homebound status (i.e., dyspnea or bowel/bladder incontinence)
Cognitive areas	Ability to learn, identified best way to learn, learned skills
	Educational background, reading ability, functional illiteracy
	Knowledge of disease and therapeutic plan
	Conceptualization, discrimination
	Decision making, time orientation, memory, attention span
Affective (emotional) areas	Definition of health/illness
	Client's and family's reactions to client's illness
	Health beliefs, values, practices
	Compliance issues, willingness to engage in care
	Readiness and motivation for learning
	Client's self-image, personality, self-value, self-discipline, acceptance of body functioning/ability

Modified from Rovinski, C.A., & Zastocki, D.K. (1989). *Home care: A technical manual for the professional nurse* (p. 7). Philadelphia: W.B. Saunders.

NURSING DIAGNOSIS PROFILE

Impaired Home Maintenance Management

Definition. The state in which an individual experiences the inability to independently maintain a safe, growth-promoting immediate environment for self or others.

Classification. Moving 6.4.1.1.

Defining Characteristics. The nurse must rely on subjective statements by the individual and family members as well as on objective observations of the household. Subjective statements may include expressions of difficulty in maintaining the home in a comfortable fashion, reports of outstanding debts or financial crisis, or requests for assistance with home maintenance. The nurse will need to use effective communication skills to gain further insight into specific areas in which assistance may be needed.

Objective observations of the household include presence of offensive odors and accumulation of dirt, food, dirty laundry, or hygienic wastes. A room temperature that is too high or too low represents a clear safety risk, as does the presence of rodents or vermin. Lack of necessary cooking or health care equipment, even with the most well intentioned family support system, will also require immediate attention. An important observation involves the health status of the household members and includes assessment of the coping skills and physical abilities of the family care giver. Examples of areas of concern include signs of anxiety, exhaustion, repeated hygienic disorders, infestations, or infections.

Sample Related Factors. Related factors include environmental and supportive elements such as unfamiliarity with neighborhood resources, insufficient family organization or planning, inadequate support systems, and decreased financial resources. Lack of knowledge, lack of motivation, and lack of role modeling can represent needs for both the individual and the family. The physiologic implications of impaired cognitive or emotional functioning, substance abuse, effects of chronic debilitating disease, and individual/family member disease or injury can result in limited home management capabilities.

Concept Description. The individual may be acutely or chronically ill, physically or mentally handicapped, frail and elderly, or a dependent child. Both the individual and the family may need additional assistance in adapting to the requirements of maintaining a safe home environment. When an individual whose previous role may have been the head of household is in a dependent role, other family members may not be aware of ways of maintaining a safe and hygienic home environment.

Comprehensive and holistic care requires that the person with unique care needs be viewed within a family that not only needs to care for the individual but also must care for its own maintenance needs.

Examples. Depending on the specific assessment data, this diagnostic category could be applicable in the following situations, among others:

▶ A person whose mental or physical health is impaired to the point at which independent maintenance of an adequate environment is not possible

For example, a middle-aged person with type II diabetes mellitus is discharged home from the acute care setting to recover from debridement of a right foot ulcer. The person has had numerous hospitalizations for complications; self-management of the diabetes regimen and the home environment seems a problem.

Diagnosis: *Impaired Home Maintenance Management* R/T the effects of chronic debilitating disease.

▶ A person whose health is adequate but who is, for a number of other possible reasons, unable to independently maintain an adequate environment

For example, an infant has been hospitalized for failure to thrive. The mother, an unwed adolescent living in an elderly sick relative's home, expresses feelings of being overwhelmed by the care of the house, her infant, and her grandmother.

Diagnosis: *Impaired Home Maintenance Management* R/T lack of knowledge of management techniques.

Related/Similar Nursing Diagnoses. *Ineffective Family Coping: Disabling* is a similar diagnosis in that it addresses a family's lack of ability. However, in ineffective family coping, the family (care giver) lacks the ability to care for *the identified client* in a family, and this impairs the client's own abilities to adapt to the health care challenge. In *Impaired Home Maintenance Management,* the family members lack the ability to manage *the home environment* in a manner conducive to healthy living.

Another similar diagnosis is Activity Intolerance. With activity intolerance, the individual is unable to complete *any required or desired tasks for the self or for others*. The person with this diagnosis might also have a diagnosis of impaired *Home Maintenance Management,* if the person were expected to maintain the home environment for self or others. Otherwise, only the diagnosis of *Activity Intolerance* would pertain.

Impaired Physical Mobility is another similar diagnosis in that it identifies a limitation or lack of ability. In this event, the lack is for independent movement. Like *Activity Intolerance,* this diagnosis could coexist with a diagnosis of *Impaired Home Maintenance Management* if the person with impaired mobility were responsible for home maintenance and unable to fulfill the role expectations because of impaired mobility. Still, the two diagnoses would be different. In such a case, the impaired mobility would serve as a related factor, supporting the diagnosis of *Impaired Home Maintenance Management.*

Functional assessment includes a focus on activities of daily living, such as when and how well the individual will bathe, toilet, dress, eat, sleep, move about, cook, clean, and communicate with care givers. The home care nurse evaluates the functional abilities by noting whether the individual is completely independent; requires use of devices, equipment, or another person; or is totally dependent.

It is useful to organize assessment findings into two groupings: strengths and limitations/deficits. Strengths such as positive family dynamics can be built on when intervention strategies are designed. Limitations or deficits must be identified before nursing care can be planned. In identifying limitations, the family's coping effectiveness must also be addressed. If a limitation is identified and the family has developed effective coping mechanisms, then nursing action may not be warranted. If a limitation is identified with which there is an inadequate coping response, the home care nurse must then evaluate whether nursing actions can effect change. For example, a person with severe lung disease may cope with anxiety by smoking cigarettes even after education and counseling sessions. The nurse would have to assume the likelihood is high that the person will continue to smoke. Skillful documentation of the individual's and family's needs and limitations forms the basis of the nursing diagnoses as well as justification for third-party reimbursement.

NURSING DIAGNOSIS

The data from the assessment phase are used to support the nursing diagnoses that communicate the individual's and family's needs. Because the basic premise of care in the home is to maximize independence, one of the most frequently encountered nursing diagnoses in home nursing is *Impaired Home Maintenance Management* (Nursing Diagnosis Profile). Other frequently encountered nursing diagnoses include those appropriate for individuals and families of all ages, at all levels of wellness. Therefore, they are quite diverse:

Constipation
Diarrhea
Pain
Health Maintenance, Altered
Nutrition, Altered
Urinary Elimination, Altered
Anxiety
Airway Clearance, Ineffective
Family Coping, Ineffective (disabling or compromised)
Individual Coping, Ineffective
Home Maintenance Management, Impaired
Knowledge Deficit
Noncompliance
Activity Intolerance, High Risk for
Skin Integrity, High Risk for Impaired
Infection, High Risk for
Injury, High Risk for

Self-Care Deficit
Self-Esteem Disturbance
Sleep Pattern Disturbance
Sexual Dysfunction

PLANNING

In planning to meet identified needs, it is important to evaluate what is realistically able to be achieved within the family system.

In this respect, the nurse must consider health values and beliefs, financial constraints, and available resources. The individual and the family should have a large measure of control. Their wishes and abilities should drive the planning of care. Members of the multidisciplinary team are guests in the recipient's home. Asking the individual and the family what they expect as outcomes of the plan of care forms the basis for a trusting professional relationship. Mutual goal setting, prioritizing the goals, and stating the outcomes in measurable behaviors allows both parties to follow the same path in outcome achievement. For example, a partial list of measurable criteria for a person at home with a urinary catheter would contain the following:

Individual or family identifies signs and symptoms of urinary tract infection in two visits.
Individual or family demonstrates appropriate daily catheter care, that is, daily soap and water cleansing, in two visits.

Establishing goals in a realistic and reimbursable manner requires a focus on "survival skills."[42] The survival skills are those essential aspects of care that are most likely to result in the individual and family being able to manage the therapeutic regimen safely within defined parameters. The survival skill approach is useful, for example, in planning to meet learning needs. Planning to give the individual and family the most comprehensive review of a topic is typically unnecessary, frequently overwhelming, and certainly not reimbursable.

Focusing content on safety and what is needed to maintain and improve health is more likely to be successful in meeting the individual's and family's needs as well as in receiving reimbursement. This approach does not compromise professional standards. On the contrary, it is the professional nurse's unique knowledge base that allows individualization of care.

NURSING INTERVENTION

Clinical Skills

Therapeutic nursing actions are based on the established plan of care and are consistent with and supportive of the medically prescribed treatment regimen.

Therapeutic nursing activities include clinical/technical skills, teaching, counseling, and coordination of care.

Direct care skill requirements vary greatly as a result of the environment, the technology being used, and the practice setting. Clinical competence in the practice setting is the responsibility of the professional nurse through continuing professional growth and education. Clinical skill application in the home requires a shift in perspective from the acute care approach. Many of the key principles are applicable in both the acute care and home care setting, whereas the equipment or procedures used may vary. For example, expensive disinfectants may be used in the hospital to disinfect equipment; in the home, the safe and acceptable practice may be to wash equipment in a chlorine bleach solution. Also, in the hospital, many supplies are sterile and the equipment is disposable; in the home, "clean technique" and reusable equipment may be needed. Individual and family willingness to reuse supplies requires skill, motivation, and extra work for cost savings to be realized.

Teaching

Teaching is focused on behavior change that is considered essential to health maintenance in the home.

Areas to consider for potential teaching opportunities include self-care skills necessary for maintenance of a new treatment regimen, body system changes as a result of a disease process, diet, medication, and activity. The teaching plan must be coordinated with all of the disciplines providing care. Teaching should follow known principles of teaching and learning, including an environment conducive to learning, the consideration of the age and readiness of the learner, and a plan that progresses from known to unknown. Teaching in the home setting allows the nurse to demonstrate and the individual/family to practice new skills with the equipment and supplies that will actually be used and in the setting in which they will be used. This realism offers an advantage over much of the teaching that can be done in an acute care setting.

Some teaching situations demand a creative approach. For example, to promote compliance with the physician's orders regarding medications, the home nurse may need to design a system to help individuals organize and remember to take their medications. For instance, a clean, empty egg carton can be labeled for various medications and for the times each is to be taken. The individual would have to agree to fill each slot in the morning with the appropriate medications and would have to be able to understand that the medication should be taken on time so that all slots are empty by bedtime. A monthly calendar can be labeled to prompt an individual to adhere to a schedule. It is important to adapt, to the extent possible, the treat-ment regimen to the individual's and family's daily routine. Insisting that the client adhere to the arbitrary medication times that are used in the acute care setting can adversely affect compliance.

Mutual goal setting and the use of contracts are successful tools for effective home care teaching.[6] Use of written material that can be left in the home promotes compliance. Written material should contain easy-to-follow directions, preferably written at no higher than the eighth-grade reading level, as well as illustrations, when possible. Figure 23–4 is an example of a standardized client instruction sheet.[42]

Counseling

Counseling the individual and family requires knowledge of family theory and of general systems theory. Most individuals exist within a family system, and the family is part of larger social and cultural systems. It is important to work with these relationships in mind. As an example, commonly encountered changes within an individual include role adjustments, issues with dependency, and feelings of loss of control, all of which can disturb previously established patterns of family functioning. Thus, the nurse may need to counsel the family as well as the individual.

As another example, beliefs and values of the individual family are most often derived from their larger social and cultural context. A review of this area can be found in Chapter 19. The health beliefs and values held by the family can be a problem when they differ from the beliefs and values held by the new practitioner. Focusing on the individual and family as people first, and on their different beliefs and values as secondary, can remove barriers to therapeutic interventions.

Coordination of Care

Coordination is essential for continuity of care.

Coordination bridges the gap between acute care and home care services; it also promotes continuity if the individual requires admission to acute care from the home setting.

Organizing the actions of the multidisciplinary team requires coordination if planned outcomes are to be accomplished. In an increasingly high technology environment, the multitude of providers, services, and equipment can easily result in duplications or omissions in the plan of care. As case manager, the home care nurse monitors and evaluates each component of the plan of care to ensure that all actions complement each other. As part of this role, the home care nurse functions as an advocate to ensure that the individual's and family's rights and confidentiality are protected.

GENERAL INFORMATION

Foot care is important, especially if you have diabetes or poor circulation. Signs to watch for are cold or swollen feet, painful, burning or tingling feelings, lack of sensation (feeling), and slow healing of sores on the feet.

GUIDELINES

Check Your Feet Daily

1. Look for any infection (redness, swelling, pus, or pain), dry skin, cracks, blisters, cuts, and any changes in skin color or temperature.

2. Look at the tops and bottoms, between the toes, and around the toenails. Use good light; a mirror or magnifying glass can be helpful.

Wash Your Feet Daily with Warm Water and Mild Soap

1. Test the water temperature with your wrist before putting your feet in the water.

2. Soaking your feet is *not* necessary. It can be harmful.

3. Dry your feet well, especially between the toes. Be gentle.

4. Use a mild lotion or skin cream daily for dry skin. You may use lanolin, vegetable oil, Crisco, Vaseline, cold cream, Nivea, and Eucerin. Do not use creams or lotions between toes or on open cuts.

5. Use a little powder for sweaty/perspiring feet. You may use nonperfumed powder, talcum powder, or cornstarch to help keep your feet dry. Do not let the powder cake, especially between toes.

6. Use a small piece of plain gauze, cotton, or lamb's wool between toes if your toes overlap or if you have trouble with wetness between toes.

Cut Your Toenails Straight Across with Nail Clippers

1. Toenails are softer after bathing.

2. Use a file (emery board) to remove sharp edges.

3. Do not treat ingrown toenails or corns yourself. Call your doctor, nurse, or foot specialist.

4. Do not use chemicals (like iodine) or corn and callus removers.

5. Do not use razor blades, scissors, or other tools to cut toenails, corns, or calluses.

Wear Proper Shoes and Socks

1. Wear shoes that are wide and long enough to allow toes to wiggle without pressure. Shoes should be comfortable, fit well, and have good support.

2. Avoid shoes with seams or buckles that rub on your feet. Open shoes and sandals should not be worn if you have foot problems.

3. Buy new shoes in the afternoon. Your feet will be larger after walking for awhile. Break new shoes in gradually.

4. Do not go barefoot, especially on hot sand or concrete.

5. Shake out shoes (to remove small objects) before putting them on.

6. Wear clean, dry socks or stockings every day. Socks should be colorfast and fit well.

7. Avoid tight socks, stockings, or garters with elastic tops.

Exercise Your Feet

1. Walking or doing other exercises your doctor or nurse has shown you can help your circulation.

2. Wear sturdy, comfortable shoes when walking.

3. Check your feet after exercise (for blisters, cuts, or redness).   *Illustration continued on following page*

▲ Figure 23–4

An example of a standardized client instruction sheet. (From Zastocki, D.K., & Rovinski, C.A. (1989). *Home Care: Patient and Family Instructions*. Philadelphia: W.B. Saunders Co.)

FOOT CARE

4. Do not walk if you have pain or an open sore that rubs the shoe.

General Reminders

1. If you need help in caring for your feet, ask family or friends for assistance.

2. Do not put heat or cold packs directly on your feet (no heating pads, hot water bottles, or ice packs). Your feet may not have enough feeling to warn you of injury. Wear extra cotton socks or use a blanket to keep your feet warm at night.

3. No smoking. It is bad for your circulation. Crossing your legs also cuts down the circulation to your feet.

4. Eat a balanced diet. Limit the amount of cholesterol, saturated fat, and caffeine in your diet.

5. First aid for minor cuts and scratches:

    a. Wash the area with warm water and mild soap.
    b. Dry your foot.
    c. Cover the area with a dry, sterile bandage.
    d. Use paper tape instead of adhesive tape.

6. Call your doctor or nurse if you have a foot infection (pain, tenderness, swelling, redness, pus, or a warm/hot area), an ingrown toenail, a problem cutting your toenails, or any foot problems or questions. Remember: early treatment can prevent major foot problems.

OTHER INSTRUCTIONS

▲ *Figure 23–4* Continued

EVALUATION

Documentation of the individual's and family's progress or lack of progress toward the established outcomes is part of the ongoing evaluation of the effectiveness of the plan of care. Accurate descriptive documentation is essential for continuity of care among health care team members; legal and professional accountability; quality assurance; and, most important in home care, reimbursement and continuation of services. The old nursing caveat "if it is not written, it is not considered done" should also include "it is not reimbursable." In documenting home care nursing, always state facts; make note of **skilled nursing** interventions—those activities within the scope and practice of the registered professional nurse such as assessment, observation, evaluation of signs and symptoms, planning of individualized goal-directed care, teaching self-care to promote independence, and using clinical skills in the application of treatments and the provision of direct care. Also describe the exact nature or circumstances of the person's condition. For example, if a person is described as "up ad lib," the homebound status may no longer be valid. However, stating that the person can walk 20 feet but then experiences extreme shortness of breath indicates why it is difficult for the person to leave the home. Examples of terminology associated with reimbursed services include "acute" instead of "chronic," "instructed" instead of "reviewed," "assessed" instead of "observed," and "unable to" instead of "has difficulty with." An example would be that the person new to insulin is "unable to self-administer insulin; lives alone."

Documentation should reveal the answers to the following questions:

▶ Why are the skills of a professional nurse necessary to meet the individual's health care needs?
▶ What are the clinical findings that demonstrate the individual's condition is not stable?
▶ Why is the individual unable to maintain the management of his or her health care needs?
▶ Why is the chosen plan of care reasonable and essential in light of the individual's medical diagnoses?[30]

During evaluation, the measurement of clinically significant changes and assessment of the individual and family stabilization are discussed with the individual and family. Although discharge planning begins during the assessment phase, preparation for discharge from home care receives increasing emphasis as outcomes near achievement. Planning for discharge from home care is just as important as it is from acute care.

Legal and ethical issues of abandonment are as relevant in home care as in acute care. The relationship that is formed between the home care nurse and the individual and family requires skillful preparation for termination, just as is true in acute care.

The Client

Cynthia Mullen is a 35-year-old female with a history of type 1 diabetes mellitus controlled by insulin. Cynthia had been performing blood glucose self-monitoring and was administering her own injections of insulin in the morning and before her evening meal. Cynthia's spouse was very supportive but was seldom available owing to long trips away from home at his job as a truck driver. Recently, Cynthia developed a right foot ulcer that required hospitalization for surgical debridement.

The stress of surgery and the right foot wound resulted in fluctuating blood glucose levels that seemed difficult to control. The physician planned to discharge Cynthia from the hospital with daily visits from the home care nurse for wound care and diabetes management by adjustment of the insulin dosage on the basis of blood glucose monitoring. Cynthia was given crutches to help her prevent weight bearing on the right foot.

In preparation for discharge, the home care coordinator met with Mr. and Mrs. Mullen to prepare for continuing care in the home. The home care coordinator then communicated with the home care nurse responsible for Cynthia's care. In addition to ensuring that the necessary supplies and equipment would be available for the first home visit, the home care nurse initiated the therapeutic relationship with a telephone call to the Mullens' home on the day of discharge, November 2, to confirm the visit time for the following day, 10 AM, November 3.

ASSESSMENT DATA

During the first home visit, the home care nurse immediately began the assessment. A partial listing of the admission assessment data included the following:

- 35-year-old well-developed white female
- Right foot wound located on the dorsum measuring 2.5 cm × 3.5 cm
- Right foot wound bandaged with dry sterile dressing
- Wound exhibits no signs of infection
- Right foot and toes warm to touch
- Blood glucose monitoring results range from 180 to 240
- Urine, free of ketones
- T 98.8°F, BP 130/74, P 74, R 18
- Height and weight: 5'7", 135 lb
- States no numbness or pain in right foot wound
- States, "I can't get my housework done when I'm on these crutches. I need to get this foot healed up. Look at this house. It's a mess!"
- Dirty dishes and pans all over kitchen counter, on table, and in sink; laundry piled up on and near washing machine in kitchen; house generally unkempt and dusty

The following represents part of a nursing care plan written for her and the current evaluation of outcomes that were expected at that time.

CARE PLAN

November 3

Nursing Diagnosis	Planning: Expected Outcomes	Implementation: Nursing Interventions	Evaluation
Home Maintenance Management, Impaired R/T effects of chronic debilitating disease, AEB foot ulcer	By November 27 ▸ Maintains adequate wound healing, without signs of infection	Teach signs and symptoms of wound infection Teach importance of maintaining dressing dry and intact and wound free from contamination Perform wound care Teach wound care techniques Assess client's ability to consistently maintain technique while performing wound care Assess stages of wound healing	November 27, 4PM Foot and toes warm to touch States no numbness or pain Wound pink with absence of redness, swelling, tenderness, odor, or purulent drainage Wound healing continues without signs of infection
	▸ Able to bear weight bilaterally without crutches	Teach when to begin weight bearing	Client able to bear weight bilaterally without crutches
	▸ States increased satisfaction with own ability to maintain home	Arrange for temporary assistance with housework (until able to bear weight bilaterally)	States, "Its so good to be up and around again. See, no more dirty dishes!"

Summary

▶ Both religious and secular groups provided home nursing care before the efforts of Florence Nightingale.

▶ The 1980s witnessed a shift from institution-based care to highly technical home-based care.

▶ Home care services include nursing care, social work, physical therapy, respiratory therapy, speech therapy, occupational therapy, registered dietitian counseling, laboratory services, and home health aide services.

▶ People of all ages and from varying socioeconomic backgrounds may need a variety of home care services.

▶ The home care nurse assumes the roles of technically skilled direct care provider, educator, advocate, collaborator, leader, and case manager.

▶ The Albrecht Nursing Model for Home Health Care assumes that individuals and their families are active and responsible participants in their care.

▶ The goals of home care nursing are to restore health and assist the person to return to an appropriate level of functioning; maintain health and preserve functional abilities and independence; promote health and minimize effects of illness; and improve health and help the person achieve a higher level of functioning.

▶ The professional nurse as the case manager collaborates and coordinates care with other members of the multidisciplinary health care team.

▶ Assessment includes biopsychosocial and environmental factors as well as functional abilities.

▶ The most frequently encountered nursing diagnosis in home care nursing is *Home Maintenance Management, Impaired.*

▶ Planning in home care requires focusing on what is realistically able to be achieved within the family system.

▶ Home care nursing interventions include clinical/technical skills, teaching, counseling, and coordination of care.

▶ During evaluation, the measurement and documentation of clinically significant changes are discussed with the individual and family.

▶ Home care implies a philosophy of promoting independence in a qualitative and cost-effective manner.

Bibliography

1. Abel, P.E. (1990). Ethics committees in home health agencies. *Public Health Nursing,* 7(4), 256–259.
2. Albrecht, M.N. (1990). The Albrecht nursing model for home health care: implications for research, practice, and education. *Public Health Nursing,* 7(2), 118–126.
3. American Nurses' Association (1986). *Standards of home health nursing practice.* Kansas City, MO: Author.
4. Arnold, L.S., & Bakewell-Sachs, S. (1991). Models of perinatal home follow-up. *Journal of Perinatal and Neonatal Nursing,* 5(1), 18–26.
5. Brent, N.J. (1991). Assessing, evaluating, and selecting patient care products. *Home Healthcare Nurse,* 9(2), 9–11.
6. Cady, C., & Yoshioka, R.S. (1991). Using a learning contract to successfully discharge an infant home total parenteral nutrition. *Pediatric Nursing,* 17(1), 67–71.
7. Caserta, J.E. (1991). Renovating a home for the aging parent. *Home Healthcare Nurse,* 9(3), 6–7.
8. Churness, V.H., et al. (1991). Home health patient classification system. *Home Healthcare Nurse,* 9(2), 14–22.
9. Cloonan, P.A., & Shuster, G.F. (1990). Care coordination: a resource-intensive component of home health nursing practice. *Public Health Nursing,* 7(4), 204–208.
10. Gaynor, S.E. (1990). The long haul: the effects of home care on caregivers. *IMAGE: Journal of Nursing Scholarship,* 22(4), 208–212.
11. Harris, M.D. (1988). *Home health administration.* Baltimore: National Health Publishing.
12. Harris, M.D. (1991). Clinical and financial outcomes in patient care in a home health care agency. *Journal of Nursing Quality Assurance,* 5(2), 41–49.
13. Harris, M.D. (1991). Structure and process criteria assist with goal attainment. *Home Healthcare Nurse,* 9(2), 12–13.
14. Helberg, J.L. (1990). Resource utilization in home care. Methods and issues. *Nursing & Health Care,* 11(9), 464–468.
15. Johnson, E.A., & Jackson, E. (1989). Teaching the home care client. *Nursing Clinics of North America,* 24(3), 687–693.
16. Johnson, J.E., & Clark, B.R. (1990). Orientation to home care: maximizing Medicare reimbursement. *Home Healthcare Nurse,* 8, 45–49.
17. Joint Commission on Accreditation of Healthcare Organizations (1991). *Accreditation manual for home care* (vol. 2). Chicago: Author.
18. Katz, K.S., et al. (1991). Home-based care for children with chronic illness. *Journal of Perinatal and Neonatal Nursing,* 5(1), 71–79.
19. Kaufman, J. (1991). An overview of public sector financing for pediatric home care, part 1. *Pediatric Nursing,* 17(3), 280–281.
20. Livengood, W.S., et al. (1983). The impact of DRGs on home health care. *Home Healthcare Nurse,* 1(1), 29–31, 34.
21. Lutz, S. (1990). Hospitals reassess home-care ventures. *Modern Healthcare,* 20(37), 23–32.
22. Lutz, S. (1991). Recuperating at home preferred. *Modern Healthcare,* 21(24), 17.
23. McNamara, E. (1982). Home care: hospitals rediscover comprehensive care. *Hospitals,* 56(21), 60–66.
24. Moore, P., et al. (1991). Collaborative model for continuing education for home health nurses. *Journal of Continuing Education in Nursing,* 22(2), 67–72.
25. Mundinger, M. (1983). *Home care controversy: Too little, too late, too costly.* Rockville, MD: Aspen Systems.
26. North American Nursing Diagnosis Association (1990). *Taxonomy 1 revised-1990 with official nursing diagnoses.* St. Louis: Author.
27. O'Hare, P.A., & Terry, M.A. (1991). Community-based care management: a framework for delivery of services. *Home Healthcare Nurse,* 9(3), 26–32.
28. O'Neill, C., & Sorensen, E.S. (1991). Home care of the elderly: a family perspective. *Advances in Nursing Science,* 13(4), 28–37.
29. O'Neill, G., & Ross, M.M. (1991). Burden of care: an important concept for nurses. *Health Care for Women International,* 12(1), 111–121.

30. Rovinski, C.A., & Zastocki, D.K. (1989). *Home care: A technical manual for the professional nurse.* Philadelphia: W.B. Saunders.
31. Saba, V.K., et al. (1991). A nursing intervention taxonomy for home health care. *Nursing & Health Care,* 12(6), 296–299.
32. Schmele, J.A. (1989). Standards: the state of the art. In Meisenheimer, C.G. (ed.). *Quality assurance for home health care* (pp. 56–64). Rockville, MD: Aspen.
33. Simmons, J. (1990). The 3 R's of discharge planning: risks, rights, realities. *Continuing Care,* February, 9(2), 18–34.
34. Smith, J.B. (1991). Competition and continuity of care in home health nursing. *Home Healthcare Nurse,* 9(1), 9–13.
35. Speigel, A.D. (1983). *Home health care: Home birthing to hospice care.* Baltimore: National Health Publishing.
36. Spradley, B.W. (ed.) (1985). *Community health nursing: Concepts and practice.* Boston: Little, Brown.
37. Stanhope, M.K. (1989). Home care past perspectives and implications for the present and future. In Meisenheimer, C.G. (ed.). *Quality assurance for home health care* (pp. 3–12). Rockville, MD: Aspen.
38. Stern, T.E. (1991). An early discharge program: an entrepreneurial nursing practice becomes a hospital-affiliated agency. *Journal of Perinatal and Neonatal Nursing,* 5(1), 1–8.
39. Stewart, J.E. (1979). *Home health care.* St. Louis: C.V. Mosby.
40. Strandell, C. (1991). Strategies for financing home healthcare. *Home Healthcare Nurse,* 9(1), 4–8.
41. Thatcher, R.M. (1989). Community support: promoting health and self-care. *Nursing Clinics of North America,* 24(3), 725–731.
42. Zastocki, D.K., & Rovinski, C.A. (1989). *Home care: Patient and family instructions.* Philadelphia: W.B. Saunders.

Part

II

▼ **Skills Basic to Nursing**

▼ Communication Skills

▼ Therapeutic Communication: The Nurse-Client Interaction

▼ *The most important thing in communication is to hear what isn't being said.*

Peter F. Drucker

▼

▼

▼

▼ **CHAPTER OUTLINE**

THE THERAPEUTIC RELATIONSHIP
    Phases of the Therapeutic
      Relationship
    Improving the Therapeutic
      Relationship Through Process
      Recordings
ELEMENTS OF THE THERAPEUTIC
  RELATIONSHIP: THE NURSE, THE
  CLIENT, AND COMMUNICATION
    Elements of Communication
    Theories Concerning the Nurse, the
      Client, and Communication
TYPES OF COMMUNICATION
    Verbal Communication
    Nonverbal Communication
FACILITATING EFFECTIVE THERAPEUTIC
  COMMUNICATION
    Nursing Attitudes that Promote
      Communication
    Action-oriented Characteristics
TECHNIQUES THAT IMPAIR THERAPEUTIC
  COMMUNICATION
TECHNIQUES THAT ENHANCE
  THERAPEUTIC COMMUNICATION

Techniques Often Helpful at the
    Beginning of an Interaction
Techniques Often Helpful as an
    Interaction Progresses
Techniques Often Helpful in
    Keeping Communication Clear
Techniques that Can Help the
    Client Gain Increased Self-
    Awareness
Techniques Helpful When Contact
    with Reality Is Impaired
Techniques Often Helpful Near the
    End of an Interaction
One Technique that Must Occur
    Throughout the Interaction:
    Active Listening
EFFECTIVE COMMUNICATION WITH
  DIFFERENT GROUPS
    Developmental Differences
    Cultural Differences
    Gender Differences
    The Hearing Impaired
    The Visually Impaired
    The Dying

▼ **KEY TERMS**

Acting-out behaviors
Active listening
Agraphia
Alogia
Aphasia
Aphemesthesia
Auditory aphasia
   (auditory amnesia,
   word deafness)
Attending behaviors
Body language
Braille
Context

Decoder (receiver)
Encoder (sender)
Feedback
Finger spelling
Global aphasia
Human reduction
Language
Message
Motor (ataxic,
   expressive) aphasia
Nontherapeutic
   communication
   techniques

Nonverbal
   communication
Open body posture
Paralanguage
Personal space
Positive listening
Process recordings
Sensory (receptive)
   aphasia
Sensory channel
Sign language
Talking
Therapeutic rapport

Therapeutic
   relationship
Therapeutic
   relationship,
   orientation phase
Therapeutic
   relationship,
   termination phase
Therapeutic
   relationship, working
   phase
Unconditional positive
   regard

Verbal communication
Verbatim notes
Visual aphasia (word
   blindness)

▼ **LEARNING OBJECTIVES**

After studying this chapter, you should be able to

1. *Identify the tasks associated with each of the three phases of the therapeutic relationship.*
2. *Describe how process recordings may benefit the student, instructor, client, and graduate nurse.*
3. *List the six elements of communication.*
4. *Identify how Peplau, Travelbee, Satir, and Watzlawick contributed to an understanding of the nurse, the client, and communication.*
5. *Contrast the four main forms of verbal communication.*
6. *Identify the elements of body language and paralanguage.*
7. *Describe the responsive characteristics (nursing attitudes) and action-oriented characteristics that facilitate effective therapeutic communication.*
8. *Contrast nontherapeutic communication techniques.*
9. *List seven guidelines for the appropriate use of therapeutic techniques of communication.*
10. *Contrast therapeutic techniques of communication.*
11. *State the nursing implications related to communication skills for different client groups.*

Jennifer was in the hospital for observation after an automobile accident and seemed to be doing well. On the evening before she was to be discharged, Jennifer told her nurse, "I'm getting married next month." Her nurse said, "That's wonderful! I hope you'll be very happy." Jennifer said, "Thank you very much." After the nurse left, Jennifer launched into an angry tirade against the nursing supervisor.

Had the nurse been more careful about her communication techniques, she might have avoided upsetting Jennifer. What did the nurse do that she should not have done? What should she have done that she did not do? What could she have done better? The answers to these questions lie in an understanding of therapeutic communication techniques.

This chapter will orient you to beginning theories, principles, and techniques of therapeutic communication related to the nurse-client interaction. Because you will be expected to use therapeutic communication techniques throughout your professional life, it is vital that you begin to learn these techniques early in your student experience. Like most skills you learn in nursing, you will continue to develop skill and will gain mastery of these techniques as you practice them in the clinical setting over time. Also like other skills, the more you understand and practice before you try them with actual clients, the more confident you will be and the better will be the outcomes.

THE THERAPEUTIC RELATIONSHIP

A **therapeutic relationship** is a helping relationship. Nurses are helpers and clients are those seeking help. A therapeutic relationship is personal, client focused, and aimed at realizing mutually determined goals.

In a therapeutic relationship, individuals who are seeking help bring their own life experiences, intelligence, achievements, values, beliefs, and motivations for change to the relationship. Nurses bring experience, understanding, and skills. The nurse and client can be viewed as unique systems that intersect on a common ground: the therapeutic nurse-client relationship.

A therapeutic relationship is not a social relationship.

Although it is true that people often help each other in social relationships, the help that occurs in social relationships differs from that occurring in therapeutic relationships. Social relationships may involve an infinite range of nonspecific helping activities such as walking the neighbor's dog or helping a person who is using a walker to cross the street safely. Social helping such as this may result in the helper deriving more satisfaction from the interaction than the person being helped. Social helping is often only a small part of the total relationship.

The help that occurs in the therapeutic relationship is the main reason for the relationship to exist. It is the central activity of the relationship. It is focused on the client and has a specific purpose.

The therapeutic relationship remains focused on eliciting the client's feelings, thoughts, and values and centers on achieving the client's goals.

Another difference between the social relationship and the therapeutic relationship is that the social relationship is more reciprocal, with both persons sharing personal beliefs, feelings, and opinions with each other. This is not true of the therapeutic relationship. Although the nurse may share some feelings with the client, this is not a reciprocal sharing and it is done only when appropriate for the benefit of the client.

For example, Mrs. Brown is 82 years old and is reminiscing about her life. Nurse Smith is listening to her. Mrs. Brown says, "I was never allowed to make my own choices because I was a woman." If Nurse Smith is truly therapeutic, which of the following replies would she make?

▶ "That's infuriating! I couldn't have lived like that!"
▶ "You felt restricted because ideas were different then than they are now?"
▶ "People were so narrow-minded then. Thank goodness we have the women's movement now!"

The first and third choices are excellent examples of social responses and represent the way people most often talk to and support each other. However, it is the second response that is focused on the client and that is attempting to elicit further information and feelings that might lead to the client being helped. In this case, there is no helpful reason for the nurse to share personal feelings with the client. Therefore, the second example is the therapeutic response.

Phases of the Therapeutic Relationship

Therapeutic relationships develop and evolve over a period of time. The time may be brief, or it may extend over weeks, months, or even years. Regardless of the length of time, there are three distinct phases to the relationship: the orientation phase, the working phase, and the termination phase. Because relationships are fluid, the phases flow into each other but each phase may be recognized by the tasks associated with it.

ORIENTATION PHASE

During the **orientation phase of the therapeutic relationship** the nurse and client make an agreement that they will be working together to solve one or more of the client's problems. This phase represents an oral contract between nurse and client. It signals the initiation of a working relationship. This part of the relationship is the basis for the work they will do together in the future.

As you enter into a relationship with a client, it is helpful to be aware of the personal feelings that can arise at these times. Both nurse and client may experience anxiety and discomfort during this phase. As the nurse, you may feel inadequate. The client may feel unsure about you and may need to know that you are willing and able to help.

A primary goal of the orientation phase is the establishment of trust. Trust is enhanced when the nurse connects with the client in a respectful and nonintrusive manner that conveys personal consideration and concern.

Your consideration and concern give the client confidence in you. It is not necessary that you know all there is to know about everything. That would be impossible. Anyone knows that no one human being knows everything. If you try to pretend that you know more than you do, you will fool no one and the client's trust in you will drop precipitously.

Honesty and enthusiasm are helpful in establishing trust. These two traits are shown in responses such as, "I don't know the answer right now, but I will ask and let you know in 1 hour" or "I can't promise I can help solve your problem but I can listen and I do care."

Trust is also promoted when the nurse establishes confidentiality as a ground rule for the relationship. However, you must be careful with promises about confidentiality. Sometimes, in a desire to have the client trust us, we are tempted to promise complete confidentiality and then are placed on the horns of a dilemma when the client confides something that must be told to others for the client's protection or for the protection of others. For example, what would you do if you pledged unconditional confidentiality to a client only to have her confide that she has a gun and is contemplating shooting her son and then committing suicide? If you do not tell someone, you are left alone to deal with the possibility of two deaths. If you do tell, you have broken your word and violated the client's trust.

Recall, from Chapter 3, that confidentiality may be regarded as an ethical obligation to share health care information about a person only with other persons who have a need to know the person's health status. The phrase "only with other persons who have a need to know the person's health status" is key.

Do not promise that you will never tell anyone about anything that occurs between you and your clients. You may safely promise that you will maintain respect for client privacy and will not share anything with anyone else unless another person has a need to know. It is important to tell your clients that you cannot maintain confidentiality if doing so would endanger the health and well-being of themselves or others.

Such a pledge should make clients feel that you will protect them and not allow them to hurt themselves or others. If clients feel safe, they will feel a sense of trust and the relationship will be reinforced.

During the orientation phase, the nurse is responsible for establishing the ground rules for the relationship. If you will be meeting with a client a number of times, it is important to specify clearly where, when, and for how long each meeting will be. For example, Mrs. Flemming, a primary nurse, might say, "As your primary nurse, I will be following your care very carefully and would like to meet with you routinely throughout your stay here in the hospital. Would you agree to meet with me every weekday for 15 minutes, between 10:15 and 10:30, here in your room? I will not be here on weekends, but Mr. Carlisle can meet with you Saturdays and Sundays at the same time."

As you establish meeting times and places, honesty and achievability are paramount. Do not promise what you may not be able to do. It is better if the client can rely on meeting with you for 15 minutes each day than for you to promise 30-minute sessions that may not be possible.

At any time after your initial contact, you may begin to feel a bond with the client. This bond, termed **therapeutic rapport,** is a special bond that exists between nurse and client because they have established a sense of trust and a mutual understanding of what will occur in their relationship with each other.

It is during the orientation phase that the nursing process begins. At this stage, the nursing process consists of collecting assessment data, making preliminary nursing diagnoses, and formulating an initial plan of care.

WORKING PHASE

Once rapport has been established with the client and the therapeutic relationship has been structured, the working phase (middle phase) of the relationship begins. In the working phase, the nurse participates actively in further client assessment and in examining and exploring data found. Covert client feelings, values, beliefs, and attitudes are sought out and examined.

Often during this phase, initial nursing diagnoses are corrected or additional nursing diagnoses are formulated. However, the **working phase of the therapeutic relationship** is mainly a time for completing nursing interventions that address expected nursing outcomes. The nurse responds to the clients. It is a time when the nurse presents information to clients and helps to validate and clarify client understandings. Rather than directing them, the nurse attempts to help them become self-directed. It is a time when clients can formulate, try, and test solutions to their emotional problems. Evaluation also occurs in this phase of the relationship and, when necessary, the plan is revised.

TERMINATION PHASE

The **termination phase of the therapeutic relationship** occurs near the end of the relationship when the work of the client and nurse is coming to a close.

The termination itself should not be abrupt and unexpected because it is acknowledged from the beginning of the relationship. Recall the example given in the orientation phase in which the primary nurse, Mrs. Flemming, said, "As your primary nurse, I will be following your care very carefully and would like to meet with you routinely throughout your stay here in the hospital." The phrase "throughout your stay here in the hospital" was not a meaningless pleasantry. It was a way of clarifying exactly when the relationship would end. The nurse did not say she wanted to meet with the client "every weekday" and leave it at that. No one should have interpreted her offer to meet with the client as extending beyond the hospital stay. Therefore, the nurse was saying, in effect, "I will be meeting with you only until you are discharged." Such communications help to set up clear expectations from the onset of the relationship.

Although the end of the relationship is planned, it is still often difficult to end a meaningful interaction. Both nurse and client understand that this phase precedes a permanent separation, and both may experience anxiety, sadness, and a sense of loss.

The client's reaction to the termination is determined by the meaning assigned to it, the length of the relationship, and how or whether outcomes were achieved. Clients may display denial and regret and may engage in **acting-out behaviors** (inappropriate or unexpected client behaviors that communicate a message to the nurse about the client's true or subconscious feelings and concerns). Acting-out behaviors frequently seen in the termination phase include refusal to talk during meetings with the nurse, missing appointments with the nurse, and increased forgetfulness. At such times, the nurse may help the client to recognize feelings about saying good-by while pointing out positive changes that have occurred during the relationship. It may be helpful to offer support and express optimism for the future. At the same time, it is important to be clear about ending the relationship without offering false hope for continuation. This is often uncomfortable for the new nurse but offers the client clear boundaries and expectations.

Improving the Therapeutic Relationship Through Process Recordings

As a student, you will be learning to interact with clients in the clinical setting. This may be in a client's home, in a hospital, or in some other setting within the community. A time-honored method of learning to master communications with clients in any setting is to complete a process recording for each interaction. **Process recordings** are written records in which the nurse writes, word for word, everything the client says and everything the nurse replies. The nurse also writes observations of nonverbal communication by both client and nurse. Because process recordings are written word for word, they are also referred to as **verbatim notes.**

Process recordings vary in format but they are frequently written in columns. They contain not only verbal and nonverbal communications but usually some method of assessing or evaluating what is going on throughout the interaction. This way the student can demonstrate to the instructor the rationale for responses to the client.

Process recordings are used to provide a record that the student can later use to help learn, for example, which communication techniques are being used most frequently, which of the techniques being used are helpful and which are not, how these might be improved on, what went wrong with a situation that allowed it to deteriorate, and many other factors about the interaction. The recordings also help the instructor, who reads them and is able to follow along and guide the student in ways to improve. Perhaps most of all, they help the client because the growth that occurs through the completion of process recordings allows the student to be more therapeutic. Sometimes, when the student experience is over and the graduate nurse is having difficulties with communications, it helps to begin process recordings again and take an objective look at the communication patterns the nurse is using. A trusted mentor can often look at the notes and give the nurse additional insight.

In addition to written process recordings, audiotaped or videotaped process recordings may be done for the same purposes. The audiotaped recordings cannot indicate nonverbal behaviors observed, and written recordings are usually necessary to accompany them and fill in this missing information. On the other hand, audiotapes provide information about tone of voice and other qualities of speech that are impossible to record adequately on paper. Videotapes are excellent at capturing the verbal and nonverbal behaviors, and they can make tremendous learning tools. However, recording with sound video cameras is more difficult and intimidating (at least at first) to both client and nurse than is true of the other two methods.

There is no perfect way to complete process recordings, but, regardless of the method used, process recordings can prove to be one of the most valuable learning experiences in any student's education. Because they are so valuable, it is sometimes tempting to share them with others beside the instructor. This would be a blatant violation of the client's confidentiality and must never be done.

To see what a page from a sample process recording looks like, let us look at one that might have been a beginning process recording for Jennifer, the young woman mentioned at the start of this chapter, if her nurse had not responded to her on a social level and instead had been therapeutic (Fig. 24–1).

ELEMENTS OF THE THERAPEUTIC RELATIONSHIP: THE NURSE, THE CLIENT, AND COMMUNICATION

There are three elements that are present in all phases of the therapeutic relationship: the nurse, the client, and communication. As an element of the therapeutic relationship, the nurse is a helper who is trained in

skills that facilitate client growth, the client is the person seeking help with personal growth, and communication is the meaningful interaction between the two that leads to growth. Before we discuss theories about the interactions among these three elements, let us discuss the elements of communication.

Elements of Communication

A widely accepted model for the communication process is depicted in Figure 24–2. This model consists of the following six elements:

▶ **Encoder (sender):** This person initiates a transaction to exchange information, convey thoughts and feelings, or engage another.
▶ **Message:** This is the content a sender wishes another person (the receiver) to receive in the process of communication. The message must be encoded in a language of symbols or cues that are understandable to both sender and receiver.
▶ **Sensory channel:** This is the means by which a message is sent. The three primary routes are the visual, auditory, and kinesthetic channels. Using these three channels, a wink, a tone of voice, and a hand gesture can all effectively convey a message without benefit of words.
▶ **Decoder (receiver):** This is the person to whom a message is aimed. This person must be able to decode the message sent so it is a clearly understood thought. If the message that the sender intends is what the receiver understands, then clear and effective communication has occurred.
▶ **Feedback:** This is the process by which effectiveness of communication is determined.
▶ **Context:** This is the condition under which a communication occurs.

Feedback is a process that is so important to communication that it deserves additional attention. There are four types of feedback: internal, external, positive, and negative.

Internal feedback is a mechanism of self-perception. When we communicate, an inner critical assessment of what we have said or done is triggered. For example, if we make a verbal blunder, we react self-consciously after realizing our mistake. If, however, we communicate clearly what we meant, we feel pleased and satisfied with the effort.

External feedback is received from another (see Fig. 24–2) or others such as an audience. The response to the message sent gives information about how effectively we transmitted the message.

Positive feedback affirms our efforts to communicate by rewarding and reinforcing successful communication. If our messages are met with a smile or exclamation of relief, we feel good and continue to use those communication behaviors.

Negative feedback is a return message that our original message was poorly transmitted or received. This feedback tells us that modification is needed. However, there is more to negative feedback than just a message telling us our original message was garbled. Negative

	CLIENT	STUDENT	NOTES
○	(In J's room. I am cleaning up her bath articles. She is in bed, combing her hair. It is 10:00 AM) I'm getting married next month.		I thought, "Oh great, she'll never have a problem to work on."
		How do you feel about it?	I said this because I thought it was therapeutic, but I really felt dumb.
	Just awful. I don't love Jimmy.		I didn't believe what I was hearing.
○		What led up to this situation?	I wanted to ask "why," but I didn't.
	I'm pregnant and my father will kill me if I end up with a baby and no husband. I'm such a disgrace. (Covered her face c̄ her hands)		She seemed to "fall apart" before my eyes.
		But Jimmy loves you and he's going to marry you. That's no disgrace.	I got on a social level and forgot all my techniques. Nontherapeutic disagreeing.
○	It's not Jimmy's baby, and Jimmy doesn't even know about it.		I thought I'd better sit down and talk more.
		(I pulled a chair up closer to the bed and sat down.) Let's start at the beginning. Can you tell me about that?	Placing the events in sequence.
	Well, it started when we moved here from Ohio. I was new at school and there was		

▲ *Figure 24–1*

Page from a sample process recording.

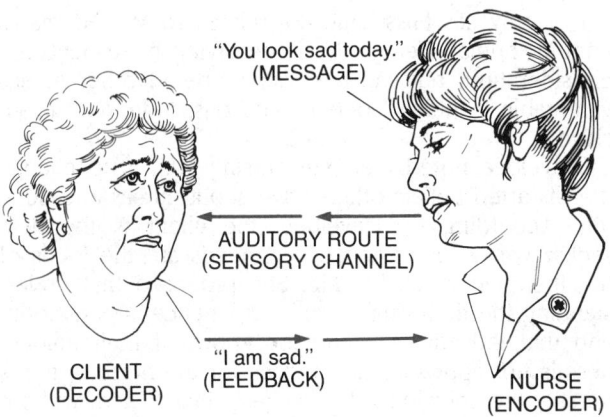

"You look sad today."
(MESSAGE)

AUDITORY ROUTE
(SENSORY CHANNEL)

CLIENT
(DECODER)

"I am sad."
(FEEDBACK)

NURSE
(ENCODER)

THERAPEUTIC RELATIONSHIP
(CONTEXT)

▲ **Figure 24–2**

The six elements of communication: the encoder (sender), the message, the sensory channel, decoder (receiver), feedback, and context.

feedback may also be judgmental and can send us a negative opinion that has resulted from the message. For example, let us compare positive and negative feedback that might be received in response to the same message:

Judy:	"I can't go to lunch with you as we had planned."
Carol:	(Providing positive feedback) "I'm sorry you can't make it, maybe some other time."
Ellie:	(Providing negative feedback) "I'm sorry you think you can never eat lunch with me again. If you were a friend, you'd find some time."

In both cases, the feedback given provides us with clear information about how the message was interpreted by the receiver.

It is important to note that both sender and receiver can seek feedback and clarify and qualify the message as necessary. For example, consider the following interaction between Mrs. Cantu and her nurse, Mrs. Schultz, as Mrs. Schultz is completing Mrs. Cantu's bed bath:

Mrs. Cantu:	"I felt so much better after my bed bath yesterday."
Mrs. Schultz:	(Insulted that her bed bath was being compared unfavorably with a bath given by another nurse and seeking clarification) "Are you saying that you feel worse today after this bath than you felt yesterday, after the bath Miss Fredericks gave you?"
Mrs. Cantu:	(Understanding that Mrs. Schultz has misunderstood) "Oh, not at all. I wasn't comparing her bath to your bath. I was comparing how I felt yesterday, before her bath, with how I felt after her bath. I had blood all over me from the accident and I felt so much better after it was cleaned off."

Had Mrs. Schultz not clarified what Mrs. Cantu meant by "better," she might have left the interaction with negative feelings about Mrs. Cantu and about her own ability to give a bath. Suppose Mrs. Schultz had not

sought clarification. The interaction might still have been saved by the process of seeking feedback. For example, it might have gone like this:

Mrs. Cantu:	"I felt so much better after my bed bath yesterday."
Mrs. Schultz:	(Obviously hurt) "I see."
Mrs. Cantu:	"What I said seems to bother you." (Seeking feedback) "Can you tell me what I said that upset you?"
Mrs. Schultz:	"When you said you felt better after Miss Fredericks gave you a bath than you feel today after your bath I guess my feelings were a little hurt. I suppose I'm being childish but I did think I had done a good job."

With the receipt of this feedback about how her message was perceived, Mrs. Cantu can clarify, as in the first interaction.

With these two examples, you can see how disruptive it could be to an interaction, and even to a relationship, if an unclear message is not clarified by seeking and receiving feedback or correction. It is unfortunate that the client had to be the one to seek feedback and to clarify in this situation, because this should be done by the nurse.

The nurse bears responsibility for keeping communications clear and therapeutic, and there are a number of ways to do this.

Theories Concerning the Nurse, the Client, and Communication

Several theorists provided us with a better understanding of the nurse, the client, and communication and of the interaction among these elements in a therapeutic relationship. Here we look only at selected examples.

HILDEGARD PEPLAU'S CONTRIBUTION

Hildegard Peplau, a psychiatric nurse and one of the first nurse theorists, identified the following six roles[24] assumed by the nurse (in relation to the client) within a therapeutic relationship:

▶ The stranger: This role is shared by both nurse and client entering into the therapeutic relationship. The nurse offers the client respect, interest, and acceptance in a nonpersonal manner. The client is assumed to be emotionally intact unless conflicting evidence arises.

▶ The resource: In the resource role, the nurse helps the consumer-client to negotiate the health care system by providing care and offering answers to specific questions.

▶ The teacher: In the role of teacher, the nurse educates the client and helps him or her understand and use experiences within the health care system.

▶ The leader: In the leader role, the nurse helps the client, as follower, to contribute to and participate in a democratic nursing process.

▶ The surrogate: As a surrogate parent figure, the nurse helps the client to resolve interpersonal problems that need to be safely worked out in the presence of an understanding other. The nurse provides the client with a corrective interpersonal experience.

▶ The counselor: In the counselor role, the nurse helps to integrate both reality and the client's emotional responses associated with illness into the total life experience.

Peplau believed that a nurse who related with a client in a healthy way could provide a corrective interpersonal experience for the client. She believed that the experience of a positive relationship with the nurse would allow for healthier relationships with others. She encouraged nurses to promote trust in their relationships by relating to their clients in an authentic manner. For Peplau, relating in an authentic manner meant sharing feelings and thoughts appropriately. For example, note how Miss Knight, a baby's nurse, shares her feelings with Mr. Little when he learns that his infant daughter has died of sudden infant death syndrome. He is red eyed and shaking but unable to verbalize his feelings.

Miss Knight: (Making eye contact with Mr. Little) "This is a hard time for you."
Mr. Little   starts to cry but remains silent.
Miss Knight: (Wiping her eyes) "I feel very sad too, Mr. Little. It doesn't seem fair to lose a baby without warning."

Peplau noted that closeness in a therapeutic relationship builds trust, increases the client's self-esteem, and leads to new personal growth for the client.[24]

JOYCE TRAVELBEE'S CONTRIBUTION

Joyce Travelbee, another noted nurse theorist, pointed out that the nurse is a human being who is vulnerable to stereotypes, labels, and generalizations. Travelbee noted that it is not possible for a stereotype (of a nurse) to relate to another stereotype (of a client) in a human way. Take, for example, Miss Lane, a nurse working with elderly clients. Miss Lane believes that older people are less mentally astute and have poorer hearing than younger people. She also thinks that nurses are poorly paid and that elderly people should be grateful for whatever nursing care they receive. Miss Lane is assigned to care for Mr. Adams, an alert 76-year-old man who is recovering from a stroke that impaired his mobility. Miss Lane enters his room and the following dialogue takes place:

Miss Lane: "Hi, Mr. Adams, it's time for us to take our walk today."
Mr. Adams: "I think I can use the walker alone this morning."
Miss Lane: (In an aside to another nurse) "This guy is crazy if he thinks I'm going to lose my license over this."
             (To Mr. Adams) "No, sweetie, I'm going to help. Now let's get this show on the road. I have eight other people to take care of this morning."

Not only has Miss Lane not related to Mr. Adams as another human being who is deserving of respect and consideration, but she has also rendered other nurses vulnerable to being labeled as callous, rude, and insensitive.

Travelbee noted that one nursing goal is to change the distorted beliefs others have about nurses and nursing. According to Travelbee, the client is the help seeker whose overt and covert needs are the focus of the therapeutic relationship. She proposed that understanding the individual client's experience is paramount and that individuals cannot be known if their uniqueness is not appreciated. The task for the nurse, then, is to see the individual "with fresh eyes" and without labeling or stereotyping.[36]

An important component of Travelbee's theory concerns the process of **human reduction**.[36] This term is synonymous with the word dehumanization. The term refers to viewing the client as other than a human being. Viewing the client as an illness ("the heart attack in 210"), a task ("the bed bath and dressing change on Team B"), or a stereotype ("all amputees") are three examples of human reduction. It is only in overcoming assigned labels that nurses and clients can relate humanly and a therapeutic relationship be established.

Like Peplau, Travelbee conceptualized the communication process as a means of fostering the development of human relationships. She believed that the human-to-human relationship allows nurses to help individuals and families cope with illness and to find meaning in the experience. She believed communication to be reciprocal, dynamic, and influential. Travelbee recognized that each interaction has differences and similarities that prohibit forming rigid rules of action but do permit the nurse to develop skill as a communicator.[36]

VIRGINIA SATIR'S CONTRIBUTION

Virginia Satir, a dynamic family therapist and expert communicator, described effective communication as a transaction in which the sender of the message makes a clear request or statement, which the receiver accurately receives. If communication is effective, what the sender intends and what the receiver receives match.

She noted, however, that communication is often unclear and believed it may be unclear because certain message senders are purposely attempting to send incorrect messages to blur the reality of their own feelings. This is dysfunctional communication and Satir[27] identified four types:

▶ The placator: This person feels vulnerable to rejection and avoids it by always seeking to please the other.
▶ The blamer: This person feels like a failure but hides it by being unreasonable and controlling as a cover.
▶ The superreasonable: This person intellectualizes events so feelings are not experienced. This refusal to feel covers inner feelings of vulnerability.
▶ The irrelevant posture: The person with this communication style demands a focus away from feelings

and current reality. By pretending a stressor does not exist, the individual can ignore feelings of alienation.

For an example of these four dysfunctional patterns, let us look at Mr. Johnson. Mr. Johnson is driving in heavy traffic, and the car in front of him stops suddenly. Mr. Johnson cannot stop his car in time and runs into the other car, causing a dent in the other car's bumper. The other driver angrily approaches Mr. Johnson. Mr. Johnson might reply in any one of the following ways, according to the four different dysfunctional patterns:

Placating:	"I'm sorry I ran into your car! Let me give you my insurance information now so you won't be inconvenienced."
Blaming:	"Where did you learn to drive? I'm calling the police to turn you in for carelessness."
Superreasonableness:	"This is a dilemma, isn't it? I guess it happens."
Irrelevant:	"Were you listening to the game on the radio? The Cubs are beating the Sox 7-0."

Each of these dysfunctional patterns of reaction results in impaired communication by relaying inaccurate information about Mr. Johnson's true feelings of concern and anxiety. With such individuals, it is necessary for the nurse to help the clients understand and communicate their true feelings before progress can be made.

PAUL WATZLAWICK'S CONTRIBUTION

Paul Watzlawick,[37] a noted communication theorist, wrote extensively about the pragmatics of communication. He believed communication to be inevitable. As he noted:

► All behavior has message value or meaning.
► We are always behaving. We cannot not behave.
► Inasmuch as we cannot stop behaving, we cannot stop communicating.
► Therefore, communication is inevitable.

TYPES OF COMMUNICATION

There are generally two types of communication: verbal and nonverbal. Each type has several components.

Verbal Communication

Verbal communication is the use of words to convey messages. This type of communication is achieved by writing or speaking in a code mutually understood by sender and receiver. The tool of verbal communication is language. Language is a set of words that have meanings that are comprehensible within a group. Because a word has a definition, however, does not guarantee that its meaning will be interpreted in the same way by all group members. For example, in the English language, the word *hot* could mean, very warm, stolen, or attractive to members of the opposite sex. It is important, therefore, to validate meaning between nurse and client.

TALKING

Talking is the act of verbalizing symbols to convey thoughts, feelings, or ideas. It is a skill so taken for granted that we feel helpless to communicate without it. Consider, for example, the plight of the client who has some form of expressive aphasia. Box 24-1 presents a list of selected forms of aphasia.

WRITTEN COMMUNICATION

Written communication transfers a thought or spoken symbol into printed form. Being able to communicate accurately and clearly in writing is critical for nurses (e.g., in documenting nursing care). It can be especially useful in communicating with clients who are unable to hear or speak clearly, if at all. If you communicate with clients by writing, you should communicate as clearly as if you were speaking to the person. For example, it is important that you use clear language, use an appropriate vocabulary, and speak at the client's level of understanding. Correct spelling is vital to clear

---

Box 24-1. Forms of Aphasia

Aphasia is the general term for several different neurologic conditions in which the client has the ability to think without a corresponding ability to exchange information with others by correctly encoding, sending, or decoding messages. Types include the following:

Motor (ataxic, expressive) aphasia: The client knows what to say and how to say it but is unable to coordinate the muscles of speech or muscles of the hand sufficiently to formulate the message in spoken or written words. Two types include alogia and agraphia. Motor aphasia may be complete or partial.

Alogia: The client is unable to speak.

Agraphia: The client is unable to write.

Sensory (receptive) aphasia: The client is unable to understand words communicated to him or her. Three types include auditory aphasia, visual aphasia, and both auditory and visual aphasia (aphemesthesia).

Auditory aphasia (auditory amnesia, word deafness): The client is unable to understand the spoken word.

Visual aphasia (word blindness): The client is unable to understand the written word.

Aphemesthesia: The client is unable to understand the spoken or the written word.

Global aphasia: The client has an inability to express or perceive words or any other form of communication.

written communication. Here are two examples of correct and incorrect written communication:

Correct: "Are you having trouble breathing?"
Incorrect: "Are your respirations labored or are you experiencing any other form of dyspnea?"
Correct: "Are you hoarse?"
Incorrect: "Are you horse?"

Obviously, in the first example, the incorrect case is at too high a level of understanding for most lay persons and could lead to a breakdown in communication. The spelling error in the second example might not only cause the message to be misunderstood, but it could also cause the client to lose faith in the abilities of a nurse who cannot spell correctly.

When communicating with clients in writing, you should ensure that your printing is large enough and dark enough to be legible, that the room lighting is conducive to reading, and that the client is wearing reading glasses, if needed. Clients with visual deficits could be completely frustrated if they cannot see, hear, or speak.

SIGN LANGUAGE AND BRAILLE

Both sign language and Braille are languages that resemble written speech in that they are composed of an alphabet with letters that can be put together to make up words and the words are used to convey messages. Thus, these are verbal means of communication.

Braille is a language used by the visually impaired to communicate by indicating letters and numbers with a series of raised dots. Usually these dots are on paper, but they may also be on other material such as plastic or metal. Braille is used to replace the written word.

Sign language is used by the hearing impaired to communicate by indicating letters and words with different positions and movements of the hands. Sign language is used to replace the spoken word.

There are several sign languages that are available to the hearing impaired. Each of these sign languages makes use of signs that stand for entire words. Therefore, a person may spell out a word by signing the individual letters, such as making eight individual signs to spell out the eight letters in the word *hospital,* or one may simply use the index and middle fingers of one hand to trace an invisible cross over the opposite upper arm at the area of the deltoid muscle. This single sign stands for the word hospital.

Obviously, signing single letters one at a time **(finger spelling)** to spell out each word is a more laborious and time-consuming task than signing entire words. In fact, those who have been signing for a time can often communicate entire sentences in sign language as fast as, or faster, than these same sentences can be communicated with spoken words. It should be understood, though, that mastery of finger spelling is the basis for learning many of the signs that stand for entire words.

As with any language, much practice is needed signing or in reading Braille before proficiency can be attained. You may want to practice with the single-hand alphabet pictured in Figure 24–3.

Do not avoid your hearing impaired or visually impaired clients because you feel you lack the ability to communicate with them. Remember that, unless impaired in some other way, visually impaired individuals should be able to hear and speak and hearing impaired individuals should be able to read and write. Hearing impaired persons may have excellent speaking and lip reading abilities as well.

OTHER FORMS OF VERBAL COMMUNICATION

We have barely scratched the surface in a discussion of the many ways that human beings have created to communicate with each other by using words. When we think about how humans may communicate words with drum beats, smoke signals, flags, dots and dashes over a wire, and so on and about how the simple turning of power off and on has led to the almost miraculous things we can now do with computers, we cannot help but feel humbled by the ingenuity of our species. Further, we must stand in awe of the intense human drive to communicate, which has resulted in the generation of so many means of doing it. It behooves us never to forget the importance of verbal communication and to keep trying during those frustrating times when our initial efforts falter or fail. At those times, one must remember that verbal communication is not the only type of communication available.

Nonverbal Communication

Nonverbal communication is the set of behaviors that conveys messages either without words or by supplementing verbal communication. Nonverbal communication consists of body language, paralanguage, and any other means by which we communicate with each other without the use of words. As health care professionals, we are mainly concerned with body language and paralanguage.

Body language refers to nonverbal communication behaviors that are accomplished by how we move our bodies or body parts, present ourselves to the world, and use the personal space around us. Thus, personal appearance; conscious and unconscious changes in facial expressions, body posture, and gestures; the distances we maintain from others; and how we touch others are among the common body language behaviors we use and observe daily. **Paralanguage** refers to nonverbal components of spoken language. These components give speech its rhythm and humanness and include stress, accent, pitch, pause, intonation, rate, volume, and quality.

As nurses, we frequently look at nonverbal behavior when we assess and evaluate our clients. Take, for example, the case of Mr. Goldberg. His body language shows that he is red faced, sweating profusely, clenching and unclenching his fists, and pacing the length of

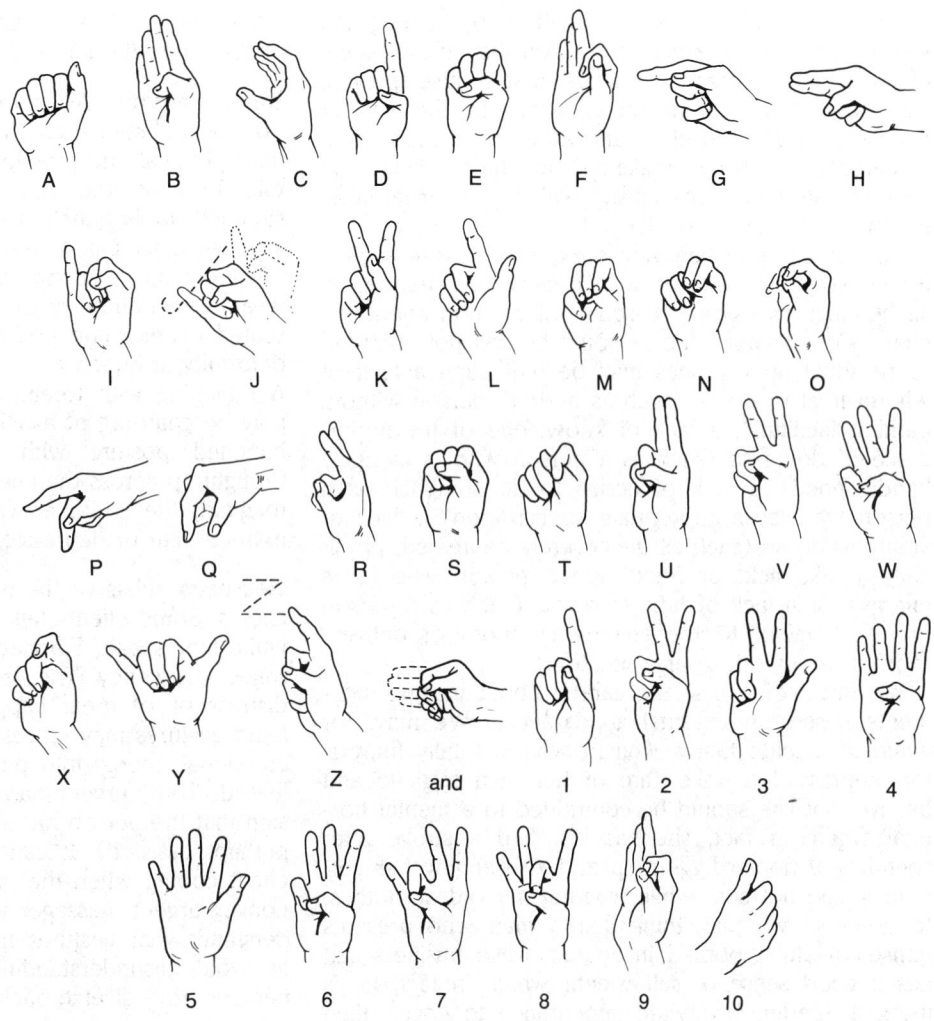

▲ *Figure 24-3*

The American Manual Alphabet. Note that the sign for the word "and" is included, as are the signs for the numbers one through ten.

the hall. His paralanguage consists of mumbling inaudibly most of the time with occasional outbursts of loud sounds resembling "Phah!" When asked what is troubling him, he shouts answers such as, "I'm fine. You don't have to concern yourself with me!" Obviously, his verbal message clashes with the way he says it and with all of his other nonverbal messages. Most nurses would surmise that this client is truly angry and agitated despite his protests. Similarly, a client who is sitting calmly and who has no readable facial expressions, but who laughingly tells you that he is "furiously angry," is providing verbal and nonverbal cues that do not match. The nurse who assesses clients who demonstrate incongruent verbal and nonverbal behaviors should make further inquiries to determine their actual emotional status.

Most nonverbal behavior is unconscious and is therefore more difficult to control than verbal communication. Because this is true, nonverbal behavior is generally considered to be a more reliable indication of a person's true message.

ASSESSING BODY LANGUAGE

Clients may communicate a great deal with body language. Messages sent by this means can be important in the overall assessment of the client. A few examples of the general areas you may assess follow.

Personal Appearance. A rapid assessment of the client's general appearance gives an initial impression of factors as varied as social standing, self-esteem, and emotional status. Because most persons are aware that they are being judged about such things, they usually take steps to alter the way they appear to others so as to make a more favorable impression. This is as true of their initial meetings with persons within the health care system as it is with other initial meetings.

It is the rare mother who has not warned her child to wear clean underwear so, in the event of an accident, the doctor in the emergency room will not think badly of the child.

Most clients prepare to meet with us by bathing and shaving appropriate areas of the skin that will be seen, cleaning out the ears that will be looked into, applying deodorant so as not to offend, grooming the hair for neatness, dressing in clean and attractive clothing, and sometimes applying make-up to hide flaws, all (consciously or unconsciously) with a goal of impressing the health care provider.

This preparatory behavior is expected in our society today. Noting whether or not the client has attended to such things can give you some information about the client. For example, the person who has not attended to personal appearances may be indicating a lack of wherewithal to do so (such as a street person without bathing facilities), a lack of knowledge of the importance of doing so (such as a person who is mentally handicapped), a lack of desire to do so (such as a person who lacks appropriate socialization), a lack of ability to do so (such as the severely depressed, physically weak, sick, or handicapped person who lacks energy), or a lack of time to do so (such as a person brought straight to the emergency room or delivery room from a work or play situation).

We must, of course, be careful about making judgments based on external appearances. We may, for example, decide that a woman who is totally filthy is too depressed to take care of her own hygiene and believe that she should be committed to a mental hospital when, in fact, she has just had a stroke after spending 9 hours digging up and rearranging her garden, in the hot sun, while wearing her oldest clothes. In contrast, we may think that a man who presents himself neatly groomed in an expensive business suit has a good sense of self-esteem when, in fact, he is using a "perfect" outward appearance to cover deep feelings of inadequacy that are paralyzing his life in all other ways. To avoid hasty judgments, it is always useful to validate impressions with additional data.

Facial Expressions. Assessing a client's eyes and facial movements can yield valuable information. When you assess these areas, note whether the movements are voluntary or involuntary (winks or smiles vs. tics or twitches). Note whether the client can focus and maintain eye contact. Observe the eyes for redness, clarity, and tearing and the face for the raising and lowering of eyebrows or the presence of a smirk, smile, or frown.

A client can communicate pain, fear, anger, sadness, happiness, contentment, or excitement with the eyes and with facial muscular activity. Do not be too quick to assign meaning to facial expressions alone, however, because reading body language is not an exact science. For example, if you note a client's eyes are red rimmed and teary and see that he has difficulty making eye contact with you, further investigation is warranted. It may be that the client is embarrassed that he has been crying, or he may be a bashful person who is suffering from a seasonal allergy. It may also be that he is from a rural area in another country where direct eye contact is considered a sign of rudeness, and perhaps smog in your city has irritated his eyes. Other possibilities exist to explain these few observations. Use your observations of facial expressions as cues to let you know where further assessment might be needed.

Body Posture. As is true of facial movement, body posture and stance can also provide cues to an individual's physical and emotional state. To assess body posture, note whether the person is standing straight, is slumped, or is hunched over. An erect posture usually signifies a feeling of fitness and confidence. A slump often occurs in persons who are physically exhausted, weak, or emotionally depressed. When a client is in a seated or reclining position, in the absence of spinal deformity, a hunch can signal a desire to be left alone. A hunching with forearms crossed over the abdomen may be guarding of a painful abdomen. An even more hunched posture with head down, with forearms brought up across the chest, and with knees brought up to guard the abdomen (a fetal position) may indicate extreme fear or depression.

Gestures. Observe the types of gestures used by your clients. Some clients talk with their hands by gesturing while they speak. Emphatic gestures often convey messages of urgency. The urgency may be expressions of distress or of great happiness or excitement. Urgent hand gestures may represent the conversion of pent-up emotional energy into physical energy that can be released. Thus, urgent hand gestures can be read as a sign that the person has strong needs to be heard (and perhaps assisted). It can also be seen as a means of client coping when the person is unable to adequately convey urgent messages verbally. It is important to understand what gestures mean within different cultures to avoid misunderstanding when communicating with persons from diverse backgrounds.

Personal Distances. We all have a **personal space** (a private zone or "bubble" around our body that we believe is an extension of ourselves and belongs to us). We carry this space with us at all times wherever we go. Except for a very select number of other persons, whom we allow to enter this space at certain times, we tend to be uncomfortable if others enter this space at all. Therefore, we behave in ways to prevent this from happening. At certain times, and in certain situations, the space grows larger and, to maintain comfort, most people must stay even farther away from us than usual.

The size of this space appears to be, at least partially, culturally determined and can vary considerably from culture to culture. Persons within each culture respect each other's personal space and use culturally determined body language signals to help maintain appropriate distances from each other. Although individuals vary in their need for space, in our own Western culture, most persons maintain similar distances from each other according to their relationships and to the activities involved. As an example, two men who are strangers on opposing teams might grapple together on a football field when they would never think of allowing their bodies to come into contact in the shower after the game. See Table 24–1 for the generally accepted levels of personal space in our culture as these might be seen in nursing situations.

TABLE 24-1. Four Levels of Personal Space

Level of Personal Space	Distance Range (feet)	Nursing Examples
Intimate (involves primarily tactile and very close communications)	0–1.5	Often used by nurses when holding infants, hugging children, lifting immobilized adults, or completing procedures or treatments that involve touching
Personal (involves most communication between nurse and client)	1.2–4	Often used for therapeutic nurse-client interactions; allows most accurate visualization and hearing; closer end of range allows nurse to reach out to touch client or, in emergency, to grasp and hold client physically if suddenly necessary to prevent a fall
Social (involves more casual, social level communications between nurse and client)	4–12	Most often used by nurses in a casual exchange of greetings such as when passing a client or family member in the hallway
Public (involves more formal contacts between the nurse and larger groups)	12 or more	May be used by nurses who work with groups such as when teaching in an auditorium or at other public speaking events; requires louder voice or microphone use

In our culture, if one person feels a second person is coming too close, the first person tends to back away to maintain the desired distance between the two. In fact, backing away should not be necessary and any subtle movement of the body in the backward direction should send the same signal, "Stop. You are getting into my bubble." The second person should read this body language, stop approaching the person, and back off slightly to adjust the distance between the two to a more comfortable level. Consider this when you approach a client who is in bed. Remember that the mattress prevents the client from backing away from you and be cognizant of subtle client movements, such as a tucking in of the chin or a tensing of the muscles, that indicate discomfort as you approach and interact with the client. Usually, the edges of the mattress are the client's outermost boundaries in such a case.

Touching. Nurse-client touching is an issue that requires much sensitivity on the part of the nurse. Because nursing is a hands-on profession, it is our daily practice to touch persons often and intimately. However, we must constantly be aware that touch has many meanings to our clients. It may indicate such things as agreement, caring, loving, or even sexual desire.

Many clients are hungry for a handclasp or other form of human touch and will demonstrate this by reaching out to you. Most desire or feel neutral about such touching as a pat on the arm during the course of normal conversation. However, clients who have been physically or sexually abused tend to see uninvited touch as a boundary violation.

If a client has not indicated a specific desire to touch or be touched, you should assess the client's feelings about touch before using it. A rule of thumb is to ask permission before touching. It is easy to ask, "May I touch your arm?", and asking can avoid possible problems. In certain settings, it is appropriate to say, "I'd like to give you a hug. May I?"

Touch may be accepted more or less readily in different situations. A nurse's hug, for example, may be greeted with relief by a family member in a hospice when support is needed most, whereas it would proba-

bly be looked on as a violation of personal space in an initial meeting with a client in a clinic. Touch has different meanings within different communications. It can soothe or disturb us to our very depths. It must, therefore, be used judiciously based on assessment of the client's needs and wishes.

ASSESSING PARALANGUAGE

Clients may communicate a great deal with verbal messages as they attempt to relate the content of their thoughts. Even better communication can occur when appropriate use is made of paralanguage. An understanding of paralanguage can help us better understand the content of the message, and it can sometimes help us tune in to the emotional component of the message: the client's mood.

Stress. Stress refers to the part of a word, phrase, or sentence that is highlighted by changing pitch or elongating the syllable. Words that are stressed are generally the more important words. For example,

"Nice to meet you" (with no particular stress),
"*Nice* to meet you,"
"Nice to *meet* you," and
"Nice to meet *you*"

all have slightly different meanings because of the way stress is used.

Accent. Accent refers to the different pronunciation of syllables used by non-native speakers of a language. Accent alone can cause a loss of clarity that can result in a breakdown in communication. Do not pretend that you understand what someone has said when you do not. Seek to clarify what has been said by asking the person to repeat what was said, say it in different words, or write out the troublesome phrase.

Pitch. Pitch refers to how high or low the voice is. Pitch results from the speed of vocal cord vibrations. Pitch is sex related in that men's voices are usually pitched lower than that of women. It is also age related in that children's voices are usually pitched higher than voices of adults. In any individual, changes in pitch can alter the meaning of the content of a message. We all know that the pitch rises at the end of a question (interrogative sentence) and stays the same or lowers when we make a statement (declarative sentence). Thus, "You have tuberculosis" and "You have tuberculosis?" are very different in meaning.

Pause. Pauses punctuate speech with periods of silence or non-word sounds, such as "Let me see . . ." or "Hmm, I believe you are right." Often a pause indicates that the person is still considering something, is considering whether to share something with you, or is considering the words to use to encode properly what is to be told to you. At other times, pauses are used for effect as part of varying intonation. In any event, the pause should be respected and the person given adequate time to complete the communication interrupted by a pause.

Intonation. Intonation is the variety of stress and pause patterns within a phrase or sentence. For example, persons often use one intonation when giving a formal speech and other intonations when communicating with a superior at work and with a close friend.

Rate. The rate of speech refers to how many syllables are spoken per unit of time. Rate also takes into account the number of pauses made. Increased rate of speed may indicate nervousness or agitation. It is sometimes possible to control anxiety by focusing on a rapid speech rate and slowing it.

Volume. Volume is the loudness and intensity associated with the speaking voice. Intensity is a measure of forcefulness and can convey a message about the speaker's emotions. Generally, a loud voice indicates anger or frustration as if the volume somehow increases the power of the words to control the listener or others. Changes in volume (either up or down) may also occur in anxiety.

Quality. Voice quality is a measure of clarity, hoarseness, or nasality of the speaker's voice. Physical and emotional conditions can cause a change in voice quality. For example, the voice often becomes husky with deeply felt emotions, harsher with anger, and more nasal with a cold.

FACILITATING EFFECTIVE THERAPEUTIC COMMUNICATION

Nursing Attitudes that Promote Communication

Before an attempt to enter into a therapeutic relationship, it is helpful to know the nursing attitudes that facilitate effective therapeutic communication. These are sometimes referred to as responsive characteristics.

AWARENESS

Awareness of clients is necessary before human relationships with them are possible. Showing awareness is acknowledging the presence of clients. It is best demonstrated by displaying attending behaviors.

Attending behaviors show that the nurse is paying attention to what the client is saying. The nurse demonstrates attending behaviors, for example, by facing the client, leaning toward the client, using appropriate eye contact, keeping eyes open with eyebrows raised, and maintaining an **open body posture,** a body position in which the arms and legs are uncrossed.

ACCEPTANCE, RESPECT, AND UNCONDITIONAL POSITIVE REGARD

Acceptance is an openness to the unique qualities and attributes of individual clients. Acceptance does not mean condoning inappropriate client behaviors. It means that clients are accepted for the persons they are, even if their behavior is undesirable.

Respect is more than an attitude of acceptance. It also includes valuing, highly regarding, or esteeming clients for what they are.

Unconditional positive regard, coined by the psychologist Carl Rogers, describes respect that is not dependent on the client's behavior. For example, as nurses, many of us can value and care for clients because their humanity warrants our care.

This is appropriate because nurses should not be critical, derogatory, or judgmental. We should understand the client's imperfections as part of the total picture, and those behaviors that are undesirable can be understood to be coping mechanisms the client needs at the time. Many clients struggle with dehumanizing aspects of illness and dependency. Nurses empower clients by showing respect, by appreciating their humanness without ridiculing or demeaning them.

Another reason why the nurse should not judge the client is simply that the client should not view the nurse as a judge. Judgment by the nurse sets up a relationship in which the client seeks to please the nurse. This diverts attention from the real business at hand, which is to focus on the client's growth.

EMPATHY

Empathy is the accurate perception of the client's feelings. It is the experience of "being in the other person's shoes" without taking on the client's feelings or thoughts. Empathy is not sympathy wherein the nurse feels sorry for the client. Rather, it is a sense of "being with" the client.

RELATEDNESS

Relatedness is the experience of recognizing similarities between nurse and client and the forging of emotional connections based on them. Relating to clients helps to establish human-to-human ties that make communication possible. Common experiences make nurse and client more easily known to one another.

CARING

Caring is feeling a personal interest in the client's welfare. By investing ourselves in the client, we consciously decide to take emotional risks and give of our skills, compassion, and experience. Such concern can be draining, and the nurse must continually assess personal psychic energy and emotional resources to prevent exhaustion.

OBJECTIVITY

Objectivity is a reality-based sense of the communication process that allows the nurse to attend to the client's thoughts and feelings over his or her own. To be truly objective does not rob the nurse of warmth or feelings for the client, but it does require the nurse to attach an evaluative component to the relationship. Thinking about the client objectively allows the nurse to understand client experiences and to identify areas of difficulty so the client can be guided toward developing appropriate problem-solving skills.

PROTECTIVENESS

Protectiveness leads the nurse to shield the fragile and vulnerable client while he or she recovers from illness. There is a fine line between protectiveness and fostering dependence. Protectiveness is a caring attitude that should be judiciously used while continuing to evaluate the client's capacity to defend the self.

GENUINENESS

Genuineness is the ability of the nurse to be honest, open, and sincere in self-presentation. The phrase "what you see is what you get" describes the demeanor of a genuine person. It is important not to confuse being genuine with being totally self-disclosing or casually spontaneous as one would be with friends or family.

OPENNESS

Being open with a client reflects the ability and willingness of the nurse to be real, genuine, and emotionally accessible. Openness does not mean that boundaries are violated. It means that the nurse chooses what to share with the client and shares it in an authentic manner. When the nurse is open with a client, the client tends to lower defenses and to relate more honestly with the nurse.

PROFESSIONAL CLOSENESS OR DISTANCE

There is a delicate balance between maintaining the objectivity and firm boundaries associated with professional distance and the warmth, openness, and availability associated with professional closeness.

Nurses should be accessible to the clients, but the therapeutic relationship is not a friendship. Friendships are social rather than therapeutic relationships. This does not mean, however, that nurses must be impersonal or treat clients with indifference.

Professional closeness and distance vary throughout the relationship as nurses and clients come together as strangers, work on mutual goals, and proceed to termination. New nurses may feel uncomfortable with attempts at maintaining professional closeness and distance. A good rule to follow is to become invested without being engulfed. This guideline translates to caring about clients and allowing yourself to know their concerns but not taking their thoughts, feelings, or attitudes as your own.

SENSE OF HUMOR

Many have questioned the appropriateness of the use of any form of humor in a therapeutic relationship. Surely, we must avoid certain types of "humor" such as material referred to as morbid humor, humor based on sarcasm, or humor that degrades anyone. This type of material is unfunny and beneath us as professionals. However, we must be open to laugh at ourselves and at the humorous situations that can arise. Being a role model of this openness and demonstrating the appropriate use of humor can be therapeutic for clients just as it is for ourselves.

Thus, appreciation of the humor in life can be a desirable attitude for the nurse. However, the ability to use humor therapeutically is a talent that not all nurses possess. Nurses who are comfortable with the sensitive use of humor can sometimes use it to put clients at ease, defuse emotionally loaded situations, or simply inject a light note into an otherwise difficult day. Such nurses must assess each client's readiness for humor. If the client will perceive any levity as a put-down, it is much better to maintain a more serious demeanor.

Although clients can appreciate wit as much as anyone, they must first feel that the nurse is trustworthy, dependable, and on their side.

Action-oriented Characteristics

In addition to the responsive attitudes discussed previously, the nurse who is to be effective in therapeutic communications must possess three action-oriented characteristics. These characteristics must be used with the responsive attitudes if they are to be effective without alienating the client.

CONCRETENESS

Concreteness refers to communicating concerns in specific and personal language. The nurses can help the client be concrete by role modeling concreteness and by asking the client to remain in the "here and now" during discussions.

The concrete nurse discourages vague or general references to events and seeks information as explicitly as possible. For example, rather than inviting a client to "tell me all about yourself," the nurse might ask the client to "tell me how that affects you personally at this time." Concreteness helps keep communications clear and helps the client cope with experiences in measurable terms.

IMMEDIACY

Immediacy requires direct attention to the specific dynamics existing within the relationship between the nurse and client. If a nurse has difficulty working with a client or if there has been tension in the relationship, it is easier to ignore the conflict and avoid the client. However, this models avoidance for the client and provides no assistance in negotiating human relationships.

To practice immediacy, the nurse speaks with the client to attempt to elicit information about what is interfering with their interactions. For instance, if the nurse had previously reminded the client that it was nearing time for terminating their relationship and the client refused to talk to the nurse after that, the nurse might say, "I've noticed that we've been pretty quiet around each other since our last meeting. I wonder what's going on between us that makes it difficult for us to talk." Note that the nurse does this without focusing on the client or the nurse. Rather the focus is on what is occurring between the two.

CONFRONTATION

Confrontation is the process in which the nurse sensitively points out inconsistencies in a client's behavior. Confrontation is not angry, attacking, or demeaning. Nor should it be used before trust is established. In a therapeutic relationship, the nurse uses confrontation to enlighten the client about inconsistencies in verbal and nonverbal behaviors. For example, the nurse might say, "Your jaw is clenched tight and you are wringing your hands but you told me you were calm. Now I am wondering what it is you really feel."

TECHNIQUES THAT IMPAIR THERAPEUTIC COMMUNICATION

Before you begin to learn about therapeutic techniques, it is imperative that you understand what not to do. This is true because there are so many ways to say things that you cannot be given specific words or phrases that will always be helpful to all people, in all situations, at all times. You can only be given generally accepted guidelines and examples, and you must practice your therapeutic techniques within these guidelines using your own words. It is difficult to know which of your own words might be hurtful, or merely less than helpful, unless you have a good grasp of what should not be done.

It is vital that you recognize nontherapeutic techniques so you can avoid them as you begin to practice using therapeutic techniques.

Nontherapeutic communication techniques impair the flow of communication in what would otherwise be a progressive movement toward client growth. Some nontherapeutic techniques thwart communication by undermining the nurse, for example, by calling into question the nurse's honesty or by diminishing trust in the nurse. Other nontherapeutic techniques thwart communication by undermining the client. Nontherapeutic techniques that undermine the client are those that are demeaning, those that reinforce or strengthen irrational ideas or beliefs, those that tend to raise client anxiety levels, and those that tend to make the client dependent on the nurse. Still other nontherapeutic techniques block the flow of ideas between client and nurse. Some nontherapeutic techniques block communication in more than one way. Brief descriptions of these techniques are listed in Table 24–2, along with selected examples that might be used with clients of different age levels.

TECHNIQUES THAT ENHANCE THERAPEUTIC COMMUNICATION

Maximizing therapeutic communication requires the use of techniques that encourage clients to open up and speak more freely. There are a number of such therapeutic techniques of communication that are generally considered helpful for nurses to use. However, inappropriate use of these techniques can turn them from therapeutic techniques to nontherapeutic techniques, so it is helpful to know what to do and what not to do when using them. Some guidelines follow.

▸ Individualize each technique to your client's level of understanding. For example, you might tell a 30-year-old man, "I'd like some private time with you to focus on some of your personal issues and concerns," whereas, you'd ask a 6-year-old boy, "Can we talk a while, Timmy?"
▸ Vary the therapeutic techniques used. Particularly avoid using any one type of technique repeatedly. For example, saying "I see" shows acceptance of what the client is saying and is therapeutic. However, saying "I see" after everything the client says will quickly show that you are not giving a thoughtful response to each utterance. Too many "I see's (or any other therapeutic technique) can be maddening.
▸ Use paralanguage appropriately to convey your intended meaning. For example, you may say something generally considered to be therapeutic, such as "I see," and say it sarcastically, icily, or in some other way so as to be nontherapeutic. Another nurse may say something generally considered to be nontherapeutic but say it so warmly and with such caring that it is actually therapeutic for the client. Two nurses may say the exact same words and one will

TABLE 24-2. Nontherapeutic Techniques of Communication

Technique	Description/Definition	Example
Reassuring	The nurse implies that the anxious client has no cause for worry or concern.	Nurse with child: "Don't cry. Mommy will come back." Nurse with adolescent: "You have nothing to worry about. Someone will come along who will love you and will make you very happy." Nurse with adult: "Of course you don't have AIDS."
Parroting	The nurse mechanically repeats the client's words without thinking, without evaluating what has been said, and without helping the client to think things through. It indicates a lack of interest, respect, and relatedness on the part of the nurse.	Child: "My puppy died." Nurse: "Your puppy died." Child: "Yes, and I was very sad and I cried. Nurse: "And you were very sad and you cried." Adolescent: "I hate you." Nurse: "You hate me." Adolescent: Yes, all you ever do is repeat what we say to you." Nurse: "All I ever do is repeat what you say to me." Adult: "She's right. All you do is talk like a parrot." Nurse: She's right. All I do is talk like a parrot."
Giving approval	The nurse provides positive sanctions for client thinking or behavior, thereby setting and maintaining standards of good and bad. The client may work to earn the nurse's praise rather than to make progress.	Nurse with child: "You are a good boy." Nurse with adolescent: "I'm happy to hear you made that choice." Nurse with adult: "Your choice was the only correct one."
Rejecting	The nurse refuses to consider, or shows contempt for, the client's thinking. Rejection closes topic to exploration.	Nurse with child: "Don't mention that to me again." Nurse with adolescent: "Don't let me hear any more about . . . " Nurse with adult: "Let's not talk about . . . "
Disapproving	The nurse makes a negative value judgment about the client's behavior or thinking.	Nurse with child: "That was bad to do." Nurse with adolescent: "Let's not have any more of that nonsense." Nurse with adult: "I'm afraid I can't approve of such behavior."
Disagreeing	The nurse opposes the client's thinking. The nurse's disagreement implies the client is wrong and must defend himself or herself.	Nurse with child: "That's not right. That's wrong." Nurse with adolescent: "You may, but I definitely don't believe that side of the story." Nurse with adult: "I don't agree with you on that point."
Advising	The nurse literally tells the client what to do. This implies that the nurse knows best and the client is incapable of independent problem solving.	Nurse with child: "Put all the blue blocks over here and the red blocks over there, and your block house will be prettier." Nurse with adolescent: "You should use acne medication and stop drinking those soft drinks." Nurse with adult: "If I were you, I'd see Dr. Peters about that rash rather than going to your family doctor."
Interrogating	The nurse bombards the client with multiple questions that do not allow the client time for a thoughtful response. The questions interrupt therapeutic communication.	Nurse with child: "Your twin brother fell? When? Where did it happen? How did it happen? Was anyone else there?" Nurse with adolescent: "How did you like your new school? Did all of the other kids dress the same as you? Do you think you were accepted well? Are you going to fit in?" Nurse with adult: "How did you feel after the surgery when they took the bandages off your face? Were you nervous? Did you dread looking in the mirror? Who was with you at the time?"

Table continued on following page

TABLE 24–2. Nontherapeutic Techniques of Communication Continued

Technique	Description/Definition	Example
Probing	The nurse digs for information or persistently questions the client even after the client indicates unwillingness to discuss the issues.	Nurse with child: "Tell me more about Mommy." Nurse with adolescent: "If you trusted me, you'd tell me about what happened on your first date." Nurse with adult: "Tell me about your history of alcohol abuse."
Challenging	The nurse insists the client provide a rational basis for irrational thinking. The client then becomes defensive, and issues are closed to exploration.	Nurse with child: "If there is a monster in the closet, why don't I see it?" Nurse with adolescent: "How can you be Elvis Presley when he is dead?" Nurse with adult: "If you really have no legs, how can you walk up here to the nurses' station?"
Testing	The nurse tests the client's capacity for insight by first assuming that the client has no insight and then expecting the client to agree.	Nurse with child: "What color do you think this red ball is?" Nurse with adolescent: "Do you know where you are yet?" Nurse with adult: "Are you still clinging to the idea that . . . ?"
Defending	The nurse protects someone or something from attack by the client, thereby implying that the client has no right to express feelings or judgments.	Nurse with child: "Your mom does the best she can." Nurse with adolescent: "Mr. Brown is a very good teacher." Nurse with adult: "This hospital has the best food in the area, no matter what people say."
Requesting an explanation	The nurse asks "why" of the client, thereby asking for a reason for feelings and behaviors when the client may not know the reason.	Nurse with child: "Why did you do that?" Nurse with adolescent: "Why are you angry?" Nurse with adult: "Why do you see it that way?"
Indicating the existence of an external source	The nurse implies that the client is compelled to think or behave in a certain way by a source outside of the client.	Nurse with child: "What made you behave so poorly?" Nurse with adolescent: "Who gave you the idea you could get away with that?" Nurse with adult: "What gave you that idea?"
Belittling feelings expressed	The nurse minimizes the degree of the client's distress or discomfort, thereby implying that the client's feelings are insignificant.	Child: "I'm very mad." Nurse: "Everybody in this room is very mad." Adolescent: "My life is over." Nurse: "Every teenager thinks that at one time or another." Adult: "I just gave up on my marriage." Nurse: "I've given up on mine a thousand times. These things happen."
Making stereotypical comments	The nurse makes empty conversation using trite phrases and clichés, thereby encouraging the client to do the same rather than honestly exploring issues.	Nurse with child: "This is for your own good." Nurse with adolescent: "Have a nice day." Nurse with adult: "Nice weather, isn't it?"
Stereotyping	The nurse reduces persons to generalized categories and ignores or minimizes their unique experiences, perspectives, and gifts. Stereotyping according to gender, race, social class, diagnosis, religion, or occupation are personal biases that offend most clients and can disrupt chances for a therapeutic relationship.	Nurse with child: "You're 6 years old and all 6-year-olds need a daily nap. Lay down and go to sleep." Nurse with adolescent: "You are just weepy; all women get that way just before that time of the month." Nurse with adult: "It is disease X that makes you so needy and demanding."
Giving literal responses	The nurse responds to the client's figurative statement as though it were factual. The nurse misses a chance to explore material with the client.	Child: "I'm a firecracker." Nurse: "It's better than being a Christmas tree." Adolescent: "There's a radio playing in my head." Nurse: "Turn it down." Adult: "Everyone is staring at me." Nurse: "Just stare back."

TABLE 24–2. Nontherapeutic Techniques of Communication Continued

Technique	Description/Definition	Example
Using denial	The nurse refuses to acknowledge that a problem exists, thereby cutting off exploration of the problem with the client and denying the validity of the client's perceptions.	Child: "My uncle does bad things to me." Nurse: "That's not possible!" Adolescent: "I'm going to be dead in the morning." Nurse: "No, you won't be." Adult: "I'm not going to be able to stop drinking." Nurse: "Of course, you will."
Rationalizing feelings expressed	The nurse provides a seemingly rational (but untrue) excuse for the client's expression of emotions in order to avoid an emotional reaction to the client's feelings or to avoid having to respond appropriately to the client. This rationalization of the feelings robs affective material shared by the client of its power.	Child with tears: "Mrs. Nurse, I just saw Bambi on TV." Nurse: "And the light from the TV in that dark room is making your eyes smart. You'd better go to bed and rest them." Nurse to adolescent with tears: "Carla, you seem overly tired. Get some sleep and I'm sure you'll feel better." Adult with tears: "I can't get over this relationship." Nurse: "You are just overly sensitive; your hormone shot is due. I'll get it for you."
Interpreting	The nurse attempts to tell the client the meaning of the client's experience by seeking to make conscious that which is unconscious.	Nurse with child: "What you wish you could say is . . ." Nurse with adolescent: "What you really believe down deep is . . ." Nurse with adult: "Subconsciously, you feel . . ."
Blaming	The nurse inappropriately expresses feelings of anger or impatience with the client as a means of faulting the client because the nurse-client relationship is not progressing well. This is a therapeutic dead-end that negates the nurse's role as a client advocate, destroys trust, and takes away client motivation to work with the nurse to identify and explore sensitive topics.	Nurse with child: "Of course, your daddy didn't come to visit. What did you expect after the way you acted last time he was here?" Nurse with adolescent: "So you have a mustache just in time for the senior prom. That's what you get for going on birth control pills." Nurse with adult: "I know the pain is bad when I have to try to turn you, but it was you who climbed up on that ladder and risked breaking a hip, not me."
Patronizing	The nurse treats the client in a condescending manner, thereby demeaning the client. This makes acceptance, respect, and mutual decision making impossible.	Nurse with child: "Okay, Mary, we all heard you spell 'cat' at least 17 times. Now go play somewhere. Nurse with adolescent: "Thank you for your insightful comments. We'll take them under advisement, dear." Nurse with adult: "You want a pass for tomorrow? Well now, we'll just have to forget that idea."
Dogmatism	The nurse offers opinionated assertions of a tenet or belief as fact and will allow no compromise with the beliefs of the client. The client must choose between obeying or defying the nurse, and the opportunity to explore feelings and choices is lost.	Nurse with girl: "Avoid all men when you grow up. None of them are any good. Just look at your father as an example." Nurse with adolescent: "Girls who wear make-up at your age are just asking for it." Nurse with adult: "I'm afraid I cannot allow your husband to visit. He abused you once and he'll do it again."
Moralizing	The nurse judges the client according to personal moral values. Because the client must feel free to discuss issues within the therapeutic relationship, this moralizing oversteps appropriate limits and places the relationship in jeopardy.	Nurse with child: "You don't go to church every Sunday? What kind of family are you from?" Nurse with adolescent: "You have smoked marijuana! And you look so sweet and innocent too." Nurse with adult: "You and your husband actually went to a nudist colony? I didn't think such evil actually existed!"

Table continued on following page

TABLE 24-2. Nontherapeutic Techniques of Communication Continued

Technique	Description/Definition	Example
Introducing an unrelated topic	The nurse changes the subject when the client brings up material the nurse prefers not to discuss.	Child: "That doctor was mean." Nurse: "What did you eat for breakfast?"
		Adolescent: "I'm not taking that pill." Nurse: "Did you talk to your girlfriend today?"
		Adult: "I wish I could die." Nurse: "What dress are you wearing today?"
Using jargon	The nurse excludes the client and makes the interaction incomprehensible by using nursing jargon (the specialized language used by a group)	Nurse with child: "Micturate before retiring to prevent enuresis."
		Nurse with adolescent: "Your neck is uncomfortable because you have a malaligned cervical vertebra that results in forward flexion and associated discomfort [crick in the neck]."
		Nurse with adult: "Ingestion of a cholecystocholangiographic medium [gallbladder pills] is necessary."

be seen as a helpful nurse, whereas the other is not. In such cases, it may be paralanguage that makes the difference.

► If you are using therapeutic techniques correctly, your client will be doing most of the talking as you listen and guide the interaction. If you find you are doing most of the talking, something is wrong and you need to pause and reflect about how to get back on track.

► You will probably make mistakes in talking with clients and say some things that are not the best possible responses. In fact, there may be times you will want to bite your tongue off because you said something so nontherapeutic. However, if you have a genuinely therapeutic relationship with the client, the relationship will be able to withstand an error or two.

► As you enter the clinical area to talk with a client for the first time, relax and realize that most clients want very much to talk to you.

► Any specific technique of communication might be used at any time, according to the client and the situation, but some techniques tend to be more helpful at the beginning of an interaction and some tend to be more helpful in the middle or at the end of an interaction.

Techniques Often Helpful at the Beginning of an Interaction

OFFERING SELF

Offering self is a technique in which the nurse offers to stay with the client and either talk or just sit quietly. In offering self, the nurse clearly establishes parameters for the amount of time offered. For example, "I have 20 minutes available to talk with you at one o'clock today" or "I'll stay with you while you wait for

the surgeon." Additional examples are found in Table 24-3.

In some cases, it is therapeutic to give the person a choice about your offer: for example, "Would you like to meet with me for 20 minutes at one o'clock today?" However, some persons, such as those who are depressed, very much need to have you with them but will tend to reject your offer. Others should not be asked to make decisions about anything because it raises their anxiety level. As you learn more and more about such persons and their individual needs, you will learn who can be asked and who should just be told that you are there for them. Until you do know, or if you are ever in doubt, it is always safe to offer without allowing a choice.

Offering self can be very helpful when you are talking with someone who seems unable to express his or her thoughts or who does not want to talk at the moment. You can say something like, "It is okay if you don't feel like talking right now. I'll just stay here with you for 10 minutes." Be sure that, if you say you will stay for a period of time, you do follow through and stay for as long as you said you would. This helps establish you as someone who can be trusted.

PROVIDING BROAD OPENINGS

Early in a meeting with a client, it may be useful to provide a broad opening. In this case, the nurse invites the client to select a topic for discussion. Here, too, it is therapeutic to set some parameters in regard to what you are willing to discuss. For example, in most instances, it would not be helpful for the client to discuss personal information about you or for you to engage in social level small talk with the client. Therefore, it is not always appropriate to say, "We can talk about anything you like." It is better to say, for example, "We

TABLE 24-3. *Therapeutic Techniques of Communication*

Technique	Description/Definition	Example
Offering self	The nurse offers to stay with the client and either talk or just sit quietly.	Nurse with child: "Let me sit with you for 15 minutes and read a story." Nurse with adolescent: "I'd like to eat lunch with you." Nurse with adult: "Let's walk to the cafeteria together."
Providing broad openings	The nurse invites the client to select a topic.	Nurse with child: "What would you like to tell me about yourself?" Nurse with adolescent: "Tell me what's been on your mind." Nurse with adult: "I'm interested in hearing about issues of concern to you."
Making an observation	The nurse acknowledges that something or someone exists or has changed in some way.	Nurse with child: "You've drawn a picture." Nurse with adolescent: "That's a new hair style, isn't it?" Nurse with adult: "I noticed on your chart that today is your birthday."
Suggesting collaboration	The nurse makes an offer to work together with the client.	Nurse with child: "Let's try to figure this out together." Nurse with adolescent: "Let's talk and see if we can work together to understand this." Nurse with adult: "Perhaps we can discuss this and see what offended you."
Providing silence	The nurse allows the verbal conversation to stop to provide a time for quiet contemplation of what has been discussed, for formulation of thoughts about how to proceed, or for tension reduction.	(Silence)
Accepting messages	The nurse acknowledges that he or she has heard and understood what the client has said.	Nurse with child: (Smiling) "Um-hmm." Nurse with adolescent: (Nodding) "I hear what you're saying." Nurse with adult: "I understand."
Providing general leads	The nurse provides brief interjections that let the client know that he or she is on the right track and should continue.	Nurse with child: "Then what?" Nurse with adolescent: "Please go on." Nurse with adult: "And . . . ?"
Exploring	The nurse asks the client to describe something in more detail or to discuss it more fully.	Nurse with child: "You said you liked Billy best. Can you tell me about Billy?" Nurse with adolescent: "You say you get more satisfaction out of helping out at the flower shop. I'd like to hear more about that." Nurse with adult: "These dreams you mentioned, what are they like?"
Focusing	The nurse selects one topic for exploration from among several possible topics presented by the client.	Nurse with child: "You said you hate all of your brothers. Tell me about Melvin first." Nurse with adolescent: "You've briefly mentioned three different suicide attempts. For now, I'd like to focus on just what was going on with you at the time of the first attempt." Nurse with adult: "Let's return to the last point you made and talk more about that."
Asking for clarification	The nurse lets the client know that what was said was unclear. If necessary, the nurse asks for clarification or provides input regarding how to make the message clearer.	Nurse with child: "I'm sorry. I can't give you a kissen because I don't know what a kissen is. Is it like a hug and kiss?" Nurse with adolescent: "I didn't understand what you meant then. Can you say that in different words?" Nurse with adult: "Let me repeat back to you what I think I heard you say."

Table continued on following page

TABLE 24-3. Therapeutic Techniques of Communication Continued

Technique	Description/Definition	Example
Restating	The nurse paraphrases what the client has said. This paraphrased message may be fed back to the client in the form of a statement or a question to provide the client the opportunity to agree or to disagree and clarify further.	Child: "Ugh! That's poo poo!" Nurse: "The medicine tastes pretty bad, huh?" Adolescent: "I called Ralph on the big white porcelain telephone." Nurse: "You vomited." Adult: "I'm down." Nurse: "You feel depressed?"
Seeking consensual validation	The nurse attempts to verify with the client that a certain term means the same thing to both parties.	Nurse with child: "You want 'moo moo'? Does 'moo moo' mean milk?" Nurse with adolescent: "When you say your brother is crazy, does the word "crazy" mean 'kind of wild'?" Nurse with adult: "Tell me if we both understand that word the same way."
Placing events in time or sequence	The nurse asks the client to explain more about when an event occurred (placing the event in time) or to explain the sequence of a series of events (placing events in sequence) to clarify for the nurse.	Nurse with child: "Were you frightened before or after the movie?" Nurse with adolescent: "Tell me what went on before the fight broke out in the gym?" Nurse with adult: "Did you go to the women's shelter after the beating but before you came to the hospital or did he find you at the shelter and beat you?"
Verbalizing the implied	The nurse voices what is understood to be the client's underlying meaning in a message.	Child: "Nobody here will want to play with me." Nurse: "Do you think they won't like you?" Adolescent: "It doesn't do any good to tell you or the doctor my problems." Nurse: "Do you think we can't help you?" Adult: "Don't bother to try to call my son and tell him I am in the hospital." Nurse: "Are you saying your son doesn't care?"
Encouraging assessment of emotions	The nurse asks the client to focus on his or her feelings to get in touch with emotions.	Nurse with child: "When that happens, do you feel good or bad?" Nurse with adolescent: "How do you feel when that happens?" Nurse with adult: "What are your feelings right now?"
Translating into feelings	The nurse translates the client's message into a verbal expression of feelings.	Child: "I feel all black inside." Nurse: "That sounds lonely and scary." Adolescent: "My life is over." Nurse: "You sound like you feel hopeless." Adult: "I'm off in outer space." Nurse: "Would you say you're feeling disconnected?"
Reflecting	The client asks a question and the nurse turns the question around and reflects it back to the client or the client makes a statement and the nurse selects one or more words to reflect back to the client for consideration. The purpose is to strengthen the client's confidence.	Child: "Should I eat peas or carrots?" Nurse: "Which would you like to eat?" Adolescent: "What would you do if your mother wouldn't let you cut your hair?" Nurse: "What do you think would be the most reasonable approach?" Adult: "What would you do in that case?" Nurse: "What would you do?"

TABLE 24-3. Therapeutic Techniques of Communication Continued

Technique	Description/Definition	Example
Encouraging comparison	The nurse asks the client to compare or contrast a certain experience with other experiences to help the client integrate a new experience into life.	Nurse with child: "How was your mom different from last time?" Nurse with adolescent: "Has this ever happened before?" Nurse with adult: "Is this marriage similar to your first one?"
Encouraging descriptions of perceptions	The nurse asks the client to describe perceptions and associated emotions. This is particularly useful in understanding a client's experiences during hallucinations.	Nurse with child: "How do you feel when you think the big ape under the bed might grab you?" Nurse with adolescent: "What did the voice tell you to do that frightened you so?" Nurse with adult: "How do you feel when you hear the voices?"
Voicing doubt	The nurse questions how something the client has misperceived could possibly be true. This is done by questioning the truthfulness of what was perceived without questioning the truthfulness of the client.	Nurse with child: "Isn't that strange?" Nurse with adolescent: "It is hard for me to imagine that." Nurse with adult: "That is something I find difficult to believe."
Presenting reality	When a client has had an unrealistic perception of reality, the nurse accepts the fact that the client has perceived something but indicates that the nurse did not have a similar perception. When something in the environment is stimulating the misperception, the nurse attempts to point this out.	Nurse with child: "I don't see any monsters in the closet." Nurse with adolescent: "No. I didn't hear a ghostly wail, but I did think I heard a train whistle off in the distance." Nurse with adult: "I didn't see a walrus in the corner. Maybe the way this blanket is draped on the chair made it look like a walrus with the light low like it is."
Encouraging formulation of a plan of action	The nurse asks the client to consider, in advance, what might be the best thing to do in a future situation should the occasion arise. The purpose of the technique is to allow the client to think things out in advance and to be prepared.	Nurse with child: "Next time you get mad, what would be a better way to let me know?" Nurse with adolescent: "What do you think might be a better way to approach your parents next time?" Nurse with adult: "If you become suicidal again in the future, how could you handle it safely?"
Summarizing	The nurse briefly states, in an orderly manner, what has been discussed. The purpose is to help ensure that client and nurse are in agreement about what went on and what decisions were made, to help ensure that nothing was omitted, and to bring the relationship to closure.	Nurse with child: "Okay, we agreed that you will take your medicine when the cartoons are over." Nurse with adolescent; "In the past half hour we have talked about several possible ways you could handle this. These are . . . " Nurse with adult: "When we first met, you were afraid you were never going to get over your depression. As we progressed, you began to take charge of your life. Now you are . . . "

can discuss any issues of concern to you." The latter is a very broad opening that still focuses on the client.

MAKING AN OBSERVATION

In making an observation, the nurse acknowledges that something or someone exists or has changed in some way. The nurse makes an observation without appearing to judge either positively or negatively. When the observation pertains to the client, this technique may be termed *giving recognition*. However, the term *recognition* is less desirable because it may be miscon-

strued to mean that the client is receiving approval or praise from the nurse. The acknowledgment made by the nurse who is making an observation should open up communication about the subject at hand but not provide the client with any specific positive reinforcement.

SUGGESTING COLLABORATION

Suggesting collaboration is a technique in which the nurse offers to work together with the client. This technique is useful in beginning a relationship with a client because it establishes that the nurse and client will work together as a team. Initially, the work may be to discuss some of the issues of concern to the client. Later, as problems are identified and nursing diagnoses made, the work may be to establish and meet client outcomes. At all times, the work focuses on the client.

Techniques Often Helpful as an Interaction Progresses

PROVIDING SILENCE

Providing silence in a therapeutic manner is allowing the verbal conversation to stop to provide a time for quiet contemplation of what has been discussed or for formulation of thoughts about how to proceed. This can also provide a time for tension reduction when the interaction has been concerned with powerful issues and when emotions have been particularly deep.

Many persons are uncomfortable with silence and will talk continuously about nothing just to break it. This is obviously not a therapeutic approach for the nurse to take. If you find that you are uncomfortable with silence, think about what is going on during the silence, and use it constructively to think about what you will say next. You will find that, with practice, you can become more and more comfortable with silence.

ACCEPTING MESSAGES

Accepting messages is a way of providing feedback to acknowledge to the client that the nurse has heard and understood what has been said. The acknowledgment is done in a manner that is neutral in tone, without the nurse agreeing, disagreeing, or providing any judgments about the message. The accepting may be done verbally or nonverbally. Your method of accepting messages should be brief and should allow the client to continue on with a train of thought without any real interruption.

PROVIDING GENERAL LEADS

In ordinary social communications, people are used to taking turns in communicating. Therefore, after your clients have spoken for awhile, they may hesitate because they are uncertain whether it is appropriate to continue, or they may try to draw you into the conversation to give you "your turn." It is the nurse's task to keep clients focused on their own issues and to ensure that they continue to feel comfortable discussing them. To do this, you may use the technique of providing general leads. General leads are brief interjections that let clients know that they are on the right track and should continue. The leads provided should not cause real interruptions in the train of thought as they urge clients forward.

EXPLORING

As clients are talking, they may mention something that you believe is significant enough to warrant further at-

tention. If they have brought the subject up and have not indicated that further discussion is undesirable, it is appropriate to attempt to delve into the matter in greater detail. To do this, the nurse uses the technique of exploring. To explore, you ask the client to describe something in more detail or to discuss it more fully.

When you use exploring with clients, be careful not to use the nontherapeutic technique of probing. That is, if your client gives any indication that further discussion is off limits, honor this and use another technique such as providing a general lead to get them to continue with what they were saying.

FOCUSING

Often as clients are talking with nurses, they will come to a point at which they provide a great deal of meaningful information in a very short amount of time. It may seem that several topics seem worth exploring, but, of course, this cannot all be done at once. In such instances, it is helpful to select one subject to explore further and to keep the other subjects in mind for future discussion. Selecting one subject for exploration from among several is termed *focusing*.

For example, an adult client might say, "My sister died when I was 7. She was only 4 years old. My alcoholic father had been drinking and killed her in an automobile accident. My mother was so grief stricken and felt so guilty that she had failed to prevent the accident that she had to have several series of electroshock treatments for depression. It seems she was always away in the hospital." How do you decide which point to explore? You may decide to focus on how the client felt about losing a sibling at the age of 7, about having a father who was an alcoholic, about the fact that the death was the father's fault, about the absences of the mother during her hospitalizations, or about how one or more of these factors affected the way the others in the family related to the client.

If you focus on any one point, you can always return to other points at a later time. You might prepare the client for this by making an observation, focusing, and then requesting further exploration in the future. For example, you might say, "You have given me a great deal to think about and much of it seems worth talking about [making an observation]. For now, I'd like to hear what went on with you at the time of your sister's death [focusing], and later on, perhaps we can explore some of the subsequent events [requesting further exploration in the future]."

Techniques Often Helpful in Keeping Communication Clear

ASKING FOR CLARIFICATION

Sometimes clients say things that lack clarity, have more than one specific meaning, or are simply vague. These types of messages can garble communication. When this is the case, a number of techniques can be used to help clarify the message for both the nurse and the client. The most straightforward technique is asking for clarification. Simply let the client know that you are not certain about what was said, and, if necessary, request that the client clarify anything that is obscure. If the client does not understand what was unclear, you may have to tell the person how it could be clarified for you. For example, if you are unsure whether the client said "The thing I liked best in that country was the prints" or "The thing I liked best in that country was the prince," you may have to ask the client to spell the word — prints or prince — or define it.

RESTATING

Another way to clarify is to use the therapeutic technique of restating. This is paraphrasing what the client has said. To do this, you take the client's words and alter them so that the meaning is the same as what you understand the client's meaning to be but you use somewhat different words. You may feed this back to the client in the form of a statement or a question, and provide the client the opportunity to agree that this was the intended message or to disagree and to clarify further.

SEEKING CONSENSUAL VALIDATION

Sometimes, when a certain term used by a client has been unclear, the nurse can use the technique of seeking consensual validation to help ensure that both client and nurse agree on the meaning of the term. For example, a female client might say, "I'm blue." The client might mean that her skin is literally blue from cold or that she is feeling sad. In such a case, the nurse might believe one meaning of the word to be the one intended and seek to verify whether this was, in fact, the client's meaning. For example, the nurse might ask, "When you used the word 'blue,' I believe that you meant 'sad' or 'depressed.' Is that correct?" The client then has the opportunity to agree or disagree and to clarify further.

PLACING EVENTS IN TIME OR SEQUENCE

Often in describing an event or a series of events, clients fail to relate the story in strict chronologic order. This can make the client's message about the occurrence difficult to follow. When this happens, the nurse can ask the client to explain more about when the event occurred (placing the event in time) or to explain the sequence of a series of events (placing events in sequence).

Techniques that Can Help the Client Gain Increased Self-Awareness

VERBALIZING THE IMPLIED

With the technique of verbalizing the implied, the nurse understands the words that the client has said but believes that the words have an underlying meaning that was hinted at but not voiced specifically. The nurse verbalizes this underlying message. The client may then verify that the message the nurse received was indeed true. This frees the client to discuss with the nurse some underlying feelings that had not been voiced before.

It is always possible, however, that the client did not mean to imply anything more than the actual words expressed. Verbalizing the implied allows the client to clarify, if the nurse has an inaccurate perception of the communication.

ENCOURAGING ASSESSMENT OF EMOTIONS

It is important for people to be in touch with their own feelings. Too often, to cope with overwhelming feelings, clients wall themselves off from all emotions. This can be very unhealthy. To help clients get back in touch with their feelings, the nurse can use the technique of encouraging assessment of emotions. To do this, the nurse asks clients to focus on their feelings and asks them how they feel.

TRANSLATING INTO FEELINGS

Sometimes clients find it difficult or impossible to express their feelings verbally using appropriate terms for common emotions. The nurse can help the client by translating their messages into verbal expressions of feelings. The nurse should always be open to correction if the client finds the translation to be inaccurate.

REFLECTING

Reflecting is a technique whereby questions and statements are reflected back to the client to assist him or her in thinking about them and coming to a conclusion. This helps the client gain confidence in making assessments and decisions and encourages the client's self-reliance.

There are two forms of reflection. One form is used when the client asks a question and the question is turned around and reflected back to the client. For example, the client might ask, "Do you think I have been making enough progress to go home for a pass this weekend?", and the nurse might reflect back with, "Do you think you have?" This shows that the nurse values the client's opinion.

The second form reflects back to the client some of the client's own words. This should not be confused with parroting, in which all of the client's words are directed back, without thought on the part of the nurse. With reflection, however, the nurse does think about the message and selects the word or words that are important for the client to think about. This requires active involvement on the part of both client and nurse. For example, the client might say, "I have always hated my brother." With parroting, the nurse would reply, "You have always hated your brother." With reflection, the nurse might reply, "Hated?" and suggest that the client think about that word and perhaps reconsider it or discuss it further. Alternatively, the nurse might reflect back with the word, "Always?" and cause the client to think back to a time when perhaps no hard feelings existed toward the brother.

ENCOURAGING COMPARISON

To help clients integrate new experiences into what they know of life and to help them learn, the nurse can encourage comparison. To do this, the nurse may ask the client to compare or contrast a certain experience with some other experiences in life.

Techniques Helpful When Contact with Reality Is Impaired

ENCOURAGING DESCRIPTIONS OF PERCEPTIONS

Sometimes clients perceive things that others do not. It is helpful if the nurse can ask the client to describe such perceptions and the emotions attached to them. This is the technique of encouraging descriptions of perceptions. This technique is suitable when working with clients who have hallucinations of various types.

It is not recommended that you attempt to communicate with a client who is actively hallucinating. If you know that this is happening, wait until the hallucination has ended.

VOICING DOUBT

Sometimes clients have a misperception of reality. You know that it is nontherapeutic to disagree with clients because it strengthens their resolve to convince you that they are correct. So what do you do when clients tell you they see something that is not there and ask whether you also see it? One thing you can do is use the therapeutic technique of voicing doubt. To do this, you do not agree or disagree. You accept the fact that they have perceived something that you have not perceived, but you let them know that you have difficulty understanding how their perception could be real. You do not doubt them, but you do doubt the reality of their perception.

For example, thousands of persons have reported seeing unidentified flying objects. Are all of these persons hallucinating? Such persons, regardless of what they have perceived, should understand that it is difficult for you to believe that flying saucers exist because you have never seen one. They should also be made to understand that, although you may question the validity of their perceptions, you still accept them as persons of worth. Therefore, it is always the reality of the perception that is questioned and never the person's truthfulness about the perception. Say, for example, "I just can't believe such a thing could be," not "I just can't believe you."

PRESENTING REALITY

When faced with situations in which clients are with you when a misperception of reality occurs, you can be the person who can help these clients identify what is

real and what is not. This is termed presenting reality. Presenting reality can be very reassuring to some persons. To use this technique, as with voicing doubt, you accept the fact that they have perceived something that you have not perceived, but you let them know that you did not have a similar perception. You might say, for example, "It must be very frightening for you to see a dead person over there on the pool table but I don't see anything there."

If something in the environment is obviously being misperceived, it is therapeutic to try to make a correction about that as well. For example, someone might hear sounds coming from a nearby room and believe that others are in there talking. You could present reality by saying, "A radio is playing in there. That might account for the voices that you heard."

Techniques Often Helpful Near the End of an Interaction

ENCOURAGING FORMULATION OF A PLAN OF ACTION

Once you are into the working phase of the relationship and you and the client have identified problems, diagnoses, and desired outcomes, you need to encourage formulation of a plan of action. Note that, in using this technique, you encourage the client to formulate the plan. It is much more therapeutic and much more likely to be successfully carried out if the plan comes from the client rather than from you or others.

To encourage formulation of a plan of action, you ask the client to consider, in advance, what might be the best thing to do in a future situation should the occasion arise. The situation that is anticipated might be one that the client has never experienced, or it might be one that the client has experienced but was not able to handle successfully. This allows the client to think things out in advance and to be prepared.

This technique may also be used near the end of a relationship in which the client has had an opportunity to try out a plan and has not been successful. After evaluating with the client what went wrong, the nurse might suggest formulation of a new plan of action. This helps the client to see that new approaches can always be tried.

SUMMARIZING

One therapeutic technique that might be done at intervals is summarizing. Most often, the nurse summarizes by briefly stating, in an orderly manner, what has been discussed. One usually thinks of this as a final activity, but if a client presents a great deal of data to you, or you and the client have discussed many options, it is often helpful to summarize briefly at opportune times. Such summaries help ensure that you and the client are in agreement about what went on and what decisions were made. They also help to ensure that you covered all of the information you both wanted to discuss. As a final activity in a longer term relationship, summarizing can help bring closure as you terminate.

One Technique that Must Occur Throughout the Interaction: Active Listening

Listening is how we receive spoken and other auditory information. Listening is an integral part of communication. **Positive listening** is simply understanding the auditory messages sent by a sender. It can be tremendously comforting to be listened to when we are lonely, frightened, and doubtful. In **active listening,** the nurse takes an active part by eliciting details from the client and by inviting the client to think more about what is being said. It is more than positive listening.

Active listening is a means of "being with" the client and indicating acceptance and agreement. It is an art. It is the key to therapeutic interaction. To use it, you must understand and use all of the other therapeutic techniques of communication. Compare the following two examples.

Passive listening:
- Client: "My mom died when I was 5."
- Nurse: "Hmm."
- Client: "I never got over it."
- Nurse: "I see."

Active listening:
- Client: "My mom died when I was 5."
- Nurse: "You were very young to lose your mother."
- Client: "I never got over it."
- Nurse: "I wonder what it was like for you."
- Client: "My father thought that trying to raise six kids was too much and that is what killed her. I was the sixth kid."
- Nurse: (With a concerned tone of voice) "Your father blamed you for killing your mother?"
- Client: "He's hated me ever since."

Note how the active listening brought out details not available to the passive listener. This is truly the basis for a therapeutic interaction.

EFFECTIVE COMMUNICATION WITH DIFFERENT GROUPS

Nurses must develop effective communication skills to enhance their work with clients of different age groups, of different cultures, and at different stages of health.

Developmental Differences

As has been mentioned, communication techniques must be appropriate for the client's stage of development, or communication can be diminished. Examples of how to apply therapeutic techniques to children, adolescents, and adults of all ages have been provided in Table 24–3. For additional information on specific developmental stages, see Chapters 12, 13, and 14.

Cultural Differences

Clients from different cultures may or may not speak a different language but will most often have differing customs, values, mores, and social structures, all of which can affect communication. Obviously, the more you understand about the culture of your client, the better you will be able to communicate. Learning crucial words and sentences can be very helpful, as can having a translator write out cards with bilingual sentences. However, understanding the non-native client requires more than just learning a few new phrases. You must be aware of any personal biases to avoid stereotyping and labeling clients. Respect for the client's experience and acceptance of the differences that exist between you can help to establish a safe, therapeutic environment in which maximum communication can occur.

Gender Differences

Men and women communicate differently, and understanding those differences enhances therapeutic relationships. Deborah Tannen, a popular author and communication expert, pointed out that men and women have different styles of intimacy and independence.[33] According to Tannen, men seek dominance in a hierarchical structure to be independent; women avoid being dependent and subordinate but do not need to dominate. Intimacy to women means a free sharing of thoughts, hopes, and feelings. Men avoid such sharing to preserve personal freedom.[33]

Tannen's theories can help the nurse to negotiate hierarchy and power issues delicately when talking with persons of both genders. For example, Tannen referred to *rapport talk* and *report talk*. Rapport talk, more comfortable to women, is a way of connecting with others and negotiating relationships. Report talk, the demonstration of knowledge and skill, is the preferred conversational style of men. Women speak to connect. Men speak to preserve status and independence.[33] The nurse must recognize the validity of both styles. A respectful awareness that gender affects style as well as a willingness to "read between the lines" promotes more effective communication with both sexes.

The Hearing Impaired

Those who are hearing impaired have special problems to be overcome. Hearing loss can range from mild to profound. Clients may be deaf or hard of hearing since birth, or they may lose all or part of their hearing at a later time as a result of trauma, illness, or aging. The greatest incidence of hearing loss occurs in individuals 65 years of age and older.

Because hearing is especially important in decoding spoken messages, its loss presents a challenge to both nurse and client. The client with a profound hearing loss may have an inability to speak clearly or may have an excellent speaking ability, usually depending on whether the hearing loss occurred before or after speech was mastered. If speech is not understandable, the nurse will also have difficulty decoding the client's messages.

If some residual hearing remains, the client will usually wear a hearing aid. To increase communications with persons with hearing aids, be certain the aid is fine-tuned to the correct volume for the client, that the batteries in the aid are fresh, and that the aid is turned on.

For either clients with aids or those who are unable to hear, even with an aid, it is helpful if the nurse follows some basic guidelines, as follows:

▶ Assess the profoundly hearing impaired client for sign language skills. If the client uses signing, ascertain whether the client needs a sign language interpreter and obtain one, if available and necessary. Hospitals should have sign language interpreters available to translate for the hearing impaired, but these persons are often volunteers who are on call and are not readily available around the clock.

▶ Ensure that the client can see you as you speak by providing adequate lighting and by standing in front of the client.

▶ As you speak, enunciate words clearly as you would for any hearing person (e.g., do not say "jeet?" when you mean "Did you eat?") but do not exaggerate lip movements.

▶ When the client cannot understand you by reading your lips, try gestures, pantomime, or writing notes.

▶ Always have plenty of paper and pens available for notes.

Do not shout at the hearing impaired. This can be painful to the ear and can actually result in additional loss of residual hearing they might have. If they have no residual hearing, they will not be able to hear you even if you do shout. Also, shouting will cause distortions in your facial features that can prevent them from reading your lips.

The Visually Impaired

Visually impaired clients receive messages via speech effectively but lose nonverbal communications such as facial expressions, body posture, hand gestures, and nods or shakes of the head. Visually impaired clients need support to negotiate new environments, and the nurse should describe new places to provide orientation.

Touch is often important to prevent feelings of isolation. Other senses should also be used as necessary to maximize communication, just as is true with sighted individuals.

Do not shout at the visually impaired. They are not hearing impaired, but your shouting could damage their hearing.

The Dying

Clients who are dying have special communication needs. Depending on the cause of the impending death and the stage of dying, the client may be fearful, in pain, and unable to communicate or totally calm, oriented, and able to participate. The situation determines the strategy.

Soft voice tones, gentle touch, and soft lighting may increase the client's comfort and reduce anxiety. It is also often comforting to have significant others near when possible and desired by the client. They may be needed to interpret for the client.

Respect, empathy, acceptance, and flexibility are particularly important qualities for the nurse to bring to the interaction. Dying is private, and the nurse should accede to the client's wishes as much as possible. Remind family members and friends that hearing is the last sense to be lost before death is final, so they may continue to speak to the client even when a response is not possible.

Summary

▶ The three phases of the therapeutic relationship are the orientation phase, the working phase, and the termination phase. Each phase has certain tasks associated with it.

▶ Process recordings are verbatim records of a nurse-client interaction. The student, the instructor, the client, and the graduate nurse may benefit by their use.

▶ The six elements of communication are encoder, message, sensory channel, decoder, feedback, and context.

▶ Theorists who contributed to an understanding of the nurse, the client, and communication include Peplau, Travelbee, Satir, and Watzlawick.

▶ Four main forms of verbal communication are talking, written communication, sign language, and Braille.

▶ Body language is a form of nonverbal communication that consists of human communication by alterations in personal appearance, changes in facial expressions, changes in body posture, use of gestures, maintenance of personal distances, and use of touching; paralanguage is a form of nonverbal communication that consists of the elements of stress, accent, pitch, pause, intonation, rate, volume, and quality.

▶ Responsive characteristics (nursing attitudes) that facilitate effective therapeutic communication include awareness, acceptance, respect, unconditional positive regard, empathy, relatedness, caring, objectivity, protectiveness, genuineness, openness, appropriate professional closeness or distance, and sense of humor; action-oriented characteristics that facilitate effective therapeutic communication include concreteness, immediacy, and confrontation.

▶ It is vital to recognize nontherapeutic communication techniques so they may be avoided while beginning to learn and practice therapeutic techniques.

▶ Inappropriate use of therapeutic communication techniques can turn them from therapeutic techniques into nontherapeutic techniques so it is important to adhere to the guidelines for their correct use.

▶ Although any specific therapeutic technique might be used at any time, according to the client and the situation, some techniques tend to be more helpful at the beginning of an interaction and some tend to be more helpful in the middle or at the end of an interaction. Nurses can prepare for therapeutic encounters by being familiar with a wide range of therapeutic techniques.

▶ Nurses must develop effective communication skills to enhance their work with different client groups such as clients of different ages, from different cultures, with different genders, and with different health problems.

Bibliography

1. Bradley, J.C., & Edinburg, M.A. (1990). *Communication in the nursing context* (3rd ed.). Norwalk, CT.: Appleton and Lange.
2. Burnside, I. (1990). Reminiscence: an independent nursing intervention for the elderly. *Issues in Mental Health Nursing*, 11, 33–48.
3. Carkhoff, R. (1969). *Helping and human relations: Vol. I*. New York: Holt, Rinehart, and Winston.
4. Carkhoff, R., & Berenson, B. (1967). *Beyond counseling and therapy*. New York: Holt, Rinehart, and Winston.
5. Carkhoff, R., & Truax, C. (1967). *Toward effective counseling and psychotherapy*. Chicago: Aldine.
6. Cassell, E.J. (1985). *Talking with patients: The theory of doctor-patient communication*. Cambridge, MA: MIT Press.
7. Crowther, D.J. (1991). Metacommunications: a missed opportunity? *Journal of Psychosocial Nursing*, 29(4), 13–16.
8. Davis, A.J. (1984). *Listening and responding*. St. Louis: C.V. Mosby.
9. Dorroh, T.L. (1974). *Between patient and health worker*. New York: McGraw-Hill.
10. Duldt, B.W., et al. (1984). *Interpersonal communication in nursing*. Philadelphia: F. A. Davis.
11. Edwardo, B.J., & Brilhart, J.K. (1981). *Communication in nursing practice*. St. Louis: C.V. Mosby.
12. Gazda, G.M., et al. (1982). *Interpersonal communication: A handbook for health professionals*. Rockville, MD: Aspen Publications.
13. Hall, E.T. (1966). *The hidden dimension*. New York: Doubleday.
14. Hays, J.S., & Larson, K.H. (1963). *Interacting with patients*. New York: Macmillan.
15. Hein, E.C. (1980). *Communication in nursing practice* (2nd ed.). Boston: Little, Brown.
16. Hotchkiss, D.R. (1989). *Demographic aspects of hearing impairment: Questions and answers*. Washington, DC: Gallaudet Research Institute.
17. King, M., et al. (1982). *Irresistible communication: Creative skills for the health professional*. Philadelphia: W. B. Saunders.
18. Kohut, H. (1984). *How does analysis cure?* Chicago: University of Chicago Press.
19. Lapp, C.A. (1991). Nursing students and the elderly: enhancing intergenerational communication through human-animal interaction. *Holistic Nurse Practitioner*, 5(2), 72–79.
20. Miller, L.E. (1989). Modeling awareness of feelings: a needed tool in the therapeutic communication workbox. *Perspectives in Psychiatric Care*, 25(2), 27–29.
21. Munn, H.E. (1980). *The nurse's communication handbook*. Germantown, MD: Aspen Publications.
22. O'Brien, M.J. (1978). *Communications and relationships in nursing*. St. Louis: C.V. Mosby.
23. Peitchinis, J.A. (1976). *Staff-patient communication in the health services*. New York: Springer.
24. Peplau, H. (1952). *Interpersonal relations in nursing*. New York: McGraw-Hill.
25. Phickhan, M.L. (1978). *Human communication: The matrix of nursing*. New York: McGraw-Hill.
26. Purtilo, R. (1990). *Health professional and patient interaction* (4th ed.). Philadelphia: W.B. Saunders.
27. Satir, V. (1971). *Peoplemaking*. Palo Alto, CA: Science and Behavior Books.
28. Satir, V., & Baldwin, M. (1983). *Satir step by step*. Palo Alto, CA: Science and Behavior Books.
29. Scott, A.L. (1988). Human interaction and personal boundaries. *Journal of Psychosocial Nursing*, 26(8), 23–27.
30. Selleck, K.J. (1991). Nurses' interpersonal behavior and the development of helping skills. *International Journal of Nursing Studies*, 28(1), 3–11.
31. Severtson, B.M. (1990). Therapeutic communication demystified. *Journal of Nursing Education*, 29(4), 190–193.
32. Stevenson, S. (1992). Heading off violence with verbal deescalation. *Journal of Psychosocial Nursing*, 29(9), 6–10.
33. Tannen, D. (1990). *You just don't understand: Women and men in conversation*. New York: Ballantine Books.
34. Thobaben, M. (1990). Evaluation of the therapeutic nurse-patient relationship. *Home Healthcare Nurse*, 9(3), 46–47.
35. Topf, M. (1988). Verbal interpersonal responsiveness. *Journal of Psychosocial Nursing*, 26(7), 8–16.
36. Travelbee, J. (1966). *Interpersonal aspects of nursing*. Philadelphia: F.A. Davis.
37. Watzlawick, P., et al. (1967). *Pragmatics of human communication*. New York: W.W. Norton.

Chapter 25

▼ *Communication Within Groups*

▼ *One of the most widespread human problems of modern society is making contact with other humans. Painfully few methods for meeting are socially acceptable, a condition that makes for much human heartbreak. . . . When the issue is learning how to join with others, several methods have proven useful.*

W. Schutz[18]

▼ **CHAPTER OUTLINE**

THE NATURE OF GROUPS
    Characteristics of Groups
    Primary and Secondary Groups
TYPES OF GROUPS FOUND IN HEALTH
  CARE SETTINGS
    Therapeutic Groups
    Task (Work) Groups
    Educational Groups
GROUP DYNAMICS AND GROUP PROCESS
    Concepts Related to Group
      Dynamics
    Concepts Related to Group Process
GROUP LEADERSHIP

    Leadership Development
    Leadership Styles
STRATEGIES FOR EFFECTIVE GROUP
  COMMUNICATION
    Barriers to Effective Group
      Interactions
    Constructive Confrontations
THE GROUP AS CHANGE AGENT
GROUP DECISION MAKING
    Decision-Making Strategies
    Steps in the Decision-Making
      Process

▼ **KEY TERMS**

Authoritarian leadership
Community support
  groups
Democratic leadership
Educational groups
Encounter groups
Group
Group cohesion
Group culture

Group dynamics
Group goals
Group membership
Group norms
Group process
Group roles
Group therapy
"Group think"
Laissez-faire leader

Leadership
Maintenance role functions
Primary groups
Secondary groups
Self-help groups
Task groups
Task role functions
Work groups

▼ LEARNING OBJECTIVES

After studying this chapter, you should be able to

1. *Define what is meant by a group.*
2. *Contrast the nature of primary and secondary groups.*
3. *Identify different types of groups used in health care settings.*
4. *Define selected concepts related to group dynamics.*
5. *Describe five phases of group development.*
6. *Contrast the three principal leadership styles.*
7. *Discuss situations in which confrontations can be constructive.*
8. *Describe Kurt Lewin's change model.*
9. *Identify different methods of decision making in groups.*

Group communication is important in nursing. Developing good group communication skills and having a basic understanding of group dynamics are critical to successful living.[11] People are social animals. Life is a cooperative enterprise involving an unending series of negotiations within and between groups. Socialization into the larger society occurs through membership in a number of different groups. Groups offer a slightly different approach to self-awareness. In a group, a person learns to combine experiences in new and different ways. Group communication provides a structural framework for many aspects of our activities of daily living. Self-esteem, social status, and work performance all reflect communication with others as a member of one or more groups. Throughout life, our values and attitudes reveal the groups to which we belong.

In health care settings, groups are essential to effective functioning. Group work with clients, other nurses, other health professionals, and families or caretakers is ongoing in the nurse's work environment. Nurses work with groups of health care workers and conduct client education groups on a regular basis. Group discussion is widely recognized as an indispensable tool for brainstorming and effective decision making in health care settings. Newer models of health care delivery (such as case management, shared governance, and managed care) all require a strong knowledge of group dynamics for successful implementation.

As beginning students, you will engage in a variety of group communication experiences, directly with forethought or indirectly as part of the educational process. Your clinical conferences and group assignments will run more smoothly with an understanding of the group dynamics and process underlying their accomplishment. As you interact with client, family, and professional groups, group communication concepts of norms, cohesion, goals, and role functions will take on new meaning. The purpose of this chapter is to provide you with a basic understanding of what makes a group a group and how you might interact with others in a group.

THE NATURE OF GROUPS

A **group** is two or more individuals who share one or more common characteristics and meet on a regular basis in face-to-face interactions to achieve a common goal. Much of what we know about group life and the impact it has on the behavior of individuals developed from the work of Kurt Lewin and his colleagues. His findings suggest that life experience, viewed in a structured setting that allows feedback, reflection, and examination by others, provides an experiential learning that is impossible individually. Lewin[12] visualized the group as a "dynamic whole" in which change in any part of the group system necessarily affects other parts. He maintained that the essential component of group effectiveness is the active interdependency of group members on one another. The value of the collective good will that emerges in the group serves as the catalyst for wanting to achieve group goals.

Characteristics of Groups

Groups differ from other combinations of unrelated people in several important ways (Box 25–1). Most important is the concept of shared purpose. People join together because of common interests in achieving similar goals. Without a common purpose in mind, the group will disintegrate because there is little reason to stay together. The group develops a **"group culture"** or set of common characteristics that help facilitate goal achievement. Shared characteristics might involve a common ethnic heritage, a similar health problem, or the need to complete a group project for a grade. Interactions occur on a regular basis. Group conversations occur within a certain format, they are related to the accomplishment of group goals, and they take place over time. In a group, members intentionally influence, and are influenced by, others in the group. There is a unity of purpose that draws individuals together in face-to-face interaction.

Box 25–1. Characteristics of Groups

Unity of purpose
Face-to-face interactions over a span of time
Shared meanings and characteristics
Interdependency of individuals
Unique role relationships and norms

During the course of the group's life, emotional bonding develops from the shared meanings. The result is that members become socially interdependent as they strive to reach common, agreed upon goals. The group is held together through these interrelated elements and by norms regulating the behaviors of group members and defining specific role relationships.

Primary and Secondary Groups

Groups are classified as primary and secondary. **Primary groups** are naturally occurring formations with informal structures. Membership is automatic or spontaneously chosen. Primary groups include family, friends, and social groups. **Secondary groups** are formations specifically developed by people for the purpose of achieving identified goals. Therapeutic groups, work groups, and educational groups are classified as secondary groups. They have a prescribed structure.

PRIMARY GROUPS

Primary groups consisting of family and close friends are the most basic group formations. These informal groups do not always have identified prescribed goals, yet in each there is a distinct unity of purpose and interdependency among its membership that has meaning and distinguishes members from nonmembers. Social groups in neighborhoods offer an example of short-term informal groups (e.g., bridge, scouting, exercise groups). They gather together for social purposes, and when the social purpose is no longer served, the group disbands. A person can be a member of several social groups simultaneously. They are an important source of social and emotional support to people.

Characterized as a long-term informal group structure, family groups exist throughout a lifetime, ideally providing nurturance and support. Membership automatically begins at birth. Older members of the family introduce the younger members of the group to the cultural heritage and social mores. Parents teach their children the group culture in a fundamental way through their overall communication style and parenting approaches. The ways in which members of family groups interact with each other significantly affect the productivity and emotional satisfaction of the family unit. Implicit and explicit social norms learned in the family group continue to operate throughout the individual's life, affecting human responses with others outside the family group. Many individual communication problems can be traced to behavioral responses originally learned within the family group that are not applicable and are poorly understood outside it.

Acknowledging the membership of an individual client within a larger family group is an important dimension of nursing care that can mean the difference between successfully achieved or failed treatment goals.

SECONDARY GROUPS

As the child's world enlarges to include more than family, socialization into the larger society becomes necessary, which stimulates the formation of secondary groups. Secondary groups have a formal structure and purpose. They meet for a variety of interpersonal and work-related goals. From a social perspective, people seek to recreate or build on the sense of belongingness a family represents in school and civic life. Sororities, fraternities, and civic groups such as the Masons or Junior Chamber of Commerce expand group memberships beyond those of the family unit.

Group membership can also serve as a buffer for unsatisfactory family relationships. When membership in a family group becomes too difficult for individual members, the alienated member often seeks membership in one or more other intimate social groups to compensate for the deficiency. As an extreme form of membership, cults effectively demonstrate the sense of belonging and loyalty to a group culture that all of us need for emotional survival. Positive use of group membership to augment or substitute for deficient family relationships includes boys' clubs, Big Sisters, and Scouts.

In therapeutic and work groups, members join together as a unit to achieve specific goals. They have a more structured format and specific, identified purposes. Group purposes relate to broadened interpersonal functioning, problem solving, information giving, or task accomplishment. Members join together as a unit to achieve specific goals. Usually, a designated leader assumes primary responsibility for the overall functioning of the group. Specified meeting times related to the achievement of objectives are identified. Members are not likely to meet on a regular basis socially outside the group experience.

Educational groups have goals related to information exchange. Some educational groups are highly structured and require mandatory attendance and participation. For example, some classes have lab groups or discussion groups as part of the course requirements. Other educational groups form spontaneously to complete a project or provide practical information and support. The purpose of the secondary group determines the structure and influences the quality and focus of group communication.

TYPES OF GROUPS FOUND IN HEALTH CARE SETTINGS

In health care settings, nurses use structured groups with clients, families, and other health care professionals to accomplish the goals of professional nursing practice. The group's purpose determines its classification.

Therapeutic Groups

Therapeutic groups include group psychotherapy, therapeutic communities in hospital and outpatient settings, encounter groups, and self-help groups. **Group therapy** is a form of psychotherapy designed to help clients gain insight into dysfunctional behaviors and develop more appropriate coping strategies. Group therapy is increasingly used to help people enhance personal growth and as a temporary resource for coping with isolated life issues such as bereavement or job searches.

Groups offer people a format for increasing self-esteem and taking charge of their lives. Through group interactions, clients learn to handle frustration, anger, and conflicts constructively in a nonthreatening environment.

Group therapy serves as a powerful antidote for the feelings of isolation, loneliness, and withdrawal associated with severe emotional stress. Peer involvement and immediate feedback overcome denial and resistance to exploring painful emotions. The opportunity to explore more effective communication strategies in a nonthreatening group often enables people to work more effectively with family, friends, and coworkers.

Special training is required for leadership of therapy groups. Membership in most therapy groups is closed (i.e., members are not free to come and go as they choose). Group therapy is conducted in a small group format to allow maximal interchange among members, usually no more than eight to ten members.

A different but related form of group therapy is the therapeutic community, an important component of treatment in many mental health and psychiatric facilities. Membership is involuntary; that is, clients and staff have no choice about becoming a member of the group. By virtue of being on an inpatient unit, clients and staff automatically become members of a therapeutic community conducted in a large group format. All of the members of the unit, including staff, have a chance to provide input into the functioning of the group. The group elects its leaders from the client group, and leadership rotates among the client members. All decisions are the responsibility of the full community. The therapeutic community helps clients build self-esteem and develop skills that will be useful in the larger community outside the hospital.

ENCOUNTER GROUPS

Encounter groups are time-bound and intense experiences designed to enhance personal awareness. They generally meet for a predetermined concentrated period of time (hours or days) and then disband permanently. The strategies used in encounter groups are often unconventional and are deliberately designed to jar conventional attitudes and behavior patterns. Encounter groups have objectives different from those of traditional therapy group formats. As a stimulus for greater personal awareness, and led by trained specialists, encounter groups are highly effective. Intended to release greater awareness in relatively stable emotional circumstances, they can be counterproductive when used with emotionally unstable individuals and in the hands of untrained professionals. Encounter groups can be threatening when there is no mechanism for working through the powerful emotions evoked with this format.

SELF-HELP (COMMUNITY SUPPORT) GROUPS

Self-help groups, or **community support groups,** have a common purpose and identity deriving from the similar life circumstances of the participants, rather than from their emotional needs. Self-help groups are less formal than therapy and encounter groups (Fig. 25-1). Although they share many common values with therapy groups, their purpose is fundamentally different. The goals of self-help groups are supportive rather than insight oriented.[16] In contrast to therapy groups, they are usually formed and led by a peer leader to provide mutual support and practical advice in dealing with a difficult situational, medical, or social problem. Group norms, which are less fixed, are centered mostly on furnishing mutual aid and support for members. Relief is often obtained from hearing the problems of others with similar issues and receiving concrete suggestions for coping. Self-help groups provide the person strug-

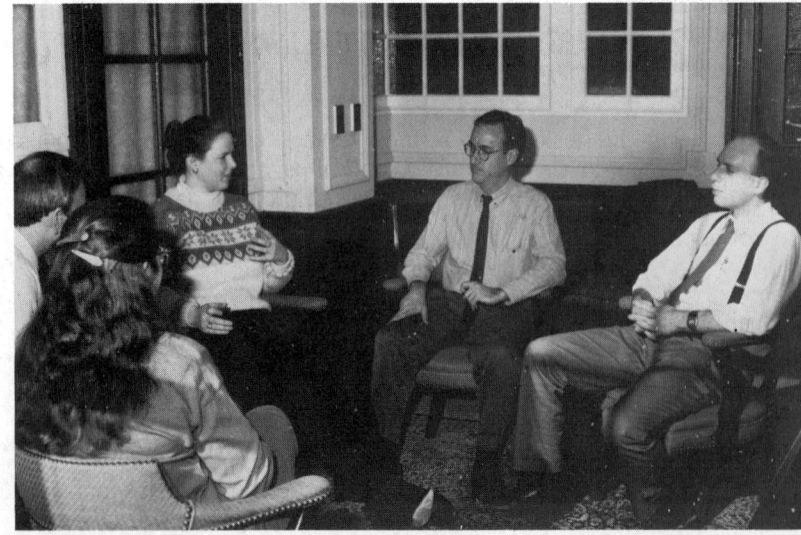

▲ Figure 25–1

Self-help groups provide support for members with a common purpose.

gling with a seemingly impossible problem with a renewed sense of identity and hope. Some of the more well known support group formats include Alcoholics Anonymous, Weight Watchers, Candlelighters, and Parents without Partners. Self-help groups have the advantage of being free or very low cost to operate. They also may be a useful adjunct to formal therapy approaches.

In a time of political activism, self-help groups often become, or are connected with, advocacy groups in the community. Collaboration with official community agencies and advocacy efforts continues for many support groups on an ongoing basis. Examples of politically active self-help groups include Alliance for the Mentally Ill, Alzheimers Association, and Association for Retarded Citizens. Created informally, or formally as an advisory committee to a larger agency or constituency, social advocacy groups provide education and information designed to focus greater attention on specific problem issues. The primary goals of social advocacy groups relate to advocating better treatment, research, or understanding of specific problems and issues in the political community.

Task (Work) Groups

Task groups, or **work groups,** are designed to further the goals of an organization. They exist as the official communication unit in many health care settings. Examples of task (work) groups within health care settings include standing committees, ad hoc task forces, and "quality circles." A standing committee is an established committee usually made up of elected members and designed to accomplish the goals of the organization. Examples of standing committees include professional standards committees and administrative councils. Ad hoc task forces are temporary committees established for the purpose of performing a certain task. Quality circles are unit-based task forces formed to resolve administrative and clinical problems.

Input from task (work) groups often forms the nucleus for important changes within a work organization. Shared governance represents a participative management approach heavily dependent on group communication. Participative management relies on group decision making for strategic planning and implementation of its goals. Health care settings using participative management in group formats experience higher levels of productivity and employee morale. With participative management, the work group functions as an integrated unit linked by shared history, vision, and values and a collective commitment to achieving tangible outcomes. Workers involved in the decision-making process in matters related to their work world feel they have the capacity to improve their immediate work environment. They are more likely to take an active interest in doing their work and to have pride in their organization. Employees actively involved in participative management report greater satisfaction with their work.[14,17]

Educational Groups

Educational groups are developed to teach participants skills and provide information. They are a modified form of the work group. Study groups, training seminars, aerobics classes, and adult education courses are examples of groups formed for educational purposes. Unlike primary groups, group meetings are scheduled, and the group life is time limited even when the group is informally structured.

GROUP DYNAMICS AND GROUP PROCESS

In the study of group life, there are two important considerations, group dynamics and group process. **Group dynamics** are the conscious and unconscious forces or emotional flow operating in a group and facilitating or impeding the group process and progression toward goal achievement. The naturally progressive phases of group development constitute **group process.** An understanding of both concepts plays an important role in determining successful group communication.

Concepts Related to Group Dynamics

Effective group dynamics depend on the establishment of clear goals, group norms that support goal achievement, a healthy balance between the group's tasks and its maintenance, and the development of group cohesion. Structural factors such as a pleasant and private environment, timing, and interpersonal sensitivity for members' needs will influence the dynamics of the group (Fig. 25–2).

GROUP GOALS

An established group goal is the foundation of the group's existence. It gives meaning and direction to the group's efforts. **Group goals** are the outcomes, or end results, the group seeks to achieve through its common effort. Group goals differ from personal goals in that they are broader. They represent a collective aim; they are not necessarily the same as the goals of individual group members. In a group, each member is expected to contribute to the overall group goal.

Group goals vary from group to group, depending on the personal and collective resources of the individuals composing the group, the nature of the group, and other external factors such as time and institutional support. Individuals join groups because they or their employers believe that certain goals can be achieved better collectively than alone. Achievable goals in line with individual values, reinforced through support and encouragement, and rewarded by those in power are likely to stimulate greater group participation. Two prerequisites for successful goal achievement are (1) that goals be clearly stated and (2) that goals be accepted by the group members as valid and achievable. The leader who allows full presentation of facts and maxi-

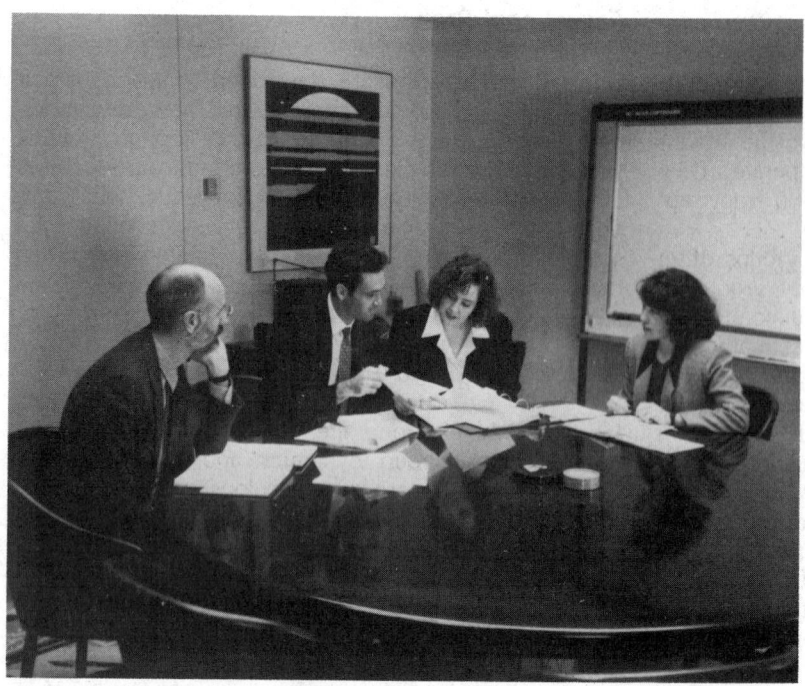

▲ *Figure 25-2*

Characteristics of effective groups: balanced role functions, clear and achievable goals, flexible leadership, and group cohesion.

mal involvement of the group members in the development of group goals is more likely to find that group members work effectively toward goal achievement.

GROUP ROLES

Group roles support the goals and affect the functioning of the group. **Group roles** are sets of behaviors that individuals display in relation to the expectations of the rest of the group members.[21] The roles people take in groups can be formal, for example, chairperson or secretary; or they can be informal, fulfilling a function needed for goal achievement.

Benne and Sheats in their classic work[3] on group role functions describe three types of informal role functions observed in group dynamics: task, maintenance, and self-centered goals. Task role functions are important because they promote task accomplishment. Maintenance roles are equally important because they support member involvement.

Group task and maintenance role functions are very much interrelated. A healthy balance between task and maintenance role functions provides a rewarding work atmosphere in which members work together to achieve common group goals. Group members assume different role functions at different times.

Task Role Functions. Task role functions are the roles of group members that facilitate group processing of ideas. Task role functions help the group stay focused on the task and directly assist the group in achieving its identified goal. Group members assuming task role functions keep the group focused on the generation of new ideas and critical thinking about the information available in the group. Examples of task role functions include initiating new ideas, clarifying ideas of others, and marking the group's progression toward goal achievement. Because task role functions are cognitive in nature, they depend on the quality of thinking that members bring to the group.

Measures of task role effectiveness include a capacity to reach identified goals, with minimal expenditure of time and energy, and satisfaction with the outcome.

Maintenance Role Functions. Group maintenance role functions relate to the interpersonal dynamics occurring in group communications. To achieve a desired result, people need to work together. Group members who do not respect each other and are unwilling to work together drain energy from the group that is needed to accomplish the group task. Group maintenance goals strengthen group participation, which thereby facilitates task accomplishment. Group **maintenance role functions** are the role functions that help build and maintain group morale. Group members assuming maintenance role functions draw attention to the relational aspects of group life needed to nourish and support members as they labor to achieve the group task. Examples of group maintenance role functions include seeking to reduce conflict, encouraging compromise, and keeping the channels of communication open among members. Because group maintenance functions relate to the emotional life of the group, they require interpersonal sensitivity and good interpersonal communication skills.

Measures of group maintenance effectiveness include observation of respect, harmony, and absence of nonproductive conflict. Expressed satisfaction with group interactions and congruence between actual and desired group relations are evidence of effective group maintenance. When there is a large discrepancy between desired and actual group interactions, group maintenance needs more careful attention. Box 25-2 summarizes the major task and maintenance role func-

Box 25-2. Tasks and Maintenance Role Functions

Task (Goal Accomplishment) Role Functions	Maintenance (Group Building) Role Functions
Initiator: Introduces new ideas	**Encourager:** Provides support for individual contributions
Information seeker: Requests clarification	**Harmonizer:** Seeks to reduce conflict between members
Information giver: Provides additional information	**Compromiser:** Provides ideas that acknowledge and incorporate other persons' contributions
Elaborator: Clarifies or expands on ideas	**Gatekeeper:** Keeps channels of communication open and encourages balanced participation
Opinion seeker: Asks for group's opinion of facts presented	**Tension releaser:** Reduces tension through humor
Opinion giver: Gives belief about ideas presented	**Standard setter:** Challenges unproductive norms or behaviors
Orienter: Keeps the group on task	**Feeling expresser:** Identifies the feeling tone of the group
Recorder: Keeps record of group progress	**Group observer:** Makes process comments about the group climate
Energizer: Spurs the group to action	**Follower:** Goes along with the majority
Consensus seeker: Asks for agreement/disagreement with proposals	

Adapted from Benne, K. D., & Sheats, P. (1948). Functional roles and group members. *Journal of Social Issues*, 4(2), 41–49.

---

tions originally described by Benne and Sheats in 1948.[3]

Self-centered Roles. Benne and Sheats[3] also identified self-centered roles that sabotage group process. Self-centered roles are not functional roles for the group. They distract from task accomplishment and group maintenance functions. Focus on self gets members mired down into resolving personal conflicts rather than attending to the meeting of group goals. Continued lack of task results can reduce interaction effectiveness and decrease morale. Self-centered roles that interfere with successful group functioning are presented in Box 25-3.

GROUP NORMS

To function successfully, every group needs to develop its own set of operating procedures. **Group norms** are standards of conduct that provide guidelines for acceptable behaviors in groups. Group norms are powerful written or unwritten laws about how members should relate with each other. Some are more impor-

Box 25-3. Self-centered Roles

Blocker: Rejects legitimate ideas; takes persistent negative stand without offering options

Aggressor: Verbally attacks or puts down other members

Dominator: Monopolizes group conversation

Recognition seeker: Continually calls group attention to personal needs

Confessor: Focuses on personal difficulties and feelings unrelated to group task

Clown: Humor that significantly damages and distracts from group goal achievement

tant than others, but once established, group norms are particularly resistant to change. The more group norms reflect and support the group goals, the more effective the group accomplishment. Basic group norms that should govern behavior in any group involve mutual aid and emotional support for other group members. Other norms relevant to group life include confidentiality, attendance, and an expectation of verbal contributions from all members.

An effective group operates with high ethical standards. When this is the norm, the leader and other group members demonstrate a respect for individual differences in people and a natural regard for the worth and significance of each group member. Operating from this perspective, the group acknowledges the positive quality of each person's contribution even when it seemingly causes the group to pause in its forward movement.

Confidentiality is a universal norm required in all groups. Group and individual member communications are held private. They are not shared outside the group without the group's permission. Confidentiality is such an important basic norm of group life that without it, the group trust needed for people to work together cooperatively simply cannot develop.

When norms are seriously in conflict with goal achievement, members recognize it unconsciously and react accordingly. Either the norm itself becomes the focus of attention for the group, or group members withdraw because of the untenable position it creates for them. People who deviate from the group norms are subject to being scapegoated, ignored, or devalued. In extreme cases, failure to observe the norms of the group can result in expulsion from the group.

GROUP COHESION

Group cohesion is an important dynamic characteristic of effective groups. The word *cohesion* is a Latin derivative of a word meaning "sticking together." **Group cohesion** refers to all of the positive values that people hold about the group experience and the reasons that prompt them to remain with the group. Some people refer to it as the group climate. A positive group climate is perceived as cooperative and ego enhancing. People are attracted to groups that provide companionship and practical or emotional support. They will choose groups in which they can have status as a member of the group and personal satisfaction with goal achievement.

Cohesion is measured by the degree to which the group satisfies an individual's need for belonging. In a group with high cohesion, members feel relaxed and are more willing to share ideas and feelings. Highly cohesive groups are characterized by a strong commitment to group goals, individual involvement in completion of assigned tasks, low absenteeism, and low membership turnover.

A lack of group cohesion decreases group productivity, satisfaction, and frequency of comments. People are afraid to express their ideas openly for fear of criticism. In groups in which there is a win-lose and competitive norm, people become guarded in their communication. Most people do not want to waste their time and effort in a competitive environment with people they dislike and at the risk of being subjected to criticism.

Lack of cohesion develops when there are unreasonable demands on individual members. This can take the form of scapegoating or forcing a quiet member to speak. Allowing dominating or blocking members to sabotage the group goals by default, that is, by not confronting their actions, prevents cohesion from developing.

Positive Group Cohesion. There are several ways to foster cohesion. Cohesion develops from a trusting relationship. Personal involvement in a group effort usually is directly related to the level of acceptance a person feels in the group. A group in which an individual's contributions are valued and accepted in a cooperative atmosphere encourages people to disclose their ideas and to commit their resources to accomplishing group goals. Ideally, the leader and other members consider the impact of their communication on the other person. They are careful not to confuse disagreement with an idea with criticism of the person presenting it.

"Group Think." It is possible for a group to become too cohesive. Carried to an extreme, it can create overt or subtle pressure on individual members to conform to ideas and decision implications that are blatantly inconsistent with their personal beliefs and values. Janis[10] describes **"group think"** as a group decision-making process in which loyalty to the group and approval of other group members take precedence over expression of personal values, ideas, and conflicting opinions. Characterized by group pressure to present an agreeable, unified front, group think decision making discourages critical evaluation of ideas on their own merits and bars alternative decision-making strategies

from consideration. The group maintains the illusion of perfect harmony at the expense of more appropriate creative problem solving, and sometimes even of morality.

With a group think mentality, members rationalize that their ideas and actions are right without any input from those affected by their decision. People within or outside of the group who disagree with the group think perceptions are stereotyped as uninformed, obstructionists, or stupid. Their ideas are excluded from consideration. Members who have contradictory information do not share it with the group for fear of criticism or ridicule. Group pressure to maintain the illusion of unanimity about a group decision further fosters this silence. Some of the atrocities committed during Hitler's regime offer an extreme example of the evil in a group think decision-making process whereby a small group of individuals implemented decisions in conflict with the law and morality in attempting to develop what they defined as the "perfect race."

Ways to counteract the development of group think include maintaining a cooperative group climate. Leadership that supports critical independent thinking and alternative problem-solving strategies as fundamental group norms creates a cooperative group climate. Deliberately playing devil's advocate regarding group decisions and looking at the consequences of their implementation reduce the possibility of group think solutions.

STRUCTURAL COMPONENTS OF EFFECTIVE GROUPS

Group structure plays an indirect but highly significant role in the group's dynamics. Certain structural characteristics, such as group size, time frame, and setting, will directly affect the communication dynamics of a group. For example, does the size of the group allow meaningful interaction; are the time and duration of group sessions compatible with other scheduling considerations; is the location of the group meeting readily accessible? Ideally, the group should meet in a setting apart from other traffic at a regularly scheduled meeting time. Sessions longer than 3 hours are tiring and usually counterproductive. People need time to reflect and to regroup. Smaller chunks of data with time in between to process them prevents informational overload.

Concerns about membership, size of the group, and environmental factors enhance or diminish the possibility of effective conversations in groups.

Membership. Group membership is an identified relationship between a person and designated other persons who make up a group. There is a shared identity simply because one is a member of the group. Membership defines who is and who is not a part of the group. There are specialized communications, expectations, and roles emerging during the life of the group; these distinguish group communication of one particular group from that of other groups.[14]

A prerequisite for membership should be the capacity to contribute to group goals. For example, placing an Alzheimer's victim in a medication group may be counterproductive for the client as well as for the group because the client's deficit may prevent full participation. Members should have enough in common to feel comfortable interpersonally. Marked differences in functional abilities and life experiences compromise member contributions and the comfort level needed to express oneself in the group.

Regardless of specific group goals, group membership offers a unique opportunity for an individual to help others and to enhance personal functioning. In the process of developing insight and gaining strength from others, or accomplishing a task, there is an increase in self-esteem. The mutual support expressed by a group of peers working through similar issues and interpersonal difficulty gives a person a special identity beyond a purely personal identity. Receiving feedback and feeling respected in an open, honest, and nonexploitative relationship with peers help a person gain self-confidence. From an experiential point of view, the individual knows that honest, open communications are possible, even about the most difficult issues. The ability to communicate directly and openly with a variety of personalities while retaining one's own unique identity is a first-time experience for many people. There is a sense of mutual accomplishment and bonding with others that is highly self-sustaining, personally energizing, and meaningful.

Size. The size of the group will influence the interpersonal dynamics. Smaller groups facilitate personal involvement and a sense of making a meaningful contribution. Thelen suggests having membership numbers depend on the "smallest groups in which it is possible to have represented at a functional level all the social and achievement skills required for the particular required activity." [19] To be effective, a group should include enough members to carry out the group objectives and to support the personal relationships needed to achieve the group goals, and no more. Usually, five is the optimal number of members for small task groups.

Therapy groups usually try to limit membership to eight to ten members. Although it may be possible to carry out group objectives with a small number of people, the emotional intensity experienced by a group that is too small may interfere with productivity. When a member is absent, group interaction suffers or ceases until full membership is restored. In groups of three, two members often form a coalition and exclude the third person, thereby affecting morale and effective decision making. Large groups also compromise productivity. Groups of more than 10 lessen the possibility of intimacy and self-disclosure needed for effective problem solving and goal accomplishment.

Environmental Factors. The nature and goals of the group determine the frequency of meetings. Once the meeting time and place are established, the leader should make every attempt to honor the commitment. It is very disconcerting to block time out for a meeting that does not take place. If the leader repeatedly rearranges meeting times, the group members receive a message that the group is of secondary importance. Beginning and ending groups on time tells individual members that the needs of the participants to honor other time commitments are respected.

If the time and extent of group meetings interfere with the legitimate activities of group members, resentment develops that affects commitment. It is difficult to concentrate on group issues when you are thinking of where you need to be next. Likewise, functional groups extended arbitrarily beyond completion of the original group tasks decrease group commitment. There is a tendency in many work settings to have a functional group take on new responsibilities once the original tasks have been completed. Within the membership, frequently there is a feeling of "bait and switch" when the original contract for group participation is extended indefinitely. Resentment develops, and people are reluctant to volunteer for other group assignments. People caught in vague or dysfunctional group dynamics will react by becoming aggressive or by leaving the group psychologically, if not physically, regardless of how worthy the group goals are. Whereas each of these factors may seem minor, failure to recognize their importance as critical variables in group dynamics can mean the difference between an effective group and one in which participation is minimal and passive.

Concepts Related to Group Process

Group process refers to "the stages of development of a group and the characteristics of each stage." [6] Many theorists believe that the group process offers a microcosm of life relationships. Groups grow and develop from simple beginnings to emerge as complex, productive forces during the middle working phase of group life and cease to exist when goals are achieved. In the process of developing, groups form their own identities.

Different theoretical models of group development are presented in Table 25–1. In each of these models, there is an initial introductory stage in which members come together and tentatively explore what membership in the group will mean for each of them. This stage is followed by a second conflictual stage marked by greater assertiveness, conflict, and the establishment of operating procedures. Once group norms are established to the satisfaction of the group, the actual work of the group on task accomplishment begins. When the group task is complete, members take stock of their achievement, determine the need for follow-up or referral, and disband.

GROUP PROCESS AS PARALLEL WITH THE NURSING PROCESS

In many ways, the group process developmentally parallels the nursing process. There is an initial assessment phase in which the group explores the nature of the problem, develops a diagnostic statement, and determines the activities necessary to resolve it. Within the group, the members plan what activities will be needed to achieve group goals and who will be responsible for

TABLE 25–1. Phases of Group Development

Theorist							
Tuckman	Forming	Storming	Norming	Performing			
Sarri and Galinsky	Origin phase	Formative phase	Intermediate phase	Revision phase	Intermediate phase II	Maturation phase	Termination
Bennis and Shepard	Dependence (authority relations) Dependence-flight Counterdependence-flight Resolution-catharsis			Interdependence (personal relations) Enchantment-flight Disenchantment-flight Consensual validation			
Yalom	**Early Formative**			**Advanced Group**			
	Orientation Hesitant participation Search for meaning		Conflict Dominance Rebellion	Development of cohesion	Recurrent problems Subgrouping Self-disclosure Conflict		Termination
			Stormy and Emotionally Intense				
Bach (analytic approach)	Members test out group situation	Look to conductor and center hopes on him	Regression—playing out family roles	Role playing becomes more fanciful	Emotional discharge results	Take more serious view of selves as group; see structure and function	Deep analytic interpretations
Schultz	Inclusion	Control	Affection				
Gibbs	**4 Modes of Activity**						
	Acceptance	Data flow	Goal	Control			

From Arnold, E., & Boggs, K. (1989). Interpersonal relationships: *Professional communication skills for nurses.* Philadelphia: W.B. Saunders.

carrying out the functions. Together, group members develop a plan of action. Although this is an informal process in many groups, the developmental process is similar to the planning phase of the nursing process. In the working or implementation phase of the group, group members implement their plan so that most of the actual interventions related to task accomplishment take place. The termination phase of group life parallels the evaluative segment of the nursing process. When the work of the group is complete, group members evaluate their progress and goal achievement, make necessary modifications, and terminate the group.

PHASES OF GROUP DEVELOPMENT

Preinteraction Phase. There is a preinteraction phase of group development in which the leader sets the stage for effective group interactions. Issues such as group composition, size of the group needed to achieve group goals, time and group setting, and preparation of group members for the experience all require attention before the group actually begins. Attention to group composition is critical to group identity and ability of members to achieve group goals. Group members who share functional similarities (i.e., they have a comparable level of functional skill) will have less of a struggle understanding one another.

During the preinteraction phase, the leader plans the steps needed for goal accomplishment. Having an overall plan of action greatly facilitates the process.

Needed equipment for work groups such as flip charts, blackboards, and handouts are prepared ahead of time. Some groups use agendas as a way of organizing discussion. Whether there is a written agenda depends on the purpose of the group. Written agendas for task groups provide the members in work groups with an opportunity to consider relevant issues. Even if there is no formal agenda, it is useful to have some overall plan in mind and some ideas to stimulate interest in the discussion. The plan should be flexible enough to withstand modification if the situation warrants it.

Introductory Phase. The first few meetings involve a getting-acquainted process. The leader identifies basic structural norms, such as expected attendance, confidentiality, how the group will function, and group goals, early in the group development. Without explicit initial directions and some systematic preparation related to what members can expect in the group process, a lack of knowledge may limit progression toward goal accomplishment.

Usually everyone, leader included, is anxious. Anxiety is natural because you do not know what to expect. Preparing ahead of time what you will say is a useful strategy. For example, as leader, you might start the group by introducing yourself, stating the purpose of the group, and identifying initial norms: "We need to respect each other's feelings; everything that is said in this room is confidential." Details such as how often the group will meet, the duration of the meeting, and how you will function as a leader provide important information for the group and increase its interpersonal safety. Having a good idea of how you will proceed also decreases the leader's anxiety. If group members are unknown to each other, the leader might ask each person to briefly introduce himself or herself. The ways in which people express themselves and the preliminary information they present give the leader and other members important information.

Communication when the group is forming is tentative, polite, and guarded. Trust is the major issue facing the group, just as it is in the initial stages of individual relationships. People need to have confidence that others in the group, and particularly the leader, will not make them look foolish if they take the risk of presenting new ideas.

A priority during the initial stages of group development is to foster member involvement and interest in achieving group goals. Helping members to clarify and refine common group goals so that they are congruent with personal values and offer a personal challenge creates deeper involvement and greater personal satisfaction. Some of the problems frequently encountered during the early stages of the group are unrealistic expectations and an unclear perception of group goals and procedures.[22] Allowing enough time for the members' concerns to be addressed and for helping members to develop realistic expectations related to goal achievement early in the group's life will prevent later frustration.

The leader assumes a more active role in the beginning stages of the group in facilitating an atmosphere in which trust can develop. Trust is earned through open nondefensive communication by the leader, who serves as a role model for the type of communication expected of group members. Clarity of group goals, tasks, and norms; an interpersonal honesty; and a genuine level of participation and involvement in the group are likely to stimulate similar behaviors in other group members. Leadership is shared once a basic level of trust develops among members and their leader.

Member attitudes are an important dynamic often overlooked by group leaders. Working through negative attitudes during the early stages of group life can be helpful. If the group leader anticipates that some people have negative attitudes or a reluctance to commit fully to the group, the leader might address the issue in the following manner:

I know that some of you have reservations about being in this group or working on this project. I'd like to tell you a little about what I hope we can accomplish with this project that may be of interest to you.

As a follow-up to the data presented, the leader would elicit concerns and answer questions. The leader might end the communication with a statement:

Now, I would like to ask you to suspend your judgment and give us your best effort in making _____ work. Can you do this?

At the end of the meeting, the leader summarizes group activities and thanks participants for coming.

Transition Phase. Once preliminary trust is established, there is a period when the differences in the members' personalities and approaches to the work of the group come into sharp focus. This stage of the group's development is uncomfortable and stormy, compared with the introductory stage. Transition is marked by the expression of strong feelings and open conflict about goals and the best way to reach them. As group members struggle with issues related to who will assume responsibility for different aspects of the task, group operating procedures, and how decisions will be made, the discussion gets lively and at times heated. Uncomfortable as it is, this stage of group development is a necessary prelude to the development of group norms required for task accomplishment. In this stage of the group's development, members are testing whether it is OK to express different opinions and have their ideas acknowledged. The leader's role during the transition stage is to keep the lines of communication open. Helping group members move beyond their immediate personal concerns toward reflection and collaborative action is essential to making the transition to the working phase.

It is not uncommon for the leader to experience intense emotions during this phase. Identifying personal reactions to challenging behaviors helps the leader maintain crucial perspective in this phase of the group's development. Consultation with a valued mentor is useful when the leader experiences a strong negative personal reaction to a person or idea.

In some groups, members handle the normal stormy phase of group development in a more passive manner. Members hold back strong feelings and seem content to stay at a superficial level. Conversation remains stilted and inconsequential, with little movement toward goal accomplishment. If this occurs, the leader might note that it seems as though the group is having difficulty moving to a deeper level and ask members if they feel this is true. Sometimes, this is all that is needed. Other times, it may be necessary to become more directive and focus members on the need to move toward goal accomplishment. During the transition stage, the leader becomes the "affirmer of standards." The leader, through words and actions, reflects a basic respect for each person's contribution and encourages risk taking by making the interpersonal environment safe for each group member.

Working Phase. The working phase is characterized by cohesion and productivity.[6] Members become actively engaged in directly achieving the group goal. Communication reflects cooperation rather than competition, and there is a psychic energy that is almost palpable. Self-disclosure is more spontaneous. Group cohesion and morale are at their highest peak. Members seek feedback, both positive and negative. Individual members assume responsibility for leadership around issues, although the leader continues to accept primary responsibility for ensuring a group structure and climate that facilitates group task and maintenance goals. During this phase of group development, the leader uses open-ended and focused questions to elicit more information from group members. The group completes the major tasks related to goal accomplishment during this stage of group development. The leader can facilitate the process by summarizing or linking main ideas and asking for agreement on key points before moving on to the next issue.

Termination Phase. In the final stages of group life, the group focuses on completing unfinished business and summarizing group achievements. The group identifies plans for group follow-up, as needed. In contrast to the working phase, the termination phase is characterized by members who seem more emotionally distant and disengaged in anticipation of the group's end. Effectively ending the group by giving members sufficient time to work through unfinished agendas or feelings can mean the difference between a member's desire or reluctance to participate in future group experiences. Need for further work is identified and referred appropriately. During this stage of group life, the leader helps members identify important elements of personal group involvement and reflect on the meaning of the group. Effective group endings are just as important as strong group beginnings.

GROUP LEADERSHIP

A leader provides guidance and direction to a group. The task of the group leader is to guide the group process by maintaining rapport and moving the group process forward to facilitate goal accomplishment. Barker et. al define **leadership** as "influential behavior, voluntarily accepted by group members, that moves a group toward its recognized goal and/or maintains the group."[2]

Leadership Development

Leadership is both a position and a role. Usually, there is a formally designated leader in charge of the group. This is the "position" aspect, and the leader is referred to as the appointed leader. Leaders also emerge within the group and are referred to as emergent leaders. Emergent leadership can be highly effective when it is shared, when it is sanctioned by the leader, and when it fits the temporary needs of the group. It can be highly disruptive when it occurs because the designated leader fails to take charge of the group or lacks the communication skills to respond effectively to the members' needs. Emergent leadership that is competitive rather than collaborative with the designated leadership can sabotage group goals.

There are several ways of viewing leadership. The first, referred to as the Great Man or trait theory, assumes that leaders are born, not made. The difficulty with this theory is that people with different personal traits are excellent leaders. Leadership can be learned, as evidenced by the fact that many individuals who were not identifiable as leaders in their youth emerge as highly effective leaders when circumstances force them to become leaders in adult life. Another way of looking at leadership is to describe different styles of leadership. Styles of leadership can vary from individual to individual and according to the situational needs of the members.

Leadership Styles

Leadership style may be described as authoritarian, democratic, or laissez faire. An **authoritarian leadership** is a leader-centered leadership style in which the leader makes the decisions and controls the conversation among group members. Agendas are predetermined by the leader and not by the needs of the group. **Democratic leadership** is a leadership style in which the leader assumes a collaborative role with other members and serves as guide while other members take steps toward accomplishing group goals. The democratic leader is likely to provide an initial overview of the tasks to be accomplished and permit more flexibility in the steps toward accomplishment (Fig. 25–3). The **laissez-faire leader** is a group leader who turns leadership over to group members and steps in only when requested to give feedback. The group members take total responsibility for group productivity. Research indicates a lower level of satisfaction and productivity in groups led by a laissez-faire leader. Passivity and resentment among group members often are products of an authoritarian leadership style.[4]

Leadership does not just happen. Effective leaders should have the training, knowledge, and experience necessary to lead the group. The group needs to know that the leader has the capacity to help the group achieve identified outcomes. Effective leaders are enthusiastic and committed to group goals. They are willing to provide competent direction to the group.

Effective leaders are flexible and able to weather conflict without becoming defensive. They are able to vary their approach depending on the needs of the group and to manage conflict when it occurs. For example, a mature group will require less structuring by the leader, and members will respond best when they can actively participate with the leader in making group decisions. A newly formed group will need far more structure and planning. At times, members will respond best to a task-oriented approach; at other times, group members will need to focus on the process aspects of their group. Sensitivity to changes in the members' needs and being able to adapt leadership style responsively to them is a communication skill that is critical to an understanding of leader-member relationships and task accomplishment. Generally, when members are feeling insecure about their abilities or demonstrate a resistance to progressing toward goal achievement, they need a more directive leadership style. Groups exhibiting these characteristics respond best when the leader provides specific instructions, clarification, close collaborative guidance, and opportunities for asking questions.

By contrast, mature groups in which the members are more confident about their ability and are able to share ideas easily react more favorably to a leadership style that invites participation in decision making and responsibility for the direction of the group.

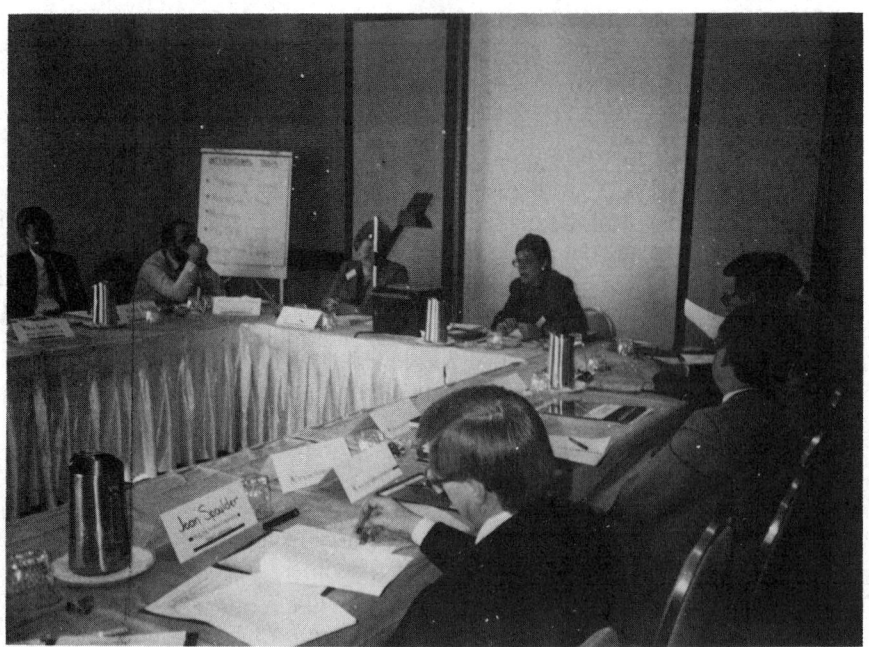

▲ *Figure 25-3*

Effective leadership is typically a collaborative process. The leader is a guide who encourages members to participate.

STRATEGIES FOR EFFECTIVE GROUP COMMUNICATION

Effective groups focus on the task, yet reflect a healthy balance between task and relationship maintenance. Goals are well defined and understood by all members. In effective groups, there is a basically cooperative atmosphere marked by open communication, respect for differences, participative management of objectives, and a sense of cohesion. Progress reports show clear progression toward stated group goals.

A cooperative group atmosphere does not develop spontaneously. It is the result of much hard work. Members of effective groups choose to develop individual goals in ways that are complementary to or compatible with the identified group goals. Team sports offer a good example. The goal of the individual team member as well as of the team as a whole is to win as many games as possible. In a cooperative group atmosphere, the norms support each participant's efforts to achieve the common goal. The teammates of the individual who makes the winning score are just as excited as if they were personally making it. The successful effort of one member brings them closer to the team goal of winning the game. Although the skills and personal resources of each individual member are judged and valued as different, they are all vitally important to the successful achievement of the whole.

The group leader can stimulate greater discussion and commitment to group goals by using focused or open-ended questions. For example, the leader might use one or more of the following comments to draw out member reactions:

We talked a great deal about _____. Which ideas seem most relevant to you?

Would anyone like to react to what Jack just said?

We've covered much ground today. Is there anything you think we haven't considered yet?

Barriers to Effective Group Interactions

Groups have identified agendas related to the accomplishment of task objectives. They frequently also have unidentified agendas that relate to the emotional aspects of task or group life. It is the unexplained agenda that consumes energy and can sabotage legitimate group goals. Unidentified agendas can relate to power, jealousy, mind reading, or overcoming personal insecurities. Such agendas can interfere with the achievement of apparently straightforward group goals. Sometimes, there is a legitimate misunderstanding of the motives of others that also needs to be clarified before the work of the group can progress.

Understanding the underlying dynamics that cause people to act in ways that are directly opposed to the goals of the group and to their own self-declared interest helps the leader.

Hidden agendas are expressed in a variety of ways. For example, silence can be productive when it occurs when people are thinking about the issue under discussion. Or the silence can be a reflection of escalating anxiety and resistive anger.

One way of determining the nature of silence is to make the observation that the group seems silent and wait for a response. If none is forthcoming, the leader might ask, "Does this mean that everyone is in agreement?" Usually, the group will respond at this point, and the points of conflict will be out on the table for group discussion and resolution.

Uncomfortable as the process of confrontation is for group members and their leader, failure to resolve important emotional responses to the group process can negatively affect group outcomes. Individual member attitudes can have an impact on group dynamics in ways that sabotage group goals.

Constructive Confrontations

Constructive confrontation of an issue interfering with goal achievement or of a person sabotaging group goals is sometimes necessary if the group process is to progress satisfactorily. Confrontations should focus on the issue or behavior rather than on the person. Delivered with forethought and compassion, they are unsettling but usually not as damaging to the person receiving them as are communications containing a value judgment about the person or the person's motivations. Objective feedback that takes into consideration the impact the communication is likely to have on the person receiving it is more likely to be heard. Strategies for handling difficult group dynamics follow.

WHEN A GROUP MEMBER IS HOSTILE

The negative, hostile group member drains energy from the group. Left unattended, the negativity becomes a focus and an underlying force that seriously compromises the work of the group. There are several ways of addressing the issue. The leader can meet with the member outside the group and explore why the person is so negative within the group. It happens that individuals sometimes are not aware of how angry their interactions appear to others. Other times, there is a lack of understanding about some aspect of the group role or purpose. The leader can ask for the individual's cooperation in working with the group to make it more mutually satisfying and productive.

If the behavior persists in the group, another strategy is to summarize the ideas of the more positive members and to turn to them more frequently with comments and questions. This strategy, although indirect, is highly effective as the group communication takes on the flavor of those members who make the most verbal comments. It is not advisable to ridicule or criticize a negative person in front of other group members. Other members perceive it as a lack of respect.

The same phenomenon occurs when a member seizes control of the group as a personal forum for expression of negative attitudes and feelings. If the leader and members do nothing to check the flow of communication, the group quickly becomes demoralized. It is a delicate balance to speak to the destructive elements present in the group dynamics without destroying the individual in the process. As a member of the group, the person has the option of joining in the group activity productively or of leaving. Group members unable or unwilling to engage productively in the group may have to leave if they cannot resolve their negativity. It is important, however, to distinguish between a destructive personal negative attitude and the conflicts that are bound to emerge in any productive group setting.

WHEN A GROUP MEMBER SEEMS RESISTANT

The resistant member differs somewhat from the hostile member in that the group member is not necessarily opposed to the group or to the group goals. Rather, it is a personal human response to being in the group and not wanting to be there; or it occurs when the person has serious reservations about some aspect of the group task that has not been resolved in the group discussion. The resistant member may have negative expectations about the group goals or feel a personal inability to participate in their accomplishment. A resistant member is likely to show through body posture or lack of communication a reluctance to become an active member of the group. Verbal resistance is demonstrated by members who repeatedly question their personal participation in the group, the group goals, or the effectiveness of the group in meeting goals. Resistant members are most likely to emerge in involuntary groups.

The leader might encourage the resistant member to discuss his or her reservations about group participation. This can occur either in the group or individually with the leader outside the group. Sometimes, resistance evaporates if the leader gives permission to the reluctant member to assume a passive role in the group until he or she feels more comfortable. The key is to provide a temporary permission. Another strategy is to go around the room and ask each member what he or she is experiencing in the group. The answers are quite revealing. Having an understanding of the resistant member's reluctance enhances the acceptance and facilitates the possibility of a compassionate response. The silent member should never be singled out to give an explanation. If the resistant member appears to share more easily with other members than with the leader, other group members can encourage and support the contributions of the more silent member. Sometimes, one or two individual sessions with the reluctant or resistant group member can be helpful.

WHEN A GROUP MEMBER MONOPOLIZES GROUP COMMUNICATION

Strange as it may seem, the monopolizer usually has a limited self-awareness of the impact of his or her rather forceful presentation of self on other group members. Often well-intentioned, the monopolizer would say that he or she plays an active role in facilitating goal accomplishment. Caught in the web of self-absorption, the monopolizer seizes attention and control in the group. Initially, other members may tolerate or even encourage the monologue because it keeps the group focused on the monopolizer and not on their own lack of participation or interpersonal difficulties. The communication approach with the monopolizer is one of firmness and compassion. The leader can acknowledge the individual's contributions but may suggest that others in the group may be able to add something to the information presented by the person who is monopolizing the conversation. For example, the leader might say, "I think that is an interesting idea, but I'd like to hear from some of the other people too." The leader then can look around the group for a response. Usually one is forthcoming. If group members seem reluctant to engage or take the power away from the monopolizer because of their feelings, the leader might turn to someone else in the group with status and ask directly, "What do you think, Jack?"

THE GROUP AS CHANGE AGENT

One of the primary purposes of group interaction is to introduce and facilitate change.

Change is difficult, even under the best of circumstances.

Resistance to change occurs when the purposes of the change are unclear, when the persons affected by the change are not consulted, when there is a vested interest in maintaining the status quo, and when the legitimate needs of the group are ignored. Lewin[12] proposed a classic three-phase model that can be used to facilitate changes in attitudes and actions. The first phase, unfreezing, focuses on motivating people to think more creatively about an idea or situation. New information and explanations are used that force a person to experience the "here and now" in a different way. The format encourages members of a group to suspend the ways they usually conduct their lives and to embrace a new and often entirely different approach. It is important for the leader to provide full disclosure about the real reasons for the change, including anticipated difficulties. Rarely is a change, particularly in attitude or action, simple. The group will have more confidence in the leader who acknowledges this fact. Questions should be encouraged and answered as directly as possible. Creating enthusiasm and encouraging participation are essential. When everyone plays a part in developing a planned change, the chances of implementing the change increase dramatically.

Once motivated, the individual group members enter into the second phase of the change model, the change phase. In this phase, group members consider all of the driving forces that will help bring the change about and the restraining forces likely to prevent change from occurring. Consider a clinical example.

Mary Porter wants to update and change entries in the procedure manual. The old procedure manual is outdated, and there are some new procedures to be included. Some of the *driving forces* likely to be present are staff interest; the possibility that a revision will save time and mistakes; the need to meet JCAOH standards; and the fact that it could be used for orientation. *Restraining forces* might include lack of staff time to work on the project; lack of motivation to take on another task; and familiarity with the old procedure manual. To complete the project successfully, Mary will need to develop strategies convincing staff that the driving forces outweigh the restraining forces.

The second phase of the process involves feedback in which the leader and other group members challenge ineffective interactions and proposals. Simultaneously, they encourage group members to experiment with a different response pattern. The third phase, refreezing, deliberately fosters continued development of new behavior patterns. Praise, a reward system for compliance

with the change, and reality testing of goal achievement all can serve to reinforce the new behaviors. Closely related to understanding the nature of the change process in groups is the need to appreciate how the decision-making process works.

GROUP DECISION MAKING

Decision-Making Strategies

Making group decisions that move the group toward goal accomplishment is an essential part of effective group dynamics. There are several decision-making strategies. Methods that involve member participation and involvement throughout the process result in greater group commitment and personal satisfaction.

Some decisions are made by default. A group member suggests an idea, and other members latch onto it for lack of anything better or because there is a lack of interest or investment in the issue. Generally, this represents a poor decision-making method. The members have no real commitment to implementing the decision. Likewise, authority rule (decisions made by one person in authority) results in little commitment to the goal unless the leader has taken into consideration the advice of the group and bases the decision on their input. In some instances, when a decision must be made quickly, there are few alternatives to decision making by authority rule.

Majority rule occurs when a group member or members propose an idea and seek agreement from the majority of members, either informally or by voting. Agreement by over half of the members present constitutes a majority. The problem with this strategy is that the minority who do not agree with the decision sometimes are left with strong objections that may impede goal attainment.

Decisions made by consensus take a much longer time and more negotiation to be achieved. With a decision made by consensus, all members fully agree with, support, and are committed to the decision. Decisions are made after lengthy discussion and exploration of enough alternatives so every member feels satisfied that the group has reached the best decision, given the circumstances and resources surrounding the decision.

A unanimous decision occurs when all members agree and fully support a decision psychologically, even if they are not fully convinced personally. The group elects to speak with one voice about their choice. In contrast to consensus decisions, unanimous decisions are evaluative more of persons than of ideas. Unanimous decisions form the basis of our judicial criminal trial system.

Decision making by a minority occurs usually as a result of a power play. An individual or small faction of the group pressures the rest of the group to make a decision in their favor. The other group members lack or perceive a lack of ability to influence the decision-making process. This type of decision making also occurs when there are time constraints and a need to make a decision quickly. Usually, it is not an effective way of making a decision because there is no real commitment to it. People find indirect ways to sabotage decisions with which they disagree.

Steps in the Decision-Making Process

There are three sequential steps in the decision-making process. The first is diagnosis of the problem in need of a solution. Accurate diagnosis of the problem serves as the foundation for assessing the resources and maturity level of the system regarding its ability to resolve the problem. This involves open discussion with the group and a climate that allows members to freely pose and answer questions. The amount of time available to resolve the problem, how important group members perceive the resolution of the problem to be, and the level of acceptance of the consequences of proposed solutions are considered.

The clarity of problem identification is significantly related to the second step in the decision-making process, identification of alternative solutions. This step can take time because it involves brainstorming ideas. All ideas are given equal weight initially, and group members are encouraged to express all of their thoughts and feelings about the problem even if they seem far-fetched. The key element is that the ideas must relate to the problem under discussion. Without this norm, group discussions can become tangential to the accomplishment of the group goal.

Once sufficient ideas have been generated, the group turns to an analysis of possible alternatives. Group members realize that there are a number of alternative solutions to the problem, but some will result in more desirable outcomes based on what is known about the problem at the time. The focus shifts from equal consideration of all ideas to further discussion of the most promising ones. The outcome of the decision-making process is the final selection of the most desirable solution and a call for commitment to its implementation. After implementation, the group can focus on further revisions and refinement of the original decision.

Summary

- Groups are composed of two or more individuals who share one or more common characteristics and meet on a regular basis in face-to-face interactions to achieve a common goal.
- Primary groups are naturally occurring group formations in which membership is automatic or spontaneously chosen; secondary groups are specifically developed by people for the purpose of achieving identified goals.
- The main types of groups encountered in health care settings are therapeutic groups, encounter groups, self-help (community support) groups, task (work) groups, and educational groups.

- Some concepts important to an understanding of group dynamics are *goals, role functions, norms,* and *cohesion.*
- Five stages of group development are the preinteraction, introductory, transition, working, and termination phases.
- The three principal leadership styles are authoritarian, democratic, and laissez faire.
- Strategies for constructive confrontations can be helpful when a group member is hostile, seems resistant, or monopolizes group communication.
- Kurt Lewin's change model includes three phases: unfreezing, changing, and refreezing group decision making.
- Group decisions may be made by default, by authority rule, by majority rule, by consensus, by unanimous decision, or by minority pressure.

Bibliography

1. Arnold, E., & Boggs, K. (1989). *Interpersonal relationships: Communication skills for nurses.* Philadelphia: W.B. Saunders.
2. Barker, L., et al. (1987). *Groups in process: An introduction to small group communication.* Englewood Cliffs, NJ: Prentice Hall.
3. Benne, K.D., & Sheats, P. (1948). Functional roles and group members. *Journal of Social Issues,* 4(2), 41–49.
4. Bernard, L., & Walsh, M. (1990). *Leadership: The key to the professionalization of nursing.* St. Louis: C.V. Mosby.
5. Budman, S.H., et al. (1989). Cohesion, alliance and outcome in group psychotherapy. *Psychiatry,* 52(3), 339–350.
6. Corey, G. (1990). *The theory and practice of group counseling* (3rd ed.). Pacific Grove, CA: Brooks/Cole.
7. Corey, G., & Corey, M.S. (1987). *Groups: Process and practice* (3rd ed.). Pacific Grove, CA: Brooks/Cole.
8. Halperin, D.A. (1989). *Group psychodynamics: New paradigms and new perspectives.* St. Louis: C.V. Mosby.
9. Harvill, R., et al. (1983). Systematic group leadership training: a skills development approach. *The Journal for Specialists in Group Work,* 8(4), 16–20.
10. Janis, I.L. (1983). *Groupthink: Psychological studies of foreign policy decisions and fiascos* (2nd ed., revised). Boston: Houghton Mifflin.
11. Johnson, D., & Johnson, F. (1989). *Joining together: Group theory and group skills* (3rd ed.). Englewood Cliffs, NJ: Prentice Hall.
12. Lewin, K. (1951). *Field theory in social science* (pp. 146–147). New York: Harper & Row.
13. Masson, R., & Jacobs, E. (1980). Group leadership: practical pointers for beginners. *Personnel and Guidance Journal,* 58(3), 52–55.
14. Napier, R., & Gershenfeld, M. (1989). *Groups: Theory and experience.* Boston: Houghton Mifflin.
15. Redland, A.R. (1988). Working effectively in groups. *Clinical Nurse Specialist,* 2(3), 131.
16. Riordan, R.J., & Beggs, M.S. (1988). Some critical differences between self help and therapy groups. *Journal for Specialists in Group* Work 13(1), 24–29.
17. Sashkin, M. (1984). Participative management is an ethical imperative. *Organizational Dynamics,* 12(4), 5–22.
18. Schutz, W. (1967). *Joy: Expanding human awareness.* New York: Grove Press.
19. Thelen, H. (1954). *Dynamics of groups at work* (p. 187). Chicago: The University of Chicago Press.
20. Tuckman, B. (1965). Developmental sequence in small groups. *Psychological Bulletin,* 63(6), 384–399.
21. Wilson, G., & Hanna, M. (1990). *Groups in context: Leadership and participation in small groups* (2nd ed., pp. 154–162). New York: McGraw-Hill.
22. Yalom, I. (1985). *The theory and practice of group psychotherapy* (3rd ed.). New York: Basic Books.

Chapter 26

▼ *Teaching and Learning*

▼ Only as we educate individuals can they become full partners in their health care.

Judy Kopper

▼ CHAPTER OUTLINE

DOMAINS OF LEARNING
    Perceptual Domain
    Cognitive Domain
    Affective Domain
    Psychomotor Domain
UNDERSTANDING THE INDIVIDUAL
  LEARNER
    Assumptions That Characterize
      Adult Learning
PRINCIPLES OF LEARNING
    Factors That Facilitate Learning
    Factors That Hinder Learning
PRINCIPLES OF TEACHING
    What to Teach
    When to Teach
    How to Teach
ASSESSMENT
    Client Characteristics
    Level of Education

    Cultural Awareness
    Psychologic/Physiologic
      Considerations
    Socioeconomic Considerations
NURSING DIAGNOSIS
PLANNING
    Planning Concepts Related to
      Learning/Teaching Theory
    Learning Objectives
    Additional Learning Objectives
NURSING INTERVENTION
    Enhancing Client's Motivation to
      Learn
    Developing Content and Learning
      Activities
EVALUATION
    Short-term Learning
    Long-term Learning

▼ KEY TERMS

Affective learning domain
Cognitive learning domain
Learning
Learning contract

Learning objectives
Perceptual learning
    domain

Psychomotor learning
    domain

Learning is an experience that encompasses a person's total being. **Learning** involves not only perceiving and acquiring new knowledge, information, and skills but also changing one's behavior. When people learn, they may change their attitudes, lifestyle, and method of solving problems as a result.

Because learning takes great energy and concentration, it is a true nursing challenge to help people to learn when they are experiencing illness, anxiety, and pain.

The whole health care team is involved in the challenge of teaching.[4]

Among members of the health care team, we, as nurses, carry the primary responsibility for health education. The nurse practice act in each state indicates that teaching is a primary role for registered nurses. Standards for nursing care, which are used to accredit hospitals, include the statement that clients and their significant others receive education specific to their health care needs throughout their stay.[29]

All disciplines will teach the clients but, as a nurse, the public sees you as a person who is knowledgeable about health and illness, and therefore they respect your opinion. Perhaps you have already been in the situation in which a person says, "My doctor told me something about the test I'm supposed to have tomorrow, but I didn't understand all that medical talk. Do you think I really need this test?" Alternatively, the spouse of a business executive says to you, "I read an article recently that said table salt isn't really that bad for you if you have high blood pressure, but sodium is harmful. I thought table salt was sodium!" In these situations, people have made their learning needs readily known, and you are in the position to facilitate learning. In so doing, you enable people to make informed decisions and to take the responsibility for their own health care.

Nurses' abilities to teach vary depending on many factors, among them nurses' understanding of the subject to be taught, nurses' accuracy of assessing client learning needs, and environmental factors such as time and place available to teach. Regardless of the situation, range of nurse abilities, type of teaching materials used, or client characteristics, there appears to be a consistent benefit to patients when health education is incorporated into the nursing process.

The teaching/learning process is an integral part of the nursing process. Each step of the nursing process —assessment, nursing diagnosis, planning, nursing intervention, and evaluation—is used in the teaching/learning process to identify the learning needs of clients and their significant others and to take appropriate actions to meet those needs.

Whether we are actively promoting wellness, helping people maintain their present level of functioning, or facilitating rehabilitation, we depend on the teaching/learning process.[31]

This process allows us to (1) communicate necessary knowledge, (2) help change unhealthy patterns of behavior, and (3) assist a person to acquire a new skill needed for effective self-care. Numerous research studies are documenting the benefits of teaching (Box 26–1).

DOMAINS OF LEARNING

According to learning theory, there are four domains of learning, each representing a broad classification of human behavior.[25] Learning domains are *hierarchical.* Thus, each category of behavior builds on the skills in the category below it. Learning domains are (1) the **perceptual learning domain,** which is the ability to perceive written or verbal information; (2) the **cognitive learning domain,** which involves the intellectual

---

Box 26–1. Benefits of Patient Education

▶ Promotes early discharge
▶ Improves client satisfaction
▶ Improves quality care
▶ Conveys respect for the client

abilities; (3) the **affective learning domain,** which includes the states of feeling and valuing; and (4) the **psychomotor learning domain,** which encompasses the manipulative and motor skills. These domains each have levels or classifications ranging from the most simplistic learning to the most complicated.

Bloom developed the latter three domains into a classification system to help educators teach more effectively.[8] He described the cognitive and affective domains in depth. The psychomotor domain, although important to nursing practice, was not emphasized for the teacher in general education. Currently, nurses are expected to integrate *all four domains* of learning into a learning/teaching plan.[7] For example, formerly, when a nurse instructed a person with diabetes to self-administer insulin, the nurse simply demonstrated the steps of the procedure and asked for a return demonstration (psychomotor domain). Today, the nurse assesses for the client's feelings or attitudes toward self-injection (affective domain) and provides information as to the importance of the medication (cognitive domain). Most recently, we have recognized the importance of first assessing the perceptual domain, ensuring the client's ability to see the syringe and recognize dosage calibrations, before instruction.

Perceptual Domain

The perceptual domain of learning was proposed in the 1970s as an important first step in teaching. Being able to perceive (see, hear, understand, and respond to) various written and spoken words, pictures, or symbols is essential to understanding information. Nurses have learned always to first determine whether the client can see and hear well. However, nurses must also assess whether the client can correctly perceive the meaning of the information given and can apply the meaning to their own situation.

Nurses may assume that the person is able to look at a picture or a printed page and to comprehend the meaning of the symbols or words that appear there. The nurse should evaluate the client's ability to perceive information in the initial assessment phase of client teaching. Any limitations that are discovered can then be incorporated into the teaching plan. For example, extra-large print might be needed for the person with visual impairment. For the profoundly hearing-impaired client, a film would probably be inadequate unless it was captioned or accompanied by printed material.

LEVELS OF PERCEPTUAL LEARNING

The classification system for the perceptual domain was developed by Moore in 1970.[41] These levels of perceptual learning are described in terms of behavior nurses can observe. They are as follows:

Level 1. The client demonstrates that information can be detected through seeing, hearing, and fine motor ability or touch. For example, does the male diabetic client see the unit marks on the insulin syringe? Furthermore, does he recognize that he must master for himself the skill of drawing up the insulin to the appropriate mark?

Level 2. The client can sense through seeing, hearing, and fine motor ability that changes have occurred in the information given. In this case, the client can detect differences in the amounts of insulin units in his syringe.

Level 3. The client responds to visual and auditory stimuli such as pictures, words, and faces (symbol recognition and figure perception).

Level 4. The client can associate symbols perceived as having significant meaning personally. For example, the diabetic client would recognize the blood sugar level number on his glucometer that is abnormal for him.

Level 5. The client's decisions have been made on the basis of accurate observations. In this example, the diabetic client would select the appropriate insulin units when the glucometer blood sugar level number has changed.

This last level of the perceptual domain may not be assessed fully until the nurse has taught in the other domains as well.

To make decisions, clients must have information and cognitive understanding. For example, the diabetic client must understand why insulin is important and how it works in the body.

Cognitive Domain

The cognitive domain encompasses knowledge, comprehension, and a person's thinking skills.

LEVELS OF COGNITIVE LEARNING

Within the cognitive domain, there are several levels at which learning occurs:

Level 1: *Acquisition of Knowledge.* This is the process of acquiring information and is the simplest, most basic level of learning. It involves obtaining information and memorizing terminology, specific facts and principles, and techniques. For example, as a beginning student of nursing, you must learn nursing/medical terminology, facts about human anatomy and physiology, principles of asepsis, trends in health care delivery, and so forth.

Level 2: *Comprehension of New Information.* When people truly comprehend new facts, they are able to repeat the content back in their own words.

Level 3: *Application of Knowledge.* This is the intellectual ability to use that information *concretely* in a variety of situations. An example is in the care of individuals and significant others.

Level 4: *Analysis.* This is the ability to (1) break down information into its component parts and (2) determine the relationship of those parts to the whole. For example, to be able to analyze a disease entity, you must be able to (1) determine the signs and symptoms that characterize the disease, (2) analyze how the data relate to each other physiologically, (3) identify how they are affecting the individual, and (4) organize the information systematically so that you can communicate the person's needs clearly to other members of the health care team. Proficiency in this area requires a higher degree of cognitive ability than simply recalling facts by rote memory.

Level 5: *Synthesis.* This is the ability to communicate an idea or concept in a way that reflects your own unique and creative perspective of that idea. For example, the diagram of the nursing process shown on the inside of the front cover of this book is a *synthesis* of those scientific concepts that provide the structure for nursing practice.

Level 6: *Evaluation.* This involves making a critical judgment about how effectively certain criteria of learning have been met. For example, when you have a clinical evaluation, your instructor evaluates how effectively you have met the behavioral objectives for clinical practice.

Synthesis and evaluation represent the highest levels of cognitive abilities. Although we expect nurses to function at these levels, this is not always appropriate or necessary for client learners. Generally, these learners need to know what caused their illness, necessary lifestyle changes to prevent complications, basic symptom management, and sometimes specific procedural skills, such as how to do a colostomy irrigation. Usually, the individuals can function when given this amount of information, although many people ask for in-depth explanations.

Be aware that the nurse and the client have different learning needs.

Affective Domain

The affective domain of learning relates to ethics or principles that guide moral behavior and to reasoning that determines right behavior. Values, beliefs, feelings, and attitudes characteristic of the affective domain provide a powerful motivation for our behavior and the choices we make.

LEVELS OF AFFECTIVE LEARNING

Within the affective domain, there are four levels of learning:

Level 1: *Receiving.* This is the process by which people begin affective learning (i.e., they become sensitive to the existence of a certain situation or condition). For example, as you begin your career in nursing, you gradually become sensitive to the need to solve problems effectively so that you may provide high-level nursing care. Initially, this may seem an unnecessary and time-consuming exercise. However, as you progress in clinical practice, you come to realize that problem solving is essential and also a time saver. Having realized the benefits, you come to value the problem-solving process in preference to the imprecise ways in which you used to solve problems.

Level 2: *Valuing.* This is the process of you choosing freely from among several alternatives to act in a certain way. You make a commitment to that pattern of behavior.

Level 3: *Organization.* This is the integration of a value into your everyday life. For example, by graduation, you should have integrated all that you have learned, and you should have come to value problem solving throughout your daily clinical practice.

Level 4: *Characterization.* This is the highest level of affective learning. At this level, the internalized values contribute to your overall philosophy of life, making it possible for you to attain self-actualization.

You can promote people's health and well-being by facilitating high-level learning in the affective domain. To illustrate, alcoholism is a disease that requires learning in the affective domain. In the rehabilitation phase, alcoholic individuals have cognitive learning needs (i.e., they must learn the facts about their alcoholism, understand its pathophysiology, and learn about the impact that alcohol abuse has on interpersonal relationships).[47] Many alcoholic persons are quite capable of recalling factual information or of stating clearly the negative physiologic and interpersonal consequences of the alcohol abuse. If your evaluation of an alcoholic client were to stop at this point, you might conclude that meaningful learning had occurred. However, if the person continues to abuse alcohol, it is probable that the underlying values, attitudes, or needs in the affective domain have not changed. By setting *behavioral learning objectives* specific to the affective domain, the person may eventually replace self-destructive behavior with health-promoting behaviors.

The challenge to you in educating people in the affective domain is threefold: (1) to know and recognize your own value system and provide information to people in such a way that your own biases are minimized; (2) to respect the validity and uniqueness of other people's value systems, especially when they are different from your own; and (3) to provide people with accurate and complete information regarding their health or illness, so that affective learning can occur.[53]

Learning specific to the affective domain is often difficult to evaluate. It may take a person years to internalize feelings and values to the extent that behavior changes. Therefore, evaluation of affective learning is an ongoing process.

Psychomotor Domain

The psychomotor domain is concerned with physical or motor skills such as giving injections. These skills may require dexterity or fine muscle coordination and the ability to manipulate equipment and objects such as syringes. Teaching and learning psychomotor skills are areas in which nurses have traditionally felt comfortable and to which they have attached a great deal of significance. Historically, we know that nurses have been exceedingly task oriented in their approach to nursing practice. It was the "technically" excellent nurse who was regarded as the expert. However, if you learn a psychomotor skill merely to obtain technical competence, you disregard the importance of the cognitive and affective learning that provides the rationale for performing the skill. Students of nursing are now being educated to be critical thinkers in addition to being proficient in psychomotor skills.

It is the integration of the perceptual, cognitive, affective, and psychomotor domains that gives meaning to learning. Therefore, to perform only the skill renders learning incomplete. Similarly, the acquisition of intellectual knowledge without the ability to perform necessary skills renders learning inadequate.

LEVELS OF PSYCHOMOTOR LEARNING

There are five levels of learning within the psychomotor domain:

Level 1: _Imitation._ The first level of the psychomotor domain begins with the learner _observing_ an expert performing a skill. This step is followed by the learner attempting to _duplicate_ the steps of the procedure. Observing young children at play imitating their parents' actions is a classic example of how imitation facilitates learning. In this early phase, imitation may lack accuracy, coordination, or association with the appropriate real-life situation. By beginning with imitation, however, the learner is soon capable of manipulation.

Level 2: _Manipulation._ This is the ability to follow directions to perform the skill. The ability to follow instructions requires a familiarity with all the parts of the whole. Recall when you first learned how to take a blood pressure measurement. Watching your teacher, it looked so easy! Then you tried it; it did not seem simple any more. However, after inspecting and handling the equipment and learning to discern the front from the back of the cuff, you grew more comfortable. Then, as your teacher explained how to apply the cuff to the arm, you were able to do so correctly. As you grew more comfortable and knowledgeable, you were able to take blood pressure readings independently of a role model or instructions. As accuracy increased, you achieved precision.

Level 3: _Precision._ This connotes the _exactness_ with which a skill is performed. Precision leads to articulation.

Level 4: _Articulation._ This is the ability to incorporate _speed_ and _timing_ while maintaining _control_ in skill performance. For example, in time and with practice,

you were able to take a blood pressure accurately and within a reasonable time. Soon you had accomplished naturalization.

Level 5: _Naturalization._ At this point, the performance of the skill has become natural, spontaneous, and automatic. When you obtain this level of proficiency, it is difficult to remember that once you did not know how to measure blood pressure!

Proficiency at each level of the psychomotor domain is necessary to master any manual skills. Once mastered, the psychomotor skill then becomes a means to an end. Thus, once you learn the technique of blood pressure measurement, _interpreting_ the reading in terms of "normal," "too high," or "too low" and _understanding_ the clinical implications of the measurement become the focus of your attention. This example illustrates why learning is incomplete if you merely take the blood pressure reading without the cognitive or affective ability to interpret the data and act accordingly.

A clear understanding of the _interdependency_ of the perceptual, cognitive, affective, and psychomotor domains of learning enables you to begin to assess your client's learning needs with confidence.

When those needs are accurately identified, learning objectives can be mutually negotiated. Together with the client, you can develop a specific teaching plan that (1) builds on the person's present knowledge base, (2) provides new information, and (3) increases the person's level of understanding regarding her or his health status.

UNDERSTANDING THE INDIVIDUAL LEARNER

Teaching and learning for adults can be fundamentally different from the teaching/learning process for children. Nurses must gear the level and amount of information they teach according to a person's cognitive level. It is especially important to use age-appropriate terms and teaching techniques. For example, young children respond well to teaching by play in which games or drawings are used,[11] whereas older adults may want simply stated facts. See Unit 3 for more specific information concerning developmental stages.

Assumptions That Characterize Adult Learning

Malcolm Knowles, a leading authority on adult learning theory, identified four assumptions that characterize adult learning.[30] These four assumptions assist nurses in planning the teaching of adults. Remember, however, that adults are highly variable and must be treated as individuals.

ADULT LEARNING IS SELF-DIRECTED

The first assumption is that, as individuals mature, they become increasingly _self-directed_ regarding learning.

Knowles identified those changes in self-concept that take the learner from a state of learning dependency to a state of increasing *self-directedness*. This self-direction is reflected in adults who first identify their learning needs and then take direct action to acquire the needed knowledge. Consider two adults who want (need) to learn how to use a computer to increase their employment potential. One enrolls in a formal course at a local junior college; the other buys a book on word processing and devises a self-study program that combines reading the book and practicing the skill at the local library using computerized instruction. Both of these adults identified their desire to learn to use the computer and chose a method of study that best suited their own learning style. They exhibited self-directed learning behavior.

PAST EXPERIENCES ENHANCE LEARNING

The second assumption is that the adult learner approaches new learning experiences in light of a *lifetime of accumulated learning*. As adults, "we are what we learn." We define or characterize ourselves in terms of our experiences. This process is quite different from children, who view experiences as something that happens *to* them. The older we become, the more varied (and ingrained) are our learning experiences. Therefore, to facilitate adult learning, we should convey respect for people by making use of their past learning and drawing on their experiences as a resource to enhance present learning.

ADULT LEARNERS AND READINESS TO LEARN

Third, the adult learner is often characterized by a *readiness to learn*. For the adult, learning becomes more meaningful as it relates to what the person needs to know to perform effectively in a social role: spouse, parent, nurse, mechanic, professor, and so forth. It is often a challenge to structure health education in terms of developmental readiness to learn. People learn more readily when the information is useful and relevant to them socially, professionally, or personally. Mutual exploration and planning enable you and the adult learner to set learning priorities.

SOLVING REAL-LIFE PROBLEMS

Closely related to readiness to learn is the fourth assumption that adult learning is based on solving *real-life problems* and the necessity for immediate results. This problem-centered orientation to learning is in contrast to the subject-centered orientation typical of a child's learning. Children study mathematics, science, and English because they must in order to pass a test or enter high school, college, or graduate school. Subject-oriented learning has a delayed application.

Adults are more inclined to spend time, effort, and money to obtain knowledge that has *immediate* application to their circumstances. Also, when adults cope ineffectively with some of life's problems, they are motivated to seek new information. People who experience angina that interferes with job performance and

---

> **Box 26–2. Methods of Facilitating Adult Learning**
>
> ▶ Recognize that adults are often self-directed.
> ▶ Integrate past learning experiences into the present learning situation.
> ▶ Be sensitive to developmental readiness to learn.
> ▶ Make learning applicable to current life problems.

activities of daily living, for example, may be motivated to learn how to modify their stress level, lose weight, and stop smoking. The executive who has hypertension may be less motivated to learn these things because the disease process does not presently interfere with job performance. Thus, to spend time performing these activities does not seem relevant to this person's present goals. Your task is to convince the person that performing the healthy behaviors will ultimately lead to a more productive life. On the other hand, the person needs to realize that, by ignoring a serious health problem, complications can develop that may impede work performance altogether (e.g., a stroke). Helping people achieve immediate short-term goals that are positively rewarded reinforces learning. In turn, this success motivates people to continue healthy behaviors.

These characteristics of the adult learner are strengths if they are integrated sensitively into the learning process. You can provide a supportive learning environment by applying these assumptions when interacting with adult learners.

PRINCIPLES OF LEARNING

To meet the challenge of teaching, you need to understand which factors facilitate learning and which factors hinder learning. Principles that can guide your decisions about teaching children, adults, families, groups, and communities are discussed next.

Factors That Facilitate Learning

EMOTIONAL AND PHYSICAL READINESS TO LEARN

The person must be *ready to learn, both physically and emotionally*. A person who is in severe pain or who is frightened, restless, or anxious is obviously not going to profit from a teaching session no matter how well it is presented. In addition, the person must be able to comprehend the information and ideas being discussed. Thus, if a person is very groggy from anesthesia, it is best to postpone teaching sessions until he or she is better able to comprehend.

Readiness to learn can be assessed in groups or in individuals by asking various questions (Box 26–3).

MOTIVATION TO LEARN

The person learns more if there is a *genuine desire to learn*. People differ greatly in the amount and type of information they can tolerate concerning their illness or behavior. Some people become anxious if they feel "in the dark" about their illness. They want to know as much as possible about its cause, prevention, and treatment. Others become extremely anxious if the nurse tries to talk with them concerning their disorder. When anxious people resist instruction, it is best not to push them into listening to information for which they are emotionally unprepared. Instead, wait until they approach you with questions about their condition. At this point, anxiety may well have lessened and they will be more receptive to new information.

ENVIRONMENT CONDUCIVE TO LEARNING

People learn best in a *warm, accepting atmosphere.* They need to feel that the nurse is genuinely interested in helping them learn. People should not be criticized if they cannot recall everything they have been taught. Remember how anxious you were during your first days in the school of nursing and how overwhelmed you felt (and may still feel) by the enormous volume of new words and concepts to learn. In this respect, clients are not different from yourself. They need time to assimilate ideas and develop new skills. They should have the right to make mistakes and even to fail at a task without losing face. Your role is to act as a facilitator and not as a judge.

Learning is facilitated in a *pleasant, quiet environment, free from distractions.* The teaching area or classroom should be well lit, comfortably warm, and (if possible) away from the hub of activity.

RELEVANCE OF CONTENT

Content is learned more easily when it is presented in a *way that has personal relevance.* You might ask a woman what she already understands about her pregnancy and what in particular she would like to learn at this time. While teaching, check that people understand the content; also validate that you are still discussing material that is relevant to them.

WELL-DEVELOPED TEACHING PLAN

The person is more successful in remembering and assimilating well-organized materials that proceed from the simple to the complex. In a well-developed teaching plan, each concept presented is based on a broader and more fundamental concept. Clearly, a person cannot understand abnormalities of function without first understanding normal function. Likewise, an individual cannot comprehend the treatment and prevention of a disease without first learning about its cause. Thus, when teaching someone about illness and therapy, begin with a broad discussion of the normal anatomy and physiology of the diseased organ or system, proceed to a description of those factors that cause the disease, and end the discussion with a presentation of how the person can assist in her or his treatment and rehabilitation program.

REWARD FOR POSITIVE BEHAVIORS

Learning is strengthened and reinforced when positive behaviors are rewarded. We are all more motivated to study and learn when we know that our efforts will be rewarded. For you, the reward may be a high grade. For ill individuals, incentives and rewards center on (1) controlling pain or other symptoms, (2) returning to a normal or near-normal lifestyle, (3) avoiding complications, and (4) pleasing the nurse or the physician. In addition, remember that, other things being equal, immediate rewards reinforce positive behaviors far more than do delayed rewards. Therefore, it is important to compliment people immediately after they ask a thoughtful question, demonstrate what they have learned about their illness, or perform a procedure satisfactorily.

ACTIVE PARTICIPATION IN THE LEARNING PROGRAM

People learn more effectively when they are encouraged to participate in their health education program. Active participation generates interest in learning, whereas absence of participation results in boredom. Who has not read an article and forgotten most of the subject matter because the passive act of reading was not supplemented with the active act of discussion? Who has not almost fallen asleep during a long, tedious lecture? Who has not doodled and daydreamed during classes conducted by teachers who never ask questions or call for a discussion? As has been said, "The more the teacher teaches, the less the student learns."

There are a number of ways to encourage participation. For instance, as you present new material, ascertain the person's understanding of the subject. Discuss all written materials and brochures.

Do not assume that if you hand people a list of instructions they will necessarily follow them.

People usually require discussion as to why those particular instructions are so important. If you demonstrate a procedure, have the person give a return demonstration as soon as possible. Better yet, if extra equipment is available, allow the person to work through each step of the procedure with you rather than waiting to demonstrate the entire procedure again later.

REPETITION OF KEY FACTS AND CONCEPTS

Repetition of key facts and concepts reinforces learning. Frequent practice reinforces the learning of skills and facilitates the performance of procedures. Reviewing materials presented earlier prepares the individual for learning new materials.

PUTTING NEW INFORMATION SKILLS INTO PRACTICE

People retain information and skills longer when they are allowed to put new information skills into practice immediately. When people cannot use their knowledge, they tend to forget quickly what they have learned. For example, in many obstetric units, it is common practice for new mothers to begin almost immediately to care for their infants. While on the unit, mothers learn, under supervision, to bathe, feed, and diaper their infants. In the past, these procedures were usually demonstrated by the nurse, but mothers had to wait until they went home to perform the care themselves. By the time of discharge, many first-time mothers had already forgotten important points about caring for their infants. Currently, new mothers are encouraged to perform a return demonstration of a learned skill almost immediately, under supervision, instead of being sent home to flounder alone.

SURMOUNTING LEARNING PLATEAUS

People occasionally reach learning plateaus. At this time, it may appear to you that the person has lost interest in learning and may even seem to be discouraged. Learning plateaus, as you know from your own educational experiences, are normal. To assist the person to surmount the plateau, you might use audiovisual aids, such as videotapes or other stimulating methods of presentation. It may help to give the person a break from structured learning until previous levels of enthusiasm return.

   If you remember these factors that facilitate learning, you can use them to motivate clients to learn.

Factors That Hinder Learning

PHYSIOLOGIC LEARNING BARRIERS

People experiencing critical illness, severe pain, restlessness, oxygen deprivation, fatigue, weakness, deafness, or visual problems have difficulty learning. These physiologic states act as barriers to learning because they reduce the individual's ability to concentrate and they deplete energy.

EMOTIONAL LEARNING BARRIERS

Psychologic stresses also interfere with one's ability to concentrate. People who feel anxious, fearful, and angry because they are ill may be too psychologically stressed to learn. Patients who are adjusting to a new diagnosis may experience denial and be unable to attend to your teaching. Clients who are grieving may not be able to learn well until they are in the stage of accepting their loss.

CULTURAL LEARNING BARRIERS

Problems in teaching/learning arise when people speak a different language from you or have differing educational backgrounds and values. Unfortunately, some nurses have been known to reject and consequently avoid teaching people who are a part of a counterculture (e.g., ex-convicts, persons with acquired immune deficiency syndrome, or members of the drug culture). Being aware of cultural differences and obtaining assistance with teaching are important.

ENVIRONMENTAL LEARNING BARRIERS

Lack of privacy, a noisy environment, and numerous interruptions tend to disrupt teaching sessions seriously. When the room temperature is too hot or cold, the client may be too uncomfortable to concentrate. Clients in a group may be distracting to one another.

INADEQUATE OR POOR TEACHING

Teaching problems that hinder a person from learning include lack of knowledge and preparation on your part, lack of planning, overuse of technical words, the delivery of poorly prepared or fragmented presentations, unwillingness to draw the person into discussion, hurried or poorly planned demonstrations, and a condescending attitude as you relate to the person.

PRINCIPLES OF TEACHING

To be effective in an educator role, you must make three important decisions: (1) what to teach, (2) when to teach, and (3) how to teach.

What to Teach

The hospitalized client and family members may be interested to learn about the following:

▶ Basic normal anatomy and physiology of the body[6]
▶ The underlying pathology causing the disease symptoms
▶ The rationale for the treatment program
▶ Complications and limitations resulting from the illness that may impose a lifestyle change
▶ The prognosis for the disease
▶ The purpose of medications, their safe administration, and any possible side effects
▶ The cost of nursing/medical care
▶ The expected duration of hospitalization—short-term or long-term care
▶ The nature of diagnostic tests and studies—the preparation for those tests and the meaning of test results

▶ Preventive and rehabilitative measures to help prevent or overcome complications
▶ The health care facility environment (e.g., the bedside equipment and how it works; the location of bathrooms, cafeteria, and chapel; hospital policies and routines)
▶ The health care facility staff; the names of the nurses caring for the client; the names of the nursing supervisor, head nurse, team leader, and dietitian; and the names and telephone numbers of the chaplain and others whose services may be desired
▶ Home care (e.g., assistance the person and family members may require on discharge; available community resources; and follow-up with personal physician, nurse practitioner, and outpatient facilities

As you continue to assess individual learning needs, you may identify other interest areas unique to that person.[17] Asking clients for input into the teaching plan helps to ensure that content is interesting and relevant to their needs.

When to Teach

Teaching occurs at any time. It can be scheduled or unscheduled. For example, instruction can be given at specific times that are formally designated and presented throughout the day or informally when a person asks questions or encounters new experiences that require explanation. In general, however, try to avoid hectic times or periods when people are distracted (e.g., during meals or after they have received a pain medication). The nurse must decide when learning will be optimum. Research studies indicate that teaching at the time when family members or significant others are available is an advantage.[2]

How to Teach

The teaching method selected depends on the subject matter and on the person's background, personality, and needs. Teaching may be in the form of formal lectures and demonstrations. Informal discussions, either individually or in a group, may often be more appropriate. Audiovisual aids and printed information often facilitate learning. Numerous technologic advances have been made in developing audiotapes and videotapes and in using in-hospital television channels for client teaching. Computer programs are also becoming available for client education. When these methods are used to teach, the nurse should be available afterward to answer questions and evaluate what clients have learned. Before using any print teaching aids, analyze the content and reading level. Typically, a fourth- to sixth-grade reading level is best.

In whatever way you decide to teach, focus your efforts on individual learning needs, and communicate accurate, current, and relevant information. Conduct your teaching/learning program according to the steps of the nursing process (Box 26–4).

Box 26–4. The Nursing Process Applied to Health Teaching

By applying the nursing process to a learning/teaching situation, a systematic approach includes the following major steps:

▶ Identify the person's learning capabilities (assessment).
▶ Identify the person's learning needs (nursing diagnoses).
▶ Develop learning goals and behavioral objectives designed to meet those goals (planning).
▶ Select the appropriate teaching strategy (intervention).
▶ Evaluating the person's progress and the effectiveness of the overall teaching plan (evaluation).

ASSESSMENT

Each client, whether young or old, will have individual characteristics or factors affecting his or her learning. Assess each client as an individual, and tailor your teaching plan to meet each person's needs.

Client Characteristics

As you prepare to teach people, incorporate your awareness of age, as well as medical diagnosis and clinical progress, into the teaching plan. Each of these factors may influence your approach to learning needs. Children and their parents may require specialized teaching approaches. Children are often receptive to instruction that involves playing games or role-playing. This type of interaction may be therapeutic and may be a vehicle for learning. Parents, on the other hand, may need affective domain assessment for their emotional reactions to their children's problems. Although you should always assess hearing and visual acuity, problems with these senses are more common in the elderly. If the person has a sensory deficit, consider this factor as you select visual aids or teaching strategies. Like age, other characteristics such as sex, religious beliefs, and cultural background may alter the learning needs of the client and therefore affect the materials you use in presenting a particular content area.

Level of Education

Level of education is determined by the highest year of formal education or reading/comprehension ability. Before beginning instruction, assess people's general health knowledge, their perception of the current disease situation, and the type of instruction that they will most easily assimilate.[18]

Do not assume that a well-educated person is a well-informed person when it comes to health education!

In addition to assessing people's educational status, determine (1) what they have been told by the physician or have gleaned from the media; (2) what they

---

Box 26–5. Sample Interview to Use in Assessing What Clients Already Know About Their Health Care

1. Can you tell me what you have learned about your illness?
2. You have had surgery before. Can you tell me what you remember from that experience?
3. When you spoke with your physician or pharmacist, what did they tell you was important to know about your medications?
4. Have you heard about your therapy from anyone else who has had your health problem?
5. Have you read or heard reports about the treatments your physician wants you to undergo?

Adapted from Smith, C. (ed.) (1987). *Patient education: Nurses in partnership with other health professionals* (p. 62). Orlando, FL: Grune & Stratton. Used with permission.

---

know about the illness in general; (3) their experience with illness, the health care system, and hospitalization (Box 26–5).

All these areas provide information and influence learning, although they may be unrelated to a person's formal education. It is in this informal educational realm that you may determine people's readiness to learn, goals for learning, and learning needs; those things you think they need to know to assume self-care.

Cultural Awareness

Every ethnic group has its own unique beliefs and practices. Many of these center around diet, nutrition, health, and illness. There may be certain forbidden foods or certain health rituals to observe. For many individuals, their religious beliefs influence their health care practices. Sometimes it is necessary to distinguish between beliefs that are a part of a tightly held value system and ideas that result from misinformation.

At all times, consider cultural or religious values in assessing overall teaching/learning needs. However, it is equally important to avoid stereotyping individuals on the basis of sex, age, race, ethnic origin, or lifestyle preferences.

The nurse must also recognize that the values she or he holds may vary from those of the client. The nurse may value self-care, whereas a client may not, and may say, "Oh, just tell my wife. She gives me all my pills." Each person must be regarded as a unique individual, and his or her instruction needs must be considered.

Psychologic/Physiologic Considerations

Attitudes change throughout the course of a serious illness and also when a person moves from wellness to

 APPLYING RESEARCH TO NURSING PRACTICE

Tailoring Your Teaching to Fit Your Clients

Grahn, G., & Johnson, J. (1990). Learning to cope and living with cancer: learning-needs assessment in cancer patient education. *Scandinavian Journal of Caring Science, 4*(4), 173–181.

 ▼ ▼ ▼

When a client is newly diagnosed with cancer, the information that can be covered in client and family education is vast. It may cover such areas as (1) the biomedical aspects of cancer, (2) treatments and their side effects, (3) nutritional needs, (4) pain management, (5) psychosocial and family concerns, (6) changes in sex life, (7) resources in society, and (8) future plans. Because client and family education after a diagnosis of cancer can span such a wide range of areas, Grahn and Johnson set out to determine specifically what clients and their families need and want to know. They also attempted to determine how effectively health care professionals match learning needs with appropriate cancer-related education. To answer those questions, researchers studied 50 clients newly diagnosed with cancer, 20 of their family members, and 30 of their nurses and physicians. The study found that between 60 per cent and 80 per cent of clients and families wanted to learn about all eight of the areas just noted. Although clients and their families expressed interest in a broad range of topics associated with cancer, staff members reported that clients and families had actually asked questions on only a narrow range of topics. The most frequently asked questions (asked by 69 per cent to 83 per cent of clients and families) were associated with treatment options and treatment side effects. Only 50 per cent of clients and families had asked questions related to nutritional needs and pain management.

Applications for Practice

In practice, encourage open communication with your clients and their families. Doing so will enable you to assess learning needs and to match your teaching to those needs.

---

illness. It is helpful to understand what the person's personality and self-image were like before the onset of the present illness. People sometimes experience a personality change as a result of a real or perceived threat to their self-esteem or present lifestyle. Many learning needs center on the person's emotional response to illness. New learning may be required to facilitate the person's adjustment to altered function or lifestyle changes. You also need to assess the entire family's response to the illness of one member. Does this illness change the roles of family members and significant others or alter their interpersonal communication? Teaching content may also be altered by the medical/nursing prognoses.

A person who is terminally ill may have different learning needs and capabilities from those of the person who is not facing death. Unfortunately, because the learning needs of the dying person are different, they are often ignored altogether. Dying people and their significant others have many question and concerns and have a right to learn the answers.

Socioeconomic Considerations

While you are teaching people about their illness and the necessary self-care, it helps to understand the home situation: living arrangements and the usual activities of daily living. Relationships with significant others are important and can provide a strong support group for the ill person. Evaluating the type of work a person does, as well as understanding related job stress and work experiences, may be useful in identifying learning needs. Knowing the person's financial situation enables you to plan cost-effective health and maintenance care when possible.

NURSING DIAGNOSIS

In planning to meet client teaching needs, *Knowledge Deficit* is the most commonly used nursing diagnosis. This is not always an accurate diagnosis. For example, nurses sometimes note that a client needs to be taught about diet or health care and write diagnoses such as *Knowledge Deficit R/T Low-Fat Diet* or *Knowledge Deficit R/T Insulin Injections*. This is an inappropriate use of the diagnosis of knowledge deficit. Remember: It is the second part of the nursing diagnosis that is the etiologic factor, and it is incorrect to think that a low-fat diet or insulin injections actually *caused* a person to have a knowledge deficit.

Several other etiologic factors better explain the client's knowledge deficit. For example, *Knowledge Deficit* R/T limited vision interfering with reading medication labels or *Knowledge Deficit* R/T situational depression interfering with a desire to learn about illness are both pertinent diagnostic statements for persons with unmet learning needs. Such etiologic factors usually interfere with the person learning anything (not just low-fat diet or insulin injections, for example). Illiteracy, substance abuse, anxiety, or pathophysiologic problems (pain, poor eyesight) may be other causes of knowledge deficit.[20] The nurse should be able to set objectives in the perceptual and affective domains that will guide interventions for such nursing diagnoses and barriers to learning.

PLANNING

It is important to remove barriers to learning that have caused knowledge deficit to occur. Only by improving the person's vision, treating the depression or anxiety, or dealing with the substance abuse, for example, will the person be ready to learn.

After barriers that cause knowledge deficit are removed, planning for client teaching begins.

Planning Concepts Related to Teaching/Learning Theory

CONCEPT OF LEARNING STYLES

Everyone has a unique learning style: a way he or she learns best. It enhances your teaching effectiveness if you discover early each person's learning style. Unfortunately, many nurse educators use a teaching strategy that is most comfortable for them rather than individualizing their strategy to accommodate the client's style of learning. Consider a class of beginning nursing students. Some students learn best by listening instead of taking notes during class; they listen intently to the discussion or lecture. Others are more comfortable taking notes, and write furiously to capture verbatim the lecture content. Still others may skip the lecture altogether, preferring to read the content in the textbook independently. The same is true for the client learner. Some do well when you simply lecture about the topic of interest. Others prefer to read a pamphlet or handout and clarify questions after their own independent study. Ask your clients how they most enjoy learning new information. Adapt your teaching strategy to their preference.

CONCEPT OF MUTUAL NEGOTIATION

By actively involving people in the decision-making process, you stimulate their motivation to learn. People are more apt to be enthusiastic about learning information that they have identified as important to them. Combining their interests with content you think they must know to accomplish self-care makes the teaching/learning process mutually gratifying!

Sometimes, however, people seem to resist learning. Perhaps they are still denying the disease process or feel angry at the adjustments they must make in their lifestyle. Until clients have accepted the fact that their health status affects them personally, they will not consider learning about it relevant to their needs. Other people resist for other reasons; for example, they "don't have time," they are presently asymptomatic, or they lack family support. For these individuals, *contracting* may be an effective way to elicit their participation. A **learning contract** is a mutually negotiated plan for health education. In a learning contract, much like any business contract, each party (you and the client) agrees to contribute certain things to the arrangement. You may promise to provide information, and the client promises to use that information. The contract helps develop learning goals to help the person achieve the desired outcomes in a learning situation. As time goes by, the client may experience the satisfaction or reward of accomplishment in learning, and the contract will no longer be necessary.

Mager stated that "instruction is effective to the degree that it succeeds in changing the learning in the desired direction."[37] If teaching (instruction) does not lead to learning or a change in behavior, then it has no effect, no power.

Learning Objectives

So how do nurses use teaching to accomplish the overall goal of changing clients' health behavior? They do so by clearly stating learning objectives. A **learning objective** describes the intended results of learning rather than the process of instruction. Objectives that describe the performance you want persons to exhibit before you consider them competent in a certain area are essential to planning. Learning objectives must be clear, realistic, and measurable. In addition, learning objectives must be client centered and stated in behavioral terms so that progress can be measured and evaluated.

Characteristics of a well-written learning objective include (1) a statement of the expected performance, (2) conditions under which the behavior is to be performed, and (3) the criterion by which the performance will be evaluated.

Consider the following objectives, one of which is vague and ambiguous and therefore difficult to evaluate, the other of which incorporates the characteristics of a well-written objective (Box 26-6).

Objective 1: Mr. Philips will understand about diabetes mellitus (a metabolic disorder characterized by elevated blood glucose resulting from an inadequate amount or lack of insulin from the pancreas and

treated by diet, insulin, and exercise) before discharge from the health care facility.

Objective 2: By the end of the second teaching session, Mr. Philips will be able to state the signs and symptoms of hyperglycemia (high blood glucose) with 100 per cent accuracy.

Objective 1 is vague and difficult to measure. Objective 2, in contrast, is specific and measurable. Do you see why Objective 2 is the clearer statement of the desired outcome? Let us identify the necessary characteristics.

Performance: The person will be able to state the signs and symptoms of hyperglycemia

Condition: by the end of the second teaching session

Criterion: with 100 per cent accuracy

Having written the objective clearly, using measurable criteria, you are able to evaluate whether the desired learning has occurred. Additionally, Mr. Philips will know what is expected of him as an outcome of the teaching sessions and will be able to focus his efforts on accomplishing that outcome. Because the management of diabetes mellitus requires a multifaceted approach to learning, you can see that several learning objectives are necessary for Mr. Philips to assume the responsibility for self-care. Examples of additional objectives might include the following:

Additional Learning Objectives

1. By the end of the first teaching session, Mr. Philips will correctly state the pathophysiology of diabetes mellitus in terminology appropriate to his level of understanding in the cognitive domain.

2. Each morning before breakfast, Mr. Philips will correctly test his own blood glucose by the finger-stick method: (1) using sterile technique, (2) using the proper equipment, (3) accurately interpreting the blood glucose measurement on the test strips, and (4) correctly recording the findings on a permanent record.

3. The day before discharge, given a list of food choices, Mr. Philips will choose appropriate foods to plan a sample breakfast, lunch, and dinner menu with 100 per cent accuracy.

Take a moment to practice writing behavioral objectives that address (1) maintenance of ideal body weight during college, (2) stress reduction exercises for students at examination time, and (3) time management in the clinical area during morning care.

NURSING INTERVENTION

Enhancing Client's Motivation to Learn

After deciding on learning goals and objectives, the next step is to enhance clients' motivation to learn. Assess the learners' determination, motivation, and desire to learn. For example, individuals seeking nutritional instruction to control obesity often state how discouraging advertising is because unrealistically thin

---

Box 26-6. Writing Learning Objectives

Behavioral Objectives to Individualize Client Teaching In Regard to a Pathologic Condition

Client and/or significant other:

1. States in simple terms what the diagnosis is and what was done to treat the problem in the hospital;
2. States what, if any, normal residual effects of the condition and subsequent procedures may be expected;
3. Lists reasons to call the nurse or physician after discharge;
4. States who or where the client should call with problems or questions between regularly scheduled follow-up appointments;
5. Explains any technologic care required;
6. Demonstrates any psychomotor skills required.

Nonbehavioral Phrases to Avoid Using When Writing Behavioral Objectives

These phrases are broad, vague, and ambiguous. They permit a variety of interpretations and do not allow for specific measurement.

to be acquainted with	to be familiar with
to understand	to sympathize with
to appreciate	to be aware of
to comprehend	to increase interest

Box 26-7. Enhancing Willingness or Motivation to Learn

1. Explore past teaching experiences that created negative attitudes toward learning.
2. Compliment individual and groups on information already learned.
3. Determine what the person wants to learn and teach this first.
4. Take steps to overcome deficiencies in perceptual skills (e.g., vision limitations, memory loss).
5. Provide counseling to reduce patient or family anxieties.

Adapted from Smith, C. (ed.) (1987). *Patient education: Nurses in partnership with other health professionals* (pp. 66–67). Orlando, FL: Grune & Stratton. Used with permission.

people are often portrayed as the ideal. This may decrease their motivation because they fear they cannot live up to this ideal. Nurses must be alert for these barriers so that past learning experiences will not interfere with current teaching. In addition to motivation, past experiences and perceptual skills are important factors to assess in determining what learning activities are best for the needs of the client (Box 26–7).

Developing Content and Learning Activities

The next intervention is developing content and learning activities. As stated earlier, the content taught and the level of its presentation depend on the person's situation as well as his or her condition, age, and prognosis. The content should incorporate the person's own objectives. In addition, it must be cost effective.[5]

Learning activities vary with the content to be taught and with the individual's learning needs and capabilities.[9]

TEACHING STRATEGIES

One-to-One Instruction. One-on-one instruction may be formal or informal. It allows you to pace the learning content and activities to people's learning rates. Also you can modify the program in keeping with client progress.

Group Instruction. Group instruction requires that you arrange for a meeting place, prepare handout materials in advance of the meeting, develop a meeting agenda and a lesson plan, arrange seating to facilitate group interaction (e.g., putting the chairs into a circle), lecture on major topics, lead a discussion, review major points covered in the discussion, and arrange for the next meeting. The two major advantages of group instruction are that (1) it is economical in terms of your time, and (2) individuals with similar problems can share experiences, viewpoints, and opinions with each other. Two disadvantages are that (1) you must pace your instruction to the level of the group rather than to an individual, and (2) some people are intimidated by a group and find it difficult to ask questions or enter into the discussion.

Lectures. Lectures are usually delivered in a group setting. This method is useful for delivering a large amount of factual information to a group.

Discussion. Discussion is an important teaching activity because it encourages people to participate actively in the health education program. Draw people into a discussion by asking for their responses to the content, for examples of ways in which the content is applicable to their lives, and for personal experiences and opinions.[21] For instance, in a class for people being treated for cancer, you might ask how they dealt with the problem of alopecia (baldness) after radiation therapy. In a prenatal class, an experienced mother might describe (for the benefit for expectant mothers) the "3-day blues" that many mothers feel after the birth of a child and the ways she coped with them.

Demonstration. Demonstrations are typically used to teach motor skills (e.g., how to give a self-injection of medication or how to transfer safely from bed to wheelchair). To prepare for a demonstration, (1) organize your notes and thoughts so that you can accompany the demonstration with a discussion of the procedure; (2) assemble the equipment and make certain that it works properly; (3) if possible, prepare a handout that outlines the procedures so that people can follow the demonstration more easily; and (4) practice the demonstration until you feel comfortable doing it. When giving the demonstration, make certain that people can see you perform each step. Proceed slowly and allow time for questions. Afterward, have people return the demonstration as soon as possible, which immediately reinforces learning.

Role-Playing. Role-playing is a creative strategy that allows the person to act out different roles (physician, nurse, spouse, employer) in a variety of real-life situations. This allows them to learn new behaviors or to problem solve. Initially, some people may feel too inhibited to role-play in a hypothetical situation. Nevertheless, this can be a very effective strategy because it enables people to glean new insights in a "safe" environment. Role-playing is often used in nursing skills classes or labs in which students role-play how to interact with different clients in a variety of situations (i.e., one student plays the client, one student plays the nurse). This allows students to experience a situation from more than one vantage point. Role-playing is often constructive for clients with mental health problems or those with chronic, irreversible diseases.

Programmed Study. Programmed study is highly effective with motivated, bright, self-directed people. It involves a prepared program of study that lists learning objectives and provides activities to meet those objectives. Often it includes a pretest and a posttest for self-evaluation. Using this method, learners can study at their own pace and proceed to more difficult concepts once basic content is well understood. You may follow up this method with discussion or a question-answer period to clarify or expound on the content in light of the learner's individual questions or needs.

Computerized Learning Packages. Computerized learning packages are similar to printed programmed studies, except that the learning package is programmed into a computer. It allows self-study and self-pacing but also provides an "interactive" component that many learners find helpful. Computerized learning packages are used at all levels of formal education and are likely to enjoy broader usage as client education software packages become more commonly used.

TEACHING AIDS

Teaching activities can be enhanced by the proper use of teaching aids. Useful teaching tools include pamphlets, hand drawings, models of organs, charts, graphs, audiotapes, a bulletin board, a blackboard, posters, pictures, overhead transparencies, slide shows, films, videotapes, closed-circuit television, flash cards, programmed instructions, and games.

RESOURCE PERSONS

Resource persons are extremely helpful adjuncts to any of these teaching activities. For example, when teaching people about a special diet, ask the dietitian to attend the session and share his or her expertise with the group. Physicians, physical therapists, and occupational therapists may all make significant contributions to a group lecture or discussion. Additional useful resources include other clients with similar health care concerns who have managed to meet their own learning needs and changed their health behavior; for example, a teenager who has managed cancer chemotherapy previously might be called on to teach youngsters in whom cancer is newly diagnosed. Most clients find teaching given by another client to be of value.

EVALUATION

The final step in the teaching/learning process is *evaluation*.

Short-term Learning

Has the person met the learning objectives that were mutually negotiated at the beginning of the teaching period? Is the person knowledgeable, demonstrating with proficiency the skills necessary to maintain self-care? Are you able to discern a measurable difference in the person's attitude about the disease process? Does the person demonstrate an ability to cope with the limitations imposed by the illness and show a willingness to make necessary lifestyle changes?[27] Do the person's significant others understand the problems, and are they supportive?

You should be asking these and many other questions to determine whether short-term learning has occurred and is being acted on.[47]

Long-term Learning

Long-term learning must be evaluated as well as short-term outcomes.[52] Nurses often focus heavily on evaluating short-term learning (i.e., what a person learns in the health care facility before discharge) and neglect the importance of long-term learning evaluation. One long-term evaluation strategy is to recommend a home health nurse to visit after discharge to evaluate and to reinforce learning or correct mistakes early. Another strategy is a follow-up questionnaire. Consider the client who, after suffering a myocardial infarction, has learned about diet, stress management, and exercise before being sent home. At the time of discharge, you may determine that significant learning has occurred and that the person appears highly motivated to change unhealthy lifestyle habits and incorporate this new learning into everyday life. However, what is actually happening 2 months, 6 months, and 1 year after the myocardial infarction? It is during this time that the change of behavior (or lack of it) becomes evident and begins to affect the person's recovery and way of life. Nurses must be able to determine the effectiveness of teaching strategies on a long-term basis. Evaluating the long-term consequences of learning is a shared responsibility. The person, the health care facility staff, the outpatient nurse, and the physician all share the responsibility for reinforcing long-term learning and evaluating learning over time.

How is long-term evaluation accomplished? Many units are sending out follow-up questionnaires at selected intervals after discharge to evaluate the effectiveness of in-hospital teaching programs. This accomplishes several things. First, the person has had the opportunity to test the learning in a real-life situation.

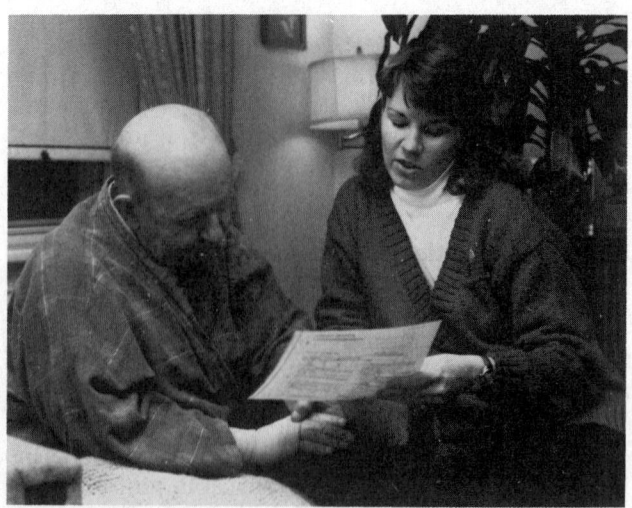

▲ **Figure 26–1**

A home health nurse can evaluate and reinforce learning.

Many times, when we are removed temporarily from the demands of everyday living (in the health care facility), it is tempting to assume that a behavioral change is easy to implement. However, the ideal is seldom encountered in the real-life (at-home) circumstance, and additional learning, problem solving, and creativity may be necessary to integrate the desired change at home.

On the other hand, in the relaxed and familiar home environment, the person may discover a readiness to learn that was not experienced during the stress of the care facility environment. In addition, new learning needs may become evident at home.

Second, short-term outcomes may differ from the long-term reality. Individuals may know what is needed at the time of discharge, but over time, if they lack support or reinforcement of the learning, some content is invariably forgotten. Long-term follow-up can be used to renew information learned in the hospital. By reinforcing what is learned in health care facility teaching programs, the primary care nurse in the community provides continuity and promotes retention of learning.

Finally, the health care facility's nursing staff benefits tremendously from feedback received from people after they have been discharged. This information allows nurses to evaluate the effectiveness of hospital teaching by identifying relevant content and effective teaching strategies. It also allows for the reevaluation and possible restructuring of teaching strategies that were not effective.

Evaluating how well you and your client have met teaching/learning goals is an important part of the total teaching/learning process. It is important to develop learning objectives in terms of behaviors and measurable outcomes before beginning the teaching/learning program. Then, after the program, you will be able to evaluate how successful you have been in teaching the individual and how successful the client has been in making positive life changes. Ideally, evaluation should determine that learning has occurred and that you were effective as a teacher. If discrepancies exist between the desired and actual outcomes, systematic problem solving can help to rectify them and strengthen the teaching/learning process.

Summary

- Nurses carry the primary responsibility for health education.
- All client outcomes depend, at least in part, on the teaching performed by nurses.
- Nurses teach in the perceptual, cognitive, affective, and psychomotor domains.
- When attempting to understand individual learners, it is important to know their developmental level and how they prefer to learn.
- Certain factors facilitate learning in most persons.
- The nurse uses principles of teaching to decide what, when, and how to teach.
- Five major factors that can help in assessing learning needs are client characteristics, level of education, cultural awareness, psychologic/physiologic considerations, and socioeconomic considerations.
- In planning to meet learning needs, the diagnosis of "knowledge deficit" is most commonly used, but this diagnosis is not always correct.
- In planning for client teaching, it is important to understand and adapt to individual learning styles and to be comfortable with mutual negotiation.
- Nursing interventions useful in teaching require the ability to motivate the learner and to develop content and learning activities.
- Short-term and long-term evaluation are both important to determine whether learning has actually occurred in relation to changes in health behaviors.

Bibliography

1. Abdellah, F. G. (1961). *Patient-centered approaches to nursing.* New York: Macmillan.
2. Agre, P., et al. (1990). How much time do nurses spend teaching cancer patients? *Patient Education and Counseling,* 16, 29–38.
3. Arakelian, M. (1990). Learned self-help response to chronic illness experience: a test to three alternative learning theories scholarly. *Inquiry for nursing practice: An International Journal,* 4(1), 23–41.
4. Barnes, L. P. (1991). Commitment to patient education. *American Journal of Maternal-Child Nursing,* 16, 17.
5. Bartlett, E. E. (1988). Which patient education strategies will pay off under prospective pricing? *Patient Education and Counseling,* 12(11), 51–91.
6. Bates, B. (1991). *A guide to physical examination* (4th ed.). Philadelphia: J.B. Lippincott.
7. Berg, B. K., et al. (1987). Patient education needs assessment: constructing a generic guide. *Patient Education Counselor,* 9, 199–207.
8. Bloom, B. S. (1956). *Taxonomy of educational objectives, book 1: Cognitive domain.* New York: Longman.
9. Boswell, E. J., et al. (1990). Training health care professionals to enhance their patient teaching skills. *Journal of Nursing Staff Development,* 6(5), 233–239.
10. Brown, C., et al. (1987). Association between type of medication instructions and patient knowledge, side effects, and compliance. *Hospital Community Psychiatry,* 38, 55–60.
11. Brown, S. (1988). Effects of educational interventions in diabetes care: a meta-analysis of findings. *Nursing Research,* 37, 223–230.
12. Byers, P. (1986). Infant crying during aircraft descent: what parents can do. *Nursing Research,* 35, 521–529.
13. Carlson, J. H., et al. (1991). *Nursing diagnosis: A case study approach.* Philadelphia: W.B. Saunders.
14. Christie, D., et al. (1988). Patient and spouse responses to education early after myocardial infarction. *Journal of Psychosomatic Research,* 32(3), 321–335.
15. Cifani, L., & Vargo, R. (1990). Teaching strategies for the transplant recipient: a review and future directions. *Focus on Critical Care, AACN,* 17(6), 476–479.
16. Cohen, N. H. (1980). Three steps to better patient teaching. *Nursing,* 80(10), 72.
17. DeMuth, J. (1989). Patient teaching in the ambulatory setting. *Nursing Clinics of North America,* 24, 645–653.
18. Devine, E. C., & Cook, T. D. (1983). A meta-analytic analysis of effects of psychoeducational interventions on length of postsurgical hospital stay. *Nursing Research,* 321, 267–274.
19. Dixon, E., & Park, R. (1990). Do patients understand written health information? *Nursing Outlook,* 38(6), 278–281.
20. Doak, C., et al. (1985). *Teaching patients with low literacy skills.* Philadelphia: J.B. Lippincott.
21. Garding, B., et al. (1988). Effectiveness of a program of information and support for myocardial infarction patients recovering at home. *Heart and Lung,* 17(4), 355–361.
22. Glaser, R. (1990). The reemergence of learning theory within instructional research. *American Psychology,* 45(1), 29–39.

23. Hathaway, D. (1986). Effect of preoperative instruction on post-operative outcomes: a meta-analysis. *Nursing Research, 35,* 269–274.

24. Helberg, J. (1990). Information needs in home care: a review and analysis. *Public Health Nursing, 2*(1), 65–71.

25. Hoffman, S. (1987). Planning for patient teaching based on learning theory. In C. Smith (ed.). *Patient education. Nurses in partnership with other health professionals.* Orlando, FL: Grune & Stratton.

26. Hyman, R., et al. (1989). The effects of relaxation training on clinical symptoms: a meta-analysis. *Nursing Research, 38,* 216–220.

27. Johndrow, P. D., & Worthington, P. (1988). Making your patient and his family feel at home with TPN. *Nursing, 18*(10), 65–69.

28. Johnson, J., et al. (1978). Sensory information: instruction in a coping strategy, and recovery from surgery. *Research in Nursing and Health, 1,* 4–17.

29. Joint Commission on Accreditation of Hospitals. (1991). Accreditation manual for hospitals, Oak Brook Terrace, IL: Authors, 131–132.

30. Knowles, M. (1980). *The adult learner: A neglected species* (2nd ed.). Houston, TX: Gulf Publishing.

31. Krathwoh, D. R. et al. (1964). *Taxonomy of educational objectives, book II: Affective domain.* New York: Longman.

32. Kruger, S. (1990). A review of patient education in nursing. *Journal of Nursing Staff Development, 6*(2), 71–74.

33. Lange, J. W. (1989). Developing printed materials for patient education. *Dimensions of Critical Care Nursing, 8*(4), 250–259.

34. Lindeman, C. (1988). Patient education. In Fitzpatrick, J. J., & Werley, H. H., (eds.). *Annual review of nursing research.* New York: Springer.

35. Lindeman, C. (1989). Patient education: part II. In Fitzpatrick, J. J., & Werley, H. H., (eds.). *Annual review of nursing research.* New York: Springer.

36. Lipetz, M. J., et al. (1990). What is wrong with patient education programs? *Nursing Outlook, 38*(4), 184–189.

37. Mager, R. F. (1975). *Preparing instructional objectives* (2nd ed.). Belmont, CA: Fearon Publishers.

38. Mazzuca, S. A. (1982). Does patient education in chronic disease have therapeutic value? *Journal of Chronic Disease, 35,* 521–529.

39. McCain, N. L., & Lynn, M. R. (1990). Meta-analysis of a narrative review: studies evaluating patient teaching. *Western Journal of Nursing Research, 12,* 347–358.

40. Miner, D. (1990). Preoperative outpatient education in the 1990s. *Nursing Management, 21,* 40–44.

41. Moore, M. R. (1970). The perceptual-motor domain and a proposed taxonomy of perception. AV Communication Review, 18, 379–413.

42. Mumford, E., et al. (1982). The effects of psychological intervention in recovery from surgery and heart attacks. *American Journal of Public Health, 72,* 141–151.

43. O'Connor, F. W., et al. (1990). Enhancing surgical nurses' patient education: development and evaluation of an intervention. *Patient Education and Counseling, 16,* 7–20.

44. Redman, B., & Thomas, S. (1992). Patient teaching in nursing interventions (2nd ed., pp 304–314). In Bulechek, G. M., & McCloskey, J. C., (eds.). Nursing interventions: Essential nursing treatments. Philadelphia: W.B. Saunders.

45. Rohret, L., & Ferguson, K. J. (1990). Effective use of patient education illustrations. *Patient Education and Counseling, 15,* 73–75.

46. Rorden, J. W. (1987). *Nurses as health teachers.* Philadelphia: W.B. Saunders.

47. Schmidt, G. L. (1988). Practical aspects of teaching home parenteral nutrition therapy. *Patient Education and Counseling, 12,* 159–165.

48. Smith, C. (1985). Legal responsibilities in patient teaching. In Ford, R. D. (ed.). *Nurse's legal handbook.* Springhouse, PA: Springhouse Corp.

49. Smith, C. (ed.). (1987). *Patient education: Nurses in partnership with other health professionals.* Orlando, FL: Grune & Stratton.

50. Smith, C. E. (1987). Patient teaching. It's the law. *Nursing '87, 17*(7), 67–68.

51. Smith, C. E. (1989). Overview of patient education. Opportunities and challenges for the twenty-first century. *Nursing Clinics of North America, 24*(3), 583–587.

52. Steele, J. M., & Ruzicki, D. A. (1987). An evaluation of the effectiveness of cardiac teaching during hospitalization. *Heart and Lung, 16,* 306–311.

53. Walsh, K. C. (1990). Communication: the heart of patient education. *Plastic Surgical Nursing, 10*(4), 171–172.

▼ **Documenting Care**

Chapter

27

▼ *It is possible to be both brief and boring but it isn't easy.*

Ed McMahon

▼ CHAPTER OUTLINE

THE CLIENT RECORD
    Historical Issues in Recording
    Purposes of the Client Record
    Guidelines for Documentation
    Current Problems in Recording
COMMON DOCUMENTATION SYSTEMS
    Narrative Charting
    Flowcharts and Other More
      Structured Formats
    The Problem-Oriented Record
      System

    FOCUS Documentation
    PIE Charting
    Charting by Exception
    CORE Documentation
METHODS OF DOCUMENTATION
    Hand-written Records
    Dictated and Recorded Records
VERBAL REPORTING
AUTOMATED INFORMATION SYSTEMS
FUTURE TRENDS

▼ KEY TERMS

Back-up	Expert system	Narrative (free-form)
CAI	Flowchart (flowsheet,	charting
Change-of-shift report	flownote)	PIE
Chart	Graphics	POMR
Charting by exception	Hard copy	PONR
(CBE)	Hardware	POR
Computer	HIS	Response time
CPU	Input device	Software
CRT	Kardex	Source-oriented systems
Cursor	LAN	Terminal
Data base	Menu	User
Documentation	MIS	User-friendly
Down time	Modem	VDT
EDP	Monitor	

THE CLIENT RECORD

Historical Issues in Recording

The recording of health care activities has been an ongoing struggle from the beginning of the development of the helping professions. In a letter written in 1855 to Mr. Sidney Herbert in the London War Office, Florence Nightingale reported a serious problem with the record keeping at the barracks hospital in Scutari during the Crimean War. She wrote, "No statistics are kept as to between what ages most deaths occur, as to modes of treatment, appearances of the body after death, etc. . . . Our registration generally is so lamentably defective that often the only record kept is—a man [sic] died—on such a day."[14]

A consistent view of the importance of documentation and record keeping continued to be an important part of the Nightingale approach to clinical care. When she founded the training school for nurses at St. Thomas' Hospital in London, written records played an important role in the curriculum. Even though she rarely visited the school, Florence Nightingale read over probationers' papers and records about the nursing care they provided. She was often critical of the lack of specific and important information in the students' descriptions of their patient-related activities. For example, in 1880, after her review of a batch of student records, Miss Nightingale wrote to Mary Crossland (who was in charge of the educational program for the student nurses). In her letter, she made the following complaints:

Another remark I would make almost universally. No one gives you the progress of the cases. . . . One cannot make out from any one's diary whether the case is going well or ill. . . . There is an immense deal of zinc rubbing but I have not met with a single observation as to whether there was danger of bed sore. . . . She washes a patient "all over" in bed—but does not describe this process. . . . These are unsatisfactory . . . where test details are omitted which they too often are. . . . It is nothing for instance to tell us that she has "taken the temperatures" which are abnormally high. . . . There is rarely or never any notice given by which one can tell whether any critical disease is doing well or ill. This is a capital fault.[40]

In short, Nightingale was looking for the following information about the nurses' clients of yesterday: progress reports, key observations, clear description, sufficient details, clear statistics and critical values, and outcome measures. These points from over 100 years ago are the same factors that nursing faculty and administrators are looking for in the health care records being created today.

Purposes of the Client Record

It is a major task of the modern nurse to help produce and maintain a record for each client. Each record must be an accurate and comprehensive depiction of the client and of events that have occurred during the course of client care. This client record is traditionally called the chart. A **chart** is a document that may consist of a single form or a number of forms compiled to provide a complete record of client care from the initial client assessment (including historical information of note) to the evaluation of the final client outcomes (including plans for follow-up by others, as needed). Although the actual form and organization of the chart usually vary among different institutions, the responsibility of the nurse remains constant: to provide data of high quality—data that can be vital to the continued care of the individual client and to the ultimate improvement of health care for society as a whole. Many of the purposes for creating and maintaining client health care records follow.

► Communication: The record provides a centralized source of information about the implementation of health care and the client's response to that care. Various members of the health care team use the written record to share pertinent data about the client with each other.
► Care planning: Written documentation of a plan enhances teamwork in assessing and modifying the treatment plan.
► Auditing: The record can be monitored to assess the health care received by the client as well as the competence of the care givers. A retrospective re-

view of the record can be conducted to determine whether care met specific predetermined standards.

▶ Research: Information from a number of records can provide a data base for researchers to use in identifying problems and tracking variables. Records also provide a rich source of statistical information.

▶ Education: Educators use case records to teach about clinical care, such as symptom recognition, clinical events, treatment responses, and evaluation. The records present a comprehensive picture of clients and their health-related problems.

▶ Legal documentation: Health care records are legal documents that may be used in court proceedings or in accident claims filed by a client.

▶ Historical documentation: Specific information entered into a client's record provides a chronologic document of each health care episode.

One of the key points to learn about health care records is that they are legal documents. The information recorded on them is used by the health care team during the treatment and intervention phases of care and is then stored in some form for later retrieval. The information may be used as evidence in a legal proceeding many months or even years after the care is administered. It is critical that the input into the record be accurate, complete, and in the correct format.

Guidelines for Documentation

The recording of information in the legal record is termed charting or documenting. **Documentation** is written evidence of nursing practice. Documentation is not an exact science, so it is not always possible for everyone to agree about exactly what to write in documenting the innumerable observations or the myriad nursing interventions that might be needed for a given individual's record. It is possible, however, to reach agreement about how these recordings should be made. It is, in fact, mandatory that all nurses adhere to legal guidelines in all of their charting activities. These guidelines are listed in Box 27–1.

Study the guidelines in Box 27–1 and keep them in mind when you are preparing to make an entry in any client's records.

Current Problems in Recording

Numerous audits of health care records have found that there are often wide discrepancies in the quantity and quality of the records produced—even within a single agency. A lack of quantity and quality in charting can cause enormous problems for clients, nurses, and other health care personnel as well as for society at large. A review of the purposes of the record (listed earlier) can help us realize why this is the case.

As a rule, charting is just not what it can and should be. If the nursing profession is to prevent problems that stem from inadequate charting, it is important that nurses identify and alleviate factors that tend to lead to inadequate charting.

Box 27–1. Legal Guidelines for Charting

▶ Communicate information in legible handwriting or printing.

▶ Use black ink when writing on client records unless directed to do otherwise. Black denotes a legal record, stands up better to photocopying, and is essential in microfilming documents.

▶ Identify the source of information for documenting that which you did not see or experience, such as "Client states that . . . "

▶ Chart only for yourself.

▶ Chart procedures or treatments after you complete them, not before.

▶ Correct errors in documentation as soon as possible.

▶ Do not erase the error or use correction fluid.

▶ Draw a single line through any erroneous information; write the words "incorrect entry," "error," or "error in charting" above it along with your name or initials (according to agency policy), and write the entry correctly.

▶ Do not leave blank spaces in your narrative; draw a horizontal line through unused space.

▶ If you document some aspect of the client's care that is clearly out of chronologic order in the record, label it "late entry" and record the date and time.

▶ Use concise descriptions instead of generalized phrases that convey little meaning, such as "Client had no complaints."

▶ Initiate each entry with the date and time. Close with your signature, including first initial, last name, and license or certification (such as R.N., L.V.N./L.P.N., S.N.).

▶ If your note is spread out on more than one page, mark each subsequent page as a continuation of the original.

▶ Do not write critical or judgmental comments about the client, family, or staff.

▶ If you question an order or seek clarification regarding the client's care, document the action.

▶ Use standard symbols and abbreviations only (Table 27–1).

▶ Use medical terminology only if you are sure of its meaning.

▶ Chart each medication, treatment, and procedure; note time, effect, and results.

▶ Chart the fact that a client has refused a medication or treatment, and state the reason why. Document any action you took as well as whom you notified.

▶ Document incidents in progress notes in addition to doing so on the appropriate incident report form.

There are many reasons for problems to occur in charting activities. One often overlooked factor is the various levels of complexity in nursing activities. Whereas it may be easy to signify precisely that a medication was given at a specific time or to record an exact number as a pulse rate, there are significant nursing activities that are more difficult to describe in words or numbers. As Masson noted, nursing is not always a chartable activity, and much of it takes place in a wordless medium.[25] She has written that "to the extent possible, I have to coax the nonverbal into

TABLE 27-1. Common Abbreviations and Symbols

Abbreviation/ Symbol	Term	Abbreviation/ Symbol	Term
Assessment Data			
abd	abdomen	neg	negative
ax	axillary	ng	nasogastric
BM	bowel movement	OTC	over-the-counter (medicine without a prescription)
BP	blood pressure	P	pulse
BSA	body surface area	PE	physical examination
bx	biopsy	PMH	past medical history
C&DB	coughing and deep breathing	R	respiration
c/o	complains of	R/O	rule out
cc	chief complaint	ROM	range of motion
DOA	dead on arrival	ROS	review of systems
dx	diagnosis	RX	treatment
F	Fahrenheit (temperature scale)	SOB	shortness of breath
h/o	history of	sx	signs; symptoms
HR	heart rate	T	temperature
in	inch	TPR	temperature, pulse, respiration
LMP	last menstrual period	VS	vital signs
LOC	level of consciousness	WNL	within normal limits
Disease-Related			
AIDS	acquired immune deficiency syndrome	fx	fracture
ASHD	arteriosclerotic heart disease	GI	gastrointestinal
BPH	benign prostatic hypertrophy	GU	genitourinary
CA	cancer	HTN	hypertension
CAD	coronary artery disease	MI	myocardial infarction
CHF	congestive heart failure	PVC	premature ventricular contraction
COPD	chronic obstructive pulmonary disease	PVD	peripheral vascular disease
CVA	cerebrovascular accident	STD	sexually transmitted disease
DM	diabetes mellitus	URI	upper respiratory infection
FUO	fever of unknown origin	UTI	urinary tract infection
Orders			
$\bar{a}$	before	OS	left eye
ac	before meals	O.T.	Occupational Therapy
ad lib	at will; as desired	$\bar{p}$	after
AMA	against medical advice	po	by mouth (per os)
bid	two times daily	post op	postoperative
$\bar{c}$	with	pre op	preoperative
CPR	cardiopulmonary resuscitation	prep	preparation
D/C	discontinue	prn	as needed; whenever necessary
D/W	dextrose in water	pt	patient
DNR	do not resuscitate	P.T.	Physical Therapy
DSD	dry sterile dressing	q	every
gtt	drop	q4h	every 4 hours
h	hour	qid	four times a day
hs	hour of sleep; bedtime	qod	every other day
I&O	intake and output	qs	quantity sufficient
IM	intramuscular	$\bar{s}$	without
IPPB	intermittent positive-pressure breathing	SC	subcutaneous (also sq)
IU	international unit	soln	solution
IV	intravenous	STAT	at once; immediately

TABLE 27–1. Common Abbreviations and Symbols Continued

Abbreviation/ Symbol	Term	Abbreviation/ Symbol	Term
Orders	*Continued*		
ko	keep open (IV)	T&C	type and crossmatch
noc	night	tid	three times a day
NPO	nothing by mouth	tpn	total parenteral nutrition
NS	normal saline	×	times
OD	right eye		
Client Activity			
ADL	activities of daily living	OOB	out of bed
AMB	ambulatory	up ad lib	up as desired
BRP	bathroom privileges	wc	wheelchair
CBR	complete bed rest		
Studies, Elements, and Measures			
ABGs	arterial blood gases	mEq	milliequivalent
BE	barium enema	Mg	magnesium
C	Celsius; centigrade	mg	milligram
C&S	culture and sensitivity	min	minute
CBC	complete blood count	mL	milliliter
Cl	chloride	mm	millimeter
cm	centimeter	MRI	magnetic resonance imaging
CO	carbon monoxide	N	nitrogen
CO_2	carbon dioxide	Na	sodium
CSF	cerebrospinal fluid	NaCl	sodium chloride; salt
CVP	central venous pressure	O_2	oxygen
ECG	electrocardiogram	oz	ounce
ECT	electroconvulsive therapy	ppm	parts per million
EEG	electroencephalogram	RBC	red blood cell
ft	foot	wk	week
gm	gram	sp gr	specific gravity
Hb	hemoglobin	spec	specimen
Hct	hematocrit	tab	tablet
Hg	mercury	tbsp	tablespoon
ICP	intracranial pressure	tsp	teaspoon
K	potassium	u	unit
Kcal	kilocalorie (food calorie)	UA	urinalysis
kg	kilogram	US	ultrasound
L	liter	WBC	white blood cell
lytes	electrolytes	wt	weight
m	meter	μ	micron
Symbols			
/	per	$\bar{c}$	with
<	less than	$\bar{s}$	without
>	more than	♂	male
≤	equal to or less than	♀	female
≥	equal to or more than	1°	primary; first-degree
≅	approximately equal to	2°	secondary; second-degree
±	plus or minus; very slight trace	3°	tertiary; third-degree

words. It requires commitment, talent, and hard work."[25]

Researchers are starting to investigate documentation activities of nursing staff members in order to learn more about the usual problems and concerns in the area of charting. One administrator looked into the factors that staff nurses acknowledged as facilitating and inhibiting their documentation of nursing practice.[38] She found that the staff nurses identified the largest deterrent to charting to be a lack of time on busy units. The majority described a dilemma they perceived between spending their time in documenting care given and spending their time actually doing something for their clients. Even when time was not a crucial factor, subjects reported that a lack of a place to think and lack of space in which to write prevented optimal charting behavior. Indistinct terminology and redundancy in the forms they were required to use were named as problems as well.

In another study, researchers looked at nurses' documentation behavior and contrasted it with their attitudes, their intentions about documenting in an optimal way, and the subjective norms in the work situation, which they defined as the influence of others in the environment.[35] The majority of their subjects were full-time employees who worked in intensive care units. Nearly half of the nurses studied had a bachelor's degree. The study assessed both the mechanics of the nurses' documentation (such as correct time and date and use of approved abbreviations) and the content of their documentation. Results showed that nurses charted an average of seven clients per shift and that only 65 per cent of what was defined as minimal documentation was found in the charts assessed. Only 13 per cent of the records noted information about the client's emotional status. Attitudes toward documentation did not significantly affect charting behavior, but the subjective norm or influence of others and the behavioral intent did. Thus, a lack of communication of high ideals for charting and a lack of expectations of important others could be factors that decrease the quality of the documentation completed by staff nurses.

One of the main problems with forms that are used is a lack of uniformity. There is no standardized client care record. Health care agencies and settings have their own variations in the way that important information is captured, reported, and filed. Diversity in agency settings, in the client populations, and in the writers of the documentation contributes to the variations in this process. Multiple variations in documentation procedures and style can even occur throughout a single institution. For example, in an article entitled "The Documentation Dilemma: A Practical Solution," Weeks and Darrah discussed the experience of nurses in a 1200-member division of nursing. They stated that seven years of experience with primary nursing resulted in an abundance of different charting systems and methods and that the quality and frequency of charting varied greatly within this large medical center.[41]

Because a multitude of different forms exist for charting client information, the beginning student can benefit more by understanding the basics of several charting systems than by studying in detail several examples of pages from one specific charting system.

COMMON DOCUMENTATION SYSTEMS

Narrative Charting

Since the time of Florence Nightingale and the beginnings of modern nursing, student nurses have been introduced to general guidelines for the content and style of hand-written nurses' notes. However, the actual notes nurses have written to document events important to client care have always been completed as a one-of-a-kind procedure.

The basic structure of the early nurses' notes is still being used today. It is termed narrative charting. **Narrative (free-form) charting** consists of paragraphs of information written sequentially and usually organized in chronologic order as a means of relating observations, interventions, and client responses to care. This type of charting is the traditional way that nurses and other health care providers have documented client care for centuries. Narrative charting is found most often in **source-oriented systems,** in which each group of health care professionals has its own portion of the chart set aside for storing information about observations and care unique to that group. With narrative charting, the information is entered into the record in an unstructured way, with each recorder making the decision about the amount and focus of the written material. For the most part, nurses provide the amount of narrative material necessary to document everything they do for the client during each shift.

By convention, the information used in narrative charting refers only to the client, unless specifically stated otherwise, so the client's name and all pronouns that would normally be used to refer to the client are omitted for the sake of brevity. All other unnecessary words are deleted as well. Thus, the nurse might chart "to operating room via stretcher" rather than "the client was taken to the operating room via stretcher."

The chief advantage of this system is that it is easy to use and provides a quick way of reviewing recent events in the client's care. It has been used in all types of clinical settings. The narrative format enables nurses to use their creativity and focus on what they view as the key observations or events to be noted, as can be seen in the first entry in Figure 27–1. Conversely, the second entry is an example of the use of "fillers" or meaningless information when pressure is exerted to document information during an uneventful period.

The chief disadvantages in using a narrative format stem from the unstructured style and fragmented location of information throughout the record. A chart may contain much important and individualized material, but the dispersion of the data often makes the tracking of client outcomes a difficult task. The variable quality and quantity of the notations in the record make comparisons and quantification difficult; the unique nature of each entry makes charting time-consuming. In addi-

NURSING NOTES

PATIENT'S NAME Irene Sullivan

ALL ENTRIES MUST BE TIMED AND SIGNED WITH STATUS

5/15/94 1600—Admission Note: Received this 64 yo. white female $\bar{c}$ diagnoses of sudden death and Rt. hip fracture

from ER via stretcher. Responsive to voice (opens eyes when name is called), follows simple commands, equal hand

grasps, pupils equal, round, reactive to light (+) 3. EKG—sinus tach $\bar{c}$ frequent PVC's, heart rate 103, peripheral

pulses palpable x 4 extremities, edema present. Capillary refill good. Orally intubated $\bar{c}$ 7.5 ET tube on Bear 5

ventilator $\bar{c}$ the following vent. settings: tidal volume—750, FiO$_2$—45%, AC-12, peep-0. Spontaneous respirations

noted. Respiratory rate—16. Lungs $\bar{c}$ occasional bibasilar crackles—otherwise clear. O$_2$ saturation 96-98% via pulse

oximeter. Bowel sounds active x 4 quadrants. Abdomen soft, nontender. Foley to gravity draining about 100cc/hr.

clear, yellow urine. Lt. PIV 0.9 NS at 75cc/hr. + Rt. PIV Lidocaine drip: 1 gm/50ccD$_5$ W at 9cc/hr. (or 3 mg/min) via

Harvard pump. Both dsgs. dry and intact $\bar{c}$ positive blood return. Lt. radial a-line intact, dressing dry, secured on

armboard. Good waveform and blood return, accurate $\bar{c}$ cuff. B/p ^{98}/$_{70}$. Afebrile. Son in waiting room. Skin warm

and dry, siderail in up position, bilateral soft wrist restraints in place to avoid possible extubation.   R. Jensen, RN

5/15/94 1800 Resting comfortably at this time. S. Clark, R.N.

▲ **Figure 27-1**

Narrative (free-form) charting.

tion, nurses sometimes complain that physicians and other health care workers often skip over the nursing narrative section when they read through the chart. This situation was highlighted further when some institutions began to discard parts of the nursing portion of the record when storage and retrieval of client records became an issue after discharge.

Flowcharts and Other More Structured Formats

To overcome some of the disadvantages of the narrative style of charting, documentation in certain sections of the record has undergone a gradual change from a free-flowing narrative style to a more structured appearance. One such change is the increased use of flowcharts. A **flowchart (flowsheet, flownote)** consists of one or more forms used to chart the flow of information concerning selected client observations and treatments that are repeated over a period of some time (as opposed to the more comprehensive narrative format used to chart a great deal of or all possible client information noted in relatively short periods of time). Flowcharts are versatile and may be used, according to agency requirements, to chart information over time periods that vary from minutes or hours (e.g., urinary output per hour during the time a client is in surgery) to months or even years (e.g., yearly results of vision examinations during a child's school years). Flowcharts have been readily adopted by health care agencies as ways of saving time when entering data, reading data, or comparing data (such as results of treatments).

Over the years, any repetitive information that could be graphed or plotted or put into a table has been gradually moved into this newer flownote format. Various types of forms are used for flownotes. For example, much numerical information has been transferred to a graphic format. One commonly encountered example of a flowchart is a graphic chart, such as that routinely used to chart vital signs (Fig. 27–2).

There are several advantages to the increased use of flowcharts and other structured forms like checklists and forms that call for open-ended responses, such as pre-set assessment forms. One advantage is the time saved by nurses, who do not have to repeatedly write out information that can simply be checked off or completed. More structured records also permit easier retrieval of information and comparison of results with external standards.

Increased use of client-based information will be possible when it is concise, accurate, and easily located.

Various other formats have been suggested as a means of saving time in the production of the charting entry as well as getting the key or meaningful points across to the busy reader. A number of suggested revisions have brought varying degrees of success in providing structure to written reports. Examples have ranged from the elaborate problem-oriented SOAP or SOAPIE method to the newer, streamlined FOCUS and charting by exception methods of documentation.

The Problem-Oriented Record System

The problem-oriented record system was originally developed for physicians by Dr. Lawrence Weed. The purpose of the system was to facilitate documentation of health care by creating integrated progress notes. The system was widely adopted by different health care providers and, when necessary, was altered to fit the needs of the diverse users. This system is also known as the problem-oriented record **(POR),** the problem-oriented nursing record **(PONR),** and the problem-oriented medical record **(POMR).** The problem-oriented record system consists of four components: a data base, a problem list, care plans, and progress notes.

THE DATA BASE

The data base consists of information collected at the time of the initial assessment. It usually includes a medical history, physical examination, and nursing history. The data base holds both subjective and objective data and provides the beginning point for development of the client's problem list.

THE PROBLEM LIST

The problem list contains a set of client problems that are prioritized and numbered. The number is useful because the entries about each particular problem can easily be identified throughout the entire chart. The problem list may contain a mixture of medical and nursing problems, and it is usually placed in the front of the chart. It is useful in providing an overview of the client's status.

THE CARE PLANS

The care plans hold information on the actions that are taken in relation to each identified problem as well as the outcome goals and expectations. Specific details about such things as procedures, interventions, and responses are tracked by means of the care plan. This plan may be stored in a location other than the chart. Often such plans are stored in a bedside information record or *Kardex* (a system used by many agencies to store 6 × 11 inch cards, each of which contains vital information about, and the nursing care plan for, a specific client.

THE PROGRESS NOTES

The progress notes contain important information about each problem on the list. The structure of the notes can vary from an organized format for entries with the use of labeled columns to an open format in which the organization is left up to the individual recorder. The usual format used in organizing the content documenting the nursing process is called SOAPIER. The acronym is explained in Table 27–2.

The POR system is useful in keeping the focus on the client's problems and on implementing a problem-solving approach. It moves away from a task-oriented ap-

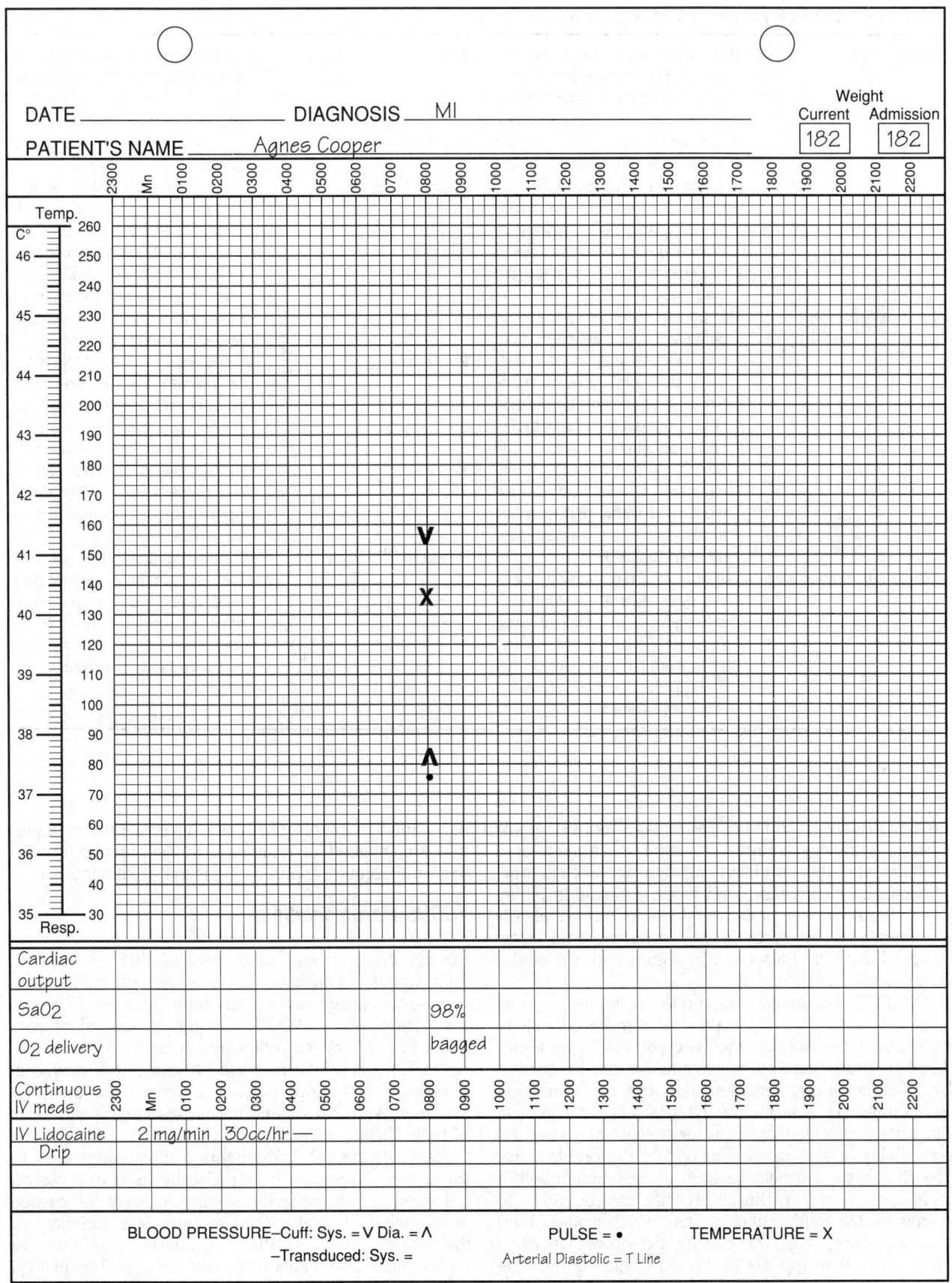

▲ **Figure 27–2**

One type of flow note.

TABLE 27–2. SOAPIER Format for Charting Client Data

Subjective data	This information provides the client's perspective of the problem. It consists of direct quotations from the individual or paraphrasing of the client's remarks. If the client is unable to provide this information directly (such as in cases involving aphasic or unconscious individuals), the section is marked to indicate that no data are available.	**P**lan	A plan of care is developed and implemented to assist each individual. The plan should include outcome criteria and a time frame for measuring progress.
Objective data	This portion of the progress notes contains data collected from non–client-related sources, such as laboratory tests, monitoring instruments, physiologic data, unbiased observations, and information from the client's family members. The information is used to document the clinical status and provides a foundation for medical and nursing diagnoses.	**I**nterventions	These actions are taken to help decrease the identified problems. The client should have input into this intervention process as much as possible. The changing status of the client will keep this section in a dynamic and ever-changing mode.
		Evaluation	An appraisal of the effectiveness of interventions by care givers is a crucial component of the nursing process. If outcome criteria or goals are not attained, the evaluation process can be the cornerstone for the development of new or different interventions.
Analysis and assessment	Use of both subjective and objective data leads to the formation of diagnoses. A constant reassessment is carried out throughout the treatment phase, making this section an ever-changing segment.	**R**evision	If the client outcome has not been met, an alteration in the plan, treatments, or interventions must be undertaken. The actions or the time line may have to be revised to provide more effective care.

proach to care.[12] Additional advantages consist of the ease in retrieving information about each numbered problem and the continuity of data about each one. This can be clearly visualized in the example in Figure 27–3. Problem interventions and resolutions are clearly documented. The problem list serves as both a reminder list of the most pressing issues and a checklist of areas needing attention.

The POR system can be applied to acute or long-term care settings, but the process is more difficult to initiate and maintain in emergency or short-term areas. Another disadvantage is that confusion can be created by divergent views regarding the type of information that should be entered on the problem list (medical diagnoses, nursing diagnoses, or both) and whose responsibility it is to revise and update the problem list. The POR system should be used in conjunction with a variety of forms or flowcharts that can be used to document the routine clinical care, which would otherwise go unrecorded. This can be a disadvantage when information that appears in the POR charting must be duplicated on the other forms (e.g., when the Demerol that is given in the example in Figure 27–3 must be charted on a medication record as well as on the form). The final disadvantage of the POR system is the

mind set that places the focus on problems or issues that are in need of treatment. Some practitioners see this as a negative approach to overall treatment.

FOCUS Documentation

FOCUS charting was developed at Eitel Hospital in Minneapolis, Minnesota, by a group of nurses who wanted to change the nurses' notes from the POR system. They used a FOCUS column in the client care notes to organize the topics documented in the nurses' notes.[12] The term *focus* is used because it is viewed in a broader and more positive context than the term *problem*. With this system, the nurses identify the focus of their nursing actions.

Although the FOCUS column is most often used to list nursing diagnoses, it may also be used to focus on a sign, symptom, behavior, significant event, or change in condition. It is also used to provide a summary of the overall client situation; a flowsheet is used to record daily treatments and interventions. The FOCUS system provides a compact record of each 24-hour period of health care treatment.

With this system, the progress notes are organized in a three-part structure known as DAR, which stands for

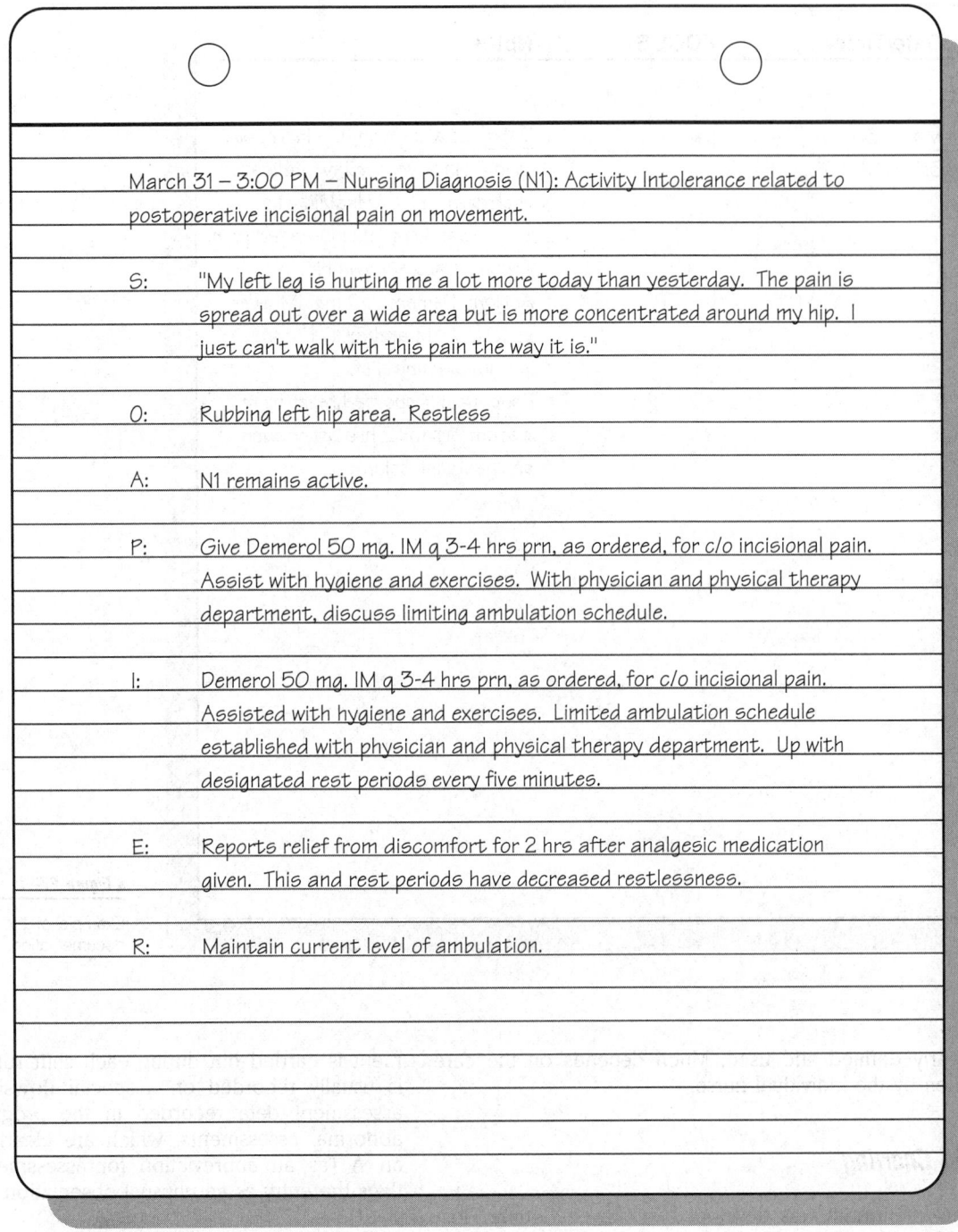

March 31 – 3:00 PM – Nursing Diagnosis (N1): Activity Intolerance related to postoperative incisional pain on movement.

S: "My left leg is hurting me a lot more today than yesterday. The pain is spread out over a wide area but is more concentrated around my hip. I just can't walk with this pain the way it is."

O: Rubbing left hip area. Restless

A: N1 remains active.

P: Give Demerol 50 mg. IM q 3-4 hrs prn, as ordered, for c/o incisional pain. Assist with hygiene and exercises. With physician and physical therapy department, discuss limiting ambulation schedule.

I: Demerol 50 mg. IM q 3-4 hrs prn, as ordered, for c/o incisional pain. Assisted with hygiene and exercises. Limited ambulation schedule established with physician and physical therapy department. Up with designated rest periods every five minutes.

E: Reports relief from discomfort for 2 hrs after analgesic medication given. This and rest periods have decreased restlessness.

R: Maintain current level of ambulation.

▲ *Figure 27–3*

Example of the POR system of documentation.

data, action, and response. The data portion describes observations and contains both subjective and objective information that led to the FOCUS. The action portion covers interventions and treatments; the response portion holds client responses to the nursing and medical care plan. The format is flexible and can be adapted to a wide range of clinical settings. Some entries may contain information on all three concepts, whereas others may have comments on only one or two of these. Figure 27–4 shows how the same information charted in the SOAPIER format would appear in the FOCUS format.

Advantages of the FOCUS documentation include its ease of use and the way that it makes information accessible to other health care professionals. It saves time by organizing each day into a summary that can be located quickly. It is a system that facilitates the recording of nursing actions and decisions.

The main disadvantage in using FOCUS documentation is that the action portion of the record may not be

Date/Time	FOCUS	Notes
March 31 3:00 PM	pain	Data: States pain has increased "a lot" since yesterday. Indicates operative hip. C/o inability to walk because of the increased pain. Restless and rubbing hip. Action: Demerol 50 mg. IM given at 10:00 AM and 2:00 PM for incisional pain relief. Response: Reported relief from discomfort for 2 hrs after each analgesia injection.

▲ *Figure 27-4*

Example of the FOCUS system of documentation.

clearly defined and used. Much depends on the care taken by the individual nurse.

PIE Charting

The PIE format was developed in Craven County Hospital in New Bern, North Carolina, in 1985. The acronym **PIE** stands for problem identification, interventions, and evaluation. This problem-oriented approach emphasizes nursing process and nursing diagnosis while incorporating the plan of care into the nurses' progress notes. The lack of the generation of a traditional care plan is a notable feature of this style of documentation.

The problem identification process begins with the initial admission assessment in which client problems, teaching needs, and discharge planning needs are identified. After completion of the initial assessment, the problems are listed as nursing diagnoses on a problem list. They are labeled with a P (for problem) and are numbered. A comprehensive physical assessment is carried out during each shift rotation, and this is usually recorded on a special flowsheet. The only assessment data recorded in the progress notes are abnormal assessments, which are clearly labeled with an A (as an abbreviation for assessment). The label flags the entry as an unusual observation or a change in status.

Intervention, the second step, is the documentation of the action that was taken for each nursing diagnosis. Interventions may be documented on the shift assessment/flowsheet form or in the progress notes. P#1 I means that the information relates to the intervention for the first nursing diagnosis, P#2 I relates to the intervention for the second nursing diagnosis, and so on.

The third step in the PIE documentation method is evaluation. Each nursing diagnosis is evaluated once each shift to determine the effectiveness of the interventions and the amount of progress that has been noted in regard to the resolution of the problem. The documentation of the evaluation component is similar to that of recording interventions. P#1 E is shorthand for the evaluation of the first nursing diagnosis, P#2 E refers to the evaluation of the second nursing diagnosis, and so forth. An example of this form of documentation can be seen in Figure 27–5.

The PIE method of documentation has the following advantages: increased time efficiency, flexibility, tie-in with the nursing process, enhanced tracking of client progress, strengthened accountability, and ease of adaptation for automated charting systems. The continuity of care is promoted by this method, and care is easily tracked. It promotes clear identification of the client's problems, the nursing interventions that were applied to the problems, and the type of progress that resulted from the care.

The key disadvantage of the PIE method is the limitation of its use to a single group of health care practitioners. The system does not lend itself to multidisciplinary use. Nurses in some clinical settings may find the lack of a traditional care plan to be a problem as well.

Charting by Exception

Charting by exception (CBE) is a system of documentation in which only exceptions to the norms or some other important or significant findings are recorded. The information in the chart identifies the variance from expected findings. This system was developed in 1983 at St. Luke's Hospital in Milwaukee, Wisconsin, as a way of decreasing duplication and repetition while streamlining the documentation process. Several authors have supported the method as a means of saving charting time and reducing accumulation of repetitive client data. In a 1989 article, Cline described the process of implementing CBE in a regional medical center in California, where it is used in all areas except critical care units. Cline detailed the lengthy process of developing the written standards used as the norms with the clients as well as the retraining of staff required to implement this system effectively.[8] Agencies using CBE in critical care areas usually devise a large series of flowcharts to cover the various contingencies in the unit.

The CBE system uses clinical standards and standardized assessments that are presented in a format in which the care giver can use a shorthand or check-off system to show that the information was within the expected range. Thus, for routine findings with a postoperative client, the nurse may place a simple check mark and the time of an assessment on a flowsheet and sign the form in the appropriate place. Provision is made for the nurse to be able to document unexpected findings as well as to track the client response in progress notes until findings return to normal limits. Exceptions are usually documented in a narrative format.

The chief advantage of this CBE system is in the reduction of time spent in charting activities. Exceptions or significant findings are highlighted for the whole team to see in a timely manner. Note the pertinent observations in the example in Figure 27–6. This CBE documentation is for the same client as in Figure 27–1 in the narrative format. Note the decrease in the amount of written material in the CBE format and how much less time it would take to read. The numerical data (such as the heart rate, ventilator settings, and oxygen saturation via pulse oximeter) are recorded on the appropriate areas of the CBE flowchart. It is less time-consuming to extract the figures from a graph or table than from a narrative description.

The primary disadvantage of CBE is the prolonged preparation time required before this system can be used effectively. The preparation time includes time for the generation of forms like flowcharts, care plans, and assessment checklists as well as time for the educational preparation of the staff.

CORE Documentation

St. Joseph's Hospital in Hamilton, Ontario, Canada, developed the CORE documentation and implemented the system as a measure of improving the documentation of nursing practice. The CORE or most important part of the documentation system is the nursing process. The client information is divided into the following areas: the data base, care plans, flowsheets, progress notes, and discharge summaries.

As soon after admission as possible, the nurse completes an assessment of the client's functional competence, including a review of systems and activities of daily living. A written summary containing nursing diagnoses and client problems is placed in the Kardex. Two care plans incorporate information from the flowsheets. One care plan is placed in the permanent record; the other is used as a work sheet. The progress notes are based on the FOCUS documentation format and thus have a three-part structure with DAE as the organizing framework. The DAE acronym stands for data, action, and evaluation.[27] The CORE documentation system uses a comprehensive discharge summary that incorporates diagnoses, client teaching, and follow-up care.

The primary advantage in this documentation system is that it promotes charting on each component of the nursing process. It also facilitates concise record keeping and the daily updating of psychosocial information. It can be used in acute care and long-term settings.

The disadvantages of the CORE documentation system relate to order and integration. It is not always possible to determine the chronologic unfolding of events, and the progress notes may not relate directly to the care plan.

METHODS OF DOCUMENTATION

Hand-written Records

Hand-written records have been the primary method of communicating client information since the beginnings of the delivery of modern health care. Despite a long and rich tradition, hand-written documents are being slowly replaced by newer methods of documentation that provide greater efficiency, increased flexibility, and

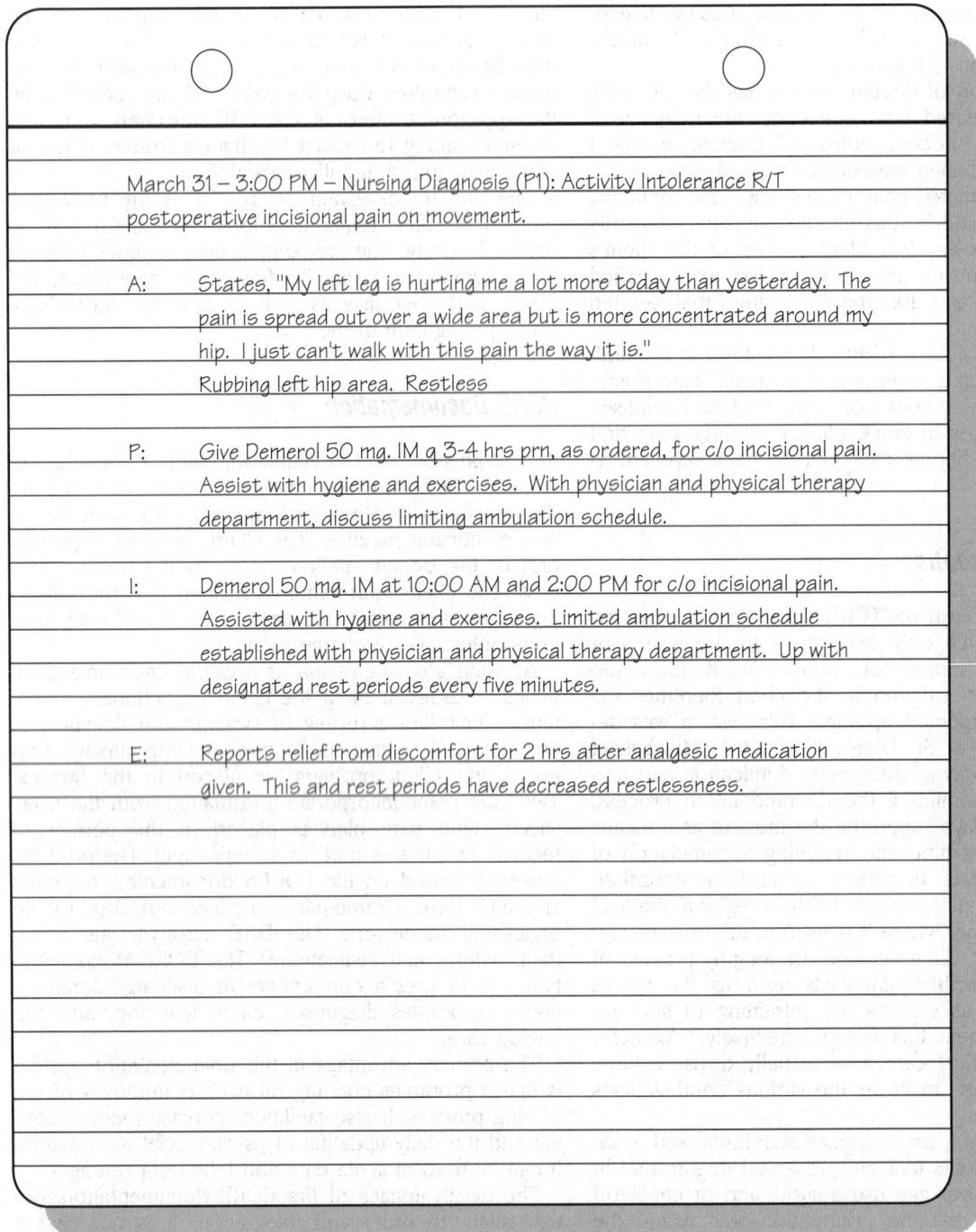

March 31 – 3:00 PM – Nursing Diagnosis (P1): Activity Intolerance R/T postoperative incisional pain on movement.

A: States, "My left leg is hurting me a lot more today than yesterday. The pain is spread out over a wide area but is more concentrated around my hip. I just can't walk with this pain the way it is."
Rubbing left hip area. Restless

P: Give Demerol 50 mg. IM q 3-4 hrs prn, as ordered, for c/o incisional pain. Assist with hygiene and exercises. With physician and physical therapy department, discuss limiting ambulation schedule.

I: Demerol 50 mg. IM at 10:00 AM and 2:00 PM for c/o incisional pain. Assisted with hygiene and exercises. Limited ambulation schedule established with physician and physical therapy department. Up with designated rest periods every five minutes.

E: Reports relief from discomfort for 2 hrs after analgesic medication given. This and rest periods have decreased restlessness.

▲ **Figure 27–5**

Example of the PIE system of documentation.

greater consistency. These newer methods make use of the technology now available in many health care agencies.

Dictated and Recorded Records

Health care practitioners make varied use of audio recording devices in constructing client records. Many examples can be cited of physicians using audio recordings to prepare such items as post-operative reports and summaries of radiologic findings. However, the dictated form of reporting has been used infrequently by nursing personnel except in settings in which a recorded end-of-shift report is an accepted custom.

The main drawback for nonmedical personnel in using audio devices has been the lack of availability of personnel for the preparation of a typed transcript. This situation may change in the near future with the refinement of voice-activated computer programs. The need has already been identified.

SHIFT ASSESSMENT

PATIENT'S NAME Irene Sullivan   **DATE** 5/15/93

04-05	05-06

24° INTAKE	
PO/NG	
IV	
BLOOD	
OR COLLOID	
OR CRYSTAL	
OTHER	
TOTAL INTAKE	

24° OUTPUT	
URINE	
STOOL	
NG	
EMESIS	
DRAINS	
DIALYSIS	
OTHER	
TOTAL OUTPUT	
I & O BALANCE	

DX TESTS	TIME
EKG:	
CXR:	
OTHER:	
OTHER:	

CULTURES SENT

BLOOD PRODUCTS

04-05	05-06

NURSING NOTES

1600. Received 64 yo white female c̄ diagnoses of sudden death and Rt hip fx from ER via stretcher. Responsive to voice. Opens eyes when name called. Follows simple commands, has equal hand grasps. Peripheral pulses palpable x 4 extremities. Capillary refill good. Lt. radial a-line intact, dressing dry. Good waveform. Siderail up position. Bilateral soft wrist restraints in place to avoid possible extubation. Son in waiting room.

R. Jensen, RN

▲ **Figure 27–6**

Example of charting by exception.

After a two-month experiment in which computers were installed to document client care at the bedside in a 30-bed orthopedic unit, nurses were asked to describe the ideal bedside system. Many suggested a small terminal with voice recognition capability so that their hands would be free to provide client care.[5]

With the development of advanced technologies, plans for implementing different methods of documentation should consider audio input as a potential area of focus.

VERBAL REPORTING

In addition to contributing written information to each individual client's chart, it is a nursing responsibility to verbally convey pertinent and timely information about each individual client to other health care professionals. One major responsibility in this respect is the **change-of-shift report,** in which one nurse sums up for one or more other nurses all the information necessary for the other nurses to safely assume responsibility for continuing care of the clients. This report has traditionally taken place three times per day at eight-hour intervals but has, in recent years, been changed to accommodate nurses on more flexible time schedules and so may be required at any number of different times.

Conveying client information verbally during the change-of-shift report is commonly done on audio tapes as well as "live." Whichever method you use, as you prepare to give a verbal report to others, you should be well aware of the following guidelines.

▶ Report essential information as quickly as possible.
▶ Be clear, concise, and accurate.
▶ Describe objective facts, measurements, and observations.
▶ Omit routine information that is readily available from other sources.
▶ Highlight recent or significant changes in the client's condition.
▶ Avoid value judgments, such as "good" or "poor," by giving specific examples.
▶ Present unbiased information that is pertinent to the client's health care.
▶ Discuss the client and family in a professional manner.
▶ Use discretion in ensuring that the discussion of confidential information is audible to professional staff only.
▶ Organize clients into a particular order for report.
▶ Give client name, room number, bed designation.
▶ Give diagnosis or reason for admission.
▶ Give tests, therapies, and results for last 24 hours.

Items on the list should be presented in the order most appropriate to your individual situation, not necessarily in the order they are listed. After giving the report, you should be ready to answer questions, as necessary.

In addition to reporting to others at the change of shift, nurses frequently report verbally to individuals concerning one or more clients. Such reports might occur on leaving the unit for a meal or when a problem is reported to a charge nurse or to the physician. Many of the guidelines pertain to reports about individual clients as well as to change-of-shift reports.

Another example of verbal reporting of client information occurs when a nurse must convey information to the physician, to another nurse, or to other members of the health care team via telephone. In using the telephone, the following guidelines should be observed.

▶ Clearly identify both yourself and the clinical site.
▶ Use a natural tone and volume of voice.
▶ Listen carefully and courteously.
▶ Write down pertinent information.
▶ Repeat important information (such as laboratory results or medication orders) to ensure accuracy.
▶ When accepting verbal orders, verify the instruction by reading it back to the physician clearly and precisely.
▶ Write the information in the appropriate location in the record and sign it.
▶ Do not divulge confidential information about the patient unless you are sure the caller has a legitimate right to access.

AUTOMATED INFORMATION SYSTEMS

Each of the methods of documentation discussed thus far consists of a system that is in effect to communicate data in the health care setting, whether by way of a hand-written notation or by way of a typed transcript of an oral recording. By convention, each of these information systems has followed a set routine, and individual practitioners have used them to make their unique contribution to the client's record. The information has been targeted on the formation of a single comprehensive chart or record for each client. This record has traditionally been housed in a central location, such as the chart rack in the nurses' station of a clinical unit. The written record has been available for use by a single member of the health care team at any one time. However, all of this has been changing with the advancement of technology.

The organization of the information systems in the health care field has been undergoing significant changes since the introduction of computer systems. The early applications of computer technology were primarily focused on business-oriented uses, such as financial management and client scheduling. This held true for all types of clinical settings. Willey and Winstead have written that from the 1970s to the mid-1980s, the majority of computer applications, even in home health care, were for insurance processing and billing.[42]

Early clinical documentation systems gained attention in the mid-1980s as they were developed and expanded throughout the various client-related departments. By 1990, over 50 per cent of the community hospitals with more than 100 beds and nearly 80 per cent of hospitals with more than 300 beds used some type of computerized client care system.[17] In contrasting the computerized clinical record systems with the old paper-based documentation systems, Zielstorff and coworkers[44] report that the automated systems are generally superior because they are better organized, more legible, more accessible, and more complete. They can also make client information available to multiple health care personnel at the same time.

The majority of the early clinical computer systems symbolically took the place of the hand-written chart in the nurses' station. These centrally located terminals were viewed as the primary input and output headquarters. Nursing departments joined in the automation process by working toward the integration of the computer into nursing service with attention on application design, system selection, and implementation procedures.[11] Many nursing administrators found that their staff nurses needed to be comfortable with computer use and familiar with basic computer terminology (such as the definitions in Box 27–2). Schools of nursing began to see the need to help student nurses become increasingly computer literate. Research into the potential uses of the computer continued.

The trend today is toward use of computers at the client's bedside. This makes sense in terms of documentation because it is estimated that over half of the information collected about clients is gathered at the bedside. Because the nurse is at the bedside so much of the time, it also makes sense to be able to access the client's record from either the client's room or the nurses' station. Access to the computer at the bedside encourages documentation and eliminates the need for notes that are hand-written at the bedside only to be copied over into a chart at a later time. Terminals, such as the one pictured in Figure 27–7, are being used for documentation of care at the time it is being performed.

The evaluation of bedside computer terminals in test sites has revealed that they improve documentation by health care personnel[17] and that they are looked at positively by clients and families.[5]

FUTURE TRENDS

A number of factors are converging together to streamline charting activities and upgrade the quality of the information. A great deal of the impetus for change in charting procedures can be attributed to preparation for the use of automated (computer) documentation systems. Changes concerning how we think about doc-

---

Box 27–2. Computer-Related Terms

Back-up A copy of a computer file placed onto a storage medium to be saved as an extra copy in case of loss or damage to the original

CAI Computer-assisted instruction

Computer Electronic device used to perform programmed activities in an efficient, accurate way

CPU Central processing unit, the main part of the computer; the part that performs calculations

CRT Another name for a computer monitor; the letters stand for cathode ray tube

Cursor A symbol visible on a computer screen; the symbol that indicates the currently active portion of the screen (often a blinking line)

Data base A program that organizes a collection of information so that it can be easily accessed or used for reports

Down time The time in which a computer is not available to users; this can be a planned break for preventive maintenance or a sudden loss of computer function (otherwise known as a "crash")

EDP Electronic data processing; using a computer to perform functions with data

Expert system A specialized computer program that aids in problem solving or decision making

Graphics Computer-produced pictures or images as opposed to written text or numbers

Hard copy A paper printout of what appears on a computer screen

Hardware The equipment or sections of a computer system that are necessary for operation of the system

HIS Hospital computerized information system; a computer is used for such functions as client billing and pharmacy orders

Input device A device used to put information into the computer system, such as a keyboard, light pen (a device used to "write" on the computer screen), touch-sensitive screen, or mouse or other pointing-and-clicking device

LAN Local area network; computers are connected to each other so they can share software or peripheral devices

Menu A list of options that a computer presents to a computer user

MIS Medical information system

Modem A device that enables computers to communicate over telephone lines

Monitor A screen used to display information from the computer

Response time The amount of time required for a computer to accept a user's input

Software Programs of instructions that tell the computer what functions or steps to perform to carry out a task

Terminal Hardware used to input or access client information; bedside terminals are usually small, hand-held computers; unit-based systems are larger and usually stationary

User Person using the computer

User-friendly Programs or equipment that is perceived as being easy to use

VDT Another name for a computer monitor; the letters stand for video display terminal

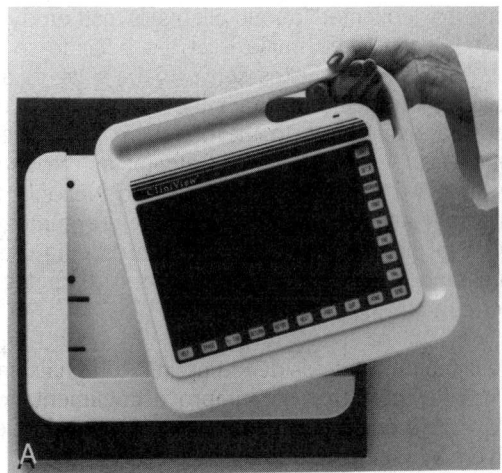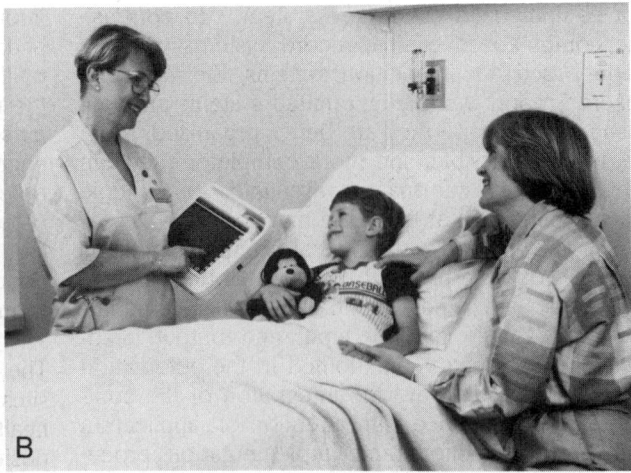

▲ *Figure 27-7*

Bedside computer terminals. *A*, The computer is portable. *B*, Example of bedside terminal being used to document nursing care. (Courtesy of CliniCom, Inc., Boulder, CO.)

umentation are occurring in two areas: how the input to the client record will be handled, and how the output available from the record will be used. The influence of computer-oriented systems has brought about a focus on the format of the information in the client record, the way it is structured, and the uniformity in what is being recorded (and eventually retrieved). Health care personnel are becoming advocates of "minimum data sets" for each discipline to ensure that nursing actions can be contrasted for diverse clients in many different types of settings. In the future, there will be increased emphasis on the assessment activities and more use of a predetermined standardized protocol for a care plan. Data entry during treatment will be recorded more frequently on flowcharts to increase efficiency and uniformity.

The retrieval of information will increase as it undergoes standardization and compression, and more focus will be placed on client outcomes and discharge planning.[19] As the style of the documentation activities becomes more focused on flowcharting, more of it will take place at the actual site of care, whether it is the bedside in preference to the nurses' station or the examining room or home as opposed to the office. The use of hand-held computers and networked systems for storing health records will speed up the trend toward efficient management of information that is already well under way.

Summary

▶ In client records, factors important to both Nightingale and present-day nursing faculty include progress reports, key observations, clear description, sufficient details, clear statistics and critical values, and outcome measures.

▶ Purposes for maintaining client records include communication, care planning, auditing, research, education, legal documentation, and historical documentation.

▶ Legal guidelines for charting concern how to write rather than what to write.

▶ Current problems in recording include a lack of quantity and quality of the records produced. This lack stems from nursing activities that are difficult to describe, lack of time for charting, lack of a place to think, lack of space in which to write, indistinct terminology and redundancy in required forms, lack of a high subjective norm or influence of others in the agency, lack of a positive behavioral intent on the part of the nurse, and lack of uniformity among different agencies regarding forms to be used.

▶ Anyone recording in a client's chart should use only standard symbols and abbreviations.

▶ Commonly used documentation systems include narrative charting with flownotes and other more structured forms, the problem-oriented record system, FOCUS documentation, PIE charting, charting by exception, and CORE documentation.

▶ Hand-written records are being slowly replaced by dictation, and voice-activated computer recording is a focus for future development.

▶ Nurses frequently give and receive verbal reports during the change-of-shift report, during individual face-to-face interactions, and during communications via the telephone. Established reporting guidelines should be followed during these events.

▶ Since their inception, computers have been used increasingly in health care agencies. Starting in the business offices of large hospitals, terminals have moved to central locations in most nurses' stations; they are expected to be used increasingly at the bedside in the future. Where they are used, computerized clinical record systems have improved record keeping because these systems are better organized, more legible, more accessible, and more complete than the old paper-based systems.

▶ Much streamlining of charting has occurred in preparation for the use of computerized documentation systems. Increased use of hand-held computers at the bedside along with networked systems for storing health records should speed up a trend toward efficient management of health care information.

Bibliography

1. Austin, J.K. (1990). Response to "The relationship of attitude, subjective norm, and behavioral intent to the documentation behavior of nurses." *Scholarly Inquiry for Nursing Practice*, 4(1), 61–64.
2. Buckley-Womack, C., & Gidney, B. (1987). A new dimension in documentation: the PIE method. *Journal of Neuroscience Nursing*, 19(5), 256–260.
3. Carpenito, L. (1991). Has JCAHO eliminated care plans? As I see it. *American Nurse*, 23(6), 6.
4. Carr, P. (1990). Visit notes. *Home Healthcare Nurse*, 8(3), 47–48.
5. Cassasa, E. (1990). Bedside computing positively impacts patient care. *Computers in Healthcare*, 11(5), 26–27, 30, 35.
6. Cassidy, D., & Friensen, M. (1990). QA: Applying JCAHO's generic model. *Nursing Management*, 21(6), 22–27.
7. Clark, L.A. (1988). Documentation: a lingering impact. *Emergency*, 20(4), 52–54.
8. Cline, A. (1989). Streamlined documentation through exceptional charting. *Nursing Management*, 20(2), 62–64.
9. Coles, M.C., & Fullenwider, S.D. (1988). Documentation: managing the dilemma. *Nursing Management*, 19(12), 65–66, 70, 72.
10. Doenges, M.E., & Moorhouse, M.F. (1991). *Nurse's pocket guide: Nursing diagnoses with interventions* (3rd ed.). Philadelphia: F.A. Davis.
11. Edmunds, L. (1984). Computers for inpatient nursing care. *Computers in Nursing*, 2(3), 102–108.
12. Fischbach, F. (1991). *Documenting care: Communication, the nursing process, and documentation standards*. Philadelphia: F.A. Davis.
13. Fuller, J., & Schaller-Ayers, J. (1990). *Health assessment: A nursing approach*. Philadelphia: J.B. Lippincott.
14. Goldie, S. (ed.). (1987). *I have done my duty, Florence Nightingale in the Crimean War, 1854–56*. Iowa City: University of Iowa Press.
15. Gruber, M., & Gruber, J.M. (1990). Nursing malpractice: the importance of documentation, or saved by the pen! *Gastroenterology-Nursing*, 12(4), 255–259.
16. Guzelaydin, S.K., & Pfoutz, S.K. (1984). Differences in documentation of nursing services according to recording format. *Classification of Nursing Diagnoses, Proceedings of the Fifth National Conference*, pp. 267–273.
17. Herring, D., & Rochman, R. (1990). A closer look at bedside terminals. *Nursing Management*, 21(7), 54–56, 60–61.
18. Hirshfield-Bartek, J., et al. (1990). Decreasing documentation time using a patient self-assessment tool. *Oncology Nursing Forum*, 17(2), 251–255.
19. Iyer, P. (1991). New trends in charting. *Nursing 91*, 21(1), 48–50.
20. Iyer, P., & Camp, N. (1991). *Nursing documentation: A nursing process approach*. St. Louis: C.V. Mosby.
21. Joint Commission on Accreditation of Hospitals (JCAHO) (1992). *Accreditation manual for hospitals*. Oak Brook Terrace, IL.
22. Kirk, R. (1990). Using workload analysis and acuity systems to facilitate quality and productivity. *Journal of Nursing Administration*, 20(3), 21–30.
23. Koska, M. (1992). Joint Commission cracks down on falsified records. *Hospitals*, 66(15), 47.
24. Lucatorto, M., et al. (1991). Documentation a focus for cost savings. *Journal of Nursing Administration*, 21(3), 32–36.
25. Masson, V. (1990). Nursing the charts. *Nursing Outlook*, 38(4), 196.
26. McMahon, R. (1990). Communication: What are we saying? . . . shift handover report. *Nursing Times*, 86(30), 38–40.
27. Montemuro, M. (1988). CORE documentation: a complete system for charting nursing care. *Nursing Management*, 19(8), 28–32.
28. Nine, S., et al. (1992). Organizing quality assurance in a maternal-child health division. *Journal of Obstetrical-Gynecological and Neonatal Nursing*, 21(1), 28–32.
29. O'Grady, B.V. (1984). Computerized documentation of community health nursing—what shall it be? *Computers in Nursing*, 2(3), 98–101.
30. Olivieri, R. (1984). Clinical recordkeeping using a personal computer, part 2: implementation. *Nurse Educator*, 9(2), 28–31.
31. Olivieri, R. (1984). Clinical recordkeeping using a personal computer, part I: preparation. *Nurse Educator*, 9(1), 43–48.
32. Owen, L., et al. (1988). A process to improve the documentation of nurses' notes. *Journal of Nursing Staff Development*, 4(3), 104–111.
33. Patterson, C. (1989). Standards of patient care: the Joint Commission focus on nursing quality assurance. *Nursing Clinics of North America*, 23(3), 625–638.
34. Regan, M.T. (1987). Documentation for the defense. *Journal of Perinatal and Neonatal Nursing*, 1(2), 49–59.
35. Renfroe, D., et al. (1990). The relationship of attitude, subjective norm, and behavioral intent to the documentation behavior of nurses. *Scholarly Inquiry for Nursing Practice*, 4(1), 47–60.
36. Scholes, M. (1989). Current issues in data protection as they affect nursing both in the United Kingdom and generally. *Medical Informatics (London)*, 14(3), 247–249.
37. Southard, P., & Frankel, P. (1989). Trauma care documentation: a comprehensive guide. *Journal of Emergency Nursing*, 15(5), 393–398.
38. Tapp, R.A. (1990). Inhibitors and facilitators to documentation of nursing practice. *Western Journal of Nursing Research*, 12(2), 229–240.
39. Taptich, B., et al. (1989). *Nursing diagnosis and care planning*. Philadelphia: W.B. Saunders.
40. Vicinus, M., & Nergaard, B. (eds.) (1989). *Ever yours, Florence Nightingale*. London: Virago Press, Limited.
41. Weeks, L.C., & Darrah, P. (1985). The documentation dilemma: a practical solution. *Journal of Nursing Administration*, 15(11), 22–27.
42. Willey, B.L., & Winstead, W.W. (1990). Computer-based charting and patient case management. *Caring*, 9(6), 44–47.
43. Willis, J., et al. (1988). Charting how-to's. *AD Nurse*, 3(4), 8–10.
44. Zielstorff, R., et al. (1990). Issues in designing an automated record system for clinical care and research. *Advances in Nursing Science*, 13(2), 75–88.

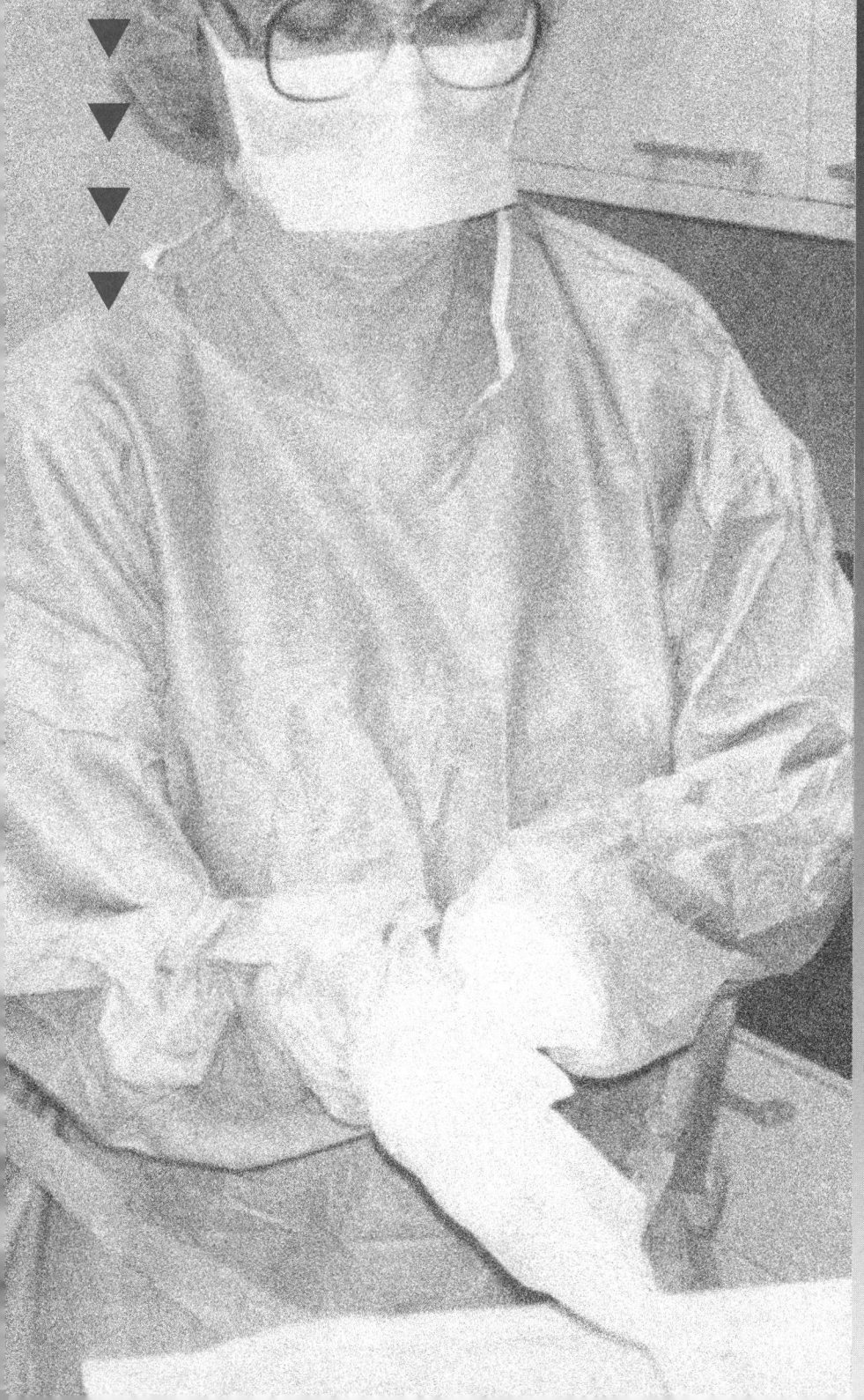

▼ **Skills Required for Safe Practice**

▼
▼
▼
▼

Chapter 28

 ## Infection Control

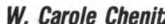

 Two years ago I donated blood during a blood drive. Ninety days later, on a cold, gray northern California day, I received a certified, registered letter.

W. Carole Chenitz

▼ **CHAPTER OUTLINE**

PROMOTING MICROBIAL SAFETY
INFECTION CONTROL IN HISTORICAL
 PERSPECTIVE
PROCESS OF INFECTIOUS DISEASE
  Infectious Agents
  Infection Risk
  Nosocomial Infections
BREAKING THE CHAIN OF INFECTION
  Infectious Agents
  Reservoir, or Source, of Infection
  Portal of Exit

Mode of Transmission
Portal of Entrance
Susceptible Host
NURSING PROCESS AND INFECTION
 CONTROL
  Assessment
  Nursing Diagnosis
  Planning
  Nursing Intervention
  Evaluation

▼ **KEY TERMS**

Antiseptics
Barrier techniques
Body substance isolation
Body substances
Category-specific CDC
 system
Chain of infection
Clean technique
Cleaning
Communicable disease
Community-acquired
 infections

Contaminated
Cross-contamination
Disease-specific CDC
 system
Disinfecting
Host
Infection
Infectious agent
Isolation precautions
Leukocytosis
Medical asepsis
Neutropenia

Normal flora
Nosocomial infections
Pathogen
Reservoir
Reverse (protective)
 isolation
Serology
Sterile technique
Sterilization
Surgical asepsis
Universal precautions
Virulence

Every year, approximately 6% of hospitalized clients contract infections *while* hospitalized. Thousands die from these infections; many thousands more become very sick, and the direct cost of these infections is between $5 and $10 billion annually.[16,35] Even if you or your family members never have a nosocomial infection, the cost of these infections affects you in increased insurance rates and taxes. Nurses have the opportunity to improve the statistics because more than one third of these infections are estimated to be potentially preventable. Nurses influence some, but not all, of these.

Preventing hospital-acquired infections is not a simple matter. To be effective, you must understand the basic concepts about infectious agents (microbes that produce disease) and factors that increase a person's risk for infection. Then you will be able to perform risk assessment and risk reduction for yourself and the people for whom you care as a nurse.

This chapter discusses the nature and means of preventing nosocomial infections in hospitalized persons and in health care workers.

PROMOTING MICROBIAL SAFETY

An **infection** is an illness produced by the invasion and multiplication of an infectious agent in body tissues. **Infectious agents** are microorganisms (bacteria, fungi, viruses, Rickettsia, and protoza) that can cause disease. Increased susceptibility to infection occurs in people with the following characteristics: (1) extreme in age (very old or very young) because of undeveloped or declining immunologic responses; (2) dysfunctioning immune systems (e.g., immature leukocytes as in leukemia or low protein level as in renal dysfunction); (3) very ill or traumatized and with invasive therapeutic devices entering and exiting the body; and (4) experiencing high levels of stress.

In health care facilities, it is essential that careful hand washing be done by all caretakers to avoid **cross-contamination,** the transmission of infectious agents from one person to another. During home care, although a person's susceptibility to infections may be increased, the actual risk of infection is less because fewer people are in the environment, with less risk of cross-contamination. Hand washing, however, is still important.

Local or systemic infection development requires (1) an infectious (causative) agent, (2) a source, or **reservoir,** of the infectious agent in which the agent lives and multiplies, (3) a mode of exit from the reservoir, (4) a mode of transmission of the infectious agent, (5) a portal of entry into the susceptible person, and (6) a susceptible person (host). This sequence in the development of infection is called the **chain of infection** (Fig. 28–1).

Protecting people from infection involves both surgical and medical asepsis. **Surgical asepsis** is the preparation and handling of materials so as to prevent the client's exposure to any living microorganisms. Nurses practice surgical asepsis through **sterile technique.** **Sterilization,** the destroying of all forms of microbial life, is the goal of surgical asepsis. **Medical asepsis** refers to practices designed to reduce the number of organisms present or reduce the risk for transmission from one person to another. Nurses practice medical asepsis through **clean technique.**

Cleaning (removing visible dust, soils, and other foreign material), **disinfecting** (killing or destroying most disease-producing microorganisms on inanimate objects), and sterilizing are activities important in ensuring microbial safety. Disinfectants are chemicals so strong that they are used only on inanimate objects. **Antiseptics,** chemicals that destroy microorganisms or inhibit their growth, are less strong and are safe enough to be used on living tissue.

Cleaning practices are important not only for reducing the numbers of microorganisms on environmental surfaces but also for aesthetic reasons. Factors involved in cleaning are chemical energy (detergent), thermal energy (temperature), and mechanical energy (friction). Examples of mechanical cleaning are

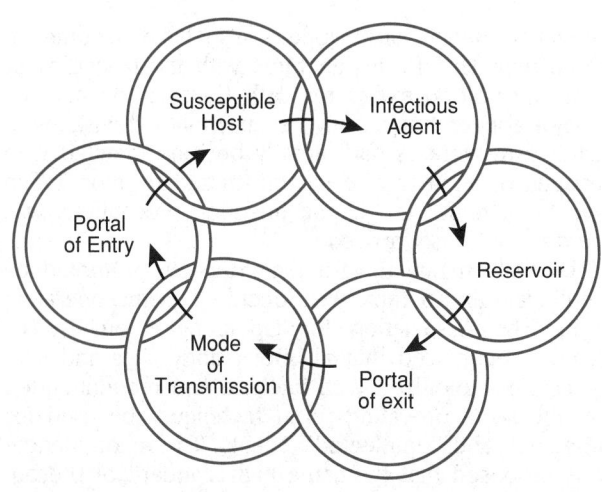

▲ *Figure 28-1*

Chain of infection. Links of the infection chain all must be present for the transmission of disease. Break the chain, and the spread of infection stops.

dishwashers, washer-sterilizers, ultrasonic cleaners, and utensil washer-sanitizers.

Disinfectants usually kill vegetative forms of bacteria, fungi, and some viruses but rarely kill spores. Factors affecting disinfectant activity are (1) disinfectant concentration, (2) type and concentration of microbial contamination, (3) cleanliness of the surface, (4) contact time, and (5) chemical and physical factors in the surrounding environment or medium being treated (e.g., temperature, water hardness). Three major methods of disinfection are pasteurization (hot-water disinfection at temperatures below 100 °C [212 °F]), liquid chemicals, and radiation.

Because sterilization kills all forms of microbial life, all bacteria, spores, viruses, and fungi are destroyed. Methods of sterilization are thermal (heat) and chemical. Heat may be moist (steam autoclave) or dry (hot-air oven). Chemical sterilization may be accomplished with liquid chemicals or ethylene oxide. Factors affecting any sterilization process are (1) time, (2) type of microorganisms present, (3) number of microorganisms present, (4) type and amount of soil present, and (5) amount of protection given by the object being sterilized to the microbes (e.g., hinges, coils). Radiation is usually not used in care facilities as a method of sterilization, but is used in manufacturing some equipment (e.g., to sterilize single-use items).

Amazingly, about 15 lb (6 to 8 kg) of solid waste is generated for each person receiving care in an acute care facility each day. Solid waste may be biologic or nonbiologic and is discarded and not intended for further use. Biologic waste results from activities related to diagnosis, treatment, and care (e.g., medical waste such as bandages, surgical and autopsy waste such as organs, and laboratory waste such as blood samples). Biologic waste may be infectious or noninfectious. Nonbiologic waste consists of food garbage, combustible (burnable) and noncombustible (nonburnable) rubbish, and ashes (residue from fires). Infectious waste is commonly rendered noninfectious by incineration or steam sterilization before disposal. Other methods are rarely used. Hazardous waste must be handled carefully and treated properly to prevent the spread of infectious agents and toxic substances within the care facility as well as to the surrounding general community.

Some people enter a health care facility specifically for treatment of known infections acquired outside a health care facility. Such infections are called **community-acquired infections.** Infections that were not present when a person entered a health care facility but instead develop after admission are called **nosocomial infections.** Whatever the source, once an infection develops, specific intervention is appropriate to control its spread.

Always remember that hand washing is the single most important activity in controlling the spread of infection.

Hands cannot be sterilized, however, and **normal flora** (microorganisms that grow abundantly as part of the body's normal defense system) on the skin can cause nosocomial infections. Still, hand washing is very effective in preventing the spread of infection.

INFECTION CONTROL IN HISTORICAL PERSPECTIVE

Practices that prevent the spread of infection have changed over the years, and in some ways, the emphasis now resembles earlier times. Ignaz Semmelweis is often referred to as the "father" of infection prevention in hospitals. In 1847, he noticed that, when physicians came directly from an autopsy and performed examinations on women who had just had or were about to give birth, "childbed fever" (puerperal sepsis) developed in the women. Careful observation confirmed that the frequency of infections declined when hand washing was instituted, and one of the first infection-control concepts became widely used. Since the time of Semmelweis, we have come to appreciate the importance of hand washing in the prevention of a number of **communicable diseases,** or illnesses caused by specific infectious agents that can be transmitted from an infected person, animal, or reservoir to a susceptible **host,** or person who then harbors the disease.

In 1863, Florence Nightingale founded a school of nursing in London. Like Semmelweis, Nightingale emphasized cleanliness, both for the personnel and for the environment. At a time when everyone believed that infection resulted from bad air (then called miasmas), Semmelweis and Nightingale based new precautions on their own accurate observations. They fostered generic practices—precautions that were to be used by all health care workers in the care for all clients. Eventually, their efforts changed some practices worldwide.[18] Unfortunately, some of their important message was lost over the following years.

As the medical profession learned more about infectious diseases, precautions became more and more focused on identifying infected persons, isolating them in special communicable disease hospitals or in isolation areas within general hospitals, and taking precautions only with their body excretions and the air they breathed out. Elaborate "isolation routines" were developed for them, and many health care workers ignored the old principle that all humans, particularly those who are sick, are likely to acquire infections if microbes are placed on their mucous membranes or nonintact skin. In other words, protection of susceptible persons by using generic standards of cleanliness was lost.

By the middle of the 20th century, immunizations had reduced the incidence of some communicable diseases, such as smallpox, and antibiotics often cured bacterial infections. Special communicable disease hospitals had been closed. Most people with community-acquired infections were cared for at home by family members with the support of public health nurses. In hospitals, infected individuals were cared for using barrier precautions consisting of different combinations of gowns, masks, and gloves as part of isolation routines. To protect the uninfected, gowns, caps, masks, and gloves were used in surgery.

Shortly after midcentury, a new wave of hospital-acquired staphylococcal infections began to appear. These infections affected healthy hosts, particularly surgical clients and newborns, and were resistant to (unaffected by) commonly used antibiotics. Health care workers often transmitted the infectious agents, either by having undiagnosed infections themselves or by transferring organisms from client to client as they provided care. The situation was alarming, and for more than a decade, efforts increased to identify and isolate those infected. Finally, with new antibiotics developed to treat the staphylococcal infections, health care facilities had no apparent reason to return to the practice of generic precautions. Isolation for infected persons was still considered most important for reducing the transmission of staphylococci, and this belief persisted even when newer microbes, including *Pseudomonas, Serratia,* and *Acinetobacter,* began to cause increasing numbers of infections in critical care units.

By the late 1970s, clinical journals were publishing the results of new research that showed that some of the older methods of infection control, such as protective isolation, were ineffective and that some of the newer methods, such as protocols for managing invasive devices, were more effective. Studies revealed that disease transmission was diminished when precautions were focused on the susceptible mucous membranes and nonintact skin and the infectious agents present in the moist body substances of all people.[20,22]

In the early 1980s, the entire world was awakened to the tragedy of the acquired immune deficiency syndrome (AIDS), an infectious viral disease transmitted by blood and some moist body substances. The disease could be transmitted by people who did not know they were infectious; in fact, about 90% of people with human immunodeficiency virus (HIV) infection do not have symptomatic AIDS and are not sick. Even in the United States, hospitalized people have acquired nosocomial HIV infection from inadequately sterilized instruments. Health care workers also have become infected with HIV from punctures with used needles or from other blood exposures. HIV transmission became a major concern, especially because many thousands of health care workers had already become infected with hepatitis B, another disease transmitted by blood. The time for a return to generic infection precautions was overdue but finally arrived.

The first change toward the concepts promoted by Nightingale and Semmelweis occurred in the operating room. The Association for Operating Room Nurses (AORN) recognized that all moist body sites and substances are colonized with bacteria and recommended that the same operating room techniques be used for "infected" and "uninfected" clients. The recommendations proposed that the same high standard of precautions be used for everyone.

In 1983, the Centers for Disease Control (CDC), the public health agency that often makes recommendations on management of nosocomial and community-acquired infections, revised its recommendations for isolation. These new recommendations reduced emphasis on isolation rituals but retained a diagnosis-based focus in which different hospital clients were to be treated with different precautions based on diagnosis.[14] In the mid-1980s, a system of generic precautions —called **body substance isolation**—based on interactions or task assessment by health care workers was published. This is a set of guidelines for caring for people with infectious disease. Body substance isolation is a system of precautions taken when in contact with all moist body sites and substances regardless of a person's diagnosis. This system is intended to reduce risk of transmission of microbes to sick people in health care facilities and also to the care givers.[23] Its basis is the probability that **body substances,** secretions or excretions that are usually moist and support the growth of microorganisms, will transmit infection.

In 1987, the CDC published recommendations to reduce risk for transmission of blood-borne pathogens to health care workers. These were called **universal precautions,**[6,7] and these guidelines require that all persons be treated as though they are infectious. Universal precautions include the use of **barrier techniques,** activities designed to prevent transmission of infectious agents from one source to another. Barrier techniques involve the use of gloves, gowns, aprons, masks, and eye shields, which create physical barriers to disease transmission. These, together with hand washing and safety with sharp objects, comprise universal precautions.

Since 1987, the combination of universal precautions, the more generic isolation practices of body substance isolation, and the older diagnosis-based isolation systems have been used concurrently.

The new emphasis is to recognize that all moist body sites and substances from all humans are potentially infectious. It is therefore important to follow appropriate infection precautions when handling any body substances. It is also essential to assess each individual's care requirements and correctly choose when to wear gloves and sometimes gowns or plastic aprons. These simple measures, accompanied by hand washing for 10 seconds, are usually sufficient to interrupt transmission of potentially infectious agents except for airborne communicable diseases.

PROCESS OF INFECTIOUS DISEASE

A spectrum illustrates the various ways infection may present itself. As Figure 28-2 shows, the diagnosis of an infection may not occur until after a person's body tissue has responded to the presence of an infectious agent. Body substances are colonized with bacterial agents, and viral agents infect cells before any clinical signs or symptoms of infection appear. Figure 28-3 uses an iceberg to represent all of the infections present around us. As you can see, most of the iceberg is hidden under the water and only the tip is apparent. In other words, most infections are not apparent to us.

Infectious Agents

Sources of infectious agents include (1) an individual's own microbial flora (normal flora), (2) colonized body substances (potentially infective materials) from other people, and (3) objects or fluids in the environment contaminated with infectious agents (occasional source).

It is important to understand all aspects of the infection cycle. Then appropriate care strategies can be used for all people requiring health care and not just for those identified as "infected."

The term **pathogen** has historically referred to microorganisms that cause disease. The term infectious agent is probably more appropriate. Because of the compromised immunity of many people requiring health care, it is unrealistic to consider some microorganisms pathogenic and others harmless.

Any microorganism has the potential to cause disease in a susceptible person and is therefore potentially pathogenic.

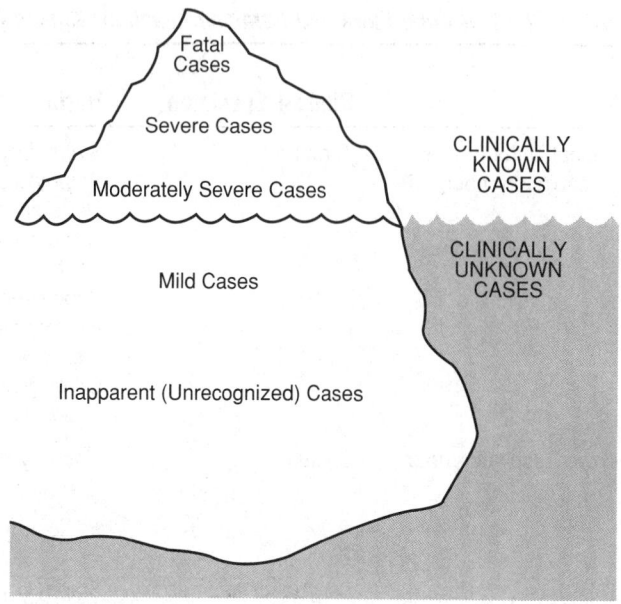

▲ *Figure 28-3*

"Iceberg phenomenon" of infectious disease. This iceberg represents the incidence of a specific disease in a population. Above the "water line" are clinically known cases of the disease. Below the water line are clinically unknown cases of the disease. Placement of the water line varies from disease to disease. More of the iceberg, however, is usually below the water line than above it. In other words, many people have infectious agents in their body substances but do not know it. They may have a mild or subclinical illness. Such people transmit the infection to others without knowing it.

Microorganisms possess various characteristics that make them able to cause infection. The term **virulence** refers to a microorganism's ability to cause infection. Microorganisms do not have equal virulence. Variables affecting a microorganism's virulence include their ability to (1) adhere to mucosal surfaces or skin, (2) penetrate mucous membranes, (3) multiply within the body, (4) secrete enzymes or toxins, and (5) resist being destroyed by white blood cells (phagocytosis).

Even those microorganisms that normally inhabit or colonize various body sites without usually producing disease may, under certain circumstances, produce in-

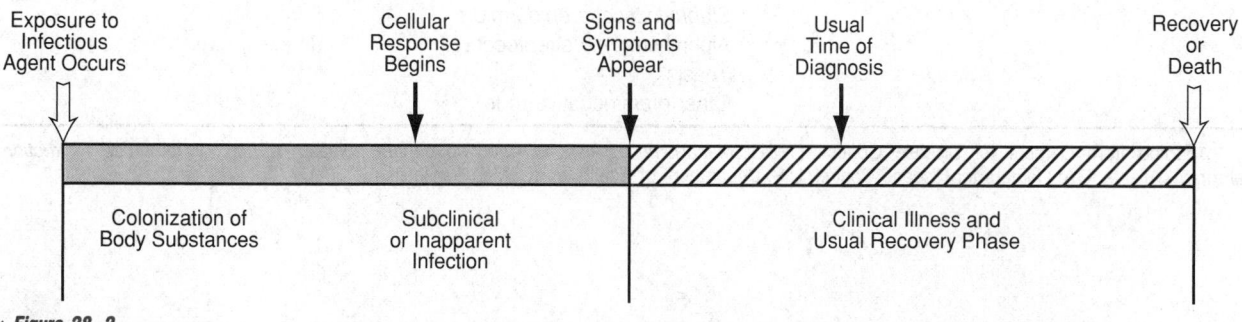

▲ *Figure 28-2*

Spectrum of infection. Transmission of bacterial organisms begins when a person's body substances are colonized sufficiently to be transmitted to another person. Transmission of viral agents usually begins at the time of cellular response. Note that both events *precede* the onset of signs and symptoms of clinical illness.

TABLE 28-1. Normal Flora and Common Infectious Agents (Pathogens) Found in Various Human Body Sites*

Site	Clinical Specimen	Normal Flora	Common Infectious Agents (Pathogens)
Nasopharynx (upper respiratory tract)	Throat	*Staphylococcus epidermidis* *Staphylococcus aureus* *Neisseria* species Alpha-hemolytic streptococci Peptococci Peptostreptococci *Haemophilus influenzae* *Klebsiella* species Other gram-negative rods (occasionally)	*Streptococcus pyogenes* (Group A)
Lower respiratory tract	Sputum	Normally sterile	*Streptococcus pneumoniae* Enterobacteriaceae group *Haemophilus influenzae* Other gram-negative rods
Skin, hair Perianal skin	Surgical or traumatic wounds, lesions, pustules Deep wound, intraabdominal abscess	*Staphylococcus epidermidis* *Staphylococcus aureus* Diphtheroids Streptococci (*viridans* group) *Enterobacter* species Other gram-negative rods Yeasts *Streptococcus* pyogenes (Group A)	*Staphylococcus aureus* *Streptococcus pyogenes* (Group A) Enterobacteriaceae group Other gram-negative rods Anaerobic gram-positive rods Anaerobic gram-negative rods
Central nervous system	Cerebrospinal fluid	Normally sterile	*Streptococcus pneumoniae* *Neisseria meningitidis* *Haemophilus influenzae* Other gram-negative rods
Small bowel and colon	Stool	*Enterobacter* family (coliforms) *Bacteroides* species *Pseudomonas* species *Streptococcus faecalis* (enterococci or Group D) *Clostridium perfringens* Yeasts	*Salmonella* species *Shigella* species *Yersinia* species *Campylobacter* species
Bladder and upper urinary tract	Urine	Normally sterile	*Escherichia coli* *Enterobacter* species Other gram-negative rods *Streptococcus faecalis* (enterococci or Group D)
Vagina (adult)	Endocervical swab	*Lactobacillus* species *Acidophilus* species *Staphylococcus epidermidis* Alpha-hemolytic streptococci Yeasts Other gram-negative rods	*Neisseria gonorrhoeae* *Chlamydia* species

* Adapted from Centers for Disease Control. (1982). *Management skills for infection control nurses—A criterion-reference instruction program.* Atlanta, GA: Centers for Disease Control, U.S. Department of Health and Human Services.

fection. Certain sites of the body normally have abundant microorganisms, which are a part of the body's normal flora. Thus, the presence of microorganisms alone does not mean that infection is present. For example, *Escherichia coli* is present in the feces of all humans. However, when this organism gets into the urinary bladder, where it is not normally found, infection may result. Normal flora are presented in Table 28-1.

Organisms that are normal flora for a person who is healthy may cause infections if immune defenses are compromised.

Infection Risk

The risk or probability that infection will occur is influenced by (1) the competence of the individual's immune system, (2) the quantity of the infectious agent, (3) the agent's virulence, and (4) the duration and intimacy of contact between individual and microorganism (Fig. 28-4).

A healthy person in the community usually has a competent immune system and has few contacts with large quantities of microorganisms. When such contacts do occur, however, they are usually short and present little risk of infection. For example, even though microorganisms are present in feces, people rarely become infected from changing an infant's diaper. Likewise, bladder self-catheterization may sometimes be done in the home setting by clients who use "clean" rather than "sterile" technique (see Chapter 44).

A person admitted to a health care facility, however, may have body defenses compromised by drugs, illness, and invasive or indwelling medical devices. For example, the intimacy and duration of contact between a person and infectious agents may be increased by devices (such as indwelling urinary catheters) left in the body for a period of time. Also the microorganisms present in hospitals may be more virulent or more multidrug resistant than those generally found in other types of care facilities or in the community.

People admitted to intensive care units are at great risk for infection. The body defenses of such people are compromised in many ways, including serious illness and the presence of numerous indwelling treatment devices. Frequently, the microorganisms present are multidrug resistant. Also the duration and intimacy of contact between the individual and infectious agents are extensive.

Nosocomial Infections

Nosocomial infections are neither present nor incubating until after admission to a care facility. Various factors increase the likelihood of the development of nosocomial infections. Severe illness may predispose people to infection. Treatment regimen may include the use of indwelling devices (e.g., urinary or intravenous

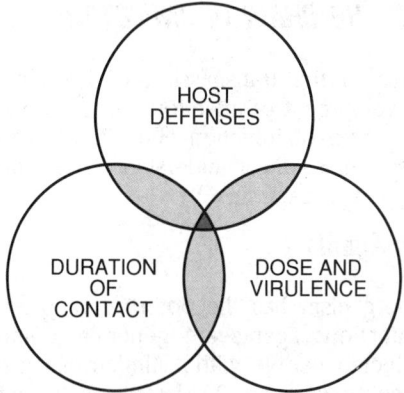

A. Healthy person in the community

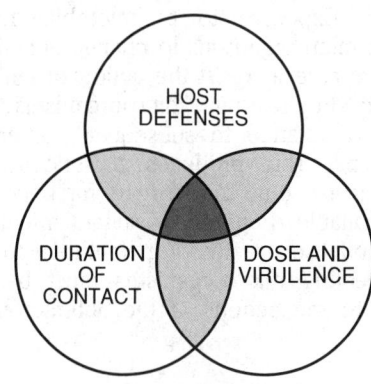

B. Hospitalized person

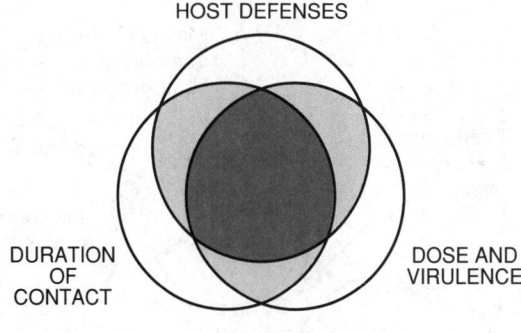

C. Person in intensive care unit

▲ *Figure 28-4*

Infection risk (areas shown in color) is greatest when a person's host defenses are compromised, when the dose and virulence of a microbial contact are increased, and when the duration of contact between microorganisms and the host is prolonged or intimate. As graphically shown, the risk of infection increases as the intersecting areas within each circle increase. *A*, In the community, the overlap among compromised host defenses, dose and virulence of a microbial contact, and duration of the contact is very small. *B*, In a hospital, infection risk is increased as illness and medical devices alter host defenses, increasing the duration of contact with microorganisms. *C*, In an intensive care unit, a person's host defenses are often severely compromised by illness, medical devices, and antimicrobial therapy, making prolonged contact with microorganisms common.

catheters) that can introduce infectious agents. Also antimicrobial and other drugs may alter an individual's immune response.

BREAKING THE CHAIN OF INFECTION

The process of the transmission of infectious agents and the development of infection can be broken at any link in the chain of infection (Fig. 28-5). To interrupt the process, nurses must understand interventions that can be applied to each link.

Infectious Agents

Any microorganism has the potential of producing infection. Infectious agents are generally controlled by treating infected people with antimicrobial medication. These products work by (1) destroying the microorganisms by disrupting their cell membranes, (2) interfering with the synthesis of proteins vital to the microorganisms, and (3) inhibiting the microorganism's reproduction. Exposure to antimicrobial medication causes some microorganisms to change genetically into forms that are able to resist the action of antimicrobial drugs. These drug-resistant microorganisms can then transmit the resistance to subsequent generations of microorganisms. This produces a serious treatment problem, because some microorganisms become resistant to all available drugs and resultant infections cannot be controlled or treated. For treatment to be effective, the infecting microorganisms must be sensitive (vulnerable) to the actions of the antimicrobial being used.

Reservoir, or Source, of Infection

Once present, infectious agents can reproduce in many reservoirs. Human tissue, colonized body substances (e.g., feces, wound drainage, sputum, saliva, and sometimes urine and blood), and some articles in the environment may all serve as reservoirs. Environmental articles that become reservoirs for infectious agents are mostly moist rather than dry. Therefore, hard surfaces such as doorknobs, table tops, and bed rails are unlikely to harbor microorganisms in the same quantity as moist or wet reservoirs. Examples of possible reservoirs in care facilities include large-volume nebulizers for ventilators, urine collection devices, and hydrometers used for measuring specific gravity. In the community, possible reservoirs include sewage, stagnant water, and improperly cooked or stored food. Some human beings may also become reservoirs for infectious agents. Human reservoirs include people ill with infectious diseases, those with unrecognized illness, and those who do not have a disease but who do have infectious agents in their body substances.

In the United States and other developed countries, even the smallest communities have sanitation measures established and usually have regulations governing their use. Safe water, sewage, and food are thus ensured. In care facilities, reservoirs for infectious agents in the environment are controlled by cleaning, disinfection, and sterilization measures.

Many human reservoirs for infectious agents are not identified. Thus, treat all body substances from all people (staff, clients, visitors) as potentially infectious.

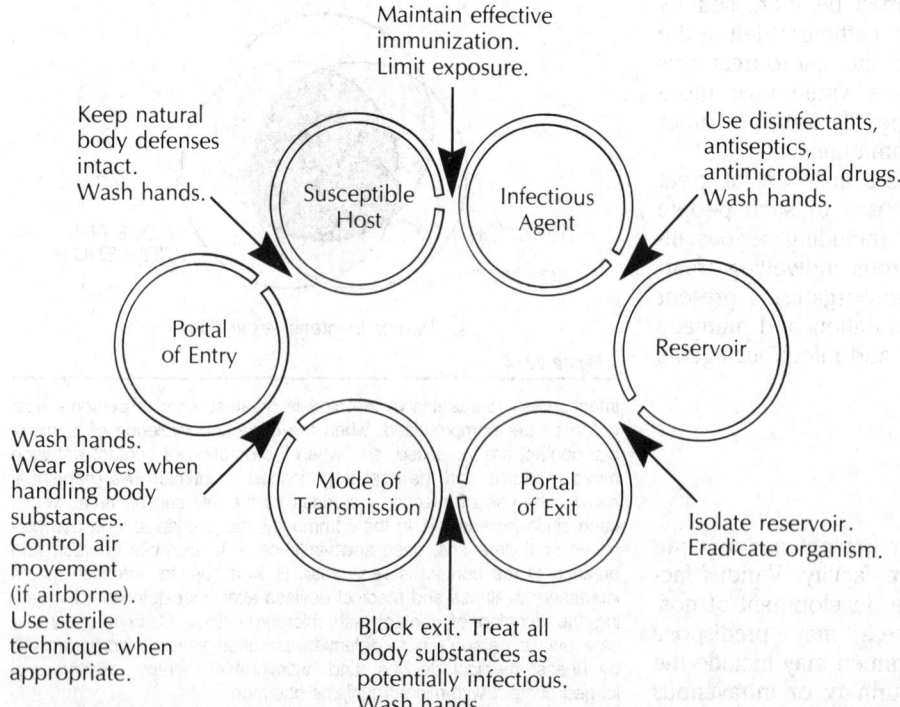

Maintain effective immunization.
Limit exposure.

Keep natural body defenses intact.
Wash hands.

Use disinfectants, antiseptics, antimicrobial drugs.
Wash hands.

Susceptible Host

Infectious Agent

Portal of Entry

Reservoir

Wash hands.
Wear gloves when handling body substances.
Control air movement (if airborne).
Use sterile technique when appropriate.

Mode of Transmission

Portal of Exit

Isolate reservoir.
Eradicate organism.

Block exit. Treat all body substances as potentially infectious.
Wash hands.

▲ *Figure 28–5*

Creating barriers to transmission of disease. Note all the actions *(arrowed points)* that can be taken to break the chain of infection.

One must direct intervention toward both recognized and unrecognized reservoirs to disrupt the chain of infection at the infectious agent link.

Portal of Exit

Potentially infectious agents leave the body in body substances (e.g., respiratory secretions, feces, urine, blood, wound drainage, and genital secretions). Sanitation measures are used to control and contain these substances as well as to eliminate environmental reservoirs or to manage them in a safe manner (e.g., sewage treatment, water chlorination, and sanitary landfills).

Mode of Transmission

Four major modes of transmission allow infectious agents to move from portals of exit in reservoirs to portals of entry in people. These include contact transmission, common-source transmission, airborne transmission, and vector-borne transmission. For each of these modes, disruption of transmission may be accomplished by scrupulous sanitation measures (e.g., hand washing) or by using gloves or gowns or both when indicated.

CONTACT TRANSMISSION

Contact transmission may be by direct contact, indirect contact, or droplet contact. Direct contact with infectious agents in moist body substances might include touching feces and then putting finger in mouth. Indirect contact occurs through an intermediate object contaminated with a moist body substance. For example, a nurse might handle an object that has been soiled by droplets and then touch his or her own eye. Infection results. Droplet contact occurs when infectious agents contained in most respiratory secretions are coughed or sneezed into the environment (usually within 3 feet). For example, one person sneezes near another person, and moist droplets touch the conjunctiva of the second person's eye.

COMMON-SOURCE TRANSMISSION

Infectious agents may be transmitted through a common source (e.g., shared food or fluids contaminated during preparation). In health care facilities, it is possible for various contaminated fluids to transmit infectious agents, resulting in outbreaks of infection. Intravenous fluid, for example, can be contaminated with gram-negative rods during manufacture, although this problem is not very common today. Outbreaks of food poisoning from food served at picnics or restaurants are another example of a common source of transmission.

AIRBORNE TRANSMISSION

The air can carry droplet nuclei, the small residue that results from evaporated fluid from droplets coughed or sneezed by an infected person. Droplet nuclei can sur-

vive suspended in air for long periods of time. Very few infectious agents can be transmitted this way, however. Tuberculosis and chickenpox are examples.

VECTOR-BORNE TRANSMISSION

Vectors include flies, mosquitos, rodents, and fleas. Transmission of infectious agents by way of vectors is unlikely to occur in modern health care facilities.

Portal of Entrance

Portals of entrance are usually the same as portals of exit. For example, agents causing gastrointestinal (GI) infection usually exit from the source or reservoir through the GI tract (i.e., in the stool) and enter the susceptible host through the GI tract (i.e., the mouth).

Susceptible Host

Many factors protect a potential host from infection. Natural barriers offer protection (e.g., unbroken skin, the protective secretions of mucous membranes, and ciliary action in the respiratory tract). Microorganisms do not penetrate intact skin. Mucous membrane secretions trap foreign particles. Cilia are hairlike processes that transport mucus and foreign particles out of the upper airway by a wavelike action. Additionally, a flushing action is provided by the flow of tears or urine, which can remove particles and bacteria.

If natural mechanical barriers fail, the body can further defend itself in several ways. These include (1) production of phagocytes, (2) production of antibodies specific to the infecting organism, and (3) an inflammatory response that increases circulation of blood and white blood cells to the infected area. An immune response is limited by malnutrition, stress, some chemotherapeutic drugs, and some diseases. One of the best ways to reduce host susceptibility to infection is to maintain good health and adequate nutrition. Immunization programs for children are a major attempt to reduce the number of people susceptible to diseases preventable by vaccination. These diseases include rubella, mumps, measles, polio, pertussis, diphtheria, and tetanus. New vaccines are being developed for *Pseudomonas* and some other nosocomial microorganisms in hospitals. Additionally, some hospital personnel are at increased risk for hepatitis B because of their unprotected contact with blood and body substances. Hepatitis B vaccine is available and is recommended for such people.

NURSING PROCESS AND INFECTION CONTROL

Using the nursing process in caring for clients with particular infections or risk for infection is a process you will learn throughout your nursing program. Infection control is so important that it is applied in every phase of nursing care. For example, the risk for infection is an important consideration when planning nursing care for clients with certain problems in urinary elimination (see Chapter 44), for clients with wounds (see Chapter 48), and for clients in the perioperative period of hospitalization (see Chapter 49).

Infection control requires you to have the knowledge and skills necessary to practice all of your nursing activities in a safe manner. This requires you to establish habits for going about all of your work; habits that you will use consistently, without even thinking; habits that will help to keep you and your clients free from unnecessary exposure to infection. Remember that failure to adhere to good practices of medical and surgical asepsis can always result in infection.

Assessment

Within health care facilities, infection-control practitioners (also called nurse or hospital epidemiologists) have a responsibility for consultation about infection control and prevention. Infection-control practitioners work with infection-control committees to assess infection risks and develop policies to reduce these risks. The committee is usually multidisciplinary and includes members of both nursing and medical personnel as well as representatives from other departments (e.g., pharmacy, dietary, housekeeping). Recommended policies, and nursing procedures for their implementation, are usually included in nursing manuals.

Physicians are usually responsible for the treatment of infections. Nurses, however, often identify the early signs of infection in people receiving health care. A careful physical assessment and review of laboratory data are helpful in identifying the presence of infection. Risk assessment and self-assessment are also important.

Physical assessment includes looking for the classic signs of inflammation—redness, warmth, swelling, and pain. The presence of any one of these signs may indicate infection. Other indications of infection include purulent discharge (pus) from a wound or natural body opening; diarrhea; cloudy urine; cough and sputum production (lower respiratory tract infection); or fever and malaise (systemic infection, which may be due to bacterial, fungal, or viral infectious agents).

Review of laboratory data about the individual is also part of a thorough assessment. Laboratory data that may indicate infection include hematologic changes (e.g., **leukocytosis,** an increase in the number of white blood cells, also termed a left shift), and abnormal urinalysis indicating the presence of white blood cells or bacteriuria. Special serologic tests (**serology** is the study of antigen-antibody reactions in the serum) may be used to identify infections (e.g., acute and convalescent sera for viral diseases). Microbiology laboratory data include Gram's stain and culture information about specific body substances or sites.

Laboratory data are correlated with physical assessment and other clinical information before it is concluded that infection is present.

Risk assessment is another part of nursing assessment. When assessing an individual's risk of infection, identify the type and number of invasive medical devices used on the person. Remember that such devices interrupt the body's natural defense system. Additionally, determine whether the person's ability to produce white blood cells is reduced. An individual with **neutropenia,** a decrease in the number of neutrophils (a type of white blood cell) is at increased risk for infection.

Also assess whether the individual may be a reservoir for infectious agents that can be transmitted to others. In other words, is the person producing body substances that may contaminate the environment? People with abundant excretions and secretions can produce more infection risks than those with minimal secretions.

For example, feces flushed down toilets present no risk. Fecal incontinence, however, requires a care giver to have direct contact with the potentially infectious agents present in feces when cleaning the individual and removing soiled linen.

Infection risk related to body substances is directly influenced by the quantity of the substances and by the extent to which they contaminate the environment in such a way that others may come in contact with the substances.

Self-assessment is also important in infection control. Health professionals (including nurses) have a responsibility to assess their own health status. When ill, do not work with others.

Nursing Diagnosis

The most pertinent nursing diagnosis regarding prevention of infection is, of course, *High Risk for Infection* (see the Nursing Diagnosis Profile in Chapter 49). Keep in mind that you and your clients always have a potential for infection because you exist in a world abundant with microorganisms. As a nurse, you must look at known risk factors that place you and your clients in particular jeopardy. These factors serve as related factors that make up the second part of a nursing diagnosis of *High Risk for Infection*. Some examples follow.

Clients with inadequate primary defenses might have nursing diagnoses such as these:

▶ *High Risk for Infection* R/T alterations in skin integrity
▶ *High Risk for Infection* R/T decrease in ciliary activity
▶ *High Risk for Infection* R/T stasis of body fluids

Clients with inadequate secondary defenses might have nursing diagnoses such as these:

▶ *High Risk for Infection* R/T leukopenia
▶ *High Risk for Infection* R/T suppressed inflammatory response

Clients and their significant others may have normal defense mechanisms and yet be at risk because they are exposed to greater than normal amounts or unusual types of infectious microorganisms. For example, clients who are hospitalized or families of infected clients in the home setting might have nursing diagnoses such as these:

▶ *High Risk for Infection* R/T increased environmental exposure
▶ *High Risk for Infection* R/T insufficient knowledge to avoid exposure to infectious microorganisms (pathogens)

Some clients are at great enough risk of infection to require some type of isolation from others or to require some other life-style change. These clients often have nursing diagnoses that are psychosocial in nature:

▶ *Anxiety* R/T high risk for infection
▶ *Fear* R/T high risk for infection
▶ *Impaired Social Interaction* R/T high risk for infection
▶ *Situational Low Self-Esteem* R/T high risk for infection

When these psychosocial nursing diagnoses apply, they are made *in addition to* the diagnosis *High Risk for Infection*. Many other nursing diagnoses frequently coexist with a nursing diagnosis of *High Risk for Infection* including, for example, *Altered Protection, Impaired Skin Integrity,* and *Impaired Tissue Integrity.* When you see such nursing diagnoses, you should automatically consider the nursing diagnosis of *High Risk for Infection.*

Planning

When a person is at high risk for infection, you will want to plan how to break at least one link in the infection chain to prevent the infection from occurring. For example, you may plan to strengthen the client's immune system. Several interventions will help you achieve this. Alternatively, you may wish to prevent microbes from entering a newly created surgical wound; a variety of interventions will do that. Whatever your plan, however, your expected outcome should be simply that the client will not become infected. You can state this outcome in a positive way and build in a number of objective criteria, but the goal is always to keep the client free from infection. Some outcomes might be stated as follows:

▶ Remains free from infection AEB, WBC count within 5–10,000 range
▶ Remains free from infection AEB, a clean surgical wound that is free of redness, heat, edema, and purulent drainage
▶ Remains free from infection AEB, vital signs within normal limits

Such outcomes provide objective evidence that the client remains free from infection. You may also include outcomes that show that learning has taken place or that the client is progressing in the ability to use preventive measures. Such outcomes as "Lists five

methods to decrease risk of opportunistic infection" or "Verbalizes understanding of methods to break the chain of infection" can be effective parts of the overall plan.

Nursing Intervention

MEDICAL ASEPSIS

A number of nursing interventions are designed specifically to prevent the spread of infection. We term these interventions *isolation precautions* when they are used with clients with known or suspected infectious diseases.

Although interventions vary according to the types of precautions required, the following guidelines always apply:

▶ Wash your hands before giving care and any time they are likely to have been soiled.
▶ Put on clean gloves just before contact with mucous membranes or nonintact skin.
▶ Put on sterile gloves for sterile procedures.
▶ Wear appropriate gloves when contact with moist body substances is likely.
▶ Wear a gown or apron when your skin or clothing is likely to become soiled with body substances.
▶ Wear a mask and protective eye wear (glasses, goggles, or face shields) when body substances are likely to spatter on your facial skin or mucous membranes.
▶ Assess each task that you are about to perform for the infection risk to the client receiving the care, to other clients, and to yourself.

Isolation Systems. Formal **isolation precautions** are systems designed to use barriers to prevent transmission of infectious agents. Systems may be category specific or disease specific and may vary among care facilities. Published isolation systems are summarized in Table 28–2. The rationale behind each of these systems is to disrupt the mode of transmission link in the chain of infection by using barrier techniques—usually gloves but sometimes gowns and face protection—between the potentially infectious material such as wound drainage and the health care worker.

The **category-specific CDC system** is a set of guidelines that groups similar infectious diseases together and describes the precautions for each category. The **disease-specific CDC system** is a set of guidelines that prescribes specific precautions to be taken for each infectious disease. The body substance isolation system bases precautions on the anticipated interaction between the care giver and the care recipient and recommends that precautions be based on the likelihood of contact with moist body sites or body substances, regardless of the diagnosis.

Always become familiar with the isolation system in the facility where you are working, and always take appropriate precautions based on your risk assessment for yourself and the person for whom you are caring.

TABLE 28–2. Summary of Centers for Disease Control Category-specific Isolation Precautions

Factor	Strict Isolation	Contact Isolation	Respiratory Isolation
Common diseases or conditions requiring the isolation precautions listed	Diphtheria, pharyngeal Varicella (chickenpox) Zoster, localized in immunocompromised person, or disseminated	Acute respiratory infections in infants/young children Herpes simplex, disseminated, severe primary, or neonatal Rubella, congenital and other Skin, wound, or burn infection, major	Measles Meningitis Bacterial Meningococcal *Haemophilus influenzae* Mumps Pertussis *Haemophilus influenzae* pneumonia in children
Room	Private indicated* Door closed	Private indicated*	Private indicated*
Masks	All persons entering room	For those who come close to infected person	For those who come close to infected person
Gowns	All persons entering room	If soiling is likely	Not indicated
Gloves	All persons entering room	For touching infective material	Not indicated
Hands	**For All Categories:** Wash hands after touching an infected person or potentially contaminated articles and before giving care to another person.		
Articles	**For All Categories:** Contaminated articles should be discarded or bagged, labeled, and sent for decontamination and reprocessing.		

Acid-fast Bacillus Isolation	Enteric Precautions	Drainage/Secretion Precautions	Blood/Body Fluid Precautions
Tuberculosis Pulmonary Laryngeal	Diarrhea, acute illness with suspected infectious cause Encephalitis Gastroenteritis Hepatitis, viral type A Poliomyelitis Typhoid fever	Abscess, minor or limited Burn infection, minor or limited Conjunctivitis Pressure sore, infected, minor or limited Skin and wound infections, minor or limited	Acquired immune deficiency syndrome Creutzfeldt-Jakob disease Hepatitis B (and HBsAg carrier) Hepatitis, non-A, non-B
Private with special ventilation* Door closed	Private only if the person's hygiene is poor†	May share room	Private only if the person's hygiene is poor†
Only if person is coughing and does not cover mouth	Not indicated	Not indicated	Not indicated
Only if needed to prevent gross soilage of clothing	If soiling is likely	If soiling is likely	If soilage with blood or body fluids is likely
Not indicated	For touching infective material	For touching infective material	For touching blood or body fluids
			Wash hands immediately if potentially contaminated by blood or body fluid

* People infected with the same organism may share the same room.
† A person with poor hygiene habits may not wash hands after touching infective material and may contaminate others.

Isolation Precautions. Most commonly, nursing decisions about isolation involve determining (1) when to wear gloves and when to change them, (2) when to wash hands, (3) whether to put on a gown to prevent clothing from becoming soiled with body substances, (4) whether to wear facial protection (mask and eye protectors), (5) who are appropriate roommates for people receiving care, and (6) how to care for and transport infected individuals and materials. These are decisions that can and should be made by all care givers, including nurses and students.

Gloves. When you wear gloves, you reduce the possibility that you will transmit infectious agents to those for whom you care and also reduce the chance that you will become infected yourself as a result of contact with body substances. For example, herpetic whitlow (an infection of the fingernail bed caused by the herpes simplex virus) will not develop on gloved hands through contact with infected oral secretions from a person with a cold sore or colonized secretions. Gloves even help reduce the risk of infection with hepatitis B or C and HIV from a puncture with a used needle. Gloves clean blood off the outside of the needle and make the dose of blood that enters from the puncture less than if gloves are not worn. Additionally, gloved hands will not become so heavily soiled that hand washing fails to remove the microbes.

To reduce risk for the people for whom you care, put on a fresh pair of clean gloves just before you touch mucous membranes and nonintact skin. Use sterile gloves for sterile procedures. To reduce risk for yourself, wear appropriate gloves whenever you are likely to have contact with body substances. Keeping a box of clean gloves at each bedside will encourage their use; if you are working in a place where gloves are inconvenient to obtain, keep spare clean gloves in your pocket.

There is no specific procedure for donning clean gloves, except to be sure that your hands are clean before putting them on. The gloves should cover your hands and wrists as well as covering the cuffs of your gown sleeves if a gown is worn. To remove the gloves after use, it is a good idea to always consider the gloves contaminated and follow the guidelines for removing a contaminated gown and gloves (see p. 534). Wash your hands after glove removal.

Hand Washing. *Everyone* should wash their hands (1) before performing invasive procedures or touching wounds or other susceptible body sites, even if gloves are worn, and (2) after it is likely that contact with body substances occurred. Good personal hygiene also suggests that you wash your hands after using the toilet, before eating, and between contacts with clients. It is always best to keep your hands away from your face, especially your eyes, nose, and mouth. See Procedure 28–1 for specific hand-washing techniques.

When washing you hands, 10 seconds of suds and friction are sufficient. Count the time out for yourself until you get used to the proper amount; many people do not wash for a long enough time. Plain soap and water are acceptable because hand washing is basically a mechanical activity, but antimicrobial soaps have a residual effect that can be beneficial, particularly if the hands have become extensively soiled. If you are working where hand washing is not possible, waterless hand cleaners containing antiseptics are effective when the skin is not visibly dirty; soilage usually is composed of protein materials such as saliva, mucous, or blood that may inactivate the germicide. When hands are extensively soiled, you need to wash your hands.

Gowns. Gowns are put on over the caregiver's clothing when soilage of the clothing is likely. Single-use gown technique (using a gown only once before it is discarded or laundered) is the usual practice in hospitals. After the gowns are worn, they are discarded (if paper) or placed in a laundry hamper, and the caregivers wash their hands before leaving the individual's room.

In the recent past, the same gown was reused by various people many times. There were specific procedures associated with donning and removing gowns. For example, neck strings and the inside of the gown were treated as "clean," and waist straps and the outside of the gown were treated as "dirty." Extreme care was used not to contaminate clean areas with dirty hands. The gowned care givers washed their hands after untying the waist and before touching the neck ties. These procedures are not necessary with single-use gowns. Multiple-use gowns should be avoided.

To don a clean gown,

▶ Put on the gown with the gown opening in the back
▶ Tie the ties at neck level
▶ Cover your uniform with the gown by overlapping completely in the back
▶ Tie the ties at the waist level
▶ Don gloves after gowning if gloves are needed

To remove a soiled gown, see the guidelines for removing a contaminated gown and gloves (see p. 534).

Masks and Protective Eye Wear. Wearing masks and protective eye wear (glasses, goggles, or masks with eye shields) may be indicated in circumstances in which body substances may splatter someone's eyes, nose, or mouth. You cannot assume, however, that a mask will interrupt transmission. Wearing a surgical mask does not effectively protect the respiratory tract of a susceptible care giver working with an individual who has an infection spread by the airborne route (e.g., chickenpox or tuberculosis). Thus, it is better if susceptible care givers are not assigned to care for such individuals.

Care givers or significant others who are immune to the specific disease in question (e.g., have had chickenpox, are tuberculin positive, or have been immunized for measles, mumps, and rubella) can safely provide

PROCEDURE 28–1

Hand Washing

Definition/Purpose. The combined use of chemical and mechanical forces removes transient microorganisms from the skin of the hands. Chemical forces include antimicrobial soap solutions and bar, leaflet, powder, or liquid soaps. Mechanical forces include friction during the washing and flushing away during the rinsing. Hand washing helps control infectious disease by decreasing the possibility of cross-contamination.

Hand washing is the single most effective means of promoting good medical asepsis.

Contraindications/Cautions. Health care workers must wash their hands so frequently that the skin can break down. It is important to wash the hands for a sufficient time to remove microbes but not to prolong the procedure unnecessarily. Likewise, cleaning under the fingernails with sharp instruments such as nail files or plastic fingernail cleaners can damage delicate tissues. Use such instruments only when visible soil has accumulated and cannot be otherwise removed. Keep fingernails short to reduce the area where microbes may harbor and thus reduce the total number of microbes on the hands.

Report to your supervisor any lesions on your hands, such as broken skin, a rash, or one or more vesicles. Such lesions are capable of harboring microbes, are potential portals of entry for pathogens, and may be made worse by hand washing.

Learning/Teaching Guidelines. Clients may be frightened of acquiring an infectious disease from health care workers. Telling them that you are going to wash your hands or, if facilities allow, actually washing your hands in their presence can be reassuring to them. Teaching them how to wash their own hands effectively may be an important part of teaching them certain types of self-care. Role modeling is a good beginning. However, clients are not the only ones who need information. When it comes to hand washing, every nurse must be a good role model for other health care workers and must teach by example.

Preliminary Activities. Long sleeves are inconvenient in the clinical area. The distal portion of the sleeves can easily be soiled during work and can get wet during hand washing. It is easier not to wear long sleeves at all, but, if worn, the sleeves must be rolled up or pushed up before each hand washing. Likewise, your wristwatch should either be worn 2.5 to 5 cm (1 to 2 in.) above the wrist at all times, or it will have to be moved up on the arm before each hand washing.

ASSESSMENT/PLANNING

Plan to wash your hands at least

► at the beginning of the work day
► before giving any nursing care
► after giving any nursing care

Also plan to wash your hands during the process of providing nursing care to an individual whenever there is a chance of transmitting pathogenic microorganisms from a potentially contaminated area to a cleaner area; for example,

► before assisting the client with eating
► before contact with mucous membranes or nonintact skin (e.g., before any invasive procedure or contact with a wound)
► after soilage of the hands with most body substances was likely to have occurred (e.g., after contact with any blood or body fluid such as might occur when assisting with client toileting, wound care, or invasive procedures, even if gloves were worn)

When not caring for clients, plan to wash your hands whenever necessary according to your own activities; for example,

► before eating
► after contaminating your hands by touching your hair, wiping your nose, or using the toilet

EQUIPMENT

► soap (liquid, leaflet, powder, or bar) or antimicrobial soap solution
► running water
► paper towels
► nail cleaner, if necessary

PROCEDURE

Actions

1. Standing well back from the sink, turn on the water and adjust the flow to a comfortable temperature: 105 °F to 110 °F (40.5 °C to 43.3 °C).

Rationale/Discussion

1. Standing close to running water exposes the uniform to splashing. Having to adjust water temperature that is too hot or too cold later (before rinsing) may require touching faucets that are considered contaminated with hands that have just been cleaned.

Procedure continued on following page

PROCEDURE 28–1 Continued

Hand Washing

Actions	Rationale/Discussion
2. Wet hands well with water before soaping them with liquid soap, a soap leaflet, powdered soap, bar soap, or an antimicrobial soap solution. If a bar soap is used, rinse it to flush away surface dirt before lathering with it and again before replacing it in the soap dish.	2. The addition of water to soap promotes the formation of suds that help to emulsify body secretions, oils, or greases that may be present on the hands and that tend to protect microbes. With some antimicrobial soaps, the addition of water reduces skin irritation. Although soap can serve as a medium for the growth of bacteria, there is no evidence that rinsing the bar is effective in reducing bacterial growth. Rather, the rinsed bar is more esthetically pleasing.
3. If it is the first hand wash of the day or if hands are grossly soiled, clean under fingernails with file or plastic fingernail cleaner, as necessary. Otherwise, clean under each fingernail with a fingernail from the opposite hand.	3. Fingernails can harbor microbes. Cleaning helps remove subungual microbes and thus decreases microbe proliferation. Sharp instruments can damage delicate subungual tissues and should be used with care and only when necessary.
4. Rub palms and fingers together using friction. Pay particular attention to places where microbes can hide (e.g., under and around fingernails and in the knuckle creases). Also give attention to the thumbs and to the lateral aspects of the hand and fifth fingers. If a ring is worn, move it enough to clean the finger under it and wash the ring with friction as well as the fingers.	4. Friction helps to loosen microbes so they can be removed. These areas are often overlooked during hand washing.
5. Continue washing for at least 10 seconds.	5. Ten seconds is the minimum acceptable time established for hand washing, but more time may be taken if required.
6. With fingernails lower than wrists, rinse hands well under running water.	6. Rinse water will flush loosened microbes away from the cleanest part of the hands (the wrists) toward the least clean part (the fingernails). Thorough rinsing removes residual soap solution that can dry the skin of the hands.
7. Thoroughly dry hands with paper towel.	7. Paper towels are disposable and are used only once, so they do not contribute to cross-contamination. Hands that are not thoroughly dried are prone to maceration.
8. Unless foot or knee controls are being used, use paper towel to turn off water faucet.	8. The towel serves as a barrier between clean fingers and contaminated faucet handles.
9. Carefully discard paper towel.	9. Touching the waste container contaminates clean fingers. Having to pick up a paper towel from the floor can contaminate clean hands and is a waste of time and energy.

FINAL ACTIVITIES

Use extra paper toweling as a barrier to protect your clean hands as you wipe up splashed water and suds as necessary to keep the work area clean and dry.

---

care for persons with that particular disease without wearing masks. Likewise, when care givers are ill with respiratory diseases, it cannot be assumed that wearing a mask will protect susceptible persons from being infected.

Although masks vary in their filtration effectiveness, single-use disposable masks are of sufficient quality to rarely require changing during a care interval. Discard masks in the trash when the episode of care is completed or if they become wet or soiled. Masks should cover both the nose and the mouth (see p. 533 for guidelines regarding donning and removing a mask).

Isolation Carts. Some hospitals use isolation carts to store gowns, masks, linen, trash bags, and other supplies for use with people requiring isolation precautions. Such carts can simplify the process of obtaining supplies provided they are kept well stocked!

Roommate Selection. Private rooms are used for many reasons and are preferred by most people admitted to health care facilities. However, most facilities do not have as many private rooms as are needed, and guidelines are usually developed for their assignment. Individuals who have infections transmitted by the airborne route require a private room. Additionally, a private room may be indicated for an individual who soils the environment with body substances (e.g., feces).

Occasionally, a private room with special ventilation is recommended for people with certain infections (e.g., active tuberculosis). However, many care facilities without such rooms still provide care for these individuals.

When it is unavoidable that an infected person share a room, it is especially important for both people to practice good personal hygiene. Individuals with the same infectious disease and sometimes people infected with the same microorganisms may share a room.

For many years, it was believed that providing a private room for neutropenic individuals was helpful. Many physicians still prefer to use this option, although its effectiveness has not been proved.[26] It is probably just as easy to transmit potentially infectious agents on the hands of personnel between people occupying adjacent rooms as it is between people in the same room. The key to interrupting such transmission is hand washing between contacts with body substances from all people.

Soiled Care Equipment and Supplies. Various personnel in care facilities handle soiled equipment and supplies. It is common practice to put soiled items in a plastic bag and tie it closed before either putting them in a trash receptacle or sending reusable items for

APPLYING RESEARCH TO NURSING PRACTICE

Double Bagging Is a Procedure of the Past

Weinstein, S. A., Gantz, N. M., Pelletier, C., & Hibert, D. (1989). Bacterial surface contamination of patients' linen: isolation precautions versus standard care. *American Journal of Infection Control,* 17(5), 264–267.

▼▼▼

Weinstein and colleagues examined the usefulness of an age-old nursing procedure: double bagging the soiled linens of clients under isolation precautions. In this procedure, one nurse, located in the isolation room, placed soiled linen into a special type of linen bag that was soluble in hot water. The nurse then dropped it into a second polyethylene bag held by a "clean" nurse standing outside the isolation room. Weinstein and colleagues removed and cultured soiled linens from 50 of these water-soluble bags used in isolation cases and from 50 polyethylene bags used in nonisolation cases. When comparing the bacteria cultured from the linens of bags used in isolation and from the linens not used in isolation, the researchers found no significant differences.

Applications for Practice

This study and others have cast considerable doubt on the need for double bagging. Eliminating the practice of double bagging saves nursing time, cuts costs, and reduces the use of nonrenewable resources.

reprocessing. Bagging is done to prevent people from inadvertently soiling their hands.

"Double bagging" is the term used to describe the practice of removing trash or used linens from an isolation room by having a "clean" nurse hold open a "clean" bag to accept a "contaminated" bag full of linen or trash that is touched only by a gowned and gloved nurse who is considered "contaminated." Double bagging is no longer recommended (see Applying Research to Nursing Practice: Double Bagging Is a Procedure of the Past).

Many pieces of equipment are supplied for single use only. These are disposed of after one use. Some items are reusable, however. Individual care facilities have specific policies and procedures for the care and handling of reusable equipment that include cleaning, disinfection, or sterilization before reuse. Familiarize yourself with the policies operating in the areas in which you work.

Disposal of "Sharps." Used "sharps" such as scalpels, broken glass, lancets, and needles are discarded into a puncture-resistant container. Do not break needles purposely or recap them using a two-handed recapping technique before disposal. (Since 1975 the CDC has recommended not to recap or cut needles after use because of the risk of puncture wounds or aerosols created by breaking the needle.) Many states have regulations about the disposal of hospital waste including needles and syringes. Acquaint yourself with appropriate regulations.

Dishes. No specific precautions are necessary for dishes, silverware, or trays unless they are visibly contaminated with infective matter. Some facilities use disposable dishes and utensils for people requiring isolation precautions even though the CDC does not recommend this practice. There is no evidence that the use of disposable dishes reduces the transmission of infection. Unfortunately, it usually results in cold, unattractively served food.

Trash. Bag all wound dressings, paper tissues, and other disposable items soiled with body substances. Dispose of the bag according to facility policy. Local regulations vary and may require special handling for hospital waste. Autoclaving or incineration is commonly required.

Thermometers. Used nondisposable thermometers should receive high-level disinfection between clients (e.g., soaking in glutaraldehyde at least 10 minutes).

Linen. Handle soiled linen as little as possible. Do not flap or shake it in the air. Place linen soiled with body substances in a laundry bag in the person's room. Tie the bag closed; then send it to the laundry according to facility policy. Some care facilities use water-soluble bags to contain contaminated linen. Using these bags means the soiled linen does not have to be touched again after placing it in the bag. The bags dissolve in the hot washing water. They can also begin to dissolve if kept in contact with damp linens for a sufficient time and so should not be used unless the soiled linens are dry.

Laboratory Specimens. Place specimens of human tissues or body substances in containers with secure lids to prevent leaking. The outside of the container should be kept clean. Procedures for transporting laboratory specimens and for handling the container and the specimen should prevent personnel from having bare-hand contact with the potentially infective material.

Transporting People with Infections. Individuals with chickenpox and other infections that may be transmitted by the airborne route should not be transported outside their rooms unless absolutely necessary. Check to see how your facility prefers to transport clients with communicable diseases. People with less transmissible infections may be moved provided precautions are taken to prevent soilage of the environment (e.g., securely cover any draining wounds). Notify personnel at the "receiving" place of any infection risk so that necessary precautions can be maintained.

Routine Cleaning. The same thorough daily cleaning procedures should be used for all rooms in a health care facility. Microorganisms may be present on walls, floors, and tabletops in the rooms occupied by people with or without infections. However, these surfaces are rarely associated with the transmission of infectious agents. Promptly clean surfaces whenever they are visibly soiled. Many health care facilities have specific policies and procedures about cleaning.

Postmortem Handling of Bodies. When handling a person's body after death, use the same precautions to protect yourself that you would use if the person were still alive. Notify morgue personnel as necessary about infections so that appropriate precautions can be maintained when the body is taken to the morgue. Local regulations may call for additional special procedures.

Infection Precautions to Protect Personnel

Epidemiology of Infections in Health Care Workers. As you carry out your nursing interventions, you should always remember your risk for infection. Health care workers are at greater risk for certain infectious diseases than people who do not work in health care settings. This is called "occupationally associated risk." Although health care workers have occupational risk for viral respiratory diseases, particularly when they work with sick children (and also for some bacterial infections), a major concern is the type of disease transmitted by blood and body fluids: viral hepatitis B, hepatitis C, and HIV infection.

Health care workers were first recognized to have occupational risk for the blood-borne viral diseases as a result of hepatitis B outbreaks among staff who worked in kidney dialysis centers. Large numbers of them became ill, and chronic liver failure or hepatic

carcinoma developed in some. By the late 1970s, studies confirmed that most risk was associated with blood exposure and that some occupations such as dentist, surgeon, emergency room nurse, and critical care nurse had very high risk.[10] The CDC estimates that approximately 12,000 health care workers develop occupationally associated hepatitis B annually and that perhaps as many as 200 die each year as a result of acute or chronic infection.[9]

Less is known about health care worker infection with hepatitis C (formerly called parenterally associated non-A, non-B hepatitis) because a test to identify this infectious agent was developed only in 1989. We do know, however, that this disease progresses to chronic infection even more frequently than is true of hepatitis B, and is as easy to transmit. In other words, hepatitis C may be as easily transmitted by a very small amount of infected blood as hepatitis B and may be even more likely to result in complications.[1]

HIV infection is transmitted by blood and body substances, as is viral hepatitis. The infection always progresses to chronic disease, but it is not as easily transmitted. When a susceptible health care worker receives a needle stick with a needle used for a person infected with hepatitis B or C, the needle stick will result in infection about 20% of the time (one time out of five). In contrast, about 1 in 250 sticks from a needle used on an HIV-infected person will result in HIV infection. As of early 1991, fewer than 100 U.S. health care workers were believed to have occupationally associated HIV infection. Several clients acquired HIV infection from a dental office, either from inadequate disinfection and sterilization of instruments or from the infected dentist.

Several factors influence the likelihood that infection will result: the amount of blood transmitted, the number of infectious particles available from the infected person, whether the exposure was superficial, such as a spatter of bloody fluid to the face, or deep, such as a deep needle stick in which some blood was actually injected.

Risk for health care workers is a major concern to the nation and also to the health care workers who are directly affected by the risk.

Reducing Risk for Blood-borne Diseases in Health Care Workers. Three important tools for reducing risk already exist: the hepatitis B vaccine, barrier precautions for blood exposure, and "sharps safety." You are already familiar with the concept of using barrier precautions when exposure to blood or body substances is likely; it is essential for safety to use the precautions for everyone, not only for those with diagnosed infections.

An excellent vaccine is available for hepatitis B, and all health care workers who are likely to have blood exposure should receive it. The Occupational Safety and Health Administration requires health care facilities to offer the vaccine at no charge to employees.

Be sure you complete your hepatitis B vaccine series (all three injections) before you begin practice in a health care facility. The vaccine will also protect you from nonoccupational exposures such as sexually transmitted hepatitis B. Unfortunately, there is still no vaccine to prevent hepatitis C or HIV infection. You must rely on assessing your own risk in every situation and then on barrier precautions and sharps safety for your protection.

Sharps safety is a term used to describe safe handling practices for the many sharp tools used in health care: lancets, needles, scalpels, and other sharp devices. The kinds of sharps that cause most injuries are needles, especially those used for intravascular access. Two-handed recapping of used needles is a major cause of punctures and should be avoided.

Syringes are available with a variety of safety devices such as needle shields (see Chapter 46) or retractable needles. Health care agencies should supply sharps containers as needed so there should be little reason to recap a used needle. However, if you must for some reason recap a needle, use a device to hold the cap or place the cap on a flat surface and then use one hand to insert the needle until the cap safely covers the needle and you can secure it. Do not have your other hand anywhere near the cap as you are inserting the needle into it.

Never recap a needle by holding the cap in one hand and inserting the needle with the other hand.

Avoid handing sharp tools to other people unless you are sure they are paying attention; sometimes it is safer for one health care worker to place a used sharp on a flat surface or in a basin rather than handing it directly to another person. Accidents are most likely to happen when personnel are rushed and inattentive to the situation or when the task is difficult, such as giving an injection to an uncooperative person or a child. Obtain help from others when necessary, and be sure you are supervised by an experienced person the first few times you perform a task that might result in injury to you or to others.

Amazingly enough, hundreds of housekeepers in hospitals are injured every year with sharps that were placed in the trash instead of in sharps containers. Also, health care workers are sometimes injured when they clean up procedure trays that were used by others who left sharps out of sight on the tray. This situation frequently injures nurses.[19] In both cases, one person places another at risk. Always avoid being the person who places others at risk, and be aware of the possibility that others might not be as careful as you are.

According to the CDC, the use of body substance isolation, universal precautions, and the hepatitis B vaccine, together with sharps safety, have brought about a significant decline in hepatitis B in health care workers since about 1985.[2] The decline is still continuing.

Reducing Risk for Airborne Communicable Diseases in Health Care Workers.
Since 1985, nosocomial transmission of measles and tuberculosis has occurred. Measles epidemics in a number of hospitals and communities have spurred increased immunization; a second dose of vaccine is indicated for all health care workers.

HIV infection and poverty, including homelessness, are associated with greatly increased risk for tuberculosis. More persons are being admitted to hospitals with tuberculosis now than at any time in the past 15 years. In some cases, the tuberculosis organism has been resistant to common drug therapy and is very difficult to treat. New types of face masks, called "personal respirators," have been developed to filter the inhaled air of the person who wears the mask; these are recommended when caring for those who have infectious tuberculosis.

Conventional surgical masks are intended only to filter the exhaled air of the person who wears one and are not effective for protecting the wearer from airborne communicable diseases.

In addition to using personal respirators, the CDC recommends that health care workers have tuberculin skin tests after unprotected exposures; in facilities in which many persons with HIV infection and tuberculosis are cared for, annual tuberculins are recommended.[8] Individuals who become infected (become tuberculin positive) are usually treated with medication to prevent them from developing tuberculosis.

Many schools with students in the health sciences offer counseling about risk for blood-borne pathogens and the airborne communicable diseases. Many also offer postexposure management. Additionally, many hospitals and sometimes other health care facilities offer these same services to personnel, including students. It is a good idea for students and their faculty to discuss the services that are available for pre- and postexposure management.

Psychosocial Aspects of Infection Control. In addition to using interventions to prevent the spread of infection, the nurse must attend to the psychosocial aspects of infection control. Perhaps the most difficult psychosocial aspect of infection control occurs when a person is required to be confined to a private room for a long period. Imposing such limitations is seldom necessary, but when such precautions are necessary, they are difficult to cope with for the person and significant others.

Isolation precautions, including a private room with the door shut and everyone entering the room wearing masks and gowns, are sometimes prescribed for people receiving bone marrow or organ transplants. This **reverse (protective) isolation** is a set of procedures intended to control a client's environment so that it is similar to an operating room. There is some question as to whether this measure is necessary even for those receiving transplants.

When it is necessary for a person to be confined to a private room (e.g., because of chickenpox), the limitations often involve children. The psychosocial impact may be significant. Confined individuals (children or adults) experience reduced stimulation and attention and describe feeling lonely and bored (see Chapter 51). In these circumstances, any of us, particularly children, might become irritable, angry, or depressed.

Always assess an "isolated" individual carefully, and be certain that the isolation precautions are indeed necessary. If the confinement produces a great deal of discomfort, alternatives other than a care facility may be considered. Early discharge from the facility may be possible, and the person may be cared for at home with the help of significant others and visiting nurses. If confinement in a health care facility is the only choice, the physical environment and everyone who goes into the room should be very supportive.

Traditionally, isolation rooms have been barren. Personal belongings were not permitted in the room because the assumption was that these articles would have to be destroyed or sterilized to prevent cross-contamination. We now know that this assumption is almost never true. Confined people greatly appreciate having their personal articles nearby and being able to arrange their own belongings. Confined people, particularly, appreciate having pictures, photographs, and other mementos in the room. Children enjoy favorite toys or blankets and can have such objects with them. Such objects do not have to be destroyed. Newspapers and magazines provide information and contact with the outside world, and confined people can have access to such items. Clocks, television, and calendars help in time orientation. Telephone calls, mail, and recorded messages from significant others may also help considerably.

For many confined people, the decrease in the quality and number of human contacts is the greatest deprivation experienced. People who are normally surrounded by others may be alone for the first time in their lives. The care of persons in isolation may require donning protective clothing such as gloves, gowns, and masks. To save time, care providers tend to "save up" several tasks and do them all at once when they do go into the room. It is important, however, to spend enough time with the person to meet psychosocial as well as physical needs. People who go into the room can introduce themselves and greet the person from the doorway before putting on a mask and gown. While in the room, be particularly sensitive to the person's feelings. Isolated people often feel personally rejected and forgotten because of the restrictions imposed on them. Children often need to be held and cuddled, and adults appreciate a friendly touch.

In most health care facilities, most people with infections are not in private rooms but may have a label or sign over their bed describing the precautions necessary in their care. A sign that says "isolation" may make a person feel dirty or uncomfortable. It is important to explain to the person and significant others why the sign is there. Some infectious diseases (e.g., hepatitis B, syphilis) rarely require care in a private room, but for some, such diseases do have a negative social stigma. Infected people may wonder what others think of them. Roommates and even friends and family members who learn of the diagnosis may become fearful and may shun such a person. Nurses can provide support, information, and reassurance to everyone in the room when such situations occur. Helpful nursing intervention is focused on acknowledging feelings, providing accurate information, and doing everything possible to affirm an individual's dignity and sense of worth.

For some people a sense of "dirtiness" or "uncleanness" is associated with having an infection. Care givers may either reinforce or reduce these impressions by what they say or do around people with infections. For example, if you had a ruptured appendix and were in the operating room, how would you feel if you overheard someone call you a "dirty case"?

People experience considerable confusion and anxiety if an infection precautions sign is put on the door or bed without adequate explanation. Likewise, if some care givers wear gloves, gowns, and masks when caring for an individual and others do not, a person's anxiety increases. The person may worry and wonder, "What can this possibly mean?"

Information that people need to know to understand their own infections and to reduce the risk of transmission is fairly simple. It can be presented clearly and logically. Allow the learners to bring up questions and concerns and discuss them carefully. After a teaching session, be sure to evaluate what has been understood (see Chapter 26). It is essential that a sick person understand that a care giver experiences more risk from handling body substances than from merely entering the room. A person who understands this distinction will understand that gloves and gowns may be used for direct-care activities but that people may come into the room to visit without them.

People who live together are often exposed to the same infectious diseases at the same time. It is not practical or necessary to try to carry out isolation precautions in the home. Basic hygiene measures, including hand washing (especially after toileting and before preparing food), are usually all that are practical.

When teaching people about their infections, use language they can understand. Include the following information:

▶ All people have infectious agents ("germs") in their body substances. There are always microorganisms in feces, sputum, and wound drainage and sometimes in urine and blood as well.

▶ The infectious agents in these substances may be transmitted to others. They may also be transported from one site to another on the same person's body. For example, drainage from a wound infection can be introduced into the conjunctiva of the eye if a person touches wound drainage and then the eye.

▶ The risk of infection is greatly reduced by careful hand washing after contact with a contaminated substance and by washing linen and household utensils after use.

▶ Care givers should wear gloves if contact with body substances is anticipated. They should wear a cover gown if their clothing is likely to be soiled. This measure may occasionally be necessary in a home situation.

▶ Infectious agents of a few communicable diseases are also transmitted by the airborne route.

▶ In health care facilities, people with communicable diseases will be placed in private rooms or with a roommate who either has the same disease or is immune to it. The door to the room may be closed.

These communicable diseases include measles, mumps, rubella, chickenpox, whooping cough, and tuberculosis. People who have communicable diseases in the community should avoid public contact until the period of infectivity is over. Isolation within the home is usually neither necessary nor effective.

Remember that providing care to anyone requires sensitivity and caring. It also requires knowledge and understanding of each person's condition. Professional nurses learn about health promotion and disease prevention. These same principles can be applied to persons at risk of infection as well as those in whom infection is already present.

SURGICAL ASEPSIS: BASIC CONCEPTS

Like medical asepsis, surgical asepsis (sterile technique) is used to prevent infection. Sterile technique, however, is used only in those special circumstances when it is necessary to prevent exposing the client to *all* living microorganisms. The goal of surgical asepsis is to prevent contamination.

It is important to understand that, when we talk about sterile technique and maintaining sterile conditions, *there are no gradations.* One object is not more or less sterile than another. Either an object is sterile, or it is not. The presence of even one living microorganism or spore render an object **contaminated,** or unsterile.

When Sterile Technique Is Used. Sterile technique is used during certain procedures in which the skin or mucous membranes are broken, resulting in hemo-access (access to blood vessels). In addition, sterile technique is always used when performing a procedure in or on any sterile body part (e.g., the urinary bladder) or cavity (e.g., the peritoneal cavity). Specific procedures requiring surgical asepsis include

▶ all surgical procedures to prevent the introduction of microorganisms into the vascular system
▶ bladder catheterization to prevent the introduction of organisms into the sterile bladder
▶ administration of injections or intravenous fluids to prevent the introduction of organisms into the subcutaneous tissues, muscles, or blood vessels
▶ dressing changes to prevent the introduction of organisms into the wound and vascular system
▶ care of people with burns to prevent infection when the skin is damaged
▶ eye treatments (although eyes are not sterile, this delicate tissue warrants the use of surgical aseptic technique) to prevent eye infection

When Sterile Technique Is Not Necessary. Nonsurgical procedures involving the mouth, ears, GI tract, vagina, and rectum generally do not require sterile technique. Such nonsurgical procedures include temperature measurement, administration of eardrops, gastric tube feedings, insertion of vaginal suppositories, and administration of enemas. Although sterile technique is not necessary, these procedures do require medical asepsis. Sometimes, equipment used for these procedures is initially sterile. If equipment is used for more than one client, it must be sterilized between clients.

Nursing Responsibilities in the Practice of Surgical Asepsis. Nurses have many responsibilities in infection control. For example, nurses

▶ practice sterile technique in the operating room (OR) and during other invasive procedures
▶ ensure that other health team members practice sterile technique. In the operating room, for example, the circulating nurse helps to make certain that all members of the scrub team, including nurses, surgeons, and surgical assistants, do not break aseptic technique. If aseptic technique is accidently broken, this nurse helps to reestablish sterility.

Make it a rule never to continue a sterile procedure with gloves, instruments, or objects (e.g., a tray or drapes) that you suspect may be contaminated. Instead, stop immediately and obtain new equipment to replace what has been contaminated.

▶ teach people and significant others how to use sterile technique at home (e.g., to change dressings or administer parenteral medications)
▶ act as infection-control practitioners to train personnel and maintain medical and surgical asepsis throughout a health care facility

Preparing Materials for Sterilization. The first step in the sterilization process is to prepare used instruments and other equipment by decontaminating them. This practice removes organic material (e.g., blood, saliva, feces) and begins the process of destroying microorganisms that are present. Decontamination does not, however, destroy all microorganisms. Therefore, sterilization must follow decontamination.

Removing heavy debris from used equipment is analogous to rinsing heavily soiled dishes before placing them in the dishwasher. Unrinsed dishes often remain dirty. Similarly, microbes can remain in debris that is not cleaned off used equipment. This debris can harbor the microbes and prevent their destruction during attempts at sterilization.

A sterilant cannot penetrate dirt, dried secretions, clotted blood, or any other substance that may coat the instrument or equipment.

Specific recommendations for decontamination procedures can be found in each agency's infection control manual. In general, however, the following guidelines prevail:

▶ All instruments used on moist body surfaces are considered contaminated and must be decontaminated before sterilization.
▶ Before decontamination, instruments that are heavily soiled with bone, dried blood, or other body tissues should be presoaked.

▶ Decontamination may be done by a washer-sterilizer, or cleaning may be completed by manual washing. The washer-sterilizer mechanically agitates water and detergent to wash the instruments and then submits them to conditions that render exposed surfaces sterile. Because only exposed surfaces are sterile, instruments that are decontaminated in a washer-sterilizer are not considered sterile. An object is not sterile unless it is free of all living microorganisms and spores. Manual washing is done by personnel in special clothing that covers the entire body, that is fluid resistant, and that includes facial protection.

▶ After initial decontamination, all instruments (unless the procedure is contraindicated by their delicate nature or by their plating) should be placed in an ultrasonic cleaner to remove any remaining organic material from unexposed surfaces (e.g., crevices, serrations, and box locks). An ultrasonic cleaner passes ultrasonic waves through a fluid to generate submicroscopic bubbles that collapse and pull tenacious dirt from the instruments by a suction-type action.

▶ After ultrasonic cleaning, instruments should be prepared for sterilization.

Methods of Sterilization. Sterilants are divided into two general classes: physical agents (e.g., dry heat, pressurized steam) and chemical agents (e.g., ethylene oxide, glutaraldehyde). Cold sterilization is another term for chemical sterilization. The type of sterilization used depends on expense, type of equipment to be sterilized, time necessary for sterilization, and organisms that may be present on equipment. Pressurized steam (autoclave) and gas (ethylene oxide) (Fig. 28-6) are the most frequently used methods of sterilization. Table 28-3 summarizes important facts about each major type of sterilant.

Note in Table 28-3 that the method of sterilization used is determined by the type of material to be sterilized. For example, although moist heat sterilizes materials more rapidly than does dry heat, it damages some materials. In these cases, dry heat or chemical sterilization is necessary.

Time is also an important variable. All sterilization procedures require that materials be exposed to the physical agent or chemical for specific periods. Length of exposure depends on such factors as (1) type of sterilant (e.g., pressurized steam achieves higher temperatures than does dry heat, thus decreasing sterilization time), (2) type of equipment, (3) type of wrapping if any, (4) amount and type of organisms present on the item, and (5) concentration, temperature, and pH of chemical sterilant.

Sterilization Indicators. Sterilization indicators are devices placed on wrappers and inside packages to indicate whether the object inside has been exposed to the sterilization process. Most indicators monitor only one part of the sterilization process. For example, some indicators are sensitive to pressure, whereas others detect exposure to proper temperatures.

Most indicators do not ensure sterility. Rather, they simply indicate that the object has been exposed to a sterilization process.

Despite these limitations, remember to check sterile packages for indicators to ensure exposure to sterilization. Many commercially prepared items do not contain indicators. Instead, they are clearly marked "sterile" on the package.

Major types of indicators are (1) glass pellet indicators, (2) chemical indicators, (3) and biologic or spore strip indicators. A glass pellet indicator is a small glass tube containing a temperature-sensitive pellet that melts and changes color when exposed to certain temperatures for specific periods. Chemical indicators are made of paper that is impregnated with a chemical dye. The dye changes color when exposure to the sterilization

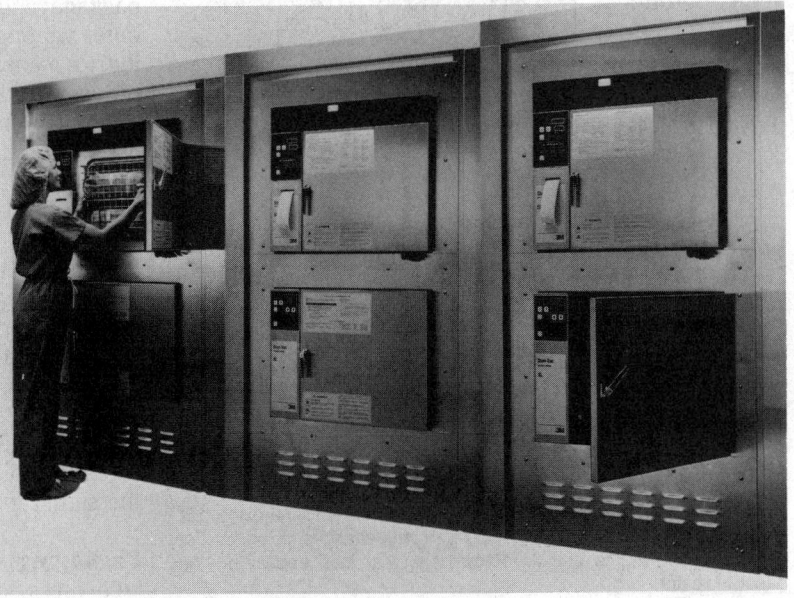

▲ *Figure 28-6*

Steri-Vac brand ethylene oxide gas sterilizers. (Courtesy of 3M, St. Paul, Minnesota.)

TABLE 28-3. Types of Sterilization

Type	Exposure Time	Advantages	Disadvantages	Comments
Physical Agents				
Heat				
Pressurized steam	Approximately 15 minutes at 121 °C (250 °F)	Economical, effective, requires less time than other sterilization methods	Impractical for plastic, rubber, or objects that are sensitive to heat	Contains heat, pressure, and humidity to kill microorganisms
Dry heat	1 hour at 171 °C (340 °F), 8 hours at 121 °C (250 °F)	Use for metals that corrode when exposed to moisture; use for sharp instruments (e.g., needles, scalpels); also use for oils, powders, and glassware	Requires longer time and higher temperatures than pressurized steam	
Chemicals				
Gas				
Ethylene oxide	3–8 hours depending on concentrations of gas, temperature, type of wrap	Use for heat-sensitive objects, instruments with lenses, thermometers	Toxic: can cause skin burns, irritation; mutagenic	Wear gloves when working with this chemical; only use in well-ventilated areas; aerate articles thoroughly after sterilization
Liquid				
Glutaraldehyde	10 hours to kill spores; 10–30 minutes for use as disinfectant	Noncorrosive; useful for instruments with lenses; has low surface tension; permits good penetration and rinsing	Irritant—must rinse articles thoroughly after sterilization	Wear gloves; use only in well-ventilated areas

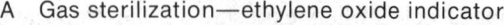

A   Gas sterilization—ethylene oxide indicator

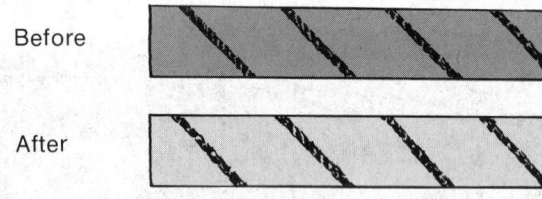

Before

After

B   Steam sterilization—autoclave indicator

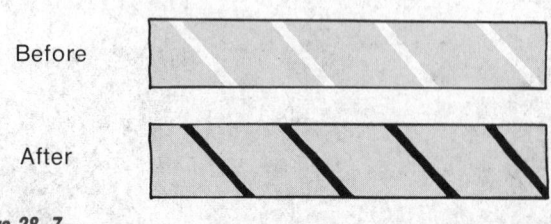

Before

After

▲ Figure 28-7

Chemical indicator tape. *A,* When all conditions for ethylene oxide gas sterilization are met, the paper tape indicator changes color. *B,* For items sterilized in the autoclave, dark diagonal lines appear on the paper indicator.

process occurs. Such paper indicators are placed inside packages in the form of a paper strip and outside the package in the form of a tape that adheres to the package and must be broken to open the package's outer wrapper (Fig. 28-7). They differ in color according to manufacturer and according to the sterilization process used (gas or steam under pressure).

Always check a sterile package for color changes on chemical indicators.

If you find a package in which the necessary color change has not taken place, do not use this item. Return it to the sterilizing area in your facility.

Spore strips differ from other indicators because they do ensure sterility. Specially prepared strips or ampules containing a known population of highly resistant bacteria are wrapped in the center of the package to be sterilized. After sterilization, they are removed and sent to a microbiology laboratory, which ascertains whether the sterilization process has killed all the bacteria.

Packaging and Storing Sterile Supplies. Once objects are sterilized, it is necessary to protect them from contamination. If properly wrapped and then stored in a clean, dry place where they are not handled excessively before use, sterile objects remain sterile for a period. However, the shelf life of some objects is shorter than others. Implantable devices, for example, may have a shelf life of a few weeks. On the other hand, properly stored sterile forceps may be used after several months.

Do not use any object for procedures requiring sterile equipment if the

▶ expiration date on the wrapper is past
▶ package or wrapper is torn, is wet, or has been opened
▶ sterilization indicator is not positive

Nursing Role in Disinfection and Sterilization. In many health care facilities, the nurse is not responsible for the sterilization of equipment. Central supply or central service personnel perform these functions. In certain settings, however, nursing personnel or technicians do sterilize equipment. These settings include some operating rooms, emergency departments, clinics, homes, and offices. In addition, the nurse may need to know and be able to perform emergency sterilization measures when equipment is needed quickly. For these reasons, become familiar with basic sterilization procedures and know under which circumstances each method is appropriate. In addition, learn about disinfection and cleaning methods because nurses often perform these procedures or supervise other health care workers in these tasks.

In the home, for instance, you may have to disinfect or sterilize materials or teach family members to do these tasks. You should understand that the most commonly used methods in the home are (1) soaking in chemical disinfectants, (2) boiling in water, and (3) using a pressure cooker. All of these methods require an initial cleaning to remove any visible soil.

Using a disinfectant requires soaking for a time indicated by the manufacturer of the chemical. Note that some disinfectants are effective only against vegetative forms of bacteria and are not effective against the spore forms. Some will kill spores but only if used for an extended period. Be sure to follow the manufacturer's directions.

Boiling in water for 10 to 20 minutes is a commonly used method to disinfect objects in the home. Depending on the microorganism involved, boiling will sterilize some items but not others.

Boiling will not kill spores.

Because the item's sterility can be questioned, this method is not considered to guarantee sterility. Altitude is an important factor when boiling supplies. At sea level, water boils at a higher temperature than it does at increased altitudes. Thus, when this method is used at higher elevations, the boiling time must be increased.

A pressure cooker improves on the basic boiling process because it operates on the same principle as an autoclave. The closed system and the higher pressure and temperature are more effective in killing microorganisms. When using a pressure cooker, place the items on a rack above the water.

Nursing Responsibilities in Maintaining Sterility

Establishing and Maintaining a Sterile Field. A sterile field is a work area in which sterility is continually maintained. A sterile field can be any size, depending on the procedure and equipment. In the operating room, the sterile field may be several large tables covered with sterile drapes. Sterile instruments are then placed on the field. At the bedside, the inside of one sterile package makes a small sterile field. You may use one or more of such small sterile fields, a larger sterile field to which you have added extra supplies, or combinations of larger and smaller sterile fields. Before attempting to establish and use a sterile field, you should be familiar with the principles listed in Table 28–4.

Usually, a sterile field is established at the client's bedside before performing a sterile procedure such as a bladder catheterization or sterile dressing change. You may be the only one to use the sterile field, or you may assist a physician who is completing a sterile procedure.

To establish a sterile field in a client's room, prepare the client for the procedure to follow. Complete necessary positioning and draping in advance as much as possible. These activities make airwaves that could contaminate your sterile field once it is opened, so they are better done in advance.

Rearrange any furniture as needed. You should plan to have your sterile field and equipment exactly where you will use it (e.g., you may want the sterile tray on the client's overbed table and sterile solutions on the bedside stand or on another table nearby). In deciding how the furniture should be arranged, keep the principles of sterile technique in mind. For example, plan so that you will not have to reach over a sterile field with a nonsterile hand, you will not have to turn your back on a sterile field, and you will not have to bring anything that is nonsterile too near a sterile field. (For example, do not place two sterile fields where you will have to walk between them.)

Once the furniture is arranged, be sure to clear enough table space to allow plenty of room to establish your sterile field. Remember that the field will enlarge as you open it. Prepare for this enlargement in advance. Be sure the work surface is clean and dry. A wet surface will contaminate your field by capillary action.

Gather your materials. Check all sterile packages for holes, tears, or stains. Note the expiration date on all sterile supplies, including bottles of sterile solutions you might use. Be sure the indicator tape has changed to the appropriate color. Place all supplies where they can be opened and used without violating principles of sterile technique.

If you will be donning sterile gloves and they are not a part of the sterile field you will be opening, wash

TABLE 28-4. Selected Scientific Principles and Related Nursing Interventions for Maintaining a Sterile Field

Principle	Nursing Interventions
Sterile objects that are out of the line of vision are considered questionable or their sterility cannot be guaranteed.	Always face the sterile field. Do not turn your back or side on a sterile field.
Waist level and table level are considered margins of safety that can be uniformly enforced and that promote maximum visibility of the sterile objects.	Keep sterile equipment above your waist level or above table level.
Microorganisms from the oral cavity are spread into the air when a person speaks or coughs and the organisms may drop onto the sterile field.	Do not speak, cough, sneeze, or laugh over a sterile field. If it is necessary to do any of these, turn your head away from the sterile field.
When a nonsterile object is held above a sterile object, gravity causes microorganisms to fall onto the sterile object.	Never reach across the sterile field. Instead (1) move yourself around the field (while continuing to face the field), (2) reach around the edges of the sterile field, or (3) cautiously turn the entire sterile field either by touching the edges of the bottom wrapper or by reaching underneath the bottom wrapper.
A sterile object becomes contaminated when touched by a nonsterile object.	Never touch a sterile field with any object that is not sterile.
A sterile field cannot be contaminated by a sterile object.	Sterile objects (or hands covered with sterile gloves) may safely touch or pass over a sterile field.
A general rule is that there is a 2.5-cm (1-in.) margin of safety around the outside edge of a sterile field. This 2.5-cm (1-in.) border is considered contaminated.	The unsterile hand may touch the edge of the sterile field if necessary to make a small adjustment.
Microorganisms are present in, and travel on, air currents.	Prevent excessive air currents around the sterile field (e.g., close the door before opening the sterile field, move slowly, minimize flapping of clothing and drapes).
Sterilization indicators are used to demonstrate whether an object has been exposed to the sterilization process.	Never assume that an object is sterile. Always check the sterilization indicators on or inside of wrappers of sterile objects.
Sterility expiration date indicates the last possible date on which the contents of the package can be assumed to be sterile.	Always check the sterility expiration date, which is clearly stated on the package.
Only intact wrappings protect sterile objects from contamination.	Always check to be sure the sterile package is intact. Look for holes, tears, watermarks, or other signs that might indicate contamination.
Any object is considered contaminated if its sterility is in question.	If the sterility of an object is in doubt, do not use it.
When a liquid connects a nonsterile surface to a sterile one, microorganisms may be transferred from the unsterile to the sterile area. Consequently, the sterile area becomes contaminated by capillary attraction.	Handle liquids cautiously near the sterile field to prevent drapes or wrappers from becoming wet. Do not allow splashing to occur.
Microorganisms do not pass easily through a dry surface; rather, they tend to move slowly along the surface.	Dry sterile objects (e.g., sterile towel) may have one surface that is contaminated and one surface that is sterile.
That which is sterile remains sterile unless contaminated, but one part of an instrument may be sterile and another part contaminated as long as there is no question about what is sterile and what is not.	A sterile object (e.g., a pair of scissors) may be picked up from a sterile field with a sterile instrument (e.g., a forceps) and touched with bare hands on parts of the object that can be contaminated (e.g., touched handles become contaminated). The tips, however, may still be considered sterile if they touch only that which is sterile (e.g., the tips may be placed within the sterile field's 2.5-cm [1-in.] border while the contaminated handles stay outside of the 2.5-cm [1-in.] border).
Fluid flows downward by gravity. Fluid that flows into a contaminated area becomes contaminated. Fluid that is contaminated can flow back into a sterile area and contaminate it.	When working with liquids on a sterile field by using forceps with contaminated handles, always be certain to keep the tips of the forceps pointed downward.

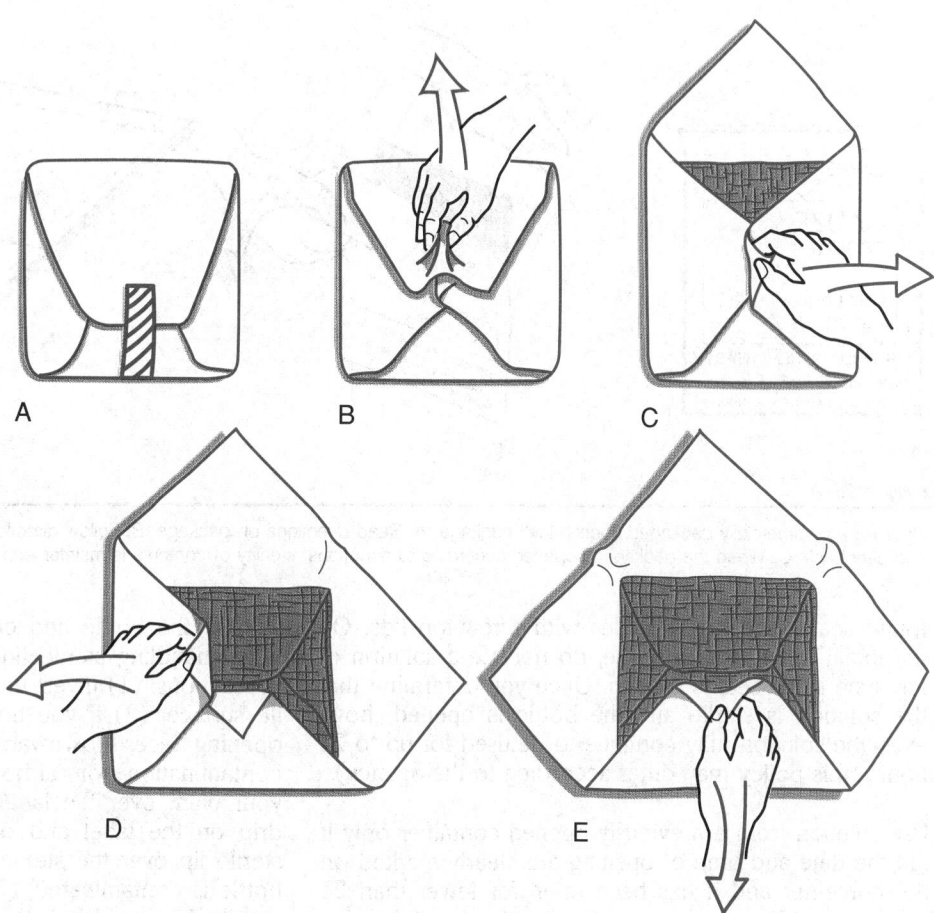

▲ **Figure 28–8**

Opening a sterile package (see text for technique).

your hands and then open your sterile field *before* you open your gloves. Open and prepare all supplies in advance so that once you have donned your gloves you will touch only the sterile insides of the packages with your gloved hands.

Handling Sterile Supplies. If you are to maintain sterility, you must be able to handle sterile supplies without contaminating them. Therefore, you must understand how supplies are packaged. For example, many agencies sterilize their own supplies, and you will find each package double wrapped in cloth or paper. To open a sterile package, remove the indicator tape and grasp the side of the wrapper that will open away from you and open it first. Note in Figure 28–8B that the nurse's hand approaches the package from behind. Thus, the wrapper can be pulled back away from the sterile package without the unsterile hand passing back over the field after opening the flap. At this time, you may note that you have misunderstood the packaging and that the flap opens toward you. If the flap opens the wrong way, leave it open and, by carefully touching only nonsterile parts of the package, turn the entire field around so that it opens away from you. Then continue as in Figure 28–8C, and open a flap to one side and then a flap to the other. If a triangular fold has been made available for you, grasp its corner (remember that a 2.5-cm, or 1-in., border around the field

is considered contaminated). The last flap should open toward you. The package inside should be wrapped in the same manner as the one you just opened, except that there will be no indicator tape. Leaving the wrapper that you just opened in place and without moving the sterile field, unwrap the second wrapper following Steps B through E in Figure 28–8. When you open the last flap toward you, the sterile field is ready for use.

Commercially packaged items are often individually wrapped, thus providing safety and convenience. One of the most commonly encountered types of commercial packaging is the peel-back package. Peel-back packages have two edges that can be separated, folded back, grasped, and pulled apart (Fig. 28–9). Once the package is opened, it is a small sterile field. To maintain its sterility, lay it on a clean, dry surface with both flaps pulled well apart so that neither flap can close up and contaminate the contents of the package. Very small packages do not have 2.5-cm (1-in.) borders that are considered contaminated. Only the parts that are grasped to peel back and the very edges should be considered contaminated.

Sterile liquids are often necessary for procedures such as catheter irrigation. They may be bottled and sterilized by the health facility or by commercial manufacturers. Health care facilities often provide glass bottles with rubber stoppers that are sealed with dated indicator tape. Commercially prepared liquids are often

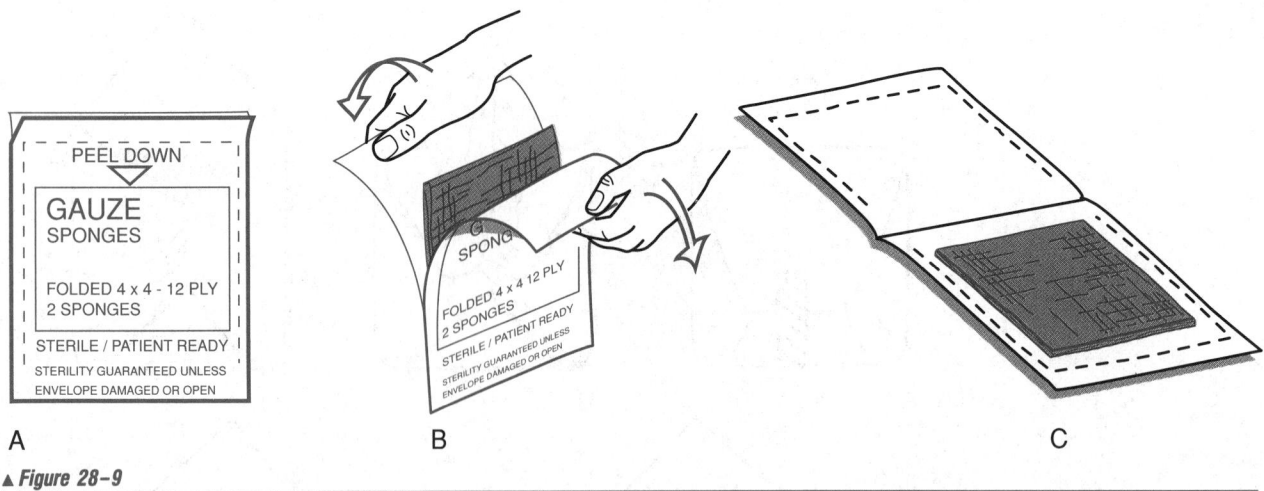

▲ *Figure 28-9*

Opening a commercially packaged "peel-back" package. *A,* Read directions on package. *B,* Follow directions and grasp flaps at top of package and peel back. *C,* When the package is opened according to directions, sterility of contents is maintained.

found sealed in plastic bottles with screw-top lids. On the initial opening of a bottle, do not use a solution of any type if the seal is broken. Once you determine that the solution is sterile and the bottle is opened, however, the solution may continue to be used for up to 24 hours (this policy may differ according to the agency).

Use solution from a previously opened container only if (1) the date and time of opening are clearly marked on the container and it has been open for fewer than 24 hours and (2) you are certain that the container or solution has not been contaminated with previous use. If you have any doubts about the sterility of the solution, do not use it!

When opening the container, remember that the inside of the bottle and cap is sterile, whereas the out-

side of the bottle and cap is considered clean. Thus, when handling sterile liquids, observe the following 6 precautions: (1) Invert the cap to place it on a nonsterile surface; (2) if you hold the cap, make certain the opening faces downward to decrease the chance of contamination from airborne microorganisms; (3) place your palm over the label so that the contents do not drip on the label and obscure it; (4) place only the sterile lip over the sterile field because the rest of the bottle is contaminated; (5) hold the container approximately 15 cm (6 in.) above the field and slowly pour the liquid to avoid splashing; and (6) do not allow the lip of the bottle to touch a nonsterile object or surface (Fig. 28-10).

Adding Sterile Supplies. Once you have opened all of your sterile materials, you may wish to add sterile

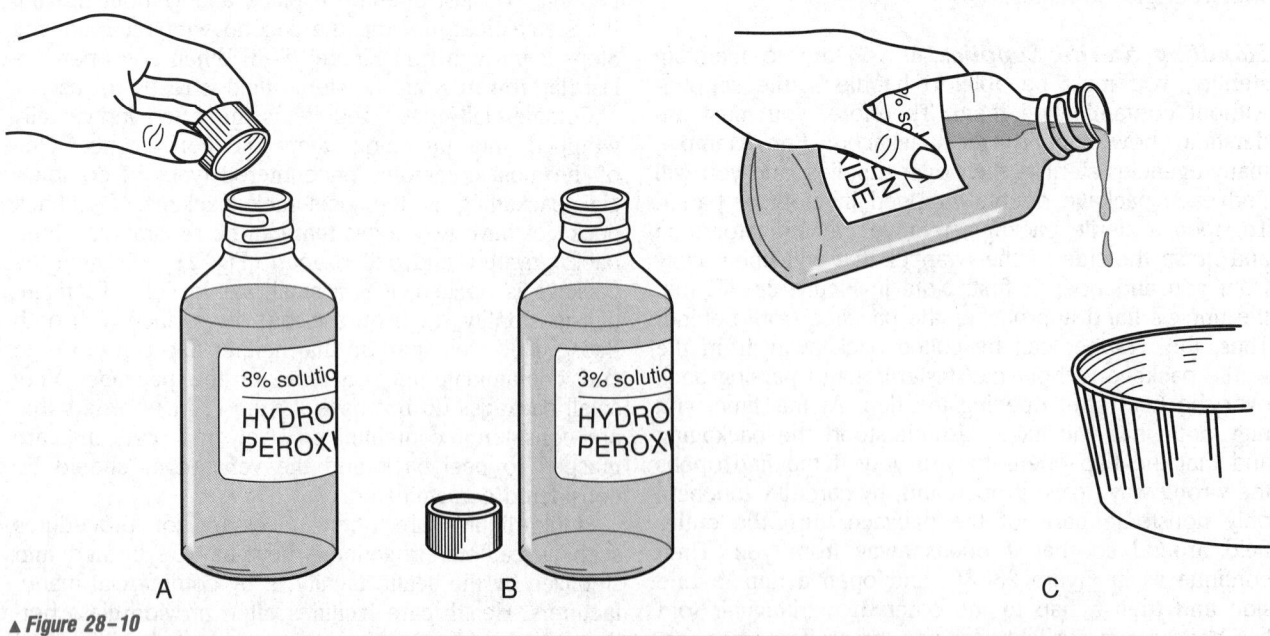

▲ *Figure 28-10*

Pouring a sterile liquid.

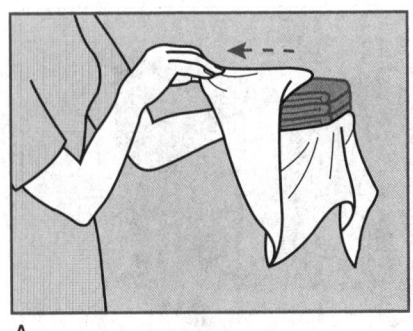 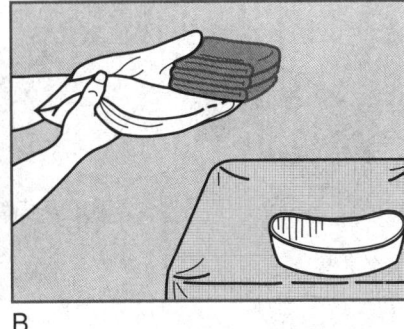 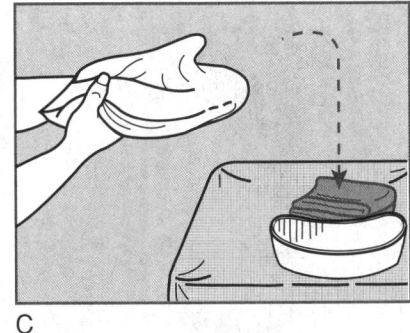

▲ *Figure 28–11*

Transferring sterile supplies to a sterile field. *A*, Holding a sterile package while unwrapping it. *B*, Securely holding the package wrapper out of the way of the sterile field while preparing to flip the sterile package contents onto the sterile field. *C*, Sterile item transferred to sterile field.

items to one or more sterile fields. When adding a sterile item to a sterile field, you may use several techniques depending on whether your hands are covered with sterile gloves. The first technique is recommended when you are initially establishing your sterile fields but have not yet donned gloves or when you are assisting a doctor or another nurse who is gloved (i.e., when you are "circulating"). The remaining three techniques are recommended when you are actually gloved and working with the supplies on the sterile field. These techniques follow:

▶ When ungloved, flip a sterile item onto the field directly from its package (Fig. 28–11).
▶ When gloved, transfer the item from one opened sterile field to another with a gloved hand.
▶ When gloved, transfer the item by using sterile forceps (Fig. 28–12).
▶ When gloved, pick the item from the sterile package that is opened and offered to you by an assistant.

When working alone, once you have independently established your sterile fields and have added all necessary items, the next step is to wash your hands and don sterile gloves.

When to Wash Your Hands and When to Complete a Surgical Hand Scrub. When you will be working in the operating room, delivery room, or other area where you will need to wear a sterile gown and sterile gloves, you must complete a surgical hand scrub before gowning and gloving. In all other cases, your routine hand-washing procedure (Procedure 28–1) is recommended before gloving.

Gloving. Sterile gloves are frequently packaged in a paper peel-back outer package. Inside this is usually another paper package that contains two gloves marked "right" and "left." This inner package is sterile and can be opened to form a sterile field. Gloves may be put on by using an open method or a closed method. The open method is used for routine sterile procedures at the client's bedside. The closed method is used in operating rooms and other areas where the nurse dons a sterile gown with the gloves.

Open Gloving Method. Follow the directions in Figure 28–13 to put on gloves using the open gloving method. This method is a very basic skill that all nurses must master. Even those who routinely use the closed method in the operating room must use the open method on occasion. It requires a good deal of practice to do it correctly every time.

Once your sterile gloves are on, you are ready to begin the sterile procedure. From this point forward, your hands must always remain in front of you and at or above table level.

If at any point you believe you might have contaminated your glove or if anyone else questions the sterility of your glove, immediately discard it and reglove.

Removing Gloves. When the procedure has been completed and you are ready to remove your gloves, consider them contaminated and make every effort to protect your bare skin and clothing from touching them (Fig. 28–14). With the finger and thumb of one hand, pinch up a bit of the glove at the inside wrist of the opposite hand approximately 2.5 cm (1 in.) below the edge of the cuff. Pull downward, inverting the glove as you go, until only the fingers and the thumb are covered. These digits are now covered by the clean inside of the glove. Use them to pinch up the opposite glove and pull it off to the same level. Then use the second glove to remove the first glove and the bare fingers to

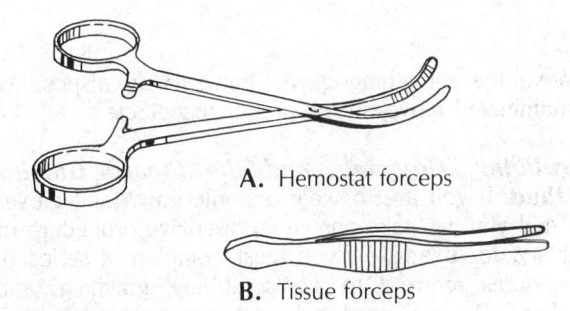

A. Hemostat forceps

B. Tissue forceps

▲ *Figure 28–12*

Examples of sterile forceps.

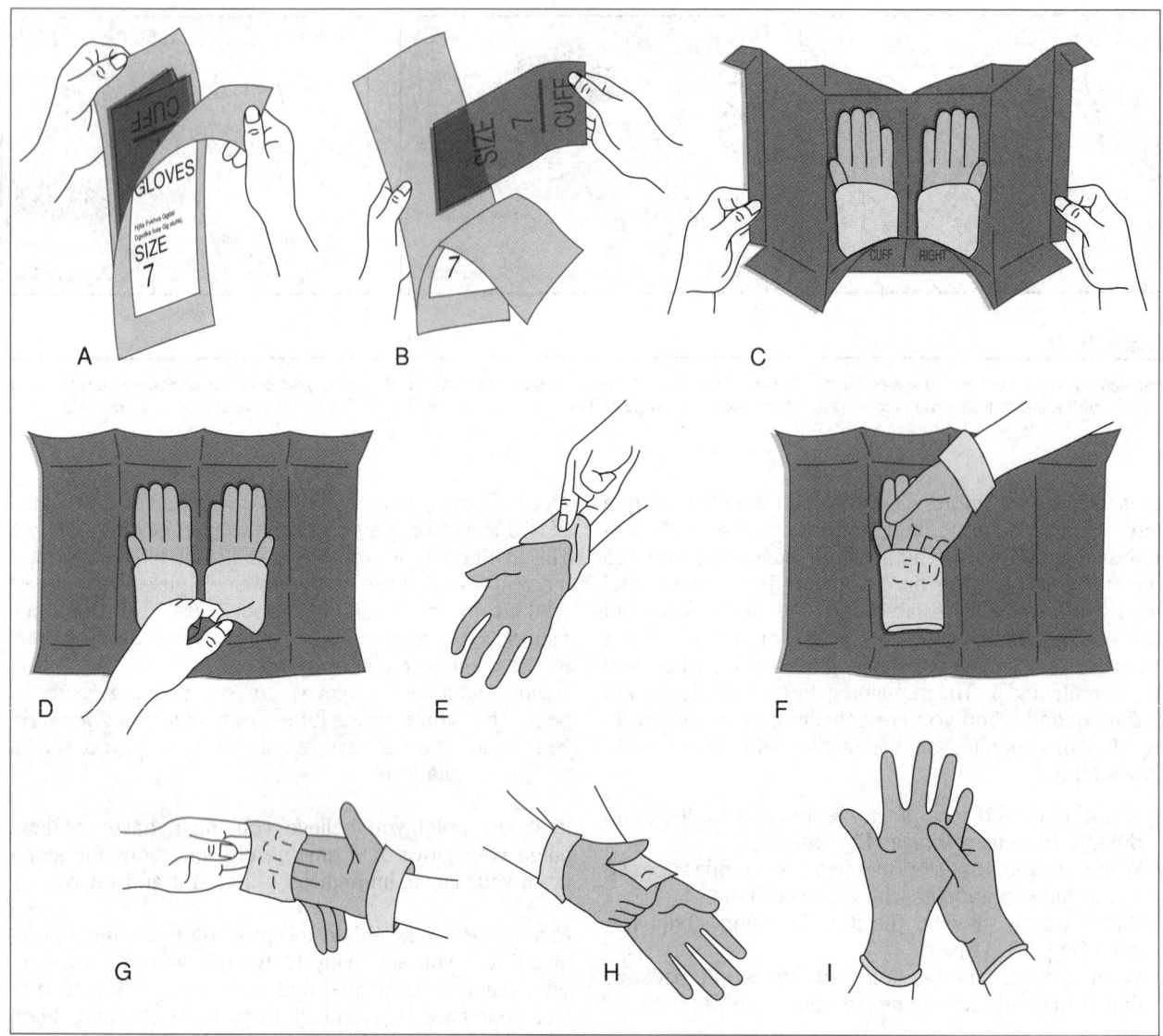

▲ *Figure 28–13*

Donning sterile gloves. *A,* First wash your hands. Then open outside wrapper by peeling down. *B,* Remove inner wrapper. *C,* Place inner wrapper on a clean, dry surface with "cuff" end facing you. Unfold wrapper to expose gloves. Hold lower corners of wrapper securely with both hands as you open both sides at the same time. Allowing either side to "flap back" will contaminate the gloves. *D,* With your nondominant hand, grasp the glove that fits your dominant hand by pinching the edge of its cuff between your forefinger and thumb, pick it up and hold it well above table level, and step back from the sterile field. *E,* Holding glove above waist level, with its fingers pointing down, carefully slip your hand inside the glove. Do not allow the fingers of the glove to touch any nonsterile surface as you work your hand into the glove. Do not adjust this glove until you have donned the second glove. *F,* Place your gloved fingers under the cuff of the remaining glove, lift it well above table level, and step back away from the table. *G,* Keep your gloved thumb abducted so it does not become contaminated as you carefully slip your ungloved hand into the remaining glove. *H,* Put cuffs up by slipping gloved fingers under them. Be careful not to touch bare skin of the arm as you put the cuff up. *I,* Adjust gloves for comfort, as necessary.

remove the remaining glove. Immediately dispose of contaminated gloves in the proper receptacle.

Scrubbing, Gowning, and the Closed Gloving Method. If you are to wear a sterile gown and gloves (so that you can take part in an operative procedure or delivery, for example), you must complete a series of procedures referred to as "scrubbing, gowning, and gloving." These procedures are longer and more intricate than the skills required for hand washing and donning gloves with the open method.

For scrubbing, gowning, and gloving, you must prepare by removing all jewelry from the arms and hands, ensuring that the skin of your arms and hands is intact (free of open lesions), ensuring that your fingernails are trimmed and free of polish, and dressing appropriately in the following items:

▶ scrub garments (to prevent shedding, a one-piece coverall suit or pants with shirt tucked in are recommended in preference to dresses)

▶ a cap to cover all hair on the head (special caps,

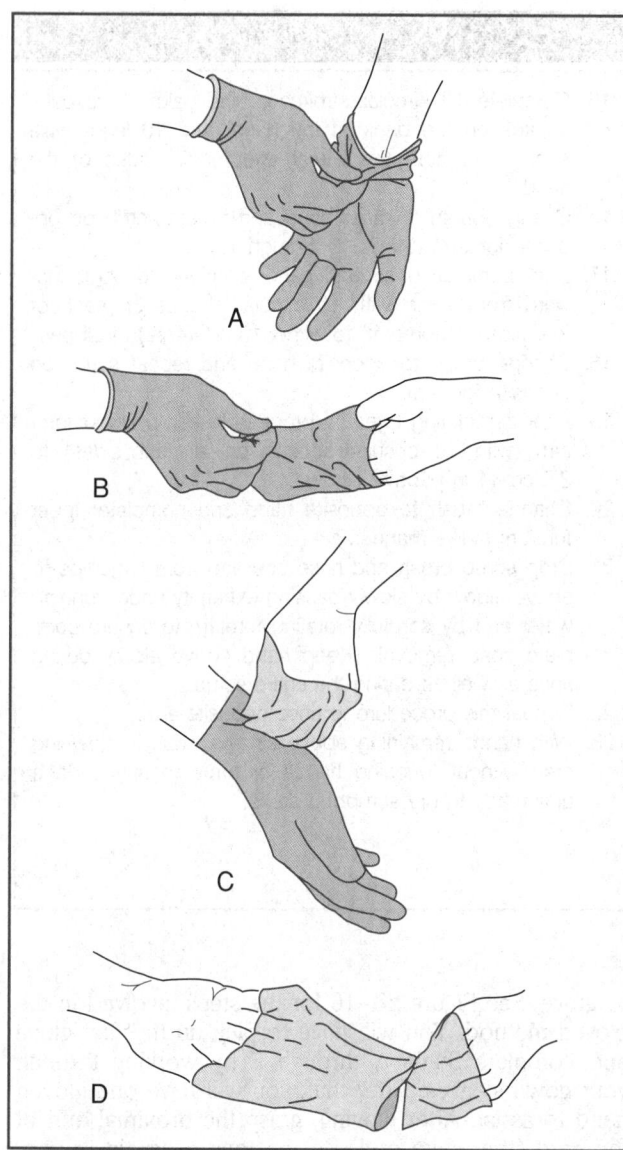

▲ *Figure 28-14*

Removing contaminated gloves.

around your head, and secure them over your occipital area by tying them in a bow. Next, bring the two lower strings around and tie them at the back of your neck. Both ties should be tight enough that the mask is secured over your mouth and nose, with no gaps around the edges through which air may vent.

Removing a Mask. To remove the mask, remember that you have been breathing into it for some time and that it has filtered many microorganisms into a concentrated mass. Try to prevent this mass from being dispersed into the air currents or touching your hands or scrub clothing. Do not tear the mask off. Instead, carefully untie the lower two strings first. Then untie the top two strings and, without letting go, bring the mask away from your face and immediately drop it into the appropriate receptacle for disposal.

It is false economy to attempt to save a mask for future use. Never let your mask hang around your neck and contaminate your scrub clothes and do not place it in your pocket!

Surgical Hand Scrub. There is no one perfect method for completing the surgical hand scrub. Several overall guidelines, however, should be followed in each agency. For example, it is important that all personnel in the agency use the same standardized scrub technique, that they use an effective antimicrobial soap or detergent, and that they include at least the following in their scrub procedure:[3]

▶ keeping the hands and forearms up and away from the scrub clothing during the procedure
▶ washing the hands and forearms to remove transient microorganisms
▶ cleaning the fingernails and subungual areas with a sterile cleaner (or file)
▶ using friction for the application of antimicrobial soap or detergent
▶ rinsing the scrubbed areas with clear water

The two general methods of scrubbing are the time method and the counted-stroke method. With a counted-stroke method, each surface is scrubbed a given number of strokes. With a timed scrub, each surface is scrubbed for a given period of time. See Box 28-1 for a method used for a counted-stroke scrub using a commercially prepared, disposable combination scrub brush and sponge that is packaged with a plastic fingernail cleaner at one side. Note that this method is merely one of a number of equally correct procedures. You will have to learn the one that is in use at your agency.

Research has been unable to identify any significant difference in efficacy between the following:

▶ a timed scrub and a counted-stroke scrub
▶ use of a brush, a sponge, or neither
▶ a 5-minute scrub and a 10-minute scrub

Drying. After the surgical hand scrub, you will have to use aseptic technique to dry your hands on a sterile

called "beard covers," are available for those with facial hair such as sideburns or beards)
▶ a mask to cover the nose and mouth
▶ eye protectors that may be prescription or regular eye goggles or protectors or eye shields that are part of the mask
▶ shoe covers

Applying a Mask. The mask is the last item of apparel that should be applied before you begin your surgical hand scrub. To apply it, take the mask from its dispenser box by grasping the strings and holding only the strings or the very edge around the mask. Do not touch the part that you will breathe through. Holding the mask by the very top, mold the metal piece inside to fit comfortably but securely over the bridge of your nose so that the mask is centered over your nose and mouth. Then take the top two strings, bring these

---

Box 28–1. Scrubbing with the Counted-Stroke Method

1. Have on correct surgical garments.
2. Have all jewelry removed.
3. Have fingernails appropriate for the scrub.
4. Apply mask.
5. Select scrub brush (Betadine-impregnated or plain brush with antimicrobial solution applied from wall dispenser).
6. Open brush, do not remove it from package, place opened package on flat surface at back of scrub sink.
7. Standing well back from sink from this point on, select desired water temperature and correct scrub cycle (standard).
8. Keeping hands well above elbows from this point on, wet hands and arms.
9. Take brush in one hand and remove fingernail cleaner from side of brush.
10. Using sponge side of brush, brush soap down ends of fingernails on both hands.
11. With fingernail cleaner, clean carefully under each fingernail on both hands and then discard fingernail cleaner.
12. Considering the fingers, thumb, hands, and arms as squares and holding the brush in one hand, begin scrubbing the opposite hand using the bristle side of the brush.
13. Begin with 10 strokes along the fingertips.
14. Follow with 10 strokes along each of the four sides of each finger and thumb.

15. Complete 10 circular strokes of the palm, 10 circular strokes on the back of the hand, and 10 lengthwise strokes on both the lateral and medial sides of the hand.
16. Change brush to other hand and repeat scrub on opposite forearm (Steps 13 through 15).
17. After completing second hand, continue to scrub upward from wrist (with 10 circular strokes on each of four sides of forearm) to within 10 cm (4 in.) of elbow.
18. Change brush to opposite hand and repeat scrub on opposite forearm.
19. After completing forearm, proceed to scrub upper forearm (with 10 circular strokes on all four sides) to 2.5 cm (1 in.) above elbow.
20. Change brush to opposite hand and complete upper forearm in like manner.
21. Drop scrub brush and rinse one arm from fingertips to above elbow by slowly passing extremity under running water and by carefully rotating forearm to ensure complete soap removal. (Keep hand above elbow during rinse as well as during the entire scrub.)
22. Repeat this procedure to rinse opposite arm.
23. With hands remaining above elbows, walk to gowning area without touching hands or arms to any surface until ready to dry scrubbed areas.

---

towel that is lying on an opened sterile field. To do this, keep your hands above your elbows and flex at your hips and knees to pick up the sterile towel. Grasp it firmly and, keeping it folded, pick it up above table level and step back away from the table. Leaning slightly forward, so as to keep the towel from touching your unsterile clothing, allow the towel to unfold by gravity until it is only doubled. Then, with one end of the towel, dry first your fingers, then your hand and forearm, and finally your upper arm, as needed. Use the opposite end of the towel to repeat the drying process on your opposite hand and arm. Discard the towel without dropping your hands below waist level.

Gowning and Using the Closed Gloving Method. To don a sterile gown, use your clean, dry hands to pick up the gown by grasping it firmly enough to prevent it from unfolding as you lift it up and away from the sterile field (Fig. 28–15). Step well back from the table and any other sterile or nonsterile surfaces. Hold the gown so that the upper half is in front of you, as it is to be worn, with sleeve openings to either side. Allow the gown to unfold by gravity as you work your arms into the sleeve openings and raise and spread your arms to assist the process.

Keep your hands within the sleeves and covered while your assistant (the circulating nurse) ties the gown at the neck and waist in the back. Before completing the gowning procedure, use the closed method

to glove. See Figure 28–16 for the steps involved in the closed method. You will have to pick up the first glove and complete Steps A through E by working through your gown sleeves. After that, you will have one gloved hand to assist. After gloving, grasp the proximal end of the card (the white end) on the long waist tie in your right hand and the distal end of the short tie in your left hand and pull the short tie away from the card. Hand the distal (red) end of the card to your circulating nurse. Pirouette counterclockwise while the circulating nurse holds the card. Pull the long tie from the card, and tie it to the short tie toward the front and side of the gown at waist level.

Removing a Contaminated Gown and Gloves. Because you work with blood and other body fluids during operative procedures, you must consider your gown and gloves contaminated. You must remove them carefully so that, in the process, you do not contaminate your skin or scrub clothing underneath. When you are wearing both gown and gloves, you can remove your own attire by untying the waist ties in the front and allowing the circulating nurse to untie or unsnap the back. With your gloves still on, grasp the gown at the shoulder area on both sides and peel it forward and off your arms so that it turns inside out as it comes off. Removing the gown in this manner will roll your glove cuffs down but your gloves will remain on your hands. Carefully roll the gown lengthwise so that the side that

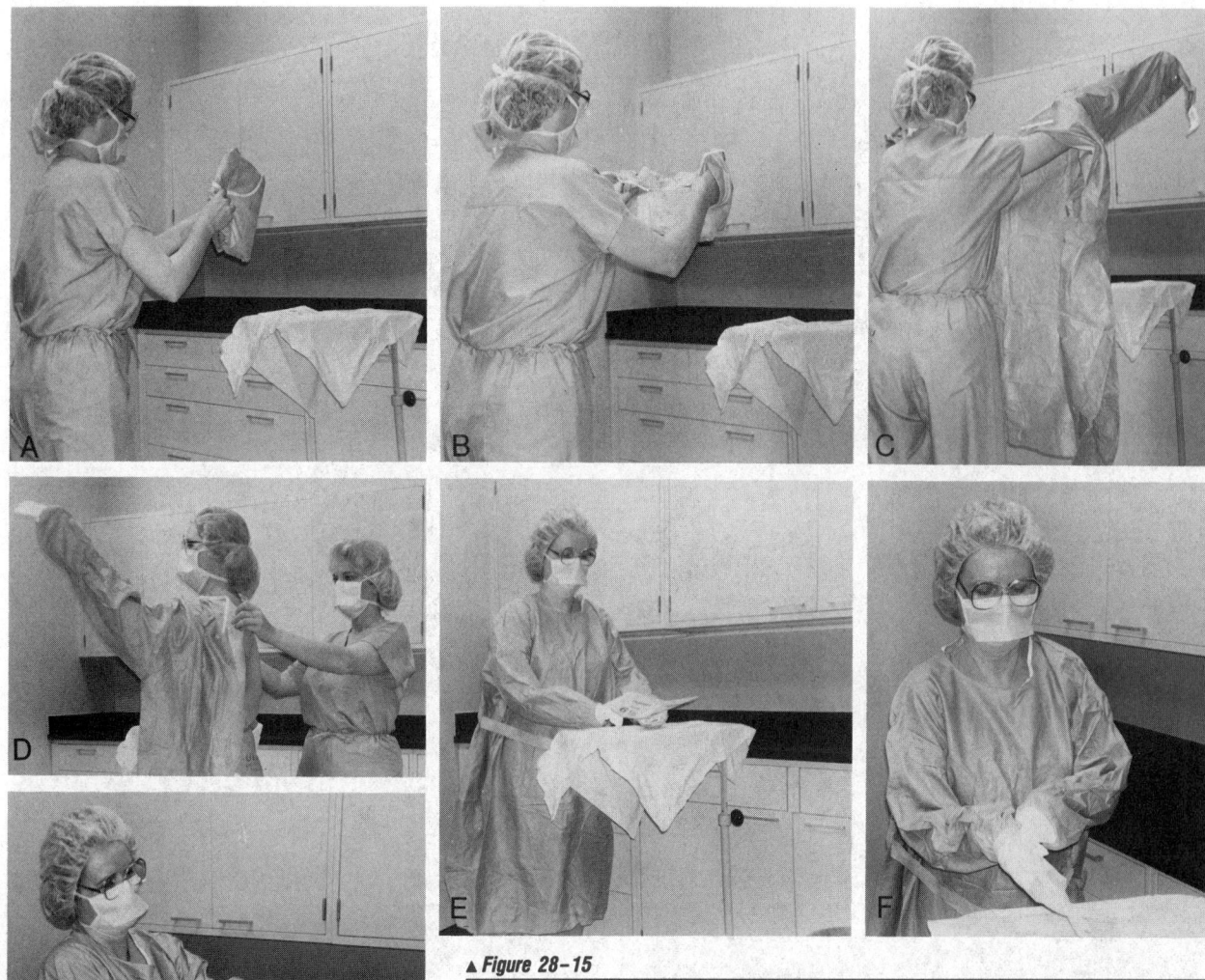

▲ **Figure 28–15**

Donning a sterile gown. *A*, Use your clean, dry hands to pick up the gown by grasping it firmly enough to prevent it from unfolding as you lift it up and away from the sterile field. *B*, Step well back from the table and any other sterile or nonsterile surfaces. Hold the gown so that the upper half is in front of you, as it is to be worn, with sleeve openings to either side. *C*, Allow the gown to unfold by gravity as you work your arms into the sleeve openings and raise and spread your arms to assist the process. *D*, Keep your hands within the sleeves and covered while your assistant (circulating nurse) ties the gown at the neck and waist in the back. *E*, Before completing the gowning procedure, use the closed method to glove. *F*, Work through the gown sleeves as you don your first glove (see Fig. 28–16 for the specific steps involved in the closed method). *G*, After donning the first glove, you will have one gloved hand to assist you in donning the second glove.

Illustration continued on following page

was toward your body (the cleaner side) is outermost and the contaminated side is contained within. Then roll the gown from top to bottom and discard it. Avoid making airwaves as you do this.

Because your glove cuffs roll when you remove your gown this way, you will have a roll to pinch up for glove removal. This roll may be used instead of pinching down about 2.5 cm (1 in.) from the cuff end. It will help protect your skin from being touched as you pinch up the glove to remove it. After pinching the roll, remove the gloves in sections, as during any glove removal, to avoid contaminating your hands.

Whether you have washed your hands and used the open method of gloving or have completed a surgical hand scrub and have donned a sterile gown and gloves by using the closed method of gloving, you did so to maintain sterile technique during a procedure, and you

did this in order to prevent infection. Removal and disposal of your equipment are also part of preventing infection, but these final procedures involve using clean technique (medical asepsis) rather than sterile technique (surgical asepsis). The use of medical asepsis, however, does not make the cleanup any less important. Never allow the chain of infection to remain intact. Do not interrupt it at one point only to allow it to come together again at another point.

Evaluation

To evaluate whether your client has achieved the expected outcome and has remained free of infection, you must, of course, look at the physical assessment and laboratory data again and compare these to the

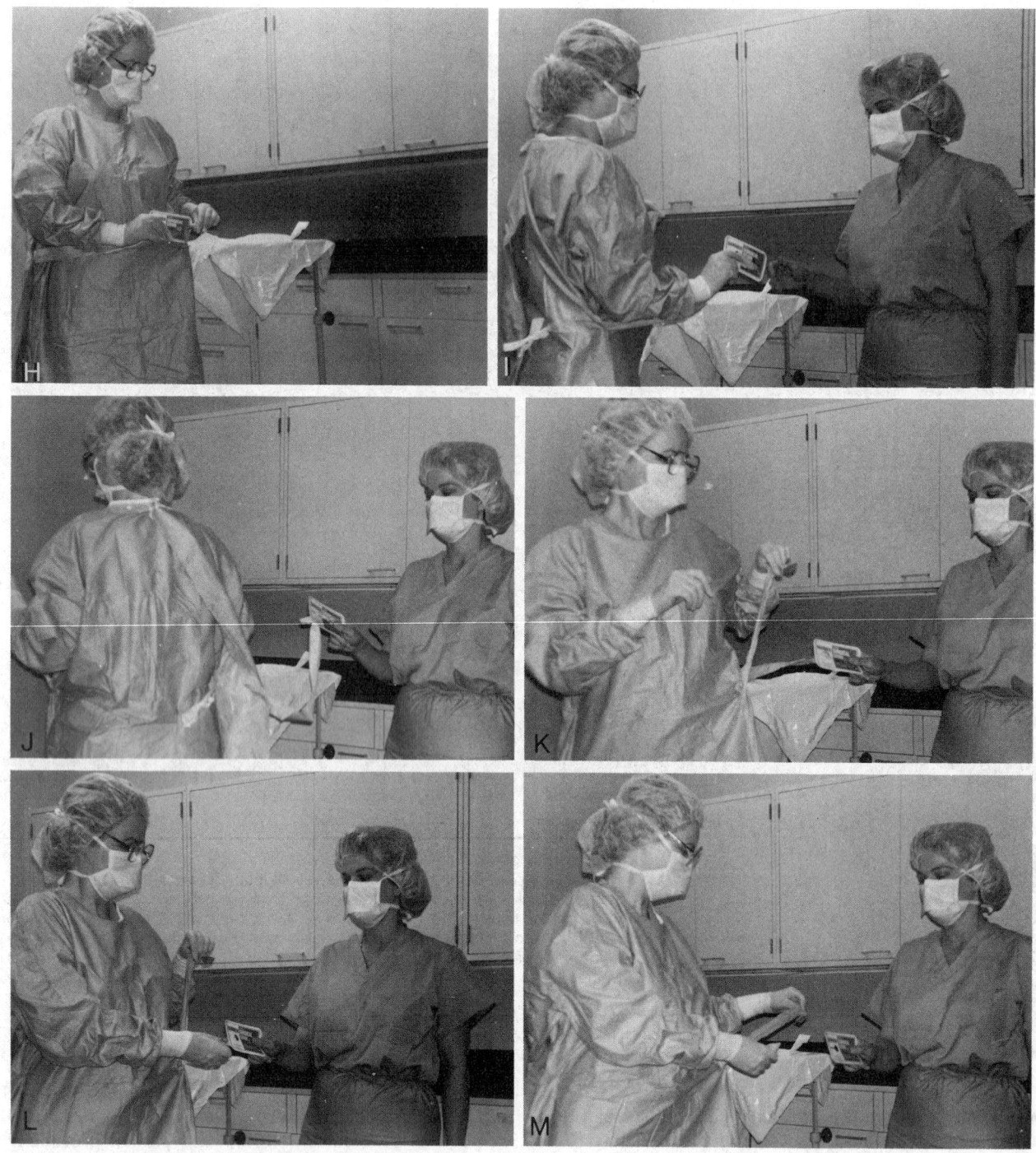

▲ **Figure 28–15** Continued

H, After gloving, grasp the proximal end of the card (the white end) on the long waist tie in your right hand and the distal end of the short tie in your left hand and pull the short tie away from the card. *I*, Hand the distal (red) end of the card to your circulating nurse. *J* and *K*, Pirouette counterclockwise while the circulating nurse holds the card. *L*, Pull the long tie from the card. *M*, Tie the long tie to the short tie (tie ties toward the front and side of the gown at waist level).

baseline values you established at your initial assessment. But, even if all signs appear to be quite positive, can you be certain that your client is truly free of infection?

It is not always easy to evaluate whether you have been successful in preventing infection. Depending on many factors, such as incubation period, the results of your actions may not be evident for a long time. The best that you can do is to maintain high standards of medical and surgical asepsis and constantly monitor the client for signs of infection. The assumption is that you have prevented infection until such time as an infection becomes evident. This assumption is akin to looking at the indicator tape on the outside of a sterile package and having faith that the package is indeed sterile when all that the tape indicates is that one of the conditions for sterility was, at one time, met. Not until you see the results of the biologic monitor are

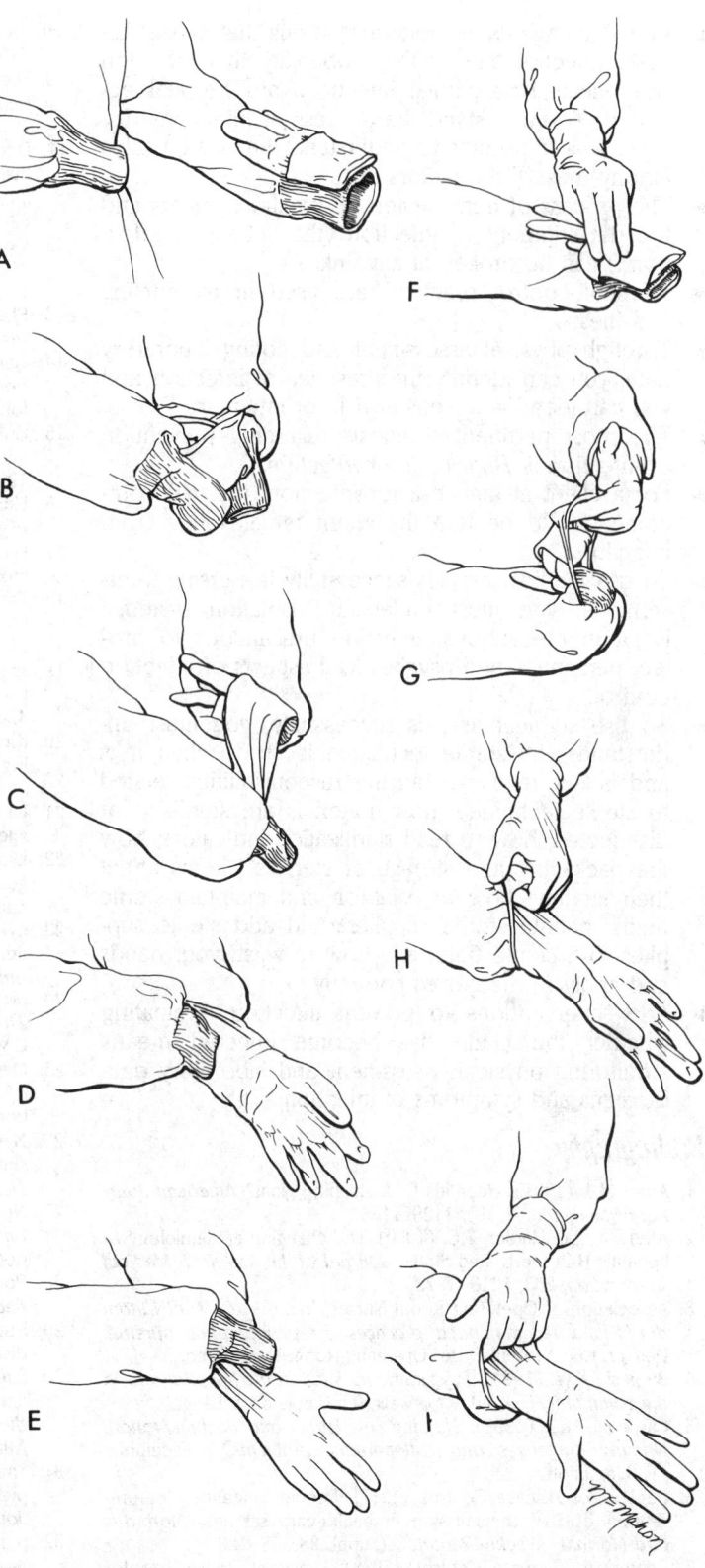

▲ Figure 28–16

Gloving—closed technique. A, Lay the glove palm down over the cuff of the gown. The fingers of the glove face toward you. B and C, Working through the gown sleeve, grasp the cuff of the glove and bring it over the open cuff of the sleeve. D and E, Unroll the glove cuff so that it covers the sleeve cuff and secure both cuffs as you slide your hand into the glove. F, G, H, and I, Proceed with the opposite hand, using the same technique. Never allow the bare hand to contact the gown cuff edge or outside of glove. (From Fuller, J.R. (1986). *Surgical technology: Principles and practices* (2nd ed.). Philadelphia: W.B. Saunders.)

you sure, and by the time you find out the results, the package may have been contaminated.

At our current state of knowledge, we can never be entirely certain that the client is free of infection. We can, and we must, however, uphold the highest standards of medical and surgical asepsis possible to prevent infection from occurring.

Summary

▶ Proper hand washing is the most important activity in controlling the spread of infection.

▶ Since the times of Nightingale and Semmelweis, the need for generic cleanliness to protect all of the sick has been overshadowed by practices aimed at isolating and treating those with known infections. This trend is now reversing.

▶ Infectious agents are microorganisms that cause disease. Infection risk is the probability that infection will occur. Nosocomial infections are hospital acquired. To understand the process of infectious disease, it is important to understand the relationships among these three factors.

▶ The process of transmission of infectious agents and the development of infection (the "chain of infection") can be broken at any link.

▶ Infection-control practices are used in all nursing activities.

▶ Through physical assessment and noting laboratory data, you can identify the presence of infection and you can identify persons at risk for infection.

▶ The most pertinent diagnosis regarding prevention of infection is *High Risk for Infection*.

▶ For a client at high risk for infection, the main outcome should be that the client remains free from infection.

▶ To use medical asepsis successfully in nursing interventions, you must understand isolation systems, isolation precautions, infection precautions to protect personnel, and psychosocial aspects of infection control.

▶ To use surgical asepsis successfully, you must understand why sterile technique is used; when it is and is not required; nursing responsibilities related to sterile technique; how materials are sterilized or disinfected; how to read sterilization indicators; how the packaging and storage of sterilized items affect their sterility; how to establish and maintain sterile fields, handle sterile supplies, and add sterile supplies to a sterile field; and how to wash your hands and apply sterile gloves correctly.

▶ After interventions to prevent infection, evaluating whether the client has become infected means monitoring physical assessment and laboratory data for signs and symptoms of infection.

Bibliography

1. Alter, M.J. (1991). Hepatitis C: A sleeping giant? *American Journal of Medicine 91*(3B), 112S–115S.
2. Alter, M.J., & Hadler, S.C. (1990). The changing epidemiology of hepatitis B in the United States. *Journal of the American Medical Association, 263,* 1218–1222.
3. Association of Operating Room Nurses, Inc. (1992). *AORN standards and recommended practices for perioperative nursing.* Denver, CO: Association of Operating Room Nurses, Inc.
4. Burgess, A.W. (1990). *Psychiatric nursing: In the hospital and in the community* (5th ed.). Norwalk, CT: Appleton & Lange.
5. Carpenito, L.J. (1991). *Nursing care plans and documentation: Nursing diagnoses and collaborative problems.* Philadelphia: J.B. Lippincott.
6. Centers for Disease Control. (1987). Recommendations for prevention of HIV transmission in health-care settings. *Morbidity and Mortality Weekly Report, 36*(Suppl. 2S), 1S–18S.
7. Centers for Disease Control. (1988). Universal Precautions for Prevention of Transmission of Human Immunodeficiency Virus, Hepatitis B Virus, and Other Bloodborne Pathogens in Health-Care Settings. *Morbidity and Mortality Weekly Report, 37,* 377–388.
8. Centers for Disease Control. (1990). Guidelines for preventing the transmission of tuberculosis in health-care settings, with special focus on HIV-related issues. *Morbidity and Mortality Weekly Report, 39*(RR-17), 1–29.
9. Department of Labor/Department of Health and Human Services. (1987, October). *Federal Register,*
10. Dienstag, J.L., & Ryan, D.M. (1982). Occupational exposure to hepatitis B virus in hospital personnel. *American Journal of Epidemiology, 115,* 26–39.
11. Doebbeling, B.N., et al. (1992). Comparative efficacy of alternative hand-washing agents in reducing nosocomial infections in intensive care units. *New England Journal of Medicine, 327*(2), 88–93.
12. Doenges, M.E., & Moorhouse, M.F. (1991). *Nurse's pocket guide: Nursing diagnoses with interventions* (3rd ed.). Philadelphia: F.A. Davis.
13. Flaskerud, J.H., & Ungvarski, P.J. (1992). *HIV: A guide to nursing/care* (2nd ed.). Philadelphia: W.B. Saunders.
14. Garner, J.S., & Simmons, B.P. (1983). *Guidelines for the prevention and control of nosocomial infections.* Atlanta, GA: Centers for Disease Control.
15. Goldmann, D., & Larson, E. (1992). Hand-washing and nosocomial infections. *New England Journal of Medicine, 327*(2), 120–122.
16. Haley, R.W. (1986). *Managing hospital infection control for cost effectiveness.* Chicago: American Hospital Publishing.
17. Hickey, P.W. (1990). *Nursing process handbook.* St. Louis: C.V. Mosby.
18. Jackson, M.M., & Lynch, P. (1985). Isolation practices: A historical perspective. *American Journal of Infection Control, 13,* 21–31.
19. Jagger, J., et al. (1988). Rates of needle stick injury caused by various devices in a university hospital. *New England Journal of Medicine, 318,* 284–288.
20. Klein, B.S., et al. (1989). Reduction of nosocomial infection during pediatric intensive care by protective isolation. *New England Journal of Medicine, 320,* 1714–1721.
21. Larson, E. (1988). APIC guideline for use of topical antimicrobial agents. *American Journal of Infection Control, 16,* 253–266.
22. Lynch, P., et al. (1990). Implementing and evaluating a system of generic infection precautions: Body substance isolation. *American Journal of Infection Control, 18,* 1–12.
23. Lynch, P., et al. (1987). Rethinking the role of isolation precautions in the prevention of nosocomial infections. *Annals of Internal Medicine, 107,* 243–246.
24. McCance, K.L., & Huether, S.E. (eds.). (1990). *Pathophysiology: The biologic basis for disease in adults and children.* St. Louis: C.V. Mosby.
25. Meeker, M.H., & Rothrock, J.C. (eds.). (1991). *Alexander's care of the patient in surgery* (9th ed.). St. Louis: C.V. Mosby-Yearbook.
26. Nauseef, W.M., & Maki, D.G. (1981). A study of the value of simple protective isolation in patients with granulocytopenia. *New England Journal of Medicine.* 304, 448–453.
27. North American Nursing Diagnosis Association. (1990). *Taxonomy I—Revised 1990.* St. Louis: North American Nursing Diagnosis Association.
28. Porth, C.M. (ed.). (1990). *Pathophysiology: Concepts of altered health states* (3rd ed.). Philadelphia: J.B. Lippincott.
29. Rutala, W.A. (1990). APIC guideline for selection and use of disinfectants. *American Journal of Infection Control, 18,* 99–117.
30. Simmons, B.P., et al. (1981). Centers for Disease Control. Guideline for prevention of intravascular infection. In *Guidelines for the prevention and control of nosocomial infections* (p. 85). Atlanta, GA.: Centers for Disease Control.
31. Smith, P.W., & Rusnak, P.G. (1991). APIC guideline for infection prevention and control in the long term care facility. *American Journal of Infection Control, 19,* 198–215.
32. Stuart, G.W., & Sundeen, S.J. (1991). *Principles and practice of psychiatric nursing* (4th ed.). St. Louis: C.V. Mosby-Yearbook.
33. Varcarolis, E.M. (ed.). (1990). *Foundations of psychiatric mental health nursing.* Philadelphia: W.B. Saunders.
34. Viall, C.D. (1990). Your complete guide to central venous catheters. *Nursing, 20*(2), 34–42.
35. Wenzel, R.P. (1988). The mortality of hospital-acquired bloodstream infections: Need for a new vital statistic? *International Journal of Epidemiology, 17*(1), 112–117.

Preventing Back Injury

While employees in occupations [such as seen in hospitals and nursing homes] . . . comprise about one-fifth of the total work-force, they report one-fourth of the injuries.

U. S. Department of Health and Human Services

Chapter
29

▼ **CHAPTER OUTLINE**

SELECTED PHYSICS PRINCIPLES
    Stability of Objects
    Use of Leverage
    Motion

GUIDELINES FOR CORRECT BODY
  MECHANICS
    Correct Body Alignment
    Effective Body Movement

▼ **KEY TERMS**

Axis	Center of gravity	Lever
Base of support	Force	Leverage
Body alignment (posture)	Friction	Line of gravity
Body mechanics	Fulcrum (axis)	Load
(biomechanics)	Inertia	Stability

Nurses frequently do lifting as part of their job activities. Lifting subjects the body to physical stresses that can result in musculoskeletal injury. Nurses are particularly at risk when the objects lifted are heavy, as when nurses lift clients who weigh as much as, or more than, they do. However, nurses need not lift heavy loads to injure themselves. Temporarily or permanently disabling injuries, particularly back injuries, can occur when nurses lift even small objects, if the lifting is done incorrectly.

Because musculoskeletal injuries are so common, most hospitals insist that nurses be trained in good body mechanics as a condition of employment. Good **body mechanics (biomechanics)** are the coordinated and efficient ways in which the body is used while moving from one position to another. Nurses are expected to come to their jobs in the hospital knowing and habitually using good body mechanics. Still, most hospitals provide a review of safe body mechanics as part of their employee orientation programs. In addition, most hospitals and nursing homes provide mechanical devices and may even provide teams of specially trained staff members to do the lifting or to assist in lifting and moving heavy loads. Employers are generally doing whatever they can to prevent musculoskeletal injuries on the job. They know that such injuries are significantly costly to their employees, to themselves, and to the clients they serve.

Try to imagine how you would feel if you were attempting to help a sick, weak person get out of bed and you hurt your back in the process. What if you could no longer hold the person up and caused a fall? How would you feel if the person broke a bone, received bruises, or suffered a head injury during the fall? Aside from your feelings, could you afford to be out of work with your back injury? Could you afford a legal defense if an injured person sued you? Would you have the means to pay if you lost a lawsuit? How would your employers feel about you dropping one of their patients? How would they feel about you causing them to be sued? Would your insurance rates go up because of such an incident? The implications of such a back injury can be enormous, particularly because musculoskeletal injuries are often preventable. And, because they are preventable, you may bear the responsibility for their occurrence.

For your own protection, as well as for the good of your clients and your employers, you must learn proper body mechanics and use them consistently in all of the work that you do. Consistently using good body mechanics will be difficult as you are learning new nursing skills.

As you learn and practice new skills, you will have to think consciously about everything you do and how you are holding your body as you do it. You will be tempted to think only of the steps of each new skill you need to master and to forget about your body. Forgetting can be a costly mistake.

This chapter will provide you with some basic principles that will help you to learn body mechanics. In addition to attending to your health and safety, these principles can be applied to help ensure the safest and easiest completion of certain tasks. In fact, these are principles you should be using, often without thinking about them, every day for the rest of your professional life. Your instructors will do their part in insisting that you follow through with good body mechanics as they observe all that you do throughout your nursing education. However, in the final analysis, it will be your own attention to forming new, and correct, habits that determines how successful you will be at preventing your own injury.

In this chapter, we focus on scientific principles that will help you to protect yourself from back injury. In subsequent chapters, these principles will be integrated into procedures you will use as you provide client care. In Chapter 35, for example, you will see many of these principles applied to the care of persons who require lifting, positioning, and moving. In Chapter 36, you will see many of them applied to the care of clients who are in need of assistance as they begin to move about after a period of dependence. You will be able to use them, for example, in teaching a client how to walk on crutches.

SELECTED PHYSICS PRINCIPLES

As a nurse, you will frequently be called on to apply principles from the sciences to your work in providing client care. In particular, three sets of scientific principles from physics will be of assistance to you in preventing musculoskeletal injuries. These include principles relating to stability, leverage, and motion.

Stability of Objects

Stability is steadiness of position. Three important principles concerning the stability of an object relate to the **base of support** (foundation on which an object rests), the **center of gravity** (center, or heaviest part, of an object), and the **line of gravity** (imaginary line

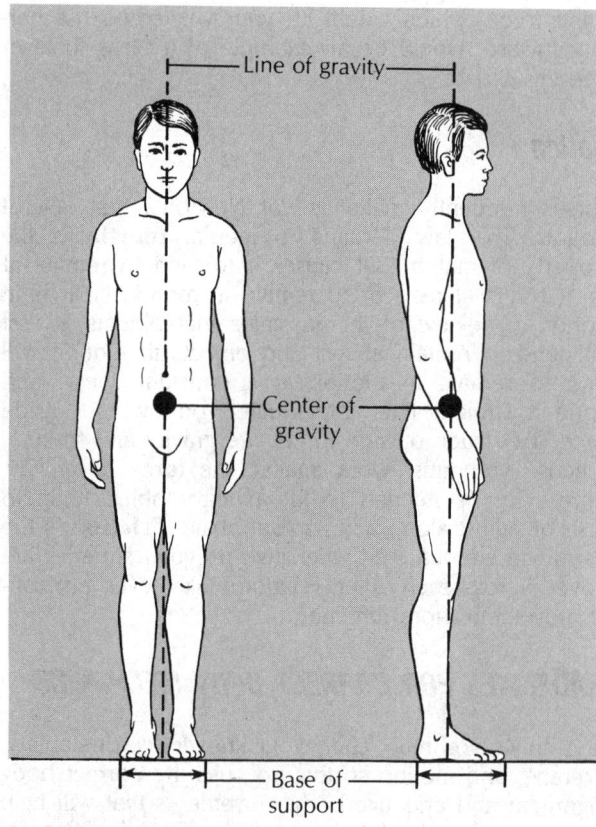

▲ **Figure 29-1**

The base of support, center of gravity, and line of gravity in a man who is in correct body alignment. The center of gravity would be slightly lower in a woman. Note how the line of gravity passes through the center of the base of support.

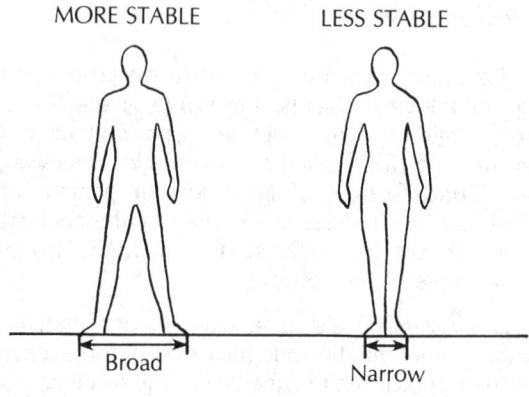

A

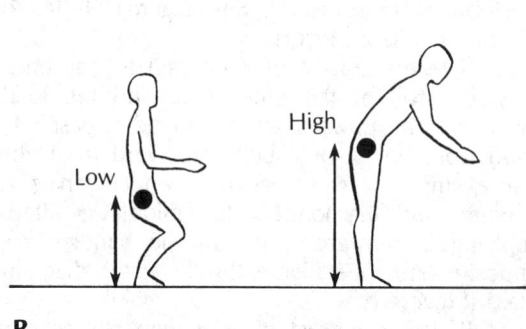

B

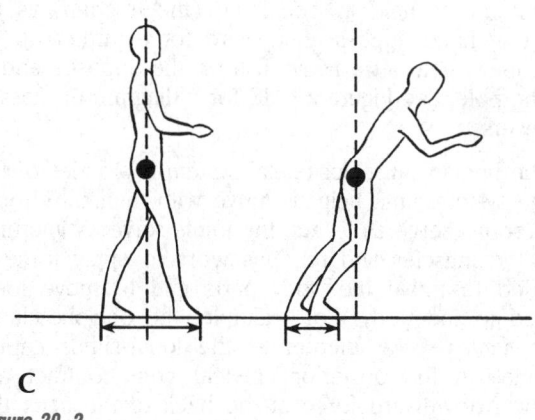

C

▲ **Figure 29-2**

Factors affecting stability. *A,* The wider the base of support, the more stable the object. *B,* The lower the center of gravity, the more stable the object. *C,* The closer the line of gravity to the center of the base of support, the more stable the object.

going straight down through an object's center of gravity). Figure 29-1 shows these areas on a human male in correct body alignment, and the three principles concerning stability are illustrated in Figure 29-2. The three principles are as follows:

▶ The wider the base of support, the more stable the object. For example, the pyramids of Egypt are very stable. A tall lamp with a small base is less stable. A typewriter is stable. A dime balanced on its edge is not. A briefcase that is standing with its handle up is less stable than when placed on its side, ready to be opened. A nurse with feet spread so as to provide a wider base of support is more stable than a nurse with feet held together (see Fig. 29-2A).

▶ The lower the center of gravity, the more stable an object. For example, when lying flat, a brick is very stable. A long pole, if placed on one end, lacks stability and can easily topple. A merry-go-round is stable. A Ferris wheel is much less stable. A heavy book is less stable when placed upright on its bottom edge than when placed flat on its side. A nurse who needs to reach down (to pick up an object, for example) is more stable if the center of gravity is lowered in a squat than if the body is bent at the hips and the center of gravity remains high (see Fig. 29-2B).

▶ The closer the line of gravity is to the center of the base of support, the more stable is the object. For example, the Eiffel Tower is stable. The Leaning Tower of Pisa is far less stable. In fact, the Leaning Tower of Pisa leans just a bit more each year, and if its line of gravity is allowed to fall too far outside of its base of support, it will surely topple. A nurse who leans too far from the base of support is much less stable than when standing upright (see Fig. 29-2C).

Use of Leverage

The wise nurse uses principles of leverage to assist in lifting and moving objects. **Leverage** is the use of a **lever** (a rigid or firm structure) supported on a **fulcrum,** or **axis** (fixed point on which a lever moves), to move a **load** (weight of an object or person, often referred to as resistance) more easily by the application of **force** (effort exerted). As Figure 29-3 illustrates, there are three classes of levers:

▶ Class I levers consist of a load on one end, a fulcrum in the middle, and downward force exerted on the opposite end of the lever. The force can be a pushing downward from above or a pulling downward from below. For example, a person pushes downward (applies force) on one end of a crowbar (lever) over a log (fulcrum) to move a heavy rock (resistance) more easily. See Figure 29-3A for a diagram of Class I levers.
▶ Class II levers consist of a fulcrum at one end, an upward effort at the other end, and the load in between. The upward effort can be a pushing upward from below or a pulling upward from above. For example, a wheelbarrow's wheel serves as a fulcrum, and the load in the middle is lifted by applying an upward force on the handles at the opposite end. See Figure 29-3B for a diagram of Class II levers.
▶ Class III levers consist of a fulcrum at one end, a load at the opposite end, and an upward (pushing or pulling) force in the middle. For example, a fishing rod is held in one hand (the fulcrum) as the other hand applies an upward force further up the pole to help lift a heavy fish on the opposite end of the pole. See Figure 29-3C for a diagram of Class III levers.

The human musculoskeletal system is a series of leverage systems that help us move with minimal effort.[12] The bones serve as levers; the joints serve as fulcrums; and the muscles and tendons work to apply force as needed to move the body parts and to move loads added to the body. For example, the occipitoatlantal joint serves as a fulcrum as the longissimus capitus muscles in the posterior cervical area contract and apply a downward force at the back of the neck that moves the posterior portion of the head downward and the anterior portion of the head (the load) upward. This movement is an example of a Class I lever (see Fig. 29-3A).

A nurse might exemplify the use of a Class II lever in lifting a client. You would begin to lift the client by putting your arms under the person's body so that your radius and ulna bones served as levers, your wrists rested on the bed to serve as fulcrums, and you applied an upward force with your entire upper body to pull your forearms (and the added weight on them) upward (see Fig. 29-3B). As you shifted the person's weight in your arms to continue with the lift, you would use your elbows as fulcrums and your forearms as levers. You also would contract your biceps muscles to apply a lifting force between elbow and wrists. This lifting force, which would lift your wrists and the person upward, would be an example of a Class III lever (see Fig. 29-3C).

Motion

Nurses frequently make use of Newton's first law of motion. This law pertains to inertia. **Inertia** is the property of matter that causes it to tend to remain at rest (if it is at rest) or to remain in motion (if it is in motion). The law of inertia states that objects at rest will tend to remain at rest and objects in motion will tend to remain in motion at a constant speed and along a straight line unless acted on by an outside force. Two such outside forces are gravity and friction. Because you must work against the force of gravity, more effort is needed to lift a heavy object than to push or pull it along a horizontal plane. **Friction** is the resistance encountered when two irregular surfaces are moved across each other. Friction makes even horizontal movement more difficult.

GUIDELINES FOR CORRECT BODY MECHANICS

As a nurse, you must apply your knowledge of stability, leverage, and motion so that you use the correct body alignment and effective body movements that will help you to prevent back injuries. Scientific principles related to these three areas are summed up in Table 29-1.

Correct Body Alignment

Body alignment, or **posture,** is the proper relationship of body parts to one another. Correct body alignment is important for proper body functioning, reduces strain, and helps maintain balance. When standing in correct alignment, as Figure 29-1 illustrates, the body is held in the following ways:

▶ back is straight
▶ head is erect, not leaning forward, backward, or sideways
▶ chin is tucked in, not jutting forward
▶ arms are at sides with elbows slightly flexed
▶ the lower abdominal area is pulled up and in
▶ buttocks are tucked under to prevent excessive curvature of the lumbar spine
▶ knees are slightly flexed
▶ toes are pointed forward

It is important to practice proper body alignment yourself and to demonstrate it to others. Also it is essential to position those people in your care in proper body alignment.

Effective Body Movement

Good body mechanics begins with proper body alignment and continues with adherence to several guidelines. These guidelines can be used in many of the

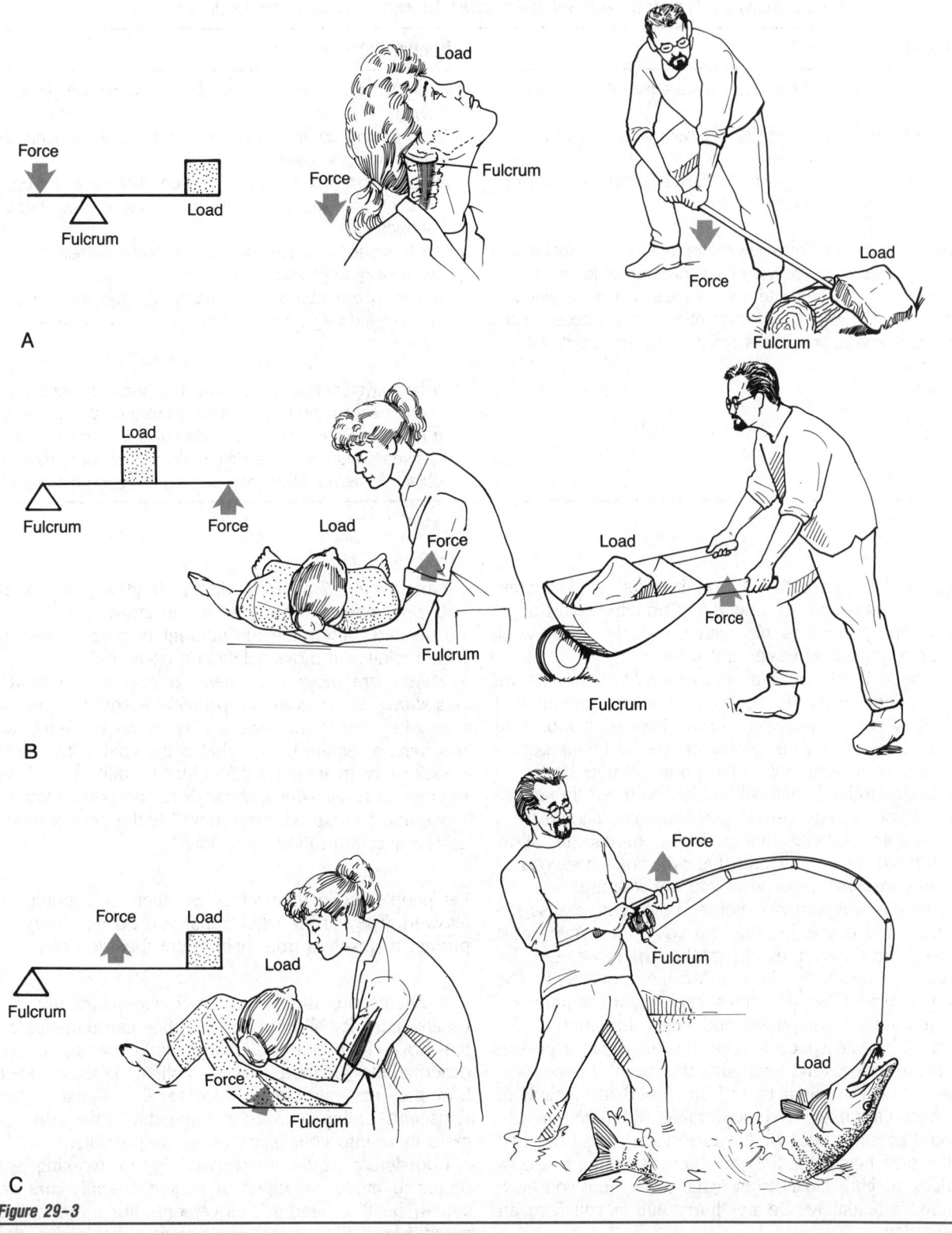

▲ *Figure 29-3*

Three classes of levers. *A,* Class I levers consist of a load on one end, a fulcrum in the middle, and downward force exerted on the opposite end of the lever (e.g., using a crowbar). The posterior cervical muscles contracting to lift the anterior head provide another example of class I levers. *B,* Class II levers consist of a fulcrum at one end, an upward or lifting effort at the other end, and the load in between (e.g., using a wheelbarrow). The use of the wrists as fulcra, the arms as levers, and an upward force on the arms to lift a helpless client provides another example of a class II lever. *C,* Class III levers consist of a fulcrum at one end, a load at the opposite end, and an upward or lifting force in the middle (e.g., a fisherman reeling in a fish). The contraction of the biceps muscles to apply a force between the elbows as fulcra and a load on the hand or lower forearm is another example of a class III lever.

TABLE 29-1. *Selected Scientific Principles and Related Nursing Interventions for Body Mechanics*

Principle	Nursing Interventions
The wider the base of support, the more stable the object.	When lifting clients or heavy objects, stand with your feet apart.
The lower the center of gravity, the more stable the object.	When picking up an object from the floor, squat rather than bend from the waist.
The closer the line of gravity to the center of the base of support, the more stable the object.	When reaching for something a short distance from you, do not let your line of gravity fall outside of your base of support
Leverage is the use of a lever supported on a fulcrum to move a load more easily by the application of force.	Use leverage whenever possible to reduce strain and prevent injury to yourself and others.
An object at rest tends to stay at rest, and an object in motion tends to stay in motion at a constant speed and along a straight line unless acted on by an outside force such as:	To turn heavy clients more easily, change the center of gravity and begin the turn that will tend to continue.
Gravity	To help overcome gravity, lower the head of clients' beds before attempting to slide them upward on the mattress.
Friction	To move a client more easily, decrease friction by applying powder to lubricate the skin, using a lift sheet to move the client, or rolling rather than pushing or pulling the client.

tasks you will have to perform in nursing. If you are able to understand the underlying principles and apply them appropriately as new situations arise, your work will be a good deal easier and safer.

Come to work dressed appropriately for lifting and moving. For example, you should wear clothing that will allow you to maintain a broad base of support and to squat to keep your center of gravity (your pelvis) low and over your base of support as necessary. Do not wear clothing that will subject you to embarrassment if you assume certain positions. You should wear comfortable clothing that is loose enough to allow freedom of movement and that will not cause you to be self-conscious about what you are wearing.

Plan your movements. Before beginning, assess the situation and determine the best (e.g., the safest, most efficient, and least difficult) method of movement. Be aware of the space allowed for the movement. The space available for the move can vary depending on the amount of equipment and other furniture in the room. Adequate space is important to move a person safely and effectively. Rearrange the room, if necessary. When moving a client to or from a bed, the height of the bed can make a considerable difference in the amount of effort you will have to make. Adjust the bed to the best height for the work you are going to do (a working height). Do not begin the move until you have planned adequately. Do not hurry unless you face an emergency.

Be realistic about your ability to lift the weight involved. Be aware of your personal abilities, muscle strength, and limitations.

Generally, nurses should not lift more than 35 per cent of their body weight without assistance. For example, a 60-kg (132-lb) nurse should not lift a load greater than 21 kg (46 lbs).[15]

Obtain help if at all in doubt about whether or not you can manage the move. If you know that help will be needed, determine the number of persons required to complete the move safely and correctly.

If you are moving a client, assess the amount of assistance the person can provide. Assess the person's strengths, limitations, and ability to move. Why does this person require help? What is the goal of the move? People vary in their weights (load), abilities, and willingness to assist with moves. Does the person want to move and to help with the move? Is the person able to understand and follow directions?

Let people move themselves as much as possible and allowed. They know what hurts; you do not. They can protect themselves from pain better than you can.

If clients are unable to move independently, it is usually safer for all concerned if they can participate in the move. To prepare clients for participation, carefully describe the planned moves to them. Discuss exactly how they can participate. Consider the clients' suggestions and preferences concerning the move and integrate them into your plans whenever possible.

Coordinate your movements. When working with others to move an object or person, identify one person to be the "leader." Movements are more coordinated when directed by one person. The leader clarifies what each person will do (e.g., "Debbie, you take his feet" or "I'll count '1-2-3-lift' and we'll all lift on the word 'lift'"). Following a leader's directions helps to ensure that the move is coordinated, with everyone beginning and moving at the same time, and that the move is safer for all concerned.

Maintain a broad base of support. Keep your feet apart to increase your stability. This stance also allows you to shift your weight readily from one foot to the other.

Keep your center of gravity low. Bending your knees while your feet are spread apart not only lowers your center of gravity but also widens your base of support to provide for extra stability and balance.

Be sure your line of gravity passes through the center of your base of support. You ensure the correct position by moving your center of gravity (pelvic area) directly over the space between your two feet. Alternatively, you can position your feet so as to widen your base of support, helping to ensure that it remains under your center of gravity. If you are shifting your weight (and center of gravity with it) as you move, you may move your line of gravity outside of your base of support unless you have planned correctly and widened your base of support before the move.

Use leverage to increase the efficiency of the energy you use. Levers help move heavy objects by decreasing the amount of force required to complete a lift and move. Nurses frequently use their elbows as fulcrums and their hands and arms as levers. To help lift a sick child and place a pad or bedpan under the child, for example, you might place your hands and forearms under the child's back and contract your biceps to lift the weight. These maneuvers use your body's natural levers.

Bring the load to be lifted or moved as close as possible to your center of gravity. Notice what happens to your body as you take a heavy bowling ball in one hand and hold it down by your side. Your head and shoulders shift and flex your spine in the opposite direction because the weight added to one side of your body by the ball has moved your center of gravity toward the ball, and you must move your body in the opposite direction to reestablish the center of gravity over your base of support. Failure to make such a

compensating move would make you unstable, and you would topple over unless you compensated in some other way (Fig. 29–4).

One way to compensate is to use your muscles to hold the ball in place at your side. This method, however, would cause a strain on your back muscles and on your leg muscles on the side holding the ball. A better way to compensate for the additional load on your body, without flexing your spine in the opposite direction, is to bring the ball as near as possible to your center of gravity by holding the ball in both hands in front of your body just below waist level. This position reestablishes your center of gravity over the center of your base of support and provides stability. However, what do you do if you cannot bring the object you want to move close to your center of gravity? For example, suppose the object to be moved is a stuck window you want to raise. In such a case, you should bring your center of gravity as close as possible to the windowsill. Even if the load to be lifted is not particularly heavy, bringing it closer to your center of gravity lessens the amount of work your muscles have to do to lift it. If you doubt this statement, try holding this textbook out at arm's length for awhile and then try holding it in, near your center of gravity. Compare for yourself which position is easier to maintain.

Move in a straight line and avoid twisting. When pushing or pulling an object or person, face the direction in which the movement will be made. Point your toes in that direction, placing one foot in front of the other to widen the base of support. Place the object in motion by exerting pressure on it as you move your body forward. For example, if you stand at the side of a person's bed and try to pull the person more toward the head of the bed, you should face the head of the bed and move toward the head of the bed. If you were to face the side of the bed and attempt to move the

▲ *Figure 29–4*

A combined center of gravity. *A,* The normal person's line of gravity runs through the center of gravity (at approximately mid pelvis) and down into the middle of the base of support. *B,* When the person picks up a heavy object, such as a bowling ball, the center of gravity of the combined person–bowling ball unit moves to a point between the person and the bowling ball. This position moves the line of gravity outside of the base of support and makes the person unstable. *C,* To reestablish stability, the person usually moves the upper body in the direction opposite the added weight. This position moves the center of gravity back and restores the line of gravity to its place at the middle of the base of support. In restoring stability, however, the person's posture has become distorted, and the back muscles have become strained.

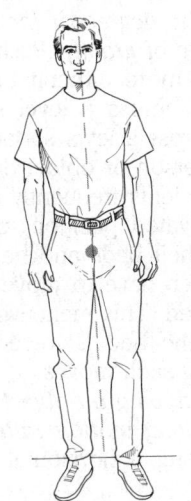
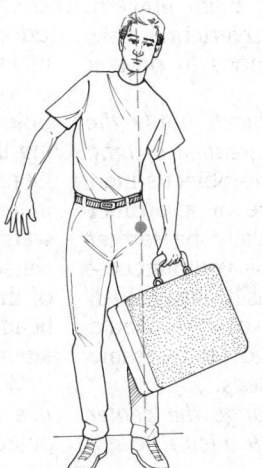
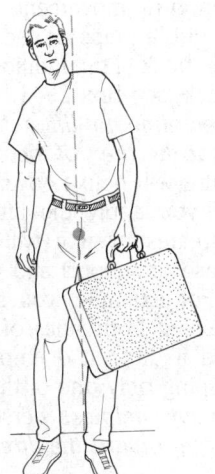

person toward the head of the bed, you might have to twist your back to complete the movement. Twisting movements can cause strains that can be severely painful and disabling.

Move heavy loads forward while maintaining a wide base of support. Once you have a good hold on a heavy object, it is close to your base of support, you are facing in the direction you wish to move, and your feet are apart with one leg in front of the other providing a wide base of support, you are ready to move. How do you move without lifting one foot to take a step (i.e., how do you lift one foot without causing the other foot to become the sole base of support)? When you do not have to move very far, you can simply shift your weight (and the weight of the load) from one foot (the one behind) closer to the other (forward) foot rather than taking a step to effect movement. Shifting your weight in such a manner avoids strain on muscles.

Use smooth, continuous, rhythmic movements. More energy is required to make many short movements than to make one continuous movement. Smooth rhythmic movements permit the efficient use of muscles by allowing more time for muscle contraction.

Use larger muscle groups, such as those in the legs and thighs, for heavier work. These muscles fatigue less quickly than smaller muscles, such as those of the arms and back. The use of long, strong muscles of the legs and thighs also helps to protect the back and prevent damage to the intervertebral disks (cushionlike structures between the vertebrae of the spinal column). These disks can be damaged when sudden or extreme force is exerted on them (e.g., by incorrectly lifting or trying to lift too heavy a weight).

Use your entire hand rather than your fingers. The hand has a broader area than individual fingers do, and hand muscles are stronger than finger muscles.

For longer tasks, change positions and alternate the larger muscle groups being used. Changing the muscles being used lessens the chance of fatigue in the muscles (e.g., bear weight more on your right leg for awhile and then shift to your left leg).

Put on your "internal girdle" before lifting and moving heavy objects. To put on your internal girdle, contract your abdominal muscles, so that you feel them move in and up, and contract your gluteal (buttocks) muscles in a firm movement, drawing them upward. The internal girdle helps protect the intervertebral disks of the lower back. For additional methods to protect the lower back, see Box 29–1.

When attempting to lift a heavy object, apply the lifting force at the area of the object's greatest weight. This procedure will help to overcome the object's inertial mass. If you apply the lifting force at any other point, the greatest weight will most likely be farther from your base of support and will cause you unnecessary strain. For example, you might easily lift a small table by grasping both sides of its top, but you would probably find it difficult or impossible to lift the same table by grasping only one of the table legs.

To roll heavy, helpless persons, change the center of gravity more toward the direction you wish it to go.

Box 29–1. Methods to Protect the Lower Back

To prevent lower back strain, keep the spine straight and prevent activities that cause an increased lordotic curvature of the lumbar spine (swayback).

▶ Avoid prolonged standing in one position. If standing is necessary, as for surgical nurses, who frequently cannot move very far during a long procedure, place one foot up on a stool to keep one hip flexed.

▶ Avoid bending forward at the hip without flexing the knees. It is especially harmful to lift something while in this position.

▶ Avoid sitting in a chair that places the knees at the level of or lower than the hips. Knees should be above hip level when seated, especially when driving.

▶ Avoid sleeping in the prone position (on the abdomen). If you must sleep in this position, place pillows below your abdomen to prevent strain on the spine. If possible, sleep on one side with hips and knees flexed or on the back with lower legs elevated on at least two large pillows.

▶ Avoid use of poor body mechanics at any time.

For example, before attempting to roll a completely helpless man to his left side, cross his right arm over his body toward the left side and cross his right leg over his left leg. The rest of his body will be easier to roll as it follows the limbs that have led the way.

To move a heavy object, rock it back and forth several times to help it gain momentum before providing the full effort necessary to move it where you want it to go. This maneuver shows that you can apply Newton's first law and start an object in motion with the understanding that it will tend to stay in motion.

Use pulling or pushing rather than lifting movements whenever possible. Pulling or pushing an object or person across a level surface uses less effort than lifting because lifting requires overcoming the effects of gravity, whereas pulling or pushing requires only overcoming the effects of friction.

When moving an object or person up an incline, change the degree of incline, if possible, to best take advantage of gravity. Pushing a person or object up an incline is more difficult than moving the same person or object across a level surface. Moving a person or object across a level surface is more difficult than sliding the person or object down an incline. For example, helpless clients frequently keep the heads of their beds in an elevated position, causing them to slide downward in their beds and be in abnormal body positions. Nurses then have to move them back toward the head of their bed. This maneuver is much easier to do if the head of the bed is lowered to a flat position before attempting such moves.

When moving an object across a horizontal surface, use a pulling motion rather than pushing. Pushing an object along a horizontal plane creates more friction

Text continued on page 554

PROCEDURE 29-1

Lifting an Object from the Floor

Definition/Purposes. Procedure enables nurses to pick up an object from floor level without self-injury. Two methods are presented.

Contraindications/Cautions. Assessment of the weight of the load is especially important. Persons with back problems should not use either of the following methods without first consulting with a physician.

Learning/Teaching Guidelines. To teach correct body mechanics to clients or to auxiliary personnel: (1) serve as a role model by always using good body mechanics, (2) carefully demonstrate the specific method to be used, (3) provide information about the correct use of muscles and ways to use leverage, and (4) supervise use of the method by those whom you have taught.

PRELIMINARY ACTIVITIES

Assessment/Planning

▶ Assess weight of the load to be lifted.
▶ Decide the lifting technique to be used.

PROCEDURE

Actions	Rationale/Discussion
1. Stand near object with feet a shoulder's width apart.	1. This stance places object nearer your center of gravity and provides a wide base of support. Line of gravity should run through center of base of support.
2. Put on internal girdle.	2. Internal girdle helps protect intervertebral disks.

Method 1	
a. Bend toward object by flexing at the hips and partially flexing at the knees. The back can be slightly curved.	a. This position lowers center of gravity.
b. Grasp object and bring it to thigh level by pulling with arm and shoulder muscles while thigh and leg muscles provide an upward thrust.	b. Muscles share the workload. Back muscles remain contracted to protect the intervertebral disks.
c. Bring object to waist level by using the leg and thigh muscles for greater thrust while beginning to straighten the back.	c. This brings load as close as possible to center of gravity.

Method 2	
a. Position feet 18 inches apart with left foot forward.	a. Position maintains wide base of support while allowing use of the left knee as a fulcrum.
b. Tuck chin in and squat down with back straight.	b. This protects intervertebral disks.
c. Grasp object with both hands, tipping it if necessary to attain balance.	c. This allows firm control of object.
d. Rest left elbow on left thigh, just above knee and apply pressure as needed to stand up. Straighten legs.	d. Position allows use of leverage.

PROCEDURE 29-2

Placing a Lift Sheet Under the Client

Definitions/Purposes. A flat sheet that has been folded into quarters and is free of wrinkles is placed under the helpless client to be used by nurses to help lift, move, and position the client as needed.

Contraindications/Cautions. Lift sheets may be left under helpless clients for future use only if they are absolutely free of wrinkles.

Procedure continued on following page

PROCEDURE 29–2 Continued

Placing a Lift Sheet Under the Client

Learning/Teaching Guidelines. Even if the client is unconscious, explain what you are going to do and why.

PRELIMINARY ACTIVITIES

Assessment/Planning

▶ Review diagnosis and activity orders.
▶ Review the chart for any contraindications to movement.
▶ Assess level of consciousness and ability to follow directions.
▶ Assess mobility level.
▶ Plan the move.
▶ Depending on the client's weight and condition, decide on the number of nurses or helpers needed and the actions of each; one person must be the leader.

Equipment

▶ one flat bed sheet
▶ firm mattress with clean, smooth, tightly tucked bottom linen
▶ side rails
▶ incontinence pad, if needed

Preparation of Person

▶ Discuss with client and helpers how the move will be accomplished.
▶ Provide privacy; avoid drafts.
▶ Adjust bed to working height to reduce back strain, lock wheels, and lower side rails.
▶ Cover client with bath blanket.
▶ Fan fold top linen to foot of bed.
▶ Provide for any tubes or attachments to the client to ensure that they are not accidently dislodged or pulled out when the client is rolled.
▶ Place mattress in level position if not contraindicated.
▶ Bathe client and change soiled linen if needed.

PROCEDURE

Actions	Rationale/Discussion
1. Fold flat sheet in quarters.	1. This provides four thicknesses of material for strength that is not possible with a draw sheet
2. Lower the side rail nearest you, and roll the client toward the opposite side rail.	2. Your body can prevent a client's fall on your side (an object in motion tends to stay in motion unless it is acted on by an outside force). Rolling overcomes friction. Rolling the person exposes the client's back and allows material to be tucked under the body more easily. The client can hold onto the opposite rail for security. The rail can also help prevent falls.
3. Fan fold half of the lift sheet by drawing it up into gathers in your hand.	3. As it is being gathered upward, the weight of the ungathered sheeting, hanging below your hands, will allow wrinkles to fall out of the material by gravity.
4. Place the fan-folded half under the client's back (between shoulders and midthighs) and smooth the other half on the bed behind the client's back.	4. Enough material must be under the client's back to reach to the other side of the bed after the client has turned back to the supine position.
5. Repeat Step 4 with an incontinence pad over the lift sheet, if needed.	5. Incontinence pads protect the bed linens in the event of involuntary loss of body excreta.
6. Roll the person back toward you, and reach over the person to pull out and smooth the lift sheet (and pad, if needed).	6. This method allows the placement of materials under the client with the least effort for client and nurse.
7. Roll the client back to the supine position.	7. Lift sheet should now be under the heaviest part of the client, free of wrinkles, and ready for use.
8. Keep a lift sheet under the client at all times for use as needed.	8. A lift sheet can assist in lifting or pulling a client to help reduce the effects of friction.

FINAL ACTIVITIES

Assess for pain or discomfort caused by the move; check client for correct body alignment; check any tubes present to be certain they are still in place and functioning correctly and secure them as necessary; check bed linen for smoothness; cover person; raise rails; lower bed; and discard soiled laundry as necessary. Document pertinent findings.

PROCEDURE 29-3

Shoulder Lift Procedure for Moving a Helpless Person in Bed

Definition/Purposes. Enables two nurses or helpers to move a dependent person to a position nearer the head of the bed.

Contraindications/Cautions. Shoulder lift procedure is not to be used to move a completely helpless client, a heavy client, or a client with injuries of (or recent surgery on) the shoulders, chest, or spine. Provide for catheters, intravenous catheters, and other tubes and attachments to the person's body by allowing enough slack to prevent anything from being dislodged by the movement.

Learning/Teaching Guidelines. To maintain or increase muscle strength, encourage clients to move themselves as much as they are able.

PRELIMINARY ACTIVITIES

Assessment/Planning

▶ Review diagnosis and activity orders.
▶ Review the chart for the presence of skin, muscle, bone, or joint lesions that would serve as contraindications for this procedure.
▶ Assess level of consciousness and ability to follow directions.
▶ Assess mobility level.
▶ Decide on the placement and actions of each nurse or helper; one person must be the leader.

Equipment

▶ Clean bed linens and gown, if needed before move
▶ Firm mattress with smooth, tightly tucked bottom linen

Preparation of Person

▶ Provide privacy; avoid drafts.
▶ Lock bed wheels.
▶ Cover client with bath blanket.
▶ Fan fold top linen to foot of bed, and provide for any tubes or attachments to the client.
▶ Move mattress to level position if not contraindicated.
▶ Bathe client, and change soiled linen if needed.
▶ Remove head pillow, and place it at the top of the bed near the headboard.
▶ Discuss with client and helper how the move will be accomplished.

PROCEDURE

Actions	Rationale/Discussion
1. Adjust height of bed to level between nurses' hips and knees if possible.	1. Height adjustment allows better leverage.
Caution Do not use this method for a completely helpless client, a heavy client, or a client with injuries of (or recent surgeries on) the shoulders, chest, or spine.	
2. With a nurse on each side of the bed, lower both side rails and assist client to a sitting position.	2. This allows proper arm placement. Nurses can prevent the client from falling.
3. Nurses stand slightly behind the client, facing the head of the bed, and place their shoulders next to the client's chest near the axillae (Fig. 29-5). Nurses' feet are apart and toes are pointing in the direction of movement. If the bed is very wide, the nurses may put their near knee (or even both knees) on the bed next to the client's hips.	3. Position places the client near the nurses' centers of gravity and the lifting force at the area of the client's greatest weight; this provides a wide base of support.
4. The client places an arm on the back of each nurse.	4. Arm placement shifts the client's weight and allows a secure hold on the client.
5. Nurses grasp each other's wrists under the client's thighs, very near the hips.	5. This step permits a stable, secure grip as close as possible to the client's area of greatest mass.
6. Nurses place their other hands on the mattress, behind the client, and keep their elbows slightly flexed. Alternatively, their hands may be placed on the headboard.	6. This step creates a fulcrum that helps shift weight effectively and allows the use of leverage.
7. Keeping their backs straight, on the count of three, the nurses lift the client between them as they shift their weight toward the head of the bed.	7. Keeping the back straight avoids strain. This step is an example of a Class II lever.
8. The helpers lower the client's upper body to the bed.	8. The client should now be at the correct place in the bed.

Procedure continued on following page

PROCEDURE 29–3 Continued

Shoulder Lift Procedure for Moving a Helpless Person in Bed

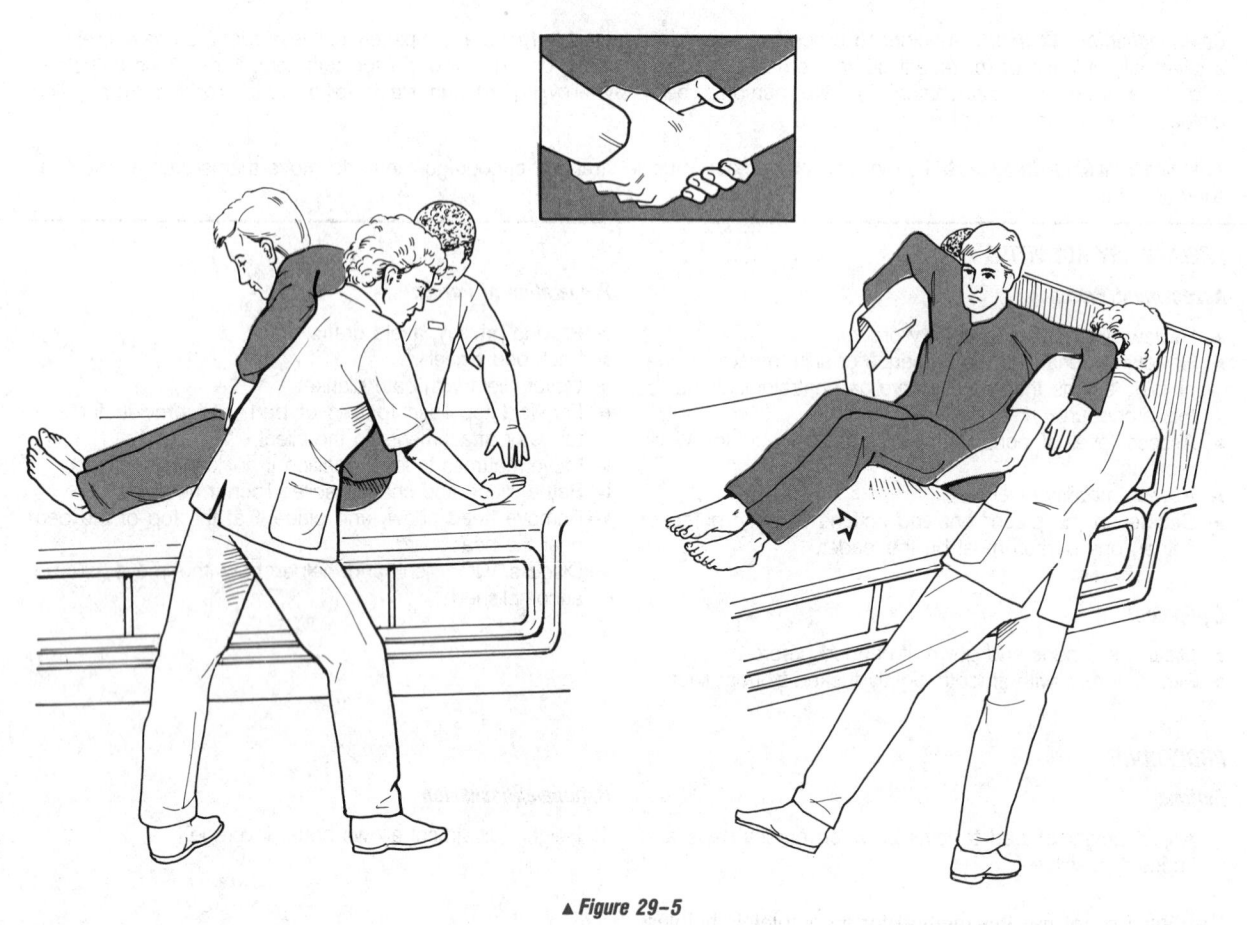

▲ Figure 29–5

FINAL ACTIVITIES

Assess for pain or discomfort caused or relieved by the move; check client for correct body alignment; check any tubes present to be certain they are still in place and functioning correctly and secure them as necessary; check bed linen for smoothness; replace head pillow and other positioning devices as needed; cover client; raise rails; lower bed. Document pertinent data.

PROCEDURE 29–4

Emergency Carries

Definition/Purposes. Enables the rapid removal of helpless people from dangerous situations (e.g., fires), without using equipment (e.g., stretchers).

Contraindications/Cautions. Persons with spinal injuries or respiratory aids cannot be safely moved by these methods. Assess the seriousness of the situation, the person's size and weight, and the number of helpers needed to move the person.

Learning/Teaching Guidelines. As time permits, (1) encourage people to move themselves if able, (2) explain method of transfer, (3) explain necessity for moving to a safer area, (4) assure persons you will stay with them until they are in a safe area.

PRELIMINARY ACTIVITIES

Assessment/Planning

Rapidly assess as time permits:

- ▶ level of consciousness
- ▶ abilities and limitations
- ▶ presence of equipment
- ▶ type and method of move
- ▶ person's comfort and safety

Preparation of Person

As time permits:

- ▶ explain move
- ▶ adjust bed to low position
- ▶ fold top linen to foot of bed
- ▶ cover with blanket

PROCEDURE

Actions	Rationale/Discussion

Blanket Drag

1. Blanket drag is done by one nurse and is the most effective one-person carry method.
  a. Lower bed to low position.
  b. Cradle person's head and shoulders in your arms and slide person to floor.
  c. Spread blanket along floor next to person. Raise person's arm beside head on side in direction of turn. Roll person onto side; slide blanket under person.
  d. Roll person back onto blanket. Place arms at sides, and wrap blanket securely around person.
  e. Grasp portion of blanket near person's head and drag to safe area (Fig. 29–6).
	1. Uses less energy to pull or slide person than to lift
	
	  a. Easier to slide person to floor
	  b. Supports head and neck; protects person from injury
	
	  c. Raising arm protects head while turning
	
	  d. Protects arms from injury during move
	
	  e. Supports head and neck

Pack-Strap Carry

2. Pack-strap carry is done by one nurse. Similar to "piggyback" carry.
 	
  a. Assist client to a sitting position on side of bed.
 	
  b. Face client. Grasp client's right wrist in your left hand and left wrist in your right hand.
  c. Pivot around, slipping under client's arm so client's chest is against your shoulders and client's arms cross over your chest (Fig. 29–7).
  d. Lean forward slightly.
 	
  e. Put one foot forward and stand up gradually.
  f. Walk to area of safety with client on your back.
	2. Assess client's weight and your strength. If client is too heavy for you to carry this way and help is not available, you must use blanket drag in extreme emergency.
	  a. If possible, allow time for adjustment to position change. This positions client for the carry.
	  b. This positions client's arms around you so they can be held to keep client on your back.
	  c. This positions client so your larger leg muscles will bear weight.
	
	  d. This helps center client's weight over your center of gravity.
	  e. This increases your base of support and stability.

Caution This is an emergency carry. The client should weigh much less than the normal adult. This carry would be most suitable for a helpless child.

Procedure continued on following page

PROCEDURE 29–4 Continued

Emergency Carries

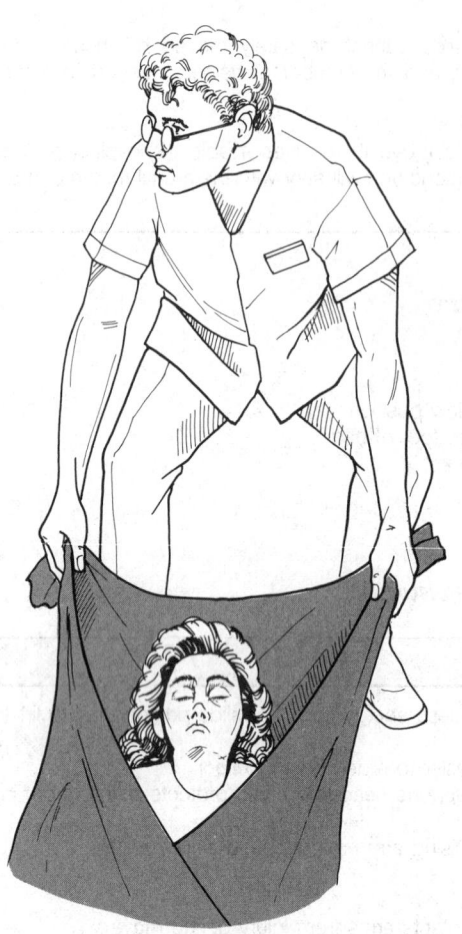

▲ *Figure 29–6*

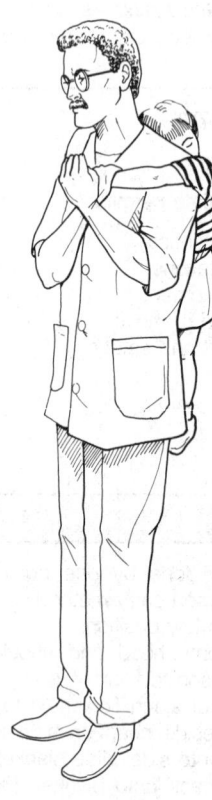

▲ *Figure 29–7*

Swing Carry

3. Swing carry is done by two nurses

   a. One nurse stands on either side of person.
   b. Place person's arms around shoulders of each nurse.

   c. First nurse places arm behind person's buttocks and grasps forearm of other nurse. First nurse grasps own forearm with other hand (Fig. 29–8).
   d. Second nurse places arm behind person's thighs and grasps forearm of first nurse. Second nurse grasps own forearm with other hand.
   e. Nurses carry person to area of safety.

3. Heavier people must be moved by two nurses. If emergency does not permit getting another helper, try to move person by blanket drag if possible.
   a. Provides stability on each side of person
   b. Helps distribute person's weight between nurses and stabilizes person onto each nurse's center of gravity
   c. Combined with Action d, forms "chair" for person to sit on

PROCEDURE 29–4 Continued

Emergency Carries

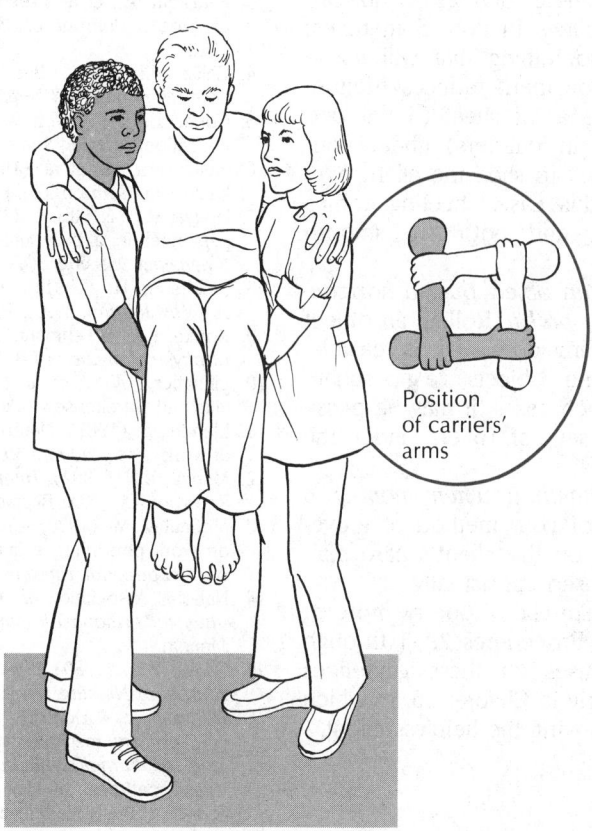

Position of carriers' arms

▲ Figure 29–8

FINAL ACTIVITIES

Leave blanket covering person, if appropriate. Assess person rescued for comfort level (was discomfort experienced during or after the move?), anxiety related to emergency transfer, body alignment (was alignment maintained during and after the move?), and safety (was the person injured during the emergency or during the move?).

than does pulling it. It is therefore easier to pull than to push.

When necessary, decrease friction before pushing or pulling an object across a surface. Decreasing friction can reduce your workload. Friction may be decreased by measures to smooth the two surfaces that will come into contact. Sometimes, cleaning, drying, or lubricating one or both surfaces reduces friction. Sometimes, covering one surface with something that will cause less resistance during the movement reduces friction. For example, you may place a lift sheet (a flat bed sheet that has been folded in quarters) under your client and pull on the lift sheet to slide the client over the surface of the bed. In this case, sheeting comes into contact with sheeting, and both are smooth enough to reduce friction.

If possible, when moving an object over a horizontal surface, roll it rather than pull it. Rolling an object creates less friction than pulling does. If it is feasible, rolling may be easier. Some objects (e.g., square boxes) do not roll well. In such cases, it may be possible to place one or more sets of rollers under the object to ease movement.

Maintain consistency of method when moving a client. Evaluate the success of your method of movement, and write the method on the client's care plan so the same method will be used consistently.

Some interventions that make use of one or more of these guidelines are given in Procedures 29–1 through 29–4. You will find more uses for these guidelines throughout the text, particularly in Chapter 35, in which we discuss positioning and moving the helpless client.

Summary

▶ For your own protection, as well as for the good of your clients and your employers, you must learn proper body mechanics and use them consistently in all of the work that you do.

▶ The stability of an object (including a nurse's body) is related to the relative positions of its base of support, its center of gravity, and its line of gravity. The correct use of leverage decreases the amount of work that must be done to move a heavy object or a person safely. The best application of Newton's first law of motion requires the nurse to understand and use methods to overcome gravity and friction.

▶ Correct body alignment is important to the safety of both nurses and clients. Good body mechanics begin with correct body alignment and continue with adherence to established guidelines for effective body movements.

Bibliography

1. Charney, W., et al. (1991). The lifting team: a design method to reduce lost time back injury in nursing. *AAOHN Journal*, 39(5), 231–234.
2. Dittmar, S.S. (ed.). (1989). *Rehabilitation nursing: Process and application*. St. Louis: C.V. Mosby.
3. Feldstein, A., et al. (1990). Evaluating the patient-handling tasks of nurses. *Journal of Occupational Medicine*, 32(10), 1009–1013.
4. Galka, M.L. (1991). Back injury prevention program on a spinal cord injury unit. *SCI Nursing*, 8(2), 48–51.
5. Gonet, L., & Kryzwon, A. (1991). Preventing back pain through education. *Nursing Standard*, 5(24), 25–27.
6. Heliövaara, M., et al. (1991). Determinants of sciatica and low-back pain. *Spine*, 16(6), 608–614.
7. Hogya, P.T., & Ellis, L. (1990). Evaluation of the injury profile of personnel in a busy urban EMS system. *American Journal of Emergency Nursing*, 8(4), 308–311.
8. Jacobson, H. (1991). Protecting the back during pregnancy. *AAOHN Journal*, 39(6), 286–291.
9. Kottke, F.J., & Lehmann, J.F. (eds.). (1990). *Krusen's handbook of physical medicine* (4th ed.). Philadelphia: W.B. Saunders.
10. Ljungberg, A.-S., et al. (1989). Occupational lifting by nursing aids and warehouse workers. *Ergonomics*, 32(1), 59–78.
11. Mandel, S. (1987). Neurologic syndromes from repetitive trauma at work. *Postgraduate Medicine*, 82(6), 87–92.
12. Marieb, E.N. (1992). *Human anatomy and physiology* (2nd ed.). Redwood City, CA: Benjamin/Cummings.
13. McCauley, M. (1990). The effect of body mechanics instruction on work performance among young workers. *American Journal of Occupational Therapy*, 44(5), 402–407.
14. National Association of Orthopaedic Nurses. (1991). *Core curriculum for orthopaedic nursing* (2nd ed.). Pitman, NJ: Anthony J. Jannetti.
15. Owen, B.D. (1980). How to avoid that aching back. *American Journal of Nursing*, 80, 894–897.
16. Piterman, L., & Dunt, D. (1987). Occupational lower-back injuries in a primary medical care setting: a five-year follow-up study. *Medical Journal of Australia*, 147(6), 276–279.
17. U.S. Department of Health and Human Services, Public Health Service. (1990). *Healthy people 2000: National health promotion and disease prevention objectives* (DHHS Publication No. PHS 91-50213). Washington, DC: U.S. Government Printing Office.
18. Venning, P.J., et al. (1987). Personal and job-related factors as determinants of incidence of back injuries among nursing personnel. *Journal of Occupational Medicine*, 29(10), 820–825.
19. Videman, T., et al. (1990). 1990 Volvo Award in Clinical Sciences. Lumbar spinal pathology in cadaveric material in relation to history of back pain, occupation, and physical loading. *Spine*, 15(8), 728–740.
20. Videman, T., et al. (1989). Patient-handling skill, back injuries, and back pain. An intervention study in nursing. *Spine*, 14(2), 148–156.
21. Walsh, N.E., & Schwartz, R.K. (1990). The influence of prophylactic orthoses on abdominal strength and low back injury in the workplace. *American Journal of Physical Medicine and Rehabilitation*, 69(5), 245–250.
22. Wollenberg, S.P. (1989). A comparison of body mechanic usage in employees participating in three back injury prevention programmes. *International Journal of Nursing Studies*, 26(1), 43–52.

▼ *Cardiopulmonary Resuscitation*

Chapter
30

▼

▼

In 1960 . . . the interaction of closed chest compression with mouth-to-mouth ventilation was developed as basic CPR, which offered hope for substantially reducing the nearly 1000 sudden deaths that occurred each day in the United States before the patients reached the hospital.

**Emergency Cardiac Care Committee and Subcommittees,
American Heart Association**

▼

▼

▼ CHAPTER OUTLINE

HISTORICAL PERSPECTIVE ON METHODS
   OF RESUSCITATION
CARDIOPULMONARY ARREST
      Normal Cardiopulmonary Function
      Failure of the Respiratory System
      Failure of the Cardiovascular
         System
      Clinical and Biologic Death
      Recognition of Cardiopulmonary
         Arrest
BASIC LIFE SUPPORT
      Sequence of Cardiopulmonary
         Resuscitation
      Two-person Rescue
      Performance Errors and Problems
         in Cardiopulmonary Resuscitation
INFANT AND CHILD RESUSCITATION
      Newborn Resuscitation

Causes of Infant and Child
         Respiratory Arrest
      Establishing an Airway
      Signs of Successful Ventilation
      Chest Compressions
      Compressions Mnemonic
COMPLICATIONS OF CARDIOPULMONARY
      RESUSCITATION
TERMINATION OF BASIC LIFE SUPPORT
ADVANCED LIFE SUPPORT
HELPING SIGNIFICANT OTHERS
SURVIVORS OF CARDIOPULMONARY
      ARREST
FOREIGN BODY AIRWAY OBSTRUCTION
      Recognition of Foreign Body Airway
         Obstruction
      Management of Obstructed Airway

▼ KEY TERMS

Acidemia
Anaerobic
Angina pectoris
Anoxia
Biologic death
Cardiac arrest

Cardiopulmonary arrest
Clinical death
Hemopericardium
Hypercarbia
Internal respiration
Intrathoracic pressure

Myocardial contusion
Myocardial rupture
Respiratory arrest
Ventilation

Maintenance of life has been a human concern throughout history. Over time, a variety of ingenious methods have been used in attempting resuscitation. Among these were burning feathers under a victim's nose, rolling a victim over a barrel, slinging victims over the backs of trotting horses, and intubating the trachea with a hollow reed and inflating the lungs with fireplace bellows.

The American Heart Association, in cooperation with the American Red Cross, the American College of Cardiology, and the National Heart, Lung, and Blood Institute, cosponsors ongoing reviews of basic life support (BLS) techniques and teaching methods. The content of this chapter is based on current guidelines. Because recommendations periodically change, however, it is a nursing responsibility to consult the American Heart Association's latest recommendations for BLS annually.

The major purpose of this chapter is to provide basic background information so that you can (1) recognize a cardiopulmonary arrest, (2) recognize people at risk for this emergency, and (3) apply the techniques of immediate life support for both adults and children. Also discussed in this chapter are the possible complications of cardiopulmonary resuscitation (CPR) and problems that may occur during basic life support.

Although this chapter presents the information necessary for successful CPR, repeated supervised practice using mannequins is essential to develop competency and to overcome a natural tendency to panic in emergencies. The American Heart Association and the American Red Cross require annual or biennial renewal of CPR certification.

Health professionals (including nurses) have a professional responsibility to be up-to-date in BLS skills and knowledge. In health care facilities, nurses often discover individuals who have had a cardiopulmonary arrest and must immediately initiate CPR. If your health care facility or school does not provide training and certification in BLS, contact your local chapter of organizations such as the American Heart Association and the American Red Cross for information.

HISTORICAL PERSPECTIVE ON METHODS OF RESUSCITATION

Modern immediate life support began in 1954 when it was discovered that mouth-to-mouth and mouth-to-nose ventilation was more effective than the back pressure methods of artificial respiration used previously. In 1960, it was found that chest compressions to circulate blood were successful. These replaced the previous method of opening the chest surgically to massage the heart. These methods have become known as CPR. CPR is now a significant part of emergency care for people experiencing **cardiopulmonary arrest** (cessation of heartbeat and respiration). Currently, health care professionals, firefighters, police officers, and rescue workers all use CPR skills.

Outside of hospitals, an estimated 76 per cent of cardiac arrests occur at home in the presence of family members who are not trained in CPR. This is unfortunate because, with proper training, anyone can perform CPR. The Medic II program instituted in Seattle, Washington, is one of the most widespread community education programs in the United States. Initially, more than 100,000 citizens were trained in CPR techniques. After training, the survival rate of people experiencing cardiopulmonary arrest rose significantly in Seattle. This and similar programs training thousands of people every year are offered in many communities. With training, immediate action is possible by people who are present when cardiopulmonary arrest occurs. Instead of waiting for emergency personnel, trained people can begin CPR immediately. Because irreversible brain damage may occur in 4 to 6 minutes, rapid response significantly increases the victim's chance of survival.

CARDIOPULMONARY ARREST
Normal Cardiopulmonary Function

The respiratory system provides the body with the oxygen (O_2) required for the normal function of every body cell. The lungs also eliminate carbon dioxide (CO_2) during cellular metabolism. The process of oxygen going into the blood and carbon dioxide coming out is called gas exchange, or respiration. In the lungs, gas exchange takes place through the alveolar capillary membrane. Normally, gas exchange is very efficient. All that is required is that ventilation and perfusion (blood flow) take place.

Ventilation is the movement of air in and out of the lungs. It is necessary for normal gas exchange but does not guarantee that effective gas exchange occurs. For example, despite adequate ventilation, gas exchange may not occur if lung tissue is diseased.

Internal respiration is a cellular process that occurs when oxygen moves from the blood into the cell and carbon dioxide leaves the cell and enters the blood to be carried back to the lungs to be expelled.

In short, the cardiovascular system is a gas-transport system that carries oxygen from the lungs to the cells and carbon dioxide from the cells back to the lungs, where it is expelled by expiration. The heart is a "pump," and the arteries, capillaries, and veins are "conducting pathways."

The respiratory and cardiovascular systems are interdependent. Consider that the heart consumes more oxygen than any other organ of the body except the brain. Consequently, when the lungs fail, the heart fails. Conversely, ventilation stops soon after the heart stops or soon after blood supply to the central nervous system is blocked. Ventilation may stop because the respiratory centers in the brain's medulla cannot function without a continuous oxygen supply, which is normally transported to them by the cardiovascular system.

Failure of the Respiratory System
ACUTE RESPIRATORY FAILURE

Acute failure of the respiratory system is marked by sudden hypoxemia (a fall in arterial oxygen, or Pao_2) and **hypercarbia** (a rise in arterial carbon dioxide, or $Paco_2$). An abrupt rise in $Paco_2$ results in respiratory acidosis, causing a fall in blood pH (acidemia). **Acidemia**, or "acid blood," is a condition caused by a disturbance in the acid-base balance of the blood, in which the blood is more acidic than normal. (Normal blood pH ranges from 7.35 to 7.45.) In this case, acidosis is due to the rapid accumulation of acids that are normally maintained at a safe level by the process of exhaling carbon dioxide.

CHRONIC RESPIRATORY FAILURE

When chronic respiratory failure occurs, the process of acid accumulation in the blood is slower, and there is time for the acids to be buffered (chemically altered to return them to a state more toward alkalinity than acidity). This buffering alters the blood pH so that the acid-base balance in the blood may be nearer to normal. The Pao_2 will remain low, however, unless treated by oxygen therapy.

RESULTS OF RESPIRATORY FAILURE

The Pao_2 is significant in either acute or chronic respiratory failure. If there is insufficient pressure of oxygen in the blood to load the hemoglobin molecules with oxygen, the content of oxygen (milliliters of oxygen/100 ml of blood) falls. Every 100 ml of blood passing through the heart normally carries 20 ml of oxygen. (The constant beating of the heart typically consumes 15 ml of this 20 ml.) When the heart fails to receive adequate oxygen, the electrical signal that causes cardiac muscle fibers to contract is disrupted and arrhythmias (variations in normal heartbeat patterns) occur.

In severe hypoxemia, **cardiac arrest** (cessation of the heartbeat) eventually occurs. This event is also called cardiac standstill or asystole.

Hypoxemia also affects all other body tissues, often causing symptoms that are noticed earlier than cardiac arrthymias. For example, confusion and disorientation are indications of cerebral hypoxia. These occur because the brain is even less tolerant of hypoxia than the heart. The brain is capable of only very limited **anaerobic** (without oxygen) metabolism. Consequently, thought processes are altered in moderate hypoxemia, and unconsciousness occurs quickly when hypoxemia is severe. When severe hypoxemia remains untreated, brain neurons begin to die. If too much brain damage occurs before hypoxemia is corrected, brain function will never again be normal. Neurons do not reproduce.

Peripheral tissues (skeletal muscles and organs) are more tolerant of hypoxemia than the heart and brain. Pyruvic acid and lactic acid, however, are produced when oxygen is insufficient for normal aerobic metabolism in peripheral tissues and organs. Thus, metabolic acidosis is added to the (usually) already present respiratory acidosis, further upsetting homeostasis. The specific respiratory and metabolic status of the body is determined by arterial blood gas (ABG) analysis.

Failure of the Cardiovascular System
SUDDEN CARDIAC ARREST

When the heart suddenly stops beating from causes other than hypoxemia (e.g., electrical shock or arteriosclerotic heart disease), the oxygen content of the blood may be normal at first. The oxygen concentration quickly changes, however. Cellular activity continues throughout the body and the oxygen in the blood is soon gone. Abrupt unconsciousness follows because of cerebral hypoxia, which is due to the lack of oxygen. Peripheral cells continue to metabolize but without oxygen, a process called anaerobic metabolism. Metabolic acidosis soon follows because the waste products of anaerobic metabolism are lactic acid and pyruvic acid.

If **respiratory arrest** (cessation of respiration) is recognized very quickly and ventilation is maintained, cardiac arrest may not occur. The respiratory center is less sensitive to hypoxia than the cerebral cortex. For instance, hypoxia of the cerebral cortex causes unconsciousness, but loss of consciousness can occur without respiratory arrest. Whether cardiac arrest occurs after respiratory arrest depends on how fast oxygen delivery is restored to the respiratory center. If oxygen delivery (through circulation) is delayed, respiratory arrest occurs and is followed quickly by respiratory acidosis because carbon dioxide is no longer eliminated by the lungs.

Because of their great interdependence, failure in one system (cardiovascular or respiratory) is soon apparent in the other. More important is the result of failure of either system on the brain, because the brain is more likely to experience permanent damage than are the systems that support it. Indications of impending arrest of the respiratory and cardiovascular systems are different, depending on which system is failing first. Failure of the respiratory system is often accompanied by confusion and delirium as a result of hypoxemia. If these symptoms are recognized and treated promptly, it may be possible to prevent the sequence of events leading to respiratory arrest. When a person exhibits abnormal or confused behavior, respiratory function (ABG levels) should be evaluated.

It can be unfortunate when abnormal or confused behavior is treated with sedatives or tranquilizers without looking for the cause of the symptoms. Often the treatment for this behavior is oxygen therapy.

Table 30–1 lists the common causes of cardiopulmonary arrest. Cardiopulmonary arrests can occur anywhere at any time—at work, at home, or on vacation.

CORONARY ARTERY DISEASE

Coronary artery disease is the most frequent cause of cardiac arrest and is also associated with an early symptom. **Angina pectoris** (also called angina) is chest pain produced by hypoxic heart muscle. In angina pectoris, hypoxia is often localized to the heart muscle itself. Hypoxia results from insufficient blood flow through narrowed or clogged vessels rather than generalized hypoxemia (low blood oxygen) caused by respiratory failure. People do not often ignore pain, so angina pectoris is usually brought to the attention of health professionals.

Clinical and Biologic Death

Clinical death occurs with cessation of blood flow or respiratory arrest. It is manifested by reversible loss of

TABLE 30–1. Events That Frequently Lead to Cardiopulmonary Arrest

Mechanism	Event
Impaired airway	Severe hypoxia
	Severe hypercarbia
	Upper airway obstruction
	Massive aspiration of gastric contents
	Near drowning
Impaired circulatory system	Air embolism
	Pulmonary embolism
	Thrombus formation
	Hemorrhage
Impaired cardiac function	Idiopathic dysrhythmias and other forms of cardiac dysfunction
	Electrical shock
Idiosyncratic reactions	Anaphylactic reaction resulting from idiosyncratic drug interactions, bee stings, allergic response to medications or anesthetics
	Overdose of barbiturates or other sedatives, tranquilizers, analgesics, or recreational drugs
Altered state of homeostasis	Electrolyte imbalance
	Severe acidosis
	Hypothermia/hyperthermia

consciousness. **Biologic death,** however, is marked by irreversible destruction of brain tissue. Prevention of biologic death is the goal of CPR. Resuscitation depends on prompt recognition of clinical death and immediate and skilled support of the respiratory and cardiovascular systems.

Cerebral ischemia lasting 3 to 4 minutes produces permanent brain damage. Cerebral ischemia that lasts for 5 to 6 minutes results in biologic death with no return to life except in rare circumstances involving hypothermia.

Figure 30–1 illustrates the bridge between life and death and the way this pathway may be reversed with CPR. Notice the importance of time in the development of brain and other organ impairment and biologic death.

Recognition of Cardiopulmonary Arrest

AN UNCONSCIOUS PERSON

A person may be unconscious for many reasons, but sudden and unexpected unconsciousness is often caused by cardiopulmonary arrest. Resuscitation usually will not hurt a person who is suddenly unconscious for reasons other than cardiopulmonary arrest. On the other hand, failure or slowness to initiate CPR can cause residual brain damage after recovery from arrest.

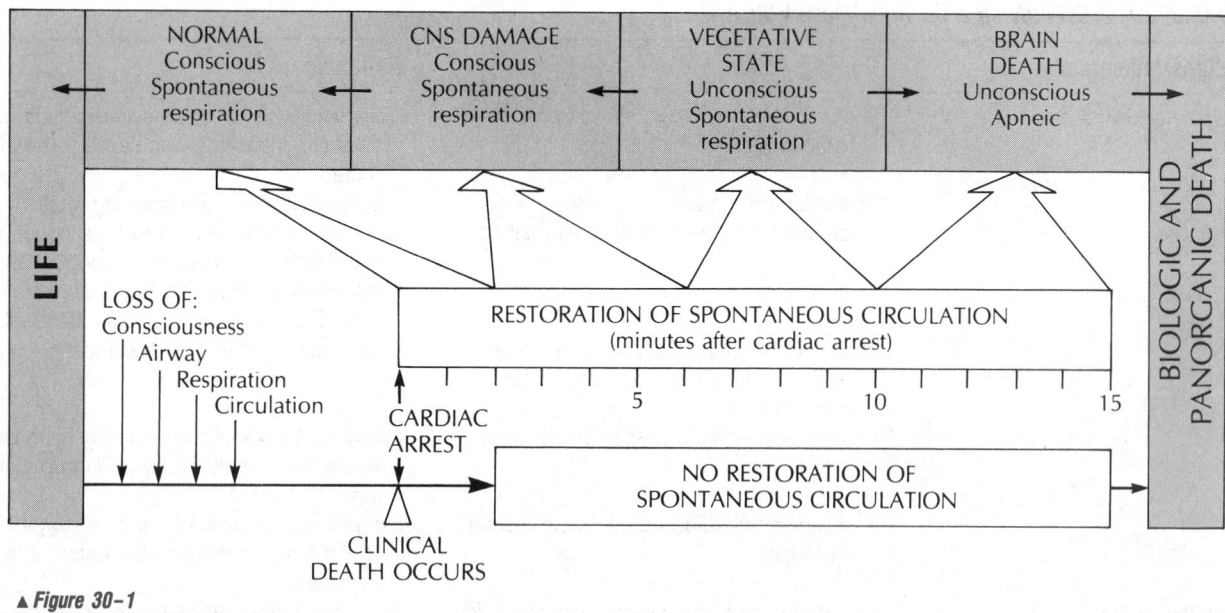

▲ Figure 30-1

Bridge from life to death and reverse pathways with resuscitation.

The most common cause of failed CPR is failure to recognize a cardiopulmonary arrest.

Table 30-2 lists the steps necessary to determine whether a cardiopulmonary arrest has occurred. Appropriate actions and their rationale are also listed. The rescuer must memorize these vital actions. There is a narrow time limit between recognition of clinical death and actual biologic death, so you must act quickly.

IMPENDING CARDIAC ARREST

Clinical indications of impending cardiopulmonary arrest are listed in Table 30-3. These may also be evidence of other problems. All indications should be carefully assessed for possible causes.

BASIC LIFE SUPPORT

CPR techniques are divided into two categories or levels. These are basic and advanced life support techniques. This chapter is concerned primarily with BLS, the "first aid" for cardiac or respiratory arrest (see Procedure 30-1). Knowledge of BLS procedures are recommended for the lay public as well as for all health care professionals.

Sequence of Cardiopulmonary Resuscitation

CPR for BLS has developed into a formal sequence of actions, simplified into the mnemonic (a group of words or letters that assist with remembering something) "ABC." This mnemonic stands for airway, breathing, and circulation, the order in which CPR ac-

tions are taken in most arrests. Table 30-2 summarizes the recognition of cardiopulmonary arrest and the initial steps in the ABC sequence (establish an *a*irway, begin rescue *b*reathing, and restore *c*irculation with cardiac compressions). Basic steps and actions must be learned and practiced repeatedly on appropriate mannequins.

An important change in the 1992 American Heart Association guidelines is that the first step in the process of the BLS protocol is to activate the emergency medical system before establishing an airway, when discovering an unconscious victim, or when witnessing a collapse.[14] In the pediatric protocol, it is still recommended to administer 1 minute of CPR before activating the emergency medical system.

The ABC sequence is carried out in this order so that oxygen is increased in the lungs and blood is then "pumped" to the brain. Air must be delivered to the lungs first to provide oxygen to the newly reestablished or artificially supported circulation as it passes through the lung.

A: AIRWAY

During cardiac arrest, all muscles are relaxed, including jaw muscles. This relaxation causes the tongue to fall back and obstruct the airway. The tongue is the most common cause of airway obstruction. Sometimes this obstruction is noticeable if the person is still trying to breathe. In such situations, retractions of the soft tissue of the chest wall will be seen in the suprasternal, supraclavicular, and intercostal areas, and abdominal muscles will contract. If food or vomitus is obviously obstructing the airway, turn the person on the back,

TABLE 30-2. Identifying a Cardiopulmonary Arrest*

Signs/Indicators	Nursing Action	Rationale
Unconsciousness	Shake victim's shoulder; shout victim's name in ear.	Determine whether unconsciousness is due to arrest. Hearing is last sense to be affected.
	Roll victim onto back.	It is easier to carry out following steps.
No respirations (apnea)	Open airway by head tilt–chin lift method.	Head tilt–chin lift method relieves upper airway obstruction caused by tongue falling into posterior pharynx. Respiratory status may return and avoid cardiac standstill.
	Lean over victim, place your cheek near victim's mouth, turn your face toward victim's chest.	Look, listen, and feel for respirations.
	Quickly bare victim's chest if easily done.	Allows better visualization of chest. Do not waste time, however, by pulling up clothing.
	If no respiratory effort noted, begin rescue breathing.	Exhaled air contains 16 per cent oxygen. Blood must be oxygenated before it is circulated.
Absent pulse	As rescue breathing begins, also check for pulse. Absent pulse indicates need for cardiac compressions. Feel for either carotid or femoral pulse.	Peripheral pulses are often absent during cardiac distress. When palpating carotid artery, palpate artery closest to you. To locate carotid artery, place two fingers gently over cricothyroid cartilage and move toward ear closest to you.
Absent spontaneous respiration or heartbeat	Institute cardiopulmonary resuscitation. Place victim on hard surface.	Resuscitative efforts must be begun within narrow time frame of clinical and biologic death to reduce irreversible effects of no oxygen or circulation on brain and other vital organs.

* Memorize these facts.

open the mouth, and scoop it out with two fingers. If the airway is not obstructed by food or vomitus, turn the person on the back, remove pillows, and then open the airway by one of the following methods:

Head Tilt–Chin Lift Method. Position yourself at the person's side. Place one hand on the person's fore-

TABLE 30-3. Indications of Impending Cardiopulmonary Arrest

Cause	Indications
Cerebral hypoxia	Confusion, disorientation, restlessness, feeling of impending doom, loss of consciousness
Ineffective cardiac output	Weak, feeble, or absent pulse; hypotension; bradycardia; ventricular arrhythmias; chest pain
Respiratory impairment	Shortness of breath, abnormal pattern of ventilation; agonal respiratory effort
Peripheral indications	Change in skin color (cyanosis); change in skin temperature (cold and clammy or cold and dry); weak peripheral pulses; decreasing urinary output

head. Place the other hand under the bony portion of the lower jaw at the chin. While pushing downward on the forehead, push upward on the chin to support the jaw and help tilt the head back (Fig. 30-2A–C). Do not press deeply into the soft tissue under the chin. The mouth should not be completely closed unless you are using mouth-to-nose breathing.

Jaw Thrust Method. The jaw thrust without head tilt is the safest first approach to opening the airway of a person who has a suspected neck injury, because the technique does not involve neck flexion. Place yourself at the person's head. Place your fingers (of both hands) behind the angle of the jaw and lift the jaw forward. Carefully support the head without tilting it backward or turning it from side to side (see Fig. 30-2D). If ventilation cannot be successfully accomplished with this modification, tilt the head back slightly and try to ventilate the person again. The priority is to not increase damage to an injured spinal cord by moving the head.

Research[14] from 1960 to 1980 has shown that the head tilt–chin lift method produces the best airway. In addition, this technique is less tiring than the jaw thrust method. Minimizing fatigue is important for a rescuer who is maintaining the airway and providing ventilation, because this position must be maintained throughout CPR, which may last a long time.

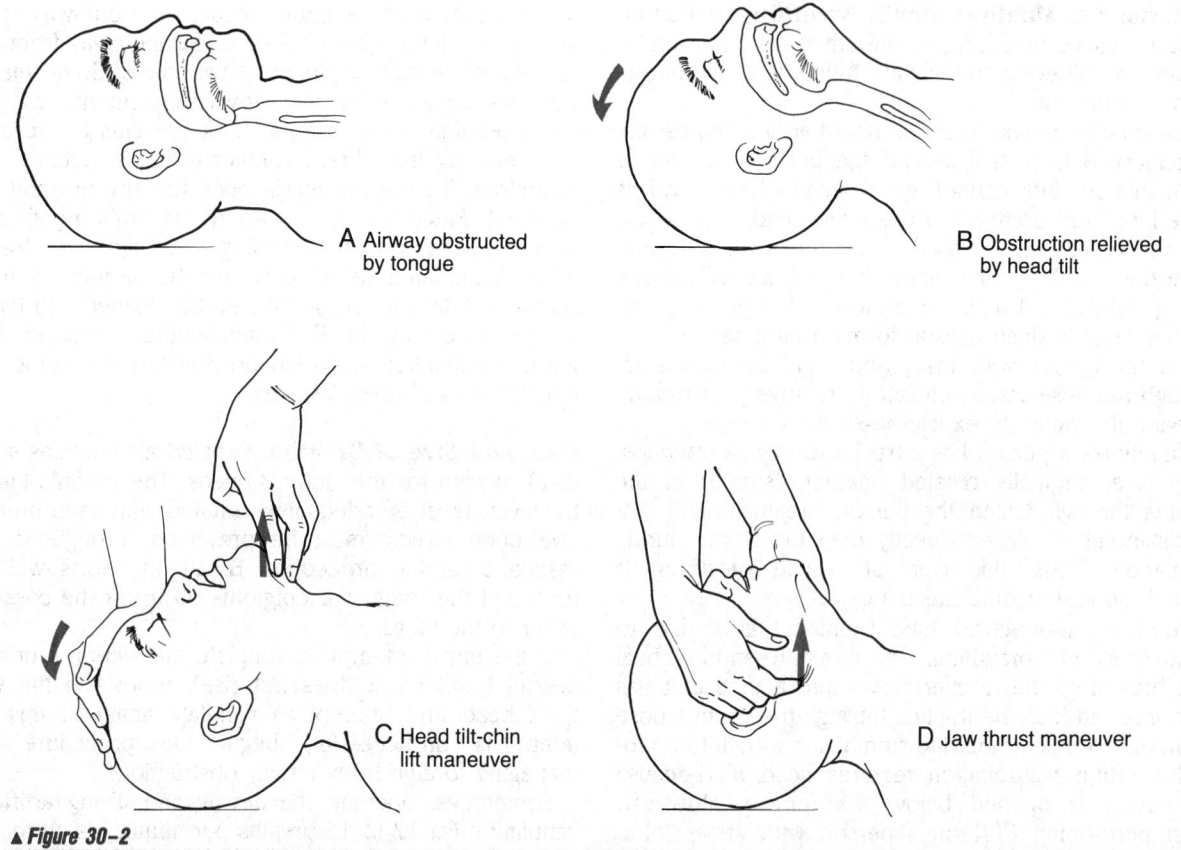

A Airway obstructed by tongue

B Obstruction relieved by head tilt

C Head tilt-chin lift maneuver

D Jaw thrust maneuver

▲ **Figure 30–2**

Opening the airway—two techniques. The tongue is the most common cause of airway obstruction. By performing one of these maneuvers, the tongue is pulled forward away from the posterior pharynx, thus opening the airway. This is the airway portion of the ABCs of CPR. Note that the jaw thrust maneuver may be performed either while tilting the head back or without head tilt, depending on the person's condition.

B: BREATHING

Immediately place your cheek close to the person's mouth so that you can feel the breath and watch the chest. If opening the airway is not promptly followed by spontaneous breathing, start artificial ventilation.

Although studies have concluded that it is unlikely that the human immunodeficiency virus may be contracted from performing mouth-to-mouth ventilations, other pathogens may be transmitted by mouth-to-mouth contact. All CPR courses should include instruction on the use of a pocket mask. An inexpensive, easy-to-carry mask prevents direct contact with the victim's oral mucosa and decreases the chance of transmission of pathogens. The Centers for Disease Control in Atlanta recommends the use of barrier devices, such as a bag-valve mask, mechanical ventilation equipment, and other resuscitation masks with valves that divert air away from the rescuer.[14] Although the effectiveness of pocket masks has not been determined, it is advisable to carry your own mask because unforeseen situations may arise at any time.[14]

Mouth-to-Mouth Breathing. The simplest and fastest way to establish ventilation is mouth-to-mouth respiration. Once you have opened the airway, using the head tilt–chin lift maneuver or jaw thrust maneuver, use your thumb and index finger (of the hand on the victim's forehead) to gently pinch the nostrils closed. Pinching the nostrils prevents air from escaping through the nose during ventilation. Take a deep breath. Create an airtight seal with your lips around the victim's mouth. Give two slow breaths lasting 1.5 to 2 seconds each. Allow exhalation to be completed between breaths. Complete exhalation should decrease the chance of gastric distention, regurgitation, and aspiration.[14]

Artificial ventilation is successful if you can (1) see the person's chest rise, (2) feel the inflation (compliance) of the lungs as they fill with air, and (3) feel the person exhale air.

Each ventilation should be of an adequate volume to make the victim's chest rise. Adequate volume is usually about 800 cc for an adult. Indicators of adequate ventilation are the rise and fall of the chest and air escaping during exhalation. You can feel and hear the air.

Rescue breathing (for both one-person and two-person CPR) is 10 to 12 breaths per minute. In one-person CPR, the rescuer pauses for two rescue breaths after the 15th compression of the chest. In two-person CPR, rescuers provide one rescue breath after the fifth compression.

Variations of Mouth-to-Mouth Breathing. Variations of basic rescue breathing are mouth-to-mouth, mouth-to-stoma, mouth-to-endotracheal tube, and mouth-to-barrier ventilation.

Use mouth-to-nose resuscitation when it is impossible to achieve a tight seal around the person's mouth or when the mouth cannot be opened. One hand is placed on the forehead to keep the head tilted back, and the other hand is used to lift the lower jaw and close the mouth. (If the mouth is open, air will escape during ventilation.) As in mouth-to-mouth breathing, the rescuer takes a deep breath, forms a tight seal around the victim's nose with the mouth, and blows the air through the nose. After ventilation, remove your mouth, allowing the victim to exhale passively.

Sometimes a person has a tracheostomy. A tracheostomy is a surgically created opening (stoma) in the trachea through which the person breathes. The rescuer's mouth is placed directly over the stoma during ventilation. Thus, this type of rescue breathing is termed mouth-to-stoma breathing.

Mouth-to-endotracheal tube breathing is similar to mouth-to-stoma breathing. In mouth-to-endotracheal tube breathing, the rescuer blows into a tube that has been inserted into the trachea through the client's nose or mouth. Neither mouth-to-stoma nor mouth-to-endotracheal tube resuscitation requires head tilt because the airway is opened below the tongue. However, when performing CPR on a person with an endotracheal tube, hold the mouth and nose closed to prevent escape of the rescuer's breath if the tube does not have an inflatable cuff.

Mouth-to-Barrier Device Breathing. The technique for mouth-to-barrier device breathing uses two kinds of barrier devices: masks and face shields. The transparent mask shown in Figure 30–3 is a type of collapsible pocket mask with a mouthpiece and a one-way valve

that is considered desirable because the one-way valve allows the victim's exhaled air to escape away from the rescuer. Face shields do not have valves. Some masks have an oxygen inlet that allows supplemental oxygen to be administered. Using a mask prevents the rescuer from coming into direct contact with the victim's oral secretions. To use the mask, open the airway using the head tilt. Place the mask over the victim's mouth and nose. Be sure you are providing an airtight seal. Ventilation is initiated using slow breaths lasting 1.5 to 2 seconds. After use, masks should be cleaned and disinfected according to the manufacturer's instructions. Further evaluation needs to be done to determine the effectiveness of these devices.

Rate and Size of Breaths. Exhaled air contains sufficient oxygen for the victim's needs. The victim's lungs, however, must be adequately inflated with each breath. The open airway must be preserved throughout the rescue breathing procedure. Breathing efforts will be useless if the tongue or epiglottis obstructs the passage of air to the lungs.

If the initial attempt to ventilate the victim is unsuccessful (e.g., chest does not rise), reposition the victim's head and attempt to ventilate again. If this attempt is unsuccessful, begin the procedure for managing foreign body airway obstruction.

Sometimes, opening the airway and giving artificial ventilation (at 12 to 15 breaths per minute) is all that is necessary to restore consciousness because the blood, although hypoxemic, is still circulating. If hypoxemia is reversed (by opening the airway and/or giving artificial ventilation) and the myocardium is reoxygenated, effective pumping action resumes before cardiac arrest occurs.

C: CIRCULATION

While opening the airway and giving the first breaths, also feel for the person's carotid pulse on the same side as the rescuer. If the pulse is absent or questionable, start external cardiac compressions (i.e., artificial circulation).

The person must be flat on the back on a hard surface for external cardiac compression to be effective.

Artificial circulation of blood is possible because closed-chest compression produces a generalized increase in **intrathoracic pressure** (pressure within the chest cavity). This increase in intrathoracic pressure is the basis for the mechanism that keeps blood flowing forward through the heart and lungs to the brain and the rest of the body.

Figure 30–4 illustrates the anatomic location of the heart in relation to the spine and the sternum. If the person sinks into a soft mattress (instead of being correctly placed on a hard surface), it is difficult to evaluate the amount of sternal depression obtained during each compression and thus the amount of the intrathoracic pressure generated. The person must be horizontal because blood pressure generated by exter-

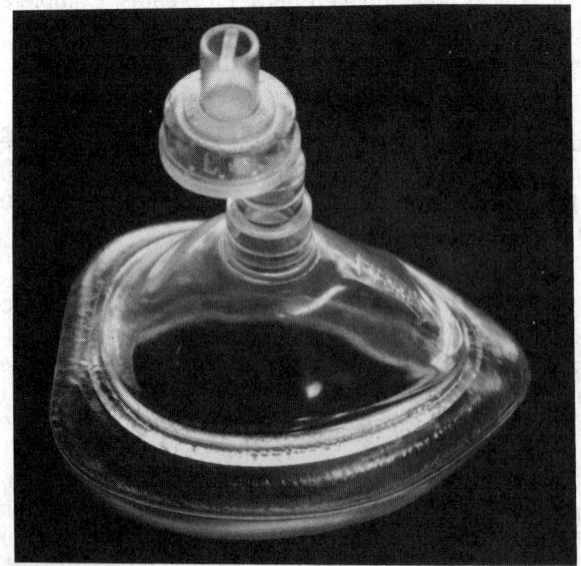

▲ *Figure 30–3*

A pocket mask.

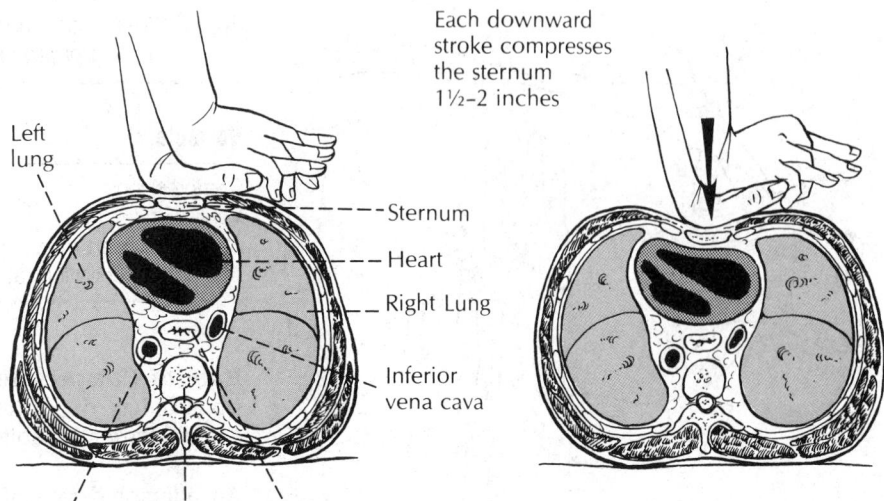

Each downward stroke compresses the sternum 1½–2 inches

Left lung — Sternum — Heart — Right Lung — Inferior vena cava

Aorta   Spine   Esophagus

▲ *Figure 30–4*

Cross section of thorax during CPR. During the chest compression phase of CPR, the sternum is depressed 1½ to 2 inches. The downward stroke of the compression should equal 50 per cent of the compression cycle. The upward, relaxation stroke equals the remaining 50 per cent of the cycle. Blood flow occurs because the intrathoracic pressure changes during the compression phase. During the relaxation phase, the heart fills with blood, ready for the next compression.

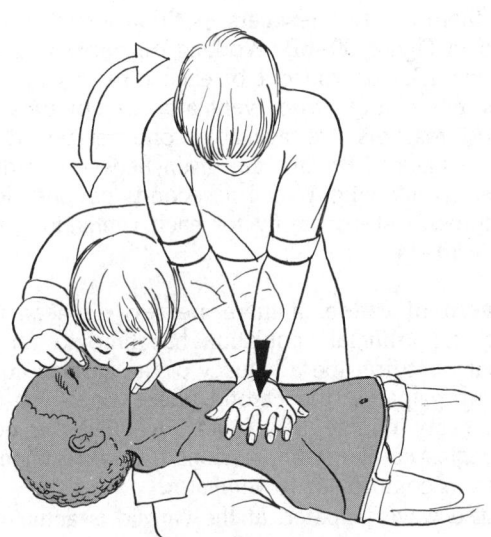

A. Single rescuer

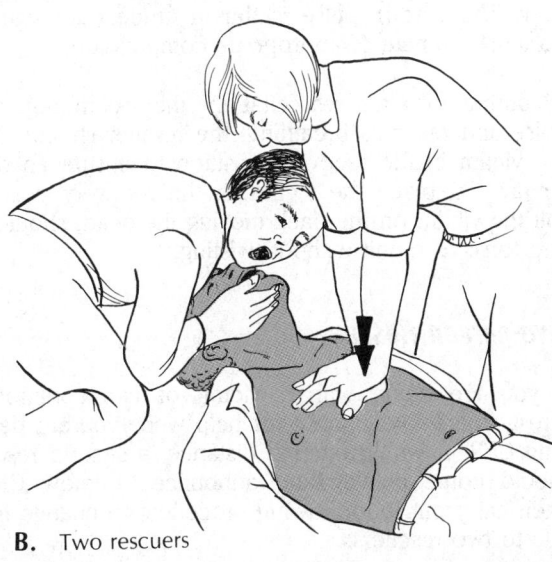

B. Two rescuers

▲ *Figure 30–5*

Positions used for CPR when there are one or two rescuers. *A,* One rescuer. Rescuer's shoulders and arms must be directly over person's sternum. This position allows best compression and is less tiring for the rescuer. The single rescuer alternates 15 chest compressions with two ventilations. *B,* Two rescuers. Positioning themselves on opposite sides of the person facilitates changing roles (as compressor or ventilator) without losing the rhythm.

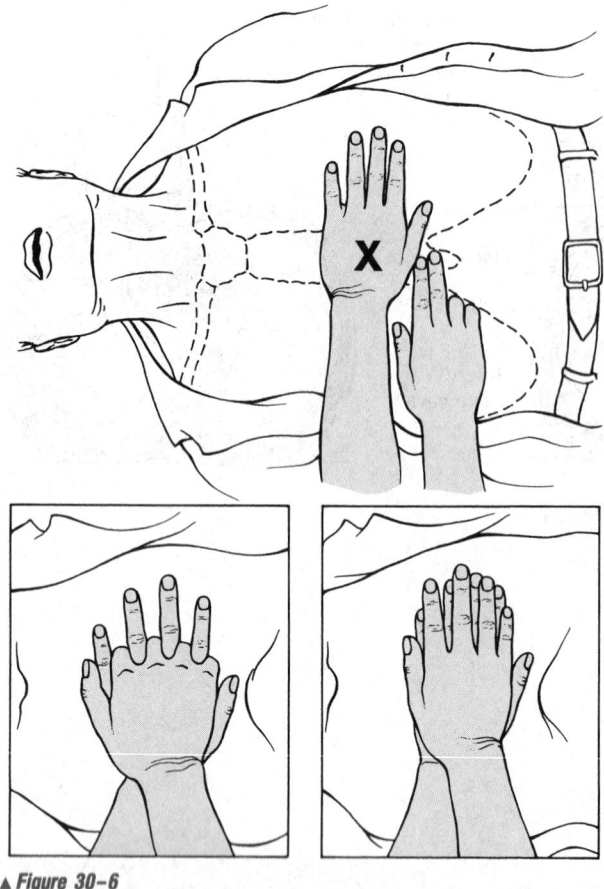

▲ Figure 30-6

Hand and finger positions for chest compressions. *A,* Thoracic landmarks used to locate correct hand position for compression. If on client's right side, slide fingers of your right hand along person's costal margin to locate the xiphoid process. Place your left hand as shown, with thumb next to fingers, on the xiphoid process. Place your right hand on top of your left hand. *B,* Fingers may be either interlaced as shown here or extended as shown in *C. C,* The force of compression must always be downward through heel of hand. Keep fingers lifted off chest.

nal compression is not adequate to pump blood up to the head when the person is seated. If the person is seated in a chair, slide the person to the floor. The position for a single rescuer is shown in Figure 30-5. If the person is in bed, quickly look for a large, firm, flat object to slip under the thorax. A food tray may serve as a temporary board. Many newer hospital beds have removable head or foot sections to use for CPR. If nothing is at hand, do not delay. Correct hand placement for cardiac compressions is important. If too low, the xiphoid process may be fractured and driven into the upper abdomen, damaging the liver, spleen, or stomach. If too high, compressions are not effective because the upper sternum is rigid and difficult to depress (Fig. 30-6A). Begin heart compressions promptly, and observe the chest carefully during compression to see whether the sternum is actually being depressed 3.75 to 5 cm (1.5 to 2 in.) with each compression.

Do not practice breathing or cardiac compressions on a living person. Use only mannequins designed for the purpose.

TABLE 30-4. Cardiopulmonary Resuscitation Compression-to-Ventilation Ratio

Variable	Single Rescuer	Two Rescuers
Compressions	15	5
Ventilations	2	1
Attempted heart rate	80–100/min	80–100/min
Attempted ventilation rate	12/min	12/min

Rate of Compression. The rate of cardiac compressions differs depending on whether one or two rescuers are present (Table 30-4).

An attempted rate of 80 to 100 compressions and 12 ventilations per minute is difficult for a single rescuer to maintain for long. Obtain help as soon as possible. Shout loudly for help, even in the quiet setting of a hospital.

When there are two rescuers, position yourselves as illustrated in Figure 30-5B. Working on opposite sides of the person keeps you out of each other's way and facilitates the change from ventilator to compressor. When two rescuers are available, one rescuer does artificial ventilation. Breaths are given between cardiac compressions allowing 1 to 1.5 seconds per inflation. The compressor stops briefly for each ventilation (see Procedure 30-1).

Assessment of Pulse. If there are two rescuers, the person giving artificial ventilation has time to assess and partially confirm the adequacy of the cardiac compression by palpating the carotid pulse. Make this assessment every couple of minutes, whenever a new rescuer begins cardiac compressions or after a change of roles from compressor to ventilator.

The pulse wave palpated at the carotid is actually a shock wave produced by cardiac compression, and it does not definitely confirm blood flow. Without such a shock wave, however, there is no possibility of blood flow. The carotid pulse is thus a crude (although important) estimate of appropriate compression.

If, during or after resuscitation, the victim regains a pulse and resumes breathing, the rescuer should place the victim in the recovery position to ensure an open airway. To place the victim in the recovery position, roll the victim on the back moving the head, shoulders, and torso as a unit without twisting.[14]

Two-person Rescue

If you are alone with a victim of cardiopulmonary arrest, immediately shout for help while you are beginning CPR. If within hearing distance, a second rescuer should come quickly and announce "I know CPR." Then carry out the following procedure to change from one to two rescuers.

Text continued on page 568

PROCEDURE 30–1

Basic Cardiopulmonary Resuscitation

Definition/Purposes. Basic cardiopulmonary resuscitation (CPR) is a series of first aid procedures, including recognition and treatment of circulatory and respiratory arrest, capable of maintaining life until advanced life support is available. CPR provides artificial ventilation and circulation to a person experiencing cardiac and respiratory arrest. Procedures are modified depending on the presence of one or two rescuers; whether the victim is an infant, child, or adult; and the nature of the arrest (e.g., respiratory arrest [without circulatory arrest]).

Contraindications. Do not resuscitate when a decision not to resuscitate has been noted in the chart. This order is often abbreviated to "DNR" (do not resuscitate), is sometimes referred to as "no code," and is now discussed with the client on admission and is referred to as "an advanced directive."

Learning/Teaching Guidelines. Because of the emergency nature of this procedure, it is seldom possible to explain the procedure to the person before its use. Significant others, however, need information. If they are present at the time of the arrest, explain (1) why the person is receiving such apparently "rough" treatment (e.g., being put on the floor); (2) the necessity of having a hard surface under the person's thorax; (3) the expected results of artificial ventilation and circulation; (4) why the rescuers are counting together; (5) why it is necessary to push "so hard" on the sternum; and (6) that struggling motions made by the victim are a good sign but do not necessarily indicate that the emergency is over. Significant others may be taught CPR if living with a person who may experience cardiac or respiratory arrest. All adults should receive CPR instruction because cardiopulmonary arrest can happen anywhere, any time.

PRELIMINARY ACTIVITIES

Assessment/Planning

▶ Know code words for cardiopulmonary arrest used in setting in which you work (e.g., "Code 99").

▶ Know locations of emergency buzzers (e.g., in client rooms and bathrooms).

▶ Know special telephone numbers for reaching the operator who calls the CPR team.

▶ Know your specific responsibility during a "code" in the health care facility.

▶ Periodically practice CPR technique with training mannequin and skilled, certified instructor.
Renew CPR certification annually or biennially as recommended by certifying agency.

▶ Clarify with nursing team members which specific persons in your care are not to have CPR if sudden cardiac arrest or respiratory arrest occurs.

▶ Determine whether client's diagnosis is frequently associated with sudden cardiac arrest or respiratory failure or whether client has a history of cardiac arrest.

Preparation of Person

▶ Not possible owing to sudden nature of cardiopulmonary arrest.

Equipment

▶ No equipment is absolutely required for effective performance of CPR. However, CPR pocket masks and Ambu bags are recommended to decrease the transmission of pathogens when carrying out the mouth-to-mouth breathing procedure.

▶ If the arrest occurs while the client is in bed, a hard, boardlike object (such as a meal tray) should be placed under the client's chest if such an object is readily available.

Procedure for Unwitnessed Cardiopulmonary Arrest

Actions

1. Quickly assess need for CPR in person who suddenly collapses or is unexpectedly found unconscious. Diagnostic actions include the following steps:
   a. Activate emergency medical system (EMS) in your area (many areas use 911 system) before assessment.
   b. Shake victim and call name loudly.

   c. Check for following signs confirming cardiopulmonary arrest:
   i. Absent or inadequate respiratory motions after clear airway has been established.

Rationale/Discussion

1. Success of CPR depends largely on speed with which basic life support (BSL) measures are effectively initiated.

   a. Quick access to EMS improves chances for survival.

   b. This helps assess state of consciousness. Do this quickly and only once while you move into position for further assessment.

   c. Prompt treatment is based on rapid, accurate recognition of respiratory or cardiac arrest.
   i. Assess ventilations first. Correction of respiratory arrest may prevent subsequent cardiac arrest.

Procedure continued on following page

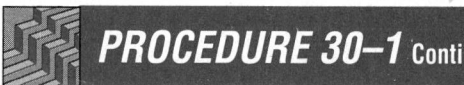
Basic Cardiopulmonary Resuscitation

Actions	Rationale/Discussion
▶ Place victim in horizontal position on firm surface.	▶ Gravity aids in circulation of oxygenated blood to all parts of the body, especially the brain. A firm surface is needed to compress heart adequately between sternum and spine.
▶ Place cheek close to victim's nose and mouth.	▶ This is done to listen for air movement and "feel" exhalations if present.
▶ Observe chest and upper abdomen for respiratory motions for a minimum of 5 seconds.	▶ Absence of motion confirms respiratory arrest.
ii. Absence of major pulses.	ii. Central pulses (i.e., pulses in large arteries close to heart) are palpable when peripheral pulses (e.g., radial) are absent.
▶ Palpate for carotid pulse in adults and older children and brachial pulse in infants. Use carotid pulse located on same side as rescuer.	▶ Carotid pulse is most easily checked because rescuer is already at victim's head (having just checked breathing). Clothing need not be removed to check carotid pulse. Loosen tight clothing at neck, however.
	▶ Absence of pulse indicates cardiac arrest.
2. Action (One Rescuer) a. Activate EMS system first.	2. a. Quick access to the EMS system improves chances for survival.
b. Roll victim horizontally and flat onto back.	b. Position is essential for airway management and external cardiac compressions.
c. Remove pillows from under head and neck.	c. Neck flexion may cause or add to upper airway obstruction.

A: Airway

d. Open airway by tilting head backward as far as possible by lifting jaw forward with one hand while pressing down on forehead with your other hand (see Fig. 30–2C).	d. Relaxed muscle tone present in loss of consciousness causes slack jaw muscles and allows tongue to fall to back of throat and obstruct airway. Correction of airway obstruction may restore spontaneous respiration and prevent subsequent cardiac arrest.
	▶ Determine whether ventilation has been restored. Can you feel victim's breath on your cheek or see chest rise?
	▶ Clear airway of obvious foreign matter (e.g., vomitus) only if obstruction has not been relieved by previous maneuvers. You may be wasting time.
e. Alternatively, open airway using jaw thrust maneuver. Place fingers under lower jaw on bony part near chin. Use thumb only to depress lower lip, not to lift chin. Lift jaw so that teeth are nearly brought together (see Fig. 30–2D).	e. Use if neck injury suspected.

B: Breathing

Actions	Rationale/Discussion
f. Begin artificial ventilation immediately by appropriate route if respirations are absent or inadequate.	f. Lack of ventilation rapidly leads to severe hypoxemia (and hypercarbia), which in turn may result in brain damage, cardiac arrest, and death. Rescuer's expired air supplies oxygen needed to support victim's requirements.
i. Mouth-to-mouth ventilation	i. Mouth-to-mouth ventilation
▶ Maintain head tilt or jaw lift.	▶ Both will keep airway open.
▶ Take a breath; just enough air to make the victim's chest rise.	▶ This prepares you to breathe this air directly into victim's lungs or use a CPR pocket mask (Fig. 30–3). Your exhaled air does not contain as much oxygen as inhaled air; thus, you need to breathe into victim a breath two or three times larger than normal. An alternative is to use an Ambu bag.

Basic Cardiopulmonary Resuscitation

Actions

▶ Use a CPR pocket mask or place your mouth tightly over victim's mouth and pinch both nostrils. Remove victim's dentures only if they interfere with seal or cause obstruction.
▶ Blow air from your lungs into victim's lungs, pausing 1.5 to 2 seconds per breath.

▶ After giving each breath, remove your mouth.

    ii. Mouth-to-nose ventilation

▶ Maintain head tilt.
▶ Place your mouth tightly over victim's nose while holding victim's mouth closed.

    iii. Mouth-to-stoma ventilation

    iv. Mouth-to-tracheostomy tube ventilation: Hold victim's mouth and nose closed when ventilating through uncuffed tracheostomy tube.

    g. Give victim two breaths, pausing 1.5 to 2 seconds per breath.
    h. Continue artificial ventilation at rate of 12 to 15 breaths per minute if respiratory arrest only.

    i. If pulse cannot be felt, begin external cardiac compression.

Rationale/Discussion

▶ This will help form a tight seal and prevent air leaks.

▶ Assess adequacy of artificial ventilation by (1) watching chest rise, (2) feeling inflation or "give" of victim's lungs as ventilation is accepted, and (3) feeling air exhaling from victim.
▶ This allows air to escape (after each breath), thereby permitting victim to artificially inhale and exhale.

    ii. Mouth-to-nose ventilation

▶ This keeps airway open.
▶ This prevents air leaks. All other steps are same as in mouth-to-mouth ventilation.

    iii. Mouth-to-stoma ventilation: Ventilation is applied directly into stoma, because upper airway (nose and mouth) is not connected to lower airway (lungs and tracheobronchial tree).

    iv. Mouth-to-tracheostomy tube ventilation: A tracheostomy tube is also ventilated directly as it by-passes upper airway. Air will escape from victim's nose or mouth unless upper airway is sealed off by inflated cuff.
    g. This step reoxygenates blood before starting artificial circulation.
    h. This rate is maintained only if external cardiac compression is not needed. Continue to assess pulse while ventilating.
    i. Compression will circulate blood.

C: Circulation

Actions

    j. Begin external cardiac compression immediately after initial two breaths.
    i. Place person on hard surface (e.g., floor), or insert hard board (e.g., tray) under person's chest. Kneel at the victim's side. With the middle and index fingers of lower hand, locate lower margin of rib cage on side next to you. Then run your fingers up along rib cage to notch where ribs meet sternum in center of lower chest (see Fig. 30–6). If victim is obese and ribs cannot be felt, locate xiphoid process and continue as follows. With one finger on notch, place other finger next to it on lower end of sternum.
    ii. Place heel of other hand on lower half of sternum above finger of palpating hand. Keep fingers and palm off chest, and apply force only with heel of hand.
    iii. Remove first hand and place it on top of hand on sternum. Both hands should be parallel and aimed away from you, with fingers extended or interlaced as long as they are kept off chest wall (see Fig. 30–6).
    iv. Straighten your arms by locking your elbows. Lean forward until your shoulders are directly over your hands. In this way, weight of back adds pressure for chest compression. Applying pressure with both hands, depress victim's sternum 3.75 to 5 cm (1½ to 2 in.) with each compression for adult patient.

    v. Release pressure on sternum quickly and completely after each compression, but do not lift your hands off chest. Fifty per cent of compression time is in downward phase and 50 per cent is in upward phase.

Rationale/Discussion

    j. Tissue hypoxia will cause irreversible brain damage if adequate circulation is not restored within 3 to 4 minutes.
    i. Sternum is flexible here, and heart lies directly below (see Fig. 30–4). External force on sternum will compress the heart only if there is a firm surface beneath it.

    iii. This provides added strength. If whole hand is flat on chest, force of compression dissipates to ribs instead of being applied directly to heart.

    iv. Circulation is maintained as blood is squeezed from heart with each compression because of changes in intrathoracic pressure brought about by cardiac compressions. (Small rescuer may have to kneel on bed beside person and exert extra pressure from shoulders.)

    v. This allows time for heart to fill with blood before next compression.

Procedure continued on following page

Basic Cardiopulmonary Resuscitation

Actions	Rationale/Discussion
k. Continue external cardiac compressions at rate of 80 to 100 per minute, giving two full breaths after every 15 compressions for adults. Maintain ratio of one breath per five cardiac compressions for infants and children.	k. Single rescuer must provide both artificial ventilation and circulation and must therefore work very rapidly.
l. Periodically assess victim's status.	l. Assessing circulation is difficult for one rescuer. Improvement of color and return of spontaneous motion are only observations possible in this situation. Never interrupt CPR for more than 5 seconds.
3. Actions (Two Rescuers)	3. Rationale—Two Rescuers
a. Give cardiac compressions at rate of 80 to 100 per minute (with only slight pauses for ventilation) for adults; 100 per minute for infants; and 80 to 100 per minute for children.	a. Uninterrupted cardiac compression provides victim with more even flow of blood.
b. Ventilation is provided by second rescuer. One breath is given to victim after every fifth cardiac compression.	b. Breath is given quickly between compressions. Compressions must not be interrupted any longer than necessary.
c. Periodically assess victim's status.	c. Assessment of victim's status is done by person ventilating. Periodically check carotid pulse and pupils.
d. Continue artificial ventilation and external cardiac compression as necessary.	d. CPR is continued until (1) effective spontaneous ventilation and circulation are restored; (2) CPR team takes over BLS or begins advanced life support actions; (3) rescuer is exhausted and unable to continue; or (4) a physician gives a medical directive to stop the procedure. (For position of two rescuers, see Fig. 30-5.)

FINAL ACTIVITIES

Change over smoothly to compression and ventilation by CPR team when they arrive or discontinue CPR if spontaneous ventilation and circulation return, positioning victim in the recovery position. In this case, the person will require close observation and frequent assessment.

DOCUMENTATION: Includes (1) time victim discovered (or if witnessed, time arrest occurred); (2) type of arrest (respiratory or cardiac or both); (3) any complication during CPR (e.g., vomiting); (4) time CPR team arrived; (5) time spontaneous ventilation or pulse returned; (6) time CPR discontinued if rescuer became exhausted; or (7) time decision was made to stop CPR because it was futile.

ROLES FOR TWO RESCUERS

The second rescuer takes a position on the opposite side of the person from the first rescuer (see Fig. 30-5). The first rescuer completes a cycle of 15 compressions, gives two breaths, and checks the person's pulse by palpating the carotid artery (for 5 to 10 seconds) to determine whether a pulse is present. The first rescuer then gives a breath, and the second rescuer begins compressions. As the two begin working together, the rescuer performing chest compressions begins the mnemonic to coordinate the compressions and ventilations to ensure an adequate rate of both: "one-and, two-and, three-and, four-and, five-and." One compression is done on each count. While counting out loud, the rescuer performing compressions depresses the sternum in a smooth manner, allowing 50 per cent of the compression to be in the downward phase and 50 per cent in the upward phase. The audible count helps maintain a compression rate of 80 to 100 per minute. It coordinates the two rescuers, prevents unnecessary fatigue, and reduces error in the compression-to-ventilation ratio.

The ventilator is responsible for interspersing a single ventilation between the *fifth* compression and the *first* compression of the next cycle. Compressions are briefly stopped to facilitate ventilations.

Delivering an effective breath requires practice on a mannequin. Before giving the breath, have the airway open, ready for ventilation. As the chest is compressed and the upward stroke begins, the rescuer providing ventilations seals the mouth tightly around the victim's mouth or around the one-way air valve on a pocket mask that is sealed around the victim's nose and mouth. Observe the effectiveness of each ventilation by watching the rise of the chest.

CHANGING RESCUER ROLES

External chest compression can be tiring for a rescuer. A tired rescuer cannot deliver compressions effectively. When two people are familiar with CPR techniques, they can switch roles. The change is done in the following order:

► The compressor gives a clear signal to change and may use a mnemonic such as "change-and, two-and, three-and, four-and, five-and . . . ."
► Compressions are performed as each phrase is said.

▶ On the fifth count, the ventilator at the head delivers one breath.

▶ The ventilator then moves to the person's chest, locating the rib notch with two fingers, and slides the second hand in next to the two fingers while the compressor gives the fifth compression, moves to the person's head, and checks for spontaneous pulse and breathing.

▶ If no pulse and no spontaneous respirations are noted, the compressor gives one ventilation and states, "No pulse. Continue CPR."

The two rescuers continue CPR at a rate of 80 to 100 cardiac compressions and 12 breaths per minute.

Performance Errors and Problems in Cardiopulmonary Resuscitation

Each step of the ABC sequence has potential problems or errors (Box 30–1). Practicing correct techniques on a resuscitation mannequin is essential in learning to perform error-free CPR. Through such practice, you develop the "feel" for each action.

Never interrupt CPR for more than 5 seconds. Waiting for special equipment, such as oxygen, self-inflating resuscitation bags or Ambu bags, endotracheal tubes, defibrillators, or suction equipment decreases the chance of survival or may result in permanent brain damage. Aesthetically, mouth-to-mouth breathing may be unpleasant for the person performing rescue breathing and may result in transmission of pathogens from the victim's oral mucosa. Use of a mask is advised. Failure to perform the vital function of rescue breathing, however, may be fatal for the victim. Rescuers are sometimes afraid of acquiring infectious diseases through mouth-to-mouth resuscitation. This fear may slow initial treatment, especially during an arrest outside a medical facility when the health status of the person is not known. Such a delay may reduce the chances of success of resuscitation efforts. It is advis-

---

Box 30–1. Performance Errors and Problems in Cardiopulmonary Resuscitation (CPR)

Error/problem	Ventilation not successful, little or no airflow with mouth-to-mouth efforts	**Comments**	Incorrect hand placement leads to ineffective compressions and greater risk of complications.
Cause	Airway not open because of obstruction from tongue in hypopharynx or from foreign material (e.g., bolus of food, vomitus, foreign body)	**Error/problem**	Chest fails to rise with artificial ventilation.
		Cause	Obstruction resulting from previously mentioned causes; failure to determine that your mask/mouth is making a tight seal; air may be coming back out of nose; victim may have a tracheostomy or laryngostomy.
Solution	Manually lift jaw forward to pull tongue away from hypopharynx. If ventilation still impaired, open mouth, "sweep" oropharynx with your fingers, and "scoop" material out. If ventilation is still impaired, perform abdominal or chest thrusts. Make certain dentures are not loose or creating obstruction.	**Solution**	Follow previous sequences for troubleshooting. Open your mouth wide, and cover victim's mouth tightly or be sure mask is sealed against skin. Pinch nostrils closed. Take a larger-than-normal breath when giving artificial respiration to an adult. Ventilate victim through stoma, if appropriate.
Comments	Continue to make efforts to ventilate victim even while clearing airway.	**Comments**	Even a partially opened airway will allow oxygen to enter victim's body. Breathe normally between rescue breathing attempts to prevent dizziness resulting from hyperventilation. Some diseases cause very stiff lungs, which require more forceful breaths to achieve minimal lung inflation (e.g., interstitial lung diseases, severe bronchospasm, pulmonary edema).
Error/problem	Inability to feel carotid pulse		
Cause	Insufficient force used for cardiac compressions; rescuer's hands in wrong position; rescuer's small body size; pressure on chest not completely relaxed between cardiac compressions, causing restriction in cardiac filling		
		Error/problem	Exhaustion of rescuer
		Cause	Incorrect techniques of compression and ventilation; if two-person rescue, failure to switch tasks before exhaustion leads to ineffectiveness.
Solution	Be certain sternum is depressed to correct depth (see Table 30–6) with each compression. Check hand placement: Rescuer's hands should be stacked one on the other, placed two fingerbreadths above xiphoid; force should be applied directly downward; arms must be extended straight, with elbows locked; fingers must be off chest wall (see Fig. 30–4B). If rescuer small, get up on bed or position up close to victim, with rescuer's body placed squarely over victim's body. When applying downward compression, avoid tendency to lean onto victim. Release pressure from sternum during upward stroke without actually removing hands from chest wall.	**Solution**	Keep arms straight and elbows locked. Breathe normally between rescue ventilations. Rescuer's body must be placed correctly next to and directly over victim. Work surface

Box continued on following page

Box 30–1. Performance Errors and Problems in Cardiopulmonary Resuscitation (CPR) (Continued)

	must be firm. Practice changing roles until it is natural, using a mannequin to gain confidence and competence. Attempt to locate help, if only one rescuer. CPR may have to be stopped if rescuer is unable to continue, unless others trained in CPR can be found.		vomiting and aspiration of stomach contents into airway.
Error/problem	Ventilation volume too great in infant or child rescue breathing	*Error/problem*	Bouncing compressions, and compressions that are too deep in infant and child resuscitation
Cause	Rescuer's anxiety, fear, and panic may cause too great a volume to be delivered into infant's or child's airway or may cause airway to be opened incorrectly, failure to recognize that infant and child lung volumes are much smaller than that of adult	*Cause*	Rescuer's anxiety, panic, or other emotions; failure to remember correct depth of sternal depression when performing chest compressions on infants and children; incorrect technique when performing chest compressions.
Solution	Try to remain calm. Do not hyperextend an infant's or child's head to same degree as you would an adult's. Do not take a deep breath before delivering rescue breath. Breathe normally and exhale in puffs for an infant, with somewhat greater volumes for a child, depending on size of child.	*Solution*	Try to stay calm. Review correct hand placement and depth of depression of sternum. Know differences between adult, child, and infant chest compression (see Table 30–6). Do not remove fingers/hands from contact with sternum. Practice on adult, child and infant mannequin until you are well established in correct technique.
Comments	Too great volumes and incompletely opened airway allow gastric distention, which may build up and restrict ventilation later or cause	*Comments*	Incorrect hand placement and compression technique lead to rib fractures or damage to liver or spleen or other internal organs. Too deep compressions may bruise heart. Bouncing causes bruises and fractures.

able to purchase an inexpensive, easy-to-carry pocket mask that will allow immediate initiation of CPR with little risk of the rescuer coming into contact with the person's oral secretions.

INFANT AND CHILD RESUSCITATION

The basic principles of infant and child resuscitation are the same as those used in adult CPR (i.e., airway, breathing, and circulation). The skills require additional practice, however. Infant and child resuscitation mannequins can help you learn the skills and make the modifications necessary to perform CPR safely and effectively on an infant or child.

Newborn Resuscitation

Resuscitation of a newborn may be necessary at delivery (1) if the infant is unable to establish a patent airway and begin effective ventilation or (2) when cardiovascular status is unstable and the circulatory system is unable to supply the brain, heart, and other vital organs with blood. Some of these problems may begin before delivery; others may arise in the period immediately after birth.

An infant's airway may be obstructed by mucus, blood, meconium, or posterior displacement of the tongue. Drugs (e.g., narcotics, sedatives, and local or general anesthetics) given to the mother during labor may depress the respiratory system. Other factors that can affect infant ventilation and create a need for resuscitation include prematurity; neurologic damage; congenital abnormalities of the heart, respiratory system, or central nervous system; compression of the umbilical cord during labor and delivery; and hemorrhage.

The first few minutes after birth require special assessment and resuscitation from specially trained health care professionals. Nursing students may be present during such an emergency and assist the resuscitation team. (For a detailed discussion of the assessment and care of newborns requiring airway management, assisted ventilation, and assisted circulation, refer to pediatric and neonatal textbooks.) Here we focus on BLS measures for infants and children.

Causes of Infant and Child Respiratory Arrest

Infants and children generally experience respiratory arrest before developing asystole. If the airway and ventilation are not reestablished quickly, however, a full cardiopulmonary arrest occurs. It is extremely important to pay close attention to airway patency and the adequacy of ventilation in infants and children.

After the perinatal period (the first 6 weeks of life), the major causes of airway obstruction, respiratory arrest, and subsequent cardiac arrest in young children include (1) aspiration of foreign bodies (toys, peanuts, chewing gum, beads); (2) asphyxia (e.g., from filmy plastic covers); (3) drowning; (4) automobile or other accidents; (5) poisoning and drug overdose; (6) smoke inhalation; (7) sudden infant death syndrome; and (8) infections (e.g., epiglottitis). Most of these are preventable.

CPR is initiated in infants and children if tactile stimulation does not produce spontaneous ventilation, if there is airway obstruction, or if the infant or child has no pulse.

Establishing an Airway

When an infant or child requires CPR, follow the action outlined in Table 30–5 and Figure 30–7. Remember to use the ABCs (airway, breathing, circulation) to help you remember the steps.

Signs of Successful Ventilation

Ventilation is effective when (1) bilateral chest movement is visible, (2) bilateral breath sounds are heard on auscultation, (3) the heart rate increases to a regular rate of 100 beats per minute or more, and (4) there is an improvement in skin color and peripheral pulses.

Chest Compressions

If the pulse rate (brachial in the infant or carotid in the child) does not improve after the establishment of a patent airway, ventilation and oxygen administration (if available) are started along with chest compressions. Table 30–6 compares compression techniques for infants, children, and adults. Adult chest compression techniques are used for children older than 8 years. Ages are a guide only. *Modify techniques according to the actual size of the child.*

A backward tilt of the head lifts the back of an infant or small child. Use a folded towel or small blanket for back support, if available. Support can also be provided by slipping one hand beneath the infant or child's back while the other hand performs chest compression.

Compressions Mnemonic

The rescuer providing compressions counts "one, two, three, four, five" for an infant (one compression for each word) and "one-and-two-and-three-and-four-and-five-and-breathe" for a child (one compression on each number). Following this mnemonic will help the rescuer achieve the correct compression rate. As with adults, ventilations are interposed between compressions.

COMPLICATIONS OF CARDIOPULMONARY RESUSCITATION

If a victim has a recent neck injury or one is suspected, hyperextension of the neck and head is contraindicated.

Neck hyperextension can damage the spinal cord by dislodging an unstable vertebra or vertebral fragment. In this circumstance, use a strong jaw thrust to open the airway (Figure 30–2D). To be effective, however, this step requires two rescuers because it is impossible for a single rescuer to keep the victim's jaw in place while compressing the chest.

During artificial ventilation, air may enter the stomach. If the amount is significant, gastric distention results. Gastric distention is a frequent problem during CPR on infants and children and can be a serious problem for several reasons: (1) It can result in a ruptured stomach (gastric rupture); (2) it often triggers vomiting, which may produce serious airway management problems both during the resuscitation and during post-CPR care; (3) if severe, it can impede movement of the diaphragm, thus compromising ventilation; and (4) it is associated with increased vagal tone, which can cause reflex bradycardia (heart rate below 60 beats per minute) and hypotension.

Severe gastric distention requiring intervention is seen as a bulge in the abdomen just below the rib cage. Gentle abdominal pressure over the stomach may cause the air to "belch" out. Be cautious when performing this maneuver, however, because gastric rupture or vomiting can occur.

Gastric distention occurs most often when (1) lungs are difficult to ventilate, (2) high inflating pressures are used in infants and children, and (3) the airway is partially obstructed. When performing rescue breathing in these situations, blow in just enough air to cause the victim's chest to rise. Gastric distention can also occur when cardiac compressions and ventilation are mistimed and occur simultaneously. If the victim's lungs are stiff with bronchospasm or if the tongue has fallen back to block the airway, the pressure to open the esophagus and cardiac sphincter can be easily exceeded. In both situations, it is easier for the air to go into the stomach than into the lungs. The stomach fills with air, and the chest fails to rise.

Aspiration can occur if vomiting occurs during CPR because the person is without a gag reflex or cough reflex. The risk of aspiration is further increased because the person is positioned flat on the back. Aspiration of gastric contents may cause immediate problems with mechanical blockage of the upper or lower airways or a later problem of aspiration pneumonia, which is particularly serious if the gastric contents have a low pH, as is usually the case.

Incorrect hand placement during CPR can cause rib and xiphoid fracture. Sometimes rib fractures occur with appropriate compressions, especially among the elderly. The fractures in themselves are often not serious, but the fractured pieces can cause serious damage

TABLE 30-5. *ABCs of Infant and Child Cardiopulmonary Resuscitation (CPR)*

Observation	Action	Rationale
Infant or child seems unresponsive	Call for help. Determine unresponsiveness by tapping feet of infant or shaking victim's shoulder.	Two-person CPR is more effective than single rescuer CPR. Diagnosis of unresponsiveness must be accurate. This is a highly charged emotional situation.
	Position victim horizontal on floor, table, or other firm surface. Support spine.	Horizontal position aids effective circulation and places victim in position for further action if needed.
No respirations, no activity, labored breathing, or abnormal color.	**A.** Open airway by tipping head back, using head tilt–chin lift method.*	Hyperextension straightens trachea, and respirations may begin spontaneously.
	Look, listen, and feel for respirations. Place your cheek down close to victim's mouth and nose. Look for rise and fall of chest.	Detection of airflow indicates that airway obstruction has been relieved at least temporarily.
Blue color of lips and mucous membranes.	If blue color is apparent, begin rescue breathing. If lip color is pink, do not begin rescue breathing. If color determination is difficult by only looking at lips, turn lower eyelid down and examine color of mucous membrane.	Blue color indicates insufficient supply of oxygen.
	B. Begin rescue breathing. Cover victim's mouth or nose, or both, with rescuer's mouth.	*Infant:* Cover both mouth and nose. *Child:* Pinch nose and cover mouth to form a tight seal.
	Give two breaths lasting 1 to 1½ seconds per breath.	Smaller lung capacity of child or infant dictates less volume and force than used for adult rescue breathing. Overinflation of lungs can lead to gastric distention and vomiting.
Apparent pulselessness.	Establish pulselessness. *Infant:* Palpate brachial pulse (inside of upper arm midway between shoulder and elbow). *Child:* Palpate carotid as on adult.	Brachial pulse is easiest to locate on infant. Infant's short, fat neck makes location of carotid more difficult.
Confirmed pulselessness	**C.** Begin cardiac compressions. *Infant:* Locate *midsternum* by drawing imaginary line between nipples. Place two or three fingers on sternum, one fingerbreadth below imaginary line.	Heart in infant and child is situated higher in chest. For *infant,* the proper area for compression is midsternum.
	Child: Locate notch where ribs join, in chest center, with middle finger. Compress area just above index finger on sternum.	Child's heart is lower than infant's but not as low as adult's.
	Infant: Compress over midsternum. Depress sternum 1.25 to 2.5 cm (½ to 1 in.) at a rate of 100 per minute. Compress with two or three fingers.	Infant requires a faster heart rate.
	Child: Deliver compressions with heel of one hand. Depth of compression for child is 2.5 to 3.75 cm (1 to 1½ in.) at a rate of 80 to 100 per minute.	Heart rate for child is higher than adult's but less than infant's.
	Maintain both ventilations and compressions.	
	Interpose a breath after every five compressions.	Ratio of compressions to ventilation is 5:1 for both two rescuers and a single rescuer.
	Infant: Give a breath every 3 seconds.	Ventilation rate of 20 per minute.
	Child: Give a breath every 4 seconds.	Ventilation rate of 15 per minute.

* Caution: Excessive hyperextension can collapse trachea or cause cervical injury.

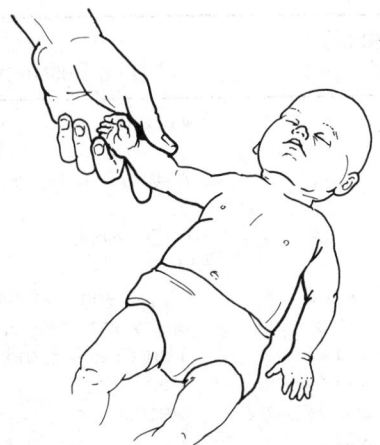

Step 1:
Determine responsiveness.

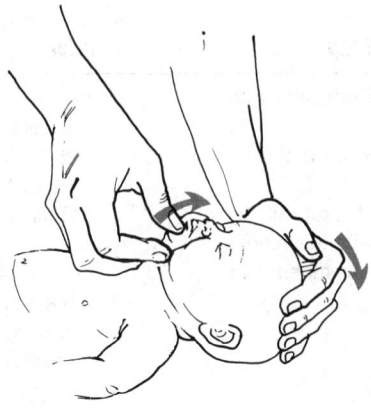

Step 2:
Chin lift-head tilt. Observe for
spontaneous respiration.

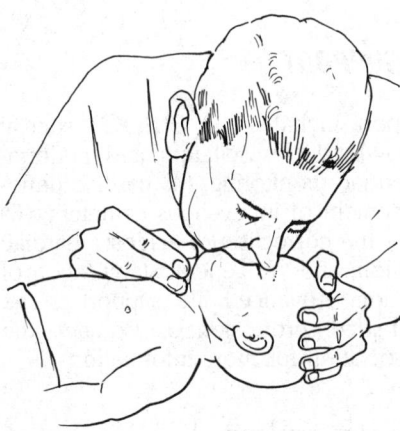

Step 3:
Begin rescue breathing by forming an
airtight seal covering victim's mouth and
nose with rescuer's mouth. Infants require
a rescue breathing rate of 20 per minute;
children require 15 breaths per minute.

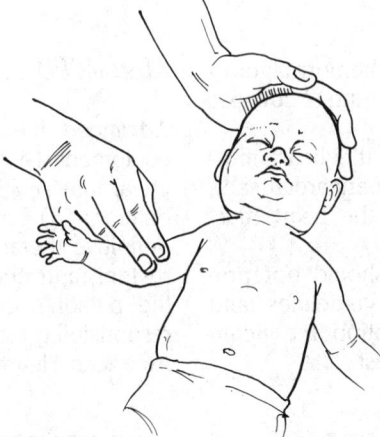

Step 4:
Palpate brachial pulse in infants; carotid
pulse in children.

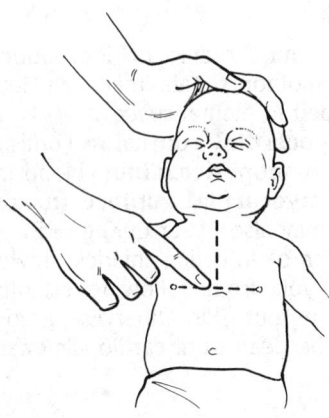

Step 5:
Locate correct landmarks for performing
chest compressions.

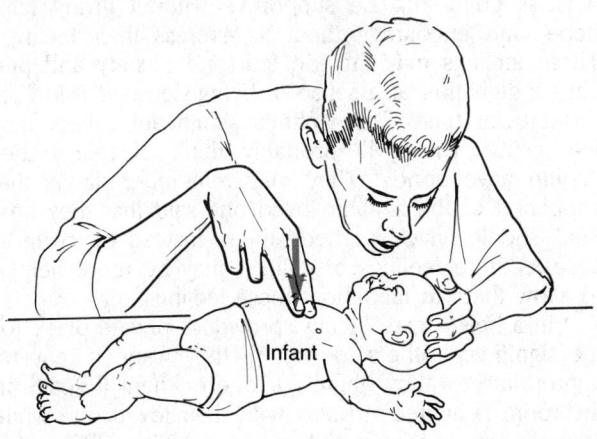

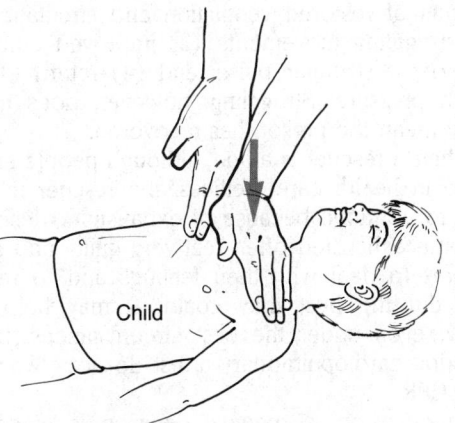

Step 6:
Perform external chest compressions at a rate of 5:1 artificial breaths.
Use finger-pressure chest compression on infants; one hand on children.

▲ *Figure 30–7*

CPR for infant and child.

TABLE 30-6. Comparing Techniques in Infant/Child/Adult Cardiopulmonary Resuscitation

Step	Infant	Child	Adult (Single Rescuer)	Adult (Two Rescuers)
Compress with . . .	Two to three fingers	Heel of one hand	Two hands	Two hands
to a depth of . . .	1.25 to 2.5 cm (½ to 1 in.)	2.5 to 3.75 cm (1 to 1½ in.)	3.75 to 5 cm (1½ to 2 in.)	3.75 to 5 cm (1½ to 2 in.)
at a rate of . . .	100/minute	80–100/minute	80–100/minute	80–100/minute
with this ratio . . .	5:1	5:1	15:2	5:1
and mnemonic . . .	"1, 2, 3, 4, 5, breathe. 1, 2, 3, 4, 5, breathe"	"1 and 2 and 3 and 4 and 5 and breathe, 1 and 2 and 3 and 4 and 5 and breathe"	"1 and 2 and 3 and 4 and 5 and 1 and 2 and 3 and 4 and 5 and 1 and 2 and 3 and 4 and 5 and breathe"	"1 and 2 and 3 and 4 and 5 and breathe, 1 and 2 and 3 and 4 and 5 and breathe"

(e.g., intrathoracic or intraabdominal hemorrhage or pneumothorax [air that can lead to lung collapse trapped in pleural space]).

Myocardial contusion (bruising of the heart muscle), **hemopericardium** (blood in the pericardial sac), and **myocardial rupture** (rupture of the heart muscle) may also occur during CPR.

Fear of inflicting injuries, however, should not prevent you from following established guidelines and carrying out CPR. Otherwise, a complication-free victim may be dead from cardiopulmonary arrest.

TERMINATION OF BASIC LIFE SUPPORT

CPR is stopped as a result of a number of circumstances; these are typically restoration of spontaneous respiration and circulation, complete rescuer exhaustion, or medical decision.

Signs of restored ventilation and circulation include (1) struggling movements, (2) improved color, (3) return of or stronger pulse, and (4) return of systemic blood pressure. Struggling, however, does not necessarily mean the person has recovered.

When a rescuer is alone, although people are seldom alone in health care facilities, the rescuer may not be able to continue because of exhaustion. Rescuers who become exhausted often feel very guilty and may need support to deal with their feelings and to realize that they did the best they could. It may help them to know, even under the best circumstances, individuals suffering cardiopulmonary arrest do not always recover after CPR.

On occasion, a medical decision is made to stop CPR without going on to advanced life support techniques. This decision is usually related to the person's underlying disease or condition. Sometimes these decisions are made in advance by the person and significant others in consultation with the physician. In these cases, CPR is *not* initiated.

ADVANCED LIFE SUPPORT

Advanced life support includes (1) BLS; (2) special equipment (e.g., bag-mask resuscitators and endotracheal tubes); (3) cardiac monitoring; (4) cardiac defibrillation; (5) establishment of intravenous catheters; (6) definitive therapy for the correction of acidosis, cardiac rhythm, and circulation; and (7) general stabilization of the person's condition. Advanced life support is the responsibility of trained professionals. Contact the American Heart Association for more information.

HELPING SIGNIFICANT OTHERS

One of the most significant contributions nurses make, after being relieved of the BLS role, is to support the person's significant others. Keep them informed about what is going on. Be supportive without giving false hope, and encourage them to express their feelings. These feelings may include fear and anxiety and perhaps indignation at a sense of being "pushed aside" at this crucial time. The victim's significant others may feel guilty. They will probably think of things they "could have done." They may remember things that happened or things their loved one said that they now think should have "warned" them. Instead of trying to absolve these feelings of guilt, it may be more helpful to allow them to talk about these feelings.

If in a health care facility, provide a private place for the significant others to wait. If they want, it may be appropriate to allow them (or one of them if space in the room is limited) to stay with their loved one while resuscitation continues, although observing CPR activities may be distressing. (Consult the hospital policy regarding this practice.) After all, if the person were not in the facility, significant others would not be separated from them. Keep them informed frequently (every few minutes) with specific details about what is happening. For example, "We are still trying to resuscitate

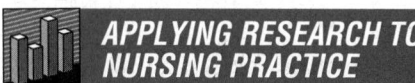

APPLYING RESEARCH TO NURSING PRACTICE

When Performing Cardiopulmonary Resuscitation, Keep Both Hands on the Bag

McCabe, S., Smeltzer, S.C. (1992). Tidal volumes delivered by 1- and 2-hand manual compressions (abstract). *Heart & Lung,* 21(3), 291.

▼ ▼ ▼

In some instances nurses provide ventilatory support by compressing a manual resuscitation bag during CPR. This is done to deliver a tidal volume—the amount of air that the client normally receives with each breath, which is usually about 10 to 15 ml of air per kilogram of body weight. During CPR, the nurse uses the manual resuscitation bag to deliver 100% inspired oxygen to the client. A common practice is to compress the bag using only one hand, while "saving" the other hand to carry out other tasks during resuscitation. However, McCabe and Smeltzer wondered whether the force exerted by one hand is sufficient to deliver an adequate tidal volume. These investigators compared differences in the effects of hand size, grip strength, and experience with manual resuscitation on tidal volume in 108 health care providers using a 1-L manual resuscitation bag. The study found that two-handed compressions delivered an average tidal volume of 827 ml, whereas one-handed compressions delivered a tidal volume of only 694 ml. The differences in tidal volume did not depend on the type of health care provider, years of clinical experience, or previous training in basic or advanced life support. Differences were found, however, in gender; the grip strength and hand size of men were greater than those of women. Men were also able to deliver higher tidal volumes.

Applications for Practice. If you have average hand size and grip strength, you can improve the effective delivery of an adequate tidal volume by using both hands to compress the manual resuscitation bag.

George" or "There are some signs that George is starting to respond."

Give information that is objective without raising false hope. Acknowledge their fear and concern with gentleness and understanding. Significant others are included in the decision-making process either to stop resuscitation attempts or to proceed with advanced life support.

If appropriate, ask those present whether there is a special friend or spiritual advisor whom they would like you to contact for them. Make a telephone available, or offer to place the call for them.

If significant others are not present, they should be notified. Give the information that their friend or relative has "taken a turn for the worse," and ask them to come to the care facility (or wherever the person is). Someone should meet them when they arrive, show them to a private area, and advise the physician or CPR coordinator that they have arrived.

If the person survives, keep the significant others informed regarding further treatment. If the person's condition is hopeful, offer this reassurance. If the person does not survive, remain with the significant others as they are told that their loved one has died.

SURVIVORS OF CARDIOPULMONARY ARREST

Surviving cardiopulmonary arrest is an emotional experience. Survivors react in a variety of ways. Denial, isolation of feelings, displacement, projection, hallucinatory or delusion behavior, and violent dreams are common during the period after a cardiac arrest. Symptoms such as insomnia, tenseness, restlessness, irritability, and memory impairment may continue for months.

Studies of people who have had near-death experiences describe a number of similar experiences. One especially significant finding for health professionals is that a considerable number of people report that they were aware of people working around them during the cardiac arrest. They were also aware of what was being said by these people. Remember that when working in emergency situations such as cardiac arrest, you should always think before speaking, especially when working on someone who is seemingly unconscious. Research suggests that hearing is one of the last senses lost before death.

After cardiopulmonary arrest, recurrence of arrest is of great concern to both the person and significant others. Emotional and educational support is important to these persons. They need information about

- signs and symptoms of arrhythmias and the necessary steps to deal with them
- other diagnostic and treatment measures that may be necessary
- follow-up services in the community

FOREIGN BODY AIRWAY OBSTRUCTION

The term *choking* is often used for difficult breathing or swallowing. This problem is caused by acute external or internal obstructions or impediments of the airway or trachea. If airway blockages are not quickly removed, a full cardiopulmonary arrest will occur. A significant number of deaths occur annually because of airway obstruction. Foreign body airway obstruction has a number of causes. In adults, the most common cause is food. A number of factors are often present when an airway is obstructed by food. These include

- large, poorly chewed pieces of food
- elevated blood alcohol levels
- poor-fitting dentures
- talking or laughing when putting food into the mouth

Many people have survived foreign body airway obstructions (choking) because someone nearby has applied the Heimlich maneuver. This technique was first described in 1973 by Dr. H. J. Heimlich. The Heimlich

---

Box 30–2. Preventing Foreign Material Airway Obstruction

- ► Cut food into small pieces.
- ► Chew slowly and thoroughly.
- ► Chew carefully if wearing dentures.
- ► Avoid laughing and talking while chewing and swallowing.
- ► Avoid excessive alcohol intake before and during meals.
- ► Stop children from walking, running, or playing while eating.
- ► Stop children from placing objects in their mouths.
- ► Keep small objects such as beads and marbles out of reach of small infants and children.

---

maneuver is a method of applying pressure to the abdomen to dislodge a bolus of food from the pharynx, larynx, or trachea. Through this technique, the upward displacement of the abdomen forces air from the lung and expels the foreign body.

Box 30–2 lists ways of preventing foreign material airway obstruction. Figure 30–8 shows the universal choking signal used to alert others to an acute airway obstruction so they can help.

Recognition of Foreign Body Airway Obstruction

Quick and accurate recognition of choking is essential to saving a person's life. It is important to determine quickly whether the person's distress is due to airway obstruction or to some other medical situation (e.g., fainting, heart attack, stroke, epilepsy, drug overdose, or other condition resulting in respiratory failure).

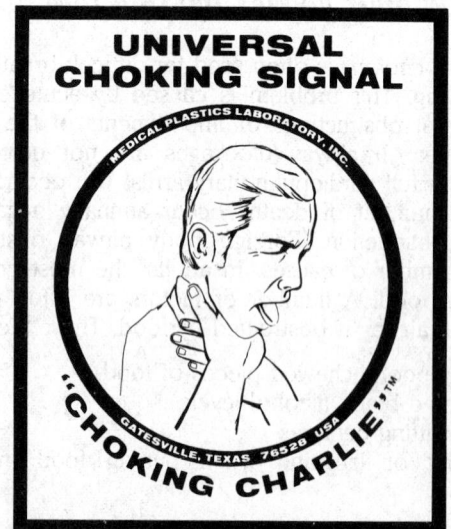

UNIVERSAL CHOKING SIGNAL

MEDICAL PLASTICS LABORATORY, INC.

"CHOKING CHARLIE"™

GATESVILLE, TEXAS 76528 USA

▲ **Figure 30–8**

Clutching the neck between the thumb and index finger is generally accepted as the universal sign for choking.

PARTIAL AIRWAY OBSTRUCTION

When an obstruction partially blocks the airway, the person may be able to generate a forceful enough cough to dislodge the material. Say to the person, "Can you speak?" If the person can speak, the airway is not completely blocked. The person who can speak only weakly can probably cough only weakly. If a person can speak strongly, a strong cough is possible. If the person can speak, encourage strong, forceful coughing to attempt to remove the obstruction. There may be wheezes between coughs because airflow is partially impeded.

Treat a person as having a complete airway obstruction if (1) the person tires, (2) speech becomes weaker or impossible, (3) the person becomes a dusky color, (4) respiratory efforts become more labored, or (5) attempts to breathe produce a high-pitched crowing sound.

COMPLETE AIRWAY OBSTRUCTION

When the airway is completely obstructed, the person will be unable to speak, breathe, or cough. The victim may clutch at the neck (see Fig. 30–8). Complete airway obstruction is an emergency because no oxygen is being exchanged for carbon dioxide. This produces **anoxia** (complete lack of oxygen), which will lead to cerebral and systemic hypoxia, unconsciousness, and death unless the condition is quickly reversed. See Box 30–3 for steps to take when complete airway obstruction is suspected.

Management of Obstructed Airway

The two techniques for relieving foreign body airway obstruction are manual chest and abdominal thrusts (Heimlich maneuver) and finger sweeps.

MANUAL THRUSTS (ABDOMINAL OR CHEST)

Thrusts to the abdomen are delivered from behind if the person is standing or sitting or from the front if the person is lying on the back (supine). Apply quick, inward thrusts to the upper abdomen between the umbilicus and the xiphoid process.

Thrusts to the lower chest are used when the person's abdominal girth is so great that it is not possible for rescuers to wrap their arms around the abdomen to perform abdominal thrusts. Chest thrusts are also appropriate when force to the abdomen would cause trauma or create complications (e.g., during pregnancy) (Fig. 30–9).

If the victim is unconscious and lying supine, the technique is somewhat different; see Figure 30–10.

FINGER SWEEPS

The finger sweep technique is what its name suggests: manually reaching for and removing foreign material that is at or above the level of the epiglottis. Before beginning the more complicated methods of relief of

Box 30–3. Action Steps for Complete Airway Obstruction

1. Conscious victim:

▶ Determine whether obstruction is complete ("Can you speak?").
▶ If obstruction is complete, apply 6 to 10 manual thrusts (chest or abdominal) (see Fig. 30–9).
▶ Repeat the 6 to 10 thrusts until they are effective or the victim becomes unconscious.

2. Conscious victim who becomes unconscious:

▶ Call for help.
▶ Open the airway.
▶ Attempt to ventilate the lungs.
▶ *Look* for the rise and fall of the chest. *Listen* for airflow. *Feel* for airflow by placing your face close to the person's mouth.
▶ If no air movement noted:
   Apply 6 to 10 manual thrusts in rapid succession (Fig. 30–10).
   Perform finger sweep of the oropharynx.
   Remove dentures only if they are loose and obstructing airflow and ventilation.
   Perform finger sweep.
   Reposition the victim's head, open the airway, and attempt ventilation.
   Repeat until the obstruction is removed.

3. Unconscious victim—cause unknown:

▶ Confirm unresponsiveness (touch the person and shout "Can you hear me?"). Call the person's name if known.
▶ Follow the ABC steps of cardiopulmonary resuscitation.
▶ If unable to ventilate, proceed as listed in Step 2.

4. Conscious victim without help:

▶ If a person chokes while alone, it may help to sit or stand close to a piece of heavy furniture (e.g., table, chest, couch, chair).
▶ Strike the chest forcefully halfway between rib cage and umbilicus against the furniture (avoid sharp edges).
▶ Repeat as often as necessary.

an airway obstruction, open the victim's mouth and inspect the oropharynx for visible material. If possible, remove it with the fingers. (Use a barrier device, if available, such as gloves to protect yourself from the victim's secretions.)

To perform a finger sweep, position the person supine (face up). Open the victim's mouth by grasping the tongue and jaw (the mandible) between your thumb and fingers. This maneuver draws the tongue forward and may partially relieve the obstruction.

If the obstruction cannot be quickly removed by a finger sweep, use thrust techniques. You may be able to use the finger sweep after a series of thrusts if the obstruction has been partially dislodged. The finger sweep is also used to remove vomitus from the mouth before CPR.

EFFECTS OF PROLONGED HYPOXIA

The longer a person is without oxygen, the more relaxed the muscles become. Your efforts, although at first inhibited by muscular opposition, may become successful as you persevere. As hypoxia worsens, however, the effects of anaerobic metabolism on the organs of the body will continue. Remember, biologic death occurs approximately 6 minutes after the beginning of a cardiopulmonary arrest.

As muscles relax and the obstruction is partially dislodged, the airway may become partially open, allowing ventilation if spontaneous ventilations do not begin. Often it is necessary to modify your exhalations (i.e., slow them down) to ventilate around the partial obstruction. When the partial obstruction is bypassed, partial ventilation and oxygenation may be accomplished. Even a reduced volume of air may be enough to keep the person alive until more sophisticated means of relieving or bypassing the obstruction are available.

POSTOBSTRUCTION REMOVAL ACTIVITIES

After removal of the obstruction, full CPR may be necessary. Always try to obtain help without leaving the victim. Memorize the telephone number in your facility or community for the emergency medical system (e.g., 911). If full CPR is necessary, you will certainly need help because you may be exhausted from airway clearance techniques and so may not have the strength to perform CPR. The victim is likely to require advanced life support measures such as oxygen, mechanical ventilation, defibrillation, intravenous medications, and other supportive therapies.

The shorter the time between CPR and advanced life support measures, the greater the person's chances for survival and viability.

FOREIGN BODY AIRWAY OBSTRUCTIONS IN INFANTS AND CHILDREN

Foreign body airway obstructions in children are often caused by inhaling small toys or other small objects such as coins, peanuts, marbles, or buttons. Infections of the upper airway such as croup and epiglottitis may also cause airway obstruction. It is very important to determine the cause of the upper airway obstruction. If techniques for removing foreign bodies are attempted when the obstruction is due to infection, effective treatment is delayed. Such delay may lead to serious complications. Infants and children with obstructed airways resulting from infection have barking coughs and fever, appear obviously ill, and exhibit signs of progressive airway obstruction (e.g., a change in color or drooling). An infant or child exhibits the same basic symptoms of partial and complete obstruction as do adults.

Infant Technique. To remove a foreign body obstruction from the trachea of an infant, straddle the infant over your forearm. Keep the head lower than the trunk.

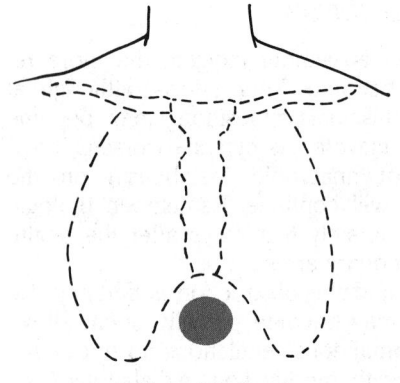

Abdominal thrust

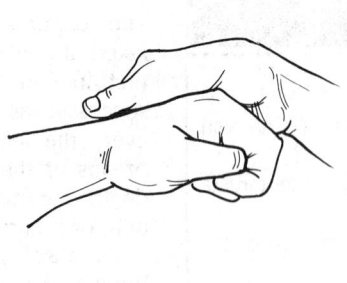

Position of hands
from rescuer's view

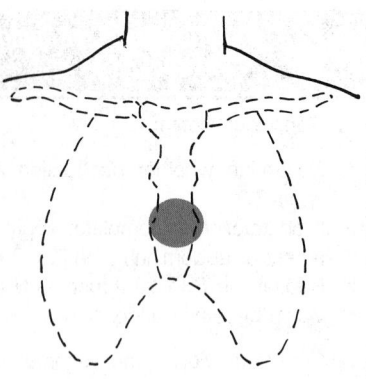

Chest thrust

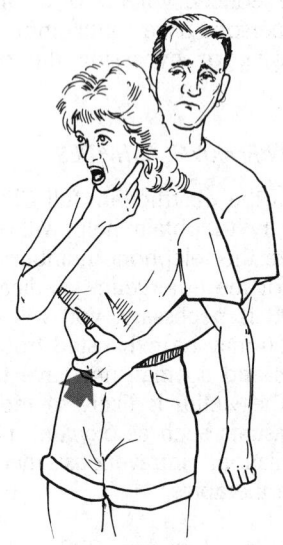

ABDOMINAL THRUST

Call for Help!!!

Stand behind victim.

Wrap your arms around victim's waist.

Make a fist.

Grasp fist with your other hand.

Place fist and hand thumb side against victim's abdomen, midline between umbilicus and rib cage.

Press fist four times into abdomen with an inward and upward motion.

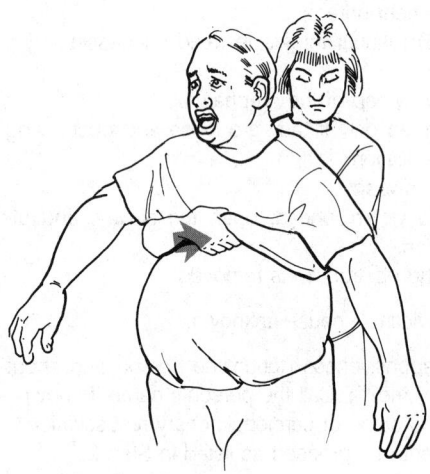

CHEST THRUST

Call for Help!!!

Stand behind victim.

Place your arms under victim's arms at level of armpits.

Encircle victim's chest with your arms.

Make a fist.

Grasp fist with your other hand.

Place thumb of fist on middle of victim's sternum, but not over xiphoid process or costal margins.

Exert four quick backward thrusts.

▲ **Figure 30–9**

Thrust techniques with the victim conscious, either sitting or standing.

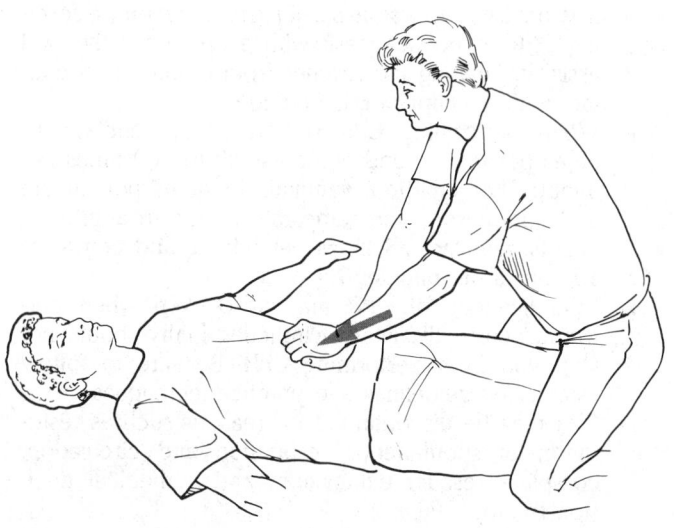

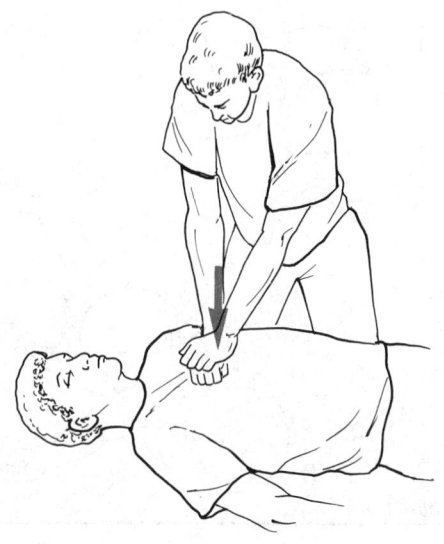

ABDOMINAL THRUST

Call for Help!!!

Position yourself either to victim's side (close to hips) or astride victim with legs over person's thighs.

Open victim's airway and turn head chin-up.

Place heel of one of your hands against victim's abdomen midline between umbilicus and rib cage.

Place heel of your second hand over the other.

Your shoulders should be directly over victim's abdomen.

Use heel of your hands to press into victim's abdomen with a fist.

Press into abdomen with four quick inward and upward thrusts.

DO NOT PRESS TO EITHER SIDE. PRESS IN DIRECTION OF CHEST AND HEAD.

CHEST THRUST

Call for Help!!!

Kneel to side of victim.

Open victim's airway and turn head chin-up.

Locate victim's rib border and follow it to xiphoid process.

Place two of your fingers over base of sternum just above xiphoid process.

Bring heel of your other hand alongside the two fingers.

Your shoulders should be directly over victim's chest, as if doing chest compressions.

Use heel of your hands to compress the sternum. Rescuer may either make a fist or use heel of hand with fingers held away from chest.

Apply four quick downward thrusts to compress chest cavity.

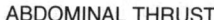

▲ *Figure 30-10*

Thrust techniques with the victim unconscious, lying supine.

Support the infant's head and neck by holding the jaw and chest. If the infant is large or the rescuer small, place your arm on your upper thigh (Fig. 30-11).

Give four back blows with the heel of the hand between the infant's shoulder blades. Use firm blows, but use caution not to exert excessive force.

Immediately after the back blows, turn the infant over (face up) onto your thigh, carefully supporting the infant's head and neck, keeping the head down so the object does not slip back into the throat or go farther down the trachea. Give four rapid chest thrusts. The technique for chest thrusts in an infant are the same as those for administering external chest compressions to an infant.

Child Technique. To remove a foreign body obstruction from the trachea of a child, roll the child onto the back on the floor or on a firm surface. Administer 8 to 10 chest thrusts in the same manner and location as for external cardiac compression techniques for a child.

Do not perform "blind" finger sweeps in infants and children because their airways are much smaller than those of adults and the risk of pushing the foreign object further into the airway is too great. After the 8 to 10 chest thrusts, lift the tongue and lower jaw forward and open the mouth. Inspect the oral cavity for a foreign object.

If the object is visible and removable, remove it with a finger sweep.

If spontaneous respirations do not return immediately after removal of the foreign object, place your pocket mask (or mouth) over the child's mouth or nose, or

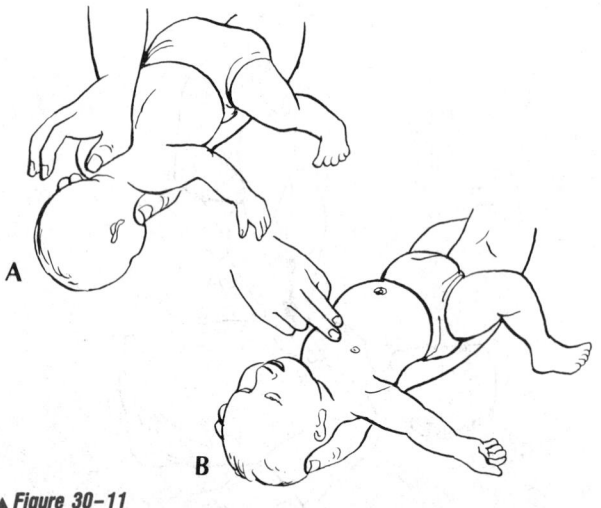

▲ *Figure 30–11*

Removal of an airway obstruction—infant technique. Removal is managed in two steps: back blows *(A)*, followed by turning the infant over to perform chest thrusts *(B)*. The technique for chest thrusts is the same as that for infant chest compressions.

both, and deliver two breaths. If the chest does not rise, repeat the series of back blows, chest thrusts, inspection, and ventilation until spontaneous respirations return or advanced life support teams arrive.

Summary

▸ Modern life support measures began in 1954, when mouth-to-mouth and mouth-to-nose ventilation was found to be effective.

▸ Cardiopulmonary arrest interrupts gas exchange and the flow of blood and oxygen to the brain, heart, and other organs. If not quickly restored, this interruption may cause brain damage or clinical or biologic death.

▸ Clinical death is manifested by reversible loss of consciousness. Biologic death is marked by irreversible destruction of brain tissue.

▸ The 1992 American Heart Association guidelines advocate activating the emergency medical system as the first step in the cardiopulmonary resuscitation (CPR) protocol when discovering an unconscious person or after witnessing a collapse. The pediatric protocol is to perform CPR for 1 minute and then activate the emergency medical system. The ABCs of CPR are airway, breathing, and circulation. These words help the rescuer remember the sequence to follow when performing CPR.

▸ The head tilt–chin lift maneuver is the preferred technique for opening the airway of an unconscious victim. If neck injury is suspected, use the jaw thrust maneuver to decrease the chance of compounding the injury.

▸ Because of the risk of contracting pathogens when coming into contact with a victim's oral secretions,

it is advisable to use a barrier device when performing CPR. A pocket mask with a one-way valve will assist in keeping the rescuer from coming into contact with a victim's oral secretions.

▸ When performing CPR on an adult, ventilate 12 times per minute and compress 80 to 100 times per minute. For children, ventilate 15 times per minute and compress at the same rate as for an adult. For infants, ventilate 20 times per minute and compress 100 times per minute.

▸ Complications of CPR may arise even when performed correctly. Fear of inflicting injury should not stop you from performing CPR. Be sure to follow established guidelines and practice techniques.

▸ CPR may be discontinued for reasons such as restoration of spontaneous respiration and circulation, complete rescuer exhaustion, and a medical decision to stop CPR.

▸ Advanced life support is the responsibility of trained professionals. In addition to performing BLS, nurses can provide support to the cardiac arrest victim's significant others. Keep them informed without giving them false hope.

▸ Survivors of cardiopulmonary arrest react in a variety of ways. A number of survivors report that they heard everything said by the staff during a resuscitation. Think before speaking in these emergencies.

▸ Manual chest thrusts and abdominal thrusts (Heimlich maneuver) are used to relieve a foreign body airway obstruction in adults. After removal of an airway obstruction, CPR may be necessary. Foreign body airway obstruction in infants and children is relieved by a combination of back blows (infant) and chest thrusts (infants and children).

Bibliography

1. Alteri, C., & Doherty, J. (1988). Current recommendations for basic life support: application of the nursing process. *Journal of Cardiovascular Nursing*, 3(1), 57–67.
2. American Heart Association. (1988). *Healthcare provider's manual*. Dallas, TX: American Heart Association, Office of Communications.
3. Britt, J. (1990). What to do when your patient codes. *Nursing*, 20(1), 42–43.
4. Criley, J. M. (1980). Coughing to keep the flow. *Emergency Medicine*, 12, 61.
5. Dierking, B. H. (1990). Reviewing basic life support for children. *Journal of Emergency Medical Services*, 15(2), 112–115.
6. Dolan, M. B. (1984). Where do you stand on . . . the coding question? *Nursing 84*, 4(3), 42.
7. Durbin, C. G. (1990). Mouth-to-mask resuscitation by lay rescuers—will they or won't they. *Respiratory Care*, 35(8), 832–833.
8. Ellstrom, K., & Bella, L. D. (1990). Understanding your role during a code. *Nursing 90*, 20(5), 49–51.
9. Ferguson, A. (1990). Cardiopulmonary resuscitation—a teaching guide. *Nursing Education Today*, 10(1), 38–48, 53, 241–244.
10. Finkelmeier, B. A., et al. (1984). Psychological ramifications of survival from sudden cardiac death. *Critical Care Quarterly*, 7(9), 71.
11. Fluck, R. R., & Sorbello, J. G. (1990). Mouth-to-mask resuscitation by lay rescuers—should they or shouldn't they. *Respiratory Care*, 35(8), 831–832.
12. Fracassi, J., & Moran, P. (1987). Cardiac arrest: when documentation is critical. *Critical Care Nurse*, 17(3), 90–93.

13. Green, E. (1990). Clues to a code: subtle signs can help you save a life. *RN*, 53(7), 26–31.

14. Guidelines for cardiopulmonary resuscitation and emergency cardiac care. (1992). *Journal of the American Medical Association*, 268(16), 2171–2197.

15. Guildner, C. W. (1980). Getting air into the lungs. *Emergency Medicine*, 12, 18.

16. Barkalow, C. E. (1975). Letter to the editors. *Heart and Lung*, 4(6), 972.

17. Heimlich, H. J., & Patrick, E. A. (1990). The Heimlich maneuver: best technique for saving any choking victim's life. *Postgraduate Medicine*, 87(6), 38–48.

18. Hess, D., & Spahr, C. (1990). An evaluation of volumes delivered by selected adult disposable resuscitators. *Respiratory Care*, 35(8), 800–805.

19. Juip, M. (1988). Giving mouth-to-mouth ventilations. *Nursing*, 3(1), 57–67.

20. Litwack, K., & Rothenberg, D. (1989). An update on basic and advanced cardiac life support. *Journal of Post Anesthesia Nursing 89*, 4(6), 377–381.

21. Luce, J., et al. (1980). New developments in cardiopulmonary resuscitation. *Journal of the American Medical Association*, 244, 1366.

22. Miracle, V. A., & Allnutt, D. R. (1990). Using a manual resuscitator correctly. *Nursing 90*, 20(5), 49–51.

23. Newman, M. (1990). CPR comes full circle: issues and trends for the 1990's. *JEMS*, 15(4), 48, 51–55.

24. O'Mara, S. R., & Summers, C. (1984). Caring for the sudden death survivor. *Critical Care Quarterly*, 7(9), 81.

25. Ornato, J. F., et al. (1990). Attitudes of BCLS instructors about mouth-to-mouth resuscitation during AIDS epidemic. *Annals of Emergency Medicine*, 10, 151–156.

26. Outwater, K. M., et al. (1989). Pediatric resuscitation. *Journal of Emergency Nursing*, 15(6), 466–474.

27. Risk of infection during CPR training and rescue: supplemental guidelines. (1989). *Journal of the American Medical Association*, 262(19), 2714–2715.

28. Rudnitsky, G. S., & Cahill, L. J. (1989). Pediatric and neonatal resuscitation. *Topics in Emergency Medicine*, 11(2), 68–76.

29. Sheard, T. (1990). Going face to face with fear. *Nursing 90*, 20(4), 43.

30. Spence, A. A., et al. (1967). Observations on intragastric pressure. *Anesthesia*, 22, 249.

31. Standards and guidelines for cardiopulmonary resuscitation and emergency cardiac care. (1986). *Journal of the American Medical Association*, 255(21), 2841–3044.

32. Stueven, H. A. (1990). Prehospital CPR: a review, in perspective. *Resuscitation*, 17, S71–77.

33. Willens, J. S., & Copel, L. C. (1989). Performing CPR on adults. *Nursing 89*, 19(1), 34–43.

34. Willens, J. S., & Copel, L. C. (1989). Performing CPR on infants. *Nursing 89*, 19(3), 47–53.

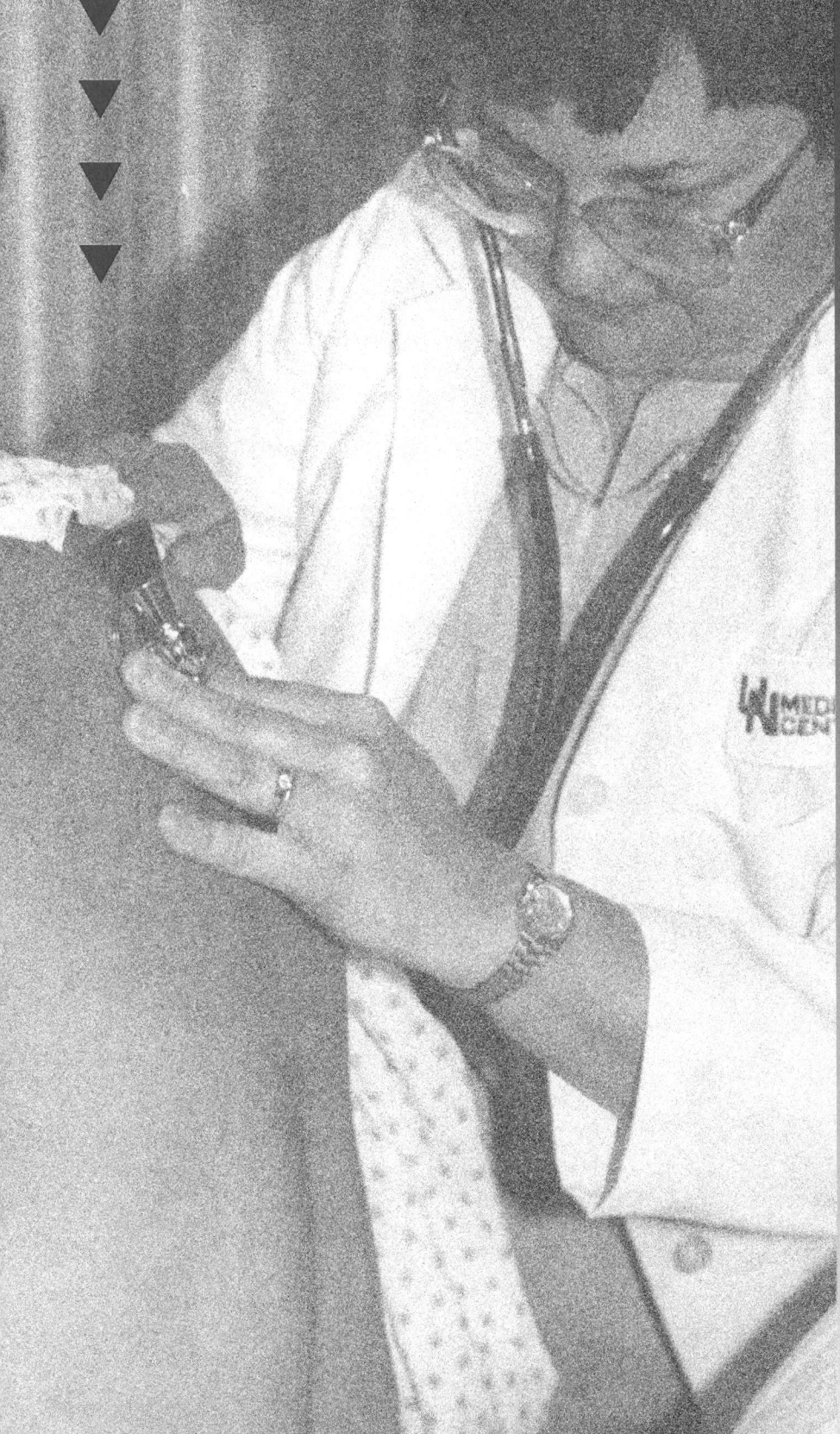

Assessment Skills

Unit 8

▼ Assessing Vital Signs

Chapter
31

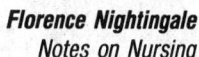

The most important practical lesson that can be given to nurses is to teach them what to observe—how to observe—what symptoms indicate improvement—what the reverse—which are of importance —which are of none. . . .

Florence Nightingale
Notes on Nursing

▼ CHAPTER OUTLINE

VITAL SIGNS AS THE BUILDING BLOCKS OF ASSESSMENT
ASSESSMENT OF TEMPERATURE
    Heat Production
    Heat Loss
    Regulation of Body Temperature
    Normal Ranges for Body Temperature
    Measuring Body Temperature
    Alterations in Body Temperature
ASSESSMENT OF PULSE
    Basic Cardiovascular Physiology
    Pulse Sites
    Pulse Rate
    Pulse Rhythm
    Pulse Force (Pulse Quality)
ASSESSMENT OF RESPIRATION
    Basic Pulmonary Physiology
    Control of Respiration
    Techniques for Assessing Respiration
    Quality of Respiration
    Rate and Depth of Respirations
    Patterns of Respiration

    Significant Characteristics in Respiratory Assessment
ASSESSMENT OF BLOOD PRESSURE
    Physiology of Arterial Pressure
    Blood Pressure Equipment
    Blood Pressure Measurement Techniques
    Blood Pressure Measurement in Infants and Children
    Errors in Blood Pressure Measurement
    Interpreting Abnormal Blood Pressure Findings
NURSING RESPONSIBILITY IN COMMUNICATING FINDINGS
SPECIAL PROCEDURES USING ELECTRONIC MONITORING
    The Cardiac Monitor
    The Doppler
    The Pulse Oximeter
    The Arterial Line
    Hemodynamic Pressure Monitoring
    Care of the Person Being Monitored

▼ KEY TERMS

Afebrile
Apnea
Apneustic respirations
Arrhythmia
Auscultatory gap
Biot's respirations

Bradycardia
Bradypnea
Central integrator
Cheyne-Stokes respirations
Core temperature

Defervescence
Diastolic pressure
Diffusion
Dyspnea
Hypercapnia
Hyperpnea

▼ *KEY TERMS* Continued

Hyperpyrexia	*Kussmaul's respirations*	*Pulse*	*Stroke volume*
Hypertension	*Orthopnea*	*Pulse deficit*	*Systolic pressure*
Hyperthermia	*Orthostatic hypotension*	*Respiration*	*Tachycardia*
Hyperventilation	*Oximeter*	*Sigh*	*Tachypnea*
Hypotension	*Paradoxical pulse*	*Sphygmomanometer*	*Vital signs*
Hypothermia	*Peripheral vascular resistance*	*Stertor*	*Wheeze*
Hypoventilation		*Stridor*	
Korotkoff sounds			

▼ *LEARNING OBJECTIVES*

After studying this chapter, you should be able to

1. *Discuss the meaning of "routine" vital signs.*
2. *Explain the importance of monitoring body temperature.*
3. *Identify the factors that affect body temperature.*
4. *List the types of thermometers and routes for measuring temperature.*
5. *List measures for nursing management of fever.*
6. *Describe the physiology of the pulse.*
7. *Explain the technique for assessment of the pulse.*
8. *Describe the mechanisms that control respiration.*
9. *Describe the assessment of respirations.*
10. *Define the term* blood pressure.
11. *State the rationale for blood pressure measurement.*
12. *Identify nursing responsibilities related to the assessment of vital signs.*
13. *Describe the role of new technologies in the assessment of vital signs.*

Temperature, pulse, respiration, and blood pressure are **vital signs,** vital because they are indispensable indicators of a person's current state of health. Even when your client seems to be in a state of high-level wellness, it is often important to assess the vital signs as a means to establish baseline data with which to judge the significance of any future deviations from what appear to be the "characteristic" or "normal." Vital signs are always assessed at the following times:

▶ During a basic screening physical examination
▶ Upon admission to the hospital or health care agency
▶ As a daily routine while hospitalized, to reveal any change in physical or psychologic status
▶ Before and after surgery or invasive diagnostic procedures
▶ While on medications that alter cardiovascular, respiratory, or temperature control status (e.g., antihypertensives, digitalis)
▶ Following nursing interventions that may affect cardiovascular status (e.g., resuming ambulation, nasotracheal suctioning)
▶ Whenever the client's perception of the health state changes (e.g., "I feel funny," or "Nurse, I'm feeling faint.")

Measuring vital signs is a basic skill on which your assessment prowess can build. Although electronic machinery is used in selected situations to help in gathering data, you have an irreplaceable role in interpreting data.

VITAL SIGNS AS THE BUILDING BLOCKS OF ASSESSMENT

"Routine" vital signs is a misnomer. Rather than a rote task performed automatically so many times a day, the accurate assessment of vital signs is an important and crucial part of nursing care. You must know how to take vital signs, interpret data, communicate them to others, and plan nursing interventions appropriately. Thus, taking vital signs is a part of the nursing process.

As you recall, the nursing process (assessment, nursing diagnosis, planning, nursing intervention, evaluation) is a deliberate problem-solving approach. Assessment is a systematic way of collecting data. It determines nursing diagnoses for development of the nursing care plan. Taking vital signs means gathering data for the data base. The more knowledge you have about vital signs, the more enriched the data base will be.

Keep the following guidelines in mind while assessing vital signs.

▶ Routine vital signs should be taken by the staff member caring for the person during that shift — *not* by one nurse assigned to take vital signs for the whole floor. In this way, the staff member who knows the person best is the one gathering the data and assessing how these data fit into the whole health picture.

▶ Know the normal range of each vital sign.

▶ Know the baseline data for each person; that is, know what is normal for each individual. What is "normal" for one person may differ from the standard range typical for that age and physical condition.

▶ Know the vital sign readings from the previous shift. In the case of seriously ill individuals, these data will help you evaluate whether the person's condition is improving or deteriorating and will give you a basis for planning nursing actions.

▶ Know the person's medical diagnosis, treatment, and medications; these factors may alter vital signs.

▶ Take the vital signs in a systematic manner. Establish routines for yourself and do not vary them, otherwise you could omit an important step. When appropriate, compare the data bilaterally (on corresponding sides of the person's body).

▶ During the shift, gather vital signs as often as you think necessary. Assessing vital signs is a *serial* process, not a single event. The establishment of trends or the comparison of changes is much more meaningful than stating one-time statistics. Do not wait for the next routine time if you suspect an untoward trend is developing. For example, after surgery, Mr. Charles J.'s order reads, "Check vital signs q 15 min × 1 hr, then q 1 hr × 4, then QID." If you note a rapid, weak pulse and blood pressure (BP) significantly below Mr. J.'s recovery room value, do not wait for another 15 minutes to elapse. Remain with Mr. J.; check his vital signs at least every 5 minutes, inspect him for signs of hemorrhage, and notify the physician. Your prompt intervention can forestall serious, perhaps fatal, consequences.

▶ Recheck the vital signs on a newly admitted person at least twice during the first 8 hours of admission. Pulse and BP measurements obtained on admission may not be reliable baseline data from which to interpret the person's subsequent physiologic status. Anxiety associated with hospital admission, nervousness, and exertion tend to distort initial vital sign readings, causing them to be higher.

▶ At the bedside, be aware of your nonverbal communication. If your facial expression and body movements contradict your verbal message, the person will believe the nonverbal message more than spoken words. Think about Mr. J. again. Assuring Mr. J. that he is fine and that his vital signs are normal is meaningless if you take the BP three or four times in a row, furrow your brow in a concerned fashion, and call in another staff member to check your findings. Mr. J. will feel much more confident in your skill and in his future if you give him some information such as, "Your blood pressure is lower than it was in the recovery room, so I am going to stay with you and check it a few more times."

▶ After checking the vital signs, put this information together with other data collected about the person. Analyze the data along with the complete health status. What relationship exists among the data? Are

any *trends* evolving? Also, consider any environmental factors that may influence the data, such as room temperature, humidity, or noise.

Vital signs are not isolated numbers. They are grouped data that reflect interrelated physiologic systems.

Once the data have been collected, analysis leads to the nursing diagnosis and to planning the nursing interventions. To analyze the data, you must know the physiology behind each of the vital signs, the variations that are normal, and the implications of abnormal vital signs. Take time now to review individually the temperature, pulse, respiration, and BP. As you proceed through the chapter, note how the vital signs relate to one another and to the person as a whole.

ASSESSMENT OF TEMPERATURE

Body temperature reflects an organism's capacity to balance heat production and heat loss. When this homeostatic mechanism goes awry, the result is an abnormally elevated body temperature, termed fever, or an abnormally low temperature, termed **hypothermia.**

The body continually produces and loses heat. A constant exchange of energy in the form of heat takes place not only between a person's body and the environment but also between compartments within the body itself. Heat exchange is influenced by such factors as ambient temperature, humidity, wind velocity, air currents, the amount of clothing worn, and body position.

Maintenance of body temperature despite variations in the environmental temperature is a homeostatic process involving the coordinated functioning of many organ systems. For body temperature to remain constant, a homeostatic balance must exist between heat production in the body (thermogenesis) and heat loss to the environment (thermolysis).

Heat Production

Heat is produced by metabolism, which is the sum of all the chemical reactions in all body cells. The minimal rate at which the body produces heat from metabolic processes is called the basal metabolic rate. In the normal adult, the heat produced under resting conditions is about 70 kilocalories (kcal) per hour.[21] The following five factors increase the metabolic rate: (1) muscular activity (exercise or shivering); (2) increased sympathetic nervous system stimulation, which in turn raises blood epinephrine and norepinephrine levels; (3) increased blood levels of thyroxine, a thyroid hormone; (4) oxidation of food; and (5) fever.

Heat Loss

The principal method for regulating heat loss is by the body varying the amount of blood flowing near the body surface, where the heat can be lost to the atmosphere. This process is accomplished by vasodilation, an increase in the size of the blood vessel lumen. A rise in body temperature stimulates vasodilation, which increases the peripheral circulation and brings blood and heat to the body surface. As a result, the skin appears flushed or pink in lightly pigmented individuals, and is warm to the touch. Under proper conditions, excess body heat is eliminated through four methods of heat loss: (1) radiation, (2) conduction, (3) convection, and (4) evaporation. The effectiveness of each method depends on the amount of heat generated by the body and on environmental conditions.

RADIATION

Radiation is the movement of heat, in the form of infrared rays, outward from a warm object to the cooler surrounding air. When a person is resting at normal room temperature, 60 per cent of heat loss occurs by radiation. In a warm environment, the amount of heat lost by radiation decreases and can even reverse; that is, heat can be gained by radiation.[21] Variables that can influence heat loss from radiation include the amount of body surface area exposed, skin and surface temperature, reflective power of the skin and clothing, radiant temperature, and the nature of the environment.

CONDUCTION

Conduction is the flow of heat from a warmer to a cooler object when the objects are in direct contact. In the body, heat is conducted from the warm internal tissues to the skin surface. It is then lost to the environment (to the air or to objects in direct contact with the body).

Some materials are better conductors than others (e.g., metal conducts better than wool or air). Layers of clothing or feathers provide good insulation. Muscle and fat are also good insulators, since they provide resistance to heat flow. Hence, a thicker layer of subcutaneous fat is advantageous in cold climates.

CONVECTION

Convection is the transfer of heat from a warmer to a cooler object by means of circulating fluid or gas. For example, the body loses excess heat as surrounding air currents carry away the heat to the cooler environment. These currents are called convection currents. Water and other fluids also serve as convection currents.

The rate of heat lost from a hotter object to a colder one is proportional to the temperature difference between the objects. The rate of heat loss by convection depends on the difference between skin and air (or water) temperature as well as air velocity or rate of water movement. If the wind velocity is high, for example, heat is lost more rapidly.

Convection also operates within the body. The transfer of heat from the bloodstream to the skin is very important. In a cold environment, vasoconstriction, a decrease in the size of the blood vessel lumen, prevents heat loss by convection. Thus, less heat reaches the body's surface to be carried away by the air. The converse is also true. In a hot environment or during increased muscular activity, vasodilation increases heat flow to the surface, increasing heat loss.

EVAPORATION

Evaporation is the transfer of heat through the conversion of water to vapor. Evaporation occurs in two ways: insensible loss and sweating. An adult loses approximately 600 ml of water per day through "insensible" water evaporation from the skin and lungs, which results in a loss of 280 to 380 kcal of heat per day. This loss occurs regardless of body temperature and does not play a major role in thermoregulation.

In contrast, evaporative sweating can greatly alter body temperature. Sweating is a major protective mechanism against overheating. Sweating occurs as a result of high skin temperature or high internal temperature, muscular activity, and emotional or mental stress. Certain types of shock activate sweating, which accounts for the cold, clammy skin observed in these conditions. In cold weather, sweat production is minimal. A person who has been exposed to hot weather for at least 1 to 6 weeks, however, becomes acclimatized and can produce as much as 1.5 L of sweat per hour!

Several factors affect the efficiency with which sweating is able to reduce body heat. Efficiency decreases when there is a reduction in air currents. The air surrounding the body becomes saturated with water vapor, which inhibits further evaporation. High humidity also interferes with evaporation. Thus, a person often feels hotter on a humid, windless day. Finally, in older adults, sweat glands decrease in number and function. Decreased response of the sweat glands to thermoregulatory demand puts the aging person at greater risk of heat stroke.

Regulation of Body Temperature

Humans and other mammals are homeothermic (warm blooded) and so have body temperatures that remain relatively stable despite variations in environmental temperatures. In homeothermic mammals, body temperature is regulated in the presence of environmental extremes by means of physiologic and behavioral control mechanisms. Physiologic regulation involves the body's involuntary responses to changes in environmental temperature. The nervous system, in particular the hypothalamus, is the principal physiologic regulator. Behavioral regulation involves voluntary responses; that is, individuals consciously control their actions to manipulate the environment.

PHYSIOLOGIC REGULATION*

Physiologic regulation refers to the involuntary responses that maintain constant body temperature. The body generally strives to maintain a temperature around 37°C (98.6°F). This critical temperature, called the set point, is optimum for the body. A shift away from the set point in either direction activates thermoregulatory mechanisms that alter heat production and dissipation in order to return body temperature to the set point. Fever results from an increase in the thermal set point.

Body temperature is primarily regulated by the nervous system. Nervous system regulation depends on (1) receptors, (2) a central integrator, and (3) effector mechanisms.

Receptors are temperature-specialized nerve endings that sense internal and external temperatures. They are located in the skin, abdominal organs, spinal cord, and hypothalamus. Receptors send information regarding internal and external environment to the integrator.

The **central integrator** is the center in the brain, located in the hypothalamus, that maintains core body temperature. The central integrator interprets data from the receptors and initiates the appropriate response. This area is often called the hypothalamic thermostat. The "thermostat" operates in much the same way as a thermostat in the home. In the body, the hypothalamic thermostat operates through negative feedback mechanisms to keep body temperature stable at the set point of approximately 37°C (98.6°F). If the thermostat detects excessive heat or cold, it sends signals to the effector organs that alter blood flow, metabolism, sweating, and insensible heat loss in order to return the body to normal temperatures.

The effectors of temperature regulation include blood vessels, skeletal muscle, and sweat glands. When the body conserves heat, superficial blood vessels constrict, thus bringing less blood to the body's surface for dissipation. Skeletal muscles contract to produce more heat (sometimes resulting in shivering), and the sweat glands are inhibited. In addition to these responses, secretion of epinephrine and norepinephrine increases in order to stimulate heat production. During periods when heat dissipation is necessary (e.g., during exercise or exposure to hot environmental temperatures), the effectors respond in a contrary manner—cutaneous blood vessels dilate, shivering is inhibited, and sweating is stimulated. Also, respirations become rapid and shallow, which slightly increases heat loss.

BEHAVIORAL REGULATION

Behavioral regulation operates in environmental extremes and is important in temperature control. When possible, humans modify their behavior in response to sensations of heat or cold. The type and extent of behavioral modification depends on (a) the thermal environment, (b) the person's ability to perceive the sensation as comfortable or uncomfortable, and (c) the person's emotional state. For example, when individuals perceive heat, they respond by shedding clothing, seeking a cooler environment, stretching out their bodies, and decreasing activity. A person responding to intense cold may curl up in a ball, move to a warmer place, increase the temperature setting on a home thermostat, or increase activity by foot stamping and jumping up and down. For humans, behavioral regulation is the only really effective mechanism for conserving body heat in severely cold environments.[21]

Behavioral modification is effective in controlling body temperature only when people can manipulate their environment and limit exposure. Modern technology allows us to adjust environmental temperatures and humidity and to wear special clothing. However, not everyone can afford adequately heated homes and warm clothing in the winter and air conditioning in the summer. Also, immobilized or elderly individuals may be unable to sense extremes of heat and cold. Consequently, they fail to recognize the need to modify environmental temperatures, body position, activity level, and clothing.

Figure 31–1 summarizes the mechanisms of thermoregulatory control.

CONSEQUENCES OF THERMOREGULATORY FAILURE

Cells, tissue, and organs of the body function best between temperatures of 36° and 38°C (96.8° to 100.4°F). However, when the homeostatic mechanisms of thermoregulation malfunction and the body temperature is either too high or too low, cell and tissue damage occurs. For short periods, people can tolerate increased temperatures of 40° to 41°C (104° to 106°F) without irreversible damage. When temperatures climb above 41° to 42.2°C (106° to 108°F), however, tissue damage results because cellular proteins are denatured or inactivated and most enzyme functions are impaired.[21,41]

Conversely, humans also do not tolerate a low body temperature, and prolonged hypothermia damages cell membranes. Crystals form as tissues freeze, causing injury. Low body temperature (hypothermia) of 21° to 24°C (70° to 75°F) may be tolerated for short periods, especially if it occurs under medical supervision.

Normal Ranges for Body Temperature

Because many factors such as age, physical activity, and circadian rhythms affect normal body temperature, it is misleading to say that 37°C (98.6°F) is the one "normal" body temperature. Actually, "normal" body temperature consists of a range of temperature readings that is relatively constant from day to day. Figure 31–2 depicts the range of body temperature in a healthy individual.

FACTORS AFFECTING BODY TEMPERATURE

External Temperature. A warm room or a hot day may increase body temperature by 1°C. On the other

---

*Homeostatic feedback mechanisms are discussed in Chapter 17. Take time to review this material before proceeding further with this chapter.

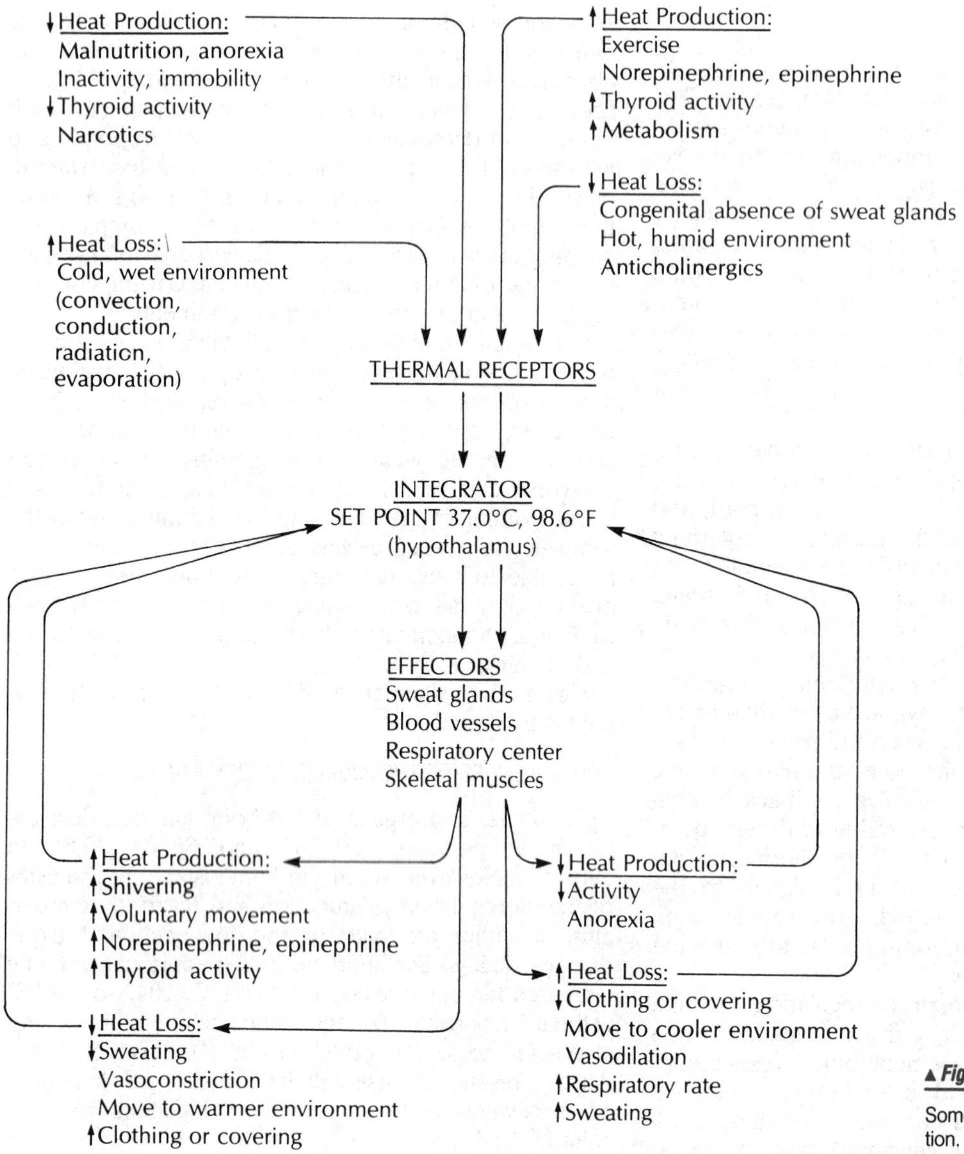

↓Heat Production: ────────────
    Malnutrition, anorexia
    Inactivity, immobility
    ↓Thyroid activity
    Narcotics

↑Heat Production: ────────────
    Exercise
    Norepinephrine, epinephrine
    ↑Thyroid activity
    ↑Metabolism

↓Heat Loss: ────────────
    Congenital absence of sweat glands
    Hot, humid environment
    Anticholinergics

↑Heat Loss:\ ────────────
    Cold, wet environment
    (convection,
    conduction,
    radiation,
    evaporation)

THERMAL RECEPTORS

INTEGRATOR
SET POINT 37.0°C, 98.6°F
(hypothalamus)

EFFECTORS
Sweat glands
Blood vessels
Respiratory center
Skeletal muscles

↑Heat Production: ◄────
    ↑Shivering
    ↑Voluntary movement
    ↑Norepinephrine, epinephrine
    ↑Thyroid activity

↓Heat Loss: ◄────
    ↓Sweating
    Vasoconstriction
    Move to warmer environment
    ↑Clothing or covering

►↓Heat Production: ────
    ↓Activity
    Anorexia

►↑Heat Loss: ────
    ↓Clothing or covering
    Move to cooler environment
    Vasodilation
    ↑Respiratory rate
    ↑Sweating

▲ *Figure 31–1*

Some mechanisms of thermoregulation.

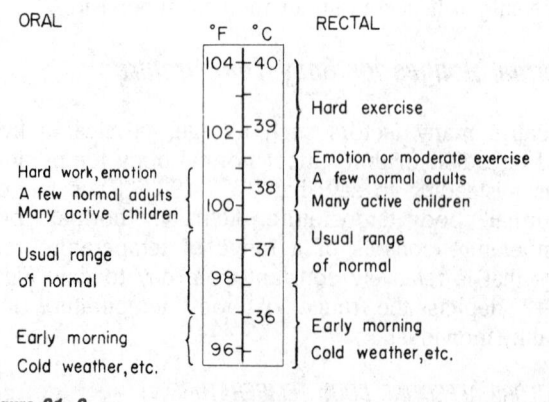

ORAL   RECTAL
                          °F   °C
                        104┬─40
                                      Hard exercise
                        102┤─39
                                      Emotion or moderate exercise
Hard work, emotion   A few normal adults
A few normal adults   100┤─38   Many active children
Many active children
                            ┤─37
Usual range   Usual range
of normal   98 ┤   of normal
                            ┤─36
                        96 ┤   Early morning
Early morning   Cold weather, etc.
Cold weather, etc.

▲ *Figure 31–2*

Estimated normal range of body temperature in healthy persons. (From DuBois, E. F. [1948]. *Fever and the regulation of temperature.* Springfield, IL, Charles C Thomas.)

hand, a cold environment usually induces little change in body temperature, although a temperature drop may occur in infants and older adults.

Age. Body temperature is generally lower in older adults than in other age groups. This difference has a variety of causes. Older adults have a decreased sensitivity to temperature changes. Many older persons have limited incomes that, coupled with high fuel costs, prevent them from heating their homes properly. Older adults often have less subcutaneous fat to provide insulation. Some aging adults are malnourished and thus more susceptible to the deleterious effects of cold environments, and some aged persons are much less active than their younger counterparts and so produce less heat for dissipation.

In contrast, infants and young children have body temperatures slightly higher than the general population norm. Also, thermoregulatory mechanisms in the neonate are not fully developed. Infants are subject to marked temperature fluctuations when exposed to very warm or very cold external conditions. Therefore, babies must be protected from excessive heat or cold.

When caring for newborns, promote temperature homeostasis by keeping them dry, adequately clothed, and protected from cold or excessively hot environments.

Internal body temperature control remains somewhat labile until children reach puberty. Normal temperature ranges in children are wider than in adults and are more influenced by external conditions and activity levels. For example, youngsters in a warm environment may experience an elevated temperature after only slight exertion.[41]

Because children have a labile body temperature, they develop high temperatures rapidly when ill, dehydrated, or exposed to hot environments.

Circadian Rhythm (Diurnal Rhythm). The core temperature in humans fluctuates rhythmically from 0.5° to 1°C (0.9 to 1.8°F) over a 24-hour period. Generally, it rises steeply from early to midmorning, rises more gradually in the afternoon, peaks between 4:00 PM and 8:00 PM, and then sharply declines. Body temperature is generally lowest between midnight and 6:00 AM. Most hospitals have a routine of checking temperatures of all people twice a day—once in the early morning and once before 5:00 PM. However, from a study of over 100 hospitalized adults, one researcher concluded that taking the temperature *once* a day between 5:00 PM and 7:00 PM during the peak of the circadian thermal rhythm is adequate to screen for fever in hospitalized adults.[47]

Hormones. In women, periodic temperature fluctuations occur in relation to the menstrual cycle. Physiologists believe that this change results from the rise of progesterone levels in the blood. Studies show that, on average, body temperature drops approximately 0.3°C (0.54°F) a few days before ovulation. Immediately following ovulation, the temperature jumps about 0.6°C (1.1°F), then falls slightly just prior to menstruation.[35]

Body temperature also becomes elevated in response to large amounts of circulating thyroid hormone and growth hormone. These hormones increase body metabolism, thus increasing heat production. The release of epinephrine from the adrenal medulla in response to cold is another example of interaction between the endocrine system and the thermoregulatory centers.

Stress. Psychologic and physiologic stressors raise body temperature by triggering neural and hormonal activity. For example, stimulation of the sympathetic nervous system results in secretion of epinephrine and norepinephrine, which in turn increases metabolic activity, thereby increasing body temperature.

Temperature Variances Between Body Core and Surface. The term *body temperature* usually refers to the temperature of the interior of the body—the **core temperature** in the thoracic and abdominal cavities and in the central nervous system. Ideally, it is the core temperature that you measure when you take someone's temperature. Core temperature is closely regulated and deviates less than 1°C (1.8°F) under normal conditions. However, surface temperature, the temperature of skin and underlying peripheral tissues, can fluctuate widely, depending on the environment. Peripheral skin, muscle, and subcutaneous fat are generally cooler than core temperatures. In general, the skin of the face, trunk, arms, and legs is warmer than that of the feet, hands, ears, and nose. Because of these differences, it is important to place the thermometer near a major artery when measuring body temperature. Otherwise, you may report surface temperatures rather than core temperatures.

Measuring Body Temperature

Body temperature is one of the oldest and most frequently used indicators of health or illness. Unfortunately, the procedure for measuring body temperature is often "ritualistic" and follows the routine of an agency rather than being performed in response to a particular clinical situation.

Take temperatures carefully and report them promptly and accurately. If you question the temperature obtained, repeat the procedure with the same or a different thermometer.

TYPES OF THERMOMETERS

Body temperatures have been recorded since the 16th century, when a precursor of the modern glass thermometer was developed. Until recently, the mercury thermometer has been the one most often used, but now many hospitals and health care agencies use electronic, disposable, or tympanic thermometers.

All thermometers are calibrated in degrees Celsius (centigrade) or Fahrenheit. In the Celsius scale, 0°C is the point at which water freezes, and 100°C is the point at which water boils. In the Fahrenheit scale, 32°F is the freezing point and 212°F the boiling point of water. Table 31–1 gives equivalents and conversion factors for Celsius and Fahrenheit readings. Familiarize yourself with both scales; you will need to be able to think in both scales without taking the time for paper-and-pencil conversions.

Glass Thermometers. Glass mercury thermometers operate on the principle of thermal expansion. Mercury expands as it is heated and contracts as it is cooled. Thus, when mercury, encased in a closed, calibrated glass tube, comes into contact with the warmer body tissues of the mouth, rectum, or axilla, it expands and registers body temperature. Glass thermometers take approximately 3 to 8 minutes to register, depending on

TABLE 31-1. Celsius and Fahrenheit Equivalents

°C	=	°F
−10		14.0
−5		23.0
0	←Freezing point of water→	32.0
1		33.8
10		50.0
13		55.4
18		64.4
20		68.0
21		69.8
24		75.2
27		80.6
28		82.4
30		86.0
34		93.2
35		95.0
36		96.8
37	←Human body temperature→	98.6
38		100.4
39		102.2
40		104.0
41		105.8
42		107.6
43		109.4
44		111.2
45		113.0
46		114.8
50		122.0
55		131.0
60		140.0
65		149.0
70		158.0
75		167.0
80		176.0
85		185.0
90		194.0
95		203.0
100	←Boiling point of water→	212.0

Conversions:

$$T_{FAHRENHEIT} = (9/5)T_C + 32$$
$$T_{CELSIUS} = (5/9)(T_F - 32)$$

---

the route (oral, axillary, or rectal). Note that different shapes of glass thermometers are used for different routes (Fig. 31-3).

One advantage of glass thermometers is that they can be reused following careful disinfection. Disadvantages of glass thermometers are that they take a significant amount of time to register and that they have a risk of breaking. A person may inadvertently break the thermometer by biting it. Biting risks lacerating the delicate mucous membranes and ingesting the mercury that leaks out of a broken thermometer, causing mercury poisoning.

Because of the potential for injury and the problem of disinfection, many hospitals have stopped using glass thermometers, although glass thermometers are still widely used in the home. In any location, to avoid a serious accident, do not use glass thermometers by the oral route for people with these problems:

▶ Severe coughing or sneezing attacks
▶ Shaking chills
▶ Convulsive disorders
▶ Severe confusion and combativeness

This route also is contraindicated in young children.

Also, use caution when taking a rectal temperature with a mercury glass thermometer. A broken rectal glass thermometer can perforate the colon and rectal wall.

Electronic Thermometers. Electronic thermometers are convenient to use, accurate, safe, and rapid in registering temperature (2 to 60 seconds). Their disposable covers save time and work and prevent contamination (Fig. 31-4). They operate on the principle that heat offers resistance to a current in proportion to its temperature. This resistance is converted to a measurement that is displayed digitally.

The electronic thermometer equipment consists of a battery pack with a probe attached and disposable probe covers. Read instructions carefully before use. Some types of electronic thermometers use the same probe for oral, rectal, or continuous temperatures, but other manufacturers supply different probes for different routes. Use of the wrong probe can result in inaccurate readings.

Disposable Thermometers. Disposable, single-use thermometers come in several types. Chemical dot

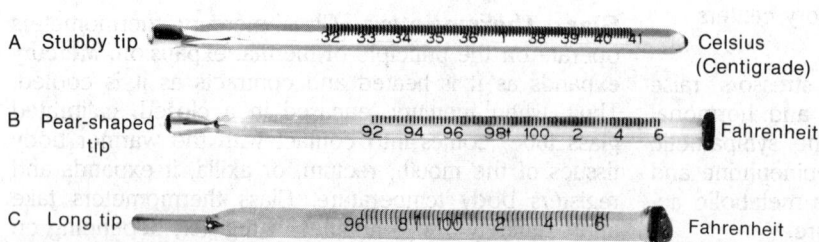

A Stubby tip · · · · · · · · · Celsius (Centigrade)

B Pear-shaped tip · · · · · · · · · Fahrenheit

C Long tip · · · · · · · · · Fahrenheit

▲ **Figure 31-3**

Oral thermometers have (A) stubby, (B) pear-shaped, or (C) long tips. Those with the stubby or pear-shaped tips are also used as rectal and axillary thermometers. All types are available in the Celsius (centigrade) scale or the Fahrenheit scale.

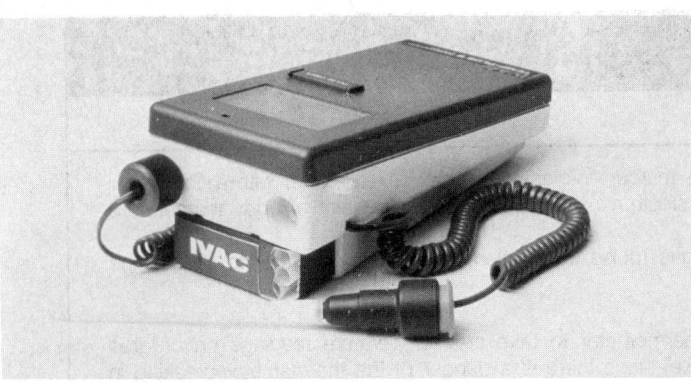

▲ **Figure 31-4**

The IVAC TEMP-PLUS II Model 2080A electronic thermometer with digital readout. Note the probe covers and the two probes, separate probes for oral and rectal temperatures. (Courtesy of IVAC Corporation, San Diego, CA.)

thermometers contain chemical units that change color at a specific temperature. Keep these thermometers in their individually sealed wrappers until they are ready for use. Place the device in the mouth under the tongue like a glass thermometer. It usually takes about 60 seconds to register a temperature. People can bite down on these devices safely. They are used for people in clinics, schools, blood banks, and in isolation rooms in hospitals.

Tympanic Thermometers. The tympanic thermometer is the newest development in temperature monitoring and one that utilizes a new route (Fig. 31-5). The thermometer senses the infrared emissions of the tym-

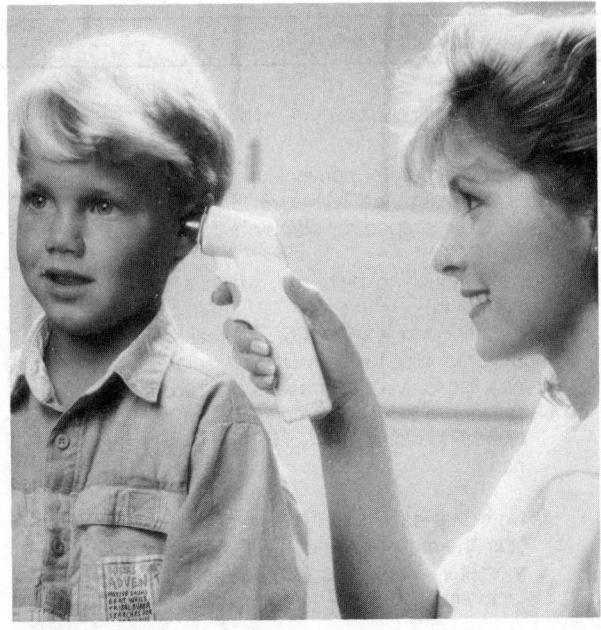

▲ **Figure 31-5**

A nurse takes a child's temperature with the IVAC CORE-CHECK tympanic thermometer. (Courtesy of IVAC Corporation, San Diego, CA.)

panic membrane in the ear and obtains a measurement of the body's core temperature. The tympanic membrane gives an accurate measurement of the core temperature because the membrane shares the same blood supply as the hypothalamus. Shinozaki and colleagues studied core temperatures measured with the Swan-Ganz catheter in the pulmonary artery near the heart and with the tympanic thermometer in the ear. Measurements of core body temperature using the Swan-Ganz catheter correlated highly with measurements using the tympanic thermometer.[49]

The tympanic thermometer is a noninvasive, nontraumatic device that is extremely quick and efficient. The probe tip has the shape of an otoscope. The probe is gently placed in the person's ear canal while the examiner pulls up and back gently on the pinna. The pinna must be tugged gently to straighten the ear canal and give the device good access to the radiations from the tympanic membrane and not the ear canal.[44] Activate the thermometer and the temperature can be read in 2 to 3 seconds! There is minimal chance of cross-contamination because the ear canal is lined with skin and not mucous membrane.

The tympanic thermometer does not seem to be affected by the presence of cerumen in the ear canal, nor does the presence of otitis media seem to affect the temperature reading to any significant degree.[6] The thermometer should not be used in persons with drainage or discharge from the ears or those who have a great deal of scarring on the tympanic membrane.[44]

This thermometer has been used successfully in critical care units, emergency departments, ambulatory care and pediatric settings, nurseries, clinics, and hospital units. Barber and Kilmon studied over 700 children and parents in a pediatric clinic and found that the nurses, parents, and children all favored the use of the tympanic thermometer over the usual rectal and oral thermometers because of its speed, convenience, and lack of invasiveness.[3]

TECHNIQUES FOR TEMPERATURE MONITORING

Temperature monitoring is a *serial* process performed to identify trends and to evaluate a person's health status and progress. Therefore, always obtain a baseline temperature to establish a value against which to compare subsequent temperature readings. Methods for monitoring temperature are described in Procedure 31-1.

The five routes for measuring temperature are oral, rectal, axillary, tympanic, and core. Each route has a place in clinical practice. Although many agencies stipulate the route and frequency of measuring temperatures, you must also use your own judgment in monitoring temperatures. Your decision concerning route and frequency of measurement should be based on careful and continuing assessment of the individual's condition.

Once a route is selected, use it *consistently* unless the person's condition changes. Avoid comparing temperatures taken via one route with those taken via another route.

Text continued on page 598

PROCEDURE 31–1

Measurement of Body Temperature

Definition/Purposes. Measurement of body temperature using a mercury-in-glass thermometer calibrated with a Celsius or Fahrenheit scale. Measurement of body temperature using an electronic thermometer. Measurement of body temperature using a tympanic thermometer.

Body temperature is used in conjunction with other vital signs (pulse, respiration, and blood pressure) to assess the person's health status.

Contraindications/Cautions. Oral: Do not use glass mercury thermometer to take oral temperature readings on children younger than 4 to 5 years or on confused or combative people, since there is a danger of the thermometer breaking in the mouth. Avoid the oral route in people with injuries or conditions that prevent them from closing their mouths fully. Do not use the oral route on individuals who are comatose, have a history of convulsive disorders, are mouth breathers, or have an oral infection (e.g., abscessed tooth). Wait at least 15 minutes after the person smokes, drinks, or eats. **Rectal:** Do not take rectal temperatures in people with rectal or perineal injuries or surgery. Lubricate the thermometer well and insert it gently to avoid damage to the mucosa or perforation of the rectum. **Axillary:** None. **Tympanic:** Insert the tip gently into the ear canal to avoid damage.

Learning/Teaching Guidelines. Provide the following information as appropriate: (1) explain the reason for monitoring body temperature; (2) teach about the types of thermometers and their use; (3) explain the factors that influence the choice of route for measurement of body temperature; (4) instruct the person not to eat, drink, or smoke for 15 minutes prior to an oral temperature reading.

PRELIMINARY ACTIVITIES

Assessment/Planning

▶ Check diagnosis.
▶ Note date and type of surgery (if applicable).
▶ Assess person's ability to follow directions.
▶ Note presence of oxygen, nasogastric tube, rectal tubes, or dressings.
▶ Check previous method of temperature determination.
▶ Check last measurement and range of temperatures.
▶ Assess need to measure temperature.
▶ Select appropriate route.
▶ Select appropriate thermometer.

Equipment

▶ Clean glass thermometer (or)
▶ Electronic thermometer and probe with disposable probe covers (or)
▶ Tympanic thermometer
▶ Paper and pencil or pen
▶ Water-soluble lubricant and disposable gloves for rectal temperature

---

Measurement of Body Temperature Using the Mercury-in-Glass Thermometer

ORAL TEMPERATURE

Actions

1. Oral temperature reading with mercury thermometer is appropriate for individuals over 4 or 5 years of age who are able to follow directions, close lips, and breathe through nose.
   a. Hold thermometer at end opposite bulb.

   b. Rinse in cold water if thermometer has been soaked in disinfectant. Dry with clean tissue, from bulb end to fingers.
   c. Read level of mercury.
      i. Hold thermometer with fingertips of right hand horizontal to floor with bulb to your left at eye level (or below head for individuals with bifocals).
      ii. Rotate thermometer with hand until you can read calibration and until silver mercury line comes into view.

Rationale/Discussion

1. Generally an accurate, convenient measurement of temperature. Normal range 36.5 to 37.5°C (97.6 to 99.4°F). Use long, pear-shaped, or stubby bulb oral thermometer (see Fig. 13–3).
   a. Prevents touching bulb end, which is placed in person's mouth.

   b. Hot water, over 41°C (106°F), breaks mercury thermometers. Disinfectants are unsafe for use on human tissue. Maintains asepsis of bulb end.
   c. Necessary to assess mercury level.
      i. Numbers would be upside down if held in left hand.

      ii. Note that each small line measure 0.1°C on Celsius thermometer and 0.2°F on Fahrenheit thermometer. Mercury is colored red by some manufacturers.

PROCEDURE 31–1 Continued

Actions

d. Shake down thermometer if mercury reads above 35.0°C (95.0°F).
  i. Grasp thermometer securely at end opposite bulb.
  ii. Stand away from walls, furniture, and equipment.
  iii. Quickly flex wrist with a snapping movement of the hand, as if cracking a whip.
e. Place plastic cover over thermometer if it is to be used for more than one person, if agency policy.
f. Moisten thermometer in cold water and/or ask person to moisten lips.

g. Place bulb of thermometer under person's tongue in the posterior sublingual area. This area is a pocket formed by frenulum of tongue, base of tongue, and floor of mouth on right or left side.
h. Tell person to close lips around thermometer and to avoid biting it.

i. Leave in place 3 to 4 minutes if person is afebrile and up to 8 minutes if febrile. (Take other vital signs during this time.) Obviously you cannot always predict if person is afebrile. Note the reading after the first 3 to 4 minutes, then reinsert the thermometer for 1 more minutes. If reading is the same, accept it. If it is rising, reinsert a third time. Continue until reading is stable.
j. Each time you remove the thermometer, grasp the end first and then ask person to open the mouth.
k. Remove plastic cover and discard. If not using plastic shealth, wipe secretions off with tissue. Wipe from your fingertips toward bulb.
l. Read thermometer measurement (see c above.).

m. Care for thermometer according to agency policy. Mallison[36] suggests washing thermometer with warm water and soap, then wiping with solution of 70 to 90 per cent isopropyl alcohol. Ideally, thermometer should be sent to central processing for disinfection and sterilization.

Rationale/Discussion

d. Reading must be below actual body temperature before use.
  i. Maintains asepsis of bulb end.

  ii. Avoids striking thermometer and breaking it.
  iii. Produces centrifugal force needed to move mercury past constriction and back into bulb.
e. Decreases contamination, and thus reduces cleaning time.
f. Dry thermometer adheres to dry mucous membranes. Danger of tearing tissue when thermometer removed.
g. ''Heat pocket'' at posterior base of tongue adjacent to molars is more accurate because of proximity of the pocket to larger blood vessels (Fig. 31–6).

Caution: Thermometer can break if bitten. Danger of lacerating mouth, lips, and gastrointestinal tract. Causes mercury poisoning if swallowed.

i. A 3- to 4-minute interval is practicable for afebrile persons,[2,17] but full registering may take up to 8 minutes when the person is febrile.[39]

j. Prevents thermometer from falling out of mouth.

k. Allows for visualization of thermometer markings and mercury. Prevents tracking microbes to your fingers.

Caution: Studies have shown that careless readings are a large source of error.

m. Glass thermometers are a source of contamination.[36] Even if you use a disposable plastic sheath covering, always wash and disinfect thermometer. Store oral and rectal thermometers separately.

RECTAL TEMPERATURE

Actions

2. Take rectal temperature in individuals for whom oral method is inappropriate (infants, small children, the comatose), who have healthy perineal tissue, and for whom axillary method is too difficult to use.
  a. Follow steps a to e in 1 above.
  b. Draw curtains, close door.
  c. Ask person to turn to side, with upper leg flexed. Assist as necessary. Place infant on side prone on your lap.

Rationale/Discussion

2. Normal range of rectal temperature is 37.0 to 38.0°C (98.6 to 100.4°F). Use pear-shaped or stubby bulb rectal thermometer.

  b. Provides privacy.
  c. Allows visualization of anus and placement of thermometer at correct angle.

Procedure continued on following page

PROCEDURE 31–1 Continued

Actions

d. Fold back bedclothes to expose anus.
e. Don disposable gloves.
f. Lubricate thermometer at bulb end with water-soluble jelly for distance of 1 cm (½ inch) for infant, 4 cm (1–1½ inches) for adult.
g. Lift upper buttock to expose anus. If orifice difficult to visualize, ask person to bear down as if moving bowels.
h. Insert bulb end of thermometer into anal orifice in direction of person's umbilicus to depth of 1 cm (½ inch) for infants and 3 to 4 cm (1–1½ inches) for adults. Slide thermometer along wall of rectum.

i. Hold in place for 2 to 4 minutes.

j. Remove thermometer along same angle as inserted.
k. Wipe thermometer with toilet tissue from fingers to bulb end, using twisting motion, or push off plastic cover. Discard tissue/cover.
l. Wipe person's anal area to remove lubricant and feces.
m. Cover person and assist to a comfortable position.
n. Read thermometer measurement.
o. Care for thermometer according to agency policy.
p. Wash hands.

AXILLARY TEMPERATURE

Actions

3. Take axillary temperature reading in infants or others who cannot have an oral or rectal temperature taken. Axilla must be accessible and tissue healthy.

a. Repeat steps a to e of 1 above.
b. Ask person to lie down in bed. Place infant in supine or prone position, or hold infant.
c. Ask person to remove arm from sleeve of gown; assist as necessary.
d. Dry axilla by patting gently with a tissue.

e. Ask person to place hand over chest and lift elbow; assist as necessary.
f. Place bulb of thermometer in axilla with bulb end pointed toward person's head. Ask person to lower elbow to bed, keeping hand in contact with chest; assist as necessary. Hold thermometer in place.

g. Leave in place for 5 to 7 minutes[4,10] (4 minutes in premature infants).
h. While continuing to hold thermometer, raise elbow.

i. Wipe thermometer dry with tissue.

Rationald/Discussion

d. Proper visualization prevents errors and maintains safety.
e. Protects fingers from contamination.
f. Prevents friction and adherence of thermometer to mucosa of anus and rectum.

g. Allows for better visualization.

h. Direction of insertion conforms to anatomy of rectum. Maintaining same depth of thermometer insertion makes possible more accurate comparisons of serial readings. Keeping thermometer on rectal wall measures body temperature and not temperature of feces.

Caution: Do not use pressure or force to insert thermometer, or thermometer may break or perforate anus or rectum.

i. Studies suggest 2 to 4 minutes is adequate for accurate rectal temperature measurement.[39,40] Holding thermometer prevents displacement and ensures accurate reading.
j. Prevents injury to rectum and anus.
k. Aids visualization of mercury. Prevents contamination of fingers.

l. Lubricant feels wet and uncomfortable.

m. Maintains comfort and privacy.
n. See 1c above.
o. See 1m above.
p. Prevents spreading contamination.

Rationale/Discussion

3. Axillary temperature measurement is superior to the rectal method for infants. Axilla is hygienic, accessible site. Some people are unable to maintain necessary position for required time. Normal range is 36.0 to 37.0°C (96.6 to 98.4°F). Use pear-shaped or stubby oral thermometer.

b. Prevents danger of dropping thermometer on floor.

c. Prevents displacement of thermometer by tight clothing; exposes axilla.
d. Do not use friction because of heat produced. Moisture cools skin.
e. This "winglike" position provides largest axillary "pocket."
f. Bulb in contact with skin over axillary artery provides airtight pocket. Prevents displacement of thermometer.

g. If thermometer moves or becomes dislodged, start again.
h. Raising elbow prevents tissue injury from friction of thermometer moving against dry skin.
i. Allows for visualization of thermometer markings.

PROCEDURE 31–1 Continued

Actions	Rationale/Discussion
j. Read thermometer measurement.	j. See 1c above.
k. Assist person with placing arm in gown and to a comfortable position.	k. Maintains comfort.
l. Care for thermometer according to agency policy.	l. See 1m above.

Measurement of Body Temperature Using the Electronic Thermometer

Actions	Rationale/Discussion
a. Remove electronic thermometer unit from charger and attach the appropriate thermometer probe if necessary.	a. Electronic thermometers need to be kept charged. The thermometer probes are not interchangeable. The major manufacturers color code the probes, e.g., blue is for oral and axillary use, red is for rectal use.
b. Remove probe from the unit and note the digital display of 34°C (94°F) on the screen.	b. The display indicates that the unit is charged.
c. Firmly insert the thermometer probe into a disposable probe cover.	c. The probe cover prevents cross-contamination.
d. Follow the steps outlined earlier for taking oral, rectal, or axillary temperature.	d. Same rationale/discussion applies to both mercury and electronic thermometers.
e. Observe the digital display until it stops flashing and the unit emits a tone.	e. The tone indicates that the maximum measurement has been met.
f. Read and note the measurement.	f. Temperature display will disappear when probe is replaced in unit.
g. Remove probe from client and discard the probe cover directly into waste receptacle.	g. Prompt disposal of the cover prevents accidental reuse.
h. Replace the thermometer probe in the unit.	h. This resets the unit for the next use and turns it off.
i. Assist in any necessary cleaning or positioning measures to complete the procedure.	i. Increases comfort.
j. Wash hands.	j. Decreases transmission of organisms.

Measurement of Body Temperature Using the Tympanic Thermometer

Actions	Rationale/Discussion
a. Remove the thermometer from base.	a. Tympanic thermometers must be kept charged. They may be used several times between charges.
b. Attach disposable probe cover.	b. The probe cover prevents cross-contamination.
c. Insert the probe gently into the ear canal while gently pulling upward and backward on the pinna of the ear.	c. Care must be taken not to insert the probe too deeply or not to grind the probe into the ear, which could scratch or damage the ear canal. Gentle pulling up and back on the ear pinna straightens the ear canal and gives the probe better exposure to the tympanic membrane.
d. Activate the thermometer.	d. Most models have a button that activates the device. Tympanic thermometers give a reading in 2 to 3 seconds.
e. Read and note the measurement.	e. Note the reading immediately to prevent relying upon memory only.
f. Dispose of the probe cover in the waste receptacle.	f. Proper disposal prevents accidental reuse.
g. Return the thermometer to the base.	g. Storing the thermometer in the base unit keeps it charged and ready for use.
h. Wash hands.	

FINAL ACTIVITIES

Tell person the temperature reading, if appropriate. Ensure comfort and safety. Evaluate temperature in light of person's appearance and other vital signs. Recheck temperature with another thermometer and/or by another route if temperature measurement is markedly different from previous readings. Follow agency policy for aftercare of equipment. *Documentation:* Chart temperature on TPR "Day Sheet," bedside vital signs sheet, and/or "Graphic Sheet" in chart. Write "A" for axillary route or "R" for rectal route. Immediately report deviations from normal to appropriate personnel.

Oral Temperatures. Body temperature usually is measured orally because the oral route is currently the most accessible and convenient. (Note: the tympanic route quickly is gaining acceptance as the preferred route in many clinical settings.) An oral temperature is accurate when the thermometer is placed under the tongue next to a major artery (Fig. 31–6). The oral route is generally safe and reliable and is more acceptable to people than the rectal route. Also, oral temperatures may be taken even with nasogastric tubes and oxygen catheters in place.[24]

Some agencies require the oral route for temperatures in people following myocardial infarction, because of the belief that insertion of a rectal thermometer can stimulate the vagus nerve, which can then trigger cardiac arrhythmias. However, research shows that the rectal route has no adverse cardiac effects.[8]

Rectal Temperatures. Rectal temperatures are taken in infants, children up to the age of 5 years, delirious individuals, or those who are unconscious or critically ill. They are also taken in people who (a) are recovering from oral surgery, (b) have respiratory difficulty, (c) must keep their mouths open, or (d) have had their jaws wired together.

Despite popular belief, a rectal temperature reading is not necessarily more accurate or desirable than an oral or axillary reading. The temperature registered depends on the proximity of the thermometer to a major artery and the location of the artery itself. Unless the thermometer is properly inserted along the wall of the rectum in the direction of the umbilicus, a rectal reading may reflect the temperature of feces or of peripheral blood returning from the legs rather than the core temperature of the body.

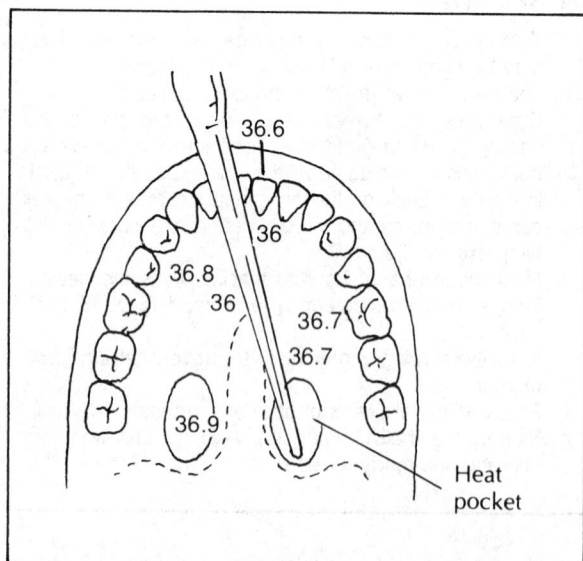

▲ *Figure 31–6*

The posterior lingual heat pocket gives the highest reading, 36.9°C (98.4°F) because of the rich blood supply. The traditional site under the tongue at the front of the mouth gives the lowest reading, 36°C (96.8°F). (Adapted from *The Guthrie Bulletin* 43:173, 1974.)

Axillary Temperatures. The axillary route is safe and noninvasive. Until the recent advent of the tympanic thermometer, the axillary route has been preferred for children because the axillary route is easily accessible and there are none of the dangers inherent in the rectal route, such as rectal perforation. Axillary temperatures previously were considered to be less accurate than the other routes, but research has dispelled that notion and has shown no clinically significant differences between rectal and axillary temperatures.[11]

The axillary route is appropriate for infants and preschoolers, those with oral disease or after oral surgery, those who are mouth breathers, and those for whom the rectal route is contraindicated.

Core Temperatures. The development of the sophisticated Swan-Ganz catheter has enabled clinicians to monitor core temperatures frequently and conveniently. The catheter contains a thermistor that can be attached to a cardiac output computer to obtain temperature readings. Insertion of a Swan-Ganz catheter is an invasive procedure; its use is limited to people in critical care units.

FREQUENCY OF TEMPERATURE MONITORING

The frequency of temperature monitoring depends on agency policy, the person's condition, and on your judgment. Many health care agencies routinely require temperature measurement two or three times a day on all clients. Recall that body temperature is influenced by normal circadian rhythms. Therefore, always take a person's routine temperature at the same time(s) every day for consistency.

In addition to routine monitoring, always take a temperature reading if you suspect a deviation.

Do not wait until the "next scheduled time" to take a temperature if the person is chilled, flushed, or hot to the touch or has other symptoms of infection.

Also, take the temperature more frequently when an individual is febrile, has an infection, or has recently had surgery.

Alterations in Body Temperature

An abnormal elevation in body temperature can result from different mechanisms. For example, an abnormally low body temperature is termed hypothermia, whereas fever represents a resetting of the set point to a higher level. A person having a fever is febrile; without a fever, a person is **afebrile.** Unlike fever, heat exhaustion and heat stroke result from high environmental temperatures, usually coupled with physical exertion. In these conditions, the body cannot adequately dissipate heat to the environment. Thus, these conditions are called heat-related disorders rather than fevers.

FEVER

Fevers can be described in numerous ways:

▶ A low-grade fever is a consistently elevated temperature above 37.1°C (99°F) but below 38.2°C (100.4°F).

▶ A high-grade fever is a temperature above 38.2°C (100.4°F).

▶ **Hyperpyrexia** or **hyperthermia** is an extremely elevated body temperature, usually higher than 40.0°C (104°F).

▶ A relapsing or intermittent fever is one in which febrile episodes alternate with periods of normal temperatures.

▶ A remittent fever occurs when body temperature is consistently elevated but fluctuates throughout a 24-hour period.

▶ Fever of undetermined origin (FUO) is a fever with no identifiable etiology. It occurs when (a) a person is febrile for an extended period (usually 3 weeks or more), with a temperature greater than 38.2°C (100.4°F), and (b) the cause of the fever cannot be deduced despite an extensive physical examination and laboratory workup.[30]

Etiology of Fever. Recall that the central integrator, or hypothalamic thermostat, operates by negative feedback to keep body temperature fairly stable at a set point of around 37°C (98.6°F). Fever results when the thermal set point is raised, causing body temperature to fluctuate around the new set point. Here is the way this happens.

First, exogenous pyrogens such as bacteria, viruses, antigens, or drugs enter the body and overwhelm its defense mechanisms (Fig. 31–7). (They are called exogenous pyrogens because they come from outside the body.) Exogenous pyrogens interact with white blood cells, which produce interleukin-1 (IL-1). IL-1 circulates

▲ **Figure 31–7**

Proposed mechanism for the generation of fever.

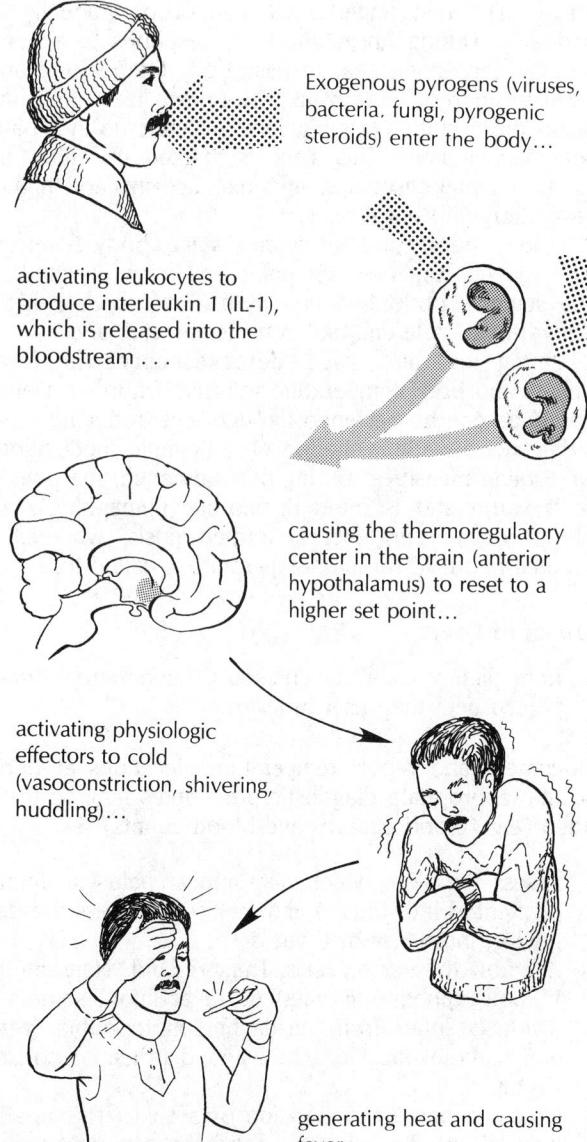

Exogenous pyrogens (viruses, bacteria. fungi, pyrogenic steroids) enter the body...

activating leukocytes to produce interleukin 1 (IL-1), which is released into the bloodstream . . .

causing the thermoregulatory center in the brain (anterior hypothalamus) to reset to a higher set point...

activating physiologic effectors to cold (vasoconstriction, shivering, huddling)...

generating heat and causing fever.

to the hypothalamus, where it alters the set point. The body then conserves heat to increase its temperature. Effectors cause the blood vessels to constrict and the person shivers and feels cold, even though the temperature is rising. These mechanisms continue until the new set point is reached and the person experiences fever. When the stimulus producing fever is eliminated, the body responds with vasodilation and sweat production. During this phase the person is diaphoretic, feels warm, and is often flushed.

Why does the body respond in this way? Many scientists think the fever response is an adaptive mechanism rather than a pathologic condition. Thus, fever is beneficial. Many bacteria, for example, thrive within a narrow range of temperatures, so a fever may hinder their proliferation in the body. Also, at higher temperatures, the body sequesters iron and zinc, minerals that bacteria require to function. Because fever is beneficial, many clinicians question whether vigorous treatment of fevers is therapeutic.

Stages of Fever. The natural course of fever has three stages. The first stage, onset, can occur gradually or suddenly. During onset, the body responds to a pyrogen by conserving heat to raise body temperature and reset the body's thermostat. The person feels cold and seeks more clothing or blankets or "curls up in a ball" to conserve heat. This stage is marked by chills, increased metabolism and muscular activity, and higher respiratory and pulse rates.

During the second, or febrile, stage, body temperature reaches the new set point and stays elevated. If the stage is prolonged and if the fever is very high, dehydration, delirium, and convulsions may occur.

During the third stage, **defervescence,** the fever abates and body temperature returns to normal. Defervescence can be hastened through fever-reducing measures such as administration of antipyretic medications or cooling measures. During defervescence, the person feels warm and is often diaphoretic (perspiring). An abrupt decline in fever is termed crisis, whereas a gradual return to normal temperature is called lysis.

Onset of Fever

▶ Immediately take the person's temperature when you suspect the onset of fever.

Document and report temperature elevations at once so that appropriate diagnostic procedures may be instituted (e.g., blood cultures and blood counts).

▶ Assess the skin, which may appear pale (in lightly pigmented individuals) and feel cool. Assess the degree of moistness or dryness.
▶ Ask how the person feels. Thirsty? Cold? Nauseated? Without appetite? Exhausted? In addition, some individuals suffer from headache, photophobia, general malaise, muscle aches, and diarrhea or constipation.
▶ Note the onset and duration of a chill (it generally lasts 10 to 30 minutes). Take the temperature at

onset and during the chill to determine the low reading and high reading.

Do not take the temperature orally during a chill. At this time, people have great difficulty in keeping the lips closed, hence the reading is inaccurate.

▶ Note when the chill ends. Take the temperature immediately. Following a chill, the temperature increases as a result of increased heat production from muscle activity and shivering.

Febrile Stage

▶ Note the pulse and respirations. Elevations in body temperature increase metabolic demands. Therefore, the heart must pump oxygenated blood to the tissues faster. The heart rate increases, as does the respiratory rate.
▶ Determine whether the person has diarrhea and vomiting, which could cause fluid and electrolyte imbalances. Begin a fluid balance record, and document imbalances. Review serum electrolyte values.
▶ Look for signs of restlessness or confusion. Is the person restless? Does the person seem unaware of the environment? Hallucinating? If so, check the temperature immediately and report your findings.

Delirium may occur in the presence of high fever (39 to 40°C [102.2 to 104°F]). Children and older adults may develop delirium at lower temperatures. Convulsions also accompany high fever (41.1°C [106°F]), especially in very young children.[35,41]

▶ Note reaction to nursing intervention. Does the temperature lower in response to medication and cooling measures?

Defervescence

▶ Assess for signs of dehydration as the temperature begins to return to normal. Note and record diaphoresis. Check for poor skin turgor. Monitor blood pressure. Is it below the person's usual reading? Note the urine specific gravity. Weigh the person. Dehydration, particularly in children, causes weight loss.
▶ Assess and record body temperature every 2 to 4 hours. Note if the condition remains stable. Report any temperature elevation.

Controversy in Treating Fever. Since fever is a beneficial response of the body to infection, should all fevers be treated? Research indicates that the treatment of low to moderate temperature elevations below 39°C (102°F) in relatively healthy individuals is *not* indicated unless the person is very uncomfortable, has other abnormal vital signs, or is unable to tolerate the fever because of other physical illness such as compromised cardiac function.[18,35,50]

You should try to reduce fever in people who are very uncomfortable, who have other abnormal vital signs, or who register above 39°C (102°F). Try tepid baths and antipyretic medication but take care not to reduce the fever too rapidly or the person may experience chilling. The goal is not necessarily to bring the temperature to normal right away but to keep the temperature under 39°C.[18] Never let the person's temperature climb too high. High fevers, as high as 41°C (105.8°F), require immediate antipyretic measures since cell damage can occur at these temperatures.

Nursing Management of Fever

▶ Reduce fever. Antipyretics (e.g., aspirin and acetaminophen) are substances used to reduce fever. They offer a fast and effective means of reducing body temperature. These drugs work by blocking prostaglandin synthesis, which affects the thermoregulatory center. Tepid water baths and cool circulating air reduce the body's surface temperature. Do not induce chills, because that would raise the temperature again.

▶ Maintain optimal nutrition. Nutritional support is important because fever is a hypercatabolic state. Ensure adequate intake of carbohydrates for energy and protein for tissue rebuilding. Also maintain sufficient intake of minerals and vitamins.

▶ Maintain fluid and electrolyte balance. Profuse diaphoresis, anorexia, and vomiting increase the risk of fluid and electrolyte imbalances. Carefully monitor intake and output and serum electrolyte and osmolality levels. Electrolytes and fluids lost through sweating must be replaced, either orally or parenterally (see Chapter 47).

▶ Promote comfort and rest. During the onset of fever, more blankets or clothing may be needed. Later, the individual may need to change clothes often to keep skin from becoming irritated by wet, sweaty clothing. Frequent bathing may increase comfort. Schedule frequent rest periods to conserve the person's energy.

▶ Eliminate the cause of fever. Antimicrobial medications combat fever due to microbial infection. Antihistamines help quell immune or allergic responses that result in fever.

▶ Provide for home management. The goals are the same whether a person is in the hospital or at home: reduction of fever, maintenance of nutrition, maintenance of fluid and electrolyte balance, and comfort and rest. Individuals and care providers must be taught how to take a temperature properly and the proper use of antipyretic drugs. Also emphasize the simple methods of fever reduction: tepid water baths and encouraging fluids.

HEAT-RELATED DISORDERS

Heat Exhaustion. Heat exhaustion is caused by excessive fluid volume depletion resulting from exposure to severe environmental heat without prior acclimatization. The person experiences thirst, dizziness, and/or syncope (fainting), and there may be nausea, vomiting, headache, and weakness. Signs include tachycardia and low blood pressure. The skin feels cool and clammy, and lightly pigmented people appear pale. Body temperature may be increased, normal, or slightly decreased.

Nursing interventions include (a) quickly moving the person out of the sun into the coolest place possible, (b) having the person lie down and rest, and (c) replacing fluids and electrolytes, especially sodium. Intravenous fluid replacement may be needed.

Heat Stroke. Heat stroke is a dangerous, life-threatening emergency. It may be preceded by heat exhaustion. The risk of heat stroke increases when humidity is 100 per cent and environmental temperature is in the thirties Celsius (nineties Fahrenheit). If a person has been exercising strenuously in a high-humidity environment, heat stroke may occur at a temperature in the twenties Celsius (eighties Fahrenheit). Those at risk for heat stroke include aging adults, the very young, those with chronic illnesses, and the young and healthy who exercise vigorously in hot, humid weather.

The onset of heat stroke is sudden. The person may initially experience headache, dizziness, nausea, confusion, and visual disturbances. Sweating and other thermoregulatory mechanisms fail. The inability to dissipate heat causes an increase in body temperature to 41°C (105.8°F) and above. Initially, the pulse is rapid and strong; the skin is hot, flushed, and dry; and blood pressure is slightly elevated. Later, blood pressure falls as the person's condition deteriorates. If untreated, heat stroke may cause delirium, coma, clotting abnormalities, seizures, cardiac arrhythmias, severe renal damage, shock, and even death.

Intervention for heat stroke must be immediate and aggressive cooling. Cooling measures include tepid water baths, fanning the body with cool, circulating air, and administration of intravenous fluids. Immersion in ice baths is contraindicated, because this could result in uncontrolled shivering, which increases heat production.[21]

HYPOTHERMIA

Hypothermia is a core body temperature that remains consistently below normal. In mild hypothermia, body temperature ranges from just below normal, 35°C (95°F) to 32°C (89.6°F). Moderate hypothermia ranges from 32°C to 26°C (78.8°F); in deep hypothermia, temperatures are below 26°C.

The pathophysiology of hypothermia involves (1) excessive heat loss, (2) decreased heat production, or (3) impaired thermoregulation as a result of severe illness (see examples in Table 31-2).

Accidental hypothermia results from unintentional exposure to a cold, wet, windy climate with an ambient temperature below 16°C (60.8°F). It also results from accidental immersion in cold water. Populations at highest risk include people engaging in cold weather sports, such as mountain climbing and cross-country skiing; older adults who may be unable to perceive changes in environmental temperature or who are confused; homeless people; infants and children with immature thermoregulatory mechanisms; and people with neurologic deficits who are unable to sense or respond to cold. In addition, alcoholics who have excessive heat loss secondary to vasodilation are at risk in cold environments.

Spontaneous hypothermia sometimes develops following a high fever. Body temperature may remain low for several days after defervescence before returning to normal. Hypothermia also can accompany cerebrovascular disease, drug toxicity (especially barbiturates or phenothiazines), severe infections, liver or renal failure, and certain endocrine disorders (e.g., myxedema).

Induced hypothermia is a carefully controlled therapeutic measure. Cold applications to specific body parts reduce swelling, alleviate fever and pain, and increase muscle tone. Whole-body hypothermia is often used in major surgery, especially cardiac and neurologic surgery. It reduces the metabolic demands of the body and lowers oxygen consumption. Cell metabolism is reduced about 15 per cent for every 1°C drop in body temperature. Induced hypothermia is used also to treat burns, reduce inflammation, and control gastrointestinal bleeding.

Nursing assessment of the person with hypothermia includes observing for the following:

▸ A feeling of being cold and chilled (early symptom of accidental or spontaneous hypothermia)
▸ **Pallor** (absence of skin color, or paleness) in lightly pigmented people; cool, waxy skin
▸ Hypotension
▸ Decreased urine output due to hypotension
▸ Decreased respiratory rate (deep hypothermia may cause respiratory arrest)
▸ Bradycardia, cardiac arrhythmias, possibly cardiac arrest
▸ Numbness of the extremities
▸ Slurred speech, decreasing level of consciousness
▸ Drowsiness progressing to coma
▸ Metabolic acidosis secondary to inadequate tissue oxygenation (see Chapter 42)
▸ Generalized edema (in severe hypothermia)
▸ Decreased reflexes with disappearance of most reflexive responses (occurs at about 24°C [75.2°F])

Nursing interventions for all types of hypothermia include rewarming. External rewarming involves placing the person in a warm, dry environment, covered with dry blankets. This is adequate for mild hypothermia. Deep hypothermia requires careful monitoring and treatment in a critical care unit. Other interventions include fluid and electrolyte replacement; administration of antibiotics (the incidence of pneumonia is high in people with accidental hypothermia); and control of shivering, which increases intracranial pressure and increases the need for oxygen.

ASSESSMENT OF PULSE

Basic Cardiovascular Physiology

The heart is a pulsatile pump that moves blood throughout the body. Approximately 60 to 100 times a minute, specialized cells in the sinoatrial (SA) node

TABLE 31-2. Causes of Hypothermia

Cause	Example
Heat loss	Exposure to low external temperatures
	Skin disorders: erythroderma, extensive burns
	Therapeutically induced hypothermia by external methods
	Paget's disease
Diminished heat production	Malnutrition
	Endocrine disorders:
	Hypothyroidism
	Hypoglycemia
	Addisonian crisis
	Hypopituitarism
	People who have poor mobility as a result of arthritis, Parkinson's disease, or paralysis
Impaired thermoregulation	Central nervous system dysfunction
	Anorexia nervosa
	Brain tumor
	Head trauma
	Wernicke's encephalopathy
	Spinal cord injury
	Stroke
	Drug-induced (impaired central and peripheral)
	Ethanol intoxication
	Narcotics (morphine)
	Barbiturates
	Tranquilizers
	Antidepressants
	General anesthetics
	Reserpine
	Atropine
	Severe illness
	Sepsis (poor prognosis)
	Hemorrhage
	Pneumonia
	Myocardial infarction
	Uremia
	Carbon monoxide poisoning
	Cirrhosis

initiate an electrical impulse. This impulse normally travels via an orderly pathway to all parts of the heart, depolarizing cardiac muscle and causing it to contract. This contraction phase of the cardiac cycle is systole. It occupies one third of the cardiac cycle and supplies the power to push blood to all parts of the body. Diastole (or relaxation) is the resting phase of the cardiac cycle. During this time the ventricles fill with blood, which is then ejected with the next contraction. Diastole constitutes two thirds of the cardiac cycle.

During systole, the left ventricle pumps an amount of blood into the already full aorta, which greatly increases aortic pressure. This pressure increase expands the wall of the aorta and generates a fluid wave, which is felt at a peripheral artery as the **pulse.**

The heart normally beats about 70 times per minute

to send approximately 5 L of blood (the cardiac output) throughout the body. This relationship is expressed as

$$CO = SV \times R$$

That is, the cardiac output (CO) equals the amount of blood ejected by the heart in each left ventricular systole (**stroke volume,** or SV) times the heart rate (R) per minute. When internal or external stressors alter either component on the right side of the equation, the other component compensates to keep the cardiac output constant. For example, when the stroke volume decreases (as in shock), the heart compensates by increasing its rate.

To determine how efficiently the heart maintains its output, you count the number of beats per minute and judge the rhythm and quality of the pulse. In addition, to assess perfusion to all parts of the body, you often check more than one pulse site.

Pulse Sites

Palpate the pulse over arterial sites that lie close to the skin and are backed by bone or other firm structures. The most common sites for routine assessment are the radial pulse in adults and children and the apical pulse in infants. Various clinical situations call for assessment of other pulse points (Fig. 31–8).

The radial pulse is the pulse site of the radial artery and is usually the most accessible for routine vital signs. The radial artery is palpated along the radius bone proximal to the thumb on the inner wrist (the flexor side).

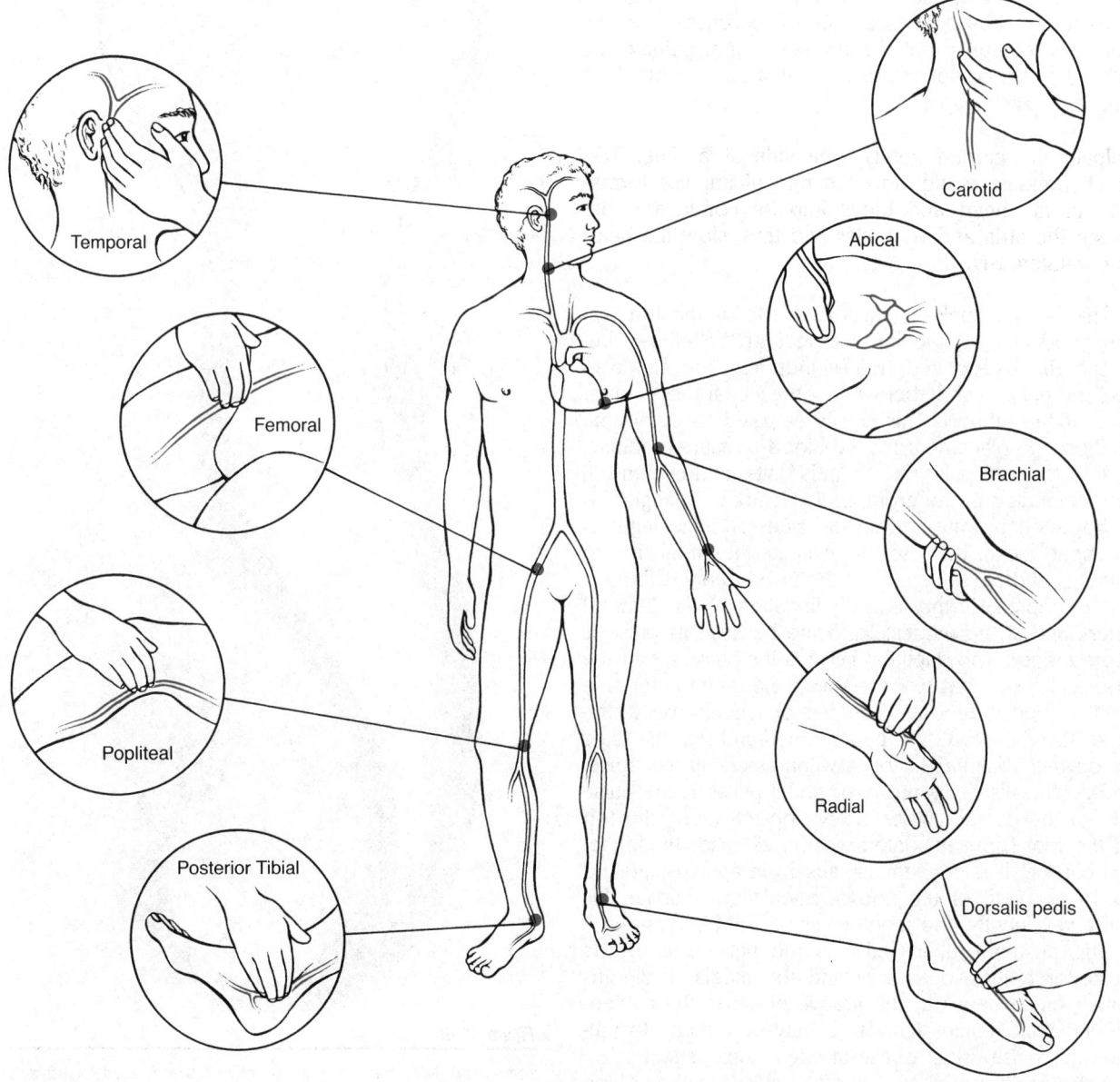

Temporal

Carotid

Apical

Femoral

Brachial

Popliteal

Radial

Posterior Tibial

Dorsalis pedis

▲ *Figure 31–8*

Pulse sites.

The apical pulse is the pulse site auscultated over the apex of the heart, in the fourth or fifth intercostal space at the left midclavicular line (halfway between the sternum and the side of the chest).

The temporal pulse is the pulse site of the temporal artery located between the eye and the hairline just above the zygomatic bone (cheekbone). The temporal pulse is a useful routine pulse site in infants and young children.

The carotid pulse is the pulse site of the carotid artery, which is located on the neck at the side of the larynx, between the trachea and the sternomastoid muscle. The carotid is a central artery, so pulsations may persist there when the stroke volume is too low for the peripheral pulses to be felt. The carotid artery is palpated in emergencies (such as cardiac arrest) because it is immediately accessible without the need to remove the person's clothing. In addition, during cardiopulmonary resuscitation (CPR), palpation of the carotid artery is used to assess the effectiveness of external chest compression. If a rescuer cannot palpate the carotid pulse, compressions are not strong enough (see Chapter 30).

Palpate the carotid gently, one side at a time. Too much pressure could slow the rate of impulse formation in the heart and block impulse conduction between the atria and ventricles and thus, slow the heart rate dangerously.

The brachial pulse is the pulse site of the brachial artery, located at the inner aspect of the elbow, between the biceps and triceps muscles. You can also feel the pulse slightly below the antecubital fossa (inner part of the elbow). This site is palpated to determine stethoscope placement for the blood pressure reading.

The femoral pulse is the pulse site of the femoral artery, located in the groin, in the femoral "triangle." It is bordered by muscles on the sides and the inguinal ligament above. It is used to evaluate the circulation to the legs and the adequacy of perfusion during CPR.

The popliteal artery is a continuation of the femoral artery and is the hardest to locate because its pulse is more diffuse. The popliteal pulse is the pulse site in the popliteal fossa (back of the knee), along the outer side of the medial tendon. The person should bend the knee slightly, or roll on the abdomen and flex the knee 45 degrees. Use a light touch when assessing this pulse.

The dorsalis pedis pulse, or pedal pulse, is the pulse site of the dorsalis pedis artery, located along the top of the foot (dorsum), lateral to the extensor tendon of the big toe. It is congenitally absent in approximately 8 to 10 per cent of the normal population. Palpate this pulse very gently; too much pressure will obliterate it.

The posterior tibial pulse is the pulse site of the posterior artery, located behind the medial malleolus (inner ankle bone) in the groove between the malleolus and the Achilles tendon. It may be difficult to palpate this pulse on an obese or edematous person.

You should assess all superficial pulses in the person having surgery, particularly for open heart or peripheral vascular operations, and for such procedures as cardiac

catheterization. It is essential to chart preoperative baseline information regarding the bilateral dorsalis pedis, posterior tibial, popliteal, femoral, radial, and brachial pulses. This information is important to nurses in the OR, recovery room, and intensive care unit (ICU) because it can be used as a standard against which to compare changes in vital signs following the procedures. Also, assess these pulses in the individual with an arterial occlusive condition such as atherosclerosis, Raynaud's disease, Buerger's disease, and aortic aneurysm. Carefully assess pulses in persons with diabetes, because they often have peripheral vascular disease.

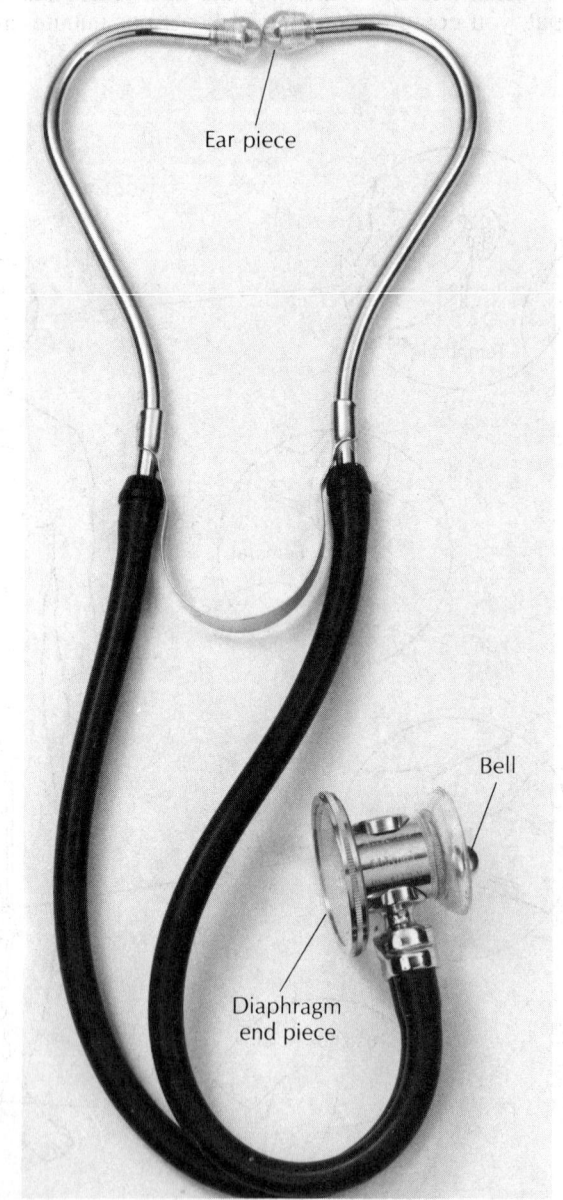

▲ *Figure 31–9*

Stethoscope. Note bell on right side of end piece, used for assessing low-frequency sounds such as heart murmurs. The diaphragm (left side of end piece) helps assess high-frequency sounds. Use this side for blood pressure and apical pulse measurement.

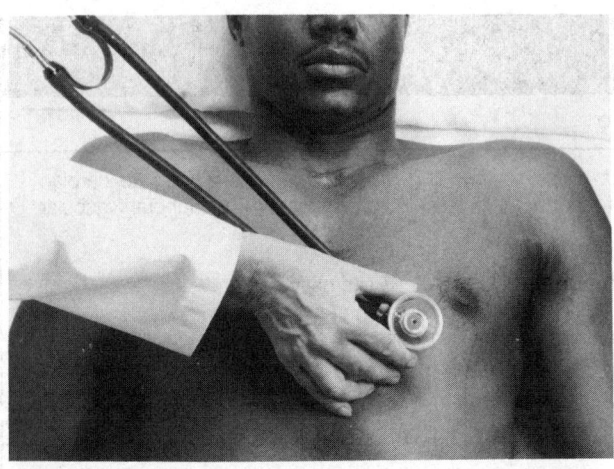

▲ *Figure 31–10*

Auscultating the apical pulse. (From Jarvis, C. [1992]. *Physical examination and health assessment*. Philadelphia: W.B. Saunders, 1992.)

To count the pulse rate on infants, auscultate the apical pulse. Use this pulse site for adults when there is an abnormality of the peripheral pulse. The apical pulse is also the site to use when assessing heart sounds.

Every normal heart beat has two components, called the first and second heart sounds, or S_1 and S_2. These sounds are caused by closure of the valves in the heart. S_1 occurs with closure of the mitral and tricuspid valves, signaling the beginning of systole. S_2 results from closure of the aortic and pulmonic valves at the end of systole. Because systole is normally only one third of the entire cardiac cycle, S_1 and S_2 sounds close together and you hear "lub-dup, lub-dup." The "lub-dup" is S_1 and S_2, and is counted as one heart beat. Because these are relatively high-pitched sounds, use the diaphragm end piece of the stethoscope to hear these heart tones (Figs. 31–9 and 31–10).

Pulse Rate

The pulse rate is the number of beats per minute. Knowing normal ranges for pulse rates allows you to identify abnormal findings.

NORMAL RANGES FOR PULSE RATES

The normal pulse rate in the resting adult is 60 to 100 beats per minute, although the American Heart Association accepts 50 to 100 as a normal range.

Women generally have a slightly faster pulse rate than men. The heart rate normally is higher in infants and children, gradually decreases as the person approaches adulthood, and increases slightly in old age (Table 31–3).

When taking a regular peripheral pulse rate, count for 30 seconds and multiply by 2. An earlier study by Jones supported the use of the 15-second interval with normal rates, and this 15-second interval is commonly

TABLE 31–3. Normal Resting Pulse Rates—Across Age Groups

Age	Average (Beats per Minute)	Normal Limits
Neonate	120	70–190
1 year	120	80–160
2 years	110	80–130
4 years	100	80–120
6 years	100	75–115
8 years	90	70–110
10 years	90	70–110
12 years		
Female	90	70–110
Male	85	65–105
14 years		
Female	85	65–105
Male	80	60–100
16 years		
Female	80	60–100
Male	75	55–95
18 years		
Female	75	55–95
Male	70	50–90
Well-conditioned athlete	May be 50–60	50–100
Adult		60–100
Aging		60–100

From Jarvis, C. (1992). *Physical examination and health assessment*. Philadelphia: W.B. Saunders.

used in clinical practice.[32] However, Hollerbach and Sneed found the 30-second interval to be the most accurate and efficient interval when heart rates are normal and rapid, and when rhythms are regular.[28] Techniques for assessing radial and apical pulses are described in Procedure 31–2.

TACHYCARDIA

Tachycardia is an abnormally rapid heart rate (over 100 beats per minute). It occurs with these conditions:

▶ Exercise and fever, when the body cells require more oxygen to meet metabolic needs. By increasing cardiac output, tachycardia results in increased oxygen to the cells.

▶ Any condition characterized by hypoxemia, which is a decreased level of oxygen in the arterial blood. One possible cause of hypoxemia is anemia, a blood disorder characterized by a deficiency in the number of red blood cells or in the amount of hemoglobin. Anemia decreases the amount of oxygen that can be carried in blood, thus resulting in hypoxemia.

▶ Congestive heart failure, a condition in which the heart becomes an inefficient pump and fluid "backs up" into the lungs and venous system instead of "moving forward" through the body. Because less oxygen reaches the cells, the heart compensates by increasing its rate.

PROCEDURE 31–2

Assessing the Radial and Apical Pulses

Definition/Purposes. *To count pulse rate per minute and assess pulse rhythm and quality.* These data indicate cardiac workload and cardiac efficiency. The presence and quality of peripheral pulses indicate status of peripheral vascular system, i.e., blood vessels in extremities.

Contraindications. Dressings, open wounds, or pain at a pulse site require the use of an alternative site.

Learning/Teaching Guidelines. Provide the following information as appropriate: (a) describe procedures regardless of the person's apparent level of consciousness; (b) as a part of discharge planning, teach the individual who has a cardiac disorder, who is taking cardiac medications, or who is monitoring progress on a cardiovascular fitness program to check the pulse.

PRELIMINARY ACTIVITIES

Assessment/Planning

▶ Schedule frequency of obtaining pulse as determined by individual's condition and physician's order.
▶ Know previous reported pulse rates.
▶ Know purpose of obtaining pulse rate, e.g., routine vital signs, post cardiac catheterization care.
▶ Choose site for obtaining pulse rate: for routine vital signs in adults, radial artery is the most accessible; take apical rate when pulse is irregular, to listen to heart sounds, before giving cardiac medications, or to assess heart rate on an infant.
▶ Obtain pulse rate of infants or young children before checking other vital signs. If child cries when temperature is taken, crying increases pulse rate and makes it harder to hear heart sounds.
▶ Postpone assessing pulse rate for a few minutes if person has just ambulated or seems very angry or anxious.

Preparation of Person

▶ Identify individual.
▶ Explain procedure and reason for obtaining pulse.
▶ Position person appropriately for site used.
▶ If using a stethoscope, request quiet during procedure so that you can hear.

Equipment

▶ Stethoscope (for taking apical pulse).
▶ Alcohol wipes (for cleaning ear tips of stethoscope).
▶ Clock or watch with second hand or digital readout.

PROCEDURE

Actions

1. Radial pulse
   a. Position person. In supine position, place forearm across chest with wrist extended, palm down. If person is sitting, bend elbow 90 degrees and support arm; extend wrist palm down.

   b. Place your first three fingers along superficial radial artery and gently press artery against radius.
   c. Avoid bracing your thumb on the back of the person's wrist at the same time.
   d. Obliterate pulsation, then gradually release pressure until pulse is again palpable.

   e. While observing a watch with a second hand, start to count rate with "zero ," then "one," "two," etc.
   f. If pulse is regular, count number of pulsations in 30 seconds and multiply by 2.
   g. If pulse is irregular, count rate for 1 full minute.

   h. Continue palpation to assess pulse volume, rhythm, and type of pulse irregularity if present.
   i. If pulse is irregular, use stethoscope to auscultate apical beat.

2. Apical pulse
   a. Expose nipple area of left anterior chest (front or belly surface of body) by raising gown to shoulders and lowering sheet.

Rationale/Discussion

a. These positions are comfortable for most people, and convenient for you. A painful position for a person may influence heart rate. An awkward position for examiner makes it difficult to concentrate on data being collected.
b. Pulsation is felt over bony prominence and is due to systolic thrust of heart's left ventricle.
c. If you use your thumb, you may feel your own pulse and confuse it with person's pulse.
d. Moderate pressure is best. Too much pressure occludes pulse; with too little pressure you will be unable to feel pulse.
e. Zero begins time interval, and next pulse felt is "one" of sequence.[23]
f. Adequate for accurate result, if rate is regular.

g. Minimal time needed to determine accurate rate of irregular pulse.
h. See text for discussion of definitions of terms and assessment of these factors.
i. Auscultate apical pulse and palpate radial pulse simultaneously to determine pulse deficit (see text for discussion).

a. Keeping shoulders covered maintains both privacy and warmth.

PROCEDURE 31-2 Continued

Actions	Rationale/Discussion
b. Rub diaphragm end piece in palm of hand.	b. Friction from rubbing warms end piece. Placement of cold end piece on person's chest is both uncomfortable and startling, and even may increase heart rate.
c. Insert ear piece tips in your ears with bend of tips pointing forward.	c. This placement matches forward slope of external auditory canal, so sound is transmitted clearly to eardrum.
d. Place diaphragm over apical area of the heart (fourth or fifth intercostal space at left midclavicular line).	d. Apical pulse is best heard in this area because heart is close to chest wall. Use diaphragm end piece for high-pitched sounds such as apical beat.
e. Listen for "lub-dup" sound.	e. There is a first *(lub)* and a second *(dup)* sound for each heart beat.
f. Count rate and note regularity, as in steps 1, e, f, g.	
g. Before and after procedure, wipe diaphragm and ear piece tips of stethoscope with alcohol sponges.	g. Prevents spread of microorganisms between people.

FINAL ACTIVITIES

Assess pulse findings in view of person's overall clinical picture. *Documentation:* Record findings. If data show a significant change in person's condition, take indicated actions, e.g., communicate findings to appropriate persons.

▶ Situations in which blood pressure falls (as in shock). The pulse increases in an attempt to maintain a stable cardiac output.

▶ Situations that stimulate the sympathetic nervous system, as when a person is in pain, or is experiencing such emotions as anger, fear, and anxiety. If you suspect that someone is experiencing these emotions, check the pulse rate later once the person has calmed down.

BRADYCARDIA

Stimulation of the parasympathetic nervous system causes **bradycardia,** an abnormally slow heart rate, below 60 beats per minute. Bradycardia may be seen in these conditions:

▶ Use of digitalis, which stimulates the vagus nerve of the parasympathetic system.
▶ Conditions that stimulate the vagus nerves, including vomiting and tracheal suctioning.
▶ Certain problems with the electrical conduction system of the heart.
▶ Increased intracranial pressure from tumor or hemorrhage.
▶ Normally, as in the well-conditioned athlete. Remember the equation CO = SV × R. In athletes, the stroke volume is increased secondary to well-developed heart muscles. For this reason, the rate can decrease and still maintain a stable cardiac output. In athletes and other physically fit people, you may count a resting heart rate of between 50 and 60, or even lower.

Pulse Rhythm

Pulse rhythm, the pattern of heart beats, should be regular. However, several types of irregularities may occur.

Sinus arrhythmia is a pulse rate that varies with respiration, increasing at the peak of inspiration and decreasing with expiration. The pulse rate increases to compensate for the decreased stroke volume that occurs during inspiration. It is common in children and young adults and requires no nursing intervention.

Premature beats occur when a pacemaker other than the usual SA node fires prematurely and initiates an early contraction. There is a decreased stroke volume with the premature beat, so you feel a pause in the rhythm.

Finally, the rhythm may feel totally irregular, which indicates a potentially serious abnormality in the heart's conduction system. If you note premature beats or other irregularities, chart this information and communicate your findings to the appropriate persons.

If you note any *irregularities,* count the pulse rate for 1 *full minute.*

A **pulse deficit** exists when the radial pulse rate is lower than the apical rate. When you note any irregularity, check carefully for a pulse deficit. Use the stethoscope to auscultate the apical beat. At the same time, palpate the radial pulse. With the aid of another nurse, take both pulses simultaneously to determine the pulse deficit. When working alone, take a serial measurement (one after the other) of apical beat and radial pulse. Doyle and Jordan found no significant difference between the use of this method by one clinician and the use of the simultaneous method by two.[9]

The usual procedure is as follows: Two nurses are positioned on either side of the person, one auscultating the apical beat, the other palpating the radial pulse. Place a watch so that both nurses can determine the count during the same time interval (Fig. 31–11). When one nurse says "Go," both nurses silently count for 1 full minute and stop when the same nurse says "Stop." Normally, the two counts should be identical. When different, the radial rate is subtracted from the apical. For example, if a person's apical rate is 96 and the radial rate is 64, report a pulse deficit of 32. If you do note a pulse deficit, take several readings to verify your findings.

A pulse deficit signals an inefficient contraction. There is not enough time for the ventricles to fill with blood between all beats. Thus, some contractions will be so weak that you will not be able to feel them when you take the radial pulse. This problem occurs with a cardiac irregularity called atrial fibrillation and with premature beats.

Pulse Force (Pulse Quality)

Pulse force or quality reflects the strength of the stroke volume. If the stroke volume decreases, as in hemorrhagic shock, you palpate a "weak, thready" pulse. If the stroke volume increases, as with exercise, anxiety, or alcohol intake, the pulse pressure (the difference between systolic and diastolic blood pressure) widens; this phenomenon is felt peripherally as an increased force. You may also feel a bounding pulse in complete heart block, anemia, hepatic failure, and aortic insufficiency.

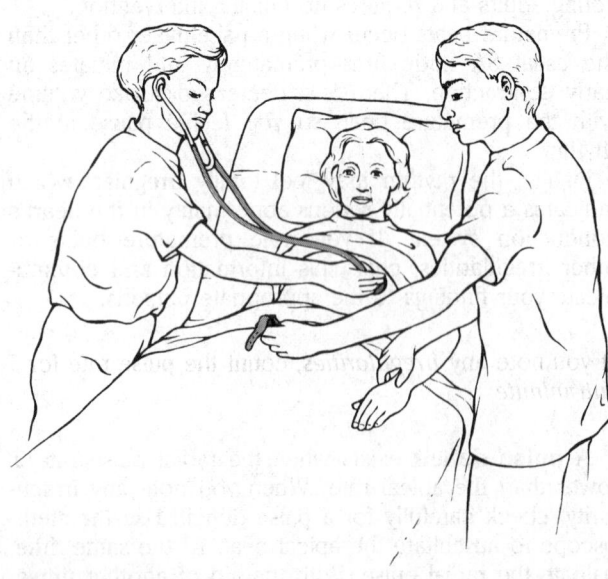

▲ Figure 31–11

Assessing the apical-radial pulse to identify a pulse deficit.

Assess and record the quality of the pulse using these terms:

▶ Bounding—strong, full force as if pounding against your fingertips
▶ Normal—easy to palpate, not easily obliterated
▶ Weak, thready—difficult to palpate and easily obliterated
▶ Absent—no palpable pulse

Some institutions use a 0 to 3+ scale, so check the policy of the agency in which you work. This assessment is subjective, and it requires clinical experience for the distinctions to be made.

ASSESSMENT OF RESPIRATION

Basic Pulmonary Physiology

The function of the lungs is to maintain homeostasis of arterial blood. By supplying oxygen (O_2) and removing excess carbon dioxide (CO_2), respiration maintains the pH of the blood, thus protecting vital tissues and nourishing the cells.

Respiration is the act of breathing, the exchange of oxygen and carbon dioxide in the lungs and tissues. Respiration refers to two processes: external respiration and internal respiration. External respiration is the act of breathing. It has four components: (1) ventilation, or the mechanical movement of air in and out of the lungs, (2) distribution of air throughout the bronchial tree; (3) diffusion of the gas molecules (O_2 and CO_2) from an area of higher concentration to an area of lower concentration across the respiratory membrane, and (4) perfusion, or the movement of blood through tissues and organs, like the lungs. Internal respiration occurs at the cellular level. Hemoglobin in the blood releases O_2 to the cell. In turn, the cell releases CO_2, a waste product of metabolism.

Any disease state that interferes with these steps results in hypoxemia. For example, a collapse or an obstruction of a lung section interferes with ventilation of those alveoli. Some diseases (pneumonia, pulmonary edema, emphysema) involve the structure of the respiratory membrane and thus block alveolar-capillary diffusion. Alternatively, the alveoli may be ventilated but not perfused with blood, as in hemorrhage, obstruction of a blood vessel by pulmonary embolism, or inadequate pulmonary blood flow due to congenital heart defects or anesthesia.

Control of Respiration

The act of breathing is automatic and involuntary, but it can also be influenced by a person's voluntary control and activities. Normally, however, our breathing pattern changes without our awareness in response to cellular demands.

The involuntary control of respirations is mediated by the respiratory center, the area of the brainstem (pons and medulla) that controls the rate, rhythm, and depth of respirations. The medulla has a basic rhythmicity that can produce repetitive inspiration and expiration. However, this rhythmicity does not produce a smooth pattern of breathing. Several feedback mechanisms work together to adjust and refine this pattern and meet the body's demands for oxygen.

The major feedback loop is humoral regulation, or the change in CO_2 and O_2 levels in the blood, and to a lesser extent, the hydrogen ion level. For most of us, the normal stimulus to breathe is an increase of CO_2 in the blood, or hypercapnia. The respiratory center senses this increase and responds by increasing the rate and depth of respirations. Hypoxemia (decreased O_2 in the blood) also increases respirations, though to a lesser degree than does hypercapnia.

Many other factors affect respiratory rate:

▶ Sudden stressful conditions may alter the respiratory rate as the body prepares for "fight or flight."
▶ Physical exercise increases the rate of metabolism, which in turn increases the oxygen requirements of the cells. The body responds to this demand through a change in the rate and depth of respirations.
▶ Environmental conditions also alter the respiratory rate. Impulses from peripheral sensory receptors in the skin run through nerves in the spinal cord and stimulate the respiratory center. Thus, temperature change (a jump into a cold shower) and pain (a slap on the skin) both change the rate of respirations.
▶ A change in altitude also affects respirations. A person first encountering the lower oxygen content at high altitudes may feel tired, weak, and short of breath and may experience "palpitations" (an awareness of heart beat). To compensate, the respiratory rate and depth increase, bringing additional oxygen to the cells.

▶ Adjustments occur to respiratory patterns to augment activities such as speaking, singing, crying, laughing, swallowing, and defecating.

In all these cases, respiratory alterations occur automatically.

Techniques for Assessing Respiration

Assess the respirations of people with acute or chronic pulmonary disease, acute heart disease, shock, or neurologic diseases each time you give them care. Also, observe the respiratory status of people who have had surgery or who suddenly experience difficulty in breathing. Know the reasons for assessing respirations for each individual, the results of previous assessments, and the current physical status. In addition to counting the respiratory rate accurately (Table 31–4), note the quality, depth, and pattern.

Assess the respirations at the same time that you observe the other vital signs. Do not tell individuals that you will be counting the breathing rate, because making them so aware may alter the results. Instead, describe the procedure for taking the other vital signs, and unobtrusively assess the respirations. A good time to do this assessment is after you obtain the radial pulse rate, while the forearm lies across the chest. For an infant or young child, obtain the respiratory rate before taking the temperature. Many babies cry when a rectal thermometer is inserted, so that respiratory data are inaccurate.

Quality of Respiration

Normal relaxed breathing is effortless, automatic, regular, and even. To determine the quality of respirations,

TABLE 31–4. Assessing Respirations

Suggested Steps	Rationale/Assessment
1. Keep fingers in place after assessing radial pulse; observe respirations.	1. Maneuver avoids calling attention to breathing, which could alter the rate
2. Observe complete respiratory cycle (inspiration and expiration), while observing for symmetric chest expansion, breathing sounds, use of accessory muscles, skin color, facial expression, level of consciousness, nasal flaring or sternal retraction in the child	2. Note indications of acute or chronic respiratory problems
3. For adults and older children, count number of respirations in 30 seconds and multiply by 2	3. Counting for only 15 seconds gives a result that can vary ±4, which is significant when working with such small numbers
4. Count infant respirations for 1 full minute	4. It is normal for infants to vary their respiratory rate and pattern
5. If respirations are abnormal, count rate for 1 full minute and note patterns, if any	5. Minimal time necessary to assess abnormal respirations
6. Note depth and rhythm of respirations	6. For complete assessment, note the character of respirations as well as the rate

uncover and observe the person's chest, maintaining the person's modesty. Does the chest expand symmetrically with inspiration? Unequal chest expansion occurs when part of a lung is obstructed or collapsed, when a person has pneumonia, and postoperatively when a person "guards" the operative side to avoid incisional pain from breathing.

Dyspnea means difficult, labored, or painful breathing. The person verbalizes a feeling of air hunger, "I can't catch my breath," and appears anxious and tired from the exertion. The person's color may be dusky, and the heart rate increases.

When a person is dyspneic, assess how much exertion it takes to produce the dyspnea. Does it result from walking to the bathroom, or is the person short of breath while just talking, pausing every few sentences to rest? Record these assessment data.

The development of noisy respirations is another noteworthy change in quality of respirations. Normal, relaxed breathing produces no noise. Recovery room nurses recognize this and have a maxim, "Any noisy breathing is obstructed breathing." Types of noisy respirations include

▶ **Stertor,** noisy respirations (e.g., snoring) that are produced by secretions in the trachea and large bronchi. Watch for this condition in people who have lost their cough reflex and their ability to handle secretions, such as neurologic or comatose persons.

▶ **Stridor,** harsh, inspiratory crowing sounds that occur with upper airway or laryngeal obstruction from laryngitis, from a foreign body, or from croup in children.

▶ **Wheeze,** high-pitched, musical, whistling sound accompanying partial obstruction in the bronchi and bronchioles. It is heard in severe emphysema and asthma.

▶ **Sigh,** a deep inspiration followed by a prolonged expiration. Occasional sighs are normal and helpful to expand alveoli. Frequent sighs may indicate emotional tension.

You do not need a stethoscope to hear these sounds. Nurses often auscultate the lungs with a stethoscope to assess the effectiveness of medication or treatment, determine the need for tracheal suctioning, or confirm suspicions of pathologic conditions such as pneumonia, atelectasis, or congestive heart failure. For additional information on assessment of breath sounds with a stethoscope, see Chapter 45.

Rate and Depth of Respirations

Normal rates are shown in Table 31–5. In adults, the normal range is 10 to 20 breaths per minute. However, in a study of the influence of different surgical procedures on breathing patterns, Zikria and colleagues noted that nursing personnel commonly believed 20 breaths per minute to be the normal value and often charted results at this figure.[51] This classic study showed a normal adult rate of 14 ± 4 breaths per min-

TABLE 31–5. Normal Respiratory Rates

Age	Breaths per Minute
Neonate	30–40
1 year	20–40
2 years	25–32
4 years	23–30
6 years	21–26
8 years	20–26
10 years	20–26
12 years	18–22
14 years	18–22
16 years	16–20
18 years	12–20
Adult	10–20

From Jarvis, C. (1992). *Physical examination and health assessment.* Philadelphia: W.B. Saunders.

ute and showed that rates of 25 to 30 per minute may indicate a significant change in respiratory status. Thus, consistent estimates of 20 per minute for a normal rate gives a falsely elevated reading and may be misleading when a true increase does occur. Several factors that normally affect the rate include age, emotions, and exercise.

Depth is the volume of air that is inhaled and exhaled with each respiration. This tidal volume is normally about 500 to 800 ml in the adult and should be constant with each breath. Although a spirometer measures the tidal volume precisely, you can make gross assessments of respiratory depth by placing the back of your hand close to the person's nose and mouth, feeling exhaled air, and observing adequate symmetric chest expansion. This technique gives you a rough estimate of tidal volume.

The following terms describe alterations in respiration. If everyone in your clinical situation is familiar with these terms, use them. If not, describe the specific character.

▶ **Tachypnea.** An increased respiratory rate (> 24 breaths/min), with respirations usually rapid and shallow. Some conditions that result in tachypnea include hypoxemia and fever. Fear can also cause tachypnea.

▶ **Bradypnea.** A decreased but regular respiratory rate (< 10 breaths/min), occurring with conditions such as depression of the respiratory center by opiate narcotics or by brain tumor.

▶ **Hypoventilation.** A reduction in the amount of air reaching the alveoli. It is characterized by a breathing pattern of slow (or irregular), shallow respirations. Overdosages of narcotics and anesthetics can cause this change. It also occurs in immobilized people and in individuals who "splint" one side of the chest to avoid postoperative pain. Hypoventilation causes excess CO_2 retention in the blood (acidosis).

▶ **Apnea.** Total cessation of breathing that may be periodic (see *Cheyne-Stokes* respirations below). Continued apnea is incompatible with life and is called respiratory arrest. Apnea may be caused by a mechanical airway obstruction (e.g., mucous plug, blood, vomitus, foreign body) or by damage to or depression of the respiratory center (e.g., head trauma, stroke, narcotic or anesthetic overdose).

▶ **Hyperpnea.** Increase in the depth of respiration. Hyperpnea normally occurs after strenuous exercise.

▶ **Hyperventilation.** An increase in both rate and depth of respirations. This condition often accompanies extreme exertion, fear and anxiety, fever, diabetic ketoacidosis (Kussmaul's respirations), aspirin overdose, and lesions of the midbrain. Hyperventilation causes decreased CO_2 in the blood, with resulting alkalosis (blood pH > 7.45).

Patterns of Respiration

The breathing pattern is normally regular and consists of inspiration, pause, longer expiration, and another pause. Some disease conditions may alter normal breathing and result in the following abnormal patterns.

▶ **Cheyne-Stokes respirations.** A cycle in which respirations gradually increase in rate and depth, then decrease with periods of temporary apnea. The respirations last 30 to 45 seconds and alternate with periods of apnea lasting up to 20 seconds. The most common cause of periodic breathing is severe congestive heart failure. Other causes include renal failure, drug overdose, increased intracranial pressure, and meningitis.

▶ **Biot's respirations.** An irregular breathing pattern in which breaths are all of the same depth rather than varying depths as in Cheyne-Stokes. The cycle length or rate is variable and may last from 10 seconds to 1 minute. This pattern accompanies spinal meningitis, encephalitis, head trauma, brain abscess, and heat stroke.

▶ **Kussmaul's respirations** (air hunger). Breathing characterized by increased depth and rate of respiration (more than 20 per minute). Kussmaul's respirations occur in metabolic acidosis (diabetic coma) and in renal failure.

▶ **Apneustic respirations.** Breathing characterized by prolonged, gasping inspiration followed by extremely short, inefficient expiration. It is often caused by lesions of the midbrain.

See Figure 31–12 for representations of some of the different breathing patterns.

Significant Characteristics in Respiratory Assessment

Change in Physical Appearance. Respiratory status is often apparent in a person's physical appearance. People with emphysema, for example, have a characteristic "barrel chest," which develops because of chronic hyperinflation.

Use of Accessory Muscles. Normally, the diaphragm is the major muscle involved in respiration. However, people experiencing respiratory difficulties or who are exercising vigorously also use accessory muscles to augment respiratory effort. These accessory muscles include the scalene, sternomastoid, and trapezius muscles of the neck and shoulders, the abdominal rectus, and intercostal muscles that line the ribs.

Change in Position. It is also valuable to note the position the person takes to breathe. People with chronic obstructive pulmonary disease (COPD), for example, sit leaning forward, arms braced against knees, chair, or bed. This position gives them leverage so that their abdominal rectus and intercostal muscles work together to force expiration. Such individuals also may

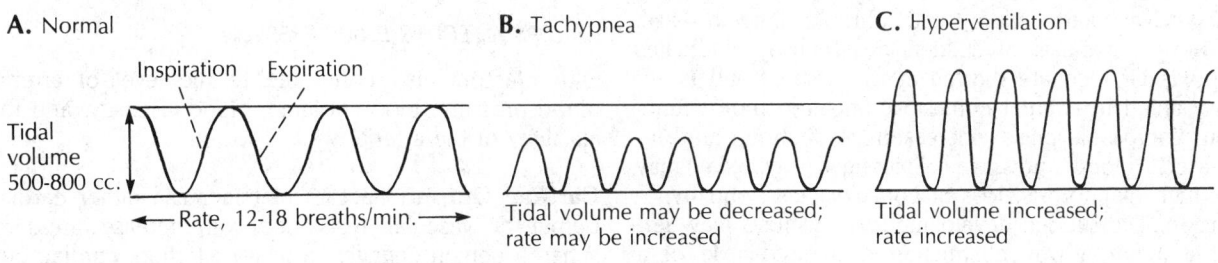

A. Normal

Inspiration   Expiration

Tidal volume 500-800 cc.

◀—— Rate, 12-18 breaths/min. ——▶

B. Tachypnea

Tidal volume may be decreased; rate may be increased

C. Hyperventilation

Tidal volume increased; rate increased

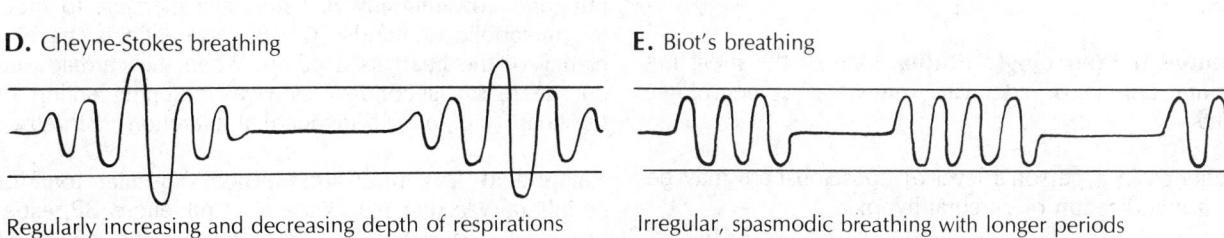

D. Cheyne-Stokes breathing

Regularly increasing and decreasing depth of respirations between periods of apnea

E. Biot's breathing

Irregular, spasmodic breathing with longer periods of apnea than breathing; tidal volume decreased

▲ *Figure 31-12*

Normal and abnormal breathing patterns.

purse their lips in a whistling position. By exhaling slowly and against a narrow opening, the pressure in the bronchial tree remains positive and fewer airways collapse. Some people must assume a sitting or standing position to breathe comfortably. **Orthopnea** is the inability to breathe except in an upright position. When charting, state the number of pillows the person uses, e.g., "two-pillow orthopnea" or "three-pillow orthopnea."

Change in Skin Color. Observe the skin for pallor or cyanosis, a bluish, mottled color of the skin and mucous membranes, especially that of sudden onset. The color of a person's lips and nailbeds varies with the skin color; therefore, do not assess color only in these areas. Instead, look under the tongue, in the buccal mucosa, or in the conjunctiva around the eyes, and be sensitive to changes in color. Realize that pallor and cyanosis are gross measures of respiratory status. For a complete assessment, you must collect additional data.

The normal pink color of mucous membranes is due to oxygenated hemoglobin in the red blood cells. Pallor indicates a diminished amount of red blood cells, or anemia. Skin pallor is best seen in the conjunctiva and mucous membranes. However, pallor is always a gross estimate of the adequacy of tissue oxygenation. A more precise measure is a laboratory analysis of a complete blood count.

Cyanosis signifies a decrease of oxygenated blood in the tissues. It is caused by reduced hemoglobin in the superficial blood vessels. Hemoglobin (the oxygen-carrying pigment of the red blood cells) is referred to as "reduced" when it is not combined with oxygen. Like pallor, cyanosis is a nonspecific sign (i.e., not diagnostic of one specific pathologic condition). Both pallor and cyanosis are produced, in part, by an inadequate peripheral blood flow or inadequate red blood cell count. They are not necessarily related to inadequacy of the respiratory tract.

Cyanosis may be a sign of congenital heart disease, congestive heart failure, and chronic lung disease. However, cyanosis of sudden onset always indicates hypoxia (inadequate oxygen in the tissues) and is accompanied by mental confusion, impaired motor function, increased pulse, increased respiration, and increased blood pressure. Prolonged hypoxia may produce diaphoresis, loss of consciousness, and hypotension. The sudden development of cyanosis may herald a major airway obstruction or the collapse of a lung.

Change in Neurologic Status. One of the most important criteria of adequate ventilation is neurologic status.

A change in a person's level of consciousness may be the *first* indication of cerebral hypoxia.

With progressive pulmonary failure, a previously alert person becomes anxious and restless, then irritable, then excessively drowsy, and finally comatose. Or,

someone who was calm and cooperative may suddenly become combative. An alert nurse will detect even subtle personality changes and intervene appropriately.

ASSESSMENT OF BLOOD PRESSURE

Physiology of Arterial Pressure

Blood pressure is the force exerted by the blood against an area of the vessel wall as measured in millimeters of mercury (mm Hg). This means that any pressure in the artery will push up a column of mercury equal to its strength. For example, 120 mm Hg means that the pressure in the artery is strong enough to elevate the mercury column to 120 mm.

The objective of the measurement is to obtain the **systolic pressure** (the maximal pressure exerted on the arteries during contraction of the left ventricle of the heart), the **diastolic pressure** (the amount of pressure exerted on the arterial walls with the ventricles at rest), and the pulse pressure (difference between the systolic and diastolic).

Blood pressure is a product of the cardiac output (stroke volume × heart rate) times the resistance to blood flow through the vessels, or the **peripheral vascular resistance.** This relationship is expressed as

$$BP = CO \times R$$

The vasomotor center in the brainstem controls BP through the autonomic nervous system. The vasomotor center receives sensory impulses from baroreceptors and chemoreceptors in the heart, aortic arch, carotid arteries, lungs, and blood vessels, and from the hypothalamus and cerebral cortex. The vasomotor center sends impulses back through the autonomic nervous system to the heart and blood vessels to alter stroke volume, heart rate, and vascular resistance in order to match BP to circulatory needs.

FACTORS AFFECTING BLOOD PRESSURE

Other factors also contribute to the level of arterial blood pressure: blood volume, blood viscosity, and the elasticity of the arterial walls.

Cardiac Output. Factors that increase either cardiac output or vascular resistance will increase pressure. When a person engages in heavy exertion, cardiac output (and consequently BP) normally increase to meet the metabolic demands. The BP also reflects the efficiency of the heart as a pump. When the cardiac output decreases secondary to weak pumping action of the heart (e.g., after a myocardial infarction), BP falls.

Peripheral Vascular Resistance. Vascular tone or peripheral vascular resistance also influences BP, especially the diastolic reading. The smaller the caliber of vessel through which the blood flows, the greater the pressure necessary to push the blood. When resistance increases (vasoconstriction), the same volume of blood is pumped into a smaller compartment; hence, BP increases. Blood pressure decreases with vasodilatation because the blood occupies a larger space and exerts less pressure on the arterial wall.

Elasticity. Blood pressure also reflects the elasticity or distensibility of the arterial walls. Atherosclerosis hardens the arteries, so that they lose their ability to stretch. The heart has to pump against a greater resistance, and so BP increases.

Blood Volume. In addition, BP reflects how tightly the blood is packed into the arterial system. Conditions causing blood *volume* to vary will affect blood pressure: BP decreases when the volume is low, as in hemorrhage; BP increases with rapid administration of intravenous fluids.

Blood Viscosity. Blood viscosity refers to thickness as determined by its cellular components. Blood pressure is higher when the blood is more viscous, as in conditions that produce increased numbers of red blood cells (polycythemia) or plasma proteins. Viscosity rises markedly when the hematocrit (the percentage of whole blood that is composed of cells) is above 50 per cent, thus elevating BP.[5]

FACTORS AFFECTING NORMAL RANGES

Average BP in the young adult is 120/80. However, a "normal" reading varies from person to person owing to many factors.

Age. Blood pressure exhibits a slow, steady rise during childhood and adulthood until age 40 to 50 years (Fig. 31–13). Blood pressure (especially the systolic reading) usually increases further into old age.

Gender. There is no difference in BP values between boys and girls until puberty. After this time, females usually have a lower BP than males of the same age, until menopause, when their pressure readings increase over men's.

Weight. Body weight makes a difference: BP is consistently higher in overweight persons than in normal-weight persons of the same age. Weight reduction usually decreases BP.

Race. Blood pressure varies with race, although the reasons for this difference are complex and involve such factors as heredity, climate, diet, and disease, as well as measuring techniques in different countries. In the United States, black adults have higher BP readings than do whites of the same age.

Climate. Climate can make a difference. Pressure norms are lower in tropical climates than in temperate zones and are highest in polar climates.

Diet. Diet plays an important role in BP control. A diet high in sodium and low in calcium may predispose a person to high BP.

Circadian Rhythm. In all persons, BP is usually lowest in the early morning, rises throughout the day to a peak in the late afternoon or early evening, and then starts to decline, falling to the lowest point during sleep.[19] This normal cyclic variation or circadian rhythm occurs every day. This daily rhythm, however, may be altered during different life stages, such as pregnancy, and during illness or hospitalization.

Exercise. Blood pressure increases with exercise, rising in proportion to the amount of activity. Therefore, it

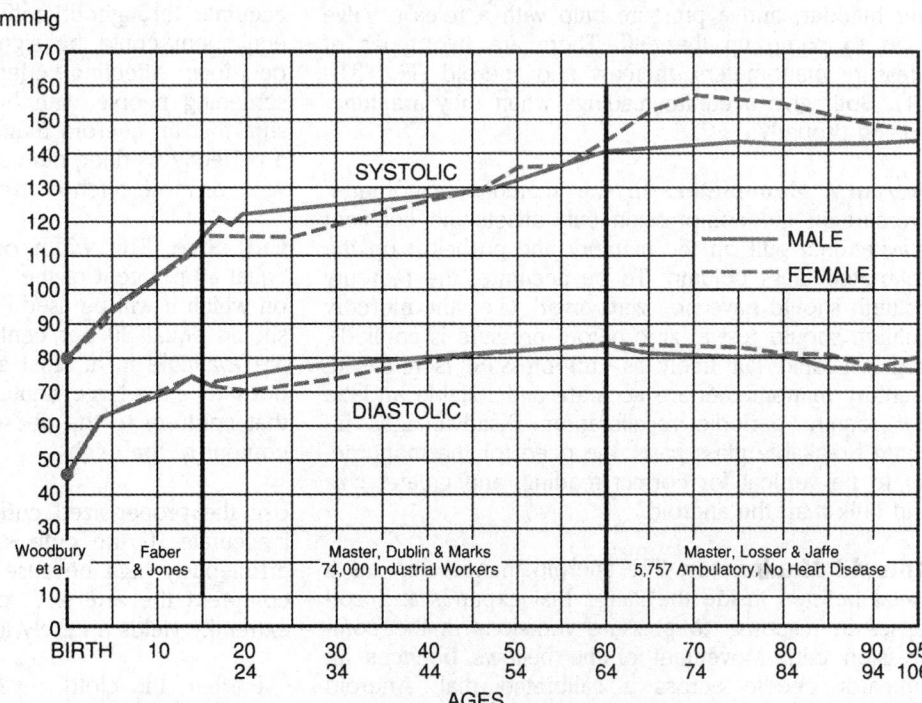

▲ **Figure 31–13**

Variations in blood pressure with age and gender. (From Master A. M. & Lasser, R. P. [1961]. Blood pressure in the elderly. In A. M. Brest and J. H. Moyer [eds.]. *Hypertension: Recent advances.* Philadelphia: Lea & Febiger.)

is advisable to refrain from taking a BP reading within 20 minutes after the person has exercised.

Stress. Blood pressure also increases with strong emotions (e.g., anger or fear) and with other physical and psychologic sources of stress.

Position. Opinions vary concerning the effect of change in position on BP. It is often stated that BP is lower when individuals are lying down than when they are sitting or standing, yet in some people it may remain the same or even decrease upon standing. A sudden decrease in blood pressure upon a person's standing is called orthostatic hypotension and is noted particularly as a side effect of antihypertensive medications, or when a person first arises after a period of prolonged immobility (see Chapter 35). Pressure also varies with different recumbent positions. Studies show that a fall in BP normally occurs in the uppermost arm when a person is turned onto the side. Systolic and diastolic pressures are significantly lower when compared with the corresponding pressures when the person is in the supine position.[7,13,38] About one fourth of the population have a difference in BP between the right and left arm, it being usually higher in the right arm. Generally this difference is transient and quite variable. The difference may range from 10 to 20 mm Hg. Finally, BP is slightly higher in the lower extremities than in the arms.

Blood Pressure Equipment

MEASURING DEVICES

The standard instrument used to measure BP is a **sphygmomanometer.** This consists of a pressure manometer, an occlusive cuff containing an inflatable rubber bladder, and a pressure bulb with a release valve used to pump up the cuff. There are two types of pressure manometers, mercury and aneroid (Fig. 31–14). Both give accurate readings when they are functioning properly.

Mercury Manometer. In the mercury manometer, pressure in the compression cuff offsets the constant gravitational pull on the mercury and pushes it up the calibrated glass column. To be accurate, the mercury column should have no "zero error" (i.e., the mercury column should rest at zero before pressure is applied), and it should fall freely as cuff pressure is released. Mercury manometers are accurate and reliable and do not require periodic recalibration. Disadvantages include breakable glass parts, the need for the manometer to be vertical for correct reading, and greater size and bulk than the aneroid.

Aneroid Manometer. The aneroid manometer has a metal bellows inside the gauge that expands and collapses in response to pressure variations in the compression cuff. Movement of the bellows bounces an indicator needle across a calibrated dial. Aneroid sphygmomanometers are portable and often easier to

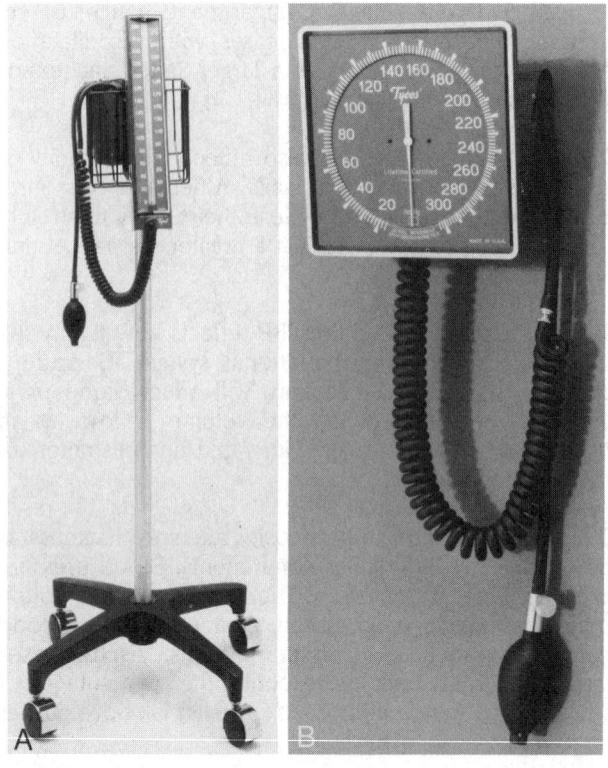

▲ *Figure 31–14*

Sphygmomanometers. *A,* A portable model with a mercury gauge. *B,* A wall-mounted model with an aneroid gauge. (Courtesy of Welch Allyn, Skaneateles Falls, NY.)

read than mercury manometers. However, the elastic properties of the metal parts make the aneroid gauge subject to drift and therefore somewhat less reliable than the mercury gauge. A needle resting at zero when the cuff is flat is no guarantee that the reading will be accurate throughout cuff deflation. Errors from faulty equipment could be significant when making clinical decisions affecting critically ill people and when screening people with hypertension. Therefore, make sure that an aneroid manometer is recalibrated against a perfectly working mercury manometer at least once a year, or more often if errors are suspected.

Cuff Size. The width of the rubber bladder should equal 40 per cent of the circumference of the extremity on which it will be used. The length of the cuff bladder should equal 80 per cent of this circumference. Cuffs are available in at least six standard sizes, from newborn to extra-large adult. Tapered cuffs are available that conform to the obese, conical arm or the natural contour of the thigh.

Use the proper-sized cuff or results will be markedly inaccurate. If the cuff is too narrow, results will be erroneously high because extra pressure is needed to compress the artery. A cuff that is too wide for the extremity yields a falsely low reading.

Further, the cloth cover for the bladder should be nonstretchable so that pressure can be distributed uniformly over the arm. The control valve on the pressure bulb must be clean and free from leaks or sticking, so that the cuff deflates evenly.

Blood Pressure Measurement Techniques

Assessment of BP combines the skills of inspection, palpation, and auscultation. Prior to measurement, try to avoid or control any factors that could influence BP: meals, smoking, exercise, pain, anxiety. Even a need to urinate can alter BP. People often are anxious at the beginning of a complete physical examination. It may be necessary to repeat the BP reading at the end of the examination, to ensure accuracy.

To decrease the person's anxiety, make certain *you* are relaxed and unhurried. The individual and significant others will watch you carefully and will be sensitive to any sign that all is not well. Explain the procedure to them. If the person asks you for the BP reading, respond honestly. First, ask to know the usual BP, so that you have an idea of the individual's level of knowledge. Then you might say, "It is 118/70 now, which is within normal limits for you," or, "It is 140/90 now, which is a little higher than your usual reading. This might have been caused by your walk down the hall, so I'll check it again in 10 minutes." Everyone should know the personal normal range. This knowledge is important for the control of hypertension, and it encourages self-care. On rare occasions, such as a sudden, dramatic increase or decrease in pressure, stating a precise number might alarm a person. Use your judgment to determine exactly what information to give. Measurement of BP at the brachial pulse site is described in Procedure 31–3.

Auscultatory Method. The auscultatory method involves (a) placing and then inflating a cuff over the brachial artery, and (b) using a properly placed stethoscope to listen for the **Korotkoff sounds,** *the sounds produced by the pressure of blood in the artery. Korotkoff sounds indicate systolic and diastolic blood pressures (Table 31–6). Inflating the cuff squeezes the tissue around the brachial artery. When that pressure exceeds the heart's systolic pressure, the brachial artery collapses and blood flow stops. Then, as cuff pressure is released, pressure on the arm tissues decreases. When pressure inside the brachial artery equals that in the compression cuff, the artery opens, a small amount of blood is pumped through with each heart beat, and you hear Korotkoff sounds.

Systolic pressure (phase I Korotkoff) is the first reappearance of clear tapping sounds. Note the sphygmomanometer reading at which you hear the tapping sound for at least *two* consecutive beats; then, the sounds increase in intensity. Phase II and phase III Korotkoff are subtle changes in the sound and are not heard.

Diastolic pressure is recorded at either phase IV or

phase V Korotkoff sound. Phase IV is the abrupt muffling or damping of sound to a soft, blowing, murmurlike quality. The sound changes in *quality,* rather than intensity. Phase V is the point at which the tapping sounds disappear completely. Phase IV is the more accurate measure of diastolic reading in children. Phase V (the last audible sound) indicates diastolic BP readings in adults.[14]

Sometimes you should note both phases IV and V, for example, 138/80/76. The difference between the fourth and fifth sounds is important for the person with a 10- to 12-mm Hg variance between phases IV and V, e.g., 138/94/80; 94 mm Hg is considered "above normal" although 80 mm Hg is within normal limits. Nursing assessment and planning for a person will differ depending on the number for the diastolic reading. Therefore, clear communication is important.

Occasionally you may notice an **auscultatory gap,** a pause in the Korotkoff sounds after the first, with the sounds resuming at a lower pressure, especially in people with hypertension. The sound is auscultated but fades out completely and is heard again 10 to 40 mm Hg lower. The pulse is palpable during this silent phase. If you do not pump the cuff high enough, you will miss the top sound and seriously underestimate the systolic pressure. To avoid this problem, always palpate the radial artery while pumping the cuff.

Palpatory Method. With the palpatory method, use your fingers rather than a stethoscope. Record that point at which you first palpate the radial artery pulsation during cuff deflation as the systolic pressure. This method is useful when a person is in shock and has a greatly reduced cardiac output. In this situation, you may be unable to auscultate the BP because the pulsations are feeble. However, you may be able to palpate the BP even when the radial pulse is weak and thready. The systolic reading is usually a few millimeters of mercury lower by palpation than by auscultation. It is difficult to palpate the diastolic reading, so this step is usually omitted. In a critically ill person, BP readings by palpation are not as accurate as the direct method using an arterial line (see section on Electronic Monitoring).

Thigh Pressure. Blood pressure readings are taken in the lower extremities to compare values with arm readings, or when arms are injured or otherwise unavailable. Position the person on the abdomen, apply the cuff to the thigh, centered over the popliteal artery in the back of the knee. Perform the procedure as you would with the arm, auscultating at the popliteal artery. If the person is unable to lie on the abdomen, use the supine position with the person's knee bent slightly. The systolic pressure may be 10 to 40 mm Hg higher in the thigh than in the arms, but the diastolic pressure will be the same in both sites.

Self-Care. You can teach people to monitor their own BP at home. Self-monitoring gives a more reliable record of the daily pattern of an individual's BP. For people with hypertension, self-monitoring may increase compliance with their diet and medication schedule.

---

* Korotkoff sounds are named for the Russian surgeon who first described them in 1905.

PROCEDURE 31-3

Measuring Blood Pressure at the Brachial Pulse Site

Definition/Purposes. *To measure systolic and diastolic blood pressure.* Blood pressure measurement reflects circulating blood volume, peripheral vascular resistance, efficiency of heart as a pump, viscosity of blood, and elasticity of arterial wall.

Contraindications/Cautions. Do not take BP reading on person's arm if arm (a) is injured or diseased, (b) is on same side of body where a female has had a radical mastectomy, (c) has a shunt or fistula for renal dialysis, or (d) is site for an intravenous infusion.

Learning/Teaching Guidelines. Provide following information: (a) describe procedure regardless of person's level of consciousness, (b) explain that inflated cuff will feel temporarily uncomfortable, and (c) instruct individual and other people in room to remain quiet during procedure so you can hear through stethoscope.

PRELIMINARY ACTIVITIES

Assessment/Planning

► Know baseline or "normal" BP for this person.
► Know reason for taking BP reading on this person (routine vital signs, postoperative care, etc.).
► Know latest series of vital sign readings for this person and be cognizant of trends.
► Postpone BP reading at least 10 minutes for a person who is angry or anxious, or who has just ambulated.
► Schedule frequency for obtaining BP readings as determined by person's condition and physician's orders.
► Postpone BP reading on a crying infant or child; it may be necessary to take it when infant is asleep.
► Choose a cuff that is appropriate for extremity used (e.g., arm or thigh) and for person's size (see discussion in text).

Equipment

► Stethoscope
► Mercury or aneroid sphygmomanometer
► Appropriate-sized cuff

Preparation of Person

► Individual should be in a stable, relaxed, sitting or lying position for 5 to 10 minutes before BP is taken.
► Permit a child to handle BP equipment before it is used, to help reduce fears.

PROCEDURE

Actions

1. Whether person is sitting or lying, position arm supported at level of heart, palm up.
2. Position yourself no more than 3 feet away from sphygmomanometer, directly in front of aneroid model and at eye level with meniscus of mercury model (Fig. 31–15). On a portable model, have mercury column vertical. (The sphygmomanometer does not have to be at heart level but the BP cuff does.)
3. If using mercury manometer, check to ensure level of mercury is at zero before cuff inflation.
4. Center arrow marking on cuff over brachial artery, located at medial side of antecubital fossa (inner aspect of elbow).
5. Expel any air in cuff, and wrap cuff evenly, with lower edge 2.5 to 5 cm above maximal brachial artery pulsation. Avoid contact with clothing.

6. Palpate radial artery (on flexor surface of wrist). Inflate cuff 20 to 30 mm Hg above the point at which radial pulsation disappears.

Rationale/Discussion

1. Arm above level of heart produces falsely low reading.

2. A position more than 3 feet away produces inaccuracies. Looking up at meniscus gives a falsely high reading. Looking down on meniscus gives a falsely low reading. If a portable mercury model is tilted on the bed, reading is falsely high.

3. Eliminating "zero error" ensures proper calibration and an accurate reading.
4. You must apply cuff pressure directly to artery to occlude blood flow.

5. An uneven or too loose cuff gives a falsely high reading because excessive amounts of pressure are needed to occlude brachial artery. Cuff edge should be high enough to avoid covering stethoscope. Accidental contact with clothing or tubing produces confusing extraneous noises.
6. Principle of counterpressure occludes blood flow. Systolic pressure is estimated to be point where radial pulsation is no longer felt. If you do not inflate high enough, you may miss true systolic pressure. Especially significant is person who has an auscultatory gap (see text). In contrast, inflating cuff too high causes unnecessary pain.

PROCEDURE 31–3 Continued

Actions	Rationale/Discussion
7. Place stethoscope end piece over brachial artery. If your stethoscope has a bell, use it. Otherwise the stethoscope diaphragm will suffice.	7. Korotkoff sounds are of low frequency, and the bell is best for low-frequency sounds.
8. Listen carefully, and release cuff at an even rate of 2 mm Hg per heart beat.	8. Deflating cuff too slowly produces venous congestion, which falsely elevates diastolic pressure. Deflating cuff too rapidly invites guessing at exact pressure. Proper deflation of cuff is especially important when pulse is irregular, as in atrial fibrillation.
9. Note manometer number at which sound first begins (Korotkoff phase I).	9. First sound is made when blood begins to flow through brachial artery again. This is called systolic pressure.
10. Continue to release cuff pressure evenly and note a "muffling" or "damping" of sound (Korotkoff phase IV).	10. Use this reading as diastolic reading in children.
11. Note final disappearance of sound (Korotkoff phase V).	11. Use this reading as diastolic pressure in adults.
12. Deflate cuff completely to zero and wait 30 to 60 seconds before taking BP again. Repeat reading if you are unsure of accuracy.	12. Occlusion of blood during pressure reading causes venous congestion in forearm. Venous blood must be allowed to drain or it will falsely elevate succeeding BP readings.
13. If unable to determine BP owing to feeble sounds, elevate person's arm and then inflate cuff. Then lower arm, deflate cuff, and listen.	13. Decreases venous pressure and makes sounds louder.
14. If still unable to hear, note palpatory systolic pressure by feeling for reappearance of radial pulse (see palpatory method, p. 615).	14. Blood pressure by palpation is a few millimeters of mercury lower than by auscultation but will still be meaningful as long as you make subsequent measurements in the same way.

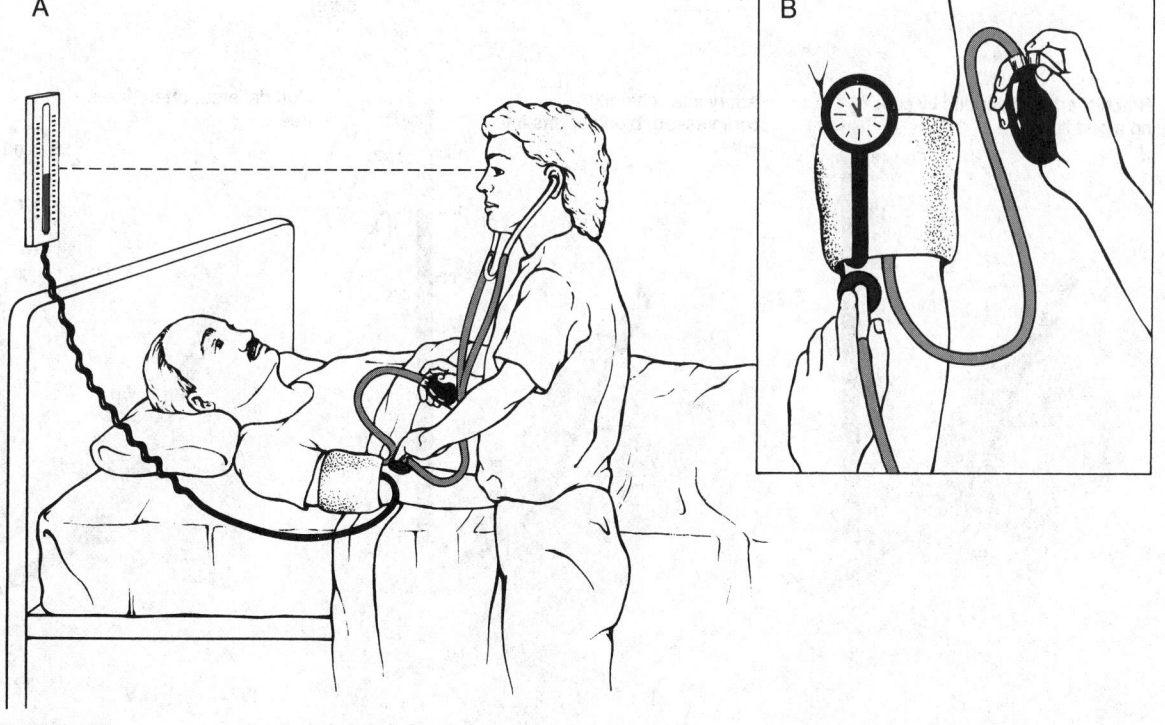

A

B

▲ *Figure 31–15*

FINAL ACTIVITIES

Assess BP findings in view of individual's clinical picture. Record findings (including individual's position) on chart. If data show significant change in person's condition, take indicated actions (e.g., communicate findings to appropriate person).

TABLE 31–6. Korotkoff Sounds

Phase	Quality	Description	Rationale
Cuff correctly in-flated	No sound		Cuff inflation compresses brachial artery. Cuff pressure exceeds heart's systolic pressure, occluding brachial artery blood flow.
I	Tapping	Soft, clear tapping, increasing in intensity	The SYSTOLIC pressure. As the cuff pressure lowers to reach intraluminal systolic pressure, the artery opens, and blood first spurts into the brachial artery.
Auscultatory gap*	No sound	Silence for 30–40 mm Hg	Sounds temporarily disappear during end of phase I, then reappear in phase II. Common with hypertension. If undetected, results in falsely low systolic or falsely high diastolic reading.
II	Swooshing	Softer murmur follows tapping	Turbulent blood flow through still partially occluded artery.
III	Knocking	Crisp, high-pitched sounds	Artery closes just briefly during late diastole.
IV	Abrupt muffling	Sound mutes to a low-pitched, cushioned murmur; blowing quality	Artery no longer closes in any part of cardiac cycle. Change in quality, not intensity. American Heart Association proposes this as most accurate level of diastolic pressure in children (Frohlich et al., 1988).
V	Silence		Decreased velocity of blood flow. Streamlined blood flow is silent. The last audible sound (marking the disappearance of sounds is adult DIASTOLIC pressure).

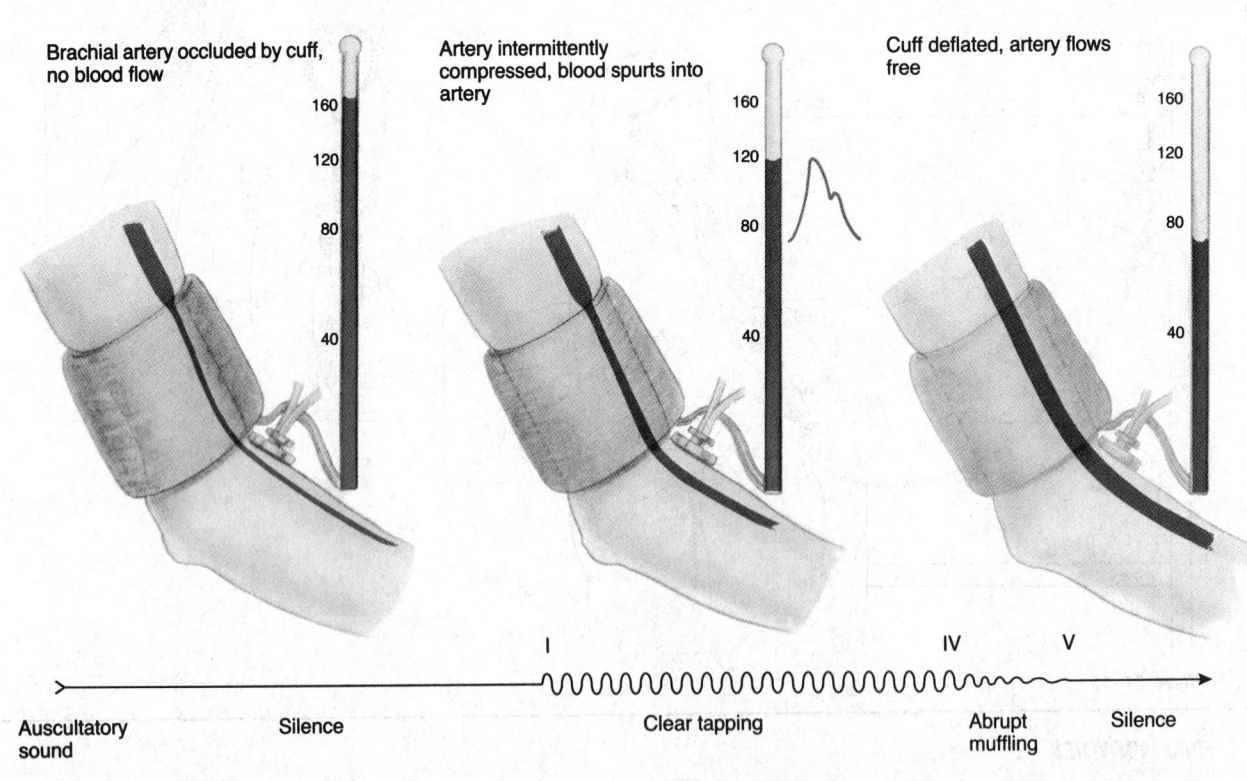

* This is an abnormal finding.
From Jarvis, C. (1992). *Physical examination and health assessment.* Philadelphia: W.B. Saunders.

Other groups in need of teaching include pregnant women and people with renal disease, renal transplants, or borderline high BP. As you teach the procedure, provide each person with complete written instructions about the method for measuring BP. During your teaching, check the person's equipment for accuracy. Monitor the person's understanding of the procedure and correct technique. Reinforce your teaching with visual teaching aids such as those available through the American Heart Association.

Equipment for a home BP kit usually includes a stethoscope, a blood pressure cuff, and an aneroid manometer. The aneroid manometer should be calibrated once a year against a standard mercury manometer using a Y-connector. Some individuals may purchase an electronic BP device that uses a digital readout instead of a stethoscope. This equipment is more expensive but is good for people who worry about their skill in measuring BP. Teach these people that the electronic BP device is very sensitive; placing the cuff incorrectly or moving the arm while measuring will produce errors.

Many people will ask you if it is all right to use the stationary automated BP machines located in many shopping centers, pharmacies, banks, airports, and workplaces. As long as this equipment is calibrated regularly, it serves in screening BP. The problem is that consumers usually have no access to the last calibration date. Advise these people to call their health care provider before they alter any treatment regimen based on a BP reading from an automated machine.

Ambulatory blood pressure monitoring is completed with a portable device worn continually for a 24-hour period. It records multiple BP readings and is used under physician supervision to help diagnose hypertension or evaluate drug treatment. The person wears a lightweight monitor on the belt and a BP cuff on the arm. The cuff inflates at preset intervals while the person performs the usual daily activities. At the end of the period, data from the monitor are transferred to a computer, and a printout is analyzed.

Blood Pressure Measurement in Infants and Children

For children, use the basic techniques described in Procedure 31–3. Make sure the child or infant has been quiet for 5 to 10 minutes before the reading. Crying can elevate the systolic reading 30 to 50 mm Hg.

The most common source of error in measuring a child's blood pressure is inappropriate cuff size.

On children, the cuff bladder width should be 40 per cent of arm circumference, and the bladder length should completely or almost completely encircle the arm without overlap.[14] Use a pediatric (small-diameter) diaphragm on the stethoscope to hear the sounds. Record the phase IV Korotkoff as the diastolic reading; children have a relatively high velocity of blood flow, which makes phase V last longer than the true diastolic value.

For children under 2 years of age, it may be difficult to hear auscultatory sounds. You can use a Doppler ultrasound device instead of a stethoscope for more accurate systolic readings. Study the technique for use of the Doppler in the section on Electronic Monitoring.

If there is no access to a Doppler, use the flush method of measuring BP in a neonate or small infant. This method gives a mean systolic-diastolic pressure. Make sure the baby is quiet. If necessary, use a bottle or pacifier. The room must be well lighted. Place the manometer gauge close to the extremity so that both can be seen at the same time. Apply the appropriate neonatal cuff around the arm or leg. Elevate the extremity and squeeze the part distal to the cuff with your hand, or wrap it tightly with an elastic bandage. These maneuvers will blanch the extremity. Pump the manometer to 120 to 140 mm Hg and lower the extremity. Release the pressure of your hand or bandage at the same time that you deflate the cuff. The rate of deflation must not exceed 5 mm Hg per second. The point at which the baby's arm or leg flushes is the mean systolic-diastolic pressure. A normal reading is 30 to 60 mm Hg for infants weighing more than 2500 gm (6.7 lb). Current standards at all weights have not been established.

The flush technique has some disadvantages. It cannot be used unless the baby is lying quietly. In addition, results are not valid for dark-skinned infants or for those with anemia, cyanosis, hypothermia, peripheral vasoconstriction, or edema. Obviously, these criteria limit the technique's usefulness. It is in just the latter instances that you need a valid BP.

Errors in Blood Pressure Measurement

Because you will make many judgments based on the results of BP determination, it is crucial to avoid errors. Haste or subconscious bias are important examples of observer error. The health professional who has a preconceived idea of what a person's BP should be may be influenced subconsciously by the person's age, weight, or diagnosis and may "hear" a value in line with what is expected for that group. Another example is "digit preference," in which the observer "hears" more values that end in zero (e.g., 140/80) than would be expected by chance alone. Box 31–1 lists other sources of error.

When you eliminate such errors—defective equipment, poor technique, haste—the results are reliable.

You must control technique and equipment to produce accurate and reliable results.

Interpretating Abnormal Blood Pressure Findings

Blood pressure determination is a part of every screening physical examination, both in the health care facil-

---

Box 31–1. Common Sources of Error in Blood Pressure Measurement

Errors That Produce a Falsely High Reading

▶ Failure to use the appropriate cuff size; a too narrow cuff gives a higher reading

▶ Wrapping the cuff too loosely or unevenly (cuff pressure must be exceedingly high to compress the brachial artery)

▶ Recording BP just after a meal, while person is smoking, or while person's bladder is distended

▶ Failure to have the mercury column vertical

▶ Deflating the cuff too slowly; this produces venous congestion in the extremity, which falsely elevates diastolic pressure

Errors That Produce a Falsely Low Reading

▶ Having the person's arm above the level of the heart (effect of hydrostatic pressure can give an error up to 10 mm Hg in systolic and diastolic pressure)

▶ Failure to notice an auscultatory gap

▶ Diminished hearing acuity of the health care professional

▶ Stethoscope that is too small or too large, or has tubing that is too long

▶ Inability to hear feeble Korotkoff sounds

Errors That Produce Either Falsely High or Low Readings

▶ Inaccurately calibrated manometer

▶ Defective equipment (valve, connections)

▶ Failure to have meniscus of mercury at eye level

▶ Performing the technique too quickly, with too little attention to details

---

ity and in ambulatory settings. Some groups of people are "at risk" and require more frequent monitoring. These groups include people with heart disease, those having surgery, those with hypertension, and those with neurologic disorders (e.g., increased intracranial pressure).

Hypotension. In adults, a reading below 95/60 represents the abnormally low BP that defines **hypotension.** In healthy adults, a persistent systolic pressure of 90 to 100 with no accompanying symptoms is not clinically significant. However, a normally hypertensive person experiences hypotension at a much higher level. You should know the *average* vital signs for each individual before you attach significance to one isolated figure.

Hypotension occurs with Addison's disease (hypofunction of the adrenal glands), hemorrhage, and vasodilation. Expect a small drop in BP when you apply blankets to warm up a postoperative person who is vasoconstricted from being in a cool operating room. The drop is not significant if the pulse remains stable. If the drop continues, if the person becomes diaphoretic, and if the pulse increases, inspect for signs of hemorrhage and notify the physician.

Hypotension also occurs with conditions of decreased cardiac output, such as an acute myocardial infarction (MI, or heart attack) or shock. In addition to low BP, the person has an increased pulse, dizziness, diaphoresis, confusion, and blurred vision. The skin feels cool and clammy because the superficial blood vessels constrict to shunt blood to the vital organs. An individual having an acute MI may also complain of crushing substernal chest pain, high epigastric pain, and shoulder or jaw pain.

Hypertension. The Joint National Committee on Detection, Evaluation, and Treatment of High Blood Pressure gives the following definitions of adult **hypertension,** or abnormally elevated BP:[31]

Range, mm Hg	Category
Diastolic:	
<85	Normal BP
85–89	High normal BP
90–104	Mild hypertension
105–114	Moderate hypertension
>115	Severe hypertension
Systolic, when diastolic BP is <90:	
<140	Normal BP
140–159	Borderline isolated systolic hypertension
>160	Isolated systolic hypertension

The Committee further defines hypertension as a *persistent* elevation of BP; that is, *a clinician cannot diagnose hypertension on the basis of one isolated high BP value.* However, one abnormal reading does indicate the need for secondary screening and follow-up.

Hypertension may be classified as primary or secondary. Most adults (about 90 per cent) with sustained high BP have essential or primary hypertension (i.e., of no known cause). Less frequently, secondary hypertension occurs as a result of conditions such as kidney disease, pheochromocytoma (tumor of the adrenal medulla), and coarctation (congenital narrowing) of the aorta. Also classified as hypertension are conditions of increased systolic but normal diastolic pressure. This phenomenon may accompany anemia, hyperthyroidism, aortic insufficiency, and atherosclerosis.

Elevated BP can signal increased intracranial pressure in the person who has had neurosurgery or brain trauma. An expanding hematoma in the brain increases the intracranial pressure and decreases blood flow. The vasomotor center in the medulla responds to the decreased O_2 and causes vasoconstriction throughout the body in an attempt to increase perfusion. The pulse rate decreases, and the respirations are Cheyne-Stokes or absent. Unfortunately, these vital signs are late consequences of increased intracranial pressure. Earlier warning signs are clouding of consciousness, hemiparesis, positive Babinski's sign, and pupil inequality (one suddenly dilated, nonreactive pupil).

You may notice other alterations in BP in your practice. A surprisingly high BP reading in the arms of the young adult or teenager may suggest coarctation of the aorta. Pressure increases as the heart works harder to pump blood through the narrowed opening. Right arm pressure always increases with coarctation. Elevation of the left arm pressure depends on the location of the stricture. In the legs, BP is much lower than normal because the blood supply to the legs is below the constriction in the aorta.

Another noteworthy alteration is **paradoxical pulse,** in which pulsations detected during blood pressure measurement decrease in volume during inspiration and increase during expiration. Paradoxical pulse may occur normally with very deep breathing; however, if it is marked (e.g., a decrease in systolic pressure more than 8 to 10 mm Hg during inspiration), it may signify *cardiac tamponade.* This is a rupture of the heart or a coronary vessel that causes blood to collect in the heart's outer lining (pericardium), thus compressing the heart. *Immediate* treatment is necessary.

NURSING RESPONSIBILITY IN COMMUNICATING FINDINGS

Analysis of data gathered during the taking of routine vital signs enables you to make nursing diagnoses and plan interventions. Integrate the data into the individual's overall clinical picture. Record the numerical data in the appropriate place on the individual's graphic sheet (Fig. 31–16). Chart other data in the progress notes. All notes concerning data must be complete and should give a total picture of the person's current status. For example, if you are caring for a person who has just had surgery, you should chart the pulse rate and characteristics (e.g., rapid, thready) as well as BP readings, skin temperature and moistness, skin color, level of consciousness, and any sign of blood loss. Similarly, charting of respiratory status should include the following: rate, pattern of respirations, comfort or pain level, and mental status.

If the data indicate a significant change, communicate the results and your interventions to the appropriate people. To make the message meaningful, you must describe all vital signs, how they have changed from previous values, how they fit into the entire clinical picture, and any interventions you have planned or have already made. Aberrant vital signs lead to a variety of nursing interventions, performed both in partnership with others on the health care team and independently. Detailed knowledge of vital signs gives you a broad base for planning care.

SPECIAL PROCEDURES USING ELECTRONIC MONITORING

Because of advances in technology, we are now able to monitor the vital signs of critically ill people continuously and accurately (Fig. 31–17).

The Cardiac Monitor

Electronic equipment may be necessary to monitor a very irregular or a very weak pulse. A person at risk of cardiac **arrhythmia** (irregular heart rhythm) requires a continuous electrocardiogram (ECG) monitor. Electrodes pasted on the chest sense the electrical impulses of the heart and transmit this pattern to a viewing screen or oscilloscope. Nurses skilled in determining arrhythmia patterns watch the person and the cardiac monitor for signs and symptoms of irregular heart beats. Persons having a myocardial infarction are particularly prone to arrhythmias that could be fatal if not detected and treated immediately.

The Doppler

In some situations, a clinician must use the Doppler ultrasonic flowmeter (Fig. 31–18) to obtain pulse and BP readings. The Doppler works by magnifying sounds produced by the heart and the blood vessels. To use the Doppler, place a drop of coupling gel (which increases sound transmission) on the end of the hand-held transducer. Then, place the transducer on the skin over an arterial pulse. Hold the probe on the skin, tilted at a 45-degree angle to the artery being monitored. Turn the device on. Locate the arterial pulsation site by listening for a pulsatile "whoosh" sound. The sound from a Doppler has a swishing, whooshing quality, rather than the tapping heard through a stethoscope. Rotate the probe, if necessary, but keep contact with the skin. Pushing too hard obliterates the pulse.

For a BP reading, inflate the cuff as you auscultate the artery. Continue inflation for another 20 to 30 mm Hg after the sound disappears. Deflate the cuff and record the first sound heard as the systolic pressure. On some newer Doppler models, the operator can sometimes hear a muffling sound that is documented as the diastolic pressure. On older Dopplers, however, the sounds never change or muffle, so it is impossible to identify the diastolic pressure.

The Doppler has many advantages: it is portable, reliable, technically easy to master, and noninvasive (i.e., there is no trauma to the vessel wall as there would be if a measuring catheter were placed directly into the artery).

You can use the Doppler to detect a weak peripheral pulse and to measure very low BP. It is also useful to monitor BP in infants or children and to obtain a lower limb BP. Some clinicians also use a Doppler to monitor BP in an obese person in whom the layers of fat muffle Korotkoff sounds. Also, an obese upper arm is conical, which makes it difficult to apply the arm cuff smoothly. To obtain a BP reading in an obese person, hold the Doppler probe over the radial artery and place the cuff below the elbow. The pressure reading with the cuff placement below the elbow equals that obtained when the cuff is in the normal position above the elbow, provided there are no abnormalities (such as occlusion) of the artery.

The Pulse Oximeter

Heralded as the "fifth vital sign,"[43] the pulse **oximeter** is a photoelectric device that measures oxygen satura-

GRAPHIC CHART

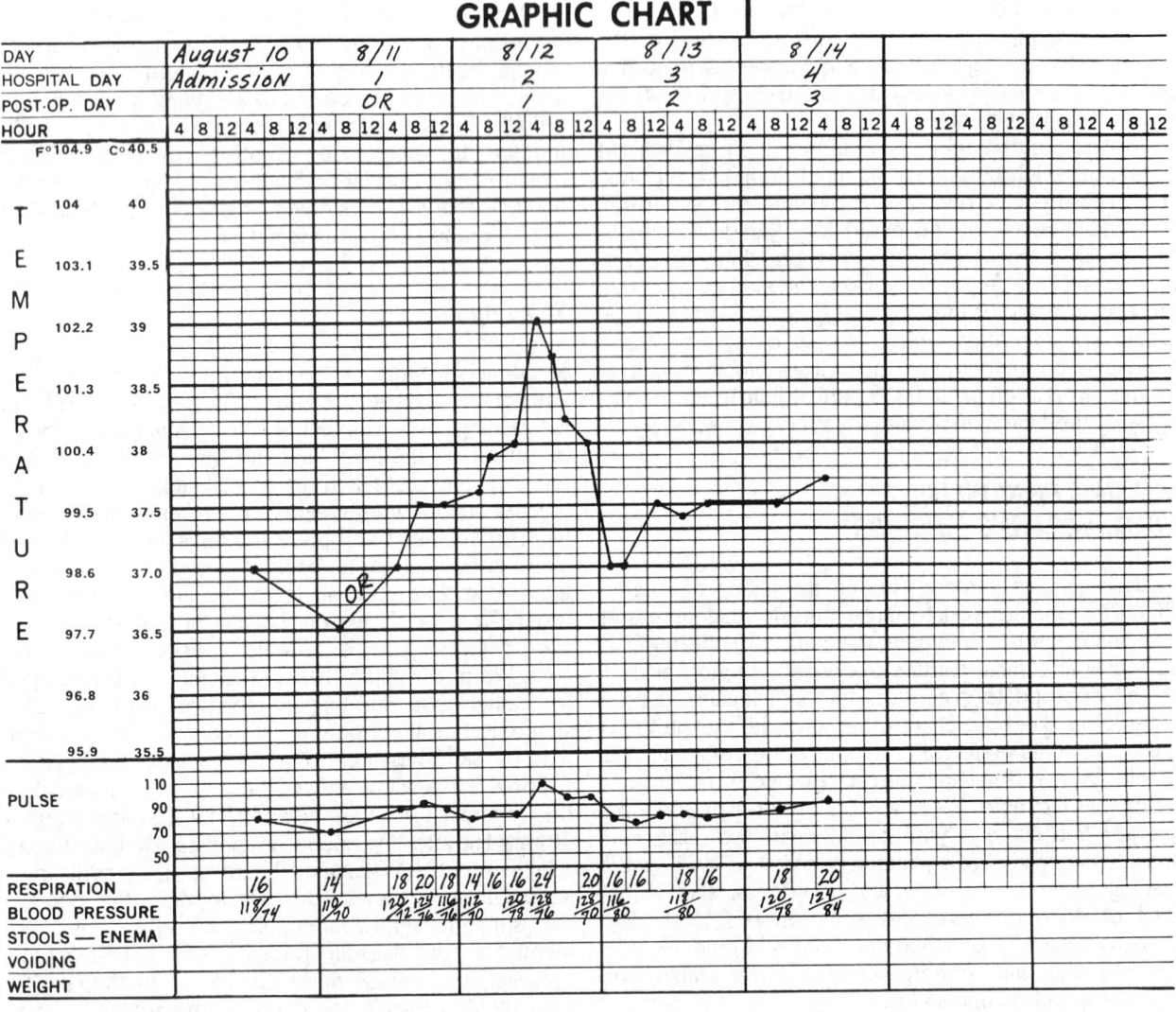

DAY	August 10	8/11	8/12	8/13	8/14			
HOSPITAL DAY	Admission	1	2	3	4			
POST-OP. DAY		OR	1	2	3			

▲ Figure 31–16

Sample of a vital sign graphic sheet. Note vital signs when this person has a fever on the first postoperative day. Also note increased frequency of measurement as the nurse suspects a developing trend.

tion of the arterial blood at peripheral sites. The oximeter recognizes lowered oxygen transport (e.g., as in shock or respiratory depression) before BP, pulse, or respiration measurements would respond.

The technique is noninvasive, easy, and rapid. A probe is attached to a finger, toe, earlobe, or the bridge of the nose. The probe contains sensors that measure the amount of oxygenated hemoglobin and reduced hemoglobin of arterial blood. An electronic "black box" interprets the ratio of these readings, determines the per cent saturation, and displays this on a visual screen.

A normal oxygen saturation is 97 to 99 per cent, indicating an intact cardiovascular and respiratory system. Values less than 94 per cent saturation suggest respiratory compromise. Values below 91 per cent saturation indicate that the person needs aggressive oxygen therapy, assisted ventilation, and possible intubation.

The Arterial Line

Direct monitoring of BP by a catheter placed within an artery is indicated in critically ill people. For example, it is appropriate after open-heart or other major surgery when moment-to-moment changes are anticipated, or in low-pressure states such as congestive heart failure and shock when cardiac output is severely decreased and peripheral vascular resistance is increased. The increased resistance impedes the already low blood flow into the arms, thus diminishing Korotkoff sounds. In these conditions, the only accurate method of BP determination is by the direct route, called an arterial line.

For this procedure, a plastic catheter is inserted into the radial artery and anchored. It is filled with heparinized fluid to prevent clotting and attached by tubing to an electronic pressure sensor or transducer. The transducer transforms mechanical energy from the pulsating

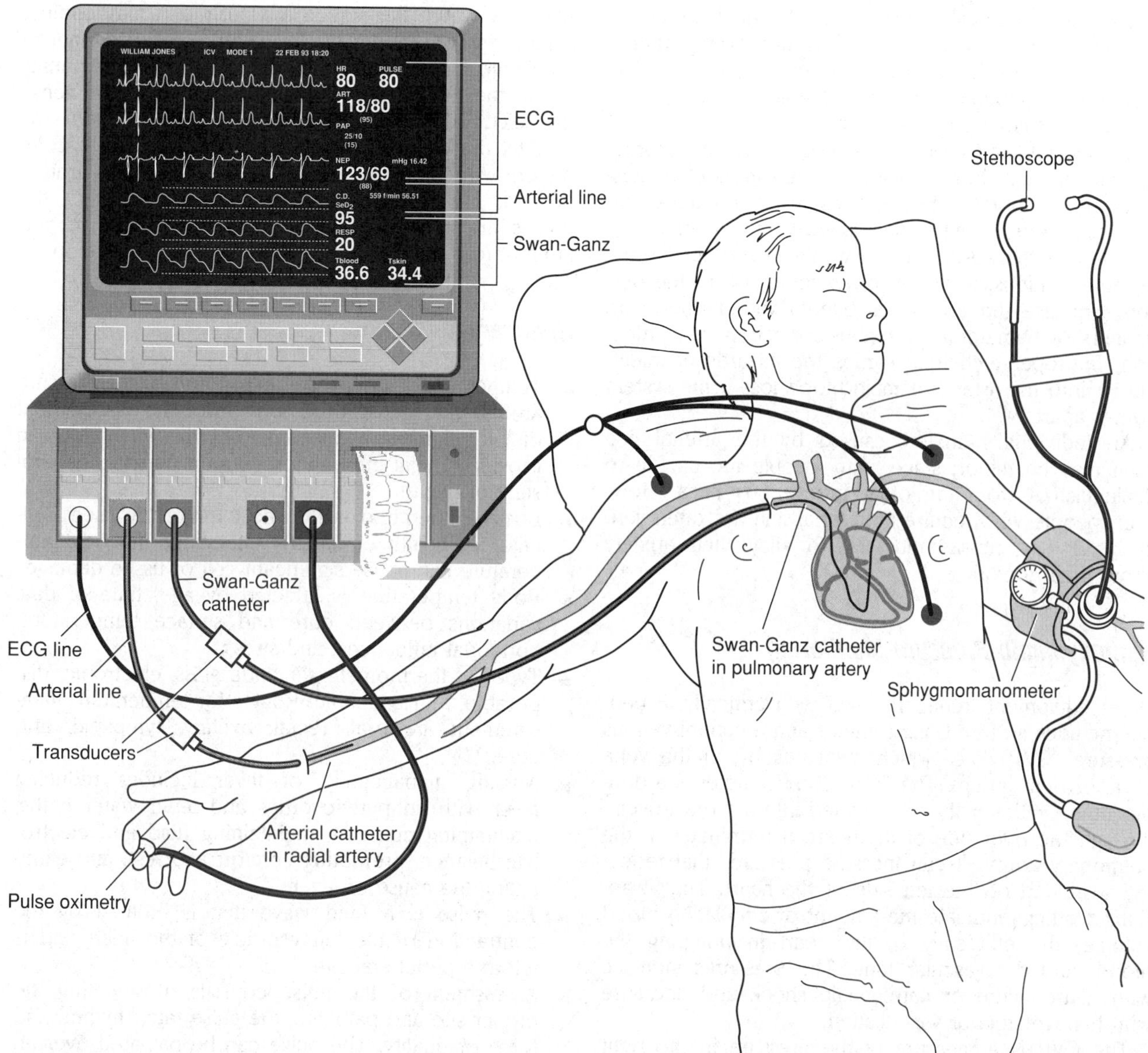

WILLIAM JONES   ICV   MODE 1   22 FEB 93 18:20

| HR | PULSE |
| 80 | 80 |

ART
118/80
(95)

PAP
25/10
(15)

NEP   mHg 16.42
123/69
(88)

C.D.   559 l/min 56.51
SeO₂
95

RESP
20

Tblood   Tskin
36.6   34.4

ECG

Arterial line

Swan-Ganz

Stethoscope

Swan-Ganz catheter

ECG line

Arterial line

Transducers

Swan-Ganz catheter
in pulmonary artery

Sphygmomanometer

Arterial catheter
in radial artery

Pulse oximetry

▲ **Figure 31–17**

Electronic monitoring of a critically ill person.

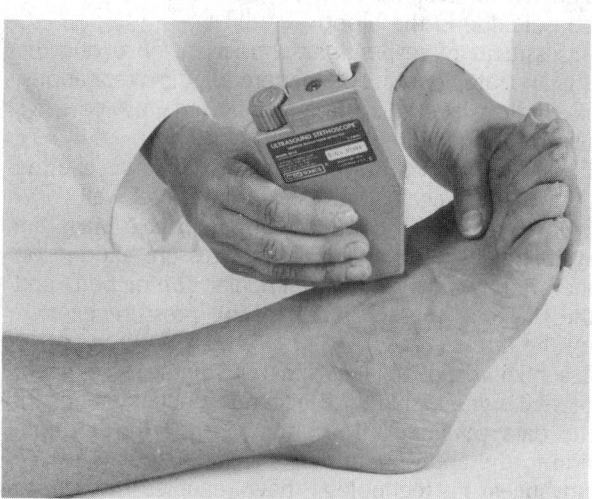

▲ **Figure 31–18**

Using the Doppler ultrasonic flowmeter. (From Jarvis, C. [1992]. *Physical examination and health assessment*. Philadelphia: W.B. Saunders.)

blood into electrical energy. The electrical pattern is transmitted as a waveform and is displayed continuously on a bedside oscilloscope (see Fig. 31–17). The electronic equipment also may display numerical systolic and diastolic pressure values.

Values obtained by intraarterial direct BP monitoring are higher than those obtained by the indirect or auscultatory method.[45] The readings are continuous and are accurate when equipment is working properly.

Although the arterial line may aid in prompt lifesaving interventions, it also involves some risk to the person. Because the artery has been invaded, there are dangers of hematoma, thrombus formation, and infection. Improper technique carries the hazards of injecting air into the artery, or rapid blood loss if the system comes apart.

An individual's anxiety caused by the arterial line itself may be minor, since many people are unable to distinguish it from the other intravenous lines. However, people who require an arterial line are often seriously ill, and nurses must try to allay their anxiety about their condition.

Hemodynamic Pressure Monitoring

Other equipment frequently used with critically ill people includes a Swan-Ganz catheter and a central venous pressure (CVP) line, which measures BP in the vena cava, or right atrium. The Swan-Ganz catheter is a double-lumen catheter that is threaded into a thoracic vein, through the right side of the heart; it terminates in the pulmonary artery. It can measure pressures that reflect the workload on the left side of the heart. The Swan-Ganz readings indicate the amount of circulating blood volume, the efficiency of the heart in pumping the blood, and the vascular tone. The pressures increase with heart failure or cardiogenic shock and decrease with hypovolemia or vasodilation.

The CVP is a measure of the pressure in the right atrium of the heart, either through a special port in the Swan-Ganz catheter, or by a CVP catheter alone, which is threaded through a vein into the superior or inferior vena cava. The CVP reflects workload on the right side of the heart. It increases with vigorous intravenous fluid infusion, with right-sided heart failure, and with peripheral vasoconstriction; it drops with hemorrhage or vasodilation.

Care of the Person Being Monitored

Although electronic monitoring is usually painless, it communicates nonverbally to individuals that they must be very sick to require such intricate machinery. In addition, this equipment is often used only in an intensive care unit, a setting that already increases anxiety. Psychologic support is paramount. Give reassurance that electronic monitoring is a preventive measure that aids the health care team in treating a possible problem before it becomes serious. Offer teaching, when appropriate. The individual on a cardiac monitor, for exam-

ple, may watch the screen anxiously and may confuse a harmless wandering of the pattern (called artifact or mechanical interference) with a serious arrhythmia. Teach the person and significant others that the sensitive electrodes pick up electrical impulses from the skeletal muscles as well as from the heart, so that the pattern will change whenever the person moves around in bed. Help significant others understand that the nurses are skilled in interpreting these patterns, and attempt to intervene *before* major problems develop.

Summary

▶ Temperature, pulse, respirations, and blood pressure are the vital signs of the body. "Routine" assessment of vital signs is a misnomer, as this vital task can provide crucial information about a person's general state of health.

▶ Body temperature is the most frequently used indicator of health or illness. Alterations in body temperature can cause significant cell or tissue damage.

▶ Body temperature is affected by age, time of day, variations between core and surface temperature, hormonal influences, and stress.

▶ Types of thermometers include glass, electronic, disposable, and tympanic. Routes for temperature measurement are oral, rectal, axillary, tympanic, and core.

▶ Nursing management of fever includes reducing fever with antipyretic drugs and tepid water baths, maintaining nutrition, maintaining fluid and electrolyte balance, promoting comfort and rest, and eliminating the cause of fever.

▶ The pulse is a fluid wave that is created by the contraction of the left ventricle of the heart and is felt at a peripheral site.

▶ Assessment of the pulse consists of selecting the proper site and palpating the pulse rate, rhythm, and force or quality. The pulse can be palpated over an artery that lies close to the skin and is backed by firm structures.

▶ Respirations are controlled by the respiratory center located in the brainstem (pons and medulla). The stimulus for respiration is an increased level of carbon dioxide in the blood.

▶ Assessment of respirations consists of observing the quality, rate, depth and pattern of the respirations. Respiratory status is often manifested in a person's physical appearance.

▶ Blood pressure is the measure of the force exerted by the blood against an area of the vessel wall.

▶ Blood pressure is measured in order to obtain the systolic pressure (the maximum pressure exerted on the arterial walls during ventricular contraction) and the diastolic pressure (the resting pressure exerted on the arterial walls).

▶ Essential responsibilities inherent in the assessment of vital signs include the accurate documentation of the data obtained and communicating the information to the appropriate persons.

▶ Advances in technology have enabled nurses to

monitor the vital signs of critically ill persons accurately and continuously.

Bibliography

1. Argondizzo, N.T. (1979). Patient assessment: pulses. *American Journal of Nursing*, 79(1), 115–132.
2. Baker, N.C., et al. (1984). The effect of type of thermometer and length of time inserted in oral temperature measurements of afebrile patients. *Nursing Research*, 33(2), 109–111.
3. Barber, N., & Kilmon, C. (1989). Reactions to tympanic temperature measurement in an ambulatory setting. *Pediatric Nursing*, 15(5), 477–481.
4. Bliss-Holtz, J. (1989). Comparison of rectal, axillary, and inguinal temperatures in full-term newborn infants. *Nursing Research*, 38(2), 85–87.
5. Burch, G.G., & DePasquale, N.P. (1962). *Primer of clinical measurement of blood pressure*. St. Louis, C.V. Mosby.
6. Chamberlain, J.M., et al. (1991). Comparison of a tympanic thermometer to rectal and oral thermometers in a pediatric emergency department. *Clinical Pediatrics*, 30(4), 24–29.
7. Clochesy, J.M. (1986). Systemic blood pressure in various lateral recumbent positions: a pilot study. *Heart and Lung*, 15(6):593–594.
8. Creative Care Unit (1977). Turnabout: rectal temperatures for postcoronary patients. *American Journal of Nursing*, 77(6), 997.
9. Doyle, M.P., & Jordan, L.E. (1968). A comparison of pulse deficit reading by serial and simultaneous measurement. *Nursing Research*, 17(5), 460–461.
10. Eoff, M.J., & Joyce, B. (1981). Temperature measurements in children. *American Journal of Nursing*, 81(5), 1010–1011.
11. Fagan, M.J. Relationship between nurses' assessments of perfusion and toe temperature in pediatric patients with cardiovascular disease. *Heart and Lung*, 17(2):157–165.
12. Fitzgerald, F.T. (1992). Hyperthermia and hypothermia. In Kelley, W.N. (ed.). *Textbook of internal medicine* (2nd ed.). Philadelphia: J.B. Lippincott.
13. Foley, M.F. (1971). Variations in blood pressure in the lateral recumbent position. *Nursing Research*, 20(1), 64.
14. Frohlich, E.D., et al. (1988). Recommendations for human blood pressure determination by sphygmomanometers. Report of a Special Task Force appointed by the Steering Committee, American Heart Association. *Circulation*, 77, 501A–514A.
15. Ganong, W.F. (1989). *Review of medical physiology* (14th ed.). Norwalk, CT: Appleton and Lange.
16. Goldstein, I.B., & Shapiro, D. (1990). The beat-to-beat blood pressure response to postural change in young and elderly healthy adult males. *Journal of Behavioral Medicine*, 13(5), 437–448.
17. Graves, R.D., & Markarian, M.F. (1980). Three-minute time interval when using an oral mercury-in-glass thermometer with or without J-temp sheaths. *Nursing Research*, 29(5), 323–324.
18. Griffin, J. (1986). Fever: when to leave it alone. *Nursing 86*, 16(2), 58–61.
19. Grossman, D.G.S. (1991). Circadian rhythms in blood pressure in school-age children of normotensive and hypertensive parents. *Nursing Research*, 40(1), 28–34.
20. Guiffre, M., et al. (1990). The relationship between axillary and core body temperature measurements. *Applied Nursing Research*, 3(2), 52–55.
21. Guyton, A.C. (1990). *Textbook of medical physiology* (8th ed.). Philadelphia: W.B. Saunders.
22. Hahn, W.K., et al. (1989). Blood pressure norms for healthy young adults: relation to sex, age, and reported parental hypertension. *Research in Nursing and Health*, 12:53–56.
23. Hargest, T.S. (1974). Start your count with zero. *American Journal of Nursing*, 74(5), 887–888.
24. Hasler, M.E., & Cohen, J.A. (1982). The effect of oxygen administration on oral temperature assessment. *Nursing Research*, 31(5), 265–268.
25. Henneman, E.A., & Henneman, P.L. (1989). Intricacies of blood pressure measurement: reexamining the rituals. *Heart and Lung*, 18(3), 263–271.
26. Hill, M.N., & Cunningham, S.L. (1989). The latest words for high BP. *American Journal of Nursing*, 89(4), 504–508.
27. Hill, M.N., & Grim, C.M. (1991). How to take a precise blood pressure. *American Journal of Nursing*, 91(2), 38–42.
28. Hollerbach, A.D., & Sneed, N.V. (1990). Accuracy of radial pulse assessment by length of counting interval. *Heart and Lung*, 19(3), 258–264.
29. Hunt, J.C., et al. (1985). Devices used for self-measurement of blood pressure. *Archives of Internal Medicine*, 145, 2231–2234.
30. Jacobs, R.A. (1992). General problems in infectious diseases. In Schroeder S.A., et al. (eds.). *Current medical diagnosis and treatment — 1992*. Norwalk, CT: Appleton and Lange.
31. Joint National Committee on Detection, Evaluation, and Treatment of High Blood Pressure. (1988). 1988 report. *Archives of Internal Medicine*, 148(5), 1023–1038.
32. Jones, M.L. (1970). Accuracy of pulse rates counted for 15, 30 and 60 seconds. *Military Medicine*, 135, 1127–1136.
33. LaDou, J., & Cohen, R. (1992). Disorders due to physical agents. In Schroeder, S.A., et al. (eds.). *Current medical diagnosis and treatment — 1992*. Norwalk, CT: Appleton and Lange.
34. Lohman, M. (1988). Fever: different types, different causes. *Nursing 88*, 18(4), 98–101.
35. McCance, K.L., & Huether, S.E. (1990). *Pathophysiology: The biologic basis for disease in adults and children*. St. Louis: C.V. Mosby.
36. Mallison, G.F. (1980). Decontamination, disinfection, and sterilization. *Nursing Clinics of North America*, 15(4), 757–767.
37. Mauro, A.M.P. (1988). Effects of bell versus diaphragm on indirect blood pressure measurement. *Heart and Lung*, 17(5), 489–494.
38. Newton, K.M. (1981). Comparison of aortic and brachial cuff pressures in flat supine and lateral recumbent positions. *Heart and Lung*, 10(5), 821–826.
39. Nichols, G.A. (1972). Time analysis of afebrile and febrile temperature readings. *Nursing Research*, 21(5), 463–464.
40. Nichols, G.A., et al. (1966). Oral, axillary and rectal temperature determination and relationships. *Nursing Research*, 15(4) 307–310.
41. Petersdorf, R.G. (1991). Hypothermia and hyperthermia. In Wilson, J.D., et al. (eds.). *Harrison's principles of internal medicine* (12th ed., Vol. 2). New York: McGraw-Hill.
42. Phoenix, J. (1990). Low blood pressure — how to investigate this ominous sign. *Nursing 90*, 20(11), 34–40.
43. Porter, R.S., et al. (1990). The fifth vital sign. *Emergency* 22(3), 37–41.
44. Pransky, S.M. (1991). The impact of technique and conditions of the tympanic membrane upon infrared tympanic thermometry. *Clinical Pediatrics*, 30(4), 50–52.
45. Rebenson-Piano, M., et al. (1989). An evaluation of two indirect methods of blood pressure measurement in ill patients. *Nursing Research*, 38(1), 42–45.
46. Rebenson-Piano, M., et al. (1987). An examination of the differences that occur between direct and indirect blood pressure measurement. *Heart and Lung*, 16(3), 285–294.
47. Samples, J.F., et al. (1985). Circadian rhythms: basis for screening for fever. *Nursing Research*, 34(6), 377–379.
48. Sheehan, M.M. (1990). Completing the picture — ambulatory blood pressure monitor. *Nursing 90*, 20(4), 79, 81.
49. Shinozaki, T., et al. (1988). Infrared tympanic thermometer. Evaluation of a new clinical thermometer. *Critical Care Medicine*, 16(2), 148–150.
50. Styrt, B., & Sugarman, B. (1990). Antipyresis and fever. *Archives of Internal Medicine*, 150(8), 1589–1597.
51. Zikria, B.A., et al. (1974). Alterations in ventilatory function and breathing patterns following surgical trauma. *Annals of Surgery*, 179, 1.

▼ *Psychosocial Assessment*

 Make no judgments where you have no compassion.
Anne McCaffrey

▼ CHAPTER OUTLINE

PURPOSE OF PSYCHOSOCIAL HEALTH
   ASSESSMENT
OBTAINING A PSYCHOSOCIAL HEALTH
   ASSESSMENT
     The Interview Process
     Data-Collecting Skills
     Components of Psychosocial Health
       Assessment

DATA ANALYSIS
   Physiologic Dimension
   Psychologic Dimension
   Social and Cultural Dimension
   Spiritual Dimension

▼ KEY TERMS

Abstract thinking	Delusions	Lability
Affect	Dysphoria	Mood
Blocking	Euphoria	Preoccupation
Blunted affect	Expansiveness	Psychosocial dimension
Circumstantiality	Flat affect	Psychosocial health
Concrete thinking	Flight of ideas	assessment
Constricted affect	Hallucinations	Psychosocial history
Defensiveness	Illusions	Rapport

After studying this chapter, you should be able to

1. Define psychosocial health assessment.
2. Describe the purpose of psychosocial health assessment.
3. Describe the essentials of conducting a successful interview.
4. Identify the skills needed to collect data for the psychosocial health assessment.
5. List the components of psychosocial history.
6. Explain the purpose of the Mental Status Examination (MSE).
7. List the components of the MSE.
8. Identify essential observations that must be made in order to assess the client's appearance, feelings, and cognitive functioning.
9. Discuss the purpose of analyzing data from the physiologic, psychologic, social, cultural, and spiritual dimensions of the client.

Successful nursing care depends as much on the alleviation of mental and emotional suffering as it does on the relief of physical suffering. A person's unmet psychologic (mental and emotional) needs can complicate an otherwise uncomplicated illness. Psychologic, social, cultural, and spiritual factors affect not only a person's physiologic well-being but also the ability to respond to treatment and recover from an illness. The connections among body, mind, and spirit are so dynamic and so vital that nurses cannot treat these dimensions of human experience as separate entities without depersonalizing the individual and fragmenting care.

Every human being is unique, and each is special. The physical structure of the body is miraculous. The interactions among cells, tissues, organs, hormones, and other chemicals is both intricate and profound. And yet a human being is much more than this marvelous physiologic structure. Heredity, learning, personality, life experiences, ethnic identity, culture, socioeconomic status, values, and beliefs are intertwined in a complex matrix that makes each person a unique whole. Sometimes, however, the latest in knowledge of human physiology, discovered through continuous advances in biomedical science and technology, is so intriguing and so captivating that health care professionals neglect to consider the person as a whole. In fact, some give only superficial attention to the person's psychologic, social, cultural, and spiritual needs. Such clinicians fail to understand that relating to another person through science and disease theory alone is impossible and inadequate.

Health care professionals claim to view every human being as whole and unique. Often, however, some do not take the time necessary to obtain a history of psychologic stressors, social and cultural background, and spiritual beliefs. As a nurse, you spend more time in direct contact with clients than does any other member of the health care team. Thus you have an excellent opportunity to assess and evaluate human responses related not only to physical needs but also to needs in other areas.

This chapter will assist you in developing psychologic, social, cultural, and spiritual assessment skills as part of a comprehensive psychosocial health assessment. To do so, the chapter builds on principles discussed earlier in the text. Although the components of a psychosocial assessment are not easily separated, you can learn to analyze them and enhance your capacity to comfort and care, which is the essence of nursing. Always remember that your most potent healing ability comes from who you are and how you relate to others.

PURPOSE OF PSYCHOSOCIAL HEALTH ASSESSMENT

The **psychosocial dimension** of a person broadly describes the psychologic (mental and emotional), social, cultural/ethnic, and spiritual components of life. These aspects or dimensions of a person combine with the physical to make up each human being. Although you will separate each of these areas for the purpose of assessing and learning, none of these elements acts independently. Instead, they interact to comprise a delicate balance. When one area is affected, this balance shifts. With systematic collection of data to determine a client's current health status,[4] the nurse conducts a **psychosocial health assessment.** With this process, you deliberately and systematically collect data to determine a client's current status in all human dimensions.

To accurately understand the concept of *psychosocial assessment,* it is helpful to view each person as a system. This analysis, a General Systems Theory (GST) approach, provides a theoretical framework for the study of organized wholes, their component parts, and the interaction of the parts with one another. This concept is discussed in detail in Chapter 15. If you view an individual as a system, you can look at the organs and physiologic processes as components, or subsystems, of the person. The family, which is greater than the individual, is part of the suprasystem.

An individual may also be seen as being made up of subsystems including physiologic, psychologic, social, cultural, and spiritual dimensions. A basic tenet of GST is that one event cannot be understood independently of the system of which it is a part. Any alteration to one component of a system affects the functioning of the entire system. Thus, whatever affects one dimension of an individual also affects the others.

A psychosocial health assessment begins with an interview process that addresses all of the dimensions of an individual. It differs from the traditional medical-surgical history in which you collect only concrete, factual information relevant to the development of symptoms and past medical-surgical conditions. In a psychosocial assessment you also strive to form a picture of the person's unique personality characteristics, including strengths and weaknesses. This picture is subjective and therefore less tangible than assessment of purely physiologic data. A **psychosocial history** is the person's own story told in the person's own words from a personal point of view. The person being interviewed is considered the primary source of data. Valuable information and insight can also be obtained from secondary data sources such as family, friends, previous records, laboratory findings, and other diagnostic tests.

The purpose of the psychosocial health assessment is to establish a data base from which you can identify specific human responses and problems, make a nursing diagnosis, and develop an appropriate nursing care plan. Much of the completeness and accuracy of the information collected depends on your ability to communicate effectively.

OBTAINING A PSYCHOSOCIAL HEALTH ASSESSMENT

The Interview Process

Because good communication skills are crucial to conducting a psychosocial history, the communication techniques discussed in Chapter 25 are important in psychosocial assessment. As in all nurse-client communications, rapport is essential. **Rapport** implies that there is a sense of understanding and trust between you and your client and that both of you have a vested interest in the client's well-being. This rapport helps the client feel more comfortable in revealing personal facts. Your ability to establish good rapport affects the quality of the psychosocial health assessment and the information that you will get throughout the interview.

In preparing for a psychosocial interview, you must consider not only the person being interviewed but also yourself and the setting in which the interview will take place. Your initial contact with a person is extremely important because it sets the tone for the development of a therapeutic relationship in all subsequent interactions. One of the goals of the psychosocial health assessment is to elicit the person's feelings, thoughts, and values in order to identify individual needs. Meeting this goal depends on your approach.

The way in which you approach a client has a direct bearing on how that person will respond to you. You give messages verbally through what you say and nonverbally through your actions and behavior. You should be aware that your appearance, the way you ask questions, and nonverbal forms of communication all contribute to the way in which another person views you. Tone of voice; choice of words; facial expression; body language, such as degree of eye contact, crossed arms, a hurried manner; and whether you stand or sit all give direct messages.

The primary goal when initiating an interview is to establish trust. Your ability to be genuine, honest, and open fosters trust. Warm human interest enhances the interview process. Without this element the interview can become a monotonous, mechanical task of little value. For many clients, talking with another person who listens with nonjudgmental understanding rather than criticizing and admonishing is a unique experience. When you focus interest and concern entirely on the client without imposing advice or control, the psychosocial health assessment can be a very positive experience.

The ideal setting for the psychosocial interview is a private office free of interruptions. This, however, is not always feasible. The interview may be conducted in a home, in a clinic examination room, at the hospital bedside, in a vehicle, or in a variety of other settings. No matter where the interview takes place, the process should have a basic structure and a quality of formality and professionalism.

You should make an effort to provide as much privacy as possible. For example, if an individual is interviewed at the bedside in a multiple-patient room, you should draw the curtains. Affording some measure of privacy indicates respect for the person being interviewed. Even this small amount of privacy may influence the person's response to your questions.

Begin the interview by introducing yourself and identifying your position. In some cases it is helpful to obtain permission for the interview from the person being interviewed. If the person is reluctant to give a history, help the person explain the reason for this reluctance. Let the person know that one of your responsibilities as a nurse is to understand how an individual feels about and reacts to illness.

You may want to assure the person that the information collected during a psychosocial health assessment is confidential within the health care team and will be used to provide more thorough and individualized care. You should explain that a client does not have to talk about anything that the person does not want to discuss. This helps decrease anxiety and gives the person a greater sense of control. If possible, it is best to sit during the interview to communicate that you are interested and have time to listen.

The person you are interviewing may reveal many aspects about lifestyle, behaviors, and attitudes during this interview process. The person also may disclose details of life that you find distressing or objectionable.

It is imperative that you maintain a nonjudgmental attitude. The purpose of the psychosocial health assessment is to obtain a data base for making judgments about health, not judgments about the lifestyles, behaviors, or attitudes of another person.

If family or significant others are present, you may ask them to step outside or wait elsewhere. If the client clearly prefers them to stay, however, respect the person's wish. Family and friends can be excellent sources of information. When others are present during the interview, you should also allow time for the client to speak with you in private. A private conference will give clients an opportunity to discuss things that they may not have wanted to talk about in front of others. In talking with persons receiving health care, it is important to speak at a level that they can understand. Therefore, it may be more appropriate to use lay terms and familiar language rather than medical jargon. Complex medical terminology and jargon can be frightening and block effective communication. Throughout the interview, you should listen for conflicting or missing information. Sometimes, you may need to rephrase a question to help the person gain a better understanding of the information you are seeking.

At the conclusion of the interview, it is always helpful if you briefly summarize or restate any major concerns. It is important to give the client a chance to ask questions, add information, and give other feedback. To make sure that the person agrees with your conclusion or understanding of the situation, it is also important for you to verify what you think you heard. At the end of the interview, you should thank the person for the time and cooperation provided. You may shake hands with the person if this step is appropriate.

Initially, you may find that conducting a psychosocial health assessment makes you uncomfortable. It takes time to develop good interviewing skills. With practice, you will become familiar with the interview process and begin to develop your own style.

Data-Collecting Skills

Three skills that will help you complete the interview in a psychosocial assessment are observing, listening, and questioning. Your own observations are important. You will learn to make deliberate, planned observations that require sensitivity to others and a capacity to see subtle changes.

When listening to what a client is saying, ask yourself if it makes sense. Can the client understand your questions? Can you understand the answers? Listen first to what the person is saying and how it is being said. Notice also what the client does not say. Are there gaps in the story?

Questioning allows you to assess specific information. For example, the questions on the Mental Status Examination (MSE) (discussed in next section) test particular areas of cognitive functioning. Questioning is an art. Sometimes it is appropriate to ask very precise questions, such as "Have you had any thoughts about harming yourself?" "Have you thought of how you might do it?" "Are you having those thoughts now?" At other times, it is better to ask open-ended questions because they allow the client to give more information than just a "yes" or "no." Examples of such questions are, "How would you describe yourself?" "Tell me

about your situation at home." "How did your illness begin?"

The following format is suggested as a guide for obtaining the data you will need to make a psychosocial health assessment. This format contains both the psychosocial history and the MSE. Remember that during the history you will be asking questions and then listening to *what* is said and *how* it is said. As part of the MSE, you will be making observations about the client's appearance, behavior, and communication, in addition to assessing the level of cognitive functioning.

Components of Psychosocial Health Assessment

The two components of the psychosocial health assessment are the history and the Mental Status Examination (MSE). Both components focus specifically on the psychologic, social, cultural, and spiritual dimensions of a person, with the physical dimension included only as a brief summary of the problems that were identified during the physical assessment. The psychosocial assessment allows you to collect data from each dimension of the client's experience and combine it with the physical dimension to form a holistic view of the person.

PSYCHOSOCIAL HISTORY

The psychosocial history consists of information given by the individual and provided by the family. The components of the psychosocial history are

1. Demographic/identifying data
2. Presenting problem
3. History of the presenting problem
4. Medical/surgical history
5. History of psychologic health problems
6. Family, social, cultural history
7. Spiritual beliefs
8. Military history
9. Educational and vocational history
10. Legal history
11. Characteristic coping mechanisms, values, beliefs, goals
12. Self-esteem/self-image
13. Current life status

A format for collecting and documenting information for a psychosocial history appears in Figure 32–1.

MENTAL STATUS EXAMINATION

The Mental Status Exam (MSE) consists of your systematic observations of clients' behaviors and responses as they interact with you throughout the entire psychosocial assessment but particularly during an examination of their cognitive function. Properly conducted, the MSE provides a detailed description of a person's cognitive functioning at a given time. The MSE helps you assess the client's ability to understand what is happening and how well the client can cooperate with the treatment plan.

1. Demographic/Identifying Data

Name _____

Age _____

Sex _____

Race _____

Marital Status   Married _____   Divorced _____   Widowed _____

　　　　　　　　Never Married _____   Separated _____

Occupation _____

Admitting diagnosis _____

Date of admission _____

Referral source _____

2. Presenting Problem

Informant; Client _____   Other _____

Problem as stated in the informant's own words. What caused you to
　　　come to the hospital, clinic, etc.?

_____

_____

Symptoms _____

Onset of symptoms _____

Duration of symptoms _____

3. History of the Presenting Problem

Previous experience with similar symptoms

_____

Previous treatment for this problem

_____

4. Medical/Surgical History

Past and present health history (summary)

_____

_____

Allergies _____

Medications being taken _____

_____

Family history of health problems (heart disease, diabetes, etc.)

_____

Use of alcohol, drugs, tobacco, caffeine

_____

_____

Most of this information will be covered in the physical assessment. It can be obtained from such sources as chart documentation and laboratory values. At this point, only a brief summary is needed. It is often very enlightening to hear the client's own version of what is happening.

▲ *Figure 32–1*

A format for documenting a psychosocial history.

Illustration continued on following page

5. History of Psychological (Emotional or Mental) Problems

Presence of emotional/psychiatric problems

Past _____   Present _____

Psychiatric diagnosis if any _____

_____

Past psychiatric admissions

Where	When (dates)

Psychiatric medications being taken _____

_____

Side effects, if any _____

Family history of mental illness. Did anyone in your family ever suffer from emotional or mental problems? If yes, whom?

_____

Suicidal or homicidal ideation - Have you ever had thoughts about hurting yourself or someone else?

_____

If yes, ask for more detail. The client may need a consult with a psychiatrist or the psychiatric nurse clinical specialist. Discuss the case with your instructor and with the nurse who has responsibility for the client.

6. Family, Social, Cultural History

Developmental history: Note any abnormalities

_____

Family background

Where reared _____

By whom? Both parents _____ One parent _____ Other _____

Ethnicity _____

Siblings _____

Birth order of client _____

Marriages _____

Children   Number _____ Sex _____ Ages _____

Level of education (client) _____

Group affiliations _____

Changes in family during the last two years

Births _____

Deaths _____

Illnesses _____

Other _____

With whom do you live now? _____

Client's role in the family _____

_____

Sexual functioning and identity _____

Information on sexual history is covered in the physical assessment. It is appropriate in this section to note how the person expresses sexuality, and if the person is comfortable in his or her sexual role (male or female). You may become aware of issues involving problems in sexual functioning, gender identity, or relationships. These should be discussed with your instructor and referred to the appropriate professional. Dealing with sexual problems can be difficult and generally requires skill and training in this specific field.

▲ *Figure 32–1* Continued

7. Spiritual Beliefs

Association with an organized religion

_____

Belief in a Higher Power _____

Sources of strength and hope _____

_____

To what extent is the client involved in religious practices?

_____

How do they affect the client's daily life?

_____

Are there any special religious practices that may need special consideration during treatment?

_____

This section can be a summary of data if previously obtained. See Chapter 53 for details.

8. Military History

Has the client had any military service? If so, branch of service?

_____

_____

    Dates _____

    Highest rank _____

    Duties _____

    _____

    Combat experience _____

    _____

    Wounds or injuries _____

    _____

This category can be extremely important if a client has had extensive military service, combat experience, prisoner of war experience, and/or wounds or injuries. These experiences or other traumas can affect an individual's life for years. For example, a client with Post Traumatic Stress Disorder (PTSD) can have an exacerbation of symptoms when a stressor such as an illness or major surgery occurs. Sometimes a person with PTSD will strike out or react violently if suddenly awakened or startled. You should be aware of these possibilities when planning nursing care.

9. Educational and Vocational History

Educational background:

    Completed High School _____ GED _____ Other _____

    Higher Education _____

    Other _____

Presently employed _____ Unemployed _____

For how long? _____

Type of work _____

Other jobs held _____

Longest job held _____

Special skills _____

_____

Hobbies / leisure activities _____

_____

▲ *Figure 32–1* Continued

Illustration continued on following page

10. Legal History

History of contact with the criminal justice system

_____

_____

_____

Types of charges _____

_____

Incarceration _____

_____

Current charges pending _____

_____

Legal charges / problems as a youth _____

_____

_____

You may find it difficult to ask questions in this area. Begin by simply asking, "Have you had any contact with the criminal justice system?" If the answer is "no" you may proceed to the next section. If "yes", you need to obtain additional information.

This area can be important. If you are caring for a client who is alchohol dependent and in denial, legal charges for driving under the influence (DUI) or alchohol intoxication (AI) can alert you to the fact that there may be a drinking problem. Pending charges can be extremely stressful even when they are minor. Certain types of legal charges such as a history of assault and battery or murder can alert you to the fact that the client may be potentially dangerous. Legal problems since childhood or as a teen can indicate extremely poor coping skills.

11. Characteristic Coping Mechanisms, Values, Beliefs, Goals

Stressors during the past 2 years

_____

How do you feel about being in the hospital, being ill, etc.?

_____

How are you dealing with it? _____

_____

How has if affected your family? _____

_____

Has it caused any changes in your life? If so, what? _____

_____

What happens when you get angry? _____

_____

How do you express your anger, e.g., yelling, cursing, hitting, other?

_____

Normal sleep pattern _____

Changes in sleep pattern _____

Recent changes in appetite _____

Weight change - loss, gain _____

Over what period of time? _____

Changes in energy level _____

Changes in desire to do things _____

Changes in enjoyment of things _____

▲ *Figure 32–1* Continued

12. Self-esteem/self-image

How do you feel about yourself? _____

_____

How would you describe yourself? _____

_____

What 3 words best describe you? _____

_____

What do you see as your strengths? _____

_____

What do you see as your weaknesses? _____

_____

Describe your ideal self. _____

_____

How do you judge yourself in relation to others? _____

_____

Your ideal self? _____

13. Current Life Status

Employed   Yes _____   No _____

Financial Status _____

Residence _____

Living arrangements _____

Presence of social support systems: Family _____ Other _____

Plans for the future _____

_____

This section is a brief summary of
the client's current social status.

▲ *Figure 32–1* Continued

Many of the elements included in the MSE are gathered through your direct observations. For example, appearance, behavior, cooperation with the interviewer, affect, and speech can be assessed just by looking and listening.

The ability to think clearly and logically affects a client's capacity to understand and cooperate with treatment. The client who is capable of **abstract thinking,** for example, has the ability to reason logically and generalize from specific instances. The person who is incapable of abstract thinking engages in **concrete thinking,** or the literal interpretation of questions or instructions.

The MSE identifies deficits such as confusion or memory impairment and bizarre or unusual thinking. Individuals who are disoriented and do not recognize anyone will require close observation and special safety measures to prevent accidents such as might occur from the client climbing out of bed and falling, getting lost on the unit, or trying to leave the hospital. Those who believe others are "out to get them" or poison their food may refuse to eat or take medication. The nursing care plan will need to be designed to deal with these special problems. A person's mental status can fluctuate throughout a 24-hour period and may need to be reassessed frequently.

As you talk with the client and take the history, observe the appearance, behavior, and communication and be sensitive to client feelings. There are two ways to assess feelings, including asking about the person's mood and monitoring the person's affect. **Mood** is a pervasive, sustained emotion. Extreme moods can color a person's entire view of life. A mood cannot be observed. The client must tell the nurse the mood being experienced. **Affect** is an external expression of emotion related to ideas or objects as the person perceives them. Through observation, the nurse infers a client's affect. Terms commonly used to identify mood and affect are defined in Table 32–1. A format for documenting observations appears in Figure 32–2.

In introducing the examination of cognitive functioning, it can be helpful to comment that you are going to ask some questions that may sound somewhat "silly" or "unusual." Explain that many of these questions are to test memory. As you talk with the client and take the history, ask questions or follow directions in Figure 32–3, which provides a format for describing cognitive functioning in the following areas:

1. Orientation
2. Memory
3. Intellectual functioning
4. Abstract thinking
5. Concentration
6. Thought—content, process
7. Perceptions
8. Social judgment[16]
9. Insight

After completing the examination of cognitive function and making your observations, you must document your findings using appropriate terminology. Terms that identify deficits in cognitive functioning are listed in Table 32–2.

Once you have completed the initial psychosocial health assessment, you may need to reassess mental status at times, especially if the person is confused or has a fluctuating mental status. A brief MSE can be used for a quick assessment. A brief MSE includes the questions shown in Box 32–1.

A client who misses more than two or three of the questions and calculations has some impairment in cognitive functioning.

TABLE 32-1. Terms Commonly Used to Describe Mood and Affect

Term	Definition
Dysphoria	Mood of disquiet, dejection, unhappiness, and dissatisfaction with oneself or life
Euphoria	Mood that is expansive or elated, with an exaggerated sense of well-being
Lability	Mood instability, with rapidly changing emotions
Blunted affect	Facial expression or emotion less than would normally be expected but not totally flat or lacking all emotion
Constricted affect	Indication of a limited range of emotional expression, with a decrease in variability of emotion and spontaneity
Flat affect	Lack of any facial expression or indication of emotion

DATA ANALYSIS

Once the history and the MSE have been completed, you must organize the data in order to assess the person's needs and inadequacies. Worksheets for compiling data can help you analyze your data, consolidate patterns of clues, and draw conclusions in a logical, concise manner. With your data analysis complete, you will be prepared to make a nursing diagnosis and develop a nursing care plan.

Because all dimensions of a person are interrelated and affect each other, the physiologic dimension must be considered along with the psychologic, social, cultural, and spiritual dimensions when you make your assessment.

Physiologic Dimension

Information relevant to the person's current physiologic state includes data obtained through a physical examination and laboratory reports. The worksheet in Figure 32–4 can be used to analyze and record data. For example, in evaluating the respiratory system, details such as skin color and rate and depth of respiration should be considered. If they are adequate, the signs and symptoms should be recorded in the "Adequacies" column. If signs and symptoms indicate a deficit in functioning, this information should be recorded in the "Inadequacies" column.

In addition, ask yourself

▶ What is the actual age, weight, height, sex, and nutritional status of the person?
▶ Are there congenital conditions, genetic endowments, or constitutional vulnerabilities that predisposed the individual to the present condition?
▶ Were physical changes, such as weight gain or loss, hypertension, or other diseases, brought about by the presenting problem?
▶ Does the individual have any habits such as smoking or substance abuse that have contributed to the present condition?

The worksheet provides space for evaluation of other physiologic body systems, which have been discussed in previous chapters. Enter the summary of physiologic findings in Figure 32–4.

Psychologic Dimension

Information relevant to the person's current psychologic state includes data indicating the current level of functioning. Psychologic findings are obtained from the MSE and the psychologic history. Results of formalized psychologic testing, if available, can be included in this section. Using your findings, record all detailed infor-

Text continued on page 643

1. General Appearance	Grooming: Neat _____ Clean _____ Unkempt _____
	Other _____
	Apparent Age: Same as stated _____
	Older _____ Younger _____
	General state of health:Excellent _____ Good _____
	Fair _____ Poor _____
	Level of conciousness:Alert _____ Lethargic _____
	Confused _____ Other _____
	Manner of dress: Streetclothes _____ PJ's and robe _____
	Other _____
	General self-care: Able to care for self. _____
	Needs some assistance _____
	Totally dependent _____
	Posture: Rigid _____ Relaxed _____
	Facial expression: _____
	Distinct physical features: _____

Additional description might include some of the following: drowsy/comatose/cheerful/tearful/grimaces in pain/average build/overweight/thin/casually dressed/wearing hospital gown and robe/three-piece suit/tattoos/handicaps/scars/edentulous.

Behavior	Behavior during interview: Appropriate _____ Other _____
	Relation to interviewer: Cooperative _____ Withdrawn _____
	Other _____
	Degree of activity: Calm _____ Restless _____ Slowed _____
	Other _____
	Eye contact: Good _____ Fair _____ Poor _____
	Other _____
	Distinctive mannerism or gestures: _____
	_____

Additional description might include some of the following: indifferent/distant/courteous/intense/jokes/answers readily/defensive/crying/hostile/wringing hands/nail-biting/rocking/agitated/aloof.

Communication	How does the client communicate with the interviewer?
	_____
	Tone of voice: _____
	Can client be understood? _____
	Choice of words: _____
	Rate of speech: _____
	Presence of abnormalities: _____
	_____
	Unusual speech patterns: _____
	_____

Additional description might include some of the following: spontaneous/expansive/vague/articulate/incoherent/stutters/speech rapid/speech slow/voice loud/voice soft/voice monotonous/client shouts.

▲ *Figure 32–2*

A format for documenting observations.

Illustration continued on following page

| 2 Feelings | Mood: | Describe the person's subjective statements about overall feeling state. Ask, "How are you feeling inside?" or "How do you feel about _____?"

 _____

 _____

 _____ |
| | Affect: | Describe the feeling state you infer on the basis of the statements, appearance and behavior of the client.

 _____

 _____

 _____ |

Mood and affect can be confusing to the beginner. Mood is often compared to overall climate, while affect is compared to weather on a certain day. Thus, depressed mood with sad affect or anxious mood with tense affect.

Additional description of mood might include some of the following: depressed/anxious/hostile/euphoric/angry/elated/labile/dysphoric. Additional description of affect might include some of the following: flat/appropriate/constricted/blunted/vacant stare/subdued/sad/tense.

▲ *Figure 32–2* Continued

1. Cognitive Functioning: Orientation	Awareness of time, place, and person. Usually an individual loses the sense of time and place before losing personal identity.	
	Time:	• Can you tell me what day of the week it is? _____ • Do you know the month and year? _____ • What is the exact date for today? _____
	Place:	• Can you tell me where we are? (Setting, type of institution, city, state.) _____
	Person:	• What is your name? _____ (Pay attention to nicknames, hesitations, or other versions of names.)

Additional description might include the following: Oriented x 3 or oriented to _____ but not to _____

▲ *Figure 32–3*

A format for documenting cognitive functioning.

2. Cognitive Functioning: Memory	Introductory questions: • Have you had any problems with your memory lately? What, if any? _____ • Have you had any problems concentrating? _____ • Can you watch a television program all the way through? _____ • Can you remember things you have read? _____ Recent memory: • When were you admitted to the hospital? _____ • Can you recall what you had for supper last evening? (Ask only if this can be verified.) _____ • Can you tell me some of the things you have seen in the news lately? _____ • I will name three items and ask you to repeat them now and in 5 minutes. (Ex: a chair, the color blue, and New York City.) Ask the client to repeat them immediately, and ask for them again in 5 minutes. _____ Remote memory: (From approximately 6 months prior to this interview to a lifetime) • What is your birthdate? _____ • What is your address and phone number? _____ • Can you recall your social security number? _____ • Can you recall who is president? _____ • Can you recall who was president just before him? Before him? Before him? _____ • What are your children's names? Ages? _____

Often recent memory will show impairment before remote. For example, the client is unable to recall foods eaten at supper yesterday but is able to recall birthdate, address, phone number, and social security number correctly.

Additional description might include the following: recent memory-intact/recent memory-impaired/remote memory-intact/remote memory-impaired/remote memory able to recall 3 of 3 items immediately and after 5 minutes, or perhaps, able to recall 3 of 3 items immediately and only 2 after 5 minutes.

▲ *Figure 32-3* Continued

Illustration continued on following page

3. Cognitive Functioning: Intellectual Functioning	General level of intellectual function: Above average _____ Average _____ Below average _____
4. Cognitive Functioning: Abstract Thinking	Abstract thinking is assessed by asking the client to analyze the meaning of simple proverbs. • Ask "Have you heard the old saying "People who live in glass houses shouldn't throw stones?" What does it mean?" or "A rolling stone gathers no moss?" (Others may be used instead.) _____ _____ _____ _____
5. Cognitive Functioning: Concentration	Is the person able to follow and carry out instructions? • Ask the client to name the days of the week backward starting with Sunday. _____ • Ask the client to perform serial 7's or 3's. "What is 7 from 100? 7 from 93, and so on?" _____ A normal pace is one minute or less in subtracting to 2 with 2 or fewer errors, not including spontaneous self-corrections.
6. Cognitive Functioning: Thought	**Content:** Note trend of thought, any particular preoccupation. Look for delusions (false beliefs that cannot be shaken with reason). Examples include the notions that someone is reading your thoughts or putting ideas into your head; the CIA is after you; and you are the all-knowing, all-powerful master of time and space. _____ _____ _____ **Progression:** Note relatedness of thoughts to each other. Are associations vague, loose, poorly organized, or do they flow from one to another in logical progression? Observe for: 1. *Circumstantiality* - providing much unnecessary detail but eventually reaching the point of the story. 2. *Blocking* - suddenly stopping in the stream of thought for no apparent reason but eventually reaching the point or goal idea. 3. *Flight of ideas* - talking in a continuous but fragmentary way with or without connections between ideas and without a logical point. _____ _____

Look for concrete, bizarre, or nonsensical interpretations. Ask yourself if the client's train of thought is logical and coherent or if it is difficult for you to understand what the client is saying. A person with concrete thinking is very literal in interpreting meaning.

An example of a concrete response to proverb number one is "Well it would break if they threw stones." An abstract response could be "Don't criticize others when you are doing some of the same things yourself."

Ordinarily you would not ask the client to work this fast or go all the way to 2 during a psychosocial assessment. If serial 7's seem too difficult for the client, try serial 3's.

Additional description might include the following: easily distracted/listless/uninterested/ unable to perform serial 7's/able to perform serial 7's without error.

Additional description might include the following: magical thinking/bizarre thinking/unusual thinking/no obsessions, phobias, delusions, or hallucinations/faulty perceptions/ flight of ideas

Additional description might include the following: Logical progression of thoughts/clear/ coherent thoughts/well-organized/ relevant/ flight of ideas/ loose associations.

▲ *Figure 32–3* Continued

| 7. Cognitive Functioning: Perceptions | Sensory awareness and interpretation of the environment. Observe for:

1. *Illusions:* Misinterpretation of external sensory stimuli. Example: Seeing a moving dust ball under a bed as a mouse or mistaking an identity of a person in the mall for a loved one who has recently died.
2. *Hallucinations:* False perceptions without any external basis. They may be visual, auditory, olfactory, gustatory, and/or tactile.

• Have you ever heard voices or sounds that other people don't hear?

_____

• Have you ever seen visions or anything like a dream when you were awake?

_____

• Have you ever felt strange sensations in your body or things crawling on you?

_____

• Have you ever had strange tastes or sensations in your mouth?

_____

• Have you ever smelled strange odors that you couldn't account for?

_____

Note: If the client denies hallucinations, certain behaviors may suggest that the person is hallucinating. Observe for return of gaze to a certain spot, sudden turning of head, staring at a particular place in the room, eyes following something moving (invisible to you), mumbling or talking with someone you cannot see. | **Additional description might include the following: denies hallucinations/hears voices talking and making derogatory remarks/ hears someone calling when no one is there/sees visions of people walking about in the house/feels snakes and spiders crawling under clothing.** |
| 8. Cognitive Functioning: Social Judgment | Can the client compare and evaluate alternatives, make and carry out reasonable decisions, and behave in an appropriate manner?

• What would you do if you found a letter with a stamp and an address on it?

_____

The usual answer is "mail it" or "drop it in a mailbox." Some people will say they would open it and look for money or give other inappropriate answers.

• What would you do if you found a purse or wallet in the street? Why should children go to school? What would you do if you won $10,000 in the lottery?

_____ | **Description of judgment might be noted as adequate/good/ impaired/limited/poor/responded appropriately to imaginary situations requiring judgment /knowledge of usual norms and expectations of society.** |

▲ *Figure 32–3* Continued

Illustration continued on following page

9. Cognitive Functioning: Insight	Client's accurate assessment and understanding of the current situation.
	• What has you caused you to be here?
	_____
	• What do you think has caused this problem/illness/ hospitalization?
	_____
	• Do you think you need treatment or medication?
	_____
	• How do you think we could help you the most?
	_____

Description of judgment might be noted as good/adequate/limited/ poor.

▲ *Figure 32–3* Continued

TABLE 32–2. Terms Commonly Used to Describe Deficits in Cognitive Functioning

Term	Definition
Blocking	Sudden interruption in train of thought
Circumstantiality	Flow of conversation made tedious by unnecessary description of details that would ordinarily be omitted
Defensiveness	Argumentative behavior to justify beliefs, thoughts, or actions
Delusions	False beliefs that are firmly maintained in spite of obvious evidence to the contrary and lack of support of others
Expansiveness	Lack of restraint in one's feelings and actions, overvaluation of one's accomplishments
Flight of ideas	Acceleration of thoughts, evidenced by rapid, pressured speech and disorganized conversation
Hallucinations	Sensory perceptions (auditory, visual olfactory, tactile, or gustatory) without a source of stimulus in the external world
Illusions	False interpretations of real sensory images
Preoccupation	Absorption in one's own thoughts that hinders effective contact with or relation to external reality

Box 32–1. Brief Mental Status Examination

1. What is the date today? Date, month, year?
2. What day of the week is it today?
3. What is the name of this place where we are? Hospital/clinic? City? State?
4. What is your full name?
5. (Name three objects and) ask the person to repeat them now.
6. Where do you live? City, street address?
7. How old are you?
8. Who is the president of the United States?
9. Name the three items mentioned earlier.
10. Subtract 3 from 20 and keep subtracting 3 from each new number all the way back to 1.

From Nurcombe, B., & Gallagher, R. M. (1986). *The clinical process in psychiatry: Diagnosis and management planning.* New York: Cambridge University.

Physiologic Dimension	Adequacies	Inadequacies
1. Respiratory		
2. Cardiovascular		
3. Integumentary		
4. Neurologic/Sensory		
5. Musculoskeletal		
6. Nutrition and Elimination		
7. Endocrine/Reproductive		
8. Sleep/Rest/Exercise		

▲ Figure 32-4

Physiologic dimension of a psychosocial health assessment.

mation relating to the person in Figure 32-5. Your questions and observations from the psychosocial assessment will help you identify adequacies and inadequacies and summarize your findings.

Social and Cultural Dimension

Information about the client's current social and cultural state helps determine whether the person is functioning adequately or inadequately within society. Cultural data also could demonstrate major influences on the present condition. For example, if a man from India has a heart attack while visiting in the United States, his cultural background will affect his perception of and his response to that event and its treatment.

Sociologic information is gathered through questioning and observing the person's interactions and relationships with others and by observing and questioning personal feelings and beliefs. Figure 32-6 can be used to help assess these data and to determine how the person is functioning in this area. The information can then be used to summarize findings. Consider the following questions:

▶ Interpersonal relationships: Does the person describe support systems such as family or significant others? Does the person participate in any group activities? How does the person interact with others?
▶ Social roles: What roles has the person assumed in society? How has the person adjusted to them?
▶ Self-concept: What is the person's view of the self?

Psychologic Dimension	Adequacies	Inadequacies

1. Appearance, behavior, communication
   a. General appearance
   b. Behavior
   c. Communication		

2. Feelings
   a. Mood
   b. Affect		

3. Orientation
   a. Time
   b. Person
   c. Place		

4. Memory
   a. Remote past
   b. Recent past
   c. Immediate past
   d. General recall		

5. Intellectual		
6. General functioning		
7. Concentration		

8. Thoughts
   a. Content
   b. Progression		

9. Perception		
10. Social judgment		
11. Insight		
12. Self-esteem		
13. Defense mechanisms and coping strategies		

▲ *Figure 32–5*

Psychologic (mental and emotional) assessment.

Sociological Dimension	Adequacies	Inadequacies
1. Interpersonal relationships		
2. Social roles		
3. Self-concept		
4. Ethnic/cultural/economic/military/legal		
5. Human sexuality		

▲ *Figure 32–6*

Social and cultural assessment.

▶ Ethnic/cultural/economic: Do any ethnic/cultural/economic/military/legal factors need consideration, such as urban/rural, origin/nationality, poverty/abundance?

Has this person been connected with military service? If so, what effect did the service have upon the person? Has this person been involved with the criminal justice system? If so, in what way has this experience affected the person?

▶ Human sexuality: How does the person express sexuality? Does the person feel comfortable in the male or female sexual role?

Spiritual Dimension

Information relevant to a person's current spiritual state is considered, including data about specific religious practices (for example, dietary restrictions, prayer rituals) that may need to be included in the nursing care plan. Data help determine whether the person is functioning adequately according to personal standards within this dimension. Adherence to correct nursing practice should prevent you from judging a person's particular religious beliefs, but you can determine whether the person has needs in this realm and can make appropriate referrals, such as to the clergy.

Beck and associates quote Clinebell as stating that some of the needs that relate to the spiritual dimension include the following:[3]

▶ A meaningful philosophy of life: What does the person value? What does the person consider to be right and wrong?

▶ A sense of the "numinous" and "transcendent:" Is the person filled with higher emotions, such as awe or reverence? Does the person have the ability to transcend the human condition? Is there evidence of hope and faith?

▶ A deep experience of trustful relatedness to God, a Supreme Being, or a universal power or force: Does the person appeal to a higher force when personal resources fail? Does the person rely on this higher power for assistance? Does the person have specific religious practices?

▶ A relatedness to people and nature: If the person does not experience a relatedness to a deity, does the person have a meaningful relatedness to other people or to nature that enables spiritual growth?

▶ Self-actualization: Has this person reached a personal highest potential? How has this process been affected by the person's present circumstances?

Figure 32–7 can be used to analyze the data and to determine how the person is functioning spiritually. Specific religious practices are noted for incorporation in the nursing care plan.

Summary

▶ The psychosocial health assessment is an interview process that considers each of the five dimensions of an individual with a focus on psychologic (mental/emotional), social, cultural, and spiritual dimensions.

▶ The purpose of the psychosocial health assessment is to establish a data base from which you can

Spiritual Dimension	Adequacies	Inadequacies
1. Philosophy of life		
2. Numinous and transcendent		
3. Trustful relatedness to God or higher power		
4. Relationship to people and nature		
5. Self-actualization		
6. Religious practices that need consideration in the nursing care plan		

▲ Figure 32–7

Spiritual assessment.

identify specific human responses that indicate a need or problem, make a nursing diagnosis, and develop an appropriate nursing care plan.

▶ A successful interview requires rapport between nurse and client, privacy for the client, and a nonjudgmental attitude on the part of the nurse.

▶ Areas covered by the psychosocial history are demographic data; presenting problem; history of the presenting problem; medical/surgical history; history of psychologic problems; family, social, cultural history; spiritual beliefs; military history; educational and vocational history; legal history; characteristic coping mechanisms, values, beliefs, goals; self-esteem; and current life status.

▶ The MSE assesses the client's level of cognitive functioning which has a direct impact on her or his ability to understand and cooperate with treatment.

▶ Components addressed in the MSE are appearance, behavior, communication, feelings, and cognitive function.

▶ Assessment of appearance, feelings, and cognitive function include making observations about mood, affect, communication, orientation, memory, intel-

lectual functioning, abstract thinking, concentration, thought, perception, social judgment, and insight.

▶ Once collected, data must be analyzed and organized into a useful form to identify human responses that indicate a need or problem, make nursing diagnoses, and develop a nursing care plan.

Bibliography

1. Barry, P.D. (1989). *Psychosocial nursing assessment and intervention: Care of the physically ill person* (2nd ed.). Philadelphia: J.B. Lippincott.
2. Beck, C.K., et al. (1988). *Mental health-psychiatric nursing: A holistic life-cycle approach*. St. Louis: C.V. Mosby.
3. Burns, P. (1991). Elements of spirituality and Watson's theory of transpersonal caring: Expansion of focus. *Anthology on Caring* (National League for Nursing Publication 15-2392, pp. 141–153). New York: National League for Nursing.
4. Carpenito, L.J. (1989). *Nursing diagnosis: Application to clinical practice* (3rd ed.). Philadelphia: J.B. Lippincott.
5. Kalman, N., & Waughfield, C.G. (1987). *Mental health conception* (2nd ed.). Albany, NY: Delmar.
6. Kaplan, H.I., & Sadock, B.J. (1991). *Synopsis of psychiatry, behavioral sciences, clinical psychiatry* (6th ed.). Baltimore: Williams & Wilkins.

7. Leigh, H., & Reiser, M.F. (1980). *The patient: Biological, psychological, and social dimensions of medical practice.* New York: Plenum Medical.

8. Lewis, S., et al. (1989). *Manual of psychosocial nursing interventions.* Philadelphia: W.B. Saunders.

9. Maurin, J.T. (1989). *Chronic mental illness: Coping strategies.* Thorofare, NJ: Slack.

10. McFarland, G.K., & Thomas, M.D. (1991). *Psychiatric mental health nursing: Application of the nursing process.* Philadelphia: J.B. Lippincott.

11. Mishel, M.H. (1990). Reconceptualization of the uncertainty in illness theory. *Image: Journal of Nursing Scholarship, 22*(4), 256–262.

12. Nurcombe, B., & Gallagher, R.M. (1986). *The clinical process in psychiatry: Diagnosis and management planning.* New York: Cambridge University.

13. Stuart, G.W., & Sundeen, S.J. (1991). *Principles and practice of psychiatric nursing* (4th ed.). St. Louis: C.V. Mosby.

14. Taylor, C.M. (1990). *Mereness' essentials of psychiatric nursing* (13th ed.). St. Louis: C.V. Mosby.

15. von Bertalanffy, L. (1968). *General systems theory: Foundations, development, and application.* New York: George Braziller.

16. Zuckerman, E.L. (1991). *The clinician's thesaurus.* Pittsburgh: Three Wishes Press.

▼ **Health Assessment**

Listen to people—they will tell you their diagnosis.

An old axiom

▼ **CHAPTER OUTLINE**

THE HEALTH HISTORY
PRINCIPLES OF HISTORY-TAKING
MAJOR COMPONENTS OF A HEALTH
   HISTORY
       Chief Complaint
       Present Illness
       Past Health History
       Family Health History
       Personal And Social History
       Systems Review
PHYSICAL ASSESSMENT
PREPARATION FOR PHYSICAL
   ASSESSMENT
       Purpose
       Equipment Needed
       Techniques
       Promoting Client Comfort During
         Physical Assessment

CONDUCTING THE PHYSICAL
   ASSESSMENT
       Vital Signs
       Height And Weight
       General Appearance
       Mental Status And Speech
       Integument
       Head And Neck
       Chest
       Abdomen
       Genitals And Rectum
       Extremities
       Motor System
       Sensory System
POSTEXAMINATION ACTIVITIES
DOCUMENTATION

▼ **KEY TERMS**

Adventitious breath
   sounds
Apical impulse
Ataxia
Auscultation
Barrel chest
Bronchial breath
   sounds
Bronchovesicular breath
   sounds
Chief complaint
Clubbing

Crackles
Cyanosis
Diaphragmatic excursion
Ecchymosis
Edema
Fasciculations
Fremitus
Friction rubs
Gait
Goiter
Heart murmur

Homan's sign
Inspection
Jaundice
Kyphosis
Lordosis
Pallor
Palpation
Pectus carinatum (pigeon
   chest)
Pectus excavatum (funnel
   chest)

▼ *KEY TERMS* Continued

Percussion	Rhonchi	Skin turgor	Stethoscope	Tuning fork
Petechiae	Scoliosis	Snellen chart	Symptom	Vesicular breath sounds
Ptosis	Sign	Speculum	Thrill	Wheezes
Reflex				

▼ **LEARNING OBJECTIVES**

After studying this chapter, you should be able to

1. Explain how to take a client's health history.
2. State how to prepare for a physical assessment.
3. Describe how to complete a physical assessment, including how to select appropriate tools and how to use maneuvers correctly.
4. Practice taking a health history, including using correct terminology to document findings.
5. Under instructor supervision, practice completing a physical assessment, including using correct terminology to document findings.

Health assessment is an increasingly important part of nursing practice. It is an activity shared with other health professionals. Although the processes are similar, each professional uses health assessment with a differing focus. For nurses, health assessment is an examination of a person's state of health rather than diagnosis of disease. It enables you to view the person holistically.

The ability to perform a health assessment can be a very exciting and challenging aspect of the learning process. As your knowledge increases regarding health assessment, so will your ability to make clinical judgments.

This chapter is an overview of health assessment skills as they relate to establishing a nursing data base. Health assessment can be performed in other settings besides the hospital unit: clinics, health fairs, physician's offices, and the home.

The person requiring health care is central to all assessment processes. It is this person alone who experiences both symptoms and assessment processes. It is this person who interacts with the people performing these processes and whose life, mind, and body are affected by them.

Health assessment, which includes the health history and the physical assessment, is a holistic assessment of an individual that identifies normal physical and psychosocial functioning and highlights deviations from normal. It also identifies individual health risks and points to preventive measures.

While assessment skills are described, it is important to remember that supervised practice is essential if you are to be accomplished. Do not perform activities for which you are not fully prepared and authorized. It is assumed that you already know basic normal human physical structure and functions.

It is important for you to understand the difference between signs and symptoms. A **sign** is an objective observation made by physical assessment. A **symptom** is a person's subjective experience that something is abnormal, e.g., pain, dizziness, nausea, fatigue, and anxiety.

▼ THE HEALTH HISTORY

Careful history-taking can provide useful information about an individual.

PRINCIPLES OF HISTORY-TAKING

History-taking is obtaining information in an organized manner. Communication skills and interviewing techniques are used to elicit pertinent information from the individual. As one prepares to obtain the client health history, communication principles must be considered. It is important to conduct the interview in a setting that will ensure the individual's privacy. If the individual is in a private room, be sure to close the door. If the individual is in a semiprivate room, be sure to draw the drapes between the beds. Try to interview the individual during a time when daily activities are at a minimum.

Be sure to obtain only information needed to support the health history. Inform the individual that all information provided will remain confidential within the health care team. The individual has the right not to answer a question if deemed inappropriate. Be sure to discuss this freedom with the individual. Offer to show the individual what is being written on the health history form.

Set a time frame for obtaining the client health history. This will allow the individual to be aware of how long the interview will take, and it will assure you of obtaining any and all needed information.

The tone of an interview is important. The first 5 minutes are probably most important in setting the tone. It is important that the person experience the interviewer as genuinely concerned, attentive, trustworthy, and skilled.

Consider what a person is concealing as well as revealing. Omissions in history are not necessarily intentional. Some details are simply forgotten. A skilled interviewer notices and assesses obvious omissions, sudden shifts of subject matter, shying away from topics, and nonverbal cues, e.g., facial expression, gestures, tone of voice.

A person's account of one's own history and symptoms is affected by (a) hopes and fears, (b) confidence in and reactions to the interviewer, (c) mental competence, (d) view of what actually is a reportable health disorder, and (e) ability to observe and describe life events (past experiences).

Try to assess a person's reliability in history reporting. This is important not only in interpreting information but also in considering how an individual may cooperate with treatment.

In addition to discussing an individual's present problem, it is also important to obtain information about the person's lifestyle, family history, and history of previous health problems. Finally, a thorough "systems review" (discussed later) is conducted to identify abnormalities in the various body systems.

MAJOR COMPONENTS OF A HEALTH HISTORY

Chief Complaint

The **chief complaint** is a person's description of the major problem he or she is experiencing. It is written in the person's own words and is contained within direct quotes. Help the person be specific. A person's main concerns are often a change in usual condition or the presence of pain or dysfunction. The chief complaint provides a broad beginning for assessment. It usually consists of one statement, containing one to two symptoms and the duration. Examples of a chief complaint are "I've been having chest pain for the last 2 days" or "I've been short of breath for 3 to 4 weeks."

Present Illness

The present illness is derived from the chief complaint. It details the course of the illness or the sequence of events leading up to the present illness. The history of the present illness usually identifies major disease mechanisms and may even establish the diagnosis when symptoms are precise.

To reconstruct the events leading up to the present illness, you must acquaint yourself with the seven variables central to obtaining pertinent information from the person:

Body Location. Pinpoint the body system or organs involved. A question you may ask is "Where does it hurt?"

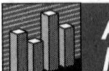

APPLYING RESEARCH TO NURSING PRACTICE

Recognizing the Importance of Subjective Data in Assessing Bronchial Asthma

Janson-Bjerklie, S., Ferketich, S., Benner, P., & Becker, G. (1992). Clinical markers of asthma severity risk: importance of subjective as well as objective markers. *Heart & Lung, 21*(3), 265–272.

▼ ▼ ▼

Bronchial asthma is a chronic lung disorder characterized by bronchial inflammation, bronchospasm, and excessive mucus production. Asthma "attacks," ranging from mild to severe and life-threatening, are signalled by signs and symptoms of wheezing, coughing, and shortness of breath. Attacks may begin in response to a wide variety of triggers. Because emotions may play a role, persons with asthma may suffer under the burden of derogatory stereotypes in emergency departments. Janson-Bjerklie and colleagues have gone a long way to challenge such stereotypes. In this study, the nurse-researchers asked asthmatic adults to measure their peak expiratory flow rates twice daily, and to keep a symptom diary. (The peak expiratory flow rate is the maximal amount of air that a person can exhale after a deep inhalation. Peak expiratory flow rates can be measured with a simple device called a peak flow meter.) Of the 95 adults studied, 19 made 29 visits to the emergency department with what they judged to be severe asthma attacks, and nine attacks were severe enough to result in admission. The researchers concluded that the subjective assessments that asthmatic clients make about the severity of their symptoms are quite accurate. Those assessments also closely match objective clinical measures of increased severity and risk of asthma attacks.

Applications for Practice

Try to recognize that asthmatic clients often have developed practical knowledge about the severity of their symptoms. The asthmatic client's statements and behavioral cues are an integral part of your assessment. When you incorporate subjective data into your health assessment, the quality, accuracy, and effectiveness of your nursing interventions will improve.

Quality. Usually a person will equate a symptom with an analogy, by stating it is "like" something. For example, "My chest pain feels like a knife is being thrust in my chest."

Quantity. You need to quantify the symptom according to the level of intensity, how it affects activities of daily living, frequency, volume, number, and size or extent of the symptom. For example, ask the person, "On a scale of one to ten with ten most severe, what is your level of pain?"

Chronology. You need to consider the symptom in relation to time. For example, when did the symptom first appear? Does the symptom begin gradually or suddenly? Does it stay the same in quality and intensity? How often does it occur? Does it wake the person from sleep?

Setting. Consider where and what the person was doing when the symptom occurred.

Aggravating or Alleviating Factors. Identify what worsens (aggravates) or relieves (alleviates) the symptom. For example, does the chest pain increase during physical activity? Does it require rest? Does emotional upset make the symptom worse?

Associated Factors. Assess the associated factors or symptoms. Some disorders produce symptoms in various body parts. For example, a person with congestive heart failure may have swollen ankles and abdomen and may experience shortness of breath. Exploration of associated factors may reveal useful information. For example, an acutely ill child may have eaten a poisonous substance, or a desperately ill adult might have been traveling recently and developed malaria or some other regional disorder.

Past Health History

The past health history reflects a chronologic review of previous disorders and contacts with health professionals. The first information you will need to obtain is a description of the person's general health immediately prior to the present illness. You may ask the person to describe health prior to this particular illness. The following are areas to be included in the past health history:

► Pediatric and adult illness: Inquire whether the person has ever had measles, mumps, chickenpox, hypertension, polio, hepatitis, pneumonia, diabetes, cancer, mental illness, scarlet fever, anemia, rheumatic fever, seizures, chronic bronchitis, heart disease, whooping cough, stroke, diphtheria, or malaria. If the person answers yes to any of these illnesses, question the person concerning the time frame and any complications resulting from the illness
► Previous hospitalizations: Obtain the date, physician, disorder, and hospital location
► Operations and injuries without hospitalization
► Immunizations
► Allergies or sensitivies, e.g., asthma, hayfever, food, skin, drugs (note drug allergies or sensitivities and manifestations)
► Transfusions
► Current medications: This should include medications prior to and during hospitalization. Remember to include prescription as well as over-the-counter medications
► Current treatments, e.g., physical or occupational therapy, respiratory therapy

Family Health History

The family health history is a past medical history of relatives. You will need to assess the person's family history with respect to the present illness and future health risks. The following are areas to be included in the family health history:

► Present status of parents and siblings: Question the person concerning the age and health status of the mother, father, and each of the siblings, or the age at death and cause.
► Medical problems: Question the person concerning the family history of disorders that may be influenced by heredity (familial disorders) or contact. Also ask about family allergies, deformities, or serious illnesses. Include the following: diabetes, hypertension, heart disease, renal disease, cancer, tuberculosis, stroke, deafness, anemia, gout, arthritis, mental illness, alcoholism, seizures, obesity.
► Similar illness or symptoms in family: Is anyone in the family experiencing an illness or symptoms resembling a person's present illness?

Personal and Social History

The personal and social history pertains to information concerning the person's personality and lifestyle. Some of the information may be emotionally charged and difficult for the person to describe. Question the person concerning the following areas (only information needed to care for the person should be obtained):

► Marital status
► Number of dependent children
► Other people in the household
► Religion
► Occupation
► Military service
► Daily routines, e.g., food intake, elimination, sleep pattern, exercise
► Habits, e.g., tobacco, caffeine, alcohol, drugs
► Pets
► Housing and living arrangements
► Family responsibilities
► Interests
► Daily activity, e.g., description of an average day
► Source of income
► Health insurance
► Travel
► Past development, e.g. childhood and adolescence, educational experiences, occupational experiences
► Patterns of interaction and communication, e.g., sexual relations, personality (mood, feelings, temperament, and general attitudes)

Systems Review

A review of systems is included in the client health history. You will be questioning the person about the structure and function of the body systems in order to identify symptoms that the person may not have previously reported. Some of the terms used will be new to you, but they are common medical terms you will have to know in your role as a nurse. You are urged to look them up and become familiar with them. The following systems should be addressed:

▶ Integument: color change, pruritus, nevi, infections, inflammations, rash, tumor, hair changes, nail changes, excessive bruising, cuts failing to heal
▶ Eyes: visual acuity, glasses/contact lenses, blurring, diplopia, pain, inflammation, excessive tearing, visual defects, date of last eye examination
▶ Ears: hearing loss, tinnitus, discharge, hearing aid, earache, vertigo, infection
▶ Nose and sinuses: frequent colds, sinusitis, epistaxis, discharge, obstruction, postnasal drip, pain
▶ Mouth and throat: gums, teeth, partial/full dentures, sore tongue, sore throat, difficulty swallowing, hoarseness, voice change, goiter, bleeding gums, date of last dental examination
▶ Neck: pain, thyroid or lymph node enlargement, limitation of motion
▶ Respiratory: cough, sputum, hemoptysis, wheezing, dyspnea, recurrent respiratory tract infections, night sweats, recent chest x-ray, pain, positive tuberculin test (date)
▶ Cardiovascular: chest pain, dyspnea, orthopnea, palpitations, murmur, hypertension, syncope, anemia, edema, varicosities, thrombophlebitis, claudication, pain
▶ Gastrointestinal: appetite changes, dysphagia, eructation, nausea, vomiting, hematemesis, pain, gas, indigestion, jaundice, change in bowel habits, food intolerance, constipation, diarrhea, stools (color, character), hemorrhoids, hernia, melena, use of laxatives, weight change, rectal itching
▶ Genitourinary/reproductive: frequency, nocturia, urgency, dysuria, incontinence, albuminuria, flank pain, venereal disease, discharge, lesions, contraception, hesitancy, hematuria, pyuria, infections, stones, glycosuria, infertility, libido, testicular mass or pain, impotence, menarche, LMP (last menstrual period), cycle, duration, regularity, dysmenorrhea, gravida, para, abortions, spotting, leukorrhea, pruritus, last pelvic examination, last Pap smear, menopause, complications
▶ Musculoskeletal: myalgia, weakness, pain, swelling, heat, limitation of motion, stiffness, redness
▶ Endocrine: sensitivity to environmental temperature, change in body configuration, changes in scalp or hair, body weight in relation to appetite, sweating, polyuria, postural hypotension, change in voice, polydipsia, polyphagia
▶ Neurologic: headache, syncope, convulsions, seizures, vertigo, diplopia, paralysis, paresis, spasm, muscle weakness, paresthesia, tremor, ataxia, memory change, unconsciousness, speech problems, coordination
▶ Psychologic: nervousness, insomnia, depression, nightmares, indecisiveness, hyperventilation, work difficulty, mood, emotional difficulty, sense of failure, social withdrawal, memory loss

A variety of printed forms are available for recording the client's health history. It is important to remember that a client health history is privileged information. Information should not be sought unless it will be used in a professional, confidential manner.

▼ PHYSICAL ASSESSMENT

PREPARATION FOR PHYSICAL ASSESSMENT

Purpose

Physical assessment is a component of the first step of the nursing process, Assessment. Data are objective because you are obtaining pertinent information from the client through the use of the senses: sight, hearing, smell, and touch. The purpose of physical assessment is to identify normal and deviations from normal. Nurses use it to identify deviations in health patterns, and they derive nursing diagnosis upon which planning, nursing interventions, and evaluation are based. Physical assessment is the key means of collecting baseline data and establishing a need for continued focused assessment. Physical assessment is done for people who are experiencing symptoms and as a health maintenance procedure for people who are well. Physical assessment often offers opportunity for health teaching —for example, breast and testicular self-examination.

Accurate assessment requires knowledge of body structure and function (anatomy and physiology), as well as pathologic changes or abnormalities. Skilled physical assessment depends on thoughtful practice and accumulated experience.

Equipment Needed

When performing a physical assessment, you will rely heavily on your senses, but in order to complete aspects of the assessment, you must use certain equipment (Fig. 33–1). This equipment is, in a sense, an extension of your senses.

▶ Stethoscope: An instrument with two earpieces connected by flexible tubing to a cone or bell, used to listen to and amplify sounds produced by internal organs, e.g., lungs, heart, intestine.
▶ Scopes: Instruments for looking inside structures; e.g., an ophthalmoscope is an instrument used to examine the interior of the eye, obtaining information about not only the eye but also the central nervous system and blood vessels; an otoscope is an instrument used to examine the external ear canal and eardrum.
▶ Speculums: Instruments used to distend or open a body orifice or cavity, permitting visual inspection of the interior. Examples include a nasal speculum and a vaginal speculum.
▶ Tuning fork: An instrument to test air and bone conduction, auditory nerve function, and vibration sensation.

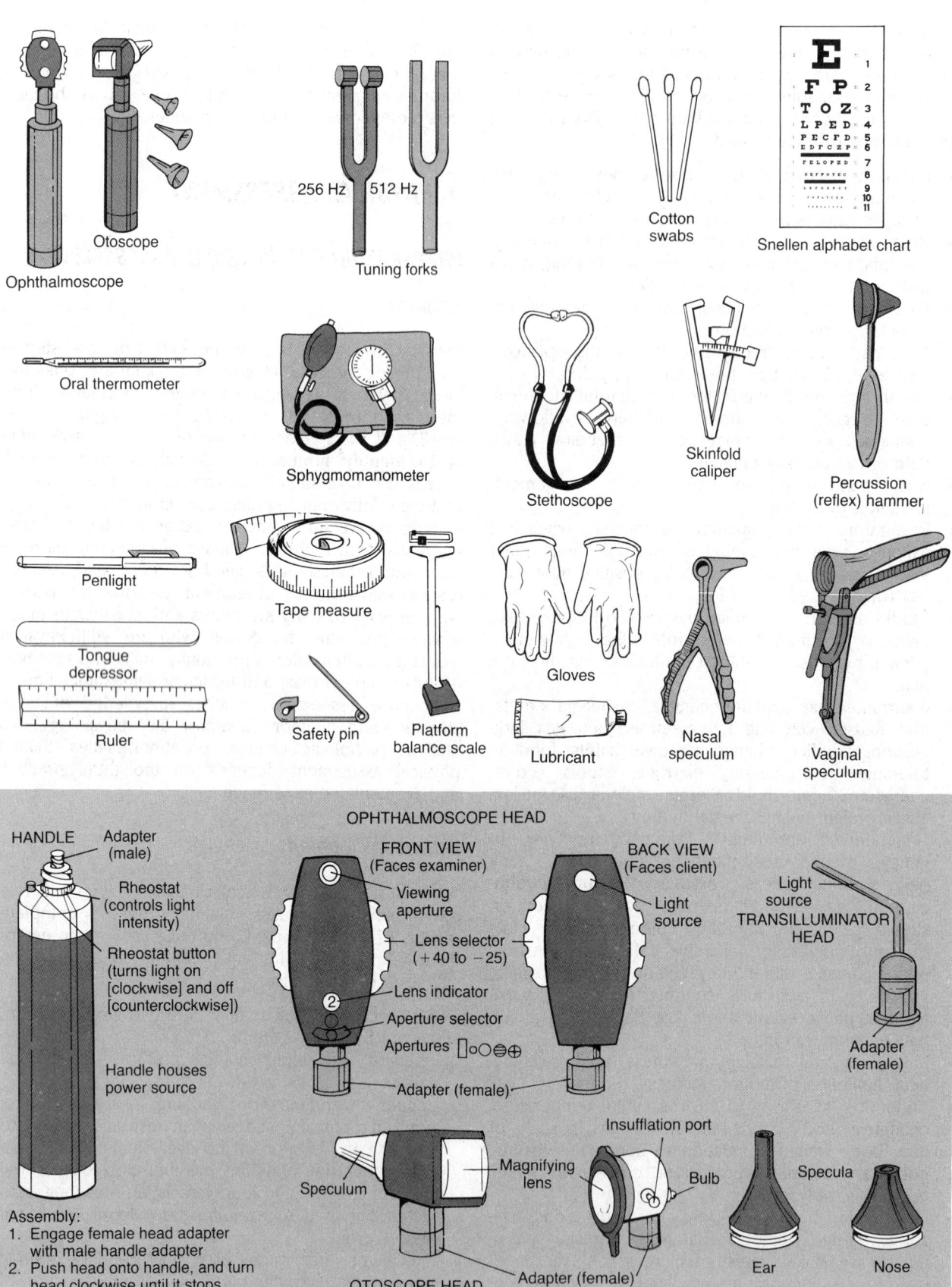

Ophthalmoscope

Otoscope

Tuning forks
256 Hz 512 Hz

Cotton swabs

Snellen alphabet chart

Oral thermometer

Sphygmomanometer

Stethoscope

Skinfold caliper

Percussion (reflex) hammer

Penlight

Tape measure

Gloves

Nasal speculum

Vaginal speculum

Tongue depressor

Ruler

Safety pin

Platform balance scale

Lubricant

OPHTHALMOSCOPE HEAD

HANDLE

Adapter (male)

Rheostat (controls light intensity)

Rheostat button (turns light on [clockwise] and off [counterclockwise])

Handle houses power source

FRONT VIEW (Faces examiner)

Viewing aperture

Lens selector (+ 40 to − 25)

Lens indicator

Aperture selector

Apertures

Adapter (female)

BACK VIEW (Faces client)

Light source

Adapter (female)

Light source
TRANSILLUMINATOR HEAD

Adapter (female)

Speculum

Magnifying lens

Insufflation port

Bulb

Adapter (female)

OTOSCOPE HEAD

Specula

Ear

Nose

Assembly:
1. Engage female head adapter with male handle adapter
2. Push head onto handle, and turn head clockwise until it stops

▲ *Figure 33–1*

Equipment used by the nurse. (Modified from Black, J.M., & Matassarin-Jacobs, E. [1993]. Luckmann and Sorensen's Medical-Surgical Nursing: A Psychophysiologic Approach [4th ed]. Philadelphia: W.B. Saunders.)

▶ Percussion hammer (reflex hammer): An instrument used to test superficial, deep tendon, and pathologic reflexes.

▶ Snellen chart: A chart used to test a person's visual acuity.

▶ Tongue depressor: A wooden stick used to aid in viewing the pharynx and stimulating the gag reflex.

▶ Safety pins and cotton swabs: Accessories used to test a person's ability to differentiate dull and sharp pain and sensitivities of touch.

▶ Penlight: An instrument used to illuminate areas for better viewing and to test pupil constriction.

▶ Instruments of measurement: examples are a scale to measure weight and a height measurement rod (often attached to the scale) to measure height. A blood pressure cuff attached to a sphygmomanometer measures blood pressure, and a thermometer measures body temperature. Pulse and respirations are counted, using a watch with a secondhand. A tape measure and small ruler may be used to make linear and circumference measurements. A special marking pen (surgical marker) may be used to mark areas on the body that require measurements.

NEUROLOGIC ASSESSMENT

Additional items are required for *neurologic* assessment.

▶ Audiometer, watch, or some other item for assessing hearing

▶ Containers of sugar and salt for testing taste

▶ Dry cotton balls for testing corneal reflex

▶ Test tubes (two) filled with cold and hot water for testing temperature sensation

▶ Vials (closed) containing fresh materials with easily recognizable odors, e.g., onion, orange extract, peanut butter, vanilla

▶ Various objects of differing, easily recognizable textures and shapes (key, paper clip, coin) for testing texture discrimination and stereognosis (ability to recognize an object by feeling it) while the individual's eyes are closed

Techniques

Inspection, palpation, percussion, and auscultation are basic maneuvers used during physical assessment. The sense of smell is also used. Figure 33–2 shows how the body can be divided into planes and subdivided for descriptions of the parts assessed.

A systematic approach to physical assessment is important to prevent omissions. The usual sequence of assessment activities is to (1) look (inspect), (2) feel (palpate), (3) tap or thump (percuss), and (4) listen (auscultate).

This sequence is not used to assess the abdomen. Instead the sequence is inspection, auscultation, percussion, and palpation. Palpation is performed last in this instance, because feeling a sensitive abdomen may

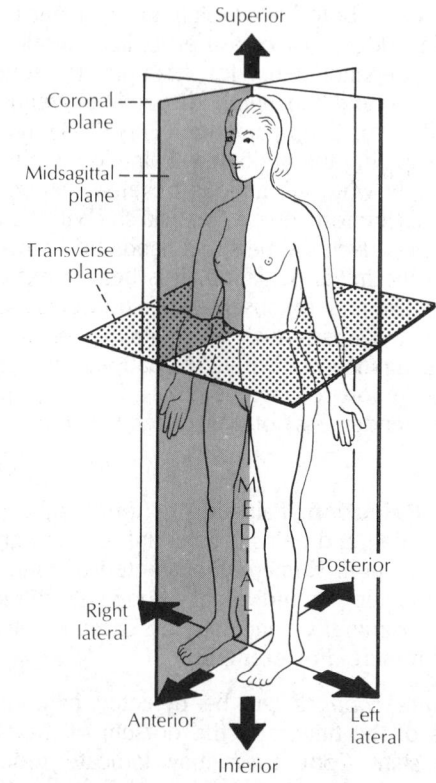

▲ *Figure 33–2*

Anatomic section and position reference terms. (Modified from Jacob, S.W., & Francone, C.A. [1989]. Elements of anatomy and physiology [2nd ed.]. Philadelphia: W.B. Saunders.)

produce additional symptoms—for example, suppress early bowel sounds, trigger painful spasms.

INSPECTION

Inspection is an assessment technique in which the examiner observes the body surface. As you inspect an area, try to develop a *visual description* of what you are seeing in your mind. Observe events (e.g., movements), colors, contours, and symmetry or asymmetry. Good lighting and adequate (but not excessive) exposure of the appropriate area facilitate proper inspection.

You must expose that which you wish to look at. You cannot inspect that which is not visible.

Whenever possible, take *measurements* (with a soft tape measure or small ruler) to quantify observations. This provides a baseline for future measurements and allows comparison with established normal ranges. Measurements are commonly made of height, weight, body temperature, and vital signs (i.e., pulse, respirations, blood pressure). Other measurements include head and limb circumference or the diameter of a lesion.

PALPATION

Technique of Palpation. Palpation is an assessment technique in which the examiner feels with his or her fingers and one or both hands. Skill and gentleness are important. The degree of pressure applied during palpation varies, depending on, for example, the tenderness of the area and the depth of palpation required. Light (Fig. 33–3) or deep palpation (Fig. 33–4) may be used when palpating the abdomen. Palpation is difficult to do on people who are anxious or tense, experiencing physical discomfort, obese, or ticklish. With ticklish or tense people, place the person's hands beneath your hands during the initial palpation. It is best to examine tender areas last and to observe the individual's face for nonverbal responses such as grimacing or smiling during the examination. During palpation, encourage the person to report feelings of discomfort (e.g., pressure, fullness, tenderness) or pain when you touch certain places.

Purpose of Palpation. Palpation confirms data gathered by inspection and helps provide information about structure or function. Numerous characteristics may be assessed by touching an individual's body with different parts of the examiner's hand and by exerting varying amounts of pressure. For example:

▶ *Temperature changes* can be detected by running the backs of the fingers or the dorsum of the hand over the skin. Cool areas may indicate reduced blood flow, and warmth may indicate inflammation.

▶ *Moisture* may be felt while lightly stroking the skin.

▶ *Events* (vibrations, such as bruits and voice sounds, crepitus, pulsations, spasticity, rigidity, elasticity, or other movements or qualities of movements occurring under the examiner's hand) can be detected by using the fingers and entire palm. Vibrations are best felt with the palm or ulnar side of the hand.

▶ *Textures* (e.g., unevenness) can be noted using fingertips. Fingertips have many nerve endings and are therefore very sensitive to touch.

▶ *Locations and dimensions or contours* are assessed by using several fingers or one or both entire hands, depending upon the size of the body part being examined. For example, swelling may be felt and organ sizes and locations assessed. Firm deep pressure is required to palpate deep organs such as the kidneys, spleen, or liver. Light touch is used to palpate the eye.

▶ *Consistencies* (hard, soft, rubbery, flaccid, tense) are determined by the fingertips.

Palpation is commonly used to take a pulse (to feel blood pulsating through arteries) and during breast examination. However, all accessible body parts may be examined by palpation, e.g., blood vessels, organs, skin, muscles, bones, glands. It is also possible to feel the vibrations of some body sounds, e.g., thrills, tactile fremitus.

Types of Palpation. Firm pressure reduces the sensitivity in an examiner's fingers, as in palpation of deep organs. To counteract this problem, use both hands when applying pressure (Fig. 33–4). Keep the lower hand (touching the individual) relaxed. Apply pressure by placing the other hand on top of the resting hand. The upper hand also directs exploratory movements of the relaxed lower hand on the person's body. Palpation of deep organs should be performed only in the presence of a qualified examiner, since injury can occur as a result of prolonged pressure.

PERCUSSION

Techniques of Percussion. Percussion is an assessment technique in which the examiner "thumps" or "taps" a body surface with a percussion hammer or the hand or fingers. Percussion assesses *density* (relative solidity, hardness, or fullness) of a cavity or organ. The location and size of underlying organs can also be determined. Diagnostic deductions can be made from the sound produced by the thumping.

Sounds of Percussion. Percussed sounds differ in various body areas, depending in part upon the density of underlying structures. The sounds produced by percussion over solid structures differ from those over hollow structures. Sounds range from *flat* (nonresonant) to *dull, resonant, hyperresonant,* and *tympanic.* Tympanic sounds occur over hollow or gas-filled organs. Flat sounds are heard over solid tissue, such as muscle or solid organs. It is possible, for example, to differentiate between normal air-filled lung tissue and diseased soli-

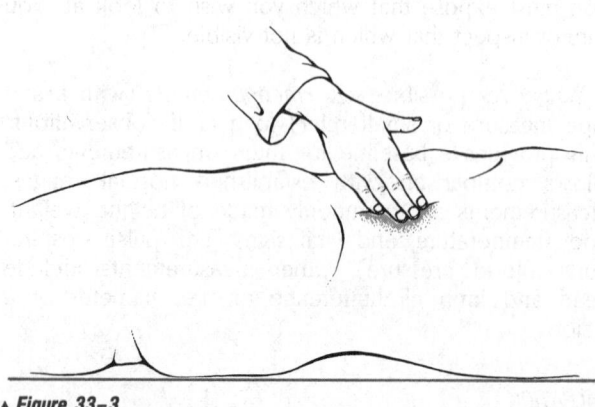

▲ *Figure 33–3*

Position of the hand during light palpation.

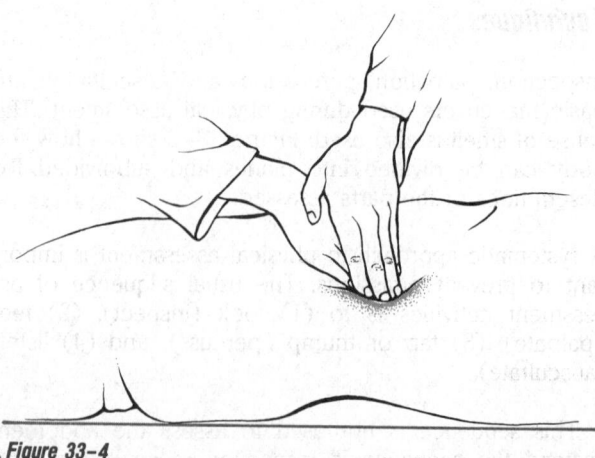

▲ *Figure 33–4*

Position of hands during deep palpation.

dified lung tissue. Nurses often percuss the abdomen to identify distention, and the urinary bladder to assess the amount of urine it contains.

Types of Percussion. Percussion may be direct or indirect. *Direct percussion* is done by the examiner's striking the fingers directly against the person's skin. With *indirect percussion,* the examiner places the first phalanx (i.e., terminal phalanx) of the middle finger of one hand (the nondominant hand) firmly against the person's skin and then strikes the phalanx (just behind the fingernail bed) with the end of the middle finger of the dominant hand (Fig. 33–5). Remember:

► Do not allow other fingers of the nondominant hand to touch the person (this will damp or suppress the percussed sound).
► Hold the forearm of the dominant arm steady and use a quick, flicking wrist action from a flexed wrist for the striking force.
► Quickly withdraw the striking finger to avoid damping the percussed sound.
► Strive for a brief, intense tap.

AUSCULTATION

Technique of Auscultation. Auscultation is an assessment technique in which the examiner listens to and assesses the sound produced by various body organs and tissues such as heart, lung, or bowel. Auscultation of the lungs and heart is routinely performed not only as a preliminary scanning procedure but also for ongoing assessment of a person receiving treatment. Auscultation of the abdomen and peripheral blood vessels is also useful. Blood vessels in the neck and head are auscultated at times—for example, if a brain aneurysm is suspected.

Sounds of Auscultation. The following are assessed by auscultation:

► *Frequency:* high pitch, low pitch
► *Intensity:* loud sounds, soft sounds
► *Quality:* differences between two sounds of equal pitch and intensity coming from differing sources, as the lungs and bowels
► *Duration* or length of the sound

Types of Auscultation. Auscultation can be performed either directly or indirectly. *Direct auscultation* (immediate auscultation) is less commonly used. The examiner places his/her ear directly against the person's body. This method is limited because the sounds are too diffuse and too soft, especially with obese people. The *indirect method* (most common) is done with a stethoscope.

A quality stethoscope (see Fig. 33–1) having both a bell and a flat diaphragm is recommended. When gently placed against a person, the bell collects low-frequency sound while permitting high-frequency sound to escape. The *flat diaphragm,* when firmly placed, excludes low-frequency sounds and picks up high-frequency sounds.

Ear pieces should fit comfortably without totally occluding the ear canals. Ear pieces should be clean to maintain unobstructed openings. The tubing should be about one foot long and free of leaks. The tubing should fit tightly on both the ear pieces and the head of the stethoscope. During auscultation, nothing should touch the tubing (otherwise, distracting noises are produced). Tell the person to remain silent unless following directions from the examiner to speak, cough, or breathe deeply through open mouth. Ask the person to turn their head away from the examiner's face and cover the mouth when coughing and deep breathing. Give the person a tissue. As with other assessment techniques, auscultation is performed systematically.

OLFACTION

Olfaction (sense of smell) may help in the diagnosis of many disorders, some of which are serious. Table 33–1 lists some characteristic odors and their possible causes.

Promoting Client Comfort During Physical Assessment

A nurse's primary responsibility is to the person receiving care.

This includes observing the person carefully and making sure comfort is maintained. The person is usu-

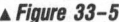
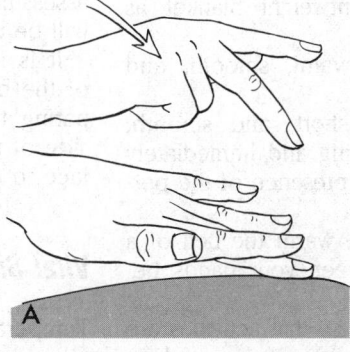
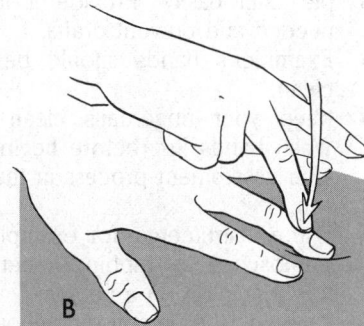

▲ **Figure 33–5**

Percussion. *A,* First phalanx of middle finger of nondominant hand is placed firmly on person's skin. *B,* Phalanx on skin is struck with end of middle finger of dominant hand.

TABLE 33.1. Characteristic Odors Detectable During Physical Assessment and Their Possible Causes

Characteristic Odor	Possible Cause
Alcohol, liquefied Sterno, lighter fluid	Intake of these substances
Ammoniac urine (ammonia-like odor)	Urinary tract infection with urea-splitting bacteria
Bitter almond odor	Cyanide poisoning
Body odor (general)	Poor hygiene; excessive perspiration (hyperhidrosis); foul-smelling perspiration (bromhidrosis)
Burnt rope odor	Marijuana
Camphor odor	Mothball ingestion
Fecal odor (in older person)	Wound infection; abscess
Feculent odor	*Bacteroides* abscess
Fetid breath	Lung abscess
Foul-smelling stools (infant)	Malabsorption syndrome, e.g., cystic fibrosis
Garlic odor	Arsenic poisoning
Halitosis ("bad breath")	Poor dental and oral hygiene
"Horsey" or musty odor (infant)	Phenylketonuria (PKU)
Ketone, acetone, sickening sweet odor	Diabetic acidosis
Musty "new-mown clover" odor (fetor hepaticus)	Liver disease, hepatic coma
Nasal malodor (foul odor from nose)	Foreign body in nose; pharyngitis; chronic postnasal drip; nasal crusts; allergic, atrophic, or chronic rhinitis
Paraldehyde odor	Acute poisoning
Stale urine odor	Uremic acidosis
Sweet, heavy, thick odor	*Pseudomonas* infection
Vaginal odor	Fungal infection; poor hygiene

ally anxious, which is uncomfortable for the person and can distort assessment findings.

Explain the assessment process to the person and the reasons it is being performed. Assure the person that appropriate draping will be provided so that there will be no unnecessary exposure of the person's body.

Before beginning the physical assessment, suggest the person go to the toilet. This helps the person relax and facilitates examination of the abdomen, male genitals, vagina, and rectum. If a urine or stool specimen is needed, you may assist the person in collecting the specimen. Promptly label the specimen with the date and time and your initials after it is collected.

Additional guidelines for promoting client comfort during the physical assessment are as follows:

▶ Keep necessary instruments and equipment assembled, close at hand, and ready for use.
▶ Keep examining area comfortable and private.
▶ Keep personal exposure to a minimum; expose only the area being examined and for only as long as necessary.
▶ Keep the person warm. Elderly, anxious, or ill people chill easily. Provide a lightweight blanket as needed and prevent drafts.
▶ Examiner's hands should be warm, smooth, and clean.
▶ Keep your fingernails clean, short, and smooth. Wash hands just before beginning and immediately after assessment process in the presence of the person.
▶ Warm instruments; for example, warm the bell of a stethoscope by rubbing it between your hands before placing it on a person.
▶ Talk with the person throughout so that activities are not unexpected. "I'm going to listen to your chest now." Give the person clear instructions: "Breathe in and out slowly and deeply through your mouth."
▶ Avoid undesirable nonverbal communication (such as frowning, looks of concern).
▶ A relaxed, friendly, yet professional attitude on the examiner's part helps put a person at ease.
▶ Help the person into required positions (Fig. 33–6). Some positions, such as lithotomy and knee-chest, are embarrassing and uncomfortable. Keep a person in these positions no longer than necessary.
▶ Initiate physical contact in nonthreatening ways. For example, inspect the hands before touching other body parts.

CONDUCTING THE PHYSICAL ASSESSMENT

When performing the physical assessment examination, you need to be well organized to ensure that no areas of the assessment are deleted. Most nurses assess according to a "head to toe" system. Working in this manner enables you to remember the order of the assessment. In this chapter, a "head to toe" approach will be used.

It is important to remember to compare both sides of the body for symmetry. For example, you are comparing the right upper extremity to the left, the right side of the thorax to the left, and the right side of the face to the left side of the face.

Vital Signs

Temperature, pulse, respirations, and blood pressure (see Chapter 31) may be measured at the beginning of

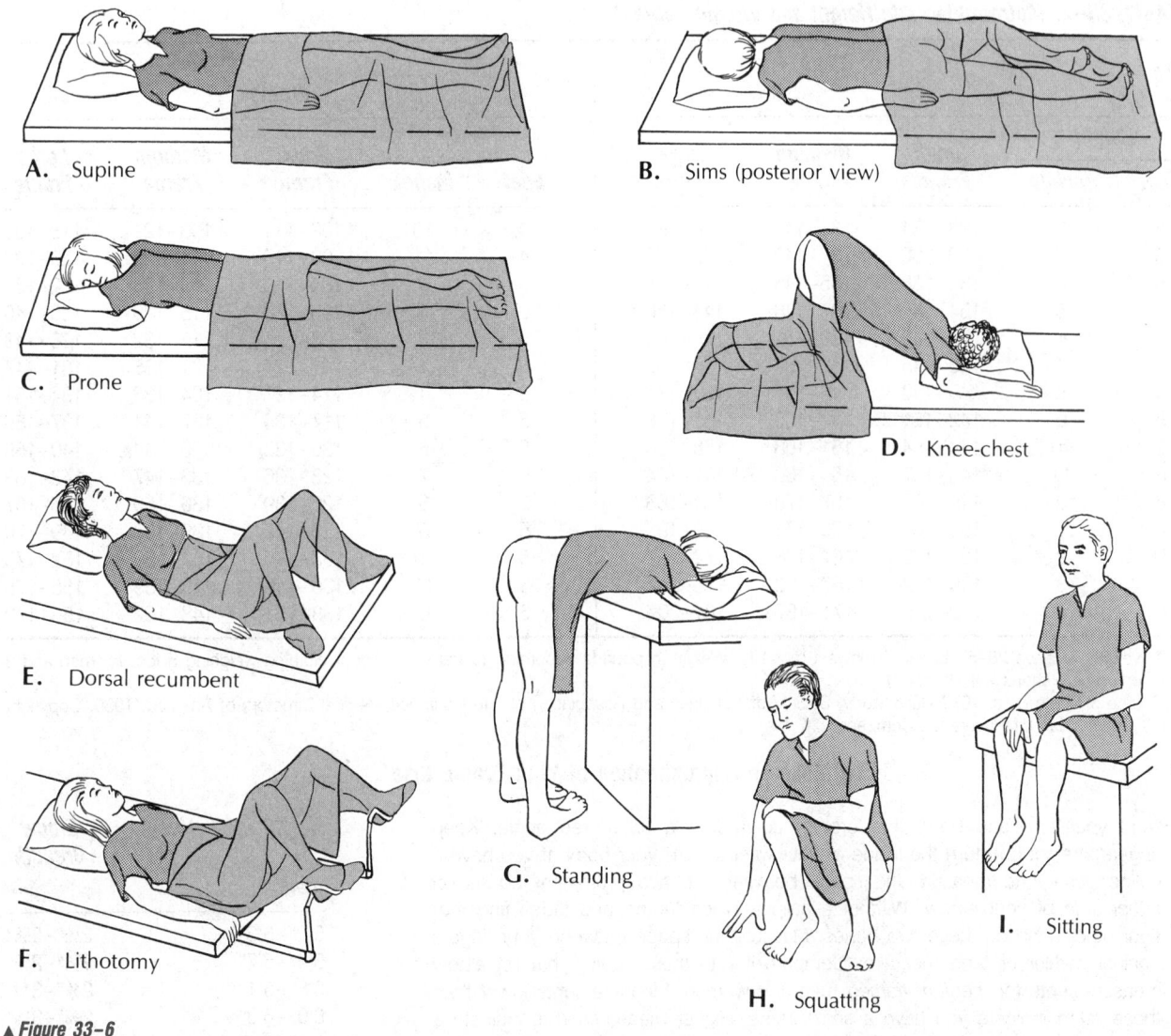

A. Supine

B. Sims (posterior view)

C. Prone

D. Knee-chest

E. Dorsal recumbent

F. Lithotomy

G. Standing

H. Squatting

I. Sitting

▲ Figure 33–6

Common examination positions.

the physical assessment examination, or you may wait to assess these during the examination of specific body systems. For example, the temperature may be obtained during assessment of the general appearance of the person, and pulse rate may be assessed during the examination of the heart. Respirations may be assessed during examination of the chest (thorax).

Height and Weight

Height and weight are important to assess to provide baseline data (Table 33–2). They also provide data regarding a person's general health and nutritional status. When assessing height, the person should be instructed to remove the shoes. A clean paper towel should be placed on the scale platform. The person is asked to turn and face the direction opposite the balance beam and stand erect on the scale platform. A height measurement rod that is attached to the scale raises up, and a level piece swings out and over the

person's head. To prevent trauma to the person, raise the measuring rod well above head level before swinging out the level piece and lowering it to the person's head. Height in inches or centimeters will be displayed at approximately eye level on the measuring rod.

Weight is also assessed while the person stands on the scale platform. Adjust the weight on the balance beam until the tip of the beam registers in the middle of the mark. Chair and stretcher scales are available for the nonweight-bearing person. Practice with this equipment before attempting to use it with clients.

General Appearance

The following areas are to be considered when assessing a person's general appearance (you may have obtained some of this information when taking the client history):

▶ Age: A person's age may influence the physical characteristics observed by the nurse. For example,

TABLE 33–2. Metropolitan Life Height and Weight Tables*

A

	Men					Women			
Height		**Small Frame**	**Medium Frame**	**Large Frame**		**Height**		**Small Frame**	**Medium Frame**	**Large Frame**
Feet	*Inches*					*Feet*	*Inches*			

Feet	Inches	Small Frame	Medium Frame	Large Frame	Feet	Inches	Small Frame	Medium Frame	Large Frame
5	2	128–134	131–141	138–150	4	10	102–111	109–121	118–131
5	3	130–136	133–143	140–153	4	11	103–113	111–123	120–134
5	4	132–138	135–145	142–156	5	0	104–115	113–126	122–137
5	5	134–140	137–148	144–160	5	1	106–118	115–129	125–140
5	6	136–142	139–151	146–164	5	2	108–121	118–132	128–143
5	7	138–145	142–154	149–168	5	3	111–124	121–135	131–147
5	8	140–148	145–157	152–172	5	4	114–127	124–138	134–151
5	9	142–151	148–160	155–176	5	5	117–130	127–141	137–155
5	10	144–154	151–163	158–180	5	6	120–133	130–144	140–159
5	11	146–157	154–166	161–184	5	7	123–136	133–147	143–163
6	0	149–160	157–170	164–188	5	8	126–139	136–150	146–167
6	1	152–164	160–174	168–192	5	9	129–142	139–153	149–170
6	2	155–168	164–178	172–197	5	10	132–145	142–156	152–173
6	3	158–172	167–182	176–202	5	11	135–148	145–159	155–176
6	4	162–176	171–187	181–207	6	0	138–151	148–162	158–179

* Weights at ages 25–59 based on lowest mortality. Weight in pounds according to frame (in indoor clothing weighing 5 lbs. for men and 3 lbs. for women; shoes with 1" heels).

Source of basic data: 1979 Build Study, Society of Actuaries and Association of Life Insurance Medical Directors of America, 1980. Copyright 1983 Metropolitan Life Insurance Company.

B **To Make an Approximation of Your Frame Size . . .**

Extend your arm and bend the forearm upward at a 90-degree angle. Keep fingers straight and turn the inside of your wrist toward your body. If you have a caliper, use it to measure the space between the two prominent bones on *either side* of your elbow. Without a caliper, place thumb and index finger of your other hand on these two bones. Measure the space between your fingers against a ruler or tape measure. Compare it with these tables that list elbow measurements for *medium-framed* men and women. Measurements lower than those listed indicate you have a small frame. Higher measurements indicate a large frame.

Height in 1" Heels	Elbow Breadth
Men	
5'2"–5'3"	2½"–2⅞"
5'4"–5'7"	2⅝"–2⅞"
5'8"–5'11"	2¾"–3"
6'0"–6'3"	2¾"–3⅛"
6'4"	2⅞"–3¼"
Women	
4'10"–4'11"	2¼"–2½"
5'0"–5'3"	2¼"–2½"
5'4"–5'7"	2⅜"–2⅝"
5'8"–5'11"	2⅜"–2⅝"
6'0"	2½"–2¾"

an elderly person may exhibit the normal physiologic changes of aging, such as loose, wrinkled skin, kyphosis (stooped posture), and a slowed, stiff gait.

▶ Race and sex: The sex of a person can influence the type of examination being performed. Sex and race can influence different physical characteristics observed by the nurse.

▶ Body type, posture, and gait: Assessment of body type, posture, and gait can provide data related to a person's general level of health. Observe a person's build as thin, average, or obese. Note whether the person assumes an erect, bent, or slouched posture. Observe the person's style of walking for smoothness and coordination.

▶ Nutritional status: A person's nutritional state can reflect the level of general health. It can also affect physical characteristics observed by the nurse.

Mental Status and Speech

The assessment of a person's mental status and speech can begin during the client health history. As you collect information concerning the history, observations can be made regarding grooming, dress, and hygiene as well as the person's judgment, orientation, memory, affect, consciousness, and speech (see Chapter 32).

To obtain a complete and detailed assessment of mental status, it will be helpful for you to remember the acronym J-O-M-A-C-S (judgment, orientation, memory, affect, consciousness, speech).

GROOMING, DRESS, AND HYGIENE

During the mental status assessment, you will be making observations regarding the person's grooming, type of dress, and hygiene. Some questions you may ask yourself are is the person clean and well-kept? Are the person's hair, skin, and nails clean and well-groomed? Is the clothing appropriate for the present weather conditions and season?

When making these observations, you must also consider the person's lifestyle, cultural orientation, peer group interaction, socioeconomic group, and age. A person may appear to have poor hygiene and grooming habits as a result of pain and weakness that may prevent normal activities of daily living, poor self-esteem, depression, or organic brain syndrome; or poor hygiene may be a result of peer group norms. Elderly individuals will wear extra clothing related to sensitivity changes in body temperature.

JUDGMENT

A person's judgment can be affected by the level of intelligence, educational level, socioeconomic level, and cultural orientation. When assessing this area you may ask the person, "What do you do at a stop sign?" "What do you wear when it is raining?" or "Who will be taking care of your children while you are in the hospital?" You can assess the person's judgment by noting the responses given to each of these questions.

To assess abstract thinking, you may ask the person to interpret a proverb. Some proverbs you might use are "Don't look a gift horse in the mouth," "A rolling stone gathers no moss," or "A stitch in time saves nine." The person who can correctly explain the meaning of "Don't look a gift horse in the mouth," for example, is capable of abstract thought. However, a person who interprets this proverb by saying "Don't look in a horse's mouth if it is a gift" is thinking on a concrete level. You need to remember that persons for whom English is a second language may translate the proverb literally and may not comprehend the abstract meaning of the proverb.

ORIENTATION

An assessment is made of a person's orientation to person, place, and time. To assess "person," you may ask the individual, "What is your name?" To assess "place," you may ask the person, "Where are you?" or "Where do you live?" To assess "time," you may ask the person, "What time of day is it?" "What day of the week is it?" or "What is the date and year?"

MEMORY

When assessing memory, you need to test the person's immediate, recent, and remote memory. Immediate memory is tested by reciting a series of seven digits and asking the person to repeat the digits back to you. Normally, a person should be able to repeat seven digits without great difficulty. Choose digits such as zip codes or telephone numbers. Make sure the digits are not in consecutive order.

Recent memory is tested by asking questions that apply to events of the day. Questions may be asked concerning what the person ate for breakfast, weather conditions of the day, and what types of tests the person had during the day. Be sure that you know the answers to each of these questions in order to check the accuracy of the person's memory.

Remote memory is tested by inquiring about past events, such as types of employment, mother's maiden name, birthday and anniversary dates, and social security number. Again, you must be sure of the accuracy of the information the person is giving you to arrive at an accurate assessment.

AFFECT

Affect is an emotional state, such as fear, anger, depression, elation, and frustration. As you observe the person, note the lack of emotional response or the presence of outward manifestations that may suggest emotion. Does the person smile, frown, exhibit anger, or cry appropriately according to the situation being discussed? Keep in mind that cultural norms may dictate one's affect.

CONSCIOUSNESS

The assessment of consciousness begins with noting whether the client is awake and alert. While communicating, note whether the person is able to answer your questions appropriately and within a reasonably quick time frame. If the person has an altered level of consciousness, assess whether the person is demonstrating obtundation, stupor, or coma.

SPEECH

Throughout the client health history and physical examination, you need to note the characteristics of the person's speech. Speech is assessed for quantity (talkative or silent), rate (fast or slow), loudness, and enunciation.

Integument

The integumentary system serves as a source of protection for the body from the environment, as a body temperature regulator, and as a sensor for temperature, pain, and touch. The layers of the skin tissue are the epidermis, dermis, and subcutaneous tissue. When assessing the skin, you may choose to assess the entire skin surface at one time or as a part of each body system. The assessment techniques used with the integumentary system are inspection, palpation, and olfaction.

Areas to consider when assessing the skin are color, temperature, texture, mobility, lesions, and vascularity. Prior to beginning your assessment, make sure that you have a good light source. Have a pair of sterile gloves ready in case you encounter a draining skin lesion, for it will require palpation. Skin odors, if any, usually will be detected in skin folds or in the axillary area.

COLOR

Inspect the skin for generalized color. Skin color will vary according to body part. A person's race will also affect skin color. The color of the skin will range from light to dark pink, light to dark brown, or yellow to olive. Assess those areas of least pigmentation for any possible color changes such as the palms, soles, sclera, and nails.

Abnormal changes in skin color include cyanosis, jaundice, and pallor. **Cyanosis,** a bluish mottled discoloration of the skin, nailbeds, and mucous membranes, caused by decreased oxygenation of the blood, can best be assessed in the legs, buccal mucosa, and tongue. In persons with darker skin tones, cyanosis may be detected better in the palms, soles, palpebral conjunctiva, and nails. **Jaundice,** a yellow discoloration of the skin resulting from an increase in bilirubin, may be assessed in the bulbar and palpebral conjunctiva, lips, hard palate, posterior aspect of the tongue, and the skin itself. **Pallor** is an absence of color in the skin, which appears whitish-gray in a light-skinned person and ashen gray or as a loss of red glow tones in a person with dark skin. Pallor is best assessed in the fingernails, lips, mucous membranes, and palpebral conjunctiva.

TEMPERATURE AND MOISTURE

Skin temperature should remain relatively the same over the entire body. When there is a change in temperature over a body area, it is an indication of a change in blood circulation to that part of the body. Palpation is the technique used in assessing skin temperature. Temperature is best assessed using the dorsum or back of the hand. Normally, the skin temperature is warm. Excessive coolness or warmth indicates a deviation from normal.

Skin moisture is assessed by inspection and palpation. Normally, the skin should be dry to touch with the exception of skin folds and the axilla, which normally are moist. Moisture refers to wetness and oiliness. Palpate the skin for temperature and moisture. Compare similar body parts in relation to temperature and moisture.

TEXTURE

The skin's texture should be smooth, soft, and flexible over the majority of the body. Normally, some areas such as the palms and the soles possess a thicker texture. The skin should be palpated to assess texture. Note the location of areas where there are irregularities in texture.

TURGOR AND MOBILITY

Skin turgor is an indication of hydration status, assessed by pinching up the skin and releasing it. It denotes the skin's elasticity. To assess skin turgor, pinch up the skin on the forehead, sternum, dorsum of the hand, or forearm, and release. You should note the speed at which the skin returns to its former state. Normally, the skin returns to its original position quickly (Fig. 33-7). Skin turgor is classified as poor when it takes 3 seconds or longer for the skin to return to its original position.

As a result of age, the elderly person loses skin elasticity. You may note upon examination that the skin turgor of an elderly person will show a delayed response. Skin turgor and mobility will be diminished when edema is present.

LESIONS

Normally, the skin should be free of lesions. Primary lesions arise from normal skin tissue. Secondary lesions occur as a result of changes in the primary lesion. If you observe a lesion on the skin, note the size in centimeters, location, distribution (localized or generalized), pattern (linear, clustered, or annular), color, and type. Palpate the lesion to denote mobility (fixed or mobile), contour (flat or raised), and consistency (soft or hard). Be sure to wear sterile gloves when palpating draining lesions. Table 33-3 summarizes some common skin lesions.

VASCULARITY

Vascularity involves the blood circulation of the skin and the appearance of superficial blood vessels. **Petechiae** (minute hemorrhages under the skin) and ecchymosis can result from abnormal vascularity. Petechiae are tiny purple or red spots on the skin. **Ecchymosis** (bruising) is a discoloration of an area of the skin. **Edema** is an accumulation of excessive fluid in the interstitial spaces. The area will appear swollen, shiny, and taut. On inspection, you should note the location and the appearance. During palpation, you should note mobility, consistency, and tenderness.

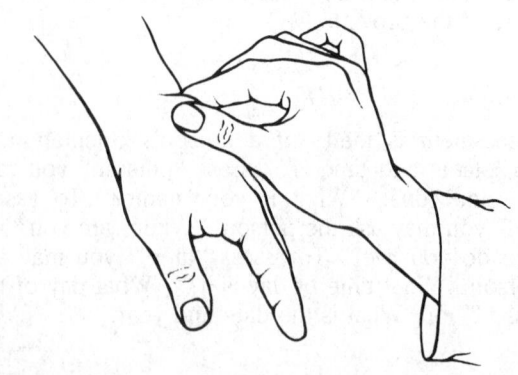

▲ *Figure 33-7*

Assessing skin turgor.

TABLE 33-3. Skin Lesions

Lesion	Characteristics	Example
Primary Lesions		
Macule	Small, up to 1 cm	Freckle, petechia
Patch	Larger than 1 cm	Vitiligo
Papule	Up to 0.5 cm	Elevated nevus
Plaque	Flat, uneven surface larger than 0.5 cm	Coalescence of papules
Nodule	0.5 cm to 1–2 cm, deeper and firmer than a papule	Wart

Table continued on following page

TABLE 33–3. Skin Lesions Continued

Lesion		Characteristics	Example
Primary Lesions			
	Tumor	Elevated and deep, larger than 1–2 cm	Epithelioma
	Wheal	Area of localized skin edema	Insect bite
	Vesicle	Contains serous fluid Up to 0.5 cm	Blister
	Bulla	Contains serous fluid Greater than 0.5 cm	Second-degree burn
	Pustule	Filled with pus	Acne
Secondary Lesions			
	Ulcer	Deep loss of skin surface	Venous stasis ulcer

TABLE 33-3. Skin Lesions Continued

Lesion		Characteristics	Example
Primary Lesions			

	Fissure	Linear crack in the skin	Athlete's foot
	Crust	Dried residue of serum, pus, or blood	Impetigo
	Scale	Thin flake of exfoliated epidermis	Dandruff, dry skin

As tissue fluid increases, pitting edema will occur. Upon palpation, you will note that your finger leaves an indention in the edematous area. To test for the degree of pitting edema, press your finger into the edematous area for 2 to 3 seconds and note the depth of the indentation. Pitting edema is described on a scale from 1+ to 4+. Table 33-4 demonstrates the degrees of edema. A measuring tape may also be used to measure edema. You would indicate the exact measure of one body part and compare it with the other body part. Both measurements would be charted.

Head and Neck

CRANIAL NERVES

The assessment of the cranial nerves is a crucial aspect of the neurologic system assessment. The cranial nerves originate from the brain stem with the exception of the olfactory nerve, which is located in the temporal lobe, and the optic nerve, which is located in the occipital lobe. Since many of the tests for cranial nerve function also measure various structures and muscles within the head and neck, assessment of cranial nerves is included in the section on head and neck.

To learn and remember the cranial nerves, you may associate the name and type of nerve with several phrases.

To remember the name of each cranial nerve, learn the following sentence: "On old Olympus' towering tops, a Finn and German viewed some hops." The first letter in each word is the same as the first letter in each of the cranial nerves. To remember the type (sensory, motor, or both) of each cranial nerve, learn the following phrase: "Some say marry money but my brother says bad business marry money." The first letter of each word represents sensory, motor, or both types. Each

TABLE 33-4. Grades of Edema

	Grade	Characteristics
	1+	Slight pit, normal contour
	2+	Deeper pit, fairly normal contour
	3+	Puffy appearance, deeper pit
	4+	Extremely deep pit, definitively swollen

Illustrations from Judge, R., et al. (1982). *Clinical diagnosis* (4th ed.). Boston: Little, Brown.

word corresponds to one cranial nerve. For example, "Some" represents the sensory function of the olfactory nerve. Table 33-5 summarizes the functions of the cranial nerves.

When assessing the head and neck, you will be using the techniques of inspection, palpation, and auscultation. Assessment of the head and neck encompasses assessment of the head, eyes, ears, nose and sinuses, mouth and pharynx, and neck.

HEAD

When assessing the head, you will be inspecting and palpating the hair, scalp, skull, and face. You will begin your assessment by asking if the person has noted any changes in relation to the hair and scalp.

Hair. Inspect the hair for quality, quantity, and distribution. The quality of the hair refers to the texture and color of the hair. Terms used to describe the texture are coarse and fine. A sudden change in texture, such as dryness, brittleness, or fragility, may indicate a bodily dysfunction. An increase in dryness and coarseness of the hair may indicate hypothyroidism, whereas an increase in silkiness and fineness may indicate hyperthyroidism. You will need to observe for nits, which are tiny, white, ovoid eggs of lice. The color of a person's hair will be significant only when there has been a sudden change in it. This may indicate nerve injury involvement.

The quantity and distribution of a person's hair will vary with age. You will need to inspect for any areas of alopecia (partial or complete loss of hair). This can be a result of normal aging, an endocrine disorder, a drug reaction, or skin disease. Also, observe for any abnormal facial hair.

Scalp and Skull. When inspecting and palpating the scalp and skull, it is important to separate the hair and take a thorough look at the skin underlying the hair. You will be observing for areas of inflammation, cysts, warts, moles, insect bites, flaking, and scaliness. If you observe any masses, be sure to describe the size, shape, consistency, and location.

Palpation of the scalp and skull involves using a rotary motion with the pads of your fingers. You will begin with the frontal region (forehead) and palpate over the entire skull to the occipital region. This includes palpating the temporal and parietal regions. You will be inspecting and palpating the skull for size, shape, symmetry, and tenderness.

Face. Inspect the face for size, shape, symmetry, and any tics or abnormal movements. A good reference point for asymmetry of the face is the palpebral fissures of the eyes and the nasolabial folds. The palpebral fissures are the spaces between the upper and lower eyelids (Fig. 33-8). They should be equal in size when comparing the right and left fissure. The nasolabial folds are creases that extend from the angle of the nose to the corner of the mouth. They should be bilaterally symmetrical.

TABLE 33–5. Cranial Nerve Functions

Cranial Nerve Number	Name	Type	Function
I	Olfactory	Sensory	Smell
II	Optic	Sensory	Visual fields
			Visual acuity
			Color discrimination
			Vision
III	Oculomotor	Motor	Pupil constriction and dilation
			Convergence
			Extraocular movement
IV	Trochlear	Motor	Extraocular movement
V	Trigeminal	Sensory and motor	Corneal sensitivity
			Sensation to skin of face
			Motor nerve to masseter and temporal muscles
VI	Abducens	Motor	Extraocular movement
VII	Facial	Sensory and motor	Facial expression
			Taste (anterior tongue)
VIII	Auditory	Sensory	Hearing
IX	Glossopharyngeal	Sensory and motor	Gag reflex
			Taste (posterior tongue)
X	Vagus	Sensory and motor	Sensation of the pharnyx
			Swallowing ability
			Vocal cord movement
XI	Spinal Accessory	Motor	Head and shoulder movement
XII	Hypoglossal	Motor	Tongue movement

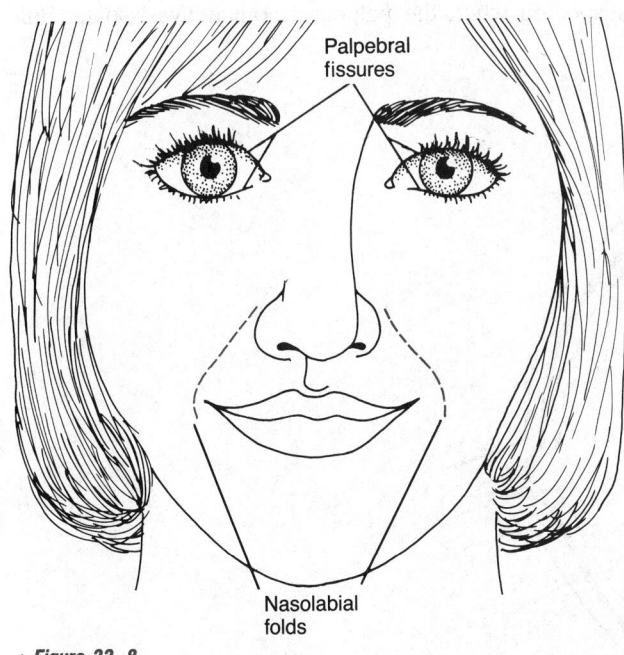

▲ **Figure 33–8**

To assess facial symmetry, observe the palpebral fissures and nasolabial folds. They should be equal bilaterally.

During the inspection and palpation of the face, test the function of the trigeminal and facial cranial nerves.

Trigeminal Nerve. The trigeminal nerve (CN V) has a motor and sensory function. The motor function of the trigeminal nerve is to innervate the muscles used in chewing. To test this function, ask the person to clench the teeth while you palpate the temporal muscles (temporal area) and the masseter muscles (jaw area). Note the strength of muscle contraction. A weakness or absence on one side may indicate a trigeminal nerve lesion.

The trigeminal nerve also innervates the nasal and oral mucosa, facial skin, and corneal reflex through its sensory branches. To test the sensory function, instruct the person to close the eyes. With a safety pin, touch the forehead, cheeks, and jaw area with the point of the safety pin, intermittently substituting the blunt end of the pin. Have the person tell you whether it is sharp or dull. Be sure to compare each side of the face. The sensory function related to the corneas will be discussed when examination of the eyes is described.

Facial Nerve. The facial nerve has sensory and motor functions. The sensory function will be discussed in relation to the mouth. To test the motor function, ask the person to smile, frown, raise the eyebrows, close the eyes tightly, and puff out the cheeks. Observe for asymmetry and weakness.

Eyes. Inspection and palpation are used to assess the eyes (Fig. 33–9). Areas to be assessed are the position and alignment of the eyes, eyebrows, eyelids, lacrimal apparatus, conjunctiva and sclera, pupils, and cranial nerves (occulomotor, trochlear, abducens, trigeminal, and optic). The desirable position for a person during the examination is sitting, if possible, looking straight ahead unless otherwise noted.

Position and Alignment. When inspecting the eyes for position and alignment, ask yourself: Are the eyes in line with the top of the ears? When you and the person look at each other, is the person's gaze focused directly on yours and do the eyes look alike? Normally, the upper quadrant of the iris cannot be seen when you are facing the person because the eyelid covers it. Any abnormal protrusion of the eyes is called exophthalmos.

Eyebrows. Inspect the quantity and distribution of the eyebrows. Ask the person if the eyebrows have been plucked. Observe for scarring, lesions, and hair loss. Hair loss may indicate a fungal infection.

Eyelids. Inspect the eyelids for symmetry, position in relation to the eyeballs, inflammation, lesions (chalazion, sty), edema, and **ptosis** (drooping of the eyelid). Drooping of the eyelid may indicate oculomotor damage because the oculomotor nerve (CN III) innervates the upper lid to open and remain open. Inspect the eyelashes, which should be full and extend outward along the entire eyelid. Crusting, scaling, and hair loss are signs of infection.

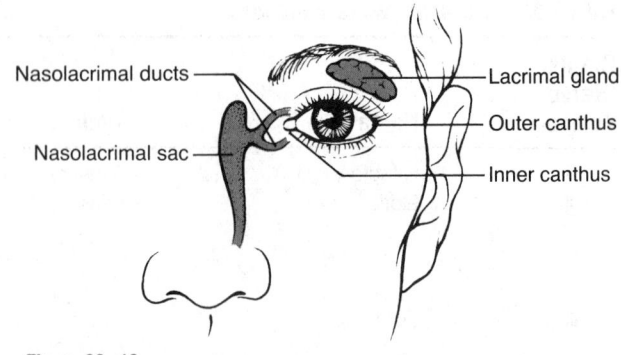

▲ *Figure 33–10*

The lacrimal apparatus.

Lacrimal Apparatus. The lacrimal apparatus comprises the lacrimal gland, sacs, ducts, and the nasolacrimal ducts (Fig. 33–10). The puncta are openings located in the inner canthus of the upper and lower eyelid. The major function of this apparatus is to create tears. Tears keep the eyes moist and clean. Upon inspection, note any excessive dryness or tearing of the eye. Gently palpate the inner canthus and observe the fluid from the puncta. A purulent fluid indicates infection.

Conjunctivae and Sclerae. The conjunctiva is a membrane that protects the outer surface of the sclera and the inner surface of the eyelids. The conjunctiva that covers the sclera is called bulbar. Palpebral conjunctiva covers the inner surfaces of the upper and lower eyelids. Inspect the palpebral conjunctiva and sclera by pulling down the lower lid while instructing the person to look up. Inspect for lesions, inflammation, and swelling. Normally, the palpebral conjunctiva is reddish in color due to tiny blood vessels. Anemia is suspected when the palpebral conjunctiva is pale. Bul-

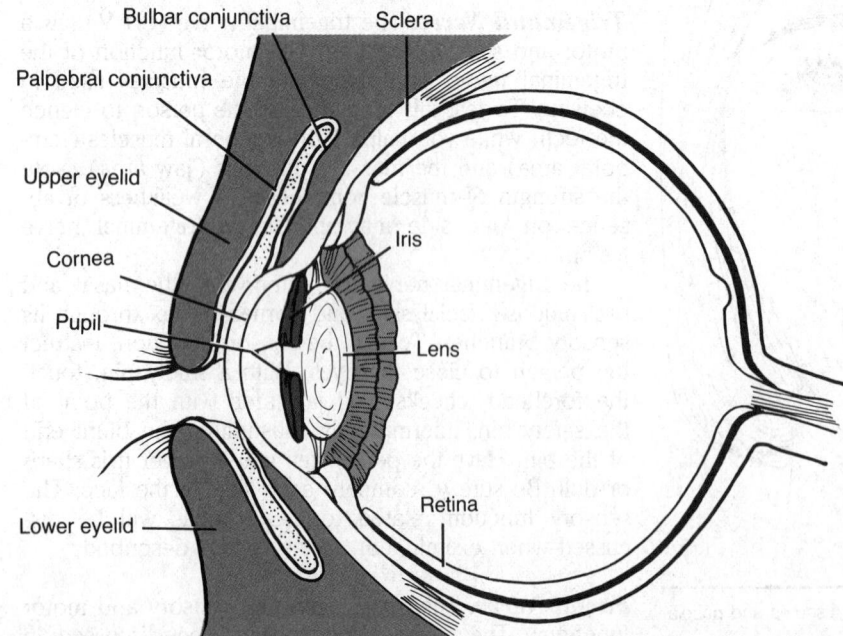

▲ *Figure 33–9*

Eye structures.

bar conjunctiva is clear but appears white due to the sclera being located beneath it. When the bulbar conjunctiva is yellow, it is indicative of jaundice. The sclera is white. You will note a yellowish color to the sclera in dark-skinned people. Because of this, you will need to ask the person if a change has been observed in the color of the sclera.

The palpebral conjunctiva of the upper eyelid is inspected when a foreign body is suspected. This requires eversion of the upper eyelid, which is an advanced skill. Therefore, it will not be discussed in this chapter.

Pupils. Inspect the pupils for equality, size, shape, reaction to light, and accommodation. The oculomotor (CN III), trochlear (CN IV), and abducens (CN VI) nerves are tested at this time because they innervate pupillary constriction. Pupillary reaction to light and accommodation test these three cranial nerves.

Normal pupillary function is documented as "PERRLA:" Pupils Equal, Round, React to Light and Accommodation.

Pupillary Reaction. Pupillary reaction to light is assessed by the direct and consensual light reflex. A penlight is used to assess this reflex. Instruct the person to focus on a distant object. This is important so that the pupils do not constrict in an attempt to focus on something close or because they are looking at you. Shine the penlight into the pupil of one eye (about 8 inches away from the eye). Observe the reaction to the light in both eyes. Normally, the illuminated pupil constricts (direct light) and the other pupil constricts simultaneously (consensual response). Test both pupils. If you should have difficulty assessing pupillary constriction, darken the room and use a bright light before making the judgment that pupillary reaction is absent. Intracranial pressure can affect the pupil's reaction to light.

Accommodation. Accommodation (eye's adaptation for near vision) is tested by asking the person to focus on a distant object, then on a near object. You may use your finger, a pencil, or an unlit penlight, holding it 8 to 12 inches from the bridge of the nose. Instruct the person alternately to look at the object and then into the distance. Normally, the pupils should converge and constrict symmetrically as the eyes focus on a near object.

Oculomotor, Trochlear, Abducens Nerves. In addition to innervating pupillary constriction (see pupils), the oculomotor, trochlear, and abducens nerves control the horizontal, vertical, and diagonal movements of the eyes. The cardinal positions test, cover-uncover test, and the corneal light reflex test are used to assess extraocular movements of the eye.

Cardinal Positions Test. To perform the cardinal positions test, hold your finger or a pencil about 6 to 12 inches from the person's eyes. Instruct the person to follow it with the eyes while keeping the head still.

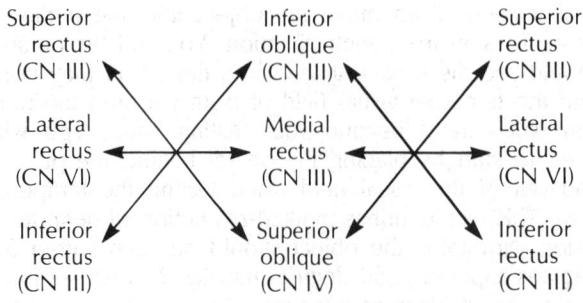

SIX CARDINAL POSITIONS OF GAZE

▲ *Figure 33-11*

Six cardinal positions of gaze.

Take the person through the six cardinal positions of gaze (Fig. 33-11). Pause at each position in order to detect nystagmus (abnormal rhythmic oscillations of the eyes).

Cover-Uncover Test. To perform the cover-uncover test, instruct the person to stare directly at an object with both eyes. Take a card and cover one eye for 10 seconds, remove it, and observe any movement in the once-covered eye as it attempts to refocus on the designated object. Repeat on the opposite eye. Normally, no movement will be noted. If movement is observed, this signifies a muscle imbalance (strabismus).

Corneal Light Reflex Test. To test for the corneal light reflex, stand about 2 feet directly in front of the person. Shine your penlight at the bridge of the nose and inspect the reflections in the person's corneas. The cornea should reflect the light in exactly the same place in both eyes. An asymmetrical reflex indicates strabismus.

Trigeminal Nerve. To assess another aspect of the sensory function of the trigeminal nerve (CN V), you will assess the corneal reflex. This is a higher level assessment skill and should not be attempted without supervision. Be sure to explain the procedure to the person before proceeding. Using a small piece of cotton, gently stroke the cornea of the eye. The normal reaction should be a blink. Test both eyes. Remember to use a separate piece of cotton for each eye to avoid cross-contamination. If the person does not have a normal response, a trigeminal lesion is suspected.

Optic Nerve. To assess the optic nerve (CN II), the person is tested for visual fields, visual acuity, color discrimination, and abnormalities of the inner eye structures (ophthalmoscopic examination).

A person's visual field is the entire area seen by the eye when it is focused on a designated point. Instruct the person to sit 2 feet in front of you. Your eyes should be at the same level as those of the person being tested. Have the person cover one eye and stare at your eye directly opposite. Close your other eye. You may use a pencil or your fingers to test the person. Instruct the person to answer when the pencil or finger is first seen. Then move the object into the person's field of vision from each direction. You and the person should see the object at the same time. You may note that the temporal visual field of both you and the person will extend beyond your testing hand. You will need to start by placing the object behind the person and out of the visual field when testing the temporal area. This test identifies marked restriction of peripheral vision. Normally, the object should be seen within 50 degrees superiorly, 60 degrees nasally, 70 degrees inferiorly, and 90 degrees temporally.

Distance Visual Acuity. A Snellen chart is a chart used to test a person's visual acuity (see Fig. 33–1). The Snellen chart has numbers at the end of each line of letters. The numerator is always 20, which is the distance in feet between the chart and the person being examined. The denominator is the distance at which a person with normal vision can read a particular line. For example, 20/30 means that a person stood 20 feet away to read a line that a person with normal vision can read at 30 feet away. As the denominator increases, the distance vision decreases. Test each eye separately by covering the other eye with the person's hand or card. Then test both eyes uncovered. If the person wears corrective lenses, the lenses may be worn for the test. Standing 20 feet away, the person is instructed to read the smallest, clearest line. A person must be able to read a line correctly with no more than two errors. The line read then indicates the person's distance visual acuity.

Near Visual Acuity. When testing near visual acuity, a newspaper with various sizes of print may be used. Hold the newspaper 6 to 12 inches from the face. Instruct the person to read several lines. Test each eye separately and then together.

Color Discrimination. To test color discrimination, have the person distinguish colors, usually red and green. You may use the Snellen chart for this test since it has various colors on it.

Ophthalmoscopic Examination. To perform the ophthalmoscopic examination, the room must be darkened. Instruct the person to stare at a designated spot. Standing in front of the person, about 18 inches away and 15 degrees to the right of the person's line of vision, shine the light of the ophthalmoscope on the pupil. To steady yourself, it might help to place your opposite hand on the person's forehead.

The ophthalmoscope should be set at 0 diopters, and your index finger should be placed on the lens selector. As the light of the ophthalmoscope enters the pupil, move the lens selector until you have the various structures in focus. Try to keep both your eyes open, as this decreases the blurriness experienced.

You should observe the following: (1) red reflex, which indicates that the lens is free of opacity (cataract) and clouding; and (2) retinal structures, which include the retinal vessels, retinal background, optic disk, and macula (Fig. 33–12). If you have difficulty finding the optic disk, look for a retinal blood vessel

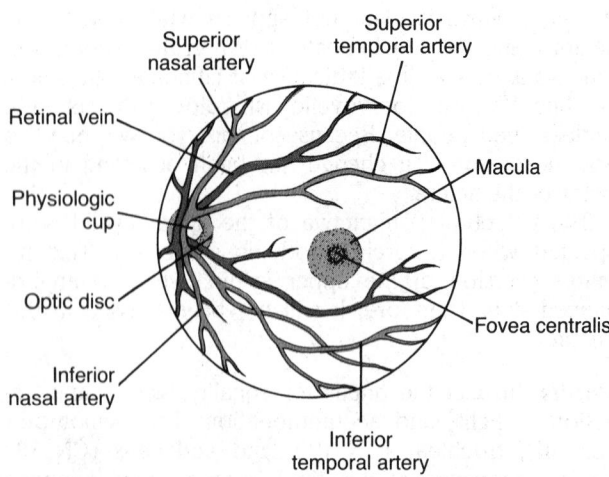

▲ *Figure 33–12*

Fundus of the eye.

and follow the vessel nasally. The vessels become larger in diameter as they enter the optic disk. Evaluate the size, shape, and arteriovenous crossing of the blood vessels. Normal arteries will not displace or indent veins. The arteries will be a light red, and the veins will be larger and darker in color. The ratio of arteries to veins is 4:5. The optic disk is a round, yellowish orange to creamy pink structure. It should be lighter than the retinal background. The macula should be examined last since it is the area of the retina with the greatest visual acuity and sensitivity to light. It is located temporal to the optic disk. When inspecting the retinal background and structures, assess any areas of hemorrhage, cotton wool patch, arteriovenous nicking, and papilledema.

Ears. Inspection and palpation are the techniques used to examine the ear. Areas to be assessed are the external ear (auricle) and ear canal, internal ear canal and tympanic membrane (by performing an otoscopic examination), and the acoustic nerve (Fig. 33–13).

Auricles. Inspect the auricle for color, size, configuration, location, and angle of attachment to the head (Fig. 33–14). The color of the ear should be the same as that of the person's skin, and the size should be in proportion to the head. The auricle should be at a level equal to the outer canthus of the eye. Inspect the external ear canal for intactness, general hygiene, a buildup of cerumen (ear wax), discharge, redness, and swelling. The normal ear canal should be clean, dry, free of lesions, and with a minimal amount of cerumen. If discharge is observed, note the color, amount, consistency, and clarity.

Palpate the external ear for nodules and tenderness. The mastoid process is also palpated for tenderness. If the person complains of pain when the auricle is moved up and down, it is indicative of an external ear infection. If palpation elicits pain in the mastoid process, otitis media is a possibility.

Otoscopic Examination. To inspect the internal ear canal and tympanic membrane, an otoscope must be

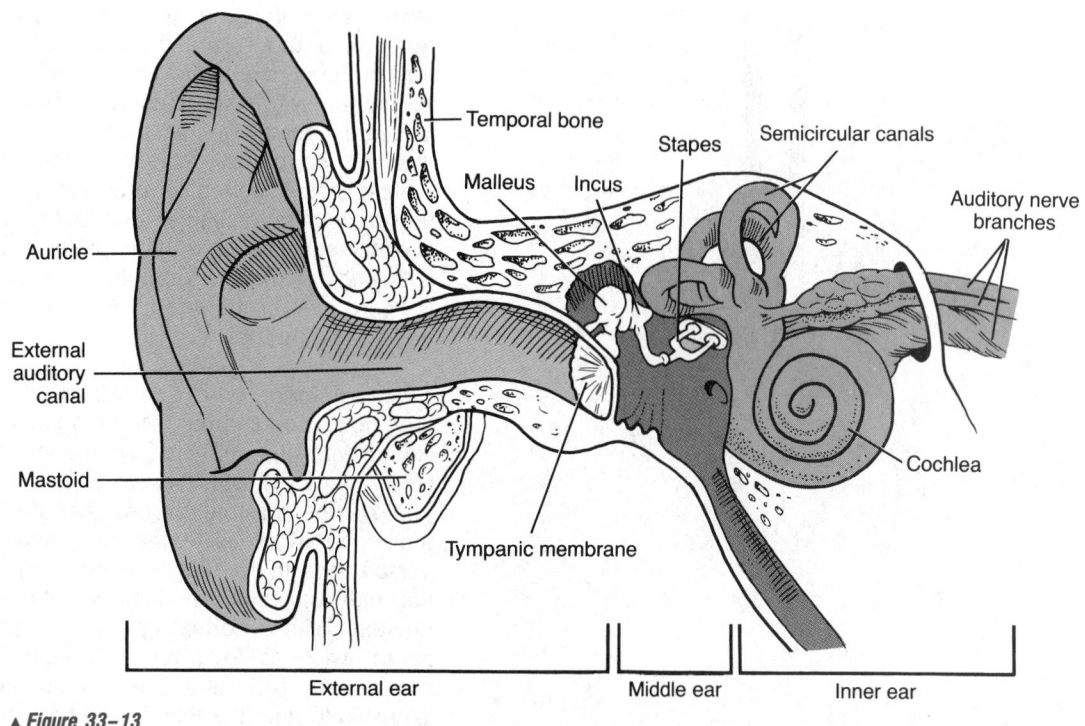

▲ *Figure 33–13*

The external, middle, and inner ear structures.

used. With your dominant hand, hold the otoscope upside down and prop your hand against the person's head. This will prevent any injury to the ear canal in case the person makes a sudden move. Use a speculum large enough to fit the ear comfortably. Instruct the person to tilt the head to the opposite shoulder. With the nondominant hand, pull the auricle up and back to straighten the ear canal. Insert the speculum slowly and cautiously.

Inspect the internal ear canal for impacted cerumen, foreign bodies, discharge, masses, redness, and swelling. Normally, you will view some cerumen, which varies in color (yellow, brown) and consistency (flaky, sticky). Inspect the tympanic membrane (Fig. 33–15), which is usually a shiny pearly gray or light pink. Note the landmarks, which include the handle and short process of the malleus, pars flaccida, pars tensa, and cone of light. The cone of light will be located at five o'clock in the right ear and seven o'clock in the left ear. Observe for perforations, altered or absent landmarks, distorted or absent cone of light, abnormal color, bulging or retraction, discharge, fluid or air bub-

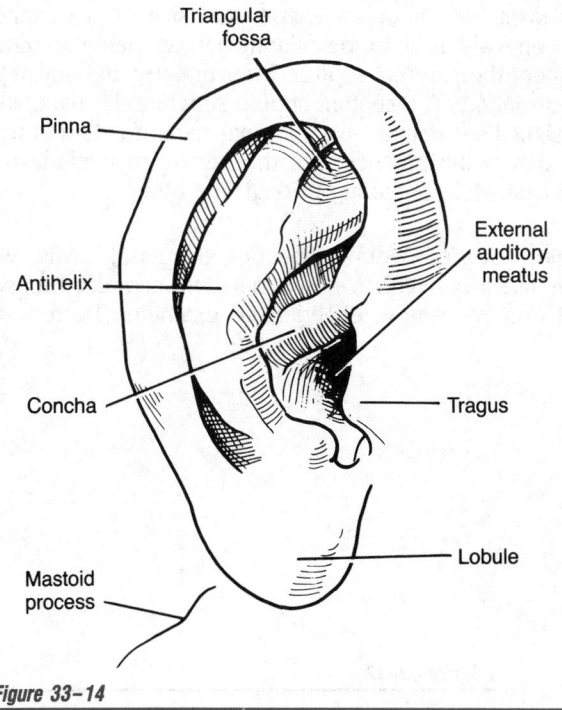

▲ *Figure 33–14*

The auricle.

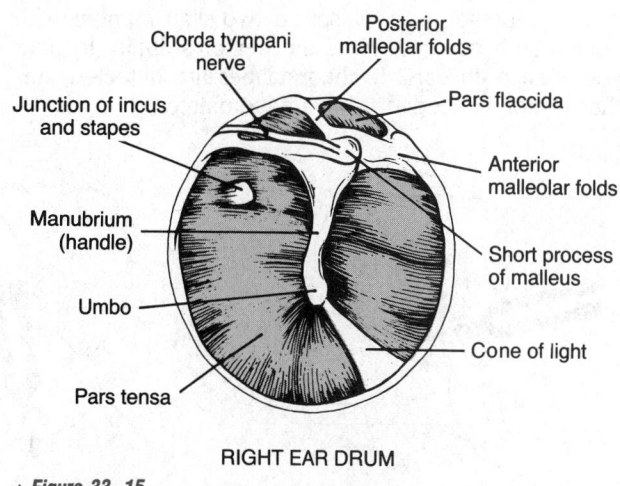

RIGHT EAR DRUM

▲ *Figure 33–15*

A normal tympanic membrane.

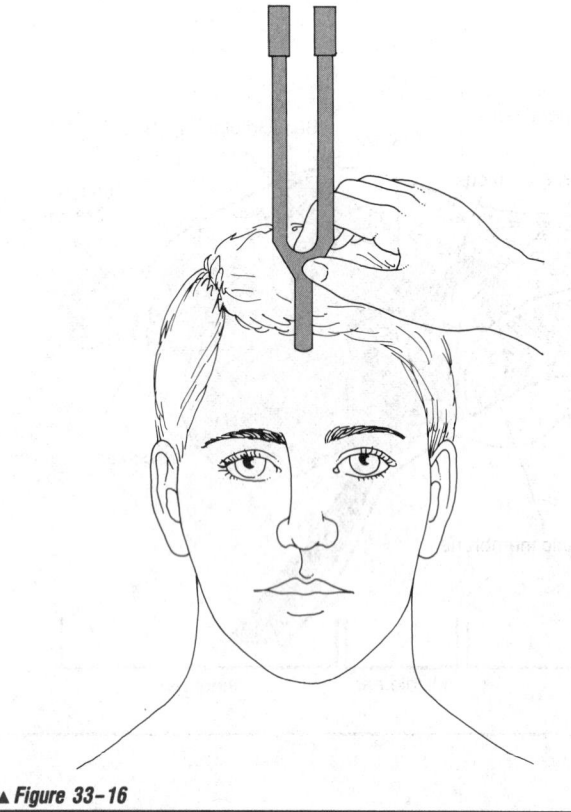

▲ *Figure 33–16*

Weber lateralization test.

bles behind the tympanic membrane, absence of normal movement, and scars.

Acoustic Nerve. The acoustic nerve is assessed by auditory acuity, Weber lateralization test, Rinne air and bone conduction test, and Schwabach test. Auditory acuity is assessed by the watch and whisper test. The watch test screens high-frequency impairment. Instruct the person to occlude one ear. Move a watch toward the person's unoccluded ear and determine the distance at which the person hears the watch. Test both ears. The whisper test is performed by having the person occlude one ear. You will stand 1 to 2 feet away from the person and whisper a two digit number with your mouth covered. Note the person's ability to hear you. Test both ears. If abnormalities are detected, further testing is needed using an audiometer.

Weber Lateralization Test. To perform the Weber lateralization test, place the stem of a vibrating tuning fork in the center of the forehead (Fig. 33–16). Ask the person where the sound is heard best. Normally, sound is heard equally well in both ears as it is conducted through the bones. Note any lateralization of sound (sound heard better in one ear than the other). A person with a unilateral conductive hearing loss will hear the sound best in the impaired ear. This can occur with otitis media, perforation, or an obstruction. Sound is heard best in the good ear with a unilateral sensorineural hearing loss.

Rinne Air and Bone Conduction Test. The Rinne air and bone conduction test compares bone-conducted sound with air-conducted sound in one ear at a time (Fig. 33–17). Place the stem of the vibrating tuning fork on the mastoid process behind the ear. Quickly move the fork beside the ear canal as soon as the person says the sound is gone from contact with the mastoid bone. Placement beside the ear tests air conduction. With a normal (positive) Rinne test, sound is heard twice as long by air conduction as by bone conduction. This finding is documented as AC > BC. You should time the length using a watch.

Schwabach Test. The Schwabach test compares the person's bone conduction with yours. Place the vibrating tuning fork on the person's mastoid process and then on your mastoid process. Continue to move the tuning fork back and forth until the sound is diminished. Normally, the bone conduction should be approximately equal between you and the person being examined.

Nose and Sinuses. The nose is assessed by inspection and palpation. Inspect the external surface of the nose for symmetry in color, shape, and size. It is common for one ala nasi to be slightly larger than the other. Inspect the external septum for symmetry and any signs of deviation. The septum should separate the nares in a straight line. Palpate the external nares for tenderness. To assess the patency, ask the person to occlude one ala nasi while breathing through the other.

Nasal Cavity. When inspecting the nasal cavity, you may use a penlight. A nasal speculum can also be used but only by a more experienced examiner. Instruct the

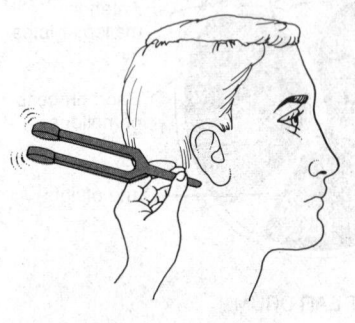
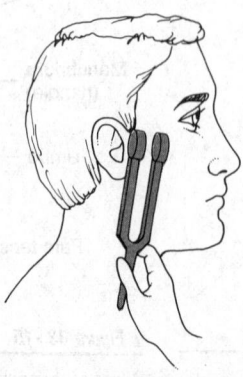

▲ *Figure 33–17*

Rinne air and bone conduction test.

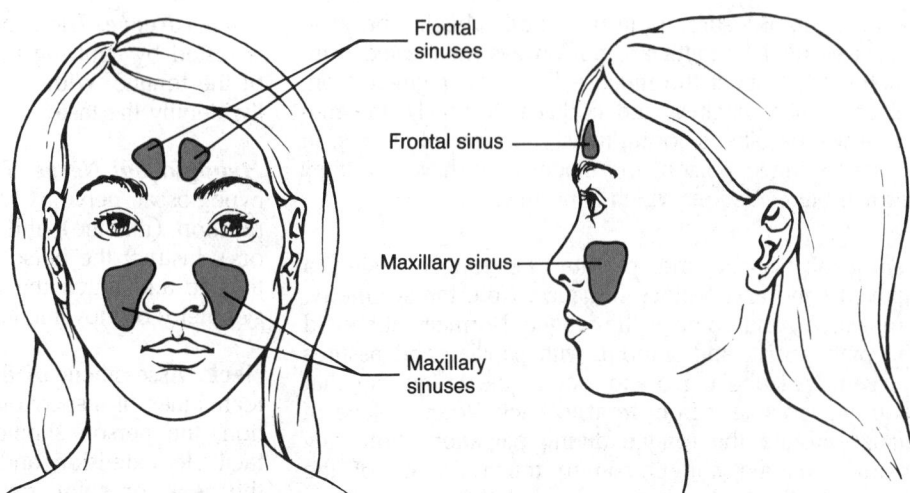

▲ Figure 33-18

Frontal and maxillary sinuses.

person to tilt the head back, then shine the penlight into the nasal cavity. Inspect the mucosa. It should be moist and pink. Note any swelling, lesions, or drainage. Inspect the middle and inferior turbinates. They should be the same color as the adjacent nasal mucosa. Note any pallor, redness, swelling, or polyps.

Frontal and Maxillary Sinuses. The frontal and maxillary sinuses are palpated for tenderness, swelling, thickening, or secretions (Fig. 33-18). Palpate the frontal sinuses by pressing up on the skull on either side of the nose under the eyebrows. Do not press on the eyes. Palpate the maxillary sinuses by pressing up over the lower part of the cheekbones on either side of the nose.

Olfactory Nerve. To assess the sensory function of the olfactory nerve (CN I), instruct the person to close the eyes and occlude one ala nasi. Provide a familiar scent such as coffee or cinnamon for the person to smell. Test both nares. An absence of the sense of smell may result from excessive smoking, cocaine use, or a sinus condition.

Mouth and Pharynx. The mouth and pharynx are assessed through inspection and palpation. Areas to be examined include the lips, buccal mucosa, gums and teeth, tongue, soft and hard palate, pharynx, and glossopharyngeal, vagus, facial, and hypoglossal nerves. A penlight, tongue blade, gauze, and a pair of gloves will be needed to complete the assessment. Remember to wear the gloves when assessing the mucosa of the mouth (Fig. 33-19).

Lips. Inspect the lips for symmetry, color, edema, and any surface abnormalities. Note that the lips are more pigmented than the facial skin. The most common lesions associated with the lips are fissures, commonly seen with chapped lips and herpes simplex (cold sores). Using a gloved hand, palpate the lips for moistness, induration, intactness, and lesions.

Gums and Teeth. Inspect the gums by placing your gloved hand on the lower lip and gently pulling it down to expose the gums. Repeat the procedure on the upper lip. Normally, the gums are pink in color and free of lesions, inflammation, and bleeding. Palpate the gums for retraction away from the teeth, lesions, swelling, and hypertrophy. If the person wears dentures, provide a paper towel and tissues for denture removal.

The teeth should be clean, white, straight, firm, evenly spaced, and free of obvious decay. Normally, there are 32 teeth. Inspect for caries, plaque, missing or loose teeth, dentures (note the fit of the denture), and color. Inspection of the teeth can also provide information regarding the person's attitude toward general hygiene.

Buccal Mucosa. When inspecting the buccal mucosa, you will need a tongue blade to displace the cheeks to the side in order to view the mucous membranes with

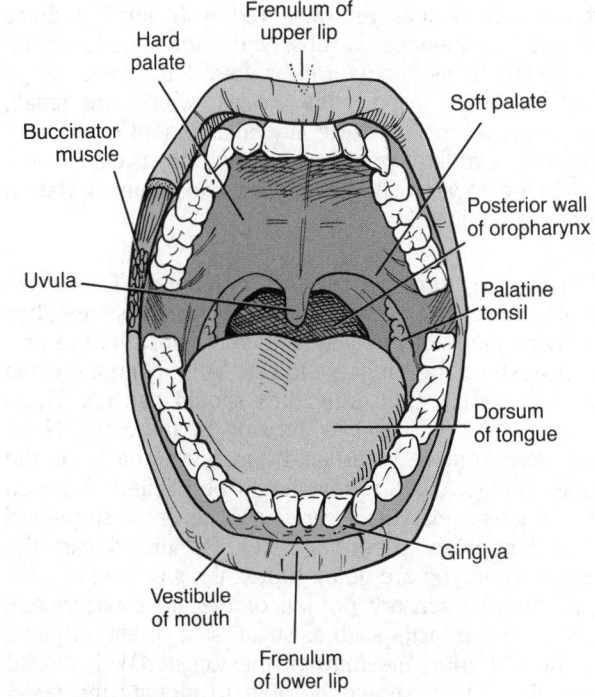

▲ Figure 33-19

Structures of the mouth.

a penlight. Be sure to inspect both cheeks, because diseases of the mouth are not always manifested symmetrically. Inspect the mucosa for color, pigmentation, ulcers, white patches, and nodules. Normally, the mucosa will be pink, smooth, moist, and free of lesions. In a dark skinned person, the mucosa will have a patchy brown pigmentation, which is normal.

Tongue. Inspect and palpate the tongue, using a gloved hand and a piece of gauze. Note the symmetry, movement, and color of the tongue. Normally, it should be pink, moist, and smooth, with papillae and fissures present. Ask the person to extend the tongue so that you may palpate it from front to back. Wrap a piece of gauze around the tongue during palpation. Note any masses. Instruct the person to touch the tip of the tongue to the top of the mouth, so that you may examine the floor of the mouth for cyanosis, pallor, and any lesions or nodules. The floor of the mouth is a common site for oral cancer.

Soft and Hard Palates. The hard palate is located in the anterior roof of the mouth. It is white or pale pink in color and firm in nature. The hard palate is where jaundice can be readily detected. The soft palate is located posteriorly and is pink in color, with a spongy texture. Inspect the hard and soft palate for lesions and asymmetry. Also, inspect for absence of elevation in the soft palate when the client says "Ah".

Pharynx. Inspect the posterior wall of the mouth with your penlight by asking the person to extend the tongue. A tongue blade may be used to press against the person's tongue for better viewing. Normally, it should be pink and free of drainage. The pharynx of a smoker will appear yellowish red with small nodules present. If drainage is observed, note the amount, color, and consistency. Unless they have been surgically removed, inspect the tonsils, which are small, pink surface growths. Note any enlargement of the tonsils with exudate present. Inspect the uvula, which should be located in the midline. Note any deviation from the midline.

Glossopharyngeal and Vagus Nerves. These two cranial nerves are usually tested together because they innervate many of the same structures. Instruct the person to extend the tongue and say "Ah." Note the uvula and soft palate. Both structures should rise up. There should be no deviation to the side by the uvula. Next, take your tongue blade and touch the back of the throat gently. A gag reflex should be elicited. A lesion of the glossopharyngeal or vagus nerve is suspected when there is an absent gag reflex. Be sure to warn the person when you are going to test the gag reflex.

To test the sensory portion of the glossopharyngeal nerve, place a taste, such as sugar, salt, or lemon juice, on the posterior one third of the tongue. With closed eyes, the person should be able to identify the taste. When applying different tastes to the tongue, use separate cotton-tipped applicators. Allow the person to drink water between tastes.

Facial Nerve. The sensory portion of the facial nerve is tested by applying a taste on the anterior two thirds of the tongue. With eyes closed, a person should readily identify the taste.

Hypoglossal Nerve. To test the motor function of the hypoglossal nerve (CN XII), observe the tongue for position (midline) and movement (smooth, no tremors). Instruct the person to move the tongue from side to side and touch the roof of the mouth. Observe for symmetry of movement.

Neck. Assessment of the neck is performed using the techniques of inspection and palpation. Upon examination, the person should be in an upright position to facilitate extension and rotation of the neck. Inspect the neck for color, symmetry, masses, enlargement of the thyroid or lymph nodes, abnormal pulsations, impaired range of motion, lesions, and scars. Palpate the neck for skin temperature and texture. Instruct the person to move the neck carefully through the entire range of motion, which includes right and left lateral, right and left rotation, flexion, extension, and hyperextension. The neck should move easily without any discomfort. The elderly person may experience some discomfort from neck movement, because of a decrease in range of motion.

Lymph Nodes. Palpate the lymph nodes, using the pads of your index and middle fingers. Instead of moving your fingertips over the skin surface, move the skin over the node area. Gently palpate in sequence bilaterally the preauricular, posterior auricular, occipital, tonsillar, submaxillary, submental, anterior cervical, posterior cervical, supraclavicular, and infraclavicular lymph nodes (Fig. 33–20).

If a node is palpated, note the location, size (in centimeters), shape (usually round), mobility (movable or fixed), consistency (soft, hard, firm), tenderness, and delimitation (discrete or matted together). If you have difficulty distinguishing an enlarged node from other structures of the neck, remember that a lymph node is able to roll up and down and side to side.

Thyroid. Inspect and palpate the thyroid gland for size, shape, symmetry, and any masses by instructing the person to swallow water while extending the neck (Fig. 33–21). Normally, the thyroid gland and the thyroid and cricoid cartilage will rise as the person swallows. An enlarged thyroid gland is called a **goiter.** You may palpate the thyroid gland by standing in front of or behind the person. Instruct the person to extend the neck as you place your fingers just below the cricoid cartilage. Ask the person to swallow. You will be able to feel the thyroid isthmus rise beneath your fingers.

Trachea. Inspect and palpate the trachea for any deviation from the midline by placing two fingers over the trachea at the suprasternal notch. Place one finger laterally to the left while placing another finger laterally to the right. Deviation of the trachea from the midline may indicate a mass or respiratory problems such as atelectasis and pneumothorax (Fig. 33–21).

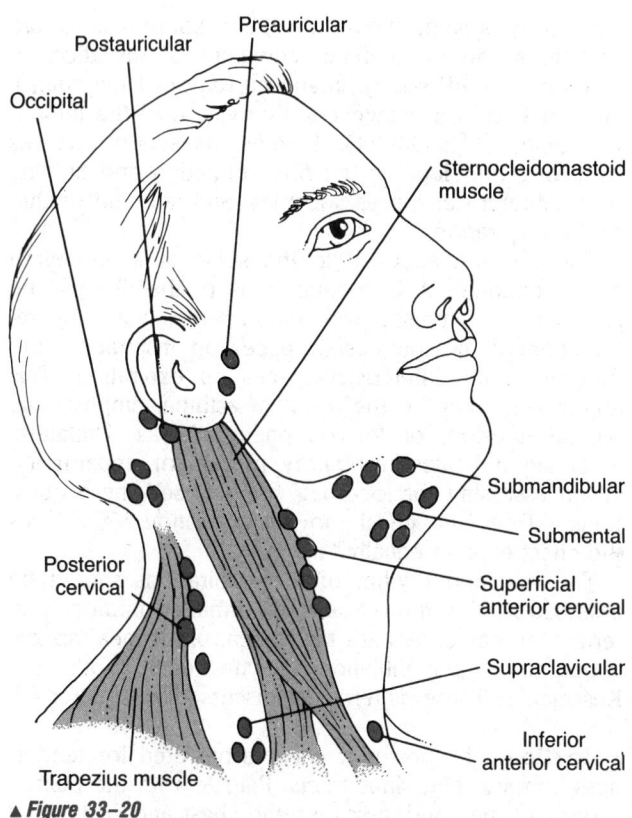

▲ Figure 33-20

Lymph nodes of the neck.

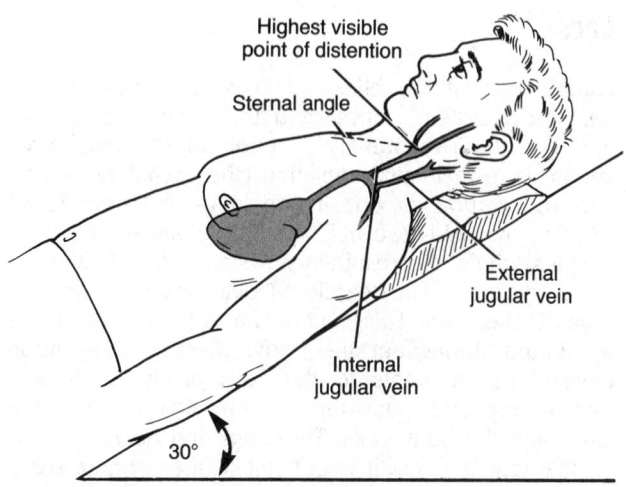

▲ Figure 33-22

Assessment of the external jugular vein.

Carotid Arteries. Inspect and palpate the carotid arteries to assess symmetry, amplitude, and rate and rhythm of the pulsations (Fig. 33-21). Palpate only one carotid artery at a time, remembering that these arteries supply essential blood to the brain. Do not press the carotid sinus (near the jaw angle) as this can cause a sudden drop in the pulse or blood pressure. Note any diminished, absent, expansile, or abnormally forceful pulsations. Auscultate the carotid artery using the bell of the stethoscope, beginning at the base of the artery and moving up toward the chin. It will be helpful if you instruct the person to hold the breath as you auscultate. Note any **bruits,** a blowing sound that indicates a distortion of a blood vessel that could interfere with blood flow.

Spinal Accessory Nerve. The spinal accessory nerve (CN XI) innervates the major neck muscles (trapezius and sternocleidomastoid) (Fig. 33-21). Assess this nerve and muscle strength by asking the person to shrug the shoulders against the resistance of your hands and to turn the head from one side to the other as you try to resist these movements.

External Jugular Veins. Inspect the jugular veins for abnormal or unusual distention. The jugular veins are not normally distended when the person sits or stands upright. However, when the person is supine and relaxed, jugular filling occurs, and the veins appear distended (not bulged) from the clavicle to the jaw's angle (Fig. 33-22).

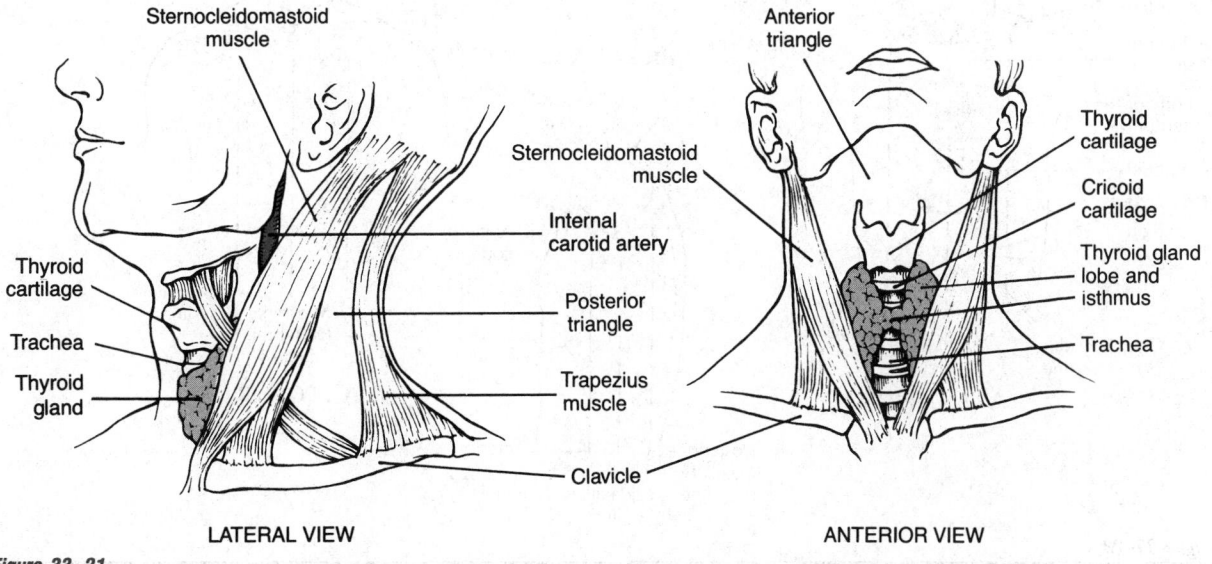

LATERAL VIEW   ANTERIOR VIEW

▲ Figure 33-21

The thyroid and surrounding neck structures.

Chest

Examination of the chest involves assessment of the respiratory system (lungs) and the cardiovascular system (heart). The primary function of the respiratory system is to maintain ventilation (the exchange of oxygen and carbon dioxide in the lungs and tissue) and regulate the acid-base balance. Any changes or abnormalities within the respiratory system will affect other body systems. The cardiovascular system's primary organ is the heart. The heart acts as a pump that moves the blood throughout the body, thereby transporting oxygen and nutrients to the cells of the body and transporting and removing carbon dioxide from the lungs and the body cells. The lungs and heart work so closely together that it is difficult to assess them separately.

A thorough examination of the chest requires you to use the techniques of inspection, palpation, percussion, and auscultation. The posterior chest is examined first, with the person in a sitting position. The anterior chest is examined with the person in either a sitting or supine position, and the examination of the heart is performed with the person in a supine position. Good lighting is imperative to assess the chest area, and the person will need to undress to the waist.

During the assessment of the thorax, bear in mind the thoracic reference lines (Fig. 33–23) and familiar landmarks—for example, ribs, sternal angle (angle of Louis), costal angle, suprasternal notch, and vertebra prominens. These make possible (a) accurate documentation of the location of findings, and (b) accurate mental visualization of underlying thoracic structures, such as lobes of lungs.

POSTERIOR CHEST

Inspection. The posterior chest is inspected for any skeletal deformities that could affect the status of the respiratory system. Some common abnormalities are **kyphosis** (an exaggerated curvature of the thoracic vertebrae), **scoliosis** (a lateral curvature of the spine), and **lordosis** (an exaggerated curvature of the lumbar vertebrae) (Fig. 33–24). Further inspection involves observing the slope of the ribs, retraction and bulging of the intercostal spaces, local lag, and rate and rhythm of the respirations.

The ribs are attached to the spine at a 45-degree angle (oblique). A horizontal slope of the ribs will be assessed on a person with emphysema. Note any retractions of the intercostal spaces on inspiration and bulging of the intercostal spaces on expiration. This abnormality may be the result of asthma, emphysema, pleural effusion, or tension pneumothorax. Unilateral local lag indicates respiratory movement impairment. When assessing for local lag, ask yourself these questions: "Does the chest move synchronously?" "Does the chest expand equally?"

The rate and rhythm of the respirations should be assessed at this time. Some abnormal respiratory patterns you may assess are tachypnea, bradypnea, apnea, hyperpnea, hyperventilation, Cheyne-Stokes, Biot's, and Kussmaul's. These patterns are discussed in Chapter 45.

Palpation. The posterior chest is palpated for tenderness, masses, and sinus tracts. Palpate with the palmar surface of the hand, assessing the chest and comparing the right side to the left (Fig. 33–25). Respiratory excursion is assessed by placing your thumbs parallel to the 10th ribs and grasping the lateral rib cage. Instruct the person to inhale deeply as you note the chest move upward and outward, and your thumbs should move apart. As the person exhales, your thumbs should return to the midline.

Fremitus is a vibration transmitted through the chest wall as the person speaks. To palpate the vibration with the palmar surface or ulnar side of the hand, ask the person to repeat the words *ninety-nine* or *one-one-one*.

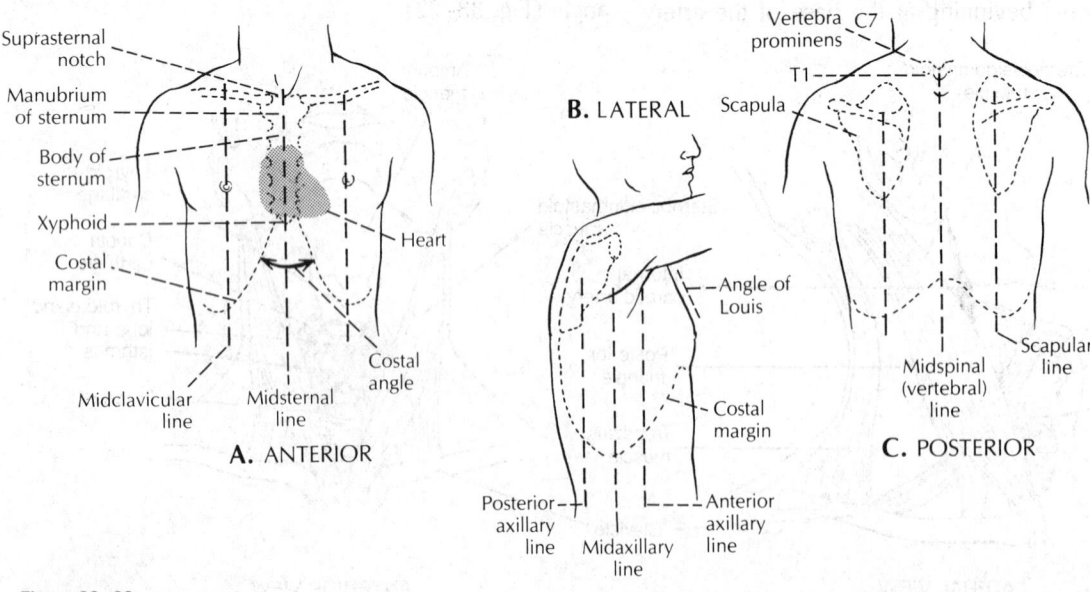

▲ **Figure 33–23**

Landmarks and reference lines on the thorax.

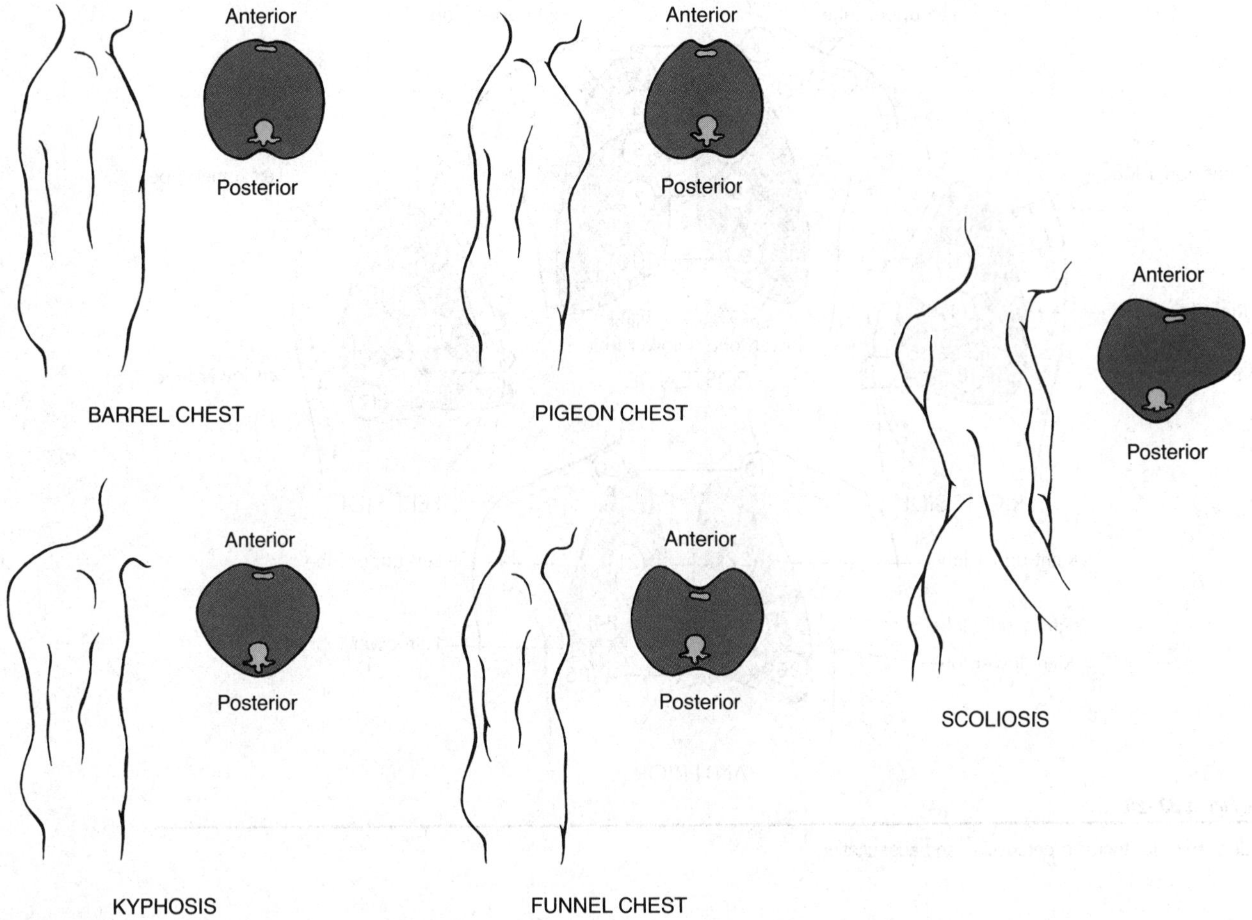

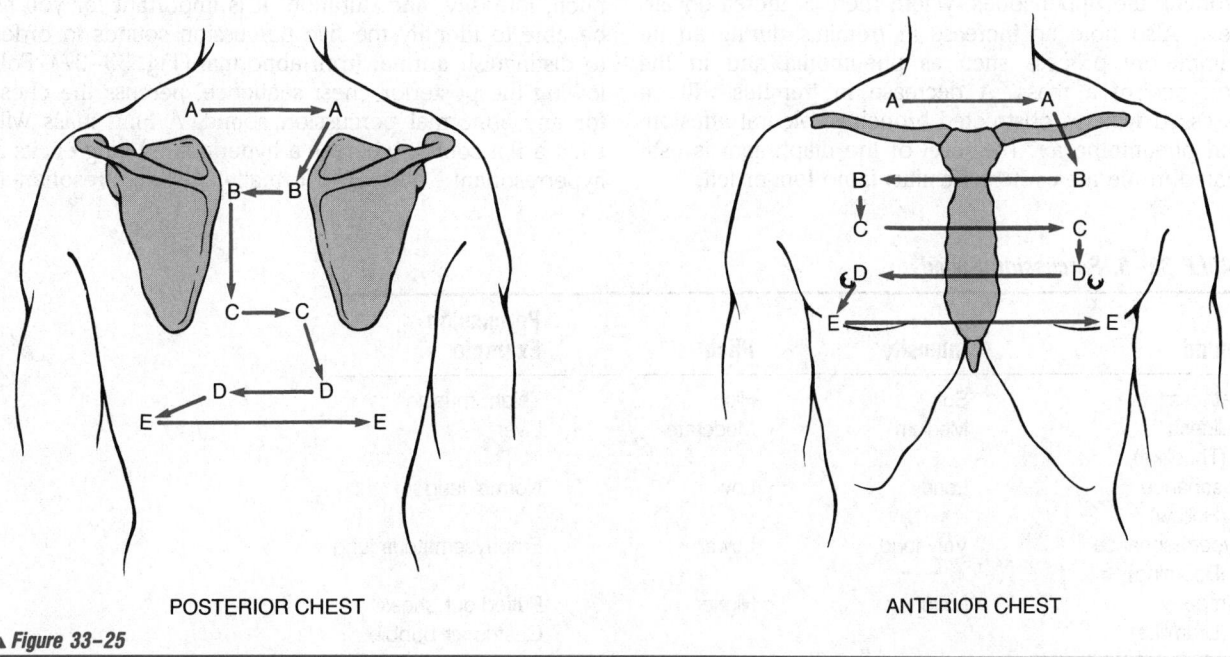

Anterior
Posterior
BARREL CHEST
Anterior
Posterior
PIGEON CHEST
Anterior
Posterior
SCOLIOSIS
Anterior
Posterior
KYPHOSIS
Anterior
Posterior
FUNNEL CHEST

▲ **Figure 33–24**

Deformities of the chest.

A
A
B
B
C
C
D
D
E
E
POSTERIOR CHEST
A
A
B
B
C
C
D
D
E
E
ANTERIOR CHEST

▲ **Figure 33–25**

Sequence for thoracic palpation.

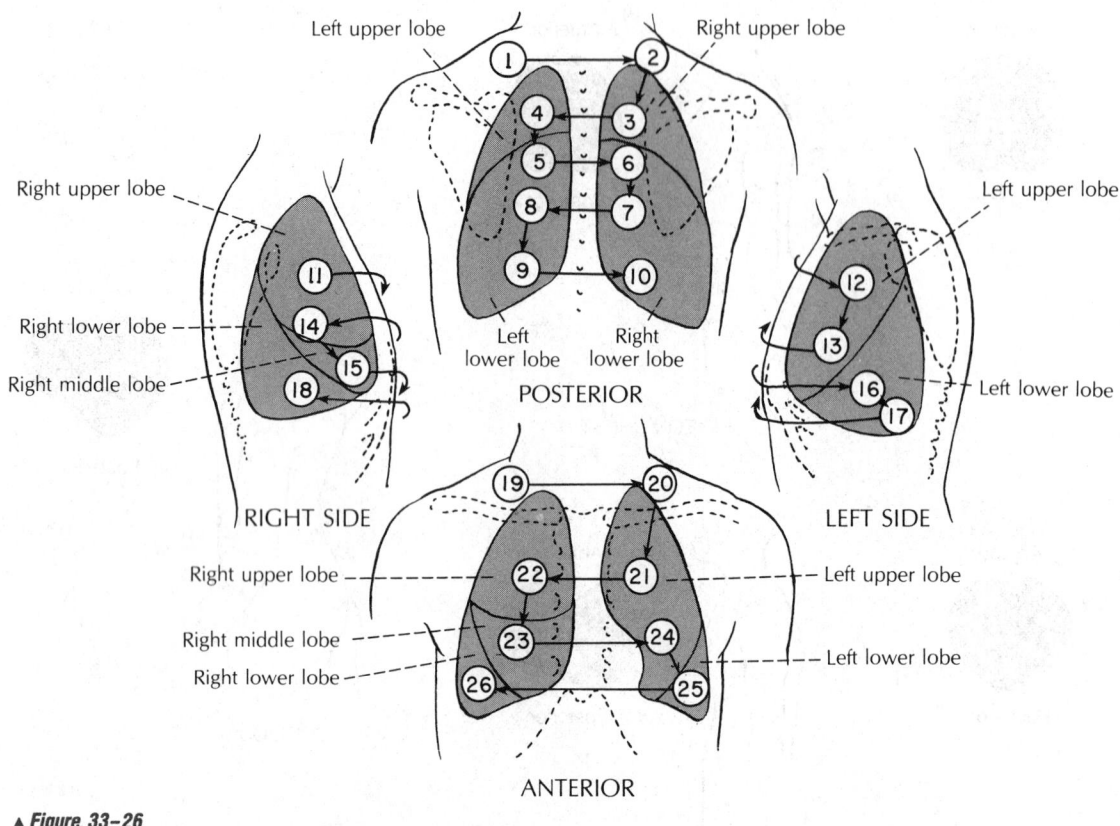

▲ Figure 33-26

Sequence for thoracic percussion and auscultation.

Use only one hand to palpate fremitus to avoid any discrepancies as a result of differing sensitivity between the hands. You will cover the entire chest, moving back and forth from one side to the other, making sure to assess the upper and lower lobes of the lungs. Expect to feel an increase in fremitus over the main stem bronchi and upper lobes, where there is increased airflow. Also note an increase in fremitus during an inflammatory process such as pneumonia and in the presence of a mass. A decrease in fremitus will be assessed with an obstructed bronchus, pleural effusion, and pneumothorax. The level of the diaphragm is estimated in the area where fremitus is no longer felt.

Percussion. The posterior chest is percussed to determine whether the underlying tissue is air filled, fluid filled, or solid (Fig. 33-26). The normal lung should be air filled, producing a resonance sound that is low pitched, of loud intensity, and of long duration. Table 33-6 illustrates other percussion sounds in relation to pitch, intensity, and duration. It is important for you to be able to identify the five percussion sounds in order to distinguish normal from abnormal (Fig. 33-27). Following the posterior chest sequence, percuss the chest for any abnormal percussion sound. A lung mass will elicit a flat sound, whereas a hyperinflated lung elicits a hyperresonant sound. Normally, when resonance

TABLE 33-6. Percussion Sounds

Sound	Intensity	Pitch	Percussion Example
Flatness	Soft	High	Thigh, muscle
Dullness (Thudlike)	Medium	Moderate	Liver
Resonance (Hollow)	Loud	Low	Normal lung
Hyperresonance (Booming)	Very loud	Lower	Emphysematous lung
Tympany (Drumlike)	Loud	Higher	Puffed-out cheek Gastric air bubble

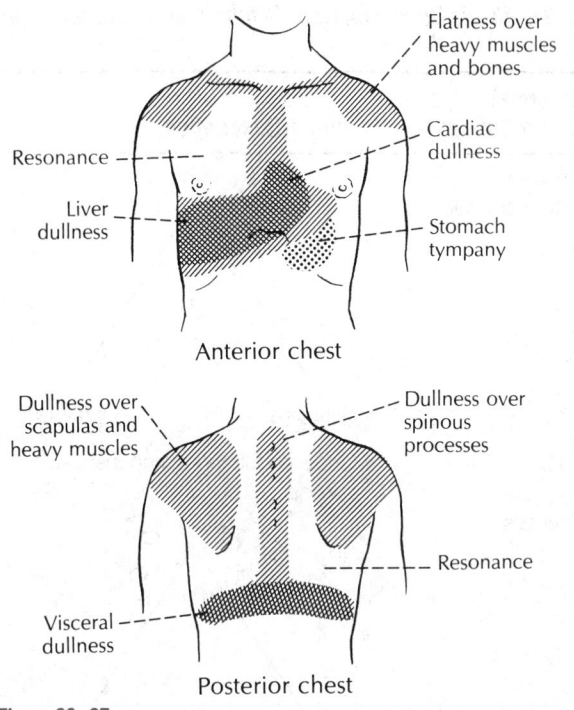

Anterior chest

Flatness over heavy muscles and bones

Cardiac dullness

Resonance

Liver dullness

Stomach tympany

Dullness over scapulas and heavy muscles

Dullness over spinous processes

Resonance

Visceral dullness

Posterior chest

▲ Figure 33–27

Percussion tones.

changes to dullness, you are at the estimated level of the diaphragm (usually at the T10 level).

Diaphragmatic excursion is movement of the diaphragm as it descends on inspiration and rises on expiration. Diaphragmatic excursion is assessed by performing the following steps:

1. Instruct the person to inhale and to hold the breath.
2. Percuss downward from the bottom of the scapulae at the midscapular line.
3. When you note the percussion sound change from resonance to dullness, mark it with your special marking pen.
4. Instruct the person to exhale and to hold it.
5. Percuss upward (beginning at your pen marking) until the percussion sound changes from dullness to resonance. Mark it with your marking pen.

The distance between the points is measured and the procedure is then repeated on the opposite side. Normally, the range in measurement is 3 to 6 cm.

Auscultation. Auscultation is useful in assessing airflow; the presence of fluid, mucus, or obstruction; and the surrounding lung and pleural spaces. When auscultating, instruct the person to take deep breaths through the mouth. Be sure to use the diaphragm of the stethoscope. Listen at least one full breath in each location following the percussion sequence (see Fig. 33–26).

Normal Breath Sounds. Normal breath sounds are vesicular, bronchial, and bronchovesicular. **Vesicular breath sounds** are soft, low-pitched, fine rustling sounds located over the periphery of the lung. If vesicular sounds are decreased over the periphery, this may indicate pneumonia, emphysema, pleural effusion, or atelectasis. Bronchial breath sounds are loud, high-pitched "tubular" sounds located over the trachea and major bronchi. **Bronchial breath sounds** are loud, high-pitched tubular sounds located over the trachea and major bronchi that are heard louder and longer during expiration. Bronchial sounds auscultated over the periphery of the lungs may indicate consolidation or atelectasis. **Bronchovesicular breath sounds** are moderately pitched sounds located between the scapulae posteriorly and on either side of the sternum at the first and second intercostal spaces anteriorly. Bronchovesicular breath sounds auscultated over the periphery of the lung may indicate consolidation. Symbols for documentation of normal breath sounds are illustrated in Table 33–7.

Adventitious Breath Sounds. **Adventitious breath sounds** are abnormal breath sounds such as crackles, wheezes, rhonchi, and friction rubs. **Crackles** (formerly known as rales) are noises created when air is traveling through vessels containing abnormal moisture. They are more pronounced on inspiration. Crackles are divided into fine and coarse. Fine crackles are soft and high pitched and sound like two hairs being rubbed together. Coarse crackles are louder and lower in pitch and have a bubbling quality. **Wheezes** are high-pitched sounds produced as air passes through a narrowed or defective vessel. They may occur during inspiration, expiration, or both. The cause may be a mucous plug, bronchospasms, or tumor. **Rhonchi** (gurgles) are coarse rattling sounds, louder and lower in pitch than crackles, caused by narrowed airways. Rhonchi are more pronounced on expiration. **Friction rubs** are crackling, grating sounds produced when two roughened or inflamed pleural spaces rub across each other during respiration. They are heard on inspiration and expiration. Note the location and the relationship in the respiratory cycle of the adventitious sounds (Table 33–8).

Spoken and Whispered Sounds. Spoken and whispered sounds are based on the principle that sound carries best through a solid, not as well through fluid, and poorly through air. Instruct the person to say "ninety-nine" while you auscultate the posterior chest. Normally, the sound should be muffled and indistinct. If the sound is clear, it is called bronchophony. Instruct the person to say "ee" while you auscultate the posterior chest. Normally the sound should be muffled and indistinct. If the sound is heard as "ay," it is called egophony. Instruct the person to whisper "ninety-nine" while you auscultate. Normally, the sound is very faint and indistinct. If the sound is louder and clear, it is called whispered pectoriloquy.

TABLE 33-7 Documentation Symbols of Normal Breath Sounds

Breath Sound	Symbol/Description
Vesicular	Inspiratory phase is approximately three times longer than expiratory phase
Bronchial	Expiratory phase is longer than the inspiratory phase at a ratio of 3:2
Bronchovesicular	Inspiratory and expiratory phases are equal

TABLE 33-8. Documentation Symbols of Abnormal Breath Sounds

Abnormal Breath Sounds	Symbol/Description
Crackles (formerly rales)	More pronounced during inspiratory phase
Wheezes	May be auscultated during inspiratory or expiratory phases or both
Rhonchi (gurgles)	More pronounced on expiration
Friction rubs	Auscultated during inspiratory and expiratory phases

ANTERIOR CHEST

Inspection. The anterior chest is inspected for any skeletal deformities. Some common abnormalities are barrel chest, pectus carinatum, and pectus excavatum. The **barrel chest** is a thoracic abnormality characterized by horizontal ribs, slight kyphosis, and a prominent sternal angle. The chest appears to be in a continuous inspiration. **Pectus carinatum (pigeon chest)** is a thoracic abnormality characterized by the forward projection of the sternum. **Pectus excavatum (funnel chest)** is a thoracic abnormality characterized by the sternum pointing posteriorly, which may cause pressure on the heart. Inspection is also performed regarding the slope of the ribs, retraction and bulging of the intercostal spaces, and local lag, as discussed in the section on the posterior chest. Some areas are inspected on the anterior chest only; this includes the anteroposterior (AP) diameter, costal angle, and use of the accessory muscles.

In a normal adult, the ratio of anteroposterior (AP) to lateral diameter is about 1:2. In an elderly person, you will observe an increase in the AP diameter, which is normal. A barrel chest and pectus carinatum will result in an increase in the AP diameter. The costal angle should be less than 90 degrees. The accessory muscles are composed of the sternocleidomastoid, trapezius, and abdominal muscles. Inspect the use of these muscles to aid in ventilation. You will observe the muscles contracting.

Palpation. The anterior chest is palpated for areas of tenderness, respiratory excursion, and fremitus (see Fig. 33–25). To assess respiratory excursion, place your thumbs along the costal margins, grasping the lateral rib cage with your hands. Slide your thumbs toward each other to raise a skin fold between the thumbs. Instruct the person to inhale deeply as you observe the divergence of the thumbs and assess the symmetry of respiratory movement.

The assessment of fremitus differs anteriorly owing to the decreased or absent vibration over the precordium (the area of the chest overlying the heart). In a woman, you will be unable to feel the vibration through breast tissue. You may have to displace the breast to complete the assessment of fremitus.

Percussion. Percuss the anterior and lateral chest (see Fig. 33–26). Normally, resonance is percussed over the entire lung area. You will percuss dullness to the left of the sternum at the third to fifth intercostal spaces as a result of the heart's presence. The liver and stomach will produce dull and tympanic sounds, respectively. Be sure that you are familiar with the location of these structures.

Auscultation. The anterior chest is auscultated using the percussion sequence (see Fig. 33–26). Auscultate for vesicular, bronchial, and bronchovesicular breath sounds. Note any adventitious sounds heard, as discussed in the section on posterior chest.

HEART

Inspection, percussion, palpation, and auscultation are the techniques used in the examination of the heart. To identify the precordial points, you must be familiar with the landmarks (Fig. 33–28). The angle of Louis is palpated as a prominence on the upper third of the sternum. Palpate this area and move the fingers laterally to identify the second intercostal space. The aortic area is located at the second intercostal space to the right sternal border. The pulmonic area is located at the second intercostal space to the left sternal border. Erb's point is located at the third intercostal space to the left sternal border. The tricuspid area is located at the fourth or fifth intercostal space to the left sternal border. The mitral (apical) area is located at the fifth intercostal space medial to the midclavicular line. The epigastric area is the area overlying the xiphoid process.

Inspection. Before beginning the assessment, position the person in a supine position or lying with the head of the bed at a 30- to 45-degree angle. The latter position will facilitate breathing for the person with heart or respiratory problems. Stand at the person's right side. This will assist you in viewing any pulsations.

Inspect the precordial points of the chest for any abnormal pulsations or lift-heaves and the apical impulse. An example of an abnormal pulsation you might observe is a pulsation located at the pulmonic area, or Erb's point, resulting from an abnormally sharp closure of the pulmonic value associated with pulmonary hypertension. Normally the only pulsation observable on the chest wall is the apical impulse. The **apical impulse** (point of maximal impulse) is a pulsation located over the apex of the heart, at the fifth intercostal space medial to the midclavicular line. If the heart is displaced or enlarged, the apical impulse may be located lateral to the midclavicular line. If this is the case, position the person in a left lateral horizontal position to observe the apical impulse.

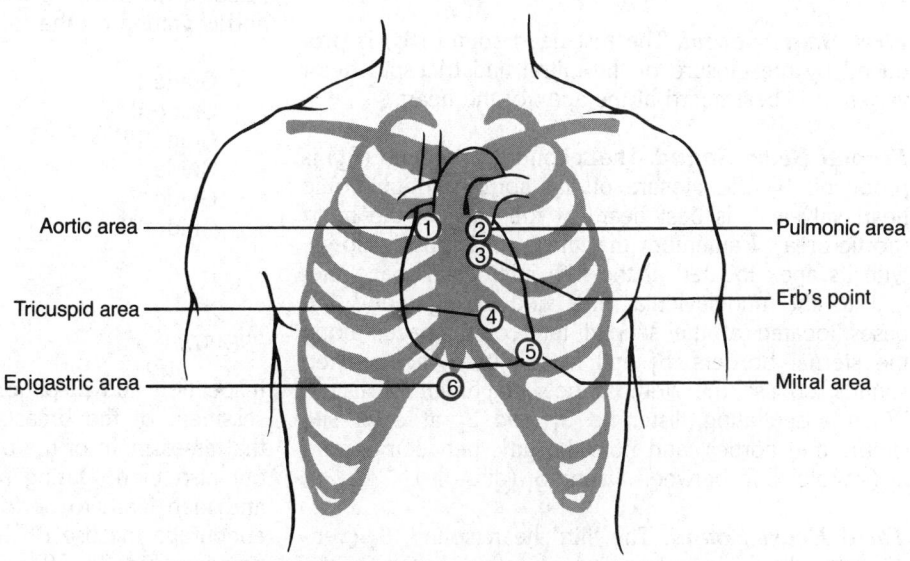

▲ *Figure 33–28*

Precordial points of the heart.

The heart's pumping action may be so forceful that you observe the chest lift or heave. A lift is a slight movement, while a heave is a more vigorous movement. Each is the result of forceful cardiac action and is considered abnormal.

Palpation. The precordial points of the chest are palpated for any abnormal pulsations, thrills, lift-heaves, apical impulses, and aortic pulsations. You may decide to palpate as you inspect each area. A **thrill** is a palpable cardiac murmur. It feels similar to the neck of a purring cat and is considered abnormal. You should not be able to palpate any pulsations at any of the precordial points except for the mitral area. To palpate the apical impulse, place the heel of the hand on the sternum with your fingers stretched across the chest, just under the breast area. After you have located the apical impulse, palpate it with your fingertips. When palpating for lifts and heaves, observe in the area at or near the sternum (right ventricular heave) and at or near the apex (left ventricular heave). The aortic pulse is palpated in the epigastric area.

Percussion. Cardiac dullness is located in the third to fifth intercostal spaces. Since chest x-ray films are much more practical and efficient in determining the size of the heart, percussion is no longer used in the assessment of the heart.

Auscultation. The auscultation technique assesses the normal heart sounds (S_1 and S_2), extra heart sounds (S_3, S_4, split S_1, and split S_2), and murmurs. Auscultate over the precordial areas (Fig. 33–28) with both the stethoscope's diaphragm and bell. Listen at each area through several breaths in and out. Instruct the person to breathe through the nose to decrease the interference of breath sounds as you are listening. Press the diaphragm firmly against the chest wall, but when auscultating with the bell hold it lightly. Describe the heart sounds according to their pitch, loudness, and timing in the cardiac cycle. Low-pitched sounds are best heard with the stethoscope bell and higher, louder sounds with the diaphragm.

First Heart Sound. The first heart sound (S_1) is produced by the closure of the mitral and tricuspid heart valves. It is best heard at the apex of the heart.

Second Heart Sound. The second heart sound (S_2) is produced by the closure of the aortic and pulmonic heart valves. It is best heard at the base of the heart (aortic area). Remember that the heart is upside down, with its apex located at the fifth intercostal space medial to the midclavicular line, and its right and left bases located at the second intercostal space, along the sternal borders. S_1 and S_2 are both high-pitched sounds, so use the stethoscope's diaphragm to listen. When auscultating, listen to S_1 and S_2 at each site (mitral and aortic), and note the time between S_1 and S_2 (systole) and between S_2 and S_1 (diastole).

Third Heart Sound. The third heart sound, S_3 (ventricular gallop), is a low-pitched sound heard in the cardiac cycle immediately after S_2 (diastole). It is normal in children and young adults. It is considered abnormal in adults over 30 years of age. It is best heard in the mitral area with the person in a left lateral horizontal position, using the bell of the stethoscope. It represents an enlarged ventricle or overly rapid ventricular filling, a sign of left ventricular failure.

Fourth Heart Sound. The fourth heart sound, S_4 (atrial gallop), is a low-pitched sound heard in the cardiac cycle just before S_1. Using the bell of the stethoscope, auscultate for S_4 in the mitral area with the person in a left lateral horizontal position. S_4 may be normal in children and trained athletes. It is considered abnormal in most adults and is associated with ischemia, coronary artery disease, and aortic stenosis.

Split First Heart Sound. A split first heart sound (split S_1) occurs when the mitral and tricuspid heart valves are not closing together. It is a high-pitched sound heard best in the tricuspid area using the stethoscope's diaphragm. It is associated with a right bundle branch block.

Split Second Heart Sound. A split second heart sound (split S_2) occurs when the aortic and pulmonic heart valves are not closing together. It is a high-pitched sound heard best in the pulmonic area with the stethoscope's bell. It is more common in children. If you auscultate a split S_2, note whether the split occurs on inspiration or expiration. A split S_2 on expiration may indicate right or left bundle branch block, atrial septal defect, or valvular problems.

Heart Murmur. A **heart murmur** is a harsh, rumbling, blowing sound caused by blood flow across a defective valve, or the shunting of blood through an abnormal passage. A heart murmur is assessed for timing, location, radiation, intensity, quality, and pitch. Timing involves determining whether the murmur occurs during diastole (between S_2 and S_1) or systole (between S_1 and S_2). Describe the location according to the precordial areas and note whether the murmur radiates. Intensity of a murmur refers to the loudness and is graded on the following scale:

Grade I	very faint
Grade II	quiet but audible
Grade III	moderately loud
Grade IV	loud
Grade V	very loud
Grade VI	very loud; may be audible with the stethoscope completely off the chest wall

BREASTS

Inspection and palpation are performed during the assessment of the breasts. It is important to remember that assessment of the breasts includes not only women but also men. During breast assessment, help women and men learn to perform breast self-examination and encourage the use of this valuable health maintenance practice (Fig. 33–29).

■ WHY DO THE BREAST SELF-EXAM?

There are many good reasons for doing a breast self-exam each month. One reason is that it is easy to do and the more you do it, the better you will get at it. When you get to know how your breasts normally feel, you will quickly be able to feel any change, and early detection is the key to successful treatment and cure.

■ WHEN TO DO BREAST SELF-EXAM

The best time to do breast self-exam is right after your period, when breasts are not tender or swollen. If you do not have regular periods or sometimes skip a month, do it on the same day every month.

Remember: A breast self-exam could save your breast—and save your life. Most breast lumps are found by women themselves, but, in fact, most lumps in the breast are not cancer. Be safe, be sure.

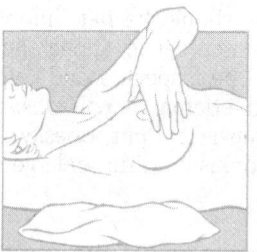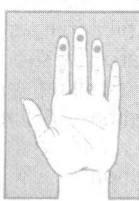

Finger Pads

■ NOW, HOW TO DO BREAST SELF-EXAM

1. Lie down and put a pillow under your right shoulder. Place your right arm behind your head.

2. Use the finger pads of your three middle fingers on your left hand to feel for lumps or thickening. Your finger pads are the top third of each finger.

3. Press firmly enough to know how your breast feels. If you're not sure how hard to press, ask your health care provider. Or try to copy the way your health care provider uses the finger pads during a breast exam. Learn what your breast feels like most of the time. A firm ridge in the lower curve of each breast is normal.

4. Move around the breast in a set way. You can choose either the circle (A), the up and down line (B), or the wedge (C). Do it the same way every time. It will help you to make sure that you've gone over the entire breast area, and to remember how your breast feels.

5. Now examine your left breast using right hand finger pads.

6. If you find any changes, see your doctor right away.

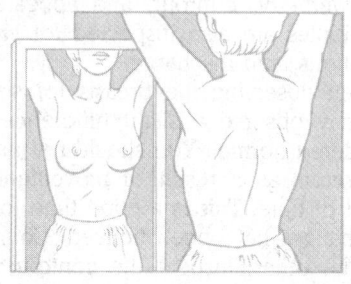

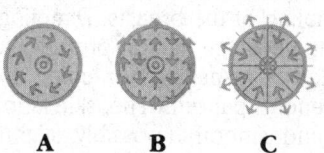

A   B   C

■ FOR ADDED SAFETY:

You should also check your breasts while standing in front of a mirror right after you do your breast self-exam each month. See if there are any changes in the way your breasts look: dimpling of the skin, changes in the nipple, or redness or swelling.

You might also want to do a breast self-exam while you're in the shower. Your soapy hands will glide over the wet skin making it easy to check how your breasts feel.

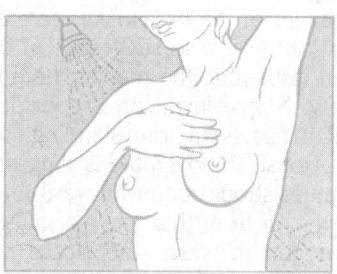

▲ Figure 33–29

A technique for self-examination of the breast. (How to Do Breast Self-Examination. American Cancer Society, 1992.)

The female breast is composed of glandular tissue, fibrous tissue, and fat. It is located between the second and sixth ribs, between the sternal edge and the mid-axillary line. It may feel soft and granular, nodular, or lumpy. Nodularity may increase prior to the menstrual period each month. This is why female breasts are examined following a menstrual period rather than just prior to one.

The male breasts should be flat, smooth, nontender, and bilaterally symmetrical in appearance. The nipple and areolae should be inspected and palpated for nodules, swelling, and edema. If you observe breast enlargement, distinguish it from obesity (soft enlargement) and gynecomastia (firm enlargement) through palpation.

Inspection. Several positions are assumed when inspecting the breasts: sitting, arms at the sides; sitting, arms raised over the head (the person may rest the arms on top of the head); leaning forward (breasts hanging down) while sitting or standing; and the hands pressed firmly on the hips or palms pressed firmly together.

The assessment begins with the person sitting and the arms at the sides. The chest area must be completely exposed in order to inspect the breast for size and symmetry, contour, and appearance of the skin. The nipples are also inspected for size, shape, rashes, ulcerations, and discharge.

When observing the breasts for size and symmetry, you may observe a slight difference in each. This is considered normal. You should not note a difference in the breasts as a result of movement, rest, or over a period of time. This is a good time to ask the person if any changes have been noticed. Comparing one breast with the other, inspect the contour, which should be smooth and convex. Observe for any masses, flattening, or dimpling of the breasts. Dimpling may be particularly evident when the person presses the hands on the hips. The skin is inspected for color, thickening or edema, and venous pattern. The skin should be intact, movable, and smooth (possibly slightly wrinkled or with striae). Redness and inflammation may indicate infection or carcinoma. Thickening or edema may be produced by lymphatic blockage. The skin that resembles an orange peel (thickened skin and large pores) suggests cancer of the breast. An increased prominence of venous pattern is also suggestive of breast cancer.

When inspecting the nipples, note that size and color may vary. Nipple inversion is considered a normal variation if it has been long-standing. Inversion occurring in a previously erect nipple is suggestive of malignancy. The nipples should point outward and downward. Note any deviation from this, since a malignancy can deviate the direction in which the nipple points. Observe for any rashes, ulcerations, or discharge. It is normal for a discharge to occur during the lactation phase of pregnancy. If discharge is present, note the odor and type of drainage (purulent, serous, or sanguineous).

Examine a large breast bimanually, with one hand under the breast to support it (Fig. 33–30). Carefully assess axillary skin folds and under pendulous breasts.

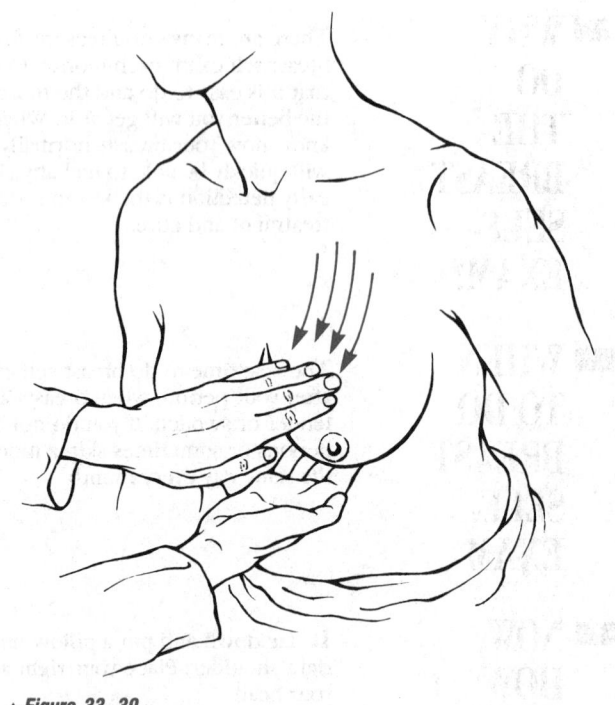

▲ *Figure 33–30*

Bimanual breast palpation.

Palpation. The person should be in a supine position with a pillow under the scapula of the side being examined. The arm should be raised above the head of the side being examined. To describe any findings, the breast should be divided into four quadrants: right upper, right lower, left upper, and left lower; or the breast should be viewed as the face of a clock (Fig. 33–31). Any abnormality will be located by the time —for example, nine o'clock— and by the distance (centimeters) from the nipple.

Palpate all four quadrants, both areolae, tails of breasts, and axillae for lumps or nodules. To palpate the breast, gently use the finger pads in a rotating movement, progressing slowly across the breast tissue until the total breast is examined (Fig. 33–32). Maintain continuous finger contact with the tissue rather than lifting the fingers up and down to change sites. If the person reports a lump, palpate the breast without the lump first, thus becoming familiar with the person's "normal" breast tissue before assessing the deviation from normal. If a nodule is detected, note the location (as described earlier), size (centimeters), shape (round, disk-shaped, oblong, tubular), consistency (soft, hard, firm), mobility (mobile, fixed), and borders (well-defined, poorly demarcated). Compress the areola and nipple of each breast with the thumb and index finger to denote any discharge. Note the amount, color, consistency, and location.

Cancerous lesions are hard, fixed, nontender, and irregular in shape.

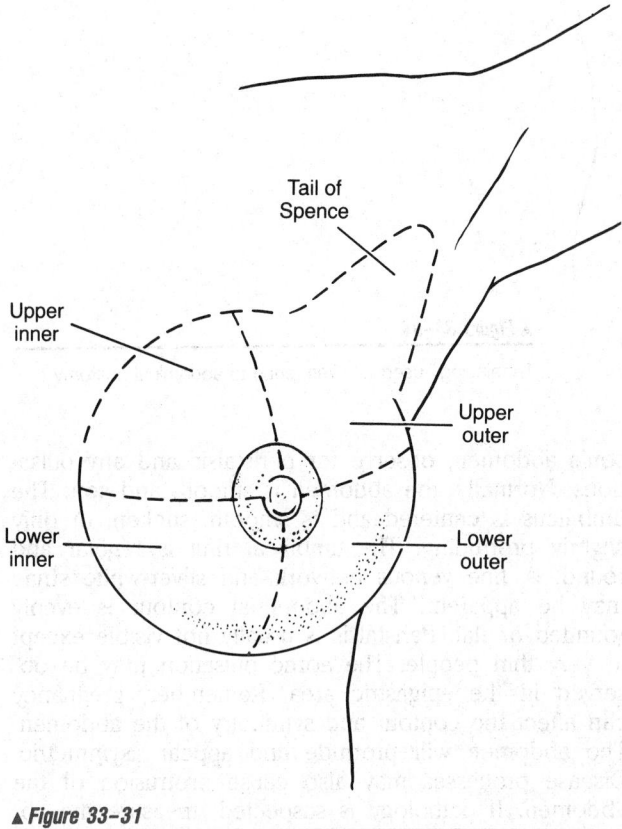

▲ Figure 33–31

Breast quadrants used for assessment.

Inspection and palpation are used to assess the axillary area with the person in a sitting position.

Inspection. Inspect each axilla for rashes, redness, infection, and unusual pigmentation. Redness and infection may originate from the sweat glands. A change in pigmentation may suggest an underlying malignancy.

Palpation. When performing palpation of the axilla, place your fingers into the apex of the axilla with the person's arm down and the wrist resting in your hand. Bring your fingers down over the surface of the ribs, compressing the nodes against the chest. Lymph nodes associated with breast lymphatic drainage are normally not palpable. Some tenderness occurs high in the axilla during palpation for lymph nodes. Assess the supraclavicular, infraclavicular, central and lateral axillary, central axillary, and pectoral lymph nodes (Fig. 33–33).

Abdomen

Assessment of the abdomen involves inspection, auscultation, percussion, and palpation. It will also include the assessment of abdominal reflexes. Remember, the order of techniques is different from the examination of other body parts. Auscultation is performed after inspection to ensure that the motility of the bowel and bowel sounds are not altered. Before you can begin the abdominal assessment, you need to be familiar with

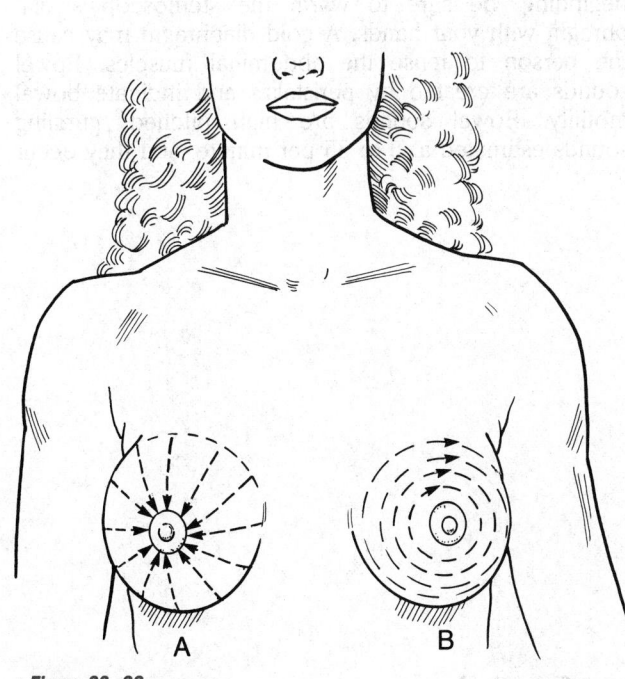

▲ Figure 33–32

Patterns of breast palpation.

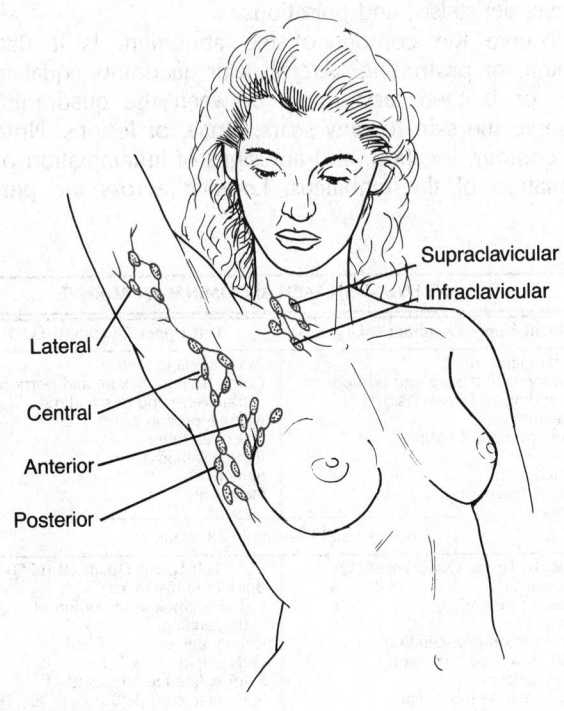

▲ Figure 33–33

Lymph nodes of the breast and axillary area.

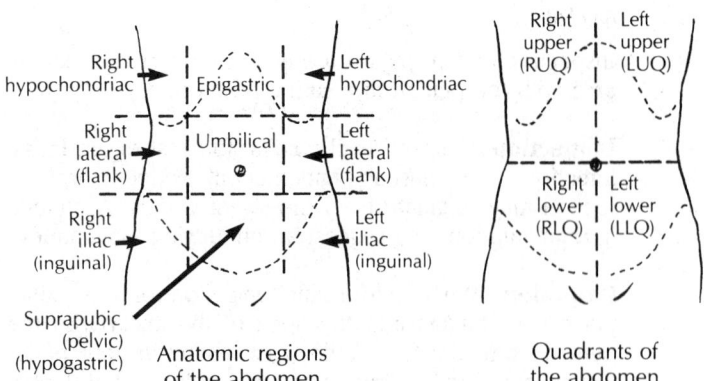

Right hypochondriac · Epigastric · Left hypochondriac

Right lateral (flank) · Umbilical · Left lateral (flank)

Right iliac (inguinal) · Left iliac (inguinal)

Suprapubic (pelvic) (hypogastric)

Anatomic regions of the abdomen

Right upper (RUQ) · Left upper (LUQ)

Right lower (RLQ) · Left lower (LLQ)

Quadrants of the abdomen

▲ *Figure 33-34*

Terminology used with reference to abdominal anatomy.

the quadrants or regions of the abdomen. The abdomen is divided into four quadrants, right upper, right lower, left upper, and left lower (Fig. 33–34). The abdomen may also be divided into nine regions. Figure 33–34 illustrates the regions of the abdomen. It is also important to know the underlying organs located in each quadrant (Fig. 33–35).

Prior to the examination, ask the person to empty the bladder. The person will assume a supine position with the arms at the side or draped across the chest. Instruct the person to flex the knees slightly. This position aids in relaxation of the abdomen. Expose the abdomen from the epigastric area to the symphysis pubis. Be sure to drape the female chest. The equipment needed for the examination will include a small ruler, marking pen, and stethoscope.

Inspection. When inspecting the abdomen, stand on the person's right side. Be sure that you have good lighting. Inspect the contour and .symmetry, skin, umbilicus, peristalsis, and pulsations.

Observe the contour of the abdomen. Is it flat, sunken, or protruding? Are all four quadrants equal in size, or is there asymmetry between the quadrants? Observe the skin for any scars, striae, or lesions. Note the contour, location, and any signs of inflammation or herniation of the umbilicus. Looking across the person's abdomen, observe for peristalsis and any pulsations. Normally, the abdomen is smooth and soft. The umbilicus is centered and is smooth, sunken, or only slightly protruding. The umbilical ring is regular and round. A fine venous network and silver-white striae may be apparent. The abdominal contour is evenly rounded or flat. Peristalsis is usually not visible except in very thin people. The aortic pulsation may be observed in the epigastric area. Remember, pregnancy can affect the contour and symmetry of the abdomen. The abdomen will protrude and appear asymmetric. Disease processes may also cause protrusion of the abdomen. If pathology is suspected, measure the abdominal girth. Dehydration may cause the abdomen to appear sunken, whereas distention, obesity, or tumors may cause a protrusion of the abdomen. Fluid (ascites), masses, or an intestinal obstruction may cause asymmetry of the abdomen.

Auscultation. The abdomen is auscultated for bowel sounds, bruits, friction rubs, and venous hums. Prior to beginning, be sure to warm the stethoscope's diaphragm with your hands. A cold diaphragm may cause the person to tense the abdominal muscles. Bowel sounds are created by peristalsis and indicate bowel motility. Bowel sounds are high pitched, gurgling sounds estimated at 5 to 35 per minute, and they occur

ORGANS FOUND IN EACH ABDOMINAL QUADRANT	
Right Upper Quadrant (RUQ)	**Left Upper Quadrant (LUQ)**
Adrenal gland (right)	Adrenal gland (left)
Colon (hepatic flexure and portions of ascending and transverse)	Colon (splenic flexure and portions of transverse and descending)
Duodenum	Kidney (portion of left)
Kidney (portion of right)	Liver (left lobe)
Liver	Pancreas (body)
Gallbladder	Spleen
Pancreas (head)	Stomach
Pylorus	
Loops of small intestine in all quadrants	
Right Lower Quadrant (RLQ)	**Left Lower Quadrant (LLQ)**
Appendix	Bladder (if distended)
Bladder (if distended)	Colon (sigmoid and portion of descending)
Cecum	Kidney (lower pole of left)
Colon (portion of ascending)	Ovary (left)
Kidney (lower pole of right)	Salpinx (uterine tube; left)
Ovary (right)	Spermatic cord (left)
Salpinx (uterine tube; right)	Ureter (left)
Spermatic cord (right)	Uterus (if enlarged)
Ureter (right)	
Uterus (if enlarged)	

▲ *Figure 33-35*

Organs found in each abdominal quadrant.

every 5 to 15 seconds. Bowel sounds within the range of 5 to 35 per minute are normal bowel sounds. Hypoactive bowel sounds are fewer than 5 per minute and indicate decreased motility. This may be seen in bowel obstruction, paralytic ileus, and peritonitis. Hyperactive bowel sounds are greater than 35 per minute and indicate an increase in bowel motility, as seen in gastroenteritis and intestinal obstruction.

Auscultate each quadrant for bowel sounds; be sure to listen at least 5 minutes before concluding they are absent. Absent bowel sounds may indicate paralytic ileus, peritonitis, or complete obstruction. Note any abnormal sounds. A high-pitched, tinkling sound may indicate fluid, whereas a rush of high-pitched sounds coinciding with an abdominal cramp may indicate an obstruction. The abdominal aorta and renal, iliac, and femoral arteries are auscultated for bruits. The aorta and renal arteries are located in the epigastric area, while the iliac arteries are located in the lower umbilical area. The femoral arteries are located in the groin area. Remember, a bruit is a low-pitched, purring sound that must be auscultated using the stethoscope bell for detection. Auscultate over the liver and spleen area for any possible friction rub. This abnormal, rough, grating sound is present during infection, malignancy, or infarction. A venous hum may be auscultated in the epigastric and umbilical area. It is an abnormal, continuous, medium-pitched sound that suggests hepatic cirrhosis.

Percussion. The percussion notes of the abdomen are dullness and tympany. Dullness is percussed over solid structures (abdominal organs), whereas tympany is percussed over air-filled areas. Prior to beginning, ask the person whether any abdominal pain is present and if so, where. Percuss this area last. Percuss all four quadrants of the abdomen, noting the change in percussion notes.

To percuss the liver borders (Fig. 33–36), start at the nipple in the midclavicular line and percuss downward from resonance to dullness. Using your marking pen, mark the area where dullness begins. This is the upper liver border. Then begin percussion at the level of the umbilicus, midclavicular line, and percuss upward from tympany to dullness. Mark the area where dullness begins. This is the lower liver border. The distance between the two markings should be 6 to 12 centimeters in an adult. Using the same procedure, percuss along the midsternal line. The distance at the midsternal line should be 4 to 8 centimeters.

The spleen is percussed at the lowest interspace in the left anterior axillary line. When the spleen is of normal size, you should elicit a tympanic note in this area. If the spleen is enlarged, tympany will be replaced by dullness. The gastric air bubble will be located between the sixth and seventh ribs on the person's left side. You will have a tympanic percussion note from this area.

Palpation. Light and deep palpation are used to examine the abdomen. Light palpation is used to assess tenderness, muscle tone, abdominal stiffening, and superficial masses. Deep palpation is used to distinguish masses, organs, and deep pain. Begin with light palpation, using the palmar surfaces of the fingertips. Depress the abdomen about 1 cm. Be sure to assess all abdominal quadrants. If the person demonstrates voluntary guarding (muscle rigidity), this usually means the person is not relaxed. Ask the person to take some deep breaths through the mouth and exhale through the nose. Involuntary guarding may indicate acute appendicitis, pelvic inflammatory disease, or acute cholecystitis. After the completion of light palpation, you may deeply palpate all quadrants. Deep palpation requires more pressure than light palpation. Therefore, you will need to proceed cautiously and with supervision when performing this form of palpation. It is sometimes easier to place one hand on top of the other. If any masses are palpated, note the size, location, contour, mobility, consistency, and tenderness.

To palpate the liver deeply, place your fingertips below the lower border of liver dullness. Ask the person to take a deep breath as you gently push inward and upward. You should be able to palpate the edge of the liver as the person inhales. The liver should feel smooth, firm, and sharp. If the liver feels hard, this may indicate cirrhosis.

The spleen is generally not palpable in an adult unless it is enlarged. To palpate, place the right hand below the left costal margin and palpate in toward the spleen.

The kidneys are usually not palpable, but you may be able to feel the lower pole of the right kidney in a thin adult. To palpate the right kidney, place your left hand on the person's back just below and parallel to the 12th rib. Place your right hand in the right upper quadrant, parallel to the rectus muscle. Instruct the person to take a deep breath. With your left hand, push the kidney upward. With your right hand push downward. You should have the kidney between your hands. Ask the person to exhale as you slowly release your right hand. If you are able to palpate, note the size, contour, and any tenderness. The left kidney is palpated by standing on the person's left side using the opposite

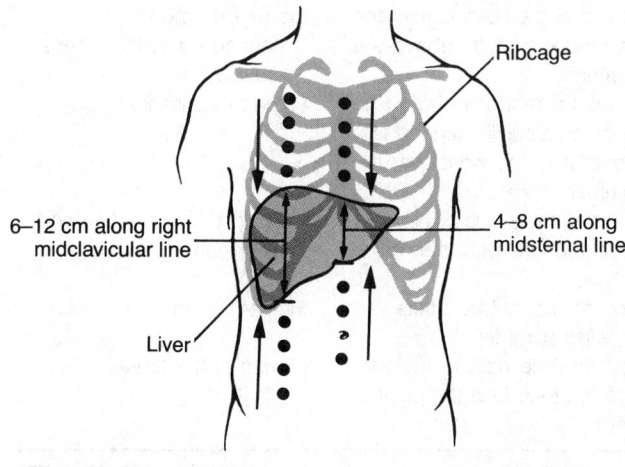

▲ **Figure 33–36**

Assessment of liver borders using percussion.

Labels on figure:
Ribcage
6–12 cm along right midclavicular line
4–8 cm along midsternal line
Liver

hands while following the same procedure as for the right kidney.

The aorta is palpated by pressing firmly into the epigastric area slightly left of the midline with your fingertips. Identify the aortic pulsation. A prominent pulsation with lateral expansion may indicate an aortic aneurysm.

Abdominal Reflex Assessment. A reflex assessment tests both sensory input and motor response. A **reflex** is an involuntary body response mediated by the spinal cord. The pathway of the reflex arc is the coordinated functioning of the horn cells at each segment of the spinal cord. Initiation of reflexes may be obtained by stimulating the skin (superficial or cutaneous reflexes) or by stimulating the tendon by tapping a tendon, bone, or muscle (deep tendon reflexes). Table 33–9 describes the procedure for eliciting the upper and lower abdominal reflexes and the cremasteric reflex.

When documenting reflexes, use a comparison chart. This may be a simple stick figure drawing with the degree of reflex activity recorded on the right and left sides, using a scale of 1+ to 4+ (Table 33–9). An alternative method is to use a simple chart such as that shown in Figure 33–37.

Genitals and Rectum

The genital and rectal areas are examined using inspection and palpation. Genital and rectal examinations

REFLEX	RIGHT	LEFT
Lower abdominal	2+	2+
Cremasteric	2+	2+

▲ Figure 33–37

A simple method for charting client reflexes.

often are anxiety-provoking for the men and women being examined. Help the person feel more comfortable by maintaining a relaxed but competent attitude. Keep the person informed of your actions. Do not make quick movements. Avoid any actions or statements that the person can interpret as sexually provocative. It may be helpful to have another health professional present during the genital/rectal examinations. Use firm touch rather than gentle stroking. If the person does become sexually stimulated, alter the examination sequence if necessary, but continue the examination in a professional manner. Enhance comfort during the genital examinations by also:

▶ providing privacy and preventing exposure, e.g., screen, door shut, drapes;
▶ not prolonging the examination unduly;
▶ warming instruments, such as vaginal speculum;
▶ using lubricants when possible to minimize discomfort during insertion, as of gloves or speculum.

TABLE 33–9. Reflex Assessment*

Reflex	Type	Procedure	Normal Response
Upper and lower abdominal	Superficial (cutaneous)	Stroke each side of abdomen above and below the level of the umbilicus, using the pointed end of the reflex hammer. Stroke toward the umbilicus	Abdominal muscle contraction and umbilicus deviation toward stimulus
Cremasteric	Superficial (cutaneous)	Stroke the inner thigh of men with the pointed end of the reflex hammer	Testes rise in the scrotum
Biceps	Deep tendon	Person's arm should be flexed with the palm down. Examiner's thumb should be placed on the biceps tendon at the antecubital space. Strike the thumb with the reflex hammer	Flexion of the elbow and contraction of the biceps muscle
Triceps	Deep tendon	Person's arm should be flexed and placed across the chest. Strike the triceps tendon directly above the elbow with the reflex hammer	Elbow extension and contraction of the triceps muscle
Supinator or brachioradialis	Deep tendon	Person's arm should rest on the abdomen with the palm down. Strike the brachioradialis tendon approximately 2 inches proximal to the wrist over the radius with the reflex hammer	Forearm supination
Knee (patellar)	Deep tendon	Person should sit with knees bent and legs hanging freely. Strike the patellar tendon with the reflex hammer	Quadriceps contraction and extension of the leg
Ankle (Achilles)	Deep tendon	Dorsiflex the person's foot at the ankle. Strike the Achilles tendon with the reflex hammer	Plantar flexion
Plantar (Babinski)	Superficial (cutaneous)	Stroke the sole of the foot from the heel to the ball, curving across the ball of the foot. Use the pointed end of the reflex hammer	Flexion of the toes

* Normal reflexes are categorized as superficial or cutaneous (elicited by stimulating the skin) and deep tendon (elicited by tapping a tendon). Reflexes are graded on a 4-point scale: 0, no response; 1+, slightly diminished; 2+, normal; 3+, brisker than normal; 4+, brisk, hyperactive. Remember to compare one side of the body with the other.

Remember to wear gloves during the genital and rectal examinations.

MALE GENITALIA

Inspection and palpation of the *male genitalia* are performed with the person in a supine position and then in a standing position.

Inspection. Inspection of the male genitalia (Fig. 33–38) includes the penis, scrotum, and inguinal ring and canal. To assess secondary sex characteristics, observe the penis and testes for size and shape, color and texture of the scrotal skin, and distribution of the pubic hair. Observe for the presence of lice or nits attached to the pubic hair.

Inspect the skin, prepuce (foreskin) if present, and the glans of the penis. Observe for any lesions, odor, discharge, or inflammation. Normally, the area should be clean. The urethra should open in the center of the glans tip. The prepuce should be retracted to observe for chancres or carcinomas. Smegma (cheesy white material) may be observed under the foreskin. This is considered normal. The urethral meatus should be observed for discharge by compressing the glans between your index finger and thumb. Inspect the scrotal skin and contours for any sores, rashes, swelling, lumps, or veins. Also inspect for any groin masses by asking the person to cough while you observe for any bulging that may indicate an inguinal hernia.

Palpation. Palpate the penis using your thumb and first two fingers. Note any tenderness or induration. The testes and epididymis of the scrotum are palpated using the thumb and first two fingers. Note size, shape, and consistency, and any tenderness or nodules. Normally, the testes feel firm (not hard), possibly spongy. Each testicle is egg (oval)-shaped, about 4 cm long and 2 to 2.5 cm wide. The testicle is descended in each side of the scrotum, with the left testicle lower than the right. The epididymis is located behind the testicles and is soft (spongy). The spermatic cords are palpated for nodules and swelling. They should be firm, smooth, and tubular. Each structure in the scrotum should be bilaterally similar.

FEMALE GENITALIA

Inspection and palpation are the techniques used to examine the female genitalia. As stated earlier, the student as well as the person being examined may experience anxiety and embarrassment thinking about the prospect of examining the genitalia as well as having one's genitalia examined. It is important for you to maintain a professional manner and be attuned to the person's fears and behaviors. Prior to beginning the examination, instruct the person to empty the bladder. If a urine specimen is needed, have the person save one at this time. The female genitalia is examined with the person in a lithotomy position. In the lithotomy position, the person is lying on the back on an examining table with the knees flexed and the feet in stirrups. Elevate the person's head slightly, as this aids in relaxing the abdominal muscles. A drape should cover the person's thighs and knees.

Be sure to explain each step of the examination. Upon palpation, touch the person's thigh prior to contact with the genitalia and avoid any sudden or unexpected movements. The equipment used during this examination includes a gooseneck lamp, vaginal speculum, water-soluble lubricant, disposable gloves, glass slides, wooden spatulas, and a specimen bottle with fixative solution. Be sure that all equipment is assembled before beginning the examination. A female student may perform the examination alone or may have another female health professional present. A male student will need to have a female present in the room during the examination.

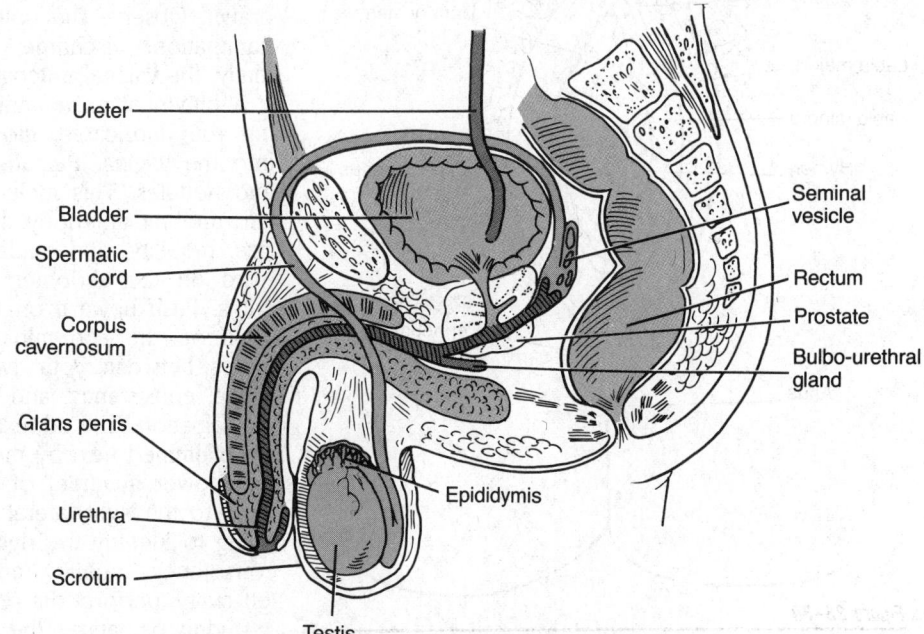

▲ *Figure 33–38*

Structures of the male urogenital tract.

Ureter
Bladder
Spermatic cord
Corpus cavernosum
Glans penis
Urethra
Scrotum
Testis
Epididymis
Seminal vesicle
Rectum
Prostate
Bulbo-urethral gland

Inspection and Palpation

External Inspection. Inspect the external genitalia (Fig. 33–39) (mons pubis, labia, and perineum). Note the character and distribution of the pubic hair. Separate the labia and inspect the labia minora, clitoris, urethral orifice, and the introitus (vaginal opening). Observe for inflammation, discharge, ulceration, and nodules. If you observe any swelling, inspect and palpate Bartholin's glands by palpating the posterior area of the labia majora with the thumb and index finger (placed near the posterior end of the introitus).

The pubic hair should be normally distributed. There should be no odor and minimal, clear discharge. No lesions should be observed. The vulva should be more darkly pigmented than the other skin. Before menopause, the labia majora are filled out and well formed. After menopause, the labia majora are thinned and eventually become atrophied. The size of the clitoris is variable, usually 3 to 4 mm. The labia minora are thinner than the labia majora and tend to lie open in women who have experienced childbirth. In a virgin, the labia minora will lie close together. The urethral orifice is located between the clitoris and the introitus. There should be no discharge from this area.

Internal Inspection. The inspection of the internal genitalia is considered an advanced assessment skill. Beginning students usually do not perform this aspect

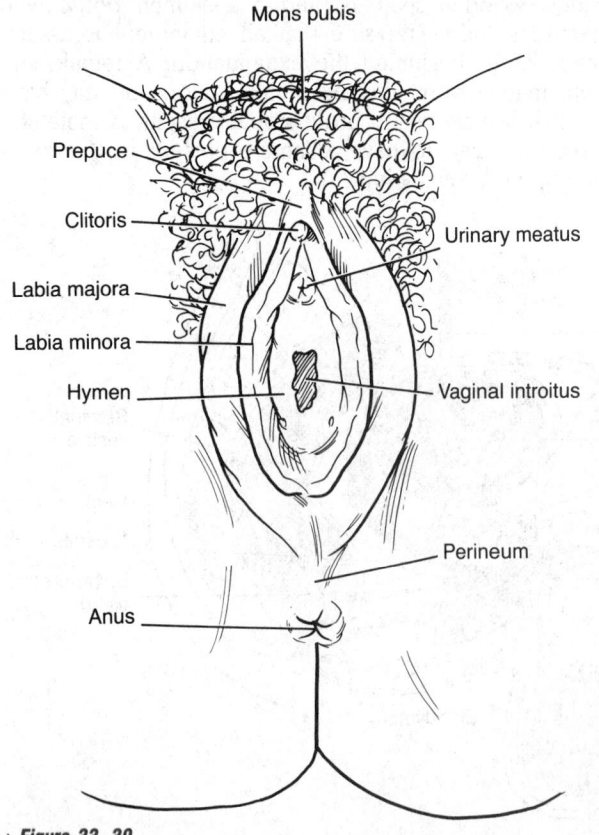

▲ **Figure 33–39**

External female genitalia.

Mons pubis

Prepuce

Clitoris

Labia majora

Labia minora

Hymen

Anus

Urinary meatus

Vaginal introitus

Perineum

of the examination. Therefore, it will be discussed briefly.

Insert your gloved index finger (lubricated with water only) into the vagina and locate the cervix. Assess the size of the introitus. This will help in deciding the size speculum you will wish to use. Next, with the labia separated, instruct the person to strain down. Observe for any bulging of the vaginal walls.

The internal genitalia (cervix and vagina) are inspected using a speculum. The speculum should be warm and lubricated with water prior to insertion. Do not use a water-soluble lubricant on the speculum because it may distort examination of the cytologic specimen. Inform the person that you are going to perform the speculum examination. Using your left index and middle fingers, depress the perineum. With your right hand, insert the speculum at an oblique angle into the introitus, passing over your left fingers. Be sure that you do not introduce the speculum vertically, as this could injure the urethral orifice and the urethra. When the speculum is completely inserted, rotate it to a transverse position and open slowly. The handle of the speculum should be pointed downward. Tighten the set screw in order to keep the speculum open. You should be able to visualize the cervix.

Inspect the cervix and os for color, position, and surface characteristics. Normally, the cervix is round, pink, and smooth. Note any ulcerations, nodules, masses, bleeding, or discharge. A cervical discharge is normally present and varies from thin and clear to thick, white, and stringy. It depends on the menstrual cycle. An endocervical swab is obtained using a cotton-tipped applicator that is inserted into the cervix and rotated. It is then removed and smeared gently on a glass slide. The slide is then placed in a fixative or sprayed with a fixative. A cervical scrape is also obtained using a wooden spatula inserted into the os. The spatula is turned and scraped in a full circle and then the specimen is placed on a second glass slide. The vaginal mucosa is inspected as the speculum is withdrawn. Observe the color of the mucosa and any inflammation, discharge, ulcerations, or masses. Normally, the vaginal mucosa is moist and pink.

A bimanual examination is performed next by placing your lubricated, gloved index and middle fingers into the vagina. Palpate the perineum for tenderness and nodules. This includes the region of the bladder and urethra, anteriorly. Palpate the cervix for position, size, mobility, and tenderness. Next, place your other hand on the abdomen slightly above the symphysis pubis. Push upward on the cervix as you push downward on the abdominal wall. Attempt to grasp the uterus between your two hands, palpating the size, shape, consistency, and mobility. Note any tenderness on palpation. The adnexa (ovaries and fallopian tubes) are examined next by moving your outside hand to the right lower quadrant of the abdomen and your inside hand to the right lateral fornix. Press in the abdomen, trying to identify the right ovary. Note the size, shape, consistency, mobility, and tenderness. To palpate the left ovary, perform the procedure on the left side.

During palpation, the normal cervix can be gently moved sideways without pain. It feels smooth and firm and lies midline usually on the anterior wall. The cervix points away from the fundus of the uterus. The uterus is usually in an anterior position but can be retroverted in some women. The rectovaginal wall is smooth, firm, and resilient when palpated. The normal ovary (4 to 6 cm) is slightly tender when palpated but should be smooth, firm, and oval. The fallopian tubes cannot be palpated.

RECTUM

Inspection and digital palpation are performed with the person in a left lateral (Sims') position. Females may be in the lithotomy position.

Inspection. The anal area is inspected by gently spreading the buttocks to expose the anus. The rectal skin should be darker than the surrounding skin. The anal and perianal surfaces should be clear and moist without hairs. Observe the anal area for hemorrhoids, rashes, inflammation, and ulcers.

Digital Palpation. Instruct the person to strain down (Valsalva maneuver). Using a gloved finger and lubricant, palpate the anus with your finger tip. When the anus is relaxed, gently insert your well-lubricated finger by turning the finger and pushing toward the person's umbilicus. Tell the person when you are going to insert your finger. Ask the person to tighten the anus around your finger. Rotate your finger to palpate all surfaces and muscles. Palpate to a depth of 6 to 10 cm. In a male, examine the prostate, feeling each lobe (Fig. 33–40). Note size, shape, nodules, consistency, and tenderness. A prostate that is tender, enlarged, soft, or hard is abnormal. Examine the stool (taken from the glove) for blood or pus. A Hemoccult test may be performed as a screening for colorectal cancer. In a woman, a vaginal/rectal palpation will be performed. This is another higher-level assessment skill that requires supervision.

Normally, the anal sphincter tone should be strong. The rectal mucosa should be smooth, without any masses. The prostate should be palpable anteriorly. The rectal-vaginal septum should be firm and smooth, and the muscles should be firm. Finally, the stool should be brown and soft.

Extremities

The upper and lower extremities are assessed by using inspection, palpation, and auscultation. As you perform this section of the examination, you will also be assessing the peripheral vascular system through assessment of pulses and the neurologic system through assessment of reflexes.

UPPER EXTREMITIES

The upper extremities are inspected beginning at the fingertips and moving toward the shoulder. The person should be in a sitting position. Observe size and symmetry, color and texture of the skin and nailbeds, venous pattern, and any edema. The nail base should be firm, with a 160-degree angle between the fingernail and the nail base (Fig. 33–41). When assessing the nailbeds, observe for any **clubbing,** an abnormality of the nail in which the nailbed appears springy (early clubbing) or swollen (late clubbing) and the angle of the nail is 180 degrees or greater. Clubbing may suggest hypoxia or lung cancer. Blanch the nailbed and note the amount of time required for capillary refill. A capillary refill occurring in less than 3 seconds is considered normal, between 3 to 4 seconds is sluggish, and greater than 4 seconds is abnormal. A prominence in venous pattern and edema may suggest a venous obstruction.

The brachial, radial, and ulnar pulses are palpated for rate, rhythm, and quality (force) (Table 33–10). Remember to compare the volume of the pulses on each arm. Attempt to palpate the epitrochlear lymph node. It is located by having the person flex the elbow to 90 degrees while you palpate the depression between the biceps and triceps muscle. Normally it is very difficult to palpate, but if present, note its size, consistency, and any tenderness.

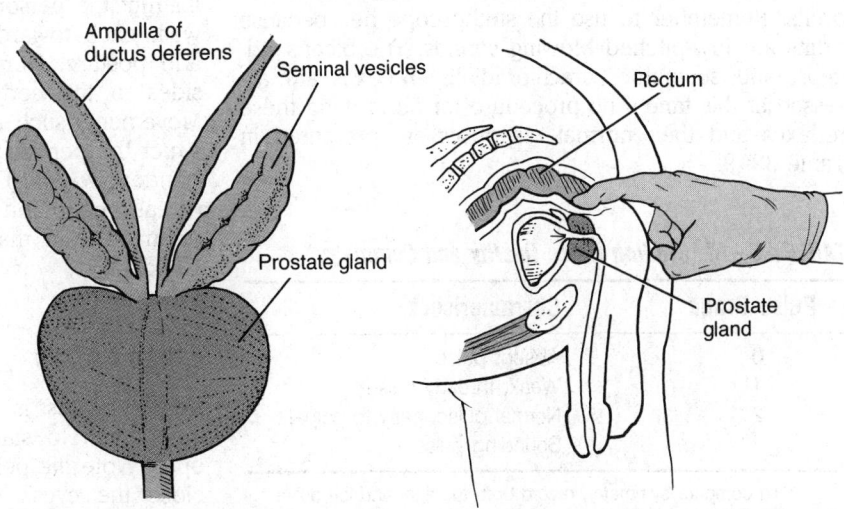

▲ **Figure 33–40**

Examining the prostate gland using palpation technique.

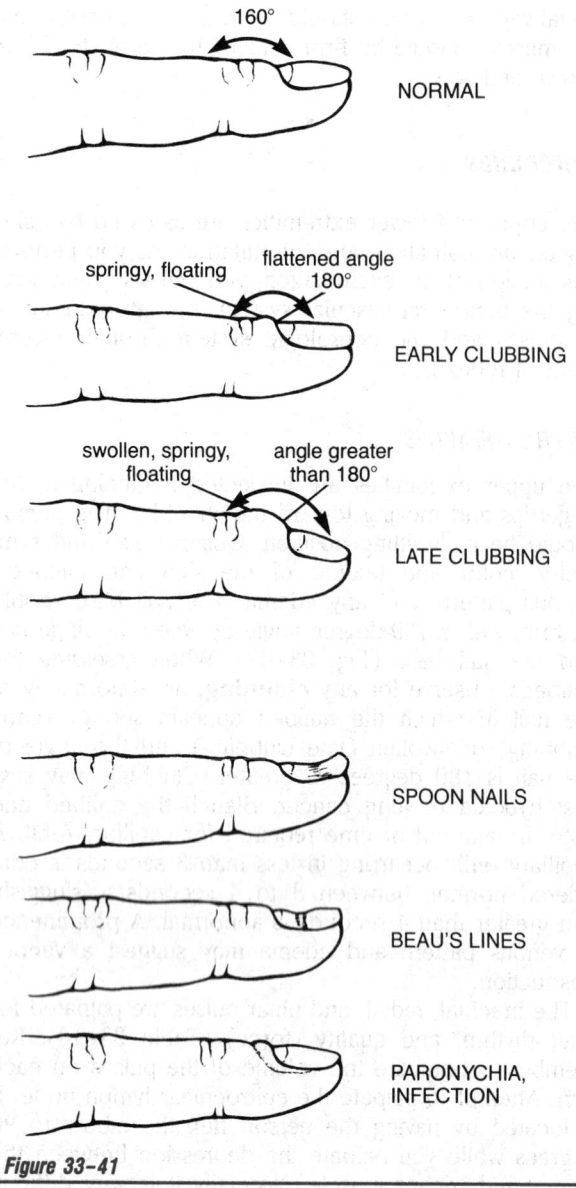

▲ **Figure 33-41**

Nail abnormalities.

Auscultate the brachial, radial, and ulnar pulses for bruits. Remember to use the stethoscope bell because bruits are low-pitched blowing sounds. The biceps, triceps, and supinator (brachioradialis) reflexes are assessed at this time. The procedure for performing these reflexes and their normal responses are presented in Table 33-9.

TABLE 33-10. Grading Pulse Quality and Symmetry*

Pulse Grade	Characteristics
0	Absent pulse
1+	Weak, thready pulse
2+	Normal pulse, easy to palpate
3+	Bounding pulse

* To compare symmetry, record both the right and left pulse quality. Example: 1+/2+.

LOWER EXTREMITIES

The lower extremities are examined with the person in a supine position, external genital area draped, and legs exposed. Inspection begins at the groin and buttock area and extends to the toes. Observe for size and symmetry, venous pattern, color and texture of the skin and nailbeds, hair distribution on lower legs, feet and toes, pigmentation, rashes, scars, ulcers, and edema. Test the toenails for capillary refill. A person experiencing arterial insufficiency will experience pain, decreased peripheral pulses, pale skin color, cool skin temperature, mild edema, thin, shiny skin, loss of hair over the feet and toes, and thickened nails. Ulcers may or may not be present.

Palpation begins by examining the superficial inguinal lymph nodes. These nodes are located horizontally and vertically to the inguinal area. Normally, you may palpate a nontender node in this area up to 2 cm in diameter. Palpate the femoral, popliteal, dorsalis pedis, and posterior tibialis pulses, comparing the volume of each pulse on each leg (Table 33-10). Test for **Homan's sign,** an indicator of deep phlebitis, in which pain and soreness are present in the calf area when the foot is dorsiflexed. The person's flexed leg is supported by the calf with your nondominant hand while you dorsiflex the foot with your dominant hand. Note any pain or soreness in the calf area. If present, this would be a positive Homan's sign, indicating the possible presence of phlebitis. The patellar, ankle, and plantar reflexes are assessed at this time in the examination.

Motor System

Inspect the voluntary muscles for atrophy, **fasciculations** (uncontrollable twitching), and involuntary movements. In addition, you will need to assess gait, Romberg's sign, muscle strength, and coordination.

GAIT

Gait is a person's style of walking. To assess gait, instruct the person to walk across the room, turn, and walk back toward you. Observe the person's balance and posture. Normally, the arms are swinging at the sides of the body and balance is easily maintained. Movements such as turns should be smooth. Next, instruct the person to walk in a straight line, heel to toe (tandem walking). Inability to do tandem walking can reveal a condition known as ataxia. **Ataxia** is an uncoordinated gait that results from cerebellar disease or intoxication.

ROMBERG'S TEST

Romberg's test is a test of sensory equilibrium. Instruct the person to stand with the feet together and eyes open. Note the person's balance. Then have the person close the eyes. Normally, you will observe minimal swaying. Stay close to the person during this test. If the person should lose balance, this is considered a "positive Romberg" and may suggest cerebellar ataxia.

TESTS OF MUSCLE STRENGTH

Muscle strength is assessed by having the person move against your resistance. All major muscle groups should be tested. Muscle strength is graded on a scale of 0 to 5 (see Chapter 35).

Flexion and extension of the elbow are tested by having the person pull and push against your hand. *Extension of the wrist* is tested by trying to pull the person's formed fist in a downward motion. *Finger abduction* is tested by instructing the person to spread the fingers while you try to force them back together. *Thumb opposition* is tested by instructing the person to touch the thumb to the little finger while you apply resistance to the thumb. *Hip flexion* is tested by applying your hand to the person's thigh and instructing the person to raise the leg against your resistance. *Abduction of the hip* is tested by placing your hand on the outside of the legs at the knee level and instructing the person to spread both legs against your resistance. *Hip adduction* is tested by placing your hands on the inside of the person's legs (knee level) and instructing the person to bring the legs together. *Knee flexion* is tested by placing one hand on the person's slightly flexed knee and your other hand behind the ankle with the person's foot resting on the examination table. Instruct the person to flex the knee against your resistance, without moving the foot. *Ankle dorsiflexion* and *plantar flexion* are tested by asking the person to pull up and push down the foot against your hand.

TESTS OF COORDINATION

Coordination is assessed using rapid alternating movements (RAM) and point-to-point testing. The person is instructed to pat the leg with the hand as rapidly as possible, to turn the hand over and back as quickly as possible, and to touch each finger with the thumb as rapidly as possible. Test each hand separately. Note smooth quick movements. Movements that are slowed and uncoordinated may indicate cerebellar dysfunction. The finger-to-nose test is performed with the person in a sitting position and the arms extended forward. Instruct the person to touch the nose with the forefinger, then return the arm to the extended position. Perform this with alternating hands. Test the person first with the eyes open and then with the eyes closed. Observe for smooth movements and maintenance of proper body posture. Cerebellar dysfunction is indicated when the person fails to perform this task.

Sensory System

The sensory system is examined through the assessment of pain, temperature, light touch, vibration, and position. The sensations are relayed through different pathways. Sensory discrimination tests, which include stereognosis, number identification, two-point discrimination, point localization, and extinction, are considered components of the sensory system. These test the ability of the cortex to analyze and interpret sensations. Prior to beginning the assessment, ask the person about any areas of numbness or unusual sensation. In each test, the person's eyes should be closed. Remember, you will be comparing both sides of the body, including arms, legs, and trunk. Note any numbness or tingling and the degree of stimulation necessary to elicit a response.

LIGHT TOUCH/SUPERFICIAL PAIN

Using a wisp of cotton and a safety pin, alternately touch the distal and proximal portions of the upper and lower extremities. Ask the person to identify the location and the type of sensation (soft or sharp). If the person exhibits an abnormal pain sensation, test the temperature sensation.

TEMPERATURE

The temperature test should be performed only when the person's perception of pain is abnormal. Fill two test tubes with water, one hot and the other cold. Touch all medial and lateral limb surfaces, while alternating symmetrical areas. Instruct the person to identify whether the sensation is hot or cold.

VIBRATION

Vibration is assessed by tapping a tuning fork and placing it firmly on the person's interphalangeal joint of the finger and great toe. Ask the person to describe the sensation (pressure or vibration) and to identify when the sensation ends. Other areas to assess are the forehead, bridge of nose, elbow, wrists, knees, and ankles. Proceed from distal to proximal areas.

POSITION (PROPRIOCEPTION)

Position is assessed by holding one of the person's fingertips between your thumb and forefinger. Slowly flex and extend the finger. Also perform the test on the great toe. Instruct the person to identify when the finger is moving and in which direction. If the person demonstrates difficulty in identifying position, proceed to the next joint and repeat the procedure.

STEREOGNOSIS

Stereognosis is the act of recognizing objects on the basis of touching and manipulating them. Place a familiar object, such as a key, paper clip, or pencil, in the person's hand and have them identify the object. The person should be able to perform this test without difficulty. If an abnormality exists, perform the number identification test.

NUMBER IDENTIFICATION (GRAPHESTHESIA)

Trace several numbers on each of the person's palms with the blunt end of a pen or pencil. The person should be able to identify the numbers.

Text continued on page 701

HEALTH HISTORY

IDENTIFYING DATA:

Initials: M.A.
Room Number: 234
Admission Date: 2/7/93
Age: 26
Ethnicity: Caucasian
Birth Place: Calgary, Alberta

HISTORICAL ASSESSMENT:

Informant: The individual

Level of Responsiveness and Reliability: Oriented to person, place, and time. Very cooperative, responding openly to questions asked.

PRESENT ILLNESS:

Chief Complaint: "I've had a really bad headache and a stopped up nose for the past two days."

Course of Illness: Individual woke up two days ago with a headache and has had it intermittently since then. It is described as a pressure around the eyes that is sometimes severe and causes the individual to become nauseated. The pressure is described as a "heavy feeling." Bending or moving the head quickly makes the headache worse. Applying a warm cloth to the face eased the headache. Nose congestion is described as an "aggravating stuffiness." The nose is draining a greenish yellow discharge. Stated that a sinus medication and antipyretic/analgesic medication are being taken.

PAST HEALTH AND ILLNESS:

Description of General Health Immediately Prior to Illness: Stated the presence of good health prior to clinic visit.

Pediatric and Adult Illness: Experienced mumps at the age of 14 and chicken pox at the age of 6, both without complications. Denied having had measles, whooping cough, scarlet fever, polio, anemia, diphtheria, rheumatic fever, diabetes, cancer, mental illness, stroke, hepatitis, malaria, seizures, chronic bronchitis, heart disease, or hypertension.

Hospitalization: Has never been hospitalized.

Operations and Injuries Without Hospitalization: Wisdom teeth removed at the age of 16 without complications. Suffered a torn ligament in the right knee at the age of 17. The knee was casted for 4 weeks. No problems with the knee since that experience.

Immunizations: All immunizations are up to date.

Allergies: No known allergies.

Transfusions: Denied any transfusions.

Current Treatment: None.

▲ *Figure 33-42*

An example of documentation of a client's health history and physical assessment.

FAMILY HEALTH AND ILLNESS:

Present Status of Parents, Siblings, and Children: *Parents are both currently healthy with no past problems. The individual has one brother and two sisters, all of whom are healthy with no past medical problems. The older sister is slightly obese. The paternal grandfather died at the age of 73 from heart disease. The paternal grandmother had breast cancer treated with a mastectomy 20 years ago. The maternal grandfather suffered from arthritis and died at the age of 70 from heart disease. The maternal grandmother suffers from hypertension. The client denies a family history of diabetes, renal disease, allergies, tuberculosis, stroke, deafness, alcoholism, or seizures.*

Similar Illness or Symptoms in Family: *Denied any knowledge of similar symptoms or illness in the family.*

PERSONAL AND SOCIAL HISTORY:

Current Situation: *Has been married for one year and does not have any children. Is of the Baptist faith and is currently a full time student. Has not had any military experience.*

A daily routine consists of the following: getting up around 6:30 a.m. and preparing for class while eating breakfast. Attends class all day, except for a lunch break, when she goes home to make supper. After cleaning up the supper dishes, she usually studies for 2 to 3 hours. Goes to bed around 11:00 p.m./midnight. Normally has a bowel movement every day. Denied any type of exercise, smoking, drug or alcohol ingestion. The husband is sole provider of income and health insurance. Denied having any pets or hobbies.

Past Development: *Childhood was a normal and happy one. Had worked since high school as an office assistant at a bakery before starting college.*

Patterns of Interaction and Communication: *Denied any problems with interaction. Described personality as basically very happy but has occasional angry outbursts and feelings of frustration when under pressure at school.*

SYSTEMS REVIEW:

Integument: *Denied color changes, pruritus, infections, inflammations, rash, tumors, nail changes, excessive bruising, or cuts failing to heal. Has moles over a good portion of her body. The client was instructed to contact a physician if there are any changes in the moles.*

Eyes: *Wears corrective lenses only for reading. Began wearing glasses at the age of 23. Last eye exam was in 1987. Complained of pain around eyes for the last two days. Described pain as a feeling of pressure and a slight feeling of puffiness. Stated that the pain at times has been severe and that it came and went depending on what she was doing. Denied any blurring, diplopia, or excessive tearing.*

Ears: *Denied any tinnitus, discharge, infection, or vertigo. Stated that she often gets an earache after flying but that it goes away by itself shortly after landing.*

Nose and Sinuses: *See Present Illness. Denied epistaxis.*

Mouth and Throat: *Denied any problems with gums, teeth, sore throat, sore tongue, difficulty swallowing, hoarseness, voice change, goiter, or bleeding gums. Does not wear dentures. Last dental exam was 3 months ago.*

Neck: *Denied any pain, limitation of movement, or thyroid/lymph node enlargement.*

Respiratory: *Denied any persistent cough, irregular sputum, hemoptysis, wheezing, dyspnea, recurrent respiratory tract infections, night sweats, pain, or positive tuberculin test. Does not remember the date of last chest x-ray.*

▲ *Figure 33-42* Continued

Illustration continued on following page

Cardiovascular: Denied any chest pain, dyspnea, PND, orthopnea, palpitations, murmur, hypertension, syncope, anemia, edema, varicosities, thrombophlebitis, claudication, or pain.

Gastrointestinal: Has had a problem with nausea in the past 48 hours. Attributed this to the headache. Stated the nausea gets better when lying down and being still. Denied any vomiting, dysphagia, eructation, hematemesis, pain, gas, indigestion, or jaundice; no changes in bowel habits, or constipation, diarrhea, hemorrhoids, or hernia; no changes in stool or bowel habits, and no weight changes or rectal itching.

Genitourinary/Reproductive: Denied any symptoms of frequency, nocturia, urgency, dysuria, incontinence, albuminuria, flank pain, venereal disease, discharge, lesions, hesitancy, hematuria, pyuria, infections, stones, glycosuria, infertility, or decrease of libido. Uses no form of birth control. Menstrual period began at the age of approximately 13. The date of last monthly period was 9/10/92. Cycle is normally 28 days. Duration of flow is usually 3 days. Periods are usually regular and very rarely cause more than a mild discomfort as well as a little irritability. Last pelvic exam was July 1991; results were normal. Last Pap smear July 1991, results were normal. Denied ever having had an abortion. Has no children and hopes to finish school before becoming pregnant. Does understand the risk of becoming pregnant since no form of birth control is being used.

Musculoskeletal: Denied any symptoms of myalgias, weakness, pain, swelling, redness, heat, limitation of motion, or stiffness.

Endocrine: Denied any sensitivity to environmental temperatures, changes in body configuration, changes in scalp or hair, sweating, postural hypotension, change in voice, polyuria, polydipsia, or polyphagia. Is comfortable with present weight in relation to body size.

Neurologic: Denied any syncope, convulsions, seizures, vertigo, diplopia, paralysis, paresis, spasms, paresthesia, tremor, ataxia, memory change, unconsciousness, speech problems, or coordination problems. See Present Illness regarding headache.

Psychologic: Denied any nervousness, insomnia, depression, nightmares, indecisiveness, hyperventilation, work difficulty, mood changes, sense of failure, social withdrawal, or memory loss. Does at times have a problem with anger and irritability during times of stress.

▲ **Figure 33–42** Continued

PHYSICAL ASSESSMENT

Vital Signs:

T: 98.6   **P:** 72 regular   **R:** 16 regular

BP: Supine: Rt. arm - 127/76   Lt. arm - 126/78
         Sitting   Rt. arm - 124/76   Lt. arm - 124/74
         Standing   Rt. arm - 122/72   Lt. arm - 122/70

Ht: 5' 4"   **Wt:** 120 lbs.

General Physical Appearance: Ms. A. is short, average weight, medium frame, middle-aged individual with a healthy appearance. The individual is cooperative, sitting comfortably on the bed with arms relaxed and shoulders slightly slouched forward. Ms. A's dress is neat, clean, and appropriate for the weather. The individual is pleasant, friendly, smiling, talking freely and intelligently.

Mental Status and Speech: Answers judgment question in realistic manner. When asked what she does at stop signs, stated that she stops. Oriented to person, place, and time. Short-term recent, and long-term memory intact. Maintains eye contact, facial expressions symmetrical and correlate with mood and topic discussed. Fully conscious, alert, remains attentive and able to focus on exam during entire interaction. Speech clear and appropriate. Follows through with train of thought. Carefully chooses words to convey feelings and ideas.

HEAD AND NECK

Hair, Scalp, Skull, Face, Skin: Head symmetrically rounded with full ROM. Hair of average texture, chin-length, black, clean, styled, evenly distributed on head. States that hair has not had any sudden changes. Scalp/skull smooth, firm, and symmetrical with no inflammation, cysts, warts, moles, lesions, or tenderness noted. Nasal labial folds, palpebral fissures equal in size and symmetrical. Face round with no tics or other abnormal movements noted. CN V (trigeminal) and CN VII (facial) intact. Skin light to dark brown with pink/red lips. Skin warm and dry to touch, smooth, soft with no diaphoresis, inflammation, edema, lesions, lumps noted. A 3 cm scar noted immediately below midline of lower lip. Intact skin turgor noted.

Eyes: Eyes symmetrical and in alignment with top of ears. Eyebrows medium with equal distribution and no scaliness, crusting, hair loss, or hordeolum noted. Lids moist, pinkish, symmetrical, without ptosis, edema, or lesions, and freely closable bilaterally. Lashes short, evenly spaced, and curled outward. Lower margin of lid at bottom edge of iris, upper margin covers upper quadrant of eye. Blinking symmetrical and involuntary. Lacrimal gland without tenderness and no exudate noted from puncta. Bulbar conjunctive is clear and palpebral conjunctive is pink.

PERRLA: CN III, IV, VI (oculomotor, trochlear, abducens) intact. Direct light revealed constricted illuminated pupils while consensual light showed a constricted pupil from each unilluminated pupil. Both eyes moved in a smooth coordinated manner through the cardinal positions with no twitching or jerking noted. Cover-uncover test revealed no evidence of nystagmus. Corneal light reflex showed the reflection of light to be located at five o'clock bilaterally. No diplopia noted CN II (optic) intact. Peripheral vision was equal to the examiners. Vision was 20/50 O.D. and O.S. Near vision revealed no hesitation, frowning, or squinting. Color discrimination intact. Ophthalmoscopic exam: Red reflex present bilaterally. Optic disc was creamy pink, round with well-defined margins. Physiologic cup occupies half of the disc. Arterioles smaller and lighter color than venules. No opaqueness, A-V nicking, hemorrhages, or exudates noted.

▲ *Figure 33–42* Continued

Illustration continued on following page

Ears: Left and right auricles without deformity, lumps, lesions, swelling, redness, discharge, cerumen buildup, nodules, tenderness. Attachment to head is anterior to mastoid process. Otoscope examination: Canal walls pink and uniform with tympanic membrane visible. Tympanic membrane shiny, pearly gray, intact. Cone of light seen at 5 o'clock in right ear and 7 o'clock in left ear. No lesions, edema, blueness (blood), pink/red (inflammation), dark shadows through oval opening (perforations), scarring, tenderness noted. CN VIII (acoustic) intact. Whisper and watch test showed no problems with the auditory acuity. Weber lateralization revealed vibration to be heard equally in both ears. Rinne test revealed a 2:1 ratio with air to bone conduction. Bone conduction was equal to the examiner during Schwabach test.

Nose and Sinuses: Nose is medium sized, symmetrical, and same color as face. External structure without lesions, nodules, erythema, discharge, crusting noted. Nasal septum midline symmetrical without bleeding, perforation, or deviation. Pink moist mucosa with uniform color with no lesions, bleeding, swelling, drainage, grayness noted. Air was felt being exhaled through opposite naris and was noiseless. Frontal and maxillary sinus palpated without tenderness. CN I (olfactory) intact: Correctly identified peppermint scent and coffee aroma.

Mouth and Pharynx: Lips symmetrical, smooth, moist with pinkish lipstick, more pigmented than facial skin, without lesions, nodules, fissures, dryness, edema, ulcerations, cyanosis, or pallor noted. Buccal mucosa pink and moist without discoloration or increased pigmentation. No ulcers or nodules. Gums pink and moist without pallor, erythemia, cyanosis, ulcers, bleeding, white patches, tenderness, inflammation. Twenty-eight shiny, pearly white teeth in good condition with few dental caries, stable with smooth surfaces and edges. Tongue midline, symmetrical, moist, pink, and with smooth movement, without dryness, ulcers, nodules, fissures, and jerky movement. Hard palate pale, soft palate pink, soft palate pink without jaundice, cyanosis, pallor, or redness. Tonsillar pillars symmetrical and without exudate, ulcers, lesions, edema, or enlargement. Uvula in midline and elevates when the individual says "ah" (CN X, vagus intact). CN IX (glossopharyngeal) and CN X (vagus) intact: Gag reflex present; successfully identified a taste on posterior third of tongue. CN VII (facial) intact: Identified sugar placed on anterior 2/3 of tongue. CN XII (hypoglossal) intact: Stuck out tongue and moved it around.

Neck: Neck is symmetrical, in upright position with smooth, controlled movement, without masses, scars, lesions, or pulsations. Preauricular, submental, submandibular, deep cervical chain, posterior auricular, occipital, superficial cervical, posterior cervical, and supraclavicular lymph nodes nonpalpable. Thyroid gland barely palpable, lobes not felt. Trachea in midline, and symmetrical. Carotid arteries equally strong and without bruits. CN XI (spinal accessory) intact: Trapezius muscles and sternocleidomastoid muscles show equal strength. No jugular distention noted.

Chest: Skin without scars, pulsations, or lesions. No hair noted. Chest symmetrical, slope of ribs at 45 degree angle, even and relaxed intercostal spaces, sternum level with ribs, without deformities, abnormal retraction or bulging of intercostal spaces during inspiration or expiration, use of accessory muscles, or local lag. AP transverse ratio is 1:2. Respirations even, unlabored, and regular at 16/min. No tenderness, masses, or sinus tracts noted. Tactile fremitus decreases below T5 bilaterally posteriorly, and 4th ICS anteriorly bilaterally which is estimated level of diaphragm. Respiratory excursion revealed equal chest expansion bilaterally both posteriorly and anteriorly. Resonance was percussed throughout chest. Diaphragmatic excursion measured 4 cm bilaterally. Bronchial, bronchovesicular, and vesicular breath sounds auscultated. No crackles, wheezes, rhonchi, or friction rubs noted. Negative for bronchophony, egophony, and whispered pectoriloquy.

Heart: No pulsations, lifts-heaves, or vibrations noted in aortic, pulmonic, Erbs, tricuspid, mitral, or epigastric area. PMI: 5th ICS to LMCL, approx. size of nickel. Apical pulse–72/min and regular. S1 auscultated loudest over mitral area with S2 being loudest over aortic area. No extra heart sounds (S3, S4, split S1, split S2, friction rubs, or murmurs) noted.

▲ **Figure 33–42** Continued

Breasts: Nontender and symmetrical. No lumps, lesions, masses, or discharge noted. No lymph nodes palpable.

Axillae: No rashes, redness, or unusual pigmentation noted. Palpation revealed no tenderness or palpable lymph nodes.

Abdomen: Abdomen round, soft, symmetrical, paler than other skin areas with approx. 10 white striae located along center of abdomen. No masses, lesions, pulsations, dilated veins, rashes, scars noted. Peristalsis noted. Abdomen free of hair, bruising, and increased vasculature. Bowel sounds audible, low pitch and gurgling in all 4 quadrants at 11/min. Aortic and renal arteries auscultated without bruit. No venous hums or friction rubs auscultated over liver or spleen. Tympany percussed over all 4 quadrants; 6 cm liver span percussed at MSL and 20 cm liver span percussed at MCL. Spleen percussed at left anterior axillary line, lateral LUQ with tympanic sound. Gastric air bubble percussed at 5th rib on left side with tympanic sound. No tenderness or masses detected with light palpation. Deep palpation not done at this time. No upper and lower abdominal reflex noted.

Upper Extremities: Arms medium, symmetrical, light brown, smooth, soft, moderate hair distribution, few moles, normal venous pattern, without edema, inflammation, scars. Short-cut nails, clear with few calcium deposits, round, medium thickness. No clubbing or Beau's lines. Nailbeds smooth, firm, pink. Brachial, ulnar, radial pulses palpable and regular. Epitrochlear lymph node nonpalpable. No bruits auscultated over arteries. Upper extremities with full ROM. Muscles moderately firm bilaterally. No deviations, inflammations, or bony deformities noted. Moves upper extremities freely against resistance. Biceps, triceps, brachioradialis reflexes eliicited bilaterally.

Lower Extremities: Medium sized legs, symmetrical, light brown, smooth, soft, few moles, without hair distribution, venous pattern, edema, inflammation, scars, rashes, ulcers. Superficial inguinal lymph node nonpalpable. No tenderness noted in region of femoral vein. Femoral pulse, popliteal, dorsalis pedis, posterior tibialis pulses palpable bilaterally. Lower extremities with full ROM. Muscles moderately firm bilaterally. No deviations, inflammations, or bony deformities. Muscles moderately firm bilaterally. Knee, ankle, and Babinski reflexes elicited bilaterally.

▲ *Figure 33–42* Continued

Illustration continued on following page

Motor Skills: Gait steady, smooth, coordinated, symmetrical bilaterally, even base, posture erect and not stooped. Romberg test revealed a minimum amount of swaying. Upper and lower extremities with full ROM and no muscle tenderness. Muscle size adequate for age with muscle tone firm at rest. Alternates finger to nose with eyes closed. Rapidly opposes fingers to thumb bilaterally without difficulty. Alternates pronation and supination of hands rapidly without difficulty. No involuntary movements noted.

Sensory System: Pain sensation intact. Superficial light touch sensation intact on arms, legs, neck, chest, and back. Vibration sensation intact on forehead, bridge of nose, elbow, wrist, knees, ankles, and hand. Position sense of fingers intact bilaterally. Discriminative sensation intact: Identified coin placed in right hand and key placed in left hand. Identified the number 4 traced in right hand and the number 7 traced in left hand; identified two-point discrimination correctly; identified point localization correctly when touched on face, hands, back, feet, chest, and forehead. Extinction discriminative sensation intact on right and left sides.

Special Maneuvers: None

PULSES:

	RIGHT	LEFT
Radial	+3	+3
Ulnar	+2	+2
Brachial	+2	+2
Femoral	+1	+1
Popliteal	+2	+2
Dorsalis pedis	+2	+2
Posterior tibialis	+1	+1
Carotid	+3	+3
Apical		+3
Temporal	+2	+2

REFLEXES:

	RIGHT	LEFT
Biceps	+2	+2
Triceps	+2	+2
Brachioradialis	+2	+2
Patellar	+2	+2
Achilles	+2	+2
Babinski	neg	neg

▲ **Figure 33–42** Continued

TWO-POINT DISCRIMINATION

When assessing two-point discrimination, touch the person alternately with one or two safety pins on a particular body part, such as the fingerpads. Ask the person if one or two sensations are felt. Find the minimal distance the person can discriminate one from two sensations. For sensitive fingerpads, the average distance is less than 5 mm.

POINT LOCALIZATION

This is assessed by touching various parts of the person's body with a wisp of cotton. The person is instructed to open the eyes after having felt the touch and point to the area.

EXTINCTION

Extinction is assessed by touching the person's skin simultaneously on opposite sides of the body with safety pins and asking the person to identify whether one sensation or two were felt. Repeat the procedure several times on different symmetric areas. Occasionally, apply only one stimulus to test the person's reliability.

POSTEXAMINATION ACTIVITIES

When the physical assessment is over, remove the drape (without exposing the individual) and help the person with clothing (and bed linens if the person is in bed). Clean rectal and perineal areas to remove lubricant or body secretions. Be sure the person is safe and comfortable. Deal with linens, pads, and equipment as appropriate and leave the examining area in order.

▼ DOCUMENTATION

Various *forms* are available for *documentation* of a client health history and a total physical assessment, or findings may be written out in a narrative, outline format. (See Chapter 27.) Also document the following: time of examination, name of examiner, observations made that may contribute to planning nursing care, specimens collected and their disposition (for example, "sent to laboratory"). An example of a written Client Health History and Physical Assessment is illustrated in Figure 33-42. This will demonstrate to you how the information provided in this chapter can be applied to the clinical setting.

Summary

▶ Correct use of principles of history-taking will assist you to understand your client's chief complaint, course of present illness, past health history, family health history, and personal and social history as well as assisting you to complete a systems review correctly.

▶ Physical assessment is the key means of collecting baseline data and requires knowledge of normal anatomy and physiology; pathology; equipment use; the four basic maneuvers of inspection, palpation, percussion, and auscultation; the use of olfaction; client preparation; and the correct procedures for completing the examination.

▶ The physical examination begins with an assessment of general parameters, including vital signs, height and weight, general appearance, mental status (JOMACS), and skin.

▶ The physical examination is completed from head to toe, bilaterally, including assessment of cranial nerves.

▶ Head-to-toe assessment includes examination of the head and neck, chest, abdomen, genitals and rectum, extremities, and motor and sensory systems.

▶ Postexamination activities include care of the client and equipment and documentation of findings.

Bibliography

1. Bates, B. (1991). *A guide to physical examination and history taking (5th ed.)*. Philadelphia: J.B. Lippincott.
2. Becker, K., & Stevens, S. (1988). Performing in-depth abdominal assessment. *Nursing*, 18, 59–63.
3. Boyd-Monk, H. (1990). Assessing acquired ocular disease. *Nursing Clinics of North America*, 25(4), 811–822.
4. Bravermun, B. (1990). Eliciting assessment data from the patient who is difficult to interview. *Nursing Clinics of North America*, 25(4), 743–750.
5. Dennison, R. (1986). Cardiopulmonary assessment: How to do it better in 15 easy steps. *Nursing*, 16, 34–40.
6. Judge, R., et al. (1982). *Clinical diagnosis (4th ed.)*. Boston: Little, Brown.
7. Kaufman, J. (1990). Assessing the twelve cranial nerves. *Nursing*, 20, 56–58.
8. Malasanos, L., et al. (1991). *Health assessment*. St. Louis: C.V. Mosby.
9. McConnell, E. (1988), Getting the feel of the lymph node assessment. *Nursing*, 18, 55–57.
10. Morgan, W.L., & Engel, G.L. (1969). *The clinical approach to the patient*. Philadelphia: W.B. Saunders.
11. Morton, P. (1990). *Health assessment*. Springhouse: Springhouse Corporation.
12. O'Toole, M. (1990). Advanced assessment of the abdomen and gastrointestinal problems. *Nursing Clinics of North America*, 25(4), 771–776.
13. Roach, L. (1977). Color changes in dark skin. *Nursing*, 7(1), 48–51.
14. Seidel, H., et al. (1991). *Mosby's guide to physical examination*. St. Louis: C.V. Mosby.
15. Stevens, S., & Becker, K. (1988). How to perform picture-perfect respiratory assessment. *Nursing*, 18, 57–63.
16. Sullivan, J. (1990). Neurologic assessment. *Nursing Clinics of North America*, 25(4), 795–809.
17. Swartz, M. (1989). *Textbook of physical diagnosis: History and examination*. Philadelphia: W.B. Saunders.
18. Willard, M., et al. (1986). The educational pelvic examination: women's responses to a new approach. *JOGNN*, 15, 135–140.

▼ *Assisting with Diagnostic Procedures*

▼
▼
▼

Closely allied to procedures carried out by the nurses is the assistance which the nurse gives the physician when examining patients, dressing wounds, giving treatments, and making tests. This is not direct service to the patient. But the purpose of assisting the physician is to save his time and render more efficient his care of the patient, so these activities are included in the hours of service given the patient.

**Florence Meda Gipe and Gladys Sellew
1949**

▼

▼ CHAPTER OUTLINE

NURSING RESPONSIBILITIES RELATED TO
  MEDICAL DIAGNOSTIC PROCEDURES
NURSING RESPONSIBILITIES BEFORE THE
  DIAGNOSTIC PROCEDURE
    Prepare the Person and Significant
      Others
    Obtain Informed Consent
    Schedule the Test
    Prepare the Person Physically
    Prepare the Equipment
    Transport the Person to the
      Examination Room and Show
      Significant Others to the Waiting
      Area
NURSING RESPONSIBILITIES DURING THE
  DIAGNOSTIC PROCEDURE
    Support the Person During
      Diagnostic Testing
    Collect Baseline Assessment Data
      and Continue to Evaluate the
      Client
    Assist with the Diagnostic
      Procedure
NURSING RESPONSIBILITIES AFTER THE
  DIAGNOSTIC PROCEDURE
    Provide Postprocedure Care and
      Comfort Measures

    Notify the Family/Significant Others
      of Procedure Completion
    Process Specimens
    Clean or Dispose of Equipment
    Document the Procedure
DIAGNOSTIC PROCEDURES ACROSS THE
  LIFE SPAN
    Diagnostic Procedures and the
      Infant
    Diagnostic Procedures and the
      Toddler
    Diagnostic Procedures and the
      Preschooler
    Diagnostic Procedures and the
      School-age Child
    Diagnostic Procedures and the
      Adolescent
    Diagnostic Procedures and the
      Adult
    Diagnostic Procedures and the
      Elderly
SPECIAL CONSIDERATIONS FOR
  DIAGNOSTIC PROCEDURES ON AN
  OUTPATIENT BASIS
ASSESSMENT BY RADIOGRAPHIC
  PROCEDURES (X-RAYS)
    Upper Gastrointestinal Series

▼ **CHAPTER OUTLINE** Continued

Small Bowel X-ray Series
Lower Gastrointestinal Series
    or Barium Enema
Cholecystogram
Intravenous Pyelogram
Angiogram
Myelogram
Bronchogram
Computed Tomography
Magnetic Resonance Imaging

ASSESSMENT BY RADIOACTIVE
    MATERIALS
ASSESSMENT BY LABORATORY STUDIES
    Blood Studies
    Specimens for Culture
    Urine Studies
    Aspiration Studies
ASSESSMENT OF ELECTRICAL IMPULSES
    Electrocardiogram
    Electroencephalogram

Electromyogram
ASSESSMENT BY ENDOSCOPY
    Bronchoscopy
    Esophagogastroduodenoscopy
    Proctosigmoidoscopy
    Colonoscopy
    Cystoscopy
ASSESSMENT BY ULTRASONOGRAPHY
ASSESSMENT BY PULMONARY FUNCTION
    STUDIES

▼ **KEY TERMS**

Amniocentesis
Angiogram
Arterial blood gas
    (ABG)
Barium enema (BE)
Biopsy
Bronchogram
Bronchoscopy
Cholecystogram

Colonoscopy
Computed tomography
    (CT, CAT, or
    CAT scan)
Cystoscopy
Electrocardiogram
    (ECG, EKG)
Electroencephalogram
    (EEG)

Electromyogram
    (EMG)
Endoscopy
Esophagogastroduo-
    denoscopy (EGD)
Fluoroscopy
Intravenous pyelogram
    (IVP)

Lumbar puncture
    (LP, spinal tap)
Magnetic resonance
    imaging (MRI)
Myelogram
Paracentesis
Proctosigmoidoscopy
Pulmonary function
    studies

Radioactive scan
Small bowel series
Specimen
Thoracentesis
Ultrasound
Upper gastrointestinal
    series (UGI)

▼ **LEARNING OBJECTIVES**

After studying this chapter, you should be able to

1. State the general purpose for carrying out diagnostic procedures.
2. Discuss general nursing responsibilities before, during, and after any diagnostic procedure.
3. Explain why a client's developmental level is important to consider when planning and carrying out diagnostic procedures.
4. Compare the nursing responsibilities for inpatient versus outpatient diagnostic procedures.
5. Identify groups of diagnostic tests that may indicate a problem in a particular organ or system of the body.
6. Describe common x-ray procedures.
7. Describe the use of radioactive materials in diagnostic procedures.
8. Identify four types of laboratory studies.
9. Describe common tests that assess electrical activity in the body.
10. State three purposes for endoscopic procedures and plan the nursing care for the person undergoing these procedures.
11. Discuss the use of ultrasonography as a diagnostic tool.
12. Discuss the assessment of pulmonary function tests to diagnose respiratory difficulties due to restrictive and obstruc-
    tive lung diseases.

Medical diagnostic procedures are used to identify "the causative agent," or source of a disorder, assess structural pathologic changes, assess physiologic responses to a disorder, and assess functional impairments related to a disorder. These examinations may be repeated during the course of a condition to assess the person's response to treatment. Diagnostic procedures investigate not only the body's systems, organs, and tissues but also its fluids, excretions, cells, and subcellular levels. Box 34–1 lists examples of diagnostic procedures by the body system they evaluate. Many of these diagnostic tests will be discussed in this chapter. You are referred to a manual of diagnostic tests for further information regarding these procedures.

NURSING RESPONSIBILITIES RELATED TO MEDICAL DIAGNOSTIC PROCEDURES

A diagnostic workup often involves specific diagnostic tests.

Nurses are involved not only in assisting the physician or technician in carrying out the tests but also in supporting and advocating for the person having the tests.

Whatever test is being done, nursing responsibilities exist before, during, and after the diagnostic procedure. General nursing responsibilities required for all tests are described next. Specific nursing responsibilities for individual tests will be discussed later in this chapter.

Box 34–1. Examples of Diagnostic Procedures by Body Systems

Cardiovascular and Hematopoietic Systems

Ballistocardiography
Blood pressure measurement
Blood tests
Bone marrow aspiration
Cardiac blood pool scan
Cardiac catheterization { intracardiac pressure / intra-arterial pressure
Circulation time
Dynamic blood flow studies (radionuclide angiography)
Echocardiography
Electrocardiogram (ECG or EKG)
Exercise tolerance
Ophthalmoscopic examination
Pericardium scan
Perthes' test
Phonocardiography
Plethysmography
Pulse assessment
Regitine test
Trendelenburg test
Tourniquet (capillary fragility) test
Ultrasound (heart; aorta)
Urinalysis
Venous pressure measurement
X-ray examinations: fluoroscopy (orthodiagraphy); intravenous angiocardiography; cardioangiography; aortography; arteriography; lymphangiography; venography (lower extremity phlebography); thoracic, abdominal, and peripheral angiography

Kidney and Urinary Tract

Blood tests
Cystometry
Cystoscopy (cystourethroscopy)
Echogram
Electronic evaluation of urinary flow rate
Kidney function tests (clearance, concentration, excretion)
Nephrotomography
Renal biopsy
Renal scan
Renogram
Urethral calibration
Urine examination
X-ray examinations: excretory urography (intravenous pyelography [IVP]); retrograde urography (pyelography); retrograde urethrography; voiding cystourethrography (VCU)

Respiratory System

Bronchoscopy (fiberoptic or rigid scope)
Blood tests
Gastric contents analysis
Lung scan
Nasal and throat swabbings for smear and culture
Pulmonary function tests (PFTs)
Respiration assessment
Skin tests
Sputum examination (smear, culture)
Thoracentesis (obtain pleural fluid for examination)
X-ray examinations: AP chest film; bronchography; fluoroscopy, tomograms

Reproductive System

Female:
  Amniocentesis
  Colposcopy
  Hysterosalpingography
  Mammography
  Papanicolaou smear (Pap)
  Placental scan
  Smear and culture
  Ultrasound
Male:
  Examination of spermatozoa
  Smear and culture

Digestive System

Feces examination (chemical, macroscopic, microscopic)
Gallbladder ultrasound
Gastric analysis (direct via nasogastric tube or indirect with dye)
Gastroenteroscopic examinations: colonoscopy with fiberoptic scope; esophagoscopy; gastroscopy with fiberoptic scope; peritoneoscopy; proctoscopy; upper GI endoscopy; sigmoidoscopy
Liver examinations: biopsy, excretory function tests; metabolic function tests, scan, serum protein tests, ultrasound
X-ray examinations: cholangiography, intravenous cholangiography (IVC), postoperative (T-tube) cholangiography, percutaneous transhepatic cholangiography; cholecystography, colon series or barium enema; endoscopic pancreatocholangiography; esophagoscopy (barium swallow); hypotonic duodenography; upper GI series (UGI) and small bowel examination

Box continued on following page

NURSING RESPONSIBILITIES BEFORE THE DIAGNOSTIC PROCEDURE

Prepare the Person and Significant Others

People are often anxious about diagnostic tests. They are concerned not only about having to undergo the procedure but also about the results of the test. Explain the test to the person and significant others. Be sure to consider the client's intellectual level and previous experience when teaching. Avoid the use of medical jargon. Tell the client exactly what will happen, where it will happen, who will do the test, who else will be there, and how long it will take. Tell the person exactly what will be expected of her or him; for example, hold breath, sit still, change body positions. Describe any sensations the person will experience. Inform the person if sedation or pain relief is available.

Box 34–1. Examples of Diagnostic Procedures by Body Systems (Continued)

Musculoskeletal System
Aspiration of synovial fluid
Biopsy (muscle)
Blood tests
Bone scan
Cultures, e.g., skin lesions
Electromyography
Knee arthrography and arthroscopy
Metabolic tests
Urine tests
X-ray examinations of bones and joints

Nervous System
Caloric test
Cerebrospinal fluid examination
Cisternal puncture
Echoencephalography
Electroencephalography (EEG)

Electromyography (EMG)
Intrathecal (subarachnoid) scan
Lumbar puncture (spinal tap)
Neurologic physical examination
Psychologic examinations
Sweat test
X-ray examinations: angiography of head and neck; cerebral angiography; computed tomography (CT scan); myelography; pneumoencephalography (PEG); ventriculography

Endocrine System
Basal metabolic rate (BMR)
Glucose tolerance test (GTT)
Pancreas scan
Spleen scan
Thyroid hormone tests
Thyroid scan

If you do not know specific information about the test, find out by checking your agency's diagnostic procedure manual or calling the department that performs the test. Allow time for the person and significant others to ask questions and express concerns. It may be helpful for significant others or the nurse to stay with the person through the diagnostic procedure. This is especially important if the person has special needs that may affect the test, such as a hearing difficulty or language barrier.

Obtain Informed Consent

Before a medical diagnostic procedure can be performed on a person, consent must be obtained from the person or someone legally authorized to provide consent for the person. Consent is the person's authorization or permission for a diagnostic procedure to be performed. Informed consent implies that the person has been given sufficient information about the diagnostic test to allow the individual to weigh the pros and cons and make a decision regarding the proposed procedure. The physician has the responsibility for providing this information, but the nurse may also be involved in teaching the person about the test and answering questions that may arise. Informed consent also implies that the person understands the explanation given about the procedure, its benefits, and its risks.

Consent without full understanding of what is being authorized does not meet the legal requirement of informed consent.

For some procedures such as drawing blood, the consent for treatment form that the person signed upon admission to the hospital may be enough. More invasive and risky procedures, such as a lumbar puncture, require the person's authorization by signature on an additional consent form. The nurse is usually the member of the health care team that obtains the person's signature on this form and also signs the form as a witness. When a person is unable to give consent, the next-of-kin or legal guardian may be asked to authorize medical care. In cases of extreme emergency, when death may be imminent, consent requirements can be waived.

Schedule the Test

After receiving a physician's order for medical diagnostic procedures, a nurse may schedule these tests with the appropriate departments of the hospital. At times the physician or a ward clerk may also be involved in scheduling diagnostic procedures. Many times several tests may be ordered at the same time. Knowledge of what is involved in each test will assist the nurse in knowing the correct order for the tests. For example, endoscopic studies of the lower gastrointestinal tract should be scheduled before contrast studies, since the contrast medium (barium) would obstruct the view of the examiner during the endoscopic procedure. Radioactive body scans should be scheduled before any radiographic procedure requiring iodine, since the presence of iodine can interfere with the body scan.

Prepare the Person Physically

Some tests require specific physical preparation, such as maintaining a fasting state, sedation, providing an intravenous line, or administering enemas. Special body positions may also be required for the test. Strive to ensure comfort and avoid embarrassment or unnecessary exposure during the test. Help the person change into a gown and remove jewelry and makeup if necessary. Be aware of how long the person is required to fast before diagnostic procedures. If tests are scheduled one after another, fasting may go on too long. Find out whether oral medications are to be given while the person is fasting.

Prepare the Equipment

Preparing the equipment is sometimes a nursing responsibility. Be sure the equipment is available and in working order before the test is scheduled. Maintain sterility of sterile equipment and supplies. Have extra lighting and drapes available if necessary.

Be sure emergency equipment is available and in working order if there is a chance that it could be needed.

Transport the Person to the Examination Room and Show Significant Others to the Waiting Area

Many diagnostic tests are carried out in specialized areas of the hospital, such as the radiology department, endoscopy department, or angiography laboratory. Arrange the appropriate form of transportation for the person. Very ill or sedated persons will require a stretcher and should be accompanied by a nurse; others may proceed to the diagnostic test center by wheelchair in the company of a transport aide.

Inform the family and significant others of available waiting rooms near the diagnostic areas of the hospital. If no waiting room is available, the family may be allowed to wait in the person's room. Advise the physician of the family's whereabouts in case a postprocedure conference is needed.

NURSING RESPONSIBILITIES DURING THE DIAGNOSTIC PROCEDURE

Support the Person During Diagnostic Testing

During diagnostic testing, the person may be cared for by a nurse or, more commonly, by a technician working in the examination room. If a nurse is not present during the procedure, good communication between the technician and nursing staff regarding the person's response to the examination is vital to delivery of the best care possible.

The nurse or technician should observe the person and communicate adverse reactions to the examiner. Pallor, pain, acute anxiety, increased or decreased pulse, and nausea should be reported. At times the test may have to be stopped for a few minutes to allow the person to become more comfortable. Interventions such as changing the person's position or administering pain relief may be needed. Tell the person what is happening throughout the procedure and describe the sensations to expect. Be sure the person is warm and protected against exposure. Encouraging the person to deep breathe will aid in promoting relaxation. Holding the person's hand or using some other form of therapeutic touch may also be effective. Remember, being an advocate for the person is a primary nursing responsibility.

Collect Baseline Assessment Data and Continue to Evaluate the Client

A baseline assessment provides information about the person's condition prior to beginning the procedure. Measure the vital signs (temperature, pulse, respirations, and blood pressure), note the level of consciousness, emotional state, and temperature and color of the person's skin. If a technician is caring for the person during the procedure, be sure the technician is aware of these baseline data. During the procedure, it is important to continue to monitor the client's vital signs and general appearance.

Since deviations from the baseline assessment may indicate a deterioration in the person's physical status, report changes immediately to the examiner.

Assist with the Diagnostic Procedure

Nursing responsibilities vary with the test and the policy of the institution. Nurses may assist with procedures by passing instruments and supplies to the examiner. Other examples of nursing responsibilities during the procedure may include positioning the person for the procedure, recording the procedure and the results in the person's medical record, processing specimens, administering medications, and assessing the person's physical and emotional status.

NURSING RESPONSIBILITIES AFTER THE DIAGNOSTIC PROCEDURE

Provide Postprocedure Care and Comfort Measures

After the test is completed, the first priority is to attend to the person first. Repeat the assessment of the individual's vital signs and general status. Observe and report any signs or symptoms that would indicate complications from the procedure, such as bleeding. Make the person comfortable and warm. If lubricants have been used, assist the person with personal hygiene. Allow the person to ask questions and talk about the experience if desired. Carry out any specific postprocedure requirements, such as encouraging or assisting person in maintaining a specific position, administering pain relief or other medications, applying pressure at puncture sites, and observing for possible complications related to the procedure. If the individual fasted before the test, check with the physician about resuming a diet. If the person can now eat, provide nourishment. Before offering food and fluids, be sure the person is fully alert, has an intact gag reflex, and can swallow and cough without impairment.

Notify the Family/Significant Others of Procedure Completion

After the test is finished, notify the family and significant others of its completion. As soon as possible after making the person comfortable and providing necessary care, allow the family or significant others to visit. Respond to any questions or concerns before allowing the person time alone with visitors.

Process Specimens

At all times during and after the test procedure it is essential to adhere strictly to universal precautions when handling blood or body secretions. Chapter 28 describes universal precautions for blood and body fluids. Follow institutional policies regarding identification and processing of potentially hazardous body fluids.

Label any specimens obtained during the test with the person's name, identification number, date, time, and type of specimen. Promptly deliver specimens to the appropriate laboratory, since undue delays in processing may alter the test results. Additional information about specimens is provided later in this chapter.

Clean or Dispose of Equipment

Postprocedure cleanup is often a nursing responsibility. Discard disposable equipment in the proper receptacle according to agency policy. Reusable equipment should be rinsed clean of body secretions, placed in a bag or other appropriate container, and clearly marked as contaminated. Send the contaminated supplies to the appropriate department for sterilization and repackaging. Be sure to wear gloves when handling contaminated equipment.

Document the Procedure

Documenting the client's preparation for and completion of the test is a legal responsibility. Figure 34–1 provides an example of charting of client preparation for one procedure. When documenting nursing activities related to a diagnostic procedure, adhere to the requirements for good documentation as outlined in Chapter 27 and follow the policies for your agency.

Document the test and the name of the examiner in the person's record. Record the time and date of the procedure and any specimens that were taken. The person's reaction to the procedure, any care given during the procedure, as well as post-test assessments and interventions, should also be recorded.

At times the chronologic order in which specimens or tests occurred may be crucial, so this should be documented clearly.

DIAGNOSTIC PROCEDURES ACROSS THE LIFE SPAN

The developmental level of a person undergoing a diagnostic workup will affect all aspects of the procedure.

1/12	0930	Scheduled for colonoscopy tomorrow at 1100. Receiving clear liquid diet. Dr. Jones in to explain procedure. Consent form signed. ———— C. Lammon RN
1/12	2000	Bisacodyl suppository given. Large amount soft brown stool expelled. —— A. Foote RN
1/13	2400	NPO for colonoscopy tomorrow. ———— M. Adams RN
1/13	0700	Two tap water enemas, 1000cc each, administered without difficulty. Small amount soft brown stool returned after first enema. Clear return of fluid after second enema. Tolerated procedure without signs of distress. —— C. Lammon RN
1/13	1030	Diazepam 10 mg IM to Rt. upper outer quadrant gluteus medius for sedation. ———— C. Lammon RN
1/13	1100	Transferred to endoscopy lab per stretcher. ———— C. Lammon RN

▲ **Figure 34–1**

Example of charting client preparation for a diagnostic procedure.

Decisions about what tests should be done, explanations of the procedure, and methods of performing the procedure may all be adjusted to accommodate varying needs across the life span.

Diagnostic Procedures and the Infant

Only essential diagnostic tests are performed on very young children. During the first 4 months, before the infant is able to selectively recognize the parents, the neonate will respond to painful procedures with a total body reaction and loud crying. Young infants can be easily distracted after the procedure is complete by holding and cuddling them. After the age of 4 to 6 months, infants will react to painful procedures with more purposeful responses, such as physical resistance, lack of cooperation, and refusal to remain still. Restraints such as a mummy restraint or papoose board may be required to restrain a child if absence of movement is essential. Since older infants will protest if separated from the parent, it may be helpful to allow the parent to remain with the child during the diagnostic test. Distraction is less effective in comforting the older infant. Attempting to prepare the infant for a procedure by allowing him or her to see the equipment is not recommended as it may actually increase the young child's fears.

Diagnostic Procedures and the Toddler

The major concerns for a toddler during diagnostic testing are separation from parents, loss of control, and pain. Toddlers will cling to parents and protest loudly if separated. If possible, allow parents to remain with the child during the test. If this is not possible, encourage the parent to provide a comfort item, such as a favorite cuddle toy, pillow, or blanket.

Toddlers are very active and autonomous. They will resist attempts to restrict their mobility by exhibiting negativism and regression in development. Encourage the toddler to talk about fears and employ measures to reduce discomfort to a minimum. To minimize worry and anxiety, give short explanations just before beginning the procedure. Offer choices when possible—for example, "Would you like to take your medicine in a cup or with a straw?" Do not ask the toddler "Would you like to take your medicine now?" The answer will be a resounding "NO!"

Diagnostic Procedures and the Preschooler

The preschooler is more mature than the toddler but still may experience separation anxiety under stressful situations such as a diagnostic test. Preschoolers have a need to be in control of what happens to them. Simple explanations of the procedure as well as role playing with the equipment will help them achieve a sense of control over the situation.

Be careful of the words you use to describe diagnos-

tic procedures to preschoolers as they are very concerned with bodily injury and mutilation. For example do not "take" the blood pressure. Preschoolers may be concerned that they are losing part of their body. Liberal use of small bandages over needle sites will also help the child maintain a sense of body integrity.

Diagnostic Procedures and the School-age Child

School-age children have a need for more detailed explanations of what is to happen to them. They will seek factual information about the nature of the procedure, such as whether it will hurt, how it will make them better, and if there are any risks involved. School-age children are aware of the concepts of disability, illness, and death. Their quest for information is an attempt to maintain control and manage fears about their condition.

Diagnostic Procedures and the Adolescent

Adolescents have the same need for information as school-age children. Often however, adolescents will portray a false attitude of calm sophistication or lack of concern to the health professional in an effort to seize control of the situation and their fears. Even though they may say they do not need you, offer appropriate information to adolescents about the procedure and provide comfort measures and reassurance during the test.

Diagnostic Procedures and the Adult

Adults will need instruction and information about the procedure they are to undergo. Before teaching, assess for prior experiences with the test, intellectual level, level of anxiety, and readiness to learn. Be sure to use language that the person can understand. Avoid the use of medical jargon and explain any medical terms that may be used regarding the individual, the test, and necessary nursing or medical care.

Diagnostic Procedures and the Elderly

Sometimes many diagnostic tests may be scheduled. For the elderly person, this can be an exhausting experience. Be sure to allow adequate time for rest when scheduling multiple procedures.

The physiologic condition of the older person may make some diagnostic procedures more difficult or dangerous. For example, drawing blood or starting an intravenous line on fragile or sclerotic veins may be difficult. Assuming the correct position for some tests may be difficult and painful for a person with contractures or joint diseases such as arthritis. In addition, when test preparations require fasting and laxatives or enemas there is a greater risk of dehydration in the elderly person.

SPECIAL CONSIDERATIONS FOR DIAGNOSTIC PROCEDURES ON AN OUTPATIENT BASIS

Many diagnostic tests that once required admission to the hospital are now performed on an outpatient basis. Diagnostic procedures are also carried out in physicians' offices, clinics, and freestanding diagnostic centers. Box 34–2 lists some common diagnostic tests that may be performed on an outpatient basis.

Preparation for outpatient procedures is usually carried out by the person at home. Since the outcome of the diagnostic test depends on correct preparation, be sure the person understands all instructions and has the ability to carry them out. Include an assessment of the home environment when taking the client history, as this information may help you anticipate problems with test preparation. Some diagnostic procedures may leave the person feeling weak and tired. Ask the person if there will be someone to provide transportation from the agency and assistance at home after the procedure, if needed. Be sure to instruct the person about signs and symptoms that would indicate complications.

Provide a phone number to call for help should complications arise once the person has returned home.

ASSESSMENT BY RADIOGRAPHIC PROCEDURES (X-RAYS)

X-rays (roentgen rays) are electromagnetic radiation with extremely short wavelengths. X-rays penetrate substances to varying depths, depending on the densities of the substances and the voltage used. X-rays pass through the body to take pictures of internal body structures. After passing through the body, x-rays affect sensitized film and produce an image. Radiologists interpret x-ray film.

Very dense or opaque structures block the passage of x-rays onto the film by absorbing more rays. Thus, film underlying bones and other dense structures, such as foreign objects, is not heavily exposed and therefore remains lighter in color. The reverse is true with less dense or more translucent structures, such as soft tissue, internal organs, skin, muscles, and body fat. X-rays easily penetrate structures of this kind and expose the underlying film, turning it darker.

Sometimes radiopaque substances are introduced into the body before x-rays are taken. Radiopaque materials block x-rays and so serve as "contrast media" by outlining the structures. Contrast medium is particularly helpful because it creates a contrast on x-ray between two equally dense structures that would otherwise be difficult to tell apart (Fig. 34–2).

There are a variety of contrast studies: gastrointestinal series, barium enema series, angiogram, intravenous pyelogram, cholecystogram, myelogram, bronchogram, and others. The contrast medium used in these studies is usually a heavy metallic salt or a gas. The medium is introduced into the body in various ways. Barium, for example, may be swallowed or given by enema. Dyes

Box 34–2. Examples of Common Outpatient Diagnostic Tests
Chest x-ray
Mammogram
Cholecystogram
Upper gastrointestinal series
Barium enema
Intravenous pyelogram
Blood studies
Lumbar puncture
Amniocentesis
Electrocardiogram
Electroencephalogram
Electromyelogram
Proctosigmoidoscopy
Ultrasound
CT scan
Magnetic resonance imaging

may be injected or swallowed in tablet form. In rare cases, air may be injected through a needle.

Fluoroscopy is the use of x-rays to study deep body structures such as joints, organs, or body systems while in motion. In a darkened room a person is positioned between a fluorescent screen and an x-ray source, and images of the moving internal structures are projected onto the screen. Often a radiopaque medium is administered to help distinguish the structure being assessed. Fluoroscopy reveals the size, shape, and movements of

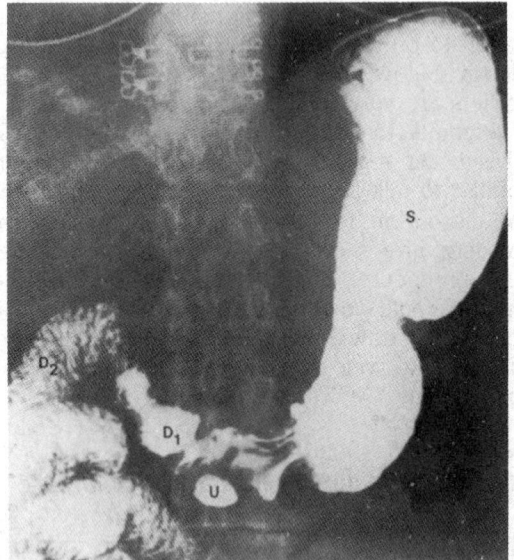

▲ *Figure 34–2*

Fluoroscopic study of the stomach (S) and duodenum shows a benign gastric ulcer (U), which appears as a rounded pool of barium surrounded by a lucent rim of edema. Also note the normal duodenal bulb (D₁) and normal descending duodenum (D₂). (From Stimac, G.K. [1992]. *Introduction to diagnostic imaging*. Philadelphia: W.B. Saunders.)

organs such as the heart, lungs, stomach, and intestines.

Table 34–1 describes the care of a person undergoing common x-ray procedures.

Upper Gastrointestinal Series

An **upper gastrointestinal series (UGI)** is a series of x-ray films of the esophagus, stomach, duodenum, and upper jejunum as the person swallows a radiopaque contrast medium such as barium sulfate or Gastrografin (diatrizoate meglumine). The radiopaque substance outlines the organs on the x-ray screen for visualization. Fluoroscopy is often done to observe the motion of the organs as the contrast medium moves through the gastrointestinal tract. This procedure is usually done in the radiology department and requires about 45 minutes to complete.

Abnormal results can reveal congenital malformations, carcinomas, polyps, diverticula, gastritis, pyloric stenosis, and hiatal hernias.

Small Bowel X-ray Series

A **small bowel series** is a series of x-rays of the esophagus, stomach, duodenum, jejunum and ileum. It is the same as an upper gastrointestinal series except the entire small intestine is examined. X-ray films are taken every 30 minutes until the contrast medium reaches the cecum. The procedure takes 2 to 6 hours to complete. Abnormal results commonly reveal tumors, active bleeding, obstruction, intussusception, and ulcerative colitis.

Lower Gastrointestinal Series or Barium Enema

A lower gastrointestinal series or **barium enema (BE)** involves distention of the colon and rectum with a barium solution that is administered through the anus as an enema. X-ray films and fluoroscopy are then used to visualize the large intestine. Careful preparation and cleansing of the bowel prior to the test are essential for a successful examination.

The barium enema is useful in detecting problems such as lesions of the colon; obstructions; inflammatory diseases such as ulcerative colitis; diverticula; polyps; carcinomas; and intussusception. The examination is usually performed in the radiology department and takes about 1 hour to complete.

Cholecystogram

A **cholecystogram** is an x-ray study to evaluate the function of the gallbladder. Filling, concentration, contraction, and emptying of bile can be assessed. The study also will reveal the presence of gallbladder diseases, such as tumors, congenital anomalies, and cystic duct obstructions, and gallstones (cholelithiasis).

TABLE 34–1. Care of the Person Undergoing X-ray Studies

| Test | Care of the Person | | |
	Before the Test	During the Test	After the Test
Upper Gastrointestinal Series (UGI)	NPO after midnight Contrast tastes chalky	Technician attends person Several films will be taken lying and standing as person swallows contrast	Provide food, drink, and rest Administer laxatives to eliminate contrast Document color and consistency of BM. (White for 72 hr) If no BM, check for impaction and notify MD
Barium Enema (BE)	Clear liquid 12–24 hr before test Stool softeners, laxatives, and enemas (3 max.) to clear bowel of fecal matter NPO after midnight No oral meds Tell person test is uncomfortable, sense of fullness, urge to defecate, and cramping Tell person toilet will be available in radiology department to expel barium after test	Technician attends person Barium will be introduced with person on side Foley catheter with balloon may be used to help person retain barium if necessary Several x-rays may be taken	Provide food, fluid, and rest Administer laxatives until stools are normal color and texture Check stools and record color and consistency for 2 days

Table continued on following page

TABLE 34–1. *Care of the Person Undergoing X-ray Studies* Continued

| Test | Care of the Person | | |
	Before the Test	*During the Test*	*After the Test*
Cholecystogram	Low-fat supper night before study Laxative after low-fat meal Assess for iodine allergy Iodine contrast capsules taken at 5-min intervals for a total of 6 capsules Take dye with full glass of water Enema (optional) Clear liquids PO only after dye administered	Technician attends person Series of three films with person lying on abdomen, with right side elevated, sitting, and standing	Offer food, fluid, rest Assess for allergy to iodine (wheezing, pruritus, change in vital signs [VS], skin rash, swollen parotid gland)
Intravenous Pyelogram (IVP)	Obtain signed consent Assess for iodine allergy NPO after evening meal No meds Laxative night before test Enema morning of test Person may have metallic taste, feel hot and flushed, and be nauseated as dye is injected. There may be a stinging at IV site	Technician attends person Observe for allergic reaction when dye is injected First x-ray supine to assure bowel is clear and not obstructing view of kidney Dye injected and series of at least three films taken Person is asked to void, then last film is taken	Provide food, fluid, rest Push PO fluids Observe for allergic reaction to iodine
Angiogram	Obtain signed consent Prep will vary with body part to be studied, i.e., renal angiography will require a clean bowel NPO after midnight Assess for allergies to iodine Tell person they will feel uncomfortable when dye is injected	Assess vital signs, cardiac rhythm Observe for allergic reaction to dye	Bed rest for several hours Pressure at arterial puncture site. Sandbag over site for several hours. Observe for symptoms of bleeding or hematoma VS every 15 min until stable Check pulses distal to puncture site Push PO fluids
Myelogram	Obtain signed consent NPO 2–6 hr before test If metrizamide is to be used, all neuroleptic drugs including phenothiazines should be D/C'd 48 hr before test Tell person tilt table will be used. Restraints will prevent person from sliding off	Technician attends person Lumbar area will be prepped and shaved Person on right side for lumbar puncture and injection of contrast Table will be tilted with person on abdomen Oil-based contrast medium will be aspirated Clean puncture site and apply small dressing	Bed rest Oil contrast: person lies prone 2–4 hr, then supine 2–4 hr Water-soluble contrast: HOB elevated 45 degrees for 8–24 hr. Person should lie quietly to prevent dye passing into head Assess urine output to check for urinary retention VS every 4 hr for 24 hr

Table continued on following page

TABLE 34-1. Care of the Person Undergoing X-ray Studies Continued

| Test | Care of the Person | | |
	Before the Test	*During the Test*	*After the Test*
Bronchogram	Obtain signed consent	Technician attends person	Restrict food/fluids until gag
	Assess for iodine allergy	Catheter will be inserted	reflex and ability to swallow
	NPO before examination to	through nose into bronchi to	return
	avoid aspiration	instill contrast	Provide rest
	Expectorants and vigorous	Films will be taken in several	Encourage cough and postural
	pulmonary toilet 2–3 days	positions	drainage
	before examination if person	Person will be asked to cough	Observe for allergic reaction to
	has cough and sputum	up contrast after test is	iodine
	Tell person not to cough	complete	Temperature may be elevated
	during test	Postural drainage will be used	2–3 days post-test
	Administer sedatives and	to drain contrast out of	Postdrainage film 24–48 hr
	anticholinergics to decrease	lungs	after test
	anxiety and secretions		
	Remove dentures		
Computed Tomography (CT)	Obtain signed consent	Technician attends person	Observe for allergic reaction to
	Assess for allergy to iodine	Client lies still on back on	iodine
	No solid food day of	narrow table	Safety measures if sedative
	examination	Table will move body part to	was given
	NPO 2 hr before examination	be examined into scanner	
	Warn person sensations of		
	flushing, warmth, metallic		
	taste, nausea may be		
	experienced when contrast		
	is injected		
	Show person pictures of		
	scanner. Discuss fears of		
	claustrophobia		
	Tell person sedatives may be		
	used to decrease anxiety		
Magnetic Resonance Imaging (MRI)	Obtain signed consent	Technician attends person	No special post-test care
	Ask person to urinate	Person will have a call button	
	Heparin lock all IVs if possible.	to talk with technician	
	If not, add two extension	Table vibrates as it passes	
	tubes and D/C IV pumps	into scanner	
	Remove all metal objects such	A loud noise will be heard	
	as jewelry, hair pins, belt	during test. Ear plugs and	
	buckles, and so on	eye shields may be used	
	Sedative may be used	Usually a family member can	
	Show picture of scanner	be with person during test	
	Discuss fears of	In cases of severe	
	claustrophobia	claustrophobia, test can be	
		stopped temporarily and	
		person removed from the	
		scanner	

An oral iodine contrast medium such as Telepaque (iopanoic acid) or Oragrafin (sodium ipodate) is taken 13 hours before the test to enhance the x-ray pictures. Be sure to assess the person for iodine allergy. This dye will be secreted by the liver into the bile, which is then stored in the gallbladder. If liver cells are diseased and unable to secrete the dye into the bile, the test will be ineffective. The examination is carried out in the radiology department and usually requires 1 hour to complete.

Intravenous Pyelogram

After injecting a radiopaque iodine contrast medium such as Hypaque (sodium diatrizoate) or Conray (*n*-methyl-glucamine iothalamate) intravenously, a series of x-ray films are made to visualize the size, shape, structure, and function of the kidneys and other structures in the urinary tract.

The **intravenous pyelogram (IVP)** is a commonly prescribed test to detect kidney disease, ureteral or bladder stones, and tumors. Renal function can be assessed by the length of time it takes the contrast material to be excreted by each kidney. This procedure is carried out in the radiology department and usually requires about 1 hour.

Angiogram

An **angiogram** is an x-ray study of the vascular system. For example, a cerebral angiogram is an x-ray of blood vessels in the brain, a pulmonary angiogram is an x-ray of vessels in the lungs, and a renal angiogram is an x-ray of blood vessels in the kidneys. Radiopaque dye is injected into an artery or vein, and x-rays are made. Because allergic manifestations include wheezing, pruritus, skin rash, swollen parotid glands, and hypotension, the client is assessed for allergy to the dye before the test is begun. Sedation is often used to make the person more comfortable and less anxious during the test. The examination is usually carried out in a specially equipped catheterization laboratory in the radiology department. The length of time for the procedure will vary with the type of study done.

Myelogram

A **myelogram** is a radiographic study of the spinal cord, nerve roots, and vertebrae. An oil-based iodine contrast medium (Pantopaque) or a water-soluble iodine contrast medium (metrizamide) is injected into the subarachnoid space in the lumbar region or into the cisterna magna to visualize the structures. The oil contrast medium must be removed by aspiration after the test is complete, but the water-soluble medium can remain in the body. The person is placed on a tilt table to maneuver the contrast medium up and down the spinal cord. Fluoroscopy is done as x-rays are taken. The test is useful in diagnosing ruptured intervertebral disks, intervertebral tumors, compression of the spinal cord, and damage to nerve roots. The examination is carried out in the radiology department and usually takes 2 hours to complete.

Bronchogram

A **bronchogram** is an x-ray examination of the bronchial tree following insertion of an iodine radiopaque contrast medium into the bronchi. This test is often done in conjunction with a bronchoscopy and can be done under local or general anesthesia. The procedure is useful in detecting bronchiectasis and bronchial obstructions such as tumors and foreign bodies. The examination is carried out in the radiology department and usually requires 45 minutes to complete.

Computed Tomography

Computed tomography (CT, CAT, or CAT scan) is an x-ray examination of a structure at varying depths so as to show sections or slices of the structure at different levels. It is a relatively recent, safe, diagnostic x-ray procedure. A machine channels x-rays through an individual at differing planes and into a computer. A 180-degree scan of the structure is made in three or four different planes. The computer records the absorption potentials of various tissues at various planes and supplies a printout, which represents the structure studied.

As mentioned earlier, body tissues vary in density. For CT computer purposes, various tissue densities are assigned numbers arbitrarily. These numbers (absorption coefficients) range from +500 (most dense) for bone, down to −500 (least dense) for air.

In addition to providing computer printouts, photographs can be taken of the image on the screen. Color photographs are possible, but most are in varying shades of gray, for example bone appears black, soft tissues are differing gray tones, and air is white. While conventional skull films are taken in lateral, anterior, or posterior views, computed tomography views cross-sections or slices of the brain and skull from the top of the head (Fig. 34–3).

X-rays taken at varying depths of the same structure produce pictures (tomograms) that visually "section" or "slice" the structure at different levels, on a horizontal plane. Tomograms make it possible to visually "slice apart" a living, intact, and functioning organ in a manner that was formerly possible only with a scalpel at autopsy.

Tomograms produced by CT are superior to those taken by conventional x-ray machines. CT is more sensitive to differences in tissue densities, thereby showing structures not seen on a standard x-ray. Sometimes dye is injected to enhance visualization.

CT scans have most commonly been used to visualize the brain, although there are now also whole-body CTs that can produce tomograms anywhere in the body. CT brain scans are replacing less safe procedures such as nuclear brain scans (with radioisotopes), cerebral angiograms, and pneumoencephalography studies. Because a CT scan uses x-rays and not radioactive tracer substances (used in nuclear brain scans), an individual receives no more radiation than is received from conventional skull x-rays.

CT scans are performed in a specially equipped area of the radiology department. A total body scan can last as long as 3 hours. During the CT scan the person lies on a table that moves through a large, doughnut-shaped machine. It is very important for the person to be motionless during the x-ray examination. Sedation may be used for persons who find it difficult to be still or for those who are very anxious or claustrophobic.

Magnetic Resonance Imaging

Magnetic resonance imaging (MRI) is a noninvasive imaging procedure that visualizes internal body structures by utilizing magnetic fields, radiofrequency waves,

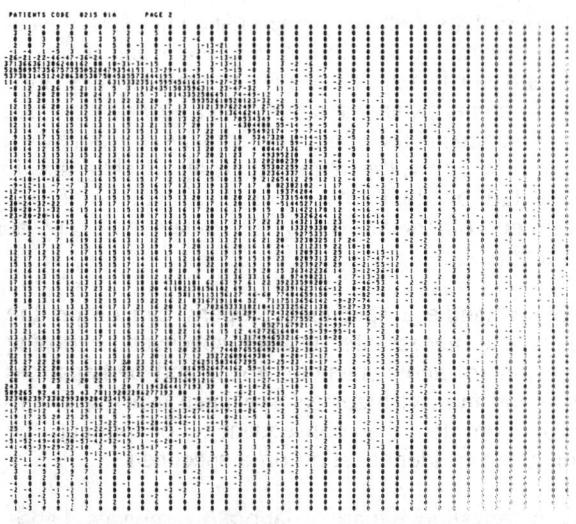

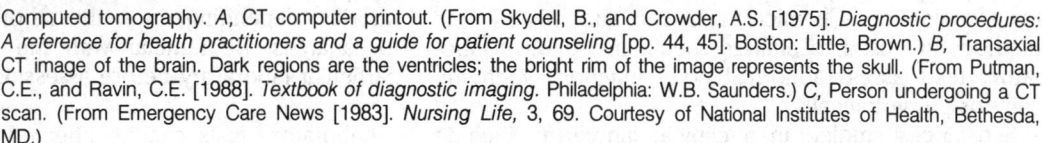

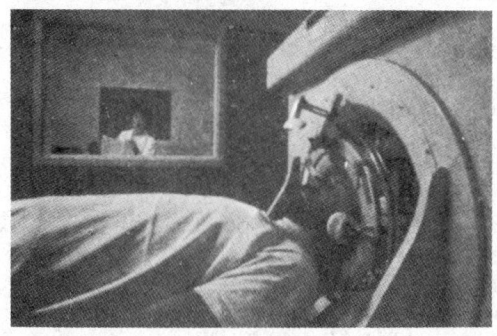

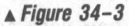

▲ **Figure 34–3**

Computed tomography. *A,* CT computer printout. (From Skydell, B., and Crowder, A.S. [1975]. *Diagnostic procedures: A reference for health practitioners and a guide for patient counseling* [pp. 44, 45]. Boston: Little, Brown.) *B,* Transaxial CT image of the brain. Dark regions are the ventricles; the bright rim of the image represents the skull. (From Putman, C.E., and Ravin, C.E. [1988]. *Textbook of diagnostic imaging.* Philadelphia: W.B. Saunders.) *C,* Person undergoing a CT scan. (From Emergency Care News [1983]. *Nursing Life,* 3, 69. Courtesy of National Institutes of Health, Bethesda, MD.)

and computers. It produces the clearest, most detailed images of body structures available today. The MRI uses no x-rays or radioactive substances. Occasionally an intravenous paramagnetic contrast medium is used to enhance the images. Paramagnetic contrast contains no iodine and reactions are rare. An MRI may be performed to study the condition of blood vessels and patterns of blood flow, as well as to diagnose tumors and other deviations from healthy tissue structure.

The person lies on a table that moves into a narrow tunnel of the scanner. It is very important for the person to be motionless during the scan. Sedation may be used for persons who find it difficult to be still or for those who are very anxious or claustrophobic.

External objects containing metal such as snaps on gowns, hair pins, or jewelry can distort the MR image and must be removed.

Internal metal objects must be evaluated for the type of metal they contain. Objects that contain iron, such as pacemakers, cerebral aneurysm clips, implanted insulin

pumps, cochlear implants, or shrapnel, will be affected by the magnet and may cause injury to the person. Persons with these devices may not be candidates for magnetic resonance imaging.

Objects made of steel, such as prostheses and dental braces, will not injure the person but may result in a less clear MR image. MRI scans usually take 45 minutes to 1 hour for each body part to be examined.

ASSESSMENT BY RADIOACTIVE MATERIALS

A **radioactive scan** is a procedure that uses radioisotope-tracer materials to test some organ functions and to locate malignancies. This is possible because radioactive isotopes (radionuclides or radiopharmaceuticals) give off radioactivity as they transform, or decay, at constant, predictable rates. A variety of radioactive tracer substances are used in diagnostic tests.

When a tracer substance has been placed in the body, some of it accumulates in specific organs or regions. Structure and function can then be assessed by placing detectors over the area of radioactive tracer accumulation and measuring radioactivity or by extracting samples (blood, urine, or stool) and measuring the sample for radioactivity.

Two types of detectors commonly used are the reticular scanner, which has a relatively small viewing field, and the gamma camera or scintillation camera, which has a larger viewing field. Both types detect emissions from a radioactive source and convert the emissions into signals that are recorded and studied. The detectors are similar to sophisticated Geiger counters.

Scanning is possible in structures and organs such as the brain, bone, lungs, liver, kidneys, spleen, pericardium, and thyroid. As the tracer substance collects in body structures, it is possible to obtain a visual representation of the distribution of the tracer. In some areas of the body the radioisotopes are more highly concentrated than in others. A skilled interpreter of nuclear scans makes assessments about an organ's size, shape, position, and function from the pattern of distribution. It is also possible to identify the presence and size of abnormalities such as malignant tumors. These examinations are usually carried out by the department of nuclear medicine.

Table 34-2 describes the care of a person undergoing a radioactive scan.

ASSESSMENT BY LABORATORY STUDIES

A **specimen** is a sample of body fluids, exudates, or excretions that may be obtained during diagnostic and treatment processes and sent to a clinical laboratory for examination. Chemical, physical, and microscopic methods are used to analyze specimens. Clinical laboratory tests assess abnormal body function biochemically or physiologically.

Substances studied in a clinical laboratory include blood, sputum, urine, feces, cerebrospinal fluid (CSF), pleural fluid, synovial fluid, amniotic fluid, peritoneal fluid, pericardial fluid, gastrointestinal secretions, and perspiration. Specimens of substances from abscesses and cysts may be obtained by aspiration. Specimens of tissue exudate, nasopharyngeal discharge, and vaginal and cervical discharge are obtained by a swab.

All specimens require proper handling. This means precise specimen collection, accurate labeling of specimens, and quick delivery of the specimen to the laboratory. In some instances, a preservative or some other agent is added to the specimen container. It is always important to know the temperature at which a specimen should be kept once it is collected. Some are refrigerated, others are iced, still others are kept at room temperature.

Failure to handle a specimen properly can distort the findings and necessitate another specimen, exposing the person to inconvenience, worry, and perhaps loss of time and money. Incorrect specimen labeling is very serious. Consider the consequences of putting the wrong name or identification on a specimen.

Computerization is part of laboratory services. Laboratory tests are commonly done as batteries rather than singly. The SMA-6 (sequential multiple analysis of six separate laboratory blood tests) is a blood test combination determining serum sodium, serum potassium, carbon dioxide combining power, serum chloride, blood urea nitrogen, and blood glucose. More detailed combinations are also available. One is the SMA-12. The results of this test are printed as a series of bar graphs. Each bar has a shaded portion that indicates normal levels. Different combinations of tests may be included among the 12 in different facilities. Batteries of tests, such as the SMA-12, are often used during hospital admission for routine screening.

Ranges of normal values can vary among clinical laboratories, depending upon the laboratory method used for analysis. Be familiar with the normal range of a particular laboratory before assessing the findings.

Laboratory tests can be affected by drugs a person has taken in the 72 hours prior to specimen collection. For example, low dosages of salicylates may elevate the blood uric acid level, and corticosteroids may elevate the white cell count, lower the sedimentation rate, and cause a diminution in the eosinophil count.

Table 34-3 summarizes care of a person undergoing laboratory studies.

TABLE 34-2. Care of the Person Undergoing a Radioactive Scan

| Test | Care of the Person | | |
	Before the Test	During the Test	After the Test
Radioactive Scans	Obtain consent Administer oral or IV radioactive substance to person Allow adequate time for radioactive material to reach body part to be scanned Tell person amount of radiation is approximately the same as with an x-ray study	Technician attends person Person may assume several positions as scan is completed	Provide nourishment and rest

TABLE 34–3. Care of the Person Undergoing Laboratory Studies

Test	Before the Test	During the Test	After the Test
		Care of the Person	
Blood Studies	NPO prior to some tests	Explain how blood is to be taken Try to decrease anxiety Sterile procedure Use universal blood and body secretion precautions	Apply pressure at puncture site until bleeding stops Apply small bandage Process specimen
Culture	Explain the test	Use sterile technique to collect the specimen Obtain the specimen on the applicator. Place specimen into the sterile tube. Crush ampule containing growth medium **OR** inoculate slide or agar plate	Label specimen Process specimen promptly to prevent overgrowth of other microorganisms Replace any dressings if necessary
Urine Studies	Explain the collection procedure	Collect urine in appropriate container Store 24-hr collection at proper temperature	Label specimen and process immediately
Lumbar Puncture (LP)	Obtain signed consent Explain the test and sensations to be felt Assess VS	Performed by physician, assisted by RN Person in side-lying position with head flexed and knees drawn up to bow the back (Fig. 34–4A), spreading the vertebrae to ease needle insertion Encourage person to relax and deep breathe Prep puncture site and drape surrounding area with sterile towels Local anesthetic injected at puncture site Spinal needle with stylet inserted. Person may feel "pop" of needle as it punctures dura mater Stylet is removed, and manometer is attached to measure CSF pressure Three specimens of CSF are removed and labeled no. 1, 2, and 3 in order Closing pressure may be recorded before needle is withdrawn Apply small sterile dressing over puncture site Process specimen immediately. Do NOT refrigerate	Person lies flat 4–8 hr to prevent spinal headache May turn side-to-side Push fluids to prevent dehydration and spinal headache. Assess neurologic status (note level of consciousness, pupils, temperature, and presence of elevated BP, irritability, or paresthesias of legs) Analgesics and bedrest if headache develops Check LP site for leakage and report any to MD

Table continued on following page

TABLE 34–3. *Care of the Person Undergoing Laboratory Studies* Continued

| Test | Care of the Person | | |
	Before the Test	*During the Test*	*After the Test*
Abdominal Paracentesis	Obtain signed consent Weigh person Measure girth of abdomen for baseline assessment Have person void Assess VS	Support client in upright sitting position (Fig. 34–4B) Prep area and drape with sterile towels Local anesthetic will be given Needle is inserted and fluid withdrawn Process specimens Apply small sterile dressing	Person usually feels better after procedure Assess for shock (pallor, elevated heart rate, decreased BP, decreased level of consciousness, clammy skin) Abdominal binder may be used Measure girth of abdomen Weigh person
Thoracentesis	Obtain signed consent Assess baseline VS X-ray study or ultrasound may be done to locate fluid or air Tell person to expect no pain during procedure other than needle prick when local anesthetic is given Person should feel better as fluid pressure is removed from lungs Warn person not to cough during test. Cough suppressants may be given 30 min before procedure. If cough is unavoidable have person warn MD first Tell person to lie still	Physician performs test, RN assists Support person in sitting position leaning forward (Fig. 34–4D) Prep site Local anesthetic administered Needle is inserted and fluid or air is withdrawn, then needle is removed Apply small occlusive dressing	Assess for shock Chest x-ray taken to assess for pneumothorax Watch for cough, dyspnea, bloody sputum
Liver Biopsy	Obtain signed consent Assess clotting factors Administer vitamin K Sedative 30 min before test NPO 2 hr before test Local anesthetic will be used Tell person to hold breath when biopsy needle is inserted Must be still Expect needle prick and pressure as biopsy is aspirated Assess VS	MD performs test, RN assists Position supine with right side of upper abdomen exposed. Raise right arm and flex over shoulder behind head Prep site Local anesthetic is administered Needle is inserted as person holds breath Specimen is aspirated and processed	Apply pressure dressing Turn person to right side with small folded towel or pillow under puncture site for 3 hr or more Observe for bleeding and report abdominal pain (may be due to bile leak) Assess VS
Bone Marrow Aspiration	Obtain signed consent Tell person test may be uncomfortable Person may hear needle as it is pushed through bone and feel pain as marrow is aspirated Administer sedative Assess VS	MD performs test, RN assists Local anesthetic administered Shave and prep area Position supine with pad between scapula for sternal puncture, prone for iliac crest puncture After aspiration, apply pressure Apply small dressing	Bed rest for 30 min, then resume normal activities Assess VS Assess for bleeding Administer medication for discomfort if needed; person may be sore for days

TABLE 34-3. Care of the Person Undergoing Laboratory Studies Continued

Test	Care of the Person		
	Before the Test	**During the Test**	**After the Test**
Amniocentesis	Obtain consent from person and husband Genetic counseling before test Ask person to void Record fetal heart tones Person may experience nausea and mild cramps during test	MD performs test, RN assists Position person on back with arms behind head Ultrasound to determine fetal position Prep abdomen Local anesthetic is given Needle is inserted and fluid withdrawn Apply small bandage	Place specimen in light-resistant container and send to laboratory Assess VS and fetal heart tones every 15 min for 1 hr Notify MD of any loss of amniotic fluid, labor, pain, bleeding, elevated temperature, chills, decreased or absent fetal activity

Blood Studies

Abnormalities of blood components or substances dissolved or carried in the blood provide valuable diagnostic information. Most diagnostic workups involve some type of blood analysis. Routine hospital admission laboratory work often includes a complete blood count (CBC), which measures levels of white cells, red cells, platelets, hemoglobin, and hematocrit, and blood chemistries such as the SMA-6, SMA-12, or SMA-18, which include electrolyte levels, enzymes, glucose levels, proteins, lipids, and hormones. Laboratory personnel usually draw blood from veins or by finger stick; however, nurses may also be called upon to draw blood specimens.

Specimens for Culture

Body secretions are commonly examined for infection with microorganisms. Specimens are commonly taken from the throat, rectum, penis, vagina, urethra, and wounds. When a culture and antibiotic therapy are ordered concurrently, it is important to obtain the specimen for culture first. This will provide the most accurate assessment of the infective organism. A long sterile applicator with a cotton tip is usually used to obtain the specimen. The tip is placed on or in the affected body area and rotated to assure contact with the secretions. The applicator is then placed in a sterile tube or used to inoculate a slide or agar plate. It is very important that you do not contaminate the specimen by touching the applicator to other objects or body surfaces. Protect yourself from contact with body secretions by wearing gloves if necessary.

Urine Studies

A urinalysis is the laboratory analysis of a specimen of urine. This is a common test that is often included as part of a routine diagnostic workup on admission to the hospital. The nurse usually collects the specimen or instructs the alert client to collect the specimen. A sample of several hundred milliliters soon after the person awakens is best.

Depending on the test to be performed, the urine may be collected in a clean or sterile container. Some tests require only a single sample, whereas others may require all urine for 24 hours to be saved.

Be sure you know whether a preservative is to be added to the urine and are aware of the temperature to store the urine. Some specimens should be stored at room temperature, whereas others should be refrigerated or iced.

Chapter 44 includes additional information on collection of urine specimens.

Aspiration Studies

Aspiration procedures involve collecting fluid or tissue from an organ or body cavity. A needle or similar instrument will be used to obtain the specimen. Aspiration procedures may provoke anxiety in the client and may be uncomfortable. Obtaining specimens by aspiration is a sterile invasive procedure and requires a signed consent from the person. The procedure may be carried out at the person's bedside or in another examination area. Common aspiration procedures will be discussed next. Some positions that the client may have to assume are shown in Figure 34-4. Table 34-3 describes care for persons undergoing aspiration studies.

LUMBAR PUNCTURE

A **lumbar puncture (LP, spinal tap)** is a procedure involving insertion of a needle into the lumbar sac of the subarachnoid space between L4 and L5 to obtain a sample of the cerebrospinal fluid (CSF). The procedure

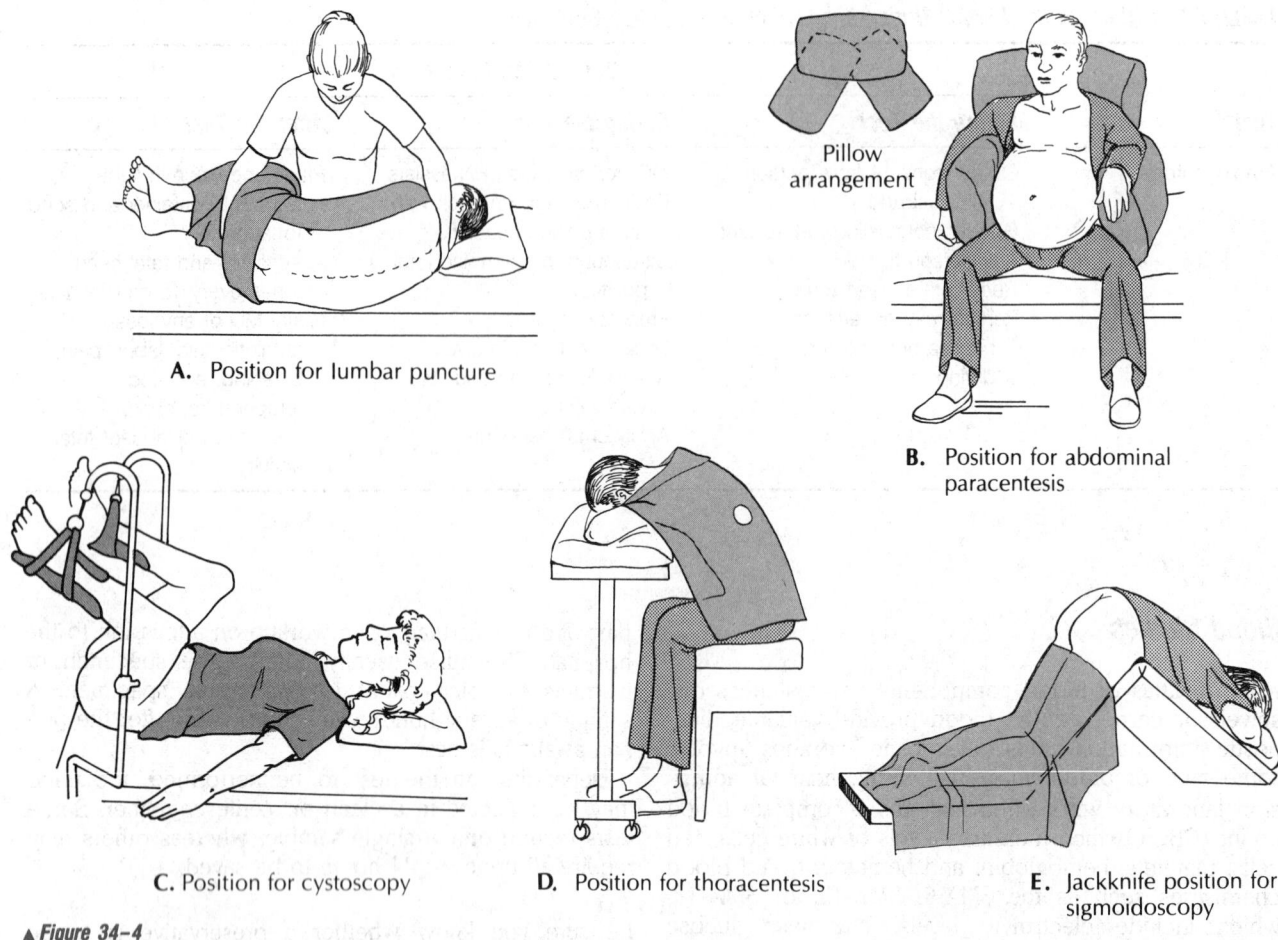

A. Position for lumbar puncture

Pillow arrangement

B. Position for abdominal paracentesis

C. Position for cystoscopy

D. Position for thoracentesis

E. Jackknife position for sigmoidoscopy

▲ *Figure 34–4*

Positions for some diagnostic tests.

is performed when infection such as meningitis is suspected or when intracranial bleeding is suspected. Normally CSF is clear and colorless and contains few cells. With the exception of chloride, which is higher, the electrolyte composition of CSF is roughly equivalent to that of serum. The specimen is analyzed in the laboratory for appearance, bacteria, cell count, proteins, chloride, and sugar.

The cerebrospinal fluid pressure can be measured by attaching a manometer to the spinal needle. This is useful in determining problems with absorption or production of CSF resulting from disorders such as hydrocephalus or increased intracranial pressure. Introcranial pressure can be lowered by removing some of the spinal fluid; however, this is dangerous and can result in herniation of the brain stem. Lumbar punctures are also performed to administer medications such as anesthetics or x-ray contrast media.

A lumbar puncture is an invasive sterile procedure and requires use of sterile technique. A signed consent form should be obtained before carrying out this procedure.

PARACENTESIS

Abdominal **paracentesis** is a sterile procedure involving the removal of fluid that has abnormally accumu-

lated in the peritoneal cavity. The fluid is analyzed for the presence or absence of malignant cells. This abnormal accumulation of peritoneal fluid, called ascites, may result in increased pressure in the abdomen causing discomfort. Respiratory distress may also occur as lung expansion is restricted by the increased abdominal pressure on the diaphragm. Performing an abdominal paracentesis gives symptomatic relief of these problems.

It is important to avoid withdrawing the fluid too rapidly, as this may produce symptoms of shock. Usually 300 to 1000 ml of fluid is slowly withdrawn during the procedure.

THORACENTESIS

A **thoracentesis** is a sterile procedure involving insertion of a needle into the pleural space to aspirate fluid or air. A thoracentesis may be done to relieve pressure, pain, or dyspnea caused by abnormal collections of fluid or air or to get specimens of pleural fluid for analysis or for pleural biopsy. Utilizing a local anesthetic, a needle is usually inserted in the upper anterior chest if air is to be removed, and the lower posterior chest if fluid is to be removed. A chest x-ray is taken after the procedure to assess for the complication of pneumothorax. A thoracentesis is usually performed at the person's bedside and takes about 15 minutes.

LIVER BIOPSY

A **biopsy** is a procedure involving removal of a tissue sample for microscopic examination. A liver biopsy, specifically, is a sterile procedure performed to obtain and examine microscopically a tissue sample for diagnosis and progress of liver disease. A needle is inserted either through the abdomen or between the two right lower ribs to obtain the specimen. Vitamin K may be administered several days before the test to improve blood clotting. Blood-clotting ability will be assessed before the procedure (prothrombin time, platelet count), since people with liver disease often have reduced blood-clotting ability.

The liver biopsy will be canceled if blood-clotting studies are abnormal.

The liver biopsy is usually done at the person's bedside and takes about 15 minutes to complete.

BONE MARROW ASPIRATION

In bone marrow aspiration, a needle is most often inserted into the bone marrow of the sternum or upper iliac crests, to obtain a sample of the marrow. The specimen is used to diagnose blood diseases such as anemia or leukemia. The procedure is usually performed under local anesthesia, and a sedative may be administered. Bone marrow aspirations are done at the person's bedside using sterile technique. The test usually takes 20 to 30 minutes to complete.

AMNIOCENTESIS

Amniocentesis is the aspiration of amniotic fluid from the amniotic sac by way of a needle inserted through the abdominal and uterine walls. This sterile procedure may be done to detect certain fetal abnormalities after the 14th to 16th week of pregnancy. Amniocentesis is also performed to determine fetal age and maturity of the lungs after the 35th week of gestation. Ultrasonography is used to guide insertion of the needle.

There is a slight risk of spontaneous abortion after the procedure.

Rh-negative mothers should receive RhoGAM after the amniocentesis to prevent Rh sensitization. The procedure takes about 20 minutes; however some test results, such as genetic studies, may take up to 4 weeks to complete.

ASSESSMENT OF ELECTRICAL IMPULSES

Electrodes can be attached to the body to record and evaluate the electrical activity in the heart, brain, and muscles. The electrical impulses can be displayed on an oscilloscope screen (monitor) or recorded on a graph.

Electrocardiogram

The **electrocardiogram (ECG, EKG)** is a recording of the electrical activity of the heart. The procedure involves placing 3 to 12 leads on the person's chest and on certain peripheral pulse sites. These leads help to measure and record the electrical activity of the heart from various angles (Fig. 34–5). The ECG is a painless, noninvasive test that gives valuable information to aid in diagnosing coronary artery disease, myocardial infarctions, dysrhythmias, and electrolyte imbalances. The 12-lead ECG takes about 10 minutes to complete. Heart rhythms can be monitored continuously in the hospital setting or recorded on paper for 24 continuous hours using a Holter monitor.

The normal heart rhythm is produced by electrical activity that originates in the sinoatrial (SA) node. The impulse travels by way of intra-atrial pathways to the atrioventricular (AV) node. The impulse is then conducted down the bundle of His to the right and left ventricles by way of the bundle branches and the Purkinje fibers (Fig. 34–6).

This electrical activity stimulates the atria and ventricle, producing contraction (depolarization) and relax-

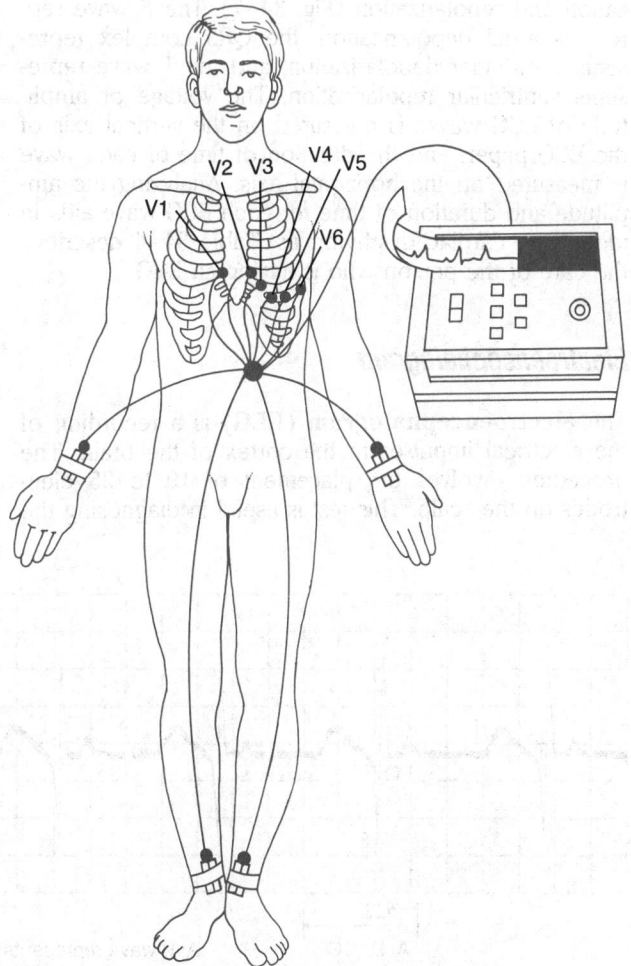

▲ *Figure 34–5*

Placement of leads for the electrocardiogram.

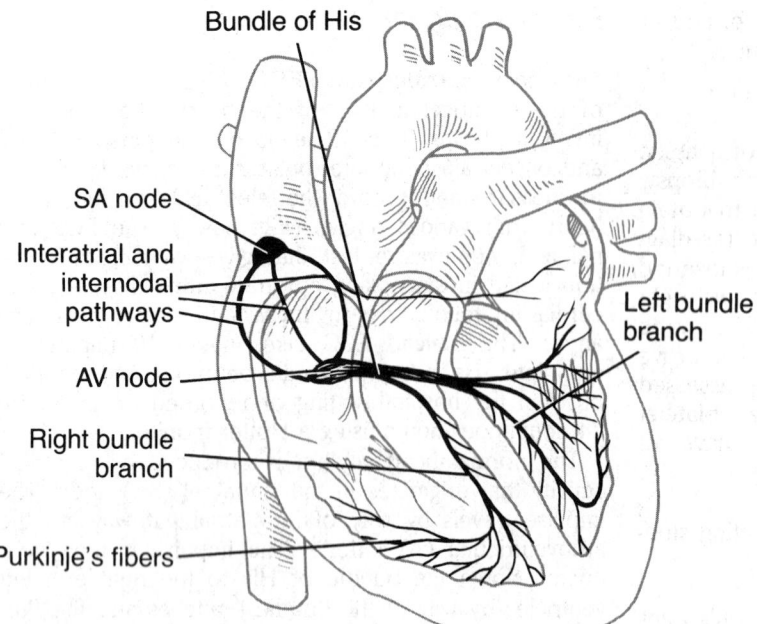

Bundle of His

SA node

Interatrial and
internodal
pathways

AV node

Right bundle
branch

Purkinje's fibers

Left bundle
branch

▲ *Figure 34-6*

Electrical conduction system of the heart.

ation (repolarization) of the myocardium. The waves of the ECG tracing are a graphic representation of the electrical activity occurring during myocardial depolarization and repolarization (Fig. 34-7). The P wave represents atrial depolarization, the QRS complex represents ventricular depolarization, and the T wave represents ventricular repolarization. The voltage or amplitude of ECG waves is measured on the vertical axis of the ECG paper, and the duration of time of each wave is measured on the horizontal axis. Analyzing the amplitude and duration of time for each ECG wave aids in identifying cardiac dysrhythmias. Table 34-4 describes the care of the person who is having an ECG.

Electroencephalogram

The **electroencephalogram (EEG)** is a recording of the electrical impulses in the cortex of the brain. The procedure involves the placement of 19 to 25 electrodes on the scalp. This test is useful in diagnosing the

absence of brain activity, or cerebral death, as well as diagnosing neurologic disorders such as epilepsy, narcolepsy, Alzheimer's disease, cerebrovascular accidents, brain tumors and abscesses, and subdural hematomas. The examination is carried out in an EEG laboratory, or it can be performed at the patient's bedside using portable equipment. Table 34-4 describes the care of the person who is having an EEG.

Electromyogram

The **electromyogram (EMG)** is a recording of nerve impulses in skeletal muscles. The procedure involves placing electrodes on the skin surface overlying muscles. Needle electrodes are placed in the muscle to record electrical activity when muscles are contracted and at rest. When muscles are stimulated, the resulting muscle activity can be viewed on an oscilloscope as well as heard on an audio recording. These tests are useful in detecting neuromuscular abnormalities, such

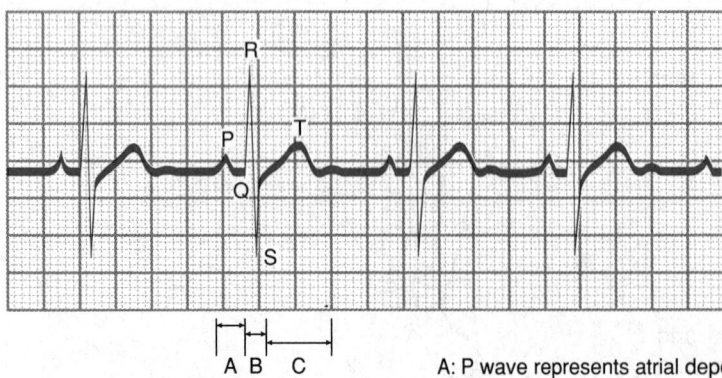

A: P wave represents atrial depolarization

B: QRS complex represents ventricular depolarization

C: T wave represents ventricular repolarization

▲ *Figure 34-7*

Graphic representation of electrical activity occurring during myocardial depolarization and repolarization.

TABLE 34-4. Care of the Person Undergoing Assessment of Electrical Impulses

Test	Care of the Person		
	Before the Test	**During the Test**	**After the Test**
Electrocardiogram (ECG)	No special preparation Tell person test is painless	Have person lie supine Prep skin with alcohol wipe. Shave any excess hair Apply leads (Fig. 34-5) using prejelled disk or ECG paste Record ECG	Remove leads Clean ECG paste from skin
Electroencephalogram (EEG)	Explain the test Check with MD regarding discontinuing drugs that interfere with test (barbiturates, anticonvulsants, tranquilizers) Client must eat before test to prevent hypoglycemia, which can alter test results No coffee, tea, or cola 8 hr before test Shampoo hair day before test to facilitate lead attachment If sleep study is to be done, deprive of sleep night before test	Technician attends person 19-25 leads are applied to scalp Conduction gel is applied to increase contact or electrodes in the form of pins are introduced through the skin Person reclines in chair or bed with eyes closed Client must be very still Person may be asked to hyperventilate or watch flashing lights to elicit seizure activity; warn person that hyperventilation may cause feelings of nausea or dizziness	Remove leads, paste, and gel Shampoo hair
Electromyogram (EMG)	Obtain signed consent Explain the test Sedation and analgesia may be given Help person into hospital gown Warn person test may be uncomfortable	Technician attends person Test has two parts: (1) Nerve conduction: test involves passing electrical current through skin electrode and observing response of muscle on oscilloscope (2) Muscle potential: needle electrodes are inserted into muscle and electrical activity is measured when person contracts and relaxes muscles	Provide analgesic and rest

as myasthenia gravis and amyotrophic lateral sclerosis. The length of time to complete the procedure varies from 1 to 2.5 hours or more. Table 34-4 describes the care of the person undergoing an EMG.

ASSESSMENT BY ENDOSCOPY

Endoscopy is a means of visualizing interior body structures using a flexible, hollow, lighted scope. Instruments can be inserted through the scopes to obtain small samples of tissue for biopsy. A biopsy is the microscopic examination of a tissue sample to identify malignancies or infection. Foreign bodies can also be removed using endoscopic equipment. Endoscopic procedures are usually carried out in a specially equipped endoscopic laboratory. Most endoscopic procedures take about 1 hour to complete. Table 34-5 describes the care of the person undergoing an endoscopic procedure.

Bronchoscopy

Bronchoscopy is an endoscopic examination of the larynx, trachea, and bronchi. During a bronchoscopy, a bronchoscope is passed into the bronchus via the mouth. A bronchoscopy is a sterile procedure.

TABLE 34-5. Care of the Person Undergoing Endoscopic Procedures

| Test | Care of the Person | | |
	Before the Test	During the Test	After the Test
Bronchoscopy	Obtain signed consent Administer anticholinergic drug such as atropine to dry secretions Sedation may be administered NPO after midnight before procedure Remove dentures and provide oral care	Local anesthetic may be sprayed on throat or gargled Procedure may be done under general anesthesia Person lies on table with neck hyperextended Person may feel short of breath; oxygen may be given by mask	No food or fluid until gag reflex returns and cough reflex is present Observe for bleeding from tissue damage Observe for edema and respiratory distress May be hoarse with sore throat after test
Esophagogastroduodenoscopy (EGD)	NPO after midnight Obtain signed consent Sedatives may be used Anticholinergic drugs such as atropine may be used to dry secretions	Anesthetic throat spray or gargle will be used to facilitate passage of scope	Same care as for bronchoscopy Observe emesis for blood
Proctosigmoidoscopy/ Colonoscopy	Obtain signed consent Clear liquid diet day before test NPO after midnight before test Laxative day before test Enemas until clear day of procedure (DO NOT give more than three enemas, to avoid water intoxication) Sedatives may be administered Void before the procedure	Person assumes knee-chest position (Fig. 34–4E) After a digital rectal examination, the scope is inserted into the anus. Person may feel need to have a BM Person may feel abdominal cramping when air is introduced into GI tract; encourage person to deep breathe	Offer nourishment and rest Take VS every 15 min for 1 hr, then every hour for 4 hr Observe and test for blood in stool for next 3 days
Cystoscopy	Obtain signed consent NPO after midnight before test Laxative or enema if IVP is to be done (see IVP prep in Table 34–1) Assess for symptoms of urinary tract infection (burning, frequency, blood) for baseline	Lithotomy position during procedure (Fig. 34–4C) General anesthetic is usual Catheters may be inserted into ureters. Dye may be introduced to outline kidneys, and x-ray (IVP) may be taken	Push PO fluid Assess urine for blood Report bright red bleeding or inability to void after 8 hr Assess for symptoms of infection

TABLE 34-6. Care of the Person Undergoing Ultrasonography

| Test | Care of the Person | | |
	Before the Test	During the Test	After the Test
Ultrasonography	NPO before abdominal ultrasound only Full bladder before pelvic ultrasound	Tell the person to lie still during the test Technician attends person	Remove ultrasound gel from person's skin

Esophagogastroduodenoscopy

Esophagogastroduodenoscopy (EGD) is an endoscopic examination of the esophagus, stomach, and duodenum. During this procedure, a gastroscope is passed through the mouth. An EGD is a clean procedure.

Proctosigmoidoscopy

Proctosigmoidoscopy is an endoscopic examination of the rectum and sigmoid colon. In this procedure, a scope is passed into the GI tract through the anus. A proctosigmoidoscopy is a clean procedure.

Colonoscopy

Colonoscopy is an endoscopic examination of the large intestine. During this procedure, a colonoscope is passed through the anus into the large intestine (colon) for visualization. The colonoscopy is a clean procedure.

Cystoscopy

Cystoscopy is an endoscopic examination of the urinary bladder. During a cystoscopic examination, a cystoscope is passed through the urethra into the urinary bladder for visualization of the interior. An intravenous pyelogram (IVP) may be done in conjunction with the cystoscopic examination. A cystoscopy is a sterile procedure. The examination may be done in a urologist's office, hospital operating room, or a radiology department.

ASSESSMENT BY ULTRASONOGRAPHY

Ultrasound is a noninvasive scan of internal structures using sound waves. It does not utilize x-rays or radioactive substances. Ultrasonic waves (sound waves too high in frequency for a human ear to detect) are used diagnostically to assess various body structures. The waves are directed at the organ or structure. As the waves vibrate back from their target, they are transduced into oscilloscope tracings.

Pathologic changes in muscles and joints may be studied by using sound. The brain (echoencephalography) and heart (echocardiography) can also be studied. Common applications for ultrasonography are to visualize a fetus to determine gestational age, to verify the presence of multiple births, and to detect certain fetal problems. An ultrasound examination usually takes 35 to 45 minutes to complete. Table 34–6 describes the care of the person undergoing ultrasonography.

ASSESSMENT BY PULMONARY FUNCTION STUDIES

Pulmonary function studies are breathing tests using a spirometer to assess the extent of dysfunction resulting from restrictive or obstructive pulmonary diseases. Common measurements include:

▶ Vital capacity (VC): maximal amount of air that can be forcefully exhaled following a maximum inspiration
▶ Tidal volume (TV): amount of air inhaled and exhaled during normal breathing
▶ Inspiratory capacity (IC): maximal amount of air that can be inspired from the end-tidal expiration
▶ Expiratory reserve volume (ERV): maximal amount of air that can be expired from end-tidal expiration
▶ Residual volume (RV): amount of gas left in the lungs after maximal expiration
▶ Total lung capacity (TLC): amount of gas in the lungs following a maximal inspiration
▶ Functional residual capacity (FRC): amount of gas in the lungs following a normal expiration

A comparison of pulmonary function tests is shown in Figure 34–8.

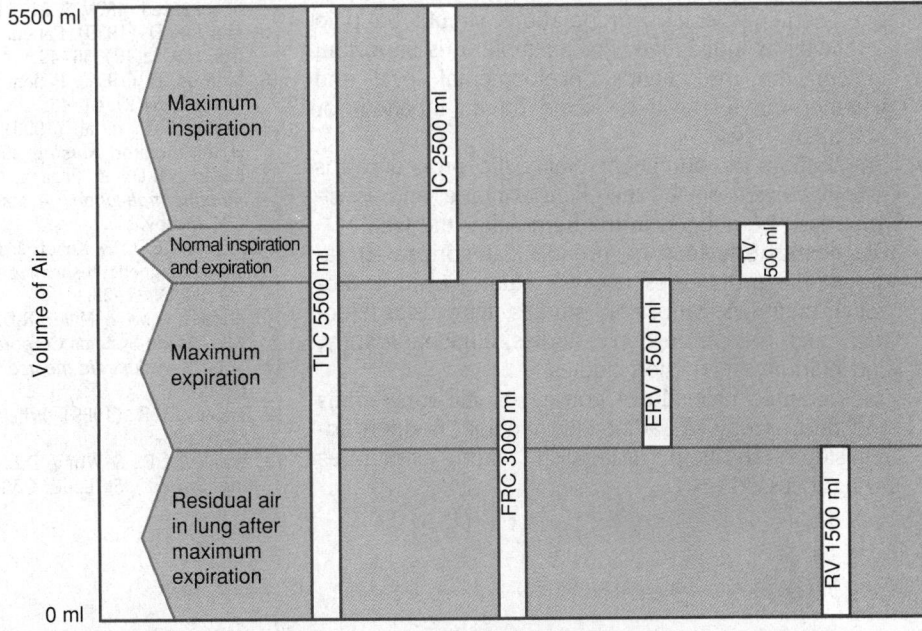

▲ **Figure 34–8**

Comparison of some pulmonary function tests.

TABLE 34-7. Care of the Person Undergoing Pulmonary Function Studies

| Test | Care of the Person | | |
	Before the Test	During the Test	After the Test
Pulmonary Function Studies	Tell to wear comfortable clothes Inform respiratory therapy department if person has had medications that affect respiratory function	Respiratory therapist conducts test Nose clip will be worn during test Person may feel suffocating sensation ABG studies may be done: person will feel pain of needle stick	Rest No special aftercare

Arterial blood gas (ABG) studies measure the pH, bicarbonate level, oxygen saturation level, and the partial pressures of arterial oxygen and carbon dioxide in arterial blood. These studies may be done in conjunction with pulmonary function tests to compare ventilation with perfusion. Pulmonary function tests may take up to 2 hours and are carried out in the respiratory therapy department. Table 34-7 describes the care of the person undergoing a pulmonary function test.

Summary

▶ Before a medical diagnostic procedure, nursing responsibilities may include scheduling the test, transporting the person to the testing area, and preparing the equipment to be used during the test, as well as preparing the person and significant others for the test.

▶ During a diagnostic procedure, nursing responsibilities may include collecting baseline assessment data and assisting with the procedure, as well as supporting and continuing to evaluate the client.

▶ After a diagnostic procedure, nursing care may include processing specimens and notifying family/significant others of procedure completion, as well as providing postprocedure care and comfort measures, cleaning or disposing of equipment, and documenting the procedure.

▶ Although diagnostic tests may be similar for everyone, certain special considerations should be paid to clients as individuals. For example, it is important to consider the client's developmental level and whether the test will be done on an inpatient or outpatient basis.

▶ Preparation for outpatient diagnostic procedures is usually carried out by the client at home, and assistance may be needed in the home after the test.

▶ Diagnostic tests may be broadly categorized as radiographic procedures (x-rays), studies using radioactive materials, laboratory studies, tests using electrical impulses, endoscopic studies, ultrasonography, and pulmonary function studies.

▶ Radiographic procedures consist of still x-ray films and fluoroscopy. A radiopaque medium is often administered to help distinguish among structures being assessed.

▶ When a radioactive substance is placed in the body, it accumulates in specific organs or regions and can be detected to test organ function and to locate malignancies.

▶ Laboratory studies consist of blood studies, specimens for culture, urine studies, and aspiration studies.

▶ Electrocardiogram, electroencephalogram, and electromyogram are three common tests that assess electrical activity in the human body.

▶ Endoscopic procedures are used to visualize internal body structures, to obtain tissue samples for biopsy, and to remove foreign bodies.

▶ Ultrasonography is a noninvasive diagnostic tool that uses ultrasound waves to assess various body structures. Commonly, it is used to assess fetal development and pathology.

▶ Pulmonary function may be assessed with breathing tests that use a spirometer and with arterial blood gas studies.

Bibliography

1. Broome, M.E., et al. (1990). Children's medical fears, coping behaviors, and pain perception during a lumbar puncture. *Oncology Nursing Forum*, 17(3), 361-367.
2. Fischbach, F. (1988). *A manual of laboratory diagnostic tests* (3rd ed.). Philadelphia: J.B. Lippincott.
3. Gipe, F.M., & Sellew, G. (1949). Ward administration and clinical teaching. St. Louis: C.V. Mosby.
4. Koss, T., & Teter, M. (1980). Welcoming a family when a child is hospitalized. *MCN*, 5, 51-54.
5. Monroe, D. (1989). Patient teaching for X-ray and other diagnostics. *RN*, 52(12), 36-40.
6. Monroe, D. (1991). Patient teaching for X-ray and other diagnostics. *RN*, 54(2), 44-46.
7. Norris, L.O., et al. (1990). Sending your patient home with a Holter monitor. *Nursing*, 20(2), 32I-32J.
8. Pagana, K.D., & Pagana, T.J. (1989). *Diagnostic testing and nursing implications: A case study approach* (3rd ed.). St. Louis: C.V. Mosby.
9. Plankey, E.D., & Knauf, J. (1990). What patients need to know about magnetic resonance imaging. *American Journal of Nursing*, 90(1), 27-28.
10. Rhodes, A.M., & Miller, R.D. (1984). *Nursing and the law*. Rockville: Aspen Systems Corporation.
11. *Taber's cyclopedic medical dictionary* (1989). Philadelphia: F.A. Davis.
12. Trasher, S.B. (1989). What I didn't know really hurt me. *RN*, 52(9), 49-50.
13. Whaley, L.E., & Wong, D.L. (1989). *Essentials of pediatric nursing* (3rd ed.). St. Louis: C.V. Mosby.

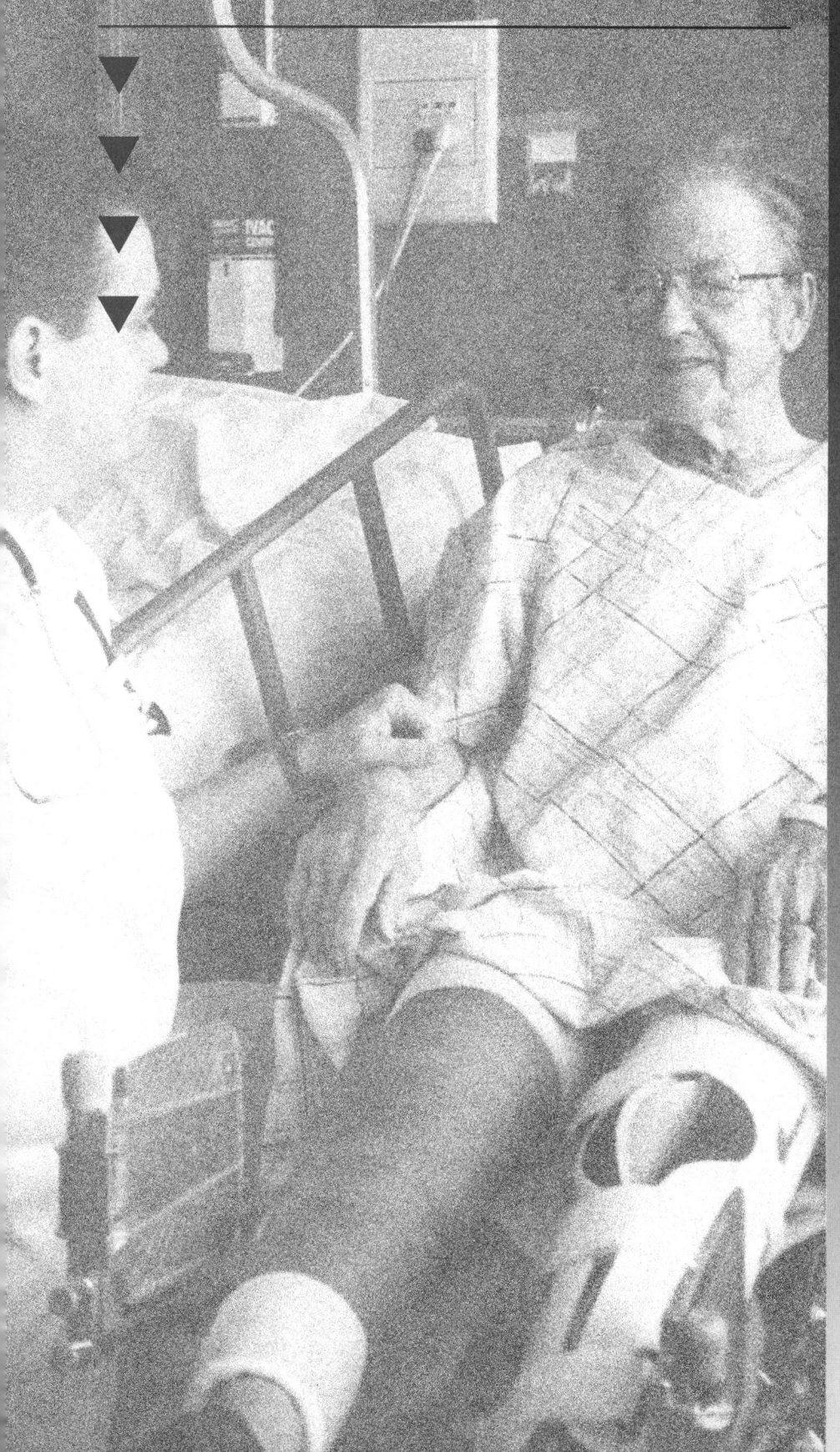

Therapeutic Skills

▼ *Preventing Complications of Immobility*

 Wherever human beings are concerned, trend is not destiny.
René Dubois

▼ CHAPTER OUTLINE

ASSESSMENT
    Review of Anatomy and Physiology
    General Mobility Level
    Range of Motion of Spine and
       Extremities
    Effects of Immobility
NURSING DIAGNOSIS
PLANNING
NURSING INTERVENTION
    Examining Bed Rest

Equipment for Positioning
Positions
Positioning the Immobilized Client
Equipment to Assist in Transferring
    the Immobilized Client
Transferring the Immobilized Client
Additional Nursing Interventions to
    Prevent Disuse Phenomena
EVALUATION
CASE STUDY

▼ KEY TERMS

Abduction
Adduction
Bone resorption
Contracture
Dangling
Dependent edema
Disuse syndrome
Edema
Erythema
Extension
External rotation
Flaccidity
Flexion
Footdrop
Horizontal abduction

Horizontal adduction
Hyperemic
Hyperextension
Hypostatic pneumonia
Ischemia
Isometric contraction
Isotonic contraction
Muscle tonus
Necrotic
Negative nitrogen balance
Nonblanchable erythema
Orthostatic (postural)
    hypotension
Osteomyelitis
Osteoporosis

Pathologic fractures
Phlebitis
Pressure-reducing device
Pressure-relieving device
Pressure ulcers
Rotation
Spasticity
Syncope
Thromboembolism
Tissue hypoxia
Tonic contraction
Tympanites
Valsalva maneuver
Venous stasis

Imagine what might happen to you if, today, you crossed the street and were hit by a fast-moving truck. Imagine yourself awakening in a hospital in some combination of casts, traction, or other immobilizing devices. Imagine yourself unable to move freely; dependent on others to help you perform even simple tasks such as feeding yourself, washing your face, turning to one side, or wiping yourself after using a bedpan. Imagine not knowing how long you would be in this state. How would you feel? How would it affect your life?

What might happen to your education? What would happen to you financially? How about your social life? What about that romantic interest? What differences would it make in your life if your immobility were prolonged?

As you think about how immobility could change your life, think about how you might feel emotionally. Would you feel anxious? Angry? Depressed? Helpless? Bored? Perhaps at various times during your illness you would feel each of these emotions and others as well.

In addition to the fact that immobility has the potential for greatly changing your lifestyle and for altering the progression of planned life events, it can cause profound physical effects. Immobility can affect every body system and can result in some life-threatening physiologic complications. In short, immobility can result in death. This chapter will review the very complex problem of immobility and will focus on preventing many potential complications. To help you focus on some of the possible complications of immobility, these complications have been indicated in italics throughout the chapter.

ASSESSMENT

Mobility requires the coordination of multiple body systems, but in assessing an individual's general mobility level, we are concerned mainly with the musculoskeletal system. Therefore, we will begin with a brief review of the anatomy and physiology of the skeletal system, articular system, and muscles.

Review of Anatomy and Physiology

SKELETAL SYSTEM

The Skeleton. The normal, adult skeleton consists of 206 bones, divided into those comprising the head and trunk (the axial skeleton) and the extremities (the appendicular skeleton) (Fig. 35–1). The skeleton functions to

▶ maintain the body's form on its supporting framework
▶ protect delicate or vital soft tissues, e.g., the brain and lungs
▶ assist in movement by providing leverage against which attached muscles may move body parts
▶ store calcium and other mineral salts for use as needed by the body
▶ manufacture and develop blood cells (hematopoiesis)

Bone. The four main types of bone are classified by shape as long, short, flat, and irregular. Table 35–1 lists the bones of the axial and appendicular skeleton, separates them by shape, and provides the number of each normally found in the adult human.

On a macroscopic level, bone tissue is of two types: (1) cortical (compact) bone that is dense, heavy, and rigid, and (2) cancellous (spongy) bone that is composed of a lattice of trabeculae that make it light and porous but very strong. The quantity of cortical or cancellous tissue varies among the different types of bones and in different parts of the same bone. Cortical bone forms the outer shaft of long bones and the hard, outer, protective layer of all other bones. Cancellous bone forms the epiphysis (end) and metaphysis (growing portion between the shaft and the epiphysis) of long bones and forms the inner portion of all other bones.

Yellow marrow fills the medullary (inner) cavity of the shaft of long bones and the small spaces in the cancellous tissue at the ends of most long bones. Red

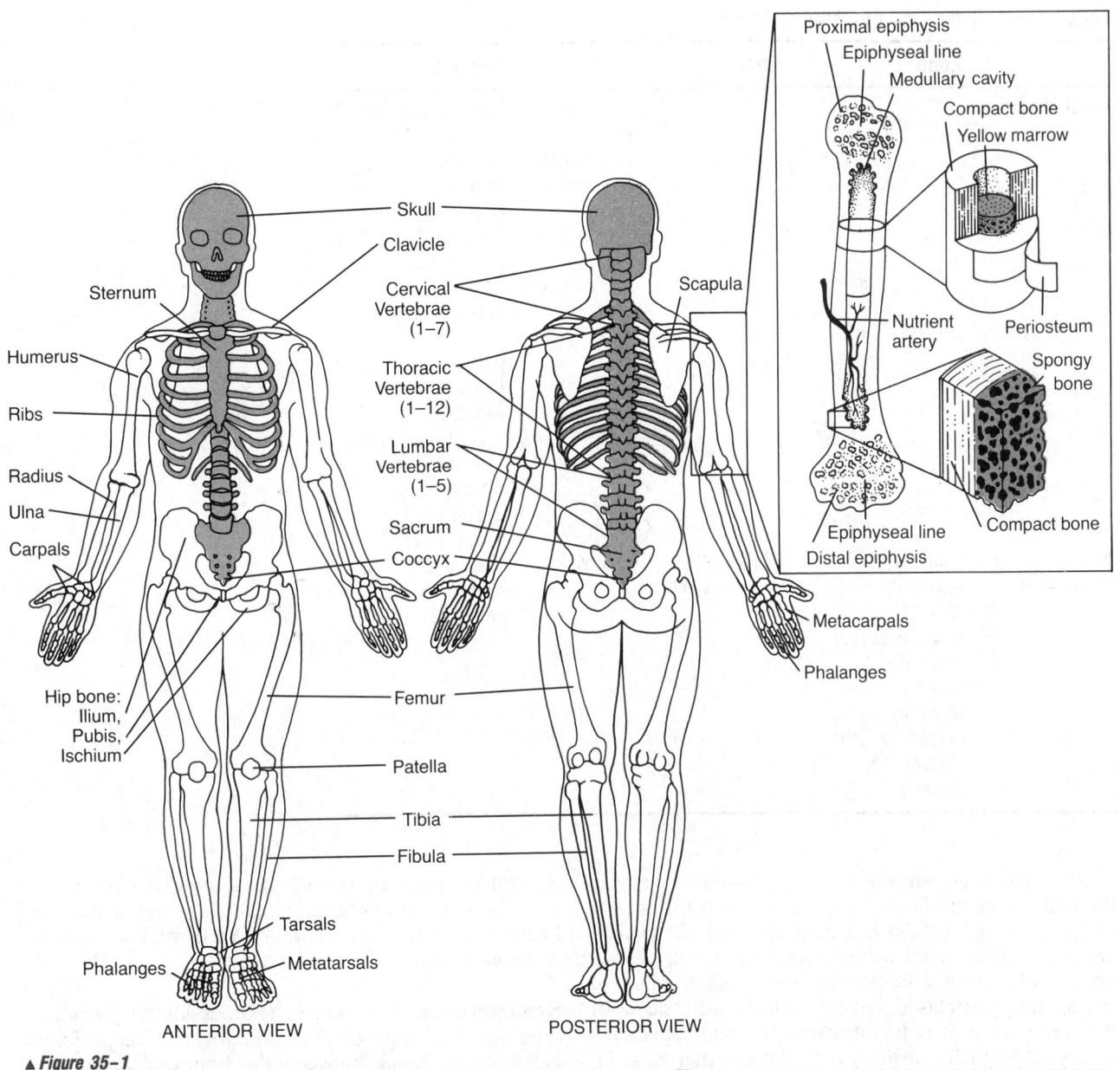

▲ *Figure 35–1*

The human skeleton consists of the axial skeleton (shown here in color) and the appendicular (extremity) skeleton. The inset shows the parts of a typical long bone.

marrow fills the spaces in the cancellous tissue in the proximal ends of the humerus and femur and in selected flat and irregular bones, e.g., the vertebrae and sternum. Red marrow is involved in the production of blood cells and hemoglobin.

The periosteum (a dense, white fibrous membrane) covers the outer surface of bones except at the articulating ends. Periosteal tissue penetrates bone tissue and supplies blood vessels for continuous nourishment of the bone cells. It also supplies osteoblasts to the bone, as needed for repair. Because its fibers penetrate the bone tissue, the periosteum is firmly anchored to the bone and provides a means for muscles, tendons, and ligaments to attach securely to the bone surface.

Cartilage. Cartilage is a specialized type of dense connective tissue that is somewhat elastic and pliable yet second only to bone in strength. Most of the fetal skeleton consists of cartilage, but this is later replaced by bone. In the adult skeleton, cartilage is normally found between the vertebral bodies, in the joints of most ribs, and covering the ends of articulating bones. It is also found in the nasal septum, external ears, eustachian tubes, larynx, trachea, and bronchi.

Cartilage cells are called chondrocytes. The chondrocytes lie in a ground substance or matrix of intercellular material that resembles a firm gel. This matrix consists of protein and mucopolysaccharides, imbedded with reinforcing collagenous and elastic fibers.

TABLE 35-1. *Types (and Number) of Bones*

	Long	Short	Flat	Irregular
Axial skeleton			frontal (1)	auditory ossicles (6)
			parietal (2)	sphenoid (1)
			occipital (1)	ethmoid (1)
			temporal (2)	maxilla (2)
			ribs:	mandible (1)
			true (14)	zygoma (2)
			false (6)	lacrimal (2)
			floating (4)	nasal (2)
			sternum (1)	turbinate (2)
				vomer (1)
				palate (2)
				hyoid (1)
				vertebrae:
				cervical (7)
				thoracic (12)
				lumbar (5)
				sacrum (1)
				coccyx (1)
Appendicular skeleton	humerus (2)	carpal (16)	scapula (2)	clavicle (2)
	radius (2)	metacarpal (14)		innominate (2)
	ulna (2)			patella (2)
	metacarpal (10)			
	femur (2)			
	tibia (2)			
	fibula (2)			
	metatarsal (10)			
	phalanx, finger (28)			
	phalanx, toe (28)			

There are three types of cartilage, differing mainly in the makeup of the fibers imbedded in their matrix: (1) elastic cartilage, (2) fibrous cartilage, and (3) hyaline cartilage. Elastic cartilage contains some collagenous fibers, but there is a preponderance of elastic fibers in the matrix. Thus elastic cartilage is the most resilient of the three types. It is found where the body structures are required to be flexible, e.g., the external ears. Fibrous cartilage consists of a matrix that contains dense masses of collagenous bundles. This gives it great tensile strength but makes it the least flexible of the three types. It is found where body structures are subject to continuous heavy stress, e.g., cushioning the joints between the vertebral bodies. Hyaline cartilage is the most abundant type found in the human body. Its matrix is imbedded with numerous fine collagenous fibers that cannot be visualized with the ordinary microscope. As a result, it appears translucent or glassy. It is strong and slightly elastic. A thin layer of hyaline cartilage covers and helps cushion the articulating surfaces of bones.

ARTICULAR SYSTEM

The articular system consists of joints. Joints function to bind bones together and to allow varying degrees of movement at the junction. When considering the degree of motion they permit, joints are classified as (1) synarthroses (immovable joints), (2) amphiarthroses (slightly movable joints), and (3) diarthroses (freely movable joints).

Synarthroses. Synarthroses (fibrous joints) provide a great deal of strength but no mobility. These joints have fibrous tissue between the bones. Examples include sutures (joints that unite bones of the adult skull) and gomphoses (joints that unite the roots of teeth and the alveolar processes in the jaw bones).

Amphiarthroses. Amphiarthroses (cartilaginous joints) provide strength and security while allowing limited motion. These joints are of two types: (1) symphyses and (2) synchondroses. The bones at a symphysis are connected by a pad of fibrous cartilage, and their articulating surfaces are covered by a thin layer of hyaline cartilage—examples are the symphysis pubis and the joints between vertebral bodies. The bones of a synchondrosis are actually joined together by hyaline cartilage, such as the costal cartilage that joins most of the ribs to the sternum.

Diarthroses. Diarthroses (synovial joints) are complex joints that provide less stability but allow more movement than do other types of joints. Most of the joints in the human body are diarthroses. Bones that articulate in a diarthrotic joint are covered with a thin, cushioning layer of hyaline cartilage at their articulating surfaces. The periosteum, near the ends of each of the articulating bones, balloons outward to form a capsule that encloses and binds together the bone ends. A synovial membrane covers the inner surface of the joint capsule and secretes a clear, colorless or pale yellow fluid the consistency of egg white. This synovial fluid moistens, lubricates, and nourishes the inner joint surfaces. Within most synovial joints, the bone ends are bound together by ligaments. These strong bands of dense, white fibrous connective tissue further strengthen the bond between the articulating bones.

Diarthrotic joints are not all equally movable. The types of movements normally possible in a synovial joint depend on the type of synovial joint. Types of synovial joints are uniaxial, biaxial, and multiaxial.

Uniaxial. Uniaxial synovial joints allow movement around only one axis and in only one plane. There are two types: hinge (ginglymus) and pivot. In *hinge (ginglymus)* joints, articulating bone ends form a hinge-shaped unit as on a door, as in elbow, knee, interphalangeal, and talocrural joints. In *pivot* joints, a ring or notch in one bone allows it to rotate around a projection on another bone, as in atlantoaxial and radioulnar joints.

Biaxial. Biaxial synovial joints allow movement around two perpendicular axes in two perpendicular planes. There are two types: saddle and condyloid. In *saddle* joints, articulating bone ends are reciprocally concave and convex—for example, the first carpometacarpal joint. In *condyloid* joints, a condyle on one bone fits into an elliptical depression in an articulating bone, as in radiocarpal, metacarpophalangeal, and metatarsophalangeal joints.

Multiaxial. Multiaxial synovial joints allow movement around three or more axes in three or more planes. There are two types: ball-and-socket, and gliding. In *ball-and-socket* joints, the rounded head of one bone (ball) fits into a cavity (socket) of another, such as the hip joint. In *gliding* joints, articulating surfaces are relatively flat, allowing very limited movement in various axes—for example, in costovertebral, sternocostal, sternoclavicular, acromioclavicular, intercarpal, tibiofibular, intertarsal, and tarsometatarsal joints.

MUSCULAR SYSTEM

The human body contains smooth muscle, cardiac muscle, and skeletal muscle. It is skeletal muscle (striated muscle, voluntary muscle) that actually contracts to maintain posture and to move the bones at the joints. Skeletal muscle contractions also help maintain total body heat.

In the adult, 40 to 50 per cent of the total body weight is derived from skeletal muscle. Look at Figure 35–2 and identify the following muscle structures as each is reviewed:

The Structure of Skeletal Muscle. Because the individual skeletal muscle cell is relatively long (approximately 50 to 200 μm in length but only 4 to 8 μm in width), it is referred to as a fiber rather than a cell. Muscle fibers normally extend the entire length of the muscle. Each fiber is ensheathed in a delicate connective tissue called endomysium. A number of fibers are bundled together into a group called a fasciculus. Each fasciculus, in turn, is ensheathed in a connective tissue called perimysium, which is visible to the naked eye. A number of fasciculi are bundled together to make up the familiar red muscle that is ensheathed in a fibrous connective tissue called epimysium (muscle fascia).

Connective Tissue and Muscle. The epimysium, perimysium, and endomysium are all continuous throughout the muscle and are also continuous with connective tissue that serves to attach the muscle to bone or to other structures. The connective tissue from the muscle, for example, may attach directly to bone or it may converge into a tendon that attaches to a bone. Alternatively, it may extend outward from the muscle in the form of a flat sheet of fibrous connective tissue (aponeurosis) that joins to bone or to other structures, including other muscles.

Muscle Fiber Patterns. Muscles may be classified by the orientation of their fibers as

► parallel—all muscle fibers are parallel to each other; an example is the rectus abdominus
► convergent—fibers converge at one end of the muscle, e.g., the deltoid
► fusiform—fibers taper inward at both ends, forming a spindle-shaped muscle like the biceps
► bipennate—muscle fibers attach to both sides of a tendon and flare outward, resembling a bird's feather; the rectus femoris is an example
► unipennate—muscle fibers attach only to one side of a tendon and flare outward, resembling half of a bird's feather, such as the palmar interossei
► sphincter—fibers form the muscle into a circular arrangement, as in the orbicularis oris

Additional information concerning the musculoskeletal system can be found throughout this chapter and in Chapter 36.

General Mobility Level

Because humans are bipedal, the spine and lower extremities provide the ability to stand, bear weight, and ambulate. This frees the upper extremities for a wider range of motion and activities. Before assessing range of motion, we will look at the ability to stand, bear weight, and ambulate.

Observe the natural posture and gait of a healthy individual walking into an examination. The person at the highest level of functioning is completely independent in ability to stand and ambulate. When walking, the face and toes point straight ahead and the arms swing freely at the sides of the body.

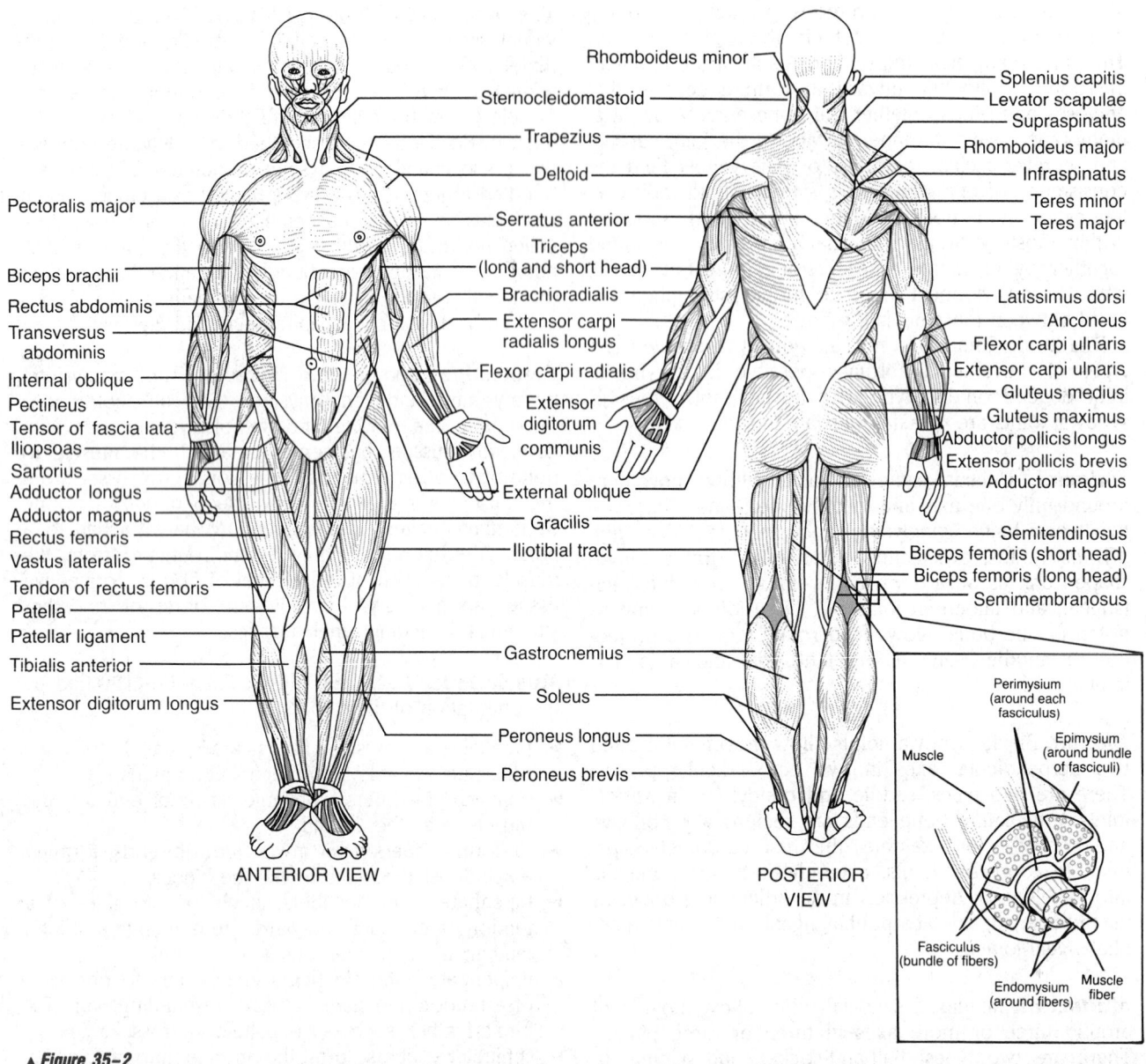

▲ Figure 35–2

Muscles of the human body. The inset shows the structure of an individual muscle.

During examination, inspection of the anterior and posterior aspects of the body should reveal bilateral symmetry and a straight spine and limbs, with body weight distributed equally on both feet. Inspection from a lateral viewpoint should show erect posture and normal spinal curves in the cervical, thoracic, and lumbar areas.

In relation to standing, bearing weight, walking, and other activities involving movement, there are different levels of functional ability. To differentiate among these different levels, it is often helpful to use the North American Nursing Diagnosis Association (NANDA) Suggested Functional Level Classification:[45]

▶ 0 = completely independent
▶ 1 = requires use of equipment or device

▶ 2 = requires help from another person, for assistance, supervision, or teaching
▶ 3 = requires help from another person and equipment or device
▶ 4 = dependent, does not participate in activity

Most of the clients we think of as immobilized are at levels 3 or 4. They are not able to stand or walk independently and may not be able to sit up, even with assistance. As they lie in bed, their body weight will be borne on their backs and heels. Their toes may point off to each side as their hip joints succumb to the effects of gravity. Raising the head of their bed may cause them to slide downward or slip to one side.

Immobilized clients may have to be placed in a better position before the assessment can begin.

Range of Motion of Spine and Extremities

For each immobilized client, it is important to know the range of motion (ROM) for all joints. ROM is the full measure of movement possible in a joint. The degree of movement may be accurately measured by use of a goniometer (Fig. 35–3A), or it may be estimated by observing the angle formed at the joint and comparing this with an angle formed within a 360-degree circle (Fig. 35–3B).

While assessing the degree of motion in a joint, it is also possible to assess a portion of the client's gross muscle strength by observing how well the muscles work to provide movement at the joints. To prevent possible joint stress and injury during assessment, begin by cautioning the client to move slowly and smoothly and not to force any movement to the point of fatigue or pain. Then, for each joint to be assessed, take the following steps:

▶ Begin by asking the person to move independently according to your verbal instructions and assess the ability to complete the movement.

▶ If the person is unable to move, provide just enough assistance to help overcome the effects of gravity.

▶ If able to complete the movement without assistance, provide slight pressure against the movement.

▶ If still able to complete the movement, provide a full measure of resistance against the movement.

Your assessment should help you quantify gross muscle strength. That is, you should be able to classify it as being at a certain point on a scale from 0 to 5, as follows:

▶ 5 = normal: very strong with ROM unimpaired against gravity and against full resistance

▶ 4 = good: adequate strength to complete ROM against gravity and against a mild-to-moderate level of resistance

▶ 3 = fair: only enough strength to complete ROM against gravity but not against any additional resistance

▶ 2 = poor: very weak, with inability to complete ROM unless gravity is eliminated by external assistance

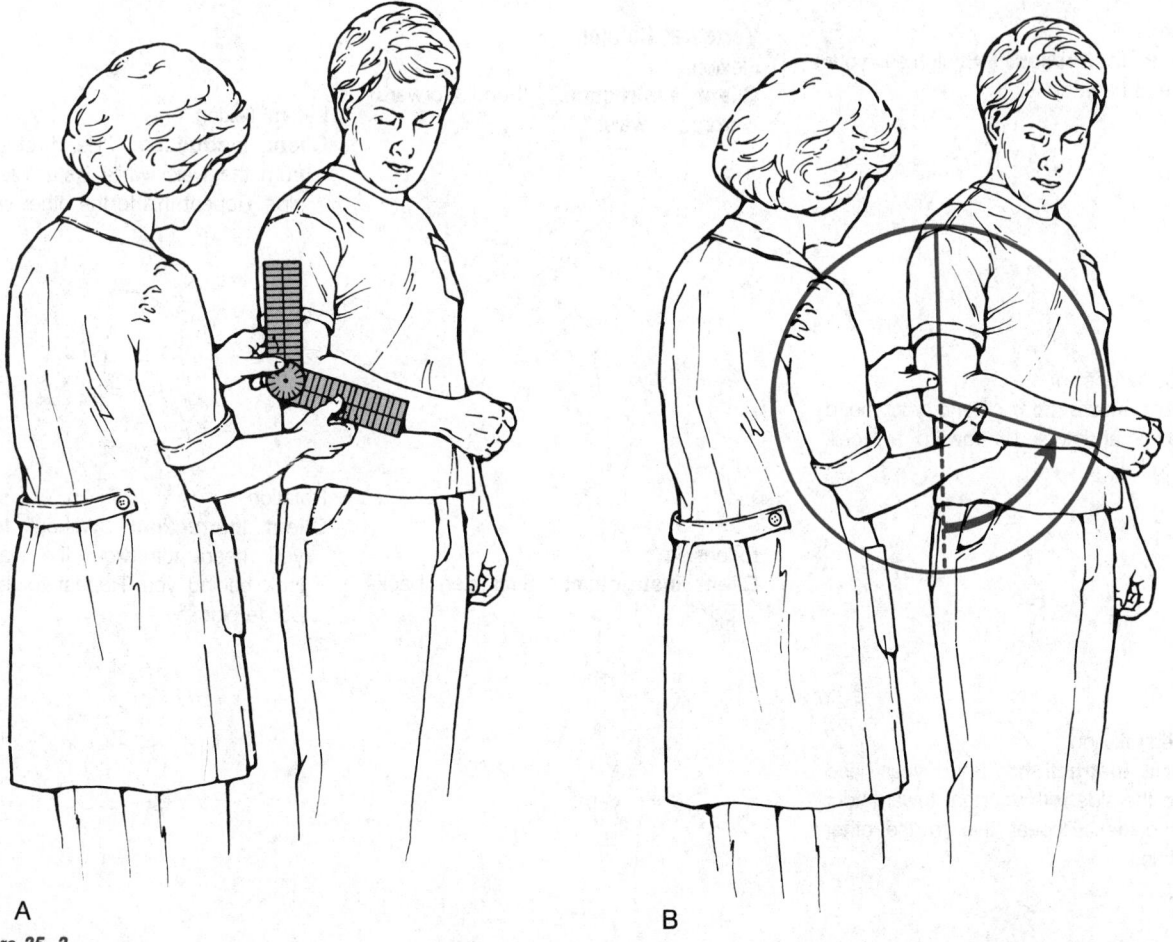

A

B

▲ *Figure 35–3*

Assessing the degree of joint movement. *A*, The nurse measures the degree of movement with a goniometer. *B*, The nurse estimates the degree of movement by thinking of the elbow as being the center point within a circle and the axes of the upper and lower arm bones as lines that form angles within the circle. In this case, the nurse starts with the arm forming a straight line and notes that the forearm moved almost one quarter of the circle, or approximately 70 degrees.

▶ 1 = trace: Unable to move at the joints, muscle shows only slight evidence of contractility

▶ 0 = zero: no evidence of muscle contractility

Table 35–2 illustrates one common sequence that may be used to assess the range of motion for each joint of the spine and extremities. This is a sequence used for mobile individuals who are able to stand. The assessment must be altered to accommodate the needs of the immobilized client. For example, if the client is unable to stand, some joints may have to be assessed in the sitting position, such as the joints of the neck, spine, and upper extremities. If the client is unable to sit up or turn to a prone position, some joints may have

Text continued on page 741

TABLE 35–2. Assessment of Range of Motion

Neck
(to be done in sitting or standing position)

Flexion

Client instruction: "Bow your head forward with your chin toward your chest."

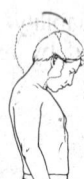

Extension

Client instruction: "Straighten your head back up."

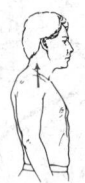

Hyperextension

Client instruction: "Bend your head back and look up toward the ceiling."

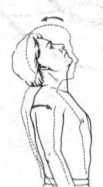

Lateral flexion

Client instruction: "Bend your head to the side with your ear toward your shoulder. Repeat this to the other side."

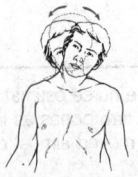

Rotation

Client instruction: "Turn your head to the side, chin toward shoulder, to look over your shoulder. Repeat this to the other side."

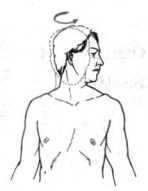

Vertebral Column

Flexion

Client instruction: "Bend forward from the waist."

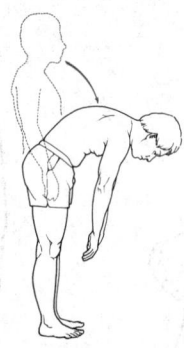

Extension

Client instruction: "Straighten back up."

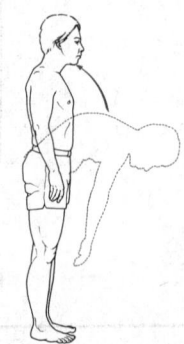

Hyperextension

Client instruction: "Keep your neck straight but bend backward from the waist while I stand beside you."

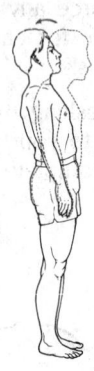

Lateral flexion

Client instruction: "Bend sideways from the waist while I stabilize your hips. Repeat this to the other side."

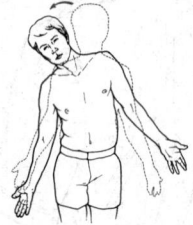

Rotation

Client instruction: "Without turning your head, turn from the waist to look behind you. Repeat to the opposite side."

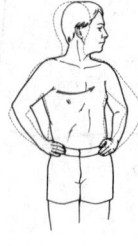

TABLE 35–2. *Assessment of Range of Motion* Continued

Shoulders

Flexion

Client instruction: "Reach both arms out in front of you and raise them straight up toward the ceiling."

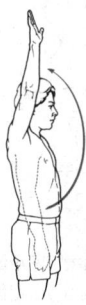

Extension

Client instruction: "Keeping them in front of you, bring them back down to your sides."

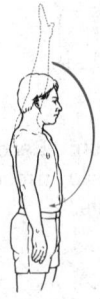

Hyperextension

Client instruction: "Continue moving them past your sides and back up behind you as far as you can reach."

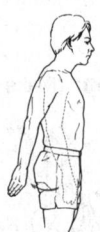

Abduction

Client instruction: "Raise your arms sideways until they point to the ceiling."

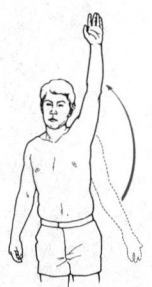

Adduction

Client instruction: "Moving them sideways, bring them back to your sides."

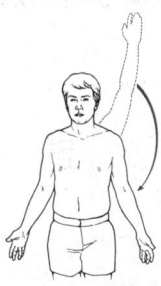

Horizontal adduction

Client instruction: "Lift your arms straight out to the side. Now, move them straight out in front of you and across your chest to your opposite side."

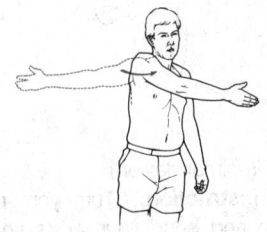

Horizontal abduction

Client instruction: "Bring them back to the beginning position, straight out to the side."

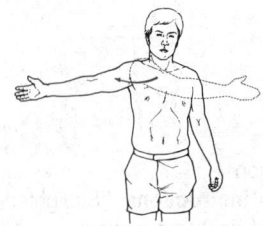

Internal rotation

Client instruction: "Bring your arms straight out to the sides and bend your elbows so your fingers point straight down."

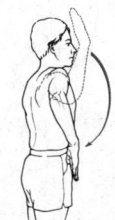

External rotation

Client instruction: "Now rotate your shoulders so your fingers point straight up."

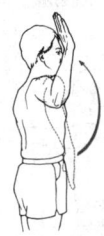

Circumduction

Client instruction: "Move each arm in a large circle."

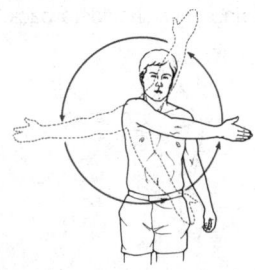

Elevation

Client instruction: "Shrug each shoulder."

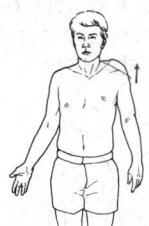

Depression

Client instruction: "Stretch your neck upward while pushing each shoulder down."

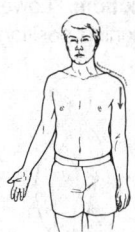

Table continued on following page

TABLE 35–2. Assessment of Range of Motion Continued

Shoulders Continued

Protraction

Client instruction: "Put your arms out straight in front of you. Now stretch them farther forward from the shoulders."

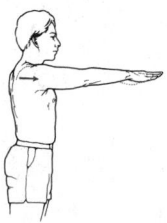

Retraction

Client instruction: "Keep your arms out, bring your shoulders back."

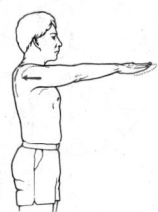

Elbows

Flexion

Client instruction: "With your arms at your sides and your palms facing forward, bring your palms up to touch your shoulders."

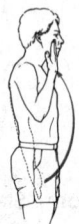

Extension

Client instruction: "Lower your palms to the beginning position."

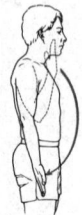

Forearms

Pronation

Client instruction: "With your arms out in front of you, rotate your forearms to turn your palms downward."

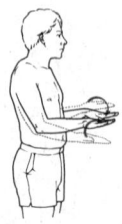

Supination

Client instruction: "Turn your palms back upward again."

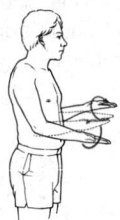

Wrists

Flexion (palmar flexion)

Client instruction: "Turn your palms down and bend your wrists so your fingers point toward the floor."

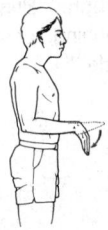

Extension

Client instruction: "Straighten your wrists back out again."

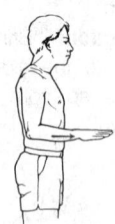

Hyperextension (dorsiflexion)

Client instruction: "Bend your wrists so your fingertips point toward the ceiling."

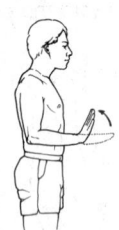

Radial flexion

Client instruction: "Bend your wrists sideways, toward your thumbs."

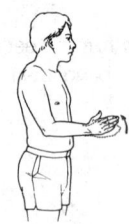

Ulnar flexion

Client instruction: "Bend your wrists in the opposite direction, toward your little fingers."

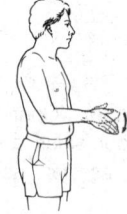

Fingers

Flexion

Client instruction: "Make tight fists."

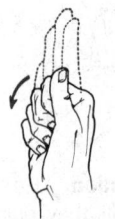

TABLE 35-2. Assessment of Range of Motion Continued

Fingers *Continued*
Extension
Client instruction: "Open your hands and straighten your fingers completely."

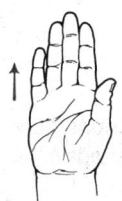

Abduction
Client instruction: "Spread your fingers and thumbs out sideways."

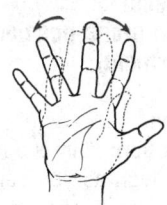

Adduction
Client instruction: "Bring them back together again so that the sides touch."

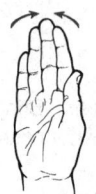

Thumbs
Flexion
Client instruction: "Try to touch the middle of each palm with your thumb tips."

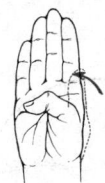

Extension
Client instruction: "Bring your thumbs back to their normal positions."

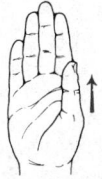

Abduction   (Tested with fingers)

Adduction   (Tested with fingers)

Opposition
Client instruction: "One at a time, touch the tip of your thumb to the tip of each of your other fingers on the same hand."

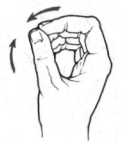

Hips
(remainder of examination to be done in bed or on examination table. Begin in supine position)
Flexion
Client instruction: "Slowly lift one leg up as high as you can toward your chest. Bring it back down on the bed and rest 5 seconds. Repeat with the opposite leg."

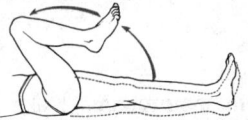

Extension
Client instruction: "Return both legs to a straightened position."

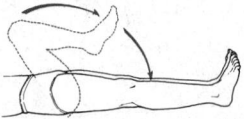

Abduction
Client instruction: "One leg at a time, move your leg out to the side as far as you can."

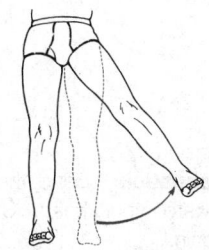

Adduction
Client instruction: "Bring the leg back in place."

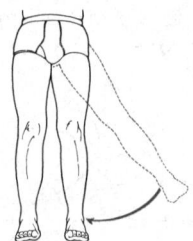

Cross-adduction
Client instruction: "Continue to carry the leg across the body to the opposite side."

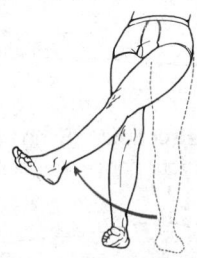

Internal rotation
Client instruction: "With your legs slightly apart, turn your toes inward, toward each other, as far as you can so that your legs roll inward."

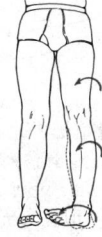

External rotation
Client instruction: "Now turn your toes in the opposite direction as far as you can so your legs roll outward."

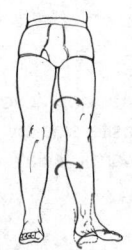

Table continued on following page

TABLE 35–2. *Assessment of Range of Motion* Continued

Hips *Continued*

Circumduction

Client instruction: "One leg at a time, move your leg in the largest circle you can."

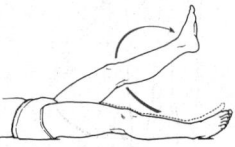

Ankles

Flexion (plantar flexion)

Client instruction: "Point your toes straight down."

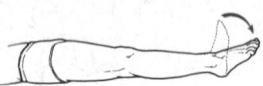

Extension

Client instruction: "Bring your feet back to your normal position."

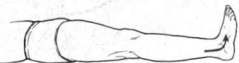

Hyperextension (dorsiflexion)

Client instruction: "Pull your toes up and backward so they point more toward your head."

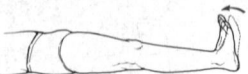

Inversion

Client instruction: "Relax your feet and ankles so the toes point upward. Then, with your feet about 6 inches apart, turn your ankles so each sole faces the other."

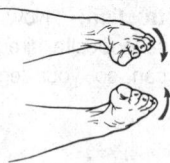

Eversion

Client instruction: "Move your ankles to the opposite side by turning your soles outward, away from each other."

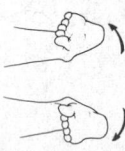

Metatarsals

Inversion

Client instruction: "While I hold your ankles still, try to turn as much of each of your soles toward the other as you can. The toe end of each foot should turn inward."

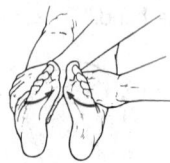

Eversion

Client instruction: "While I hold your ankles still, try to turn as much of each of your soles away from each other as you can. The toe end of each foot should turn outward."

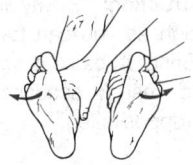

Toes

Flexion

Client instruction: "Make your toes curl up tightly."

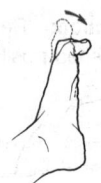

Extension

Client instruction: "Straighten them out."

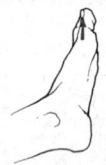

Hyperextension

Client instruction: "Bend them back and toward your head. Straighten them again."

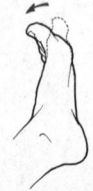

Abduction

Client instruction: "Spread them out."

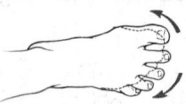

Adduction

Client instruction: "Let them come back together again."

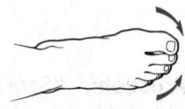

Hips and Knees
(turn client to prone position for this assessment)

Hips

Hyperextension

Client instruction: "Lift one leg up off the bed as high as you can. Rest it on the bed for 5 seconds and repeat with the other leg."

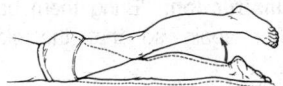

Knees

Flexion

Client instruction: "Bring your heels up toward your buttocks."

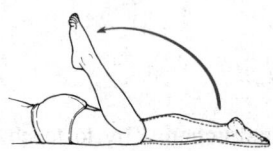

Extension

Client instruction: "Return them to the bed."

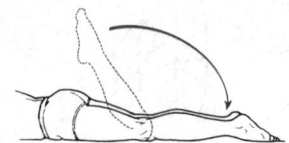

to be assessed with the client in a side-lying position, as in shoulder hyperextension. Sometimes injuries or illness will completely prevent the person from participating in a certain part of the assessment, and that part will have to be deferred. At other times the person will not have the stamina to attempt all the assessment at one time and a period of rest will be needed before continuing. Although it may be tiring, it is important that this assessment is done if possible, as the information obtained can serve as a baseline to measure the client's progress or lack of progress over the course of time.

Table 35-2 offers suggested lay terminology to use as you ask the person to perform each movement. It is also important that you become familiar with the correct medical terminology used to describe each movement, as these are the terms you will use in writing your assessment in the client's record and in reporting your findings to other members of the health care team. The general meanings of the most frequently encountered terms are listed in Box 35-1.

So far, we have been talking about the musculoskeletal system. We will examine this system in more detail later as we discuss some of the effects of immobility.

Effects of Immobility

Each body system has a unique response to the stress of immobility. The major responses of each body system will be reviewed as an introduction to the assessment of each system.

As each system is reviewed, it should be kept in mind that all body systems are related and interdependent so that what affects one system of the body will also affect other systems.

INTEGUMENTARY SYSTEM

The Formation of Pressure Ulcers. Certain local areas of the body (called "pressure points") are vulnerable to a type of *tissue breakdown* we term **pressure ulcers** (bedsores, decubitus ulcers) because (1) the skin lies over bony prominences; (2) these areas are not as adapted, as are our feet, for example, to bearing large amounts of weight for prolonged periods; and (3) a person's weight when lying down is not distributed over the entire body. Rather, it is borne specifically by the bony prominences. Figure 35-4 illustrates the major pressure points in the supine, side-lying, and prone positions.

As the name implies, a pressure ulcer often occurs as a consequence of pressure, when soft tissues of the body are compressed between the surface of the mattress on one side and the pressure of a bony prominence on the other. For example, the weight of the hip pressing down on the greater trochanter while a person is in a side-lying position (see Fig. 35-4) compresses the soft tissues between the trochanter and the mattress. This compression of the soft tissues causes **ischemia** (deficiency of blood flow to an area due to constriction or obstruction of a blood vessel). The tissues become bloodless in appearance because of **tissue hypoxia** (decreased oxygen supply to the tissues). The area may look pale or white in light-skinned persons but in persons with darker skin, it may take on a grayish hue.

If the pressure is removed and the blood flow to the area is re-established, the tissues in the area will become hyperemic (will have more blood in the area than normal). In light-skinned individuals, this will show up as erythema (reddening of the skin due to the inflow of blood). Persons with darker-pigmented skin may demonstrate underlying red tones as occurs in flushing, but the color change will be less evident. If there has been no permanent damage to the tissues, the hyperemia will disappear within one half to three fourths of the total time the tissues were compressed.[60]

If too much damage has occurred and the tissues cannot be restored, the hyperemia will not disappear. The tissues will die of anoxia (lack of oxygen); will become **necrotic** (composed of dead cells); and, over a period of days, will break down and become an open wound. See Chapter 48 for photographs of this phenomenon.

The Effects of Friction and Shearing. Friction and shearing forces also contribute to skin breakdown and the development of bedsores. Friction causes skin to break down when the skin is moved over an abrasive surface, as when a body part is pulled across a sheet. Shearing forces come into play when one layer of tis-

---

Box 35-1. Range-of-Motion Terminology

- ▶ **Flexion**—movement so as to decrease the angle formed at the joint between two body parts, bending of a straight joint; the opposite of extension
- ▶ **Extension**—movement so as to increase or straighten the angle formed at the joint between two body parts, straightening of a bent joint; the opposite of flexion
- ▶ **Hyperextension**—movement of a part beyond its straightened position in the opposite direction from flexion
- ▶ **Abduction**—lateral movement of a part away from the midline; eversion
- ▶ **Adduction**—lateral movement of a part toward the midline; inversion
- ▶ **Horizontal adduction**—movement of a part, in a horizontal plane, across the midline of the body
- ▶ **Horizontal abduction**—movement of a part, in a horizontal plane, back across and away from the midline; opposite of horizontal adduction
- ▶ **Rotation**—turning an extremity around its axis so as to turn the articulating end of the bone within the joint cavity
- ▶ **Internal rotation**—rotation toward the center of the body, medial rotation
- ▶ **External rotation**—rotation away from the center of the body, lateral rotation

SUPINE

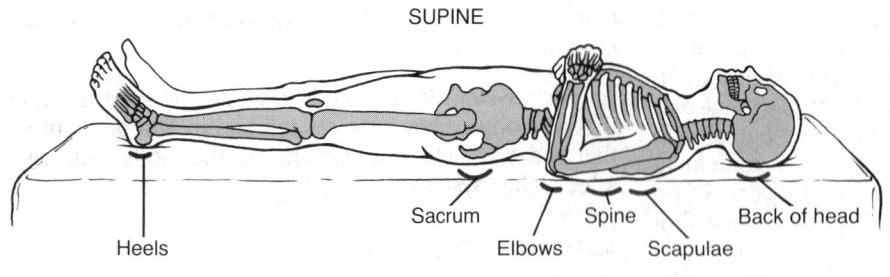

Heels   Sacrum   Elbows   Spine   Scapulae   Back of head

SIDE LYING

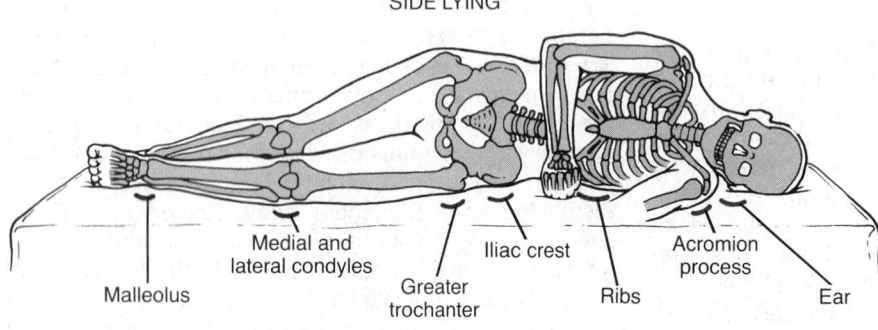

Malleolus   Medial and lateral condyles   Greater trochanter   Iliac crest   Ribs   Acromion process   Ear

PRONE

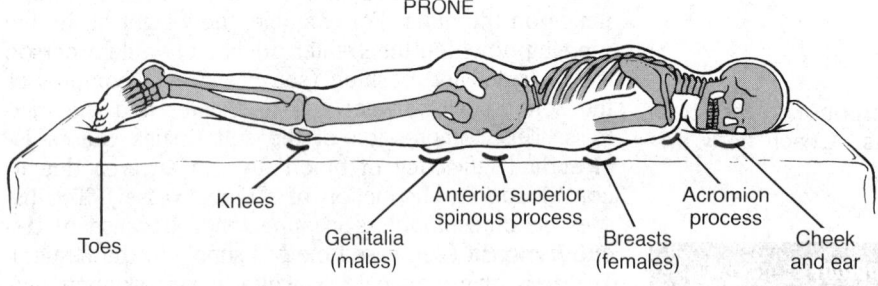

Toes   Knees   Genitalia (males)   Anterior superior spinous process   Breasts (females)   Acromion process   Cheek and ear

▲ *Figure 35–4*

The most common pressure points in supine, side-lying, and prone positions.

sue slides over another layer of tissue. This commonly occurs, for example, when the back of a hospital bed is raised more than 30 degrees and the person in bed slides downward. In such cases, the tissues next to the person's hip bone move with the bone. However, the skin and subcutaneous tissues, owing to friction between the skin and sheets, fail to move at the same rate as the deeper tissues (Fig. 35–5). Shearing forces pull these two tissue layers apart and cause damage.

Regardless of the specific cause, a pressure ulcer is a wound and, like any wound, if the skin is broken *infection* can occur. With deep decubitus ulcers, bone may be exposed to infection and **osteomyelitis** (infection of the bone and bone marrow) can result.

Assessing for Pressure Ulcers. The first step in the assessment process is to identify those who are at increased risk for developing pressure ulcers:

▶ *Elderly* persons, who make fewer spontaneous body movements
▶ *Obese* persons, whose extra weight creates additional pressure over weight-bearing areas
▶ *Emaciated* individuals, who have only a thin layer of subcutaneous tissue over bony prominences

▶ *Sedated* individuals, who consequently make fewer body movements
▶ Agitated, *restrained* persons, who cannot turn unassisted
▶ *Paralyzed* persons (e.g., paraplegics, quadriplegics, and hemiplegics)
▶ Persons with *neurologic diseases* (e.g., multiple

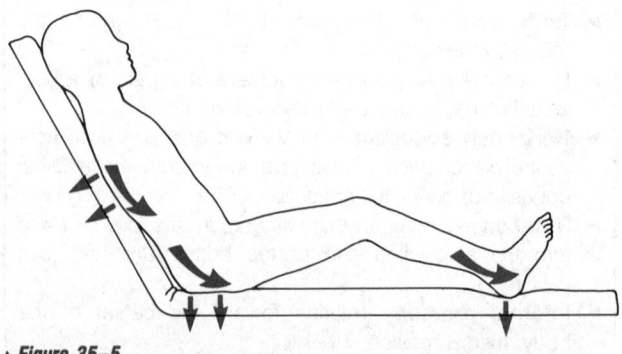

▲ *Figure 35–5*

Shearing forces pull tissue layers apart when tissues nearer the bone slide downward and forward, whereas tissue layers nearer the skin tend to be held in place by friction between skin and sheets.

sclerosis, Parkinson's disease) or persons in *coma* due to cerebrovascular accident, trauma, and the like. This category also includes people with severe mental disorders such as catatonia and people with severe mental retardation

▶ *Edematous* individuals, especially those with edema of the sacrum and buttocks
▶ *Malnourished* individuals with protein and vitamin deficiencies
▶ *Febrile* individuals, whose elevated temperature increases metabolic needs of tissues
▶ Persons in *pain* who limit activity as a means of promoting comfort
▶ Individuals who wear *braces* or *casts*
▶ Persons who are *incontinent* of feces

Caution Some of the persons in the foregoing list are at risk because of changes that do not take long and can happen during your assigned time with the client: for example, decreased level of consciousness, edema formation, and development of fever. While it is necessary to assess pressure points for all immobilized persons every 2 to 3 hours, those clients who are at increased risk should be assessed more often. Assess individuals at increased risk at least once every 2 hours.

As you assess each pressure point, observe for areas of hyperemia. Use extra care to note color changes in persons with darkly pigmented skin. Press a finger into erythemic areas, remove it, and observe for blanching (loss of color). Blanching (blanchable erythema) indicates the blood supply is still intact. **Nonblanchable erythema,** however, refers to hyperemic tissues that fail to lose their redness when subjected to pressure, and this indicates that the tissue probably cannot be saved from breakdown.

Remain alert for causes of pressure other than at bony prominences. For example, clients can develop pressure ulcers over fleshy areas if the fleshy areas are allowed to rest on drainage tubes or on objects inadvertently left in the bed.

The steps of skin assessment in the immobilized person are briefly listed in Table 35–3.

CIRCULATORY SYSTEM

Major effects of immobility on the cardiovascular system include (1) an *increased cardiac workload* leading to *diminished cardiac reserve;* (2) *cardiac strain* with use of the Valsalva maneuver; (3) *a shift of plasma to the interstitial space* resulting in *tissue edema, hypovolemia (decreased blood volume), blood hypercoagulability,* and (4) the development of *orthostatic hypotension.*

Increased Cardiac Workload. Although you might expect the opposite to be true, immobility actually leads to an *increased resting workload of the heart.* In fact, it has been accepted for some time that the supine position results in a 30 per cent increase in cardiac work load.[13] Immobility leads to *increased heart rate, increased cardiac output, and increased stroke volume* (amount of blood that the heart puts out with

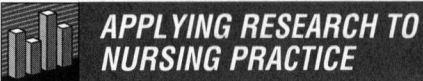

APPLYING RESEARCH TO NURSING PRACTICE
Preventing Pressure Ulcers

Pressure ulcers in adults: Prediction and prevention (1992). US Department of Health and Human Services. AHCPR Publication No. 92-0047.

▼▼▼

Nurse panel members at the Agency for Health Care Policy and Research (AHCPR) have conducted a meta-analysis (a "grand analysis") of previous research that has been done on the prevention and treatment of pressure ulcers. This analysis of more than 12,000 abstracts and 800 manuscripts was performed as a basis for national guidelines for clinical practice. The first set of guidelines applies only to adults with Stage I pressure ulcers.

The guidelines include three essential steps: (1) initial risk assessment, (2) daily systematic skin inspection and skin care, and (3) early intervention for actual Stage I pressure ulcers.

Bed-confined or chair-bound people who are unable to reposition themselves require initial risk assessments to identify factors that contribute to pressure ulcer development. Such people who may be unable to reposition themselves include the elderly, clients with fractures, quadriplegic clients, and critically ill clients. Factors that contribute to pressure ulcer development in these people include immobility, incontinence, inadequate dietary intake, and impaired mental status.

Once initial risk assessments have been conducted and at-risk populations identified, daily systematic skin inspection and skin care should be implemented. Skin care should include routine cleansing, as well as prompt cleansing at the time of soiling. Gentle cleansing with a mild agent and warm water should be followed by gentle application of a lubricant, a topical moisture barrier cream, or cornstarch to the dry skin. Although nurses commonly give backrubs to stimulate circulation, provide comfort, and protect the skin, there is evidence that massage over bony prominences in these at-risk clients may lead to deep tissue trauma.

When evidence of Stage I pressure ulcers appears, early intervention with a pressure-reducing device is essential. The type of device is not important; the timing of its use is critical.

Applications for Practice

Obtain your own copy of the guidelines by calling 1-800-358-9295 or by writing to AHCPR Publications Clearinghouse, PO Box 8547, Silver Spring, MD 20907. Then begin implementing the recommendations in your clinical practice.

each beat). This is undesirable, because an increased heart rate reduces diastolic pressure and leads to a shortening of the diastolic phase of the cardiac cycle. As a result, during diastole, a decreased amount of blood moves through the coronary vessels and into the heart muscle, diminishing cardiac reserve.

Cardiac Strain. The immobilized person may further increase cardiac workload by using the Valsalva maneuver. The **Valsalva maneuver** is the name given to the physiologic mechanism that operates when a per-

TABLE 35–3. Assessment of the Immobilized Person

Assessment	Rationale
Integumentary System	
Inspect the skin of all immobilized persons every 2 to 3 hours and the skin of persons at risk at least every 2 hours. Concentrate on pressure points	Pressure from bony prominences can result in tissue ischemia and breakdown
Compress hyperemic areas and observe for blanching of erythema	Blanchable erythema indicates tissue hypoxia can be reversed
Circulatory System	
Note the total fluid intake and output per day	Reduced intake can promote hemoconcentration and assist in clot formation
Determine baseline and daily pulse rates	Increasing pulse rates indicate a shorter diastolic phase of the cardiac cycle, with reduced coronary blood flow. This signals an increased cardiac load
Determine baseline and daily blood pressure readings	Decreased diastolic pressure may indicate reduced coronary blood flow, which could signal an increased cardiac load
Auscultate the apical pulse	The presence of a third sound may indicate early congestive heart failure. This signals cardiac strain
Observe respirations for use of the Valsalva maneuver during movement and straining	The Valsalva maneuver is often used automatically, and its use indicates a need for teaching in order to prevent cardiac strain
Inspect leg veins for venous stasis and palpate peripheral pulses	Dilated veins in edematous tissue with pulses difficult or impossible to palpate indicate increased cardiac workload
Inspect and palpate dependent tissues for edema. Include sacrum and heels in persons on bed rest	Edema indicates decreased venous return and increased cardiac workload
Inspect and palpate the calves and thighs daily for deep vein thrombosis	Redness, warmth, and tenderness indicate phlebitis may be present. These signs of injury to the vein intima, together with venous stasis and hypercoagulability, indicate a danger of developing thrombosis/thrombophlebitis
Quickly compress the calves from front to back or from side to side	Pain indicates phlebitis/thrombophlebitis may be present
Test for Homan's sign	A positive response (pain) indicates phlebitis/thrombophlebitis may be present
Measure the circumference of each calf and thigh daily	A unilateral increase in size indicates that phlebitis/thrombophlebitis may be present. A bilateral increase in size indicates the presence of edema
Compare reclining with sitting or standing blood pressure and pulse measurements	A sudden drop in blood pressure and increase in pulse, upon moving from a horizontal to a vertical position, indicates orthostatic hypotension
If the person can remain standing for more than 10 minutes, repeat blood pressure and pulse measurements	After 10 minutes in a standing position, a difference of 30 to 35 mm Hg in mean arterial blood pressure and an elevated pulse indicate orthostatic hypotension
Rapidly assess cardiopulmonary status when noting any signs of pulmonary embolism	In the event of pulmonary embolism, emergency measures will have to be taken
Pulmonary System	
Prior to the assessment:	
Note whether the person is taking medications that can affect the respiratory system	Certain medications can depress the brain's respiratory center or the brain's cough reflex center
Note the total fluid intake and output per day	Decreased fluid intake can lead to thick mucus that is difficult to expectorate
Note laboratory test results	Test results can indicate lack of oxygen or carbon dioxide retention
To begin the assessment:	
Observe body position. Note whether position is hampering the chest wall from expanding fully with each inspiration. (If necessary, reposition before continuing assessment)	Decreased chest wall expansion can inhibit ventilation
Inspect for constriction of the chest wall	A cast, bandage, or binder may constrict ventilation by inhibiting chest wall expansion
Inspect and palpate for abdominal distention	Distention may impair ventilation by interfering with the descent of the diaphragm

TABLE 35-3. *Assessment of the Immobilized Person* Continued

Assessment	Rationale
Pulmonary System *Continued*	
Assess temperature	Elevation may indicate a respiratory infection, e.g., pneumonia
Assess the pulse	A rapid pulse is one of the first signs of a lack of oxygen
Assess respirations through the full respiratory cycle	Respiratory changes can herald various problems in ventilation and gas exchange
Auscultate the lungs, including dependent areas	Decreased breath sounds on the affected side indicate atelectasis
Evaluate cough; including color, consistency, and amount of secretions	The cough and the mucus produced can indicate several problems in ventilation and gas exchange
Throughout the assessment: Assess mental status	If the person seems irritable, confused, restless, or disoriented, these problems may be signaling hypoxia
Throughout the day: Note how often the person changes position	Help with positioning may be needed to prevent pooling of lung secretions
Gastrointestinal System, Nutrition, and Metabolism	
Prior to the assessment: Review the dietary intake for types and amounts of foods. Note usual pattern	A deficient intake of dietary fiber is major etiologic factor in constipation
	Immobility often leads to anorexia, with a decreased appetite for high-protein foods, and protein-calorie malnutrition can result
Note the laboratory values for signs of negative nitrogen balance	Negative nitrogen balance means the intake of protein is insufficient for metabolic needs
Note the total fluid intake and output per day	Adequate intake of water is necessary for all metabolic functions
	Anorexia can reduce fluid intake
	Immobilized clients may also reduce fluid intake in order to avoid using the bedpan
	Decreased fluid intake can result in constipation
Note the bowel movement pattern. Compare this with the client's baseline pattern	Immobility can decrease peristalsis and promote constipation
Note color, consistency, and amount of stools	Small, frequent "diarrhea stools" may actually be fecal-stained mucus, indicating the presence of an impaction
Note whether the person is taking medications that can lead to constipation	Certain medications can increase the immobilized person's risk of constipation
To begin the assessment: Assess temperature and pulse	Elevation may indicate an infection
Assess respirations through the full respiratory cycle	Abnormal breath sounds may indicate a respiratory infection. Infections increase metabolism, and this can result in dehydration and reduced plasma volume, with compensatory mechanisms leading to constipation
Auscultate for bowel sounds	Diminished bowel sounds indicate diminished peristalsis
Inspect the abdomen for a rounded appearance with taut skin; palpate for tenderness and percuss for a tympanic sound when checking for distention	Distention can indicate the presence of excess gas or stool
Do a rectal examination if not contraindicated and impaction is suspected	If impacted and the impaction is low enough in the gastrointestinal tract, a putty-like or hardened fecal mass may be palpated. This can be manually broken up and removed
Throughout the assessment and throughout care: Assess mental status	If a confused, disoriented, retarded, or nonverbal person seems more irritable or more restless than usual, these problems may be signaling a need to move the bowels
	An anxious person may swallow excessive air and promote flatulence
Note habits	Eating rapidly, chewing gum, using a straw for drinking, and drinking carbonated beverages can increase the swallowing of air and can increase flatulence

Table continued on following page

TABLE 35–3. Assessment of the Immobilized Person Continued

Assessment	Rationale
Musculoskeletal System	
Prior to the assessment:	
Note laboratory test results	Hypercalciuria in immobilized persons can indicate bone resorption
	Slight hypercalcemia is uncommon but could increase clot formation, if present
Review the dietary intake for types and amounts of foods. Note usual pattern	A deficient intake of dietary protein in an immobilized client is one major etiologic factor in muscle catabolism
Note the overall posture and ability to maintain proper body positioning. Palpate for muscle tone. When documenting, note muscles that are flaccid (muscles with decreased tone) or spastic (muscles with increased tone)	Decreased muscle tonus can lead to inability to maintain normal physiologic positioning
	From 10 to 20 per cent of a muscle's strength can be lost for each week of immobility
Inspect the muscles for size. Compare bilaterally. Measure around the belly of major muscle groups and mark the sites of measurement	Up to 50 per cent of a muscle's mass can be lost in 2 months of immobility. A baseline will be needed to assess progress
When the client is unable to perform active range of motion, assess for contractures by noting the degree of movement and the resistance felt during range of motion	Soon after a person is immobilized, contractures can begin to form. Joints of the lower extremities are usually affected first
Urinary System	
Prior to the assessment, review chart for evidence of risk factors for stone formation	
Note urinary test results	Hypercalciuria in immobilized persons can indicate a potential for calcium kidney stone formation
	Urine pH should be low. Alkaline urine tends to promote the formation of calcium kidney stones
Note fluid intake and output	Decreased fluid intake can result in fewer voidings per day and less "flushing out" of the urinary meatus
	Decreased fluid intake with resulting concentrated urine creates a climate that supports stone formation
Note the presence of risk factors for *E. coli* infection. Female: impacted or incontinent of feces, unable to complete own perineal hygiene; both sexes: indwelling catheter	*E. coli* is the most common bacteria seen in urinary tract infection
Observe for signs of urinary tract infection	Urinary tract infection by urea-splitting organisms can raise urinary pH and promote calcium kidney stone formation
Note whether client is incontinent of urine	Incontinence may be the result of long-term distention
Note whether urination is difficult	Difficult urination can lead to urinary stasis with increased possibility of infection
Assess for urinary stasis:	
Note positions client is able to assume	A supine position promotes urinary retention and stasis, increasing risk of infection
Inspect and palpate for evidence of bladder distention as warranted	Distention can signal retention
Psychosocial Systems	
Note expressions of loss of control (powerlessness), frustration, anger, hostility, aggression, or depression	Loss of the ability to move toward, and meet, client goals commonly results in these reactions
Note expressions of loss of control with anxiety, fear, or panic	Loss of ability to move away from a perceived threat commonly results in these responses
Assess for signs of fight-or-flight response	The sympathetic nervous system is activated with certain strong emotions
Note elevated blood glucose level or stress hormones secreted in larger than normal amounts	Immobility can result in detectable chemical changes in the bloodstream
Look for changed perceptions about the self, such as alteration in body image and decreased self-esteem	Mobility is very much a part of the self
Look for changes in mental functioning, e.g., changes in cognition, judgment, problem solving, learning, memory, and alertness, or changes in perception such as paranoia or hallucinations	Sensory deprivation can result from a combination of decreased mobility and isolation. This can cause mental changes. Sensory overload can also result in behavioral and mental changes

TABLE 35–3. *Assessment of the Immobilized Person* Continued

Assessment	Rationale
Psychosocial Systems *Continued*	
Assess for isolation and for feelings of dependency	These are common interpersonal problems in immobilized persons
In children, compare the developmental level with the expected norm	Children may experience a developmental delay
In the elderly, be alert for feelings of helplessness and hopelessness that may accompany a sense of dependency	In elderly persons, opportunities to regain mobility and independence are more limited than in younger age groups

son attempts to exhale against a closed glottis and traps air in the lungs, greatly increasing intrathoracic pressure. The immobilized person most frequently uses the Valsalva maneuver when (1) using the arm and upper trunk muscles to move in bed, (2) straining during defecation, or (3) coughing, gagging, or vomiting. As a result of the increased intrathoracic pressure during the maneuver, venous blood flow to the heart slows, stroke volume decreases, the systolic blood pressure and pulse pressure drop, and the heart rate and total peripheral resistance increase.

When the person finishes moving or straining, expiration occurs, which, in turn, causes intrathoracic pressure to decrease. This causes a sudden increase in the venous blood flow to the heart and a transient but sudden and marked elevation of the stroke volume and arterial blood pressure. Because peripheral resistance is still present, the increase in arterial blood pressure causes a momentary vagal slowing of the heart rate.[52] These cardiovascular changes can cause dysrhythmias in persons with diminished cardiac reserve and may even lead to death in persons with preexisting cardiac problems.

Shift of Plasma to the Interstitial Space. Over time, immobilized individuals experience several additional cardiovascular changes. When the muscles of the legs are not being used, they no longer assist in returning venous blood to the heart. As a result, **venous stasis** or venous pooling (congestion due to slowed blood flow in the veins) occurs. This pooling of blood raises the blood hydrostatic pressure in the venous end of the capillary bed. The additional hydrostatic pressure in the venous end of the capillary bed alters the flow of blood plasma through the interstitial spaces. Normally, blood plasma moves into the interstitial fluid compartment on the arteriolar end of the capillary bed, bathes the body cells, and moves back into the bloodstream on the venous end. However, the additional pressure on the venous end of the capillary bed tends to prevent the fluid plasma from moving back into the bloodstream. As a result, excess fluid accumulates in the interstitial compartment and causes the visible swelling we term **edema.**

Edema. Because interstitial fluid builds up in areas that normally rely on muscular contraction to help move the blood back to the heart against the force of gravity,

the edema is seen in areas below heart level, such as in the distal portions of the arms and legs of individuals who are sitting or standing and in the sacral area and heels of persons lying on their backs. We refer to these areas as dependent areas and call the edema there **dependent edema.**

When plasma in dependent tissues builds up to such a degree that the cells can no longer absorb all the fluid, the excess fluid between the cells causes a specific type of edema we term pitting edema. Pitting edema occurs because the excess interstitial fluids can be moved. This fluid movement can be seen when external pressure is applied to edematous areas, as when a finger is pressed into the area and an indentation is observed to last for a period of time before the fluid redistributes in the area and restores the level contour.

Hypovolemia. Loss of plasma to the interstitial compartment leads to *hypovolemia* (decreased blood volume). Indeed, the person may sustain a decrease of 700 to 800 ml in circulating blood volume after a week to ten days of strict bed rest.[68] Loss of plasma also leads to *increased blood viscosity* (thickness) and further slows blood flow, adding to the stasis and the edema.

Blood Hypercoagulability. Venous stasis, complicated by increased blood viscosity, leads to *increased blood coagulability* and may help cause *deep vein thrombosis* (the formation of a blood clot within the deep veins). Three factors contribute to the formation of clots: (1) increased blood coagulability, (2) venous stasis, and (3) damage to the vein wall's intima (inner coat). We have seen how increased coagulability and venous stasis come about, but what causes damage to the intima in an immobilized person? We do not always know, but we do know that one causative factor is poor positioning, which can result in partial or total occlusion of blood vessels. We know that some damage has occurred to the vein wall when **phlebitis** (inflammation of the vein) is present. And we know that the longer a person is immobilized, the greater the risk of deep vein thrombosis.

The major danger from thrombus formation is **thromboembolism,** in which the clot breaks loose from the vein wall and migrates through the bloodstream to a distant site where it becomes lodged in a smaller blood vessel and blocks off the supply of oxygenated blood to tissues normally supplied by the blocked vessel. The blockage leads to tissue hypoxia and eventually to *necrosis*. Usually, an embolus is carried to the lungs, where it blocks off the blood supply to a portion of the lung tissue. In this event, it is termed a *pulmonary embolism*. If the pulmonary embolus is a small one, damage may be minimal. If the embolus blocks blood supply to a large portion of the lung, it can be fatal.

Whenever an individual demonstrates some of the common signs and symptoms of pulmonary embolism, prepare to take emergency measures.

Common signs of pulmonary embolism are:

▶ rapid onset of dyspnea with rapid, shallow breathing or wheezing
▶ a complaint of crushing or squeezing chest tightness or pain (pain may be more severe on inspiration than expiration)
▶ extreme apprehension
▶ tachycardia
▶ hemoptysis (coughing or spitting of blood)

Although lung tissue is most commonly affected, an embolus may lodge elsewhere and block blood flow to tissues other than the lungs. For example, blockage of a coronary vessel can lead to necrosis in a portion of the heart muscle. When this occurs, it is termed a *cardiovascular accident*. Similarly, blockage of circulation to a part of the brain can cause damage to brain tissue, and this is termed a *cerebrovascular accident*. A small area of tissue death, such as a spot the size of a quarter in the heart or brain, is an *infarction*. A larger area of tissue death, such as an entire foot or leg, is termed *gangrene*.

Orthostatic Hypotension. Commonly, when individuals first get up after a period of immobility, they experience weakness and dizziness. Less commonly, but more importantly, **syncope** (transient loss of consciousness, or fainting, due to a lack of circulation to the brain) may occur. Syncope results from **orthostatic (postural) hypotension,** which is a sudden drop in blood pressure caused by a reduced blood volume, decrease in venous tone, and failure of the normal peripheral vasoconstriction expected upon assuming an erect position.

Assessing for Circulatory Changes. As you begin the cardiovascular assessment, you should take the vital signs and auscultate the apical pulse. As you auscultate the apical pulse, you should be on the alert for a third heart sound at the apex, as this can indicate that the person is not able to handle the increased cardiac strain. Compare findings with the baseline findings. Assess the blood vessels in the legs by observing for distention in the veins and feeling for peripheral pulses in the arteries.

Immediately report the absence of any peripheral pulses that you know were present in a previous assessment.

Inspect and palpate the lower legs and feet for the presence of edema. If possible and not contraindicated, ask the person to turn to one side. During the turn, caution the person against using the Valsalva maneuver.

Teach the person the importance of avoiding the Valsalva maneuver by breathing normally while moving about in bed.

When the person has turned, inspect and palpate the sacrum and heels for edema. To test for pitting, firmly but gently press the fleshy part of your index finger into the edematous tissue and hold it for approximately 30 seconds. When you remove your finger, estimate the depth of any fingerprint evident in the edematous area. Rate any pitting as:

▶ 1+ only slightly observable
▶ 2+ indentation more than 1+ but no greater than 5 mm
▶ 3+ indentation 5 to 10 mm
▶ 4+ indentation greater than 10 mm

Inspect and palpate the calves and thighs. Look for color changes that indicate what would be a redness in light-skinned individuals but may not be as evident in persons with darker skin pigmentation. Feel for warmth and tenderness. Quickly compress the calves from front to back or from side to side and note whether pain is present. Test for Homan's sign (see Chapter 33). Measure the circumference of each calf and thigh daily. Take each measurement from the same point on each extremity. The measurement points should be marked on the skin of both extremities at the time of the first measurement. Usually, the thigh is measured at the midpoint whereas the calf is measured at the thickest part (approximately 10 cm below the midpatella).

If the individual is allowed out of bed, repeat the pulse and blood pressure when the client stands up, and compare findings with the reclining findings. If the pressure has dropped and the pulse has elevated, and the person feels dizzy or faint, a return to a horizontal position in bed is indicated to prevent brain ischemia. Otherwise, repeat the blood pressure and pulse determination 10 minutes later as necessary to help rule out orthostatic hypotension.

The steps of cardiovascular assessment in the immobilized person are briefly listed in Table 35–3.

PULMONARY SYSTEM

Major respiratory problems resulting from immobility include: (1) *decreased ventilation* and (2) *inadequate management of respiratory secretions*. Additional problems spring from these. To see why this is so, let us examine respiratory changes that occur when a person is immobilized.

Decreased Ventilation. Ventilation is the process of moving air in and out of the lungs. It is the mechanical phase of respiration in which the diaphragm descends and oxygenated air moves into the lungs as the chest cavity expands to accommodate it. Immobility can hinder effective ventilation when the immobilized person assumes a body position that limits chest expansion. Ventilation can also be hindered when the person is experiencing some of the more common untoward effects of immobility. For example, a person weakened by immobility has less of the muscle strength needed to breathe deeply and effectively. An individual suffering from constipation or flatulence may experience decreased ventilation because of abdominal distention (inflation) that interferes with the descent of the diaphragm. Often, the immobilized person is receiving treatments that hamper ventilation. For example, the person may be sedated with medications that depress the brain's respiratory center, or the person may be in a cast, bandage, or binder that limits chest wall expansion.

Inadequate Management of Respiratory Secretions. Normally, several forces work well together in the lungs to help manage the liquid respiratory secretions that accumulate there. Mucus is affected by gravity, so it tends to accumulate in the dependent or lowest areas of the lungs. In a sitting or standing position, this would be the base of the lungs. In a sleeping person, the lowest part would vary, depending on the different positions assumed during the night. Normal body position changes, then, help move mucus and prevent it from accumulating in any one area. Normal ventilatory movement also helps move the liquid mucus, as does an occasional deep sigh or cough. As the mucus moves, it is brought into contact with cilia that sweep it up, nearer the top of the bronchial tree, where it can more easily be expectorated (coughed up).

The immobilized individual tends to make fewer position changes. Infrequent position changes lead to accumulation or *pooling of lung secretions*. Also contributing to pooling is the fact that immobilized persons may have difficulty maintaining normal ventilations or producing an adequate cough. Often the immobilized person's intake of fluids decreases, and this results in mucus that is thick and difficult to expectorate.

The pooling of thick liquids causes a *decreased ciliary action* and a *diminished cough reflex*. When the person is finally stimulated to cough, a lack of adequate chest wall expansion can prevent an intake of air sufficient to produce a strong, effective cough. Effective coughing is also inhibited by the generalized weakness seen in many immobilized individuals and by the supine position they most often assume in bed.

Decreased ventilation and poor management of secretions produce two major complications: atelectasis (collapse of a lung or portion of lung) and **hypostatic pneumonia** (consolidation of lung tissue secondary to stagnant respiratory secretions).

Atelectasis develops when thick secretions pool in a bronchiole or bronchus and obstruct the airway, causing the *collapse of lung tissue*. Depending on the site of obstruction, the area may be a very small part of a lobe, an entire lobe, or an entire lung.

Pneumonia develops because pooled secretions provide a favorable medium for the growth of microorganisms. Pooled pulmonary secretions and inadequate ventilation both contribute to *decreased oxygen–carbon dioxide transfer* in the lungs. Ineffective diffusion of these two gases across the lung surface results in *inadequate oxygenation* and *carbon dioxide retention*.

If left uncorrected, inadequate oxygenation can produce dyspnea, tachycardia, fatigue, restlessness, and mental changes. Carbon dioxide retention can lead to *respiratory acidosis*, which in turn can cause *cardiopulmonary failure*.

Assessing for Pulmonary Changes. To assess the respiratory function of an immobilized individual, you should begin by reviewing the client's chart for factors known to affect lung expansion or gas exchange. For example, note whether the client is taking medications that affect the lungs, such as those that depress the brain's respiratory center or cough reflex center; check for evidence of decreased fluid intake, pneumonia, or fever that could lead to thickened secretions; and note the results of laboratory tests that show evidence of oxygen lack or carbon dioxide retention. For example, a decreased partial pressure of oxygen (normally 75 to 100 mm Hg) with increased partial pressure of carbon dioxide (normally 40 mm Hg) indicates decreased oxygen–carbon dioxide transfer. Another example, respiratory acidosis (plasma pH below 7.35, plasma bicarbonate above 29 mEq/L, and blood gas carbon dioxide above 40 mm Hg) indicates failure to excrete carbon dioxide.

Every 2 hours, complete an assessment of the immobilized client's respiratory status. Begin by looking for factors that affect chest wall expansion, such as improper positioning; weak muscles of respiration; constricting bandages, binders, or restraints; and abdominal distention.

Take the vital signs at least every 4 hours to look for an elevated temperature that suggests infection, such as pneumonia with thickened secretions, a rapid pulse that signals oxygen lack, or respiratory changes that herald various problems in ventilation and gas exchange. Note that

▶ Shallow respirations indicate restricted ventilation.
▶ Ineffective respirations may mean that immobility has weakened the person and that the weakness is hampering respiratory efforts.
▶ Labored, difficult breathing may indicate hypoxia or an airway blocked by mucus.
▶ Respirations that sound wet indicate that the person may be having difficulty clearing secretions.
▶ Abnormal breath sounds may also indicate a respiratory infection.

▶ Unequal expansion of the right and left chest wall indicates atelectasis in which ventilation may be seriously restricted.

▶ Severe dyspnea with cyanosis (bluish discoloration of the skin and mucous membranes) is a late sign of hypoxia and must be reported at once.

Mental changes can also indicate hypoxia. Therefore, be alert for mental changes such as irritability, confusion, or disorientation.

When assessing the respiratory system, it is imperative to auscultate the lungs, including dependent areas, and evaluate the client's cough, including color, consistency, and amount of mucus produced. In an immobilized person, a weak, ineffective cough with thin, copious mucus may indicate that the person needs help to clear the airway. A cough productive of thick mucus, however, might indicate a need for fluids to thin the mucus. Greenish-yellow sputum is one sign of pneumonia.

Throughout the day, it is important to make note of the client's spontaneous position changes. If the person is not able to independently move at frequent intervals, the nursing staff will have to assist in position changes to help prevent stasis of mucus in the client's lungs.

Assessment of the respiratory system is briefly summarized in Table 35–3.

GASTROINTESTINAL SYSTEM, NUTRITION, AND METABOLISM

In the immobilized person, the entire gastrointestinal tract seems to slow down. As a result, (1) *diminished appetite*, (2) *reduced intake*, (3) *slowed peristalsis*, and (4) *delayed defecation* occur.

Diminished Appetite. One theory accounting for anorexia (lack of appetite) is that, with reduced activity, the body's metabolic rate slows and results in a decreased need for food for energy. Whatever the trigger, we do know that anorexia occurs, and this causes a reduced intake of food.

Reduced Intake. A reduced intake leads directly to a *decrease in the consumption of calories* that may be required for healing. In particular, the desire for protein-rich foods is reduced, with a concomitant decrease in the consumption of protein. As a result of decreased consumption of protein, the person experiences hypoproteinemia (decreased protein in the blood).

Hypoproteinemia. Protein is the only nutrient that contains nitrogen, and nitrogen is essential to the body's tissue-building and repair processes. Normally, protein is taken into the body in food, metabolized, and used in fairly stable amounts as anabolic activities build and repair body tissues and catabolic activities break down tissues. Some of the end-products of protein metabolism (the nitrogenous waste products such as urea nitrogen, uric acid, and creatinine) are excreted in the urine. When there is a normal intake of protein and output of nitrogenous products, the person is said to be in nitrogen balance.

When the intake of protein is not sufficient for anabolic needs, as during periods of immobility, catabolism continues to occur. In this case, there is a greater output of nitrogenous wastes in proportion to the intake of protein, and the person is in a state of **negative nitrogen balance.** Negative nitrogen balance can cause additional anorexia and malnutrition, further debilitating the immobilized client.

Insufficient protein intake and the resultant hypoproteinemia also contribute to the formation of edema. Edema results when low levels of protein in the blood reduce the osmosis that normally helps provide for circulation of body fluids. Specifically, on the venous end of the capillary bed, hypoproteinemia reduces the return of fluid to the vascular system and promotes its retention in the interstitial tissues.

Decreased Fluid Intake. Just as anorexia causes a decrease in the intake of solid foods, it may also cause the client to take in less fluid by mouth. Another reason for *decreased fluid consumption* by an immobilized person may be anxiety about using a bedpan. Since water is needed for all metabolic activities, this is an unhealthy response.

Lack of fluid intake can cause or worsen many complications of immobility. For example, inadequate fluid intake can increase hemoconcentration and promote clot formation; add to the hypovolemia frequently seen in the immobilized; and thicken mucous lung secretions and prevent their removal.

Slowed Peristalsis. We do not know why immobilized persons are prone to have *decreased peristalsis*, but it is thought to be related to an increase in sympathetic nervous system activity. With decreased peristalsis, the contents of the gastrointestinal tract are propelled along more slowly than usual. Normally, gas forms in the lumen of the gut as air is swallowed, as the gastrointestinal contents ferment, and as gases diffuse into the gastrointestinal tract from the bloodstream. With decreased peristalsis, the slowed movement of the bowel contents may cause the accumulation of gas to become excessive. Excessive gas formation, or *flatulence*, can cause *painful cramping* as the tract stretches with **tympanites** (gaseous abdominal distention). Also, the distended abdomen can encroach upon the diaphragm and lead to a *reduced space for lung expansion*. In addition to promoting flatulence, slowed peristalsis can lead to changes in egestion (defecation).

Delayed Egestion. Egestion is the expulsion of undigested waste material (egesta) from the gastrointestinal tract. Normally, a semiliquid material termed chyme passes from the small intestine, through the ileocecal valve, into the colon. As this egesta passes through the colon, water is drawn out of it. By the time the fecal material is eliminated through the anus, it is a firm, formed stool that is moist enough for easy passage.

In immobilized persons with delayed peristalsis, the fecal material remains in the colon for prolonged periods of time. This causes an excess amount of water to be removed from the fecal material, and the stool becomes hard, dry, and difficult to pass. The client suffers from *constipation*.

Sometimes embarrassment causes immobilized persons to hold in their feces until the urge passes, rather than asking for a bedpan. Even those with a desire to defecate may find that they cannot do so on a bedpan in an unnatural position. Others find that the generalized weakness that characterizes the immobility extends to the muscles involved in defecation—the abdominal muscles and the levator ani. In these cases, too, the feces remain in the colon and the client becomes constipated.

Attempts to pass a constipated stool cause increased use of the Valsalva maneuver, resulting in increased strain on a heart that is already burdened by the effects of immobility.

Failure to pass a constipated stool leads to even more water being removed and a still drier stool that forms a putty-like plug in the gut. Proximal to the plug, more stool is retained in the colon as the plug of drier stool prevents its passage. This stool, too, becomes dry and constipated. Eventually, a large mass of dry stool becomes wedged into the colon in a condition called *fecal impaction*. A fecal impaction is difficult or impossible to pass without softening with enemas and digital removal by the nurse.

The impacted person may show signs of fecal incontinence and what seems to be diarrhea. The incontinence is due to a rectum so full of fecal material that the anal sphincter responds by becoming lax. What seems to be diarrhea is really mucus that is stimulated by the presence of the fecal mass. This mucus seeps around the mass, dissolves some of it, and is expelled frequently, in small amounts, as "diarrhea." This fecal-stained mucus can contaminate the perineum in immobilized persons.

Assessing for Gastrointestinal Changes. Begin assessment of the immobilized client's gastrointestinal status with the chart. In the chart, look for evidence of the client's pattern of intake of foods from the various food groups. Be on the alert for lack of fiber and for low protein intake. Also assess the adequacy of fluid intake. Note the color, consistency, and amount of stools and compare the pattern of bowel elimination with the client's normal pattern. Notice whether the client is taking medications that tend to cause constipation, such as certain analgesics.

Begin assessing the client by taking the vital signs. Look for elevated temperature or respiratory changes that indicate an infection. A loss of body water, with infection, can cause compensatory mechanisms to increase absorption of water from the colon and result in constipation. Question the client about symptoms of constipation and about habits that can increase the swallowing of air and lead to gas formation.

Auscultate for bowel sounds before inspecting, palpating, and percussing for abdominal distention. A rectal examination can usually be deferred but should be done if impaction is suspected and the examination is not contraindicated.

See Table 35–3 for a brief summary of elements to include in the assessment of your immobilized client's gastrointestinal system.

MUSCULOSKELETAL SYSTEM

In the musculoskeletal system, the main effects of immobility include (1) *decreased muscle contractions,* (2) *loss of muscle mass and strength,* (3) *contractures,* and (4) *osteoporosis (bone demineralization).* To review musculoskeletal changes, we will begin with changes in muscle contractions.

Decreased Tonic Contractions. At any given time within a normal muscle, a small number of muscle fibers are contracting. This **tonic contraction** is not sufficient to cause larger muscles to move but is sufficient to maintain a partial contraction referred to as muscle tonus or tone. Muscle tonus is the dynamic state of muscular tension that allows the body to be held in a normal posture or functioning position and prevents the body from collapsing into a helpless mass. Muscle tonus is maintained only by ongoing, daily muscle use as occurs through normal activities. Immobility causes decreased tonic contractions and reduced muscle tonus. Reduced muscle tonus can lead to additional problems such as the decreased muscle tension on the veins of the extremities that paves the way for venous stasis and a resulting series of untoward circulatory effects.

Decreased Isotonic Contractions. The word element *iso-* means "the same" and the element *-tonic* means "tone, tonus, or tension," so an **isotonic contraction** is one in which the muscle tonus or tension remains the same as the muscle shortens in contraction. It is the isotonic contraction of normal muscle that produces movement of body parts and that does work. During strenuous movement or work, the metabolic rate of contracting muscles can increase 50 to 100 times that of the resting rate. An increased metabolic rate requires additional oxygen for the muscles. This can result in the heart and lungs increasing the supply of oxygenated blood by 15 to 20 times the usual amount required by the muscles. Just how efficient the cardiopulmonary response is, however, depends on muscle need. In immobility, the response rate of the cardiopulmonary system decreases and muscular power declines.[33] Thus, with decreased isotonic contractions, the unused muscles become weak, and the client lacks work tolerance and endurance, which can cause problems in various body systems. For instance, the muscles of respiration can become too weak for adequate respiratory effort, leading to shallow breathing and resulting in further respiratory complications.

Decreased Isometric Contractions. The word element *-metric* refers to measurement. In **isometric contraction,** the muscle maintains the same length but its tonus increases. Although normal isometric contractions tighten a muscle, they do not produce movement or do work. They often assist other muscles to produce movement and to do work, because many body movements are completed by a combination of isotonic and isometric contractions. Isometric contraction, for example, is important in stabilizing one part of the body while another part is moved toward it, as in brushing hair when the forearm is held still by isometric contraction while the wrist is flexed by isotonic contraction. Immobility results in loss of strength and in decreased ability for isometric muscle contraction. Decreased ability for isometric contraction can lead to further problems, such as when weakened abdominal muscles fail to stabilize the abdominal wall as needed for the normal evacuation of stools and the client becomes constipated and impacted.

Loss of Muscle Mass and Strength. With immobility, muscle catabolism exceeds muscle anabolism. The reason for this is not known, but immobilized individuals are susceptible to muscle degeneration and atrophy. In fact, within 2 months of immobility, a muscle may be reduced to half its original size.

Disuse and muscle wasting cause a *reduction in muscle strength* at the rate of 10 to 20 per cent each week, so that within 2 months of immobility, over 50 per cent of a muscle's strength can also be lost.

Loss of muscle mass and strength can result in *generalized weakness; muscle pain,* including *backaches;* and *instability.* Loss of muscle strength occurs first in an immobilized person's antigravity muscles of the lower extremities and trunk and last in smaller muscles used for fine, coordinated movements such as the muscles of the hands.

Contractures. When muscles are not used to effect movement, contractures begin to occur in a fairly short period of time. A **contracture** is a condition in which the muscle is fixed, shortened, and resists stretching.

Normally, opposing muscle groups maintain a state of balance between muscles that serve to contract in opposite directions—for example, muscles that flex and extend, abduct and adduct, internally rotate and externally rotate, and so on. This state of balance is often disrupted in the muscles of immobilized clients.

Commonly, the fibers of the stronger muscles, such as the flexors, internal rotators, and adductors, remain in contraction for longer periods of time than the fibers of the weaker, opposing muscles. In muscular contractures, it is thought that it is not the muscle fibers so much as the collagen fibers in and around them that change as the contracture forms. After a muscle has remained in a shortened position for 5 to 7 days, its loose connective tissue, which normally allows full range of motion, begins to shorten and gradually changes into dense connective tissue. The joints become *stiff, painful,* and *lacking in dexterity.* After a period of time, fibrotic changes result in a contracture that limits range of motion and that is irreversible without extensive physiotherapy or surgical intervention.

Muscular contractures in immobilized individuals commonly result from muscle **spasticity** (excess tonus); paralysis with **flaccidity** (decreased tonus); or mechanical (positional) restriction of motion. Mechanical restriction of motion can be due to poor nursing care, such as when weakened, immobilized clients are left to lie supine in bed for a period of time with the weight of bed covers forcing their toes down and their ankles into a position of plantar flexion. If a contracture develops in the Achilles tendon and maintains the foot in this position, the client has **footdrop** (Fig. 35-6A).

Although most contractures occur in the hips, knees, and ankles, the long-term result of immobility is flexion of the neck and spine; adduction and internal rotation of the shoulders; flexion of the elbows, wrists, fingers (Fig. 35-6B), hips, and knees; cross-adduction of the legs; plantar flexion of the ankles; and flexion of the toes.

Without intervention, the individual assumes a fetal position from which movement is difficult or impossible.

Osteoporosis. One major change that occurs in the bones of an immobilized client is **osteoporosis,** in which there is a loss of minerals and organic materials that make up bone tissue. With osteoporosis, the bone is of its usual size, with the normal ratio of mineral to organic content, but it consists of less bone tissue than normal. The loss of bone tissue weakens the bone and makes it more susceptible to fracture. The more osteoporotic the bone becomes, the less trauma is required to cause the bone to break. For example, a severely osteoporotic individual could sneeze and fracture a vertebra. Fractures that result from very little trauma are called **pathologic fractures.**

To help in understanding disuse osteoporosis, we can look at calcium as one of the major elements of the bone. Calcium exists in two forms in the human body. Normally, 99 per cent is in the bones in the form of a mineral salt, and 1 per cent is circulating in the extracellular fluid, partially in an ionized form. The normal adult total serum calcium range is 9 to 11 mg/dl. Serum calcium levels above and below the normal range can cause dangerous changes in other body systems and can even cause death. Therefore, it is important that the body maintain normal serum calcium levels. This is accomplished through the regulation of calcium by parathyroid hormone (parathormone or PTH) and by calcitonin.

To increase blood levels of calcium, PTH can work in three ways. It can increase absorption of calcium from the small intestine (if sufficient phosphorus and vitamin D are present in the diet), increase reabsorption of calcium normally lost through the kidney, and increase bone resorption. In **bone resorption,** calcium salts leave the bone and move into the blood in an ionized form. To decrease blood levels of calcium, calcitonin decreases absorption of calcium from the gastrointestinal tract, decreases calcium resorption from the kidney, and decreases the bone resorption of calcium.

Thus, an excess secretion of PTH or a deficiency in the secretion of calcitonin can cause an excess loss of calcium from the bone to the blood. This same loss of calcium from the bones is seen in immobilized persons who lack stress on muscles, tendons, and bones, such

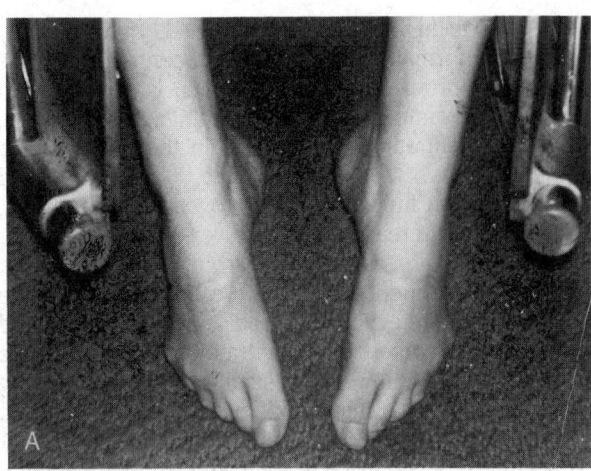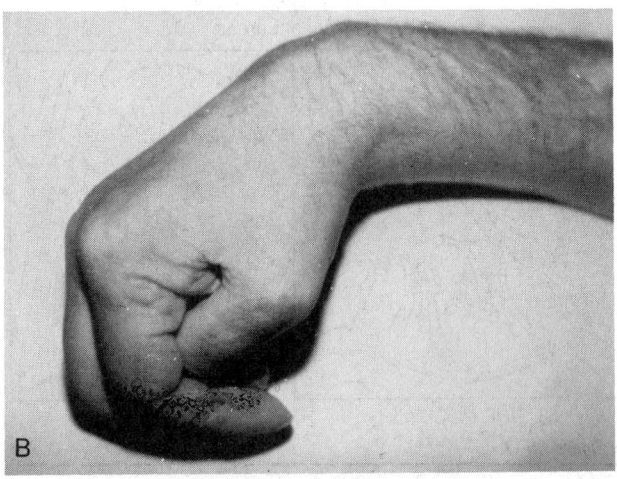

▲ *Figure 35–6*

Contractures. *A*, Footdrop. Note that the client also has flexion contractures in three toes of each foot, and her ankles are somewhat inverted. *B*, Flexion contractures of the wrist and fingers.

as occurs in the weight bearing and the muscle tension required for normal activities of daily living. Several theories have attempted to explain the relationship between immobility and bone loss, but we still do not have all the answers.

Commonly in the immobilized client, the loss of calcium from bone resorption causes disuse osteoporosis in the bone, but seldom does it cause hypercalcemia (an excess of calcium in the blood). Most often calcium blood levels are maintained within the normal or high normal range during bone resorption. This is possible because large amounts of calcium are excreted through the urine. The increased urine calcium level, or *hypercalciuria,* that occurs during bone resorption can cause an immobilized person to excrete 600 to 800 mg per day when the expected amount is only 50 to 250 mg. This excess calcium can precipitate out of the urine and form *calcium kidney stones (renal calculi).*

Osteoporosis is diffuse when the total body is immobilized, but it may be localized when only one extremity is involved. The greater the extent of immobilization, the greater the degree of osteoporosis. In total confinement to bed, the person loses bone mass at different rates, depending on such factors as age, degree of immobility, and beginning total bone mass, but the person may lose as much as 4 per cent of the total bone mass each month until 30 to 70 per cent has been lost.

Assessing for Musculoskeletal Changes. To begin the assessment of the immobilized individual's musculoskeletal system, it helps to review the chart for usual patterns of food consumption related to muscle and bone metabolism—that is, note whether dietary protein has been adequate to prevent muscle catabolism and note whether the intake of calcium, phosphorus, and vitamin D has been appropriate for the client's needs.

After your review of the chart, you should inspect the client for overall posture and ability to maintain proper body positioning. Palpate to assess muscle tension. Inspect muscles for size and bilateral symmetry.

Measure around the calves and thighs. Assess for contractures by noting the degree of movement and resistance encountered during range-of-joint-motion assessment. See Table 35–3 for a brief listing of elements to include in the assessment of your immobilized client's musculoskeletal system.

URINARY SYSTEM

In the urinary system, too, immobility takes its toll. Common disuse phenomena in this system include (1) *bladder distention,* (2) *urinary stasis,* (3) *infection,* and (4) *stone formation.*

Bladder Distention. As mentioned previously, the immobilized client may be reluctant to use a bedpan because of embarrassment or discomfort. Voluntarily holding urine in the bladder causes bladder distention. Chronic bladder distention results in excessive stretching of the detrusor muscle, which, over a long period, decreases the sensation of bladder fullness. Eventually, the person has little desire to void even when the bladder is full. Then, as pressure from urine builds, urinary incontinence sometimes occurs.

Urinary Stasis. Even if an immobilized person routinely uses the bedpan or urinal in a timely manner, problems can result. Normally, gravity assists urine to flow from the kidneys, through the ureters to the bladder, and out of the body through the urethra. In the client who is unable to attain a sitting or standing position, the flow of urine can be hampered. Note, for example, in Figure 35–7 how excess urine can accumulate in the kidney pelvis of a supine client. Excess urine can also accumulate in the bladder of an immobilized client who must attempt to void into a bedpan or urinal from a supine position. In this case, weakened abdominal muscles and incomplete relaxation of the pelvic floor can make voiding more difficult. When *incomplete emptying of the bladder* occurs, some urine is retained to become stagnant. Urinary stasis results, then, whether urinary retention is voluntary or due to an inability to sit or stand.

Stagnant areas

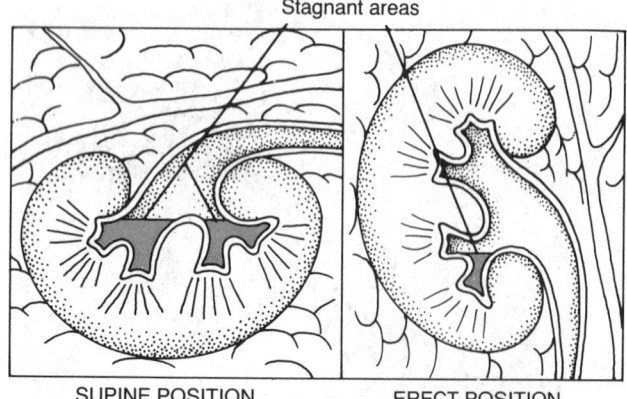

SUPINE POSITION   ERECT POSITION

▲ *Figure 35-7*

Stagnant areas of renal drainage in the erect position and the supine position.

Infection. Static urine provides an excellent medium for the growth of microorganisms, so the danger of infection is ever present. Normally, the urinary tract is sterile, but microorganisms can be easily introduced because of two factors frequently seen in immobilized females. First, the immobilized person tends to void less frequently, so there is less routine "flushing away" of microbes from the urethral meatus, a breakdown in a normal protective mechanism. Second, the client may not be receiving the best possible perineal hygiene, because cleansing of the perineal area is more difficult in a person confined to bed. Because the female urethra is very close to the anal area, it is not always easy to avoid contamination of the urinary meatus. Gross contamination, for example, is likely in the immobilized female who becomes impacted and is frequently incontinent of fecal-stained, mucus "stools."

In both the male and the female client, another common source of contamination of the urinary tract is the presence of an indwelling catheter in the urinary bladder. The indwelling catheter is usually connected to a tube that allows urine to flow by gravity into a collecting bag that is kept below the level of the bladder. As urine collects in the bag, it provides a medium suitable for bacterial proliferation. Because bacterial contamination of the contents of the bag is not at all unusual, the collected urine commonly serves as a source of infection.

If the urine collecting bag is not kept below the level of the bladder at all times, urine can flow, by gravity, back into the sterile bladder and infect the sterile urinary tract. Bacteria in the bladder may progress upward to the kidneys, causing an *ascending urinary tract infection*. Urinary tract infections may become chronic in some immobilized persons.

Stone Formation. In addition to infection, immobility increases the likelihood of stone formation in the urinary tract. Renal stones can be formed from several different materials, such as calcium, uric acid, or oxalate. Stone formation occurs when these substances are

in the urine in higher than normal levels or when they are there in normal levels that are concentrated relative to the fluid portion of the urine, which is decreased in volume. For example, in many immobilized individuals, calcium concentration is increased in the urine due to bone resorption. At the same time, the immobilized person may limit fluid intake and concentrate the urine, which further increases the relative concentration of calcium.

But even with increased urinary calcium levels, stone formation is not inevitable. An acid urinary pH created by the normal presence of citrate and other acidic substances can inhibit crystallization of stone-forming substances such as calcium. When urinary pH elevates, however, stone formation becomes more likely.

A special type of stone known as a struvite (magnesium ammonium phosphate, triple phosphate, or infection) stone can form in clients who have chronic urinary tract infections. As mentioned earlier, this can be the case in immobilized persons. When the offending microorganisms are urea-splitting bacteria, such as in a *Proteus mirabilis* infection, the microbes act on urea to produce ammonia, which raises urine pH. In the alkaline urine, struvite stones can form.

Assessing for Urinary System Changes. To begin to assess the immobilized client's urinary system, you should review the chart for evidence of risk factors for stone formation. These include high calcium levels in the urine when intake of calcium is normal, alkaline urine (high urinary pH), low fluid intake and output, and the presence of urinary tract infection. Through a combination of reviewing the chart and talking and working with the client, note evidence of risk factors for *Escherichia coli* infection. In a woman, this could include impaction, with fecal incontinence and inadequate perineal hygiene. In both sexes, it could include having an indwelling urinary catheter. Note whether the client is incontinent of urine or whether urination is difficult. Look for evidence of possible urinary stasis by noting the positions the client is able to assume. If indicated, inspect and palpate for evidence of bladder distention. See Table 35-3 for elements to include in your assessment of an immobilized person's urinary system.

PSYCHOSOCIAL SYSTEMS

Psychosocial problems that commonly occur in the immobilized person include undesirable (1) emotional responses, (2) cognitive and sensory changes, (3) interpersonal and social problems, and (4) special problems in the young and in the elderly.

Emotional Responses

Feelings of a Loss of Control. Purposeful mobility may be seen as being of two types: (1) movement toward someone or something in order to complete a task or meet a goal, and (2) movement away from someone or something that is perceived as a threat to physical or emotional well-being. With the understanding that each person is different and may respond quite differently to the same stimulus, it is still possible to say that many persons tend to respond in a similar manner when faced with the loss of these two types of movement.

The loss of ability to move toward a goal commonly results in feelings of *loss of control* and of *frustration*. Frequently, the very basic human response of *anger* results from the frustration. Anger is thought to be directed outward as *hostility* or *aggression* or to be turned inward as *depression*. The strength of these emotional responses is usually related to the desirability of the goal and how often the person has tried to reach it and failed.

The loss of ability to protect the self, by moving away from someone or something that is perceived as a threat to physical or emotional well-being, is also commonly experienced as a loss of control. In this case, though, the person most often responds by feeling *anxiety* or *fear*. The fight-or-flight response occurs, but the person is not able to fight or to flee. Stress hormones are secreted in larger than normal amounts, and, over a period of time, they can result in physical damage to the body organs. The strength and duration of the emotional and hormonal response is usually related to the degree of threat perceived. For example, the person who is totally unable to move from bed is likely to feel the extreme emotion of *panic* in the event of a fire in the building.

Changes in Self-Perception. Since we are living beings, mobility is very much a part of what we are. The loss of mobility can be perceived as a loss of part of the self. Indeed, immobilized individuals commonly experience an *alteration in body image* and a *loss of self-esteem*. However, not every immobilized person experiences these changes in self-perception. In fact, each person's emotional response to the inability to move is highly individual and is based on a number of factors, such as:

▸ societal role (e.g., student, spouse, parent) prior to the development of mobility problems
▸ occupation
▸ the probability of recovery
▸ other preexisting and coexisting health problems
▸ self-esteem and body image
▸ coping style
▸ available support systems
▸ degree of psychologic support from significant others and professionals

Cognitive and Sensory Changes. In addition to emotional responses to immobility, an individual might have cognitive changes. By themselves, neither immobility nor isolation has been shown to result in decreased cognitive ability. However, when a person is both immobilized and socially isolated, *sensory deprivation* occurs, and this can result in the deterioration of cognitive processes. It can also result in hallucinations (false sensory perceptions).

At the opposite extreme, *sensory overload* can occur in immobilized persons who cannot escape the stimulation required by treatment. For example, when the immobilized person must be physically turned by the nurse every 2 hours or so throughout the night, *sleep deprivation* can result.

Sleep deprivation and other forms of sensory overload can cause behavioral and mental changes, including hallucinations and delusions (fixed, false beliefs).

Interpersonal and Social Problems. Individuals with alterations in mobility may experience several interpersonal and social problems. One problem frequently encountered is *dependence* on another person or persons in order to meet basic needs. It is not unnatural for the immobilized person to worry about the caretaker's availability and abilities. This worry can have a definite influence on the relationship between caregiver and client. For example, the client may feel a need to please or to control the caregiver in order to assure availability. Another social problem is that immobility can easily result in *isolation*. This can have particularly devastating results; research has long shown that socially isolated clients are less likely to seek out and participate in rehabilitation measures.[33]

Special Problems in the Young and in the Elderly. Special problems can result from immobility in the young and in the elderly. Immobilized children may experience a developmental delay. This is a result of their inability to move about, explore their environment, and engage in the full range of age-appropriate play activities necessary for psychomotor, intellectual, and social growth. In immobilized elderly persons, opportunities to regain mobility and independence are more limited than are those of adults in younger age groups. The elderly may be devastated by the realization that, in becoming immobilized, they have become dependent.

Assessing for Psychosocial Changes. As you work with immobilized clients, you may note such commonly encountered emotional responses as frustration, anger, hostility, aggression, depression, anxiety, and fear. Some of these emotions cause physical changes that can be seen in the vital signs and in other physiologic responses. Some laboratory test results, such as elevated blood sugar and elevated cortisol levels, can indicate the presence of strong emotions or stress when there is no other reason for the elevations. Look for evidence of such responses.

Also, as you work with immobilized clients, look for changed perceptions about the self, such as alteration in body image and decreased self-esteem. The client may not be aware of these changed perceptions but may still react to them with a change in normal behaviors. For example, the male who feels his body image is less "manly" than previously perceived, now that he is immobilized, may unconsciously resort to proving his masculinity by "accidentally" exposing himself to the nurses.

Be alert for changes in sensory stimulation that can result in mental changes. Note whether the client is isolated from sensory input or overloaded by radio,

NURSING DIAGNOSIS PROFILE

High Risk for Disuse Syndrome

Definition. A state in which an individual is at risk for deterioration of body systems as a result of prescribed or unavoidable musculoskeletal inactivity.

Classification. Exchanging 1.6.1.5.

Defining Characteristics. Usually defining characteristics are signs and symptoms that support the conclusion that a tentative diagnosis is correct. With a high-risk diagnosis such as this one, the altered health state has not yet occurred, and there are no signs or symptoms. Instead, the defining characteristics consist of the presence of risk factors for this diagnosis. These risk factors may be identified as unavoidable inactivity or prescribed inactivity. Examples of unavoidable inactivity include paralysis, severe pain, and altered levels of consciousness. Examples of prescribed inactivity include the physician's order for immobilization: "bed rest," "no weight bearing," and so on. Examples of inactivity that is both unavoidable and prescribed include instances when the physician's prescribed treatment results in decreased ability to move. For example, a prescribed dose of medication for pain relief decreases the client's level of consciousness, or a body cast required for fracture healing prevents movement.

Sample Related Factors. The most common related factors are *Impaired Physical Mobility* and *Activity Intolerance*.

Concept Description. This diagnosis is particularly useful to nurses because it looks at the individual holistically. It says, in effect, "Because this person's ability to move is inadequate, every system in this person's body is at risk of breaking down."

The professional nurse understands all the potential disuse phenomena and is able to plan nursing care to prevent these. It is not necessary that the nurse write multiple diagnoses, such as:

▶ *High Risk for Impaired Gas Exchange* R/T impaired physical mobility
▶ *High Risk for Ineffective Airway Clearance* R/T impaired physical mobility
▶ *High Risk for Ineffective Breathing Pattern* R/T impaired physical mobility
▶ *High Risk for Infection* R/T impaired physical mobility
▶ *High Risk for Impaired Skin Integrity* R/T impaired physical mobility
▶ *High Risk for Altered Nutrition: Less than Body Requirements* R/T impaired physical mobility
▶ *High Risk for Constipation* R/T impaired physical mobility

All these diagnoses, and many more, are included in the one diagnosis of *High Risk for Disuse Syndrome*. Because you are learning about all these disuse problems and have not yet learned to synthesize your plan of care, your instructor may ask you to break down your client's diagnosis into smaller ones, as listed above. This can be very helpful when you are beginning to learn about nursing diagnoses and the nursing process.

Examples. Depending on the specific assessment data, this diagnostic category could be applicable in the following situations, among others:

▶ The person who cannot move at all because of some neuromuscular or musculoskeletal pathology. It is desirable that the person move, but the anatomic structure or function is altered so that this is no longer possible. The probability of ever regaining independent mobility is low, and any hope for improvement is based on technologic advances beyond those currently available. For such individuals, the diagnosis would be *High Risk for Disuse Syndrome* R/T impaired physical immobility.
▶ The person who is physically able to move but who is generally weak, in pain, or for some other reason is not able to move enough to prevent the possibility of disuse phenomena. The person may or may not be expected to regain some additional measure of mobility. When assessed, the person feels a greater need for rest than for movement. For such individuals, the diagnosis would be *High Risk for Disuse Syndrome* R/T activity intolerance.
▶ The person who is physically able to move but who should not do so. The person has some physical condition that could be exacerbated by movement. Movement is medically contraindicated. The person may or may not be mature enough or in sufficient contact with reality to understand that activity is harmful. Some type of immobilization device may be required to maintain the needed immobility, such as traction for a child's fractured legs or a waist restraint on a confused client who is too weak to bear weight should she get out of her wheelchair. For such individuals, the diagnosis again would be *High Risk for Disuse Syndrome* R/T impaired physical mobility.

Related/Similar Nursing Diagnoses. As mentioned in the foregoing concept description, the diagnosis of *High Risk for Disuse Syndrome* includes many other diagnoses. When making diagnoses for a client in the clinical setting, it would not be incorrect to list all the diagnoses mentioned above (and others as applicable), but it would be wasteful of the nurse's time.

High Risk for Disuse Syndrome should not be confused with *Activity Intolerance* or *Impaired Physical Mobility* but instead may be a companion diagnosis to either of these. For example, the client may have a diagnosis of *Activity Intolerance* R/T increased oxygen demands upon movement and a second diagnosis of *Potential for Disuse Syndrome* R/T activity intolerance. Likewise, a client could have a diagnosis of *Impaired Physical Mobility* R/T pain and a second diagnosis of *High Risk for Disuse Syndrome* R/T impaired physical mobility.

---

television, visitors, and ongoing activities. Look for changes in mental functioning, such as changes in cognition, judgment, problem solving, learning, memory, and alertness or alterations in perception such as paranoia or hallucinations.

Note interpersonal and social problems, such as dependency and social isolation. The client who fears dependency on the nursing staff may test the nurses, by constantly ringing the bell and making small requests, just to see if the nurses will respond.

Loss of control of the body may be manifested by the client attempting to control the nurse, others, or the environment.

In children, compare the developmental level with the expected norm. In the elderly, be especially alert for feelings of helplessness and hopelessness that may accompany a sense of dependency.

See Table 35-3 for a brief review of elements to include in the psychosocial assessment of an immobilized person.

NURSING DIAGNOSIS

The best nursing diagnosis for individuals with a decreased ability to move independently would seem to be *Impaired Physical Mobility*. This diagnosis is defined by the North American Nursing Diagnosis Association (NANDA) as "a state in which the individual experiences a limitation of ability for independent physical movement."[45] However, if we use this diagnosis, we should expect our outcomes to alleviate or to remedy the situation, and this is not always possible. Some individuals will always require assistance in moving, such as persons with a severed spinal cord. Others might be able to move by themselves but require temporary assistance with moving because movement is painful, injurious, or otherwise not medically indicated, as in a client with an unstable fracture of the pelvis.

The clients we are considering in this chapter are persons who are not able or not yet ready to attempt to regain mobility. They are individuals who are at risk for deterioration of many body systems. A better diagnosis for them is *High Risk for Disuse Syndrome*, defined as "a state in which an individual is at risk for deterioration of body systems as the result of prescribed or unavoidable musculoskeletal inactivity" (see the Nursing Diagnosis Profile for this chapter for more on this diagnosis).[45] The nursing diagnosis statement for such individuals is frequently *High Risk for Disuse Syndrome* R/T impaired physical mobility or *High Risk for Disuse Syndrome* R/T impaired physical mobility secondary to activity intolerance.

Clients with a diagnosis of *Impaired Physical Mobility* are discussed in Chapter 36. See that chapter for additional diagnoses for the immobilized client.

PLANNING

With the diagnosis *High Risk for Disuse Syndrome*, the nursing care should be directed toward preventing disuse syndrome. One way to do this is to increase the client's mobility level. Interventions that do this are covered in Chapter 36. In this chapter, we are concerned with means of preventing disuse syndrome without being able to increase the client's mobility level.

High Risk for Disuse Syndrome is what is termed a high-risk nursing diagnosis. Nursing interventions for high-risk nursing diagnoses are directed toward altering or eliminating risk factors. In this case the risk factors are "unavoidable inactivity" and/or "prescribed inactivity." Therefore, our plan should include nursing interventions that prevent disuse phenomena by altering the activity or mobility level for clients who are unable themselves to do so.

Because the diagnosis is high risk and no problem has developed, we will not be expecting the "resolution of a problem" in a given length of time, as we would with an actual diagnosis. Instead, the expected outcomes for this diagnosis are prevention of unhealthy responses, and we will not expect to see unhealthy responses (or, stated positively, we will expect to see a maintenance of healthy responses) for the full period of the nurse-client relationship. For the hospitalized client, this is for the duration of the hospital stay (DHS).

When considering outcomes, you may find it helpful to think about each body system in the order you assessed it. This should help prevent omissions. Suggested outcomes for the client with a high risk for disuse syndrome are listed in Box 35-2.

NURSING INTERVENTION

Examining Bed Rest

Most of the interventions in this chapter are intended for clients on bed rest. **Bed rest** is an ambiguous concept that can be interpreted in several ways. For example, you may see orders, written by different physicians, for "Bed rest," "Strict bed rest," "Bed rest with bathroom privileges," "Bed rest with bed side commode privileges," and "Up to chair with assistance," and find that each physician meant the same thing when the order was written. Or, you may find several doctors who have written an order for "Bed rest" and discover that each of them meant something different from the others. Differences in interpretation of the term can result in misunderstandings between staff members and can cause confusion for the client.

All members of the health care team must agree upon definitions of bed rest and strict bed rest so that everyone knows the *amount* and *type* of activity the client is allowed.

▶ Is the client allowed to perform any self-care activities in bed? If so, which?
▶ Is the client allowed out of bed to go to the bathroom or to use the bedside commode for elimination? If so, is this allowed for bladder elimination, bowel elimination, or both?
▶ If allowed to go to the bathroom for elimination, is the client also allowed to use the bathroom for other purposes while there, such as washing hands, brushing teeth, shaving, and so on?
▶ Is the client allowed to sit in a chair at the bedside? If so, how often per day and how long each time?

Rest in bed is often necessary and beneficial (see Box 35-3 for a list of the potential benefits of bed rest when it is properly prescribed and implemented).

Box 35-2. Outcomes for the Client with High Risk for Disuse Syndrome

For the duration of the hospital stay, the client:

▶ Maintains intact skin and mucous membranes with skin of normal color; free of signs of ischemia and non-blanchable erythema in pressure areas

▶ Maintains adequate circulation; without signs of edema, clot formation, phlebitis, or pulmonary embolism

▶ Maintains normal cardiac return and cardiac output; with no signs of increased cardiac workload, cardiac strain, or orthostatic hypotension

▶ Maintains normal ventilation; with no signs of carbon dioxide retention or hypoxia

▶ Maintains easily expectorated, liquid lung secretions; with no signs of thick mucus, atelectasis, hypostatic pneumonia, or lung collapse

▶ Maintains normal nutrition; without anorexia, malnutrition, muscle catabolism, or negative nitrogen balance

▶ Maintains a normal pattern of bowel movements; without decreased peristalsis, flatulence, abdominal distention, constipation, or impaction

▶ Maintains muscle mass; without signs of weakness or decreased muscle tone

▶ Maintains passive range of motion of all joints; without signs of contractures

▶ Maintains normal bone metabolism; without bone resorption, hypercalcemia, hypercalciuria, calcium kidney stone formation, osteoporosis, or pathologic fractures

▶ Maintains a normal pattern of urinary elimination; without urinary stasis, concentrated urine, urinary tract infection, bladder distention, urinary incontinence, alkaline urine, or kidney stones

▶ Copes with inability to independently complete tasks or meet goals; without excessive feelings of loss of control, frustration, anger, hostility, aggression, or depression

▶ Copes with inability to independently remove self from that which is perceived as a threat to physical or emotional well-being; without excessive feelings of anxiety, fear, or panic

▶ Maintains cognitive functions; without hallucinations or delusions

▶ Maintains healthy interpersonal relationships with caretakers; without excessive dependence or a need to please or to control the caretaker

▶ Maintains healthy social relationships; without feelings of isolation

---

However, bed rest has its hazards, as we have seen in examining the effects of immobility. Thus, bed rest is a double-edged sword. It can solve some problems but frequently creates others.

Whether the immobility is prescribed, as with bed rest, or unavoidable, as with many disorders, our task is to enhance the benefits of rest as we prevent the complications. Much of the remainder of this chapter will be devoted to interventions that will help do that. We will begin by reviewing some of the equipment that can be used to position immobilized persons so as to help prevent disuse phenomena.

Box 35-3. Benefits of Bed Rest

Bed rest can help

▶ Relieve pain by decreasing the movement that stimulates pain receptors in tissues that have been traumatized by accidents or operations or in muscle tissues that are in pain from a lack of oxygen

▶ Promote tissue repair by reducing metabolic needs

▶ Prevent the migration of microorganisms from infected tissues to healthy tissues by preserving fibrin barriers

▶ Relieve ankle edema and venous congestion by elevating the extremities above heart level

▶ Give support to weak, exhausted, or febrile persons who, because of illness, are unable to remain standing and active (e.g., those debilitated by chronic disease or incapacitating neurologic disease)

Equipment for Positioning

Over the years, many devices have been developed to help make positioning safer and more comfortable for the immobilized client and easier for the nurse. Some of the more commonly used pieces of equipment and devices are described next.

BEDS, FRAMES, AND MATTRESSES

Standard Beds. The standard hospital bed allows the client to be positioned with the bed flat or with different sections of the bed elevated or lowered according to client need. Each position has its positive points and its negative points, as summarized in Table 35-4.

The bed should always be kept at the lowest level except when the nurse is present to prevent a fall.

Side Rails. Side rails are used mainly to prevent a person from falling out of bed. They are also useful to aid in turning. Partial ("short" or "half") side rails do not provide as much protection as full-length rails, but can be helpful in reaching a sitting position or getting out of bed.

Caution Side rails can be harmful! The client who climbs over them and falls drops from a greater height than would be the case had no side rails been present at all. Use side rails only for individuals who are

▶ totally unable to climb over them, such as infants or completely immobilized persons

▶ able to *comprehend and comply with* the knowledge that side rails are in place only as a reminder that getting out of bed unassisted is not safe

▶ under constant surveillance by nursing personnel

Specialized Beds, Frames, and Mattresses. An ideal bed or frame would help prevent disuse phenomena by providing all the features listed in Box 35-4. Although some specialized hospital beds and frames have been designed to provide some of these features, no single bed or frame can provide all of them. The bed or frame selected for any particular client must provide

TABLE 35–4. Advantages and Disadvantages of Standard Bed Positions

Position	Advantages	Disadvantages	Illustration
Flat—with the mattress in a completely horizontal position	Prevents pressure on any one body area and prevents pooling of blood in any particular area	It is more difficult for the client to breathe in this position than it is with the head elevated	
Trendelenburg—with the mattress flat and the foot of the bed elevated (or the head lowered) to raise the client's heart above head level	Improves blood flow to the brain and assists with drainage of pulmonary secretions	Increases pressure on the diaphragm, making adequate lung expansion more difficult	
Reverse Trendelenburg—with the mattress flat and the head of the bed elevated (or the foot lowered)	Helps prevent reflux of gastric juices and allows adequate lung expansion	Can cause the client to slide down in bed so that shearing or friction can lead to breakdown in the tissues of the back	
Elevated foot gatch—with the legs elevated above heart level and the knee gatch elevated or not, as desired	With the head of the bed flat, improves cardiac return and reduces edema in the lower extremities	With the head of the bed elevated, causes pooling of blood in the hip region and increases pressure on tissues in the sacral area	
Elevated knee gatch—with the mattress flexed at the level of the knees and the foot gatch elevated or not, as desired	With the head of the bed raised, helps prevent client from sliding down in the bed	Places pressure on the popliteal spaces, behind the knees, and can impair circulation there, increasing the chance of clot formation	
Fowler's position—with the head of the mattress raised 30 to 90 degrees. Low Fowler's position (semi-Fowler's) is approximately 30 degrees. High Fowler's position is approximately 90 degrees. The foot of the bed or the knee gatch may or may not be elevated, as desired	Facilitates lung expansion and improves breathing	Causes the client to slide down in the bed, increasing the chances of shearing in the underlying tissues of the back	
Orthopneic position—with the head of the mattress raised 90 degrees and the client's upper body resting on pillows on an overbed table	Facilitates lung expansion and breathing	Maintains the hips in a position of acute flexion	

Table continued on following page

TABLE 35–4. Advantages and Disadvantages of Standard Bed Positions Continued

Position	Advantages	Disadvantages	Illustration
Contour position—with the head of the mattress, knee gatch, and foot gatch all slightly elevated. This is usually assumed as a position of general comfort	Assists in breathing	Causes pooling of blood in the hip area and can cause pressure on the popliteal spaces	
Hi-lo positions—with the entire bed raised to its highest level, lowered to its lowest level, or positioned somewhere in between. This refers to the height of the bed, and height adjustments may be made without interfering with the mattress positions described above	Higher levels allow the nurse to work without bending over and injuring his or her back Intermediate levels can be helpful in transferring the client to a stretcher or other device that is at a different level	Higher levels may be too high to allow the client to get into and out of bed safely. If the client were to fall out of bed, the increased distance from the floor could contribute to greater injuries than would result from a fall from a lower level	

what is most important for that person, based on individual needs. Following are some of the specialized beds, frames, and mattresses available.

Stryker Frame and Stryker Wedge Frame. The Stryker frame was one of the first successful devices used to replace a standard bed in order to assist the client in changing positions. It allowed the client to be turned to a face-down position and back to a face-up position when this would have been very difficult or impossible on a standard bed. Some Stryker frames are

---

Box 35–4. Features of an Ideal Hospital Bed

▶ All features provided by standard hospital beds
▶ Easy, comfortable movement of the client into various body positions, including the prone (face-down) position
▶ Easy movement of the client to a vertical position and assistance in maintaining standing to provide stress on muscles and bones of the legs
▶ Maintenance of the client in any required position without allowing the client to slide out of position or downward in the bed
▶ Lack of friction and shearing on the skin to prevent tissue breakdown
▶ Easy but *slow* client movement to allow for circulatory changes and to prevent orthostatic hypotension
▶ Less than 32 mm Hg pressure on soft tissues over bony prominences to prevent restriction of capillary flow and resultant tissue ischemia
▶ Solid, firm body support when needed for nursing care, medical treatments, or emergency measures, such as cardiopulmonary resuscitation
▶ Independent control by clients who have minimal mobility

---

still in use today, although many have been replaced by the Stryker wedge frame or the Stryker CircOlectric bed. To gain a basic understanding of all three of these types of beds, it helps to have an understanding of the Stryker frame.

The Stryker frame consists of two lightweight metal frames, which are covered with a strong but light material, and a metal standard that supports these two frames above the floor. The standard holds the frames only by the midpoint at each end of the frame, so the frames are free to rotate horizontally when not locked in place. Most of the time, only one frame is attached to the standard and the client lies on it in a supine (face-up) position. When ready to turn to the prone position, the second frame is firmly secured above the client so he or she is sandwiched between the material of the two frames. One or more restraining straps are belted around both frames to prevent the client from falling out from between them during the turn. Two persons work together to quickly and smoothly turn both frames and the client into a prone position. After turning, the lower frame is locked in place and the upper frame is removed from the client's back.

The Stryker wedge turning frame (Fig. 35–8) is a variation of a Stryker frame. Instead of two horizontal frames being used for a turn, the upper and lower frames are angled into a wedge shape. The wedge design allows the two frames to almost meet at one side. This is the only side that is ever turned toward the floor, so the client cannot fall out. The improved design permits one nurse to turn the frame, minimizes the client's fear of falling, decreases the need for numerous restraining straps, and allows a slower turn.

CircOlectric Bed. Like the Stryker frames, the Stryker CircOlectric bed consists of two frames that permit turning by sandwiching the client between them (Fig. 35–9). This bed is the only bed, however, that uses

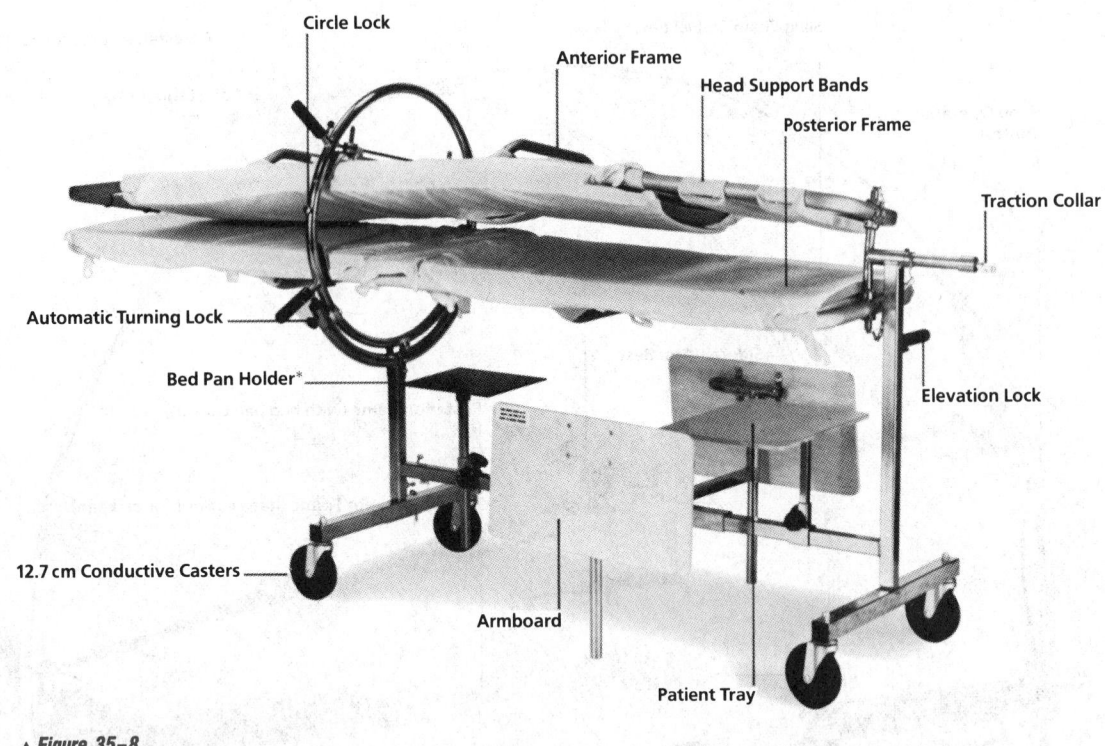

Circle Lock

Anterior Frame

Head Support Bands

Posterior Frame

Traction Collar

Automatic Turning Lock

Bed Pan Holder*

Elevation Lock

12.7 cm Conductive Casters

Armboard

Patient Tray

▲ *Figure 35-8*

Stryker wedge turning frame. (Courtesy of Stryker, Kalamazoo, MI.)

electrical power to turn the client slowly to a face-down position. It rotates the client vertically rather than horizontally and can be stopped at any point in the turn. It is particularly valuable for persons who are at risk for orthostatic hypotension and who must be trained to adjust to position changes after a period of immobility.

If the head of the bed is rotated approximately 45 degrees upward from the horizontal position, the lower, supporting frame can be adjusted to take the form of a chair and permit the client to sit for a time, if allowed. If the lower frame is kept straight and the bed is rotated 90 degrees upward from the horizontal position, it can be stopped to serve as a standing frame. A standing frame supports the client in a vertical position for as long as necessary. In this respect, the bed is well suited for persons who can benefit by increasing stress on the muscles and bones of the legs. If the client is moved 180 degrees from the horizontal back-lying position to the face-down position, the frame over the back can be loosened and raised up, away from the back, where it can be held in place by a safety bar.

This bed has much to offer, but it is not for everyone.

Caution The CircOlectric should not be used for clients with unstable spinal fractures and certain other pathologic conditions.[41]

The Stryker devices are desirable because they move the client into a prone position, but there are some negative aspects to this. One undesirable aspect is that the client often feels isolated when staring at nothing but the floor and people's feet. To counteract this, prism glasses may be worn to allow the person to see

visitors, nursing personnel, and more of the surroundings. Additionally, some persons are anxious and fear falling when first placed on these narrow frames. Armrests and restraining straps may be reassuring, especially at night.

Caution All devices that turn the client to the prone position are potentially dangerous and require careful monitoring by the nurse. After turning the client to the prone position, observe closely for signs of respiratory fatigue or complaints of dizziness, faintness, vertigo, or other unusual signs of discomfort. Should any of these occur, immediately return the client to the face-up position.[57] For some clients, a physician should be in attendance the first few times the client is turned.

ROTO REST Kinetic Treatment Table. The ROTO REST oscillating bed (Fig. 35-10) may be pre-set to rotate continuously from one side to the back, then to the other side, and back again through approximately 70 degrees of arc in each direction. The speed of oscillation is slow and safe, with 124 degrees of arc, for example, requiring 3.5 minutes. Bolster packs may be placed along the client's sides to increase stabilization. The motion can be stopped, if necessary, and each hinged section of the table may be removed for free access to all body parts for nursing care and treatments. This table is particularly valuable for preventing pulmonary complications in clients with neurologic pathology requiring immobilization of the spinal column, such as unstable fractures of the spinal column.[3,14,41]

UHI-Air-Fluidized Therapy (Clinitron Bed). The Clinitron bed was developed to reduce pressure on the client's skin (see Fig. 48-17, in Chapter 48). In it, the

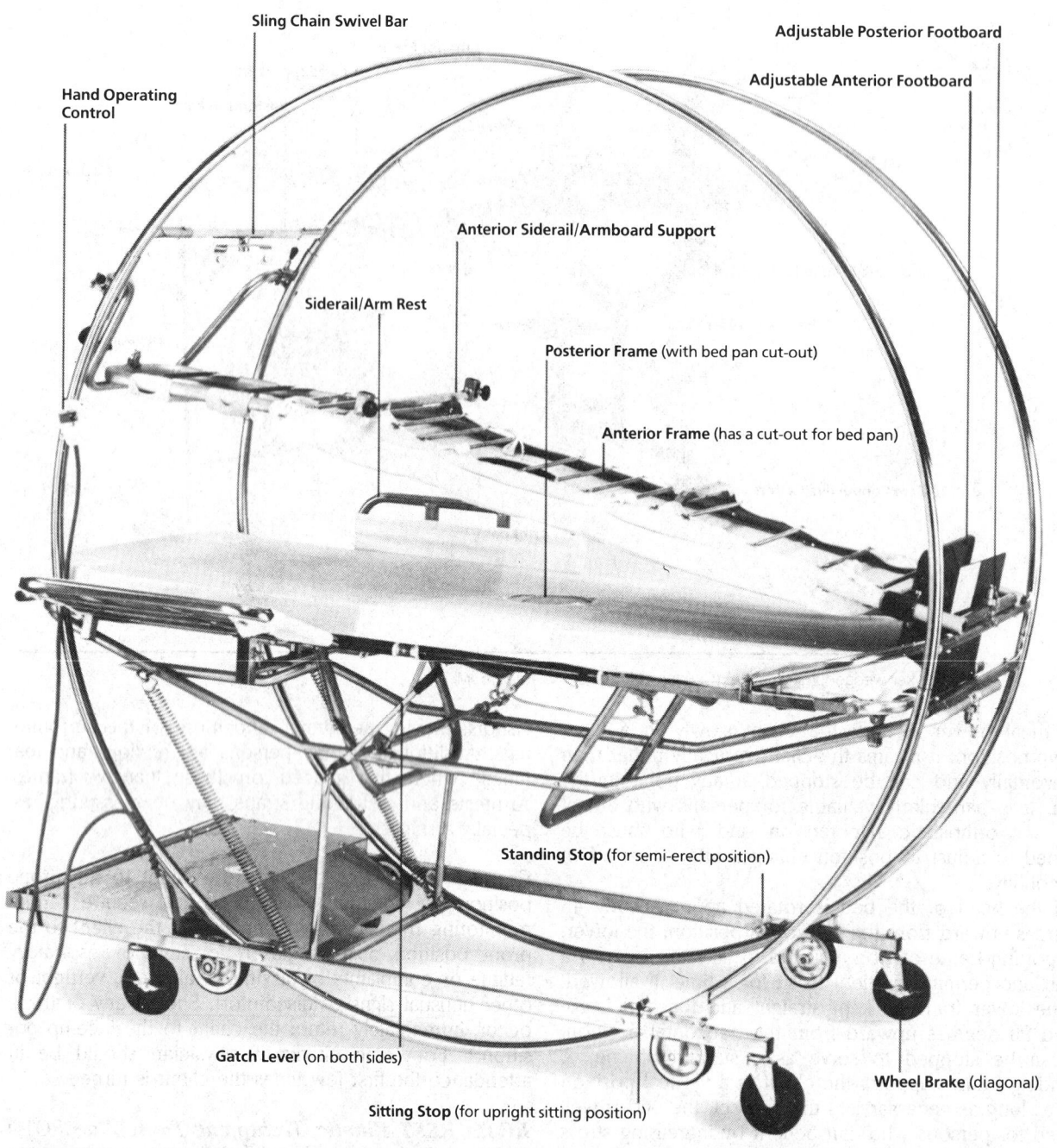

Sling Chain Swivel Bar

Hand Operating Control

Adjustable Posterior Footboard

Adjustable Anterior Footboard

Anterior Siderail/Armboard Support

Siderail/Arm Rest

Posterior Frame (with bed pan cut-out)

Anterior Frame (has a cut-out for bed pan)

Standing Stop (for semi-erect position)

Gatch Lever (on both sides)

Wheel Brake (diagonal)

Sitting Stop (for upright sitting position)

▲ **Figure 35–9**

Stryker CircOlectric bed. Both anterior and posterior frames are completely removable. (Courtesy of Stryker.)

client lies on a thin, silky, air-permeable, plasticized cover that billows upward as the air beneath it flows upward and continuously moves tiny, silicon-coated glass beads against the weight of the client's body. The movement of the air and glass beads provides comfortable flotation support that evenly distributes the body weight, as would water. Hence, the term *fluidized* in the bed's name.

The billowing, silky cover provides no friction or shearing. This is helpful in turning the client and in preventing skin breakdown, but it is more difficult to maintain the client in certain positions. Triangular foam wedges can be used to help maintain some positions,

such as sitting, but the person still tends to slide downward. The fluidization can be turned off, as necessary, to solidify the bed so that it conforms to the body contours.

Mediscus Low-Air-Loss Bed. Like the Clinitron bed, the Mediscus bed is a low-air-loss bed (as opposed to high-air-loss systems that attempt to support the client on a column of air, much like a Hovercraft). It is also considered a type of air flotation bed. The bed consists of a solid base frame that can be positioned flat, in Trendelenburg or in reverse Trendelenburg position. Over this is a hinged frame that supports a series of 21

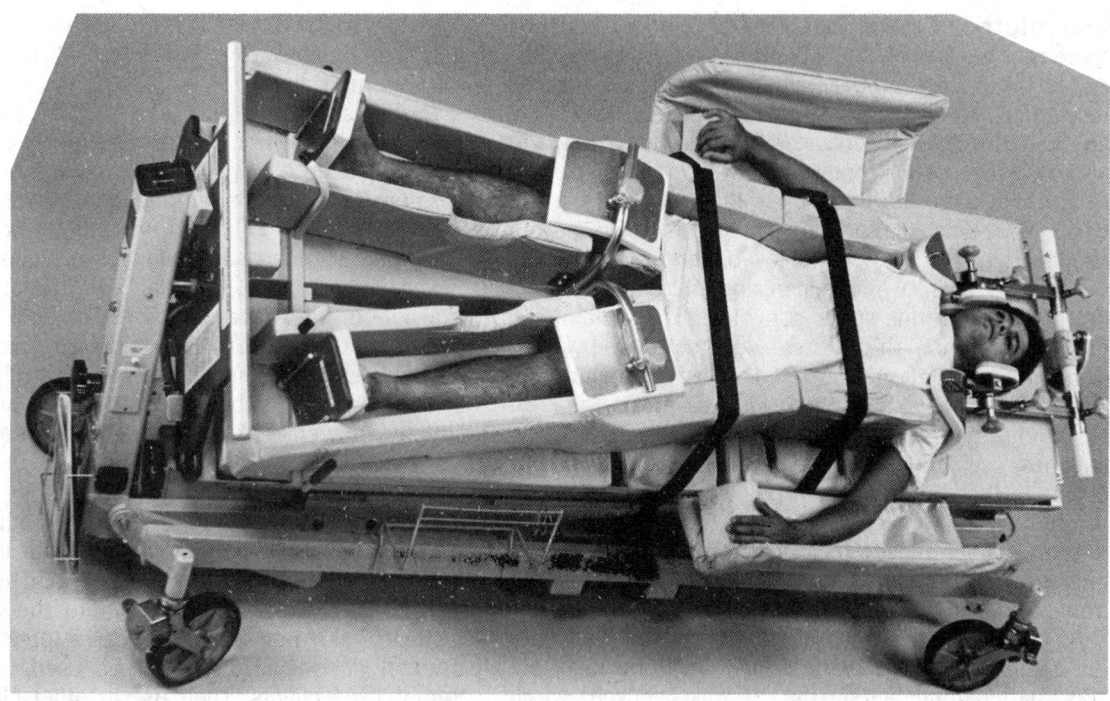

▲ *Figure 35–10*

ROTO REST kinetic treatment table. ROTO REST is Kinetic Concepts' trademark for its oscillating hospital bed. (Courtesy of Kinetic Concepts, San Antonio, TX.)

air sacs (see Fig. 48–16 in Chapter 48). The hinged frame allows the usual positioning of the upper body, knees, and feet as the client reclines on the pillow-shaped air sacs. The air sacs are divided into five sections that can be individually inflated to different pressures by a bedside air-supply system.

The bed does not exert more than 25 mm Hg of pressure on the client's skin. While it aids in preventing breakdown of the tissues, it does not assist in turning the client from side to side. It allows a sitting position to help with lung expansion, but it does not allow a vertical position to provide stress on muscles and bones. Because the client lies directly on sacs and draw sheets that are made of a low-friction material, friction and shearing are minimized.

SPECIALIZED MATTRESSES AND OTHER CUSHIONING DEVICES

Specialized mattresses and other cushioning devices are available for placement on top of a standard mattress, on a standard bed frame. They enhance comfort and help prevent skin breakdown. Some are **pressure-reducing** devices that lower the pressure on the client's skin to below the pressure that would be exerted by a standard mattress. Others are **pressure-relieving**—they actually relieve pressure by reducing the pressure to below the 32 mm Hg of pressure generally accepted as being required for capillary filling.[20] Some examples are described next.

Flotation Mattresses. Flotation mattresses contain water or a viscous gel-like substance. They may be segmented or unsegmented.

In segmented mattresses, the segments may go across the mattress or run lengthwise. Some brands are connected to electrical devices that intermittently fill and empty the different segments, alternately reducing pressure on different body parts.

Unsegmented flotation mattresses, similar to water beds used in homes, contain a water-filled bladder surrounded by a sturdy frame. With some models the frame extends above the mattress. Because of the rolling motion that occurs whenever the mattress is jostled, some people initially experience nausea or vomiting and require antiemetics.

Caution Prevent hypothermia or hyperthermia by maintaining a safe water temperature in mattresses mostly filled with water. This is especially important in persons with impaired temperature perception, that is, persons with neurologic or orientation disorders. Also use care with sharp devices that might cut an air- or fluid-filled mattress.

Air Mattresses (Alternating-Pressure Air Mattresses). Air mattresses are usually segmented, double-coiled, heavy plastic pads that may be placed on top of regular mattresses (see Fig. 48–15 in Chapter 48). They automatically rhythmically inflate and deflate to alternate pressure on body areas. Thus, prolonged pressure is minimized on the body's pressure-bearing areas. Segments may run across the mattress width or length, or the mattress may consist of small pockets or pillows that alternately inflate and deflate. Inflation is powered by a motor that is attached to the mattress by air hoses.

Convoluted Foam Mattresses and Artificial "Sheepskins." Convoluted foam mattresses are usually made of foam rubber (latex) or a synthetic material resembling foam rubber, such as polyurethane. They are called egg-crate mattresses when they have an upper surface that is convoluted with small peaks and valleys that look like the cartons that hold and cushion eggs. This type of surface was designed to protect clients from decubitus ulcers by promoting air circulation to the skin while minimizing pressure on bony prominences. In one study, convoluted foam mattresses of 2- and 4-inch thicknesses were compared with a standard, hospital mattress and other cushioning devices.[34] Only the 4-inch thickness was found to be effective in the reduction of pressure on tissues. This thickness served as a pressure-relieving device for clients in the supine position but only as a pressure-reducing device for clients in the side-lying position. Thicker, higher-density foam mattresses are more durable and provide more support than other foam mattresses.

At one time, real sheepskins were used to help cushion immobilized persons. They were soft and fluffy and contained natural lanolin that, it was believed, would help protect the skin. Today, we use artificial sheepskins made of synthetic fibers that tend to be soft, fluffy, and somewhat absorbent. They are meant to be used between the client and the bed linen to reduce pressure on bony prominences, permit air circulation to the skin, and prevent shearing when the client is moved. Although they do cushion, they have not been shown to lower pressure to below 32 mm Hg.

Convoluted foam mattresses and sheepskins have several things in common. Both are frequently supplied in a mattress size or in smaller pieces to fit under the bony prominences of the client's back while in bed, in a wheelchair, or elsewhere. Covering either device with tightly-fitted bed linens tends to flatten and decrease their cushioning effect. However, many persons are uncomfortable lying directly on these devices and prefer the feel of the usual bed linens next to their skin. Since these devices do absorb perspiration, covering them with sheeting material can help keep them fresh. Thus, a decision should be made on an individual basis concerning whether to place these devices on top of the bottom sheet, directly in contact with the client's skin, or to place them under the bottom sheet, next to the mattress.

Additional Cushioning Devices. Cushioning devices support the weight of a person seated in a chair or wheelchair or support various body parts as the client lies in bed. They are available in a variety of materials, sizes, and shapes. Usually, they are filled with air, water (or other liquid), gel, foam, or some combination of these materials. Their size and shape depend upon their intended use and the specific needs of the individual client, so they can vary considerably. They may take the form of cushions, bolsters, pillows, pads, rings, or other less common forms, such as heel and elbow protectors. Generally these devices are comfort measures that are pressure-reducing, rather than pressure-

relieving. However, a higher-density, 4-inch foam pad may lower pressure to below the 32 mm Hg required for pressure relief.

Cushions, pillows, and pads may be placed under a body area to cushion it. Bolsters, pillows, and cushions may be placed on two or more sides of a body area to cushion the surrounding area while the center is bridged (Fig. 35–11). With bridging, the area (usually a bony prominence or a wound) is not allowed to touch the mattress surface. Alternatively, the cushion may be available in the shape of a ring. The hole in the middle of the ring provides cushioning all around the supported area while the hole serves to bridge the tissues in the center. The best types of rings are those constructed of dense, 4-inch thick foam latex or polyurethane.

Caution Air-filled rings (or *any* rings other than those constructed of dense, 4-inch-thick foam latex or polyurethane), if left in place too long or if overfilled with air, can compromise circulation to the tissues in the center of the ring. This can cause pressure ulcers. If used at all, they should *not* be used in the care of immobilized clients. Their use in other clients, such as persons with perineal and/or rectal pathology, demands frequent evaluation!

Soft tissues over heels and elbows tend to break down because they lie over bony prominences. Breakdown also occurs with friction as these areas rub

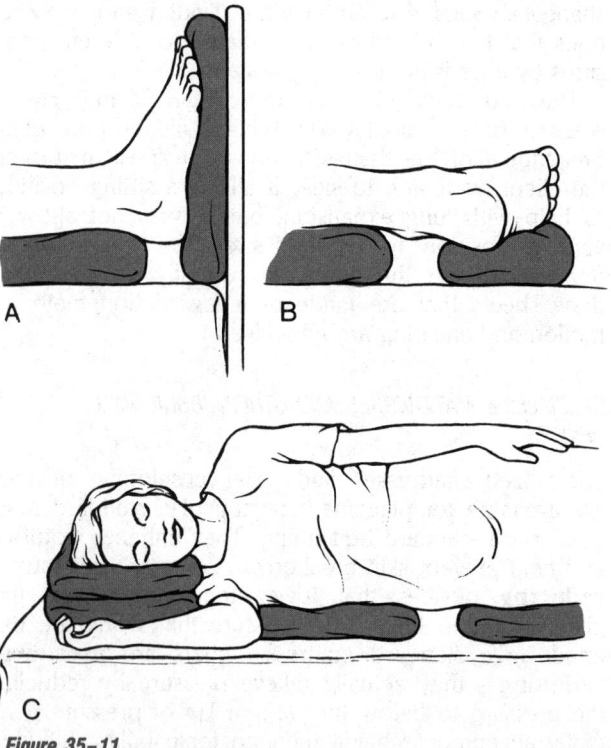

▲ *Figure 35–11*

Bridging uses bolsters, pillows, and cushions to promote comfort, distribute body weight, and maintain proper body alignment while keeping body parts supported above the mattress. *A*, Foot support while supine; *B*, foot support while side-lying; *C*, body support at hip level.

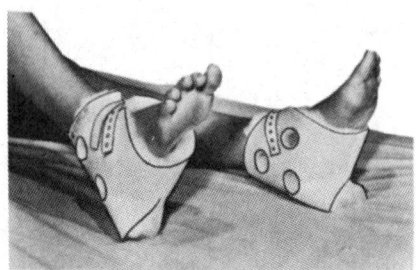

▲ *Figure 35–12*

Ventilated heel protectors. (Courtesy of J.T. Posey Company, Arcadia, California.)

against the bottom sheet and with shearing as these areas are used to "dig in" to the mattress during attempts at movement. Several styles of heel and elbow protectors are available. They all work to provide a barrier between the bed and the soft tissues and to cushion the soft tissues with various soft, fluffy materials. Some models of heel protectors provide a softly lined but rigid support for the heels, and this rigidity helps maintain the ankles at a 90-degree angle, thus assisting in the prevention of footdrop as well as helping prevent pressure ulcers (Fig. 35–12).

Caution "Donuts" (made from abdominal pads that are formed into a circle and covered with roller gauze) were used for many years in an attempt to relieve pressure at the heels and elbows. They have been found to decrease circulation and cause necrosis in the very tissues they were made to protect. Do not use these antiquated devices under any circumstances!

DEVICES TO POSITION SPINE AND EXTREMITIES

Several devices are used to help maintain the spine and extremities in the normal, functioning position and to prevent contractures in immobilized clients.

Footboards. Footboards are rigid, vertical structures that are placed at the foot of the bed to help maintain the ankles in their normal, functioning position in order to prevent footdrop. The footboard should be padded for comfort. It should be adjusted to the client's height so that the soles rest firmly against it and the ankles are maintained at 90 degrees.

Footboards are most effective when the person is supine or prone. When the client is prone, slightly elevate the lower legs on a folded towel or small pillow or extend the feet over the end of the mattress before adjusting the footboard to provide support. If a footboard is not adjustable, use a folded blanket to fill the space between the client's feet and the footboard or between the footboard and the foot of the bed (depending on the model used). In the home, improvised footboards may be made by placing a firm surface (box or piece of wood) at the foot of the bed.

Footboards may be combined with other preventive devices. For example, some footboards (Fig. 35–13) have supports on either side of the feet to prevent external rotation of the hips. If the footboard is high enough to keep the top linens off the toes, it may also serve as a bed cradle.

Bed Cradles. Bed cradles prevent the top linens from touching an area of the body, such as the toes, where the weight of the linens could promote footdrop. They may also protect a body part that is injured and cannot bear the weight of even a sheet without harming the client (Fig. 35–14). Cradles are usually made of a lightweight metal like aluminum or heavy steel wire. To be stable, they may need to be secured to the bed, beneath the mattress. For home use, bed cradles can be made from cardboard boxes that are cut out on one side.

Sandbags. Sandbags are heavy, cylindrical or rectangular sand-filled bags that range in size from a few inches to well over a foot in length. They may be as narrow as an inch or as wide as a foot. They are often used to help position body areas when other devices, such as pillows, will not work as well. For example, they may be placed along the outer aspect of the thighs to prevent external rotation of the hips for the client in the supine position. They are also useful in maintaining the feet in good alignment when the client is in a side-lying position and cannot use a footboard. Sandbags should be kept covered with clean linen, such as a pillow case. They may be padded as necessary.

Caution Sandbags can cause pressure necrosis. Use them with care.

▲ *Figure 35–13*

Adjustable footboard. Its main purpose is to maintain the feet at right angles to the legs to prevent footdrop. The client may push against the footboard for leg muscle exercise and to enhance leg circulation. (Courtesy of J.T. Posey Company.)

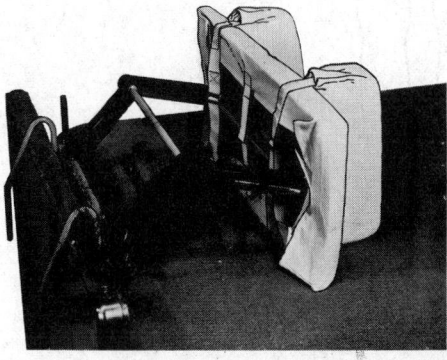
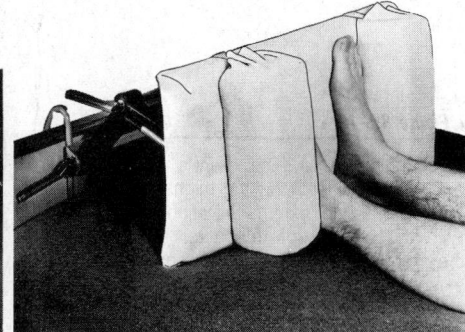

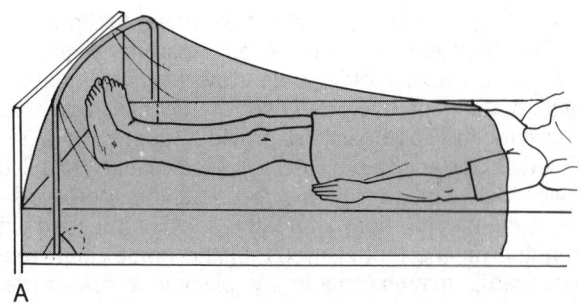

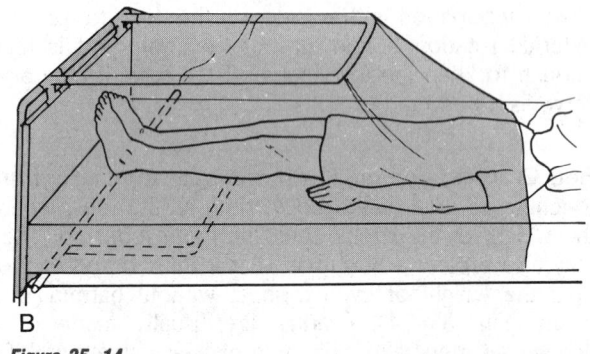

▲ *Figure 35–14*

Bed cradles.

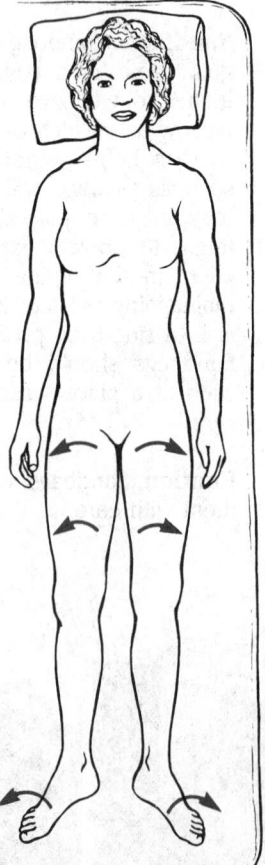

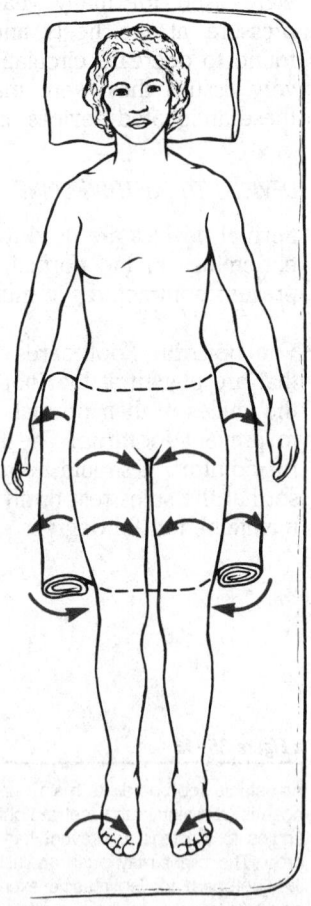

▲ *Figure 35–15*

Trochanter rolls. *A,* The client's toes point outward, following the thighs, as the hips are in external rotation. *B,* With the addition of trochanter rolls, the client's hips return to a position of extension, and the thighs, lower legs, and feet return to normal alignment with toes pointing upward.

A

B

Pillows, Bolsters, Cushions, and Pads. Pillows, bolsters, cushions, and pads not only help protect the soft tissues over bony prominences but also help maintain body parts in proper alignment. A pillow between the knees of a side-lying client helps reduce the pressure on the soft tissue over both knees as it assists in preventing the upper hip from going into a position of adduction. When the right size of cushioning device is not available, you may fashion one with the creative use of available linens; e.g., you may fold a sheet into a small square and place it in a pillow case to help maintain its shape, or you may fold a washcloth several times to make a small pad when one is needed.

Trochanter Rolls. Trochanter rolls help prevent external hip rotation in clients who are in a supine position. Trochanter rolls are made by folding a bath blanket approximately into fourths, lengthwise; centering the lengthwise blanket across the bed, under the client's hips and thighs, between iliac crest and knees; and rolling each end of the blanket under until a long, cylindrical roll of blanket is wedged under each of the client's hips (Fig. 35–15).

Hip Abduction Wedges. Hip abduction wedges are wedge-shaped devices of dense foam latex or polyurethane. The wedge fits between the client's legs and helps maintain the hips in a position of abduction (Fig. 35–16). These devices are often used after a client has a hip joint surgically replaced. In such cases, if the client were to be turned to the side and the operative leg allowed to fall into a natural position, the hip joint could adduct and cause a dislocation of the new joint. The abduction wedge helps prevent this.

Hand Rolls (Hand Grips or Palm Cones). Hand rolls are placed in the palms of the hands to help maintain the normal functioning position of the fingers. Various hand rolls are commercially available (Fig. 35–17). Or they may be easily made by taking a washcloth or abdominal dressing (ABD pad), folding it in half, rolling it into a cylinder, and maintaining it in this shape with tape or roller gauze. If necessary, secure the roll in the person's hand with roller gauze. Remove the roll several times each day for range-of-motion exercises (see Chapter 36) of the fingers and thumb and remove it during the client's bath.

Cockup Splints. Cockup splints are rigid supports that help maintain the wrists in hyperextension as a means of preventing palmar flexion contractures of the wrist (Fig. 35–18). They should be removed for bathing and for range-of-motion exercises.

OTHER EQUIPMENT TO CONSIDER IN POSITIONING

Antiembolism Hose. Antiembolism hose (thromboembolytic deterrent or TED stockings) are not posi-

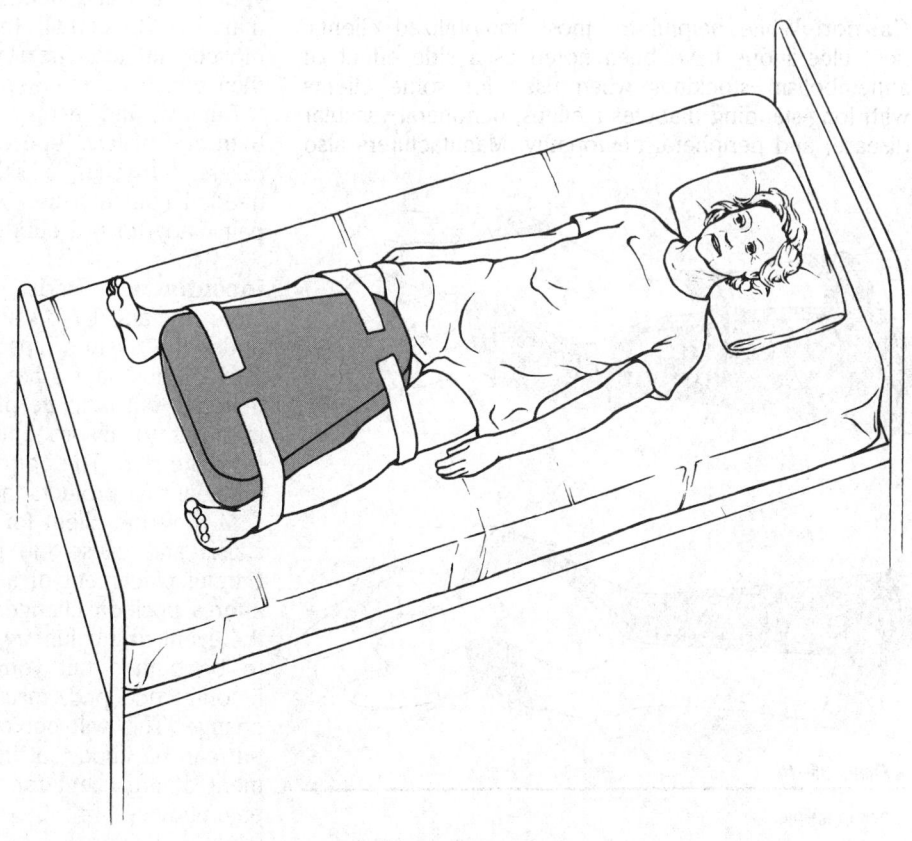

▲ *Figure 35–16*

Hip abduction wedge.

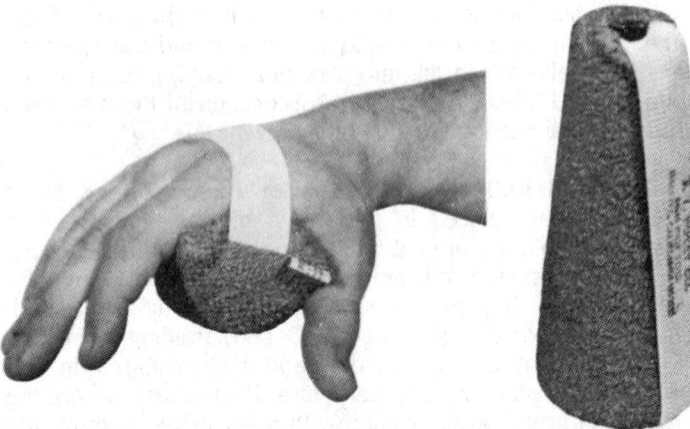

▲ *Figure 35–17*

Hand rolls. (Courtesy of J.T. Posey Company.)

tioning devices but will frequently be encountered in the care of the client who requires positioning. They should be in place before a client is positioned or their application may be difficult.

Often called "Aunty Ems" or "Teds," these firm stockings provide a great deal of support to the legs. They are available in different sizes. Lengths prescribed may be toes-to-knees, toes-to-midthighs, or toes-to-groin. TED stockings are commonly used prophylactically to prevent thrombophlebitis. They promote venous return to the heart and prevent venous pooling in the legs. They are indicated for most individuals who are immobilized but are particularly important for individuals with varicose veins, pregnant women, and individuals who have had recent surgery. An additional benefit is that they can protect the heels from friction. They are, however, not for everyone.

Caution While helpful for most immobilized clients, heel ulcerations have been noted as a side effect of antiembolism stockings when used for some clients with long-standing diabetes mellitus, peripheral vascular disease, and peripheral neuropathy. Manufacturers also warn against the use of their stockings in clients with severe arteriosclerosis.[30]

Apply the stockings initially in the morning, after the client has been in a horizontal position for several hours. Do not apply them once the client's legs have been allowed to fill with blood, as occurs upon standing or upon dangling the legs over the side of the bed. To apply them, do not gather them in a bunch, as you might do with your own socks or stockings. Instead, put one hand and arm inside and use your other hand to invert the upper part of the stocking back over its lower part. Then loosely gather the doubled stocking in your hands and guide it over the client's foot and ankle. To assist in smooth application, use powder to help decrease friction between the stocking and the skin. Pull the stocking up firmly, using the inside of your fingers and hands since fingernails can tear the material. Be certain that all wrinkles have been removed and that the stockings are not bunched up at their tops.

Remove and reapply the stockings at the time of the bath and at least one other time each day in order to assess the client's skin. Launder the stockings as needed (but at least twice weekly) and have a spare pair ready for use during laundering.

Incontinence Pads. Incontinence pads are fairly large, rectangular pads that are meant to be centered under the client's hips, between the waist and knees. The topmost layers are generally made of a soft paper material that is to be placed in contact with the client in order to absorb body fluids and draw them away from the skin. The bottom layer is usually a thin, plastic material that protects the bed linens from soiling.

Moving the client for positioning may stimulate peristalsis and cause the incontinent client to eliminate. Careful placement of an incontinence pad, during and after a position change, can protect the bed linens. In the event of involuntary elimination, the client will have to be bathed but you will only have to change an incontinence pad, instead of doing a complete linen change. This will not only save your time and energy but can be important in eliminating unnecessary movement of the client for whom each movement may be painful.

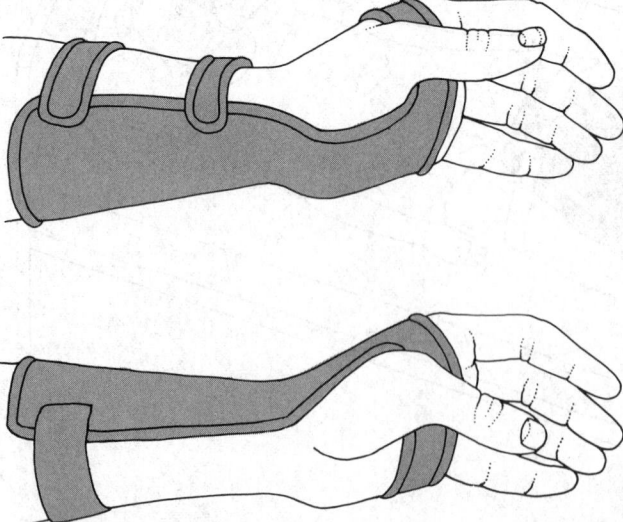

▲ *Figure 35–18*

Cockup splints.

Lift Sheets. A lift sheet should be a full-sized sheet that has been folded into quarters to quadruple its strength. This sheet is positioned under the client and left in place so it is always available to help the client move to a new position.

Positions

The usual positions accepted as safe and comfortable for most clients who can position themselves are described next. When clients are not able to independently attain and maintain these positions, you may place them in position. However, clients who cannot move themselves independently quickly become uncomfortable in any position, so they will require extra comfort measures. It will also be necessary to use additional positioning devices to help them maintain each position. See Procedure 35–2 for more details concerning each position.

SUPINE (BACK-LYING) POSITION

In the supine position, the spine is straight and parallel with the sides of the bed; the head, neck, and upper shoulders are on a pillow; the shoulders, hips, and knees are aligned at the same level bilaterally; the arms are in a position of comfort with the shoulders extended; the hips are in extension; the legs are far enough apart so that the skin between them is not touching; and the ankles are at 90 degrees with the toes pointing straight up.

ORTHOPNEIC POSITION

The orthopneic position is an upright sitting position. In this variation of the supine position, the head pillow is removed, the head of the bed is elevated to 90 degrees, and the client's head and arms are supported on pillows on an overbed table.

SIDE-LYING POSITION

The side-lying position is assumed when the client lies on either the right or the left side of the body. In this position the client lies on one side; the spine is parallel with the sides of the bed; the shoulders are aligned with the hips; the head and neck are supported on a pillow; the lower arm is in front of the body with the shoulder protracted; the lower shoulder and elbow are each flexed 90 degrees; the upper arm is supported comfortably by the body or by a pillow; the lower hips and knees may be extended or flexed; and both ankles are at 90-degree angles.

Caution The National Pressure Ulcer Advisory Panel warns against using the side-lying position for persons susceptible to the development of pressure ulcers. The "rule of thirty" states that these clients should not be turned more than 30 degrees to either side when positioned in bed. Nor should the heads of their beds be elevated more than 30 degrees. This lower head elevation helps prevent shearing, and the decrease in angle

of turn helps prevent excessive pressure from bony prominences.

PRONE (FACE-DOWN) POSITION

In the prone, or face-down, position the spine is straight and parallel with the sides of the bed; the face is turned to one side; the head is flat on the bed or supported only by a small pillow; the shoulders, hips, and knees are aligned at the same level bilaterally; the arms are in a position of comfort with the elbows flexed at 90 degrees and the shoulders both abducted and rotated 90 degrees; the hips are in extension; the legs are slightly separated; the feet either extend over the edge of the mattress or the toes are kept off the mattress by two pillows supporting the lower legs; and the ankles are at 90 degree angles.

SIMS' POSITION

Sims' position is a position between prone and side-lying. Usually Sims' position means the client is on the left side, but the same position is possible with the client on the right side. On the right, the position is correctly referred to as "right Sims'." In Sims' position the client lies on the left side; the spine is parallel with the sides of the bed; the shoulders are aligned with the hips; the body is positioned approximately halfway between that of the side-lying position and that of the prone position; the soft tissue of the face is cushioned by a small pillow; the lower arm is behind the body with the shoulder retracted and hyperextended; the elbow is comfortably flexed; the upper arm and torso are supported comfortably by a pillow; the lower hip is extended with the leg straight; the upper hip and knee are each flexed approximately 45 to 90 degrees; and both ankles are at 90-degree angles.

Positioning the Immobilized Client

To correctly position clients, you must have a clear understanding of body mechanics (if necessary, review Chapter 29). You must also understand how to move a helpless person in bed. Carefully study Procedure 35–1, and be certain you understand this material before you go on to Procedure 35–2 and learn the skill of positioning.

The positions reviewed in Procedure 35–2 are not meant to be rigid formulas that will always work for everyone. They are meant to be a starting place. If you understand the rationale, or scientific principles, behind your nursing actions, you should be able to modify your interventions according to individual client needs. Table 35–5 presents some principles to help guide your actions when positioning clients.

Equipment to Assist in Transferring the Immobilized Client

Procedure 35–1 lists several methods to move an immobilized client in bed: rolling, sliding, lifting, carrying,

Text continued on page 784

PROCEDURE 35–1

Moving a Helpless Person in Bed

Definition/Purposes. Enables one or more nurses/helpers to move a dependent person in bed. Used to correct body alignment, prepare for position change, or prevent complications of immobility.

Contraindications/Cautions. Modify steps according to the sizes of the client and the nurse(s). To maintain spinal alignment, two or more persons should move a client with spinal injuries or spinal surgery. To move a heavy client, obtain additional help and use a lift sheet. Provide for catheters, intravenous lines, and other tubes and attachments to the person's body by allowing enough play to prevent anything from being dislodged by the movement.

Learning/Teaching Guidelines. To maintain or increase muscle strength, encourage clients to move themselves as much as they are able. Even if the client is unconscious, explain how a move is to be accomplished. Teach correct body mechanics to prevent future injuries.

PRELIMINARY ACTIVITIES

Assessment/Planning

- ▶ Review diagnosis and activity orders.
- ▶ Review the chart for the presence of skin, muscle, or bone lesions.
- ▶ Assess level of consciousness and ability to follow directions.
- ▶ Assess mobility level.
- ▶ Plan the type and method of move.
- ▶ Decide upon the number of nurses/helpers needed and the actions of each; one person must be the leader.

Equipment

- ▶ Bed linens and gown, if needed prior to move
- ▶ Firm mattress with smooth, tightly tucked bottom linen
- ▶ Lift sheet (flat sheet folded into quarters)
- ▶ Side rails

Preparation of Person

- ▶ Discuss with client and helpers how the move will be accomplished.
- ▶ Provide privacy; avoid drafts.
- ▶ Adjust bed to working height to reduce back strain, lock wheels, and lower side rails.
- ▶ Cover client with bath blanket.
- ▶ Fan-fold top linen to foot of bed and provide for any tubes or attachments to the client.
- ▶ Move mattress to level position if not contraindicated.
- ▶ Change soiled linen if needed.
- ▶ Place lift sheet under client if needed.
- ▶ Place head pillow against head of bed to cushion the area in the event the client's head hits the headboard.
- ▶ Remove call signal or other items not needed for the move.
- ▶ With more than one helper, remind everyone that movement will occur on the count of "three."

One Nurse Moving Helpless Person to Side of Bed

Actions

1. Face the client's feet and lower the side rail.

2. Support client's feet and lower legs on your forearms as you pull them toward you.

3. Work your hands and forearms under the client's waist and hips and cup your fingers around the body on the opposite side. Pull this section of the body toward you.

   Alternatively, gather near side of lift sheet in your hands until your hands are very near the client's body. Stand as near to the bed as possible with one foot behind the other, and rock your weight from the forward foot to the back foot as you slowly pull the lift sheet, to slide client's torso toward you.

4. Cradle client's head, neck, and upper shoulders as you pull the upper body in line with the rest of the body.

Rationale/Discussion

1. Facing the direction of the planned movement avoids twisting your vertebral column.

2. Keeping heels off the bed during movement helps prevent friction on heels. Pulling requires less effort than lifting or pushing.

3. Supports the client's center of gravity, the heaviest part.

   Keeping the weight to be moved near your center of gravity and rocking to shift the weight toward you uses stronger leg muscles, rather than weaker muscles of the arms and back. The lift sheet decreases friction. Pulling slowly helps assure that you will not pull the lift sheet out from under the client.

4. Cradling helps avoid trauma to the client's cervical spine. This final pull completes the movement.

Caution The foregoing method will not maintain alignment of the client's spine.

PROCEDURE 35-1 Continued

Moving a Helpless Person in Bed

Two Nurses Moving Helpless Person to Side of Bed

Actions	*Rationale/Discussion*
1. One nurse places forearms under client's thighs and second nurse places forearms under client's lower legs.	1. Supporting the client's body on the nurses' forearms helps reduce friction on the client's skin during movement.
2. Standing with one foot approximately 18 inches in front of the other, on count of "three" rock backward to shift weight while pulling to move client's legs to side of bed.	2. Rocking to shift the weight uses longer, stronger leg muscles rather than weaker muscles of the arms and back.
3. Nurses position arms under client's head and trunk (Fig. 35–19). Together, on count of "three," rock back to pull client's body to side of bed, in line with legs and feet.	3. Moving the head and torso at the same time helps keep client's cervical spine straighter than when one nurse works alone but *this does not maintain complete spinal alignment.*

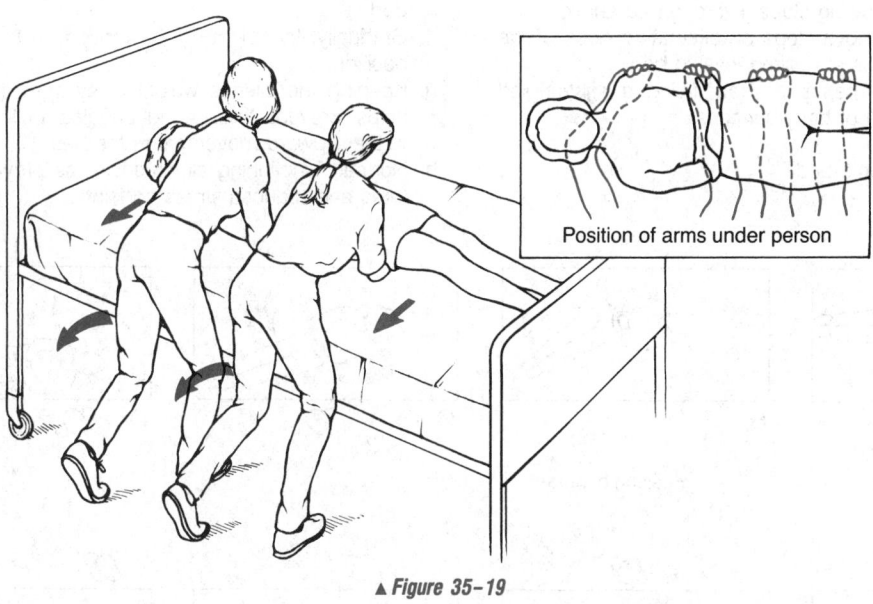

Position of arms under person

▲ *Figure 35–19*

Three Nurses Moving Helpless Person to Side of Bed

Actions	*Rationale/Discussion*
1. First nurse supports the client's head, neck, and chest; second nurse supports the hips; and third nurse supports the thighs and ankles.	1. The strongest person should be at the client's hips as this is the heaviest part of the client.
2. Standing with one foot approximately 18 inches in front of the other, on count of "three" rock backward to shift weight while pulling to move client to side of bed in one smooth motion.	2. Rocking to shift the weight uses longer, stronger leg muscles rather than weaker muscles of the arms and back. Working in unison helps reduce strain on nurses and helps maintain client's spinal alignment.

One Nurse Moving Helpless Client Up in Bed

Actions	*Rationale/Discussion*
1. Lower side rail on side nearest you and stand approximately at the level of the client's knees. Face the client's feet so you are at an angle of approxiamtely 40 degrees, in relation to the bed.	1. Facing in the direction of the planned movement avoids twisting your vertebral column.

Procedure continued on following page

PROCEDURE 35–1 Continued

Moving a Helpless Person in Bed

Actions

2. Move dependent person's body diagonally, in sections (Fig. 35–20).

   a. Pull person's legs diagonally toward head of bed as you pull them toward you.
   b. Place your forearms under the client's hips and pull in same direction as done with the feet. Use lift sheet for heavier clients.
   c. Cradle the client's head, neck, and upper shoulders as you pull the upper body in line with the rest of the body.
   d. Raise side rail and go to the other side of the bed.
   e. Repeat diagonal pull of body sections from other side of the bed, following steps 1 through 2d above.
   f. Repeat all of above steps on alternating sides of the bed until client is at desired level in bed.
   g. Pull person to center of bed, using a right-angled (90-degree) pull of body sections.

   h. Align the person's body.

Rationale/Discussion

2. Used when helpless person can easily be moved by one helper, but this method *does not maintain spinal alignment.*
   a. Pulling requires less energy than pushing.

   b. Your arms (or the lift sheet) help protect the client's skin from effects of friction.

   c. Cradling helps avoid trauma to the client's cervical spine. The final pull moves the client completely to one side and slightly upward in the bed.
   d. Side rails help prevent falls.
   e. Diagonal pulls will move the person slightly higher in bed.
   f. Gradually, the client will be moved up to the desired position.
   g. Keeping the client's weight away from the side rails helps prevent falls. A right-angled pull will prevent further upward movement in the bed.
   h. Normal, functioning alignment helps prevent contractures and reduces stress on joints.

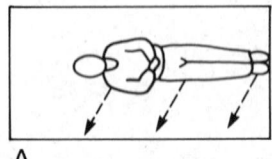

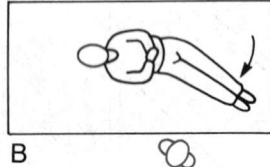

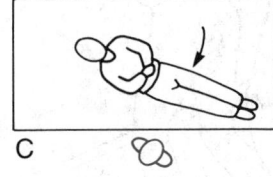

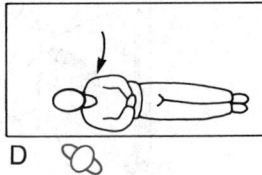

Position of nurse

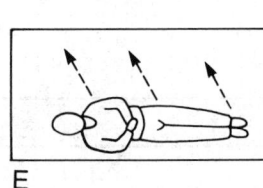

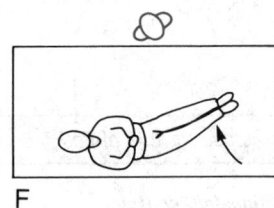

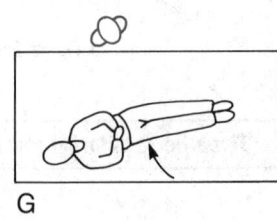

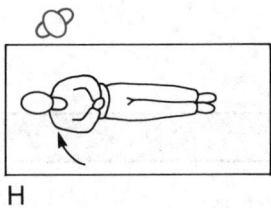

▲ *Figure 35–20*

PROCEDURE 35–1 Continued

Moving a Helpless Person in Bed

Two Nurses Moving Helpless Client Up in Bed

Actions

1. With person in supine position, nurses stand on opposite sides of the bed and lower the side rails.
2. Each nurse gathers one side of the lift sheet firmly in both hands until the hands are very near the client's body at the client's hip and shoulder level. The nurses stand as close to the bed as possible.

3. If possible, have the client grasp the headboard with both hands and flex the knees with the soles flat on the bed. Ask the client to pull with the hands and push with the feet on the count of "three."
   If the client is unable to assist, place the client's arms across the chest and flex the knees so the soles are flat on the bed.
   If the client is unable to support the neck and head, one nurse should use the arm nearest the head of the bed to cradle the client's neck and upper shoulders and the other arm to grasp the lift sheet.
4. Nurses point their feet toward the head of the bed, with one foot behind the other and the feet separated approximately 18 inches.
5. One nurse counts to three. On the word "three," both nurses lift together and rock their weight from the foot behind to the foot in front and place the lift sheet and client back down on the bed.

Rationale/Discussion

1. Both side rails may be down if nurses are on both sides of the bed to guard against falls.
2. These actions bring client's weight as near as possible to the nurses' centers of gravity. They also help assure that the lifting force will be at the area of the greatest weight. Weight should be equally distributed between the two nurses.
3. Having the client help encourages use of the arm muscles to pull and the leg muscles to push and will help decrease feelings of dependence.

   Positioning the limbs of the more dependent client prevents dragging the extremities over the sheet and creating friction on elbows and heels.
   Cradling helps protect the cervical spine from injury.

4. Facing the direction of movement avoids twisting the nurses' backs. Keeping the feet apart provides a wide base of support for stability.
5. Rocking shifts the weight forward by using the leg muscles, rather than the muscles of the arms and the back, for movement.

One Nurse Assisting Client Who Can Help Move Up in Bed

Actions

1. Face the client at approximately waist level. Lower the side rail on your side of the bed.
2. Ask the client to place both feet on the mattress, flex the knees, and grasp the headboard, trapeze, or mattress top with both hands. Ask client to pull with the hands and push with the feet on the count of "three." Remind client that the pillow at the headboard is there for protection.

3. Place your arm (the one that is closer to the head of the bed) under the client's waist. Place the other arm under the most proximal portion of the client's thighs, grasping the thigh on the far side. Move your body close to the bed.

Rationale/Discussion

1. Facing in the direction of the planned movement avoids twisting your vertebral column.
2. This encourages muscle use in arms and legs and decreases feelings of helplessness. It also helps prevent elbow and heel friction by avoiding dragging of extremities. If overhead trapeze is used, it should be high enough, toward the head of the bed, that pulling on it and flexing the elbows will indeed help the client move upward. Otherwise, the client will merely raise the torso up in the air and the actual work done to move toward the head of the bed will be done by the client's feet. This can result in shearing as client attempts to "dig into" the mattress with the heels.
3. This will place the client nearer your center of gravity for ease in lifting. Your greatest force will be exerted at the heaviest part of the client's body. Placing your arm more distally on the client's thighs and exerting pressure, when client's knees and hips are flexed, may cause you to succeed in merely increasing the angle of the client's hip flexion. At best, your arm may only provide a stable surface for client's thighs to push against while preventing straightening the knees to effect movement.

Procedure continued on following page

PROCEDURE 35–1 Continued

Moving a Helpless Person in Bed

Actions	Rationale/Discussion
4. Face the head of the bed, toes pointing forward, and feet apart.	4. Facing the direction of movement prevents twisting of the spine. A wide base of support increases stability.
5. On your count of "three," shift your weight as you help lift the client's weight up in the bed (see Fig. 35–21).	5. Shifting weight uses the long, strong muscles of the legs instead of the muscles of the arms and back.

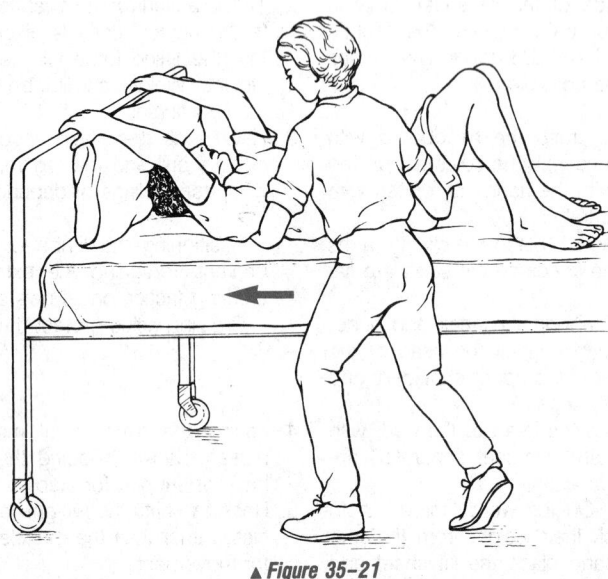

▲ Figure 35–21

FINAL ACTIVITIES

Assess client's skin condition; assess for pain or discomfort caused or relieved by the move; check person for correct body alignment; check any tubes present to be certain they are still in place and functioning correctly and secure them as necessary; check bed linen for smoothness; replace head pillow and other positioning devices as needed; cover person; replace call signal; raise rails; lower bed; discard soiled laundry. Document assessment data and teaching done.

PROCEDURE 35–2

Positioning a Helpless Person in Bed

Definition/Purposes. Places an immobilized person in a safe position with correct body alignment in order to prevent or minimize the potential complications of immobility.

Contraindications/Cautions. To move the client safely during positioning, review Procedure 35–1, as needed. Modify positions according to the individual needs of the client. Note that research studies have demonstrated that some immobilized clients must be repositioned *at least* every 2 hours, around the clock, if disuse phenomena are to be prevented. Use mechanical assistive devices according to manufacturer's instructions. Always check the client's chart for contraindications/cautions. Consult with the physician concerning any questions you may have about the client's ability to tolerate a position.

To maintain spinal alignment, two or more persons should position a client with spinal injuries or spinal surgery. To position a heavy client, obtain additional help and use a lift sheet for moving and turning. Keep sheets smooth, clean, and free of wrinkles, as an immobilized person's skin can break down easily if the weight of a body part is left over a wet spot, a wrinkle, or an object that has been left in the bed. Provide for catheters, IV lines, and other tubes and attachments to the person's body. Coil tubing loosely on the bed, allowing enough play to prevent anything from being dislodged during positioning.

Learning/Teaching Guidelines. To maintain or increase muscle strength, encourage clients to assist in moving themselves as much as they are able. Even if clients are unconscious, explain how a position is to be accomplished and explain the benefits of the planned position. Tell clients that the position of the head, arms, and legs can be adjusted for comfort. Let clients know when the next position change is planned. Encourage them to report discomfort or difficulty in breathing so you can change the position, if necessary.

PRELIMINARY ACTIVITIES

Assessment/Planning

► Review diagnosis and activity orders.
► Review the chart for the presence of skin, muscle, or bone lesions.
► Assess mobility level and limitations concerning activity.
► Assess level of consciousness and ability to follow directions.
► Review turning schedule.
► Review the record concerning the last time the client was in the planned position and how this was tolerated.
► Plan the type of position and method of moving client into it.
► Decide upon the number of persons needed and the actions of each; one person must be the leader.

Equipment

► Bed linens and gown, if needed prior to moving to new position
► Antiembolism hose, if needed
► Firm mattress with smooth, tightly tucked bottom linen
► Lift sheet (flat sheet folded into quarters)
► Side rails
► Padded footboard

► Pillows of various sizes, as needed
► Bolster, cushions, and pads, as needed
► Bath blanket
► Incontinence pad, if needed

Preparation of Person

► Discuss with client and helpers how the positioning will be accomplished.
► Provide privacy; avoid drafts.
► Adjust bed to working height to reduce back strain, lock wheels, and lower side rails.
► Cover client with bath blanket.
► Fan-fold top linen to foot of bed and provide for any tubes or attachments to the client.
► Be certain mattress is at the head of the bed.
► Move mattress to level position if not contraindicated.
► Remove call signal, pillows, and other positioning devices.
► Change soiled linen, if needed.
► Place lift sheet under client, if needed.
► Remove head pillow or place it against head of bed to cushion the area.

Supine Position

Actions

1. With client centered supine on mattress and ready to be turned, roll the client to one side and place a fan-folded incontinence pad under the hips, if needed. Place a fan-folded bath blanket, which you have prepared as a trochanter roll, between waist and knee level.

Rationale/Discussion

1. Placement of linens, pads, and so on under the client should be done first, to avoid moving the client later. Movement may stimulate peristalsis.

Procedure continued on following page

PROCEDURE 35–2 Continued

Positioning a Helpless Person in Bed

Actions	Rationale/Discussion

Actions

2. Roll the client to the other side, bring the linens through, and lift them to place a small pillow at the lumbar curvature. Smooth the linens and roll the client onto the back with the pillow in place.

3. Center the client's body with the spine straight. Align the shoulders, hips, and knees at the same level, bilaterally.

4. Roll the two ends of the folded bath blanket under, and wedge the rolls under the hips and thighs to maintain the hips in extension with the legs straight and slightly separated (Fig. 35–22).

5. Place client's head, neck, and upper shoulders on a pillow.

6. Place the upper arms on a pillow in a position of comfort, with the shoulders extended. Place the forearms and hands on one or two pillows to assure that they are higher than the upper arms.

7. Place a cockup splint on each forearm, if needed.

8. Place a handroll in each hand, if needed.

9. Place a pillow under the lower legs.

Rationale/Discussion

2. The small pillow will be on the bottom (protected by an incontinence pad, if needed) and the bath blanket should be next to the client's skin. The pillow will provide support and maintain the normal curvature of the lumbar spine.

3. Keeping the spine straight reduces strain on muscles.

4. A trochanter roll prevents external rotation of the hips. Separating the legs prevents the two skin surfaces from being in contact. The skin is an organ of excretion.

5. Pillow should be large enough to support the cervical curvature but small enough that it will not cause cervical flexion contractures.

6. This will prevent internal rotation, muscle strain, and perhaps dislocation of the shoulder joints; hyperextension of the elbow joints; and edema of the upper extremities. For adequate elevation to prevent edema, each joint should be higher than the joint proximal to it.

7. These help prevent flexion contractures of the wrists.

8. These help maintain the normal functioning position of the hands.

9. Helps prevent hyperextension of the knees and helps keep the heels off the mattress, thus preventing pressure ulcers on the heels. Also, helps prevent leg edema.

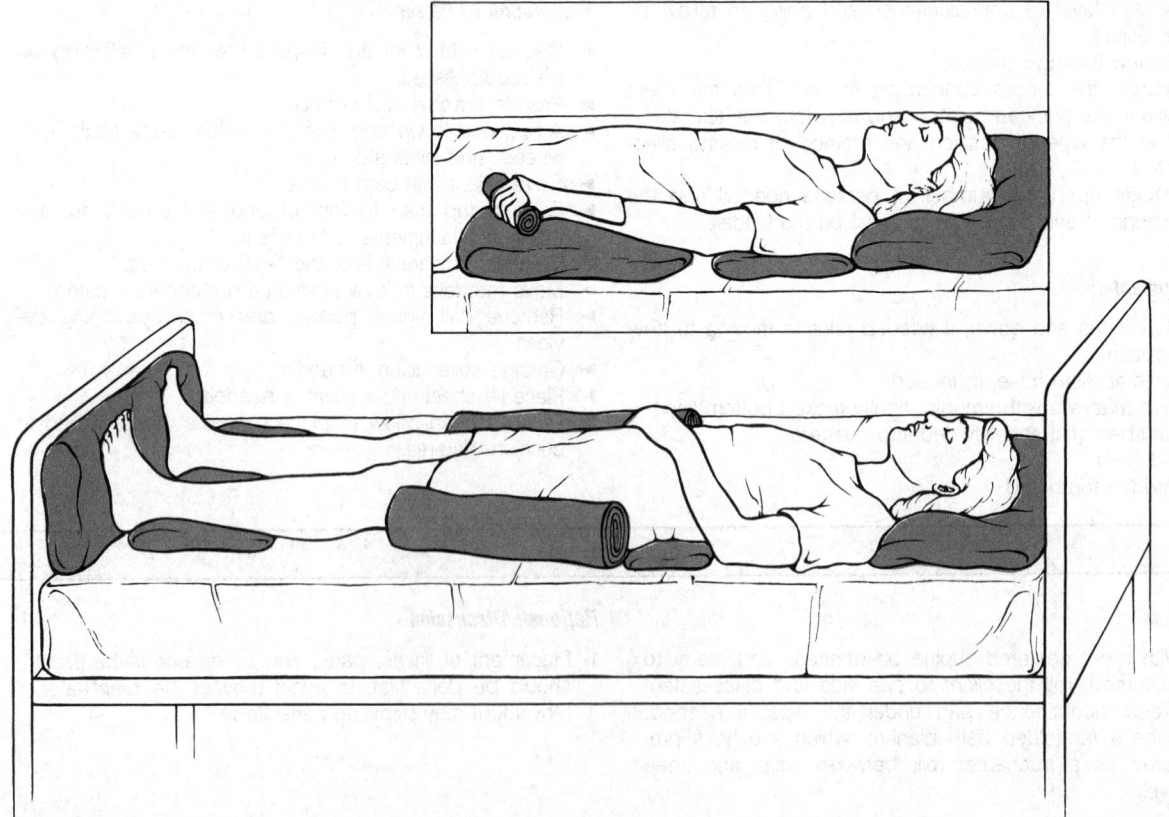

▲ **Figure 35–22**

A client in the supine position with trochanter rolls in place, with lumbar pillow visible, prior to positioning arm. Inset shows pillows for arm.

PROCEDURE 35–2 Continued

Positioning a Helpless Person in Bed

Actions	*Rationale/Discussion*
10. Place ankles at 90-degree angles, with the soles firmly against a footboard and with the toes pointing straight up.	10. Helps maintain normal ankle position and prevents footdrop.

Side-Lying Position

Caution Do not use this position for persons who are at risk for pressure ulcers.

Actions	*Rationale/Discussion*
1. With the client in supine position, remove all pillows and positioning devices. Assess the skin surfaces that are visible in this position. If a urinary drainage bag is present, clamp the tubing to prevent backflow of urine into the bladder, and move the bag to the side of the bed toward which the client will be turned.	1. Once turned, some skin surface will no longer be visible for easy assessment. Preventing backflow helps prevent infection. Moving the bag helps provide for the tubing during the turn and may improve the flow of urine after the turn.
2. Lower the side rail and move the client approximately halfway between the center of the mattress and the edge of the bed, to the side opposite the one the client will face when turned (see Procedure 35–1).	2. When turned, the client will be centered on the mattress.
3. Place a small pillow at client's waist level at the side toward which the client will turn.	3. When turned, the waist pillow will be in place to help prevent lateral flexion of the lumbar spine.
4. Place the client's head pillow so it will support only the head and neck, after the turn.	4. Helps prevent lateral flexion of the cervical spine and strain on neck and shoulder muscles.
5. Raise the side rails and go around to the opposite side of the bed. Lower the side rail. Abduct the client's shoulder nearest to you approximately 90 degrees and flex the elbow approximately 90 degrees.	5. Prevents client from rolling onto the arm during the turn.
6. Place the client's other arm and hand across the abdomen and place the far leg across the near leg. Omit this step if the spine or hips must remain extended.	6. This will facilitate the turn by shifting part of the body weight toward the direction of the turn.
7. Cup your fingers around the client's body at shoulder and hip level, unless contraindicated, and pull the client to roll toward you. Alternatively, reach over the client and gather the lift sheet toward the client where you can use it to pull the client toward you. Adjust the waist and head pillows as necessary (Fig. 35–23).	7. Pulling requires less work than pushing.
8. Gently pull the client's lower shoulder into protraction.	8. This prevents the weight of the body from pressing on the soft tissues of the arm and altering circulation or damaging nerves.
9. Place the upper arm and hand on one or two pillows with the shoulder and elbow each flexed 90 degrees.	9. Prevents cross-adduction and internal rotation of the upper shoulder joint and will place the arm in front of the client to allow for better chest expansion.
10. Place a cockup splint on each forearm, if needed.	10. These help prevent flexion contractures of the wrists.

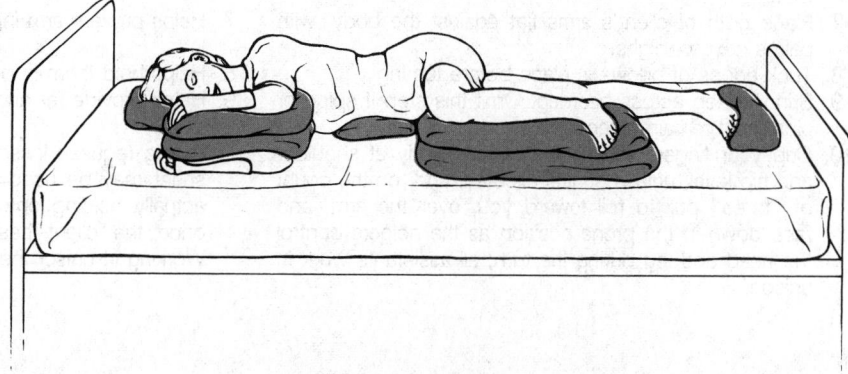

▲ *Figure 35–23*

A client in side-lying position.

Procedure continued on following page

PROCEDURE 35-2 Continued

Positioning a Helpless Person in Bed

Actions	Rationale/Discussion
11. Place a handroll in each hand, if needed.	11. These help maintain the normal functioning position of the hands.
12. Place two or more pillows under the upper leg and foot to help support the leg with the hip and knee at 45 to 90 degrees of flexion and the ankle at 90 degrees.	12. Helps prevent cross-adduction of the hip joint, reduces pressure on bony prominences at the knees, and prevents inversion and plantar flexion of the ankle.
13. Place the sole of the lower foot firmly against a sandbag that is large and heavy enough to maintain the ankle at 90 degrees.	13. Helps prevent footdrop.

Prone Position

Actions	Rationale/Discussion
1. With client in supine position, assemble nurses with at least one person on each side of the bed and another supporting the head. Remove all pillows and positioning devices. Lower the side rails. Roll the lift sheet up against both sides of the client's body and grasp firmly. With one nurse cradling the client's head and neck, on the count of "three" all nurses lift the client off the bed in unison and move toward the foot of the bed in one smooth movement. A heavy person may need to be moved in two or more stages. Position the client so the feet extend beyond the end of the mattress.	1. Use of more than one helper, use of lift sheet, and moving in stages all help prevent "dragging" the client across the sheet and help prevent skin damage due to friction. After the turn, client's toes should be well over the end of the mattress.
2. Move the client to the side of the bed opposite the direction of the planned turn (see Procedure 35-1).	2. Allows room for the client's comfort and safety after the turn.
3. Assess skin surfaces that are visible in this position. If a urinary drainage bag is present, clamp the tubing to prevent backflow of urine into the bladder, and move the bag to the side of the bed toward which the client will be turned.	3. Once turned, the anterior skin surfaces will no longer be visible. Preventing backflow helps prevent infection. Moving the bag helps provide for the tubing during the turn and may improve the flow of urine after the turn.
4. In preparation for the turn, place pillows on the bed next to the client and in line with the body as follows: a. Lower chest and abdomen for women; waist to symphysis pubis for men. b. Thighs, below hip, and above patella. c. Lower legs, below knees, and above ankles. Use two pillows here if not able to place feet over end of mattress.	4. Pillows will comfortably support body weight and help maintain normal alignment. a. Helps protect breasts and scrotum from pressure while reducing lumbar curve. b. Helps avoid pressure on patella. c. Helps prevent hyperextension of knees and lumbar spine.
5. Remove bath blanket. Adjust gown or pajama top so it is smooth over chest and loose at neck and shoulders.	5. Helps prevent the pressure of wrinkles under the person's full body weight and will avoid uncomfortable tightness at neck and axillae.
6. Stand on side of bed toward which the client will turn. Have a helper support the head and neck. An additional helper, if available, should hold the far leg and foot.	6. Additional helpers allow for safe body mechanics and enable the client to be turned as a unit.
7. Place both of client's arms flat against the body, with palms next to thighs.	7. Helps prevent arm injuries during turn.
8. Tuck edges of pillows in place before turning.	8. Helps hold them in place during turn.
9. Bring far leg across near leg. Omit this step if spine or hips must remain extended.	9. Helps provide for an easier turn.
10. Cup your fingers around the client's body at shoulder and hip level, unless contraindicated, and, on the count of "three" pull to roll toward you, over the arm, and face down in the prone position as the helpers control the head and leg during the turn; all assistants work in unison.	10. Pulling requires less work than pushing. Although a lift sheet may be used to help roll the client toward you, actually holding onto the body provides more control once the client has started to roll face downward. Working in unison helps maintain spinal alignment.

PROCEDURE 35–2 Continued

Positioning a Helpless Person in Bed

Actions	Rationale/Discussion
11. Immediately check client's nose and mouth to be certain client is breathing. Turn head if necessary or place small pillow or pad under one side of the face for comfort.	11. Helps assure that airway is not obstructed by nose or mouth pressing into mattress. A small pillow can prevent pressure from facial bones without obstructing the airway. The position should allow for drainage of secretions should any tend to accumulate.
12. Adjust the waist and leg pillows as necessary to distribute body weight evenly (Fig. 35–24.)	12. Promotes proper body mechanics and increases comfort.
13. Abduct both shoulders 90 degrees. Flex both elbows 90 degrees. Place both shoulders in external rotation, or place one in external rotation and one in internal rotation (Fig. 35–25).	13. This helps maintain normal range of joint motion by preventing adduction of the shoulder.
14. Place rolls of linen or small pillows at the angles between the lateral clavicles and axillae (see Figs. 35–24 and 35–25).	14. Shoulder rolls provide support to upper chest to facilitate expansion, and they reduce pressure on the anterior shoulders.
15. Place cockup splints on forearms, if needed.	15. Helps prevent flexion contractures of the wrists.

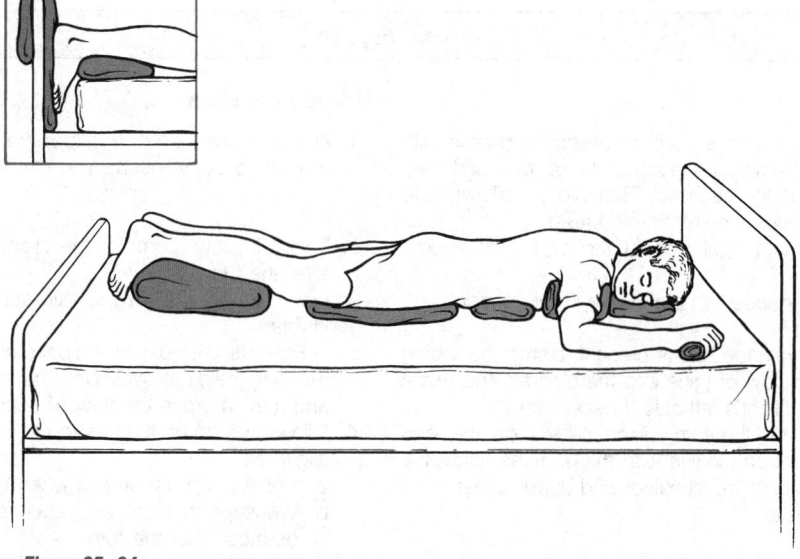

▲ *Figure 35–24*

A client in prone position.

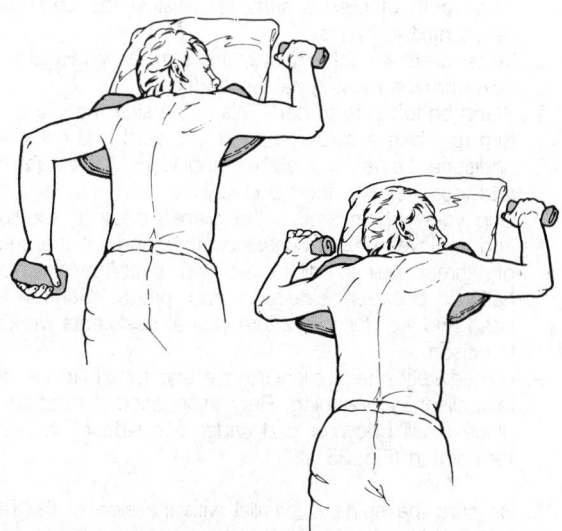

▲ *Figure 35–25*

Prone shoulder positions. *A*, One shoulder may be in internal rotation with the other in external rotation, or *B*, both shoulders may be in external rotation.

Procedure continued on following page

PROCEDURE 35–2 Continued

Positioning a Helpless Person in Bed

Actions	Rationale/Discussion
16. Place a handroll in each hand, if needed.	16. Helps maintain the normal functioning position of the hands.
17. Observe client from side and foot of bed for correct body alignment.	17. Correct alignment promotes comfort and reduces stress on muscles and joints.
18. Check that client's feet are over the end of the mattress or are supported on two pillows with the ankles at a 90-degree angle. Adjust padded footboard or pillows as necessary to achieve this angle.	18. Helps prevent footdrop.
19. Feel under all bony prominences (including under toes) for evidence of pressure. Adjust pillows as necessary for comfort.	19. Helps prevent skin breakdown.
20. Periodically change positions of arms and neck.	20. This can help maintain range of motion, decrease joint stiffness, and increase comfort.
21. To return to supine position, reverse the above procedure. Observe males for scrotal edema.	21. Scrotal edema can result from dependent edema associated with medical conditions or from pressure that obstructs circulation.

Sims' Position

Actions	Rationale/Discussion
1. With the client in supine position, assemble nurses with at least one person on each side of the bed and another supporting the head. Remove all pillows and positioning devices. Lower the side rails.	1. Use of more than one helper aids in maintaining safety with good body mechanics.
2. Move the client to right side of the bed. (See Procedure 35–1.)	2. This will allow room for the client's comfort and safety after the turn to the left.

3. Assess skin surfaces that are visible in this position.
 	
   If a urinary drainage bag is present, clamp the tubing to prevent backflow of urine into the bladder and move the bag to the client's left side if necessary.
	3. Once turned, part of the skin surface will no longer be visible.
	   Preventing backflow helps prevent infection. Moving the bag helps provide for the tubing during the turn and may improve the flow of urine after the turn.

4. In preparation for the turn, place pillows on the bed next to the client and in line with the body as follows:
  a. One to two near the shoulder and upper chest
  b. Waist to knees
 	
  c. Knee to thigh
	4. Pillows will comfortably support arms and legs in good alignment.
	  a. Will support upper arm when client is turned.
	  b. Will support thigh and knee of leg that will be uppermost after the turn.
	  c. Will be moved in place, after the turn, to support the right lower leg and foot. Right leg will be uppermost.

5. Place both of client's arms flat against the body with palms next to thighs.	5. Helps prevent arm injuries during turn.
6. Place client's right leg over left leg. Omit this step if spine or hips must remain extended.	6. Helps provide for an easier turn.
7. Stand on left side of bed. This is the side the client will turn to. Have a helper support the head and neck. An additional helper, if available, should hold the right leg and foot. Remove the bath blanket.	7. Additional helpers allow for safe body mechanics and enable the client to be turned as a unit.
8. Cup your fingers around the client's body at shoulder and hip level, unless contraindicated, and, on the count of "three" pull to roll toward you, over the arm, and halfway between side-lying and prone. Control the head and leg during the turn with all assistants working in unison.	8. Pulling requires less work than pushing. Although a lift sheet may be used to help roll the client toward you, actually holding onto the body provides more control once the client has started to roll face downward. Working in unison helps maintain spinal alignment.
9. Immediately check client's nose and mouth to be certain client is breathing. Reposition neck if needed or place small pillow or pad under one side of the face for comfort (Fig. 35–26).	9. Helps assure that airway is not obstructed by nose or mouth pressing into mattress. A small pillow can help prevent pressure from facial bones without obstructing the airway. The position should allow for drainage of secretions should any tend to accumulate.
10. Be sure the spine is parallel with the side of the bed and that the shoulders are in line with the hips.	10. Helps maintain normal body alignment and prevents strain on muscles and joints.

PROCEDURE 35–2 Continued

Positioning a Helpless Person in Bed

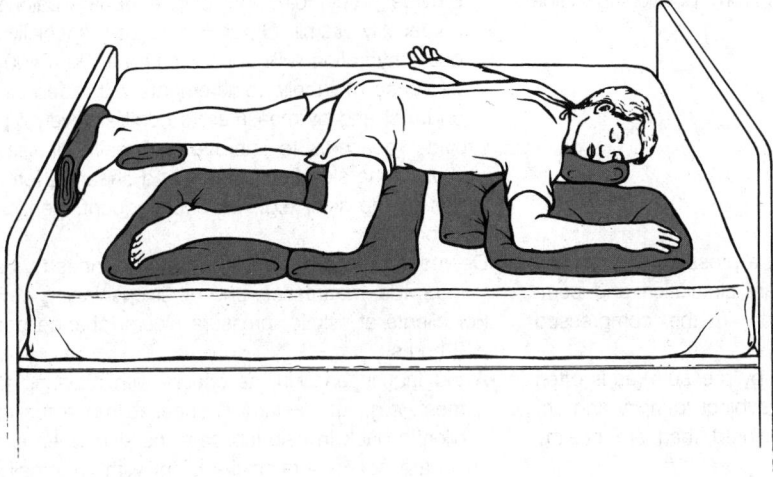

▲ *Figure 35–26*

A client in Sims' position.

Actions	**Rationale/Discussion**
11. Retract and hyperextend the lower shoulder and place the arm in a position of comfort behind the client's body.	11. Prevents the weight of the body from pressing on the soft tissues of the arm and altering circulation or damaging nerves.
12. Check that the right arm is comfortably flexed with the arm and torso supported by the one or two pillows placed before the turn. Add another pillow if necessary.	12. These pillows help prevent cross-adduction and internal rotation of the shoulder joint and prevent the torso from rolling to the prone position.
13. Place a cockup splint on each forearm, if needed.	13. These help prevent flexion contractures of the wrists.
14. Place a handroll in each hand, if needed.	14. These help maintain the normal functioning position of the hands.
15. Check that the left hip is extended, with the leg straight, and that the right hip and knee are each flexed approximately 45 degrees, with the leg and foot supported on two or more pillows.	15. Pillows help prevent cross-adduction of the hip joint, reduce pressure on the bony prominences at the knee, and prevent inversion and plantar flexion of the right ankle. The pillows also prevent the lower body from rolling into a prone position.
16. Place the sole of the left foot firmly against a sandbag to maintain it at 90 degrees.	16. Helps prevent footdrop.

FINAL ACTIVITIES

Remove bath blanket if not already removed; check for correct body alignment; check any tubes to be certain they are still in place and functioning correctly and secure them as necessary; check bed linens for smoothness; assess the skin newly exposed by the turn; assess the person's comfort level; replace covers; replace the call signal; raise the side rails; lower the bed; discard any soiled linens. Document assessment data.

TABLE 35–5. Selected Scientific Principles and Related Nursing Interventions for Positioning and Moving an Immobilized Client

Principle	Nursing Interventions
Maintaining or improving the health of tissues that will be under increased stress from positioning helps assure their survival.	Provide measures to improve the health of tissues internally, e.g., provide proper diet, including adequate calories, protein, vitamins (especially vitamin C), and minerals (especially zinc); maintain adequate hydration with approximately 1500–2400 ml of fluid per day; decrease metabolic requirements with adequate periods of activity and rest and by measures to combat fever, if present. Provide measures to improve the health of tissues externally, e.g., protect the skin from friction and shearing forces; increase circulation to the skin, e.g., provide frequent, gentle massage with mild lotions.
Compression of soft tissues at a pressure greater than 32 mm Hg prevents capillary circulation and compromises tissue oxygenation in the compressed area. Tissues that are compromised by pressure (as is often true in immobility) are more subject to injury and are less prone to heal when injured than are healthy tissues.	Decrease pressure overy bony prominences by using pressure-relieving beds, mattresses, and other cushioning devices. For clients at risk for pressure ulcers, change position at least every 2 hours. Avoid friction on skin, as occurs with shearing forces during movement, e.g., use a turning sheet to move the client or powder the client's back to help lubricate the skin when sliding is necessary. Use care not to scratch the client with fingernails, wristwatch, name pin, or other things during lifts and carrys. Position to avoid pressure on soft tissues, e.g., avoid positioning with one body part lying over another, use bridging to prevent pressure over bony prominences, elevate extremities to decrease the pressure of edema on extremity tissues. Avoid use of restraints, if possible. Avoid losing control of client and causing a fall, by always planning ahead, always having sufficient help, having the strongest person support the heaviest part of the client (under the hips), correctly using any equipment needed, and using good body mechanics.
When the hips and knees are flexed, blood pools in the hip area and increases the danger of phlebitis. Pressure can cause injury to a vein wall and result in thrombus formation in an immobilized person.	Avoid positions causing prolonged knee and hip flexion, e.g., avoid using the knee gatch when the head of the bed is also elevated. Avoid placing a pillow under the client's knees and causing pressure on the popliteal space. Avoid flexing the hospital bed mattress at the knee gatch and causing pressure on the client's popliteal space.
No organism can survive in its own excreta.	Keep skin clean and dry. Avoid two skin surfaces coming into contact for prolonged periods.
Without regular exercise, muscle fibers shorten into contractures. Larger, stronger muscle groups pull distal extremities toward them as the fibers shorten.	Use bedboards, pillows and a firm mattress to help assure good body alignment. Position to help maintain the normal, functioning position of the joints, e.g., fingers around handrolls or cones, cockup splints on forearms, pillows avoided under the knee, ankles firmly maintained by footboard.
Gravity and the weight of bedcovers assist in the formation of deformities.	Help prevent spinal and shoulder deformities by supporting in normal functioning position with pillows, cushions, or bolsters. Help prevent external rotation of the hip joints by using a trochanter roll. Help prevent footdrop by using a bed cradle with a footboard.
Adequate oxygen is necessary for human life.	Position in a manner that allows free exchange of gases through respiratory openings and that allows adequate chest expansion. Position frequently to assist in moving secretions out of the lungs and to increase peristalsis and prevent a buildup of flatus that can reduce lung expansion.

TABLE 35-5. *Selected Scientific Principles and Related Nursing Interventions for Positioning and Moving an Immobilized Client* **Continued**

Principle	Nursing Interventions
Stress on muscles and bones helps prevent formation of calcium kidney stones by decreasing the movement of calcium from the bones to the blood (and then to the kidneys).	Place the client in a standing position for at least 2 hours per day, when allowed, e.g., position vertically in CircOlectric bed. Teach isometric exercises to increase stress on muscles and bones of upper extremities. **Caution** Isometric exercises increase the blood pressure and can lead to dangerous complications in persons who have heart disease. Always consult a physician before instituting an exercise program. Encourage use of legs, e.g., pressing on footboard with feet. If unable to provide at least 2 hours' stress on muscles and bones daily, suggest a decrease in calcium intake.
The supine position results in a 30 per cent increase in cardiac workload.[13] The ideal bed or positioning device is yet to be invented.	Whenever possible, a person whose heart needs rest should rest in the sitting rather than the supine position. Carefully assess the needs of each client. Recommend the bed, mattress, and other positioning devices best suited to the individual client's needs.
In a totally helpless individual, unsupported body parts fall downward by gravity at a rate of 32.2 feet per second squared.	Always support the client's head and neck during transfer to prevent severe damage to the cervical spine. Be sure extremities are supported to prevent joint damage during transfer.
Clients immobilized with painful conditions require special consideration during movement to prevent an increase in pain.	Support weak limbs, without squeezing them, by cradling them on the flat of your hand and arm rather than grasping them from above in a pinching fashion. Instruct the person to keep a straight spine and move the body and body parts as a unit. Never allow part of a limb to drag while moving another part of the body. Move slowly and steadily when supporting an injured or painful part. Allow the person to help in the move as much as possible. Stop if the person requests it, provided it is safe to do so. Pause if muscular resistance occurs.
Tissues can be traumatized and the client's safety can be threatened if tubes are inadvertently pulled out during client movement.	Plan ahead and assure that tubes are free to move as the client moves. Assure that tubes are long enough to reach as far as necessary. If possible, coil them loosely on the bed to provide play should it be needed during the move. Always provide time and attend to tubes without rushing. Know how to move a client safely with the type of tube present or get help from someone who does know.
An object in motion tends to stay in motion.	Lock wheels to prevent the bed, stretcher, or wheelchair from beginning to move as you attempt to transfer the client. Keep side rails up or place your body against the client's body to prevent rolling farther than planned. Pad the headboard with a head pillow to prevent head trauma when moving a client up in bed.
The Valsalva maneuver increases cardiac workload and decreases coronary artery perfusion.	Teach clients with cardiac problems about the danger of using the Valsalva maneuver. Teach them to exhale when moving or straining. To prevent straining while defecating, help prevent constipation by increasing dietary fiber and by administering stool softeners, as ordered by the physician. Encourage the use of a bedside commode for defecation rather than a bedpan. The commode allows a normal sitting position, which decreases the angle between the rectum and anal canal and reduces the need to strain.

pulling, guiding, and pushing. These methods require use of the nurses' hands and arms (with or without a lift sheet) to move the client directly from one place to another in the bed. Similar hands-on methods are used to help a client transfer from one supporting surface to another, as from bed to chair and back. Additionally, some labor-saving devices have been designed not only to help transfer immobilized persons from one supporting surface to another but also to transport them from one place to another in the environment. Examples of devices that assist with client transfer are described next.

BACK (SPINE) BOARD

A back board (spine board) is a flat wooden or plastic board most often used for the emergency immobilization and transfer of injured or unconscious persons. It is used primarily to stabilize the vertebral column, facilitate safe transfer, and provide a firm surface for performing cardiopulmonary resuscitation (CPR) (see Chapter 30). The board's ends and sides have areas cut out to allow straps to be secured to immobilize the client and to allow for hand grips during carrying. Back boards may be full length (approximately 6 feet) or half-length. Half-boards may be used to move a person in a sitting position.

STRETCHER

The modern stretcher no longer consists of a canvas sling stretched between two poles. Today, stretchers (gurneys) are supported on legs with wheels to provide a smooth ride. Stretchers come equipped with padded mattresses for comfort, and they offer a variety of safety features, including a means of attaching IV poles, oxygen tanks, and drainage bags. The wheels have

brakes for use during transfer of the client from the bed to the stretcher. When the client is in place on the stretcher, side rails and safety straps help prevent falls. Some models allow multiple positions, including Trendelenburg and high Fowler's. See Procedure 35–3 for some methods of transfer from bed to stretcher.

SURGILIFT

The Surgilift resembles a stretcher (Fig. 35–27). Its purpose is to transport a client in a horizontal position. It allows this to be done by one nurse with little effort on the part of either client or nurse. The Surgilift consists of a metal frame on legs with wheels, but, instead of a mattress on a solid surface, only a strong, waterproof sheet supports the client. See Procedure 35–3 for additional details.

MULTIPLE-POSITIONING CHAIR

One type of device provides a bed-level, horizontal surface much like a stretcher but, once the client has transferred to it from the bed, the device can be lowered and adjusted to form a chair. Such a device can save nurses the work of supporting the immobilized client's weight during transfer from the bed to a standard chair when the client cannot bear weight.

MECHANICAL (HOYER) LIFT

Although several models of Hoyer mechanical lifts are available, a commonly used one is best described as a portable jack on wheels. It allows a sling support to be placed under a reclining client. The support is attached to the lift, and the nurse uses wind-up, electric, or hydraulic power to raise the sling and client easily into a sitting position, above bed level. Once the client is lifted, the Hoyer may be used to move the client as

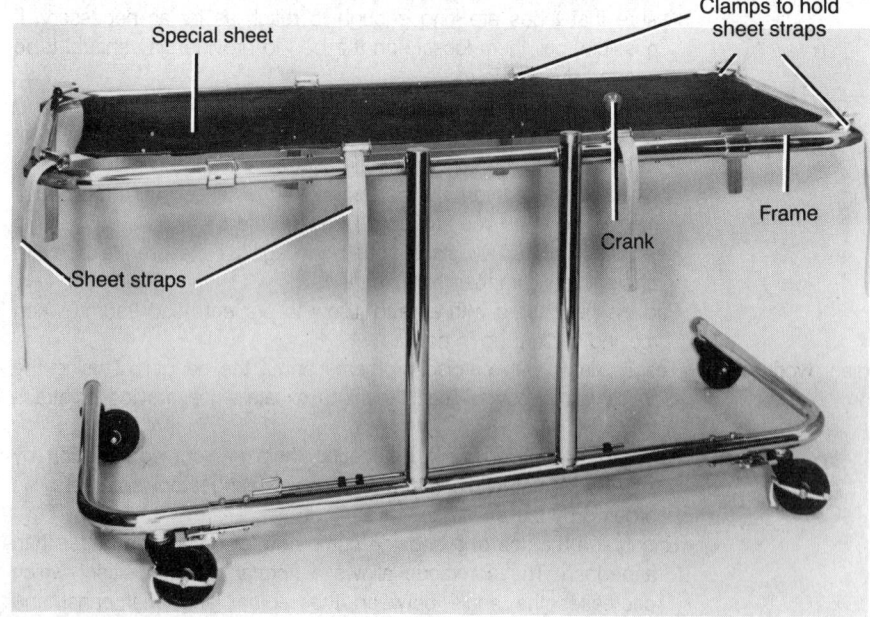

▲ **Figure 35–27**

The Surgilift.

Special sheet

Clamps to hold sheet straps

Sheet straps

Crank

Frame

Text continued on page 796

PROCEDURE 35-3

Transferring a Helpless Person from the Bed

Definition/Purposes. Enables one or more nurses/helpers to move a client out of the bed in order to be positioned in a chair or wheelchair or to be transported elsewhere. Used to prevent complications of bedrest. Used to reduce the amount of work required and to help assure safe body mechanics for client and nurse during transportation.

Contraindications/Cautions. May not be appropriate for certain individuals and therefore requires a physician's order. Each method used may be appropriate for some clients but not for others, so individualization is necessary. When using mechanical devices, be certain you are familiar with the manufacturer's recommendations and that you have received supervised practice with the equipment. Prior to transfer, be certain all wheels are locked, and then use additional measures to stabilize all equipment on wheels; for example, place your body firmly against the transporting device to keep it in contact with the bed, or place the device against a wall or other piece of furniture that can prevent rolling. Provide for all tubes and attachments to the client's body to prevent their accidental removal. When client is excessively heavy, obtain additional help.

Teaching/Learning Guidelines. To maintain or improve muscle strength, encourage clients to assist as much as they are able. Explain the use of mechanical devices. Even if the client is unconscious, explain what you are going to do and what to expect. If client is to be assisted to a standing position, teach importance of wearing shoes with nonslip soles that provide good foot support. If client must take a step and one of client's sides is stronger than the other, teach the importance of moving toward the stronger side. The stronger side will pull the weaker side along, and the weaker side will not get in the way of client movement.

PRELIMINARY ACTIVITIES

Assessment/Planning

▶ Review diagnosis and activity orders.
▶ Review the chart for presence of skin, muscle, or bone lesions.
▶ Assess level of consciousness and ability to follow directions.
▶ Assess mobility level and limitations.
▶ Plan the type and method of transfer.
▶ Decide upon the number of nurses/helpers needed and the actions of each; one must be the leader.
▶ Create working space as needed; move unnecessary furniture away from bed area, position furniture as it will be needed.
▶ Prepare mechanical devices to be used; check that they are working correctly/in safe condition to be used.

Equipment

▶ High-Low bed, if possible
▶ Footstool, if required
▶ Bath blanket
▶ Transportation device(s), e.g., Surgilift, stretcher, Hoyer lift, wheelchair, and so on

▶ Transferring equipment, e.g., lift sheet, roller, ambulation belt
▶ Shoe(s) and sock(s) for weight-bearing foot (feet), with sock or nonskid slipper on nonweight-bearing foot
▶ Paper or sheet if needed to protect bottom sheet from shoes

Preparation of Person

▶ Review equipment and the plan for the move.
▶ If client is not to sit up, cover with bath blanket or sheet.
▶ Fan-fold linen to foot of bed.
▶ If client is to sit up or stand, provide appropriate dress, including good street shoes with nonslip soles for support, as needed (place paper or sheet under person's feet to protect bed linens from shoes).
▶ Apply ambulation belt if needed.
▶ Move IV bag and urinary drainage bags so they will be in their correct places after the move; provide for all tubing to prevent its being pulled out during the move.

Using the Surgilift

Actions	Rationale/Discussion
1. Working on side of bed where Surgilift will be, lower side rail and place Surgilift sheet (Fig. 35–28) under client as you would place a lift sheet under a client (see Procedure 29–2). Assess sheet position and accessibility of straps. Keep opposite side rail raised.	1. Later, the Surgilift sheet will be needed under the client to support the body weight. The straps must be in place in order to attach the Surgilift sheet to the Surgilift frame.
2. Guard against client falling while moving Surgilift to side of bed.	2. Side rail must remain down to fit Surgilift frame close enough to client to attach Surgilift straps to it.
3. Carefully lift frame and pass it over client while positioning Surgilift base under client's bed.	3. Frame must be raised to avoid injury to client.

Procedure continued on following page

PROCEDURE 35–3 Continued

Transferring a Helpless Person from the Bed

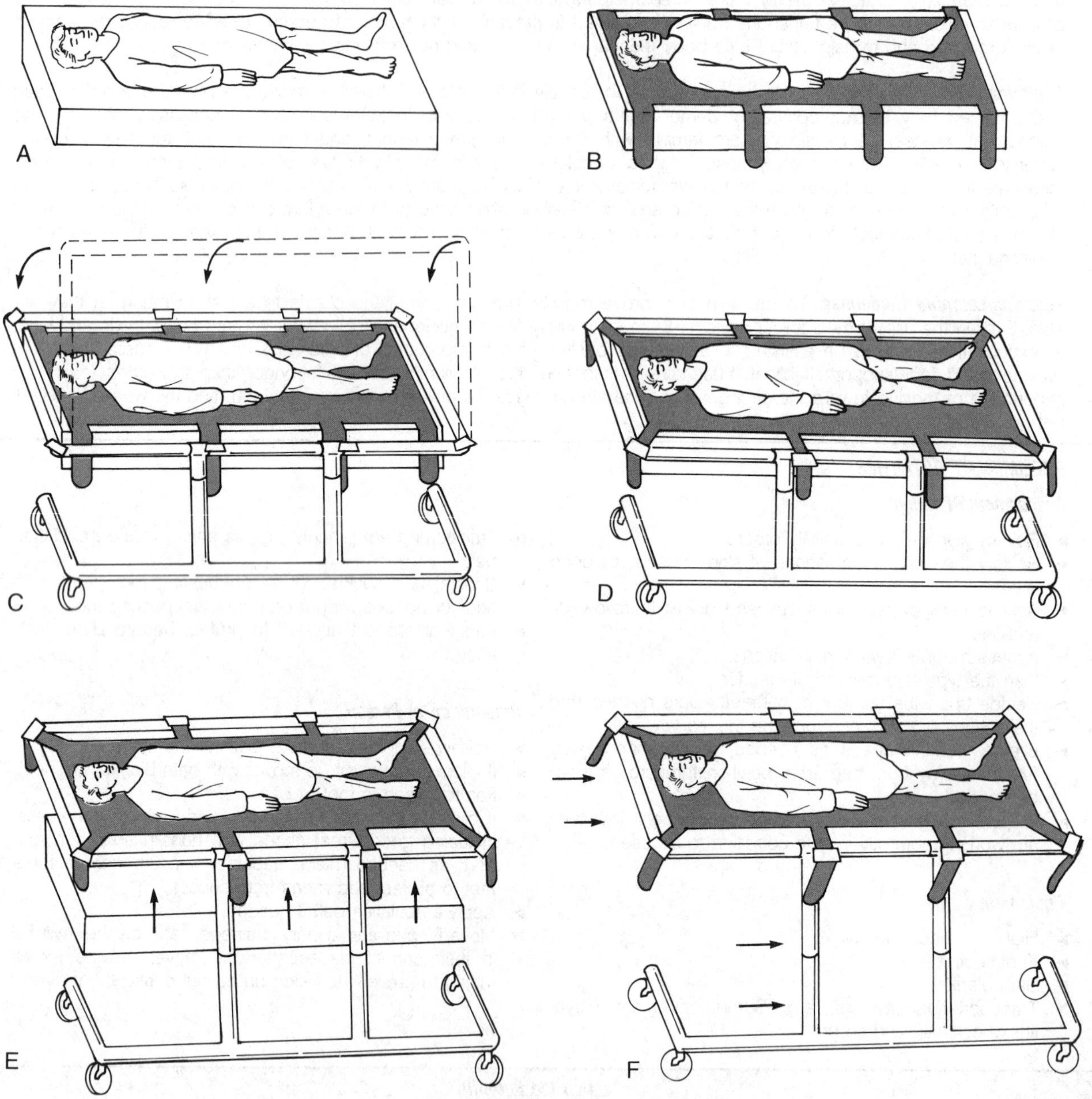

▲ Figure 35–28

PROCEDURE 35-3 Continued

Transferring a Helpless Person from the Bed

Actions	Rationale/Discussion
4. Carefully lower frame around client and secure Surgilift sheet straps to clamps on the frame. Cover client with sheet or bath blanket.	4. Avoid injuring client with frame. Blanket provides warmth, comfort, and protection from exposure.
5. Raise Surgilift by cranking handle on frame.	5. Lifts client's weight off bed and allows Surgilift to be moved without dragging client's weight over the bed surface. Tests security of clamps' hold on sheet and client while client is still over the mattress instead of being well above a hard floor.
6. Secure client with safety belt.	6. Helps prevent falling.
7. Wheel person to destination and position Surgilift over bed or table, e.g., operating room table, x-ray table, new bed.	7. Bed or table will support client.
8. Lower Surgilift by cranking as needed.	8. Person's weight must be supported on the new surface.
a. If Surgilift sheet is to be left in place, as for an x-ray, release straps, smooth sheet under client, and carefully tilt frame up, over, and away from client. When again ready to use Surgilift, repeat from steps 2 through 6 above, return client to own bed or to new destination, lower client to bed or table surface, and go on to step 8b.	a. Wrinkles are uncomfortable and cause pressure. Avoid injuring client when moving frame.
b. If Surgilift sheet is not to be left in place, remove sheet as follows: roll person to one side, gather up half of sheet into fanfolds and tuck it as far under the client's body as possible. Roll client back, over the fan-folded sheet, to the opposite side, and pull sheet out and away from client. Reposition client in correct body alignment.	b. This method is most efficient way to remove any linen from under client. Correct body alignment reduces strain on muscles.
9. Once Surgilift sheet has been removed, any further use of the Surgilift will mean following the above steps over again, beginning with number 1.	9. Clean Surgilift sheet, when finished with the move, as you would any stretcher mattress between clients. Return it to storage area.

Three-Person Carry from Bed to Stretcher

Actions	Rationale/Discussion
1. Position stretcher at right angle to head or foot of bed (Fig. 35–29).	1. Will allow for carrying the client the least possible distance.
2. Raise bed to match stretcher height and lock wheels on bed and stretcher.	2. Height allows helpers to bend no more than necessary to pick up and lower client. Locking hinders movement and helps prevent client falls.

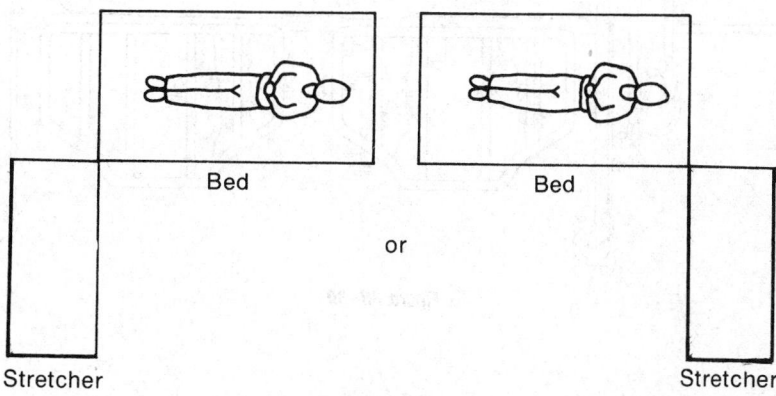

Bed   or   Bed

Stretcher   Stretcher

▲ *Figure 35–29*

Procedure continued on following page

PROCEDURE 35–3 Continued

Transferring a Helpless Person from the Bed

Actions

3. Three persons work together to move client to edge of bed (see Procedure 35–1) with arms crossed over chest.
4. Three helpers position themselves at bedside along same side of bed (Fig. 35–30). Each supports one of client's body sections: (1) head, shoulders, and chest; (2) hips; and (3) thighs and ankles. Strongest helper supports man's head and shoulders or woman's hips.
5. Helpers assume wide-based, forward-backward stances with knees flexed.

6. Helpers place their arms on bed, sliding them under client's (1) head, shoulders, and chest; (2) hips; and (3) legs. Helpers flex their fingers securely around far side of body.
7. When leader counts ''1,'' helpers simultaneously roll client to their chests, keeping their elbows on bed.
8. On count of ''2'' helpers stand, holding client securely against their chests.
9. On count of ''3'' helpers step backward, pivot toward stretcher, and walk to side of stretcher (Fig. 35–31).

10. On count of ''4'' helpers flex hips and knees (while in wide-based, forward-backward stance) to lower their elbows to stretcher edge.
11. On count of ''5'' helpers lower client to back-lying position by slowly straightening their knees and lowering their forearms onto stretcher.

Rationale/Discussion

3. Sharing reduces strain. Move brings client closer to helpers' bases of support. Crossing arms prevents dragging them during move.
4. Supports each section of client's body during transfer. Strongest helper more safely can lift heaviest body section.

5. Provides stable base in direction of motion. Flexed knees bring helpers' arms to bed level and position helpers to lift with strong leg muscles.
6. Flexing of fingers enables efficient use of force during lifting. Helpers' elbows serve as fulcrums.

7. Brings client's weight within helpers' base of support.

8. Use of strong hip and leg muscles provides safe, efficient lifting force.
9. Helpers must move in unison to maintain client's alignment and prevent injury or discomfort to client or themselves.
10. Maintains client's weight within helpers' base of support. Helpers' strong leg muscles support person's weight.
11. Controls movement of client's weight while rolling away from helpers' chests.

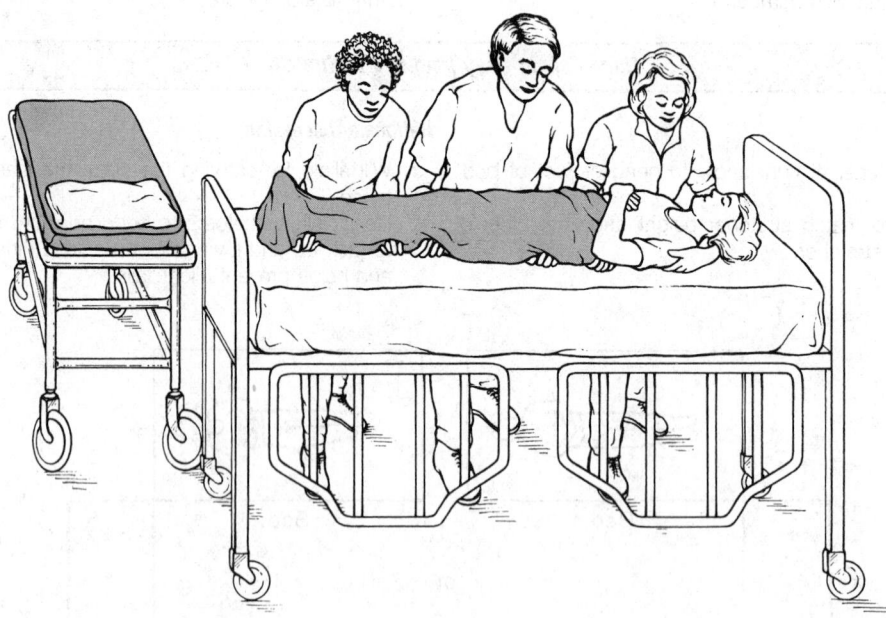

▲ *Figure 35–30*

PROCEDURE 35–3 Continued

Transferring a Helpless Person from the Bed

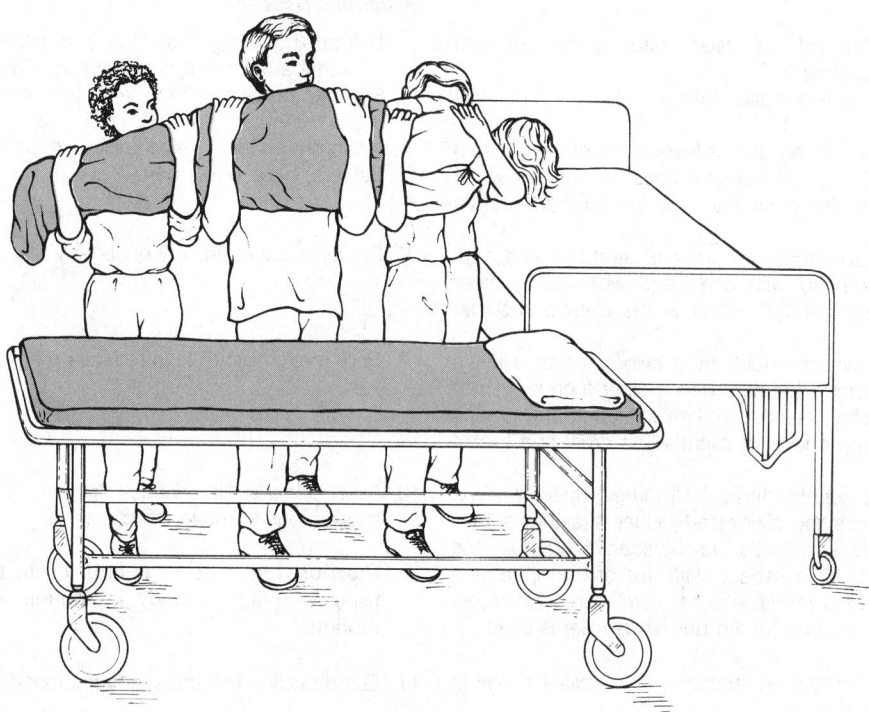

▲ *Figure 35–31*

Lift Sheet Transfer from Bed to Stretcher

Actions

1. Obtain at least three persons to help.

2. Place lift sheet under client. Roll lift sheet close to person on each side.
3. Three helpers stand at side of bed where stretcher will later be placed. Move client to edge of bed (see Procedure 35–1).
4. First helper goes to opposite side of bed and reaches across bed to hold client in place. Second and third helpers position stretcher alongside bed, near client. Lock bed and stretcher wheels.
5. Raise bed slightly higher than or equal to stretcher height (and raise head of stretcher or place pillows on stretcher equal to head elevation of bed if person requires head and chest elevation).
   a. If roller is to be used, use lift sheet to lift client just enough to get roller a few inches under side of client's back nearest to stretcher. Remainder of roller will cover gap between bed and stretcher. (Longer rollers cannot be used when the client's head must be elevated).

Rationale/Discussion

1. **Caution** Without adequate help, lift sheet transfers can injure helpers' backs, because helpers must reach beyond their base of support to lift the person's weight.

2. Lift sheet facilitates transfer.

3. Places client closer to where stretcher will be.

4. Prevent client from falling off bed by reaching across client to support arm and leg that are nearest to edge of bed. When stretcher is in place, locking wheels helps prevent movement.
5. Prevents client from having to be lifted during transfer (and head and chest elevation facilitates breathing in individuals with heart/lung disorders).

   a. Lift sheet should be on top of the roller.

Procedure continued on following page

PROCEDURE 35–3 Continued

Transferring a Helpless Person from the Bed

Actions	Rationale/Discussion
b. If no roller will be used, pad space between stretcher and bed.	b. Padding bridges surface and provides a smoother surface for sliding the client from bed to stretcher.
6. If bedding is soiled, place clean sheet over empty half of bed.	6. Protects nurse's uniform from contamination.
7. First helper kneels on bed at level of client's waist and grasps rolled lift sheet with one hand at level of client's midchest and the other hand at the level of client's hips.	7. Kneeling on bed helps assure client's weight is near helpers' base of support.
8. Second helper stands at corner of stretcher and supports client's head with one hand while using other hand to grasp rolled lift sheet at the client's shoulder level.	8. Prevents cervical injury during transfer.
9. Standing at stretcher foot, third helper moves client's legs to stretcher edge near bed. Helper then moves to side of stretcher, reaches across stretcher, and grasps rolled lift sheet at level of client's iliac crest and top of thigh.	9. Prior movement of legs reduces drag during transfer.
10. When leader counts "three," all three helpers work in unison to move the client: first helper straightens own flexed hips to lift client's weight straight up from the bed (very little lift is needed with use of roller), second and third helpers pull lift sheet toward themselves (very little effort is required for the pull when roller is used).	10. First helper's lift reduces friction. Second and third helpers pull to move the client. **Caution** Use care to control client movement when using a roller. A body in motion tends to stay in motion.
11. With client centered on stretcher, move client's legs in line with rest of body.	11. Good body mechanics reduces muscle strain.

Using the Hoyer Lift for Transfer

Actions	Rationale/Discussion
1. Center sling (with smooth side up) under client by rolling client from side to side.	1. Assess sling placement under client for (a) equal distance from side to side and (b) support of person's weight. Hems of sling are rough and cause skin abrasions.
2. Widen base with base-adjusting lever and lock the lever.	2. Lift base must be as wide as possible to maintain stability. When necessary, narrow base only temporarily, e.g., to go through narrow doorways.
3. Position lift base under bed with boom centered over sling.	3. Balances client's weight over lift's base. Line of gravity falls within base of support.
4. Lower boom far enough to attach sling by opening release valve and depressing boom manually. Do not allow boom or swivel bar to injure client.	4. Permits effortless, safe attachment of boom to sling.
5. Attach ring of webbing straps (or chains) to swivel bar with S hooks facing away from client. Shorter straps (or chains) will attach to portion of sling supporting client's back.	5. Face S hooks away from person to avoid injury. Sling support will form "bucket" seat.
6. Attach webbing straps (or chains) to sling with S hooks completely through holes in sling. Shorter portions of straps (or chains) go into holes of back support. Longer portions go into holes of seat support.	6. Assess for security of attachments and equal distance between chains or webbing straps on client's right and left sides. Client can tip/fall out of side sling if support is not even.
7. Place client's arms on chest or have grasp straps or chains.	7. Client's arms may be injured going through narrow spaces. Provides sense of security.
8. Close or tighten release valve; pump or wind jack high enough to allow sling to clear bed.	8. Assess client's weight balance in sling. If not balanced, slowly lower client to bed and readjust sling or attachment.
Valves vary in their tightness, even among similar types of lifts. Sudden release of a valve can frighten, drop, or injure the client.	**Caution** Whenever you use a particular mechanical lift for the first time or whenever a client is apprehensive, slowly lower the client to bed to demonstrate the lift's safety.

PROCEDURE 35–3 Continued

Transferring a Helpless Person from the Bed

Actions	Rationale/Discussion
9. First helper wheels lift (by holding the steering bars) while assistant guides client's legs off bed and turns person to face jack and mast (Fig. 35–32).	9. Assess for maintenance of client's weight over base of lift. In sitting slings, heels rub on bed if not supported. Protect client's feet and legs from injury. Use of two helpers ensures safety.
10. Slowly wheel lift to destination while steadying client.	10. Sling movement can frighten client. Sudden movement can unbalance lift.
	Always use an assistant to steady the client if the lift is being moved more than 10 feet.
11. First helper slowly lowers client by opening release valve (or unwinding jack) and adjusts position of lift's base to destination (e.g., chair) to compensate for boom's changing position. Simultaneously, assistant guides client to protect feet and legs and then guides client into position on chair, stretcher.	11. Client's distance from jack and mast changes when being raised and lowered. In high boom position, client is close to or touching jack and/or mast.

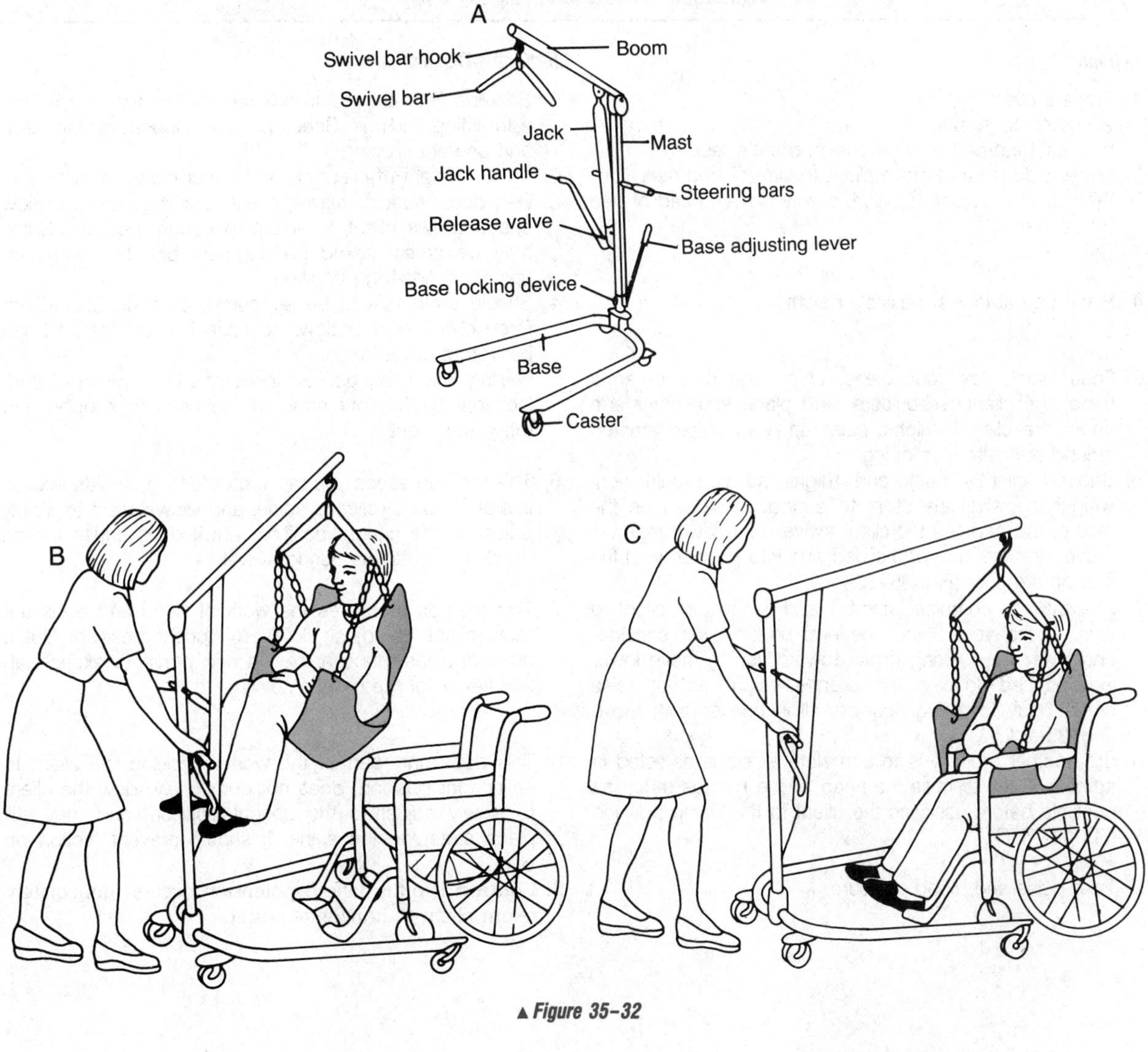

A

Swivel bar hook — Boom

Swivel bar

Jack — Mast

Jack handle — Steering bars

Release valve — Base adjusting lever

Base locking device

Base

Caster

B

C

▲ *Figure 35–32*

Procedure continued on following page

PROCEDURE 35-3 Continued

Transferring a Helpless Person from the Bed

Actions	Rationale/Discussion
12. Detach sling from straps or chains and remove lift unless continued support is necessary.	12. Support may be needed to maintain client's head above water in a bathtub.
13. *Remove sling:* (a) when client is moved to flat surface (e.g., bed, stretcher), or (b) if client can lift self to replace sling while on chair, wheelchair, or commode.	13. Do not leave client on sling. Wrinkles or seams of sling cause localized pressure on skin.
14. *Leave sling* under client when client cannot be repositioned easily on center of sling in sitting position (e.g., weak, paralyzed, or obese person). Smooth wrinkles in sling under client.	14. It is difficult to center client's sling under these individuals when sitting. Client's position may become unbalanced if sling becomes displaced. Wrinkles cause pressure on skin.
15. Position client correctly. Ensure safety, e.g., apply restraints as needed.	15. Assess client for comfort, safety, and correct body allignment.
16. Reverse steps to return client to bed.	
17. Record on care plan (if not previously recorded) lengths of chains or straps at which sling was positioned for transfer. Count loops of chain, measure straps, and record which holes are used on sling.	17. Length of chains or straps and holes of sling are adjusted for individuals. Provides for efficient, safe use of mechanical lift.

Assisting a Helpless Individual to "Dangle"

Actions	Rationale/Discussion

1. Prepare client:
  a. Take vital signs.
  b. Place appropriate footwear on client's feet.
	1. Baseline B/P and pulse will be needed for comparison with sitting findings. Shoes provide support, protect feet, and prevent slipping.

2. Lower side rail and move client to side of bed near you.	2. Moves weight of client closer to your center of gravity.
3. With client in supine position, slowly elevate head of bed 90 degrees.	3. Bed does work of raising client to sitting position. Slow speed allows client to adjust to upright position. Spine may be safely flexed 90 degrees, but this would be unsafe in side-lying position.
4. Place bed at lowest possible height.	4. Should allow feet to be supported on floor. Should not force client to step down to floor. If client falls, fall will be from a lower height.
5. Face client, flex your knees, place one of your arms under the client's shoulders, and place your other arm under the client's thighs, palm up, with fingers curved around opposite side of leg.	5. Flexing knees brings you to client's level without bending your back. Your arms will be used to support and move the client.
6. Support client's back and thighs as you shift your weight to swivel the client to a position seated on the side of the bed. As the client swivels, the lower legs will move over the side of the bed and into position with the feet on the floor (Fig. 35–33A).	6. This method saves you the work of lifting, avoids excess lateral flexion of client's spine, and allows client to slowly adjust to the upright position, but it does cause friction on skin of buttocks during swivel.
7. Alternatively, complete steps 1 and 2 and turn client to side, facing you. Place one arm under lower shoulder and lower thigh. Bring thighs toward you to move lower legs off bed (to help shift client's weight) as you raise upper body to sitting position, all in one smooth move (Fig. 35–33B).	7. This method increases the work of lifting and does not allow client to adjust slowly to upright position. But it does decrease friction to skin and prevents excess lateral flexion of the client's spine.
8. Still another method is to complete all steps as listed in number 7 but to raise the head of the bed as much as possible before assisting the client to the sitting position (Fig. 35–33C).	8. This does only part of the work of raising the client to an upright position, does not completely allow the client to slowly adjust to the upright position, and may still place strain on the spine. It should prevent friction on skin.
9. Take pulse and blood pressure.	9. **Caution** If orthostatic hypotension occurs, immediately return client to horizontal position.

PROCEDURE 35–3 Continued

Transferring a Helpless Person from the Bed

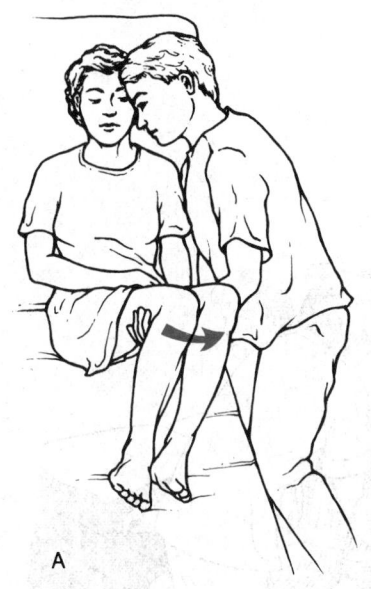
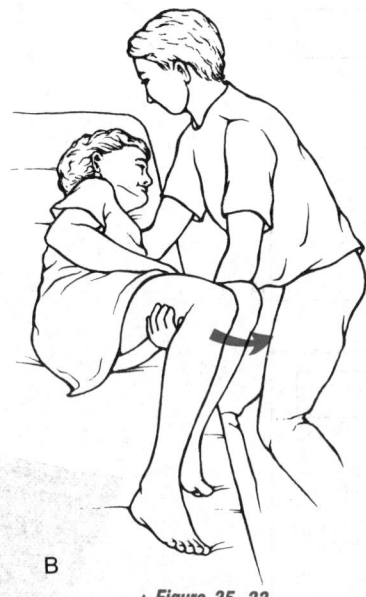
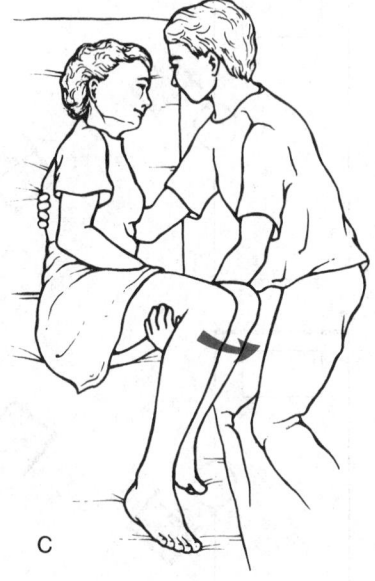

A   B   C

▲ Figure 35–33

Transfer of Person from Bed to Chair or Wheelchair

Actions

1. With bed in lowest position and chair or wheelchair at correct angle to bed, assist person to "dangle" on side of bed nearest chair (Fig. 35–34). Apply ambulation belt if indicated and not already on.

2. Assume forward-backward stance, in front of and facing client.

3. Ask client to slide buttocks close to edge of bed by shifting weight alternately from side to side, (a) pulling body forward with hands over mattress edge; (b) pushing with both fists on mattress; or (c) pushing with one fist on mattress and pulling on side rail with other hand. Assist by pulling forward alternately on right and left side of ambulation belt (or right and left upper buttock) as that side is lifted off mattress.

4. Ask client to place feet in forward-backward, wide-based position on floor (or footstool if needed), with strongest foot back slightly under bed.

Rationale/Discussion

1. Determine best side of bed for transfer by assessing placement of intravenous line, urinary drainage, room arrangement, and so on. If one side of client is stronger than the other, place chair or wheelchair so client gets out of bed toward the stronger side and moves toward the chair with the stronger side leading.

2. Position protects client from falling. Ensures your stability and correct body mechanics.

3. Positions client's trunk at edge of bed. Rocking motion lifts weight on alternate buttocks and enhances sliding by reducing friction of buttocks on sheet. Pulling with hands helps client slide. Pushing with fists (or fist and hand) reduces friction of buttocks on bed. Pull by nurse reinforces verbal instruction and helps client's weak muscles to do the work.

4. Provides wide base of support for client's weight upon standing. Back foot provides upward-forward force needed to stand up.

Procedure continued on following page

PROCEDURE 35–3 Continued

Transferring a Helpless Person from the Bed

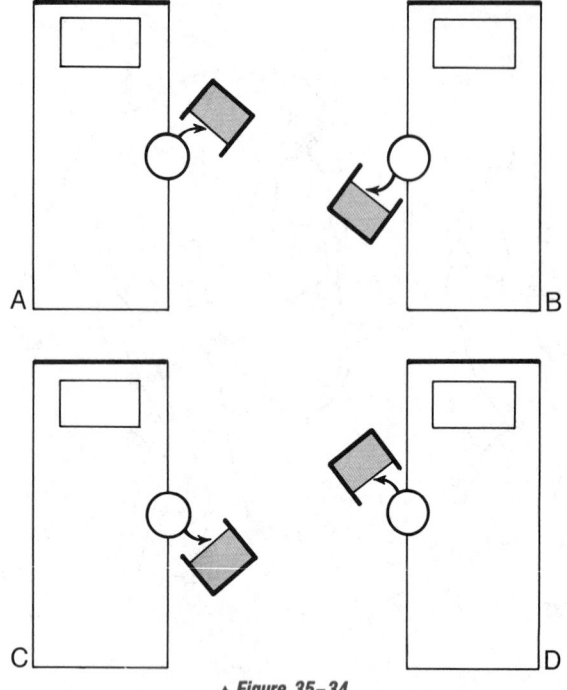

▲ *Figure 35–34*

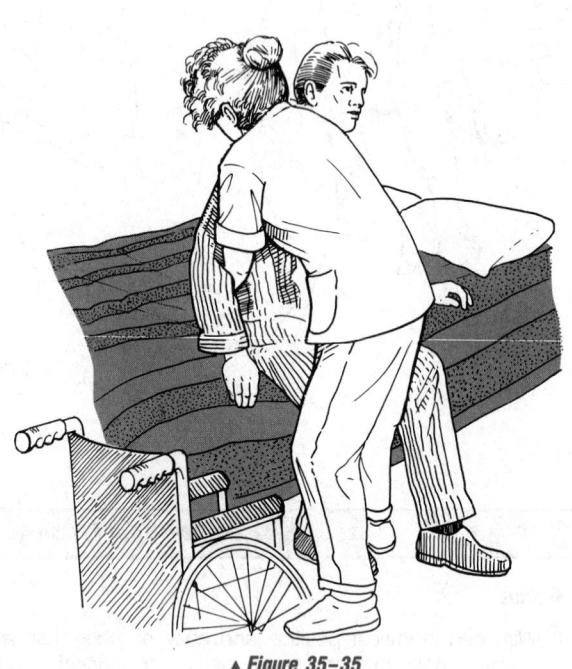

▲ *Figure 35–35*

Actions

5. Ask client to lean forward. Help pull trunk forward (a) by grasping center of belt, or (b) with your arms under client's arms and your hands clasped together just under client's shoulder blades (Fig. 35–35).

6. Ask client to push fists into edge of mattress (or grasp top of side rail with near hand) when you say "stand."

7. Ask client to stand, when directed, by simultaneously leaning forward, pushing with fists, and pushing with back foot as legs are straightened.

8. Say "stand" and shift your weight from forward to backward foot while pulling client forward and upward with belt (or with your hands on back under client's shoulder blades), or grasp transfer belt on both sides of client's waist.

9. Ask client to stand up straight and balance in standing position with hands on armchair, side rail, or mattress. Continue to face client and assist by placing one knee against client's forward knee and guide trunk by holding belt (or with hands under shoulder blades).

Rationale/Discussion

5. Brings client's trunk within base of support.

   Caution Do not support client under the armpits (axillae), since discomfort/injury to major nerves and blood vessels can occur.

6. Provides leverage for upward movement.

7. Simultaneous movements provide forward-upward force needed to stand. Leaning forward brings client's line of gravity over base of support feet provide.

8. Your action encourages client to lean forward, a difficult action to remember.

9. Your action stabilizes client's upright position by bracing one leg and pulling trunk forward. Weak individuals tend to buckle at knees. Fearful people tend to fall backward. Client's base of support is increased by holding onto chair or bed.

PROCEDURE 35–3 Continued

Transferring a Helpless Person from the Bed

Actions	Rationale/Discussion
10. Ask how client feels. Observe for indications of ortho-static hypotension. If orthostatic hypotension is present, immediately return client to bed.	10. Assess client's feelings, e.g., for lightheadedness, fainting, sweating (diaphoresis). **Caution** Do not risk danger of client's fainting and falling to floor.
11. If footstool is used, ask client to (a) place strong or dominant foot in center of footstool, (b) step to floor with other foot, and then (c) lower strong foot to floor. Use belt to assist.	11. Client's strong or dominant leg is used to provide muscle power needed to bend leg as body is lowered.
12. Ask client to place near hand on far arm of chair or wheelchair while pivoting on the balls of feet. Continue to hold belt (or clasp hands under shoulder blades). Pivot with client.	12. Holding chair gives client support to maintain balance and position body in preparation for sitting. You help maintain balance as necessary, reinforce instruction, and remain in front of client. Chair must be stable enough not to tip as client pushes down on its arm.
13. Ask client to step back until legs touch chair seat and grasp chair's other arm with other hand. Continue to hold belt (or clasp hands).	13. Client's action places feet in foward-backward stance.
14. Ask client to lean forward and lower buttocks slowly to seat by bending knees and elbows. Pull trunk forward and gradually release pressure against client's knee.	14. Maintains client's center of gravity over feet and controls movement to prevent falling back into seat.
15. Ask client to push buttocks to back of chair seat by leaning trunk forward, pushing on chair arms, and pushing against floor with feet. If necessary, pull trunk forward by pulling on shoulder blades or on belt. Simultaneously push on client's knees with your knees or hand.	15. Client's actions lift hips up, reducing friction between body and chair. Pushing on chair arms reduces amount of weight to be moved. Pushing with feet provides force for sliding back in chair. People tend to incorrectly lean *back,* thereby pushing their buttocks forward instead of backward. Do not pull on client's arms, as this can result in shoulder damage.
16. Assess client for comfort. Observe for correct sitting posture.	16. Assess body alignment, comfort, and safety.
17. Reverse procedure to return client to bed. Place the chair on the opposite side of the client to return to bed, so the person is able to "lead with the strong side." If footstool is used to return to bed, ask client to step up with dominant leg.	17. Leading with the strong side allows the stronger leg to pull the weaker leg and prevents the weaker leg from obstructing movement. Dominant leg's muscle power is needed to lift body.

desired. It may be rolled across the room and the client lowered into a chair, or it may be rolled to the bathroom and the client lowered into the bathtub. Various slings are available for different uses. Nylon or net slings are used for the bath, and canvas or nylon seats are available with openings for use with the toilet or bedside commode. Because it can be used by one person easily, this type of lift is frequently used in the home as well as the hospital. See Procedure 35–3 for more details.

WHEELCHAIR

The most commonly used model of wheelchair is the universal wheelchair (see Fig. 35–36). This model most often consists of a light-weight metal frame with a strong, slinglike seat and back that allow it to be collapsed for transportation and storage. It has two large wheels behind two smaller wheels. The large wheels may be turned by rims that are attached to them. The chair has cushioned armrests and movable legrests and

footrests. Brakes help secure the larger wheels as needed. Handles in the back allow the nurse to help hold the chair for additional security during transfers and to steer the chair when the brakes have been removed. Models can vary considerably, as they are individualized according to the needs of the owner. See Procedure 35–3 for the some methods to transfer from bed to wheelchair.

ELEVATOR CHAIR

An elevator chair is a chair mounted on an electrically operated rail or track. It can be installed in a multilevel home when needed to move a person up or down stairs. Although expensive, this chair can be extremely helpful to clients with long-term mobility problems.

AMBULATION (WALKING) BELT

In assisting a client to transfer to a chair or wheelchair, you may make use of an ambulation belt. Several models are commercially available. Walking belts are

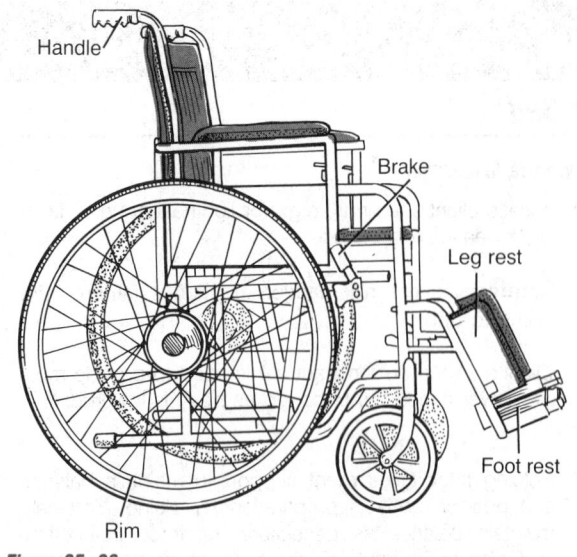

▲ *Figure 35-36*

A universal wheelchair.

commonly constructed of leather or a strong, canvas-like material, with both horizontal and vertical loops available to be used as handholds (Fig. 35-37). The belts are fastened in place around the client's waist and held securely by various combinations of closures, such as Velcro strips, buckles, and ties. They can be

used to help you maintain a safe grip on the client during transfer, but they cannot be used on everyone.

Avoid using walking belts on clients with a recent surgical incision or other pathology in the area of the belt.

ROLLER

A roller consists of a series of freely-turning rods that are secured side by side and covered with a waterproof material that rotates around the rods as the roller is used. When placed under a client's back, the rods roll to convey the client easily over the top surface of the roller and off onto another supporting surface, as from the bed, over the roller, to a stretcher. See Procedure 35-3 for more details.

Transferring the Immobilized Client

Procedure 35-3 presents selected methods for moving a helpless individual out of the bed. This series of procedures begins with transfers from bed to Surgilift, stretcher, and Hoyer lift and continues with dangling, followed by transferring a client to a chair or wheelchair.

Transfers from bed to Surgilift, stretcher, and Hoyer lift are methods to move clients who have the least mobility. As clients gain additional ability to move, they may be assisted to a sitting position on the side of the bed. This position is still referred to as **"dangling"** even though, today, clients no longer dangle their legs from hospital beds so high their feet cannot touch the

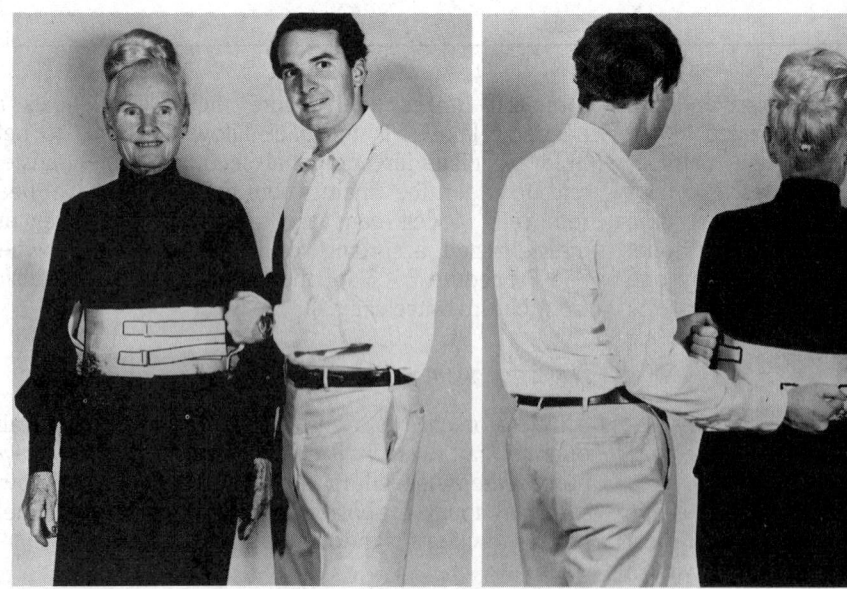

A   B

▲ *Figure 35-37*

Posey ambulation (walking) belt. (Courtesy of J.T. Posey Company.)

floor. Today, dangling is done with all body parts firmly supported, but it is still done to get the client accustomed to the vertical position after a period of lying flat. Dangling is also used as a starting point when assisting in transferring a client to a chair or wheelchair.

Additional Nursing Interventions to Prevent Disuse Phenomena

Positioning and moving are important interventions in the prevention of disuse phenomena. Repositioning the client at least every 2 hours will help prevent pressure ulcers, enhance movement of lung fluids, increase peristalsis, help keep joints mobile, and improve circulation. Positioning the client in a standing position each day (in a CircOlectric bed or standing frame) will help prevent orthostatic hypotension, bone resorption, and calcium kidney stone formation. And moving the client out of the bed will help prevent pressure ulcers and some of the negative emotional responses to immobility.

Although positioning and moving the client can prevent many untoward effects of immobility, these measures cannot do the whole job. Following are some additional nursing interventions helpful in preventing disuse syndrome. This is a beginning list and should be tailored to each client on an individual basis.

- Encourage extremity exercises to strengthen muscles and to increase venous return (see Chapter 36).
- Provide passive range-of-motion exercises to help maintain joint mobility (see Chapter 36).
- Help assure an adequate diet. For example, increase intake of fiber to prevent constipation; increase protein and calories to prevent negative nitrogen balance; assure an appropriate intake of calcium and vitamin D (increase calcium as long as the client has adequate stress on muscles and bones) to prevent bone resorption; increase acid-ash nutrients (and, if the client lacks stress on muscles and bones, decrease calcium) to prevent calcium kidney stone formation.
- Encourage fluid intake to decrease the viscosity of the blood, help keep lung secretions thin and movable, and assist in maintaining normal bladder and bowel function. When the client is on a high fiber diet to prevent constipation, increase fluid intake to 1500 to 2000 ml per day.
- Use antiembolism stockings to aid venous return to the heart and augment the vasopressor mechanism.
- Assist the person from the supine to a sitting position *slowly* to help prevent orthostatic hypotension.
- Teach to exhale when moving or straining to avoid the Valsalva maneuver.
- Encourage the client to deep breathe (see Chapter 45).
- Assist the client to cough, as necessary.

Routinely "coughing" the immobilized person is no longer recommended. But the client may be assisted to cough when necessary to clear air passages.

- Assist client, as necessary, to move toward completion of tasks or meeting of goals by helping find needed resources: rehabilitation, counseling, financial assistance, and so on.
- Assist client to withdraw strategically or to avoid persons or events as necessary for self-determination.
- Balance sensory input to prevent sensory deprivation and sensory overload.
- Use therapeutic techniques of communication to assist the client in maintaining healthy relationships with caretakers, family, friends, and others (see Chapter 24).

EVALUATION

Because disuse phenomena can occur at any time in an immobilized individual, it is important to include ongoing evaluation of all body systems as part of the plan of care. To evaluate the immobilized client, assess for evidence that the expected outcomes have been achieved. Document your findings by stating specific observations you have made. If possible, state observations in a positive way, rather than noting an absence of something. State "Skin intact and ivory in color over bony prominences" rather than "No decubitus ulcers noted." Also state the information in as specific a manner as possible so there is no question as to your meaning.

A word of caution: You may do so much work in preventing disuse phenomena that you tend to evaluate the work done, rather than the important client outcomes expected—you may want to evaluate your plan by noting whether or not you completed assessment of the client's various body systems. While it is important to make these assessments, and to document them, keep in mind that these are assessments and it is *outcomes* that need to be evaluated. Likewise, you may be tempted to evaluate whether (or how well) you completed positioning and moving; teaching; assisting with dietary intake, encouraging exercising and deep breathing; providing emotional support; and other vital nursing care. While it is important that you complete these interventions, and document them, remember that they are interventions and not outcomes.

When outcomes are not met, seek to understand why and to remedy the situation by revising the plan of care. See Table 35–6 for a brief overview of the outcomes presented earlier in this chapter; some important areas to assess when evaluating them; some measures to take to revise the plan of care if risk factors begin to be evident and expected outcomes are not being met; and examples of documentation to support the fact that outcomes are being met.

TABLE 35-6. Evaluation of the Immobilized Client

Expected Outcomes	Areas to Assess	Examples of Documentation
Maintains intact skin and mucous membranes with skin of normal color; free of ischemia and nonblanchable erythema in pressure areas	Assess entire skin surface. Describe color in general and in areas where color changes are noted. If erythema is present, state color, size, and whether it is blanchable or not. Erythema should disappear in one half to three fourths of the total time the tissues were compressed. If the time is nearing this amount, revise the plan to turn the client more often.	"Skin intact, light tan in color. Blanchable, reddened area, approximately 2" in diameter, noted over sacrum when turned from supine position. Reddened area disappeared in less than 15 minutes after client supine for 2 hours."
Maintains adequate circulation; without signs of edema, clot formation, phlebitis, or pulmonary embolism	Assess the circulation of hands and feet, bilaterally: inspect for color changes and edema, palpate peripheral pulses, feel for differences in temperature, press a nail and note the speed of capillary refill, inspect the legs for color changes and edema, measure for differences in size. Check for Homan's sign. Inspect for edema in all dependent body areas. Immediately report changes in blood supply to any body part. Elevate edematous extremities and revise plan to increase measures to enhance venous return.	"Skin warm to touch, color light tan, capillary refill less than 2 seconds, no edema noted, all pulses 2+ (unable to assess under left leg cast), thighs 15" and calves 13" bilaterally. Homan's sign negative in uncasted leg. No sacral edema noted."
Maintains normal cardiac return and cardiac output; with no signs of increased cardiac workload, cardiac strain, or orthostatic hypotension	Take B/P, pulse, and respiration measurements at rest and standing (if allowed up). Note any symptoms of hypotension upon raising head of bed or when out of bed, standing. In orthostatic hypotension, immediately return the client to bed. Revise the plan to allow for slower accommodation to the upright position. In cardiac strain, revise the plan to increase time spent with the head of the bed elevated, and take increased measures to promote circulation.	"B/P 124/74, P 72, R 20 Rt. arm reclining. B/P 128/78, P 78, R 20 Rt. arm standing."
Maintains normal ventilation; with no signs of carbon dioxide retention or hypoxia	Assess lung fields, assess respirations, note results of lab work, indicating O_2–CO_2 exchange. Report abnormal lab results. With increased retention of CO_2, revise plan to increase ventilation and gas exchange, e.g., increase position changes as well as deep breathing.	"Lungs clear. Respirations 20, clear, regular, and quiet."
Maintains easily expectorated, liquid lung secretions; with no signs of thick mucus, atelectasis, hypostatic pneumonia, or lung collapse	Assess expectorated lung secretions, assess cough, take vital signs, auscultate over lungs. If mucus thickens, revise plan to increase intake of fluids, especially water.	"Is deep breathing q2h with assistance. Coughing at approx. 1-hour intervals, expectorating small amounts clear mucus. B/P 124/74, P 72, R 20. Lungs clear."
Maintains normal nutrition; without anorexia, malnutrition, muscle catabolism, or negative nitrogen balance	Assess dietary intake, especially noting total calories, protein, fiber, calcium, and vitamin D consumption at each meal. If anorexia develops, revise plan to prevent additional anorexia that occurs with negative nitrogen balance. Increase protein intake.	"Regular diet for lunch. Ate everything on tray, including three slices of roast beef, baked potato, broccoli, salad, apple pie, and 8 oz. milk."

TABLE 35–6. *Evaluation of the Immobilized Client* Continued

Expected Outcomes	Areas to Assess	Examples of Documentation
Maintains normal pattern of bowel movements; without decreased peristalsis, flatulence, abdominal distention, constipation, or impaction	Assess bowel sounds. Monitor bowel movements. Ask about gas. If normal pattern slows, revise plan to increase fluid intake, request order for stool softener, and increase turning schedule.	"Large, brown, formed B.M. at 10:00 AM. Stated she is passing flatus. Bowel sounds all 4 quadrants. No abdominal distention noted."
Maintains muscle mass; without signs of weakness or decreased muscle tone	Take measurements to allow specific muscle groups to be compared with a baseline measurement. Assess gross muscle strength so this may also be compared with a baseline. If losses are noted, revise plan to include measures to enhance appetite and increase dietary protein and calorie intake (see Chapter 42, "Meeting Nutritional Needs"). Increase active exercises (see Chapter 36, "Meeting Mobility Needs").	"Calves 13″ bilaterally. Gross muscle strength = 5."
Maintains passive range of motion of all joints; without signs of contractures	Assess passive ROM of all joints unless contraindicated by pathology. Note any resistance present and revise the plan to increase joint positioning and movement as necessary.	"Full passive ROM of all joints noted, except unable to assess casted joints of left leg."
Maintains normal bone metabolism; without bone resorption, hypercalcemia, hypercalciuria, calcium kidney stone formation, osteoporosis, or pathologic fractures	Note amount of stress on muscles and bones each shift. If unable to place stress on muscles and bones for at least 2 hours each day, revise plan to decrease intake of calcium and increase intake of acid-ash nutrients.	"Stood with CircOlectric bed in vertical position 9:30–11:30 AM. States she is determined to prevent bone loss."
Maintains normal pattern of urinary elimination; without urinary stasis, concentrated urine, urinary tract infection, bladder distention, urinary incontinence, alkaline urine, or calcium kidney stones	Monitor fluid intake and output, inspect urine for dilution, clarity, color. Note abnormal urinalysis results. If urine becomes concentrated, revise plan to increase fluids by mouth. If necessary, revise plan to include more acid-ash nutrients (foods and fluids that are excreted in the urine as acids).	"Fluid intake and output equal at 2000 ml per day. Urine dilute, clear, and straw-colored."
Copes with inability to independently complete tasks or meet goals; without excessive feelings of loss of control, frustration, anger, hostility, aggression, depression, or loss of self-esteem	Assess emotional responses to effect of illness on goals. If untoward emotional responses are identified, revise plan to include referrals, as needed.	"States she feels sad that she can't graduate with her class but is not going to let her accident rule her life by getting depressed over it."
Copes with inability to independently remove self from that which is perceived as a threat to physical or emotional well-being; without excessive feelings of anxiety or fear, stress, or panic	Note evidence of anxiety or fear. If anxiety or fear is identified, revise plan to increase time spent with client and/or revise teaching plan, as needed.	"Stated she didn't want to have her blood drawn because she could get AIDS. Blood work delayed until she has had time to read the patient education pamphlet on AIDS transmission and have all her questions answered."
Maintains cognitive functions; without sensory deprivation, sensory overload, sleep deprivation, ICU psychosis, hallucinations, or delusions	Assess cognitive function. If decreased, report this and revise plan in order to increase or decrease sensory input, as needed.	"Oriented in all three spheres. Recent and remote memory intact. States she slept well."
Maintains healthy relationships with caretakers; without excessive dependence or a need to please, to control, or to test the caregiver	Assess interpersonal relationships. If noted to be experiencing a negative response to the need to be dependent, revise plan to help the client gain more control over own care.	"Functioning on mature level. Not happy with relying on staff but accepts the need for this."

Table continued on following page

TABLE 35-6. Evaluation of the Immobilized Client Continued

Expected Outcomes	Areas to Assess	Examples of Documentation
Maintains healthy social relationships; without feeling overly set apart, a negative body image, decreased self-esteem, or unworthy of the friendship of others	Assess social relationships. If social support system noted to be inadequate, revise plan to increase measures to increase self-esteem.	"Apparently accepting immobility in a realistic manner and maintaining self-esteem. Expressed pleasure over visitors coming."

CASE STUDY

The Client

Mr. Gary Millford, a well-developed, athletic, 41-year-old white male was admitted 2 days ago, after being found by the side of the road 1 hour after he left his home for his evening run. He was unable to remember events after leaving the house but believes he was "hit by a truck." He was admitted with multiple injuries, including fractures of the ribs, left radius, left ulna, and left tibia. His left forearm and lower leg were placed in casts and his ribs immobilized with a commercial immobilizer. A partial listing of physician's orders, on admission, included:

▶ Strict bed rest for 48 hours—then progressively mobilize
▶ Elevate left extremities on pillows at 45 degrees
▶ Regular diet as tolerated

At 4:00 PM, October 7, a partial listing of the admission assessment data included the following:

▶ 41-year-old, muscular male
▶ Chest immobilizer in place from axillae to waist

▶ Left forearm casted from hand to just above elbow; fingers and thumb freely movable
▶ Left lower leg casted from foot to just above knee; toes freely movable
▶ T 98.8° F, B/P 124/70, P 62, R 16
▶ Skin intact, ivory in color
▶ Extremities show full, passive ROM of all uncasted joints
▶ Gross muscle strength = 5
▶ Biceps 13.5″ bilaterally; right midthigh 20.5″; left midthigh 20″; right calf 15.5″; left calf casted
▶ Fingers and toes warm to touch with capillary refill less than 2 seconds, no edema observable, and pulses 2+ (unable to assess pulses under casts)
▶ States no numbness, pain, or tingling in fingers or toes

Forty-eight hours have passed since admission. The following represents part of a nursing care plan written for him shortly after admission and the current evaluation of outcomes that were expected at that time.

CARE PLAN

4:00 P.M. October 7

Nursing Diagnosis	Planning: Expected Outcomes	Implementation: Nursing Interventions	Evaluation
High Risk for Disuse Syndrome R/T unavoidable and prescribed musculoskeletal inactivity AEB casts, immobilizer, and need for bed rest	By 4:00 PM, October 9: ▶ Maintains adequate circulation; without signs of edema, clot formation, phlebitis, or pulmonary embolism AEB circulatory findings that are unchanged from baseline parameters.	Assist to change positions q2h, as follows: 6 PM—Rt. side-lying 8 PM—High Fowler's 10 PM—Rt. side-lying 12 M—Supine Assess client for spontaneous turning. If able to turn and position, do not awaken to turn at night. Continue above schedule q2h during the day.	4:00 PM, October 9: Fingers and toes warm to touch, with capillary refill less than 2 seconds, no edema observed, and pulses 2+ (unable to assess pulses under casts). States no numbness, pain, or tingling in fingers or toes. Rt. midthigh 20½″; Lt. midthigh 20″; Rt. calf 15½″; Lt. calf casted. 3-inch, blanchable, pink

CARE PLAN (Continued)

4:00 P.M. October 7

Nursing Diagnosis	Planning: Expected Outcomes	Implementation: Nursing Interventions	Evaluation
		Keep Lt. hand and foot elevated 45 degrees at all times. Keep antiembolism stocking on Rt. leg except during bath. Teach importance of moving all uncasted extremity joints, throughout the day. If unable to move by self, provide passive range-of-motion exercises 10 times to uncasted joints, q2h, on even hours.	areas noted over Rt. trochanter and Rt. tubercle after turning from Rt. side-lying position; pink areas disappear in less than 20 minutes. Homan's sign neg. in Rt. leg (unable to test in Lt. leg).
	▶ Maintains easily expectorated, liquid lung secretions; with no signs of thick mucus, atelectasis, hypostatic pneumonia, or lung collapse.	Encourage fluids to a total of 2400 ml per day by offering 240 ml of water or juice qh, between meals, until daily total reached. Measure daily fluid intake and output. Teach importance of fluids in preventing lung complications when immobilized.	Complains of rib pain upon attempts to cough. Coughing nonproductive of mucus. Upper lungs clear. Unable to assess below axillary line due to presence of immobilizer. T 98.6° F, P 70, R 22.

Summary

▶ Movement is made possible by the bones, joints, muscles, and other forms of connective tissue in the musculoskeletal system.

▶ The adult human skeleton consists of 206 bones classified as long, short, flat, or irregular and cartilage classified as elastic, fibrous, or hyaline.

▶ Joints are classified as synarthroses (immovable), amphiarthroses (slightly movable), and diarthroses or synovial joints (freely movable).

▶ Skeletal muscle is ensheathed in connective tissue that either attaches the muscle directly to the bone or is continuous with tendons or aponeuroses.

▶ In the immobilized client, the nurse should assess the general mobility level, range-of-joint motion, and status of the person relative to disuse phenomena.

▶ Assessment of the general mobility level consists of observing posture and gait and classifying functional ability level on a scale from 0 (completely independent) to 4 (dependent, does not participate in activity).

▶ Assessment of range-of-joint motion consists of observing the full measure of movement possible in each joint and classifying the client's gross muscle strength on a scale from 5 (normal: ROM unimpaired against gravity with full resistance) to 0 (zero: no evidence of muscle contractility).

▶ Assessment of the status of the person relative to disuse phenomena requires that the nurse understand how immobility affects every system of the body and how immobility has an impact on the client's psychosocial status.

▶ The main responses to immobility in each system are

integumentary system — pressure ulcers

circulatory system — increased cardiac workload, cardiac strain, and a shift of plasma to the interstitial space

pulmonary system — decreased ventilation and inadequate management of respiratory secretions

gastrointestinal system — diminished appetite, reduced intake, slowed peristalsis, and delayed egestion (defecation)

musculoskeletal system — decreased muscle contractions, loss of muscle mass and strength, contractures, and osteoporosis (bone demineralization)

urinary system — bladder distention, urinary stasis, infection, and stone formation

▶ Each of the main responses seen in each body system can lead to other untoward effects of immobility, including negative psychosocial responses as well as physical responses.

▶ Psychosocial problems that commonly occur in immobilized people include undesirable emotional responses and cognitive and sensory changes; interpersonal and social problems; and special problems in the young and in the elderly.

▶ The nursing diagnosis *High Risk for Disuse Syndrome* (a synthesis of many other high-risk nursing diagnoses) can be best understood by knowing the multiple potential effects of immobility on a person's various biologic and psychosocial systems.

▶ Planning nursing care for the client with a diagnosis of *High Risk for Disuse Syndrome* must be directed toward increasing the client's *own* activity level and using interventions that increase the client's activity level *for* the client. This chapter has focused on the latter. Chapter 36 will focus on the former.

▶ Nursing interventions for the client who is unable, or not yet ready, to increase the activity level require that the nurse be familiar with positioning and transferring equipment; with safe positioning and transferring techniques; and with additional interventions that help prevent disuse phenomena.

▶ Evaluation of the client with a diagnosis of *High Risk for Disuse Syndrome* must measure how well the client has avoided the many potential complications of immobility.

Bibliography

1. Alessi, C.A., & Henderson, C.T. (1988). Constipation and fecal impaction in the long-term care patient. *Clinics in Geriatric Medicine,* 4(3), 571–588.
2. Barker, S.M., & Crane, R. (1987). Nursing burns on special beds. *Scandinavian Journal of Plastic and Reconstructive Surgery and Hand Surgery,* 21(3), 331–332.
3. Borkowski, C. (1989). A comparison of pulmonary complications in spinal cord–injured patients treated with two modes of spinal immobilization. *Journal of Neuroscience Nursing,* 21(2), 79–85.
4. Bortz, W.M., II (1984). Commentary: The disuse syndrome. *The Western Journal of Medicine,* 141(5), 691–694.
5. Breitenbucher, R.B. (1990). UTI: Managing the most common nursing home infection. *Geriatrics,* 45(5), 68–70, 75.
6. Bucci, M.N., et al. (1989). Mechanical prophylaxis of venous thrombosis in patients undergoing craniotomy: A randomized trial. *Surgical Neurology,* 32(4), 285–288.
7. Burgess, A.W. (1990). *Psychiatric nursing: In the hospital and in the community* (5th ed.). Norwalk, Connecticut: Appleton & Lange.
8. Carpenito, L.J. (1991). *Nursing care plans and documentation: Nursing diagnoses and collaborative problems.* Philadelphia: J.B. Lippincott.
9. Clemmer, T.P., et al. (1990). Effectiveness of the kinetic treatment table for preventing and treating pulmonary complications in severely head-injured patients. *Critical Care Medicine,* 18(6), 614–617.
10. Conine, T.A., et al. (1989). The user-friendliness of protective support surfaces in prevention of pressure sores. *Rehabilitation Nursing,* 14(5), 261–263.
11. Counsell, C., et al. (1990). Interface skin pressures on four pressure-relieving devices. *Journal of Enterostomal Therapy,* 17(4), 150–153.
12. Daly, M.P. (1989). The medical evaluation of the elderly preoperative patient. *Primary Care: Clinics in Office Practice,* 16(2), 361–376.
13. Deitrick, J.E., et al. (1948). Effects of immobilization on various metabolic and physiologic functions of normal men. *American Journal of Medicine,* 4(1), 3–36.
14. Demarest, G.B., et al. (1989). Use of the kinetic treatment table to prevent pulmonary complications of multiple trauma. *Western Journal of Medicine,* 150(1), 35–38.
15. Dittmar, S.S. (ed.) (1989). *Rehabilitation nursing.* St. Louis: C.V. Mosby.
16. Doenges, M.E., & Moorhouse, M.F. (1991). *Nurse's pocket guide: Nursing diagnoses with interventions* (3rd ed.). Philadelphia: F.A. Davis.
17. Flam, E. (1990). Skin maintenance in the bed-ridden patient. *Ostomy/Wound Management,* 28, 48–54.
18. Gentilello, L., et al. (1988). Effect of a rotating bed on the incidence of pulmonary complications in critically ill patients. *Critical Care Medicine,* 16(8), 783–786.
19. Gilsdorf, P., et al. (1990). Sitting forces and wheelchair mechanics. *Journal of Rehabilitation Research and Development,* 27(3), 239–246.
20. Goode, P.S., & Allman, R.M. (1989). The prevention and management of pressure ulcers. *Medical Clinics of North America,* 73(6), 1511–1524.
21. Green, D. (1990). Symposium on immobility. Helping the handicapped. *Nursing,* 4(4), 16–18.
22. Harrell, J.S., et al. (1989). Cardiac output and associated cardiovascular responses to bedmaking. *Critical Care Nursing Quarterly,* 12(3), 19–33.
23. Herr, K.A., & Mobily, P.R. (1991). Complexities of pain assessment in the elderly: clinical considerations. *Journal of Gerontological Nursing,* 17(4), 12–19.
24. Hickey, P.W. (1990). *Nursing process handbook.* St. Louis: C.V. Mosby.
25. Hill, S.N., et al. (1987). Nursing the immobile: a preliminary study. *International Journal of Nursing Studies,* 24(2), 123–128.
26. Holm, K., & Hendricks, C. (1989). Immobility and bone loss in the aging adult. *Critical Care Nursing Quarterly,* 12(1), 46–51.
27. Huber, K.H., et al. (1988). Humoral regulation of the orthostatic reaction. *International Journal of Sports Medicine,* 9(Suppl. 2), S103–S112.
28. Jacobs, M.A. (1989). Comparison of capillary blood flow using a regular hospital bed mattress, ROHO mattress, and Mediscus bed. *Rehabilitation Nursing,* 14(5), 270–272.
29. Jay, P. (1990). Symposium on immobility. The role of community nurses. *Nursing,* 4(4), 13–15.
30. Kay, T.W.H., & Martin, F.I. (1986). Heel ulcers in patients with long-standing diabetes who wear antiembolism stockings. *Medical Journal of Australia,* 145(6), 290–291.
31. Kelley, L.S., & Mobily, P.R. (1991). Iatrogenesis in the elderly: impaired skin integrity. *Journal of Gerontological Nursing,* 17(9), 24–29.
32. Kinnunen, O., et al. (1989). Diarrhea and fecal impaction in elderly long-stay patients. *Zeitschrift fur Gerontologie,* 22(6), 321–323.
33. Kottke, F.J., & Lehmann, J.F. (eds.) (1990). *Krusen's handbook of physical medicine* (4th ed.). Philadelphia: W.B. Saunders.
34. Krouskop, T.A., et al. (1985). Effectiveness of mattress overlays in reducing interface pressures during recumbency. *Journal of Rehabilitation Research and Development,* 22(3), 7–10.
35. Levine, J.M., & Gross, J. (1989). Atypical locations of pressure sores: presentation of two cases. *Decubitus,* 2(4), 44–46.
36. Lingeman, J.E., et al. (1990). Kidney stones: identifying the causes. *Patient Care,* 24(15), 31–46.
37. Maklebust, J., et al. (1988). Pressure relief capabilities of the Sof-Care bed and the Clinitron bed. *Ostomy/Wound Management,* 21(32), 36–41, 44.
38. McCance, K.L., & Huether, S.E. (eds.) (1990). *Pathophysiology: The biologic basis for disease in adults and children.* St. Louis: C.V. Mosby.
39. McConnell, E.A. (1990). Applying antiembolism stockings. *Nursing,* 20(10), 92.
40. McConnell, E.A. (1990). Clinical do's and don'ts: placing your patient in the lateral position. *Nursing 90,* 20(7), 65.
41. McGuire, R.A., et al. (1988). Comparison of stability provided to the unstable spine by the kinetic therapy table and the Stryker frame. *Neurosurgery,* 22(5), 842–845.

42. McGuire, R.A., et al. (1987). Spinal instability and the log-rolling maneuver. *Journal of Trauma*, 27(5), 525–531.

43. Memmer, M.K. (1988). Acute orthostatic hypotension. *Heart and Lung*, 17(2), 134–143.

44. Mobily, P.R., & Kelley, L.S. (1991). Iatrogenesis in the elderly: factors of immobility. *Journal of Gerontological Nursing*, 17(9), 5–10.

45. National Association of Orthopaedic Nurses (1991). *Core curriculum for orthopaedic nursing* (2nd ed.). Pitman, New Jersey: Anthony J. Jannetti.

46. Neal, M.E. (1990). A cost-effective alternative to specialty beds for pressure relief. *Rehabilitation Nursing*, 15(4), 202–204.

47. North American Nursing Diagnosis Association (1990). *Taxonomy I—Revised 1990*. St. Louis: Author.

48. Olson, E.V., et al. (1990). The hazards of immobility: 1967 'classic article.' *American Journal of Nursing*, 90(3), 43–48.

49. Palmer, M.L., & Epler, M.E. (1990). *Clinical assessment procedures in physical therapy*. Philadelphia: J.B. Lippincott.

50. Pieper, B., et al. (1990). Visceral protein nutritional assessment of patients placed on a high or low air-loss bed. *Journal of Enterostomal Therapy*, 17(4), 145–149.

51. Pieper, B., et al. (1990). Low and high air-loss beds in acute care hospitals. *Journal of Enterostomal Therapy*, 17(3), 131–136.

52. Porth, C.M. (ed.) (1990). *Pathophysiology: Concepts of altered health states* (3rd ed.). Philadelphia: J.B. Lippincott.

53. Redfern, S. (1990). Symposium on immobility: care after a stroke. *Nursing*, 4(4), 7–11.

54. Ross, J., & Dean, E. (1989). Integrating physiological principles into the comprehensive management of cardiopulmonary dysfunction. *Physical Therapy*, 69(4), 255–259.

55. Ryan, D.W., & Byrne, P. (1989). A study of contact pressure points in specialized beds. *Clinical Physics and Physiological Measurement*, 10(4), 331–335.

56. Schmelzer, M. (1990). Effectiveness of wheat bran in preventing constipation of hospitalized orthopaedic surgery patients. *Orthopaedic Nursing*, 9(6), 55–59.

57. Schnieber, M.E. (1990). Cardiac complications of the Stryker frame. *Critical Care Nurse*, 10(8), 73–77.

58. Selikson, S., et al. (1988). Risk factors associated with immobility. *Journal of the American Geriatrics Society*, 36(8), 707–712.

59. Shannon, M.L. (1989). Pressure ulcer prevalence in two general hospitals. *Decubitus*, 2(4), 38–43.

60. Shannon, M.L., & Miller, B.M. (1988). Pressure sore treatment: a case in point. *Geriatric Nursing*, 9, 154–157.

61. Stringer, M.D., & Kakkar, V.V. (1989). Prevention of venous thromboembolism. *Herz*, 14(3), 135–147.

62. Stuart, G.W., & Sundeen, S.J. (1991). *Principles and practice of psychiatric nursing* (4th ed.). St. Louis: C.V. Mosby Year Book.

63. Travis, S.T. (1990). Personalizing self-care. *Journal of Geriatric Nursing*, 11(2), 72–73.

64. Turpie, A.G.G., et al. (1989). Prevention of deep vein thrombosis in potential neurosurgical patients: a randomized trial comparing graduated compression stockings alone or graduated compression stockings plus intermittent pneumatic compression with control. *Archives of Internal Medicine*, 149(3), 679–681.

65. Varcarolis, E.M. (ed.) (1990). *Foundations of psychiatric mental health nursing*. Philadelphia: W.B. Saunders.

66. Walsh, M., & Brescia, F.J. (1990). Clinitron therapy and pain management in advanced cancer patients. *Journal of Pain and Symptom Management*, 5(1), 46–50.

67. Walsh, M., & Judd, M. (1989). Long-term immobility and self-care: the Orem nursing approach. *Nursing Standard*, 3(41), 34–36.

68. Wenger, N., & Hellerstein, K. (eds.) (1984). *Rehabilitation of the coronary patient* (2nd ed.). New York: Wiley Medical Publications.

69. Willey, T. (1989). High-tech beds and mattress overlays: a decision guide. *American Journal of Nursing*, 89(9), 1142–1145.

Chapter 36

▼ Meeting Mobility Needs

In an aging society, the consequences of regular exercise are potentially profound—for the individual and for the society.

Eric Larson

▼ CHAPTER OUTLINE

ASSESSMENT
    Causes of Immobility
    Responses of the Body to
      Immobility
    Assessing Readiness for Mobility
NURSING DIAGNOSIS
PLANNING
NURSING INTERVENTION

    Exercises
    Progressive Mobilization
    Assistive Ambulation Devices
    Promoting Fitness for the Mobile
      Person
EVALUATION
CASE STUDY

▼ KEY TERMS

Active-assistive range-of-motion exercises
Active range-of-motion exercises
Aerobic exercise
Ambulation
Anaerobic exercises
Assistive ambulation devices
Ergometer
Flexibility exercises
Four-point gait

Isometric exercises
Isotonic exercises
Muscle-setting exercises
Orthopedics
Passive range-of-motion exercises
Prosthetic devices (prostheses)
Quad cane
Resistive range-of-motion exercises

Strength-developing exercises
Swing-through gait
Swing-to gait
Three-point gait (with partial weight-bearing on one extremity)
Tripod cane
Two-point gait

In Chapter 35, Preventing Complications of Immobility, we discussed the many ways that the human body, when immobilized, inevitably breaks down, toward ill health and death. In Chapter 35, we reviewed methods to prevent that "inevitable" course through the positioning and moving of immobilized persons and we discussed the use of the nursing process for clients who were not yet able or ready to begin the process of mobilization. In this chapter, we look at clients who <u>are</u> able and ready to increase mobility. Here we consider how to encourage them to move as independently as possible. As in Chapter 35, the nursing process will be our basis for discussing the care of clients regaining mobility.

The topics will progress (as clients so often do) from a discussion of ways to help strengthen clients before they are able to get out of bed to ways to help clients *independently* dangle and then get out of bed. The discussion will move on to consider persons who are able to walk but who require assistive devices. We will end with a discussion of clients who are independently mobile and who are seeking an even higher level of health known as fitness.

ASSESSMENT

Causes of Immobility

Clients should be assessed for impaired physical mobility when they have either a prescribed or an unavoidable decrease in musculoskeletal activity.

Unavoidable causes of immobility include

▶ pain severe enough to limit motion and curtail activity. For example, persons with diseases such as rheumatoid arthritis may be able to move joints, but severe pain causes them to limit movement. Chronic pain increases the risk of complications of immobility.
▶ impairments of motor nervous function that seriously and sometimes permanently decrease body movements. Examples of conditions in this category include progressive degenerative disorders such as

muscular dystrophy, Parkinson's disease, and amyotrophic lateral sclerosis. Paralysis from a stroke and spinal cord injury are other examples.
▶ structural problems like scoliosis (lateral deviation of the spine), degenerative joint disease, joint contractures, or osteoporosis.
▶ generalized weakness from chronic illness (e.g., cancer, anorexia with resulting malnutrition, or profound obesity).
▶ psychologic problems such as severe depression, acute confusion, and certain other mental disorders. (See Applying Research to Nursing Practice.)

Prescribed causes of immobility include

▶ orthopedic (musculoskeletal) problems that require treatment by immobilization of the spine or one or more extremities (e.g., traction or the application of a cast). **Orthopedics** is the branch of medicine that specializes in the treatment of musculoskeletal disorders.
▶ other health problems that require restriction of mobility as a part of the treatment (e.g., the person who requires restraints or bed rest).

Responses of the Body to Immobility

All body systems respond negatively to prolonged periods of immobility. Human responses to immobility, the disuse phenomena, are discussed in Chapter 35. Major complications of immobility are reviewed in Figure 36–1.

Assessing Readiness for Mobility

To assess the immobilized client's readiness for mobility, you must learn whether the person desires to increase mobility, has sufficient neuromuscular and musculoskeletal integration to complete required activities, has sufficient stamina to endure the required activities, and is able to work with you to plan and safely carry out activities as needed. To assess the client's readiness in these areas, assess the following:

APPLYING RESEARCH TO NURSING PRACTICE

Preventing Confusion to Promote Self-Care Among Hospitalized Elderly Clients

Wanich, C.K., Sullivan-Marx, E.M., Gottlieb, G.L., & Johnson, J.C. (1992). Functional status outcomes of a nursing intervention in hospitalized elderly. *Image*, 24(3), 201–207.

▼ ▼ ▼

Acute confusion is a major health problem among the hospitalized elderly. Not only is it distressing to family members, it also adversely affects the quality and scope of self-care among these clients and leads to an increased incidence of illness and death. Wanich and colleagues studied the functional status of 235 elderly subjects. A control group received standard medical and nursing care. An experimental group received nursing interventions aimed at preventing confusion and improving self-care. The nursing interventions consisted of daily ambulation, daily evaluation of medications that may contribute to delirium, early physical therapy consultation, and visits by a geriatric clinical nurse specialist to promote orientation. The nurse researchers encouraged families to visit frequently. A multidisciplinary team reviewed discharge plans weekly. Wanich and colleagues made environmental modifications to stimulate and orient the elderly clients. In addition, the clinical nurse specialists conducted an educational program designed to sensitize the nursing staff to the relationship between confusion and functional status among elderly persons.

Of the 125 clients in the experimental group, 21 per cent improved their self-care ability, and 69 per cent maintained their self-care ability. Of the 94 subjects in the control group, only 10 per cent improved their self-care ability, and 74 per cent maintained their self-care ability. Within the experimental group, the incidence of confusion was 19 per cent, compared with 22 per cent in the control group, a difference that was not statistically significant. However, those elderly clients receiving the nursing interventions were three times as likely to improve their functional status as those who did not receive the nursing interventions.

Applications for Practice

In practice, do not accept confusion as an inevitable consequence of hospitalization of elderly clients. By instituting prompt nursing interventions, you can prevent the hazards of confusion and enhance the elderly client's self-care abilities, thus helping to maintain an optimal mobility level.

▶ The client's functional level as evidenced by the ability to stand, bear weight, walk, and complete activities of daily living. Use the North American Nursing Diagnosis Association (NANDA) Suggested Functional Level Classification (see Nursing Diagnosis Profile).[44] Box 36–1 lists terms used to describe certain conditions that may be present in persons at functional levels 1 through 4.

▶ Gross muscle strength on a scale from 0 (no muscle contractility) to 5 (normal) (see Chapter 35).

▶ Body systems for the presence of conditions that would tend to make efforts at movement difficult or hazardous (e.g., pain, edema, or wounds in body parts to be moved; or dyspnea, dizziness, or lack of balance in clients who are planning to begin **ambulation** (walking).

▶ A history of angina pectoris with a particular activity indicates that the client cannot tolerate that activity. Angina pectoris is severe pain and a feeling of pressure in the heart. It occurs with exertion when there is an insufficient blood supply to the heart. Additional signs and symptoms often include pallor, dyspnea, diaphoresis (profuse sweating), anxiety, and pain that radiates down the left arm, to the back, or to the jaw.

▶ Body systems for the presence of disuse phenomena (see chapter 35). Some disuse phenomena directly hamper mobility (e.g., stiff joints, footdrop, osteoporotic bone fractures). Other disuse phenomena indirectly hamper mobility by causing pain (e.g., pressure ulcers, renal calculi), discomfort (e.g., constipation, depression), or lack of stamina (e.g., decreased O_2–CO_2 exchange, muscle atrophy). All these phenomena must be taken into consideration when planning to increase movement. Even if a particular disuse phenomenon seems to bear little relationship to the client's ability to increase movement (e.g., slight ankle edema, asymptomatic constipation), it should be noted so that it can serve as a baseline for later comparison.

▶ Emotional or psychosocial responses that could affect the desire to increase mobility (e.g., feelings of dependence or fear of falling).

▶ Cognitive ability as a way to rule out problems that could make efforts toward independent mobility unsafe (e.g., lack of ability to understand and follow directions, lack of judgment concerning own abilities).

As you assess your client in these areas, your expectations should differ according to the norm for each stage of development. The biopsychosocial stages of development are discussed throughout Unit III. Some of the major physical changes normally seen in the musculoskeletal system are listed in Table 36–1.

In addition to assessing the client, self-assessment is essential. Assess your own ability to manage the client safely (especially in the event that the client suddenly collapses and becomes totally dependent upon you for support). *Generally, you should not lift more than 35 per cent of your body weight without assistance.*

But it is not just your relative weight that is important. Are your muscles in condition for holding and lifting? Are you fit enough for the physical activity required while helping another person begin to move alone? Do you understand the principles you need to know to safely help another person lift, turn, and move? If you need equipment to help the client move, do you understand how to use it safely? Have you practiced using it under supervision?

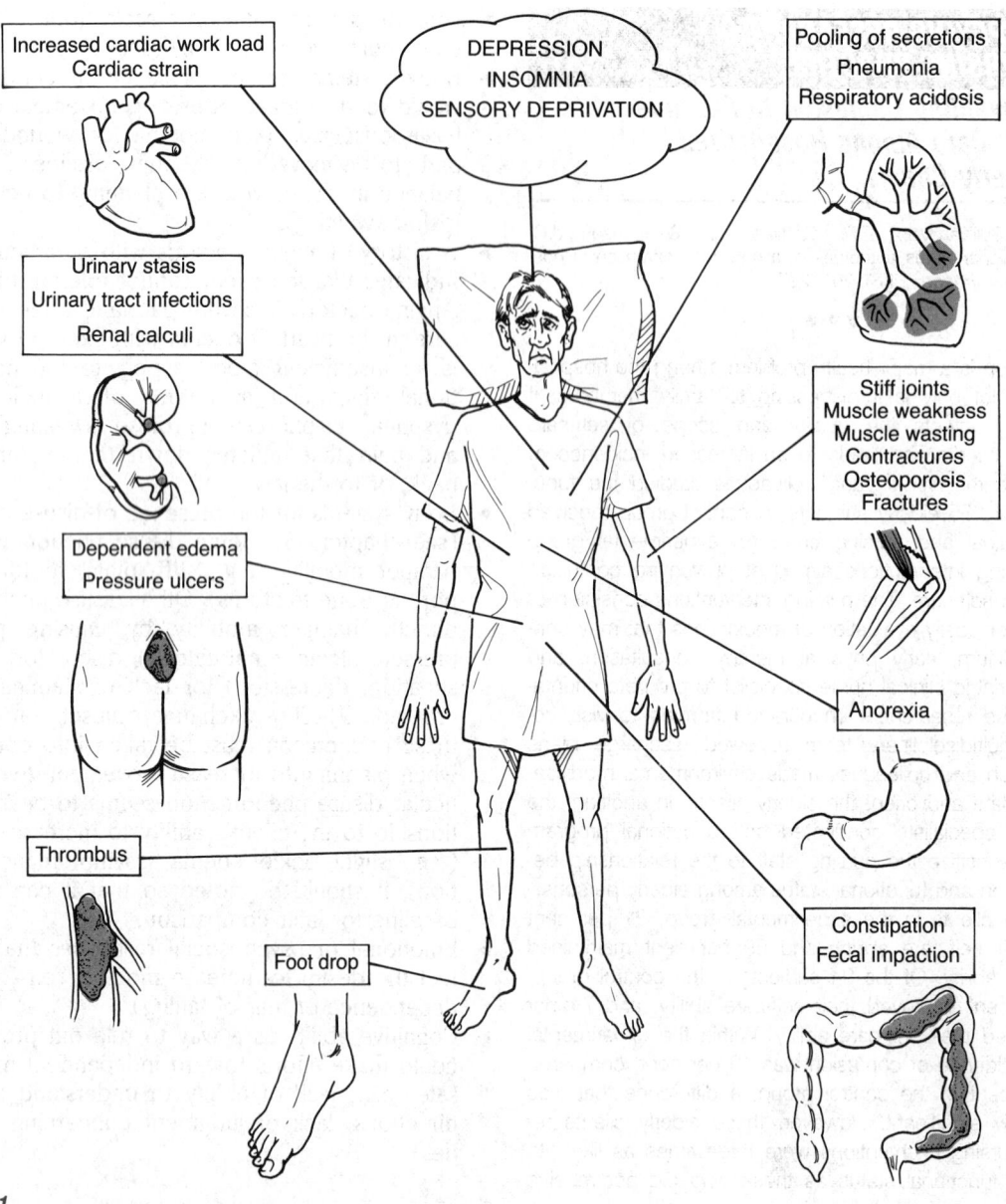

Increased cardiac work load
Cardiac strain

DEPRESSION
INSOMNIA
SENSORY DEPRIVATION

Pooling of secretions
Pneumonia
Respiratory acidosis

Urinary stasis
Urinary tract infections
Renal calculi

Stiff joints
Muscle weakness
Muscle wasting
Contractures
Osteoporosis
Fractures

Dependent edema
Pressure ulcers

Anorexia

Thrombus

Constipation
Fecal impaction

Foot drop

▲ *Figure 36–1*

Some major complications of immobility.

Box 36–1. Terms Used to Describe Selected Conditions That May Be Present in Persons at Functional Levels 1 through 4

▶ paralysis. Temporary or permanent loss of sensation and/or motor function in a part of the body

▶ hemiplegia. Paralysis of either the right or the left half of the body

▶ paraplegia. Paralysis of the lower portion of the torso and of both legs

▶ quadriplegia. Paralysis of the trunk and all four extremities

▶ paresis. Partial or incomplete paralysis

▶ hemiparesis. Partial or incomplete paralysis of one side of the body

▶ paraparesis. Partial or incomplete paralysis affecting the lower extremities

TABLE 36-1. Selected Growth and Developmental Changes in the Musculoskeletal System

Stage of Development/ Approximate Age	Usual Expectations for Able-Bodied
Prenatal Period (conception to birth):	
8 weeks	Fetus begins to move in utero.
Neonatal Period (first month of life):	Sleeps most of the time, usually in the fetal position. When awake, the neonate can kick and wiggle, but reflexes cause most movement.
Infancy (1 month to 1 year):	Reflexes replaced by learned responses:
1 month	Can turn head to one side
2 months	Fencing reflex disappears
2 months	Grasp reflex disappears
3 months	Can lift head when prone. Sits only with support. Moro reflex disappears. Can briefly hold objects and can carry them to mouth
5 months	Can reach and grasp objects. Can roll from prone to supine position and back
6 months	Can hold head steady when sitting. Can sit unaided for a brief time (allows use of both hands). Can use thumb to grasp objects
6–9 months	Babinski reflex disappears
9 months	Has good head control. Can sit alone steadily with good trunk control. Has coordinated eye-hand control
9–16 months	Is beginning to walk
12 months	Can stand while holding on. Can sit from a standing position. Handedness is determined
18 months	Can walk well and is beginning to run
Early Childhood (18 months to 6 years):	Consists of toddlerhood and preschool years. Increased coordination and physical strength develops
Toddlerhood (18 months to 3 years):	Has a particular waddling gait
By age 3 years	Can run and jump and throw and catch objects
Preschool years (3 to 6 years):	Motor skills become increasingly complex. Fine motor skills are refined
By age 5 years	Can balance on tiptoes, hop on one foot, climb, ride a tricycle. Can manipulate buttons, zippers, shoe laces, scissors, and school tools that allow pasting, coloring, and writing
School-age period (6 to 12 years):	Coordination and strength increase with increasing neuromuscular development, exercise, and training.
By age 6 years	Body proportions begin to approximate adult proportions. Rounded abdomen disappears. Back and shoulders straighten. Bones lengthen and harden as calcium is deposited. Can jump, tumble, skip, hop, and ride a bicycle
By age 12 years	Has mastered the ability to climb trees, swing from bars, ride a skateboard, and play ordinary games
10.5 to 13 years:	Time of growth spurt when adolescent may appear clumsy and uncoordinated owing to an increase in skeletal growth with a temporary delay in the development of muscle growth
10.5 to 11 years	Girls begin growth spurt
Adolescence (12 to 18 or 20 years):	A time for learning to accept one's physique and to learn to use the body effectively
12 years	Peak of growth spurt for girls
12.5 to 13 years	Boys begin growth spurt
14 years	Peak of growth spurt for boys
Adulthood (18 or 20 years to death):	Some people concentrate on exercise and physical fitness. Others do not.
Midlife (40 to 65 years)	Physical signs of aging gradually begin to appear, e.g., muscle or joint stiffness, decreased energy, weight gain. Bone density and mass decrease, particularly in women after menopause. Degenerative joint disease may occur in the back and extremity joints. Muscle tone can decrease with a lack of exercise.
Maturity (65 years to death)	Often bone mass decreases, with osteoporosis causing fractures seen as kyphosis and decreased height. Enlarged joints and flabby muscles are not uncommon

NURSING DIAGNOSIS

In this chapter, we are focusing on clients with a diagnosis of *Impaired Physical Mobility* (see Nursing Diagnosis Profile). According to NANDA, this diagnosis refers to the person who ". . . experiences a limitation of ability for independent physical movement" and whose assessment findings demonstrate one or more of the following defining characteristics:

▶ cannot move within the physical environment, including moving in bed, transferring in and out of bed, or ambulating
▶ is reluctant to attempt movement even if able
▶ has limited range of motion
▶ has impaired coordination
▶ has decreased muscle strength, control, and/or mass
▶ is under imposed restrictions of movement, including mechanical restrictions or medical protocol[44]

Very simply, the person with a nursing diagnosis of *Impaired Physical Mobility* cannot or will not move. However, not all persons who cannot or will not move should be diagnosed with *Impaired Physical Mobility*.

The diagnosis of *Impaired Physical Mobility* is not made unless the client's mobility level can be improved by nursing intervention. If the mobility level is not amenable to nursing intervention, consider the diagnosis *High Risk for Disuse Syndrome*.

The concept of *Impaired Physical Mobility* is difficult to grasp because mobility is such an important, basic need that virtually all other aspects of life relate to it in some manner or other. As a result, you will note that many nursing diagnoses include a mention of mobility (or activity) somewhere in their definition, defining characteristics, risk factors, or related factors.

Sometimes, the diagnosis of *Impaired Physical Mobility* will result from other nursing diagnoses, such as

▶ *Impaired Physical Mobility* R/T *Activity Intolerance*
▶ *Impaired Physical Mobility* R/T *Pain* (e.g., in lumbosacral area)
▶ *Impaired Physical Mobility* R/T *Fear* (e.g., of falling during ambulation)

At other times, the *Impaired Physical Mobility* will be a related factor for other nursing diagnoses, such as

▶ *Impaired Social Interaction* R/T *Impaired Physical Mobility*
▶ *High Risk for Disuse Syndrome* R/T *Impaired Physical Mobility*
▶ *Bathing/Hygiene Self-Care Deficit* R/T *Impaired Physical Mobility*

Of course, the diagnosis of *Impaired Physical Mobility* need not have a direct relationship with another nursing diagnosis. For example, when the client is restrained or when the client has beginning joint stiffness, one nursing diagnosis that might be made is *Impaired Physical Mobility* R/T the effects of musculoskeletal impairment. "Musculoskeletal impairment" is not a nursing diagnosis.

Whatever its related factor, whenever you make the nursing diagnosis of *Impaired Physical Mobility* you should also consider the possibility of an accompanying nursing diagnosis of *High Risk for Disuse Syndrome*. See Figure 36–2 for a decision tree that can help you sort out information you need about the nursing diagnosis *Impaired Physical Mobility*.

Bear in mind that persons with the nursing diagnosis *Impaired Physical Mobility* may have a number of additional nursing diagnoses that relate to the impaired mobility. Some of these are listed in the Nursing Diagnosis Profile.

PLANNING

Immobility can strike suddenly or gradually. It can be partial (e.g., the person with a broken leg who can still hobble around on crutches) or total, as with the totally paralyzed person or the unconscious client. Immobility may be caused by a temporary condition or a more permanent one. The client may be of any age and at any place along the health-illness continuum. The expected outcomes of nursing care will have to be individualized depending upon many factors.

With the diagnosis *Impaired Physical Mobility*, nursing care should be directed toward increasing the client's mobility level within the limits of the person's ability. Doing so should not only help solve the client's mobility problem but also help to prevent the complications of immobility that we term disuse syndrome. In certain cases, increasing mobility can also help increase activity tolerance.

Following correct nursing interventions, you might expect that an individual with impaired physical mobility will achieve one or more of the following outcomes. These outcomes can be modified to meet each client's specific needs and limitations as they change over time:

▶ Has measurably increased muscle mass (e.g., "measurement around largest part of biceps increases from 10 inches to 11 inches")
▶ Demonstrates measurably increased muscle strength (e.g., "completes each scheduled exercise 15 times with weights increased from 5 pounds to 7 pounds")
▶ Independently (or with minimal assistance) moves all joints through complete range-of-motion at least one time
▶ Independently (or with minimal assistance) assumes position, "dangling" at side of bed
▶ Independently (or with minimal assistance) transfers from bed to chair or wheelchair
▶ Independently (or with the use of an assistive device or with minimal assistance) walks a measureable distance (e.g., "walks from room to the end of the hall and back [50 feet]")

Planning nursing interventions begins on first contact with the client, when short-term, intermediate, and

NURSING DIAGNOSIS PROFILE

Impaired Physical Mobility

Definition. A state in which an individual experiences a limitation of ability for independent physical movement

Classification. Moving 6.1.1.1

Defining Characteristics. The main characteristic supporting this nursing diagnosis is the inability to move purposefully to the degree desired. The person may be (1) unable to move one or more individual body parts, (2) unable to move about within the physical environment (e.g., unable to ambulate, unable to transfer from the bed to a chair, unable to turn and move about within the confines of the bed), or (3) unable to move one or more body parts and unable to move about within the physical environment.

Lack of purposeful movement may be evidenced by (1) physical limitations such as reduced range of motion; decreased muscle strength, control, or mass; or impaired coordination; (2) limiting emotional states such as reluctance or refusal to attempt movement that would seem to be physically possible; or (3) mechanical restrictions such as restraints or casts or other medical treatments that result in decreased mobility, such as medications that depress the central nervous system.

For each type of desired movement, the degree to which the physical mobility is impaired may be classified according to functional level as

0—completely independent (diagnosis does not apply)
1—requires use of equipment or device
2—requires help from another person for assistance, supervision, or teaching
3—requires help from another person and equipment or device
4—dependent, does not participate in activity[44]

This diagnosis pertains to functional levels 1 through 4.

Sample Related Factors. When stating the related factor, it is not necessary to identify whether the decrease in mobility stems from unavoidable physical or emotional states or from prescribed treatments. Common related factors (whatever their source) are

▶ decreased strength and endurance
▶ the effects of neuromuscular impairment
▶ the effects of musculoskeletal impairment
▶ pain
▶ perceptual/cognitive impairment
▶ activity intolerance
▶ severe anxiety

Concept Description. This diagnosis is quite common because so many disorders affect mobility and so many treatments restrict mobility. It is appropriate for the client whose mobility level is severely restricted as well as for the client who is immobilized minimally and for only a brief period of time. This diagnosis, like all nursing diagnoses, should be used only for the client whose mobility can be improved by nursing interventions.

Examples. Depending on the specific assessment data, this diagnostic category could be applicable in the following situations, among others:

▶ The person who is physically able to move but who is generally too weak (or in too much pain) to complete purposeful movement without assistance (e.g., a person who has just awakened from general anesthesia after major chest surgery). For such persons, the diagnosis would be *Impaired Physical Mobility* R/T *Activity Intolerance* (or *Pain*).
▶ The person who is physically able to move but is unaware or unbelieving of the facts (e.g., a person with schizophrenia who believes he has no legs and who refuses to try to move). For such persons, the nursing diagnosis would be *Impaired Physical Mobility* R/T perceptual impairment.
▶ The person whose movement is temporarily limited by some type of musculoskeletal (or neuromuscular) pathology (e.g., a person with beginning joint contractures). For such individuals, the nursing diagnosis would be *Impaired Physical Mobility* R/T the effects of musculoskeletal (or neuromuscular) impairment.
▶ The person who cannot move because of extreme anxiety (e.g., a person who is afraid to attempt walking since suffering a broken hip and undergoing surgery for total hip joint replacement). For such individuals, the nursing diagnosis would be *Impaired Physical Mobility* R/T *Anxiety*.
▶ The person who is physically able to move but whose movement is restricted (e.g., a client in traction). For such individuals, the nursing diagnosis again would be *Impaired Physical Mobility* R/T the effects of musculoskeletal impairment.

Related/Similar Nursing Diagnoses. Three closely related nursing diagnoses need to be differentiated. These diagnoses may even be used concurrently for the same client. They are *Activity Intolerance, Impaired Physical Mobility,* and *High Risk for Disuse Syndrome.*

Activity Intolerance is a state in which an individual has insufficient physiologic or psychologic energy to endure or complete required or desired daily activities. With this diagnosis, the person is not physically unable to move but simply lacks the stamina or endurance to move as much as need be. *Activity Intolerance,* then, may be a related factor for *Impaired Physical Mobility.*

Impaired Physical Mobility is a state in which an individual experiences a limitation of ability for independent physical movement. This condition may be related to *Activity Intolerance* or to other factors. Whatever its contributing factor, this diagnosis can be accompanied by, and be a related factor for, a diagnosis of *High Risk for Disuse Syndrome.*

High Risk for Disuse Syndrome (see Nursing Diagnosis Profile in Chapter 35), is a state in which an individual is at high risk for deterioration of body systems as the result of prescribed or unavoidable musculoskeletal inactivity. In other words, because of the client's impaired physical mobility, the person is at risk of developing a breakdown of multiple body systems.

Nursing Diagnosis continued on following page

NURSING DIAGNOSIS PROFILE Continued

Impaired Physical Mobility

In addition to these three closely related diagnoses, the client who is immobilized may have a number of other nursing diagnoses that stem from the impaired physical mobility. These include, but are not limited to

- ▶ *High risk for injury*
- ▶ *High risk for trauma*
- ▶ *Impaired social interaction*
- ▶ *Altered role performance*
- ▶ *Sexual dysfunction*
- ▶ *Spiritual distress*
- ▶ *Ineffective individual coping*
- ▶ *Impaired adjustment*
- ▶ *Fatigue*
- ▶ *Sleep pattern disturbance*
- ▶ *Diversional activity deficit*

- ▶ *Impaired home maintenance management*
- ▶ *Self-care deficit (feeding, bathing/hygiene, dressing/ grooming, toileting)*
- ▶ *Altered growth and development*
- ▶ *Body image disturbance*
- ▶ *Self-esteem disturbance*
- ▶ *Hopelessness*
- ▶ *Powerlessness*
- ▶ *Dysfunctional grieving*
- ▶ *Anxiety*
- ▶ *Fear*
- ▶ *High risk for disuse syndrome* and other diagnoses that might be included in the disuse syndrome that often results from immobility (e.g., *Impaired tissue integrity, Constipation, Potential for infection*).

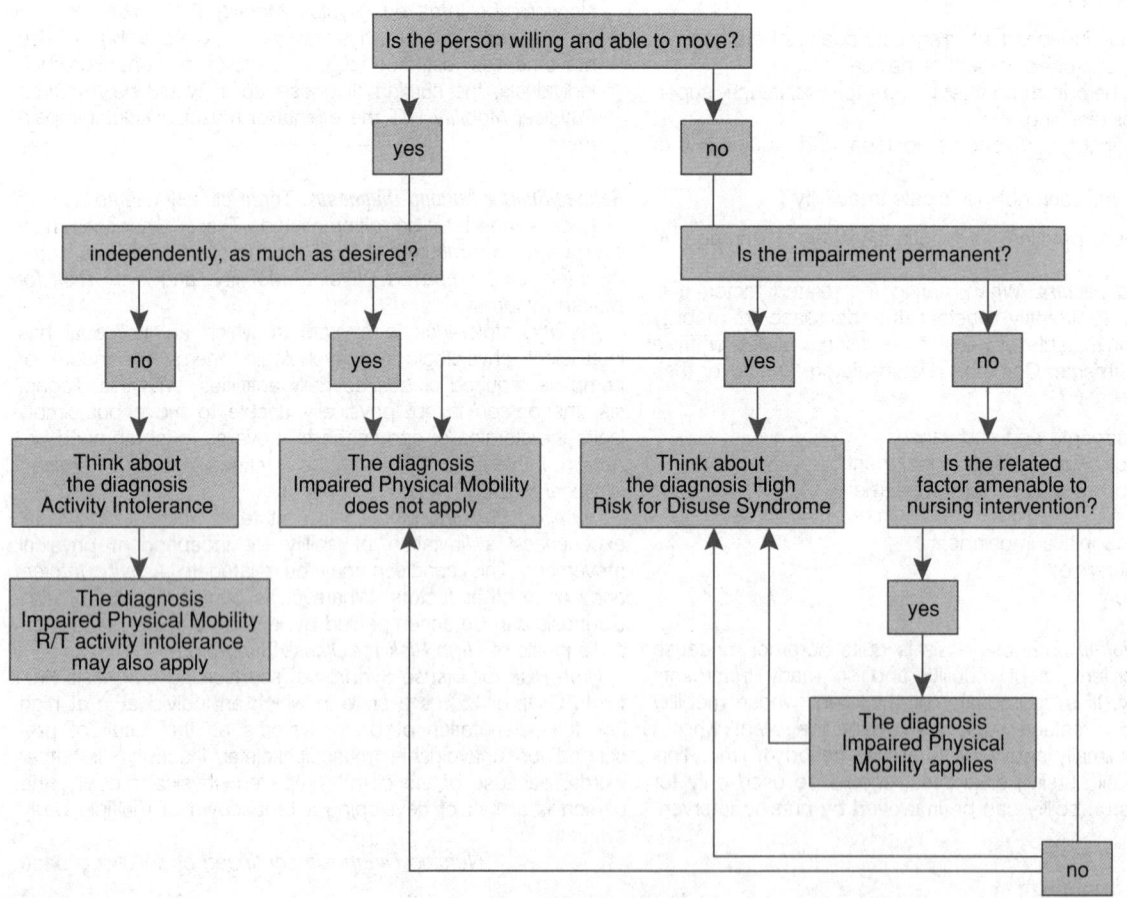

▲ **Figure 36–2**

Decision tree for the nursing diagnosis *Impaired Physical Mobility.*

long-term outcomes are identified. Often planning is done by health team members who work in collaboration and who intend to follow the client long after discharge from the health care agency. At first the focus may be on planning to strengthen the client's upper extremities so that crutch walking will be easier when the client is ready. Later, the focus may be on planning to teach and assist the client to be able to walk with crutches. After that, the focus of the plan may be to assist the client in walking without the crutches. At a future date, when independent mobility has again been achieved, the focus may be on helping the client to plan a fitness program. All of this planning is started on initial contact with the client, but the focus changes as the client progresses and achieves increasingly challenging outcomes. The main goal is, of course, optimal mobility.

NURSING INTERVENTION

Exercises

When the anticipated outcome of nursing interventions is an increase in the client's mobility level, one of the most important nursing interventions is exercise. Of course, exercise does more than increase a person's mobility level. It also helps to

▶ build muscle mass and strength
▶ promote the health of many body organs and organ systems
▶ prevent potential complications of immobility
▶ combat the negative effects of aging (Table 36–2)
▶ increase the client's sense of control and feelings of self-esteem

Caution While it is usually beneficial, exercise can cause some untoward effects too. For example, both increased cardiac workload and use of the Valsalva maneuver occur during many types of exercise, and both can be dangerous to clients who suffer from certain cardiac disorders. To prevent dangerous outcomes related to increased cardiac workload, it is essential that a physician assess each client's limitations before any exercise program is initiated. Instruct your clients to avoid the Valsalva maneuver by exhaling slowly through an open mouth during exercise.[7,36]

In addition to clients with cardiac disorders, those with certain circulatory, respiratory, neuromuscular, and musculoskeletal disorders such as osteoporosis or unstable bone fractures may be at risk for complications from exercise. Clients with these conditions need exercise to improve their health, but they can be placed in jeopardy by doing the wrong type of exercise or by doing the right type of exercise incorrectly. If in doubt about your plans for a client, verify them with the physician.

Generally, it is the physician's responsibility to specify the activity level and exercises needed for each client. Much decision making, however, is left to the judgment of the physical or occupational therapist and

the professional nurse. With no contraindications to having a client progressively building strength through exercise, how do you decide where to begin?

One common method for deciding about the amount of exercise needed is to begin by assessing what the person can reasonably do and gradually increasing the work expected. For example, if the most the person can do at one time is flex and extend the elbows five times, you might start by having the client do this five times (one set) and do perhaps two sets each day. As time passes (e.g., one to two weeks) and completing the sets becomes easier for the client, you might increase the requirements by having the client do more sets each day (say three or four sets) or increase the number of repetitions (say seven to ten repetitions per set). In some cases, you may increase both the number of repetitions per set and the number of sets per day. Use care, however, not to exhaust the person by demanding too much progress at once.

Your plan must be individualized to each client and must be reasonable.

With this general information in mind, you can consider specific types of exercises to increase a client's mobility. We are concerned, generally, with two type of exercises: those that build muscle mass and strength and those that promote range-of-joint-motion (often referred to simply as range of motion, or ROM).

BUILDING MUSCLE MASS AND STRENGTH

Isotonic Exercises. In **isotonic exercises** muscle tension remains the same while the muscles shorten in contraction as body parts move to do work. As the client flexes and extends the body parts, the muscles used increase in mass and strength.

Clients who have not started to ambulate may complete special isotonic exercises in bed. These include simpler exercises that can be done even when the person is very weak, intellectually impaired, or under the effects of medications that reduce alertness. For example, you may ask the person to flex and extend the fingers and thumbs (by repeatedly encouraging the person to "make a tight fist" or to squeeze a rubber ball or palm cone), flex and extend the elbows, wiggle the toes, flex and hyperextend the ankles, and flex and extend the knees and hips.

As the client becomes ready for more strenuous isotonic exercises, dumbbells or wrist weights may be used to increase resistance during certain exercises (e.g., while flexing and extending the elbows and shoulders). If the client is able to assume a sitting position in bed, bed push-ups may be done by pushing down on the mattress on both sides of the body in order to raise the hips from the mattress. Also in a sitting position, the client may perform bed chin-ups by pulling the body directly upward toward an overhead trapeze, until the hips are lifted off the bed. By beginning in a supine position, the client may perform bed pull-ups by pulling the torso upward toward the trapeze and into a sitting position. Figure 36–3 illustrates chin-ups and pull-ups.

TABLE 36–2. Effects of Exercise and Aging on Select Body Systems

Body System	Exercise	Aging
Circulatory		
Cardiovascular		
Maximal oxygen consumption	Increase	Decrease
Maximal heart rate	Increase	Decrease
Cardiac output	Increase	Decrease
Blood pressure	Same or decrease	Increase
Vascular resistance	Decrease	Increase
Blood components		
Serum lipids		
Total cholesterol	?*	Increase
Triglycerides	Decrease	Increase
Low-density lipoproteins	?	Increase ?
High-density lipoproteins	Increase	Decrease ?
Immune system	Increase ?	Decrease
Musculoskeletal		
Muscles		
Strength	Increase	Decrease
Endurance	Increase	Unchanged
Flexibility	Increase ?	Decrease ?
Bony structures		
Bone mineral content	Increase	Decrease
Body composition		
Lean body mass	Increase	Decrease
Adipose tissue	Decrease	Increase
Regulatory system		
Metabolic		
Basal metabolic rate	Increase	Decrease
Heat gain	Increase	Decrease
Heat loss	Increase	Decrease
Nervous		
Sleep	Increase ?	Decrease
Anxiety/depression	Decrease ?	Increase ?
Cognitive functioning	Increase	Decrease

* ? = Inconclusive or inadequate evidence.
From Schilke, J.M. (1991). Slowing the aging process with physical activity. *Journal of Gerontological Nursing* 17(6), 4–8.

When the client is ready to get out of the bed several times a day, progressively increasing the distance walked is a common practice. For example, the client moves to the bedside chair, then to the bathroom across the room, and then for longer and longer distances down the hall. Activities of daily living, too, are progressively increased. At first, you may have to do almost everything for your immobilized clients. Then, as their strength builds, you may encourage them to do more. For example, you may gather their mouth care equipment and bathing supplies so they can brush their own teeth and bathe themselves, and you may prepare the food on their trays so they can eat independently. Still later, you may stand by to observe that they can manage as they first get out of bed to stand at the bathroom sink for mouth care, as they first shower independently, and as they resume such mealtime activities as opening the milk carton, cutting meat, and feeding themselves.

Thus, in planned programs of exercise sets and in progressively increasing the client's ability to carry out activities of daily living, the client will be flexing muscles and completing isotonic exercises. Encouraging the client to complete more and more activities that promote isotonic exercise will help increase muscle mass and strength.

Isometric Exercises. With **isometric exercises,** the muscles maintain the same length, but their tension increases. This type of exercise occurs when force is exerted against a stable object so that no movement takes place and the muscles contract but do not shorten. A common example of isometric exercise is seen when nurses encourage immobilized clients to push their feet against an immovable footboard in order to prevent muscle weakness and atrophy. With isometric exercises, the client uses energy, but no work is done. Even though no work is done, isometric exercise will help build muscle mass and strength.

Isometric exercises may be compared with a person who is attempting to lift a locomotive. The person

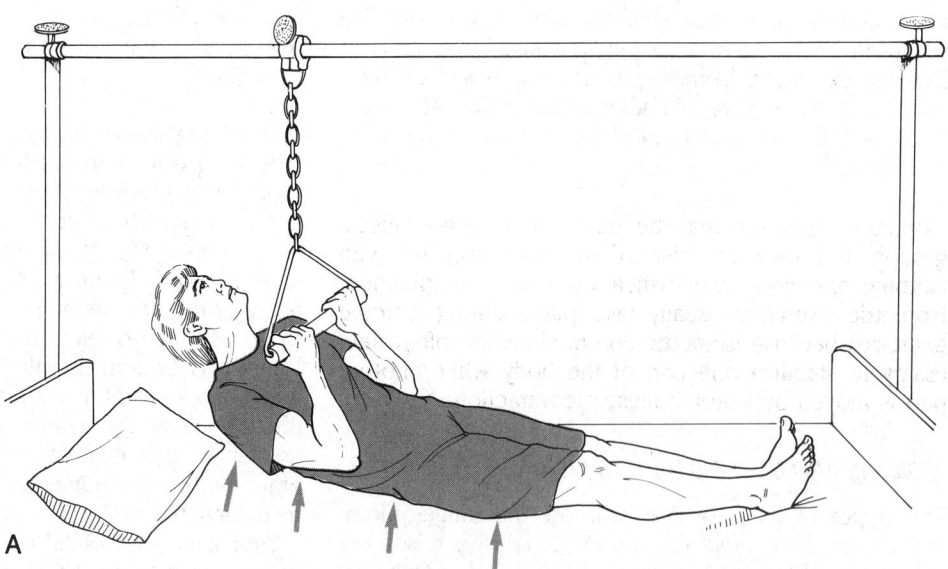

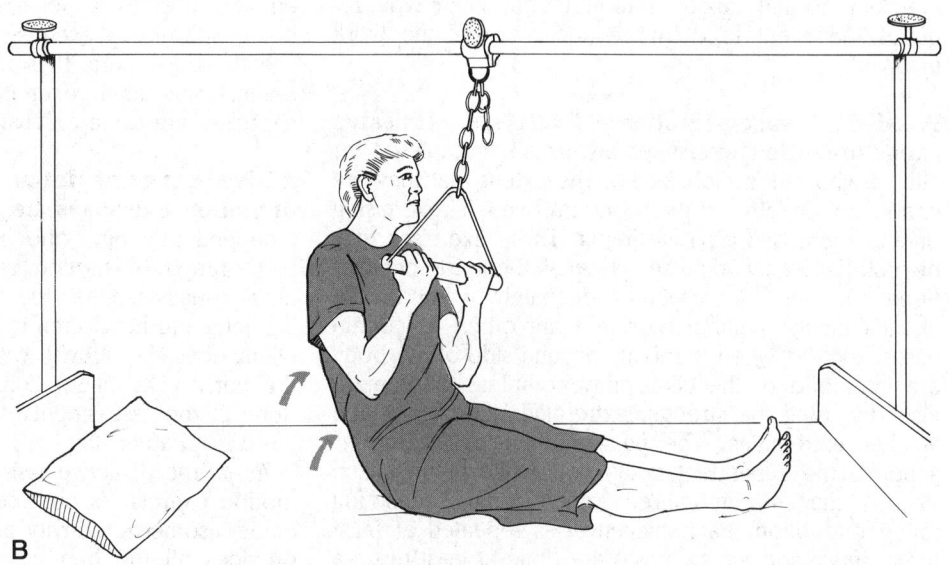

▲ *Figure 36–3*

Bed chin-ups and bed pull-ups are made possible by the overhead trapeze. The overhead trapeze can be an important piece of equipment in the exercise program as well as in encouraging increased mobility in general. *A,* Note that the trapeze has been moved nearer to the head of the bed so it is in place for the client to pull directly upward in attempts at bed chin-ups. Note, too, that the body is kept rigid so it can be lifted completely off the mattress as the heels serve as a fulcrum. *B,* For bed pull-ups, the trapeze is moved farther away from the head of the bed and its chain has been shortened, to allow the client sufficient space to pull up to it. For pull-ups, the client raises only the torso while flexing at the hips.

would use a great deal of energy but would not do any actual work. It is a physics principle that work equals force exerted times the distance that an object is moved ($W = F \times D$). Therefore, unless something is moved at least some distance, no work has been done, regardless of the amount of force (energy) expended.

Isometric exercises are also called **muscle-setting exercises.** They are frequently prescribed when the spine or an extremity is in a cast and joint movement under the cast is impossible. They are also commonly done with abdominal, quadriceps, and gluteal muscles in immobilized clients who are not in a cast. In such cases, muscle-setting exercises can help prevent muscle weakness and atrophy.

Many people have done isometric exercises or, at least, understand this term. If not, you may help them understand how to do isometric exercises, say of the gluteals, by telling them to "tighten up" the muscles and to try to squeeze their buttocks together as hard as they can for a given number of seconds. Alternatively, tell them to "make a muscle" with their biceps so they can feel what a muscle should feel like when it is in isometric contraction.

Once clients understand how to contract a muscle, they must be taught how long to hold each contraction, how many times to contract and release the muscle, and how long to rest the muscle between each contraction. One common formula for a set consists of five contractions, with each contraction held 5 seconds and with 2 minutes' rest between each contraction. The number of sets per hour or per day is variable. As with isotonic exercises, isometric exercise is based on individual tolerance. Several studies indicate that, for maximum benefit, the muscle must be worked to the point of fatigue.[26]

Isometric exercises may be done on isolated muscle groups, but they are also often done together with isotonic exercises, even when these are not planned. Isometric exercises usually take place during isotonic exercises because isometric contractions are often necessary to stabilize one part of the body while another part is moved by isotonic muscle contractions.[32]

PROMOTING RANGE-OF-MOTION EXERCISES

Four types of exercise that promote the range-of-joint motion we term range-of-motion (ROM) exercises are (1) passive ROM, (2) active-assistive ROM, (3) active ROM, and (4) resistive ROM. All four types require that one or more joints be put through the full measure of possible movements in all planes in order to help maintain normal range of motion, but each type requires the client to do more and more of the work involved.

Passive Range-of-Motion Exercises. Passive range-of-motion exercises are usually completed for clients who are immobilized to the extent that they are unable to do any of the work involved in exercising one or more of their own joints. These exercises may be completed by a nurse, physical therapist, occupational therapist, or (when adequately trained) the client's family member or significant other. In certain cases, such as when the joints on one side of the body are immobilized, the client may complete these exercises by using the stronger extremities to exercise the weaker extremities. The person doing the exercises supports the dependent body parts while putting each of the client's immobilized joints through their full range of motion. Each maneuver is repeated at least three times, and the exercises are done at least twice a day[26] (Procedure 36–1).

Passive range-of-motion exercises help to

▶ maintain joint mobility
▶ prevent shortening of muscles, tendons, ligaments, and joint capsules and thus prevent muscle contractures and joint stiffness
▶ prevent adaptive stretching or lengthening of connective tissue around joints
▶ prevent deformities that limit function
▶ stimulate circulation and sensory nerve endings
▶ restore loss of joint function
▶ increase endurance
▶ promote feelings of comfort and well-being.

Clients who require passive range-of-motion exercises are unable to independently move the body parts being exercised. The muscles of these body parts do not perform isotonic contractions. Unless isometric exercises are done, the muscles of these parts will not

increase in mass or strength. Passive range-of-motion exercises alone will not increase muscle mass or strength.[36]

Active-Assistive Range-of-Motion Exercises. Active-assistive range-of-motion exercises are also used for clients with decreased mobility in one or more body parts. The client who requires active-assistive ROM, unlike the client who requires passive ROM, is able to partially move at an affected joint, and the nurse (or other helping person) encourages the client to do as much of each particular maneuver as possible. When it is evident that the client can go no further, the nurse supports the dependent body part and completes the maneuver by passive range of motion. Each maneuver is repeated, in a like manner, at least three times before the nurse encourages the client to do the next maneuver.

Active-assistive ROM provides the same benefits to clients as passive ROM exercises, but it does even more. Active-assistive exercises increase muscle use and help build muscle mass and strength, in addition to helping to keep the joints flexible. As the client shortens the muscles to begin each movement, muscles are being isotonically exercised. The muscles used to stabilize the body parts that are not moving, however, are being isometrically exercised. Like passive ROM, these exercises are done at least three times, twice each day.

Active Range-of-Motion Exercises. Active range-of-motion exercises are exercises in which the client independently puts one or more joints through complete range of motion several times each day. The nurse usually teaches the client what to do, how to do it safely, and how often to do each maneuver. Then the client does the activity without hands-on assistance by the nurse. The client completes each maneuver as is done in the assessment of range of motion (see Table 35–2 in Chapter 35).

As is true of active-assistive exercise, active range of motion exercise is considered isotonic but actually includes isometric activity as well. Active ROM exercise provides all the benefits conferred by active-assistive ROM. The number of repetitions done each time (set) and the number of sets done each day vary according to individual tolerance, but active range-of-motion exercises are usually done more frequently than passive or active-assistive exercises.

Resistive Range-of-Motion Exercises. Resistive range-of-motion exercises are similar to active exercises except that some force is exerted to prevent easy movement of the limb during each maneuver. For example, weights may be strapped to the client's ankles to increase resistance during hip and knee exercises or the person may hold dumbbells while exercising the shoulders and elbows. Alternatively, the nurse may hold the extremity so that increased force must be used to move it in the required direction. Exercise machines are also available to provide measured amounts of resistance as the person places each joint through its full range of motion.

Text continued on page 822

PROCEDURE 36-1

Passive Range-of-Motion Exercises

Definition/Purposes. A series of maneuvers in which one or more of a client's immobilized joints are taken through complete range of motion. The primary purpose is to help maintain joint mobility.

Contraindications/Cautions. Although the client or the client's significant other may assume the task of performing passive range-of-motion exercises, it is imperative that these lay persons be taught how to complete each maneuver safely. Much joint damage can result from improper technique. *No one* should perform passive ROM without a physician's order if the client has any of the following conditions: acute arthritis, bone fracture, head injury, torn ligament, joint dislocation or subluxation, acute cardiac pathology, or thrombophlebitis.

Before beginning the exercises, caution the client to inform you if any pain is experienced. Proceed in any orderly manner, working slowly, carefully, and smoothly as you complete each maneuver in the correct plane and to the correct degree of movement. Complete all maneuvers required for each joint before proceeding to exercise the next joint, progressing systematically from head to toe. At all times, support with your hands any joint that is not supported on the bed or table.

During the exercises, note the point at which any pain is experienced and do not exceed this point as the exercises continue. Do not use force to continue a maneuver if you feel resistance. If the muscle goes into spasm because of central nervous system damage, do not use force to try to move beyond the point of spasm. The spasm will often stop if you back off on the pressure slightly and support the extremity in a functional position. You may obtain guidance from a physical therapist in working with spasms of this sort. Stop exercises if the client becomes fatigued before they are completed.

An immobilized person will begin to exhibit connective tissue changes in as brief a time as 5 days. Therefore, begin preventive passive ROM exercises as soon as possible. Complete at least three of each maneuver possible in the immobilized joint(s) at least twice daily.

Teaching/Learning Guidelines. Review with the client and significant others the purposes and the contraindications and cautions. Explain the importance of proper body positioning and teach how to achieve each required position. Teach the client to perform each maneuver correctly and how to support the extremity and protect the joint during the maneuver. Provide written instructions with illustrations to enhance understanding and for review later, as needed. Explain the importance of progression from passive to active-assistive and from active-assistive to active exercises in the restoration to mobility.

PRELIMINARY ACTIVITIES

Assessment/Planning

▶ Review chart for diagnosis and evidence of contraindications
▶ Review activity/exercise orders
▶ Check nursing orders regarding passive ROM
▶ Assess person's ability to follow directions
▶ Assess limitations of joint movement
▶ Determine joints to be exercised and positions to be used
▶ Assess need for additional assistants

Equipment

▶ Bed with firm mattress or padded table
▶ Appropriate, nonrestrictive clothing for client
▶ Bath blanket, if required for drape

PROCEDURE

Each maneuver is completed three times

Preparation of Person and Bed

▶ Explain why and how the exercises are to be performed
▶ Provide for privacy by drawing a curtain or screen or close the door to the room
▶ Raise bed to a working height and lock wheels
▶ Fan-fold top covers to the foot of the bed
▶ Dress person in pajamas or loosely fitting pants and tops; If only a hospital gown is available, use it but drape the client with a sheet or bath blanket as needed to avoid exposure. Keep feet bare.
▶ If not contraindicated, lower the mattress to a flat position and remove the pillow
▶ Caution client to let you know if the exercises cause any discomfort

Actions	Rationale/Discussion
1. With the client in supine position, face the client's head and lower side rail on side nearest you.	1. Facing the direction of planned movement avoids twisting your vertebral column.
2. Bring client's body to the side of the bed nearest you.	2. Keeping the weight to be lifted near your center of gravity helps prevent back strain.
3. Be sure the client is in good body alignment.	3. Good alignment helps assure correct movement of body parts during exercises.

Procedure continued on following page

PROCEDURE 36–1 Continued

Passive Range-of-Motion Exercises

Actions

4. Place both your hands on the client's head, slightly above and behind the client's ears (Fig. 36–4), and flex the neck by lifting the head (chin toward the client's chest) and extend it by returning it to a position flat on the bed. Repeat, *slowly,* two more times.
5. Without moving your hands, laterally flex the neck by slowly moving the head to one side (ear toward shoulder) and back three times. Repeat lateral flexion and extension to the opposite side three times.
6. Still without moving your hands, turn the head to one side (chin toward shoulder) and back, three times, to rotate the neck. Repeat, *slowly,* to opposite side three times.
7. Move your hands to each of the client's shoulders (center them approximately at midclavicular line) and cup your fingers over the shoulders, fingertips toward the scapulae.

    Carefully pull the shoulders upward and toward you as you encourage the client to relax and allow the head to fall backward into a position of hyperextension. *Do not lift the head off the bed* (Fig. 36–5).

    Allow the shoulders and neck to return to their original positions of extension. Repeat two more times.
8. Flex the client's spine by raising the head of the bed as high as it will go and then placing your hands behind the client's scapulae and pulling to curve the upper thoracic spine forward into a position of flexion (Fig. 36–6). Allow the client's torso to return to the mattress and lower the head of the bed to the flat position to extend the spine. Repeat two more times.
9. With the bed flat, laterally flex the client's spine by holding the pelvis stable with one hand over the client's far hip as you push the client's upper torso to one side by applying pressure to the client's near shoulder with your other hand (Fig. 36–7). Raising and lowering the side rails as appropriate, go to the opposite side of the bed to reverse the direction of flexion and then return to the original side for one last reversal.
10. Return the client to the supine position with spine straight. Rotate the spine by placing the flat of one hand under the client's far arm and over the scapula

Rationale/Discussion

4. This hand position will allow good control of the head. It will avoid placing pressure on the jaw and possibly dislocating it.

    Slow movement of the head helps to prevent dizziness.
5. Repeating all maneuvers possible without moving your hands allows the client to feel more secure and supported and provides for more efficiency of motion.
6. The head should not be tilted to either side but should pivot on a horizontal plane.
7. This method allows full hyperextension of the neck without turning the client to the prone position or forcing the neck into an unusual position.

    If the head does not leave the bed, the neck remains supported. Lifting the head from the bed could cause too extreme a hyperextension and result in cervical damage.
8. Spinal exercises may or may not be included as a part of the routine ROM exercises done by nurses at a given clinical facility. As is evident with this maneuver, the spine is flexed and extended to some degree each time the head of the bed is raised and lowered.
9. It is not necessary to flex the cervical spine laterally at this time because this maneuver was done with the neck exercises.
10. As you pull, rock backward from one leg to the other in order to use leverage.

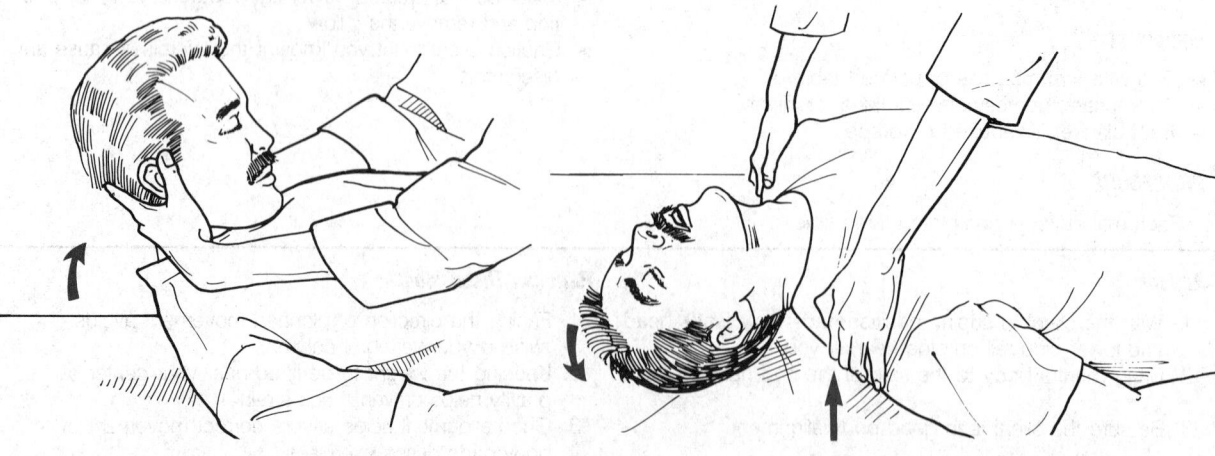

▲ Figure 36–4.   ▲ Figure 36–5

PROCEDURE 36-1 Continued

Passive Range-of-Motion Exercises

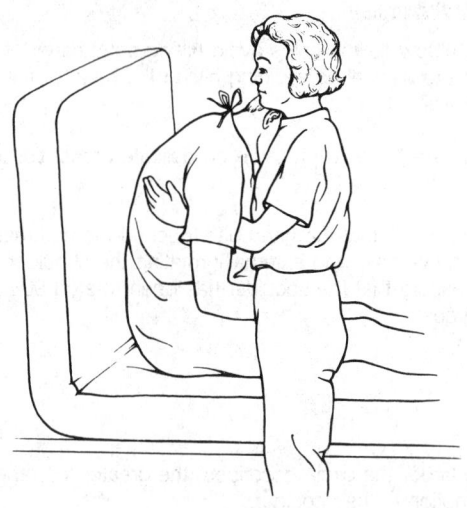

▲ *Figure 36-6*

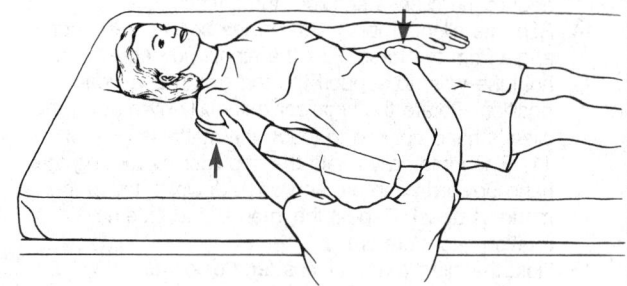

▲ *Figure 36-7*

Actions

and pulling to turn the upper part of the client's torso toward you (Fig. 36-8). Raising and lowering the side rails appropriately, go to the opposite side of the bed to rotate in the opposite direction and then return to the original side for a third rotation.

11. Move to the shoulder nearest to you. Support the client's arm with one of your hands holding the client's wrist and your other hand supporting the client's elbow as you bring the client's arm straight up 90 degrees to begin flexing the shoulder. Flex the client's elbow 90 degrees as you lower the arm toward the mattress so the client's forearm fits between the head of the bed and the client's head (Fig. 36-9). Attempt to touch the client's forearm to the mattress above the head. Return the arm to the client's side, in a position of extension. Repeat the flexion and extension two more times.

Rationale/Discussion

All neck and spinal exercises are now completed.
11. All joints not supported on the bed should be supported by the nurse's hands.

Flexing the elbow helps prevent hitting the client's forearm on the wall or head of the bed.

If the forearm touches the mattress above the client's head, you will know you have flexed the shoulder 180 degrees.

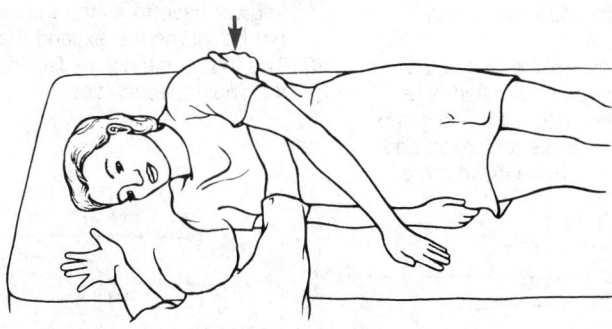

▲ *Figure 36-8*

Procedure continued on following page

PROCEDURE 36-1 Continued

Passive Range-of-Motion Exercises

Actions

12. Continuing to support the client's wrist and elbow joints with your hands, flex the elbow 90 degrees and laterally flex the client's shoulder three times to abduct it (Fig. 36–10).
13. Continuing to support the client's wrist and elbow joints, and with the client's elbow extended, cross-adduct the client's shoulder three times.
14. Rest the client's upper arm on the bed at a 90-degree angle from the torso. Flex the elbow 90 degrees and hold the wrist to support the forearm in a vertical position. Rotate the shoulder externally by moving the client's hand upward to touch the mattress (Fig. 36–11). Then internally rotate the shoulder by moving the hand upward in an arc and back down to touch the mattress again. Repeat the internal and external rotation two more times.
15. Hold the client's arm at wrist and elbow and circumduct the shoulder.
    Describing as large a circle as possible, move the arm upward from a position of extension, across the breast, above the head, out to the side of the bed, and back into place at the client's side. Repeat two more times.
16. With the arm in extension while continuing to hold the wrist and elbow, elevate and then depress the shoulder girdle three times.
17. With the elbow in extension, place one of your hands in the client's hand as if you were going to shake hands in greeting. Support the client's elbow with your other hand. Rotate the forearm into pronation and then into supination three times.
18. With the client's upper arm on the mattress and the elbow flexed 90 degrees, support the forearm in a vertical position (with one of your hands holding the forearm very near the wrist) while you use your other hand to hold the client's palm in order to flex (palmar flexion), extend, and hyperextend (dorsiflexion) the client's wrist. Repeat two more times.
19. Continuing to support the forearm in the same manner, laterally flex the wrist into radial and ulnar flexion. Repeat two times.
20. Continuing to support the elbow on the bed in the same manner as before, move both your hands to hold the four fingers as you flex them all at the same time. Roll them down so that all joints are flexed and roll them back up into extension. Repeat two more times.

Rationale/Discussion

12. The elbow flexion helps avoid hitting any nearby furniture as well as avoiding hitting the head of the bed and wall.
13. Use care to avoid pressure on delicate breast tissue.
14. By assuring that the hand has touched the mattress when internally and externally rotating the shoulder, you will assure that the shoulder has been rotated 90 degrees.
15. The larger the circle described, the greater the range of motion in the shoulder.
    Moving the arm in this direction can sweep delicate breast tissue out of the arm's way, rather than allowing the arm to come down firmly on it from above, as might otherwise occur in persons with pendulous breasts.
16. To protect the joint and the muscle from trauma, an extremity should be supported at the joints. It should not be held by grasping the belly of the muscle.
17. This hand grasp prevents you from rotating the client's arm any farther than you can rotate your own arm.
18. Holding the wrist could block full range of motion.
19. If you first lace your fingers through the client's fingers, you will have to match the client's movements and will not be inclined to exceed the normal range of motion.
20. The thumb cannot be flexed at the same time because the fingers would block its full flexion.

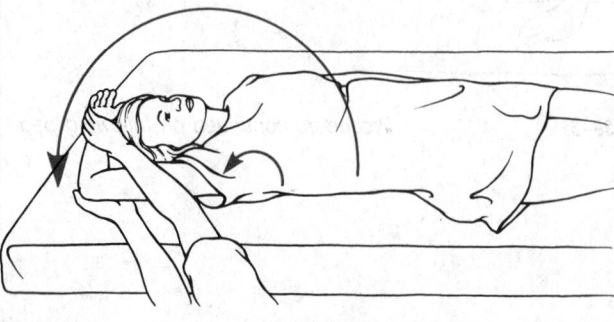

▲ *Figure 36–9*

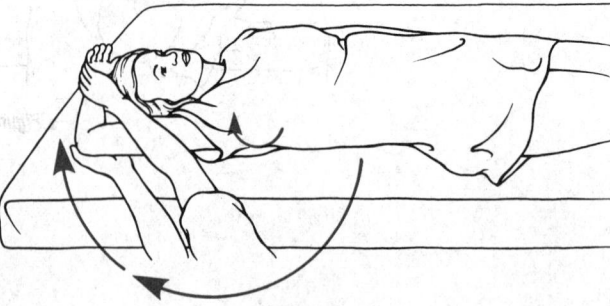

▲ *Figure 36–10*

PROCEDURE 36–1 Continued

Passive Range-of-Motion Exercises

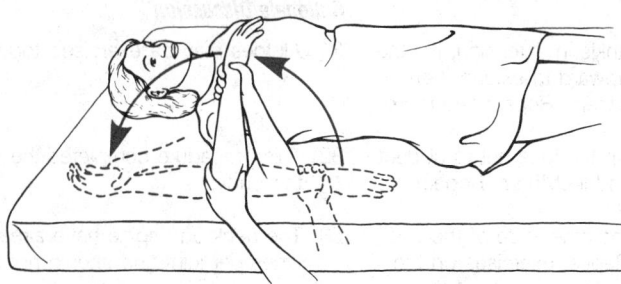

▲ Figure 36–11

Actions	Rationale/Discussion
21. While supporting the extremity in the same manner, fan out the four fingers and the thumb in order to abduct them. Return them to their natural position to adduct them. Repeat two times.	21. The thumb and fingers can be abducted at the same time.
22. Continuing in the same manner, flex the thumb across the palm and extend it. Repeat two times.	22. Be certain that both thumb joints are flexed.
23. Continuing in the same manner, touch the tip of the thumb to the tip of each finger in turn to complete thumb opposition. Repeat two times.	23. It does not matter whether you work from little finger toward index finger or proceed in the opposite direction.
24. Move to the hip. Support the lower leg by holding it below the ankle with one hand and below the knee with the other. Flex and extend the client's hip and knee at the same time (if not contraindicated). Repeat two times.	24. As you bring the knee closer to the hip, you will have to remove your hand to prevent blocking the full degree of flexion possible. To do this, slip your hand out (at the "last possible minute") and hold the side of the knee to prevent the leg from falling outward and externally rotating the hip. As you bring the leg back downward, toward extension, return your hand to its position under the knee as soon as space is available. This support at the knee is important to prevent hyperextension.
25. Establish a wide base of support and, supporting the client's leg under the ankle and knee, lift it close to your body and rock or step backward as necessary to abduct the hip. Then rock or step forward to adduct and cross-adduct it, keeping it as close to your body as possible. Repeat two more times.	25. Holding weights close to your center of gravity helps prevent back strain when lifting.
26. Lay the leg on the bed with the hip in extension. With one hand over the ankle and one hand over the knee, roll the leg inward and then roll it outward to internally and externally rotate the hip. Repeat two more times.	26. For this maneuver, the bed can support the joints and save energy expenditure.
27. Supporting the leg under the knee and ankle, circumduct the hip by describing as large a circle as possible. Repeat two times.	27. It does not matter whether the circle is clockwise or counterclockwise. What matters is that the full range of motion is achieved.
28. With the leg lying straight on the bed, support the ankle with one hand and use the other hand to move the ankle into flexion (plantar flexion) and back (through extension) into hyperextension (dorsiflexion). Repeat two times.	28. If the immobilized client is tending to develop footdrop, you may decide not to flex the ankle and to concentrate on dorsiflexion instead. If the client's ankles have been in extension against a footboard for a long time, however, both maneuvers may be important.
29. Continuing with the leg in the same position, hold the client's ankle at the lower leg and cup the other hand under the sole of the foot at the heel in order to laterally flex the ankle as you invert and evert it. Repeat two times.	29. For this exercise, the sole should remain flat as the ankle moves.
30. Continuing in the same manner, hold the ankle securely at the heel while you use your other hand to turn the distal third of the foot inward for internal metatarsal inversion and outward for metatarsal eversion. Repeat two times.	30. For this exercise, the heel should remain stable while the ball of the foot twists inward and outward.

Procedure continued on following page

PROCEDURE 36–1 Continued

Passive Range-of-Motion Exercises

Actions	*Rationale/Discussion*
31. With the leg straight and the ankle in extension, roll the toes downward to flex them, upward to extend them, and backward to hyperextend them. Repeat two more times.	31. All toes may be exercised together.
32. Continuing in a like manner, fan the toes out to abduct them and bring them back to adduct them. Repeat two more times.	32. This procedure completes the exercises for one side of the body.
33. Raise the side rail and go to the other side of the bed and move client toward you. Repeat exercises on the extremity joints as just done on the first side of the body.	33. The neck and spine have already been exercised three times per joint and should not have to be repeated.
34. When you have completed exercising all joints on the second side of the body, turn the client to the prone position, if possible.	34. Turning allows you to complete the exercises for shoulder, spine, and hip.
35. With the client's arm in extension, support the wrist and elbow as you lift the shoulder into hyperextension.	35. Most people cannot hyperextend this joint more than 45 to 60 degrees.
36. Raise the head of the bed as high as necessary to hyperextend the spine, and then lower it to the flat position. Repeat two more times.	36. This step allows the bed to do the work.
37. Supporting the leg under the knee and ankle, lift three times to hyperextend the hip.	37. For clients whose hips are contracted and in whom hyperextension is impossible, the prone position may be the most that can be accomplished.
38. Raise the side rail and go to the opposite side of the bed to repeat the exercises on the other side of the body.	38. This completes the required exercises.
39. Place the client in good body alignment, in a position that promotes comfort.	39. This will help the client rest.

FINAL ACTIVITIES

Replace covers, check vital signs, raise side rails, lower bed level, place call bell within reach. If not previously charted, document your assessment of the client's range of motion. If previously done, note any changes from the baseline data obtained. Note evidence of stiffness, pain, spasm, or other untoward effects. Chart number of repetitions completed and which joints were exercised (or omitted). State how the client tolerated the procedure. Record vital signs. List recommendations for additional exercises and/or progression to active-assistive or active exercises as needed.

This type of isotonic exercise usually requires increased stabilization of body parts by isometric contraction. Resistive exercise not only offers all of the benefits of active exercise but also helps build muscle better than the other three types. The number of repetitions per set and the number of sets per day must be individualized.

CONTINUOUS PASSIVE RANGE-OF-MOTION MACHINES

Many machines have been designed to help persons to exercise. One example is the continuous passive range-of-motion (CPM) machine (Fig. 36–12). The CPM machine supports the leg as it continuously flexes and extends the knee and hip. It can be manually stopped as desired, for example, to allow you to make the client's bed. The machine is fairly easy to learn to use and has been found to provide the desired results for the person with a knee injury who requires passive ROM exercises to maintain joint mobility.

THE EXERCISE PROGRAM

In clinical situations, the type of exercise required may vary for different body parts in the same individual, and the person's requirements may change over time. For example, consider Mr. Angelo, who suffered multiple injuries after falling three stories from a roof. He had surgery 3 days ago to place a pin in a fracture of his left femur, and he is generally weak from the trauma and the effects of surgery. Mr. Angelo needs to exercise to regain strength and prevent untoward effects of immobility. He also has a cast on his left leg and has the right leg in a continuous passive ROM machine.

He is doing isometric (muscle-setting) exercises under the cast and with the muscles of the leg that is

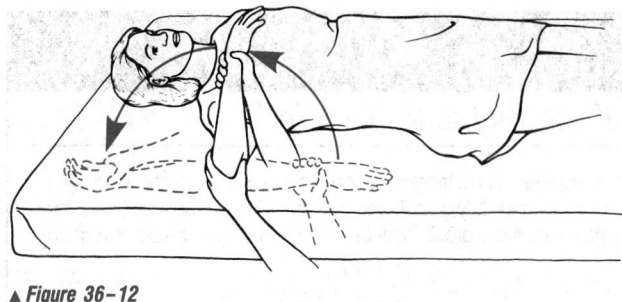

▲ *Figure 36-12*

Continuous passive range-of-motion (CPM) machine. (Courtesy of Chattanooga Group, Inc., Hixson, TN.)

in the CPM machine. The CPM machine provides continuous passive flexion and extension to the right hip and knee but restricts the hip from movement in other planes. The nurse has to take the leg out of the CPM machine to do additional hip exercises. Mr. Angelo must also do active range-of-motion exercises three times to all uninvolved joints twice a day and is expected to progress to resistive ROM of all uninvolved joints as soon as he is able. Also, because he will be on crutches when allowed out of bed in 2 more weeks, he will need to strengthen his shoulder and arm muscles. Thus, he is being encouraged to do ten bed push-ups, four times a day, in preparation for crutch walking. A program such as this is not unusual in an orthopedic unit. Can most people take this amount of exercise?

Much depends on the person's age, the person's general level of health, and other factors. For example, a 20-year-old could probably stand the exertion better than a 90-year-old, all other things being equal. A person age 90 years who is generally physically fit, however, could probably stand the exertion better than a person of age 20 years who has severe internal injuries and who has lost a lot of blood. At any age, the person who experiences a lot of pain but who has strong support systems and who is highly motivated to get well and return to usual activities could probably stand the exertion better than a severely depressed person who, for example, feels much better physically but does not want to live since being widowed 2 weeks earlier. As a nurse to such dissimilar persons, you will have much to consider as you plan for clients' exercise. It is often reassuring to know that the physician, physical therapist, occupational therapist, and client will all be working with you in planning for the exercise program.

Progressive Mobilization

The exercises we have just reviewed are nursing interventions that help meet outcomes of measurably increased muscle mass and strength and ability to independently move all joints through complete range of motion. Other outcomes important to the client with impaired physical mobility require interventions that help the client become increasingly able to move about in the environment. This increasing level of movement is termed *progressive mobilization* and includes such activities as "dangling" at the side of the bed, transferring from bed to chair or wheelchair, and walking a measurable distance.

In clients with impaired physical mobility, it is important to encourage mobilization as soon as the person can tolerate it.

The longer a person has been immobile, the longer it will take to regain strength, balance, and coordination.

Mobilization includes early efforts at positioning and moving helpless persons in beds and, possibly, "dangling" them and transferring them to a chair or wheelchair (see Chapter 35). Although immobilized clients may seem to take a fairly passive role when being helped, they are actually gaining independence and stability in sitting, pivoting, and transferring to a chair. Because exercise can be so beneficial in both increasing physical mobility and preventing disuse phenomena, however, it is vital to get clients to move with minimal or no assistance as soon as possible. Teaching is one major way to do this.

TEACHING THE PERSON TO DANGLE

Teaching clients how to sit on the side of the bed to dangle differs from assisting them to do this. For example, in assisting a client, you would make the work easier for both yourself and the client by raising the head of the bed to help move the client into a sitting position. When teaching, you want clients to do the work without your help, so they learn how to do it independently. You want them to use energy to do the work because the exercise involved will help them regain strength. You want them to learn to get out of a flat bed so they will be prepared do this when they return home and no longer have the convenience of a bed that moves into many different positions. See Procedure 36-2 for the steps in teaching a client to dangle. This procedure covers the person with generalized weakness and the person who has one-sided weakness (hemiparesis). The person with hemiparesis, for example, might have had a cerebrovascular accident (stroke) with some residual paralysis affecting one side of the body.

Whether the client is assisted to dangle or taught how to do this independently, the first time the person has assumed a position on the side of the bed, this "dangling" position should be maintained for at least 2 minutes before the person attempts to ambulate. During the time the client dangles, it is crucial that you assess for signs of orthostatic hypotension and for changes in the client's strength, balance, coordination, and pain level (see Chapter 35). If you are not convinced that the client can tolerate the ambulation to follow, a return to bed is warranted.

Text continued on page 829

PROCEDURE 36–2

Teaching a Person to Sit on the Side of the Bed and "Dangle"

Definition/Purposes. Method used to teach a client to move from a supine to a sitting position on the edge of the bed with feet supported on the floor or a footstool. May be used for a weak or partially paralyzed person. May also be used for many postoperative clients, as this method reduces stress on abdominal surgical incisions. This method helps maintain and strengthen the person's muscles.

Contraindications/Cautions. Modify the procedure to support clients when needed (e.g., assist with movements when needed, prevent falls in persons with impaired balance by supporting these clients when they are in a sitting position). For clients who have been immobilized for a time, prevent orthostatic hypotension by preconditioning and using supportive devices (e.g., place the person in a high Fowler's position for progressively longer periods of time and place T.E.D. hose on the client's legs prior to attempting sitting to dangle). If orthostatic hypotension develops, return the person to the horizontal position immediately. If the client has received medication that could impair the ability to maintain a sitting position or to understand directions, time this procedure for well before or after the medication's expected peak effects.

Teaching/Learning Guidelines. Review with the client the steps to be taken, in the order they are to be taken, before beginning the actual activity. Answer questions as needed concerning the procedure.

Bear in mind that learning self-care activities provides the person with independence and a sense of control. The responsibility for self-care is, after all, the ultimate goal for most clients.

PRELIMINARY ACTIVITIES

Assessment/Planning

- ▶ Review chart for diagnosis and evidence of contraindications
- ▶ Review activity/exercise orders
- ▶ Note presence of skin, muscle, or bone lesions
- ▶ Note presence of tubes, equipment, or devices that could make movement hazardous if not attended to
- ▶ Assess person's ability to follow directions
- ▶ Assess movement abilities and limitations
- ▶ Take blood pressure and pulse to obtain baseline readings

Equipment

- ▶ Bed with firm mattress
- ▶ Appropriate clothing for client
- ▶ Incontinence pad or other paper to protect the bed

Preparation of Person and Unit

- ▶ Explain why and how the activity will be done
- ▶ Fan-fold top covers to the foot of the bed
- ▶ Dress client in pajamas, a hospital gown, or comfortable street clothing
- ▶ Place incontinence pad or paper on foot of bed to protect linen from soil of slippers or shoes
- ▶ Place slippers or shoes on client's feet
- ▶ If present and needed, place head end of half side rail in the up position on the side of the bed upon which the client will sit
- ▶ Lower mattress to a flat position
- ▶ Lower bed to lowest height and lock wheels
- ▶ Place footstool in position (if needed)
- ▶ Provide for any tubes, equipment, or devices attached to the person's body, as needed

Usually tubes (lines) are connected to a reservoir that either supplies gases (such as oxygen) or fluids (such as infusions, transfusions, or nasogastric feedings) to the client or removes fluids from the client (such as chest drainage tubes or urinary drainage tubes). If the client will be moving away from the reservoir, the tubing may have to be clamped off and separated from its reservoir, or the reservoir will have to be made mobile enough to follow along with the client. Be certain to seek advice from your clinical instructor or appropriate agency professional before attempting to manage any tubing, equipment, or devices unfamiliar to you.

- ▶ Arrange unit furniture to provide space, as necessary
- ▶ Caution client to let you know if the activity causes any discomfort, dizziness, or unusual sensations
- ▶ Lower full side rail or foot end of half side rail on side of bed upon which the client will sit

PROCEDURE 36–2 Continued

Teaching a Person to Sit on the Side of the Bed and "Dangle"

PROCEDURE

(Person with Generalized Weakness)

Actions

1. Tell the client to remain in supine position but move to side nearest to you.
2. Stand at bedside by person's waist.

3. Ask/teach client to roll to side, facing you. During instruction, touch each body part to be moved:
   a. Ask person to move near arm so as to grasp mattress edge with near hand.
   b. Ask person to simultaneously lift far leg over near leg and reach far arm over near arm to grasp and pull on rail or mattress edge (Fig. 36–13).

4. Teach the following method for assuming a sitting position on side of bed:

   a. Ask person to prepare to slide heels off mattress edge when directed.
   b. Ask person to prepare to push fist of upper arm into mattress while grasping mattress edge with lower arm and pulling to help roll upward on lower elbow.
   c. On prearranged signal, have person push, pull, and roll upward with upper body as heels and lower legs go over mattress edge (Fig. 36–14).
5. When upright position has been attained, have person push fists into mattress to help maintain sitting position (Fig. 36–15). One hand may grasp half side rail if available.

6. Have person place both feet flat on floor or on footstool.

Rationale/Discussion

1. You will be available to assist, as needed, if you stand on the side of the bed upon which the client will sit.
2. By interposing your body, if necessary, you will be able to prevent person from rolling out of bed.
3. Rolling prevents friction on tissues. Touching body parts to be moved reinforces your verbal instruction.
   a. Will prevent rolling on near arm during turn. Will also help provide support during turn.
   b. Movement of arm and leg to opposite side of body helps shift center of gravity and provide momentum to make turn to side easier.
   Simultaneous movement helps maintain spinal alignment and minimizes stress on abdominal muscles.
4. The method minimizes stress/trauma to abdominal muscles, scrotum, ischial tuberosities, and perineal wounds.
   a. Weight of legs will act as a counterweight and will help pull trunk upright.
   b. Pushing fist into mattress allows upper shoulder to serve as a fulcrum to apply leverage to help lift the torso.

   c. Combining the counterweight of the legs with shoulder and arm leverage assists client to move trunk upward.
5. Supporting the self helps maintain stability while strengthening arm muscles. Fists maintain the wrists in a position of extension while increasing arm length. Side rail can supply support when client is not able to support full weight on fists.
6. Support for the feet helps stabilize the person. Assess popliteal spaces for pressure that could compress blood vessels and injure nerves.

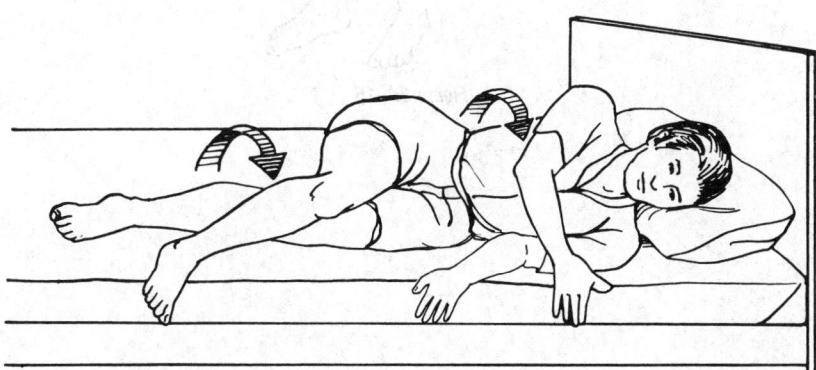

▲ *Figure 36–13*

Procedure continued on following page

PROCEDURE 36–2 Continued

Teaching a Person to Sit on the Side of the Bed and "Dangle"

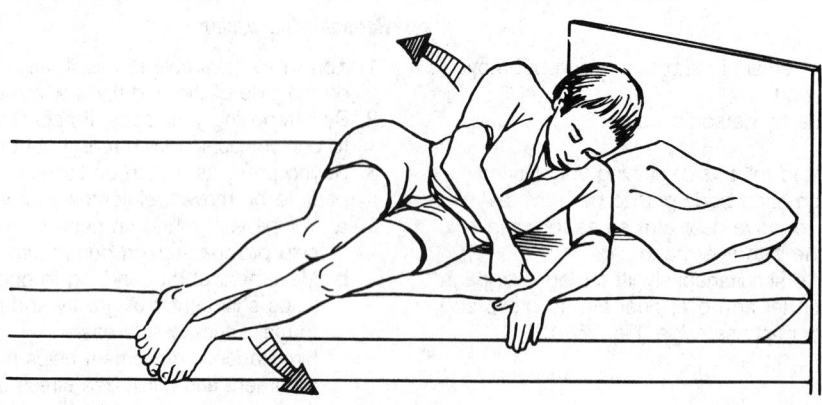

▲ Figure 36–14

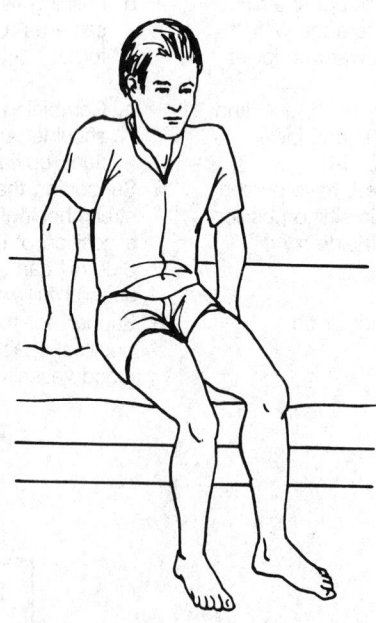

▲ Figure 36–15

PROCEDURE 36–2 Continued

Teaching a Person to Sit on the Side of the Bed and "Dangle"

Actions	Rationale/Discussion
7. Stand in front of client and assess for symptoms of orthostatic hypotension. Ask how the person feels.	7. This position will allow you to intercede if the person should begin to faint. If condition remains stable, take blood pressure and pulse and compare with baseline readings. If signs or symptoms of lightheadedness, dizziness, diaphoresis (sweating), or fainting occur, return person to horizontal position and assess blood pressure and pulse.
8. Help person put on robe or cover with bath blanket, as necessary.	8. Helps maintain body warmth.
9. Encourage person to maintain a seated position for 1 to 2 full minutes before progressing on to ambulation.	9. In clients who have been immobilized, the circulatory system tends to adjust more slowly to the upright position. Adequate time is needed for adjustment and for the foregoing assessment measures.
10. If the person is not to get up to ambulate or to move to a chair, encourage the person to maintain a seated position on the side of the bed for a given time for the initial dangling and increase the length of time for subsequent periods.	10. No specific length of time is correct for all persons. Each person should attempt to remain in the sitting position as long as possible each time dangling is done. The muscles will strengthen if used to their maximum potential, but the nurse must continually assess the person and intervene as needed to prevent exhaustion.
11. Stay with client during the entire period of dangling and instruct the person, when ready to return to bed, to return to the supine position by reversing the procedure.	11. Encouraging the client to do the work promotes independence, but you must still be readily available to provide assistance if this becomes necessary.
12. Assist the person to attain good body alignment, in a position that promotes comfort.	12. This action will help the client to rest.

(Person with One-Sided Weakness)

Actions	Rationale/Discussion
1. Stand on side of bed near client's strong side and tell client to remain in supine position but to move toward you, in sections, by a. Sliding stronger foot under weaker knee (Fig. 36–16A).	1. You will be available to assist, as needed, if you stand on the side of the bed upon which the client will sit.

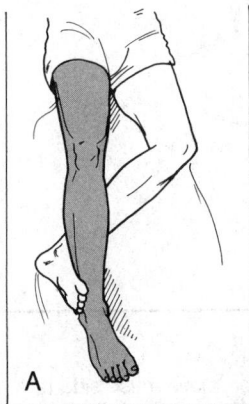
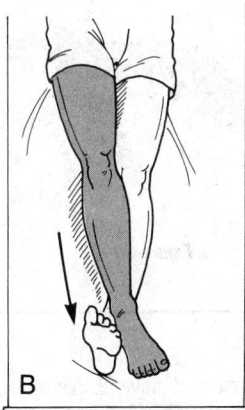
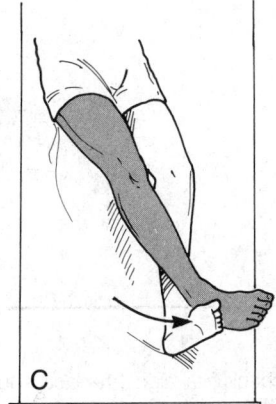

▲ *Figure 36–16*

Procedure continued on following page

PROCEDURE 36–2 Continued

Teaching a Person to Sit on the Side of the Bed and "Dangle"

Actions	Rationale/Discussion
b. Sliding stronger foot down leg and under weaker ankle (Fig. 36–16*B*).	
c. Using the stronger leg to pull the weaker leg to the side of the bed (Fig. 36–16*C*).	
d. Moving the buttocks by pushing flexed stronger leg and shoulder onto the mattress and lifting and moving lower body toward the side of the bed.	
e. Grasping side of mattress with stronger hand and pulling upper body to side of bed.	
2. Stand at bedside by person's waist.	2. By interposing your body, if necessary, you will be able to prevent person from rolling out of bed.
3. Ask/teach person to roll to side, facing you, by	3. Rolling prevents friction on tissues.
a. Grasping weaker wrist with stronger hand and bringing weaker arm toward side of bed.	a. Rolling starts the movement that will help shift weight and assist in rolling from back to side.
b. Then grasping side rail at mattress level (with stronger hand) and pushing stronger shoulder under body to help turn trunk.	b. This helps move center of gravity more toward edge of bed, further helping shift the weight from back to side to start the roll to come.
c. Finally, by placing stronger foot under weaker ankle and simultaneously pushing against mattress with stronger arm.	c. This provides the final leverage needed to roll to the side.
4. Ask the person to assume a sitting position by grasping side of mattress with stronger hand and then simultaneously using stronger leg to pull both feet off mattress edge and rolling onto elbow to get into a sitting position (Fig. 36–17).	4. Weight of legs will act as a counterweight and will help pull trunk upright. Simultaneous movement helps maintain spinal alignment and minimizes stress on abdominal muscles.
5. When upright position has been attained, have the person grasp the half side rail or push the stronger fist into the mattress to help maintain a sitting position	5. Supporting self helps maintain stability while strengthening arm muscles. The fist maintains the wrist in a position of extension while increasing arm length. The side rail can supply support when the client is not able to support full weight on the fist.
6. Follow steps 6 through 11 as for a person with generalized weakness.	

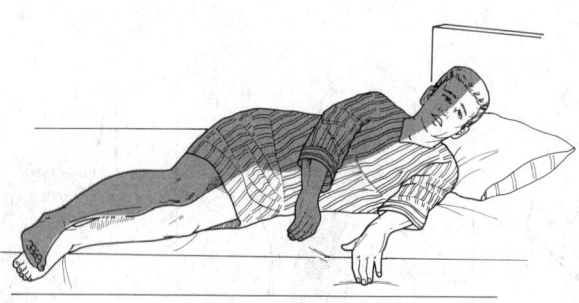

▲ Figure 36–17

FINAL ACTIVITIES

Replace covers, check vital signs, replace equipment and devices disturbed by the move, raise side rails, and assure that the call bell is within reach. Replace any furniture moved. Document your assessment of the client's ability to dangle. Record the teaching that was done and the amount of assistance that was needed. State how long the client was able to remain sitting and how the client tolerated the procedure. Record vital signs. If orthostatic hypotension has occurred, document the corrective measures taken and the effectiveness of these measures. List recommendations for progressing with activities.

ASSISTING WITH AMBULATION

If the client appears to be tolerating the dangling, use additional time, as needed, to apply the client's robe and an ambulation belt, if a belt is to be used. Make a final check of all lines and tubes to be certain they are safely provided for before assisting the person to stand. See Procedure 36–3 for guidelines in assisting with ambulation.

You should always have sufficient help to assist the client to ambulate. Most often, when you prepare well, the client will do well at ambulating a short distance, and you can walk along and provide only minimal guidance. Be ever alert, however, for those unexpected times when the client suddenly, and with minimal or no warning, becomes faint and falls. When ambulating clients, you must always be prepared for such rare events. See Procedure 36–3 for specific steps to take when fainting occurs.

Assistive Ambulation Devices

Some clients will not be able to walk without the support of **assistive ambulation devices,** aids to help the client in walking (e.g., crutches, canes, or walkers). These devices are used to support clients with long- or short-term disabilities. Their use is often taught by physical therapists while nurses reinforce the teaching. Less often, the need for an assistive device is unanticipated, as occurs in emergencies, and the teaching responsibility rests solely with the nurse. In either case, the nurse must be prepared to teach clients to use these devices.

When the need for an assistive ambulation device is anticipated, you can prepare the client in advance. Because the burden of supporting the body weight will be shifted from the lower extremities to the upper extremities, you should prepare the individual by teaching exercises to improve muscle strength of the hands, arms, and shoulders. Such exercises usually include routine isotonic exercise sets that include squeezing handgrips or rubber balls, lifting weights, and doing bed push-ups.

CRUTCHES

Types of Crutches. Three types of crutches commonly used are axillary crutches, forearm (Lofstrand) crutches, and platform crutches (Fig. 36–18). Axillary crutches have an axillary bar that fits under the client's axillae, but the client's weight is actually borne by the hands on the handgrips. Axillary crutches are most often used for short-term disabilities. Forearm crutches have no axillary bar but have a metal band that fits around the forearm to help keep the crutch in place. With these crutches too, the client bears weight on handgrips. Forearm crutches are used by persons with long-term disabilities. Platform crutches are used when the need for assistance is long-term, and weight-bearing is not feasible on the hands or wrists (e.g., when the client has hand or wrist arthritis or carpal tunnel syndrome). With platform crutches, the elbow is flexed

90 degrees and the client's weight is distributed along the forearm. In health care facilities, the need for forearm and platform crutches is usually anticipated, and teaching is arranged in advance by the physical therapy department. Here we focus on teaching the use of axillary crutches, but most of the principles involved apply to all types of crutches.

Axillary crutches, made of aluminum or wood, are usually adjustable and are sized "short" through "extra long" for both children and adults. The axillary bars and the handgrips should be covered with padding. The lower ends should be covered by rubber tips that help prevent the crutches from sliding during weight bearing.

Proper Crutch Fit. Because improper crutch fit can lead to postural changes, back pain, nerve compression, and even arm and hand paralysis, proper fit is one of the most important aspects of the use of crutches. The measurement of crutch length includes the axillary pad and rubber crutch tip. Measurements for crutches may be made in several ways:[4]

▶ Calculate 77 per cent of the client's height (height in inches or centimeters × 0.77).
▶ Calculate the client's height minus 16 inches (40.5 cm).
▶ With the person flat in bed with shoes on, measure from the axillary fold to the heel of the foot and add 2 inches (5 cm).
▶ With the person in bed or standing, measure from the axilla on the diagonal to a point 6 to 8 inches (15 to 20 cm) lateral to the heel.

With the person standing upright, in sturdy shoes and with the shoulders relaxed, there should be a space of approximately 3 fingerbreadths (2.5 inches) between the axillary fold and the top of the crutch. The crutches should extend 6 to 8 inches (15 to 20 cm) lateral to the foot. Handgrips should be adjusted so the elbows are flexed 15 to 30 degrees while the handgrips are in use (Figure 36–18A). Adjustments may be necessary as the person's posture improves and skill is gained in using crutches. Growing children may need frequent crutch adjustments.

Crutch Safety. To make sure the crutches are safe, remember the following safety measures:

▶ Fasten all bolts and wing nuts securely.
▶ Assure that crutch tips are intact (they wear through rather rapidly with use), relatively flexible (the rubber hardens with age and can cause the tips to slide), and of the correct style (with deep grooves and concave bases that are approximately 4 cm in diameter). A replacement pair should always be kept on hand. They may be purchased at some pharmacies and at most surgical supply houses.
▶ Apply new tips securely by pushing each tip on as far as possible and then placing the tip on the floor and pressing the crutch downward, with a twisting motion, into it.
▶ Pad axillary bars to prevent pressure sores where axillary bars come into constant contact with the

PROCEDURE 36–3

Assisting with Ambulation

Definition/Purposes. The procedure for helping a person walk in order to maintain or regain strength and mobility. It is often used for postoperative clients, clients who have been immobilized for a period of time, and other persons who are weak or partially paralyzed.

Contraindications/Cautions. Observe all contraindications/cautions in Procedure 36–2. Also apply an ambulation (walking) belt if indicated. Be certain to have enough help available.

Teaching/Learning Guidelines. Review with the client the steps to be taken, in the order they are to be taken, before beginning the actual activity. Explain that the client is to let you know if weakness, faintness, or other unusual sensations are experienced. Tell the client to lean against you in any of these events. Answer questions as needed concerning the procedure.

PRELIMINARY ACTIVITIES

▶ Same as for Procedure 36–2
▶ Obtain assistance as needed

Equipment

▶ Bed with firm mattress
▶ Appropriate clothing for client
▶ Shoes that provide good foot support
▶ Incontinence pad or other paper to protect the bed linens
▶ Ambulation belt, if indicated
▶ IV pole on wheels, if needed

Preparation of Person and Unit

▶ Same as for Procedure 36–2

PROCEDURE

Actions

1. Follow steps 1 through 9 in Procedure 36–2 to have the client dangle.
2. Unless contraindicated, place an ambulation belt around the client's waist (see Chapter 35).

3. Plan with client the distance that should be walked this time.

4. Ask the client to slide closer to the edge of the bed.

5. Have client place both feet on the floor in a forward-backward stance, with the stronger foot behind and slightly under the bed.

6. Holding onto the ambulation belt (see Fig. 35–37) or, if no belt is worn, placing your arms under the client's arms and your hands on the client's back, under the scapulae (see Fig. 35–35), have the client lean forward to stand up.
   If a footstool is used, have the client place the dominant foot in the center of the stool, step to the floor with the other foot, and lower the strong foot to the floor.
   Assist only as needed.

7. Ask the person to stand up straight and balance in a standing position. If necessary, have the client hold the side rail or the back of a chair for support. Assess for evidence of orthostatic hypotension.

Rationale/Discussion

1. The client must dangle before ambulating in order to become accustomed to the erect position.
2. The belt allows you to grasp the client securely by handles on the belt. Using the belt increases your control in the event the client faints, but it does not hamper the client's ability to walk independently.
3. The client who participates in the decision-making process is more likely to cooperate in the execution of the plan.
4. Moving forward reduces friction during the attempt to stand.
5. This stance provides a wide base of support. If feet are on a footstool and a wide base of support is not possible, additional assistance may be needed to help the person when it is time to stand.
6. Leaning forward assists in providing momentum. Supporting the client by the arms and pulling on the client's arms to assist in standing could result in shoulder damage.

   This sequence allows the dominant leg to provide the muscle power needed to flex the knee and lower the body.
   The more the client is able to do independently, the more benefit will accrue from the exercise involved.
7. Good posture assists the person to become stable in the standing position. Holding the rail or chair widens the base of support when the client finds it difficult to balance otherwise.

PROCEDURE 36-3 Continued

Assisting with Ambulation

Actions	*Rationale/Discussion*
8. If an ambulation belt is worn by the client, grasp the handles securely and walk slightly behind and to one side of the client as ambulation begins. If no ambulation belt is worn, walk slightly behind and to one side of the client with your arm nearest to the client around the client's waist and your other arm behind the client's nearer arm and at the client's waist on the side nearest to you. Unless it is necessary, do not grasp the client but rather allow the client to support the weight. In the event that you need to suddenly support the client's weight, however, you must be ready to grasp the client's body (with your hands around the client's waist or with the handles of the walking belt) without pulling on an arm. For clients who have a one-sided weakness, walk on the weak side but encourage the client to walk without your assistance.	8. These positions will allow you to be prepared to control the client's weight, if need be but will allow the client full freedom to walk independently, if able.
	Pulling on a client's arm to support the full body weight could seriously damage the client's shoulder joint.
	This position will promote independence while still allowing you to support the client's weak side should it become necessary.
9. While ambulating, the client may hold and push the IV pole if one is needed.	9. Holding the pole allows the client to feel more independent and still provides a small measure of security.
10. As the client walks the agreed-upon distance, check at intervals to assess the ability to continue as planned. If a feeling of weakness, dizziness, or faintness occurs, have the client sit or lie down (even if the only place to sit is on the floor).	10. The client's status could change at any time.
In the event that the client begins to lose consciousness without warning, pull the client's body toward you and physically hold it against your body as you allow it to slide to the floor. Stoop as you lower the body to the floor and cradle the client's head to prevent it from striking the hard surface of the floor.	Holding the client's body against yours will move the client's greatest weight closer to your center of gravity and will make it easier for you to control the client's descent to the floor. Stooping as you lower the weight helps maintain the weight near your center of gravity and will help prevent back injury.
11. As the client completes the agreed-upon walk and is ready to return to bed, reverse the procedure to return the client to bed. If a footstool is used, ask the person to step up with the dominant leg.	11. The dominant leg's muscle power is needed to lift the body.

FINAL ACTIVITIES

See final activities for Procedure 36-2.

---

body (rib cage, below axillae) and pad handgrips to prevent blisters and calluses on the hands. Preformed, spongy rubber pads that slip into place are available for both axillary bars and handgrips. These may be purchased at most surgical supply houses.

One of the greatest dangers of crutch use is damage to the ulnar or radial nerves. Permanent paralysis ("crutch paralysis") can occur in only a few minutes when the client leans his or her full weight on the axillary bars instead of on the handgrips.

The axillary bars are to rest against the rib cage while the client's weight is borne on the palms of the hands.

Other potential hazards of crutch use include thrombosis of the axillary blood vessels from pressure, contusions of the axillae and palms from pressure, falls from loss of balance (especially when climbing or descending stairs), falls from slipping on wet floors or pavement, back pain from poor posture and improper crutch fit, and cardiovascular complications in clients with preexisting cardiovascular problems (from the extra stress of using the crutches and particularly from rapid use).

Gaits Used in Crutch Walking. Five gaits are commonly used in crutch walking. The gait used by any individual will vary depending on (1) the pathology

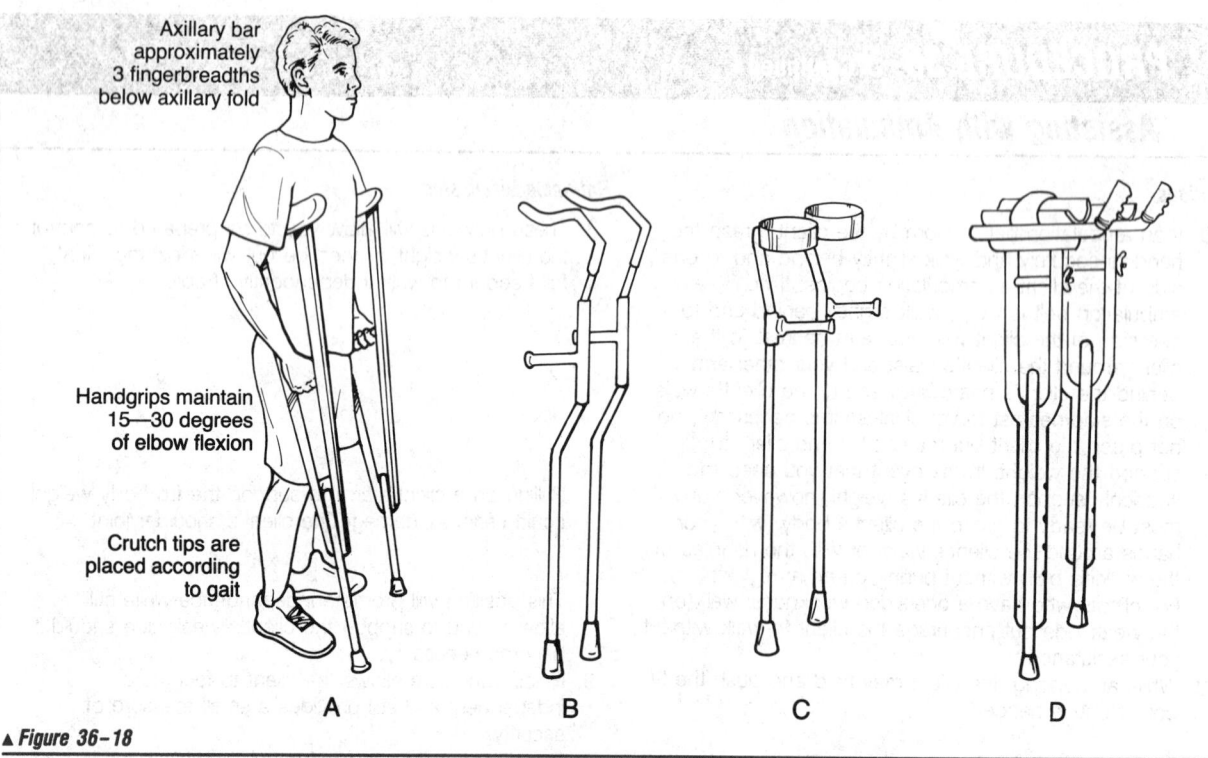

Axillary bar
approximately
3 fingerbreadths
below axillary fold

Handgrips maintain
15—30 degrees
of elbow flexion

Crutch tips are
placed according
to gait

A   B   C   D

▲ *Figure 36–18*

Various types of commonly used crutches. *A* and *B,* Two styles of axillary crutches; *C,* forearm (Lofstrand) crutches; *D,* platform crutches. *A* illustrates proper crutch fit for the axillary crutch: axillary bar approximately 3 fingerbreadths below the client's axillary fold, handgrip allowing the elbow to be flexed 15 to 30 degrees, and crutch tips 6 to 8 inches lateral to and slightly ahead of each foot. Note that crutch tips and foam padding for axillary bars and handgrips should be in place before making adjustments in crutches.

involved, (2) the weight-bearing limitations recommended by the physician, and (3) the requirements of the day-to-day circumstances encountered by the client. For example, the client may have one leg injured and may not be allowed to bear any weight on it. In such cases, one gait is usually preferred for most walking, but another gait may have to be used to climb stairs and still another to maintain stability when walking in light rain or in crowded spaces.

All crutch-walking gaits rely on each crutch to provide one point of contact and support with the floor and each weight-bearing foot to provide one point so that two, three, or four points are available for use at any given time.

Four-Point Gait. The **four-point gait** is a crutch-walking gait with four points on the floor and with one point moving at a time — crutch, opposite foot, opposite crutch, opposite foot. A four point gait is used when the client has bilateral pathology, is allowed to bear partial weight on both extremities, and requires a great deal of stability (Fig. 36–19*A*). For example, it is used by children who have bilateral, long-leg braces and who are just beginning to walk, by elderly persons who fear falling while learning to crutch walk, by weaker persons, and by others who need extra stability for safety only at certain times (e.g., on a slippery walk, in a crowd of people who are moving rapidly, or on a boat or moving train).

The four-point gait is more difficult to learn than some of the other gaits. When done correctly, it is a very slow but sure gait. It allows much safety and stability by providing a wide base of support. The gait begins with all four points on the floor, forming a square, and with the client's line of gravity running directly into the middle of the square. From this starting point, the client moves one crutch forward, followed by the opposite foot, then the second crutch followed by the opposite foot (e.g., left crutch, right foot, right crutch, left foot). This pattern is then repeated, with only one point ever leaving the floor at any given time. As the client moves each point forward, the base of support must always be maintained. To maintain the base of support, the client needs to know the following:

▶ Only one point leaves the floor at any given time
▶ Each point moves only a short distance
▶ All points move the same distance each time
▶ The client's line of gravity always remains in the center of the base of support
▶ Each time the fourth point has been moved, the four points again form a square the size of the original

Two-Point Gait. The **two-point gait** is a crutch-walking gait with four points on the floor and two points moving at a time — crutch and opposite foot together, opposite crutch and foot together. The two-point gait is a natural extension of the four-point gait (Fig. 36–19*B*).

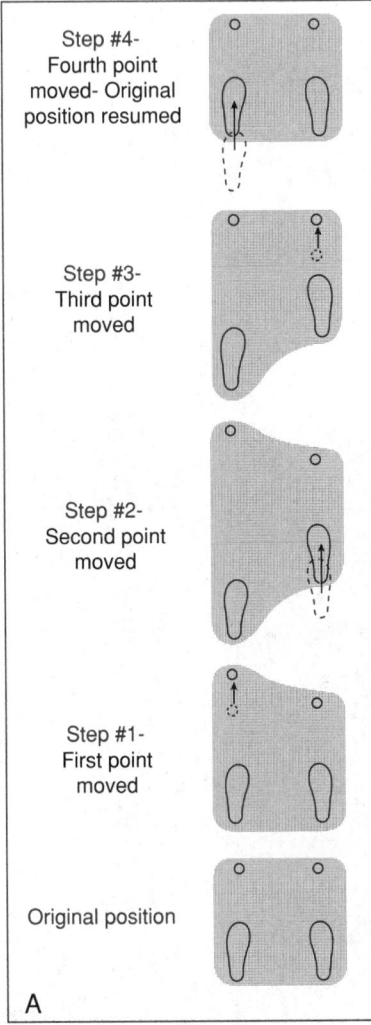

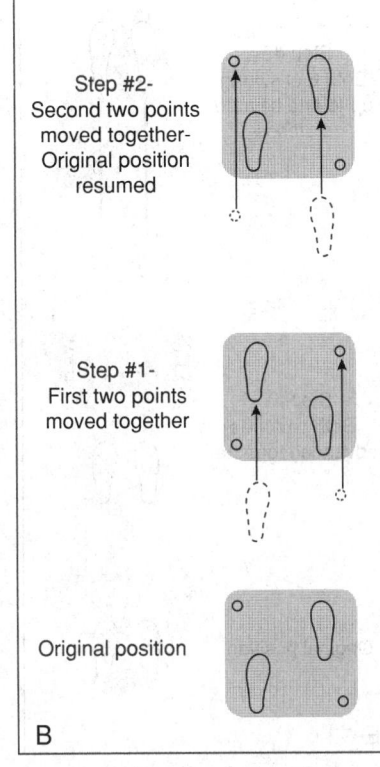

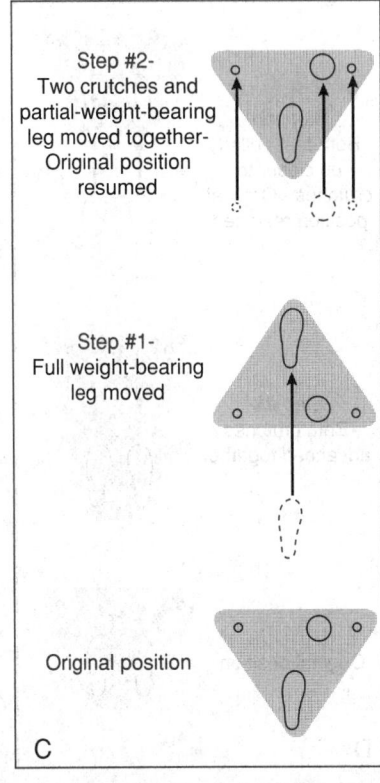

▲ *Figure 36–19*

The five main crutch gaits provide different bases of support. The areas shaded in color represent the bases of support for each gait during the starting position and after each "step," footprints indicate full weight-bearing feet, larger circles indicate the position of partial weight-bearing feet, smaller circles indicate crutch tips, and all figures drawn in dotted line indicate a previous position. *A,* The four-point gait, which offers the widest base of support at all times; *B,* the two-point gait, which is a reciprocal, "natural" gait; *C,* the three-point gait for use when partial weight-bearing is allowed on one foot.

Illustration continued on following page

The two-point gait is also used by persons who have bilateral pathology but are allowed partial weight bearing on both feet. It allows the client to move more rapidly but provides less stability than the four-point gait. The two-point gait is the most natural crutch-walking gait in that it most closely approximates the normal, unassisted gait. It is often used by the same persons who use a four-point gait after they have built up strength and confidence and are ready for more speed in walking.

The two-point gait begins with one crutch and the opposite foot, side-by-side, and the other crutch and foot, side-by-side, one step behind them. The client's line of gravity is centered in the middle of the four points. From this starting point, the client moves both the back crutch and back foot forward, together, followed by the opposite foot and crutch (e.g., left foot and right crutch together; right foot and left crutch together). This pattern is then repeated. With this gait, it is important that

▶ the foot and crutch being advanced at any one time stay together. They must be picked up together, moved forward together, and placed back on the floor together. Failure to keep the two points together can result in a confusion about the gait with a resulting loss of balance.

▶ the foot and crutch being advanced always stay in the same position relative to each other. In this gait, only two points are on the floor and providing support for the client most of the time. These two points must be on either side of the line of gravity, or the client will become unstable and fall.

▶ the foot and crutch being advanced pass through

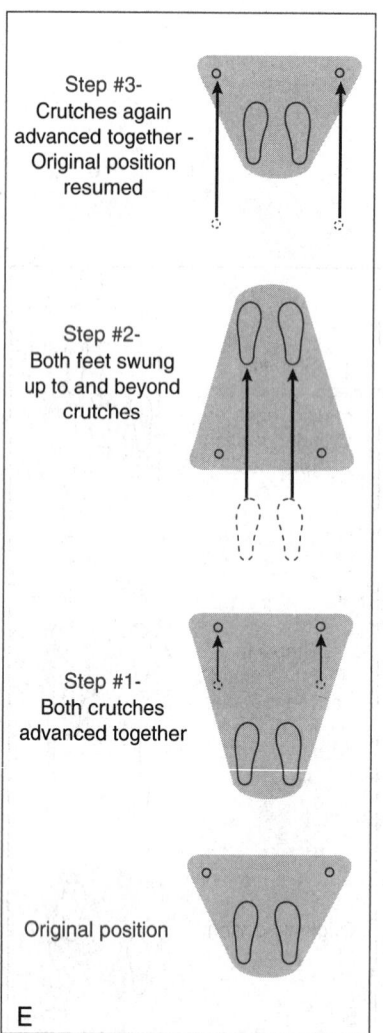

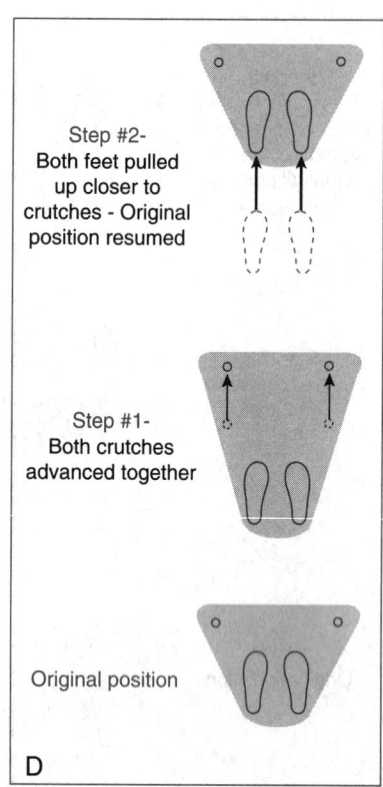

▲ *Figure 36–19* Continued

D, the swing-to gait for one unaffected foot or two weaker feet used together; *E*, the swing-through gait for the same client who uses the swing-to gait (when the person has built up strength and endurance enough to use this gait for increased speed).

and beyond the position held by the opposite foot and crutch so that a gait as near normal as possible is maintained.

► the second foot and crutch both remain firmly on the floor to provide support until the first foot and crutch have come to rest.

Three-Point Gait (with Partial Weight Bearing on One Extremity).

The **three-point gait with partial weight-bearing on one extremity** (Fig. 36–19*C*) is one type of three-point gait. This is a crutch-walking gait with three points on the floor and one injured foot bearing partial weight and therefore not counted as a point—both crutches with injured foot together, uninjured foot alone. This three-point gait is used by persons who have pathology of only one leg and who are allowed partial weight bearing on that extremity and full weight bearing on the other. It permits the client to move more rapidly than does the four-point gait but

provides less stability. This three-point gait can be used to ascend and descend stairs. It cannot be used by persons who have only one leg (amputees) or who keep both legs together to serve as a single point. In these cases, an attempt to use this gait would result in the use of the swing-to or swing-through gait (discussed later).

This three-point gait begins with both crutches and the injured leg a step ahead of the uninjured leg, so that the injured leg is supported by both crutches and the uninjured leg stands alone. Each crutch is considered to be one point, and the client's uninjured leg is considered to be the third point. The injured leg is not considered to be a point. The three points form a triangle with the client's line of gravity in the middle.

From this starting point, the client bears weight on both crutches and the injured leg while bringing the uninjured leg forward, through, and past the crutches a full step. The uninjured leg then serves as the base of support while the crutches and injured leg are brought forward together to pass the uninjured leg by a full step (i.e., both crutches and injured foot together, uninjured foot alone). This pattern is then repeated. With this type of three-point gait, it is important that

▶ the injured foot and both crutches stay together at all times. They must be picked up together, moved forward together, and placed back on the floor together. Failure to keep them together can result in a lack of support for the injured extremity, with full weight being borne on the injury and damage done as a result. It can also result in a confusion about the gait with a loss of balance as a consequence.

▶ the injured foot and both crutches always stay in the same position relative to each other. This alignment is necessary because only two points are providing support for the injured leg when the uninjured leg is in motion. If one of these two supporting points were to be moved, the client would become unstable and could fall.

▶ the injured foot and crutches being advanced pass beyond the position held by the uninjured foot and that in turn the uninjured foot passes through and beyond the crutches. Consequently, a gait as near normal as possible is maintained. This movement may not be possible at first, but the client should strive for it in order to prevent a hobbling gait.

Swing-to Gait. The **swing-to gait** is another type of three-point gait (Fig. 36–19*D*). It is a crutch-walking gait with three points on the floor and consists of two crutches and one foot (or both feet together)—both crutches together, foot (or feet) pulled nearly up to the crutches. The swing-to gait is faster and less stable than the four-point gait. It is not as fast as (but more stable than) the two-point gait. It is used by persons who have bilateral pathology and who are allowed partial weight bearing on both feet, which they keep together and use as one point. It is also used by amputees and by those who are not permitted to bear any weight at all on one foot. Thus, the swing-to gait is for those who have either one uninjured foot or two feet that are used together as one weight-bearing point. It is a gait that can be used for ascending and descending stairs.

The swing-to gait begins with both crutches forward of the client's uninjured leg (or two legs together), forming a triangular base of support with the client's line of gravity centered in the middle. From this starting point, the client bears weight on both crutches while bringing the uninjured leg or legs forward toward (but not completely up to) the crutches. The uninjured leg or legs then serve as the base of support while the crutches are brought farther forward (i.e., both crutches together, uninjured leg or legs alone). This pattern is then repeated. With the swing-to gait, it is important that

▶ the client have sufficient strength to bear the body's full weight on the arms for short periods of time. (The average load can be up to 80 per cent greater than that imposed, for example, by the two-point gait.)

▶ the injured leg or legs remain sufficiently behind the crutches so as to assure a triangular base of support at all times.

Swing-Through Gait. The swing-through gait is an extension of the swing-to gait (Fig. 36–19*E*). The **swing-through gait** is a crutch-walking gait with three points on the floor and consists of two crutches and one foot (or both feet together); the foot or feet swing through and beyond the crutches. It is used by the same persons who would use a swing-to gait but only after these clients have gained sufficient strength and confidence to be able to use it. The swing-through gait allows great speed but only at the sacrifice of some stability and a great deal of energy. Unlike the other three-point gaits, it should not be used on stairs.

Like the swing-to gait, the swing-through gait begins with both crutches forward of the client's uninjured leg (or two legs together), forming a triangular base of support with the client's line of gravity centered in the middle. From this starting point, the client bears weight on both crutches while bringing the uninjured leg or legs forward toward, through, and past the crutches one full step. The uninjured leg or legs then serves as the base of support while the crutches are brought forward together, to pass the uninjured leg by a full step, (i.e., both crutches together, uninjured leg or legs alone). This pattern is then repeated. With this gait, it is important that

▶ the client has sufficient strength to bear the body's full weight on the arms for longer periods of time and for greater distances than with the swing-to gait.

▶ the injured leg(s) remain sufficiently behind or pass sufficiently ahead of the crutches so as to assure a triangular base of support at all times.

Crutch-Walking Maneuvers. In addition to knowing the basic gaits, you should be able to teach the client who is on crutches how to stand up and sit down and how to ascend and descend stairs. Supervised practice can be very helpful, especially with stairs.

Standing Up and Sitting Down. While on crutches your client should be told to select narrow, straight-backed chairs in preference to most deep, upholstered chairs. With crutches, getting into and out of straight-backed chairs is easier.

One way to have the client stand up from a sitting position is to have the person place both crutches together on the affected side, holding them by the hand-grips (as shown in Fig. 36–20*A*) and using the opposite hand to push downward against the chair for leverage. The client should then stand by straightening the uninjured lower extremity. If the heel of the injured extremity is permitted to be placed on the floor, have the person slide the heel while rising. Have the client reverse this procedure to sit down. Remind your client that it is helpful to keep the vertebral column straight whenever changing positions.

Ascending and Descending Stairs. Climbing stairs can be dangerous for those on crutches. Several tech-

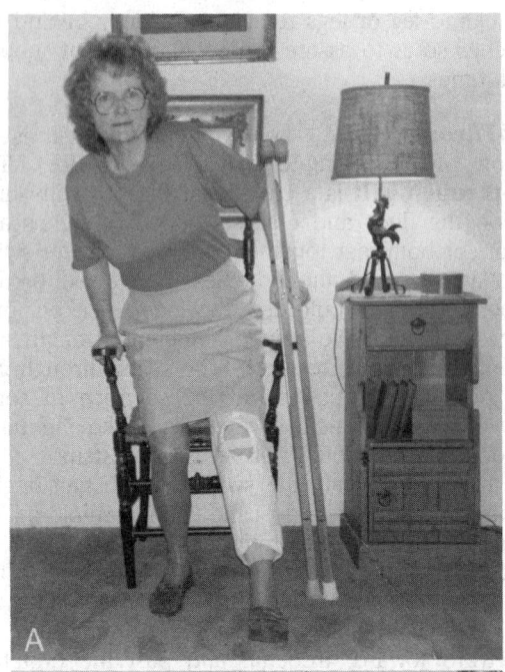

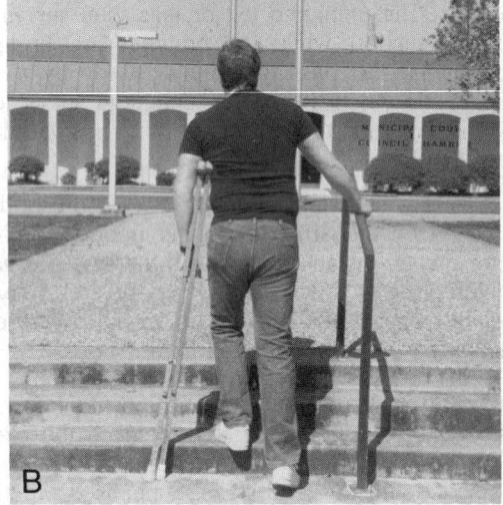

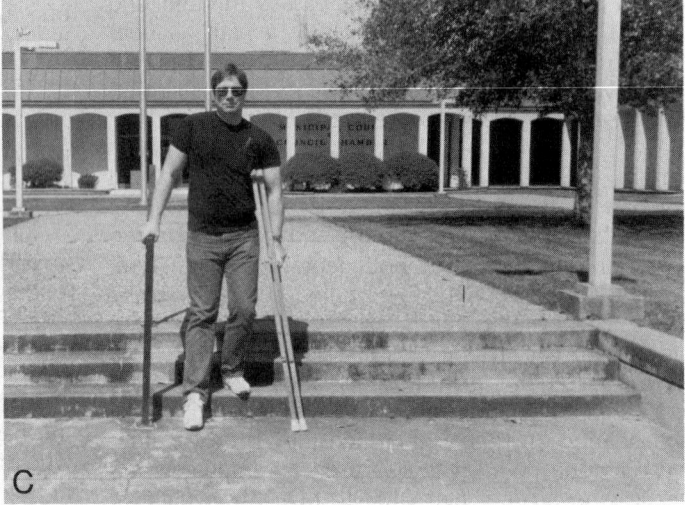

▲ *Figure 36–20*

Crutch maneuvers. *A,* Rising from a seated position; *B,* ascending stairs with a railing; *C,* descending stairs with a railing.

niques can be used to enhance safety. When there is a railing, have your client hold both crutches together under the arm opposite the railing (Fig. 36–20*B*). Have the client keep the crutches together by holding them at the handgrips. Have the client hold the railing firmly with the other hand while supporting the body weight evenly between crutch hand and railing hand. Remind the client always to keep the injured leg on the same step as the crutches (the uninjured leg does not need them). Have the client place the uninjured leg up one step and then straighten it to pull the injured leg and crutches up together. Repeat this sequence, always beginning to go upward with the uninjured leg, as this leg is stronger and can pull the rest of the body up after it. If there is no railing, have the client place one crutch under each arm and ascend the steps with the uninjured leg, followed by the injured leg and both crutches together. Repeat this sequence for each step upward.

To descend the stairs, reverse these procedures. When a railing is available, have the client place both crutches under one arm and hold the railing with the opposite hand. This time, have the client place the crutches and injured leg down one step first (Fig. 36–20*C*). Then the uninjured leg can move down to the same level. Repeat this procedure with the injured leg and crutches always leading the way. If there is no rail, use one crutch under each arm and descend by leading with the injured leg and crutches, followed by the uninjured leg alone.

Other procedures may be used for managing chairs and stairs; these are but two common examples. Consult an orthopedic nursing text or your agency physical therapists for alternatives.

If the client is too weak or too fearful to attempt to ascend or descend stairs while on crutches, it will be much safer to have the person sit on each step while ascending and descending. Lowering the center of gravity in this manner makes the client much more stable.

CANES

Canes are handgrip devices used as ambulation aids when complete weight bearing is not possible or desirable. Canes are most often made of aluminum or wood. Aluminum canes are usually adjustable, whereas wooden canes are not. Each cane consists of three parts: (1) the handle (which may or may not be covered by a rubber handgrip), (2) the shaft, and (3) the base (which is usually covered by a rubber tip). See Figure 36–21 for some variations in styles.

The cane handle is usually either straight or curved but may be individually molded to fit hand deformities. Straight handles can be easier and more comfortable for most people to grasp for support, but they lack the handy crook of the curved handle. The curved handle is more advantageous when the cane is not in use, as it can be crooked over the client's forearm, a nearby piece of furniture, a doorknob, or the back of a wheelchair that is pushed for extra support while ambulating. Canes with curved handles are less likely to fall to the floor than those that have to be propped against a wall or against a chair. To take the place of the crook, some rubber handgrips are made with a strap that can be worn around the wrist to prevent the cane from falling when not in actual use (Fig. 36–21B).

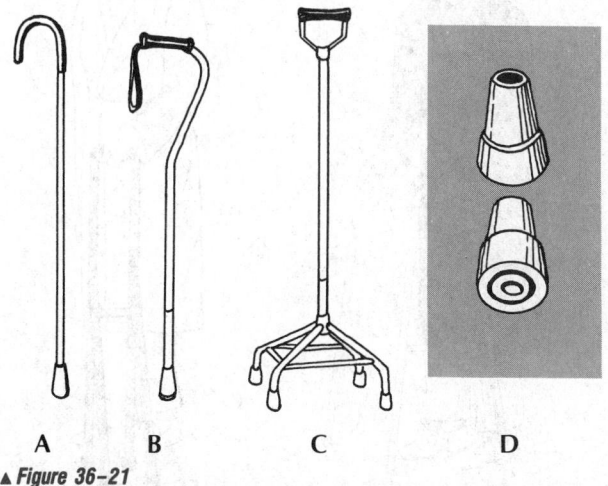

▲ *Figure 36–21*

Canes. *A,* The standard wooden cane with curved handle; *B,* the standard aluminum adjustable cane with rubber handgrip; *C,* a quad cane with a shovel-style handle; *D,* cane tips (similar to tips used for walkers). Larger tips would be used for crutches.

Retrieving fallen canes can be very difficult for some persons and impossible for others.

The shaft is usually straight for canes with curved handles and offset for canes with straight handles. The shaft must be strong enough to support twice the expected load without showing signs of deforming significantly. During normal walking, the expected load would be 25 per cent of the user's body weight. Thus, for a 200-pound man, the cane shaft should be able to support 100 pounds without too much bowing (0.25×200 lb $= 50$ lb $\times 2 = 100$ lb).

The base of the cane may come to one single foot (Fig. 36–21*A* and *B*), or it may end in a pedestal that fans outward into three smaller feet (a **tripod cane**) or four feet (a **quad cane,** Fig. 36–21*C*). Tripod and quad canes offer no additional support for the client. In fact, they may feel unstable and cause the client to feel insecure when on a hilly or uneven surface. They also take up more space than the single-footed cane does, and the client may trip over them. They do, however, have a wide enough base to allow them to stand alone. The base can prevent the cane from falling when the client needs to free a hand for some other use.

Whether the cane has one foot or three or four, each foot must be covered with a rubber cane tip (Fig. 36–21*D*). Cane tips are shaped like crutch tips but are slightly smaller (2 to 3 cm). The same safety checks needed for crutch tips apply to cane tips. Apply new cane tips in the same manner that crutch tips are applied.

The cane should be fitted to the client by assuring that the cane handle is at the level of the client's greater trochanter (or the crease in the client's wrist). This position will place the elbow at the correct angle of flexion (15 to 30 degrees) when using the cane.

The cane should be held on the side opposite the client's injured extremity (on the unaffected side).

If the cane is held on the side of the injury, the client will shift the body to one side to maintain the center of gravity between the two points that make up the base of support (the cane and the uninjured foot), with the injured foot supported between them. This position will cause poor posture as the spine curves in an awkward manner. Supporting the body with the cane on the uninjured side, however, will allow the client to maintain the body's normal center of gravity over the base of support and will help maintain correct posture and prevent back injuries.

Have your client hold the cane 6 to 10 inches to the side of, and 6 inches forward of, the foot of the unaffected leg. Using a cane in this manner can reduce the total force across the hip joint by almost two thirds.[25]

When teaching a client to use a cane for the first time, be aware that any fall will more likely be toward the affected side. Walk on the affected side and be prepared to offer physical support.

Have the client begin with cane and affected leg side-by-side and about 1 foot apart, with the unaffected leg one step (approximately 1 foot) behind (with the three points forming a triangular base of support). Have the client bear weight on the cane and affected leg while bringing the unaffected leg forward, past the cane and affected leg, and ahead approximately 1 foot. Then have the client advance the affected leg and the cane together, past the unaffected leg, and ahead approximately 1 foot. Have the client continue in this manner (i.e., cane and affected foot together, unaffected foot alone), repeating this sequence as necessary. This procedure will produce a fairly natural three-point gait (Fig. 36–22).

If the client is unable to bear sufficient weight on the affected leg to complete the gait as shown in Figure 36–22, have the person advance first the cane and then the affected leg separately, followed by the unaffected foot.[34] This sequence will produce a more hobbling gait, but it is useful when the client needs maximal support from a cane.

WALKERS

Walkers are devices used by persons unable to bear complete weight on one or both lower extremities or by those unsteady on their feet. Walkers provide a wider base of support than other assistive ambulation devices in that they surround the person on three sides and provide four points of contact with the floor.

Walkers are usually aluminum and come in various sizes, as appropriate for all clients from small children to larger adults. The standard (rigid) walker is shown in Figure 36–23. To use the standard walker, the client stands within the walker and firmly grasps the rubber handgrips. The client's line of gravity should be within the square of space outlined by the walker feet.

The client with a one-sided injury advances the walker and the injured leg together and then brings the uninjured leg up to meet the injured leg (i.e., walker and injured leg together, uninjured leg alone). This sequence is repeated as needed. It is very similar to the three-point crutch gait used with one injured leg.

The client who is allowed to bear weight on both extremities stands on both legs and advances the walker. When the walker is one pace ahead, the client takes a step to walk up to it (e.g., walker, right foot, left foot). This sequence is repeated, or it may be varied to practice a more natural gait (e.g., walker, left foot, right foot, walker, right foot, left foot).

Some of the many variations of the standard style of walker are listed in Box 36–2. No matter what the

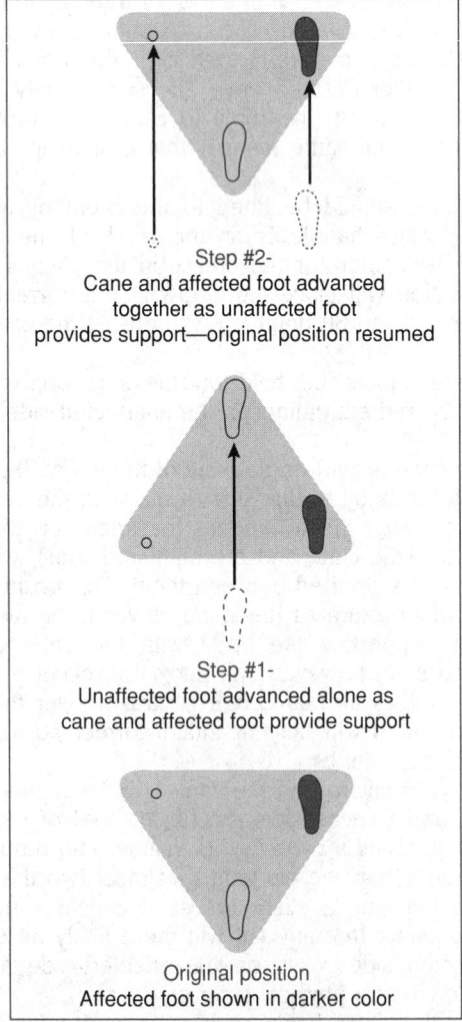

Step #2-
Cane and affected foot advanced together as unaffected foot provides support—original position resumed

Step #1-
Unaffected foot advanced alone as cane and affected foot provide support

Original position
Affected foot shown in darker color

▲ *Figure 36–22*

Cane gait.

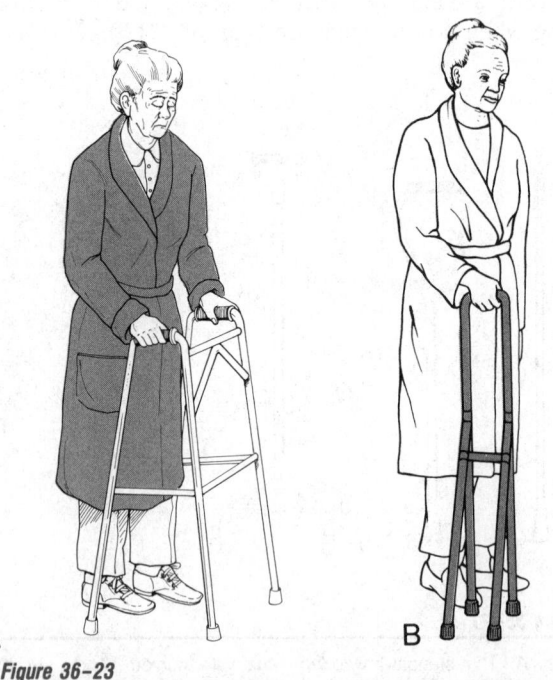

▲ *Figure 36–23*

Two walker models. *A*, The standard (rigid) walker; *B*, the side walker (quad cane).

Box 36-2. Variations of the Standard Walker

▶ Collapsible (folding) walkers are more easily transported by car or stored in narrower spaces in the home.

▶ Extra wide (both rigid and folding) walkers are wider for the client with a larger body size.

▶ Reciprocal walkers permit a two-point gait because each side can be advanced independently of the opposite side.

▶ Walkers with wheels on the two front tips assist in advancing the walker when the client needs help. When weight is borne on the walker, these wheels retract and the client again has four points of support.

▶ Walkers with platforms attached (similar to those on platform crutches) are used by clients who cannot bear weight on their wrists.

▶ Walkers with a seat that can be lowered and positioned across the walker may be used by clients who can walk only short distances before they need to sit down and rest.

▶ Walkers with a seat and four wheels instead of the usual rubber-capped tips may be used by clients who cannot stand up at all. They can sit in this model and use their feet to move it along, as desired.

▶ Side walkers are used on only one side of the body. These are really a type of quad cane. They are much more stable than a quad cane but are also more cumbersome and the client is more likely to trip over them.

style, safety considerations for walkers are similar to those for crutches and canes. For example:

▶ Be sure each foot of a walker is covered by a 2- to 3-cm rubber tip to assist with traction on the floor surface.

▶ Assist the client to maintain the line of gravity within the base of support by cautioning the client not to lean over the front of the walker and not to place the walker too far ahead of the body when advancing it.

▶ Help adjust the walker to a height that will facilitate walking and will prevent posture problems by assuring that the elbows will be flexed 15 to 30 degrees when using the walker. This position means that the walker handles are at the level of the client's trochanters (or wrist creases).

For additional considerations related to walkers, as well as the use of other assistive ambulation devices, see Table 36-3.

OTHER ASSISTIVE DEVICES

Hydraulic Chairs. Hydraulic chairs have specially designed seat cushions that can be electrically or mechanically raised and tipped forward to move the person from a sitting to a standing position. After the person has been out of the chair and is ready to return, the chair can be tipped backward and lowered to return the person to the desired sitting position. Hydraulic chairs are helpful for persons with limited motion of the knees and hips, such as occurs with arthritis, especially when these clients have weak upper extremities that limit their ability to pull themselves up.

Hydraulic chairs are most often used in the home. They are upholstered and appear similar to typical household furniture. They are more expensive, but the cost may be minimal when compared with the benefits of increased mobility. If prescribed by a licensed health care practitioner, the excess cost may be covered by insurance or may be an allowable medical deduction on the person's income tax. Hydraulic wheelchair seats are also available.

Prosthetic Devices. Prosthetic devices (prostheses) are artificial structures used to replace a natural organ, such as eyes, teeth, or limbs. When an individual has had a leg amputation, a prosthetic device can be surgically implanted in the bone so that it becomes a part of the body, or it may be worn after external application to the body. A leg prosthesis can help the person walk without the need for crutches, cane or walker. Consult a medical-surgical text or an orthopedic text for more information on leg prostheses.

Promoting Fitness for the Mobile Person

When a person has been mobilized with the use of assistive ambulation devices, you have gone a long way toward moving the person to a higher level of wellness. Some of these clients will, of course, continue to require assistive devices, while others will be able to regain complete, independent mobility. In either case, the client should strive for his or her optimal level of mobility in order to move further along the health-illness continuum toward high-level wellness. They should be ready to strive for fitness. But will they?

The human body was designed to move, yet increasingly people in industrialized countries are becoming a sedentary species. As members of a technologic society, we are not forced, like our ancestors, to move to stay alive. We no longer must spend long hours hunting for and gathering food. Water no longer must be fetched from a spring. Instead it flows from a spigot with the mere twist of a handle. Moreover, machines have eliminated many of the physical burdens of home or work: we ride instead of walk; we take elevators instead of climbing stairs; we toss clothes into dryers instead of hanging them on a line. Today, physical exertion is nearly a thing of the past.

Although many people are endeavoring to reverse this trend, most of us still do not get enough exercise. Nurses daily encounter persons who suffer from inadequate physical activity. Such inactivity ranges from complete immobilization caused by severe health problems, to a physical disability that limits movement, to mediocre fitness occasioned by casual exercise.

Physical fitness is important. Like proper diet, adequate sleep, and coping mechanisms, physical fitness contributes to high-level wellness. Today's nurses contribute to improving people's health by promoting good health habits, which include physical fitness.

TABLE 36–3. Selected Scientific Principles and Related Nursing Interventions for Assistive Ambulation Aids

Principle	Nursing Interventions
Traction decreases sliding between any two surfaces	Have all clients wear shoes that provide good support for their feet and that have nonslip soles to prevent slipping while walking with assistive ambulation aids
	Cover crutch, cane, and walker feet with rubber tips to provide traction
	Frequently check tips for signs of wear, such as cracks, loss of grooves, or decrease in concavity of the surface, all of which could decrease traction
	Replace tips that are hardened with age, as inflexible tips cause a loss of contact between tip and ground surface and decrease traction
	Caution clients with assistive devices to avoid situations in which traction can be lost (e.g., highly polished or wet floors, throw rugs, plush carpeting, and icy or wet sidewalks)
	Caution clients who will be walking outside in winter that (1) tips at room temperature can melt ice and cause a loss of traction, creating a very slippery surface; (2) tips that become cold become inflexible and cause a loss of contact between tip and ground surface
The wider the base of support, the more stable the object	For the greatest stability on crutches, teach your client to use a four-point gait
	For the greatest stability available with an assistive ambulation aid, teach your client to use a walker
	To help maintain the widest possible base of support while learning to use assistive devices, encourage clients to take short, slow steps
The closer the line of gravity is to the center of the base of support, the more stable an object	Teach clients the correct crutch-walking gait and emphasize body mechanics that will keep the line of gravity within the base of support
	Teach clients to hold a cane on their unaffected side
	Caution clients with walkers not to lean over the front of the walker and not to place the walker too far ahead of the body when advancing it
	Caution clients with walkers who must walk on grass or on soft or uneven ground to be certain that all four legs of their walker are on the ground before trusting their weight to the walker. Otherwise their base of support could suddenly shift and leave their line of gravity outside the new base of support
	Caution clients not to attempt to use a walker to climb stairs
The lower the center of gravity, the more stable an object	Clients may be able to combine their body mass with the mass of another object and rely on a low center of gravity of their "object-body unit" for stability, e.g., clients who have problems with balance and who must use a walker can benefit by lowering the center of gravity of their body and the walker (as a combined unit). Lowering may be done by hanging sand bags from the lower cross bars of the walker[25]
	Clients who are first learning to ambulate after an immobilizing illness may push a wheelchair along as they walk. In this case the wheelchair is used as an assistive ambulation aid
The normal anatomy and physiology of the upper extremities is best suited to performing a wide range of motion, whereas that of the lower extremities is best suited to weight bearing	Teach clients how to condition their upper extremity muscles to prepare them for the new tasks of weight bearing when the use of assistive ambulation aids is anticipated
	Explain to clients using assistive ambulation aids that the hands must be free to do the work of weight bearing and cannot safely be simultaneously used to carry objects
	Suggest that the client fasten a bicycle basket to the front of the walker so the client can carry a small purse or other objects as needed
	Suggest that purses with shoulder straps be worn diagonally across the body or that "fanny packs" or back packs be worn to carry light loads, as necessary
With the arm in extension, the normal human anatomy places the hand slightly below the level of the greater trochanter	The elbow should be flexed 15 to 30 degrees when using crutches, canes, and walkers
	Assure that the client's handgrips are at the level of the trochanter (or wrist crease). This position will cause the client's elbows to flex the necessary 15 to 30 degrees
Major nerves and blood vessels cross the axillae as they extend down the arm	Teach clients to avoid pressure on the soft tissues of the axillary area by not resting their body weight on the axillary bar of their crutches
	Assure that all axillary bars are padded prior to use

TABLE 36–3. Selected Scientific Principles and Related Nursing Interventions for Assistive Ambulation Aids Continued

Principle	Nursing Interventions
	Adjust assistive ambulation devices when changing from higher to lower shoe height to avoid crutches that are too high to allow a margin of safety in the axilla
Sedatives, narcotics, and alcohol all depress the central nervous system and decrease mentation, coordination, judgment, and balance	Caution clients against using CNS depressants when using assistive ambulation devices
The normal human stance is one of erect posture with eyes ahead	Adjust assistive ambulation devices when changing from lower to higher shoe height to prevent the client from stooping in order to bear weight on assistive devices
	Caution the client to avoid looking at the feet while walking with assistive devices

Physical fitness is a vital, lifelong pursuit.

When a person is physically fit, the body is able to adapt to both the usual and unusual physical demands of life. In addition, it is able to perform adequately when called upon to walk, run, jump, and so on. The person who feels physically strong and supple usually feels mentally alert and emotionally balanced as well. Some experts believe that physical exercise "drains off" excess toxins that accumulate as we react to stressors, both great and small.

There are several types of physical fitness. Passive fitness is simply the absence of debilitating disease. Muscular fitness strengthens muscle but does not necessarily improve cardiovascular or respiratory function. Similarly, flexibility fitness improves joint and muscle movements only. Endurance fitness is the most desirable form of fitness, since it improves the function of the lungs, the heart, the blood vessels, the digestive tract, and many of the body's muscles.

Endurance fitness comes with **aerobic exercise.** Literally meaning "with oxygen," aerobic exercise improves the body's capacity to consume oxygen and increases the overall amount of oxygen in the body. Oxygen is required to produce energy at the cellular level. Because it cannot be stored, oxygen must be delivered continuously to organs and tissues where energy is needed. Aerobic exercise provides this oxygen. Additionally, it conditions and strengthens the heart muscle to pump oxygen-carrying blood more efficiently throughout the body. The conditioning and strengthening then enable an individual to perform vigorous physical activity over a long period without feeling unduly fatigued. Strengthening the heart muscle also means fewer beats are required to pump blood through the body. Hence, the person who is aerobically fit usually has a lower resting heart rate.

For aerobic exercise to be beneficial, the individual must be able to sustain the chosen aerobic activity for at least 2 minutes before becoming breathless. Swimming, running or jogging, walking, hiking, bicycling, cross-country skiing, and rope-skipping are all aerobic. Bowling, golf, badminton, and sprinting are not.

Other categories of exercise include

▶ **flexibility exercises,** which lengthen, stretch, and flex muscles while enhancing balance and overall grace
▶ **strength-developing exercises** (isometric and isotonic), which contract muscles and promote their development
▶ **anaerobic exercises** ("without oxygen"), which are vigorous exercises of short duration (1 to 2 minutes) used primarily for competitive sports training. Weight-lifting is an example of anaerobic exercise

To reach and maintain adequate physical fitness, a person should perform aerobic conditioning and a combination of the other types of exercise regularly. An exercise program can begin with as little as 10 to 15 minutes of brisk walking daily. Over time, proper conditioning can

▶ enhance skills and coordination
▶ improve flexibility
▶ build muscle tone and strength
▶ help relieve tension
▶ slow the aging process or the onset of degenerative disease
▶ improve sleep and relaxation
▶ aid digestion
▶ diminish fatigue
▶ promote weight loss and weight control
▶ foster self-confidence

Exercise may also become addictive. At a certain level of fitness, most devotees report being "hooked" on exercise and feel deprived if forced to do without it. Long-distance runners, in particular, often talk about a pleasant "high." Some physiologists believe this euphoria is caused by endorphins, which are chemicals produced by the brain. When released, endorphins dull the fatigue and pain of a long run. But the "high" can be so pleasant that some runners become dependent on it. Addiction to exercise, particularly jogging, can be hazardous. The person who has an injury or is ill and continues to run jeopardizes health. Also some runners insist on jogging in very hot or cold weather. Cold weather can have dangerous consequences (e.g., falls on ice, respiratory infections). Very hot weather can result in heat exhaustion or heat stroke.

Beginning a physical exercise routine requires observing the basic tenets of moderation: go slow and easy. Remind the person that long-term improvement is the goal. One should think in terms of weeks, months, or even a full year.

Beginning an exercise program means choosing an activity that not only is appropriate for age, health status, or physical limitations but is also enjoyable enough to stick with on a regular basis. Exercise really should be fun—not like taking castor oil. To encourage regular sessions, exercise must fit easily into the person's daily routine. Otherwise the person may leave exercising until all other tasks have been completed and then be too tired to exercise. Help the person decide upon one activity or several that seem best suited. Next, encourage the individual to set up a daily or at least weekly exercise schedule. For some people an exercise class may be beneficial, because then exercise is scheduled for them.

Aerobic conditioning exercises should be done regularly because benefits are lost quickly.

Recommend exercising at least three times a week for a minimum of 20 minutes, during which time the heart rate reaches 70 to 85 per cent of its maximal capacity.

Counted in beats per minute, the maximal heart rate is best calculated as 220 minus age in years. For example, the maximal heart rate for a 32-year-old would be 188, or 220 − 32.

In remedying inadequate physical activity, the nurse is both teacher and evaluator. Monitor the person's progress through scheduled follow-up sessions. Evaluate progress on the basis of the individual's goals, history, and current physical condition. Give praise when praise is due.

As beneficial as exercise is, it is not without its hazards. To minimize the risks, instruct individuals to precede every exercise period with a warm-up of at least 5 minutes; 10 minutes are even better. Exercising makes muscles contract and sometimes shorten. Unfortunately, short, tight muscles are more susceptible to injury than loose, flexible ones. Warm-up exercises increase the flow of blood to the muscles, raising their temperature. Warm muscles are more flexible and consequently more able to stretch. Warm-ups therefore guard against injury or soreness.

Warm-up exercises can be as simple as performing a slow version of the activity. For example, joggers can start by walking 5 minutes or so, then going into a slow jog for another 5 minutes before hustling up to speed.

As warm-ups precede exercise, so should cooling down end the exercise period. Individuals should walk for 5 to 10 minutes or perform the same activity, at a slower rate, immediately after vigorous exercise. Cool-down should continue until breathing returns to normal and heart beat slows. Encourage individuals to do their cool-down exercises, even though they might be tempted to sidestep them. Cool-down exercises ensure that blood does not pool in the enlarged veins of the muscles but, rather, circulates to the brain, heart, intestine, and other organs, as necessary.

Proper nutrition is essential to maintaining sufficient energy for exercise. A well-balanced diet is a must, as is the need for adequate rest and sleep. Finally, remind individuals to begin their exercise programs slowly and build up gradually.

Pain is an indication of overuse. Instruct your clients to stop exercising at the first sign of pain.

EVALUATION

When you have completed your nursing interventions, your client should be at the highest level of physical mobility possible for that person. What is possible for each person can vary considerably, of course. Therefore, it is important that outcomes be measured against good baseline data that indicate the client's status before your interventions. Because some of the initial assessment data are subjective in clients with impaired mobility, it is preferable that the same nurse assess the client initially and at the evaluation of the outcomes.

For each of the outcomes that might be expected for an individual with impaired physical mobility, your evaluation should be carried out with minimal subjectivity. Consider the following outcomes:

▶ Client has measurably increased muscle mass. This outcome can best be determined in an extremity by measuring the circumference at the bulkiest part of the muscle mass and comparing the finding with the baseline.

▶ Client demonstrates measurably increased muscle strength. This outcome can be assessed objectively by using an **ergometer** (a device that measures work output), but these devices are not readily available in most clinical settings, so that nurses must measure muscle strength by other means. You can do this by observing the amount of work the client is able to complete (e.g., pounds of weight lifted, amount of resistance offered during resistive exercises, or strength of hand squeeze). To obtain the most reliable decision concerning possible changes in the strength of resistance or hand squeeze, it is best if the person who completes the evaluation is the same person who did the initial assessment.

▶ Client independently moves all joints through complete range of motion. This outcome is more objective in that different observers should be able to accurately estimate the degree to which any joint can be moved, in any particular plane. Use of a goniometer can make these estimates even more objective.

Additional outcomes can be objectively measured by noting whether the client can or cannot complete each activity:

▶ Independently assumes position, "dangling" at side of bed

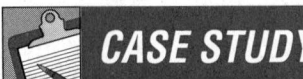

CASE STUDY

The Client

Four weeks ago, Ms. Celia Moore, a well-developed, athletic, 52-year-old white female secretary, was admitted to the emergency department after experiencing a sudden, incapacitating pain in her left ankle while playing tennis. The pain subsided, but the tenderness remaining in her ankle was of concern to her. Following medical diagnosis of second-degree strain, a splint was applied. A partial listing of the physician's orders included

- ► bed rest with bathroom privileges for 48 hours, with left leg elevated 45 degrees until edema subsides
- ► apply ice cap intermittently for 48 hours, then apply heating pad for comfort prn
- ► aspirin gr X PO, q4h prn for discomfort
- ► axillary crutches with no weight-bearing on left leg X 4 weeks
- ► regular diet as tolerated
- ► return to orthopedic clinic for evaluation in 4 weeks

At 8:00 PM, February 7, a partial listing of the nursing assessment data included the following:

- ► Alert, intelligent, 52-year-old, muscular female
- ► Left ankle splinted
- ► T 99.2 F, B/P 128/76, P 64, R 16
- ► Skin intact, ivory in color
- ► Toes of left foot edematous, freely movable, and warm to touch with capillary refill less than 2 seconds (unable to assess pulses under splint)
- ► States no numbness, pain, or tingling in toes but does complain of tenderness in left ankle
- ► Demonstrates full, active ROM of all unsplinted joints
- ► Gross muscle strength = 5

Four weeks have passed since admission to the emergency department. It is now March 9. The following represents part of a nursing care plan written for her before her discharge from emergency department, and the current evaluation of outcomes that were expected at that time.

CARE PLAN

8:00 PM, February 7

Nursing Diagnosis	Planning: Expected Outcomes	Implementation: Nursing Interventions	Evaluation
Impaired Physical Mobility R/T effects of unavoidable injury and to prescribed musculoskeletal inactivity as evidenced by left ankle strain and required splint	By 9:00 AM, February 10: Reports no increase in pain or edema. Reports no new signs or symptoms of neuromuscular or vascular compromise that could further reduce mobility	Prepare for increasing mobility in 48 hours by teaching client to 1. Rest in bed and keep left foot elevated on two pillows X 24 hours to decrease edema and pain 2. Take ordered A.S.A. gr X q4h prn to reduce pain and inflammation 3. Apply ice cap 1/2 hour on and 1/2 hour off to reduce pain and edema, as ordered 4. Call ortho clinic to report any increase in pain or edema in ankle 5. Compare toes of both feet and report any variations in temperature, color, ability to move, or sensations such as numbness, pain, or tingling	9:00 AM, February 10: No reports of increased pain or edema. No reports of symptoms of neuromuscular or vascular compromise

Care Plan continued on following page

CARE PLAN Continued

8:00 PM, February 7

Nursing Diagnosis	Planning: Expected Outcomes	Implementation: Nursing Interventions	Evaluation
	Reports no problems with or questions about crutch walking	6. Correctly walk on axillary crutches using swing-to and swing-through gaits to avoid any weight bearing. Provide for supervised practice with gaits	States, ". . . no problems with crutches"
	By 2:00 PM, March 9: Returns to ortho clinic at functional level 1, with all joints except left ankle showing full, active ROM and with gross muscle strength at level 5	7. Sit down and stand up with crutches and to use crutches safely to ascend and descend stairs. Provide for supervised practice with maneuvers	2:00 PM, March 9 Skin of toes ivory in color, warm to touch. Capillary refill less than 2 seconds No edema noted in left ankle. Pedal pulses 2+ B/P 122/70, P 68, R 16
		8. Use crutches first 48 hours only to go to the bathroom	All joints except left ankle show full, active ROM with gross muscle strength at level 5
		9. Prepare for more crutch walking, after 48 hours, by completing 10 bed push-ups per hour and squeezing firm rubber ball in each hand 20–30 times per hour, when awake	Unable to move left ankle in any plane Functional level 1, requires use of crutches Independently uses crutches with a swing-through gait
		10. Call ortho clinic with any questions or problems concerning crutch walking Give written instructions for all teaching done and include instructions for safe crutch use for client to take home with her Provide for follow-up by telephoning client 9:00 AM, February 10 Schedule for return to clinic 2:00 PM, March 9	States she is determined to prevent muscle deterioration and is eager to begin physiotherapy to restore ankle function

▶ Independently transfers from bed to chair or wheelchair
▶ Independently walks a measurable distance — for example, to the end of the hall

Summary

▶ Assessing readiness for mobility includes assessing

   ▶ functional level
   ▶ gross motor strength
   ▶ body systems for contraindications to movement

   ▶ body systems for presence of disuse phenomena
   ▶ emotional or psychosocial responses
   ▶ cognitive ability

▶ The nursing diagnosis of *Impaired Physical Mobility* is appropriate for the person who needs assistance in becoming more mobile. This nursing diagnosis should be differentiated from the nursing diagnoses of *High Risk for Disuse Syndrome* and *Activity Intolerance.*

▶ With the diagnosis, *Impaired Physical Mobility,* nursing care should be directed toward increasing the client's mobility level within the limits of the person's ability.

▶ Nursing interventions for the client who is ready to begin mobilization require that the nurse be familiar with exercises, the progressive mobilization process, assistive ambulation devices, and measures to promote fitness in the mobile person.

▶ Isotonic exercises cause muscles to shorten in contraction as body parts move and muscle tension remains the same. Isometric exercises cause increased muscle tension while muscle length remains the same.

▶ All range-of-motion exercises are done to maintain joint flexibility by putting each joint through its full range of possible movements in all planes. Passive range of motion is done by the nurse for the client. Active-assistive range-of-motion is completed by the nurse after being started by the client. Active range-of-motion is done independently by the client. Resistive range-of-motion is done by the client against a force exerted to prevent easy movement of the limb.

▶ In progressive mobilization the nurse frequently teaches the client to dangle and assists the client to ambulate.

▶ Assistive ambulation aids include crutches, canes, walkers, hydraulic chairs, and prosthetic devices.

▶ The nurse's role in promoting fitness for the mobile person involves teaching about types of exercise, the benefits of exercise, how to minimize hazards when exercising, and the importance of nutrition in maintaining fitness.

▶ Evaluation of the client with a nursing diagnosis of *Impaired Physical Mobility* can be improved when the same nurse assesses the client before and after the nursing interventions.

Bibliography

1. Allegrante, J.P., & Michela, J.L. (1990). Impact of a school-based workplace health promotion program on morale of inner-city teachers. *Journal of School Health,* 60(1), 25–28.
2. Annesley, A.L., et al. (1990). Energy expenditure of ambulation using the Sure-Gait crutch and the standard axillary crutch. *Physical Therapy,* 70(1), 18–23.
3. Basford, J.R., et al. (1990). Clinical evaluation of the rocker bottom crutch. *Orthopedics,* 13(4), 457–460.
4. Bauer, D.M., et al. (1991). A comparative analysis of several crutch-length-estimation techniques. *Physical Therapy,* 71(4), 294–300.
5. Bell, N.N. (1992). Clinical significance of ST-segment monitoring. *Critical Care Nursing Clinics of North America.* 4(2), 313–323.
6. Bhambhani, Y.N., et al. (1990). Axillary crutch walking: effects of three training programs. *Archives of Physical Medicine and Rehabilitation,* 71(7), 484–489.
7. Blaylock, B. (1991). Mobility and ambulation: not easy tasks for all older adults. *Advancing Clinical Care,* 6(6), 20–21, 41.
8. Bowers, A.C., et al. (1992). *Clinical manual of health assessment.* St. Louis: Mosby/Year Book.
9. Breslow, L., et al. (1990). Worksite health promotion: its evolution and the Johnson & Johnson experience. *Preventive Medicine,* 19(1), 13–21.
10. Burgess, A.W. (1990). *Psychiatric nursing: In the hospital and in the community* (5th ed.). Norwalk, Connecticut: Appleton & Lange.
11. Carpenito, L.J. (1991). *Nursing care plans and documentation:*

12. Crosbie, W.J., & Nicol, A.C. (1990). Aided gait in rheumatoid arthritis following knee arthroplasty. *Archives of Physical Medicine and Rehabilitation,* 71(5), 299–303.
13. Crosbie, W.J., & Nicol, A.C. (1990). Reciprocal aided gait in paraplegia. *Paraplegia,* 28(6), 353–363.
14. DeLateur, B.J., & Lehmann, J.F. (1990). Therapeutic exercise to develop strength and endurance. In Kottke, F.J., & Lehmann, J.F. (eds.). *Krusen's handbook of physical medicine* (4th ed., pp. 480–519). Philadelphia: W.B. Saunders.
15. Doenges, M.E., & Moorhouse, M.F. (1991). *Nurse's pocket guide: Nursing diagnoses with interventions* (3rd ed.). Philadelphia: F.A. Davis.
16. Ebrahim, S., et al. (1991). The valuation of states of ill-health: the impact of age and disability. *Age and Aging,* 20(1), 37–40.
17. ECRI (1991). Ambulation aids. *Health Devices,* 20(1), 5–22.
18. Evans, P.M., et al. (1990). Cerebral palsy: why we must plan for survival. *Archives of Disease in Childhood,* 65(12), 1329–1333.
19. Falconer, J., et al. (1990). Therapeutic ultrasound in the treatment of musculoskeletal conditions. *Arthritis Care and Research,* 3(2), 85–91.
20. Godin, G., et al. (1987). The impact of physical fitness and health-age appraisal upon exercise intentions and behavior. *Journal of Behavioral Medicine,* 10(3), 241–250.
21. Haywood, K.M. (1991). The role of physical education in the development of active lifestyles. *Research Quarterly for Exercise and Sport,* 62(2), 151–156.
22. Hickey, P.W. (1990). *Nursing process handbook.* St. Louis: C.V. Mosby.
23. Hjeltnes, N., & Lannem, A. (1990). Functional neuromuscular stimulation in four patients with complete paraplegia. *Paraplegia,* 28(4), 235–243.
24. Jay, P. (1990). Symposium on immobility. The role of community nurses. *Nursing,* 4(4), 13–15.
25. Joyce, B.M., & Kirby, R.L. (1991). Canes, crutches and walkers. *American Family Physician,* 43(2), 535–542.
26. Kottke, F.J., & Lehmann, J.F. (eds.) (1990). *Krusen's handbook of physical medicine* (4th ed.). Philadelphia: W.B. Saunders.
27. Lane, P.L., & LeBlanc, R. (1990). Crutch walking. *Orthopaedic Nursing,* 9(5), 31–38.
28. Larson, E.B., & Bruce, R.A. (1987). Health benefits of exercise in an aging society. *Archives of Internal Medicine,* 147(2), 353–356.
29. Levin, R.F., et al. (1989). Diagnostic content validity of nursing diagnoses. *Image—The Journal of Nursing Scholarship,* 21(1), 40–44.
30. Macera, C.A., et al. (1989). Age, physical activity, physical fitness, body composition, and incidence of orthopedic problems, *Research Quarterly for Exercise and Sport,* 60(3), 225–233.
31. Maki, B.E., et al. (1991). Fear of falling and postural performance in the elderly. *Journal of Gerontology,* 46(4), M123–131.
32. Marieb, E.N. (1992). *Human anatomy and physiology* (2nd ed.). Redwood City, California: The Benjamin/Cummings Publishing Company, Inc.
33. McCance, K.L., & Huether, S.E. (Eds.) (1990). *Pathophysiology: The biologic basis for disease in adults and children.* St. Louis: C.V. Mosby.
34. McConnell, E.A. (1991). Teaching a patient to use a cane correctly. *Nursing,* 21(9), 83.
35. Mehmert, P.A., & Delaney, C.V.W. (1991). Validating impaired physical mobility. *Nursing Diagnosis,* 2(4), 143–154.
36. Milde, F.K. (1988). Focus: Nursing diagnosis. Impaired physical mobility. *Journal of Gerontological Nursing,* 14(3), 20–24.
37. Mobily, P.R., & Kelley, L.S. (1991). Iatrogenesis in the elderly: factors of immobility. *Journal of Gerontological Nursing,* 17(9), 5–11.
38. Mol, V.J., & Baker, C.A. (1991). Activity intolerance in the geriatric stroke patient. *Rehabilitation Nursing,* 16(6), 337–343.
39. Nagy, S., & Nix, C.L. (1989). Relations between preventive health behavior and hardiness. *Psychological Reports,* 65(1), 339–345.
40. National Association of Orthopaedic Nurses (1991). *Core curriculum for orthopaedic nursing* (2nd ed.). Pitman, New Jersey: Anthony J. Jannetti.
41. Nene, A.V., & Patrick, J.H. (1990). Energy cost of paraplegic

locomotion using the ParaWalker-electrical stimulation "hybrid" orthosis. *Archives of Physical Medicine and Rehabilitation,* 71(2), 116–120.

42. Nielsen, D.H., et al. (1990). Energy cost, exercise intensity, and gait efficiency of standard versus rocker-bottom axillary crutch walking. *Physical Therapy,* 70(8), 487–493.

43. Norman, G.M., & Gibbs, J.A. (1991). Why walk when you can ride? Clinical ambulation incentives for the immobile elderly. *Journal of Gerontological Nursing,* 17(8), 28–33.

44. North American Nursing Diagnosis Association (1990). *Taxonomy 1—Revised 1990.* St. Louis: North American Nursing Diagnosis Association.

45. Olson, E.V., et al. (1990). The hazards of immobility: 1967 'classic article.' *American Journal of Nursing,* 90(3), 43–48.

46. Osterman, H.M., & Stuck, R.M. (1990). The aging foot. *Orthopaedic Nursing,* 9(6), 43–47.

47. Oullet, L.L., & Rush, K.L. (1992). A synthesis of selected literature on mobility: a basis for studying impaired mobility. *Nursing Diagnosis,* 3(2), 72–80.

48. Porth, C.M. (Ed.) (1990). *Pathophysiology: Concepts of altered health states* (3rd ed.). Philadelphia: J.B. Lippincott.

49. Redfern, S. (1990). Symposium on immobility. Care after a stroke. *Nursing,* 4(4), 7–11.

50. Sakakibara, Y., & Honda, Y. (1990). Cardiopulmonary responses to static exercise. *Annals of Physiological Anthropology,* 9(2), 153–156.

51. Schilke, J.M. (1991). Slowing the aging process with physical activity. *Journal of Gerontological Nursing,* 17(6), 4–8.

52. Steinberg, F.U., & Dean, B.Z. (1990). Physiatric therapeutics. 8. Management of the immobilized patient. *Archives of Physical Medicine and Rehabilitation.* 71(4-S), S281–282.

53. Stuart, G.W., & Sundeen, S.J. (1991). *Principles and practice of psychiatric nursing* (4th ed.). St. Louis: Mosby/Year Book.

54. Tremblay, F., et al. (1990). Effects of prolonged muscle stretch on reflex and voluntary muscle activations in children with spastic cerebral palsy. *Scandinavian Journal of Rehabilitation Medicine,* 22(4), 171–180.

55. Tursky, E.A. (1991). Muscle training physiology and practical applications of training for strength versus endurance. *Orthopaedic Nursing,* 10(2), 27–32.

56. Varcarolis, E.M. (Ed.) (1990). *Foundations of psychiatric mental health nursing.* Philadelphia: W.B. Saunders.

57. Walker, J.E., & Howland, J. (1991). Falls and fear of falling among elderly persons living in the community: occupational therapy interventions. *American Journal of Occupational Therapy,* 45(2), 119–122.

58. Whitehead, J.R., & Corbin, C.B. (1991). Effects of fitness test type, teacher, and gender on exercise intrinsic motivation and physical self-worth. *Journal of School Health,* 61(1), 11–16.

▼ *Providing Physical Protection and Body Support*

▼
▼
▼
▼

That which makes the man no worse than he was makes his life no worse; it has no power to harm, without or within.

Marcus Aurelius Antoninus
(translation by Morris Hickey)

▼ CHAPTER OUTLINE

CLIENTS WHO REQUIRE PROTECTIVE
  AND SUPPORTING DEVICES
    Clients with Orthopedic Disorders
    Clients with Neuromuscular
      Disorders
    Clients with Behavioral and
      Neurologic Disorders
ASSESSMENT
    General Considerations
    Considerations Related to the
      Application of Restraints
NURSING DIAGNOSIS
PLANNING

NURSING INTERVENTION
    Binders
    Bandages
    Antiembolism Hosiery
    Sequential Compression Devices
    Casts
    Bracing and Splinting
    Traction
    Movement Devices
    Restraints
    Suicide Precautions
EVALUATION
CASE STUDY

▼ KEY TERMS

Cerebral palsy
Cerebrovascular accident
  (CVA, stroke)
Comminuted fracture
Compartment syndrome
Complete fracture
Complicated fracture
Compound (open) fracture
Countertraction

Depressed fracture
Fracture
Greenstick (willow stick,
  hickory stick) fracture
Impacted fracture
Incomplete fracture
Multiple sclerosis
Orthopedic disorders
Parkinson's disease

Reduction
RICE
Simple (closed) fracture
Skeletal traction
Skin traction
Sprain
Strain
Traction

Mrs. Carver, a 76-year-old osteoporotic woman, was alert but in severe pain when she was admitted to the hospital with a fractured hip. She was placed in traction in an attempt to align the fractured bone fragments before surgery. During the night, she became confused and disoriented, took herself out of traction, attempted to get out of bed, and fell to the floor, fracturing her skull and left humerus.

Mrs. Carver is one of the 1.3 million Americans who will suffer unexpected disabling injuries in hospitals this year. She could be one of the 198,000 who may die as a result. Seven of 10 such iatrogenic injuries are preventable.[37a] In fact, you may be able to prevent some of these injuries. The information in this chapter describes how you might do this.

This chapter discusses the nursing care related to the immobilization of one or more body parts. Immobility can cause overwhelming health problems that must be prevented, and yet therapy for many clients is achieved by immobilization. For therapeutic purposes, immobilization may consist of bed rest, as discussed in Chapter 35, or the application of mobility-restricting devices. These devices range from centuries-old, traditional devices, such as bandages, binders, and restraints, to newer and more sophisticated devices you may not have heard of before you entered nursing. These devices have a common purpose, and that is to protect or support the client or one or more of the client's body parts. If these devices are to be maximally beneficial to the client and not contribute to the incidence of iatrogenic disorders, you must be knowledgeable about their intended therapeutic purposes and potential adverse effects so that you may ensure they are used correctly and safely.

CLIENTS WHO REQUIRE PROTECTIVE AND SUPPORTING DEVICES

Individuals who can benefit from a protective and supportive device may present with any of a variety of different medical, surgical, or psychiatric conditions. From a medical standpoint, these individuals most often include persons with certain orthopedic disorders, such as a fracture; persons with certain neuro-

muscular impairments, such as result from a cerebrovascular accident; and persons with certain behavioral or neurologic disorders, such as those who are at high risk of doing violence to themselves or to others.

Clients with Orthopedic Disorders

Orthopedic disorders are those involving the locomotion structures of the body, especially the skeleton, joints, muscles, fascia, ligaments, and cartilage. Common orthopedic disorders include fractures, sprains, and strains.

CLIENTS WITH FRACTURES

A **fracture** is a break in the continuity of the bone that usually results from traumatic injury to the body part. The injury may be from direct trauma, such as when the tibia and fibula are struck by the bumper of a speeding car, or from indirect trauma, such as when a person falls on an outstretched hand and a fracture of the clavicle results. A fracture may also be the result of sudden, violent muscle contractions, as might occur during a seizure. When the bone is healthy, a great deal of trauma is usually required to cause a fracture. However, pathologic (or spontaneous) fractures may occur with very little trauma when the bone is diseased with cancer, rickets, or osteoporosis.

Fractures may be classified as simple or compound. A **simple (closed) fracture** is a fracture in which the bone is broken but no external break in the skin is present and minimal soft tissue injury exists. A **compound (open) fracture** is a fracture in which the bone is broken and a wound extends through soft tissue and the skin. The skin may be broken either from external trauma or from penetration of the bone outward through the skin. An open fracture carries a greater risk for infection because of the break in the skin.

Fractures may also be classified according to the degree of break in the bone. A fracture may be complete or incomplete. A **complete fracture** traverses the entire bone; it may or may not require realignment of the bone fragments. An **incomplete fracture** does not traverse the entire bone. A common type of incomplete fracture is a **greenstick (willow stick, hickory stick) fracture.** This is a fracture involving only part of the thickness of a bone. The bone breaks like a green stick, bending on one side and breaking on the other. This type of fracture is seen in children because their bones are resilient and the periosteum is thicker than that in adult bones.

Still another way of classifying fractures is by the type of break. There are many different types of breaks. In a **comminuted fracture,** the bone is crushed or splintered into several bone fragments. In the **impacted fracture,** one fragment of the broken bone is wedged into the other fragment. With a **depressed fracture,** fragments of bone are forced below their normal level and below the level of surrounding portions of the bone; this type of fracture may be seen in the skull.

Fractures may be complicated. A **complicated fracture** is a fracture in which there is associated damage to an internal organ. An example might be when a depressed skull fracture results in neurologic damage or when a fractured rib penetrates the lung.

To treat a fracture, the physician must first ensure that any necessary **reduction** (realignment of the bone fragments after a fracture) is completed. Depending on the nature of the injury, the particular bone that is fractured, and the extent of soft tissue damage that may have occurred, the physician may use open reduction (in surgery, directly) or closed reduction (manually, through soft tissue). After reduction, most fractures are treated with casts in order to maintain alignment of the bone fragments while healing occurs. Reduction is sometimes achieved and maintained by the use of traction. Less often, a combination of traction and casting is used. Other devices may also be used.

CLIENTS WITH SPRAINS AND STRAINS

A **sprain** is an injury to a joint in which surrounding ligaments have been stretched or torn by a traumatic injury to the joint, such as "twisting the ankle." A **strain** is an injury in which a muscle or tendon has been damaged by overstretching or overexertion, such as might occur with a sport that involves strenuous muscle use.

Sprains and strains often result in similar symptoms, including tenderness, edema, ecchymosis, and pain. For both types of injury, the symptoms experienced depend on the degree of damage incurred.

Because treatment for sprains and strains does not completely immobilize the injured part, these soft tissue injuries may be more painful than fractures.

RICE is an acronym for a treatment that is helpful with fractures, sprains, and strains. The letters stand for *r*est (of the injured part), *i*ce (applications to reduce pain and edema), *c*ompression (applications to decrease edema), and *e*levation (of the injured part to reduce edema).

Rest for the injured part may be achieved with various types of devices, including immobilizers, bandages, slings, cervical collars, splints, and braces. Certain types of fractures may also benefit by the use of some of these devices, as may other orthopedic disorders. See an orthopedic text for complete details.

Clients with Neuromuscular Disorders

Neuromuscular disorders are disorders in which the muscles are temporarily or permanently weakened or paralyzed owing to loss of nervous system function. Major neuromuscular disorders include cerebrovascular accident, spinal cord injury, and chronic neuromuscular disorders such as multiple sclerosis, Parkinson's disease, and cerebral palsy.

CLIENTS WITH CEREBROVASCULAR ACCIDENTS

Cerebrovascular accident (CVA, stroke) is a disorder in which there is sudden loss of consciousness or loss of motor or sensory function that results from rupture or occlusion of a cerebral artery. The location and size of the cerebral artery involved determine the site and involvement of the sensory or motor loss. Whereas the resulting neurologic dysfunction may be highly variable, the client frequently suffers hemiplegia (paralysis of either the right or the left half of the body). Although it may occur at any age, cerebrovascular accident is a major cause of paralysis in elderly persons.

After a cerebrovascular accident, the individual may be on bed rest for three days or until the condition has stabilized. After this, rehabilitation begins. Protective and supportive devices, such as antiembolism hosiery, sequential compression devices, and splints, may be needed during both stabilization and rehabilitation.

CLIENTS WITH SPINAL CORD INJURIES

Paralysis due to spinal cord injury is frequently seen in the younger adult. Common causes of spinal cord injury include motor vehicle accidents and diving accidents. The vertebral level of the injury determines the level of paralysis. In general terms, cervical injuries result in quadriplegia (paralysis of the trunk and all four extremities), and lumbar injuries result in paraplegia (paralysis of the lower portion of the torso and of both legs).

If the spinal cord is completely severed, the paralysis is permanent. If the cord is damaged but not completely severed, the paralysis may be wholly or partially reversed. Spinal cord trauma is a medical emergency that requires prompt treatment in a hospital. The goal is to stabilize the fracture site to prevent further damage to the cord. This requires immobilizing the spine, and a number of devices may be used to accomplish this, for example, the Stryker wedge frame (see Chapter 35). See an orthopedic or neurologic nursing text for complete details concerning all of the specialized devices available.

At various stages after spinal cord injury, the client may have need for such protective and supportive devices as movement devices, cervical collars, antiembolism hosiery, sequential compression devices, and braces.

CLIENTS WITH CHRONIC NEUROMUSCULAR DISORDERS

Chronic, degenerative neuromuscular disorders, such as multiple sclerosis and Parkinson's disease, commonly result in progressive loss of motor function. Cerebral palsy, on the other hand, is the term for several related chronic disorders in which neuromuscular impairment is nonprogressive.

Multiple sclerosis is a chronic autoimmune disorder that involves degeneration of the myelin sheath of the white fibers in the central nervous system. The etiology may be related to both viral and genetic factors. The disease is characterized by various neurologic deficits, such as speech and vision problems, as well as by muscular weakness, paresthesias, and incoordination. Symptoms may progress steadily downward or may be marked by remissions and exacerbations. The total course of the disease may be a few months to decades before death occurs. The average span of the disease is approximately 30 years.

Parkinson's disease is a chronic, progressive disease associated with degenerative processes in the nuclear masses of the extrapyramidal system. The disorder is characterized by intermittent fine tremors of a hand or foot that spread until all four extremities are involved and the tremors are continuous. As the disease progresses, the muscles become weak; facial expression is lost so that the face becomes masklike. The client's posture is flexed forward, and the body is rigid. The gait is distinguished by small steps that become more and more rapid as the feet seem to try to keep up with the forward-inclining body. Falls often result from this gait.

Cerebral palsy is a nonspecific term for disorders of the central nervous system that result in persistent but nonprogressive bilateral, symmetric motor deficits. Deficits of sensory or intellectual function may coexist with the motor deficits. The etiology is usually related to brain damage during fetal development, at the time of birth, or in early infancy. Major classifications include the spastic type (characterized by muscle spasm and increased deep tendon reflexes), the athetoid type (characterized by uncontrollable, purposeless movements and muscle tension), and the atactic type (characterized by a staggering gait, incoordination, and poor balance).

Devices that might be used for chronic neuromuscular disorders include such supportive devices as cervical collars, splints, and braces.

Clients with Behavioral and Neurologic Disorders

CLIENTS AT HIGH RISK OF DOING VIOLENCE TO THEMSELVES OR OTHERS

Persons with certain behavioral disorders are at high risk of doing violence to themselves or to others. Such individuals may be found in psychiatric facilities, gen-

eral medical-surgical facilities, or the community. These persons are discussed in the Nursing Diagnosis Profile. Devices used to immobilize them and protect them from the consequences of their acts include a variety of restraints.

CLIENTS WITH NEUROLOGIC DEFICITS

Some persons are at increased risk of unintentionally harming themselves because they have neurologic deficits and lack the mental abilities necessary to maintain their own safety. These persons may be found in psychiatric facilities, general medical-surgical facilities, or the community. They must be watched carefully or they could harm themselves by doing any number of unsafe things. They might, for example, walk outside without adequate clothing, walk into busy traffic, attempt to walk when they are incapable of balance or coordination, disconnect themselves from medical devices (such as pulling out intravenous needles or tubes in body cavities), or fall out of bed. Such individuals can benefit from a protective environment, but sometimes an additional restraining device may be temporarily necessary.

ASSESSMENT

Clients who are expected to benefit from the use of protective and supportive devices may actually have disorders of any system of the body. In our discussion thus far, we have mentioned only some of the disorders most commonly requiring these devices. Because these devices are used for so many different disorders, it is difficult to point out specific areas that must be assessed; we must rely on the fact that a good, general assessment is completed before the initiation of these devices (see Chapters 31, 32, and 33).

General Considerations

When you are planning to use a device that restricts the client's overall mobility and disuse phenomena may result, the immobilized client should have a baseline assessment as outlined in Table 35–3. After the device has been applied, routine, ongoing assessments should be continued until the device is no longer needed.

When you are planning to use a device that restricts the mobility of an extremity and there is potential for interruption to nerve impulses or blood supply to the distal portions of the extremity, a neurovascular check (Box 37–1) should be completed to establish a baseline; these checks should be routinely completed until the device is removed.

If you are planning to use a device that restricts the torso, you should complete a baseline assessment and routine, ongoing assessments of the internal organs that will be beneath the device. For example, you should assess the bladder and bowel function of a client when an abdominal binder is needed and assess lung function when a chest immobilizer is needed.

Before applying any device to any area of the body, assess the skin of the area to be covered for breaks,

Box 37–1. Neurovascular Assessment of an Extremity

Neurovascular Checks

Neurovascular checks are brief assessments that compare an involved extremity with the opposite extremity and identify

▶ Color differences (especially lack of color or cyanosis)
▶ The presence and degree of edema
▶ Temperature differences (cool skin shows decreased circulation; warmer skin may mean inflammation)
▶ Speed of capillary refill (should be less than 2 seconds)
▶ Rate and quality of peripheral pulses

▶ The client's ability to move the extremity by moving the hand or foot in a circular motion at the wrist or ankle and by wiggling the fingers or toes (to further test for damage to specific motor nerves, see motor function tests)
▶ Complaints of numbness, pain, tingling, or any other unusual sensations (to further test for damage to specific sensory nerves, see sensory function tests)

Assessment of Function of Specific Nerves

Sensory Function

Use a pointed device, such as a straightened paper clip, to test sensation at the following sites.

Nerve	Assessment
Peroneal	On the dorsum of the foot, test the area between the great toe and the second toe

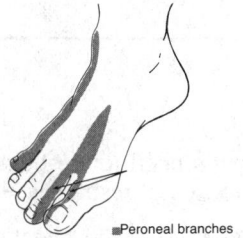

Tibial	Test toward the medial and lateral surfaces of the sole of the foot

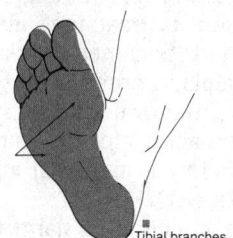

Radial	Test the webbed tissue between the thumb and index finger

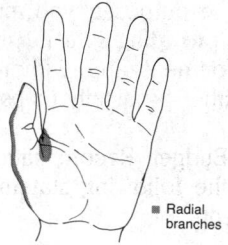

Motor Function

Ask the client to actively move the body part innervated by the following nerves.

Nerve	Assessment
Peroneal	Ask the client to dorsiflex the ankle and hyperextend the toes

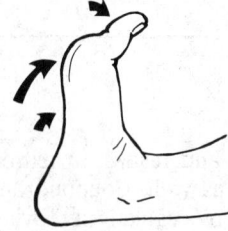

Tibial	Ask the client to plantarflex the ankle and flex the toes

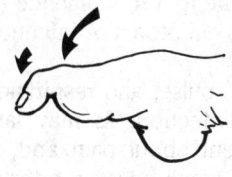

Radial	Ask the client to hyperextend the thumb or wrist

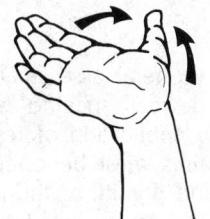

Box continued on following page

Box 37–1. Neurovascular Assessment of an Extremity (Continued)

Sensory Function

Nerve	Assessment
Ulnar	Test the distal pad of the little finger

■ Ulnar branches

Nerve	Assessment
Median	Test the distal surface of the index and middle fingers

■ Median branches

Motor Function

Nerve	Assessment
Ulnar	Ask the client to abduct and then adduct all fingers

Nerve	Assessment
Median	Ask the client to oppose the thumb and little finger and flex the wrist

signs of irritation, and rashes. In extremities, assess for signs of phlebitis as well. Continue an ongoing assessment of the skin (by regularly removing the device, if it is possible and not contraindicated). Ongoing assessment under the device is particularly important when wounds are present. If the device cannot be removed for direct assessment, use diligence in observing for indirect signs and symptoms of infection.

Body temperature, pulse, and respirations may be helpful indicators of infection, as may laboratory test results. Ask the client about pain and other sensations. Use your sense of smell because odor may be a sign of infection. It is particularly important to smell around cast edges when a wound is underneath the cast.

Considerations Related to the Application of Restraints

In addition to the general assessment considerations, which apply to all devices, specific assessments should be done before the application of restraints. Assessing the need for restraints must be done with regard for the human rights and dignity of the individual. Unnecessarily restraining a person may be construed as assault or false imprisonment if the nurse is not able to document that safe nursing care is not possible without restraints and that other avenues of providing safe care have been pursued.[19,68,70]

Assess the client's need for restraints on the basis of the following purposes of restraints:

▶ to prevent falls (assess the client's risk for falls, as outlined in Box 14–9)
▶ to prevent interruption of therapy (assess mental status on admission and as necessary to document informed consent to treatment; also assess for mental changes and document these to demonstrate need for restraints in order to carry out treatments)
▶ to prevent the removal of life support equipment (use same approach as for preventing interruption of therapy, and follow institutional and legal guidelines for your local area)
▶ to prevent the infliction of harm to self and others (again, assessment and documentation are important)

In deciding whether restraints are needed to accomplish one of these purposes, you must also think about the principle of providing safe nursing care in the least restrictive environment and without causing harm to the individual either physically or psychologically.[67]

The Omnibus Budget Reconciliation Act (OBRA) of 1987 included the following statement regarding nursing home residents:

The patient has the right to be free from any physical restraints imposed or psychoactive drug administered for purpose of discipline or convenience, and not required to treat the resident's medical symptoms.

The Omnibus Budget Reconciliation Act of 1987 became effective October 1990 as public policy.[19,68]

Standards of care for the use of restraints were set forth by the Health Care Financing Administration in 1992. The same standards apply in the acute care facility.

Any person who is dependent on the care of others is at risk for injury and has the right to safe care. You are legally responsible for any harm that comes to the person under your care. At the same time, every client has the right not to be restrained unless a court rules otherwise.

To protect yourself and your clients, try all reasonable alternatives to restraints. Assess your client for possible use of alternatives to restraints (Box 37–2). If alternatives are not the answer, follow the policy for your institution regarding the application of restraints. Institutional policy should be clear about the steps to be taken in application of restraints.[8] You should prepare to apply restraints only within the written institutional policy.

NURSING DIAGNOSIS

Common nursing diagnoses associated with the use of protective and supportive devices include diagnoses used before the application of the device in order to demonstrate that the device is needed by the client. Examples of diagnoses that demonstrate the device is needed by the client include the following.

▶ *Pain* R/T lack of support of injured body tissues. The diagnosis of *pain* might be used, for example, to show that the trauma victim at an accident site needs a safe means of immobilization in order to be transferred to a hospital. This diagnosis might also be used to show the need for a joint immobilizer for a client who is experiencing pain on the slightest movement of an injured joint. This diagnosis could also be used for a client with a recent fracture who experiences painful movement of fractured bone fragments when a cast has not yet been applied. These are but a few examples.

▶ *High Risk for Violence: Self-directed or Directed at Others* R/T toxic reactions to medication. There are many other related factors for *High Risk for Violence: Self-directed or Directed at Others,* but whatever the related factor, the diagnosis is often used to demonstrate the need for restraint use (see the Nursing Diagnosis Profile).

▶ *High Risk for Self-mutilation* R/T self-hatred. Again, there are many other related factors for *High Risk for Self-mutilation,* and this diagnosis is often used to demonstrate the need for restraint use.

Other common nursing diagnoses associated with the use of protective and supportive devices are used after

---

Box 37–2. *Alternative to Restraints*

Comfort Measures

▶ Assess for pain or other sources of discomfort
▶ Position the client with pillows or supportive devices to ensure comfort

Changes in the Form of Treatment

▶ Removing a catheter or discontinuing an intravenous line or feeding tube may be alternatives
▶ Hypodermoclysis is a method of providing fluids in the posterior thoracic subcutaneous tissue that is less accessible to the client

Psychosocial Interventions

▶ Reality orientation
▶ Remotivation therapy
▶ Behavior modification
▶ Therapeutic touch
▶ Active listening
▶ Allowance for and attention to expression of feelings or concerns
▶ Companionship and supervision

Social Interventions

▶ Activities
▶ Distraction
▶ Social-recreational-physical activity
▶ Training in activities of daily living

Environmental Manipulation

▶ Circular room arrangement around nurses' station
▶ Low beds and no wheels on chairs or beds
▶ Increased lighting
▶ Color-orienting cues
▶ Available quiet room
▶ Commode at the bedside
▶ Mattress on the floor
▶ Accessible call light
▶ Side rails down

Transfer

▶ To home or other familiar surroundings

---

the device is actually applied. These diagnoses demonstrate the nurse's awareness that these devices must be used carefully and monitored closely in order to prevent iatrogenic disorders. Examples of such diagnoses include

▶ *High Risk for Disuse Syndrome* R/T use of immobilizing device
▶ *High Risk for Peripheral Neurovascular Dysfunction* R/T use of device on extremity

NURSING DIAGNOSIS PROFILE

High Risk for Violence: Self-directed or Directed at Others

Definition. A state in which an individual behaves in a manner that is violent enough to be physically harmful either to the self or others.

Classification. Feeling 9.2.2.

Defining Characteristics. The critical defining characteristics for this diagnosis include observations of violent acts that place the self or others in jeopardy (such as uncontrolled flailing, destruction of objects in the environment) or the observed potential to commit violent acts. Examples of observations that demonstrate the potential to commit violent acts include verbalizations of hostility (threats, boasting of prior abuses) and nonverbal behavior that indicates hostility, such as hostile, threatening displays of body language (including increased body tension, clenched fists, aggressive stance), or overtly aggressive and threatening behaviors (display of knife or gun).

Sample Related Factors. Sample related factors include the effects of

- the use of toxic medications
- the excessive use of certain drugs or alcohol
- mental and physical disorders, such as antisocial personality, manic excitement, organic brain disorders, depression, schizophrenia, and temporal lobe epilepsy
- temporary emotional states, such as rage or extreme fear

Other sample related factors include a history of suicide attempts or previous spouse abuse, child abuse, elder abuse, or other acts of violence to others.

Concept Description. This diagnosis refers to the state in which a person deliberately wishes to destroy the self or to do violence to others or the state in which he or she experiences a disturbance in the ability to maintain control of his or her actions, with the result being the threat of physical harm to the self or to others.

Examples. Depending on the specific assessment data, this diagnostic category could be applicable in the following situations, among others:

- a person who feels threatened because of the effects of paranoia, delusions, or hallucinations
- a person who is escalating in irritation or agitation
- a person who is going into or coming out of a deep depression
- a person who feels that life is no longer worth living
- a person who is experiencing intense physical or emotional suffering and who is so desperate to be relieved of this that death seems preferable
- a person who feels so frustrated in reaching goals that physically attacking the person who is seen as a barrier to reaching the goals seems to be the only option
- a person who feels a need to attack another in retaliation for a perceived or actual hostile act to the person
- a person who feels powerlessness and a lack of control over life and who reaches out to fight back at anyone or anything in the environment

Related/Similar Nursing Diagnoses. This diagnosis should be distinguished from the diagnosis of *High Risk for Self-mutilation*. With the diagnosis of *High Risk for Self-mutilation*, the individual is at high risk of performing an injurious act on the self to injure but not kill. The injurious act is meant to produce tissue damage, and this tissue damage is a method of relieving tension in certain persons, such as emotionally disturbed adolescents or certain retarded or autistic children.

PLANNING

The outcomes for clients who require protective and supportive devices must be individualized to the client and to the specific device being used. The following general outcomes are commonly expected:

- Demonstrates no evidence of disuse syndrome while device is in place.
- Remains free of injury while device is in place.
- Actively participates in rehabilitation program while device is in place.
- Provides self-care while device is in place.
- Decreases use of pain medications while device is in place.

The first two outcomes relate to many devices as well as to restraints; the following pertain only to restraints:

- Remains free of harm from violence to self while restraints are in place.
- Harms no others while restraints are in place.

- Remains free of self-mutilation while restraints are in place.

NURSING INTERVENTION

Binders

Binders are pieces of material applied to the body's larger areas (e.g., chest, abdomen). They may be used to immobilize, provide comfort and support, secure dressings, or exert pressure. Materials used for binders include heavy cotton, muslin, flannel, synthetics, and sometimes disposable paper.

GENERAL GUIDELINES FOR BINDER USE AND TEACHING

Key points are as follows.

- As you apply the binder (and after application), ask the person how the binder feels. Comfort and security are important.

▶ Apply binders exerting firm, even pressure.

▶ Apply binders in a manner that does not impair neurovascular or pulmonary function.

▶ Apply binders smoothly. Wrinkles are uncomfortable and may possibly cause tissue damage.

▶ Apply binders firmly and secure them so there is no movement and friction against underlying skin.

▶ Place pins or knots away from wound edges or tender areas or where they will be lain on.

▶ Apply binders with the body part in anatomic alignment and with joints in position of function.

▶ Replace soiled or moist binders. They may promote infection over skin surfaces that are not intact.

▶ Inspect skin surfaces underneath a binder frequently.

▶ Assess the neurovascular integrity of areas distal to the binder frequently.

▶ Remove and reapply binders causing discomfort.

▶ Frequent reapplication of binders is often necessary. Because binders are not attached to the skin, they slip out of place easily.

▶ Carry out a teaching and learning program for binder self-care when appropriate. (See specific points later.)

▶ A person discharged home with a binder requires an extra binder to allow for laundering.

▶ Include in documentation: skin condition; time binder was applied and removed; skin care (e.g., cleansing, back massage); and teaching/learning activities.

TYPES OF BINDERS

In the following sections, chest, breast, straight abdominal, scultetus, and T-binders are discussed.

Chest Binders. Chest binders may provide support to the chest wall after surgery or immobilize fractured ribs. Chest binders are large, rectangular pieces of heavy muslin or flannel or pre-sized, commercially made synthetics. Chest binders are pinned in place or secured with self-adhering strips of material. Some have shoulder straps to keep them in place. Rib belts (Fig. 37–1) are modifications of chest binders. They are used primarily with rib fractures.

Complications. Major concerns in using chest binders are (1) *further impairment of traumatized lung tissue*

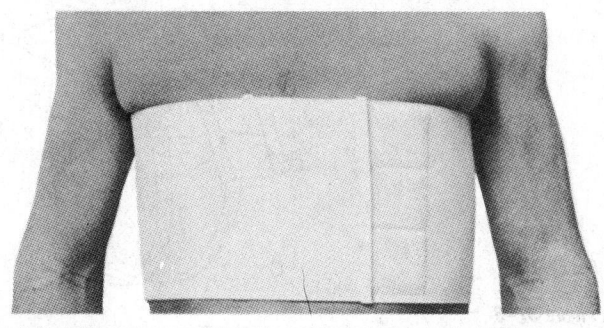

▲ *Figure 37–1*

Male rib belt, sometimes used after rib fractures. (Courtesy of DePuy, Warsaw, IN 46580.)

(respiratory insufficiency); (2) *increased pulmonary secretions* resulting from inadequate lung expansion and inadequate expectoration (coughing up) of secretions; and (3) development of *pulmonary infections* (e.g., pneumonia). These serious hazards may occur because the binder restricts chest expansion. When chest binders are prescribed for home use, it is essential that the person and significant others be taught how to watch for the preceding complications of chest binders, how to report these complications (give phone numbers), and binder removal and reapplication techniques.

Nursing Assessment. Frequently assess *chest wall excursion* by looking at the chest and by placing your hands gently on the chest to feel breathing movements. Place your hands around the chest's posterior portion at the level of the tenth rib and instruct the person to "take a deep breath."

Frequently assess *breath sounds* with and without a stethoscope to detect abnormal secretion formation. Listen for rales, rhonchi, wheezes, and rubs.

Elicit *tactile fremitus* to assess the presence of pulmonary consolidation. (Chapter 45 discusses respiratory assessment.)

Promptly report findings indicating the development of pulmonary infection and begin vigorous pulmonary hygiene measures (e.g., deep breathing, coughing, oral fluids, see Chapter 45). Remember, however, that these activities are often painful; thus, pain-reducing activities may enhance their effectiveness (see Chapter 40).

Breast Binders. Breast binders may be used to apply pressure to the breasts to decrease lactation after childbirth or to secure dressings. Breast binders look like sleeveless jackets, contoured to conform to the chest wall. However, they may need tucks pinned in them for the best fit. Apply a breast binder with the person supine to achieve maximum support. The nursing concerns and teaching requirements are the same as for chest binders.

Straight Abdominal Binders. Straight abdominal binders are used to provide support after back injury and occasionally after abdominal surgery or to secure dressings. A binder may be a large, rectangular piece of heavy cotton, muslin, or flannel pinned up the center to fit the person, or it may be a synthetic binder with adhering strips or hooks and eyes. Commercially made binders come in various sizes and may have metal stays to keep the binder in place and wrinkle free. Apply an abdominal binder with the person lying supine on the binder's center. Have the binder's lower portion extend well over the hips, but not so that it interferes with elimination or ambulation. Make sure the binder does not exert undue pressure on wound edges or interfere with respiration.

When an abdominal binder is used for postoperative support, estimate how long it may be required. Incorporate this estimate into the nursing care plan. People easily become dependent on binders and need encouragement to improve muscle tone so binders will not be needed. For individuals too large for standard binder sizes, improvise an abdominal binder from a Mayo stand cover (from the operating room or the laundry).

Scultetus ("Many-Tailed") Binders. A scultetus (many-tailed) binder is a rectangular piece of strong cloth that has many "tails" (strips of cloth) attached to its two longer sides (Fig. 37–2). It may be used as an abdominal binder to

▶ support abdominal musculature
▶ prevent wound dehiscence (opening of wound edges) and evisceration (protrusion of abdominal contents through the wound edges) after abdominal surgery
▶ secure dressings

Application. Apply a scultetus binder, with the person lying supine on the binder's center, with the tails equally extended to either side and the binder's top under the upper abdomen. Lightly powder the skin to reduce friction from the binder against the skin. (Keep powder away from the wound.) Then, starting at the binder's bottom, bring each "tail" across the abdomen, smoothing and gently pulling it taut. Overlap each succeeding tail at a slight upward angle, crossing at the midline (see Fig. 37–2B). Anchor each tail's end with your hand until securing it with the opposite tail. If tails

are too long, neatly fold them. Overlap the two top tails along a straight line and pin in place. When the binder is properly applied, there is an even pattern along the midline and a snug fit (i.e., comfortable, secure, but not tight).

Caution Chest and abdominal binders are dangerous if applied too tightly. Careful application and frequent assessment are essential.

Complications and Nursing Assessment. Potential complications and nursing assessment of chest binders have been previously discussed. Tight abdominal binders may also inhibit respiratory function. In addition, they may compress the vena cava, causing hypotension if applied with excessive pressure. Assessment of blood pressure after application of a scultetus binder is thus important. If respiratory difficulty or hypotension develops, promptly remove a binder, reapply it less tightly, and carry out follow-up evaluation.

T-Binders. T-binders (Fig. 37–3) are used primarily to secure rectal or perineal dressings. A double T-binder is used for males and the single for females. A double or single T strap is brought between the legs and pinned to the waistband in front. People usually prefer to apply T-binders themselves. It is important to explain the method of application. Most T-binders are made of washable material. Paper T-binders are available for short-term use; however, they fall apart easily. If ready-made T-binders are not available, improvise by using a sanitary belt and perineal pad or by using strips of wide roller gauze or woven gauze bandage (Kling) and pinning the pieces together to form a T. T-binders are easily soiled and need frequent changing.

SLINGS AND ARM IMMOBILIZERS

Slings are a form of arm immobilizer used to provide support and to immobilize and elevate the hand, arm, or shoulder. They are available as triangular bandages, pinned and tied according to size (Fig. 37–4), or as

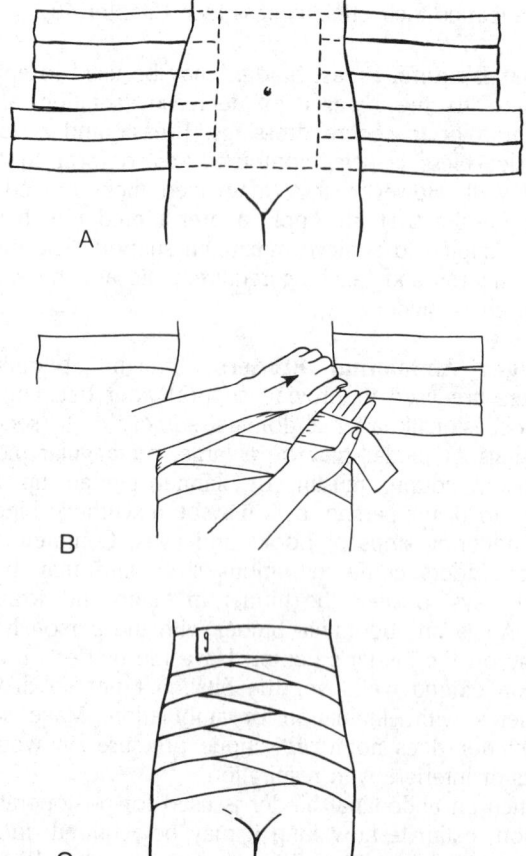

▲ *Figure 37–2*

Technique for applying a scultetus (many-tailed) binder.

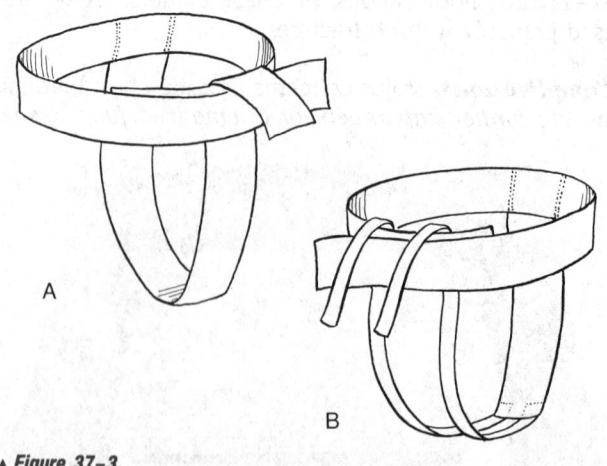

▲ *Figure 37–3*

T-binders used to secure perineal dressings. *A*, Single T-binder used for females. *B*, Double T-binder used for males. When lying flat and open, these binders form the general shape of a T.

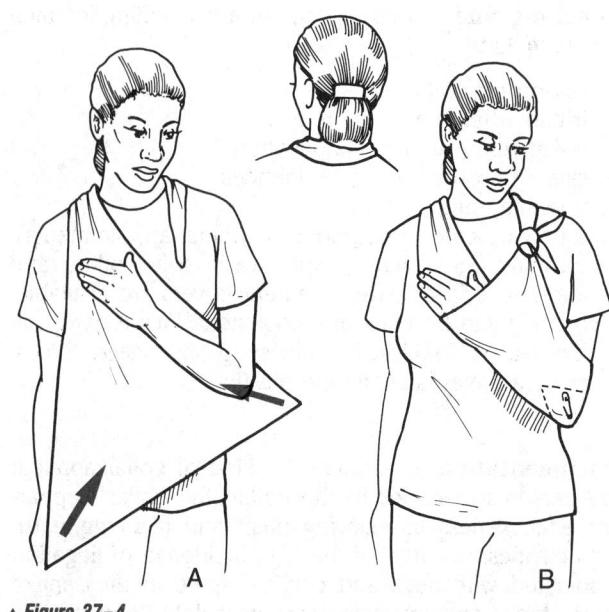

▲ Figure 37-4

Standard sling (triangular bandage). Note in *B* that the knot is placed to the front of the client and off the client's neck. This prevents pressure on the tissue overlying the cervical vertebrae.

pre-sized, contoured slings adjusted by buckles and straps. The highly versatile triangular bandage is used for various purposes, especially in first-aid situations.

Application. An arm sling is most easily applied with the person sitting with the injured arm flexed at the elbow. Place the point (apex) of the triangle at the elbow. Place one tail between the injured arm and the chest and bring it up on the shoulder on the uninjured side. Bring the other tail over the injured arm and chest and place it on the shoulder on the same side as the injury. Bring the anterior tail behind and around the neck and tie it to the other tail with a square knot at a comfortable place on the anterior chest wall, not at the neck. The movements to make a square knot are left-over-right and under, right-over-left and under. Positioning the knot away from the neck helps prevent pressure and discomfort. Fold the apex of the bandage around the elbow and pin or tuck it in place. The hand and forearm are usually positioned higher than the elbow (see Fig. 37-4).

A properly tied sling is the key to an individual's comfort. Fold a standard-size triangular bandage in half to fit a child. To apply a pre-sized sling, slide the arm into the sling, and adjust the straps to fit the sling to the person. Some pre-sized slings have an additional strap (which fits around the chest) to immobilize the shoulder (Fig. 37-5).

Complications. Complications associated with sling use may include neck discomfort and tissue damage due to incorrect knot placement; edema if the forearm and hand are dependent; wristdrop if the hand is not well supported by the sling; and immobility of the elbow and shoulder joints if the sling is worn longer than indicated.

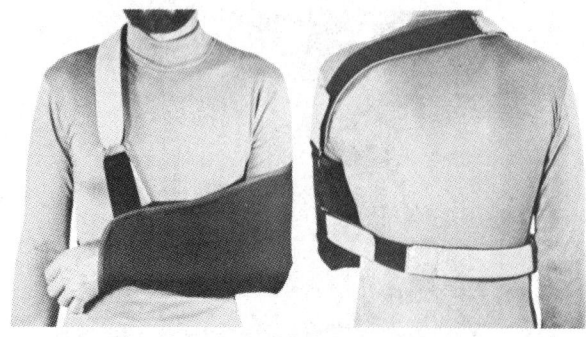

▲ Figure 37-5

Arm immobilizer. This commercially available arm immobilizer also provides support for the shoulder. (Courtesy of DePuy.)

Teaching and Learning. Important teaching/learning points include

▶ reasons for sling use
▶ when to wear the sling
▶ proper sling application and removal
▶ how to make a square knot (for easy sling removal)
▶ how long the sling is required
▶ complications associated with sling use

CERVICAL COLLARS

Cervical collars are supportive devices that are worn around the neck to immobilize a neck with suspected cervical spine fractures, relieve neck muscle spasm after trauma, and support the head if degenerative disease affects cervical vertebrae or if there has been surgery or trauma to the cervical area. Cervical collars may be soft or hard.

A soft collar (Fig. 37-6), made of foam or felt padding covered with stockinette, may be pinned in place or secured with self-adhering strips. It is for short-term or intermittent use and is relatively inexpensive.

A hard cervical collar (Fig. 37-7A), made of heavy plastic or metal, is used long term or to provide rigid support. This collar has snaps, ties, buckles, or adhering strips. A Philadelphia cervical collar (Fig. 37-7B) is a hard plastic cervical collar that rigidly supports the cervical spine. A four-poster cervical collar, often used

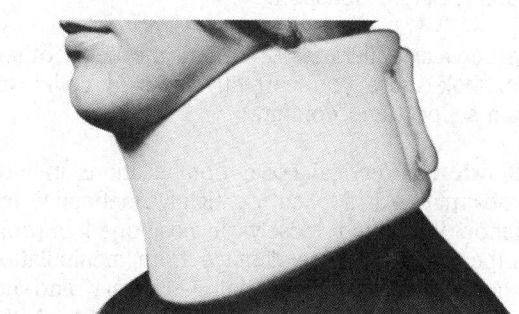

▲ Figure 37-6

Soft cervical collar. This collar provides support for the head and neck. (Courtesy of DePuy.)

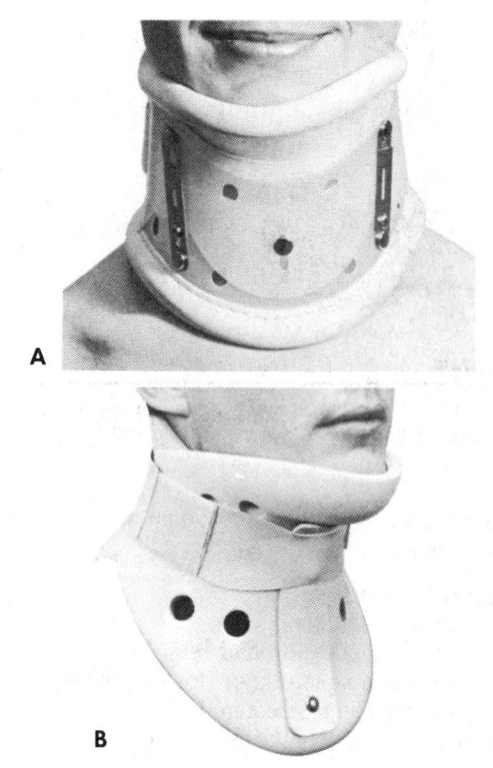

▲ *Figure 37-7*

Hard cervical collars. *A*, Standard hard collar. *B*, Philadelphia collar. (Courtesy of DePuy.)

after hospitalization for cervical spine fracture, has four steel rods in a hard collar. Cervical collars are often individually designed by a prosthetist (specialist in making and fitting prosthetic devices).

Application. Apply cervical collars with the head erect unless a cervical spine fracture is suspected. If a fracture is believed to be present, apply the collar with the neck positioned as it was found. Head traction is occasionally applied to facilitate collar application.

Caution Never move the head of a person with a suspected cervical spine fracture. Do *not* move the person until a cervical collar is applied and the person is on a spine or fracture board. Tape the person's head to the board before transport.

Some cervical collars fasten behind the neck, others in front. Make sure you correctly apply a collar for maximum support and comfort.

Complications. Cervical collar complications include airway obstruction if applied too tightly; ineffective immobilization if applied loosely or positioned improperly; further cervical spine damage from manipulation during collar placement; and pain, ischemia, and necrosis of tissues of the jaw and inner third of the clavicle. This last problem is seen more with hard collars and may be prevented by padding bony prominences.

Teaching and Learning. Important teaching/learning points include

▶ reason for collar use
▶ if and when it is to be removed
▶ collar removal and reapplication
▶ skin care over bony prominences
▶ possible complications
▶ follow-up care (e.g., phone numbers, appointments)
▶ cleaning the collar. Hand wash soft collars and allow to drip dry. Replacement covers are available, or they can be cut from stockinette. Wipe hard collars with a solution of mild soap and water. Excessive heat may damage the plastic.

Documentation. Document the kind of collar applied; the person's reactions to the collar; the collar's apparent effectiveness in relieving pain; and teaching/learning activities. Because of the high incidence of litigation associated with neck and cervical spine injuries, make your documentation accurate, complete, and legible and emphasize teaching/learning activities. Provide written and verbal instructions for people discharged home with cervical collars.

Bandages

BANDAGING MATERIALS

A bandage is a length of material applied to fit smaller parts of the body. Bandages are available in various materials, lengths, and widths. They are soft and conform to body areas. Most bandages are used to provide pressure and hold dressings in place.

Materials used for bandages include straight weave and knit weave cotton gauze (Kling, Kerlix), flannel, muslin, elasticized knit, rubberized self-adhering material (Elastoplast, Coban), elastic net webbing (Surgifix, Surgiflex), ribbed tubular cotton (stockinette), and knit tubular cotton (Tube-gauz).

Gauze is commonly used. It is absorbent yet porous, allowing air to circulate. Gauze frays when laundered, so it is usually not recycled. Flannel is sturdier, withstands repeated washings, and keeps the part warm. Muslin and flannel are less flexible than gauze. They are used to immobilize or create pressure.

Elasticized net bandages come in various sizes and shapes. Some are tubular, others are shaped like a shirt or pants. Some of these bandages are designed to keep dressings in place. Others are more constricting and apply pressure. (Bandages used to hold dressings in place are discussed with dressings in Chapter 48.)

Caution Frequently assess areas distal to bandages (see Box 37-1). Bandages may become too tight (from edema) and must be loosened or removed and replaced to prevent tissue death or gangrene. Bandages that are too tight are uncomfortable, are dangerous, and may cause permanent damage.

BANDAGE APPLICATION

Key points in bandage application are as follows:

▶ Apply bandage from most distal part toward trunk.
▶ Leave exposed, if possible, areas distal to the bandaged part (e.g., fingers, toes). Frequently assess these parts (see Box 37–1) for evidence of neurovascular impairment. Emphasize the importance of this assessment during teaching and the importance of promptly reporting abnormal findings and possibly removing the bandage.
▶ Make bandages bulky enough to be absorptive and supportive, yet not so large that they interfere with desired function.
▶ Apply bandages more loosely over wet dressings or draining wounds. The bandages may shrink during drying, causing ischemia (deficient circulation) if they are applied too tightly.
▶ Apply bandages evenly and firmly, exerting equal pressure with each turn. Avoid uneven, unnecessary overlapping.
▶ Pad bony prominences and hollows to ensure equal pressure.
▶ Apply bandage, when possible, with the body part held level to or elevated above the trunk, rather than dependent. This minimizes venous congestion and edema.
▶ Keep bandages neat, clean, durable, and functional. For esthetic and aseptic reasons, remove and reapply bandages if they do not meet these criteria.

Familiarize yourself with the use and limitations of various bandages. You can then creatively and effectively apply bandages.

ROLLER BANDAGES

Description. A roller bandage is a long strip of material (e.g., cotton gauze, elastic rubberized adhesive) wound on itself to form a roll. The roll itself is called the body of the bandage. The outside end of the bandage is the initial end, and the terminal end lies at the center inside the roll.

Application. To apply a bandage, hold the initial end in place with one hand, and pass the body of the bandage over and around the extremity being bandaged. Anchor the bandage by making two circular turns. To continue application, pass the roll from one hand to the other.

Make turns while applying equal pressure and tension. To do so, gradually unroll only small amounts of bandage. Uneven or unnecessary overlapping of turns is undesirable. Prevent this by selecting a more appropriate kind or size of bandage. When bandaging material is to be reused, rewind it as you remove it. If the bandage is to be discarded, cut along the length of the bandaged part with scissors, well away from the wound or tender areas. Then remove the bandage.

The type of turn used during bandaging depends on the body part to be bandaged and the bandage material. Turns used to apply roller bandages include the circular turn, the spiral turn, the spiral reverse turn, the figure-of-eight turn, the spica turn, and the recurrent turn.

▶ A circular turn is the simplest, most commonly used turn. It is used to bandage circumferential (circular) body parts, such as the arm. It is used when the bandage is to completely overlap the previous bandage. The initial and terminal ends are in the same location. It is used when bandaging a small part. It is also used to anchor a bandage when it is started (Fig. 37–8) and ended, such as when starting and ending a figure-of-eight (see later) or spiral bandage.
▶ A spiral turn overlaps the previous turn only partially (e.g., from half to three fourths the bandage's width). It is used most commonly to bandage cylindrical parts (Fig. 37–9).
▶ A spiral reverse turn reverses the bandage halfway through each turn. It is used to bandage circumferential areas that increase in size (e.g., forearm, leg). This turn is needed to apply inflexible bandages (e.g., roller gauze). Because more adaptable bandages are now commonly available, this turn is rarely used in health care settings (Fig. 37–10).
▶ A figure-of-eight turn overlaps turns on the oblique in an alternately ascending and descending fashion. Each turn crosses over the previous turn, forming a figure-of-eight (Fig. 37–11). It forms a herringbone appearance and is used to bandage and immobilize joints (e.g., knee, ankle, elbow).
▶ A spica turn is a variation of a figure-of-eight turn. All turns overlap at a sharp angle and alternately ascend and descend. It is used to bandage hip, thigh, groin, and thumb.
▶ A recurrent turn is used to bandage rounded areas, such as a stump after amputation, a head, or sometimes fingers (Fig. 37–12). First anchor the bandage with a few circular turns. Then place the bandage in the center of the part to be bandaged. Make a half turn and hold the material with a finger. Pass the body of the bandage back and forth over the tip of the stump or finger or the top of the head, from the superior to the inferior surfaces and back again. Hold each fold with a finger to keep it in place. Overlap the bandage from side to side until all parts are covered. Terminate with several circular turns over the folded bandage. Tape or pin the bandage in place. If the bandaged area is large, reinforce the

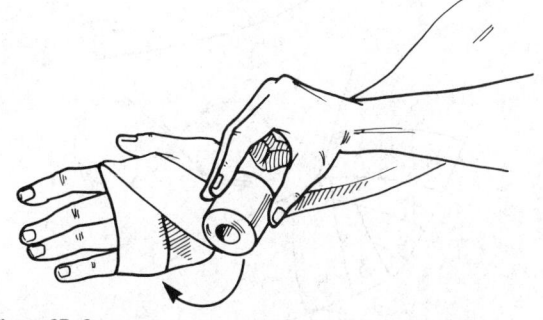

▲ *Figure 37–8*

The circular turn. This turn can be used by itself to bandage a small area, or it may be used one or two times to anchor the bandage before beginning and after ending another bandaging technique.

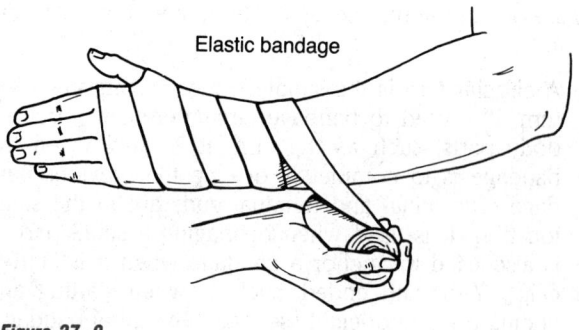

▲ **Figure 37-9**

The spiral turn.

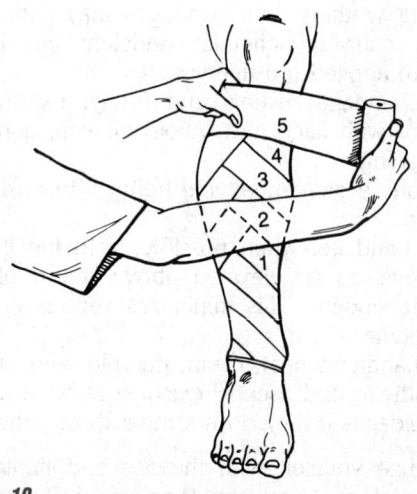

▲ **Figure 37-10**

The spiral reverse turn. One or two circular turns anchor the bandage. The bandage progresses with several spiral turns before beginning the spiral reverse turn that forms a herringbone pattern.

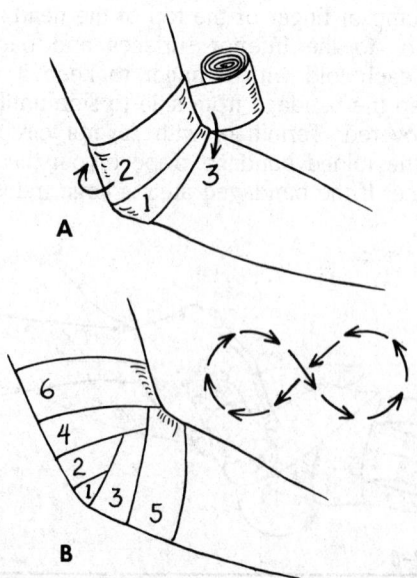

▲ **Figure 37-11**

The figure-of-eight turn is used for bandaging joints.

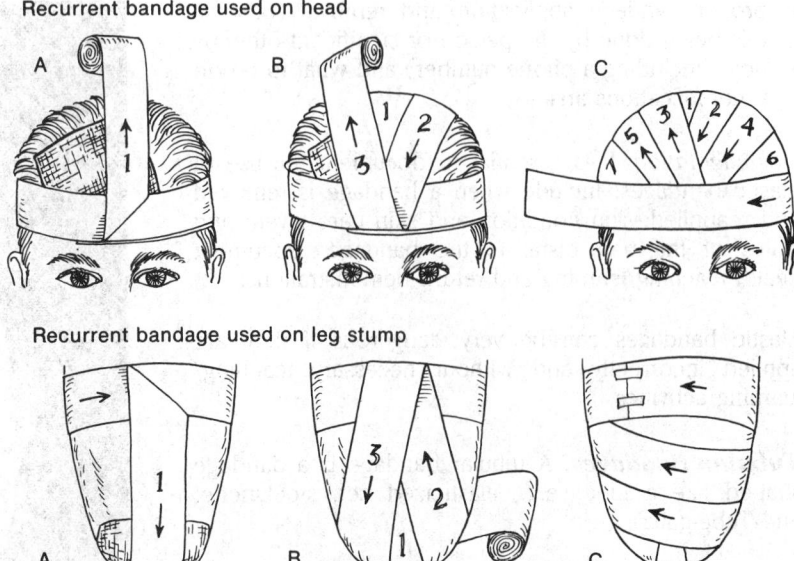

Recurrent bandage used on head

Recurrent bandage used on leg stump

▲ *Figure 37–12*

The recurrent turn is a combination of figure-of-eight and spiral reverse turns. Wrapping the amputated limb with even pressure helps shrink the swelling and shape the stump in preparation for a prosthesis.

turns with adhesive tape strips applied on the oblique (slanting).

Types of Roller Bandages. Roller bandages come in various lengths and widths. They are made of cotton gauze or rubberized or elasticized materials.

Cotton Gauze Bandages. Two major types of cotton gauze bandages are roller gauze and Kling and Kerlix.

Roller gauze is loose mesh material available in several widths. It does not conform well. When bandaging a large area with roller gauze, one must use the spiral reverse turn discussed earlier. Roller gauze is often used to secure dressings temporarily.

Kling and Kerlix are loose weave or knitted roller gauze bandages that are soft and conform easily. They are used to secure dressings, are highly absorptive, and are appropriate for bulky dressings. Apply Kling and Kerlix in a manner similar to other roller bandages. The spiral reverse turn is not needed.

Elasticized or Rubberized Adhesive. These bandages (e.g., Elastoplast and Coban) are conforming, self-clinging roller bandages used to apply firm, even pressure. They are commonly applied as an outer dressing wrap over wounds to prevent swelling (edema) or promote hemostasis (stop bleeding). When applying these adhesives as pressure dressings, relax the tension on the ends of the bandage to prevent them from curling.

The individual and significant others must understand the hazards of an adhesive roller bandage and be reliable enough to assess areas distal to the bandage for signs of impaired circulation.

Caution Elasticized or rubberized adhesive bandages applied too tightly can shut off the blood supply (cause arterial occlusion). This may result in gangrene. Radical surgery (e.g., amputation) may be needed.

Tincture of benzoin or other skin adherents are often applied to the skin to make elasticized or rubberized adhesive bandages more adherent. Individuals with allergies to perfumes may also be allergic to benzoin. It is thus important to assess allergies and do a benzoin skin test if indicated. Also, do not apply these bandages to people allergic to rubber.

Elastic (Ace) Bandages. Elastic (Ace) bandages are roller bandages made of elasticized cotton or other heavy material. They are used to support injured joints or extremities, to apply gentle pressure to minimize swelling, and to enhance venous blood return to the heart.

Application. Apply an elastic bandage in a distal to proximal direction (e.g., from the foot up the leg). Proceed toward the trunk, thus following the direction of the venous circulation. This minimizes venous congestion, stasis, and edema of the distal part. Hold the body of the bandage close to the part being bandaged. This ensures even tension and pressure.

Elastic bandages often become loose and wrinkled and need frequent reapplication. Even if they are intact and wrinkle free, remove the elastic bandages at least daily and clean and dry the underlying skin surfaces to assess them for pressure areas or lesions.

Caution Elastic bandages applied too tightly or that become too tight after "normal application" may cause neurovascular damage. Frequent assessment is essential! (See Box 37–1.)

Teaching and Learning. Key teaching/learning points include the following:

▶ complications from a tight bandage
▶ assessing neurovascular integrity in the distal part

▶ proper bandage application and removal (observe this being done by the person or significant others)

▶ how (including a phone number) and what to report if complications arise

Documentation. It is essential to document the use of elastic bandages. Include when a bandage is removed and reapplied; skin condition and skin care given; and status of the part distal to the bandage. Document health teaching/learning and return demonstrations.

Elastic bandages can be very dangerous if they are applied incorrectly and without necessary teaching/learning activities.

Tubular Bandages. A tubular bandage is a bandage shaped like a tube (e.g., elasticized net, stockinette, and Tube-gauz).

Elasticized Net. This highly adaptable net is used for a variety of purposes. There are two kinds of net with quite different uses.

One net is used to exert firm, constant pressure to decrease edema and prevent scarring and contractures. It is constrictive and is commonly used with burns or after mastectomy (breast removal) for individuals prone to the development of lymphedema (edema due to interference with lymph drainage).

The second kind of elasticized net, Surgifix or Surgiflex, is much more elastic and exerts no pressure. Holes may be cut in the net without altering its effectiveness. This net is useful in securing dressings over areas difficult to bandage, such as the head, the axilla (armpit), and joints. This kind of elasticized net is available not only in tubular form but also as pre-sized shirts and pants (Fig. 37–13). The pants are especially useful for securing perineal and buttock dressings.

Elasticized net makes frequent dressing changes easier and helps people who have lost skin from repeated adhesive removal. Elasticized net may also be used to secure intravenous catheters and tubing, armboards, splints, and ostomy bags. It is flexible, is easy to apply, and promotes healing by allowing the part to be kept dry and exposed to air. Elasticized net is economical for long-term use. It withstands repeated washings and holds its shape well. (Wash in warm, soapy water, rinse well, and drip dry.)

To determine the length of bandage needed, measure the length of the area to be bandaged and allow for any desired overlap. Then cut the same length of unstretched bandage. Place your hands inside the bandage and stretch it while applying it over the part.

Stockinette and Tube-gauz. Stockinette and Tube-gauz are stretchable cotton tubular bandages designed to cover cylindric body parts.

Stockinette may also be bias cut and used as a roller bandage. Stockinette comes in various sizes and widths. It is often used under casts to protect the skin. It may also be used as a head cap.

Tube-gauz is mainly used to secure dressings. The desired length is cut from a roll and pushed onto a

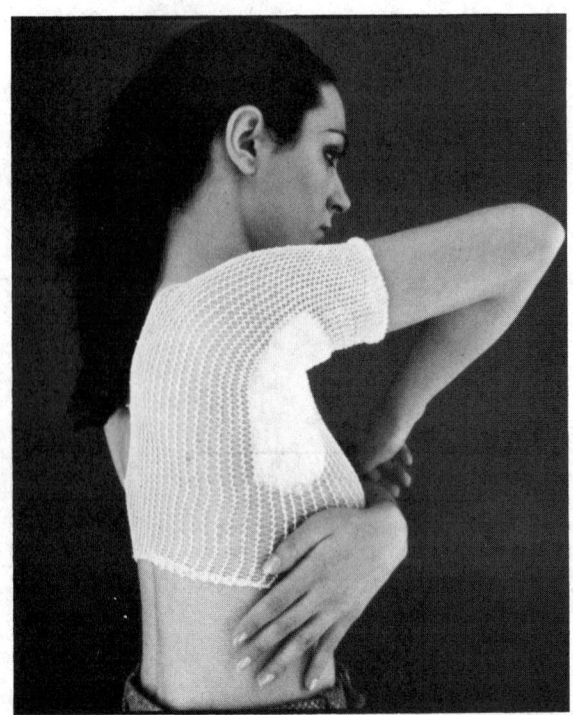

▲ *Figure 37–13*

Flexible net bandage (elasticized net) is used to secure bandages in difficult areas, such as the axilla and around joints. (Courtesy of FRA Surgifix, Inc., Elmsford, NY.)

special applicator. The gauze-covered applicator is placed over the area to be bandaged. Then some of the material is slid off the applicator onto the part and held taut. As the applicator is gradually removed, the entire length of the part is bandaged. The bandage and applicator are extended beyond the tip of the bandaged part, and the applicator is rotated 180 degrees. The applicator is again placed over the part, and the procedure is repeated until the desired thickness of bandage is achieved. The tubular gauze may then be extended several inches beyond the bandage and cut along the sides; the tails are secured around the joint. This keeps the bandage from slipping off. Tie the ends in a bow, rather than a knot, so the bandage can be quickly removed if signs of impaired blood supply develop.

Jones Dressing. A Jones dressing is a compression bandage used to immobilize and support the leg after musculoskeletal trauma. Although it is called a dressing, a Jones dressing is actually a splinted bandage. It is effective in decreasing or preventing edema and is used in place of a cast for fractures or severe sprains. A Jones dressing is left on for several days and is often replaced with a cast after swelling decreases. The dressing consists of

▶ cotton batting wrapped around the leg, from toes to knee

▶ a posterior plaster splint behind the leg

▶ bias cut stockinette or an elastic bandage wrapped around the leg, from toes to knee

Because weight-bearing is not permitted, a walking heel is not placed in the dressing. Crutches must be used when walking with the Jones dressing in place. To minimize swelling when the client is reclining, elevate the injured part at least 30.5 cm (12 in) above the heart.

During teaching, emphasize that

▶ weight-bearing is not permitted
▶ the dressing is temporary
▶ the individual must return for removal, further assessment, and possible casting
▶ elevation and application of ice are important for the first 24 hours
▶ it is essential to frequently assess neurovascular integrity (see Box 37–1) in the distal part of the injury and promptly report abnormalities. (Teach appropriate assessment measures.)

Unna's Boot. An Unna's boot is a medication-impregnated, cotton gauze, pressure bandage that contains zinc oxide and gelatin. Some brands also contain calamine lotion. It is commonly used to protect and support the lower leg and ankle in the presence of skin loss due to stasis ulcers or stasis dermatitis and for sprains or strains. Unna's boot provides medication while preventing edema and permitting ambulation (after the boot has hardened). It is packaged as a moist bandage that becomes hard and stiff when dry.

Before applying Unna's boot, clean and dry the foot and lower leg. Place the foot at a right angle to the leg. Secure the bandage with a circular turn around the foot and direct it obliquely over the heel. Then cut the bandage and smooth the edges. Repeat until the heel is covered. Apply the bandage so it is snug but not too tight. Apply more pressure distally and less as you go up the leg. If the bandage does not conform, cut it to keep it flat. Do not reverse it because this would cause ridges to form where the reverse turns are made. When the bandage hardens, these ridges cause discomfort and pressure. Overlap each turn half over the preceding one. Cover the leg three times. Finish the bandage below the knee. Cover the boot with tube gauze or a 15-cm (6-in) elastic bandage.

When the boot has hardened (about 30 minutes after application), assess capillary refill in the toes' nailbeds to make sure the boot is not too tight. If desired, apply a layer of stockinette over the dry Unna's boot to protect the person's clothing. The boot is usually removed after five to seven days and its effectiveness evaluated. Another Unna's boot may then be applied. Teaching/learning includes how to keep the bandage dry and intact, how to assess neurovascular status of the part distal to the bandage, and the importance of returning for follow-up care. The boot should be removed if the person experiences numbness, pain, sensitivity, or other adverse reactions.

Antiembolism Hosiery

Antiembolism hose are elasticized, graduated compression stockings. These devices prevent thrombophlebitis in the high-risk individual by promoting venous blood return to the right ventricle. Well-fitting stockings provide compression on the superficial and deep veins in the legs to prevent pooling of venous blood. Ambulatory pregnant women and people with varicose veins may have antiembolism hosiery recommended by the physician. For persons confined to bed rest, antiembolism hose help prevent thrombophlebitis. The stockings are available in different sizes and lengths (e.g., toes-to-knee, toes-to-midthigh, and toes-to-groin).

APPLICATION

Apply the stocking by inverting the upper part of the material back over the lower part, stretching the doubled stocking, while applying it over the foot, ankle, and lower leg and pulling the inverted part up the upper leg (Box 37–3). It is often helpful to pull it up using the palmar surface of the fingers and hands, avoiding use of fingernails, which can tear the material. Usually it is a nursing responsibility to remove and reapply elastic stockings at least twice daily to assess the condition of the skin and cleanse the legs. However, some vascular and orthopedic surgeons may prefer that hosiery not be removed for several days after the person has had lower limb surgery.

TEACHING AND LEARNING

If the person is to be discharged using antiembolism stockings, skin assessment and methods of stocking application should be taught. Because harsh detergents and hot water weaken the elastic fibers, the stockings should be washed with gentle soap, rinsed well, and dripped dry. Heat drying is not recommended. For long-term use, an additional pair of stockings is desirable. Documentation includes stocking application and removal, skin assessment and care, and teaching/learning activities.

Sequential Compression Devices

Sequential compression devices are pneumatically controlled, pressurized sleeves applied to the lower extremities to promote venous return and prevent deep vein thrombosis and resultant pulmonary embolism. Pulmonary embolism is a potentially life-threatening complication associated with immobility, vessel injury, and surgical trauma. Sequential compression devices serve the same purpose as, and are used in conjunction with, graduated elasticized compression hose.

Various styles of sequential compression devices are available; however, the basic design remains the same. Figure 37–14 provides an example of one type. Inflatable boots or sleeves, extending to or above the knee, are intermittently inflated and deflated. Compression can be applied uniformly to all parts of the extremity and then released. Compressions may also be applied in a series of intermittent wavelike compressions that facilitate distal to proximal venous return. The amount and sequence of compression is pre-set by the manufacturer but may be adjusted for individual needs. The

Box 37–3. Method of Applying Antiembolism Hosiery

1. Note the style. Hose may be knee length, midthigh length, or groin length with opening over ball of foot or over tops of toes.

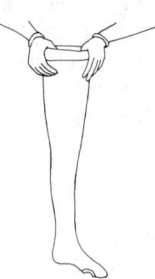

2. Invert the upper half of the stocking down so stocking is doubled and covers almost all of the foot. Leave enough of the foot visible to be able to identify toe and heel.

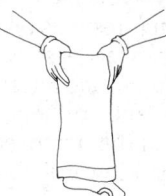

3. Gather the doubled stocking down to approximately the level of the ankle.

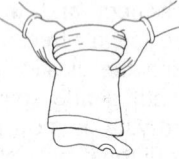

4. Work gathered stocking over the client's ankle.

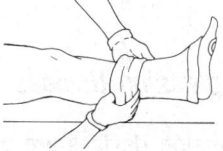

5. Pull the doubled stocking up firmly, smoothing all wrinkles in the process.

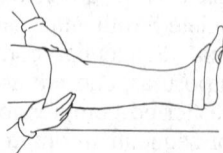

6. Pull the remaining stocking up to its full length, smoothing all remaining wrinkles from the stocking.

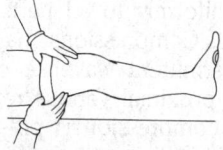

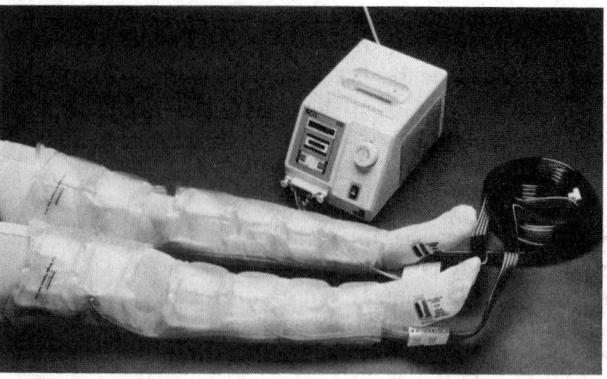

▲ **Figure 37–14**

Sequential compression system. (Courtesy of Kendall Healthcare Products Company.)

external compression simulates "normal" muscle pumping activities and, when combined with other prophylactic modalities, is highly effective in preventing deep vein thrombosis and pulmonary emboli.

GENERAL GUIDELINES

Sequential compression is indicated when the individual has experienced a lengthy surgical procedure, is or will be on prolonged bed rest, has profound venous stasis, and has a history of deep vein thrombosis. These devices are contraindicated in clients with recent (within the last six months) or acute deep vein thrombosis, severe arteriosclerosis, massive edema of the legs, pulmonary edema, or such localized skin conditions as dermatitis and gangrene that might be exacerbated by use of the sleeves.

As you assess the person, identify potential risk factors for thrombophlebitis and take action to prevent its development. Refer to Chapter 35 for risk factors of deep vein thrombosis and general measures to reduce risk.

If sequential compression devices are ordered, the specific manufacturer's instructions should be followed. General guidelines are as follows.

▶ Ensure a proper fit of the compression hose. Choose the correct size (small, medium, or large). Choose thigh, knee, or full length as appropriate to the physician's prescription.

▶ Set the machine to the correct amount and time of compression.

▶ Apply hose properly. Fit should be snug, but not tight.

▶ Assess for proper functioning of the machine. Note any alarms.

▶ Usually apply compression sleeves before surgical procedures, and continue to use them postoperatively.

▶ Use in conjunction with antiembolism hose. Avoid direct contact of the device's material with the skin; the plastic may produce an allergic reaction in some individuals.

▶ Remove the sleeves every eight hours to assess the condition of the skin. Assess for Homans' sign as an

early indicator of deep vein thrombosis.
▶ Remove only temporarily for ambulating and bathing; reapply as soon as possible.

COMPLICATIONS

You should be alert to potential complications associated with use of the sequential compression device. You must assess for pain, swelling, tenderness, and a positive Homans' sign in the lower extremities. If any symptoms of deep vein thrombosis or pulmonary emboli develop, it is essential that use of the sleeves be discontinued until these complications are ruled out.

The sleeves are constructed of a heavy vinyl material and may cause excessive heat production. The device generally has a built-in cooling element; however, you should assess the skin periodically for moisture, redness, or other evidence of tissue injury. In addition, an improperly applied sequential compression device could interfere with circulation to the extremities, cause pain, and lead to skin breakdown.

TEACHING AND LEARNING

At first glance, the sequential compression device may appear formidable and restrictive. You should explain to the individual how and why compression is being used. Describe any potential symptoms that should be reported, such as pain, tenderness, altered sensation, or excessive heat. Some persons are fearful of moving while the sleeves are in use; explain that movement is encouraged (unless it is contraindicated).

DOCUMENTATION

Key points to incorporate in documentation should include

▶ time and date of application
▶ type of sleeve used (knee or thigh length; one or both legs)
▶ concurrent use of antiembolism hose
▶ individual response to device: assessment of pain, swelling, skin condition
▶ time, date, and length of time off
▶ date and time discontinued

Casts

A cast is a temporary immobilizing and protective device made of layers of plaster or fiberglass material. Casts may be constructed to immobilize almost any body part from a forearm to an entire body. They may be of one material or may incorporate pins or braces to meet individual needs. Casts are commonly used to

▶ immobilize, support, and protect a body part during the bone healing process that follows fracture
▶ correct and prevent joint deformities
▶ apply uniform compression to soft tissue after such procedures as amputation
▶ restrict movement and support and protect a body part to facilitate healing and prevent injury in such

conditions as osteomyelitis (inflammation of the bone and bone marrow)
▶ promote early mobilization by providing support and protection to the affected body part

TYPES OF CASTS

Casts are generally made from plaster of Paris (anhydrous calcium sulfate) or from a synthetic material. The dry plaster of Paris is supplied in impregnated strips of gauze that are rolled up to form bandages of various widths. The rolls are submerged in water to activate the plaster of Paris. The wet bandage is malleable, and the material can be easily molded by the physician or technician into the desired shape by applying it as in bandaging. Additional longitudinal strips of wet plaster are added to areas, such as joints, where more reinforcement is required. Depending on the type and location of the cast, the plaster may take 24 to 72 hours to dry completely. Improper handling of the drying cast may lead to indentations that damage underlying tissue.

Synthetic casts are made from a high-density thermoplastic resin or fiberglass. These materials are strong, are lightweight, and will dry completely in about 20 minutes. Water is required to activate the fiberglass polyurethane material to allow shaping to the body part. Heat is initially generated, but the cast cools rapidly as drying occurs. Unlike the plaster casts, synthetic casts maintain their firmness even when wet. Synthetic casts are more expensive than plaster casts and more difficult to mold.

The most common types of casts are described in Table 37–1. Many adaptations may be designed from these basic casts to fulfill individual needs.

GENERAL GUIDELINES

Before cast application, you must assess the skin and neurovascular integrity of the involved body part. The affected extremity should be compared with the unaffected extremity whenever possible. You should evaluate the person's general peripheral vascular status and specifically determine the neurovascular status of the involved extremity, including temperature, capillary filling, pulses, and sensory and motor alterations.

You must also assess for the potential effects that casting, with its imposed immobilization, will have on a person's ability to carry out daily activities. For example, will the person be able to navigate the stairs at home or drive a car to work?

Casts may be applied at the hospital bedside, in the emergency department, in a specially equipped cast room, or in a physician's office or clinic. The procedure should be explained to the individual before beginning. The skin should be thoroughly cleaned before casting and any foreign material removed. You should identify and document any existing lesions.

After cleaning, the skin is usually covered with stockinette followed by a padding that is applied like roller bandage over the stockinette. Padding helps avoid injury to underlying tissue. Additional protection is provided to bony prominences, such as the styloid process of the wrist and the fibular head. These padding mate-

TABLE 37–1. Types of Casts

Cast	Location	Uses	
Upper Extremity Casts			
Short arm cast	Proximal palmar crease to below elbow	To treat stable fractures of the hand or wrist To correct and maintain correction of hand or wrist deformities To ensure correct postoperative positioning or immobilization of the hand or wrist	
Long arm cast	Hand to upper arm	To treat fractures of the forearm and elbow To correct and maintain the correction of the distal arm, wrist, and elbow To ensure correct postoperative positioning of the distal arm, elbow, or humerus	
Hanging cast	Palmar crease to distal part of upper arm	To provide traction to maintain alignment of a fracture of the humerus above the cast. Used when the client is ambulatory. Cannot be used for clients on bed rest or children under 12 years of age.	
Lower Extremity Casts			
Short leg cast	Toes to below knee	To treat fractures of the foot, ankle, and distal leg To ensure correct postoperative positioning and immobilization of the foot and ankle To treat severe sprains and torn soft tissues of the ankle To correct or maintain correction of deformities of the foot and ankle	
Long leg cast	Toes to upper thigh	To maintain reduction of fractures of the lower leg, knee, and distal femur To treat dislocation of the knee To treat torn soft tissue around the knee To ensure postoperative positioning and immobilization of the knee, distal leg, and ankle To correct or maintain correction of deformities of the distal leg and knee	
Spinal and Cervical Casts			
Body jacket	Over trunk; does not extend over the cervical area	To treat spinal injuries To correct scoliosis To ensure correct postoperative positioning and immobilization after spinal surgery	

TABLE 37–1. *Types of Casts* Continued

Cast	Location	Uses	
Minerva cast	Upper trunk; incorporates the head (with the facial area and the area over the ears cut out)	To treat cervical injuries and neck deformities	
Spica Casts			
Shoulder spica	Over the trunk, usually to the hips; incorporates the involved shoulder and the involved arm to the wrist or hand	To treat unstable fractures of the shoulder and humerus To treat shoulder dislocation To ensure correct postoperative positioning and immobilization for shoulder injury	
Gauntlet or thumb spica	From the proximal palmar crease, including the thumb, to just below the elbow	To treat fractures of the thumb, metacarpals, and carpals	
Hip spica: short leg, unilateral long leg, one-and-a-half leg	From the waist to the involved body part	To treat congenital hip dislocation (short leg cast) To provide immobilization for hip diseases To treat fractures of the femur	

rials and the plaster bandages applied over them should be smooth and wrinkle free so that skin breakdown is avoided. Loose plaster particles ("crumbs") or the sharp edges of fiberglass can damage the skin. To prevent tissue damage, the stockinette should extend beyond the length of the cast and be folded back over the cast edges to provide a nonabrasive surface against the skin.

To alleviate pain and anxiety during the manual reduction that often precedes casting, the client may require an anesthetic agent. In some cases, a general anesthetic may be administered; in others, a mild tranquilizer is sufficient.

During and immediately after cast application, the involved body part must be supported in such a way that pressure is evenly distributed. Palms of the hands (rather than the fingertips, which might cause indentations) should be used. When casting is complete, you should carefully clean the individual's skin of any excess casting material and inspect for rough edges and indentations.

After the cast is applied, the involved extremity should be elevated above heart level for the first 24 to 48 hours to prevent edema and neurovascular compromise. Ice bags that conform to the cast may be used during the first 24 hours to reduce swelling. Ice bags should be double-wrapped in plastic and applied around the cast at the site of injury. You should assess the client's neurovascular status at frequent intervals, generally at least every two hours for the first eight hours after application, if indicated. Refer to Box 37–1 for review of the assessment for neurovascular integrity. You should also observe for any drainage on the cast. Any drainage that is noted should be outlined in ink and timed and dated as a baseline for future comparisons that might be needed. Box 37–4 identifies measures that promote drying of plaster casts.

When working with the client while the cast is still damp, lift the cast by using the palms of your hands and by providing support under joints above and below the injury site to lessen stress on the cast and involved soft tissue.

Casts may be windowed or bivalved. Windowing a cast allows assessment and treatment of an underlying incision, wound, or area of pressure. The window, created by removal of a small square portion of the cast, permits a visual assessment of the underlying tissue. The piece or pieces of cast that were removed should be replaced and held in place with an Ace bandage. A cast is bivalved by splitting it along both sides to allow tissue swelling, facilitate wound care, or make a half-cast as an intermittent splint. The underlying padding is generally cut when a cast is bivalved. The bivalved cast may be reconstructed by placing the two parts together and securing them with an Ace bandage.

After an injury, particularly a fracture, a temporary plaster cast may be initially applied. The plaster material conforms more to body structure than does the synthetic material. As healing progresses and swelling decreases, the plaster cast may be removed, and a second fiberglass cast applied. When healing is complete, the cast is entirely removed. In some cases after cast removal, a bracing device may be needed to provide protection until bone and muscle have regained strength.

The cast is removed by using an electric cast cutter or vibrating cast saw. Although it makes a loud noise and causes a vibration against the skin, it does not cut the skin. The skin may be scratched if the person moves suddenly or if the saw is not removed after it cuts through the cast. The padding under the cast protects the skin.

Where the cast has been, the person generally has dry, scaly skin. The casted extremity will appear smaller than the unaffected extremity because of muscle atrophy. Pain with movement is common in the extremity and may last for several days until muscle strength improves.

COMPLICATIONS

Persons may occasionally experience complications from casts. Most complications occur because the cast is rigid, prevents movement, and may compromise circulation.

Compartment syndrome is a condition that develops in the presence of excessive swelling within the confined space of a muscle compartment. Venous pressure increases, and the arterial blood flow is compromised. The constrictive cast prevents tissue expansion, which results in increased tissue ischemia. Permanent neurovascular damage may result.

Vascular or nerve damage may be sustained during initial fracture, surgical repair, or cast application when the involved body parts are manipulated.

An infection under a cast can be a special problem because the site cannot be seen. Casts may conceal developing infections until necrosis from the infection is so severe that the extremity is in jeopardy. Other complications include skin breakdown that may occur as a result of the pressure on soft tissue under the cast. Muscles frequently atrophy because of imposed immobilization. Joints commonly become stiff and painful.

Box 37–4. Suggestions for Drying Plaster and Synthetic Casts

PLASTER CASTS

(drying of large plaster casts may take 48 to 72 hours)

► Leave the cast uncovered and open to air dry.
► Place the cast on a firm, smooth surface with a pillow (no rubber or plastic cover) to support the joints and prevent flattening of the plaster.
► When possible, reposition the client, alternating from supine to prone and side to side every 2 to 4 hours to promote even drying.
► Position fans to blow on the cast.

SYNTHETIC CASTS

(dry rapidly after application)

► Blot the cast with towels.
► Use a hand-held blow dryer on the low setting.

Cast syndrome is a complication unique to the use of a body cast. The rigid cast causes increased pressure against the abdominal walls and restricts circulation to the mesenteric arteries. This phenomenon leads to prolonged nausea and vomiting. Ongoing assessment is essential for the early identification and prevention of these complications. Table 37–2 identifies the clinical manifestations of complications of cast use.

TEACHING AND LEARNING

People are generally discharged home with their cast in place. You must provide clear and preferably written

TABLE 37–2. Clinical Manifestations of Complications of Cast Use

1. Impaired blood flow producing soft tissue ischemia (e.g., due to pressure in casted extremity). Clinical manifestations may include

   ▶ Pulselessness: slow nailbed capillary refill, as evidenced by refill greater than 3 seconds
   ▶ Skin pallor, blanching, cyanosis, or coolness
   ▶ Pain, swelling, painful edema peripheral to cast
   ▶ Paresthesias (tingling, prickling), heightened sensitivity, numbness; hypesthesia (diminished sensitivity to touch); anesthesia (numbness)
   ▶ Motor paralysis of previously functioning muscles

2. Nerve damage from pressure where a nerve passes over a bony prominence. Clinical manifestations may include

   ▶ Increasing, persistent, localized pain
   ▶ Hypesthesia (diminished sensitivity); anesthesia (numbness); paresthesias (tingling, prickling, heightened sensitivity, numbness)
   ▶ Feelings of deep pressure
   ▶ Motor weakness or paralysis not previously present

3. Infection, tissue necrosis (e.g., due to skin breakdown). Clinical manifestations may include

   ▶ Musty, unpleasant odor over cast or at ends of cast
   ▶ Drainage through cast or cast opening
   ▶ Sudden unexplained body temperature elevation
   ▶ "Hot spot" felt on cast over lesion

4. Compartment syndrome, which compromises circulation, viability, and function of tissues within the compartment. Clinical manifestations may include

   ▶ A dramatic increase in pain that is no longer controlled by analgesia
   ▶ Loss of movement
   ▶ Loss of sensation
   ▶ Pain with passive motion
   ▶ Pulselessness

5. Cast syndrome occurs with body casts and may be fatal if untreated. Possible assessment findings include

   ▶ Prolonged nausea; repeated vomiting
   ▶ Abdominal distention; vague abdominal pain

From Black, J.M., & Matassarin-Jacobs, E. (1993). *Luckmann and Sorensen's medical-surgical nursing* (4th ed.). Philadelphia: W.B. Saunders.

instructions to direct the individual in self-care to promote optimal healing and prevent complications. You should instruct the person to keep the involved extremity elevated and to be alert to symptoms of complications, including severe swelling; pain, numbness, burning, or tingling sensations; skin color or temperature changes; decreased ability to move fingers or toes; and foul odor emanating from the cast. The person should know how to clean and care for the cast and measures to take to avoid muscle atrophy and weakness. Written instructions should be provided for the client's reference; these may be needed later (Box 37–5).

You should tell the person to expect that after cast removal, the skin under the cast will be sensitive and crusted with yellow-brown scales or crusts of dead skin. The muscles will look small, and joints will ache with movement. The skin should be gently washed for several days after cast removal. Vigorous scrubbing should be avoided. Progressive exercises will gradually restore muscle strength.

DOCUMENTATION

When an individual has a cast in place, you should include the following in your documentation:

▶ type and location of cast
▶ assessment of neurovascular status and tissue integrity

Box 37–5. Client Teaching for Cast Care

▶ Avoid getting your cast wet, even if it is a fiberglass cast. If the cast becomes wet, you may use a hair dryer on the low setting to dry it.
▶ You can use plastic bags to cover the plaster cast during wet weather or bathing. Provide a secure seal around the cast.
▶ Feel and look for any skin irritation at the edges of the cast.
▶ If your skin under the cast happens to itch, *do not* attempt to put anything inside the cast to scratch. Using a blow dryer may help stop the itching.
▶ Check daily to remove any plaster crumbs or foreign objects under the edges of the cast.
▶ Avoid using lotion around the edges of the cast.
▶ Do not use lacquer or paints on the casts; they restrict air penetration.
▶ You may clean a plaster cast with cleanser or a damp cloth by gently rubbing and drying the cast well.
▶ To maintain optimal movement in your affected extremities, you should (unless your physician has directed otherwise) bend and straighten the toes or fingers of the affected extremity several times each hour. Exercise the uninvolved extremity at regular intervals.
▶ For a casted arm (unless your physician has told you otherwise), remove the supporting sling and rotate your shoulder as you would in combing your hair.
▶ For a casted leg, attempt to "tighten" your thigh muscles several times about every 2 hours during the day. Check with your physician for other specific strengthening exercises.

▶ location and amount of edema, if any
▶ individual responses to cast, including reports of pain
▶ interventions performed, including ice application
▶ elevation of affected body part

Sample Documentation

Long leg plaster cast to Rt. leg. Leg elevated on two pillows. Ice bags in place. Able to flex and extend Rt. toes. Denies pain, numbness, and tingling of Rt. foot. Brisk capillary refill. Rt. foot pink and warm to touch. States that he has had "good relief from pain."

Bracing and Splinting

Many people with orthopedic problems need braces or splinting for long-term protection and support. Splints restrict movement to provide protection and promote healing. Braces also restrict movement, but they usually do so to stabilize a body part to allow increased mobility. Braces are increasingly being employed as a means of preventing sports injuries. Knee braces are the most frequently used type. Many braces and splints are individualized for the client by an orthotist or occupational therapist. A variety of commercially prepared splints and braces are also available. Braces and splints can generally be categorized as prophylactic, rehabilitative, and functional. They may also be described as static or dynamic in function (Table 37–3).

Braces and splints are indicated when there is a need to

▶ correct or prevent anatomic deformities
▶ promote better function and prevent injury
▶ maintain or correct body alignment
▶ aid in muscle control
▶ protect in the postoperative period after surgical correction

Construction of braces and splints depends on individual need. Individuals requiring back support may use a brace constructed with metal bars and leather straps. Neck injuries may require only a cervical collar (see Figs. 37–6 and 37–7). Some painful conditions, such as rheumatoid arthritis, may necessitate specially designed cock-up splints for a functional position (see Fig. 35–18). Another brace, such as the Milwaukee brace, aids in correction of scoliosis. See Figure 37–15 for examples of braces and splints.

GENERAL GUIDELINES

Regardless of the specific orthotic device, follow these general guidelines.

▶ Provide thorough assessment before use of braces and splints, particularly including age/developmental considerations, reason for use (particular injury), knowledge of device, skin condition, neurovascular and nutritional status, and potential for compliance.
▶ Identify purpose and type of device. Determine type and amount of therapeutic activity permitted.
▶ Ensure that the device fits properly. An orthotist will specifically design some orthotic devices. Follow-up

TABLE 37–3. *Types of Braces and Splints*

Type of Brace or Splint	Uses
Braces	
Prophylactic braces	Used to prevent injury, primarily for ankle and knee support
Rehabilitative braces	After injury, can provide needed support and can be as effective as casting in certain injuries, such as knee ligament damage; also used for conservative treatment or as an alternative to plaster casts
Functional braces	Designed to provide long-term functional stability—to prevent "giving way" of a joint
Splints	
Static splints	Used to hold a body part in a functional position; static splints have no moving parts and are used primarily for the hand
Dynamic splints	Used to provide mobility to the joints and to support a body part in a functional position

assessment (long-term) is required to ensure continued fit.
▶ Monitor compliance closely, especially in those with a high potential for noncompliance, such as the adolescent.
▶ Provide teaching to promote proper use of the device.
▶ Assess for potential complications associated with orthotic devices.

Table 37–4 lists selected scientific principles and related nursing interventions for immobilizing devices like casts and braces.

COMPLICATIONS

Use of orthotic devices may lead to several complications. Immobility may develop as a result of discomfort associated with the brace or splint. Range of motion may decrease, and muscle contractures may develop as a result of wearing the device. Pathologic changes may increase when the device is not used because it feels "too heavy" or "too awkward." Some clients may feel self-conscious or embarrassed about wearing the device. Loss of skin integrity and neurovascular compromise may result from a poorly fitting device that is inadequately monitored. Deformity worsens rather than improves when the device is not fitted properly.

TEACHING AND LEARNING

Effective use of braces and splints mandates that each individual know the *why* and *how* of brace use. Generally, braces and splints are used for long-term manage-

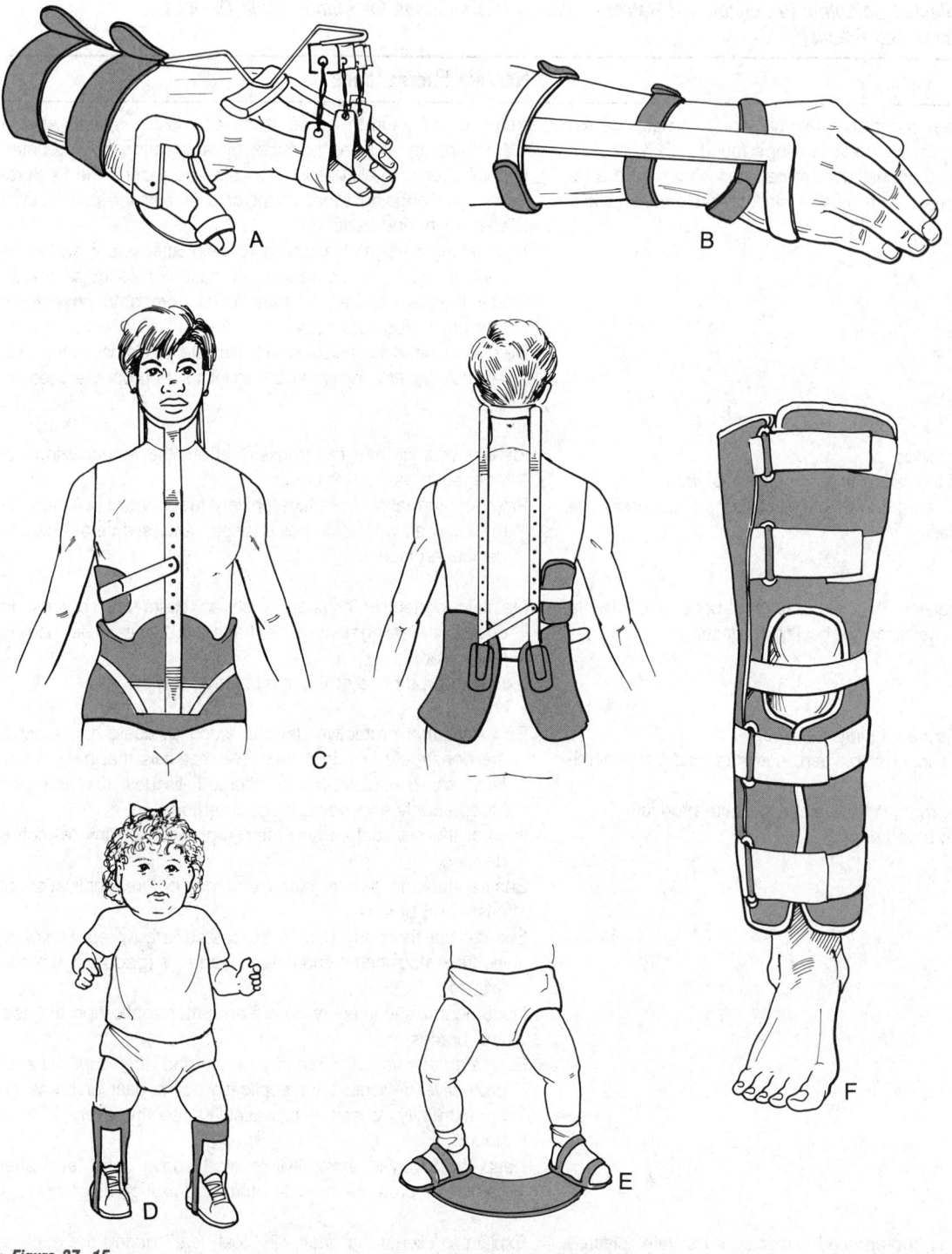

▲ *Figure 37–15*

Examples of braces and splints. *A,* Outrigger splint: dynamic hand splint. *B,* Wrist-hand orthosis: wrist stabilization. *C,* Milwaukee brace: correction of spinal scoliosis, lordosis, and kyphosis. *D,* Short-leg orthosis: maintains support and stabilizes ankle motion. *E,* Denis Browne splint: maintains hip flexion and hip abduction. *F,* Postoperative knee immobilizer.

TABLE 37–4. Selected Scientific Principles and Related Nursing Interventions for Immobilizing Devices (Casts and Braces)

Principle	Nursing Interventions
Pain stimuli include mechanical, thermal, and chemical agents; receptors for pain are nerve endings found chiefly in skin, muscles, joints, tendons, dura mater, periosteum, and arterial walls. Trauma to the musculoskeletal system stimulates pain receptors.	Remove the trauma source, such as muscle spasm after a fracture, as soon as possible by application of a counter-pulling force to alleviate the spasm and reduce the fracture Provide an ongoing assessment of pain and the pain source after injury and treatment Assess the person's response to pain after injury and intervention, such as application of cast or brace; recognize that the pain expressed may result from both physiologic and psychologic sources Determine need for analgesic to alleviate pain associated with musculoskeletal injury, and administer appropriate medication
Pain has two meanings: 1. the biologic indication that something is wrong 2. a means of communication, such as an expression of fear or distress	Identify your client's fears/anxiety about the immobilizing device, such as cast or brace Provide information to reduce anxiety/fear about application of the device, why it is being used, and self-care with the device in place
Bone healing requires that the fractured bone ends be in contact and immobilized for healing to occur	Maintain protective devices, such as casts and braces, to ensure the alignment of a fractured bone while healing takes place Explain the purpose of the immobilizing device
Maintenance of tissue integrity requires 1. a constant supply of oxygen, nutrients, and vital chemicals 2. a method of removal of metabolic waste products 3. an adequate blood supply	Be aware that protective devices, such as casts and braces, are constructed of rigid, inflexible materials that may potentially impair circulation to affected tissues (oxygen and blood supply and waste product removal) Inspect the skin before and after application of any restrictive devices Ensure that the skin is clean and dry before application of casts and braces Ensure that the body part to be casted is covered with wrinkle-free stockinette and sheet wadding (padding) for soft tissues Document tissue integrity before and after application of casts and braces Evaluate neurovascular integrity before and after application of protective devices; after application of a cast or brace on an extremity, check neurovascular integrity every 2 to 4 hours Keep the involved extremity elevated above heart level after casting to promote venous return and reduce swelling
Casting material is impregnated with calcium sulfate (plaster) or fiberglass polyurethane and reacts with water to allow molding to the desired body part. Heat is generated during this reaction Length of time for drying of cast depends on material used and amount of casting needed: plaster cast takes 24 to 72 hours to "dry"; the synthetic or fiberglass dries almost instantly	Explain to clients that they will "feel heat" during the application process Maintain body part in proper alignment during drying process; generally requires slight traction Handle "new" cast with palms of hands, never fingertips, because this would produce "molding" of cast and possible indentation on underlying tissues Promote drying of casts: turn client every 2 hours to aid drying; do not use plastic-covered pillows; provide adequate ventilation or small fans

***TABLE 37-4. Selected Scientific Principles and Related Nursing Interventions for Immobilizing Devices (Casts and Braces)** Continued*

Principle	Nursing Interventions
Bone is living tissue and requires a balance of catabolism and anabolism; associated trauma or infection increases metabolic needs	Assess nutritional status Encourage client to eat well-balanced diet with additional protein, vitamins C and B, and calories to compensate for amount lost with trauma or infection and to facilitate tissue healing; fluid intake should be 2000–3000 ml daily.
The stresses and strains of mobility and weight-bearing stimulate formation of osteoblastic cells. Bone decalcification occurs when there is immobility	Explain to the client that, when allowed, limited weight-bearing with adequate immobilization will actually encourage healing
Movement of voluntary muscles promotes venous return to the heart	Instruct client to perform active range-of-motion exercises, and perform passive range-of-motion exercises for the client within limits determined by injury and protective device; usually the uninvolved limbs should be actively exercised every 1–2 hours Assess for potential development of deep vein thrombosis

ment of specific conditions. Instructions must be specific to the device to ensure safe and effective use. You should plan to work with the orthotist (if applicable) to design a teaching plan. Be sure to include the following points in the teaching plan:

▶ purpose for and type of device
▶ complications to identify and report, such as increased pain, tissue injury, or altered sensation
▶ instructions for use of the device, such as how to apply and when to use
▶ how to care for the device, including cleaning and storage

DOCUMENTATION

Documentation should include

▶ type of orthotic device and anatomic location
▶ date and time of initial application of the orthotic device
▶ condition of the skin and neurovascular integrity relative to use of the device
▶ individual response to the device, such as pain or skin irritation
▶ time removed

Traction

Traction is a pulling force applied to a part of the body, such as an extremity. **Countertraction** is a force that pulls in the opposite direction from the force exerted by traction. Traction has many therapeutic uses, but it is most often used to realign (reduce) the broken ends of a fractured bone. Box 37-6 summarizes the uses for traction.

Application of traction requires the use of specialized equipment and bed frames (Fig. 37-16). The type of traction and length of its use are determined by the underlying problem, severity of damage, and strength of muscles and bones.

Traction can be applied manually (by pulling the body part with your hands) to provide a temporary pulling force or mechanically by exerting a pulling force on the body part with ropes and pulleys. Figure 37-17 depicts the pulling force applied to a fracture site. Mechanical traction may be applied to the client's skin. **Skin traction** is the type of traction in which the pulling force is applied directly to the skin and indirectly to underlying muscles and bones. Its use is limited by the amount of weight (less than 10 pounds) and length of time (generally no more than one to two weeks) the skin can tolerate the force. If a longer period of immobilization is anticipated or the type of injury requires a large pulling force, skeletal traction may be indicated. **Skeletal traction** is the type of traction in which the pulling force is applied directly to the bone. With skeletal traction, a steel pin or wire is inserted through the bone and is attached to the traction apparatus. Figure 37-18 demonstrates manual, skin, and skeletal traction.

Traction may be applied continuously or intermittently. In general, skin traction is designed for intermittent use whereas skeletal traction maintains a steady pulling force, but this is not always the case. It is important to understand how the traction is intended for each client.

Box 37-6. Uses for Traction

Reduction of fractures, dislocations, and subluxation
Relief of muscle spasms
Correction, reduction, or prevention of deformities and contractures
Immobilization to prevent soft tissue damage
Providing rest for diseased joints

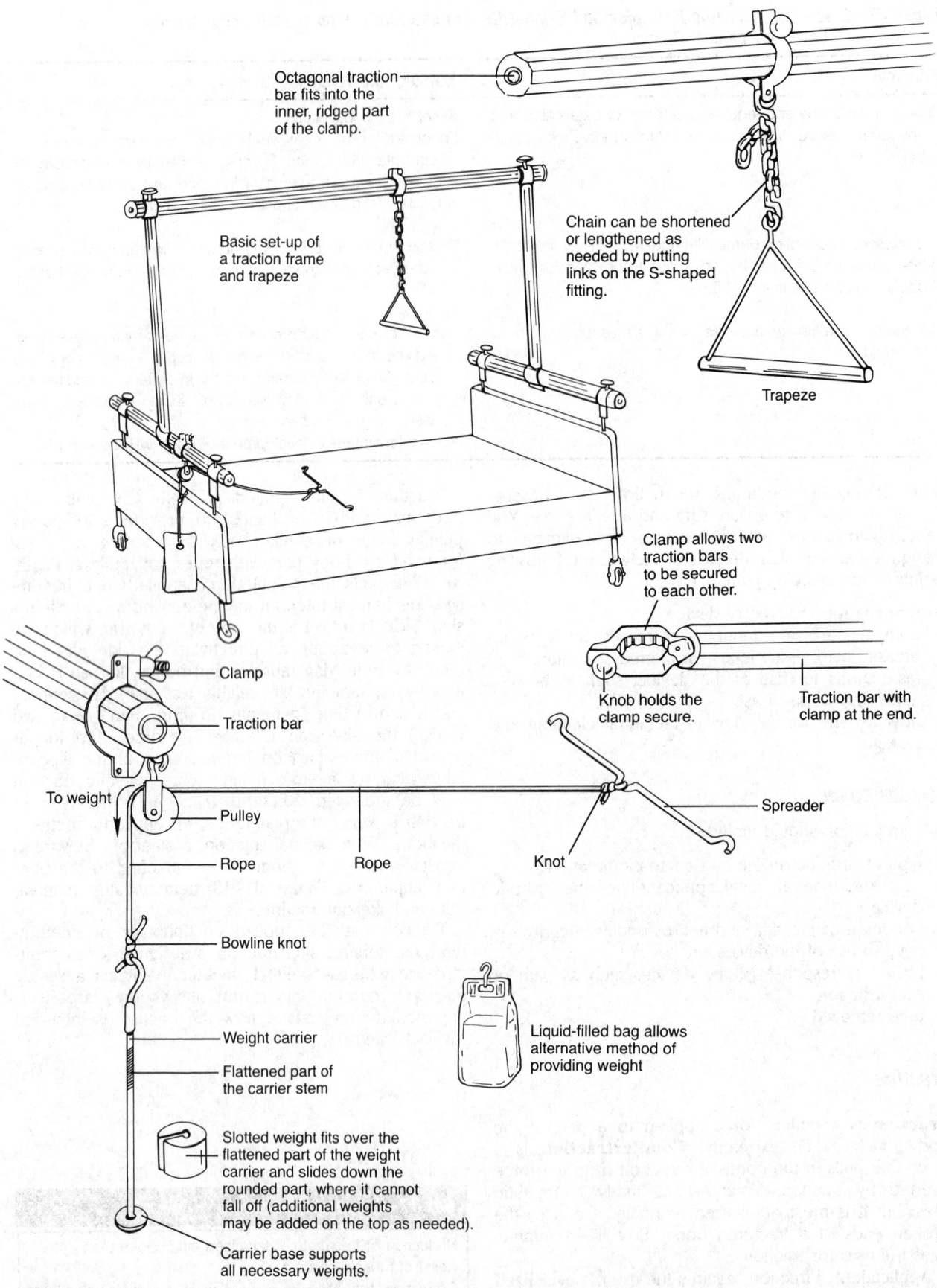

Octagonal traction bar fits into the inner, ridged part of the clamp.

Basic set-up of a traction frame and trapeze

Chain can be shortened or lengthened as needed by putting links on the S-shaped fitting.

Trapeze

Clamp allows two traction bars to be secured to each other.

Knob holds the clamp secure.

Traction bar with clamp at the end.

Clamp

Traction bar

To weight

Pulley

Rope

Rope

Knot

Spreader

Bowline knot

Weight carrier

Flattened part of the carrier stem

Liquid-filled bag allows alternative method of providing weight

Slotted weight fits over the flattened part of the weight carrier and slides down the rounded part, where it cannot fall off (additional weights may be added on the top as needed).

Carrier base supports all necessary weights.

▲ **Figure 37–16**

Bed with basic traction equipment.

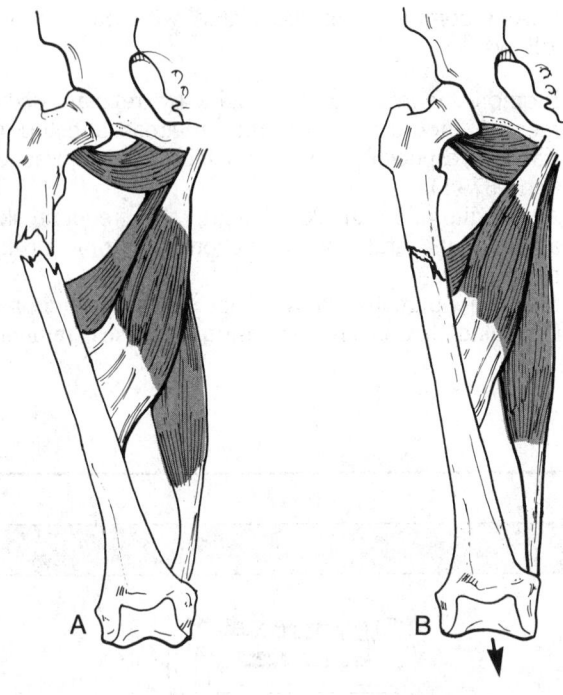

▲ *Figure 37-17*

Pulling force to fracture site. *A,* Early fracture. Note pull of muscle displacing distal fracture site. *B,* Application of traction realigns bone fragments (reduces fracture) and decreases muscle spasm.

Traction is applied by a system of weights and pulleys set at angles selected by the physician. The angle formed by the placement of the pulleys on the bed frame and the involved joints determines the line of pull. The resultant line of pull is along the long axis of the bone. Figure 37-19 gives an example of the line of pull. The addition of balanced suspension allows increased movement of the client without a change in the desired line of pull. In balanced suspension, the involved extremity is supported by a sling-type apparatus and weights that allow the extremity to "float" without altering the traction force. Table 37-5 lists major types of traction.

GENERAL GUIDELINES

Safe and effective care of the client in traction requires attention to the traction setup as well as attention to the client. Determine the type of traction and reason for its use. Maintain the line of pull once it is established.

For some traction to be effective, it must be continuous and must not be removed without a physician's order. Tissue damage could also occur if traction is removed. Before removing traction, always check the order to be certain that removal is allowed.

Countertraction is required to balance the force of traction. Insufficient countertraction, as supplied by body weight, will cause the person to slide toward the traction force. Countertraction may be increased by tilting the bed away from the traction force.

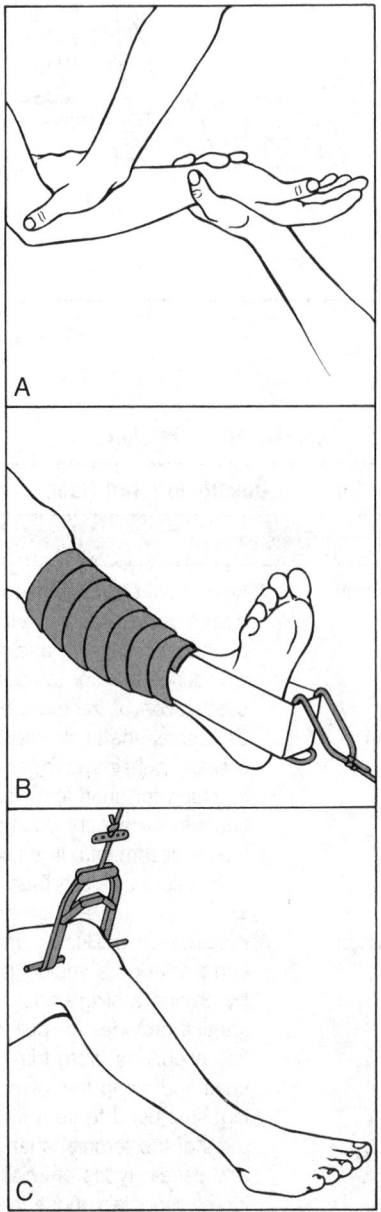

▲ *Figure 37-18*

Types of traction. *A,* Manual traction. The hands are used to exert a pulling force. *B,* Skin traction. Strips of tape, moleskin, foam boots, or some other type of commercial skin traction strips are applied directly to the skin. Skin traction is used primarily in the treatment of children's fractures and for adult fractures or dislocations that require only a moderate amount of pulling force for a relatively short period of time. *C,* Skeletal traction applies traction force directly to bone by use of pins, wires, screws, and, in the case of cervical traction, tongs applied directly to the skull. Skeletal traction allows the use of up to 20 to 30 pounds of force for as long as three to four months. (Redrawn from The Zimmer Traction Handbook [1989]. Zimmer, Inc.)

Friction reduces the effectiveness of traction and impairs the desired pulling force. Inspect traction to ensure that weights are hanging free, knots are clear of pulleys, footplates or spreaders are not touching the end of the bed, and the person's heels are not digging into the mattress.

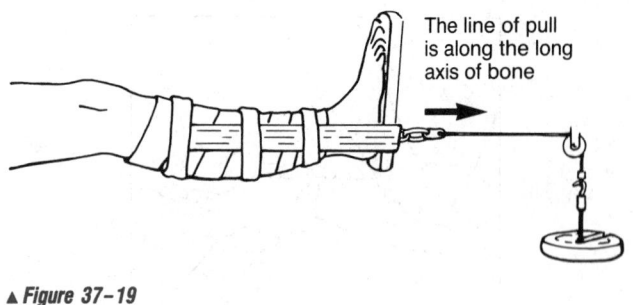

The line of pull is along the long axis of bone

▲ *Figure 37–19*

Line of pull.

Prevent complications associated with traction use, as follows.

▶ Promote neurovascular integrity by regular assessment of neurovascular status in areas affected by traction, especially hands and feet distal to traction (Box 37–1).

▶ Avoid alteration in skin integrity by frequent skin assessments and by protection of bony prominences.

▶ Maintain optimal cardiovascular status by encouraging ankle flexion and extension exercises, minimiz-

TABLE 37–5. *Major Types of Traction*

Type of Traction	Description and Uses	
Lower Extremity Traction		
Buck's extension traction	A type of skin traction used to treat muscle spasms, arthritis, hip dislocations, and pelvic injuries and for temporary stabilization of fractured hips or femoral shafts. It employs a single pulley system and is intended for short-term, continuous use except during skin assessments. It is used with weights of less than 10 lb.	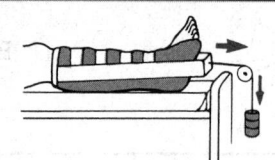
Russell's traction	A modification of Buck's traction that adds a vertical pull by placing a sling under the knee. It provides for pull in two directions (from the knee and along the lower leg). It is used to treat fractures of the femoral shaft and certain types of knee injuries, especially those involving the tibial plateau. Because of the arrangement of the pulleys, the effective traction is twice the actual weight used. Russell's traction is generally for short-term, continuous use.	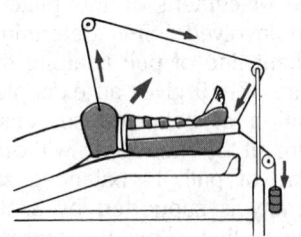
Bryant's traction	A type of skin traction that treats fractures of the femur in children up to 2 years of age. Bryant's traction provides for bilateral traction, with the hips flexed at right angles. It is for continuous, long-term use.	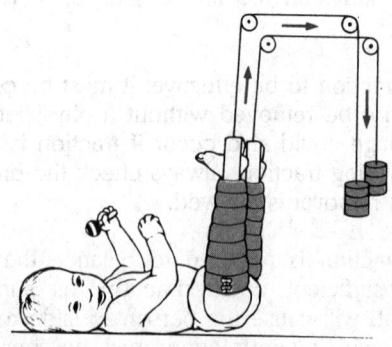

TABLE 37–5. *Major Types of Traction* Continued

Type of Traction	Description and Uses	
Balanced suspension traction with a Thomas or Brady splint	A skin or skeletal traction that treats fractures of the femoral shaft, hip, and lower leg. It is for continuous, long-term, usually unilateral use. It employs a suspension system and can be used with up to 30 lb of weight.	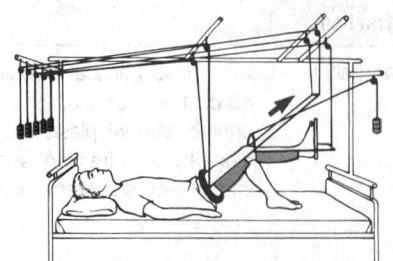
Pelvic Traction		
Pelvic belt	Used to treat ruptured discs and muscle spasms of the lower back. It is skin traction for intermittent, short-term use.	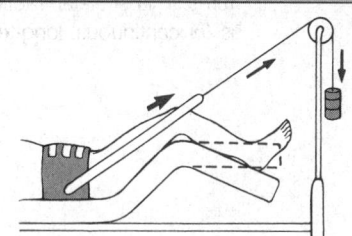
Pelvic sling	Provides continuous compression to sides of pelvis for uncomplicated pelvic fractures. It is for continuous, long-term use.	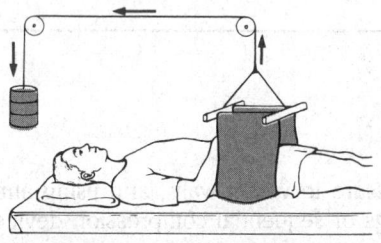
Upper Extremity Traction		
Side-arm traction	Used to immobilize or stabilize fractures, dislocations, or other injuries of the elbow, upper arm, and shoulder. It is for continuous skin or skeletal traction to the humerus with vertical suspension of the forearm.	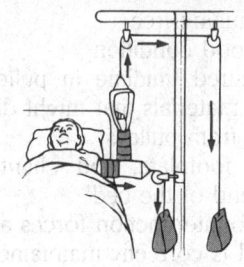
Overhead (90/90) traction	Used for the same purposes as side-arm traction. Overhead (90/90) traction is for continuous skin or skeletal traction. It employs vertical traction to the humerus, with horizontal suspension of the forearm.	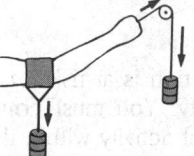

Table continued on following page

TABLE 37–5. Major Types of Traction Continued

Type of Traction	Description and Uses	
Cervical Traction		
Cervical head halter traction	Used to treat cervical myositis, dislocations, strains, sprains, arthritis, and whiplash injuries. This skin traction is for intermittent, short-term use.	
Halo traction	Used to stabilize cervical fractures. This skeletal traction is for continuous, long-term use.	

ing pressure to vessel walls, and using antiembolism stockings or sequential compression devices.

Finally, provide frequent traction checks to ensure that

▶ weights are hanging free
▶ ropes are in good condition
▶ ropes are secured, midline in pulleys, and free of linen or other materials that might disrupt the pull
▶ knots are free from pulleys
▶ the spreader, footplate, and client's feet are not touching the end of the bed
▶ traction and countertraction forces are maintained
▶ the line of pull is correctly maintained

COMPLICATIONS

The person in traction is at risk for complications from imposed immobility. You must continually take action to maintain optimal activity within the limits of traction. A priority complication is compromised circulation caused by tissue swelling and use of metallic devices that may disrupt neurovascular structures. You must perform a neurovascular assessment before and at frequent intervals after application of traction (see Box 37–1).

The person in traction is also at risk for impaired skin integrity because of pressure from traction devices. It is important that the skin be carefully assessed before application of traction and at frequent intervals while traction is in use. Bony prominences must be carefully inspected for early identification of skin breakdown.

When the client is in skeletal traction, the apparatus penetrates the skin, and risk of infection is ever-present. To prevent infection in skeletal traction, pin care is routinely done for most clients. Pin care is the prophylactic cleansing of the site of pin (or wire or other hardware) insertion with or without the application of antiseptic solutions or ointments. Pin care is done at regular intervals, such as bid or tid. Pin care requires sterile technique to prevent infection, but the actual procedures involved can vary considerably. It is necessary, therefore, that you use the procedure prescribed by the individual physician or follow your agency's procedure for this intervention. To be prepared to complete any pin care procedure, you must be familiar with the principles of aseptic technique (see Chapter 28) and wound care (see Chapter 48).

TEACHING AND LEARNING

The client is often fearful of the traction devices. The fear may arise from wondering whether movement is possible with the devices in place. You should describe the desired effect of the traction and identify what activities are permitted when the traction is in place. For example, tell the person whether he can turn, explain how high the head of the bed can be raised, and describe if and when the traction can be removed. The person should be told what symptoms to report immediately, such as a marked change in sensation or an inability to move an involved extremity.

In some situations, the person may use traction devices in the home setting. For example, a cervical strain might be treated at home with cervical traction. Home use would be determined by the type of traction needed, the home environment, and the availability of resources including family support or home health care services. When traction is used in the home setting, it is essential that instructions be given regarding

- ▶ how to set up and apply the traction
- ▶ signs and symptoms of complications (skin breakdown, neurovascular compromise, infection)
- ▶ guidelines for exercise and nutrition while using traction
- ▶ special care needs (skin, pin site care)
- ▶ pain management
- ▶ whom to call and what to report if problems develop

DOCUMENTATION

When traction is used, you must document the following information:

- ▶ type of traction in use
- ▶ amount of traction weight
- ▶ assessment of pin sites (if applicable) and skin integrity
- ▶ neurovascular and muscular assessment of involved body part
- ▶ pin care provided (if applicable)
- ▶ person's response to treatment

Sample Documentation

Buck's boot to Lt. leg c̄ 7 lb. wgt. Skin brown and intact. Brisk capillary refill, <2 seconds to Lt. toes. Able to flex and extend Lt. toes. Denies numbness, tingling, and pain in Lt. toes and foot. Denies discomfort.

Movement Devices

Movement devices facilitate transportation of injured individuals from the site of injury to the health care facility; transfer of clients to and from beds, stretchers, or diagnostic/treatment tables in the health care facility; and movement of individuals in their own beds.

Movement devices are sometimes used primarily for the safety and comfort of care providers (e.g., to move a large individual). Other times, they are used to prevent injury (e.g., vertebral column injury) or to minimize pain associated with movement (e.g., the individual with a fractured hip or arthritis).

Movement devices are discussed in general terms in Chapter 35. In this chapter, we focus on two devices that help prevent injury to the client by decreasing the amount of the client's movement necessary during transfer and transportation.

JED SLED

A JED sled (Fig. 37–20) is a device to move or turn a person. It is composed of several lightweight but rigid plastic boards and a collapsible bar. Slip the boards under the person and then secure them together by

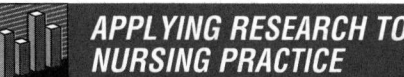

APPLYING RESEARCH TO NURSING PRACTICE

Understanding the Feelings of Clients Wearing a Halo Brace—and Helping Them to Cope

Olson, B., Ustanko, L., & Warner, S. (1991). The patient in a halo brace: striving for normalcy in body image and self-concept. *Orthopedic Nursing, 10*(1), 44–50.

▼ ▼ ▼

Although the halo brace used for treatment of cervical fractures is a remarkable device, little is known about its psychologic impact on wearers. Olson and colleagues sought to identify the psychologic concerns and needs of people using halo braces. To do so, they analyzed questionnaire responses of 38 people who had previously worn halo braces. The researchers found four types of reactions: distortion in body image, distortion in self-concept, striving for normalcy, and grieving and isolation.

A large percentage of respondents were found to have had a *distortion in body image.* Of those responding, 79 per cent reported that the halo brace affected their feelings about their appearance. They described themselves as having felt "ugly" and "terrible." Of the 38 respondents, 25 mentioned that they had suffered scars, lumps, and indentations, perhaps reflecting feelings of mutilation. Many of the respondents (17 in all) reported that they felt like a "freak," "alien," "Martian," or "R2-D2." These feelings may indicate the presence of a phenomenon called extended body image, in which a person incorporates attached equipment into the body image.

As a sequel to the distortion in body image, many of the respondents were found to have had a *distortion in self-concept,* indicated by changes in role performance and social interactions.

Striving for normalcy, another common response, is a coping method often used by persons suffering handicaps. Respondents in this study reported striving for normalcy by use of denial, rationalization, proactive coping (planning for the future), and humor.

Many of the respondents indicated that they reacted to the halo brace with *grieving and isolation* as manifested by feelings of embarrassment, depression, helplessness, fear, guilt, and anger.

Applications for Nursing Practice

In practice, recognize—and help your clients recognize—the psychologic reactions that may occur with use of the halo brace. Prepare clients going home with a halo brace by establishing trust, inspiring hope, promoting self-care, displaying nonverbal reassurance, enhancing knowledge, encouraging healthy support systems, providing encouragement and feedback, and promoting laughter and humor.

sliding the bar through loops along one side of each board. Move the person by pulling (sliding) the sled toward you. Once the desired position is obtained, pull the bar out of the loops on the boards and remove

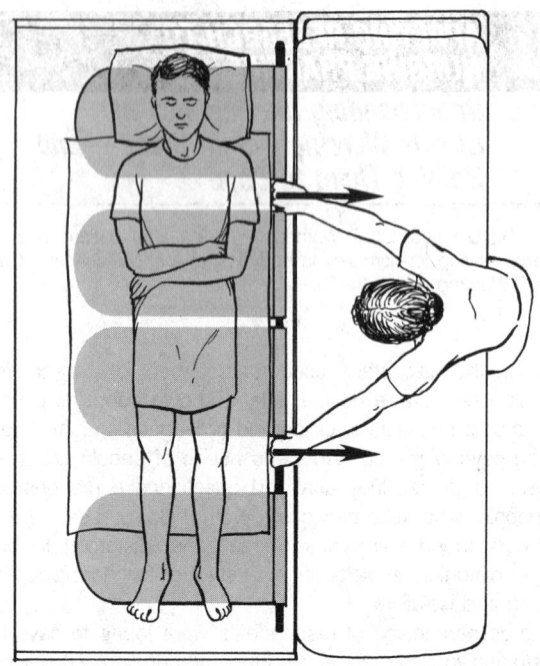

▲ **Figure 37-20**

JED sled, a device used to move people from stretchers and beds and to turn people in bed. The sleds (shown in gray) are positioned under the person, without the person having to be turned, and are secured with a pole. The pole is used to pull the person toward the health care provider.

each board separately. A JED sled cannot be used to carry a person. It helps with transfers from stretcher to bed or turning in bed.

CLAM SHELL ("SCOOP") STRETCHER

The clam shell ("scoop") stretcher is a lightweight metal frame that can be separated in half lengthwise. It is used primarily to stabilize and move injured or unconscious people who cannot be turned for backboard placement. Each half is separately placed under the person's sides. The ends are then locked together at the head and feet, producing a firm, stable frame for movement. Spinal x-ray films can be taken with the frame in place. Some clam shells have a center hinge, so the frame can be bent in half. This feature helps stabilize and move a person who is in a sitting position (e.g., automobile passenger).

Restraints

Restraints are any protective measure employed to prevent individuals from harming themselves or others and to immobilize and promote a feeling of security in a person needing control. Restraints may be environmental, chemical, or physical. Environmental restraint may be achieved with side rails, "quiet" (seclusion) rooms, plastic domes, netting, and locked wards. Chemical re-

straints include antianxiety, antipsychotic, and hypnotic medications. Physical restraints are made of linen, leather, or synthetic material with high tensile strength. Wrist, ankle, chest, waist, and total body devices are commercially available. Because suicide precautions may include the use of some form of restraints, the safety of the suicidal person is included in this discussion.

IMPORTANT CONSIDERATIONS

Your judgment is critical in the implementation of restraints that are sufficient to protect the individual without violating the person's rights. Using restraints is an emotion-laden experience; you must be aware of the feelings that may cause the error of overrestraining or underrestraining.

A person's response to being restrained is rarely submissive. A restrained person often feels like the victim of a personal physical assault and responds accordingly.[10]

Combative behavior or the effort to preserve freedom in a frightened, fearful person is *normal.*

The person may feel angry because self-control is being taken away. On the other hand, if a staff member is injured while applying restraints, the person may feel guilt.

When agitation or panic occurs, a staff member who has good rapport with the individual should converse with him or her. The person should have constant reassurance that personnel are aware of the feelings being experienced and are there to help, not punish. *Use simple terms.* Speak in a *low, calm, reassuring voice,* explaining why restraints are needed. Repeat the explanation at intervals. The possibility that organic confusion or mind-altering drugs can be affecting communication should be a reason to intensify communications and not a reason to restrain without question.

Never try to restrain a severely agitated person by yourself. Adequate personnel are needed to apply restraints safely and efficiently and to minimize potential injury to the person and staff. Psychiatric units and emergency departments[74] often have a response team that is paged when the need for physical restraint is impending. The team comes to the unit and initially remains out of the person's range but within sight. The presence of the team is sometimes enough for the person to achieve self-control of behavior. The team is trained in "holds" that can be used, if necessary, to control a person physically without injury to either the person or the staff (Fig. 37-21).

Restraining combative people is stressful for all concerned. It can be accomplished with minimal energy and anxiety by thorough preparation and communication. When it is necessary to restrain a person, make the decision quickly and carry it out promptly and quietly. The staff's indecision increases anxiety for the person and the staff. Being decisive does not mean that the decision is made lightly or that restraints are overused.

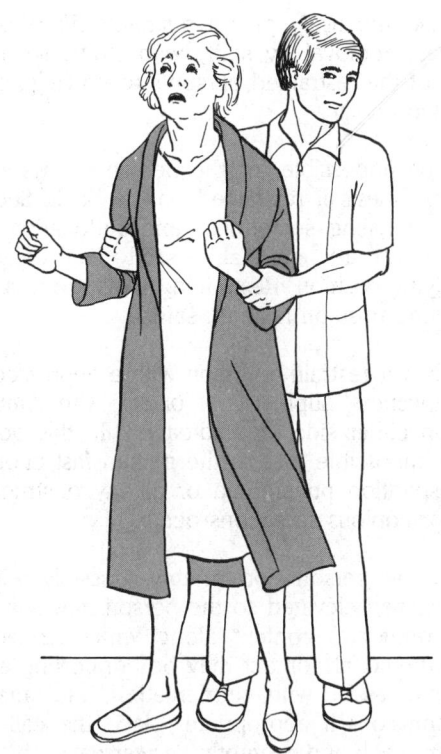

▲ *Figure 37–21*

A restraining hold enables the care giver to obtain physical control of a person who is a potential threat to self or others. The care giver stands behind and to the side of the person, with the feet separated, which provides more stability to the care giver and decreases the possibility of being kicked. The position of the care giver's right arm behind the person's back and the placement of the right hand on the upper right arm provide a base of support for the care giver and prevent movement of the person's arm forward. Likewise, the placement of the care giver's left hand on the person's left arm minimizes forward motion of the person's left hand and arm.

To act swiftly and surely with minimal confusion, the team should develop and communicate a strategy for restraint application. A designated team leader directs all activities and gives each team member a specific assignment (e.g., "restrain right wrist" or "hold shoulders"). The restraining devices should be prepared in advance and kept out of the person's sight until the individual is in a position to be restrained (e.g., sitting on the floor against a wall, or on a bed or stretcher). The team leader then signals to team members that the time to restrain is now, and a well-coordinated team movement is executed.

COMPLICATIONS AND NURSING IMPLICATIONS

The complications that may result from restraints are carefully weighed against the potential benefit. Restraints may cause as many problems as they solve. Family members may express anger about restraints, and the client may react with very strong emotions.

The following psychosocial hazards are associated with the use of restraints:

▶ Negative emotional responses, such as frustration,

stress, anxiety, fear, panic, combativeness, agitation, depression, despair, and hopelessness

▶ A sense of loss of personal control or loss of positive self-image

▶ A sense of being viewed by others as disturbed, dangerous, or mentally incompetent

▶ Sensory deprivation (see Chapter 51)

▶ Increasingly disorganized behavior

▶ Growing dependency

▶ Increased confusion from limited communication

▶ A heightened degree of disorientation

▶ Regressive behavior and withdrawal

▶ Diminished functional capacity resulting in decreased potential for rehabilitation

Other hazards are physiologic in nature. For example, one hazard is tissue damage under the restraints (e.g., from friction, pressure). Do not restrain an extremity that has an arteriovenous fistula or a Schibner shunt in it. Be very careful if restraining a limb with an intravenous infusion running. Restraints should not interfere with intravenous flow and equipment lines. If an arterial line is in place, position the restraint carefully around the armboard (not directly on the limb).

Another physiologic hazard is damage to other body parts. Shoulder dislocations can occur if the person is combative during restraint application or has a grand mal seizure while restrained. Grand mal seizures produce loss of consciousness immediately followed by generalized convulsions. Injury can occur if a restraint is tied to a movable object and the object (e.g., IV pole, light) is pulled over. Fasten restraints to the bed frame, not to side rails. This safeguard prevents injury to the person when the side rail position is changed. When changing the position of the bed or side rails of a restrained person, always check the restraint's tightness or looseness resulting from the position change.

Hypostatic pneumonia is yet another physiologic hazard of the use of restraints. The person should have frequent position changes and regular deep-breathing exercises.

Pressure areas, skin abrasions, and edema may also result from the use of restraints. These conditions can occur from the improper application of restraints, from the effects of bed rest without adequate position changes, or from the client struggling against the restraint.

Ischemia or nerve damage may result if restraints are too tightly applied or if they become constrictive after application. Restraints should be snug but not tight. They should allow as much movement as possible while restraining as necessary.

Musculoskeletal damage may result from prolonged restraint. Contractures, such as wristdrop, result from failure to put joints through range-of-motion exercises. Bone loss may result from immobility.

Aspiration pneumonia may result from the use of restraints in a manner that prevents adequate control of secretions or vomitus. Aspiration of vomitus is more likely in the presence of altered levels of consciousness. Aspiration pneumonia has a high mortality rate.

Accidental strangulation or entanglement may occur with the use of restraints. Never place restraints around the neck. Apply restraints snugly so the person cannot get out of them or become entangled in them.

Clients may also use restraints to intentionally harm themselves (e.g., suicide) or others. The use of restraints is also associated with a prolonged length of stay in the hospital or other health care facility and with an increase in death rates.

Another complication of the use of restraints is the inability to effectively resuscitate a restrained person who has a cardiac arrest because of the time needed to remove the restraints for treatment (e.g., to place the client supine on a cardiac arrest board). Finally, injury or death from fire or other disasters may occur because of the use of restraints.

The last two life-threatening situations are particularly likely to occur if linen restraints are tied in regular knots; if all staff members fail to keep a restraint key on their person at all times when locked restraints are used; or if restraint knots, buckles, or straps have been taped to secure them. Always be prepared to remove restraints quickly.

Caution To make restraints easy to remove quickly in emergencies: Tie linen restraints with a clove hitch or other appropriate knot placed out of the restrained person's reach (Fig. 37–22); do *not* use a regular knot. Have all personnel carry a key when using a locked restraint. Do *not* use tape on restraints. Face buckles up (for easy removal by staff) with straps secured in them, out of the restrained person's reach (e.g., on bed frame, behind chair).

It may be impossible for the person to swallow secretions or emesis if restrained on the back. Secretion aspiration (inhaling secretions) and suffocation (stopping breathing) are potential, possibly fatal dangers in the back-lying position. Restraining a person in a three-quarter prone position is much safer.

Caution Never restrain a person with a depressed level of consciousness supine (on back) with limbs restrained on either side (spread-eagle). In this position, it may be impossible to turn the person fast enough to prevent aspiration pneumonia or airway obstruction if vomiting or copious secretions occur.

Position the person comfortably, possibly with the head of the bed elevated so the person may see more. This environmental contact along with planned, frequent interpersonal contact may be comforting and diverting, may assist with reorientation, and may decrease confusion. If appropriate, place the call signal within easy reach and promptly answer calls.

Establish and follow a plan of nursing care for a

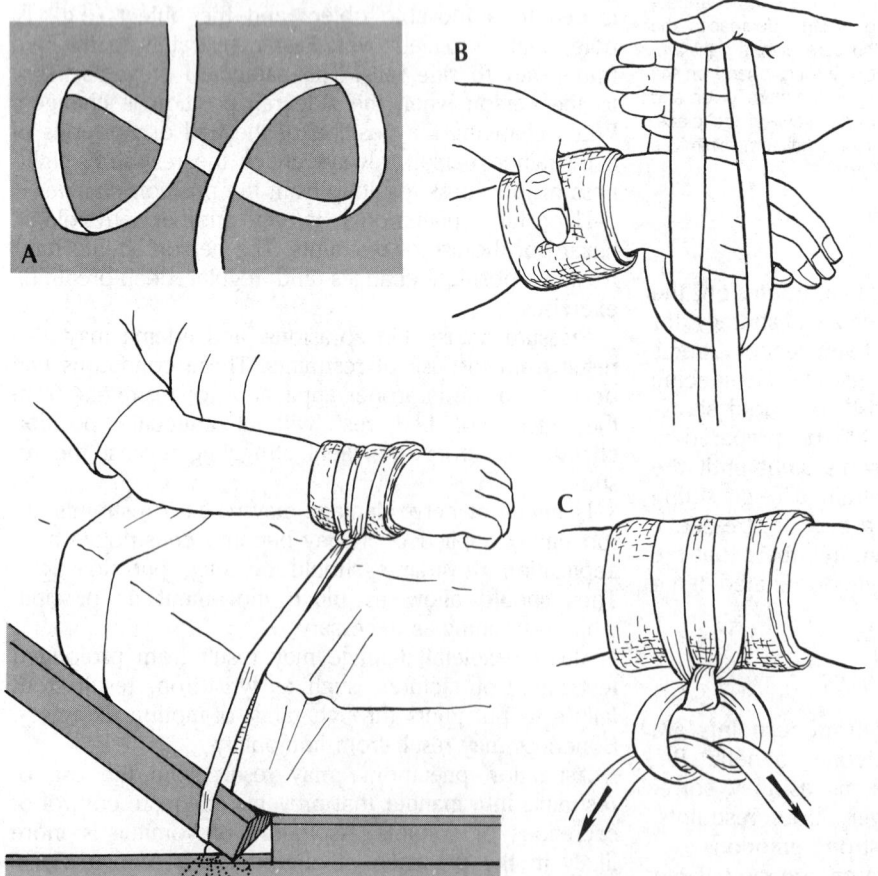

▲ *Figure 37–22*

Soft limb restraint. This restraint is applied to the wrist or ankle with a clove hitch knot (*A* and *B*). A single knot on top of the clove hitch (*C*) prevents the restraint from becoming too tight if the restrained person pulls hard against it. Note that the extremity is well padded for comfort and protection. The ends of the restraint are secured to the bed under the mattress rather than to side rails. The restraint is secured in such a way that it prevents damage to the person if the side rail position or the bed position is changed. Note that the restraint is tied with a bow knot (for quick release in an emergency) underneath the bed where the person cannot reach it.

restrained person, including scheduled visits; a regular assessment schedule (e.g., circulatory, neurologic, musculoskeletal, mental status assessments); and interventions to prevent the hazards of restraints (e.g., sensory stimulation, range-of-motion exercises, position changes, giving liquids). Change the restrained person's position often. Remove the restraints frequently (usually not all restraints are removed at once) to give care and allow the person to move.

Restrained people need to know that they are not being punished and will not be abandoned. Reaffirm the person's worth. Explain that the restraints are being used to prevent injury. When possible, use resources (e.g., significant others or volunteers) instead of restraints. Use restraints that allow the greatest freedom of motion (e.g., restrain the person at the waist rather than at all four extremities, when possible).

Use restraints therapeutically and not as "punishment" for inappropriate behavior. Never use restraints in a vindictive way (e.g., to "show the person who's boss"). Frequently reassess the need for restraints. Discontinue them as soon as possible.

Restraints can have devastating effects not only on the individual restrained but also on other clients (they may become frightened at the staff's power and fear it will be used on them, or they may feel afraid of the restrained person), visitors (they may view staff as punitive and callous), and staff (they may feel guilty, disagree with use of restraints, feel punitive).

A restrained person depends totally on care providers (e.g., for safety, fluid and food intake, hygiene, nutrition, position change, range-of-motion exercises, elimination, communication, and sensory stimulation). Observe a restrained person often (e.g., at least every 30 minutes). Think of yourself in the person's place. A restrained person is at the staff's mercy, powerless, totally dependent, possibly suffering, and needing reassurance that needs will be kindly met.

DOCUMENTATION

Because of the real possibility of being charged with false imprisonment, documentation in the clinical record is essential. Document

- ▶ the person's behavior that led to use of restraints
- ▶ the time of restraint application and types used
- ▶ the person's behavioral and physical responses to restraints
- ▶ the nursing goals, assessments, interventions, and evaluations: assessments of mental status, skin, circulation, respiration, and neurologic function; psychosocial intervention; skin care; position changes (time of change and position changed to); range-of-motion exercises, frequency and time of observations (at least every 30 minutes), and restraint removal (see later); assistance given (with food, liquids, elimination)
- ▶ every visit by a staff member, including the time

- ▶ the time of restraint discontinuance and the person's responses to being out of restraints.

Most psychiatric units use restraint records to document nursing observations.

TYPES OF RESTRAINTS

Wrist and Ankle (Limb) Restraints. Wrist and ankle (limb) restraints are used when it is necessary to significantly restrict motion of the limbs, to prevent harm to self or others, to prevent harm to the person (e.g., removal of tubes, dressings), and to immobilize a part for a procedure (e.g., wound suturing). Wrist and ankle restraints may be leather, linen, or plastic (Fig. 37–23).

Key points to remember about wrist and ankle restraints include the following.

- ▶ Protect the client from hazards, as discussed before.
- ▶ Pad skin under leather restraints well with abdominal dressings to avoid skin damage and to ensure proper fit.
- ▶ Fasten wrist straps below the person's waist and ankle straps below the knees.
- ▶ Clean and powder the wrists and ankles before applying restraints and whenever restraints are removed.
- ▶ *Always* use wrist restraints when ankle restraints are

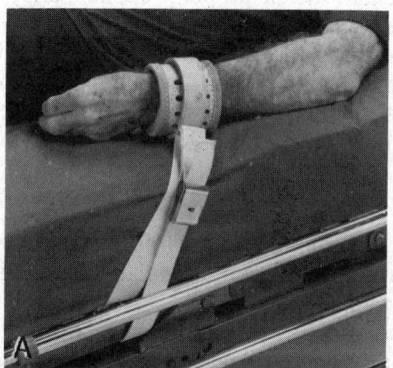
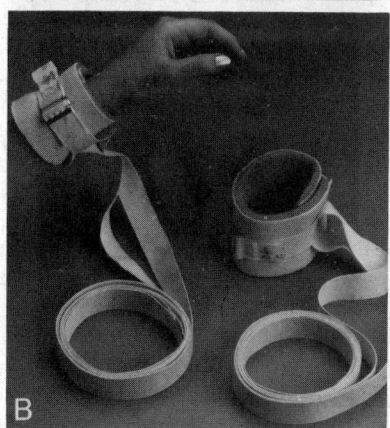

▲ *Figure 37–23*

Limb restraints. *A*, Leather. *B*, Linen. (Courtesy of J. T. Posey Co.)

used, or the person may remove the ankle restraints or commit suicide (intentional or accidental) by hanging by the heels.

▶ Allow enough slack on the straps so that the person's arms and legs can be moved if desired.

▶ Remove and reapply restraints at least every two hours during the day and every four hours at night.

▶ Remove only one restraint at a time if you are alone and if the person might harm himself or herself or others.

▶ Change the person's position at least every two hours.

▶ Frequently assess areas distal to restraints to make certain neurologic or circulatory impairment is not present.

▶ Assess a restrained individual soon after restraints are applied and reassess frequently thereafter.

▶ Assess respiratory status at least every eight hours with continuous restraint (see Chapter 45).

▶ Frequently assess the volume and nature of urine output (see Chapter 44). Muscle damage from the person pulling against restraints may cause renal failure as a result of renal tubular obstruction by large myoglobin molecules. Laboratory urinalysis for myoglobin may be indicated with prolonged restraint use when the person actively pulls against them.

Chest or Waist Restraints. Chest or waist restraints can prevent a person from getting out or falling out of bed or a chair. When properly applied, they allow full arm and leg movements and a fair degree of freedom. Waist restraint is a gentle "reminder" for mildly confused people. Chest restraints are more appropriate for agitated people. Chest and waist restraints are made of cotton, muslin, or mesh and can be washed often.

Key points to remember about chest and waist restraints include the following.

▶ Protect the client from hazards, as discussed before.

▶ Clean and dry the skin, especially the axillae, before restraint application.

▶ Make sure there are no wrinkles or bulges in the restraint that could damage skin after application.

▶ Assess the person's respiratory rate at least every hour to ensure that the restraint is not interfering with ventilation.

▶ Use a chest restraint, not a waist restraint, for restraint in a chair or wheelchair. Also, place the chair's back against a wall to prevent the chair from tipping back. Lock wheelchair wheels.

▶ Remember, pressure areas on the sacrum and buttocks may quickly develop from sitting in a chair. Use a gel-filled cushion (flotation therapy pad) or other cushion on the chair seat as needed. Do not leave people restrained in chairs for more than two hours. Some develop pressure sores in even less time (see Chapter 35).

▶ Select a sturdy, comfortable chair in which to restrain the person. Never restrain a person on a commode or rocking chair. They are hard, uncomfortable, and easily tipped over.

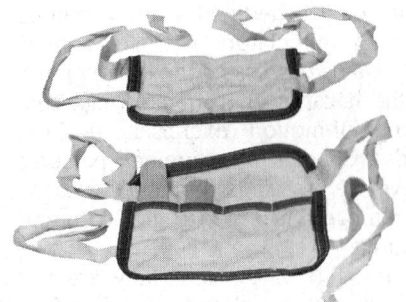
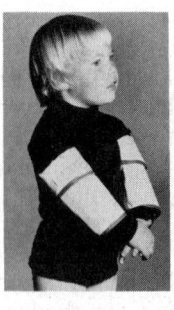

▲ *Figure 37-24*

Elbow immobilizer used to prevent flexion of the elbow. (Courtesy of J. T. Posey Co.)

Chest restraints made from sheets may be used temporarily as bed restraints but are unsafe for restraining a person in a chair. They are either too loose to be effective or too tight to be comfortable. A temporary stretcher restraint can be fashioned from a regular bed sheet. Two people grasp the sheet's two long ends and twirl the sheet until it is a tight roll. Position the roll's middle under the person's upper back and shoulders. Bring the ends under the axillae, over the anterior shoulders, and under the middle portion of the roll. Apply the sheet snugly and cross the ends under the bottom of the stretcher at the level of the head. Tie the ends in a square knot. Avoid undue pressure on the axillae.

Elbow Restraints. Elbow restraints, or immobilizers, prevent bending of the elbow and are used most often for infants and young children. Although they are available commercially (Fig. 37-24), you can make temporary elbow restraints by taping tongue blades together to form a band to secure around the elbow.

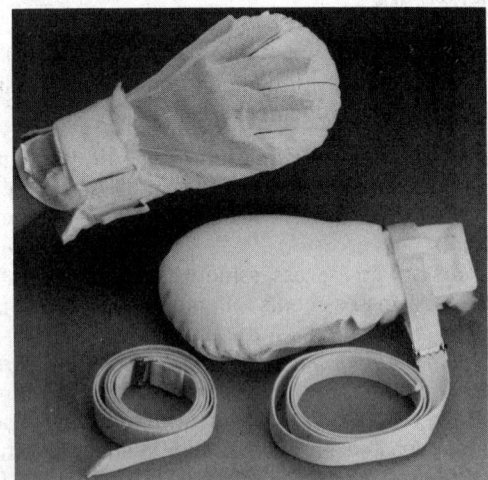

▲ *Figure 37-25*

Closed finger mitt. (Courtesy of J. T. Posey Co.)

Mitt Restraints. Mitts are devices placed over the hands to prevent removal of tubes, dressings, or appliances; trauma to tissue by scratching; or undoing of restraints. Mitt restraints are available commercially (Fig. 37–25), or they can be made from various materials.

Before applying mitts, clean and dry the person's hands. If indicated, use a hand roll to keep the fingers in a position of function. Remove and reapply mitts at least every eight hours. Clean the skin and perform range-of-motion exercises. If hand rolls or very constrictive mitts are used, provide this care more frequently. Mitts are also available with restraint straps to immobilize the limb. When these are used, nursing concerns are the same as for wrist restraints.

Body Restraints. Body restraints are used when it is necessary to immobilize all or most of the body. They are commonly used for children during procedures that require motionlessness (e.g., venipuncture or suturing) and sometimes with combative or hysterical people. Body restraints are usually linen or mesh.

The physiologic and psychologic problems associated with immobility are so great that body restraints should be used for only a short time.

Body restraints are usually used only as a final measure. Providing nursing care is difficult. Nursing concerns are the same as those for four-point (wrist and ankle) restraints.

There is often a need to completely restrain children for special procedures. This can be done in several ways. The most readily available restraint is the sheet mummy. Place the child on the center of a regular sheet folded to size. Place the child's arms against the sides of the body and straighten the legs. Bring one side of the sheet over across the body and tuck it under the body on the opposite side, encasing the arms and legs securely. Repeat with the opposite side of the sheet. The child's weight usually keeps the sheet taut, or it may be secured with pins.

A commercially made mummying device (Olympic Papoose Board) comes in three sizes for use with clients aged two years through adulthood. Three sets of closing canvas flaps fold across the body and fasten with Velcro (Fig. 37–26). Various body areas can be exposed for treatment or examination while maintaining restraint. The flaps are attached to a rigid board.

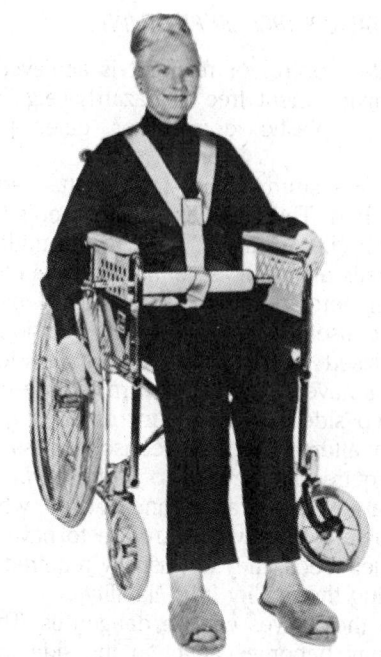

▲ *Figure 37–27*

Wheelchair safety bar. (Courtesy of J. T. Posey Co.)

Accessories for the board for young children include arm and head immobilizers.

Total body restraint of an adult is difficult without special equipment. Applying total body restraints on a combative adult client requires at least four people if other restraints are not already in place. In a disaster, immediate total body restraint of a hysterical person may have to be done without special equipment. Temporary restraint may be accomplished by sandwiching the person between two canvas litters and securing both litters with a litter strap. This is not an appropriate restraint under normal circumstances. Replace this type of restraint with other restraints or therapeutic measures as soon as possible.

Another body restraint is a wheelchair bar restraint. It is used mainly to prevent a wheelchair occupant from slipping down in the chair or falling out. It is a metal bar that slips through holes in the sides of the armrest supports after the person is seated in the wheelchair. Chest restraints may be attached to the bar (Fig. 37–27).

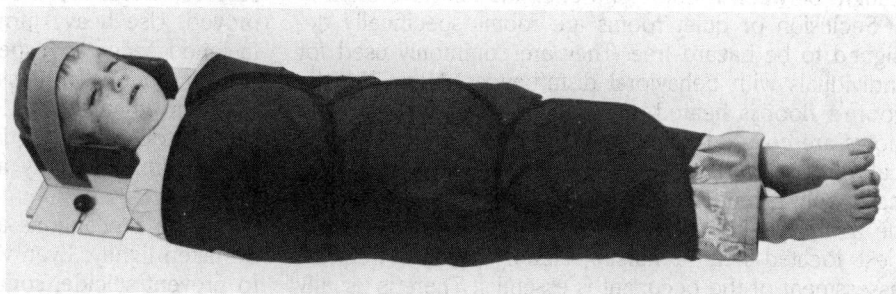

▲ *Figure 37–26*

Olympic Papoose Board with a head immobilizer on a child. (Courtesy of Olympic Medical, Seattle, WA 98108.)

ENVIRONMENTAL CONTROL OR RESTRAINT

Environmental control or restraint is achieved by providing an environment free of hazards (e.g., with side rails, netting, plastic domes, or quiet [seclusion] rooms).

Side rails are sturdy metal frames attached to both sides of the bed. They may extend the bed's full length or half length (i.e., from the head to the middle of the bed). Side rails are used as gentle reminders to prevent people from getting out or falling out of bed. (They also may be useful in turning.) The decision to keep side rails raised is usually a nursing decision. Some care facilities have guidelines governing side rail use. In general, keep side rails raised for children and for all people with altered levels of consciousness. Facilities may also require all side rails to be raised at night and possibly that they be raised and locked whenever a bed is occupied. If individuals refuse to have side rails raised on their beds, they are usually required to sign a form releasing the facility from liability.

Side rails themselves can be dangerous. The person or others may become caught in the side rails, especially folding models. Serious falls may occur if confused individuals or those unable to get attention climb over the side rails or go over the end of the bed, especially at night. Because of the increased height from the top of the side rail to the floor, it may be safer to leave side rails down. When side rails are used, inform the person that they are used to ensure safety, especially because health care facility beds and stretchers are usually much higher and narrower than beds used at home.

Safety straps can prevent falls from narrow stretchers or tables (e.g., operating room tables). Place the straps 15 cm (6 in) above the knees and at waist level. Explain the purpose of the straps.

Netting, to keep individuals in bed, is most often used on children's cribs. It ties all around the top and sides of the crib and must be secure. Be aware that children have climbed over the crib sides between the bed frame and the netting and have been caught in the netting, dying from asphyxiation. All ends of the netting must be tied securely to the frame of the bed.

Plastic domes or bubbles, used for the same reasons as netting, are rapidly replacing netting. The domes fit over a crib's top, allowing the child to stand in the crib and see more of the environment. Not all domes fit all cribs. Make sure to use the correct dome. Gaps between the dome and the crib are dangerous and must be eliminated by using the correct dome. Children caught between a dome and crib side rail have died.

Seclusion or quiet rooms are rooms specifically designed to be hazard free. They are commonly used for individuals with behavioral disturbances. Normally, the room's floor is heated, the walls are padded, any windows are covered with heavy screening, and all electrical outlets or fixtures are inaccessible. These rooms have only a mattress or no furniture at all. There may be a drain in the floor for fluids. Seclusion rooms are best located near a nursing station because frequent assessment of the occupant is essential. There is usually a heavy door that can be locked and an observation window.

Use of a quiet room may be indicated for agitated, assaultive, suicidal, or homicidal individuals. It may also be used to minimize stimuli, such as for a person in a manic state. (A manic state is characterized by increased motor activity and expansive emotional states like overtalkativeness and elation.) A quiet room is often used temporarily until medications take effect. Some individuals ask to go to the quiet room when they feel a need to gain self-control or they desire the security of a locked room.

Visit individuals in seclusion at least every half-hour. All personnel on duty must carry the key to the quiet room whenever locked seclusion is used, in case of emergency.

As with other restrained people, those in seclusion are totally dependent on care providers. It is often valuable to set a time limit on the length of stay in seclusion, especially if seclusion is not voluntary. It is essential to document the behavior that precipitated the use of seclusion, whether seclusion was voluntary or involuntary, the time seclusion started and terminated, an accurate account of the person's behavior during staff visits, the times of staff visits, and the individual's response to seclusion. (See previous discussions of documentation.)

Suicide Precautions

Suicide precautions is the term given to actions taken by the staff to prevent a person from self-harm. Care facilities often have specific guidelines identifying what suicide precautions to use. Familiarize yourself with them and with the individual's rights and related legal aspects.

Visit and assess the person at least every 15 minutes. Remove all potentially harmful objects from the person's environment. Search the person and clothes and effects for objects that could be used to inflict harm (e.g., weapons, razor blades, scissors, pencils, eating utensils, pills, anything that can be harmfully ingested). Glass in any form (e.g., bottles, light bulbs, eyeglasses, and glass from flashlights) can be broken and eaten or used to cut or puncture. Remove objects that could be used by the person for electrocution (e.g., electric cords) or hanging (e.g., shoestrings, belts, headbands, scarves, underwear). At times, bed linens are also removed. Use heavy furniture, or make sure furniture is fastened securely (especially lamps). Do not leave the person alone in an unsafe environment (e.g., examining room, room that could be jumped out of or run away from). Lock all potentially dangerous medical supplies and equipment safely away. Lock restraints if they are required.

Suicide precautions are a serious intervention not to be taken lightly. Even with a staff's most diligent efforts to prevent suicide, some individuals may still take their lives. This causes tremendous guilt feelings among staff members. These feelings may be reduced somewhat if the staff made every effort to prevent the death. There are significant legal ramifications if it can be demonstrated that staff failed to take the appropriate precautions. Documentation of all assessment and intervention (including suicide precautions) is extremely important.

EVALUATION

Evaluation of the client for achievement of the outcomes listed in this chapter requires assessing the client for evidence of disuse syndrome. Because disuse phenomena can occur in every system of the body, a thorough physical and mental assessment is required. Besides looking for evidence of disuse syndrome, the assessment should also demonstrate the absence of any history of injury during the time the device was in place. This is particularly important in view of the many possible complications that can occur with some of the assistive devices used.

In addition to noting the absence of negative findings, the final evaluation should show positive evidence that the client has been participating in a rehabilitation

CASE STUDY

The Client

Tim Worth, a 46-year-old man, was admitted to the hospital 26 days ago through the emergency department. He had attempted to kill himself and sustained a gunshot wound of the left thorax with a metal fragment 1 inch from the heart. He was in intensive care and intermediate care for three weeks before being moved to a surgical unit five days ago.

At the time of his move to the surgical unit, at 1 PM, November 4, a partial listing of the nurse's psychosocial assessment read as follows.

▶ 46-year-old white male with sad affect admitted 21 days ago with a GSW of Lt. thorax, following suicide attempt.
▶ Stated he is married and the father of two girls, ages 10 and 15.
▶ Claims affiliation with the Church of Christ but is not currently active.
▶ Recently retired after 24 years in the military and took a "highly stressful" job in a local high-school ROTC program.
▶ Admitted past history of daily alcohol use to deal with stress but denies drinking for past year. Stated he quit at wife's insistence.

▶ He and wife currently going through divorce proceedings with wife planning to move to another state with the two children.
▶ Has attended several coping and stress reduction courses presented through the army. States he found deep breathing and the use of imagery ineffective for him but has found physical exercise to be an appropriate way to relieve stress, and he likes to jog every day after work.
▶ Stated he has recently been working several 20-hour days each week, sleeping only two hours per night in order to get to work, and has been unable to do his exercises to relieve tension.
▶ Attributes his recent crisis to the divorce and to his stresses at work without the ability to exercise. States, "The depression sort of snuck up on me."

Five days have passed since this assessment by the nurse. The following represents part of a nursing care plan written for him at the time of assessment and the current evaluation of outcomes that were expected at that time.

CARE PLAN

2 PM, November 4

Nursing Diagnosis	Planning: Expected Outcomes	Implementation: Nursing Interventions	Evaluation
High Risk for Violence: Self-directed R/T recent history of suicide attempt secondary to depression and inability to cope with stresses of job and divorce	By 4 PM, November 9: ▶ Verbalizes no suicide plans.	▶ With client, establish times to sit and talk bid for 20 minutes. ▶ Attempt to draw him out so he can discuss his feelings about his life stresses and the suicide attempt.	4 PM, November 9 ▶ On November 5, talked with nurse from 9 to 9:20 AM and 5 to 5:20 PM and discussed recent feelings about his divorce and job. ▶ Stated that he is worried that he may

Care Plan continued on following page

CARE PLAN (Continued)

2 PM, November 4

Nursing Diagnosis	Planning: Expected Outcomes	Implementation: Nursing Interventions	Evaluation
		▶ Use active listening to show caring.	get depressed again and that he finds thoughts of being alone to be depressing. ▶ Did not express suicidal thoughts at this time.
		▶ Ask directly about suicidal thoughts and plans.	▶ On November 9, stated in two separate interviews that he was not inclined to commit suicide and could "never conceive of doing this again."
	▶ Verbalizes at least two healthy ways of coping with stress.	▶ Discuss with client option for dealing with stress.	▶ Client stated he will look for another job that is lower in stress and will continue to run. He may also join a health club.

program, providing self-care, and decreasing use of analgesics.

For the client who required restraints for prevention of self-mutilation or violence to self or others, it is necessary to document only the fact that the client's safety and the safety of others were maintained. However, this is a minimal expectation. It would be better to provide positive evidence that the client is making some changes away from the use of destructive behaviors toward more positive ways of coping. Examples might be documentation of the client's verbalizing thoughts and feelings instead of acting them out or documentation of the client's attendance at, and participation in, an individual or group therapy program.

Summary

▶ Many medical conditions require the use of protective and supporting devices. Examples include orthopedic disorders such as fractures, sprains, and strains; neuromuscular disorders such as CVA, spinal cord injury, multiple sclerosis, Parkinson's disease, and cerebral palsy; and behavioral and neurologic disorders such as neurologic or mental deficiencies.

▶ Before using any protective or supportive device, assess the total person in all body systems, including psychosocial assessment as a baseline for comparison with ongoing assessments.

▶ Persons requiring protective or supportive devices frequently have nursing diagnoses of *High Risk for Disuse Syndrome* and *High Risk for Violence, Self-directed or Directed at others*.

▶ Expected outcomes for clients with protective and supportive devices include safe use of the device and prevention of complications.

▶ Casts and traction are orthopedic devices used to immobilize fractured bones and joints and maintain alignment until the bone can heal. Splints and braces are used to immobilize body parts. Splints are used to decrease mobility of a part. Braces may be used to support limbs for ambulation. Braces may also be used prophylactically. Binders are devices used for support of skin and underlying structures. Binders, especially chest binders, should be used cautiously with thought to the risk of restriction of function.

▶ Restraints should be used under the guiding principle of caring for the person in the least restrictive environment that is safe for the person. Before applying restraints, you should be clear on the legality of the action under the circumstances. Institutional policy should be precisely followed. Restraints can be chemical, environmental, or physical. Alternatives to restraints should be considered and tried before restraints are employed.

▶ Evaluation includes an assessment of the client for evidence of the safe use of the protective or supportive device, including prevention of complications such as disuse phenomena.

Bibliography

1. (1992). HCFA issues rule on nurse staffing and restraints in nursing homes. *Minnesota-Nursing-Accent*, 64(4), 9.
2. Barrett, J.B., & Bryant, B.H. (1990). Fractures: types, treatment, perioperative implications. *AORN Journal*, 52(4), 755-756, 758, 760-761.
3. Bjorn, P.R. (1991). An approach to the potentially violent patient. *Journal of Emergency Nursing*, 17(5), 336-339.
4. Black, J.M., & Matassarin-Jacobs, E. (1993). *Luckmann and Sorensen's medical-surgical nursing: A psychophysiologic approach*. Philadelphia: W. B. Saunders.
5. Blakeslee, J.A., et al. (1991). Making the transition to restraint free care. *Journal of Gerontological Nursing*, 17(2), 4-8.
6. Brower, T.H. (1991). The alternatives to restraints. *Journal of Gerontological Nursing*, 17(2), 18-22.
7. Burl, M.M., et al. (1992). The effect of cervical collars on walking balance. *Physiotherapy*, 78(1), 19-22.
8. Calfee, B.E. (1991). Protecting yourself from allegations of nursing negligence. *Nursing*, 21(12), 34-40.
9. Cawley, P.W., et al. (1991). The current state of functional knee bracing research: a review of the literature. *American Journal of Sports Medicine*, 19(3), 226-233.
10. Chenitz, W.C., et al. (1991). *Clinical gerontological nursing*. Philadelphia: W. B. Saunders.
11. Condie, D.N. (1990). Lower limb orthotics. *Current Opinion in Orthopaedics*, 1(3), 462-465.
12. Craig, C., et al. (1989). Seclusion and restraints: decreasing the discomfort. *Journal of Psychosocial Nursing and Mental Health Services*, 27(7), 16-19.
13. Cutcliffe, N., & Prugger, A. (1990). Adapted clothing for patients in halo traction. *Canadian Journal of Occupational Therapy*, 57(1), 39-42.
14. Dunst, R.M. (1990). Legg-Calvé-Perthes disease. *Orthopaedic Nursing*, 9(2), 18-27, 35-36.
15. Dunwoody, C.J. (1991). Pelvic fracture patient care: reflections on the past, complications for the future. *Nursing Clinics of North America*, 26(1), 65-72.
16. Eimer, M. (1989). Management of the behavioral symptoms associated with dementia. *Primary Care: Clinics in Office Practice*, 16(2), 431-450.
17. Escher, J.E., et al. (1989). Typical geriatric accidents and how to prevent them. *Geriatrics*, 44(5), 54-56, 66-69.
18. Evans, L.K., & Strumpf, N.E. (1989). Tying down the elderly: a review of the literature on physical restraint. *Journal of the American Geriatric Society*, 37(1), 65-74.
19. Faber, H. (1990). Restraint-free care: is it possible? (editorial). *Journal of Gerontological Nursing*, 16(10), 4-5.
20. Feller, N.G., et al. (1989). Helping staff nurses become mini-specialists . . . cast care. *American Journal of Nursing*, 89(7), 991-992.
21. Fisher, F.R. (1991). Assistive devices in rehabilitation: a time for change. *Canadian Journal of Rehabilitation*, 5(2), 67-69.
22. Flenner, T.J., & Meek, M. (1991). A stump protector for the person with a lower extremity amputation. *American Journal of Occupational Therapy*, 45(2), 171-172.
23. Gerding, D.N., et al. (1991). Saving the diabetic foot. *Patient Care*, 25(4), 84-88, 90, 97-98.
24. Graebe, R. H. (1991). Comparisons of heel pressure reducing devices. *Decubitus*, 4(4), 4, 12.
25. Hall, J.K. (1990). Understanding the fine line between law and ethics. *Nursing*, 20(10), 34-40.
26. Heckman, J.D. (1991). Fractures: emergency care and complications. *Clinical Symposia*, 43(3), 2-32.
27. Hilt, N.E., & Cogburn, S.B. (1980). *Manual of orthopedics*. St. Louis: C.V. Mosby.

28. Holm, K., & Hedricks, C. (1989). Immobility and bone loss in the aging adult. *Critical Care Nursing Quarterly*, 12(1), 46-51.
29. Houston, K.A. (1990). Restraints: how do you score? *Geriatric Nursing*, 11(5), 231-232.
30. Johnson, J.C. (1990). Delirium in the elderly. *Emergency Medicine Clinics of North America*, 8(2), 255-265.
31. Johnson, R.J., et al. (1990). Management of knee injuries in athletes. *Current Opinion in Orthopaedics*, 1(3), 382-387.
32. Kallmann, S.L., et al. (1992). Comfort, safety and independence: restraint release and its challenges. *Geriatric Nursing*, 13(3), 143-148.
33. Kanak, M.F. (1992). Interventions related to patient safety. *Nursing Clinics of North America*, 27(2), 371-395.
34. Kapp, M.B. (1989). Aggressive residents and families: rights and responsibilities. *Journal of Long Term Care Administration*, 17(3), 12-17.
35. Kay, J. (1990). Trying to keep a balance . . . difficulties of being disabled. *Nursing Times*, 86(19), 37.
36. Kortman, B. (1992). Patient recall and understanding of instructions concerning splints following a zone 2 flexor tendon repair. *Australian Occupational Therapy Journal*, 39(2), 5-11.
37. Larsen, L.L. (1991). Nurses still tied in knots over restraint use. *CONA Journal ACIIO*, 13(3), 12-14.
37a. Leape, L.L., & Brennan, T. (1992). *The preventability of medical injury*. Paper delivered at a meeting of the American Academy of Arts and Sciences.
38. Malick, M.H. (1990). Upper limb orthotics. *Current Opinion in Orthopaedics*, 1(3), 450-454.
39. Marr, J., & Edmonds, V. (1990). Cervical orthoses: the issue of patient compliance. *Journal of Neuroscience Nursing*, 22(2), 104-107.
40. Martinez, A.J., & Lee, M.J. (1992). A step-by-step look at lower extremity trauma. *Journal of Emergency Medical Services*, 17(4), 42-43, 45-49, 52.
41. Masters, R., & Marks, S.F. (1990). The use of restraints. *Rehabilitation Nursing*, 15(1), 22-25.
42. McConnell, E.A. (1991). Correctly positioning an arm sling. *Nursing*, 21(7), 70.
43. Meehan, M. (1992). Nursing Dx: potential for aspiration. *RN*, 55(1), 30-35.
44. Miller, P. (1989). Safe in a cocoon . . . restraints. *Nursing Times*, 85(41), 38-40.
45. Mitchell, J., & Varley, C. (1990). Isolation and restraint in juvenile correctional facilities. *Journal of the American Academy of Child and Adolescent Psychiatry*, 29(2), 251-255.
46. Mobily, P.R., & Herr, K.A. (1992). Back pain in the elderly. *Geriatric Nursing: American Journal of Care for the Aging*, 13(2), 110-116.
47. Morrison, J., et al. (1987). Formulating a restraint use policy. *Journal of Nursing Administration*, 17(3), 39-42.
48. Mourad, L.A. (1991). *Orthopedic disorders*. St. Louis: Mosby Year Book.
49. Mourad, L.A., & Droste, M.M. (1993). *The nursing process in the care of adults with orthopedic conditions*. Albany, NY: Delmar Publishing Company.
50. Nesbitt, L. (1992). A practical guide to prescribing orthoses. *Physician and Sports Medicine*, 20(5), 76-78, 83-87.
51. North, B., et al. (1992). Living in a halo. *American Journal of Nursing*, 92(4), 54-56.
52. Ohman, K., & Spaniol, D. (1990). Halo immobilization: discharge planning and patient education. *Journal of Neuroscience Nursing*, 22(6), 351-357.
53. Palmer, P., & Simons, J. (1991). Joint protection: a critical review. *British Journal of Occupational Therapy*, 54(12), 453-458.
54. Rader, J. (1991). Modifying the environment to decrease use of restraints. *Journal of Gerontological Nursing*, 17(2), 9-13.
55. Rasin, J.H. (1990). Confusion. *Nursing Clinics of North America*, 25(4), 909-918.
56. Redheffer, G.M., & Bailey, M. (1989). Assessing and splinting fractures. *Nursing*, 19(6), 51-59.
57. Rothenberg, J.R. (1991). Innovations in treating anterior cruciate ligament deficiency part 1. *Orthopaedic Nursing*, 10(2), 17-25.
58. Salmond, S.W. (ed.). (1991). *Core curriculum for orthopaedic nursing*. Pitman, NJ: National Association of Orthopaedic Nurses.

59. *SCD compression system: Procedure guide for controller model #5325.* (Booklet.) Mansfield, MA: Kendall Healthcare Products Company.

60. Schaming, D., et al. (1990). When babies are born with orthopedic problems. *RN,* 53(4), 62–67.

61. Scherer, Y.K., et al. (1991). The nursing dilemma of restraints. *Journal of Gerontological Nursing,* 17(2), 14–17.

62. Selbst, S.M., & Henretig, F.M. (1989). The treatment of pain in the emergency department. *Pediatric Clinics of North America,* 36(4), 965–978.

63. Shurr, D.G., & Cook, T.M. (1990). *Prosthetics and orthotics.* New York: Appleton and Lange.

64. Slye, D.A., & Theis, L.M. (1991). *An introduction to orthopedic nursing: An orientation module.* Pitman, NJ: National Association of Orthopaedic Nurses.

65. Stilling, L. (1992). The pros and cons of physical restraints and behavior controls. *Journal of Psychosocial Nursing and Mental Health Services,* 30(3), 18–20, 33–34.

66. Stilwell, E.M. (1991). Nurses' education related to the use of restraints. *Journal of Gerontological Nursing,* 17(2), 23–26.

67. Strumpf, N.E., & Evans, L.K. (1991). The ethical problems of prolonged physical restraint. *Journal of Gerontological Nursing,* 17(2), 27–30.

68. Strumpf, N.E., et al. (1990). Restraint free care: from dream to reality. *Geriatric Nursing,* 11(3), 122–124.

69. Taliaferro, E.H. (1992). Coping with the violent patient. *Emergency Medicine,* 24(7), 155–156, 161–164.

70. Tammelleo, A.D. (1992). Restraints: a legal Catch-22? *RN,* 55(4), 71–72, 75–76.

71. Thackrey, M., & Bobbitt, R.G. (1990). Patient aggression against clinical and nonclinical staff in a VA medical center. *Hospital and Community Psychiatry,* 41(2), 195–197.

72. Thomas, L. (1988). Holding forth . . . the use of restraint in the care of elderly. *Geriatric Nursing and Home Care,* 8(2), 18.

73. Tinetti, M., et al. (1992). Mechanical restraint use and fall-related injuries among residents of skilled nursing facilities. *Annals of Internal Medicine,* 116(5), 369–374.

74. Wasserberger, J., et al. (1992). Violence in the emergency department. *Topics in Emergency Medicine,* 14(2), 71–78.

75. Wiest, M. (1990). The dilemma of using physical restraints. *Rehabilitation Nursing,* 15(5), 267–268.

76. U.S. Health Care Financing Administration. (1988). *Medicare/Medicaid nursing home information: 1987–1988.* Washington, DC: U.S. Government Printing Office.

77. The Zimmer Traction Handbook (1989). Warsaw, IN: Zimmer, Inc.

▼ *Promoting Hygiene*

The amount of relief and comfort experienced by the sick after skin has been carefully washed and dried, is one of the commonest observations made at a sick bed. But it must not be forgotten that the comfort and relief so obtained are not all. They are, in fact, nothing more than a sign that the vital powers have been relieved by removing something that was oppressing them.

Florence Nightingale
Notes on Nursing

▼ CHAPTER OUTLINE

HYGIENE CARE IN HISTORICAL
   PERSPECTIVE
TYPES OF HYGIENE CARE
INDIVIDUAL VARIATIONS IN HYGIENE
   PRACTICES
TERRITORIALITY
GENERAL HYGIENE CARE
   Assessment
   Nursing Diagnosis
   Planning
   Nursing Intervention
   Evaluation
ELIMINATION HYGIENE
   Bedpans and Urinals
   Assessment
   Nursing Diagnosis
   Planning
   Nursing Intervention
   Evaluation
ASSISTING WITH HANDWASHING
MAINTAINING ORAL HEALTH
   Oral Cavity Alterations
   Assessment
   Nursing Diagnosis
   Planning
   Nursing Intervention
   Evaluation
HYGIENE FOR THE EYES
   Assessment
   Nursing Diagnosis
   Planning

   Nursing Intervention
   Evaluation
HYGIENE FOR THE EARS
   Assessment
   Nursing Diagnosis
   Planning
   Nursing Intervention
   Evaluation
HYGIENE FOR THE NOSE
   Assessment
   Nursing Diagnosis
   Planning
   Nursing Intervention
   Evaluation
SKIN HYGIENE
   Skin Structure and Function
   Self-Care of the Skin
   Skin Integrity
   Assessment
   Nursing Diagnosis
   Planning
   Nursing Intervention
   Evaluation
PERINEAL CARE
   Perineal Area
   Principles of Perineal Care
   Assessment
   Nursing Diagnosis
   Planning
   Nursing Intervention
   Evaluation

▼ **CHAPTER OUTLINE** Continued

NAIL AND FOOT CARE
  Assessment
  Nursing Diagnosis
  Planning
  Nursing Intervention
  Evaluation
HAIR CARE
  Hair Structure and Function

Assessment
Nursing Diagnosis
Planning
Nursing Intervention
Evaluation
COSMETIC CARE AS HYGIENE
COMFORT AND CLEANLINESS IN BED
  Bed Linens

Assessment
Nursing Diagnosis
Planning
Nursing Intervention
Evaluation
CASE STUDY

▼ **KEY TERMS**

Alopecia	Cheilosis	Halitosis	Pediculosis pubis	Smegma
Bedside commode	Dandruff	Hygiene	Perianal area	Stomatitis
Calculus	Deciduous teeth	Pediculosis	Perineal hygiene	Tartar
Caries	Dental plaque	Pediculosis capitis	Periodontal disease	Xerostomia
Cerumen	Gingivitis	Pediculosis corporis	Sebaceous glands	

▼ **LEARNING OBJECTIVES**

After studying this chapter, you should be able to

1. Describe how to assess a client to determine specific hygiene needs and the amount of assistance needed for hygiene.
2. Identify the main nursing diagnoses related to hygiene or grooming.
3. State outcomes appropriate for specific clients with a diagnosis of Self-Care Deficit.
4. Describe nursing interventions used to meet the needs of clients with a diagnosis of Self-Care Deficit.
5. Identify methods to evaluate the client following nursing interventions for Self-Care Deficit in hygiene or grooming.
6. Describe hygiene care for the client who must use a bedpan, urinal, or bedside commode.
7. Describe oral care, including brushing and flossing teeth and care of dentures.
8. Explain eye care, including eye care for the comatose client.
9. Explain ear care, including placement and care of a hearing aid.
10. Describe nasal care, including indications and contraindications related to nasal suctioning.
11. Explain the bathing of a client who has a self-care deficit in hygiene.
12. Describe extra measures that may be necessary in the bathing of the elderly client.
13. Compare perineal care for male and female clients.
14. Describe the methods used to care for the feet and nails.
15. Explain the importance of grooming in daily nursing care.
16. Describe hair care, including shampooing and combing hair for clients.
17. Contrast procedures for bedmaking.
18. State the rationale for straightening the bed linens at several times during the day.

Hygiene is a set of practices that are conducive to the preservation of health, such as cleanliness. In normal everyday life, we meet our own needs for hygiene. During illness, however, problems such as vomiting, diarrhea, excessive perspiration, and prolonged time in bed can increase our needs for hygiene at the very time we have a decreased ability to take care of them. Good hygiene and its accompanying physical and psychologic comfort create a feeling of well-being that is very beneficial during illness. Good hygiene is also crucial to a reduction in the incidence of infection. For these reasons, assisting people with activities of hygiene has always been a fundamental part of nursing. As a nurse you will often partially or totally provide for all your clients' hygiene needs.

Assistance with hygiene is a vital nursing function that greatly contributes to the person's general well-being and recovery. Interaction with the client during hygiene activities also provides an opportunity for you to establish rapport, demonstrate caring, and explore cultural values that might affect care. Meeting hygiene needs includes any or all of the following activities: cleansing the body, including the eyes, ears, nose, and perineum; providing oral hygiene, including denture care; cleansing and grooming the hair; shaving the face or other body parts; and providing nail and foot care. Changing the bed linens is also a part of hygiene care. Most hospital beds are now changed at least once a day for every client, but because most people do not change their bed linens every day at home, this practice is being explored. Certainly, if linens are soiled with drainage, perspiration, or food, they must be changed, but it may not be cost effective to continue to change linens daily for ambulatory clients who do not have soiled sheets.

Personal hygiene practices develop during childhood and are influenced by cultural background and the teachings of significant others. Family and cultural influences have more influence on actual hygiene behaviors than do scientific principles. Nurses' attitudes about cleanliness and privacy and their teaching regarding hygiene, however, can have a positive influence on the people they care for. It is therefore vitally important that you are accepting of people in your care, regardless of their previous hygiene practices. At the same time, you must apply basic principles to meet clients' current needs for hygiene and physical comfort. As you provide for cleanliness and comfort, you can also assess the person's overall condition; teach appropriate hygiene, comfort, and self-care; and assess the person's psychosocial needs.

HYGIENE CARE IN HISTORICAL PERSPECTIVE

Historically, hygiene practices have been influenced by social norms, religious rituals, the environment (e.g., availability of water for bathing), and the evolution of hygiene aids (bathtubs, soap, and electric devices such as hair dryers and razors). Hygiene practices in health care facilities originated with the need for sanitary conditions that would promote healing and prevent the spread of disease. Unfortunately, some hygiene practices in care facilities have become ritualistic tasks, such as requiring a daily bath regardless of need.

TYPES OF HYGIENE CARE

The following terms are commonly used in health care facilities to describe hygiene care. Become familiar with them and look for their application in clinical areas.

▶ Complete morning care: Complete bath and perineal care; back massage; oral, hair, and nail care; and complete bed linen change.
▶ Partial morning care: Washing the person's face and hands, providing oral and hair care, bathing areas of the body that have the most secretions (e.g., axillae and perineum), changing soiled linens and pillow case.
▶ Early-morning care: (Often provided by the night staff to prepare people for breakfast or early-morning diagnostic tests); usually refers to refreshing comfort measures such as offering bedpan or urinal, washing face and hands, providing oral care.
▶ Hour-of-sleep care (HS care: Given in the evening just before a person retires for the night), usually involves oral care; washing face, hands; massaging the back for relaxation; and straightening bed linens and changing soiled linen and clothing as needed.

INDIVIDUAL VARIATIONS IN HYGIENE PRACTICES

We each view hygiene and comfort needs individually. We develop personal views through our life experiences (e.g., cultural and societal background, the practices of significant others, individual lifestyles, physical problems, emotional state, cost, and advertising). For example, we must respect the fact that people from some cultures do not normally use underarm deodorants and, in some cultures, it is strictly forbidden for a man to attend a woman during hygiene activities.

Illness, too, influences personal hygiene habits in various and individual ways. For example, Joe, who usually bathes daily at home, may change his personal hygiene habits in a health care facility. He may refuse to be bathed in bed because he feels dependent and embarrassed.

Illness affects a person's physical condition and may alter hygiene desires and requirements.

Emotional problems may also change hygiene practices. A depressed person may show little interest in maintaining personal hygiene.

Can you think of other reasons for variations?

TERRITORIALITY

Territory refers to the space surrounding each of us in which we satisfy our personal needs for security, fulfillment, and identity. Territory includes not only physical space but also one's own body, information about the self, and one's possessions. All species require areas of territory. Each of us identifies an area as our "own" and defends this territory from intrusion by others. It is important to take territoriality into account when planning nursing care.

Early research studies indicated that men were more anxious about territorial intrusion than were women and that people with physical limitations were more worried about territorial intrusion than were those without physical limitations. Also people with varied cultural backgrounds differed in their territoriality needs.[26,27,58]

Control over personal space (territory) is often limited when a person is in a health care facility. Respect for a person's personal space can be shown by

▶ providing privacy with sufficient screening
▶ knocking on doors before entering a person's room
▶ careful draping to minimize body exposure
▶ ensuring a person time alone with significant others
▶ providing privacy while a person uses the telephone
▶ maintaining privacy in conversation (speak low enough so that others in a multibed room cannot hear your interaction with a particular individual)

Excellent nursing care is always based on careful, individualized assessment and not on ritualized, general practices.

GENERAL HYGIENE CARE

Like all nursing care, hygiene care is based on assessment of individual needs and preferences that helps establish desired goals of care. Some goals of hygiene care include

▶ comfort and relaxation (e.g., feeling refreshed and relaxing tense muscles)
▶ stimulation of circulation (e.g., massage and friction)
▶ cleanliness (e.g., removing necrotic tissue, transient microorganisms, and secretions)
▶ improved self-image (e.g., removing unpleasant odors, enhancing appearance)
▶ skin conditioning (e.g., cleansing, stimulating circulation, minimizing dryness)

When establishing goals, it is essential to consider needs related to a person's developmental stage. The infant needs total hygiene care and must not be allowed to become chilled during bathing activities. The toddler likes to play during the bath and must have time for this. The teenager is likely to be especially modest and needs to be assured that privacy will be protected. Adults have differing skin care needs related to age and skin type. The elderly client may not be used to a daily bath and often needs special cleansing products to prevent further skin dryness.

Assessment

Assisting with daily hygiene activities provides the nurse with an excellent opportunity to learn more about the client while skillfully making observations about the person's condition. For the new nurse, it may be difficult to perform manual skills, make observations, and maintain conversation all at the same time. Communication initiated before starting hygiene care can be relaxing for the person receiving care and can allow a natural flow of interaction throughout the procedure. With increasing skill, you will be able to use your communication skills to learn more and more about the person as an individual with specific needs.

Before beginning hygiene, the following areas should be assessed:

▶ Usual preference as to type of bath and time of day for bathing
▶ Ability to perform own bath or degree of assistance needed
▶ Physician's orders regarding bathing and activity
▶ Ability to perform own grooming
▶ Cultural or other factors that might affect acceptance of hygiene assistance
▶ Developmental stage that might require alteration in usual procedure or equipment for hygiene care
▶ Determination of patient's functional level:
  0 = Independent—needs no assistance
  1 = Needs minimal assistance—for example, the person needs the nurse to provide required equipment
  2 = Needs moderate assistance—for example, the person needs the nurse to supervise the procedure and help with difficult tasks such as washing the back and providing foot care
  3 = Needs considerable assistance—for example, the person needs the nurse to provide most care, allowing person to do what can be done independently
  4 = Totally dependent—the person needs the nurse to provide total care
▶ Ability of caregiver to provide hygiene assistance in the home

Nursing Diagnosis

The nursing diagnosis for the person requiring assistance with hygiene is *Self-Care Deficit, Bathing/Hygiene* (see Nursing Diagnosis Profile). Clients at risk for a self-care deficit include those who have (1) external devices such as IV lines, drainage tubes, catheters, casts, restraints, splints, or traction in place; (2) visual impairment; (3) decreased endurance; (4) impaired mobility or dexterity; (5) pain or discomfort; (6) perceptual or cognitive impairment; (7) musculoskeletal impairment; or (8) neuromuscular disorders.

Planning

Careful planning is essential for effective, efficient provision of hygiene care. Establishing priorities is important whether you are planning care for one or for several people. Multiple factors determine priorities of nursing care:

▶ the person's general physical condition and functional level
▶ individual hygiene requirements
▶ preferences and requests from the person
▶ the number of people for whom you are caring

When caring for several people, consider each person's needs. Determine when and why care will be required. A short time spent planning can prevent many interruptions and frustrations both for you and for those in your care.

It is not always wise to be guided solely by the individual's preferences or specific requests. Before fulfilling a request, consider its therapeutic value. If necessary, discuss the request with the nurse in charge. For example, Megan may avoid oral care because of oral discomfort. She may not realize that oral care may *decrease* the discomfort of her sore mouth. Providing for personal preferences is very important, but if you cannot fulfill a preference, always gently discuss it with the person. Together you and your client can make an alternative plan.

Before beginning a task, carefully consider what equipment and items will be needed so that no more than one trip will need to be made to obtain supplies. Also consider whether there will be interruptions by other personnel for scheduled treatments or tests.

Outcomes for persons with self-care deficit generally include expectations that the person will

NURSING DIAGNOSIS PROFILE

Self-Care Deficit, Bathing/Hygiene
Self-Care Deficit, Dressing/Grooming

Definition. A state in which the individual experiences an impaired ability to perform or complete bathing/hygiene activities or dressing/grooming activities for oneself.

Classification. Moving 6.5.2 and 6.5.3.

Defining Characteristics. Whenever a *Self-Care Deficit, Bathing/Hygiene*, is present, it is usually accompanied by the diagnosis *Self-Care Deficit, Dressing/Grooming*, because the related factors contribute to both types of deficit. The specific signs that a deficit is present are

Bathing/hygiene

▶ inability to wash entire body
▶ inability to get to water source or obtain water
▶ inability to regulate temperature or flow of water
▶ inability to sit or stand while bathing

Grooming/dressing

▶ Impaired ability to obtain or replace items of clothing or toiletries
▶ Impaired ability to put on or take off clothing
▶ Impaired ability to fasten clothing
▶ Inability to maintain groomed appearance

Sample Related Factors. The most common related factors are impaired physical mobility, activity intolerance, pain, depression, severe anxiety, alteration in sensory perception, or cognitive or perceptual impairment.

Concept Description. Bathing/hygiene and dressing/grooming are considered usual activities of daily living (ADLs). These activities for self-care are learned during childhood and influenced by the teaching of parents, significant others, peers, and environmental and cultural factors. These activities become habitual in respect to how, when, where, and under what circumstances they are done. When a physical or psychologic problem interferes with an individual's ability to perform the usual ADLs, the deficit may range from one that is small and requires only minimal assistance from the nurse and other staff members to a deficit that is complete, as when the individual is in a coma and requires that all hygiene and grooming activities be performed for the client.

A disruption in the individual's ability to perform self-care means a loss of control and a threat to the person's self-concept. Signs of fear and anxiety may be displayed as an expression of feelings about becoming dependent on others.

Examples. Depending on the specific assessment data, this diagnostic category could be applicable in the following situations, among others:

▶ The person with temporary paralysis from a cerebrovascular accident, neuromuscular disorder, or spinal cord injury. The period of recovery may be lengthy, or recovery of function may be in question. For such individuals, the nursing diag-

noses would be *Self-Care Deficit, Bathing/Hygiene*, R/T impaired physical mobility and *Self-Care Deficit, Dressing/Grooming*, R/T impaired physical mobility.

▶ The person who is physically able to move but who becomes very easily fatigued, is generally very weak, has a problem with impaired gas exchange, or is in pain and cannot move about much. The person may or may not be expected to regain some ability to perform ADLs. When assessed, it is evident that this person needs to conserve energy. For such individuals, the nursing diagnoses would be *Self-Care Deficit, Bathing/Hygiene*, R/T activity intolerance and *Self-Care Deficit, Dressing/Grooming*, R/T activity intolerance.

▶ The person who is temporarily unable to move or is placed on bed rest by physician's order. Movement is medically contraindicated. The person may be immobilized by a traction device, told not to bear weight to let a wound heal, or placed on bed rest to decrease the edema of congestive heart failure. For such individuals, the nursing diagnoses would be *Self-Care Deficit, Bathing/Hygiene*, R/T impaired physical mobility and *Self-Care Deficit, Dressing/Grooming* R/T impaired physical mobility.

Related/Similar Nursing Diagnoses. Many conditions prevent individuals from performing their own hygiene self-care. If much of the nursing staff's time is spent in assisting an incapacitated individual with self-care, the diagnosis *Self-Care Deficit, Bathing/Hygiene*, or *Self-Care Deficit, Dressing/Grooming*, should be included on the nursing care plan even when other related diagnoses are present. People who only have trouble fastening clothes will require only one diagnosis of *Self-Care Deficit, Dressing/Grooming*, whereas most individuals will have deficits in both bathing and dressing/grooming.

Other nursing diagnoses that often accompany the diagnosis of *Self-Care Deficit* include

▶ *Activity Intolerance*
▶ *Impaired Physical Mobility*
▶ *Impaired Gas Exchange*
▶ *Pain*
▶ *Anxiety*
▶ *Fatigue*
▶ *Sensory/Perceptual Alteration*
▶ *Altered Thought Processes*

These diagnoses may also serve as related factors for a diagnosis of *Self-Care Deficit*. When an individual has one of these other diagnoses, the amount of time that the staff needs to spend with the client on self-care activities should be assessed and a decision made as to whether to include the diagnoses of *Self-Care Deficit, Bathing/Hygiene*, or *Self-Care Deficit, Dressing/Grooming*. Since Medicare and other insurance companies pay hospitals according to justifiable activities and time spent with the individual, it is vitally important to include these diagnoses on the care plan whenever pertinent.

▶ identify preferences regarding self-care activities.

▶ participate in hygiene activities to the greatest extent possible.

▶ demonstrate optimal hygiene after assistance with care.

▶ verbalize a sense of well-being following assistance with hygiene.

▶ resume self-care by a specified date.

Nursing Intervention

GENERAL INTERVENTIONS

Along with the specific interventions for each hygiene activity, the nurse should straighten and clean the person's environment. The bedside unit should be straightened and cleaned at the time of the daily bath. Ask the person to direct the arrangement of personal items (e.g., photos, books, flowers) so that they can be comfortably reached or viewed. Attend to an overflowing trash can and to sources of objectionable room odors. Before hygiene, clear and clean the overbed table for the procedure. When completed you can store personal items so that they are readily available. Be certain that essential items such as water, the call bell, and urinal for the male client are within the person's reach. Before leaving the unit after hygiene care, ask whether the person wants anything else.

As you focus on each individual's needs, adapt routines to suit the person's habits and preferences as much as possible. For example, if a person prefers complete hygiene care at night rather than in the morning, try to fulfill this request.

Be careful to avoid the spread of pathogenic organisms while giving hygiene care. During hygiene care (e.g., perineal care, toileting), organisms can be transmitted by body wastes or exudate (fluid draining from body orifices). Gloves are always used for perineal care and for handling body wastes.

TEACHING PRINCIPLES OF HYGIENE

Correcting misconceptions about hygiene and changing personal hygiene habits can be difficult. Hygiene practices are usually based on culture and customs, not scientific knowledge, and on habits and attitudes that become well-established are resistant to change. For example, a person with very dry skin who has used a particular soap for years may not want to change to a new soap, even if told that the old soap is harmful to the skin.

Teaching about hygiene is most successful after careful planning for teaching and learning. The following points are important in the teaching process:

▶ Know the scientific facts related to hygiene.

▶ Know theories about learning and teaching (e.g., consider the person's readiness for learning).

▶ Never tell an individual that a practice is absolutely wrong, as this judgment may reinforce the habit or make the person resistant to learning.

▶ Provide new information (e.g., explain the advantages of your recommendations).

▶ Incorporate teaching while providing hygiene care.

▶ Above all, be flexible about what is appropriate for this person (for detailed discussion of teaching and learning, see Chapter 26.)

Evaluation

To evaluate your client, you will need to determine the degree to which your client still has a self-care deficit in relation to hygiene. To determine whether outcomes have been achieved, you need to assess your client's current status. Evaluation statements might be

▶ States prefers to shower by self at night.

▶ Assisted with own bath by bathing everything except back and legs. Body clean, well rinsed, and dry.

▶ Independently completed oral hygiene when given equipment. Mouth clean, moist, and odor-free following self-care.

▶ States feels refreshed after hygiene measures completed.

▶ States will attempt own hair care tomorrow.

Document the client's ability to complete self-care. For example,

0930   Assisted with own bathing by washing face and hands. Bed bath completed. Skin intact without reddened areas. Able to brush teeth on right side of mouth. Does not wish to use deodorant.   R. Hupp, S.N.

ELIMINATION HYGIENE

The interaction between the client and the nurse during hygiene care affords an excellent opportunity to identify any problems related to bowel and bladder function. Individuals often need assistance in ambulating to the bathroom, or they require a bedpan for toileting. Dependence on others for assistance with toileting makes many people extremely uncomfortable. A gentle, kind, unhurried approach helps decrease embarrassment. Privacy and relaxation enhance the ability to eliminate.

People who are at high risk of a toileting self-care deficit are often those with impaired mobility. Thus, clients who need help with elimination are people with fractures, those with hip or knee arthroplasty, clients who have had strokes, postoperative clients, those with severe oxygenation problems, and people who are very weakened by a chronic illness. Before starting hygiene care, give the person an opportunity to defecate (have a bowel movement) or void (urinate). Offering time to use the toilet, commode, bedpan, or urinal *before* other hygiene care helps the person feel more relaxed and comfortable. Beginning care with toileting also reduces the possibility of an interruption for elimination during hygiene care. The person may need to defecate or void at any time, but the most common times are upon awakening, before and after meals, and before sleep.

Some individuals have difficulty voiding and need assistance. Measures to assist the person to void include the following:

▶ Running water in the sink so that the client can hear it.

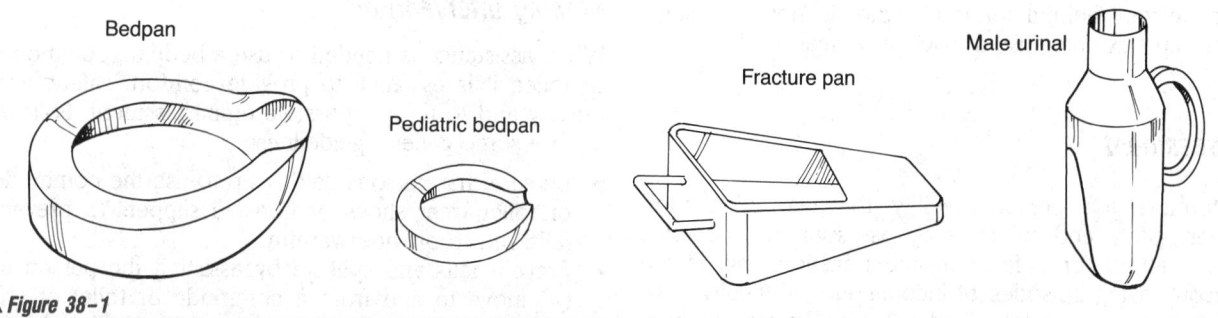

Bedpan   Pediatric bedpan   Fracture pan   Male urinal

▲ *Figure 38-1*

Elimination equipment: bedpan, pedi-pan, fracture pan, and male urinal.

▶ Warming the bedpan before use.
▶ Pouring water over the perineum slowly.
▶ Having the person assume a comfortable position by raising the head of the bed (men often prefer to stand).
▶ Providing sufficient analgesia for pain.
▶ Having the person blow through a straw into a glass of water (this tends to relax the urinary sphincter).

Bedpans and Urinals

A male confined to bed uses a bedpan for defecation and a urinal for voiding (Fig. 38-1). A woman normally uses a bedpan for both defecating and voiding. Female urinals are available but are not common.

Bedpans. Standard bedpans are available in adult and "pedi" (child) sizes and are usually made of plastic, although metal bedpans are sometimes used. Metal bedpans are quite cold unless warmed prior to use. (Put warm, not hot, water in the pan for a few minutes and empty.) A pedi bedpan is sometimes more comfortable for a thin adult or someone with small hips.

A fracture bedpan has a thinner rim than a standard bedpan. A fracture bedpan is designed to be easily placed under a person's buttocks. Be careful, however, because it is easier to spill the contents of the fracture pan. Fracture pans are useful for people who are (a) paralyzed or who cannot be turned safely (e.g., spinal injuries); (b) confined in a body or long leg cast; (c) immobilized by some types of traction; or (d) very thin or emaciated. If the individual is weak or helpless, two people are needed to place and remove the bedpan. This pan minimizes strain on the care provider's back, allows more accurate placement, and is less traumatic for the person. If a person needs the bedpan for a long time, periodically remove and replace the pan to ease pressure and prevent tissue damage. A trapeze bar over the bed is most helpful for the client who is in skeletal leg traction. The bar enables the person to lift up off the mattress so that the bedpan can be placed and removed.

When the client is finished with the bedpan, remove and cover it, carry it to the commode or dirty utility room, and empty and clean it. The bedpan should be dried before putting it in its storage location.

Bedside Commode. A **bedside commode** is a chair or wheelchair with an opening in the center of the seat (Fig. 38-2). The underside of the seat has grooves for insertion of a pail or a bedpan. A bedside commode or toilet is always preferable to a bedpan. Bedpans are uncomfortable and often embarrassing, and sitting on a bedpan in a position that facilitates defecation or urination may be difficult. Bedpans should never be used simply for the convenience of care givers. Encourage use of a bedside commode or toilet unless such activity is contraindicated. When assisting with a bedside commode, observe and dispose of excreta as with the use of a bedpan. Clean the commode after use and return it to the appropriate place.

Toilet. Many clients can use the toilet if they have assistance getting to the bathroom and back to the bed. In the home setting, a bar on one or both bathroom walls can provide a way for people to lower and raise themselves onto the toilet. A raised toilet seat can

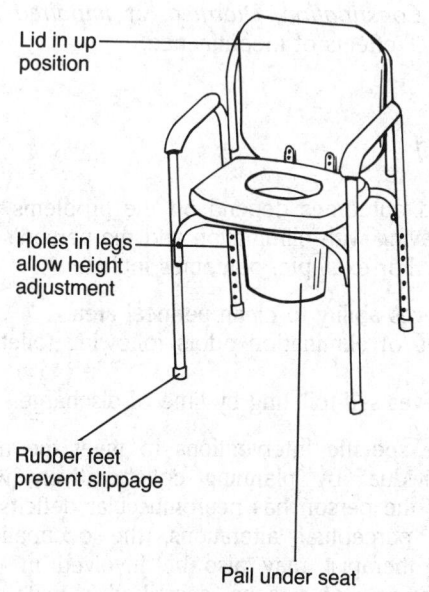

Lid in up position

Holes in legs allow height adjustment

Rubber feet prevent slippage

Pail under seat

▲ *Figure 38-2*

Bedside commode.

also be very helpful for those who do not have sufficient hip flexion to use a toilet of normal height.

Assessment

Determine the person's ability to meet elimination needs safely and privately by assessing the person's usual pattern for defecation and urination first. Is the person having episodes of incontinence, difficulty urinating, constipation, or diarrhea? Also assess the person's degree of independence (level of function) and determine how much assistance is needed. Can the person safely walk unaided to the toilet? Can the person transfer from the wheelchair to the commode? Is the height of the toilet or commode seat appropriate? Does the person experience symptoms of postural hypotension when standing up? Can the client support himself or herself in a sitting position? Does this client need to be reminded not to bear down when defecating (Valsalva maneuver) because of heart problems or increased intracranial pressure? Is a specimen of urine or stool needed? Is a measuring container ("hat") inside the toilet for measurement of output of urine, if needed? Is the urinal kept in a private but convenient spot for the male? Is sufficient toilet paper available? Do specific cultural factors make the person uncomfortable or embarrassed because the nurse must handle wastes?

Nursing Diagnosis

The general nursing diagnosis for people who need assistance with elimination is *Self-Care Deficit, Toileting*, but other, specific nursing diagnoses may apply. As you assist a client with toileting, you can collect data to support other related nursing diagnoses such as *Incontinence, Constipation, Diarrhea*, or *Impaired Skin Integrity* R/T effects of incontinence.

Planning

Expected outcomes depend on the problems the person is having with elimination and the person's level of function. For example, outcomes include

▶ Achieves ability to clean perineal area.
▶ Is free of elimination odors following toileting self-care.
▶ Achieves self-toileting by time of discharge.

Devise specific interventions to meet the needs of the individual by planning collaboratively with the client. If the person has neuromuscular deficits or sensory or perceptual alterations, the occupational or physical therapist may also be involved in planning care. A variety of devices (described in texts on rehabilitation nursing) can make toileting activities easier and safer for the person with disabilities.

Nursing Intervention

When assistance is needed to use a bedpan, commode, or toilet, it is essential to provide comfort, safety, and privacy and to reduce possible embarrassment. Following are some general guidelines:

▶ Be sure that persons getting up to use the commode or toilet wear shoes or nonskid slippers to prevent falls and to provide warmth.
▶ Prevent falls and spillage by assisting the person to (a) move to and from a commode or toilet or (b) get on or off a bedpan, commode, or toilet. Apply principles used for bed-to-chair transfer (see Chapter 35).
▶ Prevent falls by securing commode wheels as the person gets on and off the commode and by directing the client to use grab bars on the wall near the toilet, as needed.
▶ Prevent discomfort and skin breakdown by padding the bedpan or commode for thin or emaciated people.
▶ Stay with individuals who are weak or in danger of falling off the toilet, commode, or bedpan. Use safety belts as appropriate. Frequently observe a restrained person. Raise side rails as necessary.
▶ Place call signal and toilet paper within person's easy reach.
▶ Provide privacy (e.g., close bathroom or room doors, pull curtains, and close window drapes).
▶ Ensure individual's warmth (e.g., place robe or bath blanket around shoulders). Cover the person's legs with a towel or bath blanket while on commode or toilet.
▶ Observe for hypotensive episodes (sudden drop in blood pressure that can cause falls). The person may experience dizziness, appear pale, feel clammy, or have a thready pulse. Falls can usually be prevented by having the person sit on the side of the bed for a few minutes before getting up. Applying pressure on the feet during this time (e.g., by placing feet on the seat of a chair) aids venous return. Allow the body time to adjust to position change.
▶ Frequently observe individuals if elimination could cause excessive fatigue (e.g., weak people), pain (e.g., persons with kidney stones or rectal surgery), or severe complications from the strain of defecation (e.g., some persons with heart or eye problems).
▶ If possible, once the client is safely situated on bedpan, commode, or toilet, provide privacy by leaving the room and remaining outside, within calling distance.
▶ When elimination creates unpleasant odors, promptly air the room without chilling the individual. Use room deodorizers appropriately. Conduct these activities in ways that do not embarrass the person.
▶ Help the client clean the perineum and perianal area as needed (wear gloves).
▶ Assist the person with handwashing and wash your own hands. (See Chapter 28.)

Do not leave weak or helpless people on commodes or bedpans for long periods of time. Being left in this way is demeaning and uncomfortable and may promote skin breakdown by a shearing force on the buttocks (see Chapter 48).

Placing the Bedpan. Provide privacy and explain the procedure so that the person can assist. Raise the bed to a working height and assemble bath blanket, bedpan, bedpan cover, and toilet paper. Fold top bed linen out of the way and cover the client with a bath blanket so that you can see and move the person without unnecessary exposure. Raise the distal side rail (on the opposite side of the bed) for safety and as an aid when lifting or turning the person.

Two methods can be used for placing a bedpan. For either method, or any type of bedpan, the flattest part goes toward the client's head. The first method is used with the person lying on the back (Fig. 38-3*A*). Ask the person to flex the knees, push down on the mattress with the feet, and raise the buttocks. The helper uses one hand to assist in elevating the buttocks and the other hand to slide the bedpan under the person. The second method is used when the individual is turned to the side (Fig. 38-3*B*). Ask the person to turn toward the far side of the bed. Place the bedpan firmly against the buttocks. Next, place your palm firmly

against the top side of the bedpan and push downward. Roll the person back onto the bedpan, while holding the bedpan securely, by pulling the hip toward you.

After either method, elevate the head of the bed to a near-sitting position (unless contraindicated). A near-sitting position allows gravity to aid in elimination. Check that the person is correctly centered on the bedpan, so that the person is comfortable and avoids getting the bed wet. Before leaving, (a) be sure the person has easy access to call bell and toilet paper and (b) raise the side rails.

Removing the Bedpan. Put on clean gloves. Lower the head of the bed. Ask the person to push with the feet against the mattress and lift the buttocks. Slide the bedpan out. Another method is to have the person roll toward the far side of the bed. Hold the bedpan securely to prevent spillage while the individual rolls to the side.

You may need to cleanse the perineal or perianal area, because reaching this area is difficult for a person in bed. In addition to toilet paper, soap and water may be used. If the skin is excoriated, use warm water without soap. Explain to the person that you are assist-

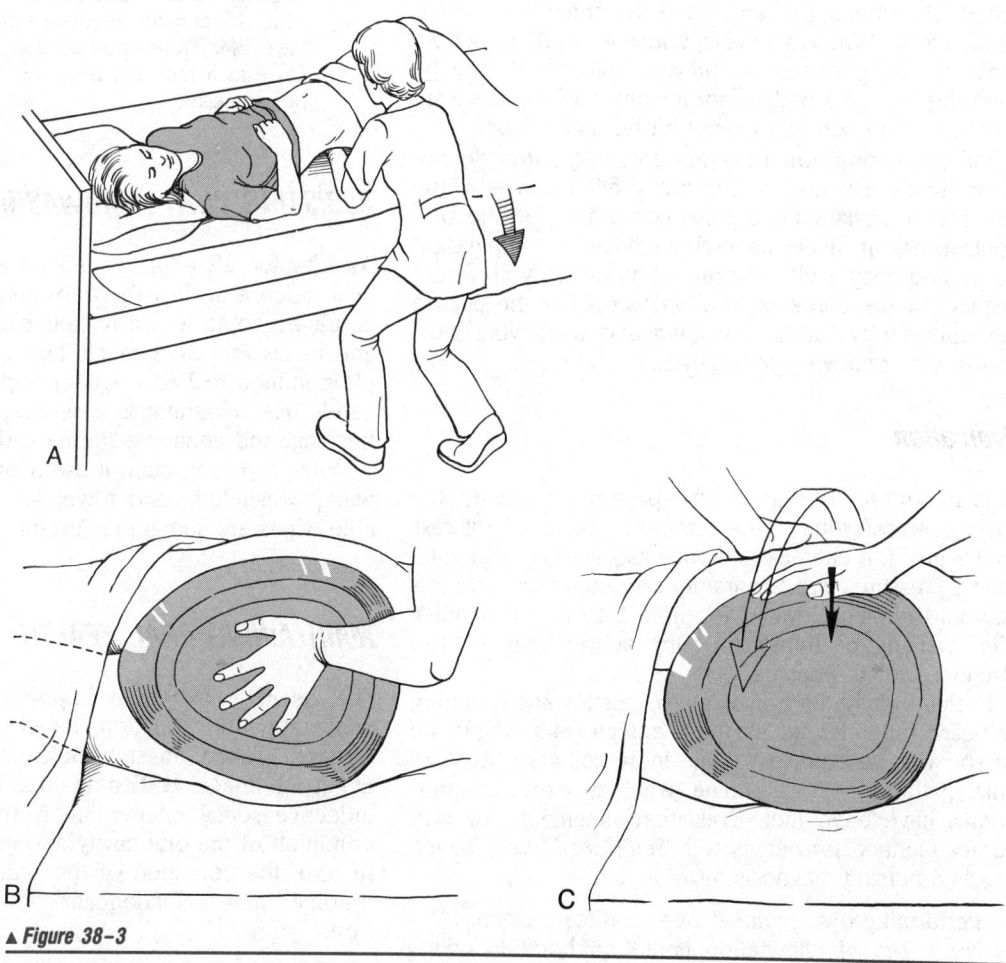

▲ *Figure 38-3*

Two methods of giving a bedpan to a person who can assist with lifting self. *A,* With person on back. *B,* With person on side. *C,* Nurse places hand on person's hip and gently pulls while rolling person onto back.

ing with this care because self-help is difficult in bed. Reposition the person for comfort, lower the bed, and provide for handwashing.

Cover the bedpan with a towel or bedpan cover and take it to the hopper, toilet, dirty utility room, or other appropriate place for disposal of excreta. Be sure to measure and record liquid waste when indicated. If the urine or feces appears abnormal, save the specimen, document your observations, and report as appropriate. Perform necessary tests on urine and feces. Document observations and findings. Clean the bedpan according to agency policy and return it to the bedside stand with a clean cover. Be sure to remove and dispose of your gloves and wash your hands after completing care.

Urinal. Urinals are usually plastic and are used by men who are unable to go to the toilet to void (i.e., urinate). If the urinal is used in bed, remind the man to tilt the urinal's closed end downward to avoid spilling. If he is unable to hold the urinal, place the urinal between his legs and position the penis in the urinal. Provide privacy by covering the person while holding the urinal in place for voiding. When assisting a man with standing to void at the bedside, use caution. He may be unsteady on his feet or may have a hypotensive episode.

A female urinal is shaped differently from a male urinal. The opening is larger, and the urinal has a wide, flat bottom. When a female urinal is used, it is held close to the perineum to prevent spillage. It may be used in place of a bedpan for a woman who has severe mobility restriction and cannot lift her buttocks.

Although some urinals have caps, they often do not close tightly. Do not leave partially filled urinals at the bedside. A partially filled urinal poses risks for infection control, has an unaesthetic appearance and unpleasant odor, and may spill. Dispose of urine as you would dispose of the contents of a bedpan. Offer the person the opportunity for handwashing and wash your own hands after removing your gloves.

Evaluation

It is important to evaluate the person walking to the toilet or transferring to the commode. Be sure to assess vital signs for alterations from baseline. If pulse rate, blood pressure, and respiratory rate increase considerably and remain elevated for more than 3 to 5 minutes after walking or transferring, the activity may be too strenuous for the person.

Evaluate daily the person's progress toward resuming self-care for toileting. As the client grows stronger, he or she will be able to resume more self-care. Analyze data gathered to determine whether expected outcomes have been met. Evaluation statements for outcomes planned for clients with *Self-Care Deficit, Toileting* as a nursing diagnosis might include

▸ Performing own perineal care, perineum clean.
▸ No odors of elimination noted on body following elimination.
▸ Able to self-toilet.

As part of your evaluation for specific nursing diagnoses you may be assessing excreta. It is a general rule that all excreta should be evaluated for signs of abnormality at the time of disposal. Note alterations in patterns of output. If urine output falls considerably, the person may be becoming dehydrated or is not taking in sufficient fluids. If no bowel movements occur for several days, the person may be constipated. Diarrhea could indicate a medication or tube-feeding reaction.

Use of the bedpan, bedside commode, or toilet should be documented. Characteristics of the excreta are also included in the charting. Note output on the intake and output record. Note complaints of dizziness, weakness, or pain. If the client is incontinent, chart the condition of the perineal area each shift. For example,

| 0630 | Assisted to the toilet after allowing to stand for a couple of minutes to stabilize BP. Voided 480 cc clear, yellow urine. Hands washed at sink; returned to bed and made comfortable. Side rails up, call light within reach.
 H. Hanna, R.N. |

| 1030 | Placed on bedpan for 5 min. for BM. Large, soft, light brown stool. Voided 275 cc. Perineum cleansed with toilet paper and warm washcloth, skin intact. States feels better. No more abdominal cramping.
 T. Page, S.N. |

| 1850 | Transferred to bedside commode; pulse 88, resp. 18. After 15 minutes requested return to bed; unable to have BM. Transferred to bed and made comfortable. Pulse at 5 min. 86, resp. 18. Given warm prune juice per request.
 R. Warren, R.N. |

ASSISTING WITH HANDWASHING

As Chapter 28 explains, effective handwashing is the best defense against the transmission of organisms. Encourage people to wash their hands prior to oral care and meals and after meals and elimination. Offer people confined to bed frequent opportunity to wash their hands. Handwashing is essential for cleanliness, is refreshing, and enhances the individual's self-esteem.

When a person cannot use a sink, provide a basin or water, washcloth, and towel for handwashing. Disposable wipes are sometimes useful.

MAINTAINING ORAL HEALTH

Oral health is extremely important. Oral problems can cause appetite reduction, localized pain, and systemic disease. Broken, absent, unclean, or crooked teeth can affect self-image. **Halitosis** (bad breath) can negatively influence social interaction. Nutrition affects both the condition of the oral cavity and general physical health. In turn, the condition of the oral cavity influences nutritional intake. Inadequate oral hygiene may result from

▸ lack of knowledge regarding effective oral hygiene practices

▶ lack of knowledge about the prevention of oral problems

▶ poor oral hygiene practices established during childhood

▶ poor nutrition and frequent snacking on "junk" foods

▶ imbalanced oral flora, allowing growth of harmful bacteria that cause dental **caries** (cavities due to tooth decay)

In spite of the importance of oral health, oral care is often neglected in everyday life. Some people neglect oral care because they believe that teeth must be removed eventually. This belief is not true. Teeth can be preserved throughout one's life with preventive dental care. Unfortunately, nurses often neglect oral hygiene. Reasons for neglecting oral care and related teaching include

▶ Assuming a person knows how to perform effective oral hygiene

▶ Limited direct observation of oral hygiene because most people do self-care

▶ Lack of assessment of the oral cavity

▶ Care giver's avoidance of oral care due to repulsion by halitosis and deteriorated oral cavities

▶ People with sore mouths refusing care because they fear discomfort

▶ Failure to understand how important oral care is to one's overall well-being

Oral Cavity Alterations

Between 5 and 8 months of age, the **deciduous teeth** (temporary teeth that are shed in childhood) begin to erupt. Between ages 6 and 25 years, these teeth are gradually lost and replaced by 32 permanent teeth. In adults, each tooth consists of three major parts: the crown, which is the exposed part of the tooth, the root, and the pulp cavity (Fig. 38–4). Enamel covers the crown, and within its covering layer is the dentin. The root of the tooth sits in the jaw bone and is covered by cementum, which holds it in place. The blood vessels and nerves are located in the pulp cavity.

A large number of young people have dental caries, mouth and gum disease, and malocclusions (malposition of the teeth interfering with chewing).

During pregnancy, the increased circulating levels of hormones cause gingival hypertrophy, which can increase the incidence of **periodontal disease** (disease of the gums and tooth-supporting structures) if good oral hygiene is not consistently practiced. Periodontal disease is common among young adults. It is often precipitated by emotional stress, which aggravates inflammatory processes. Many elderly people unfortunately have few permanent teeth left and have partial plates or full dentures. Half the people over age 65 years have no teeth. With age, the gums tend to recede and to develop a brownish pigmentation along the tooth edge. Salivation decreases, and many older people complain of a dry mouth. Tooth loss is not inevita-

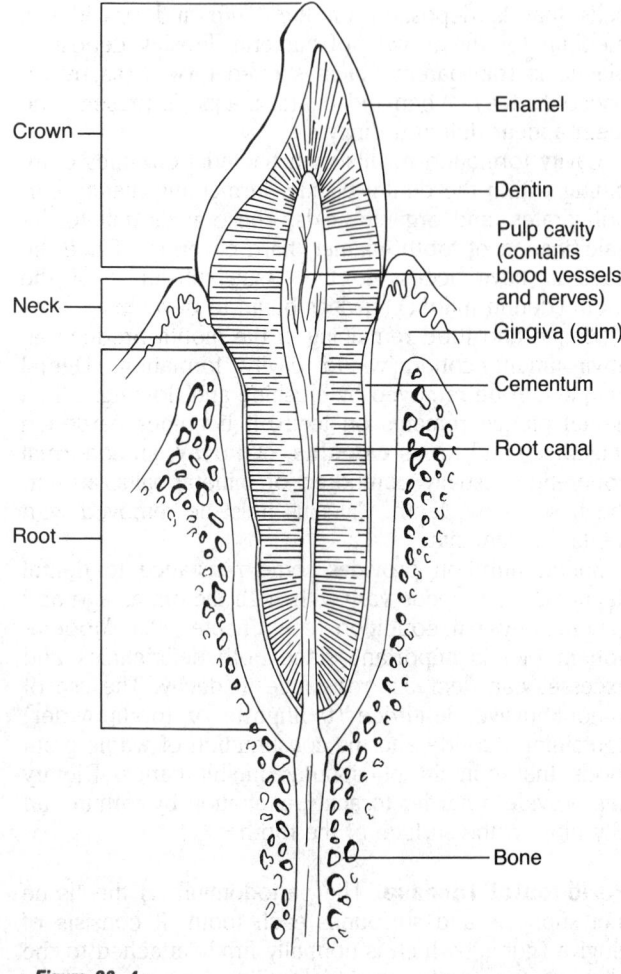

▲ **Figure 38–4**

Structures of the tooth.

ble, however, and often can be prevented with good oral care. Good oral care is necessary from the cradle to the grave if oral problems are to be prevented.

Dental caries (cavities) and periodontal disease are the two major types of oral problems. The prevention of dental caries and periodontal disease is important to prevent tooth loss.

Both dental caries and periodontal disease involve interaction among host (tooth and supporting structure), agent (dental plaque), and oral environment (e.g., amount and pH of saliva, presence of food). To break the chain of events involved in these disease processes, one must improve the resistance of the host, remove the agent, or alter the oral environment so that it is not conducive to disease.

Dental Caries. Dental caries is a disease of the calcified structure of the tooth. The agent responsible for dental caries is dental plaque. **Dental plaque** is a soft, thin film of food debris, mucin, and dead epithelial cells that is deposited on the teeth and provides a medium for the growth of bacteria. Freshly deposited plaque is transparent unless stained brown (as by tobacco or tea). When old dental plaque is present, the teeth appear dull and dingy.

Cavity formation results from bacterial enzymes combining within the dental plaque, fermenting dietary carbohydrates, and organic acids. These acids initiate decalcification of tooth enamel (hard covering). Once the bacteria have access to the tissue substance of the tooth (dentin matrix), cavities begin to develop.

Plaque and food remaining in the mouth produce an environment conducive to cavity formation. Dental plaque can be removed by brushing and flossing. When dental plaque remains on teeth, it becomes hardened (calcified) and forms **calculus, or tartar,** an abnormal concretion, usually composed of mineral salts, around the base of the teeth. Calculus must be removed with dental instruments.

Sound nutrition provides some resistance to dental decay. Dietary needs vary with such factors as age and general physical condition (see Chapter 42). Moderation in diet is important, since both deficiencies and excesses can decrease resistance to decay. The use of a nonabrasive dentifrice (toothpaste or toothpowder) containing fluoride and the consumption of whole grain foods that contain phosphorus inhibit caries. Dietary fats provide a barrier to acid penetration by forming an oily film on the surface of the tooth.

Periodontal Disease. The periodontium is the tissue that supports and surrounds each tooth. It consists of gingiva (gums), which is normally firmly attached to the neck of the tooth; gingival papilla, the projection of gingiva between the teeth; and periodontal membrane, a fibrous network that attaches the tooth to the gingiva and supporting alveolar bone. Periodontal disease is a long-term process involving destruction of the tooth-supporting structures (the periodontium). Unless treated or arrested, detachment of teeth occurs after atrophy of the periodontium.

Gingivitis (gum inflammation characterized by bleeding gums and halitosis) is an early stage of periodontal disease. Gingivitis may result from waste products and toxins from organisms in the mouth, which cause initial injury. Then, when plaque and bacteria accumulate, they form calculus, which contains more microorganisms and causes further irritation. As many as 53 per cent of children have gingivitis. Others at increased risk for gingivitis include people who breathe through their mouths, diabetics, people who use orthodontic appliances (e.g., braces), and people experiencing hormonal fluctuations (e.g., adolescents, pregnant women, and those taking oral contraceptives).[34]

Chronic gingivitis causes the inflammation to spread and destroy the underlying bone, causing periodontitis.[34] In an advanced stage of periodontal disease, the periodontium atrophies so that the gums appear to have receded completely away from the tooth. Without adequate supporting structure, the tooth becomes very loosely attached or falls out.

Good nutrition plays an important role in maintaining the tooth-supporting structures. Firm-textured foods stimulate the gingiva and are less likely to remain in the mouth. Dietary fiber helps prevent atrophy of salivary glands. A diet of only soft-textured foods increases plaque formation and leads to atrophy of the bone structure surrounding the tooth. Food debris lodged between the teeth causes inflammation.

As with dental caries, effective oral hygiene is an important factor in the prevention of periodontal disease and should be done after each meal. Tooth brushing and flossing helps remove dental plaque and favorably changes the oral environment. Flossing is particularly helpful in providing gingival stimulation for people with natural teeth. People with dentures or without teeth (edentulous) can stimulate their gingiva with gum massage. Some gingival tissue is very fragile.

Friction created by tooth brushing, flossing, and gum massage should be firm enough to stimulate gingival circulation but should not cause irritation or abrasion of the gingival tissue.

Assessment

Initial oral assessment is indicated whether a person has natural teeth, dentures, or no teeth at all. Information from assessment provides the basis for oral health care and health teaching. Before beginning an oral physical examination, talk with the individual. While talking, obtain a nursing history focused on the individual's typical oral hygiene practices and any past oral disorders. Also, assess the individual's self-care abilities and the need for health teaching.

Questions regarding oral hygiene include:

▶ How often do you brush your teeth?
▶ Do you floss? How often?
▶ Do you use a mouth wash? When?
▶ Do your gums ever bleed?
▶ Do you get sores in your mouth? When? Where?
▶ How often do you go to the dentist?
▶ How often do you have your teeth professionally cleaned?
▶ Do you have any loose teeth? Bridges? Partial plates?

For older adults, also ask:

▶ Do you have any problems with mouth dryness?
▶ What medications do you take?
▶ Can you chew all types of food?
▶ Have you noticed any change in sense of taste?
▶ Are you able to do your own mouth care?

After initial nursing assessment, determine how often subsequent assessments should be performed (e.g., once daily, twice daily). The frequency of assessments depends on the findings of the initial assessment, the need to monitor progress of oral problems, the need to reinforce teaching, and anticipated new problems.

Assessing Self-Care Abilities. This assessment goes beyond simply assessing physical abilities (flossing, cleaning dentures, mouth rinsing, teeth brushing). Also assess ambulatory skills. For example, some people can go to a sink and carry out complete oral care independently. Some people confined to bed can do self-care with assistance and need equipment placed within easy reach and removed after use. Others require total assistance. (See Box 38–1.)

Assessment of mental and emotional status is also important. A person with memory deficits may need structured verbal guidance to perform self-care. Such instructions may take more time than actually giving total care without the person's involvement. As with every activity of daily living (ADL), however, a vital part of good nursing care is to encourage people in as much self-care as possible. Failure to do so promotes dependency and undermines a person's self-concept.

To promote self-care, assess the need for health teaching. Health teaching assessment includes information from the nursing history and physical examination and direct observations of a person's oral hygiene practices.

Preparing for Oral Physical Examination. To prepare the client for oral physical examination, explain what you will be doing and how the person can assist you. Position the individual for comfort and ease of visibility, usually in a Fowler's position (nearly sitting). An oral examination provides (a) information about the condition of the oral cavity, (b) data about the effectiveness of past oral hygiene practices, and (c) clues to systemic problems.

Clients with Dentures. Remove dentures before an oral examination. Dentures prevent a thorough examination of palates and gums. Before removing a person's dentures, however, observe how well they fit. Do they adhere tightly? Do they slip and move about during talking? How easily can they be removed?

Equipment for Oral Examination. Two basic pieces of equipment are needed for oral examination:

▶ Light source (overbed light, penlight, or flashlight): must be bright enough to allow good visualization of the oral cavity.
▶ Tongue blade (tongue depressor): facilitates movement of the tongue and cheeks to see all areas of the oral cavity.

Method of Oral Examination. Wash your hands and don clean gloves. With a tongue blade in one hand and a light positioned to see clearly, you are ready to begin an oral examination. Ask the person to tilt the head back slightly and open the mouth.

Throughout the examination, assess the condition of the oral mucosa. Observe for moistness, color, inflammation, abrasions, lesions, or ulcerations of the mucous membranes.

By following the same sequence for each oral examination you perform, you will be more efficient and less likely to overlook or forget to examine an area. One suggested sequence for oral examination is

▶ Depress tongue with tongue blade while person says "Ahhhh." This procedure gives a clear view of the throat. Observe the condition of throat mucosa looking for lesions, inflammation, or white pustules.
▶ To observe the top portion of the tongue, ask the person to protrude ("stick out") the tongue (or retract the tongue for them, using a gauze sponge). Observe for moisture, color, eruptions, and adhered debris.
▶ To see the sides and underside of the tongue, use a tongue blade. With the tongue in a relaxed position, push it to one side and then the other. Note abrasions, growths, and enlarged or ruptured blood vessels. The sides of the tongue are common places for cancer to develop.
▶ For the toddler, check the number of deciduous teeth present. All 20 should have erupted by 2½ years of age.
▶ Observe the appearance of the inner aspects of the gums and teeth. Are gums inflamed, bleeding, or receding? Note any hyperplasia (increased size) of gums, as well as color and drainage between the teeth. Palpate gums if necessary. Observe the teeth for caries, calculus, debris, and erosion. If the person is edentulous (without teeth), note any atrophy of the periodontium.
▶ Look at the external aspects of gums and teeth by using a tongue blade to hold the cheek outward.

Box 38–1. Nursing Assessment of the Need for Oral Hygiene

The frequency and type of assistance needed with oral hygiene is determined by

▶ Findings from assessment (health history and physical examination) of the oral cavity. Examples of data include subjective symptoms such as unpleasant taste and objective symptoms such as excessive tartar formation on teeth; halitosis; thick oral secretions; food particles between teeth or under lips; gum disease; abnormal discharge around teeth and gums (blood, pus).
▶ Assessment of individual's self-care abilities, such as history of typical oral hygiene practices; observation of frequency and thoroughness of brushing, flossing, and rinsing of mouth when brushing is inconvenient.
▶ Assessment of health teaching needs, such as the person's understanding of the importance of oral hygiene and knowledge of preventive practices.
▶ Person's general condition (physical and mental health or impairments), such as active and self-sufficient; paralyzed on one side; confused and needing assistance, direction, and supervision.
▶ Use of treatments or substances such as oxygen, atropine, or phenytoin (Dilantin), that affect the oral status.
▶ Baseline knowledge of anatomy and normal appearance of the oral cavity.

Remember: Oral examination and the provision of oral care both require appropriate medical asepsis (see Chapter 28).

▶ Observe cheek mucosa. Note color, moisture or dryness, lumps, or lesions.

▶ Observe the floor of the mouth by asking the person to touch the roof of the mouth with the tongue. Note growths and condition of mucosa.

▶ Examine the roof of the mouth (palate) by having the person open the mouth widely and tilt the head back (hyperextending the neck). Note growths and the condition of the mucosa.

▶ Observe the inner and outer aspects of the lips. Note any dryness, lesions, or **cheilosis** (cracking or ulceration of lips and angles of the mouth).

▶ Assess neck glands and lymph nodes by palpating between the jaw and neck with your fingertips, to detect abnormal swelling.

Identifying Oral Problems. Some oral problems may develop when a person has a compromised general condition (e.g., poor nutrition, infection, irritation, drugs). More than 250 drugs decrease salivation. Drugs having this side effect include anticholinergics, antidepressants, antihistamines, antihypertensives, antipsychotics, antispasmodics, barbiturates, bronchodilators, and diuretics.[14] **Xerostomia** (dryness of the mouth from salivary gland dysfunction) combined with atrophy of the mucosal tissue in the older adult predisposes the elderly to infections such as candidiasis.

During assessment, you may find the following problems:

▶ Cheilosis can be caused by riboflavin deficiency, excessive salivation, or mouth breathing.

▶ Erosion of tooth enamel and dentin can result from chemical irritants or mechanical factors, such as hard toothbrush, abrasive dentifrices (toothpaste or toothpowder). Prolonged contact with gastric contents increases the risk of tooth enamel erosion (e.g., a bulimic person who vomits frequently over a long period is at risk for this problem).

▶ Local infections (e.g., herpes simplex) may appear as blister-like eruptions that later form crusted scabs on lip borders.

▶ Oral malignancies may appear as lumps or ulcerative areas in the mouth.

▶ **Stomatitis** (inflammation of the oral mucosa) can result from irritants such as tobacco or some drugs.

▶ Systemic diseases and the systemic side effects of drugs can cause oral problems (e.g., gingival hemorrhage, atrophy, excessive dental caries, stomatitis). Blood disorders can manifest as petechiae (tiny hemorrhagic spots) within the oral cavity. Oral problems can also cause abnormalities in other body areas (e.g., head and neck pain, enlargement of maxillary and other lymph nodes).

▶ Dry oral mucosa can be related to mouth breathing, poor function of the salivary glands, drugs, or insufficient fluid intake.

People at high risk for stomatitis and other oral problems include those undergoing drug therapy with agents that cause considerable mouth dryness, those who neglect oral hygiene, those undergoing treatment for cancer with chemotherapy or radiotherapy to the head, and those with problems of immune deficiency.

A good preventive oral hygiene program in which care is given at least four times a day appears to be the most effective in preventing stomatitis and other oral problems.[18]

Nursing Diagnosis

Nursing diagnoses following oral assessment should identify present or potential problems (e.g., altered mucous membrane) so that helpful nursing or appropriate medical or dental intervention can be planned and implemented. Oral problems often develop insidiously. A nursing diagnosis of *Altered Oral Mucous Membrane* R/T knowledge deficit is common. If inadequate oral care is caused by physical or emotional inability to perform the necessary care, use the nursing diagnosis *Self-Care Deficit, Hygiene.*

Planning

Identified problems should be discussed with the client and significant others. Together the nurse and the client establish a plan of care, including needed areas of teaching.

Plan specific interventions based on assessment findings and nursing diagnoses. For example, if a self-care deficit is present, expected outcomes would be

▶ assists with own daily oral hygiene
▶ resumes self-care for oral hygiene
▶ correctly performs oral hygiene
▶ consistently performs daily oral hygiene

If the nursing diagnosis is *Altered Oral Mucous Membrane,* expected outcomes would include "no evidence of oral infection."

Nursing Intervention

Make referrals to a physician or dentist, as appropriate. For example, poorly fitting or broken dentures need to be replaced. Abnormal lumps need investigation and possible treatment. Excessive gum disease and carious, stained, broken, loose, or heavily plaqued teeth also need attention.

Oral hygiene skills performed for dependent people frequently include refreshing and moistening the mouth (use of diluted mouthwash, moistening mouth swabs, mouth freshener), lubricating the lips, brushing and flossing natural teeth, and cleaning dentures. Clients who are not totally dependent should be encouraged to complete as much of these activities as possible.

Teaching and encouraging oral self-care are important nursing interventions. The method you use for teaching oral hygiene principles and the assistance the client needs to support and promote oral self-care are influenced by physical, mental, and emotional status.

Paralysis or a short attention span, for example, will affect a client's ability to perform self-care.

You can incorporate some planned teaching into interactions while assisting with or providing oral care. For example, encourage drinking more fluids if dryness of the oral mucosa is a concern. Also, offer appropriate information. For example, if a drug being taken has a drying effect on the oral mucosa, explain this effect to the client.

Demonstration is a good way to teach oral hygiene. Demonstrate tooth brushing and flossing techniques to increase removal of dental plaque by using a "disclosure tablet" as a teaching aid. Disclosure tablets stain dental plaque red, so that it is easy to see. Explain the activity to the individual before beginning. Then ask the person to chew a disclosure tablet for about a minute, then rinse the mouth out with water. Next have the person examine the teeth with a mirror before brushing and flossing and then again afterward, to see whether all dental plaque has been removed. Reassure the person that while some red color remains on the tongue, it is not harmful. Using disclosure tablets reinforces teaching and provides a means of evaluating the person's skill and learning.

Care for Natural Teeth. It is most important both to clean teeth thoroughly and to maintain and improve the condition of the oral mucosa. Equipment needed for providing oral care in bed includes toothbrush, dentifrice (toothpaste or toothpowder), dental floss, tissues or face towel, a cup of water, and an emesis basin.

Types of Toothbrushes. Discourage the use of frayed and uneven hard-bristle toothbrushes. They are ineffective in cleaning, cause abrasion of teeth, and traumatize the gingiva. Replace toothbrushes every 3 to 4 months.

Recommended features in toothbrush design are (1) a straight handle, (2) a size small enough to reach all areas of the mouth easily, (3) even and rounded brushing surface, and (4) soft, multitufted nylon bristles (Fig. 38-5). Rounded, soft bristles provide gum stimulation without causing abrasion. The even, multitufted design allows contact with all surfaces and is more durable. When an electric toothbrush is used, examine it for electrical hazards. An electric toothbrush should *not* be turned on until it is in the mouth.

Toothettes are pieces of foam attached to sticks. They are disposable and are sometimes used for people with very sensitive gums, after oral surgery, or temporarily when a toothbrush is not available. These sponge sticks are very good for cleaning the oral mucosa and are helpful for people with stomatitis. They are not effective for cleaning more than the middle front surface of the teeth, as the sponge cannot reach around the curves and into the crevices.[13] A combination of toothbrush and toothettes is best for the person who has stomatitis.

Dentifrices. A nonabrasive dentifrice is desirable, because long-term use of an abrasive toothpaste can damage teeth. Apply toothpaste in a thin layer and work into the toothbrush's bristles.

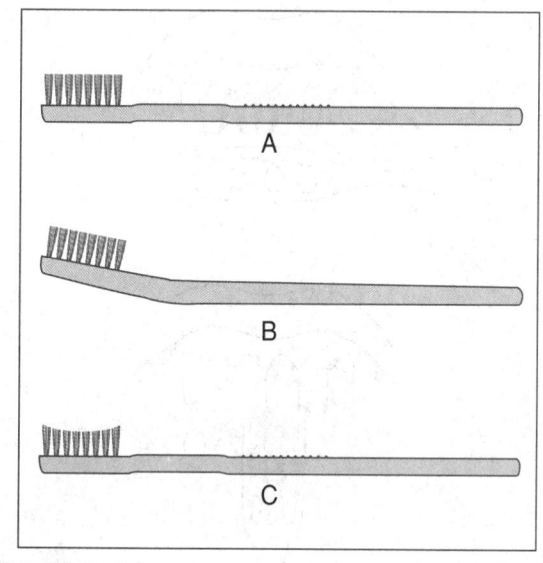

▲ *Figure 38-5*

Some common toothbrushes. Note that only type A has all recommended features.

Brushing Technique. Brushing is usually done upon arising and at bedtime, but brushing should also be done after each meal. Daily tongue brushing and teeth flossing are also recommended aspects of oral hygiene.

The recommended tooth-brushing method combines vibratory motion with gum massage.

This technique removes dental plaque from the teeth and beneath the gum margin. A soft brush is needed. For cleaning the outside surfaces of all teeth and inside surfaces of back teeth, place the bristles of the brush at a 45° angle to the teeth. Place the brush with the tips directed slightly onto the furrow surrounding a tooth (gingival sulcus). Without disengaging the brush tips, vibrate the brush back and forth with short strokes. The toothbrush will reach only two or three teeth at a time (Fig. 38-6A). After brushing one area, overlap placement with an adjacent position. For inside surfaces of front teeth, use the bristles on the end of the brush in a vibratory motion (Fig. 38-6B). To clean the chewing surfaces, brush back and forth.

After brushing the teeth, brush the tongue. Tongue brushing decreases the number of microorganisms and removes debris. When helping someone, ask the person to protrude ("stick out") the tongue. Holding the brush at a right angle to the length of the tongue, direct the bristle tips toward the throat. With light pressure, bring the brush forward and over the tip of the tongue. Then brush the tongue's sides. Now have the person thoroughly rinse the mouth. Repeat brushing and rinsing as needed until the mouth is clean. Cleanse the toothbrush under running water to remove debris. Shake out excess water and allow to dry.

Special Considerations. For people who find holding a toothbrush difficult (e.g., an arthritic person),

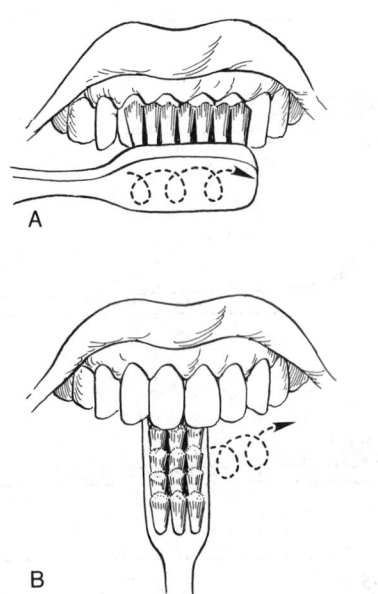

▲ *Figure 38–6*

A, Brushing outer surface of upper teeth. *B,* Clean inside surface of teeth with end of toothbrush, using vibratory motion. Hold brush at 45° angle to the teeth.

electric brushes are effective in removing plaque. They are easier to hold than a regular toothbrush, since the handle is bigger and the person does not have to move the hand as much. Other devices may be placed on a regular toothbrush to make it easier to grasp. A rubber ball, a handle grip for a bicycle, and padding attached with tape are useful devices for this purpose.

A suction apparatus may also be a part of a special toothbrush or used with a toothbrush for people unable to spit. One such device is called the ASPIR-BRUSH. A straw can be used by individuals in bed to expel water and toothpaste from the mouth.

For people who have difficulty with brushing and flossing adequately, a WaterPik device can aid in thorough cleansing of the mouth. The pressurized stream of water cleans out crevices and massages the gingival tissue.

Flossing. Brushing alone cannot completely remove dental plaque and debris around the teeth. Flossing (used correctly with tooth brushing) removes dental plaque between teeth, helps prevent periodontal disease, and helps remove oral debris (source of halitosis). Unwaxed dental floss is recommended because it is thinner, slides easily between teeth, and is more absorbent than waxed floss.

Learning to floss correctly requires instruction and practice. Children may need help with flossing until about age 10 years, depending on the child's manual dexterity.

Loosely wrap floss about 12 to 18 inches long around index or middle finger of each hand (Fig. 38–7). To floss the lower teeth, hold the floss so that the forefingers of both hands are on top of the strand. Loop the floss around a tooth and pull the ends forward to curve it into a C shape against the sides of the

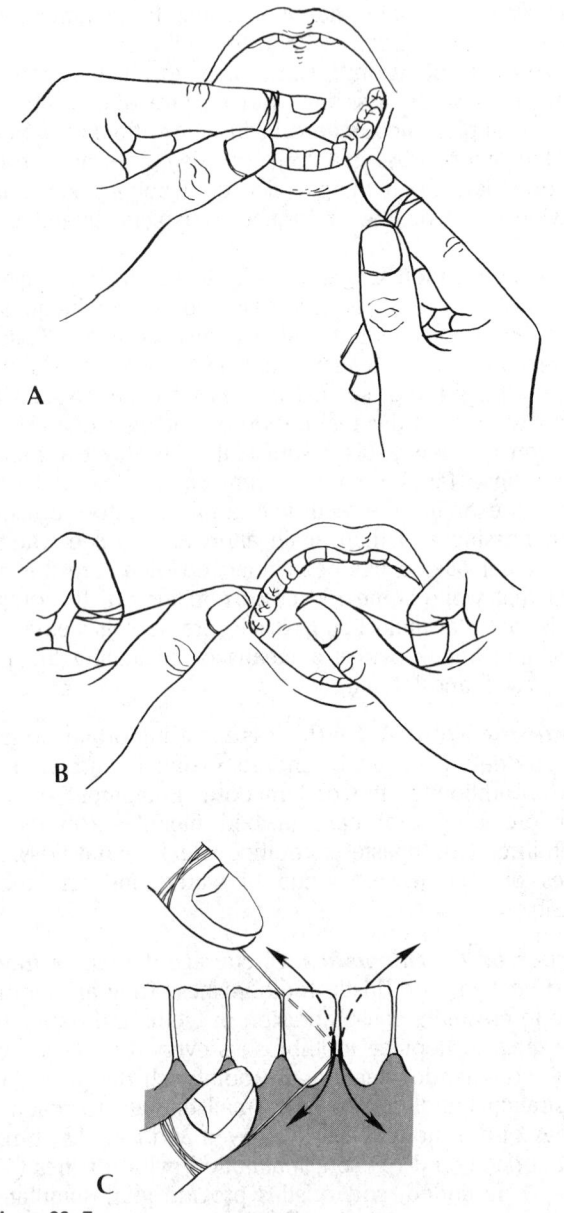

▲ *Figure 38–7*

Flossing technique. *A,* Flossing bottom teeth. *B,* Flossing top teeth. *C,* Directions of flossing. Floss should wrap around side of tooth and go between bottom of tooth and gum tissue.

tooth. Then slide the floss to the gum line. Move the floss back and forth to clean both sides of the tooth. Carefully work the floss under the gum until it meets resistance. Then bring the floss toward the biting surface.

To floss the upper teeth, hold the floss so that it is over the thumb of one hand and the forefinger of the other hand. The thumb is to the outside of the teeth to hold back the cheek. Work the floss between the teeth as done with the lower teeth.

When floss becomes soiled or frayed, move to a new section by slipping a turn of floss from the middle finger of one hand and adding a turn to the finger of the other. After flossing, rinse vigorously to remove loose debris. Although firm pressure is needed against the sides of the teeth, do not traumatize the gums.

Care for Dentures. Dentures collect debris, dental plaque, and calculus just as natural teeth do. The same type of toothbrush used for natural teeth can be used for dentures. "Denture brushes" with hard bristles wear grooves in dentures. Encourage people to wear dentures continuously during the day. This improves eating technique, speech, appearance, and contour of the mouth.

Some health professionals recommend removal of dentures at night to reduce pressure on soft tissue and bone. In care facilities, when dentures are removed from the mouth, store them in a labeled denture cup to prevent loss or breakage.

Wearing gloves, remove dentures to clean them and to provide oral care. It may be difficult to remove upper dentures. Ask the person to close the mouth and puff out the cheeks. This procedure often "breaks the seal." If the seal remains unbroken, you or the person can place a finger above the edge of the denture and exert pressure to pull it away from the gum. If the seal still remains unbroken, place one or more fingers of both hands inside the lip and over the borders of the dentures on both sides. A rocking motion breaks the seal better than pulling on both sides at the same time. Lower dentures usually come out easily. If not, place your fingers inside the person's bottom lip and grasp the denture's teeth.

After removing the dentures, (a) observe the appearance of the denture linings; (b) look for calculus, dental plaque, or food debris on the dentures; and (c) inspect them for broken or cracked areas. Then place the dentures in a denture cup to avoid dropping and breaking them as you carry them to the sink. Ideally, dentures are cleaned after each meal. Clean and massage tongue and oral mucosa at the same time.

Cleansing Agents. Many denture cleaners are available. Water with soap or a mild cleansing agent cleans dentures effectively without causing abrasion. One cleansing solution that can be prepared at home consists of 1 tsp of liquid bleach (e.g., Clorox), 2 tsp of Calgon, and ½ glass (4 oz) of warm water. Mix the solution in a clean denture cup and soak the dentures in the solution prior to brushing.

Brushing Dentures. Place paper towels and a small amount of water in a sink (towels cushion dentures if they are dropped). While cleaning, grasp dentures in the palm of one hand and brush with the other hand (Fig. 38–8). Brush all surfaces thoroughly. Rinse the dentures with cold water before replacing them in the clean denture cup to be returned to the client. The water lubricates the dentures and makes them easier to insert. For people confined to bed but capable of self-care, place an emesis basin, toothbrush, and container of water on the overbed table within easy reach and allow them to clean their own dentures.

Cleaning the Mouth. Each time dentures are removed, rinse the mouth with warm water. Use a multi-

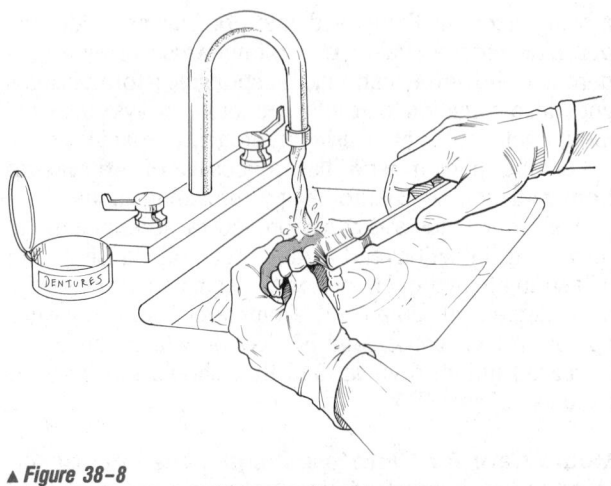

▲ *Figure 38–8*

Cleaning dentures. Place cloth or paper towel in basin for cushion in case dentures slip and fall.

tufted, soft nylon brush to clean the oral mucosa. Use long, straight strokes from the posterior to anterior surfaces of the mouth. Toothettes or gauze can be used. Remember to clean the tongue.

Massage. Massage stimulates circulation and toughens the oral mucosa, thus increasing resistance to trauma. If a toothbrush is used, apply the sides of the bristles in a vibratory motion. For digital massage, place gloved thumb and index finger over the gum's ridge. Use a press-and-release motion to massage. Rub the palate with the end of the thumb. Keep the thumbnail away from the palate to prevent mucosal trauma.

Management of Excessive Dryness or Oral Irritation. People with dry mouths or dry lips may require oral hygiene every 2 to 8 hours to improve the condition of the oral mucosa. Rinsing the mouth with water, mouthwash, or saline (water and salt solution) may be refreshing. Artificial saliva products such as Saliv-aid, Xero-Lube, or Moi-Stir can be beneficial for the person who has a very dry mouth.

Note that the use of lemon and glycerine swabs is counterproductive. The acidity of lemon juice causes irritation and decalcification of the teeth. Glycerine is hypertonic and draws moisture from the tissues, causing "reflex exhaustion of the salivation process."[13]

Mouthwashes are available in many varieties. Bactericidal mouthwashes can destroy the normal bacterial flora of the mouth, resulting in overgrowth of fungus. The astringent effect of some mouthwashes can be beneficial. Saline is easy to make and soothing for many people with mucosal irritation. For people with pain from severe stomatitis, anesthetic solutions are available. Check for allergies before using mouthwashes containing drugs such as lidocaine (Xylocaine).

A dilute solution of hydrogen peroxide can remove debris and microorganisms from coated, dry tongues and from acute necrotizing ulcerative gingivitis. By removing necrotic tissue and microorganisms, hydrogen peroxide reduces halitosis. Prolonged use of hydrogen peroxide, however, can lead to sponginess of the gums and decalcification of tooth surfaces. Always rinse the mouth with water after using hydrogen peroxide.

For the person who has mucositis or **stomatitis** from radiation or chemotherapy, providing mouth care at least four times a day has proved to be beneficial in preventing infection and further irritation. Rinsing with half-strength hydrogen peroxide seems to provide the best degree of comfort.[18] Commercial mouthwashes contain a high percentage of alcohol, which can cause increased mouth dryness, and they should not be used for these clients.[33]

Mouth Care for Comatose People. The external surfaces of the teeth of comatose people can be brushed in the usual manner (using very little liquid) after safely positioning to prevent aspiration (Fig. 38–9). To clean internal and chewing surfaces, use some means of keeping the mouth open. "Bite blocks" are commercially available in rubber or plastic, or they can be made by putting tongue blades together and covering them with gauze taped in place.

Never put your fingers in the mouth of a person with impaired awareness. Human bites can be very painful and dangerous. Serious infections may develop with broken skin and subsequent entry of organisms. Nerve sensation of the injured finger may be lost.

Put the bite block in place between the upper and lower teeth at the jaw's posterior, lateral section. Use a toothbrush, cotton-tipped applicator (see Fig. 38–9), or tongue blades covered with 4×4 gauze to clean the teeth surfaces. Clean the tongue using gauze-covered tongue blades with cleaning solution (saline, half-strength hydrogen peroxide, or diluted mouthwash). Use only a small amount of solution on the gauze and have oral suction within reach and turned on; a comatose person has a poor gag reflex and may aspirate. Use a moisturizing agent on the lips (water-soluble lu-

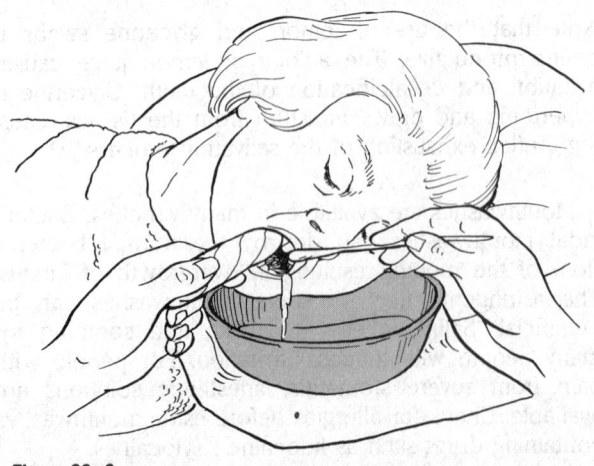

▲ *Figure 38–9*

Giving mouth care to a comatose or helpless person. Note the head is turned to the side to prevent aspiration of fluid.

bricant, lip balm, or white petroleum jelly) after completing oral hygiene.

Evaluation

To evaluate the effectiveness of care, examine the oral cavity daily. Also, periodically evaluate the progress of the person toward administering oral self-care.

For the person with a diagnosis of *Altered Oral Mucous Membrane*, evaluation statements might include

▶ Mucous membrane of oral cavity intact and moist.
▶ Lips smooth and moist.
▶ Tongue clean, pink, and moist.
▶ Gingiva not swollen or bleeding.
▶ States mouth feels clean and refreshed.

For the client with the nursing diagnosis *Self-Care Deficit, Hygiene*, the following evaluation statements might indicate that expected outcomes have been met with regard to oral hygiene:

▶ Performing own oral hygiene twice daily.
▶ Consistently performing oral hygiene correctly.

Document care given and teaching completed on activity flowsheets or in the nurse's notes in the client's chart. Examples of documentation:

0830   Oral care with tongue blade and swabs, toothbrush, and diluted mouthwash given with client in lateral position. Mouth moderately crusted from open-mouth breathing. Gums without hyperplasia. No reaction to oral care.   P. Oliver, S.N.

2100   Assisted with own oral care, able to hold toothbrush with padded handle. Can control secretions on right side of mouth. Small amount of dribbling. Has difficulty reaching all areas because of right-sided paresis. Remainder of mouth and teeth cleaned for client. Gums and mucosa pink.   S. Hanson, R.N.

HYGIENE FOR THE EYES

Heavy, crusted eye secretions make it difficult to open the eyes fully, cause eye irritation and infection, and are aesthetically unappealing. Persons at risk for crusting include people in coma, people with severe liver disease and jaundice, and those with conjunctivitis or other eye infections.

Many elderly people suffer from decreased lubrication of the eye. The resulting dryness can lead to ineffective displacement of dust and bacteria, which can predispose people to infection. Instillation of natural tear products can prevent problems in the elderly population.

Assessment

Assessment of eyes includes the entire eye orbit, eyelashes, and eyebrows (see Chapter 33). Observe for the following:

▶ Scaliness of skin underlying the eyebrows

▶ Edema, lesions, crusted secretion, inflammation of the eyelids
▶ Eyelashes turned inward that might irritate eye surface; styes
▶ Swelling of the lacrimal sac; excessive tearing or absence of tears; crusting at inner canthus
▶ Color; inflammation of the sclera or conjunctiva
▶ Pupil size, shape, and light response
▶ Eye movement; cataracts; drainage; sensations of burning; pain

Questions to ask the person include
Do you have any difficulty seeing?
Do you have any eye pain?
Do you ever have redness or swelling of the eyes?
Do your eyes water excessively?
Do you ever have any discharge or "mattering" of the eyes?
When was your vision last checked?
For the person who wears contact lenses, ask about the type of lens worn, the length of time lenses are in place, and the procedure used for cleaning the lenses. The older adult should be asked additional questions that could indicate failing vision from eye disorders such as glaucoma or cataracts:
Do you have any visual difficulty driving or using stairways?
Do you have any trouble with night vision?
Do your eyes ever feel dry or burn?
When were you last tested for glaucoma?
Do you use any eye medications?

Nursing Diagnosis

Nursing diagnoses specifically related to hygiene of the eye might be *Self-Care Deficit, Hygiene* or *Sensory/Perceptual Alteration, Visual.*

Planning

Eye hygiene outcomes for the diagnosis *Self-Care Deficit, Hygiene* might be

▶ Independently completes adequate eye hygiene.
▶ Assists with own eye care.

Expected outcomes for the nursing diagnosis *Sensory/Perceptual Alteration, Visual* might be

▶ Complains of no further loss of vision.
▶ Independently cares for eyeglasses or contact lenses.

Nursing Intervention

One major nursing intervention for eye hygiene is the routine cleaning of the eyes during bathing. When you do this procedure, be sure to clean carefully and gently from the inner to the outer canthus. This direction is the natural tract for removal of debris from eyes. Clean each eye with a separate part of the washcloth to prevent potential spread of infection from one eye to the other.

Soap causes eye irritation. Never use soap for cleaning eyes.

When crusted secretions are present, place a *wet*, warm washcloth or cotton ball over the closed eye. Leave the cloth or cotton ball in place until secretions become softened. Water or normal saline can be used. Repeat application of warm compresses until secretions are moist enough to remove easily without trauma.

Eye Care for Comatose People. A comatose person may require frequent eye care (e.g., every 4 hours), depending on the general condition of the eyes and the amount of moisture in the environment. Besides cleaning, keep eyes moist and protected from the air. If the blink (corneal) reflex is lost or decreased, the eye is lacking a normal mechanism that helps protect it. The corneal reflex is the automatic closing of the eyes in response to a sudden movement of an object toward the person's face or to the touching of the eye by a foreign object. In the comatose person, the eyes may also be at risk because they tend to remain open and become dry from the air. Dry eyes can lead to corneal ulceration and possible loss of vision. In some situations, liquid tear solution or normal saline is instilled into the conjunctival sac or eyes. If the eyes remain open or appear irritated, gently close the eyes and cover them with a protective shield.

Eyeglasses. Clean eyeglasses at least once daily. Many people do not ask to have their eyeglasses cleaned and will wear dirty glasses that impair vision. Handle eyeglasses carefully to prevent breakage. When cleaning, avoid scratching the lens. Use warm water, mild soap, and nonabrasive drying material (e.g., soft facial paper tissue) for glass lenses. Use liquid plastic lens cleaner and a similar drying material for plastic lenses. Plastic lenses scratch very easily. Label the client's eyeglass case with the person's name. When the glasses are not in use, store them in the top drawer of the bedside stand to prevent damage.

Artificial Eyes. Artificial (prosthetic) eyes are usually cared for by the client, in the same way teeth, hearing aids, and glasses are part of self-care. If a person is unconscious, paralyzed, or otherwise unable to carry out personal hygiene practices, a nurse may assist in the cleaning of an artificial eye.

To remove an artificial eye, (a) wash your hands carefully; (b) line a labeled container with gauze and fill with water (this step prevents damage to the eye); (c) have the person in a sitting or supine position; (d) pull down on the lower lid and exert slight pressure below the eyelid; (e) catch the eye in your hand and place it in the labeled container for safe storage. Another method is to apply a small suction cup to the artificial eye, depress the lower eyelid, and, using the handle of the suction cup, pull the eye out and downward to slide it out from under the upper lid.

To insert an artificial eye, (a) moisten it with saline or water, (b) hold upper lid with index finger and lower lid with thumb, (c) hold the artificial eye in the other hand with the front of the eye toward your palm, and (d) gently pull down the lower lid with the thumb and slip the eye under the lower lid and into the socket. The suction cup can also be used to hold the eye while inserting it.

To clean the socket, pull down the lower lid with the thumb and raise the upper lid with your index finger. Irrigate the socket with saline in an Asepto syringe. Direct saline from the inner canthus to the outer canthus and collect it in an emesis basin. Wash and dry the skin around the closed eyes.

Contact Lenses. Many people wear contact lenses, which are available in basically two types: hard lenses and soft lenses. Hard lenses are worn on a daily basis and need to be removed before sleeping. There are two different kinds of soft lenses: those worn on a daily basis, and those worn for extended periods.

Insertion and cleaning procedures are basically the same for all types of contact lenses. It is important to use the cleaning and wetting solutions recommended by the manufacturer. Thorough handwashing is essential before insertion or removal. After removing lenses, place them in separate containers labeled "right" and "left." Contact lenses are removed prior to surgery.

The steps for inserting contact lenses (Fig. 38–10) are the following:

► Remove the lens from its container and apply wetting solution.
► Be sure the lens is clean and undamaged (not torn or scratched).
► Place the lens on the index finger of your dominant hand.
► If the lens edges of soft lenses point outward and downward, the lens is inverted. Turn it over (Fig. 38–10*B*).
► Hold the person's upper lid with the index finger of

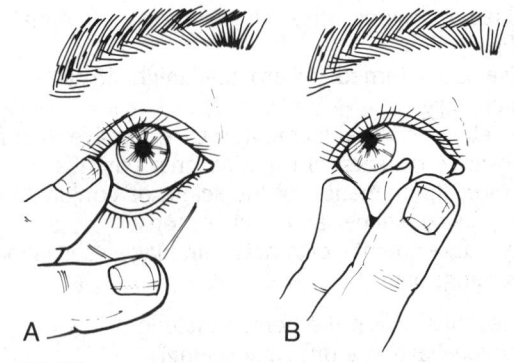

▲ *Figure 38–11*

Removal of soft lens. *A*, Pull down the lower lid with the middle finger and place your index fingertip on the lower edge of the lens. *B*, Slide the lens onto the white part of the eye; pinch lightly between the thumb and index finger to remove.

your nondominant hand. Have the person look straight ahead.
► Apply gentle downward pressure on the lower lid and place the lens directly over the iris and pupil.
► Gently rub the upper lid with your finger to remove air bubbles.
► If the person feels any discomfort, remove the lens, clean, and insert again.

The steps for removal of soft lenses (Fig. 38–11) are the following:

► Wash your hands. Ask the client to look up and to the side (laterally); with your middle finger, pull down the lower lid and place your index fingertip on the lower edge of the lens.
► Move the lens (medially) to the white part of the eye.
► Gently pinch the lens between the thumb and index finger, allowing air to go beneath the lens. The lens will double up and can be grasped for removal.

The steps for removal of hard lenses (Fig. 38–12) are the following:

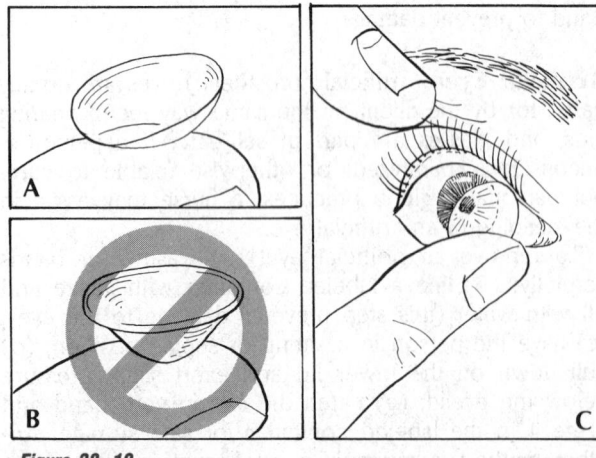

▲ *Figure 38–10*

Inserting soft contact lens. *A*, Correct appearance. *B*, Lens inside out; do not use this way. *C*, Insert by using gentle pressure on the lower lid while placing the lens over the iris.

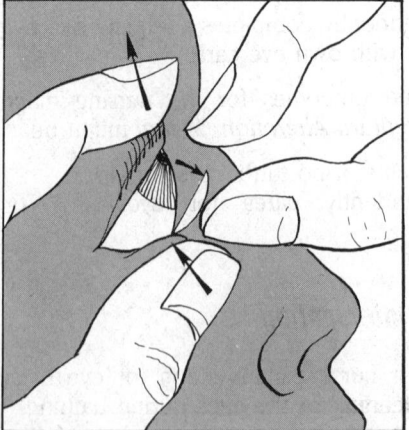

▲ *Figure 38–12*

Removal of hard lens. Apply pressure on lower edge of lens so lens will tilt out, away from eye. Grasp upper edge.

► Pull the upper and lower lids apart and to the lateral side.
► Ask the person to blink.
► Lens will fall into your hand.

An alternative method:

► Exert gentle pressure on the lower edge of the lens.
► Grasp the upper edge of the lens as it falls away from the eye.

Lack of moisture or wearing contact lenses too long can cause painful corneal abrasions.

Evaluation

The eyes of the person with a self-care deficit must be assessed each day to evaluate anticipated outcomes and to identify any signs of infection, damage, or conditions that might cause eye damage. The frequency of instilling artificial tears or cleansing the eye may need to be changed. Statements that indicate that eye hygiene outcomes for the diagnosis *Self-Care Deficit, Hygiene,* have been met include

► Independently completing own eye hygiene.
► Able to correctly clean both eyes when provided with damp washcloth.

Statements that indicate outcomes for the nursing diagnosis *Sensory/Perceptual Alteration, Visual,* have been met include

► States vision is the same or improved.
► Independently caring for eyeglasses or contact lenses.

Examples of documentation might include

0800 Crusting of eyelids present this A.M. Cleansed with warm water and fresh washcloth.   T. Parness, S.N.

1500 Natural tears instilled q2h this shift. States eyes are not so "scratchy;" redness decreased.   S. Sims, S.N.

1430 Eyes very red and irritated upon admission; contacts removed, cleansed, and stored in contact container. Placed in drawer of bedside table. Own eyedrops used per physician's instructions.   R. Richie, R.N.

HYGIENE FOR THE EARS

If the ears are not kept clean, debris accumulates behind the ear and in the anterior aspect of the external ear (see Chapter 33). Debris in and around the ears can lead to ulceration and infection.

Assessment

Assess ears by examining the anterior and posterior aspects of the external ear for dryness, crusting, debris, and drainage. Look for **cerumen** (earwax) or drainage at the entrance to the ear canal. Gently palpate the tragus (anterior external cartilage area), which is a very sensitive area. Tenderness can give clues to ear problems. Palpate lymph nodes around the ears and in the

neck for enlargement and pain. Look for tophi (hard nodules) in the helix (superior-posterior external cartilage area). Tophi are deposits of uric acid crystals characteristic of gout. Sebaceous cysts behind the ear are common. For a general, gross assessment of hearing, have the person listen to a ticking watch or whisper in the ear. Assess one ear at a time, while occluding the other ear. Assessment of the canal and tympanic membrane is done with an otoscope. Question both the individual and significant others about the quality of hearing. Often the people a person lives with will first notice hearing losses.

People who have difficulty hearing may use hearing aids. Assess the type of aid used and the person's need for assistance in care of the aid. It is important to know the basic components of hearing aids and how to care for these appliances.

Hearing aids may be worn in the ear, behind the ear, as part of the eyeglasses, in a holder on the body, or in a shirt pocket. Many aid users wear the type that is worn behind the ear (Fig. 38–13). The four basic parts to a hearing aid are (1) an earmold, which fits into the ear and directs sound toward the eardrum; (2) a tube or wire that connects the earmold to an amplifier; (3) an amplifier that makes the signals stronger; and (4) a microphone that changes the sound waves into electrical impulses.

Nursing Diagnosis

Appropriate nursing diagnoses for the person with a problem in ear hygiene would be either *Self-Care Deficit, Hygiene,* or *Sensory/Perceptual Alteration, Hearing.* The latter may be related to impacted cerumen or to inadequate use or maintenance of the hearing aid.

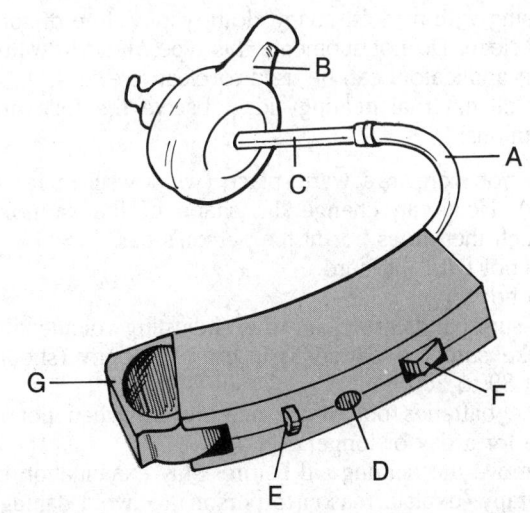

▲ *Figure 38–13*

The behind-the-ear hearing aid. A, Earhook; B, earmold; C, connecting tube; D, microphone; E, volume control; F, T/M (telephone/microphone) switch; G, battery compartment.

Planning

You may need to obtain an order for an ear irrigation to flush cerumen out of the ear. If considerable hearing loss is present and the person's hearing has not been previously evaluated, a referral for hearing tests is in order. An expected ear hygiene outcome for the diagnosis *Self-Care Deficit, Hygiene*, would be

▶ Safely completes own ear hygiene.

Expected outcomes for a nursing diagnosis of *Sensory/Perceptual Alteration, Hearing*, would be

▶ States hearing is improved.
▶ States able to hear ticking watch 1 inch from ear (or aid).
▶ Passes whisper test.

Nursing Intervention

Clean ears with several movements of a washcloth-covered finger. To remove cerumen at the entry point of the ear canal, slightly depress a washcloth-covered finger into the entrance of the ear canal. To remove cerumen from deep in the ear canal, an ear irrigation may be ordered by the physician (see Chapter 46).

Instruct people *never* to insert objects such as hairpins into the ear canal to remove earwax. Insertion of objects into the ear can cause trauma to the canal and middle ear.

To care for a hearing aid that has a removable earmold, clean the aid daily by wiping it with a soft, dry cloth. Once a week, clean the earmold and connecting tube with soap and warm water. Dry thoroughly and blow through the tube. *Do not* use a pipe cleaner or other sharp device that can damage the tube. Never use alcohol. It can dry and crack the plastic. Remove wax regularly. It builds up quickly.[29]

Cleanse "in the ear" aids by wiping them daily and cleansing with a moist soapy cloth, wiping free of soap when clean. Do not submerge this type of aid in water. Cotton applicators can be used to clean crevices.

For all external hearing aids, observe the following precautions:

▶ Do not store in a warm place (windowsill or radiator). Heat can change the shape of the earmold, which then does not fit the person's ear.
▶ Do not twist the cord.
▶ Do not drop.
▶ Be sure hands are clean when adjusting volume.
▶ Make sure the battery is inserted properly (should last 80 to 200 hours).
▶ Take batteries out of the hearing aid when not in use for a day or longer.
▶ Remove the hearing aid before x-ray examination or therapy (explain reason to person) to avoid damage from radiation.[29]
▶ Remove and store the hearing aid if a vaporizer is used, to avoid moisture's getting into the mechanism.

▶ Avoid using aerosol spray near the aid. It can clog the microphone.[24]

To insert a hearing aid, observe the following precautions:

▶ Check that the battery is operating. Hold the aid in your hand and turn up the volume. If batteries are operating, a "feedback" whistle will be heard. (Feedback is a shrill noise resulting from sound from the aid leaking out and going back through the microphones and becoming amplified.)
▶ Turn down the volume, insert the earmold into the ear canal, and secure the rest of the aid in place according to design (e.g., over the ear, in a body holder, or in a pocket of the clothing).
▶ Slowly turn up the volume while speaking to the person in a normal tone of voice. Ask the person to tell you when the volume is comfortable.
▶ If there is feedback, press in on the earmold. The earmold may be loose and need to be replaced.
▶ Be sure that the person's ear is not against the pillow in such a way that the earmold is displaced, causing feedback.

Evaluation

A statement indicating that the outcome has been met for ear *Self-Care Deficit, Hygiene*, might be

▶ Performing own ear hygiene.

Evaluation of hearing includes routine hearing reassessment. For the person with a hearing aid, evaluation should determine whether the hearing aid is being used properly and hearing is improving.

For the diagnosis *Sensory/Perceptual Alteration, Hearing*, outcome statements might include

▶ States, "I can hear much better now, thank you."
▶ Able to hear ticking watch at 2 inches from ear (or aid).
▶ Passed whisper test.

HYGIENE FOR THE NOSE

The nose provides a sense of smell and protective functions. Mucoid secretions, cilia, and specialized tissue in the nose aid in controlling temperature, humidity, and entry of foreign particles in the respiratory system. Excessive secretions can impair the sense of smell and obstruct breathing. If a person is unable to sniff or blow the nose, secretions can become crusted and may obstruct the airways or irritate nasal mucosa. If the sense of smell is impaired, inability to detect food aromas may decrease appetite.

Assessment

A history of allergies, chronic sinusitis, frequent nose bleeds, or difficulty breathing should be explored. Inspect the nasal mucosa for inflammation, moistness, or dryness, noting color, consistency, and amount of nasal discharge. Note excessive dryness of the nose or chafing and cracking from constant dripping. Frequent assessment of the condition of the nares is essential when the person has a nasogastric tube in place.

Nursing Diagnosis

The person who has severe neurologic deficits or who has a decreased level of consciousness is most likely to be at risk for *Self-Care Deficit, Bathing/Hygiene,* R/T inability to remove nasal secretions. Infants also must have their nasal secretions removed by their care givers. If secretions are copious and suctioning must be carried out frequently, a nursing diagnosis of *Ineffective Airway Clearance* is appropriate.

Planning

For small children with stuffy noses from secretions, interventions would be planned to teach them to blow the nose. For older people, the expected outcome for nasal *Self-Care Deficit, Hygiene* would be

▶ Independently completes nasal hygiene.

For all age groups with *Ineffective Airway Clearance,* the expected outcome would be

▶ Air exchange unimpaired by nasal secretions or swollen nasal mucosa.

Nursing Intervention

Adequate hygiene improves comfort and function of the nose. Liquid nasal secretions are usually removed by blowing the nose. Dry, hardened secretions are usually manually removed. Removal may be all that is needed for effective hygiene, other than cleaning the external opening during bathing. Socially appropriate ways of maintaining nose hygiene are usually taught in the home by parents. The nurse often teaches about how nose hygiene relates to health and disease.

When necessary, teach your clients that harsh nose blowing can sometimes cause problems. Nasal bleeding may occur in people with bleeding disorders and those taking drugs that increase bleeding tendencies. Some people are not permitted to blow the nose at all (such as following a head injury or brain surgery because blowing the nose increases intracranial pressure). Blowing the nose after a bleeding episode could restart the bleeding, of course. In the presence of infection, nose blowing is discouraged because it can force microbes from the throat up the eustachian tubes into the middle ear.

Some people may need help to clear congestion and protect nasal mucosa. External crusted secretions can be removed with a wet washcloth or a cotton-tipped applicator moistened with water or normal saline. Use a moisturizing lotion to keep the end of the nose from becoming dry and to prevent skin cracking. In some situations, nasal suctioning is necessary to remove congestion. See Chapter 45 for more information on suctioning.

Never suction a person without a physician's order if the person has had brain surgery or has suffered a head injury. Suctioning can increase intracranial pressure and cause brain injury.

Evaluation

An evaluation statement indicating that the expected nasal hygiene outcome has been met for the nursing diagnosis *Self-Care Deficit, Hygiene* might be

▶ Independently keeps nose free of secretions.

An evaluation statement for the nursing diagnosis *Ineffective Airway Clearance* might be

▶ No impairment to breathing through the nose is present.

Documentation indicates that interventions have been carried out. An example might read

1500   Noisy breathing; suctioned nose with bulb syringe; secretions white and copious. Breathing more quietly. Arouses with suctioning.   W. White, S.N.

SKIN HYGIENE

Skin and appendages (hair and nails) form the integumentary system. Hygiene care cleans and conditions skin so it can effectively maintain the integrity of the body. Careful skin hygiene also makes people comfortable. Bathing is the obvious way to care for skin. Hair care stimulates surrounding skin and removes sources of infection. Massage of the skin on the back and around bony prominences stimulates circulation and improves nutrition to the skin and underlying tissues (see Chapter 39 for information on massage).

Some hygiene care is directed at conditioning mucous membranes and skin around body orifices (mouth, eyes, and nose). Hygiene care of nails, feet, and the perineal area is especially important because these areas are prone to skin breakdown and infection. Bed linen can cause skin breakdown. Soiled, wrinkled sheets irritate skin and serve as sources of pressure. Heavy bed linen over sensitive, fragile skin can cause pressure that impedes circulation. In addition, various agents used in skin care can be protective or damaging to skin. Some agents cause excessive dryness, leading to breaks in the skin. (Skin care during immobility is discussed in Chapter 35.)

Skin Structure and Function

Skin, the largest body organ, has three continuous layers: epidermis, dermis, and subcutaneous tissue. The epidermis (most superficial layer) has several layers called strata. The outermost stratum contains dead cells continuously replaced by cells from deeper layers. Melanin (pigment) and keratin form in the inner cellular epidermal stratum. Melanin provides skin color and protection from ultraviolet sun rays. Keratin contributes to the skin acidity.

The dermis consists of blood vessels, dense connective tissue, nerve fibers, sebaceous (oil) glands, and hair follicles. Sebaceous glands are present on all skin surfaces except palms and soles.

Under the dermis is subcutaneous tissue, providing support and blood supply to the dermis. It consists of loose connective tissue, blood and lymph vessels, fat, sweat glands, and hair follicles.

Protection. The skin surface normally holds some bacteria (resident bacteria). On intact skin, resident bacteria prevent excess fungal growth. **Sebaceous glands** are glands that secrete sebum (an oily substance) into the hair follicles. Sebum has antibacterial and antifungal properties. Normal skin acidity inhibits growth of pathogenic organisms. Intact skin also protects underlying tissue from trauma.

Body Temperature Regulation. Many factors contribute to body temperature regulation (see Chapter 31). Skin affects body temperature through sebaceous and sweat glands. By secreting sebum, sebaceous glands provide a protective coat, preventing rapid water evaporation and skin dryness. Sweat glands (excreting sweat) regulate temperature by water evaporation from the skin surface. Heat also dissipates from the skin (lowering temperature) when cutaneous blood vessels dilate and there is more blood on the surface. Body temperature rises when cutaneous blood vessels constrict and sweat production decreases. Sweat excretion also aids in removing waste products from the body.

Sensation. Skin nerve receptors allow a sense of touch interpreted as pain, pressure, heat, and cold. Touch is a means of communicating with the external environment. Touch is important for protection and orientation.

Principles related to skin structure and function are:

▶ The intact skin and mucous membrane are the body's first line of defense against infection.
▶ Excessive skin dryness contributes to breakdown.
▶ Poor circulation impedes skin nutrition.
▶ Some bacteria are necessary to maintain a homeostatic skin surface environment.
▶ The greater the number of organisms, the greater the possibility of infection.
▶ Pathogens grow readily in warm, moist, dark environments.

Self-Care of the Skin

BATHING

Bathing (a) cleans the skin; (b) stimulates skin circulation; (c) provides exercise; (d) relaxes tense muscles;

(e) improves the sense of well-being; (f) provides physical and psychologic comfort; and (g) provides the nurse an opportunity to observe and interact with a person requiring care.

Bathing and the use of skin preparations are influenced by culture more than any other hygiene practices. In some cultures, people bathe one or more times daily, and many apply oils and other skin preparations. Such people may be compelled to bathe daily regardless of need. In other cultures, people may have different ideas about what is right and proper about bathing.

Some people bathe for reasons other than hygiene (e.g., relaxation, therapeutic baths). A warm tub bath can relax and soothe sore, tense muscles. For some people, bathing is a time for being alone to screen out external stimuli or relieve general tension. For others, bathing is a stimulant to "get started in the morning," (a cool shower to "get going.") In care facilities, whenever possible, maintain an individual's habitual bathing practices.

Guidelines applicable for all bathing are

▶ Promote safety and prevent falls.
▶ Assess psychologic and physical needs.
▶ Determine self-care abilities, know activity limitations, and encourage self-help unless contraindicated.
▶ Involve the person in the bathing process and give the person as much control as is possible.
▶ Individualize teaching according to needs.
▶ Determine the purpose of bathing.
▶ Collect all necessary items before starting care.
▶ Cleanse the skin to remove dirt, excessive oil, perspiration, transient bacteria, and dead epithelial cells.
▶ Determine effects of frequency of bathing on condition of skin.
▶ Provide frequent baths for incontinent people and those who are diaphoretic ("sweaty") or have oily skin.
▶ Immediately clean skin of body excretions (urine, feces) to prevent skin irritation.
▶ Do not apply soap to excoriated skin.
▶ Bathe from "clean to dirty" body areas (eyes, face, ears, neck, upper extremities, chest, abdomen, lower extremities, and perineum with first washcloth. Then back, followed by perianal area with second washcloth).
▶ Use friction to stimulate circulation and remove debris, unless contraindicated.
▶ Provide warmth and privacy during bathing. Cover and drape as appropriate.
▶ Use good body mechanics when assisting and bathing. Keep back straight, use legs and abdominal muscles, and maintain a wide base of support (see Chapter 29).
▶ Remember: not all people need daily baths.

Agents Used for Skin Care. Selection of an agent to clean and protect skin depends on (a) skin condition (oily, dry, intact), (b) purpose and availability of the agent, and (c) individual preferences.

Soaps. Soap lowers skin surface tension and so facilitates cleaning. Some soaps cause excessive dryness by removing too much sebum from the skin. Antibacterial soaps destroy some of the bacteria on the skin. Some people experiencing skin allergies require hypoallergenic soaps. Use plain warm water to clean excessively dry or exfoliated (loss of superficial layers) skin. Products containing a demulcent or emollient also can be used as protective skin agents.

Demulcents. Demulcents (substances that soothe and allay skin irritation) coat skin and mucous membranes. Used on abrasive areas, they prevent drying of underlying cells and protect the skin from environmental irritants.

Emollients. Emollients (e.g., lanolin and white petroleum jelly) soften skin and mucous membranes by forming an oily film that prevents evaporation of water from underlying skin layers.

Powders. Powders can prevent friction and absorb moisture. Water-absorbent powders, used sparingly, can decrease friction and retard bacterial growth. Powders should not be used on open, draining areas, since they may cake or crust, producing more irritation. Starches have a beneficial drying effect but can become doughy from absorbed moisture.

Skin Integrity

The amount of sebum on the skin surface varies. Accumulated sebum can cause skin irritation, clogged pores, or blemishes on very oily skin. Frequent bathing with a "detergent-type" drying soap conditions oily skin. Frequent bathing and thorough drying help prevent skin breakdown from moisture in diaphoretic people (those with excessive sweating).

Some people normally have dry skin; elderly people often have dry skin because of decreased secretions. Dry skin may develop from systemic changes, environmental conditions, or drug therapy. Several options are available when caring for people with dry skin: (a) bathe less frequently; (b) use plain water without soap (use soap only in those body areas that have apocrine glands); (c) use soap containing lanolin; (d) add demulcents and emollients to bath water or apply directly to skin as cleaning and protecting agents (e.g., Alpha-Keri or Septi-Soft). When these last types of products are used, do not rinse. Leave an oily film on the skin. Apply between baths as necessary.

Initiation of skin care is often an independent nursing judgment. Interventions for skin care are based on nursing assessment and nursing diagnosis. Careful skin assessment always precedes skin hygiene care. Skin care is determined by physiologic need, skin condition, personal hygiene practices, individual comfort, and psychosocial needs.

Selection of skin agents is based on thorough nursing assessment and knowledge of the purposes of various skin agents. Most health care facilities have available one or two types of soaps and some type of protective skin agent. Individual preferences are important, but discourage people from using contraindicated agents. Always explain reasons carefully. For example, encourage a person with very dry skin to use a mild soap, plain water, or a product containing a demulcent or emollient.

Assessment

Obtain information regarding the type of bath the person prefers when at home, the time of day for bathing, the type of soap and deodorant (if any), use of lotion or skin emollient, and particular preferences regarding specifics of the bath. To gauge how much assistance will be needed with skin care, note the functional level of the client.

Perform a "skin risk" assessment. People at high risk for skin breakdown are those who are edematous, malnourished, emaciated, immunocompromised, receiving radiation treatment, immobilized for any reason, or experiencing neurologic deficits of movement or sensation. People with diabetes or vascular insufficiency are also at high risk for skin problems and pressure ulcers.

The condition of the skin provides clues about a person's general health and need for hygiene. Although skin can be easily observed during hygiene care, assessment of abnormalities is difficult because the signs are often subtle. Skill in skin assessment develops through practice and by thoughtfully relating observations to knowledge of skin structure and function.

For useful assessment, have an efficient light source with nonglare daylight or 60-watt bulb. Position, environmental conditions (e.g., temperature), amount of perspiration and sebum, edema (swelling), and pigmentation patterns all affect the accuracy of skin assessment.[54]

Color. The amount of melanin varies between and within racial groups. What we may think of as black, white, yellow, brown, or red skin each contains varying shades, tones, and pigmentation patterns. Assess people with very light or very dark skin with extra care.

At first glance, a light-skinned person may appear ashen or cyanotic. A very dark-skinned person may have some conditions, such as cyanosis, that go unnoticed. Normal pigmentation in dark-skinned people includes blue lips, bluish gums, deposits of brown melanin in eyes' sclerae, and freckle-like pigmentation of gums and buccal cavity.[54]

Descriptive terms for skin color are somewhat vague: pallor (pale); cyanotic (bluish); rubra or erythema (reddish); jaundice (yellowish); and ashen (grayish). Regardless of the amount of melanin, assess the presence or absence of underlying red tones on skin surface and the color of the sclerae, conjunctivae, and mucous membranes in the oral cavity. You may be able to identify jaundice (yellow coloring) more readily on the abdomen and buttocks (areas of lighter pigmentation). Cyanosis may be detected in lips, nailbeds, conjunctivae, palms, and soles.

Assess carefully at regular intervals to notice changes. Apply light pressure to skin to create pallor. Remove pressure and watch color return. Normally, color returns in less than 1 second. If a person is cyanotic, color returns from the periphery first and color returns more slowly than normal.[54] Various types of discoloration also may be noted: ecchymosis (reddish-purple bruise); petechiae (pinpoint reddish spots); purpura (reddish-purple areas).

Temperature. The temperature of the skin gives clues to possible inflammatory and circulation problems. Assess skin temperature by touching the person's skin with the back of your fingers. Note skin color and room temperature. Skin temperature is influenced by room temperature and is correlated with skin color. Cyanosis may signal a cold environment or circulatory problems. Erythema may indicate a hot environment or an inflammation.

Suppleness. The suppleness of the skin refers to the pliability or ease of movement. Suppleness is affected by amount of moisture and oil; general texture (smooth, rough); turgor (fullness of tissue); fiber elasticity in the dermis; and edema. Lift a section of skin and observe for ease of movement and speed of return to original position. Edema (fluid in tissue) causes a change in color and a shiny appearance as the skin becomes taut.

Intactness and Lesions. Look for breaks in skin. Inspect and palpate for lesions and rashes. Skin lesions include macules (flat spots), papules (raised lesions; pimples), vesicles (fluid-filled lesions), and nodules (solid, raised lesions). Notice whether lesions are localized or generalized over the body. A macular or papular rash on arms and legs can be caused by friction of bed linens.

Sensation. Assess sensation (pressure, pain, heat, and cold) while palpating the skin for lesions. Palpate with a light but firm pressure and ask the person what is felt. Also ask the person to describe the temperature of your hands. Limited sensation of temperature, pressure, and touch may indicate generalized or localized problems (e.g., circulatory problems or calloused skin). Protect a person with altered sensations. Carefully test temperature of bath water and treatments such as warm soaks. Also protect skin while moving the person. Itching may indicate dry skin or allergies.

Cleanliness. Assess skin cleanliness by noting body odor and amount of moisture, dirt, and oil on the skin.

Nursing Diagnosis

If skin integrity is unimpaired, the nursing diagnosis for persons needing assistance with skin care is *Self-Care Deficit, Bathing/Hygiene* (see Nursing Diagnosis Profile). If skin breakdown is present, the nursing diagnoses *Impaired Skin Integrity* and *Impaired Tissue In-*tegrity are also appropriate. See Chapter 48 for information about *Impaired Tissue Integrity*.

Planning

Planning, based on the data obtained from assessment, includes working with the client and family in deciding on a schedule for bathing, the type of bath to be given, agents to be used for skin hygiene, and consideration of cultural attitudes toward these hygiene activities. Allow sufficient time to make the bath a pleasurable, relaxing event for the person. The fewer interruptions and distractions that occur, the better.

Depending on the client's functional ability level, the expected outcome might include

▶ Washes face and hands by self.
▶ Completes all hygiene care independently.
▶ Completes own bedbath except for back and perianal area.
▶ Bathes self in tub.

Nursing Intervention

METHODS OF BATHING

The bathing method and the amount of assistance needed are nursing judgments based upon assessment of benefit to the person, safety factors, individual preferences, and contraindications. Regardless of the method of bathing (shower, tub, bed), the balance between self-care and nurse assistance varies. For example, one person who showers may need assistance in back washing, or someone in bed may be able to bathe completely except for the feet or back.

In the past, many people were bathed in bed in health care facilities. Gradually more people were encouraged to bathe themselves to prevent the complications of immobility. Some people still need to be bathed in bed (those with casts, in traction, and on strict bedrest for energy conservation). Some assistive devices, such as chairs for showering (Fig. 38–14) or mechanical lifts that transfer a person into a bathtub, allow people who would otherwise be unable to take a shower or bath.

Providing for shower or tub bathing sometimes demands considerable time and energy from the care provider (e.g., getting help to transfer a person in and out of the bathtub). The physical and psychologic benefits to the person, however, take priority over care giver convenience.

MEDICATED (THERAPEUTIC) BATHS

Some people require a therapeutic bath for healing purposes. Medicated baths are used for treatment of various skin disorders. They are given (a) to clean the skin of previously applied ointments or creams; (b) to heal irritated skin; (c) to soften crusted debris for easy removal; (d) to relax the client; (e) to relieve itching; and (f) for sedative or stimulant effects. For example, agents used for a soothing effect include oatmeal, cornstarch, and sodium bicarbonate (baking soda). In a

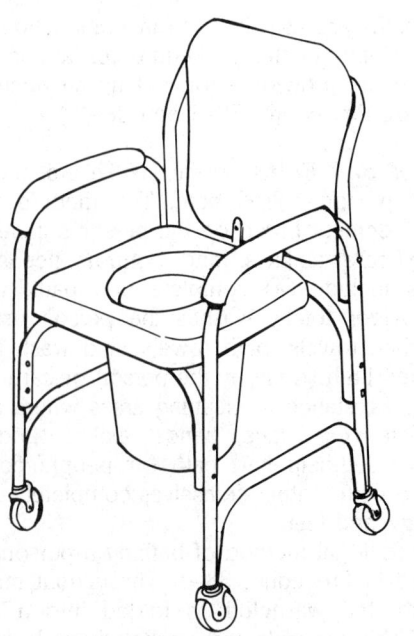

▲ *Figure 38-14*

Shower commode chair.

sense, a towel bath is a medicated (use of skin protective agent) or therapeutic bath. (For further discussion of therapeutic baths, including sitz baths, see Chapter 48.)

SHOWER OR BATHTUB BATHING

Safety is most important when assisting someone with a shower or tub bath. Base intervention on the following guidelines.

▶ Collect needed items: towel, washcloth, soap, clean gown or pajamas, personal toilet articles (deodorant, powder). Place these within easy reach to prevent possible falls from reaching for supplies.

▶ Prepare shower or tub by scheduling its use and cleaning it if necessary. Place rubber mat on bottom of shower or tub and place bath mat or towel on floor beside the shower or tub to prevent slipping. Covering the floor also prevents chilling the feet.

▶ Adjust room temperature to comfortable range.

▶ Place an occupied sign on door of bathroom for privacy. Always knock before entering an occupied bathroom.

▶ Have person wear robe and nonskid slippers en route to the bathroom. Cover with a robe or bath blanket for warmth and privacy during transportation.

▶ Assist person to bathroom as indicated to prevent falls.

▶ Explain how to use the call signal for assistance. Show the person how to use the safety grab bars when getting in and out of tub or shower to prevent falls. Remain with the individual or provide other assistance as indicated.

Instruct the person to call for help immediately if feeling weak or faint.

Faintness or weakness may be experienced during bathing because of vasodilation from hot water (blood normally flowing to the brain shifts from the central nervous system to the periphery as environmental temperature increases). Problems also can occur because of prior periods of inactivity. The body may be unable to compensate for the added physical stress, especially when showering.

▶ Adjust water temperature and pressure. Wait long enough for water temperature to stabilize at 41° to 46°C (105.8° to 114.8°F). Caution the person not to readjust the water temperature. Burns can occur when the person is unfamiliar with the faucets, or illness has altered sense of touch.

▶ Protect the person's modesty during bathing. Place a towel across the person's lap when removing the gown/robe and during bathing.

▶ After the person is finished bathing, have the bathroom cleaned. Remove soiled linen and take the occupied sign from the door.

Showering. A standing shower is usually unassisted, but the person may require help in back washing. A shower chair (Fig. 38-14) can be used for people unable to tolerate standing and for those who would otherwise need bathing in bed (e.g., confused or weak people). Often a shower chair or bathtub is most appropriate for people who can sit and have no dressings or casts. Most shower chairs have wheels and are made of plastic. A movable shower head or hand-held shower nozzle is used to direct the water at an appropriate level.

A person may be transported to the shower area in a wheelchair or in the shower chair.

If the person is confused, paralyzed, or weak, use a protective belt or other device to prevent falling or slipping out of the shower chair.

A protective device may be necessary even though someone is helping the person with the shower. Remember, when you are washing someone you may be unable to prevent the person from falling out of the chair. Once in place, set the brakes of the shower chair to keep it from rolling.

Tub Bathing. After initial preparations, half-fill the tub with water. Warn the person not to soak in the tub for longer than 20 minutes. Maximum vascular benefits are accomplished in 15 to 20 minutes. Prolonged soaking increases fatigue. Also, others may be waiting for use of the tub.

Assist a person in and out of the bathtub by giving support under the axillae. Have a chair close by for the person to sit on while drying. People capable of self-care may like or need assistance in washing their backs.

People with dressings can sometimes use a shower chair or tub if the dressings can be covered with plastic and taped to keep them dry. Sometimes a dressing is able to be wet during bathing and a dry dressing is applied afterward. Some people with casts also can be assisted into the tub or shower chair. For example, a person with an arm cast can have plastic secured over the cast and around the edges to keep it dry.

Bathing at the Sink or Side of the Bed. Sometimes the person is well enough to sit up in a chair and bathe at the sink or can sit on the side of the bed with the bath basin positioned on the overbed table. For these clients, provide privacy by closing the door and providing the top sheet or bath blanket for the person to use as a drape and for warmth. Give assistance washing the back, feet, and legs as necessary. The perineal area is often difficult or impossible to clean adequately while in a seated position. If necessary, offer the client perineal care (see page 925).

As the client bathes in a seated position, it is prudent to remain nearby in case the client needs assistance or becomes fatigued or dizzy. If the client is bathing at the sink, you may be able to change the bed linens while waiting. If the client is seated on the side of the bed, you may use the opportunity to prepare or to clean up other equipment, such as that needed for mouth or hair care.

Bathing in Bed. Bed bathing is indicated primarily for people with restricted mobility (some people with casts, traction, or back problems); limited exertion (some people with heart and respiratory problems); and often for first-day postoperative people who may experience hypotension or are very weak.

Systemic Assessment During a Bed Bath. Giving a bed bath provides nurses with excellent opportunities for communication and assessment. The following assessment can be made during bathing:

▶ Respiratory: breathing during movement and at rest (rate, quality, pattern).
▶ Cardiovascular: body temperature, color of skin, circulation to extremities and nailbeds. Note coldness and changes in heart rate (pulse).
▶ Musculoskeletal: joint mobility and muscle strength during range-of-motion (see Chapter 35); coordination; self-help abilities.
▶ Mental/emotional/social: orientation, emotional state, ability to follow directions, personal concerns, discomfort, hygiene preferences and attitudes, cultural practices, comments about social networks, and present situation.
▶ Gastrointestinal: any abdominal distention, fecal incontinence, or rectal bleeding. Ask about bowel patterns.
▶ Genitourinary: bladder distention, urinary incontinence, difficulty in voiding.
▶ Integumentary: skin intactness, general condition, and other skin factors. Assess sense of touch (temperature of water, pressure with rubbing).

Be sensitive and observant while bathing clients. Assess general physical and psychosocial needs, including learning needs. Communicate concern and care during bathing by appropriate use of touch. Caring can help establish a therapeutic relationship between a person needing care and a nurse.

Bed baths are usually done in conjunction with bed making. Combine the procedure for a complete bed bath with the procedure for making an occupied bed. (These are Procedures 38–1 and 38–2.)

Types of Bed Baths. There are several methods for giving a person a bed bath. The method used is a nursing judgment based on the person's general condition, self-care abilities, and comfort needs. Various methods include (a) complete bed bath, where the care provider totally washes the person using washcloths, face towels, bath towels, and wash basin; (b) partial bed bath (done by the person or care provider), involving assistance in cleaning areas where secretions accumulate (e.g., face, hands, axillae, and perineal area); (c) self-help bed bath for people confined to bed but able to bathe themselves completely except for back, legs, and feet.

The traditional method of bathing a person in bed is described in Procedure 38–1. Throughout most of the bed bath, the washcloth is folded into a mitt (Fig. 38–15). This prevents the washcloth ends from dragging uncomfortably over the person's body. The mitt also facilitates more effective friction in washing.

To make a mitt (Fig. 38–15):
1. Grasp edge of washcloth between thumb and base of index finger and fold one third over palm of your hand.
2. Bring remaining opposite edge across palm and hold with your thumb.
3. Bring extended end of washcloth up to palm and tuck edge under.

When using soap, always rinse thoroughly to avoid skin irritation from soap residue. Always dry skin thoroughly, especially body creases (e.g., buttocks, under the breasts, between fingers and toes). Assist people who have difficulty drying themselves (such as those

Text continued on page 923

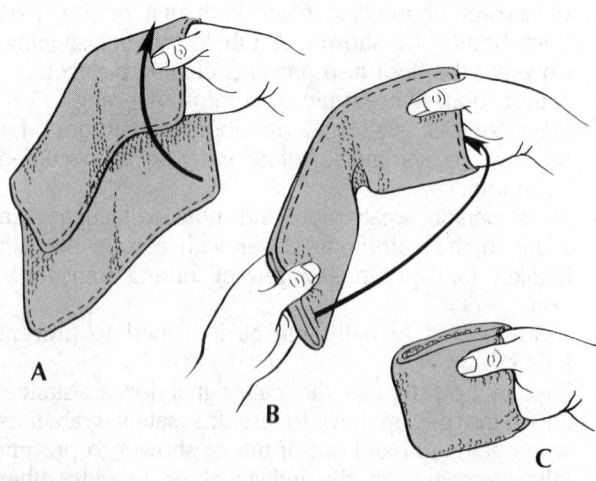

▲ *Figure 38–15*

Making a washcloth mitt for bathing. This type of bath mitt covers the ends of the fingers and protects the person from being scratched with sharp fingernails.

PROCEDURE 38-1

Complete Bed Bath

Definition/Purposes. Bathing a person in bed using a wash basin, washcloths, and towels. The purpose is to cleanse the skin of a person confined to bed and not capable of self-bathing.

Contraindications/Cautions. Keep side rail up on side away from nurse during bath to help person turn and prevent person from falling out of bed. Keep both side rails up while away from bed. Use *no* soap when washing around eyes. Assess for soap allergies. Protect casts and dressings from moisture (place plastic covering over edges of cast).

Learning/Teaching Guidelines. Present the following information as appropriate: (a) amount of participation by person that is therapeutic; (b) how energy conservation is related to individual's condition; (c) how daily bathing may contribute to dry skin; and (d) how to obtain community services if complete bathing at home is required upon discharge.

PRELIMINARY ACTIVITIES

Assessment/Planning

- ▶ Check activity orders and specific precautions for movement and positioning.
- ▶ Assess for tubes and IV line locations.
- ▶ Assess need for bathing.
- ▶ Assess person's ability to assist; plan appropriate help.

Incorporate passive range-of-motion (ROM) exercises into bed bath as appropriate.

- ▶ Assess ability to understand directions.
- ▶ Ask preference regarding hygiene aids (e.g., soap).
- ▶ Obtain hygiene aids, linen, and equipment.
- ▶ Assess room temperature and ventilation (adjust as possible); close windows and door to prevent drafts.
- ▶ Wash hands prior to obtaining linen.
- ▶ Use efficient body mechanics.

Preparation of Person and Unit

- ▶ Explain how person can assist.
- ▶ Explain sequence of activities.
- ▶ Clear work area.
- ▶ Ensure privacy.
- ▶ Place needed items on bedside stand or overbed table adjusted to comfortable height.
- ▶ Adjust bed to comfortable height with side rails up as needed.

- ▶ Place lamp away from person.
- ▶ Offer bedpan/urinal (wash hands after use).
- ▶ Position person supine if allowed.
- ▶ Make provision for tubes and IV lines to prevent their inadvertent removal.

If combining bath with occupied bed-making, note instructions for Procedure 38–2 now. Read through action 2c.

Equipment

- ▶ Wash basin
- ▶ Soap dish
- ▶ Gloves
- ▶ Linen hamper
- ▶ Laundry bag
- ▶ Bath blanket
- ▶ 2 washcloths
- ▶ 2 bath towels
- ▶ 2 face towels
- ▶ Gown
- ▶ Hygiene aids (soap, powder, deodorant, skin lotion)

PROCEDURES

Actions

1. Remove top linen. Cover person with bath blanket.
   a. Loosen top linen at foot of bed.
   b. Remove spread and blanket. If to be reused, fold while removing (see Procedure 38–2).
   c. Place one end of bath blanket at person's shoulders. Ask client to hold top edge of bath blanket in place if possible as you remove sheet.
   d. Reach under bath blanket, grasp top edge of sheet, and bring to foot of bed.
   e. Once at foot of bed, fold top sheet into bundle. Place in laundry bag or fold for replacement.
2. Position person close to edge of bed nearest you.

Rationale/Assessment

1. Use top sheet as cover if bath blanket is unavailable.

   b. Keeps linen dry for replacement.

   c. Bath blanket provides warmth and privacy. If person is unable to hold bath blanket, tuck blanket's top corners under shoulders.
   d. Keep person covered with bath blanket while removing sheet.
   e. If top sheet is clean, it may be reused as bottom sheet when bed is remade.
2. Prevents unnecessary reaching.

Procedure continued on following page

PROCEDURE 38–1 Continued

Complete Bed Bath

Actions	Rationale/Assessment
3. Remove person's gown while keeping covered with bath blanket.	3. REMOVING GOWN WITH IV RUNNING If person has IV line, remove gown from arm *without IV first*; then lower IV container and slide gown up IV tubing and over IV container. Rehang IV container and check rate of flow. See Chapter 47 for further information.
4. Place overbed table or bedside stand within easy reach and position bath basin and soap dish conveniently.	4. Prevents unnecessary twisting and reaching.
5. Remove pillow if condition permits.	5. Pillow removal simplifies washing neck and ears. Some people must have pillow (e.g., difficulty in breathing).
6. Place bath towel under head.	6. Protects bed from wetness.
7. Pull side rails up as needed for safety and obtain bath water.	7. Fill wash basin one third to one half full, with water temperature approximately 43° to 46°C (109.4° to 114.8°F). Too little water is inadequate for bathing and cools rapidly. Too much water may spill. Water too hot or too cold can cause discomfort and burns or chills. Determine water temperature by using wood-encased bath thermometer or placing your wrist in water.
8. Wash, rinse, and dry face and neck. a. Wash around eyes without soap. With your hand in mitt, place index finger at inner canthus. Then move toward outer canthus. Then use opposite corner of mitt to bathe other eye in same manner. Dry around eyes thoroughly.	8. Encourage appropriate self-help. a. Examine eyes. Using a separate section of mitt to wash each eye avoids spread of organisms. For removal of crusted secretions, see discussion of care for eyes (page 908).
	Ask person if soap is desired for bath.
b. Wash, rinse, and dry forehead, cheeks, nose, and around mouth.	b. Observe for skin eruptions, drainage from nose (note color), or parched lips. If lips are crusted, soak with wet cloth before attempting to remove secretions. This decreases tissue trauma.
c. Wash, rinse, and dry ear with cloth over hand. Place two fingers in anterior external ear and thumb behind ear.	c. One smooth motion cleans anterior and posterior ear. Examine ears for secretions. Note skin condition.
d. Wash front and back of neck. Lift person toward you, if necessary, to reach back of neck. Rinse and dry.	d. Observe for skin eruptions, scaling at hair line, and enlarged lymph nodes.
9. Remove bath towel under person's head.	
10. Wash, rinse, and dry arms. a. Place bath towel lengthwise under arm, well up under axillae (armpit).	10. a. Protects bed from wetness.
b. Grasp wrist and elevate arm.	b. Facilitates examination and range of motion (ROM).
c. Use mitt to wash and rinse arms. Use long, firm strokes in direction toward shoulder and light strokes toward hand. Cleanse axillae.	c. Smooth, continuous motion. Firmness creates friction to remove debris and stimulates circulation.
	If IV is present, (a) do not place pressure over vein or over insertion site; (b) do not dislodge needle; and (c) check IV flow after moving arm.
	Palpate for enlarged axillary nodes. Note skin eruptions, dryness. Apply lotion as indicated.
11. Wash, rinse, and dry hands.	11. To clean or clip nails, soak hands now or at end of bath.
a. Wash without mitt. b. Support at wrist joint. c. Put hands in water with bath towel under basin. Wash with cloth, using firm strokes from fingertips toward hand. Wash and dry all sides of each finger and move each finger at each joint.	a. Assess circulation by observing hands' temperature and color of hands and nailbeds. Debris between fingers may be difficult to remove. Firm strokes provide friction for debris removal and stimulate circulation. Moving joints provides ROM.

PROCEDURE 38–1 Continued

Complete Bed Bath

Actions

12. Wash, rinse, and dry chest.
   a. Place bath towel over chest and fold bath blanket down to umbilicus (navel).
   b. Hold one corner of towel up away from chest. With other hand mitted, cleanse chest using firm, long strokes. Replace towel over chest between washing, rinsing, and drying.

13. Wash, rinse, and dry abdomen.
   a. Fold bath blanket down to pubic region. Tuck sides around hips.
   b. Place bath towel lengthwise or crosswise over abdomen.
   c. Lift bath towel up with one hand. Use mitted hand to wash abdomen. Wash from side to side, using long, firm strokes.
   d. Lower bath towel to abdomen between washing and rinsing.
   e. Dry abdomen with bath towel.
   f. Remove towel(s). Reposition bath blanket at shoulder height.
14. Wash, rinse, and dry legs.

Expose one leg at a time.

   a. Begin with farthest leg. Drape leg. Slide bath blanket toward hips, keeping blanket close to leg. Bring corner of bath blanket around thigh and hip. Tuck corner under lateral thigh (Fig. 38–16).
   b. Securely position bath basin near foot to be bathed.

   c. Position your arm to cradle person's calf; grasp heel; bend leg at knee. Slightly elevate leg off mattress; slide bath towel lengthwise under leg (Fig. 38–16).

Rationale/Assessment

12.
   a. Provides warmth and avoids exposure. Keeps bath blanket dry to place over person later.
   b. Allows visualization of area being washed while covering rest of chest. Maintains privacy, warmth. Firm strokes stimulate circulation, decrease "tickling." Remember to wash under breasts. Assess condition of breast tissue, skin under breast, and nipples. Note breathing depth and rate. Possibly teach about breast self-examination.

13.
   a. Assess for abdominal distention.

   b. For a woman, place face towel across chest and bath towel across abdomen.
   c. Give special attention to cleansing umbilicus and creased folds of abdomen. Firm strokes decrease "tickling."

14.

   a. Draping prevents unnecessary exposure and drafts.

   b. Support basin with free hand while lifting foot. Prevents spilling.
   c. Cradling leg in this manner supports joints. Towel on bed protects bed from wetness.

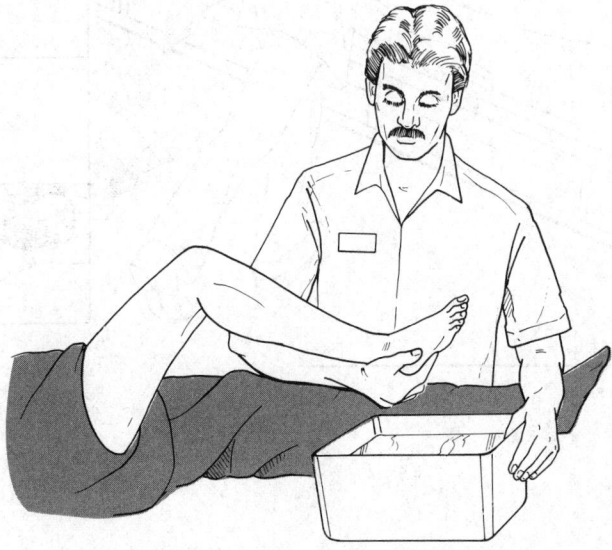

▲ *Figure 38–16*

Procedure continued on following page

PROCEDURE 38–1 Continued

Complete Bed Bath

Actions

    d. Continue supporting leg and foot. With your free hand, slide bath basin under lifted foot (Fig. 38–16). Place foot firmly on basin bottom.

    e. With mitted hand, use firm, long strokes to clean and dry leg.

    f. Open washcloth and use firm touch to wash foot.

    g. Drape and wash "near" leg and foot in the same manner as in steps a through f.

15. Obtain clean water for perineal care. (Use gloves for perineal care.) Wash, rinse, and dry perineal area.

16. Change water and washcloth.

17. Wash, rinse, and dry the back.

    a. Turn person to side-lying position while keeping covered with bath blanket (Fig. 38–17).

Rationale/Assessment

    d. Controls leg movement; prevents spilled water. Position foot to avoid pressure from edge of basin on calf of leg. Allow foot to soak while bathing leg.

    e. Aids venous return.

    f. Firm touch decreases "tickling." Wash and dry thoroughly between each toe to prevent skin breakdown. Inspect skin. Clean, clip nails as needed.

    g. For both legs and feet, assess sensation, circulation, muscle strength, and joint mobility. Provide ROM for lower extremity joints unless contraindicated.

15. For safety, raise side rails while away from bed. Check water temperature. Clean water is needed after bathing feet. Water may be soapy and cold. Assist with perineal care as needed. Discuss importance of testicle self-examination as appropriate. This step completes the bath on the anterior portion of the body.

16. Clean water and cloth are needed after bathing the perineal area.

17. Back care is especially important for clients with decreased mobility.

    a. Makes back area accessible and keeps person warm.

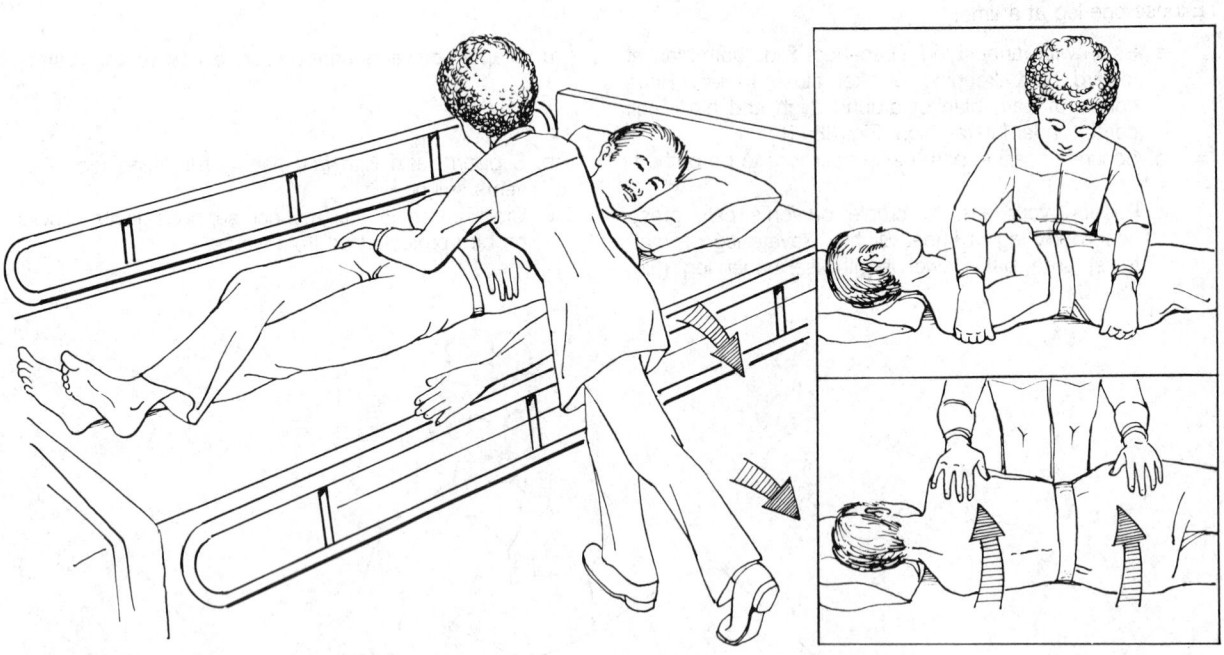

▲ *Figure 38–17*

Turning incapacitated person onto side.

PROCEDURE 38–1 Continued

Complete Bed Bath

Actions	Rationale/Assessment
b. Drape person by moving bath blanket away from back, from shoulder to thighs, and placing bath towel lengthwise over back.	b. Minimizes exposure. Assess skin, circulation, muscle tension. Watch for respiratory difficulty.
c. Use unmitted hand to hold towel away from back. Use mitted hand to wash back with continuous, long, firm strokes. Wash down from back of neck to lower border of buttocks, avoiding perianal area.	c. Promotes warmth, privacy. Bathe posterior (back) thighs, if not washed during bathing of legs.
18. Wash, rinse, and dry perianal area.	18. The perianal area is the ''dirtiest'' area and should be done last to avoid tracking microbes to cleaner areas of back.
19. Give back massage now or after bed has been completely made (see Chapter 39).	19. Back massage may be preferred in prone position.
If combining bath with occupied bed-making, apply deodorant to arm that is uppermost, apply clean gown over uppermost half of body, and refer to Procedure 38–2, steps 4–6a, to make first half of the foundation of the bed. After turning the client, apply deodorant to opposite underarm, complete dressing with the gown; continuing with client on the side, follow remaining steps of Procedure 38–2.	This sequence allows deodorant to be applied before clean gown is put on and allows gown to be put on before turning client onto clean bed linens. Once client is turned onto clean bed linens, the person should not again touch dirty linens. This sequence is most efficient of motion.

FINAL ACTIVITIES

If not yet done, offer use of personal care items (deodorant, powder, lotion). Assist with putting on clean gown. Provide hair care. For safety, replace call signal, lower bed, and replace bed cranks. Place *clean* face towel, bath towel, and wash cloth in room. If not yet done, change bed linen if damp or soiled. Care of equipment includes the following. Disinfect bath basin. Replace basin, soap, soap dish, and personal care items. Clean top of bedside stand and overbed table and position within person's reach. Dispose of soiled linen. Final interventions include the following: Position person for comfort and proper alignment. Remove unnecessary items. Leave needed items (tissues, paper bag for trash, water) within easy reach of person. Documentation requires charting the type of bath on flowsheet and noting abnormal findings on progress notes. Examples include skin breakdown, loss of motor strength, abnormal sensation, cool extremities, and respiratory distress with change of position. Note pertinent conversation, ability for self-care, and preferences in nursing care plan.

---

with physical difficulties, immobilization, stiffness, soreness, paralysis). Some people are particularly prone to skin breakdown and infection (people with diabetes mellitus or other metabolic disorders). Explain the importance of careful drying to people who do not understand that pathogenic organisms grow readily in a moist environment.

TEACHING AND LEARNING

It is effective to begin teaching/learning intervention by describing your observations to the person. For example, if you notice a person has very oily skin, you may state, "Your skin appears oily. Is this a problem for you?" The response may be, "It's not a problem when I'm able to shower every day." Or, "It's only a problem on my face." Recalling that both sebaceous and sweat glands are located in the area of the face, one expects increased secretions in that area. You might suggest that the person use soap when washing the face. In another situation, you may notice a person scratching

and may observe flaky, dry patches of skin. You may follow the same approach, offering suggestions for people with dry skin.

Some people have misconceptions about bathing. For example, some believe that bathing is harmful during illness or that chilling during bathing causes a "cold." When you discover your client has a misconception about hygiene, find out why the person believes the misconception, the significance of hygiene practices to the person, usual bathing habits, and any hygiene factors based on the individual's health status. Discuss misconceptions based on this information.

Monthly self-examination of breasts and testicles is an especially important health promotion measure appropriately taught in association with bathing.

BATHING AN INFANT

Bathing is important in caring for infants' skin. Infant bathing uses the same principles as for bathing adults.

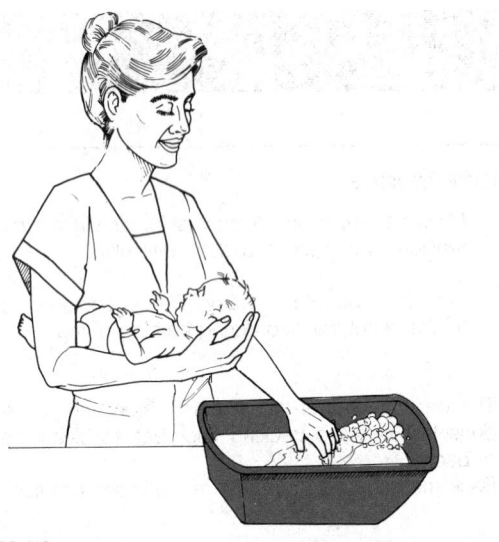

▲ *Figure 38–18*

Holding an infant in a football hold.

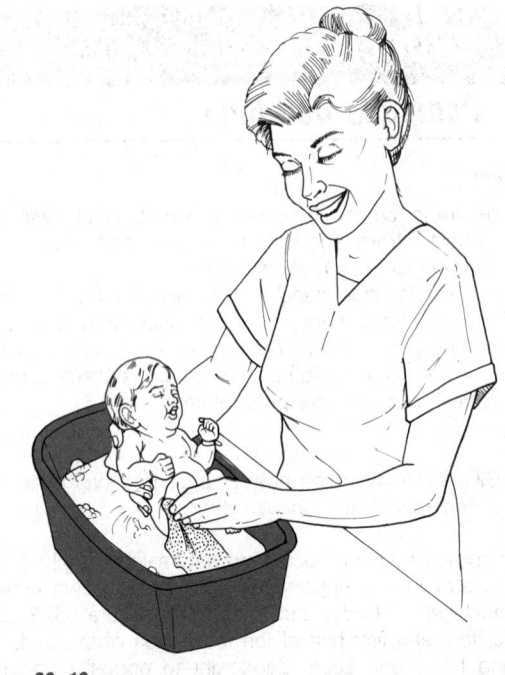

▲ *Figure 38–19*

Holding an infant in the tub. Note support of the neck and grasp of the opposite upper arm.

Safety, observation, and interaction are important. As with adults, bath time provides an opportunity for interaction. The stimulation of interaction between an infant and others is an important aspect of development. (More comprehensive information on infant bathing can be found in maternal-child nursing or pediatric nursing textbooks.)

Safety factors for infants include (a) care with water temperature, since an infant's skin is very sensitive to temperature, (b) preventing chilling since an infant may lose more heat than an adult because of the greater proportion of skin surface to body mass, (c) holding the infant securely, supporting the neck and head. An infant's muscles are not strong enough to hold the head upright (Figs. 38–18 and 38–19).

Never leave infants unattended on a surface or in the water for any reason.

Observation of an infant during the bath includes examining all areas of the skin for red or cracked areas. Closely examine the diaper area and skin creases.

Box 38–2. Infant Bathing Guide

1. Prepare bath area with all supplies and clothing to be used during the bath and clothes to be put on infant after bath.
2. Make bath water and temperature comfortable when tested with caregiver's wrist. Keep room temperature warm to avoid chilling during bath.
3. Wash around infant's eyes, moving from inner aspect of the eye toward the outer. Use a different part of washcloth for each eye to avoid possible cross-contamination. (Do not wash eyes.)
4. Wash infant's face next with clear water or a small amount of mild soap (e.g., castile).
5. Use "football" hold when washing infant's head (Fig. 33–18).
6. Gently wash fontanel ("soft spot") of infant's head.
7. Hold infant securely while in bath water (a) by the upper arm, with the caregiver's arm behind the back or (b) by reaching behind the infant's back and grasping infant's far thigh (Fig. 38–19).

8. Wash infant's body by applying soap with the hand over the entire body. Wash genital area last, either with infant next to the bath or with the infant still in bath water.
9. If the umbilical cord is still attached, opinions vary about bathing. Some believe the infant should be sponge-bathed until the cord drops off. Others think a brief tub bath (without soaking) is safe. Still others believe a tub bath is all right as long as the water does not cover the cord. Find out the policy in your care facility.
10. Dry infant thoroughly, especially in skin-fold areas (e.g., under chin, arms, and groin).
11. Carefully dry around the cord with a clean part of the towel. Some recommend the application of alcohol to the cord's base with a cotton-tipped applicator.
12. Dress the infant and place in a crib or other secure area while cleaning the bath area.

Evaluation

Statements indicating that expected outcomes for *Self-Care Deficit, Bathing/Hygiene* have been reached might include

▶ Able to wash own face and hands. Remainder of bed bath completed by nurse.
▶ Completed own bed bath except for back and perianal area.
▶ Independently bathed self in tub.

Bathing and routine skin care may be charted on an activity flowsheet rather than in the nurse's notes. Note the type of bath the client had, special skin care measures, and the time of the bath. Problems with the skin, such as reddening or breaks, or difficulty in tolerating the bathing procedure must be charted in the nurse's notes. For example,

1000   Assisted with bed bath; able to bathe upper body by self; skin over coccyx reddened with slight abrasion 1.5 × 2 cm in diameter. Cleansed with warm water and patted dry. Positioned on right side and instructed to stay off back by turning side to side q2h.
N. Harpham, S.N.

PERINEAL CARE

Perineal hygiene refers to cleaning of the external genitalia and surrounding area. Perineal hygiene is always done in conjunction with general bathing. Other indications for perineal care are genitourinary infection; incontinence of urine or feces; excessive secretions or concentrated urine, causing skin irritation or excoriation; presence of indwelling urinary (Foley) catheter; postpartum care; and care after some types of perineal surgery.

Perineal Area

The perineal area is located between the thighs and extends from the top of the pelvic bones (anterior) to the anus (posterior). The perineum contains sensitive anatomic structures related to sexuality, elimination, and reproduction.

Female Perineum. The female perineal area (Fig. 38–20) is made up of the vulva (external genitalia), including the mons pubis, prepuce, clitoris, urethral and vaginal orifices, and labia majora and minora. The skin of the vaginal orifice is normally moist. The vagina is kept moist by mucus-producing glands (Bartholin's glands) lateral to the vagina. Endocervical glands secrete an exudate that collects various cells as it moves through the vagina. The secretion has a slight odor due to the cells and normal vaginal flora. The amount of cloudy vaginal discharge (leukorrhea) varies with hormonal changes; for example, it increases during ovulation and with sexual stimulation. Vaginal secretion is slightly acid, thus inhibiting bacterial growth.

The skin of the labia majora is similar to other skin surfaces and is fairly resistant to trauma. The labia ma-

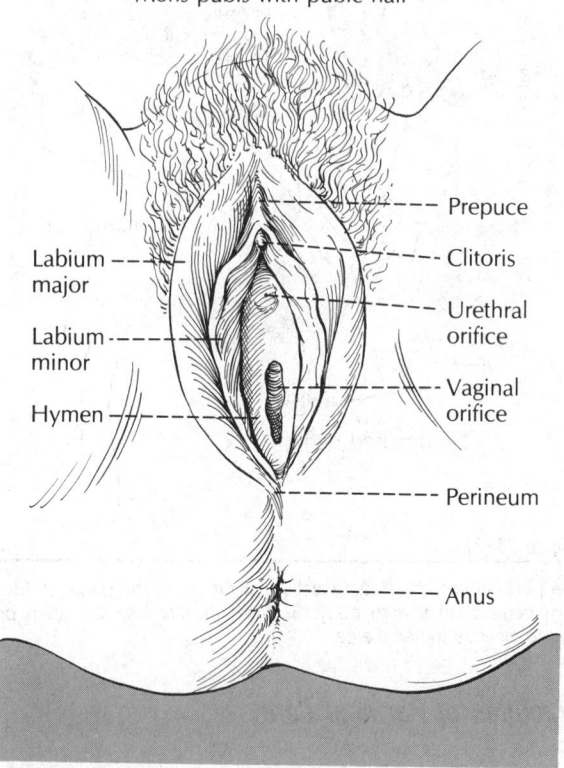

Mons pubis with pubic hair

Prepuce
Clitoris
Urethral orifice
Vaginal orifice
Perineum
Anus
Labium major
Labium minor
Hymen

▲ *Figure 38–20*

Anatomy of the female perineal area. Note that this anatomic drawing does not represent the appearance of the normal unretracted female perineum. Structures beneath the labia majora are not visible unless the labia are retracted.

jora have hair follicles and sebaceous and apocrine (sweat) glands. The clitoris consists of erectile tissue and many nerve fibers. It is very sensitive to touch. Posterior to the clitoris, the skin-fold divides to form the labia minora, which extend downward and inward to enfold the vaginal orifice. The modified skin surface is sensitive to external trauma and has only sebaceous glands.

Male Perineum. The penis contains pathways for urination and ejaculation through the urethral orifice (meatus) (Fig. 38–21). At the end of the penis is the glans covered by a skin flap (foreskin or prepuce). The urethral orifice is located in the center of the penis and opens at the tip. The shaft of the penis consists of erectile tissue bound by the foreskin's dense fibrous tissue. Skin on the penis is thin and has no hair; thus, it is easily injured. Skin on the penis is loose and allows distention. Erection is caused by engorgement secondary to stimuli.

The scrotum is located at the base of the penis. It contains testicles and a portion of the genital tract. The scrotal skin surface contains numerous apocrine glands. Because scrotal skin is thin, it is easily irritated.

The prostate is a network of glands producing prostatic secretion. The glands are embedded in muscles that contract during ejaculation to move the prostatic secretion through the ejaculatory ducts.

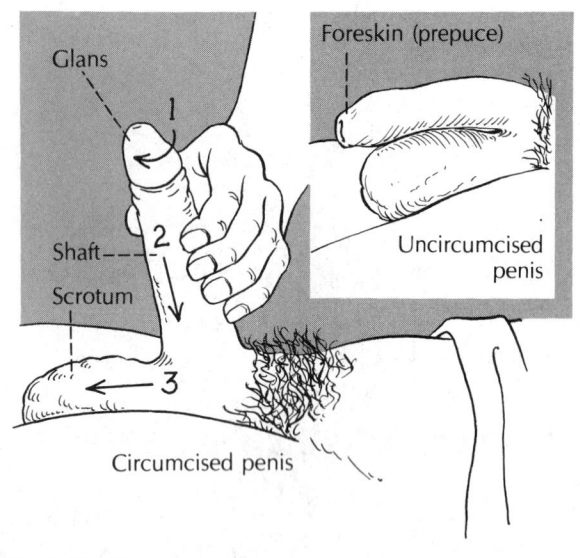

▲ *Figure 38–21*

Male perineal care. 1. Begin washing at the tip of the penis. 2. Move down penis shaft toward body. 3. Wash the scrotum last, then proceed to cleanse the anal area.

Principles of Perineal Care

Perineal care is provided in order to prevent or eliminate infection and odor, promote healing, and promote comfort. Because the perineum has several orifices, it is a common portal of entry for pathogens. The perineal area is conducive to growth of pathogenic organisms because it is warm and moist and not well ventilated. Thorough hygiene is essential to maintain skin condition and protect body integrity.

When maintaining perineal hygiene, remember that body orifices are potentially portals of entry for pathogens and that warm, moist skin is conducive to pathogenic growth. The urethral opening leads to the sterile bladder; the vaginal opening leads to the clean vagina; and the anus leads to the unclean rectum.

The urethral orifice is the "cleanest" area, and the anal orifice is the "dirtiest" area. Always stroke from front to back to wash from "clean" to "dirty" parts.

Entry of organisms from the anal orifice into the urethral orifice can cause urinary tract infections.

During perineal care, completely clean skin around the urethral orifice first. Do not clean this area after cleaning the anal orifice.

Clean gloves are essential when cleaning the perineum. Use a separate portion of the washcloth for each wipe. Because the perineal area is warm and moist, it requires frequent cleaning and thorough rinsing and drying. Because ill people have lowered resistance to infection, often spend time in bed, and get less ventilation of the perineal area, perineal skin and mucous membrane are prone to breakdown, and body integrity is jeopardized. The perineal area has hair that tends to harbor organisms.

Assessment

Assessment of the need for perineal care beyond that provided with the daily bath is based on (a) the individual's susceptibility to infection, (b) assessment of skin problems, and (c) the need to remove sources of odors. People prone to skin breakdown include those with concentrated urine, fecal or urinary incontinence, Foley (urinary) catheters; recent genitourinary or rectal surgery, diaphoresis, and metabolic disorders such as diabetes mellitus. Unpleasant odors may indicate infection or poor hygiene. Thorough perineal care and teaching the person about the importance of perineal hygiene can prevent problems.

Nurses sometimes neglect perineal assessment because of embarrassment. Deterioration of a perineal skin condition can go unnoticed when a person is doing perineal self-care. Take notice of comments about itching, burning with urination, and soreness. If the person requires help with a bedpan or urinal, observe the perineal area while assisting with this care. If you note an unpleasant odor or concentrated urine, examine the perineal area for secretions and skin irritation. Other findings can be noted by inspection and palpation. Assess for lesions; ulcers; scars; amount, color, odor, and source of drainage; tenderness; inflammation; excoriation; edema; and enlarged lymph nodes.

Nursing Diagnosis

The nursing diagnosis appropriate for the person in need of assistance with perineal care is *Self-Care Deficit, Bathing/Hygiene.*

Planning

When planning to assist the client with perineal care, take the person's feelings into account. Cultural factors are very important because in some cultures it is taboo for a member of the opposite sex other than a spouse to touch the perineum. An expected outcome for a client with a self-care deficit in perineal care is

► Able to complete own perineal care.

Nursing Intervention

Perineal hygiene is often ignored by both people receiving and those giving care because of embarrassment. A nurse's concerned professional attitude can reduce such embarrassment. Whether you are doing perineal assessment or assisting with or providing perineal care, use language the person can understand.

If you do not think that the patient has the physical capability of performing perineal care, at that point during the bath when it should be done, gently state that you will now change the water and "wash the genital area." By stating your intentions, you provide an opportunity for protest while giving yourself a chance to cleanse this area thoroughly. Many people simply cannot bend and see well enough to cleanse this area, and others are too weak or too ill. If the person realizes that perineal care would be difficult to do and that it is a normal part of the bathing routine, consent is usually given for the nurse to continue.

Wear clean disposable gloves while assisting with perineal care. Explain to the person that your purpose for wearing gloves is to prevent the possibility of carrying organisms (germs) from one person to another. Use a mild soap with warm water (43°C or 109.4°F) and clean gently. If skin is excoriated, use plain warm water only. When soap is used, be sure to rinse well to prevent skin irritation. Because the perineal area is easily traumatized by friction and retains moisture, thoroughly and gently pat dry all skin surfaces.

Positioning and Draping. Place both women and men in the dorsal recumbent position for perineal care. Provide privacy and decrease exposure by draping a person for assessment and perineal care. One method of draping is to fan-fold a bath blanket or sheet to the midthigh area. Then place a towel on the abdomen slightly above the genitalia. Have the person slightly flex the legs so that all areas can be effectively reached for cleaning.

A second method of draping, which provides a greater sense of security, involves wrapping the legs with a bath blanket. Place the bath blanket at an angle with one corner between the legs and a corner on each side of the bed. Bring one side corner around the leg and tuck under the hip. (This method is also used for leg and foot bathing, as shown in Figure 38–16.) Repeat this for the other leg. Then fold the corner from between the legs back onto the abdomen for care. Have the person slightly flex the legs so that all areas can be examined and cleaned.

Male Perineal Care. Gently retract the foreskin in uncircumcised men before starting perineal care. When perineal care is completed, pull the foreskin back over the glans. **Smegma** (a cheeselike substance that is secreted by sebaceous glands and that collects under the foreskin in males and under the labia minora in females) must be removed. Hold the shaft of the penis in one hand and the washcloth in the other (see Fig. 38–21). Start washing at the tip of the penis (cleanest area). Use a circular motion, cleaning from the center to the periphery, and use a separate section of the washcloth for each wipe. Rinse thoroughly. Wash down the shaft toward the body.

Stimulation of the glans may cause an erection. This may embarrass the man and the care giver. You might explain that this is a normal reaction and that the vasocongestion will subside once the stimulation from cleaning is complete. Verbally acknowledging this response may reduce feelings of embarrassment.

Next, wash the scrotum and perineum. Hold the scrotum so the perineum and all surfaces of the scrotal sac can be cleaned. Gently pat dry the penis and scrotum.

After perineal cleaning has been completed, you may need to clean the **perianal area** (area around the anus). To clean the perianal area, place the person in a side-lying position with buttocks toward you. To drape the buttocks, place a bath blanket or sheet over the thighs and tuck under the leg resting on the mattress. Separate the buttocks with one hand. Use the washcloth in the other hand to clean. Wash, rinse, and dry the area using strokes only toward the back.

Female Perineal Care. It is often convenient for a woman to be on a bedpan to clean and rinse the vulva and perineum. Smegma tends to collect on the inner surface of the labia. Use one hand to gently retract the labia. With the other hand, wash from front to back ("clean to dirty"). Use a separate section of washcloth for each wipe in a downward motion (Fig. 38–22). Wash from the urethral to the vaginal orifice. Then wash the labia. Next, clean the perineum. The perineum may be easier to reach while the woman is lying on the side to clean the rectal area ("dirtiest"). Rinse and gently pat dry all the skin surfaces.

Special Perineal Care. Following genital or rectal surgery, sterile supplies may be required for cleaning the operative site, e.g., sterile cotton balls to gently clean the area (see Fig. 38–22). Sometimes the operative site and perineal area are washed with plain water or an antiseptic. These fluids may sometimes be applied by squirting them on the perineum from a squeeze bottle.

If the person has a Foley catheter in place, basic hygiene care is provided, but additional precaution is needed to prevent infection (see Chapter 44).

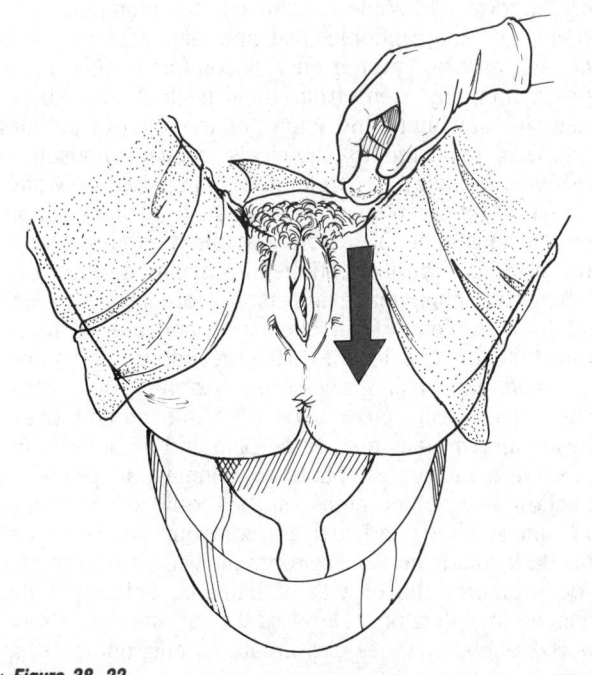

▲ *Figure 38–22*

Female perineal care. Wash from front to back, using a clean part of the washcloth for each wipe. In some circumstances sterile cotton balls are used for cleaning.

Evaluation

The state of the perineum should be evaluated daily when providing perineal care. Evaluation statements that indicate the expected outcomes have been met include

▶ Correctly performs own perineal care.
▶ Perineum is clean, without odor or abnormal secretions.
▶ States has no perineal discomfort and feels clean and refreshed after perineal care.

Document the type of care given, the solutions used, if any, and the condition of the skin and mucosa. For example,

0900   Vaginal packing removed; peri-care with half-strength povidone-iodine given. Instructed to flush perineum with iodine solution after each voiding or B.M. and then rinse with warm water using squeeze bottles. Perineal skin and mucous membrane intact with no evidence of irritation.   H. Harper, S. N.

1030   Copious foul vaginal discharge; secretions gray and foamy; c/o itching; perineum cleansed with soap and warm water. Dr. notified.   T. Tucker, S. N.

1100   Irritated reddened skin in groin and on scrotum. Washed with soap and warm water. Stated he perspired a lot yesterday. Advised to leave shorts off today. Recheck this P.M.   C. Smith, R. N.

NAIL AND FOOT CARE

Although the condition of one's nails and feet can be very important to some individuals, it is unimportant to others. For some people, nail and skin care of hands and feet may be ignored until discomfort occurs. Problems commonly stem from their neglect and abuse. Examples are biting and improper trimming of cuticles and nails, exposure to chemicals, such as household cleaners, frequent or prolonged immersion in water, trauma, ill-fitting shoes, and inadequate hygiene. Some general constitutional factors and diseases (poor nutrition, arthritis, obesity, peripheral vascular disease, and diabetes mellitus) make a person more prone to nail and foot problems. Poor circulation and altered metabolic function can lead to skin breakdown and infection, and alter nail growth and texture (e.g., brittleness). Nails easily grow into soft tissue around them. These ingrown nails may cause pain and tissue trauma.

Feet are more susceptible to trauma and prone to infection than other areas of the body. In daily life, toes get stubbed, and feet are sometimes stepped on. The dark, often moist, environment within a sock and shoe promotes the growth of bacteria, enhancing the chance of infection. Dirty socks or stockings and poorly ventilated shoes also create an environment that encourages bacterial and fungal growth.

The primary goals of nail and foot care are to enhance body image, promote self-esteem, and to prevent problems that interfere with function. These problems include infection and inflammation, trauma from ingrown nails or from long or jagged nails catching on linen or causing scratches, pressure trauma from long toenails rubbing against the end of shoes, trauma secondary to nail care (e.g., improper trimming) and accumulated debris, which causes odor and is a potential source of infection.

Assessment

Assessing nails and surrounding tissue and determining the need for care can be accomplished during general bathing, while talking with a person, or while providing other care. Assessing circulation to the hands and feet and observing for signs of inflammation and infection are important. Inspect fingernails and toenails for color, shape (contour), length, and texture (pliability, brittleness, thickness). Depress the nail plate onto the nail bed to note blanching (whitening, becoming pale) of the nail and speed of color return, which provides information regarding circulation.

Notice the condition of the skin surrounding nails; observe for edema, inflammation, calluses, abrasions, dry patches, lesions, temperature changes, and hair distribution. Temperature and hair growth indicate nutrition and circulation to the toes and fingers. Little hair grows in areas where circulation is poor. Especially observe the condition of the skin between the fingers and toes. These areas are particularly prone to moisture retention and skin breakdown.

Nursing Diagnosis

The nursing diagnosis of *Self-Care Deficit, Bathing/Hygiene,* is the appropriate nursing diagnosis for people who are unable to properly care for their feet or nails.

Planning

If the person is diabetic or has peripheral vascular disease, a physician's order will be required in most institutions before the nurse can trim toenails. If the nails are especially hard or the feet need further attention, it is sometimes best to obtain an order to call a podiatrist. Toenail care is best done during or following bathing. Although fingernails should be trimmed or filed when they are dry, toenails are much easier to cut when they have been soaked for several minutes.

Expected outcomes for foot and nail care include

▶ Correctly performs own foot and nail care.
▶ Fingernails and toenails are well groomed and smooth.
▶ Skin on feet is clean and intact.

Nursing Intervention

Foot and nail care is comforting to everyone and helps prevent problems. Basic hygiene care of nails and feet includes trimming nails, cleaning under nails, and thorough rinsing and patting dry of the skin on the hands and feet and between the fingers and toes.

Use extra care to prevent trauma when caring for people with peripheral vascular disease or diabetes mellitus. Circulatory and neurologic disorders make people very susceptible to infection and other nail and foot problems.

Infection in the toe of a person with peripheral vascular disease or diabetes mellitus can lead to gangrene (tissue death) and possible amputation of the toes, foot, or even leg. Always wear gloves when a person has open skin lesions or infections (see Chapter 28). Soaking the person's hands and feet softens skin and nails and loosens debris. Soaking aids cleaning and trimming and is comforting and refreshing.

Preparing for Care. Soaking hands and feet and trimming nails can be done at times other than during general bathing, if preferred. To organize care for several people, intersperse soaking with other care and encourage self-care. For foot care, if the person can sit up in a bedside chair, place the feet in a basin of warm water (44°C or 111.2°F). Add soap or emollient-demulcent products to the water to soften skin and nails, remove debris, and decrease odor. Then position the overbed table low and over the person's lap. Use another basin on the overbed table for soaking the hands. Place the basin so the person's arms rest comfortably on the overbed table without impeding circulation.

Cleaning and Trimming Nails. Nails do not always require soaking before trimming, but soaking softens nails, making them easier to trim. Use a nail clipper for cutting, an orange stick for cleaning under nails, and an emery board for shaping nails. Clip toenails straight across to prevent ingrowing. Do not clip nails too close to the skin. Protect your eyes from flying nail pieces as you clip. If possible, clip the cuticles around the side of the nails and push the cuticle back toward the nail root. Use a washcloth to retract the cuticle.

Appreciate the need for special attention to nail and foot care. Provide thorough hygiene. Teach about the causes and complications of nail and foot problems as well as hygiene principles to prevent these problems.

Skin Care of the Feet. Remove debris and some callous build-up on feet by vigorous scrubbing with a washcloth. Avoid friction over open skin to prevent further trauma. Never cut calloused areas. Instead, use a pumice stone to remove calluses. Cutting calluses creates scar tissue. Apply a lanolin-based lotion or petroleum jelly after foot soaks to further soften calloused areas and to moisturize dry skin. If a person has excessive foot moisture, use a small amount of water-absorbent powder between toes. Powder decreases odor and helps prevent skin breakdown.

Teaching and Assessment During Nail and Foot Care. People generally appreciate nail and foot care.

Providing this care in itself teaches the person about proper hygiene. A nurse's intervention is a model for hygiene care. Whenever possible, allow people to do at least part of the care themselves so that you can assess their knowledge and ability. For example, you might give nail care to one foot and have the individual give self-care to the other. Always explain reasons for everything you do.

Important points to emphasize about foot care are to: keep feet clean and keep areas between fingers and toes dry, prevent nail problems by properly trimming nails and avoiding injury to the skin surrounding nails, wear clean woolen socks or stockings and properly fitting shoes, eat a nutritious diet, and walk slowly using a heel-toe motion in order to promote health of the feet and nails.

Evaluation

Evaluation of teaching regarding foot and nail care can be accomplished only over a long period. Evaluation statements indicating that expected outcomes have been met include

▶ Independently performs own foot and nail care.
▶ Verbalizes importance of good nail and foot care.
▶ Skin on feet is intact, without redness, lesions, or ingrown nails.
▶ Nails are well-groomed and smooth.

Documentation regarding nail and foot care might include the following:

0900   Feet soaked for 10 min., nails trimmed straight across with toenail clippers and smoothed with emery board. Lotion applied to skin. States feet feel better. Small, 0.5-cm reddened area on superior aspect of right little toe.   P. Triste, S.N.

1000   Toenails long and jagged; requested order from M.D. for trimming. Cautioned to be careful not to cut skin on opposite leg; socks applied. Queried about usual foot care; states just showers daily. Began teaching regarding diabetic foot care.   D. Torlund, S. N.

HAIR CARE

Knowledge of various hair care practices (e.g., care of the African-American person's hair) and methods of caring for people unable to take care of their own hair is crucial to effective nursing practice. Beginning nurses sometimes do not know how to provide hair care for others, especially for people of the opposite sex or for hair different in style or texture from their own.

Hair care, however, is an important part of daily hygiene care. Clean, well-groomed hair prevents skin irritation and infection. The appearance of one's hair influences one's self-image and the reactions and opinions of others. For example, a person with dirty, unkempt hair may automatically be considered lazy and messy by others. In fact, the person may normally be meticulous about hygiene but, because of illness, may be unable to do self-care.

Hair Structure and Function

Most of the body is covered by hair. Hair serves as body insulation and acts as an organ receptor for the sense of touch. A specialized muscle (arrectores pilorum) contracts at times of stress and with changes in temperature, causing hair to stand on end, resulting in goose bumps. Most hair follicles are associated with sebaceous glands, and some sweat gland ducts open into hair follicles. Thus, the scalp becomes moist and oily, particularly in a hot environment.

Hair Growth and Loss. Hair grows in a cyclic pattern of growth, atrophy, and rest phases. This cycle partly accounts for varying rates of hair growth and hair loss. Hair growth may be affected by nutrition, hormones, or hereditary factors. Hormones influence hair growth on the trunk of the body as well as in the nasal and facial areas. One may see hereditary baldness or changes in facial and body hair growth at puberty and after menopause. The presence of body hair generally decreases with the aging process.

Excessive hair loss may occur with trauma, hormonal changes, stress, poor nutrition, and drug therapies, especially some drugs used in the treatment of cancer. Hair loss often stops when the underlying cause is corrected. **Alopecia** is hair loss of unknown cause; the condition often occurs in round patches.

Hair Care in a Health Care Facility. Hair care involves shampooing to remove dirt, dead cells, and old oils; brushing and combing to distribute oil along hair shafts and to prevent accumulation of dirt and organisms; avoiding trauma to the scalp and hair; shaving; and styling hair.

Some health care facilities have a beautician or barber available. Still, it is the nurse's responsibility to ensure that hair care is provided for the person without the individual's having to ask for it.

Assessment

Assessment of the Hair and Scalp. The condition of the hair and surrounding skin reflects general health. If a person says hair-covered areas itch, or is seen scratching, ask about the duration of the problem. Then examine the area for **pediculosis** (infestation with lice), **dandruff** (dry, white flakes that occur normally with scalp exfoliation), scaly patches, lesions or rashes, abrasion, and excoriation (abrasion of the skin surface by trauma or burns). Note whether hair is straight or curly (note extent). Observe hair for distribution, length, cleanliness, thinness or thickness, texture (coarse, fine), gloss or dullness, color, split ends, matting, and tangles. Scalp condition is easiest to examine while giving hair care.

Assessment of the Need for Hair Care Assistance. Most people can care for their own hair. Some need encouragement for self-care. Depressed or disoriented people may show little interest in hygiene, including hair care. Individuals with limited joint mobility, decreased muscle strength, or poor coordination may be unable to do their own hair. People confined to bed often need some assistance with hair care.

Ask people about their normal hair hygiene practices, including shaving of axillae and legs for women. Make arrangements to continue these usual practices as much as possible.

Self-care or having significant others provide hair care is therapeutic. Encourage these activities, without "pushing." Self-care increases range-of-motion movements and independence. Hygiene care provided by significant others allows physical contact and is a means of demonstrating care and concern.

Nursing Diagnosis

For the person who needs assistance with grooming of the hair, the nursing diagnosis is *Self-Care Deficit, Bathing/Hygiene.*

Planning

The type of hair care required depends on the condition of the hair and surrounding skin, need for washing and styling, and the individual's cultural practices, preferences, and self-care abilities. These factors are influenced by hair length and texture, length of illness or disability, imposed immobility (e.g., bed rest, arm cast), and the person's overall state of health.

Consider the type of equipment needed while planning care. Does the person usually shave with a safety or an electric razor? What type of brush, comb, or pick is usually used to style the hair? What sort of shampoo is best for this type of hair? Expected outcomes of hair care include

▶ Independently grooming own hair within 1 week.
▶ Hair clean and appropriately styled.
▶ Beard/mustache clean and well-groomed.

Nursing Intervention

Basic daily hair care consists of brushing, combing, and styling. Nurses provide or facilitate hair care at least once daily. Hair care may be done with morning care so the person feels refreshed and well-groomed for the day.

Help the person collect hair care items: comb, brush, towel, and grooming aids. Sitting is easiest for hair care. When possible, have the person sit up in a chair or in high Fowler's position in bed. Place a towel over the client's shoulders to catch loose hair and dirt, as necessary.

Brushing/Combing and Scalp Massage. Examine the brush and comb for cleanliness. Remove excess hair. If necessary, remove dirt and oil by soaking the brush in ammonia or use hot water and soap. Encourage use of blunt-toothed combs and brushes with firm (but not sharp) bristles. These prevent scratching the scalp and breaking hairs. People with coarse and curly hair need wide-toothed combs.

Brushing hair massages the scalp and distributes oil along the hair shaft more effectively than combing. Use your fingertips for scalp massage. If hair is not matted, tangled, or crinkly, start at the scalp and comb or brush toward ends of hair. If the scalp is irritated or sensitive to touch, be gentle to avoid trauma and discomfort. Ask the person how much pressure is comfortable during combing or brushing.

Grooming Hair in Bed. First brush or comb the sides. Then have the person turn the face away for doing the back of the head. Style the person's hair in a manner that prevents excessive matting and tangling and in a way that pleases the person.

Hair and Scalp Problems. For excessive flaking of the scalp, work dry patches loose with your fingertips and brush toward ends of hair. Shampooing for 5 or more minutes each day helps to decrease dandruff in some persons whether a special dandruff shampoo is used or not. Some conditioners (e.g., petroleum jelly or various oils) may help decrease itching and flaking. If the hair appears clean but oiliness irritates skin on the forehead at the scalp line, clean the forehead with a drying agent such as alcohol.

SPECIAL CONSIDERATIONS IN HAIR CARE

Hair texture, curliness, and preferred styles vary. Hair may be fine and soft, thick and coarse, straight, or tightly curled.

Very Curly Hair. Very curly hair requires more time for care to remove tangles effectively. Ask the person what equipment is needed and the style preferred. Usual equipment is a wide-toothed comb and a brush with firm bristles. If a conditioner is needed and none is available, use petroleum jelly to oil the hair.

Various methods can be used in caring for very curly hair. One method is first to divide the hair into small sections, and brush to remove some tangles and tightness. (Brushing is important for both men and women.) Then separately comb each section of hair. Comb first at ends of hair to remove tangles, and then from middle of hair shaft to the ends, and finally by stroking from the scalp to ends of hair. If the hair appears dry, apply oil at the scalp. Many African-Americans have dry hair and require oil application during basic care and after shampooing. Oil conditions the hair and makes it easy to manage. Hair that has been pressed or straightened with a hot comb returns to its natural curly state with shampooing.

Styling. When a natural, Afro, or brush style is desired, picking is done with a pick comb. Gently lift the hair out from the scalp. Then pat it gently to achieve an overall smooth contour. To prevent matting and tangling, some persons prefer to have their hair braided or placed in one or more pony tails. Some women prefer to have their hair set on regular rollers for styling later.

Wigs and Hair Pieces. Both men and women wear wigs and hair pieces. If a wig is worn, the person's natural hair and scalp need daily basic care before the wig is put on. Wigs prevent exposure of scalp and hair to the air. If a wig is not removed periodically to allow the scalp and hair to "breathe," problems may develop. Wigs may be worn because of difficulty styling hair while ill. When wearing a wig improves the person's self-image, encourage its use, particularly when illness or drug therapy has caused hair loss.

Wigs and hair pieces also need care. Ask the person about preferences. Never apply any solution to wigs and hair pieces without specific instructions from the person they belong to. Brush the person's natural hair toward top of the head prior to putting on a wig. Bobby pins, placed so they will not cause pressure, are sometimes used to hold natural hair in place, or the hair may be braided.

SPECIAL PROBLEMS IN HAIR CARE

Tangled or Matted Hair. People in bed for long periods may develop matted or tangled hair, particularly when hair is long or curly. Thorough daily hair care must be done to prevent these problems. Otherwise, hair can become so matted that little can be done other than to cut it off.

Never cut hair (e.g., to remove blood, mats, or tangles) unless the person is advised of the consequences and agrees.

Before recommending cutting, try applying water with alcohol, hydrogen peroxide, or vinegar to hair to help remove matting and tangles. Section the hair and firmly hold one section at a time between your index finger and thumb as you work with it. Brush or comb in similar manner as with curly hair. Start at the ends, with your hand just above the snarled area, and gently remove snarls. Repeat with all other sections. This procedure is time consuming, but cutting should not be needed if you persistently apply alcohol, hydrogen peroxide, or vinegar and work to remove the snarls.

Braiding hair may prevent future problems with matting and tangles. Braiding is also useful to keep hair off the neck for those who perspire heavily, as during fever. These clients frequently develop rashes as a result of hair continually rubbing and irritating moist skin. Poorly braided hair can easily tangle. Braided hair is uncomfortable for some people. Braiding is usually better using two or more braids. One braid at the back of the head can cause pressure on the scalp when the person is in bed. This pressure can lead to scalp irritation at the site of the braid. Braids that are too tight impair circulation and are painful. Undo braids at least daily and give hair care before rebraiding.

Pediculosis. Pediculosis is infestation with lice. **Pediculosis capitis** refers to infestation of the head, eyebrows, eyelashes, and beard. **Pediculosis corporis** (scabies) refers to infestation of the body. **Pediculosis pubis** refers to infestation of the perineal area. Lice are associated with poor hygiene, crowded living conditions, and exposure to others with lice. Lice live on the skin, attaching their eggs (nits) to hair. Itching and scratching are a response to lice bites. Lice are difficult to remove because the nits are attached to the hair by an adhesive substance.

Pediculosis corporis may be treated with complete bathing, application of topical medication, and washing linen and clothing in very hot water. To treat pediculosis capitis, vigorously massage the hair and scalp with gamma benzene hexachloride. Pediculosis pubis may be more resistive to treatment. The nits are difficult to remove from areas with heavy hair growth. Apply the medication to the involved area and leave it on the body 12 to 24 hours. Then bathe the person thoroughly with soap and water. Effective treatment for lice infestation requires a physician's order for medication.

Whenever lice are discovered, remove and bag clothing and linen to prevent spreading them. Assure the person that lice infestation does not necessarily mean that they are "unclean." Explain what must be done to treat the problem and prevent reinfestation. Lice can be extremely embarrassing, and the person will often need emotional support. If crab lice *(Pediculus pubis)* are found, emphasize the need for treatment of sexual partners to prevent reinfestation.

SHAMPOOING

The method of shampooing hair depends on the person's general condition and preference. Safety is a primary consideration.

Shampooing in a Sitting Position. Most people able to sit at the bedside can sit for shampooing. Three methods are possible: (1) shower chair; (2) chair at sink; (3) bedside chair with overbed table across person's lap with wash basin. With all of these methods, have shampoo items within easy reach, place a towel over the person's shoulders, and direct water away from face and shoulders. If the shower chair is used, have the person sit facing away from the shower with the head and neck hyperextended. When helping with shampooing at a sink, have the person sit facing away from the sink with the head hyperextended and resting comfortably on the sink. Place a towel over the edge of the sink for added comfort. When shampooing at the bedside, have the individual lean the head forward over the wash basin.

Shampooing on a Stretcher. People who can be moved from bed but are unable to sit can be shampooed while lying on a stretcher over a sink or shower equipped with a hand-held shower nozzle. Lock stretcher brakes to keep the stretcher from moving. Place a pillow under the shoulders to allow neck and head hyperextension. Place plastic over the end of the stretcher. Have the person's head extended slightly over the end of the stretcher to allow water to flow away from the person.

Shampooing in Bed. In some cases, it is necessary to shampoo in bed. Unless contraindicated, move the per-

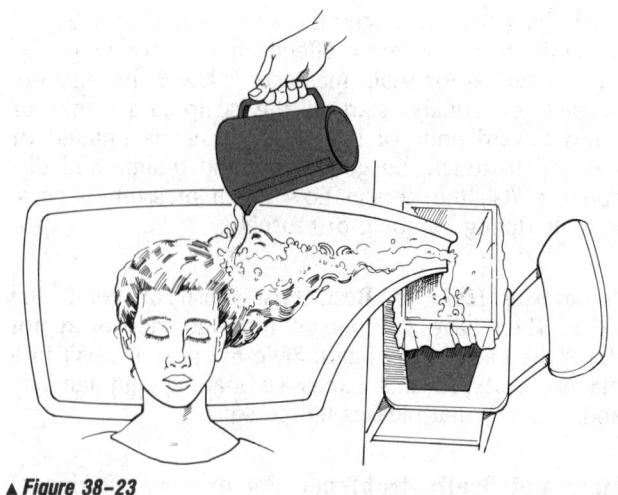

▲ *Figure 38–23*

Shampoo tray for bed shampooing.

son to the edge of the bed nearest you. Remove the pillow and place plastic under a towel under the head and neck and across the bed to protect bed linens and mattress. Most facilities have a plastic shampoo (a "bed rinser") tray with raised sides, which acts as a trough to drain off water. These may be purchased at a medical supply house, if needed for persons in the home setting (Fig. 38–23). If a trough is unavailable, improvise one out of plastic or rubber and newspapers. Roll the newspapers into a horseshoe shape, place the plastic or rubber flat on the bed, and position the rolled newspapers to form a rim on the trough. Roll edges of the plastic or rubber over the newspaper rim to facilitate drainage of water (Fig. 38–24).

Position either device toward the bedside to allow water to drain over the side of the bed and into a receptacle. Place a collecting basin or bucket on a bedside chair or table close to the bed at a height that will allow water to drain without splashing.

If a bed bath is to be given and bed linen is to be changed, do these procedures after completing the shampoo and grooming the hair. It may be necessary for the person to rest between shampoo and bath.

Shampoo Equipment and Supplies. Regardless of the shampooing method, have available two bath towels; washcloth or face towel (to protect eyes from shampoo); shampoo; hair conditioner, if necessary; comb and brush; and hair dryer, if available. Various solutions can be used to shampoo and condition the hair as desired by the client.

If the shampoo is given in bed or on a stretcher, provide a waterproof linen protector. To shampoo a person in bed or a bedside chair, you need one or two water pitchers and a water receptacle. To shampoo at a sink, a cup or pitcher usually is needed for pouring water unless the sink has a spray hose.

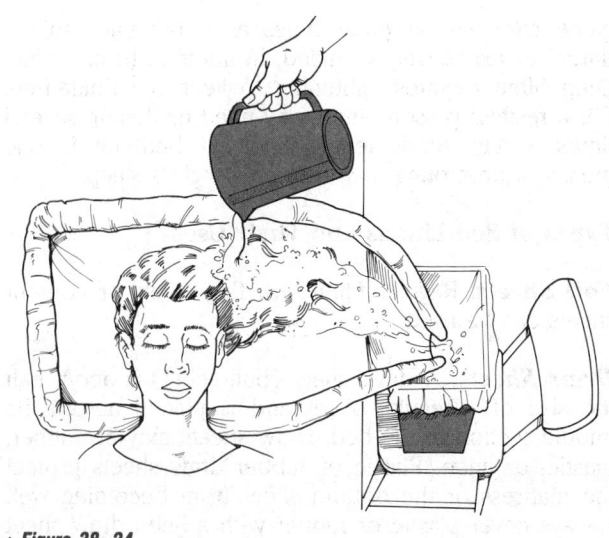

▲ *Figure 38-24*

Improvised trough for shampooing in bed.

General Shampooing Procedure. After positioning the person, providing waterproof covering, and assembling all needed items, you are ready to shampoo. Apply water until the hair is thoroughly wet. Maintain water temperature at 43° to 44°C (109.4° to 111.2°F). Although warmer water may be desired by the person, remember the scalp is easily burned. When the hair is wet, apply a small amount of shampoo and work up a lather.

Start washing at the hairline, working toward the back of the head. While washing the hair, vigorously massage all portions of the scalp by applying fingertip pressure. Long nails make it difficult to massage without scratching the scalp. Rinse thoroughly. Repeat washing and rinsing until hair squeaks when stroked between your fingers. Apply conditioner as desired. Squeeze excess water from the hair, then wrap a bath towel around the head, and use the cloth that was protecting the eyes to dry the face. When the towel is wet, remove it and use a second towel or hair dryer to dry scalp and hair thoroughly. If you use a hair dryer, check it for electrical hazards prior to use and use caution not to burn the person. Groom and style hair. Be sure the person is left in dry clothing and with dry bed linens.

Dry shampoos can occasionally be used, but some of these powder preparations irritate the scalp and do not clean the hair very well.

CARE OF MUSTACHE AND BEARD

Mustaches and beards vary in length, texture, and curliness. Keeping these areas clean and dry is important. Offer the person an opportunity to wash mustache and beard after eating. Ask the man how he usually cares for his mustache or beard. Combing is usually required at least once daily. A mustache also requires periodic trimming. Both mustache and beard need shampooing. Use a mild, nondrying shampoo, since the skin tends to become dry and flaky. Dry the area thoroughly after the shampoo.

SHAVING

Shaving is most frequently done to remove male facial hair. Because of cultural practices, women often shave their underarms (axillae) and legs. Prior to some operations, the operative site is shaved to prevent hair from contaminating an open wound. For people with heavy, long hair growth on arms, the area may be shaved prior to starting an IV infusion. Shaving prevents the discomfort of pulled hair when tape is removed following the infusion.

When shaving any area of the body, use caution not to cut the skin, especially for people prone to bleeding such as those on warfarin (Coumadin), heparin, or high doses of aspirin. An electric razor is safer for these people. Before using electric razors, check them for frayed cords and other electrical hazards.

When using a razor blade, soften the skin before shaving. Shaving the axillae and legs is best done immediately following the bath. Apply lathered soap or shaving cream before shaving. To remove male facial hair, soak the man's face with a warm-hot washcloth (be careful not to burn the face). Allow the cloth to remain on the face until the beard is soft. Then apply thick lathered soap or shaving cream. To shave the area, pull the skin taut and use short, firm (but gentle) strokes in the direction in which the hair grows. Shaving in this direction decreases skin irritation and prevents ingrown hairs.

Evaluation

Depending on the functional level of the client, evaluation statements indicating that expected outcomes have been met might include

- ▶ Assistance with grooming provided; able to comb hair on right side of head.
- ▶ Assisted to shave and groom mustache.
- ▶ Independently grooming own hair.

Grooming of the hair is usually part of daily hygiene care. Shampooing should be included in the nurse's notes or filled in on the activity flowsheet. Tending a man's beard is also considered part of daily hygiene care and is noted on the activity flow sheet. Shaving a woman's legs is usually done only for those who are in need of assistance for longer periods. Shaving her legs can greatly improve the self-esteem and feelings of well-being in the woman who has been incapacitated for more than a few days. Leg shaving should be included in the nurse's notes, as it signifies time spent in care of the person.

COSMETIC CARE AS HYGIENE

For most of us, grooming has social ramifications. We like to look good to others. Grooming aids such as cosmetics have psychologic effects on self-image, but their physical effects, ingredients, and methods of production are seldom considered. Their use is based on personal preference and moral, spiritual, and sociocultural practices.

In some cultures, deodorants are not used, whereas in others people seldom go without a daily application to prevent them from "smelling bad." Some antiperspirants or deodorants completely eliminate sweat and odor. Yet in warm climates some degree of perspiring is physiologically beneficial. Many deodorants contain chemicals irritating to skin. Feminine hygiene sprays, advertised to decrease perineal odor, may irritate skin and mucosa. Bacteriostatic deodorant soaps may eliminate odor at the expense of removing natural flora that protects skin against fungal overgrowth.

Various eye and facial make-ups may be drying and cause skin irritation. Nail polish and nail polish removers may dry nails, causing splitting and breaking. Hair sprays and permanents, when frequently used, tend to make hair dry and brittle or may irritate the scalp. Depilatory creams, used to remove hair from underarms, legs, and face, can also irritate.

Increasing numbers of people refuse to use hygiene "beauty" aids made from animals' bodies (some soaps, shampoos) or tested on animals (make-up, nail polish, perfume). Also, for religious or spiritual reasons, many people do not use products containing the bodies of creatures because these people oppose the taking of life. Some people do not use make-up.

Remember that a tactful approach is imperative in attempting to encourage or discourage the use of grooming aids.

Respect moral, spiritual, and other individual preferences concerning hygiene and "beauty" aids.

COMFORT AND CLEANLINESS IN BED

A clean, fresh, comfortable bed is very important for people who have to spend time in bed. A comfortable bed uplifts one mentally, is physically relaxing, and may prevent serious complications.

Without proper attention to the bed and bed linens, the following problems can occur:

▶ Skin irritation from laundry dyes and bleaches
▶ Abraded skin on heels from rubbing on linen, especially on seams
▶ Pressure sores from lying on wrinkled sheets
▶ Skin irritation and discomfort from wet linen

Bed Linens

Need for Linen Change. Change linen according to client need. Linen may be changed with morning hygiene care and at other times as it becomes soiled, damp, or excessively wrinkled. In addition to changing, linen often requires tightening to keep it wrinkle-free. For a restless person, linen may need tightening several times a day. Straightening linen at bedtime is one means of promoting a comfortable night's sleep.

Types of Bed Linens and Their Uses

Full Sheets. Regular full-length flat sheets or contour sheets can be used.

Draw Sheets. A draw sheet (pull sheet) is about half the size of a regular sheet and is placed across the middle section of the bed. Draw sheets may be rubber, plastic, or linen. Plastic or rubber draw sheets protect the mattress or the bottom sheet from becoming wet. Always cover plastic or rubber with a linen draw sheet to protect the person's skin and absorb moisture.

Linen draw sheets should not be relied upon for lifting (pull sheets). See Chapter 35 for the use of lift sheets.

Mattress Pads. Mattress pads are usually made of thick, soft cotton and have bound edges. When used, the pad, with or without contour corners, is placed lengthwise on the bed between the mattress and sheet. The mattress pad decreases movement of the sheet, reduces heat generated between a plastic mattress and the person's body, and absorbs moisture. All of these enhance comfort. (A bath blanket can be used in place of a mattress pad.) Change mattress pads only when excessively wrinkled, damp, or soiled.

Blankets. A bed blanket of wool, cotton, or synthetic material may be used for warmth. Thermal bed blankets are used in many facilities. These are made of a porous, synthetic material and have the advantage of being relatively lightweight yet warm. The bed blanket is usually not changed unless it becomes soiled or wet.

Bedspreads. Bedspreads are usually lightweight cotton or synthetic material. They are changed only when soiled, wet, or excessively wrinkled.

Pillow Cases. A standard pillow case is one of the most frequently changed bed linens. To reduce the need for a clean pillow case, turn the pillow over and tighten the case around the pillow with a tuck. A clean, smooth pillow case can be very refreshing.

Assessment

Nursing assessment determines whether the person will remain in bed or get out of bed while linens are changed. Some people must remain in bed during linen change because they are weak or have mobility restrictions (see Procedure 38–2). Sometimes a client on bedrest will be scheduled for a diagnostic procedure and will be taken out of the room on a stretcher for a length of time sufficient for changing the bed linen.

Text continued on page 941

PROCEDURE 38-2

Making Occupied Bed

Definition/Purposes. Enables linen change while person remains in bed. The purpose is to provide a comfortable and clean bed.

Contraindications/Cautions. Whenever condition permits, encourage the client's getting out of bed for linen change. Assess for movement limitations. Keep side rail up on side away from nurse to aid person in turning and prevent falling. Use special caution when turning people with burns, peripheral vascular disorders, or orthopedic problems. Often with traction, weights must be maintained continuously. Sterile sheets are necessary for some people with burns. Avoid shaking linen to decrease the spread of organisms. Report malfunctioning beds.

Learning/Teaching Guidelines. Provide information about the amount of participation that is therapeutic. If the client must remain in bed to conserve energy, explain how energy conservation relates to the individual's condition and how the procedure saves time and energy and promotes safety; provide information about renting hospital beds for home use.

PRELIMINARY ACTIVITIES

Assessment

- ▶ Check linen available in unit.
- ▶ Note clean linen needed.
- ▶ Identify special items needed (e.g., extra blanket, linen protectors).
- ▶ Check activity order and note movement/positioning precautions.
- ▶ Assess person's ability to assist and understand directions.
- ▶ Assess need for additional assistance.

Preparation of Person and Unit

- ▶ Explain how person can assist.
- ▶ Explain sequence of activities.
- ▶ Move furniture away from bed.
- ▶ Remove call signal if attached to bed linens.
- ▶ Place linen and laundry bag within easy reach.
- ▶ Raise side rails.
- ▶ Adjust bed to comfortable working height.
- ▶ Position person supine or as flat as possible.
- ▶ Pull curtain for privacy.

Equipment

Wash hands prior to collecting linen. For complete linen change, collect linen and stack it in reverse order of use as follows:

- ▶ Pillow case (place over your arm first)
- ▶ Bedspread (if needed)
- ▶ Blanket (if needed)
- ▶ Top sheet
- ▶ Draw sheet (if needed)
- ▶ Bottom sheet
- ▶ Mattress pad (if needed)
- ▶ Bath blanket
- ▶ Laundry bag
- ▶ Dust cloth (last item on top of pile)
- ▶ Linen hamper
- ▶ Bedside chair for placing linen in order of use
- ▶ Gloves (if bed is soiled or wet)

PROCEDURE

Actions

1. Remove *top* linen.
   a. Loosen top linens.
   b. Lower side rail by you.
   c. Remove spread and blanket and fold each separately.
      i. Fold top edge to bottom.
      ii. Fold far side to near side.
      iii. Fold again top to bottom.
      iv. Place over back of chair.
   d. Leave top sheet over person or remove and cover person with bath blanket.
2. Move mattress to head of bed if necessary. Requires two people and efficient body mechanics.

   a. Stand at side, facing head of bed, and grasp mattress at handles or each end. Have client grasp head of bed and instruct when to pull.
   b. With outside leg forward, shift weight and bend knees to move mattress on count of ''three.''

Rationale/Assessment

1.

   b. Allows better access to client.
   c. Method of folding facilitates replacement and prevents wrinkles.

   d. Provides warmth and prevents exposure (see Procedure 38-1).
2. Mattress tends to slide down when bed's head is raised. This makes it difficult to keep linen tucked in, and it is uncomfortable for the person in bed.
   a. Having client help promotes strength and independence.

   b. Using leg muscles as force saves your energy.

Procedure continued on following page

PROCEDURE 38–2 Continued

Making Occupied Bed

Actions

    c. Pull up metal bar at foot of springs to perpendicular position.

3. Position person on side on far side of bed, facing away from you. Reposition pillow under head.

4. Prepare base (foundation or bottom linen) of bed.
    a. Loosen bottom linens on your side of bed, moving from head to foot of bed.
    b. Fan-fold bottom linens (draw sheet, then bottom sheet) as close to person as possible.
    c. Fan-fold mattress pad to middle of bed if it is to be changed.

5. Make base on one side of bed.
    a. Smooth reused mattress pad *or* place clean pad with center fold at middle of bed; fan-fold top layer to person.
    b. Place clean bottom sheet even with foot end of mattress. Have center fold in middle of bed. Open sheet lengthwise (move from foot to head). Fan-fold top layer to middle of bed (Fig. 38–25).
    c. Miter bottom sheet at head of bed (Fig. 38–26).

      i. Face head of bed diagonally. Place one hand under mattress corner and lift. With other hand pull excess sheet over and under mattress head (Fig. 38–26*A*)

      ii. Face side of bed. Lift side edge of sheet to form a triangle to head of bed, with side edge hanging perpendicular to bed (Fig. 38–26*B*). Lay upper part of sheet back on bed by creasing along mattress top edge (Fig. 38–26*C*).

Rationale/Assessment

    c. Prevents mattress sliding back toward foot of bed.

3. Provides space to place clean linen. Have person use side rail for turning. Assess for comfort, ease of breathing, and alignment.

4.

It is most efficient to complete one side of bed before beginning other side.
    b. Provides maximum work area and comfort as person later rolls back over linens.
    c. Change if soiled or heavily wrinkled.

5.

    b. Most efficient to work from foot to head and back to foot. Place sheet with hem down and smooth side up toward client's body (move from head to foot).
    c. Miter holds linen firmly in place. Allows linen to fit corners. Looks neat.
      i. Secures linen.

      ii. Holds linen firmly in place.

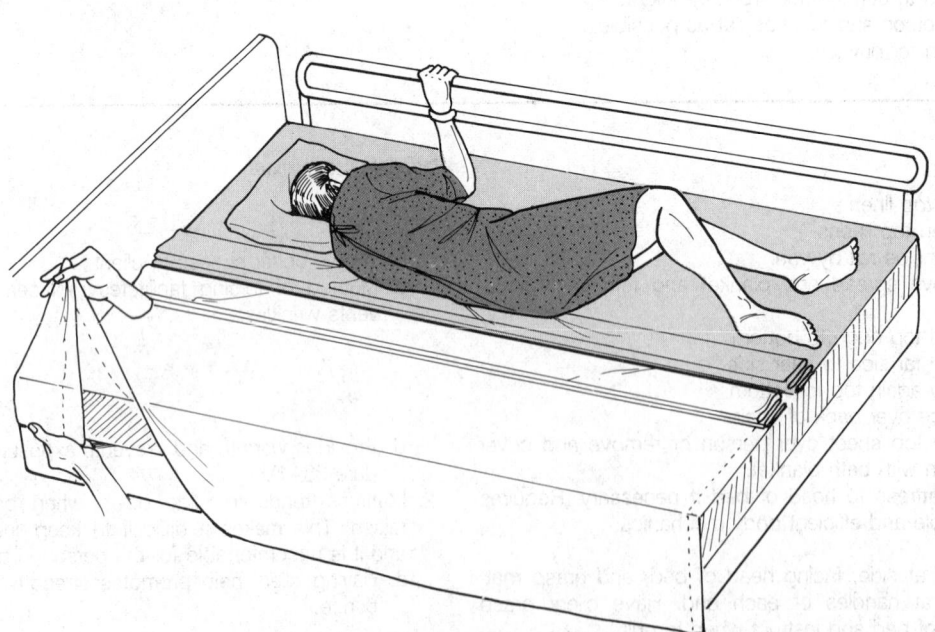

▲ *Figure 38–25*

PROCEDURE 38–2 Continued

Making Occupied Bed

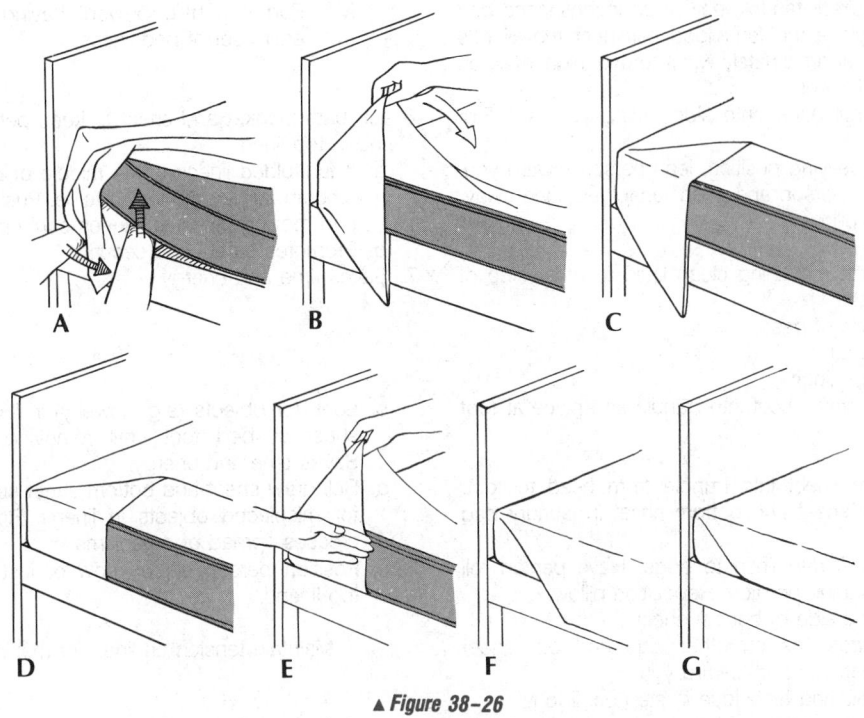

▲ *Figure 38–26*

Actions	Rationale/Assessment
iii. Tuck lower hanging portion of sheet smoothly under mattress (Fig. 38–26D).	iii. Work with palms down to protect knuckles from bedsprings.
iv. Place back side of one hand (with thumb down on palm) firmly against sheet to hold sheet against mattress. With other hand, pick up sheet corner lying on bed. Bring it down over hand against mattress edge (Fig. 38–26 E,F).	iv. Position elbow toward head of bed to allow easy removal of hand while maintaining linen position.
d. Face side of bed. Tuck side edge of sheet under mattress (Fig. 38–26G)	d. Use both hands palms down. Move smoothly from head to foot of bed.

VARIATION: If hospital policy allows, tie sheet corners at head of bed in square knot. Put sheet onto bed with knot tucked under mattress at head of bed.

Makes flat sheet into contoured sheet. Stays in place better for persons who are actively moving in bed. However, knots in linen require extra work removing them for laundering.

Actions	Rationale/Assessment
e. If needed, place draw sheet(s).	e. If both plastic (or rubber) draw sheet and linen draw sheet are to be used, place the linen draw sheet on top.
i. Identify center fold. Open draw sheet so it folds in half.	i. Usually there are only two edges with hems, and these will be tucked under the mattress. If all four sides have hems, be sure the smooth side is placed toward the client.
ii. Lay center fold of draw sheet along middle of bed.	ii. Face bedside. Grasp draw sheet at top and bottom edges of center fold. Lean across bed, bending at waist with knees flexed and back straight.
iii. Position draw sheet so that it lies under client's torso (shoulders to knees).	iii. Provides extra protection under body part most likely to soil linen.
iv. Fan-fold top layer toward person.	iv. Place cleanest part of soiled linen next to clean linen.
v. Tuck excess draw sheet smoothly under mattress. Work from center to edges.	v. Use both hands.

Procedure continued on following page

PROCEDURE 38–2 Continued

Making Occupied Bed

Actions	Rationale/Assessment
vi. If required, fan-fold half of an incontinence pad and place the fan-folded half near the client's back, approximately waist to mid-thigh level, on top of linens.	iv. Pad can help prevent having to change the entire set of bed linens.

6. Help person roll back onto side facing you (see Fig. 38–17).
  a. When in side-lying position, lean person toward you. Reach over person and push fan-folded linen away. Reposition pillow.
  b. Raise side rail.
	6. Lift bath blanket and sheet to keep person from catching in top linen.
	  a. If fan-folded linens are in middle of bed, person has smooth surface on which to lie. Pushing linens away and moving pillow enhances comfort.
	  b. Promotes safety and security.

7. Move chair with remaining clean linen to other side of bed within reach.	7. Saves time and energy.

8. Make other side of base.
  a. Lower side rail.
  b. Loosen base linens.
  c. Roll soiled draw sheet into bundle and place at foot of bed.
	8.
	
	  c. Look for objects (e.g., jewelry) in linen. Leave draw sheet at bed foot until removing bottom sheet. Saves time and energy.

d. Roll bottom sheet into bundle from head to foot. Place draw sheet and bottom sheet in laundry bag together.	d. Roll draw sheet and bottom sheet separately to look for misplaced objects in linens. Rolling linens decreases spread of organisms.
e. Smooth fan-folded linen to edge. Have person roll back into supine position. Reposition pillow.	e. Position person supine now or just before placing top linens.

f. Miter second side of bottom sheet.
    i. Lift mattress as on other side and pull sheet under mattress and toward you.
    ii. Follow mitering technique in step 5c, ii to iv.
    iii. Gather excess linen in hands.
    iv. Face bedside. Lean back and pull down to tuck excess linen under mattress.
	i. Maintain tension on linen for maximum tightness.
	
	iii. Grasp with knuckles up.

g. Tighten bottom sheet. Grasp sheet edge and gather in hands to top ridge of mattress. Lean back, pull sheet over side and tuck. Work from miter to foot, tucking excess linen under.	g. Maintain tension to keep sheet free of wrinkles. Grasp with knuckles up.

h. Tighten draw sheet.
    i. Smooth draw sheet with palms.
    ii. Gather excess linen in hands with knuckles up. Tighten and tuck middle, then top and bottom of draw sheet.
	ii. Face side of bed and lean back to tighten middle. Face foot of bed diagonally and lean back to tighten top. Face head of bed diagonally to tighten bottom.

9. Place top linens.
  a. Place clean top sheet with center fold in middle of bed. Open sheet head to foot. Then unfold sheet across person.
	9.
	  a. Leave enough linen to make a cuff at person's shoulder height. Be sure that smooth side is toward the client.

b. Ask person to hold clean top sheet or tuck around shoulders.	b. Prevents exposing individual. Encourages person's assistance.
c. Stand at foot of bed. Grasp soiled top sheet and bath blanket under clean top sheet. To remove these soiled linens, roll them into bundle while pulling toward you.	
d. If required, place folded bed blanket on person at midchest. Open blanket across person, then from head to foot.	d. Have foot end of linens hang freely over foot of bed.
e. Place and open spread as with blanket. Cuff spread under blanket. Then bring top sheet over spread as second cuff.	e. Leave enough spread to cuff under blanket at person's shoulder height.
f. Tuck top linens under mattress foot. Face diagonally to opposite corner of foot. Lift mattress corner with near hand and use other to tuck all linens under mattress.	f. When lifting, have person flex knees to decrease weight on mattress. Tucking all three layers of linen together saves time and energy.

PROCEDURE 38–2 Continued

Making Occupied Bed

Actions	Rationale/Assessment
g. Ask person to flex ankles and point toes up (dorsiflex) before tightening top linen.	g. Provides room for free movement of feet. Tight top linens can cause footdrop.
h. Miter all three layers of linen at once, while facing foot of bed diagonally.	h. Follow steps for mitering only thorugh step 5c. Top linens hang neatly together.
i. Raise side rail.	
j. Move to other side of bed. Lower side rail. Repeat steps f through h for this side of top linen. Complete cuffs as in step e.	
10. Raise head of mattress as needed.	10. Allows for comfort during change of pillow case.
11. Change pillow case.	11.
a. Remove soiled pillow case and place in laundry bag.	
b. Grasp closed end of clean pillow case at center with one hand (Fig. 38–27 A). Next, maintaining grasp, use other hand to grasp open end of case (Fig. 38–27B). Invert case over hand and forearm (at closed end) by pulling open end of case back over hand at closed end. Maintain grasp at closed end.	
c. Grasp pillow end with hand holding case (Fig. 38–27C). Maintaining grasp, use other hand to pull case down over pillow (Fig. 38–27D).	c. If a zippered plastic covering is over pillow, grasp zippered end of pillow.
d. Support person's head, lift, and place pillow under head with closed end toward door (Fig. 38–28).	
12. Adjust bed as necessary.	12. Promotes comfort and safety.

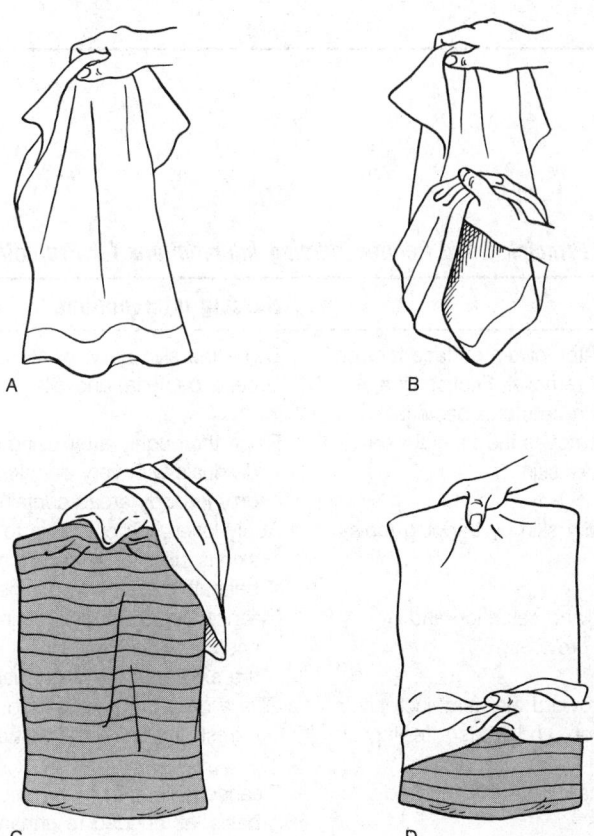

▲ Figure 38–27

PROCEDURE 38–2 Continued

Making Occupied Bed

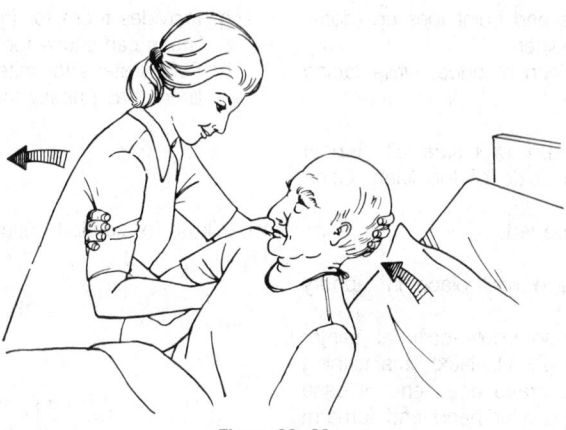

▲ *Figure 38–28*

FINAL ACTIVITIES

For safety, replace call signal; raise side rails as appropriate; lower bed to low position. If manual bed, put hand cranks in. If electric bed, be sure plug is in wall socket and cord is free of tension. Care of equipment includes the following: Replace bedside stand and overbed table within easy reach of person. Take full laundry bag to dirty utility room or linen chute. Do not return unused clean linen to linen cart, as it is now considered contaminated. Follow facility policy for use or disposal of this linen. For final assessment, assess person for correct body alignment. Leave person in position that provides comfort, ease of breathing, and good circulation. Assess person's mental/emotional status to determine need for side rail. Is bottom linen taut and wrinkle free? Are top linens off the floor and hanging evenly on both sides? Can toes move freely under top linens?

TABLE 38–1. Selected Scientific Principles and Related Nursing Interventions for Promoting Hygiene

Principle	Nursing Interventions
Washing the skin with soap and water lowers surface tension and helps emulsify oils for easier removal. Friction of a washcloth helps remove dead skin cells and bacteria.	Bathe the skin daily, or as needed, to remove dead skin cells, bacteria, and oils.
Soap lowers surface tension and removes the natural skin oils that tend to protect against dry skin.	Rinse thoroughly after using soap. For the elderly or other individuals with very dry skin, use soap every other day or only in body areas containing apocrine glands.
Demulcents and emollients soften dry skin by trapping moisture beneath them.	Apply lotion, oil, or cream to dry skin after the bath, while the skin is still slightly damp, so that moisture will be trapped beneath the oil and retained.
Body odor is caused by apocrine gland secretion and by multiplication of bacteria in body crevices.	Cleanse the axillae and groin areas thoroughly with soap, rinse, and pat dry; apply a deodorant or antiperspirant to the axillae as the individual desires.
Body cleansing using firm strokes toward the heart increases venous return, enhances circulation, and lends a feeling of well-being.	Give a daily bath using long, firm strokes toward the torso to refresh the individual as needed.
Jagged, dirty, or excessively long nails can alter the body image and lower self-esteem.	Cleanse nails, trim them, and smooth them on a regular basis, as needed to enhance appearance.

TABLE 38-1. *Selected Scientific Principles and Related Nursing Interventions for Promoting Hygiene* Continued

Principle	Nursing Interventions
Ungroomed hair becomes matted and oily, and collects bacteria. Poorly groomed hair can lower self-esteem by altering body image.	Groom hair at least once daily by thorough brushing. Shampoo every 4–7 days; according to individual preference and need.
A taut bottom sheet and tidy bed linens prevent wrinkles and creases that can cause extra pressure on the skin.	Make the hospital bed daily and straighten the linens several times a day, pulling the bottom sheet taut.
Because of pH differences and added moisture, contact with urine-soaked bed linens can cause skin excoriation.	Check incontinent clients frequently and change wet linen as soon as possible.
Dependence on others decreases self-esteem.	Encourage individual to participate in and perform as much of self-care as possible.
Bacteria proliferate in warm, moist, dark areas. Enzymes produced during the growth of bacteria can cause skin irritation.	Thoroughly dry between skin folds and between toes and inspect daily for skin irritation.
A washcloth may serve as a fomite to carry microorganisms from an infected area to a clean area, such as from one eye to the other.	Use a separate, clean corner of the washcloth to cleanse around each eye.
Two ways the body loses heat are through radiation and evaporation. Moist skin exposed to air currents decreases body temperature rapidly.	To prevent chilling, cover all body parts except that being cleansed.
Hot water can burn tissue by heat convection.	Check the temperature of the water before making it available for bathing. It should be less than 39.4°C (103°F).
Body warmth can be transferred to cooler objects by conduction.	Warm the bedpan as needed for client comfort.
Plaque builds up in the mouth after meals and contributes to cavities and periodontal disease by providing a medium for bacterial growth.	Brush teeth after meals (two to three times daily), with plaque-retarding toothpaste, flossing between the teeth.
The body's first line of defense against infection is an unbroken skin and mucous membranes.	Help keep mucous membranes intact by providing mouth care every 2 hours to the individual at risk for stomatitis or mucositis.
Bathing requires visualization of all skin surfaces. Skin assessment requires visualization of all skin surfaces.	Inspect the skin daily during the bath (see Chapter 33 for skin inspection).

For special beds such as the RotoRest or Clinitron, the manufacturer's booklet gives various tips on making linen changes easier. Each nurse should become familiar with the recommendations for linens on special beds, because the bed's effectiveness can be reduced if the manufacturer's recommendations are not followed.

If an orthopedic client is confined to bed with a cast or traction, note whether a trapeze bar is mounted above the bed. A trapeze bar allows people to lift themselves up so that the bottom sheet can more easily be changed. The client should be asked whether using the trapeze bar is possible.

Assess whether the client is warm enough with the blanket and spread provided, to determine any need for an additional blanket.

Nursing Diagnosis

Bedmaking is an expected part of the care of the hospitalized person. An appropriate nursing diagnosis for the person needing an occupied bed linen change is *Activity Intolerance* or *High Risk for Impaired Skin Integrity.*

Planning

Bedmaking is usually done during or following bath time. All linens are gathered and brought to the room before beginning the bath. The room must be warm enough; provide for keeping the person warm. If the person is to bathe sitting on the side of the bed or is to be given a bed bath, bathing is done before the bed is made. For a client with *Activity Intolerance,* the goal of bedmaking is to provide a neat, clean bed without exceeding the client's tolerance for activity. An expected outcome might be

▶ Vital signs maintained within normal limits.

For the client whose nursing diagnosis is *High Risk for Impaired Skin Integrity,* the goal is to provide a comfortable, safe bed that imposes minimal stress on the client's skin. An expected outcome might be

▶ Skin intact, without signs of discoloration.

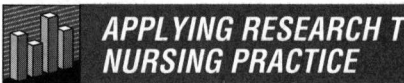

APPLYING RESEARCH TO NURSING PRACTICE
Deciding Whether to Get Post-MI Clients Out of Bed During Bedmaking

Harrell J., et al. (1992). Bedmaking in the coronary care unit (abstract). *Heart & Lung, 21*(3), 297.

▼▼▼

Physicians traditionally confine to bed clients recovering from an acute myocardial infarction ("heart attack," or MI). Nurses usually make the beds of these clients while the clients remain in bed. Recently, coronary care nurses have questioned whether mandatory bed rest for stable post-MI clients is based on scientific evidence. To study this issue, Harrell and colleagues used a noninvasive procedure to evaluate the impact of different methods of bedmaking on clients recovering from an MI. The procedure, impedance cardiography, measured cardiac performance in 20 stable clients who, on different days, sat in a chair for 5 minutes during the linen change or remained in bed during bedmaking. Whether the clients sat in a chair or remained in bed during bedmaking, the researchers found no important differences in clinical measures of the heart's performance. Cardiac contractility did decrease while the clients sat in a chair, but this measurement returned to the initial value within 2 minutes following the clients' return to bed.

Applications for Practice

If the physician allows a client to sit in a chair during bedmaking, evaluate client tolerance of this activity by monitoring blood pressure, heart rate, rate and quality of breathing, and comfort level.

Nursing Intervention

BEDMAKING

The nurse needs to know specific concepts, principles, and activities associated with bedmaking. Save time and energy by noting supplies available in the person's unit, collecting all linen before beginning and stacking it in reverse order of use and moving furniture (e.g., bedside stand and overbed table) away from bed. Have bedside chair and laundry hamper within easy reach. Work at a normal rate of speed, employing a systematic method and rhythmic movements throughout bedmaking. Provide privacy and comfort for the individual by promptly changing linens as soon as they become wet or soiled and by screening and keeping the person covered during linen change. Also remember the following principles:

▶ *Asepsis.* Prevent spread of microorganisms by handwashing as necessary (see Chapter 28). Keep linen away from your clothing, face, and hair. Shake linen minimally, and keep it off the floor.
▶ *Body mechanics.* Decrease strain and prevent back problems by facing the direction of movement. Have

your center of gravity close to your base of support, using arm and leg muscles as a force with wide base of support. Keep your back straight and knees flexed. Have the bed at working height (see Chapter 29).
▶ *Safety.* Prevent falls and injuries by appropriate use of side rails. Keep call signal within reach of the individual.

When modifying the bedmaking procedure, always consider the reasons for the variations. Individualize bedmaking according to clients' preferences and needs and facility policies.

Unoccupied Bed. When changing linen without a person in the bed, follow the principles and basic procedures used when making an occupied bed (see Procedure 38-2).

Orthopedic Bed. The bottom linen of the person who is in traction or a large cast may be more easily changed by working from top to bottom rather than from side to side. To do this, two nurses work together on opposite sides of the bed. The top covers are removed; the person is draped with the top sheet for privacy; and the bottom sheet is loosened all around the mattress so it can be removed toward the foot of the bed. The fresh sheet is positioned over the head end of the mattress, tucked under the head of the mattress, mitered on both sides (see Figure 38-26 in Procedure 38-2) and fan-folded so that it can be pulled down to the bottom of the bed. The client lifts his or her upper body using the trapeze bar or the person is lifted by the nurses while the old sheet is removed and the new sheet is simultaneously pushed under the buttocks as the nurses work from the head toward the bottom of the bed. Next, the client's hips are lifted, as if to get on a bedpan, while the nurses bring both sheets still farther toward the foot of the bed. Finally, the client's lower legs and feet are lifted to complete the linen change on the foundation of the bed. When the dirty sheet is removed and the hem of the clean sheet is in line with the mattress edge at the foot of the bed, the clean sheet is ready to be tucked in along both sides of the bed. The clean top sheet and covers are then applied, adapting them to provide warmth as necessary.

Surgical Bed. For a person returning from surgery, the bed is prepared in the usual manner, except that the pillow is removed and a draw or lift sheet and incontinence pads may be added as the need is anticipated. The top covers are fan-folded to the side or bottom of the mattress to allow for transfer of the person from the stretcher to the bed. The bed is left in the high position. An IV pole is placed at the head of the bed, and the furniture in the room is arranged to allow free passage of the stretcher. Tissues and an emesis basin are left within reach on the bedside console.

Bed Equipment. Special equipment may be placed on a bed, as indicated by an individual's condition, to prevent skin problems, promote comfort, facilitate circulation, or maintain good body alignment.

Bed Boards. A bed board may be placed between the mattress and bedsprings to provide an extra firm surface for general comfort, especially for people with back problems. Bed boards are available in several varieties: one solid piece of wood, two pieces of wood hinged together, or slats of wood encased in heavy cloth. A solid piece of wood can be used only if the bed remains flat.

When making a bed with a bed board, tuck the bottom sheet in the usual manner. It may be somewhat difficult to slide linen under the mattress. Be careful to prevent injury to your hands.

Footboards. Footboards are discussed in Chapter 35. When making a bed with a footboard, cover the footboard with a draw sheet or other linen and secure linen with tape. When making the bed, bring top linen *over* the board and then miter. The sides of the miter may need to be tucked in to prevent chilling.

Traction and Trapeze. Traction devices may restrict the ability to turn or move about in bed during bedmaking. If a traction device is attached to the bed's foot, modify top linen placement so it fits around the device and provides warmth. A trapeze bar, suspended over the head of the bed, facilitates self-care and self-movement by helping a person roll or lift off the mattress. Use of the trapeze makes it easier for care providers to place and tighten linens or for the client to use a bedpan.

Overbed Cradle. Cradles are discussed in Chapter 35.

Secure the cradle in place to maintain protection of the appropriate area of the body and to prevent the cradle from collapsing.

One method of securing a cradle is to attach one end of a piece of gauze or similar material to the sides of the cradle and the other end to the bedsprings. When making a bed with a cradle, place the top linen over the cradle. Pull the excess linen around the foot of the mattress. Bring the side edge of the sheet perpendicular to the mattress and tuck excess sheet under the mattress (as for the regular mitered corner). Complete the "modified" mitered corner by tucking the sheet sides under at the corner to prevent chilling.

Alternating-Pressure Mattress. Alternating-pressure mattresses are discussed in Chapter 35. When making a bed with an alternating-pressure mattress, place a mattress pad over the regular mattress to prevent friction, put the air mattress on top of the mattress pad, and arrange the bottom sheet in the usual manner except to modify the miter on the side with the hoses to prevent kinking the air hoses. Do not use a draw sheet because it counteracts the beneficial effect of the alternating air pressure.

Avoid puncturing the alternating-pressure mattresses with pins and other sharp objects. Check for kinks in coil and hoses. Examine the mattress for proper functioning by observing the emptying and filling of the sectioned coils.

Eggcrates, "sheepskins," and incontinence pads are all additional equipment that may be added to the bed. See Chapter 35 for a discussion of these protective items.

BED STRAIGHTENING

For continued comfort throughout the day, straighten the bed whenever necessary. Whenever the person is out of the room for a procedure or treatment, the bed should be straightened and opened to invite return. Another opportunity presents itself when the person is in the bathroom and the nurse needs to be available. The waiting time can be effectively used by straightening the bed. A straightened bed is very refreshing for the client, decreases the possibility of pressure damage from wrinkles, and conveys a sense of caring on the part of the nurse.

Evaluation

Depending upon the client's nursing diagnosis, evaluation statements indicating that expected outcomes have been met might include

CASE STUDY

The Client

Mr. Tom Horton, age 72 years, was hospitalized 4 days ago, on June 25th, after experiencing a cerebrovascular accident (stroke) that left him with paralysis of the left leg and extreme weakness of the left arm. A partial listing of physician's orders at that time included

▶ Passive ROM to joints of extremities on left side, 10× each tid; PT bid

▶ Mechanical soft diet; check swallowing before meals
▶ Bedrest
▶ V.S. and Neuro signs q2h until stable, then q4h
▶ Procardia, 30 mg tid
▶ Metamucil, 1 pkt. in juice in AM.
▶ Decadron, 4 mg po tid

Case Study continued on following page

CASE STUDY Continued

The Client

Assessment data this morning, June 26th, included

- Left leg paralysis with slight muscle spasm
- Left arm weakness
- Groggy with depressed affect
- PEARL
- Vital signs: BP 152/88, P 68, R 16, T 98.2

- Incontinent of urine during the night
- Last BM June 23rd
- Dry skin with flaking on arms and legs
- Slight difficulty swallowing

Following is part of a care plan initiated on June 26th.

CARE PLAN

9:00 AM, June 26th

Nursing Diagnosis	Planning: Expected Outcomes	Implementation: Nursing Interventions	Evaluation
Self-Care Deficit, Bathing/ Hygiene R/T inability to walk or effectively use left arm	By June 30th: Maintains personal hygiene with assistance Assists with bathing of upper body	Assist with bedbath, encouraging him to wash upper body himself.	3:00 pm, June 26th: Used right hand and washed face and upper chest: stated was too tired to do the left arm or axilla.
		Prevent fatigue by combining bedbath and occupied bed-making. Give praise for each area he washes himself.	10:30 am, June 30: Has not C/O fatigue during bath and linen change. Has washed slightly more of his own body each day. Today washed face, neck, left arm, chest, and abdomen.
	Assists with own hair care and nail care	Shave daily, encouraging participation as able.	Shaved self with electric razor; seems afraid to use safety razor as is left-handed.
		Shampoo hair q4–7 days.	Stated he will shampoo tomorrow.
		Provide grooming aids (comb, nail clippers, etc.), assist with grooming while encouraging as much self-care as possible.	Attempted to comb hair; cannot clip own nails.
	Attempts to brush own teeth	Place toothpaste on toothbrush and encourage to do own oral care.	Brushed upper teeth, but became too fatigued to finish job.

- Client able to roll independently from side to side and to maintain side-lying position as needed during linen change.
- Vital signs WNL: T 98.4, P 72, R 18, BP 118/68.
- Skin ivory in color and intact.

Summary

- Thorough assessment of the person's needs, capabilities, cultural values, and desires is essential before planning hygiene care.

- The main nursing diagnoses for persons requiring assistance with hygiene are *Self-Care Deficit, Bathing/Hygiene* and *Self-Care Deficit, Dressing/ Grooming*.
- Outcomes of hygiene care include evidence of comfort and relaxation, stimulation of circulation, cleanliness, skin conditioning, improved self-image, and ability to provide as much of the client's own self-care as possible.
- Important nursing interventions for the client with self-care deficit include oral care; skin care; bathing;

eye, ear, and nose care; perineal care; foot and nail care; hair care; and bedmaking.

▶ Evaluation of the client following nursing interventions for self-care deficit in hygiene or grooming requires determining the degree to which the client still has a self-care deficit.

▶ A matter-of-fact way of assisting with the highly personal and usually private act of toileting can decrease embarrassment.

▶ Assistance with oral care, as needed, prevents health problems and increases the appetite.

▶ Attention to eye care is essential to prevent eye injury, particularly in the care of the comatose client.

▶ Ear hygiene can help maintain the sense of hearing. Proper placement and care of a hearing aid greatly increase communication with the hearing-impaired client.

▶ Nasal suctioning is done gently and only for clients who do not have a neurologic problem that causes increased intracranial pressure.

▶ Bathing helps maintain skin integrity. It promotes circulation, removes dead skin and bacteria, and promotes a feeling of refreshment and well-being.

▶ Many elderly clients have fragile skin and need less soap and more moisturizing lotions to keep their skin supple.

▶ Both male and female perineal care should always be done at the time of the daily bath and as needed after toileting. Do not assume that all clients can perform this self-care.

▶ Care must be taken when providing nail care not to cause skin breaks. Particular care must be taken with nail and foot care in clients with diabetes mellitus or peripheral vascular disease.

▶ Grooming is considered an important part of daily care, and the nurse provides assistance with grooming activities as needed when the client has a self-care deficit.

▶ Groomed hair is essential to a good self-image for most persons. Clients' hair should be shampooed at least once a week; a bed shampoo can be given for clients on bedrest.

▶ A clean, dry, well-made bed of any type adds considerably to the comfort of the ill client and is a factor in preventing skin breakdown.

▶ Straightening the bed at various times throughout the day helps protect the client's skin from the pressure caused by wrinkles and helps demonstrate the nurse's caring.

Bibliography

1. Barsevick, A., et al. (1982). A comparison of the anxiety-reducing potential of two techniques of bathing. *Nursing Research* 31, 22.
2. Bersani, G., & Carl, W. (1983). Oral care for cancer patients. *American Journal of Nursing* 83, 533.
3. Boguslawski, M. (1980). Therapeutic touch: a facilitator of pain relief. *Topics in Clinical Nursing* 2, 27.
4. Breakey, B.M. (1982). An overlooked therapy you can use ad lib. *RN* 45, 50.
5. Brown, M.M. (1982). Nursing innovation for dry skin care of the feet in the elderly: a demonstration project. *Journal of Gerontological Nursing* 8, 393.
6. Bulechek, G.M., & McCloskey, J.C. (1992). *Nursing interventions: Essential nursing treatments* (2nd ed.). Philadelphia: W.B. Saunders.
7. Carpenito, L.J. (1992). *Nursing diagnosis: Application to clinical practice*. Philadelphia: J.B. Lippincott.
8. Casamassimo, P., & Castaldi, C. (1982). Considerations in the dental management of the adolescent. *Pediatric Clinics of North America* 29, 631.
9. Chauncey, H.H. (1982). Dry mouth in elderly patients. *American Family Physician* 26, 55.
10. Connell, M.T. (1981). Therapeutic touch: a natural potential for nurses. *New Zealand Nursing Journal* 74, 19.
11. Contact lens removal (1980). *Journal of Emergency Nursing* 6, 15.
12. Cox, H.C., et al. (1989). *Clinical applications of nursing diagnosis: Adult health, child health, women's health, mental health, home health*. Baltimore: Williams & Wilkins.
13. Crosby, C. (1989). Method in mouth care. *Nursing Times*, 35(85), 38–41.
14. Danielson, K.H. (1988). Oral care and older adults. *Journal of Gerontologic Nursing*, 11(14), 6–10.
15. Davis, M. (1977). Getting to the root of the problem. *Nursing '77*, 7(4), 60.
16. Doenges, M.E., & Moorhouse, M.F. (1991). *Nurse's pocket guide: Nursing diagnoses with interventions* (3rd ed.). Philadelphia: F.A. Davis.
17. Dossey, L. (1983). The skin: what is it? . . . The potency of touch. *Topics in Clinical Nursing* 5, 1.
18. Dudjak, L.A. (1987). Mouth care for mucositis due to radiation therapy. *Cancer Nursing*, 3(10), 131–140.
19. Fairweather, W. (1981). Care of adults with hearing loss. *Nursing* 28, 1236.
20. Fanslow, C.A. (1983). Therapeutic touch: a healing modality throughout life. *Topics in Clinical Nursing* 5, 72.
21. Fine-tooth comb for nit removal (1980). *American Journal of Nursing*, 80, 310.
22. Gannon, E.P., & Kadezabek, E. (1980). Giving your patients meticulous mouth care. *Nursing 80*, 10, 70.
23. Greifzu, S., et al. (1990). Oral care is part of cancer care. *RN*, 6, 43–46.
24. Holder, L. (1982). Hearing aids: handle with care. *Nursing 82*, 12, 64.
25. Jarvis, C. (1992). *Physical examination and health assessment*. Philadelphia: W.B. Saunders.
26. Johnson, F. (1978). Territorial behavior of nursing home residents. *Issues in Mental Health Nursing*, 1, 44.
27. Johnson, F. (1979). Responses to territorial intrusion by nursing home residents. *Advances in Nursing Science*, 1, 21.
28. Johnston, B.L., et al. (1981). Oxygen consumption and hemodynamic and electrocardiographic responses to bathing in recent post-myocardial infarction patients. *Heart Lung* 10, 666.
29. Kamenir, S., & Fothergill, R. (1982). Hands-on skills for dealing with hearing aids. *Canadian Nurse*, 78:44.
30. Kopac, C. (1983). Sensory loss in the aged: the role of the nurse and family. *Nursing Clinics of North America*, 18, 373.
31. Kreiger, D. (1975). Therapeutic touch: the imprimatur of nursing. *American Journal of Nursing*, 75, 784.
32. Lane, B., & Forgay, M. (1981). Upgrading your oral hygiene protocol for the patient with cancer. *Canadian Nurse*, 77, 27.
33. Lawson, K. (1989). Oral-dental concerns of the pediatric oncology patient. *Issues in Comprehensive Pediatric Nursing*, 12, 199–206.
34. Lesco, B.A., & Brownstein, M.P. (1982). Recognition of periodontal disease in children. *Pediatric Clinics of North America*, 29, 457.
35. Lindell, M.E. (1989). Lack of care givers' knowledge causes unnecessary suffering in elderly patients. *Journal of Advanced Nursing*, 14, 976–979.
36. Luce, M., & Sande, D. (1983). Oral health in children: prevention of dental caries. *Nurse Practitioner*, 8, 43.
37. Luckmann, J., & Sorensen, K. (1980). *Medical-surgical nursing: A psychophysiologic approach* (2nd ed.). Philadelphia: W.B. Saunders.
38. Martin, B., & Reeb, R.M. (1982). Oral health during pregnancy: a neglected nursing area. *American Journal of Maternal Child Nursing*, 7, 391.

39. Martin, B., & Reeb, R.M. (1983). The nurse as the first line of defense against periodontal disease. *Journal of Obstetric and Gynecological and Neonatal Nursing, 12,* 333.

40. McFarland, G.K., & McFarlane, E.A. (1989). *Nursing diagnosis and intervention: Planning for patient care.* St. Louis: C.V. Mosby.

41. McLaughlin, W.J. (1985). Malodorous patients. *Physician & Patient, IV,* 34.

42. McNally, J.C., et al. (1991). *Guidelines for oncology nursing practice.* Philadelphia: W.B. Saunders.

43. Meckstroth, R.L. (1989). Improving quality and efficiency in oral hygiene. *Journal of Gerontologic Nursing, 6*(15), 38–42.

44. Melamed, M. (1982). Complications of contact lenses. *Emergency Medicine, 14,* 218.

45. Meissner, J.E. (1980). A simple guide for assessing oral health. *Nursing 80, 10*(4), 84.

46. Miller, M. (1979). Recentering of displaced contact lens. *Journal of Emergency Nursing, 5,* 31.

47. Napierski, G.E., et al. (1982). Oral hygiene for the edentulous total care patient. *Special Care in Dentistry, 2,* 257.

48. National League for the Hard of Hearing. *Hearing Health Care* (pamphlet). Oticon Corporation.

49. Nightingale, F. (1969). *Notes on nursing: What it is and what it is not.* New York: Dover Publications Inc.

50. One-step brush and rinse (1980). *American Journal of Nursing, 80,* 2241.

51. Peterson, M., et al. (1982). Oral care for institutional geriatric patients. *Nursing Homes, 31,* 22.

52. Pinkerton, R.E., et al. (1981). Preventing dental caries. *American Family Physician, 23,* 167.

53. Ramos, L.Y. (1981). Oral hygiene for the elderly. *American Journal of Nursing, 81,* 1468.

54. Roach, L.B. (1977). Color changes in dark skin. *Nursing 77, 7*(1), 48.

55. Schaefer, A. (1982). Nursing measures to maintain foot health. *Geriatric Nursing, 3,* 182.

56. Schweiger, J.L., et al. (1980). Oral assessment: how to do it. *American Journal of Nursing, 80,* 654.

57. Speedie, G. (1983). Nursology of mouth care: preventing, comforting and seeking activities related to mouth care. *Journal of Advanced Nursing, 8,* 33.

58. Stillman, M.J. (1978). Territoriality and personal space. *American Journal of Nursing, 78,* 1670.

59. Tying knots in sheets (1982). *American Journal of Nursing, 82,* 295.

60. Wells, R., & Trostle, K. (1984). Creative hairwashing techniques for immobilized patients. *Nursing 84, 14,* 47.

61. Zenith Hearing Instrument Corporation. *Caring for a child's hearing aid* (pamphlet). Chicago: Zenith Corporation.

▼ Promoting Rest and Sleep

Chapter 39

Even where sleep is concerned, too much is a bad thing.

Homer (Odyssey)

▼ CHAPTER OUTLINE

NATURE OF SLEEP
    Rapid Eye Movement Sleep
    Non-rapid Eye Movement Sleep
    Sleep Cycle
    Circadian Rhythms
SLEEP DISORDERS
    Disorders of Excessive Somnolence
    Disorders of Initiating and
       Maintaining Sleep
ASSESSMENT

    Subjective Data
    Objective Data: Diagnostic Testing
NURSING DIAGNOSIS
PLANNING
NURSING INTERVENTION
    Back Massage
    Sleeping Aids
EVALUATION
CASE STUDY

▼ KEY TERMS

Arousal threshold
Cataplexy
Electro-oculogram (EOG)
Hyperpolarization
Hypersomnia
Hypnagogic hallucinations
Hypnotics
Insomnia

Narcolepsy
Nocturnal myoclonus
  (restless legs
  syndrome)
Non-rapid eye movement
  (non-REM, NREM) sleep
Pickwickian syndrome

Rapid eye movement
  (REM) sleep
Sedatives
Sleep apnea
Sleep paralysis
Somnolence
Sundowner's syndrome
Synchronization

▼ LEARNING OBJECTIVES

After studying this chapter, you should be able to

1. Discuss the nature of sleep, identifying rapid eye movement (REM) sleep, non-REM sleep, sleep cycles, and circadian rhythm.
2. Contrast disorders of excessive somnolence with disorders of initiating and maintaining sleep.
3. Explain how to assess a person's sleep pattern, including use of a sleep diary and questionnaire.
4. Describe diagnostic testing used in the measurement of sleep.
5. Contrast nursing diagnoses that are relevant to sleep disturbances and fatigue.
6. Discuss planning for the client with a sleep disorder.
7. Identify nursing interventions that promote rest and sleep.
8. State how to evaluate the individual who has received nursing care to promote rest and sleep.

Sleep is a relaxed state that is necessary to all humans. It is a universal and natural process. It is a state of composure that restores cerebral function. The brain and numerous body systems fluctuate during sleep. More than any other body part, the brain is affected by sleep. The brain is adversely affected by sleep deprivation because, during wakeful hours, the brain is constantly active. Similar to a computer on standby mode, the brain is always on alert awaiting instructions.[22] In contrast, the remainder of the body experiences a general slowing down during restful periods throughout the day. During sleep, physiologic alterations such as decreased body temperature, blood pressure, and pulse occur.

Sleep is a sensory experience. It was once thought that sleep was actually a state similar to unconsciousness. Actually, perception of and reaction to the surrounding environment decrease during sleep but the person is not comatose. The sleeping person can be aroused by tactile, auditory, and visual sensations. For example, sleep is interrupted by shaking, loud noises in the environment, and sunlight or the absence of darkness.

The sensory stimulus that awakens an individual is selective. An infant's cry will arouse its mother, whereas a telephone may not. A dog's barking may arouse its human companion, but an alarm clock may not.

Sleep is influenced by an individual biologic clock that regulates not only sleep but also levels of alertness throughout the day. Sleep is a cyclic phenomenon. Within a 24-hour period, individuals have one major sleep period and one major wake period.[15]

NATURE OF SLEEP

The brain quite naturally imposes sleep on the individual. The body adapts to progressive levels of sleep during a sleep episode. Each stage is important to the sleep episode and gradually leads to sleep that may restore the body physically and mentally.

Sleep is composed of two very distinct types of activity: **rapid eye movement (REM) sleep** and **non–rapid eye movement (non-REM, NREM) sleep.** REM sleep accounts for about 25% of a night's sleep and is characterized by REMs as detected by electro-oculograms and by intense physiologic activation.[5,9] It is often referred to as active or paradoxic sleep. NREM sleep accounts for about 75% of a night's sleep and is characterized by progressive relaxation.[5,9]

Rapid Eye Movement Sleep

REM sleep was named after bursts of extreme REMs were observed on an **electro-oculogram (EOG),** a graphic representation of the electrical activity associated with eye movements (Table 39–1). During REM sleep, the electromyogram (EMG), a graphic representation of the electrical activity associated with muscle tone, is almost flat. This shows that, during REM, neurons in the brain stem and spinal cord exhibit **hyperpolarization,** that is, overexcitement, with subsequent inability to transmit impulses. The result is immobility, much like paralysis in the large postural and skeletal muscles.[10,14] In contrast to the inactivity of the peripheral musculature, large increases in cerebral metabolic activity, and therefore cerebral blood flow, occur.

Because of all the cerebral changes occurring during REM sleep, convulsions are much more common during this stage of sleep.

In REM sleep, the electroencephalogram (EEG), a graphic representation of the brain's electrical activity, is active and closely resembles that seen in the waking state.[14,24]

Physiologically, REM is associated with activation of the sympathetic branch of the autonomic nervous system. Cardiac output, blood pressure, and heart rate can surpass waking values and may become erratic. Gastric secretion rates during REM increase. Individuals with peptic or duodenal ulcers have been shown to experience REM-induced secretions at rates 3 to 20 times that of normal individuals.[25] Respiratory rates vary greatly during REM, and self-limiting apneic (nonbreathing) episodes also occur.[17]

TABLE 39–1. Features of REM Versus NREM Activity

Feature	REM	NREM
Synonyms	Active, paradoxic sleep	Slow wave, quiet sleep (Stages 3 and 4)
Characteristics	Large-muscle immobility	Muscular relaxation
	Rapid, darting eye movements	Slow, rolling eye movements or no eye movement
Physiologic correlates	Cardiac rate increased and rhythm may become erratic; blood pressure and cardiac output increased; respiratory rate highly variable	Basal levels of cardiac and respiratory rates as well as body temperature
	Central and obstructive apneas	Obstructive apneas Central apneas ?
Hypothesized function	Mental-emotional equilibrium	Physiologic anabolism
Rebound	Yes	Stages 1, 2, and 3: None Stage 4: Yes
Dreams	Vivid, full color, and bizarre Emotionally charged	Stages 1, 2, and 3: Probably not Stage 4: Realistic, like thought process

Abbreviations: REM, rapid eye movement; NREM, non-REM.

REM sleep is also calorigenic. That is, overall oxygen consumption increases even though the postural and large skeletal muscles, which are normally a major contributor to overall oxygen consumption, are immobilized. The physiologic basis for the REM-associated calorigenesis is excessive cerebral metabolic activity.[24]

Although precise mechanisms have not been defined, REM sleep is believed to play a role in maintaining mental-emotional equilibrium.[1]

It is theorized that during REM information is processed and reviewed. Contextual and conceptual input from the previous day is sorted, selectively stored in memory, or cleared to make room for the next day's input. Evidence for this theory is largely based on the research finding that selective deprivation of REM precipitates disrupted perceptions that are manifested by disorientation, delusions, and even hallucinations.

Personality changes including withdrawal, increased suspiciousness, and paranoia have also been reported with deprivation of REM sleep.[14]

Dramatic dreams occur during REM. Described as full-color, vivid, and bizarre experiences, REM dreams often contain auditory components and frequently involve highly emotional situations. Frequently, REM dreams are associated with paralysis. Functionally, REM dreams may provide the psyche with an opportunity to deal with profound psychologic concerns from the consciousness.

Non–Rapid Eye Movement Sleep

NREM sleep is divided into four stages. NREM Stages 1 and 2 are light-sleep stages in which the individual can

be easily aroused. Stages 3 and 4 are characterized as slow-wave sleep (SWS) or quiet sleep that is deeper sleep than in Stages 1 and 2 (see Table 39–1).

STAGE 1 NREM

Stage 1 NREM is subjectively the lightest of all sleep stages. It may be most appropriately classified as a transition state between waking and sleeping. The EEG of this stage is similar to that of waking.

STAGE 2 NREM

Stage 2 NREM has been referred to as the "door" stage because it occurs both before and after REM in the characteristic cycle of sleep stages. The EEG of Stage 2 NREM is similar to that of Stage 1 NREM. However, it differs primarily in that the background wave frequency is slower and characterized by distinctive waveforms called sleep "spindles" and "K complexes."

STAGES 3 AND 4 NREM

Stages 3 and 4 NREM are associated with the appearance of very large, slow-frequency waves called delta or SWS. NREM Stages 3 and 4 differ from each other solely in the percentage of these slow waves in the EEG.[39] The **arousal threshold** (intensity of stimulus required to awaken) is typically greatest in NREM Stage 4.

Throughout NREM stages, eye movements reflected in the EOG are slow and rolling, if present at all. The EMG reveals a declining degree of muscle tone reflective of the progressive muscle relaxation characteristic of NREM. However, the EMG during NREM never

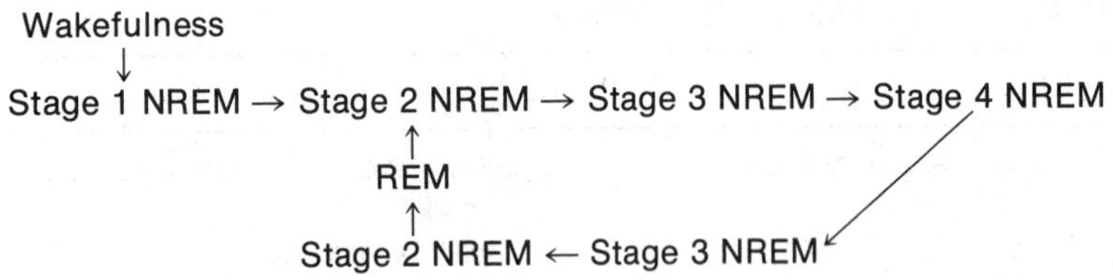

Wakefulness
↓
Stage 1 NREM → Stage 2 NREM → Stage 3 NREM → Stage 4 NREM
 ↑
 REM
 ↑
 Stage 2 NREM ← Stage 3 NREM

▲ *Figure 39–1*

The sleep cycle.

reaches levels as low as those seen in REM, in which functional immobility occurs.[39]

Dominance of the parasympathetic branch of the autonomic nervous system characterizes NREM. As a result, the degree of physiologic activation is low. Progression through NREM sleep is associated with decreases in cardiac and respiratory rates, blood pressure, metabolic rate, and body temperature. Basal levels are common.[39]

During NREM Stage 4 and probably Stage 3 as well, growth hormone is consistently secreted by the anterior pituitary.[26] Stimuli characteristically associated with growth hormone secretion include reduced availability of readily utilizable fuel for metabolic energy or increased energy demand. Because growth hormone promotes synthesis and also spares protein from breakdown and use as energy, its elevated secretion during SWS implies that NREM sleep serves an anabolic role (i.e., promotes an increase in formation as opposed to breakdown [catabolism] of body protein). This is particularly true in tissues with high protein content (e.g., cartilage and muscle).

Dream activity does occur during NREM sleep. However, NREM dreams tend to be less dramatic, more realistic, more difficult to recall, and nearer to normal thought processes than their REM counterparts[14] (see Table 39–1 for a summary of features of REM vs. NREM).

Sleep Cycle

Normally, NREM and REM occur in a specific repeating pattern or sleep cycle. With the onset of sleep, a progression through the NREM stages occurs from Stage 1 through Stage 4 and then back to Stage 2. From Stage 2, a REM period is entered. After completion of REM, Stage 2 of NREM is reentered and the cycle begins again. Figure 39–1 shows a schematic diagram of a sleep cycle. The length of a complete sleep cycle ranges from 60 to 120 minutes but averages 90 minutes.[39] The precise length of the sleep cycle is dictated by an intrinsic basic rest-activity cycle of the central nervous system.[10,27] This cycle is highly individualized. About 90 minutes elapse between the REM, or active, periods of two successive sleep cycles.

Within each sleep cycle, the proportion occupied by each stage changes as the sleep period progresses. Early, NREM Stages 3 and 4 dominate each cycle and REM periods are very brief. However, as the sleep period progresses REM periods tend to dominate, whereas NREM Stages 3 and 4 tend to shorten. Thus, most NREM typically occurs in the first half of a night's sleep, whereas most REM occurs in the second half.

Circadian Rhythms

Chronobiology is the collection of knowledge about body rhythms in health and illness. The individual biologic clock includes circadian rhythms, which are internal body rhythms that operate on a 24-hour schedule. Circadian is derived from "circa," meaning "about," and "dies," meaning "day." Knowledge of circadian rhythms is not new. It dates back to very early civilizations, when people wrote about life relating to cyclic rhythm. Some of life's most curious phenomena have been connected to circadian rhythms and body processes.[13,35] Valle and others[37] reported on the circadian influence in coronary care. The authors noted that, in recent years, heart attacks have been found to occur more frequently within the interval from 6 AM to 12 noon. This finding is unexplained physiologically; however, the influence of circadian rhythms is now being explored.

Much debate exists as to what controls circadian rhythms in the body. It is currently thought that two internal clocks are involved: one controlling sleep and wakefulness and the other controlling body temperature and physiology. It is also possible that both are part of a not-well-understood "master clock." The major function of the internal clock is to ensure optimal levels of sleep, wakefulness, alertness, and various physiologic changes such as temperature regulation.[22]

Circadian rhythms of sleeping-waking persist in environments such as a deep cave or environmentally controlled laboratories. A distinct rhythm in sleepiness was noted in the longest case of sleep deprivation on record. A 17-year-old boy stayed awake for 264 hours at which time periods of a cyclic need for sleep developed, particularly in the early morning hours of this sleep-deprivation vigil. In addition, lack of movement and stimulation brought on "extreme drowsiness" and decreased performance.[18]

Circadian rhythms can be exogenous or endogenous. Exogenous circadian rhythms stem from outside the body, and endogenous circadian rhythms originate within the body. The interaction of exogenous and endogenous rhythms is called **synchronization** and is essential to wellness. Examples of the major types of exogenous rhythms are the light and dark cycles that regulate adrenal hormones. Others are environmental temperature, precipitation, wind, and humidity. Examples of endogenous rhythms are the 28-day menstrual cycle in women, pulse rate, and blood pressure. Mental efficiency is also rhythmic, with some individuals, "night hawks," performing best mentally during the evening and others, "day larks," performing best during

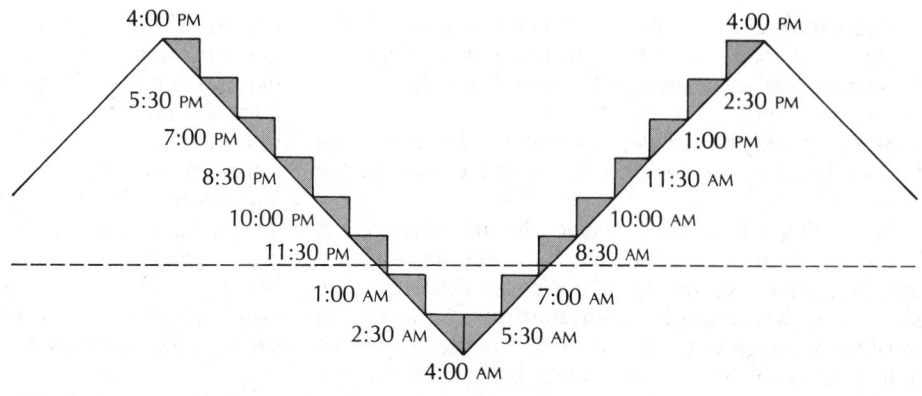

▲ *Figure 39-2*

Schematic depiction of circadian rhythm reflected by body temperature. Highest readings occur at roughly 4 PM. The lowest occur close to 4 AM. Hours falling below the dashed line (approximately 12 midnight to 8 AM) reflect the "lowest" portion of the circadian rhythm. Thus, they are the physiologically and psychologically optimal period to sleep. Hours above the dashed line correspond to the "higher" phases of the circadian rhythm, and hence those most appropriate for waking and activity. Superimposed on the overall circadian pattern are "high" (and "low") oscillations roughly every 90 minutes. Known as basic rest-activity cycles, or *BRACs (shaded areas)*, these oscillations reflect physiologic and psychologic ups and downs that occur 24 hours a day as dictated by the central nervous system. During the sleep period, each 90-minute BRAC reflects a full cycle of sleep stages, and the active or high point of each BRAC corresponds to the REM portion of each sleep cycle.

the day-time. Thus, peak alertness is a circadian rhythm with individual variation.

For optimal physiologic and psychologic function, a person's rest-activity schedule must be synchronized with the intrinsic biologic, or circadian, clock. When sleep is synchronized with the circadian rhythm, sleep activity occurs during the low phase of the physiologic and psychologic rhythm. Wakefulness and activity, on the other hand, occur during the higher phases (Fig. 39-2).

The actual number of hours a person spends sleeping reflects a balancing of external factors. Employment schedules, social commitments, and societal influences (e.g., the availability of goods and services) are all involved in determining a person's sleep-activity schedule. Once stable, acclimatization of the internal rhythm follows and circadian synchronization exists.

In contrast, attempts to sleep during hours when one is customarily awake and active or to be awake and active during hours when one is customarily asleep produce circadian desynchronization or a phase shift. Desynchronized sleep is of poor quality because the arousal threshold is known to decrease during desynchronized sleep and awakenings are more likely. Anxiety, depression, restlessness, irritability, and decreased accuracy are characteristics related to desynchronization.[7,8,11]

When the sleep schedule changes, resynchronization or internal acclimatization to the new sleep pattern must occur. Efficiency in resynchronizing varies with the individual, but the minimal time required is thought to be 3 days.[27] More commonly, the process of reacclimatization requires 5 to 12 days and is accompanied by chronic fatigue and malaise as well as a decreased ability to perform all life tasks.

SLEEP DISORDERS

Sleeplessness is common for millions of individuals. These people and others may experience **somnolence** —sleepiness, or feeling drowsy. The value of sleep has changed as a result of societal, work, and family expectations as well as other day-to-day demands. The traditional 8 to 9 hours of sleep enjoyed by families in the past has been greatly reduced because of the pace of society. The Association of Sleep Disorders Center has developed two broad categories for sleep disorders: (1) *disorders of excessive somnolence (DOES)* and (2) *disorders of initiating and maintaining sleep (DIMS)*. DOES most commonly include disorders of daytime sleepiness such as narcolepsy and sleep apnea, whereas DIMS do not describe any daytime **hypersomnia** (pathologically excessive drowsiness or sleepiness).[12] DIMS most commonly include the insomnias and the restless legs syndrome.

Disorders of Excessive Somnolence

NARCOLEPSY

Narcolepsy is a severe form of excessive daytime sleepiness (EDS) in which an individual has uncontrolled "sleep attacks" and almost immediately experiences REM sleep. It is very common among individuals between the ages of 10 and 25 years and may have a genetic cause.[3] The individual can instantly experience sleep attacks lasting for several minutes to 30 minutes at different periods throughout the day.

In addition to EDS, three classic symptoms can occur: cataplexy, sleep paralysis, and extremely vivid hallucinations.

Cataplexy is a type of muscle collapse in which the person is alert but speech is not discernible. Cataplectic attacks are associated with extreme emotions such as joy and anger.

Sleep paralysis is also an inability to move that frequently affects a person's limbs and occurs at the onset of sleep.

In fighting off a sleep attack, the narcoleptic can become extremely anxious and have intense, frightening, dreamlike experiences that can be visual or auditory called **hypnagogic hallucinations.**[38] Narcolepsy is often a dangerous sleep disorder, particularly if an individual is driving an automobile or operating heavy equipment. An accurate nursing history that focuses on age and the three classic symptoms can be helpful in formulating a nursing diagnosis.

SLEEP APNEA

Sleep apnea is a self-limiting episode of nonbreathing during sleep. Two types of apnea occur: central and obstructive.

Central Sleep Apnea. Central sleep apnea is thought to reflect some malfunction in the central nervous system. Normally, brain-stem respiratory centers control movement of the diaphragm, thus ensuring continuous breathing. In central sleep apnea, the airway remains open and the diaphragm and other chest muscles stop working. Decreasing levels of oxygen alert the brain and subsequently cause the sleeper to awaken and breathe. Central apnea is common in the elderly: One in four individuals older than 60 years experiences breathlessness to some degree. Central apnea characteristically occurs during REM sleep.[36]

Obstructive Sleep Apnea. Obstructive sleep apnea is a condition that is common in overweight individuals, often middle-age men, but it can also occur in postmenopausal women. In obstructive sleep apnea the upper airway—especially the pharynx—is obstructed, and breathing ceases momentarily. Obstruction can be related to three factors: (1) collapse of the lateral oropharyngeal walls, (2) relapse of the tongue against the soft palate and posterior pharyngeal wall, or (3) collapse of the hypopharynx.[3] Muscles of the soft palate and uvula relax and obstruct the airway. Breathing is noisy and labored, and snoring occurs. A type of "uncorking" of the airway is noted as pressure to breathe builds as a result of the muscle work of the diaphragm and chest.

During periods of breathlessness, oxygen in the bloodstream falls. Pulses are irregular, and cardiac dysrhythmias can be fatal.[15]

Periods of breathlessness last 10 to 20 seconds but in advanced cases can last up to a full minute.

Obstructive apnea ranges from a few episodes of apnea to very severe episodes called pickwickian syndrome. **Pickwickian syndrome** occurs in obese individuals and is characterized by pathologic sleepiness with severe episodes of dyspnea. The syndrome is named after a character in a Dickens novel—a young boy who was extremely obese and suffered from pathologic sleepiness. Typically, these patients weigh more than 300 pounds and complain of falling asleep during routine daily activities. Alcohol intake worsens the symptoms because of reduced muscle tone. Clinical features include obesity, excessive appetite, sleepiness, symptoms of right-sided heart failure (pedal edema; jugular vein distention; cyanosis; enlarged liver; large, brawny neck; and magnificent snoring). Laboratory values indicate low serum oxygenation and increased carbon dioxide levels.[19]

PHYSIOLOGY OF SLEEP APNEA

Arterial desaturation, hypoxemia, and systemic and pulmonary hypertension accompany both types of sleep apnea, but the degree of change in each case is consistently greater in obstructive as opposed to central apneic events.[17] The overall physiologic vulnerability associated with sleep apneas is directly correlated with the strength and frequency of apneic events. That is, individuals who have either prolonged or very repetitive apneic episodes are in the most danger. When airflow ceases, little oxygen is available to the blood passing through the pulmonary vasculature. Arterial blood thus becomes desaturated. Hemoglobin molecules bind with less oxygen, and hypoxemia results. When the blood perfusing the brain-stem respiratory centers reaches a severely decreased oxygen content, arousal is stimulated. With the transition from sleeping to waking, relaxation of the respiratory tract reverses or the diaphragm is stimulated and airflow resumes.

Sleep apnea is strongly linked to cardiovascular disorders, particularly in clients with hypertension, stroke, and congestive heart failure. Clients with severe congestive heart failure experience sleep of very poor quality. This is due to increased incidence of Cheyne-Stokes respirations (CSR), which cause significant hypoxemia during sleep. The severity of sleep disruption is related to the duration of CSR; that is, the number of arousals is due to hyperpneic phases of CSR.[20]

Disorders of Initiating and Maintaining Sleep

INSOMNIA

Insomnia is defined as difficulty falling asleep or staying asleep. In recent years, several causes and types of this sleep disturbance have been identified. Sleep disorder centers often use a classification that includes transient or situational insomnia, chronic insomnia (often of a psychiatric cause), insomnia related to the use of drugs and alcohol, and nocturnal myoclonus or restless legs syndrome.

Transient (Situational) Insomnia. Transient (situational) insomnia results from acute life changes such as recent surgery, stress, loss of a loved one, or a biologic change such as that associated with shift work or jet lag. Students, for example, often experience transient sleep loss before a difficult examination or a clinical experience. Situational insomnia typically exists for a period of 3 weeks or less and is related to significant life changes.[30] Treatment is generally symptomatic and directed at the cause. Benzodiazepines, which are short-acting, rapidly cleared **hypnotics** (medications used to induce sleep), can be effective providing that use is short term and event related.

Chronic Insomnia. Chronic insomnia is persistent and can be associated with mental disorders such as depression or mania. This type of insomnia lasts longer than weeks and can be extremely frustrating and debilitating. Often this disturbance begins with a stressful life event and develops into a persistent worry about not getting enough sleep. These individuals can also develop an expectation about sleep that is unrealistic and causes intense sleep disruption. They may feel, for example, that they must sleep 10 hours each night, not realizing that 5 hours of sleep may be sufficient for many people.

With psychiatric illness, the severity of the insomnia usually relates to the extent of the psychiatric illness. Rarely should treatment focus on the nightly use of hypnotics but rather should center on relaxation, conditioning, and removing underlying stimulus and cause.

It is also worth noting that hypnotics may be used by depressed individuals in suicide attempts and that overdose is always a possibility.[15]

Insomnia Related to Use of Drugs and Alcohol. Sleep disturbances frequently develop during and after long periods of drug or alcohol ingestion. Alcoholic individuals use alcohol to induce sleep; however, sleep fragmentation and disruption commonly result. Other drugs such as stimulants, amphetamines, and caffeinated beverages cause neural activity and sleep disturbances. Central nervous system depressants, on the other hand, will induce sleep. Authorities caution health care providers on the chronic use of depressants for this purpose. Chronic use may result in drug tolerance and eventually cause a "drug withdrawal insomnia."[15]

Nocturnal Myoclonus (Restless Legs Syndrome). Insomnia can also be associated with **nocturnal myoclonus (restless legs syndrome),** a condition in which a person feels an urge to walk in an attempt to relieve an irritating ache or "creepy" feeling in the calves and thighs. Nocturnal myoclonus is common among the elderly and can occur every 15 to 40 seconds in a sleeping state. Patterns of 300 to 1000 leg jerks a night have been reported. The cause of this disorder is not well known, and specific treatment has not been established.[15]

Sundowner's Syndrome. Finally, **sundowner's syndrome** is a common sleep disturbance most notably found among the elderly, characterized by restlessness and agitation in the late afternoon and early evening. This disorder of initiating sleep is often very upsetting to care givers in the home or nursing home setting. The syndrome is usually related to frequent daytime nap-

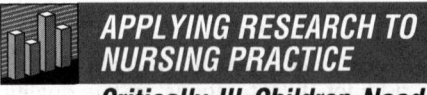

APPLYING RESEARCH TO NURSING PRACTICE
Critically Ill Children Need Their Sleep

Cureton Lane, R., & Fontaine, D. (1992). Sleep in the pediatric intensive care unit (abstract). *Heart & Lung*, 21(3), 287.

▼ ▼ ▼

The pediatric critical care unit is a brightly lighted, busy, noisy environment. These negative environmental stimuli may be quite detrimental to the rest and sleep of critically ill children. Cureton Lane and Fontaine wanted to find out just how detrimental noise and light are to the quality and quantity of sleep among critically ill children. They also sought to determine the effects of amount of care-giver contact, presence of parents, and severity of illness on sleep. These nurse researchers observed nine children in a pediatric critical care unit every 5 minutes throughout a 10-hour night. Results indicated that noise, light, and care-giver contact are the most important variables affecting the quality and quantity of sleep. The greater the noise and light and the more care-giver contact, the lower the quality of sleep and the less the amount of sleep. The average noise level in the unit studied was 55 dB, far in excess of the 45-dB limit recommended by the U. S. Environmental Protection Agency. The average sleep episode was only 28 minutes, and the total length of nightly sleep was 4.7 hours. Children awoke approximately 9 to 10 times per night.

Applications for Practice. Although the sample size was small, these findings indicate that critically ill children in pediatric critical care units may be severely sleep deprived. Sleep is a critical factor in a child's normal growth and development. The adequacy of sleep is particularly important in the child's recovery from a critical illness. In practice, you can exert control over the levels of noise and lighting in the pediatric critical care unit. Minimize unpleasant noise at the bedside, including communication with others, sounds emanating from equipment, and noise associated with treatment preparation. Dim the lights during the evening and night. Prioritize and organize the delivery of care to ensure that your pediatric clients achieve the goal of adequate rest and sleep.

ping, changes in bladder patterns, and difficulties in the evening hours. Interventions include the establishment of a bedtime routine and a quiet setting with decreased environmental stimuli.

FATIGUE

Fatigue is often experienced by clients in health care facilities. The fatigue results from frequent interruptions in sleep caused by health team members who wish to implement therapeutic measures. In addition to fatigue, sleep deprivation, sleep fragmentation, and circadian desynchronizations often occur.

SLEEP DEPRIVATION

When individuals are denied sleep, various bodily changes occur in addition to alterations in the quality of sleep. Authorities in sleep research note two types of sleep deprivation: core sleep and optional sleep. Core sleep can repair a cerebrum that works diligently in the wakeful hours. Core sleep includes the first few hours of sleep, particularly NREM Stage 4 and some of REM sleep. Optional sleep is a type of fill-in sleep that is maintained beyond the point at which core sleep declines. The combination of core and optional sleep provides the client with a level of sleep and rest needed to repair the body in a sleep-deprived state.[22]

Other bodily changes occur during sleep deprivation. Recent research has found that overall the body seems relatively unaffected by sleep loss but some changes do occur.

Humans experience a small decrease in body temperature during sleep deprivation. It was once thought that body temperature fell significantly during sleep. However, most humans do not have a serious problem with thermoregulation if sleep is deprived.

Respirations are affected by sleepiness. Yawning and sighing are two examples of respiratory changes. The immune system may also be more vulnerable in a sleep-deprived state. Cortisol depresses the immune system, and the connection among sleep loss, stress, and susceptibility to infection continues to be investigated.[22]

SLEEP FRAGMENTATION

The quality of sleep is affected by the continuity of sleep. Sleep that is fragmented is not of good quality. Sleep continuity is judged by the NREM/REM cycle that occurs. When sleep is interrupted, the sleep cycle begins all over again rather than returning to REM or a deep stage of sleep.

The fragmentation of sleep is severe in sleep apnea syndrome in which apneic episodes cause arousal responses that interrupt sleep.[34] The apneic patient is particularly vulnerable to sleep fragmentation and poor-quality sleep. Also at high risk for sleep fragmentation are clients with coronary heart disease. A large number of awakenings and significant alterations in all stages of sleep were reported by these patients. Frequent arousals resulted in fatigue, daytime sleepiness, and changes in psychologic mood.[29]

CIRCADIAN DESYNCHRONIZATION

Because treatment and monitoring may need to occur 24 hours a day, circadian desynchronization and phase shifts are often unavoidable in hospitalized persons. Circadian desynchronization also commonly occurs during long-distance air travel over several time zones, commonly called jet lag. In health care facilities, people may sleep during hours when they usually are awake and may be awake during hours when they usually sleep. Thus, much of the sleep obtained is de-

synchronized and less effective. It is also more easily disrupted because the arousal threshold is decreased by desynchronization.

Compounding the problem is the fact that resynchronization requires that a new sleep schedule be adhered to closely throughout the adjustment process.

A minimum of 3 days (often longer) is required for internal rhythms to adapt to an alteration in sleep pattern. However, care activities especially in health care facilities are rarely consistent for 1 day let alone 3 or more. Thus, chronic desynchronization is likely.

ASSESSMENT

Assessment of sleep and rest is a process of collecting detailed subjective and objective data. The first step in assessment is to identify the factors that prevent or inhibit sleep. Your goal should be to interview the client, and encourage him or her to document in a sleep diary any impediments to sleep.[36] In this way, the sleep pattern and any behaviors that impair sleep can be analyzed. Encouraging the client to develop a chart of dos and don'ts before sleep may be one method to assist the client in recognizing factors that may inhibit sleep.

Subjective Data

Assessment and facilitation of sleep are often challenging for a nurse. Key information lies within subjective data collected. Open-ended questions about sleep, rest, and relaxation patterns may provide valuable clues to sleep disturbances.

THE INTERVIEW

In the interview, the nurse can ask questions related to work schedules, possible shift rotations, daytime sleepiness, restlessness, possible causes of sleep disturbances, and factors that facilitate sleep and rest. It is also helpful to ask about customary sleep hours and the time frame in which the client sleeps best. Assessment of prebedtime food intake is also essential (e.g., noting ingestion of coffee, tea, cocoa, or other caffeinated substances that may alter sleep). Note factors that contribute to sleep disturbances such as age, physical illness, and psychiatric disorders.

Age. Table 39–2 summarizes the sleep patterns of persons at various developmental stages. As much as 60 per cent of persons 65 years of age and older have fragmented sleep patterns.[3] A change in the architecture of sleep is common in this age group. The older adult sleeps, on average, less than any other developmental age group and experiences a number of awakenings during the night. Recent research proposed that periodic leg movements during sleep and sleep apnea increase with age. Both produce sleep fragmentation and increasing daytime sleepiness.[15]

TABLE 39-2. Sleep Patterns by Developmental Stage

Developmental Stage	Sleep Pattern
Neonates	16 hours/day
Infants	14 hours/day
Toddlers	12 hours/day, with naps
Preschool children	10–12 hours/day, with nightmares
School-age children	8–12 hours/day
Adolescents	6–9 hours/day; emotions may cause sleep disturbances
Young adults	6–8 hours/day
Middle-aged adults	6–8 hours/day
Older adults	6–7 hours/day, with frequent nighttime awakenings

Physical Illness. Physical illness affects sleep. Cardiovascular and respiratory diseases may interrupt sleep because of difficulty breathing and associated pain and anxiety. Digestive acid levels also increase in the early morning hours and cause sleep disturbance. Gastric discomfort results in a need to awaken.

Psychiatric Disorders. Clients with psychiatric disorders such as depression and certain phobias and personality disorders have altered sleep patterns. It is not uncommon for these individuals to be taking psychoactive medications that, by themselves, disturb sleep.

Sleep Aids. The use of sleep aids should also be investigated in the interview. For example, certain over-the-counter sleep aids such as Nytol and Sleep-Eze are purchased at the rate of 30 million containers per year. Their effectiveness and relative safety are still uncertain. It is known that these products contain one or more antihistamines as the sedating agent. There is little evidence, however, that hypnotic effects of the drugs exist.[23]

The interview is of major importance in understanding sleep patterns and disturbances of clients. Sleep diaries and questionnaires that are self-reported can also provide valuable subjective data that may influence your plan of care.

SLEEP DIARIES AND QUESTIONNAIRES

Diaries and questionnaires are useful in identifying sleep problems that are caused by schedule alterations and changes in routines. In diaries, clients independently document activities such as meals, bedtime rituals, daytime naps, and psychologic stressors that may arouse emotions.[33] Questionnaires are also helpful in assessing sleep problems. McNeil, Padrick, and Wellman[32] developed a sleep questionnaire that systematically assists nurses in identifying sleep patterns and related problems (Fig. 39-3). The questionnaire focuses on three concepts: physiologic arousal, stimulus control, and circadian sleep-wake rhythm. For example, the client is asked about environmental stimuli, nonsleep behaviors associated with the bed or bedroom, and items related to circadian cycles. Diaries and ques-

tionnaires provide detailed assessment data about sleep habits from the perspective of the client.

Objective Data

Four instruments are used to objectively assess sleep: EEG, EOG, EMG, and Wrist Actigraph.

ELECTROENCEPHALOGRAM

The EEG measures the electrical impulses of the brain. During the EEG, electrodes are placed on the surface of the scalp with a quick-drying gel. Wires from the electrodes measure brain signals. The cerebral cortex envelopes the brain, and the electrical activity of the cerebral cortex is measured. Much of sleep can be monitored by the EEG alone.[22]

ELECTRO-OCULOGRAM AND ELECTROMYOGRAM

The transition from an alert state to a sleep state is signaled by a slowing down of EEG waves. When deep sleep or REM sleep occurs, the EOG and the EMG are used as measurement devices. The EOG incorporates the use of electrodes around the eyes to monitor electrical currents produced by eye movements. The EMG measures the electrical action of muscles. No activity can be noted in relaxed muscles at rest during REM sleep. Thus, the EMG provides direct evidence of muscle inactivity during an episode of REM.

WRIST ACTIGRAPH

A new device for measuring sleep is the wrist actigraph (Fig. 39–4). This device provides a recording of wrist activity. Actigraphs have been found to be very accurate, inexpensive, and quite simple.[2,21] The wrist actigraph monitors motor activity. A sensor housed in a 3-oz minicomputer monitors sleep and periodic awakenings in children and adults. The device fits into a wristlet and can be worn for days or weeks. Data retrieved by the minicomputer are analyzed with a software package that visually displays sleep-awake time periods.

NURSING DIAGNOSIS

The main nursing diagnoses that relate to alterations in sleep are *Sleep Pattern Disturbance* and *Fatigue*. The diagnoses are derived from assessment data that collectively indicate alterations in sleep. The causes of sleep alterations are unique to the individual and are often related to life events, changes in routine, health problems, and, at times, mental illness. A sleep care plan and related nursing diagnosis can be found in the case study for this chapter.

PLANNING

After subjective and objective assessments are made and a nursing diagnosis identified, plans should be

THE SLEEP QUESTIONNAIRE

At home, what do you do at bedtime to help you sleep? _____

Some of the statements may *appear* to be the same, but each is different and should be rated as such.*

A. I think I have difficulty with sleep
   a. in the hospital
   b. at home
B. I sleep more at home than in the hospital.
C. When I awaken in the hospital, I feel fatigued and groggy.
D. It takes me longer than 30 minutes to fall asleep in the hospital.
E. Since I've been in the hospital, I awaken frequently at night.
F. In the hospital, if I wake up in the middle of the night it takes me longer than 30 minutes to fall back to sleep.
G. It bothers me that I now go to bed at a different time than I would like.
H. It bothers me that I get up at a different time each morning.
I. Hospital staff awaken me while I'm sleeping.
J. I am awakened at night for treatments.
K. During the day, there is little time for rest.
L. At night I am awakened by noises.
M. At night I am awakened by light.
N. The mattress in the hospital bothers my sleep.
O. The pillow in the hospital bothers my sleep.
P. Having a roommate in the hospital affects my sleep.
Q. I sleep in a very warm room.
R. I have pain at night.
S. The medicines I take keep me awake.
T. My illness keeps me awake at night.

1. I drink coffee, tea, cola, or cocoa during the day.
2. I drink coffee, tea, cola, or cocoa around sleeping time.
3. I exercise during the day.
4. I exercise around sleeping time.
5. I smoke during the day.
6. I smoke around sleeping time.
7. I have unpleasant conversation during the day.
8. I have unpleasant conversation around sleeping time.
9. I have negative thoughts during the day.
10. I have negative thoughts around sleeping time.
11. I think about what happened during the day and at sleeping time plan for tomorrow.
12. I read during the day.
13. I read around sleeping time.
14. I eat around sleeping time.
15. I watch TV during the day.
16. I watch TV around sleeping time.
17. I have pleasant conversation during the day.
18. I have pleasant conversation around sleeping time.
19. I have positive thoughts during the day.
20. I have positive thoughts around sleeping time.
21. I drink alcohol around sleeping time.

*Response choices were: Never, Rarely, Sometimes, Often, Very Often.

▲ *Figure 39–3*

A sleep questionnaire. (Reprinted with permission from McNeil, B., Padrick, K., & Wellman, J. [1986.] I didn't sleep a wink. *AJN 86*[1], 26–27.)

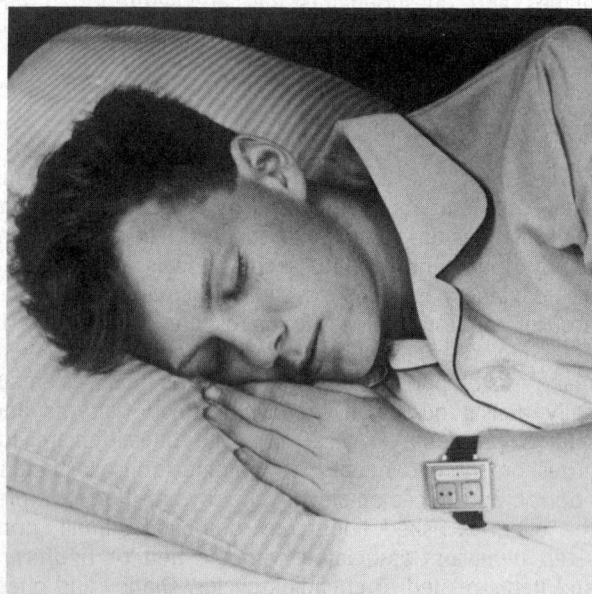

▲ *Figure 39–4*

A wrist actigraph, shown in use on a sleeping client. (Courtesy of Ambulatory Monitoring, Inc., Ardsley, NY.)

written that will assist the client in achieving outcomes that are realistic. The plan should be derived from the subjective and objective sleep assessments. For example, for the client who complains of daytime sleepiness, you should write an outcome that focuses on the client completing several sleep cycles throughout the night. You may even specify, in your goal writing, the length of time each sleep cycle should last. For example, "completes at least three sleep cycles of 90 minutes each during the 11 PM to 7 AM shift."

The plan should also be realistic for the client and should be based on information obtained from the history. The elderly client who awakens at night because of nocturia, for example, may be unable to change this behavior because of physiologic reasons. You may, however, write a realistic goal that focuses on limiting excess fluids before sleep. In this way, the periods of nocturia may not be totally eliminated but may decrease in incidence.

The plan should be individualized and client specific. The preoperative client, for example, may benefit from a therapeutic sleep aid. This may not be an appropriate plan for a client with sleep apnea, however, because of the vulnerability of this client to depressed respirations.

Finally, the plan should be specific to the developmental level of the client. Planning goals for preschoolers that focus on bedtime rituals may be very effective. Also, a night-light might help to decrease fear of the dark and prevent subsequent nightmares often experienced by this age group.

The plan of care for an individual with a *Sleep Pattern Disturbance* should be based on identification of factors that prevent or inhibit sleep (e.g., factors identified in a sleep diary).[36] Through an analysis of the sleep pattern and of behaviors that impair sleep, the nurse should assist the client in planning specific techniques to facilitate sleep.

Developing a chart of dos and don'ts before sleep is one method to assist in planning. The nurse and client must act jointly in planning care; this will ensure good communication and problem solving.

Clients experiencing *Fatigue* must understand the nature of the fatigue and seek to reduce, if not eliminate, it. The plan should encourage the client to verbalize the causes of fatigue and the effects of fatigue on his or her life. In addition, authorities recommend establishing priorities for usual activities. The client should plan participation in a balance of activities that challenge one physically, cognitively, affectively, and socially.[6] For example, participating in a social function

NURSING DIAGNOSIS PROFILE

Sleep Pattern Disturbance

Definition. Disruption of sleep time that causes discomfort or interferes with desired life style

Classification. Moving 6.2.1

Defining Characteristics. Critical defining characteristics include interrupted sleep, awakening earlier or later than desired, verbal complaints of difficulty falling asleep or maintaining sleep, and verbal complaints of not feeling well rested. Because of the sleep disturbance, each of these critical characteristics can lead to other less critical defining characteristics, including changes in behavior and performance (increasing irritability, restlessness, disorientation, lethargy, and listlessness), changes in verbal ability (thick speech with mispronunciation and incorrect word usage), and physical signs (mild fleeting nystagmus, slight hand tremor, ptosis of eyelids, expressionless face, dark circles under eyes, frequent yawning, and changes in posture).

Sample Related Factors. Sample related factors include internal sensory alterations (such as occur with illness and psychologic stress) and external sensory alterations (such as social cues and environmental changes).

Concept Description. Sleep Pattern Disturbance occurs when a disturbance of some kind causes an interruption in the person's normal sleep pattern. This disturbance results in a loss of sleep.

Examples. Depending on the specific assessment data, this diagnostic category could be applicable in the following situations, among others:

▶ A person who has experienced a change in health status that has interrupted sleep (e.g., a 20-year-old football player who has broken his leg and is disturbed at night by the pain in his leg and by the itching caused by the cast).

▶ A person who has experienced a traumatic life-style disruption (e.g., a 64-year-old woman whose daughter, and main source of support, has just been killed in an automobile accident).

▶ A person who is healthy and yet experiences internal sensory alterations (e.g., a 26-year-old female who is 8 months pregnant and who frequently experiences the need to urinate during the night).

Related/Similar Nursing Diagnoses. This diagnosis should be differentiated from the diagnosis of *Fatigue.* Although the person who experiences *Sleep Pattern Disturbance* is frequently fatigued as a result of loss of sleep, it is possible to be fatigued when the sleep pattern is not disturbed. The fatigued person feels an overwhelming, sustained sense of exhaustion and decreased capacity for physical and mental work (just as may occur as a result of *Sleep Pattern Disturbance*) but the diagnosis of *Fatigue* is used only when the person's fatigue is related to some cause other than a *Sleep Pattern Disturbance.* Such causes might be overwhelming psychologic or emotional demands, excessive social or role demands, increased energy requirements, and so on.

that also includes physical activity such as water aerobics, walking with a friend, or doing volunteer work may be beneficial, particularly for the elderly.

NURSING INTERVENTION

Many nonpharmacologic sleep aids can be used to influence sleep. For certain individuals, changes in life style or certain habits can improve sleep. For others, it may be helpful to be aware of the fact that worrying or problem solving before sleep alters sleep. The Better Sleep Council offers educators and health professionals guidance in assisting clients to facilitate sleep.[4]

You can recommend one or more of the following sleep facilitators:

▶ Avoid the use of caffeinated beverages and stimulants such as tea, cola, and chocolate and foods with tyrosine such as cheddar cheese.
▶ Keep regular hours: Stick to your usual sleep schedule on weekends and holidays as well as workdays.
▶ Exercise regularly: Exercise enhances sleep by burning off tension that accumulates during the day. A 20- to 30-minute walk, swim, or bicycle ride three times a week is helpful.
▶ Sleep on a good bed with a firm mattress.
▶ Do not smoke: Nicotine is a stronger stimulant than caffeine.
▶ Avoid the use of alcohol: Moderate drinking can suppress REM and deep NREM sleep and alter sleep stages.
▶ Get a quality sleep: Quality is more important than quantity. Six hours of sleep that is quality sleep is better than 10 hours of fragmented sleep.
▶ Set aside a time to problem solve emotional issues before going to bed at night. Pondering problems and crises in the presleep interval will disturb sleep.
▶ Do not eat a large meal before sleep. The digestive system will then work harder during a time when the body system should be relaxed and comfortable. Avoid peanuts, beans, fruits, or raw vegetables that produce gas or ice cream snacks high in fat that are difficult to digest.
▶ Develop a sleep ritual: Praying, reading, bathing, drinking warm milk, and listening to music can be soothing and can encourage a good night's sleep.

Milk contains a calming sedative-type substance called L-tryptophan that is very relaxing to many individuals. It also contains calcium, which helps to decrease nervous excitation.

Back Massage

Back massage is the purposeful manipulation of muscles and tissues to produce beneficial physiologic or psychologic effects that help the person to relax physically and mentally. When using massage, always explain the reasons. Without clear explanation, people who are not accustomed to back massage may misinterpret the actions as personal rather than therapeutic. Back massage is most effective if the person is relaxed and comfortable.

Back massage includes the area from the neck and shoulders to the lower buttocks. To give effective back massage, learn the location and directions of the major muscle groups involved: trapezius, deltoid, latissimus dorsi, external oblique, and gluteal muscle groups.

Remember the location of bony prominences to avoid direct pressure over these areas. Such pressure can damage the underlying tissue.

The major purposes of massage are to

▶ provide physical contact for physical and psychologic benefits
▶ stimulate and relax muscles
▶ increase circulation to improve cellular nutrition
▶ reduce tension, anxiety, and stress
▶ condition skin and prevent skin breakdown

Three main types of massage are straight, deep, firm strokes (effleurage); light, circular friction; and kneading (pétrissage) (Fig. 39–5). A back massage is often appropriate during morning care and when settling a person in for the night. It may be given at other times during the day or night, of course. When stimulation is desired, massage may be given after a bed bath and before changing bed linen. If massage is to promote relaxation, it is given at the end of all other hours of sleep care. Procedure 39–1 describes the purpose, procedure, contraindications, and teaching guidelines for back massage.

Sleeping Aids

Sleeping aids can be classified as either over-the-counter or prescription drugs (Box 39–1).

OVER-THE-COUNTER DRUGS

Over-the-counter drugs include certain antihistamines and alcohol. Common antihistamines sold over the counter include Nytol, Sominex, and Sleep-Eze. The effectiveness of these drugs is not well known, and many authorities question their beneficial effects. Residual difficulties such as poor coordination and memory changes are cited as reasons for avoiding their use. Other reasons include the potential for exacerbating asthma, urinary retention, and glaucoma.[16,28]

Although it causes drowsiness, alcohol interferes with the normal stages of sleep and causes sleep fragmentation.[23]

PRESCRIPTION DRUGS

While hypnotics are medications used to induce sleep, **sedatives** are medications used to reduce anxiety. Some sedatives are reduced doses of hypnotics in which enough medication is given to relax a person but

Text continued on page 962

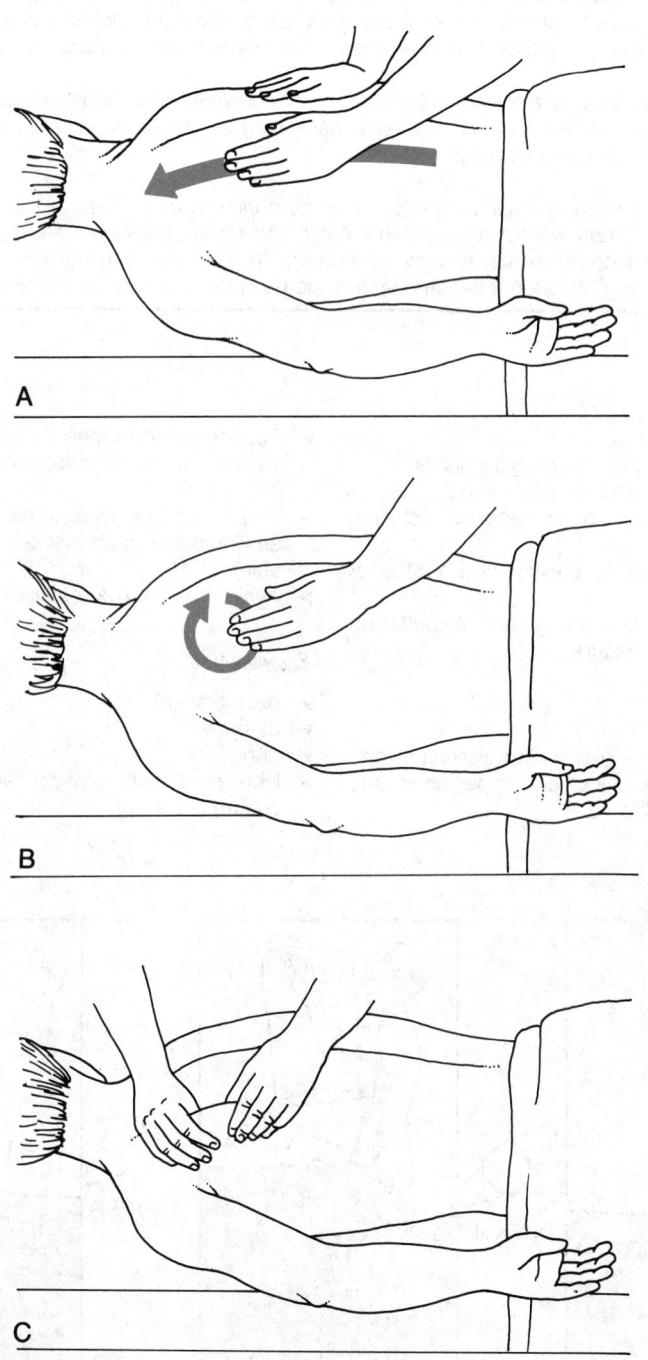

▲ Figure 39–5

Three basic types of massage. A, straight, deep, firm stroking (effleurage), B, light, circular friction, C, kneading of muscles with a lifting motion.

PROCEDURE 39-1

Back Massage

Definition/Purposes. Back massage consists of rhythmically rubbing, squeezing, and stroking tissues of the back, buttocks, neck, and upper arms. It is used to provide physical and psychologic comfort and relaxation, increase local circulation, prevent pressure ulcers, stimulate general circulation, and stimulate physical activity. Adapt procedure to individual needs.

Contraindications/Cautions. May be contraindicated in suspected or confirmed myocardial infarction (heart attack) or trauma (accidental, surgical, pressure induced, e.g., rib fractures, back surgery, incisions, skin ulcers, pressure areas showing nonblanchable erythema, and other skin lesions).

Learning/Teaching Guidelines. Present the following information as appropriate: (1) Explain indications/contraindications for massage; (2) never massage limbs without a physician's order and never massage limbs if tender areas develop after surgery or if person is on prolonged bedrest (danger of emboli); (3) use other nursing measures as indicated to relieve pressure and muscle tension (e.g., frequent position changes, padding bony prominences, proper body alignment).

PRELIMINARY ACTIVITIES

Assessment

Includes determination of

- diagnosis, activity orders, and psychosocial needs
- limitations of position and optimum position possible
- contraindications to massage or to particular massage techniques (e.g., stroking)
- purpose of massage (e.g., to prevent skin lesions or prepare for sleep)
- person's postprocedure activities (e.g., rest, ambulation)
- lubricant indicated by skin texture

Preparation of Person

- Complete preliminary care; adjust bed to working height.
- Position person with back, shoulders, upper arms, and buttocks exposed if possible.

- Position person prone if possible, otherwise side-lying or supine; when possible, move person to edge of bed (Fig. 39-6).
- Drape genitalia, legs, arms, and front torso for warmth and modesty (bath blanket conforms and feels comfortable).
- Avoid drafts; provide privacy.

Equipment

- back blanket
- bath towel
- pillows
- lubricant (lotion, powder, vegetable oil, shortening, or cream)

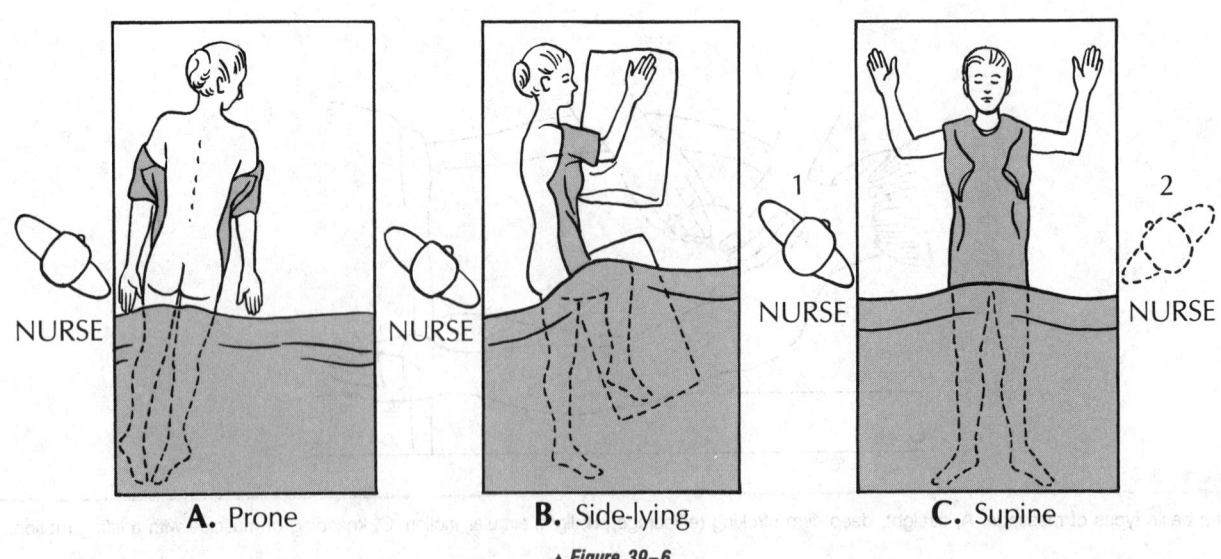

A. Prone   **B.** Side-lying   **C.** Supine

▲ *Figure 39-6*

PROCEDURE 39–1 Continued

Back Massage

INTERVENTION

Actions

1. Prone position (see Fig. 39–6A)
   a. Warm hands, warm lubricant (under warm water or in hands), and rub lubricant between hands.
   b. Tell person how lubricant will feel (e.g., cool, wet, or greasy).
   c. Gently apply lubricant to sacral area.
   d. STROKING
      i. Stroke from base of buttocks up to shoulders, over upper arms, and back to base of buttocks. Keep hands parallel to vertebrae and in contact with skin at all times.

      ii. Use palmar surface of hands for stroking.
      iii. Conform hand to body contour.
      iv. Shift body weight between heels and toes of feet (rocking motion) to achieve stroking force, rhythm, and rate. Face person's head; keep outside foot forward.
      v. Start stroking with medium upward, light downward force. Increase to firm upward stroke and medium downward stroke.

      vi. Apply firm stroke from base of buttocks parallel to vertebrae. Change to thumb strokes at cervical vertebrae, continuing up to occipital area (Fig. 39–5A). Return down to base of cervical vertebrae. Next, compress, squeeze, and lift trapezius muscle (see Fig. 39–5C). Repeat motions until relaxation is obtained.
   e. Maintain skin contact with back of one hand while adding lubricant and distributing lubricant between hands.
   f. KNEADING
      i. Knead one half of back and upper arm, starting at buttocks and moving up to shoulder; include deltoid and upper arm. Knead down or stroke down. Repeat on other half of body.
      ii. Knead by using palmar pressure with thumb abducted. Pick up tissue between thumb and fingers; release before pinching or twisting of skin (see Fig. 39–5C).
      iii. Achieve force, rhythm, and rate by shifting weight between right foot and left foot with feet perpendicular to person's body.
      iv. Begin kneading motion with second hand before release of first hand. Rhythmically alternate hands. Repeat motion until relaxation is obtained.
   g. FRICTION
      Use friction by exerting pressure in small circular motion around but not over bony prominences (see Fig. 39–5B). Exert gentle pressure with tips of second and third fingers. Do *not* massage injured tissue in pressure areas.

Rationale/Assessment

1.
   a. Cold causes vasoconstriction and muscle tension.

   b. Knowledge reduces apprehension and startle response.

      i. Long, continuous, and rhythmic rubbing is soothing. Pressure over bones (vertebrae) produces tissue injury. Rubbing skin increases circulation to superficial tissues and produces blanching followed by tissue redness (alternate emptying and filling of vessels). Oxygen and nutrients reach cells via the circulation.
      ii. Large surface contact reduces "tickle."
      iii. Continuous contact treats more tissue.
      iv. Rhythmic rubbing of body tissues is soothing and applies force in direction of motion.

      v. Use of body weight produces efficient force. Use of strong leg muscles rather than weaker arm and back muscles decreases energy use and avoids injury. Massage in direction of venous circulation and total circulation. Firm pressure reduces tickle. Assess response to pressure.
      vi. Squeezing muscle belly increases circulation, reduces tension. Assess muscle tension.

   e. This nonverbally informs person you have not completed massage or that it will not end suddenly.

      i. Kneading and squeezing at right angles to muscle fibers increase circulation to muscles.

      iii. Apply force in direction of movement. Body weight shift produces efficient force. Rhythm is soothing.

      iv. Continuous skin contact is soothing. Assess muscle tension.

   g. Assess skin for signs of tissue injury. Assess skin color and response to friction (duration of redness, response of blanched or red skin). Healthy tissue blanches with pressure and quickly returns to normal color after pressure release. Inadequate circulation is characterized by white, bluish, or reddened skin that slowly responds to pressure or does not change.

Procedure continued on following page

PROCEDURE 39–1 Continued

Back Massage

Actions	**Rationale/Assessment**

Actions

    h. Throughout massage, maintain contact with skin. Rhythmically proceed from stroking to kneading to friction. Rhythm rate varies with procedure purpose (e.g., slow, sedative massage; fast, stimulating massage).

        i. End massage with long, stroking movements. Gradually reduce pressure until massage is complete.

2. Side-lying position (alternative method) (see Fig. 39–6*B*)

    a. Position person on left side to massage right half of back. Turn person to right side to massage left half of back.

    b. If unable to turn person, support uppermost side with one hand and massage lowermost side with other hand. Use forward-backward motion for all one-handed massage movements.

    c. Flex at hips, with trunk rotated slightly toward person, to accomplish stroking and kneading movements. Place feet in forward-backward stance, advancing forward foot gradually. Maintain comfortable position with good body alignment.

    d. Proceed with massage, stroking, kneading, and friction. Avoid skin lesions.

3. Supine position (alternative method) (see Fig. 39–6*C*)

    a. With person lying in center of bed, massage one half of back at a time. Nurse moves from one side of bed to other.

    b. Lower bed level to comfortable working height.

    c. Fist of nurse's near arm depresses mattress while other hand massages closer half of back area. Stroke and knead while standing with outside foot forward. Supply force with forward-backward movements.

    d. Massage cervical areas, trapezius, and deltoid on both sides, with fingers of both hands stroking up and down cervical region. Lift and squeeze trapezius and deltoid muscles with thumb in front and fingers in back.

    e. Face person in forward-backward stance.

Rationale/Assessment

    h. Sedative effect: achieved by slow massage movements, enhanced by subdued lighting and quietness. Stimulation effect: achieved by rapid massage movements, conversation, frequent position changes.

    i. Long stroking is most soothing massage movement.

    a. Turning person exposes all skin surfaces and enables effective massage.

    b. This permits best body mechanics for nurse.

    c. See Steps iv and v in 1d. Increased pressure can be obtained by applying force to massaging hand (i.e., place one hand flat over other).

    d. Expose area during massage to avoid pressure over damaged tissue.

    a. This reduces strain on nurse's back. When possible, move person from one edge of bed to other to reduce reaching.

    b. Helps nurse maintain straight back while leaning forward.

    c. Stroking movement is not possible if person cannot be positioned to clear bed.

    e. Shift weight to obtain additional force.

FINAL ACTIVITIES

Wipe excess lubricant from back with bath towel. Tie or replace gown. Change person's position if indicated for comfort. Cover person; remove bath blanket. Aftercare of equipment: Place lubricant in bedside stand. Fold bath blanket and bath towel, or send to laundry. Store unnecessary pillows. Final assessment: Determine individual's general response to massage (e.g., relaxed, stimulated). Assess skin condition after massage (e.g., presence of blanched or reddened areas or lesions). Documentation: Document procedure, final assessment data, and teaching/learning.

---

not enough to cause sleep. These drugs should be used judiciously as a short-term intervention for sleep disturbances because of their potential for addiction as well as adverse affects. Taking sleeping pills for a short period of time may be very helpful for someone who is experiencing anxiety about a pending surgical procedure, experiencing stress, or suffering a transient type of insomnia. With a chronic sleep disturbance, the use of sleeping pills may not be helpful. In these cases, it is essential for the nurse to investigate the true cause of the problem and not just treat the symptom of the problem.

Benzodiazepines are a group of nonbarbiturate sedative-hypnotics that interfere with the transmission of nerve impulses in the brain. The benzodiazepines produce actions similar to the barbiturates. Both primarily cause sedation and sleep induction.[31] With peak blood levels of benzodiazepines, thinking is disorganized and memory is impaired. Hangover effects, nightmares, and rebound insomnia can be experienced. Physical dependence and tolerance may result if the therapeutic dose is exceeded. Common drugs in this category include diazepam (Valium), flurazepam (Dalmane), triazolam (Halcion), and temazepam (Restoril). Nursing goals include the following:

▶ Instruct client to avoid alcohol ingestion when using these drugs.
▶ Instruct users of these drugs not to drive an automobile or operate heavy equipment.
▶ Monitor for tolerance and dependence.
▶ Never increase the dose without medical supervision.
▶ Educate clients about other methods to induce sleep, such as drinking warm milk, limiting caffeine, and using environmental comforts.[23,31]

For many years, Dalmane was a very popular drug used for sedation. Studies conducted in Great Britain, however, cautioned health care providers to be aware of the prolonged influence of this drug on the individual. The day after drug ingestion, altered psychomotor function was noted as a result of the time it took for the level of the drug to reduce by half. In a normal adult, that time is 50 hours, but for the elderly population it could be twice as long.

In the 1970s, Halcion was widely used as a sleep inducer. However, it was so short acting that people felt the need to take another pill during the course of the evening. Halcion also has the potential to disrupt memory and can induce a period of amnesia.

Behavioral changes also have been associated with Halcion such as daytime anxiety, sleep walking, and hyperexcitability.[16]

The barbiturates produce central nervous system depression ranging from a mild to a severe state of sedation. The depressant effects result from interfering with the transmission of nerve impulses to the cerebral cortex, thereby inducing sleep. Gamma-aminobutyric acid (GABA), a neurotransmitter, is thought to be associated with this interference. This group of drugs also depresses the heart muscle and has the potential for abuse. In some persons, these drugs can produce an atypical excitation rather than a hypnotic effect. They

are distributed in all tissues, appear in breast milk, and can be very hazardous to the fetus because of their ability to cross the placental barrier. It is important to note that the benzodiazepines have largely replaced the barbiturates in drug therapy. Examples of barbiturates include sodium pentobarbital (Nembutal) and secobarbital (Seconal).[31]

Caution: The elderly are particularly vulnerable to the negative effects of sleeping aids. Because of liver or kidney difficulties, the elderly may clear drugs systemically at a much slower rate than is true of younger persons. As a result, the cumulative effects of these drugs can last for days. If sleeping pills are given nightly, an overabundance of the drug is circulating in the blood and the effects can be deadly. Age-related cardiac and respiratory changes can also complicate drug usage. It is essential for the nurse to monitor the use of sleeping pills in the elderly and protect these clients against indiscriminate distribution of these drugs by other nurses and health care personnel.

EVALUATION

Evaluation of care should be individual and should focus on the individual needs of the client. Basically, the questions to be asked are as follows: Is the sleep disturbance alleviated? Are the episodes of fatigue reduced or absent? Is the individual sleeping better in his or her opinion?

If the plan is not successful after adequate modifications, the nurse must recognize the importance of referral, perhaps to a sleep clinic. Explaining the significance of the referral to the client and the family is also essential. The sleep clinic can monitor the stages of sleep of the client in a laboratory setting. Sophisticated equipment used to diagnose sleep problems is available with highly competent staff who help approximately 85 per cent to 90 per cent of their clients. There are more than 170 sleep disorder centers in the United States and Canada. Several associations and foundations that may be helpful in recommending therapeutic sleep measures are listed in Box 39–2.

Box 39–1. Sleeping Aids

Over the Counter	Prescription
Alcohol	*Benzodiazepines*
Antihistamines	Diazepam (Valium)
Nytol	Flurazepam (Dalmane)
Sominex	Triazolam (Halcion)
Sleep-Eze	Temazepam (Restoril)
	Barbiturates
	Secobarbitol (Seconal)
	Sodium pentobarbitol (Nembutal)

Box 39–2. Sleep Associations

American Sleep Disorders Association, 604 Second Street SW, Rochester, MN 55902. (507) 287-6006
National Sleep Foundation, 122 South Robertson Boulevard, Suite 201, Los Angeles, CA 90048
American Narcolepsy Association, P.O. Box 1187, San Carlos, CA 94070. (415) 591-7979
National Institute of Mental Health, Public Inquiries Section, 5600 Fishers Lane, Room 15C05, Rockville, MD 20957
Canadian Sleep Society, c/o Dr. Harvey Moldothsy, Western Division of the Toronto Hospital, 399 Bathurst Street, Toronto, Ontario, Canada M5T 2S8

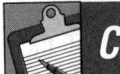

CASE STUDY

The Client

Mrs. Carmella Carole, 68 years old, visited the nurse practitioner complaining of overwhelming exhaustion and an "inability to function" in activities of daily living. She was visibly upset and chain-smoked during the entire interview. She also verbalized that her energy level had been quite low and that she had been very irritable lately. On further investigation, she complained of awakening at least five times during the night and each time had difficulty falling back to sleep. She stated that she naps at least twice a day "out of need" and denies taking any hypnotics or sedatives.

At 10:30 AM, a partial listing of Mrs. Carole's assessment data included the following:

▶ 68-year-old widow who lives alone
▶ complains of overwhelming exhaustion

▶ complains of "inability to function"
▶ states she drinks approx. 10 cups of coffee per day
▶ chain-smokes cigarettes
▶ states husband died 4 months ago
▶ complains of decreased energy level
▶ complains of awakening five times at night
▶ complains of difficulty falling asleep
▶ states she naps twice a day
▶ denies sedative or hypnotic use but states she has been "drinking a glass of wine at bedtime recently" to help her sleep.

Three days have passed since her assessment. The following represents part of a nursing care plan written for her at the time she was first seen by the nurse practitioner.

CARE PLAN

10:30 AM, October 6

Nursing Diagnosis	Planning: Expected Outcome	Implementation: Nursing Interventions	Evaluation
Sleep Pattern Disturbance R/T poor sleep hygiene practice	By 10 AM, October 9: Completes at least two sleep cycles of 90 minutes each	Encourage and teach about sleep hygiene practices: ▶ Discontinue nicotine use because of its stimulant effect ▶ Control environmental noise (i.e., close doors, turn off telephone) ▶ Promote sleep with soft music ▶ Eliminate unpleasant thoughts in the immediate bedtime hours ▶ Discontinue daytime napping ▶ Avoid consumption of foods high in tyrosine because these can impair sleep ▶ Avoid consumption of stimulants such as coffee, tea, cola, and cocoa in the evening hours because these beverages can delay sleep	10 AM, October 9: Client states she slept three 2-hour intervals last night and awakened feeling "rested and comfortable" this AM

CARE PLAN (Continued)

10:30 AM, October 6

Nursing Diagnosis	Planning: Expected Outcome	Implementation: Nursing Interventions	Evaluation
		▶ Encourage the consumption of foods high in L-tryptophan, a natural sedative, before sleep (e.g., warm milk and tuna sandwich) ▶ Discourage further alcohol use because it can promote sleep fragmentation	

Summary

▶ More than any other body part, the brain is affected by sleep.

▶ Sleep is a cyclic phenomenon; within a 24-hour period, individuals have one major sleep period and one major wake period.

▶ Sleep is composed of two very distinct types of activity: rapid eye movement (REM) sleep and non-REM (NREM) sleep.

▶ REM sleep accounts for about 25 per cent of a night's sleep and NREM, 75 per cent.

▶ REM sleep is associated with activation of the sympathetic branch of the autonomic nervous system and includes elevated cardiac output, blood pressure, and heart rate.

▶ NREM sleep is divided into four stages. Stages 1 and 2 are light-sleep stages and 3 and 4 are deeper sleep stages.

▶ REM and NREM occur in a specific pattern; a progression through the NREM stages occurs from Stage 1 through Stage 4 and then back again to Stage 2. From Stage 2, a REM period is entered.

▶ Sleep disorders are classified as disorders of excessive somnolence (narcolepsy and sleep apnea) and disorders of initiating and maintaining sleep (insomnias and restless legs syndrome).

▶ Sleep can be assessed via an interview or a sleep questionnaire. Sleep diaries and questionnaires are useful in identifying sleep problems caused by schedule alteration and changes in routine.

▶ Sleep can be measured by the electroencephalogram (EEG), electro-oculogram (EOG), and electromyogram (EMG). In addition, a wrist actigraph can be used to record motor activity and to monitor sleep and periodic awakenings.

▶ The nursing diagnoses *Sleep Pattern Disturbance* and *Fatigue* are commonly used for clients with increased needs for rest and sleep.

▶ Planning nursing care focuses on the client achieving an optimal level of sleep and completing several quality sleep cycles throughout the night.

▶ Nursing intervention for the client with sleep alterations should assist the client to increase his or her sleep by using safe therapeutic measures. Nursing interventions require that the nurse be knowledgeable about sleeping aids and hypnotic drugs.

▶ Evaluation of the client with a diagnosis of *Sleep Pattern Disturbance* or *Fatigue* must measure how well the client has improved on his or her sleep pattern.

Bibliography

1. (1985). A recipe for jet lag. *Emergency Medicine*, 17(12), 32–45.
2. Ambulatory monitoring. (1991) In *Wrist actigraph: Noninvasive, nonrestrictive*. New York: Ardsley.
3. Berman, R., et al. (1990). Sleep disorders: take them seriously. *Patient Care*, 24(11), 85–89.
4. Better Sleep Council. (1990). *The sleep better, live better guide*. Washington, CD: Better Sleep Council.
5. Biddle, C., & Oaster, T. (1990). The nature of sleep. *Journal of American Association of Nurse Anesthetists*, 58(1), 36–39.
6. Carpinito, L. (1990). *Nursing diagnosis—Application to clinical practice* (3rd ed.). Philadelphia: J.B. Lippincott.
7. Clark, R. (1989). Recognize "sleepy" workers by asking the right questions early in the rehabilitation process. *Journal of Rehabilitation*, 55(1), 9–12.
8. Coffey, L., et al. (1988). Nurses and shift work: effects on job performance and job related stress. *Journal of Advanced Nursing*, 13(2), 245–254.
9. Cutter, R.W.P. (1984). Disorders of sleep. In Rubenstein, E., & Federman, D.D. (eds). *Scientific American Medicine: Neurology* xiii (pp. 1–5). New York: Scientific American.
10. Dement, W.C., et al. (1973). Some fundamental considerations in the study of sleep. *Psychosomatics*, 14, 89.
11. Dickenson-Hazard, N. (1990). Study effectiveness: are you a 10 am or pm scholar? *Pediatric Nursing*, 16(4), 419–420.
12. Dinges, D. (1989). The nature of sleepiness: causes, contexts, and consequences. In Stunkard, A., & Baum, A. (eds.). *Perspectives in behavioral medicine: Eating, sleeping, and sex* (pp. 147–179). Hillsdale, NJ: Erlbaum.
13. Fernsebner, B. (1987). Chronobiology and institutional influences on the operating room nurse's level of wellness. *Perioperative Nurse Quarterly*, 3(3), 23–33.
14. Freemon, F.R. (1974). *Sleep research: A critical review* (2nd ed.). Springfield, IL: Charles C Thomas.
15. Gackenbach, J. (1987). *Sleep and dreams*. New York: Garland.

16. Gillin, J.C. (1990). Sleeping pills. *HMS Health Letter*, 5–8.
17. Guilleminault, C. (1980). Sleep apnea syndromes: impact of sleep and sleep states. *Sleep*, 3(3/4), 227–234.
18. Gulevich, G., et al. (1966). Psychiatric and EEG observations on a case of prolonged (264) wakefulness. *Archives of General Psychiatry*, 15, 29–35.
19. Hammond, B., & Hartzell, C. (1989). Sleeping beauty: a case of pickwickian syndrome. *Journal of Emergency Nursing*, 15(1), 8–11.
20. Hanly, P., et al. (1989). Respiration and abnormal sleep in patients with congestive heart failure. *Chest*, 96(3), 480–488.
21. Hartsell, M. (1987). New technology for safety and research. *Journal of Pediatric Nursing*, 2(3), 212–213.
22. Horne, J. (1988). *Why we sleep*. New York: Oxford University Press.
23. Institute of Medicine. (1970). *Sleeping pills, insomnia, and medical practice*. Washington, DC: National Academy of Science.
24. Kales, A. (1969). *Sleep physiology and pathology*. Philadelphia: J.B. Lippincott.
25. Karacan, I., et al. (eds.). (1974). *Sleep, stress, and the heart* (Vol. 1). Mt. Kisco, NY: Futura.
26. Kay, D.C., et al. (1976). Human pharmacology of sleep. In Williams, R.L., & Karacan, I. (eds.). *Pharmacology of sleep*. New York: Wiley.
27. Kleitman, N. (1969). Basic rest-activity cycle in relation to sleep and wakefulness. In Kales, A. (ed.). *Sleep: physiology and pathology*. Philadelphia: J.B. Lippincott.
28. Kolcaba, K., & Miller, C. (1989). Geropharmacology treatment: behavioral problems extend nursing responsibility. *Journal of Gerontological Nursing*, 15(5), 29–35, 42–43.
29. Landis, C. (1988). Arrhythmias and sleep pattern disturbances in cardiac patients. *Progress in Cardiovascular Nursing*, 3, 73–80.
30. Lareau, S., & Bonnet, M. (1985). Sleep disorders: insomnia. *Nurse Practitioner*, 10(8), 13–17.
31. Loebl, S., et al. (1989). *The nurses drug handbook* (5th ed.). New York: Wiley.
32. McNeil, B., et al. (1986). I didn't sleep a wink. *American Journal of Nursing*, 86(1), 26–27.
33. Ross, M., et al. (1986). When sleep won't come. *The Canadian Nurse*, 82(9), 14–17.
34. Rothenberg, S. (1987). Measurement of sleep fragmentation. In Peter, J., et al. (eds.). *Sleep related disorders and internal disease*. New York: Springer-Verlag.
35. Ryan, L., et al. (1987). Impact of circadian rhythm research on approaches to affective illness. *Archives of Psychiatric Nursing*, 1(4), 236–240.
36. Sleep Apnea. (1988). *Symptoms, causes, evaluation, and treatment*. Rochester, MN: American Sleep Disorders Association.
37. Valle, G., et al. (1988). Circadian influence on coronary events. *Heart & Lung*, 17(5), 586–593.
38. Walsleben, J., & Detscher, L. (1989). Disorders of excessive daytime sleepiness. *Nurse Practitioner*, 14(3), 11–16.
39. Williams, R.L., et al. (1974). *EEG of human sleep — Clinical applications*. New York: Wiley.

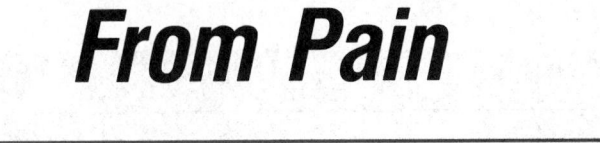 **▼ *Facilitating Relief From Pain***

 He teaches patience that never knew pain.

Proverb

▼ CHAPTER OUTLINE

WHAT IS PAIN?
    Acute Versus Chronic Pain
    Somatic, Visceral, and
        Sympathetically Maintained Pain
    Phantom Pain
    Referred Pain
    Pain and Suffering
PAIN TRANSMISSION AND PAIN
  MODULATION
    Opiate Receptors
    Endogenous and Exogenous Opioids
    Pain Modulation in the Peripheral
      Nervous System
    Early Theories of Pain Transmission
    Recent Theories of Pain
ASSESSMENT
    Assessment of Acute Pain
    Assessment of Chronic Pain
    Tolerance, Dependence, and
      Addiction
    Assessment of Pain in the Elderly
    Assessment of Pain in Children
    Sociocultural Aspects of Pain
      Assessment

    Pain Assessment Tools
NURSING DIAGNOSIS
PLANNING
NURSING INTERVENTION
    Pain and Loss of Control
    Pharmacologic Interventions
    Psychologic Interventions
    Nonpharmacologic Interventions
      Directed by the Client
    The Team Approach
    Physical Interventions
    Patient-controlled Analgesia
    Epidural Analgesia
    Transcutaneous Electrical Nerve
      Stimulation
    Alternative Routes of Opioid
      Therapy
    Other Pain-Relieving Techniques
    Interventions for Children
    Documentation of Interventions
EVALUATION
CASE STUDY

▼ KEY TERMS

Acute pain
Afferent neurons
Allodynia
Analgesia
Analgesic
Breakthrough pain
Chronic pain

Drug addiction
Drug dependence
Drug tolerance
Endorphins
Enkephalins
Epidural space
Gate control theory

Hyperalgia
Myelin
Nerves
Neural plasticity
Neuroablation
Nociception
Opiate antagonist

▼ KEY TERMS Continued

Opiate receptors	Phantom pain	Referred pain	Subarachnoid space	Visceral pain
Patient-controlled analgesia (PCA)	Placebo Psychogenic	Rescue medication Somatic pain	Sympathetically maintained pain (SMP)	Wind-up theory

▼ LEARNING OBJECTIVES

After studying this chapter, you should be able to

1. *Define pain, emphasizing the subjective aspect of pain.*
2. *Differentiate between acute and chronic pain.*
3. *Describe the pain pathways and the modulation of pain within the nervous system.*
4. *Discuss theories of pain and the use of these theories in nursing practice.*
5. *Explain how the nursing process is used to provide care for a person experiencing pain.*
6. *Identify assessment and treatment strategies for older adults in pain.*
7. *List three factors that affect the pain a child experiences.*
8. *Discuss the expression of pain by persons with different sociocultural backgrounds.*
9. *Identify pharmacologic principles for effective pain management, including those specific to cancer pain management.*
10. *Discuss some independent nursing interventions that can help relieve pain.*
11. *Describe several activities that can be directed by the client to alleviate pain.*
12. *Explain selected methods of pain management that require physician or nurse monitoring.*
13. *Explain the importance of evaluation in the management of pain.*

Pain is an elusive concept. We have all known pain in one way or another, and we have seen others in pain. Yet we have difficulty understanding exactly what another person's pain feels like, and so we should. Only the person experiencing pain can truly say what it is like. In this chapter, you will learn about acute and chronic pain and the many facets of pain that often elude even the most proficient nurse. You will find that technical skill is not as important in pain management as astute powers of observation and compassion.

Until recently, most schools of nursing and medicine gave misinformation about the dangers of addiction and excessive sedation and actually devoted very little attention to the topic of pain management.[42] When you have read this chapter, you should have replaced some of the myths of pain and pain relief with valuable information that will accompany you in any practice setting throughout your career. As you apply the nursing process to the person in pain, you may discover that facilitating pain relief is not always simple, but it is a challenge worthy of pursuit.

WHAT IS PAIN?

The International Association for the Study of Pain defined pain as "an unpleasant sensory and emotional experience associated with actual or potential tissue damage, or described in terms of such damage."[79] A more simplified definition is one given by Margo McCaffery, a nurse, who stated that "pain is whatever the person says it is, existing whenever the person says it does."[73] Both definitions remind us that pain is a subjective experience that cannot be quantified by someone *not* experiencing it. The word "pain" comes from the Greek word *"algesia."* Pain results when nerves conduct pain messages to the brain. **Nerves** are one or more bundles of fibers that connect the brain and spinal cord with other parts of the body. Individual nerve fibers are composed of neurons. If the pain message can be blocked, **analgesia,** or absence of pain, results. An **analgesic** is something (i.e., a drug or a procedure) that produces analgesia.

Acute Versus Chronic Pain

Acute pain is pain that has a sudden onset, is triggered by tissue injury, and has a healing time of less than 6 months. **Chronic pain** is pain that is persistently present and lasts longer than 6 months without healing.[38] A more specific definition is one introduced by Bonica, who described chronic pain as lasting more than a month past the usual course of an acute disease or a month past expected healing time.[11] Assessments and interventions vary in acute and chronic pain.

Somatic, Visceral, and Sympathetically Maintained Pain

Pain may also be classified according to its place of origin as somatic, visceral, or neuropathic. **Somatic pain** arises from bone and muscles; it is caused by the inflammatory process, which often results in muscle spasm. Somatic pain is aggravated by coughing, sneezing, movement, and palpation. **Visceral pain** emanates from the viscera (the abdominal organ or organs in other body cavities). Visceral pain is felt as diffuse, and poorly localized pain. It is often located near the midline because of the numerous overlapping nerves that supply this region. Pain felt in acute and postoperative situations is usually a combination of somatic and visceral pain. **Sympathetically maintained pain (SMP)** is pain associated with the sympathetic nervous system. The spontaneous firing of pain fibers without apparent stimulation constitutes sympathetic pain; the pain is perpetuated by the sympathetic nervous system despite the lack of further pain stimulus. When neural pathways are damaged, as in traumatic crushing nerve injury, healing occurs, but often the pain remains. SMP may not respond well to opioid therapy.[5]

Unfortunately, much about SMP remains unexplained.[53] Usually sympathetic pain follows tissue injury, but it may occur without any apparent cause. One example of SMP is the stabbing pain sometimes felt around an incision several months after surgery. Other sources may be less obvious; repetitive stimulus such as typing, playing tennis, operating a jackhammer, or carrying heavy objects may precipitate sympathetic pain in the arm. The pain is often accompanied by numbness and atrophy. Frequently reported sensations of sympathetically maintained pain are "burning pain," pain on light touch, extremely cold sensations in an extremity, and intense shooting or stabbing pain that cuts like a knife through the area of pain (very often an extremity). Swelling and weakness are also common signs. Sometimes a person will report that even very light tactile stimulus to the affected area (e.g., wearing a shirt) causes pain. This sensation is called **allodynia,** a sensation of pain from a stimulus that should not be painful (e.g., light touch).

Phantom Pain

Amputation of a limb most often results in postoperative pain, usually somatic pain similar to the pain that occurs after most invasive surgeries. Another type of pain, however, is not clearly somatic and may occur in the amputee. This sensation is **phantom pain,** or pain that is felt in a nonexistent extremity (or other body part) that has been amputated. If all phantom pain were relieved with opioids, we could correctly say this pain is somatic pain. Some phantom pain, however, is completely resistant to opioids but responsive to other drugs such as amitriptyline (Elavil), suggesting that it is neuropathic (the result of damage to neural pathways).[57]

Phantom pain symptoms are similar to neuropathic pain symptoms (e.g., intense burning, shooting pain). Phantom limb pain must not be confused with phantom limb *sensation*, which is quite different. Most amputees feel the sensation of the missing limb for a period of weeks to months regardless of whether they feel phantom pain.

Referred Pain

A person's pain may appear to emanate from one specific location when its source is actually very distant from the pain. Such pain is **referred pain,** pain experienced in a location different from the source, usually along the nerve path (e.g., left shoulder and arm pain during myocardial infarction). Visceral pain is the most common source of referred pain. The pain is referred from an organ through nervous pathways to areas of the skin outside the organ. For example, the pain of a myocardial infarction is often felt all the way to the fingertips of the left hand.

The sympathetic nerves are involved in visceral pain. When they are activated, a person in pain experiences autonomic nervous system responses to visceral pain such as sweating, restlessness, nausea, emesis, pallor, restlessness, and agitation. The somatic pain in muscles results in an impingement on nerves through swelling or stretching and can also refer to another location; the pain of the sciatic nerve, for example, is often felt throughout the entire leg.

Pain and Suffering

Pain is not synonymous with suffering. Suffering may include pain but is not limited to pain (Fig. 40–1). In fact, suffering may occur without the presence of pain, and so we need to make a distinction between the two. Suffering as a result of pain happens when people feel out of control from the pain, when the pain is overwhelming, when the source of the pain is unknown, or when the pain is chronic and appears hopelessly unending.[20] The more pain one feels, the more likely one is to experience suffering, but the perceived *meaning* of the pain has a great deal to do with suffering as well. For example, a person with leg pain who believes it is sciatica can endure the pain fairly well with codeine, but if it is discovered that the pain is due to cancer, much greater amounts of analgesia may be required. Suffering is surely a factor.

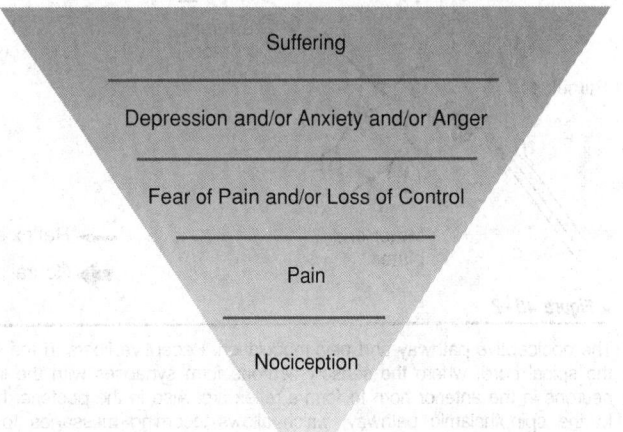

▲ *Figure 40–1*

Model of sensation from nociception to suffering. From the point of injury, nociception is transformed into pain in the brain, but other factors also affect the person in pain. Factors such as fear, anxiety, depression, loss of control, and anger may contribute to the ultimate suffering a person in chronic pain often experiences.

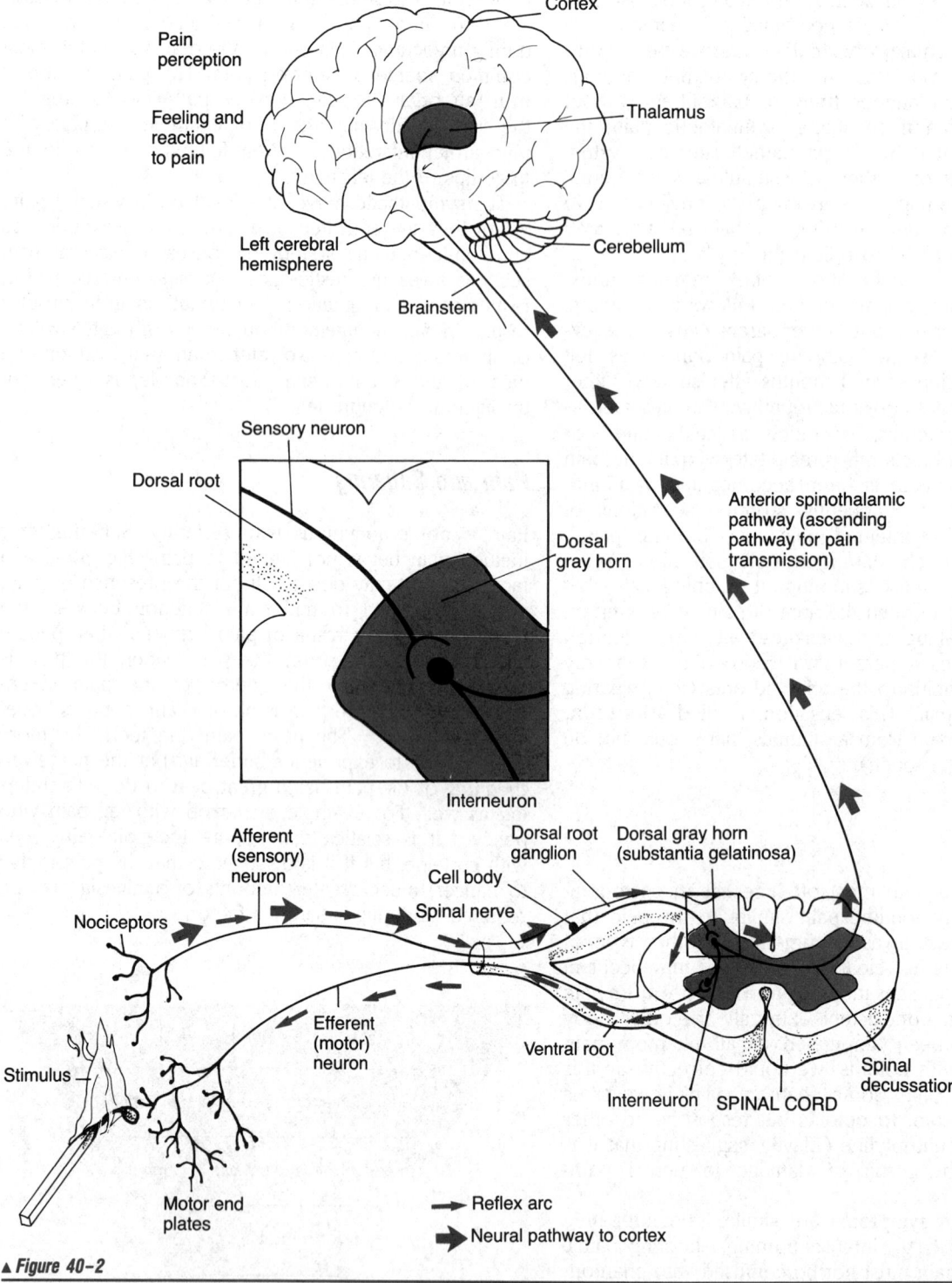

▲ *Figure 40–2*

The nociceptive pathway and pain modulation. Receptive fibers in the sensory neuron carry messages to the dorsal column of the spinal cord, where the sensory neurons form synapses with the interneuron. The interneurons form synapses with motor neurons in the anterior horn to form a reflex arc. Also in the posterior horn, sensory neurons form synapses with fibers leading to the spinothalamic pathway, which allows incoming messages to be sent to the brain, where they are perceived as sensations such as touch or pain. When certain types of touch and pain fibers in the sensory neurons are activated, interneurons in the posterior horn release enkephalins that prevent the transmission of pain and touch messages to the spinothalamic pathway. This, in turn, prevents perception of these sensations by the brain.

PAIN TRANSMISSION AND PAIN MODULATION

Knowledge of pain pathways and pain modulation is of critical importance when administering analgesics to a person in pain. The pain pathways illustrated in Figure 40–2 represent a fundamental tracing from the point of stimulation to the cerebral cortex.

The pain of somatic and visceral origin is called nociceptive pain. **Nociception** is the process by which specific receptors in the skin and other peripheral tissues respond exclusively to noxious or tissue-damaging stimuli. Quite simply, nociception is the pain message coming from the periphery into the central nervous system before the brain identifies it as pain. Nociceptive fibers are highly specific nerves that differ from other afferent fibers in that they respond only to noxious, or painful, stimuli. Nociceptors may be myelinated or unmyelinated. **Myelin** is a lipoprotein sheath surrounding a nerve fiber. Myelinated nociceptors are either A beta or A delta fibers. These fibers have a much greater conduction velocity than nonmyelinated nociceptors, called C fibers. Some C fibers are polymodal; they respond to several types of stimuli: thermal, mechanical, and chemical.[36]

The pain experience begins with tissue injury caused by disease, inflammation, accident, or surgery. Injured tissue causes cellular breakdown and the release of chemicals, referred to as excitatory amino acids, into the extracellular fluid. Excitatory amino acids include histamine, serotonin, prostaglandin, and substance P. These amino acids cause local changes and activate nociceptive nerve fibers. Nociceptive fibers in the peripheral nervous system transmit the message to the spinal cord, where they form synapses with other neurons in the dorsal horn. These nociceptive fibers are **afferent neurons,** nerves that travel toward the spinal cord and brain. In the dorsal horn of the spinal cord, these afferent neurons stimulate interneurons that incite motor reflexive responses.

If you have ever placed your hand on a hot stove by accident, you have experienced a monosynaptic motor response (a reflex arc). Instantaneously, you remove your arm without having to think. The incoming afferent nociceptor required only one synapse before a reflex response made you pull your hand away. Also in the horn, the afferent nociceptors continue to send the message to the cerebral cortex after your hand is removed.

In the cortex, the nociception is interpreted (in the hot stove example, it is usually identified as burning, throbbing, on certain fingers) and becomes pain. Excitatory amino acids are released in the central nervous system as well as at synaptic junctions. Substance P, glutamate, and aspartate play a role in the experience and modulation of pain. They may act as neurotransmitters, but even among prominent pain researchers much about the actions of these chemicals is yet to be discovered (S. Abram, personal communication, June 1992).

Opiate Receptors

Reynolds[89] demonstrated in 1969 that certain areas of the rat's brain stem could be stimulated electrically, resulting in analgesia. This finding led to the discovery of (opiate) receptors, or binding ports, which were found in abundance in the hypothalamus, the periaqueductal gray matter, the substantia gelatinosa of the dorsal horn of the spinal cord, and the gastrointestinal tract. **Opiate receptors** are molecular structures on the cell bodies of nerves. These receptors have two functions: (1) to recognize certain opiates for which they have greater affinity and (2) to bind with those opiates. When many receptors are activated by binding to opiates, analgesia results.

The word "opioid" comes from the discovery of opium in Greece more than 2000 years ago. "Opium" means "juice," referring to the juice of the poppy flower from which morphine is extracted. When it became known that morphine and other similar drugs provided analgesia by binding to the receptors in the central nervous system, the receptors became known as opiate receptors.

Endogenous and Exogenous Opioids

Animal research has shown the effects of chemicals produced by the body that decrease the pain experience.[7] These endogenous opioids are **endorphins** and **enkephalins,** neuropeptides produced by the body to provide analgesia in the nervous system by binding with opiate receptors. These chemicals are created during intense excitement, danger, and exercise and are in abundance in the midbrain and brain stem. They descend through nerve pathways where they attach to opiate receptors in the dorsal horn of the spinal cord, inhibiting the transmission of nociceptive signals through the central nervous system.

The presence of endogenous opioids has been documented in brain tissue during periods of intense stress and pain. When certain types of touch or pain fibers are stimulated in the sensory neuron, the interneurons release enkephalins, which prevent transmission of both pain and touch sensations from the dorsal horn of the spinothalamic pathway (see Fig. 40–2). Unfortunately, we do not have an endless supply of these chemicals in our bodies, hence the need for exogenous, or external, pain control.

It has long been known that morphine and opium, from which morphine is extracted, produce analgesia. We now also know that the action of this and all opioids is the same type of opiate receptor binding as occurs with endorphins and enkephalins, with a resultant decrease in pain.[111]

The drug naloxone (Narcan) is known as an **opiate antagonist** (opponent of opiate drugs such as morphine). Naloxone was developed synthetically from altered forms of opioids and is known to reverse opioid analgesia. It has a high affinity for the opiate receptors but provides *no* analgesia. Naloxone reverses the effect of endorphins, enkephalins, and most of the opiates. It competes with opiates at opiate receptor sites, thus reversing excessive sedation or any side effect caused by too much of the drug.

The fact that naloxone reverses the effects of opiates further substantiates the action of opiates in the central nervous system.

Pain Modulation in the Peripheral Nervous System

The relief of pain occurs not only in the central nervous system but also in the peripheral nervous system. When tissue is damaged, (for example, when you put your hand on the hot stove), arachidonic acid is released at the site of injury. Arachidonic acid is transformed into the compound prostaglandin, which produces **hyperalgesia** (increased sensitivity to pain), vasodilation, and edema.

Aspirin and other antiinflammatory drugs have been found to block the conversion of arachidonic acid into prostaglandin, which results in a decreased nociceptive input to the central nervous system, thus reducing pain. Now we can appreciate the pharmacologic rationale for combining aspirin or acetaminophen (e.g., Tylenol) with opioids, such as codeine or oxycodone. The pain relief is greater and is accomplished by two separate mechanisms: peripheral and central.

Early Theories of Pain Transmission

The earliest pain theory of which we have an abundance of information is that recorded by Descartes, a French scientist who identified pain as a response to excessive nerve stimulation and wrote volumes about his observations and theories in the 17th century.[27] He described pain as a specific sensation resulting from nerves leading to the brain after stimulation by a noxious stimulus (e.g., fire). Descartes's theory led to the specificity theory 200 years later.

The theory of specificity described by Schiff[91] in 1858 postulated that pain is the unique consequence of excitation of nociceptive afferent nerve fibers. These sensations are transmitted directly to the brain and constitute all pain sensations. This theory is limited in scope and has generally been abandoned.

The gate control theory was first presented in 1965 by Melzack and Wall in England. This theory explained why pain can be mediated or blocked completely by certain nerve fibers and by nerve stimulation. Although there is no actual gate in the central nervous system, the concept of a gate, open or shut, is helpful in understanding the physiology of pain at the spinal cord level.

The **gate control theory** is an explanation of pain transmission in which large myelinated nerve fibers (A beta fibers) have a low threshold for painful stimuli and, when activated, inhibit the response to other noxious stimuli, closing the gate to further painful stimuli. Tissue damage may cause small-diameter nerve fibers to be activated and to open the gate, causing pain. C fibers are nonmyelinated small-diameter nerve fibers that transmit sensations more slowly than large-diameter myelinated fibers.[103] Because they transmit more slowly than other fibers, C fiber pain messages can be blocked in the spinal cord if the gate is occupied by A beta fibers.

The hypothesis of a gate control was supported by the discovery of the phenomenon of stimulation-produced analgesia, a suppression of pain produced by electrical stimulation of discrete brain sites. Inhibitory signals also most certainly arise from the thalamus and the cerebral cortex, which in turn decrease the pain experience, closing the gate to pain.

Recent Theories of Pain

The **wind-up theory** was postulated in the early 1990s when researchers noticed that repeated noxious stimuli often produced a nociceptive response much greater than expected. The spinal cord seemed to be barraged with nociceptive input that increased even though the repeated noxious stimulus did not increase.[108] The nociceptors seemed to be *wound up* and more excitable to stimuli than they ordinarily would have been. In rat models, the pain was found to be allodynic (so that touch sensation that ordinarily would not cause pain did so). The allodynia found in rats has not been found in human models scientifically, but the concept offers an explanation of why people complain of intense pain when the noxious input is not intense but repeated.

The wind-up theory has clinical application for nurses. If wind-up can be prevented by pretreatment with a certain drug, then pain can be prevented to some extent. The excitatory amino acid glutamate is a neurotransmitter that probably plays a part in wind-up activity. Drugs that cause glutamate inhibition may impede the wind-up response, thus controlling pain before it is allowed to build. Ketamine is an anesthetic agent currently being investigated as a pretreatment for pain in humans. Preliminary data suggest that ketamine administered before the first incision is made in the operating room, then repeated before the end of the operation, may decrease the experience of postoperative pain.[34] As drugs that prevent wind-up are identified, nurses can pretreat people in anticipation of pain, possibly with a significant decrease in pain!

A related concept under current investigation is **neural plasticity,** or hyperexcitability of neurons in the dorsal horn of the spinal cord after severe pain and inflammation. Neural plasticity involves the release of excitatory amino acids (e.g., glutamate) that act at receptor sites in the dorsal horn to increase the pain. The action of plasticity and wind-up suggests that drugs with an affinity for certain receptors (not opiate receptors) could block the release of glutamate and be effective in pain control.[108] If drugs are developed that are less expensive than some of the opioids and have fewer side effects, a bright new era of pharmacotherapy could be on the horizon.

ASSESSMENT

Assessment of Acute Pain

Assessment of acute pain may be a 2-minute process or a 20-minute process. Assessment depends on the nature of the person's pain, on the nurse's understanding of pain, and possibly on the nurse's past exposure to pain, either personally or vicariously. Nurse researchers in Illinois found that nurses who had experienced intense pain themselves or who witnessed a loved one's intense pain were significantly more sympathetic to clients' pain.[51] Regardless of our past pain experience, however, we can perform appropriate and thorough pain assessments given the skills and techniques provided next.

When postoperative incisional pain is expected, we often neglect to ask the client for details about the pain. Frequently, the person's pain is not caused by the incision. The pain may be back pain from lying in bed for an extended period, arm pain from an infiltrated intravenous catheter, or throat pain from a nasogastric tube.

The following questions will guide you in the assessment of acute postoperative pain:

▶ "How intense is your pain?" (Use a scale from 0 to 10 or a 5-point scale indicating no pain, mild pain, moderate pain, severe pain, excruciating pain.)
▶ "What is the character of your pain? Is it sharp, dull, stabbing, aching, pressing, burning, or shooting?" (You may suggest words or have clients describe their pain in their own words.)
▶ "Where is your pain located? Does it travel anywhere (e.g., down the leg, across the abdomen)?"
▶ "What makes your pain worse (e.g., coughing, moving, walking)?"
▶ "What makes your pain better (e.g., rubbing the area, lying still, applying heat, taking medication)?"
▶ "What was your response to the last analgesic you received (e.g., took away all the pain, took the edge off, no difference felt)?"

In addition to the subjective assessments you elicit from the client, objective data often support the complaint of acute pain:

▶ blood pressure elevated (hypertension)
▶ heart rate increased (tachycardia)
▶ respiratory rate increased (tachypnea)
▶ diaphoresis
▶ guarding (unconsciously protecting the painful body part)

With this information, you can treat a client's pain more appropriately than if you were merely to administer analgesic medications as ordered. It might be that a warm compress to an inflamed extremity is all the person in pain needs. Alternatively, the pain might be more severe than expected, with vital signs suggesting profound pain. The physician should then be called to investigate potential surgical complications. Complica-tions of surgery with pain as the chief complaint include evisceration (extrusion of viscera through a wound), infection, and blockage of tubes or body parts.

Physiologic signs of surgical complications in which pain is the chief complaint include the following:

▶ severe stabbing pain described as "deep" in the body tissue
▶ hypotension
▶ bradycardia
▶ fever
▶ elevated white blood cell count
▶ loss of sensation in any part of any extremity

Assessment of Chronic Pain

Chronic pain may be either malignant (with cancer as the source) or nonmalignant. Assessment strategies are similar, although chronic pain related to cancer will necessitate a slightly different line of questioning. The physiologic signs seen in the sympathetic response to acute pain (tachycardia, tachypnea, and hypertension) are often absent in chronic pain. The subjective behaviors such as grimacing and crying are also often absent. Therefore, it is important to perform a thorough assessment of the chronic pain sufferer. The following questions will guide you in assessing chronic pain.

▶ "When and how did your pain begin? Was it initiated by an injury?"
▶ "Where is your pain located?" (Sometimes a person can point with one finger to the one place where the pain is the worst or may describe referred pain felt in another part of the body away from the source.) You should also ask, "Does your pain travel anywhere?"
▶ "What is the character of your pain? Is it constant, intermittent, dull, pressing, sharp, or shooting?"
▶ "What is the intensity of your pain?" Describe a scale for pain assessment and have the person respond without prompting.
▶ "How does your pain affect your activity?" (Activity patterns are especially important in persons with chronic pain because prolonged immobility may lead to physical disorders and psychologic distress.)
▶ "How does the pain affect your appetite or sleep?" (Do not lead the person toward a certain response by saying, "Are you able to sleep despite the pain?")
▶ "What does your family think (or say) about this pain (e.g., are family members supportive or critical? Are they helpful or neglectful?)"
▶ "What makes your pain worse? What makes it better (e.g., medication, heat, cold, immobility)?"
▶ "What are your expectations with regard to pain relief (e.g., to be able to walk without pain, to be pain-free, something else)?" Another way to phrase this question is, "What would you like to do that you are currently not able to do because of the pain?"

The assessment for the person with pain related to a malignancy will include these same questions with additional questions concerning specific clinical situations. For example,

▶ "Have you recently had radiation therapy?" (Post radiation pain for a period of days or weeks is common.)

▶ "Has there been a recent radiologic test performed in the area of pain?" (Metastasis is a common source of increased pain.)

▶ "If you don't take your pain medication, why not?" (Constipation, lack of alertness, gastric upset, inability to concentrate, and dry mouth are all occasional side effects of strong pain medications.)

Frequently seen physiologic signs of chronic pain are

▶ Decreased mobility/activity
▶ Easily distressed
▶ Depression
▶ Loss of appetite (but sometimes eating out of frustration or boredom)
▶ Loss of sleep
▶ Muscle atrophy
▶ Weight gain (sometimes weight loss, especially in cancer pain)

The concomitant changes in family dynamics and financial and sexual patterns of the chronic pain sufferer are often as serious and worthy of treatment as the pain itself. The head of household on whom a family depends undergoes profound loss of self-esteem and self-worth because of loss of work, loss of income, inability to care for children, and changes in intimacy. In effect, chronic pain means inability to pursue a normal life.

A combination of acute and chronic pain symptoms may further challenge the pain assessment process. We cannot assume that a person who has undergone cholecystectomy has only a gallbladder problem. This same person could have preexisting arthritis, migraines, or any number of syndromes that cause chronic pain, including cancer.

Tolerance, Dependence, and Addiction

While you are performing an assessment on someone in pain, it may occur to you that the person is using an exorbitant amount of opioid (narcotic) medications to control the pain. We often hear that a client is "addicted" to a certain drug, so that even before we see the person we have conjured up preconceived ideas and attitudes about "drug addicts." Addiction is actually a very complex problem, stemming from tolerance, physical dependence, and psychologic dependence.

Tolerance to a drug develops within several days of receiving frequent intravenous dosing.[62] **Drug tolerance** is a natural physiologic response to opiates, characterized by a markedly diminished effect with continued use of the same amount of an opiate analgesic.[8] Virtually everyone taking an opioid for a few days acquires some amount of tolerance to the drug. However, although this condition may accompany physical de-

pendence, it should not be confused with psychologic dependence.

Drug dependence is a physical or psychologic condition in which the person must continue taking a drug to avoid withdrawal symptoms. If stopping the drug suddenly causes withdrawal symptoms to occur, it is most correctly referred to as a physical condition.[14] The body has become dependent on the drug and reacts to its sudden absence. Physical dependence is associated with obvious clinical signs, whereas psychologic dependence is associated with emotional signs such as mood changes and is often associated with addiction. **Drug addiction,** or psychologic dependence, is the craving for a drug that goes beyond the physiologic need for it.

The assessment phase may require consultation with a psychologist or substance abuse specialist to differentiate between addiction and dependence. When in doubt, proceed as though the person in pain has a dependence (which is easily identified), and put aside your biases about addiction.

The assessment challenge occurs when you encounter a person with legitimate pain and an addiction to a drug. The most dangerous thing you can do for this client is to stop all opioid therapy during a period of acute pain.

It is not appropriate to wean a person off opioid analgesics during an acute pain situation. Because of the extreme tolerance, this client requires more drugs than a normal individual (often 10 times more) just to obtain some level of comfort. After the acute phase has subsided, plans can be made to control the pain with nonopioid methods. Careful and slow tapering of opioids may be initiated as other treatments are instituted by trained personnel.

Drug addiction can exist in people taking drugs on advice of a physician and in people taking illicit drugs, such as heroin or cocaine purchased illegally. You may discover that a person has an addiction of both types: prescribed drugs for chronic pain and illicit drugs purchased or stolen to further the person's sense of "freedom from pain." This sense of freedom from pain is sometimes referred to by physicians and nurses as euphoria, which has a negative connotation.[55] Keep in mind that the person with chronic pain and a street addiction has often been treated unsuccessfully with conventional analgesics. In such cases, the person frequently seeks relief on the street, and euphoria is a desired alternative to pain. There exists a real conflict, at least in the minds of many nurses and physicians, as to how to provide pain relief and control drug abuse at the same time.[70] The general consensus seems to be that using as many noninvasive or nonopioid measures as possible helps solve this dilemma.

Unfortunately some physicians believe that they are being observed by state governing agencies for the amounts of opioids they prescribe. They are therefore reluctant to increase the prescribed drug dose despite obvious tolerance and ineffective analgesia.[85] In view of this problematic pattern of practice, other resources and pain management strategies (e.g., psychiatric evaluation and assistance, muscle relaxation and biofeedback training) should be introduced. Despite these interventions, the person in pain may still require pharmacologic pain management in a carefully controlled environment.[98]

The person with malignant pain should *never* be denied effective pharmacologic pain management because of a physician's or a nurse's fears of addiction or of governing agency retributions. Your assessment can make the difference between a person obtaining adequate pain relief legally and a person having to go to the street for illegal drugs in a desperate attempt to relieve pain.

Assessment of Pain in the Elderly

It is well known that older persons' reactions to stimuli are different from those of young persons. One of the myths we hold for the elderly is that their perception of pain is diminished along with other sensations. Although senses such as sight and hearing are diminished with age, there is no clinical proof of nociceptive sensations diminishing as well. Interestingly, some researchers found that the elderly have increased pain threshold and pain tolerance, whereas others reported just the opposite.[24,48]

Clinical differences in the elderly person's pain behaviors are, however, easily detected. The elderly person may have grown up in an environment that placed great value in not complaining, in "being strong," and in not putting foreign substances into the body. The person with this background may tell you he or she feels discomfort rather than pain. A person may say "It's not too bad; I'll be fine" when the pain actually may be moderate to severe. An approach that is often successful is accepting the person's assessment of the pain but relying on nonverbal pain behaviors to dictate treatment. The elderly person is often willing to take analgesics or accept pain relief measures if offered but will not pursue this course without encouragement. You might ask the person to describe the discomfort. When prompted to describe the sensation in detail, the person may agree that it is fairly painful after all.

Metabolic changes in the elderly affect their response to opioid analgesics. Drugs are metabolized more slowly in older people, so that a drug remains longer in the bodies of older persons than it does in younger persons. Over several doses, this slower metabolism could produce excessive sedation. Studies performed on the pharmacotherapeutic nature of opioids in the elderly show that morphine given to elderly individuals may respond as though it were four times the amount given younger persons.[61] Assessment becomes particularly difficult in these clients because mental status changes might appear to be due to excessive opioids but could also be indicative of increasing severity of disease.

Some estimate that 80 per cent of the elderly (older than 65 years) suffer from at least one chronic illness.[47]

Chronic pain may be associated with the illness, which affects ability to cope, quality of life, and mortality. Age-related chronic pain syndromes such as trigeminal neuralgia, postherpetic neuralgia (after an adult herpes zoster infection), and polymyalgia rheumatica are very painful and show an increase in incidence with age. Depression and pain have been strongly correlated and may be even more evident in the elderly.[67,74] Sadly, this population tends not to be referred for more help or to seek assistance in multidisciplinary pain centers. To date, no systematic studies have been conducted to explain why this is true.

Assessment of Pain in Children

The child in pain presents some unique challenges in pain assessment. If you are performing a pain assessment that will lead to a nursing plan and intervention, you must be familiar with the developmental level of the child and the child's prior pain experiences as well as the family's coping patterns and resources available. Children's expressions of pain differ greatly from one developmental level to another. Very young children are often thought to be exempt from pain because of immature nervous systems and a lack of myelinated nerve fibers. In fact, although some myelination of nerve fibers is not complete until a child has reached the age of 2 years, the unmyelinated nerve fibers that conduct pain (C fibers) are present even in the fetus. Up until the mid-1940s, painful invasive procedures, including surgery, were performed on infants without anesthesia. Fortunately, the treatment of infants has become more humane in recent decades.

You should never assume that an infant cannot feel pain during a procedure.

Neonates, toddlers, school-age children, and adolescents all exhibit pain behaviors, although they are often discrete or unexpected.[4] Their pain experience is further influenced by family and situational variables. Behaviors ranging from stoicism to temper tantrums may indicate pain responses (see Table 40-1).

Prior medical, surgical, and/or hospital experience has an impact on the child that may be to your advantage or disadvantage. If prior experiences were positive, you have the advantage of assessing a young person who is probably not anxious or overwhelmed by new surroundings. This child also has a basic knowledge of medical terminology and can identify with words such as "IV" and "catheter." The child's experience allows you the opportunity to focus on the pain rather than describing and defining all the components of the hospital stay.

A negative prior experience means that the child enters the hospital with some trepidation. Anxiety and fear may be greater than pain, but these sensations are difficult to sort out, even for the child. Before the pain assessment, try to determine the child's situation. Is this an admission to the hospital for surgery? Is this a home visit to determine nutritional and functional status? Is

TABLE 40-1. Children's Developmental Level and Responses to Pain

Children at Developmental Stage	Indicators of Pain
Infants	Generalized body distress, crying, restlessness, flailing arms and legs
Toddlers	Clenched lips, rocking, rubbing, agitated or aggressive behavior (e.g., kicking, hitting, biting, throwing temper tantrums), running away from the pain, considering pain a "thing," more fear of pain than infants or school-age children
Preschoolers	Verbalizing the "hurt," no understanding of concept that "this shot hurts but it will make you better," ability to point to painful area
School-age children	Verbalizing pain, perhaps feeling responsible for it, connecting events without understanding relationships ("When I go here, I get a hurt"), having a passive attitude about pain ("I can't stop it")
Preadolescents and adolescents	Abstract awareness of the psychologic and emotional aspects of pain; ability to understand causes, consequences, and cures; reversion to some traits characteristic of younger age in stressful situations; perhaps withdrawing from others

Note: Regardless of the developmental level or age, children with a past experience with pain tend to rate their pain as less intense than those with no prior pain experience.[68]

this a clinic visit for chemotherapy? The child may assume the worst and be gratified to learn that the feared event may not happen at all.

Pain behaviors in the child may be similar to those of adults. Crying, grimacing, and guarding are all common behaviors, but in the child these behaviors represent more than pain; they also reflect emotional disturbances such as fear or anxiety related to hospitalization or separation from a parent. The child with positive prior experiences or coping mechanisms will probably not exhibit the same distress as the child without these experiences.[76] For example, on her eighth admission a 9-year-old with cancer may be watching television to distract herself from the pain because she has learned that this activity is helpful. Watching television is not regarded as a pain behavior, so an assessment that is visual only may lead the nurse to assume that the child is not in pain.

Children in chronic pain have been known to suffer sleep disturbances, loss of appetite, absenteeism, and personality changes. When behaviors are used to infer a child's pain, you must remember that a specific behavior may reflect anxiety or fear in one child, pain in

another, and anger in yet another. Children's pain responses also change over time. Thus, you need to collect as much data as possible at each assessment point.

A pain interview for a child should be as simple, clear, and direct as possible. One question might be, "Tell me about the hurt (pain) you have now." Have the child describe where the hurt is and how it feels. If the child needs prompting, use examples with which the child may be familiar. "Is the pain like a bee sting?" "Is it as bad as falling down?" These questions can be followed up with the question, "What would you like me to do for you to help the hurt?" If the child again needs prompting, you might suggest interventions you know you can do. These could include giving medicine (but *not* an injection), rocking the child, providing heat or ice to the painful area, giving a massage, or repositioning.

Beware of the tendency to look for a "typical" pain behavior from a child.

Infant pain behavior was studied intensely in the 1970s and 1980s, when major discoveries of pain transmission were disseminated. Crying as an infant pain behavior was the focus of most infant pain studies.[37,58,59,86] The intensity, frequency, duration, and pitch of cries have been evaluated and some commonalities reported. The initial cry after a painful stimulus tends to be high pitched and phonated (basic auditory pattern, harmonic), with a flat or slightly decreasing melody. The second cry is dysphonated (cry obscured by noise of overloading of the larynx), lasting for 16.5 to 17.5 seconds. The last cry, at 55 to 60 seconds, is lower pitched with a rising-falling rhythmic melody. More recent research focused on facial expression as an indicator of degree of pain.[45] However, there were no statistically significant findings. Further investigation regarding infant pain behaviors is necessary to determine whether other behaviors such as facial expressions or generalized physical distress can be predictable indices of pain.[6]

Pediatric assessment tools enable us to ascertain the child's level of pain in a consistent and valid manner. Tools range from the very simple—a thermometer on which the child places a mark to indicate the degree of pain (very cold = no pain; very hot = terrible pain)—to the more complex—Eland Color Scale, in which the child selects light colors for varying degrees of pain and then marks those colors on a figure of a child to indicate the location and amount of pain experienced.[33] Another tool that is less time consuming is the Wong/Baker Faces Rating Scale, consisting of six faces ranging from very happy to very sad and crying (Fig. 40-3). The child indicates which face represents how he or she feels.[110] Even young toddlers can respond to these tools, although many prefer the Hester Poker Chip Tool. In this tool, the child selects a certain amount of poker chips to represent the amount of pain he or she is experiencing. One chip indicates a tiny bit of hurt. Two chips indicate a little more hurt. Three chips mean still more hurt, and four chips represent the most hurt of all.[50] Children who cannot read and even

Explain to child that each face is for a person who feels happy because there is no pain (hurt) or sad because there is some or a lot of pain. Face 0 is very happy because there is no hurt. Face 1 hurts just a little bit. Face 2 hurts a little more. Face 3 hurts even more. Face 4 hurts a whole lot, but Face 5 hurts as much as you can imagine, although you don't have to be crying to feel this bad. Ask child to choose face that best describes own pain.

▲ **Figure 40-3**

The faces rating scale (From Whaley, L., and Wong, D.: *Nursing Care of Infants and Children.* ed. 4, 1991, p. 1148. Copyrighted by Mosby-Year Book, Inc. Reprinted by permission.)

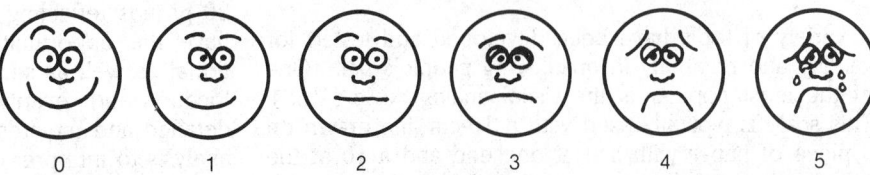

those who speak very little can usually respond to this assessment tool. The Hester Poker Chip Tool was recently translated into Spanish for use in the barrios of Los Angeles.[60]

The Agency for Health Care Policy and Research, a division of the U.S. Department of Health and Human Services, offers a quick reference guide for clinicians for infants and children in pain. The two tools suggested in this guideline are the Word-Graphic Rating Scale,[90] and the Poker Chip Tool. The Word-Graphic Rating Scale is similar to the five-point verbal pain rating scale (no pain, mild pain, moderate pain, severe pain, excruciating pain), but the words used are more appropriate for a young child (no pain, little pain, medium pain, large pain, and worst possible pain.)[3] In clinical situations, either of these tools is helpful when children deny pain verbally or when you have trouble differentiating their fear and anxiety from their pain. The guidelines also recommend that the principles in Box 40-1 be followed in the management of acute pain in the child.

Sociocultural Aspects of Pain Assessment

Observed pain behaviors may be influenced by one's culture as much as one's personality. Cultural patterns include beliefs about pain, customs, values, and accepted responses to pain. Numerous studies have been conducted on the influence of ethnicity on pain. Wolff[109] reviewed the findings of studies over the past two decades and found some interesting differences in pain threshold (the point at which one experiences pain) and pain tolerance (the amount of pain one can withstand). In his study population of Americans, the Scandinavians and Anglo-Saxons tended to have a higher pain tolerance, while Italians and Jews resembled African-Americans in their lower tolerance for pain.

In many countries, particularly throughout Asia, children are raised to be "brave," not to display weakness or pain, and not to complain of pain. This behavior becomes a problem in assessing a person in pain because often the person will deny that pain exists. Nurses must display respect and acceptance of these people's beliefs while identifying other cues that they are in fact experiencing pain. Guarding, grimacing, and immobility are all nonverbal cues that pain is present.

In other countries, exaggerated responses to stimuli are the rule. A person who is particularly expressive may cry or moan and plead for help while in pain. This behavior is accepted and routine in some European countries. Unfortunately, many care givers in America see this as "drug-seeking behavior." Your own biases need to be put aside because these people do require pain relief despite the seemingly theatric performance that may appear exaggerated.

You can *explain* sociocultural differences in pain perception, but do not *expect* them.

People in pain behave individually in ways that may or may not be associated with their sociocultural back-

---

Box 40-1. Principles of Acute Pain Management in Children*

► Unrelieved pain has negative physical and psychologic consequences. Aggressive pain prevention and control that occur before, during, and after surgery and medical procedures can yield both short-term and long-term benefits.

► Prevention of pain is better than treatment of pain. Pain that is established and severe is very difficult to control.

► A positive relationship between health care professionals and children and their families helps determine the successful assessment and management of pain. Children and their families should be informed that pain relief is important and that information about pain control options is available. They should be encouraged to discuss their concerns with the nurse or other members of the health care team.

► Children and their families should be actively involved in the assessment and management of pain.

► If all postoperative or procedure-related pain cannot be relieved, pain reduction to acceptable levels should be a goal in the majority of cases.

* Data from Agency for Health Care Policy and Research Public Health Service. (1992). *Acute pain management in infants, children, and adolescents: Operative and medical procedures. Clinical practice guideline, quick reference for clinicians* (AHCPR Pub. No. 92-0020). Rockville, MD: U.S. Department of Health and Human Services.

ground. The best assessment approach is to treat persons individually rather than stereotype them into what we have seen before from other people of their nationality or with their cultural background.

Pain Assessment Tools

A variety of tools have been developed and tested for validity and reliability in quantifying people's pain. One of the most popular is the visual analog scale (VAS). This scale is typically used with a 10-cm line drawn on a piece of paper with a 0 at one end and a 10 at the other, with 0 labelled "no pain" and 10 labeled "worst pain imaginable" (Fig. 40–4). The person in pain is instructed to put a slash mark with a pencil through the line at any point that represents how much pain they are having. The point at which the pencil mark intersects the line is measured and given a value (e.g., 7/10, with 10 being the worst pain imaginable[3]).

Pain measurement can be enormously helpful when trying different treatments or medications to facilitate pain relief. If a person reports 7/10 pain on one day (or at a certain hour) and 4/10 pain the next day (or hour), you have data to substantiate a decrease in pain. Clients who cannot write may be asked to rate their pain verbally on a scale from 0 to 10. A decrease from day to day can be seen as a positive course for both clinician and client.

Some people cannot use the VAS or choose not to respond with a number. People from foreign countries and the elderly sometimes have a difficult time with this form of quantifying pain. For this group, a five-point scale, as follows, may be more effective:

- ▶ 0 = no pain
- ▶ 1 = mild pain
- ▶ 2 = moderate pain
- ▶ 3 = severe pain
- ▶ 4 = excruciating pain

You need not mention the numerical value but merely document it on a flowsheet. The question may be asked, "Do you have no pain, mild pain, moderate pain, or severe pain?" Most people can remember these choices. Unfortunately, this smaller scale does not reveal the subtle improvements or regressions of pain relief that is evident in the scale ranging from 0 to 10.

The pain assessment tool you use is not as important as the consistency with which you use it.

Elaborate and detailed pain assessment tools are used predominantly for clients with chronic pain syndromes. Several have achieved a high degree of validity and reliability and are able to detect numerous psycho-

logic aspects of a person's pain and suffering. These tools take from 10 minutes to 2 hours to complete and should be administered by someone trained in psychologic testing. An example is the McGill Pain Questionnaire (MPQ), introduced in 1975 by Melzack.[78] This assessment tool is completed by the person experiencing the pain. Seventy-eight adjectives are arranged in 20 groups reflecting similar pain qualities. Respondents have the opportunity to describe their pain in emotional as well as sensory terms rather than in terms of location and severity of disease. The tool is extremely detailed and requires a person specifically trained in its analysis to interpret the results.

NURSING DIAGNOSIS

The nursing diagnosis *Pain* is the starting point from which to design an individualized plan for the relief of pain. *Pain* is the most common nursing diagnosis in use today, yet it is often identified without using the other components of the nursing process: assessment, planning, intervention, and evaluation of pain relief outcomes. This nursing diagnosis stems from the data gathered during the pain assessment phase.

Pain may be further described by relating it to its underlying cause. A nursing diagnosis might be *Pain* R/T the effects of abdominal surgery or *Chronic Pain* R/T the effects of tumor impingement on the spinal cord.

The most widely accepted diagnoses in this area are *Pain* and *Chronic Pain*.[83] See the Nursing Diagnosis Profiles to compare and contrast these two diagnoses.

PLANNING

The plan for facilitating pain relief may be derived from a list of desirable client outcomes such as

- ▶ reports freedom from pain
- ▶ performs daily activities without pain restriction
- ▶ requests for analgesics decrease

Sometimes, it is not possible to achieve a pain-free state. A desired outcome and plan that strive to achieve as much pain relief as possible are appropriate goals from which to initiate interventions. Chronic pain may always involve some restriction of activities related to pain, but the goal of performing activities of daily living is plausible and may be more readily achieved if the plan reflects that expectation.

Because of the subjective nature of pain, there exists a need for measurable outcomes that accompany the subjective report of pain relief. For example, "I feel less pain now" is subjective. Objective, measurable data could include the number of times the person was medicated over the past 24 hours. If that number reflects a decrease in medication, then it supports a subjective report of feeling less pain.

When the plan is well thought out, the intervention phase follows with a logical and appropriate progression and the likelihood of achieving pain relief is greater than with a nonplanned intervention. To be

No pain	Worst pain imaginable

▲ **Figure 40–4**

Visual analog scale for pain assessment.

NURSING DIAGNOSIS PROFILE

Pain

Definition. The state in which an individual experiences and reports the presence of severe discomfort or an uncomfortable sensation

Classification. Feeling 9.1.1

Defining Characteristics. The subjective complaint of pain is the most obvious characteristic of pain. If the person does not verbalize pain, the diagnosis may be made on the basis of objective observations such as guarding, grimacing, trembling, crying, clutching of the painful area, frequent requests for analgesics, changes in blood pressure, pulse, or respirations; diaphoresis; or dilated pupils.

Sample Related Factors. Inflammation, muscle spasm, obstructive processes, pressure on pressure points, the infectious process, overactivity, and experiences during diagnostic tests and treatments can all be related factors for the pain experience.

Concept Description. Pain is an emotional and physical experience, and it is not always directly observable. Pain may be of any magnitude, ranging from a twinge to incapacitating agony. It is often confused with suffering. A person in pain may not be suffering, but if suffering is present, more than the routine pain relief strategies will be necessary to improve the person's condition. Several factors contribute to one's perception of pain, notably anxiety and fear.

Examples. Depending on the specific assessment data, this diagnostic category could be applicable in the following situations, among others:

▶ A person who has very recently awakened from surgery under general anesthesia.

▶ A person whose Foley catheter tubing has become twisted and whose bladder has become distended with urine.

▶ A person who is not accustomed to exercise who has just run a mile.

Related/Similar Nursing Diagnoses. Pain and chronic pain are two different diagnoses. Pain must last longer than 6 months if it is to be diagnosed as chronic. Additionally, chronic pain may not cause the autonomic response seen in pain that is not chronic.

The nursing diagnosis *Pain* may be related to the nursing diagnosis *Noncompliance*, e.g., *Pain* R/T noncompliance with medical directive (to reduce exercise until sprain heals, for example). In such cases, noncompliance causes the pain. The nursing diagnosis *Noncompliance* might also be related to the nursing diagnosis *Pain*, e.g., *Noncompliance* R/T pain of medical regimen (prescribed medication might cause the side effect of an upset stomach so the client avoids taking the medication). In such cases, the pain causes the noncompliance. Do not confuse these two nursing diagnoses. *Pain* R/T noncompliance is very different from *Noncompliance* R/T pain!

Clients undergoing certain procedures could have a potential for developing pain, e.g., *High Risk for Pain* R/T expected effects of bone marrow aspiration. Anticipation of this pain-producing procedure is important in applying the nursing process to pain. A potential diagnosis with pain as the cause is *High Risk for Ineffective Breathing Pattern* R/T pain. The person who will not move or take deep breaths because of pain is certainly at high risk for additional respiratory problems as well.

---

truly effective, however, you should not be afraid to change plans or intervene in an unplanned manner as the situation dictates.

NURSING INTERVENTION

Pain relief is best achieved when a variety of methods are used. Your interventions will have a tremendous impact on the person in pain with regard to the person's perception of his or her environment, expectation of obtaining pain relief, and ability to manage the pain that remains.

Interventions should include teaching the client about pain "triggers" (factors that bring on the pain) and "reducers" (factors that relieve the pain). Include a brief teaching session about nonpharmacologic techniques that reduce pain. Both acute pain and chronic pain warrant a comprehensive approach that includes the most obvious interventions, such as

▶ Medicate for pain as necessary
▶ Position for comfort

and the less often enumerated but highly effective interventions, such as

▶ Perform frequent pain assessments
▶ Apply ice pack
▶ Massage painful area (unless risk of thrombosis is present)
▶ Provide distraction (through music, television, and so on)

Often the activities we must perform produce pain. Dressing changes, positioning, and even giving a bath can be very uncomfortable for someone who already has some degree of pain. Individuals who undergo painful procedures or activities develop anticipation of pain and sometimes anger at the persons causing the pain. You can improve the situation by verbally recognizing the discomfort, by offering to do something about it in anticipation of the discomfort (i.e., premedicate), and by carrying out the activities as gently and skillfully as possible. The correct use of positioning and supportive devices promotes comfort and helps prevent or reduce pain. You can also splint an area with your

NURSING DIAGNOSIS PROFILE

Chronic Pain

Definition. The state in which an individual experiences pain that continues for more than 6 months

Classification. Feeling 9.1.1.1

Defining Characteristics. Some of the characteristics for acute pain are also present in chronic pain, e.g., guarding or grimacing. In addition, chronic pain may be identified through such characteristics as fatigue, changes in posture, depression, anxiety, impaired thought processes, changes in eating habits, altered time perception, anger, altered affect, guilt, sorrow, altered libido, poor sleep patterns, family stress, and altered communication patterns.

Sample Related Factors. Most often, *Chronic Pain* is related to the effects of chronic or terminal illness, e.g., muscle spasm, chronic inflammation, pressure on pressure points for the immobilized. *Chronic Pain* may also be related to psychosocial stresses in which there is no evidence to support a physical cause for the long-lasting pain.

Concept Description. The diagnosis of *Chronic Pain* depends more heavily on the subjective report of the person than does the diagnosis of acute pain. Actual tissue damage is often documented, but because of the length of time since injury or illness, we tend to make light of persistent pain. To differentiate between acute and chronic pain, it may be more helpful to observe for pain that has remained more than a month after normal healing would have been expected to take place. The criterion of 6 months' duration is a guideline, not a research-based definition. Someone who has continued pain from a minor injury that healed a month ago should be designated as a person in chronic pain. If the physician waits for 6 months to

act, more damage may be done by not assessing the person and exploring possible interventions in a timely manner. Chronic pain, like acute pain, is a warning that something is wrong. For people in chronic pain, we sometimes know exactly what is wrong; in other situations the etiology is unclear.

Examples. Depending on the specific assessment data, this diagnostic category could be applicable in the following situations, among others:

▶ A person with continuous, chronic low back pain lasting 3 years
▶ A person who has experienced at least one headache a week for the past 15 years, since the person discovered that his father had committed suicide

Related/Similar Nursing Diagnoses. Because chronic pain can interfere with life in so many ways, the person may have several "psychosocial" nursing diagnoses, e.g., *Hopelessness, Body Image Disturbance,* and *Altered Sexuality Patterns.* These coexisting diagnoses may all be related to the chronic pain. Chronic pain can also be a related factor in "physical" nursing diagnoses such as *Impaired Physical Mobility, Feeding Self-Care Deficit,* and *Sleep Pattern Disturbance.* All of these diagnoses stem from chronic pain and would be worded, for example, *Hopelessness* R/T chronic pain or *Body Image Disturbance* R/T chronic pain. The diagnosis *Chronic Pain* would also include a related factor.

A similar diagnosis is *Pain.* To differentiate *Pain* from *Chronic Pain,* see Nursing Diagnosis Profile—Pain.

---

hands or a pillow during movement. For example, you can splint painful incisions postoperatively with your hands or a pillow while the person coughs or moves. Splinting supports abdominal contents and helps prevent them from applying pressure on the sensitive incision area.

Pain and Loss of Control

A person with chronic or acute pain usually experiences a loss of control over daily life events and decisions. This loss occurs in the hospital setting and at home. In the hospital, clients are told when they will eat, bathe, go to therapies, visit with physicians, and go for a walk. At home the situation is similar; if the pain is debilitating, they rely on someone to assist them to the bathroom, with meals, and with ambulation. Loss of control generally adds to the anxiety one has over the entire situation. Thus, if pain exists at all, the sense of having no control over it or other aspects of the environment often intensifies the person's perception of pain. Involving clients in decisions and activity times

can help them regain a sense of control and may facilitate pain relief strategies. For example, the person in pain appreciates being asked, "Would you be more comfortable if we put two pillows under your leg this time?" or "Would you prefer the dressing change before or after lunch?"

If you have an opportunity to discuss postoperative pain before surgery, you may lessen the anxiety related to fear of pain. Some people are reluctant to ask for pain medication. The person may not know what we mean if we ask "Do you want your prn medication?". The term "prn" ("pro re nata," or as necessary) is foreign to many people, yet we use this term (and others) frequently and without explanation.

Reassurance that you will provide pain relief measures swiftly and competently should decrease anxiety significantly. Explain the meanings of various medical terms your colleagues use—prn, IM injection, Foley, and so on, and inform the person that you will perform frequent pain assessments and offer medication for pain.

Always assess pain before taking action to relieve it.

Pharmacologic Interventions

Pharmacologic interventions may appear to be quite simple, yet they are often the most poorly understood and poorly followed strategies for the management of pain.[22,52,69] Nurses often have very little knowledge of the action of various analgesics and are thus reluctant to medicate adequately.[75]

TIMING MEDICATIONS

The pain cycle, seen in Figure 40–5, represents a typical time course for a person who receives prn intramuscular injections for pain. The medications ordered often do not provide analgesia for the entire time interval for which they are prescribed. For example, meperidine (Demerol) gives analgesia for about 2 hours, yet it is most often ordered "every 3 to 4 hours prn for pain." Pain relief usually occurs, but sedation follows, and pain returns before the nurse is able to administer another dose of the medication.

Opioid analgesics, whether offered on a routine basis or prn, are the mainstay of postoperative pain management (see Table 40–2 for opioid equivalencies and Table 40–3 for dosing recommendations). Other analgesics may be beneficial or even preferable in the case of hypersensitivity to opioids. Nonsteroidal antiinflammatory drugs (NSAIDs) such as ibuprofen and naproxen are particularly useful in orthopedic surgery, in which tissue inflammation around joints occurs (see Table 40–3). One powerful NSAID frequently used as an adjunct to opioids is ketorolac tromethamine (Toradol). It has been compared in potency with 12 mg of morphine but does not have the undesirable central nervous system effects such as sedation, nausea, and tolerance. Whether given intravenously, orally, or intramuscularly, its efficacy and safety are well established.[16,84]

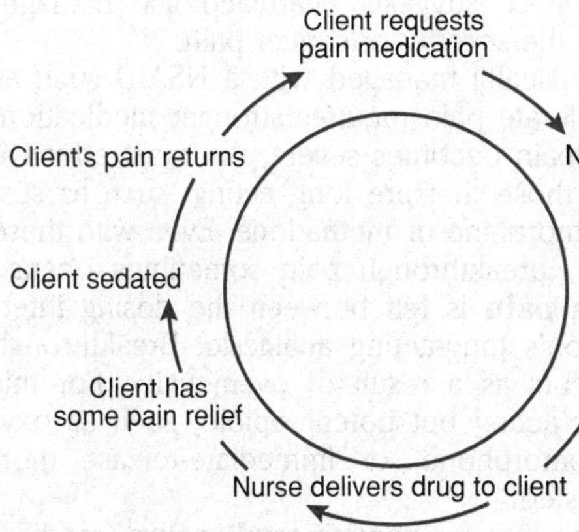

It is helpful to consider the following principles of pharmacologic pain management when formulating intervention strategies:

1. To achieve greater pain relief, offer prn analgesics routinely around the clock (ATC) rather than only when the client asks. If the drug is already ordered prn, ATC administration does not require a specific physician's order. Your assessment confirms the need to administer the drug routinely.

2. Administer adjunctive medications if ordered (for sleep, for anxiety) as necessary to augment the pain medications.

3. Combine opioid and nonopioid medications for greater analgesic effect.

4. Record response to last analgesic given. If medication was ineffective, give more next time. If medication was effective but did not last until the next dose available, decrease the time interval. If orders do not include these possibilities, consult with the physician to obtain the orders necessary to achieve greater comfort.

PRECAUTIONS WITH NSAIDs

Nonopioids such as NSAIDs may be administered to adults and children. Suggested NSAIDs are listed in Table 40–4, and there are new drugs in this category arriving on the market every month. The most common side effect of NSAIDs is gastric upset (affecting up to 20 per cent of all persons who take it). NSAIDs should not be taken on an empty stomach. Less frequent side effects (in less than 3 per cent of clients) are dizziness, headache, nervousness, tinnitus, and diarrhea. This category of drugs is contraindicated in people with bleeding disorders, past or present gastric ulcers, allergies to aspirin or other NSAIDs, or any condition that predisposes to bleeding. Nonsteroidal drugs tend to prolong bleeding time and inhibit platelet aggregation although less so than aspirin. As with most drugs, NSAIDs should be used with caution in persons with renal problems.

USE OF PLACEBOS

A **placebo** is a neutral preparation (such as a saline injection or a sugar pill) given as a medication. The person receiving it is not informed that the "medication" is actually only saline. Placebos have a role in only two areas of pain management: in clinical research as a comparison to the efficacy of a real analgesic and in situations in which there is a clearly defined **psychogenic** (of psychologic origin) component to the pain that is unresponsive to other pharmacologic interventions. Even with psychogenic pain, placebos should not be the primary treatment unless they are completely successful in relieving pain.

Placebos are rarely indicated for the treatment of pain.

As a primary pain relief method, placebos are not useful, nor are they ethical in most cases of acute or chronic pain.[15,39,41] People can usually tell when they are receiving a placebo, and they feel deceived by the care givers. No trust develops between the person in

▲ **Figure 40–5**

The pain cycle.

TABLE 40-2. Opioid Analgesics: Equivalencies*

The following opioids are equipotent to morphine, the standard of comparison. The amount required of each drug that would be equipotent to morphine, 10 mg IV or IM, is not necessarily the recommended dose of that drug.

Opioid Analgesic	Equianalgesic Oral Dose	Equianalgesic Parenteral Dose (IV or IM)
Morphine	30 mg q 3–4 hours (around-the-clock dosing)	10 mg q 3–4 hours
Meperidine (Demerol)	300 mg q 2–3 hours (not very effective orally)	100 mg q 3 hours (dangerous metabolite; normeperidine)
Levorphanol (LevoDromoran)	4 mg q 6–8 hours (long acting)	2 mg q 6–8 hours
Methadone (Dolophine)	20 mg q 6–8 hours (long half-life, never give more frequently)	10 mg q 6–8 hours (watch for cumulative effect after several days; sedation possible)
Oxymorphone (Numorphan)	Not available	1 mg q 3–4 hours
Buprenorphine (Buprenex)	Not available	0.3–0.4 mg q 6–8 hours (cannot be reversed with naloxone if excessive sedation occurs)
Butorphanol (Stadol)	Not available	2 mg q 3–4 hours
Codeine	130 mg q 3–4 hours (it would take four or five Tylenol no. 3 to equal 10 mg of morphine IM)	75 mg q 3–4 hours (this is not recommended because of probable constipation)
Oxycodone (this is the opioid in Percocet and Tylox [also available plain])	30 mg q 3–4 hours	Not available
Hydrocodone (the opioid in Vicodin, Lorcet, Lortab [also available plain])	30 mg q 3–4 hours	Not available
Pentazocine (Talwin)	150 mg q 3–4 hours	60 mg q 3–4 hours

* Data from Agency for Health Care Policy and Research, Public Health Service. (1992). *Acute pain management in adults: Operative procedures. Clinical practice guideline, quick reference guide for clinicians* (AHCPR Pub. No. 92-0019). Rockville, MD: U. S. Department of Health and Human Services.
Abbreviations: IV, intravenous; IM, intramuscular.

pain and the person administering placebos, and, of course, placebos have no true analgesic action, so the person remains in pain. Although there have been reports of postoperative pain relief as a result of placebo administration,[9,12] it appears that numerous factors influence that response, among them the client's attitude (a positive outlook increases the likelihood of a positive placebo response) and social and cultural expectations.[39] The best approach in facilitating pain relief is to intervene with methods that are effective. Placebos are not usually effective and therefore are best reserved for research or for psychogenic pain.

PHARMACOLOGIC MANAGEMENT OF CANCER PAIN

The client with cancer pain requires a more aggressive pharmacologic approach than does the client with noncancer pain. When the source of pain is known to be a tumor or metastasis, the World Health Organization ladder is usually implemented, with no great concern for addiction to opioids, in light of the client's often escalating pain and abbreviated life expectancy.[92] Side effects of the opioids are treated aggressively as well, most notably, nausea and constipation. The ladder in Figure 40–6 suggests pharmacologic management based on the severity of cancer pain.

Mild pain is usually managed with a NSAID such as ibuprofen. Moderate pain requires stronger medication, and when the pain becomes severe, the most effective analgesics are those that are long acting, such as sustained-release morphine or methadone. Even with these potent opioids, breakthrough pain sometimes occurs. **Breakthrough pain** is felt between the dosing intervals of a person's long-acting analgesic. Breakthrough pain often occurs as a result of overactivity. For this pain, a shorter acting but potent opioid, such as oxycodone, hydromorphone, or immediate-release morphine, is suggested.

It is important that the **rescue medication** (medication taken for breakthrough pain) not be so weak as to fail to provide relief during this difficult time of pain. For example, a person taking 240 mg of sustained-re-

TABLE 40-3. Opioid Dosing Recommendations*

Opioid Analgesic	Starting Dose for Adults (>50 kg in weight)		Starting Dose for Children (<50 kg in weight)	
	Oral	*Parenteral*	*Oral*	*Parenteral*
Morphine	30 mg q 3–4 hours	10 mg q 3–4 hours	0.3 mg/kg q 3–4 hours	0.1 mg/kg q 3–4 hours
Meperidine (Demerol)	Not recommended	100 mg q 3 hours	Not recommended	0.75 mg/kg q 2–3 hours
Levorphanol (LevoDromoran)	4 mg q 6–8 hours	2 mg q 6–8 hours	0.04 mg/kg q 6–8 hours	0.02 mg/kg q 6–8 hours
Methadone (Dolophine)	20 mg q 6–8 hours	10 mg q 6–8 hours	0.2 mg/kg q 6–8 hours	0.1 mg/kg q 6–8 hours
Oxymorphone (Numorphan)	Not available	1 mg q 3–4 hours	Not recommended	Not recommended
Buprenorphine (Buprenex)	Not available	0.4 mg q 6–8 hours	Not available	0.004 mg/kg q 6–8 hours
Butorphanol (Stadol)	Not available	2 mg q 3–4 hours	Not available	Not recommended
Codeine	60 mg q 3–4 hours	60 mg q 2 hours, IM or SQ route	1 mg/kg q 3–4 hours	Not recommended
Oxycodone	10 mg q 3–4 hours	Not available	0.2 mg/kg q 3–4 hours	Not available
Hydrocodone	10 mg q 3–4 hours	Not available	0.2 mg/kg q 3–4 hours	Not available
Pentazocine (Talwin)	50 mg q 4–6 hours	Not recommended IM, IV	Not recommended	Not recommended

* Data from Agency for Health Care Policy and Research, Public Health Service (1992). *Acute pain management in adults: Operative procedures. Clinical practice guideline, quick reference guide for clinicians* (AHCPR Pub. No. 92-0019). Rockville, MD: U. S. Department of Health and Human Services.

Abbreviations: IM, intramuscular; SQ, subcutaneous; IV, intravenous.

TABLE 40-4. Nonopioid Choices for Pain Control (Partial List of NSAIDs and Dosing Recommendations)*

Oral Medication	Usual Adult Dose	Usual Pediatric Dose	Comments
Aspirin	650–975 mg q 4 hours	10–15 mg/kg q 4 hours	Inhibits platelet aggregation; may cause bleeding; gastric irritation common
Acetaminophen	650–975 mg q 4 hours	10–15 mg/kg q 4 hours	Not a strong antiinflammatory
Ibuprofen (e.g., Motrin)	400 mg q 4–6 hours	10 mg/kg q 4–6 hours	Many brands, also generic; liquid available; less gastric upset than aspirin
Choline magnesium trisalicylate (Trilisate)	1000–1500 mg bid	25 mg/kg bid	Minimal antiplatelet activity; available in liquid form
Ketoprofen (Orudis)	25–75 mg q 6–8 hours	Not usually given	
Naproxen (Naprosyn)	500 mg to start followed by 250 mg q 6–8 hours	5 mg/kg q 12 hours	Available in liquid
Parenteral or oral NSAID: ketorolac tromethamine (Toradol)	30 or 60 mg IM initial dose; then 15 or 30 mg q 6 h if IM, 10 mg q 6 h if oral	Not recommended in very young children; children older than 12 years could use low adult dosages	IV route has been investigated and shown safe; awaits FDA approval; use more than 7 days not recommended (IV route; same dosage as IM)

* Data from Agency for Health Care Policy and Research, Public Health Service (1992). *Acute pain management in adults: Operative procedures. Clinical practice guideline, quick reference guide for clinicians* (AHCPR Pub. No. 92-0019). Rockville, MD: U. S. Department of Health and Human Services.

Abbreviations: NSAID, nonsteroidal antiinflammatory drug; IM, intramuscular; IV, intravenous; FDA, Food and Drug Administration.

Severe pain
(stronger opiates such as
slow release morphine,
hydromorphone,
transdermal fentanyl patch,
and NSAIDs adjuvants as
needed)

Moderate pain
(NSAIDs, weaker opioids
such as Vicodin, Percocet,
Tylenol #3, and adjuvants such
as sleeping medication and
muscle relaxants as needed)

Mild pain
(Weaker NSAIDs, such
as aspirin and acetaminophen)

▲ *Figure 40-6*

World Health Organization Ladder of Cancer Pain Management. In
Cancer Pain Relief (1986). Geneva: World Health Organization.

lease morphine every 8 hours with breakthrough pain
should never be given a Tylenol no. 3 as a rescue
medication. It simply is not strong enough for a person
who is already requiring more than 700 mg of morphine a day. A more appropriate rescue medication
would be immediate-release morphine, 75 mg. People
at home with cancer pain should have frequent assessments by a home health nurse. Ongoing assessment
will assist the client and physician in titrating the
amounts of the primary analgesic, the long-acting
opiate, and the breakthrough medication for the best
possible pain relief.

Psychologic Interventions

Divine is the work of subduing pain.

Hippocrates

Pain may be intensified by anxiety, fear of the unknown, fear of pain, and hopelessness. All these poten-
tiators can be alleviated somewhat through nursing interventions. Anxiety, to be diffused, must be identified
and acted on as early as possible. A person may be
anxious about impending surgery, with fear of disfigurement or fear of death. A poor prognosis can also
create anxiety in a person. Concern about how the
family will cope after one's death is sometimes more
worrisome than death itself. Clients with chronic pain
may feel anxious about their job, finances, sexual dysfunctions, and major changes in self-image. It is not
possible to alleviate all these anxieties in everyone with
pain, but we can recognize them and take action to do
what is possible to reduce the anxiety. We may not
relieve the pain, but we might reduce the suffering a
person is experiencing.

Spending time listening to a person with psychologic
problems can be helpful, but on occasion a profes-

APPLYING RESEARCH TO NURSING PRACTICE

Using Psychologic Preparation to Alleviate the Pain of Chest Tube Removal

Gift, A.G., Bolgiano, C.S., & Cunningham, J. (1991). Sensations during
chest tube removal. *Heart & Lung, 20,* 131–137.

▼ ▼ ▼

Your client's chest tube will be removed this morning. How will
you prepare the client for the procedure? What words will you
use to describe the sensations most likely to occur? Although
information that you and your colleagues will provide is important for promoting a favorable outcome, research-based literature on this subject is sparse. Gift and colleagues studied the
sensations that 36 clients experienced during and after chest
tube removal following thoracic surgery. Thirty-three per cent
of the clients reported a "burning" sensation, whereas 29 per
cent described the sensation as "painful" or "hurting." Approximately 20 per cent stated that chest tube removal felt like
"pulling or yanking," and 14 per cent described the sensation
as "pressure." After chest tube removal, few clients reported
any sensation, although 14 per cent complained of soreness.
Although you might expect that administration of analgesic
medication before chest tube removal would lessen the intensity of sensations experienced, analgesia did not diminish the
intensity of discomfort. However, the researchers did not study
the amount of analgesia given or the waiting period after analgesic administration before chest tube removal. In addition,
this study did not measure the levels of client anxiety before
chest tube removal.

Applications for Practice. This study gives several descriptive words reported by clients who experienced chest tube
removal. In practice, use these words in preparing your clients
for chest tube removal. Although this study suggests that analgesia may not be effective for preventing the burning sensation most often reported, keep in mind that opiate analgesia
may alleviate clients' anxiety about pain during tube removal.

sional evaluation or intervention by a psychologist or
psychiatrist is necessary. If you recognize a person's
anxieties as being beyond the scope of the current
nursing and medical staff, it is best to facilitate a referral to an appropriate specialist. You can intervene,
however, if the person has a fear or anxiety that is
within your expertise to discuss. For example, a person
afraid of postoperative pain because of a negative past
experience may need to ventilate those fears and hear
your reassurance that pain medication will be offered
frequently and that providing pain relief will be one of
your goals.

Spiritual care may be requested by a person in pain
who has cancer or another life-threatening condition. A
physician's order is not required to contact a priest,
rabbi, or pastor on behalf of the client. Many people
find spiritual intervention a great comfort. This aspect
of a person's health (or illness) should never be overlooked. Do not assume that a person will ask for the

clergy in all situations. Often the person is afraid to admit a need for spiritual attention, fearing that it is an admission of weakness or a fear of death. You can discreetly offer clients the opportunity to speak with a representative of their faith, or, if they have no religious preference, perhaps they would want to know more about a particular faith. Spiritual care may not seem directly related to pain relief, but many times pain is more than a physiologic occurrence. The spiritual and emotional health of a person affects the response to pain. Sometimes nurses are the only care providers who recognize this connection. If all you do is provide a quiet private place for the person to talk with a loved one or a pastor, you may have accomplished more than any pill could do in facilitating relief of pain.

Individuals' trust and confidence in you will greatly influence your effectiveness in relieving pain.

Nonpharmacologic Interventions Directed by the Client

Nonpharmacologic nursing interventions are often the most satisfying for both nurse and client. Some interventions are performed directly by the nurse, whereas others can be taught to the clients in pain and to family members. They are noninvasive, inexpensive, and simple to perform. These common nonpharmacologic interventions can be used for any person suffering from acute or chronic pain.

The successful use of these methods may not eliminate all the person's pain, but these interventions can act as an adjunct to other pain relief measures, such as analgesics. It is important not to promise complete pain relief with these strategies or to lead the client to believe that they are all you have to offer. If the pain is severe, these techniques may help pass the time and alleviate the pain somewhat while medication is being prepared or ordered. The techniques suggested usually alleviate pain to some degree and almost always improve the nurse-client relationship because they demonstrate your caring attitude.

CUTANEOUS STIMULATION

Massage, back rub, and applications of heat, cold, or ice are all worthwhile palliative measures to use for pain. Massage is contraindicated if the person has suspected thrombosis of the veins. The application of heat, cold, or ice may require a physician's order. The site of pain may not be amenable to the application of an ice bag, for example, but applying it "between the pain and the brain" or at a point distal to the pain is often beneficial as well.[73]

Heat can relieve pain by increasing blood flow to an area of inflammation or infection (i.e., thrombophlebitis). Heat can also reduce joint stiffness, relax smooth muscle, and reduce peristalsis. Abdominal pain often responds favorably to a heating pad, and a painful infiltrated intravenous site responds to heat or cold.

The application of cold to relieve pain has been practiced for centuries, yet we are just beginning to understand the mechanism of action in providing pain relief. Often the cold application is able to penetrate the muscles; thus, it can reduce muscle spasm and inflammation. Cold also prevents bleeding and edema through vasoconstriction. Although not the primary treatment for pain, cold compresses have been shown effective in reducing pain after orthopedic surgery.[23] Initially, cold compresses may be painful, but the area may become "numb," and pain relief can be long lasting. The effect of a cold compress lasts longer than that of a hot compress because it takes longer to heat up a cooled muscle as a result of the insulating layer of fat above the muscle.

Cold can relieve pain at a site distant from the point of application. For example, if you have a sore finger, cold applied to the wrist can relieve the sensation of pain in the finger because the cold contacts a superficial nerve coming from the painful area or the cold could be on an acupuncture point. Suggested cold packs are those in plastic containers (e.g., a plastic bag, a damp cloth placed in a freezer for a short time, a frozen bag of peas or corn that can be refrozen for reuse [but not eaten!], or a commercially purchased "instant ice" bag composed of a chemical activated by punching it with the fist). See Chapter 48 for more information on the application of heat and cold.

DISTRACTION

The purpose of distraction is to encourage the person in pain to focus on a particular image or stimulus other than the painful one. Examples used by children and adults are television, music,[40] and verbal distraction games or repetitions (e.g., counting, describing objects). This technique is more effective with mild pain than severe pain but has been used in conjunction with opioid medications to enhance pain relief. Distraction can not only decrease one's perception of pain but also can improve one's mood while giving a sense of control over the painful situation.

Teaching a person to use distraction can be accomplished in a few moments. Suggest this strategy to your client if you anticipate that the pain will be very brief (e.g., removing tape from skin) or believe distraction in conjunction with medication or other interventions can improve the pain relief for your client. The person in pain will need to be able to focus attention on something and be able to listen to you describe or suggest distraction techniques. Singing is one of the easiest distractors; whether it be Christmas carols or rock and roll music, the person can hum, whistle, or sing and even tap out the rhythm, which encourages greater concentration. The most effective distraction techniques are those that are interesting to the person in pain and that stimulate the senses. Hearing, seeing, touching, tasting, and moving activities are all useful.

While you are teaching or coaching people through distraction during a painful event, offer praise for the efforts, whether it seems to be effective or not. If someone has trouble concentrating enough to sing a song, regulated breathing may be an alternate form of distraction worth trying. The person is spoken to in a soft voice, reminded to listen and focus on breathing and hearing the air swooshing in and out of the lungs. About 9 to 12 breaths a minute is slow enough for an adult; 12 to 18 breaths a minute for a child is appropriate.

If the person has difficulty creating distraction despite your coaching, consider recorded music with earphones. The person is not required to make the music but can focus on it while tapping out the rhythm with hands or feet. Encourage the tapping out of the rhythm because this distances the person from the pain by actively doing something not at all related to the pain. Arrangements can be made with family members to bring in the person's favorite music.

Develop skill in facilitating pain relief. Your confidence helps those receiving care feel more relaxed and confident in you.

IMAGERY

People experiencing chronic pain often use imagery to displace their pain with positive images of places and things they enjoy. Nurses have taught this technique to postoperative clients and found it effective.[26] You may need to assist clients at first in reaching into their imagination to remove themselves from painful events. If they have never performed this technique before, give examples of how guided imagery is accomplished. Provide one of your own favorite images, such as a summer vacation in Hawaii or a sunset over the mountains you saw last week. You might ask them to describe their favorite vacation, encouraging details and helping them "see" themselves in that place. It must be clear that the imagery is not expected to remove all the pain but that it may help them relax, it may be a significant distraction, and thinking pleasant thoughts may be a mood elevator!

Imagery can be religious or spiritual in nature. If a person knows the Bible, for example, the 23rd Psalm may be recited, imagining that the person is walking through a beautiful field holding God's healing hand. The imagery strategy works best if it is initiated or at least designed by the person in pain; people should not be forced to imagine something they are not interested or motivated in pursuing. One way to ensure that you are not guiding people against their will is to use suggestions rather than directives. "Perhaps you see yourself in . . ." or "Maybe you'd like to imagine being . . ." Once you receive some feedback, you will be able to assist the person in obtaining the desired image and can assure the person that it is possible to call up that image again in any future painful moments and that the image will distract him or her from the pain at least momentarily.

If you find clients who value imagery as a pain-relieving technique, you will want to furnish them with additional information. Numerous audiotapes and written guidelines are available for health care professionals and lay people.[13,29]

RELAXATION TECHNIQUES

Relaxation is the antithesis of anxiety. A person in pain who becomes less anxious may perceive less pain. The relaxation techniques are active rather than the "rest and relaxation" we sometimes think of doing after a long day at school or at work. Specific strategies can be taught to people by audiotapes or videotapes or by someone familiar with the technique. The goal is to lessen tension and anxiety and provide distraction from pain. Progressive muscle relaxation is used often by people who have enough time to identify specific muscles in the body and consciously make them relax. This technique may take up to 1 hour to complete and, by the experienced client, may appear to be a form of self-hypnosis.

A less involved method of relaxing certain parts of the body can be used in any setting by adults and children. Examples of relaxation techniques are jaw relaxation; slow, rhythmic breathing; meditative relaxation; and massage. As with imagery, helpful tapes and publications can provide the client with further training to perform relaxation techniques independently.[13,73] Children who undergo repeated painful procedures secondary to cancer can particularly benefit from relaxation techniques. Specific guidelines in performing or assisting the client in progressive muscle relaxation are described in McCaffery's[73] book *Pain: Clinical Manual for Nursing Practice.*

REASSURANCE

Provide reassurance to people in pain. They need to be reminded that everything possible will be done to prevent pain and to lessen it when it does occur. Help people understand that they are not completely helpless as far as their pain is concerned. They can do a variety of things to alleviate their pain, such as splinting an incision when coughing or using progressive relaxation. Even if pain cannot be completely relieved, you can provide or help the family provide comfort measures such as back rubs, repositioning, listening, and providing privacy and quiet. You can also teach nonpharmacologic strategies to improve a person's situation.

Help people with pain gain some sense of control over their situations.

The Team Approach

A combination of noninvasive methods and pharmacologic management is usually the most beneficial approach in facilitating pain relief. Additionally, pain relief is most effective when viewed as a team approach. Nurses, physicians, social workers, and pharmacists coordinate their efforts to provide the best approach for a particular pain situation. In some instances, analgesics are withheld until a diagnosis is established, because the opioids have a tendency to mask or confuse a diagnosis. If analgesics are to be withheld, all team members must be informed of the rationale. Possible alternative pain relief strategies should be used promptly in the interim. A growing number of acute care facilities have pain management services, usually from within the department of anesthesia. A designated physician with training in acute pain management, accompanied by a clinical nurse specialist and often a pharmacist, sees all the people who need pain management after surgery.[88]

Some hospitals and medical centers have developed specialty clinics or centers for control of chronic pain. They may be psychologically based, with a core staff of psychologists, psychiatrists, and psychiatric nurses; neurologically based, with neurologists and neurosurgeons as the primary physicians; or anesthesia based, with an anesthesiologist specializing in pain assisted by other team members in a variety of fields. Probably the most comprehensive approach in dealing with chronic pain is through a multidisciplinary pain center. In this type of program, physicians from a variety of specialty backgrounds work alongside nurses with special pain training, physical therapists, occupational therapists, psychologists, and pharmacists. Together, they formulate a comprehensive plan individualized to each person who enters the center for treatment.[53] One of the few drawbacks to this type of program is the cost, which is substantial. Some insurance companies do not recognize pain management centers, whether inpatient or outpatient, to be necessary and fail to cover any costs.

Physical Interventions

Whenever possible, prevent pain-producing situations, such as

▶ local irritation or inflammation
▶ muscle spasm or muscle strain
▶ interference with local blood supply or venous and lymphatic drainage
▶ distention of hollow visceral organs

Assess each person for painful complications such as infection, thrombophlebitis, pressure ulcers, contractures, muscle strain, spasm, pulmonary congestion, impaired circulation, bladder and bowel distention, and other painful conditions (Chapter 35 discusses prevention of complications of immobility.) Prevent further damage to injured tissue. Do not drag linens over wounds or forcefully pull anything off wounds. For example, soak off adhering dressings rather than pulling them off. Do not apply irritating substances to open wounds. Protective dressings may prevent further pain. See Chapter 48 for more information on the treatment of wounds. To prevent pain or complications from drainage tubes, periodically check them to be certain they are not caught, stretched, or pulled. Be sure they are patent and securely in place.

Fatigue can lower a person's tolerance for pain. Plan rest periods throughout the day, and facilitate a good night's sleep. Repositioning a person in pain, providing quiet, and administering an ordered sleeping medication can be helpful interventions.

Elevation of a swollen part uses the force of gravity to increase venous return and reduce painful extremity swelling. Elevate edematous and casted limbs. In-

creased tissue fluid can be quite painful. Elevation promotes the drainage of fluid through lymph channels and reduces fluid production in the area of inflammation. A position of semiflexion reduces the pains of joint disorders in which increased pressure in the joint cavity increases pain (e.g., arthritis). When a joint is partly flexed, the capacity of the joint cavities is greatest. Thus, the pressure of synovial fluid in the joint is minimal.

Plan pain-producing activities such as dressing changes when analgesics have been recently administered and are at their peak of effectiveness. It is helpful for nurses on all shifts to know what procedure works best for a person's pain. You can ensure the most effective and least painful procedures for the person in pain by documenting the effectiveness of your approach.

Use pillows, braces, or splints to support painful body parts during movement to help prevent or reduce pain. You can also splint an area with your hands during movement. For example, during movements or deep-breathing exercises, splint painful incisions with hands, a folded towel, or a pillow that has been doubled over.

Massage can relieve muscle tension that causes or potentiates pain. Massage increases blood flow to the area and can be quite beneficial, although certain med-

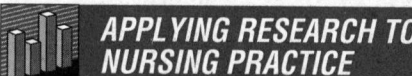

APPLYING RESEARCH TO NURSING PRACTICE

Using Swedish Massage to Relieve Cancer Pain

Weinrich, S.P., & Weinrich, M.C. (1990). The effect of massage on pain in cancer patients. *Applied Nursing Research*, 3(4), 140–145.

▼ ▼ ▼

Nurses have long recognized that analgesics do not always relieve cancer pain. For that reason, they have explored nonanalgesic alternatives for relieving cancer pain. Following in that tradition, Weinrich and Weinrich sought to evaluate the effectiveness of a 10-minute Swedish massage in decreasing cancer pain in hospitalized clients. In this study, 14 hospitalized clients with cancer pain received a Swedish massage, a type of massage based on a system of therapeutic massage and exercise for the muscles and joints, developed in Sweden in the 19th century. Fourteen other clients, serving as controls, participated in a 10-minute conversation with the researchers but received no Swedish massage. None of these clients reported significant pain relief with use of medications. Of the clients receiving Swedish massage, male clients reported high levels of pain before the massage and a significant decrease in pain immediately after the massage. The effects of massage were short term but statistically significant. Female clients, in contrast, reported pain as being less severe than that of the male clients before receiving the massage and no pain relief after the massage.

Applications for Practice. When your assessment of clients with cancer reveals pain unrelieved by medications, consider the suitability of Swedish massage, especially for male clients.

ical situations, such as deep vein thrombosis in which you would not want to dislodge a thrombus, may preclude you from performing a massage. Any person who lies in bed for a period of time is at risk for the development of blood clots in the legs, which you would not want to dislodge. Never massage the calf of the leg. Blood clots may form in that area, and massage could break them loose, possibly causing death.

Giving people information about procedures and the sensations they may experience during them reduces their anticipatory distress. Describing the sensations the person will experience during a procedure allays fears more than merely describing the procedure itself.

Patient-controlled Analgesia

Patients often feel a loss of control during hospitalization. They are told when to eat, when to bathe, and when to ambulate. The timing of medication for pain has traditionally been the responsibility of the physician and the nurse. **Patient-controlled analgesia (PCA)** is a method of pain control that allows the person in pain to self-administer analgesics at frequent, fixed intervals, usually by the intravenous route but sometimes by the subcutaneous, epidural, or oral routes. PCA provides safe and effective analgesia, with the client in control.

In contrast to conventional analgesia, administered prn by the nurse, PCA provides an analgesic the instant the person calls for it. The pain cycle in Figure 40-5 describes the waiting aspect of conventional analgesia. Another drawback to conventional prn dosing is that the person in pain is frequently sedated as a result of the intermittent intramuscular injection. The drug must be injected in enough quantity to provide analgesia for 3 to 4 hours, which unfortunately often produces sedation. The result is a person who swings from pain to sedation because of intermittent bolus dosing. These changes have been described as the peaks and troughs of conventional analgesia. In comparison, as Figure 40-7 illustrates, PCA therapy is given in small, frequent increments, allowing a constant serum level to be maintained and resulting in a more alert, comfortable client.[35]

Increasingly powerful and sophisticated PCA devices have made this modality attractive in cancer pain as well as in postoperative pain and acute medical pain. A computerized machine is connected to the client's intravenous catheter (see Fig. 40-8). The PCA device contains a vial of morphine (or meperidine or another opioid medication). The device is programmed to deliver a set amount of analgesic through the intravenous catheter whenever the client pushes a button. A programmed lock-out interval also "locks out" the person from receiving too much medication in a given time. A typical delay, or lock-out interval, is 8 to 10 minutes. During this time, no matter how often the button is pushed, the device will not deliver medication. The device may also be programmed to infuse a continuous infusion, sometimes referred to as a "basal rate." Continuous infusion is particularly helpful for the person who awakens in the night in pain because of not having used PCA for a period of time. People who have used PCA are overwhelmingly in favor of this therapy for control of acute pain.[54]

PCA has been used effectively in postoperative pain, in cancer pain, and with children.[49] Even the elderly have preferred PCA to intramuscular injections.[31] Devices range in size and capability from a 6-oz "watch" (Baxter Daywatch) to a 4-lb portable device (Abbott Pain Management Provider) to a 17-lb semiportable device with a 36-hour memory and optional printer (Abbott Lifecare Plus). In most settings, PCA is slightly more expensive than conventionally delivered analgesia, but it is most often superior in facilitating relief from pain.

Epidural Analgesia

Since the discovery of morphine action in the spinal cord in the 1970s, effective pain management by means of intraspinal opioids has been used. "Intra-

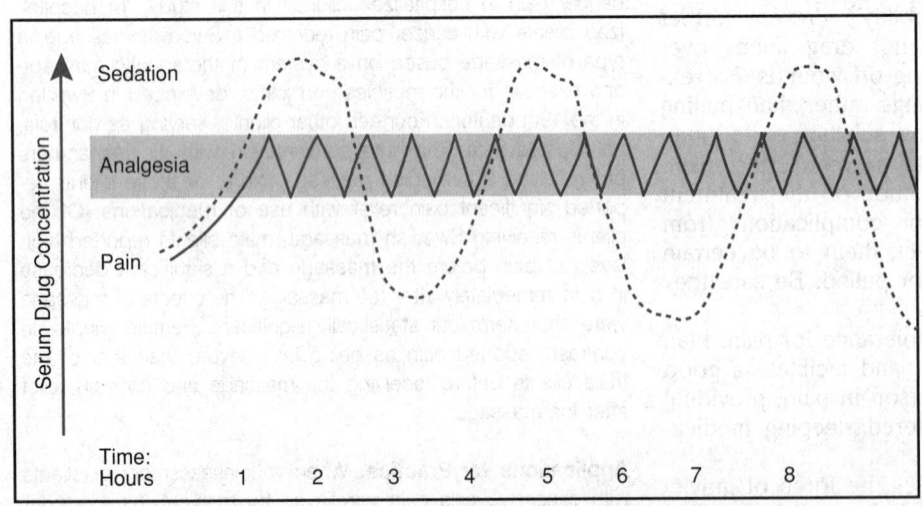

▲ **Figure 40-7**

Conventional analgesia vs patient-controlled analgesia (PCA). Frequent intermittent bolus doses, self-administered I.V., avoid the peaks and troughs of conventional analgesia delivered in intramuscular injections every 3 or 4 hours. A steady-state serum level is achieved, providing more consistent pain relief.

KEY

IM Bolus ············   PCA /\/\/\/\   Optimal Serum Concentration

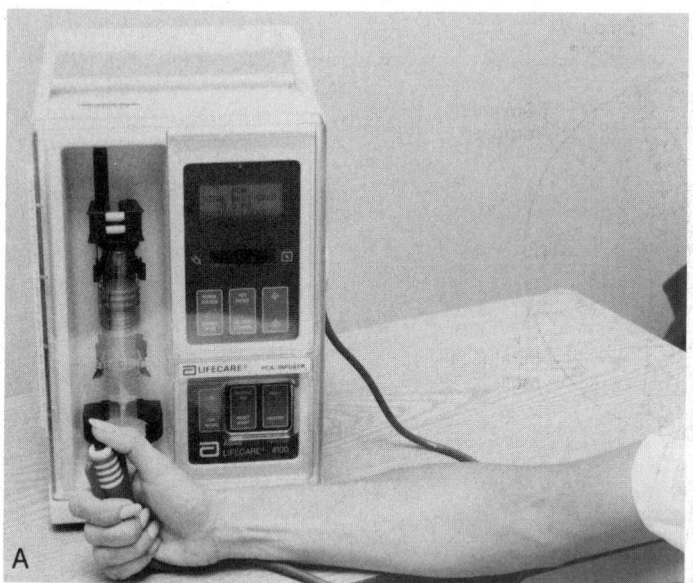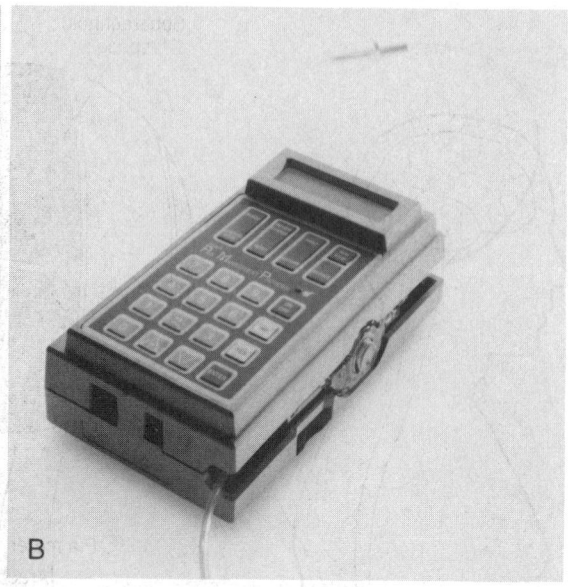

▲ *Figure 40–8*

Patient-controlled analgesia devices. A, The Abbott Lifecare Plus Infuser. B, The Abbott Pain Management Provider (B, Courtesy of Abbott Laboratories, Abbott Park, IL).

spinal" refers to both the epidural space and the subarachnoid space. The **epidural space** lies outside a dural sheath, or protective layer of tissue, surrounding the subarachnoid space. The **subarachnoid space** lies directly outside of the pia mater. This space contains cerebrospinal fluid and many opiate receptors. Drugs may be infused into either the epidural space or the subarachnoid space (Fig. 40–9), but for clients in acute pain the epidural technique is most often used.

Epidural analgesia is growing in popularity for the management of moderate to severe postoperative pain either by constant infusion or by intermittent bolus. Only a small amount of drug is necessary to achieve adequate pain control, because it is absorbed into the cerebrospinal fluid and bound to opiate receptors without first going into the plasma. This treatment regimen is usually reserved for those situations in which multiple trauma or major surgery has left the person with severe pain in which relief would be beyond the capacity of PCA.[44]

Nursing management of epidural analgesia is straightforward and founded in the basic assessment techniques that are used for anyone receiving potent analgesics for the relief of pain. The most common side effects are pruritus and nausea. These are readily treated with antipruritics and antiemetics.[99] If reasonable infusion rates of opioids are used, sedation rarely occurs. If sedation does occur, naloxone, 0.1 to 0.4 mg by IV push, reverses the effects of the opioid almost instantaneously.

The site of catheter insertion is usually the lumbar region of the spine. This area is covered with a sterile dressing, and the catheter is taped up the back or around the side, where it connects with the infusion tubing (or is capped for intermittent bolusing). The epidural catheter is marked with solid blue lines at 5-cm increments near the tip of the catheter. By examining the catheter on a daily basis, the nurse and physi-

cian are able to determine whether the catheter has slipped out of the epidural space. For example, at the time of placement the catheter may be at 11 cm at the skin. If after 2 days the catheter is only 7 cm at the skin and the client is complaining of increased pain, it is most likely due to the catheter withdrawing from the epidural space. If the catheter is dressed carefully with a sterile covering, movement of the catheter is unlikely to occur.

Rarely, the catheter comes out of the back entirely or migrates into the subarachnoid space. Both these untoward events are serious. If the catheter tip moves out of the epidural space, the person experiences increased pain and the therapy becomes completely ineffective. If the catheter tip migrates into the subarachnoid space, which contains the cerebrospinal fluid, the person becomes excessively sedated. Drug dosing in the subarachnoid space need only be one tenth of that in the epidural space.

You can help circumvent these problems by inspecting the catheter site and dressing as soon as you begin care of the client and calling the physician as necessary.

Sedation, if it occurs, necessitates prompt administration of oxygen, cessation of the epidural opioid at least temporarily, and possibly the administration of naloxone (Narcan) to reverse the effect of the opioid. Persons who are excessively sedated may have depressed respirations. Respiratory rate, however, should not be the only consideration in assessing sedation. Excessive sedation is not to be confused with respiratory depression. A depressed respiratory rate of 10 or 8 may be adequate if the person is exchanging oxygen and carbon dioxide sufficiently through deep ventilations. In contrast, a respiratory rate of 14 may be inad-

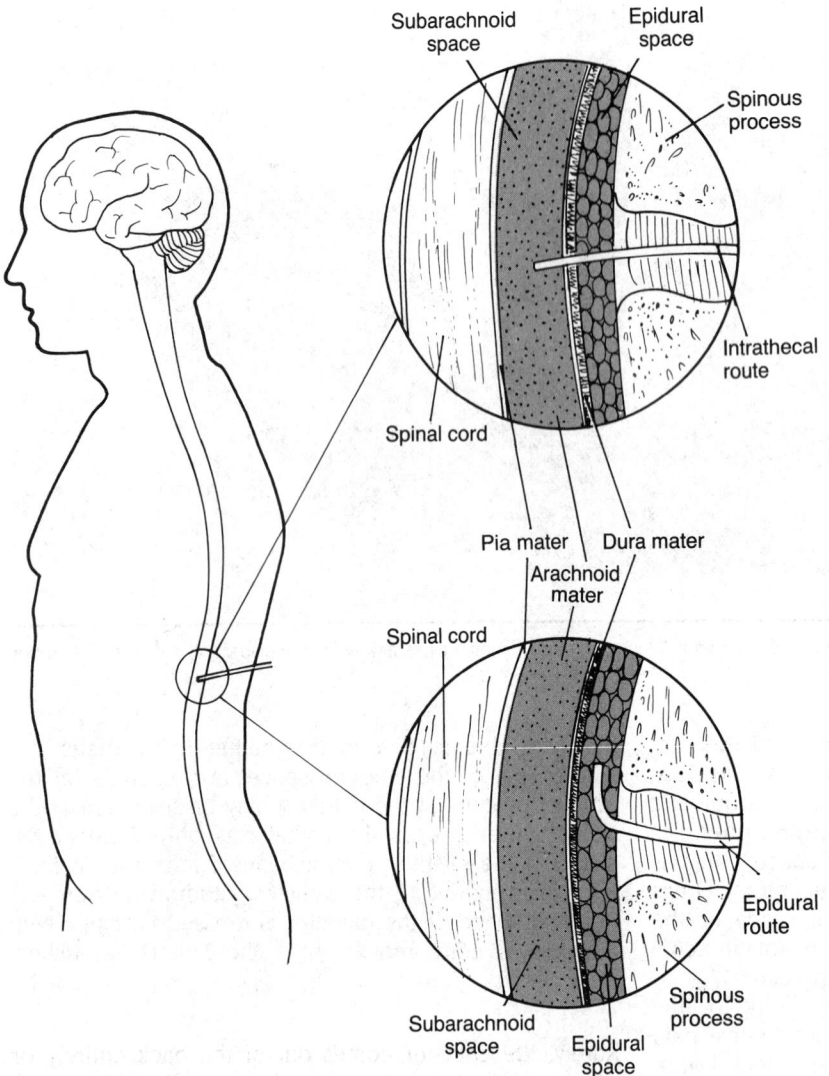

Pia mater \ Dura mater
Arachnoid
mater

▲ Figure 40-9

Epidural Anatomy and Catheter Placement. Note the distance between the epidural space and the spinal cord. The spinal cord ends at the thoracic 12-lumbar 1-vertebral level. Below this level, inadvertent puncture of the subarachnoid space does not risk injury to the spinal cord.

equate to exchange oxygen and carbon dioxide if the volume of each breath is very small. Scales have been developed to assist in determining the level of sedation without being misled by a respiratory rate alone. For example,

▶ 0 = awake, no sedation
▶ 1 = drowsy, easily aroused
▶ 2 = difficult to arouse
▶ 3 = unarousable
▶ S = normal sleep

Sedation scales are used for a number of pain treatment modalities including PCA and epidural analgesia. People with cancer pain often have respiratory rates of 10 or below while they are not excessively sedated. In this population, it is particularly helpful to use the scale.

Patient-controlled epidural analgesia (PCEA) is being researched in some areas of the United States and has become common practice in a few medical centers around the country. The self-administration aspect of PCA combined with the excellent analgesia available with epidural analgesia led clinicians to combine these

therapies. One study at the University of Kentucky Medical Center reported a high degree of clinical efficacy and safety in more than 4000 persons recovering from a variety of surgical procedures. Advantages over traditional epidural opiate infusions are that (1) the client is able to self-adjust medication, (2) the client experiences increased satisfaction (3) the client experiences decreased anxiety, and (4) there is a reduced opioid requirement.[104] The major drawback to this technique is that morphine, the most commonly used epidural opiate, has a somewhat delayed onset time (30 to 60 minutes) when administered into the epidural space because of its water solubility (the epidural space is very lipid rich, so lipid-soluble drugs diffuse much more rapidly). Drugs such as fentanyl or sufentanil are highly lipid soluble and are more appropriate for PCEA. These drugs are also extremely potent and prone to systemic absorption, so they must be used with caution.[94] When more research on the safety and efficacy of PCEA is available, PCEA will probably assume a more important role in acute postoperative pain management.

Transcutaneous Electrical Nerve Stimulation

Transcutaneous electrical nerve stimulation, or TENS, therapy is based on techniques that have been in use for centuries. Since the 1700s, electrotherapy has been used in medicine, but new-found interest in TENS came about with the 1965 publication of Melzack and Wall's gate control theory. Electrical stimulation has been studied in conjunction with exercise for the relief of back pain[28] and phantom limb pain[64] and has been an effective treatment for acute postoperative pain.[46] The pain of childbirth as well as cancer has also been found to respond well to TENS therapy.[38,95]

In the mechanism of TENS therapy, a battery-powered electrical pulse generator is connected to two electrodes (see Fig. 40–10). It sends an electrical current between the electrodes, which are placed on the skin on either side of the injured body part. This minor electrical charge activates large diameter (A beta) pain fibers that send a "pain message" to the spinal cord, although it feels to the person wearing the device merely like a vibration. The fibers activated by TENS tend to override the other pain fibers (from the injured site), thus diminishing the person's perception of pain. It has been suggested that the mechanism of action of TENS demonstrates the gate control theory of pain in that A fibers activated appear to inhibit the transmission of C fibers because of a closing of the "gate" in the dorsal horn of the spinal cord.

Obvious benefits of this therapy are that it is noninvasive and relatively inexpensive and it may lessen the need for opioid analgesics in acute and chronic pain. Its only side effects appear to be local skin irritation experienced in some people after several days with electrodes located in the same position on the skin.

It is also possible to stimulate peripheral nerves through subcutaneously implanted electrodes connected to an external control box. An even more invasive form of peripheral nerve stimulation requires the surgical implantation of the electrodes directly on the nerves causing pain. These methods are used less frequently because of the risk of further injuring the nerves, but they are plausible alternatives to opioid therapy for nonmalignant pain.

Alternative Routes of Opioid Therapy

The ability to change the route of administration of an analgesic when necessary is always advantageous. Of the 20 per cent of clients with cancer who require a change in route of therapy,[25] many can effectively be switched from oral to intravenous morphine. However, at times the intravenous route is inadvisable. It is associated with a high risk of infection; people tend to acquire a tolerance to opioids administered in this manner, and substantial monitoring is required. The rectal route has been in use for some time, but rectal irritation or bleeding may minimize its desirability.

There are several alternatives to intravenous, oral, or rectal administration of analgesics. One alternative is the transdermal fentanyl patch (Duragesic), a four-layered laminate on a protective liner that adheres to the skin. The fentanyl is contained in a drug reservoir next to the skin and is continuously released for 72 hours (Fig. 40–11). In persons with cancer or with acquired immune deficiency syndrome, this method has shown promise because of its ease of administration and apparent success.[19] For acute postoperative pain, it has shown some side effects (nausea and skin irritation) but has also been effective.[18]

Sublingual and transmucosal opioids are being studied for pediatric use. Of particular interest to researchers is the fentanyl "lollipop." The lollipop actually delivers a transmucosal dose of the fentanyl citrate under the investigatory name OTFC (oral transmucosal fentanyl citrate). It holds great promise as a premedication for painful procedures or surgery.[106] In Seattle, investigators found transmucosal midazolam as a prein-

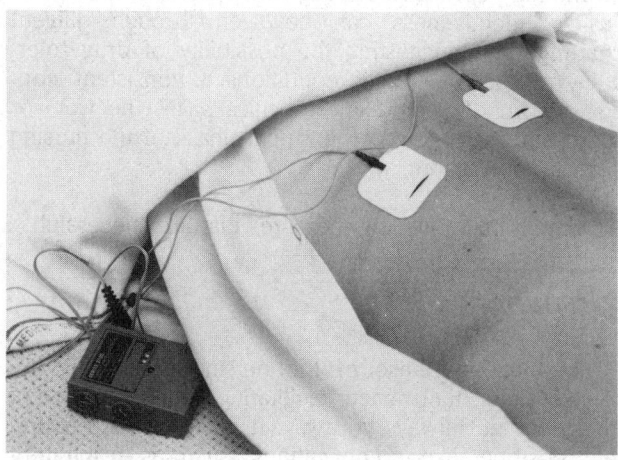

▲ Figure 40–10

Transcutaneous electrical nerve stimulator (TENS) applied to the lower back for pain relief.

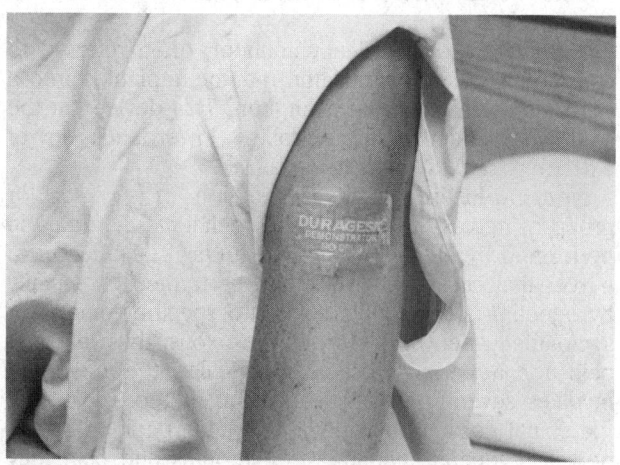

▲ Figure 40–11

Transdermal fentanyl patch (Duragesic, by Janssen Pharmaceuticals).

duction agent in pediatrics to be as effective as the nasal route and more readily accepted by children.[63]

A relatively new and effective treatment for chronic pain is the implantation of a spinal catheter into the subarachnoid space or epidural space and the constant infusion of an opioid through a reservoir implanted somewhere in the body cavity. This type of system is completely enclosed within the body. The nurse or physician refills the reservoir percutaneously (through the skin with a needle). In this manner, many different medications can be administered; chemotherapeutic agents, opioids, regional anesthetics, or insulin. It is especially useful for cancer pain when other routes are unavailable and the client has a life expectancy of a year or more. Because a spinal catheter is completely contained within the body, caring for it is relatively easy, and people with cancer pain often report an improvement in their quality of life as a result of the device.[83] Side effects are similar to those for epidural analgesia. In addition, problems with the indwelling catheter becoming kinked or the reservoir malfunctioning may need to be addressed, although in most cases the spinal catheter has been shown to be very safe for clients experiencing chronic pain.[101] The Synchromed, manufactured by Medtronic Corporation, is a computerized reservoir that receives programming messages from an external computer that can change the flow rate, direct boluses at certain times of day, and obtain information regarding what medication is used and how much is left in the reservoir.[71]

A profound increase in analgesia sometimes occurs when routes of opioid administration are changed. If one route proves ineffective, it is often well worth the effort to institute one of these techniques because they are of relatively low risk and may show surprising benefit to a person in chronic pain.[77]

Other Pain-Relieving Techniques

Biofeedback is a noninvasive technique that has shown some promise in lessening chronic pain,[10] but it requires extensive education, equipment, and practice to initiate therapy. Biofeedback techniques are covered in Chapter 16.

A spinal cord electrical stimulator, often referred to as a dorsal column stimulator, may be implanted into a person's spinal canal by a surgeon. This device can be somewhat effective in controlling lower back, lower extremity, or postamputation pain.[72]

Neuroablation is the destruction of a nerve or group of nerves. It is an invasive technique that may be performed by either chemical or surgical destruction of nerves that cause pain. It can be performed chemically by injecting alcohol or phenol into specific somatic or sympathetic nerves to destroy the axons, thus relieving pain for a period of time. Surgically, the treatment involves severing the nerves at one or more levels of the spinal cord.[97] Unfortunately, for the person in pain, nerves regenerate within 1 to 6 months and pain may return with either technique. For cancer pain, however, these rather drastic treatments may be extremely helpful.[107]

When these alternative techniques are contemplated, nurses can teach about them and help reduce anxiety. Anxiety reduction itself can help reduce pain.

Interventions for Children

Many of the treatments used for adults are applicable to children in pain. Children use PCA quite successfully.[100] They can be taught relaxation and imagery techniques, and they respond favorably to many of the independent nursing interventions used for adults. Children have been found occasionally to require enormous amounts of opioid analgesics and to tolerate them without problems and with superb pain relief.[80,81]

Whenever possible, parents should be informed of the interventions being used. If parents appear confident in these pain management strategies, analgesia is often enhanced because the child's anxiety decreases. If parents expect their children to respond to painful procedures like little adults, however (making statements such as "now that didn't hurt much, did it?"), they may make the children feel more stress because they are faced with the unrealistic expectation not to experience pain.[76]

Documentation of Interventions

Document your interventions and save yourself and others time and discomfort in the future. Legally, an intervention not documented may be said not to have occurred. Pain may recur and persist unnecessarily if you forget to chart the details of your interventions (what you did, how you did it, and whether it worked or not). The best overall strategy for providing individualized pain relief is to document what works and report it verbally to colleagues.

Documentation of the person's response to various strategies affords other care givers the benefit of knowing whether a given strategy is likely to succeed in promoting pain relief. A progressive decline in an analgesic's effectiveness can be seen through diligent charting, thus suggesting the possibility of drug tolerance or other pathologic conditions. A consistent, concise record of pain relief strategies paves the way for successful progression to the next phase of the nursing process: evaluation.

Document pain-relieving measures that are successful.

EVALUATION

The evaluation phase of the nursing process is extremely important when facilitating relief from pain. Pain does not always go away. It may, in fact, precipitate postoperative complications, such as respiratory compromise when it prevents deep breathing. Frequent and consistent evaluation of outcomes following pain relief strategies will enable you to change to another strategy promptly, if necessary. If the evaluation phase is omitted from the process, a person could suffer needlessly for several days before someone discovers that the medication was never effective in the first place.

A good approach when evaluating pain relief strategies is to give each strategy one or two tries; then if it is ineffective, change to another strategy. For example, if Demerol, 75 mg administered intramuscularly every 3 hours, does not provide effective pain relief after two doses, as reported in pain scores by the client, discuss alternative analgesics with the physician.

Nonpharmacologic techniques for relieving pain should be evaluated as well. It may be that the application of a cold compress relieves pain in an extremity, whereas a heating pad relieves pain in the lower back.

Evaluation may consist of the simple confirmation that a technique is working to achieve the desired outcome, or it may consist of the complaint of continued pain despite a specific strategy. In either case, readiness to change the approach is at the core of the evaluation phase.

CASE STUDY

The Client

Mrs. Gail Cummings, a 43-year-old obese mother of three, was diagnosed with a uterine fibroid tumor 1 week ago. She underwent removal of the uterus (hysterectomy) yesterday and returned to the floor at 4 PM. At that time, she had in place a nasogastric (NG) tube, urinary catheter, and an intravenous catheter for fluids and antibiotics. Her incision is lower midline abdominal, 10 inches long, approximated with metal staples, and covered with a sterile dressing.

A partial list of the postoperative physicians orders included

▶ turn, encourage to deep breathe every hour
▶ incentive spirometry every hour
▶ monitor intake and output
▶ up to the bathroom with assistance
▶ NPO with NG tube to low, constant suction
▶ dressing change by physician; reinforce prn

At 4 PM yesterday, March 30, a partial list of the postoperative assessment data included the following:

▶ 43-year-old obese pale female, awake, oriented, and moaning

▶ abdominal dressing in place and secure with serosanguineous drainage (approximately the size of a dime) evident on dressing
▶ temperature = 98.8°F (36.7°C); blood pressure = 156/88; pulse = 74; respirations = 22
▶ skin cool and diaphoretic
▶ moves all extremities slowly
▶ unable to turn unassisted secondary to c/o pain
▶ IV infusing dextrose 5% with 1/2 normal saline in left forearm, no signs of infiltration
▶ Foley catheter to gravity drainage, light-yellow urine in tubing
▶ NG to low, constant suction, dark-green liquid draining in tubing
▶ decreased breath sounds heard on lung auscultation
▶ C/o severe abdominal pain at this time

It is now 10:00 AM, March 31. Eighteen hours have passed since Mrs. Cummings returned to her room from surgery. The following represents part of a nursing care plan written for her shortly after her return to the floor.

CARE PLAN

4:30 PM, March 30

Nursing Diagnosis	Planning: Expected Outcomes	Implementation: Nursing Interventions	Evaluation
Pain R/T effects of surgery	By 10:00 AM, March 31: ▶ Verbalizes absence of pain or minimal discomfort ▶ Deep breathes and moves about without signs and symptoms of substantial pain	Assess pain q 1 h using any subjective pain scale (e.g., 0–10 or 0–5). When indicated, administer pain medication, as ordered, at first c/o pain. Plan painful activities during peak action of pain medication: about 45–90 minutes after medication administered.	10:00 AM, March 31: Reports of pain are 2/10 at rest, up to 5/10 on movement, which she states is satisfactory After receipt of pain meds, given at regular intervals, reports having slept well without pain Able to reposition and ambulate without c/o intolerable pain

Care Plan continued on following page

CARE PLAN (Continued)

4:30 PM, March 30

Nursing Diagnosis	Planning: Expected Outcomes	Implementation: Nursing Interventions	Evaluation
		Splint incision with pillow during coughing and moving. Provide assistance and support to prevent straining incision during repositioning. Arrange all tubing before moving client so nothing pulls unexpectedly. Keep all drainage tubes patent to prevent painful obstructions. Document and report effectiveness of pain meds and other pain relief measures.	States spontaneous coughing results in less discomfort when she uses pillow to splint incision
		Encourage client to request pain meds when uncomfortable. Encourage client to use independent pain-relieving techniques (e.g., distraction, muscle relaxation, positive imagery).	

Summary

▶ Pain is an unpleasant sensory and emotional experience, but the recognition of pain is subjective. Only the person experiencing it can truly say what it is.

▶ Acute pain is typically triggered by tissue injury, has a sudden onset, and involves a healing time of fewer than 6 months. Chronic pain is persistent, lasting longer than 6 months without healing. Acute pain and chronic pain may present different symptoms; it is important to distinguish between the two when assessing a person in pain.

▶ Knowledge of pain pathways and pain modulation in the central nervous system (by endogenous opioids such as endorphins and by exogenous opioids such as morphine) is critical nursing knowledge.

▶ Theories of pain transmission help us to understand how we respond to acute and chronic pain and why we sometimes feel more pain than at other times.

▶ The nursing process provides a systematic way of dealing with a person's pain by using a variety of tools for assessment, identifying factors that lead to the nursing diagnosis *Pain*, identifying pertinent outcomes, implementing nonpharmacologic and pharmacologic interventions, and evaluating pain relief and ability to function.

▶ Elderly clients experiencing pain require specific assessment techniques. Their treatment plan must be made by nurses who understand that elderly clients experience the same pain as others. It is a myth that the elderly have less pain than younger clients.

▶ For children in pain, numerous factors affect expression of the pain. Among them are prior experience with pain and hospitalization, parental attitudes, and developmental level.

▶ People from different socioeconomic backgrounds may respond to pain and express pain in a variety of ways.

▶ To enhance pain relief, the nurse should use principles of pharmacologic pain management when formulating intervention strategies. The client with cancer pain requires a more aggressive approach than is true of most other clients.

▶ Specific independent nursing interventions that can help relieve pain include alleviating anxiety as much as possible by interacting with the client and, if necessary, referring the client for psychologic or spiritual care.

▶ The nurse can assist the client in performing pain-relieving techniques such as cutaneous stimulation, distraction, imagery, and relaxation.

▶ Various treatment modalities that require physician and nurse monitoring can be extremely effective in pain management. These include patient-controlled analgesia (PCA), epidural analgesia, transcutaneous electrical nerve stimulation (TENS), alternative routes of opioid therapy, and other techniques. Many of the treatments used for adults are applicable to children in pain.

▶ If the evaluation phase is omitted from the process, the person could suffer needlessly for several days.

Bibliography

1. Agency for Health Care Policy and Research, Public Health Service, (1992). *Acute pain management in adults: Operative procedures. Clinical Practice Guideline, Quick Reference Guide for Clinicians* (AHCPR Pub. No. 92-0019). Rockville, MD: US Department of Health and Human Services.
2. Agency for Health Care Policy and Research, Public Health Service, (1992). *Acute pain management in infants, children, and adolescents: Operative and medical procedures. Clinical practice guideline, quick reference guide for clinicians* (AHCPR Pub. No. 92-0020). Rockville, MD: U.S. Department of Health and Human Services.
3. Agency for Health Care Policy and Research, Public Health Service, (1992). *Acute pain management: Operative or medical procedures and trauma Clinical practice guideline* (AHCPR Pub. No. 92-0032). Rockville, MD: U.S. Department of Health and Human Services.
4. Anand, K.J.S., & Carr, D.B. (1989). The neuroanatomy, neurophysiology, and neurochemistry of pain, stress, and analgesia in newborns and children. *Pediatric Clinics of North America, 36,* 795–822.
5. Arner, S., & Meyerson, B.A. (1988). Lack of analgesic effect of opioids on neuropathic and idiopathic forms of pain. *Pain, 33,* 11–23.
6. Barr, R.G. (1992). Is this infant in pain? Caveats from the clinical setting. *APS Journal, 1*(3), 187–190.
7. Bausbaum, A.I., & Fields, H.L. (1984). Endogenous pain control systems: brain stem spinal pathways and endorphin circuitry. *Annual Review of Neuroscience, 7,* 309–338.
8. Benedetti, D., & Butler, S.H. (1990). Systemic analgesics. In Bonica, J.J. (ed.). *The management of pain* (p. 1653). Philadelphia: Lea & Febiger.
9. Benson, H., & McCallie, D. (1989). Angina pectoris and the placebo effect. *New England Journal of Medicine, 300,* 1424–1429.
10. Blanchard, E.B., & Ahles, T.A. (1990). Biofeedback therapy. In Bonica, J.J. (ed.), *The management of pain* (pp. 1723–1733). Philadelphia: Lea & Febiger.
11. Bonica, J.J. (1990). Biochemistry and modulation of nociception and pain. In Bonica, J.J. (ed.), *The management of pain* (pp. 95–121). Philadelphia: Lea & Febiger.
12. Bourne, H. (1971). The placebo—a poorly understood and neglected therapeutic agent. *Rational Drug Therapy, 5*(11), 1–6.
13. Bresler, D.E. (1979). *Free yourself from pain.* New York: Simon & Schuster.
14. Brietbart, W., & Holland, J. (1990). Psychiatric aspects of cancer pain. In Foley, K., Bonica, J.J., & Ventafridda, V. (eds.). *Advances in pain research and therapy:* Vol. 16. (pp. 73–87). Philadelphia: Lea & Febiger.
15. Brody, H. (1980). *Placebos and the philosophy of medicine.* Chicago: University of Chicago Press.
16. Brown, C.R., et al. (1988). Comparison of intravenous ketorolac tromethamine and morphine sulfate in postoperative pain. *Clinical Pharmacologic Therapy, 43,* 142–145.
17. Bundsen, P., et al. (1982). Pain relief in labor by transcutaneous electrical nerve stimulation. *Acta Obstetricia et Gynecologica Scandinavica, 61*(2), 129–136.
18. Caplan, R.A., et al. (1989). Transdermal fentanyl for postoperative pain management: a double-blind placebo study. *Journal of the American Medical Association, 261,* 1036–1039.
19. Caplan, R.A., & Southam, M. (1990). Transdermal drug delivery and its application to pain control. In Benedetti, C., et al. (eds.). *Advances in pain research and therapy:* Volume 14 (pp. 233–240). New York: Raven Press.
20. Cassli, E.J. (1982). The nature of suffering and the goals of medicine. *New England Journal of Medicine, 306*(11), 639–645.
21. Chapman, C.R., et al. (1985). Pain measurement: an overview. *Pain, 22*(1), 1–31.
22. Chapman, P.J., et al. (1987). Attitudes and knowledge of nursing staff in relation to management of postoperative pain. *Australia and New Zealand Journal of Surgery, 57,* 447–450.
23. Cohen, B.T., et al. (1989). The effects of cold therapy in the postoperative management of pain in patients undergoing anterior cruciate ligament reconstruction. *American Journal of Sports Medicine, 17,* 344–349.
24. Collins, G., & Stone, L.A. (1966). Pain sensitivity, age and activity level in chronic schizophrenics and in normals. *British Journal of Psychiatry, 112,* 33–35.
25. Coyle, N., et al. (1987). *Changing pattern of pain, drug use, and routes of administration in the advanced cancer patient* (abstract). *Pain* (Suppl. 4), S339.
26. Daake, D.R., & Gueldner, S.H. (1989). Imagery instruction and the control of postsurgical pain. *Applied Nursing Research, 2,* 114–314.
27. Descartes, R. (1664). *L'Homme.* Paris: Angot.
28. Deyo, R.A., et al. (1990). A controlled trial of transcutaneous electrical nerve stimulation and exercise for chronic low back pain. *New England Journal of Medicine, 322*(23), 1627–1634.
29. Donovan, M.I. (1980). Relaxation with guided imagery: a useful technique. *Cancer Nursing, 3,* 27–32.
30. Donovan, M.I. (1987). Clinical assessment of cancer pain. In D.B. McGuire, & Yarbro, C.H. (eds.). *Cancer pain management* (pp. 105–132). Orlando, FL: Grune & Stratton.
31. Egbert, A.M., et al. (1990). Randomized trial of postoperative patient controlled analgesia vs. intramuscular narcotics in frail elderly men. *Archives of Internal Medicine, 150,* 1897–1903.
32. Eland, J., & Anderson, J. (1977). The experience of pain in children. In Jacox, J. (ed.). *Pain: A source book for nurses and other health professionals* (pp. 453–473). Boston: Little, Brown.
33. Eland, J.M. (1989). The effectiveness of transcutaneous electrical nerve stimulation (TENS) with children experiencing cancer pain. In Funk, S.G., Tornquist, E.M., Champagne, M.T., Copp, L.S., & Wiese, R.A. (eds.). *Key aspects of comfort: Management of pain, fatigue, and nausea* (pp. 87–100). New York: Springer.
34. Evans, S., et al. (1992). *The effects of intraoperative ketamine on postoperative opioid requirements: a randomized double-blind study.* Research in progress at the University of California San Diego Medical Center.
35. Ferrante, F.M., et al. (1990). *Patient-controlled analgesia.* Boston: Blackwell Scientific.
36. Fields, H.L. (1987). *Pain.* New York: McGraw-Hill.
37. Fisichelli, V.R., et al. (1974). The course of induced crying activity in the first year of life. *Journal of Pediatric Research, 8,* 921–928.
38. Fordyce, W.E. (1976). *Behavioral methods for chronic pain and illness.* St. Louis: C.V. Mosby.
39. Gaupp, L.A., et al. (1989). Adjunctive treatment techniques. In Tollison, C.D. (ed.). *Handbook of chronic pain management* (pp. 174–196). Baltimore: Williams & Wilkins.
40. Glynn, N.J. (1986). The therapy of music. *Journal of Gerontologic Nursing, 12,* 6–10.
41. Goodwin, J., et al. (1979). Knowledge and use of placebos by house officers and nurses. *Annals of Internal Medicine, 91,* 106–110.
42. Graffam, S. (1990). Pain content in the curriculum—a survey. *Nurse Educator, 15,* 20–23.
43. Green, J., & Coyle, M. (1989). Methadone use in the control of nonmalignant chronic pain. *Pain Management,* 241–246.
44. Gregg, R. (1989). Spinal analgesia. *Anesthesiology Clinics of North America, 7*(1), 79–100.
45. Grunau, R.V.E., et al. (1990). Neonatal facial and cry responses to invasive and non-invasive procedures. *Pain, 42,* 295–305.
46. Hargreaves, A., & Lander, J. (1991). Use of transcutaneous electrical nerve stimulation for postoperative pain. *Nursing Research, 38,* 159–161.

47. Harkins, S. W., et al. (1990). Pain and suffering in the elderly. In Bonica, J.J. (ed.). *The management of pain* (pp. 552–562). Philadelphia: Lea & Febiger.

48. Harkins, S.W., et al. (1986). Effect of age on pain perception: thermonociception. *Journal of Gerontology*, 41, 58–63.

49. Harmer, M., et al. (1985). *Patient controlled analgesia.* Oxford, England: Blackwell.

50. Hester, N.O., & Barcus, C.S. (1986). Assessment and management of pain in children. *Pediatrics: Nursing Update*, 1, 2–7.

51. Holm, K., et al. (1989). Effect of personal pain experience on pain assessment. *Image: Journal of Nursing Scholarship*, 21(2), 72–75.

52. Iafrati, N.S. (1986). Pain on the burn unit: patient vs. nurse perceptions. *Journal of Burn Care*, 7(5), 413–416.

53. International Association for the Study of Pain, Task Force on Acute Pain. (1992). *Management of acute pain: A practical guide.* Seattle: IASP Publications.

54. Jackson, D. (1989). A study of pain management: patient controlled analgesia versus intramuscular analgesia. *Journal of Intravenous Nursing*, 12, 42–51.

55. Jaffe, J.H. (1989). Misinformation: euphoria and addiction. In Hill, C.S., & Fields, H. (eds.). *Advances in pain research and therapy:* Vol. 11 (pp. 163–174). New York: Raven Press.

56. Jeans, M.E. (1983). Pain in children: a neglected area. In Firestone, P., et al. (eds.). *Advances in behavioral medicine for children and adolescents* (pp. 23–37). Hillsdale, NJ: Erlbaum.

57. Jensen, T.S., et al. (1985). Immediate and long term phantom limb pain in amputees: incidence, clinical characteristics and relationship to preamputation limb pain. *Pain*, 21, 267–278.

58. Johnston, C.C., & O'Shaugnessy, D. (1987). Acoustical attributes of infant pain cries: discriminating features. Pain (Suppl. 4), S233.

59. Johnston, D.C., & O'Shaughnessy, D. (1988). Acoustical attributes of infant pain cries: discriminating features. In Dubner, R., et al. (eds.). *Pain research and clinical management:* Volume 3 (pp. 336–340). Amsterdam: Elsevier.

60. Jordan-March, M., et al. (1990). Poker chip tool: Spanish instructions. In *The Harbor-UCLA Medical Center humor project for children.* Los Angeles: Harbor-UCLA Medical Center.

61. Kaiko, R.F., et al. (1982). Narcotics in the elderly. *Medical Clinics of North America*, 66, 1079–1089.

62. Kanner, R.M., & Foley, K.M. (1981). Patterns of narcotic drug use in a cancer pain clinic. *Annals of New York Academy of Science*, 362, 161–172.

63. Karl, H.W., et al. (1991, April). *Transmucosal midazolam for preinduction of anesthesia in pediatric patients: comparison of intranasal and sublingual routes.* Poster presented at the Second International Symposium on Pediatric Pain, Montreal, Quebec, Canada.

64. Katz, J., & Melzack, R. (1991). Auricular transcutaneous electrical nerve stimulation (TENS) reduces phantom limb pain. *Journal of Pain and Symptom Management*, 6(2), 73–83.

65. Keele, C.A., & Armstrong, D. (1964). Substances producing pain and itch. In Barcroft, H., et al. (eds.). *Monographs of the Physiological Society.* Vol. 12 (pp. 1–374). London: Edward Arnold.

66. Levine, J.D., & Gordon, N.C. (1982). Pain in prelingual children and its evaluation by pain-induced vocalization. *Pain*, 14, 85–93.

67. Lindsay, P., & Wyckoff, M. (1981). The depression-pain syndrome and its response to antidepressants. *Psychosomatics*, 22, 571.

68. Lollar, D.J., et al. (1982). Assessment of pediatric pain: an empirical perspective. *Journal of Pediatric Psychology*, 7, 267–277.

69. Marks, R.M., & Sachar, E.J. (1973). Undertreatment of medical inpatients with narcotic analgesics. *Annals of Internal Medicine*, 78, 173–181.

70. Max, M.B. (1989). Pain relief and the control of drug abuse: conflicting or complementary goals? In Hill, C.S., & Fields, H. (eds.). *Advances in pain research and therapy*, vol. 3 (pp. 241–246). New York: Raven Press.

71. Medtronic, Inc. (1987). *Clinical summary: The synchromed infusion system cancer pain management.* (Available from Medtronic Inc., 7000 Central Avenue N.E., Minneapolis, MN 55432. Telephone: (800) 328-0810.)

72. Meyerson, B.A. (1983). Electrostimulation procedures: effects, presumed rationale, and possible mechanisms. In Bonica, J.J., Lindblom, U., & Iggo, A. (eds.). *Advances in pain research and therapy*, vol. 5 (pp. 495–534). New York: Raven Press.

73. McCaffery, M., & Beebe, A. (1989). *Pain: Clinical manual for nursing practice.* St. Louis: C. V. Mosby.

74. McCaffery, M., & Ferrell, B. (1991). Pain control for the adult vs. elderly. Does age make a difference? *Nursing*, 21(9), 44–48.

75. McCaffery, M., et al. (1990). Nurse's knowledge of opioid analgesic drugs and psychological dependence. *Cancer Nursing*, 13, 21–27.

76. McGrath, P.A. (1990). *Pain in children, nature, assessment, & treatment* (pp. 132–172). New York: Guilford Press.

77. McQuay, H.J. (1990). The logic of alternative routes. *Journal of Pain and Symptom Management*, 5(2), 75–77.

78. Melzack, R. (1988). The tragedy of needless pain: a call for social action (IASP president's address). In Dubner, R., et al. (eds.). *Proceedings of the Vth World Congress on Pain* (pp. 1–11). Amsterdam: Elsevier.

79. Mersky, H. (ed.). (1986). Classification of chronic pain: description of chronic pain syndromes and definition of pain terms. Pain (Suppl. 3), S1–S8.

80. Miser, A.W., et al. (1983). Continuous subcutaneous infusion of morphine in children with cancer. *American Journal of Diseases of Children*, 137, 383–385.

81. Miser, A.W., et al. (1980). Continuous intravenous infusion of morphine sulfate for control of severe pain in children with terminal malignancy. *Journal of Pediatrics*, 96, 930–932.

82. North American Nursing Diagnosis Association. (1990). *Taxonomy revised, with official nursing diagnoses.* St. Louis: North American Nursing Diagnosis Association.

83. Paice, J.A. (1986). Intrathecal morphine infusion for intractable cancer pain: a new use for implanted pumps. *Oncology Nursing Forum*, 13, 41–47.

84. Peirce, J., et al. (1990). Intravenous ketorolac tromethamine morphine sulfate in the treatment of immediate postoperative pain. *Pharmacotherapy*, 10(6, part 2), 111S–115S.

85. Portenoy, R.K. (1991). Chronic opioid therapy for persistent noncancer pain: can we get past the bias? *American Pain Society Bulletin*, 1(2), 1–5.

86. Porter, F.L., et al. (1988). Newborn pain cries and vagal tone: parallel changes in response to circumcision. *Child Development*, 59, 495–505.

87. Radwin, L.E. (1987). Autonomous nursing interventions for treating the patient in acute pain: a standard. *Heart and Lung Journal of Critical Care*, 16(3), 258–266.

88. Ready, L.B., et al. (1988). Development of an anesthesiology-based postoperative pain service. *Anesthesiology*, 68, 248–252.

89. Reynolds, D.V. (1969). Surgery in the rat during electrical analgesia induced by focal brain stimulation. *Science*, 164, 444–456.

90. Savedra, M.C., et al. (1989). *Adolescent pediatric pain tool (APPT): Preliminary user's manual.* San Francisco: University of California Press.

91. Schiff, J.M. (1858). *Lehrbuch der Physiologie des Menschen I: Muskel und Nervenphysiologie.* Larh, M. Schauenburg, pp. 23–34, 253–255.

92. Schug, S.A., et al. (1990). Cancer pain management according to WHO analgesic guidelines. *Journal of Pain and Symptom Management*, 5, 27–32.

93. Shutty, M.S. (1990). Chronic pain patients' beliefs about their pain and treatment outcomes. *Archives of Physical Medicine and Rehabilitation*, 71(2), 128–132.

94. Sinatra, R. (1992, October). Research in regional anesthesia: patient-controlled epidural analgesia. *American Society of Regional Anesthesia News*, pp. 2–3.

95. Smith, C.M., et al. (1986). The effects of transcutaneous electrical nerve stimulation on post-cesarean pain. *Pain*, 27, 181–193.

96. Spross, J.A. (1992, July). *Pain management: Issues in the hospital setting.* Proceedings of the Sixth National Conference on Cancer Nursing, Seattle, WA. American Cancer Society Inc., 1992.

97. Tasker, R.R. (1990). Pain resulting from central nervous system pathology (central pain). In Bonica, J.J. (ed.). *The management of pain* (pp. 264–283).

98. Turk, D.C., & Brody, M.C. (1991). Chronic opioid therapy for

persistent noncancer pain: panacea or oxymoron? *American Pain Society Bulletin*, 1(1), 1, 4–7.

99. Turnage, G., et al. (1990). Spinal opioids: a nursing perspective. *Journal of Pain and Symptom Management*, 5(3), 154–161.

100. Tyler, D.C., & Krane, E.J. (1989). Postoperative pain management in children. *Anesthesiology Clinics of North America*, 7(1), 155–170.

101. Waldman, S.D. (1990). Implantable drug delivery systems: practical considerations. *Journal of Pain and Symptom Management*, 5(3), 169–174.

102. Wall, P. (1992). The placebo effect: an unpopular topic. *Pain*, 51(1), 1–3.

103. Wall, P., & Melzack, R. (1990). *The textbook of pain*. London: Churchill Livingstone.

104. Walmsley, P.N.H. (1992). Patient controlled epidural analgesia. In Sinatra, R.S., et al. (eds.). *Acute pain: Mechanisms and management*. (pp. 312–320). St. Louis: C.V. Mosby.

105. Warfield, C., et al. (1985). The effect of transcutaneous electrical nerve stimulation on pain after thoracotomy. *Annals of Thoracic Surgery*, 39, 462–465.

106. Weisman, S.J., et al. (1991, April). *Safety and efficacy of oral transmucosal fentanyl citrate for procedures in children*. Poster presented at the Second International Symposium on Pediatric Pain, Montreal, Quebec, Canada.

107. Whedon, M., & Ferrell, B.R. (1991). Ethical issues and high tech pain management. *Oncology Nursing Forum*, 18, 1135–1143.

108. Willis, W.D. (1992). *Hyperalgesia and allodynia*. New York: Raven Press.

109. Wolff, B.B. (1985). Ethnocultural factors influencing pain and illness behavior. *The Clinical Journal of Pain*, 1, 23–30.

110. Wong, D., & Baker, C. (1988). Pain in children: comparison of assessment scales. *Pediatric Nursing*, 14, 9–17.

111. Yaksh, T.L., & Rudy, T.A. (1978). Narcotic analgesics: CNA sites and mechanisms of action as revealed by intracerebral injection techniques. *Pain*, 4, 299.

▼ Maintaining Fluid and Electrolyte Balance

Chapter 41

> Organisms . . . live . . . relatively free and independent of changes in their external environment because of the constancy of the composition of their internal environment, their extracellular fluids.
>
> **Lawrence Sullivan**

▼ CHAPTER OUTLINE

BODY WATER
 Total Body Water
 Water Distribution
 Water Balance
 Minimal Water Requirements
ELECTROLYTES AND PLASMA PROTEINS
 Chemistry of Electrolytes and
  Plasma Proteins
 Functions of Electrolytes and
  Plasma Proteins
 Measuring Fluids and Electrolytes
 Water and Electrolyte
  Concentrations in the Body
MOVEMENT OF FLUID AND
 ELECTROLYTES
 Fluid and Electrolyte Transport
  Between the Intracellular and the
  Extracellular Fluid Compartments
 Fluid Transport Between the
  Vascular and Interstitial
  Compartments
MAJOR MECHANISMS REGULATING
 FLUID AND ELECTROLYTE BALANCE
 Neuroendocrine System as a
  Homeostatic Regulator
 Gastrointestinal Tract as a
  Homeostatic Regulator

Renal System as a Homeostatic
  Regulator
 Cardiovascular System as a
  Homeostatic Regulator
ACID-BASE BALANCE
 Mechanisms of Acid-base
  Regulation
 Failure of Acid-base Regulation
 Risk Factors for Fluid, Electrolyte,
  and Acid-base Imbalances
ASSESSMENT
 Client History
 Physical Assessment
NURSING DIAGNOSIS
PLANNING
NURSING INTERVENTION
 Recording Intake and Output
 Regulating Diet
 Regulating Oral Fluid Intake
 Administering Medications
 Administering Tube Feedings
 Monitoring Intravenous Therapy
EVALUATION
CASE STUDY

▼ KEY TERMS

Acid	Blood oncotic pressure	Extracellular fluid	Hypotonic	Nonelectrolytes
Acidosis	Body fluid	(ECF)	Hypovolemia	Osmolality
Active transport	Cation	Facilitated diffusion	Interstitial fluid	Osmolarity
Alkalosis	Colloid osmotic	Filtration	Intracellular fluid (ICF)	Osmosis
Anion	pressure (COP)	Filtration pressure	Ions	Osmotic pressure
Base	Colloids	Hydrostatic pressure	Ionization	Plasma
Blood buffer	Diffusion	Hypertonic	Isotonic	Proteinates
Blood hydrostatic	Electrolyte	Hypervolemia	Milliequivalent	Serum
pressure (BHP)		Hypoproteinemia	Milliosmole	

▼ LEARNING OBJECTIVES

After studying this chapter, you should be able to

1. Discuss water in relation to function, distribution, and balance.
2. State the average human requirements for water each day.
3. Describe the chemistry of electrolytes and plasma proteins.
4. List the functions of electrolytes and plasma protein within the body's fluid compartments.
5. Identify the units of measure used for fluid and electrolytes.
6. Describe electrolyte concentrations in the body.
7. Explain how water and electrolytes move within the body between ICF and ECF compartments and between plasma and interstitial fluid compartments.
8. Describe the neuroendocrine mechanisms that regulate fluid and electrolyte balance.
9. Describe the gastrointestinal, renal, and cardiovascular mechanisms that regulate fluid and electrolyte balance.
10. Describe respiratory and metabolic acidosis and respiratory and metabolic alkalosis.
11. Explain the four mechanisms of acid-base regulation.
12. Identify risk factors for water, electrolyte, and acid-base imbalances for which the nurse should assess.
13. Identify appropriate nursing diagnoses for persons with fluid imbalance.
14. Identify objectives of fluid replacement and fluid reduction.
15. Identify nursing interventions for fluid, electrolyte, and acid-base imbalances.
16. State the nurse's responsibilities for evaluating clients with water, electrolyte, and acid-base imbalances.

Human cells depend on an aqueous medium for sustenance and continued life much as the bodies of marine animals depend on the sea. The aqueous medium we need is the body fluid within us. Body fluid contains both water and various "salts," technically termed electrolytes. An **electrolyte** is any compound that, when dissolved in water, separates into electrically charged particles, which are termed **ions.** It is important to understand that the term **body fluid** refers to both water and electrolytes, whereas the term body water refers to water alone.

Water and electrolytes are distributed between two fluid compartments: the **intracellular fluid (ICF)** compartment, which consists of body fluid contained within cells, and the **extracellular fluid (ECF)** compartment, which consists of body fluid found outside the cells. Note in Figure 41–1 that 70 per cent of total body water is ICF, whereas 30 per cent of the total body water is ECF.

Body fluid is in a state of balance when (1) its water and electrolyte components are present in the proper proportions, (2) the distribution of body fluid between compartments is normal, (3) losses of body water and electrolytes are replaced, and (4) excesses of water and electrolytes are eliminated. For body cells to function normally, the composition of body fluids must remain constant.

Several physiologic mechanisms operate to keep the concentration of important components in body fluids within the normal range. Disturbances of these mechanisms by disease processes or even by therapeutic measures designed to treat physiologic disorders may produce water and electrolyte imbalances that range from mild to life threatening. The study of water and electrolyte balance and imbalance, therefore, has numerous practical and vital implications for nurses and the persons in their care.

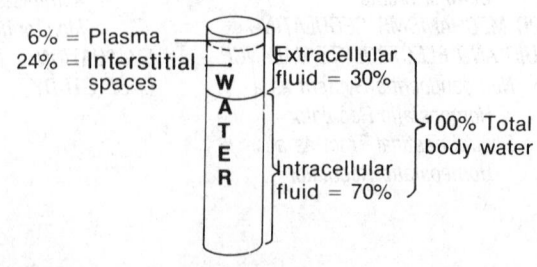

▲ Figure 41–1

Total body water distribution in the adult.

Because the outcome of a disease process can be influenced by imbalances, water and electrolyte therapy is a vital part of the total therapeutic plan. Many decisions concerning medical therapy are based on nurses' documentation of a client's assessment. Accurate assessments and documentation are therefore imperative as a basis for medical therapy as well as nursing care.

BODY WATER

Like a fish torn from the sea, a human being deprived of water cannot live for long. Without water, the skin dries and cracks, the body temperature soars, the mind deteriorates, the cells shrivel, and the body becomes as withered and dead as an ancient Egyptian mummy. What, then, is this all-important substance so absolutely vital to life? What is its chemical make-up, and what are its functions? Where is water distributed in the body, and how can it be replaced?

Total Body Water

The most abundant component of all living matter is water. Water is the major constituent of the body; the rest of the body is composed of solids. Adults vary significantly in the amount of water their bodies contain. This variance is due mainly to the amount of body fat present, because fat is essentially water free. Consequently, a thin individual will have more fluid per kilogram of weight than an overweight individual. Water makes up 60 per cent of the body of an average adult male. A woman's body contains a smaller percentage of fluid in relation to her total weight because her body contains a larger amount of fat. It is estimated that water makes up 50 percent of the average female body.

The percentage of water present in the body varies significantly with age. Table 41–1 compares the proportion of body water at different ages. Note that the

TABLE 41–1. Body Water as a Percentage of Body Weight Across the Life Span

Variable	Total Body Water (% of Body Weight)
Neonate	77
6 months	72
2–16 years	60
20–39 years	
Male	60
Female	50
40–59 years	
Male	55
Female	47
Older than 65 years	
Male	45–50
Female	45–50

percentage of water decreases with age. Also note that there are no differences in the percentage of body water between the male and female until late adolescence or early adulthood, when the female body increases in the proportion of fat.

Water balance carries important nursing implications. Water balance is more easily compromised in infants and in elderly adults than in middle-aged adults. Small imbalances in children become immediately evident, and the younger the child, the more serious the decrease or increase in body water. In addition to decreased body water, elderly adults may have altered thirst mechanisms, which places them at risk for an adequate water intake and dehydration. The decreased dry, scaly skin. Therefore, the elderly do not need to be bathed as often as younger people, and soothing skin lotions and gentle soaps should be used. Early assessment of imbalances can be vital in both the young and the old.

Water Distribution

Water and electrolytes make up the body fluids that move between the ICF and ECF compartments and, within the ECF compartment, between the interstitial fluid and the plasma. Despite the interchange of fluid among compartments, the fluid found in each compartment has its own particular function.

▶ ICF, found within all body cells, provides the cell with the internal aqueous medium necessary for its chemical functions.
▶ ECF, found outside body cells, serves as the body's transportation system. The ECF carries water, electrolytes, nutrients, and oxygen to the cells and removes the waste products of cellular metabolism.
▶ **Interstitial fluid** is the part of the ECF that lies outside the vascular system. The interstitial fluid provides the cells of the solid body tissues with an external medium necessary for cellular metabolism.
▶ **Plasma** is the part of the ECF that lies within the vascular system. Plasma is the liquid part of the blood. It contains colloids (plasma proteins) and by-products of cell function and metabolism. It helps maintain vascular volume and transport blood cells throughout the vascular system. Figure 41–1 shows the distribution of body water among the four fluid compartments.

Water Balance

Body water balance depends on a balance between intake and output of water. Water imbalance exists when water intake and output are unequal, when gains in body water exceed losses or when losses in body water exceed gains. In water imbalance, individuals can become subject to either water overload or dehydration. If overload becomes too great, the lungs fill with water, impairing carbon dioxide and oxygen exchange. If intake is less than what the body needs or is entirely lacking, dehydration occurs.

When a state of water balance exists, water intake—in ingested food and fluid resulting from oxidation of food—equals the water output through the kidneys, bowel, skin, and lungs. Accurate assessment of intake and output (I and O) must take into consideration all sources of water gains and losses. See Procedure 41–1 for the method of measuring intake and output. The 24-hour intake and output record in Table 41–2 shows an approximate intake and output necessary to maintain an adult's water balance.

Note that our greatest single source of water intake is from water or fluids ingested as beverages; our second greatest source is the "hidden" water in foods. Indeed, it may surprise you to learn that lean meats are 75 per cent water, whereas fruits and vegetables may contain an even greater percentage. If the intake of hidden water in foods and the water obtained by oxidation of foods are combined, these two sources of water exceed the beverage intake.

Next, note that the largest proportion of water is eliminated from the kidneys. Only small amounts are normally eliminated from the gastrointestinal (GI) tract. Moderate amounts are eliminated from the skin and lungs through insensible, or evaporated, water loss. Insensible water loss from the skin is not the same as visible sweating or diaphoresis. Insensible loss includes the 750 to 1000 ml of water eliminated in the moisture that constantly forms on the skin and in the vapor that is exhaled in the breath. These losses become sensible or noticeable when the body metabolism is accelerated as with fevers, when respirations are significantly increased as with pneumonia, or when a person is acclimatizing to living in a hot climate. Consequently, when calculating needs for fluid replacement, a clinician must estimate amounts of water lost through the skin and in respiration.

To assess water balance, it is important to keep an accurate record of all liquids taken into the body, such as those on a surgical or full liquid diet, and all output (e.g., urine; fluid lost through diarrheal stools, diaphoresis, hyperventilation, and other drainage).

Minimal Water Requirements

An "average" person should take in approximately 2600 ml of fluid per day to meet the body's water requirements; Box 41–1 lists the functions of water. How much water does an individual need for survival? Although a minimum of 2000 ml of fluid intake per day is recommended for fluid balance, 1500 ml per day is the basal requirement. (Basal requirements are those absolute minimums that sustain cellular activity if the individual is totally at rest.) The basal requirement of 1500 ml of fluid per day applies only if the individual is healthy, relatively inactive, and living in a temperate climate. Individuals who live in hot climates, who have high fevers with excessive perspiration, or who have rapid respiratory rates may require up to 5000 ml of water per day. When these requirements are not met, dehydration is inevitable.

How long can a person live without water? Healthy adults can live several days without water but will exhibit signs and symptoms of severe fluid deficit. The elderly and children may show signs and symptoms of fluid deficit within 2 days depending on the severity of fluid loss, the person's health state (ability of regulatory systems to compensate), and degree of fluid replacement. Extreme fluid losses such as exposure to desert conditions could cause death within hours. In other words, anyone is at risk for death from dehydration.

Initiate fluid replacement rapidly for a severely dehydrated child.

ELECTROLYTES AND PLASMA PROTEINS

In addition to water balance, homeostasis depends on the proper balance of electrolytes and plasma proteins. Thus, nurses need to consider the role of these substances in the body's physiology. This involves knowing the chemistry and functions of electrolytes and plasma proteins, including an understanding of their measurement, balance, and concentration within the body's fluid compartments.

Chemistry of Electrolytes and Plasma Proteins

An electrolyte, when placed in a solvent such as water, breaks up into separately charged particles, or ions. Positively charged ions are called **cations;** negatively charged ions are called **anions.** Important cations in body metabolism are sodium (Na^+), potassium (K^+), calcium (Ca^{++}), magnesium (Mg^{++}), and hydrogen (H^+). Important anions are chloride (Cl^-), bicarbonate (HCO_3^-), phosphate (HPO_4^-), sulfate (SO_4^-), and proteinate ($^-$).

Ionization occurs when a substance breaks apart into its positively and negatively charged particles. Electrolytes break apart in solution. To show how ionization works, let us consider sodium chloride (NaCl). If we place NaCl into solution, it will dissociate, or ionize, into the positive cation Na^+ and the negative anion Cl^- ($NaCl \longrightarrow Na^+ + Cl^-$).

Body fluid contains both anions and cations. Each cation is always balanced chemically by an anion. This relationship is expressed by Faraday's law of electrical neutrality:

The sum of the number of negative electrical charges must equal the sum of the number of positive electrical charges in a solution.

Thus, if the number of cations in a body fluid compartment increases, the number of anions must also increase; if the cations decrease, the anions must also decrease. In this way, electrolyte balance is maintained.

Not all substances dissociate in solution. Substances that do not ionize and consequently do not carry electrical charges are called **nonelectrolytes.** Glucose, a

PROCEDURE 41–1

Recording Intake and Output

Definition/Purpose. Measurement and recording of all fluid intake and output (I & O) during a 24-hour period. Fluid intake includes total fluids from oral, gastric, or intestinal feedings and parenteral solutions. Fluid output includes total output from urine (including urinary incontinence), diarrhea, vomitus, suction, wound drainage, diaphoresis, and other drainage. I & O are measured to provide a more complete and accurate assessment of a person's water, electrolyte, and acid-base status.

Contraindications/Cautions. There are no contraindications to I & O. I & O may be a physician's order or an independent nursing intervention. It should be initiated on any person at risk for water, electrolyte, or acid-base imbalance (see Table 41–3). Cautions include being certain to communicate to all staff members when a client is on I & O and to communicate all intake and output appropriately.

Learning/Teaching Guidelines. Explain to the person or significant others the following, as appropriate: (1) the purpose of monitoring I & O, (2) that accuracy in measurement is essential for both nurse and physician in planning care, (3) the importance of not discarding empty or partially empty containers until the amounts consumed are recorded, (4) the importance of saving output until recording has occurred, and (5) procedure for measuring and recording their own I & O to promote self-care.

PRELIMINARY ACTIVITIES

Assessment/Planning

▶ Check medical and nursing diagnoses and purpose of I & O.
▶ Check physician and nursing orders.
▶ Be aware of agency's guidelines for measurement and recording.
▶ Be aware of foods included in a clear or full liquid diet.

Equipment

▶ I & O forms with pencil or pen: temporary forms for placement in person's room (these include measurement equivalents consistent with the agency's fluid containers) and a permanent I & O form for chart (graphic or flow sheet) for 24-hour recording (all forms must be identified with client's name and the date)
▶ Pen with appropriate ink color for recording on permanent record
▶ Various sized measuring containers (30-ml medicine cup, 240-ml cup, and 500-ml graduated container)

▶ Elimination collection devices (fracture bedpan, regular bedpan, "hat" specimen pan for toilet or commode, urinal)
▶ Clean, disposable gloves

Preparation

▶ Place signs or notes in appropriate places to communicate to all staff members that client is on I & O.
▶ Obtain appropriate equipment.
▶ If client is receiving tube feedings or intravenous (IV) solutions, note amount left in bag at beginning of shift.
▶ Place gloves, collection devices, and measuring containers in client's room or bathroom.
▶ Review with client and family the purpose and procedure of I & O measurement.

PROCEDURE

Measuring and Recording Intake

Actions

1. Wash hands.
2. Before removing any dietary tray, check whether person is on I & O; using equivalencies on form, measure and record accurate amounts of fluid ingested, including time, type, and amount of each fluid consumed.
3. If person is on calorie count, record ingested proportion of all fluids and foods on menu according to agency policy.
4. At regular intervals, measure and record times, types, and amounts of all other fluids taken in during shift (water, clear and full liquid, foods eaten, tube feedings, IV fluid, fluids used to dilute medications).

   Ice chips are equal to one half their amount in fluid (e.g., one cup of ice chips equals one-half cup of water, if all ice chips were ingested).

Rationale/Discussion

1. This helps maintain universal precautions.
2. This helps ensure accuracy of measurement and recording without omissions or duplications.

3. This helps ensure accuracy of kilocalorie intake totals.

4. The more often the intake is recorded, the less likely will be omissions.

Procedure continued on following page

PROCEDURE 41-1 Continued

Recording Intake and Output

Actions	**Rationale/Discussion**
5. At the end of each shift, transfer fluid intake total to the permanent chart form; totals for oral, tube feedings, and parenteral fluids should be itemized separately followed by one numerical total for all the fluid intake for each shift and one for the entire 24-hour period. Follow agency guidelines as to protocol for recording the amount of IV or tube feeding fluid left to be taken in during the upcoming shift.	5. Evaluation of fluid status is based on comparison of 24-hour totals of each type of fluid intake as well as the total fluid intake. Recall that the nutrient content of fluid varies. Fluid credits must consistently be recorded by using the same method if accuracy is to be ensured.

Measuring and Recording of Output

Actions	**Rationale/Discussion**
1. Wash hands, and don clean, disposable gloves.	1. This helps maintain universal precautions.
2. Using appropriately sized measurement container, measure fluid output (30-ml container for <30-ml output, 240-ml container for <240-ml output, 500-ml container for >240-ml output); read output at eye level. Use a catheter bag with an overflow collection chamber when hourly assessments are needed.	2. This helps ensure accuracy of measurement and recording. Large graduated containers do not have enough increments for accurate measurement of small amounts such as obtained from Hemovacs or Jackson-Pratt drains.
3. Dispose of output according to agency guidelines; usually urine is emptied into agency plumbing system; if person is subject to isolation or radiation protocols, see specific agency policies. Most agency policies require that closed collection devices are marked with a pen every shift or more often to indicate output and single or double bagged before the collection device is disposed (e.g., nasogastric or chest tube collection devices).	3. This helps maintain universal precautions and radiation precautions; single or double bagging will depend on weight of bag in millimeters.
4. Rinse measuring container before disposal; place in bathroom, or return to bedside (e.g., urinal, bedpan, graduate).	4. Rinsing reduces environmental odor.
5. If output is from drainage, urinary incontinence, or diaphoresis, estimate the amount (e.g., number of incontinent pads saturated, amount of linen saturated, number and size of dressings saturated). If extreme accuracy is needed, compare weight of clean material with saturated material (difference in grams equals milliliters of output).	5. Weighing is usually indicated when fluid balance is very critical (e.g., critical care, neonate or infant [weighing of diapers]).
6. Record each output (time, amount, and type) on temporary I & O form in person's room; for output estimate, write "approximate" by output.	6. Accurate recording on temporary form helps ensure accuracy of total output.
7. Measure and record all fluid output (including measurement of diarrheal stools and estimates of loss through lungs by noting rate of respirations if tachypneic).	7. Evaluation of water and electrolyte status is based on comparison of 24-hour totals of each type of fluid output as well as the total fluid output. Recall that the source of output affects the type of electrolytes lost. The physician also uses the data to make decisions about discontinuing output collection devices (e.g., pulling drains, discontinuing a nasogastric tube).
8. At the end of the shift, transfer fluid output total to the permanent chart form, itemizing the total for each type of output separately, followed by one numerical total of all fluid output for the shift and one for the entire 24-hour period. Follow agency protocol for recording outputs obtained after totals are done (credits for the oncoming shift).	8. The I & O totals are important assessment data that belong on the permanent record.

FINAL ACTIVITIES

Record quality of output on nurse's notes or form designated by agency. Evaluate I & O based on person's metabolic state and normality of quantity and quality. The physician needs to be notified of any serious alteration from the normal (e.g., hemorrhage, marked increase in wound or gastric drainage, sudden fever, inability or refusal to drink or eat in person with high risk for complications [such as diabetes mellitus], inability to urinate after trying for 6 to 8 hours, or urinary output less than 20 to 30 ml/hour for 2 consecutive hours [unless renal failure is already diagnosed]).

Box 41-1. Basic Functions of Water

- ▶ provides aqueous medium for cellular metabolism
- ▶ transports material to and from cells
- ▶ acts as a solvent for electrolytes and other substances necessary for cell function
- ▶ helps to regulate body temperature
- ▶ maintains physical and chemical constancy of intracellular and extracellular fluid
- ▶ maintains vascular volume
- ▶ aids in digestion of food
- ▶ provides medium for waste excretion

---

nonelectrolyte, remains a nondissociated, electrically neutral molecule in body fluid. Many organic compounds are nonelectrolytes.

Proteins play a significant role in fluid and electrolyte metabolism. They are found both in cells and in plasma. Proteins within the protoplasm of cells are **proteinates,** whereas proteins in the plasma are in colloid form. **Colloids** are protein macromolecules too large to pass through cell membranes. Consequently, these plasma proteins tend to remain within the blood vessels rather than diffusing out into the tissues. Plasma proteins behave like anions and carry a negative charge. The most important plasma proteins are albumin, globulin, and fibrinogen; these colloidal substances are synthesized in the liver.

Functions of Electrolytes and Plasma Proteins

Electrolytes and plasma proteins perform important physiologic functions within the body. The interrelated functions of electrolytes include (1) promotion of neuromuscular irritability, (2) maintenance of body fluid osmolality, (3) regulation of acid-base balance, and (4) maintenance of body water distribution among the fluid compartments. Plasma proteins also play an important role in body water distribution. Basically, plasma proteins hold water within the blood vessels and promote the return of water from the interstitial spaces to the plasma.

Boxes 41-2 through 41-9 outline the basic functions of sodium, potassium, calcium, magnesium, hydrogen and bicarbonate, chloride, phosphate, and proteinate,

respectively. Table 41-3 lists the common etiologies of imbalances that can occur with each.

Measuring Fluids and Electrolytes

Correct measurement of water and electrolytes is very important. Even small errors in measurement can result in serious water and electrolyte imbalances. The most important measurements used are the following:

- ▶ Measures of volume: the liter and milliliter and cubic centimeter. For practical purposes, the milliliter and cubic centimeter are equivalent, and fluid measurements are often expressed in cubic centimeters. Intravenous (IV) solutions are always measured in liters and milliliters. For example, 1 L (1000 ml) of normal saline may be ordered for a person with a fluid imbalance.
- ▶ Units of weight: the gram and milligram; 1 gm equals 1000 mg. Serum electrolytes and plasma proteins are expressed in percentages. This measurement tells us the number of grams or milligrams of an electrolyte or colloid in 100 ml of fluid. For example, the normal plasma protein content of blood is 6 gm/100 ml, or 6 gm per cent. In other words, there are 6 gm (6000 mg) of protein in every 100 ml of plasma.
- ▶ A measure of the chemical activity or chemical combining power of an ion: the **milliequivalent.** The milliequivalent is a measure of the power of a cation to combine with an anion, thus forming a molecule. The milliequivalence makes it possible to compare one compound with another. The electrolyte content within a fluid can be most accurately expressed in milliequivalents per liter.

Although two different chemicals may have equal weights, one may have a greater chemical combining power or greater number of charges than the other chemical. For example, 23 mg of sodium, 39 mg of potassium, 20 mg of calcium, and 4140 mg of proteinate differ significantly by weight, yet each exerts only 1 mEq of chemical activity. Therefore, 1 mEq of any electrolyte acts chemically as 1 mEq of any other electrolyte, even though the weights of the two electrolytes may differ significantly. This equality is the reason that electrolytes are measured in milliequivalents rather than milligrams (i.e., according to chemical combining

---

TABLE 41-2. Body Water Balance in the Adult over a 24-Hour Period

Source	Intake	Source	Output
Oral fluids	1200 ml	Urine	1500 ml
"Hidden" water from foods	1100 ml	Water vapor (lungs)*	400 ml
Metabolic sources		Perspiration*	600 ml
Oxidation of foods	300 ml	Feces	100 ml
Protein	40 ml/100 gm		
Fat	100 ml/100 gm		
Carbohydrate	100 ml/100 gm		
Total	2600 ml	Total	2600 ml

* Insensible water loss.

Box 41–2. Basic Functions of Sodium (Na⁺) (135–145 mEq/L)

- ▶ regulates extracellular fluid volume
- ▶ increases cell membrane permeability
- ▶ maintains blood volume
- ▶ controls water distribution between extracellular fluid and intracellular fluid spaces
- ▶ provides necessary mechanism for normal nerve impulse conduction
- ▶ helps maintain neuromuscular irritability
- ▶ assists in controlling muscle contractility (e.g., myocardium)
- ▶ provides necessary mechanism for buffer system as cation that combines with bicarbonate and phosphate

---

Box 41–3. Basic Functions of Potassium (K⁺) (3.5–5.0 mEq/L)

- ▶ regulates water and electrolyte content of intracellular fluid (ICF)
- ▶ promotes nerve impulses, especially in heart muscle
- ▶ promotes skeletal muscle function
- ▶ assists in transforming carbohydrates into energy and restructuring amino acids into proteins
- ▶ provides necessary mechanism for glycogen deposition in liver
- ▶ assists in regulation of acid-base balance by cellular exchange with hydrogen

---

Box 41–4. Basic Functions of Calcium (Ca⁺⁺) (4.5–5.5 mEq/L)

- ▶ nonionized form required for building strong bones and teeth
- ▶ acts as essential component for blood coagulation
- ▶ decreases neuromuscular irritability
- ▶ promotes normal nerve impulse transmission
- ▶ strengthens and thickens cell membrane
- ▶ assists in absorption and utilization of vitamin B_{12}
- ▶ activates enzymes that in turn activate chemical reactions within body
- ▶ inhibits cell membrane permeability to sodium
- ▶ moves into cell with sodium during depolarization, binding troponin
- ▶ results in actin- and myosin-promoting muscle contraction

---

Box 41–5. Basic Functions of Magnesium (Mg⁺⁺) (1.5–2.5 mEq/L)

- ▶ affects metabolism of carbohydrates, lipids, and proteins
- ▶ activates many enzymes (B_{12} metabolism, use of potassium, calcium, protein)
- ▶ promotes regulation of calcium, phosphate, potassium
- ▶ provides essential mechanism for nerve transmission, muscle contraction (needs to be present for actin and myosin to use adenosine triphosphate), heart function
- ▶ powers sodium-potassium pump
- ▶ necessary for energy release in adenosine triphosphate $\longrightarrow$ adenosine diphosphate reaction
- ▶ inhibits smooth-muscle contraction

Box 41–6. Basic Functions of Hydrogen (H⁺)/ Bicarbonate (HCO₃⁻) (serum pH 7.35–7.45)

- ▶ Ratio of the concentration of each determines acidity or alkalinity of body fluids.
- ▶ Acid-base balance promotes efficient enzyme functioning.
- ▶ Acid-base balance is necessary for binding of oxygen by hemoglobin.

Box 41–7. Basic Functions of Chloride (Cl⁻) (98–106 mEq/L)

- ▶ regulates extracellular fluid volume
- ▶ serves as blood buffer–chloride shift
- ▶ digestion—required for secretion of hydrochloric acid (necessary for activation of protease)

> **Box 41–8. Basic Functions of Phosphate (HPO_4^-) (1.2–3.0 mEq/L)**
>
> ▶ nonionized form promotes bone and teeth rigidity
> ▶ promotes acid-base balance (buffer system)
> ▶ provides necessary mechanism for production of adenosine triphosphate

> **Box 41–9. Basic Functions of Protein (Serum Proteinate) in the Intracellular Fluid (6–8 gm/dl)**
>
> ▶ promotes tissue growth and repair
> ▶ necessary for manufacture of hormones, antibodies, and coagulation factors
> ▶ maintains colloid osmotic pressure in plasma (promotes normality of blood volume, blood pressure, and interstitial fluid levels)

TABLE 41–3. Fluids and Electrolytes: Etiologies of Imbalances

Water Deficit

1. Increased water output: vomiting, diarrhea, fever, gastric/intestinal suction, ileostomy, fistulas, burns, hyperventilation, diuretics, hyperthyroidism, hemorrhage, decreased ADH, Addison's disease, diabetes insipidus, diabetes mellitus
2. Decreased water intake: decreased level of consciousness, decreased thirst, dysphagia, unavailability of water
3. Impaired concentration of urine as in renal disease
4. Iatrogenic solute loading: excessive hypertonic IVs or tube feedings
5. Third-space loss: ascites, peritonitis, pancreatitis

Water Excess

1. Excessive intake: iatrogenic-excessive electrolyte-free IVs or excess saline IVs (osmotic pull of Na^+ causes increased water in the plasma), increased oral intake after loss of sodium-containing fluids (e.g., diarrhea, vomiting, suction)
2. Decreased excretion through the kidney: renal disease, increased ADH
3. Increased retention at the plasma level: Cushing's syndrome, hyperaldosteronism, increased venous pressure, lymphatic obstruction, congestive heart failure, excess tap-water enemas, cortisone therapy
4. Increased capillary permeability: sepsis, inflammatory responses

Saline (NaCl) Deficit (Serum Na^+ < 135 mEq/L)

1. Increased loss: vomiting, diarrhea, fistulas, wound drainage, gastric or intestinal suction, irrigating NG tube with hypotonic solution or overingestion of plain ice chips or H_2O when NG to suction, increased diaphoresis, low salt intake while on diuretics, renal disease, Addison's disease
2. Overdilution of sodium: increased ADH, excessive tap-water enemas
3. Decreased intake: low-sodium diets, excessive electrolyte-free or low-Na^+ IV solutions

Saline (NaCl) Excess (Serum Na^+ > 145 mEq/L)

1. Increased Na^+ intake: excessive salt intake in presence of renal disease, excessive IV saline solutions, hypertonic feedings
2. Diseases causing failure of homeostatic fluid regulation: heart disease, renal failure, liver disease, Cushing's syndrome, hyperaldosteronism
3. Conditions in which H_2O loss is greater than sodium: diabetes mellitus or diabetes insipidus, hyperventilation, diaphoresis
4. Decreased water intake (will also result in hemoconcentration of sodium)

Chloride Deficit (serum Cl^- < 98 mEq/L)

1. Increased loss: loss through vomiting, diarrhea, suction, diuretics, interstitial fluid loss, excess bicarbonate (UGI loss usually > LGI loss), Addison's disease

Chloride Excess (Serum Cl^- > 106 mEq/L)

1. Nonspecific: related to cation excess, usually Na^+ or K^+ imbalances; Cl^- imbalances are often listed as saline imbalances

Potassium Deficit (serum K < 3.5 mEq/L)

1. Decreased intake: alcoholism, decreased intake through diet or IV solutions without K^+ (need 40–80 mEq/day)

Potassium Excess (serum K^+ > 5.0 mEq/L)

1. Increased intake: excessive oral intake in presence of renal disease, excessive IV K^+, transfusion of stored blood (cells in blood break down over time and release the intracellular contents, including large amounts of K^+)

Table continued on following page

TABLE 41-3. Fluids and Electrolytes: Etiologies of Imbalances Continued

2. Increased loss: vomiting, diarrhea, fistulas, wound drainage, osmotic diuresis (diabetes mellitus), during severe stress/trauma/burns in healing phase (after third day), diuretic phase of renal failure, Cushing's syndrome, hyperaldosteronism, metabolic and respiratory alkalosis, high carbohydrate intake (K^+ moves into cell with increased insulin)

2. Decreased output: renal failure, postoperative oliguria, Addison's disease
3. Gain from ICF excessive cellular destruction: first 3 days after burns or severe trauma
4. Gain from intracellular movement of K^+ outward in exchange for H^+, which moves into cell: metabolic and respiratory acidosis (except diabetic acidosis)

Calcium Deficit
(serum Ca^{++} < 4.5 mEq/L)

1. Decreased intake: poor dietary intake of Ca^{++}, or vitamin D, especially when need higher (pregnancy and lactation), IV solutions without Ca^{++} after several days of infusion
2. Increased loss: diarrhea, wound drainage, diuresis, alcoholism, Cushing's syndrome, renal failure (high PO_4^-, Mg^{++}), high-protein diets
3. Decreased availability: burns (trapped in eschar), pancreatitis, metabolic alkalosis (decreased ionization), excess citrated blood (Ca^{++} binds to citrate)
4. Diminished regulatory hormone: removal or damage to parathyroids

Calcium Excess
(serum Ca^{++} > 5.5 mEq/L)

1. Increased intake: excess milk or vitamin D intake
2. Increased loss of Ca^{++} from the bone: immobilization, cancers (breast, lung, kidney, multiple myeloma, leukemia), hyperparathyroidism
3. Increased intestinal absorption and skeletal mobilization in hypophosphatemia
4. Increased ionization: metabolic acidosis (bound calcium displaced from albumin)
5. Addison's disease (decreased Na^+) mechanism uncertain[36]

Caution Abnormal serum albumin levels influence interpretation of Ca^{++} levels. When serum albumin levels are elevated, serum Ca^{++} is lower than the laboratory reading and vice versa

Magnesium Deficit
(serum Mg^{++} < 1.5 mEq/L)

1. Decreased intake: decreased diet intake, softened water, refined foods, alcoholism, IV solutions over long time without Mg^{++}
2. Increased loss: gastric suction, vomiting, diarrhea, diuretic phase of renal failure, alcoholism, diabetic acidosis, toxemia (PG)
3. Decreased absorption: Crohn's disease, celiac disease, pancreatitis, hyperparathyroidism (Ca^{++} inhibits), Cushing's syndrome, and hyperaldosteronism (Na^+ inhibits)

Magnesium Excess
(serum Mg^{++} > 2.5 mEq/L)

1. Increased intake: overdoses of Mg^{++} or ingestion of Mg^{++} in presence of renal disease
2. Decreased output: renal disease
3. Decreased opposition: Addison's disease and hypoaldosteronism (less Na^+)

Phosphate Deficit
(serum HPO_4^- < 1.2 mEq/L)

1. Decreased intake: decreased diet intake, IV solutions long term without HPO_4^-
2. Increased loss: osmotic diuresis of diabetic acidosis, malabsorption (colitis, decreased vitamin D)
3. Increased opposition: Cushing's syndrome (increased Na^+), hyperparathyroidism (increased Ca^{++}), lead poisoning
4. Chronic respiratory alkalosis (shift of phosphorus to cell occurs when $PaCO_2$ is decreased) leads to severe loss[34]
5. Metabolic alkalosis (increased renal loss of phosphate) leads to mild loss

Phosphate Excess
(serum HPO_4^- > 3.0 mEq/L)

1. Increased intake: excess dietary intake of high-phosphate foods (milk and milk products), increased absorption: excess vitamin D
2. Decreased output: renal failure
3. Decreased opposition: hypoparathyroidism (decreased Ca^{++}), Addison's disease (decreased Na^+)

Protein Deficit
(serum total protein < 6 gm/dl or decrease in any plasma proteins)

1. Decreased intake: decrease in dietary consumption
2. Increased loss: hemorrhage, draining wounds (burns, open ulcers, ascites, renal disease)

TABLE 41-3. *Fluids and Electrolytes: Etiologies of Imbalances* Continued

3. Increased utilization for rebuilding tissue (burns, trauma, fractures)
4. Increased protein catabolism: fever, increased metabolism, infection, malignancy
5. Decreased synthesis: liver disease
6. GI malabsorption

Base bicarbonate deficit in ECF (metabolic acidosis, pH < 7.35; HCO_3^- < 25 mEq/L)	**Base bicarbonate excess in ECF (metabolic alkalosis, pH > 7.45; HCO_3^- > 29 mEq/L)**
1. Increased loss of HCO_3^-: severe diarrhea, loss of biliary, pancreatic, or lower bowel fluid 2. Overproduction of metabolic acids: diabetic acidosis, shock (anaerobic metabolism increases blood lactic acid levels), starvation, prolonged fasting 3. Excessive ingestion of metabolic acids: high-fat, low-carbohydrate diets; salicylate toxicity; overingestion of certain medications cause H^+ overload Decreased ability to excrete overload of acid: renal disease 4. ease 5. Conditions leading to increase in serum K^+ as result of compensatory chloride shift (Cl^- moves out of cell to combine with K^+, HCO_3^- moves into cell)	1. Increased HCO_3^- intake: ingestion of large amounts of alkali (baking soda) 2. Loss of acid: loss of HCl acid from the stomach (by vomiting or gastric suctioning) 3. Decreased loss: diuretic therapy, can result in loss of K^+ and Cl^- with compensatory increase in HCO_3^-
Carbonic acid deficit in ECF (respiratory alkalosis, pH > 7.45; Pco_2 < 35 mm Hg)	**Carbonic acid excess in ECF (respiratory acidosis, pH < 7.35; Pco_2 > 45 mm Hg)**
Increased excretion of CO_2: hyperventilation (anxiety, hysteria, severe prolonged exercise, anoxia at high altitudes, early salicylate intoxication, oxygen lack, fever, CNS disease such as meningitis and encephalitis)	Increased retention of CO_2: breath holding, apnea during CPR, chronic respiratory conditions (asthma, bronchitis, emphysema); acute respiratory conditions (pneumonia), trauma of respiratory centers, overdose of respiratory depressants (narcotics, sedatives)

Abbreviations: ADH, antidiuretic hormone; IV, intravenous; Na^+, sodium; H_2O, water; NG, nasogastric; UGI, upper gastrointestinal; LGI, lower gastrointestinal; K^+, potassium; ICF, intracellular fluid; H^+, hydrogen; PO_4, phosphorus; PG, prostaglandin; $PaCO_2$, partial pressure of arterial carbon dioxide; GI, gastrointestinal; ECF, extracellular fluid; HCl, hydrochloric; CO_2, carbon dioxide; PCO_2, partial pressure of carbon dioxide; CNS, central nervous system; CPR, cardiopulmonary resuscitation.

power rather than weight). Moreover, the number of milliequivalents of cations in a body fluid compartment must always balance the number of milliequivalents of anions for chemical neutrality to exist (Fig. 41-2). Chemical neutrality of the body fluids is essential for the maintenance of normal neuromuscular excitability.

Water and Electrolyte Concentrations in the Body

We normally obtain water and electrolytes by dietary intake. Water and electrolytes are then distributed throughout the body's fluid compartments. The compartments contain the same electrolytes but in different amounts. Potassium is the major cation of the ICF;

phosphate is the major anion. Sodium is the major cation of the ECF; chloride is the major anion. Figure 41-3 shows the relative proportions of electrolytes for both the intracellular and extracellular compartments.

Laboratories use samples of plasma or **serum** (plasma without the clotting substance fibrinogen) to measure most electrolytes in the ECF compartment. Serum is used because the plasma has almost the same electrolyte composition as the interstitial fluid, except that plasma contains the plasma proteins (colloids). Although electrolyte concentration of the ECF is measurable, scientists are not yet able to measure the concentration of electrolytes in the ICF directly. Diagnostic tests such as the electrocardiogram (ECG) are used to evaluate the status of some intracellular ions (e.g., potassium, magnesium). (See Chapter 34 for further information related to the ECG.)

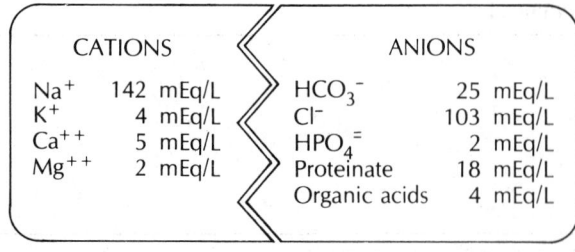

▲ *Figure 41–2*

When their combining power is expressed in milliequivalents, the cations and anions of extracellular fluid approximately balance.

The transcellular fluids (e.g., cerebrospinal fluid, bile, saliva) each have their distinct electrolyte composition, which tends to remain fairly stable in healthy individuals. When illness strikes, the transcellular fluids may also become depleted, and electrolytes are lost along with water.

Electrolytes are also dissolved in the fluid that we lose through urination, defecation, and sweating. Thus, to maintain water and electrolyte balance, whenever water is replaced, electrolytes must also be replaced, and electrolyte replacement requires water replacement. A minimal daily intake of 2400 to 2600 ml of water, 2.4 gm of sodium, 3.5 gm of potassium, and 0.08 gm protein per kilogram of body weight is required for healthy balance.

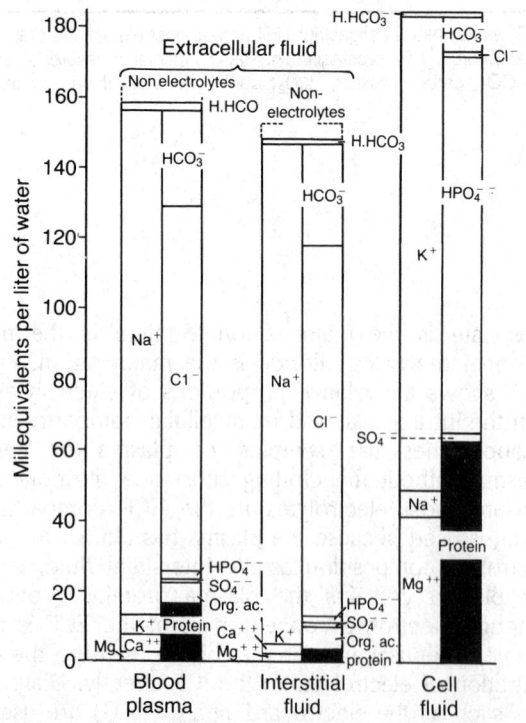

▲ *Figure 41–3*

A comparison of the electrolyte composition of the extracellular and intracellular fluid compartments. (Reprinted with permission from Guyton, A. C. [1991]. Textbook of medical physiology [8th ed]. Philadelphia: W. B. Saunders.)

MOVEMENT OF FLUID AND ELECTROLYTES

Knowledge of water and electrolyte transport and regulation is basic to an understanding of the pathophysiology of edema, dehydration, circulatory overload, water intoxication, and other water and electrolyte imbalances. To understand fluid and electrolyte movement, you must consider the transport of water and electrolytes between the ICF and ECF and the transport of fluids between the interstitial fluid compartment and vascular compartment. The flow of fluids depends on a number of physiologic mechanisms.

Fluid and Electrolyte Transport Between the Intracellular and Extracellular Fluid Compartments

Water moves from one compartment, through a semipermeable membrane, to another compartment by the processes of filtration and osmosis.

HYDROSTATIC PRESSURE AND FILTRATION

Hydrostatic pressure is pressure exerted by a liquid within a compartment. Hydrostatic pressure promotes the flow of fluid, outward, across a membrane that is permeable to the fluid. The passage of water and particles through a semipermeable membrane, assisted by hydrostatic pressure, is called **filtration.** Thus, with filtration, water is *pushed* through the membrane. **Osmosis** is a process in which water crosses a semipermeable membrane from an area of lesser concentration of particles to one of greater concentration of particles. The amount of pressure required for osmosis to occur is termed **osmotic pressure.** Osmotic pressure is determined by the concentration of the solutions (the number of dissolved particles relative to the amount of water) on both sides of a semipermeable membrane through which water will flow. A unit of osmotic pressure is a **milliosmole.**

OSMOLALITY, OSMOLARITY, AND OSMOSIS

Osmolality is a measure of the number of milliosmoles per kilogram of a fluid. Osmolality is used to compare body fluids. **Osmolarity** is a measure of the milliosmoles (unit of force/number of dissolved particles or solute) per liter of solution (solvent). Osmolarity is used to compare solutions with plasma.

When a solution has the same or approximately the same osmotic pressure as the solution with which it is compared, the solutions are said to be **isotonic.** A **hypertonic** solution has an osmotic pressure greater than that of the solution with which it is compared; in the body, a hypertonic solution is greater than 375 mEq/L. A **hypotonic** solution has an osmotic pressure lower than that of the solution with which it is compared; in the body, hypotonicity occurs at 250 mEq/L. Because water moves toward the greatest number of particles (electrolytes), the solution with the greatest osmolality (greatest concentration of dissolved particles per liter) gains water. In the same way, the solution with the lowest osmolality (lowest concentration of dissolved particles per liter) loses water. Thus, when two solutions of different osmolality are separated by a membrane permeable to water but not to particles (and therefore semipermeable), the distribution of water shifts so that the osmolalities of the two solutions equalize.

The dissolved particles within the body fluids are primarily electrolytes and colloids. Should a greater osmolality develop (more electrolytes per liter) in the ICF than in the ECF, water will shift from the ECF compartment into the ICF compartment; consequently, the cells will swell. Should a greater osmolality develop in the ECF than in the ICF, water will shift from the cells into the ECF compartment, and the cells will shrivel. Thus, osmolar changes affect cell volume.

Although osmolality controls water distribution, osmolality itself is principally regulated by water intake and output. Thirst and habit control water intake, whereas the antidiuretic hormone (ADH), kidneys, and GI tract control water loss.

The serum sodium level is used as direct measure of plasma osmolality because sodium is the major ECF ion. It is also an indirect measure of ICF osmolality because both the ICF and ECF compartments have the same osmolality. The normal serum sodium level is 135 to 145 mEq/L. When the serum sodium level rises beyond normal limits, the osmolality of the plasma, and consequently of the body, increases. When the serum sodium level is depressed below normal limits, osmolality decreases.

A person with an elevated serum sodium level as a result of water depletion suffers from a hyperosmolar imbalance. There is a decrease in water relative to particle concentration (hyperosmolality). Thus, the electrolytes are relatively concentrated. Conversely, when a person has a lowered serum sodium or an increase in body water because of water retention or overload, a hypo-osmolar imbalance has occurred, with an increase in water relative to particle concentration (hypo-osmolality). The electrolytes are thus diluted. Figure 41–4 presents concepts of hyperosmolality and hypo-osmolality.

DIFFUSION, FACILITATED DIFFUSION, AND ACTIVE TRANSPORT

Whereas filtration controls the movement of both water and ions and osmolality controls water movement and distribution, the processes of diffusion, facilitated diffusion, and active transport control the movement of ions across the cellular membrane. Most ions move by **diffusion,** the process of molecular (particle) movement from an area of higher particle concentration to an area of lower particle concentration. Larger molecules such as glucose need a carrier molecule (for glucose, the molecule is insulin) to facilitate transfer across the cell membrane from an area of higher concentration to an area of lower concentration of molecules. This process is known as **facilitated diffusion. Active transport** is the movement of ions across a cellular membrane against a concentration, chemical, or electrical

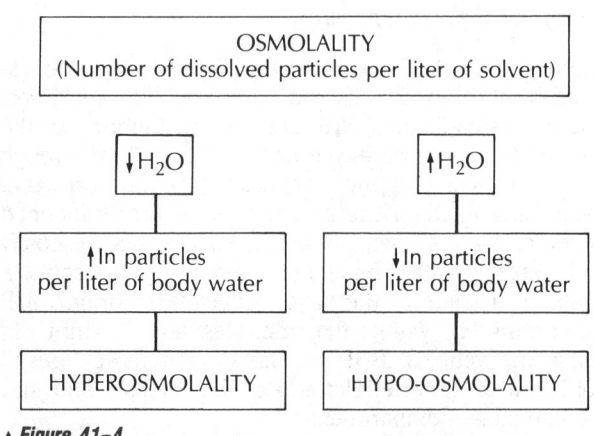

▲ *Figure 41–4*

Hyperosmolality means more than 145 mEq of Na+ per liter of body water; hypo-osmolality means less than 135 mEq of Na+ per liter of body water.

gradient. Because the ions move against a gradient, active transport requires energy.

One special type of active transport is the sodium-potassium pump. Recall that large amounts of sodium exist extracellularly and large quantities of potassium exist intracellularly. Both sodium and potassium can diffuse through the cell wall, so an active mechanism must operate to keep these ions in their respective compartments where they are needed. The sodium-potassium pump conserves intracellular potassium levels by actively excluding sodium and thereby preventing cellular swelling.

Fluid Transport Between the Vascular and Interstitial Compartments

To understand fluid exchange between the vascular (blood) and the interstitial (tissue) compartments, you need to consider the factors that contribute to the maintenance of a homeostatic state (relatively constant internal environment): (1) plasma proteins, (2) capillary permeability, (3) plasma and interstitial osmolality, (4) blood hydrostatic pressure, (5) colloid osmotic pressure (COP), (6) filtration pressure (FP), and (7) the lymphatic system.

HOMEOSTATIC STATE

Although the capillaries are freely permeable to water and to certain electrolytes, they are not freely permeable to protein. Thus, the plasma protein concentration remains high. In the normal state, plasma has a 0.5 per cent greater osmolality than interstitial fluid, so that plasma has a 0.5 per cent greater capacity than interstitial fluid to attract and to hold water. Any reduction in plasma osmolality results in swollen tissues (edema) and loss of blood volume.

Two major factors involved in maintaining the balance of water between the vascular space and interstitial space are blood hydrostatic pressure (BHP) and colloid osmotic pressure (COP). Together, these two factors help to determine filtration pressure (FP) (according to Starling's law of capillary force).

BLOOD HYDROSTATIC PRESSURE

Blood hydrostatic pressure (BHP) is the force exerted by the blood cells and plasma within blood vessels. In the capillaries, BHP depends on the level of the arterial blood pressure, the rate of blood flow through the capillaries, and the level of the venous pressure. Recall that each of these factors is in turn influenced by other factors, such as blood volume and viscosity and cardiovascular function. Figure 41–5 presents a diagram of some of the major influences. Normal BHP is 32 mm Hg within the arterioles and 12 mm Hg within the venules. BHP generally functions to "push" fluids out of the arteriolar end of the capillary and into the interstitial compartment.

COLLOID OSMOTIC PRESSURE

Colloid osmotic pressure (COP), or **blood oncotic pressure,** is the negative pressure exerted by plasma proteins. Plasma proteins work somewhat like a sponge, holding water within the vessels and pulling back water that escapes from the vessels. In the healthy state, COP within the capillary is about 22 mm Hg. Because blood vessel walls are impermeable to these proteins, they remain in the vessel and exert this pressure at a constant rate in the arteriolar end of the capillary bed, within the capillaries, and in the venous end of the capillary bed. Albumin makes up more than 50 per cent of the plasma proteins but is responsible for 80 per cent of the COP.

Filtration pressure (FP) is the pressure of blood in the blood vessels minus COP (FP = BHP − COP). Normally, FP in the arteriolar end of the capillary is +10 mm Hg (32 mm Hg BHP − 22 mm Hg BOP = +10 mm Hg FP). In the venous end of the capillary, FP is −10 mm Hg (12 mm Hg BHP − 22 mm Hg BOP = −10 mm Hg FP). These figures demonstrate that, at the arteriolar end of the capillary, BHP is greater than COP; therefore, fluid is forced out of the capillaries and into the tissues. At the venous end of the capillary, BHP is less than COP, and the water is pulled back into the vessels. Thus, filtration occurs at the arteriolar end of the vessel, and reabsorption occurs at the venous end of the capillary. Figure 41–6 represents these mechanisms.

Lymphatic filtration is yet another factor influencing fluid transport between the plasma and interstitial fluid. The lymphatic system filters interstitial fluid and removes debris. After debris is removed, the excess fluid is returned to the heart and the general circulation through the superior vena cava.

FACTORS LEADING TO EDEMA

Alterations in any of the factors that regulate fluid transport can change the pressure relationship between the intravascular and interstitial compartments. A rise in BHP on the venous end of the capillary reduces the amount of reabsorption of fluid that normally flows readily from the interstitial space to the vascular compartment. The result is edema or enlargement of the interstitial space. For example, a rise in BHP in the venous end of the capillary occurs in immobilized individuals with venous stasis.

A decrease in COP also reduces the rate of reabsorption of fluid at the venous end of the capillary. Fluid accumulates in the tissues, with resulting edema. A decrease in COP is often the result of protein depletion. See Table 41–3 for causes of **hypoproteinemia** (low levels of plasma proteins).

An obstruction in the lymphatic system can lead to fluid retention within the interstitial spaces, because fluid is blocked from returning to the venous circulation. For example, lymphedema can occur after a radical mastectomy (surgical removal of a breast), which involves removal of the lymphatic vessels from the axilla. It can also result from certain tropical infestations in which parasites block flow through the lymph nodes.

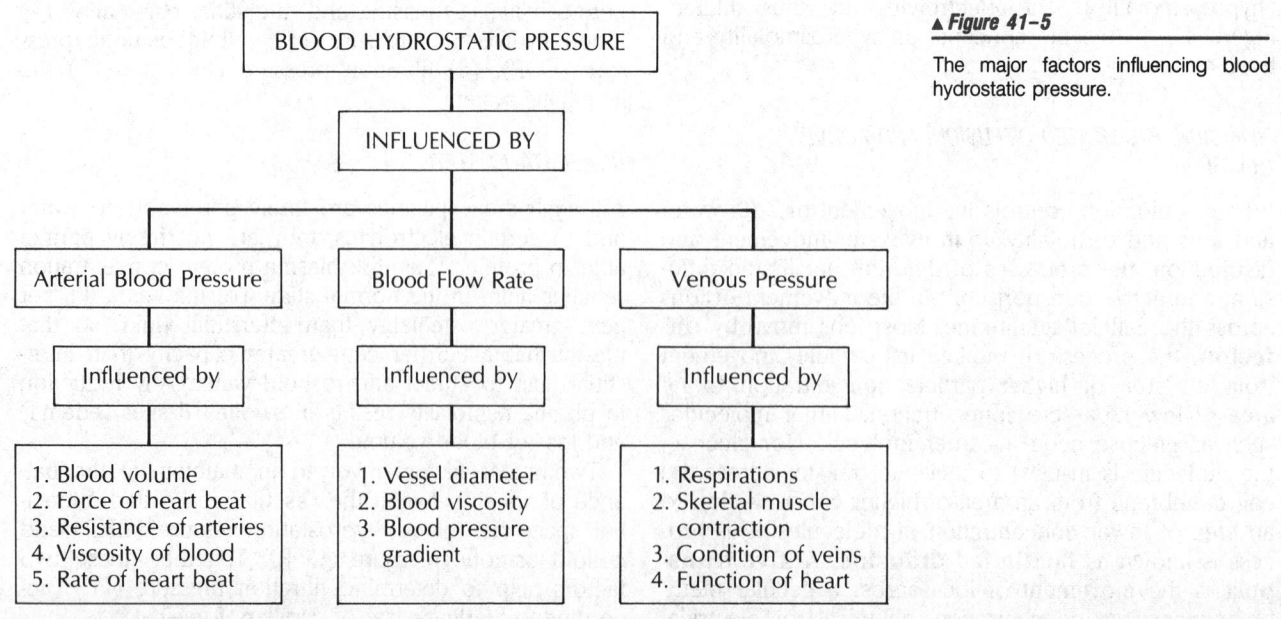

▲ Figure 41–5

The major factors influencing blood hydrostatic pressure.

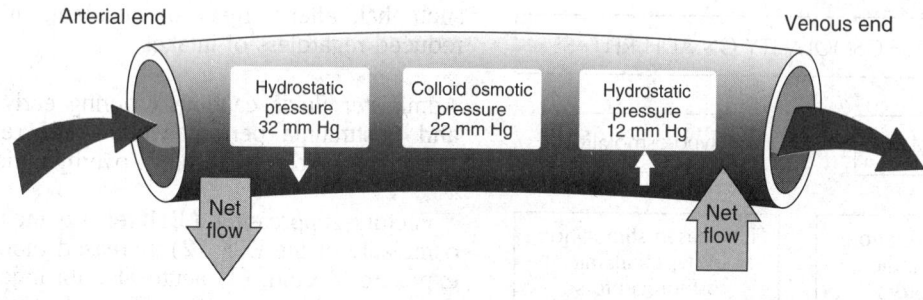

▲ *Figure 41–6*

Pressure differences within the capillary shift fluid. Fluid is pushed out of the capillary into the tissue spaces at the arteriolar end and is pulled back into the capillary from the tissue spaces at the venous end. (Modified from Black, J. M., & Matassarin-Jacobs, E. [1993]. *Luckmann and Sorensen's medical-surgical nursing: A psychophysiologic approach* [4th ed.]. Philadelphia: W. B. Saunders.)

MAJOR MECHANISMS REGULATING FLUID AND ELECTROLYTE BALANCE

Water and electrolyte balance and distribution throughout the body are homeostatically regulated by the neuroendocrine, GI, renal, cardiovascular, and respiratory systems. These body systems maintain water and electrolyte balance by regulating fluid intake and output. Even a minor breakdown in the function of any of these systems can lead to water and electrolyte imbalances.

Neuroendocrine System as a Homeostatic Regulator

The neuroendocrine system regulates fluid volume, fluid osmolality, and electrolyte balance through the production and secretion of hormones. When released into the blood, hormones act on target tissues such as the kidney and the GI tract. Hormones involved in fluid and electrolyte balance include antidiuretic hormone, aldosterone, the thyroid hormones (thyroxin, triiodothyronine, and calcitonin), and parathyroid hormone (PTH).

ANTIDIURETIC HORMONE

As its name implies, antidiuretic hormone (ADH, vasopressin), prevents the body from losing fluid. It opposes (hence the prefix "anti") fluid loss (diuresis).

The following is essential information about ADH:

► function: maintenance of osmolality within normal limits
► stimulus: increased osmolality of ECF
► synthesis: neurosecretory cells of hypothalamus
► site of release: posterior lobe of pituitary gland (neurohypophysis)
► site of action: distal renal tubules and collecting ducts
► action: increased water reabsorption

Hyperosmolality of ECF stimulates osmoreceptors in the hypothalamus, which in turn stimulate release of ADH from storage in the posterior pituitary. Thus, an increase in the osmolality of the ECF causes increased secretion of ADH. Higher blood levels of ADH cause increased reabsorption of water in the kidney and a decreased urinary output results.

The reabsorbed water decreases the hyperosmolality of the blood, and ECF osmolality returns toward normal. As ECF osmolality returns more and more toward normal, the stimulation of hypothalamic osmoreceptors occurs less and less, with ADH release decreasing as a result. Figure 41–7 is a diagrammatic summary of the effect of osmolality on ADH release and inhibition.

The following circumstances stimulate ADH production and release (with resulting water conservation):

► water loss or salt (electrolyte) gain that causes an increase in ECF osmolality
► reduced circulating blood volume
► presence of pain
► administration of certain drugs (e.g., morphine sulfate, barbiturates, anesthetic agents)
► stress: emotional and physiologic (e.g., surgical or accidental trauma, unusual and prolonged physical exertion)

The physiologic reaction to the stress of surgical or accidental trauma is to increase production and release of ADH. Excessive stress appears to activate hypothalamic centers. Consequently, both ADH and adrenocorticotropic hormone (ACTH) are released in large amounts after injury. The action of these hormones is

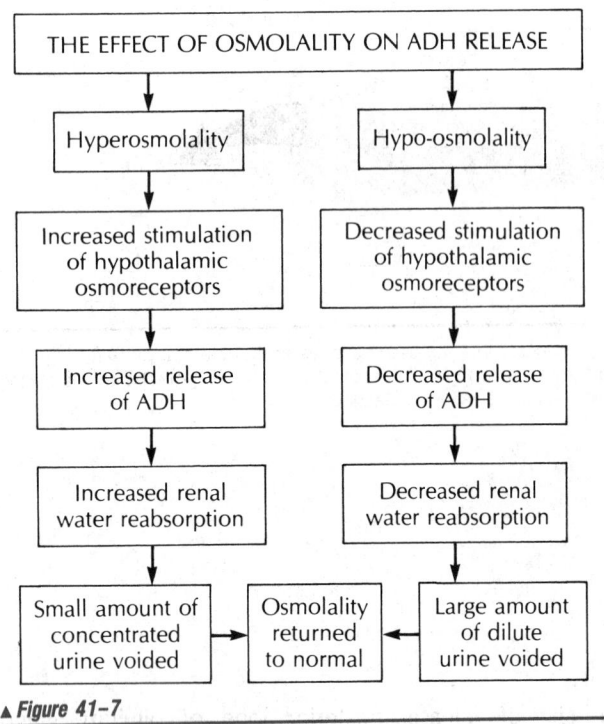

▲ *Figure 41-7*

The effect of osmolality on ADH release and inhibition.

such that, after surgery or accident, urine volume is reduced regardless of intake!

Administer fluids cautiously during early postoperative and posttrauma periods when ADH release is high. "Forcing" fluids can result in overhydration.

Factors suppressing ADH release include (1) hypo-osmolality of the ECF, (2) increased blood volume, (3) exposure to cold, (4) acute alcohol ingestion, and (5) carbon dioxide inhalation. These factors cause an increased urinary output. Diabetes insipidus is a disease caused by inadequate ADH production or secretion or renal resistance to its effect. Signs and symptoms include large amounts of very dilute urine, with resultant extreme thirst and high fluid intake. Figure 41-8 presents a diagrammatic summary of factors affecting ADH release.

ALDOSTERONE

Whereas ADH regulates water reabsorption or excretion, the hormone aldosterone regulates sodium reabsorption and excretion. Because sodium holds fluid in the body (more specifically, in the ECF), aldosterone helps maintain ECF volume. Moreover, aldosterone is a major controlling mechanism for body fluid (ECF) volume because it causes the reabsorption of both sodium

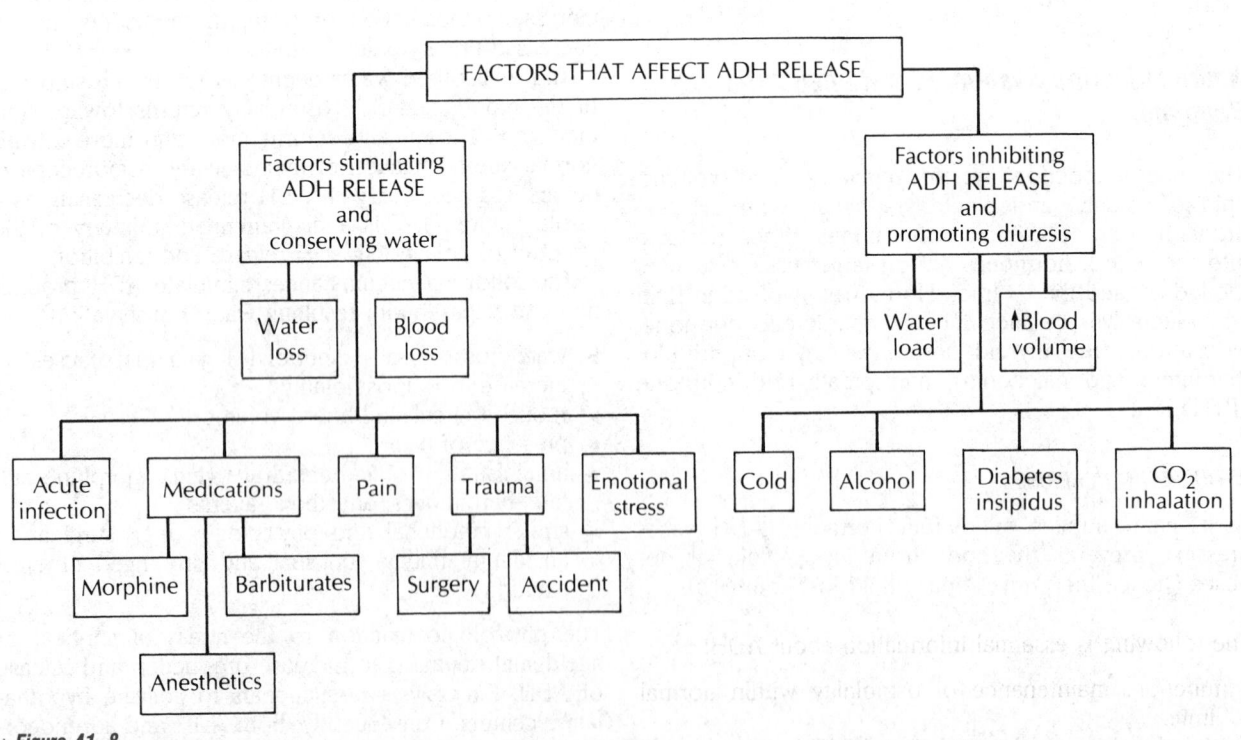

▲ *Figure 41-8*

Factors that stimulate and inhibit the release of ADH.

and water. When aldosterone secretion is increased, sodium is reabsorbed and chloride is passively reabsorbed along with the sodium and water follows along by osmosis. When aldosterone levels decrease, sodium, chloride, and water are all excreted in greater amounts.

The following is essential information about aldosterone:

▶ major function: regulation of ECF volume
▶ stimuli: principally angiotensin II and increased plasma potassium; secondarily, ACTH and decreased plasma sodium
▶ sites of formation and release: zona glomerulosa of adrenal cortex
▶ site of action: distal renal tubules and collecting ducts
▶ action: increased renal reabsorption of sodium and water, facilitation of magnesium excretion in the urine

Aldosterone secretion is stimulated primarily by the renin-angiotensin system. In response to a decrease in blood pressure, renin is secreted by the juxtaglomerular apparatus of the kidney. Renin converts angiotensinogen in the blood to angiotensin I. Angiotensin I is converted by an enzyme from the pulmonary capillaries to angiotensin II, which stimulates the adrenal gland to secrete aldosterone. The following factors stimulate renin release, with consequent formation of angiotensin II, aldosterone secretion, and renal reabsorption of sodium, chloride, and water:

▶ Decreased blood flow through the renal artery, e.g., with decreased ECF volume as during hemorrhage
▶ Decreased sodium load in the renal distal tubules as during severe hyponatremia
▶ Stimulation of renal sympathetic nerves as during a stressful situation

A second major stimulus to the secretion of aldosterone is an increase in the plasma potassium concentration. In addition to causing renal retention of sodium, chloride, and water, aldosterone increases the excretion of potassium in the urine. As aldosterone secretion increases, more potassium is excreted, and the plasma potassium returns to normal. (Remember that sodium, chloride, and water are retained in the process.)

Two minor stimuli that increase aldosterone secretion are a decrease in the plasma sodium concentration and the short-term secretion of very large amounts of ACTH as occur in conditions of severe stress (e.g., physical trauma). Figure 41–9 summarizes the causes and effects of increased aldosterone secretion. An increase in blood pressure causes decreased action of the renin-angiotensin system. Both increased blood pressure and decreased plasma potassium can suppress aldosterone secretion.

FLUID VOLUME REGULATION

Baroreceptors are special nerve endings located in the walls of the large veins, the arteries, and the atria. They

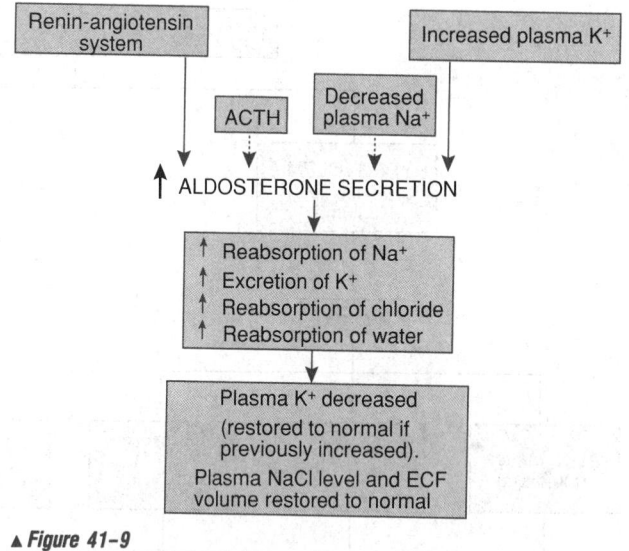

▲ *Figure 41–9*

Causes and effects of increased aldosterone secretion.

respond to changes in pressure inside the blood vessel and send information about ECF volume to certain areas of the brain.

How are these mechanisms stimulated and inhibited? Receptors in the hypothalamus are responsible for stimulating the release of ADH from storage in the posterior pituitary gland. Changes in body fluid osmolality stimulate cells in the lateral preoptic area of the hypothalamus; in turn, these cells trigger the thirst mechanism. Baroreceptor mechanisms and angiotensin II also stimulate thirst. In addition, angiotensin II stimulates the adrenal cortex to secrete aldosterone.

To understand how body fluid volume is regulated, consider the following examples of volume increase and decrease. When circulating fluid volume increases (a condition called **hypervolemia**), ADH and aldosterone secretion is inhibited. As a result, urine output increases. In addition, because the sensation of thirst is absent, the lost volume is not replaced. Thus, body fluid volume returns to normal. When circulating fluid volume decreases significantly (a condition called **hypovolemia**), ADH is released; the thirst mechanism is triggered; and aldosterone is secreted. These measures restore body fluid volume to normal. Figure 41–10 presents a diagrammatic summary of the interrelationship of ADH, aldosterone, thirst, and body fluid volume.

FLUID OSMOLALITY REGULATION

The hypothalamus is the locus of activity for the regulation of body fluid osmolality. The hypothalamus manufactures ADH, which is then stored in the posterior pituitary gland. The hypothalamus also contains osmoreceptors (specialized nerve endings that respond to changes in ECF osmolality), which signal the posterior pituitary gland to release ADH as needed. Increased ECF osmolality causes the osmoreceptors to stimulate

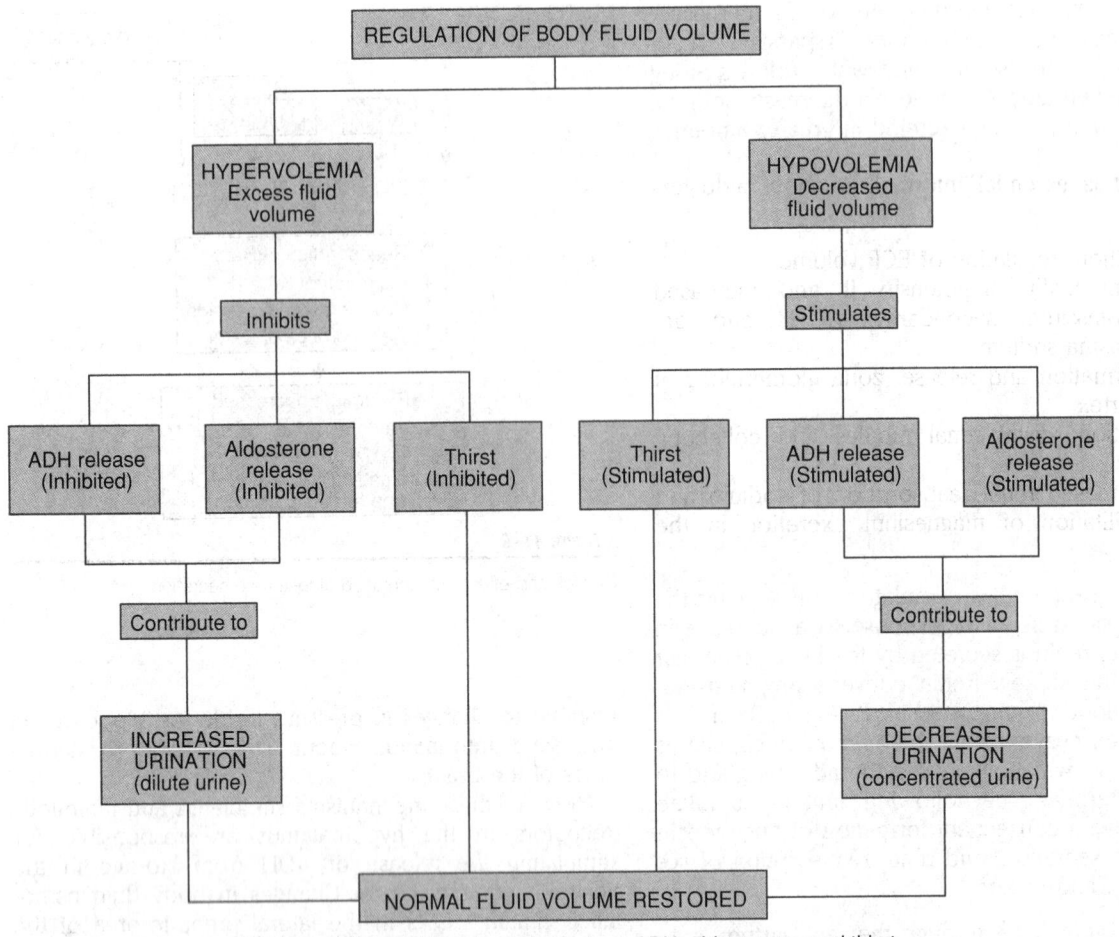

Regulation of body fluid volume depends on ADH, aldosterone, and thirst.

▲ *Figure 41–10*

Regulation of body fluid volume depends on ADH, aldosterone, and thirst.

ADH release. When ECF osmolality decreases, the osmoreceptors inhibit ADH secretion.

The thirst mechanism, a psychophysiologic phenomenon that is not fully understood, also operates to control ECF osmolality. Basically, thirst results from hyperosmolality of the ECF, hypovolemia, and dryness of oral mucous membranes. Hyperosmolality is caused by (1) low water intake, (2) excessive water loss (e.g., through sweating or bleeding), (3) excessive sodium intake, and (4) excessive IV infusion of hypertonic solutions. These changes in osmolality stimulate the thirst mechanism. The opposite set of conditions inhibit the thirst mechanism; reduced thirst is caused by high water intake, water retention, low sodium intake, and excessive infusion of isotonic or hypotonic IV solutions.

Although thirst is an important symptom, the presence or absence of thirst is not always a true indicator of fluid balance because

▶ Edematous individuals may be thirsty, although they appear to be overloaded with fluid. Thirst develops because the blood volume may actually be quite low as a result of movement of a large amount of plasma into interstitial spaces.

▶ A dehydrated person who is comatose may not experience thirst.

▶ A confused, dehydrated individual may be unaware that the urge to drink is the cause of discomfort and may show signs only of agitation.

▶ A person with hypo-osmolality of the ECF will not experience thirst even though the fluid volume of the body is low. Hypo-osmolality inhibits the thirst mechanism.

▶ Thirst may be influenced more by culture than by actual fluid requirements. An individual may be either in a state of fluid balance or in a state of fluid overload and still experience thirst. For example, in American culture, it is customary to drink socially at meals. We consider it impolite not to offer a guest a beverage. Consequently, our drinking habits may at times be more influenced by social custom than by the physiologic need for fluid.

▶ Even a healthy elderly person has a reduced thirst mechanism. This lack of thirst is only one of the contributing factors in dehydration, the most common fluid and electrolyte imbalance in the elderly population.

The neuroendocrine system regulates both body fluid volume and osmolality by means of hormonal production and secretion. Consider normal neuroendocrine response to changes in fluid volume and osmolality in a person who is vigorously exercising. This person is losing a great deal of water and some sodium in the sweat and consequently is losing a certain amount of blood volume. As a result, the receptors in the vascular system respond to the loss of blood volume and relay the message to the brain. These messages are conveyed to the hypothalamus, which then stimulate the release of ADH from the posterior pituitary gland. In this case, the plasma is more concentrated than normal, so fluid is pulled by osmosis from the interstitial and intracellular compartments into the vascular system. In addition, the hyperosmolality of the ECF stimulates osmoreceptors in the hypothalamus, which also contribute to ADH release. With the secretion of ADH, urine volume diminishes, and the urine produced is somewhat concentrated. Thirst occurs in response to a decrease in body fluid volume and an increase in osmolality. Finally, as a result of aldosterone release, any sodium that this individual ingests will be retained, and will help hold fluid within the body. Thus, this person, weary from exercise and possibly pleased with weight loss, may be found resting, having a large cold drink, eating potato chips, and rapidly regaining both fluid and weight!

Now consider someone with fluid overload, after excessive intake of very salty food followed by a great deal of water. The changes that occur in the overhydrated person are the opposite of those present after loss of fluid. In situations of fluid overload, blood and interstitial fluid volumes increase. Volume receptors respond accordingly, and the secretion of ADH and aldosterone decreases. The overhydrated person, then, who has healthy neuroendocrine and renal systems will urinate a large amount of dilute urine. Thirst is also inhibited. As a result, the blood and interstitial fluid volumes are restored to normal.

THYROID AND PARATHYROID HORMONES

The thyroid hormones tetraiodothyronine (thyroxine, or T_4) and triiodothyronine (T_3) are important for normal diuresis. These two hormones increase cardiac output sufficiently for adequate perfusion of the nephron. They also increase the volume of glomerular filtrate and hence urinary output. The hormone calcitonin (or thyrocalcitonin), also produced in the thyroid gland, helps maintain calcium balance by decreasing serum calcium levels if these levels rise.

The parathyroid gland secretes parathyroid hormone (PTH), which controls calcium and phosphate metabolism. This hormone regulates calcium and phosphate ion concentration by (1) increasing resorption of calcium and phosphate from bone, (2) increasing calcium reabsorption by inhibiting phosphate reabsorption from the renal tubule, and (3) increasing calcium and phosphate absorption from the GI tract. Thus, PTH increases serum ionized calcium and depresses serum phosphate. These ions perform many functions in the body; most notably, they maintain normal neuromuscular excitability and energy. The nonionized forms of calcium and phosphate promote rigidity of bones and teeth. The parathyroids also regulate magnesium balance by in-

creasing or decreasing renal tubular reabsorption according to body need.

Gastrointestinal Tract as a Homeostatic Regulator

Under normal conditions, the GI system is the sole route of intake for fluids and electrolytes. Therefore, the GI tract plays a very important part in maintaining fluid and electrolyte balance. The GI tract absorbs fluids from dietary intake. It also absorbs approximately 7 to 9 L of glandular and GI secretions per day. About 100 ml of water are excreted from the bowel daily; the rest is reabsorbed.

Fluids and electrolytes within the intestinal tract are subject to rapid transport across the intestinal mucosa in both directions. Approximately every 90 minutes, a volume of fluid equal to the volume of the body's plasma (approximately 3000 ml in a 70-kg person) passes through the intestinal mucosa. With such a rapid turnover of fluids, it is no wonder that even minor upsets in GI tract function precipitate fluid and electrolyte imbalance.

Renal System as a Homeostatic Regulator

The kidney, one of the most active and complex organs of the body, maintains a homeostatic internal environment by regulating water and electrolytes (including bicarbonate and hydrogen ions). The many functions of the kidney include removal of wastes, regulation of water and electrolytes, vitamin D metabolism, renin synthesis and secretion, and production of the hormone erythropoietin. These functions of the kidney are all related to regulation of fluids, electrolytes, and acid-base balance.

The kidney assists in regulating

▶ ECF volume and osmolality
▶ electrolyte concentration
▶ acid-base balance
▶ erythropoiesis and blood pressure

(For additional information related to the kidney, see Chapter 44 or consult an anatomy and physiology textbook.)

EXTRACELLULAR FLUID VOLUME REGULATION

Because aldosterone acts on the distal tubular cells to increase or decrease the reabsorption of sodium and water from the renal tubules back into the ECF, ECF volume is adjusted by changes in aldosterone secretion. Another factor that influences renal regulation of ECF volume is body posture. Changes in body posture are associated with changes in urine flow and sodium excretion. For example, when an individual first stands up after lying down, urine flow and sodium excretion decrease. If a person has been standing up and then goes to bed, both urine flow and sodium excretion increase. These changes in posture have definite implications for immobilized people. Individuals lying down may initially have a better urinary output than those standing for prolonged periods. Thus, bedrest temporarily facilitates diuresis.

EXTRACELLULAR FLUID OSMOLALITY REGULATION

ADH causes the cells in the renal distal tubules and collecting ducts to reabsorb water from the tubular fluid. Increases and decreases in ADH secretion thus influence the osmolality of ECF by adjusting the reabsorption of water without changing the reabsorption of sodium. By altering the osmolality of ECF, the kidneys indirectly affect the osmolality of ICF. The regulation of osmolality is another way in which the renal system works in conjunction with the neuroendocrine system.

ELECTROLYTE CONCENTRATION REGULATION

Many of the electrolytes that pass through the kidney's glomerulus into the renal tubules are returned to the bloodstream by the tubular cells. Some electrolytes are also secreted into the tubular fluid. By altering the amounts of electrolytes excreted in the urine, the kidney plays a major role in the regulation of electrolyte concentrations in ECF and, indirectly, in ICF as well. Many factors, including several hormones, influence electrolyte excretion by the kidneys. The kidneys (which excrete 80 per cent to 90 per cent of the potassium) conserve potassium when cellular potassium becomes depleted.

HYDROGEN/BICARBONATE ION BALANCE

One vital role of the kidney is to maintain blood at the slightly alkaline pH of 7.35 to 7.45. The kidney controls pH by controlling the rate at which hydrogen and bicarbonate ions are excreted and reabsorbed from the distal and collecting renal tubules.

Kidney function also regulates urine concentration and volume. The ability of the kidney to concentrate urine is a good indicator of both kidney function and body fluid status. Urine specific gravity measures the concentration of urine and thus the kidneys' concentrating ability. The normal range is 1.003 to 1.030. When a person has healthy renal function, the degree of dehydration or overhydration can be determined by urine specific gravity. That is, a dehydrated person will have low volume output and high specific gravity, and an overhydrated person will have high volume output and low urine specific gravity.

IMPAIRMENT OF RENAL FUNCTION

Recall that ADH normally results in the reabsorption of water after trauma or surgery. In people with certain renal, pituitary, or central nervous system diseases, this mechanism will not be operative; consequently, they may lose more fluid than they should at this critical time.

In addition to renal disease, other serious illnesses —for example, congestive heart failure, hypertension, diabetes mellitus, diabetes insipidus, and disorders of the adrenal cortex—may impair the functioning of the nephron. In diseases unrelated to the kidney, individuals may be subject to dehydration because of the kidney's inability to concentrate urine. Concentrating ability is also markedly altered in the very young and the elderly populations.

Cardiovascular System as a Homeostatic Regulator

The heart also plays an important role in the control of fluid balance. It functions as an endocrine gland by releasing a hormone known as atrial natriuretic peptide (ANP) whenever the atrial cells are distended. Conditions that cause fluid overload (e.g., congestive heart failure and liver or renal disease), vasoconstriction (e.g., hypertension, stress, pain), or direct cardiac alterations (e.g., cardiac inflammatory processes, ischemia, infarction, valve disease, atrial dysrhythmias) can increase ANP secretion. The main effect of ANP release is to oppose the effects of the renin-angiotensin-aldosterone system. The systemic results include (1) vasodilation (arterioles and venules), (2) natriuresis (sodium excretion), and (3) diuresis.[7,43]

ACID-BASE BALANCE

The cation hydrogen (H^+, the free hydrogen ion) is the active component of most acids. The greater the amount of hydrogen present in a solution, the more acidic the solution. Conversely, the lower the amount of hydrogen present in a solution, the less acidic—or more alkaline—the solution.

An **acid,** by definition, is a hydrogen ion (proton) donor. An acid loses hydrogen ions to a base, thereby neutralizing or lessening the strength of the base. On the other hand, a **base** is a hydrogen ion (proton) acceptor. A base accepts hydrogen ions from an acid, thereby causing the acid to become weaker. For example, if strong acid such as hydrochloric acid is added to a strong base such as sodium bicarbonate, the result is a weaker acid (carbonic acid) and a neutral salt (sodium chloride):

$$HCl \quad + \quad NaHCO_3 \quad \rightleftharpoons$$

hydrochloric acid   sodium bicarbonate
(strong acid)   (strong buffer base)

$$H_2CO_3 \quad + \quad NaCl$$

carbonic acid   sodium chloride
(weak acid)   (neutral salt)

Hydrogen ions, which play a vital role in the regulation of numerous biochemical and metabolic activities (see Box 41–6), are found in both ICF and ECF. Hydrogen ions are normally present in ECF in a concentration between 0.0000001 and 0.00000001 gm/L. Because hydrogen circulates in the body fluids in such minute amounts, the hydrogen ion concentration of the body fluids (and of any solution) is measured in pH values rather than in grams per liter.

pH is a measure of the acidity or alkalinity of a solution.

Technically, pH is chemical shorthand for the negative logarithm of the hydrogen ion concentration. Neutral pH is a hydrogen concentration of 0.0000001 gm/L, which is 10^{-7} gm/L, or a pH of 7. The pH scale extends from 0 to 14, with 7 being neutral. For each pH interval, there is a 10-fold difference in the concentration of hydrogen in a solution. The higher the pH, the lower the hydrogen concentration in a solution. The lower the pH, the higher the hydrogen concentration in a solution. A solution with a pH that is less than 7 is acidic; when the pH is greater than 7, the solution is alkaline.

Different body fluids have different pH values. Normal ranges for the pH of various body fluids are as follows:

Blood	7.35–7.45
ICF	6.9–7.2
Urine	averages 6.0
Cerebrospinal fluid	7.35–7.45
Gastric juice	1.0–2.0
Bile	5.0–6.0

Note that the blood and cerebrospinal fluid are slightly alkaline, whereas the urine is usually acidic. Many waste by-products formed during metabolism are acids. Excretion of these acids in the urine keeps the blood alkaline and the urine acidic. An abnormal blood pH indicates that the body is in a state of acid-base imbalance.

Acidosis exists when the blood pH drops below 7.35. The hydrogen concentration is above normal; or the base level is below normal. **Alkalosis** exists when the blood pH rises above 7.45. The hydrogen concentration is below normal, or the blood base level is above normal. The range of blood pH compatible with life is from 6.8 to 7.8 (a 10-fold difference in the number of hydrogen ions in the blood).

Because the blood must remain alkaline and because our bodies produce sizable quantities of acid, the body must be able to control hydrogen concentration and maintain pH within the narrow range that is compatible with life. Figure 41–11 shows this narrow range.

Mechanisms of Acid-base Regulation

The four regulatory systems that control pH balance are (in order of activation) (1) buffer systems, (2) lungs, (3) cells, and (4) kidneys. Buffers are usually referred to as chemical regulators; the cells are called biologic regulators; the lungs and kidneys are considered physiologic regulators. Each of these vital homeostatic regulatory systems has a specific role.

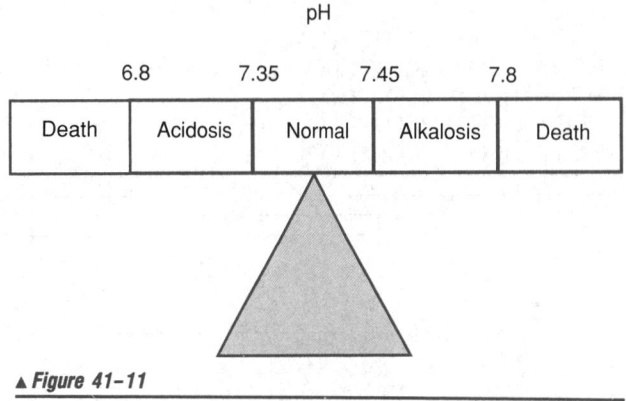

▲ *Figure 41–11*

Note the narrow range of pH—life vs. death.

BLOOD BUFFERS AS CHEMICAL REGULATORS OF ACID-BASE BALANCE

Blood buffers are chemicals that can donate or accept hydrogen ions as needed to maintain arterial blood pH between 7.35 and 7.45. This buffer action protects the body against dangerous fluctuations of hydrogen concentration when excess acids or alkali are added to body fluids. Within the body, the major buffer system is the base bicarbonate (HCO_3^-)/carbonic acid (H_2CO_3) system. This system acts to regulate hydrogen concentration of body fluids by maintaining a ratio of 20 parts base bicarbonate to 1 part carbonic acid (Fig. 41–12). If this ratio changes, acidosis or alkalosis results.

A chemical buffer system has the advantage of reacting immediately to acid or alkali excesses. Its disadvantage is that it cannot sustain regulation. For more powerful and longer lasting regulatory action, the body must rely on the lungs and kidneys to maintain acid-base balance. The lungs and kidneys act to regulate the hydrogen ions that dissociate from the body's chemical buffer system. This principle is illustrated in the following equation:

$$CO_2 + H_2O \rightleftharpoons H_2CO_3 \rightleftharpoons$$

carbon dioxide (regulated by lungs)   water   carbonic acid

$$H^+ + HCO_3^-$$

hydrogen ion   bicarbonate ion (regulated by kidneys)

Note that the lungs regulate acid by controlling carbon dioxide, whereas the kidneys normally regulate acid by controlling bicarbonate.

Other buffer systems include the phosphate buffer and protein buffer systems. Each has an acid-base component and chemically combines with a strong acid or strong base to weaken its effects, much as in the HCO_3^-/H_2CO_3 buffer system. The phosphate buffer

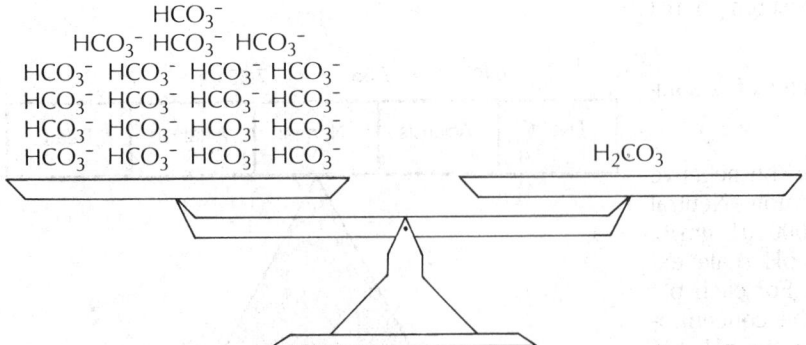

Twenty parts of bicarbonate to one part of carbonic acid in the blood are necessary to maintain normal acid-base balance.

system produces its main effect in the cell and in the tubules of the kidney. Protein buffers are found in the cell and in the plasma. Most of the protein buffering is at the cell level. The most familiar protein buffer is the hemoglobin molecule in the red blood cell (RBC). Hemoglobin promotes the movement of chloride ions across the RBC membrane in exchange for the bicarbonate ions; this mechanism is known as the chloride shift. The chloride-bicarbonate exchange is affected by oxygen levels and overall acid-base balance.

LUNGS AS PHYSIOLOGIC REGULATORS OF ACID-BASE BALANCE

The lungs constitute the second line of defense against acid-base imbalances. The respiratory system (including the neurologic centers that regulate respiration) controls the H_2CO_3 component of the HCO_3^-/H_2CO_3 buffer system. The lungs regulate the carbonic acid level by altering the rate and depth of respiration. If the blood has an acid overload, the rate and depth of respiration increase, enabling the person to "blow off" excess carbon dioxide. The weak carbonic acid dissociates into carbon dioxide, which is blown off by the lungs, and water which is excreted through the kidneys:

$$H_2CO_3 \longrightarrow CO_2 + H_2O$$

In a reverse process, a base overload causes the rate of respiration to decrease, so that carbon dioxide is retained and combines with water, which increases the carbonic acid part of the ratio:

$$CO_2 + H_2O \longrightarrow H_2CO_3$$

Healthy lungs are rapid regulators, partially correcting acid-base irregularities within minutes.

CELLS AS BIOLOGIC REGULATORS OF ACID-BASE BALANCE

The cells are capable of admitting or releasing excess hydrogen ions. For example, with the potassium buffer system, excess hydrogen ions move to the cell from the ECF. When they cross the cell membrane, they must be exchanged for ions of the same charge. Therefore, in acidosis, hydrogen ions move from the plasma into the cell and potassium moves from the cell into the plasma. The opposite occurs in alkalosis. In

this way, the cells maintain electrical neutrality. Compared with the chemical buffer systems and the lungs, the cells are slow regulators, requiring at least 2 hours to control shifts in hydrogen concentration. Because the potassium buffer alters potassium levels in the blood, this type of buffering must be limited if death from severe potassium imbalance is to be prevented. Fortunately, potassium regulation is not the last line of defense.

KIDNEYS AS PHYSIOLOGIC REGULATORS OF ACID-BASE BALANCE

The renal system constitutes the fourth line of defense against acid-base imbalance. The kidneys regulate HCO_3^- in the HCO_3^-/H_2CO_3 buffer system and HPO_4^- in the phosphate (HPO_4^-/H_2PO_4) buffer system. At the same time, they also eliminate metabolic acid (e.g., lactic acid and all acids except carbonic acid), whereas the lungs regulate carbonic acid. To compensate for acid-base imbalances, the kidneys alter the rate of excretion of hydrogen and bicarbonate ions in the urine. In alkalosis, the kidneys retain hydrogen ions and excrete bicarbonate ions. In acidosis, the kidneys retain bicarbonate and excrete hydrogen ions. The renal system is the slowest of all the regulating systems, taking from a few hours to several days to compensate for acid-base imbalances.

Failure of Acid-base Regulation

Maintenance of acid-base balance depends on the healthy functioning of the kidneys, lungs, cells, and brain. Normally, these remarkable organs can adjust swiftly and efficiently to fluctuations in hydrogen concentration. When the body is subjected to (1) unusually heavy loads of acid or alkali or (2) the development of renal, respiratory, or brain disease, however, these organs can fail to regulate acid-base balance, and imbalances result. The two major types of imbalances are acidosis and alkalosis.

Acidosis and alkalosis are further classified as metabolic or respiratory. Respiratory imbalances are caused by changes in the pulmonary system. Any imbalance not caused by the pulmonary system is a metabolic imbalance. Table 41–3 describes all four pH imbalances.

Risk Factors for Fluid, Electrolyte, and Acid-base Imbalances

Many variables, conditions, and diseases increase a person's risk for fluid, electrolyte, or acid-base imbalance.

LIFE SPAN

The fluid distribution varies across the life span (see Table 41–1). Because of their higher metabolic rate, less efficient fluid management by immature kidneys, and proportionately greater body surface area compared with body weight, children and infants are at greater risk for fluid imbalances. Hormonal changes and growth demands can challenge adolescents' fluid and electrolyte regulatory systems. Children's compensatory responses to illness are less stable; fevers tend to be higher and last longer.

Pregnancy influences the fluid and electrolyte status throughout different phases of the developing fetus. Common changes include a rise in aldosterone levels, an increase in fluid pressures, and fluid shifting. Extra fluid is retained to meet the needs of the developing fetus and to provide for amniotic fluid development, increased blood volume needs, and changes in mammillary and uterine tissues.

The elderly are at high risk for fluid deficit, fluid excess, and electrolyte imbalances. Their kidneys often lose the ability to concentrate urine, which leads to fluid losses. Even the healthy elderly experience diminished thirst, placing them at risk for fluid deficit. Higher incidences of chronic diseases also increase their susceptibility to imbalances.

BODY SIZE

Because fat cells contain little water, persons with a greater level of body fat are at a greater risk for fluid deficit. Women have proportionately more fat than men; therefore, they are at higher risk for fluid deficit.

ENVIRONMENTAL TEMPERATURE

Changes in environmental temperature and relative humidity affect fluid and electrolyte balance as a result of the body's attempt to compensate. When environmental temperatures exceed 29.7 °C, the body responds by promoting heat loss through peripheral vasodilation, sensible water loss (sweating), and increased aldosterone secretion to compensate for the fluid and sodium losses. Even water loss as minimal as 1.2 per cent has been found to impair thermoregulation. Increased heart rates, increased body temperatures, and decreased plasma volumes have been found with as little as a 2 per cent decrease in body weight secondary to fluid loss. Temperatures as low as 16.5 °C with humidity levels of 97 per cent and as high as 33 °C with humidity levels of 50 per cent have caused fatal heat strokes in high school football players.[68] Both high ambient temperatures and high humidities limit the thermoregulatory compensatory potentials.

LIFESTYLE

Lifestyle can directly or indirectly affect fluid and electrolyte balance. A person's occupation may greatly influence dietary intake through availability of healthy foods or time allotted for eating three balanced meals a day, through stress associated with the occupation, or through environmental hazards that increase risk for imbalance (e.g., working outdoors).

A balanced diet containing fluids and the recommended proportions of carbohydrates, fats, and proteins is necessary to maintain fluid, electrolyte, and acid-base balance. Alterations in intake (deficits or excesses) can place a person at risk for imbalances. Persons with altered health states (e.g., heart, kidney, lung, liver, GI, pancreatic, or pituitary disease) are even at greater risk for acid-base imbalance. Special diets predispose individuals to imbalances because they lessen intake of certain types of foods and seasonings. A low-sodium diet, for example, is often prescribed for people with cardiovascular disease or kidney disease. The diet helps control edema or hypertension, but severe sodium restriction can also result in saline deficit, especially if individuals are taking diuretics at the same time. Low-carbohydrate/high-protein diets, popular in the treatment of obesity, can result in metabolic acidosis because of the accumulation of ketones in the blood and urine. (See Chapter 42 for more information about specific foods for special dietary needs.)

Conditions resulting in stress responses precipitate sympathetic hormonal release, resulting in increased levels of epinephrine, norepinephrine, and corticosteroids. Aldosterone and ADH secretion also increase, resulting in increased sodium and water reabsorption. Exercise can be a stressor. The amount of sweat produced during exercise increases relative to work rate and expenditure of energy, the person's body weight, the amount of protective clothing, and the ambient temperature. Sweating will continue up to the point of heat stroke. The efficiency of the sweating mechanism improves with conditioning. Heat acclimatization in the adult can be achieved through 8 to 12 days of intense 30-minute exercise periods. This regimen, however, only acclimatizes the person to the temperature experienced during exercise trials. Although acclimatization reduces the risk of hyperthermic insult, it is of vital importance to ensure fluid and electrolyte balance through adequate fluid replacement.

The loss of electrolytes through sweat is the greatest during the early phase of exercise. Prolonged exercise stimulates a compensatory release of aldosterone, which decreases the amount of sodium loss. Therefore, with prolonged exercise, fluid continues to be lost, with little loss of electrolytes. Potassium and magnesium losses are insignificant, whereas sodium losses can lead to hyponatremia with extensive fluid losses (greater than 5 L per day). Hyponatremia (inadequate levels of sodium) may occur during the early stages of acclimatization or during prolonged exposure to exercise in heat or high humidity.[68]

The greatest risk factor for heat illness is, therefore, fluid loss. Rapid replacement of boluses of fluid to preexercise levels has been found to increase the amount of fluid only in the GI tract and kidneys and not in the plasma. Current recommendations to decrease the risk of heat stroke secondary to the dehydration of exercise include (1) avoiding diuretics, which predispose to fluid and electrolyte alterations, (2) wearing appropriate clothing during exercise, because excess clothing reduces the exposed evaporative surface areas, (3) following conditioning protocols (the early phases of an exercise program are a time of increased risk), (4) using more caution if obese because adipose tissues have higher tissue temperatures and obesity impairs the sweating mechanism, (5) using more caution in children because they have less efficient thermoregulation, decreased sweat output, and a slower rate of acclimatization, and (6) using more caution with clients who are taking drugs that interfere with thermoregulation (e.g., thyroid hormone, amphetamines, haloperidol, antihistamines, anticholinergics, phenothiazines, and benztropine mesylate).[68]

ALTERATIONS IN HEALTH

Diarrhea is a common problem that varies greatly in severity from mild to life threatening. The rapid movement of the fecal contents through the intestine results in poor absorption of nutrients, water, and electrolytes. Diarrhea results in serum losses of sodium (hyponatremia), chloride (hypochloremia), potassium (hypokalemia), water (dehydration), and base (acidosis). Emotional stress, intestinal infections, irritating foods (e.g., fried, greasy, or spicy), certain drugs, fecal impactions, ulcerative colitis, carcinoma, and certain neurologic diseases are among the more common causes of diarrhea.

Vomiting is another common problem that accompanies numerous disorders. Vomiting results in serum losses of chloride (greatest amount), sodium (next greatest in amount), and potassium (least in amount but greatest in importance). It can also result in dehydration and alkalosis. Causes include emotional stress, drugs (e.g., morphine sulfate, meperidine, codeine sulfate), viral infections, febrile conditions, excessive alcohol intake, pain, surgery, motion sickness, pregnancy, and obstruction of the GI tract.

A fever accompanies most infectious and toxic disorders. Fever may also complicate blood diseases (e.g., anemia and leukemia), some central nervous disorders (e.g., head and spinal cord injuries), cancerous tumors, heat stroke, serum sickness, and allergy. Furthermore, fever may be a side effect of some drugs (e.g., barbiturates, morphine, and phenytoin). Prolonged fever can result in increased fluid loss through the skin (sensible perspiration or sweating) and the lungs with rapid respirations (tachypnea).

Children and the elderly are particularly vulnerable to the rapid development of dehydration (e.g., with fever, vomiting, diarrhea). The younger the child, the greater the risk.

Edema (excess interstitial fluid) is a symptom of many common diseases, among them congestive heart failure, hypertension, preeclampsia, burns, trauma, allergic reactions, malnutrition, kidney disease, and liver disorders. Edema can result in ECF volume deficit (in the vascular compartment), or it may accompany ECF volume excess. The treatment of edema can lead to imbalances.

Third-space accumulation (third spacing) is the abnormal accumulation of fluid and electrolytes (including protein) within a body space that is not normally a fluid compartment. Ascites is an example of third spacing in the abdominal cavity. Ascites is a complication of many conditions, including cirrhosis, congestive heart failure, kidney disease, and an abdominal tumor growth. With ascites, as much as 20 L of fluid can accumulate in a person's abdominal cavity. Other examples of third spacing include fluid accumulation in the lungs (as with pneumonia) and under the skin (as with blisters).

Hemorrhage (bleeding that can result in depletion of ICF, ECF, and electrolytes) may follow severe burns, serious accidents, surgery, and childbirth. In addition, persons who suffer from peptic ulcers, cancer, tuberculosis, esophageal varices, and clotting disorders may also experience hemorrhage.

Persons with draining wounds (e.g., burns, eviscerated wounds, open pressure ulcers) can lose a considerable amount of water and electrolytes (including protein).

MEDICAL TREATMENTS

Certain medical treatments also have the potential to cause imbalances. These are iatrogenic (treatment-induced) imbalances.

Persons receiving gastric or intestinal suction, whether it is implemented to promote healing after gastric or intestinal surgery or to remove secretions because of a bowel obstruction or ileus, are at risk for water, electrolyte, and acid-base imbalances. See Table 41-4 for comparison of electrolyte composition in common secretions and excretions.

IV solutions have the potential to cause imbalances. See Table 41-5 for review of the precautions and risk factors of commonly prescribed IV solutions. Many medications can place a person at risk for imbalances. In particular, you should anticipate risk for imbalances in persons who are taking medications specifically designed to alter acid-base levels (e.g., acidifiers, antacids), to replace or alter electrolytes (e.g., sodium, chloride, potassium, magnesium, calcium, phosphate), to alter fluid excretion in the kidney (e.g., diuretics), to alter bowel elimination (e.g., laxatives, cathartics), or to alter neuroendocrine response (e.g., hormones, lithium). Other therapies may involve drugs with side effects that alter water, electrolyte, or acid-base balance. People rarely suffer from only one imbalance; most have a mixture of imbalances. Furthermore, few individuals display all the classic symptoms for each imbalance described in Table 41-6.

ASSESSMENT

Accurate diagnosis depends on a careful assessment of fluid and electrolyte status. Assessment involves data

Text continued on page 1033

TABLE 41-4. Comparison of Electrolyte Composition in Common Secretions/Excretions*

Fluid	Na⁺	K⁺	Cl⁻	HCO₃⁻	H⁺
Plasma	135–145	3.5–5.0	98–106	25–29	pH 7.35–7.45
Gastric Secretions	55–100	10–15	120	5–10	90
Pancreatic Juices	145–160	5	65–90	50–80	—
Bile	130–145	5–9	75–100	10–45	—
Ileum	125	10–80	55	60	—
Sweat					
Insensible	8	10	15	—	—
Sensible	10–80	6	5–85	—	—

Abbreviations: Na⁺, sodium; K⁺, potassium; Cl⁻, chloride; HCO₃⁻, bicarbonate; H⁺, hydrogen.
* These levels may vary depending on the physiologic state of the body.

TABLE 41-5. Commonly Used Intravenous Solutions

IV Solution	Tonicity	Rationale	Precautions/Risks
0.9% saline (NS)	Isotonic (310 mEq/L)	Adds saline in normal physiologic amounts; expands ECF without changing osmolality; to prime IV catheter before and flush after transfusion	Fluid excess
0.45% saline (half normal)/0.2% saline (quarter strength)	Hypotonic (<250 mEq/L)	Adds fluids; adds some Na⁺	Hyponatremia: water excess (give slowly to prevent sudden ICF shift)
5% Dextrose (D₅W)	Hypotonic after entry into plasma (glucose enters cells, leaving only water in plasma)	Adds water; adds only enough calories to prevent ketosis (714 Kcal/L)	Hyponatremia; hypokalemia
5% D/0.9% NS	Isotonic after entry into plasma	Adds saline without changing tonicity; adds 714 Kcal/L; expands ECF	Fluid excess
5% D/0.45% saline/ 5% D/0.2% saline	Hypotonic after entry into plasma	Adds calories, fluid, and some Na⁺	Hyponatremia; water excess
Lactated Ringer's	Isotonic	Replaces fluid loss (replaces Na⁺, K⁺, Ca⁺⁺, Cl⁻, and lactate); treats metabolic acidosis (except lactic acidosis)	Fluid excess
Ringer's	Isotonic	Replaces fluid and same electrolytes as lactated Ringer's except no lactate	Fluid excess
3% or 5% saline	Hypertonic (>375 mEq/L)	Replace severe sodium losses	Hypernatremia, ECF excess, pulmonary edema, phlebitis at IV site; give slowly to prevent cellular dehydration
IV with KCL 40–80 mEq/day >80 mEq/day		K⁺ maintenance requirement K⁺ replacement therapy	Hyperkalemia, especially in decreased renal output; if IV bag not agitated after added, can cause cardiac arrest; if small vein, phlebitis more likely to result

Abbreviations: IV, intravenous; NS, normal saline; ECF, extracellular fluid; D5W, 5% dextrose/water; Na⁺, sodium; ICF, intracellular fluid; D, dextrose; K⁺, potassium; Ca⁺⁺, calcium; Cl⁻, chloride; KCl, potassium chloride.

TABLE 41-6. Nursing Process Applied to Fluid and Electrolyte Imbalances

Assessment Data (grouped by systems)	Outcome Criteria	Nursing Interventions
Fluid Volume Deficit		

Integumentary/mucous membranes: dry mouth; dry, sticky mucous membranes; longitudinal wrinkles on tongue; poor skin turgor (see Fig. 42–13)

Cardiovascular: weak, rapid pulse; standing systolic BP lower than lying BP (difference is ≥ 10 mm Hg); peripheral vein filling > 5 seconds (see Fig. 42–14); syncope; flat neck veins in supine position

Musculoskeletal: muscle weakness

Digestive: decreased number of stools, decreased moisture in stools, nausea

Urinary: oliguria

Neurologic (if ICF deficit): thirst, headache, fever, change in cerebral function (restlessness, delirium, confusion, stupor)

General: fatigue, weight loss unless masked by third spacing or edema

Infant: depressed fontanels

Lab findings: increased urine specific gravity (1.030 or >) (accurate only if renal function normal), increased serum osmolality AEB, increased serum Na^+, increased Hct, increased Hgb

Shows improved fluid balance in 48 hours (time may vary) AEB:
1. intake and output balance within 200 ml
2. reports of decreased thirst
3. presence of moist mucous membranes
4. urinary output > 30 ml/hour
5. weight gain 1–2 lbs
6. absence of confusion
7. peripheral vein filling < 5 seconds
8. vital signs WNL for age

1. Increase fluid intake PO to meet maintenance needs (2400 ml/day) and replacement needs (replace losses).
2. Provide IV or NG fluid replacement as ordered by physician.
3. Monitor lab results: Na^+, Hgb, Hct for serum or urine osmolality; do urine specific gravity every 8 hours for urine osmolality.
4. Monitor I & O and record every 8 hours (hourly if output < 30 ml/hour).
5. Validate with person if change in thirst.
6. Assess mucous membranes every 8 hours.
7. Weigh daily: 1 kg weight change = 1 L of fluid loss or gain (1 kg = 1 L).
8. Assess level of cerebral function. If cerebral signs are present, use safety measures such as elevated side rails, low bed position, and night-lights.
9. Avoid increasing ICP if cerebral signs present (e.g., prevent hypoxia, no neck flexion, instruct not to strain at stool or hold breath).
10. Every 8 hours: Assess mucous membranes where cheeks and gums meet, assess peripheral vein filling and neck veins, and take BP lying and standing.
11. Assess vital signs every 4 to 8 hours or more often as indicated by data.

| **Fluid Volume Excess** | | |

Cardiovascular: increased BP; rapid, bounding pulse; S_3 gallop, peripheral vein emptying > 5 seconds; neck vein distention

Respiratory: rales (crackles), dyspnea, pleural effusion, pulmonary edema

Musculoskeletal: muscle weakness

Digestive: nausea, vomiting

Urinary: diuresis (unless excess is due to lack of output)

Neurologic (if ICF excess): cerebral symptoms, headache, confusion, convulsions, coma

General: edema, rapid weight gain, third spacing (ascites, pleural effusion)

Infant: bulging fontanels

Lab findings: decreased serum Na^+, decreased urine specific gravity (accurate only if renal function nor-

In 48 hours (time may vary) shows fluid volume decrease AEB:
1. leg edema decrease (e.g., from 4+ to 2+)
2. decrease in rales (crackles) to only lung bases
3. weight loss > 2 lbs
4. peripheral vein emptying ≤ 5 seconds
5. absence of confusion, seizures
6. no neck distention when HOB elevated 45 degrees
7. vital signs WNL for age
8. no dyspnea at rest or with exertion

1. Restrict fluid intake (oral and IV) to amount ordered by physician.
2. Administer diuretics as ordered.
3. Provide low-sodium diet, as ordered, if sodium is retained.
4. Administer medication as ordered to reduce workload on heart.
5. Monitor lab: Na^+, Hgb, Hct for serum osmolality; assess specific gravity every 8 hours for urine osmolality.
6. Assess dependent edema every 8 hours.
7. Assess lung sounds every 4–8 hours.
8. Weigh daily before breakfast, using same scales and clothing each day
9. Assess peripheral vein emptying every 8 hours.
10. Additional nursing interventions may in-

TABLE 41-6. Nursing Process Applied to Fluid and Electrolyte Imbalances Continued

Assessment Data (grouped by systems)	Outcome Criteria	Nursing Interventions

Fluid Volume Excess

mal), decreased serum osmolality, decreased Hct and Hgb		clude the following (depending on cause and expected outcome): a. Assess level of cerebral function. b. Provide safety measures: elevate side rails; use low bed position and night-light. If client is weak, assist with activity. c. Avoid increasing ICP if cerebral signs present. d. Provide seizure precautions: padded side rails, airway at bedside. e. Assess neck veins every 8 hours. f. Assess vital signs every 4 to 8 hours or more often as indicated by data. g. Assess heart sounds every 8 hours. h. Record I & O every 8 hours. i. Assess for dyspnea at rest or with exertion or orthopnea. j. Use IV pump or minidrip IV tubing to limit fluid intake. k. Elevate HOB 30–45 degrees if not contraindicated (improves cerebral function by increasing jugular venous return and decreases workload on heart from excess fluid by decreasing venous return) 11. Use minimal amounts of water to dissolve crushed medications.

Saline Deficit

Assessment Data	Outcome Criteria	Nursing Interventions
Cardiovascular: orthostatic hypotension; rapid, thready, weak pulse; decrease in fullness of neck and hand veins Respiratory: rapid respirations Musculoskeletal: muscle weakness Digestive: nausea, vomiting, diarrhea Urinary: oliguria, anuria Neurologic: hypothermia, absence of thirst, confusion, stupor, convulsions General: fatigue, weight loss Lab findings: $Na^+ < 135$ mEq/L, $Cl^- < 98$ mEq/L, serum osmolality < 285 mOsm/kg	In 48 hours (time may vary) saline level shows increase AEB: AEB: 1. serum $Na^+ > 135$ mEq/L 2. serum $Cl^- > 98$ mEq/L 3. serum osmolality > 285 mOsm/kg 4. strong, full regular pulse between 60 and 100 5. peripheral vein filling ≤ 5 seconds 6. vital signs WNL for age 7. weight gain 1–2 lbs 8. absence of confusion and seizures	1. Monitor person on low-Na^+ diet and diuretics very closely for this deficit. 2. Monitor labs: Na^+, Cl^-, serum osmolality. 3. Administer IVs with NaCl as ordered. 4. Irrigate NG tubes only with isotonic solutions (e.g., with .9 NS). 5. Restrict H_2O intake to level specified by physician. 6. Give ice chips (only enough to moisten mucous membranes if NG tube connected to suction; no water orally). 7. Give no more than three enemas in a row without questioning physician. 8. Assess vital signs every 4 to 8 hours. 9. Record I & O every 8 hours. 10. Weigh daily. 11. Assess peripheral vein filling every 8 hours. 12. Provide safety precautions: Monitor for confusion; use side rails, low bed positions, night-lights. If convulsions probable, use padded side rails, keep airway at bedside. If client is weak, assist with activity.

Table continued on following page

TABLE 41-6. Nursing Process Applied to Fluid and Electrolyte Imbalances Continued

Assessment Data (grouped by systems)	Outcome Criteria	Nursing Interventions
Saline Excess		
Cardiovascular: rapid, bounding pulse; S_3 gallop; increased BP; peripheral vein emptying > 5 seconds; neck vein distention Respiratory: dyspnea, rales (crackles), pulmonary edema, pleural effusion Musculoskeletal: muscular weakness Urinary: oliguria, anuria Neurologic: fever, confusion, restlessness General: pitting edema, puffy eyelids, ascites, weight gain Lab findings: Na^+ > 145 mEq/L, Cl^- > 106 mEq/L, serum osmolality > 295 mOsm/kg	In 48 hours (time may vary) shows NaCl level decrease AEB: 1. serum Na^+ < 145 mEq/L 2. serum Cl^- < 106 mEq/L 3. serum osmolality < 295 mOsm/kg 4. pulse 60–100, not bounding 5. peripheral vein emptying < 5 seconds 6. vital signs WNL for age 7. weight loss 1–2 lbs 8. absence of confusion	1. Monitor labs: Na^+, Cl^-, serum osmolality. 2. Administer hypotonic IVs as ordered. 3. Administer diuretics as ordered. 4. Replace fluid lost with hypertonic feedings by giving 1 ml fluid for every Kcal of feeding. 5. Restrict Na^+ and H_2O intake to level ordered by physician (fluids may be restricted or replaced depending on ECF status). 6. If transfusion is necessary, use fresh blood. 7. Assess vital signs every 4 to 8 hours. 8. Record I & O every 8 hours. 9. Weigh daily. 10. Assess peripheral vein emptying every 8 hours. 11. Provide safety precautions: bed rails, low bed positions, night-lights. If client is weak, assist with activity.
Potassium Deficit		
Cardiovascular: hypotension, dysrhythmias (atrial or ventricular), cardiac arrest Respiratory: respiratory muscle weakness, shallow respirations, apnea, respiratory arrest Musculoskeletal: muscle weakness Digestive: decreased GI motility-distention, paralytic ileus, anorexia, nausea, vomiting Neurologic: dysphasia, lethargy, irritability, disorientation (alkalosis secondary to cell buffer system attempting to compensate for low K^+ by releasing more K^+, H^+ moves into cell in exchange for K^+), alkalosis results in neurologic signs: hyporeflexia, tetany, paresthesias, convulsions General: malaise, fatigue Lab findings: K^+ < 3.5 mEq/L; ECG most reliable tool for ICF K^+ level; peaked P, depressed ST, flat T, U wave	In 24 hours (time should be less if level critical) shows increased K^+ level AEB 1. serum K^+ > 3.5 mEq/L 2. absence of U wave on ECG 3. less than five premature beats/minute (unless history of atrial fibrillation) 4. normoactive bowel sounds 5. absence of confusion, convulsions	1. Monitor serum K^+ and ECG. 2. Administer IVs with KCl as ordered (if crisis, may be replaced as rapidly as 10 mEq/hour if on cardiac monitor). *Ensure adequate renal function first; rapid infusion can induce acidosis.* 3. Administer oral K^+ after meals (K^+ is irritating to GI mucosa). 4. Encourage foods high in K^+ (e.g., bananas, broccoli, cantaloupe, citrus fruits, nuts, fish, whole grains). 5. Monitor for digitalis toxicity (hypolakemia increases sensitivity of myocardium to digitalis-induced dysrhythmias). 6. Monitor persons who are NPO for K^+ deficit (40–80 mEq/day needed for maintenance). 7. Give IV K^+ only in diluted forms; if added to bag, agitate solution before infusing. 8. Notify physician if hypokalemia exists preoperatively. (Surgical procedures increase the risk of K^+ loss. If already hypokalemic, extreme risk for cardiac dysrhythmia exists. General anesthesia potentiates risk of dysrhythmia associated with hypokalemia.)

TABLE 41-6. Nursing Process Applied to Fluid and Electrolyte Imbalances Continued

Assessment Data (grouped by systems)	Outcome Criteria	Nursing Interventions

Potassium Deficit

		9. Assess vital signs every 1 to 8 hours depending on severity of deficit; include apical pulses for full minute and pulse deficit if irregular.
		10. Assess bowel sounds every 4 to 8 hours.
		11. Note quantity of urinary output every 8 hours (hourly if < 30 ml/hour).
		12. Use IV pump to control flow of KCl solutions.
		13. Provide safety precautions: Anticipate risk of convulsions; elevate side rails; use low bed positions; use night-lights. If convulsions probable, use padded side rails and keep airway at bedside. If client is weak, assist with activity.

Potassium Excess

Assessment Data	Outcome Criteria	Nursing Interventions
Cardiovascular: hypotension, dysrhythmia, cardiac arrest Respiratory: dyspnea Musculoskeletal: severe weakness Digestive: nausea, intestinal colic, diarrhea Urinary: oliguria, anuria Neurologic: restlessness, dysphasia (acidosis secondary to cell buffer system attempting to compensate for high K^+, K^+ moves into cell in exchange for H^+, which moves out of cell); acidosis results in signs such as paresthesias, possible convulsions Lab findings: K^+ > 5.0 mEq/L; ECG most reliable tool for ICF K^+ level: depressed P, wide QRS, depressed ST, tall, tented T waves	In 24 hours (time should be less if level critical) shows K^+ level decrease AEB: 1. serum K^+ < 5.0 mEq/L 2. absence of tall T waves on ECG 3. less than five premature beats/minute (unless history of atrial fibrillation) 4. decrease in number of diarrheal stools	1. Monitor serum K^+ and ECG. 2. Restrict oral and parenteral foods/fluids/meds with K^+ to level prescribed by physician (low-K^+, high-CHO diet often prescribed). 3. Urgency of situation depends on cardiac status (administer IV glucose and insulin as ordered). Caution: Rapid removal may induce state of alkalosis. Give Kayexalate (a cation-exchange resin that is given by mouth or by retention enema and that exchanges Na^+ for K^+ to increase K^+ excretion as ordered. Start peritoneal or hemodialysis as ordered. 4. Assess vital signs every 1 to 8 hours depending on severity; include assessment of apical pulses and pulse deficit if irregular. 5. Assess bowel sounds every 4 to 8 hours. 6. Assess urinary output every 8 hours (hourly if < 30 ml/hour). 7. Provide safety precautions: Elevate side rails; use low bed positions; use night-light. If client is weak assist with activity.

Calcium Deficit

Assessment Data	Outcome Criteria	Nursing Interventions
Cardiovascular: palpitations, dysrhythmias, hypotension Respiratory: stridor, laryngospasm Musculoskeletal: pathologic fracture Neurologic: abdominal and muscle cramps, paresthesias, tetany, convulsions, diplopia, positive Trousseau's and Chvostek's signs General: bleeding	In 48 hours (time will vary with severity of deficit) shows Ca^{++} level increase AEB: 1. serum Ca^{++} > 4.5 mEq/L 2. absence of paresthesias 3. regular apical pulse 4. BP within normal adult ranges	1. Monitor serum Ca^{++} and ECG. 2. Administer IV calcium gluconate or oral forms of Ca^{++} as ordered. 3. Provide high-calcium diet as ordered. 4. Administer vitamin D supplements as ordered.

Table continued on following page

TABLE 41–6. Nursing Process Applied to Fluid and Electrolyte Imbalances Continued

Assessment Data (grouped by systems)	Outcome Criteria	Nursing Interventions
Calcium Deficit		
Lab findings: $Ca^{++} < 4.5$ mEq/L; ECG prolonged QT interval	5. absence of Trousseau's & Chvostek's signs 6. absence of bleeding	5. If low Ca^{++} from hypoparathyroidism, avoid high-PO_4 foods (e.g., cheese, milk-based products, milk, carbonated beverages [high-PO_4 foods inhibit absorption of Ca^{++} and vitamin D supplements. 6. Use caution if Ca^{++} and digitalis are both given (will lead to potentiation of inotropic effect; hypercalcemia also increases risk of digitalis toxicity). 7. If transfusion is necessary, use fresh blood. 8. Assess for paresthesia, Trousseau's and Chvostek's signs. 9. Assess vital signs every 4 to 8 hours; include apical pulses. 10. Assess for signs of bleeding. 11. Assess diet for adequacy of intake of Ca^{++} foods. 12. Record I & O every 8 hours. 13. Use caution when moving person (client at high risk for fracture, even when moved properly).
Calcium Excess		
Cardiovascular: dysrhythmia → cardiac arrest Musculoskeletal: bone pain; osteoporosis; osteomalacia; pathologic fractures; weak, relaxed muscles Digestive: nausea, vomiting, constipation Urinary: polyuria; if urethral calculi, flank pain Neurologic: confusion, lethargy Lab findings: $Ca^{++} > 5.5$ mEq/L, decreased PO_4	In 48 hours (time will vary with severity of excess) shows Ca^{++} level decrease AEB: 1. serum $Ca^{++} < 5.5$ mEq/L 2. regular pulse 3. reports of increased strength	1. Monitor serum Ca^{++} levels. 2. Restrict Ca^{++} intake (IV and oral) to levels ordered by physician. 3. Hydrate with IV saline solutions as ordered. 4. Force/encourage oral fluids as ordered. 5. Administer loop diuretics (no thiazides) as ordered. 6. Administer steroids as ordered. 7. Provide foods and fluids to increase urine acidity (e.g., meat, cheese, eggs, whole grains, cranberry juice, prune juice). 8. Administer etidronate sodium (Didronel) as ordered (inhibits precursors to calcium mineralization and retards hyperossification). 9. Strain all urine. 10. Assess vital signs every 4 to 8 hours (including apical pulse). 11. Assess person's level of strength. 12. Record I & O every 8 hours. 13. Encourage resistive range of motion, activity, and weight bearing to decrease Ca^{++} loss from bone. 14. Use caution when moving person because there is increased risk for pathologic fractures, even if moved correctly.

TABLE 41-6. Nursing Process Applied to Fluid and Electrolyte Imbalances Continued

Assessment Data (grouped by systems)	Outcome Criteria	Nursing Interventions
	Magnesium Deficit	
Cardiovascular: tachycardia, dysrhythmia Musculoskeletal: weakness Neurologic: muscle tremors, hyperactive reflexes, tetany, tremor, disorientation, convulsions, diplopia, nystagmus Lab findings: $Mg^{++} < 1.5$ mEq/L (serum does not usually reflect clinically important signs; often we see low K^+ and Ca^{++} with low Mg^{++}; if K^+ deficiency treated and signs/symptoms persistent, probably low Mg^{++})	In 48 hours (time may vary) shows Mg^{++} level (serum or cell) increase AEB: 1. less than five irregular beats per minute (except if history of atrial fibrillation) 2. decrease or absence of tremors 3. orientation to person, place, time 4. absence of convulsions	1. Administer Mg^{++} IV, IM, or orally (meds or diet) as ordered. 2. Monitor for low Mg^{++} when lab results indicate low K^+ or Ca^{++}. 3. Assess vital signs every 4 to 8 hours. 4. Assess for presence or change in tremors. 5. Assess level of orientation. 6. Anticipate safety needs: Elevate side rails (use padded side rails and keep airway at bedside if convulsions probable); keep bed in low position; use night-lights. If client is weak, assist with activity.
	Magnesium Excess	
Cardiovascular: hypotension, dysrhythmia → arrest Respiratory: respiratory depression → arrest Musculoskeletal: weakness, dysarthria Digestive: nausea, vomiting Neurologic: thirst, CNS depression, hyporeflexia, lethargy, coma General: flushing Lab findings: $Mg^{++} > 2.5$ mEq/L	In 48 hours (time may vary depending on severity of excess) shows Mg^{++} level (serum or cell) decrease AEB: 1. absence of flushing 2. BP within normal adult range 3. regular pulse: 60–100 beats/minute 4. deep, regular respirations	1. Administer calcium gluconate as ordered. 2. Administer thiazide diuretics as ordered. 3. Administer IV saline as ordered. 4. Question order for meds with Mg^{++}. 5. Assess for flushing in absence of fever. 6. Assess vital signs every 4 to 8 hours (including apical pulses). 7. Monitor I & O. 8. Assess deep tendon reflexes (if present, Mg^{++} levels sufficient). 9. Provide safety: Elevate side rails; use low bed positions; use night-lights. If client is weak, assist with activity.
	Phosphate Deficit	
Cardiovascular: decreased cardiac function Musculoskeletal: weakness, brittle bones, and pain Neurologic: confusion, seizures General: fatigue Lab findings: $PO_4 < 1.2$ mEq/L	In 48 hours (time may vary) shows PO_4 level increase AEB: 1. serum $PO_4 > 1.2$ mEq/L 2. vital signs within normal adult ranges 3. oriented to person, time, place 4. absence of confusion	1. Administer IV or oral PO_4 as ordered. 2. Monitor serum PO_4. 3. Assess vital signs every 8 hours. 4. Assess for changes in orientation. 5. Provide safety: Elevate side rails; use low bed positions; use night-lights; caution with movement or transfers (clients prone to fractures, even with proper techniques). If seizures probable, use padded side rails, keep airway at bedside. If client is weak, assist with activity.

Table continued on following page

TABLE 41–6. Nursing Process Applied to Fluid and Electrolyte Imbalances Continued

Assessment Data (grouped by systems)	Outcome Criteria	Nursing Interventions
Phosphate Excess		
Cardiovascular: tachycardia Digestive: anorexia, nausea, vomiting Neurologic: hyperreflexia, tetany Lab findings: $PO_4 > 3.0$ mEq/L; low serum Ca^{++}	In 48 hours (time may vary) shows PO_4 level decrease AEB: 1. serum $PO_4^- < 3.0$ mEq/L 2. absence of anorexia, nausea, vomiting 3. vital signs WNL for age	1. Limit PO_4^- intake (diet: decrease milk, cheese, eggs, fish, nuts, whole grains, carbonated beverages) to level specified by physician. 2. Administer Ca^{++} or Al products as ordered. 3. Monitor serum PO_4^-. 4. Assess for GI distress. 5. Assess vital signs every 8 hours. 6. Provide safety: Elevate side rails; use low bed positions; use night-lights. If client is weak, assist with activity.
Protein Deficit		
Cardiovascular: anemia, hypotension Musculoskeletal: weakness, loss of muscle mass and tone, delayed growth General: chronic weight loss, fatigue, pallor, mental depression, decreased resistance to infection, slow wound healing, edema, ascites Lab findings: serum albumin < 4 gm/ 100 ml, decreased Hgb, Hct, RBCs (if iron normal)	In 5 to 7 days (time may be longer) shows improved protein status AEB: 1. weight gain of 1 to 2 lbs/week in absence of edema or third spacing 2. no signs of infection (e.g., WBC normal, no fever, urine and lungs clear) 3. Hgb and Hct normal for adult range 4. BP WNL adult ranges 5. Epithelialization in wound sites	1. Monitor labs: Hgb, Hct, RBCs, WBCs, albumin. 2. Administer IV albumin as ordered. 3. Provide high-protein, high-CHO diet as ordered. 4. Weigh daily. 5. Assess vital signs every 8 hours. 6. Assess lung sounds, urine characteristics every 4 to 8 hours. 7. Measure edematous sites every day. 8. Maintain universal precautions (high risk for infection related to decreased immunoglobulins). 9. Provide for safety: Elevate side rails; use low bed positions; use night-lights. If client is weak, assist with activity.
Metabolic Acidosis		
Cardiovascular: dysrhythmia Respiratory: Kussmaul's respirations (deep, rapid); sweet, fruity, acetone breath Musculoskeletal: weakness Neurologic: disorientation → lethargy → stupor → coma Lab findings: plasma pH < 7.35, plasma $HCO_3^- < 25$ mEq/L in adults and < 20 mEq/L in child, urine pH < 6; $K^+ > 5.0$ mEq/L	In 24 hours (time may vary with severity of excess) shows blood is less acidic AEB: 1. plasma pH 7.35–7.45 2. plasma HCO_3^- 25–29 mEq/L (in adult) 3. plasma K^+ 3.5–5.0 mEq/L 4. increased level of consciousness 5. vital signs WNL for adult, absence of dysrhythmia	1. Replace fluid loss via IV or oral route as ordered by physician. 2. Follow prescribed therapy to treat underlying cause (see Table 41–3). 3. Administer HCO_3^- as ordered. 4. Provide low-protein, diet as ordered. 5. Monitor lab results: ABGs, K^+. 6. Weigh daily. 7. Record I & O every 8 hours. 8. Assess level of consciousness hourly. 9. Record vital signs every 1 to 8 hours. 10. Provide safety precautions: Elevate side rails; use low bed positions; use night-lights. If client is weak, assist with activity.

TABLE 41–6. Nursing Process Applied to Fluid and Electrolyte Imbalances Continued

Assessment Data (grouped by systems)	Outcome Criteria	Nursing Interventions
Metabolic Alkalosis		
Cardiovascular: tachycardia, dysrhythmia Respiratory: slow, shallow respirations → apnea Digestive: recent history of nausea, vomiting, diarrhea, decreased GI motility as K^+ level decreases Neurologic: irritability, disorientation, muscle twitching, hypertonic muscles, tetany, paresthesias, convulsions General: cyanosis Lab findings: plasma pH > 7.45, plasma HCO_3^- > 29 mEq/L in adults and > 25 mEq/L in child; urine pH > 6; K^+ < 3.5 mEq/L	In 24 hours (time will vary with severity of imbalance) shows blood is less alkaline AEB: 1. plasma pH 7.35–7.45 2. plasma HCO_3^- 25–29 mEq/L (in adult) 3. plasma K^+ 3.5–5.0 mEq/L 4. improved level of consciousness 5. respirations deep, regular, 16–20 6. absence of convulsions 7. fewer than five premature beats/minute	1. Replace GI fluid loss via IV or oral route as ordered. 2. Follow prescribed therapy to treat underlying cause (see Table 41–3). 3. Administer acidifying solution IV or orally as ordered. 4. Administer K^+ IV or orally as ordered to restore lost K^+. 5. Administer IV Ca^{++} gluconate as ordered if tetany occurs. 6. Monitor labs: ABGs, K^+. 7. Weight daily. 8. Record I & O every 8 hours. 9. Assess level of consciousness hourly. 10. Assess vital signs every 1 to 8 hours. 11. Provide safety precautions: Elevate side rails; use low bed positions; use nightlights. If convulsions probable, use padded side rails, place airway at bedside. If client is weak, assist with activity.
Respiratory Acidosis		
Cardiovascular: tachycardia, dysrhythmia Respiratory: hypoventilation, shallow respirations, dyspnea, wheezing Neurologic: drowsiness → disorientation → lethargy → stupor → coma General: headache, diaphoresis, cyanosis Lab findings: plasma pH < 7.35, plasma HCO_3^- > 29 mEq/L in adults and > 25 mEq in children, PCO_2 > 45 mm Hg, K^+ > 5.0 mEq/L, urine pH < 6	In 24 hours (time will vary with severity of imbalance) shows blood is less acidic AEB: 1. plasma pH 7.35–7.45 2. plasma PCO_2 35–45 mm Hg 3. plasma K^+ 3.5–5.0 mEq/L 4. dyspnea reduced to a level allowing person to progressively perform activities of daily living (e.g., hygienic self-care) 5. pulse 60–100, regular 6. increased level of consciousness	1. Follow prescribed therapy to correct or control underlying respiratory condition (see Table 42–3), including ventilation treatment, percussion and postural drainage, maintaining oral or artificial airway (endotracheostomy), and use of respirator in serious conditions. 2. Administer meds to enhance exchange of gases as ordered (e.g., bronchodilators, antibiotics). 3. Use caution with meds that cause sedation. 4. Maintain fluid needs via IV or oral route to prevent further metabolic alterations. 5. Meet nutritional needs (IV, oral, tube). 6. Monitor labs: ABGs, K^+. 7. Demonstrate deep-breathing exercises; encourage use every hour. 8. Weigh daily. 9. Record I & O every 8 hours. 10. Assess level of consciousness hourly. 11. Assess vital signs every 1 to 8 hours. 12. Provide safety precautions: Elevate side rails; use low bed positions, use nightlights. If client is weak, assist with activity.

Table continued on following page

TABLE 41–6. Nursing Process Applied to Fluid and Electrolyte Imbalances Continued

Assessment Data (grouped by systems)	Outcome Criteria	Nursing Interventions
	Respiratory Alkalosis	
Cardiovascular: dysrhythmia Respiratory: rapid respirations (sometimes related to anxiety) Neurologic: lightheadedness, tingling of fingers and toes progressing up arms and legs, muscle twitching, tetany, convulsions, unconsciousness Lab findings: plasma pH > 7.45, plasma HCO_3^- < 25 mEq/L in adults and < 20 mEq/L in children, PCO_2 < 35 mm Hg, K^+ < 3.5 mEq/L, urine pH > 7	In 24 hours (time will vary with severity of imbalance) shows blood is less alkaline AEB: 1. plasma pH 7.35–7.45 2. plasma PCO_2 35–45 mm Hg 3. plasma K^+ 3.5–5.0 mEq/L 4. respirations deep, regular, 16–20/min 5. pulse 60–100, regular 6. improved level of consciousness 7. absence of tingling, twitching, tetany, convulsions	1. Counsel to decrease anxiety as needed. 2. Provide sedation for hysteria as ordered. 3. Follow prescribed therapy to correct or control underlying conditions (see Table 41–3). 4. Provide CO_2 treatment (e.g., rebreathe own CO_2 from a paper bag). 5. Meet fluid needs (IV, oral) as ordered. 6. Meet nutritional needs (IV, oral, tube) as ordered. 7. Monitor labs: ABGs, K^+. 8. Weigh daily. 9. Record I & O every 8 hours. 10. Assess level of consciousness hourly. 11. Assess vital signs every 1 to 8 hours. 12. Provide safety precautions: Elevate side rails; use low bed positions; use nightlights. If convulsions probable, use padded side rails, keep airway at bedside. If client is weak, assist with activity.

Abbreviations: BP, blood pressure; WNL, within normal limits; PO, orally; IV, intravenous; NG, nasogastric; Na^+, sodium; Hgb, hemoglobin; Hct, hematocrit; I & O, intake and output; ICF, intracellular fluid; AEB, as evidenced by ICP, intracranial pressure; HOB, head of bed; Cl^-, chloride; NaCl, sodium chloride; NS, normal saline; H_2O, water; ECF, extracellular fluid; GI, gastrointestinal; K^+, potassium; H^+, hydrogen; ECG, electrocardiogram; NPO, nothing by mouth; KCl, potassium chloride; CHO, carbohydrate; PO_4, phosphate; Ca^{++}, calcium; Mg^{++}, magnesium; IM, intramuscular; CNS, central nervous system; Al, aluminum; RBCs, red blood cells; WBC, white blood cell; HCO_3^-, bicarbonate; ABGs, arterial blood gases; PCO_2, partial pressure of carbon dioxide; CO_2, carbon dioxide;

APPLYING RESEARCH TO NURSING PRACTICE

Accurately Detecting Dehydration in Elderly Clients

Gross, C. R., (1992). Clinical indicators of dehydration severity in elderly patients. *Journal of Emergency Medicine,* 10(3), 267–274.

▼ ▼ ▼

Quick and accurate assessment of dehydration in the elderly is critical. Therefore, Gross and colleagues sought to determine how closely the signs and symptoms commonly attributed to dehydration correlate with the severity of dehydration in elderly clients. To make that determination, these researchers studied 55 emergency department clients older than 60 years. The researchers first took a history of each client and performed physical examinations. From these histories and physical examinations, Gross and colleagues identified predictors of the severity of dehydration. These predictors included such signs as tongue dryness. Later in the clients' hospitalization, the researchers rated the severity of dehydration in each client by conducting a comprehensive chart review. The goal of the chart review was to link those predictors of the severity of dehydration identified initially in the emergency department with objective data gathered during client hospitalization, such as laboratory tests. The researchers concluded that the most significant clinical indicators of the severity of dehydration are tongue dryness, longitudinal tongue furrows, dryness of the oral mucous membranes, upper body muscle weakness, confusion, and speech difficulty. Subjective sensation of thirst did not correlate with the severity of dehydration.

Applications for Practice. To assess the fluid and electrolyte status of cognitively impaired elderly clients, you cannot rely on subjective data. Focus more closely, then, on the presence of the following objective clinical signs of dehydration: tongue dryness, longitudinal tongue furrows, dryness of the oral mucous membrane, upper body muscle weakness, confusion, and speech difficulty.

collection to identify signs and symptoms, summarized in Table 41–6, or risk factors, which might cause imbalances, as listed in Table 41–3. The assessment process involves collection of subjective data by interviewing the client and objective data from physical examination (inspection, palpation, percussion, auscultation). Other sources of assessment data are family or significant others, the chart (including laboratory/diagnostic findings), and other health team members. (See Chapter 34 for specific information related to laboratory and diagnostic testing.)

Client History

When reviewing a person's history, make special note of clues that suggest possible imbalances. Subjective reports of thirst, weakness, fatigue, nausea, dizziness, restlessness, tingling or numbness of fingers or extremities, muscle cramps, bone pain, changes in bowel pattern, or changes in body weight or swelling may indicate an imbalance. In addition to subjective symptoms, each water, electrolyte, and acid-base imbalance is characterized by many objective signs that affect almost every system in the body (see Table 41–6). Note that several imbalances may have similar symptoms and that one imbalance can trigger the onset of another (see Table 41–3). Because the manifestations of water, electrolyte, and acid-base disturbances are numerous, widespread, and interrelated, it is important to gather information in a systematic way. Table 41–7 lists common assessment data and possible associated imbalances.

TABLE 41–7. Indicators of Fluid and Electrolyte Imbalances

Assessment Data	Related Imbalance
1. Temperature	
a. Elevated temperature	a. Water deficit (ICF)
b. Subnormal temperature	b. Water excess or ECF volume deficit
2. Pulse	
a. Increased bounding pulse (not easily obliterated)	a. Fluid volume excess
b. Increased thready, weak pulse	b. Fluid volume deficit
c. Weak, irregular pulse	c. Potassium deficit or excess
d. Tachycardia	d. Water deficit, magnesium deficit, fluid volume deficit
e. Bradycardia	e. Magnesium excess
3. Respirations	
a. Deep rapid breathing (Kussmaul's respirations)	a. Metabolic acidosis, respiratory alkalosis
b. Shallow, slow respirations progressing to intervals of apnea	b. Metabolic alkalosis, respiratory acidosis
c. Shallow, slow respirations because of respiratory muscle weakness	c. Potassium deficit (severe) or potassium excess (severe)
d. Moist rales	d. Fluid volume excess
4. Blood Pressure	
a. Hypotension	a. Fluid volume deficit, magnesium excess
b. Hypertension	b. Fluid volume excess, magnesium deficit
5. Weight	
a. Rapid weight gain	a. Fluid volume excess
b. Rapid weight loss	b. Fluid volume deficit
c. Chronic weight loss	c. Protein deficit
6. Thirst	
a. Increased thirst	a. Decreased blood volume as a result of hemorrhage, water deficit resulting in hypertonic ECF
7. Appetite	
a. Loss of appetite (anorexia)	a. Potassium deficit; protein deficit
8. Urinary Output	
a. Decreased urinary output	a. Decreased blood volume resulting in increased secretion of ADH and aldosterone, water deficit, fluid volume deficit
b. Increased urinary output	b. Increased blood volume resulting in decreased secretion of ADH and aldosterone, water excess, fluid volume excess, potassium deficit
9. Stools	
a. Hard, dry stools	a. Fluid volume deficit
b. Abdominal distention with few or no stools	b. Potassium deficit
c. Abdominal cramps accompanied by diarrhea	c. Potassium excess
10. Energy and Stamina Levels	
a. Easy fatigability and loss of stamina	a. Potassium deficit, water excess, protein deficit, fluid volume deficit

Table continued on following page

TABLE 41–7. *Indicators of Fluid and Electrolyte Imbalances* Continued

Assessment Data	Related Imbalance
11. Facial Appearance	
a. Drawn facial appearance with sunken eyeballs	a. Severe fluid volume deficit
b. Full, swollen-appearing face with puffy eyelids	b. Fluid volume excess
12. Level of Consciousness (CNS Changes)	
a. Apathy, lethargy, lassitude	a. Fluid volume deficit, water excess, potassium deficit
b. Disorientation and confusion	b. Water excess (water intoxication), severe potassium deficit, magnesium deficit, metabolic or respiratory acidosis, calcium excess
c. Hallucinations	c. Magnesium deficit, water excess
d. Stupor terminating in unconsciousness	d. Profound alkalosis, profound acidosis, shock
13. Muscle Tone	
a. Flabby muscles	a. Potassium deficit, protein deficit
b. Flaccid paralysis	b. Severe potassium deficit or severe potassium excess
c. Tetany	c. Calcium deficit, metabolic alkalosis, magnesium deficit
d. Convulsions	d. Magnesium deficit, calcium deficit, water excess (water intoxication), metabolic alkalosis
14. Sensation	
a. Tingling and numbness of fingers	a. Calcium deficit, metabolic alkalosis, potassium deficit, magnesium deficit
b. Severe muscle cramps	b. Calcium deficit
c. Sensation of numbness and deadness in extremities (prelude to flaccid paralysis)	c. Potassium deficit or potassium excess
d. Numb extremities	d. Calcium deficit, potassium deficit
e. Deep, bony pain and flank pain	e. Calcium excess
15. Tissue Turgor	
a. Decreased skin turgor	a. Fluid volume deficit
b. Edema of dependent parts of body	b. Shift of fluid from vascular compartment into interstitial spaces, fluid volume excess
c. Pitting edema	c. Fluid volume excess
d. "Finger imprinting" on sternum	d. Saline deficit
e. Mucous membranes dry and sticky	e. Water deficit
f. Dry but otherwise normal axillae or groin (normally, apocrine sweat glands in axillae and groin are constantly producing moisture)	f. Severe water deficit
16. Neck Veins	
a. Flat (collapsed) neck veins	a. Fluid volume deficit
b. Distended neck veins	b. Fluid volume excess
17. Peripheral Veins	
a. Increased vein filling time (veins not apparent)	a. Fluid volume deficit
b. Increased vein emptying time (peripheral veins appear engorged)	b. Fluid volume excess, shift of fluid from interstitial spaces into vascular compartment

Abbreviations: CNS, central nervous system; ICF, intracellular fluid; ECF, extracellular fluid; ADH, antidiuretic hormone.

Physical Assessment

For physical assessment data pertinent to the client with an imblance, refer to Tables 41–6 and 41–7. Note that two important findings, which are rapidly and easily assessed, relate to the skin turgor and peripheral veins.

Skin turgor describes the elasticity of the skin. To assess skin turgor, pinch the skin inferior to the clavicle or over the sternum, dorsum of the hand, or forearm and release (Fig. 41–13). In the elderly, assess skin turgor on the inner thigh (affected less by aging). Observe how long it takes for the pinched skin to fall back to its original shape. If fluid balance is normal, the skin immediately returns to its original shape. If the skin remains elevated in a slightly pinched position for several seconds, the person may have a fluid volume deficit. Aging and recent weight loss also decrease normal skin turgor.

Assessment of the peripheral veins, specifically the speed with which they fill and empty on positional changes, also aids in identifying fluid balance status. To check peripheral vein emptying and filling, follow this simple procedure: (1) Have the individual raise a hand and hold it in an elevated position; (2) observe how many seconds it takes for the blood to empty from the hand veins; (3) have the individual lower the hand and keep it in a dependent position; (4) observe how many seconds it takes for the blood to fill the veins. Normal veins empty in 3 to 5 seconds. On lowering the hands

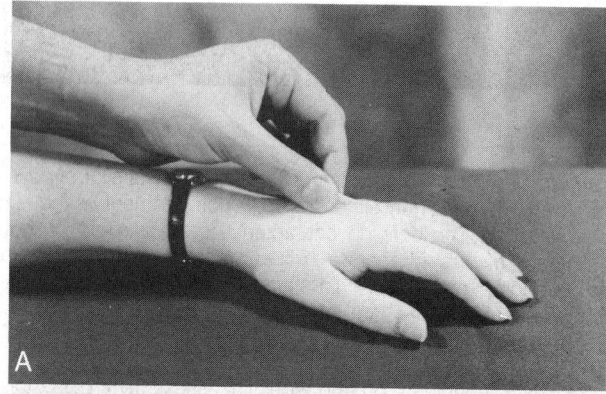

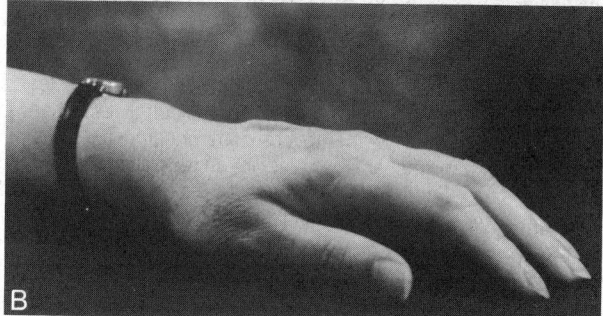

▲ *Figure 41-13*

A, The nurse tests tissue turgor by lifting the tissue of the dorsum of the hand. *B,* A closer view of the same hand shows the tissue still tented after a time lapse of 15 seconds. This is poor tissue turgor.

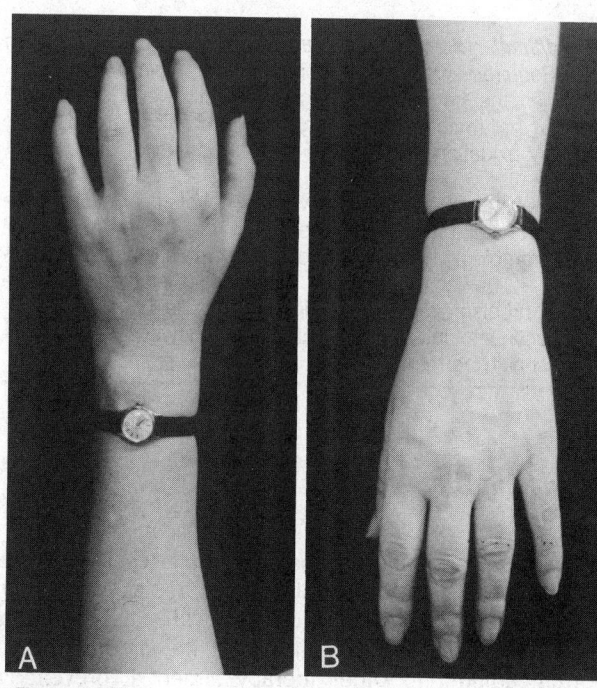

▲ *Figure 41-14*

Testing vein emptying and filling. *A,* As the hand is raised to an elevated position, note the number of seconds needed for the veins to empty. *B,* As the hand is lowered to a dependent position, note the number of seconds needed for the veins to fill. The rounded appearance assumed by the blood-filled veins is clearly visible in this closer look at the hand of a 51-year-old female client. The filled veins are usually less prominent in younger persons than in older persons and less prominent in females than in males.

into a dependent position, the veins should fill in 3 to 5 seconds (Fig. 41-14).

Veins take longer to fill when fluid volume is decreased and empty more slowly when fluid volume is excessive.

NURSING DIAGNOSIS

The North American Nursing Diagnosis Association (NANDA) recognizes three nursing diagnoses specific to altered fluid volume. These include (1) *Fluid Volume Deficit* (Nursing Diagnosis Profile), (2) *Fluid Volume Excess* (Nursing Diagnosis Profile), and (3) *High Risk for Fluid Volume Deficit.* All other water, electrolyte, and acid-base imbalances are not yet accepted as conditions that nurses treat. These other conditions include (1) hyponatremia, (2) hypernatremia, (3) hypokalemia, (4) hyperkalemia, (5) hypocalcemia, (6) hypercalcemia, (7) hypomagnesemia, (8) hypermagnesemia, (9) hypophosphatemia, (10) hyperphosphatemia, (11) hypoproteinemia, (12) metabolic acidosis, (13) metabolic alkalosis, (14) respiratory acidosis, and (15) respiratory alkalosis. These are all conditions nurses address in collaboration with physicians and other members of the health team. They are conditions nurses must understand, and they require many nursing interventions (see Table 41-6). These are also conditions that can be difficult to keep separated from the accepted NANDA diagnoses.

PLANNING

Outcomes for the diagnoses *Fluid Volume Excess, Fluid Volume Deficit,* and *High Risk for Fluid Volume Deficit* focus on reversing imbalances. Outcomes for these conditions are listed in Table 41-6. Often evidence that the outcomes have been achieved will include additional information concerning the client's water, electrolyte, and acid-base balances (see Table 41-6).

NURSING INTERVENTION

Depending on the severity of the imbalance, people with fluid disturbances may have only a few mild symptoms, or they may be desperately ill. Consequently, the various interventions used to correct fluid problems range from simple to complex. For nursing interventions related to specific fluid, electrolyte, or acid-base imbalances, see Table 41-6. Many treatments of individuals with fluid disturbances involve two approaches: (1) replacement of lost fluids and (2) reduction of excess fluids.

The three major objectives of fluid replacement are (1) to correct preexisting deficits of water and electrolytes and restore the vascular volume, thus reducing shock and dehydration, (2) to maintain the person's life-sustaining needs for water, electrolytes, and calories, and (3) to replace dynamic or concurrent losses of water and electrolytes from suctioning, vomiting, di-

NURSING DIAGNOSIS PROFILE

Fluid Volume Deficit

Definitions. The state in which an individual is experiencing vascular, interstitial, or intracellular dehydration

Classification. Exchanging 1.4.1.2.2.1

Defining Characteristics. Persons who have a urinary output greater than their intake will experience *Fluid Volume Deficit* unless this output is merely a compensatory response. Because the main source of fluid is oral intake, those individuals experiencing a decrease in intake are at high risk for this alteration unless adequate fluid is provided by another source such as intravenous (IV) solutions or tube feedings. Because fluid makes up 50 to 70 per cent of weight, it is not surprising that acute weight loss is a common finding. Homeostatic compensatory mechanisms either to replace or to conserve the fluid balance include thirst and decreased urinary output, which produces more concentrated urine. Other signs commonly present as a result of decreased fluid include hypernatremia; peripheral vein filling > 5 seconds; hypotension followed by a compensatory increase in pulse rate; a weak, thready pulse; decreased skin turgor; a change in mental state (restlessness, delirium, confusion, stupor); dry skin and mucous membranes; and weakness. Intracellular fluid (ICF) deficit will result in fever, whereas extracellular fluid deficit may result in a fever or in a subnormal temperature if the volume is so depleted that there is not enough fluid to transport heat.

Sample Related Factors. Related factors include the following:

▶ Increased fluid loss such as might occur with
vomiting or diarrhea (illness, iatrogenic factors)
abnormal drainage (wounds, burns, suction)
third spacing (inflammatory responses, ascites, blisters)
failure of regularity mechanisms that control retention of output (e.g., increased metabolic rate in illness and infancy, fever causing marked diaphoresis, and excessive urine output as during illness or during certain treatments)
▶ Decreased fluid intake such as might occur with
pain
dysphagia
failure of regulatory mechanisms that control intake (e.g., decreased thirst in old age or illness)

Concept Description. This diagnosis refers to a state of hypovolemia or dehydration in either the ECF compartment or the ICF compartment. The defining characteristics are a direct or indirect result of a rapid change in fluid output or a lack of intake without compensation by fluid shifts or by other normal regulatory mechanisms.

Examples. Depending on the specific assessment data, this diagnostic category could be applicable in the following situations, among others:

▶ A person with gastrointestinal (GI) suction who has lost a greater amount of fluid (water and electrolytes) than is being replaced by IV therapy or compensated for by regulatory mechanisms and who is in an actual state of fluid deficit, e.g., *Fluid Volume Deficit* R/T unreplaced GI fluid loss greater than compensatory efforts or replacement therapy
▶ A person with hyperosmotic tube feedings who experiences fluid deficit secondary to the increased osmolarity of the tube feeding (fluid shifts into the bowel in an attempt to decrease the osmolality of the intestinal fluid), e.g., *Fluid Volume Deficit* R/T effects of hyperosmotic tube feedings
▶ An elderly person who has decreased thirst (one of the most common changes in the aged) and who fails to drink an adequate amount each day, e.g., *Fluid Volume Deficit* R/T effects of decreased thirst mechanism.

Related/Similar Nursing Diagnoses. *Altered Nutrition: Less than Body Requirements* may be confused with *Fluid Volume Deficit.* When the person has difficulty ingesting enough food to provide the material necessary for production of adequate water by oxidation, the primary problem is that of overall nutrition.

Diarrhea may be confused with *Fluid Volume Deficit.* If the defining characteristics are specific to the bowel (abdominal pain, cramping, hyperactive bowel sounds, increased frequency in bowel movements, loose liquid stools), then the primary problem is bowel elimination, not fluid deficit. If diarrhea continues until fluid deficit occurs, however, both diagnoses should be made.

---

arrhea, or other losses. Replacement involves measures to reduce loss of water and electrolytes while increasing their intake.

The objective of fluid reduction is to prevent such problems as systemic edema, pulmonary edema, and circulatory overload. Fluids are reduced by limiting water and electrolyte intake while enhancing output.

Recording Intake and Output

Assessment of intake and output is an important nursing measure in all water, electrolyte, and acid-base imbalances. See Procedure 41-1 for details concerning recording of intake and output.

Regulating Diet

Monitoring a client's diet is important when you are attempting to promote, maintain, or replace water or electrolytes to a level consistent with health and a feeling of well-being. Regulation of the diet is an important adjunct to other therapy aimed at preventing further body insult secondary to a metabolic disorder or any other disorder that is causing or increasing the risk for water, electrolyte, or acid-base imbalance. Nutritional management is discussed in Chapter 42.

An excess or deficit of fluids and foods can compromise the person with coexisting metabolic dysfunc-

NURSING DIAGNOSIS PROFILE

Fluid Volume Excess

Definition. The state in which an individual experiences increased fluid retention and edema

Classification. Exchanging 1.4.1.2.1

Defining Characteristics. Persons who have a greater intake than output and are unable to excrete this overload because of renal disease or other metabolic dysfunctions will experience a fluid volume excess. Because most of the body is fluid, it is not surprising that fluid excess is reflected in an acute weight gain. When renal disease is the cause, signs and symptoms secondary to renal dysfunction are often seen along with fluid overload: oliguria, concentrated urine, azotemia, alteration in electrolytes, and anemia. Signs and symptoms specifically related to retention of fluids include peripheral edema, an S_3 gallop, and pulmonary congestion (rales or crackles, dyspnea, orthopnea, change in respiratory pattern, pleural effusion). The respiratory difficulty may lead to a feeling of anxiety. Signs of increased vascular volume include a bounding pulse, increased blood pressure, an increased central venous pressure, neck vein distention, peripheral vein emptying > 5 seconds, and a positive hepatojugular reflex. An ICF excess will result in changes in mental status: confusion, restlessness, lethargy.

Sample Related Factors. Related factors include the following:

▶ Increased intake such as might occur with
    excess oral or intravenous fluids
    excess tap-water enemas
    excess sodium intake
▶ Increased retention such as might occur with
    renal disease that decreases excretion
    increased secretion of antidiuretic hormone that causes increased reabsorption of water
    lymphatic or venous obstruction that interferes with transport of excess fluid resulting in increased fluid pressure in interstitial tissues
    liver disease (decreased protein that causes decreased colloid osmotic pressure, thus decreased reabsorption, increased venous pressure that causes increased hydrostatic pressure forcing more fluid into the interstitial tissues)

decreased cardiac output that interferes with filling during diastole and retrograde fluid build-up
pregnancy with increased levels of adosterone, sodium, and fluid
inflammatory processes that cause damage to capillary and cell walls and allow movement of fluid into interstitial tissues
sepsis that results in release of toxins, pH changes, cellular damage, and fluid loss to interstitial tissues

Concept Description. This nursing diagnosis refers to a state of hypervolemia or water intoxication in the vascular compartment or to the presence of edema (in the interstitial compartment). The defining characteristics are a direct or indirect result of an increase in fluid intake or decrease in excretion without compensation by intercompartmental fluid shifts or other regulatory mechanisms.

Examples. Depending on the specific assessment data, this diagnostic category could be applicable in the following situations, among others:

▶ A person with decreased water excretion secondary to decreased renal function or compensatory overflow who experiences systemic signs and symptoms of fluid overload because the kidney is the primary organ responsible for water excretion, e.g., *Fluid Volume Excess* R/T increased retention of water secondary to decreased renal function
▶ A pregnant woman with hypervolemia secondary to increased sodium retention, e.g., *Fluid Volume Excess* R/T increased sodium, aldosterone, and fluid retention secondary to pregnancy.

Related/Similar Nursing Diagnoses. *Altered Nutrition: More than Body Requirements* may be confused with *Fluid Volume Excess*. When the person has a problem with ingesting more food than the body requires, the primary problem is nutrition, not fluid.

Urinary Retention may be confused with *Fluid Volume Excess*. If the defining characteristics are specific to the bladder (bladder distention; small, frequent voidings; absence of urine output), then the primary problem is urinary elimination, not fluid excess.

---

tion or other state of imbalance. Following are some examples:

▶ Fluids and foods high in sodium are restricted in persons with congestive heart failure, renal failure, liver failure, and Cushing's syndrome. Use caution by first consulting the physician before encouraging high-sodium foods when serum sodium levels are low. IV sodium replacement is usually preferred.
▶ Foods high in potassium are restricted in persons with such metabolic dysfunctions as renal failure, early phases of traumatic injuries (e.g., burns, crushing injuries), Addison's disease, and acidosis. Foods high in potassium are encouraged for persons expe-

riencing loss secondary to upper or lower GI dysfunction, fistulas, wounds, diuretic therapy, Cushing's syndrome, hyperaldosteronism, alkalosis, or inadequate intake of potassium. Food sources high in potassium may be an adjunct to oral or IV potassium therapy.
▶ Foods high in calcium are restricted in persons with such metabolic dysfunctions as hyperparathyroidism and certain cancers (kidney, lung, bone, breast, some leukemias) that promote higher serum calcium levels. Foods high in calcium are encouraged for persons with such metabolic dysfunctions as hypoparathyroidism, pancreatitis, alkalosis, chronic renal failure, increased calcium need such as in pregnancy

and lactation, or increased loss as in diarrhea, wound drainage, or burns. Food sources may be an adjunct to oral or IV calcium therapy. Vitamin D supplements or foods high in vitamin D also may help promote return to safe calcium levels when serum levels are low.

► Foods high in magnesium are usually restricted in persons with renal failure. Foods high in magnesium are encouraged in persons with chronic alcoholism or preeclampsia and persons experiencing inadequate magnesium intake or loss secondary to upper or lower GI losses or diuretic therapy.

► Foods high in protein are encouraged for persons with protein loss secondary to certain renal diseases, certain liver diseases, hemorrhage, wound drainage, burns, severe trauma, decreased intake as in starvation or decreased GI absorption, or increased protein demand as in infections, wounds, and bone fracture healing.

► Chloride abnormalities are treated in association with other specific imbalances.

► Phosphate imbalances are usually treated with IV therapy for low phosphate levels and dialysis for high phosphate levels. See Chapter 42 for more specific nutrition information.

Regulating Oral Fluid Intake

Restricting oral intake of fluids is an important nursing measure for clients with *Fluid Volume Excess*. Similarly, increasing fluid intake (through "forcing" oral fluids) is an important nursing measure for clients with *Fluid Volume Deficit* or *High Risk for Fluid Volume Deficit*. Regulating oral intake by restricting or "forcing" fluids is discussed in Procedure 41-2.

Administering Medications

Medications may be ordered specifically to correct water, electrolyte, and acid-base balance. Medications may be ordered for some other reason, but they may <u>also</u> alter water, electrolyte, and acid-base balances as one of their side effects. In either case, the nurse must be knowledgeable about possible imbalances and ever alert to the client's water, electrolyte, and acid-base status. When you administer medications, you will be responsible for assessment (1) before giving the medication, (2) during the time the drug is acting in the body, and (3) after the client has achieved the expected response. Medication administration is discussed in Chapter 46. Following are some of the nursing interventions most pertinent to administering medications that alter water, electrolyte, and acid-base balances.

► Monitor water, electrolyte, and acid-base imbalances for persons who will be given medications known to cause imbalances. Careful monitoring will help to identify imbalances in early stages and will allow treatment before serious consequences occur.

► Record intake and output every 8 hours, and record daily weights for those at risk for fluid imbalance; record hourly output if renal function is impaired. Measuring intake and output not only helps assess imbalances but also helps ensure adequate renal function. Most medications depend on adequate renal function for excretion. If renal function is impaired, the person is at higher risk for side effects and toxicity.

► Encourage food to replace lost electrolytes only if loss of electrolytes is a side effect and not a desired outcome and only if such foods are within dietary prescriptions. Usually foods are used to replace lost electrolytes only if the serum electrolyte levels are in a low-normal or deficient state.

► Follow specific nursing interventions related to each medication as listed in your agency medication manual unless contraindicated or contrary to physician's prescription (e.g., assess and record vital signs specific to expected outcomes of medication before and after administration, such as temperature for antipyretics, blood pressure for all antihypertensive medications regardless of mode of action, apical pulse for medications affecting atrioventricular conduction or cardiac rhythm). Review lung sounds in clients taking medication affecting cardiac contractility. Check serum potassium and digitalis levels before giving digitalis derivatives, and record apical pulse before each dose.

► Digitalis derivatives act to slow the heartbeat and are not to be given if the apical pulse is less than 60. If the apical pulse is less than 60, notify the physician. The physician may want digitalis given if the pulse is above 50.

Potassium depletion sensitizes the myocardium to digitalis, resulting in risk of increased automaticity in cardiac cells. Therefore, digitalis toxicity may develop in persons with hypokalemia even when the serum digoxin concentrations are within the normal laboratory ranges.

Consult with the physician if serum potassium is low, borderline, or low normal or if serum digitalis level is at high normal or above normal before giving digitalis derivatives. Note that diuretics that alter potassium levels in the body can also cause an alteration in the effects of digitalis.

► Monitor laboratory results (electrolytes, hemoglobin and hematocrit, RBC count, liver enzymes, blood urea nitrogen [BUN], creatinine). These values not only help in identifying imbalances but also indicate liver and kidney dysfunction that may lead to imbalances when medications cannot be properly detoxified or excreted. Recall that creatinine is the best indicator of renal function (BUN is altered by many other conditions).

► Consult agency protocol or physician regarding administration of critical oral medications when client status is changed to "nothing by mouth" (NPO). Serum levels of critical medications (e.g., steroids, anticonvulsants) <u>must</u> be maintained. If agency protocol is not clear, consult with the physician (medi-

PROCEDURE 41-2

Regulation of Oral Fluid Intake (Forcing or Restricting Fluids)

Definition/Purpose. Monitoring and altering oral intake to promote, maintain, replace, or reduce fluids to a level consistent with health or feeling of well-being; regulation of oral fluid intake is important adjunct to other therapy aimed at preventing further body insult secondary to metabolic disorder or other disorder causing or increasing the risk for fluid imbalance

Contraindications/Cautions. Fluid requirement to maintain cellular function for a normal adult is 2 to 2.5 L of water per day. School-age children need 100 to 110 ml/kg/24 hours; toddlers need 120 to 135 ml/kg/24 hours; and infants need 70 to 100 ml/kg/24 hours.[15]

Restricting fluid intake to less than the age-related minimal intake or forcing liquids to more than the age-related upper limits must be based on the person's physiologic needs and capabilities. A physician, therefore, should prescribe these amounts. The nurse functions in an interdependent role with dietary staff and the person and family to facilitate limitation or increased intake of fluids and to promote teaching associated with fluid regulation. Remember that the caloric content, electrolyte content, and amount of the fluid must fit into the dietary prescription. Thus, any fluid items offered between meals are just as important in the overall fluid, electrolyte, and caloric totals as those on the meal tray. A person with diabetes mellitus must not only have the fluid and calories calculated but must also have them coordinated with prescribed glucose-lowering agents.

Use caution when interpreting physician orders. Clarify with the physician whether the prescribed restriction or increase in fluids is in reference to a total fluid intake (intravenous [IV], tube feedings, oral) or whether it is only the oral component of fluid intake.

Learning/Teaching Guidelines. Discuss with the person and significant others the following as appropriate: (1) the relationship of the fluid prescription to homeostasis, maintenance, and recovery of optimal bodily functioning, (2) the types of fluids that can be included or excluded, (3) the time the fluids will be given, (4) whether this fluid prescription is temporary or whether it requires permanent life-style changes, and (5) the importance of verbalizing concerns related to the fluid prescription.

PRELIMINARY ACTIVITIES

Assessment/Planning

- ▶ Check medical/nursing diagnoses.
- ▶ Check physician and nursing orders.
- ▶ Be aware of fluids included or excluded in prescribed diet.
- ▶ Be aware of metabolic dysfunction or circumstances that place a person at risk for *Fluid Volume Deficit* or *Fluid Volume Excess* (review Table 41–3).
- ▶ Be aware of dietary items with measurable fluid content (fluids included in a clear or full liquid diet).
- ▶ Be aware of agency's edema scale.
- ▶ Calculate the fluid intake goal per shift (approximately 3/5 for the day shift, the remainder divided among the evening and night shifts); if the fluid prescription refers to total intake, the oral fluid must be calculated taking into account all other fluid sources (e.g., IV solutions, tube feedings, fluids given with medications).
- ▶ Assess person's fluid preferences within diet prescription.

Equipment

- ▶ same as needed for recording I & O (see Procedure 41–1)
- ▶ dietary manual
- ▶ balanced weight scale

Preparation

- ▶ Remove person's bedside water pitcher if he or she is on fluid restriction.
- ▶ Place measurement devices in room, adjacent bathroom, or anteroom.
- ▶ Place explicit information related to fluid restriction or forcing of fluids in care plan (Kardex) (e.g., if person is on 1500-ml fluid restriction: days—900 ml, evenings—300 ml, nights—300 ml; if prescription is to force fluids to 3000 ml: days—1800 ml, evenings—800 ml, nights—400 ml).

PROCEDURE

Actions

1. Limit or force fluids according to care plan.

2. Offer fluids at frequent intervals according to preference; if client is on fluid restriction, also offer hard candies or lozenges between fluids if within diet prescription.

   Thirst is not a reliable indicator for the amount of necessary fluid replacement. Two per cent to 3 per cent of body weight can be lost before thirst is stimulated. Replacing fluids only until thirst is relieved can result in one half to two thirds of the fluid lost not being replaced.[68]

Rationale/Discussion

1. This helps promote return of bodily function to optimum level of well-being.

2. Providing fluids according to preference involves person in decision making, so that plan is more likely to be successful; if forcing fluids, frequent intervention increases the likelihood of meeting the desired outcome, whereas, if client is on fluid restriction, frequent fluids and candies keep the mucous membranes from becoming dry.

Procedure continued on following page

Regulation of Oral Fluid Intake (Forcing or Restricting Fluids)

Actions	Rationale/Discussion
Electrolyte and carbohydrate drinks have no advantage over water in maintaining plasma volume and electrolyte concentrations or in improving intestinal absorption but may enhance performance because of the carbohydrate component. Cold water is the preferred fluid for replacement for loss secondary to exercise.[68]	
3. Serve iced fluids, with large ice cubes, in thick glasses with large outside diameter but smaller inside diameters.	3. Cold liquids quench thirst faster than warmer liquids. Ice cubes displace fluid and make the glass appear to hold more than is the case. The thick glass makes the person believe it holds more fluid than it does, and the person feels satisfied with less to drink.
4. Assist with or encourage oral care every 8 hours and every 1 or 2 hours if client is on fluid restriction.	4. Oral care in a client with a dry mouth helps to decrease the risk of alteration in oral mucous membranes; frequency of care is increased to decrease sensation of thirst when fluid restricted.
5. Record all intake accurately (e.g., oral, including ice chips; liquid with medications; IV fluids, including piggyback medications; tube feedings) every 8 hours.	5. Physician and nursing orders are based on I & O data; accuracy is imperative to ensure that orders are therapeutic; totals must reflect all intake in order to be accurate.
6. Monitor and record all output.	6. Intake must be evaluated within the context of output as well as other assessment findings; one measurement of data is never enough on which to base intervention.
7. Assess daily weights every morning before breakfast, after voiding, using the same scale, clothing, and linens.	7. If assessed accurately, daily weights assist in evaluation of fluid balance.
8. Use pumps for delivery of IV fluids and tube feedings.	8. Pumps provide a more accurate delivery system for fluids; accuracy is essential for clients with critical fluid imbalances, for children, and for those persons with central catheters.
9. Monitor laboratory values: electrolytes, hemoglobin and hematocrit, blood urea nitrogen (BUN), creatinine, urine and serum osmolarity.	9. Monitoring laboratory values provides data to help evaluate desired outcomes related to fluid balance or imbalance, kidney function, effects of interventions; nurse is responsible for notifying physician of laboratory values; in some agencies, laboratory personnel are responsible for notifying physician of critical values.
10. Monitor response to prescribed medications (desired as well as side effects).	10. Medications can either cause or help correct fluid imbalances.
11. Teach person and family to assist with monitoring/recording of I and O if appropriate.	11. Client and family assistance increases chances of success and helps person feel more involved in own care, improves self-esteem.
12. Teach person and family about signs and symptoms of fluid imbalance in order to monitor them at home.	12. Knowledge of signs and symptoms will increase the likelihood of early detection and treatment of imbalances.
13. Teach person and family conditions that increase risk for fluid imbalance (e.g., fever, exercise, hot and dry climates, medications, vomiting, diarrhea).	13. Knowledge of risk factors will increase the likelihood of self-care interventions aimed at fluid replacement or using caution to decrease risks for fluid overload. Knowledge alone does not ensure positive health behaviors; it only increases the likelihood of occurrence as well as improves self-care potential, especially for internally motivated persons. Externally motivated persons are more likely to respond to chance or to those they consider powerful others (e.g., the physician).
14. Assist person and family in identifying risk factors and barriers that affect ability to adapt life style (e.g., changes in cooking methods, financial concerns, lack of knowledge concerning diet, medications, illness).	14. Barriers decrease the potential for successful outcomes; knowledge of these provides information necessary to adapt plan to individual needs and situations.
15. Refer to appropriate resources for assistance with lifestyle changes as necessary (e.g., nutritionist, social services department) on the basis of assessment findings; social service departments may be in charge of the referrals to Visiting Nurses Association or home health.	15. Team approach to identified problems provides more expertise and consistency in care planning and interventions.

PROCEDURE 41–2 Continued

Regulation of Oral Fluid Intake (Forcing or Restricting)

Actions	*Rationale/Discussion*
16. Provide client with needed telephone numbers (dietary, social services, nursing unit).	16. This provides person with security of knowing help is available; clients often forget to ask questions because of the stress of the situation, eagerness to go home, or lack of awareness until the person actually becomes a more active participant in self-care.

FINAL ACTIVITIES

Document the I & O, weight, other physical assessment data, teaching, referrals, medications, and person's and family's responses to each intervention on appropriate forms. Indicate need for further teaching. If fluid balance is to be monitored at home, teach person and significant other about subtle signs of fluid overload such as weight gain, edema in feet, and increased difficulty in breathing. If the person is more at risk for fluid deficit, teach about minimal fluid requirements and the importance of taking fluid every hour and to report vomiting or diarrhea that persists for more than 24 hours to the physician. Continue to offer support and guidance to the person and family.

---

cation is sometimes changed to another route or given with a sip of water).
- ▶ Be aware of the potential for undesirable medication interactions. Many medications potentiate each other (increasing the risk for side effects) or oppose each other (so that larger dosages may be needed to obtain a desired outcome). Increased awareness of these interactions leads to early detection of either effect.
- ▶ Document administration, refusal, or withholding of medication. Notify the physician if the person was unable to take the medication or refused it or if a condition change indicates a need to change the medication order. Document rationale for holding (not administering) a medication (e.g., change in condition) and notification of the physician.
- ▶ Monitor response to medications and document these data.
- ▶ Review the person's and family's understanding of medication therapy as related to water, electrolyte, and acid-base balances, and provide teaching based on identified need, including dietary component if appropriate.
- ▶ Notify the physician if the medication is not achieving the desired outcomes or if side effects or toxicity are present. The urgency of notifying the physician depends on the critical nature of the side effect or toxicity.
- ▶ Reinforce rationale and importance of ongoing assessments (e.g., pulse or blood pressure assessments) if the client is going home while taking any medications.
- ▶ Review understanding through the person's or significant other's verbal repetition of information taught or return demonstration of skills taught.

Administering Tube Feedings

Tube feedings can be used to correct water, electrolyte, and acid-base imbalances. Tube feedings can,

however, <u>cause</u> water, electrolyte, and acid-base imbalances. Therefore, monitor the person's fluid and electrolyte status while he or she is on enteral feedings. Cautions are similar to those for administering medications.

Enteral feedings are prescribed by a physician, provided by the dietary department, and initiated, controlled, and monitored by the nursing team. As a nurse administering tube feedings, you are accountable for monitoring the client's water, electrolyte, and acid-base balances before, during, and after the feedings and for consulting the physician whenever there are concerns related to the feedings. Tube feedings are discussed in Chapter 42. In relation to water, electrolytes, and acid-base balances, you should know that

- ▶ Feedings with high solute content can produce an osmotic imbalance known as hypertonic dehydration. Feedings with high osmolarity include Meritene, Carnation Instant Breakfast, Compleat Regular, Criticare HN, Pepti-2000, Travasorb STD HN-Renal and Hepatic, Reabilan, Vital HN, Vivonex HN, Vivonex TEN, Amin-Aid, Hepatic-Aid, Pulmocare, Ross SLD, Stresstein, Trauma Cal, Enrich, Sustacal, Sustacal with Fiber, Sustacal HC, Twocal, Ensure HN, Ensure Plus, Magnacal, and Isocal HCN.[8,54]
- ▶ Because the elderly are at risk for hypernatremia, the sodium content of the feeding, as well as the serum sodium levels, should be monitored.
- ▶ Lactose-based feedings should be avoided for those persons with lactose intolerance. If a person with an intolerance receives a lactose-based feeding, the resultant diarrhea could further compromise water, electrolyte, and acid-base status. Examples of lactose-based solutions include Vitaneed, Compleat B, Compleat-Modified, Carnation Instant Breakfast, and Meritene.[54]
- ▶ Persons with renal or hepatic dysfunction will have very specific fluid and electrolyte needs. Amin-Aid and Travasorb Renal provide an appropriate low-protein electrolyte source for persons with severe renal disease. Hepatic Aid and Travasorb Hepatic

provide appropriate low-protein electrolyte levels for a person with severe liver disease.[54]

▶ Glucerna is recommended for persons with diabetes mellitus because of its low-carbohydrate and high-monounsaturated fat content.[54]

▶ Examples of high-protein, low-potassium feedings for persons experiencing hypermetabolic states secondary to early stages of tissue trauma include Stresstein, Trauma Cal, Ross SLD, and Citrotein.[54]

▶ Pulmocare is often ordered for persons with chronic respiratory disease because it promotes the excretion of carbon dioxide.[8,54]

▶ Osmolarity and nutrient content of feedings vary. Isotonic feedings have an osmolarity of 275 to 295 mOsm/kg; hypertonic feedings have an osmolarity greater than 300 mOsm/kg.

▶ Check the temperature of the unit refrigerator if the formula is prepared by the dietary department. Bacteria (Clostridium difficile) growing in the feeding formula can lead to diarrhea, with resulting water, electrolyte, and acid-base imbalances.

▶ Note the expiration date on the container, or, if the can is open, use only a refrigerated source within 24 hours of the time the can is opened.

▶ When medications are changed to elixir sources, check them for a sorbitol base.[20] Sorbitol-based elixirs, which cause osmotic diarrhea, have been frequently implicated as an etiologic factor of diarrhea in clients on tube feedings. Do not assume that diarrhea is caused by the tube feeding.

General nursing interventions related to maintaining water, electrolyte, and acid-base balances in clients receiving tube feedings include

▶ consulting the physician regarding additional fluid needed when receiving a hyperosmotic feeding; 1 ml of water is required for every Kcal delivered.[54]

▶ recording intake and output every 8 hours, and recording weights daily

▶ measuring abdominal girth every 8 hours if abdominal distention occurs

▶ evaluating normality of bowel response to feedings

▶ observing for signs and symptoms of fluid, electrolyte, and acid-base imbalances (see Table 41-6)

▶ monitoring laboratory values (e.g., electrolytes, hemoglobin and hematocrit, BUN, creatinine, liver function studies, arterial blood gas values)

▶ keeping the head of the bed elevated 30 degrees at all times to assist in retention of feeding and decrease risk of aspiration

▶ documenting administration of feedings; observe the person's response to tube feedings and document findings using subjective data (e.g., presence or absence or nausea) and objective data (e.g., intake and output, weight, bowel sounds, abdominal girth, stool characteristics)

▶ explaining to the person and significant others (1) the purpose of the enteral feeding, (2) the rationale for monitoring intake and output and weight, and (3) the rationale for the skin care associated with the presence of an artificial tube.

▶ evaluating the client's and family's need for reinforcement of prior teaching; for example, if a client is going home on tube feedings, demonstrate the procedure for the care giver, and evaluate the level of performance and understanding with return demonstration.

Monitoring Intravenous Therapy

Whenever possible, fluids and electrolytes should be administered by the oral route (mouth or by tube) rather than by the IV route. Nevertheless, IV infusion is the method of choice when a person cannot receive fluids, electrolytes, or medications by other routes. Because of the risk of infection and the increased cost of the IV route, tube feeding is the route of choice for long-term therapy. More specifically, IV infusions are ordered under the following circumstances:

▶ persons in life-threatening situations (e.g., hemorrhage, shock, and severe burns); immediate plasma volume replacement is vital to life under these circumstances

▶ persons who are NPO or who are unable to ingest oral fluids because of prolonged nausea, vomiting, diarrhea, peritonitis, paralytic ileus, or fistula

▶ persons who require medications that can be given by the IV route and that would be destroyed by digestive juices or would not be absorbed by the GI tract if given orally

▶ persons unable to digest or absorb a diet administered by mouth or tube (e.g., those who do not have an anatomically or functionally intact GI tract)

The type of IV solution ordered depends on the individual's condition and the fluid and electrolyte imbalance. Many substances can be infused intravenously (carbohydrates, protein hydrolysates, electrolytes, alcohol, vitamins, water, and many medications). In addition, parenteral fluids vary in their tonicity. Thus, IV fluids may be hypotonic, isotonic, or hypertonic. Table 41-5 summarizes information and precautions about commonly used IV solutions. Because of the dangers inherent in parenteral therapy, a safe order should include the specific solutions, the additives and dose to be given, and the time schedule for each infusion. Major nursing responsibilities include knowing the uses and precautions for each solution and keeping the infusion on schedule. Correctly calculating IV flow rates using adhesive strips on the side of the IV bag or using IV infusion pumps are ways to help ensure precise fluid delivery.

Several vital assessments are required in IV therapy. Observe the individual for signs and symptoms of fluid overload (see Table 41-6) and reactions to medications or electrolytes within the infusion. Monitor urinary output; poor urinary output could lead to circulatory overload and electrolyte excesses or deficits (deficits are secondary to dilution of serum electrolytes). Assess the infusion site for signs of infiltration (tissue swelling, hardness, pain at the needle site, a feeling of coldness around injection site, evidence of tissue necrosis) and signs of phlebitis (redness, warmth, and tenderness at the puncture site or along the vein). Monitor the needle or catheter site to ensure that dressings are dry and intact and that the needle or catheter is anchored securely to decrease the risk of infection and venous trauma. Monitor the IV fluid and flow rate to make certain the IV and drip rate are accurate. Ascertain that there are no kinks in the tubing. Anticipate when the next IV will be needed, and alert the pharmacist if a bag is not already available. Assess circulation to ensure that the arm board, if required, is not occluding tissue perfusion.

Other solutions may be prescribed to meet specific metabolic deficits. For example, whole blood and packed cells may be ordered to restore blood volume after severe trauma or hemorrhage. Immunosuppressed persons may receive leukocyte-poor red blood cells. Volume expanders such as plasma, albumin, or plasma protein fractions may be ordered to restore plasma volume or replace protein losses. Persons with thrombocytopenia may receive platelet concentrations; those with fibrogen deficiencies or hemophilia may receive cryoprecipitated antihemophilic factor. Persons who are unable to meet their nutritional metabolic needs through oral or tube feeding may receive their nutritional supplementation through parenteral hyperalimentation (carbohydrate, amino acids, lipids, electrolytes, and vitamins). Each of these various fluid solutions have specific nursing responsibilities. You are responsible not only for following the specific guidelines related to each of these different solutions as addressed in the literature but also for following specific agency procedural policies governing administration, monitoring, and intervention related to development of complications. See Chapter 47 for more information related to nursing responsibilities of IV therapy.

EVALUATION

Evaluation is not a final step of the nursing process but instead an interactive component related to each of the other steps. The following list provides suggestions of evaluation categories that relate to a person with water, electrolyte, or acid-base imbalance:

▶ intake and output status (all forms of intake and output)
▶ weight loss or gain
▶ reports of or absence of "thirst"
▶ moisture level of mucous membranes
▶ time frames for peripheral vein filling and emptying
▶ presence of neck vein distention (including angle of client's head and neck)
▶ presence of edema, third spacing (e.g., ascites)
▶ quality of lung sounds; presence of adventitious sounds
▶ Rates, rhythm, and quality of vital signs (blood pressure, temperature, pulse, respirations)
▶ respiratory or cardiac distress at rest or with activity
▶ presence of paresthesias, tremors, and Chvostek's or Trousseau's sign
▶ level of consciousness (including presence of convulsions)
▶ bowel sounds or change in bowel characteristics
▶ characteristics of urinary excretion (including change)
▶ ECG findings (including changes in PQRST waves or presence of dysrhythmias)
▶ laboratory findings (including hematocrit; hemoglobin; specific gravity; serum and urine osmolalities; electrolyte levels, particularly sodium, chloride, potassium, calcium, magnesium, phosphate, and serum protein; arterial blood gases)
▶ chest x-ray findings

Your evaluation of your client's progress toward achievement of the desired outcomes should indicate improvement in water, electrolyte, or acid-base balance, but such positive changes do not always occur. Several factors may influence the achievement of the desired outcomes: The client's condition may have deteriorated; the desired outcomes or time frame may have been unrealistic; or perhaps the interventions were unsuccessful or inappropriate. A thorough evaluation of the total picture should help you revise the client's current care plan as appropriate.

CASE STUDY

The Client

Loran Lindel is a 69-year-old married father of three who drives an intercoastal semitruck for his primary occupation. His history includes hypertension and congestive heart failure. Current medications include digoxin, 0.25 mg daily, and thiazide, 25 mg twice a day. On June 15, nausea, vomiting, and diarrhea developed. Three days later, he was still experiencing the same problems and was becoming concerned about missing more work. A routine office visit led to hospital admission. On June 18, nursing and medical assessment data included the following:

▶ "I have had vomiting and diarrhea for 3 days."
▶ "I'm so thirsty, but I've been so afraid to drink, except for

my pills, because I've vomited every time I've tried."
▶ reports eight liquid stools per day for the last 3 days
▶ reports "severe weakness"
▶ reports "dizziness" when changing positions
▶ weight on admission 170 lbs; states normal weight is 178 lbs
▶ blood pressure = 102/86 standing, 80/60 lying down
▶ temperature = 37 °C; pulse = 84; weak, and slightly irregular; respirations = 24, shallow
▶ skin warm, dry; turgor 5 seconds; mucous membranes dry; tongue furrowed
▶ restless but alert and oriented to person, place, and time

Case Study continued on following page

CASE STUDY Continued

The Client

▶ lung sounds clear in all fields; denies cough; no peripheral edema, no abnormal heart sounds
▶ abdomen distended and nontender, bowel sounds hyperactive all quadrants
▶ Laboratory findings:
WBC = 15,000 with shift to left (indicates increase in immature WBCs, usually secondary to bacterial infection)
RBC = 5.0
Hgb = 19 gm/100 ml
Hct = 57%
Na+ = 120 mEq/L
K+ = 3.2 mEq/L
Cl⁻ = 85 mEq/L
BUN = 15
Creatinine = 0.8

▶ Physician's orders:
start 5% D/NS with 40 mEq KCl, infuse 150 ml/hour
CBC, electrolytes stat and daily × 3
BUN and creatinine stat
serum digoxin level (hold digoxin until lab called)
stool to lab for C & S
I and O, daily weight
clear liquid, high-carbohydrate diet; advance to full liquid if tolerated
Prochlorperazine (e.g., Compazine) 10 mg IM or supp. q 6 hours prn nausea or vomiting
Loperamide (e.g., Imodium) 4 mg stat and 2 mg q 4 hours prn diarrhea

CARE PLAN

June 18

Nursing Diagnosis	Planning: Expected Outcomes	Implementation: Nursing Interventions	Evaluation
Fluid Volume Deficit R/T excess fluid loss, decreased fluid intake secondary to nausea, vomiting, and diarrhea	By 3 pm, June 20: ▶ reports less thirst	▶ Assess for presence of thirst every 8 hours. ▶ Offer small amounts of clear fluids (1 oz) every hour while awake and on awakening at night.	3 pm, June 20: Outcomes partially met. Client has improved fluid balance AEB: ▶ Reports decreased thirst, drinks 1 oz fluid per hour
	▶ has moist mucous membranes and improved skin turgor (<5 seconds)	▶ Encourage or assist with oral hygiene every 8 hours and prn. ▶ Lubricate lips with lanolin or petroleum jelly every 2 hours. ▶ Assess skin turgor every 4 hours while awake.	▶ Oral mucous membranes moist; skin returns immediately when turgor assessed
	▶ has weight gain of 1 lb and improved I & O	▶ Weigh QD at 0600, after voiding, with same scale and clothing. ▶ Record I & O every 8 hours. ▶ Monitor IV fluids every hour. ▶ Use IV pump to regulate IV flow. ▶ Administer prochlorperazine every 6 hours prn nausea as ordered.	▶ Weight = 171.5 lbs; no vomiting, one diarrheal stool; 24-hour I & O: oral intake = 500 ml; IV = 3600 ml output: urine = 3300 ml; gastric = 150 ml; bowel = 100 ml Total: intake = 4100 ml; output = 3550 ml IV infusing as ordered without swelling or redness

CARE PLAN (Continued)

June 18

Nursing Diagnosis	Planning: Expected Outcomes	Implementation: Nursing Interventions	Evaluation
	▶ has systolic lying and standing BP within 10 mm Hg difference; pulse = 60–100, regular and strong	▶ Administer loperamide every 4 hours prn diarrheal stool as ordered. ▶ Record characteristics of vomitus and stool. ▶ Assess lying and standing BP at 0900 and 1600. ▶ Assess TPR every 4 hours, and rate, rhythm, and quality of pulse and respiration 0800, 1200, 1600, 2000, 2400, 0400.	June 20: BP lying down = 116/76, standing = 110/70; apical pulse = 86, full, regular; temperature = 36.5 °C, respirations = 18, even, deep

Summary

▶ Water is the main constituent of body fluid. With electrolytes, it is distributed between the intracellular fluid (ICF) and the extracellular fluid (ECF) compartments. The ECF compartment contains the interstitial fluid and plasma. Body water and electrolytes continually move between the ICF and ECF compartments. Water balance exists when the intake of water and electrolytes equals the output (loss) of water and electrolytes.

▶ The average adult requires 2600 ml of water per day.

▶ Electrolytes break down in water to cations and anions. Cations carry a positive charge. Anions carry a negative charge. Plasma proteins are not electrolytes, but they carry a weak negative charge and thus behave as anions.

▶ Electrolytes promote neuromuscular irritability, maintain body fluid osmolality, regulate acid-base balance, and maintain body water distribution. Plasma proteins hold water within blood vessels and promote water movement from the interstitial spaces into the plasma.

▶ Units used to measure fluid and electrolytes include the liter and milliliter, the gram and milligram, and the milliequivalent, a measure of the chemical combining power of an ion.

▶ Body fluid compartments contain the same electrolytes, but the electrolytes occur in different amounts.

▶ Processes involved in fluid and electrolyte transport between the ICF and the ECF include osmotic pressure, hydrostatic pressure, filtration, diffusion, facilitated diffusion, and active transport. Processes involved in fluid transport between the vascular and interstitial compartments include blood hydrostatic pressure, colloid osmotic pressure (also called blood oncotic pressure), filtration pressure, and lymphatic filtration.

▶ The neuroendocrine system is a major homeostatic regulator of body fluid volume and body fluid osmolality through the hormones antidiuretic hormone and aldosterone and the thirst mechanism. Other hormones aid in regulation of electrolyte balance. Disorders that affect these neuroendocrine mechanisms may disrupt fluid and electrolyte homeostasis.

▶ The gastrointestinal system is the route of intake, absorption, and rapid transport of water and electrolytes. The renal system functions interdependently with the neuroendocrine system to regulate the ECF volume. Healthy kidneys alter the volume and concentration of urine as a response to the body's requirements. Altered renal function leads to the danger of developing imbalances of ECF volume, osmolality, and electrolytes (including hydrogen and bicarbonate ions). The cardiovascular system controls fluid balance through the action of atrial natriuretic peptide.

▶ Respiratory alkalosis and respiratory acidosis result from respiratory problems. All other acid-base imbalances are metabolic in origin.

▶ Mechanisms of acid-base regulation are blood buffers, which are chemical regulators; the lungs and kidneys, which are physiologic regulators; and body cells, which are biologic regulators.

▶ Risk factors for fluid, electrolyte, and acid-base imbalances include age, with infants, young children, and the elderly at high risk; pregnancy, body size, with body fat increasing the risk for fluid deficit; heat; stress; diet; and health problems that cause diarrhea, vomiting, fever, edema, third-space accumulation, hemorrhage, and drainage wounds. Medical treatments involving infusions, suction, and some medications may also cause imbalances.

▶ Nursing diagnoses for persons with fluid imbalances are *Fluid Volume Deficit, High Risk for Fluid Volume Deficit,* and *Fluid Volume Excess.*

▶ Objectives of fluid replacement are to correct deficits and restore vascular volume, thus resolving shock and dehydration; to maintain life-sustaining needs; and to replace dynamic or concurrent losses. Objectives of fluid retention involve reversing the mechanisms of edema and circulatory overload.

▶ Nursing interventions that relate to water and electrolyte and acid-base problems include recording intake and output, regulating diet, regulating oral fluid intake, administering medications and tube feedings, and providing intravenous therapy.

▶ Nurses are ethically and legally responsible for ongoing assessment and evaluation of the client's response to nursing and physician-ordered interventions aimed at optimizing water, electrolyte, and acid-base homeostasis.

Bibliography

1. Altara, R. (1990). *Applying nursing diagnosis and nursing process: A step-by-step guide* (2nd ed.). Philadelphia: J. B. Lippincott.
2. Baer, C. L. (1990). Acute renal failure: recognizing and reversing its deadly course. *Nursing 90,* 20(6), 34–39.
3. Balistreri, W. F. (1990). Oral rehydration in acute infantile diarrhea. *American Journal of Medicine,* 88(S6A), 30S–33S.
4. Barrus, D. H., & Danek, G. (1987). Should you irrigate an occluded I.V. line? *Nursing 87,* 17(3), 63–64.
5. Barta, M. A. (1987). Correcting electrolyte imbalances. *RN,* 50(2), 30–34.
6. Binder, H. J. (1990). Pathophysiology of acute diarrhea. *American Journal of Medicine,* 88(S6A), 2S–4S.
7. Birney, M. H., & Penny D. G. (1990). Atrial natriuretic peptide: a hormone with implications for clinical practice. *Heart and Lung,* 19(2), 174–183.
8. Bowman, M., et al. (1989). Effect of tube-feeding osmolality on serum sodium levels. *Critical Care Nurse,* 9(1), 22–28.
9. Calloway, C. (1987). When the problem involves magnesium, calcium, or phosphate. *RN,* 50(5), 30–36.
10. Carpenito, L. J. (1992). *Nursing diagnosis: Application to clinical practice* (4th ed.). Philadelphia: J. B. Lippincott.
11. Chambers, J. K. (1987). Fluid and electrolyte problems in renal and urologic disorders. *Nursing Clinics of North America,* 22(4), 815–825.
12. Chambers, J. K. (1987). Metabolic bone disorders: imbalances of calcium and phosphorus. *Nursing Clinics of North America,* 22(4), 861–871.
13. Chenevey, B. (1987). Overview of fluids and electrolytes. *Nursing Clinics of North America,* 22(4), 749–759.
14. Chernow, B., et al. (1989). Hypomagnesemia in patients in postoperative intensive care. *Chest,* 95(2), 391–397.
15. Cox, H., et al. (1989). *Clinical applications of nursing diagnosis.* Baltimore, MD: Williams & Wilkins.
16. DeAngelis, R. (1991). Hypokalemia. *Critical Care Nurse,* 11(7), 71–75.
17. Deters, G. E. (1987). Managing complications after abdominal surgery. *RN,* 50(3), 27–32.
18. Dreq, D., & Schumann, D. (1986). Homogeneity of potassium chloride in small volume intravenous containers. *Nursing Research,* 35(6), 325–328.
19. Dukes, G. E. (1989). Over-the-counter antidiarrheal medications used for the self-treatment of acute nonspecific diarrhea. *American Journal of Medicine,* 88(S6A), 24S–29S.
20. Edes, T. E., et al. (1990). Diarrhea in tube-fed patients: feeding formula not necessarily the cause. *American Journal of Medicine,* 88, 91–93.
21. Eschleman, M. M. (1991). *Introductory nutrition and diet therapy* (2nd ed.). Philadelphia: J. B. Lippincott.
22. Fadnes, H. O., & Olan, P. (1989). Transcapillary fluid balance and plasma volume regulation: a review. *Obstetrical and Gynecological Survey,* 44(11), 769–773.
23. Feldstein, A. (1986). Detect phlebitis and infiltration before they harm your patient. *Nursing 86,* 16(1), 44–47.
24. Felver, L., & Pendarvis, J. H. (1989). Electrolyte imbalances: intraoperative risk factors. *AORN,* 49(4), 992–1008.
25. Friday, B. A., & Reinhart, R. A. (1991). Magnesium metabolism: a case report and literature review. *Critical Care Nurse,* 11(5), 62–71.
26. Guyton, A. C. (1986). *Textbook of medical physiology* (7th ed.). Philadelphia: W. B. Saunders.
27. Henkelman, W. J., et al. (1991). Fluid volume dynamics. *Critical Care Nurse,* 11(4), 74–76.
28. Herlihy, B. L., & Herlihy, J. T. (1987). Physiologic role and regulation of potassium. *Critical Care Nurse,* 7(5), 10–11.
29. Holtzman, G. M. (1990). Magnesium. *Critical Care Nurse,* 10(7), 81–83.
30. Jackson, M. F. (1988). High risk surgical patients. *Journal of Gerontological Nursing,* 14(1), 8–15.
31. Janusek, L. W. (1990). Metabolic acidosis. *Nursing 90,* 20(7), 52–53.
32. Jones, A., et al. (1991). Fluid volume dynamics. *Critical Care Nursing,* 11(4), 74–75.
33. Karb, V. B. (1989). Electrolyte abnormalities and drugs which commonly cause them. *Journal of Neuroscience Nursing,* 21(2), 125–129.
34. Kassierer, J. P., et al. (1989). *Repairing body fluids: Principles & practice.* Philadelphia: W. B. Saunders.
35. Keppler, A. B. (1988). The use of intravenous fluids during labor. *Birth,* 15(2), 75–79.
36. Kokko, J. P., & Tannen, R. L. (1989). *Fluids and electrolytes* (2nd ed.). Philadelphia: W. B. Saunders.
37. Kositzke, J. A. (1990). A question of balance: dehydration in the elderly. *Journal of Gerontological Nursing,* 16(5), 4–11.
38. Kuhn, M. M. (1991). Colloids vs. crystalloids. *Critical Care Nurse,* 11(5), 37–51.
39. Kurtzman, N. A. (1990). Disorders of distal acidification. *Kidney International,* 38, 720–727.
40. Lacy, J. A. (1991). Albumin overview: use as a nutritional marker and as a therapeutic intervention. *Critical Care Nurse,* 11(1), 46–49.
41. Lancaster, L. E. (1987). Renal and endocrine regulation of water and electrolyte balance. *Nursing Clinics of North America,* 22(4), 761–772.
42. Managing special patients' fluid and electrolytes. (1988). *Nursing 88,* 18(1), 64.
43. Marshall, P. (1990). The heart as a gland. *Nursing Times,* 86(7), 42–43.
44. Mathewson, M. (1989). Intravenous therapy. *Critical Care Nurse,* 9(2), 21–36.
45. Metheny, N. M. (1990). Why worry about IV fluids? *American Journal of Nursing,* 88, 50–56.
46. Meyers, K. A., & Hickey, M. K. (1988). Nursing management of hypovolemic shock. *Critical Care Nursing Quarterly,* 11(1), 57–61.
47. Millam, D. A. (1988). Managing complications of I.V. therapy. *Nursing 88,* 18(3), 34–42.
48. Mintz, P., et al. (1986). The latest protocols for blood transfusions. *Nursing 86,* 16(10), 34–41.
49. Morton, P. B. (1989). *Health assessment in nursing.* Springhouse, PA: Springhouse Corp.
50. Mueller, K. D., & Boisen, A. M. (1989). Keeping your patient's water level up. *RN,* 52(7), 65–68.
51. Pagana, K. D., & Pagana, T. J. (1990). *Diagnostic testing and nursing implications* (3rd ed.). St. Louis: C. V. Mosby.
52. Palmer, T. A. (1990). Anorexia nervosa, bulimia nervosa: causal theories and treatment. *Nurse Practitioner,* 15(4), 12–21.

53. Patterson, L. M., & Noroian, E. L. (1989). Diabetes insipidus versus syndrome of inappropriate antidiuretic hormone. *Dimensions of Critical Care Nursing,* 8(4), 227–234.

54. Petrosino, B., et al. (1989). Implications of selected problems with nasoenteral tube feedings. *Enteral Care Nursing Quarterly,* 12(3), 1–17.

55. Poyss, A. S. (1987). Assessment and nursing diagnosis in fluid and electrolyte disorders. *Nursing Clinics of North America,* 22(4), 773–783.

56. Querin, J. J., & Stahl, L. D. (1990). 12 simple sensible steps for successful blood transfusion. *Nursing 90,* 20(10), 68–81.

57. Rice, V. (1991). Shock, a clinical syndrome: an update. Part I. *Critical Care Nurse,* 11(4), 20–27.

58. Rice, V. (1991). Shock, a clinical syndrome: an update. Part 3. *Critical Care Nurse,* 11(6), 34–39.

59. Rice, V. (1991). Shock, a clinical syndrome: an update. Part 4. *Critical Care Nurse,* 11(7), 28–38.

60. Rinard, G. (1989). Water intoxication. *American Journal of Nursing,* 89, 1635–1637.

61. Rolls, B. J., & Phillips, P. A. (1990). Aging and disturbances of thirst and fluid balance. *Nutritional Reviews,* 48(3), 137–144.

62. Sands, J. M., & Kokko, J. P. (1990). Countercurrent system. *Kidney International,* 38, 695–699.

63. Sherman, J. E., & Sherman, R. H. (1989). I.V. therapy that clicks. *Nursing 89,* 19(5), 50–51.

64. Simmons, B., et al. (1990). Infection control for home health. *Infection Control Hospital Epidemiology,* 11(7), 362–370.

65. Sommers, M. (1990). Fluid resuscitation following multiple trauma. *Critical Care Nurse,* 10(10), 74–81.

66. Sommers, M. (1990). Rapid fluid resuscitation. *Nursing 90,* 20(1), 52–59.

67. Sprauve, D. (1990). Fluids, electrolytes, and acid-base balance. *Nursing 90,* 20(3), 103–106.

68. Squire, D. L. (1990). Fluid and electrolyte issues for pediatric and adolescent athletes. *Pediatric Clinics of North America,* 37(5), 1085–1101.

69. Sullivan, L., & Grantham, T. (1982). *Physiology of the Kidney* (2nd ed.). Philadelphia: Lea & Febiger.

70. Taptich, B. J., et al. (1989). *Nursing diagnosis and care planning.* Philadelphia: W. B. Saunders.

71. Taylor, D. L. (1990). Respiratory acidosis. *Nursing 90,* 20(9), 52–53.

72. Taylor, D. L. (1990). Respiratory alkalosis. *Nursing 90,* 20(8), 60–61.

73. Valle, G. A., & Lemberg, L. (1988). Electrolyte imbalances in cardiovascular disease: the forgotten factor. *Heart and Lung,* 17(3), 324–329.

74. Walpert, N. (1990). Calcium metabolism disorders. *Nursing 90,* 20(7), 60–64.

75. Woodtli, A. (1990). Thirst: a critical care nursing challenge. *Dimensions of Critical Care Nursing,* 9(1), 6–15.

76. Yarnell, R. P., & Craig, M. P. (1991). Detecting hypo-magnesemia: the most overlooked electrolyte imbalance. *Nursing 91,* 21(7), 55–57.

77. York, K. (1987). The lung and fluid-electrolyte and acid-base imbalance. *Nursing Clinics of North America,* 22(4), 805–814.

78. Young, M. E., & Flynn, K. T. (1988). Third-spacing: when the body conceals fluid loss. *RN,* 51(8), 46–48.

Chapter 42

 ## *Meeting Nutritional Needs*

 Give me a good digestion, Lord, and also something to digest.
Anonymous

▼ CHAPTER OUTLINE

BASIC CONCEPTS OF GOOD NUTRITION
    Structure and Function of the
      Gastrointestinal Tract
    Nutritional Requirements
    Calories, Body Weight, and
      Nutrients
    Recommended Dietary Allowances
      and Dietary Guidelines
POPULAR CONCERNS ABOUT DIET AND
  HEALTH
    Food Additives
    Natural and Organic Foods
    Vitamin, Mineral, and Food
      Supplements
    Special Foods
    Vegetarianism
ASSESSMENT
    Food and Dietary Records
    Physical Assessment

Feelings About Diet Changes
Factors That Influence Food Intake,
    Dietary Patterns, and Nutritional
    Status
NURSING DIAGNOSIS
PLANNING
NURSING INTERVENTION
    Managing Diet Therapy
    Maintaining or Improving the
      Appetite
    Increasing Ingestion of the
      Appropriate Diet
    Increasing Digestion
    Increasing Absorption
    Maintaining Nutrition When
      Gastrointestinal Function Is
      Impaired
EVALUATION
CASE STUDY

▼ KEY TERMS

Anorexia nervosa
Bulimia nervosa
Cachexia
Carbohydrate loading
Celiac sprue
Cellulose
Dextrins
Dietary Guidelines for
  Americans
Dysphagia
Enteral feeding

Esophagogastrostomy tube
Esophagostomy
Gastric analysis
Gastrointestinal
  compression
Gastrointestinal
  decompression
Gastrostomy tube
Gavage
Glycolipids
Gums

Hyperlipidemia
Hypoglycemia
Intubation
Jejunostomy tube
Lacto-ovovegetarian
Lactovegetarians
Lavage
Lignin
Lipoproteins
Monounsaturated fats
Mucilages

Nasogastric (NG) tube
NPO (nil per os)
Orogastric tube
Parenteral support

Pectins
Peripheral parenteral
   nutrition (PPN)

Phospholipids
Polyunsaturated fats

Recommended Dietary
   Allowances (RDAs)
Saturated fats

Unsaturated fats
Vegans
Vegetarians

▼ LEARNING OBJECTIVES

After studying this chapter, you should be able to

1. Discuss how the nurse uses the basic concepts of good nutrition to meet clients' nutritional needs.
2. Discuss popular concerns about diet and health.
3. Describe methods to assess a person's dietary intake and nutritional status.
4. Identify factors that influence food intake, dietary patterns, and nutritional status.
5. Identify special nutritional needs associated with each stage of the life cycle.
6. State how to assess a client's nutritional needs.
7. Discuss nursing diagnoses appropriate for clients with nutrition problems.
8. List expected outcomes for a client with nutritional problems.
9. Explain nutritional interventions.
10. State how to evaluate nutritional outcomes.

Good health is based on good nutrition. The person who understands the principles of good nutrition and who eats a balanced diet can more successfully meet the challenges of work and enjoy the pleasures of play. Poor nutrition, however, causes illness of body and mind. The person who suffers from long-term inadequate nutrition can develop severe deficiencies that result in disorders of bones and teeth, low body weight, anemia, weakness, apathy, faulty digestion of nutrients, and so forth. In turn, these problems create additional nutritional deficiencies due to loss of appetite or interest in food, which then compounds the original problem. Excessive ingestion of calories or certain nutrients (e.g., cholesterol) can also cause dangerous health disorders.

Today, people are more aware of the benefits of good nutrition and more concerned about the disabling effects of poor nutrition. Classes, books, magazine articles, and television programs stress ways for the average person to eat a balanced diet and thus prevent both nutritional deficiencies and excesses. Yet much in the media can lead the consumer in unhealthy directions. To help show the public the way, nurses need to support clinical programs, community activities, and media coverage that focus on improving the eating habits of people in the community and worldwide.

As a nurse, you will frequently assess a person's nutritional status. With the dietitian (nutritionist) and other members of the health care team, you will check that persons in your care are receiving adequate foods, fluids, and nutritional supplements on a regular basis. Also, you may need to orient an individual and significant others to a new therapeutic dietary regimen by explaining the specifics of the new diet, including reasons why certain foods are important and why other foods cannot be eaten. You therefore will need to know not only the theoretical aspects of nutrition but also the practical problems of helping people adjust to

changes in two basic human activities, eating and drinking.

BASIC CONCEPTS OF GOOD NUTRITION

Structure and Function of the Gastrointestinal Tract

The primary function of the gastrointestinal (GI) tract is to provide the body with nutrients, fluids, and electrolytes in a form that can be used at the cellular level. Specifically, its functions include (1) ingestion (the mechanism of taking and swallowing food), (2) digestion (the mechanical and chemical breaking down of food substances into absorbable forms), (3) absorption (the passage of absorbable food substances from the gastrointestinal tract into the blood or lymph), and (4) elimination.

Anatomically, the GI tract (also called the alimentary tract) is a continuous tube approximately 6.9 m (23 ft) in length from mouth to anus (Fig. 42–1). The GI tract includes the mouth, pharynx, esophagus, stomach, small and large intestines, and numerous accessory organs.

The mouth contains the teeth, tongue, and salivary glands. The teeth grind (i.e., masticate, or chew) food with the help of the jaw muscles. The tongue is a voluntary muscle covered with mucous membrane. It helps move food within the mouth during the processes of chewing and swallowing. Saliva is secreted into the mouth by the parotid, submandibular, and sublingual glands. Saliva contains mucus, which provides lubrication for swallowing, and a starch-splitting enzyme, salivary amylase (ptyalin). Salivary amylase begins the digestion of starches and other carbohydrates.

Ingestion and digestion begin as a bite of food is

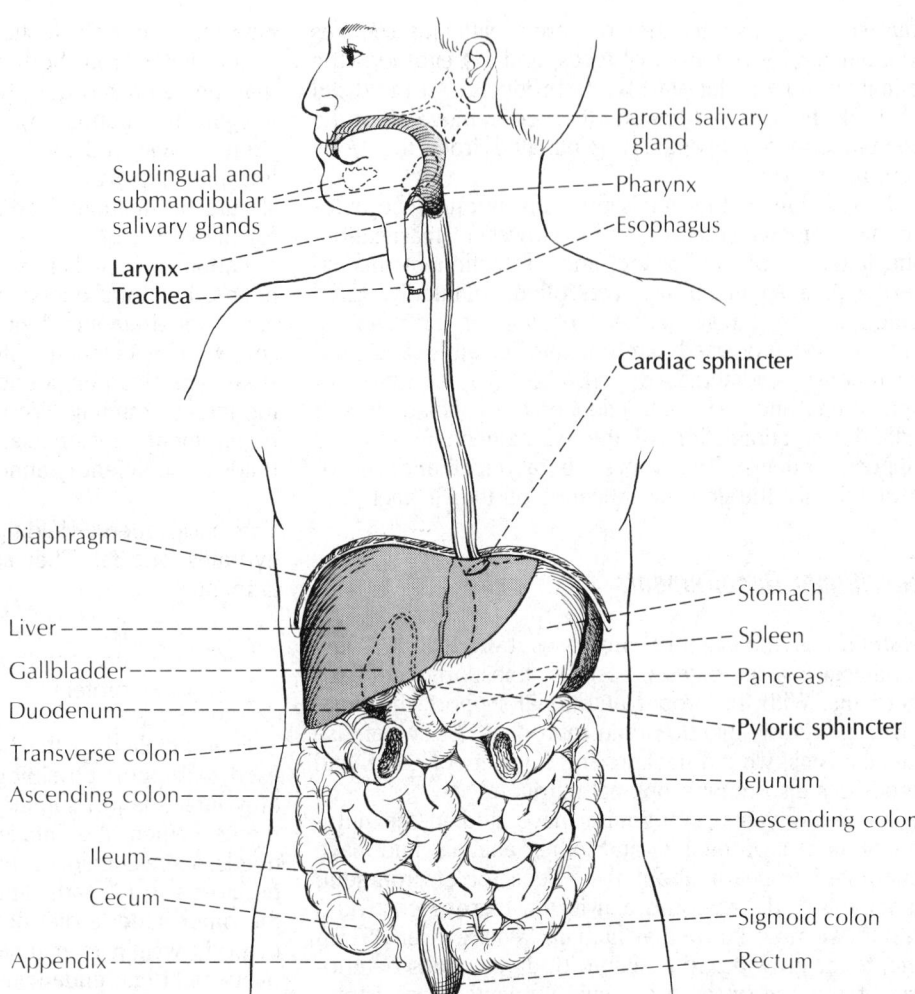

▲ *Figure 42-1*

Structure of the gastrointestinal tract.

taken into the mouth. After entering the mouth, food is chewed into smaller pieces and mixed with saliva. Saliva then lubricates the food and starts the process of digestion, and the moistened, lubricated food forms a bolus that is pushed to the back of the mouth in preparation for swallowing (deglutition).

The pharynx is the next segment of the GI tract. It serves as a common pathway for food and air. Contraction of its muscular tissue directs food and fluid into the esophagus, closing off entrances to the larynx and nasal cavities.

The esophagus is the portion of the GI tube that connects the pharynx with the stomach. This muscular, hollow tube expands and contracts rhythmically, thus propelling food down into the stomach. These rhythmic movements, called peristaltic waves, are normally present from the esophagus to the end of the GI tract.

The area of the esophagus proximal to the stomach normally remains in a state of contraction and is called the gastroesophageal, cardiac, or lower esophageal sphincter. It opens ahead of the peristaltic wave and closes behind it, preventing regurgitation.

Like the esophagus, the stomach is a muscular structure. It continues digestion by adding mucus, enzymes, and hydrochloric acid. These substances help change the consistency of the food bolus into a semiliquid

mixture called chyme. Chyme is stored for gradual release into the small intestine. Some absorption of nutrients also takes place in the stomach.

The pyloric sphincter, the distal opening of the stomach, controls the passage of chyme from the stomach into the small intestine. The small intestine is a thin tube coiled in the abdominal cavity. It is suspended from the posterior abdominal wall by the mesentery, a double-layered fold of peritoneum that protects and stabilizes the abdominal organs. The three sections of the small intestine are the duodenum (proximal portion), jejunum (middle portion), and ileum (distal portion).

In the small intestine, the chyme is churned and mixed with digestive juices from the small intestine, pancreas, gallbladder, and liver. These secretions act on starches, sugars, proteins, and fats to prepare them for absorption. Most of the products of this digestive process are absorbed into the circulation through microscopic projections of epithelial cells (villi) in the walls of the small intestine. Undigested food products are propelled into the large intestine.

The large intestine is divided into the cecum, ascending colon, transverse colon, descending colon, and sigmoid colon. The major functions of the large intestine are (1) absorption of water and remaining nutrients, (2) manufacture of certain vitamins such as vitamin K, (3) formation of feces, and (4) egestion (the elimination of undigested waste products). At the distal end of the sigmoid colon, the feces move into the rectum and are eventually eliminated from the body through the anus.

Innervation of the gut is primarily through the autonomic nervous system (ANS). However, mastication, the initiation of swallowing, and the action of the external anal sphincter are controlled voluntarily. Excitation of the parasympathetic portion of the ANS results in (a) increased parotid, gastric, and pancreatic secretions; (b) increased peristalsis; (c) relaxation of sphincters; and (d) contraction of the gallbladder and bile ducts. Stimulation of the sympathetic nerves has opposite effects. The vagus (parasympathetic) nerve probably has the greatest influence on the GI tract.

Nutritional Requirements

Nutrition is the sum of processes by which a living organism ingests, digests, absorbs, transports, and uses nutrients. With the proper nutritional support, the organism can grow, function, and reproduce. Body defense mechanisms, wound healing, and a variety of other vital processes also require optimal nutrition.

For many years, nutritionists have studied the nutritional needs of people and other animals and have attempted to learn about the effects of environment, metabolism, disease, and activity on these needs. As a result, we now know that humans require over 35 nutrients for growth and function. Body functions deteriorate if any one of these essential nutrients is consistently missing from the diet. We also know that nutritional requirements change with age, disease, activity, and stress.

The perceptive nurse identifies the nutritional requirements and problems of those needing care, seeks solutions, and incorporates the findings into the nursing care plan. To plan care, the nurse must be knowledgable about the principles of nutrition and food composition and must also be sensitive to the role food plays in the lives of individuals and groups. Knowledge combined with sensitivity will help the nurse incorporate the person's food preferences and habits into a new therapeutic dietary plan that the individual is able and willing to follow.

Calories, Body Weight, and Nutrients

All foods supply a source of energy to the body in the form of calories. A calorie is the amount of heat needed to raise the temperature of 1 gram of water 1 degree Celsius. Nutritional requirements are generally expressed in kilocalories (kcal). Caloric needs vary with age, sex, rate of growth, body size, activity level, and other factors.

The minimum energy needed by the body to maintain the circulation, respiration, muscle tone, body temperature, and other vital processes is called the basal energy requirement. This requirement is related to the amount of muscle tissue present in the body and can be predicted from body weight data. Adult basal needs may be estimated quickly by multiplying the ideal body weight (in pounds) by 10 kcal for women under 45 years of age and by 11 kcal for men under 45 years. For persons over 45 years of age, ideal body weight should be multiplied by 9 kcal for women and 10 kcal for men.[116]

People of similar size have similar basal energy needs, but total energy requirement differs greatly because requirements depend on physical activity. A person with a sedentary life style, for example, requires fewer calories per pound per day than an athlete during intense training. We meet these daily human energy requirements by regular consumption of foods and fluids in sufficient quantities.

The basic energy-yielding nutrients are protein, carbohydrates, and fat. They supply calories in the following amounts:

fat	9 kcal/gm
carbohydrate	4 kcal/gm
protein	4 kcal/gm

Fuel supplied to the body in the form of calories is used to support physiologic functions. Ideally, daily energy intake is just sufficient to meet the body's requirements. When the intake of calories exceeds energy needs, excess calories are converted into body fat to be stored in fat pads, and the person gains weight. On the other hand, a diet deficient in calories leads to loss of body weight over time. Being either underweight or overweight can endanger life and health.

CARBOHYDRATES

Carbohydrates are one of the major energy sources in the diets of all people throughout the world. Because carbohydrate is the predominant compound in grains, vegetables, fruits, and other plants, carbohydrate-containing foods are widely available. Generally such foods are low in cost and often can be easily stored for relatively long periods. In some countries, carbohydrate-rich foods make up almost the entire diet. In developed countries, about 50 per cent of the total calories are derived from this source, with the remainder coming from fats and proteins (Fig. 42-2).

The three major groups of carbohydrates are monosaccharides, disaccharides, and polysaccharides. Monosaccharides are the simple sugars: glucose, fructose, and galactose. Disaccharides are composed of two monosaccharides in combination. The major disaccharides include sucrose (glucose plus fructose), lactose (glucose plus galactose), and maltose (glucose plus glucose). Polysaccharides are complex carbohydrates made up of many units of one monosaccharide, usually glucose. Significant dietary polysaccharides include starch, **dextrins** (carbohydrates formed during the hydrolysis of starch to sugars), **cellulose** (the form of carbohydrate that constitutes the supporting framework of plants), **pectins** (purified carbohydrates extracted from citrus rinds or apple pulp), and glycogen. Most dietary carbohydrate is found in the form of polysac-

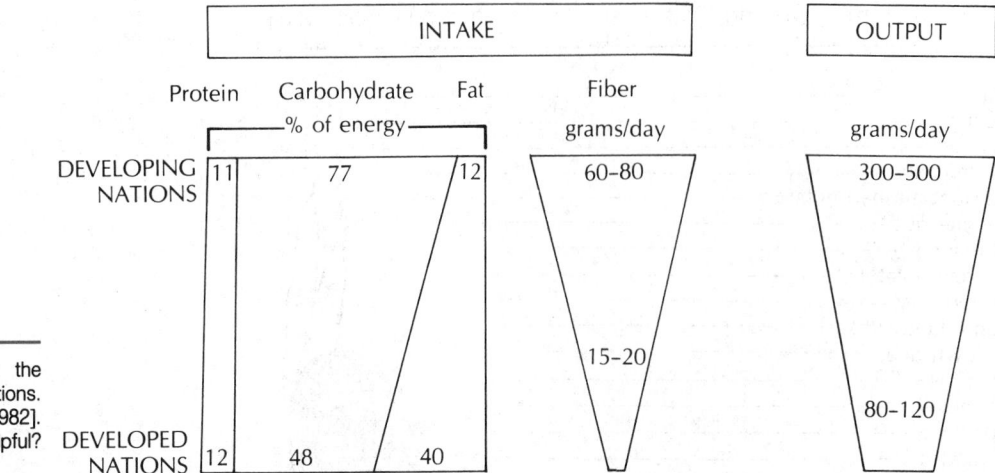

▲ Figure 42-2

Dietary differences between the developing and developed nations. (Adapted from Burkitt, D.P. [1982]. Dietary fiber: is it really helpful? *Geriatrics* 37:119.)

charides and disaccharides, but a limited number of foods contain free monosaccharides (e.g., some fruits).

Glucose is the major energy source for the body. Cells use glucose, rather than other substrates, for energy. This simple sugar is made available to body cells by being consumed as glucose in foods; released in the small intestine by digestive processes that break down polysaccharides and disaccharides into glucose and other monosaccharides; created in the liver from fructose, galactose, glycerol, and some amino acids; and released from stored glycogen found in the liver and muscle.

A sufficient level of glucose in the body depends upon normal digestion of polysaccharides and disaccharides and absorption of monosaccharides in the small intestine. If digestive enzymes such as amylase, lactase, sucrase, and maltase are absent, normal breakdown of polysaccharides and disaccharides cannot take place and dietary sources of glucose become limited.

Carbohydrate-rich foods vary substantially in their rates of digestion and absorption. The term *glycemic index* has been coined to define the speed and intensity of the blood glucose response after food is eaten. Slow releasers, which bring only moderate changes in blood sugar, have a low glycemic index. High releasers stimulate a rapid increase in glucose levels. In general, legumes and dairy products have low glycemic indices, whereas some sugars and root vegetables have high glycemic indices. These differences have relevance in some clinical nutrition settings. For example, diabetic people may be better able to regulate blood glucose by eating a diet composed of foods with low glycemic indices. Less drastic fluctuations in blood sugar may in turn reduce long-term complications from disease. Figure 42-3 provides the glycemic index for a variety of typical foods.

Since the amount of carbohydrate held in the body at any time is relatively small, regular ingestion of carbohydrate is essential. This is because several vital organs, including the heart and the brain, must receive glucose continuously in order to function adequately. Carbohydrates are also important for their protein-sparing action; that is, a sufficient intake of carbohydrate prevents significant utilization of protein for energy. This protein-sparing action of carbohydrate allows the major portion of protein entering the body to be used for its basic purposes, building lean body tissue and synthesizing enzymes, hormones, and other regulatory compounds.

In addition, carbohydrates are necessary for their valuable antiketogenic effect. Ketones, the intermediate products of fat metabolism, are normally broken down or excreted. However, in extreme conditions such as starvation or uncontrolled diabetes in which carbohydrate supply is inadequate or unavailable, ketones accumulate and produce a condition called ketosis. Left untreated, ketosis can result in coma and death.

Carbohydrates are also the source of dietary fiber. Fiber includes carbohydrates and carbohydrate-like components that our gastrointestinal tracts cannot digest. Sources of dietary fiber include cellulose, **gums** (resin-like substances derived from plants), **lignin** (a polysaccharide that combines with cellulose to form plant cell walls), **mucilages** (aqueous forms of gums), and pectin. Even though fiber is not an essential nutrient, it is known to serve an important role in the maintenance of health.[10,11,46] Fiber provides some accepted and some potential benefits. A definitive benefit of dietary fiber is relief of constipation; a probable benefit is the improved management of chronic diverticular disease. Possible benefits of dietary fiber are a mild reduction in blood cholesterol level, a mild improvement in glucose tolerance, and the increased success of reduced-calorie weight-reduction regimens. Its speculative value is that fiber might reduce the risk of colon cancer.

Dietary fiber can cause adverse effects. Possible adverse effects from increased fiber in the diet are interference with absorption of certain minerals, and flatulence and loose stools during the first few days of increased fiber intake. These consequences are minor, however, and should not be major deterrents to emphasizing fiber-rich foods in the daily diet.

FATS

Fat is a combination of fatty acids and glycerol. Its main function is to provide the body with a concentrated source of energy, providing 9 kcal/gm. Fat is also the primary storage form of energy. In fact, this

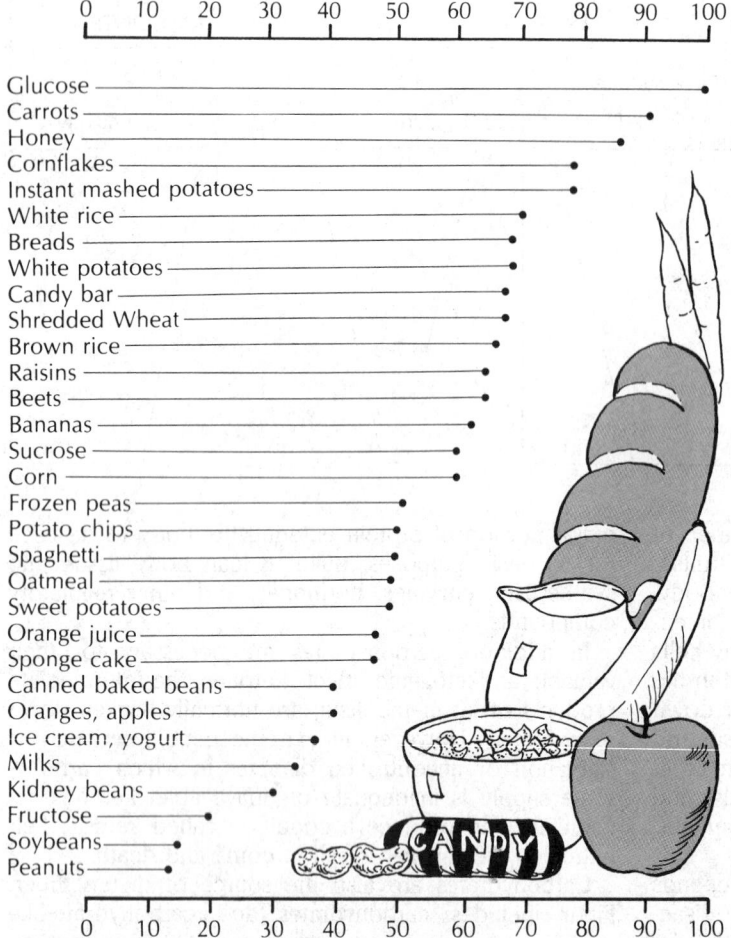

```
        0   10   20   30   40   50   60   70   80   90  100
        |____|____|____|____|____|____|____|____|____|____|
```

Glucose ——•
Carrots ————————————————————————————————•
Honey ————————————————————————————————•
Cornflakes ——————————————————————————•
Instant mashed potatoes —————————————————————•
White rice ——————————————————————•
Breads ————————————————————•
White potatoes ——————————————————•
Candy bar ——————————————————•
Shredded Wheat ——————————————————•
Brown rice ————————————————•
Raisins ————————————————•
Beets ————————————————•
Bananas ———————————————•
Sucrose ———————————————•
Corn ———————————————•
Frozen peas —————————————•
Potato chips ————————————•
Spaghetti ————————————•
Oatmeal ————————————•
Sweet potatoes ————————————•
Orange juice ———————————•
Sponge cake ———————————•
Canned baked beans ——————————•
Oranges, apples —————————•
Ice cream, yogurt —————————•
Milks ————————•
Kidney beans ————————•
Fructose ——————•
Soybeans —————•
Peanuts —————•

```
        0   10   20   30   40   50   60   70   80   90  100
        |____|____|____|____|____|____|____|____|____|____|
```

▲ *Figure 42–3*

Glycemic index of selected foods. (Data from Jenkins, D.J., et al. [1981]. Glycemic index of foods: a physiological basis for carbohydrate exchange. *Am J. Clin. Nutr.* 34:362. Copyright *Am J. Clin. Nutr.* American Society for Clinical Nutrition.)

nutrient has almost unlimited storage capacity in the body as adipose tissue. Besides these majors functions, fat also

▶ acts as an insulator for the body in the form of subcutaneous fat
▶ transports the fat-soluble vitamins, A, D, E, and K
▶ maintains cellular function in the form of the essential fatty acid, linoleic acid
▶ supplies cholesterol, which is necessary for the synthesis of adrenal and sex hormones
▶ is a vital component of cell membranes

Fats are derived from both animal and plant sources and come in many forms: hard, oily, or soft (e.g., waxes). They are all greasy to the touch and insoluble in water. Some foods such as butter, certain margarines, oil, salad dressings, bacon, and cream consist almost entirely of fat. Other foods contain substantial fat but in a form that is less obvious. Foods in this category include egg yolk, olives, and nuts. The significance of fat as an energy source in the diet varies according to country and culture.

Dietary fat comes in several chemical forms, classified as simple lipids, compound lipids, and derived lipids. Simple lipids are composed of triglycerides, which are neutral fats made up of glycerol linked to three fatty acids. Following digestion, glycerol is con-

verted to glucose, which is then used for energy. Fatty acids not used for energy in body cells are involved in the synthesis of various structural compounds or are stored as adipose tissue. Compound lipids consist of **phospholipids** (any lipids that contain phosphorus), **glycolipids** (lipids that contain carbohydrate), and **lipoproteins** (large protein molecules combined with lipid components). All these compounds play a role in proper body functioning. For example, lipoproteins transport cholesterol to and from cells. Derived lipids, such as steroids, are produced from fats and fat compounds. Steroids are important components of sex and adrenal hormones.

Another important classification system is the division of fatty acids into saturated and unsaturated forms. Fatty acids are composed of long chains of carbon atoms with attached hydrogen atoms. **Saturated fats** are fatty acids in which all the carbon atoms are connected by single bonds and which contain much hydrogen. **Unsaturated fats** are fatty acids with double bonds in the carbon chain and less hydrogen than saturated fats. Unsaturated fats are divided into two categories: monounsaturated and polyunsaturated. **Monounsaturated fats** are fatty acids with only one double bond; **polyunsaturated fats** are fatty acids with two or more double bonds. Triglycerides with unsaturated fatty acids tend to be soft or liquid substances, whereas saturated fatty acids tend to be hard and solid. Some foods that contain predominantly saturated fats include red meat, eggs, cream, butter, lard, and chocolate. Foods containing mostly polyunsaturated fats include liquid vegetable oils, peanut butter, fish, and some margarines.

Cholesterol is a major form of dietary fat and a source of controversy in the health community. A steroid compound, cholesterol is largely present in egg yolk, liver and other organ meats, and fatty dairy products such as butter. It is absorbed intact without prior digestion. In addition to dietary sources, the liver synthesizes significant amounts of cholesterol.

During transport in the bloodstream, cholesterol is carried in complexes called lipoproteins, the most significant of which are low-density lipoproteins (LDL) and high-density lipoproteins (HDL). A high level of circulating LDL indicates an increased risk of developing coronary heart disease. A high level of HDL cholesterol indicates that clearance of fatty debris from the circulation is working well. Risk of coronary artery disease is therefore relatively low.

Cholesterol is needed by the body to produce a variety of hormones, bile acids, and other structural and regulatory compounds. Because it is synthesized readily by the liver, however, cholesterol is not a required dietary component. In fact, too much dietary cholesterol can raise blood cholesterol to dangerous levels in some individuals. For this reason, a general dietary guideline for Americans is to be moderate in consumption of cholesterol-rich foods.

PROTEINS

Whereas the major role of fats and carbohydrates is to provide energy, the major role of proteins is to build tissues and aid in the manufacture of essential substances like enzymes and hormones. The amount of dietary protein varies in different cultures, but in geographic areas with adequate nutritional provisions, protein contributes about 10 to 15 per cent of the total calories.[24]

Proteins are found in most animal and plant foods. They consist of chains of amino acids. A given protein contains a specific number of individual amino acids linked in a specific sequence. Of the 20-plus amino acids, 9 cannot be synthesized by adult humans in satisfactory amounts and must be obtained from the diet. These amino acids are classified as essential amino acids. The remaining acids can be synthesized in the body and thus are called nonessential. Nonessential amino acids, despite their name, are necessary for synthesis of body proteins (Box 42–1).

Protein foods are broadly classified as complete or incomplete. Complete protein foods are those that contain all the essential amino acids in sufficient quantity and ratio to supply the body's needs. These proteins are of animal origin and include meat, milk, cheese, and eggs. Incomplete protein foods are deficient in one or more of these essential amino acids. These foods are of plant origin and include grains, legumes, seeds, and nuts. In a mixed diet, animal and

Box 42–1. Essential and Nonessential Amino Acids

Essential	Nonessential
Threonine	Glycine
Leucine	Alanine
Isoleucine	Aspartic acid
Valine	Glutamic acid
Lysine	Proline
Methionine	Hydroxyproline
Phenylalanine	Cystine
Tryptophan	Tyrosine
	Serine
	Arginine
	Histidine

vegetable proteins complement each other. In a totally vegetarian diet, plant proteins can be appropriately mixed to provide a balanced ratio of essential amino acids. It is therefore important to consider the quality and sources of protein in dietary planning.

The primary function of dietary protein is to provide necessary amino acids for growth and maintenance of proteins in body tissues. Amino acids also contribute to the body's overall energy metabolism. After removal of the nitrogenous portion (the amino group) of the amino acid, the remaining part may be converted to fat or carbohydrate. If dietary carbohydrate or fat is not sufficient for energy, then as much as 58 per cent of the total dietary protein becomes available for oxidation and energy production. Therefore, sufficient nonprotein calories are needed in the diet to ensure that protein is used for its primary tissue-building purpose and is not broken down to yield energy. Burning protein for energy, rather than carbohydrates and fats, is an expensive way to run the body.[24]

VITAMINS AND MINERALS

Many energy-producing and tissue-building processes are necessary to maintain life and health. These processes require the participation of a variety of vitamins and minerals that operate as coenzymes or cofactors. A coenzyme is an organic molecule required for activation of a basic enzyme or enzymes. A coenzyme usually contains phosphorus or a vitamin. A cofactor is a mineral needed to activate an enzyme.

A vitamin is a vital organic compound required in small amounts for coenzyme functions in biochemical pathways. Vitamins must be ingested because the human body is not able to manufacture them. Vitamins are usually classified according to their solubility in either fat or water. The fat-soluble vitamins include A,[12] D,[109] E,[15] and K. Water-soluble vitamins include vitamin C and the B-complex group. Usually, sufficient amounts of all the vitamins can be obtained in the daily diet. However, under unusual conditions (e.g., stresses such as illnesses, debilitation, alcoholism, drug therapy, severe caloric restriction), dietary vitamin sources may be insufficient, and it may be necessary to supplement the diet with appropriate vitamin preparations.[1,4] (Tables 42–1 and 42–2 and Box 42–2 contain important information about each of these vitamins.)

Minerals are inorganic elements acting in the body as control agents in a variety of processes that involve energy production as well as body building and maintenance. Although only small amounts of all vitamins and most minerals are necessary for life and health, some minerals are required in larger amounts. For example, the body of an adult weighing about 150 pounds contains about 3 pounds of calcium. On the other hand, iodine is present in very small amounts in the body. This same 150-pound adult contains only a small fraction of an ounce of this material.

The body minerals are generally classified into the two main categories of major minerals and trace elements. In addition, a third classification of minerals includes those elements whose physiologic function is not clearly understood. These three groups of minerals and their chemical symbols are listed in Box 42–3. Table 42–3 summarizes significant data about some of these minerals.

Healthy children and adults generally get all the essential vitamins and minerals by eating a balanced diet and do not require additional vitamin or mineral supplements. People with restrictive diets, however, may be good candidates for vitamin or mineral supplements. Some situations that may indicate this need are

▶ people on extreme reducing diets
▶ people with limited food preferences
▶ heavy drinkers and drug abusers
▶ "casual" vegetarians who do not systematically plan their daily diets

TABLE 42–1. Basic Information About Selected B-Complex Vitamins

Vitamin	Coenzymes: Physiologic Function	Clinical Applications	Food Sources
Thiamine (B₁)	Carbohydrate metabolism Thiamine pyrophosphate (TPP): oxidative decarboxylation	Beriberi (deficiency) Neuropathy Wernicke-Korsakoff syndrome (alcoholism) Depressed muscular and secretory symptoms	Pork, beef, liver, whole or enriched grains, legumes
Riboflavin (B₂)	General metabolism Flavin adenine dinucleotide (FAD) Flavin mononucleotide (FMN)	Cheilosis, glossitis, seborrheic dermatitis	Milk, liver, enriched cereals
Niacin (nicotinic acid, nicotinamide)	General metabolism Nicotinamide adenine dinucleotide (NAD) Nicotinamide adenine dinucleotide phosphate (NADP)	Pellagra (deficiency) Weakness, anorexia Scaly dermatitis Neuritis	Meat, peanuts, enriched grains (protein foods containing tryptophan)
Vitamin B₆ (pyridoxine, pyridoxal, pyridoxamine)	General metabolism Pyridoxal phosphate (PLP): transamination and decarboxylation	Reduced serum levels associated with pregnancy and use of oral contraceptives Antagonized by isoniazid, penicillamine, and other drugs	Wheat, corn, meat, liver
Pantothenic acid	General metabolism CoA (coenzyme A): acetylation	Many roles through acyl transfer reactions (for example, lipogenesis, amino acid activation, and formation of cholesterol, steroid hormones, heme)	Liver, egg, milk
Biotin	General metabolism N-Carboxybiotinyl lysine: CO_2 transfer reactions	Deficiency induced by avidin (a protein in raw egg white) and by antibiotics Synthesis of some fatty acids and amino acids	Egg yolk, liver Synthesized by intestinal microorganisms
Folic acid (folacin)	General metabolism Single carbon transfer reactions (for example, purine nucleotide, thymine, heme synthesis)	Megaloblastic anemia	Liver, green leafy vegetables
Cobalamin (B₁₂)	General metabolism Methylcobalamin: methylation reactions (for example, synthesis of amino acids, heme)	Pernicious anemia induced by lack of intrinsic factor Megaloblastic anemia Methylmalonic aciduria Homocystinuria Peripheral neuropathy (strict vegetarian diet)	Liver, meat, milk, egg, cheese

Modified from Williams, S.R. (1990). *Essentials of nutrition and diet therapy* (5th ed.). St. Louis: C.V. Mosby.

TABLE 42–2. Basic Information About Fat-Soluble Vitamins

Vitamin	Physiologic Functions	Results of Deficiency	Food Sources
Vitamin A Provitamin: betacarotene Vitamin: retinol	Production of rhodopsin and other light-receptor pigments Formation and maintenance of epithelial tissue Growth Reproduction Toxic in large amounts	Poor dark adaptation, night blindness, xerosis, xerophthalmia Keratinization of epithelium Growth failure Reproductive failure	Liver, cream, butter, whole milk, egg yolk Green and yellow vegetables, yellow fruits Fortified margarine
Vitamin D Provitamins: ergosterol (plants); 7-dehydrocholesterol (skin) Vitamins: D_2 (ergocholecalciferol) and D_3 (cholecalciferol)	1,25-Dihydroxycholecalciferol, a major hormone regulator of bone mineral (calcium and phosphorus) metabolism Calcium and phosphorus absorption Toxic in large amounts	Faulty bone growth: rickets, osteomalacia	Fortified milk Fortified margarine Fish oils Sunlight on skin
Vitamin E Tocopherols	Antioxidation Hemopoiesis Related to action of selenium	Anemia in premature infants	Vegetable oils
Vitamin K K_1 (phylloquinone) K_2 (menaquinone) Analog: K_3 (menadione)	Activation of blood-clotting factors (for example, prothrombin) by α-carboxylating glutamic acid residues Toxicity can be induced by water-soluble analogs	Hemorrhagic disease of the newborn Defective blood clotting Deficiency symptoms, which can be produced by coumarin anticoagulants and by antibiotic therapy	Cheese, egg yolk, liver Green leafy vegetables Synthesized by intestinal bacteria

Modified from Williams, S.R. (1990). *Essentials of nutrition and diet therapy* (5th ed.). St. Louis: C.V. Mosby.

Box 42–2. Basic Information About Vitamin C (Ascorbic Acid)

Physiologic Functions	Clinical Applications	Food Sources
Antioxidation	Scurvy (deficiency)	Fresh fruits, especially citrus
Collagen biosynthesis	Wound healing, tissue formation	

General metabolism
  Makes iron available for hemoglobin synthesis
  Influences conversion of folic acid to folinic acid
  Oxidation-reduction of the amino acids phenylalanine and tyrosine
	Fevers and infections
	Stress reactions
	Growth	

Modified from Williams, S.R. (1990). *Essentials of nutrition and diet therapy* (5th ed.). St. Louis: C.V. Mosby.

Also, pregnant or lactating women, breastfed infants, some children who eat poorly after weaning, elderly people, or those with certain diseases (e.g., malabsorption) have special dietary needs that sometimes require vitamin and mineral supplements.

FLUIDS

Maintenance of life and health demands that water balance be kept within closely defined limits at all times. Water is an essential nutrient that is basic to life. Its overall balance within the fluid compartments of the body is regulated by various complex physiologic processes. The physiology of normal fluid and electrolyte balance and imbalance is discussed in Chapter 41.

Recommended Dietary Allowances and Dietary Guidelines

In 1941, the Food and Nutrition Board of the National Academy of Sciences developed its first listing of recommendations for daily intake of specific nutrients. Since that time, these recommendations, called the Recommended Dietary Allowances (RDAs), have been revised about every 4 years to reflect new findings in nutrition research (Table 42–4).

In the judgment of the Food and Nutrition Board, the **Recommended Dietary Allowances (RDAs)** are the

Box 42-3. Minerals in the Body

Major Minerals

Calcium (Ca)
Magnesium (Mg)
Sodium (Na)
Potassium (K)
Phosphorus (P)
Sulfur (S)
Chlorine (Cl)
Fluorine (F)

Trace Minerals (Elements)

Iron (Fe)
Copper (Cu)
Iodine (I)
Manganese (Mn)
Cobalt (Co)
Zinc (Zn)
Molybdenum (Mo)
Chromium (Cr)
Selenium (Se)

Minerals Whose Function Is Poorly Understood

Aluminum (Al)
Boron (B)
Cadmium (Cd)
Vanadium (V)

levels of intake of essential nutrients considered, on the basis of available knowledge, to be adequate to meet the known nutritional needs of almost every healthy person.

Therefore, except for calories, RDAs do not represent minimal or average nutritional requirements of individuals. Instead, they designate the minimal need plus a margin of safety sufficient to accommodate the normal variations in nutritional needs observed in a healthy population.

Health professionals frequently use RDAs to assess dietary adequacy. The RDAs provide a rough standard against which one can compare an individual's or a group's dietary intake. It is essential, however, to apply common sense when using an RDA as a reference point in the overall dietary evaluation. For example, the dietary recommendations may not be adequate for individuals depleted by disease, trauma, stress, specific drug therapy, or chronic dietary deficiencies. In addition, RDAs may prove to be of limited value if the person being compared with the RDA is distinctly different anatomically or physiologically from the average, healthy person used as a standard of reference by the Food and Nutrition Board.

While RDAs provide quantitative directions for nutrient intake, they are not aimed at assisting individuals to make sensible food choices. The **Dietary Guidelines for Americans** are meant to satisfy this latter goal. They were first created in 1980 and have been modified several times since (Box 42-4). They are advice for healthy Americans aged 2 years and over and

TABLE 42-3. Basic Information About Selected Essential Minerals

Mineral	Metabolism	Physiologic Functions	Clinical Applications	Food Sources
Calcium (Ca)	Absorption according to body need; requires Ca-binding protein and regulated by vitamin D, parathyroid hormone, and calcitonin; absorption favored by protein, lactose, acidity Excretion chiefly in feces: 70%–90% of amount ingested Deposition-mobilization in bone tissue constant, regulated by vitamin D and parathyroid hormone	Constituent of bones and teeth Participates in blood clotting, nerve transmission, muscle action, cell membrane permeability, enzyme activation	Tetany (decrease in serum Ca) Rickets, osteomalacia Osteoporosis Resorptive hypercalciuria, renal calculi Hyperthyroidism and hypothyroidism	Milk, cheese Green leafy vegetables Whole grains Egg yolk Legumes, nuts
Phosphorus (P)	Absorption with Ca aided by vitamin D and parathyroid hormone as above; hindered by binding agents Excretion chiefly by kidney according to serum level, regulated by parathyroid hormone	Constituent of bones and teeth, ATP, phosphorylated intermediary metabolites Participates in absorption of glucose and glycerol, transport of fatty acids, energy metabolism, and buffer system	Growth Recovery from diabetic acidosis Hypophosphatemia: bone disease, malabsorption syndromes, primary hyperparathyroidism Hyperphosphatemia: renal insufficiency,	Milk, cheese Meat, egg yolk Whole grains Legumes, nuts

TABLE 42-3. *Basic Information About Selected Essential Minerals* Continued

Mineral	Metabolism	Physiologic Functions	Clinical Applications	Food Sources
	Deposition-mobilization in bone compartment constant		hypothyroidism, tetany	
Magnesium (Mg)	Absorption according to intake load: hindered by excess fat, phosphate, calcium, protein Excretion regulated by kidney	Constituent of bones and teeth Coenzyme in general metabolism, smooth muscle action, neuromuscular irritability Cation in intracellular fluid	Low serum level following gastrointestinal losses Tremor, spasm in deficiency induced by malnutrition, alcoholism	Milk, cheese Meat, seafood Whole grains, Legumes, nuts
Sulfur (S)	Elemental form absorbed as such; split from amino acid sources (methionine and cystine) in digestion and absorbed into portal circulation Excreted by kidney in relation to protein intake and tissue catabolism	Essential constituent of protein structure Enzyme activity and energy metabolism through free sulfhydryl group (—SH) Detoxification reactions	Cystine renal calculi Cystinuria	Meat, egg Milk, cheese Legumes, nuts
Sodium (Na)	Readily absorbed Excretion chiefly by kidney, controlled by aldosterone	Major cation in extracellular fluid, water balance, acid-base balance Cell membrane permeability, absorption of glucose Normal muscle irritability	Losses in gastrointestinal disorders, diarrhea Fluid-electrolyte and acid-base balance problems Muscle action	Salt (NaCl) Sodium compounds in baking and processing Milk, cheese Meat, egg Carrots, beets, spinach, celery
Potassium (K)	Readily absorbed Secreted and reabsorbed in gastrointestinal circulation Excretion chiefly by kidney, regulated by aldosterone	Major cation in intracellular fluid, water balance, acid-base balance Normal muscle irritability Glycogen formation Protein synthesis	Losses in gastrointestinal disorders, diarrhea Fluid-electrolyte, acid-base balance problems Muscle action, especially heart action Losses in tissue catabolism Treatment of diabetic acidosis: rapid glycogen production reduces serum potassium level Losses with diuretic therapy	Fruits Vegetables Legumes, nuts Whole grains Meat
Chlorine (Cl)	Readily absorbed Excretion controlled by kidney	Major anion in extracellular fluid, water balance, acid-base balance, chloride-bicarbonate shift Gastric hydrochloride—digestion	Losses in gastrointestinal disorders, vomiting, diarrhea, tube drainage Hypochloremic alkalosis	Salt (NaCl)
Iron (Fe)	Absorption controls bioavailability; favored by body need, acidity, and reduction agents such as vitamins; hindered by binding agents, reduced gastric HCl, infection, gastrointestinal losses Transported as transferrin, stored as ferritin or hemosiderin Excreted in sloughed cells, bleeding	Hemoglobin synthesis, oxygen transport Cell oxidation, heme enzymes	Anemia: hypochromic, microcytic Excess: hemosiderosis, hemochromatosis Growth and pregnancy needs	Liver, meat, egg Whole grains Enriched breads and cereals Dark green vegetables Legumes, nuts (Iron cookware)

Table continued on following page

TABLE 42–3. *Basic Information About Selected Essential Minerals* Continued

Mineral	Metabolism	Physiologic Functions	Clinical Applications	Food Sources
Iodine (I)	Absorbed as iodides, taken up by thyroid gland under control of thyroid-stimulating hormone (TSH) Excretion by kidney	Synthesis of thyroxine, which regulates cell metabolism, BMR	Endemic colloid goiter, cretinism Hypothyroidism and hyperthyroidism	Iodized salt Seafood
Zinc (Zn)	Absorbed with zinc-binding ligand (ZBL) from pancreas Transported in blood by albumin; stored in many sites Excretion largely intestinal	Essential coenzyme constituent: carbonic anhydrase, carboxypeptidase, lactic dehydrogenase	Growth: hypogonadism Sensory impairment: taste and smell Wound healing Malabsorption disease	Widely distributed: Seafood, oysters Liver, meat Milk, cheese, egg Whole grains
Copper (Cu)	Absorbed with copper-binding protein metallothionein Transported in blood by histidine and albumin Stored in many tissues	Associated with iron in enzyme systems, hemoglobin synthesis Metalloprotein enzymes constituent	Hypocupremia: nephrosis and malabsorption Wilson's disease, excess copper storage	Widely distributed: Liver, meat Seafood Whole grains Legumes, nuts (Copper cookware)
Manganese (Mn)	Absorbed poorly Excretion mainly by intestine	Enzyme component in general metabolism	Low serum levels in diabetes, protein-energy malnutrition Inhalation toxicity	Cereals, whole grains Legumes, soybeans Leafy vegetables
Chromium (Cr)	Absorbed in association with zinc Excretion mainly by kidney	Associated with glucose metabolism; improves faulty glucose uptake by tissues; glucose tolerance factor	Potentiates action of insulin in persons with diabetes Lowers serum cholesterol, LDL-cholesterol Increases HDL	Cereals Whole grains Brewer's yeast Animal proteins
Cobalt (Co)	Absorbed as component of food source, vitamin B_{12} Elemental form shares transport with iron Stored in liver	Constituent of vitamin B_{12}, functions with vitamin	Deficiency only associated with deficiency of B_{12}	Vitamin B_{12} source
Selenium (Se)	Absorption depends on solubility of compound form Excreted mainly by kidney	Constituent of enzyme glutathione perioxidase Synergistic antioxidant with vitamin E Structural component of teeth	Marginal deficiency when soil content is low Deficiency secondary to parenteral nutrition (TPN), malnutrition Toxicity observed in livestock	Varies with soil Seafood Legumes Whole grains Low-fat meats and dairy products Vegetables
Molybdenum (Mo)	Readily absorbed Excreted rapidly by kidney Small amount excreted in bile	Constituent of oxidase enzymes, xanthine oxidase	Deficiency unknown in humans	Legumes Whole grains Milk Organ meats Leafy vegetables
Fluorine (Fl)	Absorption in small intestine; little known of bioavailability Excreted by kidney—80%	Accumulates in bones and teeth, increasing hardness	Dental caries inhibited Osteoporosis: may help control Excess: dental fluorosis	Fish Fish products Tea Foods cooked in fluoridated water Drinking water

Modified from Williams, S.R. (1990). *Essentials of nutrition and diet therapy* (5th ed.). St. Louis: C.V. Mosby.

TABLE 42–4. Food and Nutrition Board, National Academy of Sciences—National Research Council Recommended Dietary Allowances,[a] Revised 1989[a]

Age (years) or Condition	Weight[b] (kg)	Weight[b] (lb)	Height[b] (cm)	Height[b] (in)	Energy (kcal)	Protein (g)	Fat-Soluble Vitamins				Water-Soluble Vitamins							Minerals					
							Vita-min A (µgRE)[c]	Vita-min D (µg)[d]	Vita-min E (mg α-TE)[e]	Vita-min K (µg)	Vita-min C (mg)	Thia-mine (mg)	Ribo-flavin (mg)	Niacin (mg NE)[f]	Vita-min B6 (mg)	Fo-late (µg)	Vita-min B12 (µg)	Cal-cium (mg)	Phos-phorus (mg)	Mag-nesium (mg)	Iron (mg)	Zinc (mg)	Iodine (µg)
Infants																							
0.0–0.5	6	13	60	24	650	13	375	7.5	3	5	30	0.3	0.4	5	0.3	25	0.3	400	300	40	6	5	40
0.5–1.0	9	20	71	28	850	14	375	10	4	10	35	0.4	0.5	6	0.6	35	0.5	600	500	60	10	5	50
Children																							
1–3	13	29	90	35	1300	16	400	10	6	15	40	0.7	0.8	9	1.0	50	0.7	800	800	80	10	10	70
4–6	20	44	112	44	1800	24	500	10	7	20	45	0.9	1.1	12	1.1	75	1.0	800	800	120	10	10	90
7–10	28	62	132	52	2000	28	700	10	7	30	45	1.0	1.2	13	1.4	100	1.4	800	800	170	10	10	120
Males																							
11–14	45	99	157	62	2500	45	1000	10	10	45	50	1.3	1.5	17	1.7	150	2.0	1200	1200	270	12	15	150
15–18	66	145	176	69	3000	59	1000	10	10	65	60	1.5	1.8	20	2.0	200	2.0	1200	1200	400	12	15	150
19–24	72	160	177	70	2900	58	1000	10	10	70	60	1.5	1.7	19	2.0	200	2.0	1200	1200	350	10	15	150
25–50	79	174	176	70	2900	63	1000	5	10	80	60	1.5	1.7	19	2.0	200	2.0	800	800	350	10	15	150
51+	77	170	173	68	2300	63	1000	5	10	80	60	1.2	1.4	15	2.0	200	2.0	800	800	350	10	15	150
Females																							
11–14	46	101	157	62	2200	46	800	10	8	45	50	1.1	1.3	15	1.4	150	2.0	1200	1200	280	15	12	150
15–18	55	120	163	64	2200	44	800	10	8	55	60	1.1	1.3	15	1.5	180	2.0	1200	1200	300	15	12	150
19–24	58	128	164	65	2200	46	800	10	8	60	60	1.1	1.3	15	1.6	180	2.0	1200	1200	280	15	12	150
25–50	63	138	163	64	2200	50	800	5	8	65	60	1.1	1.3	15	1.6	180	2.0	800	800	280	15	12	150
51+	65	143	160	63	1900	50	800	5	8	65	60	1.0	1.2	13	1.6	180	2.0	1200	1200	280	10	12	150
Pregnant					+300	60	800	10	10	65	70	1.5	1.6	17	2.2	400	2.2	1200	1200	320	30	15	175
Lactating 1st 6 months					+500	65	1300	10	12	65	95	1.6	1.8	20	2.1	280	2.6	1200	1200	355	15	19	200
2nd 6 months					+500	62	1200	10	11	65	90	1.6	1.7	20	2.1	260	2.6	1200	1200	340	15	16	200

a The allowances, expressed as average daily intakes over time, are intended to provide for individual variations among most normal persons as they live in the United States under usual environmental stresses. Diets should be based on a variety of common foods in order to provide other nutrients for which human requirements have been less well defined.

b Weights and heights of Reference Adults are actual medians for the U.S. population of the designated age, as reported by National Health and Nutrition Examination Survey II (NHANES II). The use of these figures does not imply that the height-to-weight ratios are ideal.

c Retinol equivalents. 1 retinol equivalent = 1 µg retinol or 6 µg β-carotene.

d As cholecalciferol. 10 µg cholecalciferol = 400 IU of vitamin D.

e α-Tocopherol equivalents. 1 mg d-α-tocopherol = 1 α-TE.

f 1 NE (niacin equivalent) is equal to 1 mg of niacin or 60 mg of dietary tryptophan.

reflect recommendations of nutrition authorities who agree that enough is known about diet's effect on health to encourage certain dietary practices.

POPULAR CONCERNS ABOUT DIET AND HEALTH

The daily consumption of foods containing appropriate amounts of vital nutrients is essential to maintenance of health and recovery from illness. In recent years, however, many people have inflated the curative or therapeutic powers of foods and vitamins. As a nurse, you will be confronted with various forms of "food faddism." Thus, you need to understand the causes of these beliefs and recognize the dangers associated with faulty eating patterns based on fads. Understanding human psychology will help you appreciate the appeal of such misinformation. In addition, your scientific background will enable you to evaluate the nutritional value of a diet and assess the untoward effects of food fads on the long-term health and well-being of people who adhere to these diets.

Current information concerning food fads is available through continuing education programs, journal articles, research reports, and resource persons in the community.

Food Additives

Food additives are substances added to foods to improve color, flavor, consistency, or stability. Additives have traditionally been used to help preserve food for future use. Today, many food additives are used for aesthetic purposes.

Some food additives have become a source of concern and have been criticized because laboratory experiments indicated that ingestion of very large amounts of these additives produced tumors in the laboratory situation. In humans, the long-term effects of small amounts of these additives are unknown, but the research suggests that gradual accumulation of large amounts of such materials in body tissues might eventually endanger health. To date, however, there is no definitive proof that additives are dangerous. While reasonable use of preservatives is necessary and beneficial for the long-term preservation of food commodities, it seems wise to avoid use of unnecessary additive chemicals in the food supply.

Natural and Organic Foods

As concern about additives increased over the past several decades, distrust of the food industry grew, and efforts to avoid "processed" foods developed. Widespread enthusiasm for "natural foods" has caused supermarkets as well as other specialty stores to stock a substantial number of whole-grain or minimally processed food products. By and large, these products are wholesome and certainly palatable. Their nutritional composition, however, may not be much different from that of products not advertised as "natural." Table 42–5 provides a comparison of the nutritive composition of two representative cereal products on the market. It is clear that in terms of the nutrients indicated on the chart, the "processed" product is, in fact, superior in many ways.

"Organic foods" have also risen to a position of substantial popularity in recent years. This movement, again, is the direct result of the popular dislike for widespread use of chemicals in food production and processing. Organic foods, by definition, are grown in the absence of "chemical" pesticides and fertilizers or animals raised without use of any "chemicals in their foods" or "injections" to promote or modify growth. Organic farming entails the use of organic fertilizers, like manure and compost. Also, no sprays or other

TABLE 42–5. Nutrient Values of a Typical "Natural" Cereal Compared with a Popular Conventional Cereal

	Quaker 100% Natural	Cheerios
Serving size	1 oz (¼ cup)	1 oz (1¼ cups)
Calories	120	110
Nutrient composition (percentage of Recommended Dietary Allowances):		
Protein	2	6
Vitamin A	*	25
Vitamin C	*	25
Thiamine (vitamin B₁)	2	25
Riboflavin (vitamin B₂)	*	25
Niacin	2	25
Calcium	2	4
Iron	2	25
Vitamin D	*	10
Vitamin B₆	†	25

* Contains less than 2 per cent of RDA.
† Value not given.

such pest control agents are employed. Fresh organic foods are often very tasty and in many cases are quite superior to "standard" fresh foods in overall aesthetic quality. Organic foods, however, are not always superior nutritionally to their comparable counterparts, and in some geographic areas their high cost and substantial deterioration and spoilage losses make it difficult to justify the purchase of these foods.

Vitamin, Mineral, and Food Supplements

Millions of people take vitamin supplements each day. When winter rolls around, some individuals stock up on vitamin C. Some consume large amounts of vitamin E in hopes of improving sexual performance or vitality. Persons with various maladies may also be unwary victims of propaganda emphasizing that vitamins are good for them. They may assume that the more vitamins they take, the better off they will be. Although vitamin and mineral supplements are indicated for some groups of people, health professionals must work to educate citizens concerning what vitamins can and cannot accomplish.[1,4]

In addition to the advertised necessity of supplements, people also need to be wary of the fallacies that lie behind the popularity of so-called natural vitamins. The first fallacy is the belief that natural vitamins (those naturally occurring in plants and animals) are superior to those synthesized by laboratories. Actually, each vitamin has a specific molecular structure that remains the same, regardless of how the vitamin is produced. The body cannot distinguish in any way between vitamin C present in oranges and vitamin C produced in a laboratory; only the wallet "knows for sure." A second misconception about natural vitamins is the belief that "natural" vitamin products do not contain synthetic ingredients. In processing tablets and capsules, for example, manufacturers of all types of vitamins must use excipients and binders such as methyl cellulose and gum.

Food supplements are often advertised as essential for good health. According to the advertisements, the normal diet is inadequate; processed foods have low nutritional value; and people are more stressed today than ever before. Consequently, the ads state, most people require nutritional supplements. Many of these products are high-protein materials with or without the added bonus of several vitamins and minerals. These items are frequently expensive, and individuals with limited financial resources may sacrifice other necessities to purchase them. It is important to understand that vitamins are by no means so benign that large amounts can be taken without fear of toxic effects. Large amounts of certain vitamins, especially the fat-soluble vitamins A, D, E, and K and possibly vitamins C, B_6, and niacin, can cause serious anatomic and physiologic damage. Table 42–6 summarizes some of the limited knowledge available about the potential undesirable effects of large doses of certain vitamins.

The truth is that most people who decide that these products are essential for their health really do not need dietary supplementation at all. This is especially true of protein. Only the rare individual in a developed society does not obtain sufficient protein in the daily diet to meet physiologic needs. If protein supplements are added to the diet when protein intake is sufficient, the extra protein (amino acids) will simply be broken down and the residual compounds burned for energy or stored as fat. The malnourished individual who does need to consume an increased amount of protein daily is best advised to select an acceptable food source of protein. Most "natural" products, therefore, are not natural at all but instead contain a number of necessary "chemical" constituents.

In some cases, supplementing the diet with iron is a wise practice,[38] especially for adult premenopausal women whose regular diets may be relatively low in calories. Even with careful planning of daily menus and responsible daily consumption of calories, these women may find it difficult to obtain the recommended

TABLE 42–6. Known Information on Vitamin Toxicity

Vitamin	Range of Toxicity	Reported Symptoms
Vitamin A	Greater than 30,000 IU daily for at least 3 months	Fatigue, lethargy, insomnia, anorexia, abdominal discomfort, weight loss, bone and joint pain, loss of body hair, headaches, liver dysfunction
Vitamin D	Greater than 2000 IU daily	Anorexia, nausea, vomiting, drowsiness, headache, pallor, diarrhea, polydipsia, polyuria, fever, hypertension, renal damage, calcium deposition in soft tissues with hypercalcemia and hypercalciuria
Vitamin C	Greater than 1000 mg daily	Rebound scurvy, inaccurate urinary glucose assay, menstrual bleeding in pregnant women, hemolytic reaction in people with G-6-P dehydrogenase deficit, oxalate kidney stones, false-negative tests for stool blood, destruction of vitamin B_{12} in food
Niacin	Greater than 1 gm daily	Flushing, itching, dermatoses, hyperbilirubinemia, liver damage, elevated blood sugar, elevated blood uric acid with gouty arthritis, peptic ulceration, cardiac arrhythmias, gastrointestinal problems
Pyridoxine (vitamin B_6)	Greater than 1 gm daily	Sensory neuropathy

TABLE 42-7. Facts About Some "Special" Foods

Food	Source	Nutritional Composition	Pertinent Information
Brown sugar	A refined sugar product with small amounts of mineral residue from the original molasses preparation	410 kcal per ½ cup 2.6 mg of iron per ½ cup	Almost identical to white sugar in nutrient content (negligible) and calories (high)
Honey	A sweet material produced by bees from the nectar of flowers	65 kcal per tbsp 0.5 mg of iron per 5 tbsp	Supplies carbohydrate largely in the form of glucose and fructose; not significantly easier to tolerate or digest than refined sugar; no special curative properties for fatigue, colic, sleeplessness, coughs, or a variety of other problems
Sea kelp/seaweed	Marine plants that grow in the sea	100 gm contains 312 kcal 756 mg calcium 7.8 mg iron Good source of iodine Fair source of some trace elements	Nutritious but has no known curative properties; for those who meet their iodine needs by use of iodized salt, expenditure for special products to obtain iodine seems wasteful
Desiccated liver	Dried and powdered form of beef liver	Excellent source of vitamin B_{12} and some other nutrients	Does not necessarily prevent or cure pernicious anemia; taken in large amounts, it might mask the hematologic signs of pernicious anemia and allow the degenerative neurologic changes to progress unnoticed
Wheat germ	The central germ portion of wheat kernels	Good source of B vitamins, vitamin E, and protein	Nutritious but unable to increase strength and endurance, prevent aging, cure muscular dystrophy or heart disease
Lecithin	A natural emulsifier found in egg yolks and soybeans	Phospholipid	Role in dissolving calcium and cholesterol plaques in blood vessels not clearly proved; in health, lecithin is produced in the body
Raw milk	Unpasteurized cow milk	Basically the same as pasteurized milk with no vitamin D; slightly higher vitamin C content	No special health benefits; may easily become contaminated if not kept in sterile containers at proper temperature
Yogurt	A fermented, cultured form of milk	Similar in composition to milk; may have considerable amount of added sugar	No special health benefits; not easier to digest; may alter gut flora favorably by supplying bacteria that produce B vitamins and vitamin K
Blackstrap molasses	Molasses syrup formed in the process of refining sugar	1 tbsp contains 45 kcal 137 mg of calcium 3.2 mg of iron	Potent-flavored concentrated calorie source with no special curative properties; good source of iron
Brewer's yeast	Byproduct of the beer-brewing industry	Good source of some B vitamins, amino acids, and some minerals 1 tbsp contains 1.4 mg of iron 1.25 mg of vitamin B_1 0.34 mg of vitamin B_2 3.0 mg of vitamin B_3	A nutritious food supplement but has no special curative properties
Gelatin	A glutinous material (colloidal protein) obtained from animal tissues	Incomplete protein	*Alone,* it is useless in building body protein; not necessary for strong nails, since nail formation is also influenced by general body nutrition, health, environment, local nail care, and many other factors

TABLE 42-7. Facts About Some "Special" Foods Continued

Food	Source	Nutritional Composition	Pertinent Information
Fertilized eggs	Eggs produced by hens kept with roosters	Similar nutritionally to unfertilized eggs	*In conjunction with other dietary amino acid sources*, it may provide useful sources of amino acids for body proteins. No special health benefits; do not contain "special hormones" that commercial eggs lack; more expensive than unfertilized eggs

15 mg of iron from their diets. The daily iron need of the individual woman relates directly to the volume of her monthly menstrual blood loss. Those women with a regular blood loss of more than 30 to 40 ml per month are good candidates for iron supplements. If iron supplementation is recommended, it is important to select an appropriate (absorbable) form of iron. The ferrous salts are more readily absorbed and thus preferable to ferric compounds.

Use of calcium supplements for prevention or amelioration of osteoporosis is indicated in some situations.[101] Osteoporosis is a condition in which reduction in bone mass leads to marked bone weakness and development of fractures and pain. This process is especially problematic in postmenopausal females, for a number of reasons: (1) Calcium intake in this group is generally lower than the RDA; (2) adult women have approximately 25 per cent less bone mass than men do; and (3) estrogen reduction at menopause promotes bone loss. Clinical studies have confirmed that calcium supplementation in young women with low dietary calcium intake may increase peak bone mass and that postmenopausally, calcium supplementation may retard the rate of bone loss.[48]

Special Foods

The idea has prevailed for years that some foods possess special preventive or therapeutic characteristics that make them especially desirable in the daily diet. Included in this category are honey, wheat germ, brewer's yeast, seaweed, lecithin, blackstrap molasses, and fertilized eggs. All these foods are nutritious and contribute significant amounts of certain nutrients to the daily diet. None, however, possesses special curative properties, and these foods are not superior to many other foods in promoting healthy digestion, absorption, or metabolism. Table 42-7 provides a listing of some of these special foods, along with data related to their derivation, nutritional composition, and role in the diet.

Vegetarianism

A vegetarian diet consists exclusively or primarily of plant foods. Many people adopt this diet for religious, philosophic, or health reasons. Others eat a vegetarian diet because quantities of meat products are not available or are too costly.

Traditionally, the term *vegetarian* encompasses two major subgroups: vegetarians and vegans. **Vegetarians** are individuals who may eat some eggs and dairy products but no flesh (animal, fowl, or seafood). Some vegetarians may be either **lacto-ovovegetarians** (people who eat dairy products and eggs but no animal, fish, or fowl flesh) or **lactovegetarians** (people who eat dairy products but no eggs or flesh). People who omit all animal products are called **vegans.**

Including some animal protein in the diet makes diet planning much easier. Planning reasonable menus is simplified by use of a four-food-group plan for lactovegetarians (Box 42-5). This plan has a protein group that includes nuts, grain, legumes, and seeds. There is also a vegetable group, a fruit group, and a milk and/or eggs group. Achieving an adequate diet is not a problem.

The vegan must do some special diet planning. Also, additional food preparation time is generally needed. Some excellent cookbooks are available to assist the meal planner in avoiding potential nutrient deficiencies. Combining vegetables to achieve a balance of essential amino acids improves overall diet quality, a special concern for young children who are raised on this restrictive food pattern (Table 42-8).

Box 42-5. A Four-Food-Group Plan for Lactovegetarians

GROUP 1	GROUP 2
Grains, legumes, nuts, and seeds	Vegetables
6 servings	3 or more servings (include one dark green leafy)
Key nutrients: protein, thiamine, niacin, vitamin B_6, folate, vitamin E, zinc, magnesium, and fiber	*Key nutrients:* vitamin A, vitamin C, and folate

GROUP 3	GROUP 4
Fruits	Milk
2 or more servings	2 or more servings
Key nutrients: vitamin A, vitamin C, and folate	*Key nutrients:* protein, riboflavin, vitamin D, vitamin B_{12}, and calcium

TABLE 42-8. Important Nutrients for the Total Vegetarian (Vegan)

Nutrient	Plant Sources
Calcium	Fortified soy milk; tofu; almonds; dry beans; some leafy vegetables; some fortified breakfast cereals, flours, and brands of orange drinks
Zinc	Whole grains, wheat germ, beans, nuts, seeds
Iron	Whole grains, prune juice, dried fruits, beans, nuts, seeds, some leafy vegetables
Vitamin D	Fortified margarines, fortified breakfast cereals
Riboflavin	Whole and enriched grains, leafy vegetables, beans, mushrooms, nuts, seeds
Vitamin B_{12}	Fortified breakfast cereals, fortified yeast, fortified soy milk

The following nutritional considerations should be observed when omitting all forms of flesh from the diet.

▶ Combine plant proteins with each other (e.g., wheat + beans) and with dairy foods (e.g., cereal + milk) to provide a complete protein.
▶ Increase intake of legumes, dried seeds, and nuts for protein and iron.
▶ Increase intake of dairy foods for calcium, protein, and vitamin B_{12}.
▶ Increase intake of whole grain breads and cereals for vitamin B.
▶ Increase intake of fruits and vegetables for vitamins A and C and minerals.
▶ Decrease intake of "empty calories" (sugars, concentrated sugars, visible fats) at least by one half.

The responsibilities of health care professionals counseling vegetarians, vegans, and nonvegetarians are the same—to promote good health through reasonable food choices. These responsibilities include doing the following with the individual or household:

▶ Support every positive aspect of the chosen food pattern
▶ Evaluate food intake to help identify those dietary ingredients that might be deficient because of food choices or food preparation methods
▶ Encourage purchasing of foods that provide the most nutrients for the money
▶ Encourage food evaluation for nutrient content, amount of excess packaging, and excess processing
▶ Help identify practices undermining satisfactory nutritional health.

ASSESSMENT

Assessment of nutritional status is an important part of the total health evaluation, and it provides essential information for differential diagnosis.[42,107] Recognition of nutritional deficits, excesses, or imbalances can be particularly important in determining the type of diet therapy needed to return the person to health as quickly as possible. The major features of nutritional assessment include: (a) obtaining dietary data, (b) performing a thorough physical assessment including noting anthropometric and biochemical measurements, and (c) noting the client's feelings about diet changes. Box 42-6 outlines one example of an assessment tool that might be used to collect data during a typical nutritional assessment.

The data that you collect with your assessment can be put together with your knowledge of good nutrition in order to diagnose and plan nursing care for your client. Your knowledge of good nutrition should include an understanding of factors that influence food intake, dietary patterns, and nutritional status.

Food and Dietary Records

The nurse or dietitian can obtain valuable quantitative data from food records or food diaries. The food record or diary provides precise information about the amounts of specific nutrients consumed daily. The food record requires the cooperation of the person in the household or institution responsible for food preparation. The person is instructed to keep a careful record of the amounts of each type of food consumed within a period of 1 to 7 days. The longer an accurate record is kept, the more valid the data, because food intake for one particular day may not reflect the typical eating habits of the person.

Upon completion of the record, it is given to a health care team member (e.g., dietitian or nurse), who determines the average daily intake of specific nutrients as reported by the person. The average daily intake of specific nutrients is then compared with the RDAs for an individual of the same age and sex. Significant deviations from the RDA may suggest inadequate nutrition.

The food record cannot be taken as an absolute indication of adequate nutrition, but such records are widely used to obtain presumptive evidence of dietary inadequacies or excesses. Information related to diet is useful in assessing the need for nutritional intervention programs or for special feeding programs within homes or entire communities. Additionally, knowledge of dietary habits is an absolute necessity if recommendations for dietary modifications are to fit comfortably and appropriately into the client's lifestyle.

In some settings, the food frequency score sheet has proved to be the most useful and rapid assessment method. This tool assesses the weekly frequency of consumption of each food on a carefully selected list of foods designed to contain all major sources of key nutrients. Data obtained are tabulated by computer to provide a rough estimate of average daily consumption of major nutrients, vitamins, and minerals.

Physical Assessment

Physical signs and symptoms of malnutrition can be valuable aids in detecting nutritional deficiencies. Table 42-9 lists physical characteristics of malnutrition. Re-

Box 42–6. Dietary Assessment

1. Dietary data
   a. Usual food patterns
      i. Duration of meal
      ii. Kinds of foods eaten
      iii. Amounts of foods eaten
      iv. Items used regularly in large amounts
      v. Times during day when eating occurs
      vi. Other pertinent features
   b. Use of dietary supplements (type, dose, time taken, specific preparation)
   c. Previous experience and success with modified diets
   d. Specific food likes, dislikes, intolerances
   e. General state of appetite
   f. Money available for food
   g. Transportation and facilities available for food purchasing, preparation, and storage
2. Health history (as a partial indicator of past nutritional status)
   a. History of current illness
   b. History of past illness and recovery from surgery
   c. History of past pregnancy and outcome
   d. History of bleeding problems
   e. Drug use (what, when taken, why taken)
3. Physical condition and anthropometric data
   a. Height, weight, skinfold thickness
   b. Muscular development
   c. Neurologic condition
   d. Status of eyes, skin, tongue, mouth
   e. Dental status
4. General biochemical measurements
   a. Urinalysis
   b. Stool assay (blood, fat, etc.)
   c. CBC, blood indices
   d. Serum proteins and lipids
   e. Serum electrolytes, blood pH
   f. Liver function studies
   g. Blood sugar, BUN, creatinine
5. Special biochemical measurements
   a. Nutrient and/or metabolic excretion after fasting or provision of test dose
   b. Concentration of nutrients in blood, plasma, RBC, WBC, or other tissue
   c. Activity of specific enzymes (which suggest availability of certain nutrients, especially vitamins)
   d. Excretion of abnormal metabolites

ANTHROPOMETRIC MEASUREMENTS

Anthropometric measurements are physical data that document the size and proportions of parts of the body.[42] The measurements of an individual are taken and compared with normative standards. Without these comparisons, anthropometric data have little meaning. Delayed growth and development of children can be determined by comparing growth data of an individual or a group with standard height and weight trends on growth charts. In adults, discrepancy in the height/weight relationship suggests malnutrition or excessive fat stores. Anthropometry also goes beyond simple measurement of height and weight, which can be misleading and does not supply adequate information on body composition, fat stores, muscle mass, and fluid volume. Additional measurements of arm circumference can supply information about muscle mass; skinfold measurements with calipers give indications of amounts of body fat. In gathering anthropometric measurements, personnel should use standardized equipment and procedures.

BIOCHEMICAL ASSESSMENT

Evaluating nutritional status by laboratory methods is usually a more objective and precise approach than food records and anthropometric measurements. Biochemical assessment utilizes biochemical tests performed in a clinical laboratory to measure levels of nutrients in biologic fluids (blood or urine), or evaluate certain biochemical functions that are dependent on an adequate supply of essential nutrients. The interpretation of laboratory data, however, is often difficult and does not necessarily always correlate with either clinical or dietary findings.

Be aware that all assessment methods are most effective when used in combination. Also remember that a deficiency in one nutrient can be considered an almost certain indicator of other nutritional inadequacies.

Obviously, the sooner the diagnosis of poor nutritional status is made in individuals and in populations, the sooner individual clinical and public health intervention programs can be put into action.

Feelings About Diet Changes

Frequently, diet assessment will show that the individual is not obtaining adequate quantity and quality of specific nutrients. The diets of some people, for example, completely exclude some types of foods or entire food groups, or the total food consumption may be inappropriately high or low. In such circumstances, the person needs to make some reasonable dietary modifications. The sensitive nurse recognizes, however, that individual eating habits are very personal and in many cases are so deeply ingrained that it may be difficult for the person to change them. If the client is to change a diet, even moderately, it is essential to introduce changes slowly. Also, the client must be convinced that

member, however, that signs of malnutrition are sometimes related to non-nutritional factors such as poor hygiene or excessive exposure to the sun and that these signs may not correlate with dietary intake data or the biochemical values for the individual or the population. Therefore, it is generally wise to consider any physical finding that suggests a nutritional abnormality as a "clue" to be pursued further rather than a "diagnosis." For example, pallor is not diagnostic of anemia, but it is a clue that could lead to laboratory confirmation of anemia.

TABLE 42-9. Physical Signs Indicative or Suggestive of Malnutrition

Body Area	Signs of Good Nutrition	Signs of Poor Nutrition
General appearance	Alert, responsive	Listless, apathetic, cachectic (emaciated, wasted)
Weight	Normal for height, age, body build	Overweight or underweight (special concern for underweight)
Posture	Erect, arms and legs straight	Sagging shoulders, sunken chest, humped back
Muscles	Well-developed; firm, good tone	Flaccid, poor tone; undeveloped; tender, "wasted" appearance; inability to walk properly
Nervous control	Good attention span; not irritable or restless; normal reflexes; psychologic stability	Inattentive, irritable, confused; burning and tingling of hands and feet (paresthesia); loss of position and vibratory sense; weakness and tenderness of muscles (may result in inability to walk); decrease or loss of ankle and knee reflexes
Gastrointestinal function	Good appetite and digestion; normal, regular elimination; no palpable (perceptible to touch) organs or masses	Anorexia, indigestion, constipation or diarrhea, liver or spleen enlargement
Cardiovascular function	Normal heart rate and rhythm, no murmurs, normal blood pressure for age	Tachycardia (heart rate above 100 beats/min), enlarged heart, abnormal rhythm, elevated blood pressure
General vitality	Good endurance, energetic, sleeps well, vigorous	Easily fatigued, no energy, falls asleep easily, looks tired, apathetic
Hair	Shiny, lustrous, firm, not easily plucked; healthy scalp	Stringy, dull, brittle, dry, thin, and sparse; depigmented; can be easily plucked
Skin (general)	Smooth, slightly moist, good color	Rough, dry, scaly, pale, pigmented, irritated; easily bruised; petechiae present; delayed wound healing
Face and neck	Skin color uniform with smooth, pink, healthy appearance; not swollen	Greasy, discolored, scaly, swollen; skin dark over cheeks and under eyes; lumpiness or flakiness of skin around nose and mouth
Lips	Smooth, good color, moist, not chapped or swollen	Dry, scaly, swollen, reddened, fissures at the corners (cheilosis)
Mouth, oral membranes	Reddish pink mucous membranes in oral cavity	Swollen, boggy oral mucous membranes; inflamed oral tissue (stomatitis)
Gums	Good pink color, healthy, red, no swelling or bleeding	Spongy, bleed easily, marginal redness, inflamed, receding
Tongue	Good pink color or deep reddish in appearance, not swollen or smooth, surface papillae present, no lesions	Swelling, scarlet and raw, magenta color, beefy (glossitis), hyperemic and hypertrophic papillae, atrophic papillae
Teeth	No cavities; no pain; bright, straight, no crowding; well-shaped jaw; clean, no discoloration	Unfilled caries, absent teeth, worn surfaces, mottled (fluorosis), malpositioned
Eyes	Bright, clear, shiny; no sores at corner of eyelids; membranes moist and healthy; pink color; no prominent blood vessels or mound of tissue on sclera; no fatigue circles beneath	Eye membranes pale (pale conjunctivas), redness of membrane (conjunctivitis), signs of infection; Bitot's spots; redness with fissuring of eyelid corners (angular palpebritis, blepharitis); dryness of eye membrane (conjunctival xerosis); dull appearance of cornea (corneal xerosis); soft cornea (keratomalacia)
Neck (glands)	No enlargement	Thyroid enlargement
Nails	Firm, pink	Spoon-shaped (koilonychia), brittle, ridged
Legs, feet	No tenderness, weakness, or swelling; good color	Edema, calf tenderness, tingling, weakness
Skeleton	No malformations	Bowlegs, knock-knees, chest deformity at diaphragm, beaded ribs, prominent scapulas

the dietary changes are absolutely necessary for better health. For ensured success, modifications must meet the client's cultural, personal, and economic needs and must be adapted to the individual's lifestyle.

Factors That Influence Food Intake, Dietary Patterns, and Nutritional Status

APPETITE

Although a wide variety of factors determines an individual's choice of foods, the sensation of hunger is certainly a basic one. The mechanisms that regulate hunger and satiety in the human body are poorly understood, but certain factors are known to play a significant part. The sense of smell is an important component of appetite. If the olfactory sense is not functioning properly, the person might experience reduced appetite.

Centers in the brain's hypothalamus regulate food intake. Experiments have shown that injury of the ventromedial part of the hypothalamus results in overeating, whereas injury to the lateral regions promotes undereating. Other factors involved in regulation of appetite include blood sugar level, gastric secretions, gastric motility, hormonal factors, and responses to the autonomic nervous system. For most people, the body adjusts ingestion of food to meet the requirements of health, proper functioning, and growth. Occasionally this homeostatic mechanism does not operate properly, and excessive or insufficient hunger develops, with obesity or emaciation as a long-term result.

FINANCIAL STATUS

The amount of money you have to spend will influence what and how much you purchase, especially for food. Families with middle or high incomes are generally able to purchase whatever they desire in the way of food items. However, the limited amount of money available for people with low or fixed incomes is often inadequate to buy enough food to prevent hunger, let alone promote good health. Thus, low-income persons commonly have difficulty meeting their nutritional needs.

GEOGRAPHY

The specific location in which an individual resides will have a distinct effect on the types of foods consumed. Location is less significant in developed societies where food preservation, packaging, and transportation are sophisticated. Even under the best circumstances, however, geographic location definitely affects the availability of many fresh food items, meats, and seafood.

CULTURE

Eating habits are generally learned in early life and very definitely reflect the cultural influences that predominated in the home at the time. In addition, child-rearing practices, eating utensils, mealtimes, and food service patterns vary from culture to culture. Eating and food patterns that are unique to a specific cultural group are difficult for a person from that specific culture to change. For example, Asian cultures rely heavily on flavoring compounds that are high in sodium, such as soy sauce and MSG. A person accustomed to these ingredients and requiring a low-sodium diet will need to be educated concerning new flavorings and cooking styles that will substitute for these high-sodium flavorings or spices.

RELIGION

Religious practices often indicate what a person will and will not eat, how food will be prepared, and when it will be eaten. The Jewish and Islamic religions, for example, are rich in food-related traditions. Those who carefully follow Jewish dietary laws and "keep a kosher kitchen" will not eat meat and dairy products together. Those who follow Islam celebrate religious holidays with long periods of fasting followed by enormous feasts.

The Seventh Day Adventists and the Church of Jesus Christ of the Latter Day Saints support the philosophy that dietary practices are an integral part of religious beliefs. Seventh Day Adventists believe that a vegetarian diet is prescribed by God. The diets of these people, therefore, are typically based on grains, fruits, vegetables, and nuts, although dairy products and eggs may also be consumed. Many religious groups eliminate tea, coffee, alcoholic beverages, and strong spices and condiments in the interest of maintaining optimal health and preventing disease.

SOCIAL CIRCUMSTANCES

In most societies, social gatherings revolve around food and drink. The items served on these special occasions are often determined by tradition or custom. Eating and drinking typically accompany social gatherings with friends and family. When opportunities for this source of enjoyment are eliminated (as may be the case for most hospitalized persons and many elderly citizens), the pleasure of eating may be greatly reduced. The result may be poor or nonexistent appetite leading to serious malnutrition.

Friends and caretakers must make an effort to provide lonely people with appropriate social contacts on a regular basis, especially during meals. This one gesture of kindness may have a sizable impact on the eventual health status and well-being of the person involved.

AGE

The age of an individual influences not only the types of foods preferred but also the amount of food and specific nutrients required on a daily basis. Persons who are growing most rapidly (i.e., infants and adolescents) have the highest nutritional demands per kilogram of body weight. Adults who are simply maintaining a stable body structure require the least nutritional support per unit of body weight. However, special conditions such as pregnancy and lactation increase nutritional requirements substantially. As the adult becomes older, calorie needs per day decrease, but the requirement for all other nutrients stays approximately the same.

Each stage of the life cycle imparts a unique set of circumstances that dictate an individual's nutritional needs. The nurse who recognizes the basis for nutritional requirements throughout the life cycle can provide appropriate guidance to people of all ages.

Infancy. During the first year of life, the infant grows rapidly. By 6 months of age, birth weight generally has doubled, and by 1 year it usually has tripled. To support this rapid rate of tissue synthesis, sufficient calorie and protein intake is critical. The other nutrients, such as carbohydrates, fat, minerals, and vitamins, also play an important role in the growth process.[80]

In most countries, a variety of milks and solid foods are available for feeding infants. The "ideal" food for young infants is breast milk, which is potentially available to 99 per cent of all babies. Breast milk contains almost all the nutrients the infant needs until about 4 to 6 months of age. In addition to a satisfactory calorie content (20 kcal/oz) and easily digestible forms of protein, carbohydrate, and fat, breast milk has a low electrolyte load, a high vitamin content (if the mother's diet is adequate), an acceptable iron content (in absorbable form), and an abundance of "protective factors" such

as immunoglobulins, macrophages, and antiviral agents. No artificial formula precisely duplicates human milk!

In addition to making good nutritional sense, breastfeeding also makes good economic sense. Breast milk is much less expensive than commercially prepared formulas. Also, evidence indicates that breastfeeding can promote healthy infant-mother bonding. Nonetheless, many mothers bottlefeed their babies. Ideally, every pregnant woman should receive sufficient information about all the options of infant feeding and be allowed to choose the method most compatible with individual circumstances, preferences, and lifestyle.

To counsel the mother who chooses to breastfeed effectively, the nurse-clinician must thoroughly understand the process of lactation and then explain it to the mother. Additionally, the nurse needs to instruct the mother in proper breastfeeding techniques and support her in her first attempts. Finally, the nurse should (a) know and be able to identify the reasons for lactation failure, and (b) be prepared to plan management strategies for the baby who fails to thrive while breastfeeding (Fig. 42–4).

For mothers who choose to bottlefeed, a variety of commercial formulas on the market are designed to resemble human milk. Most of them contain about 20 kcal/oz and provide the nutrients babies need.

It is also important to teach parents which infant foods to avoid. Some important cautions for parents:

▶ Do not prepare infant formulas in the home. These preparations, which are usually composed of evapo-

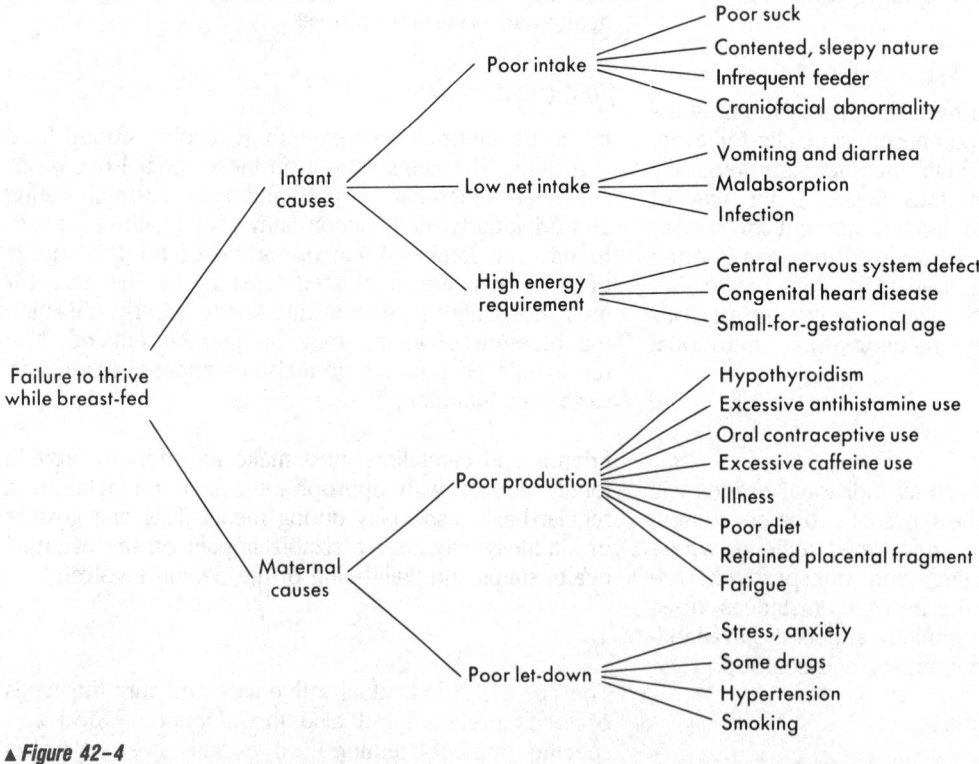

▲ **Figure 42–4**

Diagnostic flow chart for failure to thrive. (Reprinted with permission from Worthington-Roberts, B.S., et al. [1989]. *Nutrition in pregnancy and lactation* [4th ed.]. St. Louis: Times Mirror/Mosby College Publishing; modified from Lawrence, R. [1989]. *Breast-feeding: A guideline for the medical profession.* St. Louis: C.V. Mosby.)

rated milk, corn syrup, and water, are deficient in iron and vitamin C. In addition, they are inconvenient to prepare.

▶ Do not feed infants fresh homogenized milk during the first 6 months of life. Fresh cow's milk contains protein that can cause intestinal bleeding and thus may promote iron-deficiency anemia.

▶ Do not feed skim milk to infants under 1 year of age. Not only is skim milk derived from "fresh" cow milk, it also contains only 10 kcal/oz and thus cannot support optimal growth of young infants.

Advise parents to add textured foods when the baby is about 4 to 6 months of age. Most babies do not need solids before this time. Parents should introduce solid foods only when the baby needs additional calories in the diet. Iron-fortified rice cereal is a reasonable first choice. Later, they may add strained fruits and vegetables. Babies do not need commercially prepared baby foods. Parents can easily prepare suitable foods from fruits, vegetables, and other table foods. Teach parents to replace strained foods first with foods of lumpy texture and finally with fully textured foods that require considerable oral-motor manipulation.

Always encourage parents to provide infant diets that contain sufficient calories, iron, vitamin D, and vitamin C. These nutrients are essential for proper growth and development.

Unfortunately, some infants receive either excessive calories or insufficient calories. Reasons for faulty caloric intake include

▶ high or low formula concentration
▶ misinterpretation of "fussiness" to mean hunger
▶ excessive use of solids in the diet, resulting in excessive caloric intake
▶ stressful environment promoting poor appetite
▶ chronic anorexia related to disease or drug therapy
▶ excessive loss of calories by vomiting or diarrhea

Providing adequate nutrition to the small, preterm infant is a major challenge for the health care team. Preterm babies have high nutritional needs, but providing adequate nutrients is a problem because of the immaturity of the gastrointestinal tract, liver, and kidneys. In addition, regular feeding by nipple is often difficult or impossible for infants of less than 34 weeks' gestation, because sucking and swallowing reflexes are not sufficiently developed. Even tube gavage feeding for preterm babies is limited by their small stomach capacity and the poorly coordinated motility of their gastrointestinal tract; thus, gastric distention is a common problem. In turn, distention increases the risk of respiratory distress. The development of distention may also herald necrotizing enterocolitis, a potentially life-threatening breakdown of the intestinal lining. Poor cardiac sphincter function makes regurgitation with aspiration a particular hazard.

Because of these dangers, parenteral feeding may be required for a period. However, it is wise to introduce oral foods as soon as possible. Increase the volume of food slowly and monitor the infant carefully. Breast milk is the food of choice if it is available. Milk provided by mothers who deliver prematurely is more concentrated in its nutritional make-up than milk provided by mothers who deliver at term. "Fortification" of human milk with a commercial human milk fortifier augments the calorie and nutrient concentration of this already high-quality infant food. As an alternative to breast milk, special formulas are available for the preterm infant.

Preschool Age. With growth, the infant gradually becomes more capable of self-feeding.[90] The young child develops self-feeding skills through regular practice with foods and thus needs to be provided with an opportunity to finger feed and manipulate feeding utensils. As the youngster learns these necessary skills, tell the parents to anticipate spills and messes. A parent who expects the young preschooler to avoid mishaps while learning the feeding process will soon become frustrated. Teach parents that young children characteristically

▶ assert their independence increasingly as they mature
▶ tend to reject new foods at first
▶ eat less some days than other days, as adults do
▶ rebel when forced to eat
▶ learn by experience, using fingers before forks

Remind significant others that preschool children are individuals who must be allowed to develop in their own way and at their own speed. Teach parents that children typically become more independent as they grow older, even though their increasing independence may try one's patience. Preschoolers eat best when they are in a relaxed environment with minimal distractions, sit in a comfortable chair that fits them properly, are given small servings, and are free to choose some foods.

Because of an increased interest in the surrounding world, the preschool child may not demonstrate much interest in food. Refusal of food is common, as is the desire to consume the same food repeatedly throughout the day or week. Encourage parents to offer a variety of foods to their children at this age but not to be upset if the food is merely explored or nibbled. With repeated exposure, the child usually learns to accept the food.

Preschool children learn very quickly that parents can be easily manipulated if the child rejects certain foods or refuses to eat. Teach parents not to feel guilty or upset if their children will not eat. Parents soon find that if they do not respond to children's behavior by becoming upset, young children usually return to more cooperative eating habits.

The entire family influences the young child's food habits. Young children tend to imitate adults and other siblings. Consequently, youngsters often develop food preferences and eating habits by observing the significant people in their environment.

School Age. The slower growth rate demonstrated by the school-age child results in a general decline in the food requirement per unit of body weight.[80] This lower requirement continues until the onset of the adolescent growth spurt. Most food likes and dislikes manifested during this stage developed at a younger age. The eating behavior of peers and media advertisements for specific foods, however, also strongly influence the child's eating habits.

Myriad school activities exert yet another powerful influence on eating behavior. School-age children become increasingly involved in sports, school-related activities, and other social activities that compete with the dinner hour. Thus, children may rush through meals or skip them entirely. In addition, older children may often be left alone to prepare food. Consequently, snacks play a significant part in the total food intake. Encourage parents to prepare nutritious snack foods that children can eat at home or at school. Wholesome snacks contribute effectively to the child's nutritional intake.

Adolescence. To support the rapid physical growth of adolescence, caloric needs must increase to meet metabolic demands. Typically, girls require fewer calories than boys do, but the caloric needs of individual adolescents vary. And, unless a child's family is poor, an adolescent easily can meet calorie and protein needs through a balanced, daily diet.[59]

During adolescence, calcium is important for the support of long-bone calcification, and iron is critical for maintaining increased red blood cell mass. Menstrual blood losses in pubescent girls further increase iron needs and put girls at risk for iron-deficiency anemia. Young boys may suffer from the same condition if they are growing rapidly. Vitamins C and A, too, are necessary at this stage, although intake of both vitamins may be inadequate if food intake is erratic. Typically, adolescence is a time when peer group pressure often leads to increased snacking and dependence on a diet based on a limited number of foods.

Adolescents, especially females, are prone to eating disorders. Surveys of nutritional habits in developed societies indicate that adolescent girls are more vulnerable to severe eating disorders than any other members of the population. Indeed, serious and even fatal eating disorders have become more prevalent with this group during the past 20 years. The four most common eating disorders of adolescence are (1) overeating in response to stress and depression, (2) compulsive dieting due in part to society's emphasis on the "svelte" figure, (3) anorexia nervosa, and (4) bulimia nervosa (Fig. 42–5).

Overeating and subsequent obesity affect persons of all ages and can cause serious physical and psychologic problems. In particular, a teenage girl who feels socially inferior because her weight is high may eat even more to compensate for her hurt feelings.

Compulsive dieting is a special problem for the young. As a rule, adolescents long to be attractive and acceptable to their peers. Consequently, they are preoccupied with being thin almost at any cost. Teenage girls, for example, may not understand that as they grow into womanhood, fat deposits develop normally around the hips, thighs, and breasts. Believing these deposits unsightly, these young women may nearly starve themselves on self-imposed crash diets to reverse a natural evolution into adulthood. But compulsive dieting can leave the teenage girl malnourished, a condition she can ill afford at a life stage when her body is depositing bone minerals and building nutritional reserves to support the reproductive requirements of a fetus at some time in her life.

Anorexia nervosa is a serious and sometimes fatal eating disorder characterized by severe and constant dieting. Anorexia nervosa can develop at almost any age but is more common in adolescence. It has been diagnosed in boys, although female anorectics outnumber their male counterparts by an overwhelming margin of 9 to 1. Although its cause is still unknown, anorexia nervosa seems to be related to lost control:

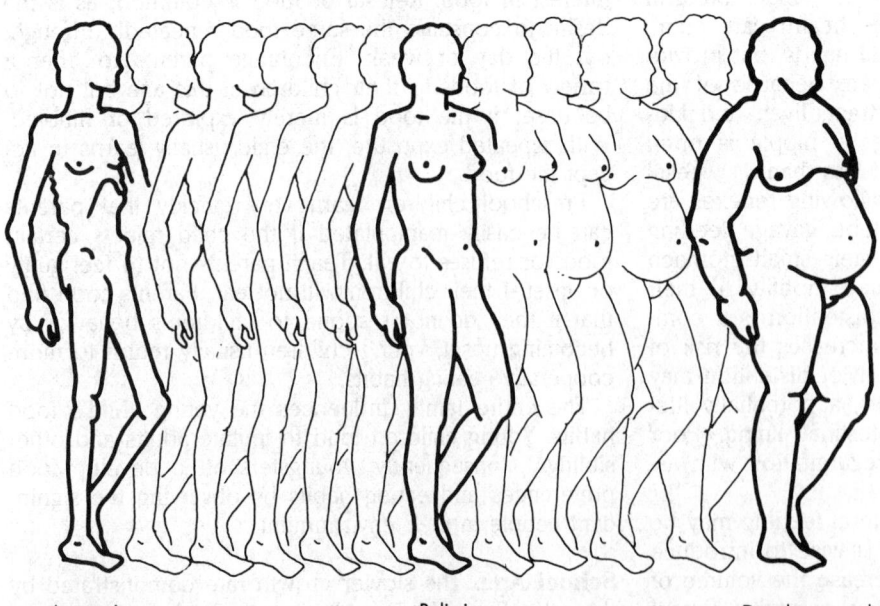

Anorexia
nervosa

Bulimia
nervosa

Developmental
obesity

▲ *Figure 42–5*

Spectrum of eating disorders. Although physical conditions vary, underlying psychologic characteristics are held in common across the spectrum. (Reprinted with permission from Mahan, L.L., & Rees, J.M. [1984]. *Nutrition in adolescence.* St. Louis: Times Mirror/ Mosby College Publishing.)

rigid dieting allows anorectics to regain and exercise control over at least one aspect of their lives (Box 42–7).

Anorectic clients frequently lose 15 to 25 per cent (or more) of their body weight, a proportion so dangerous it can lead to death. Moreover, such drastic weight loss causes victims to develop a gaunt, skeletal appearance; to exhibit a growth of fine, soft hair over their bodies; and to cease menstruating. Additionally, hypothermia, low blood pressure, edema, bradycardia (low heart rate), and disturbed sleep may develop.

Treating anorectic clients typically involves first getting them to ingest enough nutrients to restore their physiologic well-being. Gaining weight, however, is not the only answer. Integrating the anorectic's family relationships and psychologic symptoms into a care plan is necessary to achieve a long-term cure.

Bulimia nervosa is an eating disorder characterized by periodic binging and purging. Bulimics usually have unrealistic ideas about food and what constitutes "too much" food and generally are unsure about the amount of food necessary to maintain good health. These uncertainties, along with the "fear of fatness" common in developed societies, lead bulimics to deliberately vomit or purge themselves with laxatives when they feel they have eaten excessively. Nevertheless, bulimics typically remain close to their ideal body weight and rarely become seriously malnourished (Box 42–7).

Periodic vomiting, especially over time, can lead to tooth damage (erosion of the enamel), irritation of the throat and esophagus, swelling of the salivary glands caused by acidic reflux and constant stimulation, fluid and electrolyte imbalances, and, occasionally, fistulas or rupture of the upper gastrointestinal tract. Laxative abuse may further aggravate fluid and electrolyte imbalance and may cause rectal bleeding.

Because bulimics tend to binge and purge in secret, they are not easily detected. Little still is known about this disorder, but bulimia is thought to be common among college-age women. It is generally more prevalent in women than in men, with onset generally in the late teens or early adulthood.

A completely successful treatment for bulimia has yet to be developed. At present, common treatment methods include individual or group therapy with a strong behavior modification component.

To prevent these potentially dangerous eating disorders, adolescent females need appropriate and responsible dietary counseling. Discourage young women from severe dieting and exercising to maintain an unreasonably low body weight. Young women also need nutritional information that focuses on the requirements for healthy growth and development. All young women should be advised to participate in regular physical activity to balance calorie intake and output. Over time, such a program usually will result in stable, normal body weight.

Adulthood. On the basis of available research and clinical data, the "best" diet for the average adult appears to be one containing all needed nutrients and providing approximately 30 per cent of the calories from fat, 55 per cent of the calories from carbohydrate,

---

Box 42–7. Diagnostic Criteria for Anorexia Nervosa and Bulimia Nervosa

Anorexia Nervosa

1. Refusal to maintain body weight at a normal weight for age and height (e.g., weight loss leading to maintenance of body weight 15 per cent below that expected; or failure to make expected weight gain during period of growth, leading to body weight 15 per cent below that expected)
2. Intense fear of gaining weight or becoming fat, even though underweight
3. Disturbance in the way in which one's body weight, size, or shape is experienced (e.g., the person claims to "feel fat" even when emaciated, believes that one area of the body is "too fat" even when obviously underweight)
4. In females, absence of at least three consecutive menstrual cycles otherwise expected to occur (primary or secondary amenorrhea). (A woman is considered to have amenorrhea if her periods occur only following administration of a hormone such as estrogen)

Bulimia Nervosa

1. Recurrent episodes of binge eating (rapid consumption of a large amount of food in a discrete period of time)
2. A feeling of lack of control over eating behavior during the eating binges
3. The person regularly engages in self-induced vomiting, use of laxatives or diuretics, strict dieting or fasting, or vigorous exercise in order to prevent weight gain
4. A minimum average of two binge-eating episodes a week for at least 3 months
5. Persistent overconcern with body shape and weight

Eating Disorder Not Otherwise Specified

1. A person of average weight who does not have binge-eating episodes but frequently engages in self-induced vomiting for fear of gaining weight
2. All the features of anorexia nervosa in a woman except absence of menses
3. All the features of bulimia nervosa except the frequency of binge-eating episodes

Adapted from American Psychiatric Association (1987). *Diagnostic and statistical manual of mental disorders* (3rd ed.–Revised). Washington, D.C.: American Psychiatric Association.

---

and 15 per cent from protein.[72] Ideally, fat should be predominantly unsaturated fatty acids, and the carbohydrate should be predominantly complex (such as starch) rather than refined sugar. Additionally, the diet should include enough nondigestible material (fiber) to promote normal gut motility.

The total daily caloric requirement for adults depends directly on the level of physical activity in the daily routine. The moderately or highly active adult has little difficulty meeting nutritional needs, unless the person is economically deprived, but the inactive adult who consumes limited calories may not select foods that can support nutrient needs. Such individuals, especially those who chronically undertake weight reduction regimens in addition to rigorous exercise, may find themselves seriously malnourished unless they consciously monitor nutrient intake or use nutritional supplements.

Later Maturity. Although the aging process is associated with many changes in physiologic functions (Fig. 42–6), the nutritional needs of the older adult change very little.[25,69,75] By and large, the body has about the same nutritional requirements at age 70 years as it does at age 40 years, but daily calorie needs do decrease with age because older adults generally undergo a reduction in their basal metabolic rate. In addition, a decrease in activity that often accompanies aging results in lower daily calorie needs. As a rule, daily calorie requirements decrease by about 7 per cent with each decade after age 25 years, but considerable individual variation exists. Active senior citizens require more caloric support than the immobilized or inactive adult.

A major challenge for the inactive older adult is to obtain the necessary nutrients from a diet sufficiently

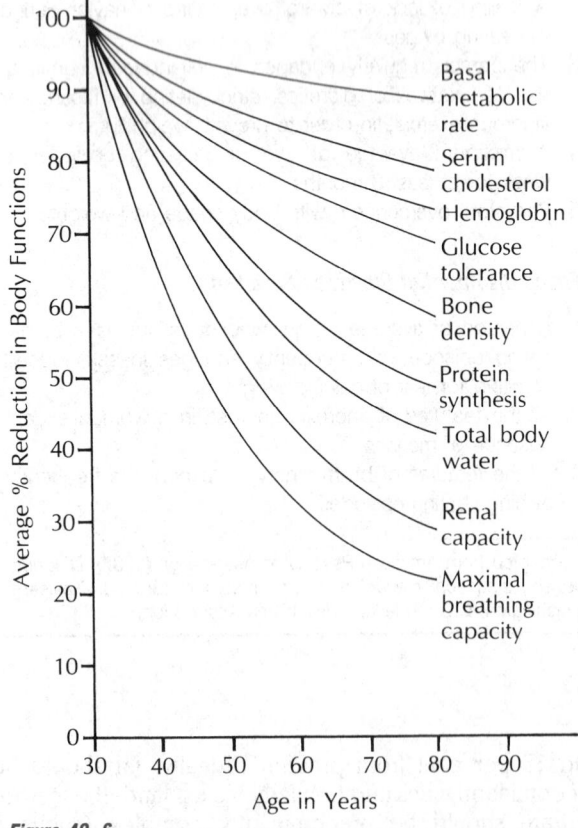

▲ *Figure 42–6*

Aging results in a reduction in body functions. A decline is evident in such areas as metabolic rate, glucose tolerance, bone density, and maximal breathing capacity. Here the average rate of decline is shown for men from 30 to 80 years of age. (Adapted from Albanese, A.A. [1980]. *Nutrition for the elderly.* New York: Alan R. Liss.)

low in calories. Such a goal can be achieved if the older person attends closely to diet planning and omits the sources of "empty calories." For some people, however, it is better to take small doses of vitamin or mineral supplements.

Insufficient intake of food may be a problem in elderly people and results from many factors. Physical incapacities may interfere with food shopping, meal preparation, and eating. Other physical problems, such as the need for dentures, may also affect the individual's ability and desire to eat. Fixed incomes may limit purchase of some food items. Loneliness or other emotional problems often result in a lack of interest regarding meals.

INDIVIDUAL PREFERENCES

Eating patterns and nutritional requirements are dictated not only by one's culture and lifestyle but also by one's individual preferences and physiologic differences. Each human being is unique in the specific nutritional requirements for optimal function. In the final analysis, choice of specific foods is an individual matter and relates to taste, texture, and flavor preferences, which are based, in turn, on experience with foods in the home and on cultural and religious traditions. Recognition and appreciation of these highly important individual characteristics are vital to providing sound dietary advice and overall high-quality health care.

PHYSIOLOGIC AND OTHER REACTIONS

Some people exhibit strong allergic responses to certain foods or food groups. The symptoms associated with these reactions include skin rash, vomiting, diarrhea, and headache. Therefore, be aware of any food allergies and make certain that those foods are specifically excluded from the person's diet.

PREGNANCY AND LACTATION

Pregnancy and lactation are associated with increased nutritional needs and frequently are accompanied by altered eating patterns. These patterns of eating may be related to specific appetite changes and food-related beliefs. Many traditions, superstitions, and prejudices determine what foods are "acceptable" for the pregnant or lactating woman in most cultures. In parts of the South Pacific, for example, pregnant women are advised not to consume shellfish so that the baby will not develop scales on the head. In some areas of Ethiopia, it is traditionally believed that eating roasted meat during pregnancy will cause spontaneous abortion. In many cultures, women may consume a variety of nonfood items (clay, dirt, starch, ashes) because they believe it will ease delivery, prevent birthmarks on the infant, or otherwise improve the health status of mother and infant before or after birth. It is important to understand the cultural basis of an unusual eating practice before formulating an approach to the situation. If the unusual practice does not appear to compromise the health of the woman involved, recommending that she discontinue the practice may be unwise.

When a woman becomes pregnant, her nutritional requirements increase.[118] For a normal, healthy pregnancy, the woman must increase her daily calorie intake by approximately 300 kcal during the second and third trimesters. She must also ingest 10 gm of extra protein and also slightly increase other vital nutrients such as calcium and iron. International studies support the view that the average woman should gain about 25 to 35 pounds during the entire pregnancy. In most cases, simple and sensible increases in daily food intake will accommodate the added nutritional needs of the pregnant woman, but iron, folic acid, or general vitamin supplements may be justified for women at risk for malnutrition. High-risk women include adolescents, women with previous pregnancy difficulties, women pregnant after a very short interconceptional period, women pregnant with more than one fetus, women from low socioeconomic levels, and women with heart disease, renal disease, diabetes, or other chronic diseases.

Prenatal nutritional counseling is a routine part of well-organized care of pregnant women. The prenatal counselor helps the woman meet her nutritional needs to fit with her culture and lifestyle.

The mother who breastfeeds usually produces about 700 to 800 ml of milk daily for her growing infant.[118] Therefore, the lactating woman should ingest an additional 500 kcal and 10 to 15 gm of protein per day. She should also moderately increase her intake of other essential nutrients, particularly vitamins. Although more studies are needed, it appears that the nutritional content of breast milk is fairly constant regardless of the mother's nutritional status. This constancy suggests that necessary protein and minerals are drawn from maternal stores. Therefore, it is the mother rather than her baby who suffers more from nutritional deficiencies.

THE MEDIA

The media have a dramatic influence on the eating patterns and supplementation regimens of people in most societies of the world. Radio, television, newspapers, magazines, and similar media often influence our food-related behaviors. Ingenious marketing techniques introduce new food products, supplements, and other innovations to the public. A listener who had no prior interest in the product and no need for the article may suddenly feel compelled to purchase the item simply on the basis of the ad. Because one nursing role is to educate the public concerning the realities of good nutrition, you need to be particularly sensitive to the seductive nature of advertising, especially when advertising claims associated with food, health, or anti-aging products are grandiose in their promises of instant health, eternal youth, unlimited vitality, and the like.

USE OF ALCOHOL AND DRUGS

Regular use of both alcohol and drugs can significantly modify appetite and food intake over time. Moderate drinking (and use of some drugs) may be accompanied by increased appetite along with an undesirable gain in body weight. On the other hand, heavy use of alcohol and some drugs may depress appetite to such an extent that malnutrition eventually develops if the drinking or drug ingestion is not controlled. Many drugs, including alcohol, damage the mucosal linings of the stomach and bowel and thus prevent efficient absorption of the limited nutrients that are consumed. In such cases, malnutrition is especially likely.

Additionally, some drugs (e.g., phenytoin, amphetamines) alter taste sensations or interfere with the proper functioning of specific vitamins and minerals. For example, oral contraceptives are folic acid antagonists, and some antibiotics decrease the synthesis of vitamin K by intestinal bacteria. Thus, it is important to include a medication history in the nutritional assessment, because many drugs can promote deficiencies even when nutritional intake may be adequate.

ILLNESS AND INJURY

Disease and trauma can markedly affect both appetite and nutritional requirements. People who are ill or who have been traumatized must receive appropriate nutritional care or their nutritional status will gradually deteriorate.

Most people who are sick or injured have a poor appetite. At the same time, nutritional needs are frequently higher than usual because of the increased metabolic work required during fever, wound healing, and combatting infection (Fig. 42–7). Nutritional needs may be further elevated by sizable losses of protein, fluid, and electrolytes in the urine or from a bleeding or draining wound.

Protein-energy malnutrition associated with serious illness or trauma is a problem in the United States as well as in the rest of the world. This kind of malnutrition occurs when lean tissue is being broken down and more nitrogen (protein) is being lost than is being laid down in new tissue. The loss of protein causes a negative nitrogen balance, and the client has a questionable prognosis unless the phenomenon can be reversed.

Also associated with serious illness or trauma is the use of certain medications that may adversely affect nutritional status. Nutrients and medications can interact in many ways:

▶ Medications can alter food intake
▶ Nutrients and foods can alter medication absorption
▶ Medications can alter nutrient absorption
▶ Nutrients can alter the intended actions of medications
▶ Nutrients can alter the metabolism and excretion of medications
▶ Medications can alter the metabolism and excretion of nutrients

To date, the number of nutrient-medication interactions is sizable, and more interactions are discovered regularly. Remembering all these interactions is difficult for any clinician. Therefore, when entering the clinical area, you should attend to the following:

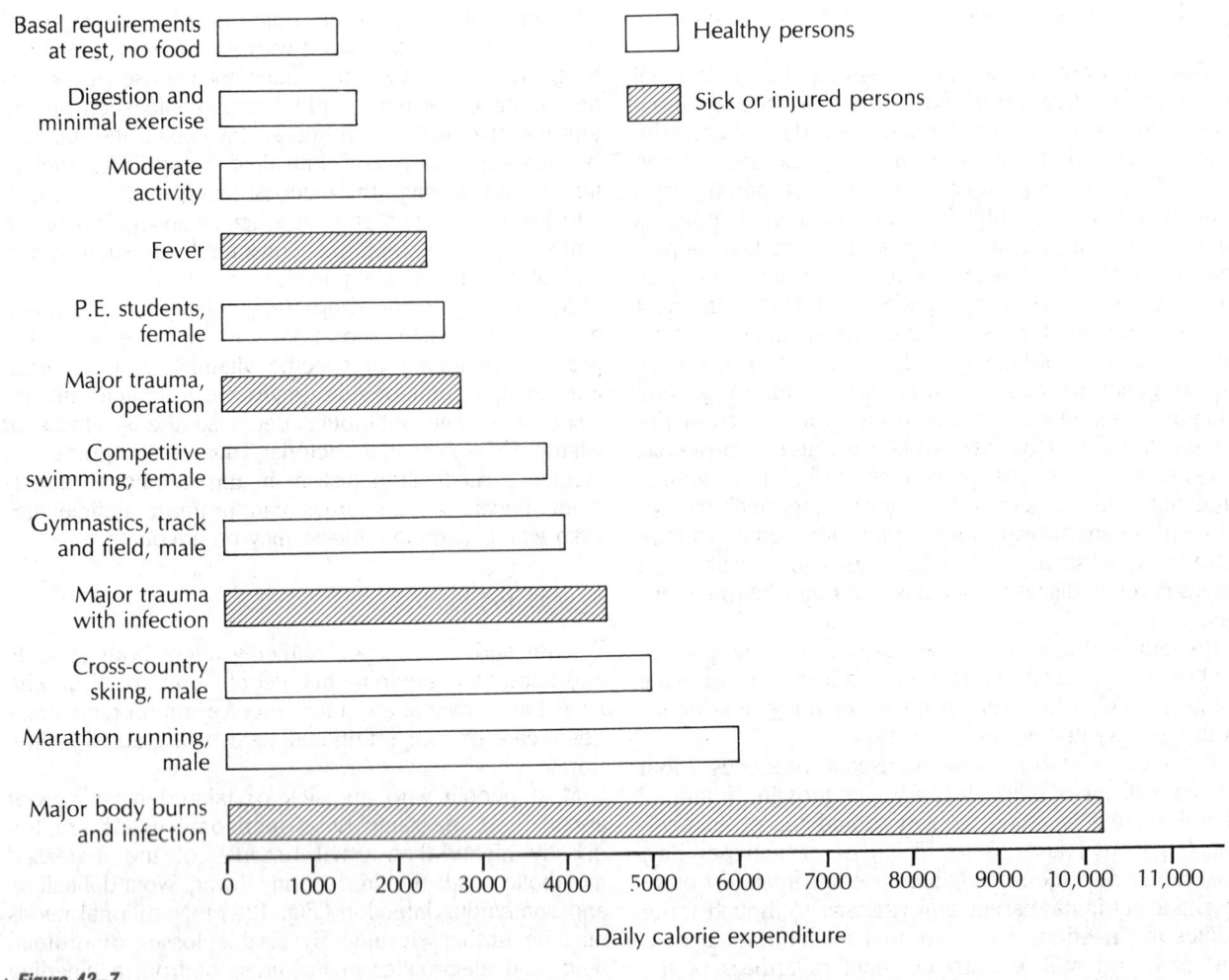

▲ *Figure 42-7*

Daily calorie expenditure. Caloric expenditure of adults at rest, during exercise, and during illness. (Data from Lieber, C.S. [1976]. The metabolism of alcohol. *Sci. Am.* 234:25; Saltin, B. [1978]. Fluid, electrolyte and energy losses and their replenishment in prolonged exercise; and Rogozkin, V.A. [1978]. Some aspects of athletes' nutrition. In Parizkova, J., & Rogozkin, V.A. [eds.]. *Nutrition, physical fitness and health.* Baltimore: University Park Press.)

▶ Be aware of people who are at risk for developing medication-related nutrient deficiencies
▶ Remember that medication interactions can and do occur
▶ Become familiar with the nutrient interactions of medications commonly used to treat the disorders of the types of clients you see
▶ Determine available laboratory tests that might allow you to explore the potential impact of a medication on your client

The health care team is responsible for assessing the ongoing condition of each person and estimating daily nutritional needs on the basis of clinical, anthropometric, and laboratory data. Nutritional support through intravenous or tube feeding may be necessary instead of or in addition to the standard oral diet.

ACTIVITY PATTERN

Individuals differ markedly in their level of physical activity each day. When participation in sports is a major commitment, daily food intake can far exceed that of the nonathletic person without resultant weight gain. When a demanding workout schedule is accompanied by adolescent growth, daily caloric intake may be exceptionally high (Fig. 42–7). If **carbohydrate loading** (eating much high-carbohydrate food to increase muscle glycogen stores) and weight management are incorporated into the training routine, the person must adjust dietary patterns.

NURSING DIAGNOSIS

Because nutrition is a basic need and because food is vital to life, nutrition is an area of possible concern for every client you may care for. Nursing diagnoses of importance to a client's nutrition are

▶ *Altered Nutrition: More than Body Requirements* (see Nursing Diagnosis Profile). Most commonly, this diagnosis is *Altered Nutrition: More than Body Re-*

quirements R/T excessive intake in relation to metabolic need.

▶ *Altered Nutrition: Less than Body Requirements* (see Nursing Diagnosis Profile). Most commonly, this nursing diagnosis is *Altered Nutrition: Less than Body Requirements* R/T inability to ingest sufficient nutrients, inability to digest sufficient nutrients, or inability to absorb sufficient nutrients.

▶ *Altered Nutrition: High Risk for More than Body Requirements* (see Nursing Diagnosis Profile). Most commonly, this nursing diagnosis is *Altered Nutrition: High Risk for More than Body Requirements* R/T dysfunctional eating pattern.

Each of these diagnoses may be secondary to biologic, psychologic, or social factors. How, for example, is your appetite and gastrointestinal function affected when you are in a great deal of pain? When you are nervous about an important test? When a big social event has you apprehensive or excited? When you act in a manner contrary to your own ethical standards or break a religious taboo? When you fall in love? Such biopsychosocial and cultural situations may be the underlying cause of a nutritional diagnosis. As you seek potential underlying causes for your client's nutritional problems, be sure to consider how the person's other nursing diagnoses may affect nutrition. Some additional nursing diagnoses that are frequently the underlying cause of nutritional problems are

▶ *Self-Care Deficit, Feeding*
▶ *Altered Oral Mucous Membrane*
▶ *Impaired Swallowing*
▶ *Ineffective Breastfeeding*
▶ *Altered Thought Processes*

NURSING DIAGNOSIS PROFILE

Altered Nutrition: More than Body Requirements

Definition. The state in which an individual is experiencing an intake of nutrients that exceeds metabolic needs.

Classification. Exchanging 1.1.2.1.

Defining Characteristics. A weight 20 per cent over the ideal for height and frame and a triceps skinfold greater than 15 mm in men or 25 mm in women are the only critical defining characteristics that support this diagnosis. Other defining characteristics include an objective physiologic measurement of weight 10 per cent over the ideal for height and frame and a reported or observed sedentary activity level or dysfunctional eating pattern. Dysfunctional eating patterns indicative of excess intake include pairing food with other activities, concentrating food intake at the end of the day, eating in response to external cues such as time of day or social situation, and eating in response to internal cues other than hunger (e.g., eating when anxious or lonely).

Sample Related Factors. The only related factor for this diagnosis is excessive intake in relation to metabolic need. You may wish, however, to specify more exactly what you believe to be the etiologic factor (e.g., lack of physical exercise, decreased activity pattern, effects of appetite-stimulating drug therapy, eating in response to stress or emotional trauma). It is important to understand that the underlying etiology may be multicausal and complex, with unconscious as well as conscious motivators operating.

Concept Description. This diagnosis refers to an excessive intake of nutrients. It does not refer specifically to calories, although calories might be the first thing to come to mind in our diet-conscious society. This diagnosis is appropriate for the individual who takes in an excessive amount of proteins, carbohydrates, or fat, even when the overall number of calories is sufficient for metabolic needs. The diagnosis also refers to nutrients such as vitamins and minerals, which may be taken in amounts exceeding metabolic requirements. Metabolic needs must be kept in mind. The person who is consuming the appropriate amounts of nutrients of all types for body height and frame might be consuming an excessive amount if the activity level is less than normal.

Examples. Depending on the specific assessment data, this diagnostic category could be applicable in the following situations, among others:

▶ A person who appears to have no health problems but whose activity level is below normal and yet the intake of various nutrients is not reduced as appropriate for the lowered metabolic needs (e.g., a professional football player in the off season who lounges around relaxing and who continues to eat at the same level as when he was much more active).

▶ A person who appears to have no health problems but who is consuming any of a number of different types of nutrients in excess of normal or even increased metabolic needs (e.g., a person who has just been divorced and who fills lonely evening hours by consuming pizza pies and chocolate cakes for consolation).

▶ A person who has a health problem that requires a decreased intake of one or more different types of nutrients but who is unable or unwilling to comply with prescribed dietary reduction (e.g., a person diagnosed with chronic renal failure who believes that eating a healthy diet will correct the condition and who tries to consume a T-bone steak and as much additional protein as possible every day).

Related/Similar Nursing Diagnoses. This diagnosis should be distinguished from the diagnosis of *Altered Nutrition: High Risk for More than Body Requirements*. The person at high risk engages in activities that demonstrate a risk of the nutrient intake exceeding the metabolic requirements. Although the high-risk diagnosis has not yet become actual, some of the observed or reported behaviors are the same. For example, with a diagnosis of high risk, the person may pair food with other activities, concentrate food intake at the end of the day, or eat in response to external cues, but these behaviors have not yet caused the client to eat more nutrients than needed by the body.

NURSING DIAGNOSIS PROFILE

Altered Nutrition: Less than Body Requirements

Definition. The state in which an individual is experiencing an intake of nutrients insufficient to meet metabolic needs.

Classification. Exchanging 1.1.2.2.

Defining Characteristics. An important defining characteristic for this diagnosis is a loss of weight with adequate food intake. Other defining characteristics that support the belief that nutrition is inadequate for metabolic needs include a body weight 20 per cent or more under the ideal for height and frame, capillary fragility, pale conjunctival and mucous membranes, poor muscle tone, and loss of hair.

The following characteristics could indicate insufficient ingestion of nutrients: reported or evident lack of food; lack of interest in food; lack of information, misinformation, or misconceptions about food or nutrition; aversion to eating; perceived inability to ingest food; sore, inflamed buccal cavity; reported altered taste sensation; reported intake of less than recommended daily allowance; and satiety immediately after ingesting food. Insufficient digestion of ingested nutrients could be indicated by weak muscles required for mastication or swallowing. The following could indicate insufficient absorption of nutrients: hyperactive bowel sounds, abdominal cramping, diarrhea, and steatorrhea.

Sample Related Factors. Related factors for this diagnosis include the inability to ingest, digest, or absorb sufficient nutrients secondary to biologic, psychologic, or social factors (e.g., economic factors). You should specify which related factor applies and indicate the underlying cause, if known (e.g., *Altered Nutrition: Less than Body Requirements* R/T inability to ingest sufficient calories for metabolic needs secondary to aversion to eating or *Altered Nutrition: Less than Body Requirements* R/T inability to absorb sufficient nutrients secondary to diarrhea).

As is true of the diagnosis of *Altered Nutrition: More than Body Requirements*, it is important to understand that the underlying etiology may be multicausal and complex, with unconscious as well as conscious motivators operating.

Concept Description. This diagnosis refers to a deficient intake of one or more nutrients, including calories, proteins, carbohydrates, fat, vitamins, or minerals. Metabolic needs must be kept in mind. The person who is consuming the appropriate amounts of nutrients of all types for body height and frame might be consuming an insufficient amount if the activity level is higher than normal.

Examples. Depending on the specific assessment data, this diagnostic category could be applicable in the following situations, among others:

▶ A person whose metabolic needs have increased but whose intake of nutrients has remained the same or decreased (e.g., a 12-year-old female with anorexia nervosa who is growing rapidly but is dieting enough to lose weight rather than gaining it at the expected rate). Another example would be a person who has just had surgery and who has an increased need for protein, vitamin C, and zinc for wound healing but who is existing on a clear liquid diet.

▶ A person whose metabolic needs have remained the same but whose intake has decreased (e.g., an elderly person of normal weight who has just been widowed and who has no desire for food).

▶ A person who attempts to ingest adequate amounts of nutrients for metabolic needs but who is unable to digest them sufficiently for absorption (e.g., the person who lacks teeth or the muscle strength to chew or who lacks hydrochloric acid in the stomach or digestive enzymes in the small intestine).

▶ A person who is able to ingest and digest sufficient nutrients for metabolic needs but whose absorbing surface is bypassed too rapidly for adequate absorption (e.g., the person with a chronic diarrheal disease).

Related/Similar Nursing Diagnoses. This diagnosis is quite clear and should not be confused with any other. However, some other nursing diagnoses may serve as etiologic factors when the client's nutrition is less than required. For example, the client may have a nursing diagnosis of *Impaired Swallowing* and a diagnosis of *Altered Nutrition: Less than Body Requirements* R/T inability to ingest sufficient nutrients secondary to impaired swallowing. In the same way, the client may have the diagnoses *Self-Care Deficit, Feeding,* and *Altered Nutrition: Less than Body Requirements* R/T inability to ingest sufficient nutrients secondary to self-care feeding deficit, or the diagnoses of *Ineffective Breastfeeding* R/T inadequate milk supply and *Altered Nutrition* R/T inability to ingest sufficient nutrients secondary to ineffective breastfeeding. In such cases, both diagnoses should be made, since the nursing interventions will differ for each diagnosis.

PLANNING

When the client's nursing diagnosis is *Altered Nutrition: More than Body Requirements*, expected outcomes should be

▶ maintains weight within the ideal range for height and frame (state actual weight expected)
▶ maintains triceps fold less than 15 mm in men and less than 25 mm in women (state actual measurement expected)

Beginning short-term outcomes that can demonstrate a movement toward achieving the above, long-term outcomes might include

▶ identifies factors that contribute to obesity
▶ identifies foods high in undesirable nutrients (state which nutrients)
▶ changes eating pattern from dysfunctional to functional (define expected behaviors)
▶ increases activity level (define the amount of activity expected) without increasing food intake

NURSING DIAGNOSIS PROFILE

Altered Nutrition: High Risk for More than Body Requirements

Definition. The state in which an individual is at risk of experiencing an intake of nutrients that exceeds metabolic needs.

Classification. Exchanging 1.1.2.3.

Defining Characteristics. Because this is a high risk diagnosis, the defining characteristics consist of the presence of risk factors for excess nutrition. The only critical risk factors are a rapid transition across growth percentiles in infants or children and reported or observed obesity in one or both parents. Other risk factors include reported use of solid food as a major food source before 5 months of age, observed use of food as a reward or comfort measure, reported or observed higher baseline weight at the beginning of each pregnancy, and dysfunctional eating patterns. Dysfunctional eating patterns predictive of excess intake include pairing food with other activities, concentrating food intake at the end of the day, eating in response to external cues such as time of day or social situation, and eating in response to internal cues other than hunger (e.g., eating when anxious or lonely).

Sample Related Factors. In high-risk diagnoses, the related factor for the diagnosis is the risk factor identified in the client. Most often the risk factor is a dysfunctional eating pattern, but a dysfunctional pattern may not be evident to the nurse until a pattern of weight gain or rapid growth begins to be evident. There may be more than one risk factor in any individual.

Concept Description. This diagnosis refers to the high risk for an excessive intake of nutrients. It is used when the nurse observes unhealthy patterns that can lead to the actual diagnosis of *Altered Nutrition: More than Body Requirements*.

Examples. Depending on the specific assessment data, this diagnostic category could be applicable in the following situations, among others:

▶ A healthy infant or child whose parents use inappropriate feeding techniques.
▶ A person who has no apparent health problem but who eats in patterns that have been associated with excessive nutritional intake.

Related/Similar Nursing Diagnoses. This diagnosis should be distinguished from the diagnosis *Altered Nutrition: More than Body Requirements*. With this high-risk diagnosis, the person engages in activities that demonstrate risk of nutrient intake exceeding the metabolic requirements. Although the high risk diagnosis has not yet become actual, some of the observed or reported behaviors are the same as those of the actual nursing diagnosis. For example, with both the high-risk and the actual diagnosis, the person may eat in response to external cues or to internal cues other than hunger.

When the client's nursing diagnosis is *Altered Nutrition: Less than Body Requirements*, expected outcomes should be

▶ maintains weight gain (specify the amount to be gained)
▶ maintains signs of good nutrition, such as body weight closer to ideal range for height and frame (specify how much closer), no signs of capillary fragility (skin and mucous membranes free of bruising and petechiae), skin pink or with red undertones, conjunctiva and other mucous membranes pink, and so forth. (See Table 42-9 for additional signs of good nutrition.)

Beginning short-term outcomes that can demonstrate movement toward achieving the above two long-term outcomes might include

▶ identifies factors that contribute to malnutrition
▶ identifies foods high in desirable nutrients (state which nutrients)
▶ increases intake of required nutrients (define expected level)
▶ demonstrates increased ability to chew and/or swallow food
▶ demonstrates increased interest in food or nutrition
▶ demonstrates increased information about food or nutrition
▶ maintains decrease in or cessation of diarrhea
▶ maintains decrease in or cessation of steatorrhea

When the client's nursing diagnosis is *Altered Nutrition: High Risk for More than Body Requirements*, the expected outcome should be

▶ changes eating pattern from dysfunctional to functional (define expected behaviors)

Beginning short-term outcomes that can demonstrate a movement toward achieving the above long-term outcome might include

▶ identifies factors that contribute to obesity
▶ identifies foods high in undesirable nutrients (state which nutrients)

NURSING INTERVENTION

In providing for the client's nutritional needs, the nurse assures that the client receives nutrition appropriate for metabolic needs in a manner consistent with optimal health promotion. This is not always easy to do. For instance, a postoperative client may not only have increased needs for certain nutrients in order to help heal the surgical wound but also could have increased metabolic needs because the surgical wound has become infected. It would seem to be a matter of simply calculating the increased need for various nutrients and calories and providing them in the diet. But suppose the client has an aversion to food, is nauseated, and vomits everything eaten? Providing all the extra protein, vitamin C, calories, and the like will be of little value because the food provided is likely to make the client sick.

In attempting to meet a client's nutritional needs, you will have to be aware of methods to enhance appetite, ingestion, digestion, and absorption, as needed.

Managing Diet Therapy

The primary objectives of diet therapy are to (a) meet the nutritional needs of the person who requires a special diet, and (b) modify that diet so that it is compatible with the individual's food tolerances and intolerances, personal dietary problems, and overall program of nursing and medical management. Therefore, the health care team must carefully assess and consider all these factors in order to prescribe a diet that is therapeutic.

It is also important to continue to assess the health status of the person and the appropriateness of the diet. Usually, the original diet order is modified over time. For example, following surgery, individuals normally receive a clear liquid diet, advance to a soft diet within a few days, and then to a regular diet. If the person cannot tolerate oral intake within a few days, it may be necessary to institute an intravenous or enteral feeding program. The best feeding regimen is based on the person's current dietary needs.

STANDARD DIETARY REGIMENS IN THE HEALTH CARE SETTING

In some cases, the nutritional needs of ill or hospitalized individuals do not differ from those of healthy people. Therefore, the routine hospital or institutional diet is designed to meet the needs of the average person and to be reasonably palatable to people from many cultural and social backgrounds.

During hospitalization, most people receive the general (house, regular) diet. In some hospitals, only one general menu is provided each day; in other hospitals, clients may select from among a number of foods in each food group on a general menu. In either case, foods can be modified for people who cannot tolerate the texture, composition, or other characteristics of the food on the menu. Routine modifications of the house diet include the soft, full liquid, and clear liquid diets (Table 42-10). The soft diet is commonly ordered for the person with problems in chewing or digesting the more complex and sometimes "rich" foods in the general house diet. Persons without teeth and those recovering from surgery are excellent candidates for the soft diet. Liquid diets may be used before and after surgery as well as in circumstances in which substantial oral or esophageal lesions make it difficult to manipulate and swallow solid foods. All types of liquids are permitted on the general or full liquid diet, whereas a clear liquid diet provides only tea, broth, gelatin dessert, and other "clear" liquid items. In addition to the modifications, diets are often altered to limit calorie or salt intake.

DIET BEFORE AND AFTER SURGERY

Surgery constitutes a major stress on the body. Therefore, people may need additional calories and nutrients before and after surgery. Also, recovery from surgery is often shorter for people who were well-nourished before the operation. For these reasons, nutritional preparation of the surgical candidate involves the correction of any existing nutrient deficits and establishes nutritional reserves that the body may draw upon during the early postoperative period. The time needed to prepare an individual is related to the degree of debilitation. In some cases, several days may be satisfactory; in others, weeks may be necessary to rectify nutritional deficiencies.

During the intraoperative period, the stomach must be empty. It is standard practice to keep the client NPO after midnight, the night before surgery. **NPO (nil per os)** means "nothing by mouth." This practice ensures that there is no food in the stomach, which may be vomited and aspirated when the person is under the effects of anesthesia. Keeping the client NPO also decreases the gastric distention that can cause postoperative pain and can impinge on full expansion of the lungs.

During the postoperative period, a major requirement for rapid healing is optimal nutritional support. The client should progress from clear to full liquids and then to a soft or regular diet as soon as possible. Nutrient stores deposited before surgery are rapidly depleted, especially if blood and fluid losses are substantial. Include adequate protein intake at this time to replace protein losses and supply increased protein demands. In addition to the protein losses from tissue breakdown, plasma protein depletion occurs through hemorrhage, wounds, and exudates. Increased metabolic losses of protein also result from inflammation, infection, and trauma.

Other important nutrients during the postoperative period include vitamin K for normal blood clotting, vitamin C and zinc for tissue repair, iron for hemoglobin production, and B-complex vitamins for carbohydrate, fat, and protein metabolism.

DIET IN THE MANAGEMENT OF OBESITY

Obesity is a serious health problem in North America and is considered one of the most important nutritional diseases among Western societies. The goal of maintaining an ideal or desirable body weight has appeared in every set of health and nutrition recommendations published from government and not-for-profit organizations.

Despite this prudent recommendation, the prevalence of obesity among Americans has remained unchanged or even increased in some demographic subgroups. Data from the second National Health and Nutrition Examination Survey (1976-1980) estimated that nearly one of four adults is overweight, and one in every ten

TABLE 42–10. Types of Hospital Diets

	Clear Liquid Diet	Full Liquid Diet	Soft Diet	Regular—House General—Full
Characteristics	Temporary diet of clear liquids without residue; nonstimulating, nongas-forming, nonirritating	Foods liquid at room temperature or liquefying at body temperature	Normal diet modified in consistency to have no roughage Liquids and semisolid food; easily digested	Practically all foods; simple, easy-to-digest foods, simply prepared, palatably seasoned
Adequacy	Inadequate: deficient in protein, minerals, vitamins, and calories	Can be adequate with careful planning: adequacy depends on liquids used	Entirely adequate liberal diet	Adequate and well-balanced
Use	Acute illness and infections Postoperatively Temporary food intolerance To relieve thirst Reduce colonic fecal matter 1- to 2-hour feeding intervals	Transition between clear liquid and soft diets Postoperatively Acute gastritis and infections Febrile conditions Intolerance for solid food 2- to 4-hour feeding intervals	Between full liquid and light or regular diet Between acute illness and convalescence Acute infections Chewing difficulties Gastrointestinal disorders 3 meals with or without between-meal feedings	For uniformity and convenience in serving hospital clients Ambulatory people Immobilized people not requiring therapeutic diets
Foods	Water, tea, coffee, coffee substitutes Fat-free broth Carbonated beverages Synthetic fruit juices Ginger ale Plain gelatin Sugar	All liquids on clear liquid diet plus: All forms of milk Soups, strained Fruit and vegetable juices Eggnogs Plain ice cream and sherbets Junket and plain gelatin dishes Soft custard Cereal gruels	All liquids Fine and strained cereals Cooked tender or puréed vegetables Cooked fruits without skins and seeds Ripe bananas Ground or minced meat, fish, poultry Eggs and mild cheeses Plain cake and puddings Moderately seasoned foods	All basic foods
Modification	Liberal clear liquid diet includes fruit juices, egg white, whole egg, thin gruels	Consistency for tube feedings: foods that will pass through tube easily	Low residue—no fiber Bland—no chemical, thermal, physical stimulants Cold soft—tonsillectomy Mechanical soft—requiring no mastication Light diet—intermediate between soft and regular *Note:* Because of trend toward more liberal interpretation of diets and foods, soft diet may be combined with light diet in some hospitals.	For a light or convalescent diet, fried foods, rich pastries, fat-rich foods, coarse vegetables, raw fruits may be omitted

From Keane, C.B. (1982). *Saunders review for practical nurses* (4th ed.). Philadelphia: W.B. Saunders.

is severely overweight. Females are more overweight than males, and black females are more overweight than white females.

The hazards associated with obesity are familiar to almost everyone. Diseases that occur more frequently in obese people include hypertension, coronary heart disease, thrombophlebitis, diabetes mellitus, gallbladder disease, osteoarthritis, and some cancers (including breast cancer). Obese individuals also are at greater risk for accidents, emotional disorders, and social discrimination. Menstrual abnormalities and ovarian dysfunction are most common in obese women, and obese women carry a greater risk of adverse course and outcome in pregnancy.

Many factors interact in the process by which an individual becomes obese and then maintains that weight. Consideration of these factors is valuable in understanding the obese person and in designing effective treatment. Note the medical diagnosis and metabolic aberrations and assess the client's history of weight gain, extent of obesity (body mass index, skinfold measurements, fat tissue biopsy, if available), family attitudes, role in the family, emotional and psychologic status (self-concept and body image, self-esteem), eating behavior (binges, night-eating, usual eating patterns, eating for emotional reasons), activity and exercise habits, social relationships, motivation, and reasons for desiring weight loss.[18]

The importance of genetics in the establishment of this problem is now widely appreciated,[104,116] but eating behavior and exercise patterns clearly modify the extent of fat deposition. While it is known that weight loss is achievable through a variety of means, it is still unclear why maintenance of weight loss is so difficult for most people. Efforts are being made to define specific metabolic differences between lean and obese individuals. Attention is also being given to identifying the means by which the "fat pad" communicates with the brain to assure that the genetically mandated level of fatness is maintained over time. Pharmaceutical companies are investing heavily in research directed toward the development of drugs that will reduce appetite effectively or otherwise prevent or treat obesity. Some experts say that by the year 2000, one or more such products may be available to the general public.

In a nutshell, our understanding of energy balance goes something like this: Energy balance depends on calorie input and calorie output; excessive input or decreased output will increase energy stores, primarily in adipose tissue. Many factors influence the desire to eat. Hunger is a signal of the physiologic drive to find and eat food; appetite represents the psychologic drive to find and eat food. When both these drives are satisfied, the state of satiety is said to exist. Centers in the brain interact with other groups of cells in the brain and liver that participate in the complicated network of messages that control hunger and satiety. When stimulated, specific sites in the brain and other organs greatly affect (increase or decrease) the desire to seek and eat food. Many hormones and hormone-like compounds have been identified as potentially influential in affecting feeding behavior and satiety.

Most adults maintain a relatively stable body weight over months and years. The mechanism by which this takes place is unknown, but the "comfort zone" for an individual has been referred to as the "set point." One hypothesis is that a compound (specifically a protein) is produced by adipose cells and the brain, allowing for body weight regulation. Sound evidence suggests that body weight is regulated. Loss of weight to a level below the set point, for example, is known to be associated with a defensive response. Basal metabolic rate goes down; adipose tissue fat-synthesizing enzyme (lipoprotein lipase) levels go up; and constant hunger sets in. Over time, these effects usually lead the client to regain the weight that was originally lost. Successful maintenance of body weight below the set point therefore is "painful" and requires much patience and perseverance.

While achieving and maintaining a reduced level of body fat is known to be difficult, it is not impossible. Success is often associated with a pattern of gradual weight loss accompanied by a strong motivation to resist caloric temptations. Most successful weight-management programs consist of three components: a sensible diet, an individualized exercise schedule, and management of food habits.

A sound weight-loss diet should include attention to a number of issues. Specifically, the diet should

▶ meet nutritional needs, except for calories
▶ allow adaptations to individual habits and tastes
▶ provide for a slow and steady weight loss
▶ minimize hunger and fatigue
▶ contain readily available foods
▶ be socially acceptable
▶ help change problem eating habits
▶ improve overall health

While moderation in total calorie intake is the primary concern, achieving this goal can usually be simplified by specific attention to moderation in consumption of fat. Not only is dietary fat calorically dense, it is also very efficiently converted into body fat; only about 3 to 5 per cent of the ingested calories are burned in the process. On the other hand, about 25 per cent of ingested carbohydrate calories are burned in the process of laying down fat.

Regular physical activity is essential in a program of weight management. Not only does exercise burn calories, it also maintains or even increases lean body mass. Lean tissue is metabolically active 24 hours per day; the larger the lean body mass (which is mostly skeletal muscle), the higher the resting metabolic rate. The significance of this augmented metabolic rate is by no means trivial. The number of calories expended meeting metabolic resting needs each 24-hour day, 365 days per year, can make a major contribution to energy expenditure.

Long-term success in managing body weight usually involves a behavior modification effort.[18,19,40] A close look at lifestyle and environment should be followed by definition of problem periods and behaviors and development of strategies to change them permanently. Psychologists use the following terms discussing behavior management:[18]

▶ Chain-breaking—breaking the link between two or more behaviors that encourage overeating, such as snacking while watching TV
▶ Stimulus control—altering the environment to minimize the stimuli for eating (e.g., removing foods from sight and storing them in kitchen cabinets)
▶ Cognitive restructuring—changing one's frame of mind regarding eating (e.g., instead of using a difficult day as an excuse to overeat, substitute other

pleasures for rewards, such as a relaxing walk with a friend)

▶ Contingency management—forming a plan to respond to an environment in which overeating is likely, such as when snacks are within arm's reach at a party

▶ Self-monitoring—a process of tracking food eaten and conditions affecting eating; actions are usually recorded in a diary, along with location, time, and state of mind. Self-monitoring is a tool to help a person understand more about personal eating habits.

Books and classes on behavior modification (specifically, food habit management) are widely available. In the end, however, dieters must analyze their own particular shortcomings and sensitize themselves to facets of their lifestyle that make dieting difficult. A written plan of action may be useful. Social support is always valuable. A system of rewards for both short-term and long-term successes may add incentive.

Even motivated dieters periodically experience a lapse in their planned weight-management routine. Such lapses should be viewed as expected and not as signals that failure is imminent. Plans for dealing with lapses can be made in advance. Encouragement from oneself and others to "stay calm" and "return to the original plan" may help prevent a true relapse in the weight control program.

While level of body fatness is a characteristic that appears to be embedded in one's genes, it is certainly possible to create a lifestyle that limits the expression of this trait. In fact, because this "gene for obesity" seems to be widespread, conscientious efforts to develop a lifestyle emphasizing wise food choices and regular aerobic exercise make much sense. Beginning in childhood to establish a "fat-minimizing" routine is in order. Aggressive thrust in this direction over the next several decades might reverse the trend toward rising adiposity.

DIET IN THE MANAGEMENT OF THE UNDERWEIGHT INDIVIDUAL

An underweight individual is more than 15 per cent below the recommended weight. Excessive weight loss can result from severe, prolonged dieting, hospitalization, immobilization, disease, or inability to obtain food. Severe emaciation and substantial weight loss are associated with the following problems:

▶ Decreased resistance to disease
▶ Impaired wound healing
▶ Retarded physical growth
▶ Reduced physical activity
▶ Increased vulnerability to environmental insults

The therapeutic goal for the underweight person is to produce a positive calorie balance gradually. The diet should contain adequate vitamins and minerals as well as additional kilocalories and protein. Without protein, the person will be unable to build body tissue. Concentrated sources of kilocalories (e.g., milkshakes, nuts) are important components of diet therapy.

DIET IN THE MANAGEMENT OF GASTROINTESTINAL DISEASE

The function of the gastrointestinal system is to accept and process food for the body's metabolic needs. Thus, disease, injuries, or surgical procedures that compromise gut integrity may necessitate a temporary "special" diet.[32,45,94] Overall, the current trend in dietary management of gastrointestinal (GI) disease is directed toward liberalization of old traditions. Health professionals now believe that individual tolerance rather than a rigid dietary rule should dictate the degree of dietary restriction. For example, a person with a peptic ulcer may tolerate spicy food without difficulty.

The specific dietary modification chosen for a person with GI disease is directly related to the type of disease present, its severity, its probable duration, and a host of other variables. A wound, lesion, or inflammatory process in the upper regions of the GI tract may require a diet that will not irritate the lesions by excessive spices, temperature, or texture. Constipation or diverticular disease may warrant a high-fiber regimen. Mucosal inflammation in the lower bowel may necessitate restriction of dietary fiber. Generally these modifications are implemented on a short-term basis, but in some cases, long-term dietary control is necessary. Table 42–11 summarizes some common GI diseases along with their "standard" dietary regulations.

DIET IN THE MANAGEMENT OF LIVER AND GALLBLADDER DISEASE

Because both the liver and gallbladder have important metabolic functions, diseases of these organs frequently require dietary management.[67]

Hepatitis. Hepatitis is an inflammation of the liver caused by various agents but most commonly by two types of virus. These agents cause diffuse injury to liver cells. In milder cases, tissue injury is largely reversible, but with increasing severity, permanent damage occurs. Consequently, clinical symptoms vary, depending on the degree of liver involvement. Jaundice (yellow pigmentation of the skin) is a common symptom, but general malaise, loss of appetite, diarrhea, headache, fever, and enlarged liver and spleen may also occur.

Treatment involves bed rest, adequate hydration, and optimal nutrition to promote recovery of the damaged liver tissue. Some authorities advocate frequent meals with high protein (75 to 100 gm/day), high carbohydrate (300 to 400 gm/day), and moderate fat (100 to 150 gm/day). The trend, however, is away from this diet and toward a general high-calorie diet. The person with hepatitis is generally permitted to eat whatever can be tolerated, provided there is no extensive liver damage. Alcohol is not allowed. When a person cannot tolerate food by mouth, it may be necessary to institute tube or intravenous feeding.

Cirrhosis. Cirrhosis is a chronic disease of the liver characterized by diffuse destruction of hepatic cells. When liver damage is severe, functional liver cells may be replaced with scar tissue.

TABLE 42–11. Dietary Management of Selected Gastrointestinal Diseases

Disease	Description	Clinical Symptoms	Diet Therapy
Peptic ulcer	Excessive acid erosion of gastric or duodenal mucosa	Increased gastric contractions with pain	Individualized; recommend regular meal consumption; avoid stomach distention; avoid drinking coffee, tea, cola, and other caffeine-containing beverages; avoid drinking alcohol; avoid hot spices in cooking; avoid foods or drinks that cause discomfort; relax while eating
Diverticulosis, diverticulitis	Small protrusions from the intestinal lumen, with or without inflammation	With inflammation; pain, tenderness, nausea, vomiting, distention, intestinal spasms, fever	Acute phase: liquid or low-residue Chronic phase: high-residue to reduce intraluminal pressure
Celiac sprue	Inherited intestinal sensitivity to the protein gluten	Diarrhea with multiple bulky, foamy, greasy stools; distended abdomen; malnutrition	Gluten-free diet (omission of wheat, oats, rye, and usually barley)
Regional enteritis	Regional inflammation and thickening of the wall with decrease in luminal diameter	Abdominal pain and diarrhea	Individualized; high-calorie; liberal in animal proteins; rich in vitamins and minerals; restriction may be required with steatorrhea; medium-chain triglycerides have been tried
Ulcerative colitis	Mucosal inflammation in the lower bowel	Pain and mucosal bleeding with frequent loose stools	Individualized; high-protein, high-calorie; vitamin and mineral supplements recommended; frequent small feedings advised
Hemorrhoids	Blockage of venous blood flow from the lower abdomen causes high portal and/or systemic venous pressure with dilatation of venous channels leading from the anus	Pain and bleeding related to defecation	Individualized; high-fiber plus 8–10 glasses of water/day to prevent constipation; in the acute phase, may require low-residue, low-fiber diet with gradual return to high-fiber regimen

Malnutrition frequently accompanies cirrhosis. In developed societies, alcoholism is often the root of the difficulty. With continuous, heavy drinking, the person with alcoholism neglects food intake. The diminished intake results in multiple nutritional deficiencies that further accelerate liver cell destruction. Early symptoms of liver damage include nausea, vomiting, loss of appetite, abdominal distention, and epigastric pain. Jaundice may eventually develop and be accompanied by weakness, edema, and ascites (collection of fluid within the peritoneal cavity). The person may also have anemia secondary to GI bleeding and iron or folic acid deficiency.

Treatment is difficult when alcoholism is the underlying problem. The individual with a severe drinking problem requires supportive psychiatric, nursing, and nutritional care. Goals of nutritional therapy are correction of fluid and electrolyte imbalances and provision of nutritional support to encourage healing and limit further damage. Dietary measures include

▶ a basic high-protein diet, if liver damage is not severe

▶ a low-protein diet when liver damage is severe. Because the liver plays a major role in protein metabolism, compromised liver function causes increased blood ammonia levels and coma can result. The amount of protein restriction will vary according to the extent of liver damage

▶ sodium restriction to 1000 to 2000 mg daily to reduce fluid retention when edema or ascites is present

▶ a soft diet if esophageal varices (enlarged veins in the esophagus) develop. Soft foods help to prevent rupture of these blood vessels

Cholelithiasis (Gallstones) and Cholecystitis (Inflammation of the Gallbladder). The gallbladder concentrates and stores bile from the liver and releases it into the small intestine when stimulated. Bile is rich in cholesterol, which normally is kept in solution by other bile components. When the surface of the gallbladder is inflamed or infected, however, the absorptive characteristics of the mucosa are altered. As a result, the solubility of the bile ingredients changes, and cholesterol may precipitate and form stones. The individual with gallbladder disease usually reports pain (sometimes severe) and a sense of fullness and distention after eating.

Low-fat diets have traditionally been prescribed for people with gallbladder disease. The basis for this recommendation was that fat in the intestine causes the gallbladder to contract and therefore causes pain. It has recently been shown, however, that the gallbladder contracts and ejects bile at the same rate after either a high-fat or a low-fat meal. Thus, the best advice for patients with gallbladder disease is not necessarily to avoid fat but to consume a well-balanced diet and avoid foods, or amounts of foods, that cause pain. Obese people should be encouraged to lose weight, especially if surgery is being considered.

DIET IN THE MANAGEMENT OF KIDNEY DISEASE

The kidney may be adversely affected by various inflammatory and degenerative diseases.[57] Such disorders disrupt the normal functions of the nephron (the functional unit of the kidneys); nephron dysfunction in turn causes disturbances in the elimination of protein, electrolytes, and water. Symptoms result from either excessive retention of wastes in the circulation or excessive loss of vital blood components (e.g., protein) in the urine. Diet therapy therefore depends upon the specific disorder.

Excessive urinary losses require dietary replacement. Impaired elimination of wastes secondary to a malfunctioning kidney requires a diet that minimizes the buildup of these compounds in the circulation. This diet is low in protein, sodium, and potassium. In addition, fluid intake is restricted.

Three kidney disorders are acute glomerulonephritis, the nephrotic syndrome, and chronic renal failure. Their clinical features and dietary recommendations are summarized in Table 42–12.

DIET IN THE MANAGEMENT OF CARDIOVASCULAR DISEASE

Several disorders involving the heart and blood vessels require diet modification as part of therapy for the condition.

Atherosclerosis. Atherosclerosis is a complex disease involving the accumulation of cholesterol and other lipid material in the arterial walls.[28,47,83,84] Scientists have not yet discovered its cause but have identified multiple risk factors that may contribute to the disease process. High cholesterol intake has been associated with higher blood cholesterol levels. Egg yolks and organ meats such as liver and kidneys are high in cholesterol. Foods containing no cholesterol include fruits, vegetables, grains, cereals, and nuts.

Large-scale studies demonstrate a definite association between dietary fat and elevations of blood lipid levels **(hyperlipidemia).** Hyperlipidemia seems to be linked to high fat intake that includes a large percentage of animal or saturated fats, which tend to raise the level of cholesterol in the blood. Saturated animal fats are found in beef, lamb, pork, butter, cream, whole milk, and cheeses made from cream or whole milk. Saturated vegetable fats are found in many solid and hy-

TABLE 42–12. Diet Therapy in Diseases of the Kidney

Disease	Basic Defect	Clinical Symptoms	Diet Therapy
Acute glomerulonephritis	Infection involving glomeruli; loss of glomerular function (especially filtration)	Blood in urine, edema, hypertension, renal insufficiency; anorexia, lethargy, nausea and vomiting	Adequate protein (unless uremia develops), adequate sodium (unless edema or hypertension becomes serious), adequate potassium (unless hyperkalemia develops); general nutritional support; water intake adjusted to output
Nephrotic syndrome	Degeneration of capillary basement membrane with creation of "pores" that allow escape of protein	Massive albuminuria, low serum protein levels, edema; sometimes hypertension and hypercholesterolemia	High-protein, high-calorie diet; moderate-to-low sodium intake
Chronic renal failure	Degeneration of renal tissue with depression of all renal functions	Anemia; weakness; weight loss; hypertension; skin, oral, and GI bleeding; muscle twitching; uremic convulsions; renal osteodystrophy (metabolic bone disease)	Protein restriction (unless dialysis is frequent), emphasis on protein sources of high biologic values; controlled intake of major electrolytes (K^+, Na^+) and water; phosphate intake kept low, calcium intake kept high (supplements often recommended)

drogenated shortenings, coconut oil, cocoa butter, and palm oil.

Substituting foods high in unsaturated fatty acids for those high in saturated fatty acids has proved effective in lowering blood lipids, especially blood cholesterol. Polyunsaturated fats are usually liquid oils of vegetable origin, such as corn, cottonseed, safflower, sesame seed, soybean, and sunflower oils.

Moderate changes in the diet usually lower the blood cholesterol level. Beneficial dietary changes include (a) cutting down on cholesterol-rich foods, and (b) reducing the saturated fat content in the diet by substituting polyunsaturated fats for saturated fats. Additional general recommendations are to

▶ restrict fat intake to no more than 30 per cent of total calories in the diet
▶ restrict cholesterol intake to less than 300 mg/day
▶ eat frequent meals of fish and poultry, which contain less saturated fat than does meat. For meals that include meat, choose lean cuts and trim the fat
▶ reduce the amount of saturated fat intake in relation to unsaturated fat intake
▶ cook with liquid vegetable oils and margarines
▶ use nonfat milk and nonfat milk products
▶ eat only two or three egg yolks per week, including those used in cooking

Atherosclerosis may progress and completely block one or more of the coronary arteries in the heart. With a blocked coronary artery, the heart's oxygen supply is compromised and chest pain (angina) occurs. If the blockage is prolonged, cardiac tissue death results. The death of cardiac tissue is termed *myocardial infarction* (heart attack). In the acute phases of a myocardial infarction (MI), the person needs additional dietary modifications. The basic therapeutic objective is to reduce the cardiac work load. Therefore, the diet may be limited to 800 to 1200 kcal daily to reduce demands on the heart resulting from high metabolic loads. During this early stage, the person needs to eat soft or easily digested foods to avoid effort in eating and chewing. Also, smaller meals served more frequently

may provide needed nutrition without causing undue strain or pressure. If the person is overweight, the dietary goals may include lifelong dietary modifications.

Congestive Heart Failure. The heart is composed of two pumps, the right and left ventricles, each of which plays a unique role in maintaining the circulation. For this reason, it is possible for the right or left pump to fail independently of the other, resulting in either right-sided heart failure or left-sided heart failure. Yet, because the circulatory system is a closed circuit and because the work of the heart depends upon the smooth functioning of both pumps together, the failure of one side of the heart is often closely followed by failure of the other side.

Typically, left-sided heart failure precedes right-sided heart failure and is a common complication of an MI (Fig. 42–8). When necrotic heart muscle compromises the left ventricle's ability to pump effectively and thereby to sustain cardiac output, blood backs up and accumulates in the pulmonary vascular system, resulting in pulmonary congestion as well as decreased output of oxygenated blood to the cells. As the right ventricle struggles to pump blood against resistance into the person's congested lungs, it also fails. Right-sided heart failure causes increased blood volume in the systemic venous circulation and various organs (e.g., liver); increased venous hydrostatic pressure and edema result. Decreased cardiac output can further complicate the picture by decreasing blood flow to the kidneys. A reduction in renal circulation causes urinary output to fall, so that the body is taxed with even more fluid. A vicious cycle thus begins.

Treatment for CHF involves various medication regimens and dietary modifications. The diet primarily involves mild, moderate, or severe sodium restriction, depending on the amount of edema. The main source of dietary sodium is sodium chloride (common table salt). Sodium is also "hidden" in many processed foods, such as soy sauce, canned soups, catsup, and gravies. Use of salt substitutes may assist in maintaining a palatable menu. It is important to observe the person

FAILURE OF RIGHT VENTRICLE

Increased volume in systemic
  venous circulation
Increased volume in
  distensible organs
Hepatomegaly, splenomegaly
Dependent edema and
  serous effusion
Expansion of blood volume
Decreased volume to lungs

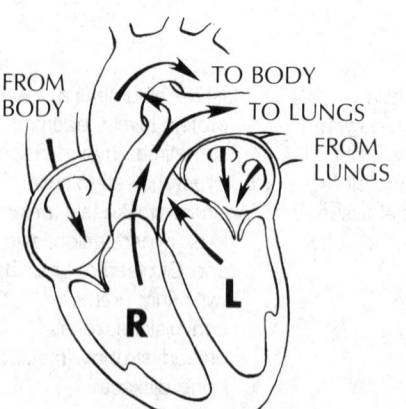

FROM BODY
TO BODY
TO LUNGS
FROM LUNGS
R   L

FAILURE OF LEFT VENTRICLE

Increased volume and pressure in
  left ventricle and atrium
Increased volume in pulmonary veins
Pulmonary edema
Decreased cardiac output
Decreased perfusion of body tissues
Decreased blood flow to
  kidneys and glands
Increased secretion of sodium
  and water-retaining hormones
Increased reabsorption of
  sodium and water
Increased extracellular fluid
  volume
Increased total blood volume

▲ *Figure 42–8*

Effects of heart failure.

Box 42–8. *Restrictions for a Mild, Low-Sodium Diet (2 to 3 gm)*

DO NOT USE

1. Salt at the table (use salt lightly in cooking)
2. Salt-preserved foods such as salted or smoked meat (bacon and bacon fat, bologna, dried or chipped beef, corned beef, frankfurters, ham, kosher meats, luncheon meats, salt pork, sausage, smoked tongue), salted or smoked fish (anchovies, caviar, salted and dried cod, herring, sardines), sauerkraut, olives
3. Highly salted foods, such as crackers, pretzels, potato chips, corn chips, salted nuts, salted popcorn
4. Spices and condiments, such as bouillon cubes,* catsup, chili sauce,* celery salt, garlic salt, onion salt, monosodium glutamate, meat sauces, meat tenderizers,* pickles, prepared mustard, relishes, Worcestershire sauce, soy sauce
5. Cheese,* peanut butter*

* Dietetic low-sodium products may be used.

on a severe sodium-restricted diet for low salt syndrome; manifestations include nausea, vomiting, and weakness. Box 42–8 summarizes a typical low-sodium regimen.

People with CHF also receive diuretic therapy, which increases urination, thus reducing volume overload. Some diuretics cause potassium depletion. Therefore, it is necessary to promote ingestion of foods containing large amounts of potassium (e.g., orange juice, bananas) or to give potassium supplements.

Hypertension. Hypertension is generally defined as persistent, elevated levels of blood pressure above 140 systolic and 90 diastolic.[33,71,102] In most cases the cause is unknown, but about 20 per cent of the United States population suffers from this disorder. It is associated with increased risk for coronary heart disease. The major therapeutic objective is to lower the blood pressure to normal levels and to prevent vascular damage. As with CHF, dietary recommendations for hypertension include moderate sodium restriction to reduce edema and potassium replacement for potassium losses secondary to diuretic therapy. In addition to these measures, a clinician may also suggest restriction of alcohol intake and encourage weight loss for the obese person.

DIET IN THE CAUSATION AND MANAGEMENT OF CANCER

Much research has been devoted to the role of dietary and nutritional factors in the development of cancer. The Committee on Diet, Nutrition, and Cancer of the National Research Council has decided that it is not yet possible to make firm scientific pronouncements about the association between diet and cancer. The committee does, however, provide the following "interim" dietary guidelines:[73]

▶ Reduce fat intake to 30 per cent of total calories in the diet
▶ Include fruits and vegetables, especially citrus fruits and carotene-rich vegetables
▶ Include whole grains in the diet daily
▶ Avoid foods preserved by pickling and smoking
▶ Avoid food contamination with carcinogens of any source (intentional additives, unintended contaminants, naturally occurring compounds)
▶ Continue efforts to identify mutagens in foods, test carcinogenic properties, and, if it can be done without reducing the nutritive value of food, remove them or limit their content in that food
▶ Avoid excessive alcohol intake

No dietary cure for cancer is available, but maintenance of good nutritional status is vital to recovery from the disease and the side effects of its treatment. This goal is difficult to attain for many reasons. First, many cancers alter taste sensations and suppress a person's appetite. Second, the disease can increase the basal metabolic rate. Also, the treatment (especially chemotherapy and radiation) often causes severe nausea and vomiting. In addition, these treatment modalities produce oral and gastrointestinal lesions that may make oral or enteral feeding difficult. In terminal cancer, the result of nutritional deficiency is often **cachexia,** a condition in which the person becomes emaciated or wasted. Nutritional support includes a high-calorie, high-nutrient diet. Also, tube feeding or intravenous nutrition is often necessary.[29]

DIET IN THE MANAGEMENT OF HUMAN IMMUNE DEFICIENCY VIRUS INFECTION

Managing clients with human immunodeficiency virus (HIV) infection has become a major challenge for health care providers. HIV attacks the immune system and results in acquired immune deficiency syndrome (AIDS). AIDS leaves the client defenseless against opportunistic infections and other disorders from which most people are protected. The serious protein energy malnutrition and wasting associated with HIV infection, much like cancer, are due to a number of factors: inadequate food intake, excessive nutrient losses, hypermetabolism, and medication-nutrient interactions. Each client is different, depending especially on the array of complications. Weight loss usually occurs in the early stages of infection and becomes more severe as the disease progresses.

While attention to nutrition cannot change the final outcome of AIDS, it is widely believed that good nutritional status can slow the progression of the disease and improve the quality of life. Immune function may be improved, and responses to medication may be better. Maintaining the best possible nutritional status may make the difference between an individual being able to stay at home or having to move to a nursing home.

Specific nutrient needs of persons with AIDS are not known. Needs probably depend on the complications experienced in each case. At least 100 per cent of the RDAs for all nutrients should be provided daily. When food intake fails to meet these needs, nutrient supplements (especially vitamins and minerals) are justified. Strategies used in working with clients who have AIDS are similar to those used with cancer. When food intake is consistently suboptimal, aggressive nutritional support should be considered. This action should be taken when a person loses 5 per cent of body weight within a month or a person has lost more than 10 per cent of body weight over the last 6 months. Enteral feeding is always preferred to parenteral feeding. Close work with the dietitian and pharmacist is essential.

DIET IN THE MANAGEMENT OF METABOLIC AND ENDOCRINE DISORDERS

Gout. Scientists have not yet determined the basic metabolic defect in gout, but abnormal purine metabolism is involved. Purines are products of the digestion of certain proteins. Breakdown of the purines adenine and guanine leads to the production of uric acid. Humans normally excrete this compound in the urine. The person with gout, however, is unable to metabolize purines, so that uric acid accumulates in the blood, causing hyperuricemia. This condition leads to the deposition of urate in joints and soft tissues, which then initiates a local inflammatory response.

Intervention for the disease requires reduction in blood uric acid by use of appropriate drugs and restriction of dietary purine. The highest level of purines is found in organ meats (e.g., liver, kidneys, sweetbreads, sardines, anchovies, and meat extracts), but other meats also contain significant amounts. It is also advisable to (a) institute a diet for weight control if obesity is a problem, (b) increase fluid intake to avoid complications from increased urinary uric acid excretion, and (c) limit alcohol consumption because alcohol inhibits uric acid excretion.

Diabetes Mellitus. Diabetes mellitus is an inherited or acquired disease in which an insulin deficiency is the primary defect.[5,113] Insulin deficiency may be due to decreased secretion of the hormone, reduction in the biologic effectiveness of the hormone, or both.

Insulin is a protein hormone formed by the beta cells of the islets of Langerhans of the pancreas. Normally, insulin is secreted into the blood, where it regulates carbohydrate, lipid, and amino acid metabolism. Impaired insulin functioning causes impaired metabolism, leading to inadequate glucose regulation. Glucose cannot move from the blood into cells and consequently remains in the bloodstream, where it draws water from the cells. Eventually, the glucose filters through the kidneys and is excreted in the urine, pulling water with it. As a result of poor glucose utilization and excessive fluid losses in the urine, the diabetic person develops increased hunger and thirst. The body begins to burn large amounts of fatty acids for energy, and ketosis (excessive accumulation of ketone bodies in the body fluids and tissues) can develop. Regulation of blood glucose level is thus a primary focus of nursing care. Regulation helps prevent acute problems (e.g., ketosis) and minimizes long-term complications (e.g., vascular disease, renal failure).

The diabetic diet is one of the essential components in the control of diabetes. Methods of dietary management differ from clinic to clinic. Generally, however, emphasis is on regulation of carbohydrate and fat intake in order to avoid large fluctuations in serum glucose levels. For this purpose, many diets use the exchange system developed jointly by the American Diabetic Association and the American Dietetic Association.[6]

The exchange system divides foods into six groups, or exchanges (Table 42–13). Foods in any one group can be substituted or exchanged for other foods in the same group. The exchanges within each group are approximately equal in amounts of calories, carbohydrates, protein, and fat. In addition, each exchange contains similar amounts of minerals and vitamins.

To obtain precise guidelines for using the exchange system, write to the American Dietetic Association, 216 West Jackson Boulevard, Suite 800, Chicago, Illinois 60606-6995.

In recent years, some authorities have proposed the high-fiber diet for control of diabetes. Although this practice is somewhat controversial, a substantial body of data supports the concept that a diet high in both carbohydrate and fiber has a beneficial impact on both carbohydrate and lipid metabolism.[11]

Hypoglycemia. The word **hypoglycemia** simply means low blood glucose. Low blood glucose levels can result in symptoms such as anxiety, confusion, tremors, and blurred vision. Generally, insulin and glucagon (a hormone that raises serum glucose levels) keep glucose relatively stable, usually between 70 and

TABLE 42–13. The Six Major Exchange Lists

Exchange List	Representative Foods
Starch/bread	Cereals, grains, pasta, dried beans, dried peas, lentils, breads, crackers, starchy vegetables
Meat	
Lean	Lean beef, pork, veal; poultry; fish, wild game, cottage cheese, diet cheeses, egg whites
Medium-fat	Most beef, pork, and lamb products, veal cutlet, chicken (with skin), domestic duck or goose, tuna or salmon canned in oil, skim or part skim cheeses, eggs, tofu, organ meats
High-fat	Most prime cuts of beef, spareribs, ground pork, lamb patties, any fried fish product, all regular cheeses, luncheon meats, peanut butter
Vegetable	Nonstarchy vegetables like asparagus and beets
Fruit	All fruits and fruit juices
Milk	All milks, yogurt
Fat	Butter, margarine, oils, salad dressings, nuts and seeds, mayonnaise, olives, cream, cream cheese, salt pork

100 mg/ml. Conditions that can cause hypoglycemia include fasting, diabetes mellitus, and liver disease.

In addition, the literature describes a syndrome in which individuals experience unstable blood sugar levels because of excessive ingestion of refined sugars. Refined sugars have a high glycemic index. Thus, after ingestion, these sugars increase blood glucose rapidly. Increased blood glucose can spark an oversecretion of insulin, which in turn depresses blood glucose below normal levels. Although the diagnosis of hypoglycemia remains controversial, the diet prescribed for people with this condition includes (1) avoidance of foods containing refined sugars, such as candy and ice cream; (2) ingestion of foods with a low glycemic index (see Fig. 42–3); and (3) the practice of eating small, frequent meals.

DIET IN THE MANAGEMENT OF SPECIAL DISEASES OF INFANCY AND CHILDHOOD

Phenylketonuria. PKU is the most widely recognized inborn error of amino acid metabolism.[37] The child with PKU is born with little or no phenylalanine hydroxylase, an enzyme needed to convert phenylalanine, an amino acid, to tyrosine in the body (Fig. 42–9). This defect results in high blood levels of phenylalanine and low levels of tyrosine, an imbalance resulting in a disruption of brain maturation with subsequent mental retardation.

Many studies have evaluated the response of phenylketonuria to dietary management. Regulation of phenylalanine intake prevents brain damage and ensures normal physical and mental development in children with PKU. Thus, it is mandatory to provide a special low-phenylalanine diet through infancy and childhood and to monitor blood phenylalanine levels at regular intervals. Current recommendations specify that the diet be maintained indefinitely, especially in girls who wish to reproduce later in life.[41]

Food Allergy. Allergy is an altered or abnormal tissue sensitivity to foreign substances. Any food substance is a potential allergen, but milk, eggs, corn, and wheat are the foods most frequently incriminated in infant allergies. Reactions to allergens are manifested in a variety of symptoms such as vomiting, colic, diarrhea, irritability, fatigue, urticaria (hives), or allergic rhinitis (inflammation of the mucous membrane of the nose). Infants are more frequently affected than are older children and adults.

Management of food allergy involves elimination of the problem foods. In children, food allergies may gradually disappear, so previously restricted foods can be successfully reintroduced into the diet at a later time.

People may also demonstrate adverse reactions to foods that immunologic testing cannot confirm as true allergies. These phenomena are called food intolerances. In many cases, their cause is unknown, but some known inducers of food intolerances include

▶ pharmacologic agents in foods, which are natural agents, such as histamine, tyramine, and phenylethylamine, or additive agents, such as monosodium glutamate (MSG), sodium nitrate, and tartrazine
▶ lactase deficiency (a genetic disorder that causes milk intolerance)[94]
▶ **celiac sprue** (a disorder characterized by gluten-induced malabsorption of essential nutrients)
▶ food toxins

Whatever the cause, therapy involves removing the problem foods from the diet.

Maintaining or Improving the Appetite

The nurse has the important responsibility of creating the physical conditions that help make eating more enjoyable. A person's appetite may improve if the environment is clean and attractive and the individual is protected from unpleasant odors and sights. Make the person comfortable before a meal is served by making sure the person has the opportunity to tend to personal hygiene and go to the bathroom, if necessary. Also, the

Metabolic Defect in Phenylketonuria

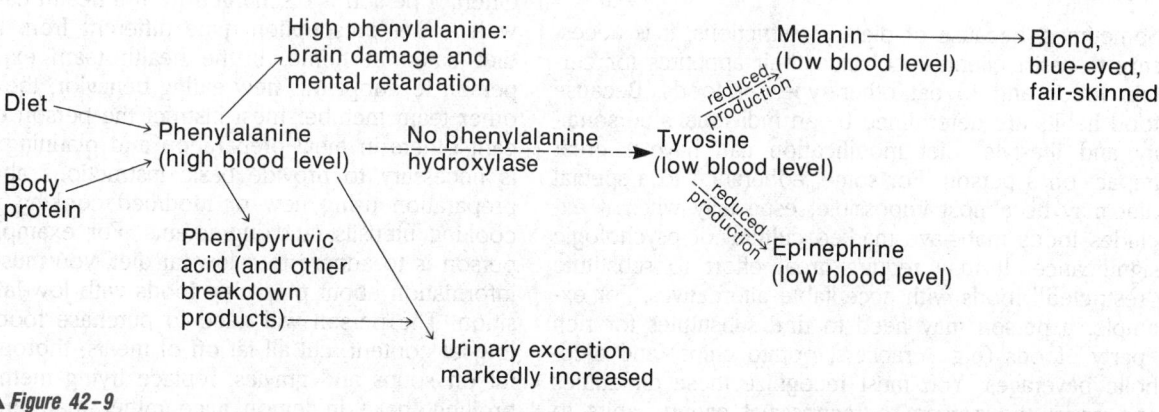

▲ *Figure 42–9*

Metabolic defect in phenylketonuria. Absence of the enzyme phenylalanine hydroxylase prevents conversion of phenylalanine to tyrosine. Blood samples reveal high phenylalanine and low tyrosine levels. Urine samples show excessive phenylalanine and its breakdown products. Production of melanin and epinephrine is decreased. Mental retardation develops owing to the toxic character of high levels of phenylalanine in the brain.

person should be in a comfortable position for eating. Assist the individual with these activities, if indicated.

NAUSEA AND VOMITING

Maintaining the appetite is particularly difficult when the client is nauseated or is subject to vomiting. To give special assistance to the person with a tendency toward nausea or vomiting:

► Avoid abrupt and unnecessary movement that might provoke nausea.
► Encourage the individual to take deep breaths when nausea occurs.
► Limit food and fluid intake when discomfort is serious; then offer small amounts of fluid (or food) as tolerated.
► Offer bland foods as opposed to those that are spicy or fatty. Liberalize the diet as the individual tolerates more food.
► Help reduce sources of stress for the person with a tendency toward vomiting.
► Administer antiemetic agents, if necessary. When possible, avoid administering nausea-producing medications near mealtime.

DISCOMFORT

Pain and other discomforts, such as intense itching, can decrease the appetite and prevent mealtimes from being as pleasant as they could be. To enhance the appetite, it is particularly important to increase comfort at mealtimes. To do this,

► Schedule painful treatments well before the meal so the client has plenty of time to recover from the treatment and to rest before the tray arrives.
► Administer medication soon enough before the tray arrives to allow for control of the symptoms of discomfort.
► Provide soothing treatments or general comfort measures, such as a back massage or linen change, immediately before the meal.

"RESTRICTED" FOODS

Sometimes, because of dietary restrictions, it is necessary to assist clients to change their appetites for certain foods and to eat other types of foods. Because food habits are determined by an individual's personality and lifestyle, diet modification can have a great impact on a person. For some, adherence to a special diet may be almost impossible, especially when it excludes foods that have marked cultural or psychologic significance. It may require great effort to substitute "restricted" foods with acceptable alternatives. For example, a person may need to find substitutes for rich "party" foods (e.g., crackers, potato chips) and alcoholic beverages. You must recognize these difficulties and assist the person to reconstruct eating habits to conform with the medical regimen while still retaining the cultural, social, and personal satisfaction associated with meals and eating.

Increasing Ingestion of the Appropriate Diet

Because food habits can be so deeply ingrained, it may not be possible to increase a given person's appetite for healthier foods and to decrease the appetite for restricted foods. Still, it is usually possible to change the person's eating habits so that the healthier foods are the foods actually ingested. This change can often be effected through education, counseling, and planning.

DIETARY COUNSELING

Helping the individual learn more about diet and nutritional needs is an important aspect of nursing care. Help the person become more aware of the role food plays in providing, maintaining, and building health and strength and in minimizing some of the discomforts of disease. Accepting diet modifications is easier if the person understands the benefits of good nutrition. If the health team is able to promote acceptance of an appropriate diet within the health care facility, the person may permanently adopt more sensible eating habits at home.

You can instruct the person about good nutrition in many ways. Arrange planned conversations with the individual during which you can discuss dietary issues. Explore the specific needs of the person and deal with questions related to the workability of a special diet. When the person makes choices from the hospital menu, provide sound guidance in appropriate meal planning. Discuss comparative food values.

Mealtime itself presents opportunities for teaching. When serving the individual the meal tray or assisting with eating, point out certain food items as examples of foods that supply specific nutrients to the body. For example, if the person requires protein to promote wound healing, you can point out the protein-containing foods on the tray. Learn to take advantage of all opportunities to assist the individual in acquiring sensible food selection patterns.

PLANNING SPECIAL MEALS IN THE HOME SETTING

Often, a person is discharged from a health care facility with a diet prescription quite different from the usual diet eaten at home. If the health team expects the person to adopt this new eating behavior, the nurse or other team member must instruct the person or significant others in meal preparation and planning. Often it is necessary to provide basic instructions about food preparation using new or modified cooking methods, cooking utensils, and ingredients. For example, if the person is to adhere to a low-fat diet, you must provide information about preparing foods with low-fat composition. The person will need to purchase foods with a low-fat content, cut all fat off of meats, thoroughly skin fat off soups and gravies, replace frying methods with broiling, bake in lemon juice rather than butter, and so on.

The hospital dietitian is generally the best source of initial information about planning the special diet.

Eventually, however, it is helpful to supply the person with printed materials to assist in special cooking modifications for a given culture and lifestyle. A variety of brochures and books relate to planning and preparing foods for special dietary regimens. Information about such publications is generally available through the nutritionist or the local branch of the American Dietetic Association. Many distributors of special food products also publish helpful tips about cooking while adhering to various dietary prescriptions.

When the dietary program requires ongoing supervision or frequent modification, the client should obtain the advice of a consulting nutritionist in the community. Consulting nutritionists are usually available on a limited outpatient basis to answer questions about special diets or food-assistance programs. Also, nutritionists in the local branches of the American Heart Association and the National Dairy Council can provide useful assistance with some problems. In addition, other nonprofit organizations throughout the world may contribute help. Each community has its own unique services, which may include health care assistance for various cultural groups and age groups. One may obtain information about local nutrition services through established dietetic associations or health care units.

SERVING FOOD AND ASSISTING WITH FEEDING

Nursing responsibilities related to food service vary from facility to facility. Most hospitals employ one or more nutritionists to organize a central food service. In general, nurses are responsible for contacting the food service to order and cancel diets, for assisting with the serving of meals, for helping people eat, and for recording information concerning the amount and type of food and fluid intake.

In most hospitals, people are served food at their bedsides. Some health care facilities, however, have cafeterias or dining rooms for clients who are ambulatory. Because mealtimes are usually considered social situations, encourage the involvement of significant others in the meal situation, whether in the cafeteria, dining room, or patient room. If friends or family members bring food to share, evaluate its suitability for the client but remember that food shared with loved ones is often much more than mere sustenance.

Obviously, the more seriously ill the person is, the more assistance is required in the feeding process. Serve trays last to those persons who need the most assistance with eating, so that you will have more time to spend with them without interruptions. Try to stay with them throughout the meal period. See Procedure 42–1 for guidance in serving food and assisting with feeding.

It is a nursing responsibility to note the amounts and types of nutrients ingested. Documentation may be more difficult when the client eats in a cafeteria because you will have to ask rather than relying on your direct observations. When foods are brought in from home, you may also have to ask for information; for example, it may be difficult to identify all the ingredients in a casserole or a salad. You will have to record intake from these sources as required for your clients.

Increasing Digestion

ENHANCING PROCESSES IN THE MOUTH

Digestion begins in the mouth as the teeth tear and grind the food taken in and the tongue and cheeks work together with salivary gland secretions to create a moist, softened bolus of food ready for deglutition (swallowing). As this mechanical breakdown begins, amylase (ptyalin) in the saliva begins to break down starches and other saccharide compounds. You can assist in this early step in digestion by helping assure that the client has adequate saliva as well as teeth and muscle strength to chew the foods provided. Saliva is reduced in clients who have insufficient intake of fluids by mouth, so you can help assure adequate saliva by helping to assure adequate fluid intake throughout the day. Giving fluids with the meal also assists with deglutition. For the client without teeth or without adequate muscle strength to chew foods well, assist with the insertion of dentures or provide a diet that is prepared in a form ready for swallowing without chewing (e.g., soft or mechanical soft).

MANAGING DYSPHAGIA

Dysphagia (difficulty or discomfort in swallowing) poses a serious threat to maintenance of nutritional status. In severe cases, tube or intravenous nutritional support may need to be instituted to provide nutrients.

Place the individual with dysphagia in a comfortable upright position in a pleasant environment. Next, instruct the individual about simple oral movements that are related to tongue and jaw movement. If the sucking mechanism is intact, you can give fluids through a straw. You can also stimulate salivation by use of tart solutions. Initiate swallowing by ensuring lip closure. Adjust the food consistency in accordance with the person's ability to swallow. If a liquid diet is required initially, strive to upgrade the texture gradually as feeding skills improve.

PROMOTING PROCESSES IN THE STOMACH AND INTESTINES

Digestion continues in the stomach and small intestine with the further mechanical and chemical breakdown of proteins, carbohydrates, and fats. Some persons lack adequate chemicals for digestion of one or more of these nutrients. The person might, for example, lack hydrochloric acid in the stomach or pancreatic enzymes in the small intestine. When replacement enzymes are ordered by the physician, it may be your responsibility to give them prior to meals. More frequently, however, you can have a positive effect on digestion by helping prevent the stimulation of the sympathetic nervous system. Provide a relaxed atmosphere rather than a stressful one.

PROCEDURE 42-1

Serving Food and Assisting with Feeding

Definition/Purposes. Enables a nurse to assist clients to eat when they are unable to feed themselves independently. Used to prevent weak clients from exerting themselves excessively or to assure adequate nutrition for clients who are totally dependent.

Contraindications/Cautions. Be certain the client receives the correct diet. Check for food allergies. Use care to prevent aspiration of food or liquid into the respiratory tree.

Teaching/Learning Guidelines. Assist the client to maintain as much independence as possible to help maintain or regain the ability to feed himself or herself. Teach or encourage practice of new skills required for eating (e.g., eating with the nondominant hand for a client who has lost the use of the dominant arm or self-feeding for the client who has recently become visually impaired). Use the mealtime to discuss dietary needs and to teach about ways to meet client's nutritional goals (e.g., identify foods high in needed nutrients and discuss client preferences to assist the client in menu selections of the next day's meals or for selection and preparation of foods after discharge from the acute-care setting).

PRELIMINARY ACTIVITIES

Assessment/Planning

- ▶ Review nutritional needs and dietary orders.
- ▶ Check the chart for the presence of food allergies.
- ▶ Assess client's level of consciousness, ability to chew and swallow, and ability to follow directions.
- ▶ Remove any unsightly or malodorous stimuli from the client's room and air it out, if necessary, to provide an atmosphere conducive to eating.
- ▶ Check the tray to be certain that
  - ▶ the name on the tray corresponds to the name on the client's identification band
  - ▶ the tray contains the type of diet ordered
  - ▶ all food, condiments, and utensils are present

Preparation of Person

- ▶ Explain that mealtime is near.
- ▶ Assist client to a chair, if possible and desired.
- ▶ If client is unable to get out of bed, adjust the bed into as near a sitting position as possible or otherwise adjust it according to client need.

- ▶ Assist the client in handwashing.
- ▶ Offer oral hygiene to enhance the flavor of the food to come.
- ▶ Be sure the client has dentures in place, if needed.
- ▶ Be sure the client has eyeglasses and hearing aid in place, if needed.
- ▶ Protect the client's gown and/or bed linens from spills by placing a napkin or towel where food might drop.
- ▶ Clear off the overbed table and place it within easy reach of the client.

Equipment

- ▶ Extra napkin or towel to protect the linens
- ▶ Overbed tray
- ▶ Ordered diet
- ▶ Condiments as allowed and desired
- ▶ Napkin, silverware, and straw

PROCEDURE

Actions

1. Place the tray on the overbed table, and remove food covers if necessary, so food is visible to the client.

2. Be sure the tray is within easy reach.
3. As much as possible, encourage the client to assist in preparing and eating the food. Allow time needed to do this.
4. When required, open milk container, butter bread, cut meat, and otherwise assist in the preparation of the food.
5. Add milk and sugar to coffee or tea, salt food, and so on, according to client preferences.
6. Tell the visually impaired where the different foods are located by comparing the plate to a clock (e.g., "The toast is between 12 and 3 o'clock; the bacon is between 3 and 5 o'clock; the two eggs are between 5 and 10 o'clock; and there is some extra jelly between 10 and 12 o'clock, if you need more").
7. For the client who must be fed and who is unable to handle utensils, encourage the holding of a piece of fruit or buttered bread or toast to be eaten at will.

Rationale/Discussion

1. The sight and smell of food stimulates the appetite and prepares the client for food ingestion and digestion by stimulating the parasympathetic nervous system.
2. Allows the client to assist in feeding self, if able.
3. Aids in maintaining a sense of independence and promotes self-esteem.

4. Some clients can feed themselves if the food is prepared for them.

5. Preparing food to client liking increases the likelihood of intake.
6. With this information, the client may more easily eat independently.

7. Finger foods are easier to manage than silverware and may allow some independent feeding.

PROCEDURE 42-1 Continued

Serving Food and Assisting with Feeding

Actions	Rationale/Discussion
8. Provide a relaxed atmosphere by sitting down, if possible, and by avoiding rushing client.	8. Meals are usually considered a social situation that should be enjoyed.
9. Before feeding the client, ascertain preferences as to the order of foods desired. For example, some persons like to eat all of one food before trying another; some want one bite of each food in a certain order; and some like to mix foods in the same forkful.	9. Eating habits are often firmly ingrained and important to the individual's enjoyment of the meal.
10. Offer liquids according to client preference. Some will want liquids more frequently than others. Liquids are usually desired every few bites throughout the meal.	10. Liquids assist in deglutition by lubricating the passageway and flushing the solid bolus of food downward to the stomach through the cardiac sphincter.
11. Provide a straw for persons unable to sip directly from a glass or cup without spilling (e.g., the client in a lateral or prone position).	11. The siphoning action with a straw overcomes gravity and allows the client to bring a controlled amount of liquid to the mouth without spilling.
12. Be certain to offer foods in manageable bites.	12. Bites of adequate size help prevent discomfort and choking.
13. Allow sufficient time for chewing and swallowing.	13. Digestion begins in the mouth with the mechanical breakdown of solids and the chemical breakdown of starches.
14. Use the napkin to wipe any spills from the client's face during the feeding.	14. Spills can be a source of embarrassment.
15. When the client is finished, assess the adequacy of the meal by determining client satisfaction.	15. Serving sizes may be increased or between-meal snacks may be provided for the client who needs additional food. Smaller, more frequent feedings may be tolerated better by the client who is not eating enough.
16. Remove tray as soon after eating as possible. Clean up any spills and change soiled linen.	16. Leaving the individual as clean and comfortable as possible will help the client associate meals with a feeling of well-being.

FINAL ACTIVITIES

After tray removal, offer oral hygiene and provide assistance as needed. Because plaque formation can be reduced if oral hygiene is completed promptly after each meal, oral care should be done within 20 minutes of finishing with the tray. Also offer assistance in washing the client's hands as needed. Position the client comfortably with the head elevated at least 30 degrees, if allowed.

Assess food and liquid intake, including time of meal and types and amounts of nutrients consumed. Take specific note of any observations that have a bearing on the individual's nutritional health. Record pertinent data in the client's record.

Increasing Absorption

It usually takes from 2 to 6 hours for partially digested food to pass from the stomach to the duodenum. During the time the food is in the stomach, very little is actually absorbed. Normally, only water and alcohol are absorbed this high in the digestive tract.

In the healthy individual, the greatest quantity of nutrients is absorbed in the small intestine. Conditions that prevent the absorption of nutrients in the small intestine usually result in the intestinal contents being passed, with little change, into the large intestine and out of the body in the feces. As a result, a fecal mass is of a larger volume and consists of more liquid than normal. Frequent passage of such stools is termed diarrhea.

Several factors can account for decreased absorption in the small intestine. Major factors include the following:

▶ *Increased intestinal motility.* As peristalsis increases, there is less time for intestinal contents to remain in contact with the mucosal surface of the intestine; as a result, less absorption occurs. Increased peristalsis can result from pathologic conditions that are treated medically or surgically (e.g., Crohn's disease, ulcerative colitis, or irritable bowel syndrome). In such cases, the role of the nurse is to carry out prescribed medical treatments and administer medications as ordered by the physician. Increased peristalsis can also result from stimulation of the sympathetic nervous system, which can occur with normal day-to-day stresses. The nurse can have an important role in reducing the stresses that can lead to diarrhea, as well as in changing how the individual responds to those stresses. See Chapter 16 for more information on stress and adaptation.

▶ *Increased intestinal secretory activity.* An increase in the amount of intestinal secretions can stimulate stretch receptors in the intestine and initiate peristalsis before the intestinal contents have been in contact with the absorbing surface for an adequate amount of time. Increased intestinal secretions may be stimulated by several pathologic conditions, such as tumors of glands that regulate secretions or the presence of bacterial enterotoxins such as those released into the intestine by the bacteria that produce cholera (*Vibrio cholerae*). The nurse can work with the rest of the health care team in treating medical diagnoses but independently can help prevent some of these conditions. For example, the nurse can counsel high-risk individuals concerning preventive health care practices.

▶ *Increased intestinal osmotic activity.* Increased osmotic activity is another process that adds fluid to the intestinal contents, increasing peristalsis and decreasing absorption. In this case, materials in the intestine draw large amounts of water into the intestine by osmosis. One example of such osmotic material is lactose (milk sugar) in lactase-deficient individuals who have insufficient lactase available to allow the normal breakdown and absorption of lactose. Another example is nonabsorbable sugar substitutes (e.g., sorbitol) that consist of large molecules of high osmolarity. These substances are present in the human gastrointestinal tract when they are ingested in some "diet" foods and beverages. In large enough quantities, they may cause diarrhea. When such osmotic materials stimulate diarrhea, other nutrients are moved through the tract too rapidly for an adequate absorption process. Therefore, the role of the nurse is teaching and counseling to assist the person to reduce the amount of osmotic materials present in the tract.

▶ *Decreased surface for absorption.* In severe malnutrition, the villi deteriorate and shrink, greatly decreasing the absorptive surface. When the individual finally receives sufficient nutrients, the intestinal wall is incapable of normal levels of absorption, and much of the food passes out of the digestive tract as diarrhea. The role of the nurse is to support the client's total nutrition by various routes until normal villi are re-established.

Maintaining Nutrition When Gastrointestinal Function Is Impaired

Ideally, a person can meet all nutritional needs with a regular, balanced diet processed through the normal gastrointestinal route. In some circumstances, however, a person cannot ingest, digest, or absorb sufficient nutrients, and nutritional requirements must be met, on either a temporary or a permanent basis, by specialized methods of feeding. Specialized methods of feeding may require bypassing normal anatomic structures in order to provide nutrients.

For a person who cannot eat solid food but who can absorb nutrients from the small intestine, enteral feeding is appropriate. **Enteral feeding** refers to a special liquid formula that can be given orally or through a tube passed through the nose or mouth into the esophagus and stomach. A tube may also be surgically implanted directly through the abdominal wall into the stomach or the small intestine (most frequently, into the jejunum) to provide enteral nutrition. For persons who cannot eat or absorb enough from the normal gastrointestinal route when fed by tubes, **parenteral support** (intravenous feedings) may be provided. This is sometimes referred to as **peripheral parenteral nutrition (PPN)**.

PARENTERAL NUTRITION

Parenteral fluids that are given to enhance nutrition are introduced directly into the venous system. These fluids usually contain glucose, amino acids, electrolytes, minerals, and vitamins. For persons in good nutritional status but with a temporary inability to absorb nutrients, solutions with amino acids and a low concentration of glucose may be administered for short periods through peripheral veins (PPN). About twice a week, lipid emulsions are given through a Y-tube connection into the intravenous line. However, in situations of major trauma or substantial damage to the gastrointestinal tract when longer-term feedings are needed, more substantial parenteral nutrition may be necessary, and a central venous catheter is placed in a large vein (usually the subclavian) that empties directly into the heart. This type of intravenous line allows the client to receive total parenteral nutrition (TPN). Total parenteral nutrition, or hyperalimentation, is the intravenous provision of total caloric needs, including both amino acids for protein building and lipid emulsions and high concentrations of glucose for calories. High risk of infection precludes using this method of feeding unless the person is unable to eat or absorb nutrients through the gastrointestinal tract.

ASSESSING THE NEED FOR SPECIAL NUTRITIONAL SUPPORT

Some institutions have nutrition teams to assess individual clients and make recommendations for nutritional support substances and methods. Teams are usually multidisciplinary and consist of a nurse, a physician, a pharmacist, and a dietitian, all of whom specialize in nutritional support. The unit staff nurse provides information about the client and assists in administering and evaluating the nutritional support provided.

A decision tree helps determine which form of nutritional support would be appropriate for the client (Fig. 42–10). The least invasive method is preferred because of the risks of infection and metabolic complications. It is less invasive, for example, to use enteral nutrition than to administer parenteral nutrition. Peripheral parenteral nutrition is less invasive than total parenteral nutrition. When the nurse has identified a nutritional deficit, the results of the assessment should be discussed with the physician. Then, interventions to help the client maintain or improve nutritional status can be started promptly.

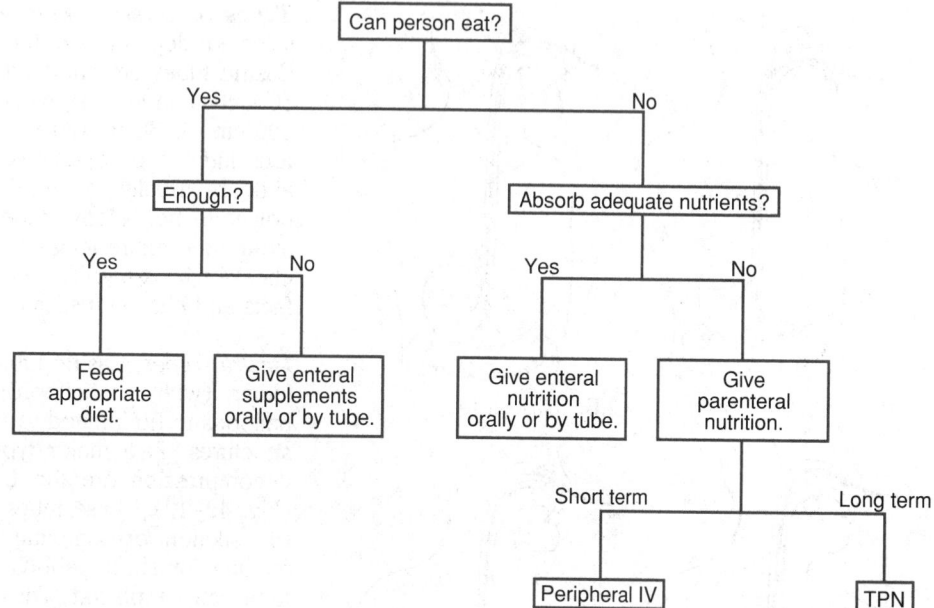

▲ *Figure 42-10*

Decision tree to help guide the nurse in providing the appropriate level of nutritional support.

ENTERAL NUTRITION

Tubes to Protect Gastrointestinal Function. When enteral feedings (tube feedings) are needed, a tube is inserted into the gastrointestinal tract as a route for the feeding solution. But gastrointestinal tubes may be placed for purposes other than feeding. Sometimes the gastrointestinal mucosa is damaged or the lumen obstructed, and a tube will be placed to remove secretions, gas, or poisons in an effort to restore the normal functions of nutrition and elimination. A tube may also be used to obtain a sample of secretions for diagnostic purposes. Gastric or intestinal **intubation** (placement of a gastrointestinal tube in the GI tract) is performed for several reasons:

▶ Decompression. **Gastrointestinal decompression** is a process of relieving pressure by removing accumulated gas and secretions from the GI tract through a tube. Tubes are usually inserted through the nose or mouth and into the GI tract for decompression when normal GI motility is slowed, usually after major surgery or trauma. It is also necessary to use decompression when an obstruction blocks some part of the GI tract.

▶ Compression. **Gastrointestinal compression** is a process of applying pressure internally using a specially designed tube with inflatable balloons. The balloons are placed at specific sites and inflated, thus applying pressure, which stops bleeding. The application of pressure is called tamponade. One of the most common uses of compression is to control bleeding of esophageal varices (varicose veins) at the gastroesophageal junction.

▶ Gavage. **Gavage** is a method of giving persons fluids and nutrients through a tube when oral intake is inadequate or impossible. Gavage is also called enteral or tube feeding.

▶ Lavage. **Lavage** is the irrigation or cleansing of an organ. For example, gastric lavage involves washing out the stomach. It is used most frequently as an emergency treatment to remove poisons. Iced water is sometimes used to constrict bleeding gastric blood vessels during GI hemorrhage. Lavage is also used to cleanse the stomach in preparation for gastric surgery.

▶ Gastric analysis. **Gastric analysis** (the laboratory analysis of stomach contents) is important in the diagnosis of gastric pathology. A tube is inserted into the stomach to aspirate gastric contents. Normal fasting contents of the stomach are clear and watery with no blood. The pH is between 1.5 and 3.5.

Routes of Gastrointestinal Tubes. Various routes are used for GI intubation (Fig. 42-11). Tubes may be placed in the gastrointestinal tract through the nose or mouth or through special surgical openings into the esophagus, stomach, or jejunum. A **nasogastric (NG) tube** is a tube that is inserted into either naris and passed through the esophagus to the stomach. An **orogastric tube** is a tube that is placed in the mouth and passed through the esophagus to the stomach. Longer intestinal tubes can be placed through either the nose or mouth into the small intestine. Sometimes these are known as nasoduodenal or nasojejunal tubes, depending upon the location of placement. An **esophagostomy** is a surgical opening into the esophagus; an **esophagogastrostomy tube** is a tube that can be passed through an esophagostomy and into the stomach. A **gastrostomy tube** is a tube that enters a surgical opening through the abdominal wall into the stomach. A **jejunostomy tube** is a tube that is inserted through a surgical opening through the abdominal wall and into the jejunum.

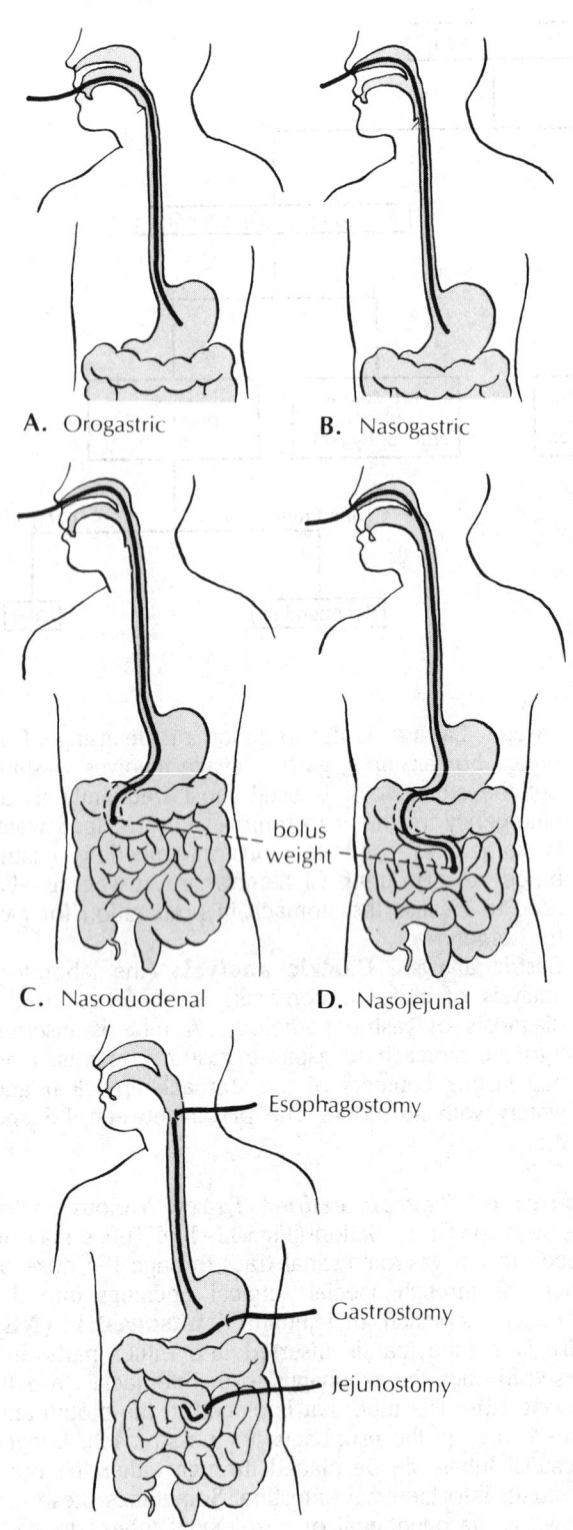

A. Orogastric

B. Nasogastric

C. Nasoduodenal

bolus weight

D. Nasojejunal

Esophagostomy

Gastrostomy

Jejunostomy

E. Others requiring surgical placement

▲ *Figure 42–11*

Routes and sites of gastrointestinal tube insertions. *A* is inserted through mouth. *B, C,* and *D* are inserted through nose. *E* shows (from top to bottom) tubes inserted externally into esophagus (esophagostomy), into stomach (gastrostomy), and into intestine (jejunostomy).

Types of Gastrointestinal Tubes. The specific tube selected depends on the purpose of the intubation. Gastric tubes are short tubes (76 to 125 cm, or 30 to 50 inches, in length), whereas intestinal tubes are 91 to 300 cm, or 36 to 120 inches long. Tubes have one to four lumens or openings, depending upon their use, and are usually made of plastic, rubber, silicone, or polyurethane. Many tubes have radiopaque stripes along their entire length so that tube placement can be checked by x-ray. Table 42–14 summarizes significant facts and characteristics of gastric and GI tubes.

Gastric Tubes. Gastric tube designs range from a single lumen (with no balloon) to a four-lumen tube with balloons to be inflated to apply pressure to surrounding structures. Two major types of gastric tubes used for decompression are the Levin and Salem sump tubes (Fig. 42–12). These tubes also serve as routes for gastric suction or sampling and can be used for tube feeding for short periods until a more pliable feeding tube can be placed. The Levin tube is a single-lumen rubber or plastic tube inserted through the nose or mouth into the stomach. The Salem sump is a double-lumen tube. The Levin tube or the larger lumen of the sump is attached to a suction apparatus to remove gastric secretions and gas. The smaller sump lumen remains unclamped and open to the atmosphere so that, as fluids and gas are removed, air can enter the stomach at atmospheric pressure. With air replacement provided by the smaller lumen, the GI mucosa is less likely to adhere to the drainage openings and become irritated by suction within the lumen.

A Levin tube can only be used with low intermittent suction, but the Salem sump tube has a second lumen and can be used with continuous suction. It is essential to keep the smaller sump lumen (also called the "pigtail") patent and open to the air. If the pigtail becomes blocked or is clamped off, the sump tube operates like a single-lumen Levin tube and may irritate the gastric mucosa.

Be sure to keep the pigtail of the sump tube unobstructed and open to the atmosphere. Otherwise, you risk gastric mucosal damage. Never clamp this lumen!

The Sengstaken-Blakemore and Minnesota tubes are used for both compression and decompression in persons with bleeding esophageal varices (Figs. 42–13 and 42–14). Both tubes have two balloons and drainage openings for removal of secretions, and the principles underlying the use of these tubes are the same. The Minnesota tube, which is newer and more sophisticated, has two balloons and several drainage openings. Once the tube is inserted and in position, the balloons are inflated to apply pressure to bleeding vessels of the esophagus and the cardiac area of the stomach. Drainage openings allow for removal of blood and secretions from the esophagus and the stomach. The Minnesota tube has four lumens, each with a specific purpose. Each lumen is individually labelled and identified to prevent accidental deflation or inflation through the wrong lumen:

TABLE 42-14. Types of Gastrointestinal Tubes

Type	Length	Size (Fr)	Lumen	Uses	Other Characteristics
Levin (gastric) (Figure 42-12A)	125 cm (50 in)	12, 16,* 18	Single	Decompression, gavage feeding, diagnostic tests	Rubber or plastic. Inserted through nose or mouth into stomach. Intermittent suction. May need irrigation. Rubber tube may need to be iced or refrigerated prior to insertion
Salem sump (gastric) (Figure 42-12B)	120 cm (48 in)	12, 14, 16,* 18	Double	Decompression of stomach	Plastic. Inserted through nose or mouth into stomach. Taped after insertion. Continuous sump suction. Radiopaque strip to use x-ray to check placement
Vivonex	88 cm (35 in)	20	Double	Decompression of stomach and esophagus	Plastic with esophageal balloon. Inserted via nose into stomach. Held in place with tension by rubber sponge at nose. Intermittent suction
Sengstaken-Blakemore (Figure 42-13)	100 cm (40 in)	20	Triple	Esophageal tamponade, compression, decompression	Rubber with gastric and esophageal balloons. Inserted through nose into stomach. Held in place by rubber sponge at nose and balloon in stomach. Intermittent suction
Minnesota (Figures 42-14, 42-15)	100 cm (40 in)	20	Quadruple	Esophageal tamponade, compression, decompression	Rubber with gastric and esophageal balloons. Inserted through nose into stomach. Held in place with tension by rubber sponge at nose and balloons. Intermittent suction
Linton	96 cm (38 in)	20, 21	Quadruple	Decompression	Rubber, gastric balloon, volume range 100-750 cc
Ewald (gastric) (Figure 42-16)	90 cm (36 in)	30	Single	Gastric washing (lavage), diagnostic tests	Rubber. Inserted through mouth into stomach. Suction provided by aspirating with Asepto syringe. May siphon with funnel
Miller-Abbott (intestinal) (Figure 42-17)	3 m (10 ft)	12, 14, 16, 18	Double	Decompression, bowel obstruction	Rubber. Balloon at distal end weighted with Hg (check balloon for leaks before inserting). Intermittent suction
Cantor (intestinal) (Figure 42-18)	3 m (10 ft)	16	Single	Decompression, bowel obstruction	Rubber. Balloon at distal end weighted with Hg (check balloon for leaks before inserting). Intermittent suction
Baker tube (intestinal) (Figure 42-19)	2.7 m (108 in)	16	Double	Decompression, prevents adhesions following surgery	Plastic. Place during surgery. Low suction
Pediatric feeding	105 cm (42 in)	8	Single	Gavage feeding	Plastic. Inserted through nose or mouth into stomach. Taped after insertion. Clamped while not in use. Water is instilled after feeding
Weighted feeding tubes (Figure 42-20)	90 cm (36 in); 109 cm (43 in)	6-18	Single	Long-term feeding	Silicone rubber or polyurethane with mercury- or tungsten-weighted tip. Inserted through nose into stomach (90 cm) or duodenum (190 cm). Smaller lumens require use of continuous feed-pump. Water is instilled after feeding if using bolus-type feeding. Clamped while not in use. Replaced every 4 weeks. Taped to nose after designated area in gastrointestinal tract is reached. Some have water-activated hydromer coating for ease of insertion. Some have radiopaque strip

Table continued on following page

TABLE 42-14. Types of Gastrointestinal Tubes Continued

Type	Length	Size (Fr)	Lumen	Uses	Other Characteristics
Gastrostomy feeding (Malecot) (Figure 42-21)	35 cm (14 in)	26, 28*	Single	Gavage feeding	Rubber or latex. Inserted directly into stomach through surgical opening in abdominal wall. Sutured to stomach wall. Clamped while not in use

*Most frequently used size for adults.

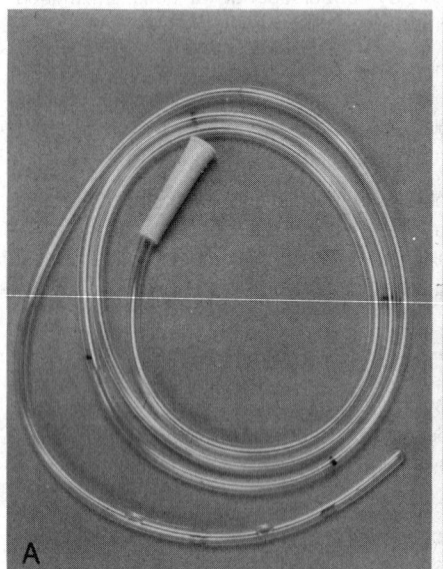
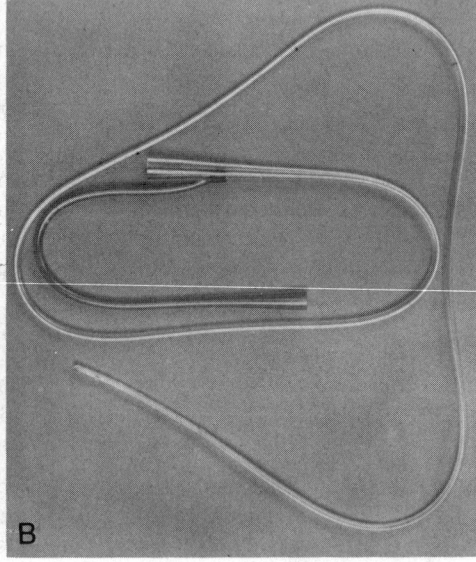

▲ *Figure 42-12*

A, The Levin tube is a single-lumen, semirigid rubber or plastic tube used for decompression, tube feeding, or gastric sampling. *B*, The Salem sump tube is a double-lumen, plastic tube and is used for decompression of stomach.

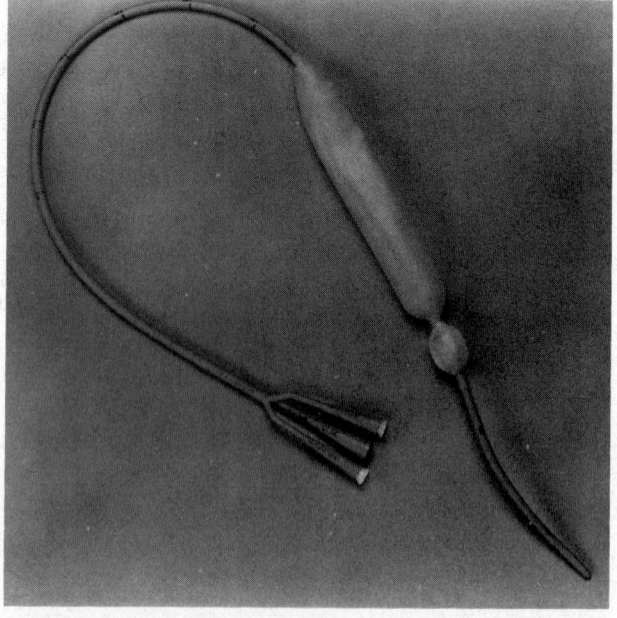

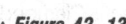
▲ *Figure 42-13*

Sengstaken-Blakemore tube has three lumens and two balloons. The long balloon controls bleeding of esophageal varices, and the small round balloon controls bleeding of gastric varices. The lumen ports provide for balloon inflation (left and right ports), and gastric aspiration, drainage, or medication instillation (center port).

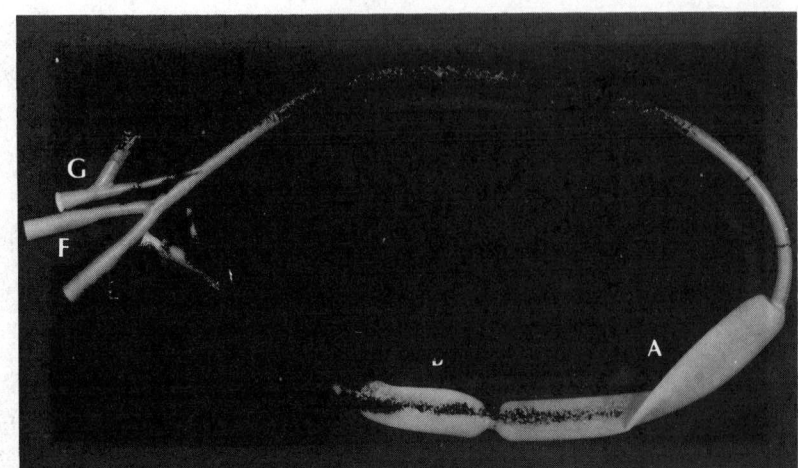

Minnesota tube for esophageal tamponade. *A,* Esophageal balloon; *B,* gastric balloon; *C,* drainage eyes; *D,* esophageal balloon lumen; *E,* gastric aspiration lumen; *F,* esophageal aspiration lumen; *G,* gastric balloon lumen. The second ports on lumens *D* and *G* are used to attach a manometer to monitor the pressure in the balloons.

▸ The esophageal balloon lumen is used to inflate the esophageal balloon (Fig. 42–14*A*). A second port on the esophageal balloon lumen allows a pressure-monitoring device to be attached to the lumen.

▸ The gastric balloon lumen (Fig. 42–14*G*) is used to inflate the gastric balloon (Fig. 42–14*B*). A pressure-monitoring port is attached to the gastric balloon lumen.

▸ The esophageal aspiration lumen (Fig. 42–14*F*) is used to aspirate secretions from the esophagus in the area above the esophageal balloon (Fig. 42–14*A*).

▸ The gastric aspiration lumen (Fig. 42–14*E*) is used to aspirate stomach contents through drainage eyes (Fig. 42–14*C*).

The Minnesota tube is held in place by a small sponge at the nose (Fig. 42–15). Sometimes the Sengstaken-Blakemore tube is stabilized by attaching that tubing to the mouthpiece of a football helmet (see Fig. 42–25*B*).

The Ewald tube is a rubber tube with a large lumen that is passed through the mouth into the stomach to remove unabsorbed stomach contents (Fig. 42–16). The Ewald tube is often used for emergency removal of blood or ingested poisons. It may also be used to administer charcoal to absorb poisons.

Intestinal Tubes. Intestinal tubes differ from gastric tubes in two important ways: (1) the greater length, and (2) the presence of a balloon at the distal end that serves as a bolus to help intestinal tubes pass through the GI tract. Miller-Abbott, Cantor, and Baker tubes are all intestinal tubes (Figs. 42–17, 42–18, and 42–19); Miller-Abbott and Cantor tubes have balloons attached to the distal end. The balloons act as a bolus and are filled with a nonpoisonous mercury to give weight and

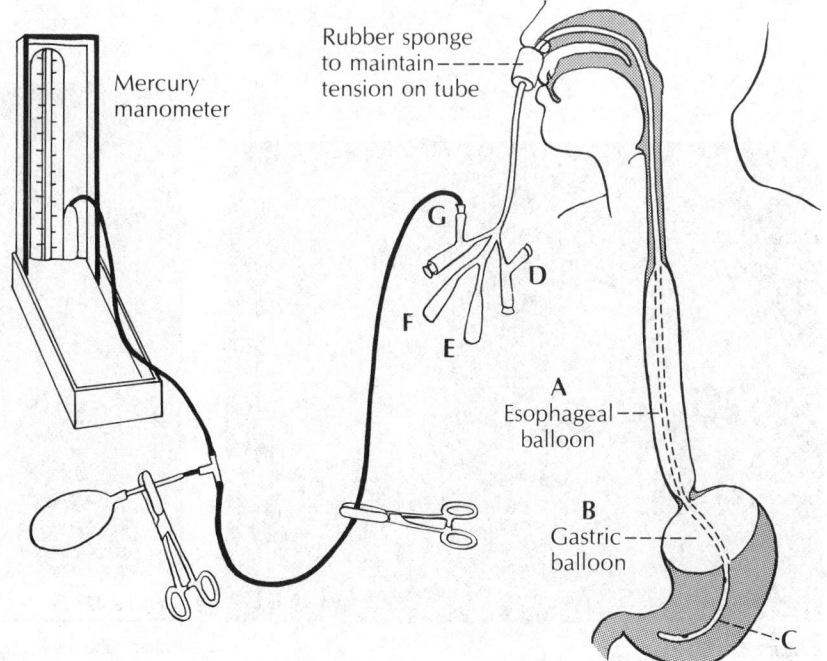

Minnesota tube in place and attached to gastric balloon pressure-monitoring equipment (see Fig. 42–14 for explanation of ports).

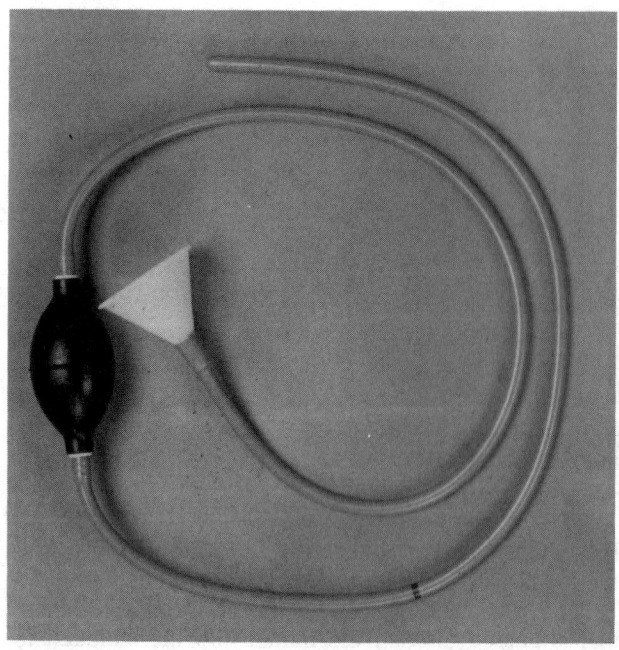

▲ *Figure 42–16*

Ewald tube for emergency removal of stomach contents.

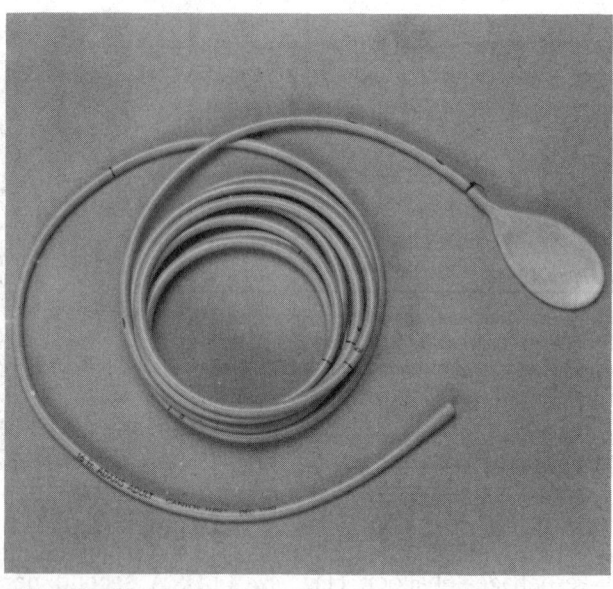

▲ *Figure 42–18*

Cantor tube. Mercury must be injected directly into balloon before tube is inserted. Used for aspirating intestinal contents.

stability. The Baker tube is not weighted but has an inflatable balloon to serve as a bolus.

Intestinal tubes differ from each other in the number of lumens. The Cantor tube has only a single lumen. Therefore, mercury must be injected, with a needle and syringe, directly into the balloon before the tube is inserted (see Fig. 42–18). The Miller-Abbott tube has two lumens, one for aspiration of intestinal secretions and gas and the other for filling the balloon. This tube is inserted into the stomach and the balloon filled with

mercury to promote passage into the intestine by gravity and peristalsis (see Fig. 42–17).

The Baker tube also has two lumens, one for balloon inflation and the other for suction (see Fig. 42–19). Miller-Abbott and Cantor tubes have been largely replaced by the Baker tube, a 270-cm (9-ft), 15-ml balloon-tipped tube used to decompress dilated bowel. The tube is usually inserted during abdominal surgery and exits the body through an abdominal wall incision. During surgery the tube will sometimes be passed into

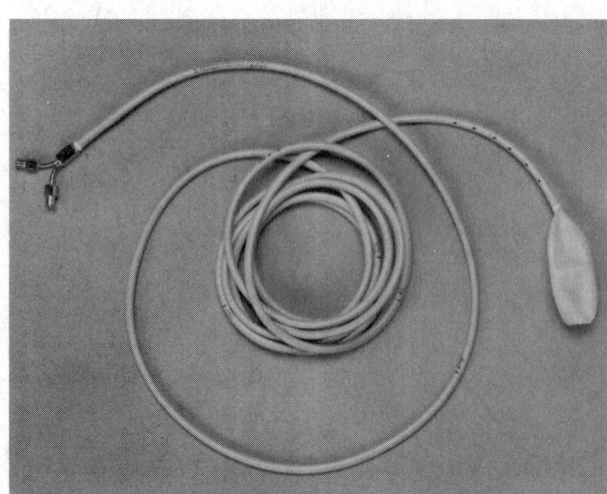

▲ *Figure 42–17*

Miller-Abbott tube for aspiration of stomach contents.

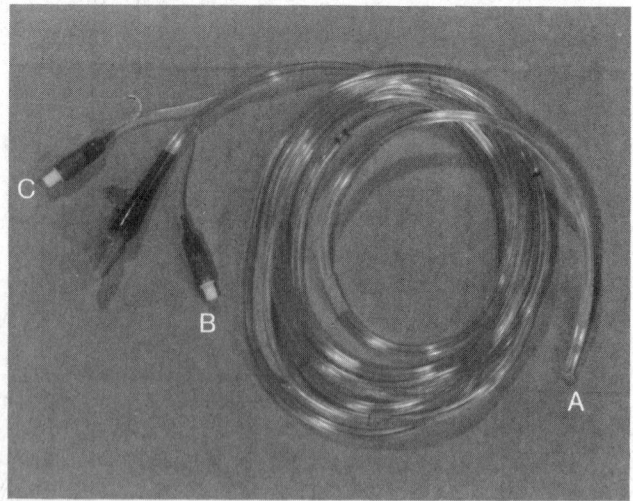

▲ *Figure 42–19*

Baker tube used for decompressing intestine and preventing adhesions following surgery. *A,* Balloon; *B,* balloon inflation lumen; *C,* drainage lumen.

the bowel through the nose. The Baker tube is often used to prevent adhesions after surgery on the bowel. The presence of the tube in the bowel keeps it from forming acute angles, so that adhesions are less likely to develop.

When caring for a person with an intestinal tube, read the instructions carefully and be certain you understand them before beginning to work with the particular tube. These tubes differ in the volume of the balloon. There are also specific requirements for the type of mercury and the size of the needle for insertion, as well as safety precautions specific for each tube.

Specialized Feeding Tubes. Feeding tubes may be placed through the nose or mouth into either the stomach or small intestine. Tubes designed for feeding are smaller and more pliable than other gastric or intestinal tubes (Fig. 42–20). Because the silicone rubber surface is less irritating to the mucosa, these tubes produce less trauma. In addition, the tubes are so small that persons can eat small bites of regular table food (if indicated) while the tube is in place. Thus the person can have the oral stimulation and satisfaction of food while meeting nutritional requirements through the formula that is fed through the tube.

Many of the feeding tubes have weighted tips, usually with tungsten or, less frequently, with mercury. Some require stylets to stiffen the tube and assist in placement. The nurse inserts a feeding tube into the stomach. The tube can be assisted to pass into the duodenum by positioning the client on the right side and allowing gravity to act. Placement into the duodenum may be done by the physician. The risk of aspiration is smaller if the tube is placed in the intestine.

Gastrostomy or jejunostomy tubes are also used for enteral feeding. These tubes have a single lumen and are surgically placed in the stomach or jejunum through an opening in the abdominal wall. They are anchored internally by a balloon or mushroom-style design and usually have a disk or plate to stabilize the tube exter-

nally and prevent displacement into the stomach (Fig. 42–21). After the tract has healed, these tubes can be removed and replaced by the nurse. Tubes that have internal disks for stabilization cannot be removed by the nurse.

Occasionally a Foley catheter will be surgically implanted in the stomach to serve as a feeding tube. Because the Foley catheter is not designed to withstand gastric acidity (pH 1.5 to 3.5) and has no external stabilizer, the physician should replace the Foley catheter with a gastrostomy tube once the tract has healed. Enteral feedings can be given either as a bolus (concentrated mass) or as an intermittent or continuous feeding.

Gastrostomy and jejunostomy tubes are flushed with water before and after feedings. The tube is clamped when not in use. Active persons who need this nutritional route can be provided with a device that has an external cap that closes flush with the abdominal wall to prevent air from entering the tube.

The Physics of Tube Drainage. Before inserting a gastrointestinal tube, you must understand the following principles of physics:

▶ Pressure difference. Pressure is equal to the amount of force per unit of area. Pressure difference is the difference between force per unit area in one area and the force per unit area in another area. Recall from physics that liquids flow readily from an area of higher pressure to an area of lower pressure. For example, when a garden hose lies on the ground, water flows out of its open end because the pressure outside the hose is considerably less than the pressure inside.

▶ Viscosity. Viscosity refers to the thickness or thinness of a fluid. The thicker, or more viscous, fluid travels more slowly through a tube. Thus, thick bloody gastric drainage will move more slowly through a Levin or sump tube than the normal clear fluid gastric secretions.

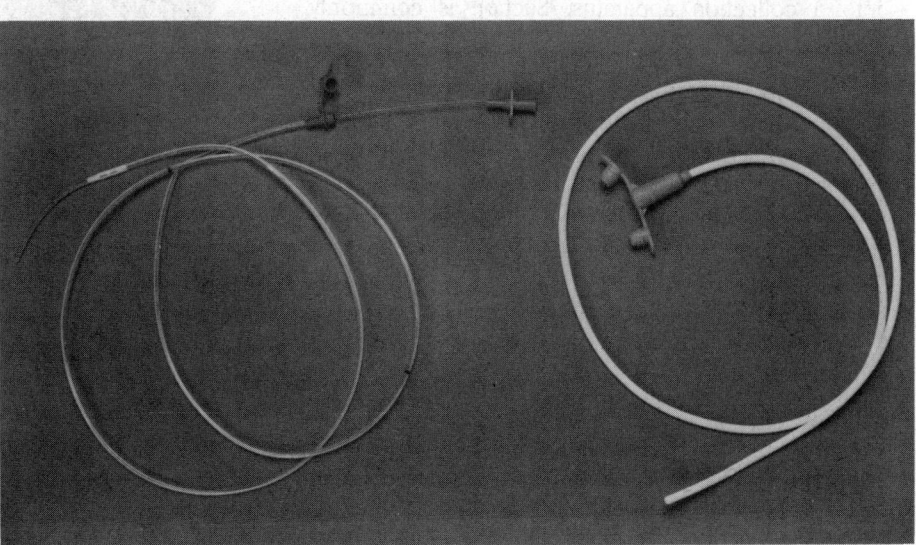

▲ *Figure 42–20*

Feeding tubes. *A,* Weighted feeding tube with stylet partially inserted. *B,* Unweighted tube with flow-through medication port.

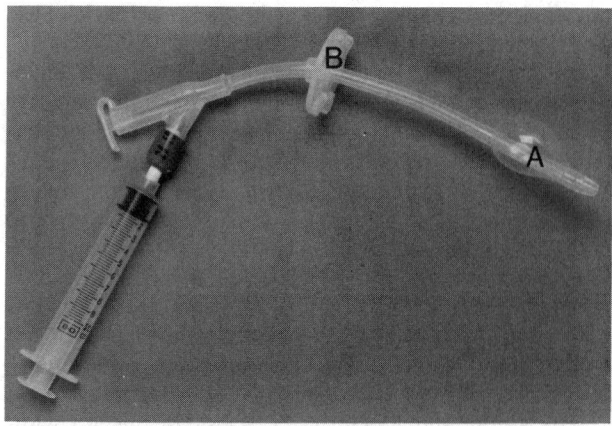

▲ *Figure 42-21*

Gastrostomy tube with syringe inserted to inflate gastric balloon. *A,* Gastric balloon. *B,* Soft plate to hold tube in place on external abdominal wall.

▶ Diameter of tube. Fluids generally move more easily through a tube with a large internal diameter (lumen) than through one with a small diameter.

The smaller the diameter of the lumen, the greater the pressure on the liquid within the tube.

Many tubes used for health care are calibrated on a French (Fr) scale. The lower the number, the smaller the external diameter and often the lumen. For example, a size 12 Fr tube has a smaller external diameter than a size 18 Fr. A tube with thin walls might have a larger internal diameter, however, even though its French size is smaller than that of another tube.

▶ Length of tube. Length is the measurement of the tube from one end to the other, usually stated in inches or centimeters. Fluid generally flows more slowly through a very long tube than through a shorter one. The slower rate is a result of friction created between fluid molecules and tube walls.
▶ Suction. Suction is the use of subatmospheric pressure (negative pressure) to pull secretions or gas into a collection apparatus. Suction is commonly used to increase the pressure difference and hence increase the rate at which a fluid will flow. When applied to GI tubes, suction may be used to (a) prevent or treat postoperative distention (particularly after surgery on the digestive tract); (b) hasten removal of dangerous substances (poison) from the stomach before absorption; (c) remove blood or secretions quickly from the GI tract; and (d) empty the stomach before surgery.

When suction is applied to GI tubes, it is important to ensure that accumulated gas and fluid are removed without traumatizing the GI mucosa. Generally, intermittent low suction may be applied safely. Use of high continuous pressure with a single lumen tube may injure the GI mucosa. A sump tube or a tube with many drainage eyes (holes) can protect the mucosa.

Most acute health care facilities have built-in wall suction units. You can select continuous or intermittent suction and high or low pressure by turning a dial to the appropriate setting. A Gomco pump is a portable electric suction apparatus used in many health care facilities (Fig. 42-22). The Gomco provides intermittent suction that can be adjusted to give high (120 mm Hg) or low (90 mm Hg) pressure. Whatever type of apparatus is used, the nurse must check the vacuum source frequently to ensure its proper function.

All principles of physics affect the flow of fluids through a GI tube. For example, a short, wide-lumen tube hooked to suction will drain faster than a narrower, longer tube that drains to gravity. Thinner or less viscous drainage will also flow faster, whereas a tube may become obstructed with very viscous drainage. The rate at which a fluid flows depends on its viscosity, the pressure differences, the diameter of the lumen, and the length of the tube through which the fluid is moving. Flow rate is described as the volume of fluid moving in a stated period of time (e.g., milliliters per hour, drops per minute, milliliters per day).

Psychologic Preparation for People Requiring Gastrointestinal Intubation. Gastrointestinal intubation is an unpleasant experience, but you can prepare a person psychologically to make the procedure more tolerable. First, assess the knowledge, feelings, and expectations each person has concerning intubation. Ask the person, "Have you ever had a tube put into your stomach through your nose (or mouth) before?" If the answer is in the affirmative, ask the person about the experience, problems encountered, and feelings about the procedure.

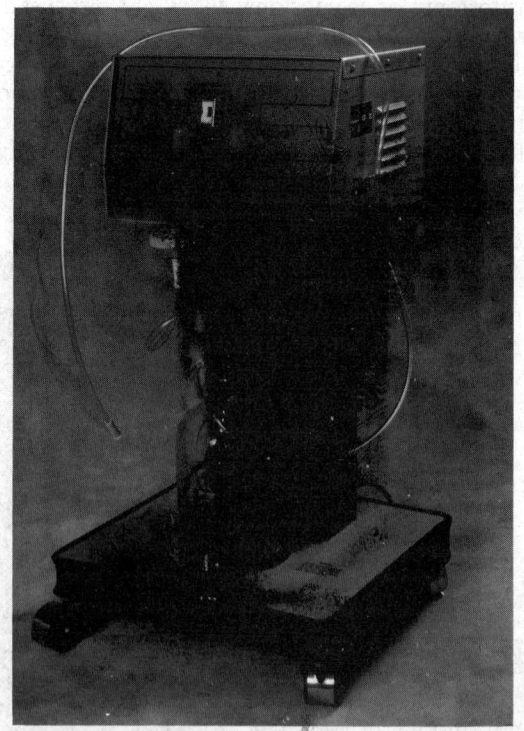

▲ *Figure 42-22*

Gomco portable suction apparatus.

Assess the person's verbal and nonverbal responses to determine knowledge and anxiety level. After this assessment, supplement the information the person already has, or correct any misconceptions. Teaching often allays anxiety and fear and can give the individual some control during the procedure.

Establish a signal for the person to use to tell you to wait a minute during tube insertion. As the tube is being inserted, reinforce participation by supportive comments such as, "You are doing very well." Demonstration of caring may also be helpful (e.g., "I will try to be as gentle as I can"). The nurse's ability to assess, inform, and support the person by confident actions helps assure the successful completion of the procedure.

Preparation of Gastrointestinal Equipment. Different equipment requires different preparation. For example, some plastic and rubber tubes should be refrigerated or placed in ice before use to stiffen them and make insertion easier. Refrigerated tubing also seems to anesthetize the nerve endings, thus facilitating passage of the tube. Large-bore plastic tubes, however, can be too stiff. These can be softened by placing them in warm water for a few minutes. An excessively stiff tube produces more trauma to the mucous membranes when inserted.

For tubes with balloons, be sure to examine the balloon for any holes or tears. Inflate the balloon with air and place it in water to double-check that it is intact. When using intestinal balloons weighted with mercury, prepare the tube according to manufacturer's instructions.

Once you have prepared the person and the equipment, you can perform the intubation as described in Procedure 42-2.

Nursing Intervention for People with Gastrointestinal Tubes. Once a client has a gastrointestinal tube in place, the nurse is responsible for emptying gastrointestinal drainage containers and recording output of drainage. Depending on the tube's purpose, the nurse may also be responsible for administering medications through gastrointestinal tubes and providing required enteral nutrition.

Emptying Gastrointestinal Drainage Containers and Recording Output. The collection apparatus is usually emptied during the end of the nursing shift, and the amount of drainage is recorded on the intake and output record. To empty the drainage canister on a Gomco or similar machine, put on clean gloves. Then clamp the tubing to prevent soiling and remove the lid from the bottle. Keep the underside of the lid clean. There is no need to turn off the suction. Empty drainage into a graduate, measure it and note the character, color, and any odor. Discard the drainage in the dirty utility room. Rinse the canister with cold water. Be sure to follow infection control (universal) precautions. Replace the lid on the drainage canister and unclamp the tube. Check that the suction functions properly. Then remove gloves and wash hands.

Drainage can also be measured by using a "time tape." For this method, place a long strip of tape vertically on the container. At appropriate intervals (e.g., every eight hours) mark the level of the drainage on the piece of tape and include the time of measurement (Fig. 42-27). Record amount on the intake and output record. This method does not allow for accurate observation of the changes in color, odor, and consistency of the drainage.

Administering Medications Through Gastrointestinal Tubes. The administration of medications through a gastrointestinal tube is an important nursing responsibility. In addition to knowing the basic principles of medication administration, you must also master specific skills related to administering through a GI tube. Refer to Chapter 46 for more discussion of this topic.

Intubation for Enteral Nutrition. Enteral hyperalimentation or enteral nutrition—also called gavage feeding or tube feeding—is the process of giving liquid nutrients through a tube into the GI tract. People who may need enteral nutrition include those who (a) are dysphagic (have difficulty in swallowing); (b) have had major oral, esophageal, or throat trauma or surgery; (c) have been unconscious for long periods; (d) have undergone GI surgery; or (e) have developed conditions such as anorexia, malabsorption syndromes, and hypermetabolism. People with chronic illnesses (e.g., cancer) may also be candidates for this therapy. Enteral hyperalimentation may supplement or replace oral intake. It may also be used to feed persons temporarily while weaning them from total parenteral nutrition to regular food.

Routes and Types of Tubes. Routes for tube feeding vary according to the person's condition. Feedings can be given via nasoenteric, nasogastric, or orogastric tubes. In addition to these routes, a physician sometimes performs surgery to place an esophageal, gastrostomy, or jejunostomy tube (see Fig. 42-11).

Types of Feedings. The physician prescribes the amount, frequency, and kind of tube feeding. For tube feedings to nourish a person adequately, the formula must contain sufficient nutrients to do the following:

▸ Meet basal requirements for calories, water, minerals, and vitamins
▸ Replace abnormal losses due to vomiting, diarrhea, or drainage
▸ Supply sufficient protein for tissue synthesis and repair
▸ Supply electrolytes and vitamins necessary for cell growth and tissue healing (e.g., potassium, magnesium, vitamin C, zinc, phosphorus)
▸ Prevent solute overload

Many commercially prepared enteral feeding formulas are available. They differ in osmolality, digestibility, caloric density, lactose content, viscosity, electrolyte content, fat content, and cost. Basic categories of

PROCEDURE 42–2

Insertion of Nasogastric or Nasoenteric Tube

Definition/Purposes. Method of inserting a tube into the stomach or intestine through the nose, for the purpose of instilling food and fluids or withdrawing fluids and gas.

Contraindications/Cautions. Know the anatomy of the GI tract. Stop the procedure and notify the physician if you meet an obstruction. Damage to tissues can result when force is used to advance the tube. Use gloves when caring for people with mouth lesions, especially those with active oral herpes. Without gloves, the nurse caring for a person with oral herpes risks developing herpetic whitlow (painful viral infection of the fingers). If you observe respiratory distress (gasping, coughing, cyanosis) during the procedure, pull the tube back to the oropharynx and wait a few moments before resuming. Have suction equipment available in case the person vomits during the procedure. Insert GI tubes cautiously in a person with myocardial infarction, aortic aneurysm, esophageal varices, thrombocytopenia, or esophageal cancer and stenosis. Many GI tubes (e.g., Sengstaken-Blakemore, Minnesota, Cantor, Miller-Abbott, Baker, and other tubes that are placed directly in the duodenum) are inserted *only* by a physician.

Learning/Teaching Guidelines. Provide the person and significant others with the following information as appropriate: (a) explain the purpose of the tube; (b) explain how the tube will be inserted; (c) tell the person that tube insertion is uncomfortable but reassure the person that you will be as gentle as possible; (d) establish a signal for the person to use to tell you to wait a minute; (e) show the person how to assist with insertion (e.g., drinking fluid through a straw, bending the head forward, swallowing on command, and avoiding touching the tube); (f) tell how long the tube will be left in place and explain how it will feel; (g) explain that the person may be thirsty while intubated and that frequent rinsing of the mouth relieves thirst and keeps the mouth clean; and (h) give information regarding dietary and fluid restrictions (sips of water are sometimes allowed).

PRELIMINARY ACTIVITIES

Assessment/Planning

- ▶ Check diagnosis and purpose of tube.
- ▶ Check physician's and nursing orders.
- ▶ Assess level of consciousness and ability to understand explanations and directions given by the nurse.
- ▶ Assess ability to move, maintain desired positions, and follow directions.
- ▶ Determine whether assistance will be required to insert tube.

Preparations

- ▶ Obtain correct equipment.
- ▶ Check that suction equipment functions properly.
- ▶ Adjust level of bed, placement of bedside stand, lighting as necessary.
- ▶ Provide privacy (pull curtains, close door).
- ▶ Provide appropriate teaching.
- ▶ Drape person's chest to protect clothing.
- ▶ Place tissues and emesis basin within person's reach.
- ▶ Prepare feeding pump if appropriate.

Equipment

- ▶ Gastric tube of appropriate size
- ▶ Water-soluble lubricant
- ▶ Linen protector and emesis basin
- ▶ Glass of cold water and straw (when person is conscious)
- ▶ Suction equipment
- ▶ Clamp
- ▶ Feeding pump when appropriate
- ▶ Basin of ice chips to stiffen rubber tube, if necessary
- ▶ Basin of warm water to soften stiff plastic tube, if necessary
- ▶ Asepto, Toomey, or catheter-tipped syringe
- ▶ Stethoscope
- ▶ Tissues
- ▶ Clean gloves
- ▶ Lidocaine (Xylocaine) jelly
- ▶ Nonallergenic tape and safety pin to secure tube
- ▶ Cotton-tipped swab (e.g., Q-tip)
- ▶ Flashlight or penlight
- ▶ Special container, if necessary

PROCEDURE

Actions

1. Place person in high-Fowler's position. If not possible, tube may be inserted with person in side-lying or supine position.
2. If right-handed, stand on right side of bed (on client's right). If left-handed, stand on left side.
3. Don clean gloves.

4. Request person to blow nose. Select a naris that is patent. Examine naris with penlight for obstruction or deformities.

Rationale/Discussion

1. Facilitates swallowing of water and movement of tube downward through GI tract.

2. Eases insertion for nurse.

3. Prevents direct skin contact with client's body fluids from the mouth and stomach.

4. Attempts to introduce a tube into an obstructed naris or previously fractured nose with deviated septum may cause discomfort and unnecessary trauma. Introduce tube through mouth if naris is obstructed.

PROCEDURE 42–2 Continued

Insertion of Nasogastric or Nasoenteric Tube

Actions	*Rationale/Discussion*
5. Measure distance on tube from tip of nose to ear lobe plus distance from ear lobe to tip of xiphoid process (NEX measurement). Mark distance on tubing with adhesive (Fig. 42–23).	5. Rough guide to determine approximate length of tube to reach stomach.
6. Twist tube in fingers until you find natural downward curve. If no natural curve found, coil tube around hand to create curve.	6. Most tubes have a natural curve when held 15 to 20 cm from tip. A curved tube follows the natural anatomy of the nasopharynx better and thus is easier to insert.
7. Apply topical anesthetic jelly with a cotton-tipped swab (e.g., Q-tip) to inside of selected naris. (First, be sure to check for allergies to anesthetic agent.)	7. Local anesthetic reduces discomfort.
8. Lubricate first 10 cm (4 inches) of tube with water-soluble jelly. If hydromer-coated, moisten first 4 inches of tube with water to activate lubrication.	8. Lubrication reduces friction between mucous membrane and tube. Never use oil: if accidentally introduced into lung, oil will cause pneumonia.
9. Have person slightly flex neck.	9. Facilitates initial insertion of tube.
10. Following natural curve of tube, gently insert it into naris (Fig. 42–24A).	10. Passage of tube is facilitated if it conforms to natural contours of nasal cavity.
11. With person's neck flexed, advance tube to nasopharynx (Fig. 42–24B).	11. Flexion of neck facilitates passage of tube to esophagus. Momentary resistance may occur as tube is passed into nasopharynx (Fig. 42–24B). Withdraw about 1 cm (¼ inch), rotate side-to-side, and gently advance tube (Fig. 42–24C).
12. When tube reaches pharynx, person may gag. Allow a few moments' rest. Tell client to take short, "panting" breaths. If gagging persists, inspect posterior cavity with flashlight for coiled tubing. (If necessary, withdraw tubing to pharynx.)	12. Gag reflex is triggered by presence of tube. Allowing a brief pause before advancing tube may prevent vomiting. Panting relaxes pharynx. Tube cannot be advanced if coiled in pharynx.

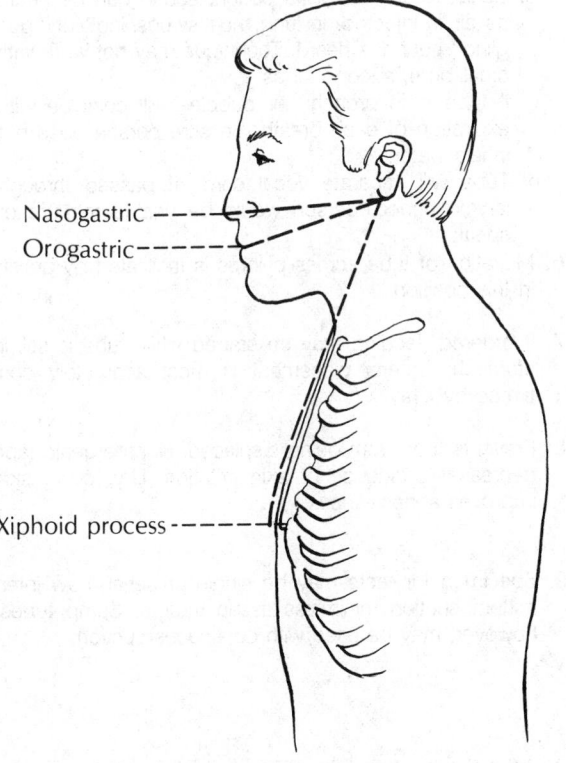

Nasogastric

Orogastric

Xiphoid process

▲ *Figure 42–23*

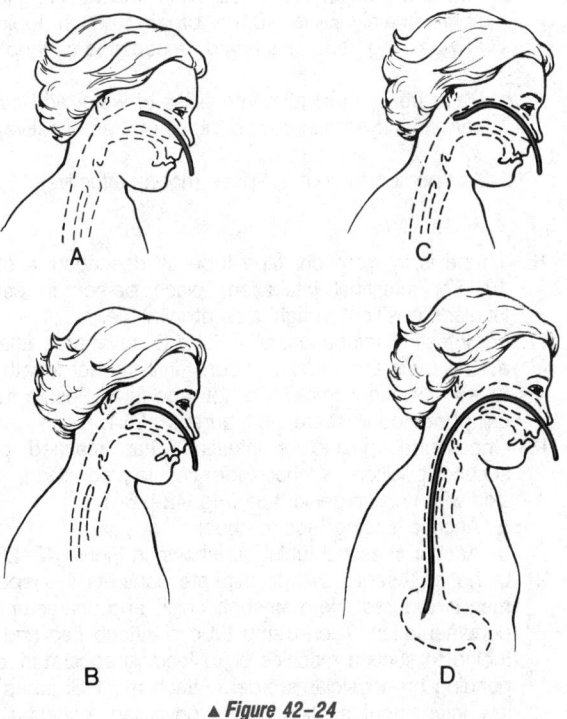

A

B

C

D

▲ *Figure 42–24*

Procedure continued on following page

PROCEDURE 42–2 Continued

Insertion of Nasogastric or Nasoenteric Tube

Actions	Rationale/Discussion
13. Have client take sips of water through straw and swallow on command. Advance tube 7.5 to 13 cm (3 to 5 inches) each time person swallows.	13. Facilitates passage of tube through esophageal sphincter. Having clients swallow on command uses physiologic action to assist in insertion process while tube is being advanced. Advance at reasonable speed to avoid prolonging process.
14. Continue to advance tube gently each time person swallows until you reach point on tube previously marked with tape (Fig. 42–24D).	14. Mark indicates tube might be in stomach.
Stop upon client's signal, or if there is marked resistance. Do not force.	**Caution** Excessive gasping, coughing, or cyanosis is a sign of respiratory distress. Immediately pull back on tube; it may be in trachea. If a small-diameter tube is used, symptoms may not be obvious.
	Caution Vapor forming in tubing may indicate that tube is in trachea.
15. Check placement of tube in stomach with at least two of the following tests:	15. Misplacement is hazardous. Therefore, use at least two tests to confirm placement. Small-bore feeding tubes and intestinal feeding tubes require placement confirmation by x-ray. An x-ray view of the kidney-ureter-bladder will be necessary to confirm tube placement since the chest x-ray film does not include the duodenum.
a. Aspirate for gastric contents with a syringe and test pH with Testape (preferred method).	a. Fluid content cannot be freely aspirated from lungs. Gastric contents will be acidic. Technique may not work with small-bore, silicone tubes.
b. Place stethoscope over stomach and rapidly inject approximately 5 to 10 ml of air through tubing. "Swooshing" sound is heard (acceptable method).	b. Because stomach is a pouch, sound can be heard as air is injected. In lung, no "swooshing" or "gurgling" sound is heard. Technique may not work with small-bore, silicone tubes.
c. Place free end of tube into glass of water and evaluate rhythm of escaping bubbles (not as effective).	c. If tube is in bronchi, air bubbles will coincide with expiration of each breath. Be sure person does not inhale water.
d. Ask person to hum or speak (not as effective).	d. Tube will separate vocal cords if passed through larynx; hence, person would be unable to hum or speak.
16. If tube is in stomach, tape tube as described in step 18. For intestinal intubation, place person in semi-Fowler's position on right side at this time.	16. Migration of tube across pylorus is facilitated by gravity in this position.
17. For intestinal intubation, allow tube to advance a little at a time over a number of hours until correct length of tube has been inserted. Do not tape tube. Secure tube using method illustrated in Figure 42–25A.	17. If ordered, feeding may be started while tube is still in stomach. Enteral placement is most accurately confirmed by x-ray.
18. Once tube (gastric or intestinal) has reached prescribed position, anchor tube securely to clean, dry skin with nonallergenic tape (Fig. 42–26A). a. Anchor feeding tube to cheek. b. Anchor intestinal tubing as shown in Figure 42–26B.	18. Prevents tube from being displaced. Nonallergenic tape decreases incidence of skin irritation. Dry, clean skin improves adhesiveness.
19. Using an Asepto syringe aspirate contents if a specimen is ordered. Note amount, color, and character for documentation. Then clamp tube or attach free end of tubing to suction machine or to feeding apparatus, depending on physician's order. Attach most GI tubes to low intermittent suction unless physician requests another type of suction.	19. Specimen for tests may be single or serial. Low intermittent suction minimizes tissue trauma. Sump tubes, however, may be used with continuous suction.
20. Place adhesive tape tab on tube at point where tube is pinned to gown.	20. Affixing tube to gown reduces "pull" and tension on nose. Tape avoids cutting or occluding tubing by safety pin.
21. Arrange excess tubing to allow person to turn and move in bed.	21. Avoids kinks in tubing and prevents person from inadvertently lying on tube and occluding it.

PROCEDURE 42–2 Continued

Insertion of Nasogastric or Nasoenteric Tube

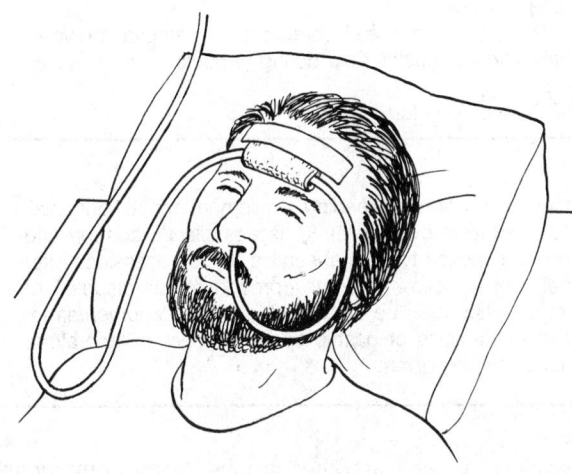

A

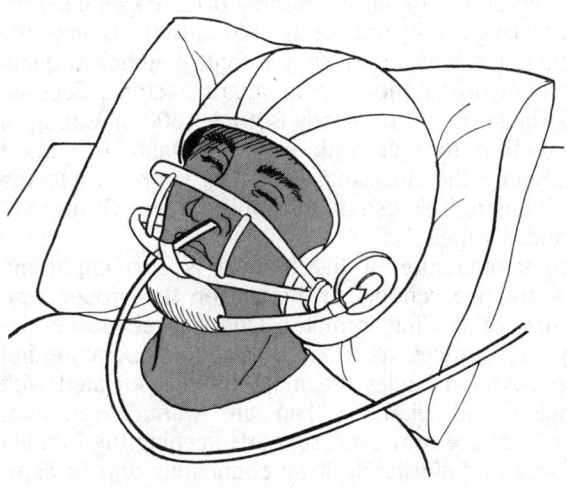

B

▲ Figure 42–25

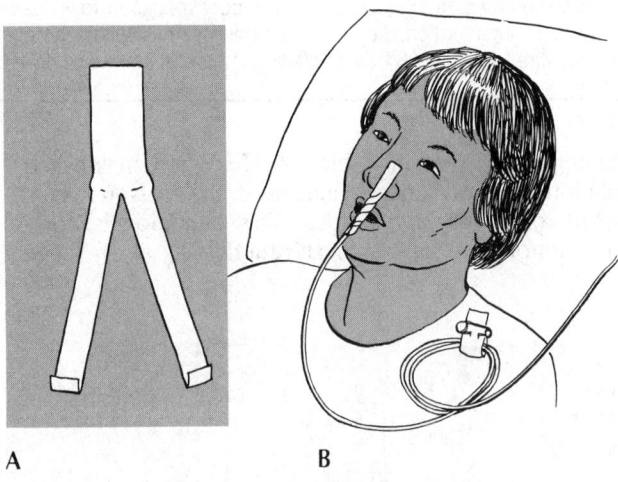

A   B

▲ Figure 42–26

Procedure continued on following page

PROCEDURE 42–2 Continued

Insertion of Nasogastric or Nasoenteric Tube

Actions	Rationale/Discussion
22. Administer oral hygiene. At nostrils, cleanse tubing of lubricant and mucus.	22. Enhances comfort. Avoids crusting of mucus on tube and naris.
23. To remove tube, discontinue suction or feeding equipment. Clamp tube.	23. Removing tube while applying suction damages mucous membranes. Clamping tube prevents escape of gastric fluid during removal.
24. Remove tape used to secure tube. Protect clothing and linen with a linen protector.	24. Tape marks may be removed with tape remover solution if necessary.
25. Request person to take a deep breath and hold it. Pull tube out with one continuous, smooth motion and wrap in towel or drape.	25. Taking a deep breath before tube removal prevents inhalation of gastric fluid during removal.
26. Give oral and nasal hygiene.	26. Enhances comfort.

FINAL ACTIVITIES

Final assessment: Position person appropriately. Check connections of suction or feeding equipment for airtight seal. Check naris for signs of pressure and excoriation. Arrange tubing to allow for movement, and assess client's comfort and safety. *Aftercare of equipment:* Discard used equipment. Send reusable supplies to central service for reprocessing. After removing a tube weighted with mercury (see section on intestinal tubes), follow agency's procedure for disposal of hazardous waste. Incineration of mercury results in toxic gases. Tungsten tips may be discarded in trash. *Documentation:* Time of intervention, person's response to intubation, amount and characteristics of gastric specimen sent to laboratory, pressure used if attached to suction machine, amount and type of tube feeding given.

---

feedings are listed in Table 42–15. When milk-based solutions are prescribed, inquire if the person has a history of lactose intolerance. This condition is common among Asians, African-Americans, and Native Americans, as well as other groups. Many commercial feeding formulas are lactose-free (see Table 42–15).

If the feeding is to be delivered directly into the small intestine, it is important first to choose a formula and method of administration that discourages bacterial growth (e.g., the predigested formulas). Unlike the stomach, the intestine does not contain sufficient quantities of hydrochloric acid to retard bacteria. Second, the formula should be nearly isotonic (300 mOsm/kg of water). If a formula with high osmolality is infused directly into the small intestine, fluid is drawn into the bowel lumen. This osmotic action produces GI discomfort and diarrhea.

The temperature of the formula is also important. There are two schools of thought on the proper temperature for feeding formulas. One side advocates delivery of formulas at room or body temperature because colder formulas are more often associated with cramping and diarrhea than are warmer formulas. Other evidence, however, supports keeping the formula iced when administering it by continuous drip so as to decrease bacterial growth in the feeding bag. With this method, the formula has attained body temperature by the time it reaches the stomach. If the person is sensitive to cold formula, administer feedings at room temperature.

Methods of Feeding. Enteral feedings may be administered through oral or nasal tubes or gastrostomy or jejusostomy tubes by several methods. For many years formulas were given by the bolus method in a belief that such practice would be similar to normal feeding

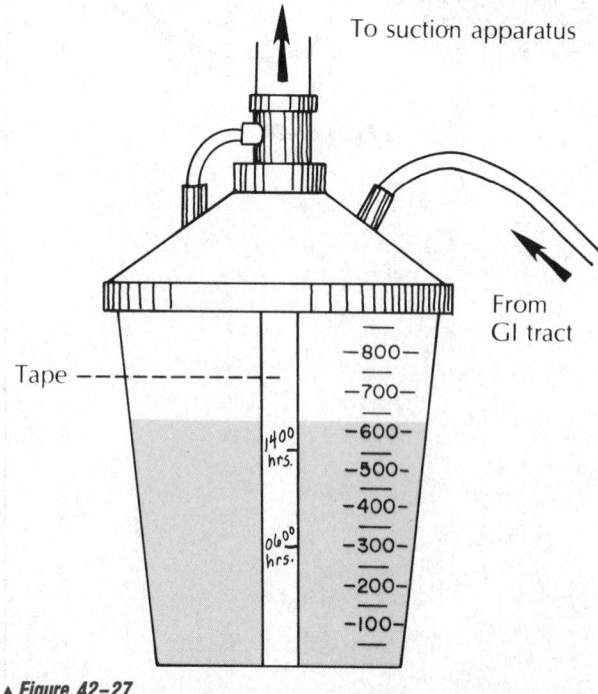

▲ **Figure 42–27**

Time-taping drainage canister. Note times marked on tape. This permits you to see how rapidly drainage accumulates.

patterns. Because a large amount of formula (often 250 to 400 ml) is given in a few minutes, this method frequently causes cramping, with diarrhea, nausea, vomiting, and possible aspiration. Either the intermittent-drip or the continuous-drip method is preferable, as these methods allow the body to adjust to the formula osmolarity.

The continuous-drip method is used if the client's GI tract will not accept a large quantity of feeding at one time. It is also the method of choice for the critically ill and for people fed through the small intestine (duodenum or jejunum). Continuous-drip feeding often prevents complications such as cramping and the dumping syndrome, a phenomenon in which fluids are drawn into the bowel lumen, resulting in massive diarrhea and weakness. The formula may be given by gravity alone or can be administered more precisely by a specialized feeding pump. A feeding pump provides formula at an even rate, which is essential to preventing diarrhea. Diarrhea prevention is particularly vital if the client is very debilitated.

For the intermittent-drip method, the feeding is given periodically, using an administration set and adjusting the drip rate to the client's tolerance. For example, a scheduled feeding of 400 ml is given four to six times a day, with each feeding being given over a period of 30 minutes. People on home tube-feeding regimens often prefer this method.

Specialized Equipment. Originally, equipment for intravenous therapy administration was adapted to provide enteral feedings. As enteral feedings have become more important in nutritional support, however, specialized equipment has been developed to make these feedings easier to administer, safer, and more effective. Some of the administration supplies are illustrated in Figure 42–28. Many of these provide greater convenience. For example, the screw top administration set (Fig. 42–28A) allows a new jar of formula to be added, eliminating the need to rinse the container before adding formula.

Although tube feedings can be given by gravity alone, electronic feeding pumps are often used to maintain a constant flow rate. One type of feeding pump is illustrated in Figure 42–28B. Tubes smaller than 10 Fr require a pump designed especially for enteral feeding to keep them patent.

Do not use IV infusion pumps to control tube feedings, because the higher pressures may damage the feeding tube. In addition, the occlusion alarms are set to be activated by the back pressure of an occluded intravenous site and would not be activated by the back pressure of a distended stomach. If the stomach were full, the IV pump would continue to operate and not sound an alarm. Thus, use of an IV pump carries a high risk of aspiration.

APPLYING RESEARCH TO NURSING PRACTICE

Can Feeding Tubes Handle Metamucil?

Davidson L.J., Belknap D.C., & Flournoy D.J. (1991). Flow characteristics of enteral feeding with psyllium hydrophilic mucilloid added. *Heart & Lung, 20* (4), 404–408.

▼▼▼

Enteral nutrition is a liquid diet that is administered to people through a feeding tube that is inserted into the stomach or duodenum. Unfortunately, diarrhea is a frequent complication of enteral feedings. Factors associated with the incidence of diarrhea include bacterial contamination of the feeding, concurrent administration of antibiotics, and the large amount of water required for the preparation of a carbohydrate-based, liquid diet. Diarrhea can lead to perianal excoriation, skin breakdown, and decubitus ulcer formation. Other complications include electrolyte imbalances that may lead to dehydration, muscle cramping, and heart rhythm irregularities.

To study one possible approach to the management of diarrhea, researchers at the University of Oklahoma mixed tube feedings with psyllium hydrophilic mucilloid (PHM) (Metamucil) in a laboratory setting and observed the flow characteristics. Since PHM binds water and congeals quickly, the problem of feeding tube occlusion had to be considered. In 72 trials, different concentrations of PHM, half- and full-strength feeding formulas, and a range of infusion rates were examined. Allowable periods of interruption of flow, and the differences between room temperature and refrigerated tube feedings, were also evaluated.

One to two teaspoons of PHM, when added to full-strength formulas, resulted in a greater number of successful trials. In contrast, PHM mixed in half-strength formula resulted in a greater number of feeding tube blockages. This may have resulted because PHM attracts water and may congeal in half-strength formulas that contain more water than do full-strength formulas. Even when the tube feeding infusion pump was interrupted for 30 minutes, the liquid feeding with the highest concentration of PHM did not affect tube feeding flow or feeding tube patency. A slower infusion rate did not disrupt successful flow or reduce tube patency. While 10 out of 17 trials with room temperature formula were successful, only one out of 12 refrigerated formula trials with PHM maintained unobstructed flow.

Applications for Practice. To prevent diarrhea in their clients who are receiving tube feedings, physicians may order Metamucil to be added to the formula. When carrying out this order, the nurse should understand that therapeutic doses of one to two teaspoons of Metamucil twice a day do not tend to clog feeding tubes as long as the Metamucil is mixed with full-strength formula that is delivered at room temperature. Following the treatment, the nurse should evaluate whether the addition of Metamucil either prevents the incidence of diarrhea or if diarrhea is present, resolves the problem.

TABLE 42–15. *Enteral Feeding Formulas*

Category/Commercial Formulas	Features	Category/Commercial Formulas	Features
Blenderized — Vitaneed (Organon), Formula 2 (Cutter), Compleat-B, Compleat-Modified (Doyle)	Mimics "home brews" of years ago. Contains ingredients such as beef purée, nonfat dry milk, and corn oil. Recommended for long-term tube feeding. May be useful for diabetic persons to manage blood sugar because of high residue content. Thicker feedings: may obstruct small-bore feeding tubes. Usually contains lactose		feeding slowly and monitor for diarrhea and glycosuria. Expensive. Low viscosity: easy administration in small-bore tubes
		Special Formulas	
		Renal — Amin-Aid (McGaw), Travasorb Renal (Travenol)	Designed for persons with severe renal disease. Provides eight essential amino acids, CHO, and fat. Restricts fluid intake. Available up to 2 kcal/cc. Electrolyte-free or low electrolytes. Expensive
Milk-Based — Meritene (Doyle), Carnation Instant Breakfast (Carnation)	High protein. Requires digestion. Contains lactose. High osmolality		
Lactose-Free — Citrotein, Precision Isotonic Diet, Precision HN Diet (Doyle), Renu (Organon), Isocal, Sustacal, Sustacal HC, Isocal HCN (Mead Johnson), Osmolite, Ensure (Ross), Travasorb Liquid, Travasorb MCT (Travenol)	Designed for persons with lactose intolerance. Available 2 kcal/cc. Higher caloric density useful for hypermetabolic states and for fluid restriction	*Hepatic* — Hepatic Aid (McGaw), Travasorb Hepatic (Travenol)	Designed for persons with chronic, severe liver disease. Formulated to improve protein intolerance in persons with this disorder
Complete Formulas with Predigested Nutrients — Standard Vivonex, High Nitrogen Vivonex (Eaton), Criticare HN (Mead Johnson), VIPEP (Cutter), Vital High Nitrogen (Ross), Travasorb HN, Travasorb STD (Travenol)	Designed for persons with malabsorption states. Contains predigested or elemental nutrients, which can be absorbed by damaged or limited intestinal surface. Hyperosmolar (460–850 mOsm/kg water). Begin	*Modular Feedings* — Microlipid (Organon), MCT Oil (Mead Johnson), Sumacal (Organon), Polycose (Ross), Controlyte (Doyle), Moducal, Casec (Mead Johnson), Pro-Mix (Navaco), Propac (Organon)	Includes single-nutrient sources of CHO, protein, and fat. Enables modification of existing formulas to meet individual needs

This table is not intended to be comprehensive.

Nursing Intervention for People Receiving Enteral Nutrition. In caring for people with tube feedings, it is the nurse's responsibility to

▸ ensure patency (see Procedure 42–3) and confirm placement of the feeding tube (see Procedure 42–2)
▸ administer the correct amount and type of feeding at the correct rate
▸ assess the client's nutritional status, including electrolyte levels
▸ promote comfort
▸ observe and document improvement in the client's condition that might allow for discontinuation of therapy and return to a normal oral intake

To administer a feeding properly, first review the type of formula; the time, frequency, and amount of feeding; and the specific directions for the individual.

Most people need time for their GI tracts to adjust to tube feeding, especially since these structures have often been dormant for days or longer. Feedings are generally started at a low rate and low concentration. If the person tolerates the feeding and does not experience cramping, diarrhea, nausea, vomiting, or hyperglycemia, it is usually safe to increase the rate slowly and then increase the concentration. A protocol for managing the rate and concentration of tube feedings for adults is illustrated in Table 42–16.

Before each feeding, explain the procedure to the person and significant others. Always check placement of the tube (Procedure 42–2). Be aware that injecting air into small-bore tubes is not always an accurate way to determine placement in the stomach. Small-bore tubes can lodge in the bronchus without causing respiratory distress. Also, you may still hear the whooshing

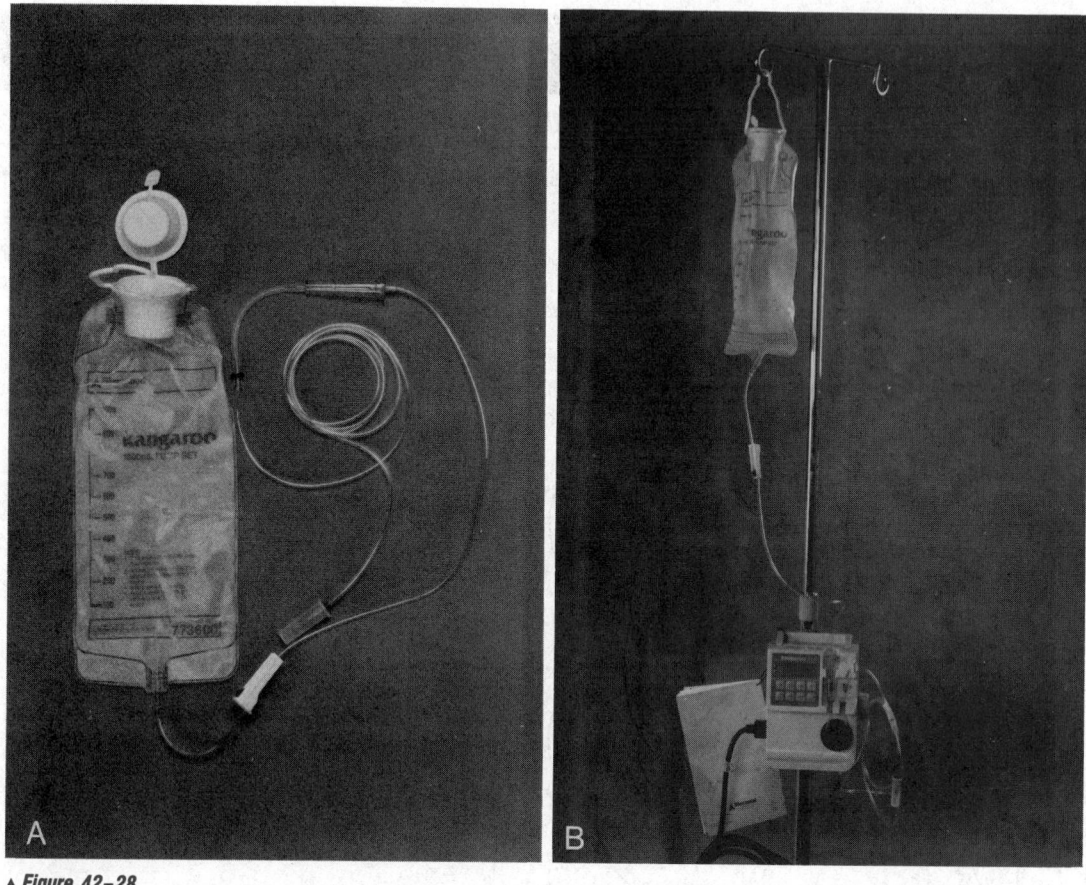

▲ *Figure 42-28*

Some administration supplies. *A*, Enteral feeding container and administration set for feeding pump. *B*, Feeding pump.

sound over the epigastric area even though the tube is not in the stomach. Therefore, gently aspirate gastric contents with a syringe. X-ray confirmation is the best way to ensure proper placement, but this method is impractical in most situations. It is used almost exclusively to confirm initial tube placement.

Check gastric residuals by aspirating stomach contents before each feeding or every 4 to 8 hours. A residual greater than 50 per cent of the previous hour's intake indicates delayed emptying. Notify the physician. Reinstill the residual feeding to prevent excessive fluid, electrolyte, and enzyme losses.

To administer the feeding, place the client in a sitting position, unless contraindicated. Wash your hands and pour the formula into the feeding bag. Attach the bag to the administration set and let the solution flow through the set to remove all air. Clamp the tubing. Connect the tubing to the feeding tube and start the feeding by releasing the clamp on the tubing. Turn on the feeding pump, if appropriate.

Observe the person's reaction to the feeding. If abdominal cramps or diarrhea develop, you should decrease the infusion rate. If the cramps continue, stop the infusion and notify the physician.

When the feeding container must be refilled with formula, clamp the feeding tube and disconnect the

bag and administration set. Rinse the bag and tubing with clear water. Refill the bag and prime the tubing before reconnecting to the feeding tube. These actions reduce the risk of infection and eliminate discomfort from air entering the stomach. Following intermittent or bolus feedings, flush the feeding tube with 15 to 30 cc of water to clear the tubing of formula before disconnecting the administration set and clamping the feeding tube.

After the feeding, encourage the person to remain in a sitting position or with head elevated at least 30 degrees for at least 30 minutes. If this position is not tolerated, place the person on the right side with the head of the bed slightly elevated to encourage gastric emptying and discourage regurgitation and aspiration of stomach contents. For continuous feedings, the person should have the head elevated at 30 degrees if the tube is placed in the stomach. A person who cannot tolerate the head elevation should have a feeding tube placed in the duodenum, or a gastrostomy or jejunostomy should be considered to reduce the risk of aspiration.

Wash reusable equipment and discard disposable equipment. Wash your hands. Make sure the person is comfortable and place the call light within easy reach. Chart the time of feeding, amount of formula and water given, amount of residual, and response to the feeding.

PROCEDURE 42–3

Irrigation of Gastrointestinal Tubes

Definition/Purpose. Process of flushing a gastric tube with solution to maintain or re-establish patency of tubing when feeding formula or drainage is thick or the tube is blocked by obstruction.

Contraindications/Cautions. Contraindicated for a person with a new gastrectomy because instillation of fluid into the gastric tube stimulates the stomach to secrete fluids, causing increased loss of electrolytes. Use gentle irrigation (under low pressure) if gastric hemorrhage has occurred. Never use syringes smaller than 50 ml. Higher pressures generated by smaller syringes may damage gastric mucosa.

Learning/Teaching Guidelines. Provide the client with the following information as appropriate: (a) the purpose of the intervention and (b) each step of the intervention if the person is to be discharged with a tube (Fig. 42–29).

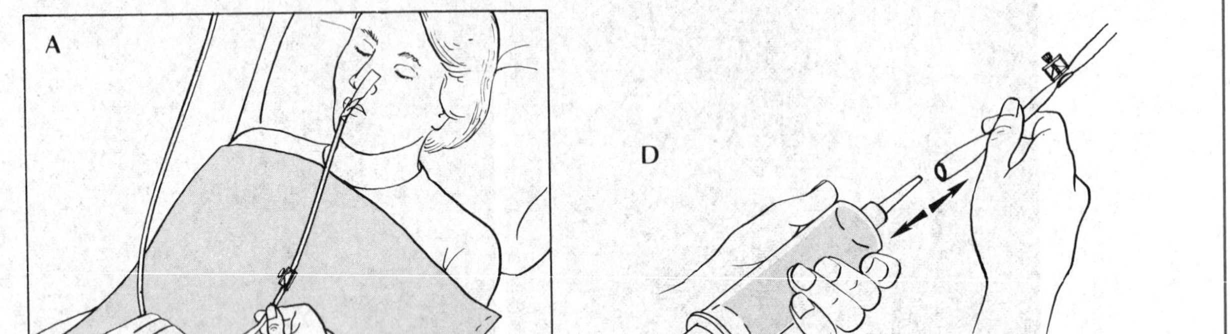

▲ Figure 42–29

PROCEDURE 42-3 Continued

Irrigation of Gastrointestinal Tubes

PRELIMINARY ACTIVITIES

Assessment/Planning

▶ Check diagnosis, date of surgery if relevant.
▶ Check type of intubation and reason for use.
▶ Assess fluid and electrolyte status.
▶ Check physician's order for irrigation and type of irrigant.
▶ Learn reason for irrigation.
▶ Obtain approval of physician for irrigation if necessary.
▶ Assemble equipment for irrigation.
▶ Pour 30 to 200 ml of irrigant into container, as ordered (usually water is used for feeding tubes and normal saline is used for decompression tubes). See Figure 42-30 for a typical container.

Equipment

▶ Disposal irrigation tray (or container for irrigation solution, catheter-tipped syringe, protective drape, antiseptic swab, drainage basin)
▶ Clean gloves
▶ Irrigant (usually isotonic saline or water)
▶ Graduate

Preparation

▶ Provide privacy.
▶ Place bed at working height.
▶ Check tubing for kinks or external pressure.
▶ Ask person to report feelings of fullness or nausea.

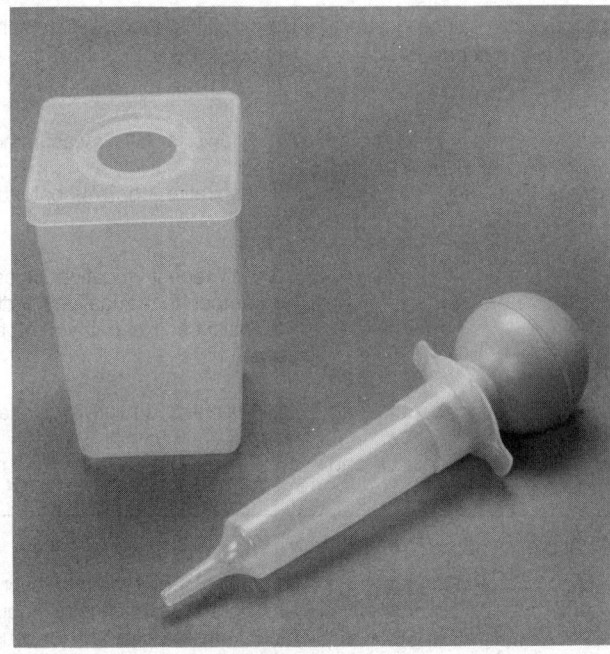

▲ *Figure 42-30*

PROCEDURE

Actions

1. Wash hands and put on clean (nonsterile) gloves.
2. Place protective drape over area of bed where tube is to be disconnected or irrigant introduced.
3. Determine correct placement of tube in stomach (see Procedure 42-2).
4. Fill syringe with amount and kind of solution ordered (usually 30 to 50 ml of water or isotonic saline).
5. Clamp tubing proximal to place where tubing is to be disconnected. Disconnect GI tube from connecting tube (Fig. 42-29A). Place a cap on connecting tubing and place end of tubing on protective drape.

Rationale/Discussion

1. Protects both client and care giver.
2. Prevents spilling of gastric drainage or irrigating solution on bed linen.
3. Prevents instillation of fluid into lungs, which could cause aspiration pneumonia.
4. Isotonic solution maintains osmotic pressure and thus reduces loss of electrolytes from GI tract.
5. Clamping prevents backflow of gastric contents. Always use rubber-shod forceps to prevent damage to tubing when clamping.

Procedure continued on following page

PROCEDURE 42–3 Continued

Irrigation of Gastrointestinal Tubes

Actions	Rationale/Discussion
6. Insert tip of syringe into main lumen of tube and un-clamp.	6. Maintains a closed system.
7. Holding syringe, inject solution slowly and gently (Fig. 42–29*B*).	7. Take care not to introduce air, which might cause gastric distention and accompanying pain.
8. If much resistance is met, check tubing again for kinks or mechanical obstruction and have person turn from side to side. If resistance persists, notify physician.	8. Instilling solution with much force may be hazardous. A sudden, forceful injection against mucosa may cause injury. Turning uses gravity to help change location of "eye" of tube.
9. If no resistance is encountered, after injecting solution into tube, release Asepto syringe bulb (or pull back on plunger, if using a Toomey syringe) to withdraw fluid from the tube (Fig. 42–29*C*).	9. Fluids flow from area of greater pressure to area of lesser pressure.
10. If no fluid returns, have person turn side-to-side, with syringe still attached. If still no return, untape tube and adjust it slightly, then retape. Notify physician if unable to aspirate or if fluid does not return.	10. "Eye" of tube may be against wall of stomach. Turning may dislodge it and allow fluid to drain. Adjust by advancing or pulling back on tube. Do not adjust position of tube after gastric surgery without consulting surgeon. Adjusting tube may damage suture lines.
Do not untape tube if placed by physician during gastrointestinal surgery. Notify the physician if patency is not restored.	Do not kink tube in stomach by advancing it too far or remove it by pulling it too far.
11. If fluid returns, collect aspirated contents in graduate as appropriate.	11. Allows for later measurement.
12. Instill and withdraw fluid several times until fluid flows freely.	12. Aspiration confirms patency.
	Do not repeat irrigation unless necessary to clear tube. Remember that irrigations further disturb fluid and electrolyte balance. Keep track of type and amount of solution used.
13. Reclamp the tubing as in step 5. Disconnect tubing from irrigator (Fig. 42–29*D*).	13. Maintains a relatively closed system.
14. Reconnect tubing to suction or feeding apparatus and release clamp (Fig. 42–29*E*).	14. Re-establishes suction or continuous feeding.

FINAL ACTIVITIES

Position person comfortably. Assess comfort and safety. *Aftercare of equipment:* Observe for proper functioning of suction or feeding equipment, and check that connections are tight. Clean irrigation equipment. Unless it is grossly contaminated or sterile equipment is required, irrigation equipment may be cleaned for reuse. Discard irrigation solution after 24 hours. *Documentation:* Time of irrigation; amount and type of solution used; color, odor, consistency, and amount (absence or excess) of drainage. Immediately report inability to irrigate tube and untoward reactions. Record amount and type of irrigant and drainage on intake and output record as appropriate.

Note whether the sputum becomes the color of the tube feeding, a sign of possible regurgitation. Return to check on the person in 20 minutes, or sooner if warranted.

Nursing management of the person receiving an enteral feeding is based upon the same principle as caring for someone with a nasal or oral tube for other purposes (Tables 42–17 and 42–18). Be alert to potential complications associated with enteral feeding. Become involved with other members of the nutritional team (e.g., the physician, pharmacist, and nutritionist) in assessing the results of the feeding program.

Nursing Intervention for People with Gastrostomy or Jejunostomy Tubes. The procedure for administering tube feedings through a gastrostomy or jejunostomy is the same as that for oral or nasogastric tube feedings. An Asepto (catheter-tip) syringe may be attached to the gastrostomy tube to administer a bolus feeding. The tube is flushed with 30 cc of water after

TABLE 42–16. Protocol for Managing the Rate and Concentration of Continuous Tube Feedings for Adults

	Strength	Rate
4–8 hr	½ strength	42 cc/hr
8–16 hr	½ strength	84 cc/hr
16–24 hr	½ strength	125 cc/hr
24 hr	¾ strength	125 cc/hr
30 hr	Full strength	125 cc/hr

The times may be increased at each step until the person adjusts to formula feeding. It is important to increase either the rate or the strength but not both at one time. Do not increase either rate or strength if the person has diarrhea or cramping.

the feeding. With the jejunostomy, a continuous-drip method should be used to prevent diarrhea or the dumping syndrome. In addition, because the jejunostomy bypasses the gastric acid barrier, the nurse must be especially careful to use infection control precautions.

The skin surrounding the tube should be washed daily and as necessary with a non-ionic cleanser such as normal saline or a commercial non-ionic cleanser. The insertion site should not be covered with a dressing but should be left open to air. A dressing would hold moisture on the skin and increase the risk of maceration and skin breakdown. For more information about appropriate cleansers and wound care, see Chapter 48.

Implementing a Home Enteral Feeding Program. Persons who require long-term enteral nutritional sup-

TABLE 42–17. Nursing Diagnoses and Interventions for Persons with Nasogastric/Enteric Tubes

Nursing Diagnosis	Nursing Interventions
Body Image Disturbance R/T anxiety over presence of tube	Establish rapport with person and family Encourage verbalization of feelings about tube Encourage participation in plan of care to increase sense of self-worth and control
High Risk for Injury R/T abdominal distention secondary to improper tube function	Monitor for indication of improper functioning of suction system: increased abdominal discomfort nausea and vomiting no drainage in collection bottle Observe for proper functioning of suction Check that tubing is patent and free from kinks Check tube position Change person's position in bed every 2 hours Irrigate tube as necessary to keep patent Observe amount, color, frequency, and odor of drainage
Altered Oral Mucous Membrane R/T dryness secondary to mouth breathing following placement of tube in nose	Apply water-soluble lubricant to lips Provide saline gargles periodically Provide mouth care with toothbrush and paste three times daily
High Risk for Impaired Skin Integrity R/T potential pressure/irritation from tube in nares	Observe nares for signs of pressure Tape tube so that pressure is not applied to nares Keep nares free from secretions Change tape when wet or soiled, and retape at different site
Sensory/Perceptual Alteration, Gustatory, R/T decreased acuity secondary to effects of NPO status	Observe oral cavity daily; if white plaques appear in throat, obtain an order for an antifungal agent as indicated (e.g., mycostatin) Provide frequent oral hygiene Give hard candy or gum if allowed, to stimulate salivary glands Encourage use of flavored mouthwash Place bed so that others cannot be observed eating at mealtimes

Table continued on following page

TABLE 42–17. Nursing Diagnoses and Interventions for Persons with Nasogastric/Enteric Tubes Continued

Nursing Diagnosis	Nursing Interventions
Impaired Physical Mobility R/T presence of equipment	Arrange tube to allow freedom of movement without pulling on tube Clamp tube or provide rolling IV pole with battery-operated feeding pump to assist ambulation Teach active or provide passive ROM as necessary Assist with frequent position changes in bed
Ineffective Airway Clearance R/T ineffective coughing secondary to tube discomfort	Encourage deep breathing, turning, and coughing every 2 hours Use lozenges or anesthetic spray as ordered and needed to decrease discomfort Monitor for increased temperature, indicating possible respiratory infection Observe color, amount, and odor of sputum
High Risk for Fluid Volume Deficit R/T possibility of removal of excessive gastric or intestinal fluids from tube during decompression*	Monitor for signs of metabolic alkalosis due to excessive loss of HCl and K^+ in gastric secretions (see Chapter 41) Monitor for signs of metabolic acidosis due to loss of base bicarbonate from intestine (see Chapter 41) Replace lost electrolytes with IV fluid or formula as ordered Irrigate tube with normal saline or commercial electrolyte solution to reduce electrolyte loss Monitor laboratory reports on client's electrolyte status Keep accurate I & O record

* Fluid balances and imbalances are discussed in detail in Chapter 41.

TABLE 42–18. Nursing Diagnoses and Interventions for Persons Receiving Enteral Feedings

Nursing Diagnosis	Nursing Interventions

High Risk for Altered Nutrition: Less than Body Requirements R/T dependence on tube feedings	Confirm tube placement periodically and when starting a new feeding
	Check gravity drip rate q 1 hour. Check pump rate q 1 hour
	Refill feeding container q 4 hours, taking care to remove air from tubing
	If pump is being used, be sure cap on feeding container is secure to prevent pumping air into stomach
	Replace weighted feeding tube every 4 weeks
	Maintain tube patency by flushing with 30 ml of water every 4 hours, before and after medications are delivered through tube, and prn
	Flush tube periodically with full-strength cranberry juice followed by water to prevent protein buildup in tube
	Monitor results of feeding program:
	    Weigh daily on same scales with same clothing, at same time of day
	    Observe laboratory reports of blood chemistries and blood counts when ordered
	    Check nitrogen balance studies when ordered

High Risk for Infection R/T possibility of bacterial contamination of formula or feeding equipment	Use medical aseptic technique with feeding equipment Change bag and tubing q 24 hours Do not allow feeding to remain in bag longer than 4 hours Do not add formula to formula in bag (rinse bag and tubing with water before refilling every 4 hours). If administration bag has ice compartment, refill as necessary

***TABLE 42-18.** Nursing Diagnoses and Interventions for Persons Receiving Enteral Feedings*
Continued

Nursing Diagnosis	Nursing Interventions
	Refrigerate and date opened formula containers. Discard unused portion in 24–48 hours
	Bring formula to room temperature before administration, if desired
	Clean spilled formula from pump as necessary
	Assess vital signs, including temperature, q 4 hours
	Observe for diarrhea, which can be caused by bacterial contamination
High Risk for Altered Nutrition: More than Body Requirements R/T potential imbalance between high glucose content of feeding and amount of insulin secreted by pancreas	Check urine sugar and acetone q 4 hours (may be discontinued in nondiabetics after 48 hours if consistently negative)
	Administer formula at constant rate to prevent imbalance between blood glucose and insulin. Do not increase rate if feeding is behind schedule; readjust to correct rate
	Observe for hypo- and hyperglycemia if feeding rate is slow or fast
	Monitor blood sugar (usually daily until stabilized)
High Risk for Aspiration R/T possibility of regurgitation of feeding	Check residual formula q 4 hours by aspirating with Asepto syringe
	Reinstill residual into tube if not excessive
	Slow the feeding rate if excess residual is observed. If residual ≥ 50% of previous hour's feeding, contact physician
	Note whether sputum becomes the color of the tube feeding—a sign of possible regurgitation
	Have suction available for persons with impaired gag reflex
	Elevate head of bed at least 30° during feeding and for 30 minutes after
High Risk for Fluid Volume Deficit R/T possible excess fluid loss or inadequate fluid intake	Monitor for dehydration (fluid loss may occur from excessive diarrhea, excessive protein intake, or osmotic diuresis)
	Monitor for changes in skin turgor, thirst, vital signs, I & O, mucous membrane moisture, level of consciousness, fever, and disorientation
	Monitor electrolytes and BUN results from laboratory
	Keep formula delivery at constant rate
	Observe for osmotic diuresis from high glucose load, particularly if rate is increased
	Record accurate I & O
	Allow extra water intake to replace insensible water loss. If water intake is inadequate, water will be pulled from tissues for excretion
	Observe for diarrhea. Dilute formula if diarrhea is due to hyperosmolar feedings
High Risk for Diarrhea R/T effects of alteration in nutrition	Inform person that decreased frequency of bowel movements is to be expected owing to low-residue feedings
	Observe for diarrhea. May be due to 　bacterial contamination of formula 　lactose intolerance 　osmotic action caused by hyperosmolar fluids 　fecal impaction 　concurrent drug therapy (e.g., antibiotics) 　low serum albumin (check laboratory reports)
	Monitor bowel sounds each shift. Report increased or decreased bowel sounds to physician

Table continued on following page

TABLE 42–18. Nursing Diagnoses and Interventions for Persons Receiving Enteral Feedings
Continued

Nursing Diagnosis	Nursing Interventions
	Discontinue feeding to prevent gastric rupture if the following symptoms are noted: increasing girth large residual (> 50% of amount received during the last hour) epigastric and left upper quadrant pain
Knowledge Deficit R/T lack of previous exposure to feeding regimen	Teach client and significant others about the feeding program and why it is necessary Involve the client and significant others in regimen as appropriate Keep the client and significant others informed of the progress of the program and any changes in the plan of care If client is to be discharged on a home feeding program, teach feeding techniques and infection control precautions to client and significant others. Provide insurance counseling to determine whether they will be able to afford cost of home feeding Encourage client and care giver(s) to practice techniques in health care facility under supervision Adapt facility techniques to use supplies commonly available in home

port but have no need for acute nursing care in the hospital are candidates for home enteral feeding programs (Fig. 42–31). The nurse or nutritionist assesses the home environment and lifestyle before planning the program. Significant others can be very supportive if they are involved in the program.

Choose the formula to fit the person's situation and lifestyle. Determine the availability of refrigeration and storage facilities as well as the ability of the person and significant others to prepare the formula. Cost considerations must be balanced with all the other factors. For example, a powdered formula may be less expensive but impossible to prepare if there is no blender. In such a case, the ready-to-feed formula would be safer and more appropriate. Consider the following questions:

► Does the client have physical, mental, and psychologic limitations that could alter the ability to maintain a home feeding program?
► What are the client's finances? Is funding available to cover the cost of a home feeding program?
► Will the client use a pump to deliver the feeding? Will the person require one that is battery operated and can be taken to a work setting?
► Must the client purchase the pump, or is a loan or rental program available?
► Does the client or significant other have the manual dexterity and eye-hand coordination to manage the feeding program?

A primary nursing responsibility is teaching the client and significant others about the feeding program. The following information should be included:

► Methods of tube maintenance (e.g., confirming tube placement, checking residual, clearing obstructions)
► Prescribed formula, including sources of supply and appropriate storage
► Feeding schedule to suit lifestyle
► Operating the pump and solving problems related to pump failure
► Complications of therapy and prevention and treatment
► Conditions under which to call the home health nurse
► Community resources

EVALUATION

In evaluating the client's response to nutritional interventions, remember to evaluate whether the planned outcomes were achieved. Recall that the expected outcomes related to the three main nutritional diagnoses are very different, depending on whether the client's nursing diagnosis is a deficit of nutrition or an actual or high risk for excess nutrition.

During evaluation, determine whether nutritional care is successful by asking whether the client

► is within the ideal weight range for height and frame
► has triceps folds within the expected norm for gender

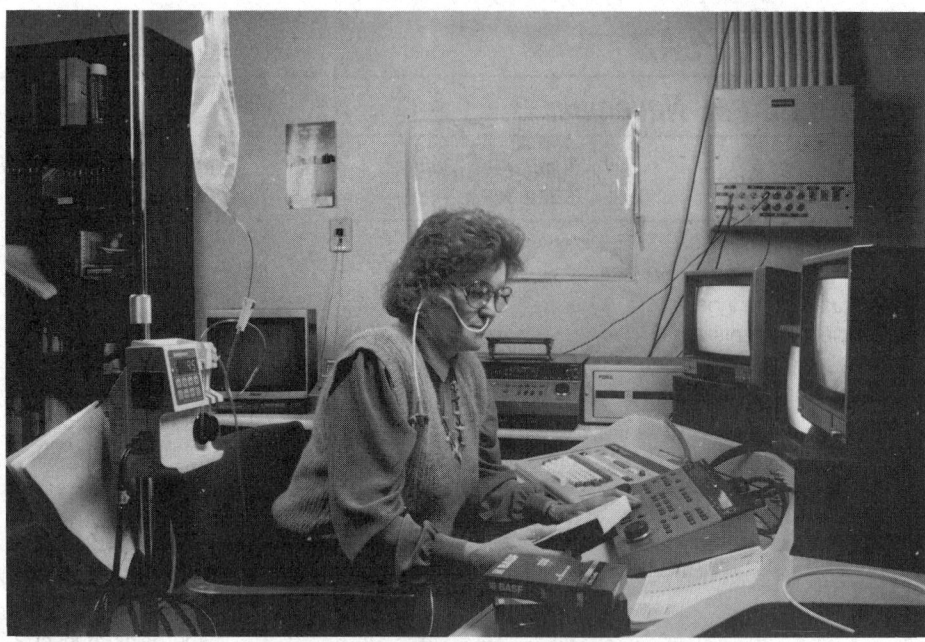

▲ *Figure 42–31*

Some persons return to work and continue tube feedings with a battery-operated pump.

▶ maintains physical signs of good nutrition (see Table 42–9)
▶ demonstrates a functional eating pattern
▶ identifies factors that can lead to poor nutrition
▶ avoids dysfunctional behaviors that can lead to poor nutrition

Of course, each person is unique and must be evaluated individually. Outcomes may not be achievable for some persons for a long time, if ever. These outcomes are, however, objective, external standards against which we are able to measure small or large steps in the right direction.

 ## CASE STUDY

The Client

Melissa Sands, a pale, emaciated, 13-year-old white female was admitted one week ago, after fainting in her exercise class. When she regained consciousness, she denied needing medical assistance, and her parents had to threaten to ground her before she would agree to come to the hospital.

Melissa admitted that she dieted and exercised strenuously and complained that she was "still fat" even though her ribs were protruding and her appearance was gaunt. Her admitting diagnosis was anorexia nervosa.

A partial listing of physician's orders, on admission, included

▶ Strict bed rest for 48 hours
▶ CBC and serum electrolytes
▶ Observe carefully at all times during meals and for 1 full hour after each meal
▶ Regular diet as tolerated with supplemental feeding at HS —monitor and record caloric intake
▶ Institute tube feedings if patient vomits or if intake below 1200 calories

At 6:00 PM, November 3, a partial listing of the admission assessment data included the following:

▶ 13-year-old emaciated female who feels "fat"
▶ Hgt. 63 inches, wgt. 87 pounds
▶ History of daily intake below 600 calories and excessive exercise in relation to caloric intake
▶ Amenorrhea past 3 months
▶ Skin intact, cool, and pale white in color
▶ T 97.4 F, B/P 86/52, P 60, R 16
▶ Parents state Melissa weighed 105 on her birthday 6 months ago

One week has passed since admission. The following represents part of a nursing care plan written for her shortly after admission and the current evaluation of outcomes that were expected at that time.

Case Study continued on following page

CARE PLAN

6:00 PM, November 3

Nursing Diagnosis	Planning: Expected Outcomes	Implementation: Nursing Interventions	Evaluation
Altered Nutrition: Less than Body Requirements R/T inability to ingest sufficient nutrients AEB body weight 20 per cent under ideal for height and age	By 6:00 PM, November 10, 1. Weighs at least 89 pounds	Discuss food preferences with client. Teach types of foods needed to meet daily requirements of a minimum of 1200 calories. Contract with client to allow her to select eating times and food to be eaten as long as she gains at least 2 pounds per week until weight is within normal limits. Closely observe and record caloric intake at and between meals. Observe closely for at least 1 full hour after each intake of food to prevent purging. Promote conservation of energy to prevent loss of calories through excess activities that raise metabolic rate. Weigh each day at 6:00 PM with same (minimal) clothing on. Check clothing for hidden weights.	6:00 PM, November 10: Weight 90 pounds
	2. Exhibits minimal untoward physical effects of nutritional deficiencies	Measure intake and output, including recording of bowel movements. Assess for water and electrolyte imbalances. Assess vital signs q AM.	Intake = output at average of 2000 cc/day Skin warm with good turgor; no muscle twitching, cramping, or weakness; daily electrolytes WNL T 98.2 F, B/P 96/68, P 68, R 18

Summary

▶ To meet clients' nutritional needs, the professional nurse must understand the relationship among gastrointestinal structure and function, nutrition, recommended dietary allowances, calories and body weight, carbohydrates, fats, proteins, vitamins and minerals, fluids, and dietary guidelines for Americans.

▶ Popular concerns about diet and health focus on the relationship between nutrition and food additives, natural and organic foods, food supplements, vitamin and mineral supplements, special foods, and vegetarianism.

▶ A client's dietary intake and nutritional status can be assessed by keeping food and dietary records, completing a physical assessment, taking anthropometric measurements, noting results of biochemical assessments, and understanding the client's feelings about diet changes.

▶ A wide range of biologic, psychologic, social, and cultural factors influence food intake, dietary patterns, and nutritional status.

▶ Special dietary needs exist during each stage of the life cycle from infancy to adulthood, during pregnancy and lactation, and in later maturity.

▶ Data collected with the nursing assessment of dietary intake and nutritional status can be put together with knowledge of good nutrition to diagnose, and plan nursing care for, the client.

▶ Nursing diagnoses appropriate for the client with nutrition problems include *Altered Nutrition: More than Body Requirements; Altered Nutrition: Less than Body Requirements;* and *Altered Nutrition: High Risk for More than Body Requirements.*

▶ Outcomes for clients with nutritional problems include achievement or maintenance of a specific weight, a specific triceps skinfold measurement, and other objective signs of good nutrition; achievement of a functional eating pattern; and movements toward achieving these outcomes.

▶ Nursing interventions include managing diet therapy; improving the appetite, ingestion, digestion, and absorption; and maintaining nutrition when gastrointestinal function is impaired.

▶ Nutritional interventions can be evaluated as successful if the client is within the ideal weight, has normal measurements for triceps skinfolds, shows physical signs of good nutrition, demonstrates a functional eating pattern, and identifies and avoids behaviors that can lead to poor nutrition.

Bibliography

1. ADA Statement (1987). Recommendations concerning supplement usage. *Journal of the American Dietetic Association,* 87, 1342–1343.
2. Adams, C.W. (1990). How tube-feeding complications can develop. *Nursing 90,* 20(3), 59.
3. Adhern, H.L., & Rice, K.T. (1991). How do you measure gastric pH? *American Journal of Nursing,* 91(5), 70.
4. AMA Council on Scientific Affairs (1987). Vitamin preparations as dietary supplements and therapeutic agents. *JAMA,* 257, 1929–1936.
5. American Diabetes Association (1987). Nutritional recommendations and principles for individuals with diabetes mellitus. *Nutrition Today,* 22, 29–35.
6. American Diabetes Association/American Dietetic Association (1986). *Exchange lists for meal planning.* Chicago.
7. American Society for Parenteral and Enteral Nutrition (1986). Guidelines for use of total parenteral nutrition in the hospitalized adult patient. *Journal of Parenteral and Enteral Nutrition,* 10, 441–445.
8. American Society for Parenteral and Enteral Nutrition (1989). Standards for nutrition support: hospitalized pediatric patients. *Nutrition in Clinical Practice,* 4(2), 33–37.
9. American Society for Parenteral and Enteral Nutrition (1991). Standards for nutrition support: hospitalized pediatric patients. *Journal of Parenteral and Enteral Nutrition,* 14(1), 33–37.
10. Anderson, J.W., & Gustafson, N.J. (1988). Dietary fiber and heart disease: current management concepts and recommendations. *Topics in Clinical Nutrition,* 3, 21–29.
11. Anderson, J.W., et al. (1987). Dietary fiber and diabetes: a comprehensive review and practical application. *Journal of the American Dietetic Association,* 87, 1189–1197.
12. Bauernfeind, J.C. (1988). Vitamin A deficiency: a staggering problem of health and sight. *Nutrition Today,* 23, 34–36.
13. Bazyk, S. (1990). Factors associated with the transition to oral feeding in infants fed by nasogastric tubes. *American Journal of Occupational Therapy,* 44, 1070–1078.
14. Benya, R., et al. (1990). Flexible nasogastric feeding tube tip malposition immediately after placement. *Journal of Parenteral and Enteral Nutrition,* 14, 108–109.
15. Bieri, J.G., et al. (1983). Medical uses of vitamin E. *New England Journal of Medicine,* 308, 1063–1071.
16. Bockus, S. (1991). Troubleshooting your tube feedings. *American Journal of Nursing,* 91(5), 24–28.
17. Bommarito, A.A., et al. (1989). A new approach to the management of obstructed enteral feeding tubes. *Nutrition in Clinical Practice,* 4, 111–114.
18. Brownell, K.D. (1984). The psychology and physiology of obesity: implications for screening and treatment. *Journal of the American Dietetic Association,* 84, 406–414.
19. Brownell, K.D. (1987). Obesity and weight control: the good and the bad of dieting. *Nutrition Today,* 23, 34–36.
20. Burkhart, K.K., et al. (1990). Whole-bowel irrigation as treatment for zinc sulfate overdose. *Annals of Emergency Medicine,* 19, 1167–1169.
21. Byrne, G. (1988). Surgeon General takes aim at saturated fats. *Science,* 241, 651.
22. Camp, D., & Otten, N. (1990). How to insert and remove nasogastric tubes quickly and easily. *Nursing 90,* 20(9), 59–64.
23. Caropreso, P., et al. (1990). Moss nasogastric tube and treatment of a perforated esophagus. *Iowa Medicine,* 80, 567–570.
24. Carpenter, K.J. (1986). The history of enthusiasm for protein. *Journal of Nutrition,* 116, 1364–1370.
25. Chernoff, R. (1987). Aging and nutrition. *Nutrition Today,* 22, 4–11.
26. Cho, S.R., et al. (1987). Inadvertent inflation of the balloon: a rare but serious complication of Miller-Abbott intubation. *British Journal of Radiology,* 60, 547–551.
27. Ciocon, J.O. (1990). Indications for tube feedings in elderly patients. *Dysphagia,* 5(1), 1–5.
28. Cleeman, J.I., & Lenfant, C. (1987). New guidelines for the treatment of high blood cholesterol in adults from the National Cholesterol Education Program: from controversy to consensus. *Circulation,* 76, 960–962.
29. Coulston, A.M., & Darbinian, J.A. (1986). Nutrition management in patients with cancer. *Topics in Clinical Nutrition,* 1, 26–36.
30. Dees, G. (1989). Difficult nasogastric tube insertions. *Emergency Medicine Clinics of North America,* 7(1), 177–182.
31. DeJonge, L., et al. (1991). Decreased thermogenic response to food with intragastric vs. oral feeding. *American Journal of Physiology,* 260, (2 Pt 1), E238–242.
32. Desai, M.B., & Jeejeebhoy, K.N. (1988). Nutrition and diet in management of disease of the gastrointestinal tract. In Shils, M.E., & Young, V.R. (eds.). *Modern nutrition in health disease* (7th ed.). Philadelphia: Lea & Febiger.

33. Disten, H.P., et al. (1988). The 1984 report of the Joint National Committee on Detection, Evaluation, and Treatment of High Blood Pressure. *Archives of Internal Medicine,* 144, 1045-1057.

34. Doenges, M.D., & Moorhouse, M.D. (1991). *Nurses pocket guide: Nursing diagnoses with interventions* (3rd ed.). Philadelphia: F.A. Davis.

35. Duke, G.J., & Harding, J. (1990). Pneumothorax from a nasogastric tube (letter). *Anesthesia and Intensive Care,* 18, 265.

36. Eisenberg, P. (1989). Enteral nutrition: indications, formulas, and delivery techniques. *Nursing Clinics of North America,* 24(2), 315-338.

37. Elsas, J.L., & Acosta, P.B. (1988). Nutrition support of inherited metabolic disease. In Shils, M.E., & Young, V.R. (eds.). *Modern nutrition in health and disease* (7th ed.). Philadelphia: Lea & Febiger.

38. Fairbanks, V.F., & Beutler, R. (1988). Iron. In Shils, M.E., & Young, V.R. (eds.). *Modern nutrition in health and disease* (7th ed.). Philadelphia: Lea & Febiger.

39. Faller, N.A. (1991). The gastro-port: an alternative to button. *Journal of Enterostomal Therapy,* 18(1), 39-40.

40. Ferguson, J.M. (1988). *Habits, not diets.* Palo Alto, California: Bull Publishing Company.

41. Friedman, E.G., & Koch, R. (1988). Report from the Maternal PKU Collaborative Study, Metabolic Study. *Metabolic Currents,* 1, 4-14.

42. Frisancho, A.R. (1988). Nutritional anthropometry. *Journal of the American Dietetic Association,* 88, 553-555.

43. Gaffney, L., & Jones, M. (1988). Knotted tubes—complication of the nasogastric tube. *Nursing Times,* 84(7), 48.

44. Glasser, S.A., et al. (1990). Intracranial complication during insertion of a nasogastric tube. *American Journal of Neuroradiology,* 11, 1170.

45. Goldsmith, G., & Patterson, M. (1985). Irritable bowel syndrome: treatment update. *American Family Physician,* 31, 191-195.

46. Greenwald, P., et al. (1987). Dietary fiber in the reduction of colon cancer risk. *Journal of the American Dietetic Association,* 87, 1178-1188.

47. Grundy, S.M., & Nestel, P.J. (1987). Fat and cholesterol, in diet and health: scientific concepts and principles. *American Journal of Clinical Nutrition,* 45(Suppl), 1037-1039.

48. Guenter, P. (1989). Percutaneous endoscopic gastrostomy feeding tube in neuroscience patients. *Journal of Neuroscience Nursing,* 21, 122-124.

49. Harkness, G.A., et al. (1990). Risk factors for nosocomial pneumonia in the elderly. *American Journal of Medicine,* 89, 457-463.

50. Harrel, J.S., & Damon, J.F. (1989). Prediction of patients' need for mouth care. *Western Journal of Nursing Research,* 11, 748-756.

51. Hecker, R.B., et al. (1990). Intra-abdominal palpation of a nasogastric tube in the stomach does not assure appropriate placement. *Southern Medical Journal,* 83, 1223-1225.

52. Herrmann, M.E., et al. (1989). Subjective distress during continuous enteral alimentation: superiority of silicone rubber to polyurethane. *Journal of Parenteral and Enteral Nutrition,* 13(3), 281-285.

53. Hickey, P.W. (1990). *Nursing process handbook.* St. Louis: C.V. Mosby.

54. Ikard, R.W., & Federspiel, C.F. (1987). A comparison of Levin and sump nasogastric tubes for postoperative gastrointestinal decompression. *American Surgeon,* 53(1), 50-53.

55. Kayser-Jones, J. (1990). The use of nasogastric feeding tubes in nursing homes: patient, family, and health care provider perspectives. *Gerontologist,* 30, 469-479.

56. Kirby, D.F., et al. (1986). Percutaneous endoscopic gastrostomies: a prospective evaluation and review of the literature. *Journal of Parenteral and Enteral Nutrition,* 10(2), 155-159.

57. Klahr, S., et al. (1988). The progression of renal disease. *New England Journal of Medicine,* 318, 1657-1666.

58. Kohn, C.L., & Keithly, J.K. (1989). Enteral nutrition: potential complications and patient monitoring. *Nursing Clinics of North America,* 24(2), 339-353.

59. Mahan, L.K., & Rees, J.M. (1984). *Nutrition in adolescence.* St. Louis: C.V. Mosby.

60. Mamer, J.J. (1987). Percutaneous endoscopic gastrostomy: a review. *Nutrition in Clinical Practice,* 10(2), 65-75.

61. Marcuard, S.P., et al. (1989). Clearing obstructed feeding tubes. *Journal of Parenteral and Enteral Nutrition,* 13(1), 81-83.

62. Martin, R.J., & Mullen, B.J. (1986). Control of food intake: mechanisms and consequences. *Nutrition Today,* 22, 4-10.

63. McKeating, J., et al. (1990). Fatal aortoesophageal fistula due to double aortic arch: an unusual complication of prolonged nasogastric intubation. *Journal of Pediatric Surgery,* 25, 1298-1300.

64. Meer, J.A. (1989). A new nasal bridle for securing nasoenteral feeding tubes. *Journal of Parenteral and Enteral Nutrition,* 13, 331-334.

65. Metheny, N., et al. (1989). Effectiveness of pH measurements in predicting feeding tube placement. *Nursing Research,* 38(5), 280-285.

66. Metheny, N., et al. (1990). Effectiveness of the auscultory method in predicting feeding tube location. *Nursing Research,* 39(5), 262-267.

67. Mezitis, N.H. (1988). Nutritional management in liver disease. *Nutrition in Clinical Practice,* 3, 108-112.

68. Moore, F.D. (1986). Current thoughts on malabsorption: parenteral, enteral, and oral feeding. *Journal of the American Dietetic Association,* 86, 1169-1170.

69. Munro, H.N. (1985). Nutrient needs and nutritional status in relation to aging. *Drug-Nutrient Interactions,* 4, 55.

70. Nash, J.D. (1987). Eating behavior and body weight: physiologic influences. *American Journal of Health Promotion,* 1, 5-12.

71. National Institutes of Health, USD-HHS (1986). *Nonpharmacological approaches to the control of high blood pressure; Final report of the Sub-committee on Detection, Evaluation, and Treatment of High Blood Pressure.* National Heart, Lung, and Blood Institute. Bethesda, Maryland: US Government Printing Office, Pub No 1986-491-292:(41147).

72. National Research Council (1989). *Diet and health.* Washington, D.C.: The National Academy Press.

73. National Research Council (1989). Executive Summary: Diet, nutrition, and cancer. *Nutrition Today,* 17, 20-25.

74. National Research Council (1989). *Recommended dietary allowances* (10th ed.). Washington, D.C.: The National Academy Press.

75. Natow, A.B., & Heslin, J.A. (1986). *Nutritional care of the older adult.* New York: Macmillan Publishing Company.

76. North American Nursing Diagnosis Association (1990). Taxonomy I—revised 1990. St. Louis.

77. Orr, M.E. (1989). Nutritional support in home care. *Nursing Clinics of North America,* 24(2), 437-445.

78. Perez, S., & Brandt, K. (1989). Enteral feeding contamination: comparison of diluents and feeding bag usage. *Journal of Parenteral and Enteral Nutrition,* 13, 306-308.

79. Pesola, G.R., et al. (1990). Hypertonic nasogastric tube feedings: do they cause diarrhea? *Critical Care Medicine,* 18, 1378-1382.

80. Pipes, P. (1989). *Nutrition in infancy and childhood* (4th ed.). St. Louis: C.V. Mosby.

81. Quill, T. (1989). Utilization of nasogastric feeding tubes in a group of chronically ill, elderly patients in a community hospital. *Archives of Internal Medicine,* 149, 1937-1941.

82. Quinless, F.W. (1988). Emergency treatment for ruptured varices: esophagogastric tamponade. *Nursing,* 18(10), 64L-64N.

83. Report (1986). Council for Agricultural Science and Technology; diet and coronary heart disease. *Nutrition Today,* 21, 26-33.

84. Report (1985). Lowering blood cholesterol to prevent heart disease, Consensus Conference. *JAMA,* 253, 2080-2086.

85. Report (1986). Sweeteners—nutritive and nonnutritive. *Food Technology,* 40, 195-200.

86. Riley, R.H. (1990). Transparent dressings for nasogastric tubes (letter). *Anaesthesia and Intensive Care,* 18, 272.

87. Roubenoff, R., & Ravich, W. (1989). Pneumothorax due to nasogastric feeding tubes. *Archives of Internal Medicine,* 149, 184-188.

88. Saini, S., et al. (1990). Percutaneous gastrostomy with gastropexy: experience in 125 patients. *American Journal of Roentgenology,* 154, 1003-1006.

89. Sands, J.A. (1991). Incidence of pulmonary aspiration in intubated patients receiving enteral nutrition through wide- and

narrow-bore nasogastric feeding tubes. *Heart and Lung,* 20(1), 75–80.

90. Satter, E.M. (1986). *Child of mine: feeding with love and good sense.* Palo Alto, California: Bull Publishing Company.

91. Shiike, M., et al. (1989). Skin-level gastrostomies and jejunostomies for long-term enteral feeding. *Journal of Parenteral and Enteral Nutrition,* 13, 648–657.

92. Short, N.M. (1989). Gastrointestinal intubation: nursing considerations. *Gastroenterology Nursing,* 12(1), 43–49.

93. Sitzmann, J.V. (1990). Nutritional support of the dysphagic patient: methods, risks, and complications of therapy. *Journal of Parenteral and Enteral Nutrition,* 14, 60–63.

94. Skinner, S., & Martens, R.A. (1985). *The milk sugar dilemma: living with lactose intolerance.* East Lansing, Michigan: Medi-Ed Press.

95. Sliwa, J.A., & Marciniak, C. (1989). A complication of nasogastric tube removal. *Archives of Physical Medicine and Rehabilitation,* 70, 702–704.

96. Smith, C.E., et al. (1990). Diarrhea associated with tube feeding in mechanically ventilated critically ill patients. *Nursing Research,* 39(3), 148–153.

97. Smith, G.M., (1990). Radiographic detection of esophageal malpositioning of endotracheal tubes. *American Journal of Roentgenology,* 154(1), 23–26.

98. Snyder, C.L., et al. (1990). Nonoperative management of small-bowel obstruction with endoscopic long intestinal tube placement. *American Surgeon,* 56, 587–592.

99. Sofferman, R.A., et al. (1990). The nasogastric tube syndrome. *Laryngoscope,* 100, 962–968.

100. Solomon, S.M., & Kirby, D.F. (1990). The refeeding syndrome: a review. *Journal of Parenteral and Enteral Nutrition,* 14, 90–97.

101. Spencer, H. (1986). Factors contributing to osteoporosis. *Journal of Nutrition,* 116, 316–319.

102. Stamler, R., et al. (1987). Nutritional therapy for high blood pressure; final report of a four-year randomized controlled trial —The Hypertension Control Program. *JAMA,* 257, 1484–1491.

103. Stern, J.S. (1986). Comparison of percutaneous endoscopic gastrostomy with surgical gastrostomy at a community hospital. *The American Journal of Gastroenterology,* 81(12), 1171–1173.

104. Stunkard, A.J., et al. (1986). An adoption study of human obesity. *New England Journal of Medicine,* 314, 193–198.

105. Swift, D.E. (1989). Misplaced feeding tube in the tracheobronchial tree. *Choices in Respiratory Management,* 19(3), 57–59.

106. Taptich, B.J., et al. (1989). Nursing diagnosis and care planning. Philadelphia: W.B. Saunders.

107. Underwood, B.A. (1986). Evaluating the nutritional status of individuals: a critique of approaches. *Nutrition Revue,* 44 (Suppl), 213–224.

108. Urschel, J.D., & Stockburger, H.J. (1990). Endoscopic extraction of an entrapped nasogastric tube. *American Surgeon,* 56, 730–732.

109. Vitamin D (1987). New perspectives. *Lancet,* 1, 1122.

110. Wake, M., et al. (1990). Effect of nasogastric tubes on eustachian tube function. *Journal of Laryngology and Otology,* 104(1), 17–19.

111. Walsh, S.N., & Banks, L.A. (1990). How to insert a small-bore feeding tube safely. *Nursing,* 20(3), 55–59.

112. Wendell, G.D., et al. (1991). Pneumothorax complicating small-bore feeding tube placement. *Archives of Internal Medicine,* 151, 599–602.

113. Wheeler, M.L., et al. (1987). Diet and exercise in noninsulin-dependent diabetes mellitus: implications for dieticians from the NIH Consensus Development Conference. *Journal of the American Dietetic Association,* 87, 480–485.

114. Wiedmann, M.A., et al. (1990). Temporary gastrostomy tubes in major gynecologic surgery. *Southern Medical Journal,* 83, 893–894.

115. Wittens, C.H., et al. (1990). Intraluminal Miller-Abbott tube stenting as treatment and prophylaxis of recurrent intestinal obstruction. *Netherlands Journal of Surgery,* 42(5), 123–127.

116. Woo, R., et al. (1985). Regulation of energy balance. *Annual Revue of Nutrition,* 5, 411–433.

117. Wood, G., et al. (1990). Ventilatory failure due to an improperly placed nasogastric tube. *Canadian Journal of Anesthesia,* 37, 587–588.

118. Worthington-Roberts, B., & Williams, S.R. (1989). *Nutrition in pregnancy and lactation* (4th ed.). St. Louis: C.V. Mosby.

Chapter 43

▼ Meeting Bowel Elimination Needs

Costiveness cannot long consist with health.
John Wesley
1764

▼ CHAPTER OUTLINE

STRUCTURE AND FUNCTION OF THE
  GASTROINTESTINAL TRACT
ASSESSMENT
    Taking the History
    Psychologic Factors Affecting Bowel
      Elimination
    Physiologic Factors Affecting Bowel
      Elimination
    Physical Assessment
    Diagnostic Tests to Locate and
      Identify Bowel Elimination
      Problems
NURSING DIAGNOSIS

PLANNING
NURSING INTERVENTION
    Bowel Management
    Stimulating Bowel Evacuation
    Constipation Management
    Impaction Management
    Diarrhea Management
    Flatulence Reduction
    Bowel Incontinence Care
    Bowel Training
    Ostomy Care
EVALUATION
CASE STUDY

▼ KEY TERMS

Acholia
Bowel incontinence
Bulk-forming laxative
Cathartic
Cleansing enema
Colostomy
Constipation
Diarrhea
Enema
Fecal impaction
Feces

Flatulence (gaseous
  distention)
Guaiac test
Ileostomy
Laxative
Lubricant
Meconium
Melena
Occult blood
Ostomy
Peristalsis

Retention enema
Return-flow enema (Harris
  flush)
Saline laxative (osmotic
  agent)
Steatorrhea
Stimulant (irritant)
  laxative
Stoma
Suppository

Elimination of wastes is one of the body's basic physiologic needs; the gastrointestinal (GI) tract serves as the major route for removal of solid wastes. This function is a relatively simple one, although it can be influenced by a number of physical as well as psychologic factors. Psychologic factors are particularly important, since many people tend to be quite bowel conscious. In working with their clients, health professionals frequently find themselves dealing with unmet bowel elimination needs as either primary or secondary problems.

The nurse is responsible for assessing clients' bowel status, helping them maintain normal bowel patterns as appropriate, collecting specimens, performing selected diagnostic tests, and working with the physician in meeting clients' bowel elimination needs. Nurses are taking the lead in basic management of bowel elimination by making nursing diagnoses, formulating nursing goals, and implementing nursing interventions.

STRUCTURE AND FUNCTION OF THE GASTROINTESTINAL TRACT

The GI tract, or alimentary canal, is a hollow, muscular tube that runs from the mouth to the anus. Figure 43–1 details the anatomy of the lower GI tract. The lower GI tract consists of the large intestine, or colon, which begins at the ileocecal valve. The lower GI tract is divided into the ascending, transverse, descending, and sigmoid colon and the rectum.[25]

The main functions of this tube are to receive fluids and nutrients, digest and absorb them, and eliminate waste products from the body. This description portrays the anatomy and physiology of the GI tract in simplest terms. These processes require a number of ancillary organs and anatomic structures, chemical substances, and physiologic processes. We are concerned with these factors as they relate to the elimination process.

The colon absorbs water, sodium, and chlorides while passing waste materials out of the body. As the digested, unabsorbed food travels through the ascending, transverse, and descending colon into the sigmoid colon, it becomes increasingly solid as the large bowel absorbs water from it.

Feces (excrement or gastrointestinal waste) moves through the large intestine by means of constant peristalsis and segmental contractions. **Peristalsis** is a propulsive movement in which a wave of smooth muscle contraction moves along an anatomical tube, forcing contents of the tube ahead of it. Although the force may propel intestinal contents in either direction, movement in the GI tract is usually toward the anus.

In addition to constant peristalsis, periods of mass peristalsis occur two or three times a day, usually following meals. Mass peristalsis is initiated primarily by the gastrocolic reflex. This movement pushes the contents along the intestine for some distance toward the sigmoid colon. The gastrocolic and duodenocolic reflexes are strongest when a person eats following a period of fasting, such as at breakfast after a night's sleep. The gastrocolic reflex occurs when the bolus of food enters the stomach and stimulates peristalsis throughout the entire GI tract. The duodenocolic reflex acts in a similar manner but is the weaker of the two reflexes.

The fecal material moves into the sigmoid portion of the colon where it is stored until eliminated from the body. Transit time through the GI tract is affected by such factors as rate of motility, amount of residue, and the presence or absence of irritating substances in the

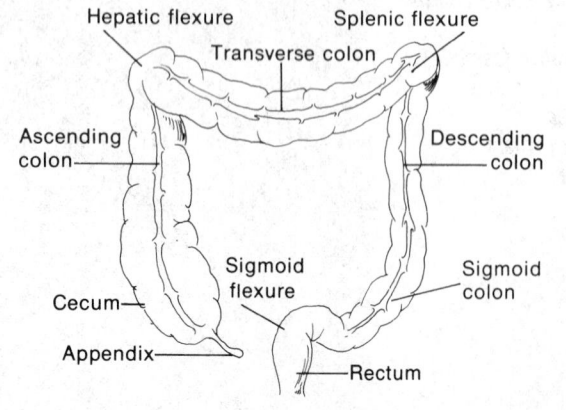

▲ *Figure 43–1*

Anatomy of the lower gastrointestinal tract.

colon. However, it usually takes from 6 to 8 hours for the contents to travel from the stomach to the sigmoid colon.

Another substance in the GI tract is gas (flatus). Flatus is formed partially from the fermentation processes in the bowel and partially from air taken in through the mouth.

The parasympathetic nerve center in the sacral segments of the spinal cord is primarily responsible for the act of defecation. To complete passage from the body, the feces and flatus move through the rectum, anal canal, and anus. This process is referred to as "having a bowel movement" and is under both voluntary and involuntary control.

The rectum usually remains empty until just before and during defecation. When the fecal mass or flatus moves from the sigmoid colon into the rectum, the defecation reflex begins. Feces enters the rectum either (a) involuntarily, as a result of a mass propulsive movement in the colon; or (b) voluntarily, by increasing the intra-abdominal pressure via abdominal muscle contraction and forced expiration with a closed glottis. This latter action (also called the Valsalva maneuver) forces the diaphragm downward, thus increasing pressure. Distention of the rectum then causes increased intrarectal pressure and the urge to evacuate the bowel.

The anal canal has two sphincters. The internal sphincter is smooth muscle and is innervated through the autonomic nervous system. Distention of the rectum causes this sphincter to relax involuntarily, to allow passage of the feces. The external anal sphincter consists of striated muscle and is under voluntary control in the healthy person who has been toilet trained. At the same time that the internal sphincter is being stimulated to relax by descending feces, so is the external sphincter. However, a person normally controls the external sphincter and thus voluntarily delays the act of defecation by constriction of the anus. If the act of defecation is stopped, the stool in the rectum remains there until the defecation reflex is again stimulated.

ASSESSMENT

Assessment of bowel status enables the nurse to identify actual and potential problems, establish nursing diagnoses, and plan appropriate nursing interventions. In assessing a person's bowel elimination needs, consider the following areas: history and physical assessment, feces characteristics, and results of diagnostic tests.

Taking the History

During the history-taking process, factors affecting normal defecation should be considered. These factors are listed in Box 43-1.

Psychologic Factors Affecting Bowel Elimination

MENTAL STATE

There appears to be a relationship between alteration of a normal defecation pattern and a person's emotional state.

It is sometimes difficult to determine which came first —the GI disturbance or the emotional condition.

Several disease processes with such severe GI disturbances as diarrhea, gaseous distention, and ulcer formation are considered to have a significant psychologic overtone. Examples include ulcerative colitis (recurrent, extensive inflammation of the colon) and Crohn's disease (inflammation of the terminal portion of the ileum, also called regional enteritis). Mental depression slows all bodily activities, thus constipation may be a presenting symptom, whereas agitation and nervousness can precipitate diarrhea. Most people have probably experienced some kind of GI disturbance when faced with a high-anxiety situation, such as a public-speaking engagement. When a person develops a GI problem, carefully assess whether a psychologic concern is precipitating or supporting it.

TOILET-TRAINING EXPERIENCE

Experiences linked with toilet training during childhood can have long-lasting effects. Helping a child learn to use the toilet takes patience, time, and understanding. A person's negative or positive attitudes toward bowel elimination sometimes can be traced back to this period. Rewards, or reinforcement, for positive behavior tend to result in continued problem-free elimination patterns. On the other hand, a person who received punishment for failures during toilet training may unconsciously transfer into adult life feelings of guilt and anxiety that are manifested in GI problems. In addition,

---

Box 43-1. Factors Affecting Normal Defecation

Psychologic Factors

► Mental state
► Toilet-training experience
► Cultural teachings
► Privacy

Physiologic Factors

► Personal habits
► Dietary intake
► Muscle tone
► Medications
► Surgical procedures
► Diagnostic tests
► Age
► Motor and sensory disturbances
► Intestinal pathology

use or nonuse of the toilet for defecation may be a means by which some children reward or punish their parents—behavior that may be manifested again in adulthood.

CULTURAL TEACHINGS

Cultural teachings significantly influence a person's defecation habits. In modern society, we are taught strict rules about when and under what conditions defecation can take place. Failure to follow these rules results in social censure and even isolation. In many societies, defecation is a private matter and we go to great lengths to ensure this privacy.

Many people avoid any discussion of bowel activity. Therefore, some individuals feel extremely anxious when forced to seek out a health professional regarding problems with bowel elimination. Even more dangerous, some people with such problems avoid seeking professional help altogether because they are too embarrassed. Such avoidance can lead to serious consequences if the problem involves undiagnosed, and thus untreated, ulcerations or cancerous growths in the bowel.

Elimination habits are different in different cultures. For example, in rural areas of South America the act of defecation is accomplished in a squatting position over a hole in the ground with no toilet or cleansing facilities. Although people in some cultures tend to be very bowel conscious, not all people will be embarrassed or reluctant to discuss bowel habits. Therefore, a person's willingness to discuss bowel function must be assessed.

Nurses, particularly at the beginning of a professional career, may also be subject to feelings of embarrassment and anxiety when dealing with clients' elimination needs. As a student, you bring to the clinical setting your own cultural background and personal experience, which may include taboos against discussion of bowel elimination. Nonetheless, you will be required to discuss elimination patterns openly with people, to make nursing diagnoses about elimination needs, and to plan and implement interventions designed to prevent and resolve elimination problems. Because elimination is a basic human need, you are required to assume this nursing responsibility very early, often in the first or second meeting with a person. Your feelings of embarrassment and anxiety will diminish with experience.

PRIVACY

When people are hospitalized and are seriously ill, they may not be able to meet their own elimination needs but must depend on others. This loss of privacy concerning a private act can be devastating. At best, some people have a private bathroom. More often the hospitalized person must share a bathroom with one or more strangers. At worst, the individual will be in a multiple-bed room and will have to use a commode or bedpan for defecation, with its accompanying sounds and odors. Because of the lack of privacy, many peo-

ple deliberately avoid having a bowel movement, which results in problems such as constipation. In turn, the constipation requires intervention and focuses even more attention on the individual's bowel habits.

Physiologic Factors Affecting Bowel Elimination

Not only psychosocial influences but also many physical factors affect elimination patterns. Bowel habits are very important. As discussed later, the bowel can be trained to evacuate at a certain time. If this pattern is followed, and all other variables remain constant, the bowel continues to empty regularly. On the other hand, if a person continually ignores the urge to defecate, no rhythmic pattern is established. Travel, which usually disrupts a person's normal schedule, is a well-known villain that often leads to constipation and sometimes to diarrhea.

PERSONAL HABITS

Along with timing, many people have other established habits related to bowel elimination, such as drinking warm or cold water, eating prunes, having a cup of coffee, or reading. Continuing these activities may trigger conscious mental stimulation of the defecation reflex.

DIETARY INTAKE

Diet strongly influences bowel habits. Fiber, or indigestible dietary residue, provides bulk in fecal material. Bulk assists peristalsis and increases the stimulation of the defecation reflex. A low-fiber, high-carbohydrate diet tends to diminish the reflex. Reduction of overall intake also directly reduces the amount of bulk present. Gas-producing foods may stimulate peristalsis by distending the intestinal walls.

How the GI tract reacts to a particular food depends on the individual. For instance, chocolate has no effect on many people, but causes constipation in some and diarrhea in others. Likewise, milk and milk products constipate some people and cause diarrhea in others. Various foods also can adversely affect defecation patterns and act as irritants. Irritants, such as spicy foods, within the GI tract usually stimulate peristalsis by local reflex stimulation. Attempt to determine how particular foods affect an individual.

The amount of water in the fecal mass affects stool consistency. The less the water content the harder the mass, and the more difficult it is to pass the mass through the anus. If the person is fluid depleted, more fluid is absorbed from the GI tract to maintain adequate hydration. Thus, dehydration can result in constipation.

MUSCLE TONE

Muscle tone affects not only the activity of the intestinal musculature but also the ability of the supporting skeletal muscles to aid the process of defecation. Weak or atrophied abdominal or pelvic floor muscles are ineffective in increasing intra-abdominal pressure or assisting the anus to control defecation. This inadequate musculature may result from lack of exercise, such as may accompany immobility; neurologic impairment; or multiple pregnancies.

MEDICATIONS

Medications administered for bowel regulation or for other purposes may alter bowel patterns. Many medications prevent or reverse constipation and diarrhea. If the dose is too large, the medication may cause the opposite disorder. For example, a drug to prevent constipation may cause diarrhea, and vice versa. In addition, overuse of laxatives can lead to physiologic and psychologic dependence on them.

Some examples of medications with side effects that alter bowel elimination are given in Table 43–1. These agents represent only a small sampling of medications that affect bowel function.

SURGICAL PROCEDURES

Surgical procedures tend to contribute to constipation. Direct handling of the bowel during abdominal surgery can cause a temporary stoppage of peristalsis called paralytic ileus. Any procedure carried out in the perineal area, such as rectal or gynecologic surgery, can affect defecation patterns through the obstructing effects of postoperative edema, through the effects of medication administered operatively and postoperatively, and through discomfort associated with distention of the traumatized tissues at the surgical site. Even surgeries at sites unrelated to the G.I. tract can result in constipation if the surgery reduces mobility for more than a few days or if the surgery requires use of pain-controlling drugs that reduce peristalsis.

Status of bowel function must be monitored postoperatively until return of the prior defecation routine.

DIAGNOSTIC TESTS

Diagnostic tests also affect defecation patterns. Many GI tests involve direct or x-ray visualization of the intestine. Prior to these examinations, the bowel is emptied of solid and gaseous contents. Bowel preparation

involves reducing oral intake and using laxatives and enemas to empty the bowel. This preparation, which is also done before surgery, reduces the amount of fecal material in the bowel and thus temporarily eliminates the need for defecation.

X-ray studies of the intestine often use a liquid contrast medium that is administered orally or rectally. This medium shows up on the x-ray film as a white area outlining the inner wall of the intestine. One commonly used contrast medium is barium. When left in the colon, barium hardens and may interfere with elimination.

AGE

Age plays a role in establishing bowel patterns. Before a child acquires bowel control through toilet training, defecation occurs whenever stool stimulates the rectum. In the elderly population, vulnerability to GI disturbances increases. Malignancies are more frequent, and motor and neurologic disturbances more prevalent. In addition, diverticulosis (an outpouching in the intestinal wall) occurs almost exclusively to people after the age of 40 years.

MOTOR AND SENSORY DISTURBANCES

Motor or sensory disturbances also affect defecation. Spinal cord injuries, head injuries, stroke, neurologic disease, and any condition causing immobility or otherwise interfering with motor activity all diminish the sensory stimulation required for defecation. Immobility also hinders the person's ability to respond to the urge to defecate. For instance, the person who is unable to walk to the bathroom or reach a call bell to summon help may (a) suppress the urge to defecate, which could eventually lead to constipation, or (b) suffer fecal incontinence.

INTESTINAL PATHOLOGY

Pathologic conditions within the intestine affect normal defecation. Bowel obstruction, as occurs with tumors or adhesions, interferes with the passage of stool, whereas inflammatory processes, such as colitis, usually speed up the movement of feces.

When completing a historical assessment of bowel elimination, questions pertinent to these latter topics are explored in depth if problems existed. Questions such as "How often do you have a bowel movement?" or "What is the color of your stool?" are appropriate starting questions for lower GI assessment.[3]

Physical Assessment

The physical assessment of the bowel system should include inspection, auscultation, percussion, and palpation of the abdomen and inspection and palpation of the anus. In the supine position, the abdomen should be inspected for peristalsis, contour, symmetry, and masses. Auscultation of bowel sounds should be completed, noting frequency and character. Percussion may elicit tympany or dullness depending on gas, normal

TABLE 43–1. Medications That May Alter Bowel Elimination

Medication	Effects
Narcotics (especially codeine and morphine sulfate)	Potent constipators
Antibiotics	Destroy normal intestinal flora and cause diarrhea
Antacids	Cause diarrhea or constipation, depending on formula
General anesthetics	Slow peristalsis by depressing CNS activity and cause susceptibility to GI disturbances

fluid, and feces in the GI tract. Palpation may elicit tenderness or masses in the abdomen. Inspection and palpation of the anus permits observation of lumps, ulcers, inflammation, rashes, or excoriation.[3]

Observation of fecal characteristics and laboratory analysis of feces give another dimension to the GI assessment. Procedures for feces collection for observation and analysis are explained next.

SPECIMEN COLLECTION

Stool Specimens. Either the individual or the nurse is responsible for specimen collection. Urination should occur before or after feces deposit, to prevent contamination, because urine kills protozoa. Stool specimens are collected in a sterile or clean bedpan or any functional receptacle, depending on the test. If the person uses a toilet, place a bedpan or liner under the seat. At home, a person can drape a piece of plastic wrap over the seat, leaving some slack so it droops in the middle. After depositing the specimen, the person then brings the corners and edges of the wrap together and twists them to form an enclosed package. If the specimen is deposited in a large container, a portion of feces is transferred to a covered specimen container with a tongue depressor. If the person cannot produce any feces, gently pass a rectal swab beyond the rectal sphincter and rotate it carefully to collect fecal material. Then place the specimen in a suitable container for transport to the laboratory. Be sure to include feces containing blood or mucus, since the greatest number of organisms are contained here.

When collecting stool specimens, one should be aware of the conditions necessary for accurate test results. In general, collect culture specimens in a sterile container and send them to the laboratory immediately, or place them in a proper medium to avoid overgrowth of the bacterial population. For example, a stool specimen to be tested for ova and parasites should be examined immediately, since the organisms die if they cool below body temperature. On the other hand, you can refrigerate specimens not needing microscopic examination if you are unable to deliver them to the laboratory right away.

Always make sure specimens are free of oil, barium, or bismuth.

Specimens from the Anal Region. Specimen collection may also be done from the anal region itself — usually to check for pinworms. For this particular specimen, a strip of nonfrosted cellophane tape is pressed, sticky side down, over and/or around the anus. It is removed immediately, placed on a glass slide, and sent to the laboratory for microscopic examination. This specimen is collected early in the morning, before the person has bathed or had a bowel movement, because the female worm deposits eggs on the perianal area during the night. The eggs may be transferred by scratching the perianal area, thus allowing specimen collection from under the fingernails.[25]

CHARACTERISTICS OF FECES

Fecal material is composed of food residues, bacteria, some white blood cells, epithelial cells, intestinal secretions, and water. The characteristics to assess to identify GI problems are

- Frequency
- Amount
- Color
- Consistency
- Shape
- Odor

Frequency of Bowel Movements. Frequency of bowel movements varies from person to person. The normal range for an adult is from two to three times per day to one to three times per week. Infants often have three to five stools per day, but for adults and older children, passing stools more than three times a day or less than once a week may indicate a problem. The frequency of bowel movements is important to many people.

An erroneous notion that a daily bowel movement is essential to healthy living is prevalent. As a result, many people worry needlessly about the frequency of their bowel movements.

Nurses should stress to people that frequency of bowel movements is individualized, and it is not necessary to have a bowel movement every day.

Amount of Stool. The amount of stool varies according to the amount and type of food ingested, fluid intake, and frequency of bowel evacuation. It is normally about 150 gm per day. Because much fecal material is not dietary in origin, the person with no oral intake still passes stool. Also, it may take several days for food to move through the entire GI tract. Therefore, the colon is not empty even if the person has not eaten for several days. Inform people of these facts to motivate them to take measures to prevent constipation. If constipation becomes complete, there is no passage of feces or gas.

Color of Stool. The normal brown color of stool is produced by bile pigments. Absence of bile causes the stool to be white, gray, or clay-colored and may indicate biliary obstruction or **acholia** — a lack of bile production. White stools also result from barium or antacid ingestion. Black stools may result from bismuth, charcoal, or supplemental iron intake. Black may also indicate upper GI bleeding, especially if the feces have a tarlike consistency. This tarry black stool is called **melena.** In newborn infants, the first stools (called **meconium**) are normally black and tarry owing to ingested amniotic fluid, epithelial cells, and bile. Red-colored stools are caused by the ingestion of beets or Povan (pyrvinium pamoate, an antiparasitic agent) or may be the result of bleeding in the lower GI tract where the red blood cells have not been hemolyzed by digestive processes in the intestine. If this red color is smeared on the surface of the fecal mass, hemorrhoids may be the source. Red blood in the stool comes from a place higher in the colon. Rifampin, an antibiotic, causes red-orange stool. Large amounts of ingested chlorophyll result in green stool.

Consistency of Stool. The consistency of stool is often a reflection of the water content, but other constituents may play a part. **Steatorrhea,** for example, is the passage of greasy stools that tend to float and are mixed with observable fat and mucus. This indicates malabsorption of fats. Abnormal water content changes consistency from formed to liquid, unformed, soft, or hard and indicates constipation or diarrhea.

Shape of Stool. The shape of the stool normally resembles that of the rectum. An abnormal finding would be that of a consistently narrowed, pencil-shaped stool, which indicates obstruction of the distal portion of the large intestine, as might occur with carcinoma.

Odor of Stool. The odor of the stool is characteristically pungent and is produced by bacterial flora present and by the food and medication ingested. Blood or infection in the GI tract causes detectable noxious changes in the normal odor.

Diagnostic Tests to Locate and Identify Bowel Elimination Problems

In addition to the history, physical, and assessment of fecal characteristics, several diagnostic tests help locate and identify problems in bowel elimination. The main categories of these tests include x-ray examination, direct visualization through scopes, and laboratory analysis. The physician may also use a surgical approach to examine the lower GI tract.

X-RAY VISUALIZATION OF THE BOWEL

X-ray examination provides information about the presence and distribution of fecal material and gas in the bowel, as well as the location and contour of the bowel and supporting structures. A flat plate of the abdomen is done without contrast material and therefore requires no pre-examination preparation. It demonstrates shadows, fluid levels, and gas.

Another common diagnostic test is a barium x-ray, usually called a "lower GI" study. The barium is a contrast medium that outlines certain areas of the bowel. Following a barium x-ray, a laxative is administered to ensure complete evacuation of barium. Barium left in the colon can cause impaction (a stool mass too large and hard to pass through the anus) and even obstruction.

The barium enema can produce anaphylactic reactions. These occur in about 1 person per 750,000 examinations.[1]

DIRECT VISUALIZATION OF THE BOWEL

Direct visualization of the lower GI tract is done by inserting fiberoptic scopes through the anus. The instrument used depends on the level to be examined. Hence, the physician may perform a proctoscopy, sigmoidoscopy, or colonoscopy. These endoscopes are hollow tubes through which the examiner visualizes the GI structures. These tubes can also be set up to clear the bowel by suction. In addition, the physician can obtain tissue for biopsy through a scope.

An explanation of the procedure is given prior to the test to allay the client's anxiety and fears. Physical preparation is also important to the success of the test. If the person's bowel has not been thoroughly cleansed, feces can interfere with fiberoptic examination. Typically, the pre-examination protocol begins 24 to 48 hours before the procedure and includes dietary and fluid restrictions, laxatives or purgatives, and/or enemas.

A method of bowel emptying using GoLYTELY (pronounced "go-lightly") solution (a polyethylene glycol-electrolyte solution) is widely used. GoLYTELY cleanses the bowel without causing the excretion or absorption of fluid and electrolytes that often occurs with traditional purgatives and enemas. This method is safer for people with congestive heart disease, chronic obstructive pulmonary disease, or controlled renal failure. The liquid is served cold and consumed at a rate of 1.2 to 1.8 liters per hour until the rectal output is clear. The process usually takes 2 to 4 hours. The solution works fast and produces diarrhea. Therefore ensure that the person has ready access to toilet facilities. Other methods for bowel preparation are the Klyx enema (a sorbitol solution) and Picolax, an oral preparation.[14]

For direct visualization, it is a nursing responsibility to assist the person into a jackknife or knee-chest position and possibly administer relaxant medication. Throughout the diagnostic procedure, provide emotional support. The embarrassment and anxiety that accompany these procedures is distressing. A continued assessment of the individual is necessary because of the positioning and medication administration. Monitor vital signs regularly during the procedure. During the procedure, assisting the physician with equipment and specimens may be necessary.

Monitor for circulatory and respiratory problems during endoscopy examination.

After direct visualization, continue to monitor vital signs and inspect frequently for fresh anal bleeding, which may indicate continued oozing at a biopsy site or bowel perforation. Bowel perforation is also accompanied by severe abdominal pain.

LABORATORY ANALYSIS OF FECES

Laboratory analysis of feces involves direct fecal examination. Stool specimens are examined for bile or bilirubin, blood, microorganisms, ova, and parasites. The presence of bacteria will be noted through cultures;

microscopic examination may reveal meat fibers and fat, indicating a malabsorption diagnosis.

Nurses often collect stool specimens to check for **occult blood** (hidden blood). Usually the nurse performs a **guaiac test,** a test that uses guaiac, a wood resin, as a reagent to detect the presence of occult blood. With most guaiac tests, a change in the reagent to the color blue manifests a positive result, which indicates the presence of blood. A variety of commercial methods are available for performing this test. Besides supplying information about a current bowel disorder, this simple test is also recommended as a screening procedure for the early detection of colorectal cancer. The American Cancer Society recommends that people over the age of 50 years have annual guaiac tests.

NURSING DIAGNOSIS

Nurses diagnose and manage many bowel elimination problems. NANDA's current list of nursing diagnoses relevant to the lower GI system include *Constipation* (Nursing Diagnosis Profile), *Perceived Constipation, Colonic Constipation, Diarrhea,* and *Bowel Incontinence.*[27]

Examples of various nursing diagnoses that are pertinent to bowel elimination are

▶ *Constipation* R/T effects of retained barium in colon
▶ *Diarrhea* R/T excessive use of laxatives
▶ *Bowel Incontinence* R/T effects of cognitive impairment
▶ *Bowel Incontinence* R/T effects of medication[27, 31]

PLANNING

Outcomes should be identified specific to the nursing diagnoses established. For the nursing diagnosis *Constipation,* an expected outcome could be:

▶ Has a normal bowel movement every morning.

Short-term outcomes that could indicate progression toward this outcome might be:

▶ Lists foods with high fiber content.
▶ Explains importance of exercise in relation to GI system activity.
▶ Identifies side effects and contraindications of laxatives.

An outcome specific to the nursing diagnosis *Diarrhea* could include the statement:

▶ Frequency and amount of stools decreased to one formed bowel movement daily.

Short-term outcomes that could indicate progression toward such an outcome might be:

▶ Remains clean and dry.
▶ Avoids foods contributing to diarrhea.

An outcome statement specific to the nursing diagnosis *Incontinence* could be:

▶ Establishes a pattern of elimination that is as near to normal as possible.

Short-term outcomes that might demonstrate progression toward this outcome could include:

NURSING DIAGNOSIS PROFILE

Constipation

Definition. A state in which an individual experiences a change in normal bowel habits, characterized by a decrease in frequency, passage of hard dry stools, or both.

Classification. Exchanging 1.3.1.1

Defining Characteristics. Objective physiologic measures of constipation include: frequency of bowel movements less than usual pattern, hard-formed stools, palpable mass, and straining at stool. Other defining characteristics are reported feeling of pressure in rectum and reported feeling of rectal fullness. Other possible defining characteristics are abdominal pain, appetite impairment, back pain, headache, interference with daily living, and use of laxatives.

Sample Related Factors. Related factors may be decreased activity, decreased fluid intake, dietary changes, and responses to various stresses. Some of these factors may be secondary to pathologic changes.

Concept Description. This nursing diagnosis refers to the state in which a person has not had normal bowel movement activity. This decreased bowel activity results in a hardened stool, causing difficulty with defecation.

Examples. Depending on the specific assessment data, this diagnostic category could be applicable in the following situations, among others:

▶ A person who is healthy until an acute illness presents and activity is restricted to bed and chair.
▶ A healthy person who begins an excessive training program to compete in sports and who becomes tense and driven about an upcoming marathon.
▶ An elderly person who consumes an inadequate amount of fluids and becomes dehydrated.

Related/Similar Nursing Diagnoses. This nursing diagnosis should be distinguished from the diagnosis of "Perceived Constipation." In "Perceived Constipation," the individual makes a self-diagnosis of constipation and treats self through medication abuse. A normal routine of bowel defecation is achieved through abnormal measures. "Constipation" should also be distinguished from the nursing diagnosis of "Colonic Constipation." With colonic constipation, related factors are similar to those of constipation, but colonic constipation can be traced directly to a delay in the passage of food residue through the gastrointestinal tract.

▶ Participates in bowel training program.
▶ Decreases incidence of incontinence.

During the planning phase of the nursing process, nursing interventions are identified to assist the client in achieving outcomes.

NURSING INTERVENTION

Nursing interventions are (1) independent, nurse-initiated actions used in response to nursing diagnoses, such as teaching clients how to improve bowel elimination; (2) dependent, physician-initiated actions used in response to medical diagnoses, such as administering enemas, laxatives, and suppositories; and (3) daily essential functions that do not relate to either nursing or medical diagnoses, such as cleaning a bedpan.[6,7]

Nursing interventions relevant to bowel elimination include: bowel management, stimulating bowel evacuation, constipation management, impaction management; diarrhea management, flatulence reduction, bowel incontinence care, bowel training, and ostomy care.[24]

Bowel Management

Bowel management is the "establishment and maintenance of a regular pattern of bowel elimination."[24] Assisting clients to attain and maintain healthy defecation habits is a goal nursing can meet through these strategies:

▶ learning/teaching activities;
▶ supporting normal bowel habits through adjustments in diet, fluids, exercise, and positioning; and
▶ providing for relaxation and privacy.

Nursing activities appropriate for this intervention are found in Box 43–2.

TEACHING/LEARNING ACTIVITIES

Health education helps people improve their bowel elimination habits. When the reasons behind therapy are understood, most individuals are more compliant if intervention becomes necessary. Helping people learn more about normal elimination is an important nursing activity. Recall the incorrect belief held by many people that it is necessary to defecate every day. If a daily bowel movement does not occur naturally, people may use over-the-counter laxatives, suppositories, and even enemas to induce a bowel movement. As described later, continued use of such measures begins a cycle that may lead to physical dependence. Because there are many other misunderstandings about defecation, nurses must give people accurate information about this normal body function.

Even those whom you assume to be knowledgeable may have misconceptions about defecation.

Box 43–2. Bowel Management

Definition

Establishment and maintenance of a regular pattern of bowel elimination

Activities

▶ Note date of last bowel movement
▶ Monitor bowel movements, including frequency, consistency, shape, volume, and color as appropriate
▶ Monitor bowel sounds
▶ Report an increase in frequency or pitch of bowel sounds
▶ Report diminished bowel sounds
▶ Monitor for signs and symptoms of diarrhea, constipation, and impaction
▶ Evaluate for fecal incontinence as necessary
▶ Note pre-existent bowel problems, bowel routine, and use of laxatives
▶ Teach clients about specific foods that assist in promoting bowel regularity
▶ Instruct client in foods that are high in fiber
▶ Instruct client/family to record color, volume, frequency, and consistency of stools
▶ Insert rectal suppository as needed
▶ Initiate a bowel-training program as appropriate
▶ Encourage decreased gas-forming food intake as appropriate
▶ Give warm liquids after meals as appropriate
▶ Evaluate medication profile for gastrointestinal side effects
▶ Guaiac stools as appropriate
▶ Refrain from doing rectal/vaginal examination if medical condition warrants

▼▼▼

From McCloskey, J.C., & Bulechek, G. (1992). *Classification of Nursing Interventions.* St. Louis: Mosby–Year Book, Inc.

BOWEL HABITS

Although defecation can occur at any time, it is best to encourage bowel movements during stimulation of the gastrocolic reflex. As described earlier, the reflex is usually strongest after breakfast. Therefore, attempts to have a bowel movement at this time are likely to be the most successful. However, other factors influence timing, such as availability of the bathroom, or personal and professional responsibilities. Assess the client's daily routine before planning a bowel program.

Help people select a time during the day when they can take their time to attend to bowel needs. As indicated, timing depends on life style and daily activities. Once the time is decided, encourage people to make this habit a daily routine. If the time selected is inappropriate, alter it until a suitable one is found. People who have little routine in their lives are a particular challenge.

In addition, hospitalization often alters established routines. During this time, ascertain what the client's patterns are and then help maintain this routine.

DIET

Dietary Fiber. Adequate dietary fiber is one of the most important factors in aiding bowel function. Dietary fiber increases fecal weight and water content and accelerates the transit of fecal mass through the GI tract.[37] The digestive system cannot break down insoluble fiber from a plant. Insoluble fibers retain water and do not break down in water. The retention of water by the fiber has the ability to soften stools and promote regularity. Supplementing diets with bran, whole grain cereals, nuts, and raw fruits and vegetables is effective in promoting normal bowel elimination.[30]

High-fiber diets may also prevent diverticular disease. A diverticulum is an outpouching of the colon that occurs as a result of weakened intestinal wall muscles. This condition can become a problem if the diverticula fill with feces, thus obstructing the colon. Perforation, ulceration, and infection can also develop. Researchers have found that diverticular disease improves with a high-fiber diet, probably because this diet produces bulkier feces, resulting in a colonic lumen with a larger diameter. Less pressure is created in a larger colon with the passage of bulkier feces. Hence, the colon muscles encounter less outward force, and fewer diverticula develop.

The National Cancer Institute recommends a daily intake of 25 to 35 gm of fiber. Meeting this goal must be done gradually; increasing the fiber in a person's diet may not be a totally benign action. For example, large amounts of dietary fiber can cause abdominal cramps, gaseous distention, and diarrhea. Slowly adding dietary fiber to the diet will allow for GI adaptation. Fulfilling this recommendation should be done with insoluble and soluble fibers from food rather than supplements that may not have necessary vitamins and minerals.[30]

Avoidance of Foods That Disrupt Bowel Function. In addition to adding fiber, people need to identify and avoid foods that cause disruptions in their bowel function. If several foods are suspect, clients should eliminate all of them from the diet and then add one at a time. Tell them to wait for several days or longer if necessary between each introduction, to see which foods cause the problem.

Fluids. Good hydration aids normal bowel function by softening stools. Although authorities differ on the amount of fluid intake necessary to maintain adequate hydration, a reasonable minimum for adults is about 1200 to 1500 ml per day. If the person has significant fluid replacement needs (as from increased sweating secondary to activity or fever), intake should be increased. Immobility also calls for increased fluid intake, since one of the normal aids to defecation—exercise—is limited.

Before instituting a plan to increase fluid intake, be certain that the person has no condition for which increased fluid would be detrimental, such as cardiac or renal disease or head injury.

Although the amount of fluid intake is the crucial element, the kind of fluids is also important. For example, milk constipates some people, whereas prune juice is a natural laxative for most people. Other fruit juices, such as apricot, cranberry, and orange, and lemonade, can also stimulate bowel activity.

EXERCISE

Exercise improves general muscle tone and strengthens the muscles used in defecation. Encourage and assist clients as necessary to take part in daily physical activity. Walking, for example, is an excellent body toner.

In addition to general exercise, teach people exercises specifically designed to strengthen the abdominal and pelvic floor muscles. Probably the most effective are isometric exercises in which a person contracts or tightens muscles as much as possible for about 10 seconds, and then relaxes them. Instruct the individual to repeat each exercise five to ten times and to perform them four times a day. Isometric exercises raise blood pressure and may cause coronary ischemia (deficient blood flow to the cardiac muscle) in persons with cardiac disease. Therefore, you should consult a physician about the person's health status before instituting an exercise program.

POSITIONING

Proper positioning promotes comfort and aids defecation by taking advantage of gravity. Also, good positioning facilitates contraction of the abdominal muscles, thereby increasing intra-abdominal pressure. Since squatting is the best position for defecation, position the person as near to this posture as possible. When the person must use a bedpan, roll the head of the bed up into a high-Fowler's position, if this is not otherwise contraindicated. If head elevation is contraindicated, use a fracture bedpan. The commode and toilet promote a natural position. Increase external pressure on the abdomen by having the person lean forward.

If the person is short, place a footstool or other appropriate device under the feet at the toilet to increase hip flexion.

Caution: Some people who have had hip surgery, especially total hip replacement, must avoid hip flexion greater than 90 degrees in order to prevent prosthesis dislocation. Some can use the toilet only when a device is attached that raises the height of the seat to decrease hip flexion. Instruct these people not to lean forward.

RELAXATION AND PRIVACY

Relaxation during attempted bowel evacuation is critical. Anxiety causes tension in the voluntary musculature, which in turn can suppress defecation. Probably the most important factor in achieving relaxation is privacy. Defecation is culturally a private affair, and the odors and sounds that naturally accompany this normal body function are easily communicated to others. Provide privacy for the person to facilitate normal defecation.

Create as private an environment as feasible. If the person must use the bedpan or commode in the room, take these measures: Ask all visitors or staff to leave the room, pull the bed curtains around the person, open the window if appropriate, and turn on the television or radio. Use room deodorizers to reduce odors.

If the person is using the bathroom, make sure that other people know the room is occupied. This practice is especially important when a bathroom has two doors opening into adjacent rooms. Be sure that the person has a way to summon you when finished, or when help is needed. Also, be aware that fainting in bathrooms is a rather frequent occurrence. Bathrooms are ordinarily warm and stuffy, and when a weakened person strains to have a bowel movement, the cardiovascular system may not be able to maintain sufficient blood flow to the brain.

In addition to providing a call light, assure people that there is no hurry. Communicate this fact by your actions as well as your words. For example, avoid interrupting people simply to see if they have finished. On the other hand, do keep careful watch on any person who is at risk for accidents such as fainting or falling.

The person may require pain relief before attempting to defecate. If you must administer narcotics, plan carefully, since they depress central nervous system function. Time medications so that the individual can attempt defecation when pain has been relieved, but before drowsiness and sleep set in.

Stimulating Bowel Evacuation

When more natural efforts to induce a bowel movement have been unsuccessful, additional actions must be taken to stimulate bowel evacuation. These actions require a physician's order and are dependent nursing actions. Such activities include administering laxatives, suppositories, or enemas (Box 43–3).

LAXATIVES AND CATHARTICS

A **laxative** is a medication used to induce emptying of the bowel. A **cathartic** is a medication that purges the bowel. It is more effective than a laxative. The two terms are often used interchangeably, although cathartics have a stronger action than laxatives. The four categories of laxatives are (1) bulk-forming, (2) lubricant, (3) saline, and (4) stimulant.

Bulk-Forming Laxatives. The **bulk-forming laxatives** are synthetic or natural polysaccharides and cellulose derivatives that absorb water and add bulk to the intestinal contents. This increased volume stretches the intestinal wall, thus stimulating peristalsis. Common examples are bran, plantago (psyllium), karaya gum, agar, and methylcellulose (Cellothyl, Cologel, or Hydrolose). Bulk-forming laxatives are the most natural and least irritating laxative preparations and are frequently used

---

Box 43–3. Agents That Stimulate Bowel Evacuation

Laxatives

Bulk-forming
Lubricants
Saline (osmotic agents)
Stimulants (irritants)

Suppositories

Glycerin
Bisocodyl

---

to wean laxative-dependent people from medication misuse. Mix bulk-forming agents with water, and follow the dose with additional fluid to make sure that none of the substance is left in the esophagus. Action usually occurs in 12 to 24 hours but may take up to 72 hours. Encourage high fluid intake to improve the action of the laxative and to avoid GI tract obstruction.

Lubricants. The three categories of lubricants are mineral oil, docusates, and poloxamers. A **lubricant** is a medication that coats the outside of the fecal mass, making it slippery and inhibiting absorption of fluid from the feces.

Mineral oil is a classic example of a lubricant laxative. It is not very palatable, but you can mask the oily aftertaste by mixing it with orange juice or root beer. Mineral oil may interfere with absorption of fat-soluble vitamins. Also, if the person has difficulty in swallowing, mineral oil aspiration can cause pneumonia. The docusates act as wetting and dispersing agents. Common examples are Colace (dioctyl sodium sulfosuccinate) and Surfak (dioctyl calcium sulfosuccinate). Poloxamers, (nonionic surfactants) are stool softeners. A common example is Poloxamer 188.[11]

Saline Laxatives (Osmotic Agents). A **saline laxative (osmotic agent)** is a medication that contains poorly absorbed salts and sugars and that, through osmotic activity, draws water into the intestine to increase bulk and lubricate feces. These drugs usually act within 1 to 3 hours and are often purgatives that empty the bowel completely. Magnesium sulfate (Epsom salt), magnesium hydroxide (milk of magnesia), magnesium citrate, and lactulose (a semisynthetic disaccharide) are osmotic agents. Lactulose causes a severe osmotic reaction and, unless dosed carefully, causes intestinal rumbling, colic, and flatulence. Because of the salts used and the severity of action, osmotic agents are usually contraindicated in people with renal, cardiac, or inflammatory bowel disease.

Stimulants (Irritants). A **stimulant (irritant) laxative** is a medication that increases peristalsis by stimulating sensory nerve endings of the colonic epithelium or by directly irritating the GI mucosa. In addition, there is evidence that some of these agents (e.g., bisacodyl) increase GI secretory activity, thus producing bulkier feces. Examples of stimulants include cascara (cascara sagrada) castor oil, senna, glycerin, and bisacodyl. Be aware that these medications are transmitted through breast milk, causing diarrhea in the nursing infant.

Laxatives are one of the most widely used and misused over-the-counter drugs. Most laxative abuse results from advertising that supports the public's misconceptions about the need for a daily bowel movement. In addition to teaching people proper use of laxatives, warn people never to take these drugs in the presence of undiagnosed abdominal pain or cramps, nausea or vomiting, or diarrhea. These symptoms may indicate appendicitis, inflammatory bowel disease, or obstruction.

Daily laxative administration is detrimental to normal bowel elimination.

SUPPOSITORIES

A **suppository** is a semisolid, cone-, or oval-shaped medication that melts at body temperature. Medicated suppositories are inserted into the rectum, where they release their active ingredients as they melt. Many types of suppositories are refrigerated because it is easier to insert a cold firm suppository than a warm one, which is soft.

Several varieties of suppositories stimulate defecation. The most frequently used are glycerin and bisacodyl. They act as a local irritant to stimulate GI mucosal secretion. Fecal softeners may also be given by suppository to moisten and lubricate the fecal mass. After administering the suppository, cleanse the anal area to remove excess lubricant. Instruct the person to retain the suppository as long as possible—at least 20 to 30 minutes. If appropriate, teach the person to self-administer the suppository.

ENEMAS

Administration of an **enema** involves the introduction of fluid into the rectum, usually for the purpose of stimulating defecation. Because this treatment is frequently administered in the home by people who have had no formal instruction in the procedure, enemas are often considered a harmless, necessary treatment for constipation. Some people even use a daily enema to prevent constipation. This can be an unsafe practice. To achieve the safest and most effective results of enema administration, it is necessary to understand and apply the scientific principles underlying enema administration.

The three types of enemas are cleansing, retention, and return-flow. A **cleansing enema** is a type of enema used to treat constipation or fecal impaction, to clean out the bowel prior to diagnostic procedures or surgery, or to help establish regular bowel function during a bowel training program. A **retention enema** is a type of enema retained in the bowel over a prolonged period. It is usually administered to lubricate or soften a hard fecal mass with oil, thus facilitating fecal expulsion through the anus. Less frequently, a retention enema is given to administer medications, to protect and soothe the mucous membrane of the intestine, to destroy intestinal parasites (anthelmintic), to relieve distention (carminative), or to administer fluids and nutrition (nutritive). A **return-flow enema (Harris flush)** relieves gaseous distention. It is described later, in the discussion of flatulence reduction.

Enemas cause bowel distention and/or irritation of the mucosal wall, both of which stimulate peristalsis. Bowel distention results from filling the colon with fluid by administering either (a) a large-volume enema, which injects large amounts of fluid into the colon

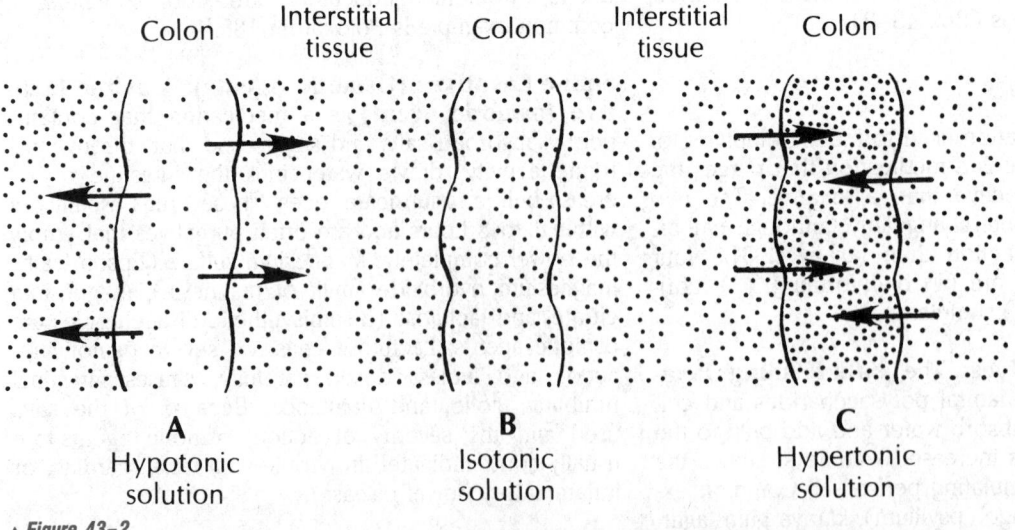

A Hypotonic solution

B Isotonic solution

C Hypertonic solution

▲ *Figure 43–2*

Concentration gradients across a semipermeable membrane. A, Hypotonic solution: Concentration is greater in interstitial tissues, so net water flow is out of colon. B, Concentration is the same on both sides of membrane, so there is no net water flow. C, Hypertonic solution: Concentration is greater inside colon, so net water flow is into colon.

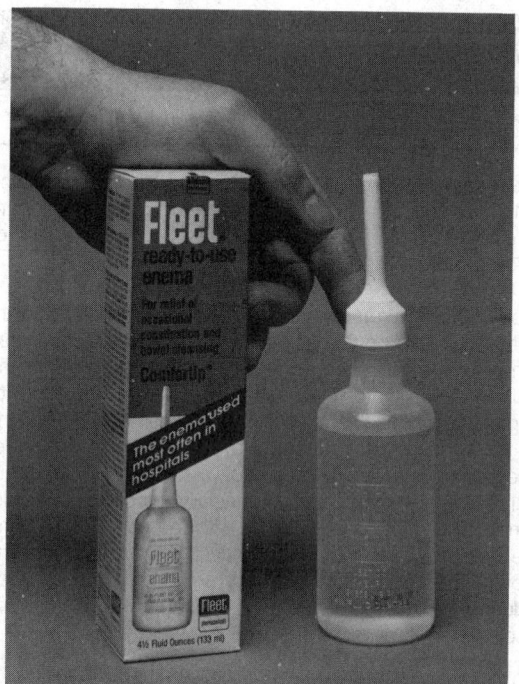

▲ *Figure 43-3*

Fleet enema. (Courtesy of the C.B. Fleet Company, Lynchburg, Virginia.)

ate colonic emptying. The large volumes, however, may present a danger to people with weakened colon walls. In addition, these enemas often require special preparation and equipment. Conversely, hypertonic enemas/small volume (120 to 250 cc) are available commercially and are easier to administer. A commonly used over-the-counter product is the Fleet enema (Fig. 43-3). It is important to avoid giving people hypertonic solutions if they have a problem with sodium retention.

A variety of enema solutions are available. One fairly common solution is a soapsuds enema in which castile soap is added to either tap water or saline solution, to cause mucosal irritation. Other enema solutions, such as milk and molasses, vegetable oils, hydrogen peroxide, and champagne, are reported in the literature. However, these types are rarely used. Various medication and nutritive formulas such as sucralfate enemas are also used, depending on the person's needs.[17]

Administration of Enemas. Box 43-4 briefly lists common nursing activities in administration of an enema (bowel irrigation). Procedure 43-1 specifically

from an external source; or (b) a small-volume enema, which draws internal fluid into the bowel. The concepts of osmosis and concentration gradient are important to an understanding of how some enemas work. Briefly, osmosis is the movement of water through a semipermeable membrane in order to equalize the concentration of particles on both sides of the membrane. Although water continuously flows back and forth across the membrane, the major net flow of water is toward the solution with a higher concentration of molecules.

Cleansing enemas utilize hypotonic, isotonic, or hypertonic solutions to distend the bowel and induce defecation. Figure 43-2 shows how solutions of different tonicity affect the net flow of water into or out of the colon.

Hypotonic solutions have a lower osmotic pressure than the fluid in the interstitial tissues, so the net flow of water is out of the bowel into the tissues. Tap water is the most common hypotonic solution. The net flow occurs slowly, however, and defecation is usually stimulated before any appreciable fluid is absorbed into the body. Significant absorption occurs if the person is fluid depleted, or if repeat enemas are given.

Isotonic solutions produce equal concentrations on both sides of the semipermeable membrane, and consequently no net water flow occurs. Physiologic saline is the isotonic enema solution.

Hypertonic solutions are of higher concentration than the interstitial fluid. Thus, with hypertonic enema solutions, the net water flow is into the colon, leading to distention that stimulates the defecation reflex.

Hypotonic and isotonic enema solutions are large-volume enemas (750 to 1000 cc) that result in immedi-

---

Box 43-4. Bowel Irrigation

Definition

Instillation of a substance into the lower gastrointestinal tract

Activities

▶ Determine reason for gastrointestinal cleansing
▶ Avoid use if client has a history of ulcerative colitis or regional enteritis
▶ Check physician order for gastrointestinal cleansing
▶ Choose appropriate type of enema
▶ Explain procedure to client
▶ Provide for privacy
▶ Inform client there may be abdominal cramping and urge to defecate
▶ Assemble equipment
▶ Position client as appropriate
▶ Protect bed linens
▶ Provide bedpan, commode as appropriate
▶ Ascertain appropriate temperature of irrigating substance
▶ Lubricate tubing prior to insertion as appropriate
▶ Insert substance in rectum, as appropriate
▶ Ascertain amount of substance return from body orifice
▶ Monitor for side effects of irrigation solution or oral medication
▶ Monitor for signs and symptoms of diarrhea, constipation, and impaction
▶ Note if returns are not clear
▶ Cleanse anal area

▼▼▼

From McCloskey, J.C., & Bulechek, G. (1992). *Classification of nursing interventions.* St. Louis: Mosby–Year Book, Inc.

Text continued on page 1142

PROCEDURE 43-1

Preparing and Administering a Normal Saline Enema (NSE)

Definition/Purposes. Injection of 500 to 750 ml (for an adult) of normal (isotonic) saline (salt) solution into the large intestine by means of a tube inserted into the anus. Fluid breaks up fecal material and stimulates peristalsis and urge to defecate by means of a tube inserted into the anus. Fluid breaks up fecal material and stimulates peristalsis and urge to defecate by distending the bowel. Used to treat constipation, empty the colon of fecal material and gas prior to surgery or diagnostic studies, relieve gas pains, and establish a bowel evacuation pattern during the bowel-training program.

Contraindications/Cautions. People with congestive heart failure or other sodium-retaining conditions may absorb sodium from enema fluid, thus disrupting fluid-electrolyte balance. Vasovagal reflexes produced by distention of the rectum may cause myocardial infarction or other severe cardiac disturbances. Therefore, avoid enemas, or administer cautiously to the elderly and to people with known heart disease. Frequent enemas may cause water intoxication, potassium depletion, or mucosal irritation, particularly in the presence of disorders that inflame the mucosa, e.g., colitis or diverticulitis. Abrasions or perforations of the anterior rectal wall can occur (a) if the rectal tip is inserted too deeply, (b) if fluid is inserted under excessively high pressure, or (c) if the enema tip is inserted while the person is in a sitting position. Anal injuries can occur when edema, hemorrhoids, or inflammation make it difficult to visualize the anus. Diseases, especially infectious hepatitis, can be transmitted by contaminated enema equipment. Therefore, never store used equipment with the person's clothing or with hygiene equipment. Fluid inserted under excessive pressure or in excessive amounts may force bacteria into the colon past the ileocecal valve into the small intestine, or it may rupture the colon. Bulb syringes are dangerous because the amount of pressure cannot be controlled. If pain is produced during the attempt to insert the enema tip, do not give the enema, since there may be a stricture, abscess, or other lesion of the anus or rectum.

Learning/Teaching Guidelines. Provide the individual and significant others with the following information, as appropriate: (a) explain the reason for the enema; (b) point out that an enema is not administered when the person is on the toilet because abrasions or perforations of the anterior rectal wall may occur; (c) explain that the enema solution should be given slowly, under low pressure (no bulb syringes) and at a lukewarm temperature, and should not cause pain or cramping; (d) teach how to prepare physiologic saline enema and explain that it is the safest, least damaging solution; (e) teach how breathing through the mouth relaxes abdominal muscles and helps avoid cramps; (f) discuss how to avoid constipation by exercise, diet modifications (especially increasing dietary fiber) and adequate fluid intake; (g) explain the need for taking adequate time to defecate; (h) teach when the enema should be used at home and how to care for equipment; and (i) explain how to recognize constipation and variance in "normal" periods between bowel evacuations.

PRELIMINARY ACTIVITIES

Assessment/Planning

▶ Check diagnosis and activity orders.
▶ Note date and type of surgery or tests.
▶ Check medical order for cleansing enema or normal saline enema (NSE).
▶ Assess person's ability to turn and ambulate and to cooperate.
▶ Note presence of skin, muscle, bone, perineal or rectal lesions.
▶ Check medical order for fecal specimen for tests.
▶ Note time and character of previous stools on record.
▶ Assess ability to retain enema solution.
▶ Gather equipment. Equipment should be disposable and used only by one person or should be sterilized between patients.
▶ Determine comfort and safety needs, e.g., need for assistance in moving to commode or toilet.
▶ Assure safe, convenient access to toilet if appropriate.

Preparation

▶ Explain that enema will be given and why, even if person is unresponsive.
▶ Explain that person is not to flush toilet or allow other personnel to empty commode or bedpan until nurse checks enema returns.
▶ Ask which bed-lying position is most comfortable.
▶ Explain that enema fluid should be retained for about 15 minutes.
▶ Provide privacy, draw curtains, close door.

▶ Cover person with bath blanket and fan-fold top covers to foot of bed.
▶ Remove pajama bottoms.
▶ Place bed at working height.
▶ Adjust IV pole or overbed table to hold enema reservoir.

Equipment

▶ Enema reservoir, i.e., fluid holder. Figure 43-4 illustrates an enema bag and bucket.
▶ Rectal tube, tubing, and clamp (usually attached to reservoir)
▶ Water-soluble lubricant (if tubing tip not prelubricated)
▶ Table salt and tap water—40.5°C (105°F) (or prepared physiologic saline solution if table salt not available)
▶ Waterproof pad
▶ Bedpan (warm a metal pan with hot water) or commode if indicated
▶ Special rubber nipple (Fig. 43-5) if person unable to retain fluid
▶ Clean gloves
▶ Bath blanket
▶ Toilet tissue
▶ Client's robe and slippers
▶ Containers for collecting specimen, if indicated
▶ Teaspoon or disposable plastic or glass medicine-measuring container, if needed
▶ Overbed table or IV pole
▶ Tubing clamp or hemostat (if clamp not attached)

PROCEDURE 43–1 Continued

Preparing and Administering a Normal Saline Enema (NSE)

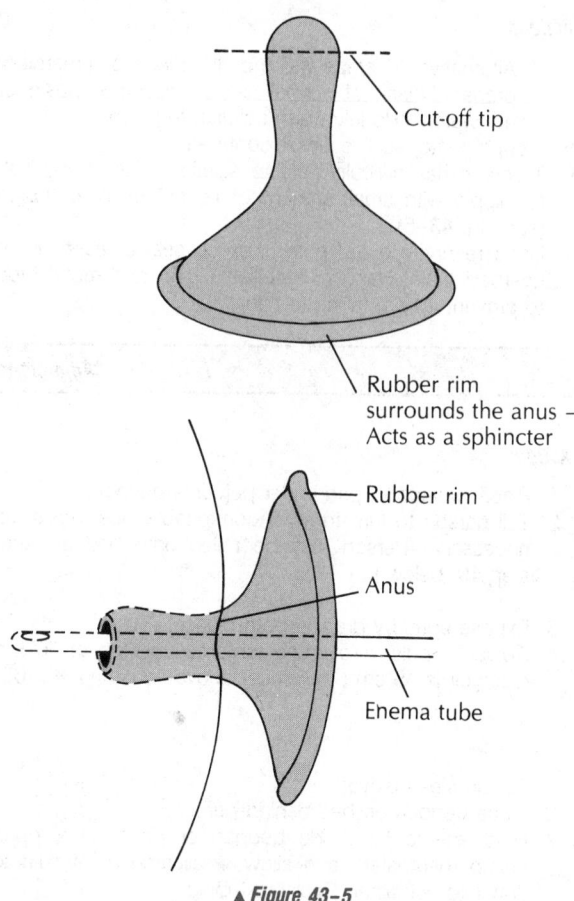

Cut-off tip

Rubber rim surrounds the anus — Acts as a sphincter

Rubber rim

Anus

Enema tube

▲ *Figure 43–5*

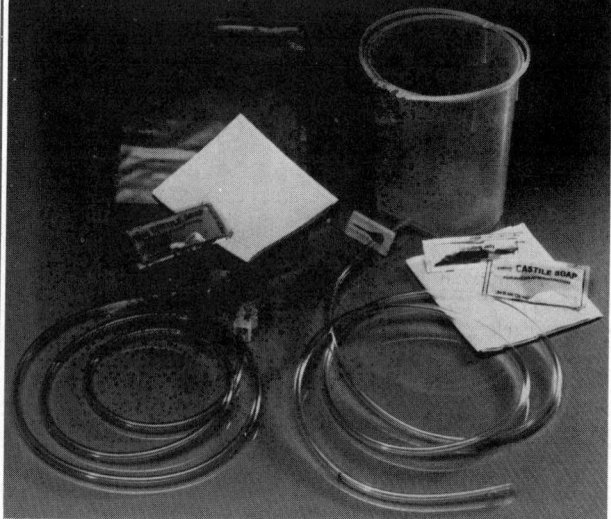

▲ *Figure 43–4*

PROCEDURE

Preparation of Saline Enema

Actions

1. Prepare solution at client's room sink or, if equipment is contaminated, in soiled utility room.

2. Attach tubing and rectal tube to reservoir if necessary.
3. Apply clamp or hemostat to tubing approximately 30 cm (12 inches) from rectal tube tip. Close clamp or hemostat.
4. Prepare physiologic saline solution:
   a. Adjust water flow at sink to lukewarm, 40.5°C (105°F).

   b. Add 1000 ml (32 oz or 1 qt) water and 2 teaspoons table salt to reservoir for adult.

Rationale/Discussion

1. Physiologic saline is solution of choice for cleansing enema unless person has sodium retention problem. Normal fecal flora contains pathogens. Previously used equipment would contaminate sink for client and personnel.
2. Completes delivery system.
3. Closing lumen of tubing prevents accidental loss of fluid. Places clamp or hemostat within easy reach during enema administration.
4.
   a. Use utility thermometer. Temperatures *above* 43°C (110°F) may injure tissues. Temperatures *below* 21°C (70°F) may produce severe cramping.
   b. Isotonic saline or physiologic salt solution is approximately 0.9 per cent salt in water. Use 500 to 750 ml (16 to 24 oz or 1 to 1.5 pints) for adults. Prepare additional amount in case some fluid is lost during administration.

Procedure continued on following page

PROCEDURE 43–1 Continued

Preparing and Administering a Normal Saline Enema (NSE)

Actions	Rationale/Discussion
c. Alternative to steps 4a and 4b: Place commercially prepared flask of normal saline solution in basin of hot water. Add lukewarm solution to reservoir.	c. This method is more expensive, and it is difficult and time consuming to bring solution to desired temperature.
5. If appropriate, seal reservoir container.	5. Prevents spillage from collapsible plastic bags.
6. If person has difficulty holding solution, place baby bottle nipple with small amount of tip cut off onto tubing (see Fig. 43–5).	6. Provides mechanical obstruction of anal canal around rectal tube when nipple is pushed up against anal sphincter to form "seal."
7. Hang reservoir on IV pole or place sealed reservoir on overbed table. Hang or stabilize tubing and rectal tube to prevent it from falling to floor.	7. Places enema equipment in position for use. Enema equipment must be kept clean and free of pathogens before use.

Administration of Enema

Actions	Rationale/Discussion
1. Place waterproof pad under person's buttocks.	1. Protects bed linen.
2. Tell person to turn to most comfortable side. Assist as necessary. (Person may be rolled onto bedpan after step 10, below.)	2. Position does not affect flow of fluid enough to be a factor in administration of enema. Enema may be given with client on bedpan and lying in supine position if client is anxious or unresponsive.
3. Expose anus by draping bath blanket.	3. Maintains warmth and prevents unnecessary exposure.
4. Adjust IV pole or overbed table so that top of fluid in reservoir is 45 cm (18 inches) above anus (Fig. 43–6).	4. Height of column of fluid produces hydrostatic pressure. Hence, fluid flows into colon. Placing reservoir higher increases pressure, thus causing pain and urge to defecate immediately. May also cause bowel rupture.
5. Put on clean gloves.	5. Protects hands from fecal contamination.
6. Place bedpan on bed behind person.	6. Bedpan is readily available.
7. Hold enema tip inside bedpan or paper cup, open clamp (hemostat), and allow small amount of fluid to flow into container. Reclamp tubing.	7. Eliminates air in tubing. Air seems to stimulate defecation reflex more than fluid does.
8. Lubricate rectal tube to 5 cm (2 inches) above tip with water-soluble lubricant if not prelubricated.	8. Reduces friction during tip insertion. Petroleum jelly (Vaseline) may be used at home.
9. Separate buttocks to visualize anus. Hold rectal tube tip against anus, pointing in direction of umbilicus (see Fig. 43–6). After anal sphincter relaxes, gently insert tip 5 cm (2 inches).	9. Stimulation of anal canal produces a protective reflex, which contracts anal sphincter. Relaxation of the sphincter usually follows the initial reflex contraction. Other methods to open or relax the anal sphincter may be used (e.g., ask person to bear down "as if moving your bowels," or to "pant like a dog") or gently insert tube while person exhales a deep breath. Forceful insertion of tip may injure anal or rectal tissue. Intended direction of rectal tip follows normal contour of colon, reducing danger of perforation.
10. *Hold enema tube in place throughout the procedure.* If the client has difficulty retaining enema fluid, use baby bottle nipple around rectal administration tube (see Fig. 43–5). Push nipple firmly against anus.	10. Presence of enema tube in anus distends anal sphincter. This causes bowel contractions, which tend to push tube out of anus. Holding tube prevents displacement. *External* placement of rubber nipple against anus prevents leakage from bowel.
11. Read level of fluid in reservoir before beginning fluid administration.	11. Remember, some solution has been used to flush air from tubing.
12. Open clamp (hemostat). Level of fluid in reservoir should fall slowly. If fluid level does not fall, briefly raise reservoir to 50 cm (20 inches) or slightly higher to increase pressure.	12. Raising reservoir increases pressure temporarily to open lumen of rectal tube if blocked by feces. If blockage remains, clamp tubing, remove rectal tube, clean lumen with toilet tissue, relubricate, and reinsert.
13. Gradually adjust height of reservoir to compensate for falling level of fluid. Goal is to keep fluid level in reservoir 45 cm (18 inches) above anus.	13. Maintains desired hydrostatic pressure.

PROCEDURE 43–1 Continued

Preparing and Administering a Normal Saline Enema (NSE)

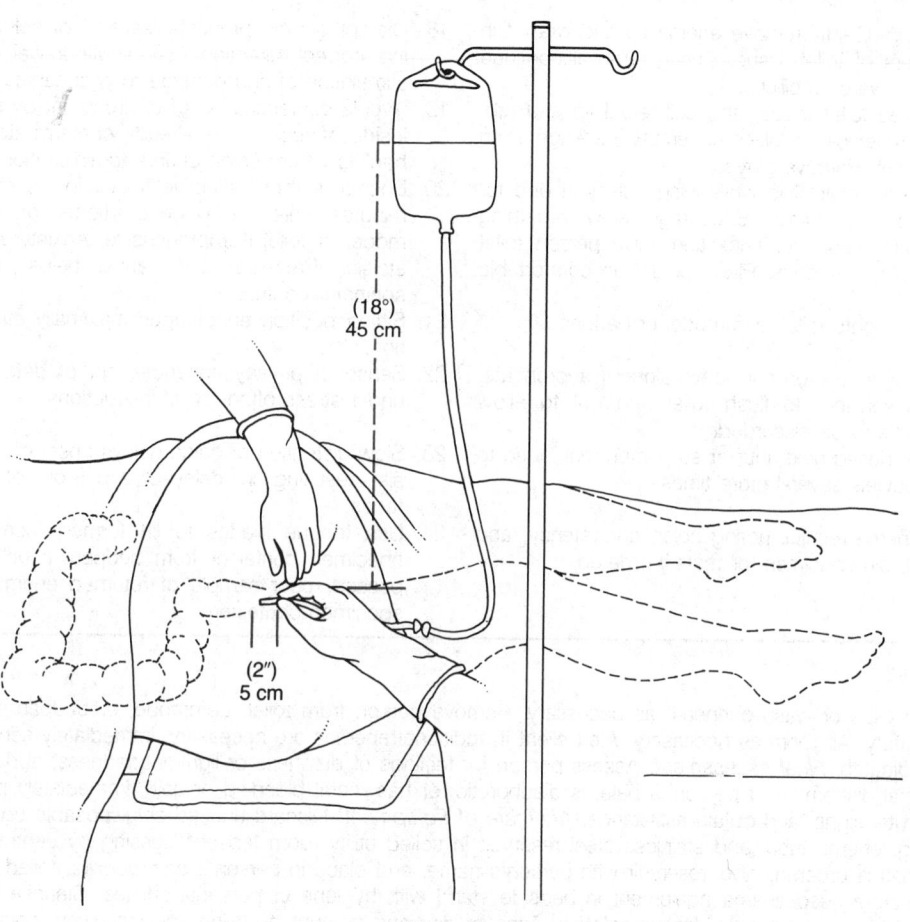

(18°)
45 cm

(2″)
5 cm

▲ Figure 43–6

Actions

14. Administer solution *slowly*. (750 ml should take 10 minutes to administer.) Remember: give adult 500 to 750 ml of solution.

15. Temporarily stop solution administration and follow step 16 until symptoms subside if:
    a. Client has urge to defecate or has abdominal cramps.
    b. Client begins to expel solution around rectal tube, or if solution level rises in reservoir. Turn bedpan on end, placing open lip of pan below anus to catch fluid. Do not remove rectal tube. Reassure person that changing bed is no trouble. Estimate amount of fluid lost.

16. During solution administration, ask person to open mouth and "pant like a dog" for short periods. Avoid hyperventilation.

17. Administer 500 to 750 ml of solution, repeating steps 15 and 16 as necessary. Do not give total amount if person is uncomfortable.

Rationale/Discussion

14. Saline enema works by causing distention of bowel (or mechanical irritation), resulting in contractions. Rapid administration of solution causes contractions of colon before desired amount is given, making retention of solution difficult.

15. Stop flow by kinking or folding tubing on itself.

    a. Distention of bowels causes discomfort; rapid closing of the tube is desirable.
    b. Removal of rectal tube stimulates defecation impulse. Anxiety increases peristalsis. Subtract amount of fluid lost from total to determine volume retained.

16. Breathing with mouth open relaxes abdominal muscles, decreasing pressure on colon. Also, distracts person enough to relax abdominal muscles.

17. Normal adult colon holds 750 ml comfortably. Large amount of feces in colon decreases volume of solution retained comfortably.

Procedure continued on following page

PROCEDURE 43–1 Continued

Preparing and Administering a Normal Saline Enema (NSE)

Actions	Rationale/Discussion
18. Clamp tubing. Gently remove enema tip and wrap it in several layers of toilet tissue. During removal continue to point tip toward umbilicus.	18. Clamping tube prevents leakage of solution. Maintaining correct direction during withdrawal of tip avoids stimulation of and damage to anal canal.
19. Discard soiled toilet tissue, and coil rectal tip and tubing inside reservoir or place in empty package from disposable set. Remove gloves.	19. Avoids contamination of environment by soiled articles. Inside of reservoir is already contaminated by solution backflow from colon during administration.
20. Ask person to retain fluid while lying quietly in bed for 15 minutes if possible. Encourage slow breathing through open mouth for relaxation. Give person toilet tissue to hold over anus. Place person in comfortable position.	20. Enema is most effective if solution is retained for 15 minutes. Person may be positioned on bedpan, commode, or toilet if apprehensive. Anxiety stimulates peristalsis. Pressure over anus helps maintain anal sphincter control.
21. Assist person onto toilet, commode, or bedpan.	21. Sitting position encourages maximally effective defecation.
22. Give call bell to person and leave alone if appropriate. Remind person not to flush toilet and not to allow enema results to be discarded.	22. Sense of privacy enhances act of defecation. People under stress often forget instructions.
23. Explain that during next hour or so person may need to evacuate bowels several more times.	23. Slow distention of colon delays onset of strong peristalsis, resulting in delayed expulsion of solution and feces.
24. Observe enema results, noting color, consistency, and amount. Obtain specimen for tests if ordered.	24. Use tongue blades to lift formed fecal material into specimen container from bedpan. If no formed feces passed, pour sample of returned enema solution into specimen container.

FINAL ACTIVITIES

Assist client to wipe or wash perineum as necessary. Remove person from toilet, commode, or bedpan. Ensure client's comfort and safety. Air room as necessary. Alert client if additional enemas are necessary. Immediately send specimen to laboratory if indicated. *Final Assessment:* Assess person for feelings of dizziness or light-headedness, abdominal cramps, nausea, or rectal discomfort. If person is pale, is diaphoretic, or has rectal bleeding or pain, immediately place in supine position, take vital signs, and obtain assistance. *Aftercare of Equipment:* Discard unused or disposable equipment. Place reusable tubing, enema tube, and stainless steel reservoir in soiled utility room for reprocessing by central services. If a series of enemas is ordered, label reservoir with person's name, and place in person's bathroom or soiled utility room for reuse. Do not store used enema equipment in bedside stand with hygiene or personal articles. Cleanse commode and bedpan, and store as appropriate. *Documentation:* Time of day and amount of saline solution given; color, consistency, amount, and time(s) of evacuation; person's reaction; time specimen sent to laboratory. Immediately report and document any untoward effects; pain, failure to expel fluid, blood or tissue expelled, change in vital signs. Record NSE on appropriate flow sheet.

describes the techniques for preparing and administering a normal saline enema. Use these methods for enemas of any volume but make any necessary changes when preparing the solution.

Administration of a Hypertonic Enema. Administration of a hypertonic enema requires several variations in the process described in Procedure 43–1, mainly because the solution comes prepackaged and ready to inject. You do not have to warm the solution, but make sure that it is at room temperature to prevent intestinal cramps. The individual may be in any position to receive this enema. However, the knee-chest position is recommended as the best way to distribute the solution throughout the colon.

To administer a commercially prepared hypertonic enema, the cap should be removed and the prelubri-

cated tip inserted into the rectum. The collapsible reservoir should be squeezed steadily until the solution is gone. The enema should be retained until the urge to defecate is very strong. People can be taught to self-administer a hypertonic enema, and they may be asked to administer one at home before x-ray studies or proctologic examinations.

Administration of a Retention Enema. Administration of a retention enema is similar to that for a normal saline enema, except that the solution must be retained over a prolonged period, usually for 1 hour at least. Some enemas (e.g., medicated or nutritive enemas) should never be evacuated. The method of solution preparation depends on what type of solution has been ordered. A smaller administration tip is used (usually a No. 14 to No. 20 French catheter for adults), to avoid stretching the sphincters, thereby diminishing stimulation of the defecation reflex. Make sure you elevate the reservoir only high enough to allow the solution to run slowly into the rectum. Administration under higher pressure distends the rectum, causing defecation. Finally, protect the bed linen in case the person cannot retain the enema. Commercially prepared retention enemas are given in the same manner as hypertonic commercially prepared enemas.

For the hazards associated with enema administration, see Box 43–5.

Dependence on Enemas. As is true of laxatives and suppositories, people can develop physical and psychologic dependence on enemas. The underlying mechanism is the same: the enema cleans the bowel so that it takes two or more days for enough fecal mass to collect again to stimulate defecation. In the meantime, the person becomes anxious because he or she does not have a bowel movement and therefore self-administers another enema. Gradually, the bowel becomes less sensitive to normal defecation reflex stimuli, and the person becomes physically dependent on bowel aids.

Constipation Management

Constipation/impaction management is the "prevention and alleviation of constipation/impaction."[24] Nursing activities appropriate for this intervention are found in Box 43–6.

Constipation is a condition characterized by a stool consistency described as excessively dry, hard, and of insufficient size. However, the term *constipation* is used by many persons to describe a decreased frequency of defecation, an increased time required for passage of the stool through the intestinal tract (intestinal transit time), and a difficulty in expelling rectal contents through the anal spincter.[22] Constipated people may also have other symptoms, such as headache, lethargy, anorexia, halitosis, furry tongue, and a bloated feeling. These discomforts are believed to be reflexes resulting from prolonged distention of the rectum.

CAUSES OF CONSTIPATION

Common causes of constipation include lack of established bowel pattern; inadequate diet, fluids, and exercise; emotional depression; weak pelvic floor muscles; and/or neuromuscular diseases. Inconvenience also is frequently a factor. When the urge to defecate is repeatedly ignored, the stool remaining in the rectum continues to lose water and stops stimulating normal reflexes. Immobilizing a person for any reason decreases the intensity of colonic propulsion and heightens the risk of constipation. Intestinal pathologic conditions, including neoplasm, stricture, hernia, megacolon (excessive dilation or stretching of the colon),

---

Box 43–5. Hazards of Enema Administration

Enema administration is not without its hazards. Complications include fluid and electrolyte imbalances, tissue trauma, vagal nerve stimulation, and dependence. Fluid imbalances usually occur because of the tonicity of the enema solution. Remember that the body absorbs water from hypotonic solutions. Use caution when administering enemas to people who are susceptible to fluid imbalance (e.g., infants or people with decompensated cardiac or kidney reserve). Water intoxication can occur. Symptoms of this condition include weakness, dizziness, pallor, sweating, and respiratory difficulties. Signs of congestive heart failure or cerebral edema may also be present. On the other hand, hypertonic solutions draw fluid from the interstitial tissues and can lead to fluid depletion, especially in children and other people who are susceptible to dehydration.

Other electrolyte imbalances may also occur. Usually, normal saline is the safest enema solution because of its isotonicity. However, in people who have problems with sodium retention (e.g., those with congestive heart failure or cirrhosis of the liver), the body absorbs sodium, which leads to saline excess and a fluid retention. Therefore, these individuals should not receive saline solutions. Depending on the contents of the enema solution, other electrolyte imbalances may also occur, such as hypokalemia, hypocalcemia, and hyperphosphatemia.

Enemas can also cause tissue trauma. The four major sources of trauma are (1) the administration tip, (2) administration of solution under high pressure, (3) a soapsuds solution, and (4) increased peristalsis. If the enema tip has any chips or broken areas, it may lacerate or abrade the rectal mucosa. High pressures or enema tips can rupture the intestinal wall. There may be no pain at the time of perforation. The first indication of rupture may be signs of peritonitis (inflammation of the peritoneum). Tissue trauma from peristalsis also occurs in people with inflammatory bowel diseases. The increased motility of the bowel enhances cramping, bleeding, and so forth.

Avoid giving enemas to people who have inflammatory bowel disease.

As stated earlier, one enema solution uses "soapsuds" and the soapsuds solution chemically irritates the mucosa. This irritation frequently leads to rectal inflammation and colitis, sometimes lasting up to 3 weeks after administration of the enema. The higher the concentration of soap in the solution, the greater is the chance of inflammation.

The practice of swirling a bar of soap or soap pieces in the enema reservoir is extremely dangerous, since it is impossible to determine the concentration. A soapsuds solution is somewhat safer if you use standardized packages of castile soap.

Box 43–6. Constipation/Impaction Management

Definition

Prevention and alleviation of constipation/impaction

Activities

- ▶ Monitor for signs and symptoms of constipation
- ▶ Monitor for signs and symptoms of impaction
- ▶ Monitor bowel movements, including frequency, consistency, shape, volume, and color as appropriate
- ▶ Monitor bowel sounds
- ▶ Consult with physician about a decrease/increase in frequency of bowel sounds
- ▶ Monitor for signs and symptoms of bowel rupture or peritonitis
- ▶ Explain etiology of problem and rationale for interventions
- ▶ Identify factors (e.g., medications, bedrest, diet) that may cause or contribute to constipation
- ▶ Encourage increased fluid intake unless contraindicated
- ▶ Evaluate medication profile for gastrointestinal side effects
- ▶ Instruct client/family to record color, volume, frequency, and consistency of stools
- ▶ Teach client/family how to keep a food diary
- ▶ Instruct client/family on high-fiber diet as appropriate
- ▶ Instruct client/family on appropriate use of laxatives
- ▶ Instruct client/family on the relationship of diet, exercise, and fluid intake to constipation/impaction
- ▶ Evaluate recorded intake for nutritional content
- ▶ Consult physician if signs and symptoms of constipation persist
- ▶ Consult physician if signs and symptoms of impaction persist
- ▶ Administer laxative or enema as appropriate
- ▶ Inform client of procedure for manual removal of stool if necessary
- ▶ Remove the fecal impaction manually if necessary
- ▶ Administer enema or irrigation as appropriate
- ▶ Weigh regularly

▼ ▼ ▼

From McCloskey, J.C., & Bulechek, G. (1992). *Classification of nursing interventions.* St. Louis: Mosby–Year Book, Inc.

diverticular disease, and painful anal lesions, all interfere with normal expulsion of the feces. Constipation frequently accompanies pregnancy, both because of hormonal changes and because of external pressure on the intestine.

Numerous medications contribute to constipation: analgesics (especially narcotics), anesthetic agents, anticholinergics, some antihypertensives, tricyclic antidepressants, calcium- and aluminum-containing antacids, iron supplements, and MAO inhibitors, which slow neural transmission and thereby slow peristalsis. Overuse of laxatives, suppositories, and enemas contributes to the problem primarily through the resulting loss of intrinsic innervation and atrophy of the smooth muscle necessary for defecation.

Disorders in body systems can also cause constipation. These problems include spinal trauma, multiple sclerosis, cerebral vascular accident (stroke), Parkinson's disease, myxedema, hypercalcemia, hypokalemia, diabetes mellitus, uremia, hypothyroidism, hyperparathyroidism, heavy metal poisoning, and pheochromocytoma.

Aging contributes to constipation, through lessened intestinal secretions for feces lubrication and through increased water absorption from the feces in the intestine because of slower peristalsis.[13]

HAZARDS OF STRAINING AT STOOL

Besides being uncomfortable, constipation can actually be hazardous for many people. To pass a hard stool, a person usually employs the Valsalva maneuver. This action can cause problems in people with cardiac disease, resulting in angina pectoris (paroxysmal chest pain) and even cardiac arrest. It also may be detrimental to people with head injuries (by increasing intracranial pressure), respiratory disease (by increasing intrathoracic pressure), and thromboembolic disorders (by causing thrombi to dislodge). Exhaling through the mouth during straining reduces the chance of increasing intrathoracic pressure, but the best precaution is to avoid constipation.

Straining to pass a stool is detrimental in other ways. Over time, it may contribute to the development of hemorrhoids. If the person has had recent bowel surgery, straining might disrupt the suture line. As a precaution, people are often given enemas preoperatively to eliminate the need for a bowel movement for several days after surgery.

INTERVENTIONS FOR CONSTIPATION

The interventions for typical constipation require all the preventive measures previously mentioned: teaching/learning activities, changes in diet, fluid intake, and exercise; and development of healthy bowel habits. Sometimes additional intervention is needed. If symptoms of constipation persist and are unresponsive to nonoperative management, surgical options are available as a last resort.[28]

Impaction Management

The prevention and alleviation of constipation prevent fecal impaction.

CAUSES OF IMPACTION

A **fecal impaction** is a collection of putty-like or hardened feces in the rectum, which usually prevents the passage of a normal stool. As the fecal mass remains in the rectum, the colon absorbs more water from it. Additional fecal material is then added to the mass as it moves down from the sigmoid colon. Eventually, the mass becomes so hard and large that it cannot pass through the anus.

ASSESSING IMPACTION

The first indication of an impaction is the client's inability to pass a normal stool. However, probably the most definitive sign is the seepage of liquid stool from the anus. Liquefaction provides the only way that fecal material can get around the impaction. Usually the liquid appears in small amounts, which helps differentiate it from diarrhea. However, bacterial action on the fecal mass sometimes causes the production of copious amounts of liquid stool.

The seepage of stool is usually uncontrolled, since the anal sphincters have become less competent, secondary to prolonged stimulation of the defecation reflex by the hardened mass.

Other signs and symptoms indicating impaction include an almost continuous urge to defecate, rectal pain, abdominal fullness, nausea and vomiting, shortness of breath, hypertension, and abdominal distention. Perform a digital examination of the rectum if an impaction is suspected. Wear a glove and liberally lubricate the forefinger, which is inserted through the anus into the rectum. If a hard fecal mass is felt, an impaction probably exists. If a mass is not felt but the symptoms are present, the mass may be higher up in the colon, out of reach.

INTERVENTIONS FOR IMPACTION

The goal of treatment for a fecal impaction is removal of the mass from the rectum. Oral laxatives or cathartics may be used to moisten and lubricate the fecal mass, although their action may be too slow. A program of enemas may be instituted, starting with the administration of an oil retention enema and followed by a volume cleansing enema. These two enemas may need to be repeated.

If the fecal mass is extremely large or the enemas are ineffective in expelling it, you will have to remove the impaction digitally. To do this, insert a gloved, heavily lubricated finger into the rectum. Remove pieces of the mass manually (have a bedpan close at hand). Even though you can use a topical anesthetic agent such as lidocaine, this intervention is uncomfortable and embarrassing for the person. Gentleness may help, but prevention is the best treatment.

Diarrhea Management

Diarrhea is the passage of liquid or unformed stool. As with constipation, some people consider the frequency of defecation as part of the definition, but consistency of the stool is the primary component. In general, diarrhea indicates increased intestinal motility, which causes GI contents to move rapidly through the tract. Because of the rapid transit time, normal amounts of water are not removed from the feces. In addition, irritation of the mucosal walls may stimulate increased secretions, which add moisture to the fecal mass. Therefore, when the feces reaches the rectum and anus, it is still liquid.

CAUSES OF DIARRHEA

The causes of diarrhea are numerous and different for acute and chronic diarrhea. Acute diarrhea may be caused by emotional states, especially anxiety; infectious organisms, such as bacteria, viruses, and parasites; alterations in diet, such as greasy or spicy foods or food to which a person is allergic; and medications, such as iron supplements, thyroid agents, magnesium-containing antacids, antibiotics, lactulose, cimetidine (an H_2 receptor antagonist), antihypertensives, colchicine (an alkaloid of colchicum autumnale), digitalis, and laxatives. Causes of chronic diarrhea have been identified as lactose-containing or hyperosmolar nutritional supplements such as those containing sorbitol or mannitol (osmotic agents); systemic diseases such as hyperthyroidism, diabetes mellitus, adrenal insufficiency, and hyperparathyroidism; inflammatory bowel diseases; cancer of the colon; gastrointestinal surgery; radiation enterocolitis; laxative abuse; alcohol abuse; and chemotherapeutic agents.[35]

ASSESSING DIARRHEA

Assessing diarrhea requires an understanding that signs and symptoms can be much more extensive than the mere passing of liquid stool. Accompanying signs and symptoms may include abdominal cramps, distention, flatus, nausea and vomiting, bleeding, anorexia, urgency, fever, malaise, and symptoms of fluid imbalance. Severe diarrhea can lead to significant fluid and electrolyte imbalance, since the body does not reabsorb water, potassium, and sodium. There is also malabsorption of other nutrients. Diarrheal stool is usually caustic and causes skin breakdown if it comes into prolonged or frequent contact with the skin. This problem is exacerbated by frequent wiping with toilet paper.

Question the individual carefully about the frequency and characteristics of the stool; the duration of the problem; the presence of abdominal cramps; recent exposure to infected people; recent travel; dietary and medication intake; and the existence of anxiety, stress, or systemic disease that might contribute to a change in elimination patterns.

INTERVENTIONS FOR DIARRHEA

Nursing activities appropriate for diarrhea management are listed in Box 43–7. As with any condition, assess the person before deciding on the appropriate intervention.

The usual treatment for diarrhea is to inhibit peristalsis, although some clinicians feel that this slows expulsion of the pathogenic organisms or irritants and may actually prolong the problem. Generally, the rule of thumb is to remove the precipitating factors first, then stop the diarrhea itself. Therefore, a person with a GI

Box 43-7. Diarrhea Management

Definition

Prevention and alleviation of diarrhea

Activities

▶ Monitor for signs and symptoms of diarrhea
▶ Instruct client to notify staff of each episode of diarrhea
▶ Observe skin turgor regularly
▶ Monitor skin in perianal area for irritation and ulceration
▶ Measure diarrhea/bowel output
▶ Weigh regularly
▶ Obtain stool for culture and sensitivity if diarrhea continues
▶ Identify factors (e.g., medications, bacteria, tube feedings) that may cause or contribute to diarrhea
▶ Notify physician of an increase in frequency or pitch of bowel sounds
▶ Consult physician if signs and symptoms of diarrhea persist
▶ Instruct in low-fiber, high-protein, high-calorie diet as appropriate
▶ Instruct in avoidance of laxatives
▶ Teach client appropriate use of antidiarrheal medications
▶ Evaluate medication profile for gastrointestinal side effects
▶ Instruct client/family members to record color, volume, frequency, and consistency of stools
▶ Teach client/family how to keep a food diary
▶ Evaluate recorded intake for nutritional content
▶ Encourage frequent, small feedings (add bulk gradually)
▶ Teach client to eliminate gas-forming and spicy foods from diet
▶ Teach client stress-reduction techniques as appropriate
▶ Assist client in performing stress-reduction techniques
▶ Suggest trial elimination of foods containing lactose
▶ Monitor safe food preparation
▶ Perform actions to rest the bowel (e.g., NPO, liquid diet)

▼▼▼

From McCloskey, J.C., & Bulechek, G. (1992). *Classification of nursing interventions.* St. Louis: Mosby–Year Book, Inc.

---

infection often receives antibiotics and possibly antidiarrheals.

For mild-to-moderate diarrhea, short-term therapy involves decreasing or eliminating food intake to reduce stimulation of peristalsis. Commonly used antidiarrheal drugs such as kaolin and pectin may also be used. These medications bind and remove irritants from the GI tract and form a soothing, protective coating on the mucosa.

Sometimes the bulk-forming laxatives hold water in the GI tract and thus reduce the fluid loss. In severe diarrhea, the physician may prescribe opiates such as paregoric or codeine, or an opiate derivative with an anticholinergic drug (such as Lomotil) to inhibit peristalsis.[11] As stated, antibiotics may be used to eliminate the cause of the diarrhea, and antibiotics can reduce or eliminate normal intestinal flora as well as pathologic microorganisms.

Normal intestinal bacterial flora can be re-established by giving the client yogurt, buttermilk, or bacillus-containing medications such as Bacid or Lactinex.

One must also manage accompanying problems. Fluid and electrolyte imbalance is a common complication of diarrhea. Infants and debilitated persons are especially susceptible to this complication. Fluid and electrolyte losses must be replaced, by either oral or parenteral (intravenous) therapy. Emphasize to the individual that decreasing fluid intake will not stop the diarrhea.

Skin care is also important for the person with diarrhea. Providing the person with soft material for wiping after each stool reduces the irritation. Washing with soap and water after each stool reduces the time that the irritating diarrhea is in contact with the skin.

The frequency and urgency of bowel movements also causes fatigue and embarrassment. Therefore, make sure that the person has quick and easy access to the bathroom, commode, or bedpan. Place the call bell near the person at all times. Provide for privacy and odor control.

Flatulence Reduction

Gas is normally found in the GI tract. Some of it is swallowed, some of it is produced by fermentation in the intestine, and some of it comes from diffusion of gases from the bloodstream. **Flatulence (gaseous distention)** is the presence of abnormally large amounts of gas within the GI tract. Symptoms include a bloated feeling, abdominal distention, cramping pains, and excessive passage of gas from the mouth (eructation) or from the anus (flatus). Respiratory distress may also occur if the distended abdomen pushes against the diaphragm. Abdominal percussion produces a tympanic sound.

Probably the most common predisposing factor in flatulence is excessive air swallowing, which results from chewing gum, drinking carbonated beverages, eating rapidly, or sucking through straws. Anxiety states and postnasal drip can also lead to excessive air swallowing.

Other causes of gaseous distention include constipation, slowed intestinal motility as may occur after abdominal surgery, bowel obstruction, medications that decrease peristalsis, decreased physical activity, and foods such as beans, cabbage, radishes, onions, cauliflower, and cucumbers.

INTERVENTIONS FOR FLATULENCE

Nursing interventions appropriate for flatulence reduction are listed in Box 43–8. The goal of therapy is to remove the gas from the GI tract.

Box 43-8. Flatulence Reduction

Definition

Prevention of flatus formation and facilitation of passage of excessive gas

Activities

▶ Teach client how flatus is produced and methods for alleviation

▶ Teach client to avoid situations that cause excessive air swallowing, such as chewing gum, drinking carbonated beverages, eating rapidly, or sucking through straws

▶ Teach client to avoid substances that cause flatulence, such as beans, cabbage, radishes, onions, cauliflower, and cucumbers

▶ Monitor for bloated feeling, abdominal distention, cramping pains, and excessive passage of gas from the mouth or anus

▶ Monitor vital signs, bowel sounds

▶ Provide for adequate exercise, e.g., ambulate

▶ Insert lubricated rectal tube about 4 inches into the rectum as appropriate, tape in place and insert distal end of tube into a receptacle

▶ Administer an enema as appropriate

▶ Monitor side effects of medication administration

▶ Limit oral intake if lower gastrointestinal system is inactive

▶ Position on left side with knees flexed, as appropriate

▶ Offer antiflatulence medications as appropriate

▼ ▼ ▼

From McCloskey, J.C., & Bulechek, G. (1992). *Classification of nursing interventions.* St. Louis: Mosby–Year Book, Inc.

Exercise. The most effective and natural way to expel the flatus is by exercise. Walking is the best method, but if this is not possible, moving around in bed will help. Exercise stimulates peristalsis, which speeds the transit time of the gas through the colon. Prevention is also important. Teach people to avoid situations and substances that cause flatulence.

Insertion of a Rectal Tube. If simple, more natural methods do not work, a rectal tube provides a passage for the gas out of the body. To insert a rectal tube into an adult, lubricate a No. 22 to No. 32 French rubber or plastic rectal tube and insert about 10 cm (4 inches) into the rectum. Place the distal end of the tube into a collecting receptacle to catch any feces that may be expelled. Tape the tube into place and leave it there for 20 minutes or less. Long periods may cause sphincter damage. Reinsert the tube every 2 or 3 hours if necessary.

Return-Flow Enema. A **return-flow enema (Harris flush)** also relieves flatulence, although this intervention is controversial because it can cause intestinal trauma. With this enema, the intestine is alternately filled and drained to move flatus through the GI tract

by stimulating peristalsis. Prepare the individual, the equipment, and the solution (tap water or saline) as in Procedure 43-1. After inserting the rectal tube, slowly infuse approximately 200 to 300 ml of fluid into the colon. Then lower the solution container 45 cm (18 inches) below the level of the anus to allow the solution and flatus to drain back into the reservoir. Expelled gas bubbles up through the solution in the container. When the return flow ceases, raise the reservoir approximately 18 inches above the anus and allow 200 to 300 ml to flow in. Repeat this process until the returned gas is minimal.

Use of Drugs to Relieve Flatulence. Several medications may help relieve flatulence. Simethicone-containing medications cause gas bubbles to coalesce, making them easier to expel. Some physicians order neostigmine to be given intramuscularly about 20 minutes before a rectal tube or return flow enema is used. Neostigmine increases GI motility and facilitates downward movement of the gas. However, this practice is controversial because of the drug's numerous side effects, such as dizziness, severe abdominal cramping, respiratory depression, and nausea and vomiting. If postnasal drip causes excessive air swallowing, a decongestant or antihistamine may prevent this cause of flatulence.

Bowel Incontinence Care

Bowel incontinence is the inability to control passage of feces and gas voluntarily. Bowel evacuation usually occurs involuntarily whenever the defecation reflex is stimulated. Lack of control is accepted during infancy and toddlerhood. However, following toilet training, continence is the norm, and any deviation meets with both personal and social disapproval.

Incontinence causes great embarrassment for the person, whose life is often arranged so as to conceal the problem from other people.

CAUSES AND CONSEQUENCES OF BOWEL INCONTINENCE

Causes of bowel incontinence are both physical and psychologic. Physical causes include anything that interferes with the integrity of sphincter function. Thus hemorrhoids, tumors, lacerations, rectal prolapse, fistulas, or loss of sensory innervation may lead to incontinence. People with explosive diarrhea may find the pressure too overwhelming to control. Psychologically, incontinence may be the result of an emotional state, as well as being itself the cause of various emotional problems. Encopresis is the socially inappropriate passage of stool when no physical reason exists to account for the behavior. It is believed to occur because of an emotional disturbance or delay in the maturational process. Sometimes a formerly continent child or adult becomes incontinent as a means of gaining attention or to express anger.

Probably the most important consequence of incontinence is the loss of self-respect, which is intensified by the reactions of significant others in the person's environment, including nurses, physicians, friends, and relatives. Also, incontinence causes skin irritation and breakdown, and soiling of clothes and linen.

INTERVENTIONS FOR BOWEL INCONTINENCE

See Box 43–9 for a list of nursing activities related to bowel incontinence.

Application of a Rectal Pouch. Application of a rectal pouch (Fig. 43–7) for the person who has bowel incontinence protects the skin and eliminates soiling of linen. The rectal pouch has a circular paper adhesive backing that adheres to the perianal skin, with a plastic bag attached that collects the feces. The adhesive opening can be altered in size to facilitate individual fitting. Perianal hair should be shaved to allow a tight fit of the adhesive back.[10]

Skin Care. Caring for the skin of an incontinent person may be a time-consuming task. The main goal is to prevent prolonged contact of the skin with fecal material, which leads to excoriation and breakdown. Wash-

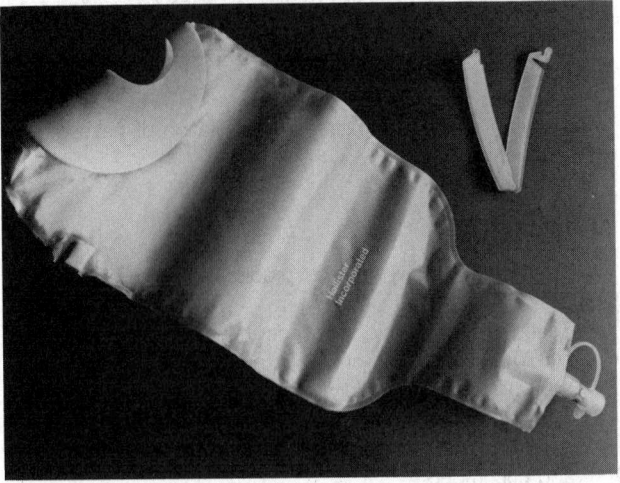

▲ *Figure 43–7*

Rectal incontinence pouch. (Courtesy of Hollister Incorporated, Libertyville, Illinois).

ing the perianal area with soap and water and drying it thoroughly after each stool keeps the skin in good condition and controls fecal odor. Nonionic detergent preparations (e.g., Peri-Wash) are even more effective than regular soap. Use powders and creams with caution since they may actually contribute to skin breakdown.

If a rectal pouch is not in use, the bed and clothing of the incontinent person must be kept clean. When using plastic or rubber sheeting to protect bed linen, make sure that it does not contact the skin, thus causing irritation.

Protection of Clothing. When incontinence is severe, the individual may need to wear waterproof undergarments to protect clothing. Adult-size disposable briefs are available with cellulose padding to draw fluid away from the skin by capillary action. However, diapers make the person feel infantile and appear to give "permission" to be incontinent, so avoid this practice whenever possible. The best way to reduce the physiologic and psychologic impact of incontinence is to reestablish bowel control.

Bowel Training

BOWEL-TRAINING PROGRAMS

Bowel-training programs are an effective method for helping people regain bowel control (Box 43–10). They require time, patience, and commitment from nursing personnel and the client, but the results are well worth the effort.

First assess and diagnose the factors causing the incontinence. Then, discuss the bowel-training program with the client and significant others, and together decide on a routine for bowel elimination. Establish the routine based upon (a) the person's previous bowel habits and (b) alterations in bowel habits that have

---

Box 43–9. Bowel Incontinence Care

Definition

Promoting bowel continence and maintaining perianal skin integrity

Activities

▶ Determine physical or psychologic cause of fecal incontinence
▶ Explain etiology of problem and rationale for interventions
▶ Determine goals of bowel management program with patient/family
▶ Discuss procedures and expected outcomes with client
▶ Instruct client/family to record fecal output, as appropriate
▶ Wash perianal area with soap and water and dry it thoroughly after each stool
▶ Use nonionic detergent preparation such as Peri-Wash for cleansing as appropriate
▶ Use rectal pouch as appropriate
▶ Empty rectal pouch as needed
▶ Place on incontinent pads, as appropriate
▶ Provide protective pants, as needed
▶ Use powder and creams on perianal area with caution
▶ Keep bed and clothing clean
▶ Implement bowel training program as appropriate
▶ Monitor for adequate bowel evacuation
▶ Monitor diet and fluid requirements
▶ Monitor for side effects of medication administration

▼ ▼ ▼

From McCloskey, J.C., & Bulechek, G. (1992). *Classification of nursing interventions.* St. Louis: Mosby–Year Book, Inc.

Box 43-10. Bowel Training

Definition

Assisting the client to train the bowel to evacuate at specific intervals

Activities

► Plan bowel program with client and appropriate others
► Consult with physician and client regarding use of suppositories
► Teach client/family principles of bowel training
► Teach client digital rectal dilatation as necessary
► Instruct client which foods are high in bulk
► Provide foods high in bulk and/or which have been identified as assistive by the client
► Ensure adequate fluid intake
► Ensure adequate exercise
► Ensure privacy
► Initiate an uninterrupted, consistent time for defecation
► Administer suppository as appropriate
► Perform digital rectal dilatation
► Evaluate bowel status regularly
► Modify bowel program as needed

▼▼▼

From McCloskey, J.C., & Bulechek, G. (1992). *Classification of nursing interventions.* St. Louis: Mosby–Year Book, Inc.

---

occurred because of illness or trauma. In addition, note when the person is most likely to be incontinent during the day.

All bowel-training programs include independent nursing measures used to aid normal defecation: diet, fluids, exercise, and maintenance of defecation patterns. Probably the most crucial element of the program is timing. The schedule for defecation is carefully determined and then strictly followed. If at all possible, position the person on the commode or toilet at the designated time to take advantage of gravity.

Bowel programs are individualized, although there are many common factors. Habit training, control of diarrhea, and biofeedback are possible strategies for bowel programming.[20]

Most programs include stool softeners to facilitate passage of feces. This intervention is especially important for people with spinal cord injuries or extreme debilitation, since they frequently cannot "bear down."

Often, suppositories are used every 1 to 3 days to stimulate evacuation. In people with spinal cord injuries, the suppository is usually followed in 20 to 30 minutes by digital stimulation of the anal sphincter to augment stimulation of the defecation reflex.

In some programs, enemas are used in place of the suppositories. Suppository or enema administration is usually discontinued as soon as bowel elimination is maintained without them.

The training program is modified until a successful routine is found. Generally, a person is kept on a particular program for at least 3 days before it is changed.

APPLYING RESEARCH TO NURSING PRACTICE

Timing Bowel-Training Programs for Clients with Strokes

Venn, M.R., Taft, L., Carpentier, B., & Applebaugh, G. (1992). The influence of timing and suppository use on efficiency and effectiveness of bowel training after a stroke. *Rehabilitation Nursing*, 17(3), 116–120.

▼▼▼

For clients who have suffered a cerebrovascular accident (a CVA, or "stroke"), restoration and control of lost bowel function is an important goal. Altered patterns of defecation following a stroke may be due to loss of sensation, confusion, decreased appetite, or difficulty in communicating the need to defecate. Venn and colleagues sought to determine whether scheduled and consistent administration of suppositories would improve the efficiency and effectiveness of bowel control in 58 clients who had had a CVA. Factors considered in this study were the timing of suppository use; food, fiber, and fluid intake; and the client's age and activity level. The researchers also investigated whether matching the timing of suppository insertion with the client's previous bowel pattern would be effective in restoring bowel function.

Those clients who received their suppositories in the morning achieved better bowel control than those receiving suppositories in the evening. Matching the timing of suppository administration with the client's previous bowel patterns was also more effective than administering suppositories on a conflicting schedule. Clients receiving suppositories on an as-needed basis did just as well as those who received them regularly, on a schedule. Although improved food and fluid intake enhanced the effectiveness of bowel training, fiber intake did not make a significant difference in this study population.

Applications for Practice

This research supports the nursing practice of assessing each client's previous pattern of bowel function to determine when to administer a suppository. If the client usually had a bowel movement in the morning, administer the suppository within 30 to 40 minutes after the client's breakfast. If the client usually had a bowel movement in the evening, schedule suppository administration for 30 to 40 minutes after the client's evening meal.

This period allows the nurse to be sure that changes are indeed necessary.

OTHER METHODS OF MANAGING BOWEL INCONTINENCE

Other methods of treating incontinence are available. Biofeedback therapy is successful for some people. Surgical intervention to create new tissue sphincters has been tried. Electrical stimulation of sphincter control has also been successful in some cases.

Ostomy Care

Yet another nursing intervention, ostomy care, is appropriate for those individuals who have a gastrointestinal tract diversion. An **ostomy** is a surgically created opening. Nursing interventions for ostomy care are listed in Box 43–11.

DIVERSION OF THE GASTROINTESTINAL TRACT

Gastrointestinal tract diversion involves channeling intestinal contents out of the body at a site other than the anus. This commonly involves an **ileostomy,** which is a surgically created opening in the ileum, or a **colostomy,** which is a surgically created opening in the large intestine. These surgical procedures establish a **stoma,** (a surgically created, mouthlike opening) on the abdominal wall through which gastrointestinal contents pass.

Ileostomy. An ileostomy may be performed because of cancer, congenital defect, or trauma, but by far the most frequent reasons are ulcerative colitis or regional ileitis (Crohn's disease). Because of the placement of the stoma in the small intestine, the flow of intestinal contents in most cases is constant and cannot be regulated. Surgical techniques do exist in which a continent ileostomy is formed by creating an internal pouch with a nipple valve that is emptied with a catheter at the person's convenience.

Colostomy. A colostomy is performed because of trauma, intestinal obstruction, a birth defect, or cancer. It may be done to the ascending (rarely), transverse, descending, or sigmoid colon. The farther down the intestine the stoma is placed, the better are the chances of regulating the bowel. Most people with a colostomy wear a pouch or bag (Fig. 43–8) that is changed periodically. Some people, however, develop such reliable bowel control that they do not wear a bag, only a small dressing to protect the stoma from irritation by clothing.

PHYSIOLOGIC PROBLEMS ASSOCIATED WITH AN ILEOSTOMY OR COLOSTOMY

Physiologic problems vary depending on the type of ostomy: ileostomy or colostomy. The major problems with ileostomies are obstruction, diarrhea, and skin irritation. These are managed as follows:

▶ *Obstruction.* Obstruction is prevented by chewing food thoroughly; it can usually be relieved by massaging the abdomen around the stoma or by gentle lavage (washing out) of the stoma with a catheter.
▶ *Diarrhea.* Diarrhea is treated as described earlier.

The person with an ileostomy is particularly susceptible to fluid and electrolyte imbalances, and therefore diarrhea must be quickly controlled.

Box 43–11. Ostomy Care

Definition

Maintenance of elimination through a stoma and care of surrounding tissue

Activities

▶ Instruct client/significant other in the use of ileostomy/colostomy equipment
▶ Assist client in providing ostomy/ileostomy self-care
▶ Have client/significant other demonstrate use of equipment
▶ Apply appropriate-fitting ostomy appliance
▶ Monitor for incision/stoma healing
▶ Encourage client/significant other to express feelings and concerns about changes in body image
▶ Encourage visitation to client by persons from such support groups as ileostomy/colostomy clubs
▶ Irrigate colostomy as appropriate
▶ Assist client in obtaining ostomy/ileostomy equipment
▶ Instruct client on mechanisms to reduce odor
▶ Instruct client/significant other in appropriate diet and expected changes in elimination function
▶ Provide support and assistance while client develops skill in caring for stoma/surrounding tissue
▶ Monitor stoma/surrounding tissue healing and adaptation to ostomy equipment
▶ Change/empty ostomy bag as appropriate
▶ Encourage participation in ostomy support groups after hospital discharge

▼▼▼

From McCloskey, J.C., & Bulechek, G. (1992). *Classification of nursing interventions.* St. Louis: Mosby–Year Book, Inc.

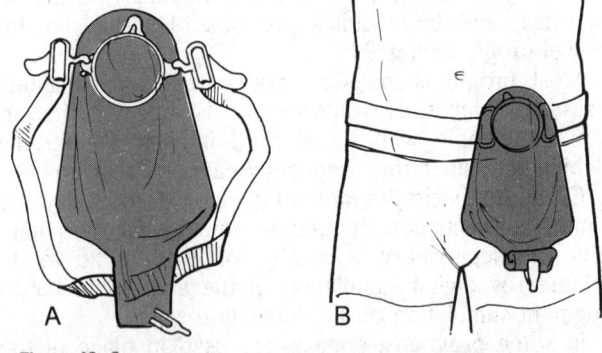

▲ *Figure 43–8*

Colostomy bag. *A,* The circular opening in the upper portion of the bag surrounds the stoma, and the firm plastic piece around the opening fastens to the ends of the belt worn around the client's waist. *B,* With the bag belted in place and folded up and clamped closed on the bottom, the colostomy opening is effectively sealed to the outside so that all fecal material will be contained within the bag.

▶ *Skin Irritation.* Skin irritation is best treated by preventive measures like proper fitting and fixation of the collection bag. If irritation does occur, the skin must be kept clean and dry, and a protective skin barrier should be used between the pouch faceplate and the skin. Use topical medications to treat severe irritation.

CARE OF AN ILEOSTOMY

Because the ileostomy (except for the continent ileostomy) is continually draining gastrointestinal contents, the person must wear a bag at all times. The pouch is emptied through an opening at the bottom whenever necessary. The person often does it at the time of urination. After stoma healing is complete, the person is fitted with a reusable appliance. The person with an ileostomy (the ileostomate) is usually very knowledgeable about changing this appliance.

CARE OF A COLOSTOMY

For the person with a colostomy, the decision about whether or not to irrigate a colostomy depends on the location of the stoma and the person's abilities and preference. A colostomy can function adequately without irrigation, but routine irrigation helps avoid fecal spillage during the day. Most persons are taught to care for their stomas and irrigate the bowel if necessary. If clients with a stoma come into the hospital, they may continue their own care if able. If not, you may temporarily take over these tasks.

Irrigation of a colostomy is very similar to the administration of a normal saline enema. The major differences are the insertion site and the fact that the person is unable to control the expulsion of the solution and fecal material, so some variation in equipment and technique is necessary. An irrigation sleeve is used to channel the expelled contents into the toilet or bedpan. The sleeve is a plastic tunnel (Fig. 43–9) that fits around the stoma and is held in place by a belt around the waist. The irrigating solution and enema equipment are prepared as they are for any volume enema. Cone-shaped irrigation tips (Fig. 43–10) are preferred to catheters, since they reduce the danger of bowel perforation. The nipple cone also seals off the stoma so that the irrigating fluid cannot leak. Be sure of the location of the stoma before inserting the cone. If using a catheter, gently insert it about 7.5 to 10 cm (3 to 4 inches). Administer the solutions as in Procedure 43–1.

When you are ready to remove the administration tip, be sure that the irrigating sleeve is well situated over the stoma, since the initial drainage may gush out. Close the top of the sleeve with clips, and allow most of the content to be expelled. This usually takes about 10 to 15 minutes. Control odor by occasionally rinsing the sleeve with water and flushing the toilet. When the person is sure that the irrigation returns have finished, the irrigation sleeve may be removed, the peristomal skin cleaned, and either a clean pouch or a dressing applied.

ODOR CONTROL

For the osteomate who wears a pouch, odor control is often a problem. Certain foods, such as cabbage, cauliflower, onions, and turnips, often increase fecal odor.

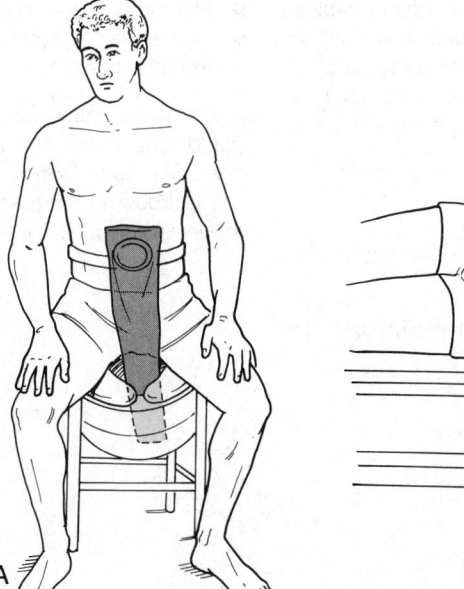
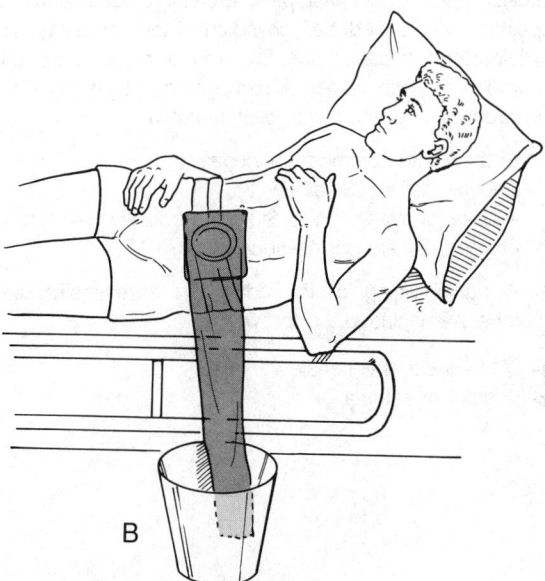

▲ *Figure 43–9*

Colostomy irrigation sleeve. *A,* When worn by the client who is able to sit up, the sleeve can drop between the legs to drain into the toilet or bedside commode. *B,* When worn by the client who is unable to sit up, the sleeve can be worn to one side so it can drain into a container at the bedside.

A

B

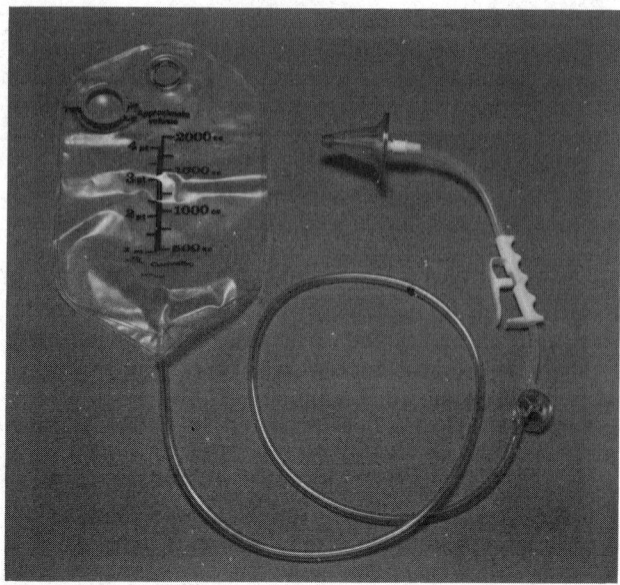

▲ **Figure 43–10**

Cone-shaped irrigation tip. (Courtesy of ConvaTec, Princeton, NJ).

Odors, which can be very distressing, can be controlled by:

► Carefully washing the appliance after use
► Placing a deodorizing agent in the pouch

► Using internal medications, such as bismuth subgallate
► Ingesting yogurt, buttermilk, parsley, green leafy vegetables, or orange juice
► Placing a few drops of Dispatch in the collection receptacle to mask the odor while emptying the pouch

Review of the new osteomate's medication regime is necessary to eliminate contraindicated medications. Diuretics, laxatives, and enteric-coated and sustained-release oral medications are usually not administered for the ileostomate and some colostomates.[16]

EVALUATION

In all nursing diagnoses related to bowel elimination, it is important to evaluate outcomes by assessing how the client's bowel elimination compares with normal, expected elimination. Ideally, following nursing intervention, the evaluation should show that the fecal contents are normal for that person and the bowel movements are on a schedule normal for that person. If the reestablishment of normal bowel elimination was not an expected outcome (as in the client with an ileostomy), it is important to assess whether the client has successfully adapted to elimination changes. Whenever elimination problems can be improved, revisions to the plan of care must be made until elimination for the client is as near normal as possible.

CASE STUDY

The Client

Mrs. Mary Colleen, a 71-year-old white woman, lived independently in an apartment of a retirement residence. She was moving a chest of drawers while cleaning and had a sudden, sharp, right-sided chest pain. Breathing became difficult and painful. She visited her physician where an x-ray study revealed three fractured ribs. She was admitted to the apartment complex's health center. A partial listing of physician's orders, on admission to the health center, included:

Bedrest with commode privileges
Regular diet as tolerated
Tylenol (acetaminophen) #3 with codeine q3–4 h prn
Oxygen, 2 liters per nasal cannula

A partial listing of the admission assessment data, November 12, included the following:

► 71-year-old, frail female
► History of asthma

► T 97.8 F, B/P 132/78, P 76, R 20
► Clear lung sounds
► States pain upon inspiration
► Independent in activities of daily living
► Attentive husband

Three days after admission, Mrs. Colleen c/o being constipated. She stated she usually moves her bowels daily. Only one small, hard, formed stool was passed since admission.

The following represents part of a nursing care plan written for her shortly after this new problem presented.

CARE PLAN

10:00 AM, November 15

Nursing Diagnosis	Planning: Expected Outcomes	Implementation: Nursing Interventions	Evaluation
Constipation R/T decreased activity	By 10:00 AM November 17: Defecates a soft, normal stool	Monitor bowel movements including frequency, consistency, shape, volume, and color Monitor bowel sounds Encourage increased intake of fluids by at least 200 additional cc/day Provide natural laxatives such as prunes, high-fiber foods Provide list of high-fiber foods	10:00 AM November 17: Defecated small, soft brown stool at 7:00 AM Reported no feeling of fullness

Summary

▶ The lower gastrointestinal tract is the main organ system responsible for the elimination of the body's solid waste. This consists of the ascending, transverse, descending, and sigmoid colon and rectum.

▶ Physiologic and psychosocial factors have a strong influence on the act of defecation.

▶ Assessment of bowel elimination needs includes noting the history of psychologic and physiologic factors affecting elimination; completing a physical assessment of the abdomen and observing the fecal characteristics; and noting the outcome of diagnostic tests completed by x-ray examination, direct visualization, and laboratory analysis.

▶ The current NANDA list of nursing diagnoses relevant to bowel elimination needs includes *Constipation, Perceived Constipation, Colonic Constipation, Diarrhea,* and *Incontinence.*

▶ Planning for clients with these diagnoses includes writing outcomes specific to resolving constipation, diarrhea, and episodes of incontinence.

▶ Nursing interventions include bowel management, stimulating bowel evacuation, constipation management, impaction management, diarrhea management, flatulence reduction, bowel incontinence care, bowel training, and ostomy care.

▶ Evaluation of outcomes should show that the fecal contents and bowel movements are as near to normal as possible for the individual or that the client has adapted successfully to elimination changes.

Bibliography

1. Al-Mudallal, R., et al. (1990). Anaphylactic reaction to barium enema. *American Journal of Medicine,* 89(2), 251.
2. Barnett, J.M., et al. (1990). Intoxication after an isopropyl alcohol enema. *Annals of Internal Medicine,* 113(8), 638–639.
3. Bates, B. (1991). *A guide to physical examination and history taking.* Philadelphia: J.B. Lippincott.
4. Battle, E., & Hanna, C. (1980). Evaluation of a dietary regimen for chronic constipation: Report of a pilot study. *Journal of Gerontological Nursing,* 6, 527.
5. Bielefeldt, K., et al. (1990). Diagnosis and treatment of fecal incontinence. *Digestive Diseases,* 8, 179–188.
6. Bulechek, G.M., & McCloskey, J.C. (1987). Nursing interventions: what they are and how to choose them. *Holistic Nursing Practice,* 1(3), 36–44.
7. Bulechek, G.M., & McCloskey, J.C. (1989). Nursing interventions: treatments for potential nursing diagnoses. In Carroll-Johnson, R.M. (ed.). *Proceedings of the Eighth Conference: Classification of Nursing Diagnoses.* Philadelphia: J.B. Lippincott.
8. Cairncross, S. (1989). Water supply and sanitation: an agenda for research. *Journal of Tropical Medicine and Hygiene,* 92, 301–314.
9. Carter, J., & Carter, R. (1987). *Everything to gain: Making the most of the rest of your life* (p. 44). New York: Random House.
10. Freedman, P. (1991). The rectal pouch: a safer alternative to rectal tubes. *American Journal of Nursing,* May, 105–106.
11. Gilman, A.G., et al. (eds.). (1990). *Goodman and Gilman's pharmacological basis of therapeutics.* (8th ed.). New York: Pergamon Press.
12. Hahn, K. (1989). When a patient's scheduled for G.I. studies. *Nursing,* 19(3), 88.
13. Hardy, M.A. (1991). Normal changes with aging. In Maas, M., et al. (eds.). *Nursing diagnoses and interventions for the elderly.* Redwood City, California: Addison-Wesley Nursing.
14. Hickson, D.E.G., et al. (1990). Enema or Picolax as preparation for flexible sigmoidoscopy? *Postgraduate Medical Journal,* 66(773), 210–211.
15. Iseminger, M., et al. (1982). Bran works! *Geriatric Nursing,* 3, 402.
16. Kuhn, J.K., & Flaherty, M.J.M. (1990). Helping ostomy patients back to independence. *Journal of Gerontological Nursing,* 16(6), 27–30.
17. Ladas, S.D., & Raptis, S.A. (1989). Sucralfate enemas in the treatment of chronic postradiation proctitis. *American Journal of Gastroenterology,* 84(12), 1587–1589.
18. Lara, L.L., et al. (1990). The risk of urinary tract infection in bowel incontinent men. *Journal of Gerontological Nursing,* 16(5), 24–26.
19. Lincoln, R., & Roberts, R. (1989). Continence issues in acute care. *Nursing Clinics of North America,* 24(3), 741–754.
20. Maas, M., & Specht, J. (1991). Bowel incontinence. In Maas, M., et al. (eds.). *Nursing diagnoses and interventions for the elderly.* Redwood City, California: Addison-Wesley Nursing.

21. Mangan, P., & Thomas, L. (1988). Preserving dignity. *Geriatric Nursing and Home Care,* 8(9), 14.

22. McClane, A.M., & McShane, R.E. (1991). Constipation. In Maas, M., et al. (eds.). *Nursing diagnoses and interventions for the elderly.* Redwood City, California: Addison-Wesley Nursing.

23. McClane, A.M., & McShane, R.E. (1992). Bowel management: controlling incontinence. In Bulechek, G.M., & McCloskey, J.C. (eds.). *Nursing interventions: Treatment for nursing diagnosis* (2nd ed.). Philadelphia: W.B. Saunders.

24. McCloskey, J.C., & Bulechek, G. (1992). *Classification of Nursing Interventions.* St. Louis: Mosby–Year Book, Inc.

25. Netter, F.H. (1975). *The CIBA collection of medical illustrations:* Volume 3, Digestive System; Part II, Lower Digestive Tract. New York: R.R. Donnelley & Sons.

26. Newman, D.K., & Smith, D.A.J. (1989). Incontinence in elderly homebound patients. *Holistic Nursing Practice,* 4(1), 52–60.

27. North American Nursing Diagnosis Association (1990). *Taxonomy I revised-1990 with official nursing diagnoses.* St. Louis: North American Nursing Diagnosis Association.

28. Orrom, W.J., et al. (1991). Rectopexy is an ineffective treatment for obstructed defecation. *Diseases of the Colon and Rectum,* 34(1), 41–46.

29. Peterson, M. (1988). Effective fecal collectors. *Journal of Enterostomal Therapy,* 15(6), 259.

30. Schwartz, R. (1991). What's the fuss over fiber? *Cooking Light,* 5(2), 42.

31. Smigielski, P.A., & Mapel, J.R. (1990). Bowel and bladder management. In Craft, M.J., & Denehy, J.A. (eds.). *Nursing interventions for infants and children.* Philadelphia: W.B. Saunders.

32. Stroh, S.E., et al. (1989). Fecal incontinence in children: a clinical update. *Maternal Child Nursing,* 14(4), 252–254.

33. Taptich, B.J., et al. (1989). *Nursing diagnosis and care planning.* Philadelphia: W.B. Saunders.

34. Tilkian, S.M., et al. (1987). *Clinical implications of laboratory tests.* St. Louis; C.V. Mosby.

35. Wadle, K. (1991). Diarrhea. In Maas, M., et al. (eds.). *Nursing diagnoses and interventions for the elderly.* Redwood City, California: Addison-Wesley Nursing.

36. Wesley, J. (1764). *The primitive physic.* Philadelphia, 1764.

37. Yaffe, B. (1991). Women should go to the bathroom more often. *Bottom Line,* 12(7), 11.

38. Yakabowich, M. (1990). Prescribe with care: the role of laxatives in treatment of constipation. *Journal of Gerontological Nursing,* 16(7), 4–11.

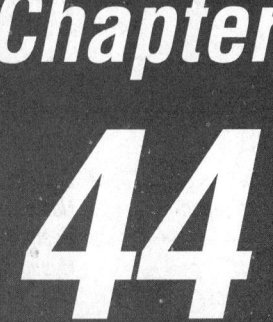

Chapter 44

▼ *Meeting Urinary Elimination Needs*

▼
    237.   *Bloody Urine*.
733. Take a quarter of a Pint of *Sheeps Milk* twice a Day:
734. Or, half a Pint of Decoction of *Agrimony*:
▼ 735. Or, of Decoction of *Yarrow*.
    238.   *Urine Drops with Heat and Pain*.
736. Drink nothing but *Lemonade*:
▼ 737. Or, beat up the Pulp of five or six rolled *Apples* with near a
    Quart of Water. Take it at lying down. It commonly cures be-
    fore Morning.
    239.   *Involuntary Urine*.
▼ 738. Ufe the *cold Bath*:
739. Or, take a Tea-fpoonful of powder'd *Agrimony* in a little Water,
    Morning and Evening.
740. Or, a Quarter of a Pint of *Allum-Poffet-Drink* every Night.
    240.   *Sharp Urine*.
741. Take two Spoonfuls of frefh Juice of *Ground-Ivy*.
    241.   *Suppreffion of Urine*.
742. Drink largely of warm *Lemonade*:
743. Or, take a Spoonful of Juice of *Lemons*, fweeten'd with Syrup
    of *Violets*:
744. Or, a Spoonful of Juice of *Radifhes*:
745. Or, two Spoonfuls of Juice of *Onions*: . . .

John Wesley
Primitive Physic (1764)

▼ CHAPTER OUTLINE

ANATOMY AND PHYSIOLOGY OF THE
  URINARY SYSTEM
    Urinary Structures and Related
      Functions
    Changes in the Urinary Tract with
      Aging
MAINTAINING NORMAL URINARY
  ELIMINATION
    Fluids and Exercise
    Urinary Elimination During Illness
    Teaching About Urinary Elimination
ASSESSMENT
    Physiologic Factors
    Personal Factors
    Psychosocial Factors
    Cultural Factors
    Medications
    Trauma
    Difficulties with Urinary Elimination
    Problems with Urinary Elimination
    Urine Characteristics

    Routine Urine Testing
    Urine Specimens
    Diagnostic Tests of Urinary
      Function
NURSING DIAGNOSIS
    Altered Urinary Elimination
    Urinary Incontinence
    Urinary Retention
PLANNING
    Altered Urinary Elimination
    Urinary Incontinence
    Urinary Retention
NURSING INTERVENTION
    Altered Urinary Elimination
    Urinary Incontinence
    Urinary Retention
EVALUATION
    Altered Urinary Elimination
    Urinary Incontinence
    Urinary Retention
CASE STUDY

Anuria	Frequency	Nephrectomy	Pyuria	Urethritis
Bacteriuria	Glycosuria	Nephrolithiasis	Residual urine	Urgency
Bladder irrigation	Hematuria	Nephrostomy tube	Retention	Urination
Calculi	Hesitancy	Nocturia	Retention with overflow	Urinary diversion
Cystitis	Hypercalciuria	Oliguria	Stent	Urinary incontinence
Diuretic effect	Lithotripsy	Polyuria	Ureters	Urolithiasis
Dysuria	Micturition	Proteinuria	Urethra	Voiding
Enuresis				

▼ *LEARNING OBJECTIVES*

After studying this chapter, you should be able to

1. *Describe the normal anatomy and physiology of the urinary system.*
2. *Discuss factors that influence the maintenance of normal urinary elimination.*
3. *List data needed to assess a person's urinary status.*
4. *Discuss common nursing diagnoses for the individual experiencing problems meeting urinary elimination needs.*
5. *Describe planning for individuals with urinary problems.*
6. *Describe nursing interventions for individuals with urinary problems.*
7. *Describe evaluation criteria for individuals with urinary problems.*

One of the body's basic physiologic needs is to rid itself of wastes. The three main routes of elimination are the respiratory, gastrointestinal, and urinary tracts. Because elimination of wastes is absolutely necessary for survival, these systems must function properly.

One body system that plays a major role in the internal environment is the urinary system. A stable internal environment is necessary to sustain life. For example, water, sodium, and potassium must be maintained in the appropriate balance to ensure equilibrium and optimal cellular function. The urinary system is largely responsible for total body water volume and electrolyte balance.

An alteration in urinary elimination may lead to destruction of renal tissue, loss of fluid and electrolyte balance, decreased excretion of wastes, and inadequate regulation of body processes. In addition to causing untoward effects on the function of the urinary system, alterations in urinary elimination can lead to social and hygienic problems as well as to changes in body image.

To meet elimination needs, people frequently need assistance from health professionals. Your role in meeting these needs involves both dependent and independent nursing actions. In either type of nursing action, sensitivity to the needs of the person with urinary elimination problems is extremely important.

ANATOMY AND PHYSIOLOGY OF THE URINARY SYSTEM

Urinary Structures and Related Functions

The urinary tract has four major structures:

▶ The kidneys, which selectively reabsorb, secrete, and excrete water, electrolytes, and other substances to maintain the body's homeostasis

▶ The **ureters,** the two tubes that carry urine from the kidneys to the bladder
▶ The urinary bladder, which stores urine until the person urinates
▶ The **urethra,** which is the conduit from the urinary bladder to the exterior of the body

Figure 44–1 illustrates the anatomy of the urinary tract.

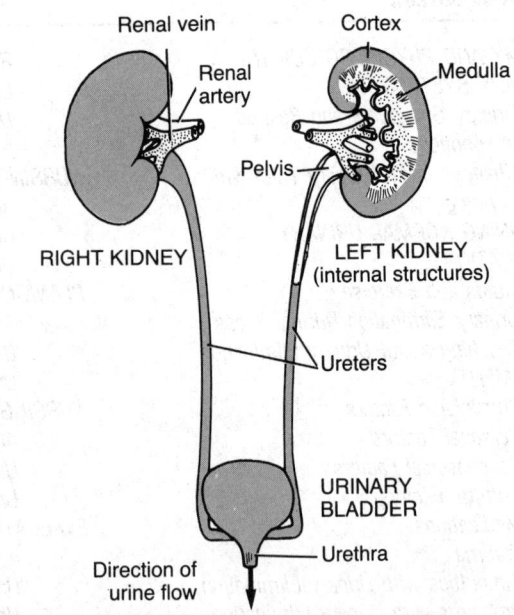

▲ **Figure 44–1**

Anatomy of the urinary tract. (From Guyton, A.C. [1991]. *Textbook of medical physiology* [8th ed.]. Philadelphia: W.B. Saunders.)

KIDNEYS

The kidneys are located retroperitoneally along the thoracolumbar spine, above the iliac crests, with the left kidney usually a little higher than the right. The kidneys are supported by a mass of adipose tissue and fibrous tissue called the renal fascia. The adrenal glands are located on the top of each kidney.

The major function of the kidney is to maintain the extracellular fluid within normal limits. To meet this goal, the kidneys (a) remove waste products from the body; (b) regulate the water, electrolyte, and acid-base balances; and (c) secrete two important hormones: renin, which indirectly increases blood volume through the renin-angiotensin-aldosterone mechanism, and erythropoietin, which causes increased red cell production.

The nephron is the functional unit of the kidney (Fig. 44–2). Each kidney contains approximately one million nephrons. These structures have two major components: the glomerulus, which is a cluster of capillaries surrounded by a Bowman's capsule, and a system of tubules. It is here in the nephron that blood is filtered, and electrolytes, water, and other substances are secreted, excreted, or reabsorbed.

The renal arteries deliver approximately 1200 ml of blood to the kidneys per minute. The blood is channeled to the glomerulus. Under high pressure, the blood (minus large-protein molecules) is filtered into Bowman's capsule and then into the tubules at a rate of about 125 to 130 ml per minute. The tubules reabsorb necessary substances such as water, sodium chloride and other electrolytes, creatinine, glucose, lactate, amino acids, and vitamin C according to body needs. Approximately 98 per cent of the glomerular filtrate is reabsorbed, so that actual urine production is about 1 to 2 ml per minute. Kidney tubules also secrete some of the same substances they reabsorb. For example, excess sodium, hydrogen, or glucose is secreted by the

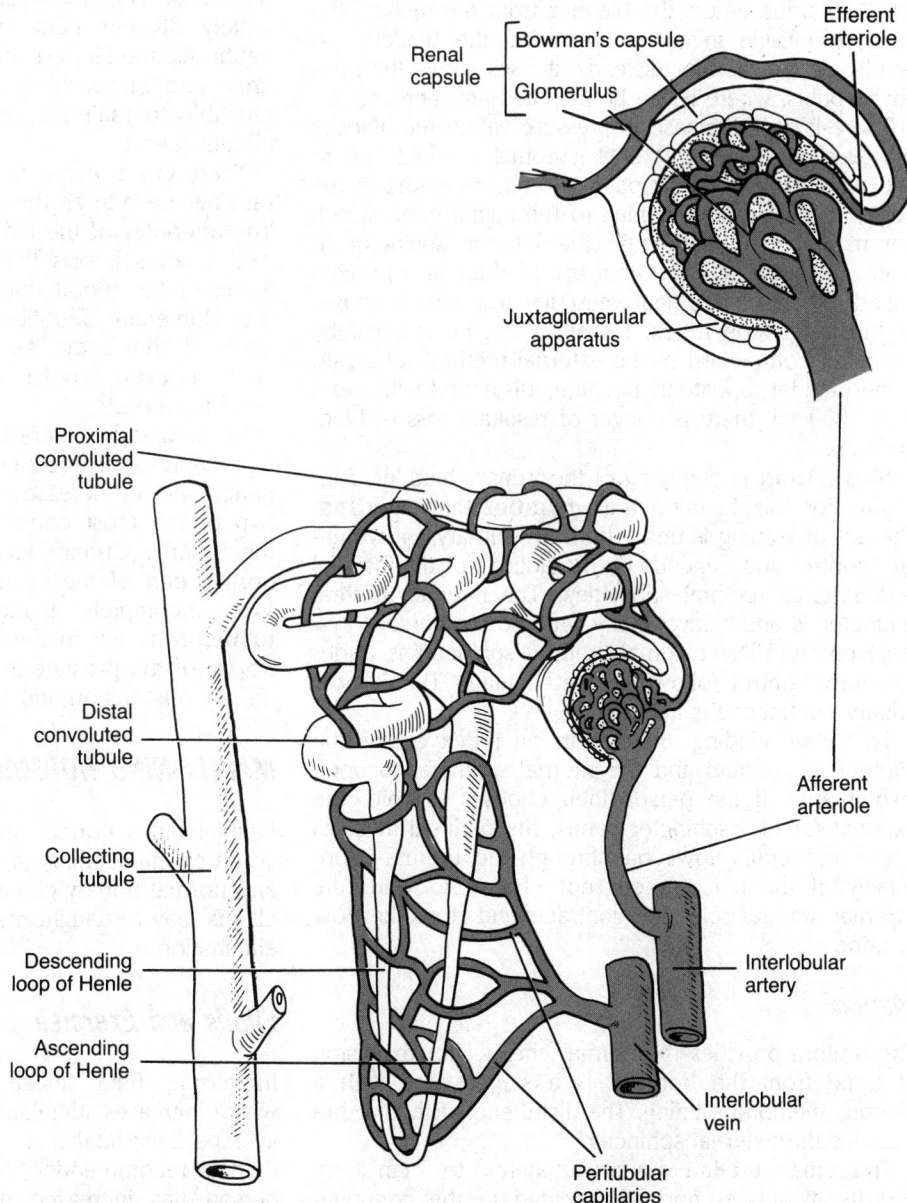

▲ **Figure 44–2**

The nephron with its blood vessels. Blood flows from the interlobular artery to the afferent arteriole to the glomerulus to the efferent arteriole. Blood then flows to the peritubular capillaries, around the tubules and venules, and into the interlobular vein.

tubules and excreted in the urine, thus maintaining fluid and electrolyte balance.

URETERS

The ureters are approximately 25 to 30 cm long in adults. They arise from the renal pelvis and enter the inferior, posterior portion of the bladder at an oblique angle. At this ureterovesical junction, there is usually an anatomic sphincter that prevents the backward flow (reflux) of urine into the kidney. Urine moves from the renal pelvis through the ureters to the bladder by gravity and peristalsis.

URINARY BLADDER

The urinary bladder is a holding vessel for urine. It is a hollow organ with three muscle layers forming its walls. These layers of smooth muscle, called detrusor muscle, come together at the base to form the internal sphincter, which is under reflex control from the spinal cord. As urine enters the bladder from the ureters, the detrusor muscle initially relaxes and the bladder expands. As the bladder distends, it rises above the symphysis pubis, where it can be palpated and percussed.

There is little increase in pressure within the bladder (intravesicular pressure) until it contains about 150 to 300 ml of urine. At this point, stretch receptors in the detrusor muscle send stimuli to the spinal cord, which returns impulses that cause the internal sphincter to open and urine to flow from the bladder in a process called urination. This neuromuscular response is known as the micturition reflex. Urination can be stopped by voluntary contraction of the external urethral sphincter. If the bladder repeatedly becomes distended with more than 1000 ml, there is danger of resultant loss of bladder tone.

Micturition is emptying of the urinary bladder. Synonyms for this function are **urination** and **voiding.** The act of voiding is under both involuntary and voluntary control and depends on the actions of the internal and external urethral sphincters. The internal urethral sphincter is under involuntary (autonomic nervous system) control. The external urethral sphincter is under voluntary control following toilet training. This is how urinary continence is achieved.

To initiate voiding, the micturition reflex causes the bladder to contract and the internal sphincter to open involuntarily. If the person then chooses to void, the external urethral sphincter opens, the perineal muscles relax, and urine flows out through the urethra. Conversely, if the person does not choose to void, the external urethral sphincter contracts and stops the flow of urine.

URETHRA

The urethra provides the normal channel for expulsion of urine from the body. It is a simple tube with a mucous membrane lining. The distal end of the urethra includes the external sphincter.

The female urethra is approximately 3 to 5 cm long, and its meatus is normally located in the perineum between the clitoris and the vagina. The male urethra is about 20 cm long and follows an S-shaped curve from the bladder neck to its meatus on the tip of the penis. The prostate gland, located below the bladder and surrounding the proximal urethra, is an important structure in the male urinary tract. Problems arise when this gland enlarges (as often occurs in older men) and partially or completely obstructs the urethra. This condition often causes urinary retention in males.

Changes of the Urinary Tract with Aging

Changes occur in both the structure and function of the urinary tract as a result of aging. These changes can lead to urinary problems such as lack of control over urinary elimination.

There is a loss of nephrons in the kidneys over the life span. By the seventh decade of life, the number of nephrons has been reduced by one third to one half.[13] In addition, some degeneration occurs in the remaining nephrons. The net weight of each kidney is approximately 30 per cent less.[2] Because of the loss of nephrons, the kidneys are less efficient in concentrating urine and reabsorbing glucose. However, the kidneys are able to maintain acid-base balance under normal circumstances.

There is a 6 per cent decrease in the renal filtration rate per decade as the general circulation decreases.[13] The arterioles of the kidneys are affected by a generalized arteriosclerosis that occurs throughout the body. Some of the blood that would normally pass through the glomerular filtration system is diverted to other parts of the body. As a result of these physiologic changes, even minor stress can cause a disturbance in renal function.[13]

In the bladder, there is a loss of muscle tone as well as a decrease in bladder capacity.[2,13,98] Urinary incontinence and an increase in nocturia can occur; these are two of the most common and annoying problems in the elderly. Urinary incontinence, however, is not a normal part of the aging process. Infection can result from incomplete bladder emptying with **residual urine,** urine left in the bladder after urination. Hypertrophy of the prostate in men, if untreated, can lead to urinary obstruction and renal failure.

MAINTAINING NORMAL URINARY ELIMINATION

Maintaining a normal urinary elimination pattern is assisted by maintaining an adequate fluid intake, exercise, and normal urinary elimination habits. When necessary, clients may be taught methods to improve their urinary elimination.

Fluids and Exercise

Increasing fluid intake increases urine production, which increases stimulation of the micturition reflex. An average daily intake of 1200 to 1500 ml of measurable fluid is recommended, with additional amounts if the person has increased demands on the body's fluid stores (e.g., through fever, hot weather, or abnormal losses from other routes). Immobilized people must maintain dilute urine to prevent urinary stones and urinary tract infection. For these people, a daily fluid intake of 2000 to 3000 ml and foods with high fluid content are encouraged, provided there are no contraindications. Caution is used with individuals who are on fluid restriction for therapeutic reasons (e.g., congestive heart failure or renal impairment).

Exercise strengthens abdominal and perineal muscles, which in turn assists urinary elimination. Strong pelvic and perineal muscles also help prevent urinary incontinence. Kegel exercises strengthen perineal muscles (Box 44–1).

Urinary Elimination During Illness

Many people develop habits that stimulate the micturition reflex. For example, most people urinate at particular times in their daily routine. Although illnesses can sometimes make it difficult, the person's normal urinary elimination pattern should be supported as much as possible.

RELAXATION AND PRIVACY

Relaxation is crucial to urination. Providing privacy is one important element in promoting relaxation. Also,

pressuring a person to void may inhibit the micturition reflexes. Individuals may not always be able to void at the time they are asked to do so. For instance, people may need to drink some fluids and relax for a few minutes before being able to supply a urine specimen. Following an operation or a vaginal delivery, people may have difficulty voiding owing to the resulting trauma. Also, they may fear that they will be catheterized if they do not urinate, which further inhibits voiding. Relief of physical discomfort can promote elimination, since pain causes increased muscle tension and reduces the mental concentration sometimes needed for urination. A warm bedpan will reduce the muscle tension caused by contact with a cold one.

POSITIONING

The normal positions for voiding are the squat position for females and the standing position for males. The recumbent position makes voiding difficult for two reasons. First, gravity cannot aid the movement of urine through the tract. Second, a person cannot increase intra-abdominal pressure as well in this position. When necessary, a male should be assisted to stand and a female to sit. Also, the person should be encouraged to lean forward or push on the abdomen with the hands to increase intra-abdominal pressure, which then increases external pressure on the bladder.

Box 44–1. Tips on Practicing Pelvic Muscle (Kegel) Exercises

How to identify the correct muscle:

1. To find the muscle, place your finger inside your vagina or rectum. Try to squeeze around your finger. That's the muscle you want to exercise. This muscle is the same one you use to hold back gas or a bowel movement.
2. Remember! Never use your stomach, leg or buttock muscles. The most common mistake is using too many muscles. To find out if you are also contracting your stomach muscles, place your hand on your abdomen while you squeeze your pelvic floor muscle. If you feel your abdomen move, then you are also using these muscles.
3. These exercises can be practiced any time, in any place. Since this muscle is internal, *no one* can see you exercising this muscle. You will build strength slowly — don't expect results right away.

Doing the exercise:

1. Squeeze the muscle that you identified earlier — squeeze and hold for a count of 10 or 10 seconds. Then relax for a count of 10 or 10 seconds. *Remember, it is just as important to relax as it is to contract this muscle.* Initially, you may not be able to hold this muscle for 10 seconds. However, slowly over a 2-week period, you will build to 10-second holds.
2. Do 15 exercises in the morning, 15 in the afternoon and 20 at night. Or else you can exercise for 10 minutes,

three times a day. Set your kitchen timer for 10 minutes, three times a day. Try to work up to doing 25 exercises at one time.

When will I notice a change?

In about 2 weeks of consistent daily exercise, you will notice fewer accidents (incontinence); in 1 month you will see an even bigger difference.

Can these exercises harm me?

No! These exercises cannot harm you in any way. Most people find them relaxing and easy. If you have back pain or stomach pain after you exercise, then you are probably trying too hard and using stomach or back muscles. Go back and find the muscle, and remember that this exercise should feel mild and easy. If you experience headaches, then you are also tensing your stomach muscles and probably holding your breath. Remember to focus on relaxation, as well as contraction, of the muscle. In time, you will learn to practice effortlessly. Eventually, work these exercises in as part of your life style, like brushing your teeth or eating a meal. This will help you remain successful for a lifetime!

From Newman, D.K., & Smith, D.A. (1989). The treatment of urinary incontinence in adults. *Nurse Practitioner: The American Journal of Primary Health Care* 14(6), 26. © The Nurse Practitioner.

POWER OF SUGGESTION

As described, micturition is a conditioned response and can be stimulated by employing various techniques. These methods do not have a sound physiologic rationale but most likely succeed through the power of suggestion. Probably the most effective measure to stimulate micturition is to run water within hearing of the person. This technique not only suggests flowing water but also masks the sound of voiding if the person finds that embarrassing. Dipping the hands in water sometimes works. Pouring warm water over the perineum or sitting in a warm bath not only appeals to the power of suggestion but also promotes muscle relaxation. Stroking the inner thighs with light pressure or applying ice to the inner thighs may also stimulate trigger points that activate the micturition reflex.

Teaching About Urinary Elimination

People who are knowledgable about normal anatomy and physiology and about health maintenance activities are better able to engage in self-care. Also, people are more likely to follow health-related advice if they understand its rationale. Information should include normal urinary tract function; factors influencing micturition; signs and symptoms of urinary elimination problems; methods to prevent or solve these problems; and self-care activities related to maintenance of normal micturition.

ASSESSMENT

To identify problems in the urinary tract and plan nursing interventions, first assess the person by taking a complete health assessment, including both physical and psychosocial data. Take into consideration factors affecting urinary elimination, urine characteristics, and results of both routine urine testing and diagnostic tests of the urinary tract. Include in your physical assessment percussion of the abdomen for the suprapubic dullness of a distended bladder, palpation of the kidneys (the normal left kidney is rarely palpable), and costovertebral angle tenderness suggesting kidney infection. (See Chapter 33, Health Assessment, for physical assessment techniques.)

Physiologic Factors

Physiologic factors that affect urinary elimination include changes with aging, motor and sensory disturbances, hormonal changes, pregnancy, and muscle tone.

AGING

Individuals are frequently unwilling to discuss the problems that may occur in the urinary system as a result of aging. Incontinence and nocturia are two of the most common and annoying problems in the elderly. Although age-related changes in urinary structure and function, as well as other physical changes (e.g., mobility and vision), can place a person at risk for the development of incontinence, it is not a normal consequence of the aging process.[2,88]

The age of onset of alterations in urinary patterns may suggest certain pathologic changes. In men older than 50 years, it may suggest hypertrophy of the prostate.

MOTOR AND SENSORY DISTURBANCES

Many disturbances that interfere with motor or sensory abilities affect urination. Factors that impede or block sensory impulses — quadriplegia, paraplegia, and multiple sclerosis — may result in ineffective or involuntary bladder emptying. People who are immobilized may have problems with urination because they are unable to get to the bathroom or to summon help when they feel the urge to void.

HORMONAL CHANGES

Urination patterns are affected by hormonal changes within the body. Hormonal changes during the menstrual cycle affect urine formation. Premenstrually, many women retain fluid, gaining up to 5 pounds. Increased urine production after the start of menstruation results in the loss of excess fluid. Postmenopausal low estrogen levels can cause atrophic vaginitis and atrophic urethritis, with urinary frequency and incontinence.[62]

PREGNANCY

Hormonal changes and the anatomic changes that occur in the body affect a woman's urination pattern. During pregnancy, the growing fetus presses on the bladder, causing increased frequency of urination and sometimes stress incontinence.

MUSCLE TONE

If there is a lack of muscle tone, a person may not be able to contract abdominal muscles effectively to increase intra-abdominal pressure. In this case, a person may be unable to void or may not completely empty the bladder. On the other hand, weakened pelvic musculature reduces the external sphincter's ability to hold back the flow of urine. This may result in involuntary discharge of urine from the bladder. Immobility often results in decreased muscle tone.

Conversely, too much muscle tone inhibits the micturition reflex. For instance, straining to void does not work. Besides being ineffective, straining blocks the passage of urine out through the meatus. Thus, the person must concentrate on relaxing.

Because the bladder is a muscle, its tone also affects micturition. Healthy bladder function depends partly on periodic activation of the micturition reflex as well as on alternate filling and emptying of the bladder. If kept continually emptied, as with catheter drainage, it loses its tone and may not function properly when the catheter is removed. Likewise, if it is continually distended, it becomes insensitive to micturition stimuli and again loses its tone. Bladder hypertonicity (the state of increased tension) can result in bladder spasms and can cause frequency and premature bladder emptying.

Personal Factors

ELIMINATION PATTERN

Many people develop a set of behaviors to help stimulate micturition. Because of the susceptibility to suggestion, often nothing more is needed for micturition than placing oneself in the appropriate environment. Some people employ additional relaxation techniques, such as reading.

Also, most people establish habits in regard to the timing of voidings. This pattern is generally subconscious and is organized around the person's normal daily routine. Typically, an adult will void first thing in the morning, at lunchtime, after work, and before going to bed at night. Variations on this pattern depend on the person's fluid intake, bladder capacity, and routine.

DIETARY INTAKE

An important factor affecting micturition is the person's fluid status. Since the kidney maintains fluid balance, the amount of urine produced depends greatly on the body's need to retain or excrete water to preserve this balance.

If all other variables of fluid balance remain constant, urine production is directly correlated with the amount of fluid intake. Concomitantly, the amount of urine produced directly influences the frequency of urination. The kind of fluid ingested is also important, because some beverages have a **diuretic effect** (increased urination) on some people. Examples include coffee, tea, and alcoholic beverages.

Timing of fluid intake may also determine or interfere with normal micturition habits. For instance, most people do not normally awaken at night to urinate unless they (a) are elderly, (b) drink a large amount of fluid just before retiring, or (c) have established this habit pattern over a period of time.

In addition to the amount and kind of fluids taken in, some foods (e.g., fruits and vegetables) have a higher fluid content than others and thus affect the total fluid intake. Caffeine, alcohol, and artificial sweeteners are known bladder irritants and cause urgency and frequency.[59]

TOILET TRAINING

Experiences during the toilet-training period in childhood affect a person's micturition pattern even in adult life. **Enuresis** (involuntary urination), for example, is sometimes caused by psychologic problems during toilet training.

Psychosocial Factors

Psychosocial factors that affect urinary elimination include power of suggestion and anxiety.

Probably the most important psychologic factor influencing micturition is the mind's susceptibility to suggestion. Micturition can be initiated by any number of auditory, visual, or somatesthetic stimuli. For example, when some people hear running water, they feel the urge to void.

Anxiety affects micturition by either initiating or hindering it. When facing a stressful situation, for example, a person often has an urge to void, even though the bladder has recently been emptied. Conversely, anxiety characterized by generalized muscle tension can interfere with urination, since relaxation of the perineal muscles is essential to micturition. Therefore anything that interferes with perineal muscle relaxation may lead to urine retention.[61,98]

Cultural Factors

Cultural teachings pass on the rules and regulations for living within a given society. Inability to follow cultural norms usually causes stress for the person involved. In many cultures, privacy during urination is the norm. Therefore, the lack of privacy (as in a public toilet or when using a bedside commode) often interferes with the ability to void.

Medications

Many medications have a direct effect on urination and can contribute to the development of incontinence. Diuretics increase urine output, which can lead to urgency and incontinence. Anticholinergics inhibit bladder contractions; hence, urgency is controlled but retention and overflow incontinence can occur. Alpha-blockers promote relaxation in the bladder neck, which can cause stress incontinence. Hypnotics and sedatives, including alcohol, decrease the awareness of the need to void. Incontinence, especially at night, can result.

Trauma

Any trauma, surgical or nonsurgical, may interfere with urinary elimination if it results in damage to the urinary structures or surrounding tissues. Edema formation can obstruct the passageways, and mucosal irritation can cause pain. Pain causes increased muscle tension and may thereby inhibit urination. In addition to edema, obstruction may be caused by tumors or scar formation.

SURGICAL TRAUMA

Surgery affects urination in several ways. Initially, most people are fluid depleted at the start of the surgical procedure, and more fluid is lost during surgery. Thus, urine production diminishes to maintain the body's fluid balance. Hormonal changes caused by the stress of surgery initially decrease urine production but later cause diuresis.

Urinary retention may be a problem following surgery. It is thought that this retention is caused by slow urine production or the inhibitory effect of the anesthetics and narcotics on the sensory and motor reflex pathways. The surgical procedure itself, if it results in damage to the urinary structures or surrounding tissues, may interfere with micturition.

NONSURGICAL TRAUMA

Renal trauma accounts for 50 per cent of all injuries to the genitourinary tract. Injuries are classified as nonpenetrating (blunt) trauma or penetrating trauma. Types of injuries include contusions, lacerations, or pedicle injury (kidney torn from its pedicle). Ninety per cent of renal injuries occur in men between 20 and 30 years of age.

Nonpenetrating or blunt renal injuries are those associated with a direct blow to the back, abdominal, or flank area. This type of injury is seen with football tackles and falls. Direct injury occurs when the kidney is crushed between an external force and the vertebra or back muscles. Indirect injuries result from the decelerating effect, often seen when the kidney is torn from its pedicle during an automobile accident.

Penetrating renal injuries are those resulting from knife and gunshot wounds. These types of penetrating injuries are rare and are most often associated with crimes of violence. In some cases, **nephrectomy** (surgical removal of a kidney) becomes necessary following nonsurgical trauma.

Difficulties with Urinary Elimination

Symptoms of urinary elimination difficulties include dysuria, frequency, hesitancy, incontinence, nocturia, retention, and urgency. Symptoms of urinary difficulties, alone or in combination, indicate a problem within the urinary system. Gathering more data about urinary symptoms can assist in the identification of the problem and initiation of treatment.

DYSURIA

Dysuria is painful or difficult urination and is described as burning on urination. It is usually associated with urinary tract infection, e.g., **cystitis** (inflammation of the bladder) or **urethritis** (inflammation of the urethra) but may also be caused by concentrated, acid urine. Frequency and urgency may also be experienced in a urinary tract infection.

FREQUENCY

Frequency is urinating at short intervals, either small or large amounts, more often than usual. The usual number of voidings during waking hours is six to

eight.[98] Several conditions can cause this number to increase above normal. Infection in the urinary tract may be the cause of frequent voiding in small amounts. Increased fluid intake or diuretic medication may be the cause of frequent voiding in large amounts. Retention of urine in the bladder with overflow may cause frequent voiding in small amounts as the person experiences discomfort and a sense of fullness in the bladder.

HESITANCY

Hesitancy is difficulty in initiating urination. It may be accompanied by a decrease in the force of the urinary stream. An enlarged prostate is the most common cause of partial obstruction in men, whereas weakened perineal muscles or meatal stenosis is the usual cause in women.

INCONTINENCE

Urinary incontinence is the involuntary loss of urine. It can be classified into two basic types: acute or chronic. Acute or transient incontinence usually results from an acute medical or surgical problem and has a sudden onset. Chronic or persistent incontinence may have a sudden onset accompanying an acute medical or surgical problem, or it may have a gradual onset with no known precipitating factors. Control can often be restored when the underlying problem is resolved.[62]

In assessing a client for transient incontinence, the acronym DRIP will help identify the possible causes.[61] These causes are listed in Box 44-2.

Persistent incontinence has been classified as stress incontinence, reflex incontinence, urge incontinence, functional incontinence, and total incontinence.[85]

NOCTURIA

Nocturia is urination during the night, which does not usually exceed two voidings.[98] If it is not associated with a large fluid intake before going to bed or taking

---

Box 44-2. Causes of Transient Incontinence

D	Delirium
	Dehydration
R	Restricted mobility
I	Inflammation
	Impaction
P	Polyuria
	Pharmaceuticals, e.g.,
	Diuretics
	Hypnotics and sedatives
	Anticholinergics
	Alpha blockers

Data from Newman, D.K., & Smith, D.A. (1989). Incontinence: the problem patients won't talk about. *RN, 52*(4), 42–45.

diuretics late in the day or at night, it could indicate the kidneys' loss of ability to concentrate urine. It is also associated with prostatic hypertrophy, congestive heart failure, or inflammation of the bladder or urethral mucosa.

RETENTION

Retention is the accumulation of an excess amount of urine in the bladder of a person with normal urine production. It is due to the person's inability to empty the bladder.

URGENCY

Urgency is the need to urinate immediately. It is usually associated with urinary tract infections and is accompanied by frequency.

Problems with Urinary Elimination

URINARY TRACT INFECTION

Urinary tract infections (UTIs) may affect any part of the urinary tract, resulting in inflammation of the kidneys, ureters, bladder, or urethra. A UTI may be ascending (coming from the exterior of the body and ascending to the bladder and kidney) or descending (coming from the kidney down through the bladder). Many ascending infections are caused by bacteria from a person's own bowel.

Many factors contribute to a UTI. Because the female urethra is shorter, women suffer more UTIs than men. Sexually active people are at risk because sexual intercourse can cause urethral inflammation. Fecal incontinence increases the risk of transmission of fecal organisms to the meatus and urinary tract. Urine reflux from the urethra into bladder, or from bladder to either ureter, puts a person at risk because organisms get washed up through the urinary tract. Obstruction secondary to anatomic abnormalities or urinary tract stones increases susceptibility to infection by causing urinary stasis. Previous urinary tract infection makes the person more vulnerable to recurrent infection. The person with a urinary catheter also has a greater chance of getting a UTI.

Symptoms of UTI vary greatly but usually include burning upon urination, urgency, and frequency. Assessment may also reveal hematuria, abdominal pain, malaise, chills, nausea and vomiting, fever, and flank pain. Some people are asymptomatic. Definitive diagnosis is based on the results of clean-catch urine cultures.

Treatment is multifaceted. Antibiotics are the mainstay of treatment. People with recurrent infections are sometimes placed on long-term prophylactic antibiotic therapy. Strictures and other anatomic abnormalities are corrected by surgical intervention.

URINARY DIVERSION

Urinary diversion is the drainage of urine from the body at a site other than the perineal meatus or tip of the penis. Urinary diversion can be either congenital or surgically created. Hypospadias is an example of a congenital diversion. In this case, the urethra opens on the underside of the penis or inside the vagina. Surgical urinary diversion is performed to treat cancer, birth defects, obstruction, or neurogenic bladder. The goal of this treatment is to assist the client to eliminate urine when part of the urinary tract must be bypassed, as Figure 44-3 illustrates.

Surgical procedures include the creation of

- an ileal conduit, which connects the distal ureters to a dissected piece of the terminal ileum, which is brought out of the body as an opening (stoma) on the abdominal wall.
- a cutaneous ureterostomy, which brings the distal end of the ureter out through an opening on the abdominal wall.
- a ureterosigmoidostomy, which connects the ureters to the sigmoid colon, allowing urine to drain out through the rectum.
- a suprapubic cystostomy, which allows the bladder to drain through an opening in the abdominal wall.
- a Kock pouch, which connects the ureters to an ileal segment and contains nipple valves created from intussuscepted portions of the ileal segment, forming the pathway from the pouch to the stoma and storing urine inside the body, thus creating a continent urostomy.[12]
- a continent Indiana reservoir, which allows storage of urine inside the body in a reservoir formed by portions of the cecum and ascending colon, with an ileum segment brought through the abdominal wall to form a stoma.[26]

In all these cases except the ureterosigmoidostomy, a stoma is created. Usually, urinary diversions with a stoma drain continually into a collection bag. The bag either is attached to the abdominal wall or is attached by tubing to a leg or Foley catheter drainage bag. The Kock pouch and continent Indiana reservoir are exceptions. They store urine inside the body and are emptied by inserting a catheter through the stoma and into the pouch. Problems resulting from these surgical procedures include (a) potential skin irritation and maceration from prolonged contact with urine and collection appliances; (b) uncontrolled odors from urine output; (c) embarrassment, feelings of dependency, damage to self-image, and lifestyle changes; and (d) lack of knowledge concerning care of the stoma and drainage devices.

URINARY TRACT STONES

Urolithiasis refers to the formation of urinary tract stones, or renal calculi in the urinary tract. **Calculi** are pathologic stones, usually composed of mineral salts, occurring in the kidneys, ureters, bladder, or urethra. The presence of stones (calculi) in the kidney is termed **nephrolithiasis.** Stones are formed by the precipitation of crystalline substances. The majority of urinary stones are formed of calcium. Other elements that form stones are oxalate, uric acid, and cystine.

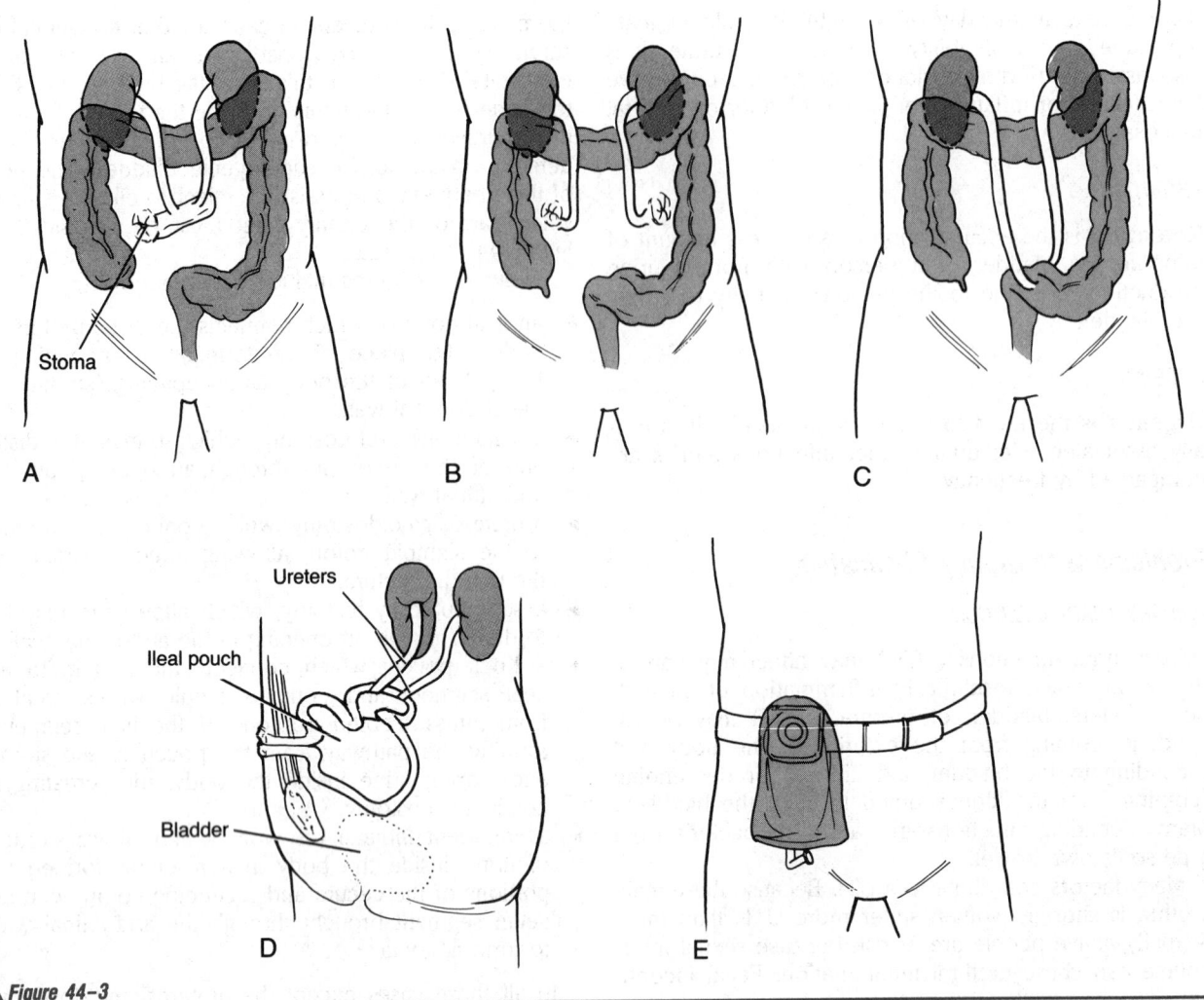

Stoma

A

B

C

Ureters

Ileal pouch

Bladder

D

E

▲ *Figure 44–3*

Methods of surgical urinary diversion. *A,* Ileal conduit. *B,* Cutaneous ureterostomy. *C,* Ureterosigmoidostomy. *D,* Kock pouch. *E,* Urinary appliance for management of urinary diversion.

Stones cause severe pain, mucosal trauma, obstruction of urine flow, and infection.

Conditions favoring stone formation include urinary stasis and **hypercalciuria** (high urinary calcium levels) from disorders such as hyperparathyroidism, excessive dietary calcium and vitamin D, and certain bone marrow diseases. Immobilized people are at risk because their condition causes urinary stasis and abnormal calcium metabolism.

Symptoms of stones include severe flank pain, nausea and vomiting, diaphoresis, pallor, fever, and hematuria. In addition to assessing for these signs and symptoms, take a complete medical and dietary history to identify risk factors. The physician orders urine studies to measure calcium and uric acid levels and to check for blood and infection. An IVP (intravenous pyelogram) or cystoscopy is often ordered to confirm the diagnosis. Also, you may be asked to assess urine for stones. To do this, collect all urine voided and pour it through at least four layers of gauze pads or through a commercial funnel-shaped urine filter, and inspect for stones. The stones can be analyzed to determine content.

URINARY RETENTION

In urinary retention, urine production is normal but accumulated urine is retained in the bladder. Retention results from mechanical or functional causes. Mechanical causes may be acquired or congenital and include calculus, trauma, and inflammation or urethral stricture, respectively. Functional causes include anxiety, decreased innervation of the bladder (neurogenic bladder), muscle tension, detrusor muscle atrophy, and medications like anesthetics, sedatives, and narcotics. Fecal impaction may cause urinary retention by applying pressure on the bladder outlet and impairing innervation of the detrusor muscle. Poor fluid intake causes retention because slow urine production in turn slows bladder filling. Hence, the detrusor muscle gradually accomodates to the increased volume without stimulating the micturition reflex. Once the detrusor muscle fibers are overstretched, they cannot contract, so micturition is further inhibited.

As the bladder fills with retained urine, it rises above the level of the symphysis pubis. As it distends, you can palpate the bladder as a tense, sensitive area. Percussion reveals a "kettle-drum" sound. The person may be uncomfortable and feel the urge to urinate. The assessment data you will collect from the person experiencing urinary retention will include voiding pattern, complaints of pain or burning on urination (indicative of UTI), frequency of voiding, volume of each void, color and clarity of urine, and comparison of intake to output. The person may also experience restlessness, lower abdominal pain or discomfort, and diaphoresis.

The cardinal sign of *Urinary Retention* is absence of urine.

Initial management involves using the independent measures described earlier: promoting relaxation, positioning, and utilizing the power of suggestion. If these actions are unsuccessful, the physician may order a cholinergic drug, such as bethanechol or neostigmine. These agents stimulate bladder contraction.

Never use cholinergic medications if mechanical obstruction is present. In this instance, intravesicular pressure increases against an obstructed outlet, which could cause urine reflux into the kidney or rupture of the bladder.

If all other measures fail to effect urination, a catheterization of the bladder may be unavoidable. Procedure 44-1 describes the technique of urethral catheterization.

Urinary Retention with Overflow. Retention with overflow is an extension of urinary retention. The individual voids frequently but in amounts that are enough only to reduce intravesicular pressure slightly. This phenomenon occurs when the bladder continues filling and the intravesicular pressure rises. In time, this pressure overcomes sphincter pressure. Hence, the person voids just enough urine to reduce intravesicular pressure to a point at which the external sphincter can control urine flow. The bladder fills again, and the cycle is repeated over and over.

The definitive sign is frequent (often more than once an hour) voiding of small amounts (usually 25 to 50 ml) of urine. The bladder remains distended since emptying is incomplete. The person feels a sense of urgency.

Management of this condition is the same as that of retention, except the likelihood of the need for catheterization is much greater.

INADEQUATE RENAL FUNCTION

Problems in renal function may develop slowly over a period of years (chronic renal failure) or rapidly in a matter of days or weeks (acute renal failure). Renal failure can result from a number of conditions. Chronic renal failure is caused by disorders that destroy the nephron, such as severe renal infections, toxemia of pregnancy, tumors, and diabetes mellitus. Acute renal failure results from sudden interruption of kidney blood flow. Interruptions in renal blood flow can be due to shock, renal vasoconstriction from drugs, surgical pro-

cedures such as open heart surgery, severe infections, toxins, and urinary tract obstructions. Acute failure is reversible in some cases, whereas chronic renal failure is progressive and irreversible.

Medical and surgical intervention includes (a) correction or control of underlying conditions (e.g., control of diabetes, removal of urinary tract obstructions), (b) dietary modifications to prevent fluid and electrolyte imbalances, (c) dialysis therapy, and (d) kidney transplantation. Nursing care of the person in chronic or acute renal failure requires advanced knowledge and nursing skills, which are too complex to describe here.

Urine Characteristics

The three principal constituents of urine are water, urea, and electrolytes, namely, sodium and chloride.[29] In addition to many other substances found in the urine are phosphoric acid, sulfuric acid, uric acid, ammonia, hippuric acid, and creatinine. Laboratory findings of glucose in the urine (**glycosuria**), bacteria in the urine (**bacteriuria**), pus in the urine (**pyuria**), blood in the urine (**hematuria**), and protein in the urine (**proteinuria**) are all indications of possible disease.

VOLUME

The amount of urine, both total daily volume and volume of each voiding, depends on a number of factors: fluid intake, fluid losses from other routes, fever, environmental temperature, age (a child excretes proportionately more than an adult), ingestion of a high-protein diet (which produces more urine), or diuretic drugs. Averages for an adult are 50 to 70 ml/hr or 1200 ml in 24 hours. Urine output less than 25 to 30 ml/hr (500 ml in 24 hours) may indicate dehydration, kidney malfunction, or urinary tract obstruction.

Total urine volume depends on urine production. **Oliguria** is the term indicating a diminished amount of urine formation (output less than 400 ml in 24 hours). Oliguria may be the result of suppression of urine formation in the kidneys or of urine retention in the bladder. **Anuria** is the term indicating complete urinary suppression or kidney failure (output less than 100 ml in 24 hours). This is associated with renal failure. **Polyuria** is excessive secretion of urine (greater than 1500 ml in 24 hours) and may indicate uncontrolled diabetes mellitus or renal disease.

The amount per voiding normally depends on the person's bladder capacity: 250 to 500 ml is an average normal voiding. Report to the physician amounts far less or much greater than this normal range.

COLOR

The normal color of urine is pale, straw colored to amber, depending on its concentration. The color of urine darkens on standing because of the oxidation of urobilinogen to urobilin.[29] This begins in 30 minutes. When there is bleeding in the upper urinary tract, the urine may be dark red or smoky. Bleeding in the lower

TABLE 44-1. Some Medications That Cause Changes in Urine Color

Medications	Urine Color Produced
Amitriptyline (antidepressant)	Blue-green
Anthraquinone laxatives (cascara, danthron, senna)	Reddish-brown in acid urine, red in alkaline urine
Chloroquine (antimalarial)	Rusty yellow
Chlorzoxazone (skeletal muscle relaxant)	Orange or purple-red
Methylene blue (diagnostic indicator dye)	Green
Phenazopyridine (urinary tract antiseptic)	Orange-brown, orange-red, or red
Phenolphthalein (ingredient in many laxatives)	Pink-red in alkaline urine
Phenytoin (anticonvulsant)	Pink to reddish-brown in freshly voided urine, iron-black or brown in urine that has been left standing
Rifampin (antibiotic)	Bright orange-red
Sulfonamides (anti-infective)	Rust yellow to brownish
Triamterene (diuretic)	Pale blue

urinary tract produces red urine. Foods that may turn the urine red are rhubarb, beets, blackberries, and red food dyes. Dark yellow urine may indicate the presence of urobilin or bilirubin. Bright yellow urine comes from ingesting large amounts of carotene (e.g., carrots or sweet potatoes). Milky white urine may be caused by pus or by fat globules released in the kidney as a result of nephrosis or severe trauma.[71] Many medications cause color changes in the urine. Table 44-1 lists some of these agents.

CLARITY

Urine is usually transparent when freshly voided. It turns cloudy on standing. Cloudiness in freshly voided urine indicates bacteria, inflammation within the urinary tract, or the presence of sperm or prostatic fluid.

ODOR

Normal, freshly voided urine is aromatic. Concentrated urine usually smells stronger than dilute urine. When urine stands, it may develop an ammonia smell due to bacterial action. Certain foods, such as asparagus, cause characteristic odor changes. Inflammatory reactions also alter the normal odor. Heavily infected urine has a particularly unpleasant odor. A sweet odor may indicate the presence of ketone bodies or acetone.

Routine Urine Testing

You will frequently perform simple, but important, diagnostic tests on urine. These tests include those for pH, specific gravity, glucose and ketone bodies, nitrites and leukocytes, and blood or hemoglobin (heme). The importance of these tests, in combination with visual examination (e.g., clarity), of the urine in reducing the number of specimens processed in the microbiology laboratory has been the subject of several recent research studies.[30,47]

One study of 418 elderly subjects compared four screening tests for bacteriuria with standard methods of bacterial culture at the inpatient unit level. As a result of the study, a suggested protocol for screening elderly people for bacteriuria was developed. It combines the visual assessment for clarity of the urine with a dipstick test for nitrites and leukocytes. Cloudy urine would be sent directly to the laboratory for urinalysis; clear urine would be sent to the laboratory only if nitrite- or leukocyte-positive.[30]

Remember to follow CDC (Centers for Disease Control) *Guidelines for Universal Precautions* and wear nonsterile gloves when performing routine urine tests and when collecting and handling urine specimens.

pH

Urine pH measures the hydrogen ion concentration in the urine, indicating its acidity or alkalinity. The normal pH of the urine is between 4.5 and 7.5. Deviations may indicate systemic acid-base imbalances. However, some foods and medications can change urine pH. A diet high in meats, eggs, cheese, whole grains, plums, prunes, and cranberries (including prune juice and cranberry juice) may decrease the pH, producing an acid urine. A diet high in vegetables, citrus fruits, and milk may increase the pH, producing an alkaline urine. Also, the urine pH may be intentionally altered to inhibit bacterial growth or urinary stone development, or to facilitate the therapeutic activity of certain medications. An acid urine should be maintained in the treatment of urinary tract infections and persistent bacteriuria and in the management of urinary calculi. Conversely, an alkaline urine should be maintained when streptomycin, neomycin, and kanamycin are used in the treatment of urinary tract infections.[29]

Measure urine pH by using a dipstick, which is a multiple reagent strip treated with chemicals. Dip the dipstick into a fresh urine specimen and compare the color change with a standardized color chart on the bottle after waiting the specified amount of time.

SPECIFIC GRAVITY

Specific gravity is a measure of the concentration of dissolved solids in the urine. The normal range is 1.003 to 1.030. If kidney function is normal, specific gravity indicates fluid status. There is usually an inverse relationship between the specific gravity and the volume of urine (i.e., the higher the volume, the less concentrated the urine and therefore the lower the specific gravity). High specific gravity in the absence of kidney failure usually indicates dehydration, whereas low specific gravity under normal circumstances reflects overhydration. Specific gravity is altered by severe kidney disease and by intravenous contrast media used during x-ray procedures. Disease processes in other parts of the body (e.g., congestive heart failure) can affect the specific gravity.

Test specific gravity by using a multiple dipstick that has a separate reagent for specific gravity or with a urinometer and urinometer cylinder. To use the dipstick, dip it into the urine specimen and compare with the standardized color strip on the bottle after the specified amount of time. When using the urinometer, fill the empty cylinder about three fourths full with urine (Fig. 44–4). Gently drop the urinometer into the cylinder to avoid splashing, and spin it between the thumb and forefinger. If the urinometer touches the cylinder when it stops spinning, spin it again; it must be floating free. Read the number on the free-floating urinometer at the level of the meniscus of the urine.

GLUCOSE AND KETONES

In persons with diabetes mellitus, the pancreas secretes an insufficient amount of insulin into the blood. Because insulin is required to transport glucose into body cells, the body cells become starved for nutrition while the glucose accumulates in high amounts in the blood. If blood levels of glucose become high enough, the glucose will begin to "spill over" into the urine, where it may be detected. If cells are deprived of glucose long enough, the body will begin to burn fat in order to provide the cells with needed energy. The end products (ketones) of this fat metabolism can also be detected in the urine.

Until the early 1980s, urine glucose and ketone tests were the only way for people with diabetes to assess their level of control of the disease. Self-monitoring blood glucose (SMBG) has since become the preferred way to monitor glucose levels and is recommended by the American Diabetes Association for all insulin-dependent diabetics.[89]

However, urine ketone tests continue to be an important part in monitoring diabetic control. Ketones in the urine indicate the burning of fat. Fat metabolism increases the acid level of the blood. Excessive ketones in urine may indicate impending ketoacidosis, which is a medical emergency. It is recommended that urine be tested for ketones during acute illness or stress, when

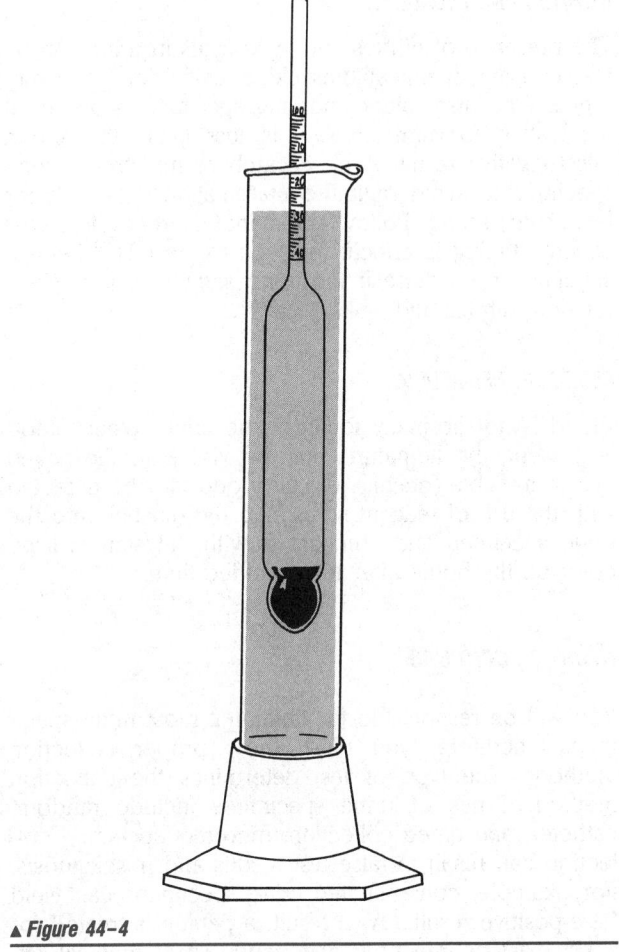

▲ *Figure 44–4*

Urinometer, used for measuring specific gravity.

blood glucose levels are greater than 240 mg/dl, during pregnancy, or in the presence of any symptoms of ketoacidosis (e.g., nausea, vomiting, abdominal pain).[89]

When not in use, the container for any tablets, tapes, or dipsticks must be tightly closed to keep the reagents dry. Incorrect results will be obtained if the reagents have absorbed moisture.

Testing the urine for glucose and ketones can be done by using reagent strips, including Clinistix, Diastix, and Tes-Tape. When you dip the strip into urine, it changes color when exposed to glucose and ketones. Compare the strip with the standardized colors on the bottle after the designated time period. Urine glucose levels can also be tested by the copper reduction test (Clinitest). When the Clinitest tablet is added to diluted urine, a heat reaction takes place, resulting in precipitation and a change in the color of the urine. The color is compared with a color chart to determine the percentage of glucose present. However, this test is nonspecific for glucose, since other substances (e.g., lactose or other sugars and chlorine) in the urine can cause the chemical reaction.[29]

NITRITES AND LEUKOCYTES

The presence of nitrites and leukocytes in urine can be tested using chemical dipsticks specific for these elements. The first voided morning specimen is preferred for testing for nitrites, as it is less likely to yield a false-negative result. A clean-catch or midstream urine specimen to avoid vaginal contamination is needed for leukocyte testing. Follow the manufacturer's directions exactly; timing is critical for accurate results.[29] Send a specimen for culture if the urine sample tests positive for both nitrites and leukocytes.[30]

BLOOD OR HEMATURIA

Blood is not normally found in the urine. When blood is present, the hematuria may be visible to the naked eye or invisible (occult). Occult blood may be detected with the use of reagent strips. Dip the dipstick into the urine specimen and compare it with the standardized color on the bottle after the specified time.

Urine Specimens

You will be responsible for obtaining most urine specimens; therefore, you must know proper collection methods. The type of test determines the collection method. Types of urine specimens include random, catheter, and timed collection. Incorrect specimen collection can result in false test results and misdiagnosis. For example, contaminated urine specimens can yield false-positive results. As a result, a person is treated for a nonexistent infection, and unnecessary medical expenses accrue. Label every specimen with the person's name, the date, and the time of collection. Replace the lid securely on the container, and place it in a plastic bag. Attach the laboratory requisition slip and send the specimen promptly to the laboratory. Check with the laboratory for any special handling or storage requirements after the specimen is collected. Remember to follow the CDC *Guidelines for Universal Precautions* when collecting and handling urine specimens.

RANDOM COLLECTION

Most urine tests, including routine urinalysis and urine culture, can be done on a single, random specimen. Random sampling means that the specimen is collected at any time; however, the time of day the specimen is collected may influence the results. The first voided morning specimen will be more concentrated and more apt to reveal abnormalities.

Urinalysis. Instruct the person to void into a clean, dry container or into a clean, dry bedpan and then transfer the specimen into a container. Usually, there is no special preparation of the person. However, advise a female to wash the perineal area to remove any vaginal debris and not to put toilet paper into the specimen. The specimen can also be collected through a Foley catheter or urinary diversion collection bag. If collecting from a Foley urinary drainage system, aseptic technique must be used, not because the urine specimen must be sterile but because the drainage system should not be contaminated.

When the specimen is obtained, label the container with the client's name, the date, and the time of collection. Place the lid tightly on the specimen container, and place it in a plastic bag. Attach the laboratory requisition slip and send the specimen promptly to the laboratory.

Urine Culture

Use sterile technique when collecting urine specimens for culture and sensitivity.

A clean-catch or midstream specimen is required for urine cultures to assess for infection. The first voided morning specimen is preferred because bacterial counts are highest at this time. Avoid contamination of the specimen by teaching clients the following procedure, and assist as necessary:

1. Instruct the person to remove the lid of the sterile collection container without touching the inside, and place the lid, inside up, on a clean surface.
2. Teach females to separate the labia, using the thumb and forefinger, and to keep them apart throughout the procedure. If a woman is menstruating, tell her to insert a tampon before specimen collection. Notify the laboratory so that results are not misinterpreted. Teach uncircumcised men to retract the foreskin before washing the penis, then to return it to its original position following urine collection.
3. Instruct the client to cleanse the perineal area or glans of the penis thoroughly with antiseptic towelettes while keeping the labia separated or continuing to hold the penis. Tell females to wash from front to back to avoid fecal contamination of the meatus. Males should wash the glans of the penis, wiping in a circular motion away from the meatus.
4. Advise the client to keep the labia separated or keep the foreskin retracted and begin voiding into the toilet, commode, or bedpan in order to wash out the distal urethra, which normally contains some bacteria. While continuing to void, and without stopping the urine stream, the person should pass the sterile container through the urine stream and collect the urine sample until the container is half full. The person should remove the container, without slowing the urine stream, and then finish voiding. The labia may be released and foreskin replaced at this time.
5. Replace the lid securely on the container. Label the container with the client's name, date, and time of collection. Place the container in a plastic specimen bag. Attach the laboratory requisition slip and send to the laboratory as soon as possible.

CATHETER COLLECTION

Collecting a sterile urine specimen by catheterization is not recommended, because the procedure increases the risk of introducing microorganisms into the urinary tract. If you must catheterize the person, follow Procedure 44–1.

A bacteriologic specimen can be collected from an indwelling (retention) catheter. It cannot be collected from a urinary drainage bag unless it is the first urine drained into a new sterile bag. Urine in drainage bags provides a medium for bacterial growth. Obtain urine from the collection port or the catheter, using the following technique:

1. Clamp the catheter distal to the collection port for about 15 to 20 minutes, to allow for accumulation of fresh, uncontaminated urine in the tubing.

2. Swab the collection port with an antiseptic swab and allow it to dry. Puncture the port with a 23- or 25-gauge needle and withdraw the urine into a sterile syringe. If there is no port, use the catheter itself just above the catheter-drainage tubing junction. Swab the aspiration site and insert the needle at a 45-degree angle to allow for resealing by the catheter when the needle is withdrawn. To avoid entering the balloon lumen by mistake, slant the needle down toward the drainage tubing.

3. Unclamp the tubing.

4. Transfer the specimen to a sterile specimen container. Label the container with the client's name, the date, the time, and the method of collection. Put the lid tightly on the specimen container, and place it in a plastic specimen bag. Attach the laboratory requisition slip and send the specimen promptly to the laboratory.

If absolutely necessary, you can obtain the specimen by disconnecting the catheter from the drainage tubing and allowing the urine to flow from the distal end of the catheter into an appropriate sterile container. This method breaks open the closed drainage system, so use aseptic technique throughout. Using friction, clean the catheter–drainage tubing junction with an antiseptic solution before separating it, and take care that neither the distal end of the catheter nor the proximal end of the drainage tubing touch anything while apart. Clean both ends again with an antiseptic solution before reconnecting them.

TIMED COLLECTION

Some diagnostic tests require a timed collection: 2-hour, 12-hour, or 24-hour specimens. Collect all these samples by means of the same basic technique. Use one container (usually a 2- or 3-liter plastic jug) for these tests. The container can be obtained from the laboratory. Label the container with the client's name and the date, time, and method of collection. Depending on the test, a preservative or other additive may be added to the container. Before beginning the collection, check with the laboratory or consult with the laboratory procedure manual for any special requirements. Use the following procedure for timed urine collections:

1. Explain the procedure and ask the client to void. Tell the client when the specimen collection will begin

and end. If necessary, instruct the client to call you immediately after each void so that the specimen can be placed in the collection container.

2. Discard the first voided specimen. This begins the test time. Collect all subsequent urine specimens, including the one at the end of the timed period. Obtain the last specimen as close as possible to the stated end of time for the test.

3. Store nonrefrigerated specimens in the person's bathroom or the dirty utility room. For specimens needing refrigeration, immediately place the specimen in a container in the refrigerator or in an iced container in the person's bathroom.

If, at any time during the timed specimen collection period, the person voids in the toilet or someone discards a specimen, begin the entire collection process again.

4. When the collection is completed, attach the requisition slip and send the labeled collection container(s) to the laboratory.

Diagnostic Tests of Urinary Function

Several diagnostic tests help identify actual and potential problems in urinary elimination. Common tests include x-ray examination (e.g., IVP and CAT scan), direct visualization (cystoscopy), and ultrasonography. Information describing the diagnostic test, its purpose, and nursing responsibilities before, during, and after the test can be found in Chapter 34, Assisting with Diagnostic Procedures.

NURSING DIAGNOSIS

Common NANDA diagnoses for the individual experiencing problems meeting urinary elimination needs include the following: *Altered Urinary Elimination, Stress Incontinence, Reflex Incontinence, Urge Incontinence, Functional Incontinence, Total Incontinence,* and *Urinary Retention.*[85]

Altered Urinary Elimination

Altered Urinary Elimination is the state in which an individual experiences a disturbance in urinary elimination. It is characterized by dysuria, frequency, hesitancy, incontinence, nocturia, retention, and/or urgency. Multiple causative factors include anatomic obstruction, sensory motor impairment, and urinary tract infection.[85] The specific types of *Altered Urinary Elimination* addressed in this chapter are urinary tract infection, urinary diversion, and urinary tract stones. Problems that can result are recurrent or complicated UTIs causing sepsis or permanent damage to the structures of the urinary tract; skin necrosis around stoma sites; and infection and structural damage with urinary tract stones.

Urinary Incontinence

STRESS INCONTINENCE

Stress Incontinence is one of five types of incontinence recognized by the North American Nursing Diagnosis Association. This diagnosis is discussed in the Nursing Diagnosis Profile.

REFLEX INCONTINENCE

Reflex Incontinence is the state in which an individual experiences an involuntary loss of urine, occurring at somewhat predictable intervals when a specific bladder volume is reached. There is no awareness of bladder filling and no urge to void or feelings of bladder fullness. There is lack of awareness of being incontinent. Usually large amounts of urine are voided. Neurologic impairment involving cerebral loss and interruption of spinal cord impulses above the level of S_3 are related factors.[85]

URGE INCONTINENCE

Urge Incontinence is the state in which an individual experiences involuntary passage of urine occurring soon after a strong sense of urgency to void. The individual is unable to get to the toilet in time after sensing the urge to void. Voiding occurs more than every 2 hours during waking hours and more than two times at night. Amounts of urine voided may be small (less than 100 ml) or large (more than 550 ml). Uncontrolled contractions of the detrusor muscle are frequently the cause. This type of incontinence is seen primarily in older adults.[85]

FUNCTIONAL INCONTINENCE

Functional Incontinence is the state in which an individual experiences an involuntary, unpredictable passage of urine. Bladder and urethral function are normal. Incontinence occurs because of factors (impaired mobility, dementia, or depression) that prevent the person from getting to the toilet.[85]

 NURSING DIAGNOSIS PROFILE

Stress Incontinence

Definition. The state in which an individual experiences a loss of urine of less than 50 ml occurring with increased abdominal pressure.

Classification. Exchanging 1.3.2.1.1

Defining Characteristics. The major defining characteristic for this condition is reported or observed urinary dribbling with increased intra-abdominal pressure. The loss of urine can occur with coughing, laughing, bending, lifting heavy objects, climbing stairs, or exercising. Minor defining characteristics can occur by themselves or may accompany the loss of urine. They include urinary urgency and frequency (voiding more frequently than every 2 hours).

Sample Related Factors. The most common related factors are degenerative changes in pelvic muscles and structural supports associated with increased age; high intra-abdominal pressure, which may be secondary to obesity or gravid uterus; incompetent bladder outlet; overdistention between voidings; or weak pelvic muscles.

Concept Description. *Stress Incontinence* occurs more frequently in women than in men. Any activity causing downward pressure on the bladder can result in an involuntary loss of urine. Urine loss occurs only with straining in the upright position. It has been attributed to weakened pelvic floor muscles associated with normal aging, childbirth, or surgical procedures (e.g., hysterectomy). The problem can be seen in men following a prostatectomy as a result of damage to the proximal urethra.

Examples. Depending on the specific assessment data, this diagnostic category could be applicable in the following situations, among others:

▶ An elderly woman who is concerned about the sudden loss of small amounts of urine when sneezing or coughing, who urinates every 3 or 4 hours during the day and once or twice during the night, but whose incontinent episodes occur only during the day. In this case the nursing diagnosis is *Stress Incontinence* R/T degenerative changes in pelvic muscles and structural supports secondary to increased age.

▶ An elderly man who had a transurethral resection of the prostate 6 months ago, who reports a sudden loss of small amounts of urine when serving in tennis and when jogging, but who has no other physical complaints and whose physical examination is unremarkable. A nursing diagnosis should be *Stress Incontinence* R/T incompetent bladder outlet.

▶ A 37-year-old woman in her third trimester of pregnancy who has had one previous vaginal birth with an episiotomy and who is experiencing small amounts of urine loss when bending to pick up her 2-year-old. She is concerned because incontinence did not occur during her first pregnancy. The nursing diagnosis should be *Stress Incontinence* R/T high intra-abdominal pressure secondary to pregnancy.

Related/Similar Nursing Diagnoses. *Stress Incontinence* must be differentiated from *Urge Incontinence*. Although urgency is commonly experienced with *Stress Incontinence*, the etiology of these two types of incontinence and the treatment differ. With *Urge Incontinence*, urine loss can occur at any time, not only with straining in an upright position.

TOTAL INCONTINENCE

Total Incontinence is the state in which an individual experiences a continuous and unpredictable loss of urine. Related causative factors include neuropathy preventing transmission of the reflex indicating bladder fullness; neurologic dysfunction causing triggering of micturition at unpredictable times; neuromuscular trauma due to surgery; trauma or disease affecting spinal cord nerves; and fistulas secondary to trauma.[85]

Urinary Retention

Urinary Retention is an accumulation of excess urine that is due to an inability to empty the bladder. Pro-longed retention, with stasis of urine in the bladder, establishes conditions that support infection. The accompanying Nursing Diagnosis Profile describes *Urinary Retention.*

PLANNING

Outcomes identified in the planning stage of the nursing process are specific to the nursing diagnosis.

Altered Urinary Elimination

URINARY TRACT INFECTION

Outcomes for the client with a urinary tract infection include voiding in normal frequency and amount with-

---

 ## NURSING DIAGNOSIS PROFILE

Urinary Retention

Definition. The state in which an individual experiences incomplete emptying of the bladder.

Classification. Exchanging 1.3.2.2

Defining Characteristics. Major defining characteristics include those signs and symptoms associated with the incomplete emptying of the bladder, such as bladder distention and either small, frequent voiding or absence of urine output. Minor defining characteristics in the individual might be a sensation of bladder fullness, dribbling, dysuria, overflow incontinence, or residual urine (more than 150 ml).

Sample Related Factors. Sample related factors include a high urethral pressure secondary to a weak detrusor muscle, inhibition of reflex arc, a strong sphincter, or blockage. Secondary etiological factors may include diminished or absent sensory or motor impulses, anxiety, the effects of medications or anesthetic agents, trauma, fecal impaction, or other physical or psychologic factors.

Concept Description. *Urinary Retention* occurs when urine is produced in the kidneys but retained in the bladder. The bladder is unable to expel urine in the normal manner. Therefore there is little or no urine output. When urine is passed, there is incomplete emptying of the bladder. Urinary retention most frequently occurs in postoperative clients who

► have had general or spinal anesthesia
► are over the age of 70
► have had total hip replacement, intra-abdominal surgery, or lower extremity surgery that required catheterization
► remain on bedrest before attempting to void
► do not attempt to void until 10 or more hours after anesthesia
► have a prolonged time interval between the last voiding preoperatively and the first attempt to void postoperatively (average 8.7 hours)
► have higher fluid intakes to compensate for blood loss during surgery
► have longer times in the operating room
► have a low fluid intake following surgery

Retention of urine following vaginal delivery is quite common and is caused by meatal swelling as a result of perineal trauma. Fecal impaction also can contribute to retention by causing pressure on the urethra and obstructing urine flow. Anticholinergic-antispasmodic, antidepressant-antipsychotic, antiparkinson, beta-adrenergic blockers, and antihypertensive drugs also interfere with the normal micturition process and result in retention. Lack of any behaviors that the individual has developed to help trigger the micturition reflex (privacy, normal position, established time for voiding) can also produce muscle tension and anxiety, resulting in retention.

Examples. Depending on the specific assessment data, this diagnostic category could be applicable in the following situations, among others:

► An elderly person who has had a knee replacement under general anesthesia. The person is unable to void 10 hours after surgery, complains of bladder fullness and discomfort, and has bladder distention. The nursing diagnosis would be *Urinary Retention* R/T inhibition of reflex arc secondary to effects of anesthesia.
► An elderly person who is living alone, who reports having been constipated for 4 days, and who now is urinating frequently in small amounts. The individual is accustomed to having a bowel movement every day and to urinating in large amounts (every 4 to 5 hours). The nursing diagnosis would be *Urinary Retention* R/T blockage secondary to fecal impaction.

Related/Similar Nursing Diagnosis. This diagnosis should be differentiated from the diagnosis *Altered Urinary Elimination.* With *Altered Urinary Elimination,* any of a number of disturbances in urinary elimination could occur, including retention of urine. In this case, urinary retention would be the related factor (e.g., *Altered Urinary Elimination* R/T urinary retention. A client with this diagnosis would also have a diagnosis of *Urinary Retention* (with its related factor). The diagnosis of *Altered Urinary Elimination* is broader than a diagnosis of *Urinary Retention* in that it does not specify exactly what the urinary alteration is. The nursing diagnosis of *Urinary Retention* is quite specific.

out pain or burning, as well as verbalizing the understanding of the disease process, methods of prevention, and follow-up instructions.

URINARY DIVERSION

Outcomes for the person with a urinary diversion include understanding the need for urinary diversion; demonstrating acceptance of the stoma; demonstrating the ability to care for the stoma as independently as possible; keeping the skin around the stoma healthy and nonirritated; and maintaining a clean, unobstructed drainage system.

URINARY TRACT STONES

Outcomes for the person with urinary tract stones include preventing infection, promoting comfort, recognizing signs of obstruction of the urine flow, and increasing fluid intake to promote passage of the stone.

Urinary Incontinence

The major goal for the person with incontinence is to achieve a reduction in incontinence or, in some instances, achieve continence. For the client with *Total Incontinence*, the goal is to maintain dry skin while using methods to contain or collect urine. Related outcomes include maintenance of skin integrity; performance of self-hygiene (to be free of urinary odor); prevention of infection; improvement of self-esteem; increased knowledge; and reduced social isolation.

Urinary Retention

Expected outcomes for the person with urinary retention are to void several times a day in volumes of 150 to 400 ml per void; maintain fluid intake of 1500 to 2400 ml per day unless otherwise restricted; and perform intermittent self-catheterization, utilizing aseptic technique, if necessary.

NURSING INTERVENTION
Altered Urinary Elimination

A variety of nursing measures can assist clients who have altered urinary elimination.

URINARY TRACT INFECTION

Intervention is multifaceted. The following nursing interventions to treat and prevent UTIs are appropriate for noncatheterized individuals. Interventions to prevent catheter-associated UTIs can be found on pages 1188 to 1191.

▶ Encourage high fluid intake to keep urine dilute and to promote natural "flushing out" of the urinary tract.

▶ Encourage clients to void when they feel the need, because drinking more fluids will increase the frequency of urination.

▶ Advise lowering the pH of the urine with a special diet, or with ordered medications, because acidic urine inhibits bacterial growth and increases the efficiency of certain urinary medications.

▶ Suggest that clients take showers instead of baths, because bacteria in the bath water can gain access to the urethra.

▶ Emphasize the importance of immediately reporting symptoms of a UTI and of getting prompt treatment.

▶ Teach the importance of taking medication for the infection exactly as ordered and taking all of the pills prescribed, even after the symptoms are gone.

▶ Teach a cardiac patient the difference between diuresis from a medication and frequency from an infection.[70]

▶ Teach methods of good perineal hygiene (i.e., wiping from front to back at all times).

▶ Suggest that women wear cotton panties, because synthetic fabrics tend to increase perineal moisture.

▶ Advise women against wearing tight slacks or pantyhose or keeping on a damp swimsuit.

▶ Recommend that women avoid the use of bubble bath, perfumed soaps, feminine hygiene sprays, or hexachlorophene.[51]

▶ Instruct women to void before and after intercourse and to use K-Y jelly as a lubricant if the vaginal epithelium is dry and causes irritation during intercourse.

▶ Suggest that sexually active women who use the diaphragm as a contraceptive acidify the urine to reduce the incidence of UTIs, because women who use the diaphragm are twice as likely as other sexually active women to get UTIs. The higher incidence suggests that the pH in the vagina of this population is more alkaline than acid.[39]

URINARY DIVERSION

Nursing care for the person with a urinary diversion is complex. For general care of the skin around the stoma, refer to Chapter 43, Meeting Bowel Elimination Needs, and Chapter 48, Caring for Persons with Wounds. A major difference between care of a urinary stoma and an enterostomal opening is that the urinary tract is sterile and, therefore, prone to infection whereas the bowel is not. Specific perioperative nursing care of clients undergoing urinary diversion procedures is beyond the scope of this chapter. However, you may be assigned to care for an individual who has a well-healed urinary diversion but who is hospitalized for some other reason. In such cases, you should have a general understanding of urinary diversion.

URINARY TRACT STONES

Nursing intervention focuses on education and prevention. Dietary changes, such as decreasing calcium, phosphorus, or purine intake, reduce high urinary excretion of these substances. High fluid intake keeps urine dilute. Altering urine pH (either alkalinization or acidification, depending on the type of stone) also inhibits calculi formation.

For the person who already has stones, provide pain relief and psychologic support. Administer analgesics, or apply hot packs to the flank areas as ordered by the physician. Prepare the person psychologically and physically for medical and surgical intervention.

Medical and surgical intervention depends on the type of stone. In general, the goal of therapy is to remove or destroy the stone. Therapy involves **lithotripsy** (crushing of a stone [calculus] in the ureter, bladder, or urethra) by percutaneous lithotripsy or extracorporeal shock-wave lithotripsy (ESWL) or removal of the stone by major surgery, especially if the stone is located in the kidney. Other therapy involves dissolving the stone by means of various chemical agents. Correcting errors in metabolism (e.g., hyperparathyroidism), if they exist, may be a type of preventive treatment.

Specific nursing care for clients undergoing these treatments is beyond the scope of this text. However, you will generally be expected to

▸ assess sensory and motor functions
▸ monitor vital signs
▸ assess surgical sites and dressings
▸ monitor respiratory and circulatory status
▸ measure intake and output
▸ provide for adequate hydration by mouth or by IV lines
▸ monitor and assess urinary output, whether by tubes or voided
▸ check for bladder distention
▸ check tubes and measure and empty drainage
▸ strain urine
▸ collect specimens

▸ observe for untoward outcomes, such as hemorrhage, infection, and allergic responses
▸ provide ordered medications, e.g., medications for control of pain, infection
▸ provide ordered treatments, e.g., warm packs
▸ teach the individual and/or family necessary self-monitoring and self-care
▸ document all care

Urinary Incontinence

Urinary incontinence can be managed and treated by interventions that not only decrease incontinence but also may restore continence. Treatment is a collaborative effort involving you, the individual, the family, the physician, and others involved with the client. Nursing interventions for the incontinent person include pelvic muscle exercises, habit training, bladder training, relaxation training, hydration therapy, bowel regimen, environmental support, skin care, collection devices, and incontinence aids.

PELVIC MUSCLE EXERCISES

Pelvic muscle exercises, or Kegel exercises, improve control of urination through active exercise of the pubococcygeus muscle (see Box 44–1 for an example of an easily understandable teaching tool that can be given to your clients to help them learn the exercises). These exercises have been found effective in reducing urinary incontinence in women of all ages who have stress incontinence; in elderly clients residing in the community and homebound persons with urge, stress,

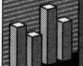

APPLYING RESEARCH TO NURSING PRACTICE

Diagnosing and Intervening for Urinary Incontinence

Pearson and Droessler screened 68 elderly women (average age of 87 years) for actual and potential problems of urinary incontinence. These nurse researchers found that 55 of the 68 elderly women were at risk for incontinence because they experienced at least one risk factor. The most frequently reported risk factors were *nocturia* and *inability to wait 15 minutes after the urge to urinate before urinating.* The researchers defined "actual incontinence" as an involuntary loss of urine at least once a month. Of the women whom they studied, the researchers found 13 to be incontinent, each of whom experienced at least four risk factors.

Following assessment, Pearson and Droessler taught the elderly women treatment strategies designed to reduce or eliminate the risk factors that they experienced.

Following these interventions, nine of the women still experienced actual incontinence. However, seven of the incontinent women eliminated one to five risk factors. Continent women who had experienced risk factors for urinary incontinence significantly increased the number of minutes they could wait following the urge to void.

Applications for Practice

In practice, you will encounter many women who assume that urinary incontinence is a normal part of aging that they must live with. Keeping in mind the reluctance of clients to discuss urinary incontinence, cautiously assess for risk factors for this common problem. Advise at-risk clients that urinary incontinence is a treatable condition — not a normal part of aging.

▼▼▼

Pearson, B.D., & Droessler, D. (1991). Problems of aging: urinary incontinence prevention. *Health Care for Women International, 12,* 443–450.

and functional incontinence; and in a long-term care population. To be effective, the exercises must be taught properly and reinforced frequently. Audio cassette tapes are available to assist individuals in practicing these exercises. These tapes provide a verbal guide through the exercise session.

HABIT TRAINING

The goal of habit training is to keep the client dry rather than to alter bladder function. Habit training involves developing a voiding schedule that is adjusted to the needs of the person. This schedule is based on the person's incontinence pattern, which is established by keeping a voiding record. Habit training is appropriate for people with functional or urge incontinence.

Have the person void at predetermined times, usually every 2 to 4 hours, even if the sensation to void is absent. Assist the person to sit on the toilet, commode, or bedpan.

BLADDER TRAINING

The goal of bladder training, or bladder retraining, is to extend the interval between voidings. The individual is taught to suppress the urge sensation by using various relaxation techniques (see Chapter 16). This breaks the habit of frequent voidings, increases bladder capacity, and lessens the urgency sensation. This intervention is appropriate for individuals with urge incontinence who are cognitively intact. It can also be effective for the physically or cognitively impaired person who has someone to assist with toileting.

Assist the person to the toilet, commode, or bedpan at prescribed times, usually every 1 to 2 hours initially, although the time span may be shorter if the bladder empties more frequently. Gradually lengthen the interval between voidings until a 3-hour interval is achieved.

RELAXATION TRAINING

Relaxation training helps the individual control the urge to void. This is an effective intervention for those diagnosed as having urge incontinence.

Teach the person relaxation techniques to use when a strong urge to urinate is felt. Techniques to use include slow, deep breathing or imagery (see Chapter 16). When the urge has been suppressed, instruct the person to walk unhurriedly to the bathroom to void.

HYDRATION THERAPY

Fluid intake should be maintained at a minimum of 1500 ml a day, unless contraindicated for therapeutic reasons (e.g., congestive heart failure or renal failure). Incontinent people often reduce fluid intake because they believe that if they drink nothing, there will be no urine to void. Explain to the client that adequate urine production is necessary to stimulate the micturition reflex. In addition, adequate fluid intake is necessary to maintain fluid and electrolyte balance.

Instruct the person to space fluid intake throughout the day and limit intake in the evening to reduce urine production during the night. Encourage the client to drink caffeine-free fluids. Observe for fluid retention and excessive weight gain.

BOWEL REGIMEN

Chronic constipation and fecal impaction are correctable causes of urinary incontinence. A diet high in fiber will relieve constipation. This can be achieved by the client's using whole, unprocessed wheat bran until having a soft, formed bowel movement every 1 to 3 days. If the person has a fecal impaction, it must be removed before beginning the bran therapy.

Instruct the client initially to mix about 1 tablespoon of bran per day into foods such as yogurt, cottage cheese, applesauce, puddings, sauces, or ice cream and to increase the bran gradually until the goal is reached. Advise the client that unprocessed wheat bran is natural to the body and superior to the use of laxatives.

Bran can cause side effects (flatulence, abdominal bloating, and cramps), but they usually disappear within 2 weeks.

ENVIRONMENTAL MODIFICATIONS

Certain environmental barriers may contribute to incontinence in the elderly (e.g., long distance to the bathroom, clutter in the path). Finding ways to increase the ease of toileting or to decrease the time needed to get to the toilet may promote continence. Assistive and collecting devices may be necessary.

Perform an environmental and functional assessment, including a mini–mental examination. Assess cognitive ability, mobility, and ability to perform activities of daily living. Install assistive devices (e.g., raised toilet seats, grab bars), provide adequate lighting, remove clutter in the pathway to the bathroom, supply assistive ambulation aids to increase support and to prevent falls, and modify clothing to facilitate toileting. Use collecting devices such as male and female urinals, bedside commodes, and fracture bedpans, if necessary.

SKIN CARE

Incontinence causes skin irritation and breakdown. Constantly moist skin becomes macerated. Also, over time, urine is converted to ammonia, which is very irritating to the skin. Skin irritation is painful and predisposes the client to developing pressure sores (decubitus ulcers).

Keep the skin clean and dry. Wash the perineum and other areas with mild soap and water after each incontinent episode. Apply body lotion to keep the skin moisturized and provide a barrier to the urine. Change any clothing or bed linens that have become wet with urine.

INCONTINENCE AIDS

Incontinence aids include both external catheters and absorbent products such as disposable briefs and absorbent pads, both of which may be either washable or disposable. These aids should not be used until the person's incontinence is thoroughly evaluated and all other appropriate methods tried.

External Catheters. External catheters, also known as condom or Texas catheters and urinary sheaths, can be used for men with all types of incontinence, particularly functional. They consist of a plastic or rubber sheath placed over the penis, with connecting tubing attached (Fig. 44–5). The tubing attaches to a leg bag or Foley catheter drainage bag.

To apply a condom catheter, don gloves and wash the penis and perineum with soap and water. Dry well. If pubic hair is excessive, shave the area first. Roll the condom sheath smoothly over the penis, leaving a 0.5- to 1-inch gap between the distal end of the penis and the connecting tube. Depending upon the kind of condom, apply a strip of elastic tape in a spiral at the top of the condom to secure it in place, or secure with a foam strip. Never completely encircle the penis with the tape, because this practice impedes circulation, especially if swelling occurs. Attach the condom to a drainage system. Be sure that the tip of the penis is not touching the condom and that the condom is not twisted. Remove your gloves. Attach the urinary drainage bag to the bed frame if the person is to remain in bed, or to the leg if ambulatory (see Fig. 44–5).

It is difficult to attach the condom securely without impairing circulation to the distal penis or damaging the skin. Therefore, apply these devices carefully!

Remove the condom at least daily to wash the penis and expose it to the air. Assess the penis for redness, edema, or excoriation. Skin sensitization has been found to be minimal, and it has been shown that it is possible to continue applying a condom catheter and even to heal sores in persons with sensitive skin.

Absorbent Products. Absorbent products protect the skin, bed linens, clothing, and furniture from urine. They are used to manage all types of incontinence. Early dependence on them may discourage continence by giving clients a sense of security and acceptance of the condition, when they might otherwise seek treatment.

Whether using briefs or pads, disposable or washable, check the individual every 2 hours for wetness and change when wet or soiled. Assess skin integrity, as a major concern is skin breakdown. One study of 276 totally incontinent persons in seven Florida nursing homes showed that the use of briefs did not increase the incidence of pressure ulcers and did not interfere with client care.[5]

These products can be purchased in surgical supply stores, supermarkets, and drugstores.

Urinary Retention

We have discussed normal micturition and helping people achieve and maintain normal urinary elimination patterns by means of adequate fluid intake, exercise,

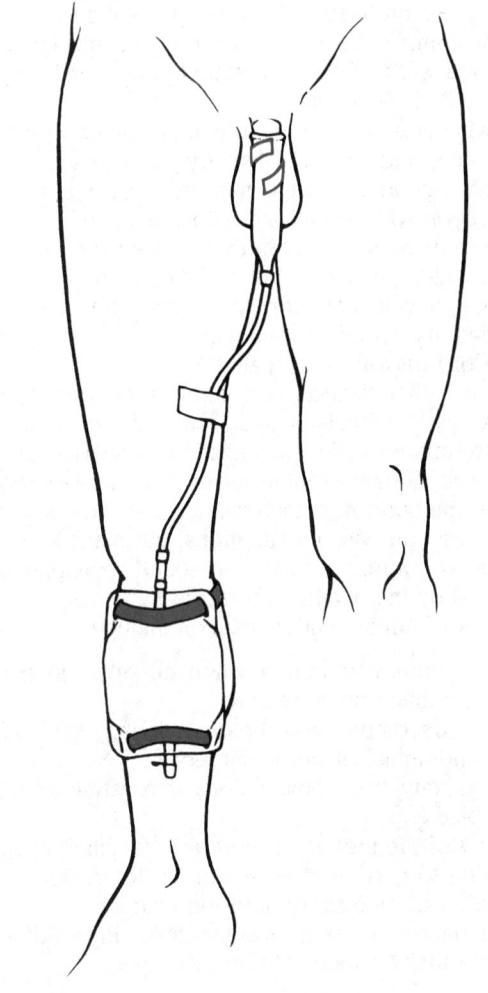

▲ *Figure 44–5*

Condom catheter with drainage bag in place.

proper positioning, and use of power of suggestion. These means are sometimes insufficient, however, and urinary catheterization is necessary.

A catheter is defined as a tubular instrument of rubber, plastic, metal, or other material, used for draining or injecting fluids or gases through a body passage. Catheterization is the process of passing a catheter into a body cavity or channel. Urinary catheterization is the introduction of a catheter via the urethra into the urinary bladder.

In the hospital and in other agencies, you will frequently care for clients who require catheterization or who have catheters in place. There is also a growing trend for hospitalized clients to return home with urinary catheters in place. In these instances, as the nurse, you will teach the individual and significant others about catheter care.

URINARY CATHETERIZATION

The nurse is responsible for (a) caring for the person with a catheter, and (b) ensuring safe and effective functioning of the drainage system. Many aspects of care involve independent nursing interventions, and many of these are directed toward prevention and mitigation of complications. At all times, the nursing care you provide will be based on sound principles from the biologic and social sciences.

You will have a primary role in catheter insertion, maintenance, and removal. Urinary catheterization is a dependent action, requiring the order of a physician. However, you will be the one who usually provides the assessment data used to identify the need for catheterization. In addition, when the catheter is in place, you will be the one to care for the person and make recommendations, based on ongoing assessment, for continuation or removal of the catheter.

Urethral catheterization is a sterile procedure. Thus, you must use surgical asepsis. The only exception is clean, intermittent self-catheterization, discussed in this chapter. The steps presented in Procedure 44–1 represent one method of catheterization. As you observe other nurses, you will see variations, but make sure the procedure you adopt is based on sound principles and is approved by the health care facility.

Purposes of urinary catheterization include

▶ relief of urinary retention when all other interventions have been unsuccessful
▶ bladder decompression before, during, and after lower abdominal or pelvic surgery
▶ lower urinary tract obstruction or paralysis (neurogenic bladder)
▶ splinting of the ureters or urethra to facilitate healing following surgery or other trauma to the region
▶ instillation of medication into the bladder
▶ determination of urinary residual following voiding
▶ accurate measurement of urinary output

Although some clinicians consider sterile specimen collection and urinary incontinence valid reasons for urinary catheterization, this practice is generally discouraged. Unless a catheter is already in place, it is generally considered acceptable practice to acquire sterile urine specimens by the midstream or clean-catch method.

The incontinent person must sometimes be catheterized to keep skin, clothing, and bed linen dry and to prevent skin breakdown, particularly if dressings or skin lesions require protection. Unfortunately, in many cases the catheter is inserted solely for the convenience of the nursing staff or the person's significant others. *This is poor practice.* The incontinent person should be catheterized *only as a last resort.* Every effort must first be made to achieve continence by carefully assessing the individual's psychophysiologic status and instituting a rigorous bladder training program, if appropriate.

Today most catheters are made of plastic or latex rubber. Glass, metal, or woven silk catheters may at times be used during diagnostic or therapeutic procedures, or when insertion of a rubber or plastic catheter into the urethra of a male client has been attempted without success.

Studies have been done to determine whether the use of specific catheter materials could reduce the incidence of bacteriuria. Although results are contradictory,

it is generally accepted that for short-term use, latex is satisfactory. However, when the catheter will be in place longer than 1 week, silicone catheters are recommended. Over time, latex tends to deteriorate and become encrusted, which results in obstruction of urine flow and irritation of the bladder and urethral mucosa.

Caution An FDA Medical Alert of March 29, 1991, warns that latex in catheters may trigger allergic reactions in sensitive people. Apparently symptoms range from contact urticaria to systemic anaphylaxis. You can protect your client from such occurrences by asking about latex sensitivity during history taking. A positive response to the question, "Do you itch, wheeze, or get a rash when you blow up a balloon?" can alert you and the person to a possible sensitivity. A medical ID bracelet might be another way to prevent problems. If an individual is sensitive to latex, consider using another type of catheter.[27]

Suprapubic Catheters. Suprapubic catheters are retention catheters inserted by a surgeon into the bladder through the abdominal wall. The incision is usually made about 3 cm above the symphysis pubis. The surgeon inserts the suprapubic catheter either during a more extensive operative procedure or at the bedside using local anesthesia. The suprapubic catheter is usually sutured in place for added security and then attached to a drainage system, as with the urethral catheter. Care of the system is similar to that of the urethral catheter, with the addition of wound care at the insertion site. There is some evidence that the suprapubic catheter reduces the incidence of urinary tract infection, and it is much more comfortable and convenient for the individual. However, there have been instances of bowel perforation during insertion, detachment of the catheter from the skin, leakage around the catheter, and hematuria resulting from the initial insertion or from irritation of the bladder mucosa by the catheter.

Stents. A **stent** is any material used to hold tissue in place or to provide support for a graft or anastomosis while healing takes place. In the urinary system, it is usually a manufactured tubular device. Red rubber, Silastic, latex Foley, or pigtail catheters are used as stents (Fig. 44–6).

Urologists use stents temporarily or permanently to divert urine flow from an area in the urinary system, to promote healing or to maintain patency of an edematous, anastomosed part of the urinary system, allowing urine to pass. Temporary stents are used to aid healing by diverting urine from the suture line of a new ileoconduit, or anastomosis. Temporary stents can enhance the healing of ureteral tears caused by trauma or accidents during surgery. Permanent stents may be inserted to maintain ureteral patency in terminally ill individuals.[38]

Nursing interventions for a person with a stent are beyond the scope of this text but generally include

▶ observing the individual for fever and purulent drainage at the insertion site or in the drainage bag

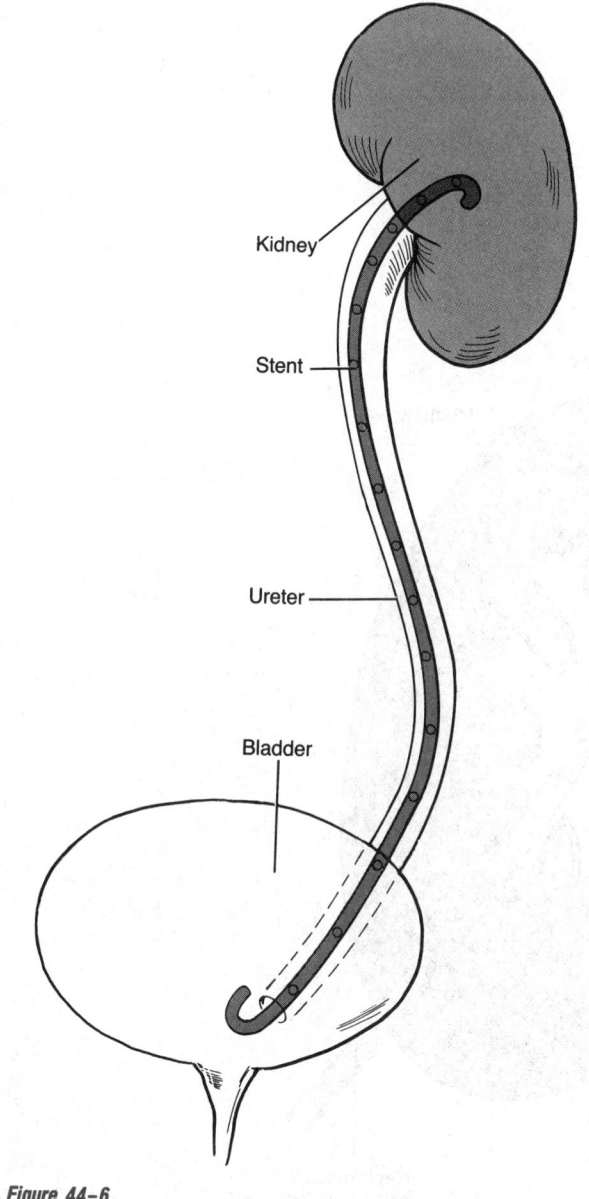

▲ *Figure 44-6*

Ureteral stent.

▶ routinely cleaning the site every 8 hours with hydrogen peroxide to decrease the chance of infection
▶ observing for urine cloudiness, brighter or darker red blood in the urine (urine should be light pink), or abnormally high or low urinary output
▶ encouraging high fluid intake to prevent infection
▶ taking daily measurements of the stent to check for placement
▶ checking the stent dressing frequently, and replacing tape as needed
▶ documenting all care as needed

Any signs of the stent becoming dislodged or plugged should be reported immediately.

Percutaneous Nephrostomy Tubes. The percutaneous **nephrostomy tube** is a tube that is implanted into the renal pelvis (Fig. 44-7). The physician inserts the tube through the skin and into the kidney, where its pigtail coils to maintain its position. The nephrostomy catheter is connected to a closed drainage system.[18,34]

Percutaneous nephrostomy tubes are used for individuals who are poor surgical candidates because they may have an infection or uremia. In people who are terminally ill, it may be used as a palliative measure to avoid prolonged hospitalizations. Other uses include removal of renal calculi or instillation of solutions that will dissolve them, brush biopsies of renal calices and ureters, introduction of a ureteral stent, pressure flow studies and other tests on the urinary system, diversion to pass a ureteral fistula, dilation of ureteral stenosis, and drainage of a renal or perirenal abscess.[18,34]

The nursing care you will provide immediately following the insertion of the percutaneous nephrostomy tube is important to prevent complications and to maintain the patency of the tube. Complications may include hemorrhage, perforation, and infection. You must be alert for signs of hemorrhage from the nephrostomy site. Frequent monitoring of blood pressure, pulse, and respirations will alert you to changes in vital signs that indicate bleeding. Perforation of a body organ by the nephrostomy tube can occur but rarely happens because soft catheters are used. If urine output decreases or if there is a sudden onset or increase in pain, notify the physician immediately. This may mean perforation has occurred. Sepsis and pyelonephritis are other complications that can result. Monitoring for an elevated temperature and cloudy urine is important, because these signs may be first indicators that the individual has an infection. Prophylactic antibiotic therapy is usually initiated, and a closed drainage system is maintained to prevent sepsis.[18,34]

Other complications associated with insertion of nephrostomy tubes are leakage around the catheter and catheter dislodgment. Leakage will occur if the catheter becomes blocked. Dressings should be checked frequently for signs of urine leakage. A sudden decrease in, or absence of, urine output may occur in individuals with catheter dislodgment. (Additional nursing care for individuals with nephrostomy tubes may be found in medical-surgical nursing texts.)

Urethral Catheters. Urethral catheters are by far the most common types of catheters. The catheter is inserted through the external meatus into the urethra, beyond the internal sphincter and into the bladder.

Catheters are sized according to the French scale. The size of the urethral catheter used depends on the size of the person. There is no rule, but a general guideline is to use size 8-10 for children, 14-16 for adult women, and 18-20 for adult men. If the catheter is too small, it is liable to curl up on itself when it meets any kind of obstruction in the urethra. Also, the smaller the catheter diameter, the more likely it is to be obstructed by blood clots or mucus plugs. On the other hand, if the tube is too large, it causes pressure on the

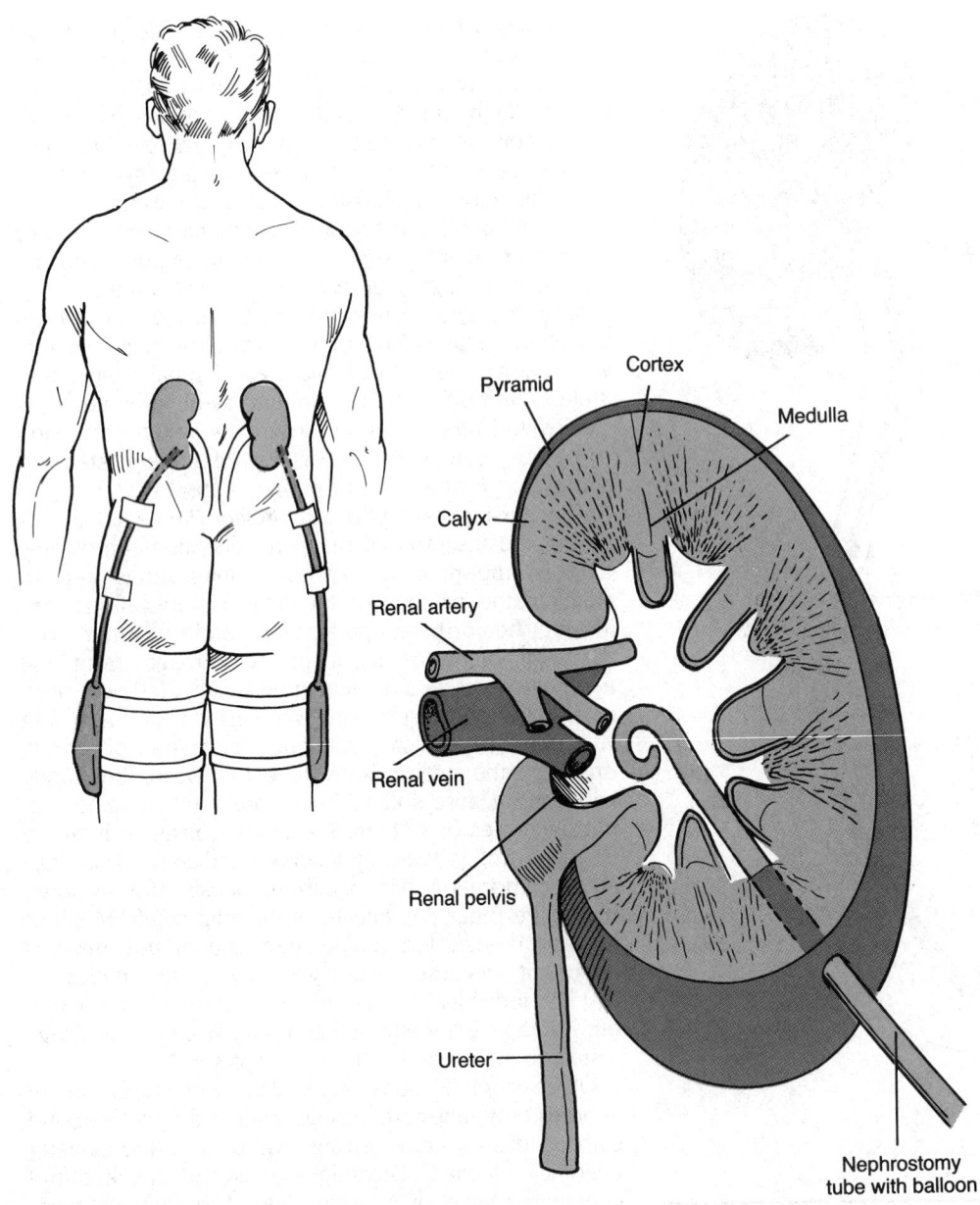

▲ *Figure 44-7*

Positioning of a percutaneous nephrostomy tube.

meatus or urethra and surrounding structures and can lead to tissue erosion.

Figure 44-8 depicts a variety of catheter configurations. The principal differences are in the shape of the catheter tip and the number of lumens within the tube. The two most commonly used catheters are the single-lumen straight catheter (Fig. 44-8A, 1) and the double-lumen, rounded-tip retention catheter (often called a Foley catheter) (Fig. 44-8B).

The shape of the tip determines catheter use. Male-cot (Fig. 44-8A, 2) and mushroom-tipped catheters (A, 3) prevent catheter dislodgment, although external fixation of the catheter tubing onto a person's leg or abdomen is still necessary. The coudé catheter (Fig. 44-8C) has a curved tip, which allows easier passage around a partial obstruction in the urethra. Rounded-tip

catheters are used for people without anatomic abnormalities or obstructions.

The number of lumens in a catheter refers to the various compartments into which the inside of the catheter tubing is divided. The urethral catheter usually contains one to three lumens, each of which has a specific purpose. In Figure 44-8, the circles at the right of the catheters illustrate the inner configuration of the tubing.

The straight, single-lumen catheter (Fig. 44-8A, 1) is used to check for residual urine, obtain a urine specimen, instill medication, and intermittently relieve bladder distention.

Figure 44-8 B and C depicts double- and triple-lumen indwelling retention catheters, which are used if the catheter must remain in place. Note that the reten-

A. Single lumen

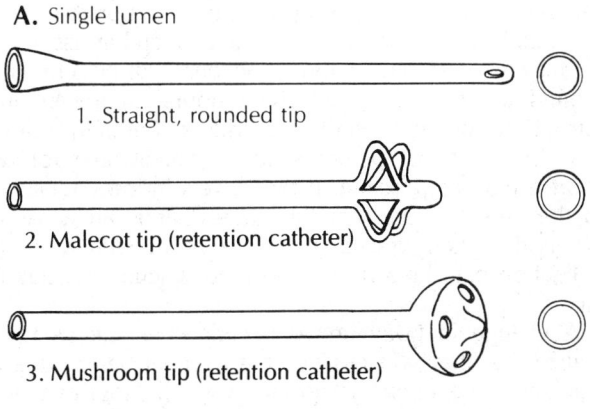

1. Straight, rounded tip

2. Malecot tip (retention catheter)

3. Mushroom tip (retention catheter)

B. Double lumen (Retention catheter with rounded tip)

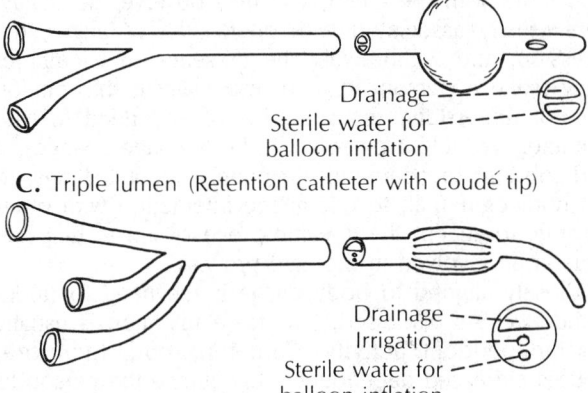

Drainage
Sterile water for
balloon inflation

C. Triple lumen (Retention catheter with coudé tip)

Drainage
Irrigation
Sterile water for
balloon inflation

▲ **Figure 44–8**

Catheter configurations.

tion catheter has an inflatable balloon. After the catheter is inside the bladder, the balloon is inflated with sterile water, using the appropriate lumen. The balloon is then too large to pass from the bladder into the urethra, thus keeping the catheter in place. The catheter is usually connected to a drainage system so that it continually drains urine from the bladder. In addition to being employed for all the reasons a straight catheter is used, a retention catheter is inserted for long-term decompression of the bladder. Observe that in the double-lumen retention catheter shown in Figure 44–8 *B*, one lumen provides for drainage of urine while the other lumen leads to a balloon located just below the drainage eye on the catheter. Figure 44–8 *C* illustrates a triple-lumen retention catheter, which can be employed for closed continuous or intermittent irrigation of the bladder or catheter. In this case, the third lumen provides a channel for irrigation fluid. The Malecot- and mushroom-tip catheters are also retention catheters but are used less frequently than the double- or triple-lumen catheters.

Determining the Need for Catheterization. The nurse frequently provides the assessment data on which the decision to use a catheter is made. As mentioned, urethral catheterization requires a physician's order.

Therefore, in many instances, you will decide on the basis of a nursing assessment that a person requires bladder catheterization. You will then communicate this information to the physician, who in turn writes the order.

Sometimes a physician writes a prn order requesting that the person be catheterized if urinary retention occurs. In this case, you must carefully assess the individual in order to make a sound judgment.

Urinary retention is a hazardous condition not only because it can lead to loss of bladder tone, but also because of its potential role in the development of UTI and renal calculi.

Studies indicate that most cases of urinary bacteriuria result from a lack of blood supply to the bladder tissue because of increased pressure within the bladder or overdistention of the bladder.[15,32] Reduced blood flow makes the tissue more susceptible to invasion by the client's own gastrointestinal bacteria, which are carried via either the blood or the lymph circulation systems. Intervene early when urinary retention develops, but suggest the use of catheterization only when absolutely necessary. Base your decision on careful assessment of each person.

Once the decision has been made to use a urinary catheter, ensure the safety and comfort of the individual by following proper techniques in catheter management. Note that the catheterization procedure itself, drainage system set-ups, and suggested care of the person with an indwelling catheter change frequently as a result of ongoing studies. Therefore, keep current with studies and findings in this area by consulting nursing journals and newsletters on a regular basis. Procedure 44–1 describes methods for both male and female catheterization.

Teaching About Catheterization. Effective instruction concerning the catheterization process reduces discomfort, anxiety, and some of the risks associated with catheters. People who have been carefully prepared and instructed about catheterization are usually more relaxed and able to cooperate in their care program. They know what to expect and how they can help alleviate the physical hazards of catheterization. As an example, many people experience a constant feeling of urgency for a time immediately after the catheter has been inserted. This discomfort is usually transient and is caused by the continuous stretching of the sphincter. Relief of this discomfort eventually comes as the sphincter adapts to the presence of the catheter. Relief may be hastened by an increased fluid intake. If the person knows to expect the sensation and realizes that it is temporary, coping with the discomfort can be easier.

You must also teach people that they can move around with a catheter in place. Many people are afraid to move, turn, or walk once the catheter has been taped into place for fear it will come out or be disconnected. Emphasize that the catheter is taped in place and that the inflated balloon keeps it in the bladder.

You must also instruct people how to move and ambulate without getting tangled in the tubing.

Also, instruct clients concerning their responsibility for (a) taking fluids, (b) performing perineal care, (c) following recommended dietary measures, and (d) taking prescribed medications. Many things interfere with the retention of information (e.g., anxiety, medications, other stimuli, and organic memory loss). Therefore, you may need to repeat basic facts over and over again. For instance, you may need to remind people that they have a catheter draining the bladder, and therefore it is not necessary to void.

Maintaining Psychologic Comfort

In addition to the physical hazards associated with catheterization, there are psychologic implications: embarrassment, body image change, and increased dependency.

Although these aspects may not be as obvious as the physical hazards, the psychologic impact of urinary catheters on people is just as important.

For many people, the act of urination is a private matter. Thus, it is not at all surprising that catheterization is charged with embarrassment, both for the individual and for the nursing student.

It is important to be cognizant of any embarrassment that might interfere with nursing care. As a beginning nursing student, you come to clinical practice with the same feelings about bladder elimination as the lay public. Suddenly, you are required to interview people about their bladder habits, to help them establish normal elimination, and ultimately to catheterize them and care for them in that state. Embarrassment is a normal response to this situation. Your embarrassment is easily transmitted to others, including those in your care. Time and experience will diminish these feelings. Soon you will be able to assess people's elimination needs and intervene effectively. However, to facilitate this period of growth, be aware of the emotions you may feel and discuss them with peers and others in the teaching/learning environment. You should also always remember the personal embarrassment you originally felt surrounding this area of nursing care. It will help you to be more sensitive to the feelings of others. Sometimes, as experienced nurses, we become so used to dealing with people's excretory needs and functions that we forget they do not share our familiarity with this basic aspect of life.

It is the nurse's responsibility to alleviate people's feelings of embarrassment as much as possible. Foremost, it is important to be sensitive, open, and honest. Acknowledge people's feelings and assure them that it is normal to be embarrassed. Explain the procedure and ways in which they can assist you. In this way, they can retain a sense of self-control and self-dignity.

Nonverbal communication is also an important means of reducing embarrassment. A matter-of-fact approach by the nurse conveys that bladder care is a normal facet of care, and that the person's needs in this area are basic to all people. Conscientiously preserving the person's privacy as much as possible also communicates awareness of potential embarrassment. During the catheterization procedure, draw curtains around the bed and shut room doors to prevent interruptions by other staff and visitors. Carefully drape the person so as to expose the perineal area for as short a time as possible. If there are windows adjacent to the bed, be sure that the drapes/blinds are closed. When the client moves from the room with a urine collection bag, help make it as inconspicuous as possible.

A change in body image occurs when clients fully realize that they will not be able to meet basic urinary elimination needs in the normal way. This loss of function may be either temporary or permanent. Loss of normal body functions commonly results in grieving. As you work with the client, you may observe the behaviors usually associated with grief, such as anger, depression, and withdrawal. The presence of a catheter may make a person agitated, especially if that person cannot understand the presence of and need for the catheter. To help a person with body image changes, it is important to communicate openly about feelings, to be nonjudgmental, to encourage interaction with other people, to accept the grieving process, and to help the person be involved in the care process.

Closely aligned to body image is the need for independence. As discussed, bladder elimination is usually an independent activity. Catheterization, therefore, causes increased dependency. Encourage the person to be as independent as possible, both in helping with urinary elimination and in other activities of daily living. In addition, keep the period of catheterization as short as possible. Remember to assess the person daily to determine the earliest possible time for catheter removal.

Maintaining Catheter Patency. For the catheter and drainage system to perform their intended function, they must be kept patent. Obstruction of the flow of urine causes accumulation of urine in the bladder. Signs of possible obstruction include decreased urine in the collection bag and symptoms of urinary retention. Sometimes the person actually voids around the catheter because of the increased intravesicular pressure.

A catheter clamp is sometimes used to interrupt the flow of urine through the system in order to collect a urine specimen or recondition the bladder after long-term catheterization. When a catheter is clamped for any reason, it is essential to remember to remove the clamp as soon as the intended purpose is achieved. Occasionally, after nurses place the clamp, they forget to remove it. This mistake can have serious consequences, leading to urinary retention and its attendant complications.

To prevent obstruction in the drainage system, place and tape drainage tubing either (a) on top of the leg, (b) under the leg, (c) between the legs, or (d) for males, taped to the abdomen. Each method has its advantages. The first method, for example, is appropri-

Text continued on page 1187

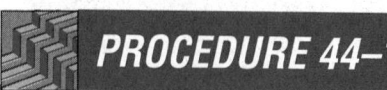

Female and Male Urethral Catheterization

Definition/Purposes. Insertion of a urinary catheter through the urethra into the bladder in order to (a) drain urine from the bladder, (b) instill medication into the bladder, (c) splint the urethra, and/or (d) prevent obstruction.

Contraindications/Cautions. Use sterile technique throughout this intervention. Review principles of surgical asepsis (Chapter 28). Arrange equipment so as to avoid breaking the sterile technique. If the client is restless or otherwise unable to cooperate, enough help must be available to ensure good visualization of the meatus and to avoid contamination of the sterile field. Also, if lighting is insufficient, another person may need to shine a light on the perineum.

Learning/Teaching Guidelines. Provide the client and significant others with information, as appropriate: (a) explain the reason for catheterization; (b) describe the procedure; (c) explain how the person can cooperate during the procedure; (d) explain that catheterization is not usually painful, but that a sensation of pressure may be experienced during insertion; and (e) emphasize how the person can turn and ambulate with an indwelling catheter.

PRELIMINARY ACTIVITIES

Assessment/Planning

▶ Check record for physician's order to catheterize.
▶ Know reason for catheterization.
▶ Assess for signs of urinary retention, if appropriate.
▶ Check record and with nursing staff to determine whether interventions have been performed to help person void (e.g., running water, pouring water over hands)
▶ Plan for assistance if client is unable to cooperate.
▶ Determine and select type of catheter needed for procedure (e.g., straight catheter, Foley catheter, and so forth).
▶ Select most appropriate position for a woman (i.e., dorsal recumbent or lateral).

Preparation

▶ Explain procedure steps to person and significant others.
▶ Position bed so you can stand on the side that puts your dominant hand toward foot end of bed.
▶ Provide for continuing privacy.
▶ Raise bed to working height; lower side rail.
▶ Place overbed table with equipment in convenient position.
▶ Move person close to your side of bed.
▶ Position a female in either dorsal recumbent or lateral position and drape appropriately.*
▶ Place a male in supine position and drape appropriately.
▶ Wash and dry perineum, if necessary.
   Focus light source correctly. Adjust gooseneck lamp or flashlight to shine on perineum.
▶ Wash your hands.

Equipment

▶ Sterile prepackaged catheter insertion kit containing
   No. 16 or 18 French Foley catheter (with 5-ml balloon if indwelling catheter required)
   Sterile drainage tubing and collection bag if using indwelling catheter. In some systems, tubing and collection bag are already connected to catheter, and therefore are included in catheterization tray. Sample port, hook for attachment, and outlet control device are parts of the drainage collection bag.
   Prep tray: water-soluble lubricant syringe or package, latex gloves (2), waterproof underpad, forceps, fenestrated drape, cotton balls (5), antiseptic cleansing solution, 10-ml syringe with sterile water to inflate balloon, if appropriate
▶ Specimen cup, cap, label (may be included in prep tray)
▶ Collection basin
▶ Tape
▶ Rubber band and safety pin, for indwelling catheter
▶ Waste bag utilized as specified by your institution and Centers for Disease Control
▶ Bath blanket to cover individual
▶ Flashlight or gooseneck lamp if needed
▶ Basin of warm water, soap, wash cloth, and towel if needed
▶ Clean pair of disposable gloves if needed to wash perineum

PROCEDURE

Actions

1. If inserting indwelling catheter that needs to be connected to drainage system:
   a. Remove drainage system from its outside container according to directions on package.

   b. Attach collection bag to bed frame near bottom of bed.

Rationale/Discussion

1.

   a. Be careful not to dislodge cap of drainage tubing. Cap ensures sterility of inside of drainage system and of connecting junction.

   b. Collection bag must remain below level of bladder to prevent backflow of urine into bladder. Urine will flow downward by gravity.

---

* Note that the position used to illustrate female catheterization is the dorsal recumbent (Figs. 44–9 and 44–10). An alternative position is the lateral (Fig. 44–11). In the lateral position, the woman lies diagonally across the bed on her side, with knees and hips flexed. The upper leg is flexed to a greater degree than the lower leg. Catheterization is carried out exactly as described, except that, instead of separating the labia with the fingers of one hand, you lift the upper labia in order to visualize the meatus. The advantages of this position include decreased embarrassment and anxiety, better body mechanics for the nurse, and better visualization. Because it is easier to hold one labia out of the field, it is less difficult to maintain aseptic technique. The lateral position is not widely used, but should be considered more frequently as an alternative.

Procedure continued on following page

PROCEDURE 44–1 Continued

Female and Male Urethral Catheterization

Actions	Rationale/Discussion

Actions

c. Bring end of drainage tubing up between side rail and mattress. Make sure side rail operates without kinking or pinching tubing.
d. Place end of drainage tubing so it is convenient to reach and will not fall off mattress during catheterization.

2. Open sterile prepackaged catheter kit according to directions on package, using sterile technique.

3. Pick up solid plastic-coated drape, stand back from table, grasp corner of drape, and allow it to fall open.

4. Place this drape, with plastic side down, on bed between person's legs. Be careful not to touch anything but the edges and bottom of sterile drape with your ungloved hands.

5. Don sterile gloves.

6. If desired, pick up fenestrated drape (with hole in center) and open it as in Step 4 above. Then place it over perineum so that hole exposes labia. For a man, place drape so that penis goes through hole. Lift penis with your nondominant hand, keeping your dominant hand sterile. Once you have touched the penis (or anything else not sterile), do not touch anything sterile with that hand.

7. Place sterile tray on sterile field between person's legs. Keep sterile objects within your line of vision at all times. Open packages and arrange so you have easy access to them as needed.

8. If obtaining urine specimen, remove lid from specimen container. Place container on end of overbed table. Set lid loosely on container. If not using container, set aside.

9. For women, lubricate about 3 to 5 cm (1.5 to 2 inches) of catheter tip with water-soluble lubricant. For men, lubricate about 17.5 cm (7 inches) of catheter tip.

10. If inserting indwelling catheter, attach prefilled syringe to balloon lumen of catheter. Inflate the balloon with appropriate amount (8 to 9 ml) of sterile water to test it. Then withdraw the solution.

11. Prepare antiseptic cleansing material as directed on package.

12. Cleanse perineal area and insert catheter.
For females:
a. Separate labia with nondominant hand to expose meatus. Place thumb and forefinger between labia minora. Separate labia, and pull up to identify urinary meatus clearly (Figs. 44–9 and 44–10).

Rationale/Discussion

c. Prevents obstruction of tube's patency and prevents tube from being in a position to be pulled out by the raising of the rail.

2. Urinary catherization requires sterile equipment and sterile technique because the bladder is a sterile body cavity that can become infected by microbes.

3. Standing back from table prevents drape from becoming contaminated by brushing against table as it opens.

4. Protects bed linen and establishes a sterile field for later placement of a sterile tray. Touching only the outer edges of the drape maintains the sterility of the more central portion of the drape.

5. Maintains surgical asepsis.

6. Although this drape is included in all commercially prepared catheterization trays, its use is optional. Its main advantage is that it provides a larger sterile field. However, many people feel that it gets in the way, thereby increasing the chance of contamination. If you decide not to use drape, pick it out of the sterile tray and drop it aside.

7. Places sterile objects close to working area. Objects out of line of vision may accidentally become contaminated.

8. Keeps container within easy reach during procedure. When needed, it should be ready to quickly collect urine as it flows from the catheter.

9. Reduces friction, thereby facilitating insertion of catheter. In some agencies, an antimicrobial lubricant is used to reduce chance of infection.

10. Most catheterization kits come with prefilled syringe. If syringe is not prefilled, draw up 8 to 9 ml of sterile water. It is best to test the balloon prior to insertion to be certain that it is functioning correctly. The balloon is inflated with 8 to 9 ml of sterile water because the balloon holds 5 ml; the extra 3 to 4 ml will fill the lumen leading to the balloon.

11. Must be prepared in advance, because once labia are separated or penis is grasped, only one hand will be available to handle sterile equipment. The perineal area must be cleansed to reduce the microbial count at meatus where passage of the catheter can track microbes into the sterile urethra. Use of nondominant hand reserves dominant hand to complete the catheterization with a sterile glove.

12.
For females:
a. Labia separation allows for good visualization. Pulling up on labia smooths out perineum. If you are catheterizing a postpartum woman with episiotomy (incision to enlarge vaginal outlet), stretching outward rather than upward prevents painful pulling on sutures.

PROCEDURE 44-1 Continued

Female and Male Urethral Catheterization

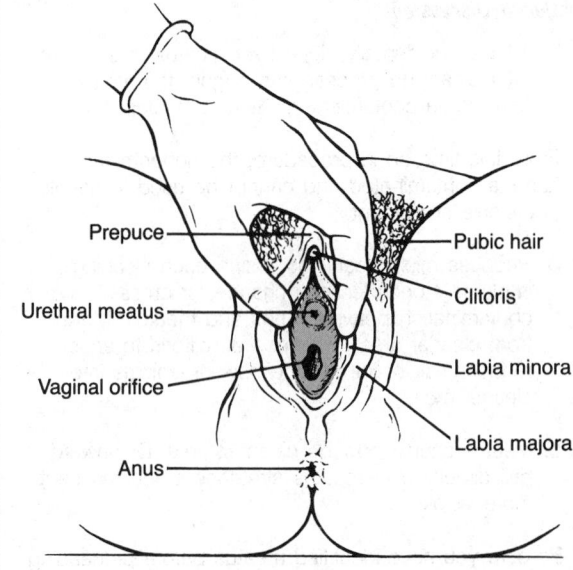

▲ Figure 44-9

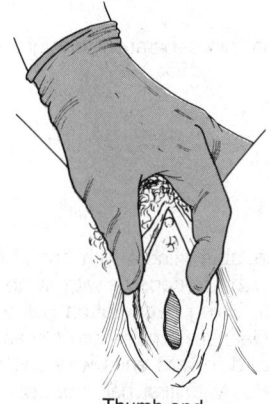

Thumb and
forefinger

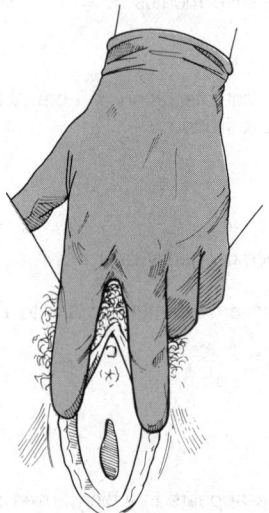

Forefinger and
middle finger

▲ Figure 44-10

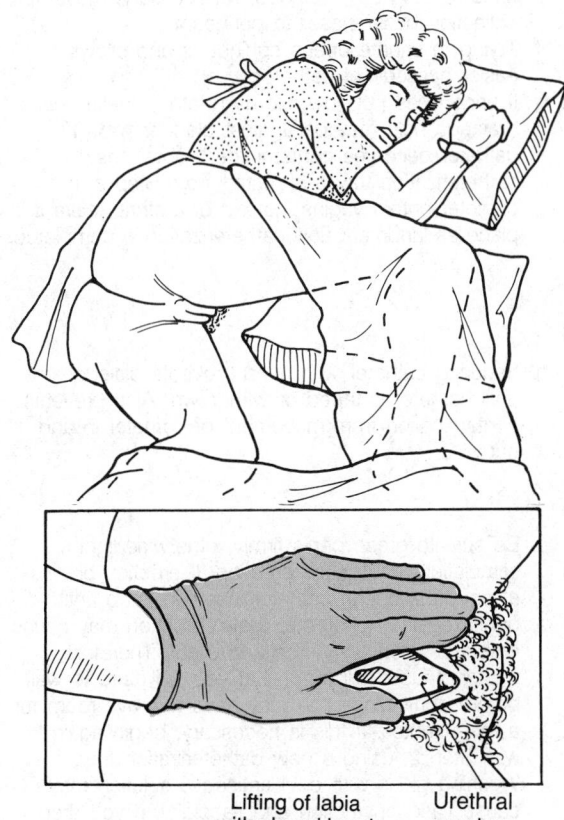

Lifting of labia   Urethral
with gloved hand   meatus

▲ Figure 44-11

Procedure continued on following page

PROCEDURE 44–1 Continued

Female and Male Urethral Catheterization

Actions	Rationale/Discussion
b. Maintain this separation throughout insertion.	b. If labia accidentally close over meatus at any time after cleansing process has begun, the area is considered contaminated. Restart at Step 12a. From this time on in procedure, the nondominant hand is contaminated and cannot be used to handle any sterile equipment.
c. Cleanse labia minora with cotton balls held securely by forceps or with swab; use antiseptic solution. Using each cotton ball or applicator only once, cleanse female from clitoris backward or downward toward anus with one stroke to one side of meatus with first ball, opposite side with one stroke with second ball.	c. Reduces microorganisms. Using each cleaning implement once lessens chance for cross-contamination between anus and meatus. Moving from cleaner area to dirtier (i.e., clitoris to anus) reduces risk of introducing new organisms into cleaner area.
d. In a likewise manner cleanse around the meatus (going from front to back), cleanse on each side, then cleanse meatus down the middle.	d. Meatus should now be cleanest area. Downward pull directly over meatus stretches it and makes it more visible. Be sure you have identified meatus before proceeding.
e. Pick up catheter about 7.5 cm (3 inches) from tip with gloved hand.	e. Allows control of tip for insertion while reducing chance of contaminating the part of the catheter that will enter the bladder. Be sure drainage end of catheter remains inside collection basin to avoid urine running out over bed. If necessary, move collection basin closer to perineum.
f. Have person gently bear down as though trying to urinate.	f. Trying to urinate opens sphincters and allows easier passage of catheter.
g. Gently insert catheter about 5 to 7.5 cm (2 to 3 inches).	g. If urine does not flow, slowly rotate catheter, since drainage hole may be against bladder wall. If catheter becomes contaminated, obtain new catheterization tray and restart from Step 2. If catheter enters vagina instead of urethra, leave it in place as landmark until catheterization is completed.

When urine appears in tubing, insert it 2 more inches to avoid inflating the balloon in the urethra.

Actions	Rationale/Discussion
h. Release labia and hold catheter securely with nondominant hand. Maintain this position until catheterization is completed or balloon or indwelling catheter has been inflated. Rest hand on person's pubis for support.	h. Securing catheter with hand prevents dislodgment until catheter is taped or withdrawn. Also prevents contamination from movement of catheter in and out of urethra.

For males:

Actions	Rationale/Discussion
a. Pick up penis with nondominant hand. Retract uncircumcised foreskin, grasp penis directly behind glans, and spread urinary meatus between thumb and forefinger.	a. Be sure to grasp penis firmly, otherwise light stimulation may cause erection. If erection occurs at any time during catheter insertion, stop until penis regains nonerectile state. Erection may cause embarrassment for nurse and client. Therefore, matter-of-factly tell client that you will need to wait before continuing. You may have to leave room for a few minutes. If this is necessary, begin again with Step 2, using a new catheterization tray. Washing glans with cool antiseptic solution may cause vasoconstriction and flaccidity. If you drop penis or release foreskin after cleansing, start this step again.

PROCEDURE 44–1 Continued

Female and Male Urethral Catheterization

Actions

b. With sterile forceps, cleanse penis, using circular motion. Start over meatus and work down toward base of glans. Cleanse to just above hand holding penis.

c. Repeat Step b twice more, using new cotton ball or swab each time.

d. With dominant hand, pick up liberally lubricated catheter at least 7.5 cm (3 inches) from distal end.

e. Draw penis upward and forward at 60° to 90° angle to legs so that it is as nearly perpendicular to body as possible.

f. Have person gently bear down as though trying to urinate. Insert tip of catheter into urethra. Gently insert 17 to 20 cm (7 to 8 inches) of tubing.

Rationale/Discussion

b. Reduces number of organisms. Moving from cleaner to dirtier areas prevents the introduction of new organisms into cleaner area.

c. Reduces chance for cross-contamination.

d. Since male urethra is longer than female urethra, grasping catheter farther down reduces chance of contaminating portion of catheter that enters body.

e. Perpendicular position straightens urethra and eases passage of catheter.

f. Trying to urinate opens sphincters and allows easier passage of catheter. If you meet resistance, stop and wait a few minutes to see whether resistance is caused by temporary spasm of sphincter. Have person take deep breaths. Change angle of penis. If there still is resistance, stop and call physician.

Because of possible strictures in male urethra, never force catheter.

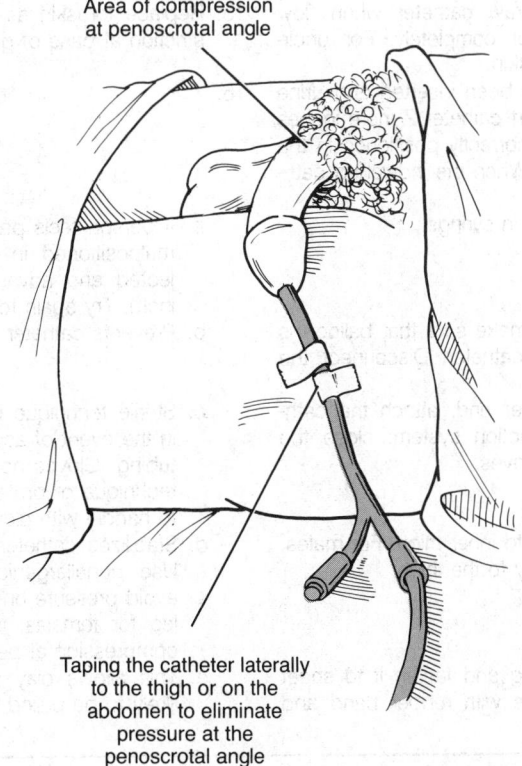

Area of compression at penoscrotal angle

Taping the catheter laterally to the thigh or on the abdomen to eliminate pressure at the penoscrotal angle

▲ *Figure 44–12*

Procedure continued on following page

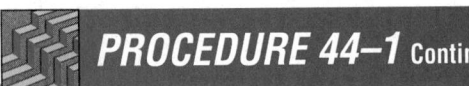

Female and Male Urethral Catheterization

Actions	**Rationale/Discussion**

Actions

    g. Lower penis to left or right side and hold securely with catheter in nondominant hand. Maintain this position until catheterization is completed or balloon on indwelling catheter has been inflated. Rest hand on client's pubis for support. Place end of catheter in collection basin.

13. Obtain specimen if needed.
    a. Remove lid from specimen container and place it top down on table.
    b. Place specimen container on bed beside collection basin.
    c. Pinch catheter with nondominant hand to stop flow of urine.
    d. Pick up drainage end of catheter and hold it over specimen container.
    e. Release pressure and allow 30 ml to drain into specimen container.
    f. Re-pinch catheter and place drainage end into collection basin.
    g. Allow urine flow from bladder to resume.
    h. With free hand, place specimen container on overbed table and secure lid.

14. Allow urine to continue flowing until bladder empties or until maximum of 1000 ml has been removed, depending on agency policy.

15. With straight catheter, withdraw catheter when flow stops. Then, remove catheter completely. For uncircumcised males, replace foreskin.

16. When indwelling catheter has been inserted and urine is seen in drainage tube, insert catheter 2 more inches to ensure that the balloon is correctly positioned in the bladder and not the urethra. When the indwelling catheter has been inserted:
    a. Inflate balloon with solution in syringe.

    b. Pull gently on catheter to make sure that balloon is inflated enough to retain catheter. Disconnect the syringe.
    c. Without contaminating either end, attach the catheter to the drainage collection system; close the drainage spout. Remove gloves.

    d. For females, tape catheter to inner thigh. For males, tape catheter tubing laterally to the thigh.

    e. Coil excess drainage tubing and fasten it to sheet on top surface of mattress with rubber band and safety pin.

Rationale/Discussion

    g. Holding prevents dislodgment. Positioning penis to either side prevents compression of penoscrotal angle (Fig. 44-12).

13.
    a. Avoids contamination of inside of sterile container.

    b. Places container within reach of catheter.

    c. Prevents urine from flowing on outside of container while moving catheter to the inside.

    d. Prepares for collection of specimen in the container.

    e. Amount of urine recommended for most laboratory tests.
    f. Prevents urine from flowing at any point, other than over a container, facilitating measurement of urine.

    h. Prevents contamination.

14. Some authorities caution against removing more than 1000 ml from bladder at any one time. They theorize that removing more than this releases pressure on pelvic blood vessels, leading to shock syndrome. However, this warning is not substantiated in the literature. Very large amounts are often removed from bladders of postpartum women without complication.[11,51]

15. Replace foreskin as quickly as possible to avoid constriction at base of glans, resulting in edema.

16.

    a. If person feels pain during inflation, balloon may be malpositioned in urethra. Withdraw all solution injected and advance catheter about 1.25 cm (0.5 inch). Try again to inflate balloon.
    b. Prevents catheter dislodgment.

    c. Sterile technique prevents contamination of bladder in the event of accidental backflow of urine from the tubing. Gloves no longer needed to maintain sterile technique or protect self from urine. Tape is difficult to handle with gloves on.
    d. Stabilizes catheter and prevents it from dislodging. Use nonallergenic tape. Leave enough slack to avoid pressure on meatus and to allow abduction of leg for females. In males, taping laterally prevents compression at penoscrotal angle.
    e. This allows play in the tubing so catheter is less likely to be pulled out.

FINAL ACTIVITIES

Wear clean gloves to wash and dry perineum. Remove perineal drapes and return client to desired position. Remove bath blanket or sheet used as drape and replace bed covers. Lower bed and raise side rail if necessary. Discard disposable equipment in proper containers. Label and send urine specimen promptly to laboratory. Record the procedure in client's chart.

ate if the person is obese and might constrict the tubing with the weight of the leg. On the other hand, the first method can cause some reflux because the urine must overcome gravity to travel up a tube taped over the leg. Hence, the second or third method is preferable. However, the second method carries the risk of tissue damage on the posterior thigh, caused by constant pressure of tubing on the skin. Pressure is usually less under the knee than under the fleshier part of the leg. The third method may be inappropriate if the person is very active, because it increases the chances of getting tangled in the tubing. Regardless of the method, make sure that nothing (e.g., side rails) kinks or pinches the drainage tubing.

Blood clots and mucus plugs may also partially or completely obstruct the drainage system. People who have had surgery of the urinary tract, such as prostatectomy, are at the highest risk for blood clots. Mucus accumulates in part from the catheter itself, which is a foreign object and thus stimulates mucus production. Mucus production also increases during UTIs. Bladder irrigation is one method to clear the catheter. It will be discussed later in some detail, since it is an important skill to learn.

To maintain good urine flow, the bag must *always,* without exception, be kept below the level of the bladder unless the tubing is clamped. When the bag is higher than the bladder, urine can flow back into the bladder, which increases the risk of infection. Also, the bag and tubing must never touch the floor or be held upside down while being emptied. These actions increase the chances for bacteria in the drainage bag to ascend the tubing and possibly to enter the bladder. Bacteria in the drainage bag can lead to UTI and subsequent increased mucus production. With moderate amounts of mucus, the likelihood of obstruction occurring is much greater.

Securing the Catheter. Once the catheter is in place, it is affixed to the body to prevent pressure and pulling on the bladder and urethra. For a woman, tape the catheter to the inner aspect of either thigh. Be sure to allow enough slack to prevent tautness when she abducts her leg. For a man, the growing practice is to anchor the catheter to the lower abdomen. This more naturally maintains the normal anatomic direction of the male urethra and avoids abscess formation at the penoscrotal junction. Use nonallergenic tape and change the tape only when it becomes soiled, wet, or nonadhesive. Shave the area first, if hair is abundant.

Alternative disposable anchoring devices are available for securing catheters. They may be used with indwelling urinary catheters, leg bag tubing, condom catheters, or urinary diversion nighttime drainage tubes. Directions for the application of these devices are product-specific.

Complications of Catheterization. The common complications seen with catheterization are urinary tract infection, retention, obstruction, and trauma. The client needs to be taught what signs indicate that complications are present, so early intervention and treatment can prevent extension of the complications. These symptoms should be reported to the physician.

Urinary tract infection (UTI) is the most frequent complication of catheterization. The elderly, the critically ill, and women seem to be most susceptible to it. It has been documented that the incidence of bacteriuria (presence of bacteria in the urine) increases in direct relationship to the length of time the catheter is left in place.[48,78,97]

In clients with catheters, signs and symptoms of urinary tract infection include discomfort, distention, markedly decreased urinary output, cloudy urine, and fever. Retention causes signs and symptoms similar to those of a urinary tract infection. Obstruction of a catheter will cause decreased or absent urine in the drainage tube. Blood in the drainage tube or at the meatus may indicate trauma. Often this is caused by the client pulling on the tube or the tube becoming entangled in the side rails of the bed.

Physicians and nurses often consider infection and bacteriuria to be of little consequence. It is true that most individuals with catheter-associated bacteriuria do recover spontaneously when the catheter is removed, and they respond to antibiotic therapy without complications. However, catheterization can lead to chronic mucosal changes, acute urinary tract infection, and tissue ischemia. Indwelling catheters are the leading cause of nosocomial infections, accounting for 53 per cent of all nosocomial infections. Of those with nosocomial infections, 66 to 85 per cent have undergone urologic instrumentation of some kind.[48,78,97] The bacteriuria can lead to gram-negative bacteremia, which is a grave complication that has an associated mortality rate of 30 to 50 per cent.[97] Also, chronic bacteriuria, acute pyelonephritis, chronic recurring pyelonephritis, hypertension, and acute and chronic renal failure can result from catheter-related infection.

Other hazards of catheterization and the use of indwelling catheters include trauma to the lower urinary tract, loss of bladder tone, bladder spasm, abscesses, strictures, fistulas, skin lesions, and inflammation of other organs near the urinary system.

Relieving Bladder Spasms. Bladder spasms are an uncomfortable side effect of catheterization. They may be caused by the underlying condition, pressure resulting from the balloon resting directly on the bladder neck, sphincter spasticity, or obstruction of the catheter. Bladder spasms cause an acute episodic pain and can thus be distinguished from bladder distention, which results in a constant dull ache.

To relieve spasms, manipulate the catheter to change the position of the balloon on the bladder neck. Increased fluid intake may also be helpful. Since the urethral and anal sphincters share common innervation from S 2–4, anal dilatation may cause a reflex relaxation of the urethral sphincter. Because of resulting vagal nerve stimulation and reflex inhibition of the heart rate, do not use this technique if the client has a heart condition. Otherwise, to perform anal dilatation, don and lubricate a finger cot and insert your finger about 2 inches into the anus. If none of these measures is effective, the physician may order medications, such as oxybutynin (Ditropan) and flavoxate (Urispas). Systemic antispasmodics, antihistamines, or narcotics may be used if necessary.

Preventing Urinary Tract Infection. The inside of the drainage system and catheter is a major pathway for access to the bladder. Whenever the catheter is disconnected from the drainage tubing, organisms may be introduced into the system. Contamination of the collection vessel usually occurs at the drainage spigot as a result of contact with (a) the floor, (b) containers used to empty the bag, and (c) urinometers and droppers used to test the urine of diabetic persons.[97] Once the drainage system is contaminated, the organisms ascend into the bladder either through their own motility or by retrograde flow of urine in the drainage system.

Another common source of drainage system contamination may be the catheter plug units. These units are used to protect the exposed end of the catheter when it must be separated from the drainage tubing.[7] Although these units are sterile initially, they are commonly saved and reused repeatedly.

In addition to contaminated equipment, another well-documented causative factor is the direct relationship between duration of catheter placement and increased incidence of urinary tract infections (UTIs). Andriole reports that, in one study, bacteriuria occurred in 50 per cent of catheterized persons after 24 hours and increased to 98 to 100 per cent after 4 days.[3]

Cross-contamination between people may also explain the high rates of UTIs. The Centers for Disease Control (CDC) recommend that handwashing be done immediately before and after any manipulation of the catheter site or drainage system. The CDC suggests that infected and uninfected persons with indwelling catheters should not share a room.

Suspect a UTI if (a) the person with a catheter reports perineal, bladder, or kidney pain; (b) the urine becomes cloudy and full of sediment; or (c) the client develops a fever. To test for UTI, obtain a sterile urine sample for culture and sensitivity studies (see pages 1168 and 1169 for that procedure).

The prevention of UTI in people who have indwelling urinary catheters is primarily the responsibility of the nurse. Although medications are sometimes used, all other interventions are within the realm of independent nursing actions.

Probably the most important weapon in the prevention of infection is conscientious handwashing by nursing and medical personnel. Hands must be washed before and after handling the catheter or drainage system of each catheterized individual.

Normally the bladder is inherently resistant to infection. This resistance is probably due to the antibacterial properties of the bladder mucosa and maybe of the urine. The mechanical action of voiding also removes organisms from the lower urinary tract.[51] Unfortunately, placement of a urethral catheter eliminates the washing action of voiding and seems to overpower the other natural defense mechanisms of the urinary tract.

The most common infecting organisms are *Escherichia coli, Proteus, Klebsiella, Aerobacter, Pseudomonas aeruginosa, Streptococcus, Staphylococcus,* and *Serratia.* Most of these organisms originate in the colon. Evidence exists suggesting that the bacteria find their way to the urethra and travel into the bladder on a thin layer of fluid that forms on the exterior of the catheter.[8,17,97]

The development of closed drainage systems has reduced infection rates.[97] A closed system is one in which the entire system, from the catheter to the collection bag, is closed to the atmosphere. Thus, it is protected from microbial invasion from the environment. The system is opened only at the emptying spout at the bottom of the collection bag.

To keep the closed drainage system protected, be careful not to allow the end of the outlet spigot to touch anything that will contaminate it when you are emptying the collection bag.

Preventing the backflow of urine stops bacteria from being carried up through the tubing and catheter into the bladder.[3] Hence, the tubing and collection bag must always be placed *below* the level of the bladder to allow gravity to drain urine. Raising the collection bag above the level of the person's bladder is a common cause of backflow. If the bag must be raised above the bladder, kink the tubing with your fingers during the transfer to prevent backflow. This hazard has prompted some manufacturers to put a one-way valve in the drainage tubing to prevent backflow. As yet there is no proof that this design is effective in reducing infection.

Loops in the tubing also increase the potential for backflow. To facilitate gravity flow, place the tubing so that the urine is in a continuous downhill stream into the collection bag. When the client is supine, all the tubing loops are to be on the bed.

Urine left sitting in the collection bag for long periods is an excellent medium for bacterial growth. Remember to empty the collection bag at least every 8 hours, and more frequently if urine output is high. Because of the danger of cross-contamination, all people with indwelling catheters should have personal emptying containers, labeled with their names. These containers should not be used for other people.

Perineal care is a crucial aspect of any catheter care program. Suggested agents and techniques are numerous, but all emphasize the need for conscientious cleanliness. The main goals of perineal care are to reduce the number of bacteria present and to remove crusts from the catheter itself, because crusts may result in tissue erosion as the catheter moves in and out of the urethra.

However, researchers have recently discovered that manipulation of the catheter during the cleansing process seems to be a significant factor in the development of bacteriuria. In several studies, people with indwelling urinary catheters who received frequent cleaning and/or application of antimicrobial substances to the meatal-catheter junction actually had higher rates of bacteriuria than did people not receiving these interventions.[14] Even when the application of antibiotic ointment to the urethral meatus resulted in a small decrease in the incidence of UTI, this benefit did not seem great enough to justify the expense. Also, there was the possibility that organisms that survived the antibiotic ointment could become resistant to antibiotics in the future.

Therefore, current recommendations of the Centers for Disease Control (CDC) are that the perineal area be gently cleansed at least daily with soap and water, but that the urethral meatus receive no special attention during this process.[97] Cleansing will be needed more often if there is fecal soiling or vaginal drainage. When providing perineal care for an uncircumcised male, be sure that the foreskin is fully retracted and the area underneath cleaned carefully. After thoroughly cleansing the perineum, rinse and dry the area. Sitz baths may also be used for cleansing, although some researchers are concerned that baths may facilitate urethral invasion by fecal microorganisms.

A high fluid intake also helps prevent infection. A continuous downward flow of urine from the kidneys to the collection bag is thought to impede ascending bacterial invasion. Urine flow rates of at least 25 ml per hour have been found to hinder the upward progress of all but 10 per cent of the bacteria.[17] Most sources recommend that in order to achieve this "internal irrigation" of the catheter and drainage system, the client should maintain a fluid intake high enough to produce at least 50 ml of urine output per hour. For most people, this goal requires about 2000 to 2500 ml of fluid intake every day. Increased fluids also aid in reducing the risk of urinary stone formation.

It is very tiring for the average person to have to drink this much fluid every day. Gentle persuasion may be needed to convince the person that a high fluid intake offers benefits that outweigh the fatigue and distaste that accompany the extra fluids.

In addition to high fluid intake, acidification of urine is also recommended, since a lower urine pH seems to inhibit bacterial growth. One method is to administer medications that decrease the pH. Ammonium chloride or large doses of ascorbic acid are administered for this reason. Dietary manipulation of urine pH through the acid-ash diet is less common, now that ammonium chloride or ascorbic acid seem to be more effective. Cranberry juice has long been touted as a cheap, safe means of lowering urine pH. However, intake of massive amounts of juice is needed to have any effect on pH.

In addition to acidifying agents, other systemic medications may be prescribed for the person with an indwelling catheter. Probably the most frequent of these are the antibiotics and urinary antiseptics. There is much controversy over the use of prophylactic antibiotic therapy to prevent UTIs in catheterized people. Although some sources advocate it strongly, others cite the cost, the development of resistant organisms, and possible adverse reactions as contraindications.[97] However, in the event of a documented UTI, there is almost universal agreement that antibiotic therapy should be started. This is usually a very effective mode of treatment.

Topical medications may be applied to the catheter or bladder, either by irrigation or instillation. A bladder instillation is done to medicate the bladder mucosa. Although this intervention helps prevent UTI, it may be performed on any person needing topical treatment for any bladder disorder.

For the medication to have its full effect, the bladder must be empty. If a catheter is not already in place, one is inserted and the bladder drained. The medication is injected with an irrigating syringe in the same way that one injects irrigating fluid. Then, instead of being drained, the medication is retained in the bladder in order to have time to exert its therapeutic effects. If the catheter is to remain in place, it is clamped off for a specified time and then reconnected to the drainage tubing, and the clamp is released. If the catheter is removed following treatment, the person is instructed not to void for a specified time so as to give the medication time to work.

The final intervention involves changing the catheter. In the past, it was common practice to remove and replace catheters on a routine schedule. However, it is now recommended that the frequency of catheter change be individualized for each person.[97] Change the catheter only when (a) it is obstructed and cannot be cleared; or (b) there is evidence of sediment in the catheter, (i.e., you feel sandlike particles when rolling the distal end of the catheter between your fingers). Change the collection bag and tubing only (a) when you replace the catheter or (b) if the drainage system is failing to function properly or is contaminated.

Preventing Tissue Trauma, Ulcer Formation, and Thrombophlebitis. Tissue trauma is probably the second most common hazard of urethral catheterization. Vigorous attempts to get past an actual obstruction during insertion may cause perforation of the urethra. Tissue necrosis is a possibility whenever (a) there is continuous pressure, such as occurs on the meatus; and (b) there is not enough slack left in the tubing between the meatus and the site of taping on the leg or abdomen. Too large a catheter may lead to tissue damage. Also, the tip of a catheter that has been in place for a long time can erode through the dome of the bladder.

Even though a retention catheter stays in the bladder, it still has the capability of movement in and out of the urethra at the distal end. This constant friction can cause tissue breakdown, and the process is aggravated if encrustation is allowed to form on the outside of the catheter.

In particular, males with indwelling catheters experience urethral irritation. Symptoms of this condition include severe burning and pain at the tip of the penis. There may also be a small amount of purulent exudate. Skin irritation can be caused by the rubber straps that hold a leg bag to the thigh. Even though the straps are applied loosely, as the bag fills up the straps tend to tighten. Other problems seen with the use of the leg bag are thrombophlebitis and ulcer formation. Thrombophlebitis results from stasis of blood and lymph circulation. Ulcer formation is caused by the straps being too tight and impeding circulation.

Individuals should be taught to remove the bag periodically to allow for normal circulation and to observe and take meticulous care of the skin under the straps. They should also be encouraged to observe for and report any redness or skin breakdown. See Table 44–2 for overall care of clients with catheters.

Removing Indwelling Catheters. Studies indicate that the less time a catheter is in place, the lower the incidence of infection.[3] Therefore, carefully assess the person daily for evidence that an indwelling catheter is no longer necessary. If strict intake and output documentation is not needed and if the individual is alert, oriented, and fairly mobile, recommend to the physician that the catheter can probably be removed.

However, there is no way to know for certain that a person is ready for catheter removal. Sometimes a catheter is removed prematurely and must be reinserted because the person is still unable to void normally.

Planned removal of an indwelling urethral catheter is usually a pain-free process as long as the person has been informed of the procedure. After you explain the procedure, position the person and drape to allow good visualization of the perineal area. Make sure you have already assembled the equipment: (a) an appropriately sized syringe, with or without a needle, depending on the kind of catheter being removed; (b) several paper towels or a small basin; (c) materials to wash and dry the perineum; and (d) clean gloves. Expose and remove the tape, freeing the catheter. Don

TABLE 44–2. Selected Scientific Principles and Related Nursing Interventions for Persons with Indwelling Urethral Catheters

Principles	Nursing Interventions
The introduction of microorganisms into a sterile body cavity promotes infection.	Follow strict sterile technique during catheterization. Only persons who know correct technique should handle catheters.
In addition to infection, catheterization places the client at risk for a number of severe complications.	Never catheterize unless it is documented as essential for therapeutic reasons, not for controlling incontinence for the convenience of staff. Do not change indwelling catheters at arbitrary, fixed intervals.
Inadequate fluid intake increases the likelihood of infection.	Encourage fluid to at least 2400 to 4000 ml per 24 hours unless the person is on fluid restriction.
Poor perineal hygiene increases the likelihood of infection, but daily meatal care with povidine iodine solution and daily cleansing with soap and water have not been shown to reduce catheter-associated urinary infection.	Maintain normal perineal hygiene with soap and water when a client has a catheter in place.
Traumatized tissues are more susceptible to infection than are healthy tissues.	Properly secure indwelling catheters to prevent movement and urethral traction. Manipulate the catheter as little as possible during daily perineal hygiene.
Retrograde urine flow increases the likelihood of infection.	Maintain unobstructed urine flow by ▶ keeping the catheter and collecting tube free of kinks. ▶ avoiding pinching the drainage tubing in the side rail or wheelchair wheels. ▶ establishing adequate internal and external irrigation to prevent catheter clogging. ▶ emptying the collection bag regularly. ▶ keeping the collection bag below the level of the bladder.
Collection bags can be a source of contamination of drainage systems.	When emptying collection bags, use a separate container for each person. Never allow the drainage spigot on the collection bag to come into contact with the nonsterile collection container.

TABLE 44–2. Selected Scientific Principles and Related Nursing Interventions for Persons with Indwelling Urethral Catheters Continued

Principles	Nursing Interventions
Interruption of a closed drainage system increases the likelihood of contaminating the system.	Maintain a sterile, continuously closed system. Do not disconnect the catheter and drainage tubing unless necessary to irrigate the catheter. If the system becomes disconnected or leaks, or if breaks in aseptic technique occur, use aseptic technique to disinfect the catheter-tubing junction or to replace the collection system.
Large catheters can cause pressure on urethral tissues and cause trauma that may lead to necrosis.	Use as small a catheter as possible, consistent with good drainage.
In all contact with body fluids, universal precautions help protect the client and the nurse from infection.	Wear clean gloves when handling a catheter or collection system. Wash hands immediately before and after any manipulation of the catheter. Assign infected persons with indwelling catheters and uninfected persons with indwelling catheters to separate rooms.
Most organisms found in urinary tract infections prefer an alkaline environment.	Acidify urine with ordered systemic and topical medications or with acid ash nutrients, as required.
Many persons are embarrassed by bodily functions.	Be sensitive to feelings and encourage verbal expression of these if client wishes. Avoid appearing embarrassed or upset. Provide as much privacy as possible.
Many persons fear their catheter will come out if they move, turn, or walk.	Teach the client and significant others what to expect, degree of mobility allowed, and the client's role in the care program.
Painful bladder spasm can result from sphincter spasticity, obstruction of the catheter, or pressure from an indwelling catheter balloon resting directly on the bladder neck.	Relieve bladder spasms by: relaxing the sphincter by anal dilatation, relieving obstruction by catheter irrigation, or manipulating the catheter to change its position.
Removal of an indwelling catheter without deflating the balloon can traumatize urethral tissues.	Protect the tube from accidental removal. Apply restraints, if necessary, to prevent confused clients from pulling on tubes.

clean gloves when removing catheters to maintain universal precautions. Insert the syringe or needle into the balloon sleeve valve and withdraw all the fluid from the balloon. With one hand, hold the paper towels or small basin near the bottom of the perineum. Have the person take a deep breath to enhance relaxation. Slowly remove the catheter, placing it in the towels or basin as it comes out. Inspect the balloon area of the catheter to be sure that it is intact and that no part of the catheter has been left in the bladder. Also, inspect the meatus for signs of infection or edema. After cleansing and drying the perineum, make the person comfortable and discard the equipment. Document the time you removed the catheter, the condition of the meatus, and the amount of urine in the collection bag.

Never try to remove an indwelling catheter by cutting off the end of the balloon sleeve with scissors. Occasionally an uninformed nurse uses this procedure to allow the water to flow out of the balloon, thereby emptying it. This method is dangerous because partial or total obstruction of the balloon lumen can occur, which then prevents the release of the solution. As a result, the balloon will not deflate. In addition, if the end of the sleeve has been cut away, it is very difficult to apply any suction or pressure on the lumen. If this problem occurs, notify the physician, who can then attempt to deflate the balloon by either (a) injecting a chemical solution such as ether or toluene into the balloon to destroy the rubber wall, (b) inserting a central venous catheter into the balloon lumen to bypass the obstruction and allow the solution in the balloon to flow out, or (c) using a stylet to puncture the balloon wall. If all else fails, the catheter will need to be removed with cystoscopy equipment, an unnecessary and painful procedure.

Following catheter removal, instruct the person to maintain a good fluid intake unless fluids are contraindicated. Inform the person that urine output will have to be measured.

The bladder should be empty when the catheter is

removed, but some people nonetheless may feel the urge to void immediately. Assure them that this feeling does not mean anything is wrong. Permit them to use a bedpan, urinal, or commode to allay anxiety. Continue to assess bladder function for approximately 24 hours to ensure that urinary retention is not developing.

If the person cannot void within a certain time period, generally 8 to 10 hours, notify the physician, who may request that you reinsert the catheter to alleviate the retention.

Sometimes unplanned catheter removal occurs. An agitated or confused person may forcibly pull out the catheter without deflation of the balloon. This is especially damaging to a man because of the length of the urethra. Usually no permanent sequelae follow this kind of catheter removal, but it is very painful, and some bleeding can be expected. In these instances, it is important to assess the amount of bleeding and the status of bladder function. Sometimes the catheter is replaced, depending on the person's needs.

Sometimes, even repetitive teaching is inadequate. If the person is continually pulling at the catheter, it may be necessary to apply restraints.

Another issue to consider in the removal of an indwelling catheter is whether or not to recondition the bladder before catheter removal, i.e., to restore its muscle tone. This is debatable. On the one hand, the bladder is a muscle and, like any muscle, it loses its tone if not used. When an indwelling catheter is in place, the bladder becomes increasingly flaccid. Like any muscle, it takes a period of reuse to regain its tone. If a catheter is removed with no bladder preparation, the person is at risk of urine retention secondary to bladder atony. The catheter may need to be reinserted to relieve distention.

One way to avoid this problem is to institute a period of bladder training. With this program, the catheter is clamped for increasing lengths of time and then released to allow drainage of the urine. A high oral fluid intake is encouraged. By following this regimen, the bladder is alternately stretched and then allowed to drain, mimicking normal function. Thus, the bladder may regain normal function and the catheter may be removed without incident.

Care for Clients Discharged with Urinary Catheters. With increasing frequency, people are discharged home with indwelling catheters. Release from the health care facility may in itself be a welcome event, but for many people the psychologic implications of an indwelling catheter—embarrassment, body image change, and dependency—are intensified in the home environment. The person's significant others may also have the same feelings of embarrassment about the drainage system and concern about how the person's increased dependency will affect their lives. Everyone involved will probably be worried about how to take proper care of the catheter and drainage system.

The nurse plays the major role in helping the person and significant others adapt psychologically to the catheter and its care. Initially, encourage all the people involved to discuss with you and with each other their concerns about the catheter and its drainage system. Try to anticipate questions and anxieties. Be prepared to discuss "sensitive" topics (e.g., prevention of odor) even if people try to avoid them, possibly through embarrassment. Be accepting and nonjudgmental in the way you pose and answer queries.

The other major responsibility in preparing the person and significant others for discharge is to help them learn how to physically care for the catheter and its drainage system. It is vital for the individual, and sometimes for at least one other person, to know how to work knowledgeably with this apparatus. Home care instructions are needed regarding where to keep the equipment, how to clean it with materials available in the home, and how to fit catheter and drainage system care into the lifestyle and daily activities of the person and significant others. An invaluable resource in this process is the community health nurse.

Remember to make referrals to the home health agency early. Ideally, the community health nurse should visit the person in the health care facility before discharge and talk to all the people at home who will be involved with the care process. This practice facilitates greater continuity of care.

Also, develop a teaching/learning plan and begin instruction of the individual and significant others before discharge. See Chapter 26 for a discussion of teaching interventions. Fashion a plan that takes into account the individual's abilities and needs. Include the following information:

▶ Physical hazards: prevention and treatment
▶ Psychologic hazards: prevention and interventions
▶ Basic catheter and drainage system care
▶ Methods of catheter insertion and removal, if necessary
▶ Methods of stabilizing the catheter, ensuring patency, and avoiding reflux
▶ Resources in the community

Some people who need long-term catheter drainage use a leg bag as a collection device. A leg bag is a small rubber or plastic bag attached to the inner thigh, usually by two adjustable rubber straps (see Figure 44–5). The catheter attaches directly to the top of this bag. A valve in the bottom of the bag allows the collected urine to be emptied into a toilet or other appropriate receptacle. This collection system grants the person much more freedom and mobility than the conventional drainage system, but it is not without its problems and risks. Because of its small capacity (200 to 300 ml), the bag must be emptied frequently. Thus, in order to sleep through the night, the person usually switches to a conventional drainage system upon retiring so as not to have to empty the leg bag. Also, because the bag is opened often and usually changed at night to another drainage system, there is increased risk of infection.

Cleanliness and odor control are also management problems in the use of leg bags. To control odor and the growth of organisms, it is usually recommended that (a) the person have two leg bags and (b) after use, each bag be carefully washed with soap and water, rinsed, and then filled with a 1 per cent acetic acid (vinegar) solution and allowed to soak until used again. This procedure is usually done on a daily basis or each night when the person switches to a conventional drainage system.

Sexuality. Another issue for people at home with long-term indwelling urethral catheters involves the resumption of sexual activity. The decision to resume sexual relations depends on the person's physical condition and the degree of sexual desire of those involved. The couple should first consult with the physician before proceeding. However, it is generally safe to have sexual intercourse with a urethral catheter in place. First, the collection bag and tubing must be drained. If the system is kept intact, it should have an antireflux valve. After the man achieves an erection, the catheter is doubled back over the penis and anchored on the abdomen, then a condom is slipped over both the penis and the catheter. For the woman, it is necessary only to tape the catheter away from the vagina. After intercourse, the drainage system should be monitored to make sure it is draining properly. The person needs to cleanse the genitals carefully and should drink extra fluids to ensure a "wash-out" of the bladder and catheter.[39]

Obtaining Catheter Supplies. At discharge, the individual should be provided with ample supplies for at least a few days. A list of names, addresses, and phone numbers of where additional supplies may be obtained should be given to the person before discharge. A written list of specific supplies needed should be provided to aid the individual. Usually, drug or surgical supply stores carry the required supplies. Many hospitals refer individuals to community health nurses, and supplies can be ordered and delivered to the home prior to the person's discharge.

Community Resources for the Clients with Catheters. The person who either requires indwelling or intermittent catheter drainage at home on a temporary or permanent basis must be able to maintain the urinary drainage system safely. Instructions and return demonstrations are necessary to teach clients to care safely for drainage systems or to catheterize themselves. The services of a community health nurse are often indicated. Referrals are made while the person is hospitalized and prior to discharge. Other important resources the individual needs to be aware of in the community are the physician and clinic or emergency room. The individual needs to be taught when to notify the physician. Also, if the catheter becomes displaced or obstructed, the individual needs to know which resource would be the most beneficial. If the tube becomes displaced, the clinic would be the likely choice. On the other hand, if the tube is obstructed, the emergency room may be the place to obtain treatment.

Intermittent Self-Catheterization. An alternative to long-term use of retention catheters is intermittent catheterization, which consists of inserting a straight urethral catheter into the bladder at specified intervals. The urine is drained and the catheter is removed immediately. With this method, the incidence of UTI is reduced, and people who need long-term catheterization (e.g., those who have atonic bladders with a large capacity) can return home and enjoy increased independence and less interference with their lifestyle. The most frequent participants in intermittent catheterization programs are those who have musculoskeletal or neurologic deficits that make normal micturition impossible (e.g., spinal cord injury or meningomyelocele).

Catheterization may be done by the individual (self-catheterization) or by anyone else in the environment who has been trained appropriately. Encourage people who require long-term catheterization to learn self-catheterization as soon as possible, since it allows for a more normal life. Table 44–3 lists principles guiding nursing interventions for people who will be performing self-catheterization.

Intermittent catheterization is either a sterile or a clean technique. For the person in a health care facility, sterile technique is advisable because of the high incidence of nosocomial infections. However, for the person at home, clean technique is adequate. Using clean technique in lieu of sterile technique is easier and less expensive for the individual, and it has not resulted in any increase in the rate of UTI.[94,99]

The purpose of clean, intermittent self-catheterization is to manage acute or chronic bladder dysfunction. Examples are acute or chronic neurogenic bladder, bladder dysfunction caused by adverse drug effects, and temporary postoperative bladder dysfunction. Insertion of the catheter requires the following equipment:

▶ Soap and water or towelette
▶ Straight catheter (rubber or plastic) No. 14 or No. 16 for an adult
▶ Water-soluble lubricant (for males only)
▶ Plastic bag for used catheter
▶ Container to collect urine if toilet is unavailable
▶ Mirror (for females)
▶ Pan for boiling water (for periodic sterilization of catheters)

Complications of Self-Catheterization. Because of repeated catheter insertion, there is a risk of infection. Also, incontinence may occur because of poor technique or bladder pathology. Urinary tract trauma, hematuria, the development of false passages, and strictures may result from poor technique. Bladder calculi occur frequently as a result of pubic hairs being inadvertently pushed into the bladder by the catheter, where they become the nidus for stones. This problem occurs more frequently in men. Psychosocial factors that interfere with an effective program include sexual concerns and lack of motivation.[13] Problems also occur when a person is not at home (e.g., at a movie) or does not have access to facilities in which the catheterization can be performed (e.g., on a plane). Under these circumstances, the person may be incontinent.

TABLE 44–3. *Selected Scientific Principles and Related Nursing Interventions for Care of Persons Who Will Self-Catheterize*

Principle	Nursing Interventions

A break in aseptic technique provides an entrance for microorganisms not normally found in the sterile GU system.	1. Prevent infections when inserting and maintaining a Foley catheter in the hospital environment.
	  a. Utilize strict handwashing prior to and after handling the catheter drainage tube.
	  b. Follow Centers for Disease Control (CDC) guidelines when caring for a person with an indwelling catheter.
	  c. Use strict aseptic technique when inserting an indwelling catheter, obtaining a specimen, irrigating a catheter, maintaining or removing a catheter.
	  d. Utilize barriers to help reduce possibility of infection by breaking chain of infection. Measures to employ include handwashing, wearing sterile gloves, environmental cleanliness, proper handling of Foley catheter, and maintaining closed sterile drainage system.

Urinary tract infection usually causes specific signs and symptoms that may be identified by the nurse.	Monitor for signs and symptoms of infection (i.e., cloudy urine, pain or burning upon urination), and elevated temperature.

Education and practice of a skill by an individual promote active participation and self-direction in care (self-catheterization).	1. Explain the reason for and intended effect of catheterization.
	2. Instruct person to increase fluid intake to about 2000 ml daily (unless on fluid restrictions).
	3. Teach basic principles of implementation of catheterization prior to skill instruction.
	4. Teach and demonstrate correct procedure for intermittent self-catheterization utilizing clean technique.
	5. Have individual practice and give return demonstrations to enhance skill development.
	6. Teach individual:
	  a. care of drainage tube system.
	  b. how to properly secure and anchor catheter.
	  c. how to maintain patency of system and empty bag.
	  d. how to use leg bag.
	  e. how to perform perineal meatus care daily.
	  f. where to obtain necessary supplies.
	  g. when to notify physician (obstruction, decreased output, change in clarity or color of urine, elevated temperature, suprapubic pain).

Teaching Self-Catheterization. When teaching an individual to perform intermittent self-catheterization, include the following:

▶ Clean technique will be taught to the individual, who will use this method at home.
▶ Strict sterile technique should be followed during catheterization when the individual is hospitalized.
▶ The catheterization schedule should be followed at all times.
▶ Medications must be taken as prescribed.
▶ Fluids should be taken at evenly spaced times between the time the person awakens and 2 hours before bedtime.
▶ Caffeine should be avoided.

▶ Calcium and phosphorus-rich foods should be limited in the diet.

▶ Extra supplies for catheterization should be available at home and work.

▶ If incontinence occurs, types, amount, and timing of fluid intake must be evaluated. (With uncontrolled urination: wash the wet skin with soap and water, dry completely, expose the skin to air, use powder sparingly, change clothing, and consider using an external device).

▶ Information must be recorded accurately on a Self-Catheterization Log.

Implementation. The clean technique involves some variations from the catheterization procedure in Procedure 44–1. The person does not wear gloves. Therefore, good handwashing is essential before beginning the procedure. Because of the natural lubrication of the female urethra, females use no lubricant on the catheter. Males use a water-soluble lubricant because of the length of the urethra, being more susceptible to traumatic urethritis.

The person may sit or stand during self-catheterization. When the female stands, she usually has one foot on the floor and places the other on a chair or the toilet seat to allow better identification of the meatus. A female may at first require a mirror to learn to locate the meatus. However, advise her not to become dependent on a mirror since she may frequently find herself in situations without one.

Teach the person, as appropriate, to perform self-catheterization in the various positions that may be necessary. A person who wears an orthopedic brace should practice both with and without the brace. The person must become sufficiently competent to handle any situation that may arise.

Self-Catheterization Procedures. Timing is the key factor in the success of intermittent catheterization programs. Catheterizations *must* be performed at specified intervals throughout the 24-hour period. The interval between catheterizations is established for each person according to the degree of continence. For adults, the initial time interval is usually every 4 hours. For a child, it is every 2.5 to 4 hours. The interval is gradually lengthened as the person progresses. People who are incapable of adhering to a schedule are not appropriate candidates for intermittent catheterization.

Fluid intake must be monitored on intermittent catheterization programs. Some people may have fluids as desired. Others must restrict fluids to varying degrees. Clinicians generally recommend that the person drink small amounts of fluid at specified times, (e.g., 250 ml or less within 2 hours for an adult). Ingestion of large amounts of fluid within a short period can cause bladder distention.

In general, intermittent catheterization seems to be a success. Although not 100 per cent effective, it can be a viable alternative to indwelling catheters. Success is measured by two main parameters: a catheter-free bladder and absence of bacteriuria. Studies report no significant bacteriuria in up to 80 per cent of the peo-

ple studied and achievement of a catheter-free bladder in 73 to 90 per cent of program participants. These results may be due to several factors, including (a) intermittent bladder distention, which stimulates the normal micturition reflex; and (b) reactivation of the bladder's normal antibacterial properties. No evidence of deterioration of renal function has been found in long-term participants who have adhered to the program.[94,99]

Other advantages of intermittent catheterization programs include increased independence, reduced incidence of complications arising from a retention catheter, better hygiene, ease of sexual relations, decreased cost, and less time devoted to bladder care.

You will teach the individual how to perform self-catheterization correctly. The steps are as follows:

1. The individual tries to urinate prior to catheterization.

2. If unable to empty the bladder, the person washes hands well with soap and water or with towelette.

3. The client organizes the equipment within easy reach.

4. The client gets into a comfortable position.

For female clients, the next steps are the following:

1. Separate the labial folds with the thumb and middle finger of the nondominant hand.

2. Wash the perineal area with warm water and soap or a moist disposable towelette. Use backward or downward strokes from the front toward the anus.

3. While keeping the labial folds separated, hold the catheter about ½ inch from the tip, in the dominant hand. Slowly insert the catheter into the urinary meatus. After urine starts to flow insert the catheter another inch or so. Allow the urine to flow into the container or toilet until flow stops. When flow stops, a change in position or straining of abdominal muscles may produce further urine flow.

4. Remove catheter slowly, pausing whenever urine flows. Hold up catheter tip as it is withdrawn to avoid dribbling urine.

For male clients, these are the steps:

1. If circumcised, wash the penis with warm water and soap or moist disposable towelette. If not circumcised, pull back the foreskin and then wash the penis as described.

2. Squeeze some of the water-soluble lubricant onto a paper towel.

3. Lubricate the catheter tip and 2 inches up from the tip by gently rolling the catheter in the paper towel.

4. Position the draining end of the catheter so that the urine flows into the toilet or collection container.

5. Hold the penis erect or at a right angle to the body.

6. Slowly insert the catheter. When urine begins to flow, insert the catheter about 2 inches more. Allow the urine to flow into the container or toilet until the flow stops. When the flow stops, a change in position, abdominal straining, or Credé's maneuver (pressure applied by the hands pressing downward on the blad-

der from just above the symphysis pubis) may produce further urine flow.

7. Remove catheter slowly, pausing whenever urine flows. Hold up catheter tip as it is withdrawn to avoid dribbling urine.

Replace the foreskin after removing the catheter.
After finishing the procedure,

1. Wash the catheter with warm water and soap, rinse with clean water, dry completely, and place catheter in a plastic bag or glass jar. When all catheters have been used, boil them for 20 minutes in water. Store in clean towels, fresh plastic bags, or clean glass jars. Replace catheters if they become hard or cracked.

2. Wash hands again with soap and water.

3. Complete the Self-Catheterization Log (record time, amount of urine obtained, and other pertinent data such as color, odor, or any problems). Keep an accurate log and adhere to the schedule at all times.

Documentation

For Catheterization. Documentation for urinary catheterization should include time, reason for catheterization, type and size of catheter used, amount and characteristics of urine removed, person's response to catheterization, any problems encountered, and whether or not a specimen was obtained.

For Indwelling Catheters at Home. Documentation for individuals preparing for discharge and going home with an indwelling catheter should include whether the person or family member knows how to maintain catheter patency, prevent urinary tract infections, maintain activity level, deal with catheter problems, obtain supplies, and continue with urologic follow-up.

For Self-Catheterization. Documentation for teaching an individual to perform intermittent self-catheterization at home should include information relative to the client's ability to perform self-catheterization, use techniques to prevent UTIs, maintain an adequate activity level, use and care for a leg bag, obtain supplies, return for necessary urologic follow-up, and use resources in the community.

BLADDER IRRIGATION

Bladder irrigation is washing out the bladder for treatment of inflammation or obstruction. Catheter irrigation is flushing out only the tube. Both can be achieved through internal irrigation with a high fluid intake or by external irrigation.

Indications for doing a prn bladder or catheter irrigation include a reduction or cessation of urine flow through the catheter of a hydrated person and increasing signs of urinary retention. Check to make sure there are no kinks in the tubing. If irrigation is necessary, look for the physician's order or obtain an order. Unless the physician orders a special irrigating solution,

review the agency's procedure manual to ascertain the kind and amount of solution to be used for routine irrigations in that facility.

Types of Bladder Irrigation. External bladder or catheter irrigation may be done using either a *closed* or *open* method. An open irrigation method is one in which the catheter drainage system must be opened to the environment with each irrigation. Conversely, a closed method does not require that the system be opened. The closed method is preferred, since it is easier to maintain asepsis and prevent infection if the system remains intact.[23] Figure 44–13 illustrates a closed irrigation system.

Techniques for Bladder Irrigation. Bladder or catheter irrigation is a sterile procedure. Therefore you will follow guidelines in Chapter 28, Infection Control. Also, you must adhere to CDC and institutional guidelines. Sterile gloves will be worn when actually performing the irrigation to prevent contamination of the system. Another important factor to remember is that the collection bag must be kept below the bladder to prevent reflux of urine, which can lead to infection.

Equipment. For closed bladder irrigation, the equipment needed is a triple-lumen catheter attached to a closed drainage system and irrigating solution (sterile saline or antimicrobial solution as ordered) in an appropriate irrigation bag or bottle.

For open bladder irrigation, equipment includes sterile solution at room temperature, container for the solution, irrigating syringe, drainage basin, two antiseptic sponges, and a covering for the drainage tubing. All this equipment, except the solution, is included in commercially prepared irrigation sets. Equipment that must be kept sterile throughout the intervention includes the solution, the tip and inside of the irrigating syringe, and the open ends of the catheter and drainage tubing.

Closed Irrigation Method. With a closed irrigation system, a three-way irrigating catheter is inserted into the bladder with one lumen attached to a bottle of irrigating solution hung above the level of the bladder, the second lumen attached to drainage, and the third lumen to the balloon. The irrigating solution may be used for either continuous or intermittent irrigation.

Closed Continuous Bladder Irrigation. When continuous irrigation is ordered, the irrigating solution flows from its bottle or bag at a specified rate of drops per minute, similar to an intravenous infusion. The fluid flows into the bladder through the irrigation lumen of the catheter and out through the drainage lumen (see Fig. 44–13).

The following steps apply to closed continuous bladder irrigation.

1. If a catheter is not already in place, insert a triple-lumen catheter using appropriate aseptic technique (see intervention for female and male urethral catheter-

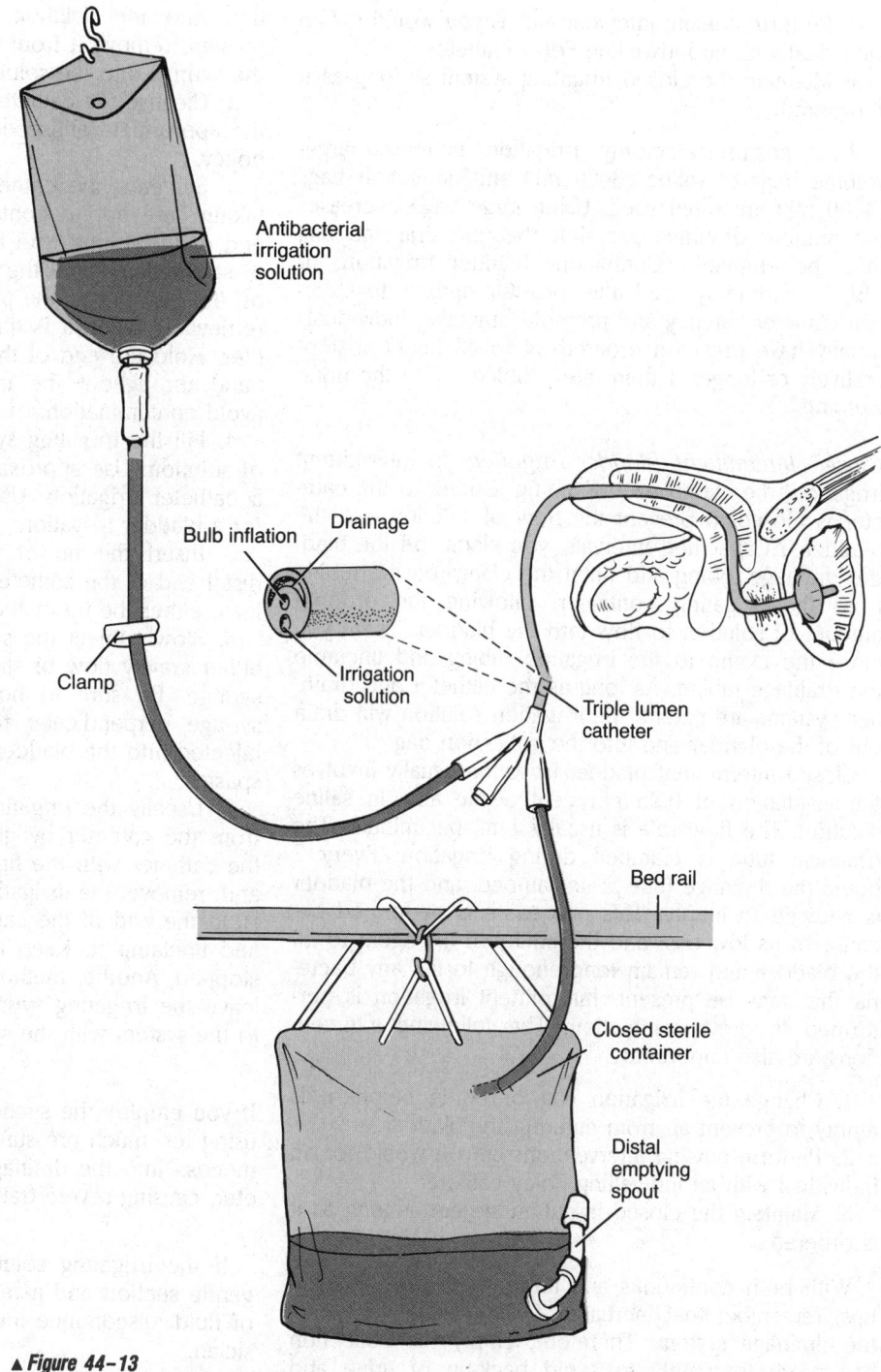

Antibacterial
irrigation
solution

Bulb inflation   Drainage

Clamp

Irrigation
solution

Triple lumen
catheter

Bed rail

Closed sterile
container

Distal
emptying
spout

▲ Figure 44–13

Closed sterile drainage system.

ization). The tubing leading from the irrigating bag or bottle should be cleared of air and attached to the irrigating lumen of the catheter prior to catheter insertion. Hang the bag or bottle on an IV pole above the level of the bladder. (Usually the catheter will already be in place following prostate surgery. The catheter may need to be taped to the thigh or abdomen as indicated. Check to see that all connections are tight.)

2. Allow the irrigation solution to flow at a specified drops-per-minute rate, as with intravenous infusion. The order often reads, "Maintain the irrigation at a rate fast enough to promote light pink to clear returns." The drops-per-minute rate will vary with different irrigation sets.

3. Change the irrigation bag or bottle before it is empty to prevent air from entering the bladder.

4. Perform nursing interventions as you would for an individual with an indwelling Foley catheter.

5. Maintain the closed irrigating system as long as it is ordered.

With postprostatectomy irrigation systems, large-volume bags of saline (3000 ml) and collection bags (4000 ml) are often used. Using large bags decreases the number of times per shift that the drainage bag must be emptied. (Continuous bladder irrigation, or CBI, is commonly used after prostate surgery to maintain catheter patency and promote drainage. Individuals usually have irrigation ordered 24 to 48 hours postoperatively or longer if there are problems with the urine clearing.)

Closed Intermittent Bladder Irrigation. In intermittent irrigation, the clamp on the tubing leading to the catheter is closed to prevent the flow of solution into the bladder. At specified intervals, you clamp off the bladder drainage tubing and open the clamp on the tubing from the irrigating container, allowing the ordered amount of solution to flow into the bladder. Then, you close the clamp to the irrigation tubing and unclamp the drainage tubing. As long as the catheter and drainage systems are patent, the irrigation solution will drain out of the bladder and into the collection bag.

Closed intermittent bladder irrigation usually involves the instillation of 0.25 per cent acetic acid in saline solution. The flow rate is usually 1 ml per minute. The drainage tube is clamped during irrigation. Every 2 hours the drainage tube is unclamped, and the bladder is allowed to empty. This procedure is performed because of its low cost and the ability of the agent to fill the bladder and remain long enough to kill any bacteria that may be present. Intermittent irrigation is performed to prevent infection. The following interventions are also important:

1. Change the irrigation bag or bottle before it is empty to prevent air from entering the bladder.

2. Perform nursing interventions as you would for an individual with an indwelling Foley catheter.

3. Maintain the closed irrigation system as long as it is ordered.

With both continuous and intermittent irrigation setups, remember that increased fluid is flowing through the drainage system. Therefore, empty the collection bag more frequently to avoid back-up of urine and fluid. You will also need to calculate the amount of irrigant added to the system and subtract it from the total urinary output to determine the exact amount of urine being produced.

Open Irrigation Method. Sometimes it becomes necessary to do an open irrigation. Use this method only if there is an obstruction. Do not use it prophylactically to prevent accumulation of debris, since open irrigation carries an increased risk of infection.

The following steps apply to open irrigation:

1. Arrange the equipment so that it can be conveniently used while maintaining sterility. Pour the solution into the solution container. If a tip guard is present, remove it from the irrigating syringe and place the syringe into the solution container.

2. Cleanse the catheter/drainage tubing junction with the appropriate antiseptic as indicated by the agency's policy.

3. Separate the catheter from the drainage tubing, taking care not to contaminate either end. Cover the end of the tubing with a sterile, dry gauze or a sterile plastic cover. Place the tubing so that it does not fall off the bed during the procedure and yet will be easily retrievable when it is time to reconnect it to the catheter. Hold the end of the catheter in the nondominant hand throughout the intervention, and take care to avoid contamination.

4. Fill the irrigating syringe with the desired amount of solution. Use approximately 30 to 50 ml of fluid for a catheter irrigation. Use approximately 90 to 400 ml for a bladder irrigation.

5. Insert the tip of the irrigating syringe into the distal end of the catheter, being careful not to contaminate either the tip or the catheter.

6. Slowly inject the solution into the catheter, using either gravity flow or slight pressure from the irrigating syringe. Be sure to hold the catheter and irrigating syringe perpendicular to the floor so that no air is injected into the bladder. Air in the bladder may cause spasms.

7. Usually the irrigating solution is allowed to drain from the catheter by gravity flow. In this case, pinch the catheter with the fingers of the nondominant hand and remove the irrigating syringe from the catheter. Hold the end of the catheter over the collection basin and unclamp it. Keep this position until the flow has stopped. Another method of removing the solution is to leave the irrigating syringe in place and apply suction to the system with the syringe.

If you employ the suction method, be careful to avoid using too much pressure, since it may suck the bladder mucosa into the drainage holes at the tip of the catheter, causing severe trauma to the bladder mucosa.

If the irrigating solution will not return, even with gentle suction and a repeated injection of 30 to 50 ml of fluid, discontinue the procedure and notify the physician.

8. Repeat steps 4 to 7, as necessary, until the debris is cleared from the lumen of the catheter.

9. When the last of the solution has drained from the catheter, put the irrigating syringe into the catheter and lay them both on the bed. This will help maintain their sterility while you retrieve the drainage tubing and remove its protective covering.

10. Cleanse the end of the catheter and the drainage tubing with antiseptic. Reconnect them, taking care to maintain sterility of the two ends. Retape the drainage tubing if necessary.

11. Discard all equipment and unused solution. Do not reuse them.

12. Make the person comfortable.

13. Continue to monitor the person's intake and output to determine whether there is an adequate output.

Complications of Bladder Irrigation. Urethral catheterization is often associated with polymicrobial bacteriuria, catheter obstruction, fever, bacteremia, urinary tract stones, and death. Periodic catheter irrigation is a common but untested management procedure intended to prevent catheter obstruction, fevers, and/or bacteremia. Often bacteria enter the bladder through the catheter lumen, caused by disconnection of the closed system at the junction between the collecting tube and the catheter or by contamination of urine in the collecting bag. The reflux of urine from a contaminated bag may occur if the bag is raised above the level of the bladder even though one-way valves or antireflux devices are used. Also, improper positioning of the bag may increase the risk of contamination. With bladder irrigations, the opening of the system may lead to contamination, even when good technique is used. Often in bladder irrigations the collecting bag is repositioned, causing reflux of urine. This can lead to infection.[15,58]

Another complication with bladder irrigations is exfoliation. This is a disruption of the inner epithial surface of the bladder, the urothelium. It has been shown that with bladder irrigations there is urothelial damage and increased shedding of abnormal cells. Irrigation might further disrupt the mucosa and thus predispose to repeated infections.

Teaching About Bladder Irrigation. It is important to teach the individual and family members the purpose for the irrigation and basic steps of the procedure. Reassure the person undergoing a continuous bladder irrigation that no discomfort should be experienced with the irrigation solution or actual instillation of fluid. For the client undergoing an intermittent bladder irrigation, you must explain that the procedure itself may be uncomfortable, but that once adequate urinary output is re-established, the general comfort level will be increased.

Documentation for Bladder Irrigation. For a continuous bladder irrigation, record carefully on the intake and output flow sheet the type and amount of irrigating fluid instilled and the total amount of output. Subtract the irrigant from the total output to determine the exact amount of urine being produced. Record the color and clarity of urine and any other pertinent observations about the catheter or drainage.

For an intermittent bladder irrigation, document the reason for the procedure, the time, amount and kind of solution used, amount and characteristics of drainage returned, results of the irrigation, and any problems encountered during the intervention. If the person is on intake and output measurement, be sure to note on the intake and output record any fluid retained or urine removed during the bladder irrigation.

EVALUATION

Altered Urinary Elimination

In evaluating outcomes of nursing care for urinary tract infection, determine whether the person is able to void without pain or burning. Can the person verbalize understanding of the disease process, the treatment, and prevention? Does the person know the follow-up instructions?

In evaluating outcomes of nursing care for urinary diversion, determine the person's understanding of the need for the urinary diversion and acceptance of the stoma. Is the person able to apply an external pouch correctly, provide skin care, and maintain the drainage system? If the person has a Kock pouch, is that person able to catheterize the stoma at appropriate intervals, using correct technique?

In evaluating outcomes of nursing care for urinary tract stones, determine the person's knowledge regarding prevention of infection and promoting comfort. Can the person verbalize understanding of the disease process, its treatment and prevention? Can the person recognize signs of obstruction and relate the importance of increasing fluid intake to promote passage of the stone and, thus, comfort?

Urinary Incontinence

In evaluating the goals for urinary *Incontinence*, assess the achievement of the outcomes identified for the client. Was urinary continence achieved? If not, was a reduction in incontinent episodes achieved? For the person with *Total Incontinence*, were ways found to contain or collect the urine to promote dryness?

Urinary Retention

In evaluating the goals for *Urinary Retention* you need to determine whether

1. the urine output is 1500 to 3000 ml daily, or equivalent to intake.

2. the client is having supra pubic discomfort.

3. the client is voiding at least 150 to 400 ml per void.

4. the client is able to perform intermittent self-catheterization if necessary due to a chronic condition.

5. the person has knowledge of causes of the health problem; signs of urinary retention and UTIs; actions, dosage, and major side effects of prescribed medications; how to prevent UTIs; and how to identify the need for and describe planned follow-up.

Your documentation includes intake and output, voiding patterns, level of comfort, discharge teaching, and the client's knowledge of the discharge plan of care.

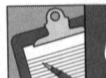

CASE STUDY

The Client

Mrs. Lynn Daro, a well-nourished 34-year-old white woman, was admitted one month ago with reports of loss of urine while standing, urgency, dribbling with coughing, and frequency every hour. She states that the vaginal delivery of her child was difficult. She sustained a second-degree laceration upon delivering her son.

A partial listing of physician's orders on admission included

▶ For cystoscopy in AM
▶ Nothing by mouth (NPO) after midnight
▶ Intake and output
▶ Acetaminophen (Tylenol), 650 mg, every 4 to 6 hours prn for discomfort

At 9:00 AM, March 10, a partial listing of the admission assessment data included the following:

▶ 34-year-old, well-nourished woman
▶ T 98.6°F, P 76, R 18, B/P 116/78
▶ Skin warm, dry, and intact, pale pink in color
▶ Abdomen soft, nontender, no distention. Bowel sounds audible in all four quadrants
▶ No bladder distention
▶ Voiding frequently in small amounts—clear yellow urine
▶ Pedal pulses palpable, no pedal edema

Thirty days have passed since admission. The following represents part of a nursing care plan written for her shortly after admission and the current evaluation of outcomes that were expected at that time. Evaluation was completed by telephone follow-up.

CARE PLAN

9:00 AM, March 1

Nursing Diagnosis	Planning: Expected Outcomes	Implementation: Nursing Interventions	Evaluation
Stress Incontinence R/T weak pelvic muscles and structural supports following pregnancy	By 1 PM March 30: States Kegel exercises have helped increase ability to retain urine Reports less dribbling with coughing and no loss of urine with standing	Describe Kegel exercises to client Give client written instructions on the exercises Encourage client to practice exercises ten times per day	1 PM, March 30: Client states that, since exercising, she is experiencing no loss of urine while standing and is only dribbling slightly with coughing

---

Summary

▶ The urinary tract is one of the three main routes of elimination of body wastes. The major structures of the urinary system are the kidneys, ureters, urinary bladder, and urethra.

▶ Maintenance of normal urinary elimination is influenced by fluid intake, exercise, and urinary elimination pattern.

▶ Assessment of the urinary system consists of a complete health assessment, including physical and psychosocial data, factors affecting urinary elimination, urine characteristics, and results of both urine testing and diagnostic tests of the urinary tract.

▶ Nursing diagnoses for the individual with urinary elimination needs focus on Altered Urinary Elimination, Urinary Incontinence, Urinary Retention, and the effects of any urinary alterations on a person's biologic and psychosocial systems.

▶ Planning nursing care for individuals with a diagnosis of Altered Urinary Elimination, Urinary Incontinence, or Urinary Retention includes identifying outcomes directed at enhancing the person's knowledge level and self-esteem as well as those designed to meet urinary elimination needs.

▶ Nursing interventions for the individual with urinary elimination needs require knowledge of urinary catheterization, bladder irrigation, and additional interventions that help prevent and/or relieve Altered Urinary Elimination, Urinary Incontinence, and Urinary Retention.

▶ Evaluation of the individual with a diagnosis of Altered Urinary Elimination, Urinary Incontinence, and/or Urinary Retention must measure how well the person has avoided potential complications and has managed self-care.

Bibliography

1. Abdellah, F.G. (1988). Incontinence: implications for health care policy. *Nursing Clinics of North America*, 23, 291–297.
2. Andresen, G. (1989). A fresh look at assessing the elderly. *RN*, 52(6), 28–40.
3. Andriole, V. (1975). Hospital-acquired urinary infections and the indwelling catheter. *Urology Clinics of North America*, 2, 451.
4. Barker, J. C., & Mitteness (1988). Nocturia in the elderly. *Gerontologist*, 28(6), 99.
5. Beber, C.R. (1980). Freedom for the incontinent. *American Journal of Nursing*, 80, 482–485.
6. Bellinger, M.F. (1989). The history of diversion and undiversion. *Journal of Enterostomal Therapy*, 16, 39–41.
7. Birum, L., & Zimmerman, D. (1971). Catheter plugs as a source of infection. *American Journal of Nursing*, 71, 2150–2152.
8. Brehmer, B., & Madsen, P. (1972). Route and prophylaxis of ascending bladder infection in male patients with indwelling catheters. *Journal of Urology*, 108, 719.
9. Brink, C.A. (1990). Absorbent pads, garments, and management strategies. *Journal of the American Geriatrics Society*, 38, 368–373.
10. Brink, C.A., et al. (1989). A digital test for pelvic muscle strength in older women with urinary incontinence. *Nursing Research*, 38, 196–199.
11. Bristoll, S.L., et al. (1989). The mythical danger of rapid urinary drainage. *American Journal of Nursing*, 89, 344–345.
12. Brogna, L., & Lakaszawski, M.L. (1986). The continent urostomy. *Journal of Enterostomal Therapy*, 13, 139–147.
13. Bullock, B.L., & Rosendahl, P.P. (1988). *Pathophysiology: Adaptations and alterations in function* (2nd ed.). Glenview, Illinois: Scott, Foresman.
14. Burgio, K.L., et al. (1986). The role of biofeedback in Kegel exercise training for stress urinary incontinence. *American Journal of Obstetrics and Gynecology*, 154, 58–64.
15. Burke, J.P., et al. (1986). Nosocomial bacteriuria: estimating the potential for prevention by closed sterile urinary drainage. *Infection Control*, 7(2), 96–99.
16. Burke, J., et al. (1981). Prevention of catheter-associated urinary tract infections: efficacy of daily meatal care regimens. *American Journal of Medicine*, 70, 655.
17. Burke, J., et al. (1983). Evaluation of daily meatal care with polyantibiotic ointment in prevention of urinary catheter-associated bacteriuria. *Journal of Urology*, 129, 331.
18. Cain, L., & Bigongiari, L.R. (1982). The percutaneous nephrostomy tube. *American Journal of Nursing*, 82, 296–298.
19. Carpenito, L. (1989). *Nursing diagnosis: Application to clinical practice* (3rd ed.). Philadelphia: J.B. Lippincott.
20. Cella, M. (1988). The nursing costs of urinary incontinence in a nursing home population. *Nursing Clinics of North America*, 23, 159–168.
21. Centers for Disease Control (1987). Recommendations for prevention of HIV transmission in health care settings. *Morbidity Mortality Weekly Report*, 36(25), 25–40.
22. Clancy, B. (1989). Continence. Bed protectors: No easy choice. *Nursing Times*, 85(33), 70–75.
23. Conti, M., & Eutropius, L. (1987). Preventing UTIs: what works? *American Journal of Nursing*, 87, 307–309.
24. Creason, N., et al. (1989). Prompted voiding therapy for urinary incontinence in aged female nursing home residents. *Journal of Advanced Nursing*, 14, 120–126.
25. Culhane, J.K. (1990). Delayed analysis of urine. *Journal of Family Practice*, 30, 473–474.
26. Davidson, M.W., et al. (1990). Continent Indiana reservoir: nursing management. *Ostomy/Wound Management*, 31(6), 50–57.
27. Dyer, J. (1991). Life-threatening reactions to latex are increasing, FDA warns. Clinical News. *American Journal of Nursing*, 91(7), 14.
28. Elliott, T.S. (1990). Disadvantages of bladder irrigation. *Nursing Times*, 86(41), 52.
29. Fischbach, F. (1988). *A manual of laboratory diagnostic tests* (3rd ed.). Philadelphia: J.B. Lippincott.
30. Flanagan, P.G., et al. (1989). Evaluation of four screening tests for bacteriuria in elderly people. *Lancet*, 1, 1117–1119.
31. Fowler, E.M., et al. (1990). Managing incontinence in the nursing home population. *Journal of Enterostomal Therapy*, 17(2), 77–86.
32. Foxman, B. (1990). Recurring urinary tract infection: incidence and risk factors. *American Journal of Public Health*, 80, 331.
33. Gallagher, E.J., et al. (1990). Performance characteristics of urine dipstick stored in open containers. *American Journal of Emergency Medicine*, 8, 121–123.
34. Ghiotta, D. (1988). A full range of care for nephrostomy patients. *RN*, 72–77.
35. Greig, B.J. (1988). You and your Kock pouch. *Urologic Nursing*, 8(4), 13–14.
36. Greig, B.J. (1990). A new option for cystectomy patients. RN, 53(5), 34.
37. Guyton, A.C. (1991). *Textbook of medical physiology* (8th ed.). Philadelphia: W.B. Saunders.
38. Hinkle, M., & Bowditch, R. (1981). The great stent mystery, can you solve it? *Nursing 81*, 11(4), 94–95.
39. Hott, J.R. (1991). Speaking of sex. *American Journal of Nursing*, 91, 28.
40. Howe, S.M., & Bates, P. (1987). The cranberry juice cure: fact or fiction? Urologic Nursing, 8(1), 13–16.
41. Hu, T.W., et al. (1989). Incontinence products: which is best? *Geriatric Nursing*, 10, 184–186.
42. Innes, B., & Bruya, M. (1977). Post-operative voiding patterns and related contributing factors. *Washington State Journal of Nursing*, 49, 13–16.
43. Iyer, P., et al. (1991). *Nursing process and nursing diagnosis* (2nd ed.). Philadelphia: W.B. Saunders.
44. Jirovec, M.M., et al. (1988). Nursing assessments in the inpatient geriatric population. *Nursing Clinics of North America*, 23, 219–230.
45. Kaltreider, D.L., et al. (1990). Can reminders curb incontinence? *Geriatric Nursing*, 11, 17–19.
46. Kidd, P. (1989). Ruptured bladder. *Nursing 89*, 19(1), 33.
47. Kiel, D.P., & Moskowitz, M.A. (1987). The urinalysis: a critical appraisal. *Medical Clinics of North America*, 71, 607–624.
48. Killion, A. (1982). Reducing the risk of infection from indwelling urethral catheters. *Nursing 82*, 12(5), 84–88.
49. Lincoln, R., & Roberts, R. (1989). Continence issues in acute care. *Nursing Clinics of North America*, 24, 741–754.
50. Madda, M.A. (1991). Helping ostomy patients manage medications. *Nursing 91*, 21(3), 47–49.
51. McConnell, E., & Zimmerman, M. (1983). *Care of the patient with urologic problems*. Philadelphia: J.B. Lippincott.
52. McCormick, K.A., et al. (1988). Nursing management of urinary incontinence in geriatric inpatients. *Nursing Clinics of North America*, 23, 231–264.
53. Miller, J. (1990). Assessing urinary incontinence. *Journal of Gerontological Nursing*, 16(3), 15–19.
54. Millette-Petit, J.M. (1988). Urinary tract infections in older adults. *Nursing Practitioner*, 13(12), 21–24.
55. Monroe, D. (1990). Patient teaching for x-ray and other diagnostics. *RN*, 53(3), 42.
56. Moriarty, M.B. (1989). The NIH puts the spotlight on incontinence. *RN*, 52(3), 44–45.
57. Morishita, L. (1988). Nursing evaluation and treatment of geriatric out-patients with urinary incontinence. *Nursing Clinics of North America*, 23, 189–206.
58. Muncie, H.L., et al. (1989). Once-daily irrigation of long-term urethral catheters with normal saline. *Archives of Internal Medicine*, 149, 441–443.
59. Newman, D.K. (1989). The treatment of urinary incontinence in adults. *Nurse Practitioner*, 14(6), 21–32.
60. Newman, D.K., & Smith, D.A. (1989). Incontinence in elderly homebound patients. *Holistic Nursing Practice*, 4(1), 52–60.
61. Newman, D.K., & Smith, D.A. (1989). Incontinence: the problem patients won't talk about. *RN*, 52(4), 42–45.
62. Newman, D.K., et al. (1991). Restoring urinary continence. *American Journal of Nursing*, 91(1), 28–34.
63. Nicolle, L.E., et al. (1988). Urine specimen collection with ex-

ternal devices for diagnosis of bacteriuria in elderly incontinent men. *Journal of Clinical Microbiology, 26,* 1115–1119.

64. O'Toole, M. (1992). *Miller-Keane encyclopedia and dictionary of medicine, nursing, and allied health* (5th ed.). Philadelphia: W.B. Saunders.

65. Palmer, M.H., (1990). Urinary incontinence. *Nursing Clinics of North America, 25,* 919–934.

66. Palmer, M.H., et al. (1989). Do nurses consistently document incontinence? *Journal of Gerontological Nursing, 15*(12), 11–16.

67. Petillo, M.H. (1987). The patient with a urinary stoma. *Nursing Clinics of North America, 22,* 263–279.

68. Petrelli, C.D., et al. (1988). Behavioral management in the inpatient geriatric population. *Nursing Clinics of North America, 23,* 265–277.

69. Pierce, S., & Campbell, M. (1988). Return of bladder function. *AORN, 47*(3), 702–712.

70. Preshlock, K. (1989). Detecting the hidden UTI. *RN, 52*(4), 65.

71. Prevention and treatment of kidney stones. (1988). *Journal of the American Medical Association, 260,* 977–981.

72. Pritchard, V. (1988). Geriatric infections: the urinary tract. *RN, 5*(5), 36–38.

73. Reilly, N. (1988). The new wave lithotripsy: implications for nursing. *RN,* 44–49.

74. Reisman, E.M., & Preminger, G.M. (1989). Bladder perforation secondary to clean intermittent catheterization. *Journal of Urology, 142,* 1316–1317.

75. Roe, B.H. (1990). Study of the effects of education on the management of urine drainage systems by patients and carers. *Journal of Advanced Nursing, 15,* 517–524.

76. Rose, M.A., et al. (1990). Behavioral management of urinary incontinence in homebound older adults. *Home Healthcare Nurse, 8*(5), 10–15.

77. Sage, S.J., & Faller, N. (1989). Managing male incontinence with external collection systems: some alternatives. *Ostomy/Wound Management, 25,* 33–40.

78. Sawyer, D.L. (1989). Potential for infection: a nursing diagnosis for the patient with an indwelling catheter. *Focus on Critical Care, 16*(1), 46–52.

79. Scheve, A., et al. (1991). Exercise in continence. *Geriatric Nursing, 12,* 124.

80. Smith, D.A.J. (1988). Continence restoration in the home bound patient. *Nursing Clinics of North America, 23,* 207–218.

81. Smith, D.A.J., et al. (1989). Managing urinary incontinence in community-residing elderly persons. *The Gerontologist, 29,* 229.

82. Squibb & Sons, Inc. (1990). *For a better way of living with a urostomy.* Princeton, New Jersey: Squibb & Sons.

83. Squibb & Sons, Inc. (1990). *Living with a urostomy the easy, the active way.* Princeton, New Jersey: Squibb & Sons.

84. Stapleton, A., et al. (1990). Postcoital antimicrobial prophylaxis for recurrent urinary tract infections: a randomized, double-blind, placebo-controlled trial. *Journal of the American Medical Association, 264,* 703.

85. Taptich, B., et al. (1989). *Nursing diagnosis and care planning.* Philadelphia: W.B. Saunders.

86. Todd, B. (1990). Treating UTIs. *Geriatric Nursing, 11,* 95–96.

87. Tunink, P. (1988). Alteration in urinary elimination. *Journal of Gerontological Nursing, 14*(4), 25–30.

88. Urinary incontinence in adults—consensus conference (1989). *Journal of the American Medical Association, 261*(18), 2685–2690.

89. Urine glucose and ketone determinations (1991). *Diabetes Care,* 39–40.

90. Voith, A.M. (1988). Alterations in urinary elimination: concepts, research, and practice. *Rehabilitation Nursing, 13*(3), 122–131.

91. Walter, F.G., & Knapp, R.K. (1989). Urine sampling in ambulatory women: midstream clean-catch versus catheterization. *Annals of Emergency Medicine, 18,* 166–172.

92. Watson, R. (1989). In praise of sheaths. *Geriatric Nursing & Home Care, 9*(3), 10–11.

93. Watson, R., & Kuhn, M. (1990). The influence of component parts on the performance of urinary sheath systems. *Journal of Advanced Nursing, 15,* 417–422.

94. Webber-Jones, J. (1991). Performing clean, intermittent self-catheterization. *Nursing 91, 21*(8), 56–59.

95. Wells, T. (1990). Conquering incontinence. *Geriatric Nursing, 11,* 133–135.

96. Whippo, C., & Creason, N. (1989). Bacteriuria and urinary incontinence in aged female nursing home residents. *Journal of Advanced Nursing, 14,* 217–225.

97. Wong, E., & Hooton, T. (1982). *Guidelines for prevention of catheter-associated urinary tract infection.* (NTIS No. P884-923402). Atlanta: US Department of Health and Human Services.

98. Wyman, J.F. (1988). Nursing assessment of the incontinent geriatric out-patient population. *Nursing Clinics of North America,* 169–187.

99. Wyndaele, J.J., & Maes, D. (1990). Clean intermittent self-catheterization: a 12-year followup. *Journal of Urology, 143,* 906–908.

100. Yu, L. (1987). Incontinence stress index. Measuring psychological impact. *Journal of Gerontological Nursing, 13*(7), 18–25.

101. Zastocki, D., & Rovinski, A. (1989). *Home care: Patient and family instructions.* Philadelphia: W.B. Saunders.

102. Zilkoski, M.W., & Smucker, D.R. (1989). Urinary tract infections in the elderly. *American Family Physician, 39*(5), 125–134.

Meeting Respiration Needs

The tepee is much better to live in: always clean, warm in winter, cool in summer; easy to move. . . . Indians and animals know better how to live than white man; nobody can be in good health if he does not have all the time fresh air, sunshine, and good water.

Flying Hawk
1852–1931
Statement in old age

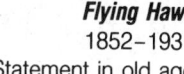

▼ CHAPTER OUTLINE

OVERVIEW OF THE RESPIRATORY
   SYSTEM
      Normal Structure
      Normal Function
      Control of Breathing
      Factors That Affect Breathing
RESPIRATORY DISORDERS
      Hypoventilation
      Hyperventilation
      Hypoxemia and Hypoxia
WORKING AS PART OF THE HEALTH
   CARE TEAM
ASSESSMENT

      Taking a Respiratory History
      The Chest Examination
      Laboratory and Diagnostic Studies
NURSING DIAGNOSIS
PLANNING
NURSING INTERVENTION
      Basic Respiratory Therapeutic
        Measures
      Measures to Maintain Airway
        Patency
EVALUATION
CASE STUDY

▼ KEY TERMS

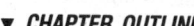

Alveoli
Atelectasis
Bronchoconstriction
Bronchospasm
Chest percussion
  (clapping)
Chest physical therapy
Chronic obstructive
  pulmonary disease
  (COPD)
Consolidation
Empyema

Endotracheal tubes
Extubation
Hemoptysis
Humidification
Hypoxemia
Hypoxia
Intubation
Mechanical ventilation
Metered-dose inhaler
  (MDI)
Nasal airway (nasal
  trumpet)

Nasotracheal intubation
Oropharyngeal airway (oral
  airway)
Pleural effusion
Pleuritic chest pain
Pneumothorax
Postural drainage
Pursed-lip breathing
Tracheostomy tubes
Vibration

Breathing is a basic human need. Like all basic needs, people are unaware of it so long as they are breathing normally. Yet the development of difficulty in breathing is one of the most frightening experiences a person can have. Acute, unexpected breathlessness may cause panic, which in turn usually makes the breathing problem worse. In contrast, long-term, unrelenting difficulty breathing may cause a person to depend on high technology for respiration needs. Faced with a sense of powerlessness, the person may give up hope for a high quality life in the future. The client may feel hopeless even though the health care team gives a good prognosis, appropriate care, and plenty of positive reinforcement. Thus, clients with respiratory problems provide ongoing challenges for nurses and other health care workers.

This chapter emphasizes the physiologic and psychosocial processes that interfere with normal gas exchange in the body. The first two sections provide an overview of the respiratory system and common respiratory alterations. The rest of the chapter prepares the student to apply the nursing process to people with the nursing diagnosis of *Impaired Gas Exchange*.

OVERVIEW OF THE RESPIRATORY SYSTEM

Normal Structure

The respiratory system is divided into two major sections: the upper respiratory tract and the lower respiratory tract. The upper respiratory tract consists of the nose and sinuses, the pharynx, and the larynx. The upper respiratory tract serves as a conducting passage for air as it enters and leaves the lungs. Its primary functions are to warm, humidify, and filter entering air and to protect the lower airway from foreign material.

The lower respiratory tract begins at the trachea, or windpipe, and ends at the **alveoli** (air sacs in the lungs where gas exchange takes place). It includes the right and left mainstem bronchi (the large airways of the lungs), the segmental and subsegmental bronchi, the

bronchioles, and the alveolar sacs (Fig. 45–1). The successive branching of the lower respiratory tract into smaller and smaller air passages gives it a treelike appearance.

Normal adult lungs weigh approximately 900 to 1100 gm. They consist of five lobes and 18 to 20 bronchopulmonary segments. Their 300 million alveoli cover an area about the size of a tennis court and are perfused by 45 square meters of pulmonary capillaries.

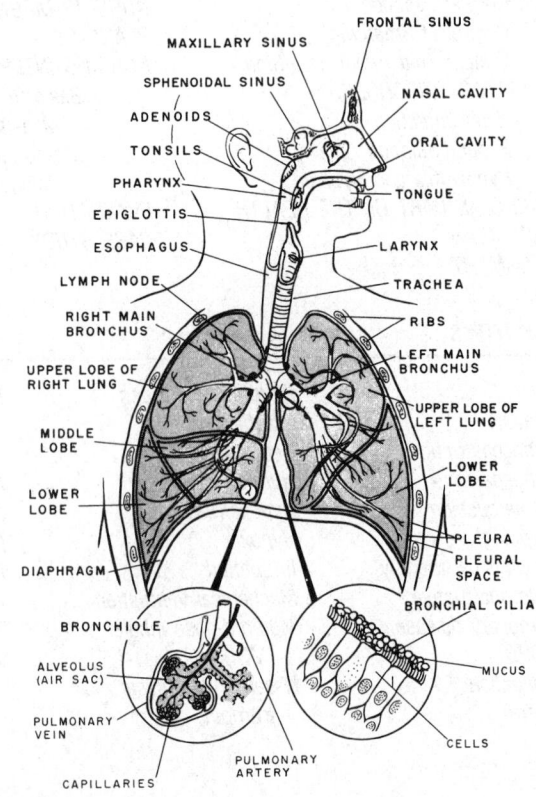

▲ *Figure 45–1*

Anatomy of the respiratory system. (Reprinted with permission from *The respiratory system*, Publication #0950 [1984]. New York: American Lung Association.)

The lungs are covered by two thin membranes: the visceral pleura, inseparably connected to the lungs; and the parietal pleura, lining the ribs and chest wall. A potential space, called the pleural space, exists between these two pleural surfaces. A thin layer of serous fluid within this space lubricates the pleural surfaces, allowing them to slide smoothly against each other while creating a cohesive force that drives the lungs to move synchronously with the chest wall during breathing.

The lungs are located within the thoracic cavity. The thoracic cavity is enclosed on the front, back, and sides by the ribs, sternum, vertebrae, intercostal muscles, and ligaments. The scalene muscles and the fascia of the neck form the top of the cavity; the diaphragm forms the bottom. The space between the lungs is known as the mediastinum. The mediastinal space contains the heart and pericardium; the thoracic aorta; the pulmonary artery and veins; the venae cavae and azygos vein; the thymus, lymph nodes, and vessels; the trachea, esophagus, and thoracic duct; and the vagus, cardiac, and phrenic nerves.

There are two entirely separate blood supplies to the lungs. The pulmonary arteries carry unoxygenated blood from the heart to the pulmonary capillaries in the walls of the alveoli. Through these capillaries, the exchange of respiratory gases takes place. The bronchial arteries are the nutrient arteries for the lung tissue and play no part in oxygenation of the blood.

Normal Function

The main function of the respiratory system is gas exchange—the intake of oxygen and elimination of carbon dioxide, the body's chief waste product. Gas exchange or respiration occurs at both the alveolar level in the lungs and at the tissue level peripherally.

In the lungs, respiration involves the exchange of gases between the circulating blood and the air. This exchange requires the movement of oxygen-rich air into the alveolar sacs (inspiration), where oxygen molecules diffuse across the alveolar-capillary membrane into the blood. At the same time, carbon dioxide molecules cross the membrane into the alveoli and are expelled during expiration.

Inspiration, the act of taking air into the lungs, involves a series of four steps. First, impulses from the central nervous system stimulate the diaphragm and external intercostal muscles to contract. As the diaphragm contracts, it descends downward. As the external intercostals contract, they raise and rotate the ribs and push the sternum forward. The net result is an enlargement of the thoracic cavity in both vertical and horizontal directions. This enlargement of the thoracic cavity causes a decrease in lung pressures. Intrapleural pressure (the pressure that exists between the two layers of pleura) lowers as the parietal pleura tends to pull away from the visceral pleura. However, because the cohesion between the two pleural layers is so great, the visceral pleura, along with the lung tissue to which it is attached, expands with the enlarging thorax. As the

lungs expand, intrapulmonic pressure (the pressure within the bronchial tree and alveoli) falls below atmospheric pressure. As a result, outside air flows into the lungs until the intrapulmonic pressure equals atmospheric pressure.

Expiration, the process of expelling air from the lungs, also involves four events. To begin, as impulses from the central nervous system cease, the diaphragm and external intercostal muscles relax. This relaxation returns the thoracic cavity to its resting size and shape. (This action is entirely passive during normal expiration.) As the thoracic cavity decreases in size, both intrapleural and intrapulmonic pressures increase. As a result, air flows out of the lungs until the intrapulmonic and atmospheric pressures equalize.

At both the alveolar and tissue level, respiration involves the diffusion of gases. In the alveoli, the concentration of oxygen in inspired air is higher than it is in the blood passing through the pulmonary capillaries. As a result, oxygen molecules diffuse from the alveoli into the blood. The oxygen binds to hemoglobin (the iron-containing protein of red blood cells), which becomes oxyhemoglobin. Some oxygen is also dissolved and carried in the plasma.

The blood then circulates throughout the body. As it reaches the peripheral tissues, where the oxygen concentration is low, oxygen molecules needed for cellular metabolism diffuse from the blood into the tissue fluid and cells.

At the same time, carbon dioxide molecules, which are more concentrated in the tissue, diffuse into the bloodstream. As the blood circulates back to the lungs, carbon dioxide diffuses across the alveolar-capillary membrane into the alveoli and is exhaled.

The movement of gas in and out of the lungs is called lung ventilation. Normal gas exchange is achieved by the proper amounts of both lung ventilation and lung perfusion (blood flow). When the ratio of ventilation to perfusion is disturbed, gas exchange is impaired, and other related respiratory problems result.

Control of Breathing

Normal involuntary respiration is regulated primarily by the medulla oblongata and the pons, both located in the brain. These respiratory centers function as a unit to regulate the rhythm, rate, and depth of respiration. Voluntary control of breathing can be attained temporarily through nerve impulses from the motor areas of the cerebral cortex. This conscious control permits such activities as speaking, singing, and swimming. However, voluntary control is limited and will be overridden by the respiratory centers to meet ventilatory needs.

Other neural reflexes and chemical changes also influence respiration. Central chemoreceptors, located in the anterior medulla, are sensitive to changes in blood carbon dioxide levels. If carbon dioxide levels rise, as with physical exertion, these chemoreceptors stimulate the respiratory centers to increase respiratory rate and depth until levels return to normal. Conversely, if blood carbon dioxide levels fall below normal, the central chemoreceptors halt breathing (apnea) until sufficient carbon dioxide levels stimulate the respiratory centers to begin again.

Peripheral chemoreceptors, located in such key areas as the aorta and carotid arteries, have an important secondary role in respiratory regulation. The peripheral receptors are primarily responsible for the secondary "hypoxic" (ventilatory) drive of respiration. They are very sensitive to decreases in the level of arterial oxygen (arterial oxygen tension). When blood oxygen levels drop, these receptors stimulate the respiratory centers to increase the respiratory rate and/or depth to introduce more oxygen into the system. The hypoxic drive is very important for individuals with certain respiratory conditions, such as emphysema, who routinely have high carbon dioxide levels. In these individuals, blood oxygen levels, not carbon dioxide levels, play the major role in regulating respiration.

The respiratory system also has a number of protective defense mechanisms. These include coughing; sneezing; the mucus blanket that lines the tracheobronchial tree; cilia (microscopic hairlike projections that help sweep particulate debris upward to be coughed or swallowed); alveolar macrophages, which engulf material; and surfactant, a phospholipid compound that maintains the surface-active forces of the lung in balance, preventing alveolar collapse.

Factors That Affect Breathing

Breathing may be affected by a number of factors. These include both internal factors (i.e., specific to the individual) and external factors (i.e., environmental factors).

Developmental stage influences respiratory rate. The respiratory rate declines throughout the life span, decreasing from 30 to 35 breaths per minute in the newborn to 12 to 20 breaths per minute in the adult. Age also influences the nature of respiratory disorders to which a person is most predisposed. For example, infants and toddlers are at high risk for upper respiratory infections; elderly individuals are more likely to develop disorders related to the structural and functional declines associated with the aging process.

Health disorders, even those that do not directly affect the respiratory system, may also affect breathing. For example, conditions leading to blood loss or anemia (decrease in number of red blood cells) affect the blood's ability to carry oxygen. Heart problems that result in reduced cardiac output also cause impairment in oxygen circulation. Nervous system disorders may hinder movement of the respiratory muscles or may interfere with neural transmissions. Thus, even when a person's medical condition is not respiratory in nature, respiration may still be affected.

Temperature, too, influences breathing. Increases in body temperature, as during fever or significant exercise, are accompanied by increases in respiratory rate. Conversely, decreased body temperature, or hypothermia, reduces the rate of respirations.

Lifestyle choices may affect respiratory status. The most obvious related factor is cigarette smoking. However, poor nutritional habits, substance abuse, and extreme anxiety may have an impact on a person's respiratory condition.

Finally, *environmental factors* can influence the respiratory system. Exposure to pollutants, in the work setting, the home, or the general atmosphere, can reduce oxygenation directly or through resultant disease. In addition, the air at higher altitudes contains lower partial pressures of oxygen. The person at high altitudes may have a higher respiratory rate and depth to help adapt to this situation.

RESPIRATORY DISORDERS

Respiratory disorders occur when the normal structure or function of the respiratory system is altered. Alterations of the respiratory system result in impairment of normal gas exchange. Three potential outcomes of respiratory disorders are hypoventilation, hyperventilation, and hypoxia. When gas exchange becomes severely impaired, respiratory failure develops. Common causes of respiratory problems are shown in Figure 45–2. Some symbols and abbreviations related to pulmonary status may be found in Box 45–1.

Hypoventilation

Hypoventilation occurs when ventilation of the alveoli fails to keep up with the body's production of carbon dioxide. Inadequate alveolar ventilation can occur as a result of

▶ decreased respiratory drive, as in some cases of drug overdose
▶ decreased ability to respond to the respiratory drive, as in cases of severe airway obstruction or massive chest trauma
▶ increased dead space ventilation (i.e., ventilation of respiratory structures that are not actively functioning in gas exchange, usually as a result of disease), as with pulmonary embolus
▶ increased carbon dioxide production, as in cases of infection or vigorous exercise (when the individual is unable to increase ventilation accordingly)

Hypoventilation is characterized by an elevated arterial carbon dioxide level. As the carbon dioxide level rises, the oxygen level falls; if hypoventilation is untreated, **hypoxemia** (insufficient oxygenation of the arterial blood) results. Acidosis (excessive acidity of body fluids) may occur as a result of increased hydrogen ion (H^+) concentrations. Retained carbon dioxide combines with water to form carbonic acid, causing an increase in H^+ content of the blood (see Chapter 41). Other effects of hypoventilation may include tachycardia, restlessness, lethargy, confusion, and coma.

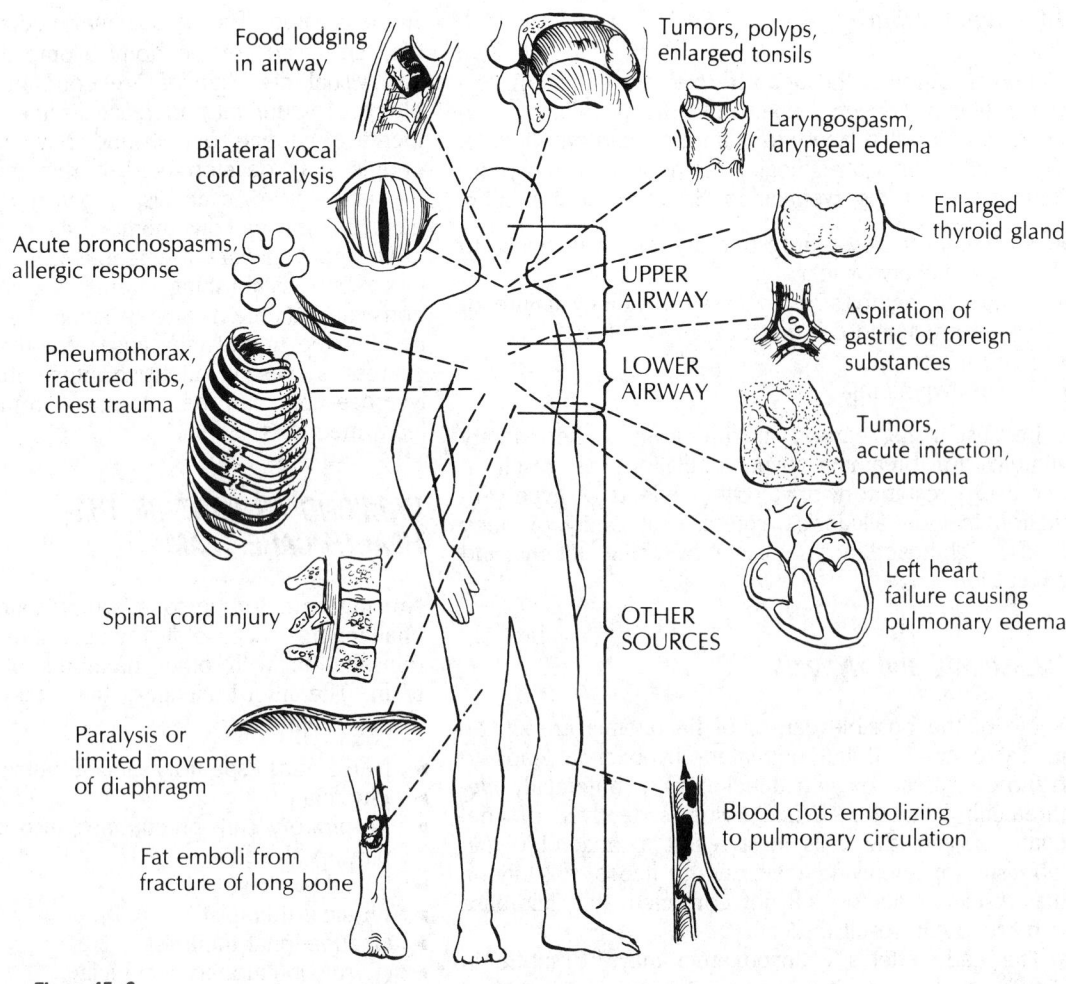

Food lodging in airway

Tumors, polyps, enlarged tonsils

Bilateral vocal cord paralysis

Laryngospasm, laryngeal edema

Enlarged thyroid gland

Acute bronchospasms, allergic response

UPPER AIRWAY

Aspiration of gastric or foreign substances

Pneumothorax, fractured ribs, chest trauma

LOWER AIRWAY

Tumors, acute infection, pneumonia

Spinal cord injury

OTHER SOURCES

Left heart failure causing pulmonary edema

Paralysis or limited movement of diaphragm

Fat emboli from fracture of long bone

Blood clots embolizing to pulmonary circulation

▲ *Figure 45–2*

Causes of respiratory disease.

Box 45–1. Pulmonary Symbols and Abbreviations

A	Alveolar	PA_{O_2}	Partial pressure of alveolar oxygen
a	Arterial	Pa_{O_2}	Partial pressure of arterial oxygen
CO_2	Carbon dioxide	Pa_{CO_2}	Partial pressure of arterial carbon dioxide
f	Respiratory rate	pH	Quantity of hydrogen ions, acid vs. base
O_2	Oxygen	PIP	Peak inspiratory pressure (on ventilator manometer)
V	Ventilation		
V_T	Tidal volume	FI_{O_2}	Fractional inspired oxygen concentration, expressed in decimal form (0.40 = 40% oxygen concentration)
$\dot{V}_E$	Minute volume		
$\dot{V}/\dot{Q}$	Ventilation/perfusion ratio		
VC	Vital capacity	SOB	Shortness of breath
FEV_t	Forced expiratory volume/time	DOE	Dyspnea on exertion
$Sa_{O_2}\%$	Percentage hemoglobin oxygen saturation		

Hyperventilation

Hyperventilation is the opposite of hypoventilation. Hyperventilation occurs when alveolar ventilation exceeds the body's need to eliminate carbon dioxide. There are many physiologic, metabolic, and psychologic causes of hyperventilation. Some of these include

▶ significant increase in respiratory rate in response to severe anxiety or fear
▶ metabolic acidosis, as in cases of kidney failure or as a complication of diabetes
▶ head injury
▶ severe hypoxemia

Because rising carbon dioxide level is the primary stimulus for breathing, hyperventilation can result in decreased respiratory drive. Other effects of hyperventilation include alkalosis (excessive alkalinity of body fluids), lightheadedness, muscle twitching, tetany, and convulsions.

Hypoxemia and Hypoxia

Some of the possible causes of hypoxemia are shown in Table 45–1. If left untreated, hypoxemia leads to **hypoxia** (tissue oxygen deficiency), a potentially life-threatening disorder. When tissue is deprived of adequate oxygen, the cells must resort to anaerobic metabolism for supplying their energy needs, a situation that results in acidosis. If not corrected, this acid-base imbalance can result in death.

The early effects of hypoxemia may be subtle in nature. As the condition worsens, however, signs and symptoms become more apparent, exhibited primarily by the respiratory, neurologic, and cardiovascular systems. Respirations become increasingly more rapid and more labored. The person may become restless, irritable, confused, or delirious. Complaints of headache and visual disturbances are common. Heart rate and blood pressure may increase as the body attempts to increase cardiac output and oxygen delivery. Some people may develop cardiac rhythm disturbances. In the late stages, cyanosis, a bluish color of the skin, nailbeds, and mucous membranes, may occur.

The goal of care for people with hypoxemia or hypoxia is reestablishing normal oxygenation. Interventions are directed at reversing the hypoxemia and treating the underlying cause. When severe respiratory distress is present, intensive interventions and supportive measures may be necessary from the health care team members.

WORKING AS PART OF THE HEALTH CARE TEAM

Nursing care for persons with respiratory problems is challenging because it requires intense and ongoing consultation with other members of the health care team. The interdisciplinary team may include the following members:

▶ Nurse and respiratory clinical nurse specialist
▶ Physician
▶ Respiratory care practitioner, also known as the respiratory therapist
▶ Social worker
▶ Physical therapist
▶ Occupational therapist
▶ (Cardio)pulmonary technician

Respiratory therapy includes a broad range of respiratory interventions, including many interventions discussed in this chapter (e.g., aerosol therapy, mechanical ventilation, and pulmonary rehabilitation). Today's respiratory care practitioners graduate from American Medical Association–accredited respiratory therapy education programs. They are either certified respiratory therapy technicians or registered respiratory therapists. A person with the registered respiratory therapist credential has passed an advanced national registry test and is the most qualified individual to practice respiratory therapy.

Because of role overlap with the respiratory care practitioner and other team members, be sure to

▶ become familiar with every agency's respiratory policies and procedures to clarify who does what
▶ regularly share respiratory assessment data with other team members
▶ involve others, as needed, in the diagnosis of respiratory problems and the planning of respiratory care
▶ negotiate responsibilities whenever roles in the clinical setting seem ambiguous

While applying the nursing process, you are encouraged to help arrange periodic informal meetings with other health care team members involved at the moment in clinical decision making. Informal meetings at the bedside, at the nurse's station, or in a conference

TABLE 45–1. Causes of Hypoxemia

Cause	Example
Inadequate inspiration of oxygen	Airway obstructed with secretions, foreign objects, or tumors; high altitude
Hypoventilation	Impaired ventilation due to disease, injury, medication effect, or anesthesia
Impaired diffusion	Interstitial lung diseases; pulmonary edema; destruction of lung tissue due to disease, e.g., pneumonia or atelectasis
Impaired perfusion and transport of oxygen	Anemia; reduced cardiac output; hemorrhage; pulmonary emboli
Altered uptake of oxygen by the tissues	Fever; carbon monoxide poisoning; cyanide poisoning; after blood transfusion

room facilitate face-to-face communication between all team members and help clarify responsibilities.

ASSESSMENT

Respiratory assessment is a vital part of nursing care. It may reveal changes in respiratory function that can threaten well-being or hinder daily activities. Early detection of such changes allows you to intervene quickly, perhaps preventing complications.

A thorough assessment of an individual's respiratory status should be performed on admission to the hospital, at regular intervals during an illness episode, and during routine health evaluations and screenings. The main components of the respiratory assessment include the nursing history, physical assessment, and review of laboratory and diagnostic study results.

Taking a Respiratory History

When preparing to take the respiratory history, try to keep the environment quiet and relaxing. Taking time and avoiding interference helps ensure a comprehensive assessment. Watch the person for signs of fatigue or increasing respiratory distress. It may be necessary to take the history in segments to avoid tiring the acutely ill individual.

Begin the history by determining the person's chief complaint. This is best elicited by directly asking, "What is bothering you?" or "What brought you here today?" The nature of the individual's complaint will help guide your line of questioning. Complete information should be obtained to verify the exact nature of symptoms such as dyspnea, cough, sputum production, hemoptysis, and pain with breathing (pleuritic pain). Try to place the development of symptoms within a time frame (e.g., months or years).

DYSPNEA

Dyspnea is the most common complaint of persons with respiratory disease. Dyspnea is the uncomfortable, distressing sensation of difficult or labored breathing. It is a subjective experience, and there is often no correlation between objective assessment of respiratory impairment and a person's perception of dyspnea. Just as some people are more able to tolerate pain than others are, so are some people less bothered by difficult breathing.

The term *shortness of breath* is often used to describe dyspnea. Other descriptions include "I can't catch my breath"; "My legs are weak, I tire easily"; "I feel as if I'm wearing a very tight jacket"; or "I'm short-winded." Many persons may appear dyspneic to the observer; but because dyspnea is subjective, the client may deny it.

Dyspnea is often apparent by the person's pattern of speech. The person takes audible, noticeable breaths at regular intervals during a conversation.

Dyspnea is also assessed by determining what activity levels produce this sensation. Ask questions that will allow an objective means of measurement. For example, "Are you short of breath when walking on level ground?" If yes, "How many blocks can you walk before stopping?" Other questions should determine whether the person feels short of breath at rest or with normal activities of daily living (e.g., during personal hygiene tasks like dressing, brushing teeth, or bathing; when making a bed; or when performing other household or yard activities). Ask if the person is able to climb stairs or hills and keep pace with other persons of the same age. Determine whether the person has had to make lifestyle changes to accommodate this respiratory impairment.

The development of dyspnea may be sudden and acute, or it may be chronic and insidious. Persons with chronic lung disorders often do not recognize respiratory impairment until their activity level has changed drastically.

COUGH AND SPUTUM PRODUCTION

Explore the report of a cough to determine its exact nature. A "loose"-sounding cough suggests mucus retention. A dry, hacking cough indicates airway irritation from an obstructive disorder. A harsh, barky cough similar to a seal's bark suggests upper airway obstruction secondary to subglottic edema. To further describe the cough, ask whether the cough is *weak* or *strong* and *productive* or *unproductive* of secretions.

Ask specifically how much mucus is expectorated per day in teaspoons, tablespoons, or cups. If aspects of sputum production seem ambiguous, you may give the person a covered sputum cup for a 24-hour sputum collection. The container is labeled with the person's name, the date, and the time of collection (e.g., 7 AM 8/19 to 7 AM 8/20). Later, the sputum is inspected for several characteristics.

Quantity of Sputum. Estimate the quantity of sputum produced. Note any increase or decrease in amount on a daily and weekly basis.

Color of Sputum. Note any change in color. The change may be from the normal anticipated sputum color (clear or slightly whitish) or from the person's particular baseline color, if the person has a chronic respiratory disorder. *Purulent* (yellow or green) mucus indicates infection (e.g., lung abscess, pneumonia). *Mucopurulent* sputum contains mucus from an airway disease (e.g., bronchitis, bronchiectasis) and pus from infection. *Blood-streaked* sputum indicates airway irritation from excessive coughing and the rupture of pulmonary capillaries from high intravascular pressures. *Pink, watery, frothy* sputum is typical of an acute episode of pulmonary edema (a symptom of left ventricular heart failure).

Consistency of Sputum. Determine whether the sputum is thick, thin, or frothy. Thick, tenacious sputum sticks to alveoli and the surfaces of airways, making expectoration difficult and predisposing the person to the problem of mucus retention. It suggests a need to increase fluid intake (provided the person is not on fluid restriction). Fluid helps to liquefy mucus and facilitate expectoration.

Odor of Sputum. Normal sputum is odorless. Purulent sputum may have a sweet, foul, or rotten, decomposed stench.

HEMOPTYSIS

Hemoptysis is the coughing up of blood. It may indicate cardiopulmonary disease or, in some cases, a potentially life-threatening bleeding problem. A small amount (e.g., 1 teaspoon or tablespoon) of frankly bloody sputum is seen in tuberculosis, bronchogenic carcinoma, and pulmonary infarction. Large amounts (e.g., ¼ cup) may be seen in persons with acute chest trauma or chronic airway disease (e.g., cystic fibrosis). Hemoptysis may occur in persons who rupture pulmonary vessels during vigorous coughing or during respiratory treatments, such as postural drainage.

PLEURITIC CHEST PAIN

Pleuritic chest pain (pain during a deep breath; associated with inflammation of the pleura or thoracic surgery) is typically described as stabbing in nature. It is usually worse with inspiration and aggravated by yawning, coughing, or sneezing. In clients who have not had surgery, it usually indicates the presence of pleural inflammation or infection but may also be due to malignant disease or pneumothorax. Pleuritic pain may be accompanied by a pleural friction rub.

ALLEVIATING AND AGGRAVATING FACTORS

In taking the nursing history, it is also important to ask the person what, specifically, makes the pulmonary symptoms better or worse. Main alleviating and aggravating factors may include health habits, especially smoking; body position in bed (e.g., supine, side-lying, prone, Fowler's or semi-Fowler's position); activity level (e.g., rest, walking, climbing stairs, performance of specific activities of daily living); and medications and respiratory treatments. Of these factors, smoking is one of the most significant factors contributing to respiratory problems.

PAST RELATED MEDICAL HISTORY

Next, obtain information about factors in the person's past history that may relate to the respiratory disorder. Ask the person about any previous incidence of respiratory diseases (e.g., pneumonia, asthma, bronchitis, emphysema, or tuberculosis), thoracic surgery, or chest trauma. Ask if the person has had any other diseases of note, particularly cardiovascular disorders, cancer, or neuromuscular problems. Find out whether the person

has any known allergies and whether there has been previous allergy testing and treatment. Chronic allergies can lead to other respiratory problems. Inquire as well about a family history of respiratory disorders, chronic allergies, or cancer.

ENVIRONMENTAL FACTORS

Question the person about home and work environments. Determine whether there has been occupational or other exposure to substances harmful to the lungs, such as chemicals, vapors, asbestos, dust, or other pollutants. Ask the person about hobbies that involve grinding, heating, sanding, or the use of chemical irritants (e.g., building models or refinishing furniture). Find out whether the person is exposed to cigarette smoke, either at home or at work. Ask about possible allergens in the house, such as pets or plants.

Whenever possible, involve the family, significant other, or other health professionals from the person's past to ensure a complete history and to check aspects of the history for accuracy. Persons with respiratory disease tend to give an incomplete history when dyspnea and associated fatigue hinder verbal communication and ongoing interpersonal involvement. Persons with chronic lung disease may deny symptoms when their low oxygen and high carbon dioxide levels interfere with their ability and desire to process information objectively. In some cases, a person may give a negative history just to prompt an early hospital discharge to a more comfortable and familiar home environment.

The Chest Examination

Physical examination of the chest is presented in Chapter 33. In the clinical setting, a quick chest examination will help you to assess persons with potential or diagnosed cardiopulmonary problems more efficiently. Use first impressions, inspection, and auscultation components of the complete chest examination.[18] Use palpation and percussion, as needed, to confirm or further describe suspected or known abnormal chest findings.

FIRST IMPRESSIONS

Note any change in vital signs, sensorium, and behavior patterns or any other readily noticeable sign that might indicate a blood gas abnormality. In addition, examine the bedside sputum cup for a change in the amount, color, consistency, and odor of the sputum. Be sure to tip the cup side to side to thoroughly assess consistency.

Cyanosis may be readily noticeable when you first approach a person for a history and physical examination. Cyanosis occurs when there is a decreased amount of oxygen in the hemoglobin of the blood. Unoxygenated hemoglobin is purple, whereas oxygenated hemoglobin is red. Cyanosis occurs when 5 gm of hemoglobin per 100 ml of blood is unsaturated (unoxygenated).

Cyanosis is not a reliable indicator of hypoxemia.

Cyanosis is a clinical observation not directly correlated with the level of hypoxemia. For example, people who are anemic may never appear cyanotic even when they are hypoxemic, simply because all of their available hemoglobin may be saturated with oxygen. The amount of oxygen available to the tissues may be inadequate, however, and hypoxemia will exist even though the saturation of hemoglobin is "normal" and no clinical evidence of cyanosis is present.

Factors that may affect your recognition of cyanosis include skin thickness, skin pigments, light in the room, color of the surroundings, and observer judgment.

INSPECTION

Use the following observation points when conducting the inspection portion of the chest examination.

Facial Features. Look for clues of respiratory dysfunction, such as circumoral (about the mouth) pallor, cyanosis of the lips and mucous membranes, flaring of the nares during inhalation, and pursed-lip exhalation. Look for hypertrophied neck muscles (indication of accessory muscle use for respiration) and distention of the neck veins.

Appearance of the Chest Wall. Note the shape, presence of surgical scars, pattern and character of superficial blood vessels, and symmetry of chest wall motion with each chest movement.

TABLE 45–2. Breathing Patterns

Type	Definition/ Graphic Representation	Significance
Normal breathing	A respiratory rate of 10–20 breaths per minute	
Tachypnea	Increased respiratory rate over 20 breaths per minute	A nonspecific finding commonly due to pain, anxiety, fever, anemia, and blood gas abnormalities
Bradypnea	Decreased respiratory rate under 10 breaths per minute or under the person's baseline rate	A nonspecific finding due to a variety of causes, including brain disorders, administration of narcotics, excessive alcohol intake, metabolic disorders, blood gas disorders, and fatigue
Apnea	Total cessation of airflow to the lungs	Normal during sleep, when less than 15 seconds in duration Called a *respiratory arrest* when longer than 2 minutes (leads to brain death) May occur from acute upper airway obstruction or damage or depression of the brain's respiratory center (e.g., head trauma, stroke, narcotic or anesthetic overdose, and alveolar hypoventilation)
Hyperpnea		Normal with strenuous exercise A nonspecific finding rarely seen without a simultaneous increase in respiratory rate
Hyperventilation		Caused by fever, low PaO_2, and other disorders causing alveolar hyperventilation

Table continued on following page

TABLE 45–2. Breathing Patterns Continued

Type	Definition/ Graphic Representation	Significance
Hypoventilation	Slow or irregular respiratory pattern with shallow respirations	Caused by depression of the respiratory system from drug overdose, anesthesia, or pain May lead to alveolar hypoventilation and ventilatory failure
Sighing respirations	Frequent sighs with a normal breathing pattern	Associated with anxiety, dyspnea, chest tightness, and tingling in the extremities (hyperventilation syndrome)
Cheyne-Stokes respirations	A cyclic pattern of progressively deeper respirations, followed by progressively shallow respirations and a period of apnea Apnea	Associated with congestive heart failure, brain disorders affecting the cerebrum, increased cerebrospinal fluid pressure, renal failure, and drug overdose
Kussmaul's respirations	Deep, regular breaths, usually at a rate greater than 20 per minute	Seen in diabetic ketoacidosis, renal failure, and other metabolic acidotic states
Biot's respirations	Irregular breaths of varying depths, interrupted by periods of apnea	Seen in spinal meningitis and other neurologic disorders
Gasping respirations	Deep breaths with spasmodic inspiratory effort	A sign of respiratory distress, commonly seen in persons experiencing severe pain, panic, acute airway obstruction, or acute pulmonary embolism
Obstructive breathing pattern	Gradual rise in the end-expiratory level during forced rapid breathing Rising end-expiratory level with forced expirations	Seen when retained secretions, bronchospasm, or other obstructive processes cause air trapping in the lungs and respiratory distress

Data from Kersten, L.D. (1989). *Comprehensive respiratory nursing: A decision-making approach.* Philadelphia: W. B. Saunders.

Respiratory Pattern. Note the rate, depth, and pattern of speech coordinated with respiration. People with impaired respiration often speak only a few words before stopping for a breath. Breathing patterns are summarized in Table 45–2. Observe the chest wall during inspiration. People with respiratory dysfunction may use muscles in the neck and shoulder girdle to assist inhalation. Retraction of the ribs and the intercostal muscles may be observed during labored breathing. Labored exhalation may be a grunting-like expiratory effort with abdominal muscle assistance or prolongation of expiratory time.

Other Inspection Points. Inspection also includes observation of

▶ the distal digits for clubbing
▶ color of nailbeds
▶ body skin color and temperature
▶ swelling in extremities or dependent body parts

► level of consciousness
► pulse rate
► presence of pulsus paradoxus (drop in blood pressure of more than 10 mm Hg during inspiration)

AUSCULTATION

Auscultate the chest in a systematic manner, proceeding downward and from side to side (see Chapter 33). Auscultation areas for a quick chest examination are shown in Figure 45-3. The black circles indicate basic areas always auscultated during any chest examination in clinic, hospital, home, and other settings. The other circles mark areas used for a more complete examination as indicated by the specific situation.

In the anterior chest, the basic area is at or slightly lateral to the midclavicular line. This location ensures detection of bronchial breath sounds from lower lobe

consolidation (replacement of air in alveoli with a liquid or solid), as in pneumonia. Ask the person to abduct the arms for auscultation of the lateral inferior area—at the level of about the sixth rib, the midaxillary line, or the posterior-axillary line for supine, critically ill persons. In the posterior chest, when you reach the last auscultation area at the lung base, ask the person to cough once or twice. This maneuver helps elicit adventitious lung sounds. The clinical implications of adventitious and other abnormal lung sounds are summarized in Table 45-3.

Laboratory and Diagnostic Studies

Complete assessment of an individual's respiratory status includes a review of the data obtained from laboratory and diagnostic studies. This information pro-

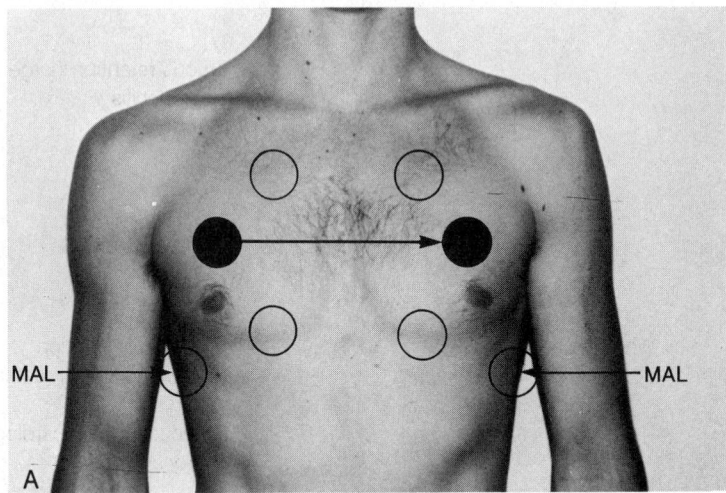

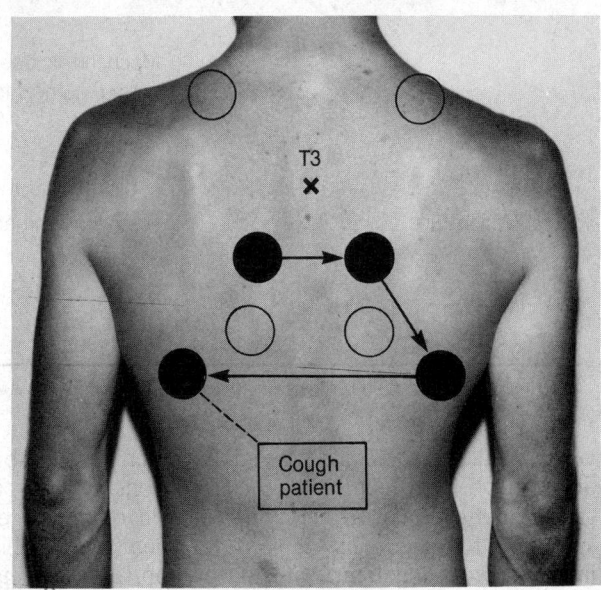

▲ *Figure 45-3*

Auscultation areas for quick examination of the anterior *(A)* and posterior *(B)* chest regions. MAL, midaxillary line; T3, third thoracic vertebra. (Reprinted with permission from Kersten, L.D. [1989]. *Comprehensive respiratory nursing: A decision-making approach.* Philadelphia: W.B. Saunders.)

TABLE 45-3. Clinical Implications of Abnormal Lung Sounds

Abnormal Sound	Associated Problems	Implications for Treatment

Absent to decreased breath sounds	Impaired ventilation
	  Hypoventilation
	  Severe atelectasis, consolidation, or compression of tissue
		More aggressive bronchial hygiene measures (e.g., coughing, deep breathing), frequent position changes, early ambulation

Bronchial or bronchovesicular breath sound	Lung consolidation or compression of tissue	

Crackles (rales)	Impaired ventilation
	  Atelectasis
	Mucus retention (small airways)
	Fluid retention (small airways)
	  Fluid overload
	  Left ventricular failure
	Interstitial fibrosis ("dry" Velcro crackles)
		More aggressive bronchial hygiene measures, frequent position changes, early ambulation
		Diuretics, fluid intake restrictions, low-salt diet, and other measures to treat heart failure
		None; sounds are from chronic disease; important only when they increase in number or become "wet"-sounding, as in early left ventricular failure

Rhonchi	Fluid retention (large airways)
	  Pulmonary edema
	
	Mucus retention (large airways)
	  Bronchitis
	  Pneumonia
		Immediate medical intervention with diuretics, cardiac drugs, morphine, aminophylline, rotating tourniquets, etc.
		Aggressive bronchial hygiene measures including postural drainage and endotracheal suctioning when ineffective cough is present
		When wheezing is also present, bronchial hygiene measures may be ineffective unless bronchodilators are given simultaneously to open airways and facilitate expectoration

Wheezes	Bronchoconstriction Bronchospasm (asthma) Bronchospasm (cardiogenic, as in pulmonary edema) Mechanical obstruction of the airway (e.g., tumor, foreign object)	Open airways with bronchodilators, relaxation exercises, psychologic support; determine etiology Give aminophylline and morphine to decrease pulmonary vascular resistance and relieve bronchospasm and anxiety; give diuretics to eliminate excess fluid in the lung Medical evaluation to determine cause; encourage deep breathing to improve lung ventilation; push fluids to liquefy secretions and facilitate their removal past constricted area
Pleural friction rub	Pleural inflammation (pleuritis)	Treat inflammatory process with antibiotics or drugs specific to underlying disease process; encourage deep breathing to keep the lung expanded and prevent atelectasis

From Kersten, L.D. (1989). *Comprehensive respiratory nursing: A decision-making approach.* Philadelphia: W. B. Saunders.

vides a fuller understanding of the person's condition and can be used to monitor the effectiveness of respiratory interventions. In addition, you will often be responsible for preparing persons for these tests. This includes providing them with the appropriate teaching and assessing their understanding.

SPUTUM EXAMINATION

Sputum examination is routinely used to assess individuals with respiratory disorders. The most commonly performed analysis is culture and sensitivity. This test is used to diagnose respiratory infection and determine the infecting organism's vulnerability to specific antibiotics. A Gram stain may be performed to determine whether the organisms are gram-positive or gram-negative. Because the results of this test can be obtained more quickly (in a few hours) than those of a culture and sensitivity study (24 to 48 hours), it is often used to select antibiotic therapy until a more definitive diagnosis can be made. An acid-fast stain, which identifies mycobacteria, may be performed when tuberculosis is suspected. Cytologic testing (examination of cells) of the sputum is done when malignancy is suspected.

Sputum is best collected early in the morning, when it is more plentiful and concentrated from pooling in the lungs overnight. If possible, the person should cough deeply and expectorate into the appropriate sterile container with lid. This should be labeled and transported immediately to the laboratory. When the person is unable to produce a specimen, sputum may be obtained through nasotracheal suctioning.

THROAT CULTURE

A throat culture may be ordered if a streptococcal infection of the throat ("strep throat") is suspected. Isolation and identification of group A beta-hemolytic streptococci allows early treatment of the disease, which prevents potential complications. Throat cultures may also be performed to screen for asymptomatic carriers of organisms such as *Neisseria meningitidis*, which causes meningitis.

To obtain the culture, have the person tilt the head back. Using a tongue depressor, swab the tonsillar areas from side to side, including any inflamed or purulent sites. Place the swab directly into the culture tube, label it appropriately, and send it to the laboratory.

COMPLETE BLOOD COUNT

The results of several blood tests may be used to assess the person's oxygenation. A complete blood cell count provides information about the oxygen-carrying capacity of the blood through measurement of the red blood cell count, the hematocrit (percentage of red blood cells in the plasma), and the hemoglobin (the component of the red blood cell that carries oxygen). The complete blood count also includes a white blood cell count, which may indicate the presence of infection if it is elevated.

ARTERIAL BLOOD GASES

Arterial blood gas analysis provides direct information about the person's ventilatory function. A sample of blood is taken from a superficial artery (usually the radial or brachial) and analyzed with precise instruments. The results of the test indicate the pH level of the blood (to determine if alkalosis or acidosis is present), the partial pressures of oxygen and carbon dioxide present, and the oxygen saturation. This information is essential for accurately evaluating gas exchange and acid-base balance and for monitoring the

TABLE 45–4. *Normal Arterial Blood Gas Values*

Value		What It Indicates
pH	7.35–7.45	Acid-base balance
$PaCO_2$	38–42 mm Hg	Level of ventilation
PaO_2	80–100 mm Hg	Level of oxygenation
HCO_3^-	24–30 mEq/L	Degree of renal function in acid-base balance
SaO_2	96% or greater	The oxygen saturation of available hemoglobin

effectiveness of respiratory therapy. The normal values for arterial blood gases are shown in Table 45–4.

PULSE OXIMETRY

Pulse oximetry is a noninvasive method of measuring oxygen saturation. The oximeter is a noninvasive device that transmits light pulses through areas with dense artery networks, such as the earlobe or finger, to measure oxygen saturation in the area (Fig. 45–4). The measurements obtained from the oximeter are not as accurate as those obtained through arterial blood testing because they may be affected by peripheral vasoconstriction or incorrect application of the probe. However, they are usually accurate enough for trends in oxygenation to be determined. Because oximetry is quick, easy, and cost effective, it is commonly used to monitor oxygenation problems and the effects of respiratory interventions in most settings, including the home.[7,30]

PULMONARY FUNCTION TESTS

Pulmonary function tests provide an indication of how well a person's chest wall, respiratory muscles, and lung tissue move gas in and out of the lungs. Lung mechanics are determined by having the person breathe through a mouthpiece; the volume of air moving in and out is measured, then various lung capacities are calculated. The relationship between lung volume and capacity is shown in Figure 45–5. Some tests also measure gas diffusion in the lungs. Parameters of basic pulmonary function tests are shown in Table 45–5.

Basic pulmonary function tests may be done in the office or at the bedside by use of a simple spirometer. More sophisticated testing requires a laboratory setting. Persons who wear dentures should have them in during testing to ensure a good seal around the mouthpiece. After testing, provide a rest period because the breathing effort required for pulmonary function tests may be tiring.

CHEST X-RAYS

Chest x-rays provide basic diagnostic information about chest disorders. They can detect such respiratory conditions as pneumonia, **pneumothorax** (the presence of air in the pleural space between parietal and visceral pleurae), **atelectasis** (collapse of all, or a portion of,

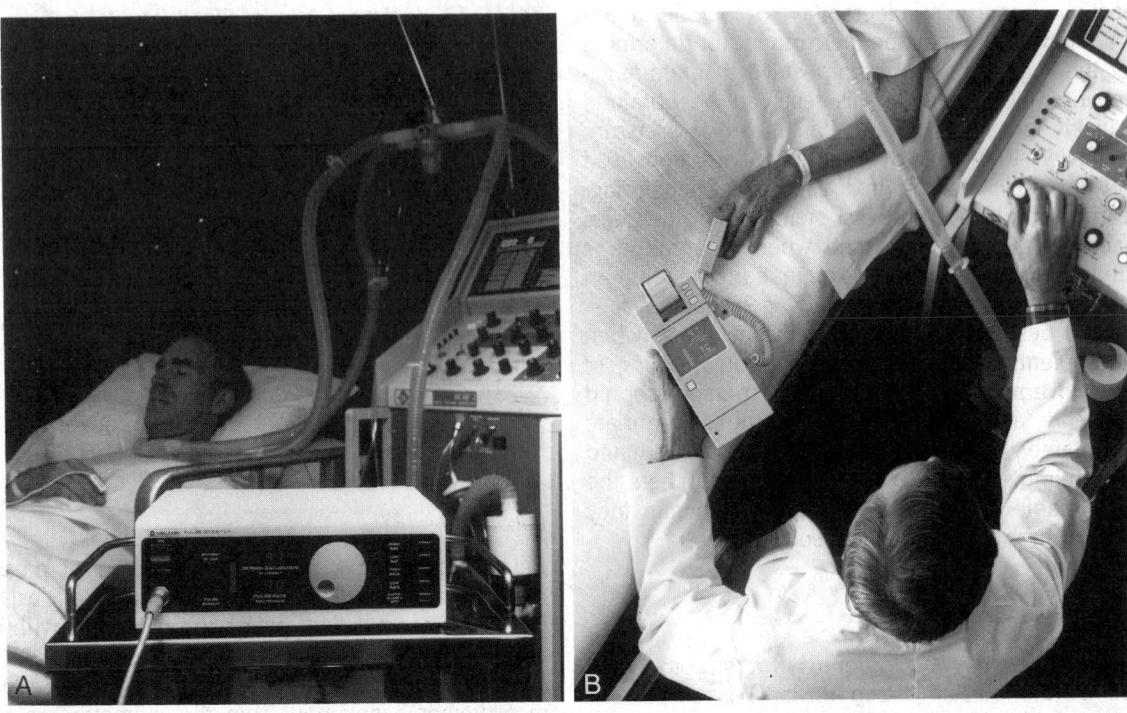

▲ *Figure 45–4*

Finger pulse oximetry. *A,* The finger oximetry unit may be used at the bedside for continuous monitoring of oxygen saturation (top digital reading) and pulse rate in beats per minute (bottom digital reading). *B,* A lightweight portable unit may be carried by the nurse for intermittent, on-the-spot checks in hospital, clinic, or home settings. This Nellcor N-10 model has both a digital display and a printer attachment that provides a copy of oximetry results for immediate interpretation. (Courtesy of Nellcor Inc., Hayward, CA.)

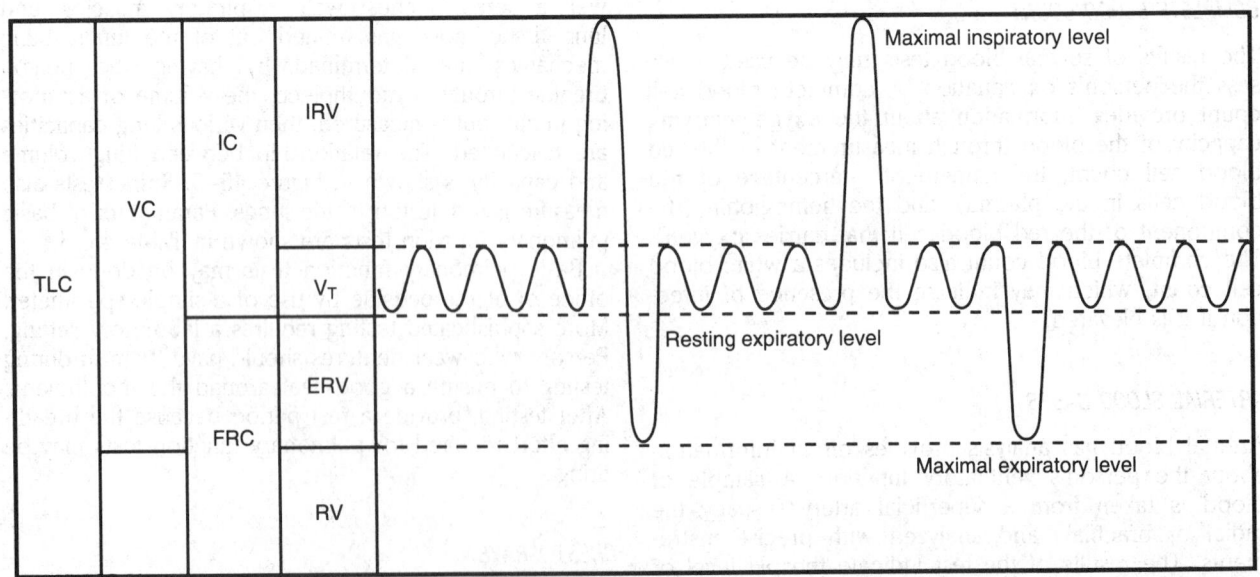

▲ *Figure 45–5*

Relationships of lung volumes and capacities. TLC, Total lung capacity; VC, vital capacity; IC, inspiratory capacity; FRC, functional residual capacity; IRV, inspiratory reserve volume; VT, tidal volume; ERV, expiratory reserve volume; RV, residual volume. (Reprinted with permission from Black, J.M., & Matassarin-Jacobs, E. (1993). *Luckmann and Sorensen's medical-surgical nursing* [4th ed.]. Philadelphia: W.B. Saunders.)

TABLE 45-5. Basic Pulmonary Function Tests

Test	Description
Tests of Lung Volume	
Tidal volume (V_T)	Volume of air inhaled or exhaled with each breath during quiet breathing
Residual volume (RV)	Amount of air that remains in lungs after a maximal exhalation
Inspiratory reserve volume (IRV)	Maximum amount of air that can be inspired after a normal inspiration
Expiratory reserve volume (ERV)	Maximum amount of air that can be exhaled after a resting expiratory level
Tests of Lung Capacity	
Total lung capacity (TLC)	Amount of air in lungs at the end of a maximal inspiration
Vital capacity (VC)	Amount of air expelled from the lungs after a maximal inhalation; the expulsion of air may be slow (slow VC) or fast (forced VC)
Functional residual capacity (FRC)	Volume of air remaining in the lungs at the end of normal expiration
Inspiratory capacity (IC)	Largest volume of air that can be inspired in one breath from the resting expiratory level
Tests of the Mechanics of Breathing	
Forced vital capacity (FVC)	Amount of air forcefully (with maximal effort) expelled from the lungs after a maximal inhalation
Forced expiratory volume in 1 second (FEV_1)	Amount of air expelled from the lungs during the first second of the FVC
FEV_1/FVC (%)	The percentage of the FVC exhaled in 1 second; commonly called the FEV_1%
Peak expiratory flow rate	The highest flow rate during FVC, measured in liters per minute

the normally aerated lung tissue), and lung tumors. They may also be used to detect broken ribs; to determine the presence and location of foreign bodies; and to check for correct placement of invasive equipment, such as endotracheal tubes (artificial airways placed in the nose or mouth and passed to just above the tracheal carina). Successive x-rays are often used to monitor the person's respiratory progress.

BRONCHOSCOPY

In certain situations, more involved techniques may be needed to visualize pulmonary structures. Bronchoscopy involves the passage of a flexible, fiberoptic tube into the tracheobronchial tree. This allows direct inspection of the larynx, trachea, and bronchi in order to locate sources of bleeding or tumors. Bronchoscopy may also be used to obtain specimens for tissue biopsy or secretion samples, to remove foreign bodies and mucus plugs, and to implant medications for tumor treatment.

Bronchoscopy is usually performed under local anesthesia with sedation. However, in some cases, general anesthesia may be required. The client should be kept NPO for at least 6 to 8 hours before the procedure. Have the person remove any dentures, and note the presence of any loose teeth. After the procedure, keep the person's head elevated. Monitor vital signs and assess breath sounds and respiratory rate and rhythm. Let the person know that fluids will be permitted after the gag and swallow reflexes return, usually about 2 hours after the procedure. Throat discomfort and temporary voice loss are common, so provide the person with paper and pencil to facilitate communication. Warm saline gargles and lozenges may help soothe the throat.

LUNG SCAN

Lung scans may be performed to evaluate perfusion or ventilation of the lungs. In a perfusion scan, a radioactive contrast agent is injected into the vein. The radioactive particles are "taken up" (retained) in the pulmonary capillary beds. The scanner can then display the distribution of blood flow through the lungs. This scan is most useful in detecting pulmonary vascular obstructions, such as pulmonary emboli. In a ventilation scan, the person inhales a mixture of radioactive gas and oxygen. The scanner then displays the air spaces in the lungs. This scan is useful in detecting regional differences in lung function. When the ventilation scan is performed together with the perfusion scan, the information obtained can be used to distinguish between different types of parenchymal disease.

THORACENTESIS

When **pleural effusion** (the presence of fluid in the pleural space) is suspected, thoracentesis may be performed to determine the cause of the effusion and to remove the fluid, if it is interfering with respiratory function. Thoracentesis involves inserting a needle through the chest wall and into the pleural space. This is usually done under a local anesthetic, with the person sitting up and leaning forward. Fluid obtained from the thoracentesis is usually analyzed to determine the cause and to check for the presence of infection. After the procedure, a chest x-ray is obtained to assess for any complications, such as pneumothorax. Watch the person closely for the development of respiratory distress.

NURSING DIAGNOSIS

Once you have analyzed the key findings from your assessment, you are ready to develop your nursing diagnostic statements. Nursing diagnoses most directly related to respiratory dysfunction are *Impaired Gas Exchange, Ineffective Airway Clearance,* and *Ineffective Breathing Pattern.* The first two are discussed in the Nursing Diagnosis Profiles for this chapter. Other nursing diagnoses commonly encountered in clients with respiratory disease include

▶ *Activity Intolerance*
▶ *Anxiety*
▶ *High Risk for Aspiration*
▶ *Body Image Disturbance*
▶ *Impaired Verbal Communication*
▶ *Ineffective Individual Coping*
▶ *Ineffective Denial*
▶ *Fatigue*
▶ *High Risk for Infection*
▶ *Knowledge Deficit*
▶ *Impaired Physical Mobility*
▶ *Altered Nutrition, Less Than Body Requirements*
▶ *Altered Oral Mucous Membrane*
▶ *Powerlessness*
▶ *Self-Care Deficit*
▶ *Sleep Pattern Disturbance*
▶ *Social Isolation*

To see how some of these diagnoses result from the clustering of data and how the diagnoses relate to health care needs, see Table 45–6.

PLANNING

You will find it helpful to identify one to three top-priority respiratory diagnoses. This approach facilitates care for the person with a respiratory disorder, who typically has multiple physical and psychosocial problems.

These three questions help in the identification and ranking of diagnoses:

▶ What are the person's most acute needs? Acute needs, such as the need to maintain a patent airway to supply oxygen, are top priorities.
▶ What is the person's overall health status? Is the health status better? Worse? Status quo? Is the person terminally ill? A deteriorating physical condition typically indicates an acute need for more aggressive respiratory interventions. For the terminally ill person, however, a deteriorating condition might suggest the need to focus on comfort measures as opposed to aggressive respiratory interventions.
▶ Which health problems are most important to the person and the family? Incorporate the person's and family's top-priority concerns into the care plan. In-

NURSING DIAGNOSIS PROFILE

Ineffective Airway Clearance

Definition. A state in which an individual is unable to clear secretions or obstructions from the respiratory tract in order to maintain airway patency.

Classification. Exchanging 1.5.1.2.

Defining Characteristics. Defining characteristics for this diagnosis include objective observations of dyspnea, abnormal lung sounds (e.g., rhonchi, wheezes, crackles), and change in the rate or depth of respiration (e.g., tachypnea). Usually, the person with this diagnosis is unable to keep the airways patent because of ineffective or marginally effective cough, with or without sputum production. Cyanosis and other signs of a blood gas abnormality develop when the airway obstruction becomes severe.

Sample Related Factors. Ineffective coughing may be related to a perceptual or cognitive impairment or to a lack of knowledge regarding proper technique. It may also be related to the pain of airway hypersensitivity or other pain on attempts to cough, to fatigue, or to blocked airways (from infection, trauma, tumor, or foreign object).

Concept Description. This diagnosis assumes airway obstruction, usually from retained secretions or aspiration of foreign material. Chest assessment findings, such as adventitious lung sounds, account for the defining characteristics. When alveoli cannot fully inflate and when secretions accumulate in the chest, the person is at risk for pneumonia or some other type of chest infection.

Examples. Depending on the specific assessment data, this diagnostic category could be applicable in the following situations among others:

▶ The person with chronic obstructive pulmonary disease (COPD)
▶ The person with an acute respiratory disorder that results in increased lung secretions, such as pneumonia.
▶ The person with pooled lung secretions due to decreased mobility secondary to orthopedic disorders, surgery, or neurologic disorders.

Related/Similar Nursing Diagnoses. Ineffective Airway Clearance must be differentiated from *Impaired Gas Exchange* and *Ineffective Breathing Pattern.* For all of these diagnoses, mucus retention or difficulties mobilizing secretions may exist to some degree. However, for *Ineffective Airway Clearance,* secretions or foreign matter is *primarily* rather than secondarily responsible for the diagnosis. The obstruction is often acute, as during the postoperative period. It may also be seen without grossly abnormal mechanics of breathing, as occurs in the person with COPD who has an ineffective breathing pattern related to lung hyperinflation and increased work of breathing. The diagnosis *Ineffective Airway Clearance* does not assume a blood gas abnormality, as in the case of the diagnosis *Impaired Gas Exchange.*

NURSING DIAGNOSIS PROFILE

Impaired Gas Exchange

Definition. The state in which the individual experiences a decreased passage of oxygen and/or carbon dioxide between the alveoli of the lungs and the vascular system.

Classification. Exchanging 1.5.1.1.

Defining Characteristics. Defining characteristics include an inability to move respiratory secretions. All other characteristics are mental and behavioral changes, such as confusion, somnolence, restlessness, general irritability, and uncooperative behavior. When these changes occur, the person may become unable or unwilling to deep breathe and participate in other respiratory therapy. Blood gas abnormalities develop, notably hypercapnia and hypoxemia with or without hypoxia.

Sample Related Factors. The only related factor for this diagnosis is ventilation/perfusion imbalance.

Concept Description. This diagnosis assumes an abnormal ventilation/perfusion ratio in the lungs and an actual or impending blood gas abnormality. In the clinic setting, the abnormality may be restricted to one region of the lung (e.g., early interstitial fibrosis) and produce no change in arterial blood gases. In most acute and home settings, the abnormality is progressive or severe enough to produce hypoxemia, a ventilatory problem (alveolar hyperventilation or hypoventilation), or both. In some cases, the diagnosis *Impaired Gas Exchange* is made when a blood gas abnormality is suspected and when the medical diagnosis and associated respiratory problems remain unknown or undetermined. An example is the person newly admitted to a health agency whose arterial blood gas analysis results are pending.

Examples. Depending on the specific assessment data, this diagnostic category could be applicable to the following situations:

▶ A person with blood gas results that show a decreased PaO_2 with increased $PaCO_2$ with the client breathing room air.
▶ A person with a medical disorder that causes an increase in lung secretions, such as recurrent pneumonia, where perfusion of gases is impaired by the secretions.
▶ A person who experienced cardiac arrest and had cardiopulmonary resuscitation.

Related/Similar Nursing Diagnoses. The diagnosis *Impaired Gas Exchange* is often made simultaneously with one or more related diagnoses, such as *Ineffective Airway Clearance, Ineffective Breathing Pattern,* or *Anxiety.* Differentiation is not difficult because this diagnosis is based primarily on results of blood gas analysis or other signs and symptoms of a blood gas abnormality.

formal discussions at the bedside or in a family conference facilitate this process.

General outcomes for common respiratory diagnoses are given in Table 45–7.

When writing outcomes, use Table 45–7 as a guide only. Outcomes must be adapted to the specific clinical setting, the person, and the family. For example, consider Mr. Tipps, a hospitalized 60-year-old man with severe emphysema (a chronic obstructive lung disease) and a nursing diagnosis of *Ineffective Breathing Pattern*. For Mr. Tipps, the general outcome listed in Table 45–7 is unrealistic. He will never have a normal breathing pattern because of his grossly abnormal mechanics of breathing. In this case, you might review the medical chart to determine Mr. Tipps' baseline respiratory rate (24/minute) and basic pulmonary function test measurements (e.g., tidal volume of 200 ml) before his acute illness. Then, in consultation with the respiratory care practitioner, clinical nurse specialist, or physician, select a reasonable outcome. The outcome should be possible by a target date, such as the date of hospital discharge or a 1-month period of time. In this example, you can see the value of reviewing past results of pulmonary function tests and consulting others to help in the determination of realistic outcomes.

Additional examples of outcomes might be the following:

▶ Demonstrates on auscultation an increase in breath sounds over the right lower lobe within the next 24 hours.
▶ Begins to express feelings relating to new tracheostomy.
▶ Maintains a PaO_2 greater than 60 mm Hg (55 mm Hg for a person with severe chronic respiratory disease) at rest, during exercise, and during sleep at night.
▶ Reports performing activities of daily living without fatigue or any increase in shortness of breath.

It is important to consider client teaching needs as you plan outcomes. When planning client teaching, a key question to ask is, What changes in this person's (family's) knowledge, skills, attitudes, and practices are needed to attain the selected outcomes? Examples of respiratory learning outcomes and associated evaluation criteria are shown in Table 45–8.

When planning education sessions, make sure each teaching/learning situation is supported by printed materials specific to the person's disease, comprehension level, cultural background, and interest. Perhaps the best source of educational materials is your local American Lung Association, which has numerous pamphlets on a variety of respiratory topics. These topics include specific respiratory diseases, smoking cessation, avoidance of second-hand smoke, flu shots, home control of allergies, oxygen therapy, requirements for traveling with oxygen, and pulmonary rehabilitation programs. Keep such pamphlets readily available in clinical areas. Ready accessibility helps you meet teaching/learning needs at the best possible time: when the person recognizes a need, feels well enough for social interaction (dyspnea under control), and indicates a willingness to learn.

NURSING INTERVENTION

Two main categories of nursing interventions for persons with respiratory disorders are basic respiratory

TABLE 45-6. Clustering Signs and Symptoms to Determine Nursing Diagnoses and Health Needs

Clusters of Signs and Symptoms	Related Factors	Nursing Diagnosis	Health Need
Cluster 1			
Wheezing and rhonchi on auscultation* Increased blood pressure, pulse, and respiratory rate No sputum production	Bronchoconstriction Mucus retention Potential chest infection	*Ineffective Airway Clearance* R/T bronchoconstriction and mucus retention	Bronchodilator medication to open airways Interventions to mobilize mucus in the chest (e.g., deep breathing, coughing, ambulation)
Cluster 2			
History of COPD Tachypnea Use of accessory muscles of respiration Dyspnea and fatigue during activities of daily living*	Increased work of breathing	*Activity Intolerance* R/T increased work of breathing	Breathing retraining to control dyspnea Energy conservation techniques to reduce work of breathing and fatigue (e.g., walking slowly instead of quickly)
Cluster 3			
Dyspnea and fatigue Decreased fluid and food intake Progressive weight loss	Poor nutrition Possible dehydration	*Altered Nutrition: Less than Body Requirements* R/T dyspnea and fatigue	Nutritional evaluation and counseling Daily intake and output determinations
Cluster 4			
History of asthma Difficulty sleeping because of wheezing* Dark circles under eyes Bronchodilator inhaler at bedside	Sleep deprivation Bronchospasm	*Sleep Pattern Disturbance* R/T bronchospasm	Further evaluation of the effectiveness of bronchodilator medications, especially the inhaler
Cluster 5			
Complains of fear of suffocation* On continuous oxygen Oximetry: SaO$_2$ = 95% Vital signs stable Recent pulmonary embolism (a restrictive disease)	Fear of suffocation Potential for hypoxemia	*Fear* R/T risk of suffocation and death	Psychologic reassurance and support Monitoring effectiveness of oxygen therapy
Cluster 6			
7-day coma* Supine position in bed* Inspiratory and expiratory snoring sounds Decreased breath sounds on auscultation	Upper airway obstruction Potential for aspiration	*Impaired Gas Exchange* R/T upper airway obstruction *High Risk for Aspiration* R/T decreased ability to manage own secretions	Position change to a side-lying position Other interventions to ensure airway patency (e.g., airway suctioning, as needed)
Cluster 7			
PaO$_2$ = 75 mm Hg*	Hypoxemia	*Impaired Gas Exchange* R/T hypoxemia	Oxygen administration

TABLE 45-6. Clustering Signs and Symptoms to Determine Nursing Diagnoses and Health Needs Continued

Clusters of Signs and Symptoms	Related Factors	Nursing Diagnosis	Health Need
Cluster 8			
$PaCO_2$ = 47 mm Hg	Alveolar hypoventilation (ventilatory failure)	*Impaired Gas Exchange* R/T alveolar hypoventilation	Ventilatory support, as indicated by the situation (e.g., airway establishment and maintenance, mechanical ventilation, as directed by physician)

* Key cues.

therapeutic measures and measures to maintain a patent (open) airway. Both of these categories require client teaching. Individuals should be taught about the nature of the respiratory disorder, preventive measures (e.g., receiving flu shots in the fall, drinking plenty of fluids), and how to implement specific interventions ordered by the physician (e.g., oxygen and medication administration).

If the person smokes, teaching efforts should also be directed at the risks of this behavior. "Stop smoking" programs, sponsored by the American Lung Association and other community organizations, provide support groups and individual "do-it-yourself" programs. Encourage smokers to become involved in such programs.

Keep in mind that *no program is effective unless the person has a desire and firm commitment to quit smoking.*[12]

TABLE 45-7. General Outcomes for Common Respiratory Nursing Diagnoses

Nursing Diagnosis	General Outcome
Ineffective Airway Clearance	Demonstrates no evidence of airway obstruction or secretion retention; resumes normal breath sounds
Ineffective Breathing Pattern	Resumes normal respiratory rate, rhythm, and depth
Impaired Gas Exchange	Shows normal blood gas levels or shows no evidence of respiratory distress
Activity Intolerance	Alters the pacing of activities of daily living to minimize dyspnea and fatigue
Ineffective Individual Coping	Identifies or implements positive strategies to manage effects of respiratory disease
Sleep Pattern Disturbance	Experiences at least 4 hours of uninterrupted sleep twice within 24 hours

You may elicit commitment by pointing out the positive benefits of smoking cessation. Benefits include reduced medical bills; reduced number of days missed from work because of illness; reduced life, automobile, and household insurance premiums; improved overall health; and sweeter-smelling breath, clothes, personal effects, and living or working areas. Even with this knowledge, however, the person may not be willing or able to break the addictive smoking behavior until after experiencing several hospitalizations for respiratory failure.

Basic Respiratory Therapeutic Measures

Respiratory therapy is concerned with the repair, maintenance, and prevention of complications of the respiratory system. Therapy is individualized and goal oriented. For one person, the goal may be to clear the airway of secretions. For another, the prevention of postoperative atelectasis may be the primary goal.

The overall goal of all respiratory therapy is to maintain lung function sufficient to support life.

Respiratory treatment modalities are used either alone or in combination. Basic measures may be grouped into eight general categories: mobilization maneuvers, hydration, chest physical therapy, oxygen administration, medication, positive-pressure breathing, respiratory exercises, and rehabilitation.

MOBILIZATION MANEUVERS

Mobilization maneuvers are intended to prevent secretion retention in the lungs and to assist spontaneous removal of secretions that are retained. The term *mobilization maneuvers* thus refers to more than attempts to get the client to move physically, although such attempts are frequently part of the approach. The term refers to the mobilization of secretions, not mobilization of the client. Unless the client's condition prohibits a specific maneuver, mobilization maneuvers should include increasing client mobility, turning and positioning, and promoting an effective cough.

TABLE 45-8. Examples of Respiratory Learning Outcomes and Evaluation Criteria

Outcomes	Evaluation Criteria
Main outcome: Administers an effective bronchodilator aerosol treatment without assistance	Main evaluation criteria: In 3 days, 1. the client reports minimal to no wheezing and no difficulty taking scheduled aerosol treatments 2. the nurse observes correct technique 3. the nurse auscultates good ventilation over all lung lobes with minimal to absent wheezing
Cognitive Outcomes	
1. States the name, dosage, therapeutic effects, and side effects of the bronchodilator medication	1. Repeats the name, correct dosage, one therapeutic effect, and three side effects of metaproterenol (Alupent) when asked by the nurse
2. States the purpose of the hand-held nebulizer used to deliver the aerosol	2. When asked by family members, explains how the nebulizer's aerosol transports the bronchodilator deep into the lungs
3. States what to do when the nebulizer does not work properly	3. Looks up the equipment vendor's name and telephone number in the telephone book when asked to do so
Psychomotor Outcomes	
4. Demonstrates correct technique for addition of medication to the nebulizer	4a. Uses a dropper to measure the correct amount of medication b. Correctly adds the medication to the nebulizer c. Holds the nebulizer so that the medication lies by the nebulizer's capillary
5. Demonstrates correct technique during aerosol delivery	5. Demonstrates a comfortable deep-breathing pattern with a 1- to 3-second end-inspiratory pause and a treatment lasting no longer than 10–20 minutes
Affective Outcomes	
6. Takes responsibility for learning and refining treatments	6. Remembers and takes his own treatments at home as reported by his wife
7. Takes responsibility for administering his own treatments at bedtime and on arising	7. Takes his treatments at the scheduled times for 1 month without fail and without assistance as reported by the client and his wife
8. Consults his wife or equipment vendor whenever equipment problems arise	8. Successfully calls the equipment vendor within 12 hours when an equipment problem arises at home

Adapted from Kersten, L.D. (1989). *Comprehensive respiratory nursing: A decision-making approach.* Philadelphia: W. B. Saunders.

Mobilization maneuvers stimulate deep breathing, facilitate the redistribution of air and blood in the lungs, aid in drainage of secretions, promote effective coughing, and aid in recirculation of blood throughout the body.

Getting a person involved in mobilization maneuvers requires teaching and encouragement to gain the person's cooperation. Significant others should be involved in the process. Simply telling someone to do certain mobilization maneuvers does not mean they will be done.

Increasing Client Mobility. Recall that immobility affects every system of the body including the respiratory system (see Chapter 35). In the respiratory system, gravity combined with immobility leads to pooling of secretions in the gravity-dependent areas of the lungs. Immobility causes the closure of some small airways and may also interfere with normal ventilation. This leads to inadequate ventilation and respiratory impairment. Hypoxemia is the end result of immobility and gravitational pooling of secretions. Hypoventilation and carbon dioxide retention result from diminished ventilation.

Many people with chronic lung disease have a predisposition to venous stasis. Prolonged inactivity promotes blood stasis in dependent limbs and increased risk of pulmonary emboli. Encourage people with a history of respiratory problems to move their toes and feet frequently, to sit with legs elevated to promote venous return, and to wear antiembolism stockings when their activity is restricted.

Some people resist physical mobilization because they fear movement will produce additional shortness of breath or pain. This is understandable, because many of these people are often fighting an exhausting battle for every breath. Be supportive and understanding while at the same time ensuring that essential mobilization activities are carried out.

Make sure that people who need oxygen administration continue to receive it during mobilization maneuvers.

Turning and Positioning. Frequent turning of people confined to bed aids the treatment of respiratory dysfunction by

▶ assisting redistribution of pulmonary blood and airflow
▶ promoting drainage of the upper lung fields
▶ preventing pooling of secretions

Turning can be hazardous, however, when lung consolidation (e.g., pneumonia) occurs and oxygenation is impaired. Such people are best positioned with the affected (consolidated) lung up so that mucus drains into major bronchi by gravity. When the affected lung is down (close to the mattress), hypoxemia is likely to occur because ventilation decreases while blood perfusion increases. However, the reduction in PaO_2 that occurs when you turn the person side-to-side is unpredictable. The PaO_2 reduction may be large (as much as 100 mm Hg in the critically ill person),[39,40] or it may be small and clinically insignificant.

As a general rule, turn all persons side-to-side, without favoring one side more than the other. For persons with pneumonia, however, you may favor positions with the consolidated lung up if it maximizes the drainage of mucus and if you occasionally turn the person to the other side, as tolerated. For all persons with unilateral lung disease, check the physician's order for any contraindication to a side-lying position. When the affected lung is down, monitor for signs and symptoms of hypoxemia. Adjust the position, whenever necessary. Persons who do not tolerate a far side-lying position (90-degree turn) may tolerate a 30-degree turn to the same side.

A cough is one of the most important protective reflexes of the respiratory system. When used with deep breathing, an effective cough clears the tracheobronchial tree of excessive secretions, particulate matter, and sometimes even large pieces of debris (e.g., food). When normal airway defense mechanisms are functioning, bronchopulmonary debris and secretions are propelled upward by ciliary action to the upper trachea. Then they are swallowed or readily expectorated. When secretions are retained or impairment of the "mucociliary escalator" occurs, a cough becomes less effective. Ineffective coughing may significantly increase the energy needed to clear the airway. Many people are afraid to cough. Fear of pain and furthering the degree of shortness of breath, pre-existing respiratory disease, and certain medications may influence a person's ability to cough effectively.

Promoting an Effective Cough. Figure 45–6 shows the anatomy of an effective cough. Interventions to assist with effective coughing are listed in Table 45–9 and illustrated in Figure 45–7. Do not expect a person to remember these instructions with one explanation. Repeated teaching/learning sessions are necessary.

1 A cough is induced voluntarily to mobilize secretions. 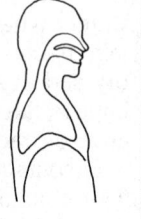	**2** The beginning of a cough starts with a deep inspiration. This distends the trachea and hyperinflates the lungs.
3 After inspiration, the glottis closes quickly and tightly while the expiratory intercostal and abdominal muscles contract forcibly. This is called the COMPRESSIVE phase because of the rise in intrathoracic and intra-abdominal pressures. 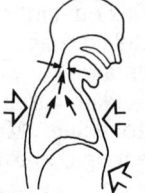	**4** After the intrathoracic pressure has reached a high level, the glottis opens slightly. Since intra-abdominal pressure is now higher than that in the thoracic cavity, the diaphragm is pushed up, producing a violent, explosive movement of air. This explosion of air is often referred to as a "pillar of air." The vital capacity must be sufficient to ensure a deep breath. If it is insufficient, the cough will be inadequate and secretions may be retained. 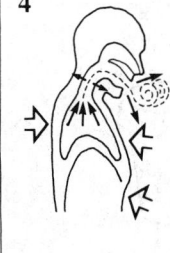

▲ *Figure 45–6*

Anatomy of a cough. (Adapted from Cherniack, R.M., & Cherniack, L. [1983]. *Respiration in health and disease* [3rd ed.]. Philadelphia: W.B. Saunders.)

TABLE 45-9. Selected Scientific Principles and Related Interventions to Assist Effective Coughing

Principle	Nursing Interventions
The movement of secretions toward the large airways stimulates irritant receptors and elicits coughing	Encourage frequent changes in body position to aid in moving secretions Increase activity level, progressing from lying to sitting to ambulation
Deep inspiration increases lung volume and widens the airway, allowing air to get behind mucus and propel it forward	Encourage slow, deep breaths before cough attempts
Forceful contraction of the expiratory muscles expels air at high flow and speed to enhance movement of mucus out of the lungs	Use thoracic splinting to assist with air expulsion; place your hands firmly along the lower lateral chest wall; while coaching a slow inhalation, begin to press against the chest wall, then squeeze during the expulsive phase of coughing For people with weak abdominal muscles or who have undergone abdominal surgery, place a pillow against the abdomen; stand behind the person, grasping the edges of the pillow; as the cough enters the expulsive phase, pull firmly to support the abdomen
Forced, harsh exhalations may collapse the airways in people with hyperreactive airway disease	Teach "huff" coughing; have person take a deep breath, then keep glottis open and cough out several times until all air is exhaled (usually 2–6 coughs); it may help to have person say the word "huff" while coughing
Prolonged exhalation aids in moving secretions more proximally	Teach persons with secretions in distal airways end-expiratory coughing; have person take a deep breath, exhale slowly, then cough once at end of exhalation

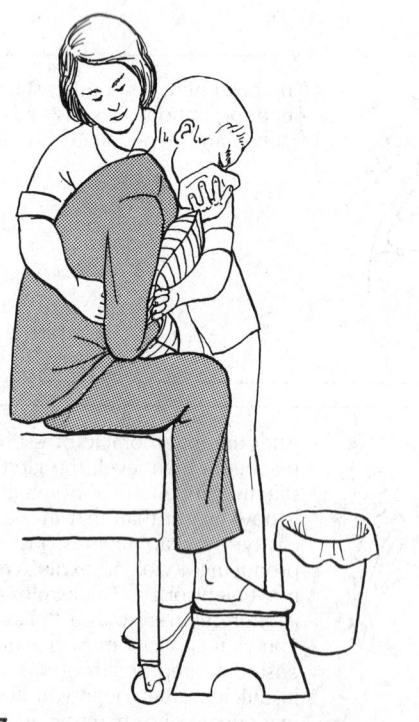

▲ *Figure 45-7*

Assisting a person to cough effectively. Use the following steps: (1) if possible, have the person sit with feet supported on a solid object; (2) support the chest and abdomen with your hands or a pillow; (3) encourage slow, deep inspiration; (4) as you hold the chest and abdomen firmly but gently, the person performs no more than two short coughing blasts per breath. Rest and encouragement between cough efforts is important.

Effective coughing may be hindered by inadequate hydration. The mucus-secreting cells normally produce 3½ ounces of mucus per day. Mucus is 95 per cent water. When there is inadequate fluid intake to maintain tracheobronchial water content, mucus becomes dry and obstructs the airway. Insufficient hydration also impairs the motility of the cilia, which aid in the clearance of tracheobronchial secretions.

Encourage people with impaired cough and those with conditions producing excess secretions to have a daily fluid intake of 2 to 4 quarts. Unless contraindicated by other medical conditions, this is an important aspect of care for people with respiratory dysfunction.

Body position influences effective coughing. Sitting is the best position, because coughing requires forward flexion motion. This is difficult to do when lying flat. Relaxed abdominal and thoracic muscles are also necessary.

Plan careful teaching/learning sessions for effective coughing. Merely telling a person to cough is not enough. The following may also be required:

▶ Pain relief with analgesics
▶ Proper body positioning
▶ Preventing hacking, ineffective, and tiring coughing
▶ Hydration
▶ Medication and treatments to help secretion removal
▶ Whole body relaxation including the abdominal muscles

Most important, remember to encourage coughing *only* when you suspect that mucus retention is a problem. In the immediate postoperative period, ask the person to take a deep breath (sustained maximal inspiration) *10 times each hour* and to cough only when he or she needs to cough up mucus.[2] This selective use of coughing is based on research findings indicating that deep breathing is the best method of preventing and treating pulmonary complications after surgery.[4,33]

HYDRATION

The human body has specific fluid requirements. Part of the total body fluid is used by the respiratory system to warm and humidify inspired air. The mucus layer of the tracheobronchial tree contains large amounts of body fluid. Many disorders affecting the respiratory system relate directly to inadequate body fluid. The respiratory system and the skin together use about 1000 ml of water per day. When physical conditions (e.g., fever, diaphoresis) or other conditions affecting fluid balance are present, the body adjusts, and supplemental fluid is necessary to maintain fluid balance. If the airway becomes dehydrated, secretions dry and increased airway resistance develops.

Hydration is supplemental fluid administration. Hydration may be done by oral (systemic) fluid administration, parenteral (intravenous) fluid administration, and topical fluid administration. Oral and parenteral hydration are discussed in Chapters 42 and 47. Topical hydration is discussed here.

The methods of topical hydration include the following:

▶ Increasing the humidity of a dry gas (e.g., with an oxygen room humidifier)
▶ Increasing room humidity (e.g., with a room humidifier)
▶ Creating an aerosol (e.g., heated nebulizers, ultrasonic nebulizers, and other types of nebulizers)

Some methods of hydration are more appropriate for home care than for acute care. Sophisticated methods of topical hydration (e.g., ultrasonic nebulizers) are used only in hospital settings unless adequate instruction, cleaning, and maintenance are available in the home.

Humidifiers. Humidifiers add water vapor to the air (increase the air humidity). Humidification equipment delivers water at room temperature, heated to body temperature, or slightly above body temperature.

Heated air is able to carry more moisture.

A humidifier is a mechanical device that delivers humidity. The most common type is a bubble-diffusion humidifier used in oxygen administration (Fig. 45–8). An impeller humidifier actually produces particles of water. These particles are too large to penetrate deeply into the tracheobronchial tree. Room humidifiers, used in many homes for upper respiratory infections, are the most common examples of this type. They require careful cleaning after use. Other, more complex forms of humidification are used with mechanical ventilators.

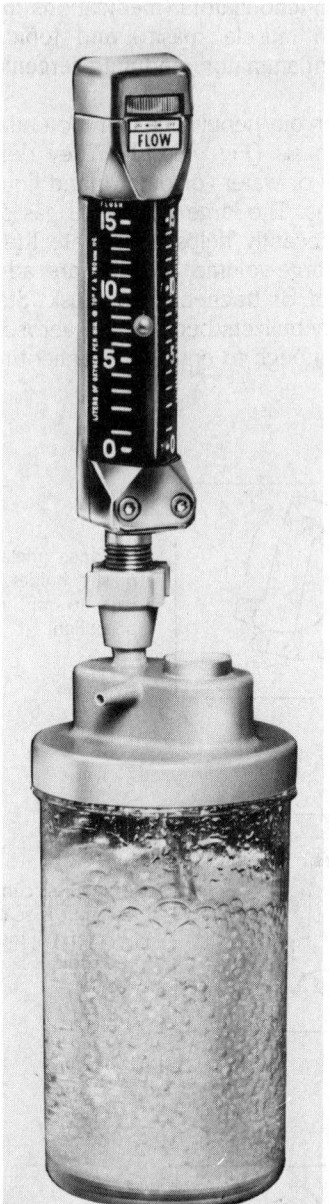

▲ *Figure 45–8*

A bubble-diffusion humidifier for use with low-flow oxygen administration devices. (Courtesy of Hudson RCI, Temecula, CA.)

Aerosolization. An aerosol is a fine suspension of a liquid or a powder carried on a stream of gas. Aerosols may be large in volume (for hydration) or may be produced in small amounts, such as dry aerosols that deliver medications topically into the airway. Devices producing an aerosol are called aerosol generators. To enter the tracheobronchial tree, a particle of liquid produced by an aerosol generator must be 1 to 3 microns in size (1 micron is equal to 3.937×10^{-5} inches).

Nebulizers produce aerosol particles of uniform size. Nebulizers may be classified as small-volume nebulizers or large-reservoir nebulizers.

Small-volume nebulizers are used for short-term or intermittent therapy and medication administration. The metered-dose inhaler is the most common type of small-volume nebulizer. It is used for topical administration of bronchodilators (medications that relax bronchial smooth muscle spasm) and topical administration of anti-inflammatory and antiallergenic medications (Fig. 45–9).

Large-reservoir nebulizers can potentially run on a continuous basis (Fig. 45–10). They deliver a dense, large volume of water (or other bland liquid) on a large volume of gas. The large volume of gas plus the dense aerosol significantly helps to hydrate the tracheobronchial tree. Large-volume aerosols are administered via either aerosol or tracheostomy mask. Sterile solutions are used in nebulizers because the aerosol particles are often small enough to enter the tracheobronchial tree.

Hazards of Hydration

Contamination. All methods of topical hydration carry a risk of contamination because all devices include a water reservoir. There is always the possibility that microorganisms may grow in the reservoir. If this occurs, microorganisms may enter the respiratory system. This hazard may be reduced or eliminated by using sterile solutions in the water reservoir and by decontaminating (sterilizing) the nebulizer and tubing every 24 hours. Decontamination is done with either cold sterilization (using a chemical solution) or ethylene oxide (gas) sterilization.

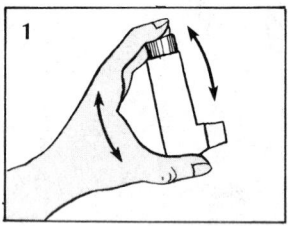

1. Place metal canister into plastic holder. Shake canister well to mix medication and propellant.

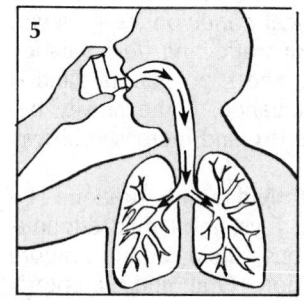

2. Depress canister if uncertain that unit is seated correctly. A full cloud of medication should be visible.

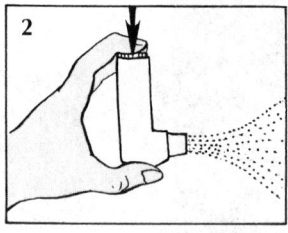

3. Exhale completely. Hold canister up to mouth.

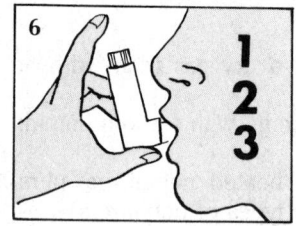

4. Open mouth. Place tip of plastic holder between the lips or 1½ inches away.

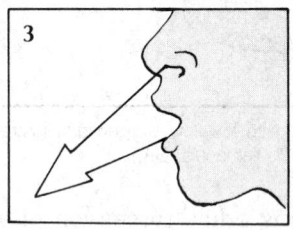

5. Depress canister into plastic holder to dispense a dose of medication. Keep mouth open, and inhale at same time as canister is depressed and medication is dispensed.

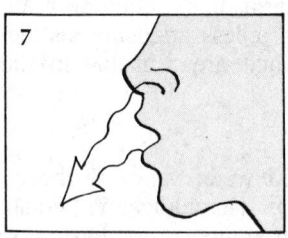

6. Hold medication in lungs for 10 seconds or as tolerated (minimum of 1 to 3 seconds).

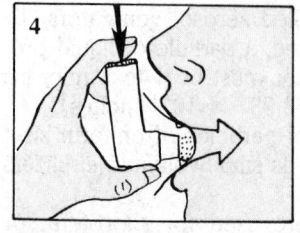

7. Exhale slowly. Wait at least two minutes before repeating steps 1 to 7. Always shake canister just before repeating steps.

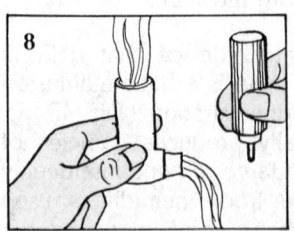

8. Wash plastic holder in warm running water at least daily. Dry and reassemble.

▲ **Figure 45–9**

Correct use of a metered dose inhaler.

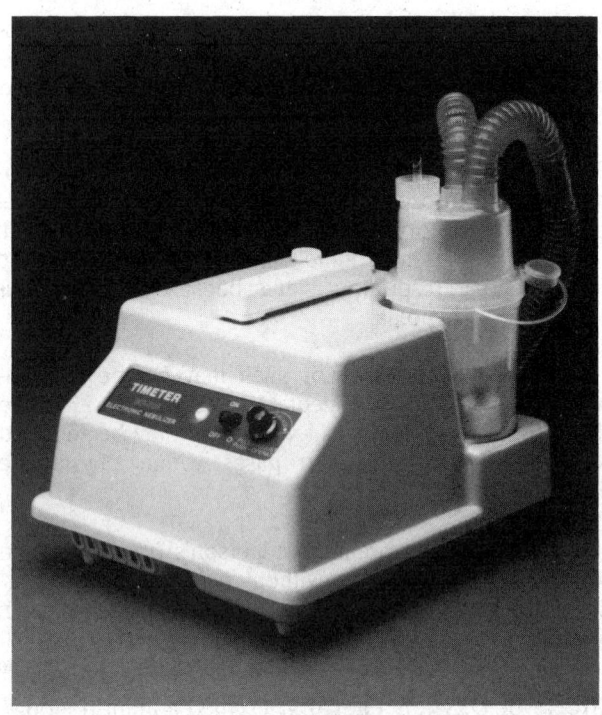

▲ *Figure 45–10*

Large-volume nebulizer. Large-volume nebulizers create a visible aerosol mist of either normal saline or distilled water. They are used for topical hydration of the airway. (Courtesy of Mistogen Equipment Co., Oakland, CA.)

Bronchospasm and Shortness of Breath. Lungs respond to irritation with spasm of the smooth muscle surrounding the airway passages. This type of spasm is called **bronchospasm.** Bronchospasm may occur during administration of any inhaled substance. Bronchospasm results in **bronchoconstriction,** or narrowing of the airway.

If sudden shortness of breath (dyspnea), cough, or audible wheeze develops while a person is receiving topical inhaled hydration, stop treatment immediately, make careful documentation, and report the incident to the physician.

Removing the source of irritation may reverse the bronchospasm. If not, parenteral and aerosolized bronchodilator agents may be required.

Overhydration. If large volumes of fluid are delivered into the tracheobronchial tree, there is a possibility of fluid overload. Overhydration is less critical in adults because the fluid is absorbed by the lungs, and excess fluid is usually carried off by the lymphatic system and drained into the circulatory system. In children, however, the balance of fluids is more critical, and respiratory system fluid overload is a greater danger.

CHEST PHYSICAL THERAPY

Hydration, aerosol medication, deep breathing, coughing, and other mobilization maneuvers may not suffi-

ciently clear retained secretions. Secretion retention is most common in gravity-dependent parts of the lungs. Secretion retention may result in serious complications (e.g., pneumonia or impaired oxygenation). If other measures are not adequate, bronchial hygiene techniques (postural drainage, chest percussion, and vibration) may be used. These techniques are usually performed by specially trained physical or respiratory therapists.

Goals of chest physical therapy include the promotion of tracheobronchial drainage, the prevention of secretion pooling, and an overall improvement in ventilation.

Chest physical therapy is a combination of postural drainage, chest percussion, and vibration. These techniques are used along with coughing, hydration, bronchodilation, and correction of improper or ineffective breathing techniques.

Postural drainage is done by placing people into specific positions to promote the gravity drainage of mucus out of the lobes of the lungs and bronchopulmonary segments and into the larger bronchi. When secretions reach upper airways, they may be coughed up spontaneously or removed by tracheobronchial suctioning (described later). Figure 45–11 shows an example of one of the postural drainage positions. Some other positions are side-to-side, supine or prone, or Trendelenburg's (i.e., the feet at a level higher than head and chest).[13]

Chest percussion (clapping) is done by rhythmically clapping on the chest with cupped hands to help loosen mucus immediately over the portion of the lung where secretions are retained. The hand should make a hollow "popping" sound as it strikes the chest wall. Chest percussion is not to be done to breast tissue, the spine, or any location off the chest wall or over a surgical incision. Done correctly, it is not painful.

Vibration is done by placing the hands flat against the chest wall and shaking (vibrating) the chest during exhalation to loosen mucus for expectoration. The shaking is done with shoulders and forearms, keeping the arms extended. Percussion and vibration help to dislodge mucus. Mechanical percussors offer the ad-

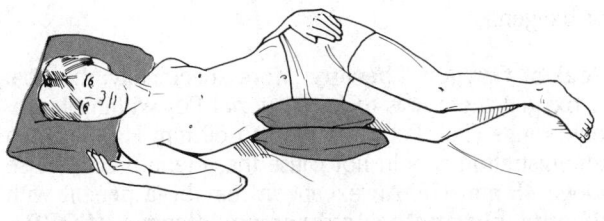

▲ *Figure 45–11*

A postural drainage position. The person is on his right side, with the left side in the upper position and the torso rotated one-quarter turn backward. The foot of the bed is elevated 14 inches, or 15 degrees. This position aids in drainage of the left upper lobe—the lingular segment. (Courtesy of Monaghan Company, Littleton, CO.)

vantages of uniform percussion and reduced therapist fatigue.

Ordered treatments are usually scheduled at these times:

► On rising in the morning (when accumulated secretions are copious)
► One hour before meals (to avoid aspiration during the treatment)
► Before sleep at night (to promote rest free of coughing and sputum production)
► Fifteen minutes after bronchodilator aerosol medication (to maximize drainage through open airways)

Chest physical therapy is not appropriate

► for people with unstable cardiovascular systems
► immediately after meals because nausea, vomiting, and aspiration of stomach contents may occur
► in people with head trauma (a head-down position increases intracranial pressure)
► for people with bone metastasis and easily fractured bones
► for people with **empyema** (pus in the pleural space)
► for people with lung tumors
► for people with hemoptysis of unknown cause

Because of the complexity of these techniques, postural drainage, chest percussion, and vibration should be done only by those specially trained in these techniques.

OXYGEN ADMINISTRATION

Oxygen administration is a common therapy for people with respiratory disorders. Oxygen is prescribed by the physician to reduce and ideally eliminate the signs and symptoms of hypoxemia and tissue hypoxia. In most situations, oxygen must be given in precise amounts. Too much may cause toxic effects. Too little may cause irreversible tissue damage. The following discussion provides general information about oxygen administration. Specific nursing interventions for administering oxygen are described in Procedure 45–1.

Oxygen is an essential and powerful substance. The goal of oxygen therapy is to achieve an optimal arterial oxygen tension by giving the lowest possible, most effective dose of oxygen while avoiding the toxic effects of oxygen.

Goal of Oxygen Therapy. More specifically, the goal of oxygen therapy is to keep arterial Po_2 within physiologic range (i.e., PaO_2 above 55 to 60 mm Hg). Oxygen administration should not cause the arterial Pco_2 to rise above 45 mm Hg. An exception may be a person with **chronic obstructive pulmonary disease (COPD).** COPD is a broad term used clinically to refer to several diseases, notably asthma, emphysema, and chronic bronchitis characterized by chronic airflow limitation. This person normally has a chronically elevated Pco_2 (above 45 mm Hg). This person's respiratory drive is a low oxygen blood level—hypoxic drive. The normal stimulus to breathe is mild **hypercapnia (hypercar-**

bia), a high $Paco_2$ level. Except in an emergency, assess the arterial blood gas status of a person before beginning oxygen therapy to determine whether there is chronic carbon dioxide retention.

People with chronically elevated $Paco_2$ may not tolerate the same doses of oxygen as people with no pre-existing respiratory disease. Administration of oxygen to these persons may inhibit their drive to breathe and further impair respiratory status because their stimulus to breathe is hypoxia.

Oxygen administration by itself may not be successful in maintaining an acceptable Pao_2. More intensive therapy (e.g., a mechanical ventilator) may be required to maintain arterial blood gases within physiologic limits.

If lack of oxygen threatens a person's immediate survival, administer oxygen without delay. Laboratory assessment of blood gases must be made after oxygen administration has been started.

Effects of Oxygen Therapy. Oxygen administration

► increases alveolar oxygen tension but may or may not increase arterial oxygen tension, depending on the cause of the hypoxemia
► reduces the work of breathing and associated fatigue
► decreases the work of the heart and vascular system

The cardiovascular system increases its workload in an attempt to compensate for hypoxemia in certain conditions (e.g., hemorrhagic shock). Table 45–10 presents some of the commonly observed signs and symptoms of hypoxemia and the observable response to oxygen administration. This is not a complete list but one that includes the obvious and frequently observed signs of hypoxemia.

The effect of oxygen therapy is assessed both by blood gas analysis and by observation of the person for improvement in the clinical symptoms of hypoxemia.

Continuous Oxygen Therapy. Oxygen is not stored in the body. Oxygen is administered continuously when acute hypoxemia is present. The tissue oxygen needs must be met at all times. Oxygen administration is never stopped until factors that caused the hypoxemia are reversed. During all phases of care, continuous oxygen administration is *never* interrupted. Sudden withdrawal of oxygen may lead to more severe hypoxemia and result in serious, possibly life-threatening cardiovascular and cerebral hypoxic effects.

Intermittent Oxygen Therapy. Intermittent use of oxygen is often of questionable value. Random "doses" of oxygen do not maintain the constant physiologic oxygen requirement of the body. Intermittent oxygen therapy may, however, be used for the relief of chest pain or other cardiopulmonary symptoms. It may also be used for the treatment of exercise-induced hypoxe-

PROCEDURE 45-1

Administering Oxygen

Definition/Purposes. Oxygen is administered for treatment of hypoxemia. Hypoxemia may be caused by breathing low concentrations (partial pressures) of oxygen (e.g., at high elevation); inadequate ventilation (hypoventilation) with an inadequate amount of oxygen supplied to the alveoli; diseases or conditions in the alveoli that interfere with the exchange (diffusion) of oxygen across the alveolar-capillary membrane; inadequate amounts of hemoglobin (anemia) resulting in insufficient amounts of oxygen circulated to the tissues; chemicals that alter the tissue's ability to accept oxygen (e.g., cyanide); and diseases or conditions that cause an imbalance in the ratio of ventilation to blood flow (perfusion) in the alveoli, with resultant atelectasis. Oxygen administration keeps the body functioning and treats the effects of hypoxemia to prevent irreversible damage (e.g., brain damage). Oxygen decreases the work of breathing; it may increase the arterial oxygen level; it will aid in the maintenance of a state of homeostasis. Oxygen administration does not treat the underlying disease. The goal of oxygen administration is to maintain the PaO_2 in the range of 80 to 100 mm Hg or at the person's baseline normal value, without causing alveolar hypoventilation (hypercapnia).

Contraindications/Cautions. Oxygen itself is not strictly contraindicated. However, caution must be observed if the ventilatory drive is due to a chronically low arterial oxygen tension (the hypoxic drive often seen with chronic respiratory disease). PaO_2 from 21 per cent oxygen (room air) below 50 mm Hg and $PaCO_2$ above 45 to 50 mm Hg usually indicate a secondary hypoxic drive. If hypoxemia persists, the lethal effects of oxygen lack may occur. More complex forms of respiratory therapy, such as mechanically assisted ventilation to maintain physiologic oxygen and carbon dioxide tension, may be required when the physical condition is too complicated for oxygen therapy alone. High concentrations of oxygen (above 50 per cent) given for long periods of time may lead to toxic effects or other problems. Oxygen administration is preceded with pretherapy measurement of arterial blood gases. Subsequent arterial blood gas analysis is done to evaluate the effffectiveness of therapy. The hazards of oxygen therapy must never prevent the administration of oxygen to a person in an acute emergency situation in which the administration of oxygen is required to maintain life.

Teaching/Learning Guidelines. There must be *no* smoking or use of combustibles, spark-producing appliances, or equipment in an oxygen-enriched environment. Administer oxygen only as prescribed and do not randomly change the dose. Administer oxygen continuously because it cannot be stored in the body. When tanks are being used, secure them to prevent their falling. Observe for the signs of hypercapnia (elevated $PaCO_2$), such as tremors, increased lethargy, somnolence, and headache; observe for signs associated with increasing hypoxemia, such as a change in pulse rate, breathlessness, or color changes.

PRELIMINARY ACTIVITIES

Assessment/Planning

▶ Check results of arterial blood gas analysis.
▶ Check prescription for liter flow delivery device, reason for therapy, additional assessment.
▶ Note significant history.
▶ Observe for physical signs of chronic respiratory dysfunction.
▶ Observe for clinical signs of hypoxemia so that reversal may then be noted and effectiveness of therapy determined.

Equipment

▶ "No Smoking" sign.
▶ Oxygen flowmeter.
▶ Oxygen connecting tube.

▶ Oxygen delivery device.
▶ Humidifier (for flow rates greater than 4 LPM).
▶ Distilled water (for humidifier).
▶ Oxygen analyzer (if applicable).

Preparation of Person

▶ Ensure electrical appliances have three-pronged or other style hospital-grade plugs and that equipment is safe for use in oxygen-rich environment.
▶ Post "No Smoking" sign on door and over bed.
▶ Inform others in room that smoking is not allowed when oxygen is in use.
▶ Remove cigarettes, matches, and other smoking equipment from room.
▶ Compare identification band with oxygen order.
▶ Place person receiving oxygen in comfortable position.

PROCEDURE

Actions

1. Assemble equipment.
   a. Fill humidifier with sterile distilled water.

   b. If HAFOE mask (Venturi style) is used, do not add humidifier.

   c. Plug in flowmeter to outlet or turn on tank valve.

Rationale/Discussion

a. Humidifier adds water vapor to dry gas (oxygen) to reduce drying and irritating effects.
b. With HAFOE mask, humidifer is resistant to efficient air entrainment, and higher than desired O_2 percentage is delivered.
c. Determine whether system is working.

Procedure continued on following page

PROCEDURE 45–1 Continued

Administering Oxygen

Actions	Rationale/Discussion
2. Adjust liter flow as ordered by physician or as required by delivery service.	2. HAFOE masks have specific liter flow for each percentage of oxygen delivered. Venturi portion of mask entrains specific amount of air to mix with oxygen so that high total liter flows of air and oxygen are delivered. Any other oxygen liter flow may not be enough to meet inspired ventilation needs of person so that percentage of oxygen remains constant. Be sure that liter flow prescribed is within acceptable range to achieve goal of treatment.
3. Apply oxygen delivery device (e.g., cannula or mask) to person; connect oxygen connecting tubing to humidifier (or flowmeter adapter if humidifier is not used). a. Make certain nothing obstructs or occludes connecting tube.	3. Device must be applied correctly to prevent hazards and discomfort and to ensure accurate flow rates of oxygen. a. Restricts or obstructs flow; stops humidifier bubbling. Characteristic audible signal is heard with some humidifiers.
4. Note effects of oxygen on person. a. *Arterial blood gas analysis* 20 to 30 minutes after initiation of oxygen or after each liter flow or change in FIO_2. b. *Respiratory rate.* Does rate improve with therapy (normal range is 12 to 20 breaths per minute for adults)? c. *Respiratory pattern.* Has oxygen therapy altered respiration pattern? d. *Level of consciousness.* Has mentation improved? Does person show signs of confusion or other changes indicating side effects of oxygen (e.g., carbon dioxide retention)?	4. Symptoms of hypoxemia should improve or disappear. Observe for signs of hypercapnia (e.g., tremors, lethargy, somnolence). a. Evaluates effect of treatment. b. Evaluates effect of treatment. c. Evaluates effect of treatment. d. Evaluates effect of treatment.
5. Do not remove oxygen unless ordered by physician and arterial blood levels show return to normal.	5. Oxygen is not stored in the body. It must be administered continuously during all activities (e.g., eating, sitting up, during transportation).

FINAL ACTIVITIES

While oxygen is flowing, continue to evaluate the effects of oxygen therapy. Check the flow rate on the flowmeter periodically. Provide oxygen during all activities. If the person is confused, raise side rails, lower bed level, and, if necessary (rare), safely place restraints to prevent tampering with equipment. (Provide other nursing interventions as needed for the confused person.) *Aftercare of equipment:* Change the delivery device, humidifier, and water reservoir daily. Discard disposable equipment as necessary. Reusable equipment must be decontaminated and stored dry. *Final assessment:* Continue to observe the effects of the therapy. Recheck liter flow and device. Take follow-up blood gas assessment. *Documentation:* Document liter flow, device used, and effects of therapy. Record positive effects of therapy (e.g., respiratory rate decreased to normal, heart rate returned to normal, breathing pattern improved, and distress relieved). Record negative effects (e.g., increased confusion, lethargy, or other signs of carbon dioxide retention). Report results of all blood gas measurements to physician immediately; enter blood gas results on a flowsheet to provide visualization of the trends of therapy. The flowsheet includes date and time; pH; PaO_2, $PaCO_2$, HCO_3^-, SaO_2; liter flow or percentage of oxygen; brief narrative of effects of or response to therapy.

mia. People with chronic lung disease may maintain marginally satisfactory PaO_2 while at rest or while performing mild activities of daily living. However, with exercise, cardiopulmonary compensatory mechanisms may be unable to maintain an adequate PaO_2. Administration of intermittent supplemental oxygen allows this person to exercise (Fig. 45–12). Intermittent oxygen may also be used to treat pulmonary hypertension and cor pulmonale. Such therapy includes 12 to 18 hours of continuous oxygen administration in every 24-hour pe-

riod. Finally, intermittent oxygen may be used after anesthesia, after cardiopulmonary arrest, in cases of reduced cardiac output, and during stressful procedures (e.g., suctioning, bronchoscopy, and cardiac catheterization).

Oxygen Dosage. Factors to consider when administering oxygen are the desired clinical effect, the past and present medical history, and the results of the arterial blood gas analysis. Oxygen delivery systems

TABLE 45-10. Commonly Observed Signs and Symptoms of Hypoxemia and Favorable Responses to Oxygen Administration

Sign or Symptom of Hypoxemia	Favorable Response After Oxygen Administration
Tachycardia	Return to normal rate
Cardiac arrhythmias	Decrease or elimination of irregularities
Increased respiratory rate and increase in work of breathing	Return to normal rate and pattern of ventilation, and reduction of excess work of breathing
Breathlessness, shortness of breath; air hunger	Return of quiet respirations that do not require conscious effort
Confusion, hallucinations, restlessness	Improved mental status
Cyanosis	Return of healthy color to skin, nailbeds, and mucous membranes

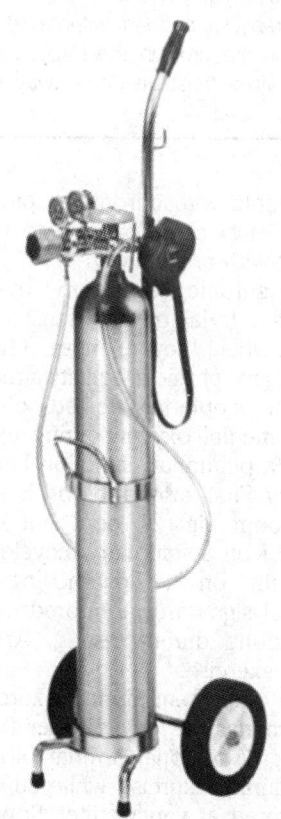

▲ *Figure 45-12*

Portable cylinder oxygen (E size). Oxygen is supplied in both large (H or K size) and small, portable (E size) cylinders. E cylinders are used during transportation and mobilization for oxygen-dependent people; they are also used by people at home. (Courtesy of Hudson RCI, Temecula, CA.)

measure the oxygen dose either as liters per minute (LPM) or as a percentage of oxygen (%) (usually expressed as the fraction of inspired oxygen, or FIO_2). Oxygen dosage is prescribed according to the appliance used and the method of measurement. For example, a prescription for oxygen might state: "Oxygen per nasal cannula at 3 LPM continuously." This means the person is to be given oxygen continuously at a rate of 3 liters per minute through a nasal cannula.

Upper respiratory passages (nose, mouth, and oral and nasal pharynx) create an anatomic reservoir for momentary "storage" of oxygen (not to be confused with storing oxygen for physiologic use) before it is inhaled into the tracheobronchial tree. This is an important concept because it dispels the belief that people receiving nasal oxygen while mouth breathing are not receiving the correct amount of oxygen. This anatomic reservoir has a capacity of about 6 liters. During inhalation, oxygen from the anatomic reservoir and the oxygen administration device are mixed with room air. The percentage of oxygen delivered by the appliance depends on the liter flow of oxygen, the respiratory rate, the pattern of ventilation, and the tidal volume of each breath.

The desired clinical effect of the dose of oxygen is monitored by observing the person for indications of

▶ improved oxygen status
▶ development of undesired effects (e.g., depression of the respiratory centers with subsequent depression of respiration and a build-up of carbon dioxide)
▶ the presence of arterial blood gas imbalances (e.g., continued hypoxemia or the development of a sudden elevation of the PCO_2)

Adjustment of the dose of oxygen depends on the disease state, degree of hypoxia, unwanted side effects, and arterial blood gas measurements. Adjustment in oxygen dosage is usually made by the physician.

Safety Considerations. Safety considerations are mandatory when oxygen is administered. Table 45-11 presents some safety considerations and nursing interventions to ensure safety.

Oxygen Humidification. Humidification of oxygen is used to prevent irritation and encrusting of the airways and to maintain an optimal environment for the normal function of the cilia. **Humidification** is the addition of water vapor to a dry gas. The addition of water vapor reduces the drying effect of oxygen on the mucous membranes, thereby making the administration of oxygen more comfortable.

Oxygen is a dry gas. Prolonged exposure to the drying effects of oxygen may cause irritation and damage to mucous membranes of the oral and nasal pharyngeal area.

Bubble-diffusion humidifiers (see Fig. 45-8) are most often used with oxygen. Oxygen is bubbled through water, which allows the molecules of oxygen to pick up molecules of water vapor. This differs from topical

TABLE 45–11. Selected Scientific Principles and Related Nursing Interventions for Safe Oxygen Administration

Principle	Nursing Interventions
Oxygen is a drug; it has beneficial as well as undesirable effects	Observe for indications of hypoxemia and hypercapnia (hypercarbia) Check the liter flow and/or analyze the FIO_2 to ascertain that the correct dose of oxygen is being administered Make certain blood gas analyses are done when ordered; correlate PaO_2 and SaO_2 with the dose of oxygen
Oxygen administration can depress respiratory drive in persons with chronic obstructive pulmonary disease (COPD).	Use caution when administering oxygen to people with COPD; observe for signs and symptoms of hypercapnia and respiratory failure; precede oxygen therapy with a baseline blood gas analysis
Oxygen has necessary physiologic effects	Do not fear psychologic dependence; physiologic need is easily determined through blood gas analysis
Oxygen is a dry gas	Humidification of inspired oxygen is necessary for nasal prong devices when the flow rate is greater than 4 LPM; observe for nasal mucosal irritation; maintain oral hydration
Oxygen supports combustion	Oxygen must not be administered where cigarette smoking, open flames, and sparks from electrical appliances, equipment, and toys may ignite; absolutely no smoking while oxygen is in use; electrical checks of all equipment must be done, and three-pronged or other hospital-grade plugs must be used to ensure safety in an oxygen-rich environment
Oxygen cannot be stored in the body	Never remove the oxygen source from a person receiving continuous therapy; a sudden withdrawal of the oxygen may cause a severe drop in the PaO_2; use portable systems when activities must be done away from the central oxygen source

hydration, in which actual droplets of water are deposited into the airway.

Oxygen Delivery Systems. Oxygen delivery devices are divided into two broad categories: high-flow oxygen systems and low-flow oxygen systems (Table 45–12). A high-flow system delivers a flow of gas that exceeds the volume of air required for the person's minute ventilation (the amount of air inhaled and exhaled in 1 minute—expressed as V̇ and measured in liters per minute). The Venturi mask is the high-flow system currently in use. Low-flow systems deliver oxygen at variable liter flows designed to add to, but not meet, the total air volume requirements. As a result, oxygen percentages in low-flow systems are variable and not as consistent as the percentages in high-flow systems. In a low-flow system, the percentage of oxygen delivered to the tracheobronchial tree is determined by the person's respiratory rate, the tidal volume, and the pattern of ventilation (deep, fast, shallow, irregular). Low-flow systems include the nasal cannula (prongs), the standard mask, and the oxygen mask with reservoir bag (nonrebreathing mask).

Oxygen and Exercise. People being treated for acute respiratory disorders and who are receiving supplemental oxygen must continue to receive oxygen during all activities. People with chronic respiratory disorders and hypoxemia must also continue to receive oxygen both at rest and with any activity.

People with chronic respiratory dysfunction who have acceptable arterial oxygen tensions at rest may require oxygen when they exercise. (In this context, exercise means any physical activity greater than lying or sitting.) Such people are tested to determine the need for supplemental oxygen during exercise. This is usually done in a pulmonary function laboratory. It is a two-step process. First, arterial blood is sampled at rest on breathing room air (21 per cent oxygen). Then exercise, whether on a stationary bicycle or walking on the level (usually on a slow-moving treadmill), is carried out. Vital signs are monitored, and an electrocardiogram is done during testing. Arterial blood is sampled during exercise.

If hypoxemia is present during exercise, the physician then determines the oxygen liter flow to be used when exercising. Additional arterial blood gas studies may be done during exercise while supplemental oxygen is administered at varying liter flows. The goal of exercise with oxygen is to maintain the PaO_2 above 55 to 60 mm Hg while eliminating the hazards of exercise with hypoxemia (e.g., cardiac dysfunction).

All people benefit from exercise. These benefits include the promotion of an improved sense of well-being and the conditioning of muscles, which allows

TABLE 45-12. Oxygen Delivery Systems

System	Description	Liter Flow/ Percentage of Oxygen Delivered	Comments
Low-flow Systems			
Nasal cannula (prongs)	Two ⅝-inch projections that fit into the entry of the nasal passages	**Flow:** 1 to 6 LPM **% Delivered:** Variable; depends on the liter flow, respiratory rate, or pattern of respiration; range: 22 to 40%	Most common device used Relatively comfortable; allows continuation of activities (e.g., eating and talking); disposable May be dislodged by restless or disoriented people Nasal passages must be patent If the person's nasal mucosa becomes dry and irritated, use a water-based lubricant on the nostrils or add humidification; humidification is recommended when the liter flow is greater than 4 LPM.[5,14]

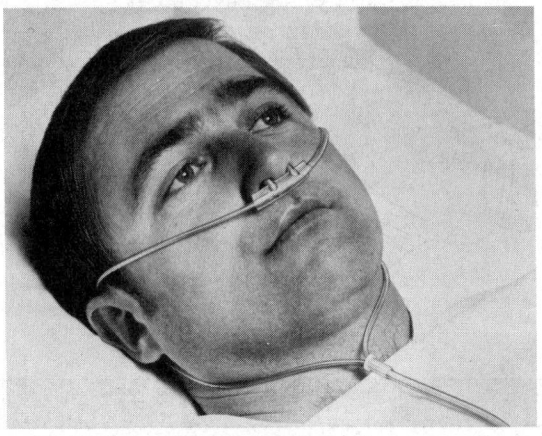

Standard mask	A clear plastic appliance that encompasses the oral and nasal cavity and creates additional area for oxygen collection (a reservoir) Exhaled air passes out small holes in the sides of the mask; the small holes also allow the entrainment of room air, which adds to the inspired oxygen flow rate to meet the person's tidal volume needs for each breath	**Flow:** 6 to 12 LPM **Caution** Must not be administered at flow rates under 6 LPM **% Delivered:** Variable; depends on the same factors listed for cannula; range: 40 to 65% (moderate range)	May cause a person to have a feeling of confinement or claustrophobia Use with caution in a person who is unable to maintain an unobstructed, patent airway or who may vomit easily and aspirate gastric contents Replace the mask with nasal prongs when eating; this may cause a reduction in the inspired oxygen concentration; reposition mask immediately on finishing meal

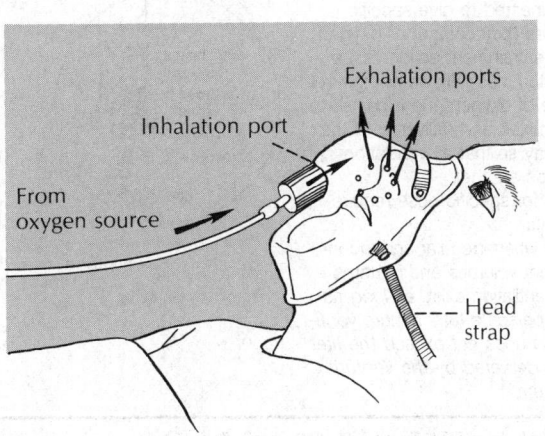

Table continued on following page

TABLE 45–12. Oxygen Delivery Systems Continued

System	Description	Liter Flow/ Percentage of Oxygen Delivered	Comments
Oxygen mask with reservoir bag (nonrebreathing mask)	A standard mask with a reservoir bag designed to give high oxygen concentration A one-way valve between reservoir bag and mask permits inspired air to come only from the reservoir bag Exhaled air exits through one-way valves at the sides of the mask	**Flow:** As required to keep the reservoir bag inflated at least one-third full during inspiration; ranges of flow rates vary from 6 to 15 LPM **% Delivered:** Variable, owing to respiratory rate, ventilatory pattern, and minute ventilation as well as the liter flow of oxygen required to keep the bag inflated; range: 60 to 90%	Useful for short-term, high concentrations of oxygen Same hazards as standard oxygen mask The fullness of the bag must be monitored; the bag must not collapse completely with each inspiration; the liter flow must be increased if this occurs

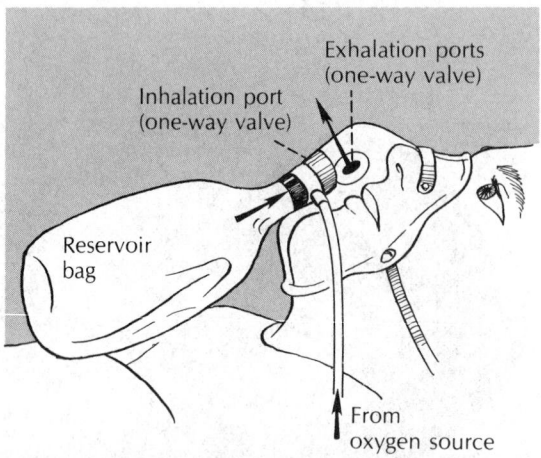

High-flow Systems

Venturi mask	A mask engineered to use the Venturi principle of high airflow oxygen enrichment (HAFOE) Oxygen moves through the connecting tube to a channel in the mask that has one diameter on the distal side and a smaller diameter on the proximal side; oxygen flows through this passage; at the point of exit, a pressure drop occurs and creates a suction or entrainment (drawing in) effect; the degree of entrainment has been engineered to give specific doses (percentage) of oxygen; the entrainment action of the Venturi mask allows a large volume of oxygen and room air to be mixed and delivered to the airway so that all ventilation needs are met Useful for specific dose requirements Useful when irregular and inconsistent volumes and patterns of ventilation exist, *as long as the person's total minute ventilation does not exceed the liter flow delivered by the Venturi system*	**Flow:** As recommended by the manufacturer **% Delivered:** Provides 24 to 50% oxygen in small increments (e.g., 24, 28, 31, etc.)	Provide supplemental oxygen by cannula during eating and other activities where the mask interferes Other equipment (e.g., nebulizers) use HAFOE or Venturi effect of air entrainment

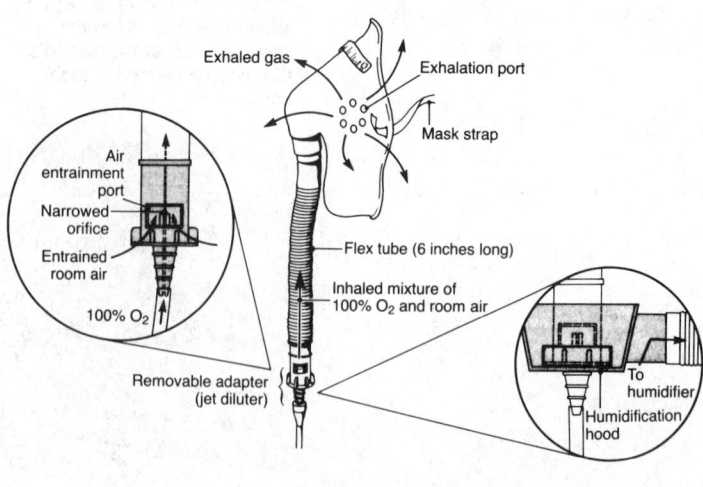

Illustration of a nasal cannula courtesy of Hudson RCI, Temecula, CA; illustration of a Venturi mask from Kersten, L.D. (1989). *Comprehensive respiratory nursing: A decision-making approach*. Philadelphia: W. B. Saunders.

optimal oxygen utilization. These are important benefits for people with chronic respiratory dysfunction.

Home Oxygen Systems. Many people with chronic lung disease exercise as part of their daily program. Regular, routine exercise is fundamental to pulmonary rehabilitation. Often, an exercise program includes the use of oxygen. Three methods of oxygen administration suitable for home use are liquid portable systems, portable cylinders of gaseous oxygen, and oxygen concentrators.

Liquid portable oxygen systems are the most versatile and suitable for people who wish to remain active. Liquid oxygen systems are composed of two parts. They have a reservoir of liquid oxygen (contained in a thermos bottle–like container), which supplies a person's stationary oxygen needs via a standard oxygen flowmeter and humidifier. The second part of the system is a portable unit for ambulatory use, which is filled with oxygen from the reservoir. When filled, the portable unit weighs approximately 9 pounds. It may be carried with a shoulder strap or pulled in a cart.

Home oxygen may also be supplied by small portable cylinders of gaseous oxygen (see Fig. 45–12). These cylinders and their larger counterparts (H and K cylinders) can be moved about on wheeled carts. Stationary oxygen is appropriate for people with severe respiratory impairment and limited mobility.

Oxygen concentrators are used when stationary, low-flow oxygen is necessary. They are often used at home by people with chronic lung disease. They do not require an oxygen source. They concentrate the air in the room into a high percentage of pure oxygen (95 per cent at 1 LPM). Liter flow rates are generally limited from ½ to 4 or 10 LPM.

Oxygen use at home depends on a number of factors:

▶ Existing medical conditions and supplemental oxygen requirements
▶ Home environment (including the physical layout)
▶ Available social support systems
▶ Geographic location
▶ Financial considerations (e.g., insurance coverage)
▶ Frequency of follow-up assessments

Provision must also be made for routine maintenance of the equipment as well as for careful instruction of the person and significant others in the care and operation of the equipment. This instruction includes safety precautions, the reason oxygen is needed, and the signs and symptoms of impaired oxygenation and carbon dioxide retention.

MEDICATION FOR PEOPLE WITH RESPIRATORY PROBLEMS

Medications injected into the bloodstream produce the most rapid effects. The second most rapid effect is achieved through the absorption of medication through the respiratory system.

Medication is delivered into the respiratory system in aerosol form. The medications administered by aerosolization may be divided into four categories: bronchodilators, mucolytics, anti-inflammatory or antiallergenic drugs, and antibiotics.

Bronchodilators open the airways by relaxing the smooth muscle of the tracheobronchial tree. All bronchodilators must be used with caution in people with known cardiac disease and hypertension. All bronchodilators may increase the heart rate and may affect the blood pressure. Always check the pulse rate before and after administering bronchodilators.

Mucolytics aid in the clearance of retained secretions by chemically altering the mucus so that it is more easily expectorated. Bronchospasm may be a side effect. Adding a bronchodilator to a mucolytic is recommended. Bronchorrhea (excessive discharge of mucus from bronchi) may also occur if the cough mechanism is weak and ineffective. Large quantities of mucus may be mobilized and may cause obstruction of the airway.

Anti-inflammatory and antiallergenic effects may both be achieved with steroids. Steroids are potent chemicals that sometimes are aerosolized for a topical effect; but during acute bronchospasm, they must also be administered systemically. Inhalation of steroids may cause an overgrowth of *Candida albicans* in the mouth; therefore, the mouth should be rinsed out after each administration. Cromolyn sodium is another drug that has both anti-inflammatory and antiallergenic effects. It is used to prevent allergic responses in the airway. It prevents the rupture of mast cells in the lung and so prevents the release of bronchoconstrictive chemicals in the lungs. It is not a steroid, nor is it a drug used during acute bronchospastic episodes. It is most effective in asthmatic children and young adults.

Antibiotics are aerosolized at times to treat pulmonary infections. Topical administration is generally less effective than systemically administered antibiotics. In the home setting, topical or intravenous antibiotics may be used to treat infection and avert hospitalization.

Most of these medications may be delivered by a nebulizer. A *nebulizer* is a device that breaks liquids into small (aerosol) particles. This *aerosolization* creates a mist that may be inhaled into the upper airways and lungs. The medication acts locally on the tracheobronchial mucosa. Systemic effects of the medication do not occur, except when the dose is large or when excessive amounts are absorbed into the bloodstream after application to the mouth and oral mucosa.

Two nebulizer devices are the hand-held nebulizer and metered-dose inhaler. They are most commonly used to deliver bronchodilators.

Hand-Held Nebulizer. *Hand-held nebulizer treatments* compose a significant portion of the respiratory care in health agencies. The nebulizer is connected to a compressed gas source, usually air or oxygen from a wall outlet next to the person's bed. In the home setting, the equipment setup is slightly different. The same type of nebulizer as that in the hospital setting is used. However, the nebulizer is connected to an air compressor machine, as shown in Figure 45–13.

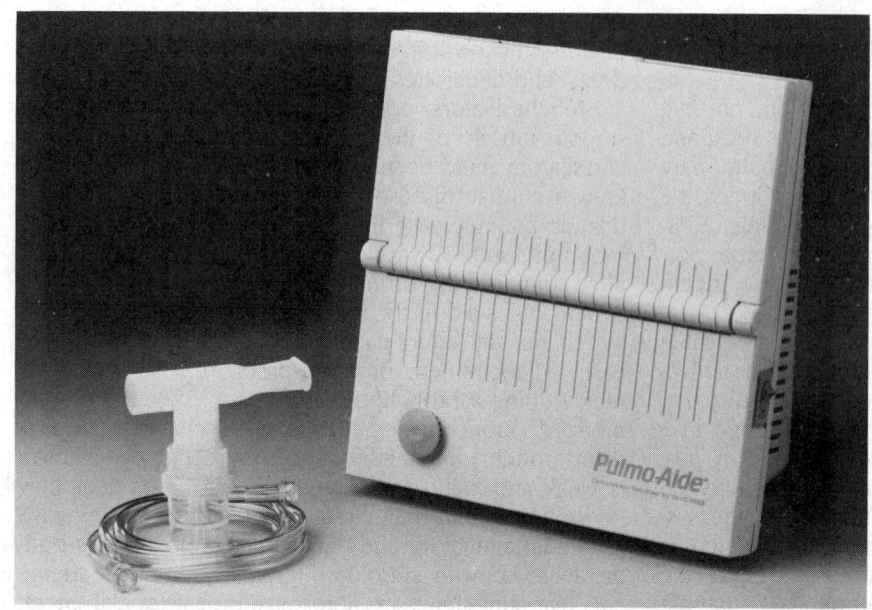

▲ Figure 45–13

A hand-held nebulizer connected to an air compressor machine in the home setting. This DeVilbiss Pulmo-Aide model has filters (in the plastic bag) for the air-inlet filter (far right knob). (Courtesy of National Medical Homecare, Sacramento, CA.)

In the illustration, when the top of the nebulizer is removed, medication is placed in the cup (above the hand) for aerosolization. The client places the mouthpiece between the teeth with the lips closed. Slow, deep breaths are taken with 3- to 5-second pauses between breaths. The pauses help the mist settle in the lungs, not in the mouth. With this technique, each treatment lasts 10 to 20 minutes. Treatments are generally ordered once, twice, three, or four or more times a day, depending on the degree of airway obstruction, severity of disease, and other factors.

In the hospital, respiratory care practitioners are responsible for the daily cleaning and gas sterilization of hand-held nebulizers and other respiratory equipment. In the home setting, people must be instructed to clean their nebulizers and other equipment daily with liquid soap and water. Equipment is disinfected with a white vinegar and water solution or as directed by the equipment company or home health agency. Failure to clean and disinfect equipment appropriately may cause a respiratory infection from the inhalation of germ-laden mist.

Metered-Dose Inhaler. **Metered-dose inhalers (MDIs)** are pocket-sized cartridges with plastic dispensers that are used to deliver bronchodilators or topically administered antiallergy or anti-inflammatory medications. They are also called metered-dose devices (MDDs). Figure 45–9 shows the correct technique for administration of medication via metered-dose inhalers. The device looks simple, but the technique requires careful instruction and practice. People who use inhalers are often not adequately instructed in the correct technique. Metered-dose inhalers are not appropriate for everyone because they require coordination of breathing and activation of the device. It is possible to get "placebo inhalers" that do not contain medication.

They may be used for practice with no danger of overmedication. Overuse, inadequate instruction, and failure to realize the potency of the medication often lead to abuse. In this situation, symptoms may worsen and harmful side effects increase (tachyphylaxis). It is often a nursing responsibility to teach a person and significant others correct use of the metered-dose inhaler. Do not assume a person knows how to use it properly just because he or she has one. Make a careful assessment and provide teaching as necessary.

POSITIVE-PRESSURE BREATHING

Positive-pressure breathing treatments are the administration of higher-than-ambient pressures to the airway to cause a flow of gas (oxygen and ambient air) into the airway and create a deep breath. Positive-pressure breathing is abbreviated IPPB (intermittent positive-pressure breathing).

IPPB may be used as follows:

▶ to stimulate and promote deep breathing in people unable to voluntarily deep breathe
▶ to mobilize secretions when simpler and more inexpensive approaches do not work (e.g., inhaler, nebulizer, or respiratory exercises)
▶ to temporarily decrease the work of breathing

IPPB was once a popular, overused form of respiratory therapy. It was used primarily to stimulate deep breathing and administer aerosolized medication. There are many undesirable physiologic effects caused by the positive pressure, however. These undesired effects (e.g., decreased venous return to the right side of the heart and overventilation) reduced the use and popularity of IPPB. It is still used in selected instances, but studies and experience show that spontaneous deep breathing is much more effective in combating atelectasis and also allows more uniform deposition of aerosol particles into the tracheobronchial tree.

RESPIRATORY EXERCISES

The most often used modality in respiratory therapy is incentive spirometry, or incentive respiratory exercises. There are many devices for this form of therapy (Fig. 45-14 is one example).

Incentive devices use a concept of sustained maximal inspiration. Each device has a means of setting an inspiratory goal. Correct use requires a spontaneous, slow, voluntary, deep breath. When full inhalation is reached, the breath is held for at least 3 seconds. This sequence is repeated 10 to 20 times an hour. Incentive exercises are most effective when used every hour while the person is awake. Visual reinforcement is provided by lights, balls rising in a column, or other indicators of success. Instruction and supervision are needed initially. The skill is quickly learned by most people.

Incentive devices provide the stimulus for a spontaneous deep breath. Spontaneous deep breathing, using the sustained maximal inspiration concept, reduces atelectasis, opens airways, stimulates coughing, and actively encourages individual participation in recovery.

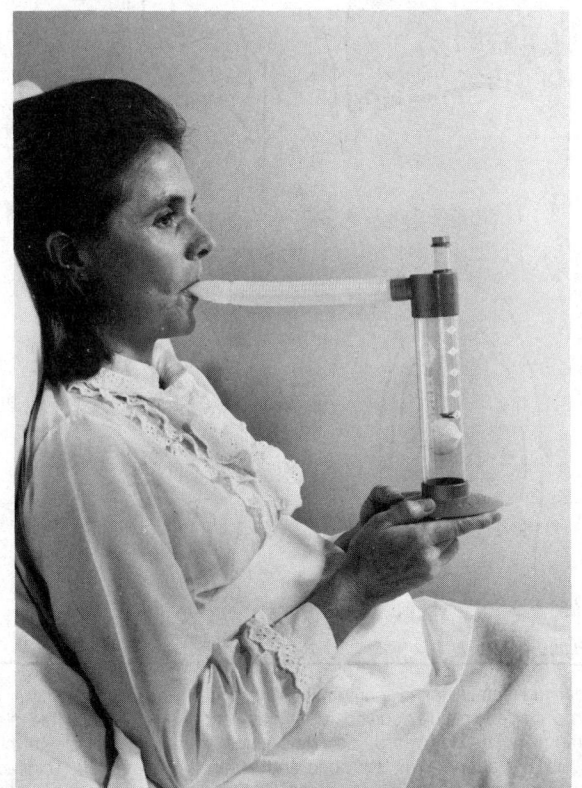

▲ Figure 45-14

Incentive spirometry device. This device is used to exercise the lungs in a goal-directed approach to promote voluntary, sustained maximal inspirations. (Courtesy of John Bunn Co., Buffalo, NY.)

Box 45-2. Basic Steps for Effective Incentive Therapy

1. Exhale to a point of comfort.
2. Place the mouthpiece between the teeth and close the lips around the mouthpiece.
3. Begin inhaling slowly and steadily.
4. Continue inhaling until the indicator on the device reaches the pre-set goal.
5. When the goal is reached, maintain the held breath, with the chest expanded for at least 3 seconds.
6. Exhale slowly.
7. Repeat steps 1 through 6 for 10 to 20 cycles or as ordered by the physician.

This form of therapy is often used postoperatively or when physical mobility is limited. It is most effectively used when people are alert, cooperative, coordinated, and motivated and have sufficient strength to generate an inspiratory flow rate that will produce a deep breath and activate the indicator on the incentive device.

Nurses often are responsible for initiating the increase of the inspiratory goal. Be familiar with the specific use instructions for each incentive device used in your clinical area. Box 45-2 lists the basic steps for an effective incentive breath. Repetitions of the deep breaths must be slow to avoid "overbreathing," which will lead to dizziness and tremors as a result of sudden lowering of the $Paco_2$.

Breathing retraining techniques are part of both in-hospital and at-home treatment of people with chronic respiratory disorders. Breathing retraining is a combination of techniques, all with the common goals of

▶ improving the quality of respiration
▶ promoting an improved mental attitude and ability to perform the activities of living
▶ conditioning muscles through exercise

Breathing retraining techniques include pursed-lip breathing (Fig. 45-15), diaphragmatic breathing (Fig. 45-16), and methods of controlling breathlessness.

Panic leads to breathlessness, which leads to more anxiety. Dyspnea is frightening in itself unless people learn to regain control of their breathing. Because people with chronic respiratory conditions have little or no pulmonary reserve (because of altered lung volumes and capacities, hypoxemia, hypercapnia, or muscle wasting), even minimal physical or emotional stress may result in a "dyspnea-anxiety-dyspnea" cycle. Even people with normal lungs or acute respiratory conditions may experience dyspnea and anxiety.

Pursed-lip breathing is a breathing technique used to increase tidal volume, decrease respiratory rate, and control dyspnea (Fig. 45-15 shows how to teach clients to do this). Box 45-3 gives details of diaphragmatic breathing. Practice these techniques yourself.

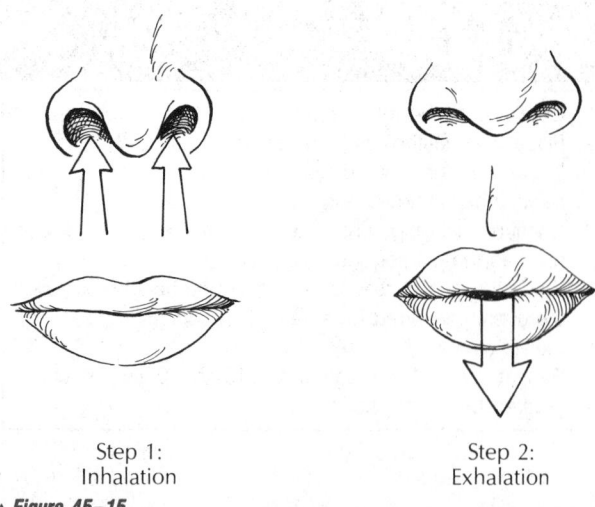

Step 1:
Inhalation

Step 2:
Exhalation

▲ *Figure 45–15*

Breathing retraining: pursed-lip breathing. *Step 1:* Inhale slowly through the nose, keeping mouth closed. Count "one and two." Pause briefly. *Step 2:* Exhale through pursed lips as if gently blowing a candle flame. Count "one, two, three, four." Allow adequate time to empty lungs and reduce air trapping. Exhalation should take at least twice as long as inhalation. Learning to breathe with this technique helps people control respiration when they are excited or anxious, exercising, or developing respiratory distress.

REHABILITATION

The damaging effects of many chronic diseases, such as emphysema, are not reversible. The disease process is slow and insidious. People whose lungs and bodies are undergoing these changes gradually alter their daily living pattern and activity level to accommodate their dyspnea. Finally, limitations are recognized either as a result of seeking medical assistance for an acute respiratory problem or when the level of disability is so great that it can no longer be ignored.

Organized formal inpatient and outpatient programs are available in most major population areas. Community education and support groups sponsored by the local American Lung Association also provide basic education courses for people and their significant others. Significant others are included because they play a major role in the outcome of these programs. Included in most programs are

▶ education concerning the respiratory system and its function
▶ the chronic disease process
▶ education about oxygen, medications, equipment, and therapeutic modalities
▶ energy conservation techniques
▶ breathing retraining
▶ supervised, individual, goal-oriented, graded exercise programs (walking, stationary bicycle, and swimming)
▶ relaxation training
▶ nutritional education
▶ psychologic and social support groups

An interdisciplinary approach (one using professionals from nursing, medicine, respiratory therapy, occupational therapy, physical therapy, and other disciplines) is generally used for formal programs.

The purpose of pulmonary rehabilitation is to promote an improved quality of life for people with chronic respiratory disease.

Objective results are not as easily measured as are the subjective results of such programs. Pulmonary rehabilitation offers a means of understanding the physical changes associated with chronic respiratory disease and provides the "tools" to cope with the disease and manage daily living. Exercise programs provide an improved sense of well-being, improved muscle conditioning, and the ability to be active again.

Pulmonary rehabilitation programs have reduced inpatient hospital time. When people are shown how to cope with chronic problems, they are much better prepared to take responsibility for their lives and less likely

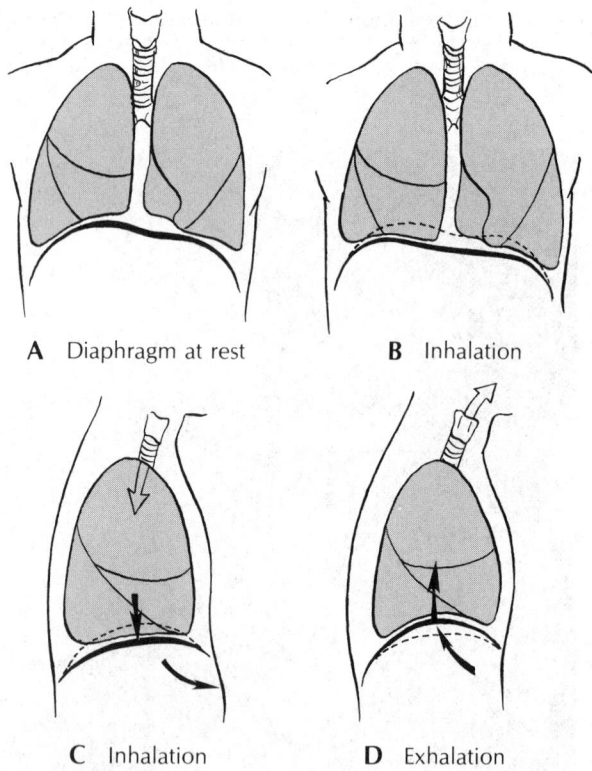

A Diaphragm at rest **B** Inhalation

C Inhalation **D** Exhalation

▲ *Figure 45–16*

Breathing retraining: diaphragmatic breathing. The diaphragm is a dome-shaped muscle, curved slightly upward at rest *(A).* As the diaphragm moves downward, air enters lungs and they expand. As this occurs, the abdomen is displaced and expands outward *(B).* To practice diaphragmatic breathing, place your hand over your abdomen, between the umbilicus and the edge of the rib cage. Inhale through your nose, relax your shoulders, and let air fill your lower chest. Feel the abdomen expand *(C).* During exhalation, pull your abdomen in toward the backbone *(D).* Abdominal muscles help move the diaphragm upward to assist exhalation.

Box 45-3. Diaphragmatic Breathing Techniques

Mechanism

The diaphragm divides the abdomen from the thorax. It is normally dome shaped and provides 80 per cent of the work of breathing. Chronic lung disease causes the diaphragm (the major muscle of respiration) to flatten and the upper chest muscles to hypertrophy and try to take over more of the work of breathing. Conscious effort to pull the diaphragm down during inhalation is needed when this occurs. This will assist in the creation of air pressure changes to improve the volume of air inhaled. By conscious pulling inward of the abdominal muscles during exhalation, a more complete volume of air may be exhaled. Avoid use of accessory muscles.

Process

1. Assume a comfortable resting position.
2. Place one hand over the upper abdomen.
3. This hand will detect diaphragmatic movement.
4. Place the other hand on the upper chest. This hand monitors accessory muscle involvement.
5. Exhale through pursed lips. Feel the inward motion of the abdominal muscles.
6. During inhalation, the abdomen expands outward.
7. Avoid overbreathing, which may lead to lightheadedness.
8. Repeat steps 5 and 6 five to 10 times. Relax after each series.
9. When coaching, speak with a calm, restful voice.

Measures for maintaining airway patency include assessing the person for signs and symptoms of airway obstruction and implementing nursing interventions, as described in Table 45-13. The goal of the interventions is to maintain adequate ventilation and oxygenation.

When reading this and other sections of the chapter, keep in mind two important points. First, *always apply universal precautions when working with the person with respiratory disorders.*

▶ Put on clean gloves when working with the person or the respiratory equipment at the bedside. Consider respiratory equipment contaminated with respiratory secretions.
▶ Wash your hands before and after each contact with the person or equipment.
▶ Follow all isolation policies on the clinical unit if the person has a specific infectious disease, such as tuberculosis or AIDS.

Second, *use all necessary attire including gown, goggles, and mask, as needed, to protect yourself from contact with airborne respiratory secretions.* People who might produce such secretions are those with a history of copious secretions or those receiving aggressive respiratory interventions, such as coughing or airway suctioning. Although the additional attire is cumbersome, it will prevent you from inhaling or coming in contact with infectious microbes, particularly when mucus is accidentally coughed or splattered in your face. Personal eyewear is an acceptable substitute for goggles, if the glasses are sufficiently protective. Place plastic wrap around the glasses for full protection. After using the required attire, dispose of it according to your agency policy.

to experience depression and the other debilitating effects of chronic respiratory disease.

Measures to Maintain Airway Patency

An unobstructed airway is essential for adequate oxygenation and ventilation.

Airway patency is affected by many factors. Techniques used for airway management vary from altering a person's position to complex actions requiring specialized equipment and procedures. Some indicators of impaired airway function are subtle, others are dramatic and obvious. It is a nursing responsibility to recognize indicators of impaired airway function and plan and implement action to correct them.

Time is often a crucial factor in the prevention of serious and sometimes lethal side effects of a poorly functioning airway. In some cases (e.g., a totally obstructed airway), establishment of an open airway must occur within 3 to 4 minutes. In other circumstances, time is less critical. However, even minor interruptions in airway patency, if allowed to go unchecked, can lead to serious and maybe permanent damage.

ARTIFICIAL AIRWAYS

Oropharyngeal Airways. An **oropharyngeal airway (oral airway)** is a curved rubber or plastic piece that inserts into the mouth and maintains a patent airway to the pharynx (Fig. 45-17). The purpose of oropharyngeal airways is to hold the tongue forward. They are placed in the mouth between the posterior pharynx and the base, or root, of the tongue.

Oropharyngeal airways are most often used for unconscious and semiconscious people. Inserting this kind of airway in a conscious person can stimulate the gagging reflex. Nausea, vomiting, and aspiration of stomach contents can result, further compromising airway patency. Remove the airway immediately if gagging occurs. An open airway can often be maintained in a conscious person by lifting the jaw forward (see Fig. 30-2).

Careful oral hygiene is essential when an oral airway is in place. Mucus and other matter may collect in the mouth, which may be aspirated into the lungs, causing pulmonary infection, interference with pulmonary gas exchange, and poor condition of the oral cavity.

TABLE 45-13. Recognition and Prevention of Airway Obstruction

Cause	Recognition	Prevention/Nursing Interventions
Loss of control of tongue and crico-pharyngeal muscles	Noisy, snoring inspiratory sound (partial obstruction) Marked inspiratory effort without ventilation; forceful contraction of thorax and neck muscles (complete obstruction)	Place person in a side-lying position with the neck extended. Insert an oral airway. Reposition as above. Insert oral airway. Auscultate chest to assess ventilation. If no ventilation, call for help (see cardiopulmonary resuscitation in Chapter 30).
Excess mucus in the airway	Wet, gurgling noise with respiration; loose, wet-sounding cough	Side-lying position to promote drainage of mucus. Suction. If thick, increase hydration.
Paralysis of vocal cords Swelling of soft tissues (laryngeal edema, epiglottitis) Tracheal tumors or strictures Swelling or tumors of oropharyngeal or of extra-airway structures (e.g., enlarged thyroid) Trauma to trachea or larynx	Stridor; impaired phonation; restlessness, dyspnea; increased anxiety; or other indications of impaired gas exchange Diminished bilateral breath sounds; when auscultating over trachea, note an increase in the degree of turbulent airflow Difficulty swallowing noted if epiglottis is swollen or if extratracheal mass impinges on the esophagus	Call to physician's attention immediately. Administer supplemental oxygen, vasoconstrictive or anti-inflammatory drugs if indicated. Place in a high Fowler's position to ensure optimal ventilation (see Table 35-4). Have emergency tracheostomy tray available. Prepare for use if respiratory arrest occurs.
Mediastinal tumors Enlarged thyroid	Tachypnea; dyspnea; inability to take a deep breath; visible swelling of thyroid gland Other laboratory and radiologic procedures required for absolute diagnosis	Report immediately. Prepare person for diagnostic and therapeutic procedures. Support respiration and oxygenation.
Aspiration of foreign object (e.g., teeth, food) Aspiration of stomach contents	Dyspnea, cyanosis; other indications of respiratory distress and hypoxemia Decreased breath sounds over affected areas, rhonchi over affected areas	Auscultate chest routinely; observe and assess respiratory status routinely. Report any change in condition immediately (fever, change in breath sounds). Prepare person for diagnostic measures (e.g., fiberoptic bronchoscopy, chest x-ray, medications). If person aspirates an object large enough to completely block airway, it is an emergency. Use abdominal thrusts (see Fig. 30-9).

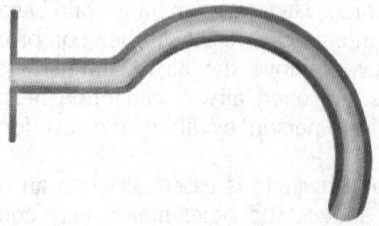

▲ **Figure 45-17**

Oropharyngeal airway. This Berman-style airway has a channel on each side to guide a suction catheter to the pharynx. (Courtesy of Hudson RCI, Temecula, CA.)

To insert an oral airway, first hyperextend (tilt backward) the neck. Carefully open the mouth and insert the tip of the airway into the mouth, turning the airway on its side (horizontal). Slide the airway along the top of the tongue until the tip of the airway reaches the posterior portion of the tongue. Rotate the airway so the curve of the airway is on a vertical axis. The curved end will hold the tongue forward. The flat portion near the lips serves as a "bite block." The mouth may bite or close around this portion.

Nasopharyngeal Airways. Nasal airways (nasal trumpets) are cuffless tubes passed through the nostrils and into the nasopharynx (Fig. 45–18). They are made of soft rubber or plastic. When inserted into the nares (nasal passage), they act as a guide for the insertion of a suction catheter. This prevents trauma to the mucous membranes of the nose. A nasal airway extends into the pharynx and is positioned at the base of the tongue. This separates the tongue from the posterior pharyngeal wall, preventing obstruction from the tongue's falling into the pharynx. The proximal end (nearest the nostrils) of a nasal airway is flared and fits against the external nares. Insertion of a large safety pin through the flared end stops the airway from slipping further into the nose or larynx.

Nasal airways are more appropriate and comfortable for conscious and semiconscious people than are oropharyngeal airways.

To insert a nasopharyngeal airway, select an airway that is slightly smaller than the nares and slightly larger than the suction catheter to be used. Observe the nose carefully. Determine which side of the nose is most open. Insert the tube in this side. If the nose is crooked, it is probably better not to use a nasopharyngeal airway. Lubricate the nares with a water-soluble jelly containing local anesthetic. (Only water-soluble substances are suitable for use in the nose. Petroleum-based substances can lead to pneumonia if they are aspirated into the trachea and lower airway.) Insert the tube with gentle, steady, upward pressure, guiding it up and over into the oropharynx.

Endotracheal Tubes and Tracheostomy Tubes. In the clinical setting, the term artificial airway usually refers to **endotracheal tubes (ET tubes)**, which are artificial tubes placed in the nose or mouth and passed to just above the tracheal carina, and **tracheostomy tubes,** which are tubes inserted into artificially created openings in the trachea. These airways are necessary when normal airway patency and protection cannot be maintained with coughing, tracheobronchial suctioning, respiratory adjuncts, or other airway clearance measures. They are also necessary when ventilation is inadequate and continuous mechanical ventilation is required. The term **intubation** refers to the placement of an artificial airway, such as an endotracheal or tracheostomy tube, into the trachea. The term **extubation** refers to the removal of an artificial airway from the trachea.

Endotracheal tubes are passed either through the nose **(nasotracheal intubation)** or through the mouth (oral tracheal intubation) and extend into the trachea. Most endotracheal tubes are made of disposable polyvinylchloride or other synthetic materials (Fig. 45–19).

Tracheostomy tubes (Fig. 45–20) are placed through a surgical incision into the trachea (Fig. 45–21). Placement of a tracheostomy tube is not usually an emergency procedure unless an immovable obstruction blocks the upper airway (e.g., a piece of food). When long-term airway management using an artificial airway is required (longer than 5 to 7 days), tracheostomy is usually chosen because oral and nasal endotracheal tubes can damage the structures of the oral and nasal pharynx, glottis, and larynx.

Most tracheostomy tubes are disposable, made of polyvinylchloride or other synthetic material, and nonreactive to human tissue. Occasionally, older-style stainless steel and silver tracheostomy tubes may be used.

Figure 45–22 shows a comparison of the endotracheal and the tracheostomy routes of artificial airway placement.

Humidification of Artificial Airways. Artificial airways bypass the normal warming, humidifying, and filtering mechanisms of the natural upper airway. Supplemental humidification is essential. Failure to provide

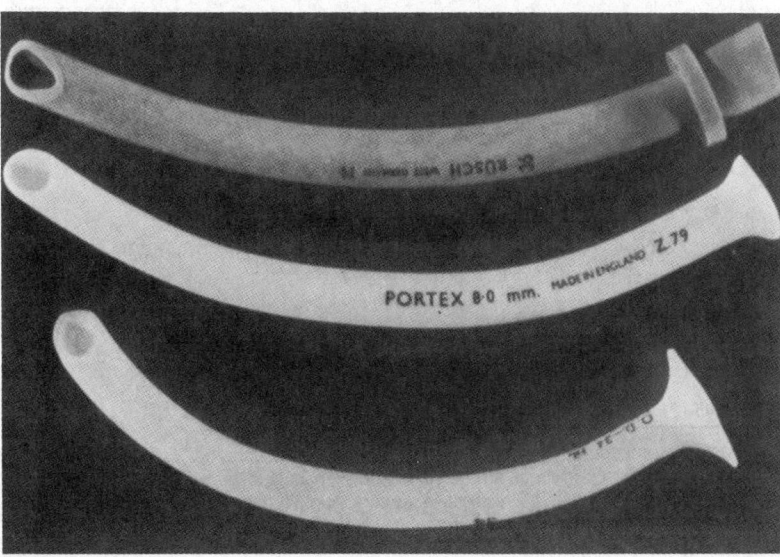

▲ *Figure 45–18*

Nasal airways. These help keep the airway open and provide a guide for insertion of a suction catheter. Suctioning through a nasal airway reduces trauma to the mucous membranes. (Reproduced with permission from Petty, T. *Intensive and rehabilitative respiratory care.* Philadelphia, Lea & Febiger; 1982.)

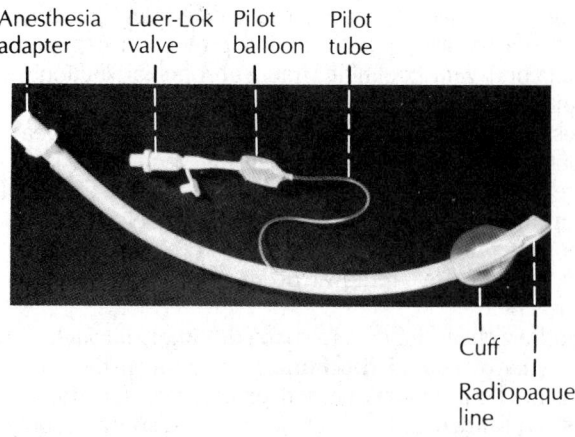

▲ **Figure 45–19**

Endotracheal tube. Air is inserted into the cuff via a pilot tube. An inflated pilot balloon shows there is air in the cuff. Add or remove air from the cuff with a 12-ml syringe via the Luer-Lok valve at the end of the pilot tube. An anesthesia (universal) adapter is connected to the proximal end of the endotracheal tube. The adapter facilitates direct attachment of the artificial airway to airway management equipment. It is important that the tip of the tube be above the carina (bifurcation of main bronchi). A radiopaque line at the distal tip enables the tube to be seen radiographically and placement to be checked. (Courtesy of Portex, Inc., Wilmington, MA.)

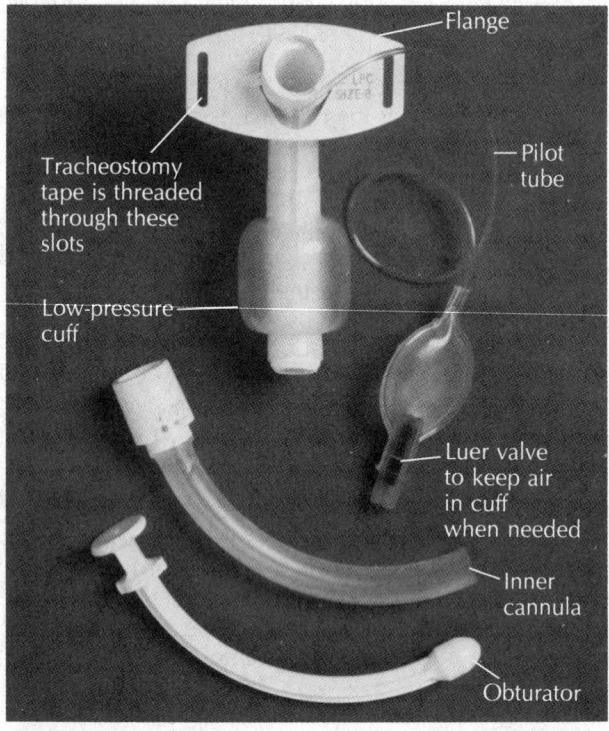

▲ **Figure 45–20**

Tracheostomy tube. Many styles are available. Here, the tube includes an inner cannula, an obturator (used when inserting the outer cannula), and an outer cannula (main tube). The cuff is inflated as it would be if the tube were inserted into a tracheostomy stoma (neck insertion site). During insertion, the cuff is deflated. (Courtesy of Shiley, Inc., Irvine, CA.)

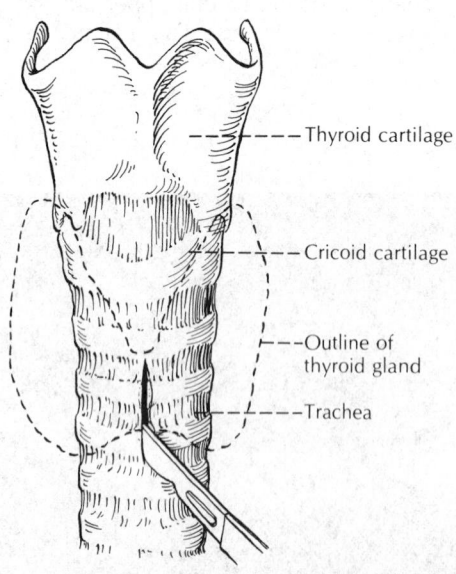

▲ **Figure 45–21**

Tracheostomy procedure. This is usually an elective procedure performed under sterile conditions. An anesthesiologist manages the airway while a surgeon makes a vertical incision through the second, third, and fourth tracheal rings. A tracheostomy tube is then inserted into the surgical opening.

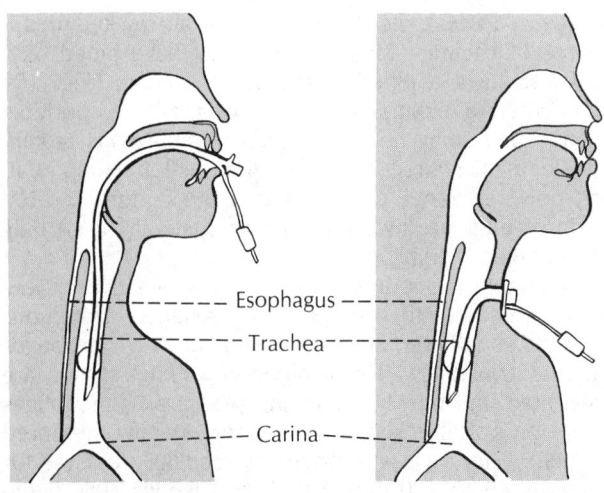

A. Endotracheal tube   **B.** Tracheostomy tube

▲ *Figure 45–22*

Endotracheal *(A)* and tracheostomy *(B)* tube placement. Note location of the trachea and esophagus in relation to the inflated cuff with both types of artificial airway. The inflated cuff can cause trauma unless precautions are taken. The tip of the tube sits above the carina. If tips are lower than shown, there is an added risk of intubating the right main bronchus only, drastically reducing ventilation of the left lung.

adequate hydration and humidification results in dried, retained secretions; increased resistance to airflow; infection; and altered respiratory gas exchange.

Various types of devices are available to provide humidification and oxygenation to people requiring artificial airways. Some provide warm (heated to body temperature) humidification, others deliver cool (room temperature) humidification. Most of these devices also provide oxygen-enriched humidification if needed. Figure 45–23 shows a tracheostomy mask. The mask fits around the neck, loosely covering the tracheostomy tube's external portion. An elastic band holds the mask

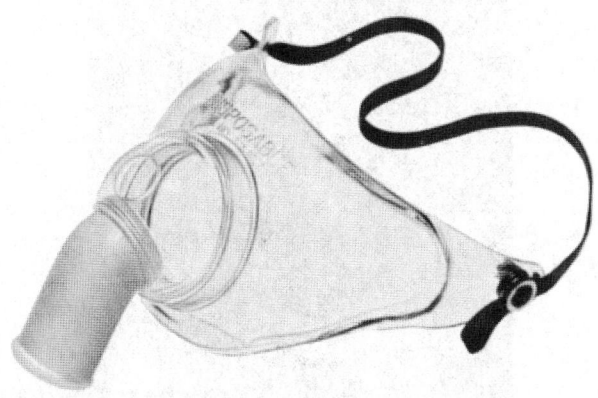

▲ *Figure 45–23*

Tracheostomy aerosol mask. This device delivers topical hydration directly to a tracheostomy. Supplemental oxygen may also be administered along with the aerosol mist. Because a tracheostomy bypasses the upper airway, humidification of inspired air is essential.

in place. Wide-bore aerosol tubing connects the mask and humidification device.

AIRWAY SUCTIONING

Choice of Suctioning Route. Secretions can be removed through the oropharyngeal route (mouth), the nasopharyngeal route (nose), or an endotracheal or tracheostomy tube. The route used depends on

▸ level of consciousness
▸ level of cooperation
▸ availability of an artificial airway
▸ type of material to be suctioned.

The thicker the material, the more difficult it is to aspirate through smaller-sized catheters.

Oropharyngeal or nasopharyngeal suctioning (aspiration) is commonly used for people unable to clear secretions from the upper airway (i.e., mouth or nose). It is often used after coughing. The same general principles apply as with lower airway (tracheobronchial) suctioning (see following section on general suctioning factors). Use attire appropriate to maintain universal precautions and sterile equipment, that is, catheters, gloves, water, or normal saline (to moisten catheter before insertion and to flush it after removal) (Fig. 45–24). Place a conscious person (with unimpaired gag reflex) in a semi-Fowler's position with the head turned toward you for oral suctioning or the neck hy-

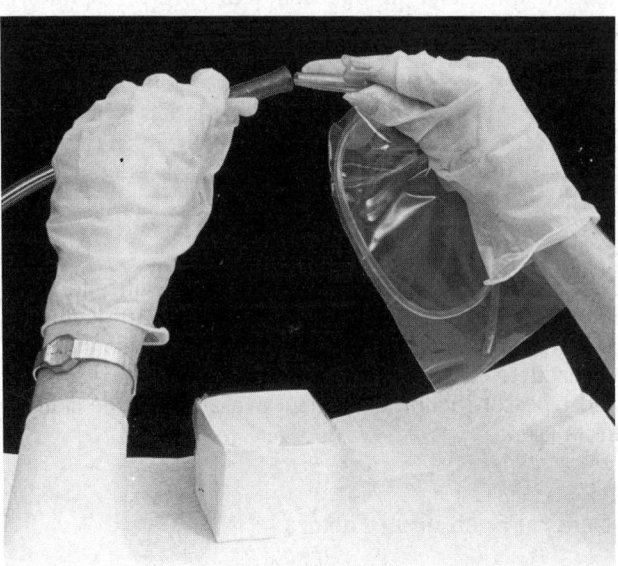

▲ *Figure 45–24*

Preparing for tracheobronchial suctioning. Rinsing solution (normal saline) is poured into the disposable cup before sterile gloves are put on. Here, the catheter is attached to the connecting tube with the dominant (right) "sterile" hand, as shown. The other (left) hand is kept "clean." Not shown, but vital to successful intervention, are collection container, source of oxygen, and (for intubated people) manual resuscitation bag for hyperoxygenation and hyperinflation before and after suctioning. (Reprinted with permission from Kersten, L.D. (1989). *Comprehensive respiratory nursing: A decision-making approach.* Philadelphia: W.B. Saunders.)

perextended (unless contraindicated) for nasal suctioning. Place an unconscious person in the lateral position. Protect the pillow and gown with towels. Use appropriate catheter and suction pressure. Throughout the procedure (Procedure 45–2), keep your gloved, dominant hand "sterile" at all times. It manages the suction catheter. Keep your other gloved hand "clean" and available for managing equipment and client needs. With the sterile hand, hold the catheter at about the same distance from the end as from the person's ear lobe to the tip of the nose. Do not insert any further than this to prevent the catheter's passing beyond the pharynx.

Complete the intervention (from insertion to removal) in less than 15 seconds. Never force the catheter. Do not apply suction during insertion. Gently enter the side of the mouth, directing the catheter into the oropharynx. Or gently enter the nostril, directing the catheter along the nasal cavity floor into the nasopharynx. During withdrawal, apply suction intermittently (to reduce trauma). Twist the catheter while withdrawing and flush the catheter to clear it. Let the person rest 20 to 30 seconds, then encourage coughing and deep breathing. Reinsert if necessary. (The same catheter can be reinserted only twice more.) Discard the catheter, gloves, and disposable attire used for precautions. Wash your hands.

Respiratory dysfunction may interfere with clearing lower airway tracheobronchial secretions. Secretions (mucus or pus) are then retained, and normal exchange of gases is impaired. Prolonged secretion retention may lead to infection and severe respiratory dysfunction.

Suctioning the tracheobronchial tree via a suction catheter is necessary for airway management when a person is unable to clear retained secretions. This includes anyone unable to cough effectively to raise secretions. Suctioning is done on an "as needed" basis. Suctioning is often needed after position changes. Excessive suctioning is dangerous and traumatic.

All health care areas must be equipped with effective, functioning equipment to clear an airway. An occluded airway is potentially life-threatening. All personnel authorized to suction must be familiar with the location and types of suction equipment available and be skilled in its use.

General Suctioning Factors

Hydration. Hydration helps liquefy secretions. Tracheobronchial secretions may be hydrated through parenteral or oral methods, aerosolization of liquid into the tracheobronchial tree to thin the mucus, and direct instillation of liquefying agents into the tracheobronchial tree. A direct relationship exists between secretion thickness or viscosity, suction catheter size, and the amount of vacuum required to remove the secretions (i.e., the thicker the secretions, the larger the size of the suction catheter required, and the higher the vacuum pressures necessary to remove them).

Vacuum Pressures. Suctioning the airway requires a source of vacuum. Most facilities that have piped oxygen also have a piped-in source of vacuum (Fig. 45–25). When a piping system is not available, portable suction units may be used. Most portable units require an electrical source to power the suction pump. Battery-powered and compressed gas Venturi-powered portable units are available but are generally used only for emergency transport.

Suctioning is accomplished by using negative or vacuum pressures to aspirate the retained secretions through a catheter and into a container. The gauges mounted on the wall in a piped-in vacuum system are calibrated in mm Hg vacuum pressure. The gauges found on portable suction units are generally measured in inches Hg. The safe range for vacuum pressures for adults is 80 to 120 mm Hg (2 to 3 inches Hg). If the catheter is too small or the secretions are too thick, excessive (higher than the safe limits) pressures may be necessary. Use a larger catheter. Additional hydration and tracheal irrigation may be required to remove tenacious secretions.

Suctioning Catheter. A **suction catheter** is a rubber or plastic tube, attached to a vacuum source, used to

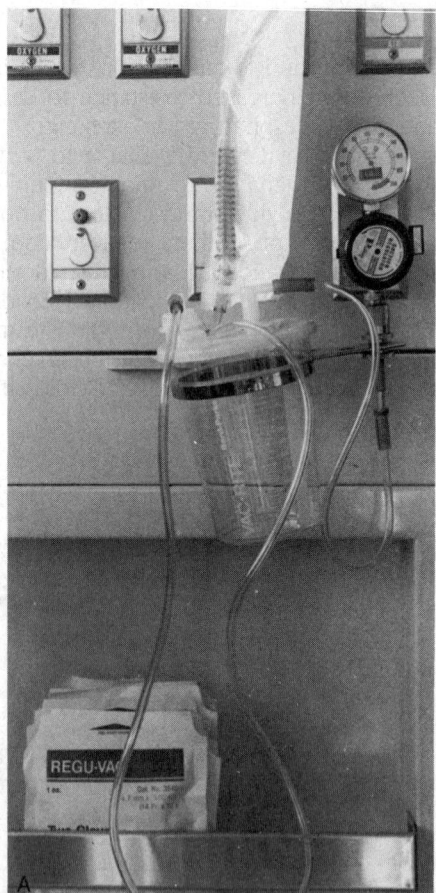

▲ *Figure 45–25*

Bedside suction canister, tubing, and tonsil tip attached to wall vacuum. (Reprinted with permission from Kersten, L.D. (1989). *Comprehensive respiratory nursing: A decision-making approach*. Philadelphia: W.B. Saunders.)

PROCEDURE 45–2

Suctioning the Tracheobronchial Tree

Definition/Purposes. To remove secretions from the tracheobronchial tree by vacuum (suction) by insertion of a sterile catheter into the airway. Suction catheters are inserted through one of three routes: nasopharyngeal route, oropharyngeal route, or endotracheal or tracheostomy tube. Purposes include (1) maintaining a patent airway by removal of retained secretions and foreign material; (2) preventing the effect of retained secretions, such as infection and atelectasis; (3) promoting improved exchange of oxygen and carbon dioxide; (4) stimulating or substituting for effective coughing when cough is impaired (e.g., by diminished mentation, progressive weakness); and (5) obtaining a tracheal aspirate specimen for laboratory analysis.

Contraindications/Cautions. Suctioning is a precise intervention requiring careful attention to safety. (See text for complications of suctioning.) Direct care toward maintaining sterility to prevent infection; avoiding traumatic vacuum pressures and mechanical trauma from suction catheter; providing oxygen administration before, during, and after intervention; hyperinflating the lungs before and after each catheter insertion by either supervising deep breathing or using an anesthesia bag or self-inflating bag if the person is unable to deep breathe independently; and using extra caution if the person has an unstable cardiovascular system.

Suctioning can produce hypoxemia and atelectasis. Insertion of the catheter into the tracheobronchial tree stimulates the vagus nerve. Vagal stimulation and hypoxemia may cause cardiac arrhythmias (e.g., ventricular tachycardia, ventricular fibrillation, and cardiac arrest).

In accordance with universal precautions, put on clean gloves before starting the suctioning procedure. After the procedure is finished, the removal of sterile gloves used for suctioning leaves you with clean gloves for promptly repositioning the person in bed or helping the person to cough up more mucus.

Always use sterile catheters. Ideally, catheters are discarded and replaced after each insertion. Some facilities change catheters after a series of tracheal insertions. Never store suction catheters in any type of solution (including antibacterial solutions).

You may use the same suction catheter to first suction the major bronchi and then the mouth or nose, as needed. However, if you suction the mouth first, you must use another sterile catheter to suction the lungs. This approach avoids contamination of the (sterile) lung with oral or nasal secretions. Catheter size should never be more than half the diameter of the airway. Safe vacuum pressures for an adult are 80 to 120 mm Hg. Apply the vacuum intermittently and as the catheter is withdrawn. An entire catheter insertion and removal sequence should not exceed 10 to 15 seconds.

Teaching/Learning Guidelines. Give clear explanations before suctioning anyone. Seek the person's cooperation. Resistance can cause trauma and introduce infection by contaminating the catheter. Reassure the person and significant others that intervention is essential and will be done as quickly and as few times as possible.

PRELIMINARY ACTIVITIES

Assessment/Planning

Determine need to suction by

- ▶ Visual assessment of respirations.
- ▶ Auditory assessment of respirations.
- ▶ Tactile assessment. Note whether vibrations from secretions are felt through chest wall.
- ▶ Auscultate chest. Determine need for suction. Locate position of secretions in tracheobronchial tree.
- ▶ Assess person's level of awareness and ability to cooperate.
- ▶ Get help as necessary to restrain person. (Careful explanation can often avoid need for restraints.)
- ▶ Get help as necessary for oxygenating person and hyperinflating lungs.
- ▶ Assemble all equipment.
- ▶ Wash hands and put on universal precautions attire.
- ▶ Test vacuum pressure—pinch off connecting tube and note amount of vacuum recorded on suction gauge. Regulate pressure as required.
- ▶ Determine route of suctioning and obtain appropriate equipment (i.e., oral and/or nasal airway, correct size catheter).
- ▶ If manual hyperinflation is not to be done, plan delivery of oxygen. Provide oxygen before and after each suction catheter insertion.

Equipment

- ▶ Vacuum gauge.
- ▶ Collection container.
- ▶ 6 to 10 feet of connecting tubing.
- ▶ Sterile straight catheter or angled catheter.
- ▶ Sterile gloves.
- ▶ Sterile solution (saline or water) to rinse catheter and tubing.
- ▶ Hyperinflation equipment (anesthesia bag or resuscitation bag).
- ▶ Oxygen administration equipment (flowmeter, tubing).
- ▶ Means for delivery of oxygen (e.g., cannula, mask).
- ▶ Sputum trap if tracheal aspirate specimen is needed.
- ▶ Oral airway for oropharyngeal suctioning (for person with diminished gag reflex).
- ▶ Nasal airway for nasopharyngeal suctioning.

Preparation of Person

- ▶ Explain intervention.
- ▶ Position correctly and comfortably. Restrain if necessary.
- ▶ Screen person for privacy.

Procedure continued on following page

PROCEDURE 45–2 Continued

Suctioning the Tracheobronchial Tree

PROCEDURE

Actions	Rationale/Discussion
1. Prepare equipment.	1. *See Chapter 28 for sterile technique.* Ready availability of equipment facilitates the quick implementation of the procedure.
a. Insert nasal or oral airway, if necessary.	a. Prevents trauma to mucosa during suctioning.
b. Open bottle of sterile rinsing solution.	b. Requires two hands, so must be done before sterile gloves are put on.
c. Aseptically open catheter, gloves, and cup.	c. These items can contaminate the lung if not kept sterile.
d. Fill sterile cup with sterile solution.	d. Solution container is not sterile, so should be done before sterile gloves are put on.
e. Put on sterile gloves.	e. Keep glove on dominant hand sterile; your other hand will be clean.
f. Attach sterile catheter to connecting tube as shown in Figure 45–24.	f. Hold catheter with sterile hand and hold connecting tube with clean hand.
2. Increase inspired oxygen concentration (Fig. 45–25) to highest possible percentage of oxygen and hyperinflate lungs with manual or spontaneous deep breaths (Fig. 45–26).	2. Best levels of oxygenation and hyperinflation are achieved with 100 per cent oxygen delivered via anesthesia bag or self-inflating bag.
a. Be aware of blood gas and cardiac status (e.g., note PO_2 on blood gas report, check pulse rate, check PaO_2 by pulse oximetry).	a. Suctioning can cause cardiac arrhythmias and increase hypoxemia. Also, it can cause airway collapse, which can increase hypoxemia and lead to atelectasis.
3. Lubricate sterile catheter with sterile rinsing solution and test patency of catheter by placing thumb of clean hand over vent in catheter.	3. Catheter will enter airway more easily. Pre-test ensures functioning of system before insertion.
4. Remove oxygen source and quickly begin to suction.	4. Oxygen is not stored. It must be supplied continuously. Maximum time oxygen may be interrupted is 10 to 15 seconds.
5. Use sterile hand to insert catheter.	5. Sterile hand prevents bacterial contamination of airway.

Suctioning via Oral Route

Actions	Rationale/Discussion
6. If oral airway is in place, slide catheter alongside it and back into pharynx. If airway is not in place, have person protrude tongue and guide catheter into oropharynx. Insert during inspiration until cough is stimulated, resistance is met, or secretions are located.	6. It is difficult to pass catheter into trachea via mouth. Oral airway helps insertion of catheter into trachea. Tongue displaced forward also helps catheter entry.
	a. *Caution:* Gag reflex may be stimulated with insertion of catheter into oropharynx, causing vomiting and aspiration of gastric contents.
	b. Oral route usually used to remove secretions from back of mouth.

Suctioning via Nasal Route

Actions	Rationale/Discussion
7. Insert and advance catheter during inhalation. Guide catheter along floor of nares, or pass catheter through nasal airway until cough is stimulated, resistance is met, or secretions are located.	7. During inhalation, epiglottis is out of way and airway is almost open. Nasal airway reduces trauma to nasal mucosa and helps insertion of catheter into trachea.
a. To suction left mainstem bronchus, turn client's head to right and align chin with right shoulder (Fig. 45–27A).	a. Facilitates passage of catheter tip to left bronchus.
b. To suction right mainstem bronchus, turn client's head to left and align chin with left shoulder (Fig. 45–27B).	b. Facilitates passage of catheter tip to right bronchus.

PROCEDURE 45–2 Continued

Suctioning the Tracheobronchial Tree

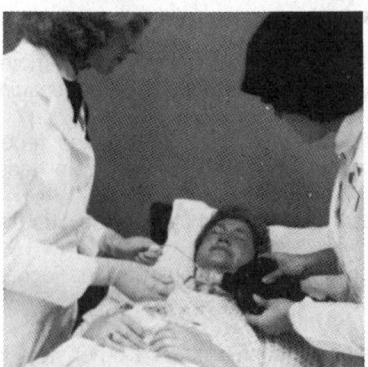

▲ *Figure 45–26*

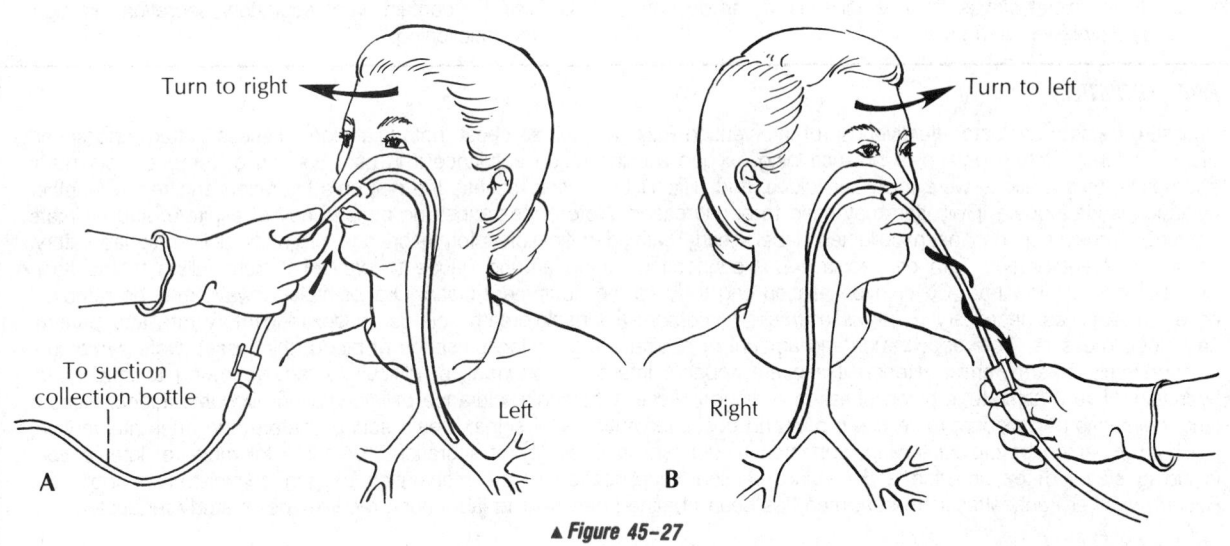

Turn to right

To suction
collection bottle

Left

A

Turn to left

Right

B

▲ *Figure 45–27*

c. Insert catheter 15 to 20 cm.

d. To remove catheter, twist rather than pulling it directly out.

c. Length required to reach desired depth in adult client.

d. Helps increase probability of catheter tip openings contacting mucus.

Suctioning via Endotracheal or Tracheostomy Tube

Actions	**Rationale/Discussion**
8. Insert catheter into airway during inhalation, not touching person or environment. Insert until cough is stimulated, resistance is met, or secretions are located.	8. Airway diameter is larger during inhalation. Never force catheter. This causes trauma.
9. Do *not* cover thumb control or apply vacuum during catheter insertions.	9. Applying vacuum during insertion dangerously increases hypoxemia and can cause atelectasis.
10. Apply *intermittent* vacuum while withdrawing catheter.	10. Intermittent vacuum reduces trauma to mucosal lining of airway. *Never* apply continuous vacuum.
a. While withdrawing, rotate catheter and/or wind it around index finger.	a. Reduces dragging of catheter along one portion of mucous membrane and controls catheter, preventing it from touching environment or person.
b. Insertions and removal of catheter should not take longer than 10 to 15 seconds.	b. Longer time increases risk of dangerous complications.

Procedure continued on following page

PROCEDURE 45–2 Continued

Suctioning the Tracheobronchial Tree

Actions	Rationale/Discussion
11. Discard catheter, glove, cup, and solution if changing routes.	11. Never use the same catheter to suction more than one route, except as described in the contraindications/cautions section.
12. Reoxygenate and hyperinflate for minimum of five breaths. Allow person to rest between insertions.	12. Reduces and corrects hypoxemia and reopens small airways that may have collapsed from vacuum pressures.
13. Assess person and repeat process if secretions are still present.	13. Unnecessary suctioning may increase side effects.
14. Use fresh catheter, glove, cup, and solution for each tracheal insertion; or after three repeated tracheal insertions; or follow facility policy.	14. Prevention of bacterial contamination. Facilities vary in policy.

15. Discard catheter, gloves, cup, solution, and (disposable) precautions attire, if no further suctioning is required.
  a. Disinfect goggles, if necessary.
  b. Put on clean gloves for final activities, if you do not already have them on.
	15. These items are contaminated. Do not store for reuse.
	
	  a. Eyewear may be nondisposable.
	  b. Risk for contact with respiratory secretions is high after suctioning.

FINAL ACTIVITIES

Reassure person. Evaluate effectiveness of intervention (e.g., auscultate chest, note vital signs, assess pattern and sound of respirations). Return person to presuctioning oxygen administration appliance if in use. Loosen or remove restraints if appropriate. If secretions were thick, tenacious, and difficult to suction, assess the person's hydration and report whether hydration is inadequate. Hydration may need to be increased. Note appearance and consistency of aspirate, and estimate amount. If specimen has been collected, label clearly with identification information and promptly deliver to laboratory. *Aftercare of equipment:* Turn off vacuum. Coil connecting tubing around gauge to prevent it from falling to the floor. Recheck oxygen flow rate. Cover hyperinflation bag to keep the equipment clean. Oral or nasal airways may be removed or left in place as necessary. *Final assessment of person:* Recheck breath sounds, pulse, respiratory rate and pattern, and blood pressure. Note appearance and amount of aspirate (e.g., color, presence of blood, thickness). Note symptoms of hypoxemia or arrhythmias. Report if aspirate appears infected, abnormal, or difficult to remove owing to inadequate hydration. Note if aspirate is blood streaked or tinged. Assess person's tolerance of intervention. *Documentation:* Record time intervention was done; route used; pre- and post-intervention vital signs; breath sounds before and after intervention; position of person before suctioning; appearance, quantity, and quality of secretions; person's tolerance of intervention, including status of oxygenation and cardiac reaction; reapplication of pre-intervention oxygen administration appliance. Record whether tracheal aspirate specimen has been obtained and sent to laboratory; record type of study requested.

---

suck secretions from the lungs, nose, and mouth. It must be made of a material that is as nontraumatic as possible. Many brands of suction catheters are designed with a smooth, rounded tip and are made from a silicone and polyvinylchloride compound. This reduces resistance and friction when the catheter is passed through an artificial airway or the nose. The end of a suction catheter has two to three "vents" (i.e., openings). This type of catheter is called the whistle-tip catheter. The vents are spaced along the lower 1½ to 2 inches on alternate sides of the catheter. This prevents the collapse of the catheter if it becomes occluded and high vacuum pressures are created. The vents also help reduce mucosal trauma by reducing the pull of the catheter against the mucosa.

The proximal end (i.e., the end closest to you) of the catheter has a port (opening) that is occluded intermittently to complete the vacuum circuit. When the port is open, air can pass in and out of the trachea.

When this port is occluded, the vacuum pressure is transmitted into the airway and secretions are removed through the catheter to the collection container.

Suction catheters are sized by the French scale. The smaller the French number, the smaller the catheter. Suction catheters generally range in size from 5 French to 18 French. Sizes 12 and 14 are most commonly used for suctioning an adult airway. Smaller catheters do not remove the secretions as effectively as larger ones do. They also tend to curl and are more difficult to direct into the airway.

An important general rule for catheter size selection: The size of the suction catheter never exceeds half the diameter of the artificial airway or the natural airway it is to enter.

When artificial airways are in place, the size of the catheter is critical. When a catheter is inserted into the

TABLE 45-14. *Indications for Suctioning*

Assessment	Indications for Suctioning
Visual	Change in respiratory pattern (e.g., increase in breathing rate, difficult or labored breathing)
Auditory	Moist, noisy, or gurgling sounds during respiration
Tactile (use flat of hand over chest wall)	Vibrations of loose secretions felt through the chest wall
Auscultation	Retained secretions sound loose, low pitched, rattling, and coarse (rhonchi); they usually disappear after suctioning
	Auscultation is an important part of assessment before and after suctioning

airway, atmospheric air must be able to pass through and alongside it, or the person will suffocate. Remember, as secretions are aspirated, air is also removed from the lungs. The larger the catheter in relation to the artificial airway, the more air will be removed from the lungs.

Assessing the Need for Suctioning. Suctioning is needed when people are unable to clear the airway by raising secretions through coughing. Retention of secretions leads to an increased risk of infection, atelectasis, and interference in the exchange of carbon dioxide and oxygen. Table 45-14 presents indicators of the need to suction. Suctioning is successful when abnormal indicators are no longer present.

Side Effects of Suctioning. Hypoxemia, alveolar collapse and atelectasis, vagal stimulation, trauma to airway mucosa, hypotension, and paroxysmal episodes of coughing may occur during tracheobronchial suctioning. Table 45-15 summarizes these effects, the causative mechanism, the means of prevention or correction, and indicators that these effects are occurring.

Oxygen cannot be stored in the body. A person must be reoxygenated between each suctioning attempt. Never suction a second time until the person has been reoxygenated for at least five breaths. Suction-induced hypoxemia may be fatal. If any cardiac irregularities are created by the suctioning, stop immediately, reoxygenate, and hyperinflate the person's lungs.

MECHANICAL VENTILATION

When respiratory problems become so severe that oxygenation and ventilation are inadequate, mechanical ventilation may be used. **Mechanical ventilation** is ventilation of the lungs by artificial means, usually by a ventilator (formerly called a respirator). The physician makes the decision to initiate mechanical ventilation on the basis of the presence of severe hypoxemia or acute

or chronic ventilatory failure, defined earlier in the chapter. Specific blood gas and pulmonary function test criteria are used to help make the decision.

Most of the time, mechanical ventilation produces highly favorable results. It rests the respiratory muscles and permits the person to recover quickly from acute respiratory disease; in the case of chronic disease, the person stabilizes into a pattern of long-term ventilation. In other cases, however, medical complications arise, especially in the person with multiple medical-surgical problems. The complications of mechanical ventilation include hypotension, decreased cardiac output, pneumothorax, oxygen toxicity, positive fluid balance, gastric distention, gastrointestinal bleeding, infection, and malnutrition.

Moreover, because of possible complications, the decision to use mechanical ventilation is not always a straightforward medical one. For example, the physician knows that when mechanical ventilation is implemented for a person with severe chronic lung disease, it is possible that the person may never get off the ventilator. Even when a large interdisciplinary team cares for the person, weaning the person off the ventilator may become impossible because of the person's poor mechanics of breathing and deteriorating condition. In this case, previous discussions with client, family, nurse, and others help the physician decide how far to go with aggressive medical therapy should acute ventilatory failure remain unresponsive to basic treatment.

Nursing management of persons on mechanical ventilation is complex and requires advanced training. To begin to learn more about monitoring these people, ask a respiratory nurse or respiratory care practitioner to share their knowledge, skill, and experience related to the topic. Whenever your client is placed on mechanical ventilation and transferred to another unit for closer monitoring, make a visit to the bedside. Observe the person and his or her ventilator setup. In addition, check the literature for details pertaining to monitoring people on mechanical ventilation.[8,11,18]

In the use of ventilators, as in all nursing interventions, scientific principles should be your guides to action. Some of the scientific principles covered in this chapter are summarized in Table 45-16.

EVALUATION

Evaluation of respiratory care consists of answering the following six important questions.

Is the person's overall condition better, worse, or status quo? If the person has achieved the agreed-on outcomes by the target date, the person's condition is considered improved.

Are respiratory interventions contributing to an improvement in the person's physical and psychosocial condition? The effectiveness of respiratory interventions may be difficult to evaluate. Subjective chest assessment findings are not always congruent with objective findings. For example, a person with chronic lung disease may deny dyspnea, but results of arterial blood

TABLE 45–15. Side Effects of Suctioning

Side Effect	Causative Mechanism	Nursing Interventions/ Prevention	Indicators
Hypoxemia	Vacuum removes oxygen; presuctioning hypoxemia is worsened; may be lethal	Give supplemental oxygen	Tachycardia; increased dyspnea; irregular heart rate; cyanosis; pallor; diaphoresis (sweating)
Alveolar collapse and atelectasis	Vacuum removes nitrogen, the "filler" gas that keeps alveoli open; high vacuum pressures collapse alveoli	Deep breathing reexpands closed alveoli	Increasing hypoxemia; chest discomfort; worsening appearance on chest x-rays
Vagal stimulation	The vagus is the major nerve supply to the trachea—a catheter may irritate or stimulate it; hypoxemia plus vagal stimulation results in cardiac arrhythmias	Suction only when needed	Bradycardia; ventricular arrhythmias; cardiac arrest
Mucosal trauma	As vacuum is applied, mucosa is pulled into the holes of the suction catheter; bleeding, edema, erosion, and increased potential for infection occur	Suction only when needed; avoid jabbing motions; lubricate catheter if mucous membranes are dry, or catheter "pulls"; use oral or nasal airway; apply suction while withdrawing catheter only	Pain; discomfort; increased difficulty breathing; bleeding
Hypotension	Caused by vagal stimulation or prolonged coughing; if this occurs, stop suctioning	Suction only when needed; maintain oxygen status	Low blood pressure readings; increased pulse; dizziness; or other signs and symptoms of reduced blood flow to the brain and heart
Paroxysmal coughing	Stimulation of carinal and tracheal cough reflexes by catheter; may seriously interrupt ventilation and cardiac output	Maintain oxygen status; limit time catheter inserted; monitor cardiac status before and after suctioning	Inadequate ventilation; gasping; change in color; hypotension; syncope; tachycardia

gas analysis and pulmonary function tests may indicate worsening of the condition. In other cases, the person may complain of dyspnea and excessive fatigue when the test results indicate an improved condition. Hence, for a thorough evaluation, evaluate subjective findings in light of laboratory and diagnostic tests.

If objective tests are not readily available, use existing resources to obtain at least one objective respiratory measurement, such as oximetry SaO_2, before evaluating therapy. Some clinical units keep an oximetry device on the unit for evaluation purposes. In other situations, you may ask the respiratory care practitioner to obtain measurements of the person's pulmonary function. Many respiratory care practitioners routinely use a portable pulmonary function test device, such as a pocket-sized spirometer (breathing test device) or peak flowmeter, to evaluate respiratory therapy. In acute settings, bedside pulmonary function test values may be charted on respiratory therapy or interdisciplinary flowsheets to facilitate evaluation by all members of the health care team.

Are the person's airways bronchodilated as much as possible? In respiratory care, perhaps the biggest problem related to pulmonary medications is undermedication. Physicians have difficulty finding the right combination of different types of bronchodilators, given in doses that maximize bronchodilation with the least side effects. In many cases, the physician prescribes adequate doses of medication; however, the person fails to take the doses on time or as needed. For these reasons, continually monitor for signs of increased bronchoconstriction and airway obstruction. If coughing or wheezing increases, or if breath sounds become progressively more distant-sounding, call the physician and check the person's medication schedule. Bronchodilators are ideally scheduled around the clock to ensure 24-hour bronchodilation. For examples, twice-daily bronchodilators are scheduled at 8 AM and 8 PM, not at 8 AM and 6 PM. Clients prescribed bronchodilators on an as-needed basis should be encouraged to use them regularly, as directed, whenever pulmonary symptoms develop.

CHAPTER 45 ▼ Meeting Respiration Needs

TABLE 45-16. Selected Scientific Principles and Related Nursing Interventions for Meeting Respiration Needs

Principle	Nursing Interventions
Normal gas exchange is achieved by the proper amounts of lung ventilation and lung perfusion	Check recent results of blood gas analysis; if results are within normal ranges, assume a normal gas exchange Check for the presence of normal breath sounds; if you auscultate them over all lung lobes, assume normal ventilation, unless blood gas results indicate otherwise
During inspiration, a slow airflow rate decreases airway resistance and promotes the even distribution of gas in the lungs	During deep-breathing maneuvers, instruct the person to take a *slow* deep breath in and hold it for at least 3 seconds before exhaling Discourage coughing and other forced expiratory maneuvers, unless the person is likely to produce mucus Encourage a deep inhalation after any forced expiratory maneuver; the breath will help prevent airway collapse and airway irritation associated with the use of frequent forced expiratory maneuvers
Droplets residing in nebulizer cups, tubing, or other pieces of respiratory equipment provide a warm, moist environment for the growth of microorganisms	Help the respiratory care practitioner or family at home change respiratory equipment setups every 12 to 24 hours, as directed by the health agency, respiratory therapy department, or home equipment company In the home setting, instruct the family to clean home equipment daily and to always start with a fresh setup in the morning
Too much oxygen may eliminate the hypoxic ventilatory drive of the person with chronic respiratory disease	When the person with chronic respiratory disease is given oxygen, monitor for signs and symptoms of hypercapnia and hypoxemia During respiratory distress, give the person with severe disease small amounts of oxygen (no more than 2 or 3 LPM of oxygen by nasal prongs), until a blood gas sample is taken and the physician adjusts the dosage and administration device
Mucus cannot drain out of the lungs without open airways	During planning, consider bronchoconstriction a top-priority problem Routinely check for signs and symptoms of bronchoconstriction (i.e., complaints of wheezing or chest tightness, wheezing or decreased breath sounds on auscultation) If bronchoconstriction is present, encourage the person to take bronchodilators, as directed, before mobilization maneuvers and other respiratory treatments

Is the person receiving the right amount of oxygen? As previously explained, the right amount of oxygen is being delivered when signs of hypoxemia and hypoxia are absent and when blood gas values remain within normal ranges. For persons with chronic lung disorders, acceptable blood gas values include a PaO_2 value greater than 55 or 60 mm Hg, or an SaO_2 value greater than 85 per cent. For persons with a hypoxic ventilatory drive, the right amount of oxygen is the amount that relieves hypoxemia *without increasing the $PaCO_2$* value.

Should any respiratory treatments be increased or decreased in intensity or frequency or both? Consult the physician, respiratory care practitioner, or physical therapist to answer this question. The challenge of respiratory care is to implement interventions, such as incentive spirometry or chest physical therapy, in the right way and at the right time. Furthermore, treatments must be spaced so that the health care team members

do not contribute unnecessarily to the person's fatigue and sleep deprivation.

Have the person and family met the learning outcomes and evaluation criteria for each respiratory intervention implemented? Examples of learning outcomes and specific evaluation criteria are provided in Table 45-8. Once you set up evaluation criteria during the planning stage of the nursing process, evaluation becomes easy. If the evaluation criteria are met, client and staff are correctly implementing the intervention. A deteriorating clinical condition may be due to faulty technique. Faulty technique may occur when the person's treatment plan is too complex or when there is inappropriate reinforcement of educational content during the early stages of the teaching/learning process.

Last, keep a family member or significant other involved in evaluation throughout all stages of the teaching/learning process. Because of complex treatment plans, persons with respiratory disease easily become overwhelmed. They have difficulties coping emotionally and physically without the support of others to help implement the plan. When personal relationships are strong, family members may help in a variety of ways. For example, they may effectively remind the person throughout the day to drink plenty of fluids to liquefy secretions. They may remind the person of other criteria, such as to use the inhaler as scheduled or to practice pursed-lip breathing with all activities of daily living.

Document the answers to these six questions in the nursing notes, in accordance with the health agency's charting protocols. Once intervention begins, evaluation and its documentation are ongoing. Initial evaluation criteria are modified on the basis of the initial response to treatment and the discovery of more sensitive indicators for progress. For example, consider Mrs. Romero, a 70-year-old woman with a history of asthma and a new fractured hip. After teaching Mrs. Romero how to deep breathe and cough effectively, your progress note in the chart might read:

Client was taught how to deep breathe and cough effectively, using the unit's printed materials for reinforcement of correct technique. On return demonstration, client met all evaluation criteria: slow inspiratory phase of respiration; 3-second pause after inspiration; and respiratory rate less than 12/minute. Coughed up 2 tsp. light yellow mucus.

On the night shift, a different nurse works with Mrs. Romero. This nurse discovers that Mrs. Romero cannot

CASE STUDY

The Client

Mrs. Mary Jones is a 59-year-old white female with a seven-year history of chronic pulmonary disease. She was seen in her physician's office with a complaint of a "cold," fatigue, loss of appetite, increased shortness of breath, and fever. Chest x-ray revealed a consolidation in the left lower lobe. She was admitted to the hospital three days ago with a diagnosis of probable pneumonia—left lower lobe. A partial listing of physician's orders on admission included:

▶ Obtain sputum for culture and sensitivity
▶ Oxygen at 2 liters/minute via nasal cannula
▶ Heated aerosol treatment every 4 hours, followed by postural drainage and chest percussion

At 8 AM, February 10, a partial listing of assessment data included the following:

59-year-old, thin female
Sitting up and leaning slightly forward onto bedside table

▶ Complains of "shortness of breath"
▶ Skin intact with slight duskiness of nailbeds
▶ T 100.8°F, B/P 120/76, P 98, R 26 and labored
▶ Breath sounds audible bilaterally—decreased in left base Rhonchi present, left > right
▶ Arterial blood gas results: PaO$_2$ 56 mm Hg   pH 7.47
                                PaCO$_2$ 52 mm Hg   HCO$_3^-$
                                                       37 mEq/L

Seventy-two hours have passed since admission. The following represents part of a nursing care plan written for her shortly after admission and the current evaluation of outcomes that were expected at that time.

CARE PLAN

4 PM, February 10

Nursing Diagnosis	Planning: Expected Outcomes	Implementation: Nursing Interventions	Evaluation
Ineffective Airway Clearance R/T excessive secretions and ineffective coughing	By 2 PM, February 13: ▶ Demonstrates improved airway clearance, AEB effective coughing techniques and breath sounds clear to auscultation	▶ Encourage client to maintain adequate hydration by: a. drinking at least 8–10 glasses of fluid/day b. increasing humidity of environmental air ▶ Teach and supervise effective coughing	2 PM, February 13: ▶ Respirations are 20/minute and slightly labored ▶ Breath sounds are clear bilaterally in the upper lobes ▶ Breath sounds over left lower lobe are slightly decreased, with some rhonchi audible

CARE PLAN (Continued)

4 PM, February 10

Nursing Diagnosis	Planning: Expected Outcomes	Implementation: Nursing Interventions	Evaluation
		techniques, including end-expiratory coughing ▶ Perform chest physical therapy, as ordered, and instruct client/significant others in these techniques ▶ Encourage position changes at least every 2 hours ▶ Assess breath sounds before and after coughing episodes	▶ Cough is productive of a moderate amount of thick, yellowish secretions

use correct deep-breathing and coughing technique because of the development of airway irritation and bronchospasm. In the following chart entry, note how the nurse documents the problem and adds more sensitive (individualized) evaluation criteria. The additions are needed to reduce airway irritation and bronchospasm during treatment.

When starting to deep breathe, client developed a nonproductive, hacking cough with wheezes on auscultation. Findings disappeared about 5 minutes after taking 2 puffs of albuterol bronchodilator inhaler. Client coughed up small amounts of mucus 15 minutes after the aerosol. *New evaluation criteria for correct deep-breathing/coughing technique:* Following 2 puffs albuterol 15 minutes beforehand, with a minimum of 2 minutes between each puff; no hacking cough or wheezes on auscultation.

Summary

▶ The upper respiratory tract consists of the nose and sinuses, the pharynx, and the larynx; the lower respiratory tract includes the trachea, bronchi, bronchioles, and alveoli.

▶ The primary function of the respiratory system is gas exchange, the intake of oxygen and the elimination of carbon dioxide.

▶ Respiration is regulated primarily by the respiratory centers of the brain. However, the central and peripheral chemoreceptors also serve as important secondary regulators, detecting changes in carbon dioxide and oxygen levels, respectively, and adjusting respiration accordingly.

▶ Breathing may be affected by a number of internal factors (e.g., developmental stage and health disorders) and external factors (e.g., environment).

▶ Hypoventilation occurs when ventilation of the alveoli fails to keep up with the body's production of carbon dioxide, with resultant increased arterial carbon dioxide, hypoxemia, acidosis, tachycardia, and changes in mentation.

▶ Hyperventilation occurs when alveolar ventilation exceeds the body's need for eliminating carbon dioxide, with resultant decreased respiratory drive, alkalosis, lightheadedness, and neuromuscular irritability.

▶ A thorough respiratory history should include a determination of the person's chief complaint, information regarding its development and what aggravates or alleviates it, past related medical history, and environmental/lifestyle assessment.

▶ In the clinical setting, the first impressions, inspection, and auscultation components of the chest examination will help you to more efficiently assess persons with potential or diagnosed cardiopulmonary problems.

▶ The data obtained from laboratory and diagnostic studies provide a fuller understanding of the respiratory condition and can be used to monitor the effectiveness of respiratory interventions.

▶ The nursing diagnoses most directly related to respiratory dysfunction are *Impaired Gas Exchange, Ineffective Airway Clearance*, and *Ineffective Breathing Pattern*.

▶ The planning of respiratory nursing care involves the identification of top-priority diagnoses; the selection of appropriate outcomes in conjunction with the individual, the family, and other health care team members; and the selection of appropriate nursing interventions, including education.

▶ Mobilization maneuvers include measures that help prevent secretion retention and assist spontaneous secretion removal.

▶ Topical hydration helps keep secretions liquid and more easily expectorated.

▶ The goals of chest physical therapy include the promotion of tracheobronchial drainage, the prevention of secretion pooling, and an overall improvement in ventilation.

▶ The goal of oxygen therapy is to achieve an optimal arterial oxygen level by giving the lowest possible, most effective dose of oxygen while avoiding the toxic effects of oxygen.

▶ Medications delivered into the respiratory system in aerosol form produce rapid effects.

▶ Positive-pressure breathing treatments help stimulate deep breathing and mobilize secretions.

▶ Respiratory exercises may be used to promote maximal inspiration or to improve the quality of respirations.

▶ Artificial airways may be used to maintain airway patency, to facilitate airway suctioning, and to attach mechanical ventilation.

▶ Suctioning the tracheobronchial tree via a suction catheter is necessary for airway management when a person is unable to clear retained secretions.

▶ Mechanical ventilation may be initiated when severe hypoxemia and acute or chronic ventilatory failure are present.

▶ Universal precautions should *always* be used in working with persons with respiratory disorders.

▶ Evaluation of respiratory nursing care involves the determination of whether client outcomes have been reached. This is not always evident strictly by objective, outward evidence.

Bibliography

1. Ahrens, T. (ed.) (1989). Advances in pulmonary care. *Critical Care Nursing Clinics of North America*, 1(4), 641–705.
2. Bartlett, R. (1984). Respiratory therapy to prevent pulmonary complications of surgery. *Respiratory Care*, 29(6), 667–677.
3. Bolgiano, C.S., et al. (1990). Administering oxygen therapy—what you need to know. *Nursing '90*, 20(6), 47–51.
4. Breslin, E. (1981). Prevention and treatment of pulmonary complications in patient after surgery of the upper abdomen. *Heart & Lung*, 10(3), 511–519.
5. Campbell, E., et al. (1988). Subjective effects of humidification of oxygen for delivery by nasal cannula—a prospective study. *Chest*, 93(2), 289–293.
6. Cherniack, R.M. (ed.) (1990). *Lung disease—State of the art*. New York: American Lung Association.
7. Ehrhardt, B., & Graham, M. (1990). Pulse oximetry—an easy way to check oxygen saturation. *Nursing '90*, 20(3), 50–54.
8. Eigen, H., & Zander, J. (1990). Home mechanical ventilation of pediatric patients [Statement of the American Thoracic Society]. *American Review of Respiratory Disease*, 141(1), 258–259.
9. Ellstrom, K., & Bella, L.D. (1990). Understanding your role during a code. *Nursing '90*, 20(5), 37–43.
10. Fedorovich, C., & Tittleton, M.T. (1990). Chest physiotherapy—evaluating the effectiveness. *Dimensions of Critical Care*, 9(2), 68–74.
11. Ferland, P. (1991). Are you ready for ventilator patients? *Nursing '91*, 21(1), 42–47.
12. Fisher, E.B., et al. (1990). Smoking and smoking cessation. *American Review of Respiratory Disease*, 142(3), 702–720.
13. Frownfelter, D. (ed.) (1987). *Chest physical therapy and pulmonary rehabilitation* (2nd ed.). Chicago: Year Book Medical.
14. Fulmer, J., & Snider, G. (1984). American College of Chest Physicians—National Heart, Lung, and Blood Institute National Conference on Oxygen Therapy. *Chest*, 86(2), 234–246.
15. Gross, N. (1990). Chronic obstructive pulmonary disease: current concepts and therapeutic approaches. *Chest*, 97(2), 19S–23S.
16. Hodgkin, J., et al. (1984). *Pulmonary rehabilitation—Guidelines to success*. Boston: Butterworth.
17. Ingersoll, G. (1989). Respiratory muscle fatigue research: implications for clinical practice. *Applied Nursing Research*, 2(1), 6–15.
18. Kersten, L. (1989). *Comprehensive respiratory nursing—A decision-making approach*. Philadelphia: W.B. Saunders.
19. Kim, M.J. (ed.) (1987). Ineffective breathing patterns and airway clearance [symposium]. *Nursing Clinics of North America*, 22(1), 121–247.
20. Konz, C.M. (1990). Action stat! Emergency intubation. *Nursing '90*, 20(2), 33.
21. Levitzky, M., et al. (1990). *Introduction to respiratory care*. Philadelphia: W.B. Saunders.
22. Lindell, K.O., & Mazzocco, M.C. (1990). Breaking bronchospasm's grip with MDIs. *American Journal of Nursing*, 90(3), 34–41.
23. Lindell, K.O., & Wesmillar, S.W. (1989). Using arterial blood gases to interpret acid-base balance. *Orthopedic Nursing*, 8(3), 31–34.
24. Make, B. (1990). Pulmonary rehabilitation—what are the outcomes? *Respiratory Care*, 35(4), 329–331.
25. Miracle, V., & Allnutt, D.R. (1990). How to perform basic airway management, *Nursing '90*, 20(4), 55–60.
26. Moody-Szymanski, E., & Scherer, Y.K. (1989). Breathing. In Dittmar, S. (ed.). *Rehabilitation nursing—Process and application* (pp. 82–119). St. Louis: C.V. Mosby.
27. Mostow, S., et al. (1990). Prevention of influenza and pneumonia [Statement of the American Thoracic Society]. *American Review of Respiratory Disease*, 142(2), 487–488.
28. Neagley, S.R. (1991). The pulmonary system. In Grif-Alspach, J. (ed.). *Core curriculum for critical care nursing*. Philadelphia: W.B. Saunders.
29. North American Nursing Diagnosis Association (1992). NANDA diagnoses: Definitions and classifications 1992. St. Louis: Authors.
30. Peters, K., et al. (1990). Increasing clinical use of pulse oximetry. *Dimensions of Critical Care Nursing*, 9(2), 107–111.
31. Petty, T. (ed.) (1990). Diagnosis and treatment of chronic obstructive pulmonary disease. *Chest* (Suppl.), 97(2).
32. Reischman, R.R. (1988). Impaired gas exchange related to intrapulmonary shunting. *Critical Care Nurse*, 8(8), 35–39, 42–44, 47–49.
33. Risser, N. (1980). Preoperative and postoperative care to prevent pulmonary complications. *Heart & Lung*, 9(1), 57–67.
34. Scanlan, C. L., et al. (1990). *Egan's fundamentals of respiratory therapy* (5th ed.). St. Louis: C.V. Mosby.
35. Sexton, D. (ed.) (1990). *Nursing care of the respiratory patient*. Norwalk, CT: Appleton & Lange.
36. Shapiro, B., et al. (1991). *Clinical application of respiratory care*. St. Louis: C.V. Mosby.
37. Siskind, M.M. (1989). A standard of care for the nursing diagnosis of ineffective airway clearance. *Heart & Lung*, 18(5), 477–482.
38. Tager, I. (1989). Health effects of "passive smoking" in children. *Chest*, 96(5), 1161–1164.
39. Tyler, M. (1982). Complications of positioning and chest physiotherapy. *Respiratory Care*, 27(4), 458–466.
40. Tyler, M., et al. (1980). Prediction of oxygenation during chest physical therapy in critically ill patients. *American Review of Respiratory Disease*, 121(4): 218.
41. Weilitz, P.B. (1991). *Pocket guide to respiratory care*. St. Louis: Mosby–Year Book.
42. West, J.B. (1987). *Pulmonary pathophysiology: The essentials* (3rd ed.). Baltimore: Williams & Wilkins.
43. Wilkins, R., et al. (1990). *Clinical assessment in respiratory care* (2nd ed.). St. Louis: C.V. Mosby.
44. Wilson, S.F., & Thompson, J.M. (1990). *Respiratory disorders*. St. Louis: Mosby–Year Book.

Chapter 46

▼ # *Administering Medications*

> It is medicine, not scenery, for which sick man must go a-searching.
>
> **Seneca**

▼ **CHAPTER OUTLINE**

GENERAL PRINCIPLES OF MEDICATION
   ADMINISTRATION
      The Responsibilities of the Nurse
      The Responsibilities of the
         Physician
      The Responsibilities of the
         Pharmacist
      Rights and Responsibilities of
         Persons Receiving Medications
      Legal and Ethical Aspects of
         Medication Administration
      Names of Medications
      Routes of Administration
      Effects of Medication
      Medication Delivery Systems
      Medication Orders
      Computing and Timing Dosages
      Safety Measures for Medication
         Administration

ASSESSMENT
      Physiologic Factors
      Psychosocial Factors
      Special Needs
NURSING DIAGNOSIS
PLANNING
NURSING INTERVENTION
      Teaching Self-care to Persons
         Receiving Medications
      Using Judgment in the
         Administration of Medications
      Administering Oral Medications
      Administering Topical Medications
      Administering Parenteral
         Medications
EVALUATION
CASE STUDY

▼ **KEY TERMS**

Adverse effects
Aerosols
Air lock technique
Ampule
Antagonistic effect
Atomization
Capsules
Creams
Dermal patches

Dorsogluteal site
Drug
Effervescence
Elixirs
Emulsions
Enteric-coated tablets
Formulary
Gels

Instillation
Local effects
Lotions
Lozenges
Medication
Mid-deltoid site
Nebulization
Ointments

▼ KEY TERMS Continued

Ommaya reservoir	Prescription medications	Solutions	Synergistic effects	Toxic effects
Oral medication	prn	Stat order	Syrups	Vaporization
Over-the-counter	Prolonged-acting tablets	Suspensions	Systemic effects	Ventrogluteal site
(OTC) medications	Quadriceps femoris site	Sustained-release	Therapeutic effects	Vials
Pharmacokinetics	Side effects	tablets	Tinctures	Volatile substance
Powders				

▼ LEARNING OBJECTIVES

After studying this chapter, you should be able to

1. Discuss the responsibilities of members of the health care team in relation to medications.
2. List the rights and responsibilities of the client in relation to taking medications.
3. Discuss legal and ethical issues that nurses face in the administration of medications.
4. Describe names of medications, routes of administration, and effects of medications.
5. Describe the common systems of medication administration.
6. List the elements of a medication order.
7. Identify the types of medication orders.
8. Describe the computation and timing of dosages.
9. Describe safety measures related to medication administration.
10. Explain general assessment criteria associated with medication administration.
11. Describe nursing measures related to medication.
12. Identify forms in which medications are available.
13. State nursing principles used for safe administration by parenteral routes.
14. Explain evaluation after the administration of medication.

Medication administration is the cornerstone in the overall plan of nursing care and medical treatment. This type of intervention is also one of the most important responsibilities borne by nurses. In practically every health care setting, nurses are responsible for (a) administering medications, and (b) assisting people to use medications safely and properly. In addition, nurses must be knowledgable concerning (a) the pharmacology of medications given, (b) the legal implications involved in the preparation and administration of medications, (c) the techniques of safe medication preparation and administration, and (d) the application of the nursing process when they are caring for individuals receiving medication.

In this chapter we discuss general guidelines for administering medications correctly and safely by the oral, topical, and parenteral (injection) routes. Because an introductory textbook cannot supply all the information necessary to give medications, however, you will need to consult other sources for reference. These include (1) pharmacology textbooks, (2) the *American Hospital Formulary* or the **formulary** (a book that provides information about medications) used in the agency in which you work, (3) nursing literature, (4) inserts provided with packaged medications, and (5) pharmacists.

This chapter focuses on the team approach to medication administration. Because the health team's goal and responsibility is optimal health care delivery, all team members (nurses, physicians, and pharmacists) must work cooperatively, realizing that each professional has special expertise and skills to contribute.

It is primarily the nurse's responsibility to ensure that medications are administered safely and that the client and significant others understand the therapy and are helped to participate, to the best of their ability, in the therapeutic program.

GENERAL PRINCIPLES OF MEDICATION ADMINISTRATION

The Responsibilities of the Nurse

Medication preparation and administration has many legal and ethical implications. Of major importance is knowledge. When you administer medications, you are responsible for developing an up-to-date knowledge base. For each medication that you administer, you should be familiar with the following:

► the generic and proprietary names
► the classification
► the normal dose or range of doses
► the route(s) of administration
► the desired action
► common side effects
► toxic and undesired effects

▶ contraindications and incompatibilities with other medications
▶ special considerations and nursing implications

To improve this knowledge base, you can record information on a medication reference card. Figure 46-1 provides a useful format for this purpose. Preprinted medication cards, in a similar format, are also available for purchase in many bookstores.

You also must be aware of the "five rights" in administering a drug. An important nursing responsibility is adhering to these "five rights." These are the

1. Right drug
2. Right dose
3. Right route
4. Right time
5. Right person

Nursing practice requires that you continue to update your knowledge base concerning medications. You are also responsible for

▶ developing skills that enable you to administer all types of medications correctly
▶ utilizing all steps of the nursing process in the administration of medications
▶ recording the medications administered (or not administered, with rationale for the omission) and documenting client responses
▶ safeguarding, storing, and caring for medications

▶ acting as a role model for the public by educating others on safe uses of medications and demonstrating these actions to the public
▶ acting as an advocate for individuals taking medications, by protecting their rights and ensuring their safety and comfort
▶ questioning an incorrect or incomplete medication order and refusing to administer one that you think is unsafe
▶ teaching clients the expected or desired outcomes, side effects, and adverse reactions related to medications

The Responsibilities of the Physician

In relation to medication, physicians are usually responsible for (a) taking a medical history and performing a physical examination, (b) diagnosing the disease, (c) prescribing medications to cure the disease or ameliorate the symptoms, (d) monitoring the response to therapy, and (e) modifying medication orders as necessary. In many settings, however, nurses and other health professionals share some of these responsibilities.

Although physicians are legally responsible for ordering medications, nurses are responsible for

▶ assessing the client on an ongoing basis and providing the physician with data that assist in establishing

DRUG: Benadryl (diphenhydramine HCl)
CLASSIFICATION: Antihistamine with anticholinergic (drying) and sedative effects
USUAL ROUTE & DOSAGE: Adults – 25 or 50 mg po TID or QID; children over 20 lbs – 12.5 to 25 mg po TID or QID or 5 mg/kg/24 hrs po
DOSE ORDERED: 50 mg po q6h prn
DESIRED ACTION:
A. General: Symptomatic relief of a variety of allergic reactions. Prevention and treatment of motion sickness. Treatment of mild parkinsonism. Treatment of mild insomnia.
B. For this person: Relief of itching from poison ivy rash.
SIDE EFFECTS: Sedation; sleepiness; dizziness; epigastric distress; dryness of mouth, nose, and throat; and thickening of bronchial secretions.
TOXIC AND UNDESIRED EFFECTS: Urticaria, drug rash, hypotension, headache, palpitations, tachycardia, hemolytic anemia, thrombocytopenia, nausea, vomiting, diarrhea, constipation, urinary frequency, urinary retention, difficult urination, confusion, insomnia, blurred vision, neuritis, convulsions.
NURSING IMPLICATIONS: Caution the person about driving or operating heavy machinary and that alcohol and other CNS depressants have an additive effect.
CONTRAINDICATIONS: Newborn and premature infants, nursing mothers, persons with lower respiratory tract symptoms, including asthma, hypersensitivity to diphenhydramine HCl and other antihistamines of similar chemical structure. Incompatible with MAO inhibitors.

▲ *Figure 46-1*

Completed medication reference card.

the diagnosis and continuing need for the medication

▶ assessing the client to be certain it is safe to administer the ordered medication each time it is to be given
▶ safely administering the ordered medication
▶ monitoring the client's individual response to the medication
▶ reporting the client's response to relevant members of the health care team

For example, if a nurse administers a narcotic to an individual and then observes that the client's respirations slow to an inadequate rate, it is the nurse's responsibility to consult with the physician concerning a possible change in dosage, route, timing, or medication.

Physicians also share with other health team members the responsibility for educating people and significant others regarding medication therapy. Physicians work with nurses and pharmacists to ensure that people have a full understanding of their therapeutic regimens. Physicians also act as resources in providing information about medication therapy to other health care providers.

The Responsibilities of the Pharmacist

Pharmacists are highly trained specialists in the area of drug chemistry, classification, action, and administration. Their work involves selecting, obtaining, and storing medications and accounting for the safe dispensing of these items. Pharmacists interpret medication orders of prescriptions, dispense medications, monitor medication usage, and educate the public concerning drug and health issues.

Pharmacists work in an agency or a community setting. In the community, pharmacists often dispense medications in a drugstore or other business. They fill prescriptions and educate individuals about medications. In addition to these responsibilities, pharmacists in some areas also act as outreach paramedics. For example, when refilling an order for antihypertensive medications, they may take the person's blood pressure.

In a health care agency, pharmacists play a slightly different role. Pharmacists maintain the complex systems required to dispense medications to large groups of individuals. These systems of dispensing medications (e.g., the unit dose systems) differ from agency to agency. Pharmacists' responsibilities include stocking the pharmacy, checking for outdated medications, and ensuring return of unused medications to the pharmacy. They also work as educators in conjunction with nurses and physicians, teaching people about medication and acting as a resource for other health care professionals.

Rights and Responsibilities of Persons Receiving Medications

Clients have rights regarding medications they are to receive. They also have responsibilities in relation to their medications. Part of promoting independence and self-care is to assist individuals and their significant others to understand client rights and responsibilities. Principal responsibilities of individuals regarding medications are to

▶ understand the therapy and to question, to the best of their ability, what they do not understand
▶ understand their role in the therapeutic regimen
▶ adhere to the regimen: to take medications at correct times and in correct amounts for as long a time as prescribed
▶ report adverse effects of medications or changes in their condition that warrant a change in therapy
▶ avoid misuse or abuse of medications
▶ store medications safely in the home

Nurses and physicians, who share responsibility for client care, also are responsible for assuring that clients' rights are not violated. People receiving medications have the right to

▶ have a complete assessment by skilled practitioners before medication is administered
▶ receive information concerning their medication, such as name, actions, and side effects
▶ receive notification if a medication is experimental. The client must be asked to give written consent before receiving an experimental medication.
▶ receive medications that are labeled or otherwise identifiable
▶ be free from unnecessary medications

Any person has a right to refuse to take any medication, and the person who refuses a medication must never be made to feel guilty or otherwise "punished" for the decision. It is far more helpful to attempt to discern the reason for the refusal and to plan with the client for a more therapeutic alternative. Refusal to take a medication must be documented in the person's chart.

Legal and Ethical Aspects of Medication Administration

Medication prescriptions and orders are written by physicians, nurse practitioners, dentists, physician's assistants, and other health care professionals. The scope of practice differs for each professional from state to state. For instance, some states have not yet granted nurse practitioners the legal authority to write prescriptions. It is essential that you know the details of your state Nurse Practice Act and follow all state rulings explicitly. Nurses are independently licensed and take full responsibility for their actions in administering medications. In all instances, nurses must protect the

APPLYING RESEARCH TO NURSING PRACTICE

Evaluating the Effect of Complex Medication Regimens on Compliance Among Elderly Clients

Conn, V.S., Taylor, S.G., & Kelley, S. (1991). Medication regimen complexity and adherence among older adults. *Image,* 23(4), 231–235.

▼ ▼ ▼

Conn and colleagues studied the impact of complex medication regimens on compliance among elderly people. The researchers rated the complexity of the regimens based on four factors:

► the number of medications
► the number of daily doses
► special instructions accompanying medications, such as the timing of dosing in relation to meals
► additional steps necessary for medication administration, such as mixing a powder in liquid

The researchers rated adherence to the regimens by asking clients what medications they had taken and by counting the pills that the clients had not taken. As expected, Conn and colleagues found clinical evidence that as the complexity of medication regimens increased, medication adherence decreased. It was surprising, however, that the effect of the complexity of the regimens was so small that it was statistically insignificant.

Applications for Practice

Although clients have a responsibility to adhere to their medication regimen, nurses have a corresponding responsibility to be on the alert for noncompliance. If complexity of the regimen is not a factor, nurses must recognize this. We must seek out other possible reasons for noncompliance and intervene appropriately.

---

individual's health by making judgments about the validity of medication orders.

If a nurse questions the validity of a physician's order, the nurse has a right and a responsibility to (a) decline to give the medication, (b) question the physician on the validity of the order, (c) document these events on the permanent record, and (d) report the matter to a higher authority, if necessary.

Because institutional policies vary, nurses must be aware of the expectations for acceptable practice in the agencies in which they work. To prevent errors, nurses must familiarize themselves with the policies for medication administration at individual health care facilities. For example, leaving medications at a person's bedside is strictly prohibited in some institutions. In others, certain medications may be left at the bedside with written permission of the physician.

LAWS GOVERNING MEDICATION ADMINISTRATION

The use and sale of medications are governed by state and federal laws. In 1938, the Federal Food, Drug, and Cosmetic Act became the major statute regulating drugs. This law also created the Food and Drug Administration (FDA) to enforce drug standards.

Medications are classified as either **prescription medications** (medications, including controlled substances, that require a physician's order) or **over-the-counter (OTC) medications** (medications that may be purchased without a physician's prescription). The FDA determines which medications require a prescription and which substances are controlled.

Prescription medications include those that (a) are habit-forming, (b) have certain potentially harmful effects, (c) must be administered under the supervision of a health care practitioner, and (d) have a strong potential for misuse and abuse (e.g., narcotics and barbiturates). Drugs that have a strong potential for misuse and abuse are classified as controlled substances because they are closely regulated by federal and state laws. OTC medications are sold without a prescription, but the FDA requires pharmaceutical companies to supply detailed information on the label.

Even though a medication is sold over the counter, it may not be completely safe. All drugs have potentially harmful effects, particularly if they are not used as recommended.

The FDA also maintains strict control of all new drugs proposed for human use. Therefore, a drug company promoting a new drug must submit its proposal to the FDA. Until controlled studies demonstrate the efficacy and the safety of a drug, its use is limited. Because of this FDA policy, certain medications available in other countries are not available in the United States. Unless a drug meets specific standards, the FDA prohibits distribution of the new product.

ETHICAL ISSUES CONCERNING MEDICATIONS

Nurses must consider a number of ethical issues when working with medications. Two important issues are drug misuse and drug dependence. Drug misuse is the improper use of prescribed or OTC medications in ways or dosages other than those recommended. A person may increase the dosage or use the medication in a way that is harmful. Drug dependence is a condition of physical or psychologic dependence that may develop with chronic use of a drug. The issue of drug dependence is complex, with many physical, psychologic, emotional, and social implications. The assessment and treatment of people who misuse or are dependent on drugs often require the combined expertise of many professionals: nurses, physicians, social workers, psychologists, biochemists, and various research scientists.

Nurses also face the ethical issue of illegal dispensing of drugs. Nurses and other health care providers have access to a variety of medications that can be abused or misused. They also have the responsibility to safeguard access to medications. Nurses must not obtain medications for their own personal or illegal use or for the illegal use of others.

Dispensing drugs illegally is a punishable offense as well as an unethical act.

Another ethical issue is the nurse's role in giving experimental drugs. Nurses must make certain that the individual's rights are protected and that the person has given informed consent before participating in the study. The rights of human subjects and the issue of informed consent are outlined in the American Hospital Association's Statement on a Patient's Bill of Rights (see Chapter 4). The American Nurses' Association delineates nurses' responsibilities in preserving the rights of individuals who serve as research subjects.

In addition, the federal government has developed strict guidelines for the use of human subjects in experiments and regulates many of the research projects involving human experimentation. Government agencies such as the National Institutes of Health (NIH), the Department of Health and Human Services (DHHS), and the FDA are also involved in the control of biomedical research programs.

Names of Medications

It is technically incorrect to use the term "drug" and "medication" interchangeably. Although all medications are drugs, not all drugs are medications. A **drug** is any substance that modifies or changes the organism's function, with or without a therapeutic effect. Drugs can be used therapeutically, as in the diagnosis, treatment, or prevention of disease, or can be abused and used illegally for nontherapeutic purposes. A **medication,** on the other hand, is a drug that is always administered with a therapeutic intent. Medications modify or change the organism to restore homeostasis.

Drugs are prescribed, administered, and sold under three different names. The chemical name identifies the particular chemical compound from which a drug is produced. The generic name is the official name of a drug, the name not protected by a trademark. The proprietary name, also known as a brand or trade name, appears as a trademark for one special product. Remember that one generic compound can be sold

under several proprietary names. For example, meperidine is the generic, or official, name of the chemical *N*-methyl-4-phenyl-4-carbethoxypiperidine. Winthrop Laboratories markets this drug under the proprietary name Demerol, whereas Wyeth Laboratories calls its meperidine product Mepergan.

Routes of Administration

Medications are administered in different ways. The most common method is oral, that is, given by mouth. Any medication given by mouth may be considered an **oral medication,** even if it is absorbed in the mouth and not in the stomach or intestine. Medications can be classified according to their method or route of administration. These classifications include

- sublingual medications: medications placed under the tongue and absorbed into the blood vessels underneath the tongue (e.g., nitroglycerin)
- buccal medications: medication held inside the mouth against the mucous membranes of the cheek (e.g., lozenges)
- topical medications: agents applied to the skin and mucous membranes for absorption or for local therapy. In addition to administration onto the skin, topical agents include optic medications (medications administered into the eye), otic medications (medications administered into the ear), nasal medications (medications administered into the nose), vaginal medications (medications administered into the vagina), rectal medications (medications inserted or instilled into the rectum), and pulmonary medications (medications inhaled into the respiratory tract)

Medications given by the sublingual and buccal routes are also sometimes classified as topical medications.

Parenteral medications are those given by injection with a needle. Parenteral medications are the most rapidly absorbed because they are administered directly into or close to the circulation or into their sites of action. Routes of administration for parenteral medications include the

- subcutaneous route: administration into the subcutaneous tissue, under the skin
- intradermal route: administration under the epidermis, into the dermis
- intramuscular route: administration into a muscle
- intravenous route: administration into a vein
- intra-arterial route: administration into an artery
- intracardiac route: administration into the heart muscle
- intraosseous route: administration into a bone
- intrathecal route: administration into the spinal canal
- epidural route: administration into the space external to the dura mater of the spinal canal

Effects of Medication

All medications have both desirable and undesirable effects. As a drug combines with cell constituents, alterations occur in cellular function. Some drugs, for example, inhibit or stimulate certain enzymes. Other drugs cause a change in cell membrane permeability or interact with body hormones. These alterations should be **therapeutic effects,** or desired outcomes. Therapeutic effects of drugs promote health (e.g., vitamin supplements), prevent disease (e.g., immunizations), alleviate discomfort or pain, or cure or control disease processes. However, **adverse effects,** or **side effects,** sometimes occur. These are unintended or harmful responses to a normal medication dose or treatment. Unfortunately, adverse effects are common.

Adverse effects occur with normal dosages, whereas **toxic effects** are adverse reactions resulting from overdose or from abnormal accumulation of a drug in the body. Adverse effects are mild, severe, or even lethal and can damage any organ system in the body.

In addition to understanding therapeutic effects and adverse effects, it is important to be aware of the sites of each medication's effects and how the effects can be altered by the ways drugs interact with each other.

Nurses must know a drug's

- **local effects:** reactions affecting only the area to which the medication is administered. For example, injections of aqueous penicillin often cause pain and erythema at the site of injection.
- **systemic effects:** effects occurring in a body organ or system distant from the site of application of a medication. For example, absorption of nitroglycerin from oral mucosa results in dilation of coronary arteries.
- **synergistic effects:** combined effects of two or more drugs given simultaneously so that the effects are greater than the sum of their individual effects. For example, a muscle relaxant combined with an analgesic results in greater pain relief than would have been achieved by the two medications separately. The term *potentiation* is sometimes used synonymously with the term *synergism.*
- **antagonistic effect:** mutual opposition or contrary action between two medications. For example, potassium speeds the heart rate, whereas digitalis slows it. Thus, when given together, potassium antagonizes digitalis.

Medication Delivery Systems

Health care agencies have developed various systems for storing and dispensing medications. Goals of any medication delivery system include (a) promotion of accurate and safe medication administration, (b) reduction of errors, (c) reduction of time involved in preparing and administering therapeutic agents, (d) cost containment, and (e) involvement of people in self-care.

The four major medication systems in current use are the stock supply system, individual cubical system, unit dose system, and self-medication.

In the stock supply system, large amounts of medications are kept available on each unit. Nurses preparing medication for administration dispense individual doses from bulk containers—that is, nurses "pour" each medication from a stock container before administration.

The individual cubicle system designates a separate container of medications for each individual. Each person's cubicle contains all the prescribed medication (except controlled substances) for that person. Each day all cubicles are refilled by pharmacy personnel.

With the unit dose system, medication is supplied in individually packaged and labeled doses. The manufacturer or pharmacy personnel package individual doses before transporting them to the nursing unit. A unit dose is the specified amount of medication normally administered to a person at one time. A single-dose package is taken to the bedside for administration.

A recently developed unit dose system consists of a cart with compartmentalized drawers for medication storage. Access to the medications is by a menu-driven computer. Each nurse has a personal code for entry. The names of the clients and the medications are listed alphabetically and entered into the computer by the pharmacy. Each medication is inventoried before and after it is removed (for a specific client) from its compartment. This kind of unit dose system also monitors narcotics and other controlled substances, which eliminates recording in a narcotic book, thereby saving much nursing time.

Self-medication systems allow clients in agencies such as hospitals to administer their own medication, thus giving them greater independence. For example, self-medication is particularly advantageous for people who have been newly diagnosed with diabetes mellitus and must learn to administer their own insulin. Others using a self-medication system include those who take nitroglycerin for angina (chest pain). Another type of self-medication is patient-controlled analgesia (PCA), in which clients administer their own pain medication intravenously through an infusion pump (see Chapter 40).

Each medication system has advantages and disadvantages. For example, unit dose medications decrease errors and reduce preparation time compared with those given from stock supplies. They are, however, more expensive than medications dispensed from bulk stock. Hospitals and agencies seek to develop systems best suited to their needs. Some agencies use more than one system.

Medication Orders

When a physician or other health care professional writes a medication order, it includes specific directives for the pharmacist filling the order, for the person taking the medication, and for the nurse administering the medication. Information includes the

- name of the person to receive the medication
- date and time the order is written
- name of the medication to be administered
- dosage
- route of administration

▶ time and frequency of administration

▶ signature of the person writing the order

The amount of information required on an order, or prescription, varies from state to state. Medication orders often contain abbreviated words. Table 46–1 lists common abbreviations that may appear on medication orders.

In the hospital setting, physician's orders are written or verbal. The physician transcribes (writes) the written order onto the client's chart, usually onto a specific order sheet. This order is signed immediately by the practitioner prescribing the medication. A verbal order (V.O.) is either stated by the physician in person or stated to a registered nurse over the telephone as a telephone order (T.O.). When accepting a verbal order, the nurse must record the date, time, medication, dosage, route, frequency of administration, and the prescriber's name and title, as well as whether the order was T.O. or V.O. The nurse must then sign the order. For example, 10/21 — 8:45 AM — Demerol 50 mg IM q4h prn for pain. T.O. Dr. J. Stern/C. Dorchester, RN.

Verbal and telephone orders must be countersigned by the prescriber as soon as possible. Because verbal communication is often misunderstood, most agencies discourage the use of verbal or telephone orders.

When accepting a verbal or telephone order, repeat to the person prescribing the medication the name, dosage, route, and frequency of administration. This verification prevents errors in communication.

Several directives are used to designate the frequency of medication administration. A single order is a directive to be followed one time only. It indicates that a medication is to be given once, often at a specified time. For example, an order for a preoperative medication is usually written as a single order. Single orders must be differentiated from other orders so that the medication dose is not repeated.

Standing orders are directives to be followed on a routine basis until canceled by another order. Standing orders are often used in special care areas where people receive very similar kinds of care (e.g., labor and delivery or coronary care units). These orders often follow an established medical protocol. For example, nurses may routinely administer certain medications, unless canceled, to individuals with designated diagnoses or health care problems without consulting with the physician each time. Like all other orders, standing orders must be written on the client's chart.

A **stat order** is a directive that is to be carried out immediately. Stat orders are often used in emergencies or when a person's condition warrants immediate attention. Medications given during a cardiac arrest or during an acute attack of asthma are ordered stat. A stat order is verbal or written. If it is written, the nurse should be alerted immediately and the medication administered promptly.

Administration of stat orders takes priority over almost any other nursing activity.

Prn is the Latin abbreviation for *pro re nata*, which translates to "as necessary." Prn medication orders are written to allow, with certain limits, the medication to be administered at the nurse's discretion. For example, a medication ordered q4h prn may be given at any time but not more frequently than at 4-hour intervals. The nurse decides whether to give or to withhold the ordered medication. A prn order is often used in the administration of analgesics for pain following surgery. The nurse assesses the person and the situation carefully and uses additional resources before administering medication. For example, the nurse consults other nurses caring for the individual and reviews the nurse's notes in the chart before making decisions about prn analgesics for postoperative pain.

Computing and Timing Dosages

Computing dosages is an important task in the administration of medications. Nurses use a variety of mathematical tools to determine safe and accurate dosages. Although health care delivery systems commonly use the metric system, medication orders can also be written in the apothecary system or in household measurements. Because all these systems are in current use, you must be able to work accurately with each one of them (Table 46–2).

Calculation errors can occur in the conversion from system to system. Learn reliable and fail-safe methods for solving dosage problems. Consult your drugs and solutions textbook. Your health agency will also have conversion charts available for reference.

TABLE 46–1. Common Abbreviations for Prescribing and Administering Medications

Abbreviation	Unabbreviated Form	Meaning
AA	ana	of each
ac	ante cibum	before meals
ad lib	ad libitum	freely
bid	bis in die	twice each day
c̄	cum	with
gtt	gutta(e)	drop(s)
hs	hour of sleep	at bedtime
ID	intradermal	into the dermis
IM	intramuscular	into muscle
IV	intravenous	into a vein
OD	oculus dexter	right eye
OS	oculus sinister	left eye
OU	oculus uterque	each eye
pc	post cibum	after meals
po	per os	by mouth
prn	pro re nata	as necessary
q	quaque	every
qid	quater in die	4 times each day
s̄	sine	without
SC, SQ	subcutaneous	beneath the skin
tid	ter in die	3 times each day

TABLE 46-2. Approximate Equivalents

Metric	Apothecary	Household
By Volume or Liquid Measure		
5 ml	60 minims	1 teaspoon
30 ml	1 oz	2 tablespoons
240 ml	8 oz	1 cup
500 ml	16 oz	1 pint
1000 ml or 1 liter	32 oz	1 quart
4000 ml or 1 liter	128 oz	1 gallon
By Weight or Dry Measure		
1 mg	1/60 gr	
60 mg	1 gr	
1 gm	15 gr	
30 gm	1 oz	
454 gm	1 pound	
1 kg	2.2 pounds	

The timing of medication administration involves the following factors:

▶ number of doses to be given in a 24-hour period
▶ pharmacokinetics of the medication, which include absorption, distribution, biotransformation, and excretion
▶ possible interactions of a medication with foods, fluids, or other types of medication
▶ scheduling of diagnostic examinations or other types of therapy
▶ needs of the individual

Although the prescriber determines the number of times a day a medication is to be given, nurses frequently decide when the medication is actually to be administered. They make that decision weighing (a) the goals of therapy, (b) the needs of the individual, and (c) the standard times used by the health care agency. For example, a physician writes an order for an antibiotic to be given four times a day without specifying whether it is to be given over a 24-hour period or during waking hours. The nurse could administer the medication at (a) 9 AM, 1 PM, 5 PM, 9 PM, or (b) 6 AM, 12 noon, 6 PM, 12 AM. Although each schedule ensures administration during a 24-hour period, each provides the person with a different circulating blood level of antibiotics. The second schedule requires that the individual be awakened to take the medication at night. Waking up interferes with the person's sleep cycle but provides the timing necessary to ensure a constant blood level of antibiotic. Therefore, the nurse must determine which schedule has the most therapeutic effect and still provides the person with sufficient uninterrupted sleep.

You need to consider other factors when timing medication administration. Some medications should always be given with meals; others must be given on an empty stomach. Certain medications are very dangerous when administered with other medications. Some medications must be withheld before certain diagnostic tests; others cannot be withheld safely. When you make

decisions about scheduling medication administration, consult with the pharmacist and other health team members.

Safety Measures for Medication Administration

Safety in medication administration is a priority. Procedures and policies have been developed to ensure safety and accuracy. To guarantee that you observe the Five Rights, remember the following precautions:

▶ Use clear and verifiable communications concerning medication.
▶ Safeguard the medication.
▶ Safeguard the individual receiving medication.

In the clinical setting, clear communications are essential to order, obtain, and deliver medication to the individual. Agency policies usually determine a system of communication. One system requires a clerk or nurse to transcribe a written order and send a carbon copy to the pharmacy, which then fills the prescription and sends the medication to the nursing unit. Under another system, the orders are also transcribed to individual medication cards (Fig. 46-2), which are then used by the nurse to administer the medication. In other agencies, the nurse or clerk transfers dosage, route, and time of administration to a medication form or other record. The nurse then uses this form or record to administer the medication and to document it. Sometimes the medication form or record is handwritten, and sometimes it is computer generated.

To ensure safety, check medication cards against the original order and against other medication records with every administration. When using a computerized form, compare it also with the original order. In agencies using a computer system, the computer-generated form will be the only record of the medications ordered. You will have to bring up the medications ordered on the computer screen to check them against the printed sheet. If you note an error on any record, report it to the appropriate person at once. In addition, if you question the order, consult the physician before administering the medication.

Because several people are involved in ordering and administering medication, the possibility of error is always present. Prevent errors by checking and double-checking the medication and order before carrying it out.

The pharmacy carefully monitors medication. On the nursing unit, keep all medications in a locked cabinet or cart until administration. When using a tray to deliver medications to individuals, do not leave it unattended at any time. Follow proper storage procedures. For example, keep medication that needs refrigeration at the recommended temperature. Discard outdated medications (check expiration dates on all medications) or return them to the pharmacy. Safeguard narcotics and other controlled substances according to agency policy by counting the number of narcotics at

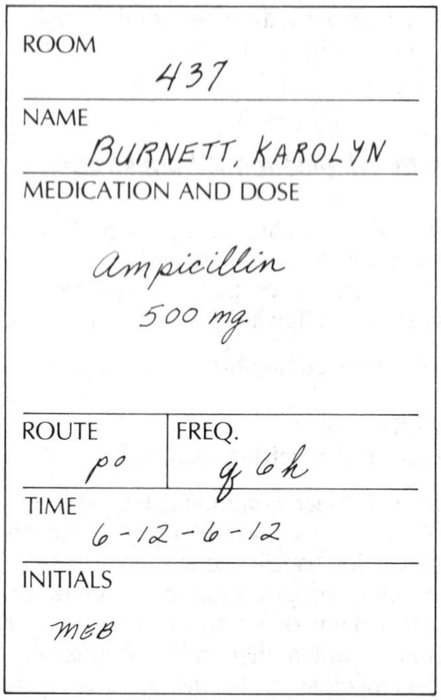

A

ROOM

437

NAME

BURNETT, KAROLYN

MEDICATION AND DOSE

Ampicillin

500 mg

ROUTE	FREQ.
po	q 6h

TIME

6 - 12 - 6 - 12

INITIALS

MEB

B

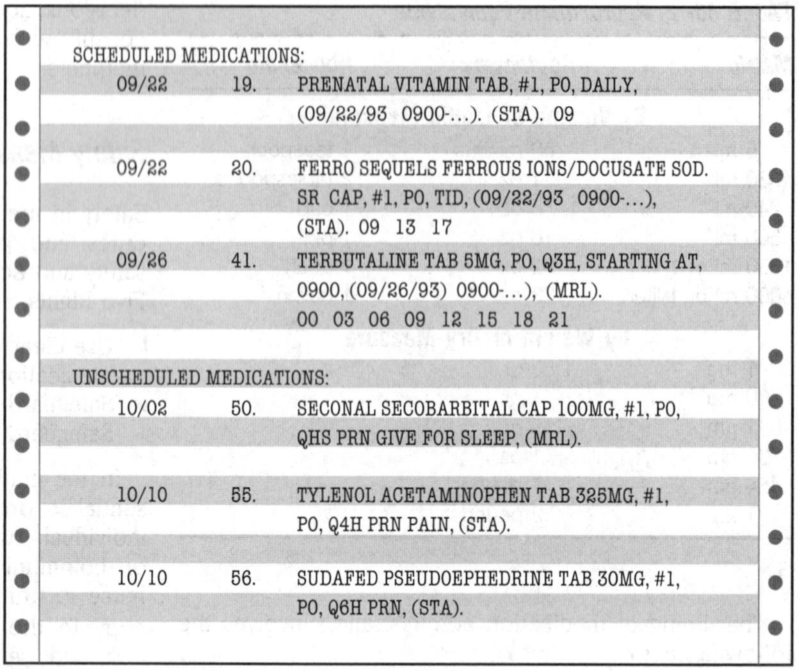

SCHEDULED MEDICATIONS:

09/22   19.   PRENATAL VITAMIN TAB, #1, PO, DAILY,
                (09/22/93 0900-...). (STA). 09

09/22   20.   FERRO SEQUELS FERROUS IONS/DOCUSATE SOD.
                SR CAP, #1, PO, TID, (09/22/93 0900-...),
                (STA). 09 13 17

09/26   41.   TERBUTALINE TAB 5MG, PO, Q3H, STARTING AT,
                0900, (09/26/93) 0900-...), (MRL).
                00 03 06 09 12 15 18 21

UNSCHEDULED MEDICATIONS:

10/02   50.   SECONAL SECOBARBITAL CAP 100MG, #1, PO,
                QHS PRN GIVE FOR SLEEP, (MRL).

10/10   55.   TYLENOL ACETAMINOPHEN TAB 325MG, #1,
                PO, Q4H PRN PAIN, (STA).

10/10   56.   SUDAFED PSEUDOEPHEDRINE TAB 30MG, #1,
                PO, Q6H PRN, (STA).

▲ Figure 46–2

A, Medication card. *B,* Computer-generated medication list. The date the order was written is at the left of the ordered medication. The date that a scheduled medication is to start is in parentheses following the order. The second set of parentheses contains the code for the physician who wrote the order. The time(s) for administration of scheduled medications follows the physician's code and is printed with reference to the 24-hour clock. Many health agencies utilize this format to avoid confusion between AM and PM.

the end of each shift and verifying the count before you remove a dose to give the client. At least two nurses must count narcotics to ensure accuracy.

Safeguard people by following established medication procedures conscientiously. For example, always check the accuracy of the dosage, check that you have the correct medication, read the individual's name band, and ask clients to tell you their names before giving medications.

Unfortunately, medication errors do occur. All agencies have a special procedure for reporting errors, which usually includes recording the error on an incident report. The report includes the names of the persons involved in the error plus a narrative of the events surrounding the incident. In addition to completing an incident report, the nurse immediately notifies the prescribing practitioner, who then decides what action to take to counteract the error.

ASSESSMENT

Assessment begins with taking a medication history in addition to the total nursing history. Recall that the nursing history should ascertain the overall needs of an individual. The medication history helps nurses obtain very specific information about the use of medication. Therefore, questions focus on the person's use and need for medications as well as on previous responses to therapy. Specialized clinics such as oncology or diabetes clinics usually adapt the basic medication history

to include even more specific questions. Do not administer any medication until these data have been gathered. Communicate the information you gather to other members of the health care team by transcribing it on the person's permanent medical record.

Communicate critical information such as allergies or previous adverse reactions to medications by noting it on the person's arm band and in a conspicuous place on the cover of the chart. Also document this information in the nursing care plan and notify the pharmacy.

Physiologic Factors

The basic considerations for a physiologic assessment are (a) age, (b) weight, (c) sex, and (d) condition of the person.

Pharmacokinetics is the way the body absorbs a drug, distributes the drug within the body, and finally inactivates it. A person's age is one of the factors that affect the pharmacokinetics of medications. For example, because of reduced circulation, absorption of medications in a 70-year-old person is generally slower than that in the body of a 20-year-old person. Age is often the determining factor in the selection of medication dosages or routes of administration. For instance, an infant may be given a small dose of antibiotic in a liquid form to simplify administration, but a school-age child can take a larger dose in chewable tablet form.

The weight of an individual is also important. Weight is obviously related to body mass, which is yet another consideration in determining the dose of medication and the route of administration. For example, the reduced muscle mass of a thin person may be a contraindication for administering intramuscular injections in certain sites. Weight also affects pharmacokinetics because the amount of body fat and rate of blood flow alter the distribution of medications.

In addition, a person's sex affects pharmacokinetics. Males and females have different body structures, tissue mass, and reproductive and hormonal systems. Some medications, such as oral contraceptives, work only in the body of a female.

Physical assessment also involves identifying alterations in a person's condition or functional abilities. In the presence of disease, certain body organs function abnormally and some illnesses affect the movement of medications through the body. Absorption and distribution may be altered by conditions involving the heart; liver disease alters biotransformation; kidney disease may result in slowed excretion of drug metabolites. Other functions to assess include nutritional and fluid status, gastrointestinal functions, and changes in activity level. Also note deficits in hearing or vision; integumentary, circulatory, gastrointestinal, and musculoskeletal systems; ability to communicate; and level of consciousness.

Continue to assess individuals throughout the therapeutic program to identify beneficial or untoward changes in physiologic functions. To make your assessment, use data gathered from laboratory tests and vital signs monitoring systems, as well as clients' objective and subjective responses.

Laboratory tests involve assaying the chemical composition of the blood, urine, and other body substances. Serum levels of medications assist physicians in deciding whether to increase or decrease dosages and in identifying overdoses. Urine levels are checked to determine the body's ability to metabolize or excrete certain medications. Chemical analysis of other body fluids also helps determine medication effectiveness. Consult specialized texts on laboratory tests to learn more about these procedures.

All persons receiving medications need to have their vital signs checked periodically. In intensive care units (ICUs), coronary care units (CCUs), and recovery rooms, these measurements must be taken at frequent intervals. Usually, special clinical settings use sophisticated monitoring systems to assess individual responses to therapy. Such monitoring systems are particularly effective in CCUs, for example, where they are used to continuously monitor changes in heart rhythms in response to cardiac medications.

In addition to physiologic monitoring, observe for and listen to the responses of people receiving medication. If they say the medication is not helping or is making them feel worse, listen carefully and take these comments seriously. Report such statements to the physician so that the medication regimen can be reevaluated. Always remember that people receiving medications are members of the health care team and that their input is a valuable part of the assessment data.

Psychosocial Factors

Always consider psychosocial factors in regard to both the administration of medications and the individual's adherence to the medication regimen. Factors you may need to assess include

▶ motivation
▶ the person's attitude toward therapy
▶ drug dependence and misuse
▶ the person's level of understanding and knowledge of a medication regimen
▶ support from significant others

These factors often determine whether the person is compliant or noncompliant with the therapeutic regimen.

Motivation greatly affects the success or failure of a medication program. Individuals' perception of a chronic illness and the need for medication vary. For example, a chronic illness such as diabetes may prompt one person to take a medication conscientiously, whereas another person may omit doses. Experience with medication often influences a person's acceptance of a regimen. For example, someone who suffers an adverse effect from one type of medication may be reluctant to take another type.

People's beliefs or attitudes about the therapeutic regimen are also important. If they think medication will help, they are likely to experience greater benefit from it. In other words, the efficacy of a medication does not depend solely on its chemical properties. As a nurse, you can increase the effectiveness of a medication by communicating a positive attitude about the therapy. For example, people receiving an analgesic may obtain better pain relief if told, "This injection will relieve your discomfort. I'll check back with you in a little while to see how you are feeling." By expressing your concern about people's discomfort and your confidence that the medication will work, you may improve their response to medication.

Another important psychologic factor is the tendency toward drug dependence and misuse. No one knows for sure why some individuals become dependent on or misuse drugs. Psychologic, sociologic, and genetic factors may all play a part. The nurse, however, needs to assess for signs of drug dependence or misuse. Consider the following questions as you assess clients:

▶ Are there physical signs of drug dependency (e.g., "track marks," dilated pupils)?
▶ Is the person under much physical or psychologic stress, and does this person use medications to cope with stress?
▶ Has the person ever abused or misused medications in the past?
▶ Does the person act anxious or upset if the medication is not administered on time?

Even if the answer to these questions is "yes," it is dangerous to assume that the person is dependent on a medication or misuses it. Drug abuse and misuse is a delicate subject and requires complex treatment using the expertise of many health care professionals. If you suspect a person has a problem with drug abuse or misuse, consult other health care providers before taking any action.

The person's understanding and knowledge concerning therapeutic intervention always influence the success or failure of treatment. People who do not adhere to the treatment plan may lack appropriate knowledge about the disease process and about the medication. They may not understand why a particular medication is necessary. Thus, the role of the nurse as educator is important.

Sometimes, a person is not able to adhere to a medication regimen without the assistance of significant others. In these instances, assess the motivation and knowledge level of significant others who may need to help the individual.

Special Needs

The nurse often encounters people who need special assistance in taking medications. People with special needs include children, disabled people, the elderly, those with neurosensory problems, and those with chronic pain. It is the nurse's responsibility to assess the needs of individuals and then assist them in taking medications safely and comfortably.

Administering medications to children requires special care. Pediatric dosage calculations are different from adult dosage calculations and are based on weight or body surface area.[23] Even though many medications are now packaged in pediatric dosages, nurses are still responsible for verifying and calculating accurate dosages. Nurses also assess the child's physiologic capacity for taking medications. Infants, for example, require liquid forms of oral medication for ease of swallowing. Nurses also determine the safest sites for parenteral medications. The use of certain injection sites such as the gluteus (hip) muscle is contraindicated for intramuscular injections in infants because of the increased danger of damaging nerves and blood vessels.

Be sure to assess children according to their developmental age group. Consider a child's needs within a particular age group when planning medication administration. An infant, for example, cannot remember the discomfort of having an injection, but a preschool child develops a fear of the experience. Therefore, plan an approach that allows the child to maintain a sense of control or security. Techniques to help children cope with injections include allowing them to cry and hold a doll during the procedure, holding and comforting them after the experience, and using a reward system to gain cooperation. Other general rules for administering medications to children include the following:

▶ Administer injections quickly, with the infant or child safely restrained by others as necessary.
▶ Improve the palatability of pediatric medications by

mixing them with foods such as applesauce or custard.
▶ Crush tablets and add them to soft foods to make tablets easier for the child to ingest.
▶ After administering medications, monitor the child closely to evaluate beneficial or side effects. Often, children cannot report reactions to medications.

Some elderly people also have special needs when taking medications. Because the process of aging changes body metabolism and organ function, older individuals often need smaller dosages of medications and require careful monitoring of their responses. In addition, elderly people often take many different medications at the same time and can experience adverse reactions from the combinations. Weakness and other physical or mental impairments require special nursing intervention.

Individuals with problems of the neurosensory system (people with impaired vision, hearing, or swallowing or alterations in mental status) require special assistance with medications. For example, a blind diabetic person needs special equipment and instruction to be able to draw up the correct dosage of insulin. A person with decreased mentation or memory loss needs increased supervision to take medication regularly. Individuals with impaired sensation of the oropharynx or impaired swallowing need special assistance to take oral medications safely. People who are unconscious must receive medications by enteral or parenteral routes.

Individuals with chronic pain that is not relieved by medical, surgical, or psychiatric interventions have complex problems that may include the long-term misuse of medications. Many types of interdisciplinary programs are available to treat chronic pain. These programs include behavior modification and other psychologic strategies (see Chapter 40 for more information on chronic pain).

NURSING DIAGNOSIS

When we talk about medication administration, we are talking about an intervention that might apply in a number of different nursing diagnoses. Whatever the nursing diagnosis, administering ordered medication will be but one of the nursing interventions in the total plan of care. None of the nursing diagnoses relates specifically to medication administration, but some nursing diagnoses often call for the administration of ordered medication. For example, in the following list, each nursing diagnosis is followed by one possible intervention:

▶ *Pain* (administration of ordered analgesics)
▶ *High Risk for Infection* (administration of ordered prophylactic antibiotics)
▶ *Constipation* (administration of ordered laxatives)
▶ *Diarrhea* (administration of ordered antidiarrheals)
▶ *Anxiety* (administration of ordered antianxiety agents)

PLANNING

When planning care for persons with the diagnoses that were previously listed, expected outcomes might be as follows:

▶ *Pain*—states pain relieved
▶ *High Risk for Infection*—WBC within normal limits (especially the differential)
▶ *Constipation*—has normal bowel movement
▶ *Diarrhea*—has a reduction in number of stools
▶ *Anxiety*—states anxiety relieved

Such outcomes are achieved through the administration of ordered medications and through other nursing interventions.

NURSING INTERVENTION

Teaching Self-care to Persons Receiving Medications

Many people who take medications at home make errors in self-administration. They fail to take medications as prescribed or misuse them in a manner that could be serious. An important part of assisting people with medication therapy is improving their self-care abilities.

Errors in taking medications occur for many reasons. People may have inadequate knowledge about the purpose of medications, inadequate social support to obtain and administer the medication, a complex daily medication schedule, or a medication regimen of prolonged duration without return to the physician to assure continuing need. Therefore, assess people's experiences with medications or explore barriers that interfere with their ability to follow the prescribed regimen. For example, lack of financial resources to purchase medications and lack of motivation to tolerate the side effects are two commonly encountered barriers.

After the assessment, develop a written teaching and learning plan. Include other health care professionals and significant others who are involved with the medication regimen. In the health care facility, learning about medication self-care begins well before the anticipated date of discharge. Use a variety of teaching methods, including verbal instruction, written instruction, reinforcement of learning through demonstration and recall, and follow-up evaluation and continued reinforcement. Suggested information components to be covered in a teaching plan include

▶ name of medication
▶ why medication is prescribed
▶ how medication works
▶ number of daily doses
▶ times of administration
▶ route of administration
▶ length of time medication is to be used

▶ proper means of medication storage
▶ possible side effects
▶ effects to be reported to physician
▶ other medications, foods, or activities to avoid while on the medication
▶ additional information pertinent to medication regimen (for additional information on teaching interventions, see Chapter 26)

Evaluation of the person's ability to self-administer medications following discharge from the health care facility is an important step to ensure lasting compliance with the regimen. Community health nurses can make follow-up home visits and phone calls. Also, people can receive more self-care instruction and reinforcement during follow-up visits to clinics or offices.

Using Judgment in the Administration of Medications

Many situations related to the administration of medications call for the use of nursing judgment. For example, you might give the ordered pain medication one half hour before dressing change, crush the ordered tablet and mix it with 1 tablespoon of applesauce, and then provide Mr. Smith with orange juice to follow his medications. In making all these decisions, you are individualizing the nursing care plan to enhance the client's care.

Administering Oral Medications

GENERAL CONSIDERATIONS FOR ORAL MEDICATIONS

Advantages and Disadvantages. The most commonly prescribed medications are oral medications. Oral medications are absorbed in the gastrointestinal (GI) tract (i.e., the mouth, stomach, and small intestine). The benefits of oral medications include reduced manufacturing costs, the ability to administer therapeutic agents without disrupting skin and mucous membrane barriers, and simplified administration. Disadvantages are limited use for individuals who cannot swallow or tolerate substances in the GI tract (e.g., the unconscious person or the person who has had abdominal surgery), unpleasant tastes of some medications, gastric side effects (e.g., gastric irritation), and alteration in absorption because of the presence or absence of food in the stomach or because of increased GI motility. The two forms of oral medications are solid and liquid. Nursing responsibilities differ slightly with each form.

Solid Forms. Solid forms of medication include tablets, capsules, and powders. Tablets are solid forms of medicinal compounds measured and shaped to a specific dosage and form by the manufacturer. **Prolonged-acting (sustained-release) tablets** are oral medications specially formulated for gradual absorption. Fast-acting tablets may contain substances such as lactose that speed absorption in the stomach. **Enteric-coated tablets** are oral medications with a hard surface that impedes absorption until the medication reaches the small intestine. Some tablets must be chewed, whereas others are swallowed whole. On the other hand, **lozenges** are tablets that should be completely dissolved in the mouth without chewing. Generally, lozenges exert their therapeutic effects directly on the oral mucosa.

Capsules are oral preparations in which one or more medicinal substances are placed inside a small shell, which is usually made of gelatin. The gelatin dissolves in the GI tract and releases the medication for absorption. Capsules are swallowed whole.

Dry medications that are mixed with liquids (water or juices) before oral administration are called **powders.** Many powders are sold in bulk and must be measured and diluted immediately before administration. Exercise care to measure proper dosages, which are calculated either by weight or by volume.

Some powders (and tablets) are supplied in effervescent forms that are also diluted just before use. **Effervescence** refers to the bubbling, hissing, and foaming that accompany the release of gases from liquid. The purpose of effervescent medication is to strengthen a therapeutic effect or to make the medication more palatable.

Liquid Forms. Liquid medications include **syrups,** medications that are blended into a sugared or thick flavored liquid. Syrups are used (a) to aid administration (e.g., in giving medication to an infant or to people experiencing difficulty in swallowing); (b) to mask an unpleasant taste; (c) to achieve a soothing effect on irritated tissues (e.g., antitussive agents); or (d) to allow for the adjustment of dosages. Be wary of using syrups for people with diabetes, because these preparations often contain sugar.

Solutions are homogenous mixtures of liquids and solids. Medications in solution are more likely to be unpalatable and may therefore need to be diluted or followed by liquids.

Suspensions are mixtures of solid particles in a liquid medium in which the particles precipitate out when the suspension is left standing. Therefore, suspensions, such as gels and magmas (thick milky suspensions of an inorganic substance), must be shaken before each administration.

Emulsions are suspensions made from fats, oils, or petrolatum suspended in a second liquid. These preparations must also be shaken before measurement and administration. Take care to avoid the client's aspiration (inhalation) of these substances, because oils and fats cause severe pneumonia if drawn into the lungs.

Elixirs are drug preparations in a solvent medium of alcohol and water (a hydroalcoholic medium). Sugar is often added to improve the taste. Like syrups, elixirs mask unpalatable medications and simplify administration.

Tinctures are also dissolved in a hydroalcoholic medium but are more potent than elixirs. Some tinctures are for topical use only, so it is important to distinguish between oral and topical tincture preparations. It is also important to use tinctures and elixirs cautiously in people who are or may be alcoholic.

Contraindications. Do not give oral medications to persons who (a) have impaired swallowing, particularly those with suspected or actual stroke, (b) are unconscious, or (c) refuse to take medications orally. In such cases, discuss the situation with the person, physician, and pharmacist as appropriate. Explore alternatives such as stopping the medication or administering medication in a more acceptable form or by an alternative route (e.g., injection or nasogastric tube).

ADMINISTRATION GUIDELINES FOR ORAL MEDICATION

Factors Affecting Oral Medication Administration. Before administering medications, review the individual's nursing and medical histories. First, carefully check the diagnosis, symptoms, and management regimen. Second, review or prepare a medication history. Third, assess environmental and dietary factors that can affect the pharmacokinetics of the medications you plan to administer. Finally, assess the person carefully for anatomic and physiologic problems that might make ingestion of medications difficult or impossible.

Environmental factors at home or in the workplace are important because they can stimulate body functions that affect the pharmacokinetics of some oral medications. For example, pesticides stimulate the activity of the liver, which in turn speeds the metabolizing of certain medications. The environmental assessment includes questions about the individual's exposure to substances such as cigarette smoke, toxic chemicals, or fumes.

The dietary assessment provides information used to prevent or reduce problems connected with medication absorption, distribution, and side effects. Be aware of the following:

▶ Some foods or food additives stimulate or inhibit certain actions of oral medications. For example, the ingestion of a tyramine-containing food such as cheese may precipitate a dangerous hypertensive crisis in an individual taking a monoamine oxidase (MAO) inhibitor.
▶ Ingestion of certain drugs can create secondary dietary problems. For example, many diuretics cause a potassium deficit.
▶ The presence or absence of food in the GI tract affects oral medication administration. The presence of food in the stomach impedes absorption of some medications. Therefore, these medications must be taken on an empty stomach. Ingesting other medications (such as certain antibiotics) on an empty stomach can cause pain or nausea.

Consult the pharmacist or drug handbook if you have questions about the potential effects of environmental and dietary factors upon the absorption, distribution, and side effects of medications you plan to administer.

Finally, determine whether the individual is able to take oral medications comfortably and safely. The GI tract should be functioning normally, with unobstructed swallowing and normal digestion. Check with the physician before giving oral medications to individuals who have experienced medical or surgical alterations of the

GI tract (e.g., gastroenteritis or gastrectomy). Review medication administration for individuals with special needs as discussed earlier.

Special Circumstances or Nursing Problems. Although most oral medications are easily administered by mouth, some people find them difficult to ingest. Reasons include partial esophageal obstruction, a dry oropharynx or esophagus, improper positioning of the individual, and unpalatability of the medication.

Some oral medications can be made more palatable by crushing them and diluting them in fluid or adding them to soft foods. First, however, determine whether a medication can be altered without changing its properties.

Some medications cannot be crushed, chewed, or dissolved in solution without changing their therapeutic value.

For example, enteric-coated tablets have a hard coating to ensure passage into the small intestine before absorption. If these tablets are crushed or diluted in liquid, the medication is introduced into the stomach, where it may be ineffective or may have undesirable effects such as damage to the mucosa.

In general, do not alter the following: (a) tablets designed to dissolve in the mouth for absorption through the oral mucosa (e.g., nitroglycerin); (b) enteric-coated tablets designed for absorption in the intestine; (c) sustained-release tablets; and (d) medications that are insoluble when mixed with other liquids. In addition, some medications should not be administered without the protective gelatin capsule because they irritate the oral or esophageal mucosa.

Before mixing or crushing an oral medication, consult the pharmacist. When mixing a medication with food or fluid to make it more palatable, use a *small* amount of the food or fluid to mix with the medication. Remaining food or fluid should *follow* that containing the medication. Otherwise, it may be difficult to get the client to take the entire dose ordered.

Assist the person who has difficulty swallowing oral medications by following these rules:

▶ Administer solid medications with at least 60 to 100 cc of fluid, if appropriate. Document the fluid you give on the fluid intake record if intake and output are being monitored.
▶ Have the person assume a standing or upright sitting position. If the person must remain lying flat, administer liquid forms of medications, if possible.

Use a variety of methods to alter and administer medications that have objectionable tastes. Administer unpalatable medications by (a) diluting them with fluids such as juices, cold carbonated beverages, or crushed ice (cold temperature numbs the taste buds and decreases unpleasant tastes); (b) placing solid medications farther back on the tongue where taste buds are less numerous; (c) mixing the medication with soft foods to mask the taste; and (d) offering flavored oral rinses, juices, or other beverages immediately after administration. You can sometimes use sweetened medications, but follow administration with good oral hygiene.

The frequent and prolonged administration of sucrose-sweetened medications may increase the incidence of dental caries among children.

Some medications, such as those that can damage or discolor the teeth, always require special administration methods. For example, always dilute acids or iron solutions with other liquids, and administer them through a drinking straw so as to avoid contact with the teeth.

Other oral medications must be administered so that they pass immediately from the mouth into the stomach. Medications such as aspirin, iron, potassium, and antibiotics damage the mucosa if they are delayed in the esophagus. This delay in transit time may be due to esophageal obstruction or dryness or improper positioning of the person. Therefore, always administer medications that cause esophageal irritation with at least 60 to 100 cc of fluid. If possible, have the person in a sitting or standing position.

When you encounter serious difficulties in administering an oral medication, notify the physician who prescribed it. An alternative route may be chosen or another medication may be substituted.

The prescribing physician must always approve and order any change in the route of administration.

Persons with nasogastric tubes can receive oral medications through the tube (refer to Chapter 42 for the procedure to ascertain proper placement of the tube prior to administering medications). Certain conditions, however, must be met. First, the medication must be in liquid form, either as ordered by the physician or as a tablet crushed and thoroughly dissolved in water. A liquid formulation will prevent medication from sticking to the tube and clogging it. Enteric-coated tablets and capsules cannot be used for crushing. Second, you need to determine whether the medication to be given can be absorbed in the presence of the tube-feeding formula. If it cannot, the medication must be given well between feedings. Third, if the person is receiving more than one oral medication at a given time, the drugs must not be mixed. Each medication should be flushed with a minimum of 30 cc of water before the next one is administered. Fourth, following administration of the last medication, the tube should be flushed with 50 cc of water. Consultation with the pharmacist would be most helpful if you have any questions.[12]

Persons with ileostomies should take all medications in the form of liquids or plain tablets that are dissolved in the stomach. Enteric-coated tablets and time-release capsules or tablets frequently pass undissolved into the ileal bag. You should advise these individuals to check the bag contents for whole tablets.

After completing the assessment and determining the best method for safe administration, prepare the medication. Procedure 46–1 outlines the principles and steps for oral medication administration.

PROCEDURE 46-1

Administering Oral Medications

Definition/Purposes. Oral medications are medications given by mouth. They are administered for their therapeutic effects on the body, such as alleviation of pain and correction of imbalances.

Contraindications/Cautions. Do not give oral medications to persons who (a) have impaired swallowing, (b) are unconscious, or (c) refuse to take medications orally. In such cases, discuss the situation with the person, physician, and pharmacist as appropriate. Explore alternative regimens, e.g., stopping medication or administering medication in a more acceptable form or by an alternative route (injection, nasogastric tube). Employ safety measures: (a) Know medication action, untoward effects, and contraindications; (b) double-check calculations for correct dosage; (c) check that you are administering medication to the right person; (d) report and document untoward effects of the medication; and (e) document whether person refused or was unable to take the medication.

Learning/Teaching Guidelines. Provide the individual and significant others with the following information, as appropriate: (a) Tell the person the name of the medication and how it works; (b) explain the need for the medication; (c) explain how often it is to be given; (d) emphasize the necessity of following the prescription; (e) explain possible side effects and encourage the person to report any that occur; (f) describe the relationship or interaction of medication with activities, rest, food, fluid intake, and the environment; and (g) emphasize the need to take medication for the duration of the prescribed time.

PRELIMINARY ACTIVITIES

Assessment

- ▶ Check medical diagnosis.
- ▶ Check age.
- ▶ Assess level of consciousness.
- ▶ Assess alterations in swallowing.
- ▶ Note nausea or vomiting.
- ▶ Assess presence of oral or esophageal lesions.
- ▶ Assess client's experience with medications (e.g., has client had previous reactions to a specific medication)?
- ▶ Determine client's knowledge of medication regimen.
- ▶ Complete special assessments required by the medication to be administered (e.g., take apical pulse and determine it is >60 before administering digitalis preparations).

Preparation of the Person

- ▶ Discuss need for medication.
- ▶ Provide information about medication.

Equipment

- ▶ Adequate lighting
- ▶ Medication references (e.g., hospital formulary)
- ▶ Medication cards, sheets, or records
- ▶ Medication tray
- ▶ Medication cups (Fig. 46–3A)
- ▶ Plastic measuring cups (Fig. 46–3B)
- ▶ Drinking water, juice
- ▶ Drinking straws

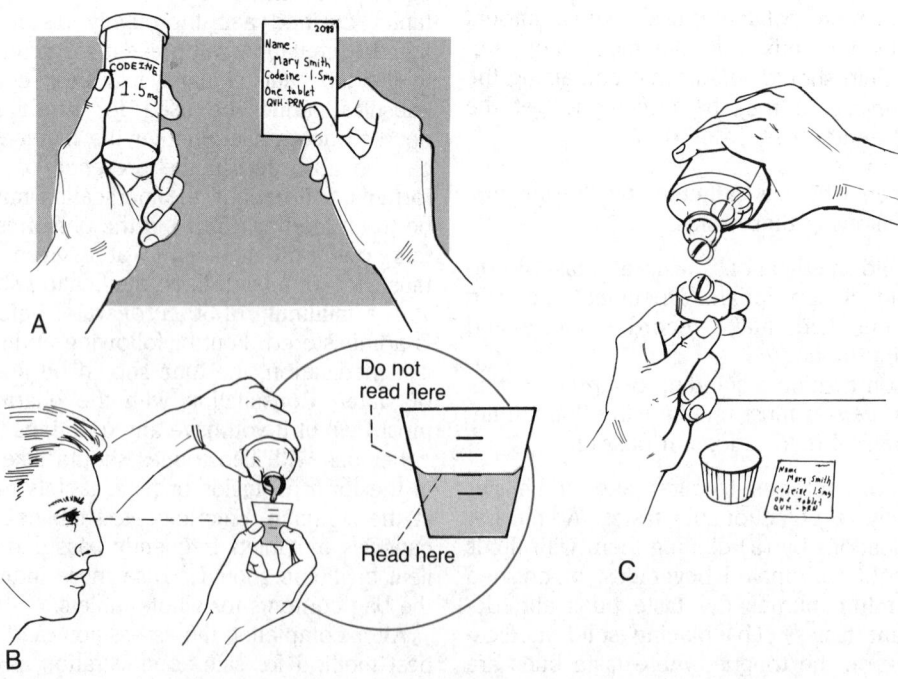

▲ *Figure 46–3*

PROCEDURE 46–1 Continued

Administering Oral Medications

PROCEDURE

Actions

1. a. Gather medication cards or sheet and check against original medication orders.

   b. Notify appropriate staff member of errors or omissions on cards or medication sheets.
   c. Correct cards and/or records if they do not match original physician's order.
2. Consult resources such as pharmacists or medication references for information on each medication to be administered.
3. Know individual's diagnosis, purpose of medication, its therapeutic effects, and possible untoward effects.
4. Wash hands.

5. Obtain access to medication storage area. Obtain key and unlock medicine drawer or cart.
6. Assemble appropriate equipment or supplies. Refer directly to medication cards and sheets for each client. Keep all medications for one person together.
7. Prepare one medication at a time.
   a. Obtain medication from drawer or closet, compare with medication card or sheet.

First safety check: Read entire label, including expiration date.

   b. Calculate dosage using a standard formula. Measure medication. Check calculations with another nurse if hospital policy requires (e.g., insulin dosages must sometimes be verified by another nurse).
      i. Pour solid medications (e.g., tablets, capsules) into cap of medicine bottle first, then into medicine cup (see Fig. 46–3). Do not use fingers to obtain medications from container cap. Discard medications that become contaminated.
      ii. Pour liquids (from side of bottle mouth opposite label) into plastic measuring cup with thumbnail at correct measurement mark on cup. Read plastic measuring cup at eye level at bottom of meniscus (Fig. 46–3). Discard excess. Wipe lip of bottle with clean paper towel before replacing cap.
      iii. If using unit dose package, leave medication in wrapper and place in medicine cup to be opened immediately prior to administration.
   c. Recheck medication label with card or medication sheet (see Fig. 46–3).

Second safety check: Make certain dose has been calculated accurately.

Rationale/Discussion

1. a. Comparison with original order identifies errors in transcription and medications that were ordered but not transcribed. Physician's orders on chart or in computer are the *only* legal source of medication prescriptions in an agency.

   When giving medications for the first time, check medication cards, sheets, and records against original order in chart or computer.

   b. Initiates action to rectify or prevent error.

   c. Eliminates errors. If administrative error does occur, document it on incident report.
2. It is nurse's responsibility to know actions, usual dosages, and therapeutic and untoward effects of each medication administered.
3. Helps nurse determine whether person is obtaining therapeutic effect from medication.
4. Medication administration is a clean procedure. Washing reduces microbes on nurse's skin, thereby reducing risk of transfer of organisms.
5. Some medications (e.g., narcotics) are safeguarded in locked cupboard or cart.
6. Use of an organized system prevents errors and saves time. Concentration on one task at a time also reduces errors.
7. Ensures accuracy and prevents errors.
   a. Comparing medication label with medication card or sheet prevents errors. Checking expiration date avoids administration of outdated medication.

   b. Accuracy of calculations.

      i. Prevents contamination of medication. Discard medications according to agency policy.

      ii. Pouring from side of bottle mouth prevents obliteration of label. Placing thumbnail at correct measurement mark maintains location of correct dose. To prevent contamination, never pour medication back into bottle. Wiping lip of bottle ensures proper resealing and protection of contents of bottle.
      iii. Maintains label with medication for an additional safety check.

   c. Guards against error.

Procedure continued on following page

PROCEDURE 46–1 Continued

Administering Oral Medications

Actions	Rationale/Discussion
d. Return medicine bottle to storage, reading label.	d. Guards against error.

Third safety check: Check card again.

Actions	Rationale/Discussion
8. Modification to step 7 to be used for narcotics: a. Before removing dose, verify count in container. b. Remove dose. c. Count remaining doses in container. d. Immediately document required information on narcotic record.	8. Narcotics require precise counts and must be documented when removed from supply.
9. Place card and medication on tray. If tray is not used, place medication with card or sheet in specified area.	9. Proper identification of each medication ensures administration of correct medication to correct individual.
10. Repeat steps 7 and 8 for preparation of each medication. Place each medication into separate cup. Unit dose medications may remain assembled with labels intact.	10. Mixing medications in a single container is hazardous. If medication spills, if person refuses mediation(s), or if one medication must be withheld, nurse is dependent on knowing color and shape of each medication in order to replace it or record the omission.
11. Lock medicine cabinet or storage area before leaving the area.	11. Ensures safe storage of medications.
12. Take medications to person at correct time.	12. Maximizes therapeutic effect. Agency policy may vary: 20 to 30 minutes before and after designated time is often accepted practice.
13. Identify person to receive medication. Use three methods of identification. a. Read name on ID band. Replace all missing name bands. b. Read name at door or bedside. c. Ask person to state name. d. Verify identification with staff member who knows person.	13. It is nurse's responsibility to identify each person properly. Agency policy often requires use of three methods of identification to prevent error. a. Most accurate identification. b. Use cautiously. Door and bed labels are not always current and accurate. c. Confused individuals may answer to another name. d. Ensures double-checking.
14. Assess person for appropriateness of medication administration (e.g., take apical pulse before administering digitalis).	14. Nursing assessment precedes administration.
15. Administer medication a. Assist person into sitting or standing position if possible. b. Administer medication according to individual's needs. i. Allow client to take tablets or capsules all at once or one at a time. Remove unit dose medications from wrapper. Place medication in client's hand or give medication cup to client. ii. Do not give the medication without checking further if the client questions the accuracy of the medication in any way (e.g., "Oh, they changed the color of my pill," "This pill looks bigger than the last time I took one," or "I thought I wasn't going to be taking this anymore"). iii. Offer fluids to moisten oral cavity. Instruct person to place medication on tongue. If person is unable to do so, pour medication into mouth directly from medicine cup or place medication in mouth with gloved hand.	15. a. Eases swallowing and prevents aspiration. b. Individuals differ in style of taking medications. Illness may require modification. Nurse may need to administer medications in special ways (e.g., by placing sublingual tablets under tongue). i. Allows person to take medication in desired number or sequence. ii. Encourage people to identify their medications and report any deviation from usual appearance or number. iii. Eases ingestion. Meets CDC guidelines related to body secretions.

PROCEDURE 46-1 Continued

Administering Oral Medications

Actions	Rationale/Discussion
iv. Have person bow head slightly and swallow medication and fluid.	iv. Flexion of neck closes epiglottis during swallowing and prevents aspiration.
v. Have person continue to swallow at least 60 to 100 cc of fluid after solid oral medication. Limit intake if on fluid restriction.	v. Prevents retention of medication in esophagus.
c. Document on intake and output record, if appropriate.	c. Helps assess water and electrolyte balance.
d. Administer liquids, lozenges, chewables, or sublingual medications separately (e.g., place sublinguals under tongue).	d. Administer as directed to ensure that person receives full therapeutic effect.
e. Administer unpalatable or difficult-to-swallow medications with juices or crushed into soft foods.	e. Masking taste eases administration.
16. Check to ensure that medications are swallowed. Ask person if medication was swallowed, or check mouth to verify. Remain with person until medication is swallowed.	16. Verifies ingestion of medication and ensures person's safety during swallowing. Verification that medication has been swallowed is necessary to document its administration.
a. Leave medications with person for self-administration if there is a written order or if person is participating in a self-medication program. Do not leave medications at bedside unless there is an order to do so.	a. Agency policies for self-medication vary. Medication left at bedside without an order interferes with safe practice.

FINAL ACTIVITIES

Provide for client's comfort and safety. Discard disposables (cups, straws). *Documentation:* Immediately on leaving client, note medication given and omitted on medication sheet and/or in computer. Cite reason for omission. Return tray or cart to storage and cleanse according to agency policy. Maintain ongoing assessment of client, monitoring for desired and adverse reaction to medications. Immediately report to appropriate person any errors, omissions, untoward reactions, or problems.

Administering Topical Medications

GENERAL CONSIDERATIONS FOR TOPICAL MEDICATIONS

Topical medications are applied to the skin or mucous membranes. Some categories of topical medications include (a) antiseptics for cleaning the skin and mucous membranes, (b) local anesthetics, (c) antipruritics, (d) moisturizers and other soothing agents, (e) antibiotics, and (f) anti-inflammatory agents. Most topical medications are given for their local effects (i.e., the medication exerts its action on the area around the administration site). Some topical medications, however, exert systemic effects—they are carried via the blood to tissues or organs located away from the area of administration. Nitroglycerin, for example, is absorbed through the skin but affects the coronary blood vessels.

Advantages and Disadvantages. The usual benefits of topical medications are

▶ local treatment of skin disease
▶ fast relief from surface itching and pain
▶ fewer systemic side effects
▶ fewer severe systemic allergic reactions
▶ added protection against local infection of injured skin and mucous membranes

The usual disadvantages of topical applications are

▶ difficulties in delivering precise dosages
▶ the possibility of staining skin, clothing, and bedding
▶ possible embarrassment to the person receiving the medication
▶ difficulties in self-administration, depending on the site
▶ unpredictability of systemic side effects

Topical Medication Preparations. Topical medications come in different forms, such as lotions, powders, and so forth. The active ingredients of a medication are suspended, dissolved, or mixed in a vehicle or base. Penetration and absorption of the medication by the skin or mucous membranes is determined by the vehicle. For example, an ointment creates a moist environment on the skin and ensures deeper penetration of the medication. A powder keeps medication on the outer skin layer and maintains a drier environment.

Lotions and creams are liquid preparations of therapeutic substances suspended in a vehicle. In general, **lotions** are suspensions of insoluble powder in water or ingredients dissolved in a thickened liquid (e.g., calamine lotion). **Creams** are oils dispersed in 60 to 80 per cent water to form a thick liquid or soft solid (e.g., antifungal cream). Both lotions and creams evaporate when applied, leaving a layer of medication on the skin. They protect and lubricate the skin without blocking evaporation of natural skin moisture. Little of the medication is absorbed.

Ointments are semisolid preparations in a fat, oil, wax, or water-soluble base. Ointments contain 25 to 50 per cent water. Petrolatum is a widely used ointment. Ointments are moderately or fully occlusive on the skin and therefore have an emollient or softening effect. Moisture retention also enhances medication absorption. Hence, ointments provide the most effective vehicle for absorption of therapeutic agents into the skin.

Powders for topical use are mixtures of chemicals in dry form that are usually dusted onto the skin. They promote dryness by absorbing skin moisture. Powders wear off easily and must be applied more frequently than other topical preparations.

Gels are semisolid mixtures that liquefy when applied to the skin. After application, gels evaporate quickly and dry to a nonocclusive film. Some corticosteroids are supplied in gel form to prevent absorption and systemic effects.

Liquids used for topical application include soaks and wet dressings. Therapeutic powders or solutions, such as salt or Burow's solution, are added to water at a controlled temperature. The person then soaks the affected body part in the solution or applies to the area compresses soaked in the solution. When the liquid evaporates, it cools and cleanses the skin, thus reducing inflammation, edema, tenderness, and itching.

Aerosols are liquid or powder medications suspended in a mist, often in an alcohol-based spray. These medications are sprayed onto a site at a controlled pressure, leaving a film of active ingredients behind. They are used to treat damaged skin and mucous membranes that are too painful to touch directly. In addition, aerosols offer a vehicle for reaching inaccessible areas, such as the mucous membranes of the respiratory tract. Local anesthetics and respiratory medications are examples of aerosols.

Dermal patches are adherent materials impregnated with measured amounts of medication that slowly pass from the patch through the skin (transdermally) as the patch is worn like a small Band-Aid. Medications used to prevent nausea, treat angina, and help people stop smoking are examples of medications frequently taken in this form.

ADMINISTRATION TO THE SKIN

The Structure of Skin. The structure of the skin influences the absorption of topical medications. Figure 46–4 illustrates a cross-section of the skin. The stratum corneum is the outermost layer of the epidermis. It is composed of a tough layer of dead cells and an insoluble protein called keratin. This layer prevents the absorption of significant amounts of topical medications, thereby limiting systemic effects. Thus, absorption of medications through the skin generally occurs through the channels created by hair follicles and sweat ducts. Absorption is enhanced when (a) the stratum corneum is well hydrated, (b) topical medications are applied in combination with a fatty substance, (c) vasodilatation increases local blood flow, and (d) the stratum corneum has been damaged (e.g., by wounds or burns).

Applications. Topical medications are frequently supplied in tubes, jars, and multiple-use containers. Re-

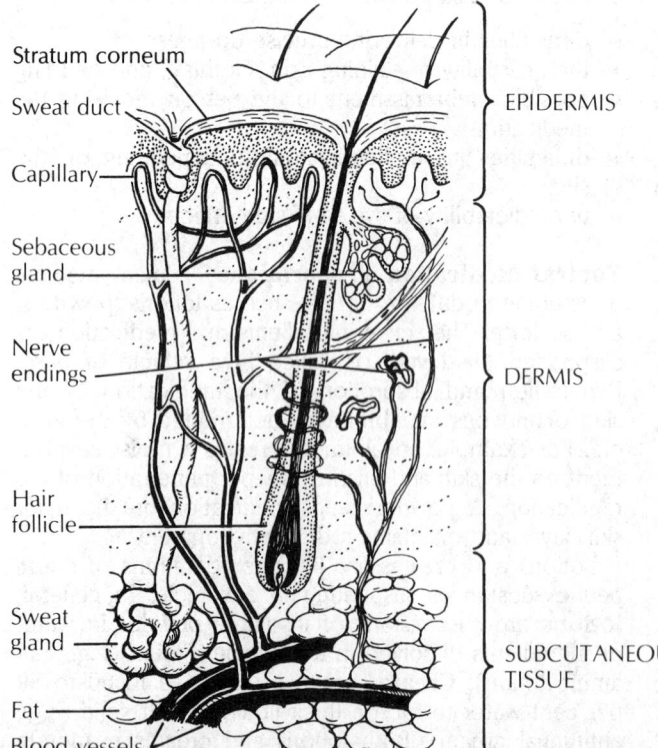

Stratum corneum

Sweat duct

Capillary

EPIDERMIS

Sebaceous gland

Nerve endings

DERMIS

Hair follicle

Sweat gland

SUBCUTANEOUS TISSUE

Fat

Blood vessels

▲ Figure 46–4

Structure of human skin.

move from the container only the quantity necessary for one application. Use a tongue blade or other clean applicator to remove the dose and prevent contamination of multiple-use containers. Prepare topical medications before taking them to the bedside, and use only medications from clearly labeled containers.

Before applying a topical medication, cleanse the skin thoroughly but gently with warm water and a non-drying soap. When skin is irritated or inflamed, omit the soap but rinse the area with water. During cleansing, assess the condition of the skin. Check color, temperature, circulation, and texture and note any changes. After cleansing, air-dry the skin or pat it dry. If moisture retention is important, apply the medication while the skin is still damp. Generally, previous doses of topical medications are removed before additional doses are applied, but consult first with the prescribing physician or pharmacist to verify the correct practice.

If previous doses of the medication have caused an adverse reaction, such as rash or irritation, consult the physician before administering the dose.

Determine whether or not to wear gloves when applying topical medications. Usually you can apply topical medications with ungloved hands, using clean technique. Ungloved hands allow you to assess changes in skin texture. The touch of your hands also communicates support, acceptance, and reassurance to the individual. In some cases, however, you must wear gloves to protect yourself from the risk of infection or to reduce the risk of transferring infectious organisms to others. Also, don gloves to protect yourself from the effects of medications. It is wise, for example, to don gloves when applying nitroglycerin, which absorbs readily and causes systemic effects. In addition, use gloves to avoid contact with irritating medications.

Wear sterile gloves and use sterile technique when treating individuals with wounds, surgical incisions, or open, draining lesions.

Apply topicals cautiously over draining tissue, proceeding carefully so as not to impede drainage.

Avoid applying certain topical medications to intertriginous skin surfaces (i.e., areas that rub together, such as the groin and axilla). The occlusive nature of petroleum-based preparations, for example, causes heat and moisture retention, with subsequent skin irritation.

Applying Lotions, Creams, Ointments, and Gels. Use similar methods to apply most topical medications to the skin. Apply lotions, creams, ointments, and gels in small amounts. A thin application of medication is necessary to ensure accurate dosages and prevent waste. Generally, you can apply these preparations with your hands. Place a small amount in the palm and rub your hands briskly together to soften the medication. Apply it with long, even strokes that follow the direction of hair growth, usually downward. This method distributes a thin coating of medication and prevents irritation of hair follicles. Avoid rubbing or patting the skin. Suspension-based lotions are applied in the same fashion with a gauze square. Drip liquid medications onto the skin and stroke gently.

Applying Powders. Apply powders to dry skin surfaces, dusting the area lightly with the surface area fully exposed. A fine layer of powder is sufficient. To prevent skin irritation, avoid applying heavy coats of powder to intertriginous areas.

Applying Aerosols. Aerosols are applied directly to skin without touching the medication. Make sure that the skin is clean and dry before applying the aerosol.

Take precautions to prevent accidental inhalation of aerosols and sprays that could irritate or damage the respiratory tract.

Turn the person's face away from the direct force of the spray. If the spray is applied near to or on the face, protect the nose and mouth with a cloth or gauze. In addition, ask the person to exhale during administration. Make certain that you do not inhale the spray.

Applying Patches. Follow the instructions on the package insert for placement of the patch to clean, dry skin. When placing or removing the patch, be careful not to touch the medicated section so that the dose will not be altered, and you will not inadvertently receive some of the medication yourself. After removing the patch, cleanse the skin to remove all traces of the medication. Cleansing is especially important if the client is to receive additional medication by this route. Place subsequent patches on other appropriate sites to prevent skin irritation, which can occur if the same site is used repeatedly.

Giving Baths and Soaks and Applying Wet Dressings. Baths are given to individuals whose entire skin surface requires therapy. Soaks are used for local therapy to a limb. When giving a bath or soak, control the temperature of the water to prevent burns. To administer a bath safely, position the client in the tub properly, and either stay with the client, if your presence is required, or make frequent checks. Guarantee the client's privacy.

Use wet dressings for smaller areas of the body or when an immersion bath is impossible. Soak the dressing in a warm solution ordered by the physician and place it on the prescribed area. Either remove the dressing after cooling, or allow it to dry in place and then remove it. Chapter 48 discusses wet dressings.

ADMINISTRATION TO MUCOUS MEMBRANES

Topical medications are most frequently administered to the mucous membranes of the mouth, vagina, rectum, bladder, and respiratory tract. The principles of administration for these mucous membranes are the same as those for the eye and the ear.

Mucous membranes are composed of thin, moist tissue layers, and they possess greater vascularity than does skin. Thus, absorption is greater on the mucous membranes than on the skin, and topical medications applied to these areas can have local and/or systemic effects. For example, analgesics or sedatives administered rectally have a systemic effect. Mucous membranes are more delicate than skin, however, and application of therapeutic agents to the mucous membranes requires extra care and gentleness.

When applying medications to mucous membranes, be aware of the systemic effects that can occur.

Insertion. The placement of medication directly onto or into mucous membranes is called insertion. Inserted medications often have systemic effects. Types of medications inserted include buccal tablets, which are placed in the cheek pouch, or sublingual tablets, which are placed under the tongue. Instruct the individual not to chew this type of tablet, because therapeutic action depends on absorption into oral mucosa.

Suppositories are another common form of inserted medication. They are generally cone-shaped or bullet-shaped and have a base such as lanolin, glycerin, or gelatin that is solid at room temperature but melts at body temperature after insertion into the vagina or rectum. Either the individual or the nurse inserts suppositories.

Rectum. To insert a rectal suppository, have the individual assume a side-lying position with knees bent. Expose the anal sphincter for good visualization. To prevent contamination of your finger, always wear a rubber finger covering (cot) or glove while inserting a rectal suppository. Clients can insert rectal suppositories without a finger covering if they are properly instructed in correct placement of the suppository within the rectum and proper handwashing technique following insertion.

Insert the suppository with the forefinger, placing medication past the internal rectal sphincter muscles to prevent inadvertent expulsion of the suppository (Fig. 46–5). Place the suppository along the wall of the rectum, in the direction of the umbilicus, thereby avoiding a possible fecal mass. Use firm, gentle finger pressure. The individual should remain lying on the side for 15 minutes to ensure medication absorption and to prevent leakage.

Vagina. Vaginal suppositories and medicated creams usually come with an inserter that allows the individual or nurse to place the suppository or cream high in the vaginal vault for maximal effect. Although the vagina normally is not considered sterile, it is important to use clean technique. Therefore, use a gloved hand for insertion, to protect the client as well as yourself, when not using an applicator.

To insert a suppository, first ask the person to assume a supine position with her feet flat on the bed or table. Insert the medication into the vagina using a down and backward motion with applicator or gloved finger (Fig. 46–6). Ask the woman to remain horizontal for at least 15 minutes to allow the medication time to absorb or cover vaginal tissue. Some suppositories and medicated creams stain undergarments, so encourage her to wear a sanitary pad for protection as necessary. Avoid tampons because they may irritate local tissue,

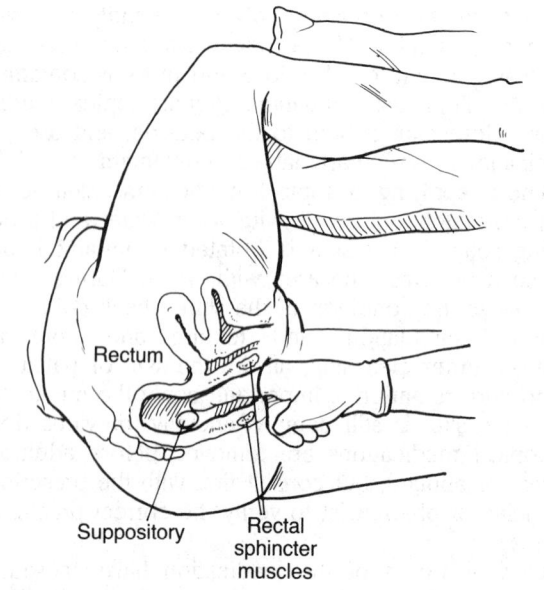

▲ *Figure 46–5*

Insertion of rectal suppository.

prevent drainage of fluids and exudates, and absorb the medication. Also caution the individual against excessive use of douches. Douches wash medication from the vagina and interfere with the treatment regimen. Douches and other vaginal medications may also alter the effectiveness of contraceptive foams and jellies. Therefore, teach women alternative forms of contraception during treatment. In many cases, sexual intercourse is contraindicated during the course of treatment with vaginal suppositories.

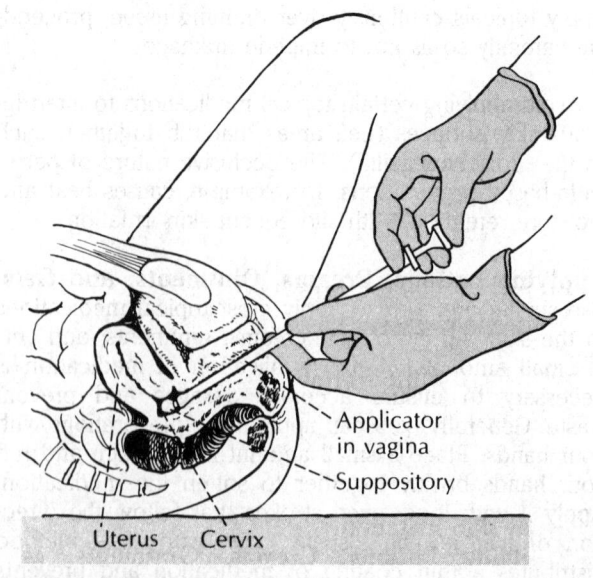

▲ *Figure 46–6*

Insertion of vaginal suppository.

Instillation and Irrigation. Instillation is the introduction of a small amount of liquid into a body cavity, drop by drop. The three most common sites are the nose, eyes, and ears. Irrigation, another topical procedure, washes or flushes out a cavity with a larger volume of therapeutic agent than is used for instillation. (Bladder irrigation is discussed in Chapter 44.)

Nose. The nose is not considered a sterile cavity. Therefore, clean technique is adequate for the instillation of nose drops, unless the sinus cavities are involved. Have the individual assume either a supine or a sitting position, with the head resting back on a pillow. Any other position allows the medication to flow out of the anterior nares. Draw up the ordered quantity of solution in the dropper and place it just inside the nares. Using a soft dropper, carefully instill the prescribed drops into the nares. To prevent contamination or stimulation of sneezing, avoid touching the nasal mucosa with the dropper tip. Instruct the person to keep the head tilted back for several minutes to maximize therapy. Because the nasal passages drain into the back of the mouth and throat, the taste of the medication may be disagreeable, causing discomfort and a desire to expectorate. Provide the individual with tissues if desired. Small children may resist therapy, so you may need help from another person.

Nasal medications are used commonly. Teach individuals to administer them safely and caution them against overuse. Systemic absorption occurs with prolonged use.

Caution people with hypertension and other cardiovascular diseases against using nasal sprays containing vasoconstrictors. These substances can cause elevated blood pressure if systemic absorption occurs.

Also, nasal decongestants used for more than 3 to 5 days cause increased congestion of the nasal membranes.

Do not instill oily solutions, such as mineral oil or other water-insoluble substances, into the nasal passages. If these solutions pass inadvertently into the respiratory tract, aspiration pneumonia results.

Nasal irrigations (washing out the nasal cavity by a stream of liquid) are ordered infrequently because of the danger of forcing purulent material into the sinuses. If irrigation is necessary, the physician usually performs the procedure.

Eyes. Although eyes are not sterile organs, health professionals advocate sterile technique when treating them. Sterile technique is preferable because of the sensitive nature of the tissue. Wash hands before administering medications. Most professionals advocate treating each eye separately, using separate solutions and equipment. This practice limits the possibility of spreading infection from one eye to the other. Discard unused portions of each dose.

When administering eye drops or ointment (Figs. 46–7 and 46–8), position the individual properly. Assist the person to sit up or lie down, and make sure the head is tilted slightly backward and to the side of the eye receiving the medication. This position will prevent inadvertent administration to the other eye. Wipe away any secretions on the lid or lashes with a sterile cotton ball.

Always wipe the eye from inner to outer canthus.

Discard the cotton ball. Hold the dropper or ointment in your dominant hand and rest this hand gently on the person's forehead for stability. Place your opposite hand on the zygomatic arch (cheek bone) and expose the lower conjunctival sac by pulling down gently. Another method is to pick up a small piece of tissue below the eye between thumb and forefinger and gently pull the tissue out. This action creates a "well" for medication deposit.

Ask the person to "look up" and then deposit the medication. This technique reduces stimulation of the corneal reflex, which could cause injury to the eye if the person startles and jerks away. Place the drop or a small ribbon of medication onto the lower conjunctiva. Close the eyelid, distributing the medication over the eye. Provide the person with tissue to wipe the cheek following instillation of drops.

▲ *Figure 46–7*

Administering eye drops. *A* shows correct method. Note that nurse's hand rests on forehead. If the person moves, the nurse's hand will tend to move also, thereby diminishing the chance that the dropper might strike the eye. Incorrect method *(B)* could result in injury to a person's eye with a sudden head movement.

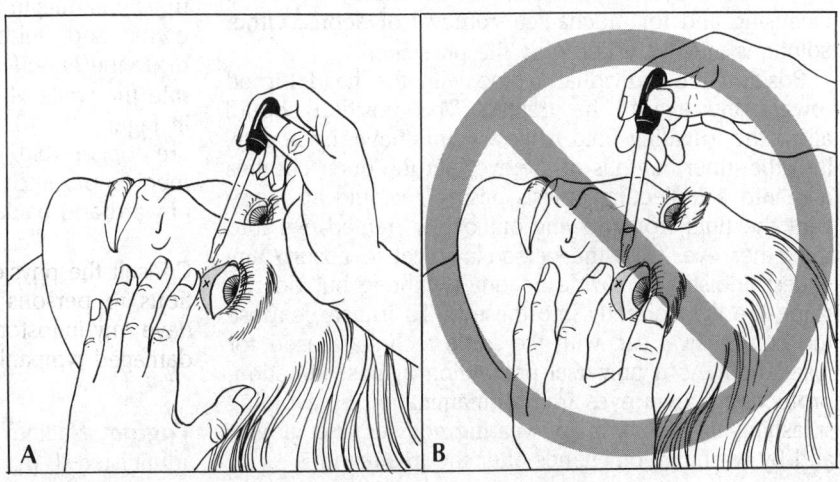

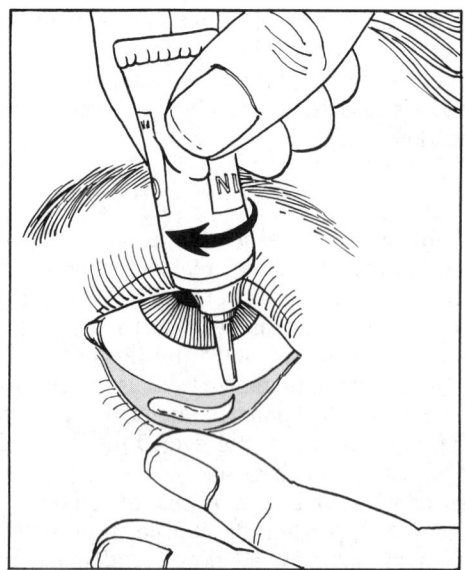

▲ *Figure 46-8*

Administering eye ointment. With nurse's hand resting on the client's forehead for support (to prevent eye damage), ointment is squeezed into the conjunctival sac. An approximately 1.3-cm (½-inch) line of medication is squeezed into the sac. With a twisting motion, the ointment tube is withdrawn. The nurse releases the conjunctival sac, and the client closes and "rolls" the eye. The ointment melts and treats the eye.

Remember these precautions when administering eye medications:

▶ Use sterile technique.
▶ Draw up only the amount of medication to be used. Discard unused medication when treatment regimen is completed.
▶ Never drop medication on the cornea.
▶ Never administer one person's eye medications to another person.

An eye irrigation washes the conjunctival sac, or sclera, with a stream of liquid. The three purposes of eye irrigation are to cleanse, remove a foreign substance, and apply a therapeutic solution for treatment of an existing eye condition. All irrigation equipment and solutions that come into contact with the eye must be sterile. Physiologic saline is commonly used for cleansing and for mechanical removal of debris. Other solutions may be ordered by the physician.

Position the individual supine with the head turned toward the eye to be treated. This position should allow the irrigating fluid to flow from above, by gravity, into the inner canthus of the eye, out the outer canthus and into a collecting emesis basin. It should also prevent the fluid from flowing out of the treated eye into the other eye. Give the person a towel to absorb any excess moisture. Provide adequate lighting but do not shine the light directly into the eye. To irrigate, expose the conjunctival sac with the same technique used for instillation. As a universal precaution against infection, protect your own eyes from contamination by avoiding splashing the solution, by wearing goggles and gloves, and by washing your hands after the treatment.

When the eye must be irrigated with copious amounts of fluid, hang a sterile intravenous bag of solution and tubing on an adjustable-height IV stand. Adjust the height of the bag low enough to create flow that does not cause pain or injury to the eye. Alternatively, you can use a hand-held bulb syringe, gently squeezing the solution from the bulb into the conjunctival sac.

Ears. To instill otic (ear) drops or to perform an irrigation of the external auditory canal, place the person in a sitting position and tilt the person's head to the side, with the ear to be treated facing up. The ear and external auditory canal are not considered sterile cavities. Therefore, use sterile solution only if there is doubt about the integrity of the tympanic membrane. A solution at body temperature is the most comfortable for the individual. Direct solutions and drops toward the side of the canal. Avoid dropping or squirting solution onto the tympanic membrane, so as to prevent damage to the structure or discomfort to the individual. After instilling medicated drops into the ear, have the person remain with the head tilted for a minute or so. This position will keep medication in the ear and increase the therapeutic effect. Following the treatment, place a cotton pledget in the external auditory canal only if ordered by the physician.

For an ear irrigation, the solution is introduced into the side of the canal, usually with a rubber ear bulb syringe. Squeeze the bulb gently (do not use force) to prevent injury to the ear, especially the tympanic membrane. Allow the solution to drain from the ear, unless the physician has ordered that a cotton pledget be placed loosely in the external auditory canal. Solution drains out of the ear when the person resumes an upright position. Therefore, have the person remain in a position with the head tilted to allow sufficient time for medication to contact the affected area. Clean and dry the outer ear and assist the person to a comfortable position. Figure 46-9 contrasts the correct and incorrect methods of administering ear drops to an adult.

When instilling medications or administering irrigations into the external auditory canal, be aware of the structural differences between the infant and adult ear. The external auditory canals of infants and toddlers are mostly cartilaginous and nearly straight. To place medication and fluids within an infant's or toddler's ear, draw the auricle (pinna) down and backward to separate the walls of the canal. This maneuver is illustrated in Figure 46-10. The external auditory canals of adults are longer and composed mostly of bone. To instill medication into an adult ear, gently pull the auricle upward and backward.

Consult the physician before administering otic medications to persons who have had a myringotomy, who have myringostomy tubes in place, or who have a damaged tympanic membrane.

Vagina. Vaginal irrigations, also called douches, are administered in health care agencies as well as at

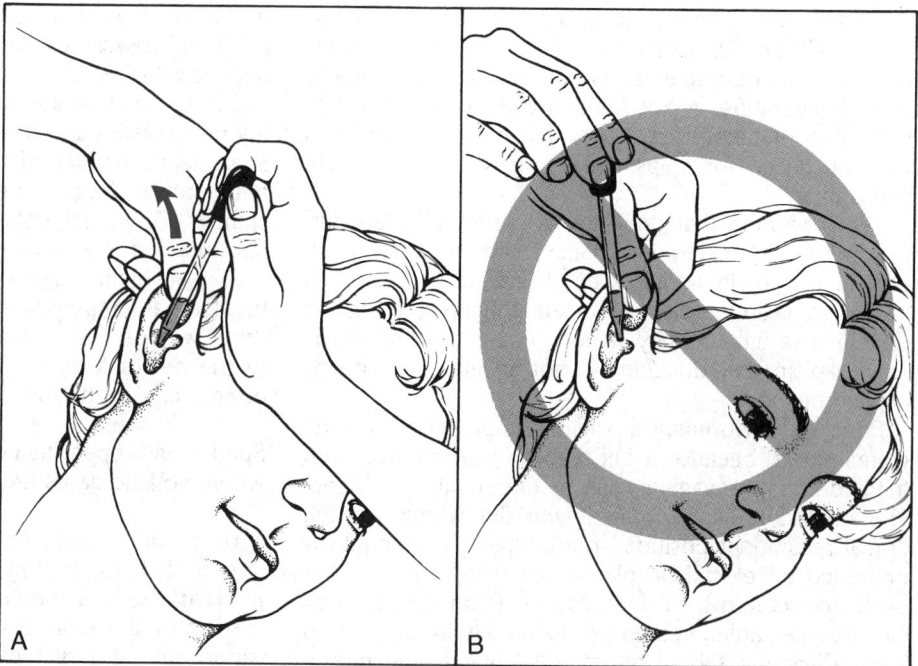

▲ *Figure 46–9*

Administering ear drops to an adult. *A* shows correct method. The nurse pulls the pinna of the ear up and back to straighten the canal. Hand rests on head. Should the client move, there is less chance that the dropper will enter and damage the ear. The method shown in *B* is dangerous, as the hand is not supported on the person's head. If the client suddenly jerks the head, the dropper could be forced into the ear canal.

home. A vaginal irrigation is a stream of tap water or medicinal solution directed into the vaginal cavity. The irrigation is used to cleanse as well as to apply heat or a medicated solution to the vaginal mucosa and cervix.

When performing or assisting with a douche, take care to protect vaginal and uterine tissues from infection. To avoid infecting the vagina, always wash away any exudate present around the labia and vulva. If you are using a douche bag, make sure you do not hang the bag more than 60 cm (23⅝ inches) above the hips.

Excessive force can injure mucosa and force infectious material into the uterus.

The condition of the vaginal tissues determines whether sterile technique is necessary or whether medical asepsis (clean technique) is sufficient. If an open wound is present in or around the vagina, use sterile technique. If vaginal tissues are intact, medical asepsis is adequate. For your protection, always wear goggles and gloves when assisting with or performing a vaginal irrigation.

▲ *Figure 46–10*

Administering ear drops to an infant or toddler. The nurse pulls the pinna of the ear down and back to straighten the canal. One hand rests on head to prevent trauma should movement occur.

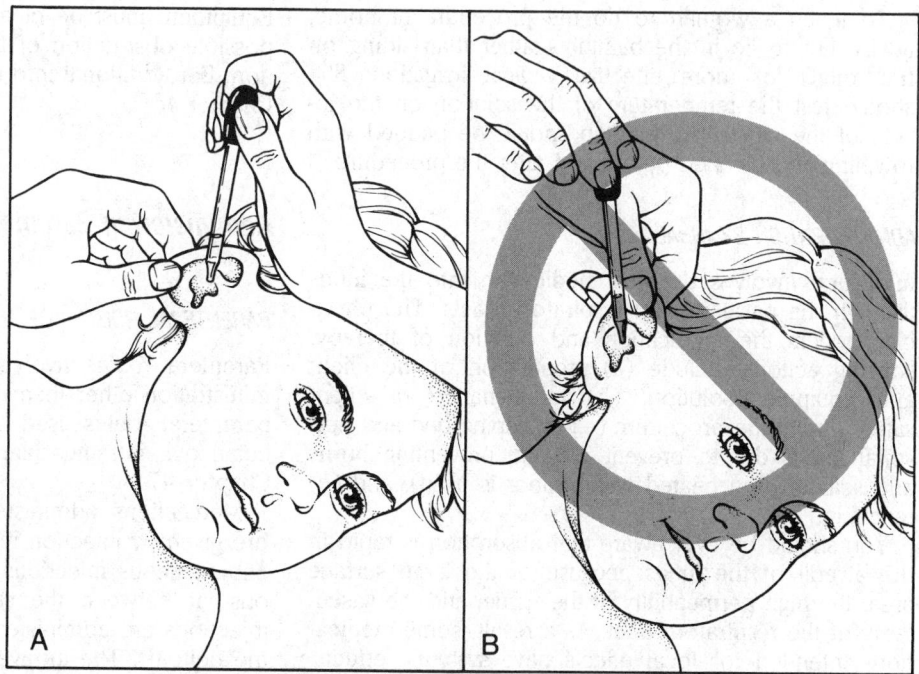

An acidified, physiologic solution is best for vaginal tissues. Check the solution on the inside of your wrist or with a thermometer to ensure that it approximates body temperature. A hot solution can easily injure delicate mucous membrane tissue. Examine the nozzle of the douche tip for chips, breaks, or cracks that might cause injury.

Teach women that douching is contraindicated during menstruation, late pregnancy, and the early postpartum period. In addition, emphasize that the normal vagina is self-cleansing and self-lubricating and that douching is unnecessary under normal circumstances. Also explain that douching is not an effective contraceptive method.

Prior to performing a vaginal irrigation, have the woman void, because a full bladder will interfere with full access to the vaginal vault by the irrigating solution. The procedure is performed with the woman in the dorsal recumbent position on a bedpan (a small pillow or folded towel can be placed under the small of her back for comfort, if needed). Put on gloves and cleanse the labia. Remember to stroke from front to back. Clear the tubing of air and lubricate the nozzle by letting some of the solution flow through it. Separate her labia with your nondominant hand and gently insert the nozzle downward and backward to conform with the anatomic position of the vagina and insert it 1.5 to 2 inches. Unclamp the tubing and allow the solution to flow. Rotate the nozzle during the procedure so that all surfaces of the vagina will be irrigated.

When the container is almost empty, clamp the tubing and remove the nozzle from the vagina. So that all the solution will be drained, raise the head of the bed to high Fowler's position and have the client lean forward. Before removing the bedpan, dry the vulva and perineum from front to back. Then apply a sterile perineal pad as necessary. Cleanse the equipment with soap and water and dry it before storing it in the bedside stand.

To teach a woman to do the procedure at home, advise her to lie in the bathtub (rather than sitting on the toilet) for more effective vaginal irrigation. She should test the temperature of the solution on the inside of the wrist. The bathtub should be padded with toweling and cleaned before and after the procedure.

ADMINISTRATION BY INHALATION

Inhalation involves drawing medication into the lungs through the nasal or oral respiratory tracts. The physician orders the medication and duration of therapy. Nursing actions include (a) preparation of the client and equipment/solution, (b) maintenance of client safety during the procedure (e.g., keeping bed and personal linens dry to prevent chilling, preventing burns and scalds when heated water vapor is used), and (c) teaching.

You should be ever aware that absorption is rapid in the alveoli of the lungs because of the large surface area, the high permeability of the tissue, and the vascularity of the respiratory tract. As a result, some medications intended for local effects have systemic effects. Observe individuals for possible side effects, including dizziness, increased heart rate, nausea, and anxiety. In addition, assess for signs of overhydration, which is also possible.

Substances that are inhaled are divided into two categories: volatile and nonvolatile. A **volatile substance** is an agent that vaporizes or evaporates easily at a low temperature (e.g., smelling salts). Nonvolatile substances, (e.g., epinephrine) do not evaporate readily and must be heated or nebulized before inhalation.

Some volatile agents are administered simply by breaking an ampule (a small, sealed glass container) or other wrapped container and holding the ampule close to the person's nostrils for inhalation. The fumes may be irritating to the eyes, so shield them.

Sparks and open flames are prohibited in the areas where volatile gases are used.

Nonvolatile medications are given by steam vaporization or by atomization and nebulization therapy. **Vaporization** is a process in which a medication is carried in a vapor or in steam. Electrically operated vaporizers are available for use in a health care agency or in the home. These are filled with water and turned on. Medication may be added, as ordered. When steam is emitted, it is directed toward the client's nose and mouth so that it may be inhaled.

Atomization and **nebulization** involve the separation of a solution into fine droplets, thus creating a mist that can be inhaled. Atomization produces larger droplets than does nebulization. Nebulization is used when therapy is directed toward the alveoli or other small areas of the lung. Teach the person to inhale deeply to achieve the maximal therapeutic effect from this therapy.

Aerosol equipment is operated electrically or by hand. Also, many nonvolatile medications are available in prepacked, hand-held nebulizers. Instruct the person in the proper handling and cleaning of equipment. Equipment must be cleaned after each use to prevent possible obstruction of the mechanisms or contamination. For additional information on respiratory care, see Chapter 45.

Administering Parenteral Medications

PARENTERAL ROUTES OF ADMINISTRATION

Parenteral routes involve all methods of medication administration other than the oral and topical. The major parenteral routes used by nurses are intradermal, subcutaneous, intramuscular, and intravenous (discussed in Chapter 47).

Medications administered by the intradermal route are given by injection into the dermal layer of the skin. Subcutaneous injections are given into the subcutaneous fat between the skin and muscle. Intramuscular injections are administered into selected muscles (e.g., the deltoid). The intravenous route is used to administer medications into the veins of the body. Figure 46–

11 shows the tissues penetrated by a needle in each of the aforementioned injection techniques.

Implantable medication delivery systems have also been developed. For example, an **Ommaya reservoir** is a container that is implanted under the skin of the scalp and connected by a tube to one of the ventricles in the brain. By puncturing the reservoir with a needle and injecting a medication (often in the course of cancer chemotherapy), one can gain access to the cerebrospinal fluid and treat areas normally inaccessible because of the blood-brain barrier. Clinical trials are also testing implantable infusion pumps. This method may have useful application in the delivery of insulin.

External infusion pump systems have been developed for the subcutaneous administration of certain medications on a continuous basis. Two such medications are insulin for people with diabetes mellitus[19] and terbutaline for women in preterm labor.

Another recently developed implantable medication system is the surgical insertion of pellets or capsules under the skin for absorption over an extended period.[18] One implantable medication is a capsule of birth control hormones. Six capsules are inserted in a fan shape in the inner aspect of the upper arm and may be left in place for up to 5 years.[17]

Giving medications by a parenteral route carries many advantages. First, the onset of the medication's effect is rapid, and the total dosage is usually absorbed. Also, you can safely give medications by injection to people who cannot take drugs orally. Those in this group include unconscious or uncooperative people and those who are unable to swallow because of neurologic or surgical alterations affecting the gastrointestinal (GI) tract. In addition, parenteral administration makes it possible to administer medications that cannot be given orally. These include drugs that are rendered inactive by the GI tract (e.g., insulin) or medications that are poorly absorbed or irritating. Finally, parenteral administration is the method of choice in emergencies because it ensures rapid, predictable absorption of medication.

The disadvantages of parenteral administration include the risk of complications, such as infection, air embolism, and tissue damage; the rapid onset of adverse reactions (e.g., severe allergic reactions) that may be difficult to treat; and possible pain and anxiety for the person receiving the medication.

ASSESSMENT FACTORS IN PARENTERAL ADMINISTRATION

Before administering parenteral medications, you need to develop special skills and knowledge. You must also

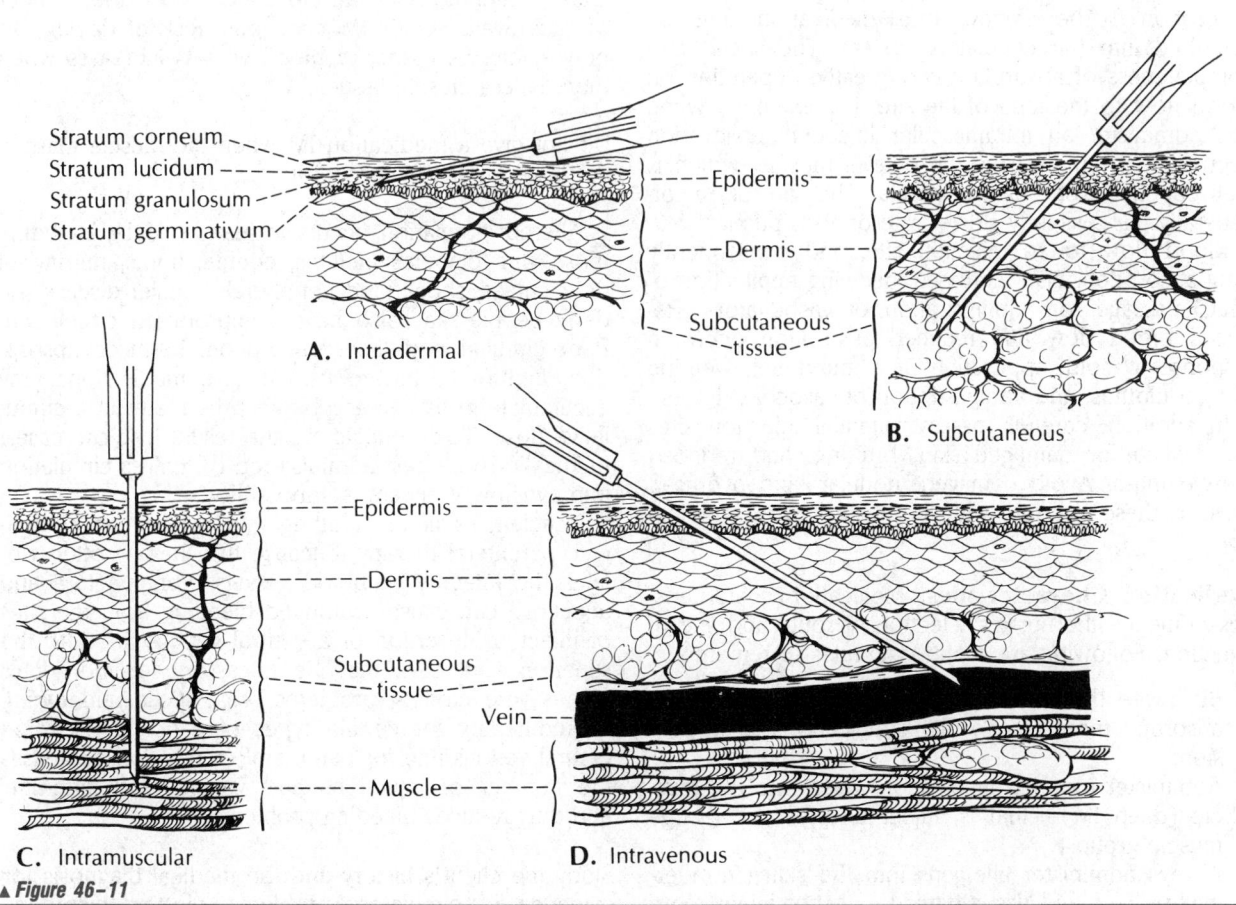

▲ *Figure 46–11*

Tissues penetrated by injections. (Note that *A* and *B* are not drawn to scale.)

be aware of the medical diagnosis and the client's current physiologic status.

Route Suitability. To assess the suitability of the route, you must understand that this is usually determined by (a) the purpose for which the medication is ordered, and (b) the rate at which medication is to be absorbed. The rate of absorption, in turn, depends on the rate of blood flow to the site.

The fastest parenteral route of administration is intravenous or intra-arterial, because medication is injected directly into blood vessels and absorbed immediately. Because of the speed of absorption, this route is most frequently used in emergencies and for people who are very ill. Because muscles are well supplied with blood vessels, absorption is also rapid following intramuscular injections. The subcutaneous route offers less rapid absorption than the intramuscular route, because subcutaneous tissues contain fewer blood vessels than muscles. Medications given subcutaneously, however, are generally absorbed more quickly than those administered orally. The intradermal area contains the fewest blood vessels and consequently results in the slowest and poorest absorption of medication. The intradermal route is most suitable for allergy testing—a situation in which rapid drug absorption is undesirable owing to the possibility of severe allergic reactions.

Potential Injection Sites. Before selecting an injection site for administering a parenteral medication, assess the potential sites for expected rate of medication absorption. To be effective, most medications must be absorbed into the circulatory system. The speed and completeness of absorption vary greatly, depending on blood flow to the area of the site. For example, when you administer an intramuscular injection, absorption occurs most rapidly from the deltoid muscle, which is well supplied with blood vessels. The gluteal region generally has a slightly slower rate of absorption.

Blood flow to an injection site, and consequently drug absorption, also increases following application of heat, massage, or administration of vasodilators. Reduced blood flow and reduced absorption occur in response to cold, application of a tourniquet, wearing of tight clothes, and administration of vasoconstrictors.

In addition, carefully assess potential injection sites for delicate or damaged skin, bruising, and reduced muscle mass. Avoid damaged, nodular, and overused sites, as these interfere with the absorption of medication.

Medication Characteristics. Medication characteristics influence the nurse's selection of route and site of injection. Following are some basic rules to remember:

▶ Be aware that medications in aqueous solution are absorbed more rapidly than medications in suspension.

▶ Administer irritating medications deep into the muscle (deep IM)—that is, inject deeply into a large muscle group.

▶ Always administer allergens into the skin (intradermally). To avoid tissue damage, do not inject more than 0.1 ml into a site. Never inject allergens into sites where absorption is rapid (muscle, vein) because of the danger of anaphylaxis (a severe, potentially deadly allergic reaction).

▶ Administer large volumes of medication (i.e., greater than 5 ml) intravenously, if possible. Alternatively, divide the dose to be given and inject it into separate muscles. Use the largest possible muscles.

▶ Check with the manufacturer's package insert or other reference for special instructions regarding a specific medication. Some medications (e.g., IV potassium) must be diluted before injection. Others are unsuitable for certain parenteral routes.

Physical Condition of Client. Although the principles of parenteral therapy are the same for everyone, some groups of people have anatomic, physiologic, and psychologic characteristics that merit special attention. Although rapid absorption of injected medications occurs when tissue is healthy and circulation is unimpaired, certain illnesses and conditions affect the absorption and distribution of medications. For example, injection pressure, hydrostatic pressure, colloid osmotic pressure, and capillary permeability all affect diffusion of a medication into the blood. A change in any of these factors affects drug absorption (see Chapter 41). Muscle mass, circulation, and skin alterations all deserve special assessment.

Reduced muscle mass often occurs in individuals who are elderly, paralyzed or immobilized, or emaciated. Alterations in muscle mass reduce the number of sites available for IM injections. Risk of damage to nerves, muscle tissue, or blood vessels increases when there is less muscle tissue.

Do not give a medication IM when the muscle mass is not large enough to accept it.

Altered circulation occurs in many people, including those with diabetes mellitus, edema, burns, nutritional deficiencies, shock, and peripheral vascular disease. Elderly people may also have compromised circulation. Poor circulation reduces absorption. Reduced absorption, in turn, is hazardous, because medications may accumulate in tissues and be absorbed later in a cumulative dose. Toxic effects are the result. In these cases, medications are best administered IV, unless circulation improves or IV access is impossible.

Deficiencies in the clotting mechanism can complicate parenteral therapy, because this therapy often violates the integrity of blood vessels. Venipuncture and injections can cause prolonged bleeding from the sites of injection. Insertion of a central venous line into the superior vena cava may be necessary for individuals with severe clotting problems (e.g., those undergoing chemotherapy for certain types of cancer). Use of a central venous line for parenteral medication decreases the number of injections and venipuncture attempts and thus reduces bleeding problems.

Study the client's history and the medical diagnosis for evidence of circulatory problems, clotting disorders, and fluid and electrolyte imbalances, all of which alter medication absorption.

People with impaired integument also require special consideration. Delicate or damaged skin is found in

▶ some elderly persons
▶ many persons with diabetes mellitus
▶ people receiving frequent injections
▶ clients with skin infections
▶ clients with certain other skin disorders (e.g., eczema, psoriasis)

Avoiding areas with skin lesions decreases pain, reduces the risk of infection, and increases absorption. Extensive skin damage may require a change in the route of administration, which, of course, requires a physician's order.

Client's Mental Attitude. Some people may wish to help with injection site selection, especially if they have been giving themselves regular or periodic injections at home, but many individuals demonstrate anxiety or fear when they are to receive injections. Some people may even refuse treatment if they think it will involve needles. These responses sometimes reflect a lack of knowledge about therapy, unpleasant experiences with parenteral therapy, anxiety associated with hospitalization or illness, or feelings of loss of control. Therefore, assess each situation individually and prepare a person psychologically before giving an injection. If you notice that the client seems apprehensive, you might ask, "What experiences have you had with injections?" "What questions do you have about this procedure?" "How can I make you feel more comfortable and less anxious?" In addition, discuss the individual's fears with the nursing and medical staffs, and document your assessment of the problem and the recommendations for solution.

Children. Parenteral medication administration to children requires special skills including the technical expertise and knowledge to administer pediatric medications safely and an understanding of the normal growth and development of children (see Chapter 12). Skillful assessment is vital. Choose and locate injection sites carefully. Infants and children have small and underdeveloped muscle tissue. Hence, the potential for tissue damage is greater than for adults. Always calculate pediatric dosages with care.

Inadvertent injection of a dose intended for an adult can be lethal in a small child or infant.

Successful administration of medications also depends on a cooperative relationship between nurse and child. First, assess the age and developmental stage of the child. Next, observe how the child is reacting during preparation for the procedure. Children often fear needles. They may feel threatened and may think that an injection is a form of punishment, and this fear can cause them to resist the therapy. You must determine whether the child should be restrained during the injection to reduce sudden movements and prevent tissue damage or needle breakage.

More than one individual may be required to restrain a child safely.

If you need to use restraints, comfort the child following the injection. If injections are made less frightening, the child may gradually come to accept them.

Elderly Clients. Assess elderly individuals receiving parenteral therapy for general physical health, alterations in circulation and sensation, skin tone and turgor, and experience with parenteral therapy. People undergo progressive tissue and muscle changes as they age. Older people may have a loss of muscle mass and altered circulation, which in turn decrease absorption of parenteral medication. Reduced liver and kidney function results in impaired distribution, biotransformation, and elimination of certain parenteral medications. These changes can make the older person prone to side effects or adverse reactions to medication.

Mental changes may also affect the ability of elderly clients to cooperate with parenteral administration. Cerebral arteriosclerosis can produce impaired memory and confusion in elderly people. Assess to what degree individuals with mental changes can understand and participate in their therapeutic program.

In some cases, you need to assess the elderly person's ability to self-administer parenteral injections. An elderly person with diabetes, for example, must learn to administer insulin injections on a daily basis. Self-administration of parenteral medications is difficult or impossible for some older individuals. Potential problems include forgetting doses or unsafely handling medications. Under these circumstances, decide whether to allow the client to administer the injection under close supervision or to teach the client's significant others to administer the injections. Also assess whether elderly individuals with loss of visual acuity or blindness or reduced peripheral sensation can safely self-administer drugs.

REDUCING DISCOMFORT AND ANXIETY DURING PARENTERAL ADMINISTRATION

Parenteral therapy causes varying degrees of discomfort for each individual. Discomfort associated with the administration of injectable medications results from physiologic and psychologic factors. Careful planning can reduce this discomfort.

The route and site of injection often determine the degree of physical discomfort. The skin and subcutaneous tissues are well innervated by pain receptors. Puncture of the skin by a needle stimulates these receptors and produces pain. Skeletal muscle is poorly innervated by pain fibers, but discomfort occurs when tissue is distended by medication deposited into the interstitial space. Reduce physical discomfort associated with injections by repositioning the individual, providing distractions, and injecting the medication quickly and skillfully.

Positioning the person in a way that relaxes the muscle is a valuable technique for reducing pain. When injecting into the dorsogluteal area, place the individual in a prone position with internal rotation of the hips (Fig. 46–12). Some individuals cannot assume a prone position but can be placed in the side-lying position with the knee and hip of the upper leg flexed and placed anterior to the lower leg.

Other techniques to alleviate the discomfort of parenteral therapy:

▶ When preparing medications drawn from a vial or ampule, change the needle after drawing up the medication. The needle point may be dulled after passing through a vial stopper. Irritating medication adheres to the outside of the needle.
▶ Select the smallest-gauge needle appropriate for the site and the medication.
▶ Carefully measure the amount of fluid you plan to insert into any one site.

▶ Do not inject more than 0.1 ml of fluid into an intradermal site (between the layers of skin).
▶ Do not inject more than 1 ml of fluid at any one subcutaneous site.
▶ Do not inject more than 5 ml into a large muscle or more than 2 ml into a small muscle.

▶ Avoid extrasensitive areas of the body, and select a site where the skin is healthy and not irritated.
▶ Allow the skin to dry after cleansing the site with antiseptic. Antiseptic causes discomfort if pushed into the tissues.
▶ Minimize puncture pain by using a smooth, quick motion to pierce the skin.
▶ Inject the medication slowly to allow it to spread into the tissue under less pressure, thus reducing tissue stretching.
▶ Hold a sterile gauze pledget firmly against the skin, close to but not touching the needle, and remove the needle quickly to eliminate discomfort associated with pulling of the tissue.
▶ Gently massage the site, unless contraindicated (e.g., heparin should not be massaged into the tissues).
▶ Rotate injection sites to avoid continual trauma to tissue.

Aside from these physiologic considerations, many individuals fear injections. Understanding why people are anxious often helps them relax. To prepare an apprehensive person for an injection, explain how and why you will administer the injection. Include in your explanation any effects, both beneficial and untoward, the person may experience. For example, you might say, "This injection will relieve your nausea," or "This medication may make your mouth feel dry." If the individual has questions about the procedure or the medication, provide an opportunity for discussion. Carefully presented information may ease anxiety and reduce discomfort. Other methods include

▶ distracting the individual by using conversation or music. This technique works especially well for children
▶ encouraging the individual to breathe deeply for a minute or so before the injection
▶ instructing the person to relax muscles located near the site for a minute or so prior to the injection
▶ giving children honest explanations, acknowledging and accepting their feelings, and performing the procedure quickly

PRINCIPLES OF PARENTERAL ADMINISTRATION

Because of the risks associated with parenteral injections, you must understand the principles of drug administration and aseptic technique and be able to translate these principles into safe practice.

Safety. It is essential to administer the correct dose of the correct medication to the correct person at the correct time by the correct route.

Once a drug is injected, it is absorbed quickly. Therefore, errors in parenteral therapy are often difficult to correct. Prevent errors by carefully calculating and double-checking the dosage, route, and site of administration. Never crush oral tablets and dissolve them for parenteral administration. Never give a parenteral medication if the solution is cloudy or contains particles.

Asepsis. The skin is the body's first line of defense against infection. Injections and venipuncture break this protective barrier, thus increasing the risk of nosocomial (hospital-acquired) infection. Infections complicate illnesses, compromise recovery, and prolong residence in the health care facility. By practicing aseptic technique when administering parenteral medications, you can prevent infection.

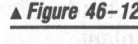 *Figure 46–12*

Positioning for dorsogluteal injection. Positioning a person prone with toes turned in will decrease dorsogluteal injection pain by relaxing the gluteal muscles.

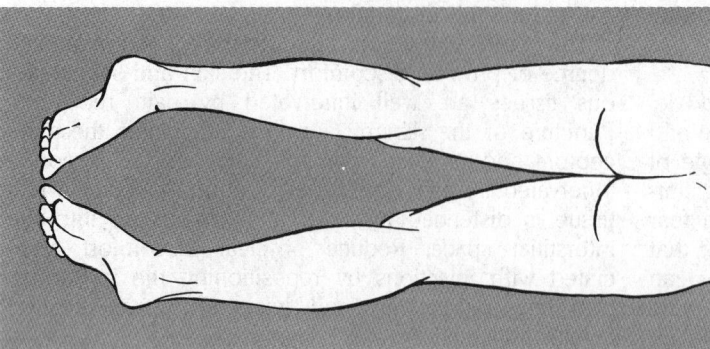

Maintain aseptic technique throughout the preparation and administration of parenteral medications.

Key activities include handwashing, maintaining sterility of equipment, and using accepted methods for cleaning the site before the injection. Be aware that breaks in technique occur easily, not only during emergencies but also during routine administration.

To prevent infection, use the following method to reduce bacteria on the skin before administering injectable medications. First, if the skin is obviously soiled (e.g., with drainage or feces), wash the area with soap and water and thoroughly dry the skin before using the antiseptic pledget. If no obvious soiling is present, cleanse the skin with a 70 per cent alcohol pledget or an iodophor pledget, using friction to remove bacteria. Cleanse the area in a circular motion from the center outward. Allow the antiseptic to dry before injection into the site. Avoid using iodophor skin preparations when injecting allergens, as this solution discolors the skin and obscures the skin reaction.

PREPARATION OF EQUIPMENT AND MEDICATIONS

Needles and Syringes. Needles come in various lengths and gauges, with different bevel types. Table 46–3 describes common sizes appropriate for intradermal, subcutaneous, intramuscular, and intravenous injections. Needle gauge is determined by the lumen of the needle. As the diameter (bore) increases, the gauge number decreases. For example, an 18-gauge needle has a larger diameter than a 22-gauge needle. Figure 46–13 illustrates a range of gauges and lengths of needles.

The bevel (slant at the tip of the needle) is designed to make a narrow, slit-type opening that closes quickly to prevent seepage of blood and medication. Needle bevels are shown in side view in Figure 46–13.

Needles usually come in sterile individual packages so that the nurse can select the appropriate size. Also, if the needle is contaminated, the nurse can change needles without having to discard the syringe.

A variety of syringes are available in both glass and plastic (mostly plastic, today). Table 46–3 describes common purposes, types, and recommended injection volumes for various injection routes, and Figure 46–14 illustrates some common syringe sizes and calibrations. Some syringes have a locking mechanism at the needle attachment (Luer-Lok); others do not (Luer-Slip). Insulin, tuberculin, and some IM syringes are often prepackaged with attached needles because the sizes are standard. To protect health care workers from accidental sticks with used needles, many syringes are available with protective sleeves that are pulled down and locked in place over the needle after the injection is given (Fig. 46–15).

Criteria for Selection. Factors to consider in choosing the appropriate needle and syringe are (1) route ordered, (2) viscosity of medication solution, (3) amount of medication to be administered, (4) muscle mass and subcutaneous fat of person, and (5) site of administration. When selecting needles, check that

▶ the needle is sharp, without burrs
▶ needle size is the smallest gauge appropriate for site and medication
▶ needle length is appropriate for site or muscle mass

In addition, check that the syringe is marked in units that will enable you to measure the dosage accurately (e.g., 100-unit insulin syringes hold 1 ml divided into 100 units, whereas 2-ml syringes hold 2 ml divided into 16 minims per milliliter). Some medications are prefilled by the manufacturer, so make sure you know what volume to administer.

Care and Handling. Syringe and needle controls are essential in health care agencies. The Joint Commission on Hospital Accreditation recommends that all needles and syringes be kept in locked drawers or cabinets to prevent theft for illegal purposes such as drug abuse. Once packages are opened, use caution in handling syringes and needles to prevent needlesticks and to

TABLE 46–3. Comparison of Parenteral Routes

	Intradermal	Subcutaneous	Intramuscular	Intravenous
Purposes	Allergy testing	Injection of many medications, e.g., insulin, heparin	For irritating medications, larger volumes that cannot be given SQ or ID	For large volumes of medication or fluid; for medications that cannot be given via any other route (e.g., some types of cancer chemotherapy); for administration of emergency medications
Syringe Type	Tuberculin, usually	Insulin, 2, 2.5, 3 ml	2, 2.5, 3 ml	Depends on dosage and type of medication
Needle Length	⅜–⅝ inch	½–⅝ inch	1–3 inches	a. "Butterfly" needle: 1 inch b. Catheter-over-needle: 1–1½ inch
Needle Gauge	26–27	25–27	20–25	a. "Butterfly": 18–21 gauge b. Plastic catheter: 14–20 gauge
Recommended Injection Volumes	≤0.1 ml	≤1.0 ml	Less than 5 ml for single injection	Any volume

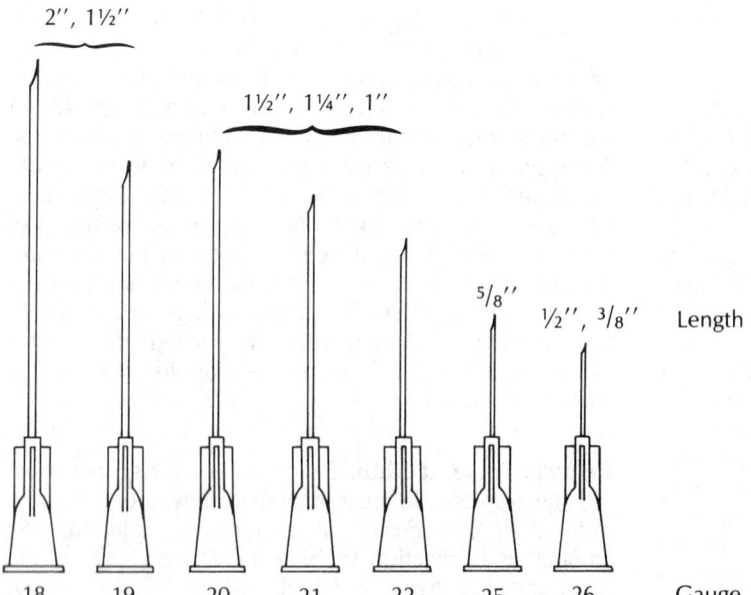

▲ *Figure 46–13*

Needle gauges and lengths. Each gauge is supplied in a limited number of lengths.

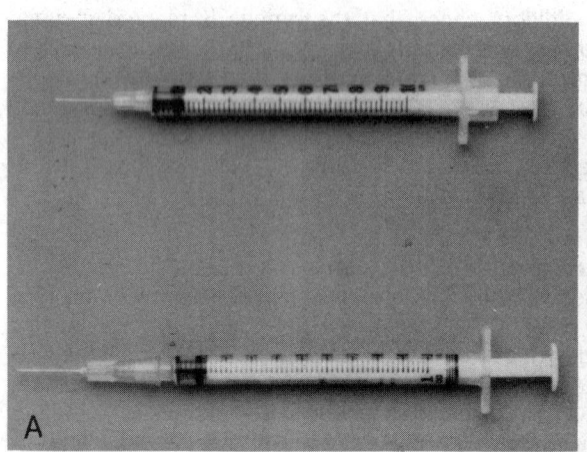

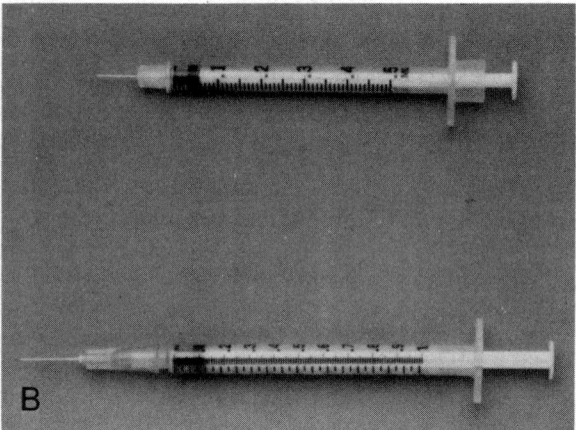

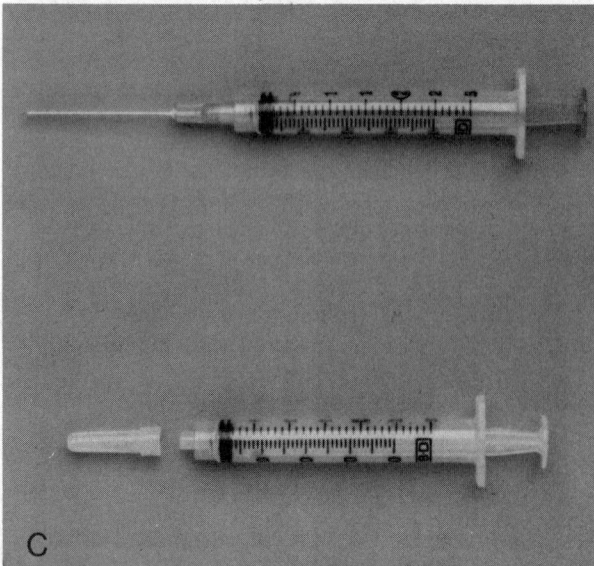

▲ *Figure 46–14*

A sampling of available syringe sizes and types. *A,* Insulin syringes. Top, 1 ml with permanently attached needle; bottom, 1 ml with detachable needle in place. *B,* Tuberculin syringes. Top, 0.5-ml with permanently attached needle; bottom, 1-ml with detachable needle in place. *C,* Standard syringes. Top, 3-ml with Luer-lock tip and detachable needle in place. Bottom, 3-ml with Luer-lock tip covered with a sterile tip shield (to protect sterility of tip until a sterile needle is prepared to be attached).

preserve sterility. Figure 46–16 shows the areas of the syringe and needle that must be kept sterile.

Take care to avoid contaminating the shaft of the needle, the area where the needle attaches to the syringe, and the plunger. If these areas do become contaminated, discard the needle and/or syringe.

Aftercare of needles and syringes differs among facilities. Guidelines from the Centers for Disease Control recommend that you discard the used syringe with attached uncapped or sleeved needle into special containers that are kept in or near the client's room. The guidelines state that you should not break the needles and plungers, nor should you recap unsleeved used needles. Most finger injuries occur during the recapping of needles for disposal. Regardless of agency policy, never discard used needles and syringes in any waste container not specifically designed for needle disposal. The risk of accidental needle puncture by housekeeping personnel is great. Always handle used equipment carefully to avoid skin puncture and risks of cross-contamination.[11]

Although most equipment is disposable, some needles and syringes (e.g., bone marrow biopsy needles) are sterilized for reuse. Often, the nurse is responsible for removing heavy debris (e.g., blood) from the instrument before sending it to central supply for reprocess-

ing. This procedure should be done with great care while wearing gloves (see Chapter 28).[11]

Medications. Parenteral medications are contained in ampules, vials, and prepackaged, prefilled cartridges and prefilled syringes (Figs. 46–17 and 46–18, Box 46–1).

Ampules. An **ampule** is a glass container of medication in solution for use as a single dose (Figure 46–17A). The glass must be broken to gain access to the medication. To prepare the medication, gently tap the stem of the ampule, so that the medication drops into the base. If the manufacturer has not scored the stem, use a file to score the glass before opening. Clean the stem by friction with an alcohol pledget. Then wrap a sterile gauze around the stem to protect fingers from laceration and to prevent contamination of the medication. Use a quick, snapping motion to open the ampule, pointing it away from your body, but never toward another person.

Once opened, the ampule is an open system. Therefore, withdraw the medication quickly to minimize airborne contamination. Withdraw the medication with the base of a large ampule on a flat surface or with a small ampule tilted in your hand (Fig. 46–19) so that you withdraw all the medication. Avoid touching the edge of the glass ampule; touching would contaminate

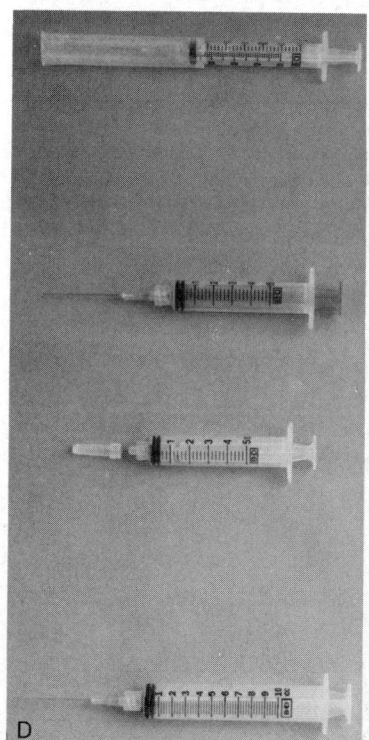
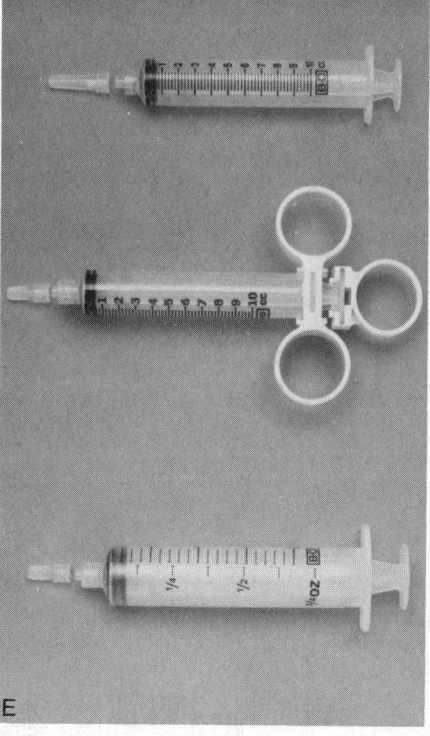
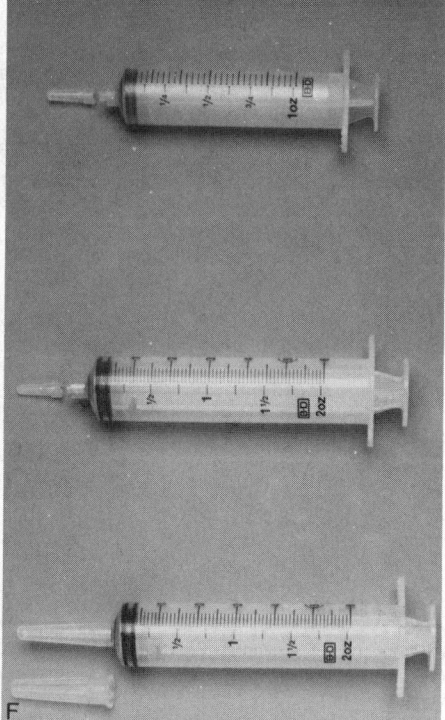

▲ **Figure 46–14** Continued

D, Standard syringes. Top to bottom: 3-ml Safety-Lok, 5-ml with Luer-lock tip and detachable needle in place, 5-ml with Luer-lock tip and tip shield, 10-ml with Luer-lock tip and detachable needle in place. E, Larger syringes. Top to bottom: 10-ml Luer-lock with tip shield, 10-ml control syringe with Luer-lock tip, 20-ml with Luer-lock and tip shield. F, Largest syringes. Top to bottom: 30-ml Luer-lock with tip shield, 60-ml Luer-lock with tip shield, 2-ounce catheter tip with tip shield nearby. (Courtesy of Becton Dickinson and Company, Rutherford, New Jersey.)

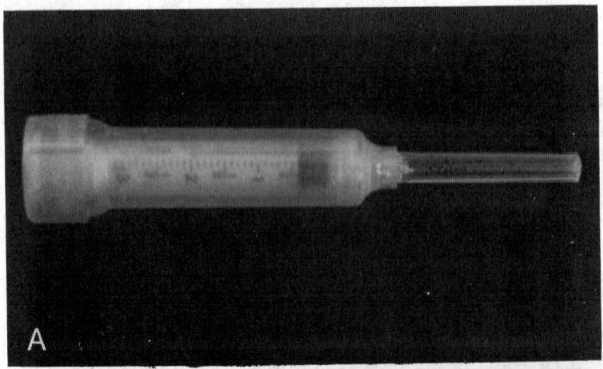

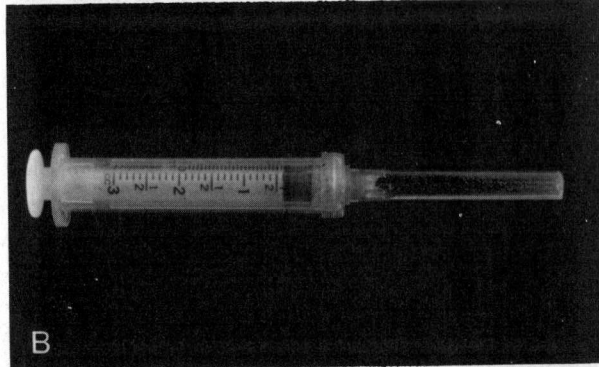

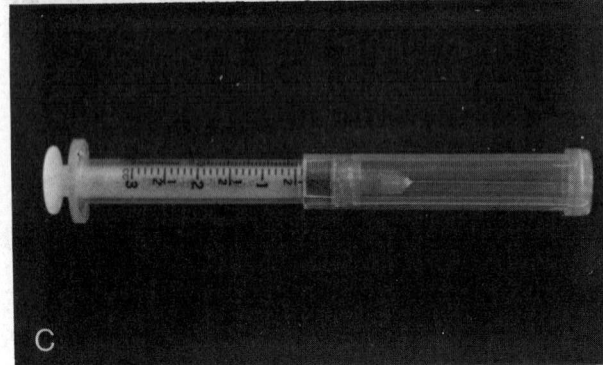

▲ **Figure 46-15**

Syringe with protective sleeve. *A,* Outer plastic cover in place before preparing medication. *B,* Outer cover removed before preparing medication. Protective sleeve covers syringe barrel. *C,* After giving medication, sleeve is moved down to cover the contaminated needle.

▲ **Figure 46-16**

Components of a syringe. Shading indicates areas that must be kept sterile before and during parenteral injections.

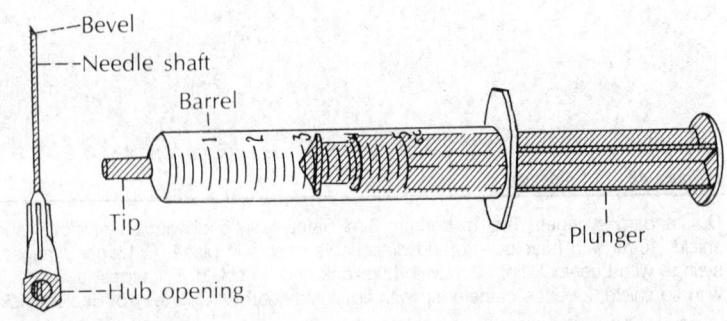

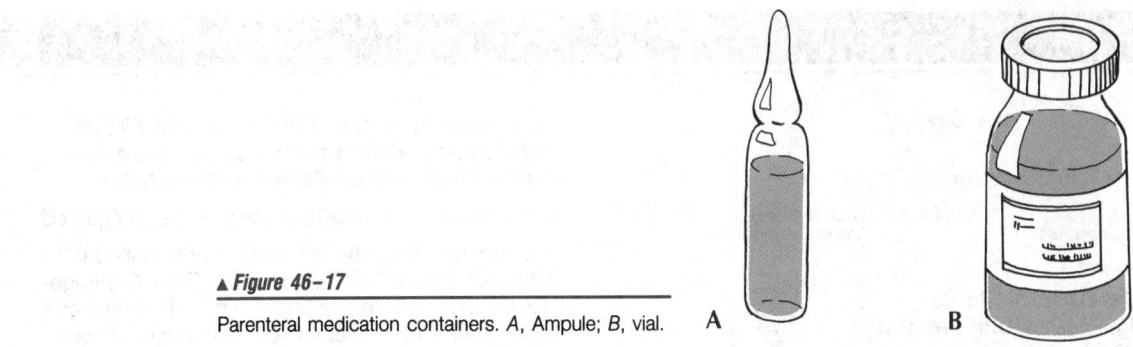

▲ *Figure 46-17*

Parenteral medication containers. *A*, Ampule; *B*, vial.

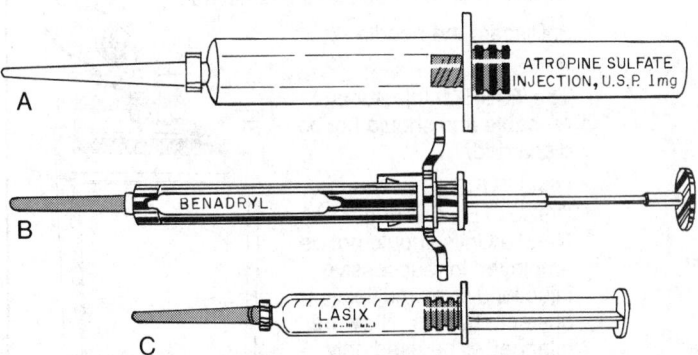

▲ *Figure 46-18*

Types of prepackaged medications. *A*, Emergency medications are available in prefilled cartridges for use with a plastic barrel and attached needle. *B*, Reusable metal or plastic syringes are used with prefilled medication cartridges. *C*, Commonly used medications are available in convenient prefilled syringes.

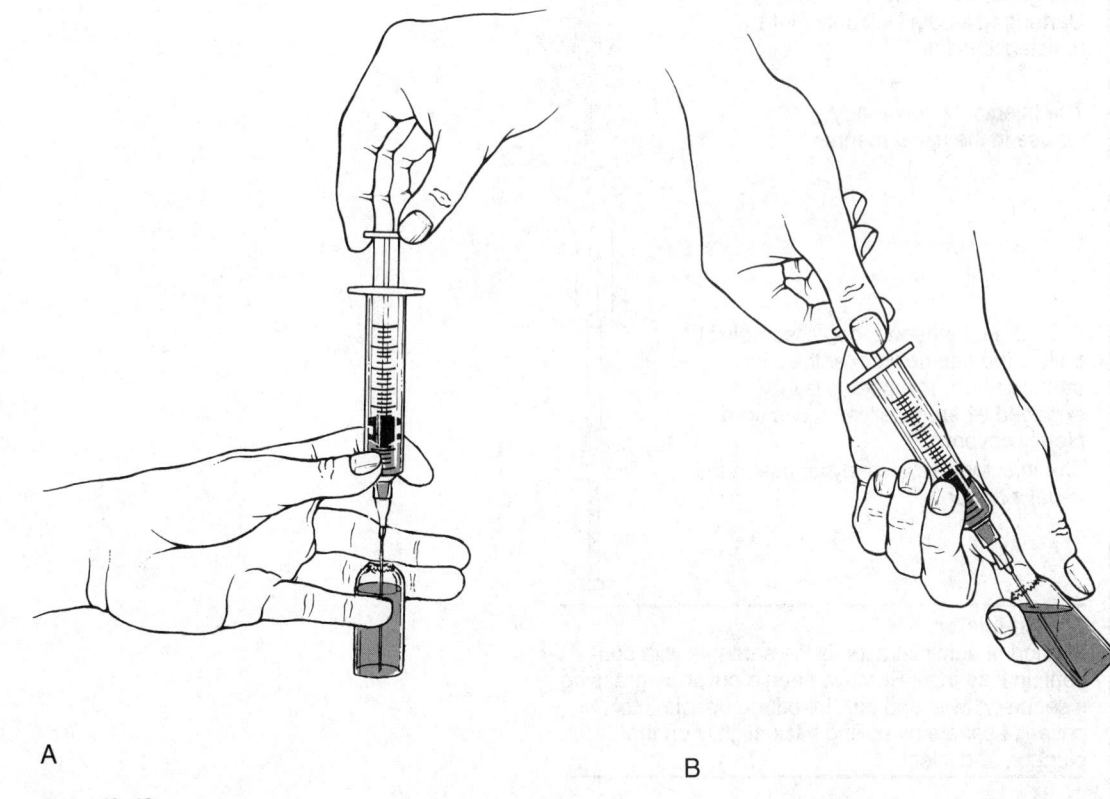

▲ *Figure 46-19*

Withdrawing medication from an ampule. *A*, Large ampule. Note position of needle—it does not touch edge of ampule where it has been opened, thereby avoiding contamination of sterile equipment. Bevel is submerged in medication to prevent air being drawn into syringe. *B*, Small ampule.

Box 46-1.

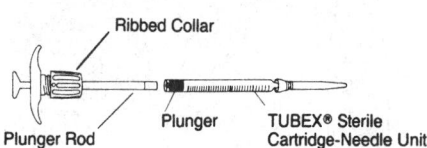

Ribbed Collar

Plunger Rod   Plunger   TUBEX® Sterile
Cartridge-Needle Unit

To load a TUBEX® Sterile Cartridge-Needle Unit into the TUBEX® Injector

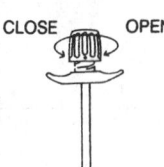

CLOSE   OPEN

1. Turn the ribbed collar to the "OPEN" position until it stops.

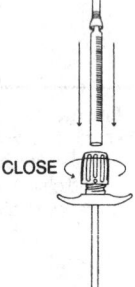

2. Hold the Injector with the open end up and fully insert the TUBEX® Sterile Cartridge-Needle Unit.

Firmly tighten the ribbed collar in the direction of the "CLOSE" arrow.

CLOSE

3. Thread the plunger rod into the plunger of the TUBEX® Sterile Cartridge-Needle Unit until slight resistance is felt.

The Injector is now ready for use in the usual manner.

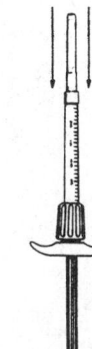

4. Engage the needle-cap assembly by pulling the cap down over the silver cartridge hub. The needle is fully engaged when the silver hub is completely covered.
The Injector is now ready for use in the usual manner.

To administer
Method of administration is the same as with conventional syringe. Remove needle cover by grasping it securely; twist and pull. Introduce needle into patient, aspirate by pulling back slightly on the plunger, and inject.

To remove the empty TUBEX® or DOSETTE® Cartridge-Needle Unit and dispose into a horizontal (mailbox) needle disposal container

1. Do not recap the needle. Disengage the plunger rod.

2. Open the horizontal (mailbox) needle disposal container. Insert TUBEX® or DOSETTE® Cartridge-Needle Unit, needle pointing down, halfway into container. Close the container lid on cartridge. Loosen ribbed collar; TUBEX® or DOSETTE® Cartridge-Needle Unit will drop into the container.

3. Discard the needle cover.

The TUBEX® Injector is reusable and should not be discarded.

Used TUBEX® or DOSETTE® Cartridge-Needle Units should not be employed for successive injections or as multiple-dose containers. They are intended to be used only once and discarded.

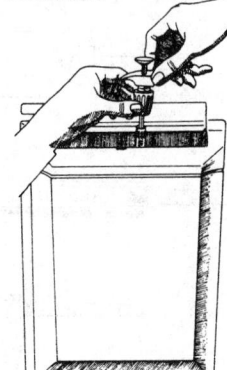

the needle. If you inadvertently get medication on yourself, wash your hands immediately to avoid skin irritation. Discard ampules (empty or not) according to agency policy. Open ampules should never be saved.

Vials. **Vials** are single- or multidose glass medicine containers (see Fig. 46–17*B*). The sterile solution (or powder requiring reconstitution) contained in the vial is protected with a rubber stopper and soft metal or plastic cap. Remove the metal or plastic cap before drawing up the medication through the rubber stopper. The rubber stopper is theoretically sterile when first opened. It is advisable, however, to cleanse the top with an alcohol pledget and friction before the first use (as well as before subsequent uses with multiple-dose vials).

Into the syringe, pull an amount of air equal to the amount of medication to be withdrawn from the vial. Turn the vial upside down and insert the needle bevel side up to avoid contaminating the vial with pieces of rubber (Fig. 46–20). Inject the premeasured air into the vial.

Be sure the bevel of the needle is above the level of fluid in the vial and that you inject air into air. This position of the bevel will prevent you from injecting air into the medication and causing the formation of bubbles.

Inject an amount of air equal to the amount of fluid to be removed. If you inject too little air, it is difficult to withdraw a sufficient dosage. If you inject too much, high pressure in the vial may cause the plunger to be ejected from the syringe. The latter case results in a loss of medication as well as contamination of equipment. After the air is injected, readjust the needle to bring the bevel to just inside the rubber stopper and withdraw all fluid.

If you need to draw medication from two vials and mix in one syringe, first inject appropriate volumes of air into each vial. Then withdraw the dosage from each vial. If using both multiple- and single-dose vials, withdraw the dose from the multiple-dose vial first to prevent possible contamination from the single-dose vial. When you need to mix regular or short-acting insulin with a long-acting insulin in the same syringe, draw up the regular insulin first. This sequence will prevent the inadvertent injection of some of the long-acting insulin into the vial of the regular insulin.

Because some medications deteriorate when mixed in a solution, manufacturers dispense them in powder form in a sterile vial. Each medication has clear directions concerning the kind and amount of solution to mix with it. Sterile normal saline and bacteriostatic water are common diluents.

Follow the dilution directions carefully to prevent overdosage or underdosage and to prevent local tissue damage from a too highly concentrated solution.

Pull the diluent into a sterile syringe and inject it into the vial containing the powder. Gently rotate the vial to

▲ *Figure 46–20*

Withdrawing medication from a vial. *A,* Inject an amount of air into the vial that is equal to the amount of medication to be withdrawn. *B,* Reposition the tip of the needle so that it is as low as possible in the fluid to be withdrawn and pull back on the plunger to withdraw medication.

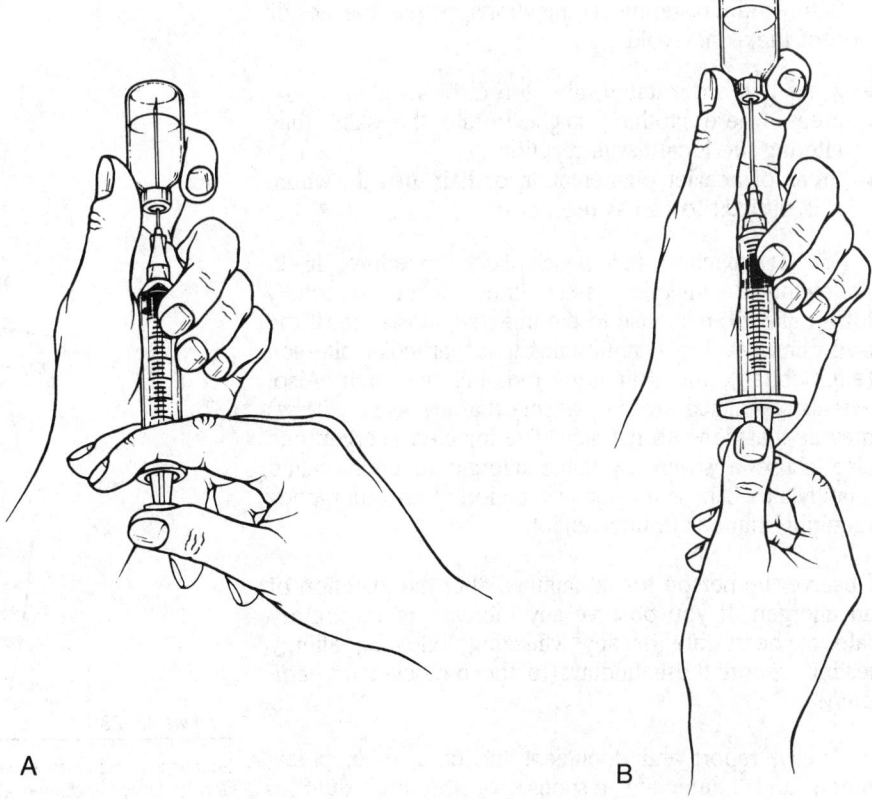

A   B

allow mixing. A thoroughly mixed solution is clear and free of lumps of medication. After reconstitution, draw up the appropriate dosage using aseptic technique. Dispose of empty glass vials according to agency policy.

Store multiple-dose vials according to the manufacturer's directions. Some must be dated and refrigerated, but others have a preservative that allows for storage at room temperature. Always mark the date of opening along with your initials somewhere on the vial label.

Prepackaged Medications. Today, many parenteral medications come in a variety of prefilled cartridges and syringes (see Fig. 46–18). Prefilled cartridges are either (a) loaded into reusable syringe holders and screwed into place, or (b) used with disposable syringes. When certain medications and dosages are ordered routinely (e.g., on a postoperative unit), prepackaged injectable medications save time and reduce errors.

INTRADERMAL INJECTIONS

Intradermal (ID) injections are administered primarily for diagnostic purposes. For example, allergy and tuberculin skin tests are administered ID. Substances used for skin testing can be potent. Therefore, the less vascular ID layer is used to retard absorption. The ventral midforearm and the scapulae are the most common ID injection sites (Fig. 46–21*A,D*). Other sites include the upper arm and upper chest (Fig. 46–21*B,C*). The upper chest site is more painful and is rarely used.

Before administering ID injections, assess the condition of the skin. Avoid

▶ areas that are irritated, discolored, or swollen
▶ areas where clothing might irritate the skin, thus altering the local tissue reaction
▶ areas of heavier pigmentation or hair growth, where it is difficult to assess reactions

For ID injection techniques, see Procedure 46–2. Following the injection, assess the individual carefully for an allergic response to the injected substance. If the body has developed antibodies to a particular allergen (e.g., pollen), the skin turns red and may itch. Also, wheals (localized areas of edema that are usually itchy) may appear beneath the skin. The injected allergen can also cause a severe systemic allergic reaction called anaphylaxis. An anaphylactic reaction is an emergency requiring immediate intervention.

Observe the person for 20 minutes after the injection of an allergen. If you observe any increase in respiratory rate or heart rate or any wheezing following allergy testing, report these findings to the physician *immediately.*

Finally, report and document the date, time, placement, and immediate response of the individual to

therapy. It is helpful to mark the site of injection with a circle of indelible ink and to note the location of the injection in the person's permanent documentation. The exact injection time is important, particularly when assessing a person's sensitivity to an allergen.

SUBCUTANEOUS INJECTIONS

Subcutaneous (below the skin; SQ, SC) tissue is used for the injection of many medications, including heparin and insulin. Subcutaneous sites lie above the muscle and are found in many areas of the body. The following sites are frequently used for SQ injections: (a) anterior thigh, (b) lower ventral abdominal wall, (c) outer aspect of upper arm, (d) flank, and (e) abdomen. Any site is acceptable if it meets the following criteria:

▶ It is not over bony prominences.
▶ It is free of large blood vessels or nerves.
▶ It is free of inflammation, excoriation, itching, tenderness, edema, and scar tissue.

Figure 46–23 illustrates preferred abdominal sites for SQ injections. Procedure 46–3 describes the technique for administering SQ injections.

Rotating-site charts are helpful for people who will be receiving or self-administering SQ injections for a prolonged time (e.g., diabetics who require insulin injections). The chart depicts the general area for injections (e.g., the abdomen), as well as the specific injec-

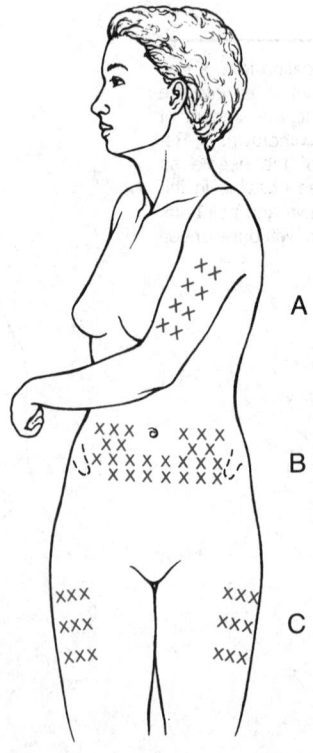

▲ *Figure 46–23*

Location of preferred subcutaneous sites for injection. *A,* Upper outer arm. *B,* Lower abdomen. *C,* Upper outer thigh.

PROCEDURE 46-2

Administering Intradermal Injections

Definitions/Purposes. Intradermal (ID) injections are medications injected "into the skin." Used for diagnostic skin tests to assess the individual's exposure to diseases (e.g., tuberculosis) or sensitivity to allergens such as grass or medications.

Contraindications/Cautions. The skin used for ID injections must be free of disease (e.g., psoriasis or eczema) and other abnormalities. Also, avoid injections into (a) hair follicles, (b) areas that have scarring or pustular eruptions, and (c) sites that could be irritated by clothing. Medications given by ID injection may cause an anaphylactic reaction. Dosages must be accurate and injected properly into the skin.

Learning/Teaching Guidelines. Provide the individual and significant others with information concerning expected reactions from ID injections and allergic reactions.

PRELIMINARY ACTIVITIES

Assessment/Planning

- ▶ Check diagnosis.
- ▶ Check physician's order.
- ▶ Assess sites available.
- ▶ Assess condition of skin.
- ▶ Select appropriate site.
  Select appropriate needle and syringe.
- ▶ Determine expected action of medication and possible side effects.
- ▶ Plan intervention if adverse effects occur.

Equipment

- ▶ Syringes (tuberculin or 1 ml)
- ▶ Needles (26 or 27 gauge, 3/8–5/8 inch in length)
- ▶ Medication card or sheet
- ▶ Alcohol pledget
- ▶ Sterile dry cotton or 2 × 2 gauze
- ▶ Disposal container for used syringe and needle

Preparation of Client

- ▶ Explain procedure to client.
- ▶ Prepare to restrain client if necessary.

PROCEDURE

Actions

1. Use aseptic technique to prepare ordered medication.
2. Identify person according to agency policy.
3. Position person with arm in relaxed position, with inner aspect of arm exposed and elbow flexed. Sit comfortably in front of person.

4. Clean skin of injection site. While skin dries (30 sec to 1 min), double-check dosage.

5. Grasp middle of forearm from underneath, pulling anterior skin taut with your thumb and fingers and, with bevel of needle facing up, insert needle almost flat against person's skin (at a 10° angle) (Fig. 46-22A). Introduce only bevel into skin (Fig. 46-22B). Bevel should be visible just under skin. Do not aspirate.
6. Inject medication slowly. You should meet some resistance. A small wheal should appear.

7. Observe person carefully for drug reaction. If an untoward reaction occurs (e.g., breathing difficulty), notify physician immediately.

Rationale/Discussion

1. Prevents infection.
2. Prevents giving medication to wrong person.
3. Intradermal injections are normally given into forearm. However, skin testing for allergies can be done on back, as well as on lateral sides of arm (Fig. 46-21).
4. Cleansing skin helps assure asepsis. Allowing skin to dry prevents injecting alcohol into tissues, which would cause irritation. Rechecking dosage prevents errors.
5. Ensures proper placement of medication or allergen.

6. Injecting slowly limits tissue damage. If you do not meet resistance, you have probably inserted needle too deeply. Deposition of drug into ID layer causes small wheal or bleb.
7. Injection of allergens can cause severe adverse reactions.

Procedure continued on following page

PROCEDURE 46–2 Continued

Administering Intradermal Injections

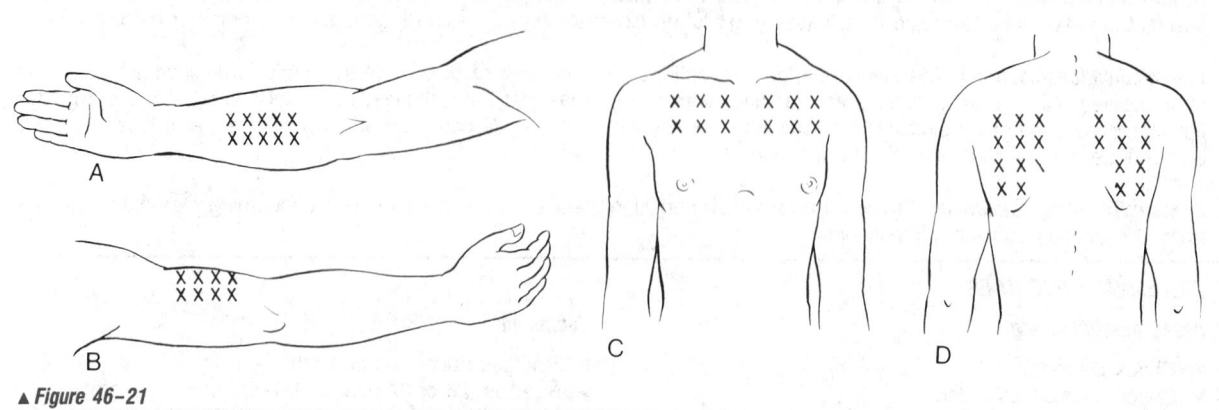

▲ *Figure 46–21*

Commonly used sites for intradermal injections. *A,* Inner surface of forearm. *B,* Lateral aspect of upper arm. *C,* Anterior upper chest. *D,* Scapular area of back.

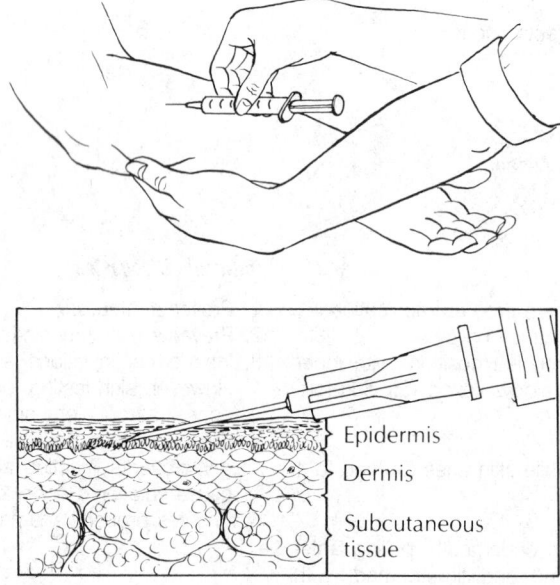

Epidermis
Dermis
Subcutaneous tissue

▲ *Figure 46–22*

Actions	Rationale/Discussion
8. Withdraw needle gently, and lightly cover site with dry sterile cotton or gauze if there is pinpoint bleeding. Do not massage or rub area.	8. Massaging is contraindicated because it increases absorption of medication or causes seepage of medication onto skin. Massaging may also alter test results.
9. Mark skin around injection site with indelible pen.	9. Allows for later assessment of local inflammatory reaction.

FINAL ACTIVITIES

Position person comfortably. Assess medication effects. Inspect injection sites for reaction. Discard disposables according to agency policy. *Documentation:* Medication name, dose, route, and site of administration. Note exact time and location of injection in chart. Report and record any adverse reactions.

tion sites within the area. Also included on the chart is a plan for rotating the injections. Rotation involves changing the site for each injection to a different area of tissue so that no one site is used excessively. Refer to the chart before choosing an injection site. After administering an injection, mark the site used on the chart. This procedure ensures that the next injection the person receives will be into a different area of tissue.

INTRAMUSCULAR INJECTIONS

Sites. Several sites for intramuscular (IM) injections are available to the nurse. Techniques for locating each site are described in Procedure 46–4.

The **ventrogluteal site** for IM injection allows deposition of medication into the gluteus minimus muscle. This site is suitable in both adults and children because no major blood vessels or nerves are located near it (Fig. 46–25). It can be used for deep IM, Z-track, and large-volume (5-ml) injections. The ventrogluteal site is accessible with the person in a supine, prone, or side-lying position.

The **dorsogluteal site** for IM injection allows deposition of medication into the gluteus medius muscle (Fig. 46–26). The gluteus medius muscle provides the slowest absorption and presents the highest risk for injury to nerves and blood vessels, e.g., the sciatic nerve and the superior gluteal artery. The risk of injury is highest among children and individuals with small muscle mass. Therefore, avoid using this site in these people.

Under no circumstances should the gluteal site be used when a person is standing or when the area cannot be fully exposed. If you cannot clearly see the area, you will not be able to locate the anatomic landmarks safely and correctly.

The **quadriceps femoris site** for IM injection allows deposition of medication into the rectus femoris or vastus lateralis muscle. Within the area between the midanterior and the midlateral thigh is a muscle group called the quadriceps femoris, which contains the rectus femoris (midanterior thigh) and vastus lateralis (midlateral thigh) muscles (Fig. 46–27). These muscles are located away from major blood vessels and nerves and are easy to locate. Because the quadriceps femoris site is the largest and most well-developed muscle mass in infants, this site is used when administering injections to infants and small children.

The **mid-deltoid site** for IM injection allows deposition of medication into the deltoid muscle. The deltoid site on the upper arm has the advantage of being easily accessible, and it does not require removal of clothing. In addition, absorption is more rapid than from the gluteal site. The disadvantages are that only a small volume (up to 2 ml) can be accommodated in an adult, and the brachial and axillary nerves and blood vessels are close to the site (Fig. 46–28). Use the mid-deltoid site for single injections only, especially in children.

Site Assessment. Before proceeding with an IM injection, determine the condition of the tissue and the suitability of the site. In assessing the tissue, make sure the skin is intact. The subcutaneous fat should not contain nodules (lumps). Remember that painful nodules may indicate that the person previously received parenteral therapy and that the medication was poorly absorbed. The proposed site should be of adequate size for the volume of fluid to be injected. If the site is too small or is "lumpy" and painful, select another site.

Special Techniques of Intramuscular Administration. Select injection sites and administer IM medications skillfully to avoid injury to tissue, nerves, and vessels and to ensure that the therapeutic effects are achieved. The general principles and steps of intramuscular injection are presented in Procedure 46–4. In addition to the basic injection technique, you must also be skilled in using the air lock technique and administering Z-track injections.

The **air lock technique** is used with most IM medications. The technique avoids leakage of medication into the needle track after the needle is withdrawn from the site, thus avoiding pain and tissue injury. The air lock technique "seals" the needle tract with a small air bubble. To provide an air lock, draw 0.2 to 0.3 ml of air into the syringe after it has been filled with medication. The bubble size is determined by the length and gauge of the needle (e.g., a 2-inch, large-bore needle requires a larger amount of air than a smaller needle). Invert the syringe and allow the air bubble to rise into the plunger end of the syringe. When the medication is administered, the air bubble enters the site last and ejects the residual medication from the needle, thus preventing medication leakage when the needle is withdrawn.

The Z-track injection also prevents the leakage of medication from injection sites. The Z-track is the displacement of tissues during intramuscular injection that helps retain the medication in the injection site when the tissues return to their normal position (Fig. 46–29). Intramuscular iron preparations are often administered using this technique. Use the Z-track method in any muscle site in which the overlying tissue can be retracted at least 1 inch, e.g., the dorsogluteal, ventrogluteal, and quadriceps femoris sites.

EVALUATION

After administering a medication, you should determine whether or to what extent your planned outcome has been achieved. For example, you will want to know whether

▶ the client who was in pain can now state that the pain is relieved
▶ the client at high risk for infection has a WBC that is within normal limits
▶ the person who was constipated has had a normal bowel movement
▶ the individual with diarrhea has had fewer bowel movements each day

Text continued on page 1303

PROCEDURE 46-3

Administering Subcutaneous Injections

Definitions/Purposes. Subcutaneous (SQ, SC) injections are medications injected into the subcutaneous tissues (below the skin). Many medications are given SQ; a common one is insulin. The absorption rate of medications given by the SQ route is generally *slower* than that of medications given intravenously or intramuscularly, but it is usually *faster* than that of medications given orally.

Contraindications/Cautions. Rotate SQ injection sites to prevent lipodystrophy (wasting of SQ fat) and excessive scar tissue. Damaged tissue hinders medication absorption. Subcutaneous injections of heparin differ in many of the actions required.

Learning/Teaching Guidelines. Provide the individual and significant others with information concerning the following as appropriate: (a) Explain and demonstrate aseptic technique, (b) show the person how to read syringe calibrations, (c) demonstrate the method for removing medications from a vial and for injecting medication into tissues, (d) teach the location and rotation of the appropriate site, and (e) explain observations pertinent to untoward reactions as well as expected effects. This information is particularly relevant to individuals with diabetes who must self-administer insulin at home.

PRELIMINARY ACTIVITIES

Assessment/Planning

▶ Check diagnosis.
▶ Check physician's order.
▶ Assess body size.
▶ Assess sites available.
▶ Assess depth of SQ tissue.
▶ Assess condition of skin.
▶ Select appropriate site.
▶ Select appropriate needle and syringe.
▶ Determine expected action of medication and possible side effects.
▶ Know and plan for appropriate interventions if adverse effects do occur.

Equipment

▶ Medication
▶ Syringe (insulin or 2.0, 2.5, or 3.0 ml)
▶ Needles (25 gauge, 1/2 to 5/8 inch in length)
▶ Medication card or sheet
▶ Alcohol pledget
▶ Sterile dry cotton or 2 × 2 gauze
▶ Disposal container for used syringe and needle

Preparation of Person

▶ Explain procedure to person.
▶ Allow for privacy.
▶ Prepare to restrain person if necessary.

PROCEDURE

Actions

1. Use aseptic technique to prepare ordered medication.
2. Identify person according to agency policy.
3. Position person according to site selected.

4. Prepare site with antiseptic and friction.
5. Check dosage against medication card or sheet. (When administering insulin, dose should have been double-checked with another nurse.)
6. Inject medication safely and at correct angle into appropriate area. Follow these steps:

   a. Compress and lift SQ tissue from muscle.
   b. Insert needle at either 90° or 45° angle. Determine angle by assessing amount of SQ fat available and by length of needle (Fig. 46-24).

Rationale/Discussion

1. Prevents infection.
2. Prevents administration of medication to wrong person.
3. Be sure that entire site is exposed and that underlying muscle is relaxed.
4. Ensures asepsis.
5. Prevents errors.

6. If injection is too shallow, injection is more painful because skin nerve endings are compressed. Also, medication is administered into incorrect tissue.

   a. Helps prevent injection into muscle.
   b. For example, for large individual, use 5/8-inch needle at 90° angle to ensure deeper penetration. For small child or emaciated adult, use 5/8-inch needle at 45° angle, or 1/2-inch needle at 90° angle (Fig. 46-24). For adult with large fat deposits, you may need to use 1/2- to 1-inch needle at 90° angle.

PROCEDURE 46–3 Continued

Administering Subcutaneous Injections

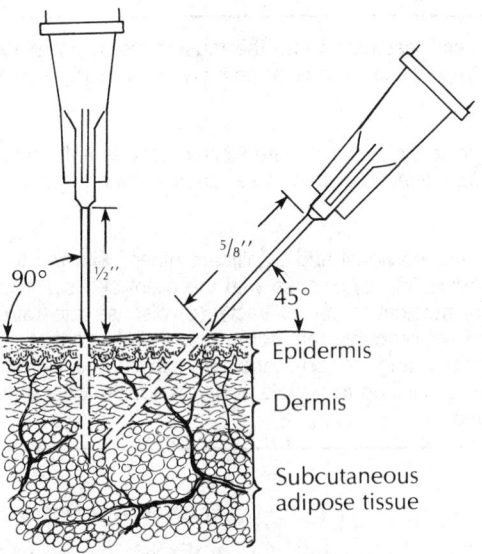

▲ Figure 46–24

Actions

7. Release pinched skin.

8. Pull back gently on plunger to aspirate. If blood appears in syringe, withdraw needle and begin procedure again. If no blood appears in syringe, inject medication slowly.
9. Remove needle along same track as inserted. Apply pressure with sterile cotton or gauze.

Rationale/Discussion

7. Prevents medication from leaking from needle tract. Also reduces pain.
8. Aspiration prevents giving medication intravascularly. Slow injection decreases pain by allowing time for absorption.
9. Careful needle removal reduces tissue damage and discomfort. Applying pressure reduces bleeding.

FINAL ACTIVITIES

Position person comfortably. Discard disposables according to agency policy. *Documentation:* Medication name, dose, route, and site of administration. Assess medication effects. Report and record any adverse reactions.

▲ Figure 46–25

Ventrogluteal injection site in a supine client.

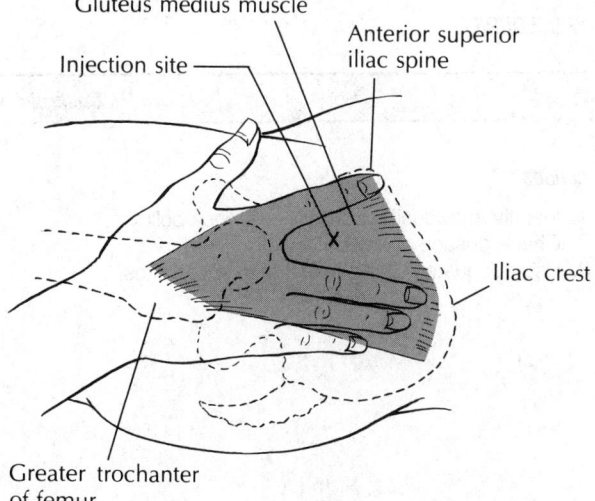

PROCEDURE 46-4

Administering Intramuscular Injection, Including Air Lock and Z-Track Techniques

Definition/Purposes. To inject a parenteral medication into the muscle, using an air lock. Deposits medication into muscle, where it is absorbed into the bloodstream. The air lock or seal prevents medication leakage and resultant pain and tissue damage.

Contraindications/Cautions. Use aseptic technique. Repeated intramuscular (IM) injections or medication leads to nodular and indurated areas. Therefore, *rotate* injection sites. Use caution when giving IM injections to children and other individuals with small muscle mass.

Learning/Teaching Guidelines. Provide the individual and significant others with the following information as appropriate: (a) Explain the actions and effects of medication, (b) discuss with the client and significant others the reason for the IM route (e.g., rapid absorption, inactivation of medication by GI tract), (c) discuss site rotation to avoid damage from repeated injections, (d) explain that the person will probably feel some discomfort but that you will use techniques to reduce this (relaxation exercises, proper positioning, and so on), and (e) explain that a relaxed muscle decreases discomfort. Encourage parents of infants and young children to cuddle, rock, or speak softly to them after the injection. Older children need explanations they can understand.

PRELIMINARY ACTIVITIES

Assessment/Planning

▶ Check diagnosis.
▶ Check physician's order.
▶ Check dosage and amount of medication.
▶ Assess muscle mass and amount of subcutaneous fat.
▶ Assess neurologic/sensory status.
▶ Assess level of cooperation.
▶ Assess previous sites of IM injections.
▶ Note areas of poor circulation due to edema or vascular problems.
▶ Note areas of painful nodular tissue due to previous injections.
▶ Select appropriate site.
▶ Select appropriate needle length, needle gauge, and syringe.
▶ Determine need for assistance if person is uncooperative.
▶ Determine expected action of medication and possible side effects.
▶ Plan intervention should adverse effects occur.

Preparation of Person

▶ Explain procedure to individual. Determine previous experience with IM injections.
▶ Provide privacy.
▶ Position individual for optimal site exposure.

Equipment

▶ Medication
▶ Medication card or sheet
▶ Needle (20 to 25 gauge, 1 to 3 inch)
▶ Syringe (1 to 5 ml)
▶ Alcohol pledget
▶ Restraining device, if necessary
▶ Bed, stretcher, or chair to provide comfortable position for person
▶ Disposal container for used syringe and needle

PROCEDURE

General Considerations

Actions

1. Identify individual according to agency policy.
2. Check dosage against medication card.
3. Use adequate lighting to locate injection sites.

Rationale/Discussion

1. Prevents errors.
2. First safety check prevents errors.
3. Allows for accurate and safe identification of anatomic landmarks.

PROCEDURE 46–4 Continued

Administering Intramuscular Injection, Including Air Lock and Z-Track Techniques

Position and Site Identification

Actions	*Rationale/Discussion*
1. Mid-deltoid site.	1.
a. Position. Have individual place arm at side and flex elbow to relax muscle. Completely expose upper arm. Person can be standing, sitting, or lying down.	a. Allows for proper exposure and identification of injection site. If air lock technique is used, person must lie on side (so that needle is perpendicular to floor).
b. Locate site. Locate triangular muscle below lower edge of acromion process (Fig. 46–28). Locate densest muscle mass by grasping area between fingers and thumb and palpating with fingers of opposite hand.	b. Mid-deltoid site is often chosen for ease of access, although this site is limited in persons with small muscle mass (e.g., children). Small muscle mass accommodates only small medication volumes.
c. Injection: For adults, spread tissue between thumb and forefinger (index finger). Insert needle at 90° angle to tissue. For children and other persons with small muscle mass, grasp muscle mass and compress between thumb and forefinger to lift muscle upward in a rounded mass. Insert needle at 45° angle.	c. Spreading the tissue compresses subcutaneous fat and helps assure that the bevel will reach well into muscle. Lifting the muscle thickens it and helps prevent contact of needle and bone under the muscle. Correct angle of injection ensures deposit of medication in densest portion of muscle.
2. Dorsogluteal site (gluteus medius muscle).	2.
a. Position. Have person lie prone (face down) with toes together (pigeon-toed) (see Fig. 46–12).	a. Internal rotation of the hip relaxes muscles. Avoid side-lying or standing position so that you can identify anatomic landmarks and avoid nerves and blood vessels.
b. Locate site. Identify greater trochanter of femur and posterior superior iliac spine. Draw an imaginary line between these two bony landmarks. Site is on upper outer quadrant of buttock, above the imaginary line, and below the iliac crest. Palpate the site to ascertain that muscle is sufficiently thick (Fig. 46–26).	b. In those with adequate muscle mass in this area, this site helps avoid the sciatic nerve. Small, undeveloped muscles make this site a dangerous one in infants and young children. Site is acceptable for child over age of 2 years who is walking and has developed good musculature.
c. Injection: Spread tissue between thumb and forefinger to make skin taut. Insert needle perpendicular (i.e., at 90° angle) to surface on which person is lying.	c. 90° angle of needle insertion prevents sciatic nerve damage.
3. Ventrogluteal site (gluteus medius and minimus muscles).	3.
a. Position person on side, supine, or prone with legs straight at the hip joints.	a. The hip may be flexed to help identify the greater trochanter but should then be placed in a position of extension for site identification.
b. Locate site. Place palm on greater trochanter and make a "V" with index and middle fingers on anterior superior iliac spine and iliac crest respectively. Switch finger position for right or left side (Fig. 46–25). Palpate site to assure adequate thickness of muscle.	b. Use care in locating site to avoid injury to veins, arteries, nerves, and bone. If you select a site too near the iliac crest, the needle could pass through the muscle and into bone.
c. Injection: In center of "V" space, spread tissue between thumb and forefinger. Inject with needle at 75° to 80° angle to skin surface, pointing toward head.	c. Deposits medication into deepest part of muscle.

Procedure continued on following page

PROCEDURE 46–4 Continued

Administering Intramuscular Injection, Including Air Lock and Z-Track Techniques

Actions	*Rationale/Discussion*
4. Quadriceps femoris site (vastus lateralis and rectus femoris muscles).	4.
a. Position. Have adult or child lie on back or maintain sitting position with knees slightly bent.	a. Exposes entire area for anatomic identification. Flexion of knees promotes muscle relaxation.
b. Locate site. For *rectus femoris,* on area of midanterior thigh, measure handbreadth below greater trochanter at proximal end, handbreadth above knee at distal end. For *vastus lateralis,* identify surface of midlateral thigh at same distance from greater trochanter and knee (Fig. 46–27). Palpate the muscle to identify the thickest part.	b. Site is relatively free of major nerves and blood vessels.
c. Injection: For adults, spread tissue taut between thumb and forefinger. Inject needle at 90° angle or pointing slightly toward the client's head. For infants and children, compress muscle to lift it away from femur. Then inject needle at 90° angle.	c. Angle of injection will deposit medication into deep muscle. Lifting tissue avoids bone, nerves, and blood vessels.

Air Lock Technique

Actions	*Rationale/Discussion*
1. Prepare syringe with proper volume of medication. After checking accuracy of dosage, draw an additional 0.2 to 0.5 ml of air into syringe to provide an air lock. Turn syringe with needle downward and tap syringe until bubble floats upward to plunger.	1. Always measure medication accurately; always double-check dosage. Drawing up 0.2 to 0.3 ml of air is usually sufficient to clear needle and its hub of medication. Up to 0.5 ml of air may be required for the air lock, however, depending on the gauge and length of the needle.
2. Place person either in prone position (using dorsogluteal site) or in side-lying position (using either mid-deltoid or ventrogluteal site). Hold syringe perpendicular to floor to keep air bubble against plunger, so that it will be injected after total dosage of medication.	2. After the injection, this air "locks" medication into muscle site, where it is absorbed. Reduces discomfort and tissue irritation. Use air lock for most IM injections. Injecting air last will help assure that the complete dose of medication has been given and the needle is cleared of the medication. This procedure will prevent tracking of medication as the needle is withdrawn from the tissues.

General Injection Technique

Actions	*Rationale/Discussion*
1. Palpate area for scarring, tenderness, nodules, or pain.	1. Individuals who receive multiple IM injections into same site may develop all these symptoms. Also, medication deposited into an overused site is poorly absorbed. Use other sites if any damage exists.
2. Check dosage in syringe against medication card. Use air lock if indicated.	2. Checking dosage prevents errors. Air lock prevents tissue damage.
3. Cleanse skin thoroughly. Allow to dry.	3. Prevents infection by ensuring clean site.
4. Hold used alcohol pledget between two fingers on nondominant hand. Make skin taut by stretching skin between forefinger and thumb. In child or adult with small subcutaneous fat and muscle mass, compress skin between fingers to lift muscle.	4. Retain pledget to apply pressure after injection. Taut skin is easier to pierce than loose skin. Compressing skin ensures deposition of medication into muscle when person is small or emaciated.
5. Prepare person for insertion of needle. Have person exhale, or ask a question; engage in conversation.	5. Diversion takes the client's mind off discomfort.
6. Pierce tissue quickly at correct angle.	6. Quick insertion reduces "drag" of needle through tissue and thus reduces discomfort.

PROCEDURE 46–4 Continued

Administering Intramuscular Injection, Including Air Lock and Z-Track Techniques

Actions	Rationale/Discussion
7. Release pressure on tissue.	7. Minimizes discomfort.
8. Aspirate for blood before injecting. If blood is aspirated into syringe, withdraw needle, eject medication, and discard syringe and needle. Replace with sterile syringe and needle and repeat from step 1. If no blood is aspirated, inject medication slowly.	8. Failure to aspirate for blood before injecting could result in intravascular administration of medication, which in turn could result in unnecessary or undesired therapy.
9. Place alcohol pledget at injection site and remove needle at same angle as inserted.	9. Removing needle at same angle prevents tearing of tissue by sharp needle bevel.
10. Apply pressure over site momentarily. If bleeding occurs, maintain pressure until bleeding stops.	10. Prevents excessive bleeding.

Z-Track Technique[7]

Actions	Rationale/Discussion
1. Z-track technique creates a zigzag needle path.	1. Prevents leakage of medication, which stains skin or irritates tissues.
a. Position. Have person prone with toes pointed inward for dorsogluteal site, prone or side-lying for ventrogluteal site, supine or sitting for quadriceps femoris site.	a. Person assumes same position for regular IM injection with air lock.
b. Prepare air lock.	b. Always use 0.3 to 0.5 cc air lock with Z-track technique. Seals medication into muscle.
c. Injection:	c.
i. Place middle finger of nondominant hand onto skin. Retract tissue laterally (to side) and downward. Do not release tissue until after you remove needle (Fig. 46–29).	i. With retraction, skin and subcutaneous tissues move; underlying muscle remains stationary.
ii. While tissue is retracted, insert 1- to 3-inch needle at 80° to 90° angle to skin surface. Support base of syringe with thumb and index finger of nondominant hand. Aspirate to avoid intravascular injection.	ii. Angle and needle length ensure deposition of medication into deep muscle.
iii. Inject medication slowly, followed by air lock. Wait 10 seconds and withdraw needle.	iii. Slow injection reduces discomfort. Waiting 10 seconds prevents medication leakage.
iv. Release skin and do not massage site.	iv. Needle track forms "Z" shape (Fig. 46–29). Massaging forces medication into tissue, causing pain.

FINAL ACTIVITIES

Position person comfortably. Assess injection sites for redness, induration, soreness. Dispose of used equipment according to agency policy. *Documentation:* Medication name, dose, route and site of administration, medication effects. Continue to monitor client for effects of medication.

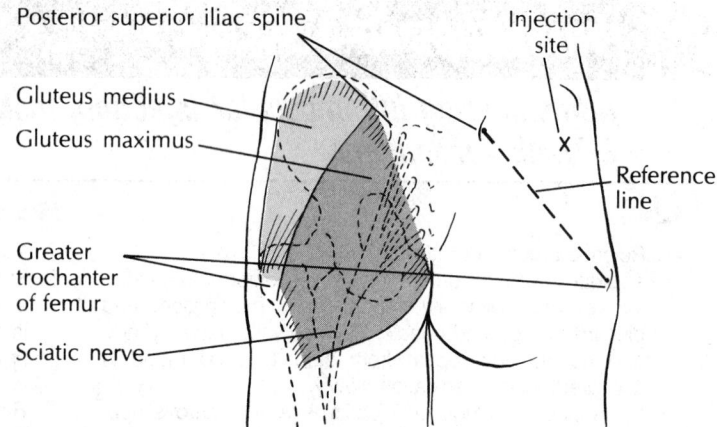

▲ **Figure 46-26**

Dorsogluteal injection site in a supine client.

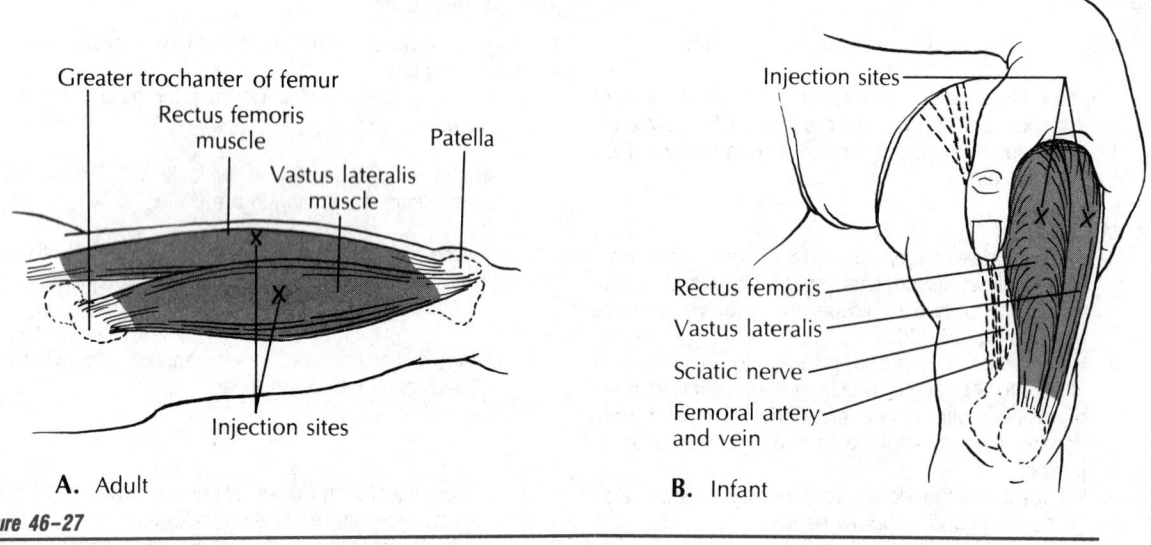

A. Adult   **B.** Infant

▲ **Figure 46-27**

Quadriceps femoris injection sites. *A*, Adult; *B*, infant.

▲ **Figure 46-28**

Mid-deltoid injection site.

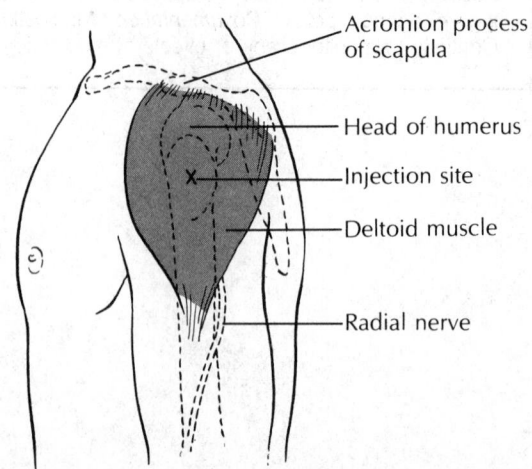

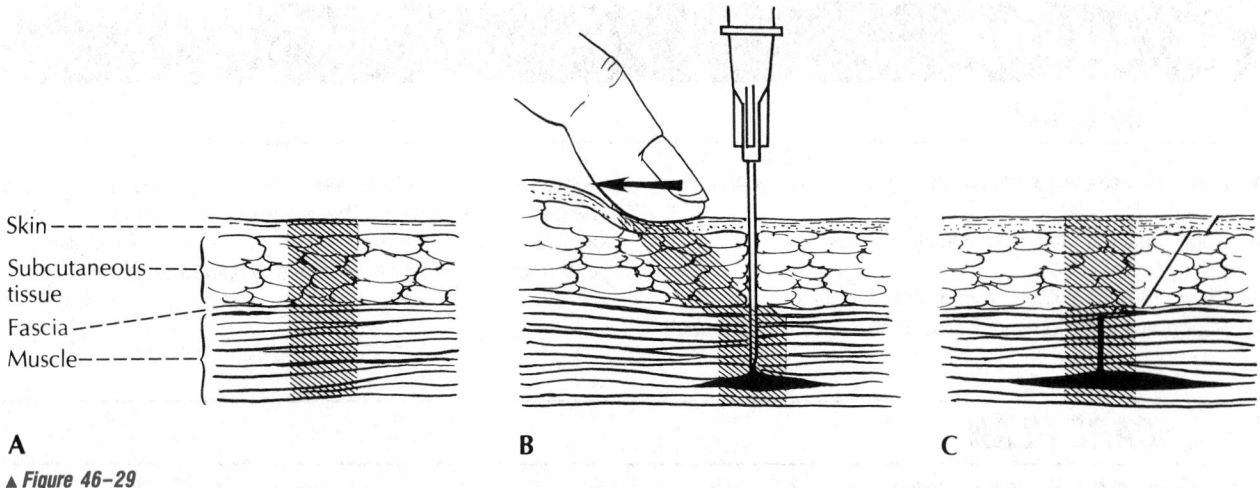

▲ Figure 46–29

Z-track technique. *A*, Normal tissue relationship prior to injection. *B*, Altered tissue relationship during injection. Retract tissue, insert needle, administer medication, wait 10 seconds, remove needle, and release tissue. *C*, Normal relationship following injection. Note angled ''Z'' track left by needle.

▶ the client who was anxious can now state that anxiety is relieved

If you want to determine how well the administration of a medication worked, you must select the best time to make the assessment. For the person who was in pain or anxious, you might expect to have results quite soon after administration of the medication. Depending on the type of medication given and such factors as the route selected, you might expect positive results almost immediately if you gave an intravenous medication, within approximately 15 minutes if you gave an intramuscular injection, within 30 minutes if you gave a subcutaneous injection, and within 45 minutes if you gave the drug orally.

For the clients who were constipated or suffering from diarrhea, the results might take 8 hours or more. The client at high risk for infection might still develop that infection several days or even weeks later, as it is not always possible to know that a prophylactic drug has completely prevented a disease until some time has passed and the client remains disease-free.

In some circumstances it takes several days or weeks of medication therapy before beneficial results are evident. Two such situations are the treatment of mental depression and Parkinson's disease. Clients with these disorders need to be assessed for some time to determine the effectiveness of the medication.

As you evaluate your planned outcomes, keep in mind that the administration of an ordered medication is but one of your responsibilities. It may seem to be of greatest importance to you now, as you are beginning to master the skills required to give the various types of medications by so many different routes, but do not let your anxiety about learning these new skills obscure the fact that there are many other interventions that your client is relying on you to implement.

CASE STUDY

The Client

On May 25 at 6:00 PM 35-year-old Jim Smith came to the emergency department with the chief complaint of an itching rash on his arms and legs. He stated that he and several of his neighbors had spent the weekend clearing brush from an empty lot in their neighborhood so that the children would have a safe place to play ball. About an hour before coming to the emergency room, he developed severe itching and noticed the rash.

A partial listing of assessment data in the emergency department included

▶ 35-year-old male
▶ T 98.4°F, P 60, R 20, BP 120/70

▶ Many areas of raised, reddened spots on forearms and lower legs, with some inflammation evident
▶ States the itching is so intense that he ''can't help scratching''
▶ No known allergies
▶ Not taking any medications at present
▶ Has not eaten any new foods recently
▶ Immunizations up-to-date
▶ Children healthy and up-to-date on immunizations

After diagnosing the rash as a reaction to poison ivy, the physician wrote the following orders:

Case Study continued on following page

CASE STUDY Continued

The Client

▶ Diphenhydramine (Benadryl) 25 mg po stat and q4h prn for itching
▶ Apply calamine lotion to affected areas stat and prn for itching
▶ Return to dermatology clinic at 2:00 PM, June 1.
▶ Report any symptoms indicating further spread of the rash

One week has passed since Mr. Smith was seen in the emergency department. The following represents a nursing care plan that was written for him at the time of his visit and the current evaluation of outcomes expected at that time.

CARE PLAN

6:00 PM, May 25

Nursing Diagnosis	Planning: Expected Outcomes	Implementation: Nursing Interventions	Evaluation
High Risk for Impaired Skin Integrity R/T to scratching of poison ivy rash	By 2:00 PM, June 1: Skin will be intact	Explain that diphenhydramine (Benadryl) will help relieve the itching Administer Benadryl, 25 mg, po stat and tell to repeat it q8h, as ordered, for itching Explain effects of Benadryl and purpose of taking drug Demonstrate how to apply calamine lotion to affected areas as ordered to decrease itching Teach client when to apply calamine lotion to himself Teach him to keep his nails short and clean, to not scratch his skin, to keep his towel and washcloth separate from other family linens, and to wash his hands before and after applying the lotion.	2:00 PM, June 1: Inspection of skin of arms and legs shows no more rash and no breaks in the skin

Summary

▶ Physicians, nurses, and pharmacists have many legal and ethical responsibilities related to medication administration.
▶ The client has both rights and responsibilities related to medication use.
▶ In order to effectively deal with the legal and ethical issues related to medication administration, nurses must be aware of federal and state laws, their state Nurse Practice Act, state rulings, and institutional policies related to medication administration.

▶ Medication may be known by a chemical name, a generic name, and several proprietary names (also called brand or trade names). Medications may be given by different routes and may have local or systemic effects. Drug effects may also be synergistic or antagonistic.
▶ The four main systems for delivery of medication are the stock supply system, individual cubical system, unit dose system, and self-medication.
▶ The amount of information required for a med-

ication order or prescription varies from state to state. Information typically includes the person's name; the date and time; the name of the medication; the dosage; the route, time, and frequency of administration; and the physician's signature.

► Medication orders may be written or verbal and may be single, standing, stat, or prn.

► Because a medication may be measured by the metric system, apothecary system, or household measurement, the nurse must be able to convert accurately from one system to the other. Although the physician orders the number of daily doses of a medication, the nurse often decides when each dose is actually to be administered.

► Safety in medication administration is a priority. Critical information such as allergies or previous adverse reactions must be communicated by noting the information on the client's armband, chart cover, and nursing care plan as well as by notifying the pharmacy.

► In relation to medication administration, the nurse must assess physiologic factors, psychosocial factors, and special needs of clients.

► Nursing interventions include teaching self-care to clients and safely administering medications orally, topically, and parenterally.

► Oral medications may be given in a variety of solid and liquid forms, including tablets, capsules, powders, syrups, solutions, suspensions, emulsions, elixirs, and tinctures.

► Topical medications include lotions, creams, ointments, powders, gels, liquid soaks and dressings, aerosols, and patches. They also may be inserted as vaginal or rectal suppositories, introduced into body cavities by instillation or irrigation, or supplied to the respiratory tract by inhalation.

► Parenteral medications may be administered by intradermal, subcutaneous, intramuscular, or intravenous routes.

► For safe medication administration, the nurse must understand principles of asepsis; know how to select equipment, prepare medications, and identify the correct site; and be able to complete the medication administration procedure.

► Evaluation of the effectiveness of medication may be completed almost immediately after the intervention or may require weeks to pass.

Bibliography

1. Carr, D.S. (1989). New strategies for avoiding medication errors. *Nursing 1989,* 19(8), 38–45.
2. Donica, S., & Ramsey, M. (1991). Hazards of reusing disposable syringes I. *Anesthesiology,* 74(4), 790–791.
3. Gibson, J. (1989). A new approach to better medication compliance. *Nursing 1989,* 20(4), 49–51.
4. Hahn, K. (1990). Brush up on your injection techniques. *Nursing 1990,* 20(9), 54–58.
5. Holdiness, M.R. (1989). A review of contact dermatitis associated with transdermal therapeutic systems. *Contact Dermatitis,* 20(2), 3–9.
6. Katz, E., et al. (1989). Successful treatment of a prolactin-producing pituitary macroadenoma with intravaginal bromocriptine mesylate: a novel approach to intolerance of oral therapy. *Obstetrics & Gynecology,* 73, 517–519.
7. Keen, M.F. (1990). Get on the right track with Z-track injections. *Nursing 1990,* 20(8), 59.
8. Kitz, D., et al. (1989). Examining nursing personnel costs: controlled versus noncontrolled oral analgesic agents. *Journal of Nursing Administration,* 19(1), 10–14.
9. McLaughlin-Hagen, M. (1991). Continuous subcutaneous infusion: new use for an old route. *Nursing 1991,* 21(7), 58–59.
10. Miccolo, M.A. (1990). Intraosseous infusion. *Critical Care Nurse,* 10(10), 35–47.
11. Millam, D. (1990). Equipment update 90: avoiding needle-stick injuries. *Nursing 1990,* 20(1), 61–62.
12. Murphy, J.I. (1990). Tube feeding problems and solutions. *Advancing Clinical Care,* 5(2), 7–11.
13. Newton, M., et al. (1992). Reviewing the "big three" injection routes. *Nursing 1992,* 22(2), 34–41.
14. Oliver, D. (1991). Syringe drivers in the community. *Practitioner,* 235(1448), 78–80.
15. Olsson, G.L., et al. (1989). Nursing management of patients receiving epidural narcotics. *Heart and Lung,* 18(2), 130–138.
16. Paice, J.A. (1991). Intraspinal drug therapy. *Nursing Clinics of North America,* 26(2), 477–498.
17. Paice, J.A. (1992). *Physicians desk reference (46th ed.).* Montvale, New Jersey: Medical Economics Data.
18. Ranade, V.V. (1990). Drug delivery systems 4—implants in drug delivery. *Journal of Clinical Pharmacology,* 30(10), 871–889.
19. Saudek, C.K. (1990). Implantable insulin pumps: a current look. *Diabetes Research & Clinical Practice,* 10(2), 109–114.
20. Stokes, D.N., et al. (1990). The Ohmeda 9000 syringe pump: the first of a new generation of syringe drivers. *Anaesthesia,* 45(12), 1062–1066.
21. Sundberg, M.C. (1989). *Fundamentals of nursing with clinical procedures.* Boston: Jones & Bartlett Publisher.
22. Williams, J.S. (1991). Disconnected epidural catheter. *Nursing 1991,* 21(8), 33.
23. Wink, D.M. (1991). Giving infants and children drugs: precision + caution = safety. *MCN, The American Journal of Maternal/Child Nursing,* 16(6), 317–321.
24. Wood, D.F., et al. (1990). Management of "brittle" diabetes with preprogrammable implanted insulin pump delivering intraperitoneal insulin. *British Medical Journal,* 301(6761), 1143–1144.

Administering Intravenous Therapy

I have heard him [William Harvey] say, that after his book of the circulation of the blood came out, that he fell mightily in his practice, and that 'twas believed by the vulgar that he was crack-brained; and all the physicians were against his opinion.

John Aubrey
Brief Lives (1690)

▼ CHAPTER OUTLINE

INDICATIONS FOR INTRAVENOUS
   THERAPY
INTRAVENOUS SOLUTIONS
   Blood Transfusions
   Parenteral Hyperalimentation
   Equipment for Intravenous Therapy
   Complications of Intravenous
     Therapy

ASSESSMENT
NURSING DIAGNOSIS
PLANNING
NURSING INTERVENTION
   Percutaneous Venipuncture
   Maintaining the IV System
EVALUATION
CASE STUDY

▼ KEY TERMS

Additive solutions
Air embolism
Bolus
Butterfly
Cannula
Central veins
Cutdown
Drip chamber
Drip rate
Drop factor
Extension hook
Flocculate
Flow rate
Hemolytic reaction
Heparin lock
Infiltration

Infusion controller
Infusion pump
Injection cap
Injection ports
Intravenous (IV) infusion
Macrodrip sets
Microdrip sets
Minidrip sets
Packed red blood cells
   (PRBC)
Parenteral
   hyperalimentation
Percutaneous
   venipuncture
Peripheral veins
Piggyback line

Plasma derivatives
Precipitate
Saline lock
Scalp vein needle
Sclerotic
Secondary IV line
Thrombophlebitis
Thrombosis
Time tape
Total parenteral nutrition
   (TPN)
Transfusions
Vasospasm
Venipuncture
Volume-control chamber
Whole blood

Intravenous (IV) infusion is the introduction of fluids into a vein. Both **central veins** (veins in the main body, as opposed to the extremities) and **peripheral veins** (veins in an extremity) may be used for this purpose (Fig. 47–1). Nurses are expected to initiate IV therapy by performing venipuncture of peripheral veins only. Although you will probably have many opportunities to care for clients receiving fluids through central veins, this chapter will concentrate on nursing responsibilities for the client receiving fluids through peripheral veins.

Venipuncture, or the introduction of a needle into a vein, is also performed for reasons other than the provision of IV therapy. These reasons include obtaining blood samples for laboratory analysis, administering blood and blood products, and administering medications. Because medications administered by this route cause an immediate response, they must be prepared and given with even greater knowledge, skill, and caution than is necessary for medications delivered through the routes discussed in Chapter 46.

INDICATIONS FOR INTRAVENOUS THERAPY

Intravenous infusion is the method of choice when a person *must* receive fluids, electrolytes, or medications swiftly or over a long period. Specifically, IV infusions are ordered under the following circumstances:

▶ People in life-threatening situations (e.g., hemorrhage, shock, and severe burns). Under these drastic conditions, IV fluids (which enter the vascular system and thereby increase plasma volume immediately) are absolutely necessary.
▶ People who may have nothing by mouth or who are unable to ingest oral liquids because of prolonged nausea, vomiting, diarrhea, or peritonitis (inflammation of the lining of the abdominal and pelvic cavities), paralytic ileus, fistula, or surgery.
▶ People who require medications that would be destroyed by the digestive juices or that would not be absorbed by the gastrointestinal (GI) tract or who require consistent therapeutic blood levels of a medication (e.g., theophylline for acute asthma).

▶ People unable to digest or absorb a diet administered by mouth or tube (e.g., those who do not have an anatomically and functionally intact GI tract). Such individuals may require administration of IV fluids over a long period.

Compared with other methods of parenteral therapy, the IV route has the advantage of providing the most rapid and complete absorption of medication. Therefore, in an emergency, medications are usually given IV. Other advantages of IV therapy are as follows:

▶ Therapeutic blood levels of medications may be maintained with continuous IV infusions.
▶ Specially prepared fluids and blood products may be administered IV to maintain fluid and electrolyte balance, to supply nutrition, or to maintain an emergency access to the vein.
▶ Intravenous therapy offers a route of fluid and medication administration for unconscious people.

Risks associated with IV therapy include (a) local and systemic infections, (b) overdosage or rapid onset of untoward effects of medications, (c) fluid overload or electrolyte imbalances associated with continuous IV infusions, and (d) damage to vessels, nerves, and other soft tissues. Prevent complications of IV therapy by using care before, during, and after administration.

Because of the rapid effect of IV medications, incorrect medications or dosages can cause significant untoward or even fatal consequences.

INTRAVENOUS SOLUTIONS

The type of IV solution ordered depends on such factors as the individual's condition or the type of fluid and electrolyte imbalance to be corrected. Many substances can be infused intravenously; these include carbohydrates, amino acids, fatty emulsions, electrolytes, alcohol, vitamins, water, and some medications. In addition, parenteral fluids vary in their tonicity, so that IV fluids may be hypotonic, isotonic, or hypertonic. For more details about IV solutions, review Chapter 41. Also be sure to read the labels on IV bags and bottles as you work with them in the clinical area.

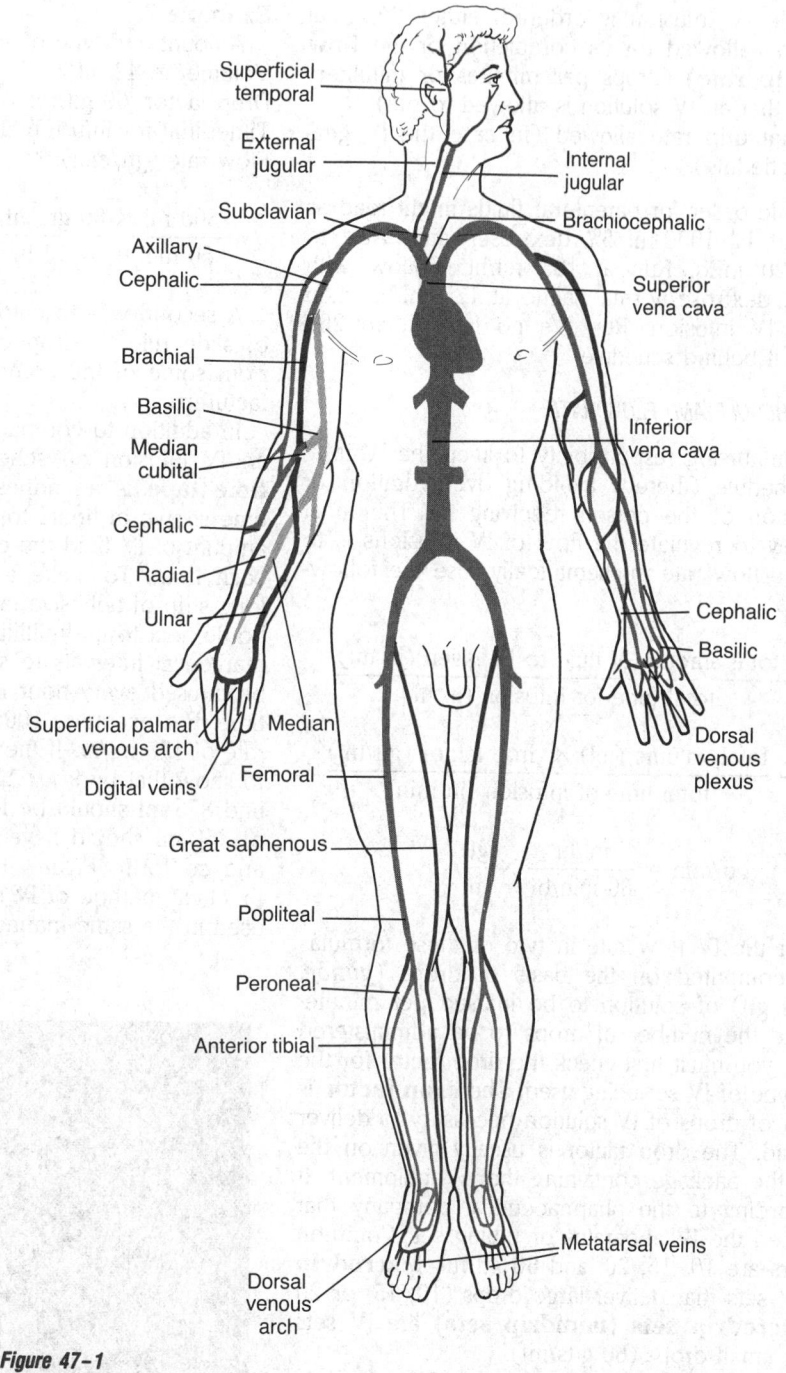

▲ *Figure 47–1*

Major veins in the body.

Because of the dangers inherent in parenteral therapy, the physician's orders for IV fluids and electrolytes must be precise and clear. A safe order for parenteral infusions should include the following items:

▶ The specific solution or solutions to be administered. If more than one bag of solution is to be given, each bag should be numbered consecutively

to assure that the correct solution is given in the correct order.

▶ The **additive solutions** (liquids added to a bag of IV fluid), if any, as well as the number of milliliters or milliequivalents to be given. The order should specify whether the solution is to be added to the bag or administered into the tubing.

▶ An estimated time schedule if more than one IV infusion is ordered.

▶ If a single IV infusion is ordered, either the total time to be allowed for its completion or the **flow rate (drip rate)** (drops per minutes or milliliters per hour that an IV solution is allowed to run).

▶ A maximal drip rate allowed (in case the IV gets behind schedule).

An acceptable order for parenteral fluids might read as follows: Start IV 1000 ml 5% dextrose/water. Add to bag—KCl 20 mEq. Run at 125 ml/hr. Follow with 1000 ml 5% dextrose/normal saline at 125 ml/hr, then discontinue IV infusion. Run IVs no faster than 200 ml/hr, even if behind schedule.

INFUSION SCHEDULE AND FLOW RATE

It is a major nursing responsibility to keep the IV infusion on schedule (thereby avoiding overhydration or underhydration of the person receiving it). The most accurate way to regulate the flow of IV infusions is to calculate the flow rate mathematically. Use the following formulas:

$$ml/hr = \frac{total\ amount\ of\ fluid\ to\ be\ given\ (in\ ml)}{total\ time\ for\ infusion\ (in\ hr)}$$

$$gtt/min = \frac{total\ volume\ (ml) \times drop\ factor\ (gtt/ml)}{total\ time\ of\ infusion\ (in\ min)}$$

$$gtt/min = \frac{ml/hr}{60\ min/hr} \times \frac{gtt}{ml}$$

Note that the IV flow rate in two of these formulas has been computed on the basis of drops (*guttae*, abbreviated gtt) of solution to be infused per minute. To compute the number of drops to be administered per minute, you must first check the drop factor for the particular type of IV set being used. The **drop factor** is the number of drops of IV solution necessary to deliver 1 ml of fluid. The drop factor is usually given on the outside of the package containing the IV equipment. It varies according to the pharmaceutical company that has produced the IV apparatus or tubing set. Common drop factors are 10, 15, 20, and 60 gtt/ml. **Macrodrip sets** are IV sets that deliver large drops (10, 15, or 20 gtt/ml). **Microdrip sets (minidrip sets)** are IV sets that deliver small drops (60 gtts/ml).

Once you have determined the drop factor, apply one of the preceding formulas to obtain the desired IV flow rate in drops per minute. Consider these two examples:

Example 1:
Amount and type of solution: 1000 ml 5% dextrose/water
Volume/hr: 125 ml
Drop factor: 15 gtt/ml
Time limit for infusion: 8 hours
Flow rate (gtt/min):

$$\frac{1000\ ml \times 15\ gtt/ml}{60\ min/hr \times 8\ hr} = \frac{15,000\ gtt}{480\ min} = 31\ gtt/min$$

Example 2:
Amount and type of solution: 500 ml 0.45% saline
Volume/hr: 42 ml
Drop factor: 60 gtt/ml
Time limit for infusion: 12 hours
Flow rate (gtt/min):

$$\frac{500\ ml \times 60\ gtt/ml}{60\ min/hr \times 12\ hr} = \frac{30,000\ gtt}{720\ min} = 42\ gtt/min$$

A second way to calculate IV flow rates is by means of slide rule IV drop calculators, which are available from some of the commercial intravenous fluid manufacturers.

In addition to computing the drip rate, you may keep an IV infusion on schedule by using a time tape. A **time tape** is an adhesive strip or printed tape with time shown in hours for the purpose of monitoring the amount of IV fluid the client receives or should receive each hour. To make a time tape, the nurse places a long strip of adhesive tape on the side of the IV bag or bottle next to the milliliter calibrations. The tape is then marked at intervals to show the amount of solution to be infused every hour in order to complete the IV on time. For example, 1000 ml is to be administered at a rate of 125 ml/hr. If the IV starts at 8 AM, mark the tape to show that by 9 AM 125 ml should have been infused and 875 ml should be left in the bag; by 10 AM a total of 250 ml should have been infused, with 750 ml left, and so forth. Figure 47–2 illustrates this simple and practical method of IV scheduling. Preprinted tapes are used in the same manner.

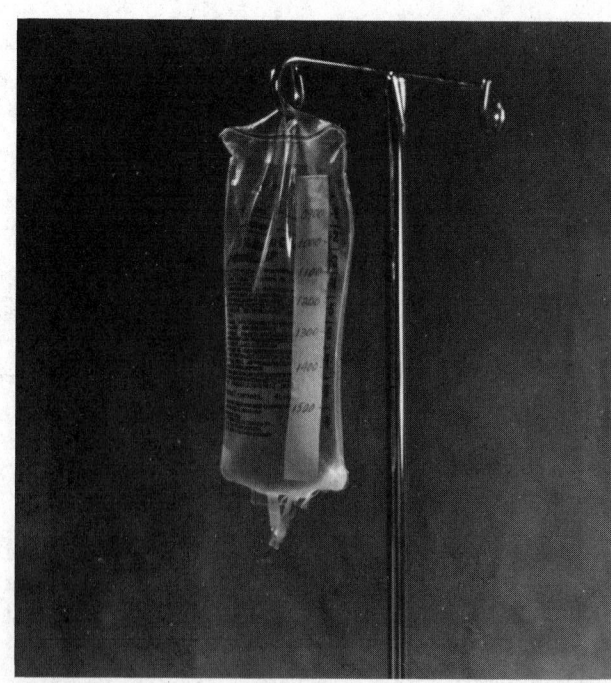

▲ *Figure 47–2*

This time-taped bag shows that 125 ml of solution should be infused each hour. The preprinted label is marked according to the 24-hour clock.

Do not use a felt-tipped pen to write on adhesive tape as some types of ink leach through the plastic and into the IV fluid.

Finally, the use of IV infusion pumps and infusion controllers helps ensure precise IV fluid delivery. An **infusion pump** is a mechanical device that monitors and uses pressure to help regulate the flow of IV fluids into a vein. An **infusion controller** is a mechanical device that monitors and helps regulate the flow of IV fluids without the use of pressure. Although these machines are usually very accurate, you should continue to check that the fluid is infusing correctly, as accurate infusion is an important nursing responsibility that helps assure client safety.

TYPES OF INTRAVENOUS MEDICATIONS

Many medications may be given through the intravenous route. Most IV medications, however, are antibiotics. A few of the other types of medication that can be given IV are certain narcotics, tranquilizers, antiemetics, antipyretics, and central nervous system depressants.

Because some medications can be given by more than one route, it is imperative that you verify on the container label that the medication is safe for IV administration.

Any medication given IV must be clear, not cloudy, and without any particulate matter in it, both before and after adding it to the IV solution. For example, when an IV drip medication of insulin is prepared, regular insulin is the only type of insulin preparation that can be used. The longer-acting insulins are in a precipitate and are cloudy. Other medications might be clear until added to an IV solution, where upon they **precipitate** (settle into solid particles within a solution) and appear cloudy, or **flocculate** (gather finely dispersed particles into larger particles that may be visible within a solution). Phenytoin (Dilantin), for example, is clear but must not be added to any IV that contains dextrose because it will flocculate. Other medications cannot be added because they change the IV fluid pH. If you are in doubt about whether or not a medication is safe for intravenous administration, consult the pharmacist.

Any additive to the bag *must* be thoroughly mixed with the IV solution before it is infused. Mixing will ensure appropriate dilution so that the client won't receive a **bolus** (concentrated mass) that could be detrimental or fatal. The bag also must be labeled with the name and dosage of the additive, along with date, time, and name of the person who prepared it.

Blood Transfusions

Blood **transfusions** (infusions of whole blood, plasma, or packed cells into a vein) are administered to restore blood volume following hemorrhage or severe trauma. Approximately 19 different types of blood

APPLYING RESEARCH TO NURSING PRACTICE

Avoiding Simultaneous Infusion of Incompatible IV Drugs

Collins, J.L. & Lutz, R.J. (1991). In vitro study of simultaneous infusion of incompatible drugs in multilumen catheters. *Heart & Lung, 20,* 271–277.

▼▼▼

Multilumen catheters are intravenous catheters that contain multiple lumens—two or more separate catheters wrapped within a larger sheath. Multilumen catheters inserted into the large central veins allow for simultaneous infusions of several drugs in separate catheters. However, it is unclear whether any significant mixing of infusion streams occurs as they exit the catheter and enter the rapidly flowing blood of the central venous circulation. Can simultaneous infusions of incompatible drugs be administered without precipitation (clumping) of these drugs in the client's bloodstream?

To test this question, a research team developed an in vitro flow system that simulates the in vivo central venous circulation. Collins and Lutz then administered phenytoin (Dilantin) and total parenteral nutrition (TPN) through both double-lumen and triple-lumen catheters, because these fluids precipitate rapidly when mixed together. In a total of ten trials using the double-lumen catheter, the researchers documented the white cloud of phenytoin precipitate on videotape. Drug assays determined that the amount of Dilantin in the white cloud was 6 per cent of the total amount of the drug. In trials using the triple-lumen catheter, the researchers observed no precipitate. However, they did document a thin white cloud at two points along the length of the catheter where infusions enter the client's venous circulation. One was at the proximal exit port (the catheter opening that is nearest to the client). The other was at the middle exit port of the catheter lumens. The distal port (the port farthest from the client) showed the least evidence of the thin white cloud. Although the total amounts of Dilantin precipitates were small in this study, the crystal particulates in the Dilantin "clouds" placed clients at risk for thrombophlebitis and emboli.

Applications for Practice

When you have a question about the compatibility of IV medications or other IV solutions, consult a drug manual or compatibility chart. In vitro systems do not precisely imitate an in vivo human state. However, the findings from this study should caution you to find alternatives to simultaneously infusing incompatible drugs through a multilumen catheter. For example, you could briefly interrupt the infusion of TPN to allow for infusion of a 50-ml solution of Dilantin.

components and **plasma derivatives** (components of the plasma, or fluid portion of the blood) may be administered. The most common type you will encounter is packed red blood cells. **Packed red blood cells (PRBC)** are red blood cells separated from the plasma of the blood. **Whole blood**, as the term implies, is blood containing all of its elements (plasma and cells).

As a student nurse you probably will not be responsible for administering blood, but you may well be providing care for clients who are receiving blood or who received blood prior to your care. The more knowledge you have concerning this procedure, the better you will be able to provide more complete nursing care for your clients.

For transfusions, it is vital that the laboratory ascertain the client's blood type and Rh factor, both of which must be cross-matched with the donor's blood for compatibility. Because other intrinsic factors may also cause incompatibility, complete cross-matching normally requires 1 to 2 hours to accomplish. In an emergency, however, a shorter cross-matching procedure can be performed.

The administration of blood components requires very specific guidelines and the use of equipment designated for that purpose. For example, the needed equipment includes a special blood administration set (tubing) that allows saline to be administered before and after the transfusion without changing the tubing. A 19-gauge or larger needle is required because of the viscosity of the blood.[15]

Nursing responsibilities before initiating the transfusion include ascertaining that all information on the bag label correlates with the accompanying bag tag and the client's ID bracelet. This correlation should be verified with another nurse. You also must obtain baseline vital signs and teach the client to tell you about any unusual reaction experienced (such as itching, a rash, or temperature change) while the transfusion is taking place. Inform the client that the transfusion will be completed within 4 hours or less.

If the blood is to be administered rapidly, it must be warmed with a special blood warmer as it is being infused. Warming the blood will prevent **vasospasm** (sudden, involuntary contraction of the vein).

During the transfusion, you must monitor the client's vital signs after the first 15 minutes and then every hour until one hour after the transfusion has been completed. Reactions can occur any time during the transfusion, but acute reactions usually occur within the first 15 to 30 minutes. Adverse effects of a blood transfusion include circulatory overload, allergic reaction, febrile episode, sepsis, or hemolytic reaction (a **hemolytic reaction** occurs when red blood cells clump together, become trapped in small vessels, and release hemoglobin into the plasma as they disintegrate). The immediate nursing intervention for each of these events is to stop the transfusion, disconnect the blood tubing from the IV needle or catheter, cover the end to preserve sterility, and keep the vein open with a new bag of normal saline and new tubing. The physician and blood bank should then be notified. Treatment will be ordered by the physician according to the type of reaction. If the transfusion must be terminated, send new blood samples and urine specimens from the client,

along with the blood that was being transfused and the used blood administration set, to the blood bank.[15]

After the transfusion is complete, you must document the type of blood product and volume transfused, the product identification (ID) number, the times the transfusion started and ended, the names of the persons verifying the client ID, the name of the person starting and ending the transfusion, and the client's immediate response — even "no apparent reaction." Delayed reactions to blood transfusions can occur any time, from days to months later. These are delayed hemolytic reaction, iron overload, graft-versus-host disease, and any one of several infectious diseases (for example, viral hepatitis, Epstein-Barr virus, cytomegalovirus, malaria, toxoplasmosis, acquired immune deficiency syndrome, syphilis). If a post-transfusion client manifests any symptoms of these disorders, the person should be investigated for a delayed reaction.

Parenteral Hyperalimentation

Parenteral hyperalimentation (total parenteral nutrition, or TPN) is a method of providing total nutrition to a person intravenously through a catheter, thus bypassing the GI tract. This therapy enables the infusion of large amounts of essential nutrients required by the body for tissue synthesis and growth. Because they must meet the individual's total nutritional needs, solutions used for parenteral hyperalimentation contain far more nutrients and calories than do ordinary IV solutions.

Solutions are composed of essential amino acids with electrolytes, vitamins, and minerals added as required for the client. Fatty emulsions (lipids) may also be added for extra calories. A prescription is written specifically for each individual so that each solution is unique. Parenteral nutrition solutions are prepared by the pharmacist, who must work within strict guidelines. Nothing may be added to the solution by the nurse, and medications may not be "piggybacked" into the TPN line.[22,23]

A hyperalimentation solution is usually administered into the subclavian vein (Fig. 47–1) because the high osmolality of the hyperalimentation solution irritates smaller veins and can cause thrombophlebitis. Intravenous catheter insertion must be performed by a physician under strict aseptic technique. This procedure is usually done in the operating room.

COMPLICATIONS OF HYPERALIMENTATION

Nurses are responsible for preventing complications in the client maintained on hyperalimentation.

Sepsis. Catheter contamination can occur during insertion. Infection may also develop around the catheter site when it is left in place for a long period. A further danger is that the IV solutions may become contaminated because of breaks in sterile technique by health care personnel. To prevent infection, change the tubing and filter daily, using strict sterile technique. Dressings over the catheter insertion site must be kept dry and occlusive. Replace them, using sterile technique, if they become moist or loose.

The most common source of central line sepsis is skin contamination.

Solutions may be prepared to be hung for as long as 24 hours. Do not allow the same bottle or bag of solution to hang beyond this expiration time.

Pneumothorax and Air Embolism. Pneumothorax (air in the pleural cavity that results in lung collapse) can occur during initial insertion or later if the catheter becomes dislodged and air is allowed to enter the thoracic cavity. To prevent pneumothorax during catheter insertion, teach the client to perform the Valsalva maneuver to increase venous filling and place the client in Trendelenburg position to dilate the vein. Use care to prevent dislodging the catheter once it is in place. **Air embolism** (air in the bloodstream) can occur if air in the IV system is allowed to enter the venous circulatory system. Use care to prevent air from entering the IV system, especially when changing tubing. If air does enter the tubing, remove it before it is infused.

Osmotic Diuresis. If the parenteral feeding is given too rapidly, the individual develops a glucose overload and consequently undergoes excessive diuresis as excess glucose in the blood spills over into the urine. As the glucose is eliminated, it pulls body water with it by the process of osmosis. If diuresis remains unchecked, extreme dehydration followed by shock and possible death will ensue. Manifestations of too rapid administration of hyperalimentation solutions include headache, nausea, lassitude, postural hypotension, and seizures.

Blood Glucose Changes. With high levels of dextrose in the IV solution or with rapid administration of the solution, the client may develop hyperglycemia. This often causes the client's pancreas to secrete additional insulin to metabolize the excess glucose. To help the client adjust, hyperalimentation should be delivered more slowly at first. It may even be necessary to administer additional insulin to help control the client's blood glucose level. With continued hyperalimentation and high insulin levels, it is necessary to slowly withdraw the infusions, because stopping them abruptly could lead to hypoglycemia. Because it is important to maintain a continuous flow rate, an infusion pump should be used to prevent blood glucose changes during hyperalimentation.

NURSING ASSESSMENT DURING HYPERALIMENTATION

When caring for people receiving parenteral hyperalimentation, use care to make the following observations:

▶ Continue ongoing monitoring of vital signs, urinary output, and daily weight.
▶ Observe for signs of dehydration or overhydration.
▶ Assess for signs and symptoms of hyperglycemia or hypoglycemia.

▶ Check blood sugar every 6 hours by fingerstick. Check urine sugar and acetone q4h according to agency policy.
▶ Assess the infusion site for signs of catheter dislodgment, infection, or inflammation.
▶ Make certain the IV infusion is flowing continuously at the ordered rate. Be certain that interruptions in the flow rate are reported so that appropriate interventions may be made to protect the client from hypoglycemia.
▶ Check that the bottle or bag does not hang for more than the recommended number of hours (usually 24).

In addition, because parenteral hyperalimentation is a hazardous procedure, the observant nurse assesses the person's condition to identify changes that allow for discontinuation of therapy and return to oral or tube feedings. With this goal in mind, note (a) the cessation of nausea and vomiting, (b) a willingness on the individual's part to drink and eat small amounts of nutrients, (c) changes in a person's mental status, such as increased alertness and orientation, and (d) increased strength.[22,23]

Equipment for Intravenous Therapy

NEEDLES AND CATHETERS

A variety of IV needles and catheters are available for starting IV infusions or administering IV medications. Insertion techniques differ, depending on the type of needle or catheter selected. For example, the small, hollow stainless steel wing-tipped needle, called the **butterfly** or **scalp vein needle** (Fig. 47–3, top), is

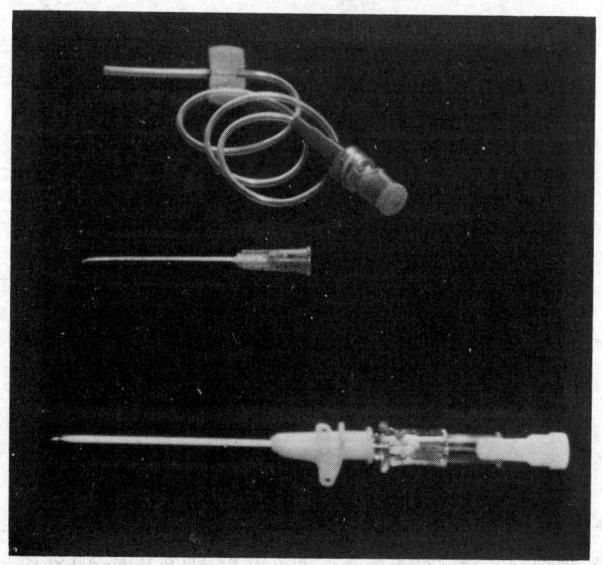

▲ *Figure 47–3*

Types of intravenous catheters and needles. Top, Butterfly infusion needle. Note rubber injection port at right side of photo, thus adapting it for use as a heparin or saline lock (frequently used for children). Middle, Stainless steel 18-gauge needle. Bottom, Indwelling plastic catheter over needle.

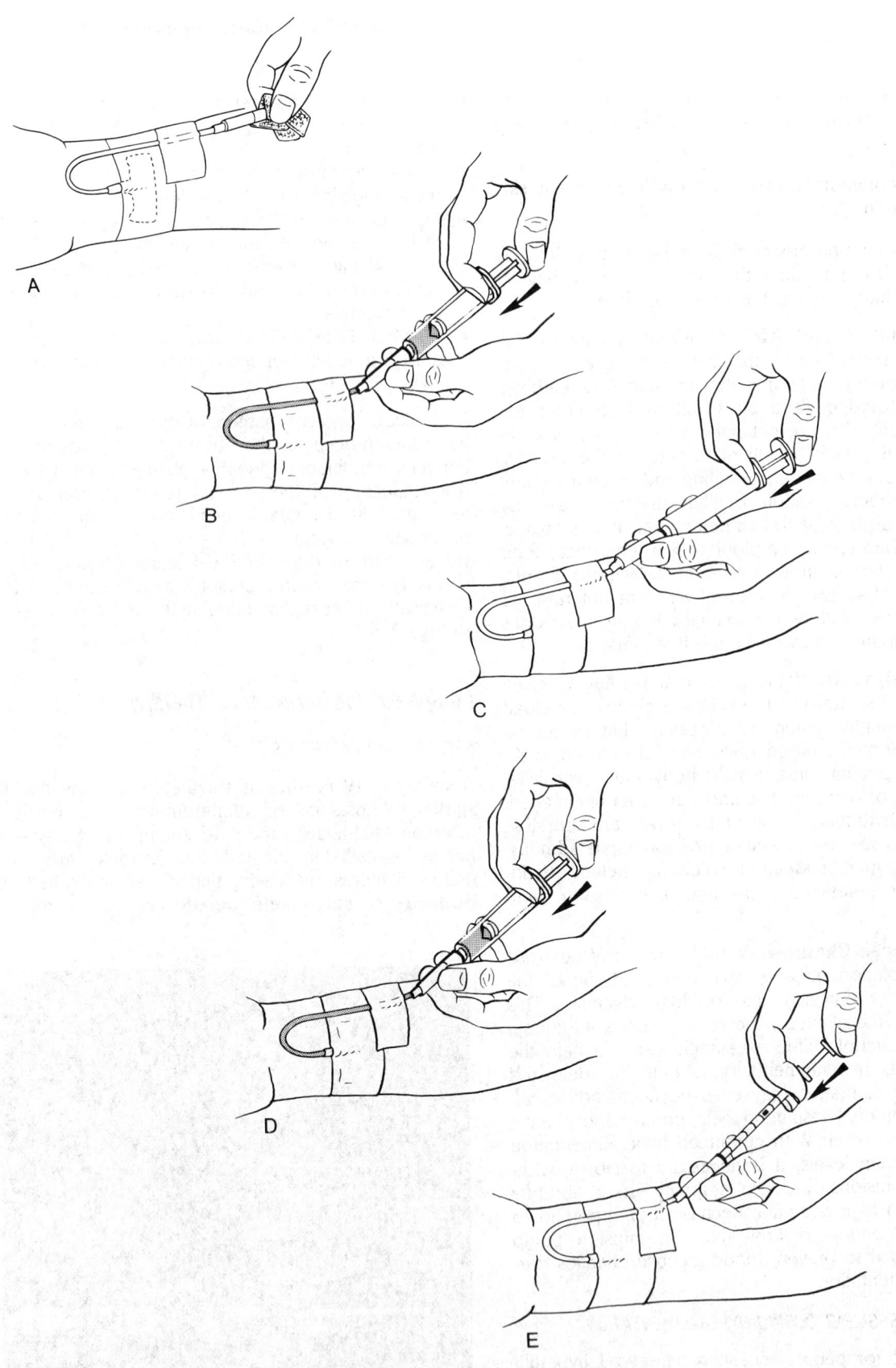

▲ Figure 47-4

Administering medication slow IV push by means of a heparin or saline lock. *A*, Wipe off injection port with sterile alcohol wipe. *B*, Verify placement of needle or catheter in vein according to agency policy. If there is no agency policy for this, flush gently with 2 ml of sterile normal saline. If resistance is felt, do *not* use force; a clot may have formed at the injection site, and the IV should be restarted in another extremity. If the line flushes easily and no blanched, puffy area appears at the site as you flush (indicating that the IV line has come out of vein), use saline to clear the line of heparin, if heparin lock. *C*, Replace saline syringe with medication syringe, using smallest-gauge needle possible to minimize damage to the port. Inject medication *slowly* (some medications require 5 minutes to administer) and remove syringe. *D*, Replace medication syringe with second saline syringe and flush medication through the line with 2 ml of saline and remove syringe. *E*, For heparin lock, attach a tuberculin syringe with the ordered amount of heparin flush and inject slowly. Remove syringe. Remember: do not recap any of the needles after use, and discard them in the appropriate receptacle according to agency policy.

employed for venipuncture of small vessels, e.g., scalp veins in children or hand veins in adults. It is frequently used for short-term or intermittent medication therapy and IV therapy in children. This needle is easily inserted, can be well stabilized, and, because it is stainless steel, is associated with a lower rate of infection. Figure 47–3, center shows a standard size, stainless steel needle (18 gauge). This can be used in larger veins in adults for short-term or intermittent medication therapy.

In contrast, indwelling plastic catheters (Fig. 47–3, bottom) are used most commonly in persons on long-term IV therapy. Indwelling catheters come in a variety of lengths and gauges. Most often, the individual catheter fits closely over a needle. The needle serves as a trocar or stylet, puncturing the vein to allow catheter insertion. After insertion, the needle is withdrawn, leaving the catheter in place to serve as a **cannula** (a hollow tube through which fluid flows after removal of a trocar or stylet). The catheter is flexible and more comfortable than a stainless steel needle.

THE HEPARIN OR SALINE LOCK

When IV therapy is intermittent and the person does not require an IV line for continuous infusion of fluids and medications, the physician may order a **heparin lock** or **saline lock.** Both are defined as a venous access device that may be a plastic, indwelling intravenous catheter or a steel butterfly needle with a short length of narrow-gauge tubing attached. The needle or catheter remains in the vein, ready to be connected to a source of IV fluid whenever necessary. On its distal end, the device is covered by an **injection cap** (a plastic fitting that keeps the heparin or saline lock sealed but that has a rubber diaphragm that can be penetrated by a needle to provide access to the vein. (Figure 47–3, top, illustrates an injection cap.) Figures 47–4 and 47–5 and Procedures 47–1 and 47–2 illustrate the methods of administering medication by means of a heparin or saline lock. After IV solution administration, the saline lock is flushed with a small amount of saline and the heparin lock is flushed with a small amount of dilute heparin (an anticoagulant) solution every 8 hours. These solutions keep blood clots from forming at the tip of the needle or catheter and clogging it.

Heparin and saline locks offer many advantages. They allow the ambulatory person more freedom of movement. They spare clients the pain of having repeated venipunctures or intramuscular injections. They allow easy collection of frequent blood samples when necessary. Finally, heparin and saline locks save valuable nursing time and are more economical because it is not necessary to set up and perform repeated injections and infusions when they are used.

Saline locks are now being used more than heparin locks. Research has demonstrated that the saline lock is just as effective as the heparin lock in providing easy access to peripheral veins when the client does not require continuous IV therapy. An added feature is its

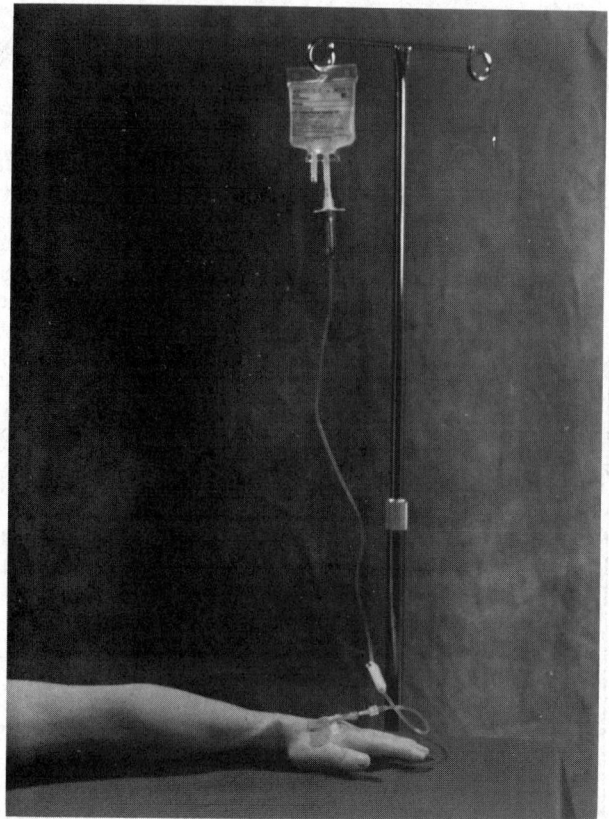

▲ *Figure 47–5*

Administering a large volume of medication through a heparin or saline lock (usually 50 to 150 ml). First, assemble equipment according to guidelines for administering medications through piggyback or secondary lines. See Procedure 47–2. Second, wipe off injection port and verify placement of needle or catheter in vein, as in Figure 47–4*A* and *B.* Third, remove saline syringe. Insert needle of tubing. Fourth, adjust flow rate with roller clamp (usual time is 30 minutes for 50 to 100 ml and 60 minutes for 150 ml). Fifth, when infusion is complete, remove needle and discard according to agency policy. Sixth, flush lock with 2 ml of normal saline, followed by heparin flush, as in Figure 47–4 if using a heparin lock. See Procedure 47–2 for details.

cost effectiveness—heparin is more expensive than normal saline.[3]

SOLUTION CONTAINERS

Practically all IV solutions today are packaged in plastic bags. Most bags hold either 1000 ml or 500 ml of solution for infusion or 50 ml or 150 ml of solution to which medication can be added as secondary infusions. All bags have entry sites that allow the attachment of tubing, and sealed **injection ports** (circular rubber dams that help keep IV bags and/or tubing intact while allowing entry of a needle when necessary to add medication to the system). Some ports are on the front of the bag, some are at the top; and some are at the bottom. Bags are safer, lighter, more compact and easier to store than glass bottles. Some solutions such as fatty emulsions must still be packaged in glass

Text continued on page 1322

PROCEDURE 47–1

Percutaneous Venipuncture (for Blood Collection, IV Infusion, and Saline or Heparin Lock) and Discontinuing an IV Line

Definition/Purposes. The percutaneous (through the skin) insertion of a plastic or metal needle into a vein to (a) withdraw blood, (b) give direct intravenous (IV) medication, (c) start IV infusion for fluid, nutrition, or blood administration. Intravenous medication and fluid administration provides rapid onset and predictable blood levels of medication as well as rapid or massive replacement of fluids. Individual agencies determine policy for venipuncture performed by a professional nurse.

Contraindications/Cautions. Individuals who have had multiple venipuncture procedures may have veins that are **sclerotic** (hardened with scar tissue) or bruised, making further venipuncture attempts difficult. A physician may have to perform a cutdown. To prevent infection, follow surgical aseptic techniques for the insertion and for the daily care of the site. Table 47–1 (page 1326) lists assessment and interventions for complications of IV therapy.

Teaching/Learning Guidelines. Explain the purpose of venipuncture. If appropriate, teach the client and significant others to observe IV equipment and infusion and to request nursing assistance if the following deviations in therapy occur: (a) fluid chamber not dripping, (b) bottle or bag of fluid nearly empty, (c) pain and discomfort at needle site or along vein, and (d) swelling of tissue around needle insertion site. Explain to all persons that they should not change flow rate.

As IV infusion therapy limits mobility, advise the client and significant others that (a) the IV line will be started, if possible, in the person's nondominant hand, (b) the arm or leg may need to be restrained by a board or dressing to safeguard the IV, (c) the person's bathing activity must be modified to keep the IV site dry, (d) the solution bag or bottle must always be kept higher than the person's extremity (even when ambulating) to allow fluid to flow into the vein, and (e) additional restraints may be necessary to prevent dislodging or removal of the IV needle or catheter.

PRELIMINARY ACTIVITIES

Assessment/Planning

- Assess medical diagnosis and activity orders.
- Check physician's order.
- Determine purpose of venipuncture (blood sample, intravenous infusion, or saline or heparin lock placement).
- Assess individual's experience with procedure.
- Assess condition of veins.
- Note presence of bruises or hematomas from previous therapy or attempts to start IV.
- Determine handedness (R or L) of individual and note any contraindications related to choice of site.
- Select an appropriate vein.
- Select needle size appropriate to type of solution to be administered (e.g., blood administration requires larger-gauge needle).
- Select and prepare necessary equipment.
- Prepare work area with necessary equipment. Adjust lighting.
- Work in a comfortable position.

Before connecting tubing to bag, check bag for leaks, check expiration date, and examine fluid for cloudiness and particulate matter.

- Prepare and label IV solution and time tape bag.

- Fill tubing with IV solution as follows before staring procedure:
  1. Clamp off tubing with roller clamp a short distance below drip chamber
  2. Remove plug or protective cap from bag of IV solution
  3. Remove protective cover from spike of IV tubing and insert spike into bag opening
  4. Hang bag on IV pole
  5. Squeeze drip chamber and fill about half-full
  6. Remove protective cap and lower distal end of IV tubing over sink or basin while slowly releasing roller clamp to clear tubing of air and to fill it with solution
  7. Reclamp tubing
  8. Replace protective cap over distal end of tubing
- Label tubing with date, time, and your initials.

Preparation of Client

- Perform procedure teaching
- Provide quiet environment
- Discuss anticipated duration of IV therapy
- If restraints are necessary, explain reason

PROCEDURE 47–1 Continued.

Percutaneous Venipuncture (for Blood Collection, IV Infusion, and Saline or Heparin Lock) and Discontinuing an IV Line

Equipment

- ▶ Tourniquet (length of rubber tubing or a strip of sturdy material with Velcro closures)
- ▶ Antiseptic solutions (e.g., 70 per cent alcohol, povidone-iodine)
- ▶ Sterile gauze pads
- ▶ Moisture-proof pad to protect bedding
- ▶ Needles: butterfly (standard), steel 14, 16, 18, 20, 21 gauge; plastic (indwelling catheter) 16, 18, 20, 21 gauge
- ▶ Restraints, if necessary
- ▶ For blood specimens: syringe or vacuum tube, proper specimen tubes and labels, requisition slips for laboratory tests
- ▶ For starting IV infusion: adhesive or paper tape to secure IV needle, tubing, and armboard. Sterile dressings for IV site. Covered arm splint/board. Prepared IV solution (in bottle or plastic container) connected to IV tubing with drip chamber

- ▶ IV pole
- ▶ Infusion pump or infusion controller, if used
- ▶ Tape or labels for marking additions to IV solution
- ▶ Medication, if appropriate
- ▶ Time tape (preprinted or adhesive)
- ▶ For inserting saline or heparin lock: venous access device (plastic indwelling IV catheter or metal butterfly needle with small length of narrow diameter tubing)
- ▶ Injection cap (to be added to the venous access device if not already part of it) that is primed (filled with normal saline)
- ▶ One syringe filled with 2 ml of normal saline
- ▶ One syringe filled with heparin according to agency directives (if needed)
- ▶ Gloves

PROCEDURE

Actions

1. Ask any visitors to step outside room while you perform venipuncture. One individual may remain to support client.

2. Place moisture-proof pad under arm.
3. Select possible vein.

4. Position client.

5. Locate vein for venipuncture.
   a. Inspect predetermined vein area.

   b. Apply tourniquet 2 to 6 inches above site chosen.

   c. If using arm, have client clench and unclench hand.
   d. Palpate vein.

   e. If arm hair is abundant and the IV needle is to be taped in place, shave area before venipuncture.

Rationale/Discussion

1. Removal of distractions aids you to insert needle quickly and safely. Also, other people may be upset by procedure. Presence of significant other, however, sometimes calms client.

2. Protects bedding from blood or IV fluid leakage.
3. For drawing blood, the median vein of the arm is commonly used, but you can also use median cubital, cephalic, and basilic veins (see Fig. 47–1) as well as other visible or palpable veins. For IV infusions, use veins on a client's nondominant hand when possible, to promote comfort and independence. Start with arm veins. Use of leg veins for IV infusions decreases a person's mobility and increases the risk of thrombophlebitis. Avoid veins near or in joints, because mobility would be decreased and the IV line could dislodge more easily.
4. Position person so that vein is readily accessible and you can work in a comfortable position.

   Never attempt to draw blood or start an IV with the client standing up. A standing position is less stable. Also, client may become faint during procedure.

5.
   a. Identify signs that contraindicate venipuncture in selected site.
   b. Tourniquet is applied with sufficient pressure to occlude venous return, without occluding arterial flow. This procedure will cause the vein to distend with blood.
   c. Activity increases blood flow to area and distends veins, thus easing visibility and palpation of vein.
   d. Aids in locating vessel and determining the presence of nodules or sclerotic (hardened) areas.
   e. Provides a better surface for tape to adhere. Also, tape removal causes less discomfort if hair is removed.

Procedure continued on following page

PROCEDURE 47–1 Continued

Percutaneous Venipuncture (for Blood Collection, IV Infusion, and Saline or Heparin Lock) and Discontinuing an IV Line

Actions	Rationale/Discussion
6. Proceed with venipuncture.	6.
a. If locating a vein has taken more than a brief moment, release the tourniquet and reapply.	a. Prolonged obstruction causes discomfort and may alter some blood chemistry values.
b. Scrub area with an antiseptic pledget in a circular motion, from center outward, using friction.	b. Removes surface bacteria by using aseptic principles. Type of antiseptic determined by agency policy.
c. Use same technique to dry area with sterile gauze or allow to air dry.	c. If alcohol enters vein, it can cause vasospasm, which decreases the caliber of the vein.
d. Don gloves.	d. To protect your hands from blood contamination.
e. Remove protective cap from sterile needle, hold needle apparatus in dominant hand, and grasp arm distal to point of needle entry with nondominant hand. Place nondominant thumb about 1 inch below expected point of entry. Pull skin toward hand.	e. Vein is held taut in this manner. Taut skin also helps locate and maintain vein in position.
f. Place needle in line with vein at a 15° to 45° angle.	f. Needle enters vein at this angle.
g. Insert sterile needle, with bevel up, through skin and into vein. Pierce skin as quickly as possible while still maintaining control. When vein is entered, decrease needle angle and prepare to thread needle approximately 1 inch into vein.	g. Less tissue damage occurs if needle is inserted with bevel up. Rapid insertion decreases discomfort. Because pressure is greater in the vein than in the needle, blood will flow into the needle when the vein is entered. Unless the angle of the needle is decreased, the needle can pass through the vein.

Blood Collection

1. If venipuncture is performed for a blood sample, collect a venous sample before removing tourniquet.	1. Blood should flow easily while the tourniquet is in place. Prolonged tourniquet placement causes venous congestion and discomfort.
2. Remove tourniquet before withdrawing needle.	2. Withdrawing the needle before removing the tourniquet causes excessive bleeding from the site.

IV Infusion

1. If venipuncture is performed with a steel needle for IV infusion, after threading needle into the vein release the tourniquet.	1. A steel needle is easier to insert but more likely to traumatize a vein if used for a long time.
2. Remove the protective cap from the IV tubing and attach IV tubing to the needle.	2. IV system is now closed.
3. Open roller clamp part way to start infusion.	3. Increases pressure in tubing over pressure in vein and allows fluid to flow into venous system.

Saline or Heparin Lock

1. If venipuncture is performed for saline or heparin lock: a. With a butterfly, when you see blood return, advance the needle to stabilize it in the vein. b. With a plastic catheter, advance the catheter approximately 1 inch while holding the needle in place. When the plastic catheter is in place in the vein, remove the steel needle.	1. a. A plastic catheter or small needle helps prevent damage to vein. b. Cannulation with a plastic catheter requires special training. With practice, these types of catheters are easy to insert, but do not attempt to do so without supervision. Once the plastic catheter is in place, the steel needle (stylet, trocar) is no longer needed.
2. Release the tourniquet.	2. Decreases venous pressure and reduces amount of blood loss.

PROCEDURE 47–1 Continued

Percutaneous Venipuncture (for Blood Collection, IV Infusion, and Saline or Heparin Lock) and Discontinuing an IV Line

Actions	Rationale/Discussion
3. Remove protective cover from injection cap and insert end of injection cap into the open end of the butterfly tubing or the indwelling plastic IV catheter to complete the saline or heparin lock.	3. This closes the system.
4. Cleanse the rubber diaphragm of the injection cap with an alcohol sponge, remove the needle cover from the syringe containing the normal saline, and inject the saline into the venous access device through the diaphragm.	4. This flushes the device to remove blood from it and fills the lock with normal saline.
5. In a like manner, inject the pre-measured dose of heparin through the diaphragm, if heparin is to be used.	5. Both normal saline and heparin solutions have been found to prevent clotting of blood within the venous access device.

Postvenipuncture Procedures

Actions	Rationale/Discussion
1. Blood collection:	1.
a. Remove needle gently.	a. Rough removal may cause damage to the vein.
b. Place a sterile pledget over the site with firm pressure for 3 minutes (longer if person's clotting mechanisms are altered secondary to disease or therapy). If site is in antecubital fossa, maintain straight arm.	b. Maintain pressure to aid in hemostasis (clotting). Maintaining a straight arm maximizes pressure.
c. Once bleeding has stopped, apply a sterile adhesive dressing and then remove gloves.	c. Dressing covers puncture site to prevent contamination.
d. Send blood sample to laboratory as soon as possible.	d. Sending an "old" blood sample sometimes alters laboratory results. Follow agency policy when preparing and transporting blood.
2. IV infusion:	2.
a. Thread needle approximately 1 inch into vein and secure IV line in place. (For proper taping method, see Figure 47–10).	a. Prevents IV from dislodging.
b. Cover IV site with sterile dressing and remove gloves.	b. Protects IV site and prevents contamination.
	Although once recommended, the application of antibiotic or other ointment to the site is now contraindicated because such ointments result in an increased incidence of allergic response to the ingredients and place the client at risk for fungal infections.
c. Secure several inches of tubing by taping it to skin (Fig. 47–10).	c. Further secures IV to prevent displacement.
d. Use armboard if position of needle is unstable (Fig. 47–10D).	d. Armboard reduces mobility of arm, thereby preventing dislodgment of needle.
e. Cover armboard and arm with stretch netting if desired.	e. Can further help protect dislodging the system.
f. Adjust fluid flow rate as ordered by physician.	f. Fluid flow rate is ordered by physician and maintained by nurse.
3. Saline or heparin lock:	3.
a. Tape the locking device securely in place (Fig. 47–4).	a. Inadvertent removal of the device would require an additional venipuncture to replace it.
b. Cover the venipuncture site with a sterile dressing and remove gloves.	b. Helps maintain sterility of site.
	The use of transparent dressings has recently come under scrutiny. There has been a higher incidence of IV site infections in some agencies but not in others. Check the policy of your agency regarding their use.[6]

Procedure continued on following page

PROCEDURE 47–1 Continued

Percutaneous Venipuncture (for Blood Collection, IV Infusion, and Saline or Heparin Lock) and Discontinuing an IV Line

Discontinuing an IV Line

Actions	Rationale/Discussion
1. Check physician's order for IV to be discontinued.	1. Discontinuing an IV before the therapy is completed would cause the client to have to undergo another painful venipuncture.
2. Explain to the client that the IV is no longer required and that it will be removed.	2. This knowledge should be a source of relief to the client.
3. Clamp off the IV tubing.	3. Stops the flow of IV fluid and prevents leakage when the needle or catheter is removed.
4. Carefully remove the tape that is securing the catheter or needle (stabilize the catheter or needle with your nondominant hand as you do so).	4. Helps prevent trauma to the vein as you free the tubing for removal.
5. Don gloves.	5. Helps prevent exposure to blood.
6. Place a sterile gauze square over the insertion site with your nondominant hand and hold it in place as you gently remove the needle or catheter with your dominant hand.	6. Confines bleeding to the gauze square and prepares you to apply pressure as soon as possible.
7. Immediately upon removal of the needle or catheter, apply firm pressure to the gauze over the site and maintain this pressure for approximately 2 minutes.	7. Stops the flow of blood and aids clotting.
8. When all bleeding has stopped, assess the site for signs of infection.	8. The site must be assessed before it is covered with a Band-Aid.
9. Cover the site with a Band-Aid.	9. This is sufficient to protect the break in the client's skin until the basal cells seal off the site.
10. Document the date and time the IV was discontinued and the amount of fluid remaining in the IV bag, if any.	10. Helps in maintaining accurate assessment of intake and output.

FINAL ACTIVITIES

Check to see that client is comfortable. Assess client for adverse reaction to therapy (e.g., signs of fluid overload, allergic reactions, or infiltration of fluid). Dispose of equipment properly. Label blood collection tubes and IV fluids appropriately. *Documentation:* If a blood sample was drawn, complete the appropriate requisition form. If IV is started, chart site, time, solution, and size and type of needle. Inform staff of progress of IV therapy: how much fluid remains in bottle and what fluids, if any, are ordered to follow fluid currently hanging. If a saline or heparin lock is inserted, chart site, time, size and type of needle, and type of lock.

PROCEDURE 47–2

Administering Intravenous Medications

Definition/Purposes. Intravenous medications are medications given into a vein. They are given to achieve rapid therapeutic blood levels in an emergency, to treat infection, to medicate a person who is NPO or unable to take oral medications, or to medicate a person when the medication cannot be given by other routes (such as when it would be destroyed by gastric secretions or would damage subcutaneous or intramuscular tissues if given in an undiluted form).

Contraindications/Cautions. Verify that the client is not allergic to the prescribed medication. Make sure that the medication can be given safely IV and that the solution is clear and without any precipitate matter or particles in it. Follow the manufacturer's instructions while preparing the medication solution for IV administration. Ascertain that the IV line is patent prior to administering the medication, to be certain that the medication will be given into the vein. Avoid infiltration since some IV medications will damage surrounding soft tissues. To prevent infection, follow surgical aseptic technique in the preparation and administration of the medication. Set the flow rate according to the physician's order or the pharmacist's instructions.

Teaching/Learning Guidelines. Provide the client and/or significant others with the following information as appropriate: (a) Explain the actions and effects of the medication, (b) the reason for the IV route (rapid therapeutic effect, person unconscious, NPO status, most appropriate route for type of medication prescribed), (c) reactions client can expect from the medication, and (d) the need to immediately report any untoward symptoms experienced or any changes in the IV system, such as fluid chamber not dripping, medication bottle or bag nearly empty, pain or discomfort at needle site or along vein, or swelling of tissue around needle insertion site.

PRELIMINARY ACTIVITIES

Assessment/Planning

▶ Check diagnosis.
▶ Check physician's order.
▶ Check medication dosage.
▶ Determine client's knowledge of medication.
▶ Plan intervention should adverse effects occur.
▶ Prepare medication, add to secondary bag, and prime tubing. (See preliminary activities for percutaneous venipuncture, Procedure 47–1.)
▶ Be sure main IV line has a backcheck valve.

Preparation of Client

▶ Explain procedure to client.

Equipment

▶ Alcohol pledgets
▶ Prepared medication from pharmacy or medication you prepared in appropriate amount of diluent as directed
▶ For piggyback administration: secondary bag and tubing with needle and IV **extension hook** (plastic or metal device to lower primary IV line while piggyback infusion is in progress)
▶ For saline or heparin lock: secondary bag and tubing with needle and extension tubing. Two syringes, each with 2 ml of normal saline and 25-gauge needle. One syringe with heparin flush for heparin lock—amount ordered by physician

IV medications that are kept refrigerated before administration must be warmed to room temperature before infusing. This procedure will prevent the occurrence of vasospasm.

PROCEDURE

Actions

1. Identify client by checking name band.
2. Piggyback infusion:
   a. Hang secondary bag of medication on IV pole.
   b. Lower primary IV infusion bag from IV pole with extension hook.

   c. Cleanse injection port on primary tubing with antiseptic.
   d. Remove needle protector and insert needle of secondary set into prepared port.
   e. Release roller clamp of secondary set.

Rationale/Discussion

1. Prevents error.
2.

   b. Pressure is greater in higher bag, allowing medication to flow while primary IV is temporarily stopped.

   Medication will flow into vein appropriately only if primary IV line has a backcheck valve. Otherwise, medication can flow down piggyback tubing and up primary tubing into IV bag.

   c. Reduces possibility of infection.

   d. Fluid will have a pathway from secondary bag into primary tubing.
   e. Fluid with medication will start to infuse.

Procedure continued on following page

PROCEDURE 47–2 Continued

Administering Intravenous Medications

Actions	Rationale/Discussion
f. With roller clamp of primary set, adjust flow rate to ordered rate for secondary medication set.	f. Medication will be infused at appropriate rate.
g. Label tubing with date, time, and your initials.	g. Tubing must be changed at least every 72 hours.
h. At conclusion of infusion of medication, clamp off secondary set.	
i. Return primary set to ordered flow rate.	
j. Remove secondary set needle from port and discard needle in appropriate receptacle.	j. To prevent needlestick.
k. Replace discarded needle with new capped needle for next infusion.	k. Keeps end of tubing sterile. Maintains setup for next dose of medication. Tubing can be flushed if next dose of medication is different.
l. Clamp piggyback line and return primary set to original position on IV pole.	l. Permits more efficient gravity flow of solution.
3. Injection cap infusion with saline or heparin lock:	3.
a. Hang bag with medication on IV pole.	a. Ease of use.
b. Cleanse injection port.	b. Reduces possibility of infection.
c. Remove protective cover from needle of syringe, insert needle through injection port, aspirate to pull blood into needle or catheter, and inject 2 ml of normal saline.	c. Ascertains patency of device. If heparin lock, it flushes heparin that may be incompatible with medication.
d. Remove protective cover and insert needle of medication tubing into port.	d. Establishes a pathway for medication from IV bag.
e. Adjust flow rate with roller clamp as ordered.	e. Maintains correct rate of flow.
f. At conclusion of infusion, clamp off tubing and remove needle from port.	f. Prevents air from entering IV line.
g. Cleanse injection port.	g. Port may have become contaminated.
h. Remove protective cap from needle of syringe and inject 2 ml of normal saline slowly, followed by heparin flush if ordered.	h. Saline assures that medication has cleared cap and maintains patency of device.
i. Remove needle from IV tubing and discard needle in appropriate receptacle.	i. Prevents needlestick.
j. Replace needle with new capped needle for next infusion.	j. Keeps end of tubing sterile. Maintains setup for next dose of medication. Tubing can be flushed if medication is different.

FINAL ACTIVITIES

Assess client for adverse reaction to medication, especially signs of allergic reaction. Dispose of equipment according to agency policy. *Documentation:* Immediately upon leaving client, note medication given on medication sheet and/or in computer. Maintain ongoing assessment of client for therapeutic and adverse reactions to the medication. Immediately report to appropriate person any untoward reactions.

bottles because they interact with the plastics available today. Figure 47–6 illustrates typical bags.

IV TUBING AND ACCESSORIES

IV tubing (an IV line) consists of a length of plastic tubing with a spike to insert into the IV bag, a **drip chamber** (an enlarged, cylindrical portion of IV tubing that allows visualization and counting of each drop of fluid that passes through the system), a roller clamp plus other clamps that control the flow of solution, and several injection ports. The distal end of tubing connects to the hub of the needle that is in the vein or is fitted into an injection cap of a heparin or saline lock (Fig. 47–7A). A **piggyback line** or **secondary IV line** may be connected to a primary IV line via a needle on the secondary line passing through an injection port in the primary IV tubing. Piggybacks are used to deliver medication at intervals, as needed, through an existing IV line (Fig. 47–7A).

Some devices may be added to IV tubing. One such device is a **volume-control chamber** (a large drip chamber that is calibrated in milliliters and placed above the standard drip chamber on some IV tubing). A clamp in the tubing above and another clamp below this large volume-control chamber allow a measured amount of solution to be drawn into the chamber to be infused over a specified period. The chamber serves as a safety feature that helps prevent overhydration or overmedication of the client. The volume-control chamber is used primarily with children and infants for

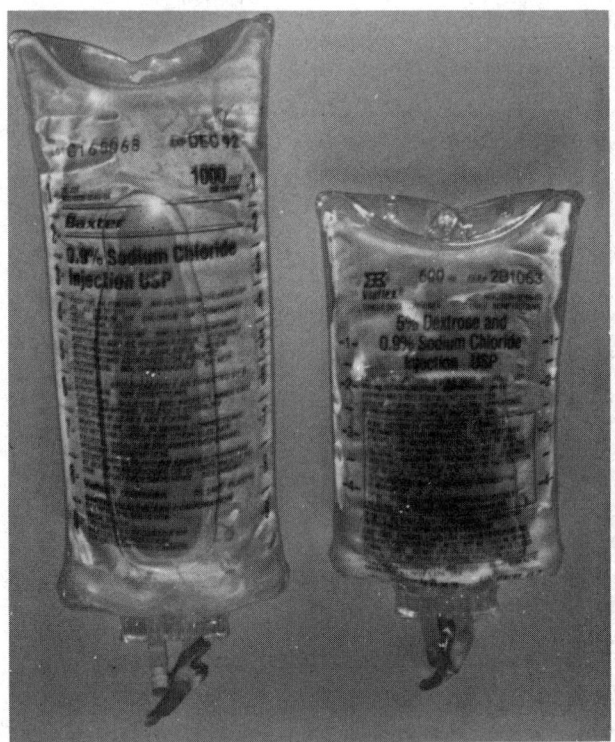

▲ *Figure 47-6*

Plastic IV bags, 1000 ml and 500 ml.

standard IV therapy and for adults who are receiving certain medications or who are in need of carefully controlled IV fluids. The chamber may be used with or without an infusion pump. It is available as one component of a complete solution administration set, or it may be added to an existing setup (see Fig. 47-7*B*).

A filter may be a part of the administration set or may be added to it. Common sizes for filters are 5 microns and 0.22 micron. Five-micron filters remove microscopic particulate matter added to the IV solution (e.g., undissolved medications, bits of rubber stoppers from medication vials, or glass from ampules). The 0.22-micron filters will remove such particulate matter and will also remove bacteria (but not viruses). These filters are useful for TPN (total parenteral nutrition) administration, as well as for administration of many medicated IV infusions. They can be obtained in models that eliminate air and help prevent air embolism.

Filters that are used with infusion pumps must be adequate to withstand infusion pump pressure without releasing the retained debris into the venous system. With or without infusion pumps, filters should be changed after at least 72 hours for peripheral lines and after at least 24 hours for central lines. Filters are always included in the drip chambers of blood transfusion tubing. The standard size is 170 microns.[15]

Another device is a short length of IV tubing that contains a built-in flow regulator instead of a roller clamp to adjust the flow rate. When added to the IV line, the flow regulator can be set to the specified milliliters per hour (Fig. 47-7*C*). The nurse still needs to count the drip rate every hour, because the rate of flow can change when the client changes positions.

Extension tubing consists of an extra length of IV tubing that can be added to the standard tubing set. Extension tubing may be added to an existing line to provide the client with more freedom of movement.

Some agencies require the addition of a T-port to IV tubing for ease in giving medications. T-ports can also be helpful in converting the IV line to a saline or heparin lock (Fig. 47-7*D*). To reduce the incidence of needlesticks from contaminated needles, many manufacturers are producing safety equipment, such as needles with protective sleeves (needle housings, as Fig. 47-7*D* shows), and needleless access devices to use for piggyback medications.

INFUSION PUMPS AND INFUSION CONTROLLERS

Many varieties of infusion pump are available for regulation of hyperalimentation and other IV solutions. Infusion pumps have the advantage of being programmed or preset to administer the solutions at the prescribed rate so that the client's IV fluid intake is more accurately controlled. Figure 47-8 shows two popular infusion pumps. Because the infusion pump is a pressure device, the rate of infusion remains constant even when the client changes position. The pressure helps prevent changes in flow rate that often happen with IVs given by gravity alone. Pumps are especially useful and safer for clients who require continuous therapy (over several days), such as those receiving TPN or a medicated drip such as insulin, aminophylline, heparin, or magnesium sulfate. Some pumps require special IV tubing designed specifically for them; others will work with standard IV tubing. Some of these pumps can also be programmed for a piggyback line. These infusion pumps will control the piggyback medication infusion and will automatically revert to the programmed primary line rate when the medication has been infused. One type of infusion pump is used to administer patient-controlled analgesia (PCA) (see Chapter 40).

Infusion controllers are devices that look very much like infusion pumps. However, they help regulate IV flow rates without the use of pressure. They may be used for chemotherapy or for IV solutions. They are *never* to be used for hyperalimentation (TPN). Figure 47-7*C* shows a drop sensor that may be used with an infusion controller or a pump.

IMPLANTABLE VASCULAR ACCESS DEVICES

A recent development in IV therapy is the use of devices that are surgically implanted under the skin. The injection port is larger than the injection port of standard IV tubing and is not visible. The exact location must be palpated before the IV is initiated with a special needle with a Huber bevel that will not core the injection port. The needle is available as either straight or angular. The 90° angle allows the hub of the needle to align with the chest wall for easy placement of a dressing at the site. These devices are used for clients who are undergoing long-term chemotherapy or antibiotic therapy (Fig. 47-9).[22, 23]

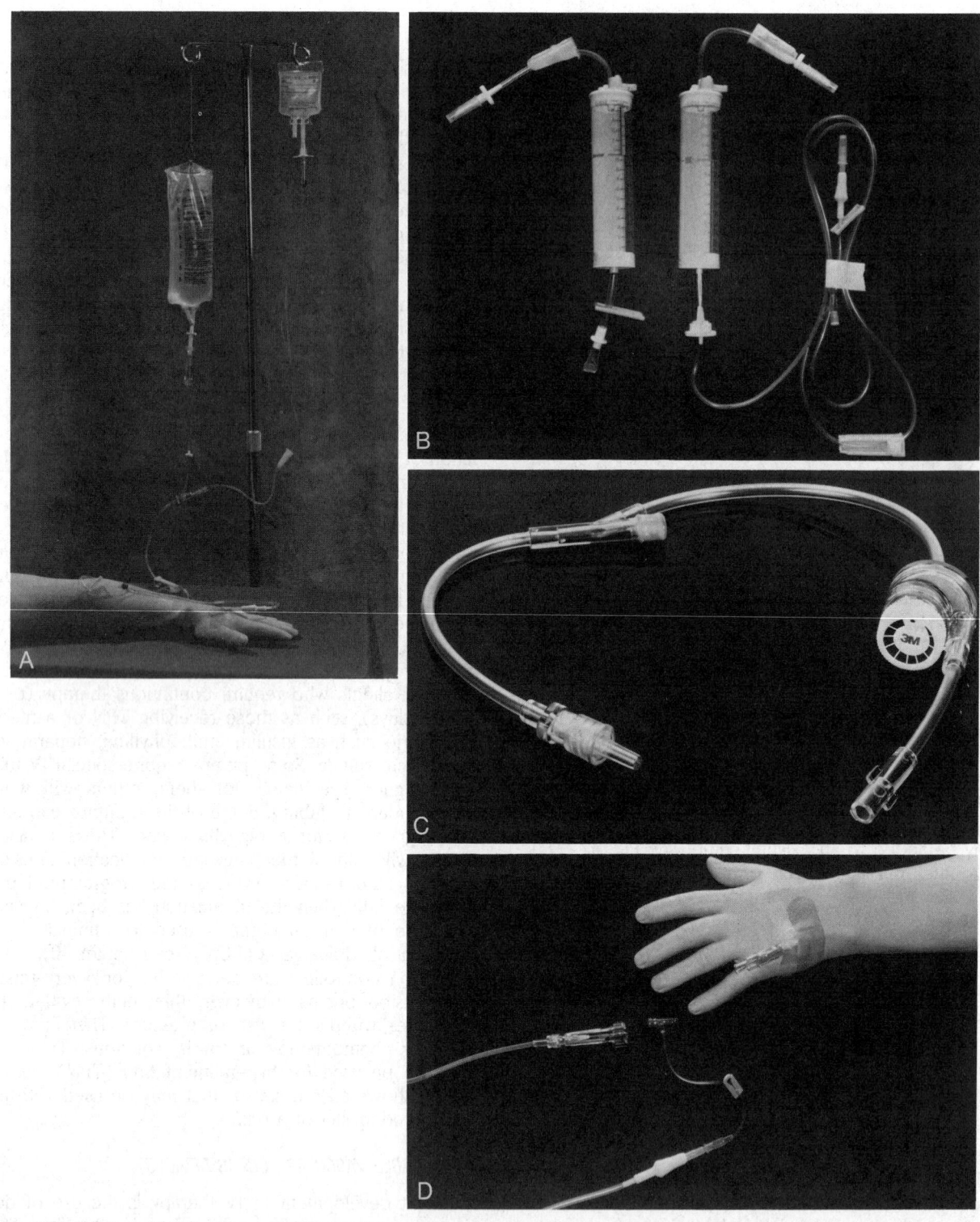

▲ **Figure 47–7**

IV tubing and accessories. *A,* Standard IV (macrodrip) tubing runs from the larger IV bag to the catheter in the client's vein. This constitutes the main (primary) line. The piggyback (secondary) line runs from the smaller IV bag to a needle that penetrates an injection port on the main line. *B,* Calibrated volume controls are available on IV tubing (right) and as a separate section that can be added to a line (left). *C,* Flow regulator. *D,* T-port and needle with protective sleeve (needle housing) for piggyback infusion. T-port (shown closest to tip of finger) inserts into catheter in the client's vein to provide a primary line for IV fluids. The needle at the end of the secondary line (shown to the left of the T-port) is surrounded by a needle housing so that the needle can be made to penetrate the rubber cap on the T-port without danger of touching the needle with a bare finger. After the secondary line is connected to the primary line, the housing is rotated to lock it into place on the T-port. (*C,* Courtesy of 3M Company, St. Paul, Minnesota.)

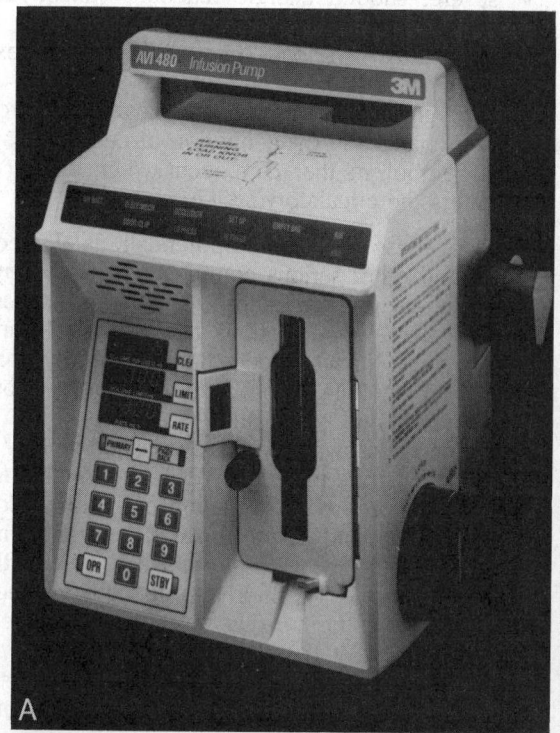

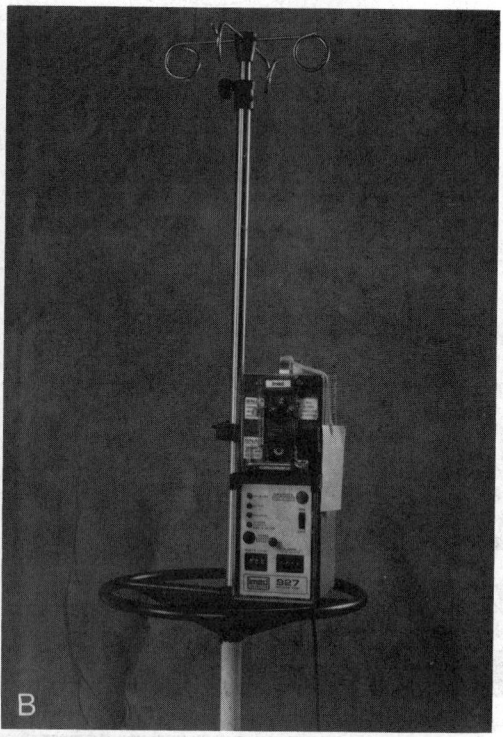

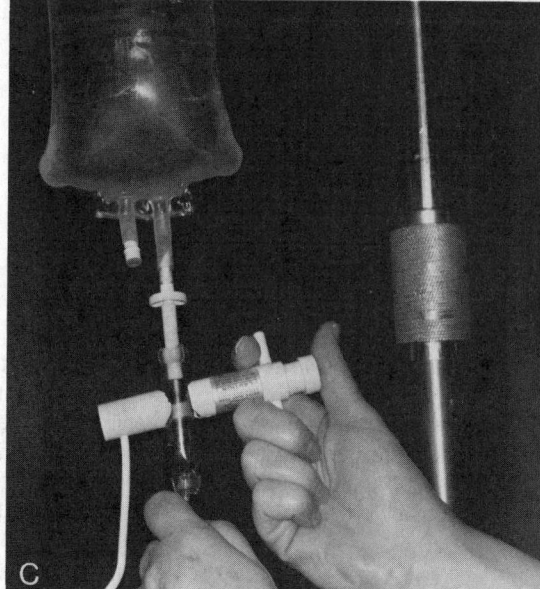

▲ **Figure 47-8**

Infusion pumps and sensor. With infusion pumps, the flow rate and infusion limit are programmed for optimal control. These pumps feature an alarm system that alerts the nurse when the infusion is complete, when tubing becomes kinked or compressed, or when air gets in the line. *A*, The AVI 480 infusion pump. *B*, The IMED 927 infusion pump, attached to IV pole. *C*, A drop sensor (an electronic eye that counts drops) in the IV drip chamber. The sensor relays information to a pump or controller that regulates the IV flow rate. These sensors are held in place by a spring. They must be placed below the source of the drops but well above the fluid level in the chamber. (*A*, Courtesy of 3M Company, St. Paul, Minnesota.)

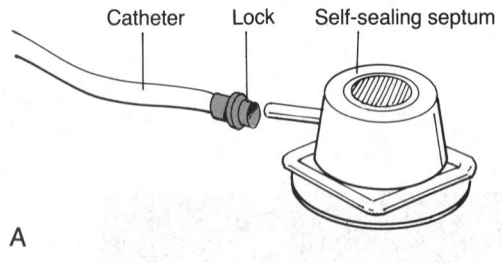

A

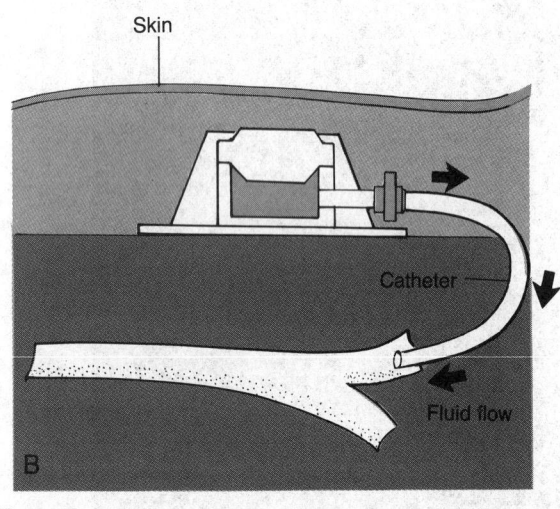

▲ Figure 47-9

Implantable vascular access device.

Complications of Intravenous Therapy

In addition to untoward effects of specific IV solutions or additives such as narcotics, severe untoward reactions to IV solutions include

▶ severe, sudden allergic reactions (anaphylactic responses) to a medication or IV fluid
▶ circulatory overload from infusion of excessive amounts of IV fluid
▶ hyperglycemia or hypoglycemia resulting from sudden changes in concentration of dextrose
▶ air embolism that can occur when air in the line enters the circulatory system

Each of these problems is potentially fatal. Because of these and other serious complications, only physicians, specially trained nurses, or closely supervised students should give IV medications and control IV infusions. Some state Nurse Practice Acts explicitly forbid the practice of certain IV procedures by anyone but registered nurses and physicians.

Common untoward effects associated with IV therapy and venipuncture include (a) phlebitis (inflammation of a vein), **thrombosis** (formation of a blood clot in the blood vessel), and **thrombophlebitis** (inflammation of a vein associated with thrombosis); (b) **infiltration** (infusion of the IV fluid into tissue surrounding the vein) because the needle or catheter has penetrated through the vein; (c) allergic reactions; and (d) infection or inflammation at the insertion site. Nursing care should prevent these complications or minimize their effects as soon as possible.

TABLE 47-1. Complications of IV Therapy

Complication	Assessment	Intervention	Prevention
Infiltration of IV solution	Infusion slows or stops when off infusion pump. No backflow of blood into needle and hub when infusion fluid source briefly lowered below IV site or IV stops dripping when tourniquet is applied. IV site edematous, blanched, painful, and cold	Discontinue IV and, if necessary, restart infusion at alternative site, preferably in another extremity. Elevate limb. Apply heat as ordered by physician	Securely tape IV at site. Avoid movement at site. Confirm placement by checking for IV patency, especially before administering IV medications. If resistance is felt when giving IV push medication, stop and reconfirm placement
Phlebitis (inflammation of vein)	Redness, pain, edema, heat at site and perhaps along vein	If necessary to continue IV, move it to another site. To avoid dislodging clots, do not massage inflamed site. Apply moist heat as ordered by physician	Use smallest-gauge needle or cannula possible to minimize mechanical trauma. Use sites that can be immobilized and table IV securely. Infuse irritating solutions slowly

TABLE 47-1. Complications of IV Therapy (Continued)

Complication	Assessment	Intervention	Prevention
Infection of site	Redness, pain, edema, heat, and perhaps a discharge at site, fever	If necessary to continue IV, move it to another site. Apply cool compress to site as ordered by physician. Elevate limb. Observe for signs of sepsis.	Use aseptic technique for all IV-related care. Keep dressing dry. Change dressing every 24 hours (or according to agency policy)
Air embolism	Drop in blood pressure, cyanosis, tachycardia, increased venous pressure, unconsciousness	Immediately turn person on left side with head down. Administer oxygen. Check vital signs. Notify physician	Remove all air from syringes and IV tubing. Secure IV connections with tape. Have person perform Valsalva maneuver or place head below heart level while changing tubing on central venous lines
Hypersensitivity reaction	Fever, redness, itching, coughing, irritability, dyspnea, cyanosis, possible convulsions, unconsciousness, death	Discontinue IV and notify physician. May require epinephrine, corticosteroids, oxygen, or artificial respiration	Check history for allergies. Monitor carefully when initiating new treatments.
Circulatory overload	Cyanosis, dyspnea, cough, diaphoresis, frothy or pinkish sputum, ascites, rapid weight gain, pitting edema, neck vein distention	Check infusion rate and amount infused. Notify physician. Diuretics and sodium restriction may be indicated	Do not make changes in infusion rate without physician approval if IV is behind schedule. Renal function is decreased at night. Avoid rapid rate increases
Hypoglycemia	Fatigue, blurred vision, diaphoresis, irritability, weakness	Check blood sugar. Check infusion solution against physician's order. Notify physician if significantly hypoglycemic	Check IV solution and infusion rate against physician's order when hanging new bag or bottle and at beginning of shift. If dextrose content $> D_5$, make any ordered changes in infusion rate slowly. Check blood glucose q6h and/or urine sugar and acetone q4h during hyperalimentation (according to hospital policy)
Hyperglycemia	Fruity breath, polyuria, excessive thirst	Check blood sugar. Check infusion rate against physician's order. Notify physician if significantly hyperglycemic	Check IV solution and infusion rate against physician's order when hanging new bag or bottle and at beginning of shift. If dextrose concentration $> D_5$, make any ordered changes in infusion rate slowly. Check blood glucose q6h and/or urine sugar and acetone q4h during hyperalimentation (according to hospital policy)

Phlebitis, thrombosis, and thrombophlebitis are caused by irritation of the vessel. Factors contributing to their occurrence include chemical irritation of tissues by IV solutions or medications, mechanical irritation of tissues by the needle or catheter during venipuncture or cannulation, and localized allergic reaction to the indwelling catheter or needle.

Infiltration occurs when a catheter or needle penetrates the vessel wall during venipuncture or later slips out of the vein and allows IV solution to flow into surrounding tissues. Infusion of fluids into the circulation is hampered or interrupted as fluid infuses into the interstitial spaces. Local tissue edema can occur. In addition, infiltration of potent or toxic medications (sometimes called vesicants) can cause severe tissue necrosis.

Always determine the patency of an IV line before administering IV medications.

One way to determine the patency of the IV line is to check for blood return. To do this, lower the IV bag or bottle below the level of the insertion site. Lowering the bag will cause the pressure in the vein to be greater than the pressure provided by the fluid in the bag or bottle, and (because fluid flows from areas of greater pressure to areas of lesser pressure) you will see back flow (blood "backing up") in the tubing. Unfortunately, this method is not a foolproof one for determining patency. An infiltrated IV line may still bring a blood return, and a patent IV needle or catheter may be lodged against the wall of the vein, thereby preventing blood return. Also, this method does not work if you are using an infusion pump, because the pump maintains pressure in the line. Nor does it work if there is a backcheck valve in the IV line that prevents back flow. Another method to determine patency is to apply a tourniquet above the IV site. If the infusion slows or stops, the line is patent. If the person is on a pump, check for infiltration q1h.

Allergic reactions may occur at the IV site. Individuals may demonstrate sensitivity to solutions used to cleanse the area, preparations (such as ointments) applied to reduce bacteria, or tape used to anchor and secure the catheter. Indwelling catheters and needles may also cause allergic reactions.

Infection or inflammation at the insertion site is most often related to catheters and catheter insertion rather than to the IV solution. Microorganisms gain access to the tissue and circulatory system through the tip of the needle or cannula device inserted during venipuncture or enter later by migration along the interface between the catheter and tissue. See Table 47–1 for assessment and interventions related to selected IV complications.

ASSESSMENT

Assessment of individuals requiring IV therapy begins before the therapy is instituted. The nurse often identifies persons who cannot take medications through the alimentary route, need rapid replacement of fluids and electrolytes, or need medications that can be given only through the IV route. During IV therapy, assess the individual's immediate response to any medications.

Make the following vital assessments throughout the period during which an IV infusion is running:

▶ Assess the individual for signs and symptoms of circulatory overload (distended neck veins, dizziness, difficult breathing) and reactions to medications and electrolytes within the infusion (e.g., K^+ excess, Ca^{++} excess).

If the vital signs or the condition of the individual changes during administration of IV medications, stop the infusion and notify the physician immediately.

▶ Assess urinary output for adequacy of renal function. Poor urinary output could cause circulatory overload and electrolyte excesses.
▶ Assess the infusion site for (a) signs of infiltration of IV fluids into tissues (swelling, hardness, pain, feeling of coldness around injection site, evidence of tissue necrosis), and (b) signs of thrombophlebitis (redness, warmth, and tenderness at or proximal to venipuncture site and along vein). Pain in the elbow or shoulder above the site may be due to a clot that has lodged in the shoulder.
▶ At the needle site, observe whether the needle is in place and attached to IV tubing. Check to see that the tape is adequately anchoring the needle or catheter to the skin. See Figure 47–10 for several methods of taping.
▶ Make certain (a) that the flow rate has been properly calculated according to the drop factor for the tubing in use, and (b) that the IV is dripping according to the scheduled number of drops per minute. To check the flow rate, count the number of drops that fall into the drip chamber for 1 minute (or count the drops for 15 seconds and multiply by four).
▶ At the beginning of your shift, note the level of fluid in the bag and note which medications have been added to the bag. Check the fluid level frequently. If more than one IV is ordered, bring the next bag to the bedside when the fluid currently running has less than 100 ml to be absorbed. Observe the height of the bag; it should be about 3 feet above the needle site.
▶ Look for kinking in the IV tubing. Kinking reduces fluid flow. Be sure that all tubing is visible so none is subjected to kinking or pressure because the client is lying on it.
▶ When using an armboard, make certain that it is positioned comfortably and that it does not impede circulation.

NURSING DIAGNOSIS

As with medication administration, when we talk about intravenous therapy, we are talking about an *intervention* that may be the basis for a number of medical and nursing diagnoses. A few examples of such nursing diagnoses include

▶ *High Risk for Fluid Volume Deficit*
▶ *Fluid Volume Deficit*
▶ *Altered Nutrition: Less Than Body Requirements*

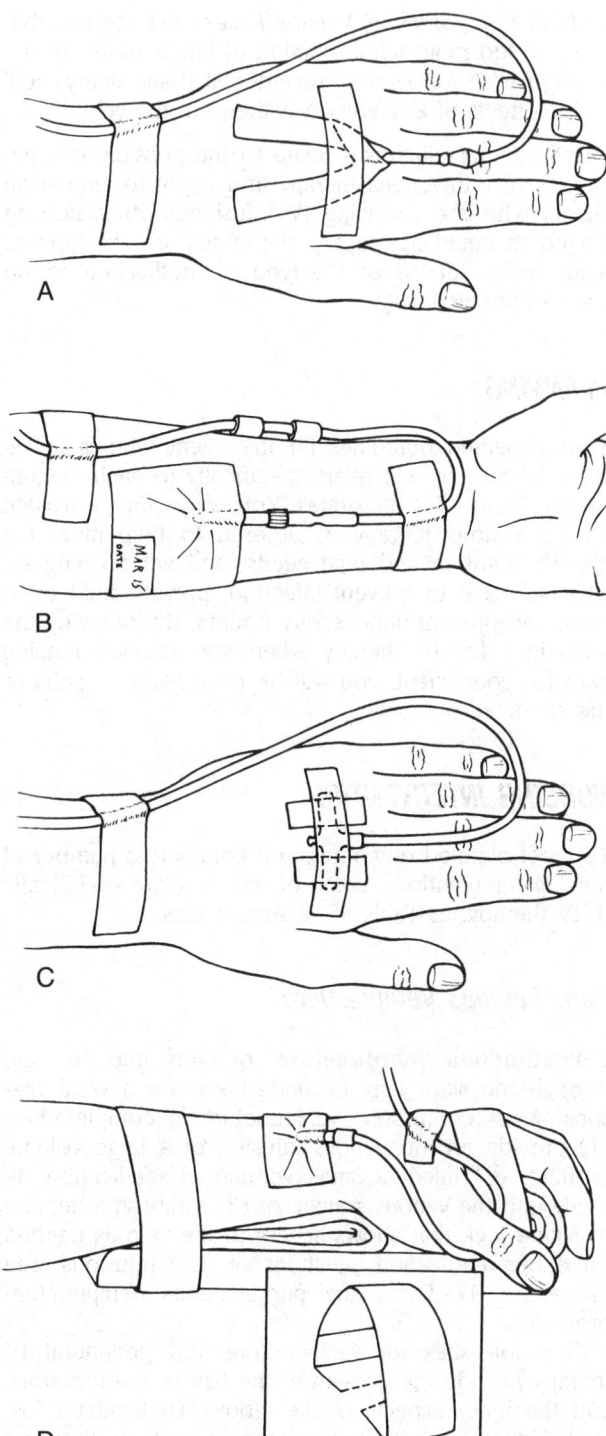

▲ Figure 47–10

Methods of securing intravenous catheters and butterfly needle. *A,* Using tape to secure catheter in hand. A 1/2-inch strip of tape is placed under the hub of the catheter, sticky side up, and then crisscrossed over the top like a chevron stripe. A small bandage is then placed over the top of the tape. The tubing is then taped at one or two places on the arm for additional security. *B,* Using transparent dressing to secure the catheter (least recommended). *C,* Using tape to secure a butterfly needle. Place one piece of 1-inch tape on each wing in line with the needle and tubing, then place a third piece of tape across the wings, forming an H, or use the chevron method as described in A, placing a piece of tape across the wings. *D,* Use an armboard to secure the catheter near a joint. Note the padding to protect the hand and arm. In the inset, note the shorter strip of tape placed in the center of the sticky side of the longer strip to prevent the longer strip of tape from adhering to hair on the arm while the sticky ends of the longer strip remain free to adhere to the armboard.

After you have assessed your client and have made these nursing diagnoses, one of your interventions is to collaborate with the physician concerning client needs. After you have conferred with the physician, another intervention might include the administration of ordered intravenous fluids or hyperalimentation.

Whenever the nursing diagnosis is *High Risk for Fluid Volume Deficit, Fluid Volume Deficit,* or *Altered Nutrition: Less Than Body Requirements,* the administration

of ordered IV fluids will be but one of the nursing interventions in the total plan of care.

Once a physician orders intravenous therapy and you begin to plan for this, a different set of nursing diagnoses will become appropriate. These nursing diagnoses include the following:

▶ *High Risk for Infection* R/T impaired tissue integrity secondary to venipuncture and the presence of a line directly into the circulatory system

▶ *High Risk for Fluid Volume Excess* R/T the possibility of too rapid administration of intravenous fluids

▶ *High Risk for Trauma* (accidental tissue injury) R/T the effects of a needle or catheter in the vein

These nursing diagnoses relate to the possible complications of intravenous therapy and apply to almost all clients who are receiving IV infusions. Other nursing diagnoses could also apply, depending on the type of fluid to be infused or the type of medication to be injected intravenously.

PLANNING

Your expected outcomes for the client who is to receive IV therapy will relate specifically to each diagnosis, as Table 47–2 illustrates. You will want to provide all intravenous therapy as ordered to help meet the client's nutrition and fluid needs, and while doing so, you will have to prevent infection, prevent fluid overload, and prevent unnecessary trauma. By following the guidelines for IV therapy when you provide nursing care for your client, you will be most likely to achieve the expected outcomes.

NURSING INTERVENTION

To meet planned outcomes, you complete a number of nursing interventions, some of which relate specifically to IV therapy, as Table 47–2 summarizes.

Percutaneous Venipuncture

Percutaneous venipuncture, or entry into the vein through the skin, may be undertaken for several reasons. Most commonly, venipuncture is completed to (1) provide an intravenous infusion of a large volume of fluid, (2) inject a small volume of medication directly into the venous system, or (3) establish a heparin or saline lock that allows access to the vein as needed for either medication injections or fluid infusions. See Procedure 47–1 for the percutaneous venipuncture procedure.

Common sites for venipuncture and peripheral IV therapy include the dorsum of the hands, the forearms, and the inner aspects of the elbows (antecubital fossae). Figure 47–1 illustrates some IV sites. In choosing a site for venipuncture or cannulation, ask yourself the following questions:

▶ Is the person in shock or circulatory collapse? If so, venipuncture may be difficult or impossible, because reduced blood causes the peripheral veins to collapse. Under these conditions, the physician will probably perform a surgical cutdown. A **cutdown** is a surgical incision made through the skin to expose a vein for venipuncture. This procedure eases the cannulation process.

▶ What type of solution is to be administered? If it is hypertonic or very irritating to the vessel, a physician should place the line into a central vein (e.g., the subclavian vein) to avoid damage to smaller, peripheral veins.

▶ What is the projected duration of therapy? If therapy is to last longer than 2 or 3 days, try to start the IV in the most distal site possible on the extremity. Then move to proximal sites later in therapy, thereby preserving the vein for long-term use.

The IV site should be changed every 2 to 3 days to reduce the risk of infection and damage to vessels.

▶ In what condition are the person's veins? In some individuals, you have little choice of IV sites. People with fragile or inaccessible veins include the elderly,[5] the obese, those who habitually use IV drugs, and those with extensive burns or skin lesions. You may also have difficulty finding suitable veins in the young child or infant.

▶ Is the individual right- or left-handed? When possible, attempt to use a vein on the nondominant arm, so as not to limit the person's independence. At certain times, dominance is not a consideration in limitation of movement. Do not, however, use the veins of the affected arm of a client with a cerebrovascular accident (CVA, stroke) or mastectomy, regardless of whether the affected arm is dominant or nondominant.

▶ Can the person cooperate during the procedure? If not, choose a vein in which a needle can be firmly stabilized. The antecubital vein, for example, requires that the arm be kept straight, in a position that can be very uncomfortable. The antecubital vein is also a poor choice in an agitated or confused person. In children, a scalp vein is often the best site because it reduces the chance that they will tamper with the IV equipment. A scalp vein is also quite often the site of choice in an infant. Use of a scalp vein may require shaving a portion of the scalp.

Once the venipuncture has been made and the IV line is established, medications may be added through it. Medications can be added by piggyback infusion or by injection through an injection port into the main IV line or into a heparin or saline lock. See Procedure 47–2 for administering intravenous medications through an existing line.

Maintaining the IV System

CHANGING THE DRESSING AT THE IV INSERTION SITE

An IV site is a potential site of infection. Routine dressing changes can decrease this potential. Agencies differ, but as a general rule, routine IV dressing changes are performed every 24 to 48 hours, with more frequent changes if dressings become damp or soiled. During the dressing change, assess the site carefully for signs of infection, infiltration, or phlebitis. The dressing itself should be dated and marked with your initials. Be sure to chart the dressing change and describe the appearance of the site.

TABLE 47-2. Expected Outcomes and Nursing Interventions Related to IV Therapy

Nursing Diagnosis	Planning: Expected Outcomes	Implementation: Nursing Interventions
High Risk for Fluid Volume Deficit	Maintains adequate fluid volume AEB vital signs within normal limits, moist mucous membranes, and sufficient urine volume, with specific gravity within normal limits	Collaborate with physician concerning the possible need for IV infusion
Fluid Volume Deficit	Resumes adequate fluid volume AEB vital signs within normal limits, moist mucous membranes, and sufficient urine volume, with specific gravity within normal limits	Administer ordered IV fluid, e.g., 1000 ml of lactated Ringer's solution at 125 ml/hr, as ordered by physician, then discontinue. Run no faster than 200 ml/hr, even if behind schedule
Altered Nutrition: Less Than Body Requirements	Restores body weight to within 20% of ideal	Administer ordered hyperalimentation, e.g., 1000 ml of prescribed solution for hyperalimentation over the next 24 hours, as ordered. Maintain uniform flow rate at no more than 40 ml/hr
High Risk for Infection	Remains free of infection AEB WBC within normal limits, vital signs within normal limits, and no redness or pain at IV site	Use aseptic technique during venipuncture and when handling all IV equipment that could place the client at risk for infection. Change IV tubing, IV site, and dressing according to agency policy. Change IV bag every 24 hours

A bag of IV solution should not infuse longer than 24 hours. Label each bag with the date and time it was hung. Changing every 24 hours helps reduce the incidence of infection. |
| *High Risk for Fluid Volume Excess* | Remains free of circulatory overload AEB weight within normal limits, no pitting edema, and clear lung sounds | Carefully calculate the required flow rate. Have another nurse check your calculations, as needed. Regulate the flow rate and check it and the amount left in the bag at intervals. Monitor the client for signs of fluid volume excess |
| *High Risk for Trauma* | Remains free of blood vessel trauma AEB no edema or pain at IV site | Select a site for the venipuncture that will be moved least by the client (e.g., avoid the antecubital space and the dominant hand in adults). After venipuncture, use care to secure the needle or catheter and tubing to the skin near the IV site. Secure the extremity to an armboard, if necessary, to reduce movement. When changing tubing or otherwise working with the IV line, use care to secure the needle or catheter as needed to prevent movement, and be careful not to move the needle or catheter any more than necessary |

Methods of applying sterile dressings are discussed in Chapter 48. Also read the procedure manual for the agency in which you work.

CHANGING THE IV TUBING AND BAG

The IV tubing is changed according to agency policy (e.g., with filters, at least every 24 hours for central lines, every 72 hours for peripheral lines). The best time to change the tubing is the point when you add a new bag of solution, so that you do not interrupt the system any more than necessary. Follow the guidelines in Procedure 47–1 for preparing the IV solution and tubing. Place a sterile 2 × 2 gauze pad under the needle or catheter to collect any fluid leakage. Put on gloves to protect your hands from potential contact with blood. Then clamp off the old tubing before care-fully removing it from the needle or catheter. To prevent trauma to the vein, stabilize the needle or catheter with your nondominant hand. Remove the protective cap from the new tubing and insert the end of the new tubing into the needle or catheter while stabilizing the hub with your nondominant hand. Unclamp the new tubing and adjust the flow to the ordered rate. Be certain that the new tubing and bag are labeled with the date, time, and your initials. Discard the old bag and tubing according to agency policy. Also document the change in the client record.

CHANGING THE TUBING WITHOUT CHANGING THE BAG

If you must change the tubing without changing the IV solution, use the roller clamp to slow the infusion to a keep-open rate (8 to 10 drops/minute), and then

CASE STUDY

The Client

Carol Brown is a 70-year-old widow who was admitted to the hospital 3 days ago (April 15) for a cholecystectomy after many years of gallbladder disease. At 2:00 PM on April 15, a partial listing of the admission assessment data included the following:

► 70-year-old thin woman
► T 98.4° F, BP 140/80, P 78, R 20
► Slow skin turgor
► Height 5'6", weight 110 lbs
► States she lives alone
► No c/o gallbladder pain at present
► States that this is her first hospitalization since the birth of her last child 40 years ago

Her surgery was performed 2 days ago (April 16). Because she continues to experience some nausea, she is still receiv-ing IV therapy and taking ice chips occasionally by mouth. She has remained in bed most of the time since the operation and has become slightly disoriented. A partial listing of the physician's postoperative orders on April 16 included

► IV of 5% dextrose in 0.9% saline with 20 mEq KCl to run at 125 ml/hour
► Ambulate in room beginning tomorrow (4/17)
► Discontinue Foley in AM
► May have clear liquids postnausea

The following nursing care plan was written April 18 (2 days after surgery), with expected outcomes to be evaluated 24 hours later.

CARE PLAN

7:00 AM, April 18

Nursing Diagnosis	Planning: Expected Outcomes	Implementation: Nursing Interventions	Evaluation
High Risk for Injury R/T presence of IV needle in right arm and to effects of slight disorientation noted recently	By 7:00 AM, April 19: Exhibits no edema or pain at IV site	Support arm with IV infusion on pillow. Teach client to be careful when moving arm. Check that needle and tubing are securely taped.	7:00 AM, April 19: Assessment of IV site reveals no edema. Client states she has no pain at site.
	IV line patent and infusion running at ordered flow rate	Monitor IV flow rate every hour to see whether it is on schedule. Assess client on orientation every hour. Check tubing for kinking every hour.	A tourniquet placed above the IV site stops infusion.

squeeze the drip chamber to fill it full. These actions will provide enough fluid to maintain patency of the IV while you prepare the new tubing. Take the IV bag off the pole and hold it upside down while disconnecting the tubing from the bag. This position will prevent loss of solution from the bag. Without touching the spike, tape the drip chamber to the IV pole to maintain the infusion. After clamping off the new tubing, insert the spike into the bag (still holding the bag upside down), hang the bag on the pole, and remove air from the tubing as in Procedure 47–1. Don gloves and move the roller clamp on the old tubing to the off position. While stabilizing the needle or catheter, remove the old tubing from it. Remove the protective cap from the new tubing and attach the end of the tubing to the needle or catheter. Adjust flow to the ordered rate with the roller clamp. Label tubing with the date, time, and your initials and discard old tubing according to agency policy. Document the tubing change in the client record.

CHANGING THE CLIENT'S GOWN WITHOUT DISRUPTING THE IV SYSTEM

Many routine nursing actions will have to be carried out while the client is receiving IV infusions or hyperalimentation. One such action is changing the client's gown. If your agency does not provide gowns with snaps or Velcro closures at the shoulder, the client will need assistance in changing the gown while receiving IV therapy. To change the gown without interrupting and possibly contaminating the IV system, first remove the sleeve from the non-IV arm, then carefully remove the sleeve from the IV arm and slip the gown over the tubing and up toward the bag (keep the client covered with the sheet or a bath blanket). Next, take the IV bag from the IV pole, keeping it above the client's arm, and slip the bag through the sleeve. While still holding the IV bag above the client's arm, place the bag and the tubing through the sleeve of the clean gown (in the same direction that you would place the arm through it) and return the bag to the IV pole. Then place the IV arm through that sleeve, using care not to dislodge the needle. Finally, place the other arm through the other sleeve.

When the IV is infusing through a pump, it is necessary to clamp off the tubing below the pump, remove the tubing from the pump, and then proceed with changing the gown, restoring the infusion as quickly as possible. If no pump is used, check the IV flow rate after the gown is changed. Movement during the change can alter the rate of flow.

EVALUATION

Evaluation of a client receiving IV therapy is an ongoing process, because complications can occur at any time during the therapy. While your client is receiving IV therapy, you should evaluate whether or not, or to what extent, your planned outcomes have been achieved in relation to preventing complications and meeting the objectives for the IV therapy.

Remember that a number of different nursing diagnoses might justify the IV therapy. Therefore, any number of specific possible outcomes might apply when you are evaluating a client.

In general, however, you should assess for the following indicators after IV therapy:

▶ Benefits of therapy. Does the individual state that symptoms are relieved? Is the condition stabilizing and improving?

▶ Untoward reactions to therapy. Have distressing side effects appeared? Is the person's condition worsening? Have any complications of IV therapy developed?

▶ Reaction of the vein and surrounding tissues. Is the area inflamed or painful? If so, the individual may be developing phlebitis. Is there drainage at the site that may indicate infection?

▶ Psychologic response to therapy. What is the person's attitude toward the therapy? Is the client apprehensive?

Carefully document your assessment in the person's record and discuss any problems and proposed changes in intervention with other health professionals.

Summary

▶ Administration of fluid by the IV route is termed intravenous therapy. IV infusions are ordered for persons who are in life-threatening situations, may have nothing by mouth, require medications that cannot be given by more convenient routes, or are unable to digest or absorb a diet given by mouth or by tube. The IV route provides the most rapid and complete absorption of medication, making this route excellent for emergencies but potentially fatal when complications occur.

▶ The physician orders the specific solution and any additive solutions to be infused. The physician may order the timing of an infusion by indicating total time the complete amount is to take to infuse, the drip rate per minute, and the maximum amount to be absorbed per hour. The nurse should know the formulas for computing milliliters per hour and drops (gtt) per minute.

▶ Because some medications can be given by more than one route, it is imperative that you verify with the container label that a medication is safe for IV administration. Always verify that the fluid is infusing correctly, even when using an infusion pump. When initiating a blood transfusion, it is vital that you assure that all information on the label of the bag correlates with all information on the accompanying tag and with the client's ID bracelet.

▶ Severe untoward reactions to IV infusions include sudden, severe allergic reactions; circulatory overload; and air embolism. Common complications of IV therapy include phlebitis, thrombosis, and thrombophlebitis; infiltration; allergic reactions; and infection and inflammation of the IV site.

► Adverse effects associated with blood transfusions include circulatory overload and reactions that may be allergic, febrile, septic, or hemolytic.

► Four major complications of hyperalimentation are sepsis, catheter dislocation, osmotic diuresis, and blood glucose changes.

► IV equipment includes a variety of needles and catheters, solution containers, types of tubing, and accessories such as infusion pumps and implantable vascular access devices.

► The nurse often identifies clients who require IV therapy. During IV therapy, the nurse assesses the client for responses to any IV medication and for signs and symptoms of circulatory overload, altered renal function, and complications at the infusion site.

► Three nursing diagnoses frequently seen in clients with IVs are *High Risk for Infection, High Risk for Fluid Volume Excess,* and *High Risk for Trauma.*

► Outcomes for these three diagnoses are all directed toward preventing commonly encountered complications of IV therapy.

► Nursing interventions include preventing complications while completing venipuncture and maintaining IV systems.

► Evaluation of the person who has received IV therapy includes assessing the benefits of the therapy, untoward reactions to the therapy, condition of the vein and surrounding tissue, and psychologic response to therapy.

Bibliography

1. Ashton, J., et al. (1990). Effects of heparin versus saline solution on intermittent infusion device irrigation. *Heart and Lung,* 19(6), 698–712.
2. Gold, C., & Morales, J. (1991). Heparin lock use. *American Journal of Emergency Medicine,* 9(1), 95–96.
3. Goode, C., et al. (1991). A meta-analysis of effects of heparin flush and saline flush: quality and cost implications. *Nursing Research,* 40(6), 324–330.
4. Gudmanm, J.T. (1991). A method to prevent tampering with an infusion pump. *Anesthesiology,* 74(6), 1159–1160.
5. Hadaway, L.C. (1991). IV tips: as veins change with age, so too must your strategies for successful venipuncture. *Geriatric Nursing,* 12(2), 78–81.
6. Hoffmann, K.K., et al. (1992). Transparent polyurethane film as an intravenous catheter dressing. *Journal of the American Medical Association,* 267(15), 2072–2076.
7. Johnson, M.S., et al. (1990). Cost and acceptability of three syringe-pump infusion systems. *American Journal of Hospital Pharmacy,* 47(8), 1794–1798.
8. Jones, L., & Brooks, J.P. (1990). The ABC's of PCA. *RN,* 53(5), 54–60.
9. Lennox, A.C. (1990). IV therapy: reducing the risk of infection. *Nursing 90,* 20(3), 60–61.
10. Lorenz, B.L. (1990). Are you using the right IV pump? *RN,* 53(5), 31–37.
11. McAfee, T., et al. (1990). How to safely draw blood from a vascular access device. *Nursing 90,* 20(11), 42–43.
12. Messner, R.L., & Pinkerman, M.L. (1992). Preventing a peripheral I.V. infection. *Nursing 92,* 22(6), 34–41.
13. Millam, D. (1990). Equipment update 90: avoiding needle-stick injuries. *Nursing 90,* 20(1), 61–64.
14. Millam, D. (1990). Controlling the flow: electronic infusion devices. *Nursing 90,* 20(8), 65–68.
15. Querin, J.J., & Stahl, L.D. (1990). Twelve simple, sensible steps for successful blood transfusions. *Nursing 90,* 20(10), 68–81.
16. Rapp, et al. (1989). Patient-controlled analgesia: a review of effectiveness of therapy and an evaluation of currently available devices. *DICP, The Annals of Pharmacology,* 23(11), 899–904.
17. Sherman, J.S., & Sherman, R.H. (1989). IV therapy that clicks. *Nursing 89,* 19(5), 50–51.
18. Southern, J.P. (1990). How to access an epidural implanted port. *Nursing 90,* 20(7), 48–51.
19. Stepura, B.A., et al. (1990). Nurses make high tech high touch. *Nursing Outlook,* 38(6), 269–271.
20. Taylor, J., et al. (1989). Heparin lock intravenous line: use in newborn infants. *Clinical Pediatrics,* 28(5), 237–240.
21. Vaida, A.J., et al. (1989). Use of an ambulatory infusion pump in a 12-year old with *Salmonella* osteomyelitis. *DICP, The Annals of Pharmacology,* 23(5), 379–381.
22. Viall, C.D. (1990). Your complete guide to central venous catheters. *Nursing 90,* 20(2), 34.
23. Whitney, R. (1991). Comparing long-term central venous catheters. *Nursing 91,* 21(4), 70–71.

▼ *Caring for Persons with Wounds*

▼

Chapter 48

Don't put any chemical into a wound that you wouldn't put into your own eye.

E. E. Peacock, Jr., M.D.

▼ CHAPTER OUTLINE

NORMAL SKIN INTEGRITY
    Layers of the Skin
    Elements of Soft Tissue
    Alterations in Skin and Soft Tissue
      Due to Aging
    Assessment of Skin and Soft
      Tissue
CLASSIFICATION OF WOUNDS
    Surgical or Traumatic Wounds
    Open or Closed Wounds
    Full-Thickness and Partial-
      Thickness Wounds
    Noninfected, Contaminated, or
      Infected (Dirty) Wounds
    Wounds and Blood-borne
      Transmissible Infectious
      Diseases
    Chronic Wounds: Pressure Ulcers
WOUND HEALING

Phases of Wound Healing
Factors Affecting Wound Healing
Local Factors in Wound Healing
Systemic Factors in Wound Healing
Wound Closure
New Therapies for Wound Care
ASSESSMENT
    Initial Assessment
    Ongoing Assessment
NURSING DIAGNOSIS
PLANNING
NURSING INTERVENTION
    Management of Wounds
    Applications of Heat or Cold
    Nursing Management in Application
      of Heat and Cold
EVALUATION
CASE STUDY

▼ KEY TERMS

Angiogenesis
Avulsions
Capillary closing pressure
Consensual response
  (consensual reaction)
Contact inhibition
Contrast baths
Conversion

Counterirritants
Dead space
Debridement
Dehiscence
Desiccation
Diathermy
Epithelialization
Eschar

Excoriation
Evisceration
Factitious wounds
Friable
Granulation tissue
Growth factors
Hypertrophic scar

▼ KEY TERMS Continued

Keloid	Necrosis	Purulent material	Serosanguineous	Tensile strength
Maceration	Nonionic cleanser	Secondary effect	drainage	Wound
Matrix	Pressure ulcers	(rebound effect)	Sitz baths	Wound exudate

---

▼ LEARNING OBJECTIVES

After studying this chapter, you should be able to

1. Define wounds.
2. State the functions of normal skin.
3. Describe effects of aging on skin.
4. Describe normal skin assessment.
5. Contrast the various types of wounds.
6. Discuss principles of prevention and management of pressure ulcers, a major type of chronic wound.
7. Describe the process of wound healing.
8. Identify factors influencing wound healing.
9. Identify signs of wound infection.
10. Describe methods of wound closure.
11. State how to assess wounds.
12. Discuss nursing diagnoses for clients with wounds.
13. Describe planning for the client with a wound.
14. Explain nursing interventions for the client with a wound.
15. Describe correct wound cleaning.
16. Contrast occlusive and nonocclusive dressings.
17. Explain the purpose of wound drains.
18. Identify appropriate action to take when wound dehiscence or evisceration occurs.
19. List mechanisms of heat and cold transfer.
20. Identify safety factors related to heat and cold therapies.

A **wound** is a disruption of soft tissue continuity. Wounds occur when an external force is greater than tissues can withstand. This tissue disruption can result in normal or abnormal repair responses. All wounds can be classified as acute or chronic. Acute wounds, such as surgical wounds, heal without significant problems and within a reasonable period. Chronic wounds do not heal as expected. These wounds may exist for weeks, months, or even years. The person with a chronic wound often has other health problems, such as infectious, metabolic, or nutritional disorders, which interfere with wound healing. Chronic wounds, such as pressure ulcers (wounds created by pressure, friction, and shear), have engendered most of the research and new products used in current wound care regimens.

More than 25 million persons per year in the United States require care for acute or chronic wounds, approximately 22 million of which are surgical wounds.[33] This figure does not take into account the increasing number of elderly and clients with acquired immune deficiency syndrome (AIDS) in the United States. These individuals are more likely to be institutionalized with a diminished ability to care for themselves, which will put them at risk for developing chronic wounds.

Wound care costs are both direct and indirect and have significant economic impact. The annual total cost of health care in the United States is approximately $550 billion.[54] Estimates suggest that wound care products (with sales of $4.8 billion in 1988[29]) account for more than 1 per cent of all health care costs.

To help control the skyrocketing cost of health care, payors (both federal and private) have tried to ensure that individuals do not remain in the hospital any longer than necessary. Consequently, wound care therapies must increasingly encourage more rapid, safe healing in the hospital whenever possible. If healing is not complete at discharge, then we must also develop safe and effective methods of caring for difficult-to-heal wounds in nonhospital settings.

NORMAL SKIN INTEGRITY

The skin is the body's largest organ. It has an average thickness of 2.5 mm. It is thickest over the palms of the hands and the soles of the feet (7 mm) and thinnest over areas such as the eyelids.[71] The stratum corneum (the external layer of skin visible to the naked eye) is thicker wherever it is exposed to repeated use, such as the hands and the feet. The dermis (layer beneath the epidermal layers) is thicker where the contact is of a more general, environmental, type as on the extensor and dorsal surfaces of the extremities.

The skin pH range is 4.2 to 5.6. The slight acidity of the skin surface is thought to discourage the growth of many bacterial species as well as fungi. The stratum corneum is impermeable to bacteria from the outside environment, and fungi can live only in its outermost layers. Bacteria reproduce most readily on moist areas of the skin. Therefore, the normal relative dryness is important in helping prevent infection. The constant turnover of cells on the skin surface also prevents many bacteria from colonizing the skin (e.g., becoming permanent skin residents).[28]

Layers of the Skin

The skin is composed of two layers: the epidermis and the dermis. The epidermis, or outer skin layer, is thin, avascular, and divided into five distinct layers:

▶ Stratum corneum, or horny layer: the tough, outer layer visible to the naked eye. It is the major chemical and mechanical barrier of the body.
▶ Stratum lucidum: the epidermal layer found just below the stratum corneum. The stratum lucidum is a thin layer and is clearly demonstrated only in the thick epithelium of the palms and soles.
▶ Stratum granulosum: the layer containing Langerhans cells, which appear to function in antigen recognition and processing. These cells are macrophages that ingest potential antigenic compounds and help prevent allergic reaction of the skin, such as contact dermatitis.
▶ Stratum spinosum: the layer made up of spinelike extensions or ''prickles'' of the basal layer.
▶ Stratum germinativum: the basal layer of the epithelium. Cells of the stratum germinativum are the parents of all the other cells in the epithelial layer. Scattered among these basal cells are the melanocytes. Melanocytes release granules of pigment called melanin, which is responsible for the color of skin and also assists in protecting the body from the harmful effects of ultraviolet radiation from the sun.

Cells formed in the stratum germinativum migrate upward through all epithelial layers to the stratum corneum layer, where they are shed by the body 26 to 28 days later. The epidermal layer of the skin is renewed on the average of once a month.

At the junction of the epidermis and the dermis lies the basement membrane. Its principal component is collagen, and it functions to provide structural support for the dermis. The basement membrane also allows the exchange of fluid and cells between skin layers.

The dermis, also called the true skin, provides strength, distensibility, and elasticity. Not as clearly layered as the epidermis, the dermis has two layers:

▶ Papillary dermis: the outer layer, which lies against the basement membrane. The papillary dermis contains collagen, elastin, and reticulin fibers.
▶ Reticular dermis: the inner layer formed of dense networks of collagen bundles that anchor the skin to the underlying subcutaneous tissue.

Fibroblasts, macrophages, and mast cells are the major cell types of the dermis. These cells are important in wound healing. Nerve endings distinguish pain, heat, cold, and touch, and pressure and lymph vessels remove excess fluid and store protein.

The major functions of the skin are regulation of body temperature and protection.[28] The skin regulates body temperature through the use of the sweat glands, alterations in blood flow, and the sensing of heat load (whether internal or external). The skin protects the body by preventing water loss and providing a barrier against pathogenic organisms. The stratum corneum is the basic barrier through which the skin prevents the penetration of chemicals and various other liquids and gases with which it comes in contact. If this layer is stripped, the skin immediately loses its impermeability. The skin is not absolutely impermeable to all agents. Certain chemicals, gases, and excess moisture may penetrate and cause injury. Because it conveys the sensations of touch, pressure, and pain, the skin also allows individual protection from noxious stimuli.

The skin also protects against the sun's harmful radiation. Sunlight, however, has a beneficial effect on the skin when exposure is kept to safe levels. As sunlight interacts with the skin, vitamin D is produced. This vitamin plays a vital part in regulating calcium metabolism in the body.

The skin is also capable of self-replication. The epidermal cells are continuously being added from the basal layer while being lost from the surface layer, the stratum corneum.

Elements of Soft Tissue

In addition to understanding the epidermal and dermal layers of the skin, you also need to know about soft tissue and its role in wound healing. Elements of soft tissue are

▶ Subcutaneous tissue, made up of dense connective tissue and varying amounts of adipose tissue. The subcutaneous tissue houses major blood vessels, lymphatics, and nerves. It acts as an insulator to retain body heat and as a shock absorber. During illness or starvation, the body draws on its fat stores for nutritional needs.
▶ Fascia, found below the subcutaneous tissue level and covering muscles, nerves, and blood vessels. The two types of fascia are superficial and deep. The superficial fascia connects the skin to its supporting tissues. The deep fascia functions as an envelope-type covering for muscles, blood vessels, and nerves. This layer has little elasticity.
▶ Skeletal and striated muscles, which form the base

for soft tissues underlying the skin. Muscles vary in thickness and function, depending on location.

Blood supply to the soft tissues is variable. In relation to metabolic needs, skin is supplied with much more blood than it needs, but the large blood supply allows the skin to dissipate body heat, if necessary. Muscle and subcutaneous fat, on the other hand, are not overly supplied with blood. Neither of these tissues tolerate ischemia (oxygen deficiency) for prolonged periods. Interruption of the blood supply to the muscle can lead to skin necrosis. Often called slough, **necrosis** is the death of a portion of tissue that is still surrounded by living tissue.

A close physiologic relationship exists between blood supply and the muscle and skin. Whereas blood supply to the soft tissues may be interrupted by various pathologic processes, including trauma, the most common disruption of blood supply to the skin in the person with impaired ability to move is external pressure from a bed or chair. The cutaneous vascular system is easily disrupted because it is predominantly a capillary system. Blood flow in the capillaries is under low pressure, compared with that of the arterial and venous systems. This low pressure allows cutaneous blood vessels to be easily occluded by externally applied pressure. Surface capillary beds are vulnerable not only to pressure but also to increased metabolic needs during wound repair. At certain stages of wound repair, particularly just after injury when metabolic demands are high, the neutrophils (a type of white blood cell) can require as much as 30 times the amount of oxygen required by resting epithelial cells.

Alterations in Skin and Soft Tissue Due to Aging

After the third decade of life, the body slowly begins to deteriorate; by the end of the sixth decade, 30 per cent of the body's cells are lost.[6] The skin of the elderly individual reflects this loss through atrophy and thinning of both the epithelial and subcutaneous layers of tissue. The collagenous attachments become less effective with aging and allow the epidermal and dermal layers of the skin to slide over each other. With minor friction or shearing force, these layers can separate from each other and tear. This type of injury is common in older clients, whose skin tends to be **friable** (easily broken or torn), and is termed skin tear. Once the skin is disrupted, the elderly person is at greater risk for infection because the immune system is no longer able to fend off attackers as readily as it once did.

The skin of older people is drier because of decreased ability to sweat and decreased sebum production. Because it is dry, the skin itches, and because of cellular loss, the skin is thinner. The elderly are more sensitive to heat and cold. Heat sensitivity results from inability to sweat effectively, and sensitivity to cold derives from the loss of insulating subcutaneous tissue and a lower metabolic rate. Elderly people will complain of cold often but rarely complain of heat because they are unaware of being too hot, largely because of hypothalamic changes associated with aging.

With aging, there is usually a loss of melanocyte production, which causes whitening of the skin in Caucasians. In general, the elderly lose body hair and develop wrinkles. Exposure to the sun is the single most important factor in producing wrinkles of the skin. In addition to environmental factors, the person's heredity and hormonal fluctuations contribute to skin changes during aging.

Assessment of Skin and Soft Tissue

Normal, intact skin should first be assessed for turgor, or tone. The skin of the healthy person should quickly return to normal when it is pinched slightly and released.

Also assess the skin for circulatory adequacy. Normal skin should have an adequate blood supply reflected by normal color and pulses. Circulatory disorders, which include both arterial and venous insufficiency, are likely to cause skin changes. In the early stages of arterial insufficiency of the lower extremities, pallor of the skin appears beyond the point of arterial obstruction. The arterial pulse may be absent beyond the obstruction. There is usually extreme pain, but it decreases if the leg is dependent. As the insufficiency progresses, the skin will break down, and an arterial ulcer will appear on the lower leg, especially the toes, the heel, or the bony prominences of the foot. The breakdown and ulceration may progress to a point at which amputation of the extremity becomes necessary if the person is not responsive to treatment.[33]

Venous insufficiency, which affects blood flow in the lower extremities, occurs because of a combination of factors, including incompetent venous valves and gravity. Elevated pressure is transmitted to the superficial veins of the lower leg. This pressure causes edema (swelling) and ulceration in the ankle region, usually just above the medial malleolus. Loss of pulsation does not usually occur, although edema may make it difficult to find the posterior tibial or the dorsalis pedis pulses. Usually the client has some degree of pain, which decreases when the leg is elevated.[33]

As you assess skin color, remember that it may vary from a flesh tone, which is slightly pink in Caucasians, to darker hues in persons of Hispanic, Asian-American, or African-American heritage. If you are assessing the color of an extremity, compare one extremity with the other. If there is a difference between the two, ask the person whether the change is a new development. If so, report it to your instructor at once and chart your findings. If it is not a new development, record this information in the person's record and advise your instructor of your finding.

If you are assessing the skin color of the entire body, look for pallor, which may be a sign of slowed circulation, anemia, or mild coldness. Look for localized areas of redness, which may indicate increased circulation, inflammation, or an impending pressure ulcer (bedsore). Look for cyanosis (blueness), which may be readily found in the nailbeds of many people on bed rest because they are cold. Both environmental temperature and inactivity associated with bed rest slows the circulation to the extremities and causes cold.

Cyanosis indicates significant oxygen problems only if it is also present centrally on the lips, on the mucous membranes of the mouth, and in the conjunctiva of the eyes. No matter what the person's skin color, cyanosis can be readily seen in these locations if it is centrally present.

Palpate the skin to assess its temperature. The skin should feel warm to the touch. Too much heat suggests increased blood flow, which may be due to inflammation, infection, or some other cause. Skin that is very cool to the touch may indicate that circulation is poor. Keep in mind that the environmental temperature may cause the person's skin to feel either warmer or cooler than expected, and compare extremities for temperature differences. The skin should feel slightly moist, neither wet nor dry.

Include the sense of touch in your assessment. Normally, the person should be able to distinguish sharp, dull, and pressure sensations. Use your fingers, a cotton-tipped applicator, or some similar instrument to check reaction to touch. Check both arms and then both legs simultaneously to see if sensation is the same in each extremity. Determine whether the person feels the identical sense of touch in both extremities or less or more in one. Ask whether the person feels unpleasant sensations when touched; individuals may suffer from hyperesthesias or paresthesias.

Immediately after admission to the institution, check for injuries, rashes, skin breakdowns, bruises, birthmarks, and nonblanching erythema (redness that does not disappear when the person is turned off of the reddened area). Note any findings on the person's record. Noted in detail are the type of finding; size, depth, and location of lesion; and the presence of any infection.

Full skin assessment should be done at regular intervals on all persons on bed rest or who are chairfast. Findings should be charted.

CLASSIFICATION OF WOUNDS

Classification is important for wound assessment because it helps the physician and the nurse anticipate likely reactions to the type of wound. Classifications are based on whether the wound is surgical (intentional) or traumatic (accidental), open or closed, full-thickness or partial-thickness, and infected or noninfected. Wounds are also classified on an etiologic basis (Table 48–1).

TABLE 48–1. Etiologic Basis of Wounds

Name	Examples	Extent of Soft Tissue Damage	Prognosis for Healing
Surgical wound		Minimal	Usually heals without problem
Mechanical wound	Auto accidents Gunshots Knifings Falls	Varying degrees of soft tissue damage Moderate to severe	May require lengthy healing period and is commonly dirty or infected
Thermal wounds Heat Cold	Burns Frostbite	Mild to severe	Healing is often lengthy; may not regain pre-injury condition
Chemical wounds	Acids Alkalis Chemotherapeutic agents	Moderate to severe	Variable; depends on nature, amount, and length of contact with the chemical agent
Radiation injury		Mild to moderate	Permanent damage of varying degrees
Vascular impairment wound	Venous stasis ulcers Arterial insufficiency ulcers Pressure ulcers	Mild to severe	Good if underlying disorder is corrected; progressive worsening if underlying disorder is not corrected
Factitious wound	Slashing of wrists	Moderate to severe	Usually heals without problem unless the person interferes with it
Battering	Burns Broken bones Severe bruising	Moderate to life-threatening	May require lengthy healing period; similar or worse wounds tend to recur if person remains in the abusive environment

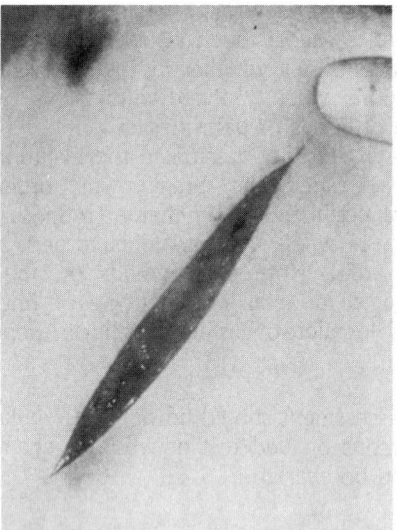

▲ *Figure 48-1*

Incised surgical wound. Note straight, clean edges. (Reprinted with permission from Westaby, S. [ed.]. [1986]. *Wound care.* London: Butterworth-Heinemann.)

Surgical or Traumatic Wounds

Surgical (intentional) wounds disrupt the skin and soft tissues under aseptic conditions and with sharp, sterile instruments that minimize skin damage. The extent of the wound is, of course, determined by the reason for which the surgery was done. Some surgical wounds can be disruptive and result in significant skin and soft tissue loss. A surgical wound has smooth, clean edges that can be readily approximated under most circumstances (Fig. 48-1). Surgical wounds usually heal quickly and with a minimum of scarring or other complications.

Traumatic (accidental) wounds occur as a result of injury. These wounds range from minor problems, such as cutting a finger, to severe injuries, such as those sustained in car accidents. Traumatic wounds differ from surgical wounds in almost all respects: they occur unexpectedly; they usually have ragged edges; they may result in considerable tissue loss; they occur under nonaseptic conditions; and they are prone to become infected. One example is an avulsion. **Avulsions** are extremely traumatic injuries characterized by forcible separation of soft tissues from the body.

Open or Closed Wounds

Open wounds are those in which the continuity of the skin is disrupted. Open wounds allow direct loss of fluid from the body and the entrance of foreign particles and potentially dangerous organisms (pathogens) into the body. Open wounds may be caused by a sharp blow or object, by projectiles such as bullets, or by surgery. Examples are seen in Figures 48-2 to 48-5.

Closed wounds cause no break in skin continuity, but they may be no less dangerous than an open wound.

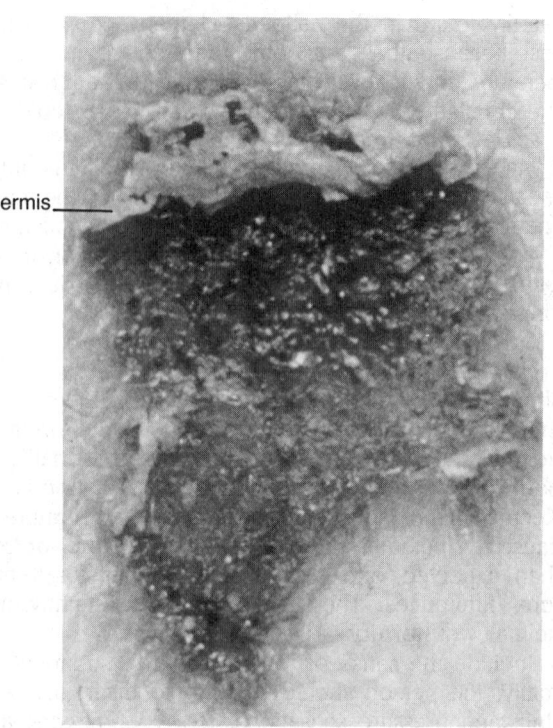

Epidermis

▲ *Figure 48-2*

Scraping abrasion. Heaping of epidermis that has been peeled back is well illustrated. (Reprinted with permission from Westaby, S. [ed.]. [1986]. *Wound care.* London: Butterworth-Heinemann.)

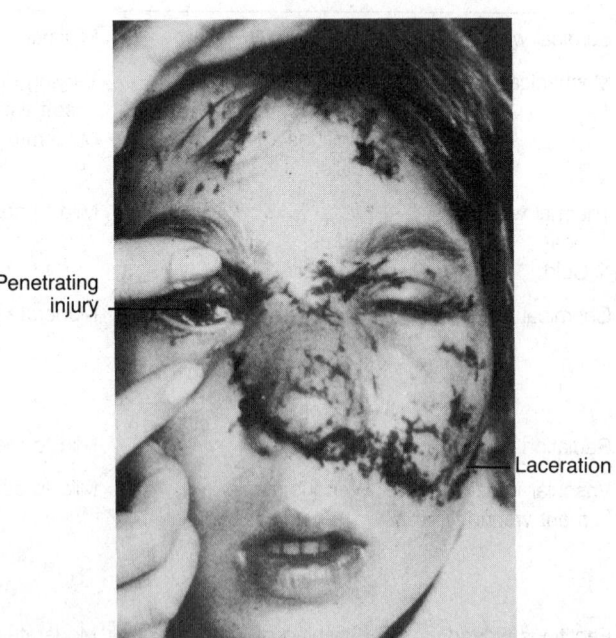

Penetrating injury

Laceration

▲ *Figure 48-3*

Injuries from a traffic accident. There is a penetrating injury of the right eye and extensive facial lacerations. (Reprinted with permission from Westaby, S. [ed.]. [1986]. *Wound care.* London: Butterworth-Heinemann.)

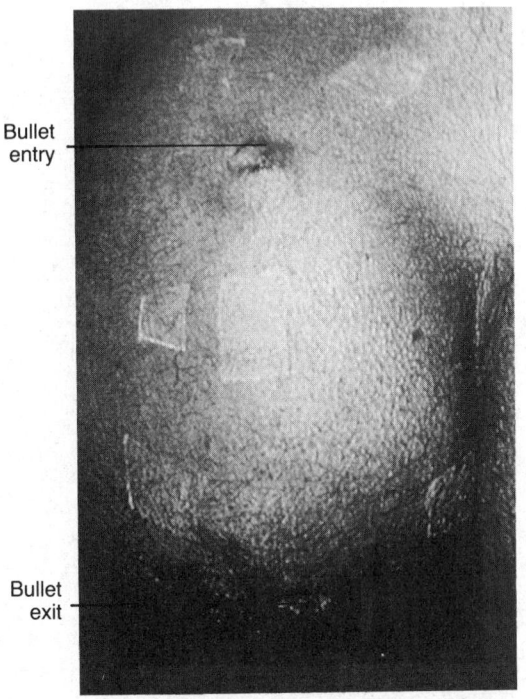

Bullet
entry

Bullet
exit

▲ Figure 48–4

Perforating wound from high-velocity bullet. Note entry and exit holes in buttock. (Reprinted with permission from Westaby, S. [ed.]. [1986]. *Wound care*. London: Butterworth-Heinemann.)

The amount of tissue damage sustained is not visible to the eye (Fig. 48–6). Closed wounds are caused by forces such as falls, direct blows, sudden deceleration, or indirect blows that often result in both soft tissue injury and broken bones. Common examples of closed wounds are injuries to internal organs, such as the liver, spleen, or bladder, as a result of car accidents; broken hips in the elderly, which result from a fall sufficient to break osteoporotic bone but not the overlying skin; fracture of the jaw suffered in a fight; and rib fractures sometimes caused by seat belts in a car crash.

Full-Thickness and Partial-Thickness Wounds

Full-thickness wounds involve total destruction or loss of the epidermis, dermis, and subcutaneous tissue (see Fig. 48–5). Muscle and bone destruction may also occur. Partial-thickness wounds involve only the epidermis or the upper portion of the dermis. An example is **excoriation** (abrasion of the epidermis by trauma, chemical burns, or other causes such as drainage from wounds, urine, or feces). These wounds heal by regeneration, without scarring or loss of function.

Noninfected, Contaminated, or Infected (Dirty) Wounds

Most wounds occurring in hospitalized clients are surgical (intentional) wounds created under aseptic conditions. These wounds are considered noninfected be-

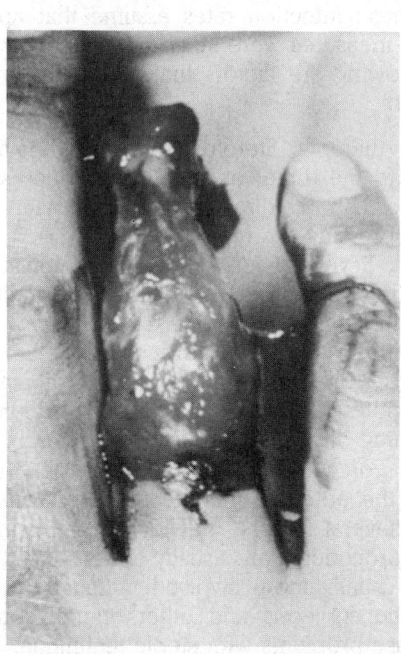

▲ Figure 48–5

Avulsion injury of ring finger; ring became entangled in moving machinery. (Reprinted with permission from Westaby, S. [ed.]. [1986]. *Wound care*. London: Butterworth-Heinemann.)

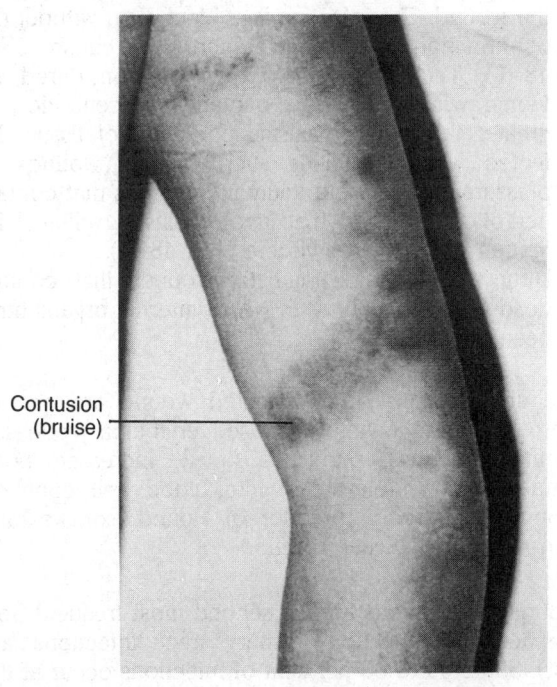

Contusion
(bruise)

▲ Figure 48–6

Contusion, a linear bruise after impact with a motor vehicle. A contusion of this origin may be the only outward sign of a possible closed fracture. (Reprinted with permission from Westaby, S. [ed.]. [1986]. *Wound care*. London: Butterworth-Heinemann.)

cause external microorganisms are prevented from entering the incision at the time that it is made. Noninfected wounds may be further classified as clean or clean-contaminated.[19] The Centers for Disease Control defines these wounds as follows.

▶ Clean wounds: uninfected operative wounds in which no inflammation is encountered, and the respiratory, alimentary, genital, or uninfected urinary tracts are not entered. Clean wounds are primarily closed and, if necessary, drained with closed drainage.

▶ Clean-contaminated wounds: operative wounds in which the respiratory, alimentary, genital, or urinary tract is entered under controlled conditions and without unusual contamination. Operations involving the biliary tract, appendix, vagina, and oropharynx are included in this category.

▶ Contaminated wounds: most chronic wounds, such as pressure ulcers, venous stasis ulcers, and arterial insufficiency ulcers. Included in this category are open, fresh, accidental wounds; operations with major breaks in sterile technique or gross spillage from the gastrointestinal tract; and incisions in which acute, nonpurulent inflammation is encountered. Contaminated wounds differ from infected wounds primarily in the quantity of bacteria found at the wound site.

All chronic wounds are contaminated; not all are infected.

▶ Infected (dirty) wounds: wounds that generally contain **purulent material** (pus), which drains from the wound. The infection is evident even without the confirmation of a positive laboratory culture (Fig. 48–7). Technically, the wound is considered infected when there is a bacterial concentration of greater than 10^5 organisms per gram of tissue. Infected wounds include such chronic wounds as pressure ulcers or old traumatic wounds that contain necrotic tissue and that involve existing clinical infection or perforated viscera (Fig. 48–8).

▶ Dirty wounds: old traumatic wounds that contain dead tissue or wounds in which internal organs have been penetrated.

The clinical signs of an infected wound are one or more of the following: increased erythema (redness), edema (swelling), purulence (pus), increased body temperature. An elevated white blood cell count, a change in the color or odor of wound exudate, and pain may also indicate infection.

Surgical infections are the second most frequent hospital-acquired infection (urinary tract infections are first). Some 60 to 80 per cent of infections occur at the site of the incision. The risk for infection is based on whether a wound is clean, contaminated, or dirty: clean wounds, 1 to 5 per cent; clean-contaminated wounds, 8 to 11 per cent; contaminated wounds, 15 to

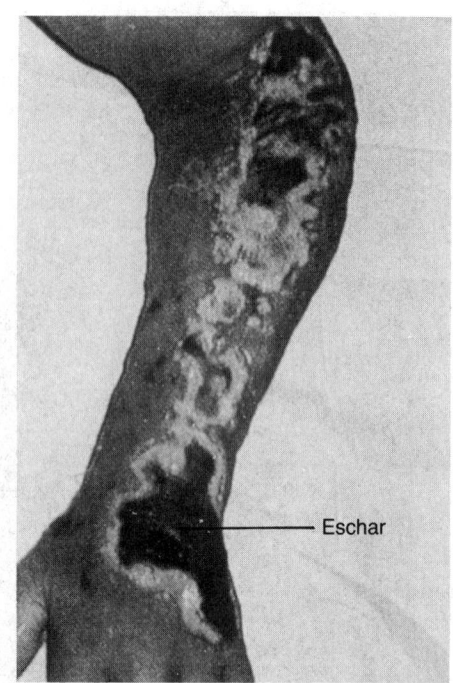

▲ *Figure 48–7*

Infected wound caused by a thorn prick on the back of the hand while gardening. Infecting organism is beta-hemolytic streptococcus type A. This type of wound is left open to heal by secondary intention. (Reprinted with permission from Westaby, S. [ed.]. [1986]. *Wound care.* London: Butterworth-Heinemann.)

17 per cent; and dirty wounds, more than 27 per cent.[102] These infection rates assume that appropriate preventive measures were taken.

The following are factors that predispose individuals to infection.

▶ Steroid therapy. Steroids suppress the host's response to the threat of infection by depressing antibody formation, diminishing phagocytic capacity, and suppressing the repair process.

▶ Obesity. Severe obesity usually prolongs surgical procedures and increases the opportunity for a breach in surgical technique.

▶ Malnutrition. Malnourished individuals are in poor general condition. The major effect of malnutrition on the potential for infection is that it depresses the functioning of the immune system.

▶ Duration of surgery. The longer surgery lasts, the greater the potential for infection. This risk may be due to several factors. Individuals having longer operative procedures are usually sicker, and the procedure is usually more involved. A fatigue factor may affect the surgeons and other operative personnel and cause problems with sterile technique.

▶ Extremes of age. Neither the infant nor the elderly individual has an immune system that protects as efficiently as that of the young to middle-aged adult.

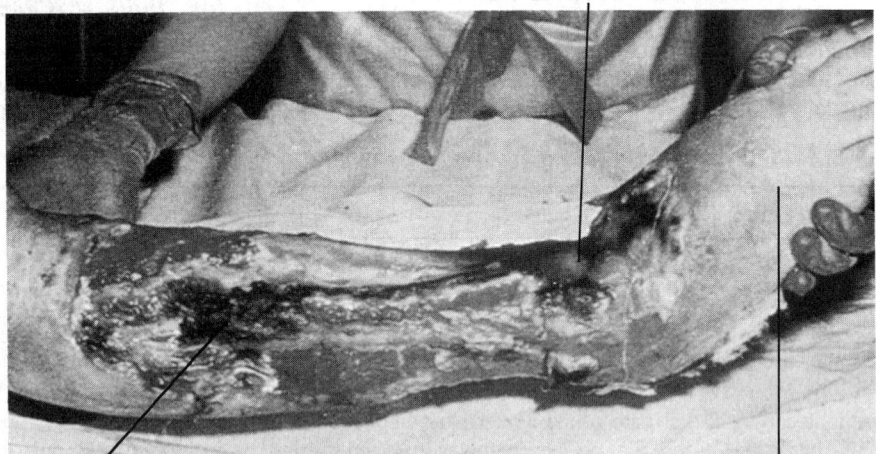

Continuing area of
tissue destruction

Continuing areas of
tissue destruction

Swollen foot

▲ Figure 48-8

Gas gangrene. Note extensive tissue destruction and swelling of the foot. Swollen tissue from gases trapped within is a characteristic finding in this condition. (Reprinted with permission from Westaby, S. [ed.]. [1986]. *Wound care*. London: Butterworth-Heinemann.)

▶ Diabetes. Because of increased blood sugar levels and reduced blood flow from atherosclerotic changes, these individuals are at greater risk.

▶ Cancer. Clients who are immunosuppressed for therapeutic reasons are at great risk for infection.

The cause of a wound (see Table 48-1) and the type (Table 48-2) may have a significant effect on both treatment and prognosis.

Although most wounds encountered in inpatient settings heal normally and cause few problems, certain

TABLE 48-2. Types of Wounds

Name	Description	Name	Description
Incisions	Usually associated with surgical wounds Edges are sharp, clean-cut, and in close approximation. Minimal skin loss (Fig. 48-1)		This type of wound can be deceptive; there is often little or no bleeding on the skin surface, but internal damage can be deadly
Abrasions	Superficial, partial-thickness wounds involving the epidermis and possibly portions of the dermis These wounds often have foreign debris contained in them; an example is a "skinned knee" (Fig. 48-2)	Penetrating	Any wound causing a skin break is a penetrating wound In clinical use, a penetrating wound involves skin, its supporting soft tissues, and possibly body organs; examples are gunshot and knife wounds
Lacerations	Torn or jagged wounds produced by such injuries as falling on broken glass (Fig. 48-3)	Perforating	A wound made by an object, such as a bullet, which enters and exits the body (Fig. 48-4)
Avulsions	Extremely traumatic injuries characterized by a tearing away or a forcible separation of tissue from the body, such as when skin is caught in a zipper or a hand is caught between two moving pieces of machinery (Fig. 48-5)	Contusions	The only type of wound in which the skin remains intact Underlying damage to blood vessels and swelling Discoloration of the skin caused by extravasation of blood into the tissues (ecchymosis) Hematomas may develop if hemorrhage into the soft tissues is localized and significant (Fig. 48-6)
Punctures	A wound produced by a sharp, pointed object, such as a knife or a nail piercing various depths into the body, leaving a small surface opening		

wounds require special knowledge and skill before you can render safe care. Some of these wounds are summarized in Table 48–3. Wounds requiring special precaution, such as those in clients with infectious processes, are frequently the responsibility of every nurse in daily practice.

Wounds and Blood-borne Transmissible Infectious Diseases

Most of the infectious diseases that were the major health problems of past years have been brought under

TABLE 48–3. Wounds Requiring Advanced Intervention

Wound	Rationale for Concern	Wound	Rationale for Concern
Abrasions	May involve large surface areas; often very painful; *Pseudomonas* infection common; often imbedded with dirt difficult to remove; dirt left in wound may cause permanent tattoo		mias (abnormal heart beat rhythms) and other organ damage may be present
Amputations	Direct care of the wound, the amputated part, and the person (amputation is emotionally traumatic); handle the part gently and prevent it from drying out; conduct wound care and handling of the part according to the agency protocol	Foreign body	Fragments of metal, wood, or other material may pierce tissues and remain in wound; wood splinters may soften, fall apart, and be difficult to remove if they become wet during wound cleaning; sewing needles may require x-ray to locate and surgery to remove; impaled objects (e.g., metal rod) may compress (tamponade) a bleeding site; thus, removal of impaled objects (e.g., pulling them out in setting other than operating room) may cause massive blood loss (exsanguination)
Bites			
Animal bite	Potential for rabies, and severe necrotizing infections with extensive tissue loss; bone fractures may occur (e.g., skull, hand); long-term fear of animals may result; incident usually reportable	Gunshot	Depending on bullet caliber, amount of tissue damage may be difficult to determine; entry wound is often smaller than exit wound; bullet pathway through tissues is difficult to determine, so organ damage is unknown; tissue damage occurs from bullet mass and also from heat and shock wave generated; these wounds require the health care professionals to report incident, document information, preserve evidence
Human bite	High risk for severe necrotizing infections; fastidious wound care essential, including careful follow-up; antibiotic therapy may be indicated; wound often not sutured because of potential infection		
Spider bite	Systemic toxin released by black widow spider, and antivenin may be indicated; extensive tissue necrosis may occur from brown recluse spider bite; anaphylaxis (severe allergic reaction) and disseminated intravascular coagulation (DIC) may result	High-pressure injuries (e.g., grease gun, paint gun)	Wound of entrance often pinpoint size; amount of actual tissue damage difficult to determine; foreign material may be directly toxic to tissues; dissects tissue planes, elevating pressures within tissue spaces; surgical wound exploration necessary to relieve pressure and determine extent of injury; complete necrosis, often resulting in amputation, not uncommon
Chain saw wound	Saw's "chewing" motion causes extensive tissue damage; wound closure may be impossible and grafts required; saw's wrenching motion may cause musculoskeletal trauma		
Chest "sucking" wound	Wound may allow air to enter pleural space, creating pneumothorax (air in pleural space); once covered, life-threatening pneumothorax may occur as large amounts of air escape through damaged lung/tracheobronchial tissue into pleural space; heart and great vessels are compressed, seriously impairing heart's output of blood (cardiac output)	Metal nail puncture	Wound edges seal off wound, promoting ideal environment for bacterial growth, especially anaerobic organisms; foreign material often present in wound (e.g., rubber from shoe sole); wound difficult to clean; bone inflammation from pus-producing organism (osteomyelitis) and bone destruction may occur
Crush injury	May cause massive tissue damage; tissue edema within closed fascial compartments may compress nerves or blood vessels, causing compartment syndrome; muscle tissue breakdown may cause myoglobinuria and renal failure	Power mower injury	Wounds sustained by objects hurled by the blades (not blade injuries) may be quite small; fractures or significant underlying tissue damage may be overlooked; the objects travel at a velocity similar to low-velocity bullets
Electrical injuries	Tissue damage magnitude difficult to determine and often minimized; cardiac arrhyth-		

TABLE 48-3. *Wounds Requiring Advanced Intervention* Continued

Wound	Rationale for Concern	Wound	Rationale for Concern
Septic wounds and necrotizing fasciitis	Serious infection, may be life-threatening; requires immediate excision of all necrotic tissue, antibiotic therapy, and frequent dressing changes		cussion of impaled objects under Foreign body wounds)
Stab wound	Size of external wound often does not indicate extent of internal damage; legally reportable; document information; preserve legal evidence if object present in wound (see dis-	Wounds from marine life, such as jellyfish, stingrays	Wounds inflicted by marine life or occurring in salt or fresh water are highly contaminated; significant infections may occur; possibility for envenomation (venom may have been injected into tissues)

control. We seldom see smallpox, diphtheria, or typhoid fever in the United States (smallpox is declared nonexistent in the world outside laboratory samples). In place of these diseases, however, are several blood-borne transmissible infectious processes, predominantly viral in origin, for which we have no current cure. The major infectious transmissible diseases are AIDS and hepatitis B and C. These three diseases are transmitted primarily by blood and by sexual contact.

When caring for individuals with any of these conditions, the nurse should be especially knowledgeable about reducing the risk to the care giver and reducing the likelihood of transmitting these organisms to other clients (see Chapter 28). Methods of reducing risk, however, should not make infected clients feel that they are not receiving the same care and consideration as others on the unit.

Blood is the single most important source of the viruses that cause AIDS and hepatitis B and C in the health care setting. The nurse must focus on preventing exposure to blood whenever possible and should receive hepatitis B immunization before assuming clinical responsibilities.

Giving wound care to clients with any of these diseases places the nurse at increased risk of exposure. Therefore, follow universal precautions as published by the Centers for Disease Control, the official United States agency responsible for research and recommendations on infectious diseases. These recommendations are continuously updated.[20-25]

The greatest risk to the nurse and other health care providers does not come from the person diagnosed with an infectious disease. The risk comes from the undiagnosed asymptomatic person. Therefore, universal precautions should be used when giving wound care to any person.

Use sterile gloves for procedures involving contact with normally sterile areas of the body, such as wounds. Use clean (unsterile or examination) gloves for procedures involving contact with mucous membranes, unless otherwise indicated, and for other client care or diagnostic procedures that do not require the use of sterile gloves. Change gloves between client contacts.

Do not become overly reliant on medical gloves to protect you from transmissible organisms. Bacteria and viruses can leak through gloves. Two per cent of all new gloves leak. Gloves that have been stressed with use have been demonstrated to leak more than 50 per cent of the time.[61] Gloves are only an additional protective barrier. To protect your client from any organisms that you might carry, wash your hands carefully before donning gloves. To protect yourself from the client's transmissible organisms, wash your hands carefully after any care procedure you perform.

The purpose of wearing gloves is to protect the health care worker and the client. Protection is possible only if clean or sterile gloves, as indicated, are put on before each client contact when the worker will be in contact with moist body surfaces and secretions.

If you suffer an occupational exposure to blood or any other body fluid that causes it to come into contact with your own blood (such as a needle stick) or mucous membranes (as by splashing of wound irrigating fluids), report the exposure at once. Reporting is especially important if the individual has known human immune deficiency virus (HIV) or hepatitis B infection.

Both the exposed worker and the source individual should be evaluated to determine the possible need for the exposed worker to receive prophylaxis. According to the guidelines of the Centers for Disease Control,

If the source individual has AIDS, is known to be HIV-seropositive, or refuses testing, the worker should be evaluated clinically and serologically for evidence of HIV infection as soon as possible after the exposure and if seronegative, should be retested periodically for a minimum of 6 months after exposure (e.g., 6 weeks, 12 weeks, and 6 months after exposure) to determine whether HIV infection has occurred.[24]

The duration of follow-up needed to detect evidence of HIV transmission is presently unknown.

Chronic Wounds: Pressure Ulcers

One chronic wound that all nurses encounter is the pressure ulcer. The National Pressure Ulcer Advisory Panel, an interdisciplinary group of experts, defines **pressure ulcers** as localized areas of tissue necrosis

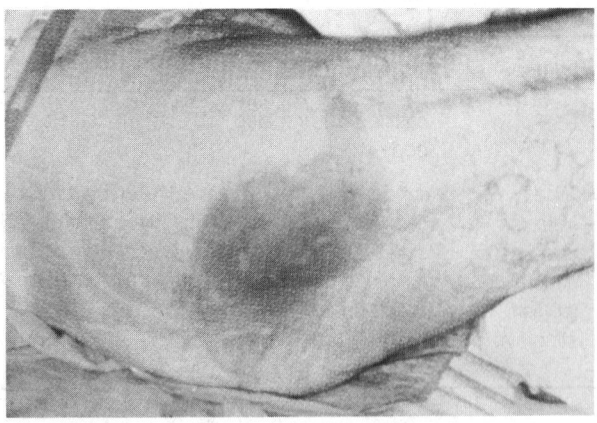

▲ **Figure 48-9**

Nonblanchable erythema. Stage I pressure ulcer. Even though unbroken, this skin is already pressure damaged and will break down within 24 to 48 hours. (Reprinted with permission from Parish, L.C., et al. [1983]. *The decubitus ulcer.* New York: Masson Publishing Co.)

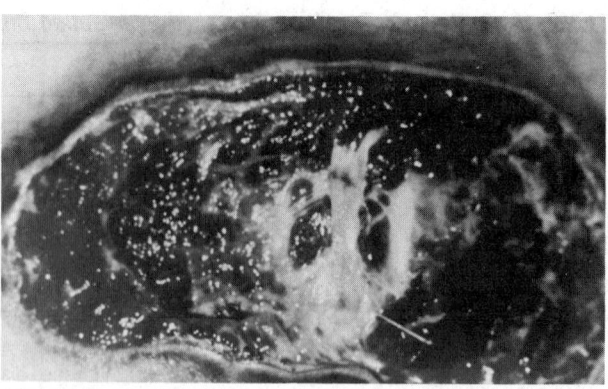

▲ **Figure 48-10**

Stage II pressure ulcer, which is healing. Tissue in the center is granulation tissue. Tissue around the wound is new epithelial cell growth. (Reprinted with permission from Parish, L.C., et al. [1983]. *The decubitus ulcer.* New York: Masson Publishing Co.)

that tend to develop when soft tissue is compressed between a bony prominence and an external surface for a prolonged period[75] (Figs. 48-9 through 48-12). This definition is consistent with that of the Agency for Health Care Policy and Research's Panel on the Prediction and Prevention of Pressure Ulcers in Adults.[1] Pressure ulcer is the preferred terminology for these skin and soft tissue wounds. Other less accurate names include "bedsore," a misnomer because many of these lesions occur as a result of sitting; "decubitus ulcer," a term deriving from the Latin word meaning to lie down or to recline; and "pressure sore," indicating that all lesions are "sore." Many clients, particularly paraplegic and quadriplegic persons, experience no sensation of discomfort at all. These people are at high risk for developing pressure ulcers, not all of which are caused by staying in bed.

Pressure ulcers represent a continuum from an erythematous soft tissue lesion to an open wound involving all of the body's tissues including the bone. The

recommended classification system appears in Table 48-4.

Nonblanchable erythema (see Fig. 48-9) is defined as erythema (redness) of the skin that persists when finger pressure is applied and then removed. For example, clients who have been lying on their backs for 1 hour will have red spots over the sacrum and other bony support surfaces when they are turned. These marks should disappear within one-half to three-fourths of the time that the individual has been lying on the area. If redness remains, then the tissue is already pressure damaged. It may be possible to prevent skin breakdown by keeping the client off the area until the skin and tissues recover. Blanchable erythema is redness that disappears within a short time when the client is turned off the spot. You can also depress the reddened spot with your finger and cause it to blanch. In nonblanchable erythema, redness does not disappear when finger pressure is removed.

Do not massage reddened areas of skin. If the skin is already injured, you will make the injury worse. If not permanently injured, skin will improve without mas-

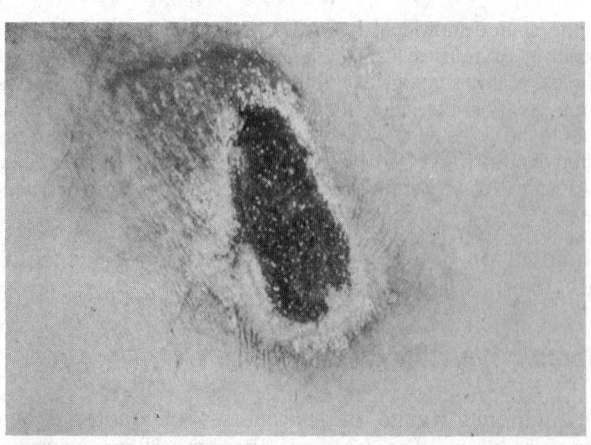

▲ **Figure 48-11**

Extensive stage III pressure ulcer down *to* but not through the fascia covering the muscle.

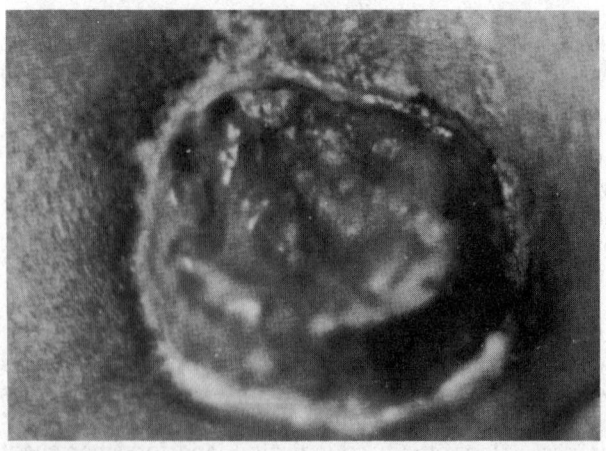

▲ **Figure 48-12**

Stage IV pressure ulcer, with full thickness of all soft tissues. Ulcers of this depth can penetrate through muscle to bone and joints.

TABLE 48-4. Pressure Ulcer Staging System

Stage	Definition
Stage I	Nonblanchable erythema of intact skin; the heralding lesion of skin ulceration (see Fig. 48-9)
Stage II	Partial-thickness skin loss involving epidermis, dermis, or both; the ulcer is superficial and presents clinically as an abrasion, blister, or shallow crater (see Fig. 48-10)
Stage III	Full-thickness skin loss involving damage or necrosis of subcutaneous tissue that may extend down to, but not through, underlying fascia; the ulcer presents clinically as a deep crater with or without undermining of adjacent tissue (see Fig. 48-11)
Stage IV	Full-thickness skin loss with extensive destruction, tissue necrosis, or damage to muscle, bone, or supporting structures (e.g., tendon, joint capsule); note: undermining and sinus tracks may also be associated with stage IV pressure ulcers (see Fig. 48-12)

As recommended by the National Pressure Ulcer Advisory Panel[75] and the Agency for Health Care Policy and Research.[1]

sage. Skin massage is a comfort measure only and should never be used on skin that is pressure damaged or skin that may be pressure damaged.[1,96]

Pressure ulcers are the most common chronic wounds found in both hospital and nursing home care settings. Studies indicate a prevalence rate (the number of old and new cases found at one point in time) in hospitals of 3 to 14 per cent, in nursing homes of 15 to 25 per cent, and in home health care settings of 7 to 12 per cent.[14,75] In projected numbers of people affected by this condition, estimates are 1.1 million to 1.8 million per year. Pressure ulcers are not a reportable condition in the United States as they are in some other countries, such as Great Britain; therefore, the United States has no national prevalence data.

No other chronic wound is as preventable as pressure ulcers are. We know the major etiologic factors: pressure, shear, and friction. We know that a number of clinical factors are implicated in a person's increased risk for pressure ulcer development: immobility, inactivity, malnutrition, fecal and urinary incontinence, decreased level of consciousness, advanced age (over 85 years carries a very high risk), fractures, and chronic systemic illness.[14,98]

PATHOPHYSIOLOGY OF PRESSURE ULCER DEVELOPMENT

Pressure exerts its influence on the capillary beds that supply the skin and soft tissues. At the arteriolar end of the capillary bed (the entering vessels), the mean pressure in normal, healthy, young adults is approximately 32 mm Hg. At the venous end of the capillary bed, it is approximately 12 mm Hg. The pressure in the midportion of the capillary bed is approximately 20 mm Hg.[59] In elderly, debilitated clients, it is probably significantly

less. The skin and soft tissues cannot tolerate pressures in excess of **capillary closing pressure** (the amount of externally applied pressure required to occlude capillary blood flow totally, generally accepted as 32 mm Hg) for long periods without sustaining damage that is often not reversible. Therefore, to prevent pressure damage to the skin and soft tissues, the individual must not be left in the same position in bed or a chair for lengthy periods.

The usual turning schedule for clients who cannot or will not turn themselves is 2 hours in any one position. No scientific data for humans validate 2 hours as the appropriate time; it is a time that has proved sufficient to protect most clients. Two hours might be too long for an elderly, debilitated client to remain in the same position without suffering skin and soft tissue damage. Sitting in chairs for long periods is also dangerous. Individuals who are able, such as paraplegics, should be taught to raise their buttocks from the chair for 10 to 15 seconds every 15 minutes (Fig. 48-13). If they are unable to raise themselves, they should not be left in the chair for longer than 1 hour and preferably less.[1] Both pressure *and* time are important in the causation of pressure ulcers.

A number of pressure-reducing beds, mattresses, mattress overlays, and chair cushions help control the pressure problem. Table 48-5 lists some of these by brand name. These devices are designed for use with clients who are at high risk for the development of

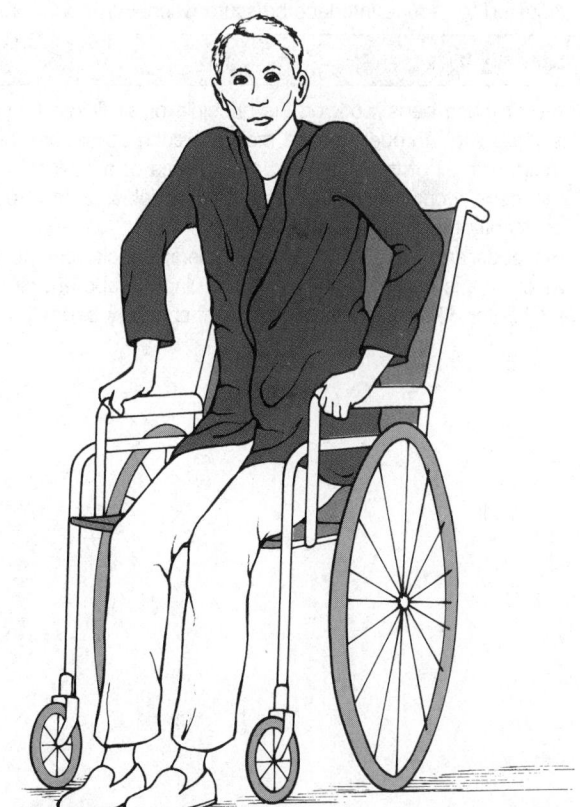

▲ *Figure 48-13*

Clients who have sufficient upper-body strength should be taught to relieve pressure over the ischial tuberosities by lifting themselves for 15 seconds, allowing blood to reperfuse ischemic areas every 15 minutes.

TABLE 48-5. *Pressure-Reducing Support Surfaces*

Classification	Example
Mattress Overlays	
These products are designed to be placed on top of the regular hospital mattress; their ability to reduce pressure to safe levels is variable	Bio Gard
	Egg Crate
Foam	geo-Matt
The thicker the foam, the better the level of skin protection; 4 inches of foam is the minimum necessary for significant pressure reduction	
Static Air	Roho
These devices contain air that moves from one place to another within the mattress or chair pad passively when the client's position changes	Sof-Care
	Sof-Care Plus
Alternating Air	AIRFLO/AIRFLO PLUS
These devices generally are connected to a mechanical motor of varying design that alternately inflates and deflates cells within the mattress or pad	Bio Flote
The thicker the air cell, the better the level of skin protection	Pillo-Pump
Gel/Water/Polymer	Action Mattress Pads (polymer)
These mattress overlays or chair pads contain one of the three substances listed	Akros DFD Gel Topper
Gels are close to the consistency of human fat; water is much thinner in its consistency, but all three substances provide protection primarily by their depth rather than their consistency	Aqua-Pedics (water)
The thicker the overlay, the better the level of skin protection	
Replacement Mattresses	**Replacement Units**
These mattresses are designed to be used in place of the regular bed mattress	Bio Gard PLUS
They may be constructed of foam, water enclosed in a vinyl shell, air contained in a vinyl shell, gel, or some combination of these elements	Century 2000
	Clinisert
Low Air Loss Bed Systems	First Step Plus
These beds are composed of air cushions that allow minimal air loss through tiny perforations in the air cushions; they are attached to a mechanical device that replaces the air lost from the cushions as needed; the client is in a bed that can be adjusted to reduce interface pressure whenever repositioning occurs	PNEU-CARE Acute
Specialty Beds	**Air Fluidized Therapy**
Some of these beds work on the principle of air fluidization (i.e., sufficient air pressure is "bubbled" through a solid medium, such as silicon spheres, to make it act as a liquid, with all of the support characteristics of a liquid)	Clinitron
	FluidAir Plus
	Skytron
Some beds work on the low air loss principles; a few (e.g., kinetic beds) work by constantly turning the client	Low air loss therapy
	Flexicair
Some beds are more effective than others; check your hospital policy manual to see which one is indicated for use in each individual client circumstance	KinAir
	Mediscus Low Air Loss System
See Chapter 35 for further description of specialty beds	PNEU-CARE Acute
	Low air loss with kinetic modalities
	BioDyne
	PNEU-CARE ICU
	Pulmonair-40
	Restcue
	TheraPulse
	Kinetic therapy without low air loss
	Keane Mobility
	RotoRest
	For the obese client
	Burke Bariatric Bed
	Magnum 800 System
	Mediscus HD System
	Pediatric use beds
	Clinitron
	Pedcare System
	PediKair
	PNEU-CARE/Pedi

Categories are listed from least expensive to most expensive. As a general rule, the most expensive are also the most effective at pressure relief. Examples listed are those commonly available in many hospitals. Not all products within a category may perform equally well. No endorsement of any product is made by the fact that it is listed.

pressure ulcers as a result of inability to move themselves because of loss of consciousness, weakness, medications, or other factors. The devices vary in their ability to reduce interface pressure (the pressure between the client's body and the surface on which the client rests) to safe levels. They will not prevent pressure ulcers from developing, but they may provide added time for clients to remain in one position safely.

Certain points on the body are more prone to pressure damage than are others. These are usually bony prominences because they support most of the body's weight. Figure 35–4 identifies these points. Most pressure ulcers occur on the lower half of the body because of the usual weight distribution in most humans. If the individual is seated in a wheelchair, gerichair, or other type of chair, then the person is likely to develop pressure ulcers over the ischial tuberosities because they are the bony prominences on which most of the body's weight rests. These people are also at risk for foot and heel ulcers as a result of pressure.

Shearing force is the second major etiologic factor in the production of pressure ulcers. It affects all tissue layers, but its primary effect is on the deeper tissues. Shear is the result of pressure, gravity, and friction acting together. In a client lying in bed, gravity pushes down on the body, causing pressure, and any attempt to move that person causes some degree of friction because the weight of the body tends to hold it in one place. The superficial skin and soft tissues are temporarily "stuck" to the bed surface while the deeper soft tissues (i.e., muscle and fascia) are more bound to the bony skeleton.

Moving the client toward the head of the bed without lifting the body causes shearing force applied to the deeper perforator blood vessels contained in the muscular layer; the result is severe angulation of those vessels and interrupted blood supply. Superficial soft tissues can be further deprived of sufficient blood supply when small thrombi form in these vessels. The eventual result is a pressure ulcer. Shear is not so much of a problem in turning the client from side to side, but it is a major problem in moving the client up in the bed. It is also a problem for those clients who continuously sit in Fowler's position in bed to watch television, talk to visitors, and eat meals. These clients tend to slide down because of gravity. The skin over the entire back, especially the sacrum, is then held in one spot while the body weight pulls the remaining soft tissues and skeleton downward. In order to minimize the effects of shear on the body, the head of the bed should never be elevated more than 30 degrees in the patient at risk. The National Pressure Ulcer Advisory Panel and the Agency for Health Care Policy and Research recommend that nursing personnel observe the "rule of 30" when caring for the person at risk for pressure ulcers:[1,75] (1) in turning clients to the side-lying position, they should be turned to only 30 degrees to help prevent trochanteric ulcers from forming; (2) in elevating the head of the bed for meals or other activities, the bed should be kept at 30 degrees or less to minimize shearing forces on the soft tissues of the back and sacrum. Lower the bed when the activity is completed.

Friction is the third factor in the production of pressure ulcers. Friction occurs because of the effects of gravity pushing down on the body while it is in contact with another surface on which it rests (bed or chair). In people who are immobile or too weak to turn without assistance, friction becomes a major factor in the production of certain types of pressure ulcers. If friction and pressure act without significant shearing force, then the pressure damage is likely to be superficial, such as is found in a "sheet burn." If significant shearing force is involved, the lesion is different.

If people are pulled rather than lifted when they are repositioned in the bed or chair, the outer protective layer of skin can be rubbed away because of friction. People who have uncontrollable spasms of extremities, such as new paraplegics, can cause a wearing away of the skin surface as well. Their legs and heels should be padded for protection. Clients who have internal fracture fixation devices, such as screws, nails, and plates, sometimes develop pressure ulcers because of the effect of the internal device rubbing the muscle that overlies it. The pressure ulcer begins in the inner tissue and will not be obvious at the skin surface until all internal layers have been affected. Pressure ulcers due to the combination of friction and pressure can be prevented by turning clients carefully and with sufficient numbers of personnel to keep from "dragging" the client over the surface.

CONTROLLING RISK FACTORS FOR PRESSURE ULCERS

Other methods for controlling the factors that have been identified as placing a person at increased risk range from simple tasks to complex or insolvable ones.

Immobility and Inactivity. Keep the person moving as much as practicable. If the person is unconscious or otherwise unable to move, use a regular turning schedule. Place a "turning clock" on the foot of the bed and on the care plan and indicate the hours to be turned and the position to which the person should be turned (e.g., supine at 2 PM, 30 degrees on right side at 4 PM). If the position is indicated for each turn, there will be no question whether turning was done at a particular time (Fig. 48–14).

Malnutrition. The person who is malnourished is at increased risk for pressure ulcers and has a much more difficult time healing those that do occur. A lack of sufficient essential body nutrients also impairs the immune system, which makes the pressure ulcer more prone to infection.

People who develop pressure ulcers are usually protein deficient, especially if the ulcer is draining; up to 30 gm of protein can be lost from one large pressure ulcer in a single day. People at risk for pressure ulcer development need to consume 0.8 gm of protein per kilogram of body weight. Those with pressure ulcers need more: 1.5 to 2 gm per kilogram of body weight. Baseline and periodic assessment of the at-risk client's protein status should be done by the physician. Serum

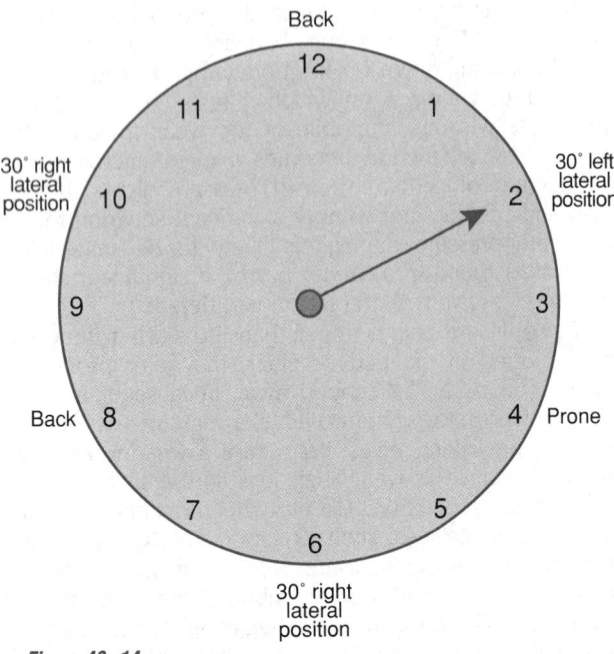

Back
12
11   1
30° right
lateral
position   10   30° left
lateral
position
2
9   3
Back   8   4   Prone
7   5
6
30° right
lateral
position

▲ *Figure 48–14*

Turning clock indicating both time of turning and the position to which the patient is to be turned. If certain positions are contraindicated, the positions on the clock can be tailored to the individual client's needs.

albumin is the test most frequently done, but it does not reflect changes in protein stores quickly. Serum transferrin has been found to be more rapidly responsive to changes in protein levels. If the serum albumin level is 3 gm/dl, the client should be considered deficient. At 2.5 gm/dl or less, there is severe protein depletion.

It is not easy to get food into the malnourished person. Favorite foods should be made available, if possible. These people should receive sufficient fluids, especially if they are in negative nitrogen balance, because fluids will assist in the elimination of large amounts of nitrogenous waste caused by protein depletion. They should also receive intravenous fluids if oral fluid intake is not sufficient. Vitamin supplements should be given. The person unable to eat enough to meet body needs should be placed on liquid nutritional supplements with high-quality protein (this is a medical responsibility and may not be possible if the person has systemic disease, such as kidney disease, that prevents using protein). Tube feedings or total parenteral nutrition may be necessary in some instances.

Fecal and Urinary Incontinence. Several large research studies indicate that fecal incontinence is much more likely to place a client at risk for pressure ulcers than is urinary incontinence alone. The reasons for this finding may be that clients with fecal incontinence are usually sicker than are those with urinary incontinence only and that feces contain a number of autolytic enzymes not present in urine.[101] It is undeniable, however, that the constant wetness caused by urinary incontinence and fecal incontinence can macerate the skin. **Maceration** is a softening of the tissues that makes them more prone to erosion.

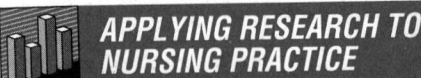

APPLYING RESEARCH TO NURSING PRACTICE

Determining Risk for Pressure Ulcers on the Basis of Nutritional Status

Ek, A-C., Unosson, M., & Bjurulf, P. (1989). The modified Norton scale and the nutritional state. *Scandinavian Journal of Caring Science, 3*(4), 183–187.

▼ ▼ ▼

Both *extrinsic* factors (those outside the client) and *intrinsic* factors (those within the client) lead to the development of pressure ulcers. We know that the primary extrinsic factors are pressure, shearing forces, and temperature. However, there has been little research on what intrinsic factors put clients at risk for pressure ulcers.

In 1960, the Norton scale was devised as a tool for predicting which clients are at risk for developing pressure ulcers. The scale included ratings (ranging from 1 to 4) of intrinsic client factors in each of the following categories: general physical condition, mental state, mobility, activity, and incontinence. Clients with low total scores have consistently been found to be more likely to develop pressure ulcers.

Other research has shown that malnutrition may be a factor leading to the development of pressure ulcers. Ek and colleagues therefore modified the Norton scale to include ratings of two new categories: food intake and fluid intake. These researchers then applied their modified Norton scale to 501 clients in a long-term care setting. They also evaluated the same clients for the presence of malnutrition on the basis of weight index, triceps skinfold thickness, arm muscle circumference, serum protein analysis, and a delayed hypersensitivity skin test. Ek and colleagues found that malnourished clients (34.8 per cent) were more likely than nonmalnourished clients (20.6 per cent) to have had pressure ulcers on admission or to develop them during the hospital stay. The researchers also found a significant correlation among malnutrition, pressure ulcers, and the following categories of the modified Norton scale: mobility, food intake, fluid intake, and general physical condition.

Applications for Nursing Practice

The results of this study suggest that you can reliably use Ek's modified Norton scale to decide which of your clients warrant special interventions for prevention of pressure ulcers.

Incontinence should be carefully managed. A simple approach in the conscious client is to ask at regular intervals (at least every 2 hours) about the need to use the bedpan or urinal. If the person is able to use these utensils without assistance, place them within easy reach. If the person is not able to make needs known, then use incontinence pads that are able to "wick" moisture away from the body. Cleanse the skin after each soiling with a nonionic cleanser and apply a skin barrier (Table 48–6).

TABLE 48–6. Wound Management Products

Classification	Example
Wound Cleansers Used to cleanse wound of foreign debris, drainage, loose necrotic tissue Should be nonionic, if possible, so that tissue regrowth is not damaged	Isotonic saline—cheap, nonionic cleanser; readily available Commercial cleansers 　Carrington Ultra Klenz 　Puri-Clens 　Saf-Clens 　Shur-Clens Hydrogen peroxide—not a nonionic cleanser but frequently used because of its efficiency in removing organic matter from a wound; it slows wound healing
Gauze Dressings Nonocclusive dressings that function to protect the wound from outside contamination or injury	Cotton mesh—in various sizes, with or without cotton filling; usual size is 4 × 4 inches Gauze wrapping—used to hold other dressings in place; wrappings may have slight degree of elasticity, which helps them conform to the body surface; examples: 　Conform 　Kling/Sof-Kling Hypertonic absorbing gauze dressing impregnated with saline —used in draining wounds, such as pressure ulcers; example: 　Mesalt
Nonadherent Dressings May be impregnated with medication or nonimpregnated Useful for skin tears, donor sites, and skin grafts Some impregnated forms contain antimicrobial agents that are cytotoxic to fibroblasts	Nonimpregnated 　Adaptic 　Release 　Telfa Impregnated 　Scarlet red 　Vaseline gauze 　Xeroflo 　Xeroform
Transparent Films Used for superficial wounds, donor sites, abrasions, burns, and autolysis of necrotic tissue Minimally absorbent and do not stay on well in high-friction areas Transmit moisture vapor from wound; semipermeable	Bioclusive OpSite Tegaderm Tegaderm Pouch
Composite Dressings Semipermeable; designed to displace wound exudate in heavily draining wounds	Airstrip Gel-Syte PolyDerm WBC POLYMEM Viasorb
Hydrocolloids Used on a wide variety of acute and chronic wounds and for autolysis of necrotic tissue Very conformable and good for hard-to-cover and high-friction spots Impermeable dressings; do not use in infected wounds	Comfeel DuoDERM Intact J & J Ulcer Dressing Restore 3M Tegasorb
Hydrogels/Gels Nonadhesive or adhesive; most can be used in both clean and infected wounds Decrease wound temperature, decrease inflammation, provide pain relief A gauze dressing and a transparent film should be used over them to hold them in place Some of these can be used on stage IV pressure ulcers	Biolex Wound Gel Carrington Spray-Gel 　Wound Dressing Geliperm Wet/Granulate IntraSite Gel NuGel Vigilon
Calcium Alginates Dry dressings that become a hydrogel when they come into contact with sodium-rich wound exudate	Algosteril Kaltostat Sorbsan

Table continued on following page

TABLE 48–6. Wound Management Products Continued

Classification	Example
Exudate Absorbers	Allevyn Cavity Wound Dressing
Dressings, beads, or pastes that absorb several times their own weight in wound exudate; used only in heavily draining wounds	Bard Absorption Dressing
	Debrisan
	Comfeel paste/powder
Autolyze necrotic tissue	DuoDERM Paste/Granules
Foams	Allevyn
Nonadhesive, nonadherent	Epi-Lock
Insulate wound and are moderately absorptive; good for leg ulcers; very comfortable	LYOfoam A (for pressure ulcers, burns, postoperative use)
	LYOfoam C (for leg ulcers, radiation injuries)
May re-injure tissue if allowed to dry before removal	Mitraflex
Carbon-Impregnated Dressings	LYOfoam C (Odor-Absorbent Dressing)
To help control wound odor	
Skin Barriers	Bard Special Care Moisture Barrier Ointment
To prevent maceration of skin from constant moisture	Barri-Care
Wound Deodorizers	Buttermilk
Internally ingested or topically applied agents to neutralize wound odor	Derifil tablets
	Medi-aire
	MetroGel
	Osto-zyme
	PALS
	Puri-Clens
	Plain yogurt
Enzymatic Debriding Agents	Biozyme-C
Special formulations of enzymes and other agents used to debride necrotic tissue in wound bed without damaging growing tissue	Elase
	Panafil Ointment
	Panafil White Ointment
	Santyl
	Travase
Stimulating Sprays	Granulex
Designed to stimulate growth of normal wound healing	Proderm
Leg Ulcer Wraps	Dome-Paste
Designed for use with venous stasis ulcers	DuoDERM Venous Ulcer Kit
	POLYMEM Roll Dressing
	Unna-Pak
	Viscopaste PB7

Not all products within a category may perform equally well. The listing of a product is not an endorsement.

Do not use incontinence pads with plastic backing that will not keep moisture "wicked" away from the client's skin surface. These products will contribute to skin maceration, not prevent it.

Decreased Level of Consciousness. If the person's level of consciousness is less than alert (e.g., if the person is on tranquilizers, sedatives, hypnotics), the person will not move as frequently as necessary to prevent skin damage. Decreased consciousness makes a person less responsive to the discomfort of remaining in one position for long periods. The person must be reminded to turn at intervals. Someone who is semi-conscious or comatose will have to be turned.

Advanced Age. Old age is the insolvable factor in controlling the risk of pressure ulcers. As people grow older, their skin becomes thinner and more atrophic. Many studies have indicated that the old-old (above 85 years) are at greatly increased risk largely because of skin changes, decreased mobility, and chronic systemic illnesses that complicate prevention. These people should be placed on bed surfaces that decrease the pressure on the body's supporting surfaces to as low a level as practicable without high cost (see Table 48–5). If the elderly client is at greatly increased risk, the pressure-reducing bed, mattress, or mattress overlay best suited to the person's needs should be used. Some of these are shown in Figures 48–15 to 48–17.

Fractures. Clients with fractures, especially those with traction devices, are at increased risk because their mobility is greatly impaired. People in traction should be placed on mattresses or mattress overlays that help decrease pressure on the body's supporting surface to less than capillary closing pressure. If they are in casts, they should be observed for signs that a cast is too tight, such as pain, discomfort, areas under the cast where the client has no sensation, or areas where "burning" pain is felt. Pressure ulcers can easily develop inside the cast. Other signs of cast tightness are decreased capillary blood flow return when the toenail

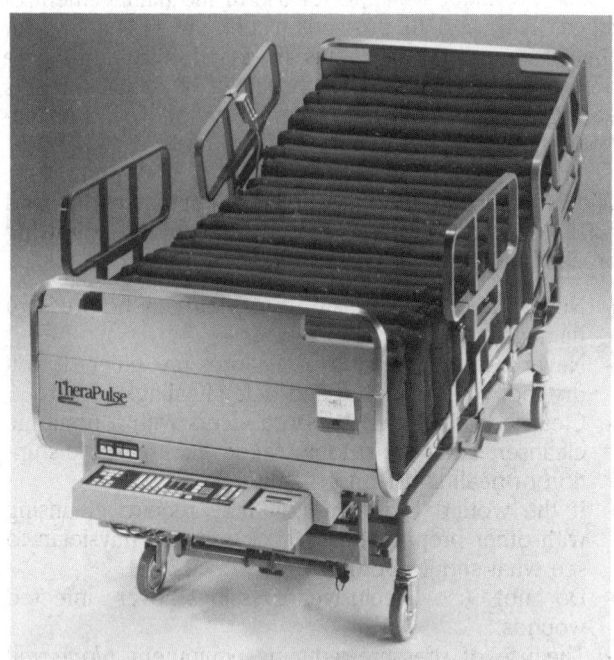

▲ *Figure 48–16*

Low air loss bed having the capability of reducing pressure on the body's support surfaces to less than capillary closing pressure. (Courtesy of Kinetic Concepts, Inc., San Antonio, TX.)

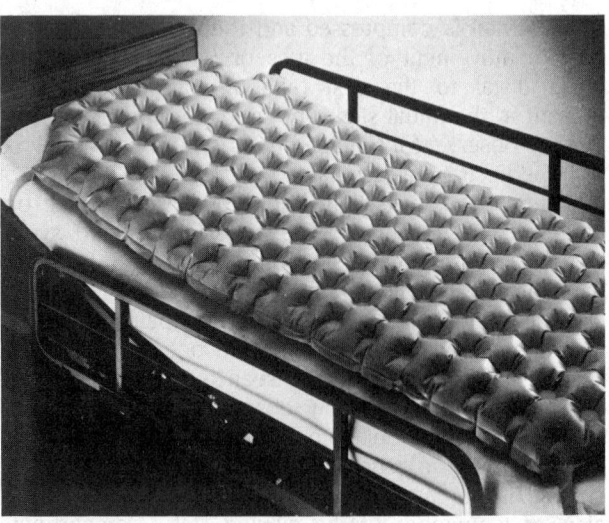

▲ *Figure 48–15*

Air mattress overlay designed to relieve pressure on the body's support surfaces. (Courtesy of Gaymar Industries, Orchard Park, NY.)

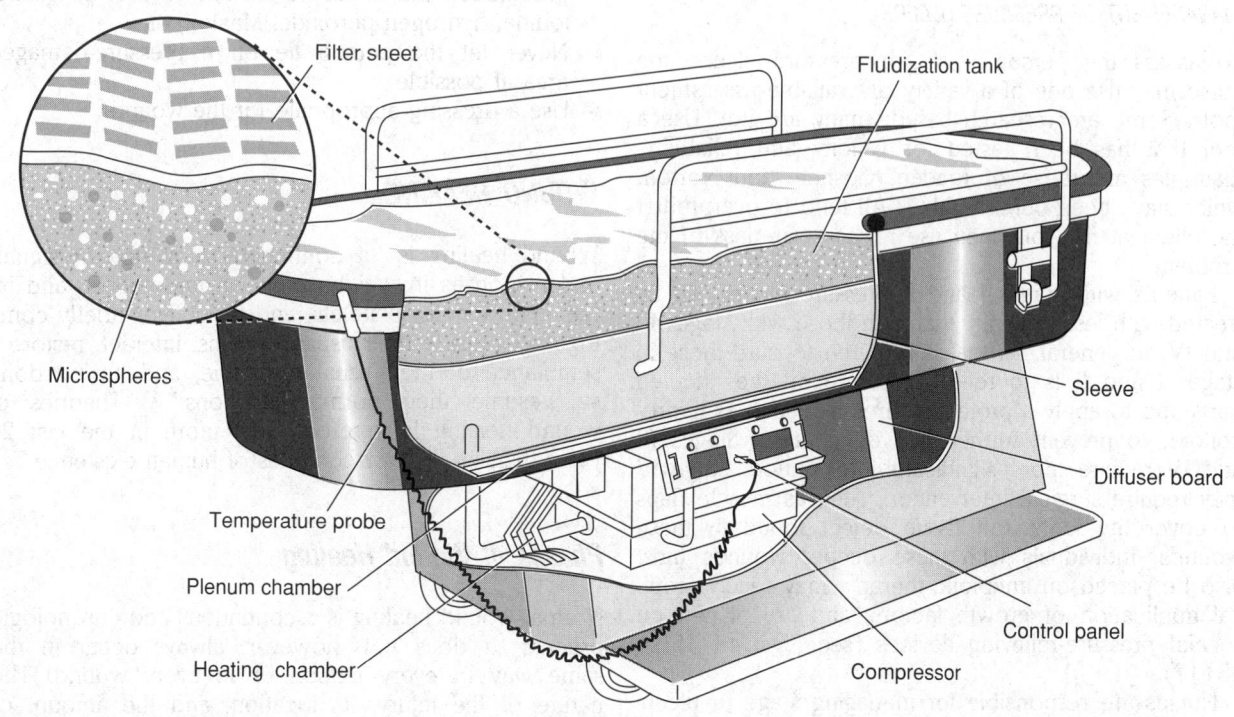

Filter sheet

Fluidization tank

Microspheres

Sleeve

Temperature probe

Diffuser board

Plenum chamber

Control panel

Heating chamber

Compressor

▲ *Figure 48–17*

Air-fluidized (Clinitron) bed that has the capability of reducing pressure on the body's support surfaces to less than capillary closing pressure. Air is "bubbled" through the microspheres (silicon granules), and the client floats on top of this air-fluidized medium. (Courtesy of Support Systems International, Inc., Charleston, SC.)

or fingernail is compressed and then released, pain on passive movement of the toes or fingers, and lack of pulse distal to the cast (although a pulse may be present in the initial stages of circulatory problems).

Also observe for compartment syndrome, a unique orthopedic trauma-associated injury due to swelling of the muscle inside its tightly adherent fascia, which occludes its blood supply. The classic signs and symptoms of compartment syndrome are the 5 Ps: pain, paresthesia (tingling sensation), pallor, puffiness (edema), and pulselessness. Of these, pain on passive movement is the most reliable and one of the earliest signs. If any of these signs is seen in the distal portion of a casted extremity, your observations should be reported at once. A delay could mean the loss of a limb. The treatment of such a finding includes immediate cutting of the cast with special equipment by the physician or a member of the nursing staff. Compartment syndrome usually occurs in extremities; it is associated with leg fractures in adults and with forearm fractures in children.

Chronic Systemic Illness. Various types of systemic illnesses place the client at greater risk for pressure ulcer development. These include cardiovascular diseases, peripheral vascular disease, diabetes, and cancer. These conditions must be treated in a satisfactory manner before the risk of pressure ulcers can be decreased. These individuals should be assessed regularly for skin problems and pressure-reduction devices used to prevent breakdown.

MANAGEMENT OF PRESSURE ULCERS

To assess the person's risk for pressure ulcers, the nurse may use one of a variety of available assessment tools. Some are research based; many are not. Use a tool that has been tested for validity and reliability. Examples are those of Braden, Gosnell, and Norton, which have been published.[1,7,39] All tend to overpredict the client at risk, but their use raises awareness of the problem.

Patients with stages I and II pressure ulcers can be treated with less difficulty than can those with stages III and IV. In general, all that is required to cure those in stages I and II is to relieve pressure on the affected parts and to apply a protective dressing, such as hydrocolloid, to prevent further skin denudation. Stages III and IV require more significant intervention. Stage IV may require surgical intervention, such as muscle flaps to cover the large soft tissue defect found in these wounds. Individuals with these deeper wounds must also be placed on antibiotic therapy, may receive topical application of growth factors, and are placed on special pressure-relieving devices (see Figs. 48–15 to 48–17).

Nurses are responsible for managing stage III ulcers with medical protocols written for the individual. Stage IV pressure ulcers are initially managed by physicians with **debridement** (removal of foreign material or dead or damaged tissue from a wound—may be done surgically, enzymatically, or with certain types of

wound dressings), systemic antibiotics, and, if possible, surgical wound closure as soon as is deemed safe. Care for these individuals so that pressure is not placed over the site of surgical repair, or it will break down again.

The products available for use in the management of stages I, II, and III pressure ulcers and indications for their use are listed in Tables 48–5 and 48–6 and Figure 48–18. You will have to consult the physician's orders about pressure ulcer management or follow the institution's protocol.

With so much misunderstanding about preventing and safely caring for pressure ulcers, keep the following precautions in mind:

▶ Never rub reddened skin. It may already be pressure damaged.
▶ Never use a heat lamp on a pressure ulcer. It will dry the wound surface and delay healing.
▶ Cleanse noninfected pressure ulcers with a nonionic cleanser, such as isotonic saline, to prevent disruption of healing. Cleanse gently.
▶ If the wound is infected, it may require cleansing with other preparations. Check with the physician to see what should be used.
▶ Do not use occlusive dressings over infected wounds.
▶ The use of pressure-reducing equipment *alone* will not prevent pressure ulcers indefinitely. Their use must be combined with good nursing care.
▶ Never put any topical preparation on a noninfected pressure ulcer that would not be safe to put in your eye. This prohibition rules out almost every favorite preparation that most nurses like to use: povidone-iodine, hydrogen peroxide, Maalox, etc.
▶ Never let the person lie on a pressure-damaged area, if possible.
▶ Use a dressing appropriate for the wound.

WOUND HEALING

Wound healing is "a continuous sequence of signals and responses in which epithelial, endothelial, and inflammatory cells, platelets, and fibroblasts briefly come together outside their usual domains, interact, restore a semblance of their usual discipline, and having done so, resume their normal functions."[44] Theories of wound healing have progressed more in the last 20 years than in all prior centuries of human existence.

Phases of Wound Healing

Normal wound healing is a continuous and chronologic process. It does not, however, always occur in the same way in every person or in every wound. The nature of the injury, its location, and the amount of tissue involved directly influence which cells predominate in the process, at what point they maximally function, and at what point they cease to function.

Three phases are usually identified in the normal healing process:[94] (1) inflammatory phase, (2) prolifer-

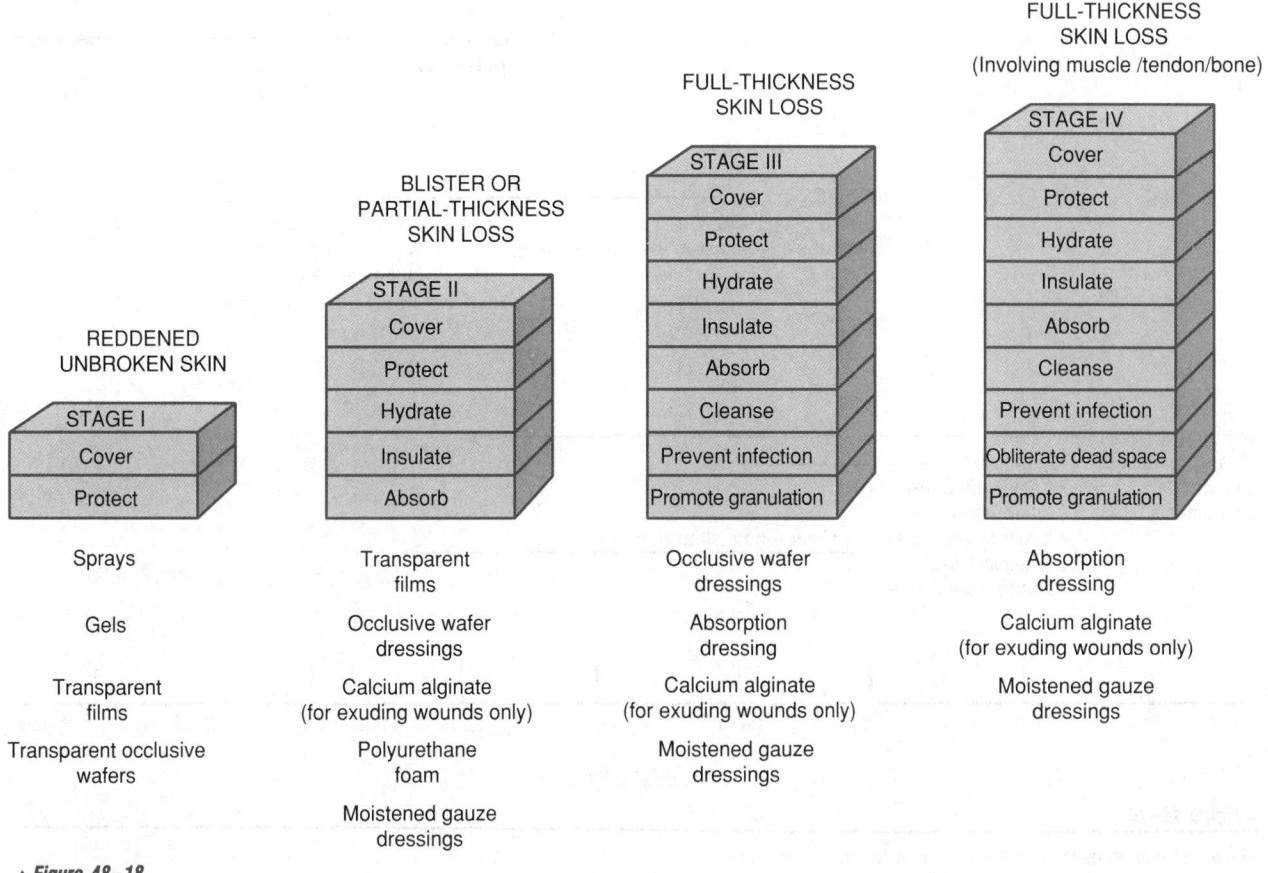

▲ Figure 48–18

Indications for wound management products. (Courtesy of Katherine F. Jeter, Spartanburg Regional Medical Center, Spartanburg, SC.)

ative phase, and (3) maturation phase. Each of these phases encompasses one or more specific processes (Table 48–7 and Fig. 48–19). These processes are coagulation, inflammation, fibroplasia, matrix deposition (often referred to clinically as collagen deposition), angiogenesis, epithelialization, contraction, and remodeling.

The inflammatory phase lasts approximately 3 days. Injury causes damage to the vessel wall and attracts platelets, which aggregate (cluster). The platelets pro-

mote formation of a fibrin clot, the function of which is to prevent bleeding at the wound site. Vasoconstriction lasts about 5 to 10 minutes. Within 10 to 30 minutes, vasodilation occurs and persists for varying amounts of time. This phase accounts for most of the signs and symptoms associated with wounds.

The cardinal signs and symptoms of inflammation are redness (rubor), heat (calor), pain (dolor), and swelling (tumor).

TABLE 48–7. Sequence of Normal Wound Healing[52,111]

Phase	Cellular Events
Inflammatory phase (lasts 3 days)	Vasoconstriction, lasts 5 to 10 minutes Vasodilation begins immediately after vasoconstriction Polymorphonuclear neutrophils appear, and the complement system is activated Monocytes become macrophages, which secrete growth factors, phagocytose bacteria, and clean wound
Proliferative phase (lasts from day 3 to day 21)	Macrophages initiate fibroplasia Matrix synthesis occurs Angiogenesis re-establishes blood flow in wound bed Epithelialization covers wound surface Contraction of wound occurs
Maturation phase (lasts from day 21 to weeks, months, or years)	Wound scar forms as a result of collagen remodeling Tensile strength increases over approximately 10 weeks; never more than 80% of pre-wound strength is regained after healing

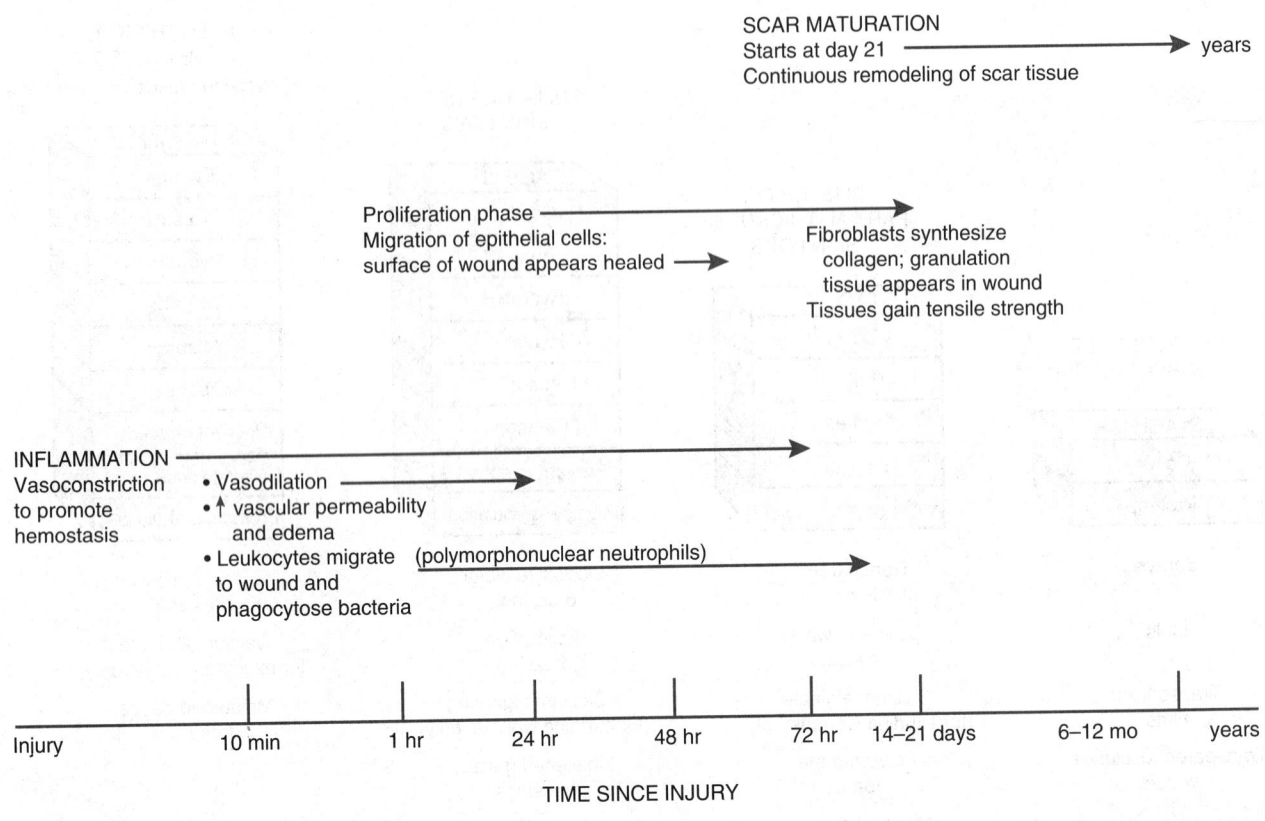

SCAR MATURATION
Starts at day 21 ⟶ years
Continuous remodeling of scar tissue

Proliferation phase
Migration of epithelial cells:
surface of wound appears healed ⟶

Fibroblasts synthesize
collagen; granulation
tissue appears in wound
Tissues gain tensile strength

INFLAMMATION
Vasoconstriction
to promote
hemostasis

• Vasodilation ⟶
• ↑ vascular permeability
  and edema
• Leukocytes migrate   (polymorphonuclear neutrophils)
  to wound and
  phagocytose bacteria

| Injury | 10 min | 1 hr | 24 hr | 48 hr | 72 hr | 14–21 days | 6–12 mo | years |

TIME SINCE INJURY

▲ *Figure 48–19*

Phases of wound healing and time frames for normal wounds.

The complement system (a series of enzymes in the serum) is activated to assist with bacteriolysis (bacterial destruction) by coating the microbial invaders (opsonization) so that the white blood cells can phagocytose them. The complement system produces the main chemoattractants for neutrophils and monocytes. The first white blood cells to appear are the polymorphonuclear neutrophils. They function largely for the first 3 days after the wound is sustained, and their job is to clear the wound of microbial invaders. The continued presence of large quantities of polymorphonuclear neutrophils after the first 3 days can be a sign of infection.

Inflammatory cells accumulate. By day 3, the presence of neutrophils is secondary to the presence of macrophages, which begin to appear in the wound at about 24 hours. They engulf bacteria, debride (clean) the wound, and secrete angiogenesis factor, which stimulates the formation of blood vessels. The macrophages, which remove dead tissue from the wound, are cells essential for healing to take place.

The proliferative phase lasts from approximately day 3 to day 21. This phase overlaps the inflammatory phase to a certain extent, and it continues until the wound is healed. Macrophages continue to be important in this phase because they are responsible for the fibroplasia occurring at this point. Fibroblasts are the major source of collagen, which repairs the injured tissue and helps return it to an approximation of its pre-injury state. These cells begin to appear in the wound about 24 hours after the injury.

Inflammation is of great importance to the establishment of fibroplasia. If there is no inflammation, it is difficult for fibroplasia to be established. Fibroblasts reproduce poorly in a wound environment that lacks oxygen, sufficient nutrition, and insulin.

At about 5 days after the injury, the fibroblast synthesis of **matrix** (the collagen and proteoglycan scaffolding that supports soft tissue repair) begins to be evident through the development of **granulation tissue** (beefy red tissue seen in a healing wound and composed of newly formed collagen and blood vessels). From day 5 to day 15, there is a progressive increase in the **tensile strength** (the wound's ability to withstand disruptive forces without rupturing) of the wound because of increased matrix production (collagen and proteoglycans). Tensile strength continues to increase with each successive day.

In a surgical wound, in which the skin is sutured together, a "healing ridge" of tissue can be felt just under the suture line. This ridge is evidence of normal matrix production. If it is not present by five to seven days after surgery, its lack is evidence that wound healing is not progressing as expected. Breakdown is a significant possibility and danger. This **dehiscence** (breaking open of a surgical incision without organ protrusion) is likely to occur between 5 and 12 days postoperatively (Figs. 48–20 and 48–21). **Serosanguineous drainage** (clear, blood-tinged serous drainage), which begins to occur on a previously intact and dry suture line, is often a sign that breakdown is about

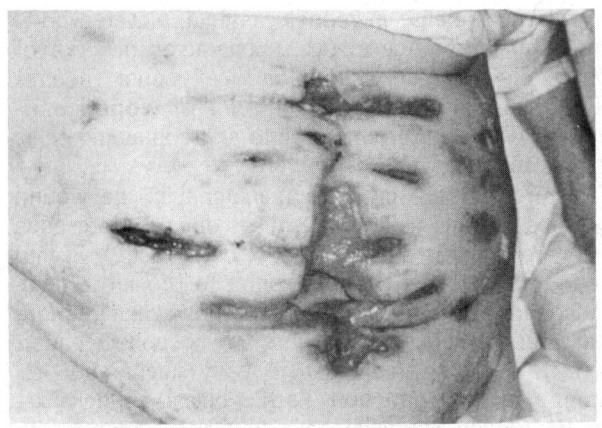

▲ *Figure 48-20*

Wound dehiscence resulting from excessively tight suturing. (Reprinted with permission from Westaby, S. [ed.]. [1986]. *Wound care.* London: Butterworth-Heinemann.)

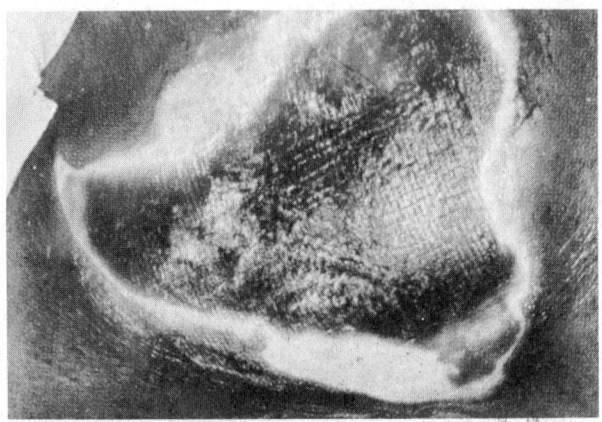

▲ *Figure 48-22*

Eschar covering wound surface. Eschar must be removed for healing to occur. Removal may be done surgically or by the use of specially formulated enzyme preparations. (Reprinted with permission from Parish, L.C., et al. [1983]. *The decubitus ulcer.* New York: Masson Publishing Co.)

to occur. It should be reported at once. The wound becomes smaller because of the influence of myofibroblasts (fibroblastic cells with contractile ability). They influence the new collagen in the wound to draw the wound margins toward the center, thus decreasing its size.

Epithelialization (the growth of epithelial cells across the surface of a wound) occurs primarily during the proliferative phase. Epithelial cells begin to migrate across the wound from its margins and from the epidermal appendages (from around any hair follicles or sweat ducts that might remain in the wound). This process continues until epithelial cells meet others that have migrated from opposite directions. When cells meet, **contact inhibition** (pressure generated between touching cells that halts their horizontal movement) occurs. Foreign material and **desiccation** (drying of body tissues) impede epithelial regeneration.[44]

Epithelial cells migrate more rapidly across a wound surface that is moist. Drying of the wound surface impedes healing.

Epithelialization will not occur completely over an infected wound. It will occur in wounds that have **eschar** (thick, leathery, fibrin-containing necrotic tissue that covers a wound surface) (Fig. 48-22), but it is much slower than when the eschar is removed by surgical debridement or by use of special enzyme preparations. Epithelialization also depends on oxygen tension in the wound. The higher the oxygen tension, the faster the rate of epithelial cell growth. Most of the wound's oxygen supply comes from the blood that perfuses it. Oxygen from the atmosphere has little or no real effect because it has no penetrating power beyond the topmost layer of cells.

The maturation phase lasts from approximately day 21 to weeks, months, or years. At the cellular level, extensive matrix formation and scar tissue remodeling occur during the maturation phase of healing. Fibroblasts leave the wound, and there is an accumulation of large fibrous bundles of collagen. Scar tissue is largely composed of collagen.

The scar possesses about 10 per cent of the skin's normal strength during the first week of its closure. By the tenth week, it has about 80 per cent, the maximum ever regained. Wounded skin is never as strong as unwounded skin. Healing of the wound may continue for a longer time than the naked eye can see, and there continues to be collagen production and breakdown until the exact amount needed for the wound is produced. Too much collagen will create a **hypertrophic scar** (excessive scarring) or a **keloid** (exuberant scar tissue that grows beyond the confines of the original wound) (Fig. 48-23). Too little collagen causes the wound to have decreased tensile strength.

Factors Affecting Wound Healing

Wound healing is affected by the overall health of the client; general good health and nutritional status contribute to efficient wound healing.

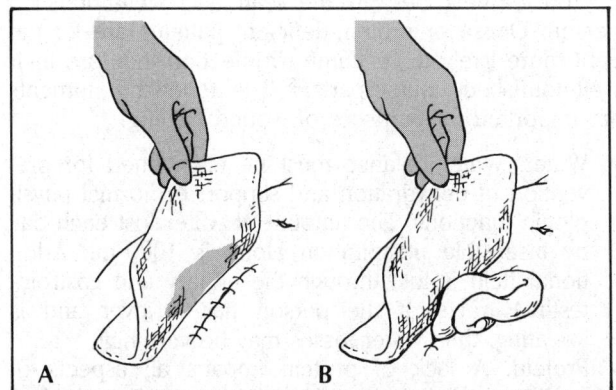

▲ *Figure 48-21*

A, Appearance of watery pink fluid on the dressing frequently precedes wound dehiscence. *B,* Evisceration may follow dehiscence and is a medical emergency.

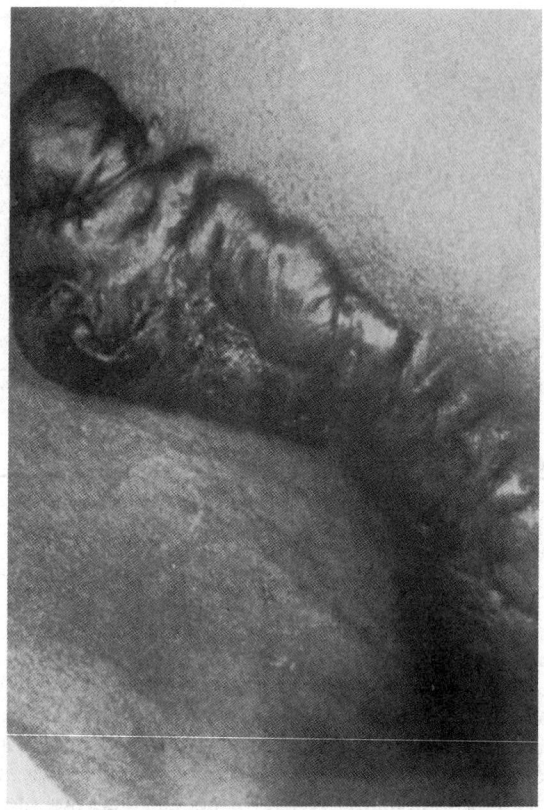

▲ Figure 48–23

Typical keloid after laceration of the anterior neck. Note exuberant growth of scar tissue that is not confined to the original wound site. (Reprinted with permission from Peacock, E. [1984]. *Wound repair* [3rd ed.]. Philadelphia: W.B. Saunders.)

The nature of the injury also affects wound healing. A surgical skin incision has clean, sharp edges that can be pulled together. These wounds have minimal tissue loss, with little need for new tissue to be synthesized. Avulsed wounds are extensive, dirty wounds that are in need of massive tissue replacement.

The amount of tissue loss also affects healing. Wounds with large amounts of tissue loss require longer to heal, are predisposed to infection, and heal with greater scarring and possible loss of function.

The amount of blood circulation affects the rate of repair and resistance to infection. The better the perfusion, the better the conditions for healing.

The location of the wound may create specific problems. For example, wounds near the nose, the vagina, or the anus are at high risk for contamination or infection. Wounds located near joints may also be subject to healing delays because of movement.

Local Factors in Wound Healing

Local factors affect wound healing in a variety of ways. Microbes are one such factor. Entrance of bacteria into wounds can result in contamination or infection. Contamination is the introduction of pathogenic bacteria into a wound but in quantities that are insufficient to overcome the body's defense system. Infection occurs when one or more of the following signs or symptoms

are present: increase in redness, edema, elevated body temperature, presence of pus, uncharacteristic odor of wound, elevation of white blood cell count (neutrophils), pain, and change in the color of **wound exudate** (fluid draining from a wound and containing cells, protein, and solid material).

The presence of any foreign material in the wound interferes with its ability to heal, as does the presence of any necrotic tissue (devitalized, dead tissue). Eschar (wound scab) is the body's attempt to provide a natural wound covering. Eschar can, however, interfere with wound healing by allowing fluid to collect underneath it, masking infection in its early stages and preventing wound contraction. Eschar delays epithelialization by forcing epithelial cells that are attempting to cover the wound surface to have to burrow beneath the eschar first (see Fig. 48–22).

Desiccation, or drying of the wound surface, also has an effect. Desiccation retards epithelialization by up to 50 per cent. Noninfected wounds heal faster in a moist environment.

Edema, another local factor, is commonly seen in wounds and probably represents the body's attempt to dilute the bacterial toxins in the area. If the amount of swelling is large, however, it will interfere with blood supply and possibly cause sutures to rupture.

Wounds require sufficient oxygen tension in the blood supply that perfuses them. They also require efficient fibrin breakdown. Fibrin is the major component of the clot that is initiated by platelets at the time of injury. After hemostasis has been attained, the clot must be broken down for wound healing to take place efficiently.

Local pressure and shear are mechanical forces that impair or occlude blood flow to the wound. Pressure and friction can also abrade superficial skin surfaces.

Systemic Factors in Wound Healing

No single factor is more important to wound healing than good nutrition. Be sure clients have the necessary reserves to combat the physiologic stresses associated with surgery, chronic wounds, and infection.

Wounds heal best in the lean and well-nourished person. Obese or protein-deficient patients are 23 per cent more likely to succumb to infection than are their well-nourished counterparts.[33] The following nutrients are important for purposes of wound healing.

▶ Water. Water balance must be maintained for prevention of dehydration and support of normal physiologic functions. The amount of water lost each day by insensible perspiration alone is 1000 ml. Additional fluid is lost through the urinary and gastrointestinal tracts. If the person has a fever and is sweating, then water losses may be very high.

▶ Protein. A lack of protein impairs all aspects of healing and impairs immune system functioning. Minimum RDA requirements for healthy adults are 0.8 gm/kg. In the person with a wound that will not heal, protein needs increase to 1.5 to 2 gm/kg.

▶ Vitamins and minerals. Vitamin C is required for the creation of normal collagen. A lack of this vitamin causes collagen instability and decreased tensile strength of the wound. Large amounts (up to 500 mg/day) may be required. Vitamin C should be given with caution in persons with gastrointestinal problems because it is caustic. It should always be followed with plenty of water (not citrus fruit juices or colas). Vitamin A is necessary for epithelialization, collagen production and stabilization, and resistance to infection. Vitamins B_6, B_{12}, and folate are important in protein synthesis. Zinc is only important if there is a deficiency of this element. If the person has a zinc level of less than 100 μg/dl, supplementation will improve healing by assisting in collagen synthesis and immunity. Iron is necessary for normal red blood cell function.

A person's vascular status is an important factor in wound healing. The inability of the body's circulatory system to deliver a sufficient quantity of adequately perfused blood to a wound directly affects healing because oxygen is necessary for healing to take place. The problem may be pathologic, such as vessel obstruction, or it may be mechanical, such as external pressure. Smoking always interferes with blood supply by causing vasoconstriction and other vascular changes.

Metabolic problems can affect wound healing. Two diseases, diabetes mellitus and renal failure, for example, can have significant effects. In diabetes mellitus, blood sugar levels that are higher than normal furnish a good medium for bacterial growth. Other changes with a direct bearing on wound healing are impaired circulation due to atherosclerotic changes (large vessel occlusive disease); reduced sensation in the feet, which makes possible injury that is not recognized; and reduced inflammatory response. Renal failure has a major effect on several body systems. Uremic patients are at increased risk of infection, delayed granulation, and wound dehiscence.

Age affects the rate of healing. Wounds heal more slowly and are less strong in the elderly (especially the old-old, 85 years of age or more) because of decreased inflammatory response, decreased collagen synthesis and breakdown, delayed epithelialization, decreased cohesion between epidermal and dermal layers, and delayed **angiogenesis** (development of blood vessels). In wound healing, angiogenesis usually means the growth of new blood vessels into the wound. Wound dehiscence is three times more likely to occur in people over the age of 60 years.

Immune system changes also affect wound healing. People at both ends of the age continuum, the very young and the very old, are at increased risk of infection because their immune systems are not as competent as those of young and middle-aged adults are. Certain diseases (e.g., AIDS) also cause severe insult to the immune system.

Clotting disorders can interfere with wound healing. Interference with platelet aggregation decreases hemostasis, release of chemotactic factors, and elaboration of growth factors. **Growth factors** are normal components of cells elaborated in response to many body needs. Growth factors are brought to the wound in response to injury. Without these factors, formation of

fibrin matrix is impaired. People with such bleeding disorders as hemophilia, hepatic disease, or thrombocytopenia or those receiving anticoagulant therapy are prone to bleed into the wound, and this delays wound healing.

Drug therapy often impairs wound healing. Glucocorticoids, given at the time of injury (or just before, as in the case of surgery), impair wound healing to a significant degree. These drugs suppress the inflammatory response, prevent normal migration of macrophages into the wound, reduce fibroblast and endothelial cell activity, and delay contraction of the wound and epithelialization. Individuals taking glucocorticoids are prone to the development of chronic wounds. Other drugs that may affect wound healing include anticoagulants, phenytoin, penicillamine, nonsteroidal anti-inflammatory drugs, and chemotherapeutic agents used in cancer.

Neurologic and psychologic health is important in wound healing. Immobility and impaired or absent sensation place paraplegic and quadriplegic persons at great risk for tissue damage from unrelieved pressure, which causes weight-bearing soft tissues to become ischemic and die. A decreased level of consciousness, such as that found in those with stroke or head injuries, predisposes the person to unrelieved pressure damage. Psychologic stress, depression, and sleep disorders have been implicated as conditions that interfere with immune responses and, therefore, with wound healing.

Wounds that, for no apparent reason, do not respond to therapy should be carefully examined for intentional causation. It is possible that they may be **factitious wounds** (tissue injuries deliberately produced by the individual). Factitious wounds are hard to diagnose at times (see Fig. 48–11). Treatment for most wounds of this type requires both wound care and psychiatric care and counseling. Have a high degree of suspicion that the wound is self-induced if the shape of the wound is unusual, if it fails to heal in spite of therapy, and if the person has minimal concern about the wound.

Wound Closure

METHODS OF WOUND CLOSURE

The method by which a wound is closed or is allowed to close is determined by the type of wound, the circumstance under which it occurred, the amount of tissue lost, and whether it is infected. All wounds are closed by one of three methods: primary closure, secondary closure, or delayed primary closure.

Primary closure is used with most surgical wounds. When the skin has been cleanly incised, the edges are closely approximated by sutures, skin clips, staples, or some other device. These wounds generally heal without complication. With little granulation tissue, there is minimal scarring. Wound closure in this manner is healing by primary intention or first intention (Fig. 48–24).

Secondary closure is the method used in open full-thickness wounds with soft tissue damage, such as lacerations or avulsions. Wounds treated in this manner

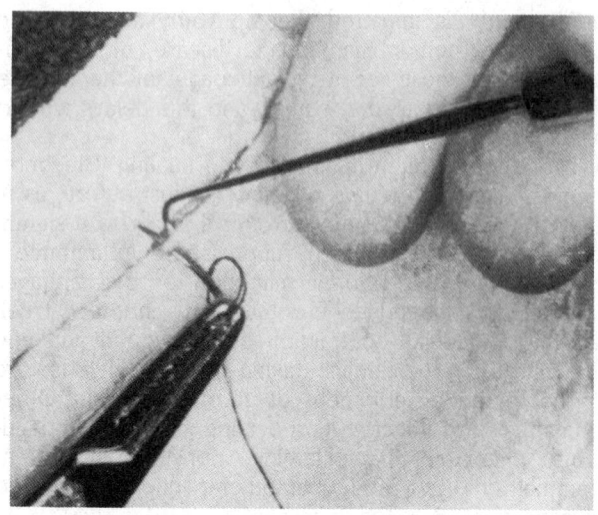

▲ *Figure 48-24*

Epidermal sutures being placed. Note curved needle used by surgeon. (Reprinted with permission from Peacock, E. [1984]. *Wound repair* [3rd ed.]. Philadelphia: W.B. Saunders.)

are contaminated or infected wounds made under nonsterile conditions. They are cleansed as necessary and allowed to heal naturally without surgical intervention. The wound heals from the bottom upward to the skin surface. Much granulation tissue is formed to fill in the wound defect, which is then followed by wound contraction and epithelialization. This process takes much longer than primary closure and leaves a larger scar. Wounds allowed to close naturally in this manner heal by secondary intention (see Fig. 48-7).

Delayed primary closure is a combination of primary and secondary methods of closure. One classic example of the delayed primary closure is a wound associated with a ruptured appendix. The surgical incision is left open until about the fifth postoperative day, and then it is sutured as in a primary closure. By delaying closure, the surgeon can determine that the healing process is progressing without abscess formation or other infection. This type of wound closure is also known as healing by third intention.[93]

APPROXIMATING TISSUE EDGES

One technique to promote optimal wound healing is approximation of tissue edges (i.e., keeping the wound edges together). Approximation may be accomplished by sutures, surgical clips and staples, or adhesive strip skin closures. The method selected depends on factors such as the tissue type, presence of or potential for infection, wound location, individual's general health and reliability, and degree of cosmesis (beauty increased or preserved) desired after healing.

SUTURES

Suture is flexible material placed through tissues (with use of a needle) to approximate (bring together) tissue edges and decrease **dead space** (space where fluids may collect in an anatomic cavity, abscess cavity, or

wound). Sutures also strengthen the wound until normal tensile strength (resistance to lengthwise stress) returns and natural support is established. Use of sutures minimizes scarring (see Fig. 48-24).

Suture material can be natural or synthetic and either absorbable (absorbed by living tissue) or nonabsorbable. Natural suture material includes silk, cotton, and surgical catgut. Synthetic fibers include nylon, polyester, polyethylene, and polypropylene. Suture material can be monofilament (single filament) or braided (Fig. 48-25). The type of suture used determines when the sutures should be removed, suture absorption time, possible effect of infection on the suture line, and appropriate nursing intervention.

Absorbable suture is generally used in areas that cannot be reached for suture removal (e.g., the abdominal cavity). It may also be used in children's skin to prevent the trauma of suture removal and in adults in areas not of high cosmetic concern. Natural absorbable sutures (animal products) tend to cause increased tissue reactivity. Their absorption varies widely in the presence of infection. Synthetic absorbable suture is replacing natural absorbable materials, and synthetic nonabsorbable suture is replacing natural fibers primarily because it is stronger than cotton or silk and because it is usually monofilament. Monofilament suture causes less tissue reactivity than braided suture does. Stainless steel, the strongest nonabsorbable suture, causes the least reaction. Nonabsorbable suture is generally used on skin.

Retention sutures, which are large and sometimes wire, are applied if a great deal of tension might be exerted on the wound or if the wound may need to be reopened. Areas of the suture lying against the skin are usually encased in sheathing material to prevent the suture from cutting the skin.

Suture may be packaged separately from a needle (to be threaded at the time of use or as "ties" or ligatures to tie off blood vessels) or already attached to a needle (swaged on the needle). During wound closure, it is important to account for all suturing materials used so none are inadvertently left in the wound.

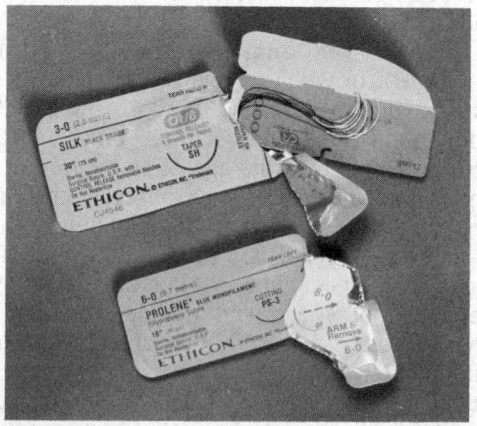

▲ *Figure 48-25*

Examples of size 3-0 black braided silk suture swedged on a curved needle *(top)* and size 6-0 polypropylene monofilament suture on a curved cutting needle *(bottom)*. Both of these sutures are nonabsorbable and must be removed when the wound is sufficiently healed.

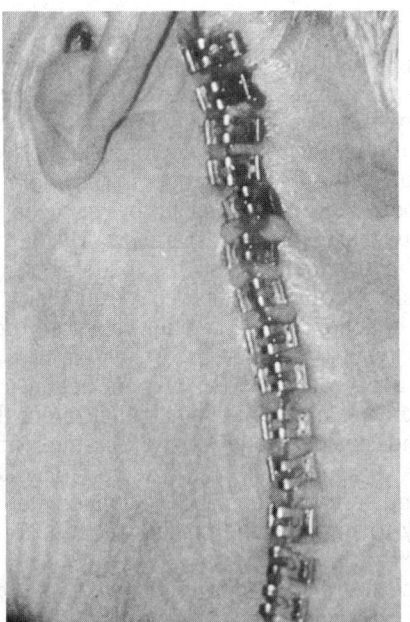

▲ Figure 48-26

Skin clips used for wound closure. These are removed by special instruments. (Reprinted with permission from Westaby, S. [1986]. *Wound care*. London: Butterworth-Heinemann.)

Suture is sized. The smaller the number, the larger the suture diameter; for example, 2-0 suture is much larger than 7-0. The suture size selected depends on characteristics of the tissue it is intended to support. For example, 2-0 suture may be used to secure intravenous catheters temporarily or to suture the sole of the foot; fine 7-0 suture is used for eye or plastic surgery.

SURGICAL CLIPS AND STAPLES

Surgical clips and staples are metal devices used to hold wound edges together. They are inserted and re-moved with special instruments. These strong devices are used like sutures, often in tissues under great tension. Some clips and staples may be used in deeper tissues and then the overlying skin sutured, and others may be used on the skin alone. Skin clips are illustrated in Figure 48-26.

ADHESIVE SKIN CLOSURES

Adhesive skin closures (e.g., reinforced adhesive strips, Clearon, Steri-Strips, skin closures) are used to approximate wound edges in areas with minimal tension on the wound (e.g., close, small wounds). These devices support a wound in which deeper structures are sutured. They are used after suture removal to support wound edges (particularly on the face), in tissues with possibly poor vascularity, in securing skin grafts, and in areas where cosmetic appearance is important. They may also be used on wounds not requiring suturing or when suturing capabilities are not available (e.g., first aid in the wilderness). No anesthesia is required to apply adhesive skin closures. Table 48-8 lists types of tape products.

Butterfly closures are pieces of adhesive tape shaped so only a thin line of adhesive bridges the wound edges while each side is supported with a wider piece of tape. Butterfly closures are available commercially or can easily be hand cut from 1/2-inch adhesive tape (Fig. 48-27).

Adhesive strips (Band-Aids) are more commonly used, often for children. These are commercially made of hypoallergenic paper tape and often reinforced with nylon threads. Some are also impregnated with an iodine solution. Strips come in various lengths and widths and are fairly easy and relatively painless to apply. They are not as strong as sutures, however, and may come off. Also, the wound edges may invert, leaving not a scar but a "dent" in the skin (dermal dent).

Key points for application and removal of adhesive tape are found in Box 48-1.

TABLE 48-8. Tape Products

Type	Purpose	Cautions
Cotton-backed adhesive tape*	Secure dressing and splints Strap joints to prevent or treat injuries Immobilize body parts, such as ribs Provide pressure Secure skin grafts Approximate wound edges	Can cause skin maceration Can cause tearing of skin or shearing on removal Can cause skin allergy or irritation
Paper, plastic, and acetate taffeta adhesive tapes*	Secure dressings Useful for small wounds where pressure and support are not primary concerns Provides greater patient comfort because they are lighter, more porous, and cause less skin irritation	Not as strong or adherent as cotton-backed tape Can cause skin irritation
Foam adhesive tape*	Used on pressure dressing or as a compression bandage	Can cause shearing of skin Can cause skin irritation

* Available in widths ranging from 1/2 to 3 inches.

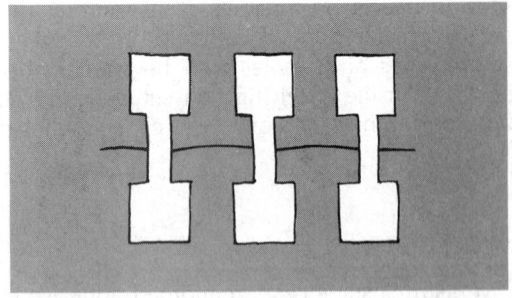

▲ Figure 48–27

Butterfly adhesive closure. This can be fashioned from 1/2-inch adhesive tape if prepackaged closures are not available. The butterfly wound closure is most often used in first-aid settings.

New Therapies for Wound Care

A number of promising new therapies are being applied to the treatment of hard-to-heal wounds. A wide variety of new dressing materials are also available.

Box 48–1. Application and Removal of Adhesive Tape

Key Points in Applying Adhesive Tape

▶ Clean, dry, and clip hair in area to be taped, if needed.
▶ Apply skin adherent (e.g., benzoin) if necessary to enhance adhesiveness.

Do not apply to wound. (Note: Adherents are not usually needed and may increase irritation.)

▶ Tape body part in position of function (use).
▶ Apply tape in strips of equal length.
▶ Allow tape to fit body contours.

Caution Taping in a continuous circle going completely around a part (e.g., arm) with inflexible adhesive tape is dangerous! It may completely shut off arterial blood flow. Always leave at least 3 cm (about an inch) of skin surface untaped (i.e., between the beginning and end of a strip).

Key Points in Removing Adhesive Tape

▶ Remove tape from end to end, rather than from side to side.
▶ Hold skin taut and push skin away from tape.
▶ Do not pull tape away from skin.
▶ Remove tape by pushing toward wound. Do not pull away from wound.
▶ Use a generic tape remover to remove adhesive tape residue from skin.
▶ Remove carefully to prevent tearing of skin.

GROWTH FACTORS

Major developments in the theory of wound healing have evolved from discoveries in cell biology and biochemistry that uncovered new information on how cells work and on the growth factors elaborated by cells important in the healing process. The more we understand about the normal healing process, the greater the possibility that clinician-researchers will be able to enhance the healing process by speeding it up, making the wound stronger as it heals, reducing the risk of wound infection, and creating a more cosmetically pleasing result. As one researcher explains, "Only in the last five years have researchers begun to work out the underlying molecular signals that direct the process of wound healing. One of the essential findings has been that a handful of growth factors play key roles in every step — from the response immediately following an injury to bringing the healing process to an orderly close."[103]

Science has shown that growth factors are made by the body and are brought to the wound in response to injury, but until recently, there has been no answer about the mechanisms that control the growth factors themselves. We have recently found that the extracellular matrix, the structure that is the framework for normal tissue, can modify the action of growth factors. It is likely that the relationship between the extracellular matrix and different growth factors lies at the heart of the wound-healing process.

More must be known about growth factors and their specific role in wound healing before they will be available for general clinical use. At present, many are in late-stage clinical trials. Certain of the 36 or more growth factors identified to date seem to be more essential to wound healing than others are. These include transforming growth factor-beta, fibroblast growth factor, platelet-derived growth factor, and epidermal-derived growth factor. A number of clinician-researchers are now using growth factors in treating human patients with nonhealing skin and soft tissue wounds, such as pressure ulcers, diabetic leg ulcers, and vascular stasis ulcers. A major assumption of these studies is that slow-healing wounds are deficient in one or more growth factors. Results have suggested improved healing. Findings have not been sufficient, however, for marketing approval to be obtained from the Food and Drug Administration, the final authority whose permission is necessary for growth factors to be made available for general use. Concerns about using growth factors in the clinical setting involve possible problems and dangers, such as how to keep these factors confined to the wound site, whether they can initiate malignant changes or cause other health problems like glomerulonephritis, and whether changing the normal mix of growth factors in a wound could alter healing in some unforeseen way.

Therefore, although externally administered growth factors appear to hold promise for wound healing, they are not without potential danger. The extent of that danger is not known at present. It is likely that there will be clear-cut indications for their uses in the next several years.

HYPERBARIC OXYGEN

When used as a local wound treatment, hyperbaric oxygen consists of more than 100 per cent surface equivalency of oxygen under pressure in a closed container sealed to a body part, such as a leg. Hyperbaric oxygen may also be systemically administered by placing the individual inside a chamber pressurized to greater than one atmosphere. The individual breathes surface-equivalent breathing mixtures in excess of 100 per cent oxygen, thus increasing oxygen perfusion through the blood to the wound.

LASERS AND ELECTROSTIMULATION

A laser is an instrument that can deliver high-energy light levels to a small area. In medicine, it can be used to cut or vaporize tissue or to coagulate small blood vessels. This is especially useful for removing tissue during debridement. Electrical stimulation of tissues with low-voltage pulsed energy has been effective in limited trials.

ASSESSMENT

Initial Assessment

The initial assessment of the client's wound must include an assessment of the client's overall status. It is important to have a health history as well as a physical, mental, and emotional baseline on which to plan your nursing interventions. If the wound is an emergency, such as hemorrhage, dehiscence (breakdown of wound incision), or **evisceration** (protrusion of body organs through the wound incision), then your first responsibility is to initiate measures to deal with the emergency (see Fig. 48–21). Obtain help and apply principles of first aid appropriate for the situation. However, most wounds are surgically created or chronic wounds that do not require emergency management. A thorough assessment, therefore, will be possible and should include psychosocial concerns (Table 48–9).

Physical assessment of systemic factors that directly affect the wound is of particular importance. In examining the wound, take into account the material listed in Table 48–10.

Charting of your assessment should include the findings obtained from your examination of the wound:

▶ Wound size and depth. Size and depth are particularly important if the wound is traumatic or chronic.
▶ Wound location. The more specific the location that you chart, the less possibility there is for misunderstanding. For example, an abdominal wound should be described with the abdominal quadrant in which it is located (e.g., left lower quadrant of the abdomen).
▶ Wound appearance. If it is a surgical wound, are the edges in close approximation without swelling or tension on the sutures? If it is a nonsurgical wound, is there evidence of normal wound healing, such as granulation tissue?
▶ Bleeding or drainage. Is there any bleeding or other drainage? How much? Describe its color and odor. How many dressings were used? What size?
▶ Sensation. Is the person complaining of pain, burning, loss of sensation, limitation of movement?
▶ Infection. Is there any evidence of wound infection?
▶ Debris. Was any foreign debris noted?
▶ Vital signs. Are vital signs within normal limits or elevated?
▶ Surrounding skin. What is the condition of the skin around the wound?
▶ Psychosocial response. What is the client's response to the wound?

TABLE 48–9. Psychosocial Concerns Associated with Wounds

Concern	Relation to the Wound
Anxiety	Distress over a real or imagined threat to the individual's well-being
Fear of pain, disfigurement, financial loss, dependence, retribution, punishment	Any of these concerns may be present, depending on the individual's greatest fears
Anger	An emotion seen in clients who feel that the wound was not their fault or that it was due to their own carelessness
Depression	A common emotion in those individuals with chronic wounds or with surgically created permanent wounds, such as colostomy (opening into colon for fecal elimination
Meaning of the injury	Implications for the person: Does the person see the injury as permanently incapacitating or one that will heal and cause no problems? Is it an accidental injury for which compensation may be given? Is it to the individual's financial benefit not to get better?
Avoidance	Unwillingness to look at the wound; the wound represents a threat to body integrity; this may occur in persons with amputations or surgically created ostomy wounds, such as colostomy, ileostomy, and ureterostomy; in the latter case, both the wound and the fact that body waste is eliminated through it are threats
Physiologic effects of psychologic responses	Effect on body function: fear, anger, and depression can affect the individual's vital signs, causing them to become elevated or decreased; fainting can occur

TABLE 48–10. Assessment of Wounds

Criterion	Nursing Response
Cause	What is the etiologic basis of the wound?
Type	Surgical or traumatic? Open or closed? Full-thickness or partial-thickness? Infected or noninfected?
Location	What is the anatomic location? Wounds near body orifices should be assessed for infection.
Extent and depth	Measure the size and depth of the wound. The larger and deeper it is, the greater the possibility for complications, such as infection, bleeding, dehiscence, or evisceration.
Presence of drainage	What type of drainage is present? Serous (clear, watery)? Sanguineous (bloody)? Serosanguineous (watery with traces of blood)? Purulent (pus containing bacteria, necrotic debris, and white blood cells)? The color of pus varies with the organism causing it. *Pseudomonas aeruginosa,* a common pathogen, typically causes blue-green pus.
Amount of drainage	Estimate by volume or by size of drainage on dressing (e.g., 2 cm × 2 cm).
Odor	Is there a strong odor to the wound? Certain types of organisms have characteristic odors, but these are variable. *Pseudomonas aeruginosa* usually has a sickly sweet odor. Odor does not always mean infection. Occlusive dressings will always create a wound odor on removal. When the wound is cleaned, the odor should disappear.
Foreign debris	Was the wound traumatic? If so, it may contain gravel, sand, wood splinters, or other foreign material. If a traumatic wound continues to have drainage, foreign debris may still be in the wound. Do not attempt to remove the foreign body. The physician will do this.
Sutures	Are all still tied and visible? Are the wound edges in close approximation? Is the skin around the sutures swollen and tight, causing sutures to cut into the tissues? Are the sutures continuous or interrupted?
Skin surrounding wound	Is the skin intact? What is its color? Is there swelling or excoriation (breaks in skin resembling an abrasion as a result of wound drainage)?
Potential complications Infection	Surgical wounds may become infected. Traumatic wounds are highly likely to have infecting organisms. To determine the bacterial source of the infection, a sample of wound drainage must be sent to the laboratory for culture and sensitivity testing. The organism will be identified by culture, and a determination of the antibiotics to which the organism is sensitive will be made.
Bleeding, hemorrhage, or excessive drainage	Is there an increased amount of bright red blood? Is there a sudden appearance of other drainage that might represent a ruptured cyst or abscess?
Dehiscence	Are wound edges widening? Have any sutures broken?
Evisceration	Has the wound broken open so that underlying tissues or organs protrude?

A sample nurse's note might look like this:

6 cm lower midline surgical abdominal incision with edges directly approximated. 12 silk sutures in place. No swelling or undue tension around sutures. Small amount dried blood present along suture line. No evidence of drainage or odor. No redness or other signs of infection. Client voices no complaint of pain. States incision is uncomfortable when she moves or coughs.

Ongoing Assessment

The frequency with which a wound is assessed is variable. For surgical wounds, the initial dressing is typically changed on the first postoperative day by the surgeon. Thereafter, the wound should be assessed at least every 24 hours until the sutures or staples are removed, unless the surgeon writes other orders. Wounds that are traumatic or infected may need to be inspected more frequently to prevent complications from developing without being recognized. Their treatment will vary, depending on the physician's plan of wound care. Continue to chart any significant findings. If a surgical wound becomes infected or any other complications occur, then inspection and dressing changes will be more frequent.

Chronic wounds such as pressure ulcers or venous stasis ulcers should be inspected daily. Developing pressure ulcers usually have an irregular shape. Chronic pressure ulcers have margins that are more regular and often circumscribed by a fibrous ring that prevents healing without intervention.

If the edges of a pressure ulcer are everted, malignant changes may have occurred.

Remember that assessment without documentation in the person's record omits important information that should be communicated to the next person caring for your client. If a legal case occurs because the client or family believes that the person did not receive safe care, the chart becomes the basis for the case.

Failure to chart observations and care in the person's record is assumed in a court of law to mean that the observations and care did not take place.

Most wounds heal without complications. But for those that do not, infection and skin breakdown around the wound are frequent occurrences. Skin breakdown around the wound occurs with chronic rather than acute wounds. Skin breakdown is common with colostomies or similar wounds. The complication is due to constant drainage that causes maceration (softening) of the skin. Wound drainage often contains autolytic enzymes that are capable of damaging skin as well. This type of complication can be prevented by applying a skin barrier (a protective substance that functions like a waterproof covering to prevent skin maceration) and an absorptive dressing to contain the drainage. These draining wounds require the attention of a nurse skilled in the art of wound management.

Excessive bleeding, or hemorrhage, is rarely seen in surgical wounds but can occur if blood vessels are not securely tied off. In traumatic wounds, hemorrhage may be more frequent if the injury involves large blood vessels, such as arteries or veins. The sudden appearance of large amounts of blood in a wound is an emergency. Place direct pressure over the wound using sterile dressings if available. If dressings are not immediately available, use the cleanest covering that you can find. Call for help using the client's call light. Do not leave the person unattended.

Wound dehiscence and evisceration are seldom seen, but both are emergencies (see Figs. 48–20 and 48–21). Dehiscence is a breaking open of a surgical incision. Underlying body organs do not protrude through the incision, but if the complication is not corrected, it will progress to evisceration. Dehiscence is seen in the obese, in people with abdominal distention, in those with wound infections, and in certain other circumstances. Evisceration is the protrusion of viscera (body organs) through a wound incision. This complication may occur in a person with wound dehiscence who suddenly coughs forcefully. In one series of 1129 major abdominal surgeries, there were 19 burst abdomens or a 1.7 per cent occurrence.[15] Should evisceration occur, do not attempt to replace the organs. Call for help at once. Place sterile, isotonic saline compresses over the wound as soon as possible and remain with the person until help comes.

NURSING DIAGNOSIS

The nursing diagnosis that best describes the client with a wound is *Impaired Tissue Integrity,* which is defined by the North American Nursing Diagnosis Association as "a state in which an individual experiences damage to mucous membrane, corneal, integumentary, or subcutaneous tissue."[77] Muscle tissue may also be involved in certain wounds, however, and should be considered when formulating nursing diagnoses (see Nursing Diagnosis Profile).

Although not all persons with the diagnosis *High Risk for Infection* have the diagnosis *Impaired Tissue Integrity,* all individuals who have the diagnosis *Impaired Tissue Integrity* should also have the diagnosis *High Risk for Infection.* Those with the diagnosis *Impaired Skin Integrity* may also have the diagnosis *Body Image Disturbance, Anxiety, Fluid Volume Deficit, Sensory Perceptual Alterations,* or *Pain.* In fact, these nursing diagnoses often result from impaired tissue integrity, and the impaired tissue integrity would be listed as a related factor in such cases. For example, *Pain R/T impaired tissue integrity* would be the diagnosis for a person who received a tissue avulsion of the finger after catching a ring in a machine at work.

On the other hand, certain other nursing diagnoses frequently lead to the diagnosis *Impaired Tissue Integrity.* These include *Impaired Physical Mobility* (which leads to pressure ulcers), *Altered Tissue Perfusion* (which leads to arterial insufficiency ulcers or pressure ulcers), *Total Incontinence* or *Bowel Incontinence*

NURSING DIAGNOSIS PROFILE

Impaired Tissue Integrity

Definition. A state in which an individual experiences damage to the structural integrity and continuity of the body's soft tissues, including skin, mucous membrane, corneal tissue, subcutaneous tissue, or muscle.

Classification. Exchanging 1.6.2.1.

Defining Characteristics. The only major defining characteristic for this nursing diagnosis is damaged or destroyed tissue of the types mentioned in the definition.

Sample Related Factors. Related factors may be any of the following:

▶ Mechanical changes secondary to surgical intervention, trauma, pressure, friction, shear
▶ Thermal changes (burns) secondary to heat or chemical injury, cold injury
▶ Chemical changes secondary to toxic injury other than heat-related chemical changes
▶ Altered circulation secondary to atherosclerosis, heart disease, peripheral vascular disease
▶ Fluid volume deficit/excess secondary to dehydration, edema
▶ Impaired physical mobility secondary to paralysis, loss of consciousness, muscle weakness, neurologic impairment, depression, certain medications
▶ Nutritional deficit/excess secondary to malnutrition, prolonged poor nutrition deficient in one or more of the essential nutritional elements, obesity
▶ Knowledge deficit concerning safety, prevention of injury, care of wound

Concept Description. This diagnosis refers to the state in which a person experiences a disruption in soft tissues that is other than damage to the oral mucous membrane and more extensive than damage to the skin alone.

Examples. Depending on the specific assessment data, this diagnostic category could be applicable in the following situations, among others:

▶ A person who is in the process of having surgery other than oral surgery
▶ A person who has had surgery (other than oral surgery) within the past 2 hours and whose surgical wound had not yet become sealed to the external environment
▶ A person who has an open soft tissue wound (other than of the oral cavity), such as a pressure ulcer, burn, abrasion, or avulsion, and whose wound affects more tissue than the skin

Related/Similar Nursing Diagnoses. This diagnosis should be distinguished from the diagnoses *Altered Oral Mucous Membrane* and *Impaired Skin Integrity*. With the diagnosis *Altered Oral Mucous Membrane*, the person experiences tissue disruption only in the oral cavity. The destruction of oral tissue may be superficial or fairly extensive. With the nursing diagnosis *Impaired Skin Integrity*, the person experiences damage only to the skin. The damage to the skin might be a disruption of the skin surface or a destruction of a layer of skin, but only the skin is involved.

(both of which lead to skin breakdown), *High Risk for Injury* (which leads to tissue trauma of various types), and *Knowledge Deficit* (which can also lead to injuries of various types). Of course, until actual tissue damage occurs, you should not give the client the diagnosis *Impaired Tissue Integrity*. Instead, the appropriate diagnosis is *High Risk for Impaired Skin Integrity*.

These are just some of the nursing diagnoses you may want to think about when assessing various types of wounds. Of greatest importance, however, is the diagnosis *Impaired Tissue Integrity*.

PLANNING

Priorities for the individual with *Impaired Tissue Integrity* depend on many factors. Is the client stable and in no immediate danger? Is the condition unstable and progressive? Care of the person's wound includes

▶ preventing further tissue damage
▶ preventing wound infection
▶ preventing injury to other body systems
▶ promoting client comfort
▶ promoting wound healing through adequate nutrition
▶ administering wound care appropriate to the wound — cleansing, medications, dressings
▶ eliminating client knowledge deficits concerning the injury
▶ promoting rehabilitation after injury
▶ assisting client to regain independence
▶ assisting client in coping with any transient or permanent alterations resulting from the wound or injury
▶ assisting client, family, or friends to attain skills necessary for safe care of wound or injury when discharged

Planning also includes client outcome criteria, which the nurse will later use for evaluating the client's health status related to the wound and readiness of the client for discharge. The client should

▶ achieve normal wound healing, as evidenced by continued decrease in size of wound, absence of drainage, absence of temperature elevation, decrease in discomfort, and improvement in subjective sense of well-being
▶ achieve acceptable nutritional status, as evidenced by normal skin turgor, weight within normal range for body build and height, and progression of wound healing
▶ progress toward attainment of pre-injury status, as evidenced by increasing participation in own care
▶ perform correct wound care technique, as demonstrated by the nurse
▶ state the signs and symptoms of wound complications, such as those of hemorrhage, infection, skin breakdown, and wound disruption, and report them to the physician if they occur

▸ report any unusual signs and symptoms to appropriate health care personnel
▸ verbalize all discharge instructions correctly

NURSING INTERVENTION

Nursing intervention for the person with a wound requires management of the wound to promote safety, comfort, and healing. Intervention includes wound cleansing, wound irrigation, wound dressing, and the application of heat and cold.

Management of Wounds

WOUND CLEANSING AND IRRIGATION

Cleansing of open, chronic wounds is safely effected by use of nonionic cleansers, which will not harm the healing environment. A **nonionic cleanser** is a wound-cleaning solution that has no electrical charge. Any charged agent is toxic to tissue. For example, hexachlorophene, chlorhexidine, povidone-iodine scrub, and hydrogen peroxide damage tissue. These agents interact with the cell membrane and cause it to lose normal permeability, which results in cell death. An additional problem with the use of hydrogen peroxide has been reported in two cases. When used as a wound irrigant under pressure in a "dirty" wound, it can produce subcutaneous gas, which spreads along fascial planes and mimics gas gangrene because it causes marked swelling, fever, and skin changes in the local area. Hydrogen peroxide under pressure should never be used as an irrigant.[95] Fibroblasts, one of the important cells in normal wound healing, are affected by these agents.[78,90,91]

Sterile isotonic saline (0.9 per cent) is one of the best cleansers for open wounds. Sterile isotonic saline will not disrupt normal cells but will reduce the number of bacteria. It is cheap and readily available, and its use in the wound bed is essentially painless. Other commercial nonionic cleansers are on the market (see Table 48–6). All manufacturers state that these agents are safe for wound healing. Some of these commercial cleansers have greater cleansing ability in the wound because they can lower surface tension more effectively than isotonic saline can. Most commercially available nonionic cleansers, however, still have sufficient reactivity to interact with cell membranes and cause problems.[90]

Cleaning a wound should be done gently unless it is grossly contaminated by foreign material, in which case more vigorous scrubbing may be needed in the first cleansing (this is usually done in the emergency department). In most instances, cleansing requires irrigation by one of several possible approaches: (1) a 30- to 35-ml piston-type syringe fitted with a 19-gauge blunt-tipped needle or angiocath (Fig. 48–28), (2) a bulb syringe, or (3) a Water-Pik. Of the three, the piston-type syringe most closely approximates the ideal pressure for flushing necrotic tissue from the wound: 8 psi (pounds per square inch). The bulb syringe generates 1

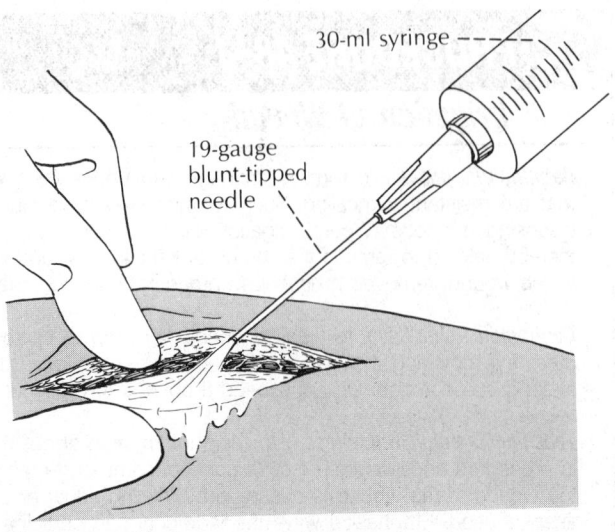

▲ *Figure 48–28*

High-pressure wound irrigation with a syringe and a large-bore, blunt-tipped needle. This type of irrigation is often used for new, accidental, or grossly contaminated wounds. If a 19-gauge blunt-tipped needle is not available, a large angiocath or a size 14 soft French catheter can be used. These devices furnish a pressure of 8 psi, which is thought to be optimal for cleansing.

psi, which is considered insufficient for cleaning. The Water-Pik delivers 50 to 70 psi (much higher than required) and may damage the wound. To be most effective, the piston-type syringe should be held with the needle tip about 1 to 2 inches from the wound surface. The needle should be carefully controlled so that it is not pushed off the end of the syringe, possibly causing injury to the individual. An angiocath can be attached to the syringe instead of the needle; the angiocath will deliver 8 psi pressure and eliminate the danger from needle stick.[71] Wound irrigation is described in Procedure 48–1.

WOUND DRESSINGS

The role of wound dressings has changed from passive (i.e., wound coverings whose function was merely to protect the wound from outside trauma and pathogens) to interactive (i.e., dressings that speed up the healing process). Alvarez[2] states that there will be much new development in dressings during the next decade:

[There is] great promise for management of internal and external wounds. Dressings that provide or create ideal environments for each of the healing phases (debridement, inflammation, angiogenesis, connective tissue repair, and epithelialization) are expected since major changes occur in the wound environment at different healing stages. Dressings will be developed that will interact with wound fluid in order to deliver a growth factor or therapeutic agent at the right stage of repair.

The major function of wound dressings is to protect the wound from microorganisms and physical injury. The dressing should also improve comfort and encourage healing. Dressings should provide absorption of wound drainage, if present. The application of dry and wet sterile dressings is described in Procedures 48–2 and 48–3.

Text continued on page 1374

PROCEDURE 48–1

Irrigation of Wound

Definition/Purposes. To remove drainage and debris from wound surface. Irrigation is commonly used in deeper wounds that are resistant to healing. Such wounds may have sinus tracks or fistulas that cannot be reached by normal wound cleansing methods. Wound irrigation allows isotonic saline or other ordered solutions to reach all parts of the wound, thereby helping to remove the source of infection. Wound irrigation is also used to deliver heat, which increases circulation to the wound, removes toxic wound products, and increases oxygenation of tissues.

Contraindications/Cautions. Irrigate wound from top to bottom to avoid contaminating areas just cleaned. Wear goggles or other eye covering if there is a likelihood of splashing. Be sure to use the proper solution at the proper temperature to avoid tissue damage. Do not exceed 8 pounds of pressure per square inch (psi) to prevent mechanical damage to tissue.

Teaching/Learning Guidelines. Providing information about the irrigation before beginning helps reduce anxiety and assists in procedure acceptance. Discuss pain concerns and measures to reduce discomfort. The individual may not want to see the wound. If the wound is observed by the individual or significant other, describe signs of healing. Explain principles of asepsis used. Emphasize ways the individual can participate. Instruct the individual to keep hands away from the wound during dressing change to prevent wound contamination.

PRELIMINARY ACTIVITIES

Assessment/Planning

Verify physician's order for irrigation.
Note individual preferences on nursing care plan.
Plan activity at least disruptive time (e.g., not just before or after meals, or when visitors are present, or late at night).
Provide privacy.
Create clean, dry work space.

Preparation of Person

Explain purposes of irrigation.
Assess with person the need for an analgesic. Allow time for analgesic to become effective before starting (e.g., 15 to 20 minutes for parenteral, 1 hour for oral).

Equipment/Supplies

Sterile gloves—1 pair
Clean gloves—1 pair
Sterile irrigation set
Prescribed irrigation solution (200 to 500 ml is usual amount), warmed to body temperature
Sterile dressing supplies
  4 × 4 gauze dressings
  Abdominal pads
  Kerlix may be needed
Sterile irrigation syringe should use a 30- to 35-ml Luer-Lok syringe with a 19-gauge blunt-tipped needle (if described needle is not available, may use angiocath or a size 14 French soft catheter)
Waterproof pad
Skin sealant if needed
Clean basin
Waterproof bag for used dressings
Tape
Gown and goggles, if needed

PROCEDURE

Actions

1. Wash hands carefully.

2. Screen, position, and drape person properly. Place waterproof pad under client to prevent irrigation solution from wetting bed. Position client so that irrigation fluid will flow vertically over the wound surface. Place clean collecting basin at the bottom of the wound, ready to contain the irrigation fluid.

3. Open waterproof bag that will contain old dressing. Fold a 1½ inch cuff. Place it near the bed.

4. If gown and goggles are needed, put them on now.

5. Don clean gloves and remove soiled dressing. Discard in waterproof bag.

6. Remove gloves and discard in waterproof bag.

Rationale/Discussion

1. Reduces microorganisms on hands. Reduces potential wound infection.

2. Provides privacy. Enhances emotional/physical comfort. Person should be comfortable, with wound site easily accessible to nurse.

3. Making a cuff will help keep the bag open and, when closed, will prevent the outside of the bag from contamination by the dressing.

4. If splashing is likely to occur during irrigation, protect eyes and clothing.

5. Gloves protect the nurse's hands.

PROCEDURE 48–1 Continued

Irrigation of Wound

Actions

7. Inspect wound. Observe for evidence of healing, such as granulation tissue. Note presence of necrosis; odor, amount, and color of drainage; and condition of skin around wound.
8. Wash hands. Open sterile supplies. Remove bottle cap from irrigation solution.

9. Open sterile gloves. Place one glove on your dominant hand. Use gloved hand to lift 35-ml syringe out of the irrigation container.
10. Place irrigation syringe on sterile field.

11. Use ungloved hand to pour sterile irrigating solution (outside of bottle is unsterile) into sterile irrigation container. Hold irrigation container with gloved hand.
12. Put on second sterile glove. Add 35-ml Luer-Lok syringe and 19-gauge blunt-tipped needle (angiocath or 14 French catheter), if needed, and assemble.
13. Fill syringe with irrigant solution.

14. Flush wound from top to bottom with prescribed solution. End of needle or catheter tip should be 1 to 2 inches from wound surface. Clean, granulating wounds should be irrigated with minimum pressure. Necrotic or heavily draining wounds should be irrigated forcefully. This requires full force to the plunger of a fully extended 35-ml syringe.
15. Wounds with sinus tracks or hard-to-reach areas are best irrigated with an angiocath or a 14 French soft catheter. These flexible tubes can be inserted to the point of resistance and then withdrawn ½ inch to prevent damage to fragile tissue.
16. Dry wound edges and surrounding skin with sterile 4 × 4 sponges. Clean from edge of wound to more distant areas.
17. Apply sterile dressings. Pack wound loosely to absorb drainage. With necrotic wounds, use Super Kerlix sponges or rolls.
18. If required, apply skin sealant to skin surrounding wound. Allow to air dry.

19. Remove and discard gloves.
20. Secure dressing with tape. If wound has mild to moderate drainage, tape edges in picture-frame style (all four sides). Write the date and your initials on the tape.

21. Assist client to comfortable position.
22. Return equipment to proper place and discard disposables in designated receptacles.
23. Wash hands. Check with client to see whether there is any discomfort or other untoward reaction.

Rationale/Discussion

7. For charting purposes.

8. Open all sterile supplies before donning sterile gloves. Once sterile gloves have been put on, another person will have to open supplies for you.
9. You will be handling both sterile and clean supplies in steps 8 to 10. One hand must remain ungloved.

10. Syringes on irrigation tray often do not allow proper control of pressure. A sterile 35-ml Luer-Lok syringe with a 19-gauge blunt-tipped needle, angiocath, or 14 French catheter is needed to provide 8 psi, which is a safe pressure.
11. Avoids contaminating glove.

12. Two sterile hands are needed for the remainder of the procedure.

13. 200 ml or more will be used to remove wound drainage and dilute bacterial toxins.
14. Delivers optimal amount of pressure; 8 psi is the optimal pressure for avoiding damage to newly forming granulation tissue. Forceful irrigation can help in mechanical debridement of necrotic tissue.

15. Flexible catheter tubing allows irrigating fluid to be directed into hard-to-reach areas.

16. Drying prevents maceration of surrounding skin.

17. Protects wound from environmental contamination and absorbs drainage.

18. If wound drainage is continuous and cannot be controlled within the confines of the wound bed, a skin sealant will help prevent maceration.

19. Gloves are no longer needed.
20. Tape dressings with nonallergic paper tape if possible to avoid further skin irritation. Dating dressing gives immediate information to the next care giver about when the dressing was last changed and by whom.

Procedure continued on following page

PROCEDURE 48–1 Continued

Irrigation of Wound

FINAL ACTIVITIES

Assess individual for comfort and safety. Make sure bed is at desirable height and position and bedside stand with personal effects is within reach. Replace side rails if indicated. Return nondisposable instruments and bowl to central service for cleaning and reprocessing. Later, return to room to assess individual and to note security and comfort of dressing. *Documentation:* wound appearance; amount, color, and type of drainage; any odor; any complaint of pain or discomfort; condition of surrounding skin; type, temperature, and amount of irrigation solution; whether a blunt-tipped needle or a catheter was used for irrigation; and what the client response was during the irrigation. Note on nursing care plan points of special importance to individual regarding dressing change.

PROCEDURE 48–2

Applying Dry Sterile Dressing

Definition/Purposes. To cover wound with a dry gauze sterile dressing, thus protecting it from environmental contaminants and the environment from wound contaminants. The procedure is done by replacing soiled dressings (usually with physician's permission) for the individual's physical and esthetic comfort. The procedure provides the opportunity to observe wound, assess healing, and remove moist dressing (thus reducing potential for wound contamination). Dressing protects skin around wound, supports or splints wound.

Contraindications/Cautions. Avoid communicating any negative personal feelings about the wound. Surgeons often want to change initial postoperative dressings. Nurses usually do subsequent dressings as needed. If dressing is soiled but cannot be changed, reinforce it to protect the wound, monitor drainage, and maintain comfort. Be gentle. Areas around the wound may be hypersensitive to touch, chemicals, and adhesives. If specific sensitivities or allergies are known, avoid precipitating agents. Wound drainage may irritate skin. Minimize drainage contact with skin.

Teaching/Learning Guidelines. Providing information about dressing change importance may promote procedure acceptance. Discuss pain concerns and measures to reduce discomfort. The individual may not want to see the wound. If the wound is observed by the individual or significant other, describe signs of healing. Explain principles of asepsis used. Emphasize ways the individual can participate. Instruct the individual to keep hands away from the wound during dressing change to prevent wound contamination.

PRELIMINARY ACTIVITIES

Assessment/Planning

Verify need for dressing change.
Check chart for orders relative to dressing change.
Note individual preferences on nursing care plan.
Plan activity at least disruptive time (e.g., not just before or after meals, or when visitors are present, or late at night).
Assess type, size, numbers of dressing needed.
Provide privacy.
Create clean, dry work space.

Preparation of Person

Explain purposes of dressing change.
Assess with person need for analgesic. Allow time for analgesic to become effective before starting (e.g., 15 to 20 minutes for parenteral, 1 hour for oral).

Equipment/Supplies

Sterile dressing tray
Additional sterile dressings of number and type needed
Solution used to clean wound should be a nonionic solution, such as isotonic saline
Tape, hypoallergenic
Clean gloves—1 pair
Sterile gloves—2 pairs
Generic tape remover, if needed
1 sterile towel
Waterproof bag to hold used dressing and used equipment
Sterile instrument dressing set, if needed, containing:
  Forceps, scissors, hemostat, 4 × 4 dressings, and cotton-tipped applicators
Ointment, if prescribed
Gauze ties, if needed

PROCEDURE 48–2 Continued

Applying Dry Sterile Dressing

PROCEDURE

Actions	*Rationale/Discussion*

1. Wash hands carefully (see Chapter 28).

2. Screen, position, and drape person properly.

3. Prepare equipment using sterile technique (see Chapter 28).
   a. Spread paper/plastic drape or double thickness of sterile towel on dry, flat surface.
   b. Open and place sterile supplies and equipment on drape or towel.
   c. Place sterile plastic tray or bowl on drape or sterile towel.
   d. Pour small amount of cleansing solution in tray compartment or bowl (if used).

4. Gently fold bedclothes and gown back, exposing dressing.

5. Loosen tape. Begin at edge away from wound center. Pull skin away from tape, moving in direction toward wound.

6. Remove soiled dressing. Use clean gloves or forceps to remove dressing. Place old dressing inside plastic bag. May use plastic bag that covered sterile dressing set.

7. If dressing adheres to wound, moisten with sterile saline until dressing lifts off easily.

8. Put on sterile gloves.

9. Thoroughly assess wound, using your eyes, nose, and gentle palpation.

10. If necessary, remove adhesive around wound with generic tape remover. Be gentle.

11. Use sterile isotonic saline (or povidone-iodine or other antiseptic) to clean wound edges and surrounding skin if necessary. Note: antiseptics should be used in the wound bed only in infected wounds and must be ordered by the physician. With each swab, clean downward with a single stroke. Clean from center of wound to periphery. Discard swab after each stroke and use a new swab.

12. Apply ointment, if prescribed.

13. Remove gloves and discard into bag with used dressing and swabs.

14. Apply sterile dressing after regloving or by using sterile hemostat or forceps. Place small dressing directly over wound. Once dressing is placed, do not reposition it. Cover with larger dressing as necessary. Place additional dressings on dependent parts to collect drainage.

15. Anchor dressing securely with tape or gauze ties.

---

1. Reduces microorganisms on hands. Reduces potential for wound infection.
2. Provides privacy. Enhances emotional and physical comfort. Person should be comfortable, with dressing site easily accessible to nurse.
3. Prevents infection.

   a. Microbes require moisture for easy mobility.

   b. Maintains dressing/equipment sterility.

   c. Keep inside of bowl sterile.

   d. Solution is sterile. Outside of bottle is not. Do not let bottle touch tray or bowl.
4. Minimize air currents. Gentleness promotes comfort.

5. Prevents wound tension. Pulling skin away (instead of tape away) prevents tearing skin. Pulling in direction away from wound edges would pull apart healing (fibrin network) wound.

6. Dressing is contaminated. Using gloves or forceps prevents organisms from transferring to nurse's hands and being spread. Gentleness and not pulling off adhering (sticking) dressing protects healing and reduces discomfort.

7. Forceful dressing removal disrupts healing process.

8. Use sterile gloves to prevent microorganisms from being introduced to the wound surface.
9. Evaluate for healing progress and complications.

10. Do not remove adhesive each time unless skin problem is present. Avoid acetone; it may chemically damage the skin or wound.
11. Consider wound line cleaner than skin area. Skin pathogens could further infect wound. Intact skin around wound usually provides barrier from infected wound.

12. Apply ointment to dressing if difficult to apply to wound.
13. Gloves are contaminated from skin cleansing.

14. Moving dressing after placement moves contaminants from skin to wound.

   Contains drainage in dressing.

15. Nonallergenic tape reduces risk of skin breakdown. For dressings needing frequent changing, use Montgomery straps and ties (see Fig. 48–35).

Procedure continued on following page

PROCEDURE 48–2 Continued

Applying Dry Sterile Dressing

Cleansing a linear wound

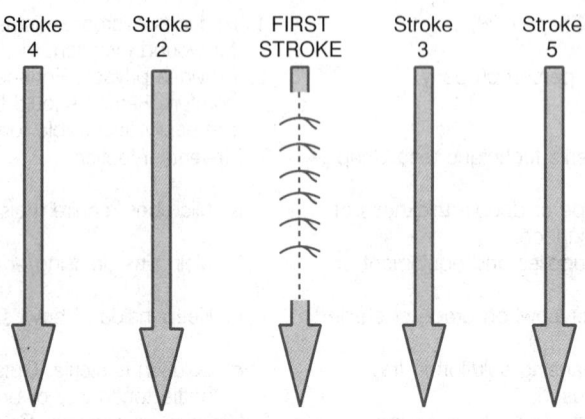

Cleansing a circular wound

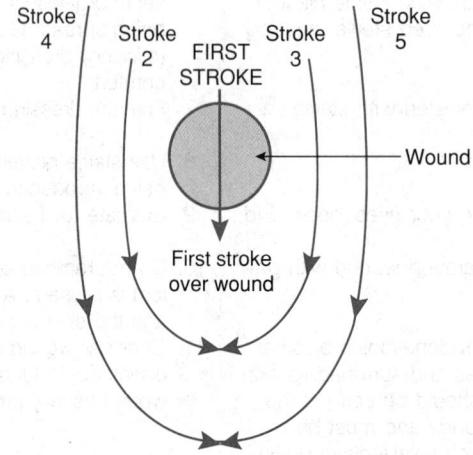

Actions

16. Replace covers over person and position as needed.
17. Collect used equipment for removal. Discard disposable equipment into waterproof bag. Wrap nondisposable equipment in sterile towel for return to appropriate area.
18. Wash hands thoroughly.

19. Gently reposition gown and bedclothes.

Rationale/Discussion

16. Increases comfort.
17. Soiled dressings and used equipment are contaminated. Prevents spread of pathogens to environment, self, and others.
18. Reduces number of microorganisms and contamination of self and others.
19. Movement of air disseminates microorganisms.

PROCEDURE 48-2 Continued

Applying Dry Sterile Dressing

FINAL ACTIVITIES

Assess individual for comfort and safety. Make sure bed is at desirable height and position and bedside stand with personal effects is within reach. Replace side rails if indicated. Return nondisposable instruments and bowl to central service for cleaning and reprocessing; discard towel in laundry. Later, return to room to assess individual and security and comfort of dressing. *Documentation:* drainage character and amount, condition of wound and surrounding tissue, person's responses to dressing change (e.g., emotional response, local pain, generalized discomfort). Note on nursing care plan points of special importance to individual regarding dressing change.

PROCEDURE 48-3

Applying Wet Sterile Dressing

Definition/Purposes. To apply moist sterile dressing to wound. This increases drainage by wick action and encourages healing. Wet sterile dressings are used to cleanse wound of debris and liquefy drainage.

Caution. Alternate wet sterile dressings with dry sterile dressings to prevent skin maceration and breakdown around wound. Some authorities believe covering a wet sterile dressing with sterile waterproof material increases the potential for skin maceration. Others believe the protection the covering gives is worth the risk. The wet dressing should be confined to the wound and should not overlap the intact skin so that the possibility of maceration is lessened. Wet dressings are ordered by the physician, who will indicate the solution to be used, duration, frequency, and temperature.

Teaching/Learning Guidelines. Explain the purpose of wet sterile dressings. Explain that this type of dressing can be considered sterile only until applied. Remember: a moist dressing brings microorganisms to the dressing surface, where they may be directly contacted. (See Procedure 48-2 for additional teaching/learning points.)

PRELIMINARY ACTIVITIES

Assessment/Planning

See Procedure 48-2.

Preparation of Person

See Procedure 48-2.
Place waterproof material in manner to protect individual and bed from moisture during procedure.

PROCEDURE

Actions

1 to 3d. See Procedure 48-2.
3e. Using sterile technique (see Chapter 28), place sterile dressing to be used in sterile container. Cover with prescribed solution.
4 to 10. See Procedure 48-2.
11. Apply dressing moistened in prescribed solution to wound. Have dressing moist but not dripping. Use instruments to twist excessive moisture out of dressing or squeeze dry with sterile-gloved hands. Wet dressings should be placed *in* the wound but not on the intact skin around it.

Equipment

Same as Procedure 48-2 plus:
   Sterile container to hold solution
   Fine-mesh gauze, 4 × 4 (without cottonfill) gauze, or
     NuGauze
   Sterile solution prescribed
   Waterproof material to protect bed from wet dressing

Rationale/Discussion

11. Moisture dripping is uncomfortable to person. Pathway is made for organism to travel to wound. Excessively wet dressing promotes skin maceration.

Procedure continued on following page

PROCEDURE 48–3 Continued

Applying Wet Sterile Dressing

PROCEDURE

Actions	Rationale/Discussion
12. Cover wet sterile dressing with dry sterile sponges or sterile waterproof material.	12. To prevent additional contamination of the wound from the atmosphere.
13. Apply outer dressing.	13. Holds dressings in place.
14. Secure dressing (see Procedure 48–2).	
15. Collect used equipment and remove (see Procedure 48–2).	
16. Wash hands thoroughly.	

FINAL ACTIVITIES

Assess individual for comfort and safety. Make sure bed is at desirable height and position and bedside stand with personal effects is within reach. Replace side rails if indicated. Return nondisposable instruments and bowl to central service for cleaning and reprocessing; discard towel in laundry. Later, return to room to assess individual and security and comfort of dressing. *Documentation:* drainage character and amount, condition of wound and surrounding tissue, person's responses to dressing change (e.g., emotional response, local pain, generalized discomfort). Note on nursing care plan points of special importance to individual regarding dressing change.

The major types of dressings are nonocclusive and occlusive. Nonocclusive dressings allow atmospheric gases to reach the wound surface. Occlusive dressings allow no exchange of gases between the wound and the outside environment.

Nonocclusive Dressings. Nonocclusive dressings are made of silk or gauze. Silk is commonly used over newly sutured wounds and donor sites. Because of its small mesh, silk does not adhere as much to the wound surface as does gauze, which is made of cotton. Gauze is the oldest of the currently used dressing materials (Fig. 48–29). Fine-mesh gauze has a slightly larger mesh size than silk and is commonly used over the donor sites of skin grafts. Coarse-mesh gauze is the most commonly used form of dry dressing. It comes in a cotton-filled version and an unfilled version consisting of gauze only.

Used primarily to cover surgical wounds closed by first intention, coarse-mesh gauze is also used by some physicians in a wet-to-dry form to debride wounds nonselectively. Wet-to-dry dressings are ordered by the physician and consist of coarse-mesh gauze pads, usually called 4 × 4s, saturated with sterile isotonic saline and then wrung out so that they are moist but not dripping. These are lightly packed into the wound. The unfilled (containing no cotton filler) gauze pads are allowed to remain in the wound until they dry out. They are then pulled off the wound surface to which they are stuck. When the gauze is removed, it debrides the necrotic tissue in the wound, but it also damages healthy tissue growing in the wound bed. Many physicians continue to order wet-to-dry dressings although less traumatic and more specific methods of debridement are available.

Wet-to-dry dressings are an outmoded method of wound debridement. Better methods of debridement are surgical removal of dead tissue, certain enzymatic preparations, and certain occlusive dressings.

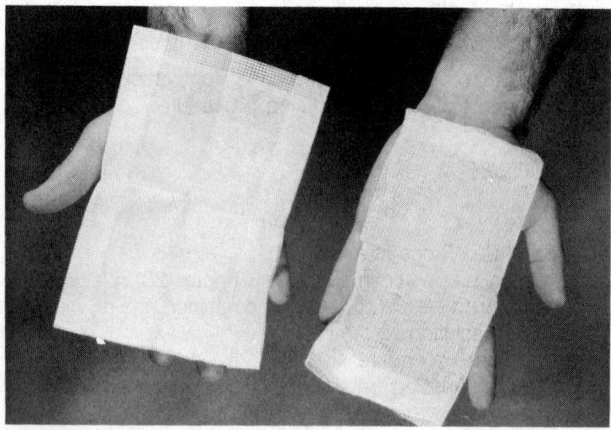

▲ *Figure 48–29*

Examples of 4 × 4 gauze dressings. The one on the left is cotton filled. The one on the right is unfilled. In wet-to-dry dressings, unfilled 4 × 4s are used.

Coarse-mesh gauze may also be used for moist soaks of uninfected wounds that do not contain necrotic tissue. For use on uninfected wounds, sterile isotonic saline is the solution of choice. Moist dressings may be used on infected wounds; the gauze may then be moistened with specifically ordered solutions, such as sodium hypochlorite (Dakin's solution), antibiotics, or acetic acid. Moistened gauze is used to promote a moist environment at the wound surface, which will encourage epithelial cell growth across the wound. It is cheaper than occlusive dressings if its use is short term, and it allows ready access to the wound surface for inspection. Be sure that the moist gauze is inside the wound bed and does not come in contact with the skin surface surrounding the wound. If intact skin remains moist for long periods, maceration will develop, and breakdown will occur. These problems can be prevented by using a commercial skin barrier if needed or a thin layer of petroleum jelly.

Moist dressings should never be allowed to dry in the wound. If they are allowed to dry, they will debride the wound surface when they are lifted.

If the dressings should dry, moisten and allow them to remain in place for several minutes before attempting to lift them.

Products made of gauze include the following:

▶ Fluffs (commonly called Toppers, their brand name). Fluffs are coarse-mesh sponges that are cotton filled. They are fluffed open to make them more absorbent and are commonly used with wounds that have large amounts of drainage (see Fig. 48–29).
▶ Abdominal pads (usually called ABDs or combines). Abdominal pads are multilayered absorbent dressings used to contain draining wounds, especially of the abdomen (Fig. 48–30). If the wound drains so much that the dressing must be changed frequently, the dressings should be held in place by Montgomery straps (Fig. 48–31). These are prepackaged adhesive straps left in place for as long as they will remain adherent to the skin. The straps have holes through which gauze strips can be placed. The strips are then laced over the abdominal pads like a shoelace and tied. Thus, they allow the abdominal pads to be removed as needed but do not require the adhesive tape to be removed each time.
▶ Gauze packing strips. Gauze strips come in a roll with a width of 1 inch or less. The gauze can be pushed gently into wounds that have tunneled or into undermined areas to eliminate dead space (i.e., that area of the wound in which fluids may collect).
▶ Roller gauze. Roller gauze may be in a flat, nonelastic form, which can be used to tie Montgomery straps, or in an unwoven, conforming, slightly elastic form, which is often called Kling (Fig. 48–32). Both forms may be used as outer wrappings for wound dressings.

Occlusive Dressings. A wide variety of occlusive dressings is available in the clinical setting. They have

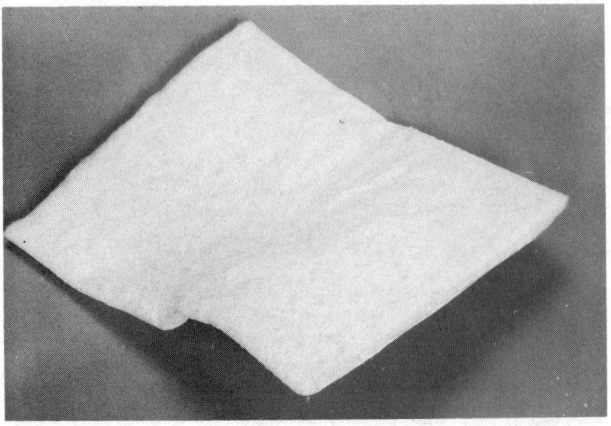

▲ Figure 48–30

Abdominal pad (also called ABD, combine, or combination pad). The heavy, thick pad is frequently used on abdominal wounds with moderate drainage. It is usually used in combination with 4 × 4s.

various properties and different indications for use. The chief property of these dressings (as opposed to nonocclusive, gauze dressings) is that they can control the wound's tissue hydration and oxygen tension. Semiocclusive dressings allow some atmospheric oxygen to penetrate; occlusive dressings allow none.

The general advantages of occlusive dressings include the following[2]:

▶ Protection from bacterial invasion
▶ Promotion of more rapid healing by keeping the wound surface moist and allowing more rapid epithelialization
▶ Debridement of necrotic material
▶ Reduction of pain by reducing drying and by insulating and protecting sensitive nerve endings in the wound that may be exposed. Some investigators believe that the ability to cool the wound surface

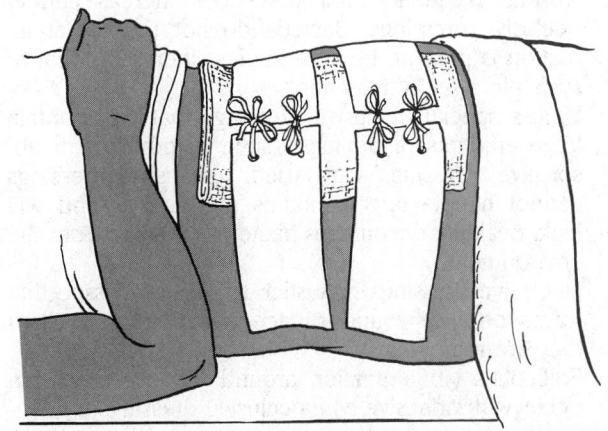

▲ Figure 48–31

Montgomery straps. These adhesive straps are made from 3-inch adhesive tape. They are tied with roller gauze.

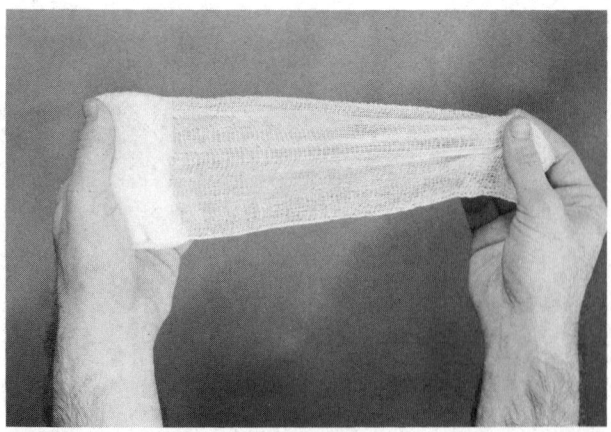

▲ **Figure 48-32**

Roller gauze with slight amount of elasticity. Also known as a Kling bandage, it is frequently used to hold dressings in place by wrapping around a body part, such as a limb. Adhesive tape is then used to secure the end of the Kling bandage to itself. This procedure avoids placing tape on the client's skin.

found with certain occlusive dressings also plays a part in relieving pain

▶ Waterproof protection to the wound surface
▶ Fewer dressing changes required than for nonocclusive dressings
▶ Cost-effectiveness for long-term use, more so than for nonocclusive dressings
▶ Ease of use for nursing and medical personnel

The potential disadvantages of occlusive dressings are as follows:

▶ Occlusive dressings should not be used on infected wounds because bacteria can multiply.
▶ If the dressing is opaque, infection may occur without the nurse's or physician's awareness. This development is termed a silent infection (i.e., one that is not clinically evident). Most infections become clinically evident in a short time (within 24 to 48 hours), but in the elderly, infection may not be obvious.
▶ Normal bacterial population does increase under occlusive dressings. Bacteria do not mean that infection is present, however, unless there are local or systemic signs of infection.
▶ Unless special occlusive dressings that can contain large amounts of drainage (such as pouches or absorptive dressings) are used, occlusive dressings cannot handle large amounts of drainage and will leak. Leakage encourages bacterial invasion from the environment.
▶ Occlusive dressings may stick to the new tissue that forms on the wound surface and disrupt it when they are removed.
▶ Folliculitis (inflammation around hair follicles) can occur with adhesive-type occlusive dressings.

Nonadherent Dressings. Nonadherent dressings do not stick to the wound surface under ordinary circumstances. They are useful for treating skin tears, donor

sites, and skin grafts. If the skin around the wound is friable (easily broken), these dressings are particularly useful. They have little absorptive ability and are applied to the wound surface and held in place by conforming roller gauze (Kling).

Polyurethane Film Dressings. Sometimes called transparent films, polyurethane film dressings have an adhesive backing that allows them to stick to dry skin. They are semipermeable and transparent. Oxygen is allowed to flow through the film, and water vapor from the wound surface is allowed to vent to the atmosphere through small pores in the material. These pores are small enough to prevent bacteria or atmospheric particles from penetrating to the wound from the outside. These dressings may be used to protect superficial wounds, intravenous sites, donor sites, abrasions, and certain other wounds. They do not have absorptive properties, and normal wound fluid builds up under them quickly. They are prone to leakage if wound fluid buildup is allowed to continue beyond their capacity to contain it (Fig. 48-33). Their use is controversial.

Polyurethane Foams. Polyurethane foams are semipermeable, nonadhesive, and nonadherent dressings. They may be either hydrophilic (absorbing fluid) or hydrophobic (not absorbing fluid). Most are moderately fluid absorbent. They create a moist wound environment and provide thermal insulation of the wound. They are designed for use with pressure ulcers, stasis ulcers, certain types of small burns, donor graft sites, postoperative incisions, and moderately exudative wounds. At least one brand adds a layer of activated carbon to the dressing to help control wound odor.

Hydrocolloids. Hydrocolloids are dressings composed of an impermeable outer polyurethane layer that covers an inner layer of gumlike materials, such as guar,

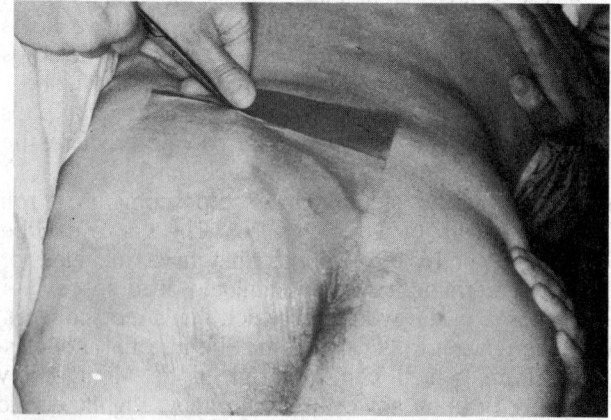

▲ **Figure 48-33**

Transparent dressing (Op-site) being placed over a stage I pressure ulcer to decrease skin abrasion from friction. There are several brands of these polyurethane dressings. (Reprinted with permission from Westaby, S. [ed.]. [1986]. *Wound care.* London: Butterworth-Heinemann.)

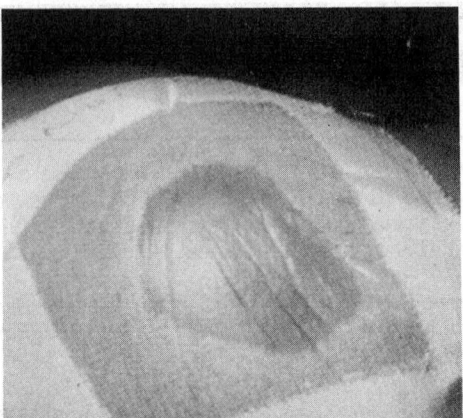

▲ *Figure 48–34*

Hydrocolloid dressing applied to pressure ulcer and "windowed" on all sides with hypoallergenic tape. Dark spot in center is typical appearance of dressing as it liquefies over wound surface to keep it moist.

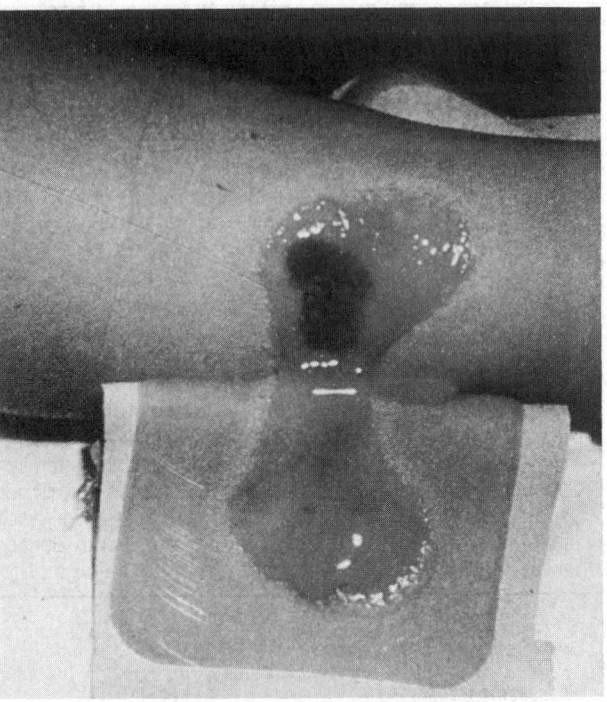

▲ *Figure 48–35*

Appearance of wound when hydrocolloid dressing is removed. This is not a sign of infection. Note that drainage is clear. There will be an odor because the dressing is occlusive. When the drainage is washed off, the odor should disappear.

karaya, gelatin, or pectin. These dressings protect the wound mechanically from injury; they prevent bacteria from entering the wound, if they are not allowed to leak; they maintain a moist wound-healing environment that allows more rapid healing; and they can be shaped to conform and seal to hard-to-cover parts of the body, such as heels, elbows, knees, and sacrum. They thermally insulate the wound as well.

Although hydrocolloids will adhere to intact skin, they must frequently be "windowed" with tape to prevent leakage if the dressing is to be left in place several days or to keep it from being pulled off of such areas as the sacrum or hips when the client is turned (Fig. 48–34). The inner layer normally liquefies over the wound surface. The yellowish mass is thick and smelly (Fig. 48–35). The dressing may be difficult at times to remove, but removal can be accomplished with sterile isotonic saline irrigations. These dressings may be used for a wide variety of wounds, both acute and chronic. They possess the ability to debride wounds of small to moderate amounts of necrotic tissue. The application of hydrocolloid dressings is described in Procedure 48–4.

Hydrogels. Hydrogels may be adhesive or nonadhesive. Most can be used in both clean and infected wounds. They do not have strong adherent properties and require that an appropriate secondary dressing be used to hold the hydrogel in place. These dressings contain a large amount of water (80 to 99 per cent). They soothe the wound surface and cool it by up to 5 degrees. They are transparent so that the wound surface can be readily observed. The frequency of change for these dressings is every one to two days. Hydrogels are used to treat wounds in people with sensitive skin and in those with significant inflammation where cooling helps relieve pain and discomfort. These dressings are absorbent, but the rate of absorption is slow.

Absorptive Products. Dressings of calcium alginate and hypertonic saline and absorptive powders, pastes, beads, and granules are designed to contain large amounts of wound drainage. Calcium alginate is made from brown seaweed. It has a high ability to absorb wound exudate, helps reduce wound odor, and activates macrophages in the wound.[26,44] Hypertonic saline–impregnated gauze dressings have the ability to "wick" away wound exudate and yet leave a moist environment at the wound surface.

The powders, pastes, beads, and granules differ somewhat in their individual properties. Most absorb wound exudate by drawing fluid away from the wound surface by osmotic action. Some have the capability of digesting necrotic tissue. In general, they form a gelatinous mass when the wound exudate is absorbed. This mass can be irrigated out of the wound with sterile isotonic saline. The major use of these absorptive products is to control the wound exudate from heavily draining wounds. As a class of products, powders, pastes, beads, and granules present certain problems. The person may complain of local stinging and pain when they are applied; some can raise the wound pH above normal levels; one has been reported to cause granulomas (a benign growth usually composed of lymphoid and epithelioid cells) if it is not washed completely out of the wound (Fig. 48–36).

Impregnated Dressings. Gauze dressings can be impregnated with antibacterial or bactericidal compounds,

PROCEDURE 48–4

Applying Hydrocolloid Dressings

Definition/Purposes. To cover chronic wounds with a nonpermeable, occlusive, sterile dressing that will provide a moist healing environment to encourage more rapid epithelialization of the wound surface. These dressings protect the wound from environmental contaminants and the environment from wound contaminants. Replace dressing as required (usually able to remain in place 2 to 7 days). Dressings are opaque and prevent wound observation without removal.

Contraindications/Cautions. These dressings are contraindicated in *infected* wounds. They are also not recommended for use in full-thickness wounds involving muscle, tendon, or bone. They are not used on clients with active vasculitis or those with third-degree burns.

Teaching/Learning Guidelines. Provide information about dressing change importance. Discuss pain concerns and reassure the person that removal of these dressings rarely causes any discomfort. The individual may not want to see the wound. If the wound will be observed by the individual or family member, prepare them for the pronounced odor that usually accumulates under these dressings; tell them it will normally disappear when the wound is cleansed of the gel-like substance that results as the dressing's interior layer dissolves on the wound surface. Prepare them also for the fact that the wound appears to increase in size and depth during the initial period of use of this dressing because it is clearing away necrotic debris. Tell them to report any feelings of fever or localized discomfort at wound site.

PRELIMINARY ACTIVITIES

Assessment/Planning

Verify need for dressing change.
Check chart for orders relative to dressing change.
Note individual preferences on nursing care plan.
Plan dressing change at least disruptive time (e.g., not just before or after meals, or when visitors are present, or late at night).
Assess type, size, numbers of dressings needed.
Provide privacy.
Create clean, dry work space.

Preparation of Person

Explain purpose of dressing change.

Equipment/Supplies

Hydrocolloid dressings of correct size
Absorptive granules or paste if needed for drainage absorption
Sterile isotonic saline
Irrigation set containing 30-ml syringe with 19-gauge blunt-tipped needle or angiocath
4 × 4 gauze sponges
Clean gloves—1 or 2 pairs
Sterile gloves—1 pair
Hypoallergenic tape
Sterile basin
Waterproof bag to contain used dressings

PROCEDURE

Actions	Rationale/Discussion
1. Wash hands carefully.	1. Reduces microorganisms on hands. Reduces potential for wound infection.
2. Screen, position, and drape person properly.	2. Provides privacy. Enhances emotional and physical comfort. Person should be comfortable, with dressing site easily accessible to nurse.
3. Put on clean gloves to remove old dressing. (Note: This step will be omitted if this is the initial application).	3. Clean gloves are primarily used to prevent contamination of the nurse's hands from handling of the old dressing.
4. Remove old dressing by pressing down on the skin with one hand and carefully lifting the edge of the dressing toward the wound. Continue lifting slowly around the wound margins until all edges are free from the skin surface. Lift carefully from the wound.	4. This allows the dressing to be removed by decreasing tension on the wound. The dressing is lifted and removed *toward* the wound. This is designed to prevent interference with new cell growth in the wound bed. Note: The wound surface under a hydrocolloid dressing will have liquefied material on it that appears purulent and has a strong odor. This is due to an interaction between the wound and the dressing and the fact that the dressing is impermeable. Both odor and drainage are normal with this type dressing.
5. Discard old dressing and gloves into plastic bag.	5. Dressing is contaminated. Gloves prevent organisms from being transferred to the nurse's hands and being spread.

PROCEDURE 48–4 Continued

Applying Hydrocolloid Dressings

Actions	Rationale/Discussion

Actions

6. Wash hands; open sterile equipment in this order—irrigation set, sterile basin, pour sterile saline into basin, open 4 × 4s and place on sterile field, open hydrocolloid dressing outer package and place dressing on sterile field. Peel back the corner of the backing paper on the granule packet (if it is to be used). Do *not* place it on sterile field, but place it closely adjacent.

7. Put on sterile gloves, if needed. (Clean gloves may be used in most chronic wounds, and clean procedure may be followed.)

8. Irrigate the wound with normal saline using a 30-ml syringe with a 19-gauge blunt-tipped needle or angiocath that furnishes the 8 psi pressure needed for safe irrigation. When a new dressing is to be applied, it is unnecessary to remove all residual dressing material from the surrounding skin.

9. Dry the skin area surrounding the wound with sterile 4 × 4s. Dry from the wound margin toward the periphery. Discard used 4 × 4s off the sterile field.

10. Assess the clean wound bed and surrounding skin for necrosis, erythema, odor, additional drainage, and changes in depth or size.

11. Select a dressing size that will cover at least 1½ inches beyond the wound margin.

12. Apply granules or paste* if wound bed is 1 cm or more into subcutaneous tissue to eliminate dead space and to absorb exudate.

13. Fill wound bed with granules* or paste only to a level that is no higher than skin level. (Gloves are no longer considered sterile at this point.)

14. Peel back inner covering of hydrocolloid dressing and discard. Do not touch inner part of dressing. Apply dressing directly over wound surface. Do *not* stretch it. Roll it from one side to the other. Smooth it gently into place. Do not hurry this procedure. Initial adhesion improves as the dressing becomes warm. Note: These dressings may be cut to conform to various body surfaces, such as the heels or elbows. If applying over sacrum, press into anal fold. Remove gloves and discard into bag with used dressing materials.

Rationale/Discussion

6. Must open all sterile equipment using sterile technique *before* putting on sterile gloves. Make sure that the hydrocolloid dressing is large enough to extend at least 1½ inches beyond the wound margin so that it can adhere to healthy skin.

7. Sterile gloves are used if wound is open and is not healing. In many chronic wounds, such as pressure ulcers, only clean technique is required.

8. Irrigation is needed to remove the liquefied wound dressing and drainage from the wound surface so that it can be inspected. The use of isotonic saline (not hydrogen peroxide) is safe for the wound surface because it does not damage granulation tissue. The mechanical action of irrigation will remove some necrotic tissue that is still loosely connected to the wound surface.

9. Drying the skin prevents maceration. It also gives the new dressing a dry surface to which it can adhere. These dressings will not stick to wet, oily, or greasy surfaces.

10. Wound surface should be clean. Because hydrocolloid dressings can debride wounds autolytically, the wound may *increase* in size and depth during the first few dressing changes. The apparent deterioration is normally accompanied by a gradual improvement in the appearance of the wound bed. However, if any of the following develops—uncharacteristic odor, change in color of exudate, fever, or cellulitis (tenderness and erythema in the area of the wound)—report this to your instructor and the physician. These may be signs of clinical infection, and the hydrocolloid dressing management will be discontinued until it resolves.

11. This will allow the dressing to adhere to healthy skin.

12. Dead space is an area of tissue destruction where fluids tend to collect and will result in abscess formation if not eliminated. Excess exudate must be absorbed to prevent leakage of the dressing.

13. This is an adequate amount to contain excess exudate or to eliminate dead space.

14. These dressings are conformable to body surfaces. They can be shaped through cutting; but if they are stretched they lose some of their adhesive qualities.

Stomahesive paste may be placed in a thin layer in the anal skin fold area at the coccyx to promote a seal and to prevent stool from getting under the dressing.

Procedure continued on following page

PROCEDURE 48–4 Continued

Applying Hydrocolloid Dressings

Actions	*Rationale/Discussion*
15. Tape all edges of the dressing with 1-inch wide hypoallergenic tape to reduce the risk of peeling.	15. "Window frame" the entire dressing with tape to secure dressing and prevent leaking.
16. Replace covers over person and position comfortably.	
17. Collect used equipment for removal. Discard disposable equipment into waterproof bag. Wrap nondisposable equipment in sterile towel for return to appropriate area.	17. Soiled dressings and used equipment are contaminated. Prevents spread of pathogens to environment, self, and others.
18. Wash hands thoroughly.	18. Reduces number of microorganisms and contamination of self and others.
19. Change dressing every 2 to 3 days or as needed if leakage occurs.	19. Frequent dressing changes during the later stages of healing should be avoided to minimize potential re-injury of the wound.

* Omit steps 12 and 13 if the wound is shallower than 1 cm and has no exudate.

FINAL ACTIVITIES

Assess individual for comfort and safety. Make sure bed is at desirable height and position and bedside stand with personal effects is within reach. Replace side rails if indicated. Return nondisposable instruments and bowl to central service for cleaning and reprocessing. Later, return to room to assess individual and security and comfort of dressing. *Documentation:* drainage character and amount, condition of wound and surrounding tissue, person's responses to dressing change (e.g., emotional response, local pain, generalized discomfort). Note on nursing care plan points of special importance to individual regarding dressing change.

---

such as scarlet red, petroleum jelly, or bismuth tribromophenate (Xeroform). Such medicated dressings, designed to be placed directly on the wound, may help control the bacterial population of the wound, but their chemical compounds may also be cytotoxic to healing cells, particularly fibroblasts (Fig. 48–37). (See Table 48–6 for a list of wound care products and Figure 48–18 for guides to their use.)

DRAINS AND SUCTION

Wound drains may be used to remove continuing wound drainage; provide an exit for unexpected bile, intestinal, or vascular leaks; provide an appropriately situated sinus track; and obliterate dead space (space where fluid may collect within an anatomic cavity, abscess cavity, or wound). A drain is placed where fluid is expected to collect (Fig. 48–38). This site is frequently in the wound or through a stab wound (separate small incision) located where drainage is expected to accumulate. The type of drain depends on its purpose (Table 48–11). A drain is removed as soon as its purpose is achieved.

When a drain is in place, anticipate drainage from it and pad the dressing accordingly. Because drainage seeks a low level, place the bulk of the dressing at the wound's lower edge.

Change dressings over drains frequently and keep an accurate record of the amount of fluid lost.

The amount of fluid lost may be estimated in two ways. The first is to record the number and size of dressings changed and describe the amount of drainage in them (e.g., one combination pad with a 4- X 12-cm area heavily saturated or a 1- X 2-cm area containing bloody drainage). The second method for estimating fluid loss is to weigh the dry dressing before application and the wet dressing after removal and then record the weight difference (this method is seldom done).

Wound drainage systems consist of wound drain and suction apparatus as one system. There are various wound drainage systems, such as Hemovac and Jackson-Pratt. A drain may be inserted with or without suction being applied.

Either a Hemovac or a Jackson-Pratt system may be used when low-pressure suction is desired. A Hemovac is a lightweight, self-contained unit composed of a closed, collapsible container attached to a drain by a

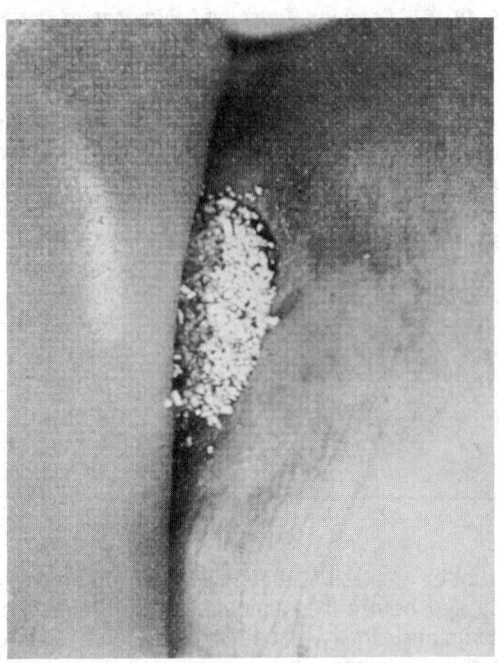

▲ *Figure 48-36*

Deep sacral pressure ulcer with wound drainage. The ulcer was treated with absorption granules to contain drainage and a hydrocolloid dressing (DuoDERM granules and dressing).

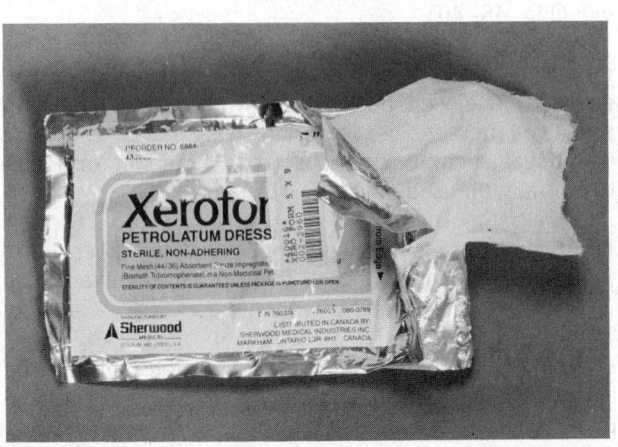

▲ *Figure 48-37*

Gauze-impregnated dressing used directly on wound surface and then covered with dry dressing material.

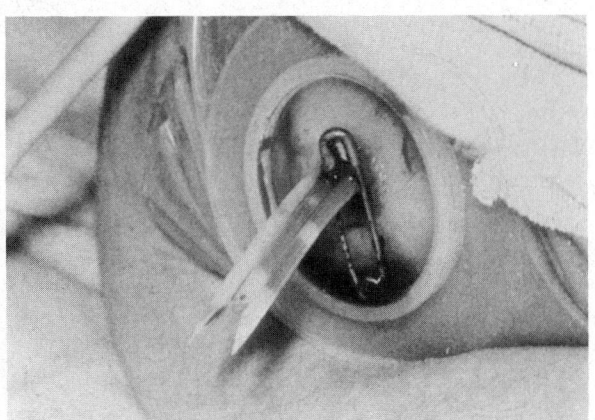

▲ *Figure 48-38*

Wound drain to the deeper layers of the abdominal wall after appendectomy. The drain allows fluid to escape and prevents abscess formation. Note safety pin to prevent the drain from being lost in the wound. (Reprinted with permission from Westaby, S. [ed.]. [1986]. *Wound care.* London: Butterworth-Heinemann.)

TABLE 48-11. Common Types and Purposes of Drains and Suction

Type of Drain	Purpose	Example
Penrose	Provide drainage track	After incision and drainage of abscess
Red rubber	Obliterate dead space	After mastectomy or chest surgery
T-tube	Vent for bile drainage	After cholecystectomy
Intracath or pediatric feeding tube	Remove continuing transudate	After paracentesis
Gauze wick, NuGauze, iodoform gauze	Keep sinus open so healing can occur from base	After hemorrhoidectomy
Jackson-Pratt	Create low suction on wounds expected to have moderate drainage	After mastectomy
Hemovac	Create low suction on wounds expected to have moderate drainage	After mastectomy
Pleur-evac	Create controlled levels of water-seal suction on wounds expected to have significant drainage	After chest or lung surgery or trauma

solid rubber or plastic tube (Fig. 48–39). The container is collapsed before it is attached to the drain. Then, as the container slowly expands, a vacuum is created within the container. This vacuum provides suction on the drain and pulls fluid from the wound into the container. Hemovac systems are used primarily in wounds with large amounts of drainage and are manufactured in sizes of 100, 400, and 800 ml. A Jackson-Pratt system is a bulb-type suction device attached to a drainage tube. It works on the same principle as the Hemovac (Fig. 48–40).

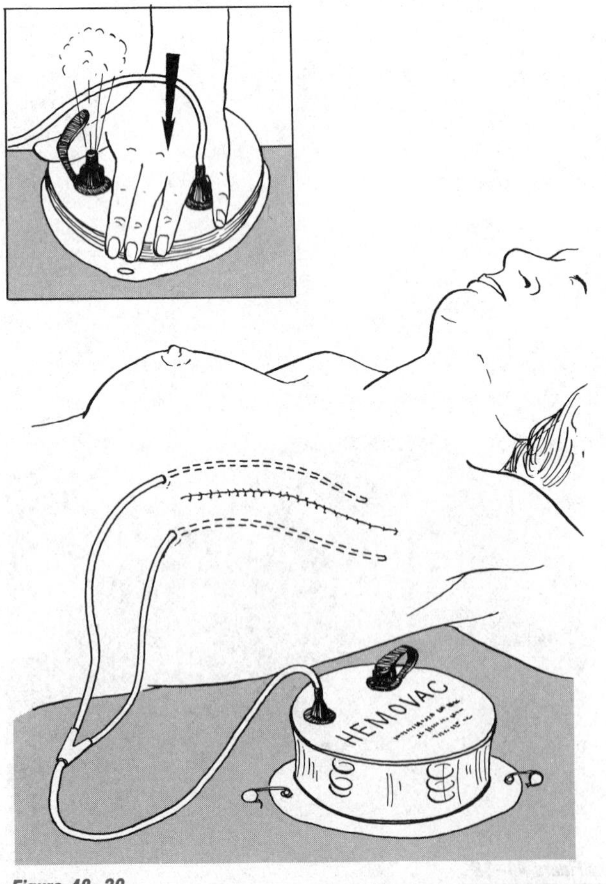

An electrical pump (Gomco) may be used when greater suction is desired. If the drainage and suction are from a closed body cavity where maintenance of negative pressure is important (e.g., the chest), a water-seal suction apparatus (e.g., Emerson or Pleurevac) may be used (Fig. 48–41).

Caution With all types of wound suction, keep tubes connecting the apparatus to the wound unkinked. Also observe drainage type and volume.

With all but electrical pump suction, the unit must be airtight to function effectively. To empty suction containers, follow equipment instructions, especially when it is necessary to maintain negative pressure within the cavity being drained.

ANTIMICROBIAL SUPPORT

Antimicrobial agents may be used therapeutically or prophylactically. They are used therapeutically to treat known or suspected infections. Therapeutic use involves using the fewest medications with the narrowest spectrum of activity that will be effective. This treatment typically continues for 7 to 10 days. Antimicrobials are used prophylactically to prevent infections. Thus, when used prophylactically, they are started before a site is contaminated with microorganisms (e.g., before surgery) and are continued for no more than 24 hours postoperatively. Because a person's normal bacterial flora changes with antimicrobial therapy, their use is discontinued as promptly as possible. Prophylaxis is usually given when a sterile area of the body is approached through an unsterile area or when implanted material (implants) will be left in the body.

Antimicrobials may be administered systemically or topically. For systemic administration, they may be given orally, intramuscularly, or intravenously. Topical administration includes skin preparations and nonab-

▲ Figure 48-39

Hemovac wound drainage and suction unit. This device is used to provide continuous low-pressure suction in wounds expected to have significant amounts of drainage. Suction is created by compressing the unit while the air vent is open. The unit is then capped and attached to the drainage tube.

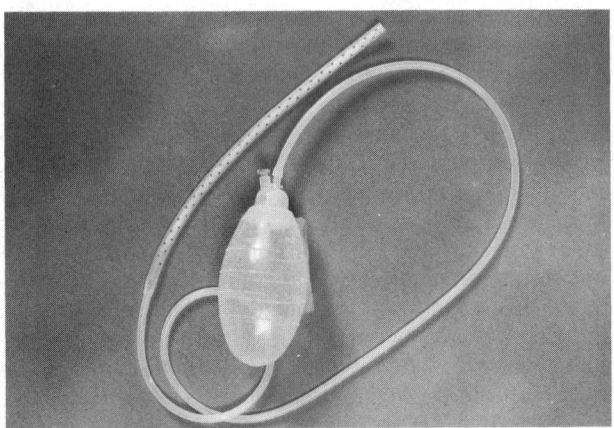

▲ *Figure 48–40*

Jackson-Pratt drainage and suction unit. The tubing's multiple openings are inserted into the wound cavity by the physician; drainage flows through them into the bulb, which is compressed while the air vent is open. The vent is then closed to create low suction. This type of drainage system is used on wounds when a moderate amount of drainage is expected that would be too great to be contained in a dressing.

sorbable agents that are effective only on the surfaces to which they are applied, such as in the gastrointestinal tract; inside the peritoneum and joint spaces; and into the spinal cord's subarachnoid space, where these agents are administered intrathecally.

There are three groups of antimicrobial agents. The first is antibacterial agents (e.g., the penicillins, tetracy-

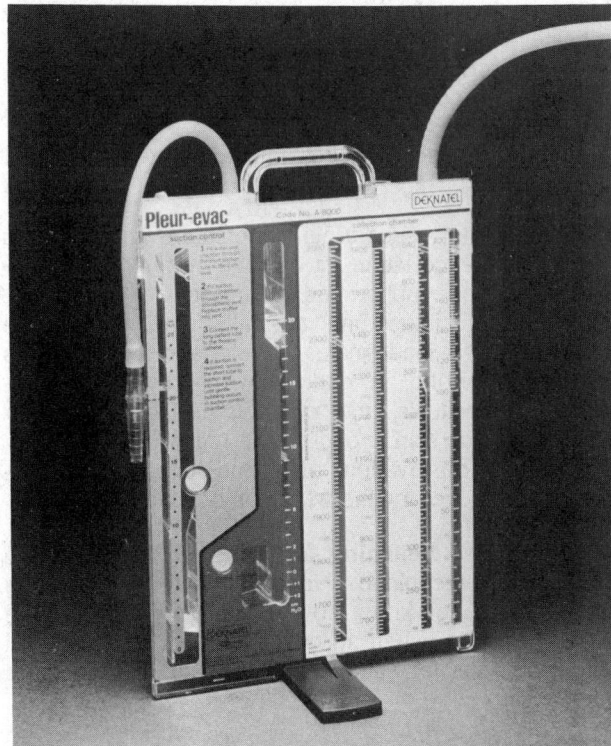

▲ *Figure 48–41*

Pleur-evac drainage system used to remove fluid from the pleural space. (Courtesy of Deknatel, Inc., Fall River, MA.)

clines, cephalosporins, and aminoglycosides). Individual agents may have a relatively narrow or broad spectrum of efficiency against specific bacteria. The second group is antifungal agents (e.g., amphotericin B, nystatin). The third group comprises antiviral agents, which include specific immune globulins and interferon.

The nurse is responsible for administering these drugs as ordered by the physician. Care must be taken to administer the correct drug in the correct dose at the correct time and to give it by the correct route to the correct client (see Chapter 46).

Remember the following guidelines for infection control during wound care:

▶ Wash hands before and after all dressing changes and wound care, even if gloves will be worn.
▶ Wear sterile gloves for contact with any wound that is not closed.
▶ Treat wounds similarly that are closed by primary intention with sutures, clips, or staples. These wounds are often left undressed, and adequate wound care is accomplished in a shower (if the wound is permitted to be wet).
▶ Ensure that sutures, clips, or staples are removed with sterile equipment.
▶ Wear clean gloves for dressing changes of closed wounds and to remove soiled dressing.
▶ Wear a mask to cover your nose and mouth for dressing changes of open wounds, plus goggles for wound irrigations in which splashing may occur.
▶ Wear a gown when your clothing is likely to become soiled with body substances. Some facilities also require gowns when caring for persons with certain infections.
▶ Wear a hair cover when caring for massive wounds (e.g., large burn wounds) where your hair could fall into the wound.
▶ Bag used dressings and disposable soiled equipment before disposing in designated container. Some facilities require autoclaving before ultimate disposal (e.g., landfill).

ODOR CONTROL

Chronic wounds, infected wounds, draining wounds, and colostomy and ileostomy wounds are capable of creating unpleasant odors. These odors are upsetting to the person, to visitors, and to health care personnel. Several types of wound deodorizers are marketed. Some commercially available wound deodorizer and cleanser combinations contain benzethonium chloride. The person can ingest oral deodorizer tablets formulated from chlorophyllin copper complex, which may help control the odor from colostomies, ileostomies, and incontinence if there is no medical contraindication. Some deodorizers are specially formulated to be added to the colostomy or ileostomy appliance. Room deodorizers are available, but they do little more than mask the wound odor. A drop or two of oil of wintergreen is often used for this purpose. Some of the newer occlusive dressings prevent wound odor or neutralize it, but remember these occlusive dressings are seldom indicated for use in infected wounds.

For clients with cancer, Welch[113] recommends using plain, room-temperature yogurt on open, superficial, nonhealing lesions that drain continuously. The wound is irrigated with isotonic saline first, followed by plain yogurt applied to the entire wound area. Follow the yogurt application by rinsing the wound with isotonic saline again, so that it is completely flushed out of the wound. Then apply a nonadherent dressing to the wound. Welch recommends that this regimen be done four times per day. Within 48 to 72 hours, the odor problem should be resolved.

If the person is about to be discharged home with a draining, odor-causing lesion, the person should be shown how to control the odor using plain yogurt. An irrigating syringe can be purchased at the drugstore, or an ordinary gravy baster can be used. The person can be instructed to use tap water or can make isotonic saline by boiling 1 liter (quart) of water and 2 tea-spoons of salt. The wound should then be covered with a nonadherent dressing. If the wound bleeds easily, a dressing coated with petroleum jelly is less likely to cause bleeding when it is removed.

Although yogurt is recommended by some nurses, especially those working with cancer patients, there are no scientific data to support its use for the purpose of wound deodorizing. Do not institute this regimen without the physician's approval first.

While the client is in the hospital, the best regimen is one that cleans the wound frequently, uses the best dressing type for the wound, and disposes of used wound dressings in the correct bags, which are then disposed of away from the person's room.

SUTURES AND STAPLES

The nursing care of individuals with sutured wounds depends on wound location, suture type, and amount of wound drainage. For example, it is important to cleanse skin around retention sutures at least daily. On the other hand, 5–0 skin sutures in a small laceration may require minimal cleansing. When physical appearance is a priority after healing, the area around the sutures may be gently cleansed (usually daily) to remove crusting, and a prescribed ointment may be applied to minimize further crusting. Wound care is often limited merely to changing dressings as needed.

Practice varies about whether to allow a sutured wound to become wet. Some practitioners allow gentle suture line washing. Others require that the area be kept dry at all times. It is important to prevent the suture line from remaining wet for a sustained period of time. Thus, after wound care, promptly dry the wound area and reapply dressings if necessary.

Monitoring Sutured Wounds. Both surgical and accidental wounds may be closed by suturing. Major areas for inspection include the sutures themselves, the wound edges, and the surrounding tissue; the presence or absence of drainage from the wound is noted.

When monitoring skin sutures, see that all the original sutures are still tied and visible. When running or continuous sutures are used, there is a knot at the incision's beginning and end. Interrupted sutures mean that each stitch is made with a separate suture and is tied individually (see Fig. 48–24). Sutures should not be so loose that the wound edges are not closed (approximated) nor so tight that they cut into the tissues. Sutures may be too tight because they were initially sewn too tightly, because the underlying structures are under great or increasing tension (e.g., as with abdominal distention after major abdominal surgery), or because the wound was sustained through blunt trauma and tissues have swollen. (Pressure dressings are usually applied to such wounds to minimize the tissue swelling. Cold application may also be ordered.)

Sutures that are too tight may cause tissue necrosis or increase the size of the scar. If the sutures are so tight that they are damaging the underlying tissue, some or all of them may be removed, even though the wound may be less than 24 hours old.

Monitor the wound edges and surrounding tissue to determine how wound healing is progressing. Ideally, newly sutured edges are everted. The wound edges are usually covered with serous material within 24 hours, and this seals the wound naturally. The serous material normally forms a small crust or scab, and small collections of serous material also may accumulate where the suture enters and exits the skin.

Note the nature of wound drainage as well as that around the sutures. Small amounts of serous or sero-sanguineous drainage are normal in a fresh wound. Gross bleeding, the presence of purulent drainage, or a large amount of drainage is not normal and should be reported and documented promptly.

In general, all wound edges should be approximated. A gap in the suture line or wound approximation may indicate developing wound dehiscence; underlying tissues may protrude through the defect in the incision, creating dehiscence.

Wound dehiscence requires immediate reporting and attention.

Examine the tissues around the suture line for signs of infection, excoriation, or damage from sutures. Monitor the blood supply and perfusion of the tissues. Well-perfused tissues are normally pink. Where the blood supply is inadequate, the skin and wound edges are pale, cyanotic, or dark brown or black. In dark-skinned individuals, the color is usually darker or grayish and the skin is cool to the touch.

Document observations of wound status until the sutures are removed or the wound is completely healed.

Teaching and Learning for Sutured Wounds. The best suturing technique is useless if the individual with sutures does not know how to care properly for the sutured wound when discharged. Key teaching and learning points for sutured wounds may include these guidelines:

▶ Keep the suture line clean and dry.
▶ Remove wound crusts and drainage using clean technique.
▶ Change dressing using clean technique.

▶ Apply topical agents if ordered.

▶ Recognize indications of infection.

▶ Splint or immobilize the wound as required.

▶ Recognize wound healing characteristics.

▶ Know how, when, and where to obtain follow-up care, including suture removal.

▶ Know strategies to protect the wound during activities of daily living. For example, use water-repellent wound covers to keep the wound dry and clean during work and bathing.

Removing Sutures. Nonabsorbable sutures are removed when wound edges are fairly well healed. If left in the wound, they may increase the risk of infection and scarring. The more distal a wound, the longer the sutures are left in place. For example, sutures of the hands or feet may be left in place for 10 to 14 days, whereas facial sutures are often removed within three to five days. Usually a wound is not completely healed when sutures are removed. Thus, adhesive skin closures (e.g., strips) help protect the wound.

DEVICES TO SECURE DRESSINGS

Dressings can be secured with adhesive tape, Montgomery straps, bandages, or elasticized net. (Binders, which can also be used to secure dressings, are discussed in Chapter 37.) The item selected to secure a dressing depends on (1) the size of the area to be dressed, (2) the frequency of dressing change, (3) the individual's activity level, and (4) the individual's location (e.g., home, hospital, wilderness).

There are several types of adhesive tapes (see Table 48–8).

Reactions to adhesive tape may be mechanical, chemical, or allergic.

Mechanical irritation to adhesive tape may appear as induced vasodilation or skin stripping. Induced vasodilation is a common, relatively brief vascular response to adhesive tape removal characterized by nontraumatic skin redness. Skin stripping is caused when skin cells are removed along with the tape (usually occlusive tape). It is characterized by prolonged skin redness (i.e., up to 24 hours).

Chemical reactions occur when components of the adhesive or backing permeate the tissues. Skin redness may be present. This reaction is also associated with occlusive adhesive tapes, which promote moisture accumulation under the tape and thus cause skin maceration and wrinkling. Such reactions may be prevented by using more porous tapes.

Caution: Severe allergic reactions may occur from the adhesive or chemical adherents used to make adhesive tapes adhere.

Allergic reactions are characterized by skin erythema (redness), edema (swelling), vesicles (blisters), and papules (small, solid, well-defined skin elevation). Allergic reactions account for only a few of the reactions to adhesive tapes. Before applying adhesive tape, ask the person or significant others about allergies to adhesives, adherents, rubber, or perfume. If such allergies may be present, a skin patch test may be indicated, or an alternative bandage (e.g., Kling bandage) may be used.

When frequent dressing changes are necessary, it is helpful to apply Montgomery straps (see Fig. 48–31) on the skin to secure dressings. With use of Montgomery straps, repeated applications and removals of adhesive tape are unnecessary, so that skin trauma is minimized. Montgomery straps are secured on the skin on either side of a wound in pairs opposite one another. Strips of gauze or material are then threaded through holes in the tape and tied over the dressings to keep them in place over the wound. Some nurses prefer instead to put a large safety pin through each hole and connect the pins to a large rubber band. This procedure holds the dressing in place and has a little elasticity as well.

When the dressing needs changing, the gauze strips or rubber bands are simply untied or released. Then the soiled dressing is removed and replaced with a fresh one, and the strips or bands are resecured over it. Montgomery straps are changed when soiled. The tie strips may be changed as needed without removing the straps. Montgomery straps are especially valuable for people with long-term dressings and those whose skin surface has been pulled off (denuded) from repeated adhesive tape removals. They are available pre-made.

Gauze or cotton dressings serve as bacterial barriers only when they are dry. Once moist, these dressings collect microorganisms and hold them close to the wound.

PREVENTION OF CHRONIC WOUNDS

Preventive devices can avert the occurrence of a wound. Obviously, traumatic wounds can be prevented only if the individual takes responsibility for safety. Surgical wounds are made in response to a pathologic condition or, perhaps, for cosmetic purposes, and so they can seldom be prevented. Prevention is therefore not as important for these wounds as it is for chronic wounds.

The chronic wounds for which most preventive devices exist are pressure ulcers (see Table 48–5 for a brief list of products available for this purpose; see also Figs. 48–15 to 48–17 for photographs of an air mattress overlay, a low air loss bed, and an air fluidized bed). Each preventive product has the capability to reduce pressure between the body and the surface on which the person rests (i.e., the interface pressure). When a person is supported on a pressure-reducing surface, the person's weight is distributed to a much greater degree than on a regular mattress.

DOCUMENTATION OF WOUND CARE

As the client's wound is assessed, a detailed description of the wound should include the specific treatment, its frequency, the progress of wound healing, any complications noted, and what was done about them. If there is any question about whether to include additional information, check with your instructor.

With pressure ulcers, be sure to include the following information.

▶ Was the wound present on admission to the agency? If so, a head-to-toe inspection of the skin must be done. If nonblanchable erythema is present, then record it as a stage I pressure ulcer present on admission.

▶ What are the wound's measurements, surface dimensions, and depth? Draw it on the nurses' notes so there will be no question about initial appearance.

▶ What is the wound's stage—I, II, III, or IV?

▶ Is there drainage from the wound? How much? What is its appearance? Does it have an odor?

▶ What is its location?

▶ Is there more than one wound? Describe each one specifically.

▶ What is the condition of the skin surrounding the pressure ulcer?

▶ How long has the patient had it? How did it start?

▶ What preventive devices were in use? What preventive devices are now in use?

▶ How frequently is the client repositioned?

▶ What dressings or other topical agents are in use? How frequently?

▶ What subjective symptoms does the person describe?

Record the progress of the pressure ulcer each time care is given.

DISCHARGE PLANNING

Meeting the individual's post-hospital needs involves planning for those needs from the moment of hospital admission. For the individual with a wound, the elements of a discharge plan include the following:

▶ The nature of the wound care that will be needed in the post-hospital setting. Will the individual be in a skilled nursing care setting, such as an intermediate care facility? If the individual goes home, will care be given on a daily basis by a home health care agency nurse? Will the client go to a nursing home? Are there family or friends who can be trained to provide the care needed at home?

▶ The need for additional teaching. If the individual is able to go home, what educational needs do the client and family have so safe wound care is provided? What information and skills need to be included? Is supervised practice of the wound care built into the educational program? (Remember that more than one return demonstration of a skill is needed to show basic mastery.)

▶ Related needs of both the client and family. Do the individual and family require additional assessment of other needs or problems that will affect wound care? For example, if the client has an infected wound and there are small children in the house-

hold, what alterations need to be made to protect both the client and the children?

▶ Psychosocial needs. Is there a need for individual or family counseling? For example, is the individual's wound so distressing to client or family that psychologic counseling is needed to deal with it? Is the family setting not conducive to recovery? Is there a need for a social worker or psychologic social worker to help in working through problems of a psychologic, financial, or social nature?

After determining the elements of the discharge plan, develop the plan using each bit of new information that can be obtained from the individual, family, friends, and health care providers. This careful process will help ensure that the discharge plan is truly tailored to the client's wound care needs. Build in coordination and implementation of the plan as well as professional follow-up to see that the wound care goals set for the client have been adequately met. Follow-up may frequently be done by phone.

HOME CARE OF WOUNDS

Clients with wounds that are difficult to heal or chronic require continued self-care or care by family, friends, or health care professionals. If the client has sufficient financial resources, there is usually no problem. More often, however, the client, family, or friends must care for the wound. It is important that they know how to care for the wound safely, what equipment is needed, what equipment can be substituted, how to use clean technique (or sterile technique if required), what the proper solutions to be used to clean the wound are, how to make isotonic saline at home, how to use the proper dressing materials correctly, and what changes in the wound are to be reported to the physician or nurse. In addition, each individual involved in wound care must be taught to protect the person's skin, to prevent pressure, and to minimize the risk of pressure ulcer development. Those caring for a person with a wound also must understand the role of nutrition in wound healing, the need for regular position changes at 1- to 2-hour intervals (if the client is unable to do this unaided), the proper use of pillows or other pressure-reducing devices, and techniques for inspecting the skin properly for changes. Table 48–12 summarizes important principles of wound care.

Applications of Heat or Cold

Applications of heat or cold are common therapeutic measures. They are often used in conjunction with other therapies for many different conditions. Heat and cold are forms of energy produced when molecules are moving. The slower the molecules move, the less heat exists.

Energy is transferred to living tissue by conduction, convection, radiation, evaporation, and conversion. Heat transfer uses the processes of conduction, conversion, radiation, and convection. Cold is transferred

TABLE 48-12. Selected Principles and Related Nursing Interventions for Care of Wounds

Principle	Nursing Interventions
A break in the integrity of skin or mucous membrane provides an entrance for microorganisms.	Plan measures to prevent infections when around individuals with wounds: ▶ Separate people with wounds from people with known infections. ▶ Provide optimal nutrition to persons with wounds so body defenses can help fight infection. ▶ Restrict people entering person's room if infection risk is high (e.g., clients with extensive burns). ▶ See Chapter 28 for additional infection control procedures.
Chemical, mechanical, thermal, and microbial agents can injure skin, mucous membranes, and deeper tissues.	For intact skin and mucous membranes, use antiseptics in safe strengths. Do not pour antiseptics into open, fresh wounds. Be gentle during wound care to avoid causing unnecessary mechanical trauma. Watch for sensitivity to adhesives (e.g., itching, redness, blisters, denuded skin). When applying heat, use safe temperatures to avoid burning tissue. Keep wound and surrounding area clean.
Skin and mucous membranes normally harbor pathogens (i.e., disease-producing microorganisms).	Practice effective infection control interventions (see Chapter 28). During wound cleansing, consider the wound itself cleanest (i.e., cleaner than skin). Hence, clean first over the wound, then clean area around wound. Discard cleaning swab after one stroke.
Microorganisms can be carried on air currents.	With clean, primary wounds, a fibrin seal develops within hours after wound closure. These wounds may be left uncovered without danger of airborne microorganisms penetrating the fibrin seal.
Respiratory tract harbors microorganisms that can enter a wound.	Masks may be worn by health care personnel when dressing large, open wounds. This reduces the number of organisms entering the wound. Avoid talking directly over wound when dressing open wounds.
Nutrients and oxygen are carried to a wound via the bloodstream and are essential for collagen formation.	Avoid constrictive measures when treating a wound. Control edema. Pressure from edema may occlude blood vessels.
Moisture facilitates the growth and movement of microorganisms.	Keep sterile fields and dressings dry. Soiled dressings provide a bridge for microorganisms to enter and leave wounds.
Fluids flow downward as a result of gravity.	Anticipate drainage at lower edge of wound. Thus, place extra dressings there if needed to collect drainage. During wound irrigation, instill solution at top of wound and collect it at lower edge.
Fluids follow the line of least resistance.	Forceful irrigation of an infected wound may push contaminated material along tissue planes, thus possibly spreading infection.
Fluids move through materials by capillary action.	Cotton between gauze layers effectively acts as a wick in dressings. Wick action carries drainage away from a wound. Penrose drains remove wound drainage by capillary action.
Obliteration of wound dead space aids healing by bringing wound edges closer together.	Drains are one method of reducing dead space. Gentle suction with a Hemovac removes wound drainage. External pressure dressings reduce dead space little but do constrict local blood vessels.

by conduction, evaporation, and convection. The following principles are important in managing heat and cold application.

▶ Conduction requires direct contact and depends on the differences between temperatures. (One example is a hydrocollator pack.)
▶ Convection occurs when energy is transferred through a liquid medium, as when drinking warm fluids.
▶ Radiation involves energy transfer through electromagnetic waves. (An example is a heat cradle.)
▶ Evaporation can produce heat loss as water is changed from a liquid to a gaseous state, as it does during sweating.
▶ **Conversion** is the change of electric energy or acoustic energy (sound waves) to heat. (One example is ultrasound.)

Skin tolerates dry applications of heat and cold better than moist applications of heat and cold.

Applications of heat and cold are often part of nursing practice. Cryotherapy (cold used locally for therapeutic purposes) and hypothermia (cold applied to the whole body for therapeutic purposes) are possibly indicated for tissue injury resulting from trauma or surgery. Cold reduces edema and inflammation, lessens pain, and diminishes bleeding and hematoma formation. Thermotherapy (heat applied locally for therapeutic purposes) relieves pain, congestion, and muscle spasm; increases mobility; and hastens the process of suppuration (pus formation) in treating infections (e.g., boils, abscesses, and wound infections).

Heat and cold applications are not usually curative, but these measures do provide relief of symptoms. They are adjuncts to other forms of treatment (e.g., physical therapy). Unless administered competently, heat and cold applications can produce complications such as frostbite, burns, tissue necrosis, or further edema.

The body's main thermoregulatory (heat-regulating) organ is the hypothalamus, situated between the brain's cerebral hemispheres and the midbrain. Throughout the body, nerve receptors respond rapidly and readily to hot and cold stimuli. Skin sensory nerve receptors (thermal receptors) consist of cold receptors; warm receptors; and two subtypes of pain receptors (thermosensitive pain receptors), cold pain receptors and warm pain receptors. Thermosensitive pain receptors are stimulated by extreme heat or cold.

Heat or cold applied to the skin initially stimulates thermal receptors strongly, but thermal perception fades in a few seconds. This response is called receptor adaptation. For example, we have all experienced getting into a very hot bathtub only to find that in a few minutes the temperature does not seem hot enough. This reaction occurs because warm receptors are initially stimulated strongly but then adapt to the temperature of the bath water. Sometimes, we then add more hot water, even exceeding the water's original temperature! The same process of receptor adaptation occurs with cold receptors. This adaptive phenomenon may cause serious problems (e.g., tissue damage) because of the inability of the body to sense the temperature.

Skin vasodilation and vasoconstriction occur in response to both systemic and local conditions. For example, if the systemic body temperature rises, the hypothalamus initiates skin vasodilation to allow heat to leave the body. Further, if a local area of skin becomes cold, vasoconstriction occurs, and heat is conserved within the body.

When cold is applied to the skin, blood vessels constrict until the skin temperature reaches 15°C. At this point, the vessels reach their maximal point of constriction. Below 15°C, the vessels dilate in a rebound effect opposite to the desired effect possibly because (1) the effect of cold paralyzes the contractile mechanism of the vessel wall, (2) cold blocks nerve impulses, and (3) cold inactivates vasoconstrictor chemicals. Between skin temperatures of 15°C and 0°C, vasodilation is at its maximal point at 0°C.

Therapeutic application of cold to the skin results in vasoconstriction. Therapeutic application of heat results in vasodilation if it is left in place less than 30 minutes.

Heating (or cooling) one part of the body produces vasodilation (or vasoconstriction) not only in the affected body part but also in other body parts. This phenomenon is called the **consensual response (consensual reaction).** The consensual response is not as strong or as fast as the direct response (at the area of application) and does not last long. For example, if heat is applied to the right arm, vasodilation occurs in the right arm. Vasodilation also occurs in the left arm for a time.

Do not make applications of heat or cold unless you are competent to do so (e.g., unless you understand the procedure thoroughly and have received proper instruction and supervised practice).

Successful heat and cold intervention demands a nurse (or other health care professional) who is skilled in the specific procedure, client assessment, and therapeutic interaction. For example, if a person has had repeated paraffin wax applications, understands the treatment, and gets pain relief from it, detailed explanation is unnecessary. Another person unfamiliar with the treatment, however, may not believe it can be helpful and may fear burns. Planning intervention for this person involves skillful communication before and during treatment.

The following are general factors important for all heat and cold interventions.

► Explain the treatment procedure to the person, indicating the reason for the treatment and the desired effect.
► Make frequent assessments.
► Give repeated and clear explanations throughout the intervention. Be willing to repeat explanations as necessary.
► Be aware of and respond to the person's verbal and nonverbal communication.
► Be patient and supportive when a person is anxious or hesitant about the treatment.
► Be sure all necessary equipment and supplies are available and in safe working condition.
► Include significant others in the intervention process, especially if others are to assume some responsibility for this or future applications. Be sure they receive clear and appropriate instructions.
► Allow significant others to be present whenever the person receiving care wants them. Despite traditional practices in health care facilities, there are few situations when this is not appropriate.

PHYSIOLOGIC EFFECTS OF LOCAL HEAT AND COLD APPLICATIONS

Heat. Application of heat produces physiologic effects, many of which can be therapeutic (Table 48–13). Therapeutic applications of heat are used in a number of situations to

► relieve pain
► decrease joint stiffness
► relieve muscle spasm

TABLE 48-13. Physiologic Effects and Therapeutic Indications for Heat

Site	Effect
Cell metabolism	Increased
Enzyme activity	Increased
Circulatory system	
Local response	Vasodilation
Capillary permeability	Increased
Cutaneous circulation	Vasodilation
Consensual response	Vasodilation
Connective tissue	Allows increased stretch
Synovial fluid	Decreased viscosity
Nerve conduction	Increased velocity
Muscles	Decreased contractility
Gastrointestinal tract	Decreased peristalsis; decreased blood flow; decreased secretion of hydrochloric acid

Symptom	Therapeutic Action
Pain	Analgesia; psychologic relaxation; increased circulation removes toxic cell metabolites, which may cause pain; relaxes muscle spasm
Inflammation	Increases blood flow and metabolism through body part; increases cell waste removal; increases phagocytosis
Muscle spasm	Relaxes muscle spasm; relieves pain
Stiffness	Reduces stiffness by allowing increased stretch of soft tissues in joint; decreases synovial fluid viscosity
Contracture	Reduces contracture and increases range of motion

Adapted from Tepperman, P.S., & Devlin, M. (1983). Therapeutic heat and cold. *Postgraduate Medicine, 73*(1), 69.

▶ increase blood flow
▶ help resolve inflammation
▶ increase the distention (ability to stretch) of connective tissue

Heat is used therapeutically for people with musculoskeletal problems (e.g., sprains and other injuries and arthritis). Both heat and cold may be used in conjunction with physical therapy to treat such conditions as contractures or low back pain.

Heat is used when increased blood flow and increased metabolism and nutrients are desired (e.g., to promote healing of wounds and ulcers and to accelerate suppuration or pus formation). Heat is also used to reduce inflammation, such as phlebitis. Heat is indicated when the treatment goal is to decrease muscle spasm and joint stiffness and to increase the ability of collagen to distend or stretch.

Heat is psychologically relaxing, and this in itself is comforting. Heat does seem to relieve pain and apparently has a sedative effect.

Therapeutic applications of heat and cold must be within prescribed ranges of temperature and duration. Extremes are dangerous.

The therapeutic temperature range for heat treatment is narrow. In general, optimal physiologic effects are achieved at a tissue temperature range of 43° to 45°C (109.4° to 113°F). Tissue damage can occur at 46°C (114.8°F). A safe time range for applications of heat is 3 to 30 minutes.

Sometimes, however, higher temperatures are prescribed. For example, dry heat is tolerated at a higher temperature than is moist heat because air is not a strong conductor of heat. Dry heat, however, should not be greater than 52°C (125°F).

Use extreme caution when administering heat at high temperatures.

Heat produces vasodilation. After prolonged application, however, vasoconstriction may occur, and tissue metabolism may decrease. As with the application of cold, this phenomenon, in which prolonged application of a thermal agent (heat or cold) causes an effect opposite to the therapeutic effect, is called the **secondary effect (rebound effect).** It should not be allowed to happen. Remove heat after 30 minutes and allow time for the tissue to recover.

Cold. The physiologic effects of cold are generally opposite those of heat (Table 48-14). The use of cold is becoming more common, especially in the treatment of sports-related injuries. Cold is most often used in young, active people. Before using it in the elderly, first carefully assess to ensure there is adequate circulation.

Because of its physiologic effects, cold is used to relieve pain and discomfort and to reduce muscle spasm. Muscle spasm can become a vicious cycle: spasm leads to ischemia (deficient blood supply to a body part), which produces more spasm and more pain. Applications of cold can help break this cycle. Cold permits increased stretching of muscles, tendons, and joints and decreases muscle contractility. These effects allow an increase in range of motion. For these reasons, applications of cold can be helpful before physical therapy for people experiencing chronic arthritic conditions.

Cold is used to treat acute traumatic tissue injury (e.g., strains, sprains, and fractures). Cold reduces inflammation and decreases capillary permeability, thus limiting post-injury swelling. When tissue is injured, the cells release enzymes and chemical substances, which brings about an inflammatory response. Serous fluid also leaks from the capillaries into the tissue, causing swelling and hematoma (localized collection of blood outside blood vessels). In these circumstances, applications of cold produce vasoconstriction, which lessens bleeding and the leaking of serous fluid and thus reduces swelling. A protocol known as ICE (ice, com-

TABLE 48-14. Physiologic Effects and Therapeutic Indications for Cold

Site	Effect
Cell metabolism	Decreased
Enzyme activity	Decreased
Circulatory system	
Local response	Vasoconstriction
Capillary permeability	Decreased
Cutaneous circulation	Vasoconstriction
Consensual response	Vasoconstriction
Connective tissue	Decreases stretch
Synovial fluid	Increases viscosity
Nerve conduction	Decreased velocity
Muscles	Decreased contractility

Symptom	Therapeutic Action
Pain	Initial discomfort followed by numbness, paresthesia
Inflammation	Decreases blood flow and metabolism through body part; decreases capillary permeability; decreases phagocytosis
Muscle spasm	Decreases muscle spasm; relieves pain
Stiffness	Increased stiffness; increases synovial fluid viscosity
Contracture	Tissue distention (stretch) can increase because of decrease in pain and increase in numbness

Adapted from Tepperman, P.S., & Devlin, M. (1983). Therapeutic heat and cold. *Postgraduate Medicine*, 73(1), 69.

pression, and elevation) is often ordered for the treatment of sprains involving ligament and soft tissue injury. However, a study by LaVelle and Snyder[64] showed that minimal cold is conducted through thick barriers, such as padded Ace bandages or other compression dressings.

Cold helps restore mobility and function. Increased movement strengthens muscles. Cold therefore helps prevent complications of acute injury, such as atrophy, adhesions, and calcification, by increasing the person's mobility. Acute injuries are painful because of (1) pressure from swelling on nerve endings, (2) other nerve ending stimulation, (3) release of certain chemical substances, and (4) muscle spasm. Cold relieves pain from all these sources.

If cold is used for the therapeutic effect of vasoconstriction, treatment should not be prolonged, or it will cause vasodilation or tissue injury.

Cold is used to reduce tissue destruction from thermal burns. Total body cooling (hypothermia) is used during brain and heart surgery to lower the body's metabolic requirements. Cold is typically applied as a mixture of ice and water at a temperature of 0°C (32°F). Skin temperature lowers quickly, but muscles take longer to cool. It takes at least 10 minutes to begin to cool muscle in a thin person and at least 30 minutes in an obese person. The effect lasts several hours.

To achieve maximal benefit, apply cold for a minimum of 10 minutes and a maximum of 20 to 30 minutes. Application of cold is then halted for 30 to 60 minutes to avoid a rebound effect (slightly longer periods may be prescribed for an obese person). An exception is treatment after severe injury when bleeding continues. In these circumstances, cold may be prescribed continuously for 4 to 6 hours or even as long as 24 to 48 hours. Frequent careful skin assessment is necessary during prolonged applications of cold so that tissue damage is avoided.

If tissue damage occurs because of incorrect application of heat or cold, nurses may be legally responsible.

See Table 48-15 for precautions and contraindications for heat and cold treatments.

TABLE 48-15. Precautions and Contraindications for Heat and Cold Treatments

Heat	Cold
Infants, children, and elderly	Infants, children, and elderly
Mental impairment	Mental impairment
Sensory impairment	Sensory impairment
Inadequate thermal regulation	Inadequate thermal regulation
Impaired circulation	Raynaud's disease
Hemorrhagic or bleeding disorders	Severe cold hypersensitivity or allergy
Noninflammatory edema	Cold hemagglutinins (a response to cold marked by renal dysfunction and hypertension)
Skin disorder (e.g., sunburn; erythema; and open, draining condition, such as blisters)	
Metallic implants (because metal is a good heat conductor and burns can result)	Cryoglobulinemia (abnormal globulin in the blood precipitated by cold)
Testes (can inhibit development of sperm)	Open wounds (can cause tissue damage)
Developing fetus (heat over the mother's abdomen may affect fetal growth or cause mutation of germinal cells)	Conditions such as rheumatoid arthritis, lupus erythematosus, and progressive systemic sclerosis in which cold causes increased stiffness and discomfort
Open wounds (tissues are more sensitive to temperature change)	
Do not apply during first 24 to 48 hours after injury; it can increase bleeding and swelling	

METHODS OF HEAT APPLICATION

Heat penetration can be superficial or deep and varies with the type of application. Superficial heat penetrates just a few millimeters under the skin.

Agents producing deep heat reach tissue deeper than the subcutaneous tissue. Ultrasound diathermy is currently the only true deep-heating agent. Mild heating produces a low degree of heat at the treated site. The temperature rise is slow, and the duration of treatment is short. Uses of mild heating include treatment of muscle spasm and other nonacute conditions. Vigorous heating produces high tissue temperatures close to the maximally tolerated level. The desired temperature is reached quickly, and the duration of the treatment is longer. Uses of vigorous heating include treatment of joint contractures with scarring and chronic pelvic inflammation. Heating increases temperature in scar tissues, and they become more extensible and less resistant to range-of-motion therapy.

Moist heat (e.g., soaks, baths) penetrates more than dry heat does, and this increases the possibility of burns.

Dry heat (e.g., lamps, heating pads) dries the skin. The possibility of burning the skin is still present. Table 48–16 summarizes the usual recommended temperature/distance and duration ranges for common heating and cooling modalities.

Dry Heat

Hot Water Bottles. Hot water bottles are not often used in health care facilities because of the danger of burns. Clients are often required to sign a "release" or "permission" form if they wish to use one.

Inspect hot water bottles for leaks before use. Use water between 46° and 52°C (115° to 125°F). Verify the temperature with a bath thermometer. Fill the hot water bottle one-half to two-thirds full and expel the air before tightly closing the cap. This procedure reduces the weight of the bottle and permits greater conformity to the body part. Place the bottle in a flannel cover to decrease the possibility of burning. Check the bottle at least every half-hour as temperature decreases. Refill with hot water as necessary. When used for general warmth, a hot water bottle can remain as long as the person wants it. Check temperature frequently. When a hot water bottle is used to relieve inflammation, a period of 20 to 30 minutes is usually prescribed. Occasionally, a longer time is ordered. In no case should it be placed *under* the person's body; burns may result. After use, empty the bottle and leave it open to dry.

Disposable Chemical Hot Packs. Disposable chemical hot packs are filled with chemical gels. Chemical hot packs are manufactured commercially. Follow the instructions on the pack carefully. The temperature from these packs is not well regulated; but in general, a hot pack ranges from 37° to 46°C (98.6° to 115°F). Although a pack retains heat for 30 to 60 minutes, it is applied for only 20 to 30 minutes. Disposable chemical hot packs are used because they are convenient and readily available.

Electric Heating Pads. Electric heating pads provide sustained heat. They are light, conform to the body, and come in various sizes. The amount of heat can be regulated, although the heat output increases with prolonged application (2 or 3 hours). They usually have three temperature settings (low, medium, and high). A medium setting usually provides heat between 46° and 52°C (115° and 125°F). Caution the person against using a higher setting. Be sure the person does not lie on the pad; lying on top of the pad increases the possibility of burns because the heat cannot dissipate.

Before using them, cover electric heating pads with flannel to decrease the possibility of burns. Use the same precautions you would use with any electrical appliance. Do not put pins through the pad. Clients must sign release forms to use heating pads in agency settings.

Aqua K Pads. Aqua K pads (also called K pads) are aquathermia pads. They come in various sizes; some can deliver moist heat through an absorbent surface, whereas others deliver only dry heat. Aqua K pads work by circulating distilled water through tubing contained within a waterproof pad applied to the client. A control unit adjusts the circulating fluid to the desired temperature (Fig. 48–42). Aqua K pads are easy to use and accurate in temperature delivery. They are most often used in acute care facilities.

Set the temperature at 40.5°C (105°F) at the control unit. Fill the reservoir two-thirds full of distilled water. Remove air bubbles in the unit and tubing by tilting the unit gently from side to side. (Air bubbles impede the equal distribution of heat and the functioning of the unit.) Close the lid tightly and then loosen it a one-quarter turn to allow heat expansion. For best performance, place the control unit level with or slightly above the body part to be treated. (This position avoids having the motor push water against gravity.) Avoid tangling or kinking the tubes. Check reservoir daily and refill as needed.

For dry heat, cover the body part with the pad. If it is on a limb, secure the pad with tape. For moist heat, place the moist surface of the pad toward the person's skin after putting it inside a pillowcase, or place a *thin* towel between the skin and the pad. The pad can be held in place with tape or gauze ties. Do not use pins because the pad will be punctured. Do not allow the person to place the pad under the body; burns are likely to result.

Careful, ongoing monitoring is essential. Check for pain and excessive skin redness throughout the first 5 minutes. If there are no signs of complications, continue the treatment for 20 to 30 minutes. After treatment, dry the skin.

Heat Cradles. A Baker heat cradle provides radiant heat. It has a metal frame containing several electric sockets in which 25-watt light bulbs are placed at a distance of at least 18 inches from the person's skin.

TABLE 48-16. Types of Therapeutic Heat and Cold Applications

Application	Temperature/Distance	Duration
Heat		
Dry Heat		
Hot water bottle	46–52°C (115–125°F)	Variable
Chemical pack	37–46°C (98.6–115°F)	Variable
Electric heating pad*	46–52°C (115–125°F)	Variable
Aqua K pad	40.5°C (115–125°F)	Variable
Baker heat cradle	25-watt bulbs: 16–18 inches from body parts	20–30 min or continuous
Irritants/counterirritants	Not measurable	20–30 min
Moist Heat		
Warm compresses	40.5–43°C (105–110°F)	15–20 min
Tub bath/soaks	32–42.5°C (90–108°F)	20 min
Sitz bath cleansing	38–40°C (100–104°F)	20–25 min
To increase circulation	43–46°C (110–115°F)	20 min
Contrast bath (alternate heat and cold)	Heat 40.6–43.3°C (105–110°F) Cold 15–20°C (59–68°F)	First 10 min in warm water, then 1 min in cold water; alternate 4 min in warm water followed by 1 min in cold water for a total of 30 min for the treatment
Hydrocollator pack	46–52°C (115–125°F)	20–30 min
Cold		
Direct		
Tepid sponge	27–37°C (80–98°F)	20–30 min
Cold compresses	15°C (59°F)	20 mins
Cold packs	0°C (32°F)	10–15 min
Ice application	0°C (32°F)	20 min
Cold soaks	15°C (59°F)	20 min
Indirect		
Ice bag	10–26°C (50–80°F)	20–30 min
Ice collar	10–26°C (50–80°F)	20–30 min
Hypothermia blanket	Ordered by physician	Variable

* Hospitals require that the client sign a release before use.

This appliance is rarely used now but may be useful if a large body area requires heat treatment. The entire cradle is placed over the body part. The cradle itself may be covered by top bedding, which adds to heat retention and provides privacy.

Infrared or Gooseneck Lamps. Other means of providing radiant heat include infrared and gooseneck lamps. These are sometimes used for healing perineal wounds after delivery of an infant. They should *never* be used on pressure ulcers. Position small lamps 18 to 24 inches and larger lamps 24 to 30 inches away from the body. Within 5 minutes after therapy is started, check to make sure there is not too much heat.

Chemical Counterirritants. Chemical **counterirritants** are agents applied locally to produce inflammatory reaction for the purpose of affecting some other part, usually adjacent to or underlying the surface irritated. Blood flow is stimulated and is redirected to the skin. Congestion is relieved. Chemical counterirritants are sometimes used for bronchitis, pneumonia, joint

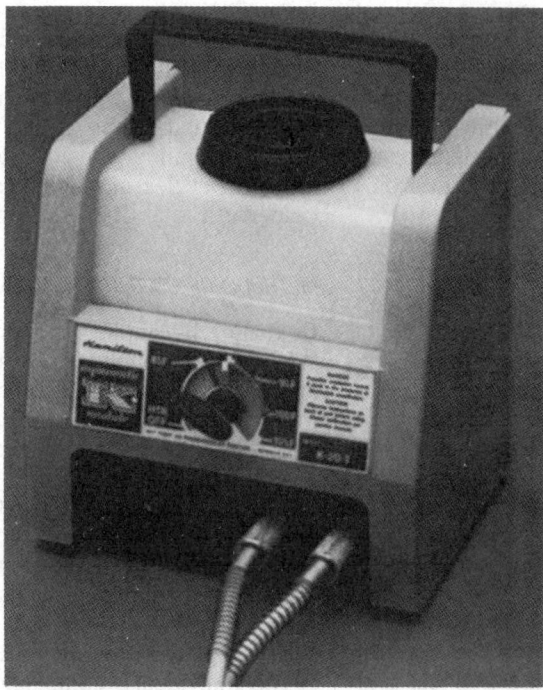
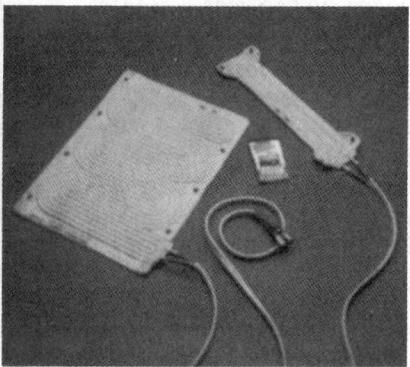

▲ **Figure 48–42**

An aquathermia pad.

pain, headache, and abdominal distention. Mustard plasters, flaxseed poultices, and liniments are examples. These products are available commercially. Apply them to the skin as directed for 20 to 30 minutes. Wash the skin carefully afterward. If the skin is red, petroleum jelly or oil may relieve the irritation.

Diathermy. **Diathermy** is the production of superficial or deep heat by converting electric and acoustic (sound) energy to heat within the body tissue. Diathermy treatments are usually administered in a physical therapy facility, without nursing involvement in delivering this treatment.

Ultrasound diathermy uses acoustic vibrations. The heat produced penetrates to a deep level. It can be used safely on people with metal implants. It is not used near the eyes.

Moist Heat

Hot Compresses. Compresses are dressings used for the application of heat or cold. Moist heat may be applied as sterile or clean hot compresses. Sterile compresses are used for open wounds, surgical incisions, or sites near the eyes. Clean compresses are appropriate when the skin is intact. To prevent burns, an insulating layer of petroleum jelly is often applied to intact skin before treatment. Petroleum jelly is not used on an open wound or near the eyes.

When continuous hot soaks are required, an Aqua K pad is placed over the compress to maintain a constant temperature. When the compresses are to be sterile, a sterile, waterproof barrier must be placed between them and the heat source.

Hydrocollator Packs. Hydrocollator packs transfer heat by conduction. They consist of a cotton bag that contains silicate gel. They are heated in a temperature-controlled water bath to extremely high temperatures (71° to 79°C [160° to 175°F]). The gel absorbs and retains heat. The pack is then wrapped in layers of terry cloth and applied to the skin. The terry cloth layers put insulation around the pack so that (1) the pack retains heat longer and (2) the skin is protected from the high temperature. (The temperature actually applied to the skin is 46° to 52°C [115° to 125°F]). The pack is light and conforms to the body.

Paraffin Wax. Paraffin wax is commonly used to relieve painful hands, especially in people experiencing chronic rheumatoid arthritis or progressive systemic sclerosis. This treatment is usually done by physical therapists.

The wax is heated in a thermostatically controlled container or double boiler to a temperature of 54.4°C (130°F). The wax mixture is then allowed to cool to 52°C (125°F) before it is applied to the body part. Two methods of application are used. For the first, the body part is dipped in and out of the wax several times to produce a glove or sleeve. This method is especially appropriate for the hands and fingers. The body part is then covered with a towel, and the heat is retained for 20 to 30 minutes. This method produces mild heating. With the second method, the body part is immersed in a bath of paraffin wax mixture for about 20 to 30 minutes. This method produces vigorous heating. With both methods, cool paraffin is easily peeled off after treatment.

Therapeutic Baths. Another way to apply moist heat is by soaking a body part in a therapeutic bath. Such baths may be administered in a whirlpool (for arms and legs) or in a Hubbard tank (for the whole body). These appliances are usually found in physical therapy facilities. They are used to treat musculoskeletal problems and to debride (remove dead tissue from) wounds and burns.

Tub Baths. Tub baths are usually administered for 10 to 30 minutes. The temperature of the solution is often 32° to 42.5°C (90° to 108°F).

Sitz Baths. **Sitz baths** are warm therapeutic baths in which the person sits. They provide moist heat to perineal and anal areas to clean, promote healing and drainage, reduce soreness, stimulate voiding, and promote relaxation. Sitz baths are used mainly (1) after rectal surgery, (2) for people with hemorrhoids, and (3) for women after pelvic surgery or the delivery of an infant.

Sitz is the German word for "seat." The word describes the bath in the sense that a person "sits in water" and is able to wash or treat the perineal and anal areas without getting the rest of the body wet. A sitz bath may be a permanent tub in some facilities. Most commonly, however, plastic disposable sitz baths are used. This type rests on the rim of the toilet bowl and is partially filled with water. The person then sits down on it, and the perineum and anus are covered with water.

To maintain temperature, a bag of warm water is hung by the toilet with its tubing end in the sitz bath. Water is dripped into the bath as the temperature cools. Water temperature depends on the purpose of the sitz bath and the condition of the person's skin. For cleaning, the temperature should be 38° to 40°C (100° to 104°F). For increasing circulation, the temperature should be 43° to 46°C (110° to 115°F). Although a person may say the water is too cool, warmer water is not used because sensitive skin and mucous membranes are easily burned.

Sitz baths are prescribed for about 20 to 25 minutes. Longer applications produce a secondary, or rebound, effect. The dilation of large pelvic blood vessels can cause sudden hypotension. Watch the person carefully. If you do not stay with the client, be sure a call light is close at hand and check frequently. Observe vital signs. If signs of faintness, shock, or severe pain develop, discontinue treatment, assist the client to a reclining position, and call for assistance. Do not leave the individual alone.

Whatever type of equipment is used, position the person's buttocks into the warm fluid without causing pressure on the area being treated or on the back of the legs. Place a bath blanket around the person for warmth and privacy. After treatment, clean the sitz bath with disinfectant and rinse thoroughly.

Contrast Baths. **Contrast baths** consist of alternately immersing body parts in basins of hot and cold water to stimulate circulation. The hot water is kept between 40.6° and 43.3°C (105° and 110°F), and cold water is kept between 15° and 20°C (59° and 68°F). These baths are often used to treat rheumatoid arthritis of fingers, feet, and ankles.

The following schedule may be used. Begin with heat. Place the limb in the hot water for 10 minutes. Follow by immersion in cold water for 1 minute. Follow with cycles of 4 minutes in hot water, 1 minute in cold, for a total of 30 minutes, counting all immersions.

METHODS OF COLD APPLICATION

Cold may be applied indirectly or directly to the skin. When cold is applied, skin temperature drops immediately, and the temperature of subcutaneous tissues follows suit. Muscle temperatures decrease more slowly and depend on the thickness of the subcutaneous fat layer. Remember that when muscle is cooled, it stays cool for a long time after the application is stopped. Subcutaneous fat is an effective insulator. Blood flow in cooled muscle is reduced, and rewarming also slows. For this reason, spasticity is reduced for long periods after cold applications, so that physical rehabilitation (e.g., range-of-motion exercises) can be carried out.

The individual's compliance or willingness to follow prescribed cold therapy is a significant factor in its effectiveness. Before beginning therapy, describe to the individual the sensations that the application of cold will produce. An uncomfortable cold sensation is initially experienced for 1 minute, followed by diffuse burning or aching lasting 2 to 7 minutes. Skin analgesia (decreased pain) occurs after about 5 minutes. Table 48–14 describes the neuromuscular response to cold or cryotherapy. These responses occur in both direct and indirect cold applications.

Moist cold (compresses, alcohol sponges) penetrates more than dry cold does, and this increases the possibility of tissue damage.

Indirect Cooling Methods

Cold Packs and Chemical Packs. Cold packs are manufactured commercially. Some varieties are reusable and contain a gel or frozen gel. Others are chemical packs or "ice envelopes." These envelopes contain chemicals that, when mixed within the package, produce a reaction that cools the pack. When the pack is cool, it is applied to the skin. Cover packs with flannel to absorb moisture and then place on the skin. There is a danger of frostbite when packs are used because the temperature is not precise and some become colder than 0°C (32°F). Packs remain cold for 10 to 15 minutes (Fig. 48–43).

Ice Bags and Ice Collars. Ice bags (Fig. 48–44) or ice collars are often used after dental or thyroid surgery. Filling an ice bag or collar is similar to filling a hot water bottle. Fill the bag two-thirds full with crushed ice. Expel air and close tightly. Cover with flannel or other absorbent material. Apply to the body part. You will sometimes see a latex or plastic glove filled with ice chips and tied shut. This is often used on small areas, such as the eyes or hands.

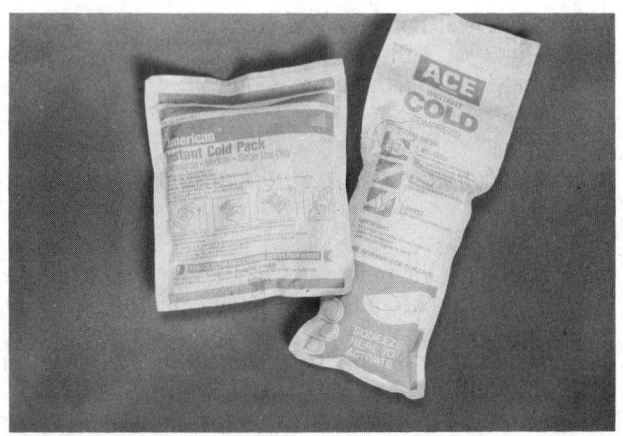

▲ *Figure 48-43*

Disposable chemical cold packs. These packs are activated by squeezing and shaking. They are not reusable.

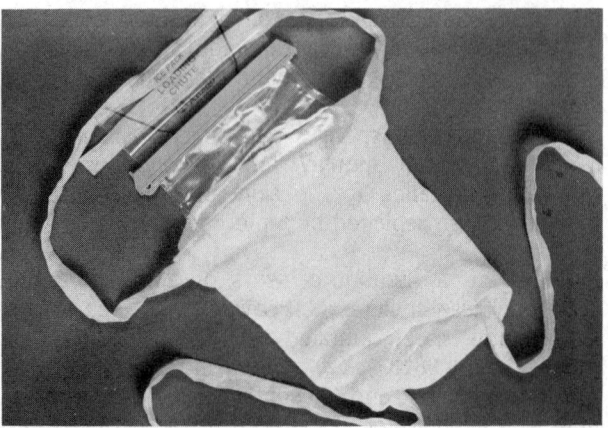

▲ *Figure 48-44*

Single-use ice pack with knitted cover.

During the first 5 to 7 minutes, take vital signs frequently. If signs of shock occur, discontinue the treatment. Remain with the person until numbness develops. Tell the person what to expect. Encourage the person to tolerate the first few minutes and remind the individual that the discomfort will pass.

After 12 to 15 minutes, the skin appears red. Assess the skin for frostbite every 10 minutes. If no complications occur, continue treatment for 30 minutes; then remove and do not reapply for 45 to 60 minutes.

Hypothermia Blankets. Hypothermia blankets are cooling blankets or mattresses. A hypothermia blanket is really a body-sized Aqua K pad. It is used to reduce high body temperature (fever). It is also used to lower metabolic activity during some surgery (e.g., heart surgery), to reduce intracranial pressure during neurosurgery, and to control bleeding and intractable pain of amputations, burns, and cancer.

A hypothermia blanket is a large pad through which cooled fluid (distilled water or distilled water and 20 per cent ethyl alcohol) circulates. A prescribed temperature is set on the control unit. It is used for both adults and children and is very effective.

Hypothermia blankets should be used with extreme caution for people with impaired circulation, because of the danger of tissue damage, and for people connected to other electrical equipment, such as electrocardiographic monitors, because of the danger of electric shock.

Monitor the person's temperature carefully. Some blankets measure temperature automatically by rectal, skin, or esophageal probes (although these are often inaccurate). The person's temperature will continue to fall about 1°C (2°F) after the blanket is removed; this trend is called downward drift. Therefore, discontinue treatment when body temperature is 1° to 1.6°C (2° to 3°F) above the desired body temperature. Take vital signs before beginning treatment. Be sure the person is not wearing clothing with metal clips or snaps (these

can cause tissue damage). Place the client in a supine position. Apply a thin layer of lotion or mineral oil to the skin to protect it and to enhance the conduction of cold. Place a cotton blanket between the hypothermia blanket and the client. The cotton blanket protects the skin and distributes the cold evenly. It also absorbs moisture and lessens the possibility of tissue damage. Place additional protection over male genitalia. Tuck the cooling blanket around the client, making sure it does not directly touch the skin. Turn the blanket on. Add additional fluid to the unit reservoir, as necessary, as the blanket fills with fluid.

Observe the client carefully. Take vital signs every 5 minutes initially and every 15 minutes if the vital signs are stable. Turn the person and massage the skin every 30 to 60 minutes to prevent tissue damage. Assess the skin for signs of frostbite or burns, especially on the hands and feet. If either frostbite or a burn is present, discontinue treatment and notify the physician immediately.

Shivering should not occur. If it does, lower the temperature of the blanket a little. If shivering continues, discontinue treatment and notify the physician. Shivering increases metabolism and so raises the temperature. Occasionally, when a person has a high temperature that needs to be reduced quickly, a lower-than-usual blanket temperature is used, and shivering may occur. The effects of the shivering (i.e., vasoconstriction) are controlled by medication (e.g., chlorpromazine), which produces vasodilation.

Direct Cooling Methods

Cold Compresses. Cold compresses consist of gauze dressings or terry cloth dipped in ice and water, wrung out, and applied to the skin. They need to be frequently dipped and reapplied or covered with an ice bag.

Tepid Baths, Tepid Sponges, and Alcohol Sponges. Cold or tepid sponge baths with water are sometimes used to bring down elevated body temperature (fever). If alcohol is added to the solution (to increase evaporation), it is called an alcohol sponge bath. A simple and effective method of bringing down high temperature in children is to place them in a tepid water bath.

Tepid baths and sponges can be conveniently used at home. Alcohol sponges are not often used now (alcohol is irritating to the skin and causes nausea); they have been replaced by tepid baths or hypothermia blankets.

There are a number of ways of applying a tepid sponge. These include (1) covering the entire body with a large sheet saturated with tepid water (27° to 37°C [80° to 98°F]), (2) placing the person in a tub full of tepid water, and (3) sponging one body part at a time with tepid water. If the third method is used, take care that the person is not chilled, because chilling can cause shivering, which would elevate the temperature. To avoid chilling, place a hot water bottle on the person's feet. An effective sequence is to sponge the person's face and extremities for 5 minutes, and then the back and buttocks for 5 to 10 minutes. While sponging, place a cool compress on the forehead, groin, and axilla.

Monitor the person's temperature every 10 minutes and continue to sponge for 20 to 30 minutes. If the temperature rises rather than falls, the person may be chilled and shivering. In this case, warm the solution a little and apply friction to the body by brisk rubbing of the arms, torso, and legs (omitting the calves). (For further discussion of temperature monitoring, see Chapter 31.)

Ice Application. Direct application of ice is an effective method of applying cold to a body part. A block of ice or ice chips in a wet towel can be applied directly to the skin. The skin may be rubbed or massaged with the ice. This procedure may be continued for 20 to 30 minutes. This method is simple, inexpensive, and convenient in home situations. A simple and effective method is to fill a Styrofoam cup with water and freeze it. When it is frozen, peel the cup back a little from the top, hold the base of the cup, invert it, and massage with the ice applied directly to the skin, using caution to prevent frostbite.

Caution The longest time ice can be held motionless in one place on the skin is typically 2 to 3 minutes, after which frostbite occurs. Signs of frostbite consist of white, pale, waxy, mottled, blue, or pulseless skin that is hard to the touch.

Immersion. If a large body part is to be cooled, immersion of the body part in a whirlpool tub filled with cold water is an effective and safe method. Treatment lasts 20 to 30 minutes.

Evaporation. Cold aerosol sprays are used to promote cooling through evaporation. Ethyl chloride or chlorofluoromethane may be used. The latter is preferred because it is less flammable. Spray the skin from a distance of 3 feet, using a sweeping or stroking motion at about 4 inches a second. Spray for a few seconds, pause, and then spray again. This method pro-

vides superficial cooling. The cold does not penetrate. The danger of skin frostbite is high. This method is appropriate for small skin areas only.

Nursing Management in Applications of Heat and Cold

Many clinical judgments are made by nurses in the application of heat and cold. Be sure there is a physician's order that indicates (1) the type of treatment, (2) the specific area to be treated, (3) the duration of treatment, (4) the time interval required between treatments, and (5) the application temperature. Remember that you are legally responsible for safely performing applications of heat and cold.

Throughout treatment, carefully assess the person's general condition, safety, and comfort.

Body Part and Condition of Skin. Monitor the body part and observe the condition of the skin. Is the skin intact? If it is not intact, use sterile asepsis and lower the temperature of the heat application. Is there a hematoma? If so, do not apply heat unless the hematoma has been present for more than 48 hours. Is edema (swelling) present? Heat may be contraindicated because it can produce more edema. If edema is due to infection, heat may be used, but observe carefully for any increase in edema.

Is there evidence of acute inflammation (redness, heat, pain, swelling)? Heat may be contraindicated, especially for such acute conditions as appendicitis and tooth abscess. Are there skin burns? If so, are they a result of previous therapy? Carefully observe the skin before and after treatment. Burns should not occur.

What is the circulatory status? Are distal pulses present? Is capillary refill brisk? If the circulation is compromised, heat or cold application may be contraindicated. Take vital signs as baseline data. Assess the affected area frequently during and after treatment to be sure that complications are not occurring.

The Individual's Overall Condition. What is the person's general condition? Assess and document vital signs to establish a baseline. What is the person's reaction to the proposed therapy? Is the person anxious? Does the person understand the reason for the therapy and how it is to be administered? Does the person know what may be experienced during therapy? Does the person agree with the type of treatment prescribed?

What are the person's underlying concerns about the therapy? Is the person afraid of burns or pain? Does the person fear that the nurse or therapist is not competent? Is the person afraid assistance will not be available during the treatment if help is needed? Has the person had previous experiences with the particular mode of treatment that might influence present reactions?

Is the person willing to cooperate with treatment? Sometimes, applications of heat, and especially of cold, are uncomfortable. Is the person willing and able to tolerate this discomfort? Is the person willing and able to provide the necessary feedback about the treatment to ensure safety?

What is the person's level of consciousness and mental status? If the person is not alert or has an impaired mental status, heat or cold therapy may be contraindicated. What is the person's age? Infants and elderly people tolerate extreme heat or cold poorly. Temperatures should not be extreme. If this therapy is used, observe closely for complications. Does the person have metallic implants or a pacemaker? If so, therapy may be contraindicated. Extreme temperatures should not be used.

Does the person have Raynaud's disease or other circulatory problems? If so, therapy may be contraindicated. Does the person have an allergy to heat or cold? If so, therapy may be contraindicated.

Significant Others. Does the person have significant others who are concerned? What are their specific concerns?

Are significant others taking some responsibility for the administration of treatment at home? If so, do they understand the purposes of treatment and the methods of administration? Do they understand the safety precautions necessary? Do they have all the requisite equipment? Do they feel able to carry out these responsibilities well?

Equipment and Supplies. Is all necessary equipment available and in working condition? Are all necessary supplies available? Is the application to be done with sterile asepsis? If so, are the additional supplies available?

EVALUATION

Nurses base evaluation on specific outcomes defined while planning interventions. Have the goals been reached? If not, why not? If goals are reached without complications, therapy has been effective. For example, if the goal of an application of heat was to relieve pain, nursing evaluation involves looking for indications that pain has, in fact, been relieved. If pain has not been relieved, look for possible reasons, and incorporate this information into further nursing planning.

As part of the nursing evaluation:

▸ Inspect the area carefully. Is there excessive redness? How long does redness remain after treatment? Is there any evidence of burns? Are there any other color changes (e.g., skin mottled, purple, or white)?
▸ Take vital signs. Do they vary from baseline recordings before intervention?
▸ If an infection is present, monitor the temperature and pulse. The desired effect is a decrease in both.
▸ Is the person experiencing pain? Is it less or more than before treatment? What kind of pain is it? Throbbing, dull, sharp?
▸ Is the person (and significant others) comfortable and relaxed?

The final evaluation defines how well the planned interventions allowed the projected outcomes to be attained. If your objective for the nursing diagnosis *Impaired Skin Integrity* is that healing of the wound will be attained by 21 days postoperatively, then your outcome criterion would be that the wound is completely covered with epithelium by day 21. However, clients seldom remain in the hospital long enough for final evaluation to be done in the hospital setting.

Ongoing evaluation is done daily. Your interventions for a client with *Impaired Skin Integrity* would include cleansing the wound daily with a nonionic cleanser and covering it with a dressing. You would inspect the wound at each dressing change for improvement in its size and appearance, and on a daily basis you would chart the improvement (e.g., "wound diameter has decreased in size to 2 cm × 2 cm from previous day's measurement of 2.2 cm × 2.2 cm, and the wound color is deeper pink").

CASE STUDY

The Client

Mrs. Kimberly Mason, a 53-year-old bank vice-president, was admitted two days ago for an abdominal hysterectomy for excessive menstrual bleeding due to multiple fibroid tumors. She has no other known health problems. Her surgery was done on the day of admission, two days ago. Her midline abdominal incision from below the umbilicus to the symphysis pubis is healing as expected. She complains of discomfort at the incision site when she moves but has no other problems. The following is a partial list of the physician's postoperative orders:

▸ May be up to bathroom ad lib.
▸ Regular diet as tolerated.

▸ Vital signs every 4 hours for 24 hours, then routine vital signs.
▸ Routine postoperative dressing change with 4 × 4s and abdominal pads daily.

It is now May 4th. At 8 AM, May 3, your assessment showed:

▸ A 53-year-old Caucasian woman
▸ Overweight (weight 152 lb, should weigh 135 lb)
▸ Voiding without difficulty
▸ Ambulates to bathroom without assistance
▸ Vital signs within normal limits for pulse, respirations, and blood pressure, temperature elevation of 1 degree

Case Study continued on following page

CASE STUDY Continued

The Client

► Complaining of abdominal discomfort at incision site.
► Midline abdominal incision, 8 cm long, extending from umbilicus to symphysis pubis
► Sutures intact—black silk interrupted sutures
► No wound odor

► Minimal swelling along suture line
► Small amount of crusted blood along incision

The following represents part of the nursing care plan written for her yesterday and the current evaluation of outcomes expected at that time.

CARE PLAN

8 AM, May 3

Nursing Diagnosis	Planning: Expected Outcomes	Implementation: Nursing Interventions	Evaluation
Impaired Tissue Integrity R/T mechanical disruption of surgery, abdominal hysterectomy, AEB ► 8″ lower midline abdominal incision with interrupted silk sutures in place ► Minimal amount of serosanguineous drainage on dressing (less than 0.5 cm in size)	By May 4: Shows wound healing without complication, AEB ► No wound drainage ► Continued decrease in swelling along incision line	► Wash hands before and after dressing change. For dressing change: Remove dressing and note type and amount of drainage and inspect wound each day. Don sterile gloves. Cleanse wound incision with sterile isotonic saline and blot dry with sterile unfilled 4 × 4s. Reapply sterile dry dressing. ► Check client's TPR at regular intervals as determined by hospital policy.	3 pm, May 4 ► 0.5 cm amount of serosanguineous drainage on dressing. ► No evidence of wound infection. Wound margins appear clean, no redness, minimal swelling around sutures noted. Wound edges approximated with crusted serosanguineous drainage along incision line as expected at this time. ► T 37.6, P 92, R 18 (temperature elevation is an expected postoperative finding).
	► No infection ► Continued decrease in incisional discomfort	► Instruct client on importance of splinting wound with small pillow when she coughs or changes position.	► No evidence of wound dehiscence.
	► Appropriate stage of healing for 72 hours after surgery	► Instruct client about the need for a dietary intake for wound healing with adequate protein, vitamins C, A, B_6, and B_{12}, iron, and folate; give examples of foods that contain these nutrients. Assist client to choose meals for May 4, e.g., Breakfast: Tomato juice Two poached eggs Whole-wheat toast with margarine Milk Coffee	► Wound at appropriate stage of healing.

CARE PLAN (Continued)

8 AM, May 3

Nursing Diagnosis	Planning: Expected Outcomes	Implementation: Nursing Interventions	Evaluation
		Lunch: Ham sandwich on whole-wheat bread with lettuce and tomato Iced tea with lemon Fruit cup Dinner: Roast beef Au gratin potatoes Green beans Garden salad Ice cream Iced tea with lemon	

Summary

▶ Wounds are disruptions of soft tissue continuity.

▶ The skin is the body's largest organ. Its functions include regulation of body temperature, protection from microorganisms, and regeneration.

▶ Aging causes drier skin, loss of cells, increased sensitivity to heat and cold, lighter skin because of decreased melanocyte production, loss of body hair, and wrinkles.

▶ Intact skin should be assessed for turgor, circulation, color, temperature, touch perception, dryness, and any unusual marks.

▶ Wounds may be classified as surgical or traumatic, open or closed, full-thickness or partial-thickness, and infected or noninfected or by etiology.

▶ Most pressure ulcers are preventable with careful nursing management. Persons who cannot move themselves without assistance should never remain in the same position in bed for more than 2 hours (in chairs, 1 hour is the maximum). Pressure-reddened skin should not be massaged. Capillary closing pressure in young, healthy adults is approximately 32 mm Hg. Above this level, capillary circulation is impaired or totally occluded. Pressure-reducing equipment that reduces interface pressures to less than capillary closing pressure helps prevent pressure ulcers. Clients at risk for pressure ulcers should not have the head of the bed elevated to more than 30 degrees or be turned to a side-lying position of more than 30 degrees.

▶ Wound healing is a process beginning with an inflammatory phase, involving a cellular response; a proliferative phase, consisting of tissue repair; and a maturation phase, involving the development of scar tissue.

▶ Wound surfaces heal best in a moist environment.

Local factors influencing wound healing include presence of microbes and foreign material; desiccation; edema; oxygen supply; fibrin breakdown; and mechanical factors, such as pressure, friction, and shear. Systemic factors influencing wound healing include nutritional, vascular, and psychologic status; age; presence of metabolic, immune, or clotting disorders; and certain drug therapies.

▶ Clinical signs of an infected wound include any of the following: increased redness, edema, an elevated body temperature, presence of pus, uncharacteristic odor of wound, change in color of wound exudate, elevated white blood cell count, and pain. Signs of infection in elderly persons may differ, and confusion, fatigue, or loss of appetite may occur in addition.

▶ Wound closure methods include sutures, surgical clips and staples, and skin adhesive closures.

▶ Wound assessment must include an assessment of the client's overall status.

▶ The nursing diagnosis that best describes the client with a wound is *Impaired Tissue Integrity*.

▶ Planning for the client with a wound should include plans for prevention of complications, promotion of comfort, promotion of wound healing, and assisting the client and significant others as needed through healing and rehabilitation.

▶ Nursing interventions revolve around management of wound care and applications of heat and cold.

▶ Wounds should be cleansed with nonionic cleansers, such as isotonic saline. Disinfectant solutions, such as hydrogen peroxide and povidone-iodine (Betadine), should only be used to clean infected wounds and must be ordered by a physician. All wounds should be cared for with use of universal precautions. Gloves provide only an additional protective barrier against microorganisms. They are *not* 100 per cent effective as a barrier.

▶ Nonocclusive wound dressings, such as gauze, allow atmospheric gases to reach the wound surface. Occlusive wound dressings allow no gaseous exchange and maintain a moist wound environment.

▶ Wound drains are used to provide a track for heavy wound drainage to be eliminated from the wound and to prevent wound complications such as abscess formation.

▶ Wound dehiscence and wound evisceration are emergencies. Call for help at once.

▶ Heat energy is transferred to living tissue by conduction, conversion, radiation, or convection. Living tissue may be cooled by conduction, evaporation, or convection.

▶ Therapeutic applications of heat and cold must be within prescribed ranges of temperature and duration for preventing injury. Skin damage occurs more quickly with moist applications of heat and cold than with dry applications.

▶ Seldom do clients with wounds remain in the hospital long enough for final evaluations, but ongoing evaluations must be done daily.

Bibliography

1. A.H.C.P.R. Panel for the Prediction and Prevention of Pressure Ulcers in Adults (1992). *Prediction and prevention. Clinical practice guideline, number 3.* AHCPR Publication No. 92-0047. Rockville, MD: Agency for Health Care Policy and Research, Public Health Service, U.S. Department of Health and Human Services.
2. Alvarez, O. (1988). Moist environment for healing: matching the dressing to the wound. *Ostomy/Wound Management, 21,* 64.
3. Arikian, V.L., et al. (1990). Education and QA: a model for continuous improvement in skin integrity. *Journal of Nursing Quality Assurance, 5*(1), 1.
4. Bale, S., & Harding, K.G. (1990). Using modern dressings to effect debridement. *The Professional Nurse, 5,* 244.
5. Barnes, S.H. (1987). Patient/family education for the patient with a pressure necrosis. *Nursing Clinics of North America, 22,* 463.
6. Baron, M., & Tafuro, P. (1985). The extremes of age: the newborn and the elderly. *Nursing Clinics of North America, 20,* 181.
7. Bergstrom, N., et al. (1987). The Braden Scale for predicting pressure sore risk. *Nursing Research, 36*(4), 205.
8. Birdsall, C. (1985). How do you handle heat loss? *American Journal of Nursing, 85,* 367.
9. Bobel, L.M. (1987). Nutritional implications in the patient with pressure sores. *Nursing Clinics of North America, 22,* 379.
10. Braden, B.J. (1989). Clinical utility of The Braden Scale for predicting pressure sore risk. *Decubitus, 2*(3), 44.
11. Brandeis, G.H., et al. (1990). The epidemiology and natural history of pressure ulcers in elderly nursing home residents. *Journal of the American Medical Association, 264*(22), 2905.
12. Branemark, P., & Ekholm, R. (1967). Tissue injury caused by wound disinfectants. *The Journal of Bone and Joint Surgery, 49,* 48.
13. Brozenec, S. (1985). Caring for the postoperative patient with an abdominal drain. *Nursing '85, 15,* 55.
14. Bryant, R., et al. (1992). Pressure ulcers. *In* Bryant, R. (ed.). *Acute and chronic wounds.* St. Louis: Mosby-Year Book.
15. Bucknall, T.E., et al. (1982). Burst abdomen and incisional hernia: a prospective study of 1129 major laparotomies. *British Medical Journal, 284,* 931.
16. Burke, M., et al. (1985). Is there a connection between cold and confusion? *American Journal of Nursing, 85,* 128.
17. Capperauld, I. (1986). Sutures in wound repair. *In* Westaby, S. (ed.). *Wound care.* St. Louis: C.V. Mosby.
18. Carlson, C.E., & King, R.B. (1990). Prevention of pressure sores. *In* Fitzpatrick, J.J., et al. (eds.). *Annual review of nursing research* (vol. 8). New York: Springer Publishing.
19. Centers for Disease Control (1985). Guideline for prevention of surgical wound infections. In *Guidelines for the prevention and control of nosocomial infection.* Atlanta: Centers For Disease Control.
20. Centers for Disease Control (1985). Guideline for handwashing and hospital environmental control. In *Guidelines for the prevention and control of nosocomial infections.* Atlanta: Centers for Disease Control.
21. Centers for Disease Control (1987). Recommendations for prevention of HIV transmission in health-care settings. *Morbidity and Mortality Weekly Report, 36,* 25.
22. Centers for Disease Control (1988). Update: Universal precautions for prevention of transmission of human immunodeficiency virus, hepatitis B virus, and other bloodborne pathogens in health-care settings. *Morbidity and Mortality Weekly Report, 37,* 24.
23. Centers for Disease Control (1989). *Guidelines for prevention of transmission of human immunodeficiency virus and hepatitis B virus to health care and public-safety workers.* Atlanta: U.S. Department of Health and Human Services, Public Health Service, Centers for Disease Control.
24. Centers for Disease Control (1990). Public health service statement on management of occupational exposure to human immunodeficiency virus, including considerations regarding zidovudine postexposure use. *Morbidity and Mortality Weekly Report, 39,* RR-1.
25. Centers for Disease Control (1991). Recommendations for preventing transmission of human immunodeficiency virus and hepatitis B virus to patients during exposure-prone invasive procedures. *Morbidity and Mortality Weekly Report, 40,* RR-8.
26. Chapuis, A., & Dollfus, P. (1990). The use of a calcium alginate dressing in the management of decubitus ulcers in patients with spinal cord lesions. *Paraplegia, 28,* 269.
27. Cooper, D.M. (1990). The physiology of wound healing: an overview. *In* Krasner, D. (ed.). *Chronic wound care.* King of Prussia, PA: Health Management Publications.
28. Cosman, B. (1971). Physiology of the skin. *In* Downey, J.A., & Darling, R.C. (eds.). *Physiological basis of rehabilitation medicine.* Philadelphia: W.B. Saunders.
29. Currents (1989). *Hospitals, 63,* 52.
30. Dembert, M.L. (1982). Medical problems from cold exposure. *American Family Physician, 25,* 99.
31. Dubin, S. (1992). The physiologic changes of aging. *Orthopaedic Nursing, 11,* 45.
32. Dyer, C., & Roberts, D. (1990). Thermal trauma. *Nursing Clinics of North America, 25*(1), 85.
33. Eaglstein, W.H. (ed.) (1990). *New directions in wound healing.* Princeton, NJ: Convatec.
34. Etris, M.B., et al. (1991). A new generation of gauze dressings. *Ostomy/Wound Management, 34,* 57.
35. Falanga, V. (1988). Occlusive wound dressings. *Archives of Dermatology, 124,* 872.
36. Fanucci, D., & Seese, J. (1991). Multi-faceted use of calcium alginates. *Ostomy/Wound Management, 37,* 16.
37. Fowler, E. (1990). Chronic wounds: an overview. *In* Krasner, D. (ed.). *Chronic wound care.* King of Prussia, PA: Health Management Publications.
38. Fowler, E., & Papen, J.C. (1991). A new hydrogel wound dressing for the treatment of open wounds. *Ostomy/Wound Management, 37,* 39.
39. Gosnell, D.J. (1987). Assessment and evaluation of pressure sores. *Nursing Clinics of North America, 22,* 399.
40. Greenhalgh, D.G., & Gamelli, R.L. (1987). Is impaired wound healing caused by infection or nutritional depletion? *Surgery, 102,* 306.
41. Hanan, K., & Schaele, L. (1991). Albumin vs weight as a predictor of nutritional status and pressure ulcer development. *Ostomy/Wound Management, 33,* 22.
42. Harding, K.G. (1990). Wound care: putting theory into clinical practice. *In* Krasner, D. (ed.). *Chronic wound care.* King of Prussia, PA: Health Management Publications.
43. Hocutt, J.E. (1981). Cryotherapy. *American Family Physician, 23,* 141.

44. Hunt, T.K. (1990). Basic principles of wound healing. *Journal of Trauma,* 30(12), Suppl. 122.

45. Hutchinson, J.J., & McGuckin, M. (1990). Occlusive dressings: a microbiologic and clinical review. *American Journal of Infection Control,* 18(4), 257.

46. Jacobson, G., et al. (1985). Handwashing: ring-wearing and number of microorganisms. *Nursing Research,* 34, 186.

47. Jeter, K.F., & Tintle, T.E. (1985). Keep the elderly cool. *Emergency Medicine,* 17, 155.

48. Jeter, K.F., & Tintle, T.E. (1991). Wound dressings of the nineties. *Clinics in Podiatric Medicine and Surgery,* 8, 799.

49. Kemp, M.G., et al. (1990). Factors that contribute to pressure sores in surgical patients. *Research in Nursing and Health,* 13, 293.

50. Knighton, D.R., et al. (1989). The use of topically applied platelet growth factors in chronic nonhealing wounds: a review. *Wounds,* premier issue.

51. Korniewicz, D.M., et al. (1991). Do your gloves fit the task? *American Journal of Nursing,* 91, 38.

52. Kottke, F.J. (1966). The effects of limitation of activity upon the human body. *Journal of The American Medical Association,* 196, 117.

53. Krasner, D. (1988). Managing draining wounds: fistulas, leaking tubes and drains. *Ostomy/Wound Management,* 19, 79.

54. Krasner, D. (ed.) (1990). *Chronic wound care.* King of Prussia, PA: Health Management Publications.

55. Krasner, D. (1991). An approach to treating skin tears. *Ostomy/Wound Management,* 32, 56.

56. Krasner, D. (1991). Product index. *Ostomy/Wound Management,* 33, 47.

57. Krasner, D. (1991). Resolving the dressing dilemma: selecting wound dressings by category. *Ostomy/Wound Management,* 35, 62.

58. Krouskop, T.A., et al. (1985). Effectiveness of mattress overlays in reducing interface pressures during recumbency. *Journal of Rehabilitation Research and Development,* 22, 7 (BPR 10–42).

59. Landis, E.M. (1930). Micro-injection studies of capillary blood pressure in human skin. *Heart,* 15, 209.

60. Landry, S.L., et al. (1989). Hospital stay and mortality attributed to nosocomial enterococcal bacteremia: a controlled study. *American Journal of Infection Control,* 17, 323.

61. Larson, E. (1989). Handwashing: it's essential even when you use gloves. *American Journal of Nursing,* 89, 934.

62. Larson, E., et al. (1986). Physiologic and microbiologic changes in skin related to frequent handwashing. *Infection Control,* 7, 59.

63. Larson, E., et al. (1989). Influence of two handwashing frequencies on reduction in colonizing flora with three handwashing products used by health care personnel. *American Journal of Infection Control,* 17, 83.

64. LaVelle, B.E., & Snyder, M. (1985). Differential conduction of cold through barriers. *Journal of Advanced Nursing,* 10, 55.

65. Lehmann, J.F., & De Lateur, B.J. (1982). Therapeutic heat. *In* Lehmann, J.F. (ed.). *Therapeutic heat and cold* (3rd ed.). Baltimore: Williams & Wilkins.

66. Lehmann, J.J., & De Lateur, B.J. (1982). Cryotherapy. *In* Lehmann, J.F. (ed.). *Therapeutic heat and cold* (3rd ed.). Baltimore: Williams & Wilkins.

67. Lehman, J.F., and De Lateur, B.J. (1990). Diathermy and superficial heat, laser, and cold therapy. *In* Kottke, F.J., & Lehmann, J.F. (eds.). *Krusen's handbook of physical medicine and rehabilitation* (4th ed.). Philadelphia: W.B. Saunders.

68. Lineweaver, W., et al. (1985). Topical antimicrobial toxicity. *Archives of Surgery,* 120, 267.

69. Lipsky, J.G. (1984). Saving the elderly from the killing cold. *Nursing '84,* 14, 42.

70. Lynch, P., et al. (1990). Implementing and evaluating a system of generic infection precautions: body substance isolation. *American Journal of Infection Control,* 18, 1.

71. Maklebust, J., & Sieggreen, M. (1991). *Pressure ulcers: Guidelines for prevention and nursing management.* West Dundee, IL: S-N Publications.

72. Mant, A.K. (1986). Some medico-legal aspects of wounds. *In* Westaby, S. (ed.). *Wound care.* St. Louis: C.V. Mosby.

73. Mertz, P.M., & Eaglstein, W.H. (1984). The effect of a semi-oc-

clusive dressing on the microbial population in superficial wounds. *Archives of Surgery,* 119, 287.

74. Mertz, P.M., et al. (1990). The wound environment: implications from research studies for healing and infection. *In* Krasner, D. (ed.). *Chronic wound care.* King of Prussia, PA: Health Management Publications.

75. National Pressure Ulcer Advisory Panel (1992). *Statement on Pressure Ulcer Prevention.* Buffalo, NY.

76. Neuberger, G.B., & Reckling, J.B. (1990). Preventing wound complications in an age of DRGS. *In* Krasner, D. (ed.). *Chronic wound care.* King of Prussia, PA: Health Management Publications.

77. North American Nursing Diagnosis Association (1990). *Taxonomy I revised–1990.* St. Louis: NANDA.

78. Oberg, M.S., & Lindsey, D. (1987). Do not put hydrogen peroxide or povidone iodine into wounds! *American Journal of Disease Control,* 141, 27.

79. Pasceri, P. (1991). Utilizing a prevention and treatment protocol for skin breakdown secondary to urinary incontinence. *Ostomy/Wound Management,* 36, 66.

80. Peacock, E.E. (1981). Control of wound healing and scar formation in surgical patients. *Archives of Surgery,* 116, 1325.

81. Peck, S. (1990). Crush syndrome. *Orthopaedic Nursing,* 9, 33.

82. Peterson, L. (1983). The psychological impact of trauma: recognition and treatment. *American Journal of Emergency Medicine,* 1, 102.

83. Pinchcofsky-Devin, G. (1990). Nutritional assessment and intervention. *In* Krasner, D. (ed.). *Chronic wound care.* King of Prussia, PA: Health Management Publications.

84. Pinchcofsky-Devin, G.D., & Kaminski, M.V., Jr. (1986). Correlation of pressure sores and nutritional status. *Journal of American Geriatrics Society,* 34(6), 435.

85. Pugliese, G., & Lampinen, T. (1989). Prevention of human immunodeficiency virus infection: our responsibilities as health care professionals. *American Journal of Infection Control,* 17, 1.

86. Ridley, M.A. (1988). Discharge planning considerations for the pressure ulcer patient. *Ostomy/Wound Management,* 19, 70.

87. Robson, M.C. (1988). Disturbances of wound healing. *Annals of Emergency Medicine,* 17, 1274.

88. Robson, M.C., et al. (1987). Principles of wound healing and repair. *In* James, E., et al. (eds.). *Principles of basic surgical practice.* Philadelphia: Hanley & Belfus.

89. Robson, M.C., et al. (1990). Wound healing alterations caused by infection. *Clinics in Plastic Surgery,* 17, 485.

90. Rodeheaver, G. (1988). Controversies in topical wound management. *Ostomy/Wound Management,* 20, 58.

91. Rodeheaver, G., et al. (1982). Bactericidal activity and toxicity of iodine-containing solutions in wounds. *Archives of Surgery,* 117, 181.

92. Ross, D. (1991). Acute compartment syndrome. *Orthopaedic Nursing,* 10, 33.

93. Rudolph, R., & Shannon, M.L. (1990). The normal healing process. *In* Eaglstein, W.H. (ed.). *New directions in wound healing.* Princeton, NJ: Convatec.

94. Rutala, W.A. (1989). Draft guideline for selection and use of disinfectants. *American Journal of Infection Control,* 17, 24a.

95. Schneider, D.L., & Hebert, L.J. (1987). Subcutaneous gas from hydrogen peroxide administration under pressure. *American Journal of Diseases in Children,* 141, 10.

96. Shannon, M.L. (1984). Five famous fallacies about pressure sores. *Nursing '84,* 14, 34.

97. Shannon, M.L. (1988). Pressure ulcers: an ounce of prevention saves millions. *The Older Patient,* 27.

98. Shannon, M.L. (1982). Pressure sores. *In* Norris, C. (ed.). *Concept clarification in nursing.* Rockville, MD: Aspen Systems Corporation.

99. Shannon, M.L., & Miller, B.M. (1988). Pressure sore treatment: a case in point. *Geriatric Nursing,* 154.

100. Shannon, M.L., & Miller, B.M. (1988). Evaluation of hydrocolloid dressings on healing of pressure ulcers in spinal cord injury patients. *Decubitus,* 1, 42.

101. Shannon, M.L., & Skorga, P. (1989). Pressure ulcer prevalence in two general hospitals. *Decubitus,* 2, 38.

102. Simmons, B.P. (1983). Guideline for prevention of surgical wound infections. CDC guidelines for the prevention and con-

trol of nosocomial infections. *American Journal of Infection Control,* 11, 133.

103. Skerrett, P.J. (1991). "Matrix algebra" heals life's wounds. *Science,* 252, 1064.
104. Stotts, N.A. (1987). Age-specific characteristics of patients who develop pressure ulcers in the tertiary-care setting. *Nursing Clinics of North America,* 22, 391.
105. Sussman, C. (1990). The role of physical therapy in wound care. *Ostomy/Wound Management,* 29, 20.
106. Sweat, E. (1990). Managing pressure ulcers in the neuroscience patient. *Journal of Neuroscience Nursing,* 22(5), 307.
107. Tepperman, P.S., & Devlin, M. (1983). Therapeutic heat and cold. *Postgraduate Medicine,* 73, 69.
108. Turner, T.D. (1990). The development of wound management products. *In* Krasner, D. (ed.). *Chronic wound care.* King of Prussia, PA: Health Management Publications.
109. Van Dover, D. (1991). To Betadine or not to Betadine. *Ostomy/ Wound Management,* 32, 40.
110. Vijswijk, L., & Cuzzell, J.C. (1991). Derm detective: managing full-thickness wounds. *American Journal of Nursing,* 91, 18.
111. Viljanto, J. (1980). Disinfection of surgical wounds without inhibition of normal wound healing. *Archives of Surgery,* 115, 253.
112. Weiss, D.S., et al. (1990). Electrical stimulation and wound healing. *Archives of Dermatology,* 126, 222.
113. Welch, L.B. (1981). Simple new remedy for the odor of open lesions. *RN,* 46, 42.
114. Westaby, S. (1986). Wound closure and drainage. *In* Westaby, S. (ed.). *Wound care.* St. Louis: C.V. Mosby.
115. Westaby, S. (1986). Fundamentals of wound healing. *In* Westaby, S. (ed.). *Wound care.* St. Louis: C.V. Mosby.
116. Whitney, J.D. (1989). Physiologic effects of tissue oxygenation on wound healing. *Heart & Lung,* 18, 466.
117. Woo, S.L., et al. (1975). Connective tissue response to immobility. *Arthritis and Rheumatology,* 18, 257.

▼ *Perioperative Nursing*

> No passion so effectively robs the mind of all its powers of acting and reasoning as fear.
>
> **Edmund Burke**

▼ **CHAPTER OUTLINE**

BASIC CONCEPTS
    Purposes and Types of Surgery
    Phases of the Surgical Experience
ROLES AND RESPONSIBILITIES OF THE
  SURGICAL TEAM
THE PERSON UNDERGOING SURGERY
    Profile of the Surgical Candidate
    Psychophysiologic Alterations from
     Surgery
    Developmental Considerations in
     Perioperative Nursing
LEGAL IMPLICATIONS OF SURGERY
PREOPERATIVE PHASE
    Admission to the Health Care
     Facility
    Assessment
    Nursing Diagnosis

    Planning
    Nursing Intervention
    Evaluation
INTRAOPERATIVE PHASE
    Assessment
    Nursing Diagnosis
    Planning
    Nursing Intervention
    Evaluation
POSTOPERATIVE PHASE
    Assessment
    Nursing Diagnosis
    Planning
    Nursing Intervention
    Evaluation
CASE STUDY

▼ **KEY TERMS**

Intraoperative phase
Nurse anesthetists
Perioperative period

Phase II recovery area
Postanesthesia care unit
  (PACU)

Postoperative phase
Preoperative phase
RN first assistant

Perioperative nursing is defined as "those nursing activities performed by the professional nurse in the preoperative, intraoperative, and postoperative phases of the patient's surgical experience."[4] The Association of Operating Room Nurses (AORN) Standards of Perioperative Nursing Practice guide the nurse throughout the perioperative period (see Box 49–1). Practice settings for perioperative nurses include hospitals, freestanding surgery centers, and physicians' offices.

More than 22.5 million surgical procedures are performed annually in the United States, 49 per cent of which are completed on an outpatient, ambulatory, or same-day surgery basis.[1] This increasing trend toward outpatient surgery reflects reimbursement changes, a focus on cost containment, advanced technology, and the development of less invasive surgical techniques. Medical costs are reduced by eliminating a hospital stay, and sophisticated equipment such as video endoscopes and lasers make less invasive surgery possible.

Regardless of the setting for surgery or the "seriousness" of the operation, the individual undergoing surgery always requires nursing assessment, care, teaching, and support. Although surgery may ultimately be beneficial, a surgical procedure, even when classified as "minor," is always traumatic for the person. Surgery invades the body and thus presents a major threat to a person's physiologic and psychologic well-being. Often the surgical staff views surgery as a procedure with intricate, well-defined steps and a predictable outcome. However, the person awaiting surgery faces the unknown. Many people do not know what to expect before, during, or after surgery, nor do they know what the staff expects of them. The sensitive nurse can help relieve anxiety by (1) providing information about perioperative events and (2) giving emotional support to the individual and support persons.

This chapter focuses on (1) the experience of the person undergoing surgery, (2) the scope of practice and activities of the nurse in assisting the individual throughout the perioperative experience, and (3) the role of the entire health team in achieving a successful surgical outcome.

Successful surgery returns the person to an optimum state of health in the shortest period with the fewest risks and complications.

BASIC CONCEPTS

Purposes and Types of Surgery

Surgery is indicated for many reasons and is classified according to (1) its purpose, (2) the degree of risk to the individual, and (3) the urgency with which it is required. These classifications offer a reasonable way to view different operative procedures. Note, however, that they are artificial divisions with overlap between categories.

Box 49–1. Standards of Perioperative Nursing Practice

Standard I

THE COLLECTION OF DATA ABOUT THE HEALTH STATUS OF THE INDIVIDUAL IS SYSTEMATIC AND CONTINUOUS. THE DATA ARE RETRIEVABLE AND COMMUNICATED TO APPROPRIATE PERSONS.

Interpretive Statement

The fundamental step of the nursing process is initiated by the operating room nurse after the individual consents to have surgical intervention. The initial collection of data may occur in a variety of settings, such as the surgical suite, the care unit, or the home or clinic. Data collection may be accomplished through diverse means, such as interview, review of records, assessment, or consultation among members of the health care team. It is a progressive and orderly process that requires the operating room nurse to possess skills necessary to gather meaningful and pertinent data relative to the surgical intervention. Priority of data collection is determined by the immediate health care problems or needs of the patient.

Box 49–1. Standards of Perioperative Nursing Practice (Continued)

Criteria

1. Health data collected is relative to the planned surgical intervention and includes, but is not limited to, the following:
   a. Current medical diagnosis and therapy
   b. Physical status and physiological responses
   c. Psychosocial status of the patient
   d. Cultural and spiritual information
   e. The individual's understanding, perceptions, and expectations of the surgical procedure
   f. Previous responses to illness, to hospitalization, and to surgery
   g. Results of diagnostic studies
2. Health data is collected by a variety of methods.
3. Health data is reported and recorded.

Standard II

NURSING DIAGNOSES ARE DERIVED FROM HEALTH STATUS DATA.

Interpretive Statement

The nursing diagnoses are judgments the operating room nurse makes based on the analysis and interpretations of data about the individual's problems and needs and health status. The nursing diagnoses are concise statements about the individual's health status and problems amenable to nursing intervention.

Criteria

1. Current health status deviations and/or problems are identified.
2. Current scientific knowledge supports the nursing diagnoses.
3. The nursing diagnoses are congruent with the diagnoses of other health professionals.
4. The nursing diagnoses are recorded and communicated.

Standard III

THE PLAN OF NURSING CARE INCLUDES GOALS DERIVED FROM THE NURSING DIAGNOSES.

Interpretive Statement

Goals for care are derived from the nursing diagnoses and are mutually formulated with the individual, significant others, and other health personnel. The goals developed must be attainable through available human and material resources. Goals direct the nursing actions to correct, alter, or maintain the nursing diagnoses. Areas for the operating room nurse to consider when formulating goals for individuals experiencing surgical intervention should include, but are not limited to, the following:

▶ Absence of infection
▶ Maintenance of skin integrity

▶ Absence of adverse effects due to proper use of safety measures related to positioning, extraneous objects, and chemical, physical, and electrical hazards
▶ Maintenance of fluid and electrolyte balance
▶ Knowledge of the patient and significant others of the physiological and psychological responses to surgical intervention
▶ Participation of the individual and significant others in the rehabilitation process

Criteria

1. Goals are clearly written as statements of outcomes.
2. The individual's present and potential physical capabilities and behavioral patterns are congruent with goals.
3. Measurable criteria for determining the attainment of the goals as a result of nursing actions are included in the goal statement.
4. Goals are prioritized.
5. Goals are recorded and communicated to appropriate persons.
6. Goals include a time estimate for attainment.

Standard IV

THE PLAN FOR NURSING CARE PRESCRIBES NURSING ACTIONS TO ACHIEVE THE GOALS.

Interpretive Statement

The goals for the nursing care become the guide for the nursing actions necessary to achieve the identified outcomes. Priorities for the provision of nursing care are established by the operating room nurse in collaboration with the individual, significant others, and members of the health care team. The plan reflects preoperative assessment, priorities for nursing action, and a logical sequence of nursing activities to attain the goals. The plan is developed with and communicated to the individual, significant others, and health care personnel as appropriate. The plan reflects consideration of the individual's rights and desires. The plan specifies nursing activities performed in the perioperative period. Examples of nursing activities performed might include, but are not limited to, the following:

▶ Assurance of information and supportive preoperative teaching specifically related to the surgical intervention and the operating room nursing care
▶ Identification of the individual
▶ Verification of the surgical site
▶ Verification of operative consent and procedure and reports of essential diagnostic procedures
▶ Positioning according to physiological principles
▶ Adherence to principles of asepsis
▶ Assurance of appropriate and properly functioning equipment and supplies for the individual
▶ Provision for comfort measures and supportive care to the individual
▶ Environmental monitoring and safety

Box continued on following page

Box 49–1. *Standards of Perioperative Nursing Practice* (Continued)

▶ Psychological and physiological monitoring of the individual

▶ Evaluation of outcomes in relation to the identified nursing activities

▶ Communication of intraoperative information to significant others and members of the health care team.

Criteria

1. Current scientific knowledge supports the plan.
2. Human and material resources are available to implement the plan.
3. The plan is written and communicated to the individual, significant others, and other appropriate members of the health care team.
4. The plan specifies the following:
   a. Nursing actions necessary to achieve the goals
   b. Priority of nursing action
   c. A logical sequencing of nursing actions
   d. How the nursing actions are to be performed
   e. When the nursing actions are to be performed
   f. Where the nursing actions are to be performed
   g. Who is to perform the nursing actions.

Standard V

THE PLAN FOR NURSING CARE IS IMPLEMENTED.

Interpretive Statement

The nursing actions performed are consistent with the plan and provide continuity of nursing care in the preoperative, intraoperative, and postoperative periods. The nursing actions are performed with safety, skill, efficiency, and effectiveness.

Scientific principles provide the basis for nursing actions. All care provided reflects the rights and desires of the individual and significant others. The nursing interventions and outcomes are documented through permanent written records, with subsequent oral or written reports to other health care providers when appropriate.

Criteria

1. Nursing actions specified in the plan are performed and documented by means of the following:
   a. Written records
   b. Observations of nursing practice
   c. Confirmation by the individual or significant others.
2. Nursing actions and patient outcomes are communicated to others as appropriate.

Standard VI

THE PLAN FOR NURSING CARE IS EVALUATED.

Interpretive Statement

Evaluation is a process the operating room nurse uses to determine the degree of goal attainment. The evaluation is

continuous and is based on the nurse's observations and the individual's responses to the nursing interventions. The operating room nurse reviews each of the formulated goals to determine the results of the individual's care. The results of the nursing actions are then compared to the desired goals to determine the degree of goal attainment. The individual, significant others, and health personnel contribute to the evaluation of goal attainment. The data collected from these sources reflect the outcomes of nursing activities.

Criteria

1. The degree of goal achievement is communicated by the operating room nurse to the individual, significant others, and health personnel.
2. The results of nursing actions are documented by written records, observations of nursing practice, and/or confirmation by the individual or significant others.

Standard VII

REASSESSMENT OF THE INDIVIDUAL, RECONSIDERATION OF NURSING DIAGNOSIS, RESETTING OF GOALS, AND MODIFICATION AND IMPLEMENTATION OF THE NURSING CARE PLAN ARE A CONTINUOUS PROCESS.

Interpretive Statement

Reassessment allows the operating room nurse to critically examine the total process from which the planned and delivered nursing interventions are derived. Implementation of the nursing process establishes a feedback to the nurse that facilitates the review of individual professional practice. The steps of the nursing process are taken concurrently and recurrently. New data and/or the degree of goal achievement are assessed and used to reconsider the nursing diagnoses, goals for individual, and plan of care. Reassessment allows the dynamics of nursing to operate in an open system whereby modification of the plan of care can be made as changes occur in the individual's internal and external environment.

Criteria

1. Review or revision of the plan of care is documented by written records, observations of patient responses, and the perception of the individual or significant others.
2. Status of the plan of care is communicated to appropriate others.

From Association of Operating Room Nurses. (1991). *AORN standards and recommended practices for perioperative nursing.* Denver, CO: Association of Operating Room Nurses.

Purposes of surgery include

▶ diagnostic or exploratory
▶ curative
▶ ablative
▶ constructive
▶ reconstructive
▶ palliative

Diagnostic surgery enables the surgeon to establish or confirm the diagnosis of an illness. By removing tissue for microscopic examination, the surgeon (and the medical pathologist) diagnoses a pathologic process. For example, a biopsy of breast tissue is used to diagnose the nature of a lesion found in the breast. Exploratory surgery is also useful in establishing a diagnosis. By exploring a body cavity or area, the surgeon is better able to determine the extent of a disease. For instance, during an exploratory laparotomy, through an incision in the abdominal wall to the peritoneal cavity, the surgeon searches the peritoneal cavity for the presence, nature, and extent of disease. In some cases, diagnostic and exploratory surgery may lead to more extensive surgery to alter the course of an illness or disease process.

Curative surgery seeks to cure illness or restore malfunctioning tissue by removing or altering diseased or damaged tissue. Removing a cancerous tumor and repairing a cleft lip are examples of curative surgery. Curative surgery may be (1) ablative, (2) reconstructive, or (3) constructive.

Ablative surgery removes diseased organs. A nephrectomy, or kidney removal, is an example of ablative surgery. Reconstructive procedures improve appearance or function through partial or complete restoration of damaged tissues (e.g., repair of a joint damaged by traumatic injury). Constructive surgery repairs congenital malformations, such as congenital facial deformities. This type of surgery improves appearance and functions.

Palliative surgery relieves the symptoms of an illness but does not result in a cure. Performing palliative surgery in the presence of a terminal or chronic disease is common. For example, a large tumor may be removed to relieve an intestinal obstruction caused by a cancerous growth, even when the cancer is beyond cure.

Surgery is classified as major or minor according to the degree of risk associated with an operation. This classification measures the hazards of the surgical procedure and the extent of physiologic alteration. Major surgery involves the highest degree of risk. It is characterized by (1) the alteration of major body organs and structures, (2) the potential for extensive blood loss, (3) the length of the procedure, and (4) the risk of complications during and after surgery. Procedures involving the chest, heart, and major abdominal organs are examples of major surgery. On the other hand, minor surgery involves the smallest combination of risks. Typically, minor surgery includes procedures that (1) are uncomplicated, (2) are of short duration, (3) have a minimal potential for blood loss, and (4) involve a low degree of risk. Breast biopsy and dental extraction are examples of minor surgery.

Minor surgery is not without the risks of surgery.

Operative procedures are also classified by the urgency and necessity for surgery. Emergency surgery is performed immediately to save a person's life, limb, or organ. Urgent or imperative surgery is not an emergency but must be performed as soon as conditions permit, usually 12 to 48 hours after determining the need for surgery. Required surgery is not urgent but is necessary for the well-being of the person. Heart valve surgery and tumor removal are examples. Elective or optional operative procedures are not required, but long-term benefits may result. For example, cosmetic facial surgery may improve a person's appearance and psychologic well-being.

Phases of the Surgical Experience

The entire surgical process is called the **perioperative period.** It consists of three phases:

▶ The **preoperative phase** begins when surgery is planned and ends when the individual is transferred to the operating room (OR) table.
▶ The **intraoperative phase** begins when the individual is transferred to the OR table and ends at admission to the **postanesthesia care unit (PACU)** or recovery room, where the client regains consciousness.
▶ The **postoperative phase** is the recovery period. It starts with the client's admission to the PACU and ends when the healing process is completed; hence, this phase may continue for weeks or months.

The nursing process and the Standards of Perioperative Nursing Practice guide the care of the individual throughout the perioperative period.

The nursing process is closely related to the AORN Standards of Practice, as Table 49-1 shows. Nursing practice in the preoperative phase may include initial assessment, explanation of perioperative events, development of nursing diagnoses and a plan of care, and initiation of discharge planning as well as physical preparation for surgery. During the intraoperative phase, nursing activities focus on ensuring safety, main-

TABLE 49-1. Relationship of Nursing Process to Standards of Nursing Practice*

Elements of Nursing Process	Standards of Nursing Practice
Assessment	Collection of data
	Formulation of nursing diagnosis
Planning	Establishment of goals
	Development of plan
Implementation	Implementation of plan
Evaluation	Evaluation of plan
	Reassessment

* From Kneedler, J. A. & Dodge, G. H. (1987). *Perioperative patient care: The nursing perspective* (2nd ed.). Cambridge, MA: Blackwell Scientific.

Box 49–2. Examples of Nursing Activities in Perioperative Nursing Practice

Preoperative Phase

Preoperative Assessment

Home/clinic

1. initiates initial preoperative assessment
2. plans teaching methods appropriate to patient's needs
3. involves family in interview

Surgical unit

1. completes preoperative assessment
2. coordinates patient teaching with other nursing staff
3. explains phases in perioperative period and expectations
4. develops a plan of care

Surgical suite

1. assesses patient's level of consciousness
2. reviews chart
3. identifies patient
4. verifies surgical site

Planning

1. determines a plan of care

Psychological support

1. tells patient what is happening
2. determines psychological status
3. gives prior warning of noxious stimuli
4. communicates patient's emotional status to other appropriate members of the health care team

Intraoperative Phase

Maintenance of safety

1. assures that the sponge, needle, and instrument counts are correct
2. positions the patient
   a. functional alignment
   b. exposure of surgical site
   c. maintenance of position throughout procedure
3. applies grounding device to patient
4. provides physical support

Physiologic monitoring

1. calculates effects on patient of excessive fluid loss
2. distinguishes normal from abnormal cardiopulmonary data
3. reports changes in patient's pulse, respirations, temperature, and blood pressure

Psychological monitoring (prior to induction and if patient conscious)

1. provides emotional support to patient
2. stands near/touches patient during procedures/ induction
3. continues to assess patient's emotional status
4. communicates patient's emotional status to other appropriate members of the health care team

Nursing management

1. provides physical safety for the patient
2. maintains aseptic, controlled environment
3. effectively manages human resources

Postoperative Phase

Communication of intraoperative information

1. gives patient's name
2. states type of surgery performed
3. provides contributing intraoperative factors (e.g., drain, catheters)
4. states physical limitations
5. states impairments resulting from surgery
6. reports patient's preoperative level of consciousness
7. communicates necessary equipment needs

Postoperative evaluation

Recovery area

1. determines patient's immediate response to surgical intervention

Surgical unit

1. evaluates effectiveness of nursing care in the OR
2. determines patient's level of satisfaction with care given during perioperative period
3. evaluates products used on patient in the OR
4. determines patient's psychological status
5. assists with discharge planning

Home/clinic

1. seeks patient's perception of surgery in terms of the effects of anesthetic agents, impact on body image, distortion, immobilization
2. determines family's perceptions of surgery

From Association of Operating Room Nurses. (1991). *AORN standards and recommended practices for perioperative nursing.* Denver, CO: Association of Operating Room Nurses. *Abbreviation:* OR, operating room.

taining asepsis, monitoring for physiologic changes, and providing emotional support. In the postoperative phase, nursing activities include communication of intraoperative information, assessment of physiologic responses to surgery and anesthesia, reinforcement of teaching, implementation of discharge planning, and evaluation of outcomes. Because the outpatient surgical experience is condensed in time, the preparation of the individual and support persons for self-care at home is accelerated.

ROLES AND RESPONSIBILITIES OF THE SURGICAL TEAM

Many health care professionals, including nurses, physicians, and technicians, attend to the person undergoing surgery. Each member of the surgical team has specialized education and training to ensure the individual's safety and well-being throughout the perioperative period.

Nurses are involved in caring for individuals through all phases of surgery. In a hospital, surgical nurses work on surgical floors; in the preoperative holding area; in the OR; in the PACU, or recovery room; in special outpatient recovery units; surgical intensive care units (SICUs); and in surgical clinics. They provide specialized care to the individual and support persons on admission to the health care facility in preparation for surgery, during surgery, and throughout the postoperative phase. Box 49–2 presents examples of nursing activities in perioperative nursing practice.

During the preoperative period, nurses working on the surgical unit or admission unit perform thorough assessments, provide physical care, give emotional support, and ensure that legal consents are in order. They also instruct the person about her or his role in promoting recovery, and they initiate discharge planning. They include support persons in planning, with the permission of the surgical candidate. During this phase, the nurse anesthetist or anesthesiologist also meets with the surgical candidate.

Operating room nurses provide specialized care during the intraoperative phase. Generally, the roles of the professional nurse in the operating room include serving as circulator, scrub person, nurse anesthetist, or first assistant. Within each of these roles, nurses may manage, educate, and engage in research. Following are the duties for each role:

▶ *Circulating nurses* (1) prepare the OR according to the individual's needs, the surgical procedure, and the surgeon's preferences; (2) receive and identify the person on arrival to the surgical area; (3) briefly orient the person to the OR and provide emotional support; (4) verify that the preoperative check list is complete and reassess the individual for allergies, skin condition, and untoward diagnostic test results; (5) help transfer and position the person on the OR table; (6) prepare the skin; (7) help the surgical team gown; (8) monitor to ensure that sterile technique and universal precautions are used by all members of the team; (9) supervise sponge, needle,

and instrument counts; (10) provide equipment, supplies, and medications needed during surgery; (11) monitor the individual undergoing a procedure under local anesthesia; and (12) make assignments and supervise client care.

▶ *Scrub persons* participate in the operative procedure. They ensure and maintain surgical asepsis during surgery, prepare and provide instruments to the surgeon, and keep accurate count of instruments, sponges, and needles used during surgery. Scrub persons may be nurses or surgical technicians with specialized training in operating room techniques.

▶ *Nurse anesthetists* are nurses with advanced training and licensure to deliver anesthesia and monitor the client during surgery and anesthesia. Nurse anesthetists work under the supervision of an anesthesiologist. (In contrast, anesthesiologists are physicians with special training in anesthesia administration.) The nurse anesthetist assesses the person before surgery, induces anesthesia, and monitors the person during and immediately after surgery.

▶ *RN first assistants* are nurses working in an expanded role with advanced, specialized education in surgical techniques and responsibilities. They assist the surgeon with the surgical procedure by helping with wound exposure, hemostasis, and suturing.[31]

During the postoperative phase, nurses again provide specialized care. For example:

▶ *PACU nurses* monitor the person during recovery from anesthesia in the immediate postoperative phase, provide comfort measures, and help to implement the discharge plan.

▶ *SICU nurses* monitor the person in a SICU after some types of major or complicated surgery (e.g., open-heart surgery).

On discharge from the PACU or SICU, surgical unit nurses continue to monitor the person and observe for complications. They assist the person during the return to normal dietary, elimination, and activity patterns. In addition, they prepare the individual and support persons for the discharge.

In some hospital and surgical facilities, perioperative nurses care for the person during all phases of the surgical experience. These nurses follow the person throughout the three phases to teach and support the individual and support persons. They also act as liaison nurses when the person is transferred from one department to another or when the person is discharged. Perioperative nursing is ideal because it allows continuity of nursing care.[28]

As members of the surgical team, nurses collaborate with surgeons and other physicians. The surgeon performs the operative procedure and is responsible for the person's medical and surgical treatment throughout the perioperative period. The person undergoing surgery may also be under the care of an anesthesiologist, who (1) determines the type of anesthesia to be administered during surgery, (2) induces anesthesia, (3) monitors the person during surgery, and (4) provides medical supervision during postanesthesia recovery. Alternatively, the anesthesiologist supervises the nurse anesthetist, who carries out many of these duties.

THE PERSON UNDERGOING SURGERY

Profile of the Surgical Candidate

People respond differently to surgery. Some recover from a major procedure with relative ease. Others experience severe complications after a minor procedure. To a great extent, the personal profile of the surgical candidate determines the person's response and thus influences the outcome of surgery. Personal factors to assess include the individual's (1) age, (2) sex, (3) level of growth and development, (4) ethnic/cultural background, (5) general health, (6) medications taken regularly, (7) mobility, (8) fluid and electrolyte status, (9) nutritional status, (10) level of knowledge regarding the surgery, (11) coping ability, (12) socioeconomic situation, (13) religious preference, (14) occupation, and (15) attitude.

Psychophysiologic Alterations from Surgery

Surgery (particularly a major procedure) can upset many aspects of a person's life. Although potentially beneficial, it poses a threat to the person's ability to meet basic physiologic and psychosocial needs. Nurses assist individuals and support persons to adapt to changes and potential or actual problems that result from surgery. Table 49–2 outlines major alterations resulting from surgery.

ACTIVATION OF THE STRESS RESPONSE

Surgery seriously upsets the body's homeostatic balance. The stress response is the body's reaction to this imbalance. It can be triggered by both psychologic and physiologic stimuli. For example, psychologic stressors include anxiety, fear of the unknown, and discomfort or pain. Physiologic stressors (e.g., anesthesia, tissue damage, blood loss, and electrolyte imbalances) result from the surgical procedure. The severity and duration of stressful stimuli determine the degree of the body's stress response. Recall from Chapter 16 that the stress response involves a complex chain of physiologic events that are controlled primarily by the neuroendocrine system.

Also recall that the stress response is an essential adaptive mechanism. The adaptive "fight or flight" mechanism occurs when the body attempts to maintain or restore its homeostatic balance. The stress response during surgery may protect the person's body from further damage caused by surgical trauma. For example, an increase in cardiac output and peripheral vasoconstriction enables the body to compensate for marked blood loss.

The body's responses to high levels of stress, however, may be maladaptive for some people undergoing surgery. In addition, certain individuals, especially the

TABLE 49–2. Psychophysiologic Alterations Resulting from Surgery

Alterations	Potential Problems
Activation of the stress response	Overwhelming stress response; failure of homeostatic mechanisms; release of excessive hormones; cardiovascular failure
Lowered defense against infection	Wound infection
Disruption of vascular system	Excessive bleeding, hemorrhage from surgical wound
Disturbed organ function	Depends on organ (e.g., gastric motility may be temporarily depressed; bladder function disrupted)
Oxygen utilization	Depression of the central nervous system (CNS) by anesthetics/analgesics alters patterns of respiration
Water and electrolyte balance	Water and electrolyte loss during surgery; acidosis or alkalosis occurs
Nutrition	Reduced intake of foods and fluids; possible nausea and vomiting
Elimination	Gastrointestinal tract function slowed; decreased renal blood flow and hormonal changes cause decreased urine output
Temperature regulation	Vasodilation from anesthetic agents; loss of body warmth in operative environment; fever secondary to infection
Sleep and comfort	Alterations in biorhythms; CNS depression; pain and discomfort
Mobility	Decrease in muscle activity from CNS depression; immobility from pain and weakness
Sensation	Alteration in sensory input; CNS depression
Body image	Loss of body part or function; invasion of body space; distortion of body image
Identity and self-esteem	Interference with role performance; interference with sexuality; threat to self-image
Safety and security	Unfamiliarity with hospital environment; disruption in normal routines and self-care

elderly or debilitated, are less able to withstand even moderate amounts of surgical stress. People with specific disorders that decrease the body's adaptive mechanisms (e.g., adrenal insufficiency, diabetes mellitus, cardiovascular disease, and psychologic disorders) are also prone to maladaptive responses to surgery. Thus, the nurse's role includes assessing and reducing stressors during the perioperative period.

PHYSIOLOGIC ALTERATIONS

Impaired Protection Against Infection. The first line of defense against bacterial invasion and infection is the skin and mucous membrane. When a surgical incision is made, this defense is destroyed. Despite surgical asepsis and sterile equipment, infection remains an ever-present danger for the person undergoing surgery.

Disrupted Vascular System. Surgical incisions interrupt blood vessels. Major vessels that are severed during surgery are clamped off and sutured or cauterized so that blood loss is controlled. Excessive blood loss can lead to hemorrhage and shock intraoperatively or postoperatively.

Disturbed Organ Function. During surgery, organs are often manipulated, which may result in a temporary disruption of function. Also some operative procedures involve the removal of tissues or organs. As a result of these more radical surgeries, the physiologic functioning of the entire body may be seriously affected.

Impaired Gas Exchange. Anesthetics and analgesics used during surgery cause central nervous system depression, which decreases respirations and interferes with oxygen-carbon dioxide exchange. Mechanical ventilation and artificial airways used during operative procedures also interfere with gas exchange. Postoperative immobility and pain produce shallow respirations, which further impair gas exchange. (Chapter 45 explains impaired gas exchange.)

Water and Electrolyte Imbalances. The loss of body fluids during surgery disturbs water and electrolyte balance. Tubes and drains inserted into the body to aid in healing also increase water and electrolyte losses in the postoperative period. Furthermore, the body's neurohormonal responses to stressors affect water and electrolyte balance. For example, secretion of antidiuretic hormone alters water balance, causing the person to retain fluids. (Chapter 41 discusses fluid balance.)

Altered Nutrition. Changes in nutritional intake occur during the perioperative period. Typically, the surgery-bound individual ingests nothing by mouth (NPO) for 8 to 12 hours before surgery. After surgery, the healing process almost doubles the basic nutritional needs of the body. Unfortunately, oral intake is usually decreased during the postoperative period, sometimes for long periods. A positive nitrogen balance is needed to enhance the healing process. Although enteric and parental nutrition can provide some nutrients, no intravenous or tube-feeding solution can totally meet increased needs (see Chapter 42). Therefore, assessment for nutritional imbalances becomes imperative after surgery.

Disturbed Elimination Patterns. Elimination patterns change secondary to decreased food and fluid intake and loss of fluids during surgery. Anesthetics and analgesics used during and after surgery depress neuromuscular functioning and slow the elimination of wastes from the body. Manipulation of abdominal organs during surgery and decreased mobility after surgery further disrupt elimination patterns (see Chapters 43 and 44).

Alterations in Body Temperature. Fluctuations in body temperature frequently occur during the perioperative period. Many anesthetic agents cause vasodilation, resulting in loss of body heat. Exposure of the skin and viscera during the intraoperative phase contributes to decreases in body temperature. Compensatory mechanisms, such as shivering, increase metabolism and rewarm the body. Later in the postoperative phase, infection may alter thermoregulation by causing elevations in temperature.

Alterations in Sensation and Mobility. Analgesics and sedatives disturb and diminish sensory input, resulting in decreased awareness. Anesthesia, pain medications, and pain reduce or eliminate the person's ability to move. Tubes and drains also limit activity. Surgical complications may necessitate bedrest or activity restrictions.

Although the need for safety and security increases with the trauma of surgery, the individual's ability to move, to protect himself or herself, and to take care of personal needs decreases with surgery. As a result of increased dependence and distortions in sensory perception, the person feels insecure and requires emotional support.

Disturbed Sleep Patterns and Comfort. Sleep disturbances are, unfortunately, very common. Alterations in normal routines and the necessity of around-the-clock monitoring disrupt an individual's ability to relax and sleep. Anesthetics, sedatives, and analgesics disrupt the quality of sleep. In addition, anxiety, stress, and discomfort interfere with comfort and sleep.

Pain results from surgical wounds, from awkward positioning during and after surgery, and from other procedures such as venipuncture and some diagnostic tests. Because pain has a strong psychologic component, anxiety and fear intensify the individual's perception of pain (see Chapter 40).

PSYCHOSOCIAL ALTERATIONS

Disturbances of Body Image, Identity, and Self-esteem. Hospitalization and surgical trauma often disrupt psychologic well-being. The invasive nature of surgery threatens body image. Surgery that results in physical changes in appearance, particularly loss of body parts or function (e.g., incisional scars or removed organs), may leave the person feeling scarred or mutilated. Such feelings can impede the individual's recovery. Moreover, loss of control, increased dependence on others, and interference with normal routines and roles can lead to a loss of identity and self-esteem.

Alterations in Lifestyle and Finances. Surgery forces some people to make radical lifestyle changes. In some cases, changes are permanent. For instance, the amputee has to learn to use an artificial limb, which requires time, effort, and money. Even with extensive rehabilitation, the person may have to curtail recreational activities or change jobs. Surgical expenses and loss of work time often upset an individual's financial status. Throughout the perioperative period, assist the person and support persons to adapt to altered lifestyles through preoperative assessment, teaching, and emotional support. When indicated, arrange appropriate referrals to other professionals and agencies.

Developmental Considerations in Perioperative Nursing

A person's age and developmental stage influence the response to surgery. A child's reactions, for example, differ from those of an adolescent. Knowledge of age and development, therefore, is important in planning for individualized care.

CHILDREN AND ADOLESCENTS

During the surgical process, children are bombarded with a host of anxiety-provoking events in unfamiliar settings. Separation from their parents or support systems, as well as the administration of parenteral medications and anesthesia, increases their fears.

Children have a limited understanding of surgery. For neonates, surgery interferes with the bonding that occurs between parents and newborns. From infancy to 4 years of age, separation from parents is the child's major concern. Thus infants and toddlers react anxiously to being separated from their parents and familiar objects.

Preschool children may accept parental separation, but fears of pain and mutilation are typical. Similar fears are shared by school-age children, who may develop new interpretations of surgery and hospitalization that may be more frightening than reality. For example, a school-age child may perceive anesthesia administration by mask as a form of suffocation. Words should be chosen carefully; for example, children remember sick animals who have been "put to sleep."

For adolescents, the surgery means a hospital stay that separates them from their peers. This age group is acutely aware of body image and physical attractiveness. Thus, teenagers are often anxious about possible disfigurement from surgery.

ADULTS

Adults also have developmental needs. Hospitalization may be a new experience, or surgery may be the result of a first major illness. Fear of the unknown and separation from support systems are common concerns for this age group. Dependence and loss of control with impending surgery and hospitalization are other developmental concerns for adults. Middle-aged adults may have concurrent medical problems. They may worry that a more extensive problem, such as cancer, will be discovered during surgery. They may fear a disruption in career goals, family living patterns, and financial status. Older adults may fear dying from surgery.[30]

NURSING APPROACHES BASED ON DEVELOPMENTAL LEVEL

The developmental needs and responses of the individual determine the nursing intervention. For both children and adolescents, you can help alleviate anxiety and reduce the trauma associated with surgery. Nursing intervention in these age groups begins with assessment of (1) the level of understanding of surgery, (2) the level of anxiety, and (3) attitudes toward surgery. Provide information to help children or support persons cope successfully with the surgical experience. Tours of the OR have been highly successful with both children and their parents. Role-playing with puppets and dress-up in surgical attire can decrease the anxiety of children and parents. Also teach parents about their children's surgery, and encourage them to stay with their infants or children as much as possible throughout the perioperative period. Reassure children that they will see their parents again. Allow children to make choices so they feel a sense of control. Minimize anxiety and potential trauma by providing a quiet, pleasant environment, using frequent physical touch, and explaining procedures. As you work with children, avoid detailed descriptions of risk and possible complications.[6,24]

Adolescents facing surgery need to talk about their anxieties and fears. When supplied with clear information, adolescents can cope better with potential changes in body image. Adolescents need the acceptance and support of others, particularly their peers. Thus, encourage friends and family to visit during the perioperative period.

Encourage adults to discuss their fears and anxieties. Assess the quality of support systems, and involve support persons in the plan of care. Offer to make arrangements for referral to spiritual support persons. Be sensitive to sensory limitations in the older adult. Provide clear information, and assist adults with potential or actual changes associated with surgery.

LEGAL IMPLICATIONS OF SURGERY

Informed consent is a basic legal consideration for individuals undergoing surgery. The person's right to self-determination is protected by informed consent, that is, the right to decide whether surgery is in one's best interest.

Every person having surgery, no matter how minor the procedure, must give *written* consent. Consent must be obtained *before* administration of preoperative medications or anesthesia. Informed consent for surgery is the responsibility of the surgeon.

The surgeon is responsible for obtaining informed consent after a complete and comprehensible explanation of the proposed procedure, risks, and potential complications to the person or legal guardian. This legal document records that the transaction of information concerning the surgery occurred and that the person consented to the procedure as an informed party.[32-34]

Often nurses are asked to witness the signing of the consent. When you act as a witness, make certain that the person is informed before you sign the document. Also ensure that the signed document is affixed to the person's record and that it accompanies him or her to the operating room.

Nurses also act as advocates to ensure that surgical candidates fully understand the implications of surgery and are aware of their legal rights. Persons who do not understand the implications of surgery must have their questions and concerns answered before giving consent and undergoing surgery. An individual has the right to refuse surgery even after giving informed consent. For additional information on informed consent, see Chapter 4.

PREOPERATIVE PHASE

You will recall that the preoperative phase begins when surgery is planned and ends when the individual is transferred to the OR table.

Admission to the Health Care Facility

The period before surgery is a difficult one. The transition from home, work, or school to the unfamiliar setting of the care facility is discomforting. Worry and fear are common. During admission, create an atmosphere of trust and open communication with the individual and support persons. As you greet and orient the individual to the physical environment and routines of the facility, allay anxiety and build confidence. Try to address the person's initial concerns as you begin preoperative nursing assessment and care.

Assessment

The nursing activities of the preoperative phase begin with assessment. This fundamental step of the nursing process is initiated by the nurse after the individual consents to have surgical intervention. The initial collection of data may occur in a variety of settings, such as the surgical suite, care unit, home, or clinic. Data collection may be accomplished through diverse means, such as interview, review of records, physical assessment, or consultation among members of the health care team. It is a progressive and orderly process that requires the OR nurse to possess skills necessary to gather meaningful and pertinent data relative to the surgical intervention. Priority of data collection is determined by the immediate health care problems or needs of the client.[4] Examples of assessment criteria are given in Table 49-3.

Text continued on page 1419

TABLE 49-3. Competency Statements in Perioperative Nursing

Competency Statements	Measurable Criteria	Examples
Assessment		
I. Competency to assess the physiologic health status of the patient	1. Verifies operative procedure	1.1 Consent form 1.2 Patient's statement 1.3 Surgeon's verification
	2. Notes condition of skin	2.1 Rashes 2.2 Bruises 2.3 Lesions 2.4 Previous incisions
	3. Determines mobility of body parts	3.1 Patient's statement 3.2 Range of motion 3.3 History and physical
	4. Reports deviation of diagnostic studies	4.1 Laboratory values 4.2 X-ray results
	5. Checks vital signs	5.1 Blood pressure 5.2 Temperature 5.3 Pulse 5.4 Respiration
	6. Notes abnormalities, injuries, and previous surgery	6.1 Loss of extremity or body part 6.2 Congenital anomalies

Table continued on following page

TABLE 49-3. Competency Statements in Perioperative Nursing Continued

Competency Statements	Measurable Criteria	Examples
	7. Identifies presence of internal and external prostheses/implants	7.1 Pacemakers 7.2 Harrington rods 7.3 Joint prostheses
	8. Notes sensory impairments	8.1 Hearing deficit 8.2 Visual deficit 8.3 Tactile deficit
	9. Assesses cardiovascular status	9.1 Pulse alteration 9.2 Arrhythmias 9.3 Edema 9.4 Electrocardiogram 9.5 Arterial lines
	10. Assesses respiratory status	10.1 Skin color 10.2 Breath sounds 10.3 Arterial blood gases 10.4 Chest tubes
	11. Assesses renal status	11.1 Intake and output 11.2 Urinalysis 11.3 Renal function studies
	12. Notes nutritional status	12.1 Nothing by mouth 12.2 Weight 12.3 Hyperalimentation line
	13. Verifies allergies	13.1 Medication 13.2 Food 13.3 Chemical
	14. Screens for substance abuse	14.1 Skin changes 14.2 Patient's statement 14.3 History and physical
	15. Communicates physiological data relevant to planning patient's discharge	15.1 Home health service 15.2 Community service
	16. Communicates/documents physical health status	16.1 Verbal reports 16.2 Written records
II. Competency to assess the psychosocial health status of the patient/family	1. Elicits perception of surgery	1.1 Patient's statement 1.2 Overreaction
	2. Elicits expectation of care	2.1 Perceived outcomes 2.2 No identified outcomes
	3. Determines coping mechanisms	3.1 Seeking information 3.2 Denial
	4. Determines knowledge level	4.1 Lack of relevant information 4.2 Well-informed
	5. Determines ability to understand	5.1 Language barrier 5.2 Lack of comprehension
	6. Identifies philosophic and religious beliefs	6.1 Blood transfusions 6.2 Sacrament of the sick 6.3 Symbols
	7. Identifies cultural practices	7.1 Disposition of limbs 7.2 Family member in constant attendance
	8. Communicates psychosocial data relevant to planning	8.1 Support group 8.2 Counseling service 8.3 Social work service

TABLE 49-3. Competency Statements in Perioperative Nursing Continued

Competency Statements	Measurable Criteria	Examples
	9. Communicates/documents psychosocial status	9.1 Verbal reports 9.2 Written records
III. Competenency to formulate nursing diagnosis based on health status data	1. Interprets assessment data	1.1 Selects pertinent data 1.2 Sets priorities for data
	2. Identifies patient problem/nursing diagnosis pertinent to surgical procedure	2.1 Actual patient problems 2.2 Potential patient problems
	3. Supports nursing diagnosis with current scientific knowledge	3.1 Theoretical base 3.2 Rationale for diagnosis
	4. Communicates/documents nursing diagnosis to health care team	4.1 Verbal reports 4.2 Written records
Planning		
IV. Competency to establish patient goals based on nursing diagnosis	1. Develops outcome statements	1.1 Patient is free from infection 72 hours postoperatively 1.2 Maintenance of skin integrity after discharge from OR
	2. Develops goals that are congruent with present and potential physical capabilities and behavioral patterns	2.1 Realistic 2.2 Attainable
	3. Develops criteria for measurement of goals	3.1 Signs and symptoms 3.2 Laboratory data
	4. Sets priorities for goals based on needs	4.1 Mutually set 4.2 Maslow's hierarchy of needs
	5. Communicates/documents goals to appropriate persons	5.1 Verbal reports 5.2 Written records
V. Competency to develop a plan of care that prescribes nursing actions to achieve patient goals	1. Identifies nursing activities necessary for expected outcomes	1.1 Specific positioning aids 1.2 Patient teaching
	2. Establishes priorities for nursing actions	2.1 Immediate 2.2 Long term
	3. Organizes nursing activities in logical sequence	3.1 Dispersive pad placement before draping 3.2 Functional suction before induction
	4. Coordinates use of supplies and equipment for intraoperative care	4.1 Instrument availability 4.2 Scheduling conflicts
	5. Coordinates patient care needs with team members and other appropriate departments	5.1 Patient transfer 5.2 Equipment needs
	6. Controls environment	6.1 Temperature 6.2 Sensory stimuli 6.3 Traffic 6.4 Noise level
	7. Assigns activities to personnel based on their qualifications and patient needs	7.1 Categories of personnel 7.2 Demonstrated competencies
	8. Prepares for potential emergencies	8.1 Cardiopulmonary resuscitation certified 8.2 Disaster plan
	9. Participates in planning for discharge	9.1 Patient/family education 9.2 Referral services

Table continued on following page

TABLE 49–3. Competency Statements in Perioperative Nursing Continued

Competency Statements	Measurable Criteria	Examples
	10. Communicates/documents patient's plan of care	10.1 Verbal reports 10.2 Written records
Implementation		
VI. Competency to implement nursing actions in transferring the patient according to the prescribed plan	1. Confirms identity	1.1 Patient's statement 1.2 Identification bracelet
	2. Selects personnel for transportation as determined by need	2.1 Sufficient number 2.2 Patient acuity
	3. Determines appropriate and safe method according to need	3.1 Stretcher/bed 3.2 Support measures
	4. Provides for the emotional needs during transfer	4.1 Comfort measures 4.2 Touch
	5. Communicates/documents patient's transfer	5.1 Verbal reports 5.2 Written records
VII. Competency to participate in patient/family teaching	1. Identifies teaching needs	1.1 Surgical routines 1.2 Coughing/deep breathing techniques 1.3 Discharge instructions
	2. Assesses readiness to learn	2.1 Attention span 2.2 Anxiety level
	3. Provides instruction based on identified needs	3.1 Post anesthesia recovery routine 3.2 "Splinting" techniques 3.3 Coughing and deep-breathing
	4. Determines teaching effectiveness	4.1 Return demonstration 4.2 Patient verbalization
	5. Communicates/documents patient/family teaching	5.1 Verbal reports 5.2 Written records
VIII. Competency to create and maintain a sterile field	1. Uses principles of aseptic practice in varying situations	1.1 Skin scrub for colostomy 1.2 Clean vs sterile field
	2. Initiates corrective action when breaks in technique occur	2.1 Changing gown and gloves 2.2 Surgical conscience
	3. Inspects sterile items for contamination before opening	3.1 Intact package 3.2 Sterile indicator
	4. Maintains sterility while opening sterile items for procedure	4.1 Delivery to field 4.2 Pouring solutions
	5. Functions within designated dress code	5.1 Hair covered 5.2 Scrub attire
	6. Communicates/documents maintenance of sterile field	6.1 Verbal reports 6.2 Written records
IX. Competency to provide equipment and supplies based on patient needs	1. Anticipates the need for equipment and supplies	1.1 Electrosurgical equipment 1.2 Prosthetic devices
	2. Selects equipment and supplies in an organized and timely manner	2.1 Preoperative 2.2 Intraoperative
	3. Assures all equipment is functioning before use	3.1 Mechanical equipment checked 3.2 Pressure-powered equipment checked
	4. Operates mechanical, electrical, and air-powered equipment according to manufacturer's instructions	4.1 Tourniquet 4.2 Electrosurgical unit

TABLE 49–3. Competency Statements in Perioperative Nursing Continued

Competency Statements	Measurable Criteria	Examples
	5. Removes malfunctioning equipment from OR	5.1 Light sources 5.2 OR bed
	6. Assures emergency equipment and supplies are available at all times	6.1 Defibrillator/monitor 6.2 Emergency drug and supply cart
	7. Uses supplies judiciously and in a cost-effective manner	7.1 Lost charge 7.2 Excess suture use
	8. Communicates/documents provision of equipment and supplies	8.1 Verbal reports 8.2 Written records
X. Competency to perform sponge, sharps, and instrument counts	1. Follows established policiies and procedures for counts	1.1 Sponges/sharps/instruments 1.2 Hospital's policies and procedures
	2. Initiates corrective actions when counts are incorrect	2.1 Surgeon notification 2.2 Risk management
	3. Communicates/documents results of counts according to facility policy	3.1 Verbal reports 3.2 Written records
XI. Competency to administer drugs and solutions as prescribed	1. Administers medication according to hospital policy	1.1 Administration route 1.2 Dosage 1.3 Patient identification 1.4 Drug reaction 1.5 Complications/contraindications
	2. Communicates/documents administration of drugs and solutions	2.1 Verbal reports 2.2 Written records
XII. Competency to physiologically monitor the patient during surgery	1. Assists/monitors physical symptoms	1.1 Skin color 1.2 Electrocardiogram
	2. Assists/monitors behavioral changes	2.1 Restlessness 2.2 Level of consciousness
	3. Calculates intake and output	3.1 Fluid intake 3.2 Blood loss
	4. Operates monitor equipment according to manufacturer's instruction	4.1 Automatic blood pressure monitor 4.2 Temperature probe
	5. Initiates nursing actions based on interpretation of physiologic changes	5.1 Surgeon notification 5.2 Crash cart
	6. Communicates/documents physiologic responses	6.1 Verbal reports 6.2 Written records
XIII. Competency to monitor and control the environment	1. Regulates temperature and humidity as indicated	1.1 Patient need 1.2 Staff need
	2. Adheres to electrical safety policies and procedures	2.1 Hazard identification 2.2 Line isolation monitor
	3. Monitors sensory environment	3.1 Noise levels 3.2 Noxious odors
	4. Maintains traffic patterns	4.1 Hospital's policies and procedures 4.2 Unobstructed corridors
	5. Adheres to OR sanitation policies and procedures	5.1 "Confine and contain" 5.2 Waste disposal
	6. Communicates/documents environmental controls	6.1 Verbal reports 6.2 Written records

Table continued on following page

TABLE 49–3. Competency Statements in Perioperative Nursing Continued

Competency Statements	Measurable Criteria	Examples
XIV. Competency to respect patient's rights	1. Demonstrates awareness of the individual rights of the patient	1.1 American Hospital Bill of Rights 1.2 American Nurses' Association Code for Nurses
	2. Provides for privacy through maintaining confidentiality	2.1 Communication 2.2 Documentation
	3. Provides for privacy through physical protection	3.1 Examination 3.2 Positioning
	4. Identifies ethnic and spirtual beliefs	4.1 Pastoral counseling 4.2 Communion
	5. Communicates/documents provisions for patient's rights	5.1 Verbal reports 5.2 Written records
Evaluation		
XV. Competency to perform nursing actions that demonstrate accountability	1. Exercises safe judgment in decision-making	1.1 Thorough assessments 1.2 Past experience
	2. Demonstrates flexibility and adaptability to changes in nursing practice	2.1 Change agent 2.2 Professional associations
	3. Responds in a positive manner to constructive criticism	3.1 Self-evaluation 3.2 Peer review
	4. Demonstrates tact and understanding when dealing with patients, team members, members of other disciplines, and the public	4.1 Team negotiation 4.2 Family interaction 4.3 Consumer awareness
	5. Practices within ethical and legal guidelines	5.1 Nurse Practice Act 5.2 Legal statutes 5.3 American Nurses' Association Code for Nurses
	6. Seeks opportunity for continued learning	6.1 Continuing education 6.2 Inservice education
	7. Communicates/documents nursing actions	7.1 Verbal reports 7.2 Written records
XVI. Competency to evaluate patient outcomes	1. Develops outcome critiera for goal measurement	1.1 Signs and symptoms 1.2 Laboratory data
	2. Measures degree of goal achievement	2.1 Nurse's observation 2.2 Patient's responses
	3. Communicates/documents degree of goal achievement	3.1 Verbal reports 3.2 Written records
XVII. Competency to measure effectiveness of nursing care	1. Establishes criteria to measure quality of nursing care	1.1 Nursing audit 1.2 Peer review
	2. Assesses the patient postoperatively	2.1 Patient interview 2.2 Questionnaire 2.3 Physical examination
	3. Compares results of nursing actions to desired patient goals	3.1 Appropriateness of nursing actions 3.2 Realistic goals
	4. Communicates/documents results of nursing care	4.1 Verbal reports 4.2 Written records

TABLE 49-3. *Competency Statements in Perioperative Nursing* Continued

Competency Statements	Measurable Criteria	Examples
XVIII. Competency to continuously reassess all the components of patient care based on new data	1. Reassesses health status	1.1 Physiological 1.2 Psychosocial
	2. Refines nursing diagnosis	2.1 Changes in health status
	3. Reestablishes goals	3.1 Changes in signs and symptoms 3.2 Changes in laboratory data
	4. Revises plan of care	4.1 Revised priorities
	5. Implements revised plan of care	5.1 Revise nursing actions
	6. Reevaluates outcomes	6.1 Patient responses 6.2 Outcome criteria
	7. Comunicates/documents reassessment process	7.1 Verbal reports 7.2 Written records

From Association of Operating Room Nurses. (1991). *AORN standards and recommended practices for perioperative nursing.* Denver, CO: Association of Operating Room Nurses.

During the preoperative phase, collect subjective and objective data from the individual and support persons. Establish a baseline of information that will assist you to formulate nursing diagnoses, develop a plan of perioperative care, and evaluate the person's responses to nursing intervention during the postoperative period.

Preoperative nursing assessment consists of (1) the nursing interview, (2) the physical assessment, and (3) the assessment of surgical risk. Collect data from many sources—the person, support persons, health team members, and health records such as medical data and diagnostic reports.

THE NURSING INTERVIEW

During your initial interview, obtain a health history and assess the individual's perceptions, expectations, and knowledge of surgery. Ask clear questions. Establish an atmosphere of trust and support, and allow the person to express concerns. Remain alert to nonverbal communication that may provide useful data for assessing psychologic status (e.g., facial expressions, body gestures, and muscle tension).

The health history includes questions about previous medical illness and surgery, current use of medications, substance abuse, and known allergies to food or medications. Also assess

▶ occupation: effect of surgery on the individual's job performance
▶ financial concerns: health insurance, potential loss of job
▶ support systems: family, friends, clergy
▶ spiritual needs: religion, concerns about death
▶ personal habits: patterns of elimination, sleep, personal hygiene, and eating
▶ cultural beliefs: attitudes and values associated with illness or surgery
▶ mental status: level of consciousness, comprehension of events related to surgery
▶ level of anxiety: feelings concerning surgery, coping mechanisms

PHYSICAL ASSESSMENT

In addition to the nursing interview, assess the person's physiologic functioning. Include a systematic physical examination and observations of the person's appearance. Be sure to take an accurate measurement of height and preoperative weight. Also record baseline vital signs. Refer to Unit 8 for a review of the physical and psychosocial assessment.

ASSESSMENT OF SURGICAL RISK

Identifying risk factors helps determine the plan of care. People with risk factors have a statistically greater chance of the development of intraoperative and postoperative complications (e.g., cardiac disturbances). These individuals also tend to recover more slowly from anesthesia.

Age. Surgical risks are greatest among the very young and elderly. Neonates have less capacity to endure surgical trauma. Elderly persons often have multisystem impairments such as reduced cardiac reserve, decreased respiratory capacity, or chronic illness.

General Health. Surgical risks increase when the person has an infection or chronic illness. Cardiovascular disease, diabetes mellitus, blood disorders, and renal or pulmonary dysfunction are examples of illnesses that increase surgical risks.

Medications. Some people take prescribed or nonprescribed medications that can increase surgical risks. Anticoagulants, for instance, impair blood clotting during surgery. Table 49-4 lists the effects of certain medications that increase surgical risk.

Mobility. Limitations in mobility are significant concerns for the OR nurse in planning positioning for the individual on the OR table. Also people with poor muscle tone, limited range of motion, or impaired mobility are at risk because it is more difficult for them to move

TABLE 49-4. Medications Associated with Increased Surgical Risk

Medication	Discussion
Anticoagulants	May cause increased blood loss as a result of lack of hemostasis during and after surgery
Antibiotics	May increase neuromuscular effects of some anesthetics; may predispose to renal insufficiency
Anticonvulsants	May increase metabolism of anesthetic agents
Antihypertensives	May cause hypotension after anesthesia
Corticosteroids	Impair body's neurohormonal response to stress
Insulin	Predisposes person to hypoglycemia during periods of reduced oral intake
Monoamine oxidase inhibitors	May precipitate hypertensive crisis when given with sympathomimetic agents
Phenothiazines	Enhance hypotensive effects of other medications
Thiazide diuretics	May result in potassium deficiencies, which interfere with cardiac functioning

and ambulate during the postoperative period. Decreased movement increases vulnerability to postoperative complications.

Nutritional Status. Major preoperative nutritional problems that increase risk include (1) deficiencies in protein, vitamin, and mineral intake, (2) malnutrition, and (3) obesity. Suspect nutritional deficiencies or malnutrition among the elderly, individuals who are chronically ill, persons who are attempting to lose weight with crash diets, and others who rely on fast-food sources for daily nutrition. Anorexia and bulimia may be suspected in undernourished adolescents and young adults.

Obese people are at risk because they are more subject to complications. An overweight body places an additional workload on the cardiovascular system and decreases the pulmonary system's efficiency. Difficulty in performing postoperative deep-breathing and in correct coughing may lead to hypoventilation and pulmonary complications. Hypertension and increased cardiac workload are also major concerns. The technical difficulty of surgery is compounded by excess adipose tissue; for example, incisions are larger than normal, there is increased bleeding in adipose tissue, and wound healing may be complicated by poor circulation and infection.

Water and Electrolyte Balance. Maintenance of homeostasis during surgery is aided by normal blood volume and electrolyte balance. Cardiac function, muscle tone, and oxygen utilization are affected by imbalances of potassium, calcium, magnesium, and acid-base (pH). Water and electrolyte imbalances often occur after surgery, and preexisting problems exacerbate this postoperative complication. Individuals who may suffer from water and electrolyte abnormalities include people taking diuretics that cause hypokalemia (low serum potassium), people who have been vomiting or sweating profusely before surgery, and unconscious people who cannot drink voluntarily.

Psychosocial Condition. Psychosocial well-being influences the outcome of surgery. Surgical risks increase

when people approach an operation with fear and anxiety.[30] Moreover, extraneous concerns—financial worries, lifestyle changes, inadequate support systems—reduce an individual's ability to cope with surgery. Assist people to acknowledge and express their concerns. Identify effective ways to help them cope. For example, provide pertinent information or arrange referrals to other professionals such as social workers and spiritual support persons. Always take the person's concerns seriously, even though their fears may seem exaggerated or inappropriate to you. Establishing a therapeutic relationship is an important part of nursing care.

Risk Factors Related to the Disorder. Surgical risk also depends on the following factors:

▶ Nature of the disease: Risk increases when a major organ or limb must be removed.
▶ Location of the disease: Surgical risk decreases in descending order in the following sites: heart, thorax, esophagus, brain, rectum, colon, and stomach.
▶ Duration of the disorder: The longer the person has had the disorder, the greater the risk. Chronicity increases risk because chronic conditions are usually debilitating.
▶ Extent of the required surgical procedure: Operative risk increases proportionately to the magnitude of the operation.[28]

Nursing Diagnosis

Common nursing diagnoses for the surgical candidate in the preoperative phase include

▶ *Fear* R/T impending surgery with possible pain, loss of control, disfigurement, knowledge deficit, and unfamiliarity with the surgical process (see Nursing Diagnosis Profile).[29]
▶ *Knowledge Deficit* R/T lack of exposure to the surgical experience.[26]

NURSING DIAGNOSIS PROFILE

Fear

Definition. Feeling of dread related to an identifiable source that the person validates

Classification. Feeling 9.3.2.

Defining Characteristics. Defining characteristics of fear are categorized as subjective or objective behaviors or signs and symptoms. Subjective characteristics include expressions of increased tension, apprehension, impulsiveness, decreased self-assurance, and feelings of being afraid, scared, terrified, panicked, frightened, or jittery. Objective characteristics are direct observations of increased alertness, concentration on source of fear, being wide eyed, the use of attack behavior, a focus on "it's out there," fight behavior (aggression), flight behavior (withdrawal), and sympathetic stimulation such as cardiovascular excitation, superficial vasoconstriction, and pupil dilation.[26] The person must be able to identify the object of fear.

Sample Related Factors. *Fear* may be related to a number of identifiable factors such as changes in sensory perception, knowledge deficit, loss of support system, pain (not fear of pain but fear of a situation that causes pain), and threat of death (whether actual or perceived).

Concept Description. *Fear* encompasses expressed subjective feelings as well as observable "fight or flight" responses. *Fear* is a universal emotion that may be called anxiety, terror, dread, or some similar term, but it is a specific emotion that involves the urge to flee when the "fight or flight" response occurs (rather than the urge to fight as with the emotion of anger).

Examples. Depending on the specific assessment data, this diagnostic category could be applicable in the following situations, among others:

▶ A person who is scheduled for an emergency cholecystectomy clearly verbalizes feelings of panic and fear of having surgery. This person asks numerous questions about what will occur, how much pain there will be, what will relieve it, what the scar will look like, and so forth. Physical assessment of the individual reveals a rapid pulse, dilated pupils, and cool skin. The individual is extremely alert, and the eyes are open wide.

▶ A person arrives in the preoperative holding area with a wife who is talking loudly and is clinging to the stretcher as the surgical client clings to her.

Related/Similar Nursing Diagnoses. *Fear* must be distinguished from *Anxiety* and *Powerlessness. Anxiety* is defined as a vague, uneasy feeling, the source of which is often nonspecific or unknown to the individual. In contrast, *Fear* implies that the source of the feeling is known and is validated by the individual. *Anxiety* and *Fear* share several subjective and objective defining characteristics; the significant point of differentiation is the individual's ability to identify the source of the threat when experiencing fear.[43]

Powerlessness describes a perception of lack of control, an inability to influence the outcome of a situation. *Powerlessness* is a subjective experience, whereas *Fear* has an observable physiologic characteristic of the sympathetic "fight or flight" response.

Both these diagnoses could be made for either inpatients or outpatients.

Planning

Outcomes for care are derived from each nursing diagnosis and are mutually formulated with the individual, significant others, and health care personnel.[4] For example, in the preoperative phase, outcomes for the nursing diagnosis *Fear* may be stated as follows:

▶ verbalizes specific fears relating to surgery[29]
▶ verbalizes realistic perception of danger[29]
▶ states own coping ability[29]
▶ states need for assistance

Outcomes for the nursing diagnosis of *Knowledge Deficit* may be stated as follows:

▶ states the physiologic responses to surgical intervention
▶ demonstrates actions to prevent untoward physiologic responses

Can you think of other outcomes for these two nursing diagnoses?

Nursing Intervention

Nursing actions to achieve the outcomes for the preoperative diagnoses of *Fear* and *Knowledge Deficit* are principally teaching activities.

PREOPERATIVE TEACHING

Preoperative teaching improves the individual's coping skills by enhancing a sense of personal control. Effective preoperative teaching helps reduce postoperative anxiety and discomfort. Preoperative teaching is also a cost-effective nursing intervention that speeds surgical recovery and shortens hospitalization.[28] The well-informed individual knows what to expect throughout the perioperative period and thus participates more fully in interventions designed to speed postoperative recovery.

Before instituting a teaching plan, assess the person and support persons. In this way, you can individualize your teaching to make it more effective. Consider the person's (1) knowledge of surgery, (2) level of anxiety and adequacy of coping skills, (3) ability to participate in the teaching plan, and (4) the involvement of support persons. Assess the person's readiness to learn. Before beginning instruction, provide psychologic support and establish an atmosphere of trust and acceptance. As you teach, continue to assess the person and adjust your teaching methods accordingly.

Begin teaching as soon as the person is admitted to the health care facility. Sometimes (e.g., with outpatient surgery) the teaching process begins in a physician's office, in a clinic, or at home. Remember to continue your instruction throughout the perioperative period. Continued teaching reinforces learning and adds information as appropriate.

Information included in a teaching program differs according to the surgical procedure, the risk factors, and the person's ability and motivation to learn. Some common basic components are outlined in Box 49–3. As you can see, preoperative instruction generally includes teaching the person exercises and the use of special aids that prevent postoperative complications and speed recovery. Figure 49–1 depicts (1) deep breathing exercises, (2) correct splinting while coughing, and (3) range-of-motion exercises of the hip, knee, and ankle. Teach the person these maneuvers, and teach them how to move and ambulate after surgery.

Deep-breathing Exercises. General anesthesia, central nervous system depressants, and immobility increase the risks of postoperative respiratory complications (e.g., atelectasis and pneumonia). These complications can be prevented by deep-breathing exercises. Periodic deep breathing aerates the lungs, inflating alveoli and maintaining normal respiratory function.

To teach people diaphragmatic-abdominal deep breathing, have them assume a supine, side-lying, or sitting position with knees flexed. Tell them to relax the abdominal muscles and slowly to inhale air through the nose. The abdomen should distend as the lungs are inflated. Have clients hold their breath for at least 3 seconds and then exhale slowly through the mouth, while placing the hands below the ribs. This will allow them to feel the distention and then contraction of the abdomen while contracting the abdominal muscles (Fig. 49–1*A*). This maneuver is performed as frequently as 5 to 10 times an hour for at least 48 hours postoperatively.

Coughing. Coughing mobilizes mucus in the lungs and helps prevent postoperative pulmonary complications. When the cough reflex is stimulated, the lungs are aerated and mucus is cleared from the bronchi. Teach effective coughing by demonstrating the technique. Inhale deeply three times, hold the breath briefly, then exhale through the mouth, and attempt to cough. The use of the chest muscles is important to ensure deep coughing that will raise mucus from the bronchial passages.

If the surgery involves a chest or abdominal incision, show the person how to "splint" the incision when coughing. Splinting reduces pain and discomfort by applying counterpressure during coughing. Have the individual splint the incision with hands interlaced and held tightly across the area or by holding a pillow firmly

---

Box 49–3. Guidelines for Preoperative Assessment and Learning Teaching

Introduce yourself.
Identify your purposes:
   to obtain information that will be helpful in planning care
   to answer questions and concerns about surgery
Determine the person's knowledge of the intended surgery
   and the need or desire for additional information.
Explain the routine for the day of surgery:
   absence of food or fluid
   premedication
   transportation to operating room
   location of and anticipated length of wait before surgery
   special skin preparations
Familiarize the person with the operating room environment:
   operating room lights and table
   accessory equipment
   intravenous fluids
   blood pressure cuff
   electrocardiogram monitoring
   anesthesia induction
Tell the significant others:
   time to arrive at the hospital
   location of waiting area during surgery
   anticipated time in operating room and recovery room
   what to expect when person returns to unit
Explain the postanesthesia care:
   location of recovery room
   purpose of recovery room

   routine of postanesthesia care (e.g., measuring vital signs, checking dressings)
   anticipated dressings, drains, catheters, casts
Discuss medications available for postoperative pain and teach relaxation techniques (e.g., guided imagery, progressive muscle relaxation).
Discuss relevant physical problems with the person (e.g., visual or hearing alterations, joint or muscle immobility).
Demonstrate and evaluate person's performance of:
   deep-breathing exercises and coughing
   turning and movement
   extremity exercises
   any special transfer procedures or aids (e.g., crutches) required after surgery
Other considerations:
   Establish an atmosphere of confidence, support, and acceptance.
   Allow person opportunity to ask questions and to discuss concerns.
   Involve significant others in teaching/learning and associated activities.
   Evaluate person's level of knowledge, and document all teaching/learning activities.

Adapted from Groah, L. K. (1983). *Operating room nursing: The perioperative role.* Reston, VA: Reston Publishing Co.

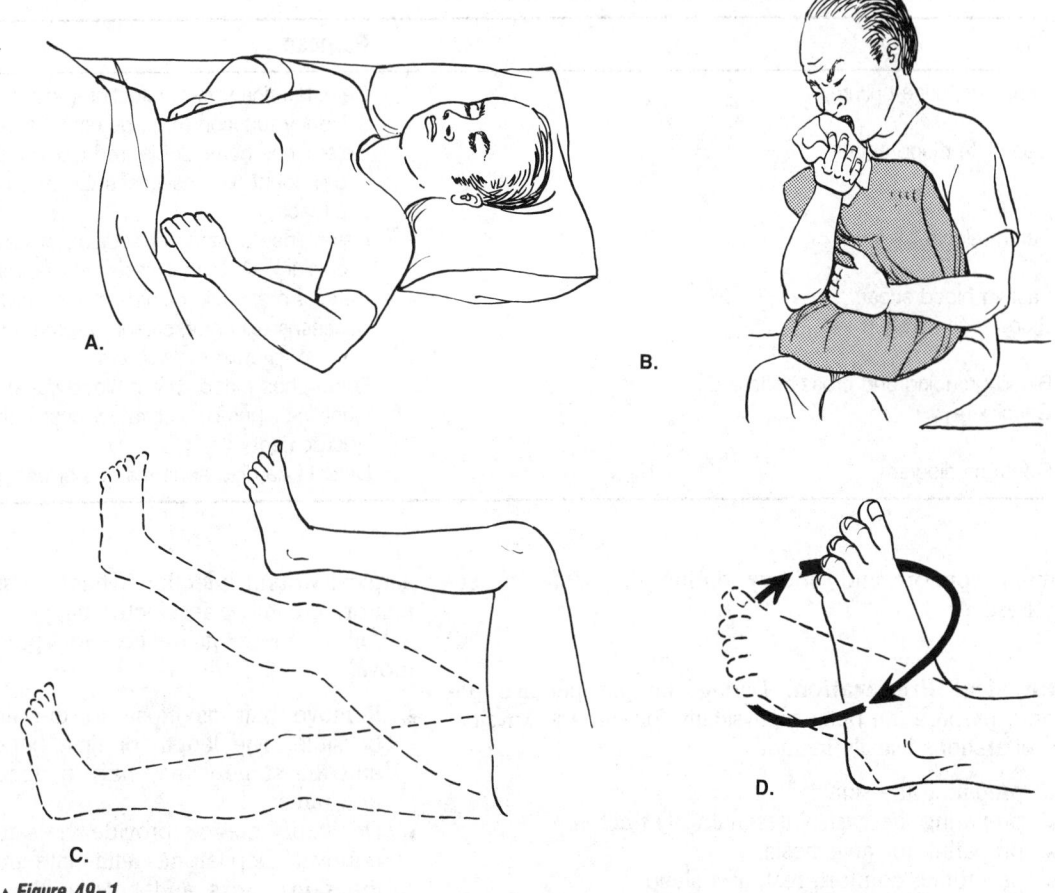

▲ **Figure 49-1**

Prevent postoperative complications by having the person perform deep breathing and extremity exercises frequently and by teaching the person how to support the incision when coughing. *A*, Deep breathing; *B*, splinting the abdomen with a pillow to reduce incisional discomfort during coughing; *C*, exercising the ankle, knee, and hip; *D*, making circles with the toes in order to flex, extend, evert, and invert the ankles.

against the incision (Fig. 49-1*B*). The abdomen should also be splinted after rectal or perineal surgery. This splinting helps prevent the forceful, downward pressure of the abdominal contents on the painful surgical area during coughing.

The person must *not* cough after certain procedures (e.g., ophthalmic, cranial, and spinal surgery, tonsillectomy).

Extremity Exercises. Frequently moving the extremities helps prevent postoperative circulatory complications (e.g., thrombophlebitis). Teach the person (1) to flex and extend the hip, knee, and ankle (Fig. 49-1*C*), (2) to move each foot in a circular motion at the ankle to provide flexion, extension, inversion, and eversion (Fig. 49-1*D*), and (3) to wiggle toes. Postoperatively, each set of extremity exercises must be performed at least five times an hour.

Movement and Ambulation. Postoperative immobility leads to venous stasis, pulmonary congestion, gastric distention, and loss of muscle tone as well as other complications. Turning and moving in bed and early ambulation help to prevent these complications. If possible, encourage and assist the person to turn from side to side at least every 2 hours during the postoperative period. If this is not possible, check with the physician to determine alternatives (e.g., side to back to side again). Reassure the individual that you will assist with turning and ambulation. Teach maneuvers such as "dangling" and special transfer techniques before surgery (see Chapters 35 and 36). Consult the nursing care plan and postoperative orders for special restrictions or guidelines for ambulation.

PHYSICAL PREPARATION OF THE PERSON FOR SURGERY

Preoperative Diagnostic Procedures. Preoperative preparation often includes diagnostic tests and procedures. Baseline information from various tests (e.g., urinalysis or chest x-ray) helps pinpoint problems before surgery. Tests appropriate to the person's age, condition, and surgical procedure are ordered. Table 49-5 outlines common preoperative diagnostic tests.

Diagnostic testing may add to the person's anxiety about the surgery. Discuss tests and procedures, and listen to the person's concerns about them to help alleviate anxiety. Assist the individual by ensuring opti-

TABLE 49-5. Common Preoperative Diagnostic Procedures

Test	Purpose
Urinalysis, urine culture	Detects urinary tract infections; estimates metabolic and kidney function (e.g., detects diabetes mellitus)
Complete blood count	Determines hemoglobin, red blood cell and white blood cell count (i.e., assesses the blood's oxygen transport capacity)
Serum electrolytes	Determines balance of sodium, potassium, magnesium, calcium, and other essential electrolytes
Fasting blood sugar	Detects metabolic disorders (e.g., diabetes mellitus)
Blood urea nitrogen	Assesses urinary excretion of urea, the breakdown product of protein metabolism
Blood grouping and cross-matching	Establishes blood type if blood transfusion is needed
Chest x-ray	Identifies signs of respiratory dysfunction and cardiac enlargement
Electrocardiogram	Detects cardiac abnormalities or arrhythmias

mum comfort and privacy during diagnostic procedures.

Physical Preparation. During the preoperative period, prepare the person physically for surgery. Physical preparations usually include

▶ preparing the skin
▶ preparing the gastrointestinal (GI) tract
▶ preparing for anesthesia
▶ promoting comfort, rest, and sleep

These activities are usually performed on the evening before surgery. Persons undergoing outpatient surgery complete some of the preparations at home.

Preoperative Skin Preparation. Wound infections lead to lengthy and costly hospitalization and increase the risks of illness or death. Preventing microbial contamination of the surgical wound reduces the risk of wound infection. One of the most important ways to prevent contamination is to reduce the number of bacteria on the skin.[5,12,19]

Surgical skin preparation (called a "prep") includes cleansing the skin and, usually, removing hair from areas surrounding the operative site. The skin prep is performed according to the health care facility policy. In some facilities, only specially trained personnel prep the skin. In others, the staff nurses perform the preps. Skin prep may include a shower or bath with an antimicrobial agent either the evening before or the morning of surgery. Additionally, the person may be required to wash and scrub the surgical area with an antimicrobial agent several times beginning 1 to 2 days before surgery. The mucous membranes often require no special preparation. However, preps for gynecologic surgery may include hair removal, douching, and the insertion of vaginal suppositories.

Hair removal from the surgical site is controversial. Shaving the hair the evening before surgery has long been the standard practice. However, research indicates razor shaving contributes to increased rates of surgical wound infection. Thus, we suggest using a depilatory cream or an electric clipper.[5,12,42]

Follow these guidelines for preoperative hair removal:

▶ Remove hair as close to the time of surgery as possible. The length of time between hair removal and the surgery may have a direct effect on infection rates.
▶ Depilatory creams provide the safest method of hair removal. Depilatories eliminate traumatic cutting of the skin. Nicks and cuts in the skin act as entry points for bacteria. Perform a skin sensitivity test before application of a depilatory cream according to the manufacturer's guidelines.
▶ The site of the incision and the nature of the surgical procedure determine the area to be prepared. Prepare a wide area around the incision.
▶ Maintain the person's privacy and comfort during skin prep. Provide adequate lighting for good visualization. Check the skin before and after for abnormal skin conditions (e.g., lesions, irritations, cuts), and document them in the permanent record.
▶ If using a razor, use the wet method of shaving, which eases removal, minimizes skin trauma, and prevents hair and skin debris from becoming airborne. Lather the skin well, hold it taut, and shave in the direction of hair growth to avoid cutting the skin. When finished, rinse the area well to remove loose hair and soap or cream residues. Properly dispose of or clean items used in the prep.[5,12,19,42]

Preparing the Gastrointestinal Tract. The GI tract is emptied or cleansed before surgery to (1) reduce the risk of vomiting and aspiration during anesthesia, (2) prevent contamination of the operative site from fecal material during bowel surgery, and (3) reduce postoperative nausea and vomiting, gastric distention, or bowel obstruction.

Restricting foods and fluids during the preoperative phase prevents vomiting. An empty stomach lessens the risk of aspirating vomitus into the lungs during anesthesia. Food and fluid are usually prohibited for 8 to 10 hours before surgery. Hospitalized persons are usually NPO after midnight. When surgery is scheduled for the afternoon, the person may eat a light breakfast but then remain NPO until surgery. Because infants and small children are prone to dehydration, intake of foods and fluids usually is restricted no more than 4 hours before surgery. Children or adults who are dehydrated or malnourished may need intravenous infusions to guarantee proper hydration while NPO.

Teach the person and support persons about the need to restrict oral intake. Remove food and fluid from the person's bedside to prevent inadvertent intake. Place an "NPO" sign on the person's door, and make a notation in the nursing care plan. Remind the person not to swallow water when brushing teeth or rinsing the mouth.

If a person accidentally eats or drinks before surgery, immediately inform the surgeon and anesthesiologist.

Bowel preparation is essential for surgical procedures involving the GI tract or abdomen. Cleansing the colon prevents contamination of the peritoneal cavity by spillage of fecal material during surgery. Depending on the person's condition and type of surgery, the physician may order preoperative administration of an enema or rectal suppository. Oral antibiotics may be ordered for 2 or 3 days before surgery to reduce the number of bacteria in the bowel. The insertion of gastric and intestinal tubes may be necessary to remove GI contents by suction.

Preparation for Anesthesia. Before surgery, the anesthetist or anesthesiologist visits the person to assess the person's physiologic condition related to the safety of anesthesia (e.g., smoking history, upper respiratory tract infection, cardiopulmonary dysfunction). The anesthetist or anesthesiologist explains the type of anesthesia, the method of administration, and the associated risks and describes the recovery period. Finally, the physician or nurse anesthetist may write orders for preoperative medications, if indicated.

Promotion of Rest and Sleep. The surgery-bound individual needs adequate rest before the operation. Promote rest by ensuring physical and emotional comfort. Give a back rub to aid relaxation. Encourage the person to discuss concerns or questions. Be supportive, interested, and helpful. Your manner can help the person feel safe and cared for and thus promote rest. If the person is still restless and cannot sleep, administer a sleeping medication if ordered. If there is no order, contact the physician.

PREPARING THE PERSON ON THE DAY OF SURGERY

If the person spent the previous night in the care facility, the nurse performs additional preoperative procedures on the day of surgery. These interventions include

- administering morning care
- making certain the consent form is signed

- administering preoperative medications
- ensuring that the preoperative check list and chart are in order
- providing support to the individual and support persons
- arranging transport to surgery
- preparing the person's room for postoperative care

Morning Care. Measure and record the individual's vital signs for use as a baseline to evaluate the person's condition after surgery.

Immediately report to the physician elevations in temperature or profound changes in heart rate and blood pressure.

In addition to taking vital signs, complete the physical preparations. Have the person

- Shower or bathe if required
- Complete dental care, including removing dentures or removable bridgework, if appropriate
- Put on a clean hospital gown (certain religious garments may also be worn)
- Remove all undergarments
- Empty the urinary bladder (void)
- Remove hairpins to prevent accidental scalp injury during surgery; hair also may be covered, if appropriate
- Remove all cosmetics and nail polish (the anesthetist or anesthesiologist observes the nail beds and skin to determine the adequacy of oxygenation of the person while under anesthesia) if directed by facility policy
- Remove all jewelry and store according to agency policy; some facilities allow special items to be worn (e.g., wedding rings and religious medals if properly taped and secured in place)
- Remove eyeglasses, contact lenses, hearing aids, and other prostheses; store these items according to agency policy (if prostheses are worn to the operating room, document their presence)

Check the person's identification band to be certain it is correct and secure. Accurate identification is essential for individuals undergoing sedation, anesthesia, and surgery. Many agencies also require arm bands indicating allergies and blood recipient information. Complete any special preoperative orders, such as administering antibiotics, eyedrops, or other medications.

Most care facilities require nurses to complete a preoperative check list (Fig. 49-2). Complete each activity, and check it off the list. This practice reduces errors or omissions in preoperative preparations. The preoperative check list accompanies the person to the operating room with the signed operative permit and the person's record.

Preoperative Medications. These medications (1) sedate or tranquilize the person, (2) provide analgesia, (3) decrease respiratory tract secretions, (4) reduce nausea and prevent vomiting, and (5) reduce gastric acid production. Most hospitalized persons receive an

Complete all items for patients going to SURGERY or SPECIAL PROCEDURES. DATE: _____ INITIAL FOR PROCEDURE DONE.

GENERAL	NURS. UNIT	HOLD. AREA	OR
ID Bracelet (location) _____			
Allergy Bracelet (location) _____			
Blood ID Bracelet ID # _____			
ALLERGIES			
Drugs _____			
Solutions _____			
Dyes _____			
Tape _____			
Other _____			
CORRECT & SIGNED CONSENTS			
General _____			
Blood Refusal _____			
Surgical _____			
Other _____			
LAB/DIAGNOSTIC TESTS			
CBC _____			
Chemview _____			
CXR _____			
EKG _____			
T&C _____ # Of Units _____			
UA _____			
Other _____			

PERSONAL	IN	OUT			
Contacts _____					
Bridge/Caps/Partials/Dentures _____					
Hearing Aid _____					
Prosthesis _____					
Rings off____ on____ taped _____					
Undergarments off____ on _____					
Other _____					
PREPARATIONS					
Enema given _____					
Gown on _____					
Last BM _____					
NPO____ Since _____					
Prep/Shave _____					
Voided _____					
Valuables: To whom given _____					

Disposition of: _____

INITIALS	NURSE SIGNATURE & TITLE

8-5410-63-0   12/86

Harris Methodist Fort Worth

1301 Pennsylvania Avenue
Fort Worth, Texas 76104

PRE-SURGICAL CHECK LIST

PRE OPERATIVE MEDICATIONS IS NOT GIVEN UNLESS FOLLOWING DONE:	YES	NO
1. H&P dictated/recorded _____		
2. Prep-op diagnosis & operative procedure recorded _____		
3. Lab results recorded _____		
4. Pre-anesthesia evaluation recorded _____		

NOTIFY SURGEON & SURGERY IF ABOVE NOT AVAILABLE.

PRE-OP MEDICATION, TIME GIVEN _____
See Graphic Record.

HEIGHT _____ WEIGHT _____

Nursing Unit: B/P____ T____ P____ R____

Holding Area: B/P____ T____ P____ R____

PRE-OPERATIVE TEACHING INTERVIEW BY O.R. RN:
_____ DATE: _____

ADDITIONAL COMMENTS: (circle) CAD HTN COPD/ASTHMA DIABETIC INSULIN/STEROID DEPENDENT SPEAKS NO ENGLISH ARTHRITIS EPILEPTIC IMPAIRED: HEARING VISION DEAF BLIND OTHER _____

PRE-OP DIAGNOSIS _____

PROCEDURE _____

PATIENT UNDERSTANDING OF PROCEDURE _____

SURGICAL HISTORY _____

COMMENTS: _____

▲ *Figure 49-2*

Preoperative checklist. (Courtesy of Harris Methodist Fort Worth, Fort Worth, TX.)

---

intramuscular injection or intravenous or oral premedication before transport to the operating room. Individuals undergoing ambulatory surgery are not routinely given preoperative medications. This practice facilitates speedy anesthesia recovery and discharge on the same day as surgery.[23]

The type of premedication depends on the person's age and condition and the anesthetic agent to be administered. The following pharmacologic agents typically are used for premedication:

▶ Barbiturates: Pentobarbital sodium and secobarbital sodium promote sleep, decrease anxiety, and reduce the amount of anesthesia required during surgery.

▶ Tranquilizers and nonbarbiturate sedatives: Chlorpromazine, promethazine, hydroxyzine, droperidol, chlordiazepoxide, lorazepam, diazepam, and midazolam reduce anxiety, decrease motor activity, and promote rapid induction of anesthesia.

▶ Narcotic analgesics: Morphine sulfate, meperidine hydrochloride, and fentanyl reduce pain, relax the individual, reduce anxiety, and reduce the amount of anesthesia required.

▶ Anticholinergics: Atropine sulfate and scopolamine

INSTRUCTIONS AND INFORMATION REGARDING PREPARATION FOR SURGERY

CIRCLE MATERIAL COVERED	Init.	INSTRUCTIONS GIVEN	VERBALIZES DEMONSTRATES CORRECTLY	COMMENTS
NEUROLOGICAL Neuro Vital Signs				
SENSORY Noise; alarms; lights; Shivering; cold; Pain medication; PCA pump				
RESPIRATORY Airway, O_2 face tent, IPPB Rx.; Nasal cannula; ETT; Ventilator; Suctioning; chest tube; Deep breathe; cough Incentive spirometer				
CARDIOVASCULAR Vital signs; B/P cuff; EKG monitor; Art. lines; CVP line IV				
GASTROINTESTINAL Diet; NPO; bowel sounds; NG tube; Nausea				
RENAL Void pre-op; catheters Irrigations				
MUSCULOSKELETAL Turning; leg exercises; Anti-embolic stockings; Cast; traction; immobilizers				
EDUCATION Evening routine, anesthesia evaluation; Shave/prep; surgery time; Holding Area; Operating room; waiting area; phone no.; Destination post-op; ICU				
ESS Emotional status				
OTHER Dressings; tubes; drains; hemovac				

DATE	INITIALS	NURSE SIGNATURE & TITLE	DATE	INITIALS	NURSE SIGNATURE & TITLE

12/86

Harris Methodist
Fort Worth

SURGICAL PATIENT
TEACHING RECORD

1301 Pennsylvania Avenue
Fort Worth, Texas 76104

▲ *Figure 49–2* Continued

reduce tracheobronchial secretions, dry out mucous membranes, interrupt vagal stimulation, and produce sedation and amnesia.

▶ Antinausea agents: Hydroxyzine reduces nausea, prevents vomiting, and provides mild relaxation.

▶ Antacid or H_2 receptor blockers: Cimetidine and ranitidine reduce gastric acid production, decrease acidity of gastric contents if aspirated, and are often given with oral premedications.[16,23]

Premedication may be ordered for a specific time or "on call" before transport to the OR. At the appropri-

ate time, administer preoperative medications and place the person in a comfortable position with adequate covering. Raise the bed side rails, place the bed in the lowest position, and caution the person not to try to smoke, drink anything, or get up without assistance and to ask for any help needed. Place the call light within easy reach. Explain that the medication will cause sleepiness, dizziness, dryness of the mouth, and so on. Continue to observe and assess the person for side effects or untoward reactions to the premedication (e.g., increased heart rate, decreased blood pressure, and respiratory depression). Notify the physician if any significant reactions occur.

Transport to Surgery. After completing preoperative routines and administering the premedication, arrange to have the individual transported to the OR. To begin the transportation (1) check and verify the person's identification and (2) check and secure all treatment devices (e.g., urinary drainage bags, intravenous solution containers, and gastric tubes). Stabilize the stretcher and the bed, then cover and assist the person safely onto the stretcher, being careful not to dislodge any tubes during movement. Arrange the cover and provide an extra cover if needed to maintain warmth. Secure the safety straps, and place the rails upright for safe transport. Avoid rapid movement and weaving motions during transport to prevent nausea, dizziness, or disorientation. Be quiet (but warm and supportive) to enhance the effect of the preoperative medication. On arrival at the OR, place the person in a waiting area under observation of the nurse in the area. Review the permanent record, signed consent, appropriate laboratory work, and preoperative check list with the nurse in the holding area.

Preparing the Room for Postoperative Care. To prepare the person's room for postoperative care, make the surgical bed with the top covers fan folded to one side or to the foot of the bed, according to hospital policy or to the dictates of the planned surgical intervention (e.g., foot surgery will require the foot to be observed frequently, so the foot end of the top linens should not be tucked in and the top linens should be fan folded to the side). Place the bed in the highest level position with the mattress flat and the pillow removed or placed on its edge at the head of the bed. Place an incontinence pad on the bed at the place where drainage might occur postoperatively. Place an emesis basin, blood pressure equipment, intravenous pole, respiratory and suction equipment, and extra pillows in the room. Make sure the call light is within reach of the person. Check the facility's procedure manual for room preparation for specific types of surgery.

Evaluation

Evaluation of the preoperative outcomes will be based on the results of the nursing actions designed to achieve the outcomes. Did the individual express his or her fears relating to surgery? Does the person acknowledge the risks and potential complications associated with the procedure? Can the individual demonstrate deep-breathing exercises and correct coughing? Can the person explain expected preoperative events?

INTRAOPERATIVE PHASE

The intraoperative phase begins when the individual is transferred to the OR table and ends at admission to the PACU. During this phase, the nurse protects the individual from injury and maintains a therapeutic environment. For example, the operating room nurse should

▶ Create a calm, quiet environment, especially before the person is given anesthesia
▶ Use touch and eye contact to reduce anxiety
▶ Quietly keep the person informed of what is happening
▶ Maintain the person's dignity (e.g., prevent unnecessary exposure)
▶ Treat each person as an individual (e.g., always refer to the person by name)
▶ At frequent intervals, communicate the individual's status in surgery to the support persons in the surgical waiting area
▶ Prevent injury (e.g., ensure well-planned, careful transfers from stretchers to the operating table and vice versa, maintain the person's body alignment and proper positioning during anesthesia, and protect the individual from biologic hazards by maintaining surgical asepsis; see Chapter 28)
▶ Recognize and correct breaks in sterile technique
▶ Document details of the intraoperative phase for the legal record and for reporting to other nurses caring for the person postoperatively

Assessment

Assessment in the intraoperative phase should begin with a focused review of the preoperative assessment from several data sources to include

▶ nursing documentation of the preoperative assessment data
▶ verbal reports
▶ medical data (i.e., history and physical)
▶ preoperative diagnostic testing results
▶ the individual's and significant other's statements

In the preoperative holding area or the surgical suite, the OR nurse's initial assessment should focus on those specific data elements that are imperative in the development of nursing diagnoses, goal setting, and an individualized care plan. Refer to Table 49–3 for a review of specific assessment criteria expected of the surgical nurse.

Nursing Diagnosis

Examples of common nursing diagnoses for the surgical candidate in the intraoperative phase may include but not be limited to

▶ *Potential for Infection* R/T possible transfer of microorganisms during invasive procedure (see Nursing Diagnosis Profile)
▶ *Potential for Impaired Skin Integrity* R/T pressure on bony prominences during surgery
▶ *Potential for Injury* R/T transfer and positioning on the OR table when consciousness decreased or absent

NURSING DIAGNOSIS PROFILE

High Risk for Infection

Definition. The state in which an individual is at increased risk for being invaded by pathogenic organisms

Classification. Exchanging 1.2.1.1

Defining Characteristics. *High Risk for Infection* is determined by the presence of risk factors such as inadequate primary defenses (broken skin, traumatized tissue, decrease in ciliary action, stasis of body fluids, change in pH of secretions, altered peristalsis), inadequate secondary defenses (e.g., decreased hemoglobin, leukopenia, suppressed inflammatory response, immunosuppression), inadequate acquired immunity, tissue destruction and increased environmental exposure, chronic disease, invasive procedures, malnutrition, pharmaceutical agents and trauma, rupture of amniotic membranes, and insufficient knowledge to avoid exposure to pathogens.

Sample Related Factors. The risk factors, listed above, for infection are also the related factors for this diagnosis.

Concept Description. *High Risk for Infection* is a concept that predicts an individual or situational risk of infection occurring because of either preexisting conditions (such as leukopenia) or the event itself (such as an invasive procedure).

Examples. Depending on the specific assessment data, this diagnostic category could be applicable in the following situations, among others:

▶ A person with acquired immune deficiency syndrome (AIDS) who is scheduled for an emergency appendectomy: Because the person has two risk factors present, a nursing diagnosis of "*High Risk for Infection* R/T broken skin during surgery and inadequate immunity secondary to AIDS" would be made.

▶ A person who has been involved in a motorcycle accident with a compound fracture of the tibia and fibula: In this case, also, two risk factors are present, and a nursing diagnosis of *High Risk for Infection* R/T tissue destruction and increased environmental exposure would be made.

Related/Similar Nursing Diagnosis. In the surgical candidate, potential for infection must be differentiated from *Impaired Skin Integrity* and *Impaired Tissue Integrity*.

In a planned surgical event, *impaired skin integrity* and *impaired tissue integrity* at the operative site are expected. Infection is not necessarily expected but is possible. Breaks in the primary defense mechanism can lead to infection and are therefore related factors in the diagnosis of *High Risk for Infection*. Thus, a diagnosis of *High Risk for Infection* R/T impaired skin (or tissue) integrity secondary to surgery would mean that a person had impaired skin or tissue integrity and a diagnosis of *Impaired Skin Integrity* or *Impaired Tissue Integrity* would also be required. Conversely, when a diagnosis of *Impaired Skin Integrity* or *Impaired Tissue Integrity* is made, a diagnosis of *High Risk for Infection* should also be made.

▶ *Potential for Injury* R/T possible presence of retained foreign body secondary to open body cavity
▶ *Potential for Fluid Volume Deficit* R/T possible excess blood loss during surgery[39]

Planning

During the intraoperative phase, the nurse plans interventions that will prevent complications and minimize the risks of surgery. Stated outcomes are listed in Table 49–6. Each outcome provides both a basis for nursing interventions and a criterion for evaluation.

Nursing Intervention

The main intraoperative nursing interventions may be broadly described as actions that are directed toward (a) maintaining a sterile field, (b) transferring and positioning the person, and (c) caring for the person during anesthesia.

MAINTAINING A STERILE ENVIRONMENT

Surgery requires a sterile environment. As discussed earlier, a surgical incision is a potential entryway for

microorganisms. The person must be protected from contamination to prevent infection. Any nurse who works in surgery must be well aware of the principles of surgical asepsis (see Chapter 28).

During surgery, all members of the surgical team who come in contact with the surgical field must wear appropriate surgical attire including scrub clothing covered with a sterile gown, sterile gloves, hair covering and face mask, and protective eye wear. Shoe covers are worn to protect the shoes from contamination from blood or body fluids. Any item that comes in contact with the sterile field must be sterile. All drapes, instruments, sutures, and dressings are sterile and are handled using sterile technique. Nurses in ORs must be constantly aware of what is occurring in and around the sterile field. Violations of sterile technique must be prevented, or serious postoperative infection may result. Controlling traffic in and out of the OR and the use of universal precautions and "confine and contain" procedures are also important responsibilities of the OR nurse in infection prevention.[4,12,13,19]

TRANSFERRING AND POSITIONING THE PERSON

To prepare a person to receive anesthesia, carefully transfer and position the individual on the OR table, ensuring adequate assistance to support the person

TABLE 49–6. Common Intraoperative Nursing Interventions

Nursing Diagnoses	Outcomes	Nursing Actions
High Risk for Infection R/T possible transfer of microorganisms during invasive procedure	The individual is free from infection.	Establish and maintain a sterile field.
High Risk for Impaired Skin Integrity R/T pressure on bony prominences during surgery	The individual's skin integrity is maintained.	Adequately pad occiput, sacrum, elbows, and heels for supine position.
High Risk for Injury R/T transfer and positioning on operating room table when consciousness decreased or absent	The person is free from injury related to transfer and positioning.	Use four operating room personnel to transfer individual from locked stretcher to locked operating room bed by lifting with a sheet while supporting the head and extremities.
High Risk for Injury R/T possible presence of retained foreign body secondary to open body cavity	The person is free from injury by foreign body.	Perform sponge, needle, and instrument counts before procedure, before closing peritoneal cavity, and before closing skin.
High Risk for Fluid Volume Deficit R/T possible excess blood loss during surgery	The individual's fluid and electrolyte balance is maintained.	Monitor the amount of blood loss (i.e., in sponges and suction container) and urinary output; communicate to physician. Work as a team to provide hemostasis as efficiently as possible (e.g., have sufficient sterile clamps and suture ready to pass to surgeon and assistant without delay).

APPLYING RESEARCH TO NURSING PRACTICE

Preventing Complications of the Lithotomy Position

Graling, P.R., & Colvin, D.B. (1992). The lithotomy position in colon surgery. *AORN Journal*, 55(4), 1029–1039.

▼ ▼ ▼

Graling and Colvin studied the incidence of complications in 60 clients who had been in the lithotomy position for 2 or more hours during colon surgery. Postoperative complications occurred in 20 of the clients studied. Complications included postoperative leg swelling (edema); leg, hip, and back pain; changes in sensation; diminished pedal pulses; and impaired ambulation. All clients who were kept in the lithotomy position for 6 hours or longer experienced complications.

Applications for Practice. This study contributes to nursing knowledge by estimating the incidence of postoperative complications associated with the lithotomy position. The researchers did not monitor the actual methods of placing clients into the lithotomy position, so it is unclear whether the development of complications was due to the lithotomy position per se or to incorrect placement into the lithotomy posi-

tion. As you observe perioperative nurses at work, watch how they focus on the prevention of complications of the lithotomy position. Before induction of anesthesia, two clinicians should assist the client to move the buttocks to the edge of the break in the operating table. They should very slowly raise the client's legs simultaneously, keeping them together, and flexing the knees and hips in 90 degree angles. The perioperative nurse should adequately pad the stirrups and position the client in correct body alignment. The perioperative nurse should pay particular attention to the alignment of the hips, knees, and feet, avoiding external rotation. During the surgery, operating room personnel should not lean on the inner aspects of the client's thighs. Avoiding leaning on the thighs prevents external rotation of the hip joints. During the surgical procedure, the circulating nurse should frequently assess the stability of the client's position, the status of potential pressure points, and the vascular status. On completion of surgery, two clinicians should simultaneously remove the client's feet from the stirrups, very slowly lower the legs, and extend the client's knees and hips.

safely. Careful positioning (1) sustains circulatory and respiratory functions (e.g., prevents venous stasis, allows diaphragmatic movement), (2) prevents damage to neuromuscular structures (e.g., avoids twisting muscles or impinging on nerves), and (3) promotes comfort. In addition, proper positioning should provide (1) the best exposure of the surgical site, (2) the best body alignment individualized to the person's needs, (3) access to the individual for administration of intravenous fluids, medications, and anesthesia, and (4) safe function of body systems during the surgery.[22]

Anesthesia is initiated with the person in a supine, dorsal recumbent position. However, different types of surgery require repositioning after anesthesia induction to allow adequate exposure and access to the surgical site (Fig. 49–3). The OR nurse must be familiar with the various positioning devices and padding available to position and protect the individual correctly.

Remember that a person under anesthesia cannot feel or report pain or discomfort. Therefore, the person's position and alignment must not cause undue strain or pressure on body parts. Serious musculoskele-

tal and neurologic damage can occur if a person is not correctly positioned.

CARING FOR THE PERSON DURING ANESTHESIA

An anesthetist or anesthesiologist administers anesthetic agents and supervises anesthesia care. The type of anesthesia given depends on the person's general condition, the extent and type of surgery, and the person's experience with anesthesia. Nurses need to be aware of anesthesia side effects, contraindications, and implications for nursing care.

Anesthesia care is classified as (1) local, (2) monitored, (3) regional, or (4) general. Local anesthesia blocks transmissions of stimuli through peripheral nerve endings. Local anesthetics are either applied to the surface of a mucous membrane (topical) or injected in the vicinity of nerves to be blocked (infiltration). For example, the intracutaneous injection of anesthetic allows painless suturing of a minor laceration. In monitored anesthesia care, the local anesthetic may be sup-

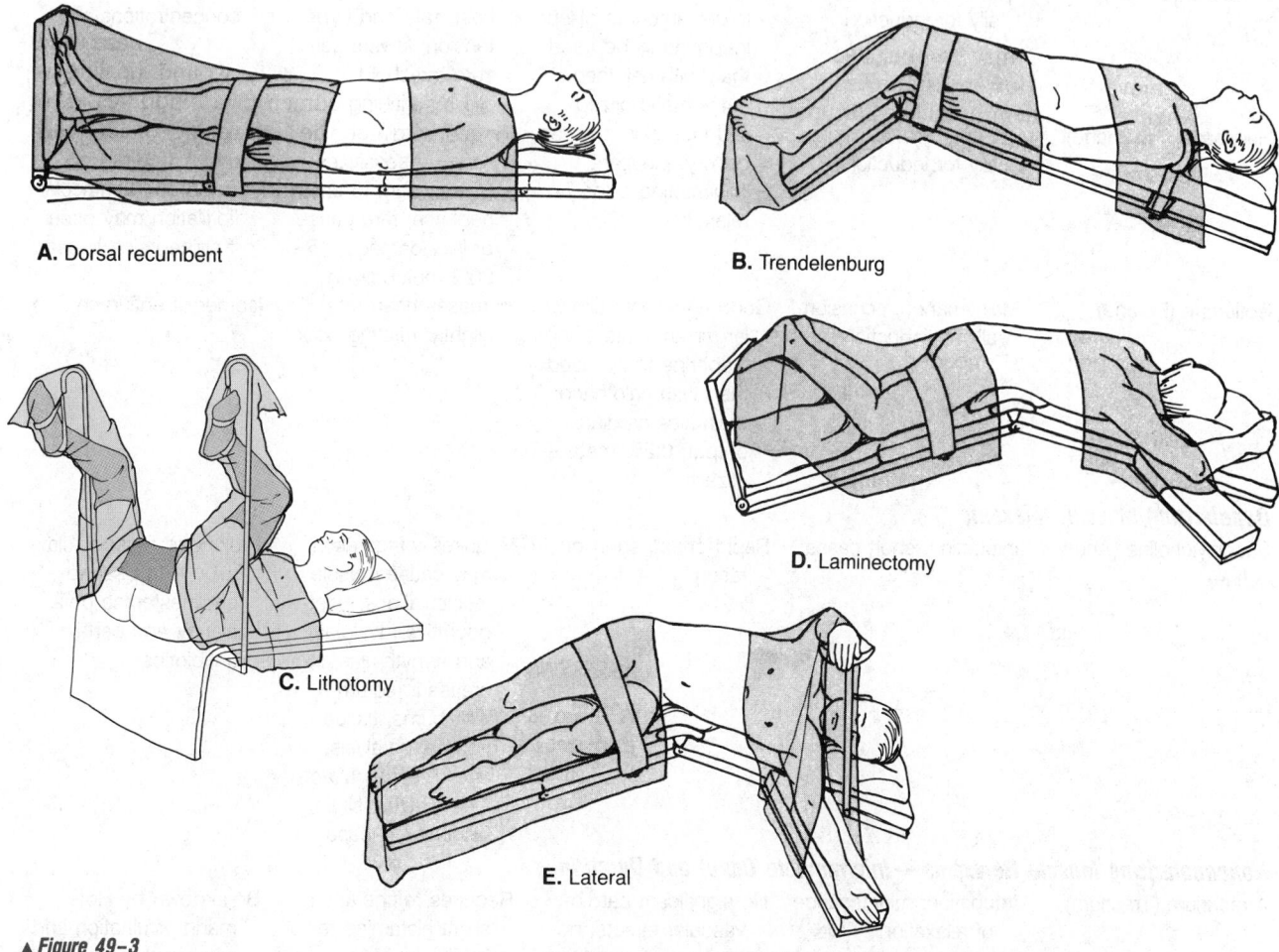

A. Dorsal recumbent

B. Trendelenburg

C. Lithotomy

D. Laminectomy

E. Lateral

▲ *Figure 49–3*

Five surgical positions. (Modified from Black, J.M., Matassarin-Jacobs, E. [1993]. *Luckmann and Sorensen's Medical-surgical nursing: A psychophysiologic approach* [4th ed.] Philadelphia: W.B. Saunders.)

plemented with an intravenous medication to provide analgesia and sedation while the person is monitored by the anesthetist or anesthesiologist. Regional anesthesia blocks nerve transmission in a large area of the body. For example, spinal anesthesia blocks sensory and motor nerves of the lower regions of the body. General anesthesia affects the brain and causes unconsciousness and widespread muscle relaxation, which usually requires endotracheal intubation. General anesthetics are usually administered by inhalation or by intravenous line. General and spinal anesthesias are useful for major, prolonged surgery.[23] Table 49–7 summarizes commonly used anesthetic drugs.

Evaluation

Evaluation and reassessment occur continuously during the intraoperative phase as planned nursing interven-

TABLE 49–7. Commonly Used Anesthetic Drugs

	Common Use	Advantages	Disadvantages	Comments
Inhalational Agents				
Oxygen (O_2)	Essential for life	Can slightly increase amount available to tissues in low cardiac output states	Can cause retinopathy in premature infants	High concentrations hazardous with lasers in surgery of head and neck and pulmonary areas
Nitrous oxide (N_2O)	Maintenance; occasionally for induction	Rapid induction and recovery; additive effects to other anesthetics	No relaxation; can depress myocardium	Hypoxia if overdose given
Enflurane (Ethrane)	Maintenance; occasionally for induction	Good relaxation; allows larger amounts of epinephrine to be used than with halothane; 2.4% metabolized	Can cause increased heart rate and hypotension; lowers seizure threshold; slightly irritating odor	Abnormal EEG at high concentrations
Halothane (Fluothane)	Maintenance; occasionally for induction	Rapid induction and recovery; pleasant, nonirritating odor, fair relaxation	Narrow margin of safety—sensitizes myocardium to epinephrine; rare cause of liver damage; 15–20% metabolized	May cause bradycardia and hypotension; PVCs and ventricular fibrillation may occur if epinephrine is used
Isoflurane (Forane)	Maintenance; occasionally for induction	Good relaxation; allows larger amounts of epinephrine to be used than with halothane; maintains cardiac output; 0.2% metabolized	Increases heart rate; slightly irritating odor	Isomer of enflurane
Depolarizing Muscle Relaxants				
Succinylcholine (Anectine)	Intubation; short cases	Rapid onset; short duration	Requires refrigeration; may cause muscle fasciculations, postoperative myalgias, and arrhythmias; increase in serum K^+ with burns, tissue trauma, paralysis, and diseases affecting muscles; slight histamine release	Prolonged muscle relaxation with pseudocholinesterase deficiency and certain antibiotics
Nondepolarizing Muscle Relaxants—Intermediate Onset and Duration				
Atracurium (Tracrium)	Intubation; maintenance of relaxation	No significant cardiovascular effects; no cumulative effects; good with renal failure	Requires refrigeration; slight histamine release	Breakdown by Hofmann elimination and ester hydrolysis

TABLE 49–7. Commonly Used Anesthetic Drugs Continued

	Common Use	Advantages	Disadvantages	Comments
Vecuronium (Norcuron)	Intubation; maintenance of relaxation	No significant cardiovascular effects; no cumulative effects and no histamine release	Requires mixing	Mostly eliminated in bile, some in urine

Nondepolarizing Muscle Relaxants—Longer Onset and Duration

	Common Use	Advantages	Disadvantages	Comments
d-Tubocurare (Curare, tubocurarine)	Maintenance of relaxation		May cause histamine release and transient ganglionic blockade	
Metocurine (Metubine)	Maintenance of relaxation	Good cardiovascular stability	Slight histamine release	Large bolus may cause hypotension
Pancuronium (Pavulon)	Maintenance of relaxation		May cause tachycardia and hypertension	Mostly dependent on renal elimination

Intravenous Anesthetics

	Common Use	Advantages	Disadvantages	Comments
Etomidate (Amidate)	Induction	Good cardiovascular stability; fast, smooth induction and recovery	May cause pain with injection and myotonic movements	
Diazepam (Valium)	Amnesia; hypnotic; preoperative medication	Good sedation	Prolonged duration	
Ketamine (Ketalar)	Induction, occasional maintenance (IV or IM)	Short acting; patient maintains airway; good in small children and burn patients	Large doses may cause hallucinations and respiratory depression	Need darkened quiet room for recovery; often used in trauma cases
Midazolam (Versed)	Hypnotic; anxiolytic sedation often used as adjunct to induction	Excellent amnesia; water soluble (no pain with IV injection); short acting	Slower induction than thiopental	
Propofol (Diprivan)	Induction and maintenance	Rapid onset; awakening in 4 to 8 min.	May cause pain if injected in small vein	Short elimination half-life (34 to 64 min)
Sodium methohexital (Brevital)	Induction	Ultrashort-acting barbiturate	May cause hiccups	Can be given rectally
Thiopental sodium (Pentothal)	Induction	Fast, smooth induction and recovery	Large doses may cause apnea and cardiovascular depression	May cause laryngospasm; can be given rectally

Local Anesthetics

	Common Use	Advantages	Disadvantages	Comments
Bupivacaine (Marcaine, Sensorcaine)	Epidural, spinal, or local infiltration	Good relaxation; long acting	Overdose can cause cardiac collapse	Maximum dose: 200 and 150 mg/70 kg with and without epinephrine, respectively
Chloroprocaine (Nesacaine)	Epidural anesthesia	Ultrashort acting; good relaxation	May cause neurotoxicity if injected into CSF	Maximum dose: 1000 and 800 mg/70 kg with and without epinephrine, respectively
Lidocaine (Xylocaine)	Epidural, spinal, peripheral, IV blocks and local infiltration	Short acting; good relaxation; low toxicity	Overdose can cause convulsions	Also used for ventricular dysrhythmias; maximum dose: 7 and 5 mg/kg with and without epinephrine, respectively
Tetracaine (Pontocaine)	Spinal anesthesia	Long acting; good relaxation		Maximum dose: 1–1.5 mg/kg (epinephrine rarely used)

Table continued on following page

TABLE 49-7. *Commonly Used Anesthetic Drugs* Continued

	Common Use	Advantages	Disadvantages	Comments
Anticholinergics				
Atropine	Blocks effects of acetylcholine; decreases vagal tone; reverses muscle relaxants; treats sinus bradycardia	Increases heart rate; suppresses salivation, bronchial and gastric secretions	Depresses sweating; may cause dry mouth, flushing, dizziness, CNS symptoms	Quite selective at muscarinic receptor in smooth and cardiac muscle and exocrine glands
Glycopyrrolate (Robinul)	Similar to atropine	Small increase in heart rate; does not cross blood-brain barrier; can raise gastric pH more than atropine	Prolonged duration of effects	Lower incidence of dysrhythmias than atropine

From Meeker, M. H., & Rothrock, J. C. (1991). *Alexander's care of the patient in surgery* (9th ed.). St. Louis: Mosby-Yearbook.
Abbreviations: EEG, electroencephalogram; PVCs, premature ventricular contractions; K+, potassium; IV, intravenous; IM, intramuscular; CSF, cerebrospinal fluid; CNS, central nervous system.

tions are carried out. Ongoing evaluation cannot be overemphasized. The person is usually unconscious and unable to let others know that problems are present. It is up to the nurse to be ever alert to the client's status. The final evaluation of the intraoperative care plan occurs at the completion of the intraoperative phase and is documented and communicated to the PACU or SICU nurse by the circulating nurse. Reassessment most desirably occurs by collaboration of the OR nurse and the PACU nurse on admission to the PACU, to ensure continuity of care.

POSTOPERATIVE PHASE

After surgery, the person is transferred immediately from the OR to the PACU or SICU. During transport, the individual is closely monitored. The anesthesiologist or nurse anesthetist and circulating nurse generally accompany the person to the PACU. Keep side rails up and safety belts secure, and observe other safety precautions during transport. Keep the person warm, and avoid hurried movements or rapid changes in the person's position during transfers from stretchers to beds. Handle the person gently to prevent hypotension and incisional strain.

The PACU is an area designed for postanesthesia care. After surgery, the person remains in the recovery room until criteria for discharge are met (see Box 49-4). A recovery room contains monitors, equipment, medication, and supplies needed for supportive and emergency care. Because numerous complications and problems may occur during the postanesthesia recovery period, PACU nurses monitor the individual continuously during this stage. Significant others may usually visit at specified intervals in the PACU, according to agency policy.

Assessment

On arrival in the PACU, begin baseline admission assessment by (1) measuring blood pressure, (2) measuring heart rate and evaluating quality and rhythm of pulse, (3) measuring depth and rate of respirations, and (4) evaluating skin color and tissue integrity and perfusion. Also assess the level of consciousness of the person and the presence of reflexes, and note intravenous sites, dressings, drains, and special equipment. The OR nurse will provide an evaluation of intraoperative care and achievement of desirable outcomes. Also read the operative report. This report includes such information as (1) type and extent of surgery, (2) anesthetic agent, medications, and intravenous fluids administered, (3) location of dressings, catheters, and drains, (4) respiratory or cardiovascular dysfunction, and (5) other pertinent factors, such as sensory impairments, anxiety level before administration of anesthesia, and primary language. Box 49-5 presents assessment factors and guidelines for nursing care after anesthesia.

Nursing Diagnosis

For examples of the common nursing diagnoses in the postoperative phase, refer to Box 49-5, which summarizes standards of care in the PACU. Nursing interventions are then planned to address these nursing diagnoses, which are determined by the person's condition and postoperative status.

Planning

In general, the desirable outcome of postanesthesia nursing care is that the person will return to a safe physiologic level after excreting the anesthetic.[15] A nursing care plan to accomplish this goal is outlined in Box 49-5.

Box 49-4. Postanesthetic Recovery Score

A. Purpose

1. To be used as a guideline for the evaluation of the postanesthetic patient
2. To provide set criteria that the postanesthetic patient should meet before discharge from the PACU
3. To provide objective information of the physical condition of patients arriving in the PACU after anesthesia

B. Scoring System

1. Activity. The muscular activity is assessed by observing the ability of the patient to move his limbs either spontaneously or on command.
   a. Ability to move all four extremities scores 2.
   b. Ability to move two extremities scores 1.
   c. Unable to move any extremity scores 0.
2. Respiration. No complicated apparatus or sophisticated physical tests are used.
   a. Ability to deep breathe and cough scores 2.
   b. Limited respiratory effort (i.e., splinting) or dyspnea scores 1.
   c. No evident spontaneous respiratory effort scores 0.
3. Circulation. This is the most difficult sign to evaluate by a simple method. Changes in the arterial blood pressure from the preanesthetic level were chosen because it is reliable, it is monitored throughout the anesthetic period, and it is one of the first signs taken on arrival in the PACU.
   a. Systolic arterial blood pressure 20% ± preanesthetic level scores 2.
   b. Systolic arterial blood pressure 20% to 50% ± preanesthetic level scores 1.
   c. Systolic arterial blood pressure 50% ± preanesthetic level scores 0.
   (Note: Great differences in diastolic blood pressure should be noted.)
4. Consciousness. Ability of patients to answer simple questions and follow verbal commands. Only verbal stimuli are to be used.
   a. Full alertness with ability to answer question scores 2.
   b. Patient arousable by calling his name scores 1.
   c. Auditory stimuli fail to elicit any response scores 0.
5. Color. Patients are to be scored on their color in the PACU, whether this skin color was present before surgery or not (example: jaundiced preoperatively and postoperatively).
   a. Obviously normal or pink skin color scores 2.
   b. Any alteration from the normal pink, but not cyanotic; for example: pale, dusky, blotchy, jaundiced scores 1.
   c. Cyanotic nailbed, lips, and skin scores 0.
   (Note: Check patient oral mucosa if any questions.)

C. Results of Postanesthetic Recovery Score

1. Optimum score is 10. Patient may be discharged from the PACU with scores of 8, 9, or 10. Nursing judgment must be used since this scoring system is not infallible.
2. Patients who had scores of 10 preoperatively but received scores less than 8 during the postoperative state require more constant observation and may need a specialized nursing care area, such as the intensive care unit.
3. Chronically debilitated, senile, or paralyzed patients may never receive an optimum score. Each patient must be treated individually and discharged from the PACU at the discretion of the attending anesthesiologist.
4. There are variables that may influence patient's emergence from anesthesia and thus his score. These include the following:
   a. Type of anesthetic agent used
   b. Use of paralyzing drugs and narcotics during surgery
   c. Type of surgery performed
   d. Duration of surgery and anesthesia

From Frost, E. A. M. (1990). *Postanesthesia care unit: Current practices* (2nd ed.). St. Louis: C. V. Mosby.
Abbreviation: PACU, postanesthesia care unit.

Nursing Intervention

CARE DURING THE IMMEDIATE POSTOPERATIVE STAGE

Immediate postoperative care includes systematic assessment and maintenance of

- respiratory function: ensuring patent airway, preventing respiratory distress, promoting adequate oxygen exchange
- cardiovascular function: preventing hypotension, shock, and cardiac arrest and promoting adequate cardiac functioning
- neurologic and sensory function: assessing level of consciousness, reorienting the person as he or she regains consciousness
- water and electrolyte balance: monitoring intake and output of fluids, restoring water and electrolyte balance
- safe, comfortable physical and psychologic environment: maintaining body temperature, relieving discomfort, and promoting relaxation, providing support and reassurance

While the individual is in the PACU, continue to assess and document respirations, heart rate and rhythm, blood pressure, and level of consciousness at 15-minute intervals. Measure body temperature on admission and at least every 1 to 2 hours thereafter. Continuously assess the person's response to analgesic medication, provide comfort measures such as repositioning and warm blankets, and encourage use of relaxation techniques to augment medications. Most PACUs have standing orders and use a standardized

Box 49-5. Guidelines for Standards of Care in the Postanesthesia Care Unit

I. Assessment

Health status data are collected. These data are recorded, retrievable, continuous, and communicated. Data are obtained by physical exam, review of records, and consultation.

1. Assessment factors include but are not limited to:
   a. relevant preoperative status, including electrocardiogram, vital signs, radiology findings, laboratory values, allergies, disabilities, drug use, physical or mental impairments, mobility limitations, prostheses (including hearing aids)
   b. anesthesia technique (general, regional, local), effect of preop medications
   c. anesthetic agents, muscle relaxants, narcotics, and reversal agents used
   d. length of time anesthesia administered
   e. type of surgical procedure
   f. estimated fluid/blood loss and replacement
   g. complications occurring during anesthetic course, treatment initiated, response
2. Initial physical assessment to include the documentation of:
   a. vital signs
      1. respiratory rate and competency, airway patency, type of artificial airway, mechanical ventilator and settings
      2. blood pressure—cuff or arterial line
      3. pulse—apical—peripheral—cardiac monitor pattern
      4. temperature—oral—rectal—axillary—digital through dermal sensors
   b. pressure readings—central venous—arterial blood—pulmonary artery wedge
   c. position of patient
   d. condition and color of skin
   e. circulation—peripheral pulses and sensation of extremity(ies) as applicable
   f. condition of dressings
   g. condition of suture line, if dressings are absent
   h. type and patency of drainage tubes, catheters, and receptacle
   i. amount and type of drainage
   j. muscular response and strength
   k. fluid therapy, location of lines, type and amount of solution infusing (including blood)
   l. level of consciousness
   m. level of comfort
3. Numerical score if used

II. Nursing Diagnosis

Nursing diagnosis is a concise statement and represents a decision based on analysis of the data collected during the assessment phase.

1. Nursing diagnosis is consistent with current scientific knowledge
2. Nursing diagnoses are based on identifiable data as compared to established norms or previous conditions

3. Nursing diagnoses include but are not limited to:
   a. altered level of consciousness
   b. alterations in comfort
   c. anxiety
   d. alterations in cardiac output
   e. alterations in fluid volume (both excess and deficit)
   f. impairment of mobility (including decrease in muscle strength)
   g. potential for physical injury
   h. respiratory dysfunction
   i. impairment of skin integrity
   j. abnormal tissue perfusion
   k. alterations in urinary elimination

III. Care Plan

The plan for nursing care describes a systematic method for achieving the goal of postanesthesia nursing care—to assist the patient in returning to a safe physiologic level after an anesthetic.

1. The plan includes setting priorities for appropriate nursing actions
2. The plan is based on current scientific knowledge
3. The plan is developed with and communicated to the patient, family and/or significant others, and appropriate health care team personnel
4. The plan is formulated in conjunction with preoperative, intraoperative, and current postanesthetic health status assessments
5. The plan includes but is not limited to the following nursing actions:
   a. identification of the patient
   b. monitor, maintain, and/or improve respiratory function
   c. monitor, maintain, and/or improve circulatory function
   d. promote and maintain physical and emotional comfort
   e. receive report from operating room nurse, anesthesiologist, and/or anesthetist
   f. monitor surgical site
   g. interpret and document data obtained during assessment
   h. document nursing plan, action, and/or interventions with outcome
   i. notify family and/or significant others of patient's arrival and discharge from PACU
   j. notify patient care unit of any needed equipment
   k. notify patient care unit when patient is ready for discharge from PACU
   l. outpatient surgicals—discharge planning with patient and family

IV. Implementation

The plan for nursing care is implemented to achieve the goal as stated under care plan.

1. Nursing actions remain consistent with the written plan to provide continuity of care in accordance with established policy and procedure

Box 49–5. Guidelines for Standards of Care in the Postanesthesia Care Unit (Continued)

2. Comfort, safety, efficiency, skill, and effectiveness are reflected in nursing actions
3. Nursing decisions and actions regarding patient care reflect upholding the dignity of the patient and family
4. The plan may be altered to meet the changing needs of the patient

V. Evaluation

The plan for nursing care is evaluated.

1. Current assessment data are collected and recorded to evaluate the patient's status for discharge:
   a. airway patency and respiratory function
   b. stability of vital signs, including temperature
   c. level of consciousness and muscular strength
   d. mobility
   e. patency of tubes, catheters, drains, intravenous lines
   f. skin color and condition
   g. intake and output
   h. comfort

2. The nurse informs the family and/or significant others and health care team personnel of the patient's status

VI. Discharge

The postanesthesia nurse shall discharge the patient in accordance with written policies set forth by the Department of Anesthesia and also in accordance with the criteria and data collected through use of the nursing process. A final nursing assessment and evaluation of the patient's condition will be performed and documented. If a numerical scoring system is used, the discharge score will be recorded to reflect the patient's status. The postanesthesia nurse arranges for the safe transport of the patient from the PACU to his or her room.

Adapted from Drain, C. B., & Cristoph, S. S. (1987). *The recovery room: A critical approach to post anesthesia nursing* (2nd ed.). Philadelphia: W. B. Saunders.
Abbreviation: PACU, postanesthesia care unit.

---

form to document and evaluate postanesthesia recovery.

The surgeon and anesthesiologist write postoperative orders. Carrying out these orders might involve administering analgesics and other special medications or monitoring for particular changes in the person's condition. Immediately report to the physician significant vital sign changes or other unusual developments. Once the person's condition stabilizes and orientation returns, the person is returned to the surgical unit for continued postoperative care.

People who have ambulatory surgery require the same monitoring and support during the immediate postoperative stage as inpatients. After such surgery, the individual remains in the recovery room until fully awake. A special observation unit, or **phase II recovery area,** may be provided for an additional 1 to 4 hours of recovery to ensure that all criteria for discharge are met.

Make certain the person who has had ambulatory surgery understands what to do after surgery, knows when and how to seek help for problems that may develop, and has a responsible adult to go home with him or her. Instructions should be shared verbally with the individual and support persons and provided in writing.

CARE DURING THE INTERMEDIATE POSTOPERATIVE STAGE

The intermediate postoperative stage begins when the person is discharged from the PACU and generally ends 48 to 72 hours later. During this period, the person remains at risk for postoperative complications, including respiratory, circulatory, or gastric dysfunction.

The Surgical Unit. The person returns to the surgical unit after stabilization in the recovery room. Maintaining safety and constant monitoring continue during transfer. The nurse on the surgical unit receives a complete report from the PACU nurse about the surgery, the person's course during surgery, postanesthesia recovery, and nursing and medical interventions.

When you are assigned to a client in the intermediate phase, review the record and begin a baseline assessment. (Follow the same assessment guidelines used in the immediate postanesthesia recovery stage.) Spend time talking quietly with the person and allaying anxiety. Check dressings, drainage tubes, and equipment for proper functioning. Position the person comfortably in bed according to the type of surgery (e.g., side lying with knees slightly flexed after abdominal surgery). Ensure that the person's room or unit is quiet. Turn down lighting to promote sleep. Review and implement postoperative orders.

Note whether the person requires medication for pain. Is the person restless? Are vital signs fluctuating? Does the individual state that he or she is uncomfortable? If the person is experiencing pain, check the physician's order and give analgesia as necessary. In some health care facilities, individuals are able to relieve their own pain by means of patient-controlled analgesia. This computer-regulated and client-controlled method of intravenous medication administration is discussed in Chapter 40.

Notify the physician immediately if untoward changes occur (e.g., increased bleeding, reduced urine output, changes in vital signs, severe pain unrelieved by analgesia).

Notify support persons of the individual's return to the surgical unit. Discuss the person's condition and appearance as well as routines of postoperative care. Provide support to them and to the client.

TABLE 49-8. Prevention of Postoperative Complications: Intermediate Stage

Potential Complication	Assessment	Prevention and Nursing Intervention	Expected Evaluation of Outcome
Atelectasis: Alveoli collapse from hypoventilation during anesthesia and immobility; increased respiratory secretions, decreased respirations Potential onset: in first 48 hours	Increased temperature, restlessness, dyspnea, tachycardia, altered breath sounds	Encourage coughing, deep breathing, turning, ambulation, hydration. Avoid respiratory depression during use of narcotic analgesics.	Chest movements during respiration are deep, bilateral. Vital signs normal. Discomfort is controlled.
Pneumonia: Inflammatory process in the lungs with collection of fluid and respiratory secretions Potential onset: in first 36 hours	Increased temperature; dyspnea; tachycardia; thick, viscous sputum; altered breath sounds	As above; may require nasotracheal suctioning to stimulate cough: Administer ordered antibiotics and antipyretics. Provide mouth care.	As above; respiratory secretions normal.
Gastric distention: Peristalsis slowed by anesthesia; accumulation of gas in intestines Potential onset: in first 24–36 hours	Abdominal discomfort, fullness, "gas pains," enlarged abdomen, decreased bowel sounds, vomiting	Encourage turning, ambulation; NPO or reduced oral intake; maintain hydration with parenteral fluids; insertion of nasogastric or rectal tube.	Bowel sounds are normal; passage of flatus; reduced abdominal girth; reduced discomfort.
Ileus:[9] Absence of peristalsis as result of manipulation of bowel during surgery or hypokalemia Potential onset: in first 24–36 hours	Decreased or absent bowel sounds, abdominal and gastric distention, vomiting, constipation	As above; maintain fluid and electrolyte balance.	As above; bowel movement is normal.
Urinary retention: Depression of urinary bladder tone by anesthesia; spasm of bladder sphincter Potential onset: in first 6–8 hours	Restlessness, bladder discomfort, inability to void or voiding frequently in small amount, bladder fullness, high fluid intake and low urine output	Provide privacy during urination (normal position for urination). Provide analgesics to decrease discomfort and promote sphincter relaxation. Encourage early ambulation. Maintain hydration.	Client urinates easily, empties bladder. Fluid intake equal to output.
Postoperative pain:[15] Response to surgical trauma; accentuated by visceral distention, anxiety, tension, past experience Potential onset: in first 6–8 hours	Restlessness, facial grimacing, clenched fists, subjective reports of pain, fluctuations in vital signs; assess sociocultural beliefs and attitudes about pain	Provide comfort measures (e.g., change positioning, back rub), quiet, subdued atmosphere. Reduce anxiety; encourage ventilation. Administer analgesics in dose and frequency to reduce pain and prevent respiratory depression.	There is subjective report of improved comfort, reduced evidence of tension, anxiety.
Wound infection:[19] Break in surgical asepsis with contamination of site during surgery, wound care, or dressing changes Potential onset: in 24–72 hours (longer if drain in place or wound otherwise not intact)	Pain, swelling, warmth, redness in incisional area; purulent, foul drainage; increased temperature; increased heart rate	Use strict aseptic technique during surgery and wound care. Monitor tubes, drains, dressings. Report early signs of infection. Maintain nutrition, hydration, mobility. Administer antibiotics and special wound care as ordered.	No signs or symptoms of wound infection; vital signs normal.

TABLE 49–9. Prevention of Postoperative Complications: Extended Stage

Potential Complication	Assessment	Prevention and Nursing Intervention	Expected Evaluation of Outcome
Thrombophlebitis: Inflammation of vein with clot formation as result of vessel injury, venous stasis Potential onset: in 7–14 days	Localized pain, redness, tenderness, induration of superficial vein; deep muscle tenderness, warmth and swelling of leg or calf; massive swelling, pain, tenderness, cyanosis of lower extremity	Encourage extremity exercises, early ambulation, possible use of elastic stockings. Prevent pressure on legs or legs in dependent position. Avoid restrictive dressings. Provide adequate hydration. If occurs: Local, moist heat, bedrest with legs elevated. Monitor during administration of anticoagulant or fibrinolytic therapy. Teach person about therapy.	Negative Homans' sign; no evidence of local inflammatory response in legs.
Pulmonary embolism:[9] Migration of foreign object (e.g., clot) to branch of pulmonary artery; massive embolism causes pulmonary hypertension, right-sided heart failure, cardiac arrest Potential onset: in 7–10 days	May be associated with thrombophlebitis (see above); sudden chest pain, dyspnea, cough, hemoptysis, restlessness, increased heart rate, increased respiratory rate, altered breath sounds	As above; avoid massage to suspected area of thrombophlebitis. Reduce anxiety; administer oxygen as ordered. Monitor during administration of anticoagulant or fibrinolytic therapy.	As above. Oxygenation is adequate; respirations within normal limits.
Dysfunctional grieving:[25] Exaggerated response to loss or change associated with surgery Potential onset: in intermediate to extended postoperative stage	Passivity, depression, reduced involvement in self-care; sleep disturbance; increased pain and use of analgesics; hyperactivity and sense of well-being inappropriate to reality of loss; onset of stress-related symptoms (e.g., gastrointestinal dysfunction)	Involve person and significant others in discussion of anticipated changes. Encourage expression of feelings. Provide empathetic listening. Reassure normalcy of grieving process. Arrange support groups and/or community referrals for person.	Person and family express feelings of loss; normal sleeping and comfort; no evidence of stress-related illness; self-care activities. Grieving process completed in 6–12 months.
Wound dehiscence:[9] Separation of wound margins; usually abdominal incision affected, caused by increased intraabdominal pressure (e.g., excessive coughing or vomiting, especially with obese persons or those with infected abdominal incisions) Potential onset: in 5–8 days	Appearance of staining or gush of serosanguineous fluid onto dressing; person feels something "give way" during coughing or vomiting	Splint wound during vigorous coughing or movement. Prevent wound infection. Maintain abdominal binder on obese persons who have had abdominal surgery. Maintain adequate nutrition, hydration, and mobility to aid healing. If occurs, protect wound with sterile dressing; notify physician.	Intact wound. Wound infection prevented if dehiscence occurs.
Wound evisceration:[9] Separation of wound margins and protrusion of abdominal viscera Potential onset: in 5–8 days	As above. Abdominal organs are visible or protrude through incision; assess for symptoms of shock	As above; if occurs, notify physician immediately. Cover area with sterile dressings or towels soaked in sterile saline. Prevent further increase of intraabdominal pressure. Position person in low Fowler's position with knees flexed. Monitor vital signs. Offer reassurance and support. Prepare person for surgery.	Wound intact. If evisceration occurs, signs and symptoms of shock do not occur. Wound infection and damage to visceral organs prevented. Wound heals normally after surgical correction.

Once the person is stabilized, encourage the performance of activities learned during preoperative teaching (e.g., deep-breathing and coughing exercises, extremity exercises, turning, and ambulation). Evaluate and document the person's responses to nursing and medical interventions. Involve support persons whenever possible.

Preventing Intermediate Postoperative Complications. Preventing postoperative complications is an important goal of the intermediate postoperative stage. Table 49–8 outlines potential postoperative complications and nursing interventions related to each complication. Use these guidelines and other resources to develop the postoperative care plan.

CARE DURING THE EXTENDED POSTOPERATIVE STAGE

A person enters the extended postoperative stage 2 to 3 days after surgery. Recovery progresses and the individual approaches discharge. Continue to intervene to meet the needs of the person and support persons, to promote self-care, and to prepare the person for discharge.

During the extended postoperative stage, the wound continues healing and the person resumes some normal routines. Healing requires additional energy. Balanced nutrition is important during recovery. Ambulation, pulmonary exercises, and physical activity aid healing and reestablish normal physiologic patterns (e.g., oxygen exchange, cardiovascular functioning, and elimination). During this phase, the individual and support persons may come to realize fully the implications of the surgery. This realization may be upsetting, even overwhelming. The sensitive nurse is available to give appropriate psychosocial care as needed.

Preventing Long-term Postoperative Complications. From 3 to 10 days after surgery, the person remains in an acute phase of recovery. Preventing complications during the extended postoperative stage continues. Use Table 49–9 as a guideline to assess and prevent postoperative complications during long-term recovery.

Preparation for Discharge. As the trend toward earlier discharge continues, the necessity for thorough discharge planning and teaching increases. Collaborative planning and follow-up with the individual, support persons, and agency/community resources prevent long-term complications and maximize the person's self-care ability.

Begin discharge planning early in the perioperative period. Throughout hospitalization, assess the quality of the person's support system (e.g., involvement of support persons in care). Evaluate the individual's ability to learn and perform self-care activities. Assess the person's psychophysiologic condition at discharge. Consider these factors when making a discharge plan. Some people may require additional assistance at home. If needed, arrange referrals to community agencies and resources (e.g., home health agencies, mental health facilities). Ensure continuity of care by communication with community resources.

Discharge teaching is extremely important. Include support persons in the teaching/learning plan whenever possible. Discharge teaching includes clear instruction, reinforcement, and evaluation of learning. Include clear guidelines on self-care skills, life-style changes, environment modification, and follow-up care. Provide instruction on diet, medications, exercise tolerance, possible complications, and referrals. Reinforce teaching with written guidelines to which the individual can refer while at home.

Evaluation

Evaluation and reassessment in the postoperative phase are continuous. Specific criteria for discharge from the PACU must be met before the transfer of the individual to the surgical unit or phase II recovery area for outpatients (see Box 49–4).[15,18,27] Ideally, the PACU nurse and the surgical unit or phase II recovery nurse collaborate in the evaluation phase as the individual is transferred for extended recovery or observation.

Surgery alters the body systems and basic needs (see Table 49–2). Personality, age and development, surgical risks, preoperative condition, and extent of surgery are some factors that determine a person's response after surgery. Evaluate by comparing data gathered in the preoperative phase with those from the intraoperative and postoperative periods. Knowing the preoperative baseline levels helps you assess changes and problems and plan appropriate interventions.

CASE STUDY

The Client

Ms. Jerry Hayes is a 38-year-old, well-nourished Caucasian who has been admitted through the emergency department with acute abdominal pain, which began 24 hours before admission. The abdominal pain is intermittent in the midepigastric area and radiates to her right shoulder. Ms. Hayes has experienced nausea and vomiting for the past 12 hours. She denies having diarrhea and indicates her last bowel movement was 3 hours before admission. Ms. Hayes indicates she has been in good health with no previous surgery.

A diagnosis of acute cholecystitis with cholelithiasis is made. Ms. Hayes is scheduled for an emergency cholecystectomy at 4:00 PM.

CASE STUDY Continued

The Client

ASSESSMENT DATA

- 38-year-old, well-nourished female
- Height 5'5", weight 138
- Midepigastric pain, 24-hour duration
- Nausea and vomiting, 12-hour duration
- Skin and sclera slightly jaundiced; skin dry, flaky, intact
- States no diarrhea, last BM 8:00 AM today, clay-colored stool
- Temperature = 38.2 °C, blood pressure = 135/80, pulse = 100, respiration = 40

- Pupils dilated bilaterally
- Verbalizes "afraid of being put to sleep and having surgery"
- Abnormal lab values include
  - Total bilirubin = 2.4
  - White blood cell count = 15,000
- States no known allergies

CARE PLAN

2:00 PM, March 23

Nursing Diagnosis	Planning: Expected Outcomes	Implementation: Nursing Interventions	Evaluation
Fear R/T hospitalization with impending emergency surgery (cholecystectomy) and anesthesia	By 4:00 PM, March 23, ► expresses explicit sources of fear related to impending surgery and anesthesia, perception of danger, own coping ability, and need for support	Use therapeutic communication skills to encourage expression of subjective feelings, perception of own coping ability, and perceived need for support and by whom (family, nursing, and so on).	2:30 PM, March 23: verbalized fear of anesthesia/surgery related to grandmother's death under anesthesia at age 75. Expressed understanding that hypertension and cardiac disease contributed to deceased grandmother's heart failure and that client shows no symptoms of same. Stated spouse is strongest support.
	► use appropriate coping mechanisms	Provide explanation of all procedures, sequence of surgical events, and OR, PACU, and unit environment. Initiate teaching and return demonstration of coughing, deep-breathing, and leg exercises and specifics of cholecystectomy, postoperative expectations regarding pain, wound care, home self-care. Request preoperative anesthesia consultation. (Communicate client's fear.)	Spouse included (with permission) in preoperative preparation and teaching. Provided return demonstration and acknowledged understanding. 3:00 PM: requested clergy visit; Pastoral Services contacted for preop visit in holding area. CRNA with client and spouse for preoperative consult.
	► verbalize diminished fear	Involve support persons (with client's permission)	3:30 PM: transported to preop holding area via

Care Plan continued on following page

CARE PLAN Continued

2:00 PM, March 23

Nursing Diagnosis	Planning: Expected Outcomes	Implementation: Nursing Interventions	Evaluation
		in teaching so they can share diminished fear and provide support. Arrange for spouse to accompany to preop holding area and remain until transported to surgery. Offer comfort measures (i.e., touch, clergy visit if desired, keeping wedding ring on [taped in place]). Observe status of fear continuously; report progress toward resolution to anesthesiologist/surgeon. Postoperatively, communicate preop nursing diagnoses to PACU nurse for reassessment of fear after emergence from anesthesia and reinforcement of preop teaching.	stretcher with spouse accompanying. Verbalized diminished fear and positive attitude about surgical outcome. 3:40 PM: received in preop holding area via stretcher from ER, accompanied by spouse. Clergy visited, stated calm and comfortable, vital signs: T = 38.2 °C, BP = 130/80, P = 80, R = 40. Wedding ring taped in place.
High Risk for Infection R/T effects of invasive procedure (cholecystectomy)	By 2:00 PM, March 25 shows no signs of infection AEB: ▶ Temperature below 37.4 °C; other VS WNL ▶ WBC WNL ▶ Incision is free of signs and symptoms of infection (i.e., no redness, swelling, tenderness, warmth, foul odor, purulent drainage) ▶ Wound edges closed, no tissue bulging	Preoperatively in OR: ▶ Identify and communicate abnormal lab values, skin condition, and vital signs. ▶ Ensure operating room cleanliness. ▶ Establish sterile field. ▶ Ensure integrity of sterile supplies before opening. ▶ Use aseptic technique when opening sterile items. ▶ Maintain temperature/humidity in OR according to protocol. ▶ Adhere to protocols for sterilization and disinfection for supplies/instruments. ▶ Ensure proper OR attire of personnel. ▶ Ensure proper surgical hand scrub technique and hand washing.	2:00 PM, March 25: ▶ Operative site clean and dry; no signs or symptoms of infection ▶ Wound edges closed; adhesive strips in place ▶ T-tube secure, minimal serosanguineous drainage around tubing ▶ States no tenderness at operative site ▶ Vital signs: T = 37.1°C, R = 25, P = 65, BP = 125/80

CARE PLAN (Continued)

2:00 PM, March 23

Nursing Diagnosis	Planning: Expected Outcomes	Implementation: Nursing Interventions	Evaluation
		▶ Ensure proper skin preparation of operative site. ▶ Ensure proper gowning, gloving, and draping technique. Intraoperatively in OR: ▶ Continuously monitor sterile field. ▶ Monitor traffic flow in and out of OR; keep OR doors closed to maintain positive pressure. ▶ Implement corrective action for any breaks in aseptic technique.	

Summary

▶ Perioperative nursing is defined as "those nursing activities performed by the professional nurse in the preoperative, intraoperative, and postoperative phases of the patient's surgical experience."[4]

▶ Surgery may be performed for diagnostic, curative, ablative, constructive, reconstructive, and palliative purposes. Surgery is classified as major or minor depending on the degree of risk associated with the operation.

▶ The preoperative, intraoperative, and postoperative phases are the three phases of the perioperative experience.

▶ Surgical nurses work on surgical floors, in the preoperative holding area, in the operating room, in the postanesthesia recovery unit, in phase II recovery units, in intensive care units, and in surgical clinics. Other members of the surgical team include physicians, surgeons, anesthesiologists, nurse anesthetists, and technicians.

▶ Surgery poses many threats to psychophysiologic functioning. Threats may be related to physiologic or psychosocial alterations.

▶ Children undergoing surgery may be anxious about separation from parent figures and familiar objects, possible pain and mutilation, and their own misinterpretations of reality. Adolescents are likely to be anxious about separation from their peers and fear possible disfigurement. Adults fear the unknown, are anxious about separation from support systems, are concerned about dependence and loss of control, and fear that more extensive health problems will be discovered during surgery or that they will die.

▶ Different nursing interventions may be appropriate in relieving anxiety of clients at different developmental levels.

▶ Nurses act as client advocates to ensure that surgical candidates fully understand the implications of surgery and are aware of their legal rights.

▶ In the preoperative phase, nurses meet the client in the admission period, interview the client, and complete a physical assessment that includes identifying risk factors. Nurses diagnose and plan preoperative nursing interventions that often include preoperative teaching, physical preparation, and preparing the person on the day of surgery. Nurses maintain client safety in the intraoperative period and continue to apply the nursing process during postanesthesia care, intermediate postoperative care, and extended postoperative care.

Bibliography

1. American Hospital Association. (1989). *AHA guide.* Chicago: American Hospital Association.
2. Association of Operating Room Nurses. (1987). *Ambulatory surgery anthology.* Denver, CO: Association of Operating Room Nurses.
3. Association of Operating Room Nurses. (1990). *Perioperative nursing documentation.* Denver, CO: Association of Operating Room Nurses.
4. Association of Operating Room Nurses. (1991). *AORN standards and recommended practices for perioperative nursing.* Denver, CO: Association of Operating Room Nurses.
5. Association of Operating Room Nurses. (1991). Recommended practices for preoperative skin preparation of patients. In *AORN standards and recommended practices for perioperative nursing.* Denver, CO: Association of Operating Room Nurses.
6. Avigne, G., & Phillips, T.L. (1991). Pediatric preoperative tours: successful hospital program expands to community. *AORN Journal, 53*(6), 1458–1465.

7. Bailes, B.K. (1989). Perioperative nursing research: part IV: intraoperative phase. *AORN Journal,* 49(5), 1397–1417.

8. Ball, K. (1990). *Lasers: The perioperative challenge.* St. Louis: C.V. Mosby.

9. Black, J.M., & Matassarin-Jacobs, E. (1993). *Luckmann and Sorensen's Medical-surgical nursing: A psychophysiologic approach* (4th ed.). Philadelphia: W.B. Saunders.

10. Carmody, S., et al. (1991). Perioperative needs of families: results of a survey. *AORN Journal,* 54(3), 561–567.

11. Carr, T., & Webster, C.S. (1991). Recovery care centers: an innovative approach to caring for healthy surgical patients. *AORN Journal,* 53(4), 986–995.

12. Centers for Disease Control. (1985). *Guidelines for the prevention and control of nosocomial infections.* Atlanta: Centers for Disease Control.

13. Centers for Disease Control. (1991). Recommendations for preventing transmission of human immunodeficiency virus and hepatitis B virus to patients during exposure-prone invasive procedures. *Morbidity and Mortality Weekly Report,* 40(RR-8), 1–9.

14. Cox, H.C., (1989). *Clinical applications of nursing diagnosis.* Baltimore, MD: Williams & Wilkins.

15. Drain, C.B., & Christoph, S.S. (1987). *The recovery room: A critical approach to post anesthesia nursing* (2nd ed.). Philadelphia: W.B. Saunders.

16. Dripps, R.D., et al. (1988). *Introduction to anesthesia: The principles of safe practice* (7th ed.). Philadelphia: W.B. Saunders.

17. Felver, L., & Pendarues, J.H. (1989). Electrolyte imbalances: intraoperative risk factors. *AORN Journal,* 49(4), 992–1008.

18. Frost, E.A.M. (1990). *Postanesthesia care unit: Current practices* (2nd ed.). St. Louis: C.V. Mosby.

19. Garner, J.S., & Schultz, J.K. (1987). Absence of infection. In Kneedler, J.A., & Dodge, G.H. (eds.). *Perioperative patient care: The nursing perspective* (2nd ed.). Boston: Blackwell Scientific.

20. Gordon, M. (1991). *Nursing diagnosis: Process and application* (3rd ed.). New York: Mosby-Yearbook.

21. Groh, L.K. (1983). *Operating room nursing: The perioperative role.* Reston, VA: Reston Publishing.

22. Gruendemann, B.J. (1987). *Positioning plus.* Chatsworth, CA: Devon Industries.

23. Hoffer, J.L. (1991). Anesthesia. In Meeker, M.H., & Rothrock, J.C. (eds.). *Alexander's care of the patient in surgery* (9th ed., pp. 146–174). St. Louis: Mosby-Yearbook.

24. Holt, L., & Maxwell, B. (1991). Pediatric orientation programs: hospital tours allay children's fears. *AORN Journal,* 54(3), 530–540.

25. Iyer, P., et al. (1991). *Nursing process and nursing diagnosis.* Philadelphia: W.B. Saunders.

26. Kim, M.J., et al. (1991). *Pocket guide to nursing diagnoses.* St. Louis: Mosby-Yearbook.

27. Kitz, D., et al. (1988). Discharging outpatients: factors nurses consider to determine readiness. *AORN Journal,* 48, 87–91.

28. Kneedler, J.A., & Dodge, G.H. (1987). *Perioperative patient care: The nursing perspective* (2nd ed.). Boston: Blackwell Scientific.

29. McFarland, G.K., & Mock, V.L. (1991). In Kim, M.J., McFarland, J.K., & McLane, A.M. (eds.). *Pocket guide to nursing diagnosis.* St. Louis: Mosby-Yearbook.

30. Meeker, M.H., & Rothrock, J.C. (1991). *Alexander's care of the patient in surgery* (9th ed.). St. Louis: Mosby-Yearbook.

31. Moss, R.C. (1986). Overcoming fear. *AORN Journal,* 43(5), 1107–1114.

32. Murphy, E. (1988). Informed consent: part I. *AORN Journal,* 47(4), 1012–1016.

33. Murphy, E. (1988). Informed consent: part II. *AORN Journal,* 47(5), 1268, 1294–1298.

34. Murphy, E. (1988). Informed consent: part III. *AORN Journal,* 47(6), 1466–1471.

35. National Certification Board: Perioperative Nursing. (1990). *CNOR study guide.* Denver, CO: National Certification Board: Perioperative Nursing.

36. North American Nursing Diagnosis Association. (1992). *Taxonomy I revised — 1992.* Kansas City, MO: North American Nursing Diagnosis Association.

37. Rothenburger, R.L. (1990). Transcultural nursing: overcoming obstacles to effective communication. *AORN Journal,* 51(5), 1349–1363.

38. Rothrock, J.C. (1989). Perioperative nursing research: part I: preoperative psychoeducational interventions. *AORN Journal,* 49(2), 597–619.

39. Rothrock, J. (1990). *Perioperative nursing care planning.* St. Louis: Mosby-Yearbook.

40. Siefert, P.C., & Grandusky, R.J. (1990). Nursing diagnosis: their use in developing care plans. *AORN Journal,* 51(4), 1008–1021.

41. Smith, K.A. (1990). Positioning principles on anatomical review. *AORN Journal,* 52(6), 1196–1208.

42. Tollerud, L. (1987). Maintenance of skin integrity. In Kneedler, J.A., & Dodge, G.H. (eds.). *Perioperative patient care: The nursing perspective* (pp. 201–211). Boston: Blackwell Scientific.

43. Yocum, C.J. (1984). The differentiation of fear and anxiety. In Kim, M.J., McFarland, G.K., & McLane, A.M. (eds.). *Classification of Nursing Diagnosis: Proceedings of the Fifth National Conference* (pp. 352–355). St. Louis: C.V. Mosby.

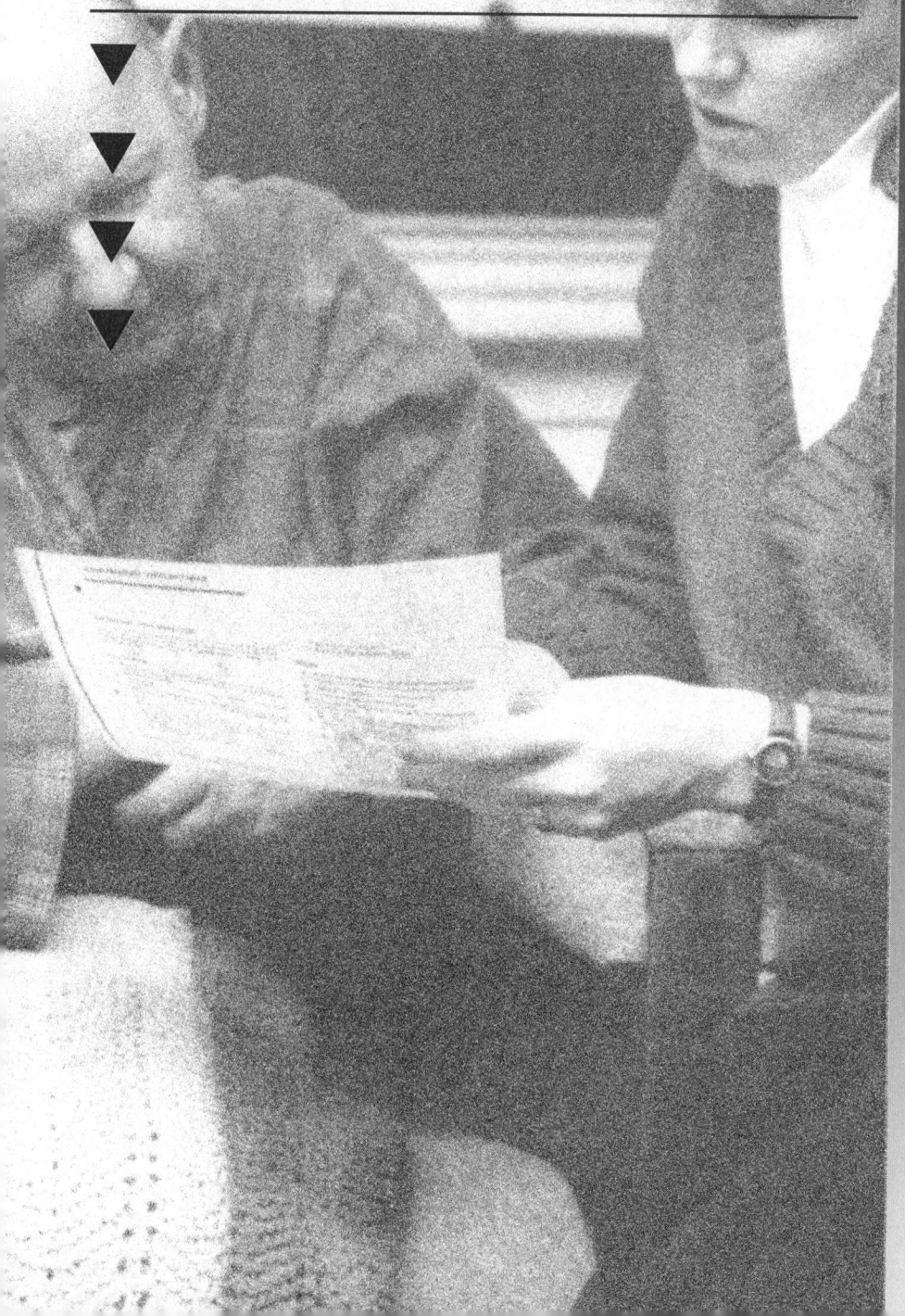

▼ **Applying Nursing Skills to Meet Psychosocial Needs**

▼ Enhancing Self-Concept

Chapter 50

▼ *What concerns me is not the way things are but rather the way people think they are.*

Epictetus

▼ CHAPTER OUTLINE

THEORIES OF SELF-CONCEPT AND SELF-ESTEEM
    Historical Overview of the Concept of Self
    Contemporary Theories Concerning Self-Esteem
RESEARCH ON SELF-CONCEPT
    Early Research
    Relationship Between Illness and Care Givers
    Problems with Research on Self-Esteem
A FAMILY SYSTEMS NURSING APPROACH TO SELF-ESTEEM
SELF-CONCEPT ACROSS THE FAMILY LIFE CYCLE
    Adults
    Families with Infants and Young Children
    Families with School-Age Children
    Families with Adolescents
    Middle-Aged Families
    Aging Families
ASSUMPTIONS ABOUT THE NURSING CARE OF PEOPLE WITH LOW SELF-ESTEEM
ASSESSMENT
    Assess the Problem of Low Self-Esteem
    Assess the Impact of Low Self-Esteem
    Assess the Context in Which Low Self-Esteem Occurs

Assess Beliefs Related to Self-Esteem
Assess Solutions Attempted to Enhance Self-Esteem
Assess Exceptions to the Problem of Low Self-Esteem
Rating Scale Assessment Questions
NURSING DIAGNOSIS
PLANNING
NURSING INTERVENTION
    Validating and Affirming the Client's Experiences
    Commending the Client
    Providing Advice and Information to the Client
    Redefining Normality to Highlight the Client's Strengths
    Normalizing the Client's Responses to Events
    Asking Future-Oriented Questions
    Implementing Bibliotherapy
    Making Behavioral Assignments
    Conducting "Research" on Self-Esteem
    Implementing "Pretending Interventions"
    Narrative Tasks
    Promoting Positive Self-Talk
EVALUATION
CASE STUDY

▼ *KEY TERMS*

Beliefs	Circularity	Future-oriented questions	Normalizing	Self-efficacy
Bibliotherapy	Circular pattern diagrams	Global self-esteem	Reciprocity	Self-esteem
Circular causality	Discounting	Linear causality	Self-concept	Specific self-esteem

---

▼ *LEARNING OBJECTIVES*

After studying this chapter, you should be able to

1. *Define self-concept and self-esteem.*
2. *Discuss theories of self-concept and self-esteem.*
3. *Describe problems with research in the area of self-concept.*
4. *Explain the family systems nursing approach to self-esteem.*
5. *Describe the consequences of high self-esteem in persons across the different stages of the family life cycle.*
6. *Discuss three assumptions and their implications regarding the nursing care of persons with low self-esteem.*
7. *List six areas important to consider while assessing a person with a self-esteem disturbance.*
8. *Discuss the three NANDA-approved nursing diagnoses related to self-esteem.*
9. *Identify two situations in which nursing intervention is contraindicated in a self-esteem disturbance.*
10. *State the focus of planning for the client with low self-esteem.*
11. *List ten interventions that may be helpful in the nursing care of persons with low self-esteem.*
12. *State how to evaluate nursing care for individuals with low self-esteem.*

On a scale of 1 to 10, with 10 being the most confident, how might you rate your own self-concept? If you were asked to rate your self-concept six months ago, would you choose the same rating or a different rating? If you were asked to predict a rating of your self-concept a year from now, which rating would you select? It is very possible that you might choose different ratings over time, depending on the context. Self-concept does not exist in isolation but rather is determined by your context, your beliefs about your capabilities, how you perceive yourself, and how you believe others perceive you. Based on this information, you then develop ideas about yourself and your capabilities. **Beliefs** are the ideas, expectations, attitudes, and opinions held by an individual or family. Your beliefs about self-concept affect virtually everything you think, say, and do. Self-concept affects how you view the world and your place in it. It influences how others view and behave toward you. It affects the choices you make about everything. As noted American feminist Gloria Steinem says, "Self-esteem isn't everything; it's just that there's nothing without it."[33]

You are not born with all the different beliefs you now possess that determine your self-concept. Many of the beliefs that influence your self-concept were acquired prior to adulthood; many other beliefs are constructed as you interact with your environment on a daily basis. Some beliefs may reflect positive images you hold about yourself, whereas others might describe negative ones. Some of these beliefs might be helpful, others unhelpful. Some beliefs actually may constrain you from behaving in different and new ways, because we all have a tendency to behave in accordance with our perception of ourselves.

Your self-concept also influences how you nurse. Your beliefs about your self-concept in relation to yourself as a nurse might be helpful or unhelpful, empowering or constraining.

Your self-concept influences all your interactions with the people with whom you work, and the people for whom you care. Your self-concept is very powerful.

THEORIES OF SELF-CONCEPT AND SELF-ESTEEM

Although the literature on self-concept is enormous, there is no clear definition of self-concept. Many constructs related to categorizing self-concept have evolved, all reflecting the theoretical presuppositions of their authors. The terms *self-concept* and *self-esteem* are often used interchangeably in the literature and will be used interchangeably in this chapter as well. More precisely, however, **self-concept** is an attitude, feeling, or evaluation about oneself, and **self-esteem** is the affective component of the self-concept that describes an attitude, feeling, or evaluation of self-worth.[5,7,24,32]

Maslow, known well to nurses, categorizes self-esteem, not surprisingly, as a need. Other theorists categorize self-esteem as an attitude,[7] a consequence of competence,[3,4] a necessary condition for achievement,[7] and the main purpose of all human activity.[12]

All theorists believe that self-esteem is a component of personality and is probably influenced by all psychologic events.[4] In the tradition of the interactionists, self-concept is believed to be constructed through social interaction from the time of birth to the present.[6,39]

You observe the responses of others toward you, and your perceptions of others' responses to you greatly influence how you construct your self-concept.[5]

APPLYING RESEARCH TO NURSING PRACTICE

Enhancing Self-Concept by Helping Clients Work with the Patterns of a Chronic Illness

Gulick, E.E. & Bugg, A. (1992). Holistic health patterning in multiple sclerosis. *Research in Nursing & Health,* 15, 175–185.

▼ ▼ ▼

To enhance the self-concept of clients diagnosed with a chronic disease, nurses need to understand the expected course of the illness. Armed with that understanding, nurses can teach these clients what to expect at different stages of their illness. Unfortunately, the courses of some chronic diseases, such as multiple sclerosis, have not been well identified. Gulick and Bugg sought to identify patterns in the development of the symptoms of multiple sclerosis, which include extremity weakness, spasms, tremors, problems with balance, blurred and double vision, difficulty in swallowing, forgetfulness, pain, burning sensations, numbness, and "pins and needles" sensations. Loneliness, depression, and anxiety are common emotional symptoms. The researchers also wanted to examine how symptoms affected self-care activities.

Over a 5-year period, these nurse researchers evaluated the health patterns of 211 clients with multiple sclerosis. All the subjects reported a decline in fine and gross motor abilities and in intimate relationships. Those who were alive 5 years after diagnosis reported the greatest surge in symptoms, such as leg weakness and loss of balance. These clients also experienced the sharpest decrease in fine and gross motor self-care abilities and a greater decline in intimate relationships. The older the client was at the time of diagnosis, the worse the decline in all areas of self-care activities. One important exception to this general decline was the preservation of communication abilities, such as reading, writing, and using the telephone. All clients in the study reported anxiety, depression, and loneliness, and these symptoms had not changed from year to year.

Applications for Practice

Teach clients newly diagnosed with multiple sclerosis the reasons for their symptoms and for the consequent decline in self-care abilities. Stress the relationship between successful achievement of self-care activities and enhancement of self-concept. As the client experiences deficits in self-care, teach the client about the use of assistive devices to help with declines in mobility. To combat social isolation and promote self-care, encourage the client to read, write, and communicate by mail or telephone.

by persons diagnosed with cancer and the amount of social support they enjoy.

The ability of individuals to change their self-concept depending on the context is of particular interest to persons diagnosed with cancer. Some researchers believe that individuals devalue the competencies they no longer perform well, as occurs in the case of debilitat-

ing illness, in an attempt to maintain high self-esteem.[21] This ability is also known as **discounting.** Discounting may be an important predictor of long-term adjustment.

IMPORTANCE OF ENHANCED SELF-ESTEEM TO CARE GIVERS

Most primary care givers of elderly persons are middle-aged, female family members. Those care givers who receive affection, affirmation, and assistance from their social network have higher self-esteem than those who do not. Those care givers with lower self-esteem reported losing a greater number of important relationships in the past year, usually by death or from relocation.

In this study by a nurse researcher, the type of network, the number of relationships, the frequency of contact, or the duration of these relationships did not matter. What did matter was that the care givers received love, validation, and help from other family members and friends. These findings suggest that self-esteem is important to cultivate in care givers as well as in those receiving care. Care givers must see themselves as valuable and worthy of meeting their own needs in order to give care.[27] Nurses need to be aware of losses experienced by care givers that have the potential for decreased social support and losses in self-esteem.

Problems with Research on Self-Esteem

Kersten, a nurse researcher from California, points out problems related to the study of self-esteem and self-concept.[14] First, self-concept is a more difficult construct to measure than anxiety or depression or other more clearly defined psychosocial behaviors. Second, Kersten suggests that no agreement exists about what self-concept should be at different developmental stages. In her work she was referring to stages of pulmonary rehabilitation, but her thesis could apply to stages of growth and development, chronic illness, or life-threatening illness.

Curbow, also a nurse researcher, and her associates suggest that the many self-esteem and self-concept measuring instruments are too global to be sensitive to the differences and similarities of experiences of individuals with certain types of cancer.[8] For example, women with breast cancer might place more value on sexuality, whereas this might not be as valued in persons receiving bone marrow transplants.

Many of the self-esteem and self-concept instruments cannot measure the construct in relation to specific populations. Curbow calls for the development of new instruments that can focus on aspects of self-concept and self-esteem in specific populations.

Another criticism of current self-esteem instruments relates to gender bias. As you might guess, what one researcher thinks important to measure when studying self-esteem might be very different from what another researcher thinks important. Often the items being measured reflect the beliefs and culture of the researcher. Many scales emphasize the importance of competitiveness and independence, which are traits usually valued by Western male society. It is not surprising that men often score higher on these self-esteem measures than women do. This may have more to do with the design of the scale than with self-esteem.[26] Again, a call is made for development of gender-sensitive measures of self-esteem and self-concept.

A FAMILY SYSTEMS NURSING APPROACH TO SELF-ESTEEM

A family systems nursing approach assumes that behavior does not occur in isolation: All behaviors are understood within an individual's relational context. This is the difference between a family systems nursing approach and a more traditional approach. The traditional approach focuses on the individual, whereas a family systems nursing approach focuses on the context in which such symptoms as low self-esteem occur. A family systems nursing approach can be useful in your work with individuals, their families, and their health problems. *How* you conceptualize the problem influences your nursing assessment and interventions, not the number of people in the interview or hospital room.

Dr. Lorraine Wright and her colleagues at The University of Calgary's Family Nursing Unit have been employing a family systems nursing approach in their clinical work with individuals, couples, and families with health problems. Wright and Leahey studied trends in the nursing of families and found that the use of family systems nursing is increasing. Family systems nursing is the integration of nursing theory and practice, systems theory, cybernetics, and family therapy theories and practice.[43]

Dr. Wendy Watson and Dr. Janice Bell, also of The University of Calgary, recently documented their clinical work that illustrated the relationship between self-esteem and marital identity.[39] One partner's low self-esteem became better understood by exploring the relationship between that partner's low self-esteem and the context of the marital relationship. It is not surprising that the wife's low self-esteem influenced the couple's identity as a couple and vice versa. It became impossible to conceptualize the wife's low self-esteem without considering the marital relationship. The interrelationship between self-esteem and context is one marked by circular causality. More complicated than **linear causality** (the process of one event causing another, as in A → B), **circular causality (reciprocity or circularity)** is the process of one event or behavior affecting another event or behavior, and then the second event or behavior influencing or affecting the first event or behavior, as in A → B → A.

The reciprocity between self-esteem and context can be pictorially represented by a circular pattern diagram, as developed by Dr. Karl Tomm of The University of Calgary.[35] **Circular pattern diagrams** (CPDs) are schematic representations of reciprocal interaction patterns. CPDs graphically depict the reciprocal influence

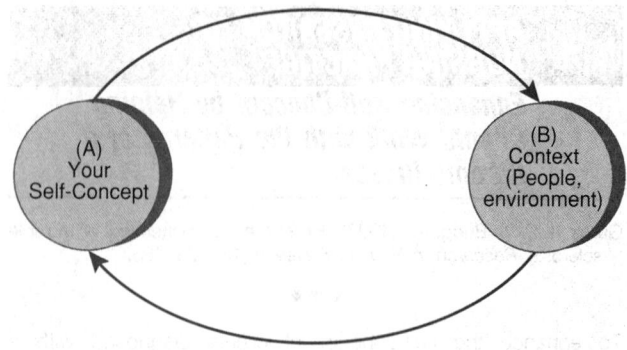

▲ *Figure 50–1*

Circular pattern diagram (CPD) of the reciprocal relationship between self-concept and context. Your self-concept *(A)* influences context *(B)*; conversely, context *(B)* influences your self-concept *(A)*. If your context is supportive, chances are that your self-esteem will be enhanced and that you will invite the people in your environment to continue to be supportive. In other words, Event A influences Event B, which influences Event A.

of behaviors and inferences or interpretations (cognitive, affective, or both). They can be used to illustrate the influence of self-esteem on context, and the reciprocal influence of context on self-esteem.

Interactional patterns can represent either vicious (negative) or virtuous (positive) patterns of interaction.[37,41]

Figure 50–1 illustrates the reciprocal relationship between self-concept and context.

SELF-CONCEPT ACROSS THE FAMILY LIFE CYCLE

The family life cycle, like other developmental frameworks, maps out stages and phases of development for family members. Unlike individual life cycle theories, family life cycle theory recognizes the contributions of all family members who may be at different individual developmental stages of family functioning. Like individual life cycle frameworks, the family life cycle delineates tasks that the family must negotiate successfully in order to reach the next developmental stage.[41] The focus of the following discussion of the family life cycle is limited to the positive and negative consequences of high self-esteem during these stages as well as strategies on how family members can be helpful to other members in fostering increased levels of self-esteem.

Adults

The positive consequences of high self-esteem in adults have been well documented and are listed in Box 50–3.

In a couple, one partner's self-esteem influences the self-esteem of the other partner, and ultimately the partnership. This is the reciprocal influence that underpins a family systems nursing approach to self-esteem.

Families with Infants and Young Children

INFANTS

As mentioned in the earlier discussion of psychodynamic theories of self-esteem, infants who learn to trust that their environment will provide for their basic needs reap the benefits of a solid foundation of self-esteem. During an infant's second year, several developmental milestones are reached related to mobility, speech, and bowel and bladder control. Each of these events offers opportunities for children to increase their competence in mastering the world. As can be expected, if the family responds with encouragement and validation, infants will come to trust their competence. Conversely, if the family responds with impatience or discipline, children learn to mistrust their capabilities for competency and may even experience shame and guilt.[10] Infants do not, of course, have the ability to evaluate themselves. It is the care giver's responsibility to lay a firm foundation for the child's future self-esteem.

TODDLERS

Self-esteem in toddlers is heavily influenced by parental influences and by the toddlers' growth and development.[30] At this stage in the family life cycle, toddlers require encouragement and limit setting, which contribute to developing competencies.

PRESCHOOL CHILDREN

One of the most critical milestones in the self-esteem development of preschoolers includes references to "I." This signals beginning self-awareness. Children at this stage start to understand that they are no longer omnipotent. Their world expands to include their siblings and peers, whereas it previously consisted of themselves and their parents.[30]

Although young children do not have the ability to verbalize their concept of their own self-worth, this does not mean that young children do not possess a sense of self-esteem. They show their self-esteem as they continually master new behaviors within their behavioral repertoires.[18]

Families with School-Age Children

School-age children, for the first time, start comparing themselves with their peers. The self-esteem of school-age children is determined by an assessment of their own abilities and what they believe others judge them to be. Self-esteem determines the variety of new experiences a child might attempt. School-age children can clearly differentiate five specific domains on most self-esteem instruments: academic competence, athletic competence, peer acceptance, behavioral conduct, and physical appearance.[18]

The positive consequences of high self-esteem in children are listed in Box 50–3. Box 50–4 lists strategies parents can use to foster self-esteem in their school-age children.

Sieving and Zirbel-Donisch, pediatric nurse practitioners, emphasize the importance of nurses assessing that the parents' expectations of their child are attainable, age-appropriate, and developmentally appropriate.[30]

If the parents' expectations are too high, too low, or age-inappropriate, review of developmental milestones and child growth and development patterns by the nurse is indicated.

Small observed that mothers with high self-esteem perceive their children to be independent and responsible.[31] These children perceived their mothers to be less controlling than the mothers with lower self-esteem levels. These children were also more likely to report that they had greater input in decision-making, a practice related to increasing children's competence, independence, and responsibility. One of the explanations for this observation is that mothers of independent children may feel better about themselves, possibly because they derive some satisfaction from what they perceive as positive and desirable behavior in their more independent children.

Families with Adolescents

In addition to the five specific domains that school-age children can clearly differentiate, adolescents can also differentiate the three domains of friendship, romantic appeal, and job competence. Although close friendship is comprehended by school-age children, they cannot differentiate it from more general peer acceptance, suggesting that the distinction between popularity and close friendship does not emerge until early adolescence.[20]

A study of 400 adolescents produced several interesting observations.[15] First, younger adolescents have higher self-esteem than older adolescents. Self-esteem seems to decline when children leave elementary school and enter high school. Second, young adolescent boys are more likely than adolescent girls to be influenced by friends' opinions of them. Young adolescent girls are more likely to be influenced by teachers' opinions of them. However, as adolescents develop, both peers and teachers influence boys and girls equally. Third, parents' views of adolescents continue to influence adolescent self-evaluation. This is contrary to popular belief, which had suggested that as children enter adolescence, their parents' "window of influence" closes to make room for peers' influences. It now seems that both parents and peers influence adolescents' self-concept. Fourth, the perceived evaluation of friends has the greatest influence on older adolescent girls' self-esteem, whereas the perceived evaluation of their father has the greatest influence on older adolescent boys' self-esteem.

Another study found that it is the perception that an adolescent ascribes to a life event as being either positive or negative that primarily contributes to self-esteem, not the event itself. This occurs regardless of how stressful the event may seem to have been.[44]

Small[31] conducted one of the more interesting studies that illustrates the reciprocal relationship between parents' sense of self-worth and how parents interact with their adolescents. He studied the relationship between parental self-esteem and various aspects of parent-adolescent interaction and adolescent behavior. One trend he observed was that adolescents of mothers with lower self-esteem perceived their mothers as more controlling and constraining than adolescents of mothers with higher self-esteem. If the father's self-esteem was also lower, there was a greater likelihood that an adolescent reported being struck by the father.

Small offers two possible explanations for the finding that parents with lower self-esteem are more likely to discipline with corporal control and to allow their adolescents less autonomy and room for decision-making. First, parents who are low in self-esteem may feel powerless and ineffectual in general. They may hang on more tightly to those areas of their life, such as parenting, in which they feel they still have some control. Second, parents with low self-esteem may be more distracted by their own worries and problems and, consequently, be less sensitive to the needs and desires of their children. From a family systems nursing perspective, this parental behavior might invite adolescents to demand more support from their parents than they are currently receiving. The adolescents' behavior might then make their parents realize that they are not responding to their children's needs, thus making the parents feel more ineffective and contributing to lower self-esteem. The reciprocal relationship between parental behaviors and adolescent behaviors is illustrated in Figure 50-2. As you can see, parental and adolescent behaviors reciprocally influence the self-esteem of each other.

Middle-Aged Families

Contrary to popular opinion, self-esteem in parents does not decline as their children leave home. Self-esteem and marital satisfaction usually increase among couples at this stage of the family life cycle. Middle-aged families are often called the "sandwich generation" as they strive to meet the demands of their elderly family members and the launching activities of their young adults. McCrae observed differences in the prominence of certain aspects across developmental stages.[21] Young adults describe themselves more in terms of routine tasks, personal relationships, personality traits, and family roles. Older adults describe themselves more in terms of life circumstances, interests, beliefs, and hobbies. As mentioned earlier, the primary care givers of elderly persons are usually female family members at this stage of development.

Aging Families

Atchley reports that four of five elderly persons have high self-esteem.[1] This finding should debunk popular

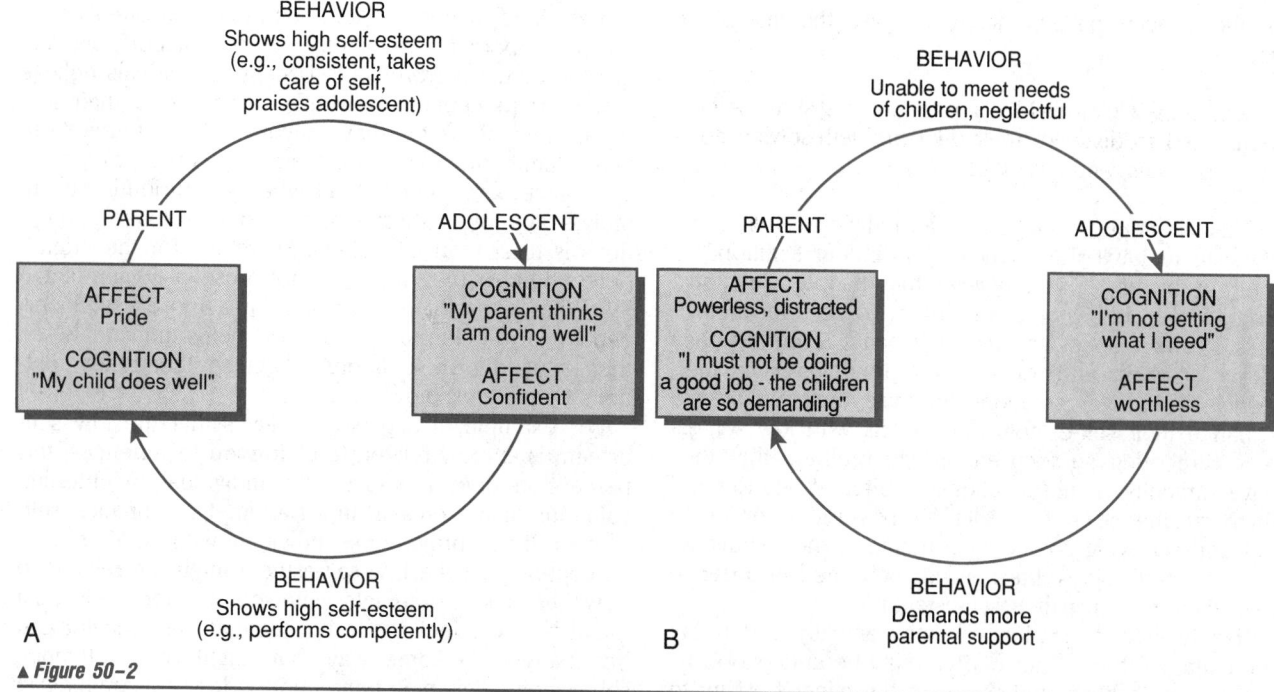

▲ *Figure 50–2*

A, Circular pattern diagram (CPD) illustrating positive (or virtuous) reciprocal relationship between parental behavior and adolescent behavior.
B, Circular pattern diagram (CPD) illustrating negative (or vicious) reciprocal relationship between parental behavior and adolescent behavior.

myths about the low self-worth that elderly persons are purported to have.

Aging can be a time of loss. Deteriorating health, loss of function, reduced independence, retirement, and deaths of friends, relatives, and partners all influence self-esteem. Those elderly persons who have the ability to anticipate death as an inevitable component of life usually continue to esteem themselves through this stage of the family life cycle.[32]

ASSUMPTIONS ABOUT THE NURSING CARE OF PEOPLE WITH LOW SELF-ESTEEM

The purpose of all nursing assessments and interventions is change. In this chapter, obviously, the goal of all assessments and interventions is the enhancement of self-concept for those individuals who identify poor self-esteem as a problem. It is helpful if you consider the following assumptions when you use the nursing process to assess, plan, intervene, and evaluate a plan of care for persons with self-esteem disturbances.

Assumption #1: Low self-esteem is best understood and treated from a circular rather than a linear perspective.

Leahey and Wright believe that this assumption is the most important assumption to use when employing a family systems nursing approach to all psychosocial problems.[17] Circularity refers to the reciprocal influence between two events or behaviors. Understanding the impact that low self-esteem has on individuals and their families is just as important as understanding the influence individuals and/or families might also have on self-esteem. A family systems nursing approach to self-esteem does not aim to find a cause-and-effect relationship for *why* a person shows low self-esteem. Rather, a family systems nursing approach aims to identify and interpret the patterns of interaction that contribute to and maintain low self-esteem. This is much different from a linear perspective of self-esteem that attempts to assign blame in a more traditional cause-and-effect model of understanding psychosocial problems. A family systems nursing approach is more interested in assessing the influence of both self-esteem and the context in which low self-esteem is maintained in order to develop useful nursing interventions.

Circular pattern diagrams are helpful in depicting interactional patterns of low and high self-esteem. Interactions, as mentioned previously, can be either vicious or virtuous. Vicious patterns are those interactions that require nursing assessment and intervention. Virtuous interactions are commendable, are adaptive, and do not require intervention.[35,37,41] Refer back to Figure 50–1 to see a circular pattern diagram of a virtuous circle of interaction.

Circular pattern diagrams include behaviors and interpretations regarding meaning. The interpretations typically include affective and cognitive components. Affective interpretations refer to feelings ("What do you *feel* when you see a particular behavior?"). Cognitive interpretations refer to thoughts or beliefs ("What do you *think* when you see a particular behavior?"). Affect and cognition influence behavior, and conversely, behavior influences affect and cognition. Each component of the circular pattern diagram drives the interactive pattern.

Assumption #2: Individuals experiencing low self-esteem need to discover their own problem-solving abilities, resources, and strengths.

This assumption suggests that individuals with low self-esteem have the capacity for finding solutions to their problems. If you believe that people can solve their own problems, you will not try to do it for them.[17] This shows respect for the skills and resources they already possess and use to solve problems. Help individuals rediscover solutions and use their abilities to enhance their self-esteem. Individuals with low self-esteem are often so focused on the problem that they have difficulty seeing solutions or alternatives. Remind them of the skills they already possess in order to develop satisfying solutions. Sometimes, these individuals have capabilities that need to be honed in order to help them enhance their self-esteem.

If you are too helpful, you may actually undermine the client's efforts. Your efforts might be understood by a client as lack of confidence in the client's ability to independently engage in activities. A circular pattern diagram of this kind of interaction between a nurse and a client is depicted in Figure 50–3.

Assumption #3: Often an individual's ability to enhance self-esteem depends upon the person's ability to alter the perception of the problem.

Leahey and Wright offer this third assumption regarding the very important variable of *perception* in enhancing self-esteem.[17] According to much of the research cited in this chapter, self-esteem is often determined by perceptions or expectations of performance, not the actual performance. Usually, individuals believe that their perception of what contributes to their low self-esteem is truer than anyone else's perception. Other family members, and the nurse as well, may have alternative perceptions about what is contributing to an individual's low self-esteem, but none of these perceptions is truer than the others. Searching for the "right" perception, or the "truth," is not a useful nursing activity. What is useful is searching for a more useful perception or an alternative truth that helps individuals see their situations in a different light so that other solutions become visible.[17]

For example, if a person believes that the low self-esteem is entirely related to childhood experiences, this perception does not invite the individual to entertain solutions in the present in an attempt to enhance self-esteem. If you provide this individual with an alternative perception that the low self-esteem might be related to how the client interacts with others, the individual might be more inclined to believe that the behavior can be changed in some way that might then influence self-esteem. This new perception is less constraining: it opens up possibilities that did not exist with the initial perception.

ASSESSMENT

Assess the Problem of Low Self-Esteem

Obtain a clear behavioral definition of what it means to the client to have low self-esteem. If other family members are available, obtain their perspective regarding when they notice the client showing low self-esteem.

Many clients will tell you that they want to "feel better about themselves." This description of the problem is simply not good enough when working with persons with self-esteem disturbances.

To obtain a clear behavioral description of the problem, ask the client to give you a "videotape description" of what it means to have low self-esteem. When asking for a videotape description, invite the client to describe situations in which he or she shows low self-esteem. The client will usually describe concrete events. The videotape description will help you and the client collaborate to develop attainable goals for change. Obtaining a description of what it means to have low self-esteem also includes determining when the client first noticed this was a problem, how often it occurs, and who else notices that self-esteem is a problem for this client.

Another way to obtain a clear behavioral description of what it means to have low self-esteem is to ask clients how they *show* their low self-esteem. Using the verb "show" also invites the client to describe the self-esteem disturbance in behavioral terms. Asking a family member how the client *shows* low self-esteem will usually elicit a behavioral description of the problem.

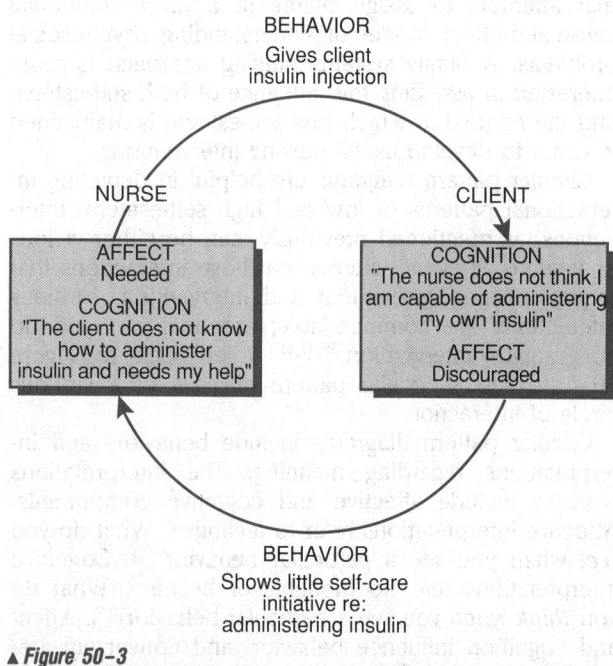

▲ **Figure 50–3**

Circular pattern diagram (CPD) of an unhelpful interaction between a nurse and a client.

The following questions may be useful as initially you assess a person with low self-esteem:

Ask the client:

▶ What is your concern about your self-esteem?
▶ When did you first notice this was a problem?
▶ Who else notices that low self-esteem is a problem for you?
▶ Could you please give me a "videotape description" of what it means for you to have low self-esteem?
▶ How do you show your low self-esteem?
▶ To whom do you mostly show your low self-esteem?

Ask the family:

▶ How does the client show low self-esteem to you?

Assess the Impact of Low Self-Esteem

Assessing the impact of low self-esteem leads to an understanding of *how* this is a problem for the client and also sets the stage for assessing the reciprocity between self-esteem and context. A self-esteem disturbance usually influences several aspects of a person's life. Low self-esteem may affect a person's self-concept, relationships with others, abilities to interact, abilities to perform a job, and virtually everything else. For some people, low self-esteem is a problem in only some of these areas, whereas for others it may affect all areas. Assessing *how* low self-esteem affects an individual in areas of a person's life will help you and the client understand the influence and power of this problem.

The following questions may be useful as you assess the impact of low self-esteem on a client's life:

▶ What is the impact of low self-esteem on your life?
▶ How does low self-esteem influence your relationships with your family?
▶ How does low self-esteem affect your marriage?
▶ How does low self-esteem affect how you perform at work?
▶ How does low self-esteem affect how you manage your illness?
▶ What does low self-esteem prevent you from doing?
▶ How does low self-esteem prevent you from trying new behaviors?

Assess the Context in Which Low Self-Esteem Occurs

If you believe that self-esteem is best understood and treated from a family systems nursing, or circular, perspective, assess the context in which low self-esteem occurs.

You will have collected some of the assessment data related to context by this time. Determine when a person most often shows low self-esteem and how this influences his or her life. This will give you a beginning understanding of the reciprocity between self-esteem and context. The knowledge you already have about growth and development and the family life cycle will assist you in assessing context. Consider, for example,

an adult daughter who believes that her aging mother has low self-esteem. When you ask the daughter for evidence about how she arrived at this assessment, she replies that she notices that when she visits her mother in the mother's home, she usually finds her mother sitting in the dark with the drapes drawn. The adult daughter concludes that her mother must be feeling poorly about herself and may even be depressed. You know that one of the physiologic changes of aging is decreased tolerance for bright lights. It may be that the mother is simply avoiding bright daylight because it bothers her eyes. Share this fact with the daughter. You may alter the daughter's perception that her mother is suffering from low self-esteem.

Assessing context may also involve assessing other people's responses to a person with low self-esteem. Ask questions to track the sequence of events surrounding a situation in which a person is showing low self-esteem. For example, ask parents what they do when their child shows low self-esteem behavior to determine how the parents' behaviors influence or maintain the child's low self-esteem. If a teenager laments that she or he cannot self-administer the necessary insulin, the parent may perform this task, thus reinforcing the teenager's belief that the teenager is not capable of doing it. The parent is then convinced that the adolescent's inability to give the insulin is related to low self-esteem. Obtaining this sort of information is valuable for planning nursing interventions. Assessing an individual's self-esteem without considering the context can prove costly to a nurse attempting to develop interventions targeted at enhancing self-concept. Circular pattern diagrams are useful in depicting the relationship between self-esteem and context. Share the beginning sketch of a circular pattern diagram with a client so you can co-construct the diagram in its entirety, leading to the development of interventions.

The following questions may be helpful in assessing the context related to self-esteem disturbance:

▶ When you show low self-esteem, what do your parents do? What do you do? What do they do? And then what happens?
▶ What do you think when you see your parents make all your decisions for you? How do you feel?
▶ What do you think your parents are thinking when you state you don't know what to do about your health problem? What do you think they feel?
▶ How do you think your parents might interpret your actions?

Assess Beliefs Related to Self-Esteem

Beliefs about the cause, consequence, and cure of low self-esteem affect the way an individual performs. As with all psychosocial problems, it is important to assess beliefs, since the meaning an individual and family members assign to low self-esteem may determine the nursing intervention.[17]

Individuals who believe that their low self-esteem is amenable to change will be managed differently from individuals who believe that they have no control over enhancing their low self-esteem.

Ask individuals what they believe will happen if things stay the same or if their current level of self-esteem does not change. Responses to this question usually elicit fears. By overtly acknowledging these fears, it is sometimes possible to move forward instead of remaining stuck with the belief that change is impossible. For example, a never-married client believed that if she did not enhance her self-esteem, she might never marry, and marriage represented a desirable goal for this woman. She might view the task of enhancing her self-esteem as enormous because the desired outcome seems unattainable. Although enhancing self-esteem in order to find a partner is a noble and worthwhile goal, it might also seem formidable because of its magnitude. Identifying an individual's beliefs regarding the perceived consequences of low self-esteem will assist you and the client in formulating more attainable goals, such as practicing asking for a date, which eventually might lead to enhanced self-esteem and mate selection.

Some individuals have very clear ideas of what they believe needs to happen in order for them to enhance their self-esteem. Ask individuals about their belief regarding a "cure" to obtain valuable assessment data about what the client believes would be helpful. Very often clients know exactly what they need to do but do not know how to do it. This is an invitation for you to develop interventions designed specifically for that individual.

Beliefs and expectations about beliefs are very powerful, as indicated in the research section of this chapter. Often a person's belief or expectation about self-concept determines performance, not actual ability.

The following questions may be helpful in assessing beliefs related to self-esteem:

▶ What is your belief about why you are not able to show higher levels of self-esteem?
▶ What do you believe will happen if your self-esteem does not change?
▶ What do you believe will happen if you enhance your self-esteem?
▶ What do you believe is the cure to your particular self-esteem problem?
▶ What do you believe you need to do to enhance your self-esteem?
▶ What gets in your way of doing the things you believe you need to do to enhance your self-esteem?

Assess Solutions Attempted to Enhance Self-Esteem

Assessing solutions that the client has attempted in order to enhance self-esteem provides information not only about what strategies have been unsuccessful, but also those that have been successful. Assessing unsuccessful solutions also helps you understand what *not* to do when designing an intervention.

For example, clients who tell you that they have tried reading five self-help books on how to enhance their self-esteem and have not found these books helpful are also telling you that reading self-help books is not a useful strategy for them. Do not prescribe more reading to such a client. If clients tell you that they used self-talk successfully in the past to encourage themselves to act more confidently, find out more about this particular strategy. Encourage clients to do more of this behavior since it has a good track record.

Asking clients about strategies they have previously used highlights the resources and strengths they possess in relation to problem-solving. Usually, a client has tried several different strategies before bringing the problem to a health care professional such as a nurse. You just might be impressed with all the solutions tried in the past! Start by asking general questions and progress to more specific questions in order to identify the most effective and least effective strategies. Include queries about when these strategies were used.[37,42]

In addition to assessing the solutions a person has attempted to increase self-esteem, assess specific advice that an individual or family receives from other family members, friends, and health care professionals.[17] Solutions are often embedded in other people's advice. An individual or family will assign some sort of value either to the advice itself or to the people who proffer it. For example, good advice may come from someone whose opinion is not valued by an individual, so the person is less likely to follow it. On the other hand, inaccurate information or advice might be offered by a source the family esteems. Assess the relative value an individual assigns to either the advice or the advisors.

The following questions may be helpful in assessing attempted solutions:

▶ What have you done so far to increase your low self-esteem?
▶ What strategies have you used to enhance your self-esteem in the past?
▶ What is the most effective strategy you have used so far to enhance your self-esteem?
▶ What is the least effective strategy you have used so far to enhance your self-esteem?
▶ Have you received any advice from anyone about how to enhance your self-concept?
▶ What is the most useful piece of advice you have received about enhancing your self-esteem?
▶ Who gave you this piece of advice?
▶ What is the least useful piece of advice you have received about how to enhance your self-esteem?
▶ Who gave you this piece of advice?

Assess Exceptions to the Problem of Low Self-Esteem

Regardless of the magnitude or chronicity of problems people experience, there are always situations in which for some reason the problem does not happen.[25] Assessing exceptions to the problem, or noting when self-esteem is not a problem, is just as valuable as assessing when it is. The exceptions to the problem offer valuable information about what is needed to solve the problem. If a person wants to have higher levels of self-esteem, you need to help assess what is different about the times the person finds that self-esteem is *not* a problem.[25]

Asking clients about exceptions often takes them by surprise. Their experience in dealing with health care professionals, including nurses, usually involves great interest in exploring only the problem. When asking about exceptions to the problem, attempt to temporarily redirect an individual's attention from the problem to what is already working. No one can suffer from low self-esteem 24 hours a day, 7 days a week, 365 days a year. A person who did could never leave home or perform any task. Ask questions about when clients show higher levels of self-esteem, to invite them to disclose strategies they may not have thought were connected to the problems of low self-esteem and their solutions. For example, if a client complains of poor self-esteem at work but admits to being able to lead a Girl Scout or Girl Guide troop competently, explore how the client manages to feel confident in this context.

The ultimate goal of this line of questioning is to discover the skills and resources that currently exist in the client's behavioral repertoire and to attempt to apply them to problem situations. Exploring with the client how she manages to feel confident with scouting activities might lead to solutions useful in other contexts. Clients might say they are able to show confidence because of their detailed preparations. Increasing organizational skills in preparation for other activities might be a useful solution to clients in other situations.

Use careful wording when assessing exceptions to the problem. Do not ask, "Have there been times when you feel more confident?" This question sets the context for an individual to deny that there ever are times when he or she feels more confident. Instead, ask, "What is it like when you show higher levels of self-esteem?" This wording presupposes that there are times when clients do not suffer from low self-esteem. It does not matter how brief or how slight the exception seems. Once an individual reports even a fleeting moment when he or she felt more confident, ask some of the following questions that may be helpful in assessing exceptions to the problem:

▶ Tell me about the times when you show higher self-esteem (or more confidence in yourself).
▶ What is different about these times than when you show low self-esteem?
▶ How do you manage to show more confidence in these particular situations?
▶ How does it make your day go differently when you have more confidence?
▶ Who else notices when you have more confidence?
▶ In what way could you tell that they noticed? What did they do or say?

Rating Scale Assessment Questions

Use rating scale assessment questions to assess the client's and other family members' perceptions of the severity of the problem and change over time. Ask, "On a scale of 1 to 10, with 10 being the most confident, where would you rate your self-esteem today?" This question invites the client to select a definite number on a 10-point scale. If other family members are accessible, ask them how they would rate the client's self-confidence on the same scale. Any discrepancy between the client's rating and a family member's rating is fodder for a therapeutic conversation. If the client rates herself as a 3 on a scale of 1 to 10 and her spouse rates her as a 5, show curiosity about the difference. Ask the following questions:

▶ How might I understand the difference between these two ratings?
▶ Of the two of you, who is most surprised about the difference?
▶ How does your spouse show you that he or she is a 5 on a 10-point scale and not a 3?

Rating scale questions provide helpful assessment data for the setting of reasonable goals. For example, asking the aforementioned client who rated herself as a 3 on a 10-point scale to change her behavior to reflect a person with a rating of 10, a 70 per cent improvement, will seem impossible! Rather, ask the client to entertain the idea of a 10 per cent improvement or to *act as though* the self-esteem is at a rating of 4 instead of 3. This smaller request for change may seem more achievable. To invite a client to improve self-esteem by 10 per cent, ask:

▶ What would it take to change your self-esteem rating from a 3 to a 4 on the 10-point scale?
▶ What would you do differently?

Rating scale questions also invite the client to consider making small steps toward increasing self-concept:

▶ On a scale of 1 to 10 with 10 being the most confident, how would you rate your self-esteem?
▶ On the same scale, how would you rate your self-esteem 1 week ago?
▶ On the same scale, how would you predict you might rate your self-esteem 1 year from now?
▶ At what rating would you be satisfied?
▶ Recognizing that things are never perfect, where on the scale would you be when things are satisfactory?

NURSING DIAGNOSIS

Currently NANDA has approved three nursing diagnoses related to self-esteem:[34]

▶ *Self-Esteem Disturbance*
▶ *Chronic Low Self-Esteem*
▶ *Situational Low Self-Esteem* (see Nursing Diagnosis Profile)

The characteristics that appear in all these nursing diagnoses include

▶ self-negating verbalization
▶ expressions of shame or guilt or both
▶ evaluation of self as unable to deal with events[34]

NURSING DIAGNOSIS PROFILE

Situational Low Self-Esteem

Definition. The state of negative self-evaluation or negative feelings that develops in response to a loss or change in an individual who previously had a positive self-evaluation.

Classification. Perceiving 7.1.2.2.

Defining Characteristics. Individuals who suffer from *Situational Low Self-Esteem* typically have experienced a life event that has negatively influenced their previous positive self-evaluation. Usually these individuals talk about how helpless, useless, and powerless they feel. They may also have difficulty making decisions, believe that they are unable to handle situations or events they previously would have handled, and may also express feelings of shame or guilt because of their perceived incompetence.

Sample Related Factors. The precipitating experiences usually involve loss or change, such as:

▶ illness
▶ loss of function due to illness
▶ alteration in body image
▶ loss of spouse, child, parent, or other significant person
▶ role change
▶ role loss
▶ loss of status
▶ violence
▶ psychologic trauma
▶ stressful change

These life experiences may contribute to lowering an individual's level of self-esteem.

Concept Description. One part of a 1985 clinical validation study conducted by Norris and Kunes-Connell,* clinical nurse specialists in psychiatric mental health nursing, identified characteristics and explored situations and factors that contribute to *Situational Low Self-Esteem.*

The researchers categorized subjects as suffering from a functional or temporary disturbance in self-esteem resulting from a loss or change. They also observed a functional self-esteem disturbance in individuals whose behavior was inconsistent with their beliefs and values, as in the case of stealing money to purchase drugs or becoming violent when inebriated.

Examples. Depending on the specific assessment data, this diagnostic category could be applicable in the following situations, among others:

▶ The person who experiences a traumatizing life event, such as rape or violence. Women who experience violence often believe they contributed to the event or were powerless to stop it, and the cycle of self-blame begins.
▶ A person who suffers a recent loss, such as the loss of status, as in a person who is laid off from a prestigious position. These persons may believe that their global self-esteem is related to their success in the work force.
▶ A person who experiences an illness or health event that now limits function. These persons may have believed that their self-concept was intimately tied to how they performed activities of daily life or to their appearance.

Related/Similar Nursing Diagnoses. The diagnosis of *Situational Low Self-Esteem* must be distinguished from the diagnoses of *Chronic Low Self-Esteem* and *Self-Esteem Disturbance.* *Situational Low Self-Esteem* differs from *Chronic Low Self-Esteem* and *Self-Esteem Disturbance* because of the presence of a prior high self-esteem level in the client. Clearly, a precipitating event such as a loss can be identified in clients diagnosed with *Situational Low Self-Esteem.*

In the nursing diagnoses *Self-Esteem Disturbance* and *Chronic Low Self-Esteem,* the longevity of exposure to either repeated negative messages or dysfunctional behaviors, such as abuse or alcoholism, determines the appropriate diagnosis. There are some differences in the defining characteristics as well. The diagnosis of *Chronic Low Self-Esteem* is made when the problem has a long-standing history. Defining characteristics specific to *Chronic Low Self-Esteem* include frequent lack of work or social services, overly conforming behavior, passive or nonassertive behavior, and excessive reassurance-seeking.

The diagnosis of *Self-Esteem Disturbance* may or may not have a long-standing history, and a clear precipitating factor or loss *cannot* be identified as in *Situational Low Self-Esteem.* In addition, the client may also deny problems obvious to others, project blame (responsibility for problems) onto others, rationalize personal failures, be hypersensitive to criticism, and be grandiose. These defining characteristics are not found in clients with a diagnosis of either *Chronic Low Self-Esteem* or *Situational Low Self-Esteem.*

---

* Norris, J., & Kunes-Connell, M. (1985). Self-esteem disturbance . . . nursing diagnoses. *Nursing Clinics of North America,* 20(4), 745–761.

The diagnoses of *Self-Esteem Disturbance* and *Chronic Low Self-Esteem* also share the following defining characteristics:

▶ Rejection of positive feedback and exaggeration of negative feedback
▶ Hesitation to try new things or situations[34]

The distinction between *Self-Esteem Disturbance* and *Chronic Low Self-Esteem* lies in the history of the problem. Although both diagnoses describe states in which individuals have negative self-evaluations or feelings about themselves and their capabilities, these states are of much longer standing in the diagnosis of *Chronic Low Self-Esteem.*[34] The precipitating factors are not as clear as the losses or changes that contribute to *Situational Low Self-Esteem*. Exposure to messages that reinforce negative aspects of self-concept or exposure to extreme dysfunctional forms of behavior such as sexual, physical, or verbal abuse or alcoholism may contribute to states described by either *Self-Esteem Disturbance* or *Chronic Low Self-Esteem*. The duration of the self-esteem disturbance determines whether a diagnosis of *Chronic Low Self-Esteem* or *Self-Esteem Disturbance* is warranted.

Clients who warrant the nursing diagnosis of *Situational Low Self-Esteem* are usually responding to an identified loss or change that now contributes to low self-esteem. These clients had a previous positive self-image. Refer to the Nursing Diagnosis Profile.

When all the assessment data have been collected and analyzed, decide whether or not to intervene. This decision is based on consideration of the individual's or family's level of functioning, the nurse's skill level, and other resources available.[41]

Intervention is recommended under the following circumstances:

▶ An individual identifies self-esteem disturbances or low self-esteem as a problem.
▶ An individual's self-esteem has an obvious detrimental effect upon other family members. For example, a parent's self-esteem is so low that the person cannot provide basic care and nurturing for children.
▶ Other family members contribute to an individual's self-esteem disturbance or low self-esteem. For example, a parent undermines an overweight adolescent's attempts to lose weight.

Wright and Leahey suggest that nursing intervention is not always appropriate or required.[41] They suggest that nursing intervention is contraindicated when the client requests no intervention or when the client states a preference to work with another health care professional. Usually, these contraindications become obvious to the nurse during the nursing assessment.

PLANNING

The most important aspect of the planning stage of the nursing process is to identify client outcomes related to enhancing self-esteem. Identifying client outcomes is a negotiable process between the client and the nurse. Some clients identify outcomes that are unattainable and unmeasurable. If clients state that they simply wish to feel better about themselves, help them identify measurable and attainable goals or changes that eventually will contribute to enhanced self-esteem. Ask the following questions to start the process of negotiating what the desirable outcomes might be:

▶ What is the *smallest* amount of change that would indicate to you that you are making progress in enhancing your self-esteem?[37]
▶ What would be the very first sign that things are starting to be on the right track in regard to enhancing your self-esteem?[25]

A client might respond, "Speaking up in class twice a week," or "Calling a friend tonight." These outcomes are much more attainable and measurable than "Feeling better about myself." Although this client's ultimate goal might be to be the life of the party, these smaller changes might be the first sign that the client is on the road to achieving the more ambitious goal.

The negotiation process between the nurse and the client is essential if treatment outcomes are to be accomplished. Individualize all outcomes to the specific client's situation and goals. What low self-esteem and desired outcomes mean to one person may mean something very different to another. General client outcomes related to self-esteem might include those listed in Box 50–5.

NURSING INTERVENTION

You must design specific nursing interventions for each individual with a self-esteem disturbance. This section presents interventions that are based upon research and clinical practice and that seem the most useful in enhancing self-concept.

Validating and Affirming the Client's Experiences

Validating and affirming an individual's experiences is an important place to start when attempting to intervene.

Disqualifying an individual's fears, reluctance, or ambivalence about the difficulties of changing maladaptive

---

Box 50–5. General Client Outcomes Related to Self-Esteem

▶ Client identifies exceptions to the problem
▶ Client identifies how and when he or she is able to show enhanced self-esteem
▶ Client attends to personal hygiene and appearance more than previously
▶ Client shows more self-confidence by initiating conversations with others
▶ Client shows more decision-making ability by deciding to . . .
▶ Client shows more assertive behavior by taking a position on . . .
▶ Client believes in own ability to manage medication administration
▶ Client shows 10 per cent more self-confidence in the interval between meetings with the nurse by . . .
▶ Client makes plans to enroll in a course, go away for a weekend, or perform other behaviors that the client believes show high levels of self-esteem
▶ Client convenes family to discuss issues of help to client and family

behaviors to more adaptive ones is disrespectful of that person's experience. Affirm the importance of going slowly and of waiting until the client is ready to make any change. At the same time, affirm for clients that when the time is right for a change, they will know it. The nurse should also affirm that change *will* occur when the client is ready by using the term *when* rather than *if*.[22] For example, ask the client, "When do you think you will be ready to change? How will you know when you are ready to change?"

Commending the Client

Take every opportunity to highlight individual and family strengths.

Offer commendations throughout your meeting with the client, or reserve them until the end of the meeting. Individuals who report low self-esteem or self-esteem disturbances frequently label themselves as failures because they are not more successful in one part of their life. It is common for these individuals and families to focus on problems; rarely does one compliment them on their strengths or acknowledge their resources.[17]

If you have assessed exceptions to the problem, the client's willingness to change, and attempted solutions, you probably have a number of commendations to offer the client and the family. Preface your commendations with, "I am impressed with how you . . ." and then present three or more compliments.[25,38] For example, commend a client who believes that low self-esteem prevents him or her from attending a staff celebration, but who shows competence as a valued employee of the company, in this way: "I am impressed with how open you are when you talk about your concerns regarding low self-esteem, how you are aware of the impact of low self-esteem on your social relationships, and how much competence you show at work, as evidenced by the comments that appeared on your most recent performance appraisal." This commendation sets the stage for the client to realize that competency and self-confidence are apparent to you. It also invites the client to consider completing any homework you might assign in the form of behavioral tasks in an effort to change behavior to a new direction.

All commendations must be well grounded upon evidence provided to you by the client or family during the nursing assessment. It is not good enough simply to say that you are impressed with a person's abilities in other areas of life. Be as specific as possible, using examples that the person provided during the interview. Clients typically respond positively to commendations. They expect health care professionals to focus solely on pathology. Note that offering commendations to a person with a self-esteem disturbance is different from simply telling or encouraging a person that he or she can do better. Such comments belong in the class of traditional verbal interventions, which Bandura[2] and Bednar and associates[3,4] believe are not helpful in enhancing self-concept.

Providing Advice and Information to the Client

Individuals with low self-esteem sometimes find advice and information helpful. Information regarding growth, development, and family life cycle theory is often appropriate to share with individuals. Recall the example of the adult daughter worrying about her aging mother's self-esteem because she sat in a darkened room. Providing this adult daughter with information about physiologic alterations in aging now gives new meaning to the mother's changed behavior. By understanding the meaning of the mother's behavior through new information, the daughter might focus less on her mother's self-esteem and more on other events of daily living.

Assessing parents' expectations of their children may also lead to a nursing intervention involving information giving. If the parents' expectations of their 2-year-old are age-inappropriate, sharing information about toddlers' growth and developmental stages can prove valuable. Parents who expect a 2-year-old to be fully toilet-trained may begin to believe that they are failures for not ensuring that their child's bowel and bladder functions are under control, and they may also convey the message, directly or indirectly, that the child is not performing well. Both behaviors contribute to decreased self-esteem in the parents and the toddler. Giving parents information that not all 2-year-olds have the physiologic or psychologic ability to control their bladder and bowel functions is indicated in this situation.

Share with clients and their families circular pattern diagrams of interaction between self-esteem and context. Diagramming a vicious or negative pattern of interaction may invite the individual to interrupt the circle by doing something different. Sharing this kind of information usually results in behavior change.

Redefining Normality to Highlight the Client's Strengths

Myers-Avis suggests relabeling as strengths what an individual regards as deficits, deviances, or pathology.[22] With a woman who suffered physical abuse, marvel at the incredible strength she must have had to survive and the strength she must have had to help her children survive under such devastating circumstances. This nursing intervention targets constraining beliefs that an individual may have about his or her perceived low self-esteem. Instead of being a victim, a label that connotes powerlessness, reframe her behavior as that of a survivor, a much more positive and empowering connotation.

Normalizing the Client's Responses to Events

You can also intervene by normalizing responses to events when warranted, especially in the case of *Situational Low Self-Esteem*, in which the *Self-Esteem Disturbance* is usually temporary and is a response to a loss or change. **Normalizing** is a nursing intervention in which the nurse assures the client and family that their response to a situation (e.g., the death of a child) is expected or typical or normal. This intervention may relieve some of the grief and emotional pain and conveys that the situation is not permanent.

Asking Future-Oriented Questions

Nurses usually ask questions to obtain assessment data. Questions can also be interventive when the intent is to introduce new information to the client or family that may be helpful in the search for solutions. One type of interventive question is the **future-oriented question,** which is used to invite clients and their families to imagine situations in the future so as to encourage visualization of details that contribute to desired outcomes.[25] Future-oriented questions are particularly useful when working with persons who identify low self-esteem as a problem. Ask a person who complains of low self-esteem these future-oriented questions:

▶ How would your life be different if you had more self-esteem?
▶ Who else would notice the self-confidence you feel?
▶ What will be the impact of enhanced self-esteem on your marriage? on your family? on your relationships with your friends?
▶ When do you think you will be ready to show more self-esteem?
▶ How will you know you are ready to show more self-esteem?[23]

Of course, the actual wording of any future-oriented questions you ask a client varies depending on the client's situation. Each question must "fit" the client's experience, as must all interventions.

Implementing Bibliotherapy

Bibliotherapy—therapeutic reading to enhance one's skills and knowledge or to solve problems—is a useful intervention if you have assessed that the individual is capable of reading books, articles, or magazines. Provide the client with readings on enhancing self-esteem if this particular intervention fits with the learning style of the client. Alternatively, direct the client to one of the many self-help bookstores available in most cities and towns. There, the client can select readings from the many publications available on the subject. To increase concentration, assign a task for the client to perform prior to the reading of any publication. One task might be for the client to identify in the reading three points that were found to be interesting, salient, or helpful. Another task might be for clients to identify one piece of advice they think may be helpful to their own situation. Following up on the assignment within a reasonable time frame is important, as it is with all interventions.

Making Behavioral Assignments

Behavioral assignments may be one of the most potent nursing interventions to use to enhance self-concept.

If you refer back to the section on research in this chapter, you will recall that Bandura[2] discovered that actual performance is more effective than traditional verbal interventions in increasing self-esteem. Asking clients to role-play situations or, better still, to experiment with new behaviors in real-life situations, should result in enhanced self-esteem.

Asking clients to make behavioral changes is best if you frame the changes as an "experiment." If you simply advise clients that all they need to do is to change their behavior to show more self-confidence, they may feel monumental performance pressure, which probably will influence negatively their competency in accomplishing this task. Alternatively, ask the client to try an experiment of a behavioral nature over the next couple of days or week. The client might be more willing to change behavior for a specified period of time. When the behavioral task assignment is framed as an experiment, the client feels less performance pressure, since the behavioral change is time limited. This reduces the risk of failure.

Frame your request to the client to try an "experiment" in the following manner:

▶ Would you be willing to try an experiment that might increase your self-esteem?
▶ Could you show more self-esteem by initiating a conversation twice this week with friends (or accepting an invitation to lunch with colleagues twice this week)?

You and the client would then assess the impact of these behaviors on the client's self-esteem.

Conducting "Research" on Self-Esteem

Some persons might be very willing to engage in a homework task of conducting "research" about self-esteem. Assign the task of observing those people who the client believes have high self-esteem, and ask the client to note what those persons say and do while they are exhibiting high self-esteem. The client will then have a list of behaviors from which to choose and possibly experiment with. Invite clients to select the one behavior they would be most willing to perform for a limited period of time in order to note its effect on other people. This is much more respectful than directing the client to perform a behavior of your choice.

Another variation on this nursing intervention has been documented by Leahey and Wallace in their work with strategic self-esteem groups.[16] They ask clients to notice the differences in affect, cognition, and behavior between people who they believe have low self-esteem and people who they believe possess high self-esteem. By drawing a distinction between these two groups, an individual again has the opportunity to become familiar with behaviors characteristic of persons with higher self-esteem. This focus on noticing how people with high self-esteem behave is similar to the psychologic intervention of visualization.

Implementing "Pretending Interventions"

Bandura's research on the importance of actual performance[2] underlies Madanes' idea of the "pretend intervention."[19] Madanes suggests that when people pretend to change a behavior, changes in their beliefs and thoughts may follow, as well as changes in their interactions with others. By asking clients to *act as though* they have more self-confidence than they believe they actually do, the context for change is set that contributes to changing their beliefs about their expectations and performance in this area. Ask clients to try an experiment in which they might *act as though* or *pretend* that they have 10 per cent more self-confidence on at least two occasions during the next week. The circularity of self-esteem and context will immediately be operational.

As you can imagine, when a person pretends to be more self-confident, others respond as if they believe that individual is competent. A client who perceives that others see him or her as competent is encouraged to continue doing more of the same. This is one of the best illustrations of reciprocity or circularity between self-esteem and context.

Try to diagram this pattern of interaction in a circular pattern diagram.

Asking a person to act as though there is 10 per cent more self-esteem intentionally leaves the amount of change in the control of the client. Clients ask, "How much is 10 per cent?" Suggest that the client will *know* how much this is. If the client reports that several behaviors were changed in the interim between meetings, compliment the fact that the 10 per cent quota was exceeded. Also compliment the client on possibly acting *as though* there was maybe 50, 60, or 80 per cent more self-esteem. This is another opportunity for the nurse to offer the client commendations on progress.

Narrative Tasks

Asking your client to read or write is useful only if you have assessed his or her literacy level. Asking an illiterate client to write a list of strengths or to read a self-help book will not enhance self-concept. Only after assessing the literacy level might you suggest a task in the narrative mode.

People with problems tend to focus only on problems. Ask clients to write a list of what they value about themselves to highlight competent parts of themselves.[26] Asking other family members or friends also to document the strengths of the clients is a helpful way to involve significant others. Suggest that clients collect these lists and other documents, such as letters of ref-

erence and positive performance appraisals, in a special folder or envelope to review on a "prn basis."

Draw a distinction between a client's "old story" of incompetence and low self-esteem and the desired "new story" of competency and increased self-esteem.[40] Asking individuals to write a "new story" lends legitimacy to the narrative as it is penned on paper. Future therapeutic conversations include categorizing all self-esteem behaviors as belonging to the "new story" or the "old story." If the client shows the kind of self-esteem more characteristic of the "old story" of incompetence, ask:

▶ What do you need to do to kick the "old story" out of your life and make room for the "new story" of increased self-confidence and competence?

By having the client write the "new story," the desired outcomes are available and accessible.

Promoting Positive Self-Talk

Some clients report that self-talk is helpful in enhancing self-esteem. These clients report that it is often useful to tell themselves to perform a behavior they would usually feel constrained from performing because of their belief about their low self-esteem and expectations. Encourage individuals who have successfully used this strategy in other parts of their life to do more of the same when they need to show more confidence in their abilities.

EVALUATION

Evaluation of the success of the prescribed nursing interventions as related to enhancing self-concept is a mutually collaborative process between the nurse and the client. To lend legitimacy to any of the prescribed nursing interventions, follow up on any homework assigned to the client during the previous meeting. If you do not check whether the homework was done, the client might infer that the prescribed nursing interventions were not to be taken seriously.

Even when individuals and families do not follow through with planned interventions, consider this to be useful assessment and evaluative data. The intervention may have been poorly designed and may not have "fit" the particular style of the client. For example, without an accurate assessment of the client's literacy skills, a bibliotherapy intervention may exacerbate rather than enhance the problem of low self-esteem.

Wright and Leahey caution against labeling individuals and families as "resistant" when they do not perform prescribed interventions as planned.[42] A client's decision not to perform a particular behavioral task may not be due to pathology but, instead, may be from lack of an adequate nursing assessment or lack of adequate interaction between the client and the nurse.

A small change is all that is necessary[25] to influence future behaviors in the direction of positive change.

Once a small, positive change is made, people feel optimistic and more confident about making more changes. Use the metaphor of a snowball rolling down a mountain to describe the importance of small changes for the client. If the client shows even 5 per cent more self-confidence than usual, show that you have confidence in the client's ability to continue making changes. This reciprocal interaction between client and nurse is essential to setting the context for further change.

CASE STUDY

The Client

Edna Plank, a single parent, requested to speak to the nurse on behalf of herself and her 14-year-old daughter Jacey. Jacey had been hospitalized recently in an attempt to confirm a medical diagnosis of lupus, which had been preceded by 6 months of fatigue. Lupus is an inflammatory disease that can cause deterioration of the connective tissues of muscles and bones in various parts of the body. Ms. Plank was most concerned about her daughter's recent periods of low self-esteem and sadness, her continual verbalizations that she was not any good any more, her reluctance to join friends in typical teenage activities, and her difficulty in making decisions about school and play. Jacey corroborated her mother's concerns and said simply, "I want to feel better about myself."

At 7:30 PM, March 14, a partial listing of the assessment data made on the third day of hospitalization included the following:

▶ A 14-year-old, slightly overweight female adolescent
▶ All developmental milestones of infancy and childhood reached successfully
▶ Mother and daughter agree that Jacey's self-esteem decreased in the half-year prior to the diagnosis of lupus

▶ Jacey unable to participate fully in grade 9 studies and in activities with friends for the past 6 months
▶ Mother and daughter report they feel relieved that Jacey's fatigue is now explained by lupus
▶ Jacey reports she feels worst about herself when she is alone, when her friends do not contact her, and when her mother works night shift
▶ Jacey has not been accepting calls or visits from friends since her hospitalization because she believes she needs "quiet time" for her recovery
▶ The more Jacey refuses calls or visits from friends, the less her friends attempt to initiate contact; Jacey reports she feels angry toward her "fair weather" friends
▶ Jacey rated her current level of self-esteem as a 2 on a 10-point scale; she retrospectively rated her self-esteem as an 8 a year ago before problems with fatigue and subsequent medical diagnosis of lupus
▶ Mother believes Jacey needs to focus more on the positive aspects of her life; Jacey agrees but admits to not knowing where to start
▶ Jacey tried reading a self-help book on enhancing self-esteem but this was not helpful as she tires easily

CARE PLAN

7:30 PM, March 14

Nursing Diagnosis	Planning: Expected Outcome	Implementation: Nursing Interventions	Evaluations
Situational Low Self-Esteem R/T perceived loss of friends secondary to impact of illness (lupus)	By 7:30 PM, March 17: Breaks the vicious pattern of interaction between herself and her friends by initiating contact with at least one friend on one occasion (current interaction pattern contributes to client's decreased self-esteem)	Share circular pattern diagram illustrating vicious circle (Fig. 50–4) Invite client to hypothesize about what her friends think and feel when she refuses their calls Invite client to "experiment" with breaking circle "by doing something different" as attempted solution of disallowing friends to visit seems unsuccessful	9:30 PM, March 14: Client hypothesized that her behavior of not accepting calls from friends may contribute to friends' decreasing frequency of contacts 7:30 PM, March 17: Client reported she contacted one friend by telephone Saturday; friend eagerly offered to visit client in hospital

Care Plan continued on following page

CARE PLAN (Continued)

7:30 PM, March 14

Nursing Diagnosis	Planning: Expected Outcome	Implementation: Nursing Interventions	Evaluations

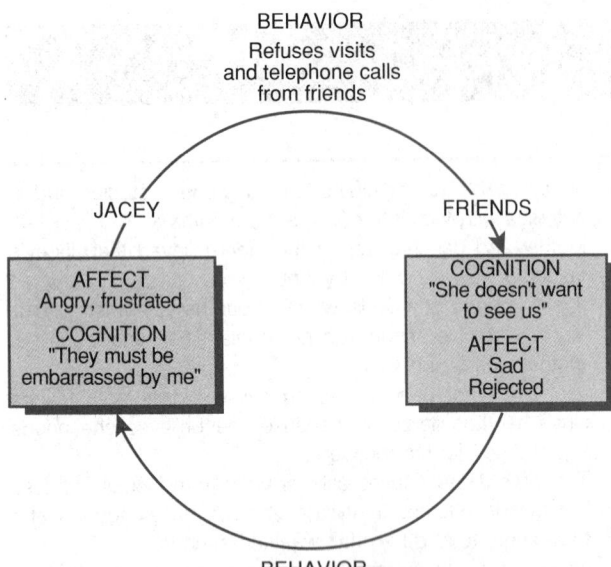

BEHAVIOR
Refuses visits
and telephone calls
from friends

JACEY

AFFECT
Angry, frustrated

COGNITION
"They must be
embarrassed by me"

FRIENDS

COGNITION
"She doesn't want
to see us"

AFFECT
Sad
Rejected

BEHAVIOR
Decreases /stops
frequency of visits
and telephone calls

▲ *Figure 50–4*

Circular pattern diagram (CPD) of a vicious circle between client and friends that contributes to decreased self-esteem (see Case Study).

	Ask client to notice friends' response to her new behavior to highlight impact of her behavior on others	Client noticed that when she initiated contact, friend was receptive Client reported she enjoyed visit with friend, and planned another visit for the next day
	Commend client for attempts to break vicious circle	Vicious pattern broken
"Acts as if" her self-esteem rating has increased to 3 from 2 on the 10-point scale on two occasions	Ask client to "act as if" her self-esteem rating increased by 10 percent (from 2 to 3 on the 10-point scale) Show confidence in client's ability to make change Assure client that requested change is an "experiment"	Client reported she "acted as if" she had more self-esteem on *three* occasions: 1. she initiated a call to a friend 2. she visited with friend in hospital; and, 3. she accepted invitation to a party for next weekend
	Ask client to notice impact on herself, family, and friends of "acting as if" her self-esteem were increased Positively commend client on any changes, however small	Client rates her self-esteem as a 6! Client noticed impact of engaging in above activities as contributing to enhancing her self-esteem

Summary

▶ Self-esteem is the affective component of self-concept, which describes an attitude, feeling, or evaluation regarding self-worth.

▶ Self-concept is influenced by context, which includes interactions with others.

▶ Global self-esteem refers to how much value you assign to yourself in total; specific self-esteem refers to how much value you assign to specific aspects of yourself.

▶ Factors that contribute to self-esteem in children are parents' acceptance of their children, clear limits regarding behavior, respect for individual action within limits set by parents, and high parental self-esteem.

▶ Expectations for success may be the most influential variable in determining capabilities.

▶ Performance accomplishments are more influential in enhancing self-esteem than are traditional verbal interventions, such as offering encouragement.

▶ Current self-esteem measuring instruments are often not sensitive to gender or to differences in various clinical populations.

▶ A family systems nursing approach focuses on the reciprocity between self-esteem and context, which can be illustrated by circular pattern diagrams.

▶ Adults with high self-esteem are more satisfied with jobs, relationships, and parenting; accept positive feedback and reject negative feedback but can acknowledge failure; have little need for social approval; are comfortable with intimacy and self-disclosure; and have better mental health.

▶ Children with high self-esteem participate in groups, show initiative, make independent judgments, take leadership roles, assert themselves at risk of disapproval, perform better academically and socially, have better mental health, and have a lower likelihood of delinquency.

▶ Low self-esteem is best understood from a circular rather than a linear perspective.

▶ Individuals experiencing low self-esteem need to discover their own problem-solving abilities, resources, and strengths.

▶ Often an individual's ability to enhance self-esteem depends upon the person's ability to alter the perception of the problem.

▶ Assessment of the person with low self-esteem should focus on problem identification, impact of low self-esteem on the client and family, context, beliefs, attempted solutions, and exceptions to the problem.

▶ The nursing diagnoses *Self-Esteem Disturbance, Chronic Low Self-Esteem,* and *Situational Low Self-Esteem* are all characterized by self-negating verbalizations, expressions of shame and/or guilt, and evaluation of self as unable to deal with events; the history of the duration of the problem and the presence of a prior positive self-image determine which diagnosis is more appropriate.

▶ Intervention is contraindicated when the client requests no intervention or when the client states a preference to work with another health care professional.

▶ Planning nursing care for the client with low self-esteem must focus on identifying attainable and measurable client outcomes with the client.

▶ Nursing interventions for the client with low self-esteem must be designed specifically for individual clients and might include validation and affirmation, commendations, advice and information, redefining normality to highlight strengths, normalizing, future-oriented questions, bibliotherapy, behavioral assignments, conducting ''research'' on self-esteem, pretending, narrative tasks, and self-talk.

▶ To evaluate the nursing care of the client with low self-esteem, the nurse must follow up on homework assigned to the client and recognize that any change, however small, influences future behaviors in the direction of continued positive change.

Bibliography

1. Atchley, R. (1982). The aging self. *Psychotherapy: Theory, Research and Practice,* 19, 388–396.
2. Bandura, A. (1977). Self-efficacy: toward a unifying theory of behavioral change. *Psychological Review,* 84, 191–215.
3. Bednar, R., et al. (1989). *Self-esteem: Paradoxes and innovations in clinical theory and practice.* Washington, D.C.: American Psychological Association Press.
4. Bednar, R.L., et al. (1991). Self-esteem: a concept of renewed clinical relevance. *Hospital and Community Psychiatry,* 42(2), 123–125.
5. Campbell, J.D., & Fehr, B. (1990). Self-esteem and perception of conveyed impressions: is negative affectivity associated with greater realism? *Journal of Personality and Social Psychology,* 58(1), 122–133.
6. Cooley, C.H. (1902). *Human nature and the social order.* New York: Charles Scribner's Sons.
7. Coopersmith, S. (1967). *The antecedents of self-esteem.* San Francisco: Freeman.
8. Curbow, B., et al. (1990). Self-concept and cancer in adults: theoretical and methodological issues. *Social Science and Medicine,* 31(2), 115–128.
9. Epictetus. Cited in von Oech, R. (1990). *A whack on the side of the head: How you can be more creative.* (revised ed., p. 162). Stamford, Connecticut: US Games Systems, Inc.
10. Eriksen, E.H. (1950). *Childhood and society.* New York: Norton.
11. Fitts, W. (1965). *Tennessee self-concept scale manual.* Nashville, Tennessee: Counselor Recordings and Tests.
12. Hayakawa, S. (1962). *Symbol, status and personality.* New York: Brace & World.
13. James, W. (1890). *The principles of psychology.* London: Macmillan.
14. Kersten, L. (1990). Changes in self-concept during pulmonary rehabilitation, part 1. *Heart and Lung,* 19(5), 456–462.
15. Lackovic-Grgin, K., & Dekovic, M. (1990). The contributions of significant others to adolescents' self-esteem. *Adolescence,* 25(100), 839–846.
16. Leahey, M., & Wallace, E. (1988). Strategic groups: one perspective on integrating strategic and group therapies. *Journal for Specialists in Group Work,* 13(4), 209–217.
17. Leahey, M., & Wright, L.M. (1987). *Families and psychosocial problems.* Springhouse, Pennsylvania: Springhouse Book Company.
18. LeGreca, A.M. (1990). *Through the eyes of the child.* Boston: Allyn & Bacon.
19. Madanes, C. (1981). *Strategic family therapy.* San Francisco: Jossey Bass.
20. Maslow, A. (1954). *Motivation and personality.* New York: Harper.

21. McCrae, R.R., & Costa, P.T. (1988). Age, personality, and the spontaneous self-concept. *Journal of Gerontology: Social Sciences.* 43, 5177–5185.

22. Myers-Avis, J. (1991). Power politics in therapy with women. In Goodrich, T.J. (ed.). *Women and power: Perspectives for family therapy* (pp. 183–200). New York: Norton.

23. Norris, J., & Kunes-Connell, M. (1985). Self-esteem disturbance . . . nursing diagnoses. *Nursing Clinics of North America,* 20(4), 745–761.

24. Norris, J., & Kunes-Connell, M. (1988). A multimodel approach to validation and refinement of an existing nursing diagnosis . . . self-esteem disturbance. *Archives of Psychiatric Nursing,* 2(2), 103–109.

25. O'Hanlon, W.H., & Weiner-Davis, M. (1989). *In search of solutions: A new direction in psychotherapy.* New York: Norton.

26. Raudsepp, E. (1991). Boost your self-confidence. *Nursing 91,* 21(2), 74.

27. Robinson, K. (1989). The relationship between social skills, social support, self-esteem and burden in adult caregivers. *Journal of Advanced Nursing,* 15, 788–795.

28. Robson, P.J. (1988). Self-esteem: a psychiatric view. *British Journal of Psychiatry,* 153, 6–15.

29. Rosenberg, M. (1965). *Society and the adolescent self-image.* Princeton, New Jersey: Princeton University Press.

30. Sieving, R.E., & Zirbel-Donisch, S.T. (1990). Development and enhancement of self-esteem in children. *Journal of Pediatric Health Care,* 4(6), 290–296.

31. Small, S.A. (1988). Parental self-esteem and its relationship to childrearing practices, parent-adolescent interaction, and adolescent behaviour. *Journal of Marriage and the Family,* 50, 1063–1072.

32. Stanwyck, D.J. (1983). Self-esteem through the life span. *Family and Community Health,* 6(2), 11–28.

33. Steinem, G. (1992). *Revolution from within: A book of self-esteem.* Boston: Little, Brown.

34. Taptich, B.J., et al. (1989). *Nursing diagnosis and care planning.* Philadelphia: W.B. Saunders.

35. Tomm, K. (1980). Towards a cybernetic systems approach to family therapy at the University of Calgary. In Freeman, D. (ed.). *Perspectives on family therapy* (pp. 3–18). Vancouver: Butterworth & Co.

36. Tschirhart Sanford, L., & Donovan, M.E. (1984). *Women and self-esteem.* New York: Penguin Books.

37. Watson, W.L. (Producer) (1988). *Fundamentals of family systems nursing* [Videotape]. Calgary: The University of Calgary.

38. Watson, W.L. (Producer) (1989). *Family systems interventions* [Videotape]. Calgary: The University of Calgary.

39. Watson, W.L., & Bell, J.M. (1990). Who are we? Low self-esteem and marital identity. *Journal of Psychosocial Nursing,* 28(4), 15–20.

40. White, M., & Epston, D. (1989). *Literate means to therapeutic end.* Adelaide, Australia: Dulwich Centre Publications.

41. Wright, L.M., & Leahey, M. (1984). *Nurses and families: A guide to family assessment and intervention.* Philadelphia: F.A. Davis.

42. Wright, L.M., & Leahey, M. (1987). *Families and chronic illness.* Springhouse, Pennsylvania: Springhouse Book Company.

43. Wright, L.M., & Leahey, M. (1990). Trends in nursing of families. *Journal of Advanced Nursing,* 15, 148–154.

44. Youngs, G.A., et al. (1990). Adolescent stress and self-esteem. *Adolescence,* 25(98), 333–341.

▼ *Meeting Sensory/ Perceptual Needs*

Chapter 51

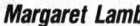

▼ *Our very hold on reality is basically dependent on us receiving a continual and uninterrupted flow of sensory stimulation from our environment.*

Margaret Lamb

▼ **CHAPTER OUTLINE**

SENSATION/PERCEPTION
    Neurophysiology of Sensation/
      Perception
    Factors Affecting Sensation/
      Perception
    Alteration in Sensory Stimuli
    Alteration in Perception
ASSESSMENT
    Persons at Risk for Sensory/
      Perceptual Alteration
    Nursing History
    Physical Assessment of Sensory
      Deficit
    Symptoms of Sensory/Perceptual
      Alterations

NURSING DIAGNOSIS
PLANNING
NURSING INTERVENTION
    Sensory Deficits
    Preventing Sensory/Perceptual
      Alterations in the Hospitalized
      Child
    Sensory Deprivation
    Sensory Overload
    Communication with a Client with
      Sensory/Perceptual Alteration
EVALUATION
CASE STUDY

▼ **KEY TERMS**

Altered thought processes
Confusion
Delusional thinking
Perception

Response
Sensation
Sensory deficit
Sensory deprivation

Sensory overload
Sensory/perceptual
    alteration
Somesthetic

After studying this chapter, you should be able to

1. Differentiate between sensation and perception.
2. Identify factors that affect sensory perception.
3. Differentiate among sensory deficit, sensory overload, and sensory deprivation.
4. Differentiate among confusion, delusional thinking, illusion, and hallucination.
5. Describe assessment findings indicating sensory/perceptual alterations.
6. Describe assessment findings indicating altered thought processes.
7. List nursing diagnoses that relate to sensory/perceptual alterations and the client's response to sensory/perceptual alterations.
8. List outcomes for a person who is responding to a sensory deficit in vision, hearing, taste, smell, touch, and proprioception.
9. Describe nursing interventions to maintain a safe environment for persons with sensory deficits.
10. Discuss specific communication techniques appropriate for persons with Sensory/Perceptual Alteration.
11. Describe evaluation of the person with a sensory/perceptual alteration.

What would you do if you suddenly found yourself without the use of one of your sense organs? Suppose you could not see a thing? How would it affect your life if you could not hear? What if you lost the sense of touch or the sense of your position in space? How would you cope? If you had to select which sense you could do without, what would your choice be? Perhaps something "less important" such as your sense of taste or smell? Surely losing your sense of smell could not affect your life very much, or could it?

Consider the case of Orpha Barnes. After suffering from the flu, she was left without a sense of smell, which greatly affected her sense of taste. With these senses diminished or absent, she found herself unable to tell when the food she was cooking tasted "just right" or when a certain spice had to be added. Even worse, she was not always sure when the food was done, and she found herself burning things on occasion. Surely this was not as bad as, say, being struck blind, and yet cooking was such a large part of her life that it affected her a great deal.

Her grandchildren will tell you that Grandma Barnes was, hands down, the best homemaker in the world, and what made her so extra special was her ability to cook. Why, she made a banana cream pie that would make grown men . . . Ah, but according to Grandma Barnes, all that was in the days before that case of the flu. Afterward, things changed. But did they change all that much? In fact, she survived her sensory alteration and adapted to it fairly well, but she would tell you that her cooking was never the same afterward, or, if it was, she could never be sure of it.

Indeed, how can you be sure of anything if you cannot trust your own senses? What are those senses anyway, and what happens to us when they change? That is what this chapter is all about.

SENSATION/PERCEPTION

As human beings, we are all dependent on a continual flow of sensory stimulation from our internal and external environments. Sensory stimulation is actually a process that has three components: sensation, perception, and response.

Sensation is the reception of stimulation through receptors of the nervous system. There are several types of somesthetic receptors, including visual (sight), auditory (sound), gustatory (taste), tactile (touch), olfactory (smell), and proprioceptive (position sense). **Somesthetic** pertains to sensations and sensory structures of the body. Minute by minute, these receptors are taking in tremendous amounts of information, and yet all that they take in is useless unless we are able to perceive it. **Perception** is the ability to receive input from the senses, interpret the information in the brain, and correlate it in a meaningful way. The ability to give meaning to incoming stimuli is learned from past experiences. A **response** is the action taken by the person after meaning has been given to the sensation. For example, Harry may be reading a book when he begins to feel certain sensations in his gastrointestinal tract. Because he has experienced these particular sensations before, he is able to interpret them as hunger pangs. He looks at the clock and sees that it is 2 hours past his usual lunch time and decides that it is time to eat. He then responds to the sensation of hunger by cooking lunch.

Neurophysiology of Sensation/Perception

Peripheral sensory receptors are located throughout the body, not just in sense organs. Each of these receptors transmits specific types of stimuli and may be classified as (1) *exteroceptors*, which are stimulated by touch, light pressure, pain, temperature, odor, sound, and light; (2) *proprioceptors*, which convey a sense of position, movement, and muscle coordination; (3) *interoceptors*, which provide visceral information regarding pain, cramping, and fullness; and (4) *chemoreceptors*, which are stimulated by various chemicals.[10]

Sensory transmission begins when peripheral receptors pick up a wide variety of stimuli and send impulses by means of afferent (sensory) nerve fibers from peripheral nerve endings to the posterior horn in the gray matter of the spinal cord. Inside the gray matter, the impulse can travel in two directions: (1) across the interneuron connection to the anterior horn of the gray matter, then to the efferent (motor) neurons, and back to the muscles of the periphery to cause movement and (2) up the spinal cord to predetermined areas of the brain, where perception is possible (Fig. 51–1).[21]

To perceive and react consciously to stimuli, the brain must be alert or aroused. Arousing the brain is the purpose of the *reticular activating system (RAS).* The RAS is located in the midbrain and thalamus and controls the sleep-wake cycle, the level of consciousness, the ability to direct attention to specific tasks, and the perception of sensory input that might alter behavior. When the RAS receives an adequate amount of sensory stimuli from the periphery, the person is aroused and alert, and perception and adaptive responses are able to occur. When an inadequate amount of sensory stimulation is received by the RAS, the person may experience confusion, boredom, and drowsiness.

Factors Affecting Sensation/Perception

Sensory/perceptual alteration is a state in which a person experiences a change in the amount, patterns, or interpretation of incoming stimuli by receptors for sight, hearing, taste, touch, smell, or body position. A number of factors can contribute to sensory/perceptual alterations. See Box 51–1 for examples of factors you may frequently see as you continue your career in nursing. Study this box well because it will assist you in identifying those persons at risk for alterations in sensory perception and allow you to intervene to prevent these alterations.

Alteration in Sensory Stimuli

It can be harmful if a person is exposed to too much or too little sensory stimulation. How each person responds to any given level of stimuli will depend on the person's usual exposure level. An amount of stimulation that is overwhelming for one person may be the usual daily fare for another. For example, Mr. Struthers, who

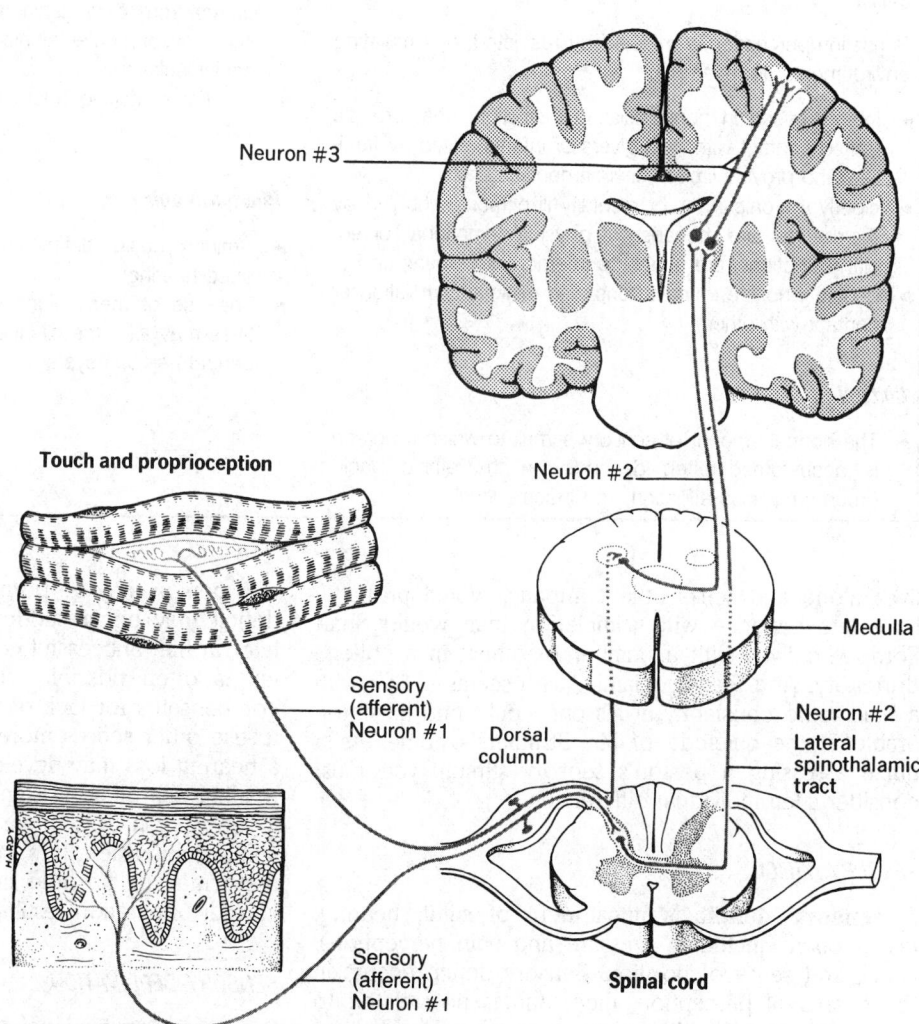

▲ *Figure 51–1*

Diagrammatic representation of the decussation (crossing) of ascending tracts. First-order neurons for touch and proprioception ascend in the dorsal columns to the medulla. Here they synapse with second-order neurons that cross to the opposite side before ascending to the thalamus. First-order neurons for pain and temperature enter the dorsal gray matter of the cord. Here they synapse with second-order neurons that cross to the opposite side and ascend in the lateral spinothalamic tract to the thalamus. Third-order neurons connect the thalamus with the cerebral cortex. (Modified from Hudak, C. M., Gallo, B. M., & Benz, J. J. [1990]. *Critical care nursing: A holistic approach* [5th ed.]. Philadelphia: J. B. Lippincott, p. 505.)

Touch and proprioception

Pain and temperature

Neuron #3

Neuron #2

Medulla

Neuron #2

Lateral spinothalamic tract

Sensory (afferent) Neuron #1

Dorsal column

Sensory (afferent) Neuron #1

Spinal cord

Box 51-1. Factors Affecting Sensation/Perception

Developmental

▶ Vision in a newborn continues to develop during the first year. Visual acuity in the newborn appears to be in the range of 20/100 to 20/400.[24]

▶ Visual acuity generally decreases after the age of 60 years as a result of presbyopia or a loss of accommodation resulting from lens rigidity. A yellowing of the lens can cause problems with glare and with color discrimination.[12] The elderly person frequently has a decrease in visual fields and an impairment in night vision, color vision, and depth perception.[27]

▶ Hearing is most acute at 10 years of age. By the age of 65 years, about 55 per cent of the population has some hearing loss. With advancing age, there is often a loss of response to high-pitched sounds and a progressive sensorineural loss. Some elderly persons may have difficulty discriminating between the sounds *sh* and *ch* or *t* and *p*.[12]

▶ Most persons older than 60 years have some loss of taste.[27]

▶ There is a decline in smell after the age of 70 years.[27]

Social

Sensation/perception is affected by restricted, unstimulating environments; for example,

▶ infants raised in nonstimulating institutions that provide limited contact with care givers or infants raised by families who provide limited environmental stimuli;

▶ elderly, chronically ill, or mentally ill persons who live by themselves and, because of physical, emotional, or social restrictions, are unable to interact with others; and

▶ people who live in institutions with minimal stimulation or contact with others.

Cultural

▶ The normal amount of sensory stimuli to which a person is accustomed often depends on the ethnic background, religious affiliation, and income level.

Occupational

▶ Many persons are subject to inordinately high levels of sensory stimulation as part of their work environment. Classic examples are air traffic controllers and those working in certain manufacturing areas that are subject to high noise levels.

Pathologic

▶ Clients with diabetes mellitus may experience an alteration in vision or peripheral neuropathy that predisposes them to injury.

▶ The presence of visual, auditory, olfactory, gustatory, or tactile sensory deficits may cause a decrease in sensory stimuli.

Therapeutic

▶ Excessive environmental stimuli in the intensive care unit (ICU) setting from unfamiliar sights, sounds, and smells can lead to sensory overload and cause confusion and disorientation.

▶ Clients who are in isolation to protect themselves or others from pathogenic organisms may experience limited environmental stimuli, which predisposes them to social isolation.

▶ Restricted visiting hours in the ICU limit social interaction.

Pharmacologic

▶ Aminoglycoside antibiotics may cause ototoxicity and reduce hearing.

▶ The use of medications such as analgesics and sedatives may alter the client's perception by depressing the central nervous system.

---

lives alone and seeks little company, would probably have less patience with stimulation than would Shari Ford, who lives with a number of others in a college dormitory. And teen-age Jamie, who seems to live with a loud radio constantly at his ear, could find life intolerable in the quietude of Mr. Struthers's home. As a nurse assessing a person's sensory stimuli, you must consider such individual differences.

SENSORY DEFICIT

A **sensory deficit** is impairment of sight, hearing, taste, touch (including pressure and pain perception), smell, and sense of position. Sensory deficit occurs in the organs of perception, then, and is not related to how much or how little stimulation is available in the environment.

A person may be born with a sensory deficit, or the deficit may occur suddenly or gradually at some time later in life. Successful compensation for a sensory deficit is often possible, such as when a blind person compensates for lack of vision by developing an ability to use other senses more fully. Likewise, a person with a hearing loss may develop compensating skills such as reading lips or using sign language. The gradual loss of a sense such as sight or hearing makes compensation somewhat easier. If a sensory deficit occurs quickly, there may be so little time for compensation that severe disorientation results.

SENSORY DEPRIVATION

Sensory deprivation occurs from inadequate reception or perception of environmental stimuli. The cause may be physiologic, such as sensory deficit, or it may be due to an inadequate amount or inadequate variety of sensory stimuli in the environment. An example of inadequate variety in environmental stimuli is a radio that is left on to play "elevator music" continuously in a client's otherwise silent room. An example of an inadequate amount of environmental stimuli might be the same room without any radio at all. Persons deprived of sensory stimulation may experience central nervous system changes such as impaired judgment, inability to solve problems, confusion, disorientation, and even hallucinations and delusions.

SENSORY OVERLOAD

When stimuli in the environment are excessive or beyond the person's ability to absorb or comprehend, the person can experience **sensory overload.** People in hospitals may be at risk for sensory overload. The hospital environment is filled with sights, sounds, smells, and tactile sensations that are unfamiliar to most persons. A person who is not used to much environmental stimulation may be hospitalized with a painful condition and may seek little more than rest and quiet only to find himself or herself in a room with a talkative roommate near a busy nurse's station, with a nearby elevator bell ringing every time the door swishes open. Add to this picture the sound of a jackhammer outside of the person's window as the hospital begins to construct a new wing, and you can see how such a person might have difficulty giving meaning to all of the incoming stimuli and handling this overload of sensation in a normal manner.

Alteration in Perception

A person with an alteration in perception has problems discriminating among sensory stimuli and has problems organizing and giving meaning to incoming stimuli. This may occur as a result of sensory deficit, sensory deprivation, sensory overload, or a pathologic process in the brain. Some alterations in perception are: confusion, delusional thinking, illusion, and hallucination.

CONFUSION

Confusion is a disturbance of consciousness in which the person feels distracted and anxious. A confused person cannot correctly respond to normal stimuli and may experience an altered awareness of person, place, time, or events. Confusion is often transient. A state of confusion may last for hours, days, or even years. Confusion can be a sign of a mental or physical disorder. See Box 51–2 for common causes of confusion.

If you believe a person to be confused, you might ask him or her some of the following questions to help assess the person's level of orientation. Note that these questions avoid the possibility of "yes" or "no" answers. Observe the client's verbal and nonverbal responses as you ask them.

Box 51–2. Common Causes of Confusion

Pathophysiologic

- ▶ Autoimmune: temporal arteritis, systemic lupus erythematosus
- ▶ Degenerative: Alzheimer's disease, Huntington's chorea, Parkinson's disease
- ▶ Infections: bacterial, fungal, or viral
- ▶ Metabolic alterations: diabetes, electrolyte imbalances, hormonal disturbances, thyroid dysfunction, and vitamin deficiencies (B_{12})
- ▶ Neoplasms: tumors either in the brain or metastasis to the brain
- ▶ Seizures
- ▶ Trauma: mechanical injury to the brain
- ▶ Vascular: transient ischemic attacks, cerebrovascular accident (stroke), ruptured aneurysm

Treatment Related

- ▶ Side effects of drugs: antiparkinsonian drugs, steroids, narcotics, sedatives
- ▶ Electroconvulsive (shock) therapy

Situational (Personal or Environmental)

- ▶ Psychiatric: depression, schizophrenia
- ▶ Sensory impairment: sensory deficit, sensory deprivation, sensory overload
- ▶ Toxins: carbon monoxide, alcohol, metal poisoning

- ▶ "What is your last name?"
- ▶ "Who is this person?" (Point to a person who should be known to the client.)
- ▶ "Where are you now?"
- ▶ "What city is this?"
- ▶ "What day, month, and year is it?"
- ▶ "What holiday did we just celebrate?"
- ▶ "Who is the president of the United States?"

As you assess the client's accuracy when answering these questions, be aware that many factors may interfere with a person's response. For example, you should consider the following:

- ▶ Does the person understand and speak your language?
- ▶ Can the person speak at all?
- ▶ Can the person hear you?
- ▶ Has the person been isolated, and is he or she unaware of current affairs?
- ▶ Is your question realistic and appropriate for the person's level of education?

When documenting your assessment of a confused person, descriptions are more useful than labels. Describe how the person appeared. State which assessment questions were asked and how the person responded. For example, do not state, "Appears confused." State instead, "Wandering down the hall, wearing only a patient gown, and carrying a bedpan. When asked where she was going, replied 'I have to feed the chickens.' When questioned further, stated her correct name but said the president of the United States is Theodore Roosevelt and 'This must be some kind of school but I don't know which one.'"

DELUSIONAL THINKING

Delusional thinking is an intellectual mechanism that helps a person maintain a sense of power and control when security is threatened. Delusions are fixed, false beliefs. That is, these beliefs have little or no basis in reality, and the person who holds them cannot be corrected by being presented with logic, reason, or argument. Delusions guide the client's interpretation of events and help him or her make sense out of disorder in life. Delusions may be comforting or threatening, but they always provide structure for what otherwise might be unmanageable. For example, take Fred Silvers, who has just been fired from his job as a middle-level manager. Fred is unable to make his house payments and argues with his wife over how the bills will be paid. Fred has developed a belief that his co-workers were "out to get" him, told lies about him, and had him fired (threatening thoughts) because they were jealous of his superior intelligence and talents on the job (comforting thoughts). Neither his former boss and co-workers nor his wife can talk him out of this fixed, false belief. The presence of delusional thought is an indication of mental illness.

ILLUSION

An illusion is a disorder of perception. It is a visual misinterpretation of a physical or environmental stimulus. That is, the person sees something that actually exists but thinks that what is seen is something else. A classic example is the person who sees small, black cracks that are present in the ceiling and interprets them to be spiders. Another example is the person who sees a dress hanging on the back of a door and interprets it as a ghost. Obviously, in both examples, there is a connection between what was seen and how it was interpreted. This is true of illusions. They are mistakes that anyone might make. It is not a sign of mental illness to have an illusion (although those who are mentally ill may also experience illusions). You may differentiate an illusion from a delusion if you explain the facts to the person ("Those are just cracks on the ceiling," "That is just a dress hanging there"). The person who is having an illusion will accept your explanation and see the true state of things. The person who is delusional cannot be talked out of his or her belief.

HALLUCINATION

Hallucinations are also disorders of perception. A hallucination is a sensory perception that has no physical or environmental stimulus. Any of the senses can be affected so that the person who is experiencing a hallucination may see, hear, smell, taste, or feel stimuli that are not actually present in the physical world. Hallucinations are sensations that arise from within a person. A man who sees spiders on the ceiling when, in fact, there is nothing there is experiencing a hallucination. With help, the person who experiences hallucinations can understand that these perceptions are not real, but this understanding does not change the perception. That is, he will continue to receive the false perception. He will, for example, continue to hear a voice in his head that calls his name and tells him he is evil and should punish himself.

Unlike the person with a delusion, who *believes* something that is not true, the person with a hallucination *perceives* something that is not real. Neither can be successfully dealt with simply by being told the true state of affairs. The person with an illusion *misconceives* something that is real and interprets it as something else. This person can easily be shown the true state of reality.

ASSESSMENT

When you identify clients at risk for sensory/perceptual alterations, your task is to identify the existence of sensory/perceptual problems by completing a health history, performing a physical assessment of the six senses to identify deficits, observing for symptoms of sensory/perceptual alterations, and noting how the person responds to any alterations identified.

Persons at Risk for Sensory/Perceptual Alterations

Of the persons you are most likely to encounter in your role as a nurse, perhaps those at highest risk for sensory/perceptual alterations are the elderly, hospitalized persons, those with occupational risks, and those with a sensory deficit.

The elderly are at risk for sensory/perceptual alterations as a result of many of the normal physiologic changes that occur to all of us with the aging process. Recall that all of our senses tend to gradually lose their acuity as we age. Although there is usually no abrupt awareness of sensory loss, over time (even with compensations) gradual changes in sensory organ function may decrease our awareness of and responses to environmental stimuli.

As previously discussed, hospitalized clients are at risk for sensory/perceptual alterations because of an increase in the amount and type of environmental stimuli. Hospitalized persons may also be at risk for sensory deprivation. For example, consider Mark, a leukemic client who has recently received chemotherapy and who has a suppressed immune system. Mark will be placed on special precautions to protect him from the environment. He will be placed in a private room, with traffic in and out of the room kept to a minimum. As a result, he may feel socially isolated. Clients in isolation, such as Mark, often experience a decrease in environmental stimulation that can lead to sensory/perceptual problems (Fig. 51-2).

It is fairly common knowledge that clients in an intensive care setting may experience sensory/perceptual alterations because of the massive amount of environmental stimuli they receive. However, even some medical professionals are unaware that nurses working in an intensive care unit may also be affected by the environmental stimuli and experience sensory overload. This is but one example of an occupational risk.

We know that persons with a sensory deficit may be at risk for a sensory/perceptual alteration. We should also understand that these persons (even though they have adapted to the deficit and are functioning well in the home environment), when placed in an unfamiliar environment such as a boarding school, hospital, or nursing home, may experience sensory deprivation or overload.

See Box 51-1 for more factors to consider regarding clients with potential risk for sensory/perceptual alterations.

Nursing History

When obtaining a nursing history for a person at risk for sensory/perceptual alteration, assess for the presence of factors known to affect sensory perception (see Box 51-1), for symptoms of alterations, and for the client's response to the symptoms. When asking about symptoms, be sure to elicit information about precipitating and aggravating factors, frequency, duration, and relief measures.

For example, you might find that Maria Estevez came from a large, close-knit family and was used to much noise and color in her daily life in Mexico. For 6 months now, she has been living in the United States, away from her family and friends, and she finds herself mostly alone. She works for a quiet, elderly couple, who have provided her with one room, with only a bed and dresser to hold her few belongings. Two weeks ago, Maria noted a hearing loss and, as a result of her sensory deprivation, has had transient episodes of confusion. This has left her anxious and depressed. She feels helpless and longs to return home to her family and friends. When you question her about her hearing loss, you find that the loss seemed to be manifested by a bilateral decrease in hearing that has not changed, no matter what she has done. She says she cannot afford to see a physician and has been trying various home remedies. Her employers gave her some medicine "awhile back" when she had an infection in her foot and it seemed to help the infection, but nothing she has tried has helped the hearing loss.

If Maria had not been asked about what she was doing for relief measures, it might not have come to light that she had been taking her employer's medicine for an infection. With this information, the nurse should suspect an ototoxicity from an antibiotic as the possible reason for the hearing loss. In any event, the nurse needs to gather more data and refer Maria to a physician to evaluate the hearing loss further.

Physical Assessment of Sensory Deficit

Nursing assessment of each of the senses provides the nurse with specific information concerning possible sensory deficits. See Box 51-3 for areas to assess in each of the six senses.

Symptoms of Sensory/Perceptual Alterations

Whether sensory/perceptual alterations result from sensory deprivation or sensory overload, the symptoms experienced may be emotional lability, alteration in thought processes, and impaired communication patterns.

Emotional lability may be expressed as mood swings, irritability, anxiety, apathy, and fear. **Altered thought processes** are demonstrated in the inability to differentiate one's thoughts and feelings from actualities of the outside world. Altered thought processes may present as auditory or visual hallucinations; illusions; delusional thinking; inability to concentrate; memory deficits; or disorientation to person, place, or time. *Impaired communication patterns* usually result from an altered thought process. For example, the person who is confused will not be able to communicate effectively with another person. The person who is ac-

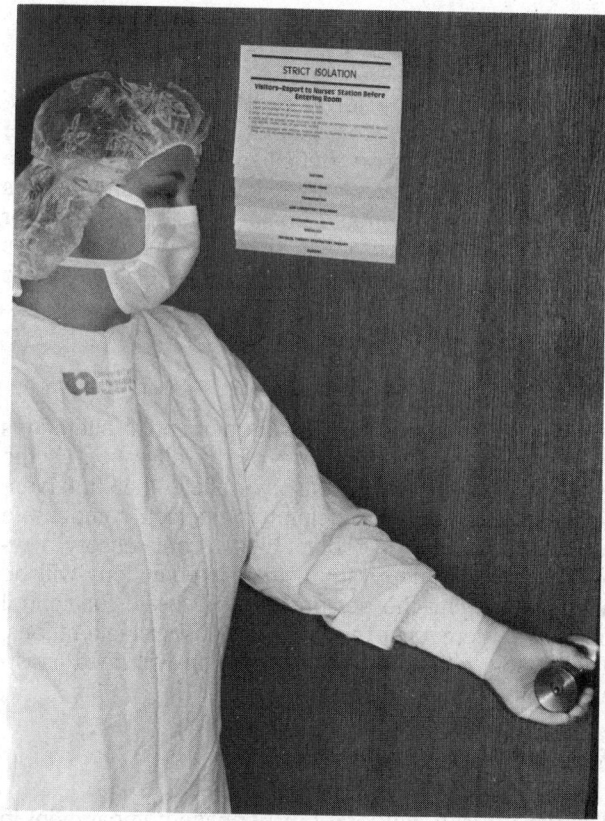

▲ *Figure 51-2*

Immunosuppressed clients in protective isolation are at risk for social isolation.

Box 51–3. Sensory Assessment

Vision

- ▶ Assess visual acuity using a Snellen chart.
- ▶ Assess visual fields.
- ▶ Assess the distance the client holds reading material.
- ▶ Assess for squinting.
- ▶ Assess presence of corneal reflex.
- ▶ Ask whether the client has experienced blurred or double vision, halos around objects, blind spots, or floaters.

Hearing

- ▶ Assess hearing acuity with normal conversation, whisper, ticking watch, or tuning fork.
- ▶ Assess speech and language development in children.
- ▶ Ask whether the client has experienced tinnitus (ringing in the ears).
- ▶ Ask the parent or significant other whether client responds inappropriately, daydreams, or is withdrawn.

Taste

- ▶ Assess the client's ability to taste.
- ▶ Ask whether the client has experienced a decrease in appetite, difficulty swallowing, or an increased use of seasoning.

Touch

- ▶ Assess the client's ability to distinguish between sharp and dull sensations.
- ▶ Assess the client's ability to feel light touch.
- ▶ Assess the client's ability to differentiate temperatures.
- ▶ Ask whether the client has experienced numbness, tingling, or prickling sensation.

Smell

- ▶ Assess the client's ability to distinguish different odors.
- ▶ Ask whether the client has noticed a decrease in ability to smell food.

Position Sense

- ▶ Assess the client's ability to walk a straight line.
- ▶ Ask whether the client has experienced dizziness, motion sickness, nausea, change in steadiness of gait, or falls.

---

tually hallucinating may be so frightened that effective communication is impossible.

When you have completed the history and assessed the person for sensory deficits and for sensory/perceptual alterations, you are not yet finished with the assessment. You still must assess the person's response to any alterations you have discovered. Remember that it is the person's responses to alterations in health that you will use as the basis for your nursing diagnosis.

NURSING DIAGNOSIS

The nursing diagnosis of Sensory/Perceptual Alterations describes a change in perception of the amount or pattern of incoming stimuli accompanied by a diminished, exaggerated, distorted, or impaired response to such stimuli (see Nursing Diagnosis Profile). The diagnosis should specify one of the following six subcategories related to specific sensory deficits: visual, auditory, kinesthetic, gustatory, tactile, and olfactory. For example, Maria Estevez's diagnosis would be *Sensory/Perceptual Alterations* R/T auditory deficit. Although she probably experienced a general sensory deprivation from lack of input of all types, it was the hearing deficit that finally resulted in the symptoms that brought her to the hospital for help.

You must also identify the client's responses to any specific sensory deficit. These responses can suggest accompanying diagnoses. Examples of nursing diagnoses that frequently accompany specific sensory deficits can be found in Table 51–1.

Also note the client's responses to sensory/perceptual alteration. Responses here may suggest additional nursing diagnoses. For example, a sensory/perceptual alteration that results in confusion, delusional thinking, illusions, or hallucinations suggests an additional diagnosis of altered thought processes.

The diagnosis of *High Risk for Injury* is appropriate for any person who experiences a sensory/perceptual alteration.

PLANNING

The outcome criteria for a client experiencing a sensory/perception alteration should be specific for (1) the response to the sensory deficit experienced or (2) the response to the sensory/perceptual alteration. Examples of outcome criteria should be specifically identified for each client in relation to the situation. Broad examples of outcome criteria for these nursing diagnoses are listed in Table 51–2.

NURSING INTERVENTION

Nursing interventions for sensory/perceptual alterations vary depending on the cause of the alteration. If the problem stems from a sensory deficit, then interventions will be directed at helping the person compensate for the deficit. If the problem stems from sensory overload or sensory deprivation, then interventions will be aimed at helping the person to compensate for central nervous system changes and psychosocial alterations. The person with an altered perception will need assistance with effective communications.

Sensory Deficits

The person with temporary or permanent impairment in vision, hearing, touch, taste, smell, or position sense is

NURSING DIAGNOSIS PROFILE

Sensory/Perceptual Alterations (specify Visual, Auditory, Kinesthetic, Gustatory, Tactile, Olfactory)

Definition. A state in which a person experiences a change in the amount, patterning, or interpretation of incoming stimuli accompanied by diminished, exaggerated, distorted, or impaired response to such stimuli.

Classification. Perceiving 7.2.

Defining Characteristics. The defining characteristics may be divided into major and minor criteria. The major criteria include an inaccurate interpretation of environmental stimuli or a change in the amount or pattern of incoming stimuli. One or both of these criteria must be present when a person experiences an alteration in sensory perception.[3]

The minor criteria include the signs and symptoms that a person experiencing an alteration in sensory perception may exhibit. At times, the symptoms may be subtle, such as a feeling of apathy, anxiety, fear, irritability, and restlessness, or the person may have difficulty in problem solving or in making decisions. At other times, the symptoms may be quite obvious such as a disorientation to person, place, or time. The person may experience auditory or visual hallucinations.

Sample Related Factors. Related factors may include excessive or insufficient environmental stimuli (as occurs in a therapeutically restricted environment such as a hospital or with changes in occupational environment); altered sensory reception (as occurs in a sensory deficit); altered sensory transmission or integration (as occurs with pathology in the nervous system); chemical alterations (as occurs with changes in certain intracellular and extracellular electrolytes and with some medications that alter nervous system function); or psychologic stress (as occurs with both internal and external factors stimulating the individual).

Concept Description. The nursing diagnosis of alteration in sensory perception is used for individuals who experience a change in reception, awareness, or interpretation of incoming stimuli. Sensory perception may be affected by pathophysiologic, psychosocial, or treatment-related factors.

Examples. Depending on the specific assessment data, this diagnostic category could be applicable in the following situations, among others:

▶ A usually pleasant elderly person who has become irritable and who has difficulty following directions. Recently, the person stated that other people are talking about him. A hearing examination reveals a decrease in hearing acuity as a result of cerumen impaction.
▶ A critically ill person who is in an intensive care unit and is exposed to a massive amount of unfamiliar environmental stimuli. The person is attached to and monitored by many highly technologic pieces of equipment with safety alarms. The atmosphere is very fast paced, with nurses and physicians performing life-saving procedures.
▶ A young soldier who is serving on the front lines during a war. Bullets fly constantly overhead. Incoming missiles scream at irregular intervals. Buddies are hit, injured, and die. The days are hot. The nights are cold. Parasites infest his body. He begins to babble incoherently.

Related/Similar Nursing Diagnosis. Because a person with a sensory/perceptual alteration may experience altered thought processes the diagnosis of *Sensory/Perceptual Alteration* must be differentiated from *Altered Thought Processes. Sensory/Perceptual Alteration* describes a person with a problem related to a sensory deficit or to inappropriate stimuli from the environment. *Sensory/Perceptual Alterations* can lead to *Altered Thought Processes.* Thus, *Sensory Perceptual Alterations* can serve as a related factor for *Altered Thought Processes.* A client with *Altered Thought Processes* experiences a disruption in cognitive operations and activities such as perception, reality, orientation, memory, comprehension, reasoning, and judgment. This is not always true of a person with *Sensory/Perceptual Alteration.*

---

most often at risk for injury, self-care deficit, impaired nutrition, and sensory deprivation. Nursing interventions are thus directed at preventing injury, maintaining independence, improving nutrition, and providing diversional activities.

VISION

Nursing care for the person with impaired vision is aimed at preventing sensory deprivation, promoting self-care, and providing a safe environment.

Sensory Deprivation. To help prevent sensory deprivation,

▶ Speak when you enter the room
▶ Obtain large-print or recorded books
▶ Give necessary instructions in large print, or provide them on a cassette recording
▶ Spend time talking with the person

Promoting Self-care. The person with a visual deficit may need assistance with such self-care tasks as feeding, bathing, dressing, and toileting. Nursing interven-

TABLE 51-1. Diagnoses that Frequently Accompany Specific Sensory Deficits

Sense	Diagnoses
Vision	Self-Care Deficit
	High Risk for Injury
Hearing	Impaired Verbal Communication
	Impaired Social Interaction
	Social Isolation
	High Risk for Injury
Taste	Altered Nutrition
Touch	High Risk for Injury
Smell	Altered Nutrition
	High Risk for Injury
Position sense	High Risk for Injury

tions that can help promote self-care in the visually impaired are listed in Box 51-4.

Providing a Safe Environment. The person with a visual deficit will need to arrange the environment to prevent injury. Furniture should be arranged so the person will not bump into or fall over it. The furniture should not be rearranged without letting the person know about the change. The visually impaired person and significant others should be taught about safe illumination, reduction of glare, and use of contrasting colors to assist with visual discrimination.

Adequate lighting should be provided in all rooms during the day, and soft lighting should be provided at night. The light switch should be easily accessible. Interventions to reduce glare include avoiding all glossy surfaces (e.g., glass and highly polished floors), using shades to provide diffuse light, wearing sunglasses or a hat with a brim when outside, and avoiding looking at bright lights (e.g., headlights). Providing color contrast aids visual discrimination and promotes safety. Methods to provide color contrast include marking edges of steps with colored tape; avoiding white walls, floors,

and counter tops; using smoked glass instead of clear glass; choosing objects colored black on white; and painting doorknobs a bright color.

HEARING

Providing a safe environment for a person with a hearing impairment is important to prevent injury. Visual aids and aids to enhance hearing are helpful. Examples of visual aids include a light that blinks when the doorbell or telephone rings, an alarm clock that flashes a light to awaken the person, flashing lights to warn of fire, and extra mirrors on the automobile to enhance vision in several directions. Aids to boost residual hearing include using telephone amplifiers and leaving the automobile window partially open and setting the air conditioner, heater, or radio on low so outside noises such as sirens and other warning signals can be heard.

A person with impaired hearing is at risk for social isolation. Nursing interventions should be directed toward promoting communications to increase social interaction. When communicating with hearing-impaired persons who can read lips, face them and be sure you have their attention before speaking. Try not to speak too rapidly, but do not slow your rate of speech below that appropriate for normal conversation. Speak clearly and simply. Do not shout or exaggerate lip movements. Use appropriate gestures to aid in the understanding of what is being said, just as you would with a hearing person. Do not draw letters in the air or make similar gestures.

If the person has residual hearing, try lowering the pitch of your voice. This often helps in communicating with the elderly hearing-impaired person because the ability to hear high-pitched sounds is often diminished in the elderly. Turn off the radio or television so that background noise does not interfere with the person's ability to hear.

For the profoundly deaf person who cannot read

TABLE 51-2. Nursing Diagnoses and Expected Outcomes

Nursing Diagnosis	Expected Outcomes
High Risk for Injury	Does not experience a fall or injury.
	Uses sensory aids (eyeglasses, hearing aid, or walker) to ensure safety.
	Demonstrates the use of a nurse call light for assistance.
Altered Nutrition	Identifies methods to increase the taste of foods.
Impaired Verbal Communication	Demonstrates an improved ability to communicate.
Social Isolation	Identifies appropriate diversional activities.
Self-care Deficit	Demonstrates the ability to use adaptive devices.
	Participates in own care.
Impaired Social Interaction	Initiates verbal communication with significant others.
Altered Thought Processes	Is oriented to person, place, time, and events.
	Communicates clearly with significant others.

<table>
<tr><td>

Box 51−4. Nursing Interventions for Promoting Self-care in the Visually Impaired Person

Feeding

▶ Describe the location of utensils and food on the tray or table using the clock as a reference (e.g., coffee, 1 o'clock; meat, 6 o'clock; potatoes, 3 o'clock).

▶ Describe food to stimulate an appetite.

▶ Place food in the person's field of vision if he or she has a visual field defect. Once client has accommodated, encourage him or her to scan the area.

▶ Encourage eating of finger foods to promote independence.

▶ If perceptual deficit, choose different-colored dishes to help distinguish items (e.g., red tray, white plates).

Bathing

▶ Verbally announce yourself before entering or leaving bathing area.

▶ Provide privacy.

▶ Place bathing equipment in location within easy reach.

▶ Place bathing equipment in person's field of vision if he or she has a visual field defect. Once client has accommodated, encourage him or her to scan the area.

▶ Observe the person's ability to reach bathing equipment.

▶ Observe the person's ability to perform hygiene tasks of bathing, shaving, brushing teeth, and combing hair.

▶ Provide clean clothing within easy reach.

▶ Place call light within reach if person is to bathe alone.

Dressing

▶ Allow the person to identify the most convenient location for clothing.

▶ Adapt the environment for the person's ease of dressing.

▶ Place clothing in the person's field of vision if he or she has a visual field defect. Once the client has accommodated, encourage him or her to scan the area.

Toileting

▶ Place call light within easy reach.

▶ Place toilet tissue within easy reach.

▶ Place bedpan or urinal in person's field of vision if he or she has a visual field defect. Once the person has accommodated, encourage him or her to scan the area.

▶ Observe the person's ability to reach the bedpan or urinal.

▶ Provide privacy.

▶ Provide a safe, clear path to the bathroom.

</td></tr>
</table>

lips, supply plenty of paper and pencils for notes. Obtain a sign language interpreter as needed.

TOUCH

A decrease in sensitivity to touch places a person at risk for injury. Teach the person to use a bath ther-

mometer to assess the temperature of bath water rather than relying on testing it with an extremity. Teach the person to assess the extremities daily for signs of undetected injuries.

TASTE AND SMELL

An alteration in taste and smell places the person at risk for impaired nutrition. Because the appetite is enhanced by smell and taste, it is important that food be flavorful. The use of spices, vinegar, and lemon juice can improve the flavor of food. Special attention should be given to the aesthetics of food preparation and serving to appeal to the person's visual sense. Frequent mouth care may also help increase taste and improve appetite.

A loss of smell can place the person at risk for injury. Smoke detectors should be installed and batteries checked regularly. Gas appliances should be monitored frequently for leaks. Foods that are prone to lose their freshness quickly should be dated and discarded before spoilage occurs.

POSITION SENSE

The person with vertigo or dizziness is experiencing an alteration in position sense and has a potential for injury. Orthostatic hypotension (the decrease of blood pressure on standing) is the most common cause of dizziness. There are numerous contributing factors for dizziness, such as cardiac dysrhythmias, dehydration, medication side effects, prolonged recumbent position, and a sudden change in position.

The person with dizziness should be taught to change position slowly and to move from a reclining to an upright position in stages, with a few minutes between each stage. A chair, walker, cane, or other assistive device should be placed nearby to steady the person when getting out of bed. The person should be taught to prevent dehydration by increasing fluid intake when excessive fluids are lost during exercise and when perspiring during hot weather.

Preventing Sensory/Perceptual Alterations in the Hospitalized Child

The strange and unfamiliar environment of the hospital may lead to sensory overload or to sensory deficit in children as well as in adults. You play a key role in preventing these sensory/perceptual alterations. There are special nursing actions you can take to help prevent them in children. See Box 51−5 for a list of these actions.

Sensory Deprivation

People need an adequate amount of sensory stimulation for normal growth and development. To prevent

---

Box 51-5. Nursing Interventions for Hospitalized Children

▶ Arrange the environment so children can look outside.
▶ Place children of similar ages together, and encourage socialization.
▶ Talk to and touch children gently and calmly.
▶ Explain what you are doing as you do it, even to small children or infants.
▶ When changing clothes, exercise their legs gently.
▶ Talk about different sensations (e.g., wet and dry or warm and cold).
▶ When bathing, allow them to play safely in the water. Provide toys that float and sink, and talk about what happens to the toys.
▶ While feeding, provide extra spoons and cups so the children can help feed themselves. Provide a variety of flavors, textures, and colors in foods.
▶ During treatment, distract children with toys.
▶ Encourage parents to visit and participate in their children's care.

---

sensory deprivation, nursing interventions should aim at providing an adequate amount of sensory stimulation without providing too much.

Sensory deprivation occurs when clients have little or no contact with other people, when the environment is dull and unstimulating, when they are exposed to excessively long periods of quiet, and when there is little opportunity to exercise.

Nursing interventions should provide a variety of environmental stimuli. Family and friends should be encouraged to visit and share useful information with the client. Do not try to "protect the person from overexcitement" by withholding family news. When inside rooms lack access to a window, vary the lighting to simulate night and day. When a window is available, try to position the client so he or she can see the view from it.

Numerous diversional activities are available, but they should be chosen carefully to ensure that they provide meaningful stimuli to the client. You might collaborate with an occupational therapist to plan diversional activities for your client. Family members might also be consulted because they know the person and know what he or she usually likes to do. For example, you may wish to play music to your comatose client. The family can tell you what type of music the person likes best, and they may even be able to bring in the person's own cassette tapes or compact disks as well as the playing device. The television and radio should not be left on continually but should be tuned in to stations the person prefers so he or she can enjoy favorite programs. Be sure the video is in focus and the sound is clear and at an appropriate level to be heard without straining.

To promote orientation or reorientation, place a clock and a calendar within the client's view. Be sure the client has clean eyeglasses and a properly working hearing aid, with working batteries, if needed. Address the person by name, introduce yourself frequently, and identify the place and time in a casual manner (e.g., "Isn't this a cool morning for the first of May?" or "Just two more days till New Year's Day. I bet you can hardly wait!" Advertise holidays with cards or decorations. Cut out and pin on a red heart for Valentine's Day. It helps if you can speak the person's predominant language. If you cannot, it is still helpful to try to communicate with the person. Encourage visitors who can speak the person's native language, and try to find an interpreter.

Sensory Overload

Ill people, especially those who are seriously ill, are at risk for sensory overload. Physiologic and psychosocial disturbances may result.

Factors that cause or contribute to sensory overload include an unfamiliar routine or environment, excessive light or noise, an altered sleep or rest pattern, and pain. In the hospital intensive care setting, nurses can reduce the stimulation of illumination by dimming lights at night, covering nonessential blinking lights, and encouraging the use of a sleep mask at night. Excessive noise may be reduced by shutting off nonessential alarms or reducing the volume of an alarm while keeping it at a safe level. It also helps to move noisy equipment away from the client's head and to avoid nonessential conversation at the person's bedside. Unfamiliar sights, sounds, and equipment should be discussed with the client.

If the person has become disoriented by sensory overload, reorientation activities are similar to those used to orient persons with a sensory deficit. Explain everything to the person in terms the person can understand.

To enhance rest and sleep, encourage client participation in activities of daily living, such as assisting with hygiene, and plan with the physical therapist the best methods for promoting mobility. See Chapters 35 and 36 for nursing activities related to decreased mobility. If the client requires restraints, remove them at least every 2 hours and provide range-of-motion exercises before replacing them. See Chapter 37 for additional nursing care related to restraints. Also see Chapter 39 for additional methods to promote rest and sleep. Do not be afraid to administer pain medications as ordered by the physician. See Chapter 40 for a discussion of pain control.

Communication with a Client with Sensory/Perceptual Alteration

Persons with sensory/perceptual alterations are at risk for impaired communication patterns. This is particularly true of clients who are confused, aphasic, delusional, or struggling with illusions or hallucinations.

THE CONFUSED CLIENT

Nursing interventions for the confused client are directed toward reorientation and prevention of injury. When communicating, speak slowly so the person has time to think about what is being said and to ask questions. If the client misunderstands, briefly attempt to clarify. Do not contribute to misunderstanding by agreeing with the misunderstanding. Do not argue with the client. Remain patient, and try to understand what the client is saying. When necessary, correct the client gently and refocus the conversation as needed. For example, if the client asks, "Aren't you Mary?", you can say, "No, Mary is the art therapist. I am Jane, one of the nurses here at University Hospital. I'll be helping you with lunch today. Are you hungry?"

Before speaking to a confused client, look into his or her eyes and speak clearly and in an appropriate tone and volume. Direct your comments at a level appropriate for the person's chronologic age. Sit or stand where the person can see your face. Avoid talking to coworkers about other topics in the client's presence.

When working with a confused person, focus on reorientation, as is done with clients with sensory deprivation. Have a family member bring in a favorite pillow or stuffed toy. These things can be helpful in reorienting a confused client.

The confused client is at risk for injury. Restraints are usually not appropriate because they increase confusion and impair reality testing and communication. It is more helpful to have someone with the client at all times to prevent injury. If possible, enlist the aid of a family member or friend to watch the person during times the person is confused. If restraints are necessary, use the least restrictive type possible. For example, if the client is pulling out tubes, use mitts instead of wrist restraints. Use a vest restraint that allows the client to sit up and roll from side to side.

THE APHASIC CLIENT

Aphasia is the general term for several different conditions in which the client has the ability to think without a corresponding ability to exchange information with others. Aphasia is a very common communication disorder for the client who has experienced cerebrovascular accident (stroke).[21] There are two main types of aphasia: receptive and expressive. The client with *receptive aphasia* cannot understand messages. He or she may fail to recognize speech or the written word. It is as though he or she is in a foreign land and cannot understand the language and yet is able to speak to you. The client may recognize objects and their use but not be able to understand what you say about them. For example, you may ask, "Would you like a glass of prune juice?" and the person will not be able to comprehend your question at all. However, you may give

the person a glass of prune juice and he or she will be able to say "Thank you very much" or "Could I have milk instead?"

The client with *expressive aphasia* can understand written and verbal communications but cannot organize words into meaningful expressions and thus cannot respond to your messages. The person who needs a bedpan very badly may wave at you frantically and say "Umbrella, umbrella, umbrella" and then begin to cry in frustration because she cannot say the words she so desperately wants to say. How do you communicate with persons with aphasia? Some interventions that have been found to be helpful are as follows:

▸ Ask questions that can be answered with a nod or by blinking an eye (once for yes, twice for no)
▸ Allow time for comprehension
▸ Talk to the person as though he or she understands you
▸ Only one person should speak at a time
▸ Position yourself so you can see each other
▸ Accompany words with visual cues such as pictures, objects, and gestures
▸ Use a normal voice level; do not shout
▸ Do not rush speech
▸ Use short phrases
▸ Adhere to familiar subject matter
▸ Keep conversation brief
▸ Keep conversation on a subject of interest to the person
▸ Organize surroundings and provide care in a predictable way

THE CLIENT WITH DELUSIONAL THINKING

Earlier, when we discussed delusions, we were discussing a particular type of delusion called a fixed delusion. Another type of delusion is a fleeting delusion. *Fixed delusions* are beliefs that have been held by the client for a long time and have repeatedly been reinforced. These usually cannot be corrected without therapy. *Fleeting delusions* are recent and usually arise from conditions or situations that can be corrected. The two most common causes of fleeting delusions are the effects of medications and a perceived loss of control over life.

When communicating with any client who has delusional thinking,

▸ Acknowledge the delusion and look for a cause
▸ Listen to the person talk about the delusion and determine whether it is fixed or fleeting
▸ Avoid agreeing or disagreeing with the person
▸ Avoid indicating the existence of an external, controlling force (e.g., do not use wording such as "What makes you . . . ?" or "Whatever possessed you to . . . ?")
▸ Give a brief explanation before doing anything to the person
▸ Do not put medicine in food or beverages

TABLE 51–3. Evaluation of Expected Outcomes

Expected Outcomes	Evaluation
High Risk for Injury	
Does not experience a fall or injury.	The client is free from any falls or injury.
Uses sensory aids (eyeglasses, hearing aid, or walker) to ensure safety.	The client uses eyeglasses, hearing aid, or walker.
Demonstrates use of the nurse call light for assistance.	The client is able to use the nurse call light for assistance to the bathroom.
Altered Nutrition	
Identifies methods to increase the taste of foods.	The client uses spices, vinegar, and lemon juice for taste.
Impaired Verbal Communication	
Demonstrates an improved ability to communicate.	The client is able to communicate with another person through the use of a hearing aid, pencil and paper, or a sign language interpreter.
Social Isolation	
Identifies appropriate diversional activities.	The client identifies senior citizen centers and church groups as possible diversional activities.
Self-care Deficit	
Demonstrates the ability to use adaptive devices.	The client is able to feed self after being oriented to the tray, using the face of a clock for orientation.
Participates in own care.	The client washes face and hands as part of hygiene care.
Impaired Social Interaction	
Initiates verbal communication with significant other.	The client wears a hearing aid to hear and understands communication with significant other. The client initiates communication.
Altered Thought Processes	
Is oriented to person, place, time, and events.	The client can correctly state name, place, time, and current events.
Communicates clearly with significant other.	The client and significant other are able to understand each other, and communication is clear.

THE CLIENT WITH ILLUSIONS

Because illusions are mistaken impressions of reality, clients with illusions may be as normal in their thinking as you are, or they may be quite out of contact with reality. If your client is functioning normally, a simple explanation is all that is necessary. For example, "Yes, that shadow on the wall does look like dirt, doesn't it? But you can tell it isn't dirt if you watch it. It moves as the sun moves." If your client is confused, highly anxious, delusional, hallucinating, or otherwise not in a position to accept a simple dose of reality, you will have to use great care in dealing with illusions. To communicate best with such clients,

▶ First, identify the object that triggered the illusion
▶ If possible, remove the object that triggered the illusion
▶ Explain what the object actually is without saying that it is not what the client thinks
▶ When the client is calm, let him or her handle the object

For example, suppose a client whispers, "Be quiet, don't move. There's a snake in my bed!" The nurse on duty would look under the cover sheet and find a Foley catheter connected to tubing that leads to a drainage bag hanging on the side of the bed. Because the object (the tubing) cannot be removed, the nurse would pick up the drainage bag enough so the client could see it and say, "This is your drainage bag. See how the tubing runs from this bag up into your bladder? It helps drain your urine." This should help the person calm down.

If the person continues to insist that there is a snake in the bed and points to a spot where there is nothing remotely like a snake, the client is having a hallucination, not an illusion.

THE CLIENT WITH HALLUCINATIONS

Recall that, when a person is having a hallucination, he or she is seeing, hearing, or otherwise experiencing something that is not present in objective reality. To communicate with a hallucinating person therapeutically,

▶ Identify yourself and let the person know you are a nurse and want to help
▶ Acknowledge that the person is experiencing some-

thing that you are not experiencing (e.g., "I know you see a snake there but I don't see it")

▶ Acknowledge the person's emotional response to the perception (e.g., if the person continues to insist that there is a snake, say, "It must be very frightening for you. I'll stay with you")

▶ Do not challenge the hallucination as unreal

▶ Do not leave the client alone while the hallucination is being experienced or immediately afterward; stay with the client but do not try to talk while he or she is actively hallucinating

▶ Avoid sedatives or hypnotics

EVALUATION

Evaluation of the person with a sensory/perceptual problem includes assessment of the client to ascertain whether outcomes have been met. In particular, the expected outcomes for a client experiencing a sensory/perception alteration would measure whether the client has achieved an improved response to the sensory deficit experienced or to the sensory/perceptual alteration. Outcomes that were listed in Table 51–2 are evaluated in Table 51–3.

Summary

▶ Sensation and perception are processes that require sensory nerve receptors to convey stimuli to the brain, where they are perceived and interpreted. The person then responds to the stimuli.

▶ Sensory deficit occurs when one of the senses is impaired and stimuli are not conveyed to the brain for perception.

▶ Sensory deprivation occurs when the brain receives too little incoming stimuli, and sensory overload occurs when the brain receives too much stimuli.

▶ Alterations in perception can result in confusion, delusional thinking, illusion, or hallucination.

▶ Many persons are at risk for sensory/perceptual alterations.

▶ The nurse can assess a client for sensory/perceptual alterations by taking the client's history, completing a physical assessment of the client's senses, noting symptoms of sensory/perceptual alterations, and noting responses to sensory deficits or sensory/perceptual alterations.

▶ The nurse should be able to differentiate between the diagnoses of *Sensory/Perceptual Alteration* and *Altered Thought Processes*.

CASE STUDY

The Client

Ms. Sarah Jane Jacobson, a 78-year-old Caucasian, was admitted 6 days ago after a motor vehicle accident. Ms. Jacobson immigrated to the United States from Germany 40 years ago with her husband and does not speak fluent English. Her husband passed away 1 year ago, and she now lives with her daughter. She was admitted with multiple injuries including a left clavicle fracture, left femur fracture, and multiple rib fractures. The chest x-ray showed a pneumothorax (collapse of the lung) from one of the rib fractures. A partial listing of physician's orders, on admission, includes the following:

▶ Bedrest
▶ 20 lbs skeletal traction to left leg
▶ Immobilize left arm in a figure-of-eight bandage
▶ Left chest tube to 20 cm of suction
▶ Foley catheter to dependent drainage
▶ IV—D5 1/2NS at 125 cc per hour
▶ Demerol, 50–75 mg IM q 3–4 hours

Forty-eight hours after admission, the night nurse stated that Ms. Jacobson had become confused, was oriented to person only, and pulled out her Foley catheter and intravenous (IV) catheter. These were replaced by the night nurse.

ASSESSMENT DATA

A partial listing of assessment data at 7:00 AM on December 14 follows.

▶ 78-year-old female with left leg in 20 lbs of skeletal traction and left shoulder in a figure-of-eight bandage
▶ temperature—36.5°C, blood pressure—132/78, pulse—72, respirations—18
▶ oriented to person only
▶ agitated, restless, and combative
▶ only speaking German
▶ pulling at IV, Foley catheter, and chest tube
▶ Foley to dependent drainage
▶ left chest tube to 20 cm of suction
▶ dorsalis pedis and posterior tibial pulses 2+ bilaterally
▶ radial and brachial pulses 2+ bilaterally
▶ capillary refill brisk
▶ movement and sensation intact in left lower extremity
▶ states she has pain in the ribs and left leg

Four days have passed since Ms. Jacobson became confused. The following represents part of a nursing care plan written then and the current evaluation of outcomes that were expected at that time.

Case Study continued on following page

CARE PLAN

7:00 AM, December 14

Nursing Diagnosis	Planning: Expected Outcomes	Implementation: Nursing Interventions	Evaluation
Sensory/Perceptual Alterations R/T an unfamiliar environment and an insufficient amount of meaningful stimuli	By 7:00 AM, December 18: ▸ answers questions demonstrating that she is oriented to person, place, time, and client role responsibilities	▸ Introduce self to client. ▸ Orient client to room and ongoing procedures. ▸ Orient client to setting by using voice, touch, and visual cues. ▸ Everytime you enter the room, orient the client to time. ▸ Teach the client and daughter the meaning of environmental stimuli. ▸ Make frequent meaningful contacts with the client. ▸ Place calendar in view of client. ▸ Decrease number of continuous and intermittent noises, lights, or noxious odors.	7:00 AM, December 18 Client is oriented to person, place, and time. Client is not pulling at IV, Foley, or chest tubes.
	▸ Interacts with family, friends, and hospital personnel	▸ Teach client and daughter importance of visitors. ▸ Speak slowly. ▸ Allow time for client to express herself in English. ▸ Encourage daughter to visit and communicate with the client in a language she can understand. ▸ Encourage daughter to bring in personal items from home. ▸ Provide communication board with pictures to facilitate interaction with hospital personnel.	Client actively interacts with daughter. Client and hospital personnel have developed effective communications. Client is able to communicate her needs to hospital personnel.

▸ The outcome criteria for a client experiencing sensory/perceptual alteration should be specific for (1) the response to the sensory deficit experienced or (2) the response to the sensory/perceptual alteration.

▸ Nursing interventions for persons with a sensory deficit are directed toward helping the persons compensate for the deficit, whereas nursing interventions for persons with sensory overload or sensory deprivation are directed toward helping the

persons to compensate for central nervous system changes and psychosocial alterations.

▸ When communicating with persons with different types of altered perceptions, the nurse must use different approaches.

▸ Evaluation of the person with a sensory/perceptual problem requires noting whether the client has shown an improved response to the sensory deficit experienced or to the sensory/perceptual alteration experienced.

Bibliography

1. Barrie-Shevlin, P. S. (1987). Maintaining sensory balance for the critically ill patient. *Nursing*, 3(16), 597–601.
2. Carpenito, L. J. (1985). Altered thoughts or altered perceptions? *American Journal of Nursing*, 85(11), 1283.
3. Carpenito, L. J. (1989). *Nursing diagnosis: Application to clinical practice* (3rd ed.). Philadelphia: J. B. Lippincott.
4. Clark, B. (1984). What to do when your patient lets slip his grip on reality. *Nursing*, 14(7), 50–56.
5. Dootson, S. (1990). Critical care: Sensory imbalance and sleep loss. *Nursing Times*, 86(35), 26–29.
6. Easton, C., & MacKenzie, F. (1988). Sensory-perceptual alterations: delirium in the intensive care unit. *Heart and Lung*, 17(3), 229–237.
7. Ebersole, P., & Hess, P. (1990). *Toward healthy aging: Human needs and nursing response* (3rd ed.). St. Louis: C. V. Mosby.
8. Gates, S. J. (1984). Helping your patient on bedrest cope with perceptual/sensory deprivation. *Orthopaedic Nursing*, 3(2), 35–38.
9. Hahn, K. (1989). About sensory loss. *Nursing*, 19(2), 97–99.
10. Hickey, J. V. (1985). *The clinical practice of neurological and neurosurgical nursing* (2nd ed.). Philadelphia: J. B. Lippincott.
11. Hudak, C. M., et al. (1990). *Critical care nursing: A holistic approach* (5th ed.). Philadelphia: J. B. Lippincott.
12. Kee, C. C. (1990). Sensory impairment: factor X in providing nursing care to the older adult. *Journal of Community Health Nursing*, 7(1), 45–52.
14. Kopac, C. A. (1983). Sensory loss in the aged: the role of the nurse and the family. *Nursing Clinics of North America*, 18(2), 373–384.
15. Lamb, M. (1969). *Pyschology as applied to nursing*. London: S. Livingston.
16. MacKinnon-Kesler, S. (1983). Maximizing your ICU patient's sensory and perceptual environment. *Canadian Nurse*, 79(5), 41–45.
17. Matteson, M. A., & McConnell, E. S. (1988). *Gerontological nursing: Concepts and practice*. Philadelphia: W. B. Saunders.
18. McGonigal, K. S. (1986). The importance of sleep and the sensory environment to critically ill patients. *Intensive Care Nursing*, 2(2), 73–83.
19. Moore, T. (1989). Sensory deprivation in the ICU. *Nursing*, 3(36), 45–47.
20. Porth, C. M. (1990). *Pathophysiology: Concepts of altered health states* (3rd ed.). Philadelphia: J. B. Lippincott.
21. Riegel, B., & Ehrenreich, D. (1989). *Psychological aspects of critical care nursing*. Rockville, MD: Aspen Publishers.
22. Rogers, J. C., et al. (1987). Maude: a case of sensory deprivation. *American Journal of Occupational Therapy*, 41(10), 673–676.
23. Rose, M. A. (1986). Sensory loss simulation use in nursing education. *Journal of Gerontological Nursing*, 12(7), 22–24.
24. Sherwin, L. N., et al. (1991). *Nursing care of the childbearing family*. Norwalk, CT: Appleton & Lange.
25. Taptich, B. J., et al. (1989). *Nursing diagnosis and care planning*. Philadelphia: W. B. Saunders.
26. Wyness, M. A. (1985). Perceptual dysfunction: nursing assessment and management. *Journal of Neurosurgical Nursing*, 17(2), 105–110.
27. Zegeer, L. J. (1986). The effects of sensory changes in older persons. *Journal of Neuroscience Nursing*, 18(6), 325–332.

▼ *Promoting Sexual Health*

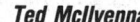

> There is no gift like sexuality. . . . We cannot fully understand
> sexuality without looking at it as a natural functioning of the body.
> Our sexuality is not something which is optional—it is a part of
> who and what we are.
>
> **Ted McIlvenna**

▼ CHAPTER OUTLINE

SEXUAL GROWTH AND DEVELOPMENT
    Physiology and Sexuality
    Psychosocial Development and
      Sexuality
    Cultural Components of Sexuality
SEXUAL FUNCTION
SEXUALITY AND SEXISM IN NURSING
    Nurse-client Relationships
    Interprofessional Relationships
SEXUALITY AND THE CLIENT'S HEALTH
  STATUS
ASSESSMENT
    General Physical Assessment
    Assessment of the Client's Sense
      of Self as a Sexual Being

    Assessment of the Client's Sexual
      Roles and Relationships
    Assessment of Sexual Function
    Gathering the Sexual History
NURSING DIAGNOSIS
PLANNING
NURSING INTERVENTION
    Culturally Sensitive Interventions
    Problems that Can Interfere with
      Sexuality
EVALUATION
CASE STUDY

▼ KEY TERMS

Androgeny   Homophobia   Sexual orientation
Gender role   Sexism   Sexuality
Gonadal sex   Sexual function

In 1975, the World Health Organization promoted the importance of sexuality as a vital component of health care and established parameters for educating health professionals about sexuality. Before that time, although nurses applied the concept of sexuality in health teaching and in the nursing care of clients, they professed limited knowledge, sophistication, and comfort in attending to clients' sexuality and sexual health needs.[38] Sexuality is a vital component of holistic nursing care, and students of nursing have an obligation to be informed and comfortable in relating to health care consumers about this sensitive topic.

Sexuality is the state or quality of being sexual. It refers to the collective characteristics that mark the differences between the male and the female. Holistically, the term sexuality has had two meanings:

▶ the pursuit of sexual pleasure, reproduction, and the need for love and personal fulfillment
▶ awareness and feelings of being male or female (referred to as gender identity)

Sexuality has biologic, psychologic, social, and cultural dimensions.[24]

Sexual health is the integration of somatic, emotional, intellectual, and social aspects of sexual being in ways that are enriching and that enhance personality, communication, and love (World Health Organization). As a nurse, you will constantly confront one or more of the sexuality dimensions because, first, you are a sexual being; second, illness, health promotion, and disease and injury prevention are likely to involve aspects of one's sexuality; and third, nursing involves the most intimate care of another sexual being. This chapter discusses major aspects of the concept of sexuality as it applies to the nurse and to the nurse's care of clients.

SEXUAL GROWTH AND DEVELOPMENT

We are unsure about the extent to which biologic influences are altered by psychologic, social, and cultural variables that result in typical male or female sexuality. Conflicting information exists, and further study is needed. Human physiology not only determines male and female physical sex characteristics (gender) but also exerts some influence on human sexual behavior, including but not limited to sexual response.

Physiology and Sexuality

CHROMOSOMAL LINKAGE

Human sexuality is based on the genetic determination of gender at the moment of conception when either the X or the Y chromosome in the sperm unites with the X chromosome of the egg; the XX chromosomal combination produces a female and the XY combination is the male. The chromosomal linkage, the establishment of genetic sex, is the first of three stages in the process of sexual differentiation. Hormonal action has an effect on genetic programming. Sometime between the fourth and eighth week after conception, testosterone (the male sex hormone) is secreted by the embryo's rudimentary testes. If it is not secreted, the embryo will develop as a physical female despite the presence of the male chromosome.[22,32]

ESTABLISHMENT OF GONADAL SEX

The second stage of sexual differentiation, the establishment of **gonadal sex** (genital sex), occurs by about the 10th to the 12th week of gestation. All fetuses, at conception, are considered dimorphic: in essence, having both female and male rudimentary elements or gonads and the potential to develop as either sex. The male determining factor in the Y chromosome leads to the development of the internal testes from the gonad medulla; without the male factor, there is development of the internal ovary from the gonad cortex.[5] The Y chromosome also directly influences body growth, skeletal muscle maturation, dental development, and the slower growth rate in boys.[25]

ESTABLISHMENT OF PHENOTYPIC SEX

The third stage is the establishment of phenotypic sex, when the additional internal and external genital organs develop[25] and result in the actual characteristics of biologic sex. This is a critical time in sexual differentiation because each fetus develops both the wolffian and müllerian genital duct systems, one of which must de-

velop and the other regress to produce actual male or female external genitalia. The wolffian duct system in the presence of testosterone gives rise to the epididymis, the vas deferens, and the seminal vesicles in males. The müllerian duct gives rise to the female fallopian tubes, the uterus, and the upper part of the vagina. Figure 52–1 illustrates the differentiation of the internal genitalia, and Figure 52–2 illustrates the differentiation of the external genitalia. Prenatally, sexual and body structure development proceeds through a complicated series of events that are dependent on continuous feedback between the production of sex hormones by the ovaries and testes and the adrenal cortex and the control in the brain by the hypothalamus and the pituitary gland.[25]

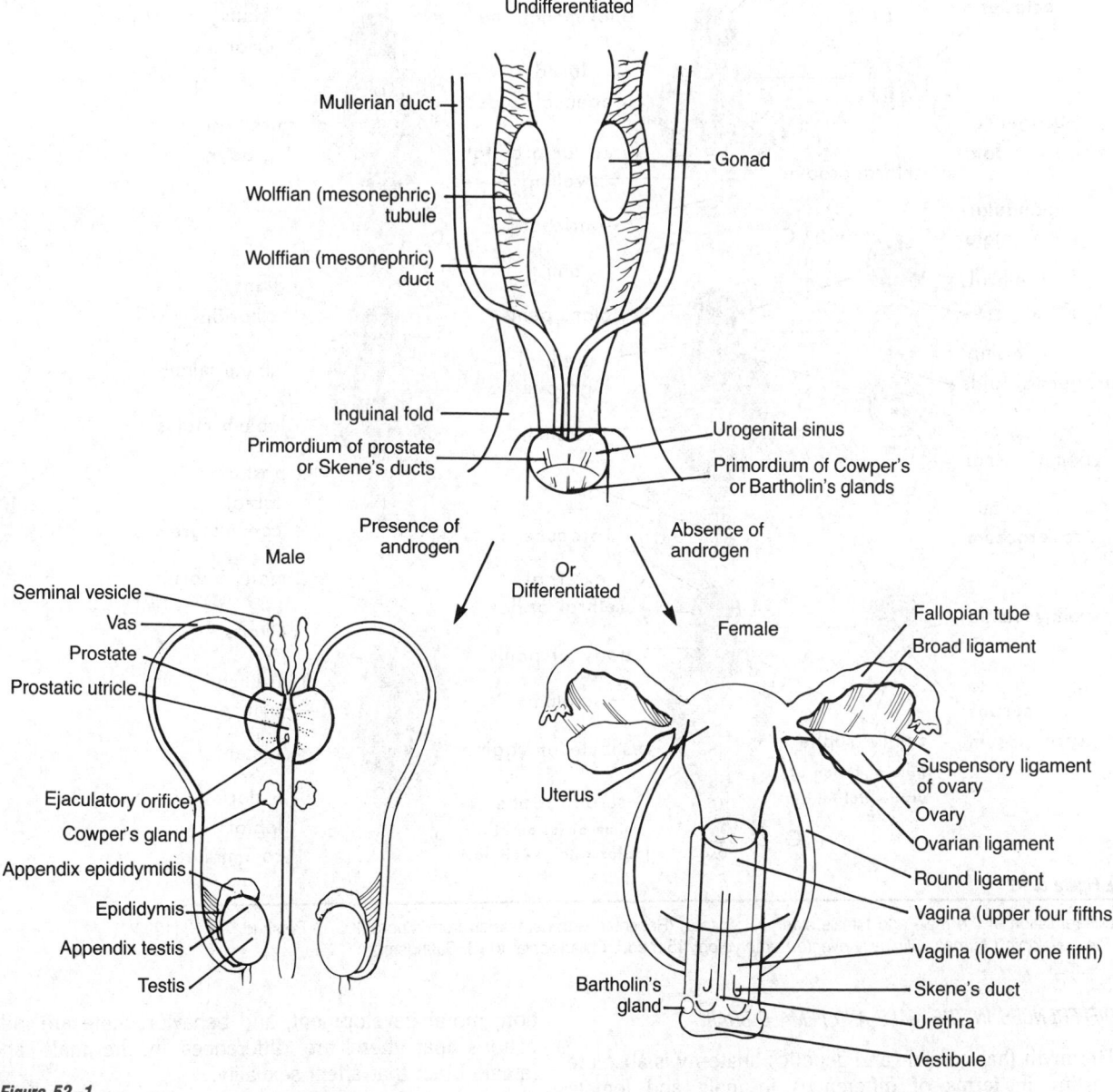

▲ *Figure 52–1*

Differentiation of the male and female internal genitalia. (Reprinted with permission from McCary, S.P., & McCary, J.L. [eds.] [1984]. *Human sexuality* [3rd brief ed.] Belmont, CA: Wadsworth Publishing Company.)

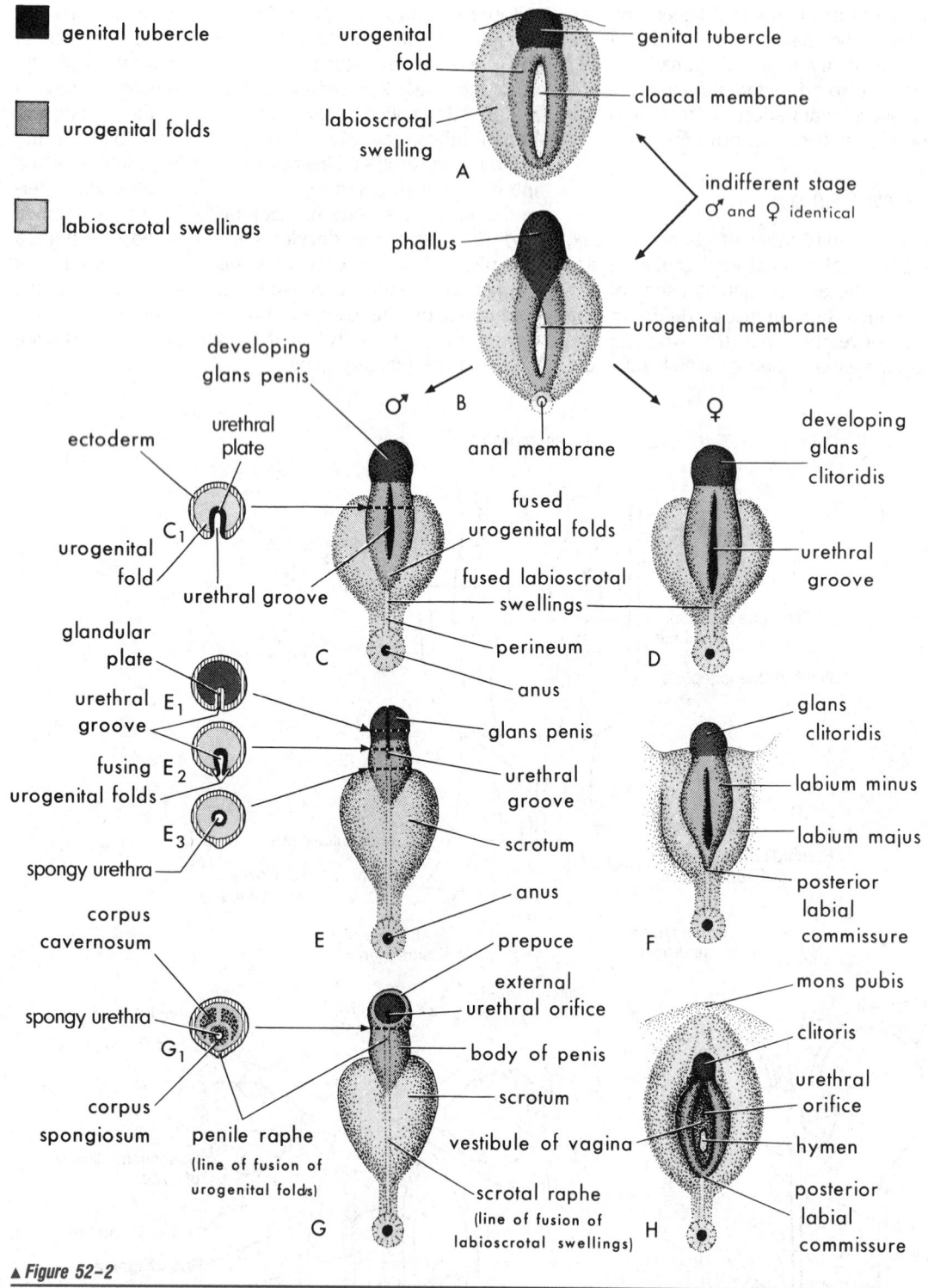

▲ *Figure 52–2*

Differentiation of the male and female external genitalia. (Reprinted with permission from Moore, K.I., & Persaud, T.V.N. [1993]. *The developing human. Clinically oriented embryology* [5th ed.]. Philadelphia: W. B. Saunders.)

DIFFERENCES IN THE MALE AND FEMALE BRAIN

The myth that genital (and genetic) anatomy is absolute destiny in terms of differences in male and female development and manifestations of later gender behavior has been fairly well dispelled. However, on the basis of findings in animal brain research and identifiable gender differences in human intelligence, cogni-tion, moral development, and behavior, there are indications that there are differences in the male and female brain that affect sexuality.

Similar to genital dimorphism, the human brain is dimorphic in the developing fetus, and it is speculated that the brain of the fetus is female unless influenced by the male hormones.[19,25] Thus, sex hormones biochemically influence the brain as to male-female differentiation and differences in gender-typical behavior.

Another difference between the male brain and the female brain is the functional asymmetry of the cerebral hemispheres, which accounts for dominant sidedness in individuals. In their review of the research literature, Kahn and Cataio[25] reported significant differences between the sexes in the lateralization of cognitive functions. In the adult female brain, language and nonverbal functions are represented in both hemispheres, but in adult males both functions occur in only the left hemisphere of the brain; thus, language and spatial functions are more one sided and localized in males. What tends to be associated with the right-left brain function is the difference between male and female typical response styles. The most enduring difference is in the greater male aggressiveness (potential and actual) that even exists cross-culturally.[5,25] Although these differences between the sexes are a result of both cerebral hemispheric difference and the influence of testosterone in males, many of the differences are eliminated or at least become closer in similarity through learning and socialization that ignores sex stereotyping.

PUBERTY

Many of the processes of biologic sex occur prenatally and again during the second stage of physiologic sexual differentiation that occurs in puberty. Once the child is born, physical sex characteristics, and the male and female reproductive systems, continue to mature along with other structures and systems of the body.

For development to progress, the individual must maintain a state of good health within an environment that ensures the meeting of basic needs necessary for all growth and development.

Puberty refers to the hormonal and physical changes leading to maturation of reproductive capacity[13] with physical maturation of secondary sex characteristics. The onset of puberty for females occurs at about 10 to 12 years of age, and for males, at about 12 years of age or later. Not only do external bodily changes take place, but there is a flurry of internal hormonal activity that often underlies the "storminess" of temperament so typically seen in adolescent behavior.

Physiologically, this is a stressful time for adolescents. The internal and external environments of adolescents are both extremely important. Adequate nutrition, good hygiene, exercise, and ample rest are important ingredients to maintain the body's energy in the physiologic processes of sexual development.

Puberty in Females. In females the pituitary gland causes a sudden rise in the sex hormone follicle-stimulating hormone (FSH). In turn, FSH acts on the ovaries in the production of estrogen. Estrogen production results in the beginning of breast development, the internal growth of the uterus and vaginal canal, and the enlargement of the labia and clitoris. The pituitary also secretes adrenocorticotropic hormone (ACTH), which stimulates the production of small amounts of androgen (male sex hormones) by the adrenal gland and results in the appearance of pubic and axillary hair. The accompanying growth spurt in girls is seen in the widening of the hips, development of the buttocks, and an increase in height. The most definitive and mature stage of uterine development is menarche (onset of menstruation) and occurs after the peak of the female growth spurt, typically anytime from 10 to 14 years. When the menses is eventually accompanied by ovulation, the female reaches full reproductive capacity.

Puberty in Males. Male puberty begins with an increase in the growth rate of the testes and scrotum and the development of pubic hair. A marked increase in gonadotropic hormones causes an increase in the growth of the penis and testes, an increase in body height, and breast and nipple sensitivity, which are the events that lead to sexual maturation. At this stage, androgens are most important for males because testosterone is necessary for activating the prenatal masculinization of the brain. Boys' growth spurt, beginning at about 13 years of age, includes increased height and weight, body hair, alteration of body contour and facial features, and muscular strength. This spurt progresses unevenly for about 2 to 3 years, is the cause of lack of coordination, and is often a source of embarrassment to boys. The onset of nocturnal emissions (wet dreams) follows the maturation of the prostate gland and seminal vesicles. Box 52–1 summarizes female and male secondary sex characteristics.

Box 52–1. Female and Male Secondary Sex Characteristics

Female Characteristics

Acne
Underarm hair
Development of breasts
Rounding of body contours
Pubic hair
Enlargement of clitoris, labia, and uterus
Beginning of menstruation

Male Characteristics

Facial hair
Acne
Changes in voice
Underarm hair
Chest hair
Enlargement of breasts
Development of muscles
Pubic hair
Enlargement of penis, scrotum, prostate, testes, and seminal vesicles
Beginning of ejaculation

Psychosocial Development and Sexuality

The psychosocial theories of sexual development and the influences of culture facilitate our understanding of the complex events that lead to gender-typical behaviors. The individual integration of psychologic make-up and social processes is what constitutes each person's response style as a sexual being. Several concepts relevant to sexuality are elaborated here to make the comprehension of theoretical premises clearer.

SELF-CONCEPT AND BODY IMAGE

Self-concept (how one perceives oneself as well as the internalized appraisals of others) and body image (the mental picture one has of his or her body) are both important concepts to sexual health. Central to self-concept is acceptance of gender role[17] and the concomitant behaviors the individual views as acceptable for oneself as a sexual being.

Positive self-concept is essential to a healthy sexual being, and a negative self-concept is likely to interfere with the establishment of effectual sexual behaviors and responses. A positive and intact image of one's body is crucial to sexuality during adolescence and early adulthood.

This is particularly true given Western culture's emphasis on physical attractiveness in relationships between the sexes. As Fogel[17] reported, women's sexuality is especially affected by self-concept because a poor body image may result in negative responses to sexual arousal. Conversely, a woman who feels good about and is comfortable with her body is much freer to engage in, and enjoy sharing herself more openly in, social interactions with both sexes. Western society's preoccupation with physical beauty also affects older women when numerous bodily changes (e.g., wrinkling and dry skin) take place during menopause and aging.

Men are typically less preoccupied with their bodies than are women, and a comfortable body image is one that reflects muscularity and virility, those qualities typically associated with masculinity. In terms of body image, most men are concerned about penis size, erection, and "staying power."[17]

GENDER IDENTITY

Gender refers to[34] "socially learned responses, meanings, and cues that are taken as reflections of society's conceptions of masculinity and femininity". The general assignment of gender begins at birth on the basis of observation of the external genitalia of the child, and the first stage of the gender concept is established by 15 to 18 months of age.[6] According to Bee,[6] the second stage is gender stability or the understanding that one stays the same gender throughout life. Gender stability occurs by 4 years of age. The third stage, at 5 or 6 years of age, is gender constancy, and this is similar to gender stability. It involves the recognition that even though a person is either masculine or feminine throughout life, he or she may dress or engage in behaviors that are more assigned to the opposite gender.

Gender identity, as distinguished from body-linked biologic sex, is a series of meanings regarding definitions of the self and behavior toward others.[34]

GENDER ROLE

Gender role consists of appearance and behaviors that demonstrate maleness and femaleness and what one presents according to a specific culture's consideration of masculine or feminine. Gender role is learned and typically congruent with gender identity and may or may not be congruent with biologic sex.

A more contemporary concept regarding gender is androgyny. **Androgyny** is an anthropologic term meaning that any one individual exhibits characteristics of both male and female sexes. Androgyny relates to both gender identity and role; for example, women known traditionally as "feminine" for their dependent identity and expressive role behaviors would be androgynous in becoming more independent and instrumental or active in shaping their own destinies. Acceptance of this concept is exemplified by young women choosing careers that were formerly only for males and by their being more aggressive. It is also shown by men taking more responsibility for household and child care activities and by their being more compassionate.

A growing body of literature reports that those persons who are more androgynous in their behaviors are better adjusted, although not always comfortable, in terms of a sexual self-concept compared with people who hold rigidly to the more traditional masculine/feminine role behaviors.[36]

SEXUAL ORIENTATION

Sexual orientation is the preference, as well as the physical and emotional attraction, that one develops for a partner. Although the norm in Western society is still heterosexual orientation, homosexuality (lesbians and gay males) does exist and is considered a normal variant of sexual behavior.

The origins of sexual orientation are elusive, and much of the research leads to acceptance of an interaction model; in essence, sexual preference emerges because of the mutual influence of biologic, psychologic, and sociologic factors.[33]

PSYCHOSEXUAL DEVELOPMENT AND GENDER DIFFERENCES

Freudian Theory. Freudian psychoanalytic theory is the most pervasive in terms of explaining psychosexual development. This theory integrates physiologic, psychologic, and social factors that influence behavioral differences in males and females throughout the developmental cycle. Freud postulated that all behavioral development — cognitive, interpersonal, and social — is motivated by two basic instinctual drives: self-preservation (an aggressive drive) and species preservation (a love, affectional, or binding together drive).[16] Psychic energy (known as libido) is the driving force toward individual fulfillment of both aggressive and affectional needs.

The psychoanalytic approach emphasizes critical events as influencing sexuality in the early stages of life. The resolution of conflict in the genital stage of development is particularly crucial to a sense of sexual identity. It is said that the male develops an incestuous craving for the mother and is resentful of the father as a rival for the mother's attention (Oedipus complex). The female has a sense of symbiosis with her mother, which is broken as she finds a love object in her father (Electra complex), who tends at this stage of development to be warm and affectionate toward her. The erotic feelings and fantasies each child has in relation to taking the place of the same-sex parent causes him or her a certain amount of conflict and concomitant anxiety. As parents maintain their parenting role, the child accepts the basic relational bond between the parents, and feelings of jealousy are shifted to an identity with the same-sex parent. The Oedipus/Electra conflict is thus resolved, and the children's masculine and feminine identities emerge.[28]

Separation-Individuation. More contemporary interpreters of Freudian psychology refer to the process of separation-individuation that occurs in the pre-oedipal phase of development as important to gender-typical behaviors. This is an object relations point of view and indicates that as the developing child interacts with people and objects in the environment, he or she forms loving or hostile mental images regarding these experiences.[26,27,35] Later, during separation-individuation, the child establishes a whole person identity separate from others and comes to accept others as having both positive and negative interaction characteristics. The relevance to healthy sexuality of this separation-individuation process is the ability of the individual to form friendly and loving bonds with others with a minimum of hostility and to sustain those relationships over time with little mutual hostility.[7]

Another important factor in object relations theory, directly relevant to gender-typical feelings and behaviors, is the mothering role universally assumed by women. The process of separation-individuation for females is within an ongoing relationship, and the female child does not separate completely from attachment to the mothering person to establish her identity. In experiencing themselves like their mothers, there is fusion of the experience of attachment with the process of identity formation.[14] The female then emerges from this process with a capacity for empathy (a strong basis for experiencing another's needs and feelings) as a primary aspect of self-definition.

For the male child, there is complete separation from the mother in order to establish a masculine identity, which breaks the primary love and sense of empathic tie. The result is a clearer sense of individuation and ego boundaries that are defensive (against the primary attachment to the mother). The profound effects of these different separation processes, as reported by Gilligan,[20] relate to gender-typical behaviors in relationship and dependency issues. Because feminine gender identity is not dependent on separation (from the mother) or on the progress of individuation, female gender identity is threatened by separation and independence, and the female experiences difficulty with individuation. The consequences to women are great because most developmental achievements in our society depend on increasing separation and independence; thus, problems with separation become perceived as failures and perpetuate the myth that females are inferior. For men, masculine gender identity is dependent on separation: therefore, they feel threatened by intimacy, closeness, and dependency and experience difficulties in forming close relationships with both sexes.

Activities and Events Critical to the Development of Healthy Sexuality. There are important observable activities and events for the development of healthy sexuality that occur throughout the developmental cycle.

Activities and Events in Infancy. In infancy, one develops a sense of self through interactions with another by touch, such as sucking and being cuddled, and through exploration with the eyes. In a nurturing and safe environment, the infant gains a sense of contentment as well as trust in another through getting needs met. Because the infant's environment is not gender neutral, he or she is the passive recipient of interactions with parents and others who influence gender-typical responses. For example, Belsky[8] reported that mothers tend to talk to and look at girls and respond to their crying more immediately than they do boys. Also by age 6 months, boys are touched less frequently, played with more roughly, and are generally encouraged to be more independent, in keeping with the stereotypical view of males.

Activities and Events in Early Childhood. In early childhood, autonomy and a continuing sense of separate identity are established through walking, through talking and being responded to verbally, and through touch. Further sexual identity is manifested in touching and exploration of the genitals, pelvic thrust movements, and even sexual arousal and orgasm that parallel adult sexual behavior. If allowed, these activities are more pleasurable and sensuous to the child than erotic.[23,29] If such self-stimulating behaviors are responded to negatively or stopped by the nurturing persons, the child may experience feelings of discomfort and shame. With increased mobility and the development of language and cognitive skills at about 4 to 5 years of age, children test boundaries more aggressively and have active imaginations. They begin to know their own bodies and become aware of sex differences; also they take pride in their genitals, and fondling becomes more purposeful. Masturbation is a natural phenomenon at this stage. In healthy sexual development, it is important that the child learn appropriate language for body parts, including the genitals.

Activities and Events in School Age. During the school-age years, sexual differentiation is further learned through role-playing that emulates both verbal and nonverbal behaviors of the same-sex adult. This may be a time when boys begin to get an adverse message about the display of affectionate behaviors if they do not witness loving behaviors between parents or receive affection themselves through touch, especially from their fathers; in essence, "boys do not hug or get hugged." There is some variability in sex-typical behaviors during this time, reported by Macoby and Jacklin:[30] Females exhibit greater sensitivity to touch, greater timidity or anxiousness, and more compliant and nurturing behavior. Males tend to be more active, competitive, and concerned with dominance in their relationships. Our society may be becoming more androgynous in planning and encouraging females in sports, such as soccer, during the school-age years, so that they learn teamwork and the abilities to compete and to resolve disputes.

Activities and Events in Preadolescence. Preadolescent years are extremely important in terms of establishing reciprocal relationships, beginning with a chum of the same sex and then "hanging around" in groups in which children observe and learn about all kinds of heterosexual and same-sex interactions of peers. They also learn "street language": labels both for genitals and for various sexual activities. A positive or negative view of sex and individual sexuality is learned depending on how influential adults respond to their use of such labels. If a boy naively calls a girl a whore, and that term is not clarified at that time as being derogatory to females and why, he may feel it is okay to continue that behavior.

Activities and Events in Adolescence. It is during adolescence that individuals solidify the sociocultural meanings of sexuality and gender identity. Physiologic development and expectations that adolescents grow and progress toward adult competencies pose some conflicts. One role socialization process in adolescence centers around dating in preparation for selecting a mate, and yet sexual intimacy is a moral taboo. Currently, engaging in sexual intercourse, especially with multiple partners, is also a health hazard that is potentially life threatening because of sexually transmitted diseases, primarily acquired immune deficiency syndrome (AIDS).

Gender and occupational identities are critical issues in adolescent sexual development. The energy for females is focused toward an expressive role of achieving interpersonal skills, including acceptance, security, and support with an identity linked to intimacy. The male focus of energy is on an identity linked to separation. Independence and achievement, autonomy from parents, and conformity to peer group values are instrumental in leading males to an occupational identity.[13]

Gender roles for both males and females are becoming less rigid, and lifestyle patterns are being established more on individual preferences and less on societal expectations of what men and women ought to do. For example, in Western society, many women are choosing to establish themselves in careers before or in place of marriage and motherhood. Both sexes are entering occupations that were previously deemed sex typical; for example, increasing numbers of men are entering the profession of nursing. Changes in society toward greater technology and more androgynous interpersonal values pose dilemmas for both men and women who have been socialized within traditional sex-stereotyped roles. Women struggle with independence and autonomy, and men may feel that their power, aggressiveness, and "sexual prowess" are being threatened.

Activities and Events in Early Adulthood. Woods[42] described adulthood as a time of maximum sexual self-consciousness, with primary tasks centering on developing a satisfactory life style and social relationships. Continued healthy sexual development includes forming stable and meaningful relationships, changing the ways sexual behaviors fit into people's lives, and understanding sex as a medium for expressing love and intimacy. Schwartz[37] indicated that mature love must transcend sex role values; that is, it involves sharing and meeting of psychosexual needs based on positive self-esteem and includes, for both sexes, characteristics of openness to tenderness, nurturing, assertion, passion, and empathy.

Activities and Events in Middle Adulthood. In middle adulthood, developmental literature refers to stage-related crises in sexuality that both men and women encounter.[10] These crises revolve around losses resulting from awareness of aging, the death of someone significant such as a parent or favorite aunt or uncle, and thoughts about one's own mortality. Biologic changes take place that lead to health risks as well as a decline in sexual functioning. Menopause in women involves a lower amount of estrogen secretion, with atrophy of the breasts and genitalia. In men, the decline is more insidious in that the decrease in androgen-dependent tissues results in changes in the penis and scrotum. Sexual response capacity is also altered.

Because physiologic changes are highly individual for both men and women, psychosocial dimensions of middle-adulthood sexuality must be considered along with them. In contemporary society, both men's and women's roles are in a state of flux, and many configurations of intimate relationships exist (e.g., blended, childless, single parent, and families with homosexual parents). Roles continue to be influenced by the expectations of society, and differences between individual and societal preferences and values are continually reconciled throughout adulthood. The greatest difficulty people encounter in relation to healthy sexuality is denial that differences and crises exist. As Davis[15] pointed out, middle-age transitions that are met by recognizing realities, confronting issues in manageable parts, taking respite as needed, discerning facts, avoiding blame of others, and accepting help from others make them much less traumatic and perhaps less interfering with healthy sexual relationships.

Activities and Events in Older Adulthood. The issue of sexuality in older adulthood has become increasingly important in Western society because technology and improvement in health status have led to an increase in the elder population. Because aging has been viewed in terms of negative qualities, there are many myths surrounding sex and sexuality in older adults. For example, sex (intercourse) is only for the young, sexual activity for older persons is immoral, or sexual desire ceases with menopause.[1] Buczny[12] stated that even professionals' perspective of impotence in older men was in the area of witchcraft until recently. It is true that in many, physiologic processes, sensory perception, and general well-being decline throughout aging.

As a result of numerous losses, both physiologic and personal, elders often experience the most insults to their sexuality, which may underlie their being perceived as "sexless" (which is also a myth).

Physiologically, atrophy of sexual organs and decline in sexual response lead both sexes to experience a gradual diminishing in intensity and duration of response to sexual stimuli. General physical health is very influential in the sexuality of older persons because elders are often more vulnerable to illness and recover more slowly when illness does occur. There is a wide variation in individual experiences, but sexual desire, physical love, and sex continue to be integral parts of the lives of elders. Because physical qualities of sexuality, such as attractiveness in women and strength and virility in men, are more difficult to sustain in aging, sexual roles and relationships take on different qualities in older age than in younger years. In addition, the qualities of gentleness and caring, such as closeness, touching, and body warmth, are equally or more important in loving activities of older people.[41]

In summary, both physiologic and psychosocial development are different for males and females. For each individual you encounter in carrying out nursing care, you will need to act on the basis of such knowledge as how both men and women develop and view their own sexuality, how it is they understand and act in interactions with the opposite sex, and the ways in which sexual expression and response enhance or inhibit their sexual health.

Cultural Components of Sexuality

In their classic cultural studies, Ford and Beach concluded that "in human beings, more than in any other species, sexuality is structured and patterned through learning."[18] In every culture, specific teachings form the beliefs, values, and rules of sex and sexuality.

There is great diversity in cultural dictates, but most transmit messages regarding the nature of sex and beauty; the acceptability of specific sexual behaviors; the relationship of sex and love; pre-, extra-, and postmarital sexual behavior; homosexuality; and the appropriateness of specific sex roles.[11]

Your understanding of specific cultural influences on sexuality can be enhanced through reading current sociologic and anthropologic studies as the need arises for individual clients. The degree of restrictiveness or permissiveness that exists within a culture regarding sexual values and practices is an important aspect of cultural knowledge. Such information will guide the extent to which the client is willing to discuss aspects of sexuality. For example, the cultural heritage in Western society is Victorian-Puritan, in which there is a relationship between sexuality (referring more specifically to sexual response) and morality; that is, the conceptualizing of one's sexuality is in terms of religious standards.[34] The studies of Masters and Johnson and Kinsey have broadened the scope of sexuality to incorporate a scientific ideology applicable to the whole range of human sexual behavior and permitting more latitude for exploration of numerous sexual issues. Other cultural divergences occur in sexual relationships (polygamous, monogamous, and so on), puberty rituals and rites (female circumcision), openness or secrecy in sexual discussions with children and adolescents, and the purpose of marriage (mating).

Currently, in American culture, sexuality is an individual concern, and the emphasis in sexual relationships is on individual rights and consent.[39]

All cultures have rules and practices regarding sexuality, and the nurse has an obligation to be informed as to what they are to avoid cultural bias and prejudice in promoting sexual health. Such information will be helpful in understanding cultural values and beliefs, but carrying out culture-specific nursing care will be difficult unless you identify, explore, and clearly understand your own sociocultural learning and concomitant feelings about sex and sexuality.

Often your beliefs and values about sexual experiences will conflict with those of clients, and you may need to work through these differences with a trusted peer or colleague to be objective and empathic in interacting with clients.

SEXUAL FUNCTION

Sexuality and sexual health include the client's ability and desire to engage in sexual activity. Sex or **sexual function** refers to the biologic aspects of sexual response. There are several patterns of sexual activity, but the most common is heterosexual genital intercourse, which involves penile-vaginal penetration. Coitus and copulation are also appropriate terms for this activity. Other forms of intercourse are anal intercourse and a variety of activities such as oral sex, manual sex, and body rubbing and are engaged in by both heterosexual and homosexual couples.

Individuals are capable of sexual arousal in the presence of diverse and various physical and psychologic stimuli (e.g., kissing, fondling the genitals, viewing naked bodies, listening to sensual music).

Human sexual response requires that body systems — nervous, endocrine, genitourinary, and cardiovascular — be intact and functional. Further, sexual response is influenced by mental and emotional states. The number of factors that influence human sexual response make clients very vulnerable to sexual dysfunction.

Masters and Johnson's classic research provides specific knowledge regarding the ways in which the body responds during sexual arousal. Their four-phase sexual response cycle is a widely accepted concept used to analyze sexual response and formulate treatment for sexual dysfunction. Table 52–1 gives a brief perspec-

TABLE 52–1. Physiologic Changes in the Four Phases of Human Sexual Response

Male	Female
Excitement Phase	
1. Penile erection (within 3 to 8 seconds) as phase is prolonged.	1. Vaginal lubrication (within 10 to 30 seconds) as phase is prolonged.
2. Thickening, flattening, and elevation of scrotal sac.	2. Thickening of vaginal walls and labia.
3. Partial testicular elevation and size increase.	3. Expansion of inner two thirds of vagina and elevation of cervix and corpus.
4. Nipple erection (in about 30 per cent of men).	4. Tumescence of clitoris.
	5. Nipple erection (in all women).
	6. Sex flush (in about 25 per cent of women).
Plateau Phase	
1. Increase in penile coronal circumference.	1. Orgasmic platform in outer one third of vagina.
2. Testicular tumescence (50 to 100 per cent enlarged).	2. Full expansion of vagina.
3. Full testicular elevation and rotation (orgasm inevitable).	3. Uterine and cervical elevation.
4. Purple hue to corona of penis (inconsistent).	4. Discoloration of labia minora.
5. Mucoid secretion (perhaps from Cowper's glands).	5. Mucoid secretion (perhaps from Bartholin's glands).
6. Sex tension flush (in 25 per cent of men).	6. Withdrawal of clitoris.
7. Carpopedal spasm.	7. Sex flush (in 75 per cent of women).
8. Generalized muscular tension.	8. Carpopedal spasm.
9. Hyperventilation.	9. Muscular tension.
10. Tachycardia (100 to 160 bpm).	10. Hyperventilation.
11 Increased blood pressure (20 to 80 mm Hg systolic; 10 to 40 mm Hg diastolic).	11. Tachycardia.
	12. Increased blood pressure (20 to 60 mm Hg systolic; 10 to 20 mm Hg diastolic).
Orgasmic Phase	
1. Ejaculation.	1. Pelvic response.
2. Contraction of accessory organs of reproduction (vas deferens, seminal vesicles, ejaculatory duct).	2. Contraction of uterus from fundus toward lower uterine segment.
3. Relaxation of external bladder sphincter and contraction of internal bladder sphincter.	3. Minimal relaxation of external cervical os.
4. Contractions of penile urethra (0.8-second interval for three to four contractions).	4. Contractions of orgasmic platform (0.8-second interval for 5 to 12 contractions).
5. Anal sphincter contractions.	5. External rectal sphincter contraction.
6. Specific skeletal muscle contractions.	6. External urethral sphincter contractions.
7. Hyperventilation (up to 40 breaths/minute).	7. Hyperventilation (up to 40 breaths/minute).
8. Tachycardia (up to 180 bpm).	8. Tachycardia (up to 180 bpm).
9. Increased blood pressure (40 to 100 mm Hg systolic; 20 to 50 mm Hg diastolic).	9. Increased blood pressure (30 to 80 mm Hg systolic; 20 to 40 mm Hg diastolic).
Resolution Phase	
1. Refractory period with rapid loss of pelvic vasocongestion.	1. Ready return to orgasm with retarded loss of pelvic vasocongestion.
2. Loss of penile erection is a two-stage response: 50 per cent loss rapidly; gradual loss of rest of erection.	2. Loss of flush in labia minora and orgasmic platform (rapid).
3. Sweating reaction (30 to 40 per cent of men).	3. Remainder of pelvic vasocongestion slow.
4. Hyperventilation.	4. Loss of clitoral tumescence.
5. Tachycardia decreases.	5. Sweating reaction (30 to 40 per cent of women).
	6. Hyperventilation.
	7. Tachycardia decreases.

Sources: Masters and Johnson, 1966; Fogel and Woods, 1981; Woods, 1984.
From Fogel, C.I., & Lauver, D. (eds.). (1990). *Sexual health promotion.* Philadelphia: W. B. Saunders.
Abbreviation: bpm, beats per minute.

tive on this cycle. If you need more in-depth information about the response cycle (for teaching or informing patients), refer to Masters and Johnson's *Human Sexual Response*[31] or to current texts or articles in which the physiologic response cycle is summarized.

SEXUALITY AND SEXISM IN NURSING

Nurse-Client Relationships

THE NURSE'S REACTIONS TO INTIMATE PHYSICAL CARE

Probably the first experience to confront the nurse's sexuality in professional education will be the intimate care (bathing or other procedures or treatments that involve genital exposure) of a client of the opposite sex. One female student who was assigned to give an elderly man a bed bath refused, stating that her father would never allow her to do such a thing. This reaction seems a bit extreme and naive about what is nursing care but not unusual when one has not examined his or her own sexual learning and moral principles. A second female student, also assigned to give an elderly man a bed bath, was found wandering in the hall an hour after the assignment and had not yet started care. When approached by the faculty as to what the dilemma was, the student replied, "I have never seen a naked man before." In these early skills experiences, both students had not yet developed a clear concept of professional relating and were most likely functioning in regard to what they knew as appropriate social relating to a member of the opposite gender.

It is imperative to discuss personal reactions to intimate physical care, such as bathing a client, at the time the skill is learned. It is also important to appreciate that your experiences with sexuality are unique. Given our currently "enlightened" society, you may be embarrassed to admit to naiveté and inexperience, which may then contribute to avoidance of aspects of sexuality. In the skills lab, it may be helpful to take a good look at the genital areas of the practice mannequins of the opposite sex and be aware of what kinds of thoughts and feelings are aroused. It may also help to talk with instructors about your fears and concerns. Discuss your own ideas about social caring and touching, and compare these with what you understand to be professional behaviors. Any further discomfort in the clinical situation may be worked through with a peer partner by sharing feelings and influences about sexuality with each other.

Any exercise that serves to raise the nurse's sexual consciousness and clarify individual values is helpful in maintaining a professional stance and overcoming barriers in intimate caring for clients.

Andrist[2] suggested consulting current literature on women's and men's sexuality as well as self-study books. She further discussed a desensitization technique in which participants in a peer group brainstorm various terms on any aspect of sexuality and discuss ways in which each person relates to them. A values clarification exercise that can be done in small groups is to discuss your thoughts and feelings about sexual behaviors such as extramarital sex, abortion, and masturbation by an elderly woman. Role-playing interactions with clients about sexual needs and concerns that arise is an excellent way to increase awareness of your areas of conflict.

CLIENT ATTACHMENT OR ATTRACTION TO THE NURSE

It is not unusual for clients to feel attached or attracted to their nurses, and this may be expressed very genuinely in an overt ("I really appreciate your caring for me") or covert (soft, lingering eye contact) manner. When these gestures are responded to meaningfully by the nurse, it can be very therapeutic for the clients.

THE SEDUCTIVE CLIENT

A different experience that nurses frequently encounter is the seductive acting out of clients. One female student who had privately contracted to give morning and evening care to a 37-year-old quadriplegic man in his home experienced the following: As the client was being transferred from bed to wheelchair, his hands rubbed the back of her neck and occasionally fell to her chest area. As time went on, comments with sexual overtones were added. The student was aware that both behaviors were inappropriate but was at a loss as to how to handle the client without alienating him. Unknown to the student at the time, several other students had cared for this man and had quit working with him because of similar inappropriate behaviors. This student was clearly comfortable with her own sexuality and astute enough to recognize his behaviors as manifestations of unmet sexual needs and realize she was not an appropriate source of fulfillment no matter how covert the behavior. Therefore, she sought consultation as to how to handle the situation, maintain a therapeutic relationship with the client, and assist him to explore and resolve his need.

In the *American Journal of Nursing* (April 1983), Jane Assey and Joan Herbert[4] discussed the seductive client. They described potential problems in female nurse–male client interactions and ways to handle them effectively. Using a definition of seductive behavior as any behavior that the nurse perceives as an intention to attract her, usually for the purpose of sexual activity, the authors described suggestive comments and other incidents of seduction by male clients toward female nurses. The nurse's perception of the behavior as seductive will lead her to react as though it *is* seductive, regardless of the client's intentions.

To compound the situation, the nurse's own sexual feelings may be aroused and may be particularly distressing because nurses are "not supposed to have these feelings about clients," and other staff members may become accusatory toward the nurse as having encouraged seduction. The nurse must keep in mind that because sexual feelings are aroused, it does not mean that she desires a sexual relationship with the client (i.e., thoughts are not actions).

The nurse's lack of understanding of her own feelings of embarrassment, fear, anger, anxiety, guilt, or confusion may result in physically fleeing from the client, avoiding him, criticizing him, or continuing to provide care while stammering or blushing. Understanding personal feelings as normal and being aware of the client's situation will facilitate a more therapeutic response. Hospitalization severely limits most forms of affection and sexual gratification, including hugging and kissing. As a result, clients may be experiencing loneliness and isolation, and their behavior may be a plea for warmth from the care givers.

Seductive behavior is also a way of getting the nurse's attention or of demonstrating anger toward a nurse who is condescending and aloof. Hospitalized clients may also feel insecure about their sexuality, and the seductive behavior may be a plea for reassurance of attractiveness or for recognition as sexual human beings; this is especially true for clients who are disfigured or paralyzed.

Assey and Herbert suggested further guidelines for understanding the client's behaviors by knowing what might be occurring at each stage of illness. In the early phase, clients commonly experience apprehension regarding their sexual attractiveness and functioning and show this by extreme concern for all bodily functions. The greatest concerns about sexuality occur during convalescence; for example, it is in this stage that spinal cord injury clients rate the resumption of previous sexual ability as second only to the ability to walk. Clients also assess their sexuality in two stages: subjective appraisal and validation. In the process of subjective appraisal, the person begins to confront issues such as himself or others being repulsed by his own appearance and ability to perform sexually. Validation comes about as thoughts, fears, and suspicions are tested on others: spouse, friend, and even the nurse. Thus, that testing may be in the form of seductive behavior.

Box 52–2 presents Assey and Herbert's suggestions for constructive responses to client's seductive acting out. For the most part, these actions will resolve the seductive behavior, increase your comfort level, and perhaps even lead to more appropriate self-disclosure and assessment. Although the authors addressed the seduction of the female nurse by the male client, the converse most definitely can happen. Male nurses should be alert to the flirtatiousness of clients and use the same self-explorations and strategies for interacting with clients in a professional manner.

Remember that both nonattention to seductive behavior and reacting inappropriately are not helpful; both are likely to increase the client's behavior and both have the potential to destroy the therapeutic value of your relationship with the client.

THE SEXUALLY DIVERSE CLIENT POPULATION

Clients coming to your care may be very diverse in their sexual identity and expression. Common diversities are homosexuality—gay men and lesbians—and bisexuality. There are a number of people who experience **homophobia,** that is, fear or threat that is expe-

---

Box 52–2. Assey and Herbert's Suggestions for Constructive Responses to Seductive Clients*

▶ Take time for introspection: Be clear about your own responses and why they occur.

▶ Obtain objective feedback from a trusted and objective co-worker.

▶ Discuss your feelings.

▶ Monitor yourself: Increase your awareness of any signals you may be sending that you do not realize. Attend to positioning, body language, and fit of uniform.

▶ Ask staff members for their observations of your behavior. The advantage of being this open with your peers invites everyone's learning and not criticism.

▶ Confront the client: Confrontation is a technique in which you point out the specific behavior to the client and tell him or her your thoughts and feelings about it. Therapeutic confrontation takes skill and practice; the client needs to know that it is the behavior that is inappropriate and not the client. (For example, "I am uncomfortable with your comments, and that makes it most difficult for me to carry out your morning care.")

▶ Set limits: Within an attitude of client acceptance, inform him or her of the consequences of continuing seductive behavior. This tactic is not to promote discussion: Discussion has failed; it is a matter-of-fact statement that you are unable to complete the nursing task because of the behavior and that someone else will be caring for him or her.

* Data from Assey, J.L., & Herbert, J.M. (1983). Who is the seductive patient? *American Journal of Nursing,* 83(4), 530–532.

---

rienced by heterosexuals in relation to homosexuals. This fear, if unrecognized, results in rejection of the homosexual, who then experiences alienation and damaged self-esteem.[21] If this response occurs in the nurse who is assigned to care for a known homosexual, the strategies of self-analysis and values clarification previously discussed will assist in clarifying the issues and in facilitating the nurse's accepting attitude toward homosexuality as an alternative life style. When a person talks about his or her partner, the nurse can use gender-neutral terms such as "that person," which avoids sex bias in communication. Nettles-Carlson[33] suggested other needs of homosexuals in the health care setting, including honoring confidentiality, using appropriate words and not slang terms, gaining as much knowledge as possible about various life styles, and making no assumptions when interviewing.

Many homosexuals feel that if they reveal their gender preference they will not be treated as equals; thus, their dilemma is between becoming known and risking unequal treatment or remaining hidden and risking misunderstanding.

THE SEDUCTIVE NURSE

One principle of professional ethics is to do no harm to the client. Both ethically and morally, a nurse's seduction of a client has potential to do harm. In social situations, deliberate enticement can occur. Similar behaviors do occur in the nurse-client relationship and are grounds for disciplinary action and perhaps even legal action. More subtle means of seduction by nonverbal behaviors, verbal innuendos, and too tight or revealing clothing may also tempt the client. You can avoid being in a vulnerable position by being continually alert to your own actions and what they might mean to the client.

Interprofessional Relationships

Sexism is the exploitation and social domination of members of one sex by the other. Nursing continues to be a female-dominated profession; in 1992 only 3% of registered nurses were men (about 7% of nursing students are men, so numbers are growing).[40] Although there is a shift away from viewing females as inferior sexual beings, there continue to be many instances in which sexism is pervasive, especially against women in the workplace. In addition, the profession of nursing was developed under the male-dominated commands of physicians on one hand and hospital administrators on the other. This heritage continues to plague the nursing profession in various ways, including but not limited to gender issues. An example is a student nurse who, while working as an extern in an intensive care unit, assessed a terminally ill male client to be severely enough depressed to warrant a psychiatric consultation. The supervising nurse (a female) stated "Dr. Jones [a male] would never consent to that." The student, feeling powerless by being a student and a female, dropped the issue while still feeling strongly about the client's need and continuing to do her inexperienced best to attend to that need. This and other examples of ways in which nurses subordinate their nursing judgment to the dictates of physicians are not only gender issues but may become serious ethical conflicts as well, particularly because the expanded scope of nursing practice blurs responsibilities between nurses and physicians.[9]

Male nurses are not immune to sexism.

The same situation could have been experienced by a man in nursing who felt dominated by a female nurse supervisor as well as a female physician. Although the women's movement of the 1970s has been of some assistance in changing the subordinate, handmaiden image of nurses, both male and female, there are no clear guidelines for resolving what may be gender conflicts. Suggestions are for the nurse to

► Gain increasing competence and confidence in using nursing knowledge and skills; speak with physicians and colleagues from a professional stance rather than from a gender stance
► Speak with all professional colleagues as equals: adult to adult communication style
► Engage physicians (and other professionals) in a collaborative effort on behalf of the client; in essence, be assertive through tone of voice, posture,

and command of professional language in sharing concerns about a client
► Participate in activities that are supportive and empowering of yourself as a professional nurse

In addition, nurses need not automatically defer to physicians when there is concern about clients needing attention beyond the expertise of the general nurse clinician. Consulting with other nurses who are specialists in an area relevant to a client's need may be a preferred nursing action and, even though there may be a gender difference between consulting nurses, the nursing bond will, it is hoped, decrease a feeling of intimidation.

SEXUALITY AND THE CLIENT'S HEALTH STATUS

Any illness, injury, or surgical procedure incurred by an individual will impact on some aspect of his or her sexuality. Emotional stress, mental and physical illness, infections, some types of medications, and sexually transmitted diseases may alter sexual functioning.

The complex of physical and psychosocial factors associated with the sexual response cycle may lead to sexual dysfunction. In the course of health care, physical or psychologic insults to an individual's body are likely to occur. Alertness to cues that warrant your attending to the client's sexuality, which may be blatant or very subtle, is very much a part of your nursing responsibility. A large part of sexual health care, especially nursing care in sexual dysfunction and impaired sexuality related to psychopathologic processes, requires advanced nursing knowledge and expertise.

ASSESSMENT

Any time the nurse is engaging the client in a dialogue about sexual issues, the environment is important and can make the difference in both nurse and client comfort. Planning a time for discussion would be ideal. However, whenever sexuality concerns are brought up spontaneously by the client, to put discussion off for a planned time may be seen by the client as the nurse's unwillingness to respond. In discussion sessions, make any possible adjustments in physical space to maintain privacy (e.g., moving client to an interview room, talking with client when the roommate is out of the room, putting up a sign on the door to prevent interruption). An emotional environment may be created by sitting as close to the client as comfortable and in a position to establish eye contact easily. The nurse's own comfort will display interest and caring. If the relevance of a discussion about sexuality to the client's condition is not clear, this should be communicated when the planned time is established.

Assessment of sexual health will include some or all of the following:

► information about clients' sexual attitudes, behaviors, feelings, and beliefs

► clients' current mental and emotional status (especially the ability to be clear about sexual issues and problem solving as well as to determine the extent to which emotional status may interfere with sexual well-being)
► illness (including medication) data pertinent to sexual well-being
► family, social, and cultural data

General Physical Assessment

You should conduct a general physical assessment of the client's sexual anatomy by inspecting genitalia and secondary sex characteristics as a part of the overall physical assessment or at any time you are bathing the client or performing other procedures that provide the opportunity to observe. Following are observations that may warrant further questioning, examination, or reporting:

► variations in development of genitalia and breasts
► abnormalities in the skin such as lesions, ulceration, unusual lumps
► foul-smelling or unusual discharges from orifices, including nipples
► evidence of poor hygienic practices

Assessment of the Client's Sense of Self as a Sexual Being

Be aware of the client's sense of self as a sexual being by attending to verbal and nonverbal clues in any interactions with the client. Observe the ways in which the client refers to himself or herself verbally through choice of words (e.g., using "I" statements), using clear and audible voice tone and eye contact. Can the client acknowledge any discomfort or ask for care from the same-sex professional if desired (as opposed to just refusing care from the opposite-sex professional without giving a reason)? Is the client "appropriately" modest nonverbally? (For example, the client does not expose sexual organs unnecessarily for the care being given or, just the opposite, does not allow the nurse to see or touch private body parts for cleansing when it is clear the client is unable to do for himself.) To the extent that self-care is possible, how does the client display masculinity or femininity in dress, grooming, and posture? Does the client interact with the nurse in a manner respectful to both their sexual beings; for example, each addresses the other by name rather than derogatory terms such as "dear" or "nursey."

Assessment of the Client's Sexual Roles and Relationships

The nurse will also know something about the client's sexual roles and relationships from the personal-social history (e.g., marital status [wife-husband role] and work status [gender-typical or non–gender-typical role]). During care, you could encourage the client to elaborate on family and work roles to learn about the client's views about these roles. All of these assessment data, in the context of the client's developmental level, offer the nurse a beginning framework for more formal sexual history taking or interviewing about specific sexual issues related to the client's condition.

Assessment of Sexual Function

The need for assessment of sexual function may be manifested by clients in a number of ways. The client may ask direct questions about sexual activity in relation to a medical/surgical condition or prescribed medication, express concern about sexual deprivation (while hospitalized), or even discuss feelings of being sexually disinterested or inadequate. More subtle cues are references to rigid upbringing, judgmental attitudes about sex (e.g., intercourse as "duty"), or more simply stating a feeling of unattractiveness in relation to a surgical scar.

Gathering the Sexual History

Gathering formal data about the client's sexuality is indicative that it is a legitimate aspect of health. Typically, sexual health information is obtained in the context of the client's basic history. However, a sexual history may be done anytime the nurse assesses a need for clarity about the client's sexual health. The purposes of a sexual history are to

► Determine how illness or injury impacts on the client's sexual health
► Facilitate the client in addressing concerns about sexuality and health
► Initiate education toward the client's understanding and self-help

You should be well informed about the client's medical history and current need for sexual health care. Specifically, you may need information to intervene in body image and gender identity issues or in problems with sexual functioning. An effective initiation of the interview is to restate the relevance of sexuality to the client's health status. Assessment may have a therapeutic value because you may use this time to validate your perception of client concerns or to answer questions.

In talking with the client, follow the general framework for interviewing in history taking.

Present questions and statements from general to specific, and proceed from the least sensitive to the more sensitive topics. Use appropriate language, which may be difficult because of the client's lack of understanding of appropriate or medical terminology.

He or she may substitute slang terms that are uncomfortable for the nurse to hear. If the client's slang term means the same thing as the proper term, for example, "dick" for penis, just acknowledge that the client is correct and continue on. When a client is too uncomfortable to respond to a question, accept that behavior and do not press for a response. If the answer is absolutely necessary for the client's welfare, perhaps the answer can be written out or be told to another professional.

A sexual history may be fairly comprehensive or brief. Table 52–2 gives an overview of topics and sample questions to be covered in a comprehensive review from the least to the most sensitive topics. One or several interviews may be necessary to complete the history. A brief history consists of the following:

▶ What does the client perceive as concerns about sexuality?
▶ When did the concerns begin, and what has changed since that time?
▶ What situation or events preceded the concern, or what does the client understand as the cause for concern?
▶ What has the client done to alleviate the concern?
▶ What would the client like to do or have happen about his or her concern at this time (intervention goals)?

NURSING DIAGNOSIS

Sexuality-related, NANDA-approved nursing diagnoses are *Altered Sexuality Patterns* (see Nursing Diagnosis Profile) and *Sexual Dysfunction*. In relation to human sexuality, the beginning student will primarily be concerned with these two diagnoses. In addition, other diagnoses pertinent to the broad definition of sexuality relate to psychosocial or emotional issues such as identity or roles or to ethical and moral attitudes. For example, *Altered Body Image* R/T the effect of surgical invasion or *Knowledge Deficit* (about sexual development or safe sexual practices) R/T no previous teaching in these areas each warrants assessment and intervention.

Anything affecting one's physical being, emotional comfort, sociocultural mores, or moral and ethical attitudes may threaten some aspect of sexuality and result in a nursing diagnosis.

TABLE 52–2. Topics to Be Covered in a Comprehensive Sexual History

Area of Inquiry	Sample Questions
Sexual knowledge	"Tell me what you learned when your periods began." "What did you understand was happening when wet dreams occurred?"
Client's perception of his or her sexual health status or current problems, if any	"What about your sexuality poses a problem for you at this time?" "In what way has your current illness (or injury) affected your sexuality, . . . image or concept of yourself, . . . sexual expression?"
Life cycle influences on sexuality	"What do you recall as significant influences on being a man or a woman (boy or girl) at a particular time in life?" "How do you now view yourself as a male or female?" "What were your primary sources of sex education."
For females: menstrual history; menopause	"Tell me about your first experiencing menopause?"
Values and standards about sexuality	"Is there anything you wish to share that would make your care more individualized?"
Religion or culture	"What should I know about your religion [culture] to assist me in being more sensitive to your sexual needs?"
Sexual function	"Are there any recent changes in your sexual activity?" If yes, ask the following: "What is the change due to?" "What contraceptive methods, if any, are you currently using?" "Do you ever experience painful intercourse?"
Knowledge of (or history of) sexually transmitted diseases	"When you became sexually active, what did you understand about sexually transmitted diseases?" "Have you ever had a foul-smelling discharge from your vagina [penis]?"
General closing questions	"Are you experiencing any interferences with a sexual relationship at present?" "What do you think the interference is due to?" "What, if any, uncertainty do you now have as a result of information you have received about sexuality?" "Is there anything else that you think I, as your nurse, should know?" "In what ways do you think I may be of further assistance to you?"

NURSING DIAGNOSIS PROFILE

Altered Sexuality Patterns

Definition. The state in which an individual expresses concern regarding his or her sexuality

Classification. Relating 3.3.

Defining Characteristics. Reported difficulties, limitations, or changes in sexual behaviors or activities are all major defining characteristics.

Sample Related Factors. The related factors may be divided into those that are health or disease oriented and those that are psychosocial in nature. Those that are health or disease oriented include knowledge/skill deficit about alternative responses to health-related transitions such as altered body function or structure, illness, or medical treatment; fear of pregnancy; and fear of acquiring a sexually transmitted disease. Those that are psychosocial in nature include lack of a significant other, lack of privacy, ineffective or absent role models, conflicts with sexual orientation or variant preferences, and impaired relationship with a significant other.

Concept Description. This diagnosis refers to the state in which a person either fears or actually experiences a disturbance in his or her usual patterns of sexual behavior. In order for the diagnosis to be made, the client must actually express a concern about his or her sexuality. If the person does not express concern but there is reason to believe that the concern exists, a diagnosis of *High Risk for Altered Sexuality Patterns* might be made instead.

Examples. Depending on the specific assessment data, this diagnostic category could be applicable in the following situations, among others:

▶ A female of childbearing age who has not been able to find birth control measures that are correct for her and who is unable to engage in sexual intercourse as frequently as she has been accustomed to because she feels all sexual intercourse might result in an unwanted pregnancy
▶ A male who has had a colostomy and who is experiencing alterations in body image so that he avoids reaching out to his wife for fear that she will reject his sexual advances
▶ A person who has just been divorced and who has not yet found a new partner

Related/Similar Nursing Diagnoses. This diagnosis should be distinguished from the diagnosis of *Sexual Dysfunction*. *Sexual Dysfunction* is a state in which an individual experiences a change in sexual function that is viewed as unsatisfying, unrewarding, or inadequate. With this diagnosis, the person does maintain the usual patterns of sexual expression, but there is a lack of pleasure in the sexual acts. This is not the case with *Altered Sexuality Patterns,* in which the pattern is disturbed but the pleasure is not.

Realizing that both men and women may feel vulnerable in relation to their sexuality should increase your awareness of the importance of a sensitive nursing diagnosis. Currently, treatments for many illnesses through the use of high-technology equipment have an impact on one's sexuality. Major deficits are frequently in the areas of knowledge and attitudes, because there are still numerous myths and fears that are associated with sexuality despite the wealth of research information.

PLANNING

From the assessment data, determine the client's category of need as well as your level of competence to intervene. The client's needs may be classified as being due to anatomic disruptions, physiologic alterations, pharmacologic interference, life cycle issues, emotional alterations, or environmental influences. Categorizing will facilitate your planning according to physical skill needs or teaching and counseling needs. Planning to have a pain medication administered to the postoperative client who has had a bowel resection before catheterizing him indicates sensitive physical care. Facilitating an illustrated talk to a local parent-teacher association (PTA) about sexually transmitted diseases demonstrates excellent planning.

Your plan should also demonstrate respect for the client as a sexual being by preparing for care that minimizes exposure of pelvic and breast areas. Your client may appreciate your planning to be available for support during "rounds," when a number of physicians and medical students examine him or her.

Your level of competence is determined by the accuracy and depth of your information about human sexuality, awareness of your own value system, level of comfort in communicating about sexuality, and interpersonal skills. You might anticipate that clients will want to discuss fears, for example, of sexual inadequacy after a prostatectomy. Plan first to just listen so that you can be prepared for the next encounter with some resource materials if necessary. A part of your plan may necessitate the inclusion of other professionals as consultants, either for yourself or the client.

Your nursing care plan needs to be within the context of the client's values and beliefs. For example, in client teaching, you will need to be accepting of the client's standards and impart information that is congruent with them. Although you may know something from general conversations or religious preference, you may need to ask specific questions about what behaviors and types of sexual interactions are acceptable to the client; in essence, develop your plan in collaboration with the client or validate your plan with him or her before implementation.

Client outcomes will depend on the assessment data. Some outcomes for the client who is experiencing altered patterns of sexuality may include the following:

▶ lists sexual developmental differences in men and women
▶ discusses sexuality without demonstrating a belief in sexual myths, stereotypes, or misconceptions
▶ discusses male and female sexual expression
▶ states achievement of healthy and satisfying sexual practices
▶ demonstrates the integration of a positive sense of self, sexual identity, sociocultural beliefs, and present situational realities

NURSING INTERVENTION

Intervention for altered sexuality patterns and sexual dysfunction is an integration of physical and psychosocial care. Changes in sexual functioning are due to both physiologic dysfunction that impairs physical processes and to psychologic processes such as self-image, self-esteem, or body image disturbances that contribute to physical dysfunction. A priority is to establish good rapport not only with the client but with the physician to encourage teamwork in sexual health care. Often the client is not comfortable sharing concerns involving intimacy with the physician. You may assist the client in this regard by encouraging the client to speak up, assisting the client to problem solve how to approach the physician (e.g., contract with the physician for a special private time to talk), and helping the client clarify the major issue.

A universally applied behavioral intervention for sexual dysfunction, which can be used for altered sexuality patterns as well, is the PLISSIT model, developed by Annon.[3]

This is a model of progressive intervention and can be used by nurse generalists in relation to a variety of client sexual needs.

PERMISSION

The first step is permission. Clients are often hesitant about initiating conversation about sexual concerns. Through your skillful communication with the client, offer him or her the opportunity to discuss bothersome sexuality issues surrounding the medical condition. Assist the client to understand further the relationship of a particular condition, such as cardiac status, to continuing a particular sexual life style. Permission to continue as before or with specific modifications may be the intervention needed.

Other permission giving may consist of assurance of normalcy. For example, a young, single, adult woman who is not in a stable relationship with a man may prefer masturbation as a sexual outlet rather than heterosexual coitus with multiple partners. She needs not only the assurance of normalcy but feedback that her judgment is decreasing her risk of sexually transmitted diseases. Offering permission to talk about sexuality often leads to the client's exposing anxieties and myths to which you can respond with factual information or resource material. An example might be a preadolescent boy who allowed his penis to be fondled by a male chum as they were exploring each other's sexual organs and who is afraid of getting AIDS from that experience. The wide scope of religious practices and

---

APPLYING RESEARCH TO NURSING PRACTICE

Promoting Sexual Health After Ostomy Surgery

Gloeckner, M. (1991). Perceptions of sexuality after ostomy surgery. *Journal of Enterostomal Therapy*, 18(1), 36–38.

▼ ▼ ▼

Ostomy surgery creates a surgical opening in the ileum (ileostomy) or in the large intestine (colostomy) and connects the intestinal lumen to an opening (stoma) on the abdominal wall. People who have undergone ostomy surgery may experience many uncomfortable emotions in learning to manage their ostomies and incorporate stoma care into their lives. Nurses can provide emotional support, counseling, and educational information to help these clients respond to ostomy surgery. In particular, clients with ostomies may experience alterations in body image that interfere with their postoperative sexual adjustment. To help nurses understand the experiences of those who have undergone ostomy surgery and its effect on sexual health, Gloeckner interviewed 24 men and 16 women. This researcher explored three dimensions of sexual adjustment: the physical, the psychologic, and the interpersonal. Most of the men and women in this study had had a colostomy or an ileostomy, and a smaller number had had a urinary diversion or Kock pouch, for at least 1 year. The primary problem for men was impotence, either temporary or permanent. Temporary impotence lasted from 3 to 12 months. The major physical problem experienced by the women was dyspareunia (discomfort during intercourse) associated with scar tissue formation and a reduction in vaginal lubrication. Gloeckner found that in preparation for sexual activities, subjects of both sexes used underpants (with the crotch fabric removed) to

conceal their ostomies. Several also wore a T shirt or nightgown. Many also relied on pouch covers and opaque pouches. Postoperatively, most subjects initially felt shock and repulsion in response to the stoma. However, after the first year, 68% stated that they had begun to feel more attractive. Those who had had surgery for inflammatory bowel disease were more likely to view themselves as sexually attractive than those who had had ostomy surgery for cancer. When asked about their partner's reaction to the first sexual experience after ostomy surgery, 46% stated that their partners had reacted positively, 30% stated that their partners had reacted negatively, and 30% stated that their partners had responded with caution. Many partners had expressed fear about hurting the stoma. Most couples expressed that their relationship had positively changed and become more intimate than it had been before surgery. Although most subjects designated the physician as the most common source of sexual information and printed materials as the second most common source, 97% stressed that either the physician or the enterostomal nurse should discuss issues of sexuality with the client having ostomy surgery.

Applications for Practice. Use the sensitive and practical information in this study to help clients preparing for and recovering from ostomy surgery. Be sensitive to the client's responses to illnesses; teach and counsel accordingly. Use the PLISSIT model discussed in this chapter as an intervention guide if you are concerned with the amount of involvement you should have with clients experiencing sexuality problems.

the general complexity of sexuality issues can combine to elicit some fairly bizarre ideas. The literature indicates that accurate information not only enhances knowledge but alters attitudes as well.

LIMITED INFORMATION

In the PLISSIT model, the second step, limited information, relates to sharing factual knowledge, especially of anatomy and physiology, body functions, developmental issues, and the impact of illness on one's sexual health. Providing visual aids is an excellent means of imparting information. For example, giving Mr. Whipple, a 67-year-old, an article about sexual adequacy after a prostatectomy to read at his convenience can help him prepare for his planned surgery. Offer to discuss the article with him to clarify any misunderstandings. Statistics are sometimes helpful to the client (e.g., about sexual function and certain diseases or specific sexual practices). This information should help the client put his or her own dilemma into some perspective. However, the information should never be used to convince the client to feel or stop feeling a certain way or that he is not as important as a "statistic."

Many diseases result in temporary or permanent alterations in sexual function or patterns. Temporary issues can be alleviated by giving adequate information as to what to expect and ways the client can facilitate a return to normal. A young, newly married woman experiences dyspareunia (painful intercourse) and is diagnosed as having an infection. Important information for her to understand is that abstention is necessary for a brief period of time until the infection clears. She may also desire to have her husband temporarily use a condom and lubrication when sexual activity is resumed. This can promote comfort and help prevent furthering the infectious process.

For long-term problems, timing of information is extremely important. A client may be struggling with the impact of a diagnosis that potentially alters his lifestyle, including sexuality issues, or may even be denying aspects of the illness. Providing information under these circumstances would be ineffective and may also be detrimental. As the client begins to seek information, a combination of information giving and assessment of the client's receptiveness to what he is hearing is an appropriate intervention. For example, "Mrs. Hillary, you are looking tired. I feel I have given you enough information to think about for now. When you feel more rested, I will return to see whether you have any further concerns or if you wish to discuss any thoughts and feelings."

SPECIFIC SUGGESTION

The next step in the PLISSIT model is specific suggestion and, from your own factual knowledge or information given to you by other clients or experts, you may give the client guidelines and strategies to prevent or alleviate a specific sexuality problem. Guiding the client in a discussion of any sexual problems anticipated as a result of a specific disease or injury may be necessary. Client teaching is an appropriate means of specific sug-

gestion, especially regarding what is known about specific disease or injury processes and sexuality or sexual function. Teaching about good hygienic practices is important, particularly when there has been surgical intervention affecting the sexual organs (e.g., hysterectomy, prostatectomy). Specific suggestion may also consist of alternative positions for intercourse or even alternative forms of sexual expression.

Few generalist nurses will be able to intervene at this level for client's sexual dysfunctions. Specific suggestion may consist of providing referrals to good resources. Some professional resources include clinical nurse specialists, psychologists, sex therapists, and mental health professionals. The nurse who has specific knowledge of the areas of expertise of referral sources will be extremely helpful to clients, especially in attempting to match the problem to the resource.

INTENSIVE THERAPY

The last step in the PLISSIT model is intensive therapy, and again only a qualified expert will use this intervention. In all of these phases, the client will likely be more receptive to your guidance if he or she feels accepted and treated with dignity and if the focus has been on the ideas, experiences, and feelings of the client.

Culturally Sensitive Interventions

Culturally sensitive interventions take into consideration the standards, norms, and values for a specific client. You will need to expand your repertoire of interventions to respect and protect each person's cultural variables. For example, a woman whose culture requires her to keep her femininity hidden with non–form-fitting clothing and veils may even be uncomfortable with a female nurse giving her a bed bath. An appropriate intervention is to explain the necessity of hygiene and inspection (after her vaginal infection), speaking in consideration of, and with respect for, her cultural beliefs.

Problems that Can Interfere with Sexuality

Numerous physical and psychologic problems can interfere with the client's sexuality. Examples include some medications as well as physical conditions that can affect sexual performance, ignorance (which makes one vulnerable to sexually transmitted diseases), and guilt (which may cause unnecessary abstinence in a particular sexual encounter). In summary, interventions that promote sexual health will be based on the client's need and the nurse's knowledge and comfort levels. For the most part, clients will rarely react with shock to sexual discussions and will appreciate the nurse's caring regarding this sensitive topic.

EVALUATION

Evaluating the effectiveness of sexual health care depends on the specific goals to be achieved. One way of evaluating your effectiveness is noting whether the client expresses comfort or displays relief after your intervention. For example, Mr. Whipple thanks you for discussing the implications of his prostatectomy and he genuinely looks much less anxious than before the discussion. In another example, after your presentation about preadolescent behavior at a PTA meeting, a mother confides that before this meeting she had worried that her son's increased closeness to his longtime male friend was an indication of homosexual activity.

If clients can repeat to you what they have learned, you will know your teaching intervention has been effective.

Evaluation should be done in the context of the developmental level of clients. Addressing the sexuality concerns of adolescent cancer patients through an adolescent oncology support group may be evaluated by attendance and the genuineness of communication among the group members. An elderly couple may express relief that their conscious decision to decrease the frequency of their intercourse does not signify they are abnormal. They may state that the nurse's acceptance of and feedback about what sexual expression means to them was very helpful.

Nurses need to expect initial anxiety in performing sexual health care. Be reassured that greater ease and comfort come with experience. The attention to and sensitive care of all clients experiencing some problems involving their sexuality can be a very challenging but rewarding experience.

CASE STUDY

The Client

Audrey Ellis is a 39-year-old woman who was admitted to the hospital after a clinic visit 2 days ago. Two weeks ago, when she was performing self-breast examination, she discovered a lump in her left breast. Her hospitalization is for a lumpectomy.

Audrey was divorced from her husband a little over a year ago. She has no children; other relatives live in another state. She is a social worker, currently working on the psychiatric unit of the medical center hospital, and supports herself totally. After her divorce, Audrey participated in 6 weeks of supportive psychotherapy because she experienced some mild depression, lack of closure on the relationship, and some low self-esteem. For the past several months, she has been happy with her life, enjoying numerous activities with close friends and beginning to date.

After her clinic visit, she had tests and x-rays to assess the nature of the lump and additional bodily involvement. A partial list of the physician's orders, on admission, included

▶ Up ad lib
▶ Regular diet—NPO after 10 PM Sept. 10

▶ Preoperative shower
▶ Scheduled for surgery—11 AM Sept. 11

At 3:00 PM, September 10, a partial list of the admission assessment data included the following:

▶ 39-year-old female in no acute distress
▶ temperature 36.9°C, pulse-68, respiration-16, blood pressure-110/88
▶ 5′7″ tall; weight, 145; engages in regular exercise
▶ brief history and physical assessment reveal normal function in all bodily systems
▶ no breast tenderness in right breast; lump in left breast about 4 mm left of nipple and slightly tender on palpation; no discoloration noted
▶ LMP August 27; states normal flow of 4 days
▶ states not currently sexually active; enjoyed a positive and active sexual life during 14-year marriage
▶ flat affect in tone of voice in answering questions

Following is a nursing care plan written for her at 3 PM, September 10, and evaluated at 10:30 that evening.

CARE PLAN

Nursing Diagnosis	Planning: Expected Outcomes	Implementation: Nursing Interventions	Evaluation
High Risk for Altered Sexuality Patterns R/T anxiety over planned altered body structure	By hs, Sept. 10: ▶ relates concerns about surgical procedure in relation to her sexuality	▶ Contract with client for a time to talk, undisturbed, after evening meal. ▶ Share and validate with client the perception that she seemed indifferent during physical assessment.	10:30 PM, Sept. 10: ▶ Client selected time to meet; during meeting, acknowledged feeling apathetic to avoid sadness. ▶ Client stated that she felt very uncertain about procedure being a lumpectomy versus mastectomy.

Care Plan continued on following page

CARE PLAN (Continued)

Nursing Diagnosis	Planning: Expected Outcomes	Implementation: Nursing Interventions	Evaluation
		► State willingness to listen to specific concerns she has about her sexuality and the surgery.	Had been "unscarred" all of her life; wondered how disfiguring the incision would be.
	► States knowledge of the surgical procedure, process for informing her of any change in plans once biopsy is completed, and options for treatment	► Ask client what she has been told by the physician. ► Assess her understanding, and provide information as needed. ► Elicit her thoughts about treatment options.	► Client knew to expect a simple excision of the lump unless biopsy was negative; would then be awakened to affirm consent for more extensive surgery. ► Showed nurse a picture the physician had drawn to illustrate incision. ► Client stated she would agree to further surgery as opposed to jeopardizing health.
	► Discusses the relationship of surgical procedure to her sexuality and status as a single woman	► Use open-ended questions to explore reactions to breast lump and surgery. ► Observe verbal and nonverbal expression of feelings. ► Acknowledge feelings. ► Dispel myths (i.e., correct erroneous information).	► Client stated she had begun to live again after divorce; looked forward to meeting new men and the potential to remarry; stated she wondered whether a man would find her less appealing with the breast scar and whether she would feel less sexually aroused by breast stimulation. ► Client responded more hopefully when told about others' positive experiences.
	► States adequate relaxation and peace of mind to be able to sleep	► Check with client after shower to assess for decreased anxiety. ► Seek information from client about comfort level as well as need for further discussion. ► Ask client whether she would like sedative as ordered.	► Client's facial expression looked relaxed. ► Client asked to have sleeping medication only if she woke up during night and could not go to sleep. ► Client turned out light about 10:15 PM after making phone call to a friend. ► Client thanked nurse for listening.

Summary

▶ In 1975, sexuality was promoted by the World Health Organization as a vital component of health care. Sexuality is a term used broadly to mean the state or quality of being sexual.

▶ Gender is genetically determined through the XX (female) or XY (male) chromosomes. The differences in male and female functioning are due to numerous factors and not merely to sexual anatomy; right-left brain function is associated with the difference between male and female response styles. Puberty in adolescence is associated with development of secondary sex characteristics.

▶ Socialization processes occurring after birth contribute significantly to differences in men and women. Self-concept and body image develop as one internalizes the appraisals of others.

▶ Gender identity, gender role, and sexual orientation are important aspects of sexuality.

▶ Individuals express and reflect their sexuality in different ways throughout the developmental cycle.

▶ All cultures have rules and practices regarding sexuality.

▶ Sexual function is the biologic aspect of sexual response and is a vital component of healthy sexuality.

▶ Sexuality and sexism affect nurses in many aspects of their practice. Nurse-client relationships are professional, not social. Effective responses to clients regarding sexuality depend on the nurse's clarification of values. Interprofessional relationships must be based on competence and confidence in nursing knowledge, not on female subordination and male dominance. Any illness, injury, or invasive procedure will impact on some aspect of the client's sexuality. Sexual health care is a part of holistic care of the client.

▶ Assessment may include brief observations and discussions regarding clients' sexual concerns as well as including comprehensive sexual histories.

▶ Two nursing diagnoses for clients with sexual alterations are: *Altered Sexuality Patterns* and *Sexual Dysfunction.*

▶ Planning includes determining clients' category of need as well as nurses' level of competence to intervene.

▶ Intervention integrates physical and psychosocial care. The PLISSIT model is a universally accepted intervention model.

▶ Evaluation is based on outcomes and can be discerned through client expression of comfort, increased knowledge, and decreased anxiety.

Bibliography

1. Allen, M.E. (1987). A holistic view of sexuality and the aged. *Holistic Nursing Practice*, 1(4), 76–83.
2. Andrist, L. (1988). Taking a sexual history and educating clients about safe sex. *Nursing Clinics of North America*, 23(4), 959–973.
3. Annon, J. (1976). The PLISSIT model: a proposed conceptual scheme for the behavioral treatment of sexual problems. *Journal of Sex Education and Therapy*, 2(1), 1–15.
4. Assey, J.L., & Herbert, J.M. (1983). Who is the seductive patient? *American Journal of Nursing*, 83(4), 530–532.
5. Bancroft, J. (1983). *Human sexuality and its problems.* New York: Churchill Livingstone.
6. Bee, H. (1983). *The developing child.* New York: Harper & Row.
7. Bellak, L., et al. (1973). *Ego functions in schizophrenics, neurotics and normals: A systematic study of conceptual, diagnostic and therapeutic aspects.* New York: Wiley.
8. Belsky, J., et al. (1984). The Pennsylvania infant and family development project: I. Stability and change in mother-infant interaction in a family setting at one, three, and nine months. *Child Development*, 55, 692–705.
9. Benjamin, M., & Curtis, J. (1986). *Ethics in nursing.* New York: Oxford University Press.
10. Berger, K. (1988). *The developing person through the life span.* New York: Worth Publishers.
11. Brink, P.J. (1987). Cultural aspects of sexuality. *Holistic Nursing Practice*, 1, 12–20.
12. Buczny, B. (1992). Impotence in older men: a newly recognized problem. *Journal of Gerontological Nursing*, 18(5), 25–30.
13. Chilman, C.S. (1983). *Adolescent sexuality in a changing American society.* New York: Wiley.
14. Chodorow, N. (1978). *The reproduction of mother.* Berkeley, CA: University of California Press.
15. Davis, A.E. (1980). Whoever said life begins at 40 was a fink or those golden years-phooey. *International Journal of Women's Studies*, 3, 583–589.
16. Eagle, M.N. (1984). *Recent developments in psychoanalysis.* New York: McGraw-Hill.
17. Fogel, C.I. (1990). Sexual health promotion. In Fogel, C.I., & Lauver, D. (eds.). *Sexual health promotion* (pp. 1–18). Philadelphia: W.B. Saunders.
18. Ford, C.S., & Beach, F.A. (1951). *Patterns of sexual behavior.* New York: Harper.
19. Gagnon, J.H. (1977). *Human sexualities.* Chicago: Scott, Foresman.
20. Gilligan, C. (1982). *In a different voice.* Cambridge, MA: Harvard University Press.
21. Govoni, L.A. (1988). Psychosocial issues of AIDS in the nursing care of homosexual men and their significant others. *Nursing Clinics of North America*, 23(4), 749–765.
22. Hines, M. (1982). Prenatal gonadal hormones and sex differences in human behavior. *Psychological Bulletin*, 92, 56–80.
23. Hogan, R. (1980). *Human sexuality: A nursing perspective.* Norwalk, CT: Appleton & Lange.
24. Jones, K.L., et al. (1985). *Dimensions of human sexuality.* Dubuque, IA: William C Brown.
25. Kahn, A.U., & Cataio, J. (1984). *Men and women in biological perspective.* New York: Praeger.
26. Klein, M. (1948). *Contributions to psychoanalysis, 1921–1945.* London: Hogarth Press.
27. Klein, M. (1957). *The psycho-analysis of children.* London: Hogarth Press.
28. Lidz, T. (1968). *The person.* New York: Basic Books.
29. Lion, E. (1982). *Human sexuality in the nursing process.* New York: Wiley.
30. Macoby, E., & Jacklin, C. (1974). *The psychology of sex differences.* Stanford, CA: Stanford University Press.
31. Masters, W., & Johnson, V. (1966). *Human sexual response.* Boston: Little, Brown.
32. Money, J. (1968). *Sex errors of the body: Dilemmas, education, counselling.* Baltimore, MD: Johns Hopkins University Press.
33. Nettles-Carlson, B. (1990). Gay and lesbian lifestyles. In Fogel, C.I., & Lauver, D. (eds.). *Sexual health promotion* (pp. 117–132). Philadelphia: W.B. Saunders.
34. Petras, J.W. (1978). *The social meaning of human sexuality.* Newton, MA: Allyn & Bacon.
35. Rubin, L.B. (1984). *Intimate strangers.* New York: Harper & Row.
36. Rynerson, B.C. (1990). Sexuality throughout the life cycle. In Fogel, C.I., & Lauver, D. (eds.). *Sexual health promotion* (pp. 53–86). Philadelphia: W. B. Saunders.
37. Schwartz, A.E. (1979). Androgyny and the art of loving. *Psychotherapy, Theory, Research and Practice*, 16, 405–408.

38. Simmons, S. (1984). Emotional aspects of the nurse/client relationship. *The Kansas Nurse*, 59(10), 16–17.

39. Smith, L.S. (1990). Human sexuality from a cultural perspective. In Fogel, C.I., & Lauver, D. (eds.). *Sexual health promotion* (pp. 87–96). Philadelphia: W. B. Saunders.

40. *The American Nurse.* (1992). p. 24.

41. Weg, R.B. (1983). *Sexuality in later years, roles and behavior.* New York: Academic Press.

42. Woods, N.F. (1984). *Human sexuality in health and illness.* St. Louis: C. V. Mosby.

▼ *Promoting Spiritual Health*

Chapter 53

 ▼ *As you ought not to attempt to cure the eyes without the head, or the head without the body, so neither ought you attempt to cure the body without the soul . . . for the part can never be well unless the whole is well.*

Plato

▼ CHAPTER OUTLINE

CONCEPTS OF SPIRITUALITY AND
   SPIRITUAL CARE
      Holistic Care
      Nurse's Role in Spiritual Care
UNIVERSALITY OF SPIRITUALITY
      Historic Perspectives
      Cultural Factors
      Societal Influences
SPIRITUALITY AND RELIGION
SPIRITUAL NEEDS
      Need for a Sense of Meaning and
        Purpose
      Need for Love and Relatedness
      Need for Forgiveness
      Need for Hope
SPIRITUAL DEVELOPMENT THROUGHOUT
   THE LIFE SPAN
      Religious Development
      Psychosocial Development
      Faith Development
      Developmental Stages
MAJOR WORLD RELIGIONS
      Hinduism
      Judaism

      Christianity
      Buddhism
      Islam
NEW AGE SPIRITUALISM
AGNOSTICISM AND ATHEISM
RESOURCES FOR CLIENTS NEEDING
   SPIRITUAL CARE
      Prayer
      Sacred Writings
      Clergy
PRACTICES TO PROMOTE YOUR OWN
   SPIRITUAL HEALTH
      Know Yourself
      Recognize the Role of Faith
      Meditate
      Practice Guided Imagery
      Pursue Aesthetic Experiences
ASSESSMENT
NURSING DIAGNOSIS
PLANNING
NURSING INTERVENTIONS
EVALUATION
CASE STUDY

▼ KEY TERMS

Abstract (transcendent)
  hope
Agnosticism
Atheism
Clergy
Concrete hope
Eucharist
Extreme unction

Faith
Hope
Horizontal relationship
Monotheism
Pluralism
Prayer
Religion

Spiritual care
Spiritual health
Spiritual needs
Spirituality
Theism
Transcendent values
Vertical relationship

▼ *LEARNING OBJECTIVES*

After studying this chapter, you should be able to

1. *Describe the concepts of spirituality and spiritual care.*
2. *Contrast spirituality and religion.*
3. *Describe spiritual development in individuals throughout the life span.*
4. *Identify basic beliefs of major world religions.*
5. *Identify spiritual care resources.*
6. *State how to assess a client's spiritual needs.*
7. *Discuss the nursing diagnosis of spiritual distress.*
8. *List outcomes for a person with a nursing diagnosis of spiritual distress.*
9. *Describe nursing interventions appropriate for the client in spiritual distress.*
10. *Describe the evaluation of the person with a diagnosis of spiritual distress.*

Surrounded by high technology, we tend to focus on physical care, with its complex procedures and intricate machines, and pay less attention to the spiritual aspects of an individual's care. Client care, moreover, has moved from caring for the individual out of love and duty to caring for the individual as an economic activity.[44] Scientific medicine demands information that can be quantified and models of treatment that can be scientifically evaluated. Therefore, the spiritual needs of clients often go unrecognized and unmet. Recognizing clients' spiritual needs begins with knowing that nursing care must expand beyond biologic needs and into the realm of spiritual needs. Most nurses need to expand their concept of spiritual care and their knowledge of various religious traditions so they are able to give spiritual care to clients with diverse beliefs and philosophies. This is what this chapter is designed to help you to do.

CONCEPTS OF SPIRITUALITY AND SPIRITUAL CARE

Spirituality is the life principle that pervades a person's entire being: a person's physical, emotional, intellectual, moral, ethical, and volitional (power of choosing and decision making) dimensions. This life principle of spirituality generates a capacity for **transcendent values,** or values beyond ordinary values and limits, and beyond material values. For example, the value of a home is more than the dollars implied in a real estate valuation; its transcendent values include feelings of belonging, comfort, and love for people in the home.

Spiritual care involves caring not only for and about clients but also assisting them in finding meaning in life experiences such as crises and suffering.

Holistic Care

Recent trends in health care have been moving toward each nurse caring for the whole client rather than fragmenting care among many specialty health care workers. Holistic nursing care is concerned with care of the whole person: the biologic, the psychologic, and the spiritual. This means you must be prepared to assist the individual client, the family members, and the significant others in coping with the client's illness and suffering, and you must also help them find meaning in these experiences.[47] The search for meaning is a part of everyone's life, but this search can become intensified when an individual meets a health crisis, such as acute illness, loss of a loved one, or onset of a lifelong disability. Thus, a physical or emotional crisis can precipitate a spiritual need or crisis. To treat the individual holistically, you must provide spiritual care as well as physical and psychosocial care.

It may not be easy to provide spiritual care because nurses generally face two barriers: (1) They do not realize that a particular client has an unmet spiritual need (clients can be reluctant to express their spiritual needs because they consider spirituality to be a socially taboo topic); (2) they do not know how to help with spiritual needs (nursing literature reflects the values of scientific medicine and generally overlooks spirituality in discussing crises, illness, and treatment).

Spiritual health in a person is a state of balance that transcends physical and material things. It indicates receptiveness to a greater power as defined by the individual. For most people, the greater power is defined as a supernatural force or God, as conceived of according to religious beliefs. For others, however, the greater power may be "the natural order of things": science, fate, or even great wealth.

The relationship among physiologic health, psychologic health, and spiritual health is intricate. Although this relationship varies among individuals, it is generally true that spiritual health may affect physical or mental health, and, conversely, a physical or mental crisis may create a spiritual crisis. An example of the first statement is a client who feels spiritually empty and who, as a result, develops a physical problem such as nausea or weight loss or a mental problem such as feelings of low self-esteem. An example of a physical or mental crisis creating a spiritual problem is a man whose family was killed in an automobile accident, whose legs had to be amputated as a result of injuries from the accident, and who begins to doubt the presence of a greater power or God or anyone or anything to which he can turn for support. In meeting client needs holistically, all dimensions of health (physiologic, psychologic, and spiritual) must be addressed if balance is to be restored.

Nurses' Role in Spiritual Care

Providing holistic care requires nurses to identify spiritual needs and to intervene effectively. The identification of spiritual needs can be facilitated by assisting the client in expressing them directly. This can best occur in an atmosphere that shows client acceptance and support. Such an atmosphere exists when the client understands that you have respect for the ideas expressed by the client and that you will maintain confidentiality concerning all client communications.

Effective intervention can begin when the nurse understands that suffering and crisis can be dehumanizing and takes steps to prevent this. Thus, attention to the spiritual well-being of clients requires attention to those psychologic forces such as depression, low self-esteem, and feelings of helplessness that can diminish the spirit. In addition, it requires attention to those physiologic forces such as pain and body alterations that can result in depression, low self-esteem, and feelings of helplessness in the first place. In short, spiritual care cannot be divorced from physical and psychologic care.

Nurses, being primary care givers and having almost unlimited access to the client and the family, have a unique role and responsibility. They can create a sense of wholeness for a client living through the experience of a chaotic hospitalization. When assistance is needed, they can help the client find meaning in the experience.

Fulfilling the nursing role in relation to spiritual care requires that you understand human spirituality and that you are aware of some of the religious beliefs and practices that are often a part of a client's spirituality. Box 53–1 summarizes some suggestions for career-long development in the area of spirituality.

Box 53–1. Suggestions for Career-long Development in the Area of Spirituality

▶ Maintain respect for every individual's religious beliefs and practices.

▶ Refrain from judging others' religious beliefs as right or wrong as based on your interpretation and knowledge.

▶ Keep an open mind; do not deny the value of any religion on the basis of personal bias.

▶ Continue to develop knowledge about all religions.

▶ Attend continuing education programs that relate to spiritual care.

▶ Implement knowledge about your client's religious beliefs to aid in more effective health care.

UNIVERSALITY OF SPIRITUALITY

Spirituality is a part of every person. It is the totality of an individual's being and is expressed or revealed in numerous ways. Examples of the expression of spirituality include the things a person values and the ways a person acknowledges others, treats others, takes care of the self and others, and uses time. The realms of intellect, emotion, and physical state are all part of the individual's spirit. Spirituality has been described as the basic quality of a person's nature—what the person is and what the person does.[33] All individuals have their own spirituality and spiritual needs.

Historical Perspectives

In the 1800s, Florence Nightingale recognized that "the needs of the spirit are as critical to the health as those of the individual organs that make up the body."[44] Now, near the end of the 20th century, medicine has become fragmented into numerous specialties, each with health care workers who were taught to be scientific, objective, and detached.[33] Since Nightingale's era, as medical and nursing technology became more complex, spirituality and spiritual care have tended to recede into obscurity. Only recently have spiritual aspects of a client's well-being again been recognized as an important area for nurses to address.

Cultural Factors

In our multicultural world, clients of diverse backgrounds, beliefs, philosophies, ethnic groups, and religions are offered health care by a variety of care givers who also are of varying backgrounds. Clients in any care setting may be from a variety of cultures and religious backgrounds. For example, a Vietnamese Buddhist may be sharing a hospital room with an American Christian; an Orthodox Jew with a Catholic; an African-American Baptist with an Indian Hindu. These clients may all be cared for by a health care team consisting of a Jewish physician, an Indian laboratory technician, and an assortment of nurses who are Christian, Hindu, and agnostic. How is it possible for nurses of such different backgrounds to provide spiritual care to such a diverse population of clients? The answer lies in the commonalities among these people in relation to their spirituality.

The concept of spirituality (the totality of an individual's being) is widely accepted in the world's religions and beliefs. Compassion and concern are a common thread among the various religious beliefs and spiritual inclinations. The nurse, to be an effective care giver, should be aware of the unique religious tenets and cultural background of each client. This knowledge should enable the nurse to provide compassionate, individualized care that addresses possible concerns relating to a client's cultural, ethnic, and religious affiliations.

Societal Influences

North Americans come from a variety of religious and ethnic traditions and thus make up a pluralistic society. **Pluralism** is defined as a state of society in which members of diverse ethnic, racial, religious, and social groups maintain an autonomous participation in and development of their traditional culture or special interests within the confines of a common civilization. Pluralism is a strength of a society that provides for individual, political, and religious freedom in that it allows for various interpretations and tolerances of a person's behaviors and beliefs. However, pluralism also results, at times, in health care workers and their clients embracing different ideologies, and this can become problematic in client care. For example, the nurse cannot categorize or make assumptions regarding a client's needs based merely on the client's culture or religion (i.e., persons from India may not be Hindu but Christian). Likewise, the Roman Catholic client may or may not eat meat on Fridays. Therefore, nurses must expand their knowledge of spiritual care concepts sufficiently to embrace a variety of client backgrounds. The more nurses expand their knowledge of spiritual care concepts and specific spiritual and religious traditions, the more effective they will be in dealing with clients of diverse spiritual backgrounds.

SPIRITUALITY AND RELIGION

Although there is overlap in the concepts of spirituality and religion, they are not the same thing. Nurses must make a distinction between these two concepts. **Religion** is a set of beliefs, values, codes of conduct, and rituals that answer the question of what it means to be human in relation to self, others, and a greater power. The greater power is defined by the individual. A greater power is an entity that has power beyond an individual's personal strength and is frequently identified as God. Belief in a god is known as **theism.** The greater power need not necessarily be considered a spiritual entity.

Nurses must not confuse religious and spiritual needs. If the nurse thinks that meeting religious needs is the total basis for spiritual care, some of the client's most important needs may be overlooked. However, religion may be an important aspect of an individual's spiritual care.

Religion may serve as a vehicle for expression of spirituality. In fact, most people satisfy spiritual needs through a particular religion and related religious practices that provide comfort through rituals and belief.

Some common examples of religious rituals include the following:

▶ The partaking of bread and wine in commemoration of the death of Christ during the sacrament of Holy Communion (the **Eucharist**)
▶ The act of prayer, which may be performed in a vast number of physical positions (lying prostrate, kneeling, sitting, or even driving a car)
▶ The act of confession, which is associated with certain religions and may provide spiritual satisfaction

It is possible, however, for spiritual satisfaction to be achieved without the use of religious rituals. For example, achieving personal insight into an individual's own behavior may provide satisfaction for that individual whether or not the insight is related to a religious belief or experience.

Spirituality is a much broader concept than religious affiliation or practice. The spiritual dimension of a person is that dimension that transcends physical and psychosocial dimensions; it is life giving and integrating. A spiritual issue may be a need for understanding or an attempt to make sense of what is happening or has happened to an individual. Spirituality is an aspect of every person regardless of that individual's religious affiliation or lack thereof.

SPIRITUAL NEEDS

Spiritual needs are those variables that inspire us to transcend the material world. Spiritual needs focus on finding meaning and purpose in life, illness, and life situations; giving and receiving of love and feelings of relatedness; experiencing forgiveness; and experiencing hope.

Need for a Sense of Meaning and Purpose

An individual's need for a sense of meaning and purpose in life, or need to have a meaning ascribed to life experiences including illness, is a spiritual need. All individuals review their life situations and realize that their lives have meaning and purpose. For instance, a recent graduate of an institution of learning may assign his or her personal worth according to the value of that educational experience; thus, personal meaning and purpose in that person's life includes his or her achievements and mission in life. Likewise, a client with a terminal illness may review his or her life and develop personal conclusions about the meaning of certain experiences or about the meaning of the illness itself. The realization that life has meaning and purpose and the subsequent search for a specific meaning and purpose in each individual's life is a spiritual quest.

Need for Love and Relatedness

The spiritual needs for love and relatedness can be experienced in either of two dimensions: horizontal or vertical. In a **vertical relationship,** a greater power and related values (not necessarily defined by a specific religion) guide an individual's life. For example, a person's feeling of being forgiven by a higher power and the desire to please that higher power and thus receive continued forgiveness would guide an individual in his or her daily life. In a **horizontal relationship,** other persons and the environment influence an individual's life.[5] A person's interactions with other people and the influence exerted by other people and the environment are considered to be horizontal in nature. Membership in a particular group is considered to be a horizontal relationship. In this sense, an individual's spirituality is two dimensional and interrelated: The vertical relationship with supreme values and the horizontal (psychosocial) interactions with others both influence the individual's life. How people interact on a psychosocial level may be a reflection of their relationship with the higher power. For instance, persons who remain cheerful and respectful of others may be reflecting the love and acceptance they feel from their higher power.

All individuals have the need to feel loved and to experience relatedness. Love and relatedness can be experienced through human relationships (the horizontal dimension) and through an individual's belief in a greater power as a source of love (the vertical dimension).

Need for Forgiveness

As persons search for meaning in their life experiences, they may experience guilt because they may assign personal liability to their situations. Guilt may occur as unfulfilled expectations or as acts of omission or commission toward others or themselves become evident.[6]

The need to be relieved of guilt is a spiritual need. In order for the guilt to be relieved, the individual must experience forgiveness in the vertical or horizontal dimension or both.

Need for Hope

To **hope** is to desire or long for something, accompanied by an expectation of fulfillment. Hope has long been recognized as necessary for life. As Simsen stated, "without hope we begin to die."[44] Hope connotes the possibility of future good. To be helpful for the individual expressing the spiritual need for hope, the hope must be based on a realistic assessment of the past and the present. Two kinds of hope are recognized: concrete hope and abstract hope.

The objects of **concrete hope** are those within the individual's experience, such as freedom from pain or other physical symptoms, or the ability to perform certain tasks.

Abstract (transcendent) hope is defined as a desire or expectation extending beyond the usual limits of ordinary experience and knowledge, beyond material existence. It is characterized by more abstract goals and tends to incorporate religious or philosophic meanings that extend the individual beyond concrete hope. An example of abstract hope is demonstrated in the terminally ill client's expression of belief in some type of spiritual existence after death. The client who does not believe in the afterlife may express abstract

hope by wishing to be remembered for his or her good works or individuality.

Usually an individual experiences both concrete and abstract hope. However, sometimes concrete hope fluctuates and fails, and the individual must modify the objects of hope. The modification of concrete hope usually results in abstract hope. An example of modification of concrete hope is when a client's physical condition continues to deteriorate toward death. The client may modify the concrete hope of physical recovery to a transcendent hope of living in a spiritual realm after death.

SPIRITUAL DEVELOPMENT THROUGHOUT THE LIFE SPAN

Spiritual growth continues throughout the life span as the individual develops and increases his or her awareness of the meaning, purpose, and values in life. Spiritual development may occur in a number of ways: by religious development (the vertical relationship), by psychosocial development (the horizontal relationships), and by faith development.

The ways that an individual develops spiritually have been studied by various theologians and theorists. The current discussion of spiritual development is limited to theories relevant to religious development, psychosocial development, and faith development.

Religious Development

Religious development depends on the acceptance of a particular system of beliefs, values, rituals, and rules for conduct as prescribed by a specific religion. Some people develop their own system from a variety of philosophic and religious traditions.

Religious development ideally leads to spiritual development; however, a person can strictly adhere to the tenets of a particular religion and practice the related rituals and yet never examine or internalize the symbolic meaning behind the rituals and religious activity. In this situation, spiritual growth and development may not occur.[5]

Psychosocial Development

As individuals develop relationships with others and the environment, they may ascribe meaning to their experiences. Individuals who do not develop a relationship with a higher being or God may yet consider themselves to be very spiritual in terms of their horizontal relationships with others. Because psychosocial relationships can have a great influence on physical and emotional health and because physical health and emotional health are so related to spiritual health, it is necessary to examine psychosocial issues to identify clients' needs and potential for spiritual growth.

Faith Development

Faith is a belief in or acknowledgment of something unable to be physically seen; however, some individuals may place faith on tangible items. For example, some sailors may place their faith in their sailboat itself and have faith that it will not sink. Other sailors will place their faith in a greater power to calm the wind and water so the boat will not sink. The definition of faith can be expanded to represent a way of being, living, or imagining.[20]

Faith is considered to be universally present in both nonreligious and religious persons.[20] It is the quality that offers meaning to life and offers individuals the ability to have and maintain meaning in life. Faith can be religious in nature or centered on the self, success, money, career, or other tangible objects of the individual's choosing. In this manner, faith can be related to vertical or horizontal facets of spiritual development. It is, however, an integral part of spirituality.

Developmental Stages

Crucial to the understanding of spiritual development across the life span is an examination of the stages of human development and the related psychosocial and faith-related tasks appropriate to the specific stages of development. The reader can refer to Unit 3 for a thorough discussion of growth and development.

INFANCY

Infants are born without religious belief or values and do not have a defined spiritual self. However, the period of infancy has significance in the development of trust and hope. Ideally, the infant begins to develop trust, primarily as a result of reliance on the significant care giver. If the relationship with the care giver is warm and consistently caring, the infant anticipates that the care giver will continue to provide for his or her needs; Erikson[15] postulated that, in this process of trusting the significant care giver, the infant begins to develop hope. If the care giver is inadequate, it is postulated that the infant will not develop trust and hope.

The development of trust is basic to the development of a relationship with a greater power.[20]

PRESCHOOL

In early childhood, the child begins to develop a sense of self-worth. According to Erikson, a lack of self-worth at this stage will affect an individual's capacity to accept love, including the love of God. Lacking the capacity to accept love will affect psychosocial relationships and the ability to participate meaningfully in an organized religious faith.[15]

The child's faith is influenced by the role models that are provided by parents and the church and by stories that assist with the development of ideas and images.

Children of preschool age have images and perceptions of God and religion. These have been provided by the family.

The ability to follow rules and an understanding of God as rewarding good behavior and punishing bad behavior indicate that religious and spiritual development has begun.

SCHOOL AGE

During school age, mastering tasks instills a sense of competence. If children do not acquire feelings of competence, they are left with feelings of inferiority. This inferiority can affect the ability to relate to others as well as to a greater power.[15]

School-age children begin to exhibit faith by copying the outward actions of the religious practices of their families. Children who are a part of a family that practices a particular religion may begin to feel that they truly are a part of the religion. For example, Roman Catholic children who attend mass with the family may begin to incorporate the rituals of the mass into their own expressions of spirituality and thus identify religious practices as fulfillment of spiritual need. They may believe in God at this time;[5] however, they describe God in concrete terms because they have not yet developed a capacity to understand abstract concepts. For example, a young child may describe God as a man who has a beard, eats with a fork, and stomps his feet when He gets angry because the child has not yet developed an ability to discuss abstract concepts.

ADOLESCENCE

Adolescence is a time of conflict as the individual strives to achieve a sense of identity. Erikson stated that the development of personal identity is necessary if the adolescent is to develop fidelity.[15]

Fidelity implies faithfulness or loyalty to personal decisions. In this light, before an adolescent can be true to a religious ideology, to a higher power, to another person, or to the self, a sense of identity (self) must have developed.

This means that adolescents must arrive at some concepts, personal decisions, and values that will remain unchanged in the face of contradiction or questioning. While attempting to achieve a sense of identity, adolescents may be confused about their identity and the beliefs and values to which they commit themselves.

During this time of rebellion, the adolescent may reject parental values, including religious values. Paradoxically, adolescents at the same time ask themselves about their personal meaning and purpose in the world; answering this question is the spiritual task for this life stage.[5]

Adolescents experience conflict about values and beliefs and thus begin a stage of faith development that continues until they become independent from their parents.[20] Adolescents experience conflict when min-gling with groups of people with different values (e.g., belonging to a group of friends from the local church youth group, which stresses family cohesion, while also belonging to a sports team that stresses healthful habits, and yet spending some time with school classmates who are actively engaged in premarital sex and neighborhood acquaintances who use illicit drugs. At this time, the adolescents' developmental task is to examine their values and beliefs and to define a personal value system.

YOUNG ADULTHOOD

Young adults who have found answers in the search for identity during adolescence are now ready to commit themselves to an intimate relationship. According to Erikson, love results when the individual achieves a healthy balance between intimacy and isolation.[15] Love is a quality of both the vertical and horizontal dimensions of spirituality.[5] For example, the love experienced from a higher power (vertical dimension) may influence and be demonstrated in loving psychosocial relationships (horizontal dimension).

The result of young adults examining their view of the world and religious beliefs is an autonomous self that can be given to a supreme being.[5,20] This means that the autonomous person can now remain independent but place dependence on God through faith and trust. Carson stated that "in general, it would seem that psychosocial development must progress to a point where the individual is able to sacrifice self, to love, and to focus on the needs of others ahead of the needs of self before making a personal commitment to a supreme being" and "with increasing age, the capacity for commitment to God increases."[5]

MIDDLE ADULTHOOD

The task of adulthood is the achievement of a healthy balance between generativity and stagnation or of being productive, constructive, responsible, and offering guidance to others versus being self-centered and lacking interest in the welfare of others. Caring about others as well as the self is the resultant virtue.[13] For many individuals, generativity includes teaching the next generation to meet life's challenges. How the adult has completed tasks and resolved issues in former life stages influences the directions offered to the next generation.

Faith at this stage acknowledges that the views and beliefs of other persons may also be valid, that personal views and beliefs may be only a partial view of the truth. The result is that individuals become more open to accepting life's paradoxes and more able to recognize the necessity for interdependence.[20]

LATE ADULTHOOD

The final psychosocial task, according to Erikson, is to achieve a balance between ego integrity and despair,[15] or feelings of self-acceptance with a sense of worth and adaptation to life versus a sense of helplessness, hopelessness, and meaninglessness, with inability to satisfy the self with satisfying activities. The virtue achieved in this process is wisdom.[5]

At this later point in life, individuals review their lives, looking at accomplishments, failures, and disappointments. Ideally, they view their lives as having meaning. The individual's life need not have been 100 per cent successful, because even failures and disappointments can add depth to a life that has been full.

It is important to keep in mind that not all individuals achieve the state of maturity. Some continue to try to meet the aspirations of idealized youth; some focus on the less favorable outcomes and do not develop appreciation for the joys and successes; and some become negative and bitter.

During maturity, the individual may reach the final stage of faith, one in which the individual feels a responsibility for universal needs.[20] This includes a sense that all of humanity has a responsibility to respond to the needs of all creatures.

MAJOR WORLD RELIGIONS

To provide holistic client care, which includes spiritual care, nurses must begin by becoming familiar with the major world religions, including their major tenets and the differences among their religious practices. Nurses should also become familiar with the ways that clients personally apply religious beliefs and practices to their situation. A good knowledge base of various religions will assist nurses in relating to their clients' spiritual needs. The following section is a brief overview of the major world religions as they relate to client care.

Hinduism

Hinduism is the primary religion in India. The recent influx of Indians to North America provides American and Canadian nurses with the opportunity to provide care for Hindu clients.

In caring for the Hindu client, it is helpful to know that Hindus believe in only one supreme being; the many gods of the religion are only aspects of a supreme unity. Life in all of its forms is an aspect of the divine, but life appears as a separation from the divine, a cycle of birth and rebirth determined by the purity or impurity of past deeds (karma). The aim of every Hindu is to grow spiritually by improving one's karma.

Nursing care for the Hindu should take into account the possibility that the client may minimize bodily ills. Yoga training, emphasizing self-control, and devotion to God through reading and meditation may cause a Hindu to seek help from inner resources and the literature of Hinduism rather than from medication or consultation with staff. Provision of an atmosphere conducive to this practice is appreciated by Hindu clients.[26]

In the Hindu religion, there are many dietary restrictions that conform to individual sect doctrine. Generally, a vegetarian diet is acceptable; however, no definite rules regarding diet should be implemented until the client is questioned regarding personal practices.

Other major health beliefs reflect acceptance of modern medical practices; however, artificial insemination is not accepted because sterility reflects divine will. The Hindu may bear illness with resignation, viewing death and rebirth as synonymous.

Judaism

The practice of Judaism is almost worldwide, with concentrations in Israel and the United States. Judaism consists of a spectrum of practices from ultraconservative to ultraliberal. Distinctions depend primarily on how closely the person observes the many prescribed duties and prohibitions in daily life, particularly dietary and Sabbath regulations.

Judaism emphasizes ethical behavior (and, among the observant, careful ritual obedience) as the true worship of one God. It is a form of **monotheism**—the belief that there is one God. Sabbath, the time for spiritual refreshment, is from sundown on Friday to shortly after sundown on Saturday.

Dietary laws may be an important consideration in client care. Orthodox and Conservative Jews adhere strictly to dietary laws and consume only a kosher diet, which prohibits pork, shellfish, and the eating of meat and milk products at the same time. Meats approved are from those animals that are ruminants (cud chewing) and have divided hooves. For example, cows and sheep are acceptable; pigs are not. Fish approved must have both fins and scales. Acceptable fish are trout, bass, cod. Also the animals used for food must be healthy and slaughtered in a prescribed manner.

A person of the Jewish faith, when dying, should not be left alone. Whenever possible, the family and rabbi should be present when a client seems ready to expire. If a Jewish person dies on the Sabbath, the body cannot be moved, except by a non-Jew, until sundown.[26] Please refer to Table 53–1 for additional information regarding Jewish beliefs and practices affecting health care.

TABLE 53–1. Jewish Beliefs and Practices Affecting Health Care

Religious Group	Beliefs and Practices
Observant Jews (Orthodox Judaism and some Conservative Jewish groups)	*Birth:* For observant Jews, babies are named by the father. Male children are named 8 days after birth, when ritual circumcision is done. A mohel performs the circumcision. Circumcision may be postponed if the infant is in poor health. Female babies are usually named during the reading of the Holy Torah. Nurses need to be sensitive to the wishes of the parents when caring for babies who have not yet been named.
	Care of women: A woman is considered to be in a ritual state of impurity whenever blood is coming from her uterus, such as during menstrual periods and after the birth of a child. During this time, her husband will not have physical contact with her. When this time is completed, she will bathe herself in a pool called a mikvah. Nurses need to be aware of this practice and be sensitive to the husband and wife because the husband will not touch his wife. He cannot assist her in moving in the bed, so the nurse will have to do this. An Orthodox Jewish man will not touch any women other than his wife, daughters, and mother. Home health care workers need to be aware of these practices.
	Dietary rules: (1) Kosher dietary laws include the following: No mixing of milk and meat at a meal; no consumption of food or any derivative thereof from animals not slaughtered in accordance with Jewish law; use of separate cooking utensils for meat and milk products; if a client requires milk and meat products for a meal, the dairy foods should be served first, followed later by the meat. (2) During Yom Kippur (Day of Atonement), a 24-hour fast is required, but exceptions are made for those who cannot fast because of medical reasons. (3) During Passover, no leavened products are eaten. (4) May say benediction of thanksgiving before meals and grace at the end of the meal. Time and a quiet environment should be provided for this.
	Sabbath: Observed from sunset Friday until sunset Saturday. Orthodox law prohibits riding in a car, smoking, turning lights on and off, handling money, and using television and telephone. Nurses need to be aware of this when caring for observant Jews at home and in the hospital. Medical or surgical treatments should be postponed if possible.
	Death: Judaism defines death as occurring when respiration and circulation are irreversibly stopped and no movement is apparent. (1) Euthanasia is strictly forbidden by Orthodox Jews, who advocate the strict use of life-support measures. (2) Prior to death, Jewish faith indicates that visiting of the person by family and friends is a religious duty. The Torah and Psalms may be read and prayers recited. A witness needs to be present when a person prays for health so that if death occurs God will protect the family and the spirit will be committed to God. Extraneous talking and conversation about death are not encouraged unless initiated by the patient or visitors. In Judaism, the belief is that people should have someone with them when the soul leaves the body, so family and/or friends should be allowed to stay with patients. After death, the body should not be left alone until buried, usually within 24 hours. (3) When death occurs, the body should be untouched for 8 to 30 minutes. Medical personnel should not touch or wash the body but allow only an Orthodox person or the Jewish Burial Society to care for the

TABLE 53-1. *Jewish Beliefs and Practices Affecting Health Care* Continued

Religious Group	Beliefs and Practices
	body. Handling of a corpse on the Sabbath is forbidden to Jewish persons. If need be, the nursing staff may provide routine care of the body, wearing gloves. Water in the room should be emptied, and the family may request that mirrors be covered to symbolize that a death has occurred. (4) Orthodox Jews and some Conservative Jews do not approve of autopsies. If an autopsy must be done, all body parts must remain with the body. (5) For Orthodox Jews, the body must be buried within 24 hours. No flowers are permitted. A fetus must be buried. (6) A 7-day mourning period is required by the immediate family. They must stay at home except for Sabbath worship. (7) Organs or other body parts such as amputated limbs must be made available for burial for Orthodox Jews, since they believe that all of the body must be returned to earth.
	Birth control and abortion: Artificial methods of birth control are not encouraged. Vasectomy is not allowed. Abortion may be performed only to save the mother's life.
	Organ transplant: Donor organ transplants generally are not permitted by Orthodox Jews but may be allowed with rabbinical consent.
	Shaving: The beard is regarded as a mark of piety among observant Jews. For the very Orthodox, shaving should not be done with a razor but with scissors or electric razor, since a blade should not contact the skin.
	Head covering: Orthodox men wear skull caps at all times, and women cover their hair after marriage. Some Orthodox women wear wigs as a mark of piety. Conservative Jews cover their heads only during acts of worship and prayer.
	Prayer: Praying directly to God, including a prayer of confession, is required for Orthodox Jews. Nurses should provide quiet time for prayer.
Reform Jews	*Birth:* Reform Jews may or may not adhere to the practices referred to for observant Jews. They favor ritual circumcision, but it is not imperative.
	Care of women: Reform Jews do not observe the rules against touching.
	Dietary rules: Reform Jews usually do not observe kosher dietary restrictions.
	Sabbath: Usually worship in temples on Friday evenings. No strict rules.
	Death: Advocate use of life support without heroic measures. Allow for cremation but suggest that ashes be buried in a Jewish cemetery.
	Organ transplants: Donation or transplantation of organs allowed with permission of a rabbi.
	Head coverings: Generally pray without wearing skull caps.

From Carson, V. B. (1989). *Spiritual dimensions of nursing practice.* Philadelphia: W. B. Saunders.

Christianity

One third of humanity adheres to Christianity, making it the largest religion in the world.[5,26] It is also the most diverse of all religions, with followers in Roman Catholicism, Eastern Orthodoxy, and a variety of Protestant faiths.

Christians believe in one God as a Trinity—Father, Son, and Holy Spirit, the latter providing a spirit of love and truth. Ethically, Christianity represents the binding of all humanity and the belief that individuals have an immortal soul accountable to God.[26]

Because there are so many Christian religions, the nurse should become familiar with the particular client's faith to provide care. Most Christian clients express the need for nurses to provide spiritual care in their practice of caring and in shared prayer.[7] Included in Table 53-2 are examples of a number of Christian beliefs and practices that affect health care.

Buddhism

Buddhism is practiced throughout Asia from Ceylon to Japan. The recent influx of Asian people into the

United States and Canada is giving the North American nurse increasing exposure to Buddhist clients.

The practice of Buddhism varies widely. Different sects range from austere meditation to magical chanting and elaborate temple rites. Many of the practices of Buddhism had their beginnings in Hinduism.

The Buddhist believes that life is misery and decay, and there is no ultimate reality in it or behind it. The cycle of endless birth and rebirth continues because of desire and attachment of the unreal "self." Right meditation and deeds will end the cycle and allow the person to achieve Nirvana, the void, the nothingness. The Buddhist religion teaches a way to overcome fears, anxieties, and apprehension. It teaches that the individual can purify himself or herself of all desires and thus do away with evil and suffering.

Beliefs related to health care are largely in harmony with modern science. There is no divine punishment; every occurrence depends on the law of causality, so illness is a trial to aid the development of the soul. The Buddhist client feels that recovery is largely dependent on family ties. Therefore, if illness or impending death causes hospitalization, family members should remain close by to offer emotional support.[26]

Text continued on page 1522

TABLE 53–2. Roman Catholic, Eastern Orthodox, Protestant, and Selected Western Religious Groups' Beliefs and Practices Affecting Health Care

Religious Group	Beliefs and Practices
Roman Catholic	*Birth:* Since Roman Catholics believe that unbaptized children are cut off from heaven, infant baptism is mandatory. For newborns with a grave prognosis, stillborns, and all aborted fetuses (unless evidence of tissue necrosis and prolonged death is present), emergency baptism is required. The nurse calls a priest to perform the baptism unless the death might occur before the priest arrives. In that case, anyone can baptize by pouring warm water on the infant's head and saying, "I baptize you in the name of the Father, of the Son, and of the Holy Spirit." All information about the baptism is recorded on the chart, and the priest and family notified. *Holy Eucharist:* For clients and health care givers who are to receive communion, abstinence from solid food and alcohol is required for 15 minutes (if possible) prior to reception of the consecrated wafer. Medicine, water, and nonalcoholic drinks are permitted at any time. If a client is in danger of death, the fast is waived since the reception of the Eucharist at this time is very important. *Anointing of the sick:* The sacrament of **extreme unction** is the act of anointing the body as a rite of consecration. The priest uses oil to anoint the forehead and hands and, if desired, the affected area. The rite may be performed on any who are ill and desire it. Persons receiving the sacrament seek complete healing, and strength to endure suffering. Prior to 1963, this sacrament was only given to persons at time of imminent death, so the nurse must be sensitive to the meaning this has for the client. If possible, the nurse calls a priest before the client is unconscious but may also call when there is sudden death, since the sacrament may also be given shortly after death. The nurse records on the care plan that this sacrament has been administered. *Dietary habits:* Obligatory fasting is excused during hospitalization. However, if there are no health restrictions, some Catholics may still observe the following guidelines: (1) Anyone 14 years or older must abstain from eating meat on Ash Wednesday and all Fridays during Lent. Some older Catholics may still abstain from meat on all Fridays of the year. (2) In addition to abstinence from meat, persons 21 to 59 years of age must limit themselves to one full meal and two light meals on Ash Wednesday and Good Friday. (3) Eastern Rite Catholics are stricter about fasting and fast more frequently than Western Rite Catholics, so it is important for the nurse to know if a client is Eastern or Western. *Death:* Each Roman Catholic should participate in the anointing of the sick as well as the Eucharist and penance before death. The body should not be shrouded until after these sacraments are performed. All body parts that retain human quality must be appropriately buried or cremated. *Birth control:* Prohibited except for abstinence or natural family planning. Referral to a priest for questions about this can be of great help. Nurses can teach the techniques of natural family planning if they are familiar with them; otherwise, this should be referred to the physician or to a support group of the church that instructs couples in this method of birth control. Sterilization is prohibited unless there is an overriding medical reason. *Organ donation:* Donation and transplantation of organs are acceptable as long as the donor is not harmed and is not deprived of life. *Religious objects:* Rosary prayers are said using rosary beads. Medals bearing the images of saints, relics, statues, and scapulars are important objects that may be pinned to a hospital gown or pillow or be at the bedside. Extreme care should be taken not to lose these objects, since they have special meaning to the client.
Eastern Orthodox	*Birth:* The child must be baptized within 40 days after birth. If sprinkling or immersion into water is not possible, baptism is performed by moving the baby in the air in the sign of the cross. An ordained priest or a deacon must be notified for this. *Holy Eucharist:* The priest is notified if the client desires this sacrament. *Anointing of the sick:* The priest conducts this in the hospital room. *Dietary habits:* Fasting from meat and dairy products is required on Wednesday and Friday during Lent and on other holy days. Hospital clients are exempt if fasting is detrimental to health. *Special days:* Christmas is celebrated on January 7 and New Year's on January 14. This is important to the care of a client who is hospitalized on these days. *Death:* Last rites are obligatory. This is handled by an ordained priest who is notified by the nurse while the client is conscious. The Russian Orthodox Church does not encourage autopsy or organ donation. Euthanasia, even for the terminally ill, is discouraged, as is cremation. *Birth control:* This as well as abortion is not permitted.
Assemblies of God (Pentecostal)	*Baptism:* Water baptism by complete immersion is practiced when an individual has received Jesus Christ as Savior and Lord based on Acts 2:38.

TABLE 53-2. Roman Catholic, Eastern Orthodox, Protestant, and Selected Western Religious Groups' Beliefs and Practices Affecting Health Care Continued

Religious Group	Beliefs and Practices
	Holy Communion: Notify clergy if the client desires.
	Anointing of the sick: Members believe in divine healing through prayer and the laying on of hands. Clergy is notified if client or family desires this.
	Dietary habits: Abstinence from alcohol, tobacco, and all illegal drugs is strongly encouraged.
	Death: No special practices.
	Other practices: Faith in God and in the health care providers is encouraged. Members pray for divine intervention in health matters. Nurses should encourage and allow time for prayer. Members may speak in "tongues" during prayer.
Baptist (more than 27 different groups in the United States)	*Baptism:* Do not practice infant baptism.
	Holy Communion: Clergy should be notified if the client desires.
	Dietary habits: Total abstinence from alcohol is expected.
	Death: No general service is provided, but the clergy does minister through counseling, prayer, and Scripture as requested by the client or family, and the client is encouraged to believe in Jesus Christ as Savior and Lord.
	Other practices: The Bible is held to be the word of God, so the nurse should either allow quiet time for Scripture reading or offer to read to the client.
Christian Church (Disciples of Christ)	*Baptism:* Do not practice infant baptism but have dedication service. Believers are baptized by immersion.
	Holy Communion: Open communion is celebrated each Sunday and is a central part of worship services. The nurse notifies the clergy if the client desires it, or the clergy may suggest it.
	Death: No special practices.
	Other practices: Church elders as well as clergy may be notified to assist with meeting the client's spiritual needs.
Church of the Brethren	*Baptism:* Do not practice infant baptism but have dedication service.
	Holy Communion: Usually received within church, but clergy will give it in the hospital when requested.
	Anointing of the sick: Practiced for physical healing as well as spiritual uplift and held in high regard by the church. The clergy is notified if the client or family desire.
	Death: The clergy is notified for counsel and prayer.
Church of the Nazarene	*Baptism:* Parents have the choice of baptism or dedication for their infant. Emphasis is on the believer's baptism, which is regarded as a symbol of the New Covenant in Jesus Christ.
	Holy Communion: Pastor will administer if the client wishes.
	Dietary habits: The use of alcohol and tobacco is forbidden.
	Death: Cremation is permitted, and term stillborn infants are buried.
	Other practices: Believe in divine healing but not to the exclusion of medical treatment. Clients may desire quiet time for prayer.
Episcopal (Anglican)	*Baptism:* Infant baptism is practiced and is considered urgent if the infant is critically ill. The priest is notified to administer the sacrament. Lay persons may baptize in an emergency.
	Holy Communion: The priest is notified if the client wishes to receive this sacrament.
	Anointing of the sick: Priest may administer this rite when death is imminent, but it is not considered mandatory.
	Dietary habits: Some clients may abstain from meat on Fridays. Others may fast before receiving the Eucharist, but fasting is not mandatory.
	Death: No special practices.
	Other practices: Confession of sins to a priest is optional; if the client desires this, the clergy should be notified.
Lutheran (10 different branches)	*Baptism:* Baptize only living infants any time, but usually 6 to 8 weeks after birth. Adults are also baptized, and modes of baptism as appropriate include sprinkling, pouring, or immersion.
	Holy Communion: Notify the clergy if the client desires this sacrament. Clergy may also inquire about the client's desire.
	Anointing of the sick: The client may request an anointing and blessing from the minister when the prognosis is poor.
	Death: A service of Commendation of the Dying is used at the client's or family's request.
Mennonite (12 different groups)	*Baptism:* No infant baptism, but the child may be dedicated if requested by the parents.
	Holy Communion: Served twice a year, with foot washing as part of ceremony.
	Dietary habits: Abstinence from alcohol is urged for all.
	Death: Prayer is important at time of crisis, so contacting a minister is important.

Table continued on following page

TABLE 53-2. *Roman Catholic, Eastern Orthodox, Protestant, and Selected Western Religious Groups' Beliefs and Practices Affecting Health Care* Continued

Religious Group	Beliefs and Practices
	Other practices: Women may wear head coverings during hospitalization. Anointing with oil is administered in harmony with James 5:14 when requested.
Methodist (over 20 different groups)	*Baptism:* Notify the clergy if the parent desires baptism for a sick infant. *Holy Communion:* Notify the clergy if a client requests it prior to surgery or another health crisis. *Anointing of the sick:* If requested, the clergy will come to pray and sprinkle the client with olive oil. *Death:* Scripture reading and prayer are important at this time. *Other practices:* Donation of one's body or part of the body at death is encouraged.
Presbyterian (10 different groups)	*Baptism:* Infant baptism is practiced by pouring or sprinkling. Immersion is also practiced at times for adults. *Holy Communion:* Given when appropriate and convenient, at the hospitalized client's request. *Death:* Notify a local pastor or elder for prayer and Scripture reading if desired by the family or client.
Quaker (Friends)	*Baptism and Holy Communion:* Since Friends have no creed there is a diversity of personal beliefs, one of which is that outward sacraments are usually not necessary since there is the ministry of the Spirit inwardly in such areas as baptism and communion. A few Friends baptize with water. *Death:* Believe that the present life is part of God's kingdom and generally have no ceremony as a rite of passage from this life to the next. Personal beliefs and wishes need to be ascertained, and the nurse can then act upon the client's wishes. *Other practices:* The name of the Quaker infant is recorded in official record books at the local meeting.
Salvation Army	*Baptism:* No particular ceremony, but they do have an Infant Dedication ceremony. *Holy Communion:* No particular ceremony. *Death:* Notify the local officer in charge of the Army Corps for any soldier (member) who needs assistance. *Other practices:* The Bible is seen as the only rule for one's faith, so the Scriptures should be made available to a client. The Army has many of its own social welfare centers, with hospitals and homes where unwed mothers are cared for and outpatient services provided. No medical or surgical procedures are opposed, except for abortion on demand.
Seventh-Day Adventist	*Baptism:* No infant baptism is practiced, but have dedication services. *Holy Communion:* Although this is not required of hospitalized clients, the clergy is notified if the client desires. *Anointing of the sick:* The clergy are contacted for prayer and anointing with oil. *Dietary habits:* Since the body is viewed as the temple of the Holy Spirit, healthy living is essential. Therefore the use of alcohol, tobacco, coffee, and tea and the promiscuous use of drugs are prohibited. Some are vegetarians, and most avoid pork. *Special days:* The Sabbath is observed on Saturday. *Death:* No special procedures. *Other related practices:* Use of hypnotism is opposed by some. Persons of homosexual or lesbian orientation are ministered to in the hope of correction of these practices, which are believed to be wrong. A Bible should always be available for Scripture reading.
United Church of Christ	*Baptism:* Practice infant and adult baptism. Three modes are used as appropriate: pouring, sprinkling, and immersion. *Holy Communion:* Clergy is notified if the client desires to receive this sacrament. *Death:* If the client desires counsel or prayer, notify the clergy.

Selected Western Religious Groups

Christian Science	*Birth:* Use physician or nurse midwife during childbirth. No baptism ceremony. *Dietary habits:* Since alcohol and tobacco are considered drugs, they are not used. Coffee and tea are often declined. *Death:* Autopsy is usually declined unless required by law. Donation of organs is unlikely, but is an individual decision. *Other practices:* Do not normally seek medical care, since they approach health care in a different, primarily spiritual, framework. They commonly utilize the services of a surgeon to set a bone but decline drugs and, in general, other medical or surgical procedures. Hypnotism and psychotherapy are also declined. Family planning is left to the family. They seek exemption from vaccinations but obey legal requirements. Report infectious diseases and obey public health quaran-

TABLE 53–2. Roman Catholic, Eastern Orthodox, Protestant, and Selected Western Religious Groups' Beliefs and Practices Affecting Health Care Continued

Religious Group	Beliefs and Practices
	tines. Nonmedical care facilities are maintained for those needing nursing assistance in the course of a healing. The *Christian Science Journal* lists available Christian Science nurses. When a Christian Science believer is in the hospital, the nurse should allow and encourage time for prayer and study. Clients may request that a Christian Science practitioner be notified to come.
Jehovah's Witnesses	*Baptism:* No infant baptism is practiced. Baptism by complete immersion of adults is done as a symbol of dedication to Jehovah, since Jesus was baptized. *Dietary habits:* Use of alcohol and tobacco is discouraged, since these harm the physical body. *Death:* Autopsy is a private matter to be decided by the persons involved. Burial and cremation are acceptable. *Birth control and abortion:* Use of birth control is a personal decision. Abortion is opposed based on Exodus 21:22-23. *Organ transplants:* Use of organ transplant is a private decision and if used must be cleansed with a nonblood solution. *Blood transfusions:* Blood transfusions violate God's laws and are therefore not allowed. Clients do respect physicians and will accept alternatives to blood transfusions. These might include use of nonblood plasma expanders, careful surgical techniques to decrease blood loss, use of autologous transfusions, and autotransfusion through use of a heart-lung machine. Nurses should check unconscious clients for Medic Alert cards that state that the person does not want a transfusion. Since Jehovah's Witnesses are prepared to die rather than break God's law, nurses need to be sensitive to the spiritual as well as the physical needs of the client.
The Church of Jesus Christ of Latter-Day Saints (Mormons)	*Baptism:* If a child over the age of 8 is very ill, whether baptized or unbaptized, a member of the church's priesthood should be called. *Holy Communion:* A hospitalized client may desire to have a member of the church priesthood administer this sacrament. *Anointing of the sick:* Mormons frequently are anointed and given a blessing before going to the hospital and after admission by laying on of hands. *Dietary habits:* Abstinence from the use of tobacco; beverages with caffeine such as cola, coffee, and tea; alcohol and other substances considered injurious. Mormons eat meat but encourage the intake of fruits, grains, and herbs. *Death:* Prefer burial of the body. A church elder should be notified to assist the family. If need be, the elder will assist the funeral director in dressing the body in special clothes and will give other help as needed. *Birth control and abortion:* Abortion is opposed except when the life of the mother is in danger. Only natural means of birth control are recommended. Artificial means can be used when the health of the woman is at stake (including emotional health). *Personal care:* Cleanliness is very important to Mormons. A sacred undergarment may be worn at all times by Mormons and should only be removed in emergency situations. *Other practices:* Allowing quiet time for prayer and the reading of the sacred writings is important. The church maintains a welfare system to assist those in need. Families are of great importance, so visiting should be encouraged.
Unitarian Universalist Association	*Baptism:* Infant baptism is unnecessary and if used at all is without trinitarian formula. Usually dedicate their children. *Death:* Cremation is often preferred to burial. *Other practices:* Use of birth control is advocated as part of responsible parenting. Strong support for a woman's right to choice regarding abortion is maintained. Unitarian Universalists advocate donation of body parts for research and transplants.
Unification Church	*Baptism:* No baptism. *Special days:* Sunday mornings are used to honor Reverend and Mrs. Moon as the true parents, and members get up at 5:00 A.M., bow before a picture of the Moons three times, and vow to do what is needed to help the Reverend accomplish his mission on earth. *Death:* Believe that after death one's place of destiny will depend on his or her spirit's quality of life and goodness while on earth. In the afterlife, one will have the same aspirations and feelings as before death. Hell is not a concern, since it will not be a place as heaven grows in size. Persons who leave the Unification Church are warned that Satan may try to possess them. *Other practices:* All marriages must be solemnized by Reverend Moon in order to be part of the perfect family and have salvation. The church supplies its faithful members with life's necessities. Members may use occult practices to have spiritual and psychic experiences.

From Carson, V. B. (1989). *Spiritual dimensions of nursing practice.* Philadelphia: W. B. Saunders.

Islam

Islam is practiced from the west coast of Africa to the Philippines across a broad band that includes Tanzania, southern Russia, and western China, India, and Indonesia. It is the youngest of the major world religions[31] and is one of the largest and fastest growing religions in the world.[5] Islam serves as a bridge between Eastern and Western religions.

Islam belief is strictly monotheistic; God, known as Allah, the creator of the universe, is omnipotent, just, and merciful. It is believed that those who sincerely submit to God return to a state of sinlessness. In the end, the sinless go to paradise, a place of physical and spiritual pleasure, and the wicked burn in hell. All Muslims are supposed to pray five times a day, give a regular portion of their goods to charity, fast during the day during the month of Ramadan (according to the

Muslim calendar), and make at least one pilgrimage to Mecca if possible.

The Muslim client's dietary restriction includes refraining from pork and pork products and intoxicants. The family is a great source of comfort, and praying with a group is strengthening, but the Muslim has no priest; his or her relationship is directly with God.[26] Please refer to Table 53–3 for additional information regarding Islamic beliefs and practices affecting health care.

NEW AGE SPIRITUALISM

In contemporary society, spirituality seems to be growing in importance but not necessarily in relation to organized religion. The themes of peace, love, and forgiveness are common to all religions; however, tradi-

---

TABLE 53–3. *Islamic and Muslim Beliefs and Practices Affecting Health Care*

Religious Group	Beliefs and Practices
Islam	*Birth:* A baby is bathed immediately after birth, before giving it to the mother. The father (or mother if the father is not available) then whispers the call to prayer in the child's ears so that the first sounds it hears are about the Muslim faith. Circumcision is culturally recommended before puberty. A baby born prematurely but at least 130 days gestation is given the same treatment as any other infant.
	Dietary habits: No pork is allowed, nor alcoholic beverages. All halal (permissible) meat must be blessed and killed in a special way. This is called zabihah (correctly slaughtered).
	Death: Prior to death, family members ask to be present so that they can read the Koran and pray with the client. An Imam may come if requested by the client or family but is not required. Clients must face Mecca and confess their sins and beg forgiveness in the presence of their family. If the family is unavailable, any practicing Muslim can provide support to the client. After death, Muslims prefer that the family wash, prepare, and place the body in a position facing Mecca. If necessary, the health care providers may perform these procedures as long as they wear gloves. Burial is performed as soon as possible. Cremation is forbidden. Autopsy is also prohibited except for legal reasons, and then no body part is to be removed. Donation of body parts or organs is not allowed, since according to culturally developed law persons do not own their body.
	Abortion and birth control: Abortion is forbidden, and many conservative Muslims do not encourage the use of contraceptives since this interferes with God's purpose. Others feel that a woman should only have as many children as her husband can afford. Contraception is permitted by Islamic law.
	Personal devotions: At prayer time, washing is required, even by those who are sick. A client on bed rest may require assistance with this task before prayer. Provision of privacy is important during prayer.
	Religious objects: The Koran must not be touched by anyone ritually unclean, and nothing should be placed on top of it. Some Muslims wear taviz, a black string on which words of the Koran are attached. These should not be removed and must remain dry. Certain items of jewelry such as bangles may have religious significance and should not be removed unnecessarily.
	Care of women: Since women are not allowed to sign consent forms or make a decision regarding family planning, the husband needs to be present. Women are very modest and frequently wear clothes that cover all of the body. During a medical examination, the woman's modesty should be respected as much as possible. Muslim women prefer female doctors. For 40 days after giving birth and also during menstruation, a woman is exempt from prayer since this is a time of cleansing for her.
American Muslim Mission	*Baptism:* No baptism is practiced.
	Dietary habits: In addition to refusing pork, many will not eat traditional black American foods such as corn bread and collard greens.
	Death: The family is contacted before any care of the deceased is performed. There are special procedures for washing and shrouding the body.
	Other practices: Quiet time is necessary to permit prayer. Members are encouraged to use black physicians for health care. Since these clients do not smoke, their request for a nonsmoking roommate should be honored.

From Carson, V. B. (1989). *Spiritual dimensions of nursing practice.* Philadelphia: W. B. Saunders.

tional religions are not recognized as adequate by many people. "New Age" spiritualism seems, in fact, largely different from traditional religions.

In attempting to explain these differences, one must keep in mind that the traditional religions via churches and forms of worship developed as ways to express themes of love, peace, and forgiveness. The New Age spiritualism likewise expresses the same themes but does so in the context of our rapidly changing contemporary world. With New Age spiritualism, a growing number of people are organizing in informal services.

An enhanced sense of spiritualism provides the capacity to recognize all religions, tolerate and accept those persons with beliefs different from one's own beliefs, and focus on the commonalities among beliefs, such as peace, love, and forgiveness. In this sense, all religions yield to a discovery of spirituality and vitality that provides the basis for all religions and that founded the various religions originally. With such a focus, the person who possesses a sense of enhanced spirituality may recognize that the major points on which to focus are the principles or the fundamental truths in all religions rather than the rituals. In this way, New Age spiritualism and traditional religions become alike, and the various approaches to either serve to satisfy spiritual issues in a larger portion of humanity.

AGNOSTICISM AND ATHEISM

Agnosticism is the belief that the existence of any higher power such as a god cannot be known. **Atheism** is denial of the existence of God. It is important to understand that these terms are not synonymous. Whereas the atheist usually shuns religious activities, the agnostic may or may not engage in religious rituals. Both the atheist and the agnostic have spiritual natures, and you should consider their spiritual needs when planning their care. Whether these spiritual needs can, in part, be met by religious activities, however, is a question to be answered on an individual basis, just as it is with clients who believe in a god.

RESOURCES FOR CLIENTS NEEDING SPIRITUAL CARE

It is important to keep in mind that, just as total health care cannot be provided by one specialty or one person, spiritual care cannot be provided by the nurse alone, nor can it be provided by *any* specific resource by itself. The nurse rarely will be the client's primary spiritual care giver. The nurse in most instances will serve as an advocate for the client; this includes recognizing and referring the client's needs to others who can best provide what is identified as the appropriate resource.

No single approach to spiritual care is satisfactory for all clients. Many kinds of resources are needed.

Following are some resources that seem to be the most useful to clients in need of spiritual care.

The client's quest for spiritual expression and care is often tied to religious practices and beliefs. It is of paramount importance, then, for the nurse to be familiar with the variety of religions and related practices that may assist in meeting the client's spiritual needs. Fairly universal religious practices include prayer, reading of sacred writings, and acts performed by the clergy or religious advisors.

Prayer

Prayer is defined as communication with a higher power. It is probably the most commonly used spiritual intervention. In one survey, most of the clients interviewed said that their major spiritual need was for prayer.[7] Prayer serves the purpose of counteracting loneliness by offering the client an individual intimacy with God. Likewise, "shared prayer can be a means of bringing love, both human and divine, to the client."[6] Prayers convey to the client that he or she is loved and understood.

When deciding which type of prayer could most benefit a client, consider the type of prayers that have been helpful to the client in the past.[18] For example, the client who practices spontaneous, unstructured prayer may find more meaning in shared spontaneous prayer rather than recitation of memorized prayers such as the Lord's Prayer or the 23rd Psalm.

Prayer is similar to meditation in that it may involve contemplation or reflection. Prayer may differ from meditation in that, unlike some meditation, prayer is not a mindless repetition of a sound, word, or thought on which one focuses to induce a calm physiologic state.

Sacred Writings

Clients may refer to the writings of their particular religion for support, or they may have other books or religious materials to which they refer for guidance. Many clients are comforted with special passages of the Bible (in Christianity) or passages from the sacred writings of their particular faith. Examples of sacred books in other religions are the Koran in Islam, the Book of Mormon and Pearl of Great Price in Mormonism, the Veda and Bhagavad-Gita in Hinduism, the Tripitaka in Buddhism, and the Torah and Talmud in Judaism.

The importance of choosing the correct time for the nurse to use written material or special passages is a major consideration, for, as Fish and Shelly stated, "right answers about God given at the wrong moment are of little therapeutic value."[18] For example, to have a nurse recite the 23rd Psalm when a client requests an explanation of a medication would not assist his or her understanding of medical treatment. Likewise, to ignore clues for the need for prayer could thwart further expression of the client's spiritual or religious needs.

Clergy

Many religious acts can be performed only by the **clergy** — persons ordained to the service of God. Clients may prefer to share certain intimacies with their religious counselor rather than with the nurse. In the eyes of many clients, the spiritual need of forgiveness can best be met by clergy.

The chaplain, local clergy, or other appropriate religious advisor should be included in client care as needed. In some settings, the chaplain confers regularly with the nursing staff. A shared relationship between the ministerial department and nursing is an asset to quality care and should be initiated by the nurse if the client expresses a desire or readiness to see a religious representative. For example, the client may ask to be visited by the clergy, or the nurse may call the clergy or chaplain as he or she identifies spiritual needs in the client. In many institutions a department of ministry makes regular rounds of client units to seek those in need of their caring. The clergy in such a department frequently request assistance from nurses in identifying clients with issues of a spiritual nature.

PRACTICES TO PROMOTE YOUR OWN SPIRITUAL HEALTH

Personal spiritual health is a requisite for nurses who wish to meet spiritual needs of their clients. Nurses must be aware of resources for personal spiritual growth, support, and renewal. The following discussion provides suggestions for promoting personal spiritual health.

Know Yourself

A primary principle in developing spiritual health is to "know thyself." Nurses who have attempted to recognize and gain insight into their personal spiritual needs are better equipped to assist clients with their own spiritual needs.

Recognize the Role of Faith

In the practice of nursing and in examining personal spiritual needs, nurses must recognize the role that faith plays. Faith has great potential for promoting health. "Faith, in relation to health, is the belief in the curative nature of an object or the healing ability of a person."[27] In this respect, nurses must possess faith as an attitude of trust, as well as demonstrate it in their caring treatment of clients. In the practice of adhering to a cause or purpose in caring for clients, nurses exercise faith.

Meditate

Meditation — reflection and purposeful contemplation — provides an opportunity to retreat within oneself and to achieve a sensation of inner peace. It also is a mechanism for gaining insight into oneself that can often assist the individual to ascribe meaning to one's situation. Meditation can be used by nurses to focus on getting to "know thyself," which in turn can enable them to meet clients' needs more fully.

Practice Guided Imagery

Guided imagery enables an individual to relax and can be a source of comfort to those who are at ease about using it (see Chapter 16). During guided imagery, suggested mental images are constructed that serve to relax the individual visualizing the images. An example of guided imagery is responding to a practitioner's suggestion to visualize taking oneself to a favorite place and lingering in this visualized place to partake of all the pleasant sights, sounds, odors, and feelings. The result should be enhanced comfort and relaxation for the responding client. Nurses who use guided imagery themselves are more acquainted with the process and benefits of using it in the care of clients.

Pursue Aesthetic Experiences

Aesthetics and spirituality are related in that spirituality pervades a person's entire being and generates a capacity for transcendental values. Experiences that have to do with artistic perceptions, such as reading and art or music appreciation, also can be used to enhance spirituality.

READING

Reading may be a source of relaxation or spiritual support. Religious and inspirational materials are used to develop refreshment, personal insight, and diversion. Poetry may be inspirational if one enjoys the beauty of the poetic rhythm or the message conveyed by the verse. Nurses who enjoy the written word for personal relaxation or inspiration are often inspired by what they read and are better equipped to confront everyday crises as they appear in client care.

ART APPRECIATION

Art appreciation can be a valuable asset in promoting relaxation or in developing insight into the self as well as in attempting to understand what the artist is trying to convey. Nurses may find a heightened awareness of client concerns through the appreciation of art (e.g., clients may use drawings or colors to depict their feelings), and the nurse who is familiar with the effect of color and art expression can facilitate clients to express themselves through artworks.

MUSIC APPRECIATION

Likewise, an appreciation of music can be an effective way to promote personal spiritual health. The nurse who has learned to appreciate and enjoy music can be more effective in encouraging clients to gain spiritual experiences and express emotions and moods through the use of music.

PHYSICAL ACTIVITY

Healthful physical activities are a mechanism to maintain spiritual stability and health. Examples of these activities are exercise, bicycle riding, swimming, and walking. Physical activity allows the nurse to develop and maintain stamina. It also provides an outlet for frustration and anxiety. Thus, physical activity assists nurses in dealing better with clients because it sustains the nurses' strength.

Client spiritual needs can be identified or met more effectively if the nurse has met his or her own personal needs relating to the life principle that pervades each being.

RELAXATION

The art of relaxation is an invaluable asset that promotes and maintains spiritual health because it allows a person to focus on tasks with reduced anxiety, thus rendering the individual more effective at whatever is undertaken. Relaxation in the form of hobbies and other diversional interests can serve as tremendous outlets for the individual. Nurses who practice relaxation and develop hobbies and outside interests are most likely more relaxed and more able to provide effective client care. They are better equipped to meet spiritual care needs of others because they have met their personal needs and can be more effective in assisting clients by not being distracted with personal issues.

ASSESSMENT

A thorough assessment is necessary if the nurse is to attempt to meet spiritual needs. An assessment of the client's affect and attitude, behavior, communication, interpersonal relationships, and environment provides strong clues to spiritual needs. A baseline physical assessment will provide information that is relevant to meeting spiritual needs. For example, a client with limited mobility, vision, or hearing may be limited in his or her participation in activities that would assist in meeting spiritual needs.

Observe the client, noting his or her affect and attitude. Does the person appear lonely, depressed, angry, anxious, agitated? Also note the client's behavior. Has the client been observed in prayer, reading religious literature, saying grace, complaining frequently, needing increased dosages of sedation, pacing the halls, joking inappropriately?

Observe the environment. Does the client display a picture of family or significant others? Do you see keepsakes, a Bible or other sacred book, a prayer book, or devotional literature? Are religious objects present, such as medals, a rosary, or a yarmulke? How about religious get-well cards or church bulletins?

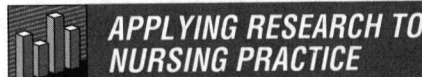

APPLYING RESEARCH TO NURSING PRACTICE

Matching Spiritual Care to Spiritual Needs

Reed, P. (1991). Preferences for spiritually related nursing interventions among terminally ill and nonterminally ill hospitalized adults and well adults. *Applied Nursing Research*, 4(3), 122–128.

▼▼▼

In this study, Reed interviewed and discussed spiritual needs with 100 hospitalized adults who had incurable cancer and who were aware of the nature of their illness. For comparison, this nurse researcher also interviewed 100 hospitalized adults who did not have a serious illness and 100 nonhospitalized healthy adults.

Adults in all three groups preferred two types of spiritually related nursing care: (1) helping to arrange visits with clergy; and (2) ensuring that private time is allowed for spiritual activities, such as prayer and family participation in spiritual readings. Most terminally ill clients also wanted nurses to read with them or to them and to provide special time for family spiritual activities. Hospitalized clients who did not have a critical illness offered negative remarks about nursing staff being too busy for spiritual care or being unable to intervene in spiritual needs. However, neither healthy adults nor terminally ill clients made such remarks.

Applications for Practice. Be sure to incorporate spiritual needs into your client assessments. When terminally ill clients cannot leave the hospital room to visit the chapel, you may arrange for a visit from clergy. Provide terminally ill clients with a period of time free of interruptions for listening to spiritual concerns. You may also organize nursing care to allow time for reflective talk with the family, for personal prayer, and for spiritual readings.

Observe interpersonal relationships. Note who visits the client, and how he or she responds.

Communicate with the client, and note spiritual needs expressed. Does he or she mention God, prayer, faith, church, or religious topics? Does the client request that clergy visit, discuss spiritual or religious topics, ask the meaning of his or her suffering, or express fear of death? In talking with the client, it may be helpful to inquire whether there is anything or anyone on whom the client can rely to help in coping.

As you observe and communicate with the client, try to identify client strengths as well as spiritual needs. Keep in mind the negative signs indicating need, but also note the positive aspects of the person's attitude and affect that could help the person to regain or maintain hope and strength. A client's spiritual state is not always a problem or a deficit. It may be providing the stability for everything else that is changing.

Summarize the client's beliefs. To what extent is the client involved in religious faith? Does the client have religious practices that serve as resources for faith, and do they affect his or her daily life? What are the client's sources of hope and strength? At this point, you can begin to create a tentative nursing diagnosis based on your assessment. Allow the client to validate or correct your perceptions of his or her needs.

NURSING DIAGNOSIS

A spiritual care diagnosis is infrequently based on stated client needs. There is seldom a clear set of signs and symptoms that pertain exclusively to a spiritual need. Accurate diagnosis requires a sensitive ear and the ability to respond to tiny clues such as a tear, anxiety, or uncharacteristic silence on the part of the client. It is necessary to observe the client carefully for small clues concerning attitude, affect, behavior, and issues discussed as well as those not discussed by the client. Ask questions about the observations you have made. Data then can be organized around issues you have identified.

The most commonly encountered spiritual diagnosis is spiritual distress. Nursing Diagnosis Profile: Spiritual Distress (Distress of the Human Spirit) discusses this diagnosis. Other diagnoses may be related to unmet spiritual needs (e.g., decisional conflict relating to unclear personal values or noncompliance related to conflicting spiritual values).

PLANNING

Taking time accurately to assess, to diagnose needs, and to plan nursing care should result in more effective and meaningful nursing care. In planning spiritual care, there are two principles to keep in mind.[18] First, a client's relationship with a higher power is individual and complex; therefore, every client must be approached on an individual and unique basis in light of his or her own needs. Second, nurses must be aware of their own spiritual beliefs because this may affect their care of clients.

In planning for a diagnosis of spiritual distress, the following outcomes might be expected:

▶ actively seeks relationships
▶ discusses beliefs and values
▶ verbalizes hope

Some persons will take longer to reach these outcomes than others. Individualize your plan by using a realistic time frame for each client.

NURSING INTERVENTION

Bear in mind that clients do not expect you to solve their religious dilemmas and spiritual problems for them. It is the very nature of spiritual growth that demands that they work through their own problems and grow from the experience.

Although they may ask very difficult questions aloud, these questions are most often rhetorical, and they do not actually expect you to respond. In fact, any attempt to answer shows only that you do not truly understand their plight. Indeed, how do you answer questions such

NURSING DIAGNOSIS PROFILE

Spiritual Distress (Distress of the Human Spirit)

Definition. Disruption of the life principle, which pervades a person's entire being and which integrates and transcends one's biologic and psychosocial nature.

Classification. Valuing 4.1.1

Defining Characteristics. The only critical defining characteristic for this diagnosis is a client's expression of concern with the meaning of life or death or concern with belief systems. Concern may be expressed verbally as inner conflicts about beliefs or about the relationship with one's deity; questions about the meaning of suffering, the meaning of one's own existence, or the implications of the therapeutic regimen; expressions of anger toward one's God or religious representatives; client's complaints that he or she is unable to participate in the usual religious practices or that he or she is having nightmares or sleep disturbances; and requests for spiritual assistance. Concern may also be expressed verbally or nonverbally through an alteration in behavior/mood in which the client shows evidence of gallows humor, anger, hostility, preoccupation, anxiety, crying, apathy, withdrawal, and so forth.

Sample Related Factors. In this spiritual diagnosis, the related factors are "separation from religious/cultural ties" or "challenged belief and value system."

Concept Description. This diagnosis refers to the state in which a person experiences a disturbance in his or her personal value system or religious beliefs or in his or her relationship with a higher power.

Examples. Depending on the specific assessment data, this diagnostic category could be applicable in the following situations, among others:

▶ A female of childbearing age who must have radiation treatments that will make her sterile when her religious beliefs have always been that sterilization procedures are a disobedience to God's directive to humankind to "go forth and multiply"
▶ A person who is experiencing intense suffering and who questions the existence of a deity who would allow this to happen at the very time he or she needs to believe in God as possibly the only source of relief from the suffering.

Related/Similar Nursing Diagnoses. This diagnosis should be distinguished from the diagnoses of *Hopelessness* and *Powerlessness*. In *Hopelessness*, the individual sees limited or no alternatives or personal choices available and is unable to mobilize energy on his or her own behalf. In *Powerlessness*, the person perceives that his or her own actions will not significantly affect an outcome. It is a perceived lack of control over a current situation or immediate happening. With a diagnosis of *Spiritual Distress*, the person may feel hopeless or helpless, but there is additional distress in that the person feels a disruption in the life principle that binds together his or her entire nature. With spiritual distress, the person may not only feel helpless and powerless to act alone but may even feel that he or she can receive no help from others or from God.

as, "Why was I ever born if all I ever get out of life is misery?", "Why does God take the lives of innocent babies?", or "Why must I suffer so? Why can't Jesus take me now?"

In relation to spiritual care, what clients want from their nurse is someone to:

▶ Take care of their physical needs or help them to take care of themselves
▶ Help relieve their pain and suffering
▶ Accept them as persons of worth
▶ Care about them
▶ Value them
▶ Affirm them
▶ Treat them with dignity and respect
▶ Help them to meet their religious needs on occasion

You can do many of these things just with simple acts, including spending time with them; listening to them; using therapeutic communication techniques to help them express themselves; or using religious resources such as prayer, religious readings, or acts by the clergy.

Spending time with your clients shows interest in them as persons. It demonstrates caring and says, "You are of value." It is a reaffirmation of their worth and dignity. The time may be spent talking with them, listening to them, reading to them, working on a diversional activity with them, praying with them, or just sitting with them in quiet contemplation.

Of particular importance is the art of listening to the client as you spend time together. Listening allows you to obtain valuable data that can help you better care for the client, but it also conveys to the client that he or she is valued as a person. Listening communicates respect. It affirms the client's worth and ability to make decisions. It allows the client time to work through problems and to make adjustments. For example, taking time to listen to a male client's numerous discussions about his pending hospital discharge may assist him in making decisions concerning situations he may encounter when he gets home. The practice he gets in decision making strengthens his decision-making skills. Thus, by listening to him as he makes decisions, you may actually be helping him to regain (or to maintain) skills that he can use as tools to meet his own needs, including spiritual needs.

Using therapeutic techniques of communication helps you remain in the helping role as you assist the client in communicating with you. This can allow you to gather data for a more accurate assessment and to evaluate the client after nursing care has been given. However, it can also be a nursing intervention in that it can help the client to talk out and work through some of his or her spiritual problems.

When a client asks some of the types of questions just posed, you can use therapeutic techniques of communication to help him or her find answers. For example, suppose your 13-year-old client, Darcie (who is in a body cast and cannot attend her eighth-grade graduation party) asks, "Why was I ever born if all I ever get out of life is misery?" You should realize that Darcie wants to tell you how miserable she feels. She wants you to listen and understand. She is crying out for you

to respond, "You sound so very sad, Darcie. Tell me what led up to your feeling so miserable." She does not want to hear a literal response to her question, such as, "All God's children were placed on this earth for a purpose and ours is not to reason why; ours is but to . . ." Darcie would most likely tune your answer out after approximately three words. Darcie needs to know you will listen and you will care. Then, when Darcie knows that you do care, she will trust you as she begins to talk about the deeper thoughts that trouble her, and you can use therapeutic techniques to help her think through her own problems. Thirteen years of age is generally a turbulent time in relation to spiritual development, and Darcie can use a sounding board as she thinks about different spiritual questions.

Suppose, for example, that one day, while just talking about general things, Darcie asks, "Why does God take the lives of innocent babies?" You might clarify to be certain she is not referring to any one particular infant but is just questioning life in general. Then, if you want to assist Darcie in her own spiritual development, you might reflect the question back to her by asking her, "What are *your* thoughts about the answer to that question, Darcie?" Listening to some of her alternative answers could truly help you to understand Darcie and where she is in her spiritual development. Listening could also provide you the opportunity to praise Darcie for her depth of caring about others and to question her further about how infant deaths might be prevented. Take such opportunities to show you value her and find her ideas worthwhile.

Three rooms down the hall from Darcie is Mrs. Johnson, who is in severe pain. As you turn her to one side to help another nurse bathe her back and change her linen, she cries with pain, clutches her Bible in one hand and your arm in the other, and asks, "Why must I suffer so? Why can't Jesus take me now?" Although it may seem so, she is not asking you to tell her why she must suffer or why she cannot be put out of her misery. She is asking for comfort. She needs a pain shot, a position change, guidance in relaxation techniques, diversion, a hand to hold, an arm around her shoulders. When you have done all that you can do to relieve her pain, you might try to comfort her spiritually by offering yourself with, "Would it help if I read to you from your Bible? Or would you like me to pray with you? Or could I call your minister or someone else to help comfort you?"

In using therapeutic techniques to assist the client in expressing his or her spiritual needs and to help work them out, it is imperative that you keep the conversation centered on the client and that you never intrude with your own thoughts, values, or advice. Doing so is not only nontherapeutic, but it is denying the client the opportunity to grow spiritually.

As previously discussed, resources for meeting religious needs are abundant. These include prayer, religious readings, and acts by the clergy.

The nurse can help with prayer, or meditation, by offering to schedule a quiet time alone. The nurse can also offer to pray with the client or to pray for him or her.

Likewise, religious readings may be best read in solitude, and this can be arranged by the nurse. Many clients cannot read because they are illiterate, because they have a pathologic problem that prevents it, or because they are taking medications that cause blurry vision or drowsiness. Some would merely prefer the nurse to read to them. Offering to read to the client can be a meaningful intervention whether the reading is religious in nature or not. It demonstrates that you are willing to spend time with the client and conveys all that that implies.

If the client wishes to see a member of the clergy, contact the department of ministry within your hospital or contact clergy from outside of the institution according to hospital policy. Most hospitals maintain regular contact with local religious institutions, groups, and leaders in the community and call on these resources to help meet clients' religious or spiritual needs as requested. Many clients will express a preference for a member of the clergy from their own religion, but some clients have no preference and still would like to talk with a spiritual advisor. You can help arrange the meeting and help to provide privacy as clients receive these visitors.

With this intervention and all other interventions related to religious rituals, be certain to validate, with the client, the appropriateness of your intervention. Asking directly is the best policy when unsure. For example, when asked to pray for a client, you might ask, "Would you like me to say the Lord's Prayer for you or would you prefer something less structured?" When asked to read from the Bible, you might ask, "Would it be helpful to hear the 23rd Psalm?" or "Do you have any special verse you prefer?"

Do not let nursing interventions for spiritual care overwhelm you. Clients do not have grandiose expectations. Dettmore[7] stated that "their requests are simple: that you listen, that you recognize spiritual needs enough to call a chaplain, and that you pray with or for them."

EVALUATION

The effectiveness of spiritual care may be indirectly determined by noting changes in the client's attitude; for instance, a decreased need for attention from the nursing staff may indicate resolution of a spiritual need. Alternatively, the client may directly express feelings about a new ability to face either the disease process or life, or the client may discuss the meaning of his or her illness. People may say, "I learned a lot about myself during that illness" or "that illness brought out strengths I never knew I had." Such statements should be charted as evidence that the client has progressed in resolving the spiritual need.

As each nurse evaluates the effectiveness of spiritual care, the need for further development of the nurse's abilities may be identified. Continued development of each nurse's education in the areas of spiritual care is crucial to holistic client care. Beginning nursing students, as well as veteran nurses, may be uncomfortable dealing with the spiritual realm when caring for clients. An understanding of the dimensions of spirituality and possibilities for nursing interventions should alleviate much of the anxiety experienced by nurses. A willingness to become involved, which is a reason most nurses become nurses in the first place, is a requisite in spiritual care. That initial step is the beginning of the development of a nurse who can effectively provide spiritual care. The nurse who is a client advocate may need to assume a leadership role in coordinating effective resources for spiritual care. As stated by Peterson,[37] "sharing in people's lives is still one of the greatest privileges and responsibilities of nursing and it should never be sacrificed for anything else that we must do . . . [Spiritual care] allows the nurse an opportunity to be involved in the deepest aspects of an individual's life, and has the potential for providing the nurse with deep and lasting rewards."

Your development as a nurse should not only address human spiritual dimensions but also provide freedom and support for you to explore and attempt to meet the deepest human spiritual questions and needs. Ongoing spiritual education and growth should be a personal priority for each nurse. It should also be a part of the interdisciplinary approach to client care.

Evaluation may also result in the identification of important gaps in nursing's knowledge base in relation to spiritual care.

Research about spiritual care is needed to create a foundation of knowledge that will enrich and increase the possibilities for spiritual aspects of client care. For example, studies suggest that nurses with higher levels of spiritual well-being have a more positive attitude toward providing spiritual care for clients and view potential intervention as appropriate for meeting the spiritual needs of their clients.[45]

Suggestions for research on aspects of spiritual care include clients' use of resources to meet spiritual needs, clients' spiritual coping strategies, effective interdisciplinary approaches, the development of additional assessment strategies, and continued identification of factors that influence both nurses and clients in dealing with spiritual concerns.

CASE STUDY

The Client

Rose Green, a 47-year-old Caucasian female, was admitted to the hospital 17 days ago through the emergency room. She had been sexually assaulted, shot in the abdomen, and left for dead by two men who had robbed her and her husband in the convenience store that they owned. Her husband, Sam, had also been shot, but he did not survive. When the mental health clinical specialist visited Mrs. Green last week, Mrs. Green stated that she could have stood the robbery and might even have eventually gotten over the brutal assault and the fact that she was left with a colostomy from the abdominal wound, but she felt she could never go on without her husband of 20 years. The loss of her major support in life was more than she could "ever hope to bear." She asked the nurse, "Where was God when I needed Him? What did I ever do to deserve such a dreadful, lonely punishment as this? Can there really be a God so unjust as to allow this to happen to me?"

At 2:00 P.M., April 4, a partial list of the nurse's spiritual assessment read:

▶ 47-year-old, Caucasian female with sad affect admitted 10 days ago after robbery, sexual assault, and GSW of Abd
▶ Stated husband died of GSW during the robbery
▶ Stated husband was major support in life for past 20 years
▶ Questioned existence of a God, who could allow the loss of her husband

▶ Stated she was Episcopalian but did not attend services because she was needed in the store on Sunday mornings; has not belonged to a church for more than 20 years; has not read any religious writings since early in her marriage; knows no clergy in the area
▶ Did admit that, in the past, whenever she was feeling overwhelmed with worries, it was silent prayer that brought her comfort; now states that she "can't even try to pray"
▶ Nurses who have worked with her say she is beginning to get up and around and is learning to care for her colostomy but that she cries and remains silent most of the time
▶ When asked about sources of support in coping, she replied she had no relatives or children and that her husband had been everything to her; they worked such long hours in the store that they had little time to make friends outside of the business
▶ Cards have poured in by the hundreds from customers and those who heard about the robbery in news reports
▶ States she and her husband had been saving money to retire somewhere in the sunbelt but now she does not even look forward to retirement

One week has passed since her assessment by the nurse. The following represents part of a nursing care plan written for her at the time of assessment and the current evaluation of outcomes that were expected at that time.

CARE PLAN

4:00 PM, April 4

Nursing Diagnosis	Planning: Expected Outcomes	Implementation: Nursing Interventions	Evaluation
Spiritual Distress R/T challenged belief and value system secondary to intense suffering	By 4:00 PM, April 11: ▶ Discusses beliefs and values	With client, establish times to sit and talk bid x 30 minutes. If client does not wish to talk, just sit with her to show caring. Without pressing her, try to draw her out so she can discuss her feelings of distress, her beliefs, and values. Use active listening to show caring.	4:00 PM, April 11: On April 5, client talked with nurse from 10–10:30 AM and 6–6:30 PM and opened up and discussed her values and beliefs. Client stated that she feared being alone in her older years. She admitted that many of her customers have often shown her they want to be her friends but that she was too shy to reach out to them and depended only on her husband for friendship and emotional support. Client does value friendship.

Care Plan continued on following page

CARE PLAN Continued

4:00 PM, April 4

Nursing Diagnosis	Planning: Expected Outcomes	Implementation: Nursing Interventions	Evaluation
	▶ Verbalizes hope	Draw out regarding possible hopes for future.	Client stated she hopes to return to the store to the work she loves but does not know whether she can do it without Sam.
			Client stated she hopes she can go on without Sam.
	▶ Discusses possible relationships to seek out	Draw out regarding acquaintances that could be support systems.	By April 10, client admitted that there were two customers she had wanted to befriend in the past but said she felt inadequate and "embarrassed" to pursue them as friends.
			By April 8, client said she had prayed and felt so comforted that she slept with ease.
			Client is no longer in spiritual distress; is in expected stage of normal grief process.

Summary

- Spirituality is the life principle that pervades a person's entire being: a person's physical, emotional, intellectual, moral, ethical, and volitional dimensions.
- Spiritual care involves not only caring for and about clients but also assisting them in finding meaning in life experiences such as crises and suffering.
- Spiritual health in a person is a state of balance that transcends physical or material things. It indicates receptiveness to a greater power as defined by the individual.
- In meeting client needs holistically, all dimensions of health (physiologic, psychologic, and spiritual) must be addressed.
- Assisting the client in expressing spiritual needs directly can best occur in an atmosphere that shows the client acceptance and support.
- Fulfilling the nursing role in relation to spiritual care requires that you understand human spirituality and that you are aware of some of the religious beliefs and practices that are often a part of a client's spirituality.

- Spirituality is a much broader concept than religious affiliation or practice.
- Spiritual needs focus on finding meaning and purpose in life, illness, and life situations; giving and receiving of love and feelings of relatedness; experiencing forgiveness; and experiencing hope.
- Spiritual growth continues throughout the life span as the individual develops and increases his or her awareness of the meaning, purpose, and values in life.
- Religious development, psychosocial development, and faith development are three ways that an individual develops spiritually.
- Major world religions include Hinduism, Judaism, Christianity, Buddhism, and Islam.
- "New Age" spiritualism tends to focus on the fundamental truths of love, peace, and forgiveness present in all religions rather than focusing on rituals.
- Prayer, sacred writings, and religious acts performed by the clergy may be of comfort to persons from various religious backgrounds.
- The nurse may promote personal spiritual growth through self-examination; faith as an attitude of trust;

meditation; guided imagery; aesthetic pursuits such as reading or art and music appreciation; physical activity; and relaxation.

▶ Assessment includes directly observing the client as well as eliciting communications regarding spiritual needs.

▶ The most commonly encountered spiritual diagnosis is spiritual distress.

▶ Outcomes for the diagnosis of spiritual distress include (1) actively seeks relationships, (2) discusses beliefs and values, and (3) verbalizes hope.

▶ Interventions include spending time with clients; listening to them; using therapeutic techniques of communication; and using religious resources such as prayer, religious readings, and acts by the clergy.

▶ Evaluation of spiritual care includes observing for a change in client attitude as well as noting the client's direct expressions of feelings.

▶ Ongoing spiritual education and growth should be a personal priority for each nurse.

Bibliography

1. Amenta, M. (1988). Nurses as primary spiritual care workers. *Hospice Journal*, 4(3), 47–55.
2. Bailey, S., et al. (1990). Assumptions and principles of spiritual care. *Death Studies*, 14(1), 75–81.
3. Burnard, P. (1988). Discussing spiritual issues with clients. *Health-Visitor*, 61(12), 371–372.
4. Burnard, P. (1988). Spiritual care: searching for meaning. *Nursing Times*, 84(37), 34–36.
5. Carson, V.B. (1989). *Spiritual dimensions of nursing practice*. Philadelphia: W.B. Saunders.
6. Conrad, N.L. (1985). Spiritual support for the dying. *Nursing Clinics of North America*, 20(2), 415–426.
7. Dettmore, D. (1984). Spiritual care: remembering your patients' forgotten needs. *Nursing*, 14(10), 46.
8. Dobmeier, T. (1990). Professionalizing spiritual care. *Journal of Christian Nursing*, 7(1), 32.
9. Doenges, M.E., & Moorhouse, M.F. (1991). *Nurses pocket guide: Nursing diagnosis with intervention* (3rd ed.). Philadelphia: F.A. Davis.
10. Donovan, C. (1988). Working with sorrow and hurt. *Oklahoma Nurse*, 33(2), 8–9.
11. Eaton, S. (1988). Spiritual care: the software of life. *Journal of Palliative Care*, 4(1–2), 91–93.
12. Ebmeier, C., et al. (1991). Hospitalized school-age children express ideas, feelings, and behaviors toward God. *Journal of Pediatric Nursing*, 6(5), 337–349.
13. Ellis, C. (1987). Teaching spiritual care of patients. *Journal of Nursing Staff Development*, 3(1), 43–44.
14. Emblen, J. (1992). Religion and spirituality defined according to current use in nursing literature. *Journal of Professional Nursing*, 8(1), 41–47.
15. Erikson, E.H. (1963). *Childhood and society*. New York: Norton.
16. Feinstein, A. (1967). *Clinical Judgements*. Baltimore, MD: Williams & Wilkins.
17. Ferszt, G.G., & Taylor, P.B. (1988). When your patient needs spiritual comfort. *Nursing*, 18(4), 48–49.
18. Fish, S., & Shelly, J. (1988). *Spiritual care: The nurses' role* (3rd ed.). Downer's Grove, IL: Intervarsity Press.
19. Forbis, P.A. (1988). Meeting patients' spiritual needs: helping patients to fulfill their spiritual needs is part of the nursing process. *Geriatric Nursing*, 9(3), 158–159.
20. Fowler, J. (1981). *Stages of faith*. San Francisco: Harper & Row.
21. Francis, B. (1990). Patient care—the spiritual dimension. *Advancing Clinical Care*, 5(5), 7–8.
22. Granstrom, S.L. (1985). Spiritual nursing care for oncology patients. *Topics in Clinical Nursing*, 7(1), 39–45.
23. Handzo, G.C. (1990). Spiritual care: talking about faith with children. *Journal of Christian Nursing*, 7(4), 17–20.
24. Henderson, K.J. (1989). Dying, God, and anger: comforting through spiritual care. *Journal of Psychosocial Nursing and Mental Health Services*, 27(5), 17–21.
25. Highfield, M.F., & Cason, C. (1983). Spiritual needs of patients: are they recognized? *Cancer Nursing*, 6(3), 187–192.
26. Hopkins, V.L. (1990). *The spiritual dimension of total patient care*. Unpublished syllabus, University of Texas School of Nursing at Galveston.
27. Kennison, M.M. (1987). Faith: an untapped health resource. *Journal of Psychosocial Nursing and Mental Health Services*, 25(10), 28–30, 32–33.
28. Krohn, B. (1989). Spiritual care: the forgotten need. *Imprint*, 36(1), 95–96.
29. Kwon, H.J. (1989). Perceptions of spiritual nursing care nurses and nursing students. *Kanho Hakhoe Chi Journal of Nurses Academic Society*, 19(3), 233–239.
30. Labun, E. (1988). Spiritual care: an element in nursing care planning. *Journal of Advanced Nursing*, 13(3), 314–320.
31. Lee, Y.H. (1988). Patient care for the long term illnesses. Spiritual care. *Korean Nurse*, 27(1), 21–27.
32. Lescohier, D. (1989). The spiritual care nemesis (editorial). *American Journal of Hospital Care*, 6(5), 7.
33. Ley, D.C.H., & Corless, I.B. (1988). Spirituality and hospice care. *Death Studies*, 12(2), 101–110.
34. Maslow, A.R. (1968). *Toward a psychology of being* (2nd ed.). New York: D. Van Nostrand.
35. McGregor, B. (1989). Natural therapies and nursing: the step beyond. *Lamp*, 46(3), 17–19.
36. North American Nursing Diagnosis Association. (1990). *Taxonomy I—Revised 1990*. St. Louis: North American Nursing Diagnosis Association.
37. Peterson, E.A. (1985). The physical . . . the spiritual . . . can you meet all of your patient's needs? *Journal of Gerontological Nursing*, 11(10), 23–27.
38. Peterson, E.A., & Nelson, K. (1987). How to meet your clients' spiritual needs. *Journal of Psychosocial Nursing and Mental Health Services*, 25(5), 34–40.
39. Piles, C.L. (1989). Putting spiritual care into the curriculum. *Journal of Christian Nursing*, 6(3), 18–21.
40. Piles, C.L. (1990). Providing spiritual care. *Nurse-Educator*, 15(1), 36–41.
41. Salladay, S.A., & McDonnell, M.M. (1989). Spiritual care, ethical choices, and patient advocacy. *Nursing Clinics of North America*, 24(2), 543–549.
42. Sardana, R. (1990). Spiritual care for the elderly: an integral part of the nursing process. *Nursing Homes*, 39(1), 30–31.
43. Sims, C. (1987). Spiritual care as part of holistic nursing. *Imprint*, 34(4), 63–67.
44. Simsen, B. (1988). Nursing the spirit . . . meeting patients' spiritual needs. *Nursing Times*, 84(37), 31–33.
45. Soeken, K.L., & Carson, V.J. (1987). Responding to the spiritual needs of the chronically ill. *Nursing Clinics of North America*, 22(3), 603–611.
46. Swaffield, L. (1988). Spiritual care: religious roots. *Nursing Times*, 84(37), 28–30.
47. Travelbee, J. (1977). *Interpersonal aspects of nursing* (2nd ed.). Philadelphia: F.A. Davis.
48. Wald, F.S. (1989). The widening scope of spiritual care. *American Journal of Hospice Care*, 6(4), 40–43.
49. Wilson, D.R. (1989). The chaplain as a resource to families of patients in I.C.U. *Canadian Critical Care Nursing Journal*, 6(1), 10–12.
50. Wilson, E.D. (1988). Spiritual care. Helping a guilt-ridden patient. *Journal of Christian Nursing*, 5(2), 10–13.
51. Windau, V., & Dewitt, P.J. (1988). Emergency baptism by nurses in an NICU: answering a spiritual need. *Journal of Neonatal Nursing*, 7(1), 57–62.

Chapter 54

▼ Coping With Loss and Grief

> The Bustle in a House
> The Morning after Death
> Is solemnest of industries
> Enacted upon Earth—
> The Sweeping up the Heart,
> And putting Love away
> We shall not want to use again
> Until Eternity.
>
> **Emily Dickinson**
> (1866)

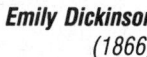

▼ CHAPTER OUTLINE

GRIEF AND LOSS
    Definitions
    Forms of Loss
    Physiologic Effects of Grief
    Developmental Perspectives on
        Loss and Grief
    Cultural Perspectives on Loss and
        Grief
THEORIES OF DYING AND GRIEF
    Theories of Death and Dying and
        the Hospice Movement

Theories of Grief and Grieving
    Cautions About Stage and Phase
        Theories
THE NURSE AND LOSS AND GRIEF
ASSESSMENT
NURSING DIAGNOSIS
PLANNING
NURSING INTERVENTION
EVALUATION
CASE STUDY

▼ KEY TERMS

Asynchronous response
Bereavement
Connecting
Doing for

Empowering
Finding meaning
Grief

Livor mortis
Loss
Rigor mortis

▼ **LEARNING OBJECTIVES**

After studying this chapter, you should be able to

1. *Discuss the concepts of loss and grief, including physiologic, developmental, and cultural perspectives.*
2. *Discuss theories related to death and dying and grief and grieving.*
3. *List ways in which the nurse may experience and cope with grief.*
4. *Describe how to assess the client and family who are attempting to cope with loss and grief.*
5. *Contrast nursing diagnoses appropriate for the client and family during loss and grief with those for the terminally ill client.*
6. *State how to plan care for an individual and family experiencing loss and grief.*
7. *Describe appropriate nursing interventions at the time of death.*
8. *Identify means of evaluating the client and family who have been cared for during a period of loss and grief.*

Grief and loss are an integral part of life. As such, both nurses and the clients for whom they care are touched by these at various points in life. The loss can be major and quite obvious, such as the loss of a loved one or a body part, or it can be subtle and less obvious, such as the loss of important roles, even temporarily, as with hospitalization. Each change encountered by an individual can bring with it an element of loss as old ways must be changed. Even happy changes entail the loss of some aspect of a familiar way of life and of separation. For instance, marriage, although generally considered a happy event, also signifies the loss of a former way of single life, elements of which may be grieved to some extent.

However, dealing with loss and grief can provide an opportunity to grow. Growth occurs as the child learns to deal with separation as part of the normal developmental process. It occurs as well when a widow finds a self-sufficiency and strength in coping with the loss of her spouse. Individuals facing terminal illness can find new insights in life that enhance the final days of their lives and leave a lasting legacy of strength and hope to their survivors. A number of studies have examined positive factors such as hope and optimism as influencing the course of a stressful situation such as bereavement or terminal illness.[1,34,47,65,76]

Above all, the response to loss is highly variable and uniquely individual. No two people will face loss in the same way or go through the grieving process on the same time schedule. In fact, the same individuals will not respond to different losses in the same manner across their life spans. Developmental level, context, meaning of the loss, available support, personality, coping abilities, and many other factors influence the manner of dealing with a loss and affect the outcome of the grieving process. All of these factors become important to the nurse in caring for persons experiencing loss and in assessing their individual needs.

Finally, the nurse, as a human being, is not immune to loss and grief. These are experienced at both the personal level and the professional level. At the personal level, the nurse is likely to lose someone close and to grieve that loss. The nurse may also grieve the loss of clients for whom he or she has cared as well as the loss of self-esteem that may occur when a desired position is lost or a serious medication error is made.

While grieving an important loss, the nurse too will experience the psychologic and physiologic effects of grieving, including the potential for growth that exists with any change.

GRIEF AND LOSS

Definitions

LOSS

Loss can be defined as the removal or absence of an important object or subject from an individual's life. The loss that is felt is believed to be related to the degree of attachment the individual had for the lost object.[8] Therefore, the response to a loss can vary from individual to individual depending on the significance of the loss to that person. Loss is both common and unique.[7] It is common in that all people undergo separations and losses yet is unique in that each individual has a distinct life history with which each new loss is approached.[7] Loss usually precipitates a change in an individual's life. The change may be major or minor or somewhere in between depending on the complex interaction of multiple factors. The impact experienced and adaptation required by any given loss vary from person to person; the more major losses represent turning points in people's lives. These turning points lead to new perspectives on the meaning of what is important in living.[7]

GRIEF, MOURNING, AND BEREAVEMENT

The terms grief and mourning are sometimes used synonymously and sometimes differently. When differentiated, **grief** is defined as the normal response to and personal experience of loss, and mourning indicates the process that occurs after loss.[18] The definition of grief can be further specified as the "multifaceted physical, emotional, and behavioral responses of an individual to the death of a significant other."[18] Mourning and grieving both denote the processes by which adaptation and reorganization occur during the period after a loss. Mourning has been defined as "the response following the death of a meaningful figure."[73]

Still another definition addresses bereavement behavior as "the total response pattern, psychologic and physiologic, displayed by an individual following the loss of a significant object."[4] In this definition, bereavement has two components: grief and mourning. Grief is a set of psychologic and physiologic reactions, whereas mourning includes the behaviors that are determined by cultural mores and custom.[4] Bowlby,[8] a prominent psychiatrist who studied loss and attachment, defined mourning as the psychologic processes that are set in motion by the loss of a loved object and grief as the sequence of subjective states that follow loss and accompany mourning. Although there are some inconsistencies in the definitions in the literature of grief and mourning, it is clear that both terms refer to the response and process that occur after loss.

Bereavement is yet another term used in relation to the period after loss. One definition states that "bereavement refers to all the physiological, psychological, behavioral, and social responses displayed by an individual following the loss of a significant person."[35] **Bereavement** most often denotes the period during which the grief process unfolds, ending with the reorganization of the individual's life. This period of time has traditionally been thought to be 1 year. However, studies have shown that the bereavement period can vary a great deal among individuals and many times extends well beyond the 1-year time period. Indeed, there is some suggestion that the effects of a major loss remain with the individual for the rest of her or his life.[9,31,35,60,77,84,92,101]

The definitions of grief, mourning, and bereavement are summarized in Table 54–1.

Forms of Loss

Loss can take a number of different forms. Benoliel,[7] a nurse researcher, identified three forms that are relevant to nursing practice. The first is personal loss,

TABLE 54–1. Definitions of Grief, Mourning, and Bereavement

Term	Definitions
Grief	A normal response to loss
	A set of psychologic and physiologic reactions
	A process of adaptation after loss
	A sequence of subjective states after loss
Mourning	Adaptation and reorganization after loss
	A response after the death of a significant other
	Behaviors determined by cultural mores and customs
	Psychologic processes set in motion by loss
Bereavement	A total response pattern (psychologic and physiologic) to the loss of a significant object
	The period during which the grief process unfolds

TABLE 54–2. Forms of Loss

Forms of Loss	Definition
Personal	Leads to destruction of personal integrity (i.e., loss of body part, death of loved one)
Group	Loss experienced by a group (i.e., family loss of a significant member)
Multiple	A number of losses occurring simultaneously or within a short period of time (i.e., a natural disaster)

which is any loss experienced by the individual as a destruction of personal integrity. This can result from the loss of a significant person, the loss of a body part, or the diagnosis of a life-threatening illness. The complex adaptation to this type of loss involves all aspects of an individual's life situation, because it often requires the development of a new pattern of living.

A second form of loss is group loss. This may occur concurrently with personal loss and involves loss experienced by a group of people such as when a family loses a significant member. It is also seen in a group of nurses when they lose a favorite client or when they struggle to care for many dying clients. The loss experienced does not necessarily have to be a death but may be the loss of potential that is unfulfilled in a child born with a severe handicap or in a parent with the diagnosis of Alzheimer's disease.

Finally, multiple losses occurring within a short period of time can greatly tax both individual and group coping resources. The elderly are particularly vulnerable, because they have accumulated a lifetime of losses and continue to face losses of close friends, siblings, and spouse. Natural and unnatural disasters often inflict multiple losses on survivors, leaving them highly vulnerable to psychologic and physiologic sequelae of conflicted or prolonged grief.[7,54] Forms of loss are briefly summarized in Table 54–2.

Physiologic Effects of Grief

Studies in psychoneuroimmunology indicate that loss and grief can have a profound impact on an individual's physical health.

Widowers have a higher rate of morbidity and mortality during the first year of bereavement, and divorced women have a lowered immune response immediately after separation.[3,71,89] A study of widows and widowers in Boston indicated that there was an increase in both psychologic and physical symptoms during the first year of bereavement.[71] The bereaved in this group also showed more disturbances in sleep, appetite, and weight, and they increased their consumption of alcohol, tobacco, and tranquilizers.[71] Such effects occur because grief is a total response involving complex reciprocal physiologic interactions. The bereaved appear to be particularly vulnerable to cardiovascular disease and infectious diseases along with a general increased susceptibility to illness.[42,50,71,89] This has important implications for nurses caring for individuals who may be experiencing loss, because client behaviors that are not conducive to good health may be increased, and the bereaved individual may be more vulnerable both physiologically and psychologically.

Developmental Perspectives on Loss and Grief

INFANCY

Experiences with separation and loss begin very early in life, perhaps even at birth. Part of the infant's development comes through learning to deal with separation. It is during this very early childhood time that the individual's patterns of adapting to loss are developed. As the individual matures, this pattern becomes more complex, encompassing coping mechanisms that are biologic, psychologic, sociocultural, and existential. As children develop language and symbolic thinking, they begin to attach meaning to people and events. This fosters the emergence of such complicated emotions as sadness, hate, love, and joy.[7] For most children between 6 months and 6 years of age, merely being separated from home and mother, such as during hospitalization, is enough to elicit grief.[22]

CHILDHOOD

Before 5 years of age, death is seen as reversible, a separation or departure. The permanence of death is not realized until approximately age 6 years. From 6 to approximately 9 or 10 years, the child views death as an inevitable, external process most often resulting from the actions of others and as a punishment for bad thoughts or deeds. After about 10 years of age, death is seen as an internal process that is universal to all life including the self. Concurrent with these conceptions, children seem to move from separation anxiety as the response to loss in the preschool child to fear of mutilation in the young school-age child to death anxiety in the older child and adolescent.[43] Young children can be vulnerable to guilt feelings when a fatal illness of a sibling or parent is seen as punishment for their "bad behavior" or if they have even wished the sibling or parent ill.[18] Young children may have their first experiences with grief through the death of a grandparent or the loss of a pet. How this is handled can set the tone for later coping with loss.

ADOLESCENCE

Adolescents move from concrete thinking in the early teen-age years to more abstract and future-oriented thinking in later adolescence. Death very often is seen to be in the distant future. It is not an immediate personal concern at this time in life. It is also a time when the young person is concerned with personal identity, independence, and separation from parents.

YOUNG ADULTHOOD

Age 20 generally serves as the entrance into young adulthood. This is a time at which tasks revolve around completing one's education, deciding on and embarking on one's life's work, finding a mate, and starting a family.[23] The major issues during this period of life revolve around intimacy and isolation.[23] Typical losses during young adulthood can involve relationship breakups and career disappointments. It may also be a time when a parent is lost.

THE 30s

The 30s represent the next developmental phase in which individuals begin to examine what they are doing in life. A sense of urgency creeps in as new choices are made or a recommitment is made to old ones. There is a desire to broaden life, and the notion of generativity starts to come into play because there may be an increased sense of urgency to bear children if this has not yet occurred or to carve out a life that contributes to future generations.[85,87] The major adaptive strength to emerge during this time is a widening concern for what has been generated.[23] As choices and recommitments are made, there may be a sense of grief for opportunities missed. Parents may be aging, and the loss of one or both parents may occur. Often, the loss of the second parent can be particularly painful because one feels a sense of aloneness at now being the older generation and no longer having a parent.

THE 40s

The 40s bring what has been popularly called midlife crisis. Death is becoming more real and personal as a heightened sense of mortality is felt. At this point, there is a recognition that the amount of time remaining in one's life is limited. Now time is considered as time left to live rather than as time since birth, which is a major transition for the individual.[62] This may be seen by some as the last chance to bear children. Women may be starting or anticipating menopause, which can bring either grief or relief depending on the meaning of the event for the individual. With a sense of time running out, there may be a major appraisal of one's life. If this reappraisal proves unsatisfactory, major life changes may be undertaken such as career switches, divorces and remarriages, or a total change in lifestyle. All of these changes involve elements of loss both of time gone and missed opportunities. If successfully negotiated, this phase can set the stage for the development of a sense of integrity in later life. Again, individuals may be facing the aging and loss of parents. Additionally, they may begin to experience the loss of contemporaries to cardiovascular disease or cancer, and children may be starting to leave home.

THE 50s

The transition in the 50s brings about minor changes in life structure as the individual approaches late adulthood.[87] Then, somewhere after the 50s, one enters late adulthood. It is not clear when midlife ends and late life begins. It may be heralded by retirement or by the last child leaving home, both of which entail a major loss and transition for most people. Employment is a large part of identity and worth. When this ends with retirement, the individual may grieve the loss of the roles and relationships that were part of the work life. The same can be true when the last child leaves home. For others these changes are welcomed as the opportunity to have time to do the things that they had wanted to do but delayed because of work and parenting responsibilities. Other losses may be experienced in the continuing loss of friends and perhaps siblings to a variety of illnesses.

OLDER ADULTHOOD

As one advances in age, there may be concerns about declining physical health, dependency, loneliness, finances, and the loss through death or abandonment of loved ones. The individual is challenged to accept the inevitability of death and the physical restrictions that may be experienced.[62,90] The major adaptive strength identified during this time is wisdom as a detached concern with life itself in the face of death itself.[23] Through the development of integrity over despair, the person copes with the loss of bodily abilities by maintaining a sense of personal integrity. The life cycle is now far more completed than yet to be lived. Reminiscing may be seen as a possible response to the biologic and psychologic fact of death. It provides an opportunity to survey and reintegrate past life experiences in assigning meaning to the life that has been lived.[62] Satisfaction at this point derives from an acceptance of the past and a recasting and reintegrating of experiences into a satisfactory overview of the life cycle.[23] The elderly may almost involuntarily think about death and illness and are challenged to counterbalance this with life-affirming involvement. Many turn to religion and experience an increase in religious feelings that provide a sense of continuity.[62] The sense of continuity across generations through children, grandchildren, and even great grandchildren can contribute to a sense of immortality necessary to transcend the despair of impending death.[23] By late life, the individual has undoubtedly experienced many major losses. At this point, the death of one's spouse is likely to be experienced in addition to the continuing loss of friends and siblings. Personal death is seen to be near and is welcomed by some and feared by others.

THE DEATH OF CHILDREN

The timing of a loss, particularly the death of a loved one, can have an impact on the meaning and effect of that loss. The death of an elderly parent, although deeply felt and mourned, is usually considered to be an "on-time" loss, as is retirement at age 65 years. However, the death of a child or young adult can be considered an "off-time" loss, as is early retirement forced by disability. These off-time losses are more difficult to deal with.

A particularly difficult loss is that of a child by a parent regardless of whether the child is young or an adult.[22,57,58,67,80,84] Several studies showed that bereaved parents have more physiologic and psychologic symptoms than those grieving other losses.[57,67,80] When a child dies, parents and family members experience very painful and difficult emotions that last for months and even years. A child represents the future with all of its hopes and dreams for the parents and even represents a sense of immortality. Therefore, the loss of a child, infant, or even pregnancy can mean the loss of a hoped-for future for the parents. Also the death of a child can leave the parents with a sense of helplessness and guilt in not having been able to protect their child. Grandparents too experience deep grief at the loss of a grandchild. Not only are they mourning the loss of the child, but they may feel responsible for helping their own child deal with grief.[58]

Caring is the most important need of parents and grandparents during this time. Nonverbal communication is very important, with an open acknowledgment of their pain and sorrow. When parents ask about the events surrounding their child's death, they need to know that everything possible was done. Some parents may remain numb and silent, whereas others may openly express rage and hostility. One must remember that both are in deep pain and that it is important to stay with them and support them in a gentle manner.

Many parents need to see their child after death before leaving the hospital. This helps them to face the reality and say good-by. However, the needs of the parents who cannot face seeing their child after death should be respected and supported also. The nurse must be aware of whether the parents need to have this time alone with their child or if they need to have someone with them. If necessary, the nurse must prepare the parents for the child's appearance. Finally, leaving the hospital after a child's death is particularly difficult for parents, especially after a long illness. It may represent the final reality of the child's death and may be eased somewhat if someone they trust can accompany them to the door.[58]

Cultural Perspectives on Loss and Grief

The coping mechanisms that people develop relative to loss are heavily influenced by the society and culture in which they live. This can be seen in the variety of practices related to the loss occasioned by death described in cross-cultural studies.[44,45] Indeed, within the United States, there is wide cultural variation regarding the appropriate response to loss. In some settings, the expectation is that people are very vocal in expressing their grief, whereas in other groups quiet endurance of the loss is the norm. In Western society, the prevalent attitude seems to be to view loss and death (the ultimate loss) as dreaded enemies to be fought and postponed. However, this attitude is not necessarily seen in other cultures in which losses, including death, are considered to be a part of the natural cycles of life.[7,44]

Death and loss are social matters as well as personal ones. It has been said that "society prescribes standards for grief and mourning, and each individual grieves not only from personal sorrow, but in a style which is the product of early socialization and later social dictates."[45] In the United States, there is a wide variety of ethnocultural backgrounds, each with its own views and practices regarding death and loss. The nurse needs to be cognizant of these differences in providing appropriate care to the individuals experiencing loss.

AMERICANS OF EUROPEAN DESCENT

Western Caucasian culture has greatly separated death from life. Death is less visible because most individuals die in hospitals and nursing homes. With the drastic decrease in infant mortality and the development of life support technology, death in many cases has been removed from the realm of everyday family life. In fact, some view death as an enemy to be held off indefinitely. Once death occurs, the body is tended and prepared by professionals from the hospital nurse to the mortician. The family has little involvement with the bathing and dressing of the body. Everything is taken care of out of sight. Even cemeteries have become less visible. They are now memorial parks with small ground-level plaques rather than the personalized headstones of the past. Indeed, the true nature of these parks may not be obvious to passers-by. The funeral rites and formal mourning activities have become much less time consuming. No longer does the widow wear black for a specified time period to signify her status. Many would say that Western culture has become a death-avoiding society, and this does tend to create a dread of death and of the dying.[44]

AMERICANS OF AFRICAN DESCENT

African-Americans have historically had a more intimate relationship with death and loss than have Americans of European descent. From the ravages of slave ships and the perils of living in slavery to an unhealthy existence in the ghettos of modern America, death has been a frequent, visible, and even violent companion to many unfortunate African-Americans.

In many African-American communities, such as inner-city ghettos and small rural areas of the South, the church plays a large role in funeral rites, which tend to be more ceremonial, a means of offering final elegance to what may have been a bare life. When an African-American is dying, it is not unusual for a family member to be at the bedside continuously. Religion often plays an important role in giving meaning to loss in the African-American community. The burial ceremony can be a very emotional occasion with much crying and vocal grieving, after which mourners gather together to share food and drink provided by the deceased person's relatives.[45] Because of increased contact with death at all ages, some authors contend that

African-Americans may be more prepared to accept death and cope with losses.[44]

AMERICANS OF MEXICAN DESCENT

The Mexican-American culture has a large interest in death in contrast to the Caucasian avoidance of death. The funeral can be the most important family event, surpassing even weddings and christenings. Grief is expressed publicly and vocally, with wailing as an expected behavior. The use of professional wailers may be found in some traditional Mexican-American communities. People of all ages, including young children, participate in these funerals. Children become familiar with death rituals and customs, and it is expected that the dying will be attended by family members. This may come into direct conflict with some institutional policies.[44] Mexican-Americans tend to carry a respect for the dead into bereavement, visiting the grave site frequently and behaving in ways deemed appropriate for those in mourning, including wearing black and curtailing social activities. Death is very much a family event for Mexican-Americans. Both physically and psychologically, a death may pull together geographically separated family members as no other event can.[45]

AMERICANS OF JAPANESE DESCENT

Culturally, Japanese-Americans come from a background in which emotional expression is controlled, particularly if it is viewed as being upsetting to others. There is also a strong work ethic, which makes debilitation in progressive illness or advancing age particularly distressful to Japanese-Americans. In fact, funerals are held in the evening so that attendees do not have to miss work. Death is accepted quietly and resolutely.[45]

It should be remembered that there are many cultures and subcultures, each with its own beliefs and practices. Also, as people of different backgrounds assimilate and westernize, there is a blending and blurring of cultural differences combined with each person's individual differences. Therefore, while being aware of cultural backgrounds in assessing persons dealing with loss, you still must not stereotype grieving persons but must treat each as an individual.

THEORIES OF DYING AND GRIEF

Theories of Death and Dying and the Hospice Movement

GLASER AND STRAUSS'S THEORY

There are primarily two types of theories of death and dying. One deals with the awareness of dying and its trajectory. The other deals with stages of death and dying.

Glaser and Strauss[29,30] described four trajectories of dying (Box 54–1). The first is certain death at a known time, when the individual is given a relatively definite prognosis, such as when a client with cancer is told he or she probably has less than 6 months to live. Another trajectory is when death is certain but the time is unknown. The individual's life expectancy is shortened, but the extent to which it is shortened is unknown. An example is a client who has a progressive neuromuscular disorder that is characterized by exacerbations and remissions but for which the rate of progression is not known. A third trajectory involves uncertainty as to whether the current situation is life threatening but there is a known time for obtaining the answer. The diagnostic and staging periods of a life-threatening illness are prime examples of this trajectory. It is a time of tremendous anxiety when waiting becomes almost unbearable and time drags painfully. Individuals often describe waiting for test results as "the longest 24 hours of my life." The final trajectory is characterized by Glaser and Strauss[30] as uncertain regarding both death and a time for knowing. This can be exemplified by situations in which the individual knows that something is quite wrong, but a diagnosis cannot be made. This high degree of uncertainty can be quite distressing.

PATTISON'S THEORY

Several researchers formulated phase/stage theories for the dying period. According to Pattison,[72] the knowledge of death precipitates a crisis in that the trajectory of the individual's life is suddenly changed. Activities must be reevaluated and rearranged. Once initiated, there are three phases in the altered trajectory. Initially, during the acute phase, anxiety rises to a peak. It may be experienced as though life is standing still.[72] The next phase begins as the anxiety levels off and then begins to decline somewhat. In this chronic living-dying period, a number of fears emerge. There is a fear of loneliness and a sense of isolation, including a fear of sorrow related to potential losses of friends, family, job, future plans, strength, and ability. People in this phase fear loss of control mentally and physically, with attendant loss of self-esteem and integrity. They fear suffering and pain along with loss of identity and regression and withdrawal into the self.[72] It can be seen that this phase is characterized by multiple actual and potential losses with which the dying individual must come to terms. Entrance into the terminal phase ends the living-dying phase and begins as the person starts to withdraw from the people, objects, and events of the outside world.

KÜBLER-ROSS'S THEORY

Kübler-Ross's stages of death and dying are probably the best known of the theoretical frameworks of death

and dying. This theory focuses on the dying person as facing the loss of all that is important. According to this model, the terminally ill individual moves from denial and anger to bargaining to depression and finally to acceptance.[51]

Denial. For many individuals faced with terminal illness, denial serves as protection from constantly being confronted with a very painful reality. Thus, denial enables them to continue to live their lives. Therefore, care must be taken in assuming that an individual must be moved out of denial to move through the expected stages. Careful assessment must be made as to the function that denial is playing in the individual's coping and living before insisting on acknowledgment of a poor prognosis. As Glaser and Strauss[29] discovered, most people are aware that they are dying even when not told directly. They then have to handle that knowledge as best they can. For some, that entails escaping, from time to time, from the reality of impending death. This may be seen in individuals when at one point they discuss a grave prognosis and its ramifications even to the extent of making funeral arrangements and then at another time talk of an event, such as a child's graduation, as if there were nothing wrong. After having dealt with the grim realities of the situation, the individual may need to push that aside to remain involved in life. On the other hand, denial can be problematic when it causes an individual to delay seeking medical attention. For example, a woman finding a lump in her breast may deny its possible implications and avoid seeing her physician, believing that it will disappear. For others, denial may lead them to shop around for a physician who will give them a better diagnosis, feeling that their diagnosis has been made in error. This can delay treatment, rendering it less effective when obtained. This can be frustrating for nurses caring for these individuals, but care must be taken not to inflict guilt on the person for the delay. The nurse can present and reinforce information as directly and gently as possible, but it is ultimately the individual's decision as to what he or she will do with that information.

Anger. The response of anger is very often hardest on family and caregivers. Although they are not the source of the anger, they are very often the targets when it occurs, because the source—the terminal illness—is not as easily targeted. One's religious beliefs may be another area on which the dying person vents anger and frustration.

In this stage, the nurse may see an individual who has usually been polite, cooperative, and friendly lash out at a spouse with an angry tirade. The spouse will likely be confused by this seemingly unprovoked outburst. The same thing may happen when the nurse walks into the room with the client's medication. The nurse may be met with a hostile verbal barrage for being late (when in fact this is not the case), for the abominable hospital food, or for the stain on the sheet. Anger may also be expressed at God or a convenient representative, the person's clergy. Sometimes those who have attempted to live a very religious life feel a great deal of anger that their God could let this happen to them. The dying person needs to be able to express this anger without fear of losing those who are important to him or her. Therefore, it is important for the nurse to be accepting of the anger, perhaps gently assisting the individual to redirect it toward the situation but above all to be available as support and not avoiding the person.

Bargaining. According to Kübler-Ross,[51] bargaining is a way of trying to postpone the inevitable. Bargaining can take a number of forms such as shopping around for medical treatment again. The person may in essence be looking for a physician or treatment that will give a better bargain: life. The bargain may be with caregivers to control the timing of medication or the promise to be cooperative with a treatment regimen if allowed to go home for the weekend. It is seen in the individual who bargains with God for more time, to see the youngest child married, for example, in exchange for living a better life. However, if the bargained-for milestone is reached, another bargaining point may be found. According to this theory, however, the person reaches the point at which he or she realizes that the inevitable cannot be postponed. This leads the individual into the next stage: depression.

Depression. The period of depression through which terminally ill individuals go is a very realistic period of grieving for all that is about to be lost as well as for the losses that have already occurred. During this period, the individual tends to withdraw from the world. Appetite may decrease, and sleep patterns may be altered. It is not uncommon to see the person lying or sitting with his or her back to the door, dismissing relatives and caregivers by turning away from them. During this time, it may be difficult for others to remain with the client but it is a time when the client needs quiet assurance that he or she will not be abandoned. The nurse can ease this time by providing physical care in a timely and gentle manner and by checking in on the client frequently but not requiring verbal exchange. If the depression is severe, prolonged, or interfering with the ability to achieve and maintain pain control, the physician may order antidepressant medication.

Acceptance. Finally, if attained, acceptance is seen as a detached peacefulness.[51] This may actually be disconcerting to care givers, family and professionals alike, because the individual may show very little emotional expression and begin to withdraw from involvement in life. Some may misinterpret this as "giving up the fight." During this period the individual realizes and accepts the full implications of the prognosis. There is a sense of closure on and satisfaction with the life that has been lived. Unfinished business has been completed, and it is a time when final good-bys are said. This is a time of growth for the individual who has been able to come to terms with the situation.[52] Acceptance is exemplified by the person who accepts that the remaining time is short, makes the decision to go home from the hospital to spend that time in quiet contemplation, and leaves those closest to him a legacy of warmth and peace.

THE HOSPICE MOVEMENT

Although not a theory of death and dying, the hospice movement grew out of the concern for the care of the dying generated by the research of Kübler-Ross and others and by a dissatisfaction with the technological approach being used at this stage of life. It was felt, by some, that the technological imperative to maintain life as long as possible by any means available, along with an avoidance of individuals who are dying, deprived the dying of the opportunity for dignity and peace. Furthermore, these two forces deprived the dying of the opportunity to finish important issues in life.

With the founding of St. Christopher's Hospice in England by Dr. Cicely Saunders, hospice care became an alternative to hospitalization as a form of care for the dying. The hospice offered care rather than cure. Within the hospice, the client and family are considered the unit of care, and it is recognized that their needs are inextricably intertwined. The management of pain and maintenance of comfort receive highest priority, and the client and family are an integral part of the ongoing care planning process. In addition to physical comfort, hospice provides psychologic, financial, social, and spiritual comfort by using a team approach. The typical hospice team includes the client and family's nurse, a physician, a social worker or psychologist, and a pastoral person of the client's choosing. The goal is to assist the client and family to work through this difficult time and to be able to live it to the fullest. After the death, a hospice will typically follow the bereaved family members for a year to assist in their reorganization of life.

Finally, in order for growth and resolution to occur during the dying period, it is important for the client and family to find meaning in the experience and to maintain hope in varying forms. The individual who is newly diagnosed with a life-threatening illness, such as cancer, is confronted with his or her own mortality and seeks to make sense of the situation so that it can be fit into the context of his or her life.[65] Hope is considered to be essential to the search for meaning in life-threatening illness and is defined as "the expectation of achieving a future good which seems realistically possible and personally significant."[65] For the dying individual, hope may be for a peaceful death or that, through his or her having undergone an experimental treatment, others in the future may benefit. One nurse author contended that "hope is so vital to life that its loss is equated with loss of life itself."[34] Hope in our culture is future oriented: Individuals who have a terminal illness may need to change the form of their hope to maintain it or put aside the constant awareness of imminent death.[34] Sources of hope for the individual can include family, friends, health professionals, religious beliefs, and a positive attitude.[34,65,76] The nurse can assess and support those sources of hope available to the individual client in her or his struggle to find meaning and maintain hope.

Theories of Grief and Grieving

LINDEMANN'S THEORY

Death and grief have been themes for much classic literature and art over the centuries. However, the subject of grief did not enter the scientific literature until Lindemann's classic 1944 study of acute grief.[54] In this study, survivors of the disastrous Coconut Grove fire were interviewed at different points in time after the incident and a common pattern of grief was identified. This pattern included six reactions: somatic distress, preoccupation with the image of the deceased, guilt, hostile reactions, loss of patterns of conduct, and appearance of traits of the deceased.

Somatic Distress. Lindemann identified specific somatic symptoms of distress in the persons interviewed. He noted that these symptoms occur in waves that last from 20 minutes to an hour. The symptoms include a feeling of tightness in the throat, choking with shortness of breath, an empty feeling in the abdomen, lack of muscle power, and an intense subjective distress likened to tension or mental pain. These waves of discomfort can be brought on by visits, by mention of the deceased, and by expressions of sympathy from others. Many tend to avoid anything that might precipitate these waves. Some individuals show a marked tendency toward sighing, especially when discussing their grief. Some describe feeling profound exhaustion or digestive disturbances such as anorexia or feeling as though everything is slowed in the stomach.[54]

Preoccupation with the Image of the Deceased. Commonly, the bereaved experience a sense of unreality with a feeling of increased emotional distance from others. Also there is an intense preoccupation with images of the deceased. Very often the person who has died will seem to appear as if still alive or as if calling to the survivor. For some, this is very disturbing because they feel that it indicates approaching mental illness when, in actuality, it is a normal reaction.[54]

Guilt. This is prominent in the reactions of some. When guilt occurs, the bereaved will search the time preceding the death for evidence of having failed to do something or see something that might have prevented the death. This is particularly painful for parents who feel they could have done something to prevent the death of a child or for bereaved persons who had a disagreement with the deceased before the death and had no opportunity to make amends.

Hostile Reactions. The bereaved are often disconcerted by their own hostility and lack of warmth toward others. There is a tendency to be irritable and to wish not to be bothered at a time when friends and relatives are making a special effort to extend support. Some expend great effort to control these feelings, resulting in stiff social interactions, whereas others fear their feelings are a sign of mental imbalance.

Loss of Patterns of Conduct. Lindemann noted that the patterns of daily life become very disrupted for the acutely bereaved. Many demonstrate a restlessness and inability to sit still or concentrate. Such individuals often move around aimlessly, searching for something to do and are unable to initiate and maintain organized patterns of activity. Many bereaved go through customary daily routine in an automatic, unenthusiastic manner, with a sense of loss of the meaning of life.[54]

Appearance of Traits of the Deceased. Finally, Lindemann noted that the bereaved may take on traits of the deceased. For example, if the deceased individual suffered from an illness before death, the bereaved person may show symptoms of that illness. Also the bereaved individual may show mannerisms of the deceased: He or she may, for example, copy the way the person walked or spoke. The bereaved one may change activities such as hobbies to ones similar to those of the deceased as a way to identify with the deceased.

Lindemann contended that, with intervention by a psychiatrist, it is possible to settle an uncomplicated grief reaction in a period of 4 to 6 weeks. The duration of the grief reaction depends on the success of the individual's grief work. Successful completion of grief work includes emancipation from ties to the deceased, readjustment to the environment without the deceased, and the formation of new relationships. Major obstacles to completing grief work successfully include avoidance of expression of emotions and intense distress connected with grief.[54]

BOWLBY'S THEORY

Another early theorist, John Bowlby,[8] using a Freudian perspective, likened mourning to the basic separation of child from mother. He theorized that grief responses are rooted in the basic biologic instinct for attachment.

In discussing the stages of the grief process, Bowlby stated that "both behavior and feeling oscillate violently, especially in the early stages: yearning, protest, and rage alternate with blank mute despair."[8]

Bowlby noted that normal grief follows a discernible trend toward resolution. This trend goes through three stages. The first is an urge to recover the lost person. This is experienced as a searching for and intense missing of the deceased. The second stage is disorganization of adaptive processes in an attempt to find a way to cope with the loss. Finally, a reorganization of adaptive processes is made and new attachments can be formed.[8]

ENGEL'S THEORY

George Engel, like the first two theorists, likened grief to wound healing in proposing that successful grief and grieving follow certain more or less predictable steps.[22]

Shock and Disbelief. Initially, according to Engel,[22] the individual experiences shock and disbelief on learning of a death. It is very common to hear someone exclaim, "No! It can't be!" This may be followed by a stunned, numb feeling in which the individual does not permit him- or herself to actually feel the reality of the death. It may be difficult to gain the bereaved individual's attention at this time as the person goes about ordinary daily activities in an automatic manner or sits motionless.

According to Engel, this initial phase can last minutes, hours, or days, alternating with flashes of anguish as the reality of the loss briefly penetrates into consciousness.[22] This initial response is more pronounced with sudden, unexpected death, but it can also be seen when death has been expected.

Developing Awareness. The second phase is that of developing awareness. This can begin within minutes to hours. In this phase, the meaning of the death begins to penetrate awareness, bringing with it feelings of anguish and painful emptiness. The mourner may experience anger toward those held responsible for the death, including the bereaved him- or herself. It is a time when despair is expressed within the limits of the individual's cultural pattern and crying is seen.[22]

Restitution. This phase includes the time of funeral rituals. These rituals emphasize the reality of the death, and this realization is necessary if recovery from the loss is to take place. The group aspect of these activities allows sharing of feelings and mutual support. The religious aspects offer the comfort of a higher power and the hope of a reunion with the lost loved one after death.[22]

In the restitution phase, the bereaved one is occupied with thoughts of the deceased and of his or her personal loss. The bereaved may experience a variety of bodily sensations and pains. Often the discomforts experienced are similar to symptoms that had troubled the deceased person before death. In the bereaved, the duration of these symptoms is usually brief.

Also in this phase, the bereaved tends to repress any negative and hostile feelings toward the deceased in a process called idealization. The process of idealization allows the bereaved to establish a distinct image of the lost person and to relive happy memories associated with the deceased. The bereaved may also start to take on admired qualities of the deceased or carry out his or her goals and ideals. Over a time span of many months, the bereaved person gradually becomes less and less preoccupied with thoughts of the deceased. During this time, thoughts of the deceased become less painful and the survivor turns more toward life.[22]

According to Engel, successful mourning takes a year or more, and the clearest evidence of a successful outcome is the ability to remember, comfortably and realistically, both the pleasures and the disappointments of the lost relationship.

A variety of factors affect the outcome of mourning, including the importance of the lost person to the bereaved, the age of the deceased, the age of the mourner, the amount of support available, the amount of preparation for the death, and the physical and emotional health of the mourner.[22]

PARKES'S THEORY

In his work on grief, Parkes,[68] a psychiatrist and prominent researcher on grief, stated that grief is a complex process that is individual, social, interactional, physical, emotional, and environmental in nature. Parkes theorized that the grieving process is a major life transition manifested by numbness, yearning, disorganization, and reorganization. According to this theory, the numbness is an initial response to loss. This response allows the bereaved individual to move through the first several days seemingly little affected by the loss, such as the widow who calmly and methodically makes funeral arrangements for her deceased husband and sees to accommodations for out-of-town family members. When the numbness wears off, the individual feels an intense yearning for the deceased. This is a very painful time and leads to a period of disorganization of daily life. During this time, the bereaved person feels disrupted and uncertain. Finally, reorganization begins, and the individual begins to structure a new life pattern with the deceased no longer present.[68] Parkes acknowledged that individuals vary in the way they move through this process.

MARTOCCHIO'S THEORY

Martocchio,[56] a nurse researcher, defined grieving as the process of moving through the pain of loss. She noted that this process involves complex, bewildering emotions and thoughts. The process is seen as a normal response to loss and as a time for healing, adaptation, and growth. Martocchio did not present a stage theory per se. Instead, she identified manifestations of grief as a series of clusters that describe the nature of the grieving process. She stated that these clusters have neither discrete boundaries nor any particular expected order.[56] The clusters are shock and disbelief; yearning and protest; anguish, disorganization, and despair; identification in bereavement; and reorganization and restitution (Fig. 54–1).

Contrary to the popular belief that grief is resolved in 1 year, Martocchio asserted that periods much shorter and much longer can still be normal. The symptoms of grief do not simply stop at a designated point in time. The individual may have periods of depression and periods of well-being as life begins to be reorganized. Life may be restabilized, but the loss remains for a lifetime. Reactions of loss may continue to recur at times when the individual is particularly reminded of the deceased, such as anniversaries or holidays.[41,56]

According to this framework, the goal of successful grief work is "to remember the loved one without major emotional pain and to reinvest emotional energy

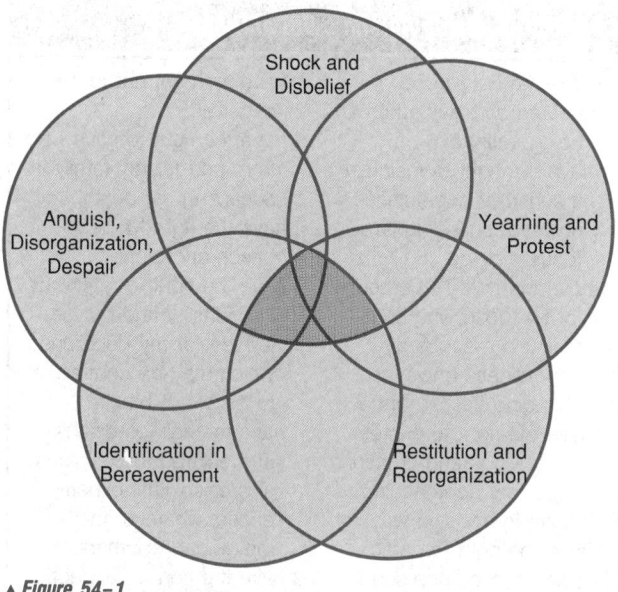

▲ *Figure 54–1*

Martocchio's clusters.

in life so that the capacity to love is not lost."[56] The time frame for successful resolution is given as 2 to 5 years for most individuals,[56] which is quite longer than proposed in other theories.

Martocchio[56] further identified four elements of grief work related to the final resolution of the grieving:

▶ emancipation from the bondage to the deceased, which involves finishing unfinished business and finding a new identity

▶ readjustment to an altered environment, which refers to such behaviors as again participating in activities once shared with the loved one

▶ development of new or renewed relationships, which occurs when the bereaved is able to invest emotionally in another person

▶ learning to live in a comfortable fashion with memories of hurt, happiness, suffering, and joys associated with the deceased, which requires a letting go of the deceased while treasuring, but not living, these memories.

According to Martocchio, factors that can affect the individual's grief response include the nature of the relationship, the quality of the relationship, the mode of death, characteristics of the survivor, the acceptability of the individual's grief responses in the social environment, and the presence of survivor risk factors as follows:[56]

▶ low socioeconomic status
▶ poor health
▶ sudden death or short illness
▶ perceived lack of available social support
▶ lack of support from religious beliefs
▶ lack of a supportive family or a family who actively discourages grief expressions

▶ strong tendency to cling to the person before death or preoccupation with the image of the deceased
▶ strong reactions of distress, anger, and self-reproach
▶ history of psychiatric illness or suicidal ideation.

Cautions About Stage and Phase Theories

Although the models just presented suggest common responses to major loss, the nurse must remember that each person experiencing a loss is unique and will respond somewhat differently from others experiencing the same loss. Indeed, for some, a particular event usually associated with loss may not be experienced as such.

People do not pass through stages in any particular order or on a set time schedule. All individuals adapt to loss in their own way and in their own time. There are many variations. Always bear this in mind when assessing any individual experiencing loss, and use these theories as guides to some potential responses, without expecting any one individual to fit any one specific theory. Also be aware of the physiologic and emotional vulnerability that occurs as bereaved persons integrate their loss into their lives.

THE NURSE AND LOSS AND GRIEF

As stated earlier in this chapter, the nurse is not immune to loss and grief. The nurse needs to be aware of this and to allow him- or herself the opportunity to grieve when needed to maintain a healthy self and to be able to provide effective care to clients.

Just like their clients, nurses are raised in a culture that helps determine attitudes toward death and appropriate expressions of grief. Also, the nurse is socialized into the biomedical culture through education and orientation into the work world. A belief held by this culture is that death represents medical failure. If this is believed, it is uncomfortable to be around the dying or the bereaved. In the past, this discomfort has led to isolation of the dying in rooms at the end of the hall or avoidance of their rooms by nursing staff.[29,75] In the belief that individuals should not know of a grave prognosis, communication with the dying and their families was often guarded and less than honest. This led to a "double-bind" situation that was uncomfortable for all.[24] It is hoped that this situation has changed with the belief that people have a right to information regarding their diagnosis and prognosis. However, the nurse may still encounter situations in which clients have not been told of their diagnosis and prognosis but indicate an awareness that something is wrong. For the new nurse, this is a situation that needs to be discussed with a more experienced nurse, such as an immediate supervisor, because resolution may require intensive discussions with family and physician, perhaps including input from a social worker or clergy. The nurse also needs to be aware of any discomfort that he or she may have in dealing with death-related issues and should seek help if needed in resolving this discomfort.

By its very nature, care involves some feeling. Therefore, nurses who care for clients will feel loss when a client dies or has a poor outcome. It is neither necessary nor desirable to deny these feelings. Indeed, it has become recognized that nurses in high-stress areas such as hospice, oncology, and critical care settings, where death and loss are common occurrences, need to grieve and to renew themselves to grow in these settings.[33,79] Some settings, hospice in particular, make provision for nurses to renew themselves. This may take the form of "mental health days," a quiet room to sit and contemplate, retreats, and regular staff sessions for mutual support, which are sometimes facilitated by a psychologist. There are times when it is appropriate for the nurse to attend a funeral of a client with whom he or she has been particularly close. This can provide closure for the nurse as well as support for the nurse and the client's family. Above all, the nurse needs to recognize and accept his or her feelings.

Assessment

The assessment portion of the nursing process is particularly important for individuals who are experiencing grief and loss because of the high degree of variability found among individuals in their responses to this experience.

To formulate a truly relevant care plan for the person, the nurse must very carefully assess the meaning of the loss being experienced by that person within the context of the individual's current situation and cultural orientation, taking into consideration previous experiences.

ASSESSING THE INDIVIDUAL AND FAMILY COPING WITH TERMINAL ILLNESS

The dying client is facing what may be the greatest of all losses: everything that has been experienced in life. The individual and family are concurrently dealing with the physiologic effects of the illness and its treatment and with any stigma that may be associated with a particular diagnosis, such as acquired immune deficiency syndrome (AIDS). The needs of these people are many, varied, and changing. Some of these needs were initially made clear to all members of the health professions when corresponding rights were established in the dying person's bill of rights, a now historic document you may review by referring to Box 54-2. Obviously, a thorough, ongoing assessment by the nurse is essential to meeting the changing needs of dying individuals and their families.

Assessing Comfort Status. For any individual in the terminal phase of an illness, the assessment priority is the individual's comfort status. This encompasses physical, psychosocial, and spiritual assessment. As can be recalled from earlier sections of this chapter, the dying portion of life can be a time of growth for both the

---

Box 54-2. Dying Person's Bill of Rights*

I have the right to be treated as a living human being until I die.

I have the right to maintain a sense of hopefulness however changing its focus may be.

I have the right to be cared for by those who can maintain a sense of hopefulness however changing this might be.

I have the right to express my feelings and emotions about my approaching death in my own way.

I have the right to participate in decisions concerning my care.

I have the right to expect continuing medical and nursing attention even though "cure" goals must be changed to "comfort" goals.

I have the right not to die alone.

I have the right to be free from pain.

I have the right to have my questions answered honestly.

I have the right not to be deceived.

I have the right to have help from and for my family in accepting my death.

I have the right to die in peace and dignity.

I have the right to retain my individuality and not be judged for my decisions which may be contrary to beliefs of others.

I have the right to discuss and enlarge my religious and/or spiritual experiences, whatever these may mean to others.

I have the right to expect that the sanctity of the human body will be respected after death.

I have the right to be cared for by caring, sensitive, knowledgeable people who will attempt to understand my needs and will be able to gain some satisfaction in helping me face my death.

This Bill of Rights was created at a workshop on "The Terminally Ill Patient and the Helping Person," in Lansing, MI, sponsored by the Southwestern Michigan Inservice Education Council and conducted by Amelia J. Barbus, associate professor of nursing, Wayne State University, Detroit.

*From Donovan, M. I., & Pierce, S. G. (1976). *Cancer care nursing.* New York: Appleton-Century-Crofts, p. 33.

---

client and the family. However, for this to occur, the individual must be comfortable and the family supported.

It is important to determine whether and to what degree the individual has physical discomfort. Discomfort can be nausea, fatigue, itching, constipation, and stiffness as well as pain. Each of these kinds of discomfort can take a number of forms and vary in pattern, duration, and intensity. Knowledge of the client's disease process and treatment is one aspect of assessing an individual's comfort status. The physiologic changes brought about by these can be one factor in any discomfort that is being experienced.

Through an understanding of the pathophysiologic process of the disease, along with the physiologic and biochemical effects of various modalities used to treat a particular diagnosis, the nurse is better able to anticipate potential sources of discomfort. This knowledge also better enables the nurse to provide anticipatory guidance to the client and family members.

Observation of the client can give clues to any discomfort. Individuals may be seen holding their bodies in positions that indicate discomfort or guarding of a painful body area. Some individuals may be very rigid when in pain, fearing movement. Others may pace restlessly when experiencing discomfort. Facial expression may be tight with grimacing, indicating pain. Some people may moan and express their discomfort vocally, whereas others suffer in silence. Some knowledge of cultural background can be useful to the nurse in assessing the client's expression of discomfort because the style of expression is very often strongly influenced by the individual's upbringing and the meaning that the situation has for the individual. The person experiencing a great deal of discomfort will probably not want to engage in much social interaction, although for a moderate degree of pain, distraction may be helpful. The nurse observing a change in a client's interactional pattern may use this in assessing comfort/discomfort. The individual's color and skin moisture, along with vital signs, can further contribute to the nurse's assessment of physical discomfort. Pallor and diaphoresis may accompany sudden acute pain, whereas an ashen color combined with diaphoresis may be seen with nausea. The person who is greatly fatigued may show signs of great effort such as increased heart rate and respiratory rate with minimal exertion. Individuals who have lived with chronic pain and discomfort may show minimal physiologic signs of discomfort, even when in a great deal of pain. Finally, the nurse needs to remember that there can be sources of discomfort other than the disease process. The client may have been positioned uncomfortably, and pressure sores can be painful, so that assessment of skin integrity and mobility is important for the dying individual. Constipation can be very uncomfortable, and a decreased mobility level and an analgesic medication regimen can leave these individuals vulnerable to constipation. Therefore, careful assessment of bowel status is vital to maintaining physical comfort for the dying individual. As the disease process progresses, symptoms change and fluctuate, making the continuous assessment and maintenance of physical comfort an ongoing challenge for the nurse.

The nurse must bear in mind that the behaviors and expressions of discomfort observed are not always in direct correspondence with the degree of discomfort being experienced by the client. The nurse is making assumptions based on his or her cultural background and knowledge, whereas the client's expressions are based on his or her background. When these two are different, there is the danger of inaccurate assessment. Therefore, the nurse's communication skills are as important as his or her observational skills in assessing comfort status. The nurse should verify the assessment with the client. It is important to ask the client to describe his or her discomfort as thoroughly as possi-

ble. This includes location, intensity, onset, duration, precipitating and relieving factors, and daily patterns. For instance, if an individual indicates that she or he is having pain, the nurse should probe further. It may be that the person has an ordinary headache that can be relieved by two acetaminophen tablets rather than an injection of morphine. Another client may be experiencing abdominal pain and nausea. Without careful, overall assessment, the nurse may not discover that this person has recently decreased activity because of increased pain, has been started on codeine for the pain, has not had a bowel movement for 4 days, and is now eating or drinking very little because of the abdominal discomfort. On the other hand, the occurrence of discomfort in between prescribed medication intervals may indicate the need to reassess the medication regimen and can be an indicator of changing disease status.

Many times, the individual will be able to tell the nurse factors that precipitate or worsen the discomfort or identify times of the day when the discomfort is better or worse. By the same token, the client may have found ways to relieve and cope with various discomforts. It is important to ascertain what these comfort measures are because they will have implications for developing a truly individualized care plan.

Finally, the nurse must assess the impact that discomforts have on the individual's life and ability to do what is important. Different individuals with a similar physiologic status experience different degrees of pain and other discomforts. Also an individual who appears to tolerate a high amount of pain may not be able to bear a relatively small amount of nausea. Therefore, the nurse must identify which symptoms are the most distressing to the individual, and which interfere the most with the quality of living. This comes from active listening, attentive observation, and a knowledge of the individual that grows over time.

The provision of physical comfort can present the opportunity to deal with clients' and families' emotional and spiritual comfort issues that can emerge during the dying period. Nurses' provision of comfort is often the greatest source of well-being that can be afforded to clients and families at this time because it frees them to attend to unfinished business. However, some clients may need additional assistance in this area as problems become discovered through the assessment process. There are times when physical discomfort cannot be relieved by usual methods. In this case, part of the assessment includes examining emotional and spiritual issues in addition to the physical care regimen.

Assessing Spiritual Needs. Spiritual and existential issues commonly arise during the dying period, when clients are searching to make sense of their situation and to solidify their relationship with their god and the universe. Although the nurse may not feel comfortable dealing with these issues directly, he or she needs to be alert to questions centering on the meaning of life and the existence of an afterlife, because these can be important observations to make while assessing clients. Additionally, the nurse should be alert to clients' indications that they may need to see or talk to a particular individual to attend to concerns that had been neglected and that have become urgent with impending death. Isolation and loneliness may be greatly feared by dying individuals, and sometimes frequent requests for medication and various activities are attempts to prevent being alone. Being present and using active listening are the nurse's best tools for assessment of these aspects.

The nurse needs to be aware of any advanced directives, such as a living will, that the client may have.

Assessing Family Needs. Caring for the family is an integral part of caring for the dying individual. Thorough assessment cannot occur without the inclusion of the family in the assessment process, because the client does not exist in isolation. The nurse needs to be observant of the interactions occurring when family members are present. Are communications open or strained? Is the client tense or calm and relaxed after visits? Is there any pattern of pain or discomfort that emerges around visits? Do some visitors seem reluctant to go into the client's room? Does the client turn certain or perhaps all people away? Some people are uncomfortable with individuals who are dying and are uncomfortable with open acknowledgment of dying. If this is occurring with people important to the client, it can impede discussion of concerns that the client may need to have with these individuals. If the nurse assesses this to be the case, he or she can plan for appropriate measures to assist all involved.

Family members may experience anticipatory grief. This is when the grieving process begins before the actual death. When this happens, visits to the client may lessen in frequency and duration as one or more persons withdraw from the dying individual. This can be painful and puzzling for both the client and the family members. Again, it is something that ought to be assessed in order that it be addressed for both the comfort of the client and the avoidance of excessive guilt by the family members after the client's death. If appropriately handled, anticipatory grief can prepare the family members somewhat for bereavement as they prepare for life after the loss has occurred.[100]

Asynchronous response (differing response patterns that may be in conflict) can occur between family and client, such as when the client is accepting and the family is denying. Therefore, the nurse needs to assess not only the client's response but the family member's response and to compare the congruence or discordance between the two. If the client and important family members are out of sync, intervention may be necessary.

Assessing the Client with AIDS. When the dying individual has a diagnosis of AIDS, there are specific social issues that must be incorporated into the nurse's understanding to assess both the individual's and important other's response. Whether a homosexual lover, a heterosexual lover, or a spouse, the significant other may be dealing with concerns related to being actually or potentially HIV positive as well as dealing with the loss of the loved one. The social stigma associated with

AIDS makes it difficult for client and family alike to share their feelings and receive the support from others so needed during this time. Indeed, for many, there may be a sense of shame connected with this diagnosis. Also, the client and significant other are likely to be dealing with multiple recent and concurrent losses related to AIDS. The nurse must be aware of these issues in order to appropriately assess responses of individuals affected by AIDS.[10,40,88,93]

Assessing the Ability of Family Members to Provide Care. For some family members, spouses and parents in particular, being able to assist with and participate in caring for their loved one is important in easing a sense of helplessness and uselessness. Additionally, the family member knows the client better than the nurse in terms of what may be most comfortable for the client. Nursing assessment can be enhanced when the nurse obtains information that families can provide. When the family desires to be involved in the client's care, the nurse needs to consider the extent to which they wish to be involved. A family member may be more comfortable with certain aspects of care, such as moving and positioning the client, but not with others, such as toileting. The nurse also needs to be aware of when a family member may need a break from any caregiving they may be doing. Also there are individuals who are not at all comfortable with any aspect of physical care or who may be worn out from having born the burden of care for a period of time at home. The need to be relieved of the responsibility of care should be considered in assessing family response.

Assessing the Needs of Children. Children are an important part of a client's family. The nurse should assess client and family concerns related to children in order to be able to plan for guidance in assisting adults to help children deal with the death in an age-appropriate manner. It can be painful for a hospitalized parent or grandparent not to be able to see their children or grandchildren. If this is a concern for a particular client, it should be assessed and incorporated into the care plan.

Assessing for Signs of Imminent Death. There are signs that may indicate death is imminent. Recognition of these signs is helpful in reprioritizing the care plan and providing anticipatory guidance to the family. Five major changes in body function occur as death nears. There is a loss of muscle tone, slowing of peristalsis, slowing of circulation, changing respiration, and decreasing sensation. With loss of muscle tone, the nurse will observe increased weakness, decreased movement, incontinence from loss of sphincter control, inability to maintain a comfortable position without support, decreasing ability to swallow, gradual loss of gag reflex, and sagging of the jaw, with flaccid lips and cheeks. As peristalsis slows, the person will have a further diminished appetite, increased flatus and distention, constipation, and dry mouth and slight fever from dehydration. Slowed circulation can result in a mottling and cyanosis of the extremities, cool and clammy feeling of extremities, perspiration, picking at the bed clothes, and poor absorption of medications. Respirations may be slowed, labored, or irregular, with a possibility of increased secretions. This may produce very noisy respirations that have been called a "death rattle." This occurs usually very near to death and can be quite disturbing to family members. Sometimes medication to decrease secretions will be prescribed if this is very upsetting. As sensation decreases, there may be an altered level of consciousness, possible mental cloudiness, changes in pain intensity (either increased or decreased), possible blurring of vision with the client turning toward light and with accumulation of secretions on eyelids, and an altered sense of hearing. Although many individuals slip into death from a state of unconsciousness, there are some who are very alert up until the moment of death.

The nurse also must be aware that hearing is the last sense to be affected, so that there may be a sense of awareness even after the ability to respond has been lost.

When death is quite imminent, the individual's pupils will become fixed and dilated; pulse will be faster, weaker, and sometimes irregular; respirations will fall into a Cheyne-Stokes pattern; blood pressure will drop; reflexes will be absent; and the person will be unable to move. Just before death, respirations and heartbeats can become widely spaced until, finally, there is no next breath and heartbeat. As the nurse assesses that death is imminent, he or she can apprise the family of what is happening. The nurse can help to make it less frightening to the family, who, in turn, can provide comfort to the client.

As a result of careful assessment, the nurse will be aware of some of the family's needs after the death. This may include a need to have some time alone with the deceased before the body is removed from the room. The nurse needs also to assess whether the family is having difficulty leaving and needs gentle support to do so.

If autopsy is to be requested or there has been a desire expressed for organ donation, the nurse can play an important role in assessing appropriate timing to present these issues as guided by his or her assessment of the family's response at the time.

ASSESSING THE BEREAVED CLIENT IN THE CLINICAL SETTING

Besides providing support to a bereaved family of a deceased client, the nurse will be caring for bereaved individuals and people grieving losses in a variety of other situations. You will recall that bereaved people have an increased rate of illness and, therefore, this may result in their need for nursing care. Part of the assessment of any client should include ascertaining whether they have experienced a major loss in their lives. If so, the nurse needs then to determine how recent the loss has been and the impact it has had in the individual's life. This includes changes in patterns of

daily living that can affect the individual's health such as appetite, sleep, smoking, drinking, and social interaction. A widow may not be eating a nutritious diet or maintaining her diabetic diet because she is not motivated to eat alone or has lost concern with her own care. In anticipation of postdischarge needs, the nurse needs to assess what supports are available to the bereaved individual.

Clients in medical-surgical settings may be responding to losses also. The nurse must assess the responses of individuals who have had mastectomies or amputations or who have received a diagnosis of a chronic or progressive illness. Although not necessarily facing imminent death, these individuals are coping with the loss of a part of the self. This can be an actual loss of a body part with an attendant change in body image, or it can be a perceived loss. With chronic illness, for example, the individual will need to grieve the loss of the perception of the self as a healthy individual, the loss of the ability to perform customary roles, such as parent, in the accustomed ways, and loss of the future as it had been previously envisioned. The grief process accompanying these losses can be very painful and must be incorporated into the nurse's assessment along with the other aspects of care in the medical-surgical setting. Grief, as a response to loss, is an integral part of responses observed by nurses in all clinical settings. Therefore, it must be considered in any nursing assessment.

Nursing Diagnosis

With a thorough assessment, the nurse will be able to formulate nursing diagnoses appropriate for the particular client. These potential diagnoses are many and involve incorporating the physical, psychologic, social, and spiritual areas. Table 54–3 lists a number of the North American Nursing Diagnosis Association (NANDA) diagnoses that are appropriate for the terminally ill cancer client. With different medical problems, there may be different or additional nursing diagnoses specific to the particular issue.

Family members may be diagnosed by the nurse as experiencing *Anticipatory Grieving* or *Dysfunctional Grieving*. The Nursing Diagnosis Profiles in this chapter describe these two NANDA diagnoses. These diagnoses may be appropriate for individuals who are anticipating or have experienced the loss of a body part or important life role as well as those facing or experiencing the loss of a loved one.

Planning

Because dying and grieving are processes that cause the client to change over time, it is essential to incorporate ongoing, continuous assessment into the care plan. Planning must be dynamic to truly meet the changing needs of these clients experiencing loss.

Part of planning is prioritizing the care to be given. With the dying client, comfort measures receive the highest priority. If the individual is in pain, in most

TABLE 54-3. Nursing Diagnoses and Desired Outcomes for a Client with Terminal Cancer

Nursing Diagnosis	Desired Client Outcomes
Ineffective Breathing Pattern R/T decreased energy, effects of medications, fatigue, immobility, inactivity, pain, tracheobronchial obstruction	Rate, rhythm, and depth of respiration normal for client; no evidence of aspiration throughout hospitalization
High Risk for Aspiration R/T reduced ability to manage own secretions secondary to reduced level of consciousness, depressed gag and cough reflexes, impaired swallowing	No evidence of aspiration throughout hospitalization
Fluid Volume Deficit R/T loss of body fluids or electrolytes, altered mental status, excessive drainage, difficulty swallowing or eating, nausea or vomiting	Within 72 hours, normal skin turgor, stable BP and P, balanced I & O
Chronic pain R/T effects of terminal illness, muscle spasm, inflammation	Expresses comfort within _____ minutes after initiation of comfort measure
High Risk for Impaired Skin Integrity R/T altered nutritional state, altered oxygen transport, decreased circulation, edema, excretions, secretions, infection, skeletal prominence, immobility	No evidence of skin breakdown throughout hospitalization
Altered Oral Mucous Membrane R/T dehydration, effects of chemotherapy, medication, radiation to head/neck, immunosupression, mouth breathing, malnutrition, vomiting	Moist, pink mucous membrane without further evidence of cracking or ulceration throughout hospitalization
Impaired Physical Mobility R/T fatigue, decreased strength and endurance, intolerance of activity, pain, side effects of narcotics, depression, severe anxiety, fear of movement	During hospitalization, achieves maximum mobility within limitations of terminal state
Self-Care Deficit R/T effects of illness, fatigue, pain, side effects of medications, presence of external devices, immobility, depression, anxiety, grieving, surgery, loss of limb	During hospitalization, performs self-care activities within physical limitations and accepts assistance when necessary
Colonic Constipation R/T less than adequate fluid intake, less than adequate dietary intake, less than adequate physical activity, immobility, lack of privacy, stress, change in daily routine, metabolic problems, side effects of narcotics	During terminal phase of illness, achieves bowel routine that provides optimum comfort
Bowel Incontinence R/T impaction, diarrhea, depression, severe anxiety, effects of medication, physical or psychologic barriers that prevent access to an acceptable toileting area	Experiences absence or decreased episodes of incontinence q 24 hours
High Risk for Disuse Syndrome R/T effects of pain, immobility, altered level of consciousness	No evidence of body system deterioration during hospitalization other than that imposed by terminal illness
Sleep Pattern Disturbance R/T side effects of medication, pain, inactivity, incontinence, nausea, life-style disruptions, fear, anxiety, depression, unfamiliar environment, circadian rhythm disturbances	Experiences at least _____ hours of uninterrupted sleep/rest q 24 hours
Altered Nutrition: Less than Body Requirements R/T impaired absorption, alteration in taste or smell, dysphagia, dyspnea, stomatitis, nausea and vomiting, fatigue, decreased appetite, effects of cancer, decreased level of consciousness, stress	Consumes maximum amount of calories that is comfortable
Anxiety R/T loss of possessions, loss of significant others, threat to or change in health status, threat to or change in role functioning, threat to or change in self-concept, threat to or change in interaction, situational crisis, unmet needs, threat of death, unconscious conflict about essential values and goals of life, lack of knowledge, loss of control.	During hospitalization, client and family verbalize decreasing anxiety
Altered Thought Processes R/T side effects of narcotics, sleep deprivation, psychologic conflicts, depression, anxiety, social isolation, fear of the unknown, negative reactions from others, loss of control, loss of familiar surroundings, loss of significant other	Identifies correct time, place, and person

TABLE 54-3. Nursing Diagnoses and Desired Outcomes for a Client with Terminal Cancer Continued

Nursing Diagnosis	Desired Client Outcomes
Dysfunctional Grieving R/T effects of loss of a body part, absence of anticipatory grieving, thwarted grieving in response to a loss, actual or perceived loss of significant other, health or social status or valued object, multiple losses or crises, lack of resolution of previous grieving response, ambivalent feelings toward loss, changes in life style, decreased support system	Before death, client and family verbalize feelings about death
Ineffective Individual/Family Coping R/T effects of terminal illness, loss of control over body part or body function, lack of support systems, separation from or loss of significant other, low self-esteem, major changes in life style, unrealistic perceptions, situational crisis, knowledge deficit regarding prognosis, knowledge deficit regarding disease process, knowledge deficit regarding therapeutic regimen, recent or impending death of family member, lack of support for family members, temporary disorganization, and role changes	Before death, client and family verbalize effective coping strategies and identify support systems
Impaired Adjustment R/T effects of terminal illness or disability requiring change in life style, incomplete grieving, inadequate support systems	Before client's death, family verbalizes positive strategies to facilitate adjustment
Family Coping: Potential for Growth R/T family's basic needs being sufficiently gratified and adaptive tasks being adequately addressed to allow goals of self-actualization to surface	During hospitalization, family's adaptive coping will continue
Body Image Disturbance R/T effects of loss of body part, or loss of body function	Before death, client verbalizes positive feelings about self
Powerlessness R/T immobility, difficulty in performing self-care, illness-related regimen, social isolation, cultural role, communication barriers, loss of financial independence, health care environment	Verbalizes increasing feelings of control of own response to disease process before death
Altered Family Processes R/T situation transition or crisis precipitated by client's dying	Before client's death, family identifies actual role changes and suggests alternatives within family system
Fear R/T high risk for pain secondary to disease process, threat of death, loss of significant other	Verbalizes decreased feelings of fear before death
Spiritual Distress R/T separation from religious/cultural ties, response to loss of significant other, challenged belief or value system, effects of personal and family disasters or major life changes	Verbalizes alternative methods of completing spiritual practices and states feelings of decreased distress before death
High Risk for Trauma R/T fatigue, pain, side effects of medications, weakness, confusion	Throughout hospitalization, no evidence of accident or injury
High Risk for Infection R/T effects of inadequate primary defenses, decreased hemoglobin, leukopenia, suppressed inflammatory response, terminal illness, immunosuppression, malnutrition, invasive treatments or procedures	Before death, no evidence of infection avoidable within the constraints of comfort
Knowledge Deficit R/T effects of medication, information misinterpretation, denial, unfamiliarity with knowledge resources	Describes disease process, discusses prognosis, identifies available personal/community support systems, describes action, dosage, and major side effects of prescribed pain medications

Adapted from Taptich, B. J., Iyer, P. W., & Bernocchi-Losey, D. (1989). *Nursing diagnosis and care planning.* Philadelphia: W. B. Saunders, pp. 212–214.

NURSING DIAGNOSIS PROFILE

Anticipatory Grieving

Definition. A state in which an individual experiences responses to an actual or perceived loss of a person, relationship, object, or functional ability before the loss occurs

Classification. Feeling 9.2.1.2

Defining Characteristics. A nursing diagnosis of *Anticipatory Grieving* is appropriate for any individual who is expecting a loss. Such an individual may show an altered affect and express anger, guilt, or sorrow. He or she may directly express distress at the potential loss or may experience choked feelings. The potential loss may be denied by some. Libido may be altered in *Anticipatory Grieving,* and the affected individual may experience changes in activity levels, sleeping, or eating habits. Crying may be seen along with altered communication patterns. Because grief is a highly individual response, anticipatory grief may be manifested as one, some, all, or none of these characteristics and may vary over time.

Sample Related Factors. The primary related factor is the actual or potential loss of a significant other, health status, social status, or valued object.

Concept Description. This diagnosis is useful to nurses in multiple settings because all individuals anticipate and experience loss. This often becomes prominent in health care settings because most clients there are experiencing a temporary or permanent threat to their health status. The grief response is one of the whole person. It is physiologic, psychologic, social, and cultural in nature. When grief is in anticipation of a loss, it is the beginning of preparing for life without what is to be lost.

Examples. This diagnostic category could be applicable in the following situations, among others:

▶ A person who has received a diagnosis of cancer and a prognosis of 6 months or less. This person experiences anticipatory grieving for the loss of his or her own life. The probability of cure or of ever regaining any health is absent. Indeed, deterioration ending in death is the most likely scenario. Profound anticipatory grieving can be expected as part of the response to dying.

▶ A person who has become aware that a loved one is dying. This person will likely experience anticipatory grief at some point. If he or she does not, the person will be at higher risk for dysfunctional grief after the death.

▶ The woman who must undergo a mastectomy or the man with diabetes who must undergo a leg amputation. Both will be grieving the loss of the body part as well as dealing with an altered body image and loss of function.

▶ The parents of an infant born with a major defect. The parents will grieve in anticipation of the loss of dreams and hopes that they had held for a healthy child.

▶ The executive facing retirement who grieves in anticipation of the loss of role identification and status that his or her current position affords.

Related/Similar Nursing Diagnoses. This diagnosis should be distinguished from a diagnosis of *Dysfunctional Grieving.* The main difference between these two diagnoses is that with a diagnosis of *Anticipatory Grieving* the loss has not yet occurred, whereas it has occurred with a diagnosis of *Dysfunctional Grieving.*

Another important difference between these two diagnoses is that *Anticipatory Grieving* is a normal process that may or may not occur when a person is faced with a loss. However, *Dysfunctional Grieving* is a diagnosis that recognizes that the normal process of grief has become pathological (usually because it is prolonged). In fact, if normal anticipatory grieving does not take place before a loss, the bereaved person is much more likely to experience dysfunctional grieving after the loss has occurred.

Also note that *Anticipatory Grieving* may be an appropriate related factor for a number of other nursing diagnoses. A few selected examples include the following:

▶ *Anxiety R/T Anticipatory Grieving*
▶ *Sleep Pattern Disturbance R/T Anticipatory Grieving*
▶ *Spiritual Distress R/T Anticipatory Grieving*
▶ *Impaired Social Interactions R/T Anticipatory Grieving*
▶ *Altered Family Processes R/T Anticipatory Grieving*

As you review the accepted North American Nursing Diagnosis Association (NANDA) nursing diagnoses, you will note many more that are appropriate.

---

instances relief will be the first concern. In addition, the care plan developed must reflect the priorities that the client and family identified during assessment. Priorities are likely to change as an individual nears death or moves through the grief process, although comfort will always remain high. Also priorities may be different for family members than for the client. For instance, comfort measures to promote a dignified and peaceful death may be the priority for the client, whereas measures that promote the mobilization of social resources for support may be the priority for individuals facing bereavement.

It may not be possible to complete all aspects of the care plan during the time of hospitalization. Therefore, the plan should include appropriate referrals for those assessed needs with which the nurse does not deal

directly. For instance, you may plan for referral to clergy for the client who has expressed spiritual concerns or to an oncology nurse clinician for difficult pain management issues. Incorporating referrals to meet postdischarge needs is essential for continuity of client care. This may include planning to refer the family to bereavement services after the client's death. In caring for individuals when several disciplines are involved, it is helpful to plan for periodic team meetings to reassess and update the care plan. Additionally, accurate recording of the care plan and subsequent updates are essential to facilitating a consistent, efficient, appropriate approach to care for any given client by all involved with her or his care. See Table 54–3 for examples of outcomes for nursing diagnoses for clients with terminal cancer. Outcomes for the diagnosis of

NURSING DIAGNOSIS PROFILE

Dysfunctional Grieving

Definition. The state in which an individual experiences an exaggerated response to an actual or perceived loss of a person, relationship, object, or functional ability

Classification. Feeling 9.2.1.1

Defining Characteristics. Grieving may be diagnosed as dysfunctional when the individual who has experienced an actual or potential loss loses weight, experiences amenorrhea, shows changes in sleep patterns, and experiences a decreased activity level. The person may also feel anger, guilt, worthlessness, denial, or sorrow. There is a decreased interest in personal appearance or interference with life functioning. There may be difficulty in expressing the loss, and there may be a reliving of past experiences. Alterations in concentration, developmental regression, hyperactivity, fear of the future, absence of emotion, suicidal thoughts, and social withdrawal are other manifestations that may be seen.

Sample Related Factors. There are many related factors. Some of the most common include effects of loss of function or body part; absence of anticipatory grieving; thwarted grieving in response to loss; actual or perceived loss of significant other, health status, social status, or valued object; multiple losses or crises; lack of resolution of previous grieving response; ambivalent feelings toward loss; changes in life style; and lack of support system.

Concept Description. This can be a particularly difficult diagnosis because of the highly individual nature of the grief response. Because of differences in personal or cultural response patterns, what is exaggerated for one individual may not be for another. However, you can consider grief to be dysfunctional when the individual is unable to incorporate the loss into his or her life and resume functioning at what the individual considers to be an acceptable level. You will note that many of the characteristics of *Dysfunctional Grieving* are those of normal grief. It is the intensity and duration that determine whether the response is dysfunctional or normal. The line between the two can be very fuzzy.

Examples. This diagnostic category could be applicable in the following situations, among others:

▶ A woman who has initiated divorce proceedings and then learns that her husband has died suddenly of a massive heart attack. She feels deep remorse and is obsessed with the thought that she caused the fatal heart attack. She also feels terribly guilty because part of her is relieved by the thought that her husband's death will free her of the long and difficult divorce process.

▶ A 6-year-old whose sibling has just died of leukemia. He is fearful to have his mother out of his sight now, fearing that she too will disappear forever. He also feels that he caused his sister's death because he had mean thoughts about her when she was getting all of the attention.

▶ A young man who has just lost his lover to AIDS. In the last 6 months, he has seen five of his close friends die of AIDS, and he, himself, has tested positive for the human immunodeficiency virus. In addition, his parents have rejected him because of his homosexual life style and have denied his request to come home. He alternates between locking himself in his apartment and crying for days at a time and going out to drink, dance, and laugh merrily as he "thumbs his nose at death."

Related/Similar Nursing Diagnoses. See the Nursing Diagnosis Profile for *Anticipatory Grieving*. Also note that the diagnoses listed there, with *Anticipatory Grieving* as the related factor, may also be listed here with *Dysfunctional Grieving* as the related factor. For example,

▶ *Anxiety R/T Dysfunctional Grieving*
▶ *Sleep Pattern Disturbance R/T Dysfunctional Grieving*
▶ *Spiritual Distress R/T Dysfunctional Grieving*
▶ *Impaired Social Interactions R/T Dysfunctional Grieving*
▶ *Altered Family Processes R/T Dysfunctional Grieving*

The similarities in related diagnoses are not accidental. They occur because the person with either *Anticipatory Grieving* or *Dysfunctional Grieving is* grieving. Just how that grief is expressed is a highly individualized matter in dysfunctional grief, just as it is in normal grief. However, we can look for the presence of commonly agreed on signs and symptoms of normal grief and expect that, if they are present, they will be exaggerated, prolonged, or otherwise inappropriately displayed in the person with dysfunctional grief.

Anticipatory Grieving include verbalization of effective coping strategies and identification of support systems before the anticipated loss. For *Dysfunctional Grieving*, an appropriate outcome would be the verbalization of feelings about the death or the meaning of the loss.

Nursing Intervention

INTERVENTIONS FOR DYING CLIENTS

Once developed, the care plan serves as a guide to the nursing interventions for the dying client. Implementing

a plan of care will include connecting, empowering, finding meaning, and doing for.[64] In implementing a care plan, the nurse will be preserving the integrity of the client and of him- or herself.[64]

Connecting. Connecting means forming a bond with the client.[64] Connecting begins to occur as the nurse meets the client and assesses needs. It will be enhanced by the inclusion of the client and his or her family in all aspects of the nursing process. With the connecting comes trust that the nurse will meet needs in the best possible way. Connecting is essential for both the client and family to feel comfortable in the hospital setting. Establishing trust results from letting the client and family know what to expect, being timely with medications and answering requests, providing honest answers to questions, touching, and listening actively to concerns and fears. The presence of the nurse or the nurse's gentle hand on the client's shoulder can be comforting once the nurse has established a sense of connection with the dying individual and her or his family. Connecting can also be a source of satisfaction for the nurse.

Empowering. Empowering is assisting clients to find or build strengths within themselves.[64] Like connecting, empowering begins during the assessment phase when the nurse elicits the client's thoughts and then incorporates them into the plan. Giving information when the client is lacking it or has misinformation is an important way of empowering. This can include informing the client and family of hospital routine, giving them information about medication and treatments, and reinforcing medical information that they have received. In this way, the client can have the knowledge needed to make informed choices regarding care and, for the dying client, regarding how to live out his or her remaining life. Empowering for the physically debilitated client can mean something as simple as giving him or her a choice of the side to which he or she would like to be turned. Family members can be encouraged to keep the dying client involved in family matters by keeping the client informed of activities and consulting the client when decisions are made. For the bereaved, empowering can entail referral to outside support resources such as a widows group for a bereaved spouse or a bereaved parent group for parents who have lost a child. The information the nurse gives the client in the hospital about maintaining health and about procedures to be done at home empowers the client to be independent. Expressing confidence that the client is capable and encouraging him or her to try are also empowering activities done by the nurse. Assisting a dying parent to make a tape recording to leave for his or her children or to express special wishes to important others can be empowering acts by the nurse. Skillfully managing uncomfortable symptoms and pain can empower the client to attend to other needs.

Finding Meaning. Finding meaning means helping individuals make sense out of what is happening.[64] As O'Connor and colleagues[65] showed, finding meaning is an important spiritual activity for those dealing with life-threatening illness (see Chapter 53). Accepting feelings and helping the client to cope with feelings are supportive of finding meaning. If the person is having a difficult struggle with this, referral and consultation with clergy or a psychologist, as appropriate, can be useful. Sitting with the client, listening, and reflecting feelings being expressed are techniques the nurse can use to assist the client who is searching for meaning. The bereaved individual is also searching for the meaning of life without the lost loved one and will be supported too by these same kinds of activities.

Doing For. The term **doing for** refers to the provision of care and technological intervention. It is an integral part of supportive care and can help the client by being empowering, by helping to find meaning, and by being connecting.[64] Pain management, symptom control, and comfort measures are the major nursing activities for the dying client.

Pain Management. This starts with careful assessment and involves continuous ongoing assessment. Medications play an important role in the pain management program for the dying client. The nurse must be familiar with analgesics being administered, including their effects, side effects, and particular effects in a given individual. It is important for the nurse to know the onset, peak, and duration of analgesics being used in order to better evaluate the effectiveness of each dose of the medication regimen and the presence of breakthrough pain. If the nurse observes that pain relief is incomplete with the prescribed dose or that breakthrough pain (pain occurring between scheduled doses of pain medication) occurs, he or she needs to consult with the client's physician for a modification in the regimen. This is also true if the client experiences unpleasant sensations from a particular medication.

Administration of medication for pain control in the terminally ill individual is usually best done on a regular schedule rather than as occasion requires. It is much easier to maintain good pain control by preventing pain than by trying to reduce it once it occurs. This also relieves the client of watching the clock to see when she or he can ask for the next dose of pain medication. When narcotics are necessary for control of pain, fear of addiction is not a concern in the dying client. Many people receive inadequate pain control because they are afraid to take the medication necessary to relieve their pain or because care givers are afraid to give it to them. When the narcotic dose has been titrated to the most effective dose and then increased gradually as needed to maintain pain control, there is minimal risk of such untoward effects as respiratory depression.

As tolerance develops for the analgesic effect of the drug, so does tolerance for other effects. Therefore, the individual who is receiving a narcotic on a regular basis can tolerate dosages of the drug that cannot be tolerated by others.

For some clients, patient-controlled analgesia (PCA) is an effective method of pain control. This will require prescription and institutional approval and policy. Most PCA is delivered intravenously, but exactly when the dose is delivered is determined by the client, who has a button he or she can push when medication is needed. The device is programmed with the dose to be delivered and a lock-out time during which another dose cannot be delivered. The nurse must still continuously assess the effectiveness of the medication, dose, and interval with PCA.

To help manage pain, the nurse may also use nonpharmacologic techniques in conjunction with the medication regimen. For some clients, guided imagery and relaxation techniques are useful adjuncts in managing pain. Not all individuals are comfortable with these techniques, so the need for their implementation will be determined by the nursing assessment. The use of transcutaneous electrical nerve stimulation (TENS) is another method of nonpharmacologic pain control that is helpful for some individuals and gives them some control of their pain management. To achieve maximum relief, the client controls the amplitude and frequency of a small electrical current delivered through electrodes around the painful area. This will require a physician's order and is often set up by a physical therapist. The nurse supports the client in its use and assesses effectiveness in consultation with the physical therapist as needed. PCA, imagery, and TENS are not appropriate for everyone. An individual who does not wish control of his or her treatment regimen or who is unable to perform the techniques should not be burdened with unwanted responsibility. If an individual is using one of these techniques and his or her health declines, the nurse must be ready to institute other measures to maintain pain control.

Other Comfort Measures. As with pain, the nurse will be implementing measures to control other distressing symptoms. The nurse will implement and maintain a bowel routine to prevent constipation. Hydration must be maintained as long as possible. However, if intake of fluids is no longer possible and intravenous fluids are not desired, careful attention must be given to mouth care and to lubrication of the skin. The maintenance of skin integrity and comfort through meticulous skin care and gentle, well-supported positioning is essential to the implementation of effective care for the dying client. The nurse assists the client in maintaining as much activity as is comfortable while remembering that the focus is now on comfort and not maintenance of long-term function. If nausea is a problem, the nurse will implement measures to relieve and control it. These usually include administration of antiemetics, provision of foods and fluids that appeal to the client, and restructuring of activities to accommodate the individual's comfort. If the nausea is related to an intestinal obstruction, for which surgery or radiation is not going to be done, the insertion of a nasogastric tube to low suction may relieve the nausea by maintaining decompression of the stomach. Uncomfortable respiratory symptoms such as dyspnea may be relieved by positioning, oxygen administration, and suctioning secretions that the client is unable to clear on his or her own. The aches and discomforts of fever in the dying client can be relieved by acetaminophen even if the decision has been made not to treat an underlying infection if one exists. Finally, when death is imminent, implementation of nursing measures will include sitting quietly with the client and family, gently touching the client, and assisting the family to say their good-bys.

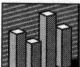

APPLYING RESEARCH TO NURSING PRACTICE

Helping Families Cope with Sudden Death in the Emergency Department

Mian, P. (1990) Sudden bereavement: nursing interventions in the ED. *Critical Care Nurse,* 10(1), 30–41.

▼▼▼

Unexpected death is a daily event in the emergency department. Meeting the special needs of bereaved family members requires special attention and structured intervention. Some emergency departments have therefore developed programs to support bereaved family members who are suddenly told their loved one has just died. In this article, Mian reported on the results of such a bereavement program, called Acute Grief Intervention, developed in a large metropolitan emergency department. The program consisted of a series of family nursing interventions by a designated nurse while the family member was undergoing emergency resuscitation. If the family member being resuscitated died unexpectedly, the nurse supported the family in a special grieving room, accompanied them to view the deceased, and returned with them to the grieving room to provide further emotional support. Mian telephoned 55 families 3 to 4 weeks after the death of their loved one to inquire how each family was managing. Mian also asked what supportive resources were available to the family and which nursing interventions they perceived as helpful. Twenty families reported that emotional support from staff, family, and friends was helpful. Sixteen of these families specifically cited the presence and caring of nurses as having been the most helpful. One third of the families reported having felt reassured that everything possible was being done to save the life of their loved one. Accurate information and honest answers to questions helped families understand what was happening to their loved one despite the hectic atmosphere of the emergency department. Twenty-nine per cent of families said that they had appreciated being able to view the loved one's body, to say good-by, and to perceive the reality of the death. Twenty-four per cent of the families said that they had valued privacy during the waiting period in the emergency department. Families also reported having appreciated being able to leave the hospital with personal items from the deceased, such as a wedding ring or a lock of hair.

Applications for Practice. Be sure to support grieving family members with privacy, information, active listening, and the opportunity to be with the deceased and take home some personal items.

INTERVENTIONS FOR GRIEVING FAMILIES

Nursing interventions for family members may focus on the diagnosis of *Anticipatory Grieving*. The loss or impending loss of a spouse or child can be particularly difficult for the family member. The nurse must remember that experiencing such loss can affect the family members' physical and psychologic well-being. Active listening and careful observation of family members and their interactions with the client are important nursing activities. Recall that the client and family may be at different points in the grieving process, which can lead to misunderstanding and confusion. An appropriate nursing intervention is to verbalize this observation to the family and client to enable them to understand the other's response better. Referral to appropriate support groups can be another helpful nursing intervention for grieving individuals. If the individual is ready, the nurse may help the person facing loss to begin to formulate a plan for his or her life after the loss, including the identification of resources. If the nurse observes family members neglecting their own health to stay with the dying client, the nurse may need to give them permission to take breaks from the bedside to attend to their own needs and to provide reassurance that the loved one will be well cared for in the family members' absence. Another intervention might involve assisting one family member to work out a plan with other family members and friends to stay with the client in shifts so that all may get adequate rest and nutrition. In some instances, referral to a psychologist, clergy, or social worker may be appropriate. Once again, one of the most powerful sources of comfort that the nurse can offer to the individual grieving a loss is a quiet, gentle presence.

POSTMORTEM CARE

After death, the care of the body will be the final nursing care measure to be implemented. The family may need some time with their loved one before the body is moved to the morgue. The nurse should facilitate this as needed. Postmortem care is done with respectful handling of the body. If the family wishes to participate in this care, they can be assisted to do so. The nurse needs to be aware of any defense mechanisms such as laughter, rough handling, and joking that can be particularly distressful to observers.

It is important to make the environment around the deceased as esthetically acceptable as possible for the family. If the client has died quietly and comfortably, this is not a difficult task. If there have been resuscitative efforts before the death, it will be necessary to remove equipment and clean any blood and secretions. Also the nurse should remove any tubing such as intravenous equipment, catheters, and the like. The body should be placed on clean bedding in a natural position and with absorbent pads placed under the body to absorb leakage of urine or feces, which can occur as sphincter muscles relax. The nurse needs to be aware that, on moving the body, the last bit of air in the lungs may be expelled and cause a sound like a sigh, which can be disconcerting to those present if they are not expecting it.

The best position is most often supine with arms at the side or folded across the chest. Eyes should be closed and dentures replaced if the jaw has not yet stiffened. If there is any resistance, leave the dentures for the mortician because forcing can leave marks that cannot be easily covered. The lower jaw should also be supported in a natural manner with a soft, folded towel under the chin. Do not tie the jaw closed with gauze because this too can leave disfiguring marks. The positioning needs to be done before the onset of **rigor mortis,** or stiffening of the dead body as a result of chemical changes occurring in the muscle protein. It is apparent first in the muscles of the jaw and progresses downward toward the legs. The feet are the last to be affected. Rigor mortis usually begins to appear 2 to 3 hours after death and is completed in 6 to 8 hours.

Another process that occurs after death is **livor mortis,** which is the appearance of purple blotches on dependent areas of the body 20 to 30 minutes after death and is caused by the effect of gravity on noncirculating blood. Place the client in the supine position promptly to prevent livor mortis on the face. A pillow placed under the head will promote drainage so the face will not become discolored. It also helps to give the appearance of comfort, and this can be helpful for family members.

Postmortem care done in a respectful and gentle manner is another method of providing comfort for the grieving family and can be a means of putting closure on the relationship for the nurse.

Finally, as mentioned earlier, the family may need gentle assistance in leaving their loved one and the hospital after death. This may include calling another family member to assist those who have been at the hospital to go home or perhaps walking to the hospital door with the family member with a gentle arm on the shoulder.

Evaluation

For the dying client, evaluation will center on how effectively nursing measures are at maintaining comfort. It can be helpful to the evaluation process to hold periodic team meetings at which the effectiveness of the care being given can be evaluated by those involved. Finally, it is important to make the client a partner in the evaluation because it is her or his comfort that is the goal of care.

Evaluation of care for individuals experiencing grief either from the loss of a loved one or loss of previous abilities will center on nursing measures that provide comfort, referral, and support to plan life in the face of the loss being experienced. It may not be possible to evaluate fully the outcomes of these interventions in the hospital setting because the resolution of grief is a long-term process. However, the nurse may evaluate the outcome of nursing intervention as successful when the individual anticipating loss verbalizes awareness that he or she is grieving the expected loss and begins to identify resources to assist in developing a plan to live with that loss or when a grieving family member expresses thoughts and feelings regarding his or her loss. Facing an important loss is a very difficult experience, but skilled and sensitive nursing care can make it a little less difficult.

CASE STUDY

The Client

Jay Benson's wife, Jean, a 28-year-old mother of two children 6 and 4 years of age, was admitted to the hospital 4 days ago when her pain could no longer be controlled at home. Mrs. Benson is being treated for a diagnosis of recurrent breast cancer for which she underwent a mastectomy and intensive chemotherapy last year. Despite treatment, the disease recurred and is now metastatic. Jean and Jay have been told that there is nothing more that can be done medically to stop the disease progress and that Jean has a life expectancy of months. Jean is emaciated and pale. Her sister and mother have been taking turns staying with her in the hospital while another sister is caring for the children at home. At the time of admission, a partial list of the physician's orders for Jean included the following:

▶ morphine, 8 mg sc, every 4 hours around the clock
▶ Percocet, 2 tablets, every 4 hours prn for breakthrough pain
▶ activity as tolerated
▶ regular diet as tolerated

At 1:00 PM, July 21, 48 hours after admission, a partial list of Jean's nursing assessment data included the following:

▶ 28-year-old emaciated female
▶ no longer diaphoretic when assisted out of bed

▶ moves freely
▶ no longer observed to moan when moving
▶ states movement is no longer painful and that she is able to find comfortable positions
▶ states that she seldom experiences pain between medication doses and that, if she does, the nurse gives her the prescribed prn dose, which prevents the pain from becoming severe
▶ B/P 136/82, P88 and regular, R22 and regular
▶ husband in to visit only 5 minutes per day since her admission
▶ has been observed watching the door during visiting hours
▶ at admission, husband stated that he could not stand the thought of losing his wife and did not know how he was going to manage with the children
▶ client's sister stated that the husband has been very tired looking recently and is irritable with the children
▶ husband gives work and child care responsibilities as reasons for short visits with client

Four days have passed since Jean's hospital admission. It is now July 23. The following represents part of a nursing care plan written on July 21, for Jay Benson, by the hospice nurse who was called in to follow the family and the evaluation of outcomes that were expected at that time.

CARE PLAN

1:00 PM, July 21

Nursing Diagnosis	Planning: Expected Outcomes	Implementation: Nursing Interventions	Evaluation
Anticipatory Grieving R/T potential loss of wife AEB client's avoidance of wife and display of signs of fatigue	By 1:00 PM, July 23: ▶ Verbalizes feelings about wife's impending death.	▶ In private setting, reflect observations of client's behavior to him and allow opportunity to express feelings.	7:00 PM, July 21 ▶ Client verbalized distress at the anticipated loss and said he had been avoiding her because of this. 5:30 PM, July 23 ▶ Client stated he had called the group and would be attending a meeting in 2 more days.
	▶ Contacts local support group.	▶ Provide name, address, and telephone number of local support group and encourage client to contact them.	

Care Plan continued on following page

CARE PLAN (Continued)

1:00 PM, July 21

Nursing Diagnosis	Planning: Expected Outcomes	Implementation: Nursing Interventions	Evaluation
	▶ Client and children visit. ▶ States he is resting adequately.	▶ Obtain administrative permission for children to visit daily. ▶ Inquire about client's sleep patterns. ▶ Explore routines that may assist with sleep.	▶ Client and children visited for 45 minutes. ▶ Client stated he is still unable to sleep more than 3 hours without waking.

Summary

▶ Grief and loss are an integral part of life.

▶ Loss, grief, mourning, and bereavement have overlapping definitions, but grief and mourning are generally considered to be the process of response to loss with mourning inclusive of cultural mores. Bereavement is the period of time over which the process unfolds.

▶ Loss can occur in several forms: personal, group, and multiple.

▶ Grief has been shown to have physiologic as well as psychologic effects. Bereavement is a time of increased health risk.

▶ Grief is viewed differently across different periods of the life span. Age is a factor influencing response to loss.

▶ Attitudes toward death and the expression of grief are heavily influenced by cultural mores and societal customs. Western culture tends to be death avoiding.

▶ The major theoretical framework for response to dying is Kübler-Ross's stages of death and dying.

▶ There are a number of grief theories. Most are stage theories, except for Martocchio's framework using clusters of typical responses rather than stages.

▶ Stage/phase theories run the risk of creating an expectation that all people will progress through stages in a sequential and predictable manner. Practice and research have shown that this is not necessarily the case.

▶ The nurse faces loss and grief both personally and professionally and must learn to deal with the associated feelings in a healthy manner. This means identifying personal feelings of grief, allowing the grieving process to occur, and providing for self-renewal.

▶ Because of the individuality of the responses to loss, and because the needs of the dying are many, varied, changing, and ongoing, nursing assessment is critical to planning comprehensive care for the individual client. Major areas of assessment for dying individuals are comfort and spiritual needs. Major areas of assessment for the family members are interactions among the family members and the client, stages of grief, and the possibility of asynchronous response.

▶ Many nursing diagnoses may be made for dying clients and for their families. *Anticipatory Grieving* and *Dysfunctional Grieving* are diagnoses specific to loss and grief.

▶ In planning care for the terminally ill client, comfort usually receives highest priority. In planning care for individuals facing bereavement, the priority might be the mobilization of social resources for support.

▶ Nursing interventions are individualized to the particular person and are focused on maintaining comfort and dignity for the client while providing support for the family.

▶ The outcomes of nursing interventions may be evaluated as successful when individuals anticipating a loss verbalize awareness of their grieving of the expected loss and identify resources to assist in developing a plan to live with the loss, or when individuals who have experienced a loss express thoughts and feelings regarding their loss.

Bibliography

1. Aber, C.S. (1992). Spousal death, a threat to women's health: paid work as a "resistance resource." *Image*, 24(2), 95–99.
2. Allan, J.D., & Hall, B.A. (1988). Between diagnosis and death: The case for studying grief before death. *Archives of Psychiatric Nursing*, 2(1), 30–34.
3. Andrianopoulos, G.D., & Flaherty, J.A. (1991). Bereavement: effects on immunity and risk of disease. In Plotnikoff, N., (eds.). *Stress and immunity*. Boca Raton, FL: CRC Press.
4. Averill, J. (1968). Grief: its nature and significance. *Psychological Bulletin*, 70, 721–748.
5. Baker, J.E., et al. (1992). Psychological tasks for bereaved children. *American Journal of Orthopsychiatry*, 62(1), 105–116.
6. Barrett, C.J., & Schneweis, K.M. (1980). An empirical search for stages of widowhood. *Omega*, 11(2), 97–104.
7. Benoliel, J.Q. (1985). Loss and adaptation: circumstances, contingencies, and consequences. *Death Studies*, 9, 217–233.
8. Bowlby, J. (1961). Process of mourning. *Journal of Psychoanalysis*, 42, 317–339.
9. Brock, A.M. (1984). From wife to widow: a changing lifestyle. *Journal of Gerontological Nursing*, 10(4), 8–15.

10. Carmack, B.J. (1992). Balancing engagement/detachment in AIDS-related multiple losses. *Image*, 24(1), 9–14.

11. Carter, S.L. (1989). Themes of grief. *Nursing Research*, 38(6), 354–358.

12. Clayton, P.J. (1990). Bereavement and depression. *Journal of Clinical Psychiatry*, 51, 30–40.

13. Cody, W.K. (1991). Grieving a personal loss. *Nursing Science Quarterly*, 4(2), 61–68.

14. Constantino, R.E. (1981). Bereavement crisis intervention for widows in grief and mourning. *Nursing Research*, 30(6), 351–353.

15. Cooley, M.E. (1992). Bereavement care: a role for nurses. *Cancer Nursing*, 15(2), 125–129.

16. Cowles, K.V., & Rodgers, B.L. (1991). The concept of grief: a foundation for nursing research and practice. *Research in Nursing and Health*, 14(2), 110–127.

17. Davidhizar, R., & Ciger, J.N. (1991). When the nurse faces separation and loss. *Advances in Clinical Care*, 8(5), 10–21.

18. Demi, A.S., & Miles, M.S. (1985). Parameters of normal grief: a Delphi study.

19. Dimond, M. (1981). Bereavement and the elderly: a critical review with implications for nursing practice and research. *Journal of Advanced Nursing*, 6, 461–470.

20. Donovan, M.I., & Pierce, S.G. (1976). *Cancer care nursing*. New York: Appleton-Century-Crofts.

21. Downey, A.M. (1983). Living, loving, and losing: implications for health and well-being. *Health Values: Achieving High Level Wellness*, 7(1), 7–14.

22. Engel, G.L. (1964). Grief and grieving. *American Journal of Nursing*, 64, 93–98.

23. Erikson, E.H., et al. (1986). *Vital involvement in old age*. New York: W.W. Norton.

24. Erickson, R.C., & Hyerstay, B.J. (1980). The dying patient and the double-bind hypothesis. In Faush, R.A. (ed.). *Death, dying and transcending*. Farmingdale, NY: Baywood Publishing.

25. Feifel, H. (ed.). (1959). *The meaning of death*. New York: McGraw-Hill.

26. Fisher, M. (1991). Can grief be turned into growth? Staff grief in palliative care. *Professional Nurse*, 7(3), 178–182.

27. Fitzpatrick, J.J., et al. (1980). Experience of time during the crisis of cancer. *Cancer Nursing*, 3, 191–194.

28. Garfield, C.A. (1979). *Stress and survival: The emotional realities of life-threatening illness*. St. Louis: C.V. Mosby.

29. Glaser, B.G., & Strauss, A.L. (1965). *Awareness of dying*. Chicago: Aldine.

30. Glaser, B.G., & Strauss, A.L. (1968). *Time for dying*. Chicago: Aldine.

31. Glick, L.O., et al. (1974). *The first year of bereavement*. New York: Wiley.

32. Goodman, M., et al. (1991). Cultural differences among elderly women in coping with the death of an adult child. *Journal of Gerontology*, 46(6), 8321–8329.

33. Grassman, D. (1992). Turning personal grief into personal growth. *Nursing*, 22(4), 43–47.

34. Hall, B.A. (1990). The struggle of the diagnosed terminally ill person to maintain hope. *Nursing Science Quarterly*, 3(4), 177–184.

35. Hauser, M.J. (1983). Bereavement outcomes for widows. *Journal of Psychiatric Nursing and Mental Health Services*, 2(9), 22–31.

36. Hegge, M. (1991). A qualitative retrospective study of coping strategies of newly widowed elderly. Effects of anticipatory grieving on the caregiver. *American Journal of Hospice Palliative Care*, 8(4), 28–34.

37. Hinton, J.M. (1963). The physical and mental distress of dying. *Quarterly Journal of Medicine*, 32, 1–21.

38. Hoagland, A.C. (1983). Bereavement and personal constructs: old theories and new concepts. *Death Education*, 7(2/3), 175–193.

39. Hogan, N.S., & Balk, D.E. (1990). Adolescent reactions to sibling death: perceptions of mothers, fathers, and teenagers. *Nursing Research*, 39(2), 103–106.

40. Houseman, C., & Pheifer, W.G. (1988). Potential for unresolved grief in survivors of persons with AIDS. *Archives of Psychiatric Nursing*, 2(5), 296–301.

41. Jacob, S.R. (1991). Preholiday grief. *Journal of Psychosocial Nursing and Mental Health Services*, 29(11), 20–24.

42. Jacobs, S., & Douglas, L. (1979). Grief: mediating process between loss and illness. *Comprehensive Psychiatry*, 20(2), 165–176.

43. Kalish, R.A. (1980). *Caring relationships: The dying and the bereaved*. Farmingdale, NY: Baywood Publishing.

44. Kalish, R.A. (1980). *Death and dying: Views from many cultures*. Farmingdale, NY: Baywood Publishing.

45. Kalish, R.A., & Reynolds, D.K. (1976). *Death and ethnicity*. Los Angeles: University of Southern California Press.

46. Kastenbaum, R.J. (1981). *Death, society, and human experience*. Columbus, OH: Charles E. Merrill.

47. Kastenbaum, R.J., & Aisenberg, R.B. (1972). *The psychology of death*. New York: Springer.

48. Klass, D. (1987). John Bowlby's model of grief and the problem of identification. *Omega*, 18(1), 13–31.

49. Klein, R. (1971). A crisis to grow on. *Cancer*, 6, 1660–1664.

50. Kraus, A.S., & Lillienfield, A.M. (1968). Some epidemiologic aspects of the high mortality rate in the young widowed group. *Journal of Chronic Disease*, 10, 207–217.

51. Kübler-Ross, E. (1969). *On death and dying*. Englewood Cliffs, NJ: Prentice Hall.

52. Kübler-Ross, E. (1975). *Death: The final stage of growth*. Englewood Cliffs, NJ: Prentice Hall.

53. Lev, C.L. (1991). Dealing with loss: Concerns of patients and families in a hospice setting. *Clinical Nurse Specialist*, 5(2), 87–93.

54. Lindemann, E. (1944). Symptomatology and management of acute grief. *American Journal of Psychiatry*, 10, 141–148.

55. Maddison, D., & Agnes, V. (1968). The health of widows in the year following bereavement. *Journal of Psychosomatic Research*, 12, 297–306.

56. Martocchio, B.C. (1985). Grief and bereavement: health through hurt. *Nursing Clinics of North America*, 20(2), 327–341.

57. Miles, M.S. (1985). Emotional symptoms and physical health in bereaved parents. *Nursing Research*, 34(2), 76–81.

58. Miles, M.S. (1985). Helping adults mourn the death of a child. In Scipien, G. M., & Barnard, M.U. (eds.). *Issues in comprehensive pediatric nursing*. Washington, DC: Hemisphere.

59. Miles, M.S., & Demi, A.S. (1991). Historical and contemporary theories of grief. In Corless, I., Germino, B., & Pittman-Lindeman, M. (eds.). *Dying, death, and bereavement*.

60. Murphy, S.A. (1983). Theoretical perspectives on bereavement. In Chinn, P.L. (ed.). *Advances in nursing theory development* (pp. 191–203). Rockville, MD: Aspen Systems.

61. Murphy, S.A. (1988). Mental distress and recovery in a high-risk sample three years after untimely death. *Nursing Research*, 37(1), 30–35.

62. Neugarten, B.L. (1968). *Middle age and aging*. Chicago: University of Chicago Press.

63. North American Nursing Diagnosis Association. (1992). NANDA nursing diagnoses: Definitions and classifications 1992. St. Louis: Author.

64. O'Berle, K., & Davies, B. (1992). Support and caring: exploring the concepts. *Oncology Nursing Forum*, 19(19), 763–767.

65. O'Connor, et al. (1990). Understanding the cancer patient's search for meaning. *Cancer Nursing*, 13(3), 167–175.

66. Osterweis, M., et al. (eds.). (1984). *Bereavement: Reactions, consequences, and care*. Washington, DC: National Academy Press.

67. Owen, G., et al. (1982–1983). Death at a distance: a study of family survivors. *Omega*, 18(3), 191–226.

68. Parkes, C.M. (1979). *Bereavement: Studies of grief in adult life*. Madison, CT: International Universities Press.

69. Parkes, C.M. (1985). Bereavement. *British Journal of Psychiatry*, 146, 11–17.

70. Parkes, C.M. (1987–1988). Bereavement. *Omega*, 18(4), 365–375.

71. Parkes, C.M., & Brow, R.J. (1972). Health after bereavement. *Psychosomatic Medicine*, 34(5), 449–460.

72. Pattison, E.M. (1977). *The experience of dying*. Englewood Cliffs, NJ: Prentice Hall.

73. Pollock, G.H. (1961). Mourning and adaptation. *Journal of Psychoanalysis*, 42, 317–339.

74. Pollock, G.H. (1962). On death, time and immortality. *Psychoanalytic Quarterly*, 40, 435–446.
75. Quint, J.C. (1966). Obstacles to helping the dying. *American Journal of Nursing*, 66(7), 1568–1571.
76. Raleigh, E.D.H. (1992). Sources of hope in chronic illness. *Oncology Nursing Forum*, 19(3), 443–448.
77. Raphael, B. (1983). *The anatomy of bereavement*. New York: Basic Books.
78. Repetti, R.L. (1992). Social withdrawal as a coping response. In Friedman, H. S. (ed.). *Hostility, coping, and health*. Washington, DC: American Psychological Association.
79. Rushton, C.H. (1992). Care-giver suffering in critical care nursing. *Heart and Lung*, 21(3), 303–306.
80. Sanders, C.M. (1979–1980). A comparison of adult bereavement in the death of a spouse, child, and parent. *Omega*, 10(4), 303–320.
81. Schneidman, E.S. (1984). *Death: Current perspectives*. Los Angeles: Mayfield Publishing.
82. Schuchter, S.R. (1986). *Dimensions of grief: Adjusting to the death of a spouse*. San Francisco: Jossey-Bass.
83. Shanfield, S.B. (1981). Illness and bereavement: unrecognized implications for prevention. *Arizona Medicine*, 38(6), 444–446.
84. Shanfield, S.B., et al. (1984). Parents' reactions to the death of an adult child from cancer. *American Journal of Psychiatry*, 141(9), 1092–1094.
85. Sheehy, G. (1976). *Passages: Predictable crises of adult life*. New York: E.P. Dutton.
86. Small, M., et al. (1991). Saying goodbye in the intensive care unit: helping caregivers grieve. *Pediatric Nursing*, 17(1), 103–105.
87. Smesler, N.J., & Erikson, E.H. (1980). *Themes of work and love in adulthood*. Cambridge, MA: Harvard University Press.
88. Sowell, R.L., et al. (1991). The lived experience of survival and bereavement following the death of a lover from AIDS. *Image: Journal of Nursing Scholarship*, 23(2), 89–94.
89. Stein, M. (1985). Bereavement, depression, and immunity. In Guillemin, R., et al. (eds.). *Neural modulation of immunity*. New York: Raven Press.
90. Stevens-Long, J. (1979). *Adult life developmental processes*. Los Angeles: Mayfield Publishing.
91. Taptich, B.J., et al. (1989). *Nursing diagnosis and care planning*. Philadelphia: W.B. Saunders.
92. Teel, O.S. (1991). Chronic sorrow: analysis of the concept. *Journal of Advanced Nursing*, 10(11), 1311–1320.
93. Ufema, J. (1990). AIDS: time to grieve. *Nursing*, 20(11), 90.
94. Vachon, M.L.S., et al. (1982). Correlates of enduring distress patterns follow bereavement: social network, life situation, and personality. *Psychological Medicine*, 12, 783–788.
95. Weisman, A.D. (1972). *On dying and denying*. New York: Behavioral Publications.
96. Weisman, A.D. (1974). *The realization of death*. New York: Jacob Aronson.
97. Weisman, A.D. (1979). *Coping with cancer*. New York: McGraw-Hill.
98. Weisman, A.D. (1986). *The coping capacity: On the nature of being mortal*. New York: Human Sciences Press.
99. Weisman, A.D., & Worden, J.W. (1976). The existential plight in cancer: significance of the first 100 days. *International Journal of Psychiatry in Medicine*, 7(1), 1–15.
100. Worden, J.W. (1982). *Grief counseling and grief therapy*. New York: Springer.
101. Wortman, C.B., et al. (1992). Stress, coping, and health: conceptual issues and directions for future research. In Friedman, H.S. (ed.). *Hostility, coping, and health*. Washington, DC: American Psychological Association.
102. Yalom, I.D., & Lieberman, M.A. (1991). Bereavement and heightened existential awareness. *Psychiatry*, 54(4), 334–345.
103. Zisook, S., & Shuchter, S.R. (1991). Early psychological reaction to the stress of widowhood. *Psychiatry*, 54(4), 320–333.

Appendix 1

▼ *Universal Precautions*

Universal precautions are intended to prevent parenteral, mucous membrane, and nonintact skin exposures of health care workers to blood-borne pathogens. Universal precautions apply to blood and to other body fluids containing visible blood, semen, vaginal secretions, cerebrospinal fluid, synovial fluid, pleural fluid, peritoneal fluid, pericardial fluid, and amniotic fluid. Universal precautions do not apply to feces, nasal secretions, sputum, sweat, tears, urine, and vomitus unless they contain visible blood.

Barrier Guidelines

1. Disposable gloves (vinyl, latex) should be worn when in contact or when there is potential for contact with blood, body fluids, or other fluids that may contain human immunodeficiency virus (HIV). Gloves should be removed after each client contact. Rubber gloves can be used for equipment cleaning.
2. Hands should be washed between clients, after any exposure, and after removal of gloves.
3. Protective eyewear, face shields, and/or masks should be worn during procedures that may aerosolize blood.

4. Impervious gowns should be worn when there is potential for exposure to large quantities of blood, such as in the labor and delivery area or emergency room.

Needle Precautions

1. Needles should never be recapped after use; keep in mind that most needlesticks are the result of missed needle recapping.
2. Do not cut, break, or bend needles after use; this may release aerosolized blood from the needle shaft.
3. Do not leave used needles lying around.
4. Do not dispose of needles in ordinary receptacles; instead, use appropriately labeled, impermeable needle containers.

Adapted from the Centers for Disease Control (1988). Update: Universal precautions for prevention of transmission of human immunodeficiency virus, hepatitis B virus, and other bloodborne pathogens in health-care setting. *Morbidity and Mortality Weekly Report, 37*(3), 377–388.

Appendix 2

▼ *American Nurses' Association*
Standards of Clinical Nursing Practice

STANDARDS OF CARE

Standard I. Assessment

THE NURSE COLLECTS CLIENT HEALTH DATA.

Standard II. Diagnosis

THE NURSE ANALYZES THE ASSESSMENT DATA IN DETERMINING DIAGNOSES.

Standard III. Outcome Identification

THE NURSE IDENTIFIES EXPECTED OUTCOMES INDIVIDUALIZED TO THE CLIENT.

Standard IV. Planning

THE NURSE DEVELOPS A PLAN OF CARE THAT PRESCRIBES INTERVENTIONS TO ATTAIN EXPECTED OUTCOMES.

Standard V. Implementation

THE NURSE IMPLEMENTS THE INTERVENTIONS IDENTIFIED IN THE PLAN OF CARE.

Standard VI. Evaluation

THE NURSE EVALUATES THE CLIENT'S PROGRESS TOWARD ATTAINMENT OF OUTCOMES.

STANDARDS OF PROFESSIONAL PERFORMANCE

Standard I. Quality of Care

THE NURSE SYSTEMATICALLY EVALUATES THE QUALITY AND
EFFECTIVENESS OF NURSING PRACTICE.

Standard II. Performance Appraisal

THE NURSE EVALUATES HIS/HER OWN NURSING PRACTICE IN
RELATION TO PROFESSIONAL PRACTICE STANDARDS AND
RELEVANT STATUTES AND REGULATIONS.

Standard III. Education

THE NURSE ACQUIRES AND MAINTAINS CURRENT KNOWLEDGE IN
NURSING PRACTICE.

Standard IV. Collegiality

THE NURSE CONTRIBUTES TO THE PROFESSIONAL DEVELOPMENT
OF PEERS, COLLEAGUES, AND OTHERS.

Standard V. Ethics

THE NURSE'S DECISIONS AND ACTIONS ON BEHALF OF CLIENTS
ARE DETERMINED IN AN ETHICAL MANNER.

Standard VI. Collaboration

THE NURSE COLLABORATES WITH THE CLIENT, SIGNIFICANT
OTHERS, AND HEALTH CARE PROVIDERS IN PROVIDING CLIENT
CARE.

Standard VII. Research

THE NURSE USES RESEARCH FINDINGS IN PRACTICE.

Standard VIII. Resource Utilization

THE NURSE CONSIDERS FACTORS RELATED TO SAFETY,
EFFECTIVENESS, AND COST IN PLANNING AND DELIVERING CLIENT
CARE.

Appendix 3

▼ *Nursing's Agenda for Health Care Reform*

▼ EXECUTIVE SUMMARY

America's nurses have long supported our nation's efforts to create a health care system that assures access, quality, and services at affordable costs. This document presents nursing's agenda for immediate health care reform. We call for a basic "core" of essential health care services to be available to everyone. We call for a restructured health care system that will focus on the consumers and their health, with services to be delivered in familiar, convenient sites, such as schools, workplaces, and homes. We call for a shift from the predominant focus on illness and cure to an orientation toward wellness and care.

The basic components of nursing's "core of care" include:

▶ A restructured health care system which:
—enhances consumer access to services by delivering primary health care in community-based settings.
—fosters consumer responsibility for personal health, self-care, and informed decision making in selecting health care services.
—facilitates utilization of the most cost-effective providers and therapeutic options in the most appropriate settings.

▶ A federally defined standard package of essential health care services available to all citizens and residents of the United States, provided and financed through an integration of public and private plans and sources:
—A public plan, based on federal guidelines and eligibility requirements, will provide coverage for the poor and create the opportunity for small businesses and individuals, particularly those at risk because of preexisting conditions and those potentially medically indigent, to buy into the plan.
—A private plan will offer, at a minimum, the nationally standardized package of essential services. This standard package could be enriched as a benefit of employment or individuals could purchase additional services if they so choose. If employers do

not offer private coverage, they must pay into the public plan for their employees.

▶ A phase-in of essential services, in order to be fiscally responsible:
—Coverage of pregnant women and children is critical. This first step represents a cost-effective investment in the future health and prosperity of the nation.
—One early step will be to design services specifically to assist vulnerable populations who have had limited access to our nation's health care system. A "Healthstart Plan" is proposed to improve the health status of these individuals.

▶ Planned change to anticipate health service needs that correlate with changing national demographics.

▶ Steps to reduce health care costs include:
—required usage of managed care in the public plan and encouraged in private plans.
—incentives for consumers and providers to utilize managed care arrangements.
—controlled growth of the health care system through planning and prudent resource allocation.
—incentives for consumers and providers to be more cost-efficient in exercising health care options.
—development of health care policies based on effectiveness and outcomes research.
—assurance of direct access to a full range of qualified providers.
—elimination of unnecessary bureaucratic controls and administrative procedures.

▶ Case management will be required for those with continuing health care needs. Case management will reduce the fragmentation of the present system, promote consumers' active participation in decisions about their health, and create an advocate on their behalf.

▶ Provisions for long-term care, which include:
—public and private funding for services of short duration to prevent personal impoverishment.
—public funding for extended care if consumer resources are exhausted.
—emphasis on the consumers' responsibility to plan financially for their long-term care needs, including

new personal financial alternatives and strengthened private insurance arrangements.

▶ Insurance reforms to assure improved access to coverage, including affordable premiums, reinsurance pools for catastrophic coverage, and other steps to protect both insurers and individuals against excessive costs.

▶ Access to services assured by no payment at the point of service and elimination of balance billing in both public and private plans.

▶ Establishment of public/private sector review—operating under federal guidelines and including payers, providers, and consumers—to determine resource allocation, cost reduction approaches, allowable insurance premiums, and fair and consistent reimbursement levels for providers. This review would progress in a climate sensitive to ethical issues.

Additional resources will be required to accomplish this plan. While significant dollars can be obtained through restructuring and other strategies, responsibility for any new funds must be shared by individuals, employers, and government, phased in over several years to minimize the impact.

▼ NURSING'S AGENDA FOR HEALTH CARE REFORM

Nurses provide a unique perspective on the health care system. Our constant presence in a variety of settings places us in contact with individuals who reap the benefits of the system's most sophisticated services, as well as those individuals seriously compromised by the system's inefficiencies.

More and more, nurses observe the effects of inadequate services and of the declining quality of care on the nation's health. Firsthand experience tells us that the time has come for change. Patchwork approaches to health care reform have not worked. While preserving the best elements of the existing system, we must build a new foundation for health care in America. It is this realization that drives *Nursing's Agenda for Health Care Reform.*

Nursing's plan for reform converts a system that focuses on the costly treatment of illness to a system that emphasizes primary health care services and the promotion, restoration, and maintenance of health. It increases the consumer's responsibility and role in health care decision making and focuses on partnerships between consumers and providers. It sets forth new delivery arrangements that make health care a more vital part of individual and community life. And it ensures that health services are appropriate, effective, cost efficient, and focused on consumer needs.

▼ A Health Care System in Crisis

The strengths and weaknesses of our nation's health care system are well documented. Every day, many Americans profit from the system's technological excellence, extensive medical research, well-educated health professionals, diverse range of providers, and myriad of facilities. Millions of people live longer lives because of the care they receive.

But America's health care system is also very costly, its quality inconsistent, and its benefits unequally distributed. Although the system provides highly sophisticated care to many, millions of Americans must overcome enormous obstacles to get even the most elementary services. In short, health care is neither fairly nor equitably delivered to all segments of the population.

As caregivers in a diversity of settings, responsible for providing care and coordinating health care services 24 hours a day, nurses clearly understand the implications of the system's failings. The more than 2 million nurses in America are at the front lines—in hospitals, nursing homes, schools, home health agencies, workplaces, community clinics, and managed care programs. And what nurses see are the alarming effects of a system that has lost touch with the communities it is supposed to serve:

▶ More and more people must overcome major barriers to gain access to even the most elementary services.

▶ Too many Americans receive treatment too late because they live in inner cities or in urban or rural areas where service levels are inadequate.

▶ People enter hospitals daily in advanced stages of illness, suffering from problems that could have been treated in less costly settings or avoided altogether with adequate disease prevention and health promotion services.

▶ The lack of access to prenatal care contributes to an alarming number of infant deaths and low birthweights each year.

▶ Obstacles to obtaining fundamental services, such as childhood immunizations, are largely responsible for a resurgence in preventable diseases.

▶ Disproportionate amounts of resources are used for expensive medical interventions, which all too often provide neither comfort nor cure.

▶ Every year, expensive nursing home care impoverishes an alarming number of residents and their families.

Major changes in the health care system can no longer be put on hold. Further analysis and investigation will neither change the facts nor diminish the problems.

Today, more than 60 million Americans are either uninsured or underinsured. This fact alone cries out for health care reform. Now, the system's inability to contain costs is placing more and more Americans with "adequate" insurance coverage at risk of hardship when major illnesses do occur. Employers and employees alike are desperately seeking solutions to the dual problems of rising health care costs and increased premium rates that threaten basic coverage for most American workers and their dependents.

Americans cannot afford to sit idly and do nothing. Health care costs are approaching 12 per cent of the gross national product (GNP). Health care is expected to cost over $756 billion in 1991.[1] If nothing is done to control expenditures, health care spending is expected to reach $1.2 to $1.3 trillion by 1995—an increase of some $500 billion in less than 5 years. At this rate, if the system remains unchanged, spending will reach between $2.1 and $2.7 trillion by the year 2000.[2]

▼ The Framework for Change

Nurses strongly believe that the health care system must be restructured, reoriented, and decentralized in order to guarantee access to services, contain costs, and ensure quality care. Our plan—the product of consensus building within organized nursing—is designed to achieve this goal. It provides central control in the form of federal minimum standards for essential services and federally defined eligibility requirements. At the same time, it makes allowances for decentralized decision making that will permit local areas to develop specific programs and arrangements best suited to consumer needs.

Nursing's plan is built around several basic premises, including the following:

▶ All citizens and residents of the United States must have equitable access to essential health care services (a core of care).

▶ Primary health care services must play a very basic and prominent role in service delivery.

▶ Consumers must be the central focus of the health care system. Assessment of health care needs must be the determining factor in the ultimate structuring and delivery of programs and services.

▶ Consumers must be guaranteed direct access to a full range of qualified health care providers who offer their services in a variety of delivery arrangements at sites which are accessible, convenient, and familiar to the consumer.

▶ Consumers must assume more responsibility for their own care and become better informed about the range of providers and the potential options for services. Working in partnership with providers, consumers must actively participate in choices that best meet their needs.

▶ Health care services must be restructured to create a better balance between the prevailing orientation toward illness and cure and a new commitment to wellness and care.

▶ The health care system must assure that appropriate, effective care is delivered through the efficient use of resources.

▶ A standardized package of essential health care services must be provided and financed through an integration of public and private plans and sources.

▶ Mechanisms must be implemented to protect against catastrophic costs and impoverishment.

The cornerstone of nursing's plan for reform is the delivery of primary health care services to households and individuals in convenient, familiar places. If health is to be a true national priority, it is logical to provide services in the places where people work and live. Maximizing the use of these sites can help eliminate the fragmentation and lack of coordination that have come to characterize the existing health care system. It can also promote a more "consumer friendly" system in which services such as health education, screening, immunizations, well-child care, and prenatal care would be readily accessible.

At the same time, consumers must be the focus of the health care system. Individuals must be given incentives to assume more responsibility for their health. They must develop both the motivation and capability to be more prudent buyers of health services. Promotion of healthy lifestyles and better informed consumer decisions can contribute to effective and economical health care delivery.

Finally, in implementing reforms, attention must be directed to the unique needs of special population groups whose health care needs have been neglected. These individuals include children, pregnant women, and vulnerable groups such as the poor, minorities, AIDS victims, and those who have difficulty securing insurance because of preexisting conditions. Lack of preventive and primary care for this sector has cost the nation enormously—both in terms of lives lost or impaired and dollars spent to treat problems that could have been avoided or treated less expensively through appropriate intervention.

Access to care alone may not be sufficient to resolve the problems of these vulnerable groups. For those individuals whose health has been seriously compromised, a "catch up" program characterized by enriched services is justified. Coverage of pregnant women and children is critical. This first step represents a cost-effective investment in the future health and prosperity of the nation.

It is this set of values that distinguishes nursing's plan from other proposals and offers a realistic approach to health care reform.

▼ A Plan for Reform

Nursing's plan for health care reform builds a new foundation for health care in America. It shifts the emphasis of the health care system from illness and cure to wellness and care. While preserving key components of the existing system, it sets forth new strategies for guaranteeing universal coverage; making health care a more vital part of community life; and ensuring that the health care services provided are appropriate, effective, and cost efficient.

The following pages provide a general overview of nursing's vision for a better health care system.

UNIVERSAL ACCESS TO A STANDARD PACKAGE OF ESSENTIAL SERVICES

Nursing's plan envisions a new and bold approach to universal access to a standard package of essential health care services and the manner in which these services are delivered.

The federal government will delineate the essential services (core of care) that must be provided to all U.S. citizens and residents. This standard package will include defined levels of:

▶ Primary health care services, hospital care, emergency treatment, inpatient and outpatient professional services, and home care services.
▶ Prevention services, including prenatal and perinatal care; infant and well-child care; school-based disease prevention programs; speech therapy, hearing, dental, and eye care for children up to age 18; screening procedures; and other preventive services with proved effectiveness.
▶ Prescription drugs, medical supplies and equipment, and laboratory and radiology services.
▶ Mental health services and substance abuse treatment and rehabilitation.
▶ Hospice care.
▶ Long-term care services of relatively short duration.
▶ Restorative services determined to be essential to the prevention of long-term institutionalization.

By taking this approach, traditional illness services are balanced with provisions for health maintenance services that prevent illness, reduce cost, and avoid institutionalization. Thus, hospital services and emergency care are covered, as are such services as immunizations, physical examinations, and prenatal and perinatal care.

The creation of federal minimum standards for essential services will necessitate modifications in existing public programs. The ultimate goal will be, over time, to merge all government-sponsored health programs into a single public program.

Coverage Options

Universal coverage for the federally defined package of essential services will be accessed through an integration of public and private plans and resources.

▶ A public plan, administered by the states, will provide coverage for the poor (those below 200 per cent of the federal poverty level), high-risk populations, and the potentially medically indigent. Any employers or individuals will also have the option of buying into this plan as their source of coverage.
▶ Private plans (employment-based health benefit programs and commercial health insurance) will be required to offer, at a minimum, the nationally standardized package of essential services. This package could be enriched as a benefit of employment, or individuals could purchase additional services from commercial insurers if they so choose.

All citizens and residents will be required to be covered by one of these options. Under both the public plan and private plans, no one will be denied insurance because of preexisting conditions. If employers do not offer private coverage, they will be required to pay into the public plan for their employees. Employer payments will be actuarially equivalent to the costs of employee and dependent coverage. Financial relief will be made available to small businesses (25 employees or less) for whom this provision would not be feasible. Individuals with no source of private coverage could also buy into the public plan. To assure universal access to essential services, systems will be developed to identify the insurance option through which each individual's needs are met.

Premiums and Payment Rates

Access to health care services will be enhanced by offering insurance premiums that the public can afford and payment rates to providers that are equitable and inclusive.

Both the public and private plans will utilize deductibles and copayments to ensure that beneficiaries continue to pay for a portion of their own care and, therefore, have financial incentives to be economical in their use of services. Deductible amounts and copayment rates, however, will never serve as barriers to care. Provisions will be made to waive or subsidize deductions and copayments for households with incomes below 200 per cent of the federal poverty level. Deductibles for certain types of programs and services (e.g., health promotion, such as well-child care, immunizations, and mammograms; and managed care plans) will be held to a minimum to encourage wider use of cost-efficient, wellness-oriented options.

Public and private payers will be required to offer fair and consistent rates of payment to providers. To protect access to care, providers will not seek payment at the point of service; nor will they be permitted to engage in balance billing. Because providers will be reimbursed fairly through insurance and the problems of uncompensated care will be largely eliminated, there will be no need for providers to charge consumers amounts above the established rate. Consequently, the consumer's financial responsibility for health care services will be more predictable.

To make insurance more affordable to individuals and to reduce costs to insurers and employers, nursing's plan calls for reforms in the private insurance market. These reforms may encompass a variety of strategies, including:

▶ Community rating for all insurers.
▶ A cap on the out-of-pocket expenses individuals must pay for catastrophic care, including nursing home and other long-term care.
▶ State reinsurance pools to protect insurers and consumers against the high costs of insuring a broader range of patients.

Special Programs for Vulnerable Groups

Countless individuals suffer from long-term health problems associated with inadequate access to basic health services over time. Often, the poor and many members of minority groups are in this category. Special programs will provide services and outreach to vulnerable populations in order to compensate for formerly inadequate care and its consequences.

For infants and children (e.g., low birthweight babies, battered and neglected children, pregnant teenagers, children who abuse drugs, and young victims of violence and homelessness), such programming could be viewed as a health service ("Healthstart") equivalent to the Headstart Program for those who are educationally disadvantaged. An expanded version of the Women's, Infants and Children (WIC) Program may be needed to produce quality outcomes in maternal-child health for poor and minority populations. Other special population groups also may warrant compensatory health programs beyond the scope of essential health benefits and services.

It is important to note that the ultimate goal of improved health is not achievable exclusively within the confines of the health sector. Social failures also have serious health consequences. Improvements in the broader environment have a major impact on health status and health care costs. While the focus of this plan is on the health care system, nursing's long-term policy agenda for the nation is much broader. National health reform must also consider the interrelationships between health and such factors as education, behavior, income, housing and sanitation, social support networks, and attitudes about health. Better health cannot be the nation's only goal when hunger, crime, drugs, and other social problems remain. Consequently, nursing is committed to pursuing reform in other areas affecting health. Discussion of such reform, however, is beyond the scope of this paper.

Long-Term Care

The high costs of long-term care often threaten to impoverish patients and their families. Nursing's plan seeks to prevent impoverishment and the potential loss of dignity by recognizing both public responsibility for long-term care and continued personal commitment to planning for such care. Financing arrangements will provide "front-end" coverage for chronic care and long-term care services of short duration through a variety of public and private options.

Beyond addressing short-term needs, individuals will be expected to assume personal responsibility for long-term care through strengthened private insurance programs and a variety of innovative financing arrangements. Such strategies will include privately purchased long-term care insurance, new savings and tax incentives, and home equity conversion opportunities. Such steps are essential to prevent individuals and their families from becoming impoverished by necessary care that can be anticipated and planned for. Emphasis on personal responsibility, however, does not ignore the fact that there will always be some individuals who will be left without resources and who must reach out for public assistance.

Catastrophic Expenses

Length and/or intensity of illness may generate catastrophic costs. Given this fact, limits will be placed on individuals' out-of-pocket payments for catastrophic health care expenses. Costs to insurers or individuals that exceed preset limits will be covered through a state reinsurance pool, to which all insurers must contribute. Under nursing's plan, insurers will tap into the pool when their total costs or costs per patient exceed preset limits. When costs decline, they will resume normal financing.

Decentralized Delivery System

Although standards for essential health services and eligibility requirements are to be mandated at the federal level, delivery mechanisms for health services will be decentralized in terms of planning and administration to foster greater consumer orientation. Because local needs differ, states will have the authority to modify implementation in order to reflect geographical diversity.

To promote greater use of disease prevention and primary health care, services will be delivered, whenever possible, in convenient, familiar sites readily accessible to households and individuals. Maximizing the use of local settings, including schools, homes, places of work, and other community facilities, will help reduce the fragmentation of primary health care delivery and promote a more consumer-friendly system.

COST-EFFECTIVE, QUALITY CARE

By properly balancing individual health needs and self-care responsibilities with provider capabilities, care can be provided in a more efficient and coordinated manner. It can be more effectively directed at health promotion activities that will ultimately improve outcomes and reduce costs. Nursing's plan for reform is designed to achieve such a balance.

Provider Availability

Financial and regulatory obstacles, as well as institutional barriers, that deny consumer access to all qualified health professionals will be removed. The wider use of a range of qualified health professionals will increase access to care, particularly in understaffed specialties, such as primary health care, and in underserved urban and rural geographical areas. It will also facilitate selection of the most cost-effective option for care.

Under this arrangement, health providers must be reasonably and fairly compensated for their services. Where fee-for-service payment arrangements continue, payments for patient services must be made directly to providers.

Consumer Involvement

Consumers will be encouraged to assume more responsibility for their own health. Health professionals will work in partnership with consumers to evaluate the full range of their needs and available services. Together, the consumer and the health professional will determine a course of action that is based on an understanding of the effectiveness of treatment.

Outcome and Effectiveness Measures

Development of multidisciplinary clinical practice guidelines is essential to the proper functioning of the health care system. These guidelines will be used to sensitize providers and others to the proved effectiveness of practices and technologies. With clear-cut information on the value of various procedures, payers, providers, and consumers can work together to eliminate wasteful and unnecessary services. Moreover, increased dissemination of research findings regarding health care outcomes will enhance provider and consumer involvement in making the most effective choices about care and treatment. By taking this approach, the likelihood of serious disputes or litigation over appropriateness of care will be minimized. Likewise, the need for defensive practices designed to protect providers against malpractice suits will be greatly reduced.

Practice guidelines and directives derived from research, while providing an element of control, will be supportive of innovation. Coverage will be extended to procedures shown to be significantly more effective and less costly than existing approaches, and/or useful in improving patient outcomes and quality of life. At the same time, an effort will be made to weigh carefully new therapeutic approaches with high start-up costs that ultimately may be less expensive than present methods.

Use of advancements in clinical practice and technology will be conditioned on satisfying criteria related to cost efficiency and therapeutic effectiveness. Such an approach will not deny people essential services. It will, however, carefully assess the appropriateness of providing high-tech curative medical care to those who simply require comfort, relief from pain, supportive care, or a peaceful death.

Review Mechanisms

State and local review bodies—representative of the public and private sectors and composed of payers, providers, and consumers—will be established. These groups, operating under federal guidelines, will determine resource allocation, cost reduction approaches, allowable insurance premiums, and fair and consistent reimbursement levels for providers. Such review will be sensitive to ethical issues.

Managed Care

Managed care will be instituted both to reduce costs and to assure consumer access to the most effective treatments. Nursing's plan envisions managed care as organized delivery systems that link the financing of health care to the delivery of services—serving to maximize the quality of care while minimizing costs. To promote the use of managed care, enrollment in approved provider networks will be a requirement for those covered by the public plan. Managed care will also be encouraged for recipients of private coverage through reductions in deductibles and copayments.

In the past, managed care has been used, in many instances, to protect the pocketbooks of insurers rather than the rights of consumers. Managed care must be restructured to retain the maximum possible consumer choice and to place a premium on services that address the health of consumers.

Case Management

In contrast to managed care systems, case management is rooted in the client-provider relationship. Case management services will be used to integrate, coordinate, and advocate for people requiring extensive services. The aim of case management is to make health care less fragmented and more holistic for those individuals with complex health care needs. A variety of health care professionals are qualified to provide this service. The first allegiance of these providers will be to their clients. Acting as advocates, they will provide direct care and negotiate with systems on behalf of their clients. They will be authorized to access services for a given client.

Both case management (provider) and managed care (delivery systems) models are important to the smooth functioning of the health care system.

A REALISTIC PLAN OF ACTION

Under nursing's plan, universal coverage will be achieved through implementation of both the public and private plan options. Employers will be motivated to collaborate with employees in shaping private plans that best satisfy their needs. At the same time, as larger numbers of more diverse groups participate in the public plan, the attractiveness of this option in terms of cost, quality, and image will be enhanced.

While the public and private sector plans can move forward simultaneously, it may be necessary to expand coverage to segments of the population in sequential steps. These steps would be introduced at an acceptable and financially reasonable rate until the ultimate goal of universal coverage is achieved. This approach would avoid excessive shocks to the health care system and allow the public to adjust to changing patterns of service.

Given this perspective, the first targeted population would include all pregnant women, children under age 6 years, and those individuals who demonstrate a health status seriously compromised by a history of inadequate care. Improvements in coverage and benefits for these groups will have the greatest impact on the nation's future health and productivity.

As expeditiously as possible, other segments of the population would be covered. These groups might be targeted as outlined below; this sequence, however, is not necessarily intended as a rigid order:

▶ All children and young people, ages 6 to 18 years.
▶ All those above age 18 years with incomes below 100 per cent of the federal poverty level.
▶ All employees and dependents.
▶ All those with incomes below 200 per cent of the federal poverty level.

The process will culminate with the merger of all entitlement plans into a single public program to provide coverage to all citizens and residents who do not have or cannot obtain coverage through a private plan.

THE FISCAL IMPLICATIONS OF REFORM

It is impossible to predict the dollar amount that will be associated with the expansion of services or the efficiencies in nursing's plan. It is predictable that additional funding will be necessary to support start-up costs and transition. It is also possible that such expenditures will be recaptured over time.

A number of proposals for reform have been introduced. Among those proposals with cost estimates, additional health care costs range from $60 to $90 billion.[3,4] While nursing's plan for expanded coverage is similar in a number of ways to some of these proposals, offsetting proposed efficiencies integral to the plan will create significant dollars for reallocation. These resources will be directed to areas currently underfunded or excluded, including long-term care and primary care services.

While precise financial estimates are not possible at this time, several general observations can be made.

Cost Impact

Extension of coverage for essential services to the uninsured and underinsured will result in the dedication of more dollars. One source estimated that such coverage, if provided in 1990, would have added approximately $12 billion to health spending.[5]

It will also be necessary to dedicate more dollars to the expansion of long-term care services. Cost estimates for improved long-term care coverage vary. One 1990 study suggests that provision of comprehensive long-term care services, if implemented in 1990, would have cost $45 billion — $34 billion of which would have been new costs.[6] Nursing's plan, however, calls for more limited coverage supported through a combi-

nation of public dollars and enhanced personal responsibility.

In the initial phases of nursing's health care reform, the emphasis on preventive services will require dollars. Over time, however, improved health resulting from the availability of comprehensive primary health care services will produce a cost-reducing "health dividend." By placing greater emphasis on health promotion and disease prevention in community-based settings, the system will reach out aggressively to individuals and households to foster an increased commitment to healthy lifestyles, prevention of disease, periodic screening for early detection of illness and earlier treatment, and promote informed decision making by the consumer. All this will contribute to cost-effective, early interventions which, over time, will reduce the need for more costly care.

Cost Savings

New costs associated with nursing's plan will be offset to a considerable degree by the following cost-saving initiatives:

▶ Required usage of managed care in the public plan and encouraged use in private plans.
▶ Incentives for consumers and providers to utilize managed care arrangements.
▶ Controlled growth of the health care system through planning and prudent resource allocation.
▶ Assurance of direct access to a full range of qualified providers.
▶ Development of health care policies based on effectiveness and outcomes research.
▶ Incentives for consumers and providers to be more cost efficient in selecting health care options.
▶ Elimination of unnecessary bureaucratic controls and administrative procedures, through such measures as standardized billing, simplified utilization review, streamlined administrative procedures, regulatory reforms, and consolidation of plans.

Sources of Revenue

To the extent that any additional dollars are needed, sources can be found. Responsibility for financing health care reform must be distributed equitably among individuals, employers, and government.

Individuals will continue to pay a portion of health costs through copayments by households and individuals with incomes above 200 per cent of the poverty level, and through reduced copayments for those whose incomes are 100 to 200 per cent of the poverty level.

Employers will provide private health insurance that meets or exceeds minimum federal standards for their employees and dependents, or will provide coverage through the public plan. Accommodations will be made to provide small businesses with the necessary financial relief to meet this obligation.

State governments currently pay a portion of health care expenses for the poor and fund certain other health programs. Nursing's health care reform plan calls for consolidation of existing government health plans into a single public program. When this occurs, all states will contribute revenues to the program through maintenance-of-effort arrangements.

Revenues to pay for any increased costs could be derived from some combination of higher tobacco and alcohol taxes, additional payroll taxes, higher marginal income tax rates, and the increase or elimination of the income ceiling for FICA tax collection. A value-added tax (similar to a national sales tax) could also be considered.

A Look Toward the Future

The existing health care system stands as evidence of the futility of patchwork approaches to health care reform. America's nurses say it is time to frame a new vision for reform—time for a bold departure from the present. Reform of any single component of the system will not do the job. Insurance reform alone will not guarantee access to care if the health care delivery system is not restructured. Conversely, many people will remain unserved or underserved if health care services are so costly that millions of Americans cannot afford to purchase care.

To be most effective, a health care system must do more than provide equipment, supplies, facilities, and manpower. It must guarantee universal access to an assured standard of care. It must use health resources effectively and efficiently—balancing efforts to promote health with the capacity to cure disease. It must provide care in convenient, familiar locations. And it must make full use of the range of qualified health professionals and diverse settings for care. It is this insight that underlies nursing's plan for reform—making it the most viable solution to the nation's health care crisis.

Sources

1. U.S. Department of Commerce (1991). *U.S. Industrial Outlook 1991* (Chapter 44, Health and Medical Services, pp. 1–6).
2. National Leadership Coalition for Health Care Reform (1991). *A Comprehensive Reform Plan for the Health Care System* (p. 2).
3. The Pepper Commission (1990). *A Call for Action: Final Report* (p. 137).
4. Battle, Mark G. (January 8, 1991). Remarks during National Association of Social Workers National Health Care press conference.
5. Lewin/ICF estimates (1990). *To the Rescue: Toward Solving America's Health Care Crisis* (p. 13). Families USA Foundation.
6. Pepper Commission, p. 151.

▼ Glossary

Numbers following definitions indicate the chapter(s) in which the term is defined.

Abduction: Lateral movement of a body part away from the midline, eversion. (35)

Abstract (transcendent) hope: Desire or expectation extending beyond the usual limits of ordinary experience and knowledge, beyond material existence. (53)

Abstract thinking: The ability to reason logically and generalize from specific instances. (32)

Acculturation: The degree to which one culture has adopted the traditions, customs, and beliefs of another culture, thereby increasing the similarities between the two cultures. (19)

Acholia: Lack of bile production. (43)

Acid: Proton or hydrogen ion donor. (41)

Acidemia: Condition caused by a disturbance in the acid-base balance of the blood, in which the blood is more acid than normal. (30)

Acidosis: Condition in which the blood pH drops below 7.35. (41)

Acting-out behaviors: Inappropriate or unexpected client behaviors that communicate a message to the nurse about the client's true or subconscious feelings and concerns. (24)

Active-assistive range-of-motion exercises: Exercises done to maintain joint flexibility by putting each joint through its full measure of possible movements in all planes. These exercises are used for clients with decreased mobility in one or more body parts. The nurse encourages the client to do as much of a particular maneuver as possible, and, when the client can go no further, the nurse completes the maneuver for the client. (36)

Active involuntary euthanasia: Performing an act that results in the death of a person without his or her consent. (4)

Active listening: Listening in which the nurse takes an active part by eliciting details from the client and by inviting the client to think more about what is being said. (24)

Active range-of-motion exercises: Exercises done to maintain joint flexibility by putting each joint through its full measure of possible movements in all planes. With active range-of-motion exercises, the client independently exercises one or more of the joints several times each day. (36)

Active transport: Movement of ions across a cell membrane against a concentration, chemical, or electrical gradient. (41)

Active voluntary euthanasia: Performing an act at a person's request that results in the death of the person. (4)

Acupressure: A noninvasive technique that applies the pressure of the practitioner's fingers to acupuncture sites in order to cure or ameliorate diseases. (2)

Acupuncture: A technique based on an ancient Chinese belief that the entire universe is composed of two types of energy: the positive yang, which contracts and stimulates, and the negative yin, which sedates and expands. Disease is believed to result from an imbalance of yang and yin in the ch'i. Acupuncture is believed to restore balance. Long, fine needles are introduced through the skin at specific acupuncture sites. (2)

Acute pain: Pain with a sudden onset, triggered by tissue injury, with a healing time of less than 6 months. (40)

Adaptation: The adjustment of an organism to changes in its environment. (16)

Adaptive model: A model that defines health as the greatest ability to adapt to stressors in the internal and external environment. (2)

Additive solutions: Liquids added to a bag of IV fluid. (47)

Adduction: Lateral movement of a body part toward the midline, inversion. (35)

Administrative law: Rules and regulations of federal or state agencies effective only after a process of review and comment by affected persons or groups. (3)

Advance directive: A written document expressing a person's wishes about use of life-sustaining measures or appointing a surrogate decision-maker when a person can no longer make decisions. Some advance directives serve both purposes. (4)

Adventitious breath sounds: Abnormal breath sounds such as crackles, wheezes, rhonchi, and friction rubs. (33)

Adverse effects: Unintended or harmful responses to a normal medication dose or treatment. (46)

Aerobic exercise: Exercise that increases the overall amount of oxygen in the body and improves the body's capacity to consume oxygen. (36)

Aerosols: Liquid or powder medications suspended in a mist, often in an alcohol-based spray. (46)

Afebrile: Without fever. (31)

Affect: An external expression of emotion related to ideas or objects as perceived. (32)

Affective learning domain: The learning domain that relates to states of feeling and valuing. (26)

Afferent neurons: Nerves that travel toward the spinal cord and brain. (40)

Ageism: Discrimination that often accompanies old age. (14)

Agency: See Health care organization.

Aggregate: A group of people sharing one or more common characteristics. (20)

Agnosticism: Belief that the existence of any higher power such as a god cannot be known. (53)

Agraphia: The inability to write. (24)

Air embolism: Air in the bloodstream. (47)

Air lock technique: Method of IM injection that requires drawing air into the syringe. The technique avoids leakage of medication into the needle track after the needle is withdrawn from the site. (46)

Alkalosis: Condition in which the blood pH rises above 7.45. (41)

Allodynia: A sensation of pain from a stimulus that should not be painful (e.g., light touch). (40)

Alogia: The inability to speak. (24)

Alopecia: Hair loss of unknown cause; the condition often occurs in round patches. (38)

Altered thought processes: Thoughts that demonstrate an inability to differentiate one's thoughts and feelings from actualities of the outside world, e.g., experiences as manifested through auditory or visual hallucinations; illusions; delusional thinking; inability to concentrate; memory deficits; or disorientation to person, place, or time. (51)

Alveoli: Air sacs in the lungs where gas exchange takes place. (45)

Ambulation: Walking. (36)

Ambulatory care center: See Clinic.

American Nurses Association: The national professional organization for registered nurses in the United States. (1)

Amniocentesis: The aspiration of amniotic fluid from the amniotic sac by way of a needle inserted through the abdominal and uterine walls. (34)

Ampule: A glass container of medication in solution for use as a single dose; the glass must be broken to obtain access to the medication. (46)

Anaerobic: Without oxygen. (30)

Anaerobic exercises: Vigorous exercises of short duration (1 to 2 minutes) used primarily for competitive sports training. (36)

Analgesia: The absence of pain. (40)

Analgesic: Something (i.e., a drug or a procedure) that produces analgesia. (40)

Androgyny: An anthropologic term meaning that any one individual exhibits characteristics of both male and female sexes. (52)

Angina pectoris: Chest pain produced by hypoxic heart muscle. Hypoxia results from insufficient blood flow through narrowed or clogged vessels rather than generalized hypoxemia. (30)

Angiogenesis: Development of blood vessels. In wound healing this usually means the growth of new blood vessels into the wound. (48)

Angiogram: An x-ray of the vascular system. (34)

Anion: Negatively charged ion. (41)

Anorexia nervosa: A serious and sometimes fatal eating disorder characterized by constant dieting. (42)

Anoxia: Absence of oxygen in the tissues. (30)

Antagonistic effect: Mutual opposition or contrary action between two medications or treatments. (46)

Antiseptics: Chemicals that destroy microorganisms or inhibit their growth. (28)

Anuria: Complete urinary suppression, or kidney failure. (44)

Anxiety: Apprehension, dread, foreboding, or uneasiness that is not related to an identifiable source of danger. (16)

Aphasia: The general term for several different neurologic conditions in which the client has the ability to think without a corresponding ability to exchange information with others by correctly encoding, sending, or decoding messages. (24)

Aphemesthesia: Aphasia in which the client is unable to understand the spoken or the written word. (24)

Apical impulse (point of maximal impulse): A pulsation located over the apex of the heart, at the fifth intercostal space medial to the midclavicular line. (33)

Apnea: Total cessation of breathing that may be periodic. (31)

Apneustic respirations: Prolonged, gasping inspiration followed by extremely short, inefficient expiration. (31)

Apocrine sweat glands: Exocrine glands that become functional only during puberty and secrete sweat that has a strong, characteristic odor. (13)

Arousal threshold: The intensity of stimulus required to awaken. (39)

Arrhythmia: Irregular heart rhythm. (31)

Arterial blood gases (ABG): A measure of pH, bicarbonate level, oxygen saturation level, and the partial pressures of oxygen and carbon dioxide in arterial blood. (34)

Assault: The act of threatening when one apparently has the capability of carrying out the threat. (3)

Assent: The agreement of a child to participate in research based on the child's understanding of the purpose, risks, and benefits of the research. (4)

Assessment: The organized, systematic, and continuous process of collecting data from a variety of sources to analyze a person's health status. (6)

Assimilation: The process in which individuals from a subculture adopt the dominant culture. (19)

Assistive ambulation devices: Aids to help the client in walking (e.g., crutches, canes, walkers). (36)

Asynchronous response: Differing response patterns that may be in conflict. (54)

Ataxia: An uncoordinated gait that results from cerebellar disease or intoxication. (33)

Atelectasis: Collapse of all, or a portion of, the normally aerated lung tissue. (45)

Atheism: Denial of the existence of God. (53)

Atomization: The separation of a solution into fine droplets, thus creating a mist that can be inhaled. Atomization produces larger droplets than nebulization. (46)

At-risk aggregate: A subgroup of a community or population that is at increased risk of illness because of some variable. (20)

Attending behaviors: Behaviors that show that the nurse is paying attention to what the client is saying. Examples include facing the client, leaning toward the client, using appropriate eye contact, keeping eyes open with eyebrows raised, and maintaining an open body posture. (24)

Auditory aphasia (auditory amnesia, word deafness): Aphasia in which the client is unable to understand the spoken word. (24)

Auscultation: An assessment technique in which the examiner listens to and assesses the sound produced by various body organs and tissues, such as heart, lung, or bowel. (33)

Auscultatory gap: Pause in the Korotkoff sounds after the first, with the sounds resuming at a lower pressure. (31)

Authoritarian leadership: A leader-centered leadership style in which the leader makes decision and controls the conversation among group members. (25)

Autonomic nervous system (ANS): A portion of the nervous system consisting of parasympathetic systems and primarily controlling involuntary body functions. (17)

Autonomy: The ethical principle upholding the exercise of personal choice. (3)

Avulsions: Extremely traumatic injuries characterized by forcible separation of soft tissues from the body. (48)

Axis: See Fulcrum.

Ayurveda (a 4,000-year-old Sanskrit word meaning *the science of life*): An ancient tradition of Indian medicine derived from a belief that the body is created from the flow of the mind. In this tradition, each cell of the body contains intelligence and the mind has control over all diseases. (2)

Back-up: A copy of a computer file placed onto a storage medium to save as an extra copy in case of loss or damage to the original. (27)

Bacteriuria: Bacteria in the urine. (44)

Barium enema (BE): Distention of the colon and rectum with a barium solution that is administered through the anus as an enema. X-ray films and fluoroscopy are then used to visualize the large intestine. (34)

Barrel chest: A thoracic abnormality characterized by horizontal ribs, slight kyphosis, and a prominent sternal angle. (33)

Barrier techniques: Activities designed to prevent transmission of infectious agents from one source to another. Barrier techniques involve the use of gloves, gowns, aprons, masks, and eye shields. (28)

Base: Proton or hydrogen ion acceptor. (41)

Base of support: Foundation on which an object rests. (29)

Battery: Unwanted touching. (3)

Bedside commode: A chair or wheelchair fitted with an opening in the center of the seat. The underside of the seat has grooves for insertion of a pail or bedpan. (38)

Behavioral ethnicity: A term that refers to situations in which ethnic customs are practiced systematically, and members are well socialized into the traditional customs and values of the ethnic group. (19)

Beliefs: Ideas, expectations, attitudes, and opinions held by an individual or family. (50)

Bellevue Training School: One of the first three U.S. training schools for nurses. (1)

Beneficence: The ethical principle of upholding doing good; sometimes beneficence incorporates avoidance of harm. (3)

Bereavement: The period during which the grief process unfolds, ending with the reorganization of the individual's life. (54)

Best interests: A term that means that the benefits of a decision outweigh the burdens. (4)

Bibliotherapy: Therapeutic reading to enhance one's skills and knowledge or to solve problems. (50)

Biofeedback training: A process that involves using feedback methods to teach individuals to be sensitive and aware of body cues so that they can cognitively control certain involuntary physiologic functions. (17)

Biologic death: Death that is marked by irreversible destruction of brain tissue. (30)

Biomechanics: See Body mechanics.

Biopsy: A procedure involving removal of a tissue sample for microscopic examination. (34)

Biopsychosocial model of disease: A recognition that the mind and body continuously interact with each other; that the total person interacts with the external, social environment; and that an illness in the biologic, psychologic, or social realm can cause disease in the other realms as well. (2)

Biot's respirations: Irregular pattern of breathing in which all the breaths are the same depth. (31)

Bladder irrigation: Washing out the bladder for treatment of inflammation or obstruction. (44)

Blended family: A married man and woman who have children from previous marriages and who have their own biologic children, all living together. (18)

Blocking: Sudden interruption in train of thought. (32)

Blood buffer: Chemical that can donate or accept hydrogen ions as needed to maintain arterial blood pH between 7.35 and 7.45. (41)

Blood hydrostatic pressure: Force exerted by the blood cells and plasma within the blood vessels. (41)

Blood oncotic pressure: See Colloid osmotic pressure.

Blunted affect: Facial expression or emotion less than would normally be expected but not totally flat or lacking all emotion. (32)

Body alignment: The proper relationship of body parts to one another. (29)

Body fluid: Aqueous medium containing both water and electrolytes. (41)

Body image: The dynamic, personal picture of one's own body or physical being. (21)

Body language: Nonverbal communication behaviors that are accomplished by how we move our bodies or body parts, present ourselves to the world, and use the personal space around us. (24)

Body mechanics: Coordinated and efficient ways in which the body is used while moving from one position to another. (29)

Body Substance Isolation: A set of guidelines for providing care for people with infectious diseases. In this system, precautions are taken when in contact with all moist body sites or substances, regardless of the specific diagnosis. (28)

Body substances: Secretions or excretions that are usually moist and support the growth of microorganisms. (28)

Bolus: Concentrated mass. (47)

Bone resorption: A condition in which the bone is losing minerals and organic material to the blood. (35)

Boston Training School: One of the first three U.S. training schools for nurses. (1)

Bowel incontinence: Inability to control passage of feces and gas voluntarily. (43)

Bradycardia: Abnormally slow heart rate, below 60 beats per minute. (31)

Bradypnea: Decreased but regular respiratory rate, less than 10 breaths per minute. (31)

Braille: A language used by the visually impaired to communicate by indicating letters and numbers with a series of raised dots. Braille is used to replace the written word. (24)

Breakthrough pain: Pain felt between the dosing intervals of a person's long-acting analgesic. (40)

Bronchial breath sounds: Loud, high-pitched tubular sounds located over the trachea and major bronchi that are heard louder and longer during expiration. (33)

Bronchoconstriction: Narrowing of the airways. (45)

Bronchogram: An x-ray examination of the bronchial tree following insertion of an iodine radiopaque contrast medium into the bronchi. (34)

Bronchoscopy: An endoscopic examination of the larynx, trachea, and bronchi. (34)

Bronchospasm: Spasm of the smooth muscle surrounding the airway. (45)

Bronchovesicular breath sounds: Moderately pitched sounds located between the scapulae posteriorly and on either side of the sternum at the first and second intercostal spaces, anteriorly. (33)

Bruit: A blowing sound that indicates a distortion of a blood vessel that could interfere with blood flow. (33)

Bulimia nervosa: An eating disorder characterized by periodic binging and purging. (42)

Bulk-forming laxative: A synthetic or natural polysaccharide and cellulose derivative that absorbs water and adds bulk to the intestinal contents. The increased GI volume stretches the intestinal wall and stimulates peristalsis. (43)

Burnout: A condition of physical and emotional exhaustion experienced as a result of job stressors related to caring for the ill and the troubled. (16)

Butterfly: A small, hollow stainless steel winged-tip needle. (47)

Cachexia: Condition in which a person becomes emaciated and wasted. (42)

CAI: Computer-assisted instruction. (27)

Calculi: Pathologic stones, usually composed of mineral salts, occurring in the kidneys, ureters, bladder, or urethra. (44)

Calculus: An abnormal concretion, usually composed of mineral salts, around the base of the teeth. (38)

Canadian Nurses Association: The national organization of Canadian nurses, a federation of 11 provincial or territorial member associations. (1)

Cannula: A hollow tube through which fluid flows after removal of a trochar or stylet. (47)

Capillary-closing pressure: The amount of externally applied pressure required to occlude capillary blood flow totally, generally accepted as 32 mm Hg. (48)

Capsules: Oral preparations in which one or more medicinal substances are placed inside a small shell that is usually made of gelatin. (46)

Carbohydrate loading: Eating much high-carbohydrate food to increase muscle glycogen stores. (42)

Cardiac arrest: Cessation of the heart beat. (30)

Cardiopulmonary arrest: Cessation of heart beat and respiration. (30)

Caries: Cavities due to tooth decay. (38)

Case law (common law): Judge-made law. (3)

Case management: A method of delivering care that focuses on achievement of timely client outcomes. The case management plan is a standardized care plan that consists of nursing diagnoses, outcomes, deadlines, nursing interventions, and physician interventions. (9)

Case (one-to-one) method: A method of providing nursing care in which one nurse provides total, comprehensive nursing care to one or more clients. (22)

Cataplexy: A type of muscle collapse in which the person is alert but speech is not discernible. (39)

Category-specific CDC system: A set of guidelines that groups similar infectious diseases together and describes precautions for each disease category. (28)

Cathartic: A medication that purges the bowel; more effective than a laxative. (43)

Cation: Positively charged ion. (41)

Celiac sprue: A disorder characterized by gluten-induced malabsorption of essential nutrients. (42)

Cellulose: The form of carbohydrate that constitutes the supporting framework of plants. (42)

Center of gravity: Center, or heaviest part, of an object. (29)

Central integrator: Center in the brain, located in the hypothalamus, that maintains core body temperature. (31)

Central veins: Veins in the main body, as opposed to the extremities. (47)

Cerebral palsy: A nonspecific term for disorders of the central nervous system that result in persistent but nonprogressive bilateral, symmetric motor deficits. Deficits of sensory or intellectual function may coexist with the motor deficits. The etiology is usually related to brain damage during fetal development, at the time of birth, or in early infancy. (37)

Cerebrovascular accident (CVA, stroke): A disorder in which there is a sudden loss of consciousness or loss of motor or sensory function that results from rupture or occlusion of a cerebral artery. The location and size of the cerebral artery involved determine the site and involvement of the sensory or motor loss. (37)

Certification: The process of review to determine whether a care facility meets standards of care at a level sufficient to qualify for payment by Medicare or Medicaid. (4)

Cerumen: Earwax. (38)

Chain of infection: The sequence in the development of infection, including an infectious (causative) agent, a source or reservoir of the infectious agent, a mode of exit from the reservoir, a mode of transmission of the infectious agent, a portal of entry into a susceptible person, and a susceptible person. (28)

Change agent: A person who facilitates planned change with an individual or group or within an institution. (20)

Change-of-shift report: A report in which one nurse sums up for one or more other nurses all of the information necessary for the other nurses to safely assume responsibility for continuing the care of the clients. (27)

Chaplains: Pastoral care providers who offer spiritual support for clients and their families. (5)

Chart: A document that may consist of a single form or a number of forms that are compiled to provide a complete record of client care from the initial client assessment (including historical information of note) to the evaluation of the final client outcomes (including plans for follow-up by others, as needed). (27)

Charting by exception (CBE): A system of documentation in which only exceptions to the norms or some other important or significant findings are recorded. (27)

Cheilosis: Cracking or ulceration of lips and angles of the mouth. (38)

Chest percussion (clapping): Rhythmically clapping on the chest with cupped hands to help loosen mucus. (45)

Chest physical therapy: A combination of postural drainage, chest percussion, and vibration. (45)

Cheyne-Stokes respirations: A cycle in which respirations gradually increase in rate and depth, then decrease with periods of temporary apnea; commonly found in severe congestive heart failure. (31)

Chief complaint: A person's description of the major problem he or she is experiencing. It is written in the person's own words and is contained within direct quotes. (33)

Chiropractic treatment: A system of healing that is based on the belief that malalignment of the spinal column causes the vertebral bones to place pressure on nerves and cause symptoms such as pain and loss of function. Treatment consists of spinal manipulations (adjustments), spinal traction, and applications of heat to the spinal area. (2)

Cholecystogram: An x-ray study to evaluate the function of the gallbladder. (34)

Chronicity: The long-term nature of an illness. (21)

Chronic obstructive pulmonary disease (COPD): A broad term used clinically to refer to several diseases, notably asthma, emphysema, and chronic bronchitis, and characterized by chronic airflow limitation. (45)

Chronic pain: Pain that is persistently present, lasting more than 6 months without healing. (40)

Chronobiology: The study of internal rhythms, or ''body clocks,'' of organisms from single cells to human beings. (17)

Circadian rhythms: Rhythms with a frequency of approximately 24 hours. (17)

Circannual rhythms: Rhythmic cycles that occur over a period of a year. (17)

Circular causality: The process of one event or behavior influencing or affecting another event or behavior, and then the second event or behavior influencing or affecting the first event or behavior, as in A → B → A. Also known as circularity or reciprocity. (50)

Circularity: See Circular causality.

Circular pattern diagrams (CPDs): Schematic representations of reciprocal interaction patterns. CPDs graphically depict the reciprocal influence of behaviors and inferences or interpretations (cognitive, affective, or both). (50)

Circumstantiality: Flow of conversation made tedious by the unnecessary description of details that would ordinarily be omitted. (32)

Civil law: The ordering of relationships among persons and groups whose violation results in monetary damages or the obligation to take or refrain from a specific action. (3)

Cleaning: Removing visible dust, soils, and other foreign material. (28)

Cleansing enema: A type of enema used to treat constipation or fecal impaction, to clean out the bowel prior to diagnostic procedures or surgery, or to help establish regular bowel function during a bowel training program. (43)

Clean technique: The practice of medical asepsis. (28)

Clergy: Persons ordained to the service of God. (53)

Clinic: Traditionally, a place where a group of physicians worked together to study and treat persons who were admitted for medical and/or surgical care. Currently the term refers to a place where outpatients come for brief treatments or follow-up observations by a group of physicians and other health team members. Hence, such places are now most often called ambulatory care centers. (22)

Clinical death: Death that occurs with the cessation of blood flow and/or respiratory arrest. It is marked by reversible loss of consciousness. (30)

Clinical nurse specialists: Nurses who are prepared at the master's level and who possess expertise in specific clinical specialties (e.g., oncology, critical care). (10)

Clubbing: An abnormality of the nail in which the nail bed appears springy (early clubbing) or swollen (late clubbing) and the angle of the nail is 180 degrees or greater. It may suggest hypoxia or lung cancer. (33)

Cognitive learning domain: The learning domain that encompasses intellectual activities. (26)

Collaborative problems: Certain physiologic complications that nurses monitor to detect their onset or changes in status. (8)

Colloid osmotic pressure: Negative pressure exerted by plasma proteins. (41)

Colloids: Protein macromolecules in the plasma that are too large to pass through a cell membrane. (41)

Colonoscopy: Endoscopic examination of the large intestine. (34)

Color therapy: A therapy, dating back to ancient Egypt, in which colored light is used to treat disease. (2)

Colostomy: A surgically created opening in the large intestine. (43)

Comminuted fracture: Fracture in which the bone is crushed or splintered into several bone fragments. (37)

Common law: See Case law.

Communicable disease: Illness due to a specific infectious agent that can be transmitted from an infected person to a susceptible host. (28)

Community: A specific population living in a defined area and having shared institutions, values, and problems. (20)

Community-acquired infections: Known infections acquired outside a health care facility. (28)

Community support groups: See Self-help groups.

Compartment syndrome: A condition that develops in the presence of excessive swelling within the confined space of a muscle compartment. (37)

Complete fracture: A fracture that traverses the entire bone and may or may not require realignment of the bone fragments. (37)

Compliance: A person's behavior or willingness to follow the advice or prescription of the health care provider. (21)

Complicated fracture: A fracture in which there is associated damage to an internal organ. (37)

Compound (open) fracture: A fracture in which the bone is broken and a wound extends through soft tissue and the skin. (37)

Computed tomography (CT, CAT, CAT scan): An x-ray examination of a structure at varying depths so as to show sections or slices of the structure at different levels. (34)

Computer: An electronic device that is used to perform programmed activities in an efficient, accurate way. (27)

Conceptus: The products of human conception. (12)

Concrete hope: Hope in which the desired objects are within the individual's experience, such as freedom from pain or other physical symptoms, or the ability to perform certain tasks. (53)

Concrete thinking: Literal interpretation of questions or instructions. (32)

Confusion: A disturbance of consciousness in which the person feels distracted and anxious. A confused person cannot correctly respond to normal stimuli and may experience an altered awareness of person, place, time, or events. (51)

Connecticut Training School for Nurses: One of the first three U.S. training schools for nurses. (1)

Connecting: Forming a bond with the client. (54)

Conscious: Feelings and thoughts of which a person is aware. (12)

Consensual response (consensual reaction): The process whereby heating (or cooling) one part of the body produces vasodilation (or vasoconstriction) not only in the affected body part but also in other body parts. (48)

Consolidation: Replacement of air in alveoli with a liquid or solid. (45)

Constipation: A condition characterized by stool described as excessively dry, hard, and of insufficient size. (43)

Constitutional law: The body of law defining and limiting government powers and protecting the rights of citizens. (3)

Constricted affect: Indication of a limited range of emotional expression, with a decrease in variability of emotion and spontaneity. (32)

Contact inhibition: Pressure generated between touching cells that halts their horizontal movement. (48)

Contaminated: Unsterile. (28)

Context: The conditions under which a communication occurs. (24)

Contract: An offer to provide goods or services and an acceptance of the offer by another in return for some sort of consideration, usually monetary payment. (3)

Contracture: A condition in which the muscle is fixed, is shortened, and resists stretching, limiting the full passive range of motion of a joint. (35)

Contrast baths: The process of alternately immersing body parts in basins of hot and cold water to stimulate circulation. (48)

Conversion: The change of electrical energy or acoustical energy (sound waves) into heat. (48)

Coping: Adjusting to or solving internal and external challenges. (16)

Core temperature: Temperature of the interior of the

body in the thoracic and abdominal cavities and in the central nervous system. (31)

Cost containment: A variety of measures designed to reduce health care costs. (5)

Counterirritants: Agents that are applied locally to produce inflammatory reaction for the purpose of affecting some other body part, usually adjacent to or underlying the surface irritated. (48)

Countertraction: A force that pulls in the opposite direction from the force exerted by traction. (37)

CPU: Central processing unit—the main part of the computer, the part that performs calculations. (27)

Crackles (formerly known as rales): Noises created when air is traveling through vessels containing abnormal moisture. They are more pronounced on inspiration. (33)

Creams: Oils dispersed in 60 to 80 per cent water to form a thick liquid or soft solid. (46)

Criminal law: A type of law that punishes behavior that threatens the integrity of society and that may warrant the deprivation of personal liberty. (3)

Crisis: A disequilibrium in a steady state, occurring when usual problem-solving strategies are ineffective. (16)

Cross-contamination: The transmission of infectious agents from one person to another. (28)

CRT: Another name for a computer monitor. The letters stand for cathode ray tube. (27)

Cues: Subjective or objective pieces of information obtained through assessment. See Diagnostic cues. (8)

Cultural adaptation: Adjustment of an individual's behavior to the concepts, ideas, traditions, and institutions of a culture. (16)

Cultural competence: Being knowledgeable about health practices, beliefs, values, culture, and ethnicity within and between different groups and being able to provide health services that are acceptable to these groups. (19)

Cultural diversity: A term used to convey that there are differences among cultures as well as between subcultures and the dominant culture. (19)

Cultural sensitivity: Awareness of cultural generalizations and intragroup differences, as well as the avoidance of stereotypes. (19)

Culture: The accumulation of human experiences that evolve into a way of life for a group of people. (19)

Cursor: A symbol visible on a computer screen, the symbol that indicates the currently active portion of the screen (often a blinking line). (27)

Cutdown: Surgical incision made through the skin to expose a vein for venipuncture. (47)

Cyanosis: A bluish, mottled discoloration of the skin, nail beds, and mucous membranes caused by decreased oxygenation of the blood. (33)

Cystitis: Inflammation of the bladder. (44)

Cystoscopy: Endoscopic examination of the urinary bladder. (34)

Dandruff: Dry, white flakes that occur normally with scalp exfoliation. (38)

Dangling: Assisting the client to a position sitting on the side of the bed. Contrary to its name, the posi-

tion assumed does not allow the client's legs and feet to hang loosely over the side of the bed. (35)

Data base: A series of pieces of information about an individual and significant others that is used to identify strengths and unmet needs and to establish the plan of care. (7); a program that organizes a collection of information so that it can be easily accessed or utilized for reports. (27)

Data gathering: Gathering of information about a person; includes information from nursing interview, medical history, health care documents, physical and psychosocial assessment, other health care professionals, and review of the literature. (7)

Dead space: Space where fluids may collect within an anatomic cavity, abscess cavity, or wound. (48)

Debridement: The removal of foreign material or dead or damaged tissue from a wound. This may be done surgically, enzymatically, or with certain types of wound dressings. (48)

Deciduous teeth: Temporary teeth that are shed in childhood. (38)

Decoder (receiver): The person to whom a message is aimed. This person must be able to decode the message sent so it is a clearly understood thought. (24)

Defamation: Intentional use of the spoken or written word to injure the reputation of another. (3)

Defense mechanisms: Unconscious psychologic and behavioral strategies that help protect a person from anxiety. (16)

Defensiveness: Argumentative behavior to justify beliefs, thoughts, or actions. (32)

Defervescence: The period in which a fever abates and the temperature returns to normal. (31)

Defining characteristics: Clinical cues that cluster as manifestations of a nursing diagnosis. (8)

Dehiscence: A breaking open of a surgical incision without organ protrusion. (48)

Delusional thinking: An intellectual mechanism that helps a person maintain a sense of power and control when security is threatened. (51)

Delusions: False beliefs that are firmly maintained in spite of obvious evidence to the contrary and lack of support from others. (32)

Democratic leadership: A leadership style in which the leader assumes a collaborative role with other members of the group and serves as a guide while other members take steps toward accomplishing group goals. (25)

Dental plaque: Soft, thin, film of food debris, mucin, and dead epithelial cells that is deposited on the teeth and provides a medium for the growth of bacteria. (38)

Dependent edema: The buildup of interstitial fluid in areas that normally rely on muscular contraction to help move the blood back to the heart against the force of gravity; edema in areas below heart level, e.g., in the distal portions of the arms and legs of standing or sitting individuals and in the sacral area and heels of persons lying on their backs. (35)

Depressed fracture: A fracture in which fragments of

bone are forced below their normal level and below the level of surrounding portions of the bone. (37)

Dermal patches: Adherent materials impregnated with measured amounts of medication that slowly pass from the patch through the skin (transdermally) as the patch is worn like a small bandage. (46)

Desiccation: Drying of body tissues. (48)

Development: A set of processes through which physical, cognitive, and psychosocial properties of the individual interact with the environment to produce both constancy and change in the person over the life span.

Dextrins: Carbohydrates formed during the hydrolysis of starches to sugar. (42)

Diagnosis: Establishment of the cause and nature of a disease. (2)

Diagnosis-related groups: Categories that represent all known disease entities classified according to medical diagnosis. (5)

Diagnostic cues: Clinical evidence that describes a cluster of behaviors or signs or symptoms that represent a diagnostic label. Diagnostic cues are concrete and measurable through observation or client/group reports and are separated into major and minor. (8)

Diaphragmatic excursion: Movement of the diaphragm as it descends on inspiration and rises on expiration. (33)

Diarrhea: Passage of liquid or unformed stool. (43)

Diastolic pressure: The amount of pressure exerted on the wall of the arteries when the ventricles are at rest. (31)

Diathermy: The production of superficial or deep heat by converting electric and acoustic (sound) energy within the body tissue. (48)

Dietary guidelines for Americans: Advice for healthy Americans aged 2 years and over that reflects recommendations of nutrition authorities who aim to assist individuals to make sensible food choices. (42)

Dietitians: Experts about the way diet (oral or intravenous) may affect a client's recovery and promote and maintain health; also called nutritionists. (5)

Diffusion: Process of molecular (particle) movement from an area of higher to an area of lower concentration. (41)

Discharge planning: A process of anticipating and planning for changing client care needs as the client moves from one level of care to another. (22)

Discounting: The ability of individuals to devalue competencies they no longer perform well, as occurs in the case of debilitating illness, in an attempt to maintain high self-esteem. (50)

Disease-specific CDC system: A set of guidelines that prescribes specific precautions to be taken for each infectious disease. (28)

Disinfecting: Killing or destroying most disease-producing microorganisms on inanimate objects. (28)

Dispensary: A place that dispenses free or low-cost medications or medical treatments. (22)

Disuse syndrome: A group of disorders caused by immobility; complications of immobility. (35)

Diuretic effect: Increased urination. (44)

Diurnal rhythm: See Circadian rhythms.

Documentation: Written evidence of nursing practice. (27)

Doing for: Provision of care and technologic intervention. (54)

Dorsogluteal site: An intramuscular injection site that allows the deposition of medication into the gluteus medius muscle. (46)

Down time: The time in which a computer is not available to users. This can be a planned break for preventive maintenance or a sudden loss of computer function—otherwise known as a "crash." (27)

Drip chamber: An enlarged, cylindrical portion of IV tubing that allows visualization and counting of each drop of fluid that passes through the system. (47)

Drip rate: See Flow rate.

Drop factor: Number of drops of IV solution necessary to deliver 1 ml of fluid. (47)

Drug: Any substance that modifies or changes the organism's function, with or without a therapeutic effect. (46)

Drug addiction: Psychologic dependence; craving for a drug that goes beyond the physiologic need for it. (40)

Drug dependence: A physical or psychologic condition in which the person must continue taking a drug to avoid withdrawal symptoms. (40)

Drug tolerance: A natural physiologic response to opiates, characterized by a markedly diminished effect with continued use of the same amount of an opiate analgesic. (40)

Durable power of attorney for health care: A written document that gives power to another person—generally a trusted friend or family member—to make health care decisions for a person when the person becomes incapable of making health care decisions. (4)

Duty-oriented ethical theory: A system of ethical thinking having the concept of duty or obligation as a foundation. (3)

Dysphagia: Difficulty or discomfort in swallowing. (42)

Dysphoria: Mood of disquiet, dejection, unhappiness, and dissatisfaction with oneself or life. (32)

Dyspnea: Difficult, labored, or painful breathing. (31)

Dysuria: Painful or difficult urination. (44)

Earned right: A right that stems from the performance of certain activities. (4)

Ecchymosis: A discoloration of an area of the skin, commonly known as bruises. (33)

Ecological approach: The study of living things as they exist in their natural environment. (2)

Edema: An accumulation of excessive fluid in the interstitial compartment. (33)

EDP: Electronic data processing. Using a computer to perform functions with data. (27)

Educational groups: Groups developed to teach participants skills and provide information. (25)

Effervescence: The bubbling, hissing, and foaming that accompanies the release of gases from liquid. (46)

Ego: That part of the personality that operates according to the reality principle and that helps the individual survive by negotiating among the demands of the id, the moralistic judgments of the superego, and the realities of the situations of life. (12)

Egocentricity: The feeling that a person is "the center of the universe" and that everyone is looking, listening, and paying attention to the person. (12)

Ego integrity: Accepting one's life as meaningful and whole. (14)

Electrocardiogram (ECG, EKG): A recording of the electrical activity of the heart. (34)

Electroencephalogram (EEG): A recording of the electrical impulses in the cortex of the brain. (34)

Electrolyte: Any compound that, when dissolved in water, separates into charged particles termed ions. (41)

Electromyogram (EMG): A recording of nerve impulses in skeletal muscles. (34)

Electro-oculogram (EOG): A graphic representation of the electrical activity associated with eye movements. (39)

Elixirs: Drug preparations in a solvent medium of alcohol and water (a hydroalcoholic medium). (46)

Empowering: Assisting clients to find or build strengths within themselves. (54)

Empty nest syndrome: Feelings of depression, sadness, and loss when children leave home. (14)

Empyema: Pus in the pleural space. (45)

Emulsions: Suspensions made from fats, oils, or petrolatum suspended in a second liquid. (46)

Encoder (sender): The person who initiates a transaction to exchange information, convey thoughts and feelings, or engage another. (24)

Encounter groups: Time-bound and intense group experiences designed to enhance personal awareness. (25)

Endocrine system: Body system consisting of several glands and other tissues that discharge their hormone secretions directly into the bloodstream. While each hormone-secreting gland or tissue is separate and has its own unique function, they also can act interdependently as an organ system. (17)

Endorphins: Neuropeptides produced by the body to provide analgesia in the nervous system by binding with opiate receptors. (40)

Endoscopy: A means of visualizing interior body structures using a flexible, hollow, lighted scope. (34)

Endotracheal tubes: Tubes placed in the nose or mouth and passed to just above the tracheal carina. (45)

Enema: Introduction of fluid into the rectum, usually for the purpose of stimulating defecation. (43)

Enkephalins: Neuropeptides produced by the body to provide analgesia in the nervous system by binding with opiate receptors. (40)

Enteral feeding: A special liquid formula that can be given orally or through a tube passed through the nose or mouth into the esophagus and stomach. (42)

Enteric-coated tablets: Oral medications with a hard surface that impedes absorption until the medication reaches the small intestine. (46)

Enuresis: Involuntary urination. (44)

Epidural space: The space that lies outside the dural sheath, or protective layer of tissue, surrounding the subarachnoid space. (40)

Epithelialization: The growth of epithelial cells across the surface of a wound. (48)

Ergometer: Device that measures work output. (36)

Erythema: Reddening of the skin due to the inflow of blood. (35)

Eschar: Thick, leathery, fibrin-containing necrotic tissue that covers a wound's surface. (48)

Esophagogastroduodenoscopy (EGD): Endoscopic examination of the esophagus, stomach, and duodenum. (34)

Esophagogastrostomy tube: A tube that can be passed through an esophagostomy and into the stomach. (42)

Esophagostomy: A surgical opening into the esophagus. (42)

Ethgender: The combination of race and gender effects. (13)

Ethical right: A right based in a particular ethical framework. (4)

Ethics: A system or code of morals; a discipline that seeks to formulate and systematically justify responses to moral dilemmas. (3)

Ethnic humanism: A humanistic perspective that focuses on strengths and resources of all ethnic groups, on the blending of traditional and Western healing practice, and on client participation in health care. (19)

Ethnicity: A term used to describe a group of people within a larger society who share a social and cultural heritage that is passed on from generation to generation. (19)

Ethnic pluralism: The term used to describe a larger culture within which several different ethnic groups have maintained distinct subcultures. (19)

Ethnocentrism: The belief that one's own ethnic beliefs, customs, and attitudes are the correct ones and are better than those of others. (19)

Ethnoscience: A scientific method of studying the unique ways of life of particular cultural groups. (19)

Eucharist: Holy Communion; partaking of bread and wine in a commemoration of the death of Christ. (53)

Eudaemonistic model of health: A model that defines health as an ideal state of vibrant, exuberant well-being in which the person experiences such positive effects as happiness, good concepts of the self, sound relationships with others, and an optimum ability to think and act. (2)

Euphoria: Mood that is expansive or elated, with an exaggerated sense of well-being. (32)

Evaluation: Making judgments about the results of the plan of care and the person's progress toward outcomes; evaluation also indicates those areas in which the person's care needs to be reappraised and modified. (6)

Evaluation, performance: A set of measurable, observable statements used to determine how a student or graduate nurse compares with the expected standard. (11)

Evisceration: Protrusion of the viscera (body organs) through a wound incision. (48)

Evolutionary model: A model that defines health as the greatest ability to survive long enough to pass along one's genes. (2)

Excess mortality: The differences between the number of deaths observed in a group, such as a particular ethnic group, and the number of deaths that would have occurred in that group if it experienced the same death rates for each age and sex as occurred in the general population. (19)

Excoriation: Abrasion of the epidermis by trauma, chemicals, burns, or other causes such as drainage from wounds, urine, feces. (48)

Expansiveness: Lack of restraint in one's feelings and actions; overvaluation of one's accomplishments. (32)

Expert system: A specialized computer program that aids in problem solving or decision making. (27)

Extended-care facility: An agency that provides long-term medical, rehabilitative, or custodial care (care that focuses on observing and protecting a person, rather than providing for a cure). (22)

Extended family: Husband, wife, children, grandparents, and other blood relatives such as aunts, uncles, and cousins who may or may not live together but who often provide other family members with emotional support, child care, and financial assistance. (18)

Extension: Movement so as to increase or straighten the angle formed at the joint between two body parts; straightening of a bent joint, the opposite of flexion. (35)

Extension hook: Plastic or metal device to lower a primary IV line while piggyback infusion is in progress. (47)

External rotation: Rotation away from the center of the body, lateral rotation. (35)

Extinction: Stopping the reinforcement of a behavior in order to stop the behavior. (12)

Extracellular fluid (ECF): Body fluid found outside the cells. (41)

Extreme unction: The act of anointing the body as a rite of consecration. (53)

Extubation: Removal of an artificial airway from the trachea. (45)

Facilitated diffusion: Process in which a carrier molecule facilitates transfer of a larger molecule across the cell membrane from an area of higher to an area of lower concentration of molecules. (41)

Factitious wounds: Tissue injuries deliberately produced by the individual. (48)

Faith: A belief in or acknowledgment of something unable to be physically seen. (53)

False imprisonment: The unlawful detention of a person. (3)

Family: The basic social unit in which human behavior occurs in relation to health. (18)

Family of origin: The family into which a person is born. (13)

Fasciculations: Uncontrollable twitching. (33)

Fecal impaction: A collection of putty-like or hardened feces in the rectum, which usually prevents the passage of a normal stool. (43)

Feces: Excrement, or gastrointestinal waste. (43)

Feedback: A process that feeds some of the output of a system back into the system as input. This input of information then influences the behavior of the system and its subsequent output. (17); the process by which effectiveness of communication is determined. (24)

Fidelity: The ethical principle of upholding commitment or the keeping of promises. (3)

Filtration: Passage of water and particles through a semipermeable membrane, assisted by hydrostatic pressure. (41)

Filtration pressure: Blood hydrostatic pressure minus colloid osmotic pressure (FP = BHP − COP). (40)

Finding meaning: Helping individuals make sense out of what is happening. (54)

Finger spelling: Signing single letters one at a time in order to spell out words in sign language. (24)

Flaccidity: Decreased tonus that results in a relaxed, flabby muscle. (35)

Flat affect: Lack of any facial expression or indication of emotion. (32)

Flatulence (gaseous distention): The presence of abnormally large amounts of gas within the gastrointestinal tract. (43)

Flexibility exercises: Exercises that lengthen, stretch, and flex muscles while enhancing balance and overall grace. (36)

Flexion: Movement so as to decrease the angle formed at the joint between two body parts; bending of a straight joint, the opposite of extension. (35)

Flight of ideas: Acceleration of thoughts evidenced by rapid, pressured speech and disorganization of conversation. (32)

Flocculate: To gather finely dispersed particles into larger particles that may be visible within a solution. (47)

Flow chart (flowsheet, flownote): One or more forms used to chart the flow of information concerning certain selected client observations and treatments that are repeated over a period of some time (as opposed to the more comprehensive narrative format used to chart a great deal of or all possible client information noted in relatively short periods of time). (27)

Flow rate: Drops per minute or milliliters per hour that an IV solution is allowed to run. (47)

Fluoroscopy: Use of x-rays to study deep body structures, such as joints, organs, or body systems, while in motion. (34)

Footdrop: Contracture of the Achilles tendon that maintains the foot in a position of plantar flexion. (35)

Force: Effort exerted. (29)

Formulary: A book that provides information about medications. (46)

For-profit agency: Health care organization that may distribute profits to partners or shareholders; also called a proprietary agency. (5)

Four-point gait: A crutch-walking gait with four points on the floor and with one point moving at a time—crutch, opposite foot, opposite crutch, opposite foot. (36)

Fracture: A break in the continuity of the bone that usually results from traumatic injury to the body part. (37)

Fremitus: A vibration transmitted through the chest wall as the person speaks. (33)

Frequency: Urinating at short intervals, either small or large amounts, more often than usual. (44)

Friable: Easily broken or torn. (48)

Friction: Resistance encountered when two irregular surfaces are moved across each other. (29)

Friction rubs: Crackling, grating sounds produced when two roughened or inflamed pleural spaces rub across each other during respiration. (33)

Fulcrum: Fixed point on which a lever moves. (29)

Functional health patterns: As defined by Gordon, describes client strengths. Also, a model for organizing nursing diagnoses into 11 categories. (6)

Functional method: A method of providing nursing care in which one nurse is assigned to do specific tasks for a large number of clients rather than being assigned to complete all tasks for a smaller number of clients. (22)

Fundamental right: A basic right shared by all human beings; for example, rights to food, clothing, and shelter. (4)

Future-oriented questions: An interventive question that is used to invite clients or their families to imagine situations in the future so as to encourage visualization of details that contribute to desired outcomes (e.g., "What would your life be like *if* you found a solution to your problem of low self-esteem?"). (50)

Gait: Style of walking. (33)

Gastric analysis: The laboratory analysis of stomach contents. (42)

Gastrointestinal compression: A process of applying pressure internally by using a specially designed tube with inflatable balloons. (42)

Gastrointestinal decompression: A process of relieving pressure by removing accumulated gas and secretions from the GI tract through a tube. (42)

Gastrostomy tube: A tube that enters a surgical opening through the abdominal wall into the stomach. (42)

Gate control theory: Explanation of pain transmission in which large, myelinated nerve fibers (A beta fibers) have a low threshold for painful stimuli and, when activated, inhibit the response to other noxious stimuli, closing the gate to further painful stimuli. Tissue damage may cause small-diameter nerve fibers to be activated, which opens the gate, causing pain. (40)

Gavage: A method of giving persons fluids and nutrients via a tube when oral intake is inadequate or impossible. (42)

Gels: Semisolid mixtures that liquefy when applied to the skin. (46)

Gender role: Appearance and behaviors that demonstrate maleness and femaleness and what one presents according to a specific culture's consideration of masculine or feminine. (52)

General systems theory (GST): Use of a hierarchical method of studying and talking about phenomena. (15)

Generativity: Being productive and creative for one's self as well as others. (14)

Germ theory: The belief that microorganisms cause infectious diseases. (2)

Gingivitis: Gum inflammation characterized by bleeding gums and halitosis. (38)

Global aphasia: Aphasia in which the client has an inability to express or perceive words or any other form of communication. (24)

Global self-esteem: A measure of how much one approves of one's perceived self in its entirety. (50)

Glycolipids: Lipids that contain carbohydrate. (42)

Glycosuria: Glucose in the urine. (44)

Goal-oriented ethical theory: A system of ethical thinking having the concept of maximizing the overall good as its foundation. (3)

Goiter: An enlarged thyroid gland. (33)

Gonadal sex: Genital sex. (52)

Granulation tissue: Beefy red tissue seen in a healing wound and composed of newly formed collagen and new blood vessels. (48)

Graphics: Computer-produced pictures or images as opposed to written text or numbers. (27)

Greenstick (willow stick, hickory stick) fracture: A fracture involving only part of the thickness of a bone. The bone breaks like a green stick, bending on one side and breaking on the other. This type of fracture is seen in children because their bones are more resilient and their periosteum thicker than in adults. (37)

Grief: The normal response to and personal experience of loss. (54)

Group: Two or more individuals who share one or more common characteristics and meet on a regular basis in face-to-face interactions to achieve a common goal. (25)

Group cohesion: All of the positive values that people hold about the group experience and the reasons that prompt them to remain with the group. (25)

Group culture: A set of common characteristics that help facilitate goal achievement. Shared characteristics might involve a common ethnic heritage, a similar health problem, or the need to complete a group project. (25)

Group dynamics: The conscious and unconscious forces or emotional flow operating in a group and facilitating or impeding the group process and progression toward goal achievement. (25)

Group goals: The outcomes, or end results, the group

seeks to achieve through its common effort. Group goals represent a collective aim that may or may not be the same as the goals of individual group members. (25)

Group membership: An identified relationship between a person and designated other persons who make up a group. (25)

Group norms: Standards of conduct that provide guidelines for acceptable behaviors in groups. Group norms are powerful written or unwritten laws about how members should relate with each other. (25)

Group process: The naturally progressive phases of group development. (25)

Group roles: Sets of behaviors that individuals display in relation to the expectations of the rest of the group members. (25)

Group therapy: A form of psychotherapy designed to help clients gain insight into dysfunctional behaviors and develop more appropriate coping strategies. (25)

"Group think": A group decision-making process in which loyalty to the group and approval of other group members take precedence over expression of personal values, ideas, and conflicting opinions. (25)

Growth: Primarily, physical changes that result from the proliferation of cells, growth of cells, and maintenance or replacement of cells. (12)

Growth factors: Normal components of cells elaborated in response to many body needs. They are brought to the wound in response to injury. (48)

Guaiac test: A test that detects the presence of occult blood in the stool. (43)

Gums: Resin-like substances derived from plants. (42)

Halitosis: Bad breath. (38)

Hallucinations: Sensory perceptions (auditory, visual, olfactory, tactile, or gustatory) without a source of stimulus in the external world. (32)

Hard copy: A paper printout of what appears on a computer screen. (27)

Hardware: The equipment or sections of a computer system that are necessary for operation of the system. (27)

Health (World Health Organization definition): A state of complete physical, mental, and social well-being and not merely the absence of disease or infirmity. (2)

Health belief model: A model used for predicting human behavior in relation to health. The model is based on the assumption that several factors contribute to a person's taking a recommended action. (2)

Health Care Financing Administration (HCFA): A federal cost-containment agency created to administer the Medicare and Medicaid programs. (5)

Health care organization (agency): A structural and functional unit of personnel who provide health services to individuals, families, groups, and/or society. (22)

Health education: Education promoting wellness behaviors and the prevention of disease, often focusing on groups and communities. (20)

Health-illness continuum: A range of well-being from excellent health through wellness and illness to death. (2)

Health Maintenance Organizations (HMOs): Networks or groups of providers who agree to provide certain basic health care services for a single predetermined yearly fee. (5)

Health promotion model: A model used to predict the likelihood of a person's engaging in health-promoting behaviors. (2)

Heart murmur: A harsh, rumbling, blowing sound caused by blood flow across a defective valve, or the shunting of blood through an abnormal passage. (33)

Hematuria: Blood in the urine. (44)

Hemolytic reaction: Red blood cells clump together, become trapped in small vessels, and release hemoglobin into the plasma as they disintegrate, a reaction that occurs with blood incompatibility. (47)

Hemopericardium: Blood in the pericardial sac. (30)

Hemoptysis: The coughing up of blood. (45)

Henderson, Virginia: One of the first nurse theorists to write a generally accepted definition of nursing and a framework for nursing care. (1)

Heparin lock: A venous access device that may be a plastic, indwelling intravenous catheter or a steel butterfly needle with a short length of narrow-gauge plastic tubing attached. The needle or catheter remains in the vein ready to be connected to a source of IV fluid whenever necessary. On its distal end, the device is covered by an injection cap. The device is kept patent by heparin that is flushed through it to prevent clotting. (47)

Herbalism: The use of bark, leaves, flowers, stems, and/or roots of plants to heal illness. (2)

Hesitancy: Difficulty in initiating urination. (44)

Hierarchy: A grading or ranking of members of a group in order of relative importance. (15)

High-level wellness: Defined by Halbert Dunn as ". . . an integrated method of functioning which is oriented toward maximizing the potential of which the individual is capable, within the environment where he is functioning." (2)

High risk nursing diagnosis: A clinical judgment that an individual, family, or community is more vulnerable to develop the problem than others in the same or similar situation. High risk nursing diagnoses are supported by risk factors that guide nursing interventions to reduce or prevent the occurrence of the problem. There are no signs or symptoms for high risk diagnoses. (8)

HIS: Hospital computerized information system. A computer is used for such functions as client billing and pharmacy orders. (27)

Holistic nursing care: The provision of biologic, psychologic, and sociocultural care to persons so that they are treated as a human whole. (15)

Holistic view of humans: The view that the human person is a whole with at least biologic, psychologic, and social parts and that the whole is more than the sum of its parts. (2)

Homan's sign: An indicator of deep phlebitis in which pain and soreness are present in the calf area when the foot is dorsiflexed. (33)

Home care: Services for individuals and families in

their place of residence for the purpose of treatment of illness, restoration of health, rehabilitation, and health promotion. (23)

Home health agency: An agency that provides certain types of health care in the home setting. (22)

Homeopathy: A system of treatment based on the belief that large doses of drugs that produce symptoms of a disease in healthy individuals will cure the same symptoms when administered in minute amounts to sick persons. (2)

Homeostasis: Self-regulation processes and negative feedback systems, which work together to produce compensatory and anticipatory adjustments in maintaining the constancy of the internal environment. (17)

Homeostatic mechanisms: Processes of self-regulation that preserve an organism's ability to adapt to stressors while maintaining inner balance. (17)

Homophobia: Fear or threat that is experienced by heterosexual beings in relation to homosexuals. (52)

Hope: To desire or to long for something, accompanied by an expectation of fulfillment. (53)

Horizontal abduction: Movement of a body part, in a horizontal plane, back across and away from the midline, opposite of horizontal adduction. (35)

Horizontal adduction: Movement of a body part, in a horizontal plane, across the midline of the body. (35)

Horizontal relationship: A relationship in which other persons and the environment influence an individual's life. (53)

Hormones: Chemical substances secreted by endocrine glands or tissue directly into the bloodstream to act as messengers linking one body system with another, thereby regulating and integrating many body functions. (17)

Hospice: An agency that provides palliative and supportive care for the dying and support for their families. In medieval times, hospices were guest houses or places of shelter for wayfarers such as pilgrims. (22)

Hospital: An agency that provides medical and/or surgical care and treatment for the sick and injured and/or obstetrical care for healthy women who are giving birth. (22)

Host: A person who harbors a disease. (28)

Human need theory: The doctrine that all persons have certain requirements essential for maintaining life and health. (15)

Human reduction (dehumanization): Viewing the client as other than a human being. (24)

Humidification: The addition of water vapor to a dry gas. (45)

Humoral theory of medicine: A belief that the four humors (body liquids or semifluids) were phlegm, blood, black bile, and yellow bile and that these humors corresponded with the four qualities of cold, heat, dryness, and moisture. These vital elements existed in various quantities in the body, and when the equilibrium among them was disrupted, disease resulted. (2)

Hydrostatic pressure: Pressure exerted by a fluid within a compartment. (41)

Hygiene: A set of practices that are conducive to the preservation of health, such as cleanliness. (38)

Hyperalgia: Increased sensitivity to pain. (40)

Hypercalciuria: High urinary calcium levels. (44)

Hypercapnia: See Hypercarbia.

Hypercarbia: A rise in arterial carbon dioxide ($PaCO_2$). (30)

Hyperextension: Movement of a body part beyond its straightened position in the opposite direction from flexion. (35)

Hyperlipidemia: Elevations of blood lipid levels. (42)

Hyperpnea: Increase in the depth of respirations. (31)

Hyperpolarization: Overexcitement of neurons with subsequent inability to transmit impulses. (39)

Hyperpyrexia: An extremely elevated body temperature. (31)

Hypersomnia: Pathologically excessive drowsiness or sleepiness. (39)

Hypertension: Abnormally elevated blood pressure. (31)

Hyperthermia: An extremely elevated body temperature. (31)

Hypertonic: Having an osmotic pressure greater than that of the solution with which it is compared; more than 375 mEq/liter in the body. (41)

Hypertrophic scar: Excessive scarring. (48)

Hyperventilation: An increase in both rate and depth of respirations. (31)

Hypervolemia: Increased circulating fluid volume. (41)

Hypnagogic hallucinations: Intense, frightening dreamlike experiences that can be visual or auditory and that occur just before sleep. (39)

Hypnotics: Medications used to induce sleep. (39)

Hypoglycemia: Low blood glucose. (42)

Hypoproteinemia: Low levels of plasma proteins. (41)

Hypostatic pneumonia: Consolidation of lung tissue secondary to stagnant respiratory secretions. (35)

Hypotension: Abnormally low blood pressure. (31)

Hypothermia: An abnormally low body temperature, sometimes induced for therapeutic purposes. (31)

Hypotonic: Having an osmotic pressure lower than that of the solution with which it is compared; less than 250 mEq/liter in the body. (41)

Hypoventilation: Reduction in the amount of air reaching the alveoli. (31)

Hypovolemia: Decreased circulating fluid volume. (41)

Hypoxemia: Insufficient oxygenation of the arterial blood. (45)

Hypoxia: Tissue oxygen deficiency. (45)

Id: That part of the personality that is governed by the pleasure principle; that is most influential in the earliest developmental stages of childhood; and that is manifest through thoughts, desires, and sensations. (12)

Ideal cultural behavior: A set of behavioral patterns that people in the culture believe to be desirable but do not practice. (19)

Ideologic ethnicity: The voluntary rather than systematic practice of ethnic customs. (19)

Ileostomy: A surgically created opening in the ileum. (43)

Illusions: False interpretations of real sensory images. (32)

Impacted fracture: A fracture in which one fragment of the broken bone is wedged into the other fragment. (37)

Implementation: Putting the nursing care plan into action; carrying out nursing actions or interventions that focus on assisting the person to cope successfully with problems and achieve outcomes. (6)

Incomplete fracture: A fracture that does not traverse the entire bone. (37)

Inertia: The property of matter that causes it to tend to remain at rest (if it is at rest) or to remain in motion (if it is in motion). (29)

Infection: An illness produced by the invasion and multiplication of an infectious agent in body tissues. (28)

Infectious agent: Any microorganism (bacterium, fungus, virus, Rickettsia, and protozoan) that can cause a disease. (28)

Inferencing: Assigning meaning to a cue or cluster of cues. (8)

Infiltration: Infusion of IV fluid into tissue surrounding the vein. (47)

Infirmary: A place where the infirm (the sick, weak, or feeble) are treated. This term may refer to a hospital or to an area within another institution, such as a school or prison, set aside for the infirm. (22)

Informed consent: The process of providing clients information about (1) the nature and purpose of a treatment or procedure, (2) the expected outcomes and probabilities of success, the material risks, the benefits, and the consequences, (3) alternatives to the procedure and supporting information, and (4) the effect of no treatment or no procedure, including the effect on the prognosis and material risks associated with no treatment. (4)

Infradian rhythms: Rhythmic cycles longer than 24 hours, such as the menstrual cycle. (17)

Infusion controller: A mechanical device that monitors and helps regulate the flow of IV fluids without the use of pressure. (47)

Infusion pump: A mechanical device that monitors and uses pressure to help regulate the flow of IV fluids into a vein. (47)

Injection cap: A plastic fitting that keeps a heparin or saline lock sealed but that has a rubber diaphragm that can be penetrated by a needle to provide access to the vein. (47)

Injection ports: Circular rubber dams that help keep IV bags and/or tubing intact while allowing entry of a needle when necessary to add medication to the system. (47)

Input: The general systems theory term for the movement of matter, energy, or information from the environment into a system. (15)

Input device: A device used to put information into the computer system, such as a keyboard, light pen (a device used to "write" on the computer screen), touch-sensitive screen, or mouse or other pointing-and-clicking device. (27)

Insomnia: Difficulty falling asleep or staying asleep. (39)

Inspection: An assessment technique in which the examiner observes the body surface. (33)

Internal respiration: Cellular process that occurs when oxygen moves from the blood into the cell and carbon dioxide leaves the cell and enters the blood to be carried back to the lungs to be expelled. (30)

Internal rotation: Rotation toward the center of the body, medial rotation. (35)

International Council of Nurses: An organization that meets every 4 years in order to foster international relationships and provide a forum for international concerns to be aired. (1)

Interstitial fluid: The part of the extracellular fluid that lies outside the vascular system. (41)

Interventions, dependent: Nursing actions that are based on the physician's orders. (10)

Interventions, independent: Nursing actions that are based on the nursing diagnosis and that nurses are qualified to use without a physician's order. (9)

Interventions, interdependent: Nursing actions that are performed in collaboration with other members of the health care team. (9)

Intracellular fluid (ICF): Body fluid contained within the cells. (41)

Intraethnic variation: Existence of cultural differences within groups. (19)

Intraoperative phase: The phase of surgery that begins when the individual is transferred to the operating room table and ends at admission to the postanesthesia care unit. (49)

Intrathoracic pressure: Pressure within the chest cavity. (30)

Intravenous (IV) infusion: The introduction of fluids into a vein. (47)

Intravenous pyelogram (IVP): A commonly prescribed test to detect kidney disease, ureteral or bladder stones, and tumors. (34)

Intravenous route: Administration into a vein. (46)

Intubation: Placement of a gastrointestinal tube in the GI tract. (42); placement of an artificial airway, such as an endotracheal or tracheostomy tube, into the trachea. (45)

Intuitionist ethical theory: A system of ethical thinking that balances goals, rights, and duties according to the situation. (3)

Ion: An electrically charged particle. (41)

Ionization: The breaking apart of a substance into its positively and negatively charged particles. (41)

Invasion of privacy: Making public the private affairs of a person without the person's consent. (3)

Ischemia: Deficiency of blood flow to an area due to constriction or obstruction of a blood vessel. (35)

Isolation precautions: Systems designed to use barriers to prevent transmission of infectious agents. Systems may be category specific or disease specific. (28)

Isometric contraction: Contraction in which the muscle maintains the same length but its tonus increases. (35)

Isometric exercises: Exercise in which the muscles maintain the same length, but their tension increases. (36)

Isotonic: Having the same or approximate osmotic pressure as the solution with which a solution is compared. (41)

Isotonic contraction: Contraction in which the muscle tonus or tension remains the same as the muscle shortens in contraction. (35)

Isotonic exercises: Exercise in which muscle tension remains the same while the muscles shorten in contraction as body parts move. (36)

Jaundice: A yellow discoloration of the skin resulting from an increase in bilirubin. (33)

Jejunostomy tube: A tube that is inserted through a surgical opening in the abdominal wall and into the jejunum. (42)

Jet lag syndrome: A complex of symptoms that occurs after jet travel across four or more time zones when a traveler attempts to adapt too rapidly to the new time zone with its different light-dark cycle and time of social activities. (17)

Justice: The ethical principle of upholding giving people their due and treating them fairly. (3)

Kardex: A system used by many agencies to store 6 × 11 inch cards in which each card contains vital information about, and the nursing care plan for, a specific client.

Keloid: Exuberant scar tissue that grows beyond the confines of the original wound. (48)

Korotkoff sounds: The sounds produced by the pressure of blood in the artery. (31)

Kussmaul's respirations: Breathing pattern characterized by increased depth and rate of respiration. (31)

Kyphosis: An exaggerated curvature of the thoracic vertebrae. (33)

Lability: Mood instability with rapidly changing emotions. (32)

Laboratory technologists: Personnel who handle client specimens such as blood, sputum, feces, urine, and body tissues to be examined for cancer or other abnormalities. (5)

Lacto-ovovegetarian: Person who eats dairy products and eggs but no animal, fish, or fowl flesh. (42)

Lactovegetarian: Person who eats dairy products but no eggs or flesh. (42)

Laissez-faire leader: A group leader who turns leadership over to group members and steps in only when requested to give feedback. (25)

LAN: Local area network. Computers are connected to each other so they can share software or peripheral devices. (27)

Language: A set of words that have meanings that are comprehensible within a group. (24)

Lavage: The irrigation or cleansing of an organ. (42)

Law: According to Webster, "a body of rules or principles prescribed by authority or established by custom, which a state, community, society or the like

recognizes as binding on its members"; law is the force that orders relationships in a society. (3)

Laxative: A medication used to induce emptying of the bowel. (43)

Leadership: Influential behavior, voluntarily accepted by other group members, that moves a group toward its recognized goal and/or maintains the group. (25)

Learning: A process that involves perceiving and acquiring new knowledge, information, and skills, and subsequently changing one's behavior. (26)

Learning contract: A mutually negotiated plan for health education. (26)

Learning objective: Statement that describes the intended results of learning rather than the process of instruction. It should be clear, realistic, client-centered, and measurable. (26)

Legal guardian: A person appointed by a court to make decisions about personal or financial affairs of a person when clear and convincing evidence demonstrates that the person is unable to do so for himself or herself. (4)

Legal right: A claim one person has to a responsibility or duty on the part of another person that is enforceable by law. (4)

Leukocytosis: Increase in the number of white blood cells. (28)

Lever: A rigid or firm structure supported on a fulcrum or axis. (29)

Leverage: Use of a lever supported on a fulcrum to move a load more easily by the application of force. (29)

Liability: A legal obligation to pay damages, perform or refrain from a specific action, or suffer a criminal penalty. (3)

Libel: A written communication intended to injure the reputation of another; written defamation. (3)

Libido: The motivating force of all positive behavior; often associated with sexual drives. (12)

Licensure: A statutory based privilege to practice a profession intended to protect the public from harm as well as establish an exclusive practice area for that profession. (3); a process of review to determine whether a long-term care facility meets standards of care at a level sufficient to continue operation regardless of source of payment. (4)

Lignin: A polysaccharide that combines with cellulose to form plant cell walls. (42)

Linear causality: The process of one event causing another, as in A → B. (50)

Line of gravity: Imaginary line going straight down through an object's center of gravity. (29)

Lipoproteins: Large protein molecules combined with lipid components. (42)

Lithotripsy: Crushing of a calculus (stone) in the ureter, bladder, or urethra. (44)

Living will: A written document that states a person's own wishes regarding use of life-sustaining measures when the person becomes incapable of expressing his or her wishes. (4)

Livor mortis: Appearance of purple blotches on dependent areas of the body 20 to 30 minutes after death (caused by the effect of gravity on noncirculating blood). (54)

Load: Weight of an object or person, often referred to as resistance. (29)

Local effects: Reactions affecting only the area to which a medication or treatment is administered. (46)

Lordosis: An exaggerated curvature of the lumbar vertebrae. (33)

Loss: The removal or absence of an important object or subject from an individual's life. (54)

Lotions: Suspensions of insoluble powder in water, or ingredients dissolved in a thickened liquid. (46)

Lozenges: Tablets that should be completely dissolved in the mouth without chewing. (46)

Lubricant: A medication that coats the outside of the fecal mass, making it slippery and inhibiting fluid absorption from the feces. (43)

Lumbar puncture (LP, spinal tap): A procedure involving insertion of a needle into the lumbar sac of the subarachnoid space between L4 and L5 to obtain a sample of the cerebrospinal fluid. (34)

Maceration: A softening of the tissues that makes them more prone to erosion. (48)

Macrodrip sets: IV sets that deliver large drops (10, 15, or 20 gtts/ml). (47)

Magnetic resonance imaging (MRI): A noninvasive imaging procedure that visualizes internal body structures utilizing magnetic fields, radio frequency waves, and computers. (34)

Maintenance role functions: The role functions that help build and maintain group morale. Group members assuming maintenance role functions draw attention to the relational aspects of group life needed to nourish and support members as they labor to achieve the group task. (25)

Malpractice: The term for professional negligence. (3)

Manifest cultural behavior: Behavioral patterns that can be readily observed and identified by individuals who are considered to be outsiders. (19)

Material culture: The sum of the tangible items produced by people in a cultural group, such as tools, equipment, furniture, and clothes. (19)

Matrix: The collagen and proteoglycan scaffolding that supports soft tissue repair. (48)

Maturational crises: Predictable, stressful events that occur during a person's developmental process and for which the person has no coping skills. (16)

Mechanical ventilation: Ventilation of the lungs by artificial means, usually by a ventilator (formerly called a respirator). (45)

Meconium: The first stools of newborn infants. (43)

Medicaid: Title XIX of the Social Security Act, a group of jointly funded federal-state health insurance programs for low-income, elderly, blind, and disabled individuals. (5)

Medical asepsis (clean technique): Practices designed to reduce the number of microorganisms present or reduce risk of transmission from one person to another. (28)

Medical model: The belief that diseases can be understood merely as physiologic processes. (2)

Medicare: Title XVIII of the Social Security Act, a nationwide federal health insurance program established in 1965. Medicare is available to people aged 65 years and over, regardless of the recipient's income. (5)

Medication: A drug that is always administered with a therapeutic intent. (46)

Melena: Tarry, black stool. (43)

Menarche: The beginning of cyclic menstrual function. (13)

Menu: A list of options that a computer presents to a computer user. (27)

Message: The content a sender wishes another person (the receiver) to receive in the process of communication. (24)

Metered dose inhaler (MDI): Pocket-sized cartridge with a plastic dispenser that is used to deliver bronchodilators or topically administered anti-allergy or anti-inflammatory medications; also called a metered-dose device (MDD). (45)

Microdrip sets: IV sets that deliver small drops (60 gtts/ml). (47)

Micturition (urination, voiding): Emptying of the urinary bladder. (44)

Mid-deltoid site: An intramuscular injection site that allows the deposition of medication into the deltoid muscle. (46)

Milieu intérieur: Internal milieu or environment. (17)

Milliequivalent: A measurement of the chemical activity or chemical combining power of an ion. (41)

Milliosmole: Unit of measurement of osmotic pressure. (41)

Minidrip sets: See Microdrip sets.

MIS: Medical information system. (27)

Mnemonics: Skills to improve the efficiency of memory, such as grouping numbers, using rhymes and jingles, and associating items or characters. (14)

Modem: A device that enables computers to communicate over telephone lines. (27)

Monitor: A screen used to display information from the computer. (27)

Monotheism: The belief that there is one god. (53)

Monounsaturated fats: Fatty acids with only one double bond. (42)

Mood: A pervasive and sustained emotion that, when extreme, can color one's entire view of life. (32)

Moral right: A claim one person has to a duty or responsibility on the part of another person that is more likely to be honored when both persons base their actions in the same ethical theory or system. (4)

Morals: The ethical customs of a society or ethical habits of a person. (3)

Motor (ataxic, expressive) aphasia: Aphasia in which the client knows what to say and how to say it but is unable to coordinate the muscles of speech or hand sufficiently to formulate the message in spoken or written words. Motor aphasia may be complete or partial. (24)

Mucilages: Aqueous forms of gums. (42)

Multiple sclerosis: A chronic autoimmune disorder that involves degeneration of the myelin sheath of the white fibers in the central nervous system. The etiology may be related to both viral and genetic factors. (37)

Muscle-setting exercises: Isometric exercises most frequently done with abdominal muscles, quadriceps muscles, and gluteal muscles. (36)

Muscle tonus: The dynamic state of muscular tension that allows the body to be held in a normal posture or functioning position. (35)

Myelin: A lipoprotein sheath surrounding a nerve fiber. Myelinated fibers conduct more rapidly than non-myelinated fibers. (40)

Myelogram: A radiographic study of the spinal cord, nerve roots, and vertebrae. (34)

Myocardial contusion: Bruising of the heart muscle. (30)

Myocardial rupture: Rupture of the heart muscle. (30)

Nägele's rule: A common method of estimating the expected date of birth: take the first day of the last menstrual period, subtract 3 months, and add 7 days. (12)

Narcolepsy: A severe form of excessive daytime sleepiness in which an individual has uncontrolled "sleep attacks" and almost immediately experiences REM sleep. (39)

Narrative (free-form) charting: Paragraphs of information that are written sequentially and are usually organized in chronological order as a means of relating observations, interventions, and client responses to care. (27)

Nasal airway (nasal trumpet): Cuffless tube passed through the nostril and into the nasopharynx. (45)

Nasogastric (NG) tube: A tube that is inserted into either naris and is passed through the esophagus to the stomach. (42)

Nasotracheal intubation: The passage of a tube through a nostril and into the trachea to maintain a patent airway. (45)

National League for Nursing: A nonprofit national coalition of individuals and agencies working to improve nursing education and practice so that the quality of health care throughout the nation will be enhanced. (1)

National Student Nurse Association, Inc.: The national organization for students enrolled in schools of nursing. (1)

Naturopathy: A system of healing that does not use drugs or other unnatural treatments. Naturopathy relies on cleansing and restoration of the body through the use of natural forces such as air, light, heat, water, and massage. (2)

Nebulization: The separation of a solution into fine droplets, thus creating a mist that can be inhaled. Nebulization produces smaller droplets than atomization. (46)

Necrosis: Death of a portion of tissue that is still surrounded by living tissue. Often called "slough." (48)

Necrotic: Composed of dead cells. (35)

Need: A requirement or lack. (15)

Negative feedback: Feedback that leads to the initiation of a series of changes that negate and attempt to correct any radical change from the norm, either toward excess or deficiency. Negative feedback thus inhibits further change from the norm. (17)

Negative nitrogen balance: A condition in which the output of nitrogenous wastes is greater than the intake of protein. (35)

Negligence: The unintentional tort of acting or failing to act as an ordinary, reasonable, prudent person with resulting harm to the person to whom a duty of care is owed. (3)

Nephrectomy: Surgical removal of a kidney. (44)

Nephrolithiasis: The presence of stones (calculi) in the kidney. (44)

Nephrostomy tube: A tube that is implanted into the renal pelvis. (44)

Nerves: One or more bundles of fibers that connect the brain and spinal cord with other parts of the body. Individual nerve fibers are composed of neurons. (40)

Neural plasticity: Hyperexcitability of neurons in the dorsal horn of the spinal cord after severe pain and inflammation. Neural plasticity involves the release of excitatory amino acids (e.g., glutamate) that act at receptor sites in the dorsal horn to increase the pain. (40)

Neuroablation: The destruction of a nerve or a group of nerves. It may be performed by either chemical or surgical destruction of nerves that cause pain. (40)

Neutropenia: Decrease in the number of neutrophils (a type of white blood cell), which causes an individual to be at increased risk for infection. (28)

Nightingale, Florence: The founder of modern nursing and a prolific writer on the subject. (1)

Nightingale School at St. Thomas Hospital, London: The prototype for the earliest training schools for nurses. (1)

Nociception: The process by which specific receptors in the skin and other peripheral tissues respond exclusively to noxious or tissue-damaging stimuli. (40)

Nocturia: Urination during the night, which does not usually exceed two voidings. (44)

Nocturnal myoclonus (restless legs syndrome): A condition in which a person feels an urge to walk in an attempt to relieve an irritating ache or "creepy" feeling in the calves and thighs. (39)

Nonblanchable erythema: Hyperemic tissues that fail to lose their redness when subjected to pressure, indicating that the tissue probably cannot be saved from breakdown. (35)

Nonelectrolyte: Substances that do not ionize in solution and consequently do not carry electrical charges, e.g., glucose, urea, creatinine. (41)

Nonionic cleanser: A wound-cleaning solution that has no electrical charge. (48)

Nonmaleficence: The ethical principle of not inflicting harm on a person. (3)

Nonmaterial culture: The sum of the intangible products of a cultural group, such as religion, legal systems, values, and attitudes. (19)

Non–rapid eye movement (non-REM, NREM) sleep: A type of sleep accounting for about 75 per cent of a night's sleep, characterized by progressive relaxation. (39)

Nontherapeutic communication techniques: Techniques that impair the flow of communication in what would otherwise be a progressive movement toward client growth. (24)

Nonverbal communication: The set of behaviors that conveys messages either without words or by supplementing verbal communication. (24)

Normal flora: Microorganisms that grow abundantly as a part of the body's normal defense system. (28)

Normalizing: A nursing intervention in which the nurse assures the client and/or family that their response to a situation (e.g., death of a child) is expected or typical or normal. (50)

North American Nursing Diagnosis Association (NANDA): An organization formed in the 1980s to promote the development of and education about nursing diagnoses. (8)

Nosocomial infections: Infections that were not present at the time an individual entered a care facility, but instead develop after admission. (28)

Not-for-profit agency: Health care organization that uses profits to pay personnel, improve services, advertise services, provide educational programs, or otherwise contribute to the mission of the agency. (5)

NPO (nil per os): Nothing by mouth. (42)

Nuclear family: A married man and woman and their biologic children. (18)

Nurse anesthetists: Nurses with the advanced training and licensure to deliver anesthesia and monitor the client during surgery. Nurse anesthetists work under the supervision of an anesthesiologist. (49)

Nursing: The diagnosis and treatment of human responses to actual or potential health problems (American Nurses Association definition). (1)

Nursing care plan: A written plan that communicates the nursing diagnoses, outcomes, and nursing interventions. (9)

Nursing diagnosis: A clinical judgment about individual, family, or community responses to actual and potential health problems/life processes. Nursing diagnoses provide the basis for selection of nursing interventions to achieve outcomes for which the nurse is accountable. (6)

Nursing interventions: Nursing actions that focus on assisting people to cope successfully with problems and to achieve outcomes desired. (6)

Nursing process: A series of steps directed toward meeting the needs and solving the problems of people and their significant others; systematic, scientific problem solving in action. (6)

Nursing standards: Authoritative statements by which the nursing profession describes the responsibilities for which its practitioners are accountable. (1)

Nutritionist: See Dietitian.

Nutting, Mary Adelaide: One of the nurses in the vanguard during the formative stages of modern nursing. (1)

Occult blood: Hidden blood. (43)

Occupational therapists: Professionals who work with physical therapists to develop plans to assist clients in resuming the activities of daily living after illness or injury. (5)

Ointments: Semisolid preparations in a fat, oil, wax, or water-soluble base. (46)

Oliguria: Diminished amount of urine formation. (44)

Ommaya reservoir: A container that is implanted under the skin of the scalp and connected by a tube to one of the ventricles in the brain. (46)

One-to-one method: See Case method.

Open body posture: Body position in which the arms and legs are uncrossed. (24)

Opiate antagonist: Opponent of opiate drugs such as morphine. (40)

Opiate receptors: Molecular structures found on the cell bodies of nerves. These receptors have two functions: (1) to recognize certain opiates for which they have greater affinity and (2) to bind with those opiates. When many receptors are activated by binding to opiates, analgesia results. (40)

Oral medications: Medications given by mouth. (46)

Orogastric tube: A tube that is placed in the mouth and is passed through the esophagus to the stomach. (42)

Oropharyngeal airway (oral airway): Curved rubber or plastic piece that inserts into the mouth and maintains a patent airway to the pharynx. (45)

Orthopedic disorders: Disorders involving the locomotion structures of the body, especially the skeleton, joints, muscles, fascia, ligaments, and cartilage. (37)

Orthopedics: The branch of medicine that specializes in the treatment of musculoskeletal disorders. (36)

Orthopnea: The inability to breathe except in the upright position. (31)

Orthostatic (postural) hypotension: A sudden drop in blood pressure caused by a reduced blood volume, decrease in venous tone, and failure of the normal peripheral vasoconstriction expected upon assuming an erect position; postural hypotension. (35)

Osmolality: A measure of the number of milliosmoles per kilogram of fluid; used to compare body fluids. (41)

Osmolarity: A measure of the number of milliosmoles per liter of fluid; used to compare solutions. (41)

Osmosis: Movement of water across a semipermeable membrane from an area of lesser to greater concentration of particles. (41)

Osmotic pressure: Amount of pressure required for osmosis to occur. It is determined by the concentration of the solutions (the number of dissolved particles relative to the amount of water) on both sides of a semipermeable membrane through which water will move by osmosis. (41)

Osteomyelitis: Infection of the bone and bone marrow. (35)

Osteopathy: A system of medicine, founded by Dr. Andrew Taylor Still (1828–1917), based on the belief that health depends on the body's ability to rectify itself against toxic conditions when it has satisfactory nourishment and favorable environmental circumstances. Osteopathic physicians use manipulation to restore the body's structural and functional balance, and they use medicine and surgery to repair any internal or external abnormalities of the system. (2)

Osteoporosis: A condition in which there is an excess loss of minerals and organic materials that make up bone tissue. (35)

Ostomy: A surgically created opening. (43)

Outcomes: Observable, measurable client behaviors that are used to evaluate the effectiveness of the plan of care. (6)

Output: The general systems theory term for the movement of matter, energy, or information out of a system and into the environment. (15)

Overshoot: To overcompensate during attempts at system self-correction. (17)

Over-the-counter (OTC) medications: Medications that may be purchased without a physician's prescription. (46)

Oximeter: Photoelectric device that measures oxygen saturation of the blood at peripheral sites. (31)

Packed red blood cells (PRBC): Red blood cells separated from the plasma of the blood. (47)

Pallor: An absence of color in the skin, which appears whitish-gray in a light-skinned person and ashen gray or as a loss of red glow tones in a person with dark skin. (33)

Palpation: An assessment technique in which the examiner feels with his or her fingers and one or both hands. (33)

Paracentesis: A sterile procedure involving the removal of fluid that has abnormally accumulated in the peritoneal cavity. (34)

Paradoxical pulse: Pulsations detected during blood pressure measurement that decrease during inspiration and increase during expiration. (31)

Paralanguage: Nonverbal components of spoken language. These components give speech its rhythm and humanness and include stress, accents, pitch, pause, intonation, rate, volume, and quality. (24)

Parentalism: An exaggerated form of beneficence that achieves good at the expense of autonomy. (3)

Parenteral hyperalimentation: A method of providing total nutrition to a person intravenously through a catheter, thus bypassing the gastrointestinal tract. (47)

Parenteral support: Intravenous feeding. (42)

Parkinson's disease: A chronic, progressive disease associated with degenerative processes in the nuclear masses of the extrapyramidal system. The disorder is characterized by intermittent fine tremors of a hand or foot that spread until all four extremities are involved and the tremors are continuous. (37)

Passive range-of-motion exercises: Exercises done to maintain joint flexibility by putting each joint through its full measure of possible movements in all planes. Passive range of motion is used for clients who are immobilized to the extent that they are unable to do any of the work involved in exercising one or more of their own joints. (36)

Passive voluntary euthanasia: Withholding life-sustaining measures at a person's request. (4)

Pathogen: A microorganism that causes disease. (28)

Pathologic fractures: Fractures that result from very little trauma. (35)

Patient-controlled analgesia (PCA): A method of pain control that allows the person in pain to self-administer analgesics at frequent fixed intervals, usually by the IV route but sometimes by the subcutaneous, epidural, or oral routes. (40)

Patient privilege: The statutory protection and restriction of communication of personal health care–related information. (3)

Pectins: Purified carbohydrates extracted from citrus rinds or apple pulp. (42)

Pectus carinatum (pigeon chest): A thoracic abnormality characterized by the forward projection of the sternum. (33)

Pectus excavatum (funnel chest): A thoracic abnormality characterized by the sternum pointing posteriorly, which may cause pressure on the heart. (33)

Pediculosis: Infestation with lice. (38)

Pediculosis capitis: Pediculosis infestation of the head, eyebrows, eyelashes, and beard. (38)

Pediculosis corporis: Pediculosis infestation of the body. (38)

Pediculosis pubis: Pediculosis infestation of the perineal area. (38)

Perception: The ability to receive input from the senses, interpret the information in the brain, and correlate it in a meaningful way. (51)

Perceptual learning domain: The ability to perceive written or verbal information. (26)

Percussion: An assessment technique in which the examiner "thumps" or "taps" a body surface with a percussion hammer or the hand or fingers. (33)

Percutaneous venipuncture: Entry into the vein through the skin. (47)

Perianal area: The area around the anus. (38)

Perineal hygiene: Cleaning of the external genitalia and surrounding area. (38)

Periodontal disease: Disease of gums and tooth-supporting structures. (38)

Perioperative period: The entire surgical process. The perioperative period consists of the preoperative, intraoperative, and postoperative phases of surgery; it commences when surgery is planned and ends when the healing process is completed. (49)

Peripheral parenteral nutrition (PPN): See Parenteral support.

Peripheral vascular resistance: Resistance to blood flow through the vessels. (31)

Peripheral veins: Veins in an extremity. (47)

Peristalsis: A propulsive movement in which a wave of smooth muscle contraction moves along an anatomic tube, forcing contents of the tube ahead of it. (43)

Personal space: A private zone or "bubble" around our bodies that we feel is an extension of ourselves and belongs to us. (24)

Petechiae: Minute hemorrhages under the skin. (33)

Phantom pain: Pain that is felt in a nonexistent extremity (or other body part) that has been amputated. (40)

Pharmacist: Professionals who prepare and dispense medications, instruct clients and other health workers about medications, monitor the use of controlled substances such as narcotics, and work to reduce medication errors. (5)

Pharmacokinetics: The way the body absorbs a drug, distributes the drug within the body, and finally inactivates it. (46)

Phase II recovery area: A special observation unit for ambulatory surgical clients. It is used for an additional 1 to 4 hours of recovery following discharge from the PACU. Time is spent in this unit to ensure that all criteria for discharge are met. (49)

Phlebitis: Inflammation of the vein. (35)

Phospholipids: Any lipids that contain phosphorus. (42)

Physiatrist: A physician who specializes in physical medicine. (2)

Physical therapists: Professionals who assist clients in regaining the maximum possible physical activity and strength, also called physiotherapists. (5)

Physiologic homeostasis: The maintenance of a relatively stable and constant internal dynamic equilibrium. (17)

Pickwickian syndrome: A syndrome, occurring in obese individuals, characterized by pathologic sleepiness with severe episodes of dyspnea. (39)

PIE: Problem identification, interventions, and evaluation. (27)

Piggyback line: A secondary IV line that is connected to a primary IV line via a needle of the secondary line passing through an injection port in the primary IV tubing. (47)

Placebo: A neutral preparation (such as a saline injection or a sugar pill) given as a medication. (40)

Placenta: The vital link between the mother's system and the unborn child. (12)

Planning: A process of setting priorities, identifying achievable outcomes, developing strategies designed to support healthy responses, and prevent, minimize, or correct unhealthy responses identified in the nursing diagnosis. (6)

Plasma: The part of the extracellular fluid that lies within the vascular system. (41)

Plasma derivatives: Components of the plasma, or fluid portion of the blood. (47)

Pleural effusion: The presence of fluid in the pleural space. (45)

Pleuritic chest pain: Pain during a deep breath; associated with inflammation of the pleura or thoracic surgery. (45)

Pluralism: A state of society in which members of diverse ethnic, racial, religious, or social groups maintain an autonomous participation in and development of their traditional culture or special interests within the confines of a common civilization. (53)

Pneumothorax: The presence of air in the pleural space between the parietal and visceral pleurae. (45)

Polyunsaturated fats: Fatty acids with two or more double bonds. (42)

Polyuria: Excessive secretion of urine. (44)

POMR: Problem-oriented medical record. (27)

PONR: Problem-oriented nursing record. (27)

POR: Problem-oriented record. (27)

Positive feedback: A response to stimuli that results in intensifying the initiating stimuli, leading the organism away from the normal state. (17)

Positive listening: Simply understanding the auditory messages sent by a sender. (24)

Postanesthesia care unit (PACU): Recovery room, where the client regains consciousness after surgery. (49)

Postoperative phase: The phase of surgery that commences with the admission to the postanesthesia care unit and continues until the healing process is complete. (49)

Postural drainage: Placing people into specific positions to promote gravity drainage of mucus out of the lobes of the lungs and bronchopulmonary segments and into the larger bronchi, where it may be coughed up spontaneously or removed by tracheobronchial suctioning. (45)

Postural hypotension: See Orthostatic hypotension.

Posture: See Body alignment.

Powders: Dry medications that are usually dusted onto the skin for topical administration or that are mixed with liquids (water or juices) before oral administration. (46)

Powerlessness: The state in which an individual experiences the perception that one's own actions will not significantly affect an outcome; a perceived lack of control over a current situation or immediate happening. (21)

Practice guidelines (protocols): Documents that specify nursing management of broad clinical issues, phases of hospitalization, or interdependent clinical issues. (9)

Prayer: Communication with a higher power. (53)

Precipitate: To settle into solid particles within a solution. (47)

Preferred provider organizations (PPOs): Groups of physicians or institutions to which insurance companies direct their policyholders for care. (5)

Preoccupation: Absorption in one's own thoughts that hinders effective contact with or relation to external reality. (32)

Preoperative phase: The phase of surgery that begins when surgery is planned and ends when the individual is transferred to the operating room table. (49)

Prescription medications: Medications, including controlled substances, that require a physician's order. (46)

Prescriptions: Orders for medications and treatments or procedures. (2)

Pressure-reducing device: A mattress, pad, or other cushioning device that lowers the pressure on the client's skin to below the pressure that would be exerted by a standard mattress. (35)

Pressure-relieving device: A cushioning device that actually relieves pressure by reducing the pressure on the skin to below the 32 mm Hg of pressure generally accepted as being required for capillary filling. (35)

Pressure ulcers: Localized areas of tissue necrosis

that tend to develop when soft tissue is compressed between a bony prominence and an external surface for a prolonged period. These wounds are often referred to as bedsores or decubitus ulcers. (48)

Presumed consent: A method of increasing donation of organs by assuming a person wishes to donate organs unless the person has clearly expressed a desire to the contrary. (4)

Prima facie case: Facts establishing the legal elements necessary to a lawsuit. (3)

Primary care: Services provided at the point at which a client first enters the health care system. (5)

Primary care method: A method of providing nursing care in which one nurse takes responsibility for making the initial assessment, making all nursing diagnoses, planning all nursing care, and ensuring the implementation of the plan for a group of clients, 7 days a week, 24 hours a day. The primary nurse is also responsible for evaluating the outcomes of client care. (22)

Primary groups: Naturally occurring group formations with informal structures. Membership is automatic or spontaneously chosen. (25)

Primary prevention: Strategies used for persons who are considered to be free from disease. The main goal of primary prevention is to prevent illness. (2)

Privacy: The right to be free from intrusion into one's personal affairs. (3)

prn: An abbreviation for the Latin term *pro re nata*, which means "as necessary." When referring to medications and treatment, prn means, with certain limits, that the directive is to be administered at the nurse's discretion. (46)

Procedural law: The type of law that governs the legal process. (3)

Process recordings: Written records in which the nurse writes everything the client says and everything the nurse replies, word for word. The nurse also writes observations of nonverbal communication by both client and nurse. Because process recordings are written word for word, process recordings are also referred to as verbatim notes. (24)

Proctosigmoidoscopy: Endoscopic examination of the rectum and sigmoid colon. (34)

Professional review organizations: Agencies that oversee and review every Medicare hospital admission to be sure clients meet the criteria for hospitalization. (5)

Prognosis: A prediction of the probable outcome of a disease. (2)

Prolonged-acting tablets: Oral medications specially formulated for gradual absorption. (46)

Proprietary agency: See For-profit agency.

Proprioceptive stimuli: Sensations from within body tissues (mainly muscles, tendons, and the neural labyrinth) that provide information about the body's position and movement. (21)

Prosthetic devices (prostheses): Artificial structures used to replace natural organs, such as eyes, teeth, or limbs. (36)

Proteinates: Anionic proteins within the protoplasm of cells. (41)

Proteinuria: Protein in the urine. (44)

Protocols: See Practice guidelines.

Psychogenic: Of psychologic origin. (40)

Psychologic homeostasis: A state of equilibrium characterized by a satisfying self-concept, emotional balance, and harmonious interactions with the environment. (17)

Psychomotor learning domain: The learning domain concerned with manipulative and motor skills. (26)

Psychosexual theory: The Freudian belief that individuals are motivated by the two basic instincts of eros (sex, love, self-preservation, unity with others) and destruction (aggression, hate, death); the idea that sexual instincts are present in young children and are prime motivators of human development. (12)

Psychosocial dimension: The psychologic (mental and emotional), social, cultural/ethnic, and spiritual aspects of a person that combine with the physical to make up a human being. (32)

Psychosocial health assessment: A process used to deliberately and systematically collect data to determine a client's current psychologic (mental and emotional), social, cultural, and spiritual health status. (32)

Psychosocial history: The person's own story told in the person's own words from a personal point of view. (32)

Ptosis: Drooping of the eyelid. (33)

Pubescence (puberty): A 2-year span that marks the physical changes that accompany the beginning of sexual maturity. (13)

Public health nursing: Population-focused activities designed to improve the quality of life, including physical, mental, and social well being; prevention of disease; promotion of health; and control of communicable disease consistent with available knowledge and resources at a given time and place. (23)

Pulmonary function studies: Breathing tests using a spirometer to assess the extent of dysfunction resulting from restrictive or obstructive pulmonary diseases. (34)

Pulse: Fluid wave, created by the contraction of the left ventricle of the heart, which is felt at a peripheral artery. (31)

Pulse deficit: Condition in which the radial pulse rate is lower than the apical pulse rate. (31)

Punishment: An aversive event that follows a behavior and decreases the likelihood that the behavior will be repeated. (12)

Pursed-lip breathing: A breathing technique used to increase tidal volume, decrease respiratory rate, and control dyspnea. (45)

Purulent material: Material that contains pus. (48)

Pyelography: X-ray examination of a renal pelvis and ureter. (44)

Pyuria: Pus in the urine. (44)

Quad cane: A cane that ends in a pedestal that fans outward into four smaller feet. (36)

Quadriceps femoris site: An intramuscular injection site that allows the deposition of medication into the rectus femoris or the vastus lateralis muscles. (46)

Quality improvement (QI): A systematic approach

for improving the effectiveness of an organization while reducing costs. (11)

Quality of life: The degree to which an individual's continued existence is of significant value to that person. (21)

Racism: The belief in the superiority of one's own race over other races. (19)

Radioactive scan: A procedure that uses radioisotope-tracer materials to test some organ functions and to locate malignancies. (34)

Radiologic technologists: Personnel who perform procedures for taking x-rays and other images for diagnostic purposes. (5)

Radiopaque: Any substance, such as a contrast medium, that blocks x-rays. (34)

Rapid eye movement (REM) sleep: A type of sleep accounting for about 25 per cent of a night's sleep, characterized by rapid eye movements as detected by electro-oculograms and by intense physiologic activation. (39)

Rapport: A sense of understanding and trust that exists between two persons. (32)

Readiness: Physiologic, cognitive, or emotional preparedness for some task, such as learning. (12)

Rebound effect: See Secondary effect. (48)

Reciprocity: See Circular causality.

Recommended Dietary Allowances (RDAs): The levels of intake of essential nutrients considered, on the basis of available knowledge, to be adequate to meet the known nutritional needs of almost every healthy person. (42)

Reduction: Realignment of the bone fragments after a fracture.

Referred pain: Pain experienced in a location different from the source, usually along the nerve path; for example, left shoulder and arm pain during myocardial infarction. (40)

Reflex: An involuntary body response mediated by the spinal cord. (33)

Reflexology (zone therapy): A therapy developed by Dr. William Fitzgerald in approximately 1913 and reminiscent of the ancient Chinese treatment of acupressure. Reflexology relies on the application of pressure to certain body parts to relieve symptoms at distant sites and in specific organs. Pressure points used in reflexology are primarily in the hands and feet. (2)

Rehabilitation: Services that help restore the client to the fullest possible level of function and independence after injury or illness. (5)

Reinforcer: An event that follows a behavior and increases the likelihood that the behavior will be repeated. (12)

Related factors: Conditions or circumstances that can cause or contribute to the development of a diagnosis. (6)

Religion: A set of beliefs, values, codes of conduct, and rituals that answers the question of what it means to be human in relation to self, others, and a greater power. (53)

Required request: An approach to encouraging organ donation that mandates that health care facilities develop a process for requesting organ donation from appropriate family members at the time of the potential donor's death or when death is anticipated. (4)

Rescue medication: Medication taken for breakthrough pain. (40)

Reservoir: Source of infectious agent in which the agent lives and multiplies. (28)

Residual urine: Urine left in the bladder after urination. (44)

Resistive range-of-motion exercises: Exercises done to maintain joint flexibility and help the client build muscle strength by putting each joint through its full measure of possible movements in all planes against resistance by an external source (e.g., another person or weights). (36)

Respiration: The act of breathing; the exchange of oxygen and carbon dioxide in the lungs and the tissues. (31)

Respiratory arrest: Cessation of respiration. (30)

Respiratory technologists: Personnel who carry out procedures and operate equipment that assists clients in breathing. (5)

Response: The action taken by the person after meaning has been given to a sensation. (51)

Response cost: Refers to the removal of a pleasant reinforcement. (12)

Response time: The amount of time required for a computer to accept a user's input. (27)

Responsibility: A duty or obligation of one person with respect to another person. (4)

Retention: The accumulation of an excess amount of urine in the bladder of a person with normal urine production. It is due to the person's inability to empty the bladder. (44)

Retention enema: A type of enema retained in the bowel over a prolonged period. It is usually administered to lubricate or soften a hard fecal mass with oil, thus facilitating its expulsion through the anus. (43)

Retention with overflow: Extension of urinary retention. The individual voids frequently but in amounts that are enough only to reduce intravesicular pressure slightly. (44)

Return-flow enema (Harris flush): A type of enema that relieves gaseous distention. (43)

Reverse (protective) isolation: A set of procedures intended to control a client's environment so that it is similar to an operating room. (28)

Rhonchi (gurgles): Coarse, rattling sounds, louder and lower in pitch than crackles, caused by narrowed airways. Rhonchi are more pronounced on expiration. (33)

RICE: An acronym for a treatment that is helpful with fractures, sprains, and strains. *R*est (of the injured part), *i*ce (applications to reduce pain and edema), *c*ompression (applications to decrease edema), and *e*levation (of the injured part to reduce edema). (37)

Right: A claim one person has to a responsibility or duty on the part of another person. (4)

Rights-oriented ethical theory: A system of ethical thinking having the concept of rights as the foundation. (3)

Rigor mortis: Stiffening of the dead body due to chemical changes occurring in the muscle protein. (54)

Risk factors: Behaviors, conditions, or circumstances that render an individual, family, or community more vulnerable to a particular problem than others in the same or similar situation. (8)

RN first assistants: Nurses working in an expanded role with advanced, specialized education in surgical techniques and responsibilities. They assist the surgeon with the surgical procedure. (49)

Robb, Isabel Hampton: One of the nurses in the vanguard during the formative stages of modern nursing. (1)

Role performance model: A model that defines health as the greatest ability to perform one's expected activities. (2)

Rotation: Turning an extremity around its axis so as to turn the articulating end of the bone within the joint cavity. (35)

Routine inquiry: A method of encouraging donation of organs that calls for inquiry on hospital admission as to whether the person has indicated the desire to be an organ donor. (4)

Saline laxative (osmotic agent): A medication that contains poorly absorbed salts and sugars and that, through osmotic activity, draws water into the intestine to increase bulk and lubricate feces. (43)

Saline lock: A venous access device identical to a heparin lock that is kept patent by saline, rather than by heparin. (47)

Sandwich generation: Middle-aged generation who are caregivers to their parents as well as their children. (14)

Saturated fats: Fatty acids in which all the carbons are connected by single bonds and which contain much hydrogen. (42)

Scabies: See Pediculosis corporis.

Scalp vein needle: See Butterfly.

Sclerotic: Hardened with scar tissue. (47)

Scoliosis: A lateral curvature of the spine. (33)

Sebaceous glands: Glands that secrete sebum (an oily substance) into the hair follicles. (38)

Secondary care: Prevention of complications from disease, treatment of temporary dysfunction requiring hospitalization, evaluation of long-term care for clients who may need treatment changes, and counseling and therapy not available in primary care settings. (5)

Secondary effect: An effect that occurs with prolonged application of heat or cold wherein an effect that is opposite to the therapeutic effect takes place. For example, heat normally produces vasodilation but when left in place for more than 30 minutes it can produce vasoconstriction. (48)

Secondary groups: Group formations specifically developed by people for the purpose of achieving identified goals. (25)

Secondary IV line: See Piggyback line.

Secondary prevention: Strategies used for people in whom disease is present. The goal of secondary prevention is to halt or reverse the disease process to prevent further disability or death. (2)

Sedatives: Medications used to reduce anxiety. (39)

Self: The union of all of the elements that comprise a person's individual and particular make-up. (15)

Self-actualization: The highest state of being, the full realization of the individual's potential. (15)

Self-care: Actions or choices individuals make to promote their own health. (20)

Self-concept: An attitude, feeling, or evaluation about oneself. (50)

Self-efficacy: Level of competence of an individual. (50)

Self-esteem: The affective component of self-concept that describes an attitude, feeling, or evaluation of self-worth. (50)

Self-help groups: Groups having a common purpose and identity deriving from the similar life circumstances of the participants, rather than from their emotional needs. The goals of the self-help groups are supportive rather than insight oriented. (25)

Self-perception: The way one, correctly or incorrectly, believes oneself to be. (15)

Sensation: The reception of stimulation through receptors of the nervous system. (51)

Sensory (receptive) aphasia: Aphasia in which the client is unable to understand words communicated to him or her. Three types include auditory aphasia, visual aphasia, and both auditory and visual aphasia (aphemesthesia). (24)

Sensory channel: The means by which a message is sent. The three primary routes are the visual, auditory, and kinesthetic channels. (24)

Sensory deficit: Impairment of sight, hearing, taste, touch (including pressure and pain perception), smell, or sense of position. (51)

Sensory deprivation: A condition that occurs because of inadequate reception or perception of environmental stimuli. The cause may be physiologic, such as a sensory deficit, or it may be due to an inadequate amount or variation of sensory stimuli in the environment. (51)

Sensory overload: Sensory changes experienced when stimuli in the environment are excessive or beyond the person's ability to absorb and/or comprehend. (51)

Sensory perceptual alteration: A state in which the person experiences a change in the amount, patterns, or interpretation of incoming stimuli by receptors for sight, hearing, taste, touch, smell, or body position. (51)

Serology: The study of antigen-antibody reactions in serum. (28)

Serosanguineous drainage: Clear, blood-tinged serous drainage. (48)

Serum: Plasma without the clotting substance fibrinogen. (41)

Set point: The optimal level or concentration above or below which the negative feedback system will inhibit or enhance the output. (17)

Sexism: The exploitation and social domination of members of one sex by the other. (52)

Sexual function: The biologic aspects of sexual response. (52)

Sexuality: The state or quality of being sexual; the collective characteristics that mark the differences between the male and the female and the constitution and life of the individual as related to sex; the pursuit of sexual pleasure, reproduction, and the need for love and personal fulfillment; awareness and feelings of being male or female (referred to as gender identity). (52)

Sexual orientation: The preference as well as the physical and emotional attraction one develops for a partner of a particular gender. (52)

Shiatsu: An ancient Japanese therapy based on maintaining and restoring the flow of energy (ki) in the human body. Like acupressure, shiatsu (literally "finger pressure") uses the application of rhythmic pressure at certain points along the body meridians to relieve symptoms of disease. (2)

Sick role: A pattern of behavior that society generally expects from ill people. (21)

Side effects: See adverse effects.

Sigh: A deep inspiration followed by a prolonged expiration. (31)

Sigma Theta Tau: An international nursing honor society committed to excellence in nursing. (1)

Sign: An objective observation made by physical assessment. (33)

Sign language: A method used by the hearing impaired to communicate by indicating letters and words with different positions and movements of the hands. Sign language is used to replace the spoken word. (24)

Simple (closed) fracture: A fracture in which the bone is broken but no external break in the skin is present and minimal soft tissue injury exists. (37)

Single-parent family: A family of children headed by only one parent. (18)

Situational crises: Usually sudden, unexpected stressful events that happen to an individual at any point in life and that cannot be controlled by the individual. (16)

Sitz baths: Warm therapeutic baths in which the person sits. (48)

Skeletal traction: The type of traction in which the pulling force is applied directly to the bone. (37)

Skilled nursing: Activities within the scope and practice of the registered professional nurse, such as assessment, observation, evaluation of signs and symptoms, planning of individualized goal-directed care, teaching self-care to promote independence, and using clinical skills in the application of treatments and the provision of direct care. (23)

Skin traction: The type of traction in which the pulling force is applied directly to the skin and indirectly to underlying muscles and bones. (37)

Skin turgor: An indication of hydration status assessed by pinching up the skin and releasing it. (33)

Slander: An oral communication intended to injure the reputation of another; oral defamation. (3)

Sleep apnea: A self-limiting episode of nonbreathing during sleep. (39)

Sleep paralysis: An inability to move that frequently affects a person's limbs and occurs at the onset of sleep. (39)

Small bowel series: A series of x-rays of the esophagus, stomach, duodenum, jejunum, and ileum. (34)

Smegma: A cheeselike substance that is secreted by sebaceous glands and that collects under the foreskin in males and under the labia minora in females. (38)

Social adaptation: The adjustment of an individual's actions and conduct to the norms, conventions, beliefs, and pressures of various groups. (16)

Social cognitive theory: A theory formulated by Bandura and stating that all behavior changes depend on a person's belief in self-efficacy (the ability to successfully perform the new behavior). (2)

Socialization: A particular form of learning by which people learn the rules, attitudes, and norms of the social group in which they live (society). (12)

Social support: Actions to promote one another's health by sharing emotional support, ideas, information, and assistance. (20)

Social worker: Professional specifically educated to assist clients and their families with social challenges. (5)

Software: Programs of instructions that tell the computer what functions or steps to perform to carry out a task. (27)

Solutions: Homogeneous mixtures of liquids and solids. (46)

Somatic pain: Pain that arises from bone and muscle; it is caused by the inflammatory process, which often results in muscle spasm. (40)

Somesthetic: Pertains to sensations and sensory structures of the body. (51)

Somnolence: Sleepiness, or feeling drowsy. (39)

Source-oriented systems: Charting systems in which each group of health care professionals has its own portion of the chart set aside for storing information about observations and care unique to that group. (27)

Spasticity: Excess muscle tonus. (35)

Specific self-esteem: A measure of how much one approves of a specific part of oneself. (50)

Specimen: A sample of body fluids, exudates, or excretions that may be obtained and sent to a clinical laboratory for examination during diagnostic and treatment processes. (34)

Sphygmomanometer: The standard instrument used to measure blood pressure. (31)

Spiritual care: Not only caring for and about clients but also assisting them to find meaning in life experiences such as crisis and suffering. (53)

Spiritual healing: The use of prayer and/or other religious rituals such as the "laying on of hands," visiting of shrines, or bathing in holy waters to promote healing. (2)

Spiritual health: A state of balance that transcends physical or material things. (53)

Spirituality: The life principle that pervades a person's entire being: a person's physical, emotional, intellectual, moral, ethical, and volitional (power of choosing and decision making) dimensions. (53)

Spiritual needs: Those variables that inspire us to transcend the material world. (53)

Sprain: An injury to a joint in which surrounding ligaments have been stretched or torn by a traumatic injury to the joint, such as "twisting the ankle." (37)

Stability: Steadiness of position. (29)

Standard of care: What a reasonable, prudent practitioner with similar education and experience would do or not do in similar circumstances. (3)

Stat order: A directive that is to be carried out immediately. (46)

Statutory law: Law created by state legislatures or the United States Congress. (3)

Steatorrhea: The passage of greasy stools that tend to float and are mixed with observable fat and mucus. (43)

Stent: Any material used to hold tissue in place or to provide a support for a graft or anastomosis while healing takes place. (44)

Sterile technique: Practices aimed at achieving surgical asepsis. (28)

Sterilization: Destroying all forms of microbial life. (28)

Stertor: Noisy respiration produced by secretions in the trachea and large bronchi. (31)

Stimulant (irritant) laxative: A medication that increases peristalsis by stimulating sensory nerve endings of the colonic epithelium or by directly irritating the gastrointestinal mucosa. (43)

Stoma: A surgically created mouthlike opening. (43)

Stomatitis: Inflammation of the oral mucosa. (38)

Strain: An injury in which a muscle or tendon has been damaged by overstretching or overexertion, such as might occur with a sport that involves strenuous muscle use. (37)

Strength-developing exercises: Isotonic and isometric exercises that contract muscles and promote their development. (36)

Stress: The process of adjusting to circumstances that disrupt, or threaten to disrupt, a person's equilibrium. (16)

Stressors: Agents or factors that challenge the adaptive capacities of an organism or person. (16)

Stress responses: Physiologic and psychologic reactions to stress. (16)

Stridor: Harsh inspiratory crowing sounds that occur with upper airway or laryngeal obstruction. (31)

Stroke volume: Amount of blood ejected by the heart in each left ventricular systole. (31)

Subarachnoid space: The space directly outside the pia mater. This space contains cerebrospinal fluid and many opiate receptors. (40)

Subconscious: Thoughts and feelings that the person is not aware of at the moment but that can easily be brought to awareness. (12)

Subculture: A smaller group within a culture. (19)

Substantive law: The legal theory under which a case is brought to court (e.g., tort or contract law). (3)

Subsystem: A subset of a system; a set of integrated, interacting parts that, together with one or more other subsystems, makes up a system. (15)

Suction catheter: A rubber or plastic tube, attached to a vacuum source, used to suck secretions from the lungs, nose, and mouth. (45)

Sundowner's syndrome: A common sleep disturbance found most notably in the elderly, characterized by restlessness and agitation in the late afternoon and early evening. (39)

Superego: The last part of the personality to develop; the conscience; the moral dimension of the personality. (12)

Suppository: A semisolid cone, or oval-shaped medication, that melts at body temperature. Medicated suppositories are inserted into the rectum, where they release their active ingredients as they melt. (43)

Suprasystem: A collection of two or more systems into a larger system. (15)

Surgical asepsis (sterile technique): The preparation and handling of materials so as to prevent the client's exposure to any living microorganisms. (28)

Surrogate: The term used for a substitute decision-maker. (4)

Suspensions: Mixtures of solid particles in a liquid medium in which the particles precipitate out when the suspension is left standing. (46)

Sustained-release tablets: See Prolonged-acting tablets.

Swing-through gait: A crutch-walking gait with three points on the floor and consisting of two crutches and one foot or both feet together; the foot (feet) swing through and beyond the crutches. (36)

Swing-to gait: A crutch-walking gait with three points on the floor and consisting of two crutches and one foot or both feet together; both crutches together, foot or feet pulled up nearly to the crutches. (36)

Sympathetically maintained pain (SMP): Pain associated with the sympathetic nervous system. (40)

Symptom: A subjective indication of organic or psychic malfunctioning, or a change in a person's condition that indicates some physical or mental states of disease. (21)

Synchronization: Interaction of exogenous and endogenous circadian rhythms that occur within the body. (39)

Syncope: Transient loss of consciousness, or fainting, due to a lack of circulation to the brain. (35)

Synergistic effects: Combined effects of two or more drugs or treatments that are given simultaneously, so that the effects are greater than the sum of the individual effects. (46)

Syrups: Medications that are blended into a sugared or thick, flavored liquid. (46)

System: A set consisting of integrated, interacting parts that function as a whole. (15)

Systemic effects: Reactions occurring in a body organ or system distant from the site of application of a medication or treatment. (46)

Systolic pressure: Maximal pressure exerted on the

arteries during contraction of the left ventricle of the heart. (31)

Tachycardia: Abnormally rapid heart rate, over 100 beats per minute. (31)

Tachypnea: Increased respiratory rate over 24 breaths per minute, with respirations usually rapid and shallow. (31)

Talking: The act of verbalizing symbols in order to convey thoughts, feelings, or ideas. (24)

Target tissues: Specialized cells that have specific receptors for particular hormones that are carried to them by the circulating blood. (17)

Tartar: See Calculus.

Task groups: Groups designed to further the goals of an organization (e.g., standing committees, ad hoc task forces, and "quality circles"). (25)

Task role functions: The roles of group members that facilitate group processing of ideas. Task role functions help the group stay focused on the task and directly assist the group to achieve its identified goal. (25)

Team method (team nursing): A method of providing nursing care in which groups of nurses and ancillary staff (teams), led by RN team leaders, provide nursing care to groups of clients. (22)

Tensile strength: The wound's ability to withstand disruptive forces without rupturing. (48)

Terminal: Hardware used to input or access client information. Bedside terminals are usually small, hand-held computers; unit-based systems are larger and usually stationary. (27)

Tertiary care: Services provided to acutely ill patients, those requiring long-term care, and those needing rehabilitation. (5)

Tertiary prevention: Strategies used to restore the physically or emotionally disabled person to the highest level of physical and mental health possible for that individual. (2)

Theism: Belief in a God. (53)

Therapeutic effects: Desired outcomes of a medication or treatment. Therapeutic effects promote health, prevent disease, alleviate discomfort or pain, or cure or control disease. (46)

Therapeutic rapport: A special bond that exists between nurse and client because they have established a sense of trust and a mutual understanding of what will occur in their relationship with each other. (24)

Therapeutic relationship: A helping relationship. (24)

Therapeutic relationship, orientation phase: A time when the nurse and client make an agreement that they will be working together to solve one or more of the client's problems. This phase represents an oral contract between nurse and client. It signals the initiation of a working relationship. This part of the relationship lays the groundwork for the work they will do together in the future. (24)

Therapeutic relationship, termination phase: The time near the end of the relationship when the work of the client and nurse is coming to a close. (24)

Therapeutic relationship, working phase: Mainly a time for completing nursing interventions that address expected nursing outcomes. (24)

Therapeutic touch: A method used to diagnose and relieve symptoms in ill persons by using the hands, much like the ancient Christian "laying on of hands." (2)

Third-party reimbursement: Payment from sources other than the person receiving care, such as insurance companies or the federal government programs of Medicare and Medicaid. (23)

Thoracentesis: A sterile procedure involving insertion of a needle into the pleural space to aspirate fluid or air. (34)

Three-point gait with partial weight-bearing on one extremity: A crutch-walking gait with three points on the floor and one injured foot bearing partial weight and therefore not counted as a point —both crutches with injured foot together, uninjured foot alone. (36)

Thrill: Palpable cardiac murmur. (33)

Thromboembolism: A condition in which a blood clot migrates through the bloodstream to a distant site. (35)

Thrombophlebitis: Inflammation of a vein associated with thrombosis. (47)

Thrombosis: Formation of a blood clot in the blood vessel. (47)

Time tape: Adhesive strip or printed tape with time shown in hours for the purpose of monitoring the amount of IV fluid the client receives or should receive each hour. (47)

Tinctures: Medications, more potent than elixirs, dissolved in a hydroalcoholic medium. (46)

Tissue hypoxia: Decreased oxygen supply to the tissues. (35)

Tonic contraction: The ongoing contraction of a small number of muscle fibers insufficient to cause the larger muscle to move but sufficient to maintain a partial contraction known as muscle tonus or tone. (35)

Tort law: That area of substantive law that recognizes that individuals, in their relationships with each other, have a general duty to take care to avoid injuring others. (3)

Total parenteral nutrition (TPN): See Parenteral hyperalimentation.

Toxic effects: Adverse reactions resulting from overdoses or from abnormal accumulation of a drug in the body. (46)

Tracheostomy tubes: Tubes inserted into artificially created openings in the trachea. (45)

Traction: A pulling force applied to a part of the body such as an extremity. (37)

Transcendent values: Values beyond ordinary values and limits, and beyond material values. (53)

Transfusions: Infusions of whole blood, plasma, or packed cells into a vein. (47)

Tripod cane: A cane that ends in a pedestal that fans outward into three feet. (36)

Two-point gait: A crutch-walking gait with four points

on the floor and two points moving at a time: crutch and opposite foot together, opposite crutch and foot together. (36)

Tympanites: Abdominal or intestinal distention caused by the buildup of gas. (35)

Ultradian rhythms: Rhythmic cycles shorter than 24 hours, such as sleep cycles. (17)

Ultrasound: Noninvasive scan of internal structures using sound waves. (34)

Unconditional positive regard: A term coined by the psychologist Carl Rogers to describe respect that is not dependent on the client's behavior. (24)

Unconscious: Thoughts and feelings that are unavailable to awareness, such as those that are repressed. (12)

Universal precautions: Guidelines requiring that all persons be treated as though they are infectious. Universal precautions include barrier techniques, handwashing, and safety with sharp objects. (28)

Unsaturated fats: Fatty acids with double bonds in the carbon chain and less hydrogen than saturated fats. (42)

Upper gastrointestinal series (UGI): A series of x-ray films of the esophagus, stomach, duodenum, and upper jejunum as the person swallows a radiopaque contrast medium such as barium sulfate or Gastrografin (diatrizoate meglumine). (34)

Ureters: Two tubes that carry urine from the kidneys to the bladder. (44)

Urethra: The conduit from the urinary bladder to the exterior of the body. (44)

Urethritis: Inflammation of the urethra. (44)

Urgency: The need to urinate immediately. (44)

Urinary diversion: The drainage of urine from the body at a site other than the perineal meatus or tip of the penis. (44)

Urinary incontinence: The involuntary loss of urine. (44)

Urination: See Micturition.

Urolithiasis: The formation of urinary tract stones or renal calculi in the urinary tract. (44)

User: A person using a computer. (27)

User-friendly: Programs or equipment that are perceived as being easy to use. (27)

Valsalva maneuver: The physiologic mechanism that operates when a person attempts to exhale against a closed glottis and traps air in the lungs, greatly increasing intrathoracic pressure. (35)

Values: An individual's personal assignment of worth to an action or idea. (3)

Vaporization: A process in which a medication is carried in a vapor or steam. (46)

Vasospasm: Sudden involuntary contraction of the vein. (47)

VDT: Another name for a computer monitor. The letters stand for video display terminal. (27)

Vegan: Person who omits all animal products from his or her diet. (42)

Vegetarian: Person who may eat some eggs and dairy products but no flesh (animal, fowl, or seafood). (42)

Venipuncture: Introduction of a needle into a vein. (47)

Venous stasis: Congestion due to slowed blood flow in the veins; venous pooling. (35)

Ventilation: The movement of air in and out of the lungs. (30)

Ventrogluteal site: An intramuscular injection site that allows the deposition of medication into the gluteus minimus muscle. (46)

Verbal communication: The use of words to convey messages. This type of communication is achieved by writing or speaking in a code mutually understood by sender and receiver. (24)

Verbatim notes: See Process recordings.

Vertical relationship: A relationship in which a greater power and related values influence an individual's life. (53)

Vesicular breath sounds: Soft, low-pitched, fine rustling sounds located over the periphery of the lung. (33)

Vials: Single or multidose glass medicine containers. The sterile solution (or powder requiring reconstitution) contained in the vial is protected with a rubber stopper and soft metal or plastic cap. (46)

Vibration: Placing the hands flat against the chest wall and shaking (vibrating) the chest during exhalation to loosen mucus for expectoration. (45)

Virulence: A microorganism's ability to cause infection. (28)

Visceral pain: Pain emanating from the viscera (the abdominal organs or organs in other body cavities). (40)

Visual aphasia (word blindness): Aphasia in which the client is unable to understand the written word. (24)

Vital signs: Temperature, pulse, respirations, and blood pressure, which are indispensable indicators of a person's current state of health. (31)

Voiding: See Micturition.

Volatile substance: An agent that vaporizes or evaporates easily at a low temperature. (46)

Volume control chamber: A large drip chamber that is calibrated in milliliters and placed above the standard drip chamber on some IV tubing. (47)

Wellness diagnosis: A clinical judgment about an individual, family, or community in transition from a specific level of wellness to a higher level of wellness. It is a one-part statement beginning with "Potential for enhanced." (8)

Western medicine: Modern, scientific medicine usually practiced according to the biomedical model. (2)

Wheeze: High-pitched musical whistling sound heard accompanying partial obstruction in the bronchi and bronchioles. (31)

Wheezes: High-pitched sounds produced as air passes through a narrowed or defective vessel. They may occur during inspiration, expiration, or both. (33)

Whole blood: Blood containing all of its elements (plasma and cells). (47)

Wind-up theory: A theory postulated in the early 1990s suggesting that the nociceptors seemed to be *wound up* and more excitable to stimuli than they ordinarily would have been. (40)

Workers' compensation: A system that varies from state to state but generally insures only workers who are injured on the job. (5)

Work groups: See Task groups.

Wound: A disruption of soft tissue continuity. (48)

Wound exudate: Fluid draining from a wound and containing cells, protein, and solid material. (48)

Xerostomia: Dryness of the mouth from salivary gland dysfunction. (38)

Yoga: A term derived from the Sanskrit *yuj* for yoking or joining. A way of life that combines mental and physical exercises to bring the mind and body into balance and prepare the person for union with the higher spiritual power in an ultimate state of being. (2)

▼ *Index*

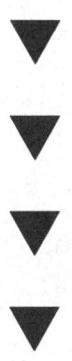

Note: Page numbers in *italics* refer to illustrations; page numbers followed by t refer to tables.

A

Abbreviations, used in charting, 486–487t
  used in prescribing and administering
    drugs, 1262t
Abdomen, anatomy of, 686, *686*
  assessment of, 685–688
  auscultation of, 686–687
  palpation of, 687–688
  percussion of, 687, *687*
  reflexes of, assessment of, 688, *688*, 688t
Abdominal binders, nursing considerations
  with, 855–856
Abdominal pads, 1375, *1375*
Abdominal thrust, for airway obstruction,
  576, *578–579*
Abducens nerve, assessment of, 669
Abortion, Canadian law on, 76
  counseling on, 76
  in Jewish faith, 1517t
  law on, 76
  spontaneous, 191
Abrasions, *1340*, 1343t, 1344t
Absorption, of drugs, 1282
  of food, 1093–1094
Abuse. See also *Substance abuse.*
  of alcohol. See *Alcohol, abuse of.*
  of children. See *Child abuse.*
  of drugs, 222, 242–243, 350, 974–975,
    1265
    in adolescents, 214
    in pregnancy, 77
  of older adults, 239
  spouse, 231–232
Acceptance, as coping mechanism in dying
  people, 1540
Accidents, in adolescents, motor vehicle,
  219, 225
  in middle-aged adults, 235
  in school-age children, 204, 205
  in young adults, 223
Acclimatization, fluid and electrolyte imbalances and, 1021
Accommodation, in Piaget's theory of development, 187, 188t

Accommodation *(Continued)*
  of pupils, 669
Accountability. See also *Nurses, responsibilities of.*
  documentation of standard of care and, 53
  evaluation process and, 166
  in ANA Code of Ethics, 48
  progress notes and, 169
Accreditation, of nursing programs, 60
Acetylsalicylic acid, action of, 872
Acholia, 1130
Acid-base balance, 1018–1022. See also *Acidosis; Alkalosis; pH.*
  failure of, 1009t, 1020
    risk factors for, 1021–1022
  in respiratory failure, 557
  mechanisms of, 1019–1020
Acidemia, 557
Acidosis, definition of, 1019
  metabolic, 557, 558
    causes of, 1009t
    outcome criteria and nursing interven-
      tions for, 1030t
  respiratory, 557, 558
    causes of, 1009t
    outcome criteria and nursing interven-
      tions for, 1031t
    with hypoventilation, 1206
Acids, function of, 1018–1019
Acne, in adolescents, 211
Acoustic nerve, testing of, 672, *672*
Acquired immune deficiency syndrome
  (AIDS), as reportable condition, 57
  assessment of, 1546
  CPR and, 561
  dietary management of, 1087–1088
  home health care for, 11–12, 404–405
  in adolescents, 215, 218
  in health care workers, 57, 521
  in young adults, 223
  prevention of, 218, 224
  spread of, 508
  stigma with, 1544, 1546
  testing for, controversies concerning, 57
  transmission of, in hospitals, 522

Acquired immune deficiency syndrome
  (AIDS) *(Continued)*
  work-related injuries and, 59
  wound care and, 1345
ACTH (adrenocorticotropic hormone), 307,
  308, 1491
Activation-Deactivation Adjective Checklist,
  316
Active transport, of ions across cell membrane, 1011
Activities of daily living, assessment of, 409
Activity. See also *Exercise; Immobility; Mobility.*
  food intake and diet and, 1076
  in young adults, 224
Activity-exercise pattern, nursing diagnoses
  in, 135
Acupressure, 38t
Acupuncture, 38t
Adaptation, and stress, 267–298
  characteristics of, 278–279
  concept of, 276–279
  definitions of, 276–277
  disease process and, 273–274
  homeostasis and, 178
  in growth and development, 182
  in Piaget's theory of development, 187, 188t
  levels of, 277–278
  of living systems, 251–253
Addiction, to drugs, 974–975
  to exercise, 841
Adhesive tape, 1385
  allergies to, 1385
  for wound closure, 1361t, 1361–1362,
    1362
    application and removal of, 1362
    products available for, 1361t
Administrative law, 51
Administrative support personnel, training
  and responsibilities of, 94
Admission to hospital, client's orientation to
  nursing unit and, 389–392, *390*
  documentation of, 394
  information required for, 394
  orientation to hospital room and, 392

Admission to hospital *(Continued)*
  prevention of liability and, 393–394
Adolescents, 210–220
  abortion laws and, nurses' responsibility
    and, 77
  acquired immune deficiency syndrome in,
    215, 218
  adult role and, 212
  as fathers, counseling for, 214
  body image and, 371
  causes of death in, 214
  cognitive and intellectual development in,
    212
  community roles of, 213
  contraceptives for, 77
  decision making about health care and, 70
  depression in, 215–216
  diagnostic procedures in, 709
  eating disorders in, 215, 1072–1073
  experiences with loss and grief in, 1536
  food intake and diet in, 1072–1073
  health concerns in, 214–215
  health education in, 216–220
  moral development in, 213
  musculoskeletal development in, 809t
  nurse's role with, 215–220
  perioperative nursing approaches to, 1412
  physical development of, 210t, 210–211
  pregnancy in, 214
  psychosocial development of, 211–213
  puberty in, 1491
  self-concept in, 1454, *1455*
  sexual development in, 1494
  sexually transmitted diseases in, 215, 216
  spiritual growth in, 1514–1515
  substance abuse in, 214
  suicide in, 215
  tobacco use in, 215
  values and beliefs of, 213
Adrenal glands, in growth and development,
    182
  in regulation of homeostasis, 302, *303*
Adrenocorticotropic hormone (ACTH), 307,
    308, 1491
Adult education, for middle-aged adults,
    231–232
Adults, chronic illness in, family stress and,
    326
  diagnostic procedures in, 709
  food intake and diet in, 1073–1074
  learning in, assumptions characterizing,
    471–472
  middle-aged, 228–235
    cognitive and intellectual development
      in, 230–231
    experiences with loss and grief in,
      1536–1537
    major health concerns of, 233–234
    nurse's role with, 234–235
    physical development in, 228, 229t
    psychosexual development in, 228–229,
      1494
    psychosocial development in, 229–233
    relationships of, 231–232
      with aging parents, 232
      with children, 231
      with community, 232
      with grandchildren, 232
      with spouse, 231–232
    self-concept and self-esteem in, 229–
      230, 1454
    values and beliefs of, 233
  musculoskeletal development in, 809t
  older, 235–243. See also *Elderly.*
    abuse of, 239
    causes of death in, 241

Adults *(Continued)*
    cognitive and intellectual development
      in, 237–238
    depression in, 241–242
    drug use and misuse in, 242
    environmental problems in, 242
    experiences with loss and grief in, 1537
    food intake and diet in, 1074
    health problems in, 241–242
    institutionalization of, 239
    lifestyle in, 242
    living arrangements of, 239–240
    nurse's role with, 242–243
    personal losses in, 241
    physical development and change in,
      235, 236t
    psychosexual activity in, 236–237, 1495
    psychosocial development in, 237–240
    psychosocial losses in, 241
    relationships and roles in, 238–240
    risk factors for falls in, 241
    self-concept and self-esteem in, 237,
      1452–1455
    spiritual growth in, 1515
    values and beliefs in, 240
  perioperative nursing approaches to, 1412
  self-esteem in, consequences of, 1452,
    1453
  young, 220–225
    developmental tasks of, 220
    experiences with loss and grief in, 1536
    health concerns in, 222–223
    health education of, 224–225
    health screening of, 223–224
    major health concerns in, 222–223
    moral development in, 222
    nurse's role with, 223–225
    physical development in, 220
    psychosexual development in, 220, 1494
    psychosocial development in, 220–222
    spiritual development in, 222, 1515
    values and beliefs in, 222
Advance directives, 1546
  decision making about life-sustaining mea-
    sures and, 74–75
  patients' right to, 67, 68
Advanced life support measures, 574
  following airway obstruction removal, 574,
    577
Advertising, food intake and, 1075
Advocacy, 365
  by nurse, 340
  self-help groups and, 455
Aerosolization, 1225–1226, 1235, 1274, 1275
Aesthetic appreciation, spiritual health and,
    1524–1525
Affect, 635, 636t
  format for documentation of, *637–638*
  in mental status assessment, 661
African-Americans, access to and use of
    health care services among, 339
  chronic diseases among, 337
  coping methods with loss and grief in,
    1538
  families of, 322
  health care disparities and, 348–349
  life expectancy in, 337–338
  mental disorders in, 338
  mortality in, 337
  older adults among, 240
  racism toward, 335
  self-concept and self-image in, in early
    childhood, 200
Age and aging, 240
  blood pressure and, 613, *613*
  body image and, 371

Age and aging *(Continued)*
  body temperature and, 590–591
  bowel elimination and, 1129
  child abuse and, 206
  communication and, 447
  constipation and, 1144
  food intake and diet and, 1069–1074
  musculoskeletal developmental changes
    with, 809t
  negative attitudes toward, 240
  perioperative nursing approaches and,
    1412
  pharmacokinetics and, 1264
  physical assessment and, 659–660
  physiologic changes with, 228, 235, 236t,
    814t
  pressure ulcers and, 1352
  reactions to illness in, 367
  respiratory changes with, 1206
  sexual development with, 1493–1495
  skin changes with, 1338
  sleep patterns with, 954, 955t
  soft tissue changes with, 1338
  stress and, 273
  surgical risk and, 1419
  urinary elimination and, 1158, 1160, 1173
  wound healing and, 1342, 1359
Aggregates, in community, 347
Agnosticism, 1523
Agraphia, 429
AIDS. See *Acquired immune deficiency syn-
    drome (AIDS).*
AIDS-related complex, as reportable condi-
    tion, 57
Air, in stomach, in CPR, 571
  swallowed, 1146
Air embolism, hyperalimentation and, 1313
  intravenous therapy and, 1327t
Airway, artificial, 1239–1243
    humidification of, 1241, 1243
    nasal, insertion of, 1241, *1241*
      suctioning of, 1246
    oropharyngeal, 1239–1240, *1240*
      suctioning of, 1246–1248
    endotracheal, suctioning of, 1246–1248
  in cardiopulmonary resuscitation, 559–
    560, *561*, 566
    head tilt–chin lift method, 560, *561*, 566
    in infants and children, 571, 572t, *573*
    jaw-thrust method, 560, *561*, 566
  ineffective clearance of, profile of, 1218
  obstruction of, 1239–1249
    in children, 579–580
    in infants, 577, 579, *580*
    management of, 576–577, *578–579*
    prevention of, 576, 1240t
    recognition of, 576, 1240t
  patency of, maintenance of, 1239
  suctioning of, 1243–1249
    assessment of need for, 1249, 1249t
    catheters used for, 1244, 1249
    general aspects of, 1244
    hydration and, 1244
    preparation for, *1243*
    procedure for, 1245–1248
    route of, 1243–1244
    side effects of, 1249, 1250t
    vacuum pressures for, 1244
Albrecht Nursing Model for Home Health
    Care, 405, *406*
Albumin. See also *Protein.*
  serum, pressure ulcers and, 1350
Alcohol, abuse of, health risks and, 233, 350
  in adolescents, 214, 219
  in ethnic groups, 338
  in young adults, 222, 225

Alcohol *(Continued)*
  motor vehicle accidents and, 225
    confidentiality vs. patient privilege and, 57
  use of, food intake and diet and, 1075
    in pregnancy, 191
    insomnia and, 953
    on self-care assessment test, 354
Alcohol sponge baths, 1395–1396
Aldosterone, basic data on, 1015
  factors influencing secretion of, 307, *1015*, 1015
  fluid and electrolyte balance and, 1014–1015
  fluid volume regulation and, 1016, *1016*, 1017
  hemorrhagic shock and, 309
Alertness, stress response and, 283
Alimentary tract. See *Gastrointestinal tract.*
Alkalosis, definition of, 1019
  metabolic, causes of, 1009t
    outcome criteria and nursing interventions for, 1031t
  respiratory, causes of, 1009t
    outcome criteria and nursing interventions for, 1032t
Allergies, at admission, 394
  food intake and diet and, 1074, 1089
  to adhesive tapes, 1385
Allodynia, 969, 972
Alogia, 429
Alopecia, 931
Alveoli, 1204
  drug absorption by, 1280
  in gas exchange, 1205
Ambulation. See also *Exercise.*
  assistance with, devices for, 829, 831–839
    canes, 837–838
    crutches, 829, 831–837
    hydraulic chairs, 839
    nursing interventions for, 840t–841t
    principles of use of, 840t
    prostheses, 839
    walkers, 838–839
  procedure for, 819–831
  preoperative teaching of, 1423
Ambulation belt, 795, 796, *796*
Ambulatory care centers, as primary care agencies, 91
  nursing practice in, 11
Ambulatory Monitoring Actigraph, 316
American Academy of Pediatrics, Baby Doe regulations and, 51
American Association of Superintendents of Training Schools for Nurses, 18, 19
American Heart Association, basic life support techniques of, 556
  1992 changes in, 559
American Hospital Association, challenge of infant care treatment decisions by, 51
  Patient's Bill of Rights of, 67–69, 1260
American Journal of Nursing, 18
American Medical Association, Baby Doe regulations and, 51
American Nurses' Association, 18, 21, 1260
  code of ethics of, 47–48, 67
  definitions of nursing by, 7, 347
  Model Practice Acts of, 60
  professional liability insurance and, 54
  standards of, 15
    for assessment, 126
    for evaluation, 170
    for implementation, 163
    for nursing care plan, 148
    for nursing diagnoses, 141
    for outcome identification, 146

American Nurses' Association *(Continued)*
  legal aspects of, 170–171
American Red Cross, Rural Nurse Service of, 11
American Society of Superintendents of Training Schools for Nurses, 21
Americans with Disabilities Act (1990), 59
Amino acids, essential and nonessential, 1055
  excitatory, pain conduction and, 971
Amniocentesis, 721
  care of person undergoing, 719t
Amphiarthroses, 732
Amputation, body image and, 371, 373
  grief process with, 1547
Anal region, bowel specimens from, 1130
Anal sphincter, dilatation of, for relief of bladder spasm, 1189
Analgesia, 968
  epidural, 988–990, *990*
  narcotic, for dying person, 1552
    premedication with, 1426
  nonpharmacologic techniques of, for dying person, 1552–1553
  opioid. See *Opioid analgesics.*
  patient-controlled, 988, *988–989*
    epidural, 990
    for dying person, 1552
Anatomy, section and position reference terms for, *655*
Androgens, in male sexual development, 1491
Androgyny, sexual health and, 1492
Aneroid manometer, for blood pressure measurement, 614
Anesthesia, drugs used for, 1432t–1434t
  nursing care during, 1431–1432
  preoperative preparation for, 1425
  types of, 1431
ANF (atrial natriuretic factor), fluid balance and, 1018
  in homeostasis regulation, 303
Anger, as coping mechanism in dying people, 1539
  as reaction to confirmed illness, 368
  immobility and, 755
Angina pectoris, activity and, 807
  cardiac arrest and, 558
  signs of, 807
Angiogenesis, in elderly clients, 1359
Angiography, 712t, 714
Angiotensin, aldosterone secretion and, 1015
  in hemorrhagic shock, 309
Angle of Louis, 681
Ankle, dorsiflexion and plantar flexion of, 693
  functional assessment of, 851, *851*
  range of motion of, 740t
    passive exercise of, 821
  restraints for, 883
Anorexia, in immobilized persons, 750
Anorexia nervosa, as psychologic adaptation, 277
  diagnostic criteria for, 1073
  in adolescents, 215, 217, 1072–1073
Anoxia, pressure and, 741
  with complete airway obstruction, 576
Anthropometric measurements, in nutritional assessment, 1067
Antibiotics, action of, 512
  for diarrhea, 1146
  for respiratory problems, 1235
  for urinary tract infection, 1190
  for wound care, 1382–1383
  types of, 1383
Anticholinergics, for anesthesia, 1434t

Anticholinergics *(Continued)*
  premedication with, 1426
Anticipatory grief, 1546, 1550, 1554
Anticipatory guidance, for adolescents, 216
Antidiuretic hormone, basic data on, 1013
  factors affecting release and inhibition of, 1013, *1014*, 1014
  in fluid and electrolyte balance, 1013–1014
  in fluid volume regulation, 1015–1016, *1016*, 1918
  osmolality and, 1013, *1014*
Anti-Dumping Act (1986), 67
Antiembolism hosiery, 767–768
  application of, 863, 864
  teaching and learning about, 864
  uses of, 863
Antimicrobials. See also *Antibiotics.*
  action of, 512
  types of, 1383
Antinausea agents, premedication with, 1427
Antipyretics, for fever, 601
Anuria, 1165
Anxiety, as reaction to confirmed illness, 367
  as response to stress, 283–285, *285*
  assessment of, 285
  characteristics of, 284, 286, 287
  defense mechanisms and, 271
  during injections, methods of reducing, 1284
  in group introductory phase, 460
  levels of, 285, 286t
  nursing diagnoses and, 286–288
  of client in hospital, 388–389
  somatic symptoms of, 285
  urinary elimination and, 1161
  vs. fear, 284, 287
Apgar scale, 195, 195t
Aphasia, forms of, 429
  nursing interventions for, 1481
  receptive and expressive, 1481
Aphemesthesia, 429
Apnea, 610–611
  pattern of, 1211t
  sleep, 952
Apocrine sweat glands, in adolescents, 211
Aponeurosis, 733
Appearance, assessment of, 123, 659–660
  personal, as body language, 431–432
  respiratory status and, 611
Appetite, food intake and, 1069
  in immobilized persons, 750
  in sick or injured, 1075
  methods of improving, 1089–1090
Aqua K pads, 1391, *1393*
Arm, assessment of, 691–692, *692*
  casts for, 866, *866*
  immobilizers for, complications with, 857
    uses and application of, 856–857, *857*
  passive range of motion exercise of, 819–820, *819–820*
Army School of Nursing, 16
Arrhythmias, cardiac, cardiac monitors for, 621, *623*
Arterial line, for blood pressure monitoring, 622, *623*, 624
Arteries, carotid, 604, 675
  coronary, disease of, 558
Articular system, 732–733
Artificial insemination, 190
Ascites, 720
Asepsis. See also *Sterile technique; Sterilization.*
  during bedmaking, 942
  medical, 506

Asepsis *(Continued)*
   in removal and disposal of sterile attire, 535
   surgical, 506
      basic concepts of, 524–535
      methods of achieving, 525
      need for, 524
      nursing responsibilities in, 524, 527, 528t, 529–535
      nursing role in, 527
   with parenteral administration of drugs, 1284–1285
Asian-Americans, chronic diseases among, 337
   older adults among, 240
Aspartate, 971
Aspiration, in cardiopulmonary resuscitation, 571
   of airway, 1243–1244
   studies of, 719–721
      positions required for, *720*
Aspirin, action of, 972
Assault, as intentional tort, 56
Assessment, 117–127, 649–701
   admission, 392–393
   as part of nursing process, 144, 160, 168. See also *Nursing process.*
   at midlife, 234
   body systems approach to, 122, 123
   cultural and ethnic factors in, 341
   data base for, 118–119
   definition of, 118
   for drug administration, 1264–1266
   for infection, 514
   functional health patterns approach to, 122, 124
   human needs theory and, 254, 255
   human response patterns approach to, 124–126
   in home care nursing, 407, 407t, 409
   measurement criteria for, 126
   methods of, 121–127
   of anxiety, 285, 286t
   of bowel status, 1127–1132
   of cardiovascular system, 676–685
   of electrocardiogram, 721–723
   of family, 326
   of fluid and electrolyte status, 1022, 1033, 1033t–1034t, 1034–1035, *1035*
   of growth and development, in adolescents, 215–216
      in infants, 198
      in neonates, 196t
         Apgar score for, 195t
         Brazelton Neonatal Behavioral scale for, 195
      in older adults, 242–243
      in school-age children, 204, 205t
      in young adults, 223–224
      in young children, 202t
   of head and neck, 665–675
   of hygiene needs, 894
      bedmaking procedure and, 935, 941
      ears, 911
      elimination, 898
      eyes, 908–909
      hair care, 931
      nail and foot care, 929
      nose, 912–913
      oral health, 902–904
      perineal care, 926
      skin care, 916
   of individual health promotion behaviors, 353–356
   of learning abilities, 475–477
   of loss and grief, 1544–1547

Assessment *(Continued)*
   of mobility, 733–734, 806–807
   of mouth, 903–904
   of need for intravenous therapy, 1328
   of need for therapeutic immobilization, 850–853
   of normal homeostasis, 315
   of nutritional status, 1066–1067, 1068t, 1069–1076
      diet and food records and, 1066
      physical examination and, 1066–1067
      tool used for, 1067
   of pain, acute, 973
      addiction and, 974–975
      chronic, 973–974
      dependence and, 974–975
      tolerance and, 974–975
   of respiratory status, 1209–1217
   of self-concept and self-esteem, 1456–1459
   of sensory/perceptual alterations, 1474–1476
   of sexuality, 1499–1501
   of skin, 1338–1339
   of sleep and rest, 954–955
   of soft tissue, 1338–1339
   of spiritual health, 1525
   of stressors and stress responses, 281–288
   of total human system, 252–253
   of urinary elimination, 1160–1169
   of vital signs, 585–625
   of wound healing, 1363–1365
   perioperative, in intraoperative phase, 1428
      in postoperative phase, 1434, 1436
      in preoperative phase, 1413, 1413t–1414t, 1419–1420
   physical, 122, 124
      client comfort during, 657–658
      documentation of, example of, *697–700*, 701
      equipment needed for, 653, *654*, 655
      formats for, 122–126
      general appearance in, 659–660
      height and weight in, 659, 660t
      measurements in, 655
      mental status in, 660–661
      positions for, *659*
      postexamination activities and, 701
      preoperative, 1419
      preparation for, 653–658
      purpose of, 653
      speech in, 660–661
      techniques of, 655–657
      vital signs in, 658–659
   prenatal, 191
   psychosocial, 627–647
      components of, 630
   pulmonary function tests for, *725*, 725–726
   purpose of, 118
   racial factors in, 341
   tools used for. See *Assessment tools.*
   ultrasonography for, 724t, 725
   vs. evaluation, 166
Assessment tools, 122–126
   Activation-Deactivation Adjective Checklist, 316
   Apgar score, 195t
   Beck Depression Inventory, 215
   Blaylock Risk Assessment Screen (BRASS), 392–393, *393*
   Brazelton Neonatal Behavior Assessment Scale, 195
   Denver Developmental Screening Test, 198, 202

Assessment tools *(Continued)*
   Fitts' Tennessee Self-Concept Scale, 1450
   for homeostasis, 315–316
   for nutritional status, 1067
   for pain, 978, *978*
      in children, 976–977, *977*
   Hester Poker Chip tool, 976–977
   McGill Pain Questionnaire, 978
   Rosenberg'a Self-Esteem Scale, 1450
   Self-Test for Health Style, 353–355
   Social Readjustment and Rating Scale, 274
   Wong/Baker Faces Rating scale, 976, *977*
Assimilation, in Piaget's theory of development, 187, 188t
Association of Operating Room Nurses, infection control precautions recommended by, 508
   Standards of Perioperative Nursing Practice of, 1404–1406
Asthma, bronchial, subjective data on, 651
Ataxia, assessment of, 692
Atelectasis, 1215
   in immobilized persons, 749
Atheism, 1523
Atherosclerosis, dietary management of, 1085–1086
Athletes, well-conditioned, bradycardia and, 607
Atomization, 1280
Atrial natriuretic factor (ANF), fluid balance and, 1018
   in homeostasis regulation, 303
Attitudes. See also *Beliefs; Values.*
   healthy behavior and, 349–351
   illness and, 364
   of nurse, in encouraging therapeutic communication, 434–435
   respiratory rate and, 609
   toward drug administration, 1265, 1283
Auricle, examination of, 670, *671*
Auscultation, of abdomen, 686–687
   of chest, 1213, *1213*, 1214t
      anterior, 681
      posterior, *678*, 679, *680*
   of heart, 682
   sounds of, 657
   stethoscope use in, 657
   technique of, 657
   types of, 657
Auscultatory gap, in blood pressure measurement, 615, 618t
Automated information systems, for documentation, 498–499
Autonomic nervous system. See *Nervous system, autonomic.*
Autonomy, as ethical principle, 46–47
   in young children, 200–201
   self and, 259
Autopsy, 1547
Avulsions, 1340, *1341*, 1343t, 1358
Awareness, encounter groups and, 454
   in theories of development, 185
Axillae, assessment of, 685, *685*
Ayurveda, 38t

B

Baby Doe regulations, 51
Back injuries, in health care workers, prevention of, 539–554
      center of gravity and, 540–541, *541*
      leverage and, 542, *543*, 544t, 545
      physics principles and, 540–542, 544t
      stability and, 540
   prevention of, 546

Back injuries *(Continued)*
　workers' compensation for nurses with, 59
Back massage, for sleep facilitation, 958, *959*
　procedure for, *959–960*, 960–962
　types of, 958
Back (spine) board, 784
Bacteriuria, 1165
Bag-valve masks, in cardiopulmonary resuscitation, 561
Baker intestinal tubes, 1097t, 1099–1101, *1100*
Bandages. See also *Dressings*.
　application of, 859, *859–861*
　cautions with, 858
　for Jones dressing, 862–863
　hazards with, 858, 861–862
　Kling, 1375, *1376*
　materials used for, 858
　roller, 859
　　circular turn with, 859, *859*
　　cotton gauze, 861
　　elastic (Ace), 861–862
　　　application of, 861
　　　documentation of, 862
　　elasticized or rubberized, 861
　　figure-of-eight turn with, 859, *860*
　　recurrent turn with, 859, *861*
　　spica turn with, 859
　　spiral reverse turn with, 859, *860*
　　spiral turn with, 859, *860*
　　types of, 861–862
　　stockinette, 862
　triangular, as arm immobilizer, 856–857, *857*
　tubular, *862*, 862–863
Bandura, Albert, theory of, 40, 189–190
Baptism, Christian beliefs about, 1518t–1521t
Baptists, beliefs and practices of, 1519t
Barbiturates, as sleeping pills, 963
　premedication with, 1426
Bargaining, as coping mechanism in dying people, 1540
Barium study, of bowel, 711, 711t, 1131
Baroreceptors, regulating fluid volume, 1015
Barrel chest, 680
Barrier techniques, 508, 513, 521. See also *Isolation precautions*.
　in cardiopulmonary resuscitation, 561, 562, *562*, 566
Basal energy requirement, 1052
Base(s), bicarbonate as, causes of imbalance of, 1009t
　function of, 1018–1019
Basement membrane, 1337
Basic life support techniques, 559–570. See also *Cardiopulmonary resuscitation (CPR)*.
　American Heart Association guidelines for, 556
　　1992 changes in, 559
　historical review of, 556
　single-person rescue using, *563*, 564–567
　termination of, 574
　two-person rescue using, 564–569
Basic metabolic rate, factors increasing, 587
Bathing, assistive devices for help with, 916, *917*
　by visually impaired clients, encouraging self-care for, 1479
　guidelines for, 914
　methods of, 916
　nursing assistance with, at sink, 918
　　in bed, 918–923
　　in shower, 917
　　in tub, 917–918
　nurse's reactions to, 1497
　of infants, 923–924, *924*

Baths, bed. See *Bed baths*.
　contrast, 1394
　medicated (therapeutic), 916–917
　methods of giving, 914, 916–918, 1275
　sitz, 1394
　tepid, 1395–1396
　tub, 917–918, 1394
Battery, as intentional tort, 56
　informed consent and, 70
Beard, care of, 934
Beck Depression Inventory, 215
Bed(s), changing linens of, for clients after myocardial infarction, 942
　orthopedic, 942, 943
　specialized, 941, 943
　surgical, 942
　while occupied, procedure for, 936–941, *937, 938, 940–941*
　while unoccupied, 942
　chin-ups and pull-ups in, 813, *815*
　comfort and cleanliness in, 935, 941–944
　designation of, 385
　made up for postoperative care, 1428
　specialized, 758, 760–763
　　cautions with, 761
　　Mediscus low-air-loss, 762–763
　　pressure-reducing, 1347, 1348t
　　　air fluidized, 761–762, 1347, 1348t, *1353*
　　　Clinitron, 761–762, 1347, 1348t, *1353, 1363*
　　　low air loss, 762–763, 1347, 1348t, *1353*
　　ROTO REST oscillating, 761, *763*
　　Stryker CirOlectric, 760–761, *762*
　　Stryker frame and wedge frame, 760, *761*
　　UHI-air-fluidized therapy, 761–762
　standard hospital, 389–390, *390*, 758
　　electric, 390
　　hydraulic, 390
　　ideal features of, 760
　　manually operated, 389–390
　　positions of, 759t–760t
　　side rails of, 390, *390*, 758, 886
　straightening linens of, 943
　transfer of client to or from, movement devices for, 879–880, *880*
Bed baths, bathing mitt for, 918, *918*
　procedure for, 918–923
　systemic assessment during, 918
　types of, 918
Bed boards, 943
Bed cradles, 765, *766*
　bedmaking and, 943
Bed linens, 935. See also *Bed(s), changing linens of*.
Bed rest, benefits of, 758
　definitions of, 757
　hazards of. See under *Immobility*.
Bedpans, guidelines for use of, 898–900, *899*
　types of, 897, *897*
Bedside commode, 897, *897*
Bedside stand, hospital, 390–391
Bedsores. See *Pressure ulcers*.
Behavior, acting-out, in therapeutic relationship, 424
　attending, of nurse, 434
　conditioning of, 189
　coping. See *Coping behavior*.
　disorders of, risk of violence to self or others with, 850
　encouraging changes in, 40–41, *41*
　extinction of, 189
　health belief model of, 32, *33*, 34

Behavior *(Continued)*
　health promotion and protection and, 349–350
　healthy, models of, 32, *33*, 34, 350–353
　home care nursing and, 410
　ideal cultural, 333
　illness and, 364
　in stress response, 283
　manifest cultural, 333
　modification of, 189
　　for health promotion, 356–358, 358t
　　for low self-esteem, 1463
　　in learning, 470
　　principles of, 358t
　　weight-loss diets and, 1082–1083
　motivation and, 182
　of mentally ill, nurses' responsibilities and, 81
　psychosocial theories of, development of, 184–190
　punishment and, 189
　reinforcers of, 189
　response cost and, 189
　self-esteem and, 1449–1450, 1463
　　reciprocity between, 1452–1456
　social learning theory of, 189–190
　temperature regulation by, 589
Behavioral theories, of development, 189
Beliefs. See also *Attitudes; Values*.
　about death and dying, 1543
　about health, health promotion and, 40–41, *41*
　　in ethnic groups, 339–340
　about self-concept, 1448
　home care nursing and, 410
Bellevue Training School, 16
Beneficence, as ethical principle, 47
Benzodiazepines, as sleeping pills, 962–963
　for insomnia, 953
Bereavement, definition of, 1535, 1535t
Bernard, Claude, ideas on homeostasis, 300
Bertalanffy, Ludwig von, 250
Bibliotherapy, 1463
Bicarbonate-carbonic acid system, as regulator of acid-base balance, 1019, *1020*
Bile, electrolyte composition of, 1023t
　stool color and, 1130
Biliary system, in homeostasis regulation, 302
Bill of Rights, abortion law and, 76
　in U.S. law, 49
　of dying person, 1544
　of patients (American Hospital Association), 67–69
Binders, abdominal, 855–856, *856*
　breast, 855
　cervical collars, 857–858, *857–858*
　chest, 855, *855*
　scultetus (many-tailed), 856, *856*
　slings, 856–857, *857*
　T type, 856, *856*
　types of, 855–858
　use of, 854–858
　　guidelines for, 854–855
Biochemical tests, in nutritional assessment, 1067
Biofeedback. See also *Feedback*.
　for chronic pain relief, 992
　in stress management, 290
　training in, 315
Biologic rhythms, 311–314
　nursing implications for, 314–318
　nursing research on, 316
Biomechanics, during bedmaking, 942
　for prevention of back injury, 540
　guidelines for, 542, 544t, 544–546
Biopsychosocial model of disease, 30

Biot's respirations, 611, *611*
  pattern of, 1212t
Birth, complications with, neonatal death
  and, 195
Birth control, Christian beliefs about, 1518t–
  1521t
  Jewish beliefs about, 1516t–1517t
Bite blocks, 908
Bites, human, 908
Bladder. See also *Urinary elimination.*
  aging and, 1158
  anatomy and function of, 1158
  distended, in immobilized client, 753
  function of, hygiene care for, 896, 897,
    899
  irrigation of, 1196–1199
    closed method of, 1196–1198, *1197*
    complications of, 1199
    documentation of, 1199
    open method of, 1198–1199
    teaching about, 1199
  spasm of, with urinary catheterization,
    1187–1188
  training of, 1174
Blanching, in erythematous areas, 743
Blanket drag, 551, *552*
Blaylock Risk Assessment Screen (BRASS),
  392–393, *393*
Bleeding disorders, wound healing and, 1359
Blood, aging and, 814t
  arterial, homeostasis of, 608–609
  buffer system of, 1019, *1020*
  coagulation of, disorders of, wound heal-
    ing and, 1359
    hypercoagulability of, in immobilized
      persons, 747
    liver biopsy and, 721
    parenteral administration of drugs and,
      1282
  collection of, venipuncture for, 1316–1320
  complement system of, in wound healing,
    1356
  components used in transfusions, 1311–
    1312
    packed red cells, 1311
    whole, 1311–1312
  exercise and, 814t
  gas exchange in, 1205, 1206, 1210
    arterial analysis of, 1215
    in pulmonary function tests, 726
    oxygen therapy and, 1228
  immobilization and, 747
  infectious viral disease carried by, wound
    care and, 1344–1345
  occult, in stool, 1132
  occupational exposure to, 1345
  serum of, 1009
  studies of, 719
    care of person undergoing, 717t
    complete blood count, 1215
  viscosity of, blood pressure and, 613
    in immobilized persons, 747
  volume of, blood pressure and, 613
  whole, 1311–1312
Blood flow, in hemorrhagic shock, 309
Blood glucose, changes in, hyperalimentation
  and, 1313
  self-monitoring of, 1167
Blood loss, in hemorrhagic shock, 309
Blood plasma, in interstitial space, in immobilized persons, 747
Blood pressure, arterial, physiology of, 612–
  614
  assessment of, 612–624
  circadian rhythm of, 312
  diastolic, 612
  factors affecting, 612–613

Blood pressure (*Continued*)
  filtration, fluid transport and, 1012, *1013*
  formula for, 612
  hydrostatic, 1011–1012, *1012, 1013*
    in body fluid transport, 1010
    in immobilized persons, 747
    in hemorrhagic shock, 309
    low, tachycardia and, 607
  measurement of, abnormal, interpretation
    of, 224, 607, 619–621
    ambulatory device for, 619
    equipment for, 614, *614*
      cuff size of, 614
    errors in, 619, 620t
    in adolescents, 210t
    in infants and children, 619
    in young adults, 224
    technique(s) of, 615–619
      arterial line, 622, *623*, 624
      auscultatory method, 615, 618t
      central venous pressure, *623*, 624
      Doppler device for, 619
      flush method (infants), 619
      palpatory method, 615
      procedure for, 616–617, *617*
      self-care method, 615, 619
      Swan-Ganz catheter, *623*, 624
      thigh pressure, 615
  normal ranges of, factors affecting, *613*,
    613–614
  oncotic, 1012, *1013*
  osmotic, fluid transport and, 1012
  paradoxical pulse in, 621
  peripheral vascular resistance and, 612
  self-monitoring of, 615, 619
  stress response and, 283
  systolic, 612
Blood supply, skin assessment and, 1338
  to soft tissues, 1338
Blood transfusions, adverse reactions to,
  1312
  blood components used for, 1311–1312
  typing and cross-matching for, 1312
Blood vessels, homeostatic state of, 1011
  interstitial fluid and, fluid transport be-
    tween, 1011–1013
  temperature regulation and, 589
Blood-Borne Pathogen Standard (BBPS),
  OSHA guidelines on, 59
Blue Cross/Blue Shield, 95
Body alignment, correct, *541*, 542
Body fluid, 1000–1002, 1015, 1019. See also
  *Fluid and electrolyte balance; Fluids,
  body.*
Body image, altered, adaptation to, 372–373
  assessment of, 373
  client teaching for, 373
  examples of, 372t
  illness experience and, 370–373
  in surgical patients, 1411
  nursing interventions for, 373
  reactions to, 371–373
  support for, 373
  urethral catheterization and, 1188
  development of, 371
  sexual health and, 1492
  situations affecting, 371
Body language, 430–433
Body mechanics, during bedmaking, 942
  for prevention of back injury, 540
  guidelines for, 542, 544t, 544–546
Body restraints. See *Restraints.*
Body size, fluid and electrolyte imbalances
  in, 1021
Body substances, infection risk and, 508,
  512, 514
Body support, provision of, 847–890

Body systems approach, in health history,
  652–653
  to nursing assessment, 122, 123
Body temperature. See *Temperature, body.*
Body type, physical assessment and, 660
Body water. See *Water, body.*
Boiling, for sterilization, 527
Bonding, in neonates, 194–195
Bone(s), anatomy and physiology of, 730–
  731
  cancellous, 730–731
  cortical, 730–731
  loss of, immobility and, 752–753
  of head, in neonates, 192, *192*
  of skull, in infants, 196
  periosteum of, 731
  resorption of calcium by, 752
  types and numbers of, 732t
Bone conduction, in ears, testing of, 672,
  672
Bone marrow, 731
  aspiration of, 721
    care of person undergoing, 718t
Boston Training School, 16
Bowel, direct visualization of, preparation
  for, 1131
  physical assessment of, 1129–1131
  preoperative preparation of, 1425
  radiographs of, 1131
Bowel elimination, 1125–1154
  assessment of, 1127–1132
  care plan for, 1153
  case study of, 1152
  evaluation of, 1152
  hygiene care for, 896, 897, 899
  in toddlers, 1148–1149
  measures stimulating, 1135t, 1135–1137
  physiologic factors affecting, 1128–1129
  problems with, constipation, 1143–1144
    diagnostic tests for, 1131–1132
    diarrhea, 1145–1146
    establishment of proper habits, 1133–
      1135
    flatulence control, 1146–1147
    impaction, 1144–1145
    incontinence, care for, 1147–1148
      causes of, 1147
      consequences of, 1147–1148
      training programs for, 1148–1149
    nursing diagnoses of, 1132
    nursing interventions for, 1133–1152
    ostomy care, 1150–1152
    planning for, 1132–1133
    stimulation of bowel evacuation, 1135–
      1143
  urinary incontinence and, 1174
Bowel movements, amount of, 1130
  characteristics of, 1130–1131
  frequency of, 1130
Bowel sounds, 686–687
Bowel training, programs for, 1148–1149
Bowlby, John, 1541
Bowman's capsule, 1157, *1157*
Braces, complications with, 870
  Milwaukee, *871*
  teaching and learning about, 870, 873
  types of, 870t
  use of, 870–873
    documentation of, 873
    guidelines for, 870
    principles of, 872t–873t
Bradycardia, conditions associated with, 607
Bradypnea, 610
  pattern of, 1211t
Braille, 430
Brain. See also *Hypothalamus.*
  cardiovascular arrest and, 557, 558

Brain *(Continued)*
damage to, cerebral ischemia and, 558, *559*
male and female, differences in, 1490–1491
Brain death, definition of, and anencephalic infants as organ donors, 83
Brain scans, with CT, 714
Brazelton Neonatal Behavioral Assessment Scale, 195
Breast binders, uses and application of, 855
Breast milk, for infants, 1070
Breastfeeding, failure of infants to thrive with, 1070, *1070*
nutritional requirements for, 1075
Breasts, anatomy of, 684
assessment of, 682
inspection of, 684
palpation of, 684, *684–685*
self-examination of, 682, *683*
Breath sounds, absent to decreased, 1214t
adventitious, 679, *680*, 1214t
bronchial, 679, 1214t
bronchovesicular, 679
documentation of, 679, *680*
normal, 679, *680*
vesicular, 679
Breathalyzer tests, 57
Breathing, 1203–1254. See also *Respiration; Respiratory system.*
auscultation of, 1213, *1213*, 1214t
control of, 1205–1206
deep, coughing and, 1225
exercises for, 1422, *1423*
diaphragmatic, 1237, *1238*, 1239
factors affecting, 1206
in cardiopulmonary resuscitation, 561–562, 566–567
mouth-to-barrier device, 562, 566
mouth-to-mouth, 561–562, 566
rate and size of breaths in, 562, 566
normal, 1211t, 1211–1213
obstructive, pattern of, 1212t
patterns of, 1211t–1212t, 1212
positive-pressure, 1236–1237
pursed-lip, 1237, *1238*
retraining techniques for, 1238, *1238*
Brewster, Mary, 11, 400
Bronchial asthma, subjective data on, 651
Bronchodilators, 1235
use of, *1226*
Bronchography, 713t, 714
Bronchophony, 679
Bronchoscopy, 723, 724t, 1217
Bronchospasm, 1235
hydration measures and, 1227
Brophy case, 74
Bruit, abdomen, 687
carotid artery, 675
Buccal mucosa, assessment of, 673
Buccal tablets, insertion of, 1276
Buddhism, beliefs and practices affecting health care in, 1517
beliefs of, 1517
Bulimia nervosa, in adolescents, 215, 217, 1073
Burnout, in nurses, 294–295
signs of, 294

C

Cadet Nurse Corps, 16
Calcitonin, calcium regulation and, 752
Calcium, deficit of, outcome criteria and nursing interventions for, 1027t–1028t
dietary, regulation of, 1037

Calcium *(Continued)*
requirements for, 1058t
in adolescents, 1072
sources of, 1058t
supplements of, 1056–1057, 1065
excess, outcome criteria and nursing interventions for, 1028t
functions of, 1006t, 1058t
imbalance of, 1008t
metabolism of, 1058t
regulation of, immobility and, 752–753, 754
Calcium alginates, for wound care, 1351t
Calculi, renal, 753–754, 1163–1164
Call light, in hospital client rooms, 391
Calories. See also *Diet; Food(s); Nutrition.*
body weight and nutrients and, 1052
daily expenditure of, during exercise and illness, *1076*
faulty intake of, in infants, 1071
Canada, abortion law in, 76
administrative law in, 51
health care goals in, 348
health care system of, vs. United States' health care system, 102t–103t
legislative process in, 51
licensure of nurses in, 61
malpractice insurance for nurses in, 54
poverty in, health care access and, 348
Canadian Charter of Human Rights, 49
Canadian Nurses' Association, 21
code of ethics of, 48, 49
definitions of nursing by, 347
nursing defined by, 7
Cancer, dietary management of, 1087
homeostatic mechanisms and, 310, *310*
in young adults, warning signs of, 224
odor-causing lesions with, odor control with, 1384
pain with, implantable spinal reservoir for relief of, 992
pharmacologic management of, 982, 984, *984*
Swedish massage for relief of, 987
self-concept and, 1450–1451
teaching clients with, 476
terminal, desired outcomes for, 1548t–1549t
nursing diagnoses for, 1548t–1549t
wound infection and, 1343
Canes, types of, 837, *837*
use of, 837–838, *838*
Cannon, Walter, ideas on homeostasis, 300
Canterbury v. Spence, 71
Cantor intestinal tubes, 1097t, 1099–1101, *1100*
Capillaries, fluid shifts in, 1011–1012, *1013*
homeostatic state of, 1011
pressure ulcers and, 1347
Caplan, Gerald, 279
Caput succedaneum, in neonates, 192
Carbohydrates, 1052–1053
Carbon dioxide. See also *Gas exchange.*
pulmonary transport of, 1205
retention of, in immobilized persons, 749
Cardiac arrest, 557
sudden, 557–558
Cardiac monitor, 621, *623*
Cardiac output, blood pressure and, 612
in immobilized clients, 743
Cardiac tamponade, with paradoxical pulse, 621
Cardiopulmonary arrest, 556–559
causes of, 558t
impending, 560, 561t
recognition of, 559–560, 560t
sudden, 557–558

Cardiopulmonary arrest *(Continued)*
unwitnessed, resuscitation procedure for, 565–568
Cardiopulmonary function, normal, 557
Cardiopulmonary resuscitation (CPR), 555–581
basic life support system of, airway in, 559–560, *561*, 566
breathing in, 561–562, 566–567
circulation in, 562–564, 567–568
carotid artery palpation in, 604
complications of, 571, 574
following airway obstruction removal, 577
historical review of, 556
in adults, vs. in children, 574t
in infants and children, 570–571, 572t, *573*, 574t
manual resuscitation bag compression in, 575
performance errors in, 569–570
procedure for, 565–568
refusal of, 74
sequence of steps in, 559–564
survivors of, 575
Cardiovascular disease, dietary management of, 1085–1087
Cardiovascular system, assessment of, 123, 676–685, 743, 744t, 747–748
failure of, 557–558
in adolescents, 210t
in homeostasis regulation, 302
in immobilized clients, assessment of, 743, 744t, 747–748
physiologic data base of, 602–603
Care givers, self-esteem and, 1451
Careers, at midlife, 232
in young adults, 221
Caries, dental, 901–902
Carotid arteries, assessment of, 675
Carotid pulse, *603*, 604
Cartilage, anatomy of, 731–732
hyaline, 732, *733*
types of, 732
Case law, 50
Case management, nursing care plan in, 151, *152*, 154
Cast syndrome, 869, 869t
Casts, application of, 868, 872t
body, cast syndrome with, 869
complications with, 868–869, 869t
documentation of, 869–870
guidelines for use of, 865, 868
principles of use of, 872t
removal of, 868
teaching and learning about, 869
types of, 865, 866t–867t
uses of, 865
windowing or bivalving of, 868
Cataplexy, 952
Cathartics, 1135
Catheters, See also *Self-catheterization.*
epidural, for epidural analgesia, 989, *990*
Foley, as feeding tube, 1101
hyperalimentation, 1312–1313
indwelling, as cannulas, *1313*, 1315
spinal, for pain relief, 992
urinary, 1190t–1191t
intravenous, methods of securing, *1329*
suctioning, 1244, 1248
urethral, 1177–1179, *1179*
urinary, 1175–1180, 1187–1199
as stents, 1176–1177, *1177*
complications of, 1187–1190
documentation for, 1196
external, for incontinence, 1175, *1175*
for specimen collection, 1168–1169
home care of, 1192–1193
documentation for, 1196

Catheters *(Continued)*
  indwelling, nursing interventions for, 1190t–1191t
    principles related to, 1190t–1191t
  infection and, 754, 1189–1191
  insertion of, procedure for, 1181–1182, *1183*, 1184–1186
  intermittent self-insertion of, 1193–1196
    documentation of, 1196
  materials for, 1176–1177
  method of securing to body, 1187
  nephrostomy, 1177, *1178*
  patency of, 1180, 1187
  psychologic comfort and, 1180
  purposes of, 1176
  removal of, 1190–1192
  retention, configuration of, 1179
    need for, 1179
  supplies for, with home care, 1193
  suprapubic, 1176
  teaching about, 1179–1180
  with closed drainage systems, 1190
CBE charting, 495, *497*
Celiac sprue, 1089
  dietary management of, 1084t
Cells, acid-base balance regulated by, 1020
  division of, circadian rhythms in, 313
Cellulose, 1052
Center of gravity, in prevention of back injury, 540–541, *541*, 544t, 545, *545*
Centers for Disease Control, infection control precautions recommended by, 508
  isolation precautions of, category specific, 516t
Central venous pressure, *623*, 624
Cephalohematoma, in neonates, 192
Cerebral ischemia, brain damage and, 558, *559*
Cerebral palsy, physical protection and support needed for, 850
Cerebrospinal fluid, from lumbar puncture, 719–720
  pressure of, 720
Cerebrovascular accidents, 748
  physical protection and support needed for, 849
Cerumen, 911
Cervical collars, complications with, 858
  uses and applications of, 857–858, *857–858*
Cervix, assessment of, 690
Chairs, elevator, 795
  hydraulic, 839
  in hospital client rooms, 391
  multiple-positioning, 784
Change agents, groups as, 465
  nurses as, 353, 356
Chaplains, training and responsibilities of, 93–94
Charting, 484. See also *Documentation*; *Record, client.*
  abbreviations and symbols used in, 486t–487t
  methods of, by exception (CBE system), 495, *497*
  diagnostic procedure, 708, *708*
  FOCUS, 492–494, *494*
  narrative (free-form), 488, *489*, 490
  PIE, 494–495, *496*
  SOAPIER format, 490, 492, 492t
  of findings on examination of wounds, 1363
Cheilosis, 904
Chemical counterirritants, 1392–1393
Chemical hot packs, 1391
Chemoreceptors, 1470
  respiratory control by, 1205–1206

Chest, anterior, assessment of, 680–681
  assessment of, 676–685
  auscultation of, 1213, *1213*, 1214t
  barrel, 680
  compression of, in cardiopulmonary resuscitation, 562, *563*, *564*, 564, 566, 574t
    in adults, 574t
    in infants and children, 571, 572t, 574t
    mnemonic for, 571, 574t
  examination of, 676, 678, 679, 1210–1213
  funnel, 680
  percussion of, 678, 678t, *678–679*
    therapeutic, 1227
  physical therapy measures for, 1227–1228
    contraindications to, 1228
  pigeon, 680
  pleuritic pain in, 1210
  posterior, abnormalities of, 676, *677*
    auscultation of, *678*, 679, *680*
      spoken and whispered sounds and, 679
    examination of, 676, 678, 679
    inspection of, 676
    palpation of, 676, *677*, 678
    percussion of, 678, 678t, *678–679*
  radiographs of, 1215, 1217
  restraints for, 884
  vibration of, therapeutic, 1227–1228
Chest binders, uses and complications with, 855, *855*
Chest thrust, for airway obstruction, 576, *578–579*
Cheyne-Stokes respirations, 611, *611*
  pattern of, 1212t
  sleep apnea and, 952
Chief complaint, 651
Child abuse, 205–208
  reporting of, 57, 207
  results of, 206
  risk factors for, 206, 207
  sexual, 206–207
  substance abuse in pregnancy and, 77
  warning signs of, 207
Child Abuse and Prevention Act, withholding of treatment and, 72
Children. See also *Adolescents*; *Infants.*
  adult, and older family members, 231, 238
  blood pressure measurement in, 619
  body restraints for, 885, *885*
  body temperature in, 590–591
  cardiopulmonary resuscitation in, 570–571, 572t, *573*, 574t
  chronically ill, family stress and, 326
  death of, parents' response to, 1537
  decision making about health care and, 69, 70
  dehydrated, 1002, 1022
  diagnostic procedures in, 709
  drug administration and, 1266
    parenteral, 1283
  fluid and electrolyte imbalances in, 1000, 1021
  growth and development in, 177–208
  high-risk, social policies for, 104
  hospitalized, family stress and, 325–326
    in pediatric critical care units, sleep in, 953
    sensory/perceptual alterations in, 1480
  immobility and, 755
  in human research, informed consent process and, 73, 73t
  interpersonal relationships of, 184, 204
  loss and grief in, 1536
  musculoskeletal development in, 809t

Children *(Continued)*
  pain in, assessment of, 975–977, 976t, *977*
    principles of management of, 977
    relief measures for, 992
  perioperative nursing approaches to, 1412
  poor, access to health care and, 348
  prenatally drug-exposed, nursing care for, 13
  related to dying person, 1546
  rights of, in organ donation and transplantation, 82
  school age, cognitive and intellectual development in, 203–204, 206t
    communication in, 203–204
    food intake and diet in, 1071–1072
    growth and development in, 202–205
    major health concerns in, 204, 205
    relationships of, 204
    self-concept in, 203
    self-image in, 203
    sexual development in, 1494
    values and beliefs in, 204
  school nursing care for, 12–13
  self-concept in, 199–200, 203, 1453–1454
  sexual development in, 1493–1494
  socialization of, 189, 204
  spiritual growth in, 1514
  vital signs in, 193t
  with disabilities, abuse and, 206
  young, autonomy in, 200–201
    causes of death in, 201, 202
    cognitive and intellectual development in, 200, 202t
    communication abilities in, 200
    day care issues and, 201, 202
    diagnostic procedures in, 709
    eating patterns in, 199, 1071
    gender identity in, 200
    growth and development in, 198–202
    health problems in, 201–202
    initiative in, 201
    motor skills in, 199
    nurse's role with, 201, 202, 202t
    physical development in, 193t, 199, 202t
    play in, 200
    psychosocial development in, 199–201, 202t
    self-concept and self-image in, 199–200
    self-control in, 201
    sleep patterns in, 199
    toilet training in, 199
    values and beliefs in, 201
    weight gain in, 199
Chills, and fever, 600
Chin-ups and pull-ups, in bed, 813, *815*
Chiropractic treatment, 38t
Chloride, functions of, 1006t
  imbalance of, causes of, 1007t
  in gastrointestinal function, 1017
Chlorine, metabolism, functions, and sources of, 1059t
Choice, consumer rights and health care providers' responsibilities and, 68–79
Choking, management of, 576–577
  in children, 579–580
  in infants, 577, 579, *580*
  prevention of, 576
  recognition of, 576, *576*
Cholecystitis, dietary management of, 1084–1085
Cholecystogram, 711, 712t, 713
Cholelithiasis, dietary management of, 1084–1085
Cholesterol, atherosclerosis and, 1085–1086
  dietary changes affecting, 1086
  function of, 1055

Chondrocytes, 731–732

Christian churches, beliefs and practices affecting health care of, 1518t–1521t
 Assemblies of God, 1518t–1519t
 Baptist, 1519t
 Church of Jesus Christ of Latter Day Saints, 1069, 1521t
 Church of the Brethren, 1519t
 Church of the Nazarene, 1519t
 Disciples of Christ, 1519t
 Eastern Orthodox, 1518t
 Episcopal, 1519t
 Lutheran, 1519t
 Mennonite, 1519t
 Methodist, 1520t
 Presbyterian, 1520t
 Quaker, 1520t
 Roman Catholic, 1518t
 Salvation Army, 1520t
 Seventh-Day Adventist, 1520t
 United Church of Christ, 1520t

Christian groups, beliefs and practices affecting health care of, Christian Science, 1520t
 Jehovah's Witnesses, 1521t
 Mormons, 1521t
 Unification Church, 1521t
 Unitarians, 1521t

Christianity, beliefs and practices affecting health care in, 1517, 1518t–1521t
 beliefs of, 1517
 of various churches and groups, 1518t–1521t

Chromium, metabolism, functions, and sources of, 1060t

Chromosomes, gender differentiation and, 1488
 growth and development and, 181

Chronic obstructive pulmonary disease (COPD), oxygen therapy for, 1228
 position for breathing and, 611–612
 self-concept and, 1450

Chronobiology, 311–314. See also *Circadian rhythms.*
 clinical applications of, 314
 sleep and, 950–951, *951*

Chronopharmacology, 314

Church of Jesus Christ of Latter-Day Saints (Mormons), beliefs and practices of, 1521t
 food intake and diet and, 1069

Church of the Brethren, beliefs and practices of, 1519t

Church of the Nazarene, beliefs and practices of, 1519t

Chyme, 1050

Cigarette smoking. See *Smoking.*

Circadian rhythms, 311–314
 blood pressure and, 613
 body temperature and, 591
 desynchronization in, 954
 disruption of, 313
 exogenous and endogenous, 951
 measurement of, 316
 nursing interventions and, 317
 nursing research on, 316
 sleep and, 950–951, *951*

Circulation. See also *Blood vessels.*
 altered, parenteral administration of drugs and, 1282
 exercise and aging and, 814t
 heat or cold application and, 1396
 in cardiopulmonary resuscitation, 562–564, 567–568
 cardiac compression for, 562, *563–564,* 564, 566

Circulation *(Continued)*
 pulse assessment in, 564, 568
 rate of compression used, 564t
 skin assessment and, 1338

Circulatory overload, intravenous therapy and, 1327t

Circumcision, in infant Jews, 1516t
 in neonates, 193

Cirrhosis, dietary management of, 1083–1084

Civil law, 51

Civil Rights Act, equal employment opportunites and, 59

Civil service employment, for nurses, 58

Civil War, nursing education and, 16

Claims-made insurance, 54

Clam shell ("scoop") stretcher, for movement of injured clients, 880

Clean technique, 506

Cleaning practices, 506–507, 521

Clergy, 1524

Client, involvement of, in health care, 163

Client record. See *Record, client.*

Clients, anxiety of, 388–389
 aphasic, communication with, 1481
 as candidates for home care, 404–405, *405*
 as research subjects, rights of, 1260
 as surgical candidates, 1410
 preoperative preparation of, on day of surgery, 1425–1428
 physical, 1423–1425
 psychophysiologic changes from surgery in, 1410t, 1410–1412
 assault and battery by, 56
 bereaved, care for, 1547, 1554–1555
 characteristics of, learning abilities and, 478–479
 teaching approach and, 475–477
 communication with, 422–425, 427–429, 448, 1481–1483
 confused, communication with, 1481
 dying, communication with, 448
 educational level of, teaching approach and, 475–476
 expectations of nurses and, 388
 hospitalized, 388–392
 hospital designation of, 385
 orientation of, 389–392
 risk of sensory/perceptual alterations in, 1474
 identification of needs of, 173
 immobile, movement of, specific techniques for, 547–549, *550,* 551t, *552–553*
 transfer from bed to chair, 793–795, *794*
 transfer from bed to stretcher, 785–795, *796*
 assistance with dangling and, 792, *793*
 Hoyer lift used for, 790–792, *791*
 lift sheet transfer for, *789,* 789–790
 three-person carry for, 787–788, *787–788*
 in bed, lift sheet placed under, procedure for, 547t–548t
 lifting or moving of, 544–546, 554
 shoulder lift procedure for, 549t, *550*
 specific procedures for, 547–549, *550,* 551t, *552, 553*
 in decision making about life-sustaining treatment, 74–76
 instruction sheet for, *411–412*
 interaction with nurse, 421–449
 involvement of, in plan of care, 145, 146, 161, 163, 168

Clients *(Continued)*
 quality assurance programs and, 55–56
 rights and responsibilities of, 67–69, 1257, 1258, 1544. See also *Rights.*
 seductive behavior of, nurse's responses to, 1497–1498
 sexual orientation of, nurse's reaction to, 1498
 socioeconomic status of, teaching approach and, 477
 therapeutic relationship with nurse, communication in, 422–425, 427–429, 448, 1481–1483
 with delusional thinking, 1481
 with hallucinations, 1482–1483
 with HIV-positive status, controversies about, 57
 with illusions, 1482

Climate, blood pressure and, 613

Clinic, definition of, 383

Clinical nurse specialists, consultation with, 162

Clinitest, 1167

Clinitron bed, 761–762, 1347, 1348t, *1353*

Clothing, protective. See also *Gloves; Gowns; Masks.*
 with respiratory disorders, 1239

Clubbing, of fingernails, 691, *692*

Cobalt, metabolism, functions, and sources of, 1060t

Cocaine exposure, health risks and, 350
 in infants, 77
 in neonates, 194
 in young adults, 222, 224
 prenatal, 191

Cockup splints, 767, *768*

Coercion, ethical aspects of, 47

Cognitive and intellectual development, at midlife, 231–232
 in adolescents, 212
 in early childhood, 200, 202t
 in infants, 196
 in neonates, 194
 in older adults, 237–238
 in school-age children, 203–204, 206t
 in young adults, 220
 theories of, 186–187, 188t, 189

Cognitive function, client learning and, 470–471
 deficits in, 642t
 gender differences in, 1491
 impaired, in clients with delusions, 1474, 1482
 in clients with hallucinations, 952–955, 1474, 1483
 in clients with illusions, 1474, 1482
 in confused clients, 1473–1474, 1481
 in Lazarus' model of stress and coping, 274–276
 mental status examination for, 635, 636
 documentation of findings on, *638–642*
 of nurse, 158, 159
 with immobility, 755

Cognitive-perceptual pattern, in nursing assessment, 124
 nursing diagnoses in, 135

Cold application, evaporation and, 1396
 for pain relief, 985
 indications for, 1389–1390
 methods of, 1394–1396
 cold packs and chemical packs, 1394, *1395*
 compresses for, 1395
 direct, 1395–1396
 hypothermia blankets, 1395
 ice, 1396

Cold application *(Continued)*
   ice bags, 1394, *1395*
   ice collars, 1394
   immersion, 1396
   indirect, 1394–1395
   tepid baths and sponge baths, 1395–1396
   nursing management of, 1396–1397
   physiologic effects of, 1389–1390, 1390t
   precautions and contraindications for, 1390t
   principles of, 1386–1388
   purpose of, 1388
Collaboration, as leadership trait, 462
   by home care nurse, 404, 407
   in case management care plans, 154
   on interdependent interventions, 147
   problems with, nursing management of, 140–141
   with other professionals, for health promotion, 358
   in implementation of care, 162
Collagen, in wound healing, 1357
Collars, cervical, uses and complications of, 857–858, *857–858*
   ice, 1394
Collective bargaining, nurses' rights in, 58
Colloids, 1005
   osmotic pressure of, fluid transport and, 1012
Colon. See also *Bowel elimination*; *Intestines.*
   structure and function of, 1051, *1126*, 1126–1127
Colonoscopy, 724t, 725
Color discrimination, testing of, 670
Color therapy, 38t
Colostomy, care of, *1150–1151*, 1150–1152
Comatose patients. See also *Unconsciousness.*
   eye care for, 909
   health care decision making and, 69
   oral hygiene care for, 908, *908*
Communication, 261, 262, 340
   Braille as, 430
   cultural differences in, 447
   developmental differences in, 447
   in early childhood, 200
   in infants, 196–198
   in neonates, 194
   elements of, 425, *427*
   feedback in, 425, *427*
   gender differences in, 447
   in groups, 451–466, *461*
   barriers to, 463–465
   strategies for, 463–465
   in nurse-client therapeutic relationship, 261–262, 425, 427–429
   with aphasic clients, 1481
   with clients with hallucinations, 1483
   with clients with illusions, 1482
   with clients with impaired cognition, 446
   with confused clients, 1481
   with deluded clients, 1482
   with dying clients, 448
   with impaired senses, 430, 1475, 1481–1483
   in systems, 251
   model for, 425, *427*
   nontherapeutic techniques of, 436, 437t–440t
   nonverbal, 430–434
   body language as, 430–433
   paralanguage as, 430, 431, 433–434
   sign language as, 430

Communication *(Continued)*
   therapeutic techniques of, 436, 440, 441t–443t, 443–447
   active listening as, 447
   at beginning of interaction, 440, 443–444
   encouragement of, 434–436
   for clarification, 444–445
   for clients with impaired sense of reality, 446, 1481–1483
   for increased self-awareness, 445–446
   in ongoing interaction, 444
   near end of interaction, 446
   theories of, 427–429
   types of, 429–434
   verbal, 429–430
   talking as, 429
   writing as, 429–430
Community, body system and, 252
   definition of, 347
   groups and aggregates in, 347
   health promotion in, 345–362, 360, 556
   health services in, 352–353
   midlife adult role in, 232–233
   nursing practice in, 11–13
   terminology of, 401
   older adults in, 239–240
   policies affecting health care and, 105
   resources in, for clients with urethral catheters at home, 1193
   for control of stress, 288
   for older adults, 240
   referral to by home care nurse, 403–404
   support groups in, 352, 454–455
   young adult roles in, 221
Community Health Accreditation Program, 404
Compartment syndrome, casts and, 868, 869t
   signs of, 1354
Compensatory mechanisms, homeostatic, 304–305
Complement system, in wound healing, 1356
Compliance, in home care nursing, 410
   powerlessness and, 370
   with drug regimens, in elderly people, 1259
Computed tomography, 713t, 714
   mechanism of, 714, *714*
   uses and advantages of, 714
Computers, bedside use of, 499, *500*, 500
   terminology related to, 499
Conception, extrauterine, 190
   new methods of, 190
   process of, 190
Conceptus, 190
Condom catheter, for urinary incontinence, 1175, *1175*
Condoms, adolescents and, 215, 216, 218
Conduction, heat loss by, 588
CONFHER model, of cultural profile for assessment, 341
Confidentiality, as ethical principle, 47
   as group norm, 457
   in ANA Code of Ethics, 48
   in human research, 72
   in therapeutic relationship, 423
   patients' right to, 67, 68, 79–80
   vs. patient privilege, 57
Confusion, 1473–1474
   as sign of cardiovascular failure, 557, 558
   causes of, 1473
   fever and, 600
   nursing interventions for, 1481
   self-care and, 807
Congestive heart failure, dietary management of, 1086–1087

Congestive heart failure *(Continued)*
   sleep apnea with, 952
   tachycardia and, 605
Conjunctivae, assessment of, 668
Connecticut Training School for Nurses, 16
Connecting, with dying client, 1551–1552
Consciousness. See also *Comatose patients.*
   cerebral hypoxia and, 612
   decreased, pressure ulcers and, 1352
   in application of heat or cold, 1397
   in mental status assessment, 661
   respiratory status and, 612
Consensual response, 1388
Consent, informed. See *Informed consent.*
Constipation, 1143–1144
   as nursing diagnosis, 1132
   causes of, 1143–1144
   hazards of, 1144
   in immobilized persons, 751
   management of, 1143–1144
   urinary incontinence and, 1174
Constitutional law, 49
Consultation, in nursing assessment, 126
Consumers. See also *Clients.*
   classification of nursing care needs of, 98
   decision making about life-sustaining treatment and, 74–76
   of health care, contracts made by, 57–58
   rights of, 84–85
   and personal choice, 68–77
   statutory and professional statements of, 67–69
   to organ transplantation, 81–83
Contact lenses, care of, *910*, 910–911
Continuous quality improvement, evaluation process and, 171, 173
Contraception, in adolescents, 219
   law on, 77
Contract law, 57–59
Contracts, employment, for nurses, 58
Contrast media, in radiography, 710–711, 713–714
Contusions, 1341, *1341*, 1343t
Convalescence, in illness experience, 365
Convection, heat loss by, 588
Conversation, nursing actions based on, 53
Cooley, C. H., 1449
Coopersmith, S., 1449
Coordination, tests of, 693
COPD. See *Chronic obstructive pulmonary disease (COPD).*
Coping behavior. See also under *Crises*; *Stress.*
   definition of, 271
   for crisis management, 292
   for hospitalized person, 292
   models of, 271
   reactions to illness and, 367
   stress response and, 282
   Lazarus model of stress and, 274–276, *276*
   types of, 271
   with loss and grief, cultural influences on, 1537–1538
Coping–stress tolerance pattern, in nursing assessment, 124
Copper, metabolism, functions, and sources of, 1060t
CORE documentation, 495
Corneal light reflex test, 669
Coronary artery disease, cardiac arrest and, 558
Corticotropin-releasing hormone, in regulation of cortisol secretion, 307, *308*
Cortisol, blood levels of, circadian rhythms in, 312–313

Cortisol *(Continued)*
  normal values of, 313
  regulation of, 307, 308, *308*
Cosmetics, as part of hygiene care, 935
Costs, of chronic illness, 326
  of health care, 95–96
    containment of, 97–98
    methods of payment of, 96–97
    of Medicare and Medicaid, 97
    patients' right to information about, 67, 69
  of home care nursing, 403–404
  of nursing care, 98–99
  of surgery, 1412
Cough reflex, in immobilized persons, 749, 750
Coughing, effects of, 1223, *1223*
  in respiratory history, 1209
  preoperative teaching of, 1422–1423, *1423*
  promotion of, 1223–1224, *1224*, 1224t
Counseling, 163. See also *Teaching.*
  in home care nursing, 410
  nursing goals and, 258
  on diet, 1090
    of adolescents, 216–217
Countertraction, 873, 875
Cover-uncover test, of eyes, 669
CPM machine, 822–823, *823*
CPR. See *Cardiopulmonary resuscitation (CPR).*
Crackles, 679, *680*, 1214t
Cramping, in immobilized persons, 750
Cranial nerves, assessment of, 665–666
  functions of, 667t
  mnemonic for, 665
Creams, 1273–1275
Criminal law, 51
Crises, characteristics of, 280–281
  concept of, 279–281
  coping with, 281, *282*
  definition of, 279
  developmental phases of, 280, *281*
  in chronic illness, 375
  intervention for, 281, 292
  maturational, 280
  reactions to, 281
  situational, 280
Crisis centers, as primary care agencies, 91
Critical path, in case management care plan, *152*, 154
Crohn's disease, ileostomy for, 1150
Cromolyn sodium, 1235
Cross-contamination, definition of, 506
Crossland, Mary, 484
Crutches, gaits used with, 831–832
  four-point, 832, *833*
  swing-through, *833*, 835
  swing-to, *833*, 835
  three-point, *833*, 834–835
  two-point, 832–834, *833*
  maneuvers with, managing stairs, *826*, 835–837
  standing and sitting down, 835, *836*
  proper fit of, 829
  safety measures with, 829, 831
  types of, 829, *832*
Cruzan decision, state and federal legislation after, 75
Crying, in cocaine-exposed babies, 194
  in neonates, 194
Cultural competence, 339–340
Cultural factors, diversity of, 333
  health risks in midlife and, 234
  in elimination patterns, 1128
  in interventions for promoting sexual health, 1504

Cultural factors *(Continued)*
  in learning abilities, 474
  in loss and grief responses, 1537–1538
  in nurse-patient communication, 447
  in psychosocial assessment, 643, *645*
  in sexual development, 1495
  in spirituality, 1511
  in teaching approach, 476
Culture, acculturation and, 333
  assimilation and, 334
  characteristics of, 333
  ethnicity and, 331–342
  food intake and diet and, 1069, 1074
  health status and, 336–338
  material and nonmaterial, 333
  sensitivity and stereotyping and, 334
  socialization and, 333
  subcultures and, 333
Cultures, specimen collection for, 719
  care of person undergoing, 717t
  urine, 1168–1169
  throat, 1215
Cushioning devices, 764–765. See also *Bed(s), specialized; Mattresses.*
  air-filled rings, 764
  bridging with, 764, *764*
  "donuts" 765
  for heels, 765, *765*
  pressure-reducing, 1347, 1348t
  use of, 767
Customers. See *Clients.*
Cyanosis, 1208, 1338–1339
  assessment of, 662
  hypoxia and, 612
  interpretation of, 1210–1211
  respiratory status and, 612
Cystitis, 1162
Cystoscopy, 724t, 725
Cytotoxic agents, handling of, OSHA guidelines on, 59

D

Dalmane, as sleeping pill, 963
Dandruff, 931
Danforth Amendment, 75
Dangling, 792, *793*, 796–797
  teaching of, preoperative, 1423
  procedure for, 824–828
    to client with general weakness, *825–826*, 825–827
    to client with one-sided weakness, 827–828, *827–828*
  vs. assisting client, 823
Data, analysis and interpretation of, in diagnostic process, 131
  changes in, computer use and, 500
  confidentiality of, 120
  reliability of, 120
  sources of, 119–120
  subjective and objective, 119
  validation of, 119
Data base, factors influencing, 120–121
  for nursing assessment, 118–119
  for problem-oriented record system, 490
  types of data included in, 118–119
Data collection, development of skills in, 630
  in nursing assessment, 110, 119
  in preoperative phase, 1413, 1419
Date rape, in young adults, 223
Dating, in adolescents, 211–212
Daughters of Charity, nursing and, 9
Day care centers, as primary care agencies, 91
  for toddlers, 201–202

Death. See also *Dying person; Grief and grieving.*
  asynchronous response to, 1546
  biologic, 558, *559*
  cardiopulmonary resuscitation as bridge from, 558, *559*
  causes of, at midlife, 233
    in adolescents, 214
    in older adults, 241
    in school-age children, 204, 205
    in young adults, 222
  Christian beliefs about, 1518t–1521t
  clinical, 558, *559*
  imminent, signs of, 1546–1547
  in Jewish faith, 1516t–1517t
  in neonates, 195
  of child, effect on parents of, 1537
  postmortem care and, 1554
  rates of, in various ethnic groups, 348–349
    poverty and, 348
  sudden, family coping with, 1553
Debridement, 1342
Decision making, about forgoing life-sustaining measures, 74–75
  about health care, 68–70
  in groups, 465–466
Decontamination, sterilization and, 524–525
Decubitus ulcers. See *Pressure ulcers.*
Deep vein thrombosis, in immobilized persons, 747
  sequential compression devices and, 864
Defamation, as intentional tort, 56
Defecation, 1127. See also *Bowel elimination.*
Defendant, 51
Defense mechanisms, 185, 271–272, 272t, 273t
  physiologic and psychologic, stress and, 269, *270*
Dehiscence, in wound healing, 1356, *1357*, 1365
Dehydration. See also *Fluid and electrolyte balance; Fluids.*
  fever and, 600
  hypertonic, 1041
  in elderly clients, 1032
  objective clinical signs of, 1032
Delirium, fever and, 600
Delusions, 1474
  immobility and, 755
  nursing interventions for, 1481
Dementia, health care decision making and, 69
Demulcents, 915
Denial, as reaction to confirmed illness, 366, 368
  of illness experience, 366
Denis-Browne splint, *871*
Dental caries, 901
  causes of, 901–902
Dentures, assessment of, 903
  care of, 907, *907*
Denver Developmental Screening Test, 198, 202
Deodorants, 935
Deodorizers, for wound care, 1383–1384
Dependence, immobility and, 755
Depression, as coping mechanism in dying people, 1540
  as reaction to confirmed illness, 369
  in adolescents, 215–216
  in immobilized clients, 755
  in older adults, 241–242
  in spouse care givers, 239
Dermal patches, 1274, 1275
Dermis, layers of, 1337

Descartes, theory of disease of, 29
Desiccation, in wound healing, 1357, 1358
Development. See also *Growth and development.*
    definition of, 179
    delays in, school nursing care for, 13
    physiologic, principles of, 180–181
    psychosocial, 179–180
    social, 180
    stages of, communication and, 447
    types of, 179–180, *180*
Dextrins, 1052
Diabetes mellitus, blood glucose regulation and, 310
    dietary management of, 1088
    nail and foot problems in, 930
    urinary glucose and ketones in, 1167
    wound infection and, 1343
Diagnosis. See *Nursing diagnoses.*
Diagnosis-related groups, as cost-containment method, 97, 98
    home care nursing and, 402
Diagnostic cues, 131
Diagnostic procedures, assistance with, 703–726
    at various ages, 708–709
    baseline assessment data for, collection of, 707
    chronobiology and, 314
    documentation of, 708, *708*
    equipment for, disposal and cleaning of, 708
        preparation of, 707
    examples of, 705t–706t
    for bowel elimination problems, 1129, 1131–1132
    notification of family about, 707–708
    nursing responsibilities with, after procedure, 707–709
        before procedure, 705–707
        during procedure, 707
    outpatient, 710
    preoperative, 1423–1424, 1424t
    preparation of client for, 706–707
    processing and delivery of specimens for, 708
    provision of care and comfort during, 707
    radiographic, 710–711, 711t–713t, 713–715
    scheduling of, 706
    transportation of client to examination room for, 707
Diaphragm, breathing from, 1237, *1238*, 1239
    excursion of, 679
Diarrhea, 1145–1146. See also *Fluid and electrolyte balance.*
    causes of, 1145
    fluid and electrolyte imbalances and, 1022
    interventions for, 1145–1146
    signs and symptoms of, 1145
    with enteral feeding, prevention of, 1109
Diarthroses, 732–733
Diary, food, 217, 357, *357*
Diastix, 1167
Diathermy, 1393
Dickens, Charles, image of nursing portrayed by, 8
Diet. See also *Food(s); Nutrition.*
    as therapy, 35
    before and after surgery, 1080
    blood pressure and, 613
    bowel elimination and, 1128
    calcium in, 1037–1038
    Christian beliefs about, 1518t–1521t
    counseling for, 216–217, 1090
    dental caries and, 902

Diet *(Continued)*
    diary for self-monitoring of, 217, *357*, 357, 1066
    differences in, between developed and undeveloped nations, *1053*
    drug administration and, 1268
    emotional reactions to changes in, 1067, 1069
    fiber in, adverse effects of, 1053
        bowel elimination and, 1134
        function of, 1053
        recomendations for, 1134
    fluid and electrolyte balance and, 1021, 1036–1038
    fluid and electrolyte imbalances and. See also *Fluid and electrolyte balance; Fluids.*
    guidelines for, 1062t
    health risks and, 233, 234, 349
    Hindu beliefs about, 1515–1516
    in adolescents, 216–217
    in adults, 224, 242
        health risks in midlife and, 233, 234, 349
        ideal, 1073–1074
    increasing intake of, 1090–1091
    influences on, 1069–1076
    Jewish beliefs about, 1516, 1516t
    magnesium in, 1038
    NPO and, 1080
    on self-care assessment test, 354
    popular concerns about, 1062t–1065t, 1062–1063, 1066
    potassium in, 1037
    protein in, 1038
    recommended daily allowances for, 1057–1058, 1061t, 1062
    records of, 217, 357, *357*, 1066
    sodium in, 1037
    special, fluid and electrolyte imbalances and, 1021
        for congestive heart faliure, 1086–1087
        for diabetes management, 1088
        for lactovegetarians, 1065
        for obesity control, 1080–1083
        for prevention of disuse syndrome, 797
        nutritional consultation for, 1036–1038, 1091
    standard hospital, 1080, 1081t
        clear liquid, 1081t
        full liquid, 1081t
        soft, 1081t
    stress management and, 290
    urinary elimination and, 1161, 1174
Dieting, compulsive, in adolescent girls, 215, 217, *1072*, 1072–1073
Dietitians, nutritional consultation with, 1091
    training and responsibilities of, 93
Diffusion, of ions across cell membrane, 1011
Digestion, promotion of, 1091
Digitalis, bradycardia and, 607
    precautions with, 1038
Disabilities, health care facilities for, rights and responsibilities of, 78, 80, 81
    health promotion and, 347
    school nursing care for children with, 13
Disbelief, with grief, 1542
Discharge, from home care, 412
    from hospital, preparation for, 1440
    from PACU, criteria for, 1435
    planning for, at admission, 395
        Blaylock Risk Assessment Screen for, 392–393, *393*
        components of, 395
        for clients with wounds, 1386

Discharge *(Continued)*
    in assessment data base, 118
    process of, 395–396
Disciples of Christ, beliefs and practices of, 1519t
Discomfort, appetite and, 1090
    during injections, methods of reducing, 1283–1284, *1284*
    in dying person, assessment of, 1544–1545
    care measures for, 1553
Disease. See also *Health; Illness.*
    biofeedback training and, 315
    causes of, theories of, 27–29
    chronic. See *Illness, chronic.*
    chronobiology and, 314
    communicable, 507
    concepts of, 25–42
    definitions of, 26–27, 27t
    issues in, 26
    models of, 27–30
        current, 29–30
        historical, 27–29
    prevention of, 30–31, 31t
        primary methods of, 32, 33t, 34
        secondary methods of, 34, 34t, 35–37
        tertiary (rehabilitation) methods of, 37, 39, 39t
        vs. health promotion, 31, 31t, 32t
    surgical risk and, 1420
    systemic, oral problems with, 904
    terminology in, 25
Disinfectants, and antiseptics, 506
    factors affecting, 507
    use of, 527
Dispensary, definition of, 383
Distraction, for pain relief, 985–986
Disuse osteoporosis, 752–753
Disuse syndrome, high risk for, 756, 850
    outcomes for, 758
        vs. impaired physical mobility, 810
    mobility assessment and, 807
    prevention of, evaluation of, 797, 798t–800t
    nursing interventions for, 797
Diuretics, potassium levels and, 1087
Diurnal rhythm. See also *Circadian rhythms.*
    body temperature and, 591
Diverticular disease, dietary management of, 1084t, 1134
Diving, safety measures for, in adolescents, 219
Divorce, in midlife, 231
Dix, Dorothea, 16
Dizziness, 1480
DNA, growth and development and, 181
Dock, Lavinia, 18
Documentation. See also *Charting; Record, client.*
    abbreviations and symbols used in, 486t–487t
    common systems of, charting by exception (CBE), 495, *497*
    CORE method of, 495
    flowcharts (flowsheets, flownotes), 490, *491*
    FOCUS charting, 492–494, *494*
    lack of uniformity in, 488
    narrative form, 488, *489*, 490
    PIE charting, 494–495, *496*
    problem-oriented system, 490, 492, 492t, *493*
    SOAPIER method, 490, 492t
    computerized, 499–500
    future trends in, 499–500
    guidelines for, 485

Documentation *(Continued)*
  in home care nursing, 412
  methods of, automated information systems, 498–500, *500*
    change-of-shift report, 498
    dictated or recorded notes, 496, 498
    hand-written notes, 495–496
    verbal, 498
  of abdominal reflexes, 688, *688*, 688t
  of admission, 394
  of bedpan use, 900
  of bladder irrigation, 1199
  of blood transfusions, 1312
  of breath sounds, *680*
  of cervical collar use, 858
  of cognitive functioning, 636, *638–642*
  of diagnostic procedures, 708, *708*
  of disuse syndrome prevention, 798t–800t
  of drug administration, 1041
  of evaluation of outcome achievement, 169, 170
  of examination of wounds, 1363, 1365
  of information given to client about use of life-sustaining measures, 76
  of interventions and outcomes for mentally ill, 81
  of modifications in nursing care plan, 169
  of nail and foot care, 930
  of nursing interventions, 163
  of observations on mood and affect, *637–638*
  of pain relief measures, 992
  of perineal care, 929
  of psychosocial history, *631–635*
  of urethral catheterization, 1196
  of use of restraints, 883, 888
  of use of seclusion rooms, 886
  of use of sequential compression device, 865
  of wound care, 1385–1386
  progress notes and, 169
  standard of care and, 53
Doppler ultrasound device, for blood pressure measurement, 619
  uses of, 621, *623*
Double bagging, 520
Douches, 1276, 1278–1280
Down's syndrome, informed consent for treatment and, 71–72
Drains and drainage, from wounds, 1380, *1381*, 1382, 1382t, *1382–1383*
  serosanguineous, 1356
Dreams, in REM sleep, 949
Dressings. See also *Bandages.*
  application of, dry, procedure for, 1370–1373, *1372*
    hydrocolloid, procedure for, 1378–1380
    nonocclusive, *1374*, 1374–1375
    wet, procedure for, 1373–1374
  at IV insertion site, changes of, 1330, 1332
  devices for securing, 1385
  for wounds, 1351t
  gauze, 1374–1375
  moist, 1375
  occlusive, 1375–1376
    absorptive, 1377, *1381*
    advantages and disadvantages of, 1375–1376
    hydrocolloids, 1376–1377, *1377*
      procedure for application of, 1378–1380
    hydrogels, 1377
    impregnated, 1377, 1380, *1381*
    nonadherent, 1376
    polyurethane film, 1376, *1377*
    polyurethane foam, 1376

Dressings *(Continued)*
    types of, 1376–1377, *1377*, 1380
  wet-to-dry, 1374–1375
Driving, accidents and, 219, 225
  alcohol use and, 225
    patient privilege and confidentiality and, 57
Drugs, abbreviations for prescribing and administering, 1262t
  absorption of, client's condition and, 1282
  abuse of, 222, 242–243, 350, 974–975, 1265. See also *Substance abuse.*
    in pregnancy, 77
  administration of, 1255–1306
    assessment for, 1264–1266, 1281–1283
    care plan for, 1304
    case study of, 1304
    chronobiology and, 314
    compliance with, among elderly, 1259
    documentation of, 1041
    dosages of, computing of, 1262–1263, 1263t
      timing of, *981*, 981, 1263
    errors in, 1263–1264, 1267
    ethical aspects of, 1258–1259
    evaluation of, 1297, 1303
    experimental, 1260
    general principles of, 1256–1264
    judgment in, 1267
    legal aspects of, 1258–1259
    medication history for, 1264
    medication orders for, 1261–1262
    oral, 1260, 1267–1269
      advantages and disadvantages of, 1267
      contraindications to, 1268
      crushing or chewing of, 1266, 1269
      effervescence medications, 1268
      enteric-coated, 1267–1269
      general considerations with, 1267–1268
      guidelines for, 1268–1269
      liquid, 1268
      powders, 1268
      procedure for, 1270–1273
      special problems with, 1269
      tablets, 1267–1268
      taste of, 1269
      through gastrointestinal tube, 1103
      through nasogastric tube, 1269
      types of drugs used for, 1267–1268
    parenteral, 1260, 1280–1297
      ampules, 1287, *1289*
      assessment of, 1281–1283
      implantable, 1281
      intradermal, 1291–1294
      intravenous, compatibility of, 1311
        procedure for, 1321–1322
      prepackaged, *1289–1291*, 1292–1293
      preparation of equipment and drugs for, 1285, 1285t, *1286–1289*, 1287, 1290–1292, *1292*
      principles of, 1284–1285
      reducing discomfort and anxiety during, 1283–1284
      routes of, 1280–1281, *1281*
      self-administration and, 1283
      site and route of injection and, 1282
      vials, *1289*, 1291, *1291*, 1292
    physiologic factors and, 1264–1265
    policies governing, 1263–1264
    routes of, 1260
    safety of, 1263–1264
    scientific principles of, 1260
    self-care in, 354, 1267, 1283
    special needs with, 1266
    topical, 1260, 1273–1280

Drugs *(Continued)*
    advantages and disadvantages in, 1273
    general guidelines in, 1273
    inhalation of, 1280
    procedures for, 1275
    to mucous membranes, 1275–1280
    types of, 1273–1274
  anesthetic, 1432t–1434t
    anticholinergics, 1434t
    inhalational agents, 1432t
    intravenous, 1433t
    local, 1433t
    muscle relaxants, 1432t–1433t
  antiallergenic, 1235
  anti-inflammatory, 1235
  as therapy, 35
  belonging to client, disposal of at admission, 394
  bowel elimination and, 1129, 1129t
  client's rights and, 1257
  constipation and, 1144
  controlled substances and, 1259
  definition of, 1260
  delivery systems for, 1261
  dependence on, 974, 1260, 1265–1266
  dispensing of, 1260
  effects of, on fluid and electrolyte balance, 1038, 1041
  types of, 1260–1261
  Food and Drug Administration control of, 1259
  food intake and diet and, 1075
  for flatulence reduction, 1147
  for pain, 981–984
    timing of, 981, *981*
  for prevention of UTI with indwelling catheters, 1190–1191
  for respiratory problems, 1235–1237
  for sleep promotion, 958, 962–963
  in adolescents, 214, 219
  in older adults, sexual activity and, 236
  use and misuse of, 242–243
  informed consent and, 71
  insomnia and, 953, 958, 962–963
  interactions of, 1041
    with intravenous therapy, 1311
    with nutrients, 1075–1076
  nurse's responsibilities with, 71
    medication reference cards and, 1257, *1257*
  oral problems due to, 904
  over-the-counter, 958, 962–963, 1259
    in young adults, 224
  pharmacokinetics of, 1264–1266
  prenatal exposure to, 191
  preoperative, 1425–1427
  prescription, 958, 962–963, 1259
  psychotropic, rights of mentally ill and, 81
  "recreational," 222
  surgical risk and, 1419, 1420t
  tolerance to, 974
  urinary elimination and, 1161
  urine color changes and, 1166t
  wound healing and, 1359
Dubos, Rene, ecological model of disease causation, 29, *30*
Dunn, Halbert, wellness model of health and, 29, *30*
Duodenocolic reflex, 1126
Duties, in ethical theories, 45–46
Dying, theories of, 1538–1540
Dying person, assessment of, 1544–1547
  bill of rights of, 1544
  communication with, 1543
  evaluation of care for, 1554–1555

Dying person *(Continued)*
  isolation of, 1543
  nursing interventions for, 7, 1551–1554
  planning care for, 1547, 1550, 1551
  referrals for care of, 1550
  teaching approach and, 476–477
Dysphagia, management of, 1091
Dyspnea, 610, 1237
  hydration measures and, 1227
  in dying person, care measures for, 1553
  in respiratory history, 1209
Dysuria, 1162

E

Ears, anatomy of, *671*
  assessment of, 670–672
  auricle of, 670, *671*
  ear drops instilled into, 1278, *1279*
  hygiene for, 911–912
  irrigation of, 1279
  otoscopic examination of, 670–672
Eating disorders. See also *Food(s)*; *Nutrition.*
  in adolescents, 215, 217, *1072*, 1072–1073
Eating patterns, in early childhood, 199
Ecchymosis, skin, 662
Ecological model of disease, 29, *30*
Edema, dependent, in immobilized persons,
    747
  factors leading to, 1012
  fluid and electrolyte imbalances and, 1022
  fluid transport and, 1012
  in immobilized persons, 747, 750
  in wound healing, 1358
  pitting, 665, 666t
    classification of, 748
    in immobilized persons, 747
    testing for, 748
  skin, 662, 665, 666t
  venous insufficiency to legs and, 1338
  with use of restraints, 881
Education. See also *Learning*; *Teaching.*
  about health, in adults, 231–232
    in school-age children, 205
    nurses' roles in, 94
  of nurses, advanced, 17–18
    baccalaureate degree in, 17–18
    continuing, 18
    early history of, 15–17
    types of, 17–18
  of patient, assessment of need for, 118
    benefits of, 468
  of staff, in risk management programs, 55
Educational groups, 453, 455
Effectors, thermal, 589, *590*
Egestion, delayed, in immobilized persons,
    750
Ego, 185
  in adolescents, 212
  in older adults, 236
Egophony, 679
Eiseley, Loren, 260
Elbow, flexion and extension of, 693
  range of motion of, 738t
    passive exercises for, 819–820, *819–820*
  restraints for, 884, *884*
Elderly. See also *Adults, older.*
  body temperature in, 590–591
  compliance with drug regimens in, 1259
  confusion in, prevention of, 807
  dehydration in, 1032
  diagnostic procedures in, 709
  drug administration in, parenteral, 1283
    special needs for, 1266

Elderly *(Continued)*
  fluid and electrolyte imbalances in, 1000,
    1021
  food intake and diet in, 1074
  home care services and, 404
  immobility in, 755. See also *Immobility*;
    Mobility, impaired.
  Medicare insurance for, 95–96
  pain in, assessment of, 975
  self-esteem in, 1454–1455
  sensory/perceptual alterations in, 1474,
    1478
  sexual development in, 1495
  sleeping pills and, 963
  spiritual growth in, 1515
  thirst mechanism in, 1016
  urinary incontinence and, 1173
Electra complex, 1493
Electric heating pads, 1391
Electrical outlets, in hospital client rooms,
    391
Electrocardiogram, 721–722, *721–722*
  assessment of, 721–723
  cardiac arrhythmias monitored by, 621, *623*
  care of person undergoing, 723t
Electroencephalogram, 722
  care of person undergoing, 723t
  sleep and, 948, 955
Electrolytes, 1000. See also *Fluid and elec-
    trolyte balance* and names of specific
    electrolytes.
  chemistry of, 1002, 1006t–1009t
  concentration of, in body fluid compart-
    ments, 1009–1010
    renal regulation of, 1018
  functions of, 1005, 1006t–1009t
  in body fluid lost, 1010
  in common body secretions, 1023t
  ionization of, 1002
  volume of, circadian rhythms in, 313
Electromyogram, 722–723
  care of person undergoing, 723t
  sleep and, 948, 955
Electronic monitoring, of vital signs, 621–624
  psychologic support and, 624
Electro-oculogram, sleep and, 948, 955
Electrostimulation, in wound healing, 1363
Elevator chair, 795
Elimination needs. See also *Bowel elimina-
    tion*; *Urinary elimination.*
  hygiene care for, 896–900
    equipment needed for, *897*, 897–898
  in surgical patients, 1411
  pattern of, in nursing assessment, 124
  nursing diagnoses with, 135
Elixirs, 1268
Embryo, 191
Emergency care, laws governing, 53, 58
Emergency carriers, 551t–552t, *552, 553*
Emergency departments, protocols in, 151
Emergency Medical Treatment and Active
    Labor Act of 1986, 67
Emollients, 915
Emotions, expression of, in clients with sen-
    sory/perceptual deficits, 1475
  in hospitalized clients, 292
  in immobilized clients, 754–755
  in infants, 197
  with use of restraints, 880
  homeostasis of, 301
  of nurses, about loss and grief, 1544
  self-concept and, 261
  stress-related, 276, 283, 284, 289
Employee health clinics, as primary care
    agencies, 91

Employees, nurses as, 58–59
  nursing care for, 12
Employment, at will, 58
  civil service, 58
  equal opportunity in, 59
  in unionized settings, 58
  personal contract, 58
Empty nest syndrome, 231
Empyema, 1228
Emulsions, 1268
Encopresis, 1147
Encounter groups, 454
Endocervical glands, 925
Endocrine glands, characteristics of, 304
Endocrine system, disorders of, dietary man-
    agement of, 1088–1089
  in growth and development, 182, *183*
  in homeostasis regulation, 302–304, *303*
  nervous system and, 304
Endomysium, 733
Endorphins, pain and, 971
Endoscopy, assessment by, 723, 725
  care of person undergoing, 724t
  of bowel, preparation for, 1131
Endotracheal tubes, insertion of, 1241, *1243*
  suctioning of, 1246
  types of, 1241, *1242*
Enemas, barium, 711, 711t
  cleansing, 1136
    administration of, 1137, 1142
      procedure for, 1138–1142
  dependence on, 1143
  Fleet, *1137*, 1137
  for bowel elimination, 1136–1137
  hazards of, 1143
  hypertonic, administration of, 1142
  in bowel training programs, 1149
  mechanism of, *1136*, 1137
  retention, 1136
    administration of, 1142–1143
  return-flow (Harris flush), 1136
    for flatulence reduction, 1147
  saline, equipment for, *1139*
    procedure for, 1138–1142, *1141*
Energy, and self-actualization, 260
  balance of, obesity and, 1082
  required nutrients for, 1052
Engel, George, 1541–1542
Enkephalins, pain and, 971
Enteral nutrition, 1094–1118
  administration of, continuous infusion of,
    1110–1111, 1115t
    nursing considerations with, 1110–1111,
      1114
  formulas for, 1103, 1108, 1110t
  gastrostomy or jejunostomy tubes for, me-
    tamucil in, 1109
    nursing considerations with, 1114–1115
  home feeding program with, implementa-
    tion of, 1115, 1118, *1119*
  intubation for, 1103, 1108–1111, 1114–
    1115
  methods of feeding with, 1108
  nursing diagnoses with, 1116t–1118t
  nursing interventions with, 1116t–1118t
  routes and types of, 1103
  specialized equipment needed for, 1109,
    1111
Enuresis, 1161
Environment, internal, equilibrium of, 301
  of older adults, 242
  restrictive, as treatment for mentally ill, 81
Environmental factors, children's safety and,
    197, 201
  drug administration and, 1268

Environmental factors *(Continued)*
  effects on health, 348–349, 352
  growth and development and, 181, 182
  in assessment data base, 118
  infant safety and, 197
  learning ability and, 474
  prenatal development and, 191, 191t
    risk histories of, 191
  relocation stress syndrome and, 316–318
  respiratory status and, 609, 1206, 1210
  urinary incontinence and, 1174
Environmental stimuli, deficit of, 1474
  excess of, 1475
  immobilized clients and, 755
  promotion of, 1480
Enzymes, replacement, for enhancement of
    digestion, 1091
Epidermis, layers of, 1337
Epidural analgesia, 988–990, *990*
  patient controlled, 990
Epinephrine, body temperature and, 589, 591
Episcopal church, beliefs and practices of,
    1519t
Epithelialization, in wound healing, 1357,
    1358
Equipment, for home care, 403
  for neurologic assessment, 655
  for physical assessment, 653, *654*, 655
  for transfer of immobilized clients, 769,
    784, 796, *796*
  soiled, disposal of, 520–521
    double bagging of, 520
Ergometer, 842
Erikson, Erik, developmental theory of, 185–
    186, 186t, 237
Erythema, blanchable, 743, 1346
  nonblanchable, 743, *1346*, 1346
  pressure and, 741
Eschar, in wound healing, 1357, 1358
Esophagogastroduodenoscopy, 724t, 725
Esophagus, anatomy and function of, 1051
Estrogen, production of, 1491
Ethgender, and self-concept in adolescents,
    212
Ethical issues, in drug administration, 1259–
    1260
  in home care nursing, 407
  in nurse-client therapeutic relationship, 423
Ethics, codes of, 47–49
  definition of, 44
  dilemmas in, 44
    decision making and, 48
    examples of, 45, 48
  in donor organ allocation, 83
  law and, 45, *45*
  principles of, 46–47
  theories of, 44
    duty-oriented, 45, 48
    goal-oriented, 46
    intuitionist, 46
    rights-oriented, 45–46
    types of, 44–46
Ethics committees, conflict resolution about
    health care decisions and, 70
Ethnic groups, conflicts among, 334–335
  health beliefs among, 339–340
  health care disparities in, 348–349
  health status in, 234, 336–338
  older adults and, 240
  teaching approach and, 476
  variations among, 334
Ethnic humanism, 332
Ethnic pluralism, 334
Ethnicity, 334–335
  behavioral, 334

Ethnicity *(Continued)*
  help-seeking behaviors and, 338
  ideologic, 334
  poverty and, 336
  self-awareness and, 339
Ethnocentrism, 334
Ethnoscience approach to nursing, 332
Eudemonistic model of health, 29–30
Euthanasia, active voluntary, 76
  passive voluntary, 76
Evaluation, 165–174
  definition and purposes of, 112, 166
  homeostatic mechanisms and, 318
  in home care nursing, 412
  in nursing process, 111–112, 168
  malpractice suits and, 170–171
  nursing research and, 171, 173
  of bowel elimination problems, 1152
  of care for dying or bereaved clients,
    1554–1555
  of clients with low self-esteem, 1464–1465
  of family problems, 329
  of fluid and electrolyte balance, 1043
  of hygiene self-care deficit, 896
    bedmaking and, 943–944
    ears, 912
    elimination needs and, 900
    eyes, 911
    hair care, 934
    nail and foot care, 930
    nose, 913
    oral hygiene, 908
    perineal care, 929
    skin care and, 925
  of infection control, 535–537
  of intravenous therapy, 1333–1334
  of medication administration, 1297, 1303
  of mobility status, 797, 798t–800t, 842–
    843
    need for therapeutic immobilization and,
      887–888
  of nursing care plan, 168
  of nutritional interventions, 1118–1119
  of pain relief measures, 992–993
  of performance evaluations, 171, *172*
  of preoperative care, 1428
  of respiratory care, 1249–1252, 1251t
  of response to health promotion programs,
    361
  of sensory/perceptual alterations, 1483
  of sexual health interventions, 1504–1505
  of sleep problems, 963
  of spiritual health care, 1528
  of teaching-learning process, 480–481
  of urinary elimination, 1199
  of wound care, 1397
  perioperative, intraoperative, 1432–1434
    postoperative, 1437, 1440
    preoperative, 1418t–1419t, 1428
  quality improvement and, 171, 173
  standards for (ANA), 170
  steps in, 166–170
  types of, 166
  vs. assessment, 166
Evaporation, cold treatment and, 1396
  heat loss by, 588
Evidence, in civil and criminal law, 51
Evisceration of wounds, 1363, 1365
Ewald gastric tube, 1097t, 1099, *1100*
Exclusion, as social adaptation, 278
Excreta, assessment of, 900
Exercise. See also *Activity*; *Mobility*.
  addiction to, 841
  aerobic, 841
  anaerobic, 841

Exercise *(Continued)*
  as therapy, 35–36, 37
  benefits of, 813, 841
  bowel function and, 1134
  caloric expenditure with, *1076*
  deep-breathing, preoperative teaching of,
    1422, *1423*
  developing a program for, 822–823, 841–
    842
  disuse syndrome prevention with, 797
  effects on body systems of, 814t
  endurance, 841–842
  flexibility, 841
  fluid and electrolyte imbalances and,
    1021–1022
  food intake and diet and, 1076
  for fitness, in mobile clients, 839, 841–842
  for flatulence reduction, 1147
  hazards of, 813, 842
  health risks with, 349
  in adolescents, 217–218
  in clients with impaired physical mobility,
    782t, 813–816, 822–823
  in middle-aged adults, 235
  in older adults, 242–243
  in self-care assessment test, 354
  in young adults, 224
  isometric, bowel function and, 1134
    in clients with impaired mobility, 814–
      816
  isotonic, 813–814, *815*
  Kegel, 1159, 1164, 1173–1174
  muscle-setting, 815
  oxygen administration and, 1232, 1235
  pain and, 842
  pelvic muscle, 1173–1174
  preoperative teaching of, 1423, *1423*
  range of motion. See also *Range of mo-
    tion.*
    active, 816
    active-assistive, 816
    in immobile clients, 816, 822–823
    passive, 816, 822
      example of program for, 822–823
      machines for, 822, *823*
      procedure for, 817–821
    resistive, 816, 822
  respiratory status and, 609, 1237, *1238*
  strength-developing, 841
  tachycardia and, 605
  warm-up and cool-down for, 842
  weight-loss diets and, 1082
Exocrine glands, in adolescents, 211
Expiration, steps in, 1205
Extended care facility, definition of, 383
  nursing care in, 12–13
Exteroceptors, 1470
Extracellular fluid, 1000, *1000*. See also
    Fluid and electrolyte balance; *Fluids.*
  distribution of, 1001t
  electrolytes in, 1009, *1010*
  fluid and electrolyte transport in, 1010–
    1011
  hyperosmolality of, fluid volume regulation
    and, 1016, *1016*
  osmolality of, renal regulation of, 1017
  volume of, renal regulation of, 1017
Extreme unction, Christian beliefs about, 1518t
Extremities. See also *Arm*; *Legs.*
  assessment of, 692
  neurovascular check of, immobilization de-
    vices and, 850–852, *851–852*
  positioning devices for, 765, *765–766*,
    767–768
    cockup splints, 767, *768*

Extremities (Continued)
  hand rolls, 767, *768*
  hip abduction wedges, 767, *767*
  trochanter rolls, *766*, 767
  range of motion of, 735–736, 736t–740t, 741
Exudate absorbers, for wound care, 1352t
Eye wear, protective, infection control and, 517, 519
Eyebrows, assessment of, 668
Eyeglasses, care of, 909
Eyelids, assessment of, 668
Eyes, anatomy of, *668*
  artificial, care of, 909–910
  assessment of, 668–670
  conjunctivae of, 668
  contact lenses for, care of, *910*, 910–911
  eye drops instilled into, 1277–1278, *1277–1278*
  fundus of, 670, *670*
  hygiene for, 908–911
  in comatose people, care of, 909
  irrigation of, 1278
  lacrimal apparatus of, *668*
  ophthalmoscopic examination of, 670, *670*
  position and alignment of, 668
  protective eye wear for, 517, 519
  pupils of, 669
  sclerae of, 668–669
  visual acuity of, 670

F

Face, assessment of, 666–667, *667*
  expression of, as body language, 432
  respiratory distress and, 1211
Facial nerve, assessment of, 667–668, 674
Faith, as part of spirituality, 1514
  development of, 1514–1515
  power of, 1524
Falls, in older adults, 241
False imprisonment, as intentional tort, 56
Family, 321–330
  African-American, 322
  altered processes of, as nursing diagnosis, 327, 328
  anticipatory grieving in, 1554
  as caregivers, 239
  as primary group, 453
  as system, 323
    self-esteem and, 1451–1452
  bereaved, care for, 1547
  blended, 322
  body system and, 252
  characteristics of, 322
  child abuse and, 206
  coping abilities of, home health care and, 409
  definition of, 322
  diversity of, 179, 322–323
  extended, 322
  frameworks for understanding, 323–325
  functioning of, 359
  genogram of, 326, *327*
  health history of, 652
  health promotion and, 325, 358–359
  heat or cold application and, 1397
  Hispanic, 322
  influence of, on adolescents, 212–213
    on infants, 197
    on middle-aged adults, 231–232
    on neonates, 194–195
    on older adults, 238–239
    on school-age children, 204
    on young adults, 220–221
Family (Continued)
  involvement in setting outcomes, 146
  nuclear, 322
  nursing theories of, 324t, 324–325
  of dying person, assessment of, 1546
    assistance with care giving and, 1546
  responses to illness by, 325–326, 376
  self-concept development and, 1452–1455
  single-parent, 322
  stages of growth in, 359
  sudden death and, coping abilities of, 1553
  types of, 179, 322–323
Family leave policy, 104
Fascia, 1337
Fasciculations, 692
Fasciculus, 733
Fatigue, sleep patterns and, 953, 957–958
Fats, dietary, atherosclerosis and, 1085–1086
  derivation and forms of, 1054
  function of, 1053–1055
  health risks and, 349
  saturated and unsaturated, 1054
  weight-loss diets and, 1082
Fear, as nursing diagnosis, 286–287
  profile of, 1421
  as reaction to confirmed illness, 369, 369t
  immobility and, 755
  in hospitalized persons, 292
  self-esteem and, 1450
  vs. anxiety, 284, 287
Fecal impaction, 1144–1145
  in immobilized persons, 751
  urinary incontinence and, 1174
Feces, characteristics of, 1130–1131
  laboratory analysis of, 1131–1132
  movement through colon, 1126–1127
  pressure ulcers and, 1350, 1351t–1352t
Federal agencies, services offered by, 90
Feedback. See also *Biofeedback*.
  in communication, 425, 427
  in stress management, 290
  mechanisms of, 252, 305
  negative, 305, *305*, *306*
    blood glucose levels and, 307
    blood hormone levels and, 307
    body weight and, 307
    hemorrhagic shock and, 309
    rangelike, 307
    temperature and, 305, *306*, 307
  positive, 307–308, *308*
    in complete heart failure, 310
  set point and, 305
  training in, 315
Feeding, assistance with, 1091
  enteral, 1094. See also *Enteral nutrition*.
  in visually impaired clients, self-care for, 1479
  of neonates, 193
  problems with, in preterm infants, 1071
Feeding tubes, 1098t, 1101, *1101–1102*
Feet, plantar flexion of, in immobilized clients, 752
  skin care of, 929–930
Felony, 57
Fentanyl, in transdermal patch, 991, *991*
  transmucosal "lollipop" of, 991
Fenwick, Mrs. Bedford, 21
Fetal membranes, 190
Fetus, development of, 190–191
  human research and, 73
  viability of, 191
Fever, 587
  causes of, *599*, 599–600
  fluid and electrolyte imbalances and, 1022
  stages of, 600
Fever (Continued)
  tachycardia and, 605
  treatment of, controversy in, 600–601
    nursing management of, 601
  types of, 599
Fiber, dietary, adverse effects of, 1053
  bowel elimination and, 1134
  function of, 1053
  recommendations for, 1134
Fiberoptic examination, of bowel, preparation for, 1131
Fibroplasia, in wound healing, 1356
Fidelity, as ethical principle, 47
  development of, 1514
Fight-or-flight response, 283, *284*, 303
Financial aspects. See also *Costs*.
  of chronic illness, 326
  of food intake, 1069
  of health care, 95–96
    patient's right to information about, 67, 69
  of home care nursing, 403–404
  of nursing care, 98–99
  of surgery, 1412
Finger spelling, 430
Finger sweeps, for airway obstruction, 576–577
Fingernails, clubbing of, 691, *692*
Fingers, abduction of, 692
  functional assessment of, 852, *852*
  range of motion of, 738t–739t
  passive exercise of, 820–821
Fissures, palpebral, 666
Fitts' Tennessee Self-Concept Scale, 1450
Fitzgerald, Dr. William, 38t
Flatulence, management of, 1127, 1147
Fleet enema, 1137, *1137*
Flossing, technique of, 906, *906*
Flowcharts (flowsheets, flownotes), 490, *491*
Fluffs, 1375
Fluid and electrolyte balance, 997–1047
  assessment of, 1022, 1033, 1033t–1034t, 1034–1035, *1035*
  care plan for, 1044–1045
  case study of, 1043–1044
  diarrhea and, 1146
  failure of, causes of, 1007t–1009t
    indicators of, 1033t–1034t, 1034–1035, *1035*
  nursing process applied to, 1024t–1032t
  risk factors for, 1021–1022
  fever and, 600, 601
  in client history, 1033
  in surgical patients, 1411
  intravenous therapy and, 1042–1043
  measures of, terms used for, 1005, 1009
  mechanisms regulating, 1013–1018
    cardiovascular system as, 1018
    gastrointestinal system as, 1017
    kidneys as, 1017–1018
    neuroendocrine system as, 1013–1017
  medications and, 1038, 1041
  movement of, 1010–1013
    between fluid compartments, 1010–1011
    between vascular and interstitial compartments, 1011–1013
  surgical risk and, 1420
  tube feedings and, 1041–1042
Fluids, body, anions and cations in, 1002
  balance of, 1000
  pH of, 1019
  requirements for, 1057
  third space accumulation of, 1022
  volume of, deficit, 1024t

Fluids (*Continued*)
    excess, 1024t–1025t
    outcome criteria and nursing interventions for, 1024t–1025t
    regulation of, 1015, 1017
  bowel function and, 1128, 1134
  dietary requirements for, 1057
  extracellular, 1000, *1000*, 1001. See also *Extracellular fluid.*
  intake of, and output records for, 1036
    digestion and, 1091
    effective coughing and, 1224
    in immobilized persons, 750
    in prevention of disuse syndrome, 797
    intermittent self-catheterization and, 1195
    oral, regulation of, 1038–1041
    preoperative restriction of, 1424–1425
    regulation of, dietary, 1036–1038
      objectives for, 1034–1035
    respiratory status and, 1225–1227
    urinary elimination and, 1158–1159, 1161, 1174
    urinary tract infection and, 1190
  interstitial, 1001, 1001t, 1011–1013
    in immobilized persons, 747
  intracellular, 1000, *1000*, 1001, 1009–1011, *1010*
  lost through wound drainage, 1380
  overload of, with intravenous therapy, 1042
Fluorine, metabolism, functions, and sources of, 1060t
Fluoroscopy, 710, *710*, 711
Flurazepam (Dalmane), as sleeping pill, 963
Foams, for wound care, 1352t
FOCUS charting, 490, 492–494, *494*
Foley catheter, as feeding tube, 1101
Folk remedies, 36
Follicle-stimulating hormone, 1491
  positive feedback and, 307–308
Fontanelles, in neonates, 192, *192*
Food additives, 1062
Food allergies, management of, 1089
Food and Drug Administration, 1362
Food diaries, 217, 357, *357*, 1066
Food intolerances, 1089
Food(s). See also *Diet; Nutrition.*
  assistance with serving and feeding, 1091
    procedure for, 1092–1093
  bowel function and, 1134
  intake of, eating disorders and, 215, 217, *1072*, 1072–1073
    in infants, *1070*, 1070–1071
    influences on, 1069–1076
    pressure ulcers and, 1350
    reduced, in immobilized persons, 750
  natural and organic, 1062t, 1062–1063
  restricted, management of diet with, 1090
    preoperative, 1424–1425
  special or "therapeutic," information about, 1064t–1065t, 1065
  supplements of, 1063, 1065
Foot care, patient instruction sheet for, *411–412*
Footboards, 765, *765*
  bedmaking and, 943
Footdrop, with immobility, 752, *753*
Ford, Loretta, 20
Forearms, range of motion of, 738t
Foreign body, airway obstruction by, complete, 576
  in children, 579–580
  in infants, 577, 579, *580*
  management of, 576–577, *578–579*
    by finger sweeps, 576–577

Foreign body (*Continued*)
    by manual thrusts, 576–577, *578–579*
    partial, 576
    prevention of, 576
    recognition of, 576
Forgiveness, need for, as spiritual need, 1513
Formulary, 1256
Formulas, for enteral feeding, 1103, 1108, 1110t
Fowler's position, pressure ulcers and, 1349
Fracture bedpan, 897
Fractures, comminuted, 849
  complete, 848
  complicated, 849
  compound (open), 848
  depressed, 849
  greenstick, 849
  hickory stick, 849
  impacted, 849
  incomplete, 848–849
  pathologic, 752
  pressure ulcers and, 1352, 1354
  reduction of, 849
  simple (closed), 848
  types of, 848–849
  willowstick, 849
Fremitus, 676, 678, 681
Freud, Sigmund, 182, 185, 272, 1449
  psychosexual theories of development of, 1492–1493
Friction, 542, 544t, 554
  effects on skin of, 741–742, *742*
  pressure ulcers and, 1349
  traction and, 875
Friction rub, 679, *680*
  pleural, 1214t
Functional health patterns, in nursing assessment, 122, 124
  in nursing diagnoses, 134–136
Funds, of long-term care residents, law governing, 78, 79
Funeral rituals, 1542
Funnel chest, 680
Furniture, in hospital client rooms, 390–391

G

Gait, assessment of, 692
  observation of, 733
  used with crutches, 831–832, *833*, 834–835
Gallbladder disease, dietary management of, 1083–1085
  gallstones with, dietary management of, 1084–1085
Gamma-aminobutyric acid, 963
Gangrene, 748
  due to tight bandages, 858, 861
Gas exchange, hypoventilation and, 1206
  impaired, profile of, 1219
  in lungs, 1205
  in surgical patients, 1411
Gas (flatus), in intestines, 1127, 1146–1147
Gas gangrene, *1343*
Gases, for therapy, 36
Gasping respirations, pattern of, 1212t
Gastric distention, in cardiopulmonary resuscitation, 571
  in immobilized persons, 750
Gastric secretions, electrolyte composition of, 1023t
Gastric tubes, 1096, 1097t, *1098–1100*, 1099
Gastrocolic reflex, 1126
Gastrointestinal system, disease of, dietary management of, 1083, 1084t

Gastrointestinal system (*Continued*)
  dysfunctional, maintenance of nutrition with, 1094–1118
  homeostasis regulation in, 302
  in adolescents, 210t
  in immobilized clients, assessment of, 745t, 750–751
  nursing assessment of, 123
Gastrointestinal tract, compression of (tamponade), 1095
  decompression of, 1095
  diversion of, with ostomies, 1150
  intubation of, for gastric analysis, 1095
    for gavage, 1095
    for lavage, 1095
    reasons for, 1095
    routes used for, 1095, *1096*
  preoperative preparation of, 1424–1425
  structure and function of, 1050–1052, *1052*, *1126*, 1126–1127
Gastrostomy tube, feedings with, administration of, 1114–1115
Gauze, for dressings, 1374–1376, *1374–1376*
Gay and lesbian partners, among older adults, 238
Gaze, cardinal positions of, 669, *669*
Gels, dermal, 1274, 1275
  for wound care, 1351t
Gender, adolescent moral choices and, 213
  blood pressure and, 613, *613*
  brain differences with, 1490–1491
  chromosomal basis of, 1488
  communication and, 447
  gonadal sex establishment and, 1488–1489
  pharmacokinetics and, 1265
  physical assessment and, 660
  psychosexual development and, 1492–1495
  puberty and, 1491
  secondary sex characteristics and, 1491
  sexual organ development and, 1489, *1489–1490*
Gender bias, in self-esteem research, 1451–1452
Gender identity, conflict resolution and, 1493
  development of through lifespan, 200, 1493–1495
  mothering role and, 1493
  separation-individuation process and, 1493
  sexual health and, 1492
General adaptation syndrome, 273–274, *274*
  in physiologic response to stress, 283, *284*
  stages of, *284*
General systems theory, 250–251
  family in, 323
  psychosocial assessment and, 628–629
Genetic factors, health risks in midlife and, 233
  in growth and development, 181–182
Genitals, assessment of, 688–689
  female, 689–691, *690*
    bimanual examination of, 690–691
    internal and external, development of, 1489, *1489–1490*
  male, 689, *689*
Genogram, family, 326, *327*
Geographical location, food intake and diet and, 1069
Germ theory of disease, 29
Gestures, as body language, 432
GI Bill, nursing education and, 16–17
Gingivitis, 902
Girdle, internal, 546
Glands, adrenal, 182, 302, 303
  endocervical, 925

Glands *(Continued)*
  endocrine, 304
  exocrine, 211
  parathyroid, 182, 302, *303*
  pineal, 302, *303*
  pituitary, 304
  prostate, *691*, 691, 925, 1158
  sebaceous, 914
  thyroid, 182, 302, *303*, 591, 674, 1017
Glaser, B.G., theory of dying of, 1538–1539
Glomerulus, 1157, *1157*
Glossopharyngeal nerve, assessment of, 674
Gloves, contaminated, removal of, 531, 532, *533*, 534–535
  infection control and, 517, 523, 1345
  purpose of, 1345
  sterile, closed method of donning, 534, *537*
    open method of donning, 531, *532*
Glucocorticoids, wound healing and, 1359
Glucose, 182
  blood levels of, glycemic index and, 1053, *1054*, 1089
    in diabetes mellitus, 310, 1088
    in hypoglycemia, 1088–1089
    negative feedback and, 307
    stress response and, 283
  digestion and metabolism of, 1053
  urine tests of, 1167
Glutamate, 971
  pain modulation and, 972
Glycemic index, 1053, *1054*, 1089
Glycolipids, 1054
Glycosuria, 1165
Goiter, 674
Goldmark Report, 17
GoLYTELY solution, for bowel preparation, 1131
Gomco suction pump, 1102, *1102*, 1382, *1383*
  emptying drainage canister from, 1103, *1108*
Gonadotrophic hormones, in male sexual development, 1491
Gonads, in establishment of sexual differentiation, 1488–1489
  in growth and development, 182
Goniometer, 735
Good Samaritan laws, and standard of care, 53
Goodrich, Annie, 16
Gordon, Marjorie, 122
Gout, dietary management of, 1088
Government, role in health care policies of, 105
Gowns, hospital, changes in patients receiving intravenous therapy, 920, 1333
  surgical, clean, donning of, 517
    contaminated, removal of, 534–535
    infection control and, 517
    sterile, donning of, 534, *535–536*
Graham, Sylvester, 37
Grandchildren, and older family members, 238
Grandparents, 232
  and kinds of relationships with grandchildren, 232
Granulation tissue, in wound healing, 1356, 1360
Graphesthesia, test of, 693, 701
Grief and grieving. See also *Death; Dying person; Loss.*
  anticipatory, 1546
    in family members, 1554
    nursing diagnosis of, 1550
  assessment of, 1544–1547

Grief and grieving *(Continued)*
  care plan for, 1555–1556
  case study of, 1555
  coping with, 1533–1558
  cultural perspectives on, 1537–1538
  definition of, 1534–1535, 1535t
  developmental aspects of, 1536–1537
  dysfunctional, nursing diagnosis of, 1551
  evaluation of care for clients with, 1554–1555
  factors affecting outcome of, 1542, 1543
  nursing diagnoses of, 1547, 1548t–1549t, 1550, 1551
  physiologic effects of, 1535–1536
  theories of, 1541–1543
    cautions about, 1543
  with sudden death, coping with, 1553
Grievances, right to, of long-term care residents, 80
Grooming, 930–934
  in mental status assessment, 661
  in visually impaired clients, self-care for, 1479
Group therapy, 453–454
"Group think," 458
Groups, as change agents, 465
  at risk, health teaching in, 360
  characteristics of, 452–453
  communication in, 463–465
  confrontation in, 463–465
    constructive handling of, 464–465
  decision-making in, 465–466
  dynamics of, 455–459
    cohesion in, 457–458
    goal establishment and, 455–456
    norms in, 457
  educational, 453, 455
  encounter, 454
  group culture in, 452
  group process in, 459–462
    models of, 459, 460t
    nursing process and, 459–460
    phases of, 460–462
  "group think" in, 458
  health promotion in, 359–360
  hidden agendas in, 463
  instruction in, 479
  leadership in, 462
    styles of, 462
  phases of development of, 460t, 460–462
    introductory phase, 460–461
    preinteraction phase, 460
    termination phase, 462
    transition phase, 461
    working phase, 461–462
  primary, 453
  roles in, maintenance role functions, 456–457
    self-centered role functions, 457
    task role functions, 456, 457
  secondary, 453
  self-help (community support), *454*, 454–455
  social, 453
  structural components of, 458–459
    environmental factors, 459
    membership, 458–459
    sessions, 458
    size, 459
  therapeutic or work-related, 453–455
  types of, in health care, 453–455
Growth, compensatory, 304–305
  definition of, 179
Growth and development. See also *Development.*

Growth and development *(Continued)*
  disabilities in, health care facilities for, responsibilities of, 78, 80, 81
  "normal" variations in, 179
  of musculoskeletal system, by age, 809t
  of sexuality, 1488–1495
  physical, in early childhood, 193t, 199, 202t
    in infants, 196
    in midlife, 228, 229t
    in neonates, normal ranges of, 193t
    in older adults, 235, 236t
    in school-age children, 202, 206t
    in young adults, 220
  physiologic, cephalocaudal, 180
    maturation of general to specific skills in, 180
    maturational and learning factors and, 181
    patterns of, 181
    proximodistal, 180
    rate and timing of, 181
    readiness and, 181
    sequence of, 181
    stages of, 181
    systems regulating, 181–182
  principles of, 179–180
  sleep patterns and, 954, 955t
  stages of, conception, 190
    early childhood, 198–202
    embryonic, 191
    fetal, 191
    germinal, 190–191
    infants, 196–198
    neonates, 192–196
    prenatal, 190
    school-age children, 202–205
  theories of, 179
    behavioral, 189–190
    cognitive, 186–187, 188t, 189
    family in, 324
    psychosocial, 179–180, 184–190, 190
Growth factors, in wound healing, 1359, 1362
Growth hormone, body temperature and, 591
  in NREM sleep, 949
Growth spurt, in adolescents, 210, 210t
Guaiac test, of stool, 1132
Guided imagery, 290–291, 986, 1524
  for dying person, 1552–1553
Guilt, with grief, 1541
Gums, 1053
  assessment of, 673
Guns, safety measures for, in adolescents, 219
Gunshot wounds, reporting of, 57

H

Habits, in urinary elimination, 1101, 1174
Hahnemann, Samuel, 37
Hair, assessment of, 666, 931
  care of, 930–934
    brushing, 931–932
    shampooing, 933–934, *933–934*
    special considerations in, 932
  growth and loss of, 931
  removal of, preoperative, 1424
  shaving of, 934
  structure and function of, 931
Halcion, as sleeping pill, 963
Halitosis, 900
Hallucinations, 1474
  hypnagogic, 952

Hallucinations *(Continued)*
  immobility and, 755
  nursing interventions for, 1482–1483
Halo brace, *878*, 878t
  psychologic impact of, 879
Hand rolls, 767, *768*
Hand washing, 507
  assistance with, 900
  for infection control, 507–509, 517, 518t, 519t, 523, 1189, 1345
  procedure for, 518t, 519t
  sterile technique and, 531
  surgical hand scrub, procedure for, 533, 534
Handguns, safety measures for, 219
Hand-held nebulizer, 1235–1236, *1236*
Handicaps, in infants, informed consent for treatment and, 71–72
Hands, restraints for, *884*, 885
Havighurst, Robert, developmental theory of, 186, 187t
Head, and neck, physical assessment of, 665–675
  assessment of, 666–674
  in neonates, 192, *192*
  passive range of motion exercise of, 818, *818*
Head tilt–chin lift method, of airway control, 560, *561*, 566
Health, beliefs about, in ethnic groups, 339–340
  definitions of, 26–27, 27t
  factors influencing, attitudes and beliefs as, 349–350
    environmental, 348–349
    external, 348–349
    internal, 349–350, 1450
  holistic, 358, 359t
  models of, 29–30
  perceptions of, 353, 356
  physiologic, and spiritual health, 1510
  promotion of. See *Health promotion.*
  sexual health and, 1499
  surgical risk and, 1419
  terminology used for, 25
  vs. wellness, 346
Health belief model, of disease prevention, 32, *33*, 34, 351
Health care, access to, 84, 99, 348
    consumer rights and health care provider responsibilities and, 84
    ethnicity and, 234, 332, 333, 339
    response to illness and, 366
  agencies and personnel in, 89–95
  challenges for, 352
    strategies for achieving, 352–353
  changing concepts of, 25–42
  continuity of, patients' right to, 67, 69
  costs of, 95–99
    containment of, 97–98
    Medicare and Medicaid, 97
    methods of payment of, 96–97
    patients' right to information about, 67, 69
  cultural diversity and, 234, 332, 333
  decision making about, 68–70
  delivery of, 88–95. See also *Health care facilities; Health care workers.*
    comparison of national systems of, 100t–103t
    policy and politics relating to, 99–105
    strategies of provision of, 30–31, 31t, 32t
    types of services offered, 88–89
  distribution of, ethical questions about, 47
  goals for, 347–348

Health care *(Continued)*
  insurance coverage for, 95–96
    private, 95
    public, 95
    retrospective reimbursement and costs, 95–96
  issues in, 26
  national systems of, comparison of, 100t–103t
  patients' right to request for, 67, 68
  policy and politics of, 99–105
  preventive, under HMOs, 98
  previous experience with, response to illness and, 366
  reform of, social and cultural dilemmas with, 99
  statistics on, 95
Health care consumers. See *Consumers.*
Health care facilities, business relationships of, patients's right to know, 67, 69
  classifications of, 382–383
  conflicts of interest with, patients with advance directives and, 75
  contracts made by, with consumers, 58
    with nurses, 58
  decisions about health care and, 70
  definition of, 383
  extended care facilities as, 12–13
  for mentally ill, rights and responsibilities of, 78, 80, 81
  hospital structure in, 92
  level of services provided by, 90–91
    primary care, 90–91
    secondary care, 90–91
    tertiary care, 91
  personal liability insurance and, 54
  personnel in, 92–95
  policies and procedures of, standard of care and, 53
  public, services offered by, 90
  quality improvement and, 171, 173
  responsibilities of, consumer rights and, 77–81
  in long-term care facilities, 77–78
  risk management and quality assurance programs in, 54–56
  source-oriented, charting in, 488
  type(s) of, 383
    government (public), 89–90
    not-for-profit, 90
    profit and nonprofit, 383
    proprietary (for profit), 90
    voluntary (private), 90, 383
Health Care Financing Administration, 97
Health care providers, responsibilities of, 84–85
  and personal choice, 68–77
  organ transplantation and, 81–83
Health care workers, back injury in, prevention of, 539–554
  infection in, 521–522, *522*
  risk of, 508
  teams of, for care of respiratory disorders, 1208
  for rehabilitation, 39t
  members of, 92–95
  quality improvement and, 173
  with HIV-positive status, controversy over, 57
Health education, of adolescents, 216–220
  of middle-aged adults, 234–235
  of older adults, 242
  of school-age children, 205
  of young adults, 224–225
Health history. See *History.*
Health maintenance organizations, 98

Health maintenance organizations *(Continued)*
  as primary care agencies, 91
Health Omnibus Programs Extension Act of 1988, 83
Health perception–health management pattern, in nursing assessment, 124
  nursing diagnoses in, 135
Health prevention, challenges for, 352
Health promotion, activities used for, 39–40
  attitudes and, 350–351
  behavior modification and, 40–41, 356–358, 358t
  definition and examples of, 347
  environmental factors and, 348–349
  ethnic groups and, 348–349
  evaluation of response to, 361
  in adolescents, 219–220
  in community, 345–362
  in families, 325, 358–359
  in individuals, 353
  in people with disabilities or illnesses, 347
  mechanisms for, 352
  models for, 40–41, *41*, 350–353, *352*
  nurse's role in, 39–40
  nursing activities aiding, 39–40, 347, 353, 356–358
    collaboration with other health care providers and, 358
  poverty and, 348
  priorities for, 356
  public policy and, 361
  services available for, 88, 89, 404
  settings for, 347
  vs. disease prevention, 31, 31t, 32t
Health protection, definition and examples of, 346, *346*
  environmental factors and, 348–349
  health belief model and, 351
  strategies for, 350, 350t
Health screening, at midlife, 234
  of adolescents, 215–216
  of individuals, 353, *356*, 356
  of older adults, 242
  of school-age children, 204
  of young adults, 223–224
Health-illness continuum, 27, *28*
Health-seeking behaviors, as nursing diagnosis, 360
  examples of, 360
Healthy People 2000, 99, 348
  objectives for illness prevention at age levels, 350, 350t
Hearing, defective, communication with clients with, 447–448
  nursing care for, 1478–1479
  in dying person, 1547
Hearing aids, cleaning of, 912
  insertion of, 912
  parts of, 911
  precautions with, 912
  types of, 911, *911*
Heart. See also *Cardiac* entries; *Cardiopulmonary resuscitation (CPR); Cardiovascular system.*
  apical impulse of, 681
  assessment of, *681*, 681–682
  atria of, in homeostasis regulation, 303
  auscultation of, 682
  cardiac cycle of, 602–603
    heart sounds and, 605
  cardiac output of, 603
  contusion of, in cardiopulmonary resuscitation, 574
  disease of, in young adults, 224
  electrical activity in, 722, *722*

Heart (*Continued*)
   heart sounds in, 605, 682
   precordial points of, *681*
   premature beats of, 607
   rupture of, in cardiopulmonary resuscitation, 574
   sinus arrhythmia of, 607
   stroke volume of, 603
   thrill in, 682
   workload on, in immobilized persons, 743, 747
Heart failure, effects of, *1086*
   homeostatic breakdown and, 310
Heart murmurs, 682
Heart rate, stress response and, 283
Heat, application of, 1389
   method(s) of, 1391, 1392t
      Aqua K pads as, 1391
      chemical counterirritants as, 1392–1393
      diathermy, 1393
      disposable chemical hot packs as, 1391
      dry, 1391–1393
      electric heating pads as, 1391
      heat cradles as, 1391–1392
      hot compresses as, 1393
      hot water bottles as, 1391
      hydrocollator packs as, 1393
      infrared or gooseneck lamps as, 1392
      moist, 1393–1394
      paraffin wax, 1393
      therapeutic baths for, 1394
   nursing management of, 1396–1397
   physiologic effects of, 1388–1389, 1389t
   precautions and contraindications for, 1390t
   principles of, 1386–1388
   purpose of, 1388
   rebound effect of, 1389
   therapeutic temperature range for, 1389
   as therapy, 35–36
   for pain relief, 985
   loss of, 587–588
   production of, 587
Heat cradles, 1391–1392
Heat exhaustion, 601
Heat illness, fluid and electrolyte imbalance and, 1021–1022
Heat stroke, 601
   dehydration of exercise and, 1022
Height, assessment of, 659, 660t
Heimlich maneuver, 575–576, *578–579*
Helmets, in adolescents, 219
Helsinki Agreement, 72
Hematuria, 1165
   urine testing for, 1168
Hemoglobin, as buffer of acid-base balance, 1020
Hemolytic reaction, to blood transfusion, 1312
Hemopericardium, in CPR, 574
Hemoptysis, in respiratory history, 1210
Hemorrhage, fluid and electrolyte imbalances and, 1022
   in wounds, 1365
Hemorrhagic shock, homeostatic fluctuations in, 309
Hemorrhoids, dietary management of, 1084t
Hemovac wound drainage system, 1380, *1382*, 1382t
Henderson, Virginia, 7
Henry Street Settlement, 18, 20, 400
   visiting nurse project at, 11
Heparin lock, advantages of, 1315
   in intravenous therapy, *1313–1315*, 1315, 1321–1322

Heparin lock (*Continued*)
   procedure for, 1316–1320
Hepatic dysfunction, tube feedings and, 1041
Hepatitis, dietary management of, 1083
Hepatitis B, 508
   in health care workers, 521
   vaccines for, 513, 521
   wound care and, 1345
Hepatitis C, in health care workers, 521
   wound care and, 1345
Herbal remedies, 36, 37, 38t
Herbert, Sidney, 484
Hester Poker Chip tool, 976–977
Hierarchy, in systems theory, 251
Hinduism, beliefs and practices affecting health care in, 1515–1516
   beliefs of, 1515–1516
Hip replacement, body position and, bowel function and, 1134
Hippocrates, ideas on homeostasis, 300
Hips, abduction wedges for, *767*, 767
   movement of, 693
   range of motion of, 739t–740t
      passive exercise of, 821
Hispanics, chronic diseases among, 337
   health care disparities and, 348–349
   mental disorders in, 338
   mortality in, 337
   older adults among, 240
History, bowel status in, 1127
   components of, 651–653
   documentation of, example of, *694–696*, 701
   family, 652
   fluid and electrolyte imbalances in, 1033
   medication, 1264
   method of taking, principles of, 650–651
   nursing, formats for, 122–126
      functions of, 122
      goals of, 122
      in nursing assessment, 121–122
   past, 652
   preoperative, 1419
   respiratory, 1209–1210
   sensory/perceptual alteration in, 1475
   sexual, 1500–1501, 1501t
   social and personal, 652
   systems review in, 652–653
Holistic care, 1510–1511
   model of health and disease and, 30, 32, 358, 359t
   nurse's role in, 1511
Holmes, Thomas, theories of stress and illness of, 274
Holy Communion, Christian beliefs about, 1519t–1521t
Holy Eucharist, Roman Catholic beliefs about, 1518t
Homan's sign, 692
Home care, Albrecht Nursing Model for Home Health Care and, 405, *406*
   assessment in, 407, 407t, 409
   case management in, 405–406
   case study in, 413
   coordination of, 410
   costs of, 403–404
   discharge planning in, 412
   documentation in, 412, 1196
   drug self-administration and, teaching about, 1267
   enteral feeding program in, 1115, 1118, *1119*
   for evaluation of long-term learning, 480–481
   for fever, 601
   goals of, 405

Home care (*Continued*)
   high tech equipment in, 402, *403*
      care givers and, 402
   history of, 400–401
   individuals needing, 404–405, *405*
   interventions in, 409–412
   legal and ethical issues in, 406–407
   nebulizer use and, 1236
   nursing care plan for, 413
   nursing diagnoses relating to, 408, 409
   oxygen administration and, 1235
   planning in, 409
   practice of, 11–12, 405–407
   reimbursement and, 409, 412
   scope of, 402–405
   services needed for, 404
   social and regulatory developments in, 401–402
   special diets in, teaching about, 1090–1091
   technical skills in, 409–410, 412
   terminology used for, 401, 412
   thermal therapy in, 1397
   traction in, teaching about, 879
   types of providers of, 402–404
   types of services available for, 402–404
   urethral catheters in, 1192–1193, 1196
   wounds in, 1386
Home health care agencies, accreditation of, 404
   as primary care agencies, 91
   definition of, 383
Homeopathy, 37, 38t
Homeostasis, 299–311
   adaptation and, 178
   compensatory, in heart failure, 310
   definition of, 300
   failure of, 304
   in living systems, 251–253
   nursing care and, 252–253, 314–318
   physiologic, 301
      failure of, 310–311
      maintenance of, 301–302
      mechanisms of, 304–309
         compensation, 304–305
         complementary processes with, 308
         failure of, 310–311
         fluctuations in, 309
         in hemorrhagic shock, 309
         limitations of, 309
         normal deviations in, 308
         of arterial blood, 608–609
         self-regulation of, 305–308
      regulators of, 302–304, *303*
   psychologic, 301
   theories of, 300–301
   unmet needs and, 256, *256, 257*
Homophobia, 1498
Homosexuality, in adolescents, 211
   nurse's reactions to, 1498
Hope, in dying people, 1540
   need for, 1513
Hormones, adaptive, 273–274
   blood levels of, negative feedback and, 307
   body temperature and, 591
   circadian rhythms in, 312–313
   definition of, 303
   functions and characteristics of, 303–304
   gonadotrophic, in male sexual development, 1491
   in growth and development, 182
   in homeostasis regulation, 302–304, *303*
   in stress response, 283, *284*
   target tissues of, 304
   urinary elimination and, 1160

Hospice movement, 1540
  definition of, 383
Hospital Stress Rating Scale, 292, 293t
Hospitalization, circadian rhythm disruption
    and, 314
  defense mechanisms and, 271
  mood swings and, 369
  of children, nursing interventions for, 1480
    parental role in, 205
    preparation for, 205
  sensory deprivation or overload with,
    1480-1481
  stress due to, in family members, 325-326
    nursing role and, 292, 293t, 294
  urinary elimination and, 1159-1160
Hospitals, admission to and discharge from,
    381-397
  business relationships of, patients's right to
    know, 67, 69
  charges of, patients' right to know, 67, 69
  client orientation in, 387-392
  client rooms of, furnishings and equipment
    in, 389-392, *390*
  definition of, 383
  infection risk in, 511, *511*
  military and veterans, 90
  nursing care models in, 385-388
  nursing practice in, 10-11
  nursing schools in, 16
  organization of, 92, 383-385
    administrative, 383, *384*
    functional, 383-384
    structural, 384-385
  rules and regulations of, patients' right to
    know, 68, 69
  value of nursing care to, 99
Host, susceptible to infection, 507, 513
Hostile reactions, with grief, 1541
Hot compresses, 1393
Hot water bottles, 1391
Hotlines, as primary care agencies, 91
Housing, for older adults, 239-240
Hoyer mechanical lift, 784, 790-792, *791,*
    795
Human immunodeficiency virus infection.
    See *Acquired immunodeficiency syn-
    drome (AIDS).*
Human needs, 253-255
  during illness, 377, 378t, 379t
    esteem, 379t
    for intimacy, 379t
    safety, 378t
    self-actualization, 379t
    stimulation, 378t
    survival, 378t
  theories of, 253-255
  unmet, nursing interventions and, 257-258
    problems with, 256, *256, 257*
    reasons for, 256
Human response patterns approach, in nurs-
    ing assessment, 124-126
  in nursing diagnoses, 132-134
Human rights. See *Rights.*
Humidification, of artificial airways, 1241,
    1243, *1243*
Humidifiers, 1225, *1225*
  with oxygen administration, 1231-1232
Humor, in therapeutic relationship, 435
Humoral theory, of disease, 28-29, 36
Hydration, airway suctioning and, 1244
  for urinary incontinence, 1174
  hazards of, 1226-1227
  respiratory status and, 1225-1227
  topical, 1225-1227
Hydraulic chair, 839
Hydrocollator packs, 1393

Hydrocolloids, dressings of, 1376-1377, *1377*
    procedure for application of, 1378-1380
  for wound care, 1351t
Hydrogels, dressings of, 1377
  for wound care, 1351t
Hydrogen bicarbonate, functions of, 1006t
Hydrogen ions. See also *Acid-base balance;
    pH.*
  function of, 1018-1019
Hydrogen peroxide, 1367
  for oral care, 907-908
Hydrogen-bicarbonate ion balance, renal
    regulation of, 1018
Hygiene, care plan for, 944
  case study in, 943-944
  client's functional level and, 894
  cosmetics and, 935
  elimination, 896-900
  for ears, 911-912
  for eyes, 908-911
  for hair, 930-934
  for nails and feet, 929-930
  for nose, 912-913
  for skin, 913-925
  general nursing care for, 892-896, 940t-
    941t
  handwashing and, 900
  in mental status assessment, 661
  individual variation in, 893
  influences on, 893
  oral, 900-908
    assessment of self-care of, 902-904
    reasons for neglect of, 900-901
  perineal, 925-926, 927-928
  principles of, 896, 940t-941t
  terminology for, 893
  territoriality and, 893-894
Hyperalgesia, 972
Hyperalimentation, 1094
  infusion pumps for, 1323
  parenteral, 1312-1313
    complications of, 1312-1313
    nursing management during, 1313
Hypercalciuria, 753, 754, 1164
Hypercapnia, oxygen therapy and, 1228
Hypercarbia, 557
Hypercholesterolemia, in various ethnic
    groups, 337
Hyperglycemia, hyperalimentation and, 1313
    intravenous therapy and, 1327t
Hyperlipidemia, atherosclerosis and, 1085
Hypernatremia, in elderly, 1041
Hyperosmolality, of extracellular fluid, fluid
    volume regulation and, 1016, *1016*
Hyperpnea, 611
  pattern of, 1211t
Hyperpolarization, in REM sleep, 948
Hyperpyrexia, 599
Hypersensitivity reaction, intravenous therapy
    and, 1327t, 1328
Hypertension, causes of, 620-621
  classification of, 620
  definitions of, 620
  dietary management of, 1087
Hyperthermia, 599
  consequences of, 589
Hyperuricemia, in gout, 1088
Hyperventilation, 611, *611,* 1208
Hypervolemia, 1015
Hypnotics, as sleep aids, 958, 962
Hypoglossal nerve, assessment of, 674
Hypoglycemia, dietary management of,
    1088-1089
  intravenous therapy and, 1327t
Hypoproteinemia, colloid oncotic pressure
    and, 1012

Hypoproteinemia *(Continued)*
  in immobilized persons, 750
Hypotension, blood pressure measurement
    of, 620
  orthostatic, dizziness and, 1480
    in immobilized persons, 748
  signs of, 620
  with bedpan use, 898
Hypothalamus, biologic rhythms and, 311
  blood cortisol levels regulated by, 307,
    308
  central integrator in ("thermostat"), for
    temperature regulation, 589, *590,*
    1388
  fluid and electrolyte balance and, 1013,
    1015
  food intake and, 1069
  interaction with pituitary (hypophysis), 304
Hypothermia, 587, 601-602
  accidental, 601
  causes of, 601, 602t
  cold water immersion and, 601
  consequences of, 589
  indications for, 1390
  induced, 602
  nursing assessment for, 602
  spontaneous, 602
  whole-body, 602
Hypothermia blankets, application of, 1395
Hypoventilation, 610, 1206
  pattern of, 1212t
Hypovolemia, 1015
  in immobilized persons, 747
Hypoxemia, 557, 1206
  causes of, 1208, 1208t
  lung function and, 608-609
  signs and symptoms of, 557, 558, 1208
    oxygen administration and, 1231t
  tachycardia and, 605
  with exercise, 1232
Hypoxia, 1208
  cerebral, level of consciousness and, 612
    with cardiac arrest, 557-558
  effects of, 577
  tissue, 741
Hypoxic drive, 1206

I

Ice, application of, 1396
  methods of, 1394, 1395, *1395*
Icterus neonatorum, in neonates, 192
Id and ego, 185
Idealization, 1542
Identity. See also *Body image; Self-concept;
    Self-image.*
  changes in, in surgical patients, 1411-1412
  in adolescents, 211-212, *213*
  in young adults, 220
Ileal conduit, 1163, *1164*
Ileostomy, care of, 1150-1152
  oral medications and, 1269
  physiologic problems with, 1150-1151
Ileum, electrolyte composition of, 1023t
Illness. See also *Disease; Health.*
  chronic, 374-376
    contemporary trends in, 375t
    family reaction to, 325-326
    family support during, 376
    grief process with, 1547
    in ethnic and racial groups, 336-337
    in older adults, 241
    pressure ulcers and, 1354
    responses to, 374-375
    stress-related, 273-274, 292

Illness *(Continued)*
  confirmed, reactions to, 367–373
    altered body image, 370–373
    anger, 368
    anxiety, 284–288, 286t, 367
    denial, 366, 368
    depression, 369
    fear, 286–287, 369, 369t, 1421
    information seeking, 368
    isolation, 368–369
    mood swings, 369
    powerlessness, 369–370
    shame, 368
    shock, 367
    uncertainty, 367
  defense mechanisms and, 271
  experience of, 363–380
    bibliography on, 364
    stages of, 365
  family reaction to, 325–326
  food intake and diet and, 1075, *1076*
  health promotion and, 347
  in adolescents, 214
  in infants, 198
  in older adults, 236, 241
  in school-age children, 205
  in young adults, 222
  mind and body relationship and, 364
  pharmacokinetics and, 1265
  prevention of, services available for, 88–89
  psychosomatic, 252
  respiratory changes in, 1206
  response to, 365–366
    previous illness and, 367
    psychosomatic context and, 366–367
    role playing and, 373–374
    seeking assistance for, 365–367
    self-concept and, 1450–1451
    symptoms and, 366
    vacillation and, 365
  sleep patterns and, 955
  somatopsychic, 252
  strategies for prevention of, 350, 350t
  terminal, advance directives and, 75
    assessment of patient and family with, 1544–1547
    response to, methods of coping with dying and, 1538–1540
Illusions, 1474
  nursing interventions for, 1482
Imagery, for pain relief, 986
  guided, in spiritual development, 1524
  in stress management, 290–291
Immersion, for cold treatment, 1396
Immobility. See also *Mobility; Mobility, impaired.*
  assessment of, 733–734, 744t–746t, 850–853
  bed rest and, 757, 758
  bowel elimination and, 1129
  cardiovascular system and, 743, 744t, 747–748
  care plan for, 800–801, 887–888
  case study of, 800, 887
  causes of, prescribed, 806. See also *Immobilization, therapeutic.*
    unavoidable, 806
  circulatory system and, 743, 744t, 747–748
  complications with, *808*
    traction and, 878
  musculoskeletal system and, 751–753, *754*
  nursing diagnoses for, 756, 757
  planning for, 757
  positioning and, equipment useful for, 758–769, 784, 796, *796*
    moving client in bed, 769, 770–774

Immobility *(Continued)*
    lift sheet place under, 547t–548t
    shoulder lift procedure for, 549t, *550*
    specific techniques for, 547–549, *550*, 551t, *551–553*
  of client in bed, 775–781
  principles and nursing interventions for, 782t–783t, 872t–873t
  transfer from bed to chair, 793–795, *794*
  transfer from bed to stretcher, 785–795, *796*
    assistance in dangling and, 792, *793*
    Hoyer lift for used for, 790–792, *791*
    lift sheet transfer for, *789*, 789–790
    three-person carry, 787–788, *787–788*
  turning client in bed, 1223, 1347
  pressure ulcers and, *1347*, 1347, 1349
  psychosocial system and, 754–755, 757
  pulmonary system and, 744t–745t, 748–750, 1222–1223
  responses to, 754–755, 806, *808*
  skin and, 741–743, 744t
  terminology related to, 808
  urinary system in, 753–754, *754*, 1159–1160
Immobilization, therapeutic. See also *Immobility; Mobility.*
  clients requiring, 848–850
  evaluation of, 887–888
  general considerations with, 850, 852
  neurovascular check for, 850–852, *851–852*
  nursing diagnoses for, 853
  nursing interventions for, 854–887
  planning for, 854
Immunity, as physiologic adaptation, 277
  wound healing and, 1359
Immunization, for infection, 513
Immunosuppressive therapy, federal funding for, 83
Impaction, fecal, 1144–1145
  causes of, 1144–1145
  in immobilized persons, 751
  interventions for, 1145
  urinary incontinence and, 1174
Impaired home maintenance management, as nursing diagnosis, 408, 409
  profile of, 408
Impaired role, 374
Implementation, 157–164. See also *Nursing interventions.*
  as part of nursing process, 160, 168
  measurement criteria for, 163
  responsibilities involved in, 158–163
  skills used in, 158–159
  standard for (ANA), 163
Imprisonment, false, as intentional tort, 56
Incident reports, in risk management programs, 55
Incisions, 1343t. See also *Wounds.*
Incontinence, bowel, management of, 1147–1148
  fecal, pressure ulcers and, 1350, 1351t–1352t
  urinary, 1158
    catheterization and, 1177–1178
    causes of, 1162
    evaluation of, 1199
    functional, 1170
    nursing interventions for, 1173–1175
    planning outcomes for, 1172
    pressure ulcers and, 1350, 1351t–1352t
    reflex, 1170
    stress, 1170
    total, 1171
    urge, 1170
Incontinence aids, 1174–1175

Indemnification, 54
Independent practice organizations, as primary care agencies, 91
Indian Health Service, 90
Indiana reservoir, continent, 1163
Industrial nursing, 12
Inertia, 542, 544t
Infant care review committees, 51
Infants. See also *Neonates.*
  anencephalic, as organ donors, 83
  assessment of, 198, 198t
  bathing of, 923–924, *924*
  blood pressure measurement in, 619
  body temperature in, 590–591
  cardiopulmonary resuscitation in, 570–571, 572t, *573*, 574t
  causes of death in, 198
  diagnostic procedures in, 709
  drug administration in, 1266
  ear drops instilled into, 1278, *1279*
  failure to thrive in, 1070, *1070*
  food intake and diet in, *1070*, 1070–1071
  foreign body obstruction in, 577, 579,
  growth and development in, 196–198
  health problems in, 198
  loss and grief experiences in, 1536
  musculoskeletal development in, 809t
  nurse's role with, 198
  pain behavior in, 976
  physical development in, 193t, 196
  preterm, feeding problems in, 1071
  psychosocial development in, 196–197
  pulse in, 605
  relationships and role of, 197
  self-concept in, 1453
  sexual development in, 1493
  spiritual growth in, 1514
  treatment of, informed consent and, 71–72
  values and beliefs of caretakers and, 198
Infarction, 748
Infection, 505–538
  airborne, 513, 522
  barriers to, 508, 513, 521. See also *Isolation precautions.*
  casts and, 868, 869t
  chain of, 506, *507*, 512–513
  community-acquired, 507
  contact transmission of, 513
  control of, 507–509
    assessment in, 514
    guidelines for, 515
    historical aspects of, 507–509
    in wound care, 1383
    isolation precautions for, 508, 515, 516t, 517–521. See also *Isolation precautions.*
    nursing diagnoses relating to, 514–515
    nursing interventions for, 515–537
    parenteral administration of drugs and, 1284–1285
    planning for, 515
    psychosocial aspects of, 522–524
  definition of, 506
  host defenses to, 513
  "iceberg" phenomenon of, *509*
  immobility and, 754, 852
  in health care workers, 521–522
  intravenous therapy and, 1327t
  laboratory data indicating, 514
  nosocomial, 507, 511–512
    control of, 507–508
  of wounds, *1342–1343*, 1342–1345, 1358, 1383
    factors affecting, 1342–1343
    oral, 904
  process of, 509, *509*, 511–512

Infection (*Continued*)
  risk of, 511, *511*
    as nursing diagnosis, 514–515, 1429
    assessment of, 514
    skeletal traction and, 878
  signs and symptoms of, 514
  staphylococcal, 508
  teaching about, 523–524
  terminology related to, 506–507
  transmission of, 513
  urinary tract, 1163
    catheterization and, 1189
      causes of, 1189
      prevention of, 1189–1191
    in immobilized client, 754
    nursing interventions for, 1172
  vector-borne, 513
Infectious agents, 509, 510t, 511
  control of, 512
  definition of, 506
  host susceptible to, 513
  mode of transmission, 513
    common sources and, 513
  portals of exit and entrance of, 513
  reservoirs of, 512–513
  sources of, 509
Infirmary, definition of, 383
Inflammation, as adaptive response, 279
  clinical signs of, 1355
Information, about organ donors and
    donees, 82
  patients' right to, 67, 68
  provided by nurses, informed consent and,
    71
  search for, as reaction to confirmed ill-
    ness, 368
Informed consent, 70–73, 84, 706
  obtainment of, 706
  patients' right to information needed for,
    67, 68
  to research on human subjects, 72–73
  to surgery, 1412–1413
  to treatment, 70–72
    components of, 70
    legal standards for, 70–71
  treatment of infants and, 71–72
  withdrawal of, 71, 72
Infrared lamps, for heat, 1392
Infusion pumps, for enteral therapy, 1109
  for intravenous therapy, 1323, *1325*
Inhalation therapy, 36
  in adolescents, 214
  metered dose inhalers for, *1226*, 1236
  of topical medications, 1280
Injections. See also *Drugs, administration of,
    parenteral.*
  in children, 1266
  intradermal, 1292–1293, *1294*
    procedure for, 1293–1294
  intramuscular, 1295, *1302–1303*, 1303
    procedure for, 1298–1301
    special techniques used for, air-lock,
      1297, 1300
    Z-lock, 1297, 1301
  sites of, 1282, 1295, 1299–1300, *1302–
    1303*
  subcutaneous, 1292, 1295, *1295*
    procedure for, 1296–1297
Injuries. See also *Wounds.*
  food intake and diet and, 1075–1076,
    1076
  preexisting, at admission, 394
  risk of, with use of restraints, 881
  sports, in adolescents, 217
  tissue, with urethral catheterization, 1189–
    1190
  urinary elimination and, 1162

Injuries (*Continued*)
  work-related, reporting of for workers
    compensation, 59
Insomnia, 952–953. See also *Sleep, disor-
    ders of.*
  chronic, 953
  drugs and alcohol and, 953
  restless legs syndrome and, 953
  sundowner's syndrome and, 953
Inspection, technique of, 655
Inspiration, in incentive spirometry devices,
    1237
  steps in, 1205
Institutional review boards, role in research
    on human subjects, 72–73
Institutions, involuntary commitment to, 80, 81
  residents of, circadian rhythm disruption
    and, 314
Insulin, 182
  deficiency of, in diabetes, 1088
  in intravenous solutions, 1311
Insurance, cost containment methods and,
    97–98
  federal programs for, 97–98
  private programs for, 98
  health care costs and, 95–96
  private, 95, 96–97
  professional liability, obtainment of, 54
    types of, 54
  prospective payment of, 97
  public, 95
    Medicaid, 96
    Medicare, 96
  retrospective reimbursement for health
    costs by, 95–96
  workers' compensation, 96
Integument. See *Skin.*
Intellectual development, Piaget's theory of,
    187, 188t
Intelligence, in older adults, 237
  in Piaget's theory, 187
Intensive care units, infection risk in, 511, *511*
  nursing practice in, 11
Interactional factors, in growth and develop-
    ment, 182–184
Interleukin-1, 599
Intermittent positive-pressure breathing
    (IPPB), 1236–1237
International Council of Nurses, 19, 21
  code of ethics of, 48
Interoceptors, 1470
Interpersonal relationships, in adolescents,
    211–212
  in children, 184
Interstitial fluid, distribution of, 1001t
  exchange of with blood vessels, 1011–1013
    in immobilized persons, 747
Interview, about pain, in children, 976
  about sleep patterns, 954–955
  for health history, 650–651
  for psychosocial history, 629–630
    format for documentation of, *631–635*
  in nursing assessment, 121
  preoperative, 1419
Intestinal tubes, 1097t, 1099–1101, *1100*
Intestines, disease of, bowel elimination and,
    1129
  innervation of, 1052
  large, structure and function of, 1051,
    1126, 1126–1127
  small, decreased absorption in, 1093–1094
    increased motility of, 1093
    increased osmotic and secretory activity
      of, 1093–1094
    structure and function of, 1051
Intimacy, in young adults, 220
Intracellular fluid, 1000, *1000*

Intracellular fluid (*Continued*)
  distribution of, 1001
  fluid and electrolyte transport in, 1009–
    1011, *1010*
Intracranial pressure, in neonates, 191
Intradermal injections, 1292
Intramuscular injections, *1293–1294*, 1295,
    1297, 1302–1303
Intrathoracic pressure, in cardiopulmonary
    resuscitation, 562, *563, 564,* 564, 566
Intravenous pyelogram, 712t, 713–714
Intravenous therapy, advantages of, 1308
  assessment of patients needing, 1328
  care plan for, 1332
  case study of, 1332
  changing dressing at insertion site of,
    1330, 1332
  complication(s) of, 1326, 1326t–1327t,
    1328
    air embolism as, 1327t
    circulatory overload as, 1327t
    hyperglycemia as, 1327t
    hypersensitivity reaction as, 1327t, 1328
    hypoglycemia as, 1327t
    infection of site as, 1327t
    infiltration of solution as, 1326t
  discontinuing IV line with, 1320
  drop factor in, 1310
  equipment needed for, 1313–1315, *1313–
    1315, 1323–1325*
    catheters, *1313,* 1315
    filters, 1323
    flow regulator, 1323, *1324*
    heparin or saline lock, *1313–1315,*
      1315, 1321–1322
    implantable vascular access devices,
      1323, *1326*
    infusion pumps and controllers, 1311,
      1323, *1325*
    needles, 1313, *1313,* 1315
    safety devices, 1323, *1324*
    solution containers, 1315, 1322, *1323*
      changes of, 1332–1333
    time tape, 1310, *1310*
    T-ports, 1323, *1324*
    tubes and accessories, 1322–1323, *1324*
      changes of, 1332–1333
  evaluation of, 1333–1334
  heparin or saline lock for, *1313–1315,*
    1315, 1321–1322
  procedure for, 1316–1320
  indications for, 1042–1043, 1308
    enteral feeding, 1109
    specific metabolic deficits, 1043
  medications used with, administration of,
    1321–1322
    compatibility of, 1311
    types of, 1311
  monitoring of, 1042
  physician's order for, 1309–1310
  risks of, 1308
  schedule and flow rate for, 1320–1321
  solutions used with, 1308–1328
    fluid and electrolyte imbalances and,
      1022
    precautions and risks with, 1023t
  time tape for, 1310, *1310*
  tubes and accessories for, 1322–1323, *1324*
Introspection, 260–261
Intuition, in ethical theory, 46
Iodine, metabolism, functions, and sources
    of, 1060t
Ions, 1000
  hydrogen, function of, 1018–1019
  movement across cellular membrane, 1011
Iron, metabolism, functions, and sources of,
    1059t

Iron (Continued)
  requirements in adolescents, 1072
  supplements of, 1063, 1065
Irrigation, 1277
  nasal, 1277
  of ears, 1279
  of eyes, 1278
  vaginal, 1278-1280
Ischemia, from pressure, 741
  with use of restraints, 881
Ischial tuberosity, as pressure point, 1349
Islam, beliefs and practices of, 1522, 1522t
Islets of Langerhans, in homeostasis regula-
    tion, 302, 303
Isolation, as infection control measure, 508-
    509
  as reaction to confirmed illness, 368
  immobility and, 755
  in chronic illness, prevention of, 375
  of body substances, 508
  psychosocial effects of, 522-523
  reverse (protective), 522-523
Isolation carts, 519
Isolation precautions, 515, 516t, 517-521
  for postmortem handling of bodies, 521
  for routine cleaning, 521
  for soiled equipment disposal, 520-521
  for transportation of people with infec-
      tions, 521
  gloves as, 517
  gowns as, 517
  hand washing as, 517, 518t, 519t
  isolation carts as, 519
  masks as, 517, 519
  protective eye wear as, 517, 519
  roommate selection as, 519-520

J

Jackson-Pratt wound drainage system, 1380,
    1382t, 1383
Japanese-Americans, coping methods with
    loss and grief in, 1538
Jaundice, assessment of, 662
  in neonates, 192
Jaw thrust method, of airway control, 560,
    561, 566
JED sled, use of, 879-880, 880
Jehovah's Witnesses, beliefs and practices of,
    1521t
Jejunostomy tube, feedings with, 1114-1115
Jet lag syndrome, 313
Jewish communities, older adults among, 240
Jews, beliefs of, 1516, 1516t-1517t
Jim Crow laws, 335
Joint Commission on Accreditation of
    Health-care Organizations, 404
Joints, anatomy of, 732-733
  ball-and-socket, 733
  condyloid, 733
  gliding, 733
  hinge (ginglymus), 733
  pivot, 733
  saddle, 733
  synovial, 732-733
Jones dressing, uses of, 862-863
Judaism, beliefs of, 1516, 1516t-1517t
Judgment, in mental status assessment, 661
Justice, as ethical principle, 47

K

K pads, 1391, 1393
Kalish, Richard, human needs theory of, 253,
    254
Kardex, with nursing care plans, 148

Kaspers, Karl, 262
Kegel exercises, 1173-1174
  urinary production and, 1159
Keloid, in wound healing, 1357, 1358
Ketamine, pain modulation and, 972
Ketones, urine tests of, 1167
Ketorolac tromethamine, as adjunct to
    opioids, 981
Ketosis, 1053, 1088
Kidney stones, 753, 1163-1164
  calcium, 753, 754
  in immobilized clients, 754, 783t
  kinds of, 754
  struvite, 754
  symptoms of, 1164
Kidneys, acid-base balance and, 1019, 1020
  anatomy of, 1156, 1156-1157, 1157
  disease of, dietary management of, 1085,
      1085t
  fluids and electrolytes regulated by, 1017
  function of, 1157, 1157
    fluid balance and, 1018
    inadequate, 1165
  homeostatic regulation by, 302
  palpation of, 687
  transplantation of, donor organ allocation
      for, 83
  trauma to, 1162
King, theory of, family in, 324t, 325
Kling bandage, 1375, 1376
Knee immobilizer, 871
Knees, flexion of, 693
  range of motion of, 740t
Knights Hospitaliers, nursing and, 9-10
Knowledge deficit, as nursing diagnosis, 477
Knowles, Malcolm, 472-473
Kock pouch, 1163, 1164
Kohlberg, Lawrence, theory of moral devel-
    opment of, 187, 188t, 189
  controversy about, 189
Korotkoff sounds, in blood pressure mea-
    surement, 615, 618t
Kriegler, Delores, 39t
Kubler-Ross, Elizabeth, theory of dying of, 7,
    1539-1540
Kussmaul's respirations, 611
  pattern of, 1212t
Kyphosis, 676, 677

L

Labor unions, employment contracts of, 58
Laboratory specimens, transportation of, 521
Laboratory studies, chronobiology and, 314
  diagnostic tests with, 716
    care of person undergoing, 717t-719t
  drug administration and, 1265
  in diagnosis of infection, 514
  in nutritional assessment, 1067
Laboratory technologists, training and re-
    sponsibilities of, 93
Lacerations, 1340, 1343t
Lacrimal apparatus, assessment of, 668, 668
Lactation, food intake and diet and, 1074-
    1075
Lactose, intolerance of, tube feedings and,
    1041
  osmotic activity in small intestine and,
      1094
Language. See also Communication.
  body, 430-433
  development of, problems with, in school-
      age children, 204
Lanugo, in neonates, 192
Lasers, in wound healing, 1363

Latex, in catheters, 1178
Law(s). See also under Legal.
  administrative, 51
  affecting nurses as employees, 58
  case, 50
  civil rights, equal employment opportuni-
      ties and, 59
  common, 50
  constitutional, 49
  contract, 57-59
  creation and passage of, 50-51
  definition of, 48-49
  ethics and, 45, 45
  federal, Cruzan decision and, 75
    for Medicare and Medicaid, 78-80
    on health care consumers' rights, 67
  Good Samaritan, and standard of care, 53
  on abortion, 76-77
  on contraception, 77
  on drug administration, 1259
  on emergency care of individuals, 53, 58
  on forgoing life-sustaining measures, 74
  on informed consent, 70-71
  on licensure, 59-61
  on organ transplantation and donation,
      81-83
  on regulation of facilities for mentally ill
      and developmentally disabled, 78, 80,
      81
  on regulation of long-term care facilities,
      77-78
  on reporting data, controversies in, 57
  on sterilization, 77
  on substance abuse in pregnancy, 77
  overview of, 50
  sources of, 48-51
  state, about decision making for minors,
      70
    Cruzan decision and, 75
    on abortion, 76
    on decision making about forgoing life-
        sustaining measures, 74-76
    on health care consumers' rights, 67
    on informed consent, 71
    on organ donation and transplantation,
        81, 82
  statutory, 50-51
  types of, 51-61
    civil and criminal, 51
    contract law, 57-59
    licensure laws, 59-61
    procedural and substantive, 51-59
    tort law, 52-57
Lawsuits, 53-56
  minimizing risk of, 55
  practices controlling, 54-56
  steps in, 53, 54
Laxatives, 1135
  for diarrhea, 1146
  types of, 1135-1136
Lazarus model of stress and coping, 274-
    276, 276
Lead exposure, equal employment opportu-
    nities and, 59
Leadership, in groups, 462
Learning. See also Teaching.
  ability for, in older adults, 237-238
  active participation in, 473
  adult, assumptions characterizing, 471-472
  affective, levels of, 470
  benefits of, 468
  cognitive, levels of, 469-470
  computerized packages of, 480
  contract for, 477
  definition of, 183
  disabilities in, in school-age children, 204

Learning (Continued)
  domain(s) of, 468–471
    affective, 470
    cognitive, 469–470
    perceptual, 469
    psychomotor, 470–471
  environmental factors in, 473
  factors hindering, 474
  in growth and development, 179, 182–183
  in Piaget's theory of development, 187,
    188t
  long-term, 480–481
  motivation for, 472–473, 478–479
  nursing goals and, 257
  objectives for, 478
  perceptual, levels of, 469
  principles of, 472–474
  putting new skills into practice and, 474
  readiness for, 472
  relevance of content to learner and, 473
  repetition in, 474
  rewards for, 473
  short-term, 480
  styles of, 477
  surmounting plateaus of, 474
  teaching plan and, 473
Lectures, in teaching process, 479
Leg bag, with urethral catheters, 1192
Legal aspects, of client record, 485
  of drug administration, 1258–1259
  of nursing diagnoses, 138, 141–142
  of nursing standards, 170–171
  of surgery, 1412–1413
Legal guardians, for health care decision
    making, 69, 70, 74, 75
Legal issues, in home care nursing,
    406–407
Legislative process, in U.S. and Canada, 50–
    51
Legs, casts for, 866, *866*
  exercises of, preoperative, 1423, *1423*
  neurovascular check of, with immobiliza-
    tion devices, 850–852, *851–852*
  passive range of motion exercise of, 821
  positioning devices for, cockup splints,
    767, *768*
    hip abduction wedges, 767, *767*
    trochanter rolls, 766, *767*
  range of motion of, 735–736, 736t–740t,
    741
Leininger, Madeline, 332
Leukocytes, in urine, 1168
Leukocytosis, 514
Leukorrhea, 925
Leverage, in prevention of back injury, 542,
    543, 544t, 545
Levin sump tube, 1096, 1097t, *1098*
Lewis, Keefa, 13
Lewis, Kurt, 452
Liability, prevention of, during admission
    process, 393–394
Liability insurance, types of, 54
Libel, 56
Libido, 185
Lice, 931–933
Licensure, current concerns in, 60
  dual roles of, 60
  for Medicare and Medicaid, 77–78
  in Canada, 61
  laws on, 59–61
  mandatory, 60
  permissive, 60
  state action against, and judicial appeal of,
    61
Life expectancy, in ethnic and racial groups,
    337–338

Lifestyle, fluid and electrolyte imbalances
    and, 1021–1022
  health promotion and protection and,
    349–350
  in midlife, 233
  in older adults, 242
  in young adults, 222
  respiratory status and, 1206
  surgery and, 1412
Life-sustaining measures, forgoing of, 74–76,
    84
  assisted suicide and, 76
  decision makers in, 74–75
  laws on, 74–75
  nurses' responsibilities in, 76
Lift sheet, use of, *789*, 789–790
Light reflex, corneal, 669
  direct and consensual, 669
Lights, in hospital client rooms, 391
Lignin, 1053
Lindeman, E., 1541
Linen. See also *Bed(s), changing linens of.*
  soiled, disposal of, 520
Lipids, 1054
Lipoproteins, 1054
Lips, assessment of, 673
Listening, active and passive, 447
Literature review, in nursing assessment,
    126–127
Lithotripsy, for urinary tract stone removal,
    1173
Liver, biopsy of, 721
  care of person undergoing, 718t
  disease of, dietary management of, 1083
  palpation of, 687
  percussion of borders of, 687, *687*
Living wills, 1546
  decision making about life-sustaining mea-
    sures and, 74–75
Livor mortis, 1554
Local adaptation syndrome, 274
Log, for self-monitoring, 357, *357*
Loneliness, in older adults, 243
Long-term care facilities, residents of, need
    for restraints in, 852–853
  rights and responsibilities of, 77–80
  services offered by, 12–13, 89
Lordosis, 676, *677*
Loss. See also *Death; Dying person; Grief
    and grieving.*
  coping with, 1533–1558
  cultural perspectives on, 1537–1538
  definitions of, 1534, 1535t
  developmental aspects of, 1536–1537
  forms of, 1535, 1535t
  of a child, 1537
  of control, with immobility, 755
Lotions, 1273, 1275
Love and relatedness, need for, as spiritual
    need, 1512
Lower gastrointestinal series, 711, 711t
Lubricants, for bowel stimulation, 1135
Lumbar puncture, 719–720
  care of person undergoing, 717t
Lung scans, 1217
Lungs. See also *Pulmonary; Respiratory* en-
    tries.
  acid-base balance regulation by, 1019,
    1020
  auscultation of, 1213, *1213*, 1214t
  blood supply to, 1205
  consolidated, 1213, 1223
  normal function of, 1205
  physiologic data base of, 608–609
  structure of, 1204
  volume vs. capacity, *1216*, 1217t

Luteinizing hormone, positive feedback and,
    307–308
Lutheran Church, beliefs and practices of,
    1519t
Lymph nodes, epitrochlear, palpation of, 691
  of neck, assessment of, 674–675, *675*
  superficial inguinal, 692
Lymphatic system, filtration of interstitial
    fluid of, fluid transport and, 1012
  obstruction of, edema and, 1012

M

Maceration, pressure ulcers and, 1350
Macula densa, 670
Magnesium, deficit of, 1029t
  dietary, regulation of, 1038
  excess, 1029t
  functions of, 1006t
  imbalance of, 1008t
  metabolism, functions, and sources of,
    1059t
Magnetic resonance imaging, 713t, 714–715
  mechanism of, 714–715
Malnutrition. See also *Diet; Food(s); Nutri-
    tion.*
  in older adults, 243
  physical signs of, 1066–1067, 1068t
  pressure ulcers and, 1349–1350
  protein-energy, 1075
  wound infection and, 1342
Malpractice suits, evaluation and, 170–171
  patient privilege in, 57
  tort law and, 52
Managed care centers, as primary care agen-
    cies, 91
Manganese, metabolism, functions, and
    sources of, 1060t
Manipulation, ethics of, 47
Marijuana, in adolescents, 214
  in young adults, 222, 224
Marriage, decision making about, 221
Martocchio, B. C., 1542, 1543
Masks, infection control and, 517, 519
  pocket, in cardiopulmonary resuscitation,
    561, *562*, 562, 566, 567
  protective effect of, 522
  surgical, application of, 533
  tracheostomy, 1243, *1243*
Maslow, Abraham, human needs theory of,
    253, 254, 1448
Mass media, food intake and diet and, 1075
  health promotion in groups and, 359
Massage, back, for sleep facilitation, 958,
    959, 960, 960–962
  contraindications to, 987–988
  for pain relief, 985, 987–988
  of oral mucosa, 907
  Swedish, for relief of cancer pain, 987
Masturbation, in adolescents, 211
Matrix, in wound healing, 1356
Mattresses, alternating pressure, bedmaking
    and, 943
  overlays for, pressure-reducing, 1347,
    1348t, *1353*
  pads for, 935
  replacement, pressure-reducing, 1347,
    1348t
  specialized, 763–765
    air, 763
    artificial sheepskins, 764
    convoluted foam (egg crate), 764
    flotation, 763
Maturation, definition of, 179
May, Rollo, 261

Mayo, Ada, 12
McDermott, Katherine C., 20
McGill Pain Questionnaire, 978
Meaning, for dying clients, 1552
    sense of, as spiritual need, 1512
Measles, in hospitals, 522
Measurements, in physical assessment, 655
Mechanical ventilation, 1249. See also *Ventilation.*
Meconium, 1130
Median nerve, testing of, 852, *852*
Mediastinum, 1205
Medic II program, 556
Medicaid, beginnings of, 95
    coverage and costs of, 96, 97
    donor organ protocols and, 82
    Health Care Financing Administration and, 97
    home care nursing and, 401–402
    long-term care facilities and, certification of, 77–78
        rights of residents in, 78–80
    Medicare and, 97t
Medical model of disease, 29
Medical record. See also *Record, client.*
    documentation in, 53, 163
        on use of life-sustaining measures, 76
    in nursing assessment, 121
    patient's right to review of, 67, 68
Medicare, beginnings of, 95
    coverage and costs of, 96, 97
    diagnosis-related groups and, 98, 402
    Health Care Financing Administration and, 97
    home care nursing and, 401–402
    length of hospital stay under, 98
    long-term care facilities and, certification of, 77–78
        rights of residents of, 78
    Medicaid and, 97t
    organ transplantation and, 82, 83
Medicated baths, 916–917
Medication errors, risk management and, 55
Medication orders, 1261–1262
Medication reference cards, 1257, *1257*, 1263, *1264*
Medicine, alternative methods of, and traditional medicine, 37, 38t–39t
    types of, 38t–39t
    early methods of, 36–37
    humoral theory of, 28–29
    physical, 35–36
    recent advances in, 35
    Western methods of, 36
Medicus low-air-loss bed, 762–763
Medulla oblongata, 1206
Melena, 1130
Memory, in early childhood, 200
    in mental status assessment, 661
    in neonates, 194
    in older adults, 238
Men, as widowers, 239
    psychosexual changes in, at midlife, 229
Menarche, 1491
    in adolescents, 211
Mennonite church, beliefs and practices of, 1519t
Menopause, 228–229
Menstrual cycle, body temperature and, 591
    in Jewish faith, 1516t
Mental health, defense mechanisms and, 271
    in middle-aged adults, screening for, 234
    in older adults, 243
    services for, use in ethnic groups, 338
Mental illness, decision making about life-sustaining measures and, 74, 75

Mental illness *(Continued)*
    health care facilities for, involuntary commitment to, 80, 81
        rights and responsibilities of, 78, 80, 81
    in ethnic groups, 338
Mental retardation, health care decision making and, 69, 75
    health care facilities for, involuntary commitment to, 80, 81
        rights and responsibilities of, 78, 80, 81
Mental status, acronym for, 661
    examination for, brief form of, 642
        components and goals of, 630, 635–636
    in assessment data base, 118
    parenteral administration of drugs and, 1283
    physical assessment and, 660–661
Mercury manometer, for blood pressure measurement, 614
Metabolic acidosis, causes of, 1009t
Metabolic alkalosis, causes of, 1009t
Metabolic disorders, dietary management of, 1088–1089
    wound healing and, 1359
Metabolic rate, factors increasing, 587
Metabolism, anaerobic, with respiratory arrest, 557, 558
    heat production and, 587
    in immobilized clients, assessment of, 745t, 750–751
Metal, internal, magnetic resonance imaging and, 715
Metamucil, in enteral feeding tubes, 1109
Metatarsals, range of motion of, 740t
Metered-dose inhaler, *1226*, 1236
Methodists, beliefs and practices of, 1520t
Metropolitan Life Insurance Company, home nursing services offered by, 400
Mexican-Americans, coping methods with loss and grief in, 1538
Microbes, resistance of, 29
Microorganisms. See also *Infectious agents.*
    infectious, control of, 512
    reservoirs of, 512–513
    normal and pathogenic, in human body sites, 510t
    virulence of, 509, 511
Micturition, 1158
Midlife. See *Adults, middle-aged.*
Milia, in neonates, 192
Milieu interieur, 300, 301
Milk, cow's, for infants, 1070–1071
Miller-Abbott intestinal tubes, 1097t, 1099–1101, *1100*
Milwaukee brace, *871*
Mind-body dichotomy, 29
Minerals, body requirements for, 1056, 1058t–1060t
    functions and sources of, 1058t–1060t
    supplements for, 1056–1057, 1063, 1065
    wound healing and, 1358–1359
Minerva casts, 867, *867*
Minnesota gastric tube, 1096, 1097t, *1099*
Minorities, 335–336. See also *Ethnic groups.*
    health care disparities and, 348–349
    health risks in midlife and, 234
Miscarriage, 191
Mitt, bathing, 918
Mobility. See also *Exercise; Immobility.*
    angina pectoris and, 807
    assessment of, 733–734, 806–807
        and self-assessment by nurse, 807
    evaluation of, 842–843
    functional levels of, 811
        conditions accompanying, 808
        NANDA classification of, 734

Mobility *(Continued)*
    impaired. See also *Immobility; Immobilization, therapeutic.*
        care plan for, 843–844
        case study of client with, 843
        decision tree for, *812*
        elimination hygiene and, 896
        factors related to, 811
        nursing diagnosis for, 810–812
        nursing interventions for, 823, 829
            teaching client how to "dangle," 824–828
        planning for, 810, 813
        suggested outcomes for, 810
        vs. activity intolerance, 811
        vs. high risk for disuse syndrome, 810, 811
    in surgical patients, 1411, 1419–1420
Mobilization, maneuvers for, in respiratory therapy, 1221–1225
    progressive, in clients with impaired mobility, 823, 829
        nursing interventions for, 823, 829
        teaching client to "dangle," 824–828
Moisture, skin, 662
Molybdenum, metabolism, functions, and sources of, 1060t
Mongolian spots, in neonates, 192
Montag, Mildred, 17
Montefiore Hospital, home care nursing program of, 401
Montgomery straps, 1375, *1375*, 1385
Mood, 635, 636t
    format for documentation of, *637–638*
    reaction to confirmed illness and, 369
Moral development. See also *Ethics; Values.*
    in adolescents, 213
    in early childhood, 201
    in school-age children, 204
    in young adults, 222
    Kohlberg's theory of, 187, 188t, 189
Morals, definition of, 44
Mormons, beliefs and practices of, 1521t
Morphine, action of, 971
Mortality. See *Death; Loss.*
Motherhood, surrogate, 190
Mothering role, gender identity and, 1493
Motion(s), body, for prevention of back injury, 542, 544–546
    Newton's law of, in prevention of back injury, 542, 544t
    used in moving heavy objects, 544–546, 554
Motivational factors, in growth and development, 182
Motor system, assessment of, 692–693
    documentation of, *700*
    development of, in early childhood, 199
    in infants, 196, 197t
Moulder, Betty, 12
Mourning, definition of, 1535, 1535t
Mouth. See also *Oral hygiene.*
    anatomy and function of, *673*, 1050
    digestion and, 1091
    dry or irritated, care of, 907
    examination of, *673*, 673–674, 903–904
    hygiene of, 900–908
Mouthwashes, 907
Movement devices, 879–880
Mucilages, 1053
Mucolytics, 1235
Mucosa, buccal, assessment of, 673–674
    dry or irritated, 907–908
Mucositis, mouth care for, 908
Mucous membranes, infection and, 508
    respiratory status and, 612

Mucous membranes *(Continued)*
 topical medication administration to,
  1275–1280
Mucus. See also *Sputum.*
 coughing and, 1224
Mullerian duct, development of, 1489, *1489*
Multiple sclerosis, physical protection and
  support needed for, 850
 self-concept and, 1451
Multiple-positioning chairs, 784
Murmurs, heart, 682
Muscle(s), accessory, respiratory status and,
  611
 as soft tissue, 1337–1338
 blood supply to, 1338
 connective tissue and, 733
 contractures of, with immobility, 752, *753*
 fiber patterns of, 733
 flaccidity of, 752
 isometric contractions of, for strength
   building, 814–816
  immobility and, 751–752
 isotonic contractions of, for strength building, 813–814, *815*
  immobility and, 751
 skeletal, structure of, 733, *734*
  temperature regulation and, 589
 spasticity of, 752
 strength of, classification of, 735–736
  evaluation of, 842
  in immobilized clients, 751–752
  isometric exercises for, 814–816
  isotonic exercises for, 813–814, *815*
  testing of, 693
Muscle mass, in immobility, 752
 isometric exercises for, 814–816
 isotonic exercises for, 813–814, *815*
 measurement of, 842
 parenteral administration of drugs and,
  1282
Muscle tone, bladder, catheter removal and,
  1192
 bowel elimination and, 1128–1129
 immobility and, 751
 urinary elimination and, 1160
Musculoskeletal system, anatomy of, 733, *734*
 changes in, in adolescents, 210, 210t
 developmental changes in, with age, 809t
 effects of exercise and aging on, 814t
 in immobilized clients, assessment of,
  746t, 751–753
 in nursing assessment, 123
 in young adults, 220
 use of restraints and, 881
Muslims, beliefs and practices of, 1522, 1522t
Mustache, care of, 934
Myelin, 971
Myelography, 712t, 714
Myocardial contusion, in CPR, 574
Myocardial infarction, dietary management
  of, 1086
 effects of, *1086*
 recovery from, bedmaking considerations
   with, 942
Myocardial rupture, in CPR, 574
Myoclonus, nocturnal, insomnia and, 953

N

Nagele's rule, 190
Nails, care of, 929–930
 cleaning and trimming of, 930
Naloxone (Narcan), action of, 971–972
NANDA. See *North American Nursing Diag-
  nosis Association (NANDA).*

Narcolepsy, 951–952
Narcotic analgesics, premedication with,
  1426
Narcotics, for dying person, 1552
Nasal airway, insertion of, 1241, *1241*
 suctioning of, 1246
Nasogastric tubes, nursing diagnoses and in-
  terventions with, 1115t–1116t
 oral medications given through, 1269
Nasolabial folds, 666
National Federation of Specialty Nursing Or-
  ganizations, 105
National Home Caring Council, 404
National Institutes of Health, 90
National League for Nursing, 18–19, 21
 accreditation function of, 60
 Community Health Accreditation Program
   of, 404
National Organ Transplant Act of 1984, 82
National Research Act, 67, 72
National Student Nurse Association, 22–23
Native Americans, life expectancy in, 338
 mental disorders in, 338
 mortality in, 337
 racism toward, 335
Naturopathy, 38t
Nausea, in dying person, care measures for,
  1553
 management of, 1090
Near-death experiences, 575
Nebulization, of topical agents, 1280
Nebulizers, 1225–1226, *1226, 1227*
 abuse of, 1236
 at home, 1236
 drugs delivered through, 1235–1236
 hand-held, 1235–1236, *1236*
 metered-dose, use of, *1226*, 1236
Neck, anatomy of, *675*
 assessment of, 674–675
 hyperextension of in CPR, spinal cord
   damage with, 571
 range of motion of, 736t
Necrosis, 1338
 in healing wounds, 1358
 in immobilized persons, 748
 pressure and, 741
Needle sticks, reporting of, 1345
 workers compensation for nurses with, 59
Needles, butterfly, 1313, *1313*
  methods of securing, *1329*
 for intravenous therapy, 1313, *1313*, 1315
 for parenteral administration of drugs,
   1285, 1285t, *1286*
  care and handling of, 1285, 1287, *1288*
  selection of, 1285
 indwelling plastic catheters and, 1313, *1313*
Needs. See *Human needs.*
Neglect, statutes on, substance abuse in
  pregnancy and, 77
Negligence, professional liability insurance
  and, 54
 under tort law, 52
Neighborhood health centers, as primary
  care agencies, 91
Neonates. See also *Infants.*
 body temperature in, 591
 cardiopulmonary resuscitation in, 570
 cognitive and intellectual development in,
  194
 crying patterns in, 194
 deaths in, 195
 developmental tasks of, 192
 growth and development in, 192–196, 193t
 head and body in, *192*, 192–193
 health concerns in, 195
 musculoskeletal development in, 809t

Neonates *(Continued)*
 nurse's role with, 195, 196t
 nursing care of, 193
 psychosocial development in, 194
 reflexes in that normally disappear, 193,
  193t
 self-concept in, 194
 shaking of, 191–192
 vital signs in, 193t
Neostigmine, for flatulence reduction, 1147
Nephrectomy, 1162
Nephrolithiasis, 1163–1164
Nephrons, aging and, 1158
 anatomy of, 1157, *1157*
Nephrostomy tube, percutaneous, 1177, *1178*
Nerve fibers, pain conduction and, *970*, 971
 pain modulation and, 972
Nerve receptors, to heat and cold, 1388
Nerves, abducens, assessment of, 669
 acoustic, testing of, 672, *672*
 cranial, 665–666
  functions of, 667t
  damage to, casts and, 868, 869t
 facial, 667–668, 674
 glossopharyngeal, 674
 hypoglossal, 674
 median, testing of, 852, *852*
 oculomotor, 669
 of extremities, testing of, 851–852, *851–
   852*
 olfactory, testing of, 673
 optic, 669–670
 peroneal, testing of, 851, *851*
 radial, testing of, 851, *851*
 spinal accessory, 675
 tibial, testing of, 851, *851*
 trigeminal, 667, 669
 trochlear, 669
 ulnar, testing of, 852, *852*
 vagus, 674
Nervous system, autonomic, blood pressure
   and, 612
  gastrointestinal tract and, 1052
  homeostasis regulation and, 302, *303*
 disorders of, physical protection and support needed for client with, 849–850
 endocrine system and, 302–304, 1013–
  1017
 exercise and aging and, 814t
 in growth and development, 182
 in nursing assessment, 123
 pain and, 969, *970*, 971–972, 992
 parasympathetic, gastrointestinal tract and,
  1052
  homeostasis regulation and, 302, *303*
  in NREM sleep, 950
 peripheral, pain modulation in, 972
 respiratory status and, 612
 sympathetic, body temperature and, 591
  homeostasis regulation and, 302, *303*
  in heart failure, 310
  in hemorrhagic shock, 309
  in REM sleep, 948
  pain and, 969, 992
  tachycardia and, 607
 temperature regulation by, 589
 urinary elimination and, 1160
 wound healing and, 1359
Netting, for children's cribs, 886
Neuman, theory of, family in, 324, 324t
Neuroablation, for pain relief, 992
Neuroendocrine system, fluid and electrolyte
   balance regulation by, 1013–1017
  homeostasis regulation and, 302–304, *303*
Neuromuscular disorders, requiring protection and support, 849–850

Neurons, afferent, pain conduction and, 971
  ascending, anatomy of, *1471*
Neurosensory system, impairment of, drug
  administration and, 1266
Neurotransmitters, 971
  pain modulation and, 972
Neurovascular function, of extremities, immobilization devices and, 850–852,
  851–852
  traction and, 878
Neutropenia, 514
New Age spiritualism, beliefs and practices
  of, 1522–1523
New York Blue Cross, home care nursing
  program of, 401
New York City Mission, 400
Newborn. See *Neonates.*
Niacin, toxicity of, 1063t
Nicotine, prenatal exposure to, 191
Nightingale, Florence, 347
  achievements of, 6–8
  cleanliness and, 507
  home care nursing and, 400
  image of nursing and, 8–9
  nursing education and, 15
  on keeping records, 484
Nightingale School at St. Thomas Hospital, 9,
  15
Nipples, inspection of, 684
Nitrites, in urine, 1168
Nitrogen balance, in immobilized persons,
  750
Nociception, pain and, *969–970*
Nocturia, 1162–1163
Nocturnal myoclonus, insomnia and, 953
Noise, control of, 1481
Nonelectrolytes, 1002, 1005
Nonmaleficence, as ethical principle, 47
Nonsteroidal antiinflammatory drugs, contraindications to, 981
  for pain, 981
  precautions with, 981
  recommended doses of, 983t
  side effects of, 981
Norepinephrine, body temperature and, 589,
  591
Normalization, of daily life, 376, 1463
North American Nursing Diagnosis Association (NANDA), definition of nursing
  diagnosis by, 130
  founding of, 112
  functional level classification of, 734
  Taxonomy I and II of, 132
  Taxonomy IR, 133–134
  use of diagnoses approved by, 131–132
Nose, assessment of, 672–673
  decongestants for, 1277
  hygiene for, 912–913
  instillation of nose drops into, 1277
  irrigation of, 1277
NSAIDs, contraindications to, 981
  for pain, 981
  precautions with, 981
  recommended doses of, 983t
  side effects of, 981
Nuclear medicine, 36
Nuremberg Code, 72
Nurse administrators, personal contract employment of, 58
Nurse practice acts, ANA Code of Ethics
  and, 48
  common features of, 60
  disclaimers in, controversy about, 60
  intravenous therapy and, 1326
  provisions for substance abuse in, 61
  state regulation of, 60–61

Nurse practice acts (Continued)
  violation of, 60–61
Nurse practitioners, licensing laws and, 60
  pediatric, 20
Nurses, burnout in, 294–295
  characteristics and qualities of, action-ori-
    ented, 435–436
    advocacy in, 94–95, 242, 340, 365,
      1413
    communication in, 340, 425, 427–429
    cultural competence in, 339–341
    empathy in, 340
    knowledge in, 121, 158–159, 161–162,
      339–340
  district, 400
  functions of, 35
  in hospitals, organization of, 92
  interprofessional relationships of, 1499
  loss and grief and, 1543–1555
  performance evaluations of, 171, *172*
  perspective of, 121
  responsibilities of, in administration of
    drugs, 1256–1258
    in ANA Code of Ethics, 48
    in blood transfusions, 1312
    in child abuse reporting, 207
    in communicating findings on vital signs,
      621, 622t
    in facilities for mentally ill and develop-
      mentally disabled, 81
    in hyperalimentation, 1313
    in implementation of care, 158–163
    in informed consent, 71–72
      involving human research subjects,
        73, 1260
    in long-term care facilities, 78, 80
    in organ transplantation, 83
    in perioperative role. See *Perioperative
      nursing.*
    in reproductive decisions, 77
  roles of, 10–13
    as administrators, 20–21, 58, 101
    as advocates, 81, 94–95, 242, 340, 365,
      1413
    as care givers, 94
    as change agents, 94, 353, 356
    as collaborators, 94
    as counselors, 94
    as educators, 94
    as employees, civil rights laws and, 59
      legal aspects of, 58–59
      safety standards for, 59
      types of contracts governing, 58–59
      unemployment compensation for, 59
    as executives, 92
    as health care team member, 94–95,
      1208
    as managers, 92
    as role models, 353
    as subjects of human research, 73
    as teachers, 356
    as witnesses to informed consent, 1413
    expanded, 19–20
    in health promotion activities, 39–41
    in managed care, 94
    in medication administration, 1256–
      1257
    in spiritual care, 1511
    in stress management, 288
    referral, 365
    with adolescents, 215–220
    with care of neonates, 195, 195t, 196t
    with infants, 198
    with middle-aged adults, 234–235
    with older adults, 242–243
    with school-age children, 204–205, 206t

Nurses (Continued)
    with young adults, 223–225
    with young children, 202
  shortages of, 13, 16, 17
  skills of, cognitive, 121, 158, 159
    interpersonal, 158, 159
    selection of intervention and, 161–162
    technical, 158, 159
  therapeutic relationship with client, atti-
    tudes toward client and, 434–435
    communication in, 425, 427–429
    encouragement of, 434–436
    sexuality and, 1497–1499
  therapeutic relationship with client and,
    422–425
  types of, licensed practical, 17
    licensed vocational, 17
    perioperative, 1409. See also *Periopera-
      tive nursing.*
    registered, 17–18, 92
    visiting, 11–12, 400
Nurses' Associated Alumnae, 18, 19, 21
Nurses' notes, 169
Nursing, as art, 250
  as profession, 18–23
    organizations promoting, 21–23, 58
  community, 400–401
    care for family caregivers and, 239
  contemporary, settings of, 10–13
    society's perception of, 10
  definitions of, 6–7
  goals of, 252
  health promotion activities of, 347, 353,
    356–358
  history of, 5–24
    early collaborative efforts in, 18
    early educational efforts in, 16–17
    images of, 7–10
  legal and ethical aspects of, 43–63
  military, 13
  model(s) of, Albrecht Nursing Model for
    Home Health Care as, 405, *406*
    case method as, 385, *386*
    functional method as, 386, *386*
    in hospitals, 385–388
    primary care method as, 387–388, *388*
    team method as, 387, *387*
  perioperative. See *Perioperative nursing.*
  physicians and. See *Physicians.*
  public health, 400–401
  quality of life issues and, 377
  specialization in, 13–14, 20
    organizations promoting, 23
  standards of care in, 14–15, 170–171
    beneficence and, 47
    components of, 52–53
    documentation of, 53
    Good Samaritan laws and, 53
    of American Nurses' Association, 15
      for assessment, 126
      for evaluation, 170
      for implementation, 163
      for nursing care plan, 148
      for nursing diagnoses, 141
      for outcome identification, 146
      legal aspects of, 170–171
    OSHA guidelines and, 59
    policies and procedures relating to, 53
    quality assurance programs and, 55
    sources of, 52
    state nurses associations vs. trade ser-
      vice unions and, 58
    tort law and, 52–53
  terminology used for patients in, 15
Nursing care plans, 147–154
  computerized, *153*, 154

Nursing care plans (*Continued*)
definition of, 147
evaluation of, 168
for case study of stress, 295–296
for problem-oriented record system, 490
formats for, 148
in case management system, 151, *152,* 154
in home care nursing, 413
individually developed, 148, 149t
measurement criteria for (ANA), 148
modifications in, 169, 170
documentation of, 169, 170
practice guidelines for, 151
purposes of, 147–148
samples of, 149t, 150t, *152, 153*
standardized, 148, 149t, 151, 154
student, 148
teaching, *150,* 151
Nursing diagnoses, 129–142, 286–287
actual, documentation of, 134
interventions and, 161
American Nurses' Association standard for, 141
at admission, 395
classification of, 112
collaborative problems in, 140–141
components of, *136,* 137t, 161t
defining characteristics of, 134
definition of, 130
documentation of, 134
drug administration and, 1266
evaluation of, 171
for altered family processes, 327, 328
for altered health maintenance, 353
for altered nutrition, high risk for more than body requirements, outcomes for, 1079
profile of, 1079
less than body requirements, expected outcomes for, 1079
profile of, 1078
more than body requirements, expected outcomes for, 1078
profile of, 1077
for altered sexuality patterns, 1501
profile of, 1502
for altered urinary elimination, 1169
for anxiety, 286–288
for bowel elimination problems, 1132
for clients needing intravenous therapy, 1328–1330
for constipation, profile of, 1132
for family unit problems, 326–328
for fear, profile of, 1421
for fluid volume deficit, profile of, 1036
for fluid volume excess, profile of, 1037
for grief and grieving, 1547, 1548t–1549t, 1550, 1551
for high risk for disuse syndrome, 757
outcomes for, 758
profile of, 756
vs. impaired physical mobility, 810
for high risk for infection, 514–515
profile of, 1429
for high risk for self-mutilation, use of restraints and, 853
for high risk for violence: self-directed or directed at others, profile of, 854
for impaired gas exchange, profile of, 1219
for impaired home maintenance management, 408, 409
profile of, 408
for impaired physical mobility, 757
decision tree for, *812*

Nursing diagnoses (*Continued*)
discussion of, 810
profile of, 811–812
for impaired tissue integrity, 1365–1366
profile of, 1366
for ineffective airway clearance, profile of, 1218
for infection, 514–515
for pain, 978–979
need for restraints and, 853
profile of, 979, 980
for relocation stress syndrome, 316–317
for respiratory problems, 1218, 1220t–1221t
clustering signs and symptoms with, 1220t–1221t
for self-care deficit, bathing/hygiene, 904
profile of, 927
dressing/grooming, profile of, 895
toileting, 898
for self-esteem problems, 1459–1461
profile of, 1460
for sensory/perceptual alterations, 1476
examples of, 1478t
profile of, 1477
for sleep pattern disturbance, profile of, 957
for sleep problems, 955, 957
for spiritual distress, profile of, 1526
for spiritual health, 1526
for stress incontinence, profile of, 1170
for surgical candidates, 1420–1421
for urinary elimination problems, 1169–1171
for urinary incontinence, 1170–1171
for urinary retention, profile of, 1171
for wound healing, 1365–1366
functional health patterns approach to, 134–136
handbooks of, 131
health-seeking behaviors, 353, 360
high-risk type, 136–137
interventions for, 161
historical overview of, 112
homeostatic mechanisms and, 316–317
human response pattern of, 133–134
immobility and, 810–812
in evaluation process, 169
in home care nursing, 409
in nursing process, 110, 144, 160, 168
legal aspects of, 141–142
nursing interventions and, 147, 161
of hygiene needs, 894
bedmaking procedure and, 941
ears, 911
elimination, 898
eyes, 909
hair care, 931
nail and foot care, 929
nose, 913
oral, 904
perineal care, 926
skin care, 916
perioperative, in preoperative phase, 1415t
intraoperative, 1428, 1429
postoperative, 1434, 1436
PES format of, 134
planning care and, 144–145. See also *Planning.*
priority rankings of, 144
process of, 130–132
critical thinking in, 141
determining the defining characteristics, 131, 132
documentation of, 132

Nursing diagnoses (*Continued*)
errors in, 141
identification of related factors in, 131–132
using the definitions, 131
related factors in, 134, 138, 139, 161. See also subheading *profile of* under specific diagnoses.
role of inferences in, 131
suggested qualifiers for, 136
teaching needs and, 477
types of, 130, 136–137, 137, 137t
vs. medical diagnosis, 130, 139–140
wellness type, 137
interventions with, 161
writing of, 134, 138–140
Nursing education, 15–18
Nursing history, formats for, 122–126
functions of, 122
goals of, 122
in nursing assessment, 121–122
Nursing homes. See *Long-term care facilities.*
Nursing interventions. See also *Implementation; Procedures.*
acceptability to client, 161
at admission, 395
capabilities of nurse and, 161–162
characteristics of, 147
choice of, 159–162
collaboration with other team members on, 162
counseling and, 163
definition of, 110–111, 147
delegation of, 162, 162t
dependent, 162–163
development of, 159, 160
direct, 162–163
documentation of, 163
drug administration and, 1267–1269, 1273–1297
evaluation of, nursing research and, 171
for bowel elimination problems, 1133–1152
for clients with impaired mobility, assisting ambulation in, 829–831
assistive ambulation devices for, 829, 831–839, 840t–841t
bed rest, 757, 758
exercises for, 813–816, 822–823
positioning and moving, 782t–783t
positioning equipment for, 758–759, 767–769, 784, 796, *796*
procedures for moving in bed, 769, 770–774
procedures for positioning in bed, 775–781
procedures for transfer from bed, 785–795
progressive mobilization for, 823, 829
teaching "dangling" to, 824–828
for clients with normal mobility, promoting fitness in, 839, 841–842
for clients with therapeutic immobilization, antiembolism hosiery for, 863, 864
bandages for, 858–863
binders for, 854–858
braces or splints for, 870–873
casts for, 865–870
compression devices for, 863–865
movement devices for, 879–880
restraints for, 880–886
suicide precautions for, 886–887
traction for, 873–879
for dying clients, 1551–1554
for family problems, 327–328
for fever, 601

Nursing interventions *(Continued)*
  for fluid and electrolyte imbalances, 1023t–1032t, 1035–1043
  for heat exhaustion, 601
  for heat stroke, 601
  for hypothermia, 602
  for infants, 198
  for infection control, 515–537
    general guidelines for, 515
    in maintaining sterility, 527–535
    medical asepsis, 515–524. See also *Asepsis, medical.*
    surgical asepsis, 524–535. See also *Asepsis, surgical.*
  for intravenous therapy, 1330, 1331t, 1332
  for low self-esteem, 1461–1464
  for meeting hygiene needs, 896, 940t–941t
    bedmaking procedure, 942
    ears, 912
    elimination, 898–900
    eyes, 909–911
    hair care, 931–934
    nail and foot care, 929–930
    nose, 913
    oral, 904–908
    perineal care, 926, 928
    skin care, 916–924
      bathing at sink, 918
      bathing of infants, 923–924
      bed baths, 918–923
      showers, 917
      tub baths, 917–918
  for neonates, 196t
  for nutritional needs, 1079–1118
    administering tube feedings, 1095–1118
    dietary therapies for specific needs, 1080–1089
    improving appetite, 1089–1090
    increasing absorption, 1093–1094
    increasing digestion, 1091
    increasing intake of appropriate foods, 1090–1091
  for pain relief, 979–992. See also *Pain.*
  for prevention of disuse syndrome, 797
  for respiratory problems, 1219, 1221
    basic measures for, 1221–1239
    measures for maintaining airway patency, 1239–1249
  for school-age children, 206t
  for sensory/perceptual alterations, 1476–1483
  for sexual health problems, 1503–1504
  for sleep-related problems, 958, 962–963
  for spiritual health needs, 1526–1528
  for stress-related problems, 288–291
  for urinary elimination problems, 1172–1199
  for wound healing, 1367–1397
  for young children, 202t
  homeostatic mechanisms and, 317–318
  human need priorities and, 254, 255
  identification of, 146–147
  in home care nursing, 409–412
  interdependent, 147
  learning and teaching, 163, 478–480. See also *Learning; Teaching.*
  referrals as. See *Referrals.*
  research base and, 161
  review of, 159
  scheduling and organization of, 162
  standing orders and, 163
  supervision of, 162
  types of, 146–147
Nursing process, 109–115
  AORN Standard of Nursing Practice and, 1407t

Nursing process *(Continued)*
  attributes of, 112–113
  chronobiologic rhythms and, 314–318
  definition of, 110
  diagram of, *111*
  example of application of, 112
  fluid and electrolyte imbalances and, 1024t–1032t
  group phase development and, 459–460
  health teaching and, 475
  homeostatic mechanisms and, 314–318
  human needs and, 250, 254
  infection control and, 513–537
  scientific method of problem solving and, 113–114
  steps of, 110–112
    assessment, 110. See also *Assessment.*
    diagnosis, 110. See also *Nursing diagnoses.*
    evaluation, 111–112, 168. See also *Evaluation.*
    implementation, 111, 157–164. See also *Implementation; Nursing interventions.*
    planning, 110–111, 143–145. See also *Planning.*
Nursing research, evaluation process and, 171, 173
  historical, 11
  on circadian rhythms, 316
  on cocaine exposure in neonates, 194
  on compliance among elderly with drug regimens, 1259
  on effect of nutritional status on pressure ulcers, 1350
  on effectiveness of incentive spirometry, 1237
  on high tech home care and care givers, 402, *403*
  on interpersonal relationships of children, 184
  on lithotomy position in surgery, 1430
  on metamucil in enteral feeding tubes, 1109
  on pressure ulcers, 743
  on prevention of confusion among elderly clients, 807
  on risk of loneliness in visually impaired elderly, 1478
  on self-image in adolescents, 217
  on sexual health following ostomy surgery, 1503
  on spiritual needs matched to spiritual care, 1525
  on subjective data in bronchial asthma, 651
  on timing of suppository administration, 1149
  on urinary incontinence, 1173
Nursing unit, client's orientation to, 389
Nursing's Agenda for Health Care Reform, 10, 12, 20, 105, 347
Nutrients, carbohydrates, 1052–1053
  fats, 1053–1055
  fluids, 1057
  minerals, 1056, 1058t–1060t
  needed for vegans, 1066, 1066t
  proteins, 1055
  required, 1052–1057
  required for infants, 1071
  vitamins, 1055–1056, 1056t–1057t
Nutrition, 1049–1123. See also *Diet; Enteral nutrition; Food(s).*
  as therapy, 35
  assessment of, 1066–1067, 1068t, 1069–1076

Nutrition *(Continued)*
  in immobilized clients, 745t, 750–751
  in older adults, 243
  tool used for, 1067
  with impaired gastrointestinal function, 1094, *1095*
  at midlife, 234, *235*
  basic concepts of, calories and body weight as, 1052–1057
    recommended dietary allowances and guidelines as, 1057–1058, 1061t, 1062
    structure and function of gastrointestinal tract as, 1050–1052, *1051*
  dental caries and, 902
  in adolescents, counseling about, 216–217
  influences on, 1069–1076
  maintenance of, with impaired gastrointestinal function, 1094–1118
  periodontal disease and, 902
  popular concerns about diet and, 1062t–1065t, 1062–1063, 1066
  requirements for, 1052
    at midlife, 234, *235*
    in adolescents, 217
    in infants, 1070–1071, *1071*
    in school-age children, 1071–1072
    in young adults, 224
    in young children, 1071
  total parenteral, 1312–1313
Nutritional status, care plan for, 1120
  case study of, 1119
  evaluation of, 1118–1119
  in surgical patients, 1411
  nursing assessment and, 124
  nursing diagnoses and, 135
  physical assessment and, 660
  surgical risk and, 1420
  wound healing and, 1358–1359
Nutritional support, for fever, 601
  removal of, decisions about, 74
Nutritionists, training and responsibilities of, 93
Nutting, Mary Adelaide, 15, 18, 22

O

Obesity. See also *Weight.*
  dietary management of, 1080–1083
  hazards of, 1081–1082
  health risks of, 349
    in adolescent girls, 1072
    in midlife, 233, 234
    in various ethnic groups, 337
  influences on, 1082
  wound infection and, 1342
Occupational Safety and Health Act (1970), 67
Occupational Safety and Health Administration (OSHA), 59, 223, 521
Occupational therapists, training and responsibilities of, 93
Occurrence insurance, 54
Oculomotor nerve, 669
Odor(s), in assessment, 657, 658t
  in wounds, control of, 1383–1384
  of urine, 1166
  ostomy, 1151
Oedipus complex, 1493
Ointments, 1274, 1275
  eye, administration of, 1277, *1278*
Olfaction, assessment of, 657, 658t
  deficit in, nursing care for, 1479
  food intake and, 1069
Olfactory nerve, testing of, 673

Oliguria, 1165
Ommaya reservoir, 1281
Omnibus Budget Reconciliation Act, 67, 78–80, 852–853
Ophthalmoscope, 653
Ophthalmoscopic examination, 670, *670*
Opiate receptors, for pain, 971
Opioid analgesics, 981
   addiction to, 974–975
   alternative routes of, 991–992
   equivalent doses of, 982t
   for diarrhea, 1146
   in elderly, 975
   recommended doses of, 983t
Opioids, endogenous and exogenous, 971–972
Opium, action of, 971
Optic nerve, assessment of, 669–670
Oral hygiene. See also *Mouth.*
   assistance with, 900–908
   causes of problems with, 904
   for comatose people, 908
   for people with dentures, 907
   for people with dry or irritated mucosa, 907–908
   for people with natural teeth, 905–907
   need for, 901–902
   neglect of, 900–901
   physical examination for, 903–904
Oral mucosa, dry, 904
   care of, 907–908
Orem, Dorothea, 253–255
Organ procurement organizations, 82, 83
Organ transplantation, allocation of, 83
   approaches to increasing organ donation, 82
   Christian beliefs about, 1518t–1521t
   consumer rights and health care provider responsibilities for, 81–83
   distribution and financing of, 82–83
   ethical concerns about, 83
   information sharing about donor and donee and, 82
   Jewish beliefs about, 1517t
   law on, 81–82
Organ transplantation and donation, 1547
Organs, changes in, in surgical candidates, 1411
Orientation, in mental status assessment, 661
   promotion of, 1480–1481
Oropharyngeal airway, 1239–1241, *1240*
   suctioning of, 1246
Orthopedic disorders, fractures, 848–849
   sprains and strains, 849
Orthopedics, definition of, 806
Orthosis, short-leg, *871*
   wrist-hand, *871*
Osmolality, antidiuretic hormone regulation and, 1013, *1014*
   osmolarity and osmosis and, 1010–1011
   regulators of, 1015–1017
Osmolarity, in tube feedings, 1041
   osmolality and osmosis and, 1010–1011
Osmoreceptors, for regulation of fluid osmolality, 1015
Osmosis, in small intestines, 1094
   in transport of body fluid, 1010
Osmotic agents, for bowel elimination, 1135
Osmotic diuresis, hyperalimentation and, 1313
Osteopathy, 38t
Osteoporosis, calcium supplements for, 1065
   immobility and, 752–753
Ostomy, care of, 1150–1152
   sexual health and, 1503
Otoscope, 653

Otoscopic examination, 670–672
Outcomes. See also *Planning.*
   acceptable, 146
   choice of intervention and, 160
   consistent, 146
   definition of, 110
   development of, in planning stage, 145–146
   evaluation process and, 166, 167t, 167–171
      documentation of, 169
   measurement criteria for (ANA), 146
   of home care services, 404
   realistic, 145
   reasons for failure to achieve, 169
   time frames for achieving, 146
      critical paths and, 154
   verification of, 145
Outrigger splint, *871*
Ovaries, in homeostasis regulation, 303, *303*
Overbed table, hospital, 391
Overhydration, hydration measures and, 1227
Overuse syndromes, in adolescents, 218
Oxygen. See also *Gas exchange.*
   administration of, 36, 1228–1235
      at home, 1235
      continuous, 1228
      delivery systems for, 1232, 1233t–1234t, *1233–1234*
      dosage of, 1230–1231
      effects of, 1228, 1231, 1231t
      exercise and, 1232, 1235
      goals of, 1228
      humidification and, 1231–1232
      intermittent, 1228, 1230, *1231*
      procedure for, 1229–1230
      safety considerations and, 1231, 1232t, 1235
   hyperbaric, in wound healing, 1363
   outlets for, in hospital client rooms, 391
   portable cylinder of, *1231*, 1235
   pulmonary transport of, 1205
   saturation of, pulse oximeter measurement of, 621–622
Oxygen tension, wound healing and, 1357
Oxygenation, in immobilized clients, 749, 750, 782t
   in REM sleep, 949
   in respiratory failure, 557
   respiratory status evaluation and, 1251
   suctioning and, 1248–1249

P

Pacemakers, in biologic rhythms, 311
Pack strap carry, 551, *552*
Padding, absorbent, for urinary incontinence, 767–768, 1175
Pain, acute, assessment of, 973
   vs. chronic, 968
   appetite and, 1090
   as nursing diagnosis, 853
   assessment of, acute, 973
      chronic, 973–974
      in children, 975–977, 976t, *977*
      physiologic signs of, 974
      questions relating to, 973–974
      sociocultural aspects of, 977–978
      tools used for, 978, *978*
   breakthrough, 982
   cancer, drugs for, 982, 984
      relief of, implantable spinal reservoirs for, 992
      Swedish massage for relief of, 987

Pain *(Continued)*
   chronic, assessment of, 973–974
      drug administration and, 1266
      specialty clinics for control of, 987
   cycle of, *981*
   drugs for, 981–984
      addiction to, 974–975
      placebo use and, 981–982
      principles of administration of, 981
   exercise and, 842
   in children, assessment of, 975–977, 976t, *977*
      management of, 977
   in dying clients, 1552–1553
   in elderly, assessment of, 975
   in immobilized clients, 783t
   loss of control and, 980
   malignant, 975
   nature of, 968–970
   need for restraints and, 853
   phantom, 969
   pleuritic chest, 1210
   referred, 969
   relief of, *970*, 971–972
      analgesia for, epidural, 988–990
         patient-controlled, 988, *988–989*, 990
      bowel function and, 1135
      care plan for, 993–994
      case study of, 993
      documentation of, 992
      evaluation of, 992–993
      implantable spinal reservoirs for, 992
      in peripheral nervous system, 972
      interventions for, nonpharmacologic, 163, 985–986
         physical, 987–988
         psychologic, 984–985
      reassurance for, 986
      team approach to, 986–987
      transcutaneous electrical nerve stimulation for, 991, *991*
      transdermal fentanyl patch for, 991–992
   rescue medication for, 982
   somatic, 968
   suffering and, 969
   superficial, test of, 693
   sympathetically maintained, 969, 992
   transmission of, *970*, 971–972
      theories of, 972
         gate control theory, 972, 991
         neural plasticity and, 972
         wind-up theory, 972
   visceral, 968
   with casts and braces, 872t
Palates, soft and hard, 674
Pallor, 1338
   assessment of, 662
   testing of, 916
   with hypothermia, 602
Palm cones, 767, *768*
Palpation, of abdomen, 687–688
   purpose of, 656
   technique of, 655–656, *656*
   types of, 656, *656*
Pancreatic juices, electrolyte composition of, 1023t
Pap smear, 224
Paracentesis, abdominal, 720
   care of person undergoing, 718t
Paraffin wax, 1393
Paralysis, physical protection and support needed for, 849–850
Paramedical personnel, training and responsibilities of, 93
Paraplegia, 849

Parathyroid glands, in growth and development, 182
  in homeostasis regulation, 302, *303*
Parathyroid hormone, calcium regulation and, 752
  fluid and electrolyte balance and, 1017
Parentalism, as ethical principle, 47
Parenteral nutrition, 1094
  peripheral, 1094
  total, 1094
Parenting, decision making about, 221
Parents, adolescent, responsibility in, 219
  aging, relationships with, 232
  as decision makers about health care for children, 69–70
  death of child and, 1537
  during hospitalization of children, 205
Parkes, C. M., 1542
Parkinson's disease, physical protection and support needed for, 850
Pathogens, 509
Patient privilege, vs. confidentiality, 57
Patient Self-Determination Act, 75, 76
Patient's Bill of Rights, 1260
Pattison, E.M., theory of dying of, 1539
Pavlov, Ivan, theory of, 189
Pectins, 1052
Pectoriloquy, 679
Pectus carinatum, 680
Pectus excavatum, 680
Pediculosis, 931–933
Peer assistance programs, for substance abusing professionals, 61
Peer relationships, in adolescents, 213
  in school-age children, 204
Pelvic muscle exercises, 1173–1174
Pender, Nola, health promotion model of, 40–41, *41*
Penis, 925
Penlight, 655
  in examination of eyes, 669
  in nasal examination, 672–673
Peplau, Hildegard, 427–428
Peptic ulcer, dietary management of, 1083, 1084t
Perception, 1470–1474. See also under *Sensory.*
  alterations in, 1473–1474
    confusion, 1473–1474
    delusional thinking, 1474
    hallucinations, 1474
    illusions, 1474
  factors affecting, 1471, 1472
  neurophysiology of, 1470–1471
Percussion, hammer for, 655
  of abdomen, 687, *687*
  of chest, 678, 678t, *678–679*, 681
    therapeutic, 1227–1228
  technique of, 656–657, *657*
  types of, 657, *657*
Performance evaluations, of nurses, 171, *172*
Perianal area, cleansing of, 927
Perimysium, 733
Perineal care, urinary tract infection and, 1190
Perineal hygiene, documentation of, 929
  evaluation of, 929
  female, 927, *927*
  male, 927
  need for, 926
  principles of, 916
  special considerations with, 927
Perineum, female, 925, *925*
  male, 925, *926*
Periodontal disease, causes of, 901–902
Perioperative nursing, approach to patient based on developmental level, 1412

Perioperative nursing *(Continued)*
  basic concepts of, 1404, 1407–1409
  nursing interventions in, intraoperative, 1429–1432, 1430t
    during anesthesia, 1431–1432, 1432t–1434t
      patient positioning, 1429, 1431
      sterile field maintenance, 1429
    postoperative, 1435–1440, 1436t–1437t
    preoperative, 1416t–1418t, 1421–1428
      on day of surgery, 1425–1428, *1426–1427*
  nursing positions in, 1409
    anesthetists, 1409
    circulating, 1409
    first assistants, 1409
    intensive care unit, 1409
    postanesthesia recovery unit, 1409
    scrub, 1409
  planning in, intraoperative, 1429
    postoperative, 1434, 1436
    preoperative, 1415t, 1421
  responsibilities of, 1409–1410
Periosteum, bone, 731
Peripheral vascular resistance, blood pressure and, 612–613
Peristalsis, 1126
  in immobilized persons, 750
Peroneal nerve, testing of, 851, *851*
Personal appearance, as body language, 431–432
Personal distance, as body language, 432–433, 433t
Personality, illness and, 364
PES format, of nursing diagnosis, 134
Petechiae, skin, 662
pH, 1019, *1019.* See also *Acid-base balance.*
  of different body fluids, 1019
  of skin, 1337
  of urine, measurement of, 1166–1167
  renal regulation of, 1018
Pharmacists, role in medication administration, 1258
  training and responsibilities of, 93
Pharynx, anatomy and function of, 1051
  assessment of, 674
Phenylalanine hydroxylase, 1089
Phenylketonuria, dietary management of, 1089, *1089*
  metabolic defect in, *1089*
Phenytoin, added to intravenous solution, 1311
Phlebitis, deep, 692
  in immobilized persons, 747
Phosphate, as buffer of acid-base balance, 1019
  deficit of, 1029t
  excess, 1030t
  functions of, 1007t
  imbalance of, 1008t
Phospholipids, 1054
Phosphorus, metabolism, functions, and sources of, 1058t
Photographs, invasion of privacy and, 56
Physiatrist, 35–36
Physical activity, health risks and, 349
  spiritual health and, 1525
Physical assessment. See *Assessment, physical.*
Physical development. See *Growth and development.*
  of adolescents, 210, 210t
Physical examination. See *Assessment, physical.*
Physical fitness, exercises promoting, 839, 841–842

Physical protection, provision of, 847–890
Physical therapists, functions of, 35–36
  training and responsibilities of, 93
Physical therapy, of chest, as respiratory therapy, 1227–1228
Physicians, as primary care agencies, 91
  dominance of nursing by, 1499
  functions of, 35
  on hospital medical staff, organization of, 92
  orders of, for intravenous therapy, 1309–1310
    for medications, 1261–1262
    on admission assessment, 392
  responsibilities of, in informed consent, 71–72
    in medication administration, 1257–1258
  training and responsibilities of, 92–93
  value of nursing care to, 99
Physics, principles of, back injury prevention and, 540–542, 544t
Physiologic factors, hindering learning, 474
  stress and, 269, 283, *284*
  in surgical candidates, 1410
  teaching approach and, 476
Physiologic functions, adaptation and, 277
  biofeedback training and, 290
  complications in, collaborative problems and, 140–141
  nursing goals and, 257
  pharmacokinetics and, 1265
  regulation of, biofeedback training for, 315
    homeostatic, 304–309
Piaget, Jean, theories of cognitive development of, 187, 188t, 212
Pickwickian syndrome, 951
PIE charting, 494–495, *496*
Pigeon chest, 680
Piggyback line, 1322
Pillows, use of, 767
Pineal gland, in homeostasis regulation, 302, *303*
Pituitary gland, hormones of, 307
  in growth and development, 182
  in homeostasis regulation, 302, *303*
  interaction with hypothalamus, 304
Placebo, use of, 981–982
Placenta, 190
Plaintiff, 51
Planning, 143–155. See also *Outcomes.*
  as part of nursing process, 110, 144, 160, 168
  discharge. See *Discharge, planning for.*
  drug administration and, 1267
  for bowel elimination problems, 1132–1133
  for care of dying patient, 1547, 1550, 1551
  for clients needing therapeutic immobilization, 854
  for family diagnoses, 327
  for fluid volume imbalances, 1023t–1032t, 1035
  for group goal accomplishment, 460
  for hygiene needs, 894–895
    bedmaking procedure and, 941
    ears, 912
    elimination, 898
    eyes, 909
    hair care, 931
    nail and foot care, 929
    nose, 913
    oral, 904
    perineal care, 926
    skin care, 917
  for immobilized clients, 757, 758

Planning *(Continued)*
  for impaired physical mobility diagnosis, 810, 813
  for infection control, 515
  for intravenous therapy, 1330, 1331t
  for low self-esteem, 1461
  for nutritional status, 1078–1079
  for pain relief, 978–979
  for respiratory problems, 1218–1219, 1221t, 1222t
  for sensory/perceptual alterations, 1476, 1478t
  for sexual problems, 1502
  for sleep problems, 955, 957–958
  for spiritual health needs, 1526
  for stress-related problems, 287–288
  for urinary elimination problems, 1171–1172
  for wound healing, 1366–1367
  homeostatic mechanisms and, 317
  identification of interventions in, 146–147
  in home care nursing, 409
  in perioperative nursing, 1415t, 1421, 1429, 1434, 1436
  learning-teaching and, 477–478
  outcome development in, 145–146. See also *Outcomes.*
  priorities in, 144–145
  purposes of, 144
  relation to assessment and diagnosis, 144
  time frames in, 146
Plasma, derivatives of, 1311
  distribution of, 1001t
  electrolyte composition of, 1023t
  interstitial fluid and, fluid transport between, 1011–1012, *1013*
Plasma proteins, 1005
  functions of, 1007t
Plastic domes, for children's cribs, 886
Play, for hospitalized children, 205
  in early childhood, 200, *201*
Pleura, chest pain in, in respiratory history, 1210
  friction rub in, 1214t
  parietal, 1205
  visceral, 1205
Pleural effusion, thoracentesis for, 1217
Pleural space, 1205
PLISSET model, of intervention for sexual dysfunction, 1503–1504
Pluralism, 1512
  ethnic, 334
Pneumonia, hypostatic, in immobilized persons, 749, 750
  use of restraints and, 881
Pneumothorax, 1215
  hyperalimentation and, 1313
Point localization, 701
Policies, and politics, 104–105
  of health care facilities, standard of care and, 53
  public, definition of, 99, 103
    kinds of, 99, 103
Politics, advocacy work and, 340
  and policy, 104–105
  definitions of, 103–104
  health care access and, 353
  health care disparities and, 348–349
  health promotion and, 348, 361
  nurses' attitude toward, 99
  self-help groups and, 455
Pollutants, environmental, and young adults, 223
Polyuria, 1165
Pons, respiratory control by, 1206
Position sense, alteration in, 1479

Position(s), blood pressure and, 614
  bowel function and, 1134
  common, 769
    orthopneic, 759t, 769
    prone, 769
      for helpless person in bed, 778–780, *779*
    side-lying, 769
      for helpless person in bed, *777*, 777–778
      pressure ulcers and, 769
    Sims', 769
      for helpless person in bed, 780–781, *781*
    supine, 769
      for helpless person in bed, 775–777, *776*
      for immobilized clients, 783t
  during physical examination, *659*
  for aspiration studies, *720*
  for injections, 1284, *1284*
  Fowler's, pressure ulcers and, 1349
  in postural drainage techniques, 1227, *1227*
  intraoperative, 1429–1431, *1431*
  lithotomy, 1430
  of extremities, devices for, 765, *765–766*, 767–768, *767–768*
  of immobilized clients, equipment useful for, 758–759, 767–769, *769*, 784, 796, *796*
    principles and nursing interventions for, 782t–783t
    procedure for moving helpless person in bed, 769, 770–774
    procedure for positioning helpless person in bed, 775–781
    procedure for transferring helpless person from bed, 785–795
  of spine, devices for, 765, *765–766*, 767
  of standard beds, 759t–760t, 760t
    Fowler's, 759t
    orthopneic, 759t
    reverse Trendelenburg, 759t
    Trendelenburg, 759t
  respiratory status and, 611, 1223, 1224
  rule of thirty and, 769, 1349
  urinary elimination and, 1159
Positive-pressure breathing, 1236–1237
Postanesthesia care unit, discharge from, criteria for, 1435, 1437
  nursing care in, 1434–1440
    guidelines for, 1436t–1437t
  protocols in, 151
Postmortem care, 1554
Postural drainage, 1227, *1227*
Posture, as body language, 432
  correct, *541*, 542
  in stress response, 283
  observation of, 733
  of nurse, therapeutic communication and, 434
  renal regulation of ECF volume and, 1017
Potassium, aldosterone secretion and, 1015
  deficit of, 1026t–1027t
    digitalis toxicity and, 1038
  dietary, regulation of, 1037
  excess, 1027t
  functions of, 1006t
  imbalance of, 1007t
  in sodium-potassium pump, 1011
  metabolism, functions, and sources of, 1059t
Poverty, community health services for, 352–353
  ethnic groups and, 336

Poverty *(Continued)*
  food intake and, 1069
  health care access and, 348
  health promotion and, 348
  Medicaid coverage and, 96
Powders, dermal, 1274, 1275
  skin, 915
Power of attorney, decision making about life-sustaining measures and, 74–75
  for health care decision making, 68–69
Powerlessness, as reaction to confirmed illness, 369–370
  causes and indicators of, 370
  compliance with therapy and, 370
Prayer and meditation, 1523
  as therapy, 37
  in Jewish faith, 1517t
Preferred provider organizations, 98
  as primary care agencies, 91
Pregnancy, estimating date of, 190
  fluid and electrolyte imbalances in, 1021
  human research and, 73
  in adolescents, 214
    prevention of, 218–219
  in young adults, 221
  nutritional requirements for, 1074–1075
  preventive health care in, 191
  stages in, 190
  substance abuse and, 77
  urinary elimination and, 1160
Pregnancy Discrimination Act, 59
Premature beats, 607
Prenatal period, care during, vs. postnatal care in intensive care units, 104
  development in, 190
  environmental influences in, 191, 191t
  health concerns in, 191
  musculoskeletal development in, 809t
  nurse's role in, 191
Prenatally drug-exposed (PDE) children, school nursing care for, 13
Prepuce, 925
Presbyterians, beliefs and practices of, 1520t
Pressure, filtration, 1012, *1013*
  injury from, in immobilized clients, 782t
  osmotic, in body fluid transport, 1010
  skin blood supply and, 1338
  used for airway suctioning, 1244
Pressure cooker, for sterilization, 527
Pressure points, 741, *742*, 1349
  with use of restraints, 881
Pressure ulcers, 741, *742*
  air-filled rings and, 764
  assessment of, 742–743, 1365
  definition of, 1336, 1345–1346
  formation of, 741–743, *742*
  management of, 1354
    documentation of, 1386
    precautions for, 1354
    products available for, 1348t, 1351t–1352t, 1354, *1355*
  pathophysiology of, 1347–1349
  persons at risk for, 742–743
  prevalence of, 1347
  prevention of, 743, 1349–1350, 1352–1354, 1385
  side-lying position and, 769
  staging system for, 1347t
Prima facie case, 50
Prisoners, human research and, 73
Privacy, ANA Code of Ethics on, 48
  as ethical principle, 47
  during psychosocial interview, 629
  elimination patterns and, 1128
    bowel function and, 1134–1135
    urinary elimination and, 1159

Privacy (Continued)
for older adults, sexual activity and, 237
invasion of, and reporting laws, 57
as intentional tort, 56
patients' right to, 67, 68
abortion law and, 76
for long-term care residents, 79–80
response to illness and, 366–367
urethral catheterization and, 1188
Private duty nursing, 11–12, 19–20. See also
Home care.
Problem-oriented record system, 490, 492,
492t, 493
disadvantages and advantages of, 492
Problem-solving, and nursing process, 114t
and scientific method, 113
methods of, 113
Procedural law, 51–52
Procedures, for administering medications,
intradermal injection, 1293
intramuscular injections, 1298–1301
intravenous route, 1321–1322
oral route, 1270–1273
subcutaneous injections, 1296–1297
for administering oxygen, 1229–1230
for airway suctioning, 1245–1248
for applying wound dressings, dry, 1370–
1373, 1372
wet, 1373–1374
for assessing pulse rates, radial and apical,
606–607
for assisting with ambulation, 829–831
for assisting with food service, 1092–1093
for back massage, 959, 959–962, 961
for blood pressure measurement, 616–
617, 617
for cardiopulmonary resuscitation, 565–
568
for complete bed bath, 919–923
for hand washing, 518–519
for inserting nasogastric or nasoenteric
tube, 1104–1108, 1105, 1107
for making occupied bed, 936–941, 937–
938, 940–941
for moving or lifting clients, for transferring helpless person from bed, 785–
795
in emergency carriers, 551t–552t, 552–
553
lifting object from floor, 547
moving helpless person in bed, 770–774
placing lift sheet under client, 547–548
positioning helpless person in bed, 775–
781
shoulder lift for helpless person in bed,
549t, 550
for performing passive range of motion exercises, 817–821
for recording fluid intake and output,
1003–1004
for teaching client how to "dangle", 824–
828
for temperature measurement, axillary,
596–598
oral, 594–595, 598, 598
rectal, 595–596, 598
with electronic thermometer, 597
with glass thermometer, 594–597
with tympanic thermometer, 597
for urethral catheterization, female and
male, 1182–1187, 1184, 1186
for venipuncture, for blood collection or
IV infusion, 1316–1320
for wound irrigation, 1368–1370
Process recordings, in therapeutic relationship, 424–425, 426

Proctosigmoidoscopy, 724t, 725
Professional organizations, for nurses, 21–23,
58
for review of research or conduct, 97–98
policies affecting health care and, 105
rights of health care consumers and, 67–
69
Programmed study, 479–480
Progress notes, 169
for problem-oriented record system, 490
Projection, 185
Proprioception, 1470
test of, 693
Prostate gland, 925
palpation of, 691, 691
urethral blockage by, 1158
Prostatectomy, bladder irrigation following,
1198
Protein, as buffer of acid-base balance,
1019–1020
complete and incomplete, 1055
deficiency, pressure ulcers and, 1349–1350
deficit, 1030t
dietary, regulation of, 1038
function of, 1007t, 1055
loss of, colloid oncotic pressure and, 1012
plasma, 1005, 1007t
imbalance of, 1009t
wound healing and, 1358
Proteinates, 1005
Proteinuria, 1165
Protocols, development and use of, 151
Psychiatric disorders, sleep patterns and, 955
therapy for, 36
Psychoanalysis, 185
Psychodynamic theories, of growth and development, 184–185
Psychologic activity, in older adults, 243
Psychologic adaptation, 277–278
Psychologic aspects, of application of heat
or cold, 1396–1397
of bowel status, 1127
of gastrointestinal intubation, 1102–1103
of pain relief, 984–985
of psychosocial assessment, 636, 643, 644
of spiritual care, 1511
of urethral catheterization, 1181, 1188
of wound healing, 1359
Psychologic needs, nursing goals and, 257
Psychologic responses, to stress, 269, 283–
285, 285
in surgical candidates, 1410
learning and, 474, 476
Psychomotor skills, in learning, 470–471
of nurse, 158, 159
Psychophysiologic disorders, stress-related,
285–286
Psychosexual development, at midlife, 228–
229
Freud's theories of, 185, 186t
gender differences and, 1492–1495
in adolescents, 211
in older adults, 236–237
in young adults, 220
Psychosocial aspects, of illness, 366–367
of infection control, 522–523
of sexual development, 1492–1495
of wearing a halo brace, 879
Psychosocial development, assessment of,
627–647
components of, 630
data analysis for, 636, 643, 645
data collection for, 630, 631–635, 635,
636
physiologic dimension of, 636, 643
psychologic dimension of, 636, 643, 644

Psychosocial development (Continued)
social and cultural dimension of, 643, 645
at midlife, 229–233
history of, components of, 630
interview for, 629–630, 631
in adolescents, 211–213
in early childhood, 199–201, 202t
in infants, 196–197
in neonates, 194
in older adults, 237–240
in school-age children, 203–204, 206t
in young adults, 220–222
Kohlberg's theory of, 187, 188t, 189
theories of, 184–190
Psychosocial status, assessment of, in immobilized clients, 746t–747t, 754–755, 757
drug administration and, 1265–1266
in nursing assessment, 126
spiritual growth and, 1513
surgical risk and, 1420
Psychosocial theories, of growth and development, 190
Psychosomatic illness, 252
Psychotropic medications, rights of mentally
ill and, 81
Ptosis, 668
Puberty, 1491
in adolescents, 211
Pubescence, 211
Public health, departments of, services offered by, 89–90
nursing practice in, 11–13
Public policy, definition of, 99, 103
kinds of, 99, 103
Pulmocare, 1042
Pulmonary embolism, in immobilized persons, 748
signs of, 748
Pulmonary function tests, 1215, 1216, 1217t
assessment by, 725, 725–726
care of person undergoing, 726t
common measurements included in, 725–
726
in respiratory care evaluation, 1249
Pulse, apical, 603, 604, 605, 605
procedure for assessing, 606–607
pulse deficit and, 607–608, 608
assessment of, 602–608, 691–692
documentation of, 700
brachial, 603, 604, 691–692
blood pressure measurement at, 616–
617, 618
carotid, 603, 604
deficit of, 607–608, 608
dorsalis pedis, 603, 604
femoral, 603, 604
force of (quality), 608
grading of, 692t
paradoxical, 621
physiologic data base of, 602–603
popliteal, 603, 604
posterior tibial, 603, 604
radial, 603, 603, 691–692
procedure for assessing, 606–607
rate of, 605, 605t, 607
normal ranges of, 605, 605t
rhythm of, 607–608
sites of, 603, 603, 604–605
temporal, 603, 604
ulnar, 691–692
Pulse oximeter, use of, 621–622, 1215, 1216
Punctures, 1343t
Pupils, assessment of, 669
Purine metabolism, in gout, 1088
Pursed-lip breathing, 1237, 1238
Pus, in wounds, 1342

Push-ups, in bed, 813
Pyridoxine, toxicity of, 1063t
Pyrogens, exogenous, 599
Pyuria, 1165

Q

Quadriplegia, 849
Quakers, beliefs and practices of, 1520t
Quality assurance programs, evaluation process and, 171, 173
 for long-term care residents, law on, 78–80
 in health care facilities, 55–56
Quality improvement, evaluation process and, 171, 173
Quality of life, 376–377, 377t
Queen Victoria Jubilee Institute, 400
Questionnaires, about sleep problems, 955, *956*
 for evaluation of long-term learning, 480–481
Quickening, 191
Quiet rooms, 886
Quinlan, Karen Ann, 74

R

Race, 335
 as concept, 335
 blood pressure and, 613
 death rates and, 337
 health status and, 336–338
 in donor organ allocation, 83
 physical assessment and, 660
 poverty and, 336
 self-concept and self-image and, 200
 socioeconomic aspects of, 335
Racial prejudice, 335
Radial nerve, testing of, 851, *851*
Radiation, heat loss by, 588
Radiation treatment, 36
Radioactive scans, diagnostic tests with, 715–716
 care of person undergoing, 716t
Radiography, diagnostic procedures with, 710–711, 711t–713t, 713–715
 angiography, 712t, 714
 bronchography, 713t, 714
 care of person undergoing, 711t–713t
 cholecystogram, 711, 712t, 713
 computed tomography, 713t, 714
 intravenous pyelogram, 712t, 713–714
 magnetic resonance imaging, 713t, 714–715
 myelography, 712t, 714
 of chest, 1215, 1217
 of gastrointestinal tract, barium enema series, 711, 711t
 lower GI series, 711, 711t
 small bowel series, 711, 711t
 upper GI series, 711, 711t
Radiologic technologists, training and responsibilities of, 93
Radios, in hospital client rooms, 392
Rahe, Richard, theories of stress and illness of, 274
Range of motion, assessment of, in immobilized person, 735–736, 736t–740t, 741
 of spine and extremities, 735–736, 736t–740t, 741
 definition of, 735
 exercises for, 816
 in immobile clients, 816, 822–823

Range of motion *(Continued)*
 procedure for, 817–821
 terminology relating to, 741
Rape, date, in young adults, 223
Rathbone, William, 401
Receptors, for fluid osmolality regulation, 1015
 for heat and cold, 1388
 opiate, 971
 sensory, 1470–1471
 thermal, 589, *590*
Recommended dietary allowances, 1057–1058, 1061t, 1062
Record, client. See also *Charting; Documentation.*
 abbreviations and symbols used in, 486t–487t
 as legal document, 485
 current problems in, 485, 488
 formatting information in, computer systems and, 500
 guidelines for documentation in, 485
 historical aspects of, 484
 purposes of, 484–485
Recovery room, care in, 1434–1440
Rectal pouch, 1148, *1148*
Rectum, assessment of, 691
 during defecation, 1127
 suppositories for, 1276, *1276*
Red Cross Nursing Service, 16
Referrals, by home care nurse, 403–404
 for crisis management, 291
 for depression, 216
 for dying person, 1550, 1552
 for learning disabilities in children, 204
 nursing goals and, 257
 to sleep clinic, 963
Reflexes, abdominal, 688, *688*, 688t
 assessment of, 688, *688*, 688t
 documentation of, *700*
 cough, in immobilized persons, 749, 750
 duodenocolic, 1126
 gastrocolic, 1126
 micturition, 1158
 neonatal, 193, 193t
Reflexology (zone therapy), 38t
Regional enteritis, dietary management of, 1084t
Registered care technicians, 105
Regression, 185
 behavioral, during hospitalization, 205
Regulations, administrative law and, 51
Rehabilitation, 89
 for disease prevention, 37, 39
 health care team members needed for, 37, 39, 39t
 nursing goals and, 257
 pulmonary, programs for, 1238–1239
Rehabilitation Act, 59
 infant care treatment decisions and, 51, 72
Relatedness, therapeutic communication and, 434–435
Relationships. See also *Family.*
 marital, in older adults, 238
 therapeutic, 422–425. See also *Communication, therapeutic techniques of.*
 elements of, 425, 427–429
 encouragement of, 434–436
 phases of, 423
 process recordings in, 424–425, *426*
 theories of, 427–429
 vs. social relationships, 422–423
Relaxation, in middle-aged adults, 235
 spiritual health and, 1525
 techniques for, for pain relief, 986
 for urinary incontinence, 1174

Relaxation *(Continued)*
 in stress management, 290
Religion(s), food intake and diet and, 1069
 in young adults, 222
 of world, Buddhism, 1517
 Christianity, 1517, 1518t–1521t
 Hinduism, 1515–1516
 Judaism, 1516
 beliefs and practices affecting health care, 1516t–1517t
 spirituality and, 1512
Religious development, 1513
Religious orders, nursing and, 9–10
Relocation stress syndrome, 316–317
 as nursing diagnosis, 317
 evaluation of, 318
 interventions for, 317–318
 outcomes for, 317
Remarriage, 231
Renal system. See also under *Kidneys; Urinary tract.*
 in nursing assessment, 123
Renin-angiotensin, aldosterone secretion and, 1015
Reporting laws, controversies in, 57
 covering nurse practice act violations, 61
Repression, 185
Reproductive rights, 76–77
Reproductive system, at midlife, 228–229
 in adolescents, 211
 in nursing assessment, 123
 in young adults, 220
Research, human subjects for, 84
 exempt from institutional review board process, 72
 rights of, 67, 69, 1260
 risk categories of and informed consent process for, 72–73, 73t
 women, 104
 nursing. See *Nursing research.*
Respect, due to patients, 67, 68
 therapeutic communication and, 434
Respiration, 1203–1254. See also *Breathing.*
 apneustic, 611
 assessment of, 608–612, 676
 techniques for, 609, 609t
 Biot's, 611, *611*, 1212t
 changes in, 610–611
 notable signs with, 611–612, 952, 1212t
 Cheyne-Stokes, 611, *611*, 952, 1212t
 control of, 608–609
 definition of, 608
 internal, 557
 Kussmaul's, 611, 1212t
 noisy, 610
 patterns of, 611, *611*
 quality of, 609–610
 rate and depth of, 610t, 610–611
 rate of, 609
 sleepiness and, 954
Respirator, removal of, decisions about, 74
Respiratory arrest, 558
 in infants and children, 570–571
Respiratory exercises, 1237, *1238*
Respiratory secretions, pooling of, in immobilized persons, 749
Respiratory system. See also *Breathing; Cardiopulmonary arrest; Cardiopulmonary resuscitation.*
 anatomy and function of, *1204*, 1204–1205
 assessment of, 123, 676–685
 chest examination for, 1210–1213
 history for, 1209–1210
 laboratory and diagnostic studies for, 1213–1217
 defense mechanisms of, 1206

Respiratory system (Continued)
  disorders of, 557, 1206–1208, 1207
    care plan for, 1252–1253
    case study of, 1252
    causes of, 1207
    evaluation of, 1249–1252, 1251t
    hyperventilation, 611, 611, 1208
    hypoventilation, 1206, 1212t
    hypoxemia, 557–558, 608–609, 1206, 1208, 1208t
    hypoxia, 557–558, 577, 1208
    principles of, 1251t
  in adolescents, 210t
  in homeostasis regulation, 302
  in immobilized clients, 744t–745t, 748–750
  overview of, 1204–1206
  pulmonary symbols and, 1207
  therapy for, 36, 1251t
    chest physical therapy, 1227–1228
    hydration, 1225–1227
    medications for, 1235–1236
    mobilization maneuvers, 1221–1225
    oxygen administration, 557, 1228–1235. See also Oxygen, administration of.
    positive-pressure breathing, 1236–1237
    respiratory exercises, 1237–1239
Respiratory technologists, training and responsibilities of, 93
Responsibilities, and rights, 66–67
  of health care consumers, 68, 69
  of health care providers, 65–86, 84–85
    and personal choice, 68–77
    in organ transplantation, 81–83
  of nurses. See Nurses, responsibilities of.
Restitution, with grief, 1542
Restless legs syndrome, insomnia and, 953
Restraints, application of, 882
    alternatives to, 853
    assessment of need for, 852–853
    general considerations with, 852
  documentation of, 883
  effects of, 883
  emotional reactions to, 880
  environmental control used for, 886
  false imprisonment and, 56
  hazards of, 882, 882
  law on, 78–80
  nursing guidelines for use of, 880, 883–884
  of long-term care residents, 78–80
  standard of care and, 53
  types of, body, 885, 885
    chest, 884
    elbow immobilizer, 884, 884
    mitt, 884, 885
    mummying device, 885, 885
    waist, 884
    wheelchair bar, 885, 885
    wrist and ankle, 883, 883–884
  use of, 879–886
    by teams, 880–881
    complications of, 881–883
Restrictive environment, as treatment for mentally ill, law on, 81
Resuscitation. See Cardiopulmonary resuscitation.
Reticular activating system, 1471
Retirement, for older adults, 240
Rhonchi, 679, 680, 1214t
Rhythms, biologic, 311–314
    cycles and frequencies of, 311, 312t
    nursing implications for, 314–318
  circadian, 311–314
    disruption of, 313–314

Rhythms (Continued)
  circannual, 311
  infradian, 311
  ultradian, 311
Rib belt, 855, 855
Rib fracture, in CPR, 571
Ribs, assessment of, 676
RICE, for treatment of orthopedic injuries, 849
Rights, and responsibilities, 66–67
  conflicts in, ethical theories and, 44, 46
  definitions of, 66–67
  in constitutional law, 49
  of health care consumers, 65–86, 84–85
    and personal choice, 68–77
    statutory and professional statements of, 67–68
    to organ transplantation, 81–83
  of human subjects in research projects, 67, 69, 72–73, 73t, 104, 1260
  of mentally ill, 78, 80, 81
  of residents of long-term care facilities, 78–80
  reproductive, 76–77
Rigor mortis, 1554
Rinne air and bone conduction test, 672, 672
Risk, assessment of, for infection, 514
  Blaylock Risk Assessment Screen (BRASS), 392–393, 393
  control of, 55
  definition of, 347
  from transmissible viral disease, wound care and, 1345
  management of, in health care facilities, 54–55
  surgical, 1419–1420
Robb, Isabel Hampton, 15, 18, 19
Roe v. Wade, 76, 84
Rogers, Carl, 324t, 325, 434
Role-playing, for teaching, 479
Role-relationship pattern, in nursing assessment, 124
  in nursing diagnoses, 135
Roller, in transferring helpless patients, 789, 796
Romberg's test, 692–693
Romeo v. Youngberg, 81
Roommate, selection of, for infection control, 519–520
Rosenberg's Self-Esteem Scale, 1450
Rosenstock, Irwin, health belief model of, 32, 33, 34
ROTO REST oscillating bed, 761, 763
Roy, 324t, 324–325
Rule of thirty, 769
  pressure ulcers and, 1349
Rust v. Sullivan, 76

S

Sacred writings, 1523
Safety, during bedmaking, 942
  environmental, for infants, 197, 924
    for visually impaired clients, 1479
    for young children, 197, 201
    in adolescents, 219
    in middle-aged adults, 235
    in older adults, 243
    in young adults, 225
    for long-term care residents, law on, 78–80
  in planning home care, 409
  of drug administration, 1263–1264, 1264
  of workers, guidelines for, 59
  on self-care assessment test, 355

Safety (Continued)
  seat belt use and, 219, 350
    with oxygen administration, 1231, 1232t, 1235
    with parenteral administration of drugs, 1284–1285
    with shower or tub bathing, 917
Salem sump tube, 1096, 1097t, 1098
Saline, deficient, 1025t
    excessive, 1026t
    imbalance of, causes of, 1007t
    sterile isotonic, 1367
Saline lock, advantages of, 1315
    in intravenous therapy, 1313–1315, 1315, 1321–1322
    procedure for, 1316–1320
    vs. heparin lock, 1315
Saliva, artificial, 907
    digestion and, 1091
    role in digestion, 1050
Salvation Army, beliefs and practices of, 1520t
Sandbags, 765
Satir, Virginia, 428–429
Saunders, Cicely, 1540
Scabies, 932
Scalp, assessment of, 666, 931
    dry, 932
    massage of, 931–932
Scar, hypertrophic, 1357
School age children. See Children, school age.
Schools, AIDS information in, 218
    nursing in, 12–13
    of nursing, early, 15–16
Schwabach test, 672
Scientific method, and nursing process, 114t
    modified form used by health care professionals, 113–114
Sclerae, assessment of, 668–669
Scoliosis, 676, 677
Scrotum, 925
Scultetus binders, uses and applications of, 856, 856
Seat belt use, health risks and, 350
    in adolescents, 219
Sebaceous glands, 914
Sebum, 914, 915
Seclusion, as treatment for mentally ill, laws on, 81
    rooms for, 886
Sedation, excessive, vs. respiratory depression, 989–990
    scales for, 990
    with epidural analgesia, 989
Sedatives, as sleep aids, 958, 962
Selenium, metabolism, functions, and sources of, 1060t
Self, and other selves, 261–262
    autonomy and, 259
    characteristics of, 258
    emotional conflict and, 261
    individual and universal, 263–264
    introspection and time and, 260–261
    knowledge of, 258–259, 263
    nursing care and, 264
    personal integration and, 258–259
    public and private, 262–263
    self-actualization and, 260–261
    sexual, assessment of, 1500
    significant others and, 264
    understanding of, 258–264
    values and, 259–260
Self-actualization, 253, 258, 260–261
Self-awareness, ethnic groups and, 339

Self-care, as health promotion mechanism, 352
  assessment of, 118, 353, 354, 355
  deficit in, bathing/hygiene, profile of, 927
    dressing/grooming, profile of, 927
    toileting, 898
  in adolescents, 219–220
  in elderly clients, confusion and, 807
  in young adults, 225
  Orem's needs theory and, 253–255
Self-catheterization. See also *Catheters*.
  intermittent, 1193–1196
    complications of, 1193–1194
    documentation for, 1196
    implementation of, 1195
    principles related to, 1194t
    procedure for, 1195–1196
    teaching of, 1194–1195
Self-concept, 262–263, 1447–1468
  and health, 1450
  assessment of, 1456–1459
  body image and, 370
  defense mechanisms and, 271
  historical overview, 1449
  in adolescents, 211–212
  in families, 1452–1455
  in growth and development, 184
  in infants, 196
  in middle-aged adults, 229–230
  in older adults, 237
  in young adults, 220
  reactions to illness and, 367
  research on, 1450–1452
  sexual health and, 1492
  theories of, 1448–1450
Self-efficacy, 1449–1450
Self-esteem, assessment of, 1456–1459
  behavior and, 1449–1450, 1452–1456
  context and, 1452
  family systems approach to, 1451
  global vs. specific, 1449
  in care givers, 1451
  in groups, 459
  in surgical patients, 1411–1412
  low, beliefs related to, 1457–1458
    care plan for, 1465–1466
    case study of, 1465
    context of, 1457
    evaluation of, 1464–1465
    exceptions to, 1458–1459
    impact of, 1457
    nursing care and, 1455–1456
    nursing interventions for, 1461–1464
    parental discipline and, 1454
    planning for, 1461
    rating scale questions about, 1459
    situational, 1460
    solutions attempted for, 1458
  nursing diagnoses for, 1459–1461
  nursing goals and, 258
  research on, problems with, 1451–1452
  theories of, 1448–1450
Self-help groups, *454*, 454–455
Self-image, emotional equilibrium and, 301
  in adolescents, 211–212, 213, 217
  in hospitalized persons, 292
  in middle-aged adults, 229–230
  in older adults, 237
  in young adults, 220
Self-monitoring blood glucose tests, 1167
Self-mutilation, high risk for, as nursing diagnosis, 853
Self-perception, 262–263
  changes in, with immobility, 755
  nursing assessment of, 124
  nursing diagnoses with, 135

Self-Test for Health Style, 353–355
Selye, Hans, 251, 268
  general adapatation syndrome of, 283, *284*
  The Physiology and Pathology of Exposure to Stress, 272
  theories of stress of, 272–274
Semmelweis, Ignaz, 507
Sengstaken gastric tube, 1096, 1097t, *1098*
Sensation, 1470–1474
  alterations in. See also *Sensory deficit*; *Sensory deprivation*; *Sensory overload*.
    nursing interventions for, 1480
    urinary elimination and, 1160
  assessment of, 693, 701, 916, 1339
  factors affecting, 1471, 1472
  in skin, 914, 916
  in surgical patients, 1411
  neurophysiology of, 1470–1471
  transmission of, 1470–1471, *1471*
Sensory deficit, 1472
  nursing intervention for, 1476–1480
  situations fostering, 1475
Sensory deprivation, 1479–1480
  immobility and, 755
  situations fostering, 1472–1474
Sensory overload, 1473, 1480
  situations fostering, 1475
Sensory system, assessment of, 693, 701, 916, 1339, 1474–1476
  documentation of, *700*
  tests of, light touch/superficial pain, 693
    number identification, 693, 701
    position (proprioception), 693
    stereognosis, 693
    temperature, 693
    vibration, 693
Sensory/perceptual alteration, assessment of, 1474–1476
  care plan for, 1484
  case study of, 1483
  communication with clients with, 1480–1483
  evaluation of, 1483
  in hospitalized children, prevention of, 1479
  nursing history of, 1475
  persons at risk for, 1474–1475
  physical assessment of, 1475, 1476
  symptoms of, 1475–1476
Separation anxiety, in infants, 196
Sepsis, hyperalimentation and, 1312–1313
Sequential compression devices, complications with, 865
  documentation of use of, 865
  guidelines for use of, 863–865, *864*
  teaching and learning about, 865
Serologic tests, 514
Seventh Day Adventists, beliefs and practices of, 1520t
  food intake and diet and, 1069
Sex, phenotypic, establishment of, 1489, *1489–1490*
Sexism, 1499
Sexual abuse, of children, 206–207
  warning signs of, 207
Sexual activity, in adolescents, safety and, 218
  in older adults, 236–237
  in young adults, 223
  indwelling urethral catheters and, 1193
Sexual harassment, examples of policies set for, 99, 103
Sexual health, 1495–1497
  after ostomy surgery, 1503
  assessment of, 1499–1501
  care plan for, 1505–1506

Sexual health (*Continued*)
  case study of, 1505
  evaluation of, 1504–1505
  nursing interventions for, 1503–1504
  problems with, 1504
  promotion of, 1487–1508
Sexual orientation, 1492
Sexual response, physiologic changes during, 1496t
Sexuality, altered patterns of, nursing diagnosis of, 1501–1502
  planning care for, 1502
  and long-term indwelling urethral catheters, 1193
  assessment in, 1499–1501
  client's health status and, 1499
  cultural components of, 1495
  development of, at midlife, 228–229
    gender differences in, 1492–1495
    in adolescents, 211
    in older adults, 236–237
    in young adults, 220
  growth and development of, 1488–1495
  nurse-client relationships and, 1497–1499
  physiologic growth of, 1488–1491
  psychosexual theories of, 1492–1493
    conflict resolution and, 1493
    mothering role and, 1493
    object relations theory and, 1493
    separation-individuation and, 1493
  psychosocial development and, 1492–1495
Sexuality–reproductive pattern, in nursing assessment, 124
  nursing diagnoses in, 136
Sexually transmitted diseases, in adolescents, 215, 216, 218
  in young adults, 224
Shame, as reaction to confirmed illness, 368
  body image changes and, 372
Shampoo, procedure for, 933–934, *933–934*
Sharps, disposal of, 520
  safe handling of, 522
Shaving, for hygiene needs, 934
  in Jewish faith, 1517t
Shearing force, effects on skin of, 741–742, *742*
  pressure ulcers and, 1349
Shiatsu, 38t
Shift rotation, circadian rhythms and, 313–314
Shock, as reaction to confirmed illness, 367
  hemorrhagic, homeostatic fluctuations in, 309
  with grief, 1542
Shoulder, range of motion of, passive exercise of, 819–820, *819–820*
Shoulder lift procedure, for moving helpless person in bed, 549t, *550*
Shoulders, in prone position, *779*
  range of motion of, 737t–738t
Showering, assistance with, 917
Shyness, in adolescents, 218
  and drug abuse, 214
Siblings, influence on school-age children, 204
  of hospitalized children, 205
  of older adults, 238
Sick role, 374
Side rails of beds, use and hazards of, *390*, 390, 758, 886
Sighing, pattern of, 610, 1212t
Sigma Theta Tau, 21–22
Sign language, 430
Significant others, and anxiety, 288
  support for, during cardiopulmonary resuscitation efforts, 574–575

Sims' position, 769
  for helpless person in bed, 780–781, *781*
Sinus arrhythmia, 607
Sinuses, assessment of, 672–673, *673*
  frontal, 673, *673*
  maxillary, 673, *673*
Sitz bath, 1394
Skeleton, anatomy and physiology of, 730–732, *731*
Skin, after cast removal, 868–869
  aging and, 1338
  assessment of, 123, 661–662, 663t–665t, 915–916, 1338–1339
    before injections, 1285
    immobilizing devices and, 744t, 850, 852
  blood supply to, disruption of, 1338
  body temperature regulation by, 914
  care of, 913–925
    agents used for, 914–915
    bowel incontinence and, 1148
    by client, 914–915
    diarrhea and, 1146
    interventions for, 916–918
    on feet, 930
    urinary incontinence and, 1175
    with casts and braces, 872t
    with ileostomy, 1151
    with wounds, 1352t
  cleanliness of, 916
  color of, 915–916, 1338–1339
    respiratory status and, 612
  dermal patches for, 1274, 1275
  dry, 915, 1337, 1338
  effects of immobility on, 741–743
    assessment for, 744t, 850, 852
  excoriated, 915, 931
  friable, 1338
  in dying person, care measures for, 1553
  integrity of, 915
    damaged, 916
      infection and, 508
      parenteral administration of drugs and, 1283
      with traction, 878
    normal, 1336–1339
  irritation of, urethral catheterization and, 1191
  layers of, 1337
  lesions of, 662, 663t–665t, 916
  preoperative preparation of, 1424
  response to heat or cold, 1388, 1396
  stimulation of, for pain relief, 985
  structure and function of, 913–914, *1274*, 1274, 1337
    protection, 914, 1337
    sensation, 914, 916
  suppleness of, 916
  temperature of, 916
  topical medication administered to, 1274–1275
  turgor of, 662, *662*, 1034, *1035*, 1338
  vascularity of, 662
Skin barriers, for wound care, 1352t
Skinner, B.F., 182, 189, *189*
Skull, assessment of, 666
  in infants, 196
  in neonates, 192, *192*
Slander, 56
Sleep, assessment of, 954–955
  circadian rhythms and, 313–314, 950–951, *951*
  disorders of, 951–954
    care plan for, 964–965
    case study of, 964
    circadian desynchronization, 954
    fatigue, 953

Sleep *(Continued)*
    insomnia, 952–953
    narcolepsy, 951–952
    organizations treating, 963
    sleep apnea, 952
    sleep deprivation, 313, 954
      immobility and, 755
    sleep fragmentation, 954
  in children in pediatric critical care units, 953
  in older adults, 243
  in surgical patients, 1411
  nature of, 948–951
  non-rapid eye movement (NREM), stages of, 949–950
  objective measurement of, 955, *956*
  optional and core, 954
  patterns of, 124, 135
    in early childhood, 199
    in infants, 196
    in neonates, 194
  preoperative preparation for, 1425
  promotion of, 958, 962–963, 1481
    back massage, 958–962, *959*, *961*
    drugs for, 958, 962–963
  rapid eye movement (REM), 948–949
    vs. NREM, 949t
  types of, 313
Sleep apnea, central, 952
  obstructive, 952
  physiology of, 952
Sleep diaries, 955
Sleep paralysis, 952
Slings, uses and application of, 856–857, *857*
SMA-12, 716
Smegma, cleaning of, 927
Smell. See *Olfaction.*
Smoking, health risks and, 233, 349–350
  health risks in midlife and, 233
  in older adults, 242
  in stress management, 290
  in various ethnic groups, 337
  log or diary for, 357, *357*
  on self-care assessment test, 354
  teaching about, 1221
Snellen chart, 655, 670
Snoring, 952
Snuff, in adolescents, 215
Soaks, method of giving, 1275
SOAPIER format, in problem-oriented nursing record system, 490, 492, 492t, *493*
Soaps, 915
Social advocacy. See also *Advocacy.*
  self-help groups and, 455
Social circumstances, at midlife, 232–233
  food intake and diet and, 1069
  in young adults, 221–222
Social factors, in psychosocial assessment, 643, *645*, 645
  spiritual care and, 1512
Social learning theory, of behavior, 189–190
Social Readjustment Rating Scale, 274
Social Security Act, 240
Social support, and anxiety, 288
  as health promotion mechanism, 352
Social workers, training and responsibilities of, 93
Socialization, 333
  in growth and development, 183–184
Sociocultural adaptation, 278
Sociocultural aspects, in assessment data base, 118
  of pain assessment, 977–978
Socioeconomic status, child abuse and, 206
  reactions to illness and, 367
  teaching approach and, 477

Sodium, dietary, regulation of, 1037
  restriction of, 1086–1087
  functions of, 1006t
  in tube feedings, 1041
  metabolism, functions, and sources of, 1059t
  regulation of fluid and electrolyte balance by, 1014
  retention of, in hemorrhagic shock, 309
  serum, as measure of plasma osmolality, 1011
    normal values of, 1011
Sodium-potassium pump, as active transport, 1011
Soft tissue, aging and, 1338
  assessment of, 1338–1339
  elements of, 1337–1338
Solutions, added to IV solutions, 1309
  drug, 1268
  for total parenteral nutrition, 1312
  hypotonic vs. hypertonic, enemas and, *1136*, 1137
  intravenous, 1308–1328
    containers for, 1315, 1322, *1323*, 1332–1333
  osmotic pressure of, 1010–1011
Somatic distress, with grief, 1541
Somatopsychic illness, 252
Sorbitol, osmotic activity in small intestine and, 1094
Spasm, bladder, with urinary catheterization, 1189
Spasticity, 752
Specimens, bowel, collection of, 1130
  examples of, 716
  handling of, 716
  urine, collection of, 1168–1169
Speculums, 653
Speech, in infants, 196–197
  in school-age children, 204
  in young children, 200
    normal, 201, 202t
  physical assessment and, 660–661
Sphincters, anal, 1127
  gastroesophageal, 1051
  pyloric, 1051
  urethral, 1158
Sphygmomanometer, for blood pressure measurement, 614, *614*
  homeostatic responses and, 316
  in hospital client rooms, 391
Spica casts, 867, *867*
Spinal accessory nerve, 675
Spinal catheter, indwelling, for pain relief, 992
Spinal cord injuries, physical protection and support needed for, 849–850
Spine, casts for, 866–867, *866–867*
  passive range of motion exercise of, 818, *819*
  positioning devices for, 765, *766*, 767
    bed cradles, 765, *766*
    footboards, 765, *765*
    sandbags, 765
  range of motion of, 735–736, 736t–740t, 741
Spiritual care, 1510
  matched to spiritual needs, 1512–1513, 1525
  need for research on, 1528
  nurse's approach to, 1511, 1528
  resources for clients needing, 1523–1524
Spiritual dimension, of psychosocial assessment, 645, *646*
Spiritual distress, as nursing diagnosis, profile of, 1526

Spiritual health, 38t, 1509–1531
  assessment of, 1525–1526
  care plan for, 1529
  case study of, 1529
  definition of, 1510
  evaluation of, 1528
  nursing diagnosis of, 1526
  nursing interventions for, 1526–1528
  of nurses, 525, 1511
Spiritual needs, in dying person, assessment of, 1545, 1546
Spirituality, 1510
  development of, 1513–1515
    stages of, 1514–1515
  in adolescents, 213
  religion and, 1512
  universality of, 1511
Spirometry, 725
  incentive, 1237, *1238*
    effectiveness of, 1237
Spleen, percussion of, 687
Splints, cockup, 767, *768*
  Denis-Browne, *871*
  documentation of use of, 873
  for pain relief, 987
  knee immobilizer, *871*
  outrigger, *871*
  principles of use of, 872t–873t
  short-leg orthosis, *871*
  types of, 870t, *871*
  use of, 870–873
  wrist-hand orthosis, *871*
Sports injury, in adolescents, 217
Spouses, abuse of, 231–232
  at midlife, 231
Sprains, 849
Sputum, characteristics of, 1209–1210
  in respiratory history, 1209–1210
  laboratory examination of, 1214–1215
St. Thomas Hospital, Nightingale School at, 9, 15
Standing orders, evaluation of, 163
  for drugs, 1262
Staphylococcal infections, 508
Staples, in wounds, care of, 1384–1385
  surgical, 1361
Starling's law of capillary force, 1011
Stat orders, for drugs, 1262
State health agencies, services offered by, 90
State laws, *Cruzan* decision and, 75
  on abortion, 76
  on decision making about forgoing life-sustaining measures, 74–76
  on decision making for minors, 70
  on health care consumers' rights, 67
  on informed consent, 71
  on organ donation and transplantation, 81, 82
State nurses' associations, vs. trade service unions, role in negotiations on practice standards, 58
States, regulation of nursing by, nurse practice acts and, 60–61
Statutory law, 50–51
Steatorrhea, 1131
Stents, urinary, 1176–1177, *1177*
Stereognosis, test of, 693
Sterile field, establishment and maintenance of, 527, 528t, 529, 1429
Sterile supplies, opening packages and bottles of, 529, *529*, 530, *530*
  packaging and storing of, 526–527
  transferring to sterile field, 530–531, *531*
Sterile technique, 506
  gloves and, contaminated, removal of, 531, 532, *533*, 534–535

Sterile technique (*Continued*)
    open gloving method and, 531, *532*
  gloves in, closed gloving method, 534, *537*
  gowning for, 524, *535–536*
  masking for, 533
  nursing responsibilities in, 527–535
  procedures requiring, 524
  removing contaminated gown and gloves, 531, 532, *533*, 534–535
  scrubbing for, 533–534
Sterilization, 506. See also *Sterile supplies.*
  indicators of, 525–526, *526*
  law on, 77
  methods of, 507, 525, *525*, 526t
  nursing responsibilities in, 527, 528t, 529–535
  nursing role in, 527
  preparation of materials for, 524–525
  types of, 526t
Steroids, for respiratory problems, 1235
  wound infection and, 1342
Stertor, 610
Stethoscope, *604*, 605, 653
  use in auscultation, 657
Still, Dr. Andrew Taylor, 38t
Stimuli, proprioceptive, 370
Stockinette bandages, 862
Stockings, thromboembolytic deterrent (TED), 767–768, 863, 864
Stoma, ostomy, 1150
Stomach, air in, in cardiopulmonary resuscitation, 571
  anatomy and function of, 1051
Stomatitis, 904
  mouth care for, 908
Stones, renal. See *Kidney stones.*
  urinary, 1172
    nursing interventions for, 1172–1174
Stool. See also *Bowel elimination*; *Feces.*
  characteristics of, 1130–1131
  specimens of, collection of, 1130
  straining at, 1144
Strains, 849
Strangulation, with use of restraints, 881
Strauss, A.L., theory of dying of, 1538–1539
Stress, 289
  adaptation and, 267–298, *279*
  antidiuretic hormone and, 1013
  assessment of, 281–286
  blood pressure and, 614
  body temperature and, 591
  case study of, 295–296
  change and, 274, *275*
  defenses against, 269, *270*
  definitions of, 268, 273
  evaluation of, 291–292
  hospitalization and, 292, 293t, 294
  in family members, 239, 325
  in midlife, 233, 235
  in nurses, 294–295
  in young adults, 223
  management of, 288–291
    biofeedback training and, 290
    crisis intervention and, 292
    general principles of, 290
    guided imagery and, 290–291
    professional help for, 292
    relaxation techniques for, 290
  models of, 272–276
    of Holmes and Rahe, 274
    of Lazarus, 274–276, *276*
    working, *270*, 281–282
  nursing care and, 252
  nursing diagnosis of, 286–288
  nursing interventions for, 288–291
  nursing role and, 292–295

Stress (*Continued*)
  on self-care assessment test, 354–355
  respiratory rate and, 609
  responses to, 268–269
    definitions of, 269
    disease and, 273–274
    fluid and electrolyte imbalances and, 1021
    in surgical candidates, 1410
    psychologic, 283–285, *285*
    psychophysiologic disorders due to, 285–286
  self-help for, 288–291
  stressors and, 268–272
Stressors, assessment of, 281–288
  defenses against, present status of, 283–288
    professional help, 292
    self help for, 288–291
  definitions of, 269
  examples of, 269
  identification of, 289
  physiologic responses to, 283, *284*
Stretcher, 784
Stridor, 610
Stroke, physical protection and support needed for, 849
Stroke volume, in immobilized persons, 743, 747
Structural-functional theory, family in, 323–324
Stryker CircOlectric bed, 760–761, *762*
Stryker frame, 760
Stryker wedge turning frame, 760, *761*
Subarachnoid space, 989, *990*
Subcultures, 333
Subcutaneous injections, 1292, *1292*, 1295
Sublimation, 185
Substance abuse, criminalization of, controversy on, 77
  in adolescents, 214, 218
  in assessment data base, 118
  in young adults, 224
  nurse practice act provisions on, 61
  pregnancy and, 77
Substance P, 971
Subsystems, in systems theory, 251–252
Suction, gastric or intestinal, fluid and electrolyte imbalances and, 1022
  Gomco pump for, 1102, *1102*, 1382, *1383*
  in gastrointestinal tubes, 1102
  of drainage from wounds, 1380, *1381–1383*, 1382, 1382t
Suction outlets, in hospital client rooms, 391
Suctioning, airway, 1243–1249
  assessment of need for, 1249, 1249t
  catheters used for, 1244, 1248
  hydration and, 1244
  preparation for, *1243*
  procedure for, 1245–1248
  route of, 1243–1244
  side effects of, 1249, 1250t
  vacuum pressures used for, 1244
Suffering, and pain, 969, *969*
Suicide, assisted, 76
  in adolescents, 215–216
  in ethnic groups, 338
  nursing precautions against, 886–887
    care plan for, 887–888
    case study of, 887
Sulfur, metabolism, functions, and sources of, 1059t
Sundowner's syndrome, insomnia and, 953
Sunlight, skin functions and, 1337
Superego, 185
Support groups, 91, 454–455
Suppositories, 1136

Suppositories (*Continued*)
  rectal, in bowel training programs, 1149
    insertion of, 1276, *1276*
    timing of, 1149
  vaginal, insertion of, 1276, *1276*
Suprachiasmatic nucleus, of hypothalamus, in
  biologic rhythms, 311
Suprasystems, in systems theory, 251
Surgery, ablative, 1407
  bowel elimination and, 1129
  care plan for, 1441–1443
  case study in, 1440–1441
  curative, 1407
  diagnostic, 1407
  duration of, surgical risk and, 1420
    wound infection and, 1342
  informed consent for, 1412–1413
  intraoperative phase, assessment in, 1428
    nursing activities in, 1408t
    nursing diagnoses in, 1428–1429
    nursing interventions in, 1429–1432
    planning in, 1429
    responsibilities of nurse in, 1428
  legal aspects of, 1412–1413
  major or minor, 1407
  palliative, 1407
  postoperative phase, assessment in, 1434
    evaluation in, 1440
    nursing activities in, 1408t
    nursing diagnoses in, 1434
    nursing interventions in, 1435–1440
    planning in, 1434, 1435
  preoperative phase, admission to health
    care facility and, 1413
    assessment in, 1413, 1413t–1414t,
     1419–1420
    nursing activities in, 1408t, 1413
    nursing diagnoses in, 1420–1421
    nursing interventions in, 1421–1428
    planning in, 1421
  purposes and types of, 1404, 1407
  recent advances in, 35
  risk with, 1419–1420
  transport of client to operating room for,
    1428
  urgency or necessity of, 1407
  urinary elimination and, 1161–1162
Surgical attire. See also *Gloves*; *Gowns*;
  Masks.
  preparation for donning, 532–533
  protective, with respiratory disorders, 1239
Surgical clips, 1361, *1361*
Surgical hand scrub, procedure for, 533, 534
  sterile technique and, 531
Surgical team, roles and responsibilities of,
  1409–1410
Surgilift, 784, *784*
  use of, 785, *786*, 787
Surrogate, definition and types of, 68–69
Suspensions, drug, 1268
Sutures, 1360–1361
  care of, 1384–1385
  looseness or tightness of, 1384
  materials used for, 1360, *1360*
  removal of, 1385
Swallowing, difficulty with, 1091
  oral medications and, 1269
Swan-Ganz catheter, *623*, 624
  core body temperature measured with,
    593, 598
Sweat, electrolyte composition of, 1023t
  fluid and electrolyte imbalances and, 1021
  heat loss by, 588
Sweat glands, function of, 914
  in adolescents, 211
Swing carry, 552t, *553*

Symbols, used in charting, 486t–487t
Symptoms, in chronic illness, 375
  in illness experience, 365
  seriousness or visibility of, 366
Synarthroses, 732
Synchromed, 992
Synovial fluid, 733
Syringes, for parenteral administration of
  drugs, 1285, 1285t, *1286–1288*
    care and handling of, 1285, 1287, *1288*
    Luer-Lok, 1285, *1286–1287*
    protective sleeves for, 1285, *1288*
    selection of, 1285
  for wound cleansing, 1367, *1367*
Syrups, 1268
Systems, definition of, 251, *252*
  goals of, 251
  input and output in, 251
  living, and adaptation, 251–253
    internal and external milieus of, 251
  types of, 251, *252*

T

Tablets, enteric-coated, 1267–1268
  lozenges, 1268
  prolonged acting (sustained release), 1267
Tachycardia, conditions associated with, 605,
  607
Tachypnea, 610, *611*
  pattern of, 1211t
Tail policy, in claims-made insurance, 54
Tannen, Deborah, 447
Tape recordings, use of, invasion of privacy
  and, 56–57
Target tissues, of hormones, 304
Task Force on Organ Transplantation, 82
Task (work) groups, 455
Taste, deficit in, nursing care for, 1479
Taxonomy, uses of in nursing diagnostic process, 132, 134
T-binders, uses and application of, 856
Teaching, 163. See also *Health promotion*.
  about bladder irrigation, 1199
  about bowel management, 1133
  about diet, 1090–1091
  about home enteral feeding program, 1118
  about hygiene principles, 896
  about incentive spirometry, 1237
  about medication self-care, 1266
  about oral self-care, 904
  about skin care, 923
  about smoking, 1221
  about sutures, 1384–1385
  about traction, 878–879
  about urinary catheterization, 1181
  about urinary elimination, 1159
  about wellness and health promotion, 356
  aids for, 480
  and learning, 467–482
  content of, 474–475
  evaluation of, 112
  for clients with cancer, 476
  for discharge, 1440
  group, 359–360, 479
  in home care nursing, client instruction
    sheets for, 410, *411–412*
  methods of, 475, 479–480
  nurses' roles in, 94, 356, 475
  nursing goals and, 257
  one-on-one, 479
  preoperative, 1421–1423, 1422t, *1423*
  principles of, 474–475
  problems with, hindering learning, 474
  programmed study for, 479–480

Teaching (*Continued*)
  resistance to, 477
  resource persons for, 480
  role-playing for, 479
  timing of, 475
TED stockings, 767–768, 863, 864
Teeth, assessment of, 673
  brushing of, 905–906, *905–906*
  calculus (tartar) on, 902
  care of, 900–908
    gingival tissue and, 902
  decay of, 901–902
  dental plaque on, 901–902
  erosion of enamel from, 904
  flossing of, 906
  structure of, *901*, 901
Telephones, in hospital client rooms, 392
Television, in hospital client rooms, 392
Temperature, assessment of, 587–602
  body, axillary, 596–598
    circadian rhythm of, 311–312, *312*, *951*
    core, 593, 598
     vs. surface, 591
    factors affecting, 589–591
    in surgical patients, 1411
    measurement of, 591–598, *593–598*
     Celsius scale for, 591, 592t
     changes in, 598–602
     Fahrenheit scale for, 591, 592t
     frequency of, 598
     procedures for, 594–597
     with fever, 600
    normal ranges of, 589, *590*
    oral, 594–595, *598*, 598
    rectal, 595–596, 598
    regulation of, 304, 307, 587, 588–589,
     1337
     behavioral, 589, *590*
     failure of, 589
     physiologic, 589, *590*
     skin's role in, 914
    respiratory changes in, 1206
    rhythmic variation in, 311–312, *312*
    sensory test of, 693
    set point of, 589, *590*
  environmental, body temperature and,
    589–590
    fluid and electrolyte imbalances and,
     1021
    skin temperature and, 1339
  of enteric feeding formula, 1108
  set point of, 599
  skin, 916, 1339
    assessment of, 662
TENS, for pain relief, 991, *991*
Teratogens, in pregnancy, 191
Tes-Tape, 1167
Testes, in homeostasis regulation, 303, *303*
Theism, 1512
Therapeutic baths, 916–917
Therapeutic touch, 39t
Therapists, training and responsibilities of, 93
Thermometers, calibration of, 591, 592t
  disposable, 592–593
  disposal of, 520
  electronic, 592, *593*, 597
  glass, 591–592, *592*, 594–597
  oral, 591–592, *592*, 594–597
  tympanic, 593, *593*, 597
  types of, 591–593
Third space fluid accumulation, fluid and
  electrolyte imbalances and, 1022
Third-party reimbursement, 58
  for home care nursing, 404
Thirst, in elderly, 1016
  in fluid volume regulation, 1016, *1016*

Thomson, Samuel, 37
Thoracentesis, 720–721, 1217
 care of person undergoing, 718t
Thoracic cavity, 1205
Thorax. See also *Chest* entries.
 auscultation of, *678,* 679, *680*
 landmarks and reference lines of, 676, *676*
 palpation of, 676, *677,* 678
 percussion of, 678, 678t, *678–679*
Thought processes, abstract vs. concrete, 635
 altered, with sensory/perceptual deficit, 1475
Throat culture, 1215
Thromboembolism, in immobilized persons, 747–748
 sequential compression devices and, 864
Thromboembolytic deterrent (TED) stockings, 767–768, 863, 864
Thrombophlebitis, intravenous therapy and, 1326, 1326t
 with urethral catheterization, 1189–1190
Thrombosis, intravenous therapy and, 1326
Thumbs, functional assessment of, 851, *851,* 852, *852*
 opposition of, 693
 range of motion of, 739t
 passive exercise of, 820–821
Thyroid gland, assessment of, 674
 in growth and development, 182
 in homeostasis regulation, 302, *303*
Thyroid hormones, body temperature and, 591
 fluid and electrolyte balance and, 1017
Tibial nerve, functional assessment of, 851, *851*
Time, adaptation and, 279
 management of, in chronic illness, 376
 relation to self, 262
Time tape, for intravenous infusion, 1310, *1310*
 for measuring drainage from gastrointestinal suction apparatus, 1103, *1108*
Tinctures, 1268
Tissues, changes in, in surgical candidates, 1411
 damage to, with use of restraints, 881
 hyperemic, 741
 hypoxia of, from pressure, 741
 in immobilized persons, 748
 subcutaneous, 1337
 trauma to, with urethral catheterization, 1191
Tobacco, in adolescents, 215
 use in pregnancy, 191
Toddlers. See *Children, young.*
Toes, functional assessment of, 851, *851*
 range of motion of, 740t
 passive exercise of, 822
Toilet, modifications of, 897–898
Toilet training, elimination patterns and, 1127–1128
 in early childhood, 199
 urinary elimination and, 1161
Toileting, in visually impaired clients, self-care for, 1479
Tomography, computed, 713t, 714, *714*
Tongue, anatomy and function of, 1050
 assessment of, 674
 in cardiac arrest, 559, *561,* 566
Tongue depressor, 655
Toothbrushes, types of, 905, *905*
Tophi, 911
Topical medications, administration of, 1273–1280
Tort law, 52–57
 intentional torts, 56–57

Tort law *(Continued)*
 in nursing practice, 56–57
 lawsuits brought under, 53–56
 standard of care and, 52–53
 unintentional torts, 52–56
Total quality management, evaluation process and, 171, 173
Touch, assessment of, 1339
 deficit in, 1479
Touching, as body language, 433
Trachea, assessment of, 674
Tracheostomy tubes, placement of, 1241, *1242–1243*
 suctioning of, 1246
 types of, 1241
Traction, application of, 873, *874–875,* 875
 general guidelines for, 875, *876,* 878
 at home, teaching about, 879
 balanced suspension with Thomas or Brady splint, *877,* 877t
 bedmaking considerations with, 942, *943*
 Bryant's, *876,* 876t
 Buck's extension, *876,* 876t
 cervical head halter, *878,* 878t
 complications with, 878
 definition of, 873
 documentation of, 879
 Dunlop's, *877,* 877t
 equipment needed for, *874*
 for head, *878,* 878t
 for lower extremity, 876t–877t, *876–877*
 for pelvis, *877,* 877t
 for therapeutically immobilized clients, 873–879
 for upper extremity, *877,* 877t
 halo, *878,* 878t
 hazards of, 875
 major types of, 876t–878t, *876–878*
 overhead, *877,* 877t
 Russell's, *876,* 876t
 side-arm, *877,* 877t
 skeletal, 873, *875*
 bedpan use and, 897
 pin care with, 878
 skin, 873, *875*
 teaching and learning about, 878–879
 uses of, 873
Tranquilizers, premedication with, 1426
Transcutaneous electrical nerve stimulation, for dying person, 1553
Transdermal fentanyl patch, for pain relief, 991–992
Transportation, for older adults, 240
Trapeze bar, bedmaking and, 941–943
 bedpan use and, 897
Trash, disposal of, 520
Trauma. See *Injuries.*
Travelbee, Joyce, 428
Treatment, alternative methods of, 36–37
 biomedical model of, 35–36
 inhalation (respiration), 36
 invasive, informed consent and, 70
 nutritional (diet), 35
 pharmaceutical, 35
 physical medicine for, 35–36
 psychiatric, 36
 purposes of, 34t
 radiation and nuclear medicine, 36
 types of, 34, 34t, 35–37
Triazolam (Halcion), as sleeping pill, 963
TriCouncil for Nursing, 105
Trigeminal nerve, assessment of, 667, 669
Triglycerides, 1054
Trochanter rolls, *766,* 767, *776*
Trochlear nerve, assessment of, 669
Trust, development of, 1514

Trust *(Continued)*
 in children, 197, 200–201, 205
 during psychosocial interview, 629
 in groups, 461
 in therapeutic relationship, 423
Tub baths, 917–918, 1394
Tubal ligation, state law on, 77
Tube feedings, administration of, 1041–1042
 fluid and electrolyte balance and, 1041–1042
 through gastrostomy tube, 1114–1115
Tube-gauze bandages, 862
Tuberculosis, in hospitals, 522
Tubes, endotracheal, 1241, *1243*
 insertion of, 1241, *1243*
 suctioning of, 1246
 types of, 1241, *1242*
 gastrointestinal, drainage from, emptying of, 1103, *1108*
 physics of, 1101–1102
 for enteral nutrition, *1096,* 1103
 insertion of, 1104–1108, *1105, 1107*
 irrigation of, 1112–1114
 medications administered through, 1103
 metamucil in, 1109
 nasogastric, nursing diagnoses with, 1115t–1116t
 nursing interventions with, 1115t–1116t
 oral medications with, 1269
 nursing interventions with, 1103, 1115t–1116t
 preparation of, 1103
 psychologic preparation of client needing, 1102–1103
 reasons for, 1095
 routes of insertion of, 1095, *1096*
 esophagogastrostomy, 1095, *1096*
 esophagostomy, 1095, *1096*
 gastrostomy, 1095, *1096*
 jejunostomy, 1095, *1096*
 nasogastric, 1095, *1096*
 orogastric, 1095, *1096*
 sizes of, 1102
 suction in, 1102
 types of, 1096, 1097t–1098t, *1098–1102,* 1099–1101
 gastric, 1096, 1097t, *1098–1100,* 1099
 intestinal, 1097t, 1099–1101, *1100*
 special feeding, 1098t, 1101, *1101–1102*
 in immobilized clients, 783t
 intravenous, 1332–1333
 types and accessories for, 1322–1323, *1324*
 percutaneous nephrostomy, *1179,* 1179–1180
 rectal, for flatulence reduction, 1147
 tracheosotomy, 1241, *1242–1243*
Tuning fork, 653
Turning, of patient, for relief of pressure, 1347
 respiratory status and, 1223
 preoperative teaching of, 1423
Turning clock, 1349, *1350*
Two-point discrimination, 701
Tympanic membrane, 671, *671*
Tympanites, in immobilized persons, 750

U

UHI-air-fluidized therapy bed, 761–762
Ulcerative colitis, dietary management of, 1084t

Ulcers, decubitus. See *Pressure ulcers.*
  formation of, with urethral catheterization, 1189–1190
  pressure. See *Pressure ulcers.*
Ulnar nerve, testing of, 852, *852*
Ultrasonography, care of person undergoing, 725t
  mechanism of, 725
Umbilical stump, 193
Unconditional positive regard, of nurse, therapeutic communication and, 434
Unconsciousness. See also *Comatose patients.*
  airway obstruction and, management of, 577
  cardiopulmonary arrest and, 559–560
  health care decision making and, 69
Understaffing, handling of, 55
  risk management and, 55
Underweight. See also *Weight.*
  dietary management of, 1083
Unemployed, Medicare insurance for, 95
Unemployment compensation, for nurses, 58–59
Ungvarski, Peter, 14
Unification Church, beliefs and practices of, 1521t
Uniform Anatomical Gift Act, 81–82
Unitarian Universalist Association, beliefs and practices of, 1521t
United Automobile Workers v. Johnson Controls, 59
United Church of Christ, beliefs and practices of, 1520t
United Network for Organ Sharing, 82
United States, Department of Health and Human Services, objectives for health promotion of, 348
  health care system of, policy and politics relating to, 99–105
    vs. Canada's health care system, 102t–103t
    vs. other national systems, 100t–101t
  home care nursing in, 400–401
United States Public Health Service, 90, 99
United States Supreme Court, abortion law and, 76
  Cruzan decision and, 75
Universal precautions, 224, 508, 708, 1345
  for urine tests, 1166
  respiratory disorders and, 1239
Unna's boot, application of, 863
Upper gastrointestinal series, 711, 711t
Ureterosigmoidostomy, 1163, *1164*
Ureterostomy, 1163, *1164*
Ureters, anatomy of, *1156*, 1158
Urethra, anatomy of, *1156*, 1158
Urethral catheter, 1177–1179, *1179*
Urethritis, 1162
Uric acid, blood, in gout, 1088
Urinal, guidelines for use of, 900
Urinalysis, 719
  specimen collection for, 1168
Urinary diversion, 1163, *1164*
  nursing interventions for, 1172
  planning outcomes for, 1172
  types of, 1163, *1164*
Urinary elimination, 1155–1202
  altered, as nursing diagnosis, 1169
    nursing interventions for, 1172–1174
    planning for, 1171–1172
  assessment of, 1160–1169
  care plan for, 1200
  case study of, 1200
  cultural factors affecting, 1161

Urinary elimination *(Continued)*
  evaluation of, 1199
  factors affecting, 1160–1161
  in hospitals, 1159–1160
  medications and, 1161
  normal, 1158–1160
  problems with, causes of, 1163–1165
    diagnostic tests for, 1169
    nursing interventions for, 1172–1199
    symptoms of, 1162–1163
  teaching about, 1160
  trauma and, 1161–1162
Urinary incontinence, 1162, 1199
  aids for, 1175, *1175*
  nursing interventions for, 1173–1175
  nursing research on, in elderly women, 1173
  planning for, 1172
Urinary retention, 1164–1165, 1177–1180, 1187–1199
  as nursing diagnosis, 1171
  catheterization for, 1181–1182, *1183*, 1184–1186. See also *Catheters, urinary.*
  evaluation of, 1199
  planning for, 1172
  with overflow, 1165
Urinary stasis, in immobilized client, 753, *754*
  kidney stones and, 1164
Urinary tract, aging and, 1158
  anatomy and physiology of, *1156–1157*, 1156–1158
  catheterization of. See *Catheters, urinary.*
  in adolescents, 210t
  in immobilized clients, 746t, 753–754, *755*
  infection of, 1163
    nursing interventions for, 1172
    planning for, 1171–1172
    with catheterization, 1188–1189
      causes of, 1189
      prevention of, 1188–1189
  stones in, 1163–1164. See also *Kidney stones.*
    nursing interventions for, 1172–1174
    planning for, 1172
Urine, acidification of, 1190
  assessment of, for stones, 1164
  characteristics of, 1165–1166
  culture of, specimen collection for, 1168–1169
  pressure ulcers and, 1350, 1351t–1352t
  residual, 1158
  retention of. See *Urinary retention.*
    with overflow, 1165
  routine testing of, 1166–1168
    care of person undergoing, 717t
    drug administration and, 1265
    for hematuria, 1168
    glucose in, 1167
    ketones in, 1167
    leukocytes in, 1168
    nitrites in, 1168
    pH, 1166–1167
    specific gravity, 1018, *1167*, 1167
  specimens of, collection of, 1168–1169
    clean-catch, 1168–1169
    24-hour or 12-hour, 1169
  volume of, circadian rhythms and, 313
Urolithiasis, 1163–1164

V

Vaccines, for hepatitis B, 521
  for infection, 513

Vagina, 925
  assessment of, 690
  irrigation of, 1278–1280
  suppositories for, 1276, *1276*
Vagus nerve, assessment of, 674
  bradycardia and, 607
Valsalva maneuver, cardiac conditions and, 743, 747, 813
  constipation and, 1144
  defecation and, 1127
  in immobilized clients, 783t
Value-belief pattern, nursing assessment and, 124
  nursing diagnoses in, 136
Values. See also *Attitudes; Beliefs.*
  and politics, 103–104
  conflicts in, 45
  definition of, 44
  health promotion and protection and, 40–41, *41*, 349–350
  home care nursing and, 410
  in adolescents, 213, 1514–1515
  in infancy, 198
  in learning, 470
  in middle-aged adults, 233
  in neonates, 195
  in older adults, 240
  in school-age children, 204
  in young adults, 222
  self and, 259
  teaching approach and, 476
  transcendent, 1510
Vaporization, 1280
Variance reports, in risk management programs, 55
Vascular disorders, peripheral, nail and foot problems in, 930
Vascular resistance, peripheral, blood pressure and, 612–613
Vasodilation, heat loss and, 588
Vassar Training Camp, 16
Vegetarianism, 1065–1066
  diet plan for lactovegetarians, 1065
  nutrients needed for vegans, 1066, 1066t
Veins. See also *Vessels.*
  external jugular, assessment of, 675, *675*
  for venipuncture, *1309*, 1330
  peripheral, filling and emptying of, 1034, *1035*
  subclavian, *1309*, 1312
Venipuncture, for blood collection or IV infusion, procedure for, 1316–1320
  for intravenous therapy, choice of site for, 1330
  reasons for, 1308
Venous insufficiency, skin assessment and, 1338
Venous stasis, in immobilized persons, 747
Ventilation, 557
  in cardiopulmonary resuscitation, successful, 571, 574
  in immobilized persons, 749
  mechanical, 1249
Veracity, as ethical principle, 47
Verbatim notes, in therapeutic relationship, 424–425, *426*
Vernix caseosa, in neonates, 192
Vertebral column, range of motion of, 736t
Vertigo, 1480
Vessels. See also *Blood vessels; Veins.*
  damage to, casts and, 868, 869t
  elasticity of, blood pressure and, 613
  response to cold, 1388
  wound healing and, 1359

Vibration, test of, 693
Vibrio cholerae, 1094
Videotapes, use of, invasion of privacy and, 56–57
Violence, risk of, 850
  as nursing diagnosis, 853–854
Visitation rights, right to, of long-term care residents, 80
Visiting Nurse Association, 402–403
Visiting Nurse Service of New York, 400
Visiting nurses, 11–12
Visual acuity, testing of, 670
Visual field, 669–670
Visual impairment, communication with clients with, 448
  loneliness and, 1478
  nursing care for client with, 1477–1479
  self-care with, 1479
Vital signs. See also specific signs (e.g., *Temperature*).
  assessment of, 123, 586–587
    guidelines for, 586–587
  definition of, 586
  drug administration and, 1265
  during blood transfusions, 1312
  electronic monitoring of, 621–624
  in children, 193t
  in immobilized persons, 749
  in infants, 193t
  in neonates, 193t
  nursing responsibility in communicating findings in, 621, 622t
Vitamin A, function and sources of, 1057t
  requirements in adolescents, 1072
  toxicity of, 1063t
  wound healing and, 1359
Vitamin B₆, toxicity of, 1063t
Vitamin C, function and sources of, 1057t
  requirements in adolescents, 1072
  toxicity of, 1063t
Vitamin D, 1337
  function and sources of, 1057t
  toxicity of, 1063t
Vitamin E, function and sources of, 1057t
Vitamin K, function and sources of, 1057t
Vitamins, B-complex, function and sources of, 1058t
  body requirements for, 1055–1056, 1056t–1057t
  fat-soluble, functions and sources of, 1057t
  natural, 1063
  supplements for, indications for, 1056–1057
  supplements of, 1056–1057, 1063
  toxicities of, 1063t
  wound healing and, 1358–1359
Voiding, 1158
Volunteer work, by adolescents, 213
  by middle-aged adults, 232
  by young adults, 221
Vomiting, fluid and electrolyte imbalances and, 1022
  in bulimics, 1073
Vulva, 925

W

Waist, restraints for, 884
Wald, Lillian, 11, 20, 105, 400
Walkers, types of, *838*, 838–839
  use of, *838*, 838–839
Walking (ambulation) belt, 795–796, *796*
Walsh, M.B., nursing interventions and human needs and, 255

Wars, and nursing education, 16–17
Waste, solid, from health care facilities, 507
Water, body, 1001–1002
  as percentage of body weight, 1001t
  balance of, 1001–1002, 1005t
    hyper and hypo-osmolality and, 1011, *1011*
  deficit of, 1007t
  distribution of, 1001
  excess of, 1007t
  functions of, 1005
  loss of, routes of, 1002
  total, 1001
  wound healing and, 1358
  intake and output, body water balance and, 1001–1002, 1005t
    measurements of, 1002, 1005t
    procedure for, 1003–1004
  minimal requirements for, 1002
Water safety, in adolescents, 219
Watson, John, behavioral experiments of, 189
Watzlawick, Paul, 429
Weapons, safety measures for, in adolescents, 219
Weber lateralization test, 672, *672*
Weed, Lawrence, 490
Weight. See also *Obesity*.
  body, assessment of, 659, 660t
    blood pressure and, 613
    calories and nutrients and, 1052–1057
    fluid and electrolyte imbalances and, 1021
    in early childhood, 199
    in young adults, 224
    pharmacokinetics and, 1265
    regulation of, 307, 1082
  lifting of, back injury and, 544
    procedure for, 547
  pushing or pulling of, 546, 554
  rolling of, 546, 554
Wellness, adolescent, 219–220
  high-level, 29, *30*
  in health-illness continuum, *28*
  vs. health, 346
Wesley, John, 36
Wet dressings, application of, 1275
Wheelchair, 795, *796*
  restraining bar for, 885, *885*
Wheezing, 610, 679, *680*, 1214t
WIC program, 195
Widows and widowers, 238–239
Wolffian duct, development of, 1489, *1489*
Women, as caregivers, 239
  as heads of single-parent families, 322
  as subjects of research, 104
  as widows, 238–239
  in Jewish faith, 1516t
  menopause in, 228–229
  nursing profession and, 7–10
  older, sexual activity among, 236–237
  pulse rate in, 605
Women, Infants, and Children (WIC) program, 195
Wong/Baker Faces Rating scale, 976, *977*
Word-Graphic rating scale, 977
Work experience, and adolescents, 212
Work groups, 455
Workers' compensation, 59
  health care coverage by, 96
Workplace, health risks in midlife and, 233
  policies affecting, 104–105
Wounds. See also *Pressure ulcers*.
  assessment of, 1363t, 1363–1365, 1364t

Wounds *(Continued)*
  care of, advanced interventions for, 1344t–1345t
    antimicrobial support and, 1382–1383
    at home, 1386
    care plan for, 1398–1399
    case study of, 1397–1398
    cleansing of, 1367
      products used for, 1351t, 1367
    costs of, 1336
    documentation of, 1385–1386
    drains and suction used for, 1380, *1381*, 1382, 1382t, *1382–1383*
    dressings used for, 1367, 1374–1377
      adhesive methods for, 1385
      procedures for, 1370–1374, 1378–1380
    evaluation of, 1397
    infection control for, 1342–1345, 1358, 1365, 1383
    irrigation of, 1367, *1367*
      procedure for, 1368–1370
    odor control in, 1352t, 1383–1384
    principles of, 1387t
    products used for, 1351t–1352t, 1367
  causes of, 1339t
  chronic, pressure ulcers as, 1345–1354, *1346*
    prevention of, 1385
  classification of, 1339t, 1339–1354
  clean, 1342
  clean-contaminated, 1342
  closure of, 1359–1362
    adhesive skin closures used for, 1361t, 1361–1362, *1362*
    approximation of tissue edges for, 1360
    methods of, 1359–1360, *1360*
    surgical clips and staples used for, 1361, *1361*
    sutures used for, 1360–1361
  contaminated, 1342
    closure of, 1360
  definition of, 1336
  dehiscence and evisceration of, 1365, 1384
  dirty, 1342
  discharge planning for, 1386
  drainage of, 1365
    fluid and electrolyte imbalances and, 1022
  exudate from, infection and, 1358
  factitious, *1346*, 1359
  full-thickness or partial-thickness, *1340–1341*, 1341
  healing of, assessment of, 1363t, 1363–1365, 1364t
    factors affecting, 1357–1358
    local, 1358
    systemic, 1358–1359
    phases of, 1354–1357, 1355t, *1356*
  hemorrhaging and, 1365
  infected, *1342–1343*, 1342–1344, 1358, 1365
    closure of, 1360
      growth factors for, 1362
      hyperbaric oxygen for, 1363
      lasers and electrostimulation for, 1363
    factors affecting, 1342–1343
    signs of, 1342
  noninfected, 1341–1342
  open or closed, 1340–1341, *1340–1341*
  penetrating, *1340–1341*, 1343t
  perforating, *1341*, 1343t
  psychologic factors in, 1363t
  skin breakdown and, 1365

Wounds *(Continued)*
  staples in, care of, 1361, 1384–1385
  surgical, *1340*, 1340, 1356–1358
  sutures in, care of, 1360–1361, 1384–1385
  traumatic, 1340, *1340*
  types of, 1343t
Wrist, flexion and extension of, 693
  functional assessment of, 851, *851*, 852,
    852
  range of motion of, 738t
    passive exercise of, 820
  restraints for, 883, *883*
Wrist actigraph, sleep and, 955, *956*

X

Xerostomia, 904
Xiphoid fracture, in CPR, 571
X-rays, action of, 710

Y

Yale University, school of nursing at, 17
Yoga, 39t
Yoghurt, for odor control, 1384
Young children. See *Children, young.*

Yura, H., nursing interventions and human
  needs and, 255

Z

Zeitgebers, 311
Zinc, metabolism, functions, and sources of,
  1060t
Zygote, 190

COMMON ABBREVIATIONS AND SYMBOLS

Abbreviation/ Symbol	Term	Abbreviation/ Symbol	Term
Assessment Data			
abd	abdomen	neg	negative
ax	axillary	ng	nasogastric
BM	bowel movement	OTC	over-the-counter (medicine without a prescription)
BP	blood pressure	P	pulse
BSA	body surface area	PE	physical examination
bx	biopsy	PMH	past medical history
C&DB	coughing and deep breathing	R	respiration
c/o	complains of	R/O	rule out
cc	chief complaint	ROM	range of motion
DOA	dead on arrival	ROS	review of systems
dx	diagnosis	RX	treatment
F	Fahrenheit (temperature scale)	SOB	shortness of breath
h/o	history of	sx	signs; symptoms
HR	heart rate	T	temperature
in	inch	TPR	temperature, pulse, respiration
LMP	last menstrual period	VS	vital signs
LOC	level of consciousness	WNL	within normal limits
Disease-Related			
AIDS	acquired immune deficiency syndrome	fx	fracture
ASHD	arteriosclerotic heart disease	GI	gastrointestinal
BPH	benign prostatic hypertrophy	GU	genitourinary
CA	cancer	HTN	hypertension
CAD	coronary artery disease	MI	myocardial infarction
CHF	congestive heart failure	PVC	premature ventricular contraction
COPD	chronic obstructive pulmonary disease	PVD	peripheral vascular disease
CVA	cerebrovascular accident	STD	sexually transmitted disease
DM	diabetes mellitus	URI	upper respiratory infection
FUO	fever of unknown origin	UTI	urinary tract infection
Orders			
$\bar{a}$	before	OS	left eye
ac	before meals	O.T.	Occupational Therapy
ad lib	at will; as desired	$\bar{p}$	after
AMA	against medical advice	po	by mouth (per os)
bid	two times daily	post op	postoperative
$\bar{c}$	with	pre op	preoperative
CPR	cardiopulmonary resuscitation	prep	preparation
D/C	discontinue	prn	as needed; whenever necessary
D/W	dextrose in water	pt	patient
DNR	do not resuscitate	P.T.	Physical Therapy
DSD	dry sterile dressing	q	every
gtt	drop	q4h	every 4 hours
h	hour	qid	four times a day
hs	hour of sleep; bedtime	qod	every other day
I&O	intake and output	qs	quantity sufficient
IM	intramuscular	$\bar{s}$	without
IPPB	intermittent positive-pressure breathing	SC	subcutaneous (also sq)
IU	international unit	soln	solution
IV	intravenous	STAT	at once; immediately
ko	keep open (IV)	T&C	type and crossmatch
noc	night	tid	three times a day
NPO	nothing by mouth	tpn	total parenteral nutrition
NS	normal saline	×	times
OD	right eye		